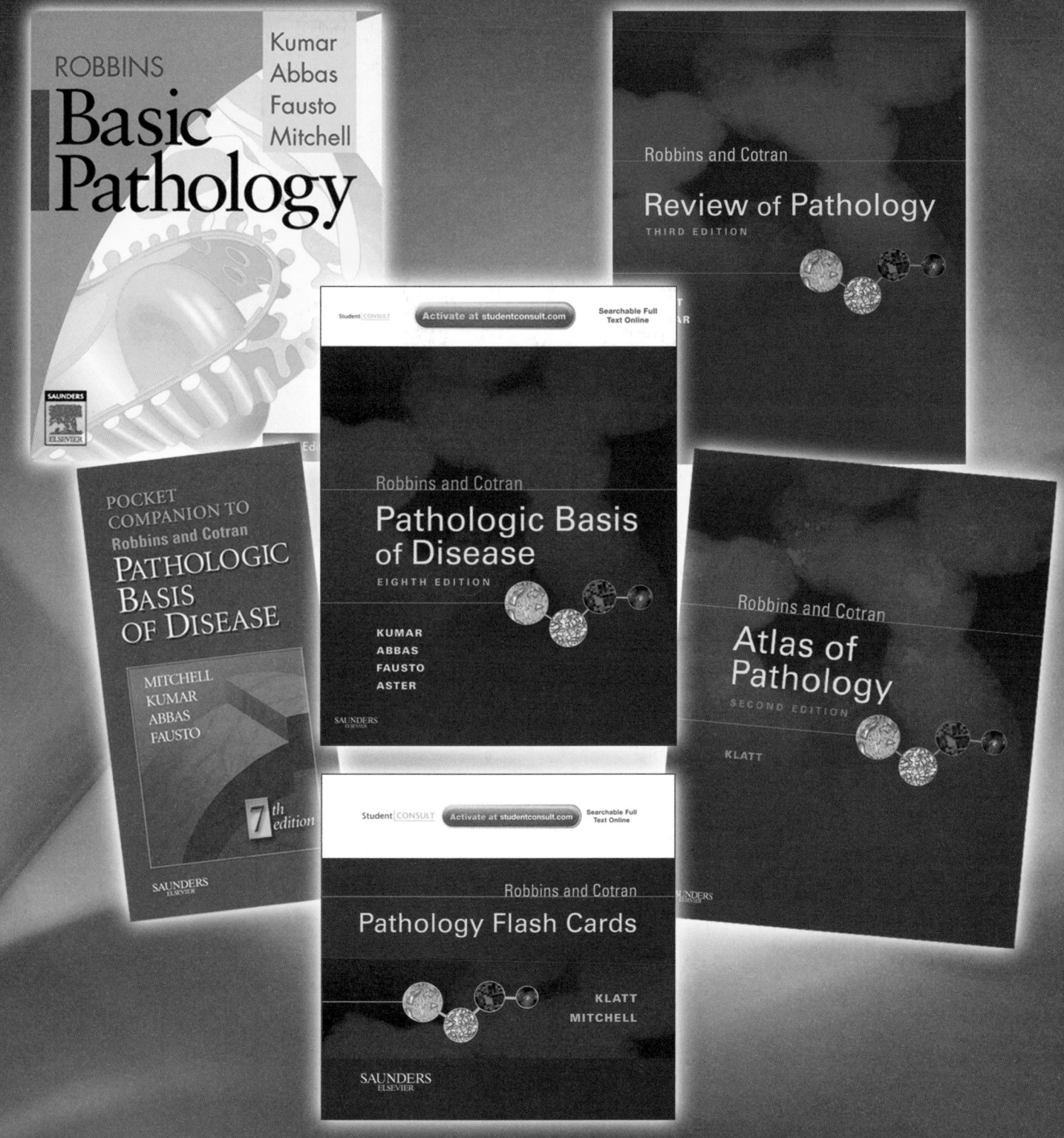

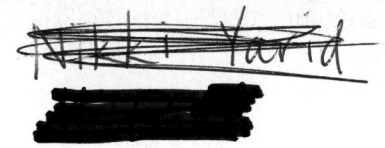

Robbins and Cotran
Pathologic Basis of Disease

Robbins and Cotran
Pathologic Basis of Disease

Eighth Edition

VINAY KUMAR, MBBS, MD, FRCPath
Alice Hogge and Arthur Baer Professor
Chairman, Department of Pathology
Executive Vice Dean, Division of Biologic Sciences and
The Pritzker School of Medicine
The University of Chicago
Chicago, Illinois

ABUL K. ABBAS, MBBS
Professor and Chairman, Department of Pathology
University of California, San Francisco
San Francisco, California

NELSON FAUSTO, MD
Professor and Chairman, Department of Pathology
University of Washington School of Medicine
Seattle, Washington

JON C. ASTER, MD, PhD
Professor of Pathology
Harvard Medical School
Brigham and Women's Hospital
Boston, Massachusetts

With Illustrations by
James A. Perkins, MS, MFA

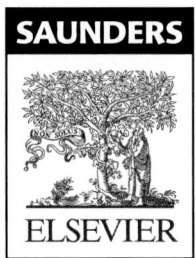

SAUNDERS
ELSEVIER

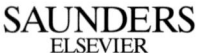

SAUNDERS
ELSEVIER

1600 John F. Kennedy Blvd.
Ste 1800
Philadelphia, PA 19103-2899

ROBBINS AND COTRAN PATHOLOGIC BASIS OF DISEASE, 8/E   ISBN: 978-1-4160-3121-5
Copyright © 2010 by Saunders, an imprint of Elsevier Inc.   International Edition ISBN: 978-0-8089-2402-9
Professional Edition ISBN: 978-1-4377-0792-2

Notice

Neither the Publisher nor the Editors assume any responsibility for any loss or injury and/or damage to persons or property arising out of or related to any use of the material contained in this book. It is the responsibility of the treating practitioner, relying on independent expertise and knowledge of the patient, to determine the best treatment and method of application for the patient.

The Publisher

Previous editions copyrighted 2004, 1999, 1994, 1989, 1984, 1979, 1974

Library of Congress Cataloging-in-Publication Data

Robbins and Cotran pathologic basis of disease. – 8th ed. / Vinay Kumar
. . . [et al.] ; with illustrations by James A. Perkins.
     p. ; cm.
   Includes bibliographical references and index.
   ISBN 978-1-4160-3121-5
   1. Pathology.   I. Robbins, Stanley L. (Stanley Leonard), 1915-   II. Kumar, Vinay, 1944-   III. Title:
Pathologic basis of disease.
   [DNLM: 1.   Pathology.   QZ 4 R6354 2010]
   RB111.R62 2010
   616.07–dc22

                                                2008007812

Executive Editor: William Schmitt
Managing Editor: Rebecca Gruliow
Publishing Services Manager: Joan Sinclair
Design Direction: Ellen Zanolle

Printed in China

Last digit is the print number: 9 8 7 6 5 4 3 2

With gratitude and affection to

Raminder Kumar
Ann Abbas
Ann DeLancey
Erin Malone

Contributors

Charles E. Alpers, MD
Professor of Pathology, Adjunct Professor of Medicine, University of Washington School of Medicine; Pathologist, University of Washington Medical Center, Seattle, WA

The Kidney

Douglas C. Anthony, MD, PhD
Professor and Chair, Department of Pathology and Anatomical Sciences, University of Missouri, Columbia, MO

Peripheral Nerve and Skeletal Muscle; The Central Nervous System

James M. Crawford, MD, PhD
Senior Vice President for Laboratory Services; Chair, Department of Pathology and Laboratory Medicine, North Shore–Long Island Jewish Health System, Manhasset, NY

Liver and Biliary Tract

Umberto De Girolami, MD
Professor of Pathology, Harvard Medical School; Director of Neuropathology, Brigham and Women's Hospital, Boston, MA

Peripheral Nerve and Skeletal Muscle; The Central Nervous System

Lora Hedrick Ellenson, MD
Weill Medical College of Cornell University, Professor of Pathology and Laboratory Medicine; Attending Pathologist, New York Presbyterian Hospital, New York, NY

The Female Genital Tract

Jonathan I. Epstein, MD
Professor of Pathology, Urology, and Oncology; The Reinhard Professor of Urologic Pathology, The Johns Hopkins University School of Medicine; Director of Surgical Pathology, The Johns Hopkins Hospital, Baltimore, MD

The Lower Urinary Tract and Male Genital System

Robert Folberg, MD
Dean, Oakland University William Beaumont School of Medicine, Rochester, MI; Chief Academic Officer, Beaumont Hospitals, Royal Oak, MI

The Eye

Matthew P. Frosch, MD, PhD
Associate Professor of Pathology, Harvard Medical School; Director, C.S. Kubik Laboratory for Neuropathology, Massachusetts General Hospital, Boston, MA

Peripheral Nerve and Skeletal Muscle; The Central Nervous System

Ralph H. Hruban, MD
Professor of Pathology and Oncology, The Sol Goldman Pancreatic Cancer Research Center, The Johns Hopkins University School of Medicine, Baltimore, MD

The Pancreas

Aliya N. Husain, MBBS
Professor, Department of Pathology, Pritzker School of Medicine, The University of Chicago, Chicago, IL

The Lung

Christine A. Iacobuzio-Donahue, MD, PhD
Associate Professor of Pathology and Oncology, The Sol Goldman Pancreatic Cancer Research Center, The Johns Hopkins University School of Medicine, Baltimore, MD

The Pancreas

Alexander J.F. Lazar, MD, PhD
Assistant Professor, Department of Pathology and Dermatology, Sections of Dermatopathology and Soft Tissue Sarcoma Pathology, Faculty of Sarcoma Research Center, University of Texas M.D. Anderson Cancer Center, Houston, TX

The Skin

Susan C. Lester, MD, PhD
Assistant Professor of Pathology, Harvard Medical School; Chief, Breast Pathology, Brigham and Women's Hospital, Boston, MA

The Breast

Mark W. Lingen, DDS, PhD
Associate Professor, Department of Pathology, Pritzker School of Medicine, The University of Chicago, Chicago, IL

Head and Neck

Chen Liu, MD, PhD
Associate Professor of Pathology, Immunology and Laboratory Medicine; Director, Gastrointestinal and Liver Pathology, The University of Florida College of Medicine, Gainesville, FL

Liver and Biliary Tract

Anirban Maitra, MBBS
Associate Professor of Pathology and Oncology, The Johns Hopkins University School of Medicine; Pathologist, The Johns Hopkins Hospital, Baltimore, MD

Diseases of Infancy and Childhood; The Endocrine System

Alexander J. McAdam, MD, PhD
Assistant Professor of Pathology, Harvard Medical School; Medical Director, Infectious Diseases Diagnostic Laboratory, Children's Hospital Boston, Boston, MA

Infectious Diseases

Richard N. Mitchell, MD
Associate Professor, Department of Pathology, Harvard Medical School; Director, Human Pathology, Harvard-MIT Division of Health Sciences and Technology, Harvard Medical School; Staff Pathologist, Brigham and Women's Hospital, Boston, MA

Hemodynamic Disorders, Thromboembolic Disease, and Shock; Blood Vessels; The Heart

George F. Murphy, MD
Professor of Pathology, Harvard Medical School; Director of Dermatopathology, Brigham and Women's Hospital, Boston, MA

The Skin

Edyta C. Pirog, MD
Associate Professor of Clinical Pathology and Laboratory Medicine, New York Presbyterian Hospital-Weil Medical College of Cornell University; Associate Attending Pathologist, New York Presbyterian Hospital, New York, NY

The Female Genital Tract

Andrew E. Rosenberg, MD
Professor, Department of Pathology, Harvard Medical School; Pathologist, Massachusetts General Hospital, Boston, MA

Bones, Joints, and Soft Tissue Tumors

Frederick J. Schoen, MD, PhD
Professor of Pathology and Health Sciences and Technology, Harvard Medical School; Director, Cardiac Pathology and Executive Vice Chairman, Department of Pathology, Brigham and Women's Hospital, Boston, MA

Blood Vessels; The Heart

Arlene H. Sharpe, MD, PhD
Professor of Pathology, Harvard Medical School; Chief, Immunology Research Division, Department of Pathology, Brigham and Women's Hospital, Boston, MA

Infectious Diseases

Thomas Stricker, MD, PhD
Orthopedic Pathology Fellow, Department of Pathology, Pritzker School of Medicine, The University of Chicago, Chicago, IL

Neoplasia

Jerrold R. Turner, MD, PhD
Professor and Associate Chair, Department of Pathology, Pritzker School of Medicine, The University of Chicago, Chicago, IL

The Gastrointestinal Tract

Preface: The Golden Jubilee Edition

As we launch the 8th edition of *Pathologic Basis of Disease* we pause to look back 50 years ago, when the first edition of this book, entitled "Pathology with Clinical Correlations" was published. (For those who may not know, the first three editions were published under this name and so the current "8th edition" is really the 11th edition of this book.)

In the preface of the first edition, Stanley Robbins wrote:

- "But the study of morphology is only one facet of pathology. Pathology contributes much to clinical medicine. The pathologist is interested not only in the recognition of structural alterations, but also in their significance, i.e., the effects of these changes on cellular and tissue function and ultimately the effect of these changes on the patient. It is not a discipline isolated from the living patient, but rather a basic approach to a better understanding of disease and therefore a foundation of sound clinical medicine."
- "The why's and how's are as important as the what's."

In today's vocabulary, what Robbins said in 1957 was that pathology is the study of the mechanism of diseases and morphology is a tool (the only one available at that time) to gain insight into pathogenesis and clinical correlations. Over the past 50 years, this focus has not changed and it remains the guiding principle for the current edition. The main difference is that now we have many more tools to supplement morphology, including molecular biology, genetics, and informatics, to name a few. Indeed, it might be said that this book presents the molecular basis of human disease with clinical correlations. This edition, like all previous ones, has been extensively revised, and some areas have been completely rewritten. A few examples of significant changes are as follows:

- Chapter 1 has been completely reorganized to include the entire spectrum of cellular responses to injury, from adaptations and sublethal injury to cell death.
- Chapter 3, covering tissue repair and wound healing, has been extensively revised to include new and exciting information on stem cell biology, growth factor signaling, and the mechanisms that underlie fibrosis.
- Chapter 5 includes a completely rewritten section on molecular diagnosis that reflects rapid advances in DNA sequencing technology. The principles of genome-wide analysis, now becoming a powerful tool in the study of

complex human diseases like cancer and diabetes, have also been added.
- Chapter 9 has been completely revised and reorganized in view of the increasing importance of environmental factors in human diseases.
- Chapter 17 has been completely rewritten and highlights new insights into the pathogenesis of inflammatory bowel disease and gastrointestinal cancers.
- Chapter 22, covering diseases of the female genital tract, includes discussion of the molecular basis of cancer, endometriosis, and preeclampsia.
- In addition to the revision and reorganization of the text, many new photographs and schematics have been added and a large number of the older "gems" have been enhanced by digital technology. Thus, we hope that even the veterans of *Robbins Pathology* will find the illustrations and figures sparkling and fresh.

Wherever appropriate, we have blended new discoveries into the discussion of pathogenesis and pathophysiology, while never losing sight that the "state of the art" has little value if it does not enhance the understanding of disease mechanisms. As in the past, we have not avoided discussions of "unsolved" problems because of our belief that many who read the text might be encouraged to embark on a path of discovery.

Despite the changes highlighted above, our goals remain the same as those articulated by Robbins and Cotran over the past many years.

- To integrate into the discussion of pathologic processes and disorders the newest established information available— morphologic as well as molecular.
- To organize information into logical and uniform presentations, facilitating readability, comprehension, and learning.
- To maintain the book at a reasonable size and yet provide adequate discussion of the significant lesions, processes, and disorders. Indeed, we have reduced the girth and the weight of this book by trimming out about 80 pages (making it less useful for weight lifting).
- To place great emphasis on clarity of writing and proper use of language in the recognition that struggling to comprehend is time-consuming and wearisome and gets in the way of the learning process.

● To make this first and foremost a student text—used by students throughout all years of medical school and into their residencies—but, at the same time, to provide sufficient detail and depth to meet the needs of more advanced readers.

We have been repeatedly told by readers that up-to-datedness is a special feature that makes this book very valuable. We have strived to remain current by providing new information and references from recent literature, many published in 2008 and some from the early part of 2009. However, older classics have also been retained to provide original source material for advanced readers.

We are now into the digital age and so the text will be available online to those who own the print version. Such access gives the reader the ability to search across the entire text, bookmark passages, add personal notes, and use PubMed to view references, and has many other exciting features. In addition, also available online are case studies, previously available separately as the Interactive Case Study Companion devel-oped by one of us (VK) in collaboration with Herb Hagler, PhD, and Nancy Schneider, MD, PhD, at the University of Texas Southwestern Medical School in Dallas. The cases are designed to enhance and reinforce learning by challenging students to apply their knowledge to solve clinical cases. A virtual microscope feature enables the viewing of selected images at various magnifications.

This edition is also marked by the addition of a new coauthor, Jon Aster. All four of us have reviewed, critiqued, and edited each chapter to ensure the uniformity of style and flow that have been the hallmarks of the book. Together, we hope that we have succeeded in equipping the readers with the scientific basis for the practice of medicine and in whetting their appetite for learning beyond what can be offered in any textbook.

VK
AKA
NF
JCA

Acknowledgments

The authors are grateful to a large number of individuals who have contributed in many ways toward the completion of this textbook.

First and foremost, all four of us offer thanks to our contributing authors for their commitment to this textbook. Many are veterans of previous editions; others are new to the eighth edition. All are acknowledged in the table of contents. Their names lend authority to this book, for which we are grateful.

Many colleagues have enhanced the text by reading various chapters and providing helpful critiques in their area of expertise. They include Drs. Michelle LeBeau, Jerry Krishnan, Julian Solway, Elyssa Gordon, Ankit Desai, Sue Cohen, Megan McNerney, Peter Pytel, and Tony Chang (at the University of Chicago); Dr. Serdar Bulun (at Northwestern University, Chicago); Drs. Steven Deeks, Sanjay Kakar, Zoltan Laszik, Scott Oakes, Jay Debnath, and Michael Nystrom (at the University of California San Francisco); Dr. Lundy Braun at Brown University and Dr. Peter Byers at the University of Washington; Drs. Frank Bunn, Jeffery Kutok, Helmut Rennke, Fred Wang, Max Loda, and Mark Fleming (at Harvard Medical School); and Dr. Richard Aster (at the Milwaukee Blood Center and Medical College of Wisconsin). Special thanks are due to Dr. Raminder Kumar for updating clinical information and extensive proof-reading of many chapters. Many colleagues provided photographic gems from their collections. They are individually acknowledged in the text.

Our administrative staff needs special mention since they maintain order in the chaotic lives of the authors and have willingly chipped in when needed for multiple tasks relating to the text. At the University of Chicago, they include Ms. Valerie Driscoll and Garcia Wilson; at The University of California at San Francisco, Ms. Ana Narvaez; at the University of Washington, Seattle, Greg Lawrence, Joscelyn Rompogren, Stephanie Meleady-Brown, and Jane Norris; at the Brigham and Women's Hospital, Deborah Kutok and Muriel Goutas. Ms. Beverly Shackelford at the University of Texas Southwestern Medical School at Dallas, who has helped one of us (VK) for 26 years, deserves a gold star since she coordinated the submission of all manuscripts, proofread many of them, and maintained liaison with the contributors and publisher. Without her dedication to this book and her meticulous attention to detail, our task would have been much more difficult. Almost all of the graphic art in this book was created by Mr. James Perkins, Assistant Professor of Medical Illustration at Rochester Institute of Technology. His ability to convert complex ideas into simple and aesthetically pleasing sketches has considerably enhanced this book.

Many individuals associated with our publisher, Elsevier (under the imprint of W.B. Saunders), need our special thanks. Outstanding among them is Ellen Sklar, Production Editor, supervising the production of this book. Her understanding of the needs of the authors and the complexity of publishing a textbook went a long way in making our lives less complicated. Mr. William Schmitt, Publishing Director of Medical Textbooks, has always been our cheerleader and is now a dear friend. Our thanks also go to Managing Editor Rebecca Gruliow and Design Manager Ellen Zanolle at Elsevier. Undoubtedly there are many other "heroes" who may have been left out unwittingly—to them we say "thank you" and tender apologies for not acknowledging you individually.

Efforts of this magnitude take a heavy toll on the families of the authors. We thank our spouses, Raminder Kumar, Ann Abbas, Ann DeLancey, and Erin Malone for their patience, love, and support of this venture, and for their tolerance of our absences.

Finally, Vinay Kumar, Abul Abbas, and Nelson Fausto wish to express their deep appreciation to Jon Aster for joining the team. Jon has proved his excellence as a contributor for many years, and now he adds luster to the entire book. Despite differences in our vantage points, opinions, and individual styles, our common vision shared with the late Drs. Stanley Robbins and Ramzi Cotran, has made this an exciting and rewarding partnership.

VK
AKA
NF
JCA

Contents*

General Pathology

1   Cellular Responses to Stress and Toxic Insults:
    Adaptation, Injury, and Death   3

2   Acute and Chronic Inflammation   43

3   Tissue Renewal, Repair, and Regeneration   79

4   Hemodynamic Disorders, Thromboembolic Disease, and Shock   111
    Richard N. Mitchell

5   Genetic Disorders   135

6   Diseases of the Immune System   183

7   Neoplasia   259
    Thomas P. Stricker • Vinay Kumar

8   Infectious Diseases   331
    Alexander J. McAdam • Arlene H. Sharpe

9   Environmental and Nutritional Diseases   399

10 Diseases of Infancy and Childhood   447
    Anirban Maitra

Systemic Pathology: Diseases of Organ Systems

11 Blood Vessels   487
    Richard N. Mitchell • Frederick J. Schoen

12 The Heart   529
    Frederick J. Schoen • Richard N. Mitchell

13 Diseases of White Blood Cells, Lymph Nodes, Spleen, and Thymus   589

* Chapters without any listed contributors have been written by the editors.

14   **Red Blood Cell and Bleeding Disorders**   639

15   **The Lung**   677
Aliya N. Husain

16   **Head and Neck**   739
Mark W. Lingen

17   **The Gastrointestinal Tract**   763
Jerrold R. Turner

18   **Liver and Biliary Tract**   833
James M. Crawford • Chen Liu

19   **The Pancreas**   891
Ralph H. Hruban • Christine Iacobuzio-Donahue

20   **The Kidney**   905
Charles E. Alpers

21   **The Lower Urinary Tract and Male Genital System**   971
Jonathan I. Epstein

22   **The Female Genital Tract**   1005
Lora Hedrick Ellenson • Edyta C. Pirog

23   **The Breast**   1065
Susan C. Lester

24   **The Endocrine System**   1097
Anirban Maitra

25   **The Skin**   1165
Alexander J.F. Lazar • George F. Murphy

26   **Bones, Joints, and Soft Tissue Tumors**   1205
Andrew E. Rosenberg

27   **Peripheral Nerve and Skeletal Muscle**   1257
Douglas C. Anthony • Matthew P. Frosch • Umberto De Girolami

28   **The Central Nervous System**   1279
Matthew P. Frosch • Douglas C. Anthony • Umberto De Girolami

29   **The Eye**   1345
Robert Folberg

Index   1369

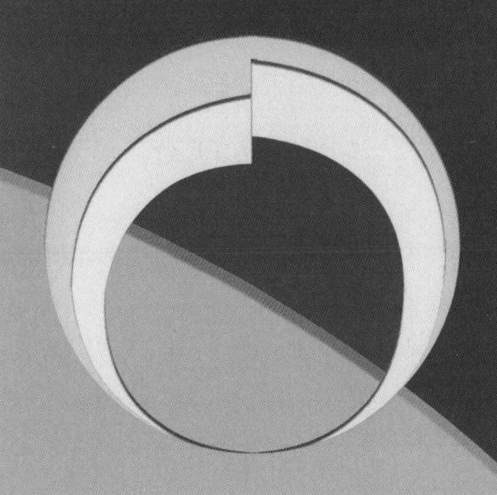

General Pathology

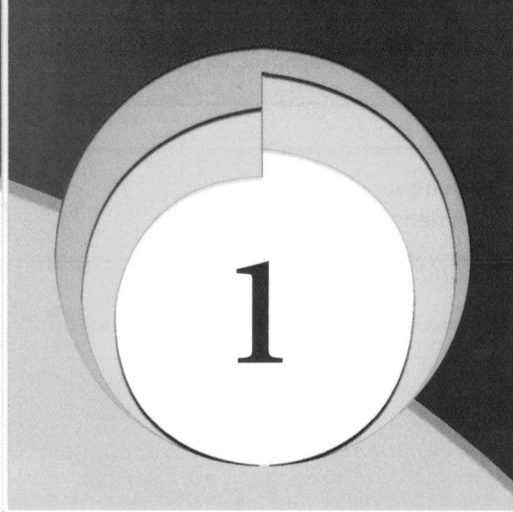

Cellular Responses to Stress and Toxic Insults: Adaptation, Injury, and Death

Introduction to Pathology

Overview: Cellular Responses to Stress and Noxious Stimuli

Adaptations of Cellular Growth and Differentiation
Hypertrophy
Mechanisms of Hypertrophy
Hyperplasia
Physiologic Hyperplasia
Pathologic Hyperplasia
Mechanisms of Hyperplasia
Atrophy
Mechanisms of Atrophy
Metaplasia
Mechanisms of Metaplasia

Overview of Cell Injury and Cell Death

Causes of Cell Injury

Morphologic Alterations in Cell Injury
Reversible Injury
Necrosis
Patterns of Tissue Necrosis

Mechanisms of Cell Injury
Depletion of ATP
Mitochondrial Damage
Influx of Calcium and Loss of Calcium Homeostasis
Accumulation of Oxygen-Derived Free Radicals (Oxidative Stress)
Defects in Membrane Permeability
Damage to DNA and Proteins

Clinico-Pathologic Correlations: Selected Examples of Cell Injury and Necrosis
Ischemic and Hypoxic Injury
Mechanisms of Ischemic Cell Injury
Ischemia-Reperfusion Injury
Chemical (Toxic) Injury

Apoptosis
Causes of Apoptosis
Apoptosis in Physiologic Situations
Apoptosis in Pathologic Conditions
Morphologic and Biochemical Changes in Apoptosis
Biochemical Features of Apoptosis
Mechanisms of Apoptosis
The Intrinsic (Mitochondrial) Pathway of Apoptosis
The Extrinsic (Death Receptor–Initiated) Pathway of Apoptosis
The Execution Phase of Apoptosis
Removal of Dead Cells
Clinico-Pathologic Correlations: Apoptosis in Health and Disease
Examples of Apoptosis
Disorders Associated with Dysregulated Apoptosis

Autophagy

Intracellular Accumulations
Lipids
Steatosis (Fatty Change)
Cholesterol and Cholesterol Esters
Proteins
Hyaline Change

Glycogen
Pigments
  Exogenous Pigments
  Endogenous Pigments

Pathologic Calcification
  Dystrophic Calcification
  Metastatic Calcification

Cellular Aging

Introduction to Pathology

Pathology is the study *(logos)* of disease *(pathos)*. More specifically, it is devoted to the study of the structural, biochemical, and functional changes in cells, tissues, and organs that underlie disease. By the use of molecular, microbiologic, immunologic, and morphologic techniques, pathology attempts to explain the whys and wherefores of the signs and symptoms manifested by patients while providing a rational basis for clinical care and therapy. It thus serves as the bridge between the basic sciences and clinical medicine, and is the scientific foundation for all of medicine.

Traditionally the study of pathology is divided into general pathology and systemic pathology. The former is concerned with the reactions of cells and tissues to abnormal stimuli and to inherited defects, which are the main causes of disease. The latter examines the alterations in specialized organs and tissues that are responsible for disorders that involve these organs. In this book we first cover the principles of general pathology and then proceed to specific disease processes as they affect particular organs or systems.

The four aspects of a disease process that form the core of pathology are its cause *(etiology)*, the mechanisms of its development *(pathogenesis)*, the biochemical and structural alterations induced in the cells and organs of the body *(molecular and morphologic changes)*, and the functional consequences of these changes *(clinical manifestations)*.

Etiology or Cause. The concept that certain abnormal symptoms or diseases are "caused" is as ancient as recorded history. For the Arcadians (2500 BC), if someone became ill it was the patient's own fault (for having sinned) or the effects of outside agents, such as bad smells, cold, evil spirits, or gods.[1] We now recognize that there are two major classes of etiologic factors: genetic (e.g., inherited mutations and disease-associated gene variants, or polymorphisms) and acquired (e.g., infectious, nutritional, chemical, physical). The idea that one etiologic agent is the cause of one disease—developed from the study of infections and single-gene disorders—is not applicable to the majority of diseases. In fact, most of our common afflictions, such as atherosclerosis and cancer, are multifactorial and arise from the effects of various external triggers on a genetically susceptible individual. The relative contribution of inherited susceptibility and external influences varies in different diseases.

Pathogenesis. Pathogenesis refers to the sequence of events in the response of cells or tissues to the etiologic agent, from the initial stimulus to the ultimate expression of the disease. The study of pathogenesis remains one of the main domains of pathology. Even when the initial cause is known (e.g., infection or mutation), it is many steps removed from the expression of the disease. For example, to understand cystic fibrosis is to know not only the defective gene and gene product, but also the biochemical and morphologic events leading to the formation of cysts and fibrosis in the lungs, pancreas, and other organs. Indeed, as we shall see throughout the book, the molecular revolution has already identified mutant genes underlying a great number of diseases, and the entire human genome has been mapped. Nevertheless, the functions of the encoded proteins and how mutations induce disease—the pathogenesis—are still often obscure. Technologic advances are making it increasingly feasible to link specific molecular abnormalities to disease manifestations and to use this knowledge to design new therapeutic approaches. For these reasons, the study of pathogenesis has never been more exciting scientifically or more relevant to medicine.

Molecular and Morphologic Changes. Morphologic changes refer to the structural alterations in cells or tissues that are either characteristic of a disease or diagnostic of an etiologic process. The practice of diagnostic pathology is devoted to identifying the nature and progression of disease by studying morphologic changes in tissues and chemical alterations in patients. More recently the limitations of morphology for diagnosing diseases have become increasingly evident, and the field of diagnostic pathology has expanded to encompass molecular biologic and immunologic approaches for analyzing disease states. Nowhere is this more striking than in the study of tumors; breast cancers that look morphologically identical may have widely different courses, therapeutic responses, and prognosis. Molecular analysis by techniques such as DNA microarrays (Chapter 5) has begun to reveal genetic differences that predict the behavior of the tumors as well as their responsiveness to different therapies. Increasingly, such techniques are being used to extend and even supplant traditional morphologic analyses.

Functional Derangements and Clinical Manifestations. The end results of genetic, biochemical, and structural changes in cells and tissues are functional abnormalities, which lead to the clinical manifestations (symptoms and signs) of disease, as well as its progress (clinical course and outcome).

Virtually all forms of disease start with molecular or structural alterations in cells, a concept first put forth in the nineteenth century by Rudolf Virchow, known as the father of modern pathology. We therefore begin our consideration of pathology with the study of the causes, mechanisms, and morphologic and biochemical correlates of *cell injury*. Injury to cells and to extracellular matrix ultimately leads to *tissue and organ injury*, which determine the morphologic and clinical patterns of disease.

Overview: Cellular Responses to Stress and Noxious Stimuli

The normal cell is confined to a fairly narrow range of function and structure by its state of metabolism, differentiation, and specialization; by constraints of neighboring cells; and by the availability of metabolic substrates. It is nevertheless able to handle physiologic demands, maintaining a steady state called *homeostasis*. *Adaptations* are reversible functional and structural responses to more severe physiologic stresses and some pathologic stimuli, during which new but altered steady states are achieved, allowing the cell to survive and continue to function (Fig. 1–1 and Table 1–1). The adaptive response may consist of an increase in the size of cells (hypertrophy) and functional activity, an increase in their number (hyperplasia), a decrease in the size and metabolic activity of cells (atrophy), or a change in the phenotype of cells (metaplasia). When the stress is eliminated the cell can recover to its original state without having suffered any harmful consequences.

If the limits of adaptive responses are exceeded or if cells are exposed to injurious agents or stress, deprived of essential nutrients, or become compromised by mutations that affect essential cellular constituents, a sequence of events follows that is termed *cell injury* (see Fig. 1–1) Cell injury is *reversible* up to a certain point, but if the stimulus persists or is severe enough from the beginning, the cell suffers *irreversible injury* and ultimately *cell death*. *Adaptation, reversible injury*, and *cell death* may be stages of progressive impairment following different types of insults. For instance, in response to increased hemodynamic loads, the heart muscle becomes enlarged, a form of adaptation, and can even undergo injury. If the blood supply to the myocardium is compromised or inadequate, the muscle first suffers reversible injury, manifested by certain

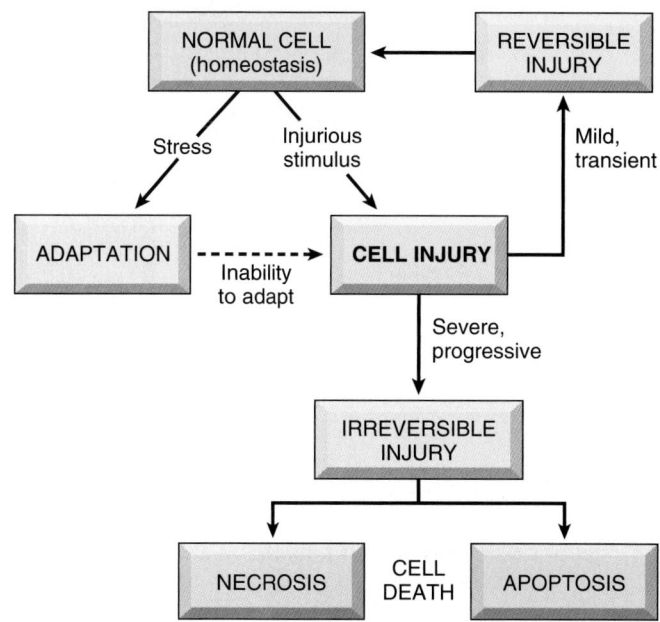

FIGURE 1–1 Stages of the cellular response to stress and injurious stimuli.

cytoplasmic changes (described later). Eventually, the cells suffer irreversible injury and die (Fig. 1–2).

Cell death, the end result of progressive cell injury, is one of the most crucial events in the evolution of disease in any tissue or organ. It results from diverse causes, including ischemia (reduced blood flow), infection, and toxins. Cell death is also a normal and essential process in embryogenesis, the development of organs, and the maintenance of homeostasis. There are two principal pathways of cell death, *necrosis* and *apoptosis*. Nutrient deprivation triggers an adaptive cellular response called *autophagy* that may also culminate in cell death. We will return to a detailed discussion of these pathways of cell death later in the chapter.

Stresses of different types may induce changes in cells and tissues other than typical adaptations, cell injury, and death (see Table 1–1). Metabolic derangements in cells and sublethal, chronic injury may be associated with *intracellular*

TABLE 1–1 Cellular Responses to Injury	
Nature of Injurious Stimulus	**Cellular Response**
ALTERED PHYSIOLOGICAL STIMULI; SOME NONLETHAL INJURIOUS STIMULI	**CELLULAR ADAPTATIONS**
• Increased demand, increased stimulation (e.g., by growth factors, hormones) • Decreased nutrients, decreased stimulation • Chronic irritation (physical or chemical)	• Hyperplasia, hypertrophy • Atrophy • Metaplasia
REDUCED OXYGEN SUPPLY; CHEMICAL INJURY; MICROBIAL INFECTION	**CELL INJURY**

• Acute and transient
 	
 • Progressive and severe (including DNA damage)
	• Acute reversible injury
	   Cellular swelling fatty change
	 • Irreversible injury → cell death
	   Necrosis
	   Apoptosis

METABOLIC ALTERATIONS, GENETIC OR ACQUIRED; CHRONIC INJURY	**INTRACELLULAR ACCUMULATIONS; CALCIFICATION**
CUMULATIVE SUBLETHAL INJURY OVER LONG LIFE SPAN	**CELLULAR AGING**

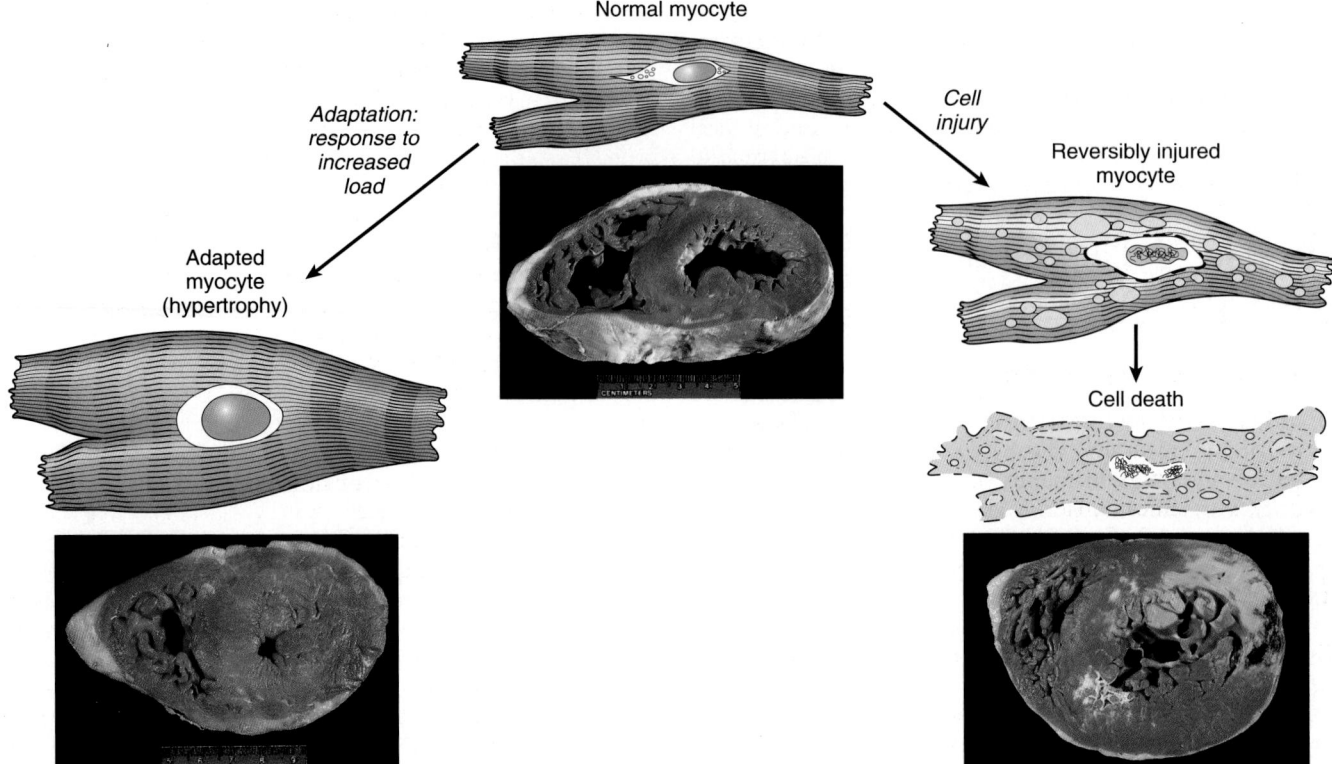

FIGURE 1–2 The relationship between normal, adapted, reversibly injured, and dead myocardial cells. The cellular adaptation is myocardial hypertrophy *(lower left),* caused by increased blood flow requiring greater mechanical effort by myocardial cells. This adaptation leads to thickening of the left ventricular wall to over 2 cm (normal, 1–1.5 cm). In reversibly injured myocardium (illustrated schematically, *right*) there are generally only functional effects, without any readily apparent gross or even microscopic changes. In the specimen showing necrosis, a form of cell death *(lower right),* the light area in the posterolateral left ventricle represents an acute myocardial infarction caused by reduced blood flow (ischemia). All three transverse sections of the heart have been stained with triphenyltetrazolium chloride, an enzyme substrate that colors viable myocardium magenta. Failure to stain is due to enzyme loss following cell death.

accumulations of a number of substances, including proteins, lipids, and carbohydrates. Calcium is often deposited at sites of cell death, resulting in *pathologic calcification.* Finally, the normal process of *aging* itself is accompanied by characteristic morphologic and functional changes in cells.

In this chapter we discuss first how cells adapt to stresses, and then the causes, mechanisms, and consequences of the various forms of acute cell damage, including reversible cell injury, and cell death. We conclude with three other processes that affect cells and tissues: intracellular accumulations, pathologic calcification, and cell aging.

Adaptations of Cellular Growth and Differentiation

Adaptations are reversible changes in the size, number, phenotype, metabolic activity, or functions of cells in response to changes in their environment. Such adaptations may take several distinct forms.

HYPERTROPHY

Hypertrophy refers to an increase in the size of cells, resulting in an increase in the size of the organ. The hypertrophied

organ has no new cells, just larger cells. The increased size of the cells is due to the synthesis of more structural components of the cells. Cells capable of division may respond to stress by undergoing both hyperplasia (described below) and hypertrophy, whereas in *nondividing cells* (e.g., myocardial fibers) increased tissue mass is due to hypertrophy. In many organs hypertrophy and hyperplasia may coexist and contribute to increased size.

Hypertrophy can be *physiologic* or *pathologic* and is caused by increased functional demand or by stimulation by hormones and growth factors. The striated muscle cells in the heart and skeletal muscles have only a limited capacity for division, and respond to increased metabolic demands mainly by undergoing hypertrophy. *The most common stimulus for hypertrophy of muscle is increased workload.* For example, the bulging muscles of bodybuilders engaged in "pumping iron" result from an increase in size of the individual muscle fibers in response to increased demand. In the heart, the stimulus for hypertrophy is usually chronic hemodynamic overload, resulting from either hypertension or faulty valves (see Fig. 1–2). In both tissue types the muscle cells synthesize more proteins and the number of myofilaments increases. This increases the amount of force each myocyte can generate, and thus increases the strength and work capacity of the muscle as a whole.

The massive physiologic growth of the uterus during pregnancy is a good example of hormone-induced increase in the size of an organ that results mainly from hypertrophy of muscle fibers (Fig. 1–3). The cellular enlargement is stimulated by estrogenic hormones acting on smooth muscle estrogen receptors, eventually resulting in increased synthesis of smooth muscle proteins and an increase in cell size.

Although the traditional view of cardiac and skeletal muscle is that in adults these tissues are incapable of proliferation and, therefore, their enlargement is entirely a result of hypertrophy, there is now accumulating evidence that even these cell types are capable of some proliferation as well as repopulation from precursors, in addition to hypertrophy (Chapter 3).[2]

Mechanisms of Hypertrophy

Hypertrophy is the result of increased production of cellular proteins. Much of our understanding of hypertrophy is based on studies of the heart. Hypertrophy can be induced by the linked actions of mechanical sensors (that are triggered by increased work load), growth factors (including TGF-β, insulin-like growth factor-1 [IGF-1], fibroblast growth factor), and vasoactive agents (such as α-adrenergic agonists, endothelin-1, and angiotensin II). Indeed, mechanical sensors themselves induce production of growth factors and agonists (Fig. 1–4).[3-5] These stimuli work coordinately to increase the synthesis of muscle proteins that are responsible for the hypertrophy. The two main biochemical pathways involved in muscle hypertrophy seem to be the phosphoinositide 3-kinase/Akt pathway (postulated to be most important in physiologic, e.g., exercise-induced, hypertrophy) and signaling downstream of G protein-coupled receptors (induced by many growth factors and vasoactive agents, and thought to be more important in pathologic hypertrophy). Hypertrophy may also be associated with a switch of contractile proteins from adult to fetal or neonatal forms. For example, during muscle hypertrophy the α isoform of myosin heavy chain is replaced by the β isoform, which has a slower, more energetically economical contraction. In addition, some genes that are expressed only during early development are re-expressed in hypertrophic cells, and the products of these genes participate in the cellular response to stress. For example, the gene for atrial natriuretic factor (ANF) is expressed in both the atrium and the ventricle in the embryonic heart, but it is down-regulated after birth. Cardiac hypertrophy, however, is associated with reinduction of ANF gene expression. ANF is a peptide hormone that causes salt secretion by the kidney, decreases blood volume and pressure, and therefore serves to reduce hemodynamic load.

Whatever the exact cause and mechanism of cardiac hypertrophy, it eventually reaches a limit beyond which enlargement of muscle mass is no longer able to compensate for the increased burden. At this stage several regressive changes occur in the myocardial fibers, of which the most important are lysis and loss of myofibrillar contractile elements. In extreme cases myocyte death can occur by either apoptosis or necrosis.[5,6] The net result of these changes is cardiac failure, a sequence of events that illustrates how *an adaptation to stress can progress to functionally significant cell injury if the stress is not relieved.*

Although hypertrophy usually refers to increase in size of cells or tissues, sometimes a subcellular organelle may undergo selective hypertrophy. For instance, individuals treated with drugs such as barbiturates show hypertrophy of the smooth endoplamic reticulum (ER) in hepatocytes, which is an adaptive response that increases the amount of enzymes (cytochrome P-450 mixed function oxidases) available to detoxify the drugs. Over time, the patients respond less to the drug because of this adaptation. Adaptation to one drug may result in an increased capacity to metabolize other drugs. For instance, alcohol intake causes hypertrophy of the smooth ER and may lead to reduced levels of available barbiturates that are being taken at the same time. Although P-450-mediated modification is often thought of as "detoxification," many compounds are rendered *more* injurious by this process. In addition, the products formed by this oxidative metabolism include reactive oxygen species, which can injure the cell. Normal genetic variations (polymorphisms) influence the activity of P-450, and thus the sensitivity of different individuals to various drugs.[7]

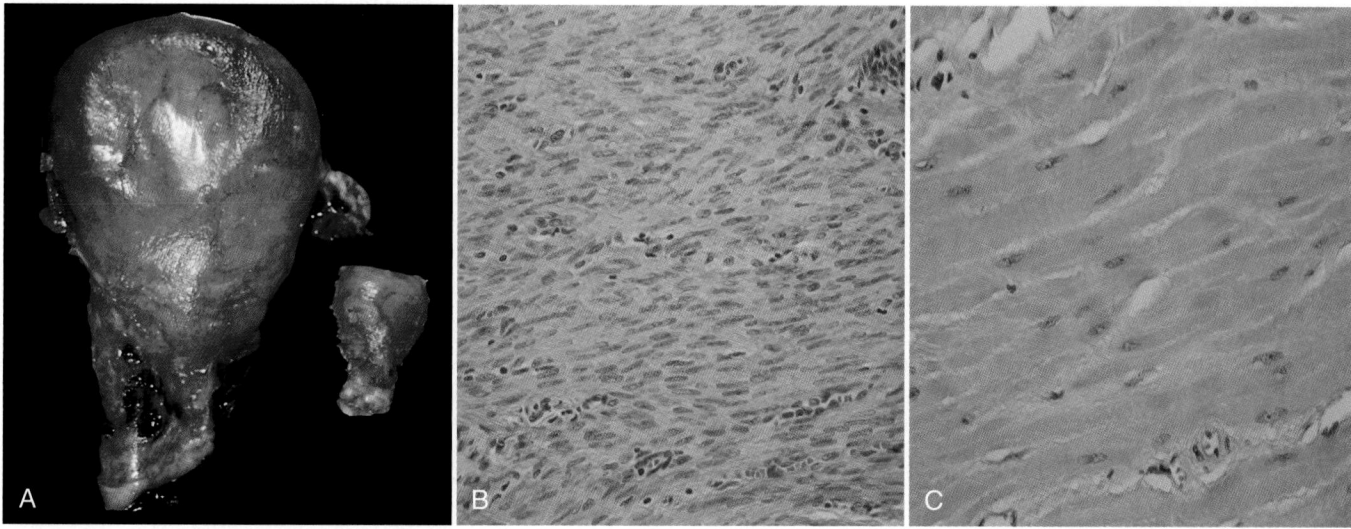

FIGURE 1–3 Physiologic hypertrophy of the uterus during pregnancy. **A,** Gross appearance of a normal uterus *(right)* and a gravid uterus (removed for postpartum bleeding) *(left)*. **B,** Small spindle-shaped uterine smooth muscle cells from a normal uterus, compared with **C,** large plump cells from the gravid uterus, at the same magnification.

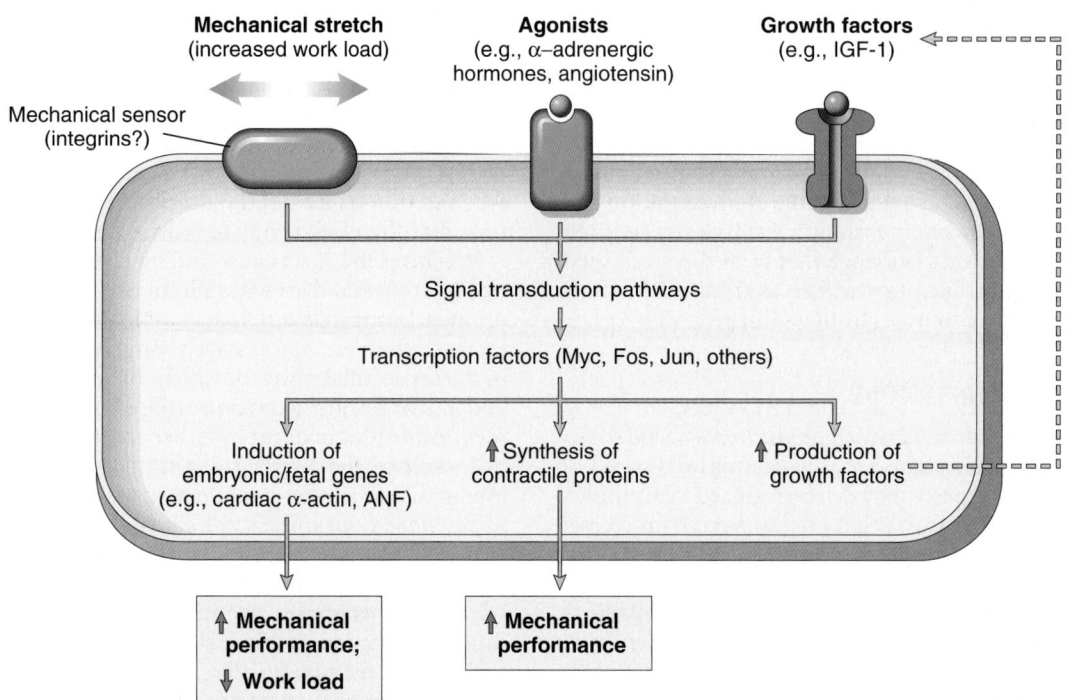

FIGURE 1–4   Biochemical mechanisms of myocardial hypertrophy. The major known signaling pathways and their functional effects are shown. Mechanical sensors appear to be the major triggers for physiologic hypertrophy, and agonists and growth factors may be more important in pathologic states. ANF, atrial natriuretic factor; IGF-1, insulin-like growth factor.

HYPERPLASIA

Hyperplasia is an increase in the number of cells in an organ or tissue, usually resulting in increased mass of the organ or tissue. Although hyperplasia and hypertrophy are distinct processes, frequently they occur together, and they may be triggered by the same external stimulus. Hyperplasia takes place if the cell population is capable of dividing, and thus increasing the number of cells. Hyperplasia can be physiologic or pathologic.

Physiologic Hyperplasia

Physiologic hyperplasia can be divided into: (1) *hormonal hyperplasia*, which increases the functional capacity of a tissue when needed, and (2) *compensatory hyperplasia*, which increases tissue mass after damage or partial resection. Hormonal hyperplasia is well illustrated by the proliferation of the glandular epithelium of the female breast at puberty and during pregnancy, usually accompanied by enlargement (hypertrophy) of the glandular epithelial cells. The classical illustration of compensatory hyperplasia comes from the myth of Prometheus, which shows that the ancient Greeks recognized the capacity of the liver to regenerate. As punishment for having stolen the secret of fire from the gods, Prometheus was chained to a mountain, and his liver was devoured daily by an eagle, only to regenerate anew every night.[1] In individuals who donate one lobe of the liver for transplantation, the remaining cells proliferate so that the organ soon grows back to its original size. Experimental models of partial hepatectomy have been very useful for defining the mechanisms that stimulate regeneration of the liver[7] (Chapter 3).

Pathologic Hyperplasia

Most forms of pathologic hyperplasia are caused by *excesses of hormones or growth factors* acting on target cells. Endometrial hyperplasia is an example of abnormal hormone-induced hyperplasia. Normally, after a menstrual period there is a rapid burst of proliferative activity in the epithelium that is stimulated by pituitary hormones and ovarian estrogen. It is brought to a halt by the rising levels of progesterone, usually about 10 to 14 days before the end of the menstrual period. In some instances, however, the balance between estrogen and progesterone is disturbed. This results in absolute or relative increases in the amount of estrogen, with consequent hyperplasia of the endometrial glands. This form of pathologic hyperplasia is a common cause of abnormal menstrual bleeding. Benign prostatic hyperplasia is another common example of pathologic hyperplasia induced by responses to hormones, in this case, androgens. Although these forms of hyperplasia are abnormal, the process remains controlled because there are no mutations in genes that regulate cell division, and the hyperplasia regresses if the hormonal stimulation is eliminated. As is discussed in Chapter 7, in cancer the growth control mechanisms become dysregulated or ineffective because of genetic aberrations, resulting in unrestrained proliferation. *Thus, hyperplasia is distinct from cancer, but pathologic hyperplasia constitutes a fertile soil in which cancerous proliferation may eventually arise.* For instance, patients with hyperplasia of the endometrium are at increased risk for developing endometrial cancer (Chapter 22).

Hyperplasia is a characteristic response to certain *viral infections,* such as papillomaviruses, which cause skin warts and several mucosal lesions composed of masses of hyperplastic epithelium. Here, growth factors produced by viral genes or by infected cells may stimulate cellular proliferation (Chapter 7).

Mechanisms of Hyperplasia

Hyperplasia is the result of growth factor–driven proliferation of mature cells and, in some cases, by increased output of new cells from tissue stem cells. For instance, after partial hepatectomy growth factors are produced in the liver that engage receptors on the surviving cells and activate signaling pathways that stimulate cell proliferation. But if the proliferative capacity of the liver cells is compromised, as in some forms of hepatitis causing cell injury, hepatocytes can instead regenerate from intrahepatic stem cells.[8] The roles of growth factors and stem cells in cellular replication and tissue hyperplasia are discussed in more detail in Chapter 3.

ATROPHY

Atrophy is reduced size of an organ or tissue resulting from a decrease in cell size and number. Atrophy can be physiologic or pathologic. *Physiologic atrophy* is common during normal development. Some embryonic structures, such as the notochord and thyroglossal duct, undergo atrophy during fetal development. The uterus decreases in size shortly after parturition, and this is a form of physiologic atrophy.

Pathologic atrophy depends on the underlying cause and can be local or generalized. The common causes of atrophy are the following:

○ *Decreased workload (atrophy of disuse).* When a fractured bone is immobilized in a plaster cast or when a patient is restricted to complete bedrest, skeletal muscle atrophy rapidly ensues. The initial decrease in cell size is reversible once activity is resumed. With more prolonged disuse, skeletal muscle fibers decrease in number (due to apoptosis) as well as in size; this atrophy can be accompanied by increased bone resorption, leading to osteoporosis of disuse.

○ *Loss of innervation (denervation atrophy).* The normal metabolism and function of skeletal muscle are dependent on its nerve supply. Damage to the nerves leads to atrophy of the muscle fibers supplied by those nerves (Chapter 27).

○ *Diminished blood supply.* A decrease in blood supply (ischemia) to a tissue as a result of slowly developing arterial occlusive disease results in atrophy of the tissue. In late adult life, the brain may undergo progressive atrophy, mainly because of reduced blood supply as a result of atherosclerosis (Fig. 1–5). This is called *senile atrophy*; it also affects the heart.

○ *Inadequate nutrition.* Profound protein-calorie malnutrition (marasmus) is associated with the use of skeletal muscle as a source of energy after other reserves such as adipose stores have been depleted. This results in marked muscle wasting (*cachexia*; Chapter 9). Cachexia is also seen in patients with chronic inflammatory diseases and cancer. In the former, chronic overproduction of the inflammatory cytokine tumor necrosis factor (TNF) is thought to be responsible for appetite suppression and lipid depletion, culminating in muscle atrophy.

○ *Loss of endocrine stimulation.* Many hormone-responsive tissues, such as the breast and reproductive organs, are dependent on endocrine stimulation for normal metabolism and function. The loss of estrogen stimulation after menopause results in physiologic atrophy of the endometrium, vaginal epithelium, and breast.

○ *Pressure.* Tissue compression for any length of time can cause atrophy. An enlarging benign tumor can cause atrophy in the surrounding uninvolved tissues. Atrophy

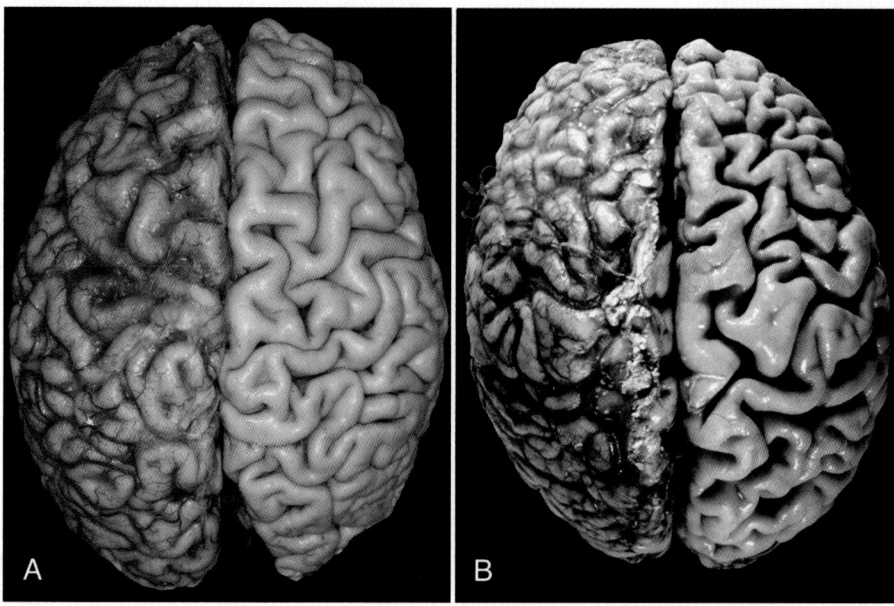

FIGURE 1–5   Atrophy. **A,** Normal brain of a young adult. **B,** Atrophy of the brain in an 82-year-old male with atherosclerotic cerebrovascular disease, resulting in reduced blood supply. Note that loss of brain substance narrows the gyri and widens the sulci. The meninges have been stripped from the right half of each specimen to reveal the surface of the brain.

in this setting is probably the result of ischemic changes caused by compromise of the blood supply by the pressure exerted by the expanding mass.

The fundamental cellular changes associated with atrophy are identical in all of these settings. The initial response is a decrease in cell size and organelles, which may reduce the metabolic needs of the cell sufficiently to permit its survival. In atrophic muscle, the cells contain fewer mitochondria and myofilaments and a reduced amount of rough ER. By bringing into balance the cell's metabolic demand and the lower levels of blood supply, nutrition, or trophic stimulation, a new equilibrium is achieved. *Early in the process atrophic cells may have diminished function, but they are not dead.* However, atrophy caused by gradually reduced blood supply may progress to the point at which cells are irreversibly injured and die, often by apoptosis. Cell death by apoptosis also contributes to the atrophy of endocrine organs after hormone withdrawal.

Mechanisms of Atrophy

Atrophy results from decreased protein synthesis and increased protein degradation in cells. Protein synthesis decreases because of reduced metabolic activity. The degradation of cellular proteins occurs mainly by the *ubiquitin-proteasome pathway.* Nutrient deficiency and disuse may activate ubiquitin ligases, which attach the small peptide ubiquitin to cellular proteins and target these proteins for degradation in *proteasomes.*[3,9,10] This pathway is also thought to be responsible for the accelerated proteolysis seen in a variety of catabolic conditions, including cancer cachexia.

In many situations, atrophy is also accompanied by increased *autophagy,* with resulting increases in the number of *autophagic vacuoles.* Autophagy ("self eating") is the process in which the starved cell eats its own components in an attempt to find nutrients and survive. Autophagic vacuoles are membrane-bound vacuoles that contain fragments of cell components. The vacuoles ultimately fuse with lysosomes, and their contents are digested by lysosomal enzymes. Some of the cell debris within the autophagic vacuoles may resist digestion and persist as membrane-bound *residual bodies* that may remain as a sarcophagus in the cytoplasm. An example of such residual bodies is the *lipofuscin granules,* discussed later in the chapter. When present in sufficient amounts, they impart a brown discoloration to the tissue *(brown atrophy).* Autophagy is associated with various types of cell injury, and we will discuss it in more detail later.

METAPLASIA

Metaplasia is a reversible change in which one differentiated cell type (epithelial or mesenchymal) is replaced by another cell type. It may represent an adaptive substitution of cells that are sensitive to stress by cell types better able to withstand the adverse environment.

The most common epithelial metaplasia is *columnar* to *squamous* (Fig. 1–6), as occurs in the respiratory tract in response to chronic irritation. In the habitual cigarette smoker, the normal ciliated columnar epithelial cells of the trachea and bronchi are often replaced by stratified squamous epithelial

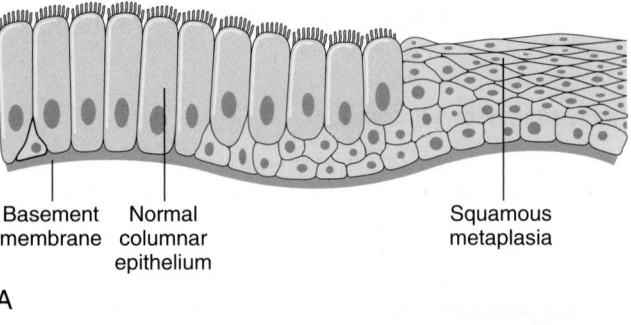

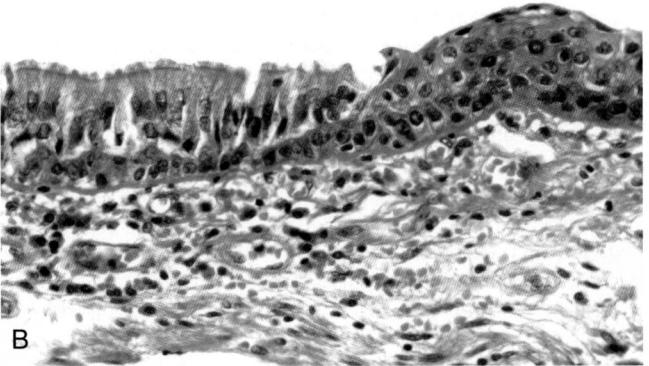

FIGURE 1–6 Metaplasia of columnar to squamous epithelium. **A,** Schematic diagram. **B,** Metaplasia of columnar epithelium *(left)* to squamous epithelium *(right)* in a bronchus.

cells. Stones in the excretory ducts of the salivary glands, pancreas, or bile ducts may also cause replacement of the normal secretory columnar epithelium by stratified squamous epithelium. A deficiency of vitamin A (retinoic acid) induces squamous metaplasia in the respiratory epithelium (Chapter 9). In all these instances the more rugged stratified squamous epithelium is able to survive under circumstances in which the more fragile specialized columnar epithelium might have succumbed. However, the change to metaplastic squamous cells comes with a price. In the respiratory tract, for example, although the epithelial lining becomes tough, important mechanisms of protection against infection—mucus secretion and the ciliary action of the columnar epithelium—are lost. Thus, epithelial metaplasia is a double-edged sword and, in most circumstances, represents an undesirable change. Moreover, *the influences that predispose to metaplasia, if persistent, may initiate malignant transformation in metaplastic epithelium.* Thus, a common form of cancer in the respiratory tract is composed of squamous cells, which arise in areas of metaplasia of the normal columnar epithelium into squamous epithelium.

Metaplasia from squamous to columnar type may also occur, as in *Barrett esophagus,* in which the esophageal squamous epithelium is replaced by intestinal-like columnar cells under the influence of refluxed gastric acid. Cancers may arise in these areas; these are typically glandular (adeno)carcinomas (Chapter 17).

Connective tissue metaplasia is the formation of cartilage, bone, or adipose tissue (mesenchymal tissues) in tissues that normally do not contain these elements. For example, bone formation in muscle, designated *myositis ossificans,* occasionally occurs after intramuscular hemorrhage. This type of metaplasia is less clearly seen as an adaptive response, and may be a result of cell or tissue injury.

Mechanisms of Metaplasia

Metaplasia does not result from a change in the phenotype of an already differentiated cell type; instead it is *the result of a reprogramming of stem cells that are known to exist in normal tissues, or of undifferentiated mesenchymal cells present in connective tissue.* In a metaplastic change, these precursor cells differentiate along a new pathway. The differentiation of stem cells to a particular lineage is brought about by signals generated by cytokines, growth factors, and extracellular matrix components in the cells' environment.[11,12] These external stimuli promote the expression of genes that drive cells toward a specific differentiation pathway. In the case of vitamin A deficiency or excess, it is known that retinoic acid regulates gene transcription directly through nuclear retinoid receptors (Chapter 9), which can influence the differentiation of progenitors derived from tissue stem cells. How other external stimuli cause metaplasia is unknown, but it is clear that they too somehow alter the activity of transcription factors that regulate differentiation.

Overview of Cell Injury and Cell Death

As stated at the beginning of the chapter, cell injury results when cells are stressed so severely that they are no longer able to adapt or when cells are exposed to inherently damaging agents or suffer from intrinsic abnormalities. Injury may progress through a reversible stage and culminate in cell death (see Fig. 1–1).

- *Reversible cell injury.* In early stages or mild forms of injury, the functional and morphologic changes are reversible if the damaging stimulus is removed. The hallmarks of reversible injury are reduced oxidative phosphorylation with resultant depletion of energy stores in the form of adenosine triphosphate (ATP), and cellular swelling caused by changes in ion concentrations and water influx. In addition, various intracellular organelles, such as mitochondria and the cytoskeleton, may also show alterations.
- *Cell death.* With continuing damage the injury becomes irreversible, at which time the cell cannot recover and it dies. *There are two principal types of cell death, necrosis and apoptosis, which differ in their morphology, mechanisms, and roles in physiology and disease.*[13–15] When damage to membranes is severe, lysosomal enzymes enter the cytoplasm and digest the cell, and cellular contents leak out, resulting in *necrosis.* In situations when the cell's DNA or proteins are damaged beyond repair, the cell kills itself by *apoptosis,* a form of cell death that is characterized by nuclear dissolution, fragmentation of the cell without complete loss of membrane integrity, and rapid removal of the cellular debris. *Whereas necrosis is always a pathologic process, apoptosis serves many normal functions and is not necessarily associated with cell injury.* Cell death is also sometimes the end result of

autophagy. Although it is easier to understand these pathways of cell death by discussing them separately, there may be many connections between them. Both apoptosis and necrosis may be seen in response to the same insult, such as ischemia, perhaps at different stages. Apoptosis can progress to necrosis, and cell death during autophagy may show many of the biochemical characteristics of apoptosis.

In the following sections we discuss the causes, morphologic features, and mechanisms of cell injury and its common end point, necrosis, with selected illustrative examples. We conclude with a discussion of the unique pattern of cell death represented by apoptosis, and then a brief description of the process of autophagy and how it may progress to cell death.

Causes of Cell Injury

The causes of cell injury range from the external gross physical violence of an automobile accident to subtle internal abnormalities, such as a genetic mutation causing lack of a vital enzyme that impairs normal metabolic function. Most injurious stimuli can be grouped into the following broad categories.

Oxygen Deprivation. *Hypoxia* is a deficiency of oxygen, which causes cell injury by reducing aerobic oxidative respiration. Hypoxia is an extremely important and common cause of cell injury and cell death. *Causes of hypoxia* include reduced blood flow (celled *ischemia*), inadequate oxygenation of the blood due to cardiorespiratory failure, and decreased oxygen-carrying capacity of the blood, as in anemia or carbon monoxide poisoning (producing a stable carbon monoxyhemoglobin that blocks oxygen carriage) or after severe blood loss. Depending on the severity of the hypoxic state, cells may adapt, undergo injury, or die. For example, if an artery is narrowed, the tissue supplied by that vessel may initially shrink in size (atrophy), whereas more severe or sudden hypoxia induces injury and cell death.

Physical Agents. Physical agents capable of causing cell injury include mechanical trauma, extremes of temperature (burns and deep cold), sudden changes in atmospheric pressure, radiation, and electric shock (Chapter 9).

Chemical Agents and Drugs. The list of chemicals that may produce cell injury defies compilation. Simple chemicals such as glucose or salt in hypertonic concentrations may cause cell injury directly or by deranging electrolyte balance in cells. Even oxygen at high concentrations is toxic. Trace amounts of *poisons,* such as arsenic, cyanide, or mercuric salts, may destroy sufficient numbers of cells within minutes or hours to cause death. Other potentially injurious substances are our daily companions: environmental and air pollutants, insecticides, and herbicides; industrial and occupational hazards, such as carbon monoxide and asbestos; recreational drugs such as alcohol; and the ever-increasing variety of therapeutic drugs.

Infectious Agents. These agents range from the submicroscopic viruses to the large tapeworms. In between are the rickettsiae, bacteria, fungi, and higher forms of parasites. The ways by which these biologic agents cause injury are diverse and are discussed in Chapter 8.

Immunologic Reactions. The immune system serves an essential function in defense against infectious pathogens, but immune reactions may also cause cell injury. Injurious reactions to endogenous self-antigens are responsible for several autoimmune diseases (Chapter 6). Immune reactions to many external agents, such as microbes and environmental substances, are also important causes of cell and tissue injury (Chapters 2 and 6).

Genetic Derangements. As described in Chapter 5, genetic abnormalities may result in a defect as severe as the congenital malformations associated with Down syndrome, caused by a chromosomal anomaly, or as subtle as the decreased life span of red blood cells caused by a single amino acid substitution in hemoglobin in sickle cell anemia. Genetic defects may cause cell injury because of deficiency of functional proteins, such as enzyme defects in inborn errors of metabolism, or accumulation of damaged DNA or misfolded proteins, both of which trigger cell death when they are beyond repair. Variations in the genetic makeup can also influence the susceptibility of cells to injury by chemicals and other environmental insults.

Nutritional Imbalances. Nutritional imbalances continue to be major causes of cell injury. Protein-calorie deficiencies cause an appalling number of deaths, chiefly among underprivileged populations. Deficiencies of specific vitamins are found throughout the world (Chapter 9). Nutritional problems can be self-imposed, as in anorexia nervosa (self-induced starvation). Ironically, nutritional excesses have also become important causes of cell injury. Excess of cholesterol predisposes to atherosclerosis; obesity is associated with increased incidence of several important diseases, such as diabetes and cancer. Atherosclerosis is virtually endemic in the United States, and obesity is rampant. In addition to the problems of undernutrition and overnutrition, the composition of the diet makes a significant contribution to a number of diseases.

Morphologic Alterations in Cell Injury

It is useful to describe the basic alterations that occur in damaged cells before we discuss the biochemical mechanisms that bring about these changes. All stresses and noxious influences exert their effects first at the molecular or biochemical level. There is a time lag between the stress and the morphologic changes of cell injury or death; the duration of this delay may vary with the sensitivity of the methods used to detect these changes (Fig. 1–7). With histochemical or ultrastructural techniques, changes may be seen in minutes to hours after injury; however, it may take considerably longer (hours to days) before changes can be seen by light microscopy or on gross examination. As would be expected, the morphologic manifestations of necrosis take more time to develop than those of reversible damage. For example, in ischemia of the myocardium, cell swelling is a reversible morphologic change that may occur in a matter of minutes, and may progress to irreversibility within an hour or two. Unmistakable light microscopic changes of cell death, however, may not be seen until 4 to 12 hours after total ischemia.

The sequential morphologic changes in cell injury progressing to cell death are illustrated in Figure 1–8. Reversible injury

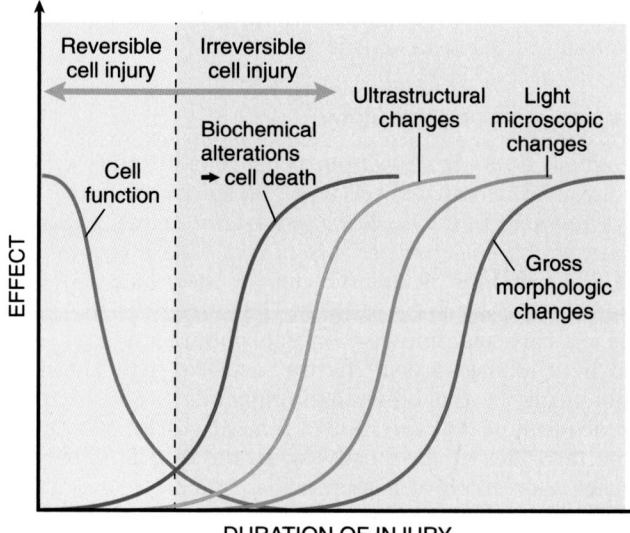

FIGURE 1–7 Sequential development of biochemical and morphologic changes in cell injury. Cells may become rapidly nonfunctional after the onset of injury, although they are still viable, with potentially reversible damage; a longer duration of injury may eventually lead to irreversible injury and cell death. Note that irreversible biochemical alterations may cause cell death, and typically this precedes ultrastructural, light microscopic, and grossly visible morphologic changes.

is characterized by generalized swelling of the cell and its organelles; blebbing of the plasma membrane; detachment of ribosomes from the ER; and clumping of nuclear chromatin. These morphologic changes are associated with decreased generation of ATP, loss of cell membrane integrity, defects in protein synthesis, cytoskeletal damage, and DNA damage. Within limits, the cell can repair these derangements and, if the injurious stimulus abates, will return to normalcy. Persistent or excessive injury, however, causes cells to pass the rather nebulous "point of no return" into irreversible injury and *cell death*. Different injurious stimuli may induce death by necrosis or apoptosis (Fig. 1–8 and Table 1–2). Severe mitochondrial damage with depletion of ATP and rupture of lysosomal and plasma membranes are typically associated with necrosis. Necrosis is the principal outcome in many commonly encountered injuries, such as those following ischemia, exposure to toxins, various infections, and trauma. Apoptosis has many unique features, and we will describe it later in the chapter.

REVERSIBLE INJURY

Two features of reversible cell injury can be recognized under the light microscope: *cellular swelling* and *fatty change*. Cellular swelling appears whenever cells are incapable of maintaining ionic and fluid homeostasis and is the result of failure of energy-dependent ion pumps in the plasma membrane. Fatty change occurs in hypoxic injury and various forms of toxic or metabolic injury. It is manifested by the appearance of lipid vacuoles in the cytoplasm. It is seen mainly in cells involved in and dependent on fat metabolism, such as hepatocytes and myocardial cells. The mechanisms of fatty change are discussed later in the chapter.

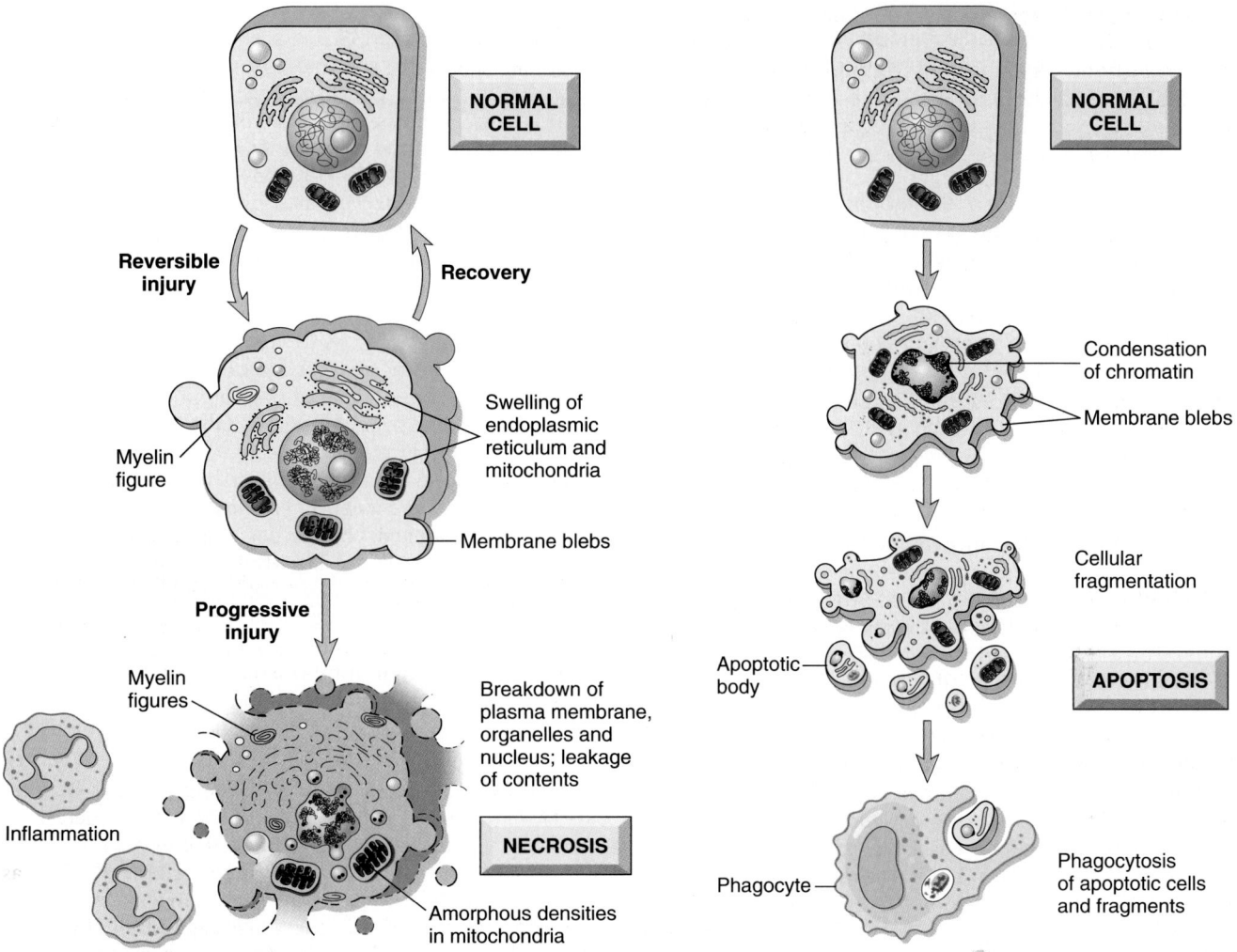

FIGURE 1–8 Schematic illustration of the morphologic changes in cell injury culminating in necrosis or apoptosis.

Morphology. Cellular swelling is the first manifestation of almost all forms of injury to cells (Fig. 1–9B). It is a difficult morphologic change to appreciate with the light microscope; it may be more apparent at the level of the whole organ. When it affects many cells, it causes some pallor, increased turgor, and increase in weight of the organ. On microscopic examination, small clear vacuoles may be seen within the cytoplasm; these represent distended and pinched-off segments of the ER. This pattern of nonlethal injury is sometimes called hydropic change or vacuolar degeneration. Swelling of cells is reversible. Cells

TABLE 1–2 Features of Necrosis and Apoptosis		
Feature	**Necrosis**	**Apoptosis**
Cell size	Enlarged (swelling)	Reduced (shrinkage)
Nucleus	Pyknosis → karyorrhexis → karyolysis	Fragmentation into nucleosome-size fragments
Plasma membrane	Disrupted	Intact; altered structure, especially orientation of lipids
Cellular contents	Enzymatic digestion; may leak out of cell	Intact; may be released in apoptotic bodies
Adjacent inflammation	Frequent	No
Physiologic or pathologic role	Invariably pathologic (culmination of irreversible cell injury)	Often physiologic, means of eliminating unwanted cells; may be pathologic after some forms of cell injury, especially DNA damage

may also show increased eosinophilic staining, which becomes much more pronounced with progression to necrosis (described below).

The ultrastructural changes of reversible cell injury (Fig. 1–10B) include:

1. **Plasma membrane alterations,** such as blebbing, blunting, and loss of microvilli
2. **Mitochondrial changes,** including swelling and the appearance of small amorphous densities
3. **Dilation** of the ER, with detachment of polysomes; intracytoplasmic myelin figures may be present (see later)
4. **Nuclear alterations,** with disaggregation of granular and fibrillar elements.

NECROSIS

The morphologic appearance of necrosis is the result of *denaturation of intracellular proteins and enzymatic digestion of the lethally injured cell* (cells placed immediately in fixative are dead but not necrotic). Necrotic cells are unable to maintain membrane integrity and their contents often leak out, a process that may elicit inflammation in the surrounding tissue. The enzymes that digest the necrotic cell are derived from the lysosomes of the dying cells themselves and from the lysosomes of leukocytes that are called in as part of the inflammatory reaction. Digestion of cellular contents and the host response may take hours to develop, and so there would be no detectable changes in cells if, for example, a myocardial infarct caused sudden death. The only circumstantial evidence might be occlusion of a coronary artery. The earliest histologic evidence of myocardial necrosis does not become apparent until 4 to 12 hours later. However, because of the loss of plasma membrane integrity, cardiac-specific enzymes and proteins are rapidly released from necrotic muscle and can be detected in the blood as early as 2 hours after myocardial cell necrosis.

Morphology. Necrotic cells show **increased eosinophilia** in hematoxylin and eosin (H & E) stains, attributable in part to the loss of cytoplasmic RNA (which binds the blue dye, hematoxylin) and in part to denatured cytoplasmic proteins (which bind the red dye, eosin). The necrotic cell may have a more glassy homogeneous appearance than do normal cells, mainly as a result of the loss of glycogen particles (Fig. 1–9C). When enzymes have digested the cytoplasmic organelles, the cytoplasm becomes vacuolated and appears moth-eaten. Dead cells may be replaced by large, whorled phospholipid masses called **myelin figures** that are derived from damaged cell membranes. These phospholipid precipitates are then either phagocytosed by other cells or further degraded into fatty acids; calcification of such fatty acid residues results in the generation of calcium soaps. Thus, the dead cells may ultimately become calcified. By electron microscopy, necrotic cells are characterized by discontinuities in plasma and organelle membranes, marked dilation of mitochondria with the appearance of large amorphous densities, intracytoplasmic myelin figures, amorphous debris, and aggregates of fluffy material probably representing denatured protein (see Fig. 1–10C).

Nuclear changes appear in one of three patterns, all due to nonspecific breakdown of DNA (see Fig. 1–9C). The basophilia of the chromatin may fade **(karyolysis),** a change that presumably reflects loss of DNA because of enzymatic degradation by endonucleases. A second pattern (which is also seen in apoptotic cell death) is **pyknosis,** characterized by nuclear shrinkage and increased basophilia. Here the chromatin condenses into a solid, shrunken basophilic mass. In the third pattern, known as **karyorrhexis,** the pyknotic nucleus undergoes fragmentation. With the passage of time (a day or two), the nucleus in the necrotic cell totally disappears.

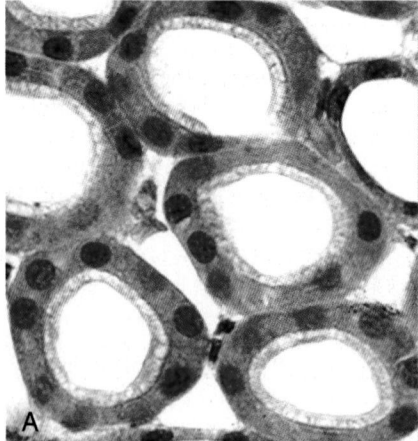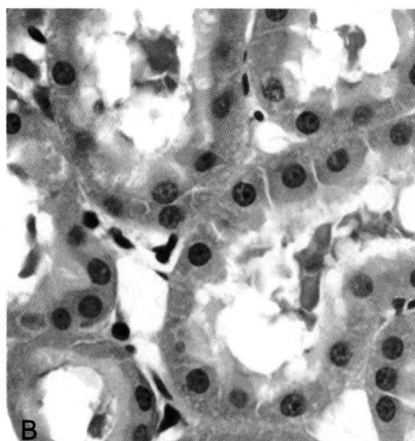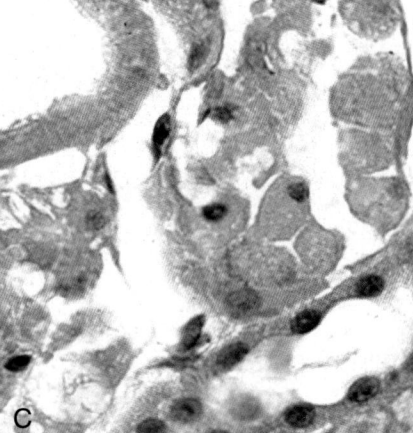

FIGURE 1–9 Morphologic changes in reversible cell injury and necrosis. **A,** Normal kidney tubules with viable epithelial cells. **B,** Early (reversible) ischemic injury showing surface blebs, increased eosinophilia of cytoplasm, and swelling of occasional cells. **C,** Necrosis (irreversible injury) of epithelial cells, with loss of nuclei, fragmentation of cells, and leakage of contents. The ultrastructural features of these stages of cell injury are shown in Figure 1–10. (Courtesy of Drs. Neal Pinckard and M.A. Venkatachalam, University of Texas Health Sciences Center, San Antonio, TX.)

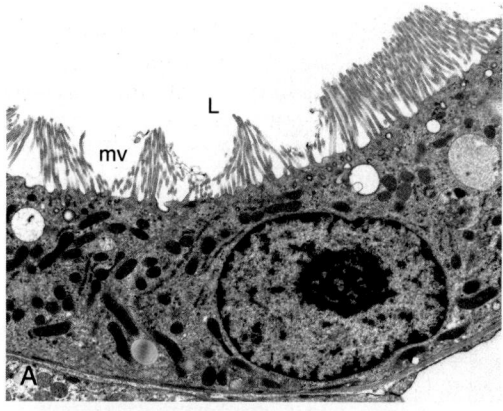

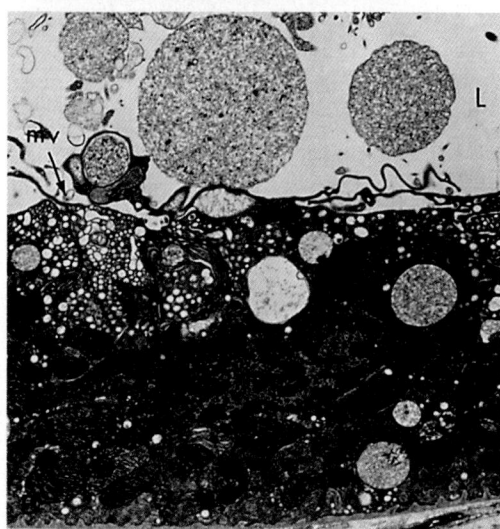

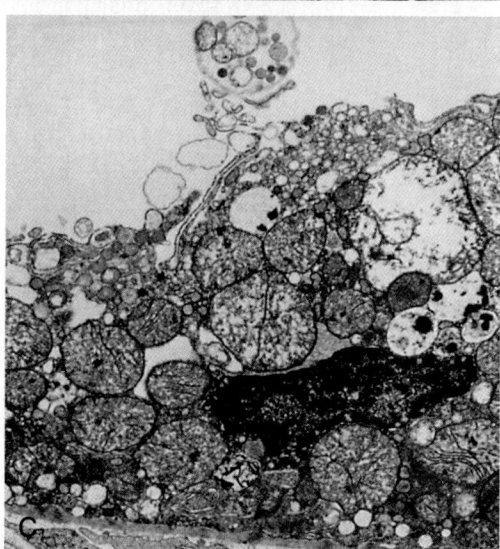

FIGURE 1–10 Ultrastructural features of reversible and irreversible cell injury (necrosis) in a rabbit kidney. **A,** Electron micrograph of a normal epithelial cell of the proximal kidney tubule. Note abundant microvilli (mv) lining the luminal surface (L). **B,** Epithelial cell of the proximal tubule showing early cell injury resulting from reperfusion following ischemia. The microvilli are lost and have been incorporated in apical cytoplasm; blebs have formed and are extruded in the lumen. Mitochondria would have been swollen during ischemia; with reperfusion, they rapidly undergo condensation and become electron-dense. **C,** Proximal tubular cell showing late injury, expected to be irreversible. Note the markedly swollen mitochondria containing electron-dense deposits, expected to contain precipitated calcium and proteins. Higher magnification micrographs of the cell would show disrupted plasma membrane and swelling and fragmentation of organelles. (**A,** Courtesy of Dr. Brigitte Kaisslin, Institute of Anatomy, University of Zurich, Switzerland. **B, C,** Courtesy of Dr. M.A. Venkatachalam, University of Texas Health Sciences Center, San Antonio, TX.)

they may provide clues about the underlying cause. Although the terms that describe these patterns are somewhat outmoded, they are used often and their implications are understood by pathologists and clinicians.

> **Morphology. Coagulative necrosis** is a form of necrosis in which the architecture of dead tissues is preserved for a span of at least some days (Fig. 1–11). The affected tissues exhibit a firm texture. Presumably, the injury denatures not only structural proteins but also enzymes and so blocks the proteolysis of the dead cells; as a result, eosinophilic, anucleate cells may persist for days or weeks. Ultimately the necrotic cells are removed by phagocytosis of the cellular debris by infiltrating leukocytes and by digestion of the dead cells by the action of lysosomal enzymes of the leukocytes. Ischemia caused by obstruction in a vessel may lead to coagulative necrosis of the supplied tissue in all organs except the brain. A localized area of coagulative necrosis is called an **infarct**.
>
> **Liquefactive necrosis**, in contrast to coagulative necrosis, is characterized by digestion of the dead cells, resulting in transformation of the tissue into a liquid viscous mass. It is seen in focal bacterial or, occasionally, fungal infections, because microbes stimulate the accumulation of leukocytes and the liberation of enzymes from these cells. The necrotic material is frequently creamy yellow because of the presence of dead leukocytes and is called **pus**. For unknown reasons, hypoxic death of cells within the central nervous system often manifests as liquefactive necrosis (Fig. 1–12).
>
> **Gangrenous necrosis** is not a specific pattern of cell death, but the term is commonly used in clinical practice. It is usually applied to a limb, generally the lower leg, that has lost its blood supply and has undergone necrosis (typically coagulative necrosis) involving multiple tissue planes. When bacterial infection is superimposed there is more liquefactive necrosis because of the actions of degradative enzymes in the

Patterns of Tissue Necrosis

The discussion of necrosis has focused so far on changes in individual cells. When large numbers of cells die the tissue or organ is said to be necrotic; thus, a myocardial infarct is necrosis of a portion of the heart caused by death of many myocardial cells. Necrosis of tissues has several morphologically distinct patterns, which are important to recognize because

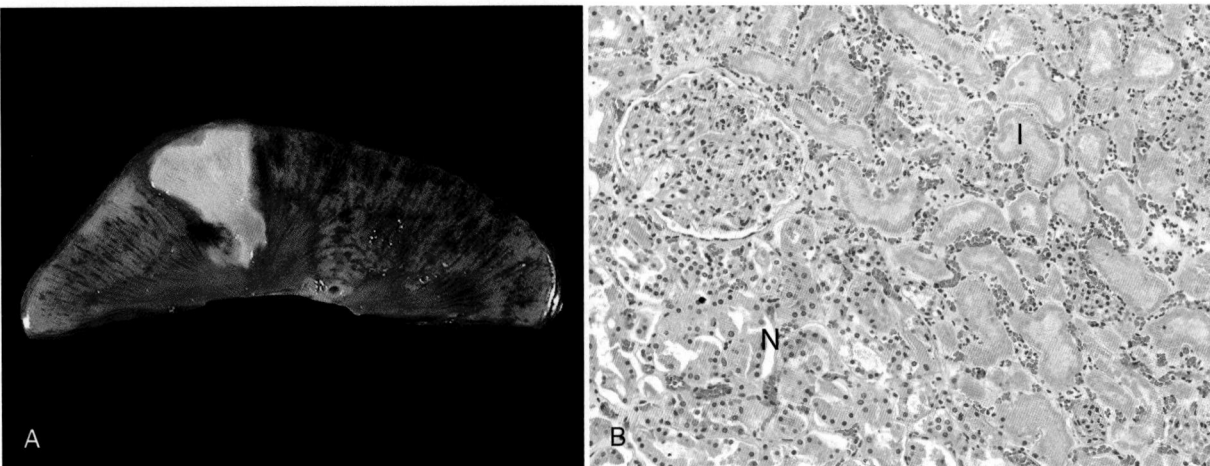

FIGURE 1–11 Coagulative necrosis. **A,** A wedge-shaped kidney infarct (yellow). **B,** Microscopic view of the edge of the infarct, with normal kidney (N) and necrotic cells in the infarct (I) showing preserved cellular outlines with loss of nuclei and an inflammatory infiltrate (which is difficult to discern at this magnification).

bacteria and the attracted leukocytes (giving rise to so-called **wet gangrene**).

Caseous necrosis is encountered most often in foci of tuberculous infection (Chapter 8). The term "caseous" (cheeselike) is derived from the friable white appearance of the area of necrosis (Fig. 1–13). On microscopic examination, the necrotic area appears as a collection of fragmented or lysed cells and amorphous granular debris enclosed within a distinctive inflammatory border; this appearance is characteristic of a focus of inflammation known as a **granuloma** (Chapter 2).

Fat necrosis is a term that is well fixed in medical parlance but does not in reality denote a specific pattern of necrosis. Rather, it refers to focal areas of fat destruction, typically resulting from release of activated pancreatic lipases into the substance of the pancreas and the peritoneal cavity. This occurs in the calamitous abdominal emergency known as acute pancreatitis (Chapter 19). In this disorder pancreatic enzymes leak out of acinar cells and liquefy the membranes of fat cells in the peritoneum. The released lipases split the triglyceride esters contained within fat cells. The fatty acids, so derived, combine with calcium to produce grossly visible chalky-white areas (fat saponification), which enable the surgeon and the pathologist to identify the lesions (Fig. 1–14). On histologic examination the necrosis takes the form of foci of shadowy outlines of necrotic fat cells, with basophilic calcium deposits, surrounded by an inflammatory reaction.

Fibrinoid necrosis is a special form of necrosis usually seen in immune reactions involving blood vessels. This pattern of necrosis typically occurs

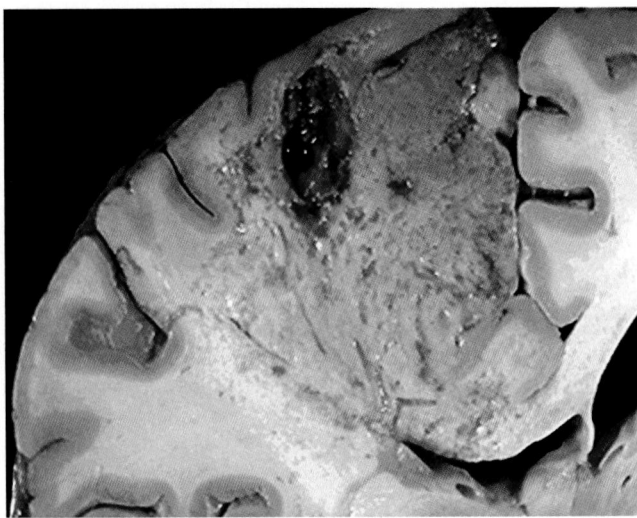

FIGURE 1–12 Liquefactive necrosis. An infarct in the brain, showing dissolution of the tissue.

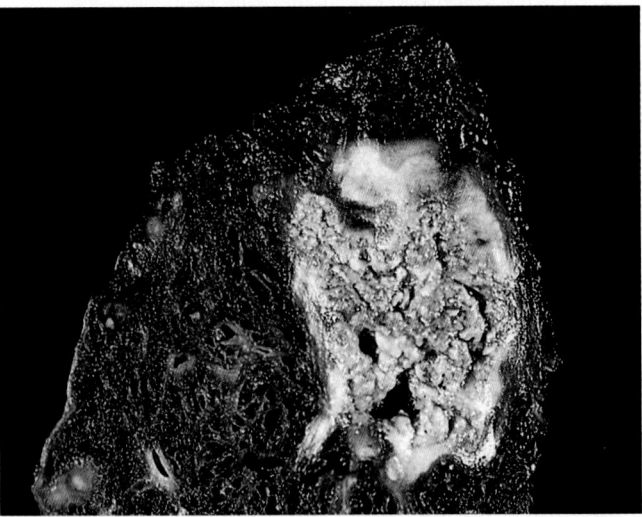

FIGURE 1–13 Caseous necrosis. Tuberculosis of the lung, with a large area of caseous necrosis containing yellow-white and cheesy debris.

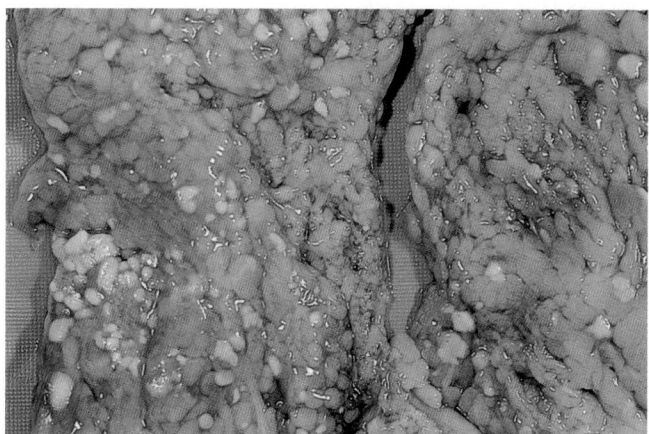

FIGURE 1-14   Fat necrosis. The areas of white chalky deposits represent foci of fat necrosis with calcium soap formation (saponification) at sites of lipid breakdown in the mesentery.

when complexes of antigens and antibodies are deposited in the walls of arteries. Deposits of these "immune complexes," together with fibrin that has leaked out of vessels, result in a bright pink and amorphous appearance in H&E stains, called "fibrinoid" (fibrin-like) by pathologists (Fig. 1-15). The immunologically mediated vasculitis syndromes in which this type of necrosis is seen are described in Chapter 6.

Ultimately, in the living patient most necrotic cells and their contents disappear by phagocytosis of the debris and enzymatic digestion by leukocytes. If necrotic cells and cellular debris are not promptly destroyed and reabsorbed, they tend to attract calcium salts and other minerals and to become calcified. This phenomenon, called *dystrophic calcification*, is considered later in the chapter.

Mechanisms of Cell Injury

The discussion of the cellular pathology of cell injury and necrosis sets the stage for a consideration of the mechanisms and biochemical pathways of cell injury. The mechanisms responsible for cell injury are complex. There are, however, several principles that are relevant to most forms of cell injury:

○ *The cellular response to injurious stimuli depends on the nature of the injury, its duration, and its severity.* Small doses of a chemical toxin or brief periods of ischemia may induce reversible injury, whereas large doses of the same toxin or more prolonged ischemia might result either in instantaneous cell death or in slow, irreversible injury leading in time to cell death.

○ *The consequences of cell injury depend on the type, state, and adaptability of the injured cell.* The cell's nutritional and hormonal status and its metabolic needs are important in its response to injury. How vulnerable is a cell, for example, to loss of blood supply

and hypoxia? When the striated muscle cell in the leg is deprived of its blood supply, it can be placed at rest and preserved; not so the striated muscle of the heart. Exposure of two individuals to identical concentrations of a toxin, such as carbon tetrachloride, may produce no effect in one and cell death in the other. This may be due to genetic variations affecting the amount and activity of hepatic enzymes that convert carbon tetrachloride (CCl_4) to toxic by-products (Chapter 9). With the complete mapping of the human genome, there is great interest in identifying genetic polymorphisms that affect the responses of different individuals to injurious agents.

○ *Cell injury results from different biochemical mechanisms acting on several essential cellular components* (Fig. 1-16). These mechanisms are described individually below. The cellular components that are most frequently damaged by injurious stimuli include mitochondria, cell membranes, the machinery of protein synthesis and packaging, and the DNA in nuclei.

○ Any injurious stimulus may simultaneously trigger multiple interconnected mechanisms that damage cells. This is one reason why it is difficult to ascribe cell injury in a particular situation to a single or even dominant biochemical derangement.

In the following section we describe the biochemical mechanisms that may be activated by different injurious stimuli and contribute to cell injury.[16] Our focus here is on reversible injury and necrosis, and the special cases of apoptosis and autophagy are best discussed separately.

DEPLETION OF ATP

ATP depletion and decreased ATP synthesis are frequently associated with both hypoxic and chemical (toxic) injury (Fig. 1-17). ATP is produced in two ways. The major pathway in mammalian cells is oxidative phosphorylation of adenosine diphosphate, in a reaction that results in reduction of oxygen by the electron transfer system of mitochondria. The second

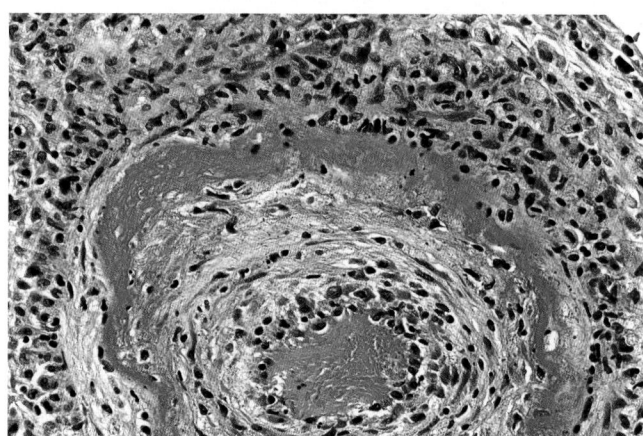

FIGURE 1-15   Fibrinoid necrosis in an artery. The wall of the artery shows a circumferential bright pink area of necrosis with inflammation (neutrophils with dark nuclei).

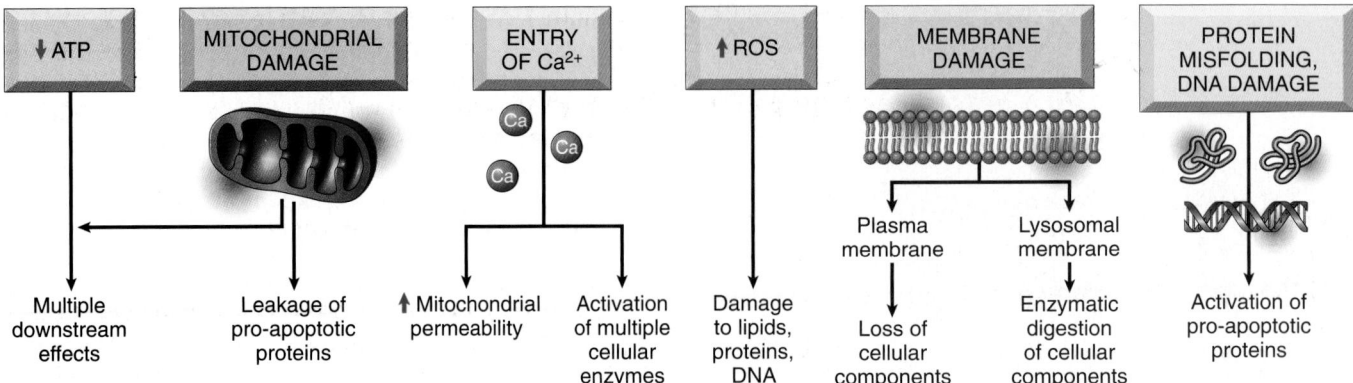

FIGURE 1–16 The principal mechanisms of cell injury, and their biochemical and functional effects, are shown. These are described in detail in the text.

is the glycolytic pathway, which can generate ATP in the absence of oxygen using glucose derived either from body fluids or from the hydrolysis of glycogen. *The major causes of ATP depletion are reduced supply of oxygen and nutrients, mitochondrial damage, and the actions of some toxins (e.g., cyanide).* Tissues with a greater glycolytic capacity (e.g., the liver) are able to survive loss of oxygen and decreased oxidative phosphorylation better than are tissues with limited capacity for glycolysis (e.g., the brain).

High-energy phosphate in the form of ATP is required for virtually all synthetic and degradative processes within the cell. These include membrane transport, protein synthesis, lipogenesis, and the deacylation-reacylation reactions necessary for phospholipid turnover. *Depletion of ATP to 5% to 10%*

Ischemia

Mitochondrion

↓ Oxidative phosphorylation

↓ATP

↓Na⁺ pump   ↑ Anaerobic glycolysis   Detachment of ribosomes

↑Influx of Ca²⁺
H₂O, and Na⁺   ↓Glycogen ↑Lactic → ↓pH
↑Efflux of K⁺   acid   ↓**Protein synthesis**

**ER swelling
Cellular swelling
Loss of microvilli
Blebs**   **Clumping
of nuclear
chromatin**   **Lipid
deposition**

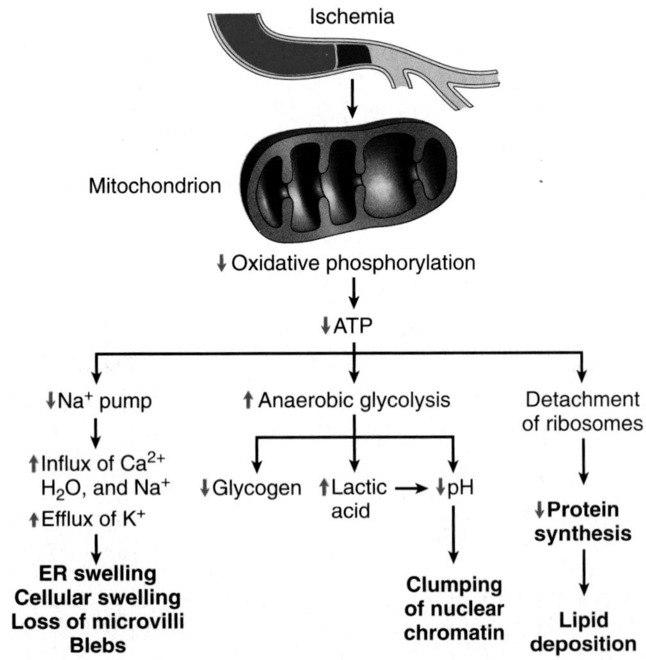

FIGURE 1–17 Functional and morphologic consequences of decreased intracellular ATP during cell injury. The morphologic changes shown here are indicative of reversible cell injury. Further depletion of ATP results in cell death, typically by necrosis. ER, endoplasmic reticulum.

of normal levels has widespread effects on many critical cellular systems:

- The activity of the *plasma membrane energy-dependent sodium pump* (ouabain-sensitive Na⁺, K⁺-ATPase) is reduced. Failure of this active transport system causes sodium to enter and accumulate inside cells and potassium to diffuse out. The net gain of solute is accompanied by isosmotic gain of water, causing *cell swelling*, and dilation of the ER.

- *Cellular energy metabolism is altered.* If the supply of oxygen to cells is reduced, as in ischemia, oxidative phosphorylation ceases, resulting in a decrease in cellular ATP and associated increase in adenosine monophosphate. These changes stimulate phosphofructokinase and phosphorylase activities, leading to an increased rate of *anaerobic glycolysis*, which is designed to maintain the cell's energy sources by generating ATP through metabolism of glucose derived from glycogen. As a consequence *glycogen stores are rapidly depleted.* Anaerobic glycolysis results in the accumulation of *lactic acid* and inorganic phosphates from the hydrolysis of phosphate esters. This reduces the intracellular pH, resulting in decreased activity of many cellular enzymes.

- Failure of the Ca²⁺ pump leads to influx of Ca²⁺, with damaging effects on numerous cellular components, described below.

- With prolonged or worsening depletion of ATP, structural disruption of the protein synthetic apparatus occurs, manifested as detachment of ribosomes from the rough ER and dissociation of polysomes, with a consequent *reduction in protein synthesis.*

- In cells deprived of oxygen or glucose, proteins may become misfolded, and misfolded proteins trigger a cellular reaction called the *unfolded protein response* that may culminate in cell injury and even death. This process is described later in the chapter.

- Ultimately, there is irreversible damage to mitochondrial and lysosomal membranes, and the cell undergoes *necrosis.*

MITOCHONDRIAL DAMAGE

Mitochondria are the cell's suppliers of life-sustaining energy in the form of ATP, but they are also critical players in

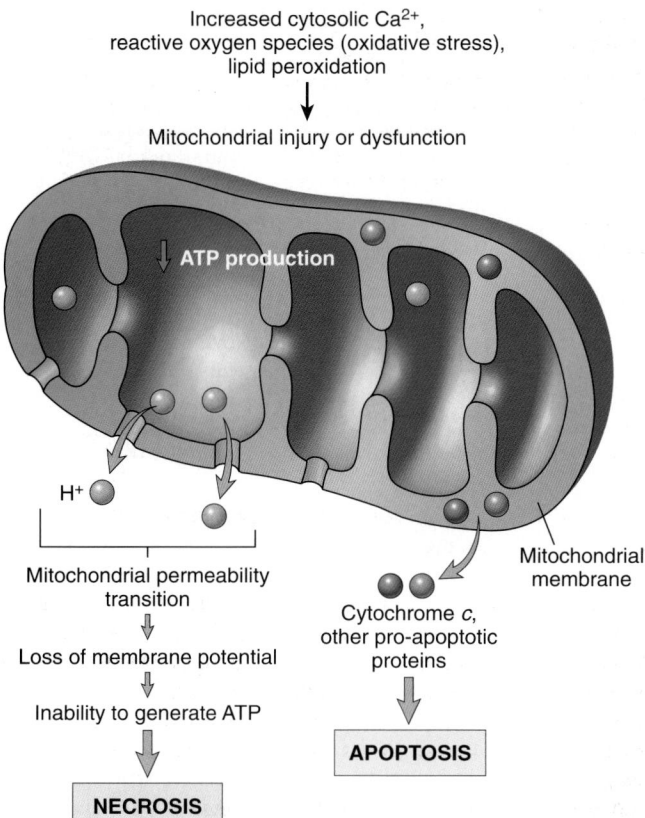

FIGURE 1–18 Consequences of mitochondrial dysfunction, culminating in cell death by necrosis or apoptosis.

cell injury and death.[17] Mitochondria can be damaged by increases of cytosolic Ca^{2+}, reactive oxygen species (discussed below), and oxygen deprivation, and so they are sensitive to virtually all types of injurious stimuli, including hypoxia and toxins. In addition, mutations in mitochondrial genes are the cause of some inherited diseases (Chapter 5).

There are two major *consequences of mitochondrial damage.*

○ Mitochondrial damage often results in the formation of a high-conductance channel in the mitochondrial membrane, called the *mitochondrial permeability transition pore* (Fig. 1–18).[18] The opening of this conductance channel leads to the loss of mitochondrial membrane potential, resulting in failure of oxidative phosphorylation and progressive depletion of ATP, culminating in necrosis of the cell. One of the structural components of the mitochondrial permeability transition pore is the protein cyclophilin D, which is a target of the immunosuppressive drug cyclosporine (used to prevent graft rejection). In some experimental models of ischemia, cyclosporine reduces injury by preventing opening of the mitochondrial permeability transition pore—an interesting example of molecularly targeted therapy for cell injury (although its clinical value is not established).

○ The mitochondria also sequester between their outer and inner membranes several proteins that are capable of activating apoptotic pathways; these include cyto-

chrome *c* and proteins that indirectly activate apoptosis-inducing enzymes called caspases. Increased permeability of the outer mitochondrial membrane may result in leakage of these proteins into the cytosol, and death by apoptosis (discussed later).

INFLUX OF CALCIUM AND LOSS OF CALCIUM HOMEOSTASIS

The finding that depleting calcium protects cells from injury induced by a variety of harmful stimuli indicates that calcium ions are important mediators of cell injury.[19] Cytosolic free calcium is normally maintained at very low concentrations (~0.1 μmol) compared with extracellular levels of 1.3 mmol, and most intracellular calcium is sequestered in mitochondria and the ER. Ischemia and certain toxins cause an increase in cytosolic calcium concentration, initially because of release of Ca^{2+} from intracellular stores, and later resulting from increased influx across the plasma membrane (Fig. 1–19). Increased intracellular Ca^{2+} causes cell injury by several mechanisms.

○ The accumulation of Ca^{2+} in mitochondria results in opening of the mitochondrial permeability transition pore and, as described above, failure of ATP generation.

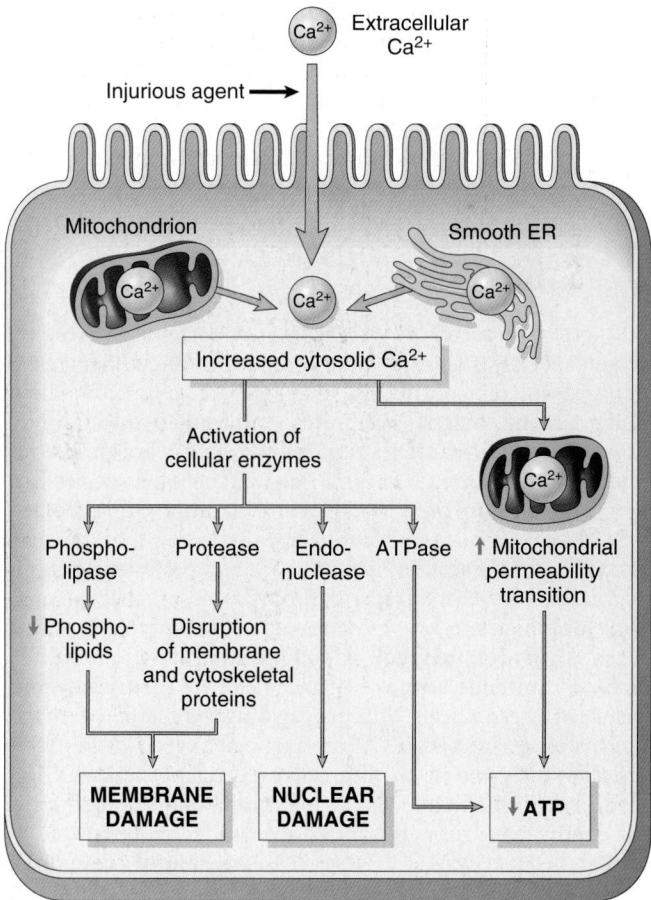

FIGURE 1–19 The role of increased cytosolic calcium in cell injury. ER, endoplasmic reticulum.

TABLE 1–3 Properties of the Principal Free Radicals Involved in Cell Injury			
Properties	**$O_2^{\cdot-}$**	**H_2O_2**	**$^{\cdot}OH$**	**$ONOO^-$**
MECHANISMS OF PRODUCTION	Incomplete reduction of O_2 during oxidative phosphorylation; by phagocyte oxidase in leukocytes	Generated by SOD from $O_2^{\cdot-}$ and by oxidases in peroxisomes	Generated from H_2O by hydrolysis, e.g., by radiation; from H_2O_2 by Fenton reaction; from $O_2^{\cdot-}$	Produced by interaction of $O_2^{\cdot-}$ and NO generated by NO synthase in many cell types (endothelial cells, leukocytes, neurons, others)
MECHANISMS OF INACTIVATION	Conversion to H_2O_2 and O_2 by SOD	Conversion to H_2O and O_2 by catalase (peroxisomes), glutathione peroxidase (cytosol, mitochondria)	Conversion to H_2O by glutathione peroxidase	Conversion to HNO_2 by peroxiredoxins (cytosol, mitochondria)
PATHOLOGIC EFFECTS	Stimulates production of degradative enzymes in leukocytes and other cells; may directly damage lipids, proteins, DNA; acts close to site of production	Can be converted to $^{\cdot}OH$ and OCl^-, which destroy microbes and cells; can act distant from site of production	Most reactive oxygen-derived free radical; principal ROS responsible for damaging lipids, proteins, and DNA	Damages lipids, proteins, DNA

HNO_2, nitrite; H_2O_2, hydrogen peroxide; NO, nitric oxide; $O_2^{\cdot-}$, superoxide anion; OCl^-, hypochlorite; $^{\cdot}OH$, hydroxyl radical; $ONOO^-$, peroxynitrite; ROS, reactive oxygen species; SOD, superoxide dismutase.

○ Increased cytosolic Ca^{2+} activates a number of enzymes, with potentially deleterious cellular effects. These enzymes include *phospholipases* (which cause membrane damage), *proteases* (which break down both membrane and cytoskeletal proteins), *endonucleases* (which are responsible for DNA and chromatin fragmentation), and *ATPases* (thereby hastening ATP depletion).

○ Increased intracellular Ca^{2+} levels also result in the induction of apoptosis, by direct activation of caspases and by increasing mitochondrial permeability.[20]

ACCUMULATION OF OXYGEN-DERIVED FREE RADICALS (OXIDATIVE STRESS)

Cell injury induced by free radicals, particularly reactive oxygen species, is an important mechanism of cell damage in many pathologic conditions, such as chemical and radiation injury, ischemia-reperfusion injury (induced by restoration of blood flow in ischemic tissue), cellular aging, and microbial killing by phagocytes.[21] *Free radicals* are chemical species that have a single unpaired electron in an outer orbit. Energy created by this unstable configuration is released through reactions with adjacent molecules, such as inorganic or organic chemicals—proteins, lipids, carbohydrates, nucleic acids—many of which are key components of cell membranes and nuclei. Moreover, free radicals initiate autocatalytic reactions, whereby molecules with which they react are themselves converted into free radicals, thus propagating the chain of damage. *Reactive oxygen species (ROS)* are a type of oxygen-derived free radical whose role in cell injury is well established. ROS are produced normally in cells during mitochondrial respiration and energy generation, but they are degraded and removed by cellular defense systems. Thus, cells are able to maintain a steady state in which free radicals may be present transiently at low concentrations but do not cause damage. When the production of ROS increases or the scavenging systems are ineffective, the result is an excess of these free radicals, leading to a condition called *oxidative stress*. Oxidative stress has been implicated in a wide variety of pathologic processes, including cell injury, cancer, aging, and some degenerative diseases such as Alzheimer disease. ROS are also produced in large amounts by leukocytes, particularly neutrophils and macrophages, as mediators for destroying microbes, dead tissue, and other unwanted substances. Therefore, injury caused by these reactive compounds often accompanies inflammatory reactions, during which leukocytes are recruited and activated (Chapter 2).

In the following section we discuss the generation and removal of ROS, and how they contribute to cell injury. The properties of some of the most important free radicals are summarized in Table 1–3.

Generation of Free Radicals. Free radicals may be generated within cells in several ways (Fig. 1–20):

○ *The reduction-oxidation reactions that occur during normal metabolic processes.* During normal respiration, molecular O_2 is reduced by the transfer of four electrons to H_2 to generate two water molecules. This conversion is catalyzed by oxidative enzymes in the ER, cytosol, mitochondria, peroxisomes, and lysosomes. During this process small amounts of partially reduced intermediates are produced in which different numbers of electrons have been transferred from O_2, these include superoxide anion ($O_2^{\cdot-}$, one electron), hydrogen peroxide (H_2O_2, two electrons), and hydroxyl ions ($^{\cdot}OH$, three electrons).

○ *Absorption of radiant energy* (e.g., ultraviolet light, x-rays). For example, ionizing radiation can hydrolyze water into $^{\cdot}OH$ and hydrogen (H) free radicals.

○ Rapid bursts of ROS are produced in activated leukocytes during *inflammation*. This occurs by a precisely controlled reaction in a plasma membrane multiprotein complex that uses NADPH oxidase for the redox reaction

(Chapter 2). In addition, some intracellular oxidases (such as xanthine oxidase) generate $O_2^{\cdot-}$.

- *Enzymatic metabolism of exogenous chemicals or drugs* can generate free radicals that are not ROS but have similar effects (e.g., CCl_4 can generate CCl_3, described later in the chapter).
- *Transition metals* such as iron and copper donate or accept free electrons during intracellular reactions and catalyze free radical formation, as in the Fenton reaction ($H_2O_2 + Fe^{2+} \rightarrow Fe^{3+} + OH + OH^-$). Because most of the intracellular free iron is in the ferric (Fe^{3+}) state, it must be reduced to the ferrous (Fe^{2+}) form to participate in the Fenton reaction. This reduction can be enhanced by $O_2^{\cdot-}$, and thus sources of iron and $O_2^{\cdot-}$ may cooperate in oxidative cell damage.
- *Nitric oxide* (NO), an important chemical mediator generated by endothelial cells, macrophages, neurons, and other cell types (Chapter 2), can act as a free radical and can also be converted to highly reactive peroxynitrite anion ($ONOO^-$) as well as NO_2 and NO_3^{-}.[22]

Removal of Free Radicals. Free radicals are inherently unstable and generally decay spontaneously. $O_2^{\cdot-}$, for example, is unstable and decays (dismutates) spontaneously into O_2 and H_2O_2 in the presence of water. In addition, cells have developed multiple nonenzymatic and enzymatic mechanisms to remove free radicals and thereby minimize injury (see Fig. 1–20). These include the following:

- *Antioxidants* either block the initiation of free radical formation or inactivate (e.g., scavenge) free radicals. Examples are the lipid-soluble vitamins E and A as well as ascorbic acid and glutathione in the cytosol.
- As we have seen, *iron* and *copper* can catalyze the formation of ROS. The levels of these reactive metals are minimized by binding of the ions to storage and transport proteins (e.g., transferrin, ferritin, lactoferrin, and ceruloplasmin), thereby minimizing the formation of ROS.
- A series of *enzymes* acts as free radical–scavenging systems and breaks down H_2O_2 and $O_2^{\cdot-}$.[21,23] These enzymes are located near the sites of generation of the oxidants and include the following:
  1. *Catalase,* present in peroxisomes, decomposes H_2O_2 ($2H_2O_2 \rightarrow O_2 + 2H_2O$).
  2. *Superoxide dismutases* (SODs) are found in many cell types and convert $O_2^{\cdot-}$ to H_2O_2 ($2O_2^{\cdot-} + 2H \rightarrow H_2O_2 + O_2$). This group includes both manganese–SOD, which is localized in mitochondria, and copper-zinc–SOD, which is found in the cytosol.
  3. *Glutathione peroxidase* also protects against injury by catalyzing free radical breakdown ($H_2O_2 + 2GSH \rightarrow GSSG$ [glutathione homodimer] $+ 2H_2O$, or $2OH + 2GSH \rightarrow GSSG + 2H_2O$). The intracellular ratio of oxidized glutathione (GSSG) to reduced glutathione (GSH) is a reflection of the oxidative state of the cell and is an important indicator of the cell's ability to detoxify ROS.

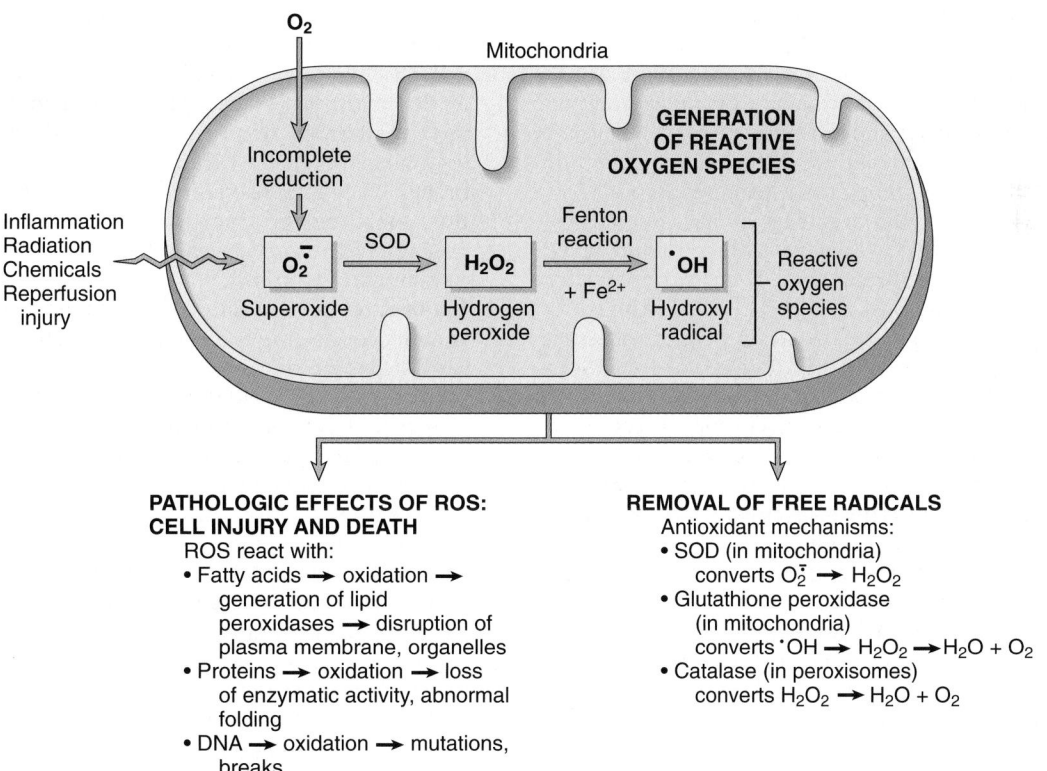

FIGURE 1–20   The role of reactive oxygen species (ROS) in cell injury. O_2 is converted to superoxide ($O_2^{\cdot-}$) by oxidative enzymes in the endoplasmic reticulum (ER), mitochondria, plasma membrane, peroxisomes, and cytosol. $O_2^{\cdot-}$ is converted to H_2O_2 by dismutation and thence to $\cdot OH$ by the Cu^{2+}/Fe^{2+}-catalyzed Fenton reaction. H_2O_2 is also derived directly from oxidases in peroxisomes (not shown). Resultant free radical damage to lipids (by peroxidation), proteins, and DNA leads to injury to numerous cellular components. The major antioxidant enzymes are superoxide dismutase (SOD), glutathione peroxidase, and catalase.

Pathologic Effects of Free Radicals. The effects of ROS and other free radicals are wide-ranging, but three reactions are particularly relevant to cell injury (see Fig. 1–20):

○ *Lipid peroxidation in membranes.* In the presence of O_2, free radicals may cause peroxidation of lipids within plasma and organellar membranes. Oxidative damage is initiated when the double bonds in unsaturated fatty acids of membrane lipids are attacked by O_2-derived free radicals, particularly by ·OH. The lipid–free radical interactions yield peroxides, which are themselves unstable and reactive, and an autocatalytic chain reaction ensues (called *propagation*), which can result in extensive membrane damage.

○ *Oxidative modification of proteins.* Free radicals promote oxidation of amino acid side chains, formation of protein-protein cross-linkages (e.g., disulfide bonds), and oxidation of the protein backbone. Oxidative modification of proteins may damage the active sites of enzymes, disrupt the conformation of structural proteins, and enhance proteasomal degradation of unfolded or misfolded proteins, raising havoc throughout the cell.

○ *Lesions in DNA.* Free radicals are capable of causing single- and double-strand breaks in DNA, cross-linking of DNA strands, and formation of adducts. Oxidative DNA damage has been implicated in cell aging (discussed later in this chapter) and in malignant transformation of cells (Chapter 7).

The traditional thinking about free radicals was that they cause cell injury and death by necrosis, and, in fact, the production of ROS is a frequent prelude to necrosis. However, it is now clear that free radicals can trigger apoptosis as well.[24] Recent studies have also revealed a role of ROS in signaling by a variety of cellular receptors and biochemical intermediates.[25] In fact, according to one hypothesis, the major actions of O_2^- stem from its ability to stimulate the production of degradative enzymes rather than direct damage of macromolecules. It is also possible that these potentially deadly molecules serve important physiologic functions.[26]

DEFECTS IN MEMBRANE PERMEABILITY

Early loss of selective membrane permeability leading ultimately to overt membrane damage is a consistent feature of most forms of cell injury (except apoptosis). Membrane damage may affect the functions and integrity of all cellular membranes. Below we discuss the mechanisms and pathologic consequences of membrane damage.

Mechanisms of Membrane Damage. In ischemic cells membrane defects may be the result of ATP depletion and calcium-mediated activation of phospholipases (see below). The plasma membrane can also be damaged directly by various bacterial toxins, viral proteins, lytic complement components, and a variety of physical and chemical agents. Several biochemical mechanisms may contribute to membrane damage (Fig. 1–21):

○ *Reactive oxygen species.* Oxygen free radicals cause injury to cell membranes by lipid peroxidation, discussed earlier.

○ *Decreased phospholipid synthesis.* The production of phospholipids in cells may be reduced as a consequence of

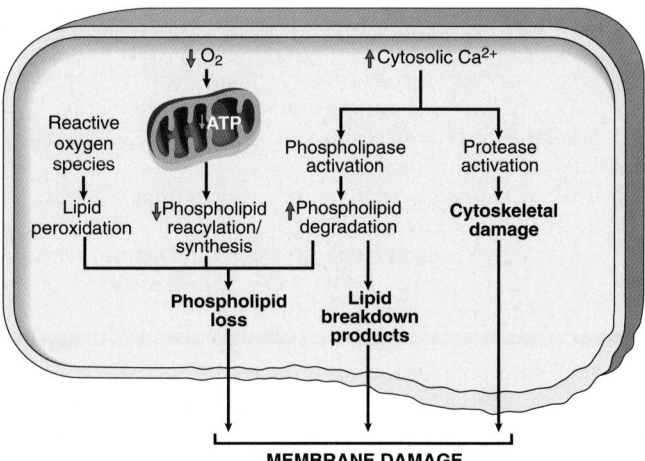

MEMBRANE DAMAGE

FIGURE 1–21 Mechanisms of membrane damage in cell injury. Decreased O_2 and increased cytosolic Ca^{2+} are typically seen in ischemia but may accompany other forms of cell injury. Reactive oxygen species, which are often produced on reperfusion of ischemic tissues, also cause membrane damage (not shown).

defective mitochondrial function or hypoxia, both of which decrease the production of ATP and thus affect energy-dependent enzymatic activities. The decreased phospholipid synthesis may affect all cellular membranes, including the mitochondria themselves.

○ *Increased phospholipid breakdown.* Severe cell injury is associated with increased degradation of membrane phospholipids, probably due to activation of endogenous phospholipases by increased levels of cytosolic and mitochondrial Ca^{2+}.[19] Phospholipid breakdown leads to the accumulation of *lipid breakdown products*, including unesterified free fatty acids, acyl carnitine, and lysophospholipids, which have a detergent effect on membranes. They may also either insert into the lipid bilayer of the membrane or exchange with membrane phospholipids, potentially causing changes in permeability and electrophysiologic alterations.

○ *Cytoskeletal abnormalities.* Cytoskeletal filaments serve as anchors connecting the plasma membrane to the cell interior. Activation of proteases by increased cytosolic calcium may cause damage to elements of the cytoskeleton. In the presence of cell swelling, this damage results, particularly in myocardial cells, in detachment of the cell membrane from the cytoskeleton, rendering it susceptible to stretching and rupture.

Consequences of Membrane Damage. The most important sites of membrane damage during cell injury are the mitochondrial membrane, the plasma membrane, and membranes of lysosomes.

○ *Mitochondrial membrane damage.* As discussed above, damage to mitochondrial membranes results in opening of the mitochondrial permeability transition pore leading to decreased ATP, and release of proteins that trigger apoptotic death.

○ *Plasma membrane damage.* Plasma membrane damage results in loss of osmotic balance and influx of fluids and ions, as well as loss of cellular contents. The cells may also leak metabolites that are vital for the reconstitution of ATP, thus further depleting energy stores.

○ *Injury to lysosomal membranes* results in leakage of their enzymes into the cytoplasm and activation of the acid hydrolases in the acidic intracellular pH of the injured (e.g., ischemic) cell. Lysosomes contain RNases, DNases, proteases, phosphatases, glucosidases, and cathepsins. Activation of these enzymes leads to enzymatic digestion of proteins, RNA, DNA, and glycogen, and the cells die by necrosis.

DAMAGE TO DNA AND PROTEINS

Cells have mechanisms that repair damage to DNA, but if this damage is too severe to be corrected (e.g., after exposure to DNA damaging drugs, radiation, or oxidative stress), the cell initiates a suicide program that results in death by apoptosis. A similar reaction is triggered by improperly folded proteins, which may be the result of inherited mutations or external triggers such as free radicals. Because these mechanisms of cell injury typically cause apoptosis, they are discussed later in the chapter.

Before concluding our discussion of the mechanisms of cell injury, it is useful to consider the possible events that determine when reversible injury becomes irreversible and progresses to cell death. The clinical relevance of this question is obvious—if we can answer it we may be able to devise strategies for preventing cell injury from having permanent deleterious consequences. However, the molecular mechanisms connecting most forms of cell injury to ultimate cell death have proved elusive, for several reasons. The "point of no return," at which the damage becomes irreversible, is still largely undefined, and there are no reliable morphologic or biochemical correlates of irreversibility. *Two phenomena consistently characterize irreversibility—the inability to reverse mitochondrial dysfunction* (lack of oxidative phosphorylation and ATP generation) even after resolution of the original injury, and *profound disturbances in membrane function.* As mentioned earlier, injury to lysosomal membranes results in the enzymatic dissolution of the injured cell that is characteristic of necrosis.

Leakage of intracellular proteins through the damaged cell membrane and ultimately into the circulation provides a means of detecting tissue-specific cellular injury and necrosis using blood serum samples. Cardiac muscle, for example, contains a specific isoform of the enzyme creatine kinase and of the contractile protein troponin; liver (and specifically bile duct epithelium) contains an isoform of the enzyme alkaline phosphatase; and hepatocytes contain transaminases. Irreversible injury and cell death in these tissues are reflected in increased levels of such proteins in the blood, and measurement of these biomarkers is used clinically to assess damage to these tissues.

Clinico-Pathologic Correlations: Selected Examples of Cell Injury and Necrosis

Having briefly reviewed the causes, morphology, and mechanisms of cell injury and necrotic cell death, we now describe some common and clinically significant forms of cell injury that typically culminate in necrosis. These examples illustrate many of the mechanisms and sequence of events in cell injury that were described above.

ISCHEMIC AND HYPOXIC INJURY

This is the most common type of cell injury in clinical medicine and has been studied extensively in humans, in experimental animals, and in culture systems. Hypoxia, referring to reduced oxygen availability, may occur in a variety of clinical settings, described earlier. In ischemia, on the other hand, the supply of oxygen and nutrients is decreased most often because of reduced blood flow as a consequence of a mechanical obstruction in the arterial system. It can also be caused by reduced venous drainage. In contrast to hypoxia, during which energy production by anaerobic glycolysis can continue, ischemia compromises the delivery of substrates for glycolysis. Thus, in ischemic tissues, not only is aerobic metabolism compromised but anaerobic energy generation also stops after glycolytic substrates are exhausted, or glycolysis is inhibited by the accumulation of metabolites that would have been removed otherwise by blood flow. For this reason, *ischemia tends to cause more rapid and severe cell and tissue injury than does hypoxia in the absence of ischemia.*

Mechanisms of Ischemic Cell Injury

The sequence of events following hypoxia or ischemia reflects many of the biochemical alterations in cell injury that have been described above. As the oxygen tension within the cell decreases, there is loss of oxidative phosphorylation and decreased generation of ATP. The depletion of ATP results in failure of the sodium pump, with loss of potassium, influx of sodium and water, and cell swelling. There is also influx of Ca^{2+}, with its many deleterious effects. There is progressive loss of glycogen and decreased protein synthesis. The functional consequences may be severe at this stage. For instance, heart muscle ceases to contract within 60 seconds of coronary occlusion. Note, however, that loss of contractility does not mean cell death. If hypoxia continues, worsening ATP depletion causes further deterioration. The cytoskeleton disperses, resulting in the loss of ultrastructural features such as microvilli and the formation of "blebs" at the cell surface (see Figs. 1–9 and 1–10). "Myelin figures," derived from degenerating cellular membranes, may be seen within the cytoplasm (in autophagic vacuoles) or extracellularly. They are thought to result from unmasking of phosphatide groups, promoting the uptake and intercalation of water between the lamellar stacks of membranes. At this time the mitochondria are usually swollen, as a result of loss of volume control in these organelles; the ER remains dilated; and the entire cell is markedly swollen, with increased concentrations of water, sodium, and chloride and a decreased concentration of potassium. *If oxygen is restored, all of these disturbances are reversible.*

If ischemia persists, irreversible injury and necrosis ensue. Irreversible injury is associated morphologically with severe swelling of mitochondria, extensive damage to plasma membranes (giving rise to myelin figures) and swelling of lysosomes (see Fig. 1–10C). Large, flocculent, amorphous densities develop in the mitochondrial matrix. In the myocardium, these are indications of irreversible injury and can be seen as early as 30 to 40 minutes after ischemia. Massive influx of calcium into the cell then occurs, particularly if the ischemic zone is reperfused. Death is mainly by necrosis, but apoptosis also contributes; the apoptotic pathway is probably activated by release of pro-apoptotic molecules from leaky mitochondria. The cell's components are progressively degraded, and there is widespread leakage of cellular enzymes into the extracellular space and, conversely, entry of extracellular macromolecules from the interstitial space into the dying cells. Finally, the dead cells may become replaced by large masses composed of phospholipids in the form of myelin figures. These are then either phagocytosed by leukocytes or degraded further into fatty acids. *Calcification* of such fatty acid residues may occur, with the formation of calcium soaps.

As mentioned before, leakage of intracellular enzymes and other proteins across the abnormally permeable plasma membrane and into the blood provides important clinical indicators of cell death. For example, elevated serum levels of cardiac muscle creatine kinase MB and troponin are early signs of myocardial infarction, and may be seen before the infarct is detectable morphologically (Chapter 12).

Mammalian cells have developed protective responses to hypoxic stress. The best-defined of these is induction of a transcription factor called *hypoxia-inducible factor-1*, which promotes new blood vessel formation, stimulates cell survival pathways, and enhances anaerobic glycolysis.[27] It remains to be seen if understanding of such oxygen-sensing mechanisms will lead to new strategies for preventing or treating ischemic and hypoxic cell injury.

Despite many investigations in experimental models there are still no reliable therapeutic approaches for reducing the injurious consequences of ischemia in clinical situations. The strategy that is perhaps the most useful in ischemic (and traumatic) brain and spinal cord injury is the transient induction of hypothermia (reducing the core body temperature to 92°F). This treatment reduces the metabolic demands of the stressed cells, decreases cell swelling, suppresses the formation of free radicals, and inhibits the host inflammatory response. All of these may contribute to decreased cell and tissue injury.[28]

ISCHEMIA-REPERFUSION INJURY

Restoration of blood flow to ischemic tissues can promote recovery of cells if they are reversibly injured. However, under certain circumstances, when blood flow is restored to cells that have been ischemic but have not died, injury is paradoxically exacerbated and proceeds at an accelerated pace. As a consequence, *reperfused tissues may sustain loss of cells in addition to the cells that are irreversibly damaged at the end of ischemia.* This process, called *ischemia-reperfusion injury*, is clinically important because it contributes to tissue damage during myocardial and cerebral infarction and following therapies to restore blood flow (Chapters 12 and 28).

How does reperfusion injury occur? The likely answer is that *new damaging processes* are set in motion during reperfusion, causing the death of cells that might have recovered otherwise.[29] Several mechanisms have been proposed:

- New damage may be initiated during reoxygenation by increased generation of *reactive oxygen and nitrogen species*

from parenchymal and endothelial cells and from infiltrating leukocytes.[30,31] These free radicals may be produced in reperfused tissue as a result of mitochondrial damage, causing incomplete reduction of oxygen, or because of the action of oxidases in leukocytes, endothelial cells, or parenchymal cells. Cellular antioxidant defense mechanisms may be compromised by ischemia, favoring the accumulation of free radicals. Other mediators of cell injury, such as calcium, may also enter reperfused cells, damaging various organelles, including mitochondria, and increasing the production of free radicals.

- Ischemic injury is associated with *inflammation* as a result of the production of cytokines and increased expression of adhesion molecules by hypoxic parenchymal and endothelial cells, which recruit circulating neutrophils to reperfused tissue.[32] The inflammation causes additional tissue injury (Chapter 2). The importance of neutrophil influx in reperfusion injury has been demonstrated experimentally by the ability of anti-inflammatory interventions, such as treatment with antibodies that block cytokines or adhesion molecules, to reduce the extent of the injury.

- Activation of the *complement system* may contribute to ischemia-reperfusion injury.[33] The complement system is involved in host defense and is an important mechanism of immune injury (Chapter 6). Some IgM antibodies have a propensity to deposit in ischemic tissues, for unknown reasons, and when blood flow is resumed, complement proteins bind to the deposited antibodies, are activated, and cause more cell injury and inflammation.[34]

CHEMICAL (TOXIC) INJURY

Chemical injury remains a frequent problem in clinical medicine and is a major limitation to drug therapy. Because many drugs are metabolized in the liver, this organ is a frequent target of drug toxicity. In fact, toxic liver injury is perhaps the most frequent reason for terminating the therapeutic use or development of a drug.[35] The mechanisms by which chemicals, certain drugs, and toxins produce injury are described in greater detail in Chapter 9 in the discussion of environmental diseases. Here we will describe the major pathways of chemically induced injury with selected examples.

Chemicals induce cell injury by one of two general mechanisms[36]:

- Some chemicals can injure cells *directly* by combining with critical molecular components. For example, in mercuric chloride poisoning, mercury binds to the sulfhydryl groups of cell membrane proteins, causing increased membrane permeability and inhibition of ion transport. In such instances, the greatest damage is usually to the cells that use, absorb, excrete, or concentrate the chemicals—in the case of mercuric chloride, the cells of the gastrointestinal tract and kidney (Chapter 9). *Cyanide* poisons mitochondrial cytochrome oxidase and thus inhibits oxidative phosphorylation. Many antineoplastic chemotherapeutic agents and antibiotic drugs also induce cell damage by direct cytotoxic effects.

- Most toxic chemicals are not biologically active in their native form but must be converted to reactive toxic metabolites, which then act on target molecules. This modification is usually accomplished by the cytochrome P-450 mixed-function oxidases in the smooth ER of the liver and other organs. The toxic metabolites cause membrane damage and cell injury mainly by formation of *free radicals* and subsequent lipid peroxidation; direct covalent binding to membrane proteins and lipids may also contribute. For instance, CCl_4, which was once widely used in the dry cleaning industry, is converted by cytochrome P-450 to the highly reactive free radical $\cdot CCl_3$, which causes lipid peroxidation and damages many cellular structures. Acetaminophen, an analgesic drug, is also converted to a toxic product during detoxification in the liver, leading to cell injury. These and other examples of chemical injury are described in Chapter 9.

Apoptosis

Apoptosis is a pathway of cell death that is induced by a tightly regulated suicide program in which cells destined to die activate enzymes that degrade the cells' own nuclear DNA and nuclear and cytoplasmic proteins. Apoptotic cells break up into fragments, called apoptotic bodies, which contain portions of the cytoplasm and nucleus. The plasma membrane of the apoptotic cell and bodies remains intact, but its structure is altered in such a way that these become "tasty" targets for phagocytes. The dead cell and its fragments are rapidly devoured, before the contents have leaked out, and therefore cell death by this pathway does not elicit an inflammatory reaction in the host. The process was recognized in 1972 by the distinctive morphologic appearance of membrane-bound fragments derived from cells, and named after the Greek designation for "falling off."[37] It was quickly appreciated that apoptosis was a unique mechanism of cell death, distinct from necrosis, which is characterized by loss of membrane integrity, enzymatic digestion of cells, leakage of cellular contents, and frequently a host reaction (see Fig. 1–8 and Table 1–2). However, apoptosis and necrosis sometimes coexist, and apoptosis induced by some pathologic stimuli may progress to necrosis.

CAUSES OF APOPTOSIS

Apoptosis occurs normally both during development and throughout adulthood, and serves to eliminate unwanted, aged or potentially harmful cells. It is also a pathologic event when diseased cells become damaged beyond repair and are eliminated.

Apoptosis in Physiologic Situations

Death by apoptosis is a normal phenomenon that serves to eliminate cells that are no longer needed, and to maintain a steady number of various cell populations in tissues. It is important in the following physiologic situations:

- *The programmed destruction of cells during embryogenesis,* including implantation, organogenesis, developmental involution, and metamorphosis. The term "programmed cell death" was originally coined to denote death of specific cell types at defined times during the development of an organism.[38] Apoptosis is a generic term for this pattern of cell death, regardless of the context, but it is often used interchangeably with "programmed cell death."
- *Involution of hormone-dependent tissues upon hormone withdrawal,* such as endometrial cell breakdown during the menstrual cycle, ovarian follicular atresia in menopause, the regression of the lactating breast after weaning, and prostatic atrophy after castration.
- *Cell loss in proliferating cell populations,* such as immature lymphocytes in the bone marrow and thymus that fail to express useful antigen receptors (Chapter 6), B lymphocytes in germinal centers, and epithelial cells in intestinal crypts, so as to maintain a constant number *(homeostasis).*
- *Elimination of potentially harmful self-reactive lymphocytes,* either before or after they have completed their maturation, so as to prevent reactions against one's own tissues (Chapter 6).
- Death of host cells that have served their useful purpose, such as neutrophils in an *acute inflammatory response,* and lymphocytes at the end of an *immune response.* In these situations cells undergo apoptosis because they are deprived of necessary survival signals, such as growth factors.

Apoptosis in Pathologic Conditions

Apoptosis eliminates cells that are injured beyond repair without eliciting a host reaction, thus limiting collateral tissue damage. Death by apoptosis is responsible for loss of cells in a variety of pathologic states:

- *DNA damage.* Radiation, cytotoxic anticancer drugs, and hypoxia can damage DNA, either directly or via production of free radicals. If repair mechanisms cannot cope with the injury, the cell triggers intrinsic mechanisms that induce apoptosis. In these situations elimination of the cell may be a better alternative than risking mutations in the damaged DNA, which may result in malignant transformation. These injurious stimuli can cause apoptosis if the insult is mild, but larger doses of the same stimuli may result in necrotic cell death.
- *Accumulation of misfolded proteins.* Improperly folded proteins may arise because of mutations in the genes encoding these proteins or because of extrinsic factors, such as damage caused by free radicals. Excessive accumulation of these proteins in the ER leads to a condition called *ER stress,* which culminates in apoptotic cell death. Apoptosis caused by the accumulation of misfolded proteins has been invoked as the basis of several degenerative diseases of the central nervous system and other organs.
- *Cell death in certain infections,* particularly viral infections, in which loss of infected cells is largely due to apoptosis that may be induced by the virus (as in adenovirus and HIV infections) or by the host immune response (as in viral hepatitis). An important host response to viruses consists of cytotoxic T lymphocytes

specific for viral proteins, which induce apoptosis of infected cells in an attempt to eliminate reservoirs of infection. During this process there can be significant tissue damage. The same T-cell-mediated mechanism is responsible for cell death in *tumors* and cellular rejection of *transplants*.

○ *Pathologic atrophy in parenchymal organs after duct obstruction*, such as occurs in the pancreas, parotid gland, and kidney.

MORPHOLOGIC AND BIOCHEMICAL CHANGES IN APOPTOSIS

Before discussing the mechanisms of apoptosis, we describe the morphologic and biochemical characteristics of this process.

Morphology. The following morphologic features, some best seen with the electron microscope, characterize cells undergoing apoptosis (Fig. 1–22, and see Fig. 1–8).

Cell shrinkage. The cell is smaller in size; the cytoplasm is dense (Fig. 1–22A); and the organelles, though relatively normal, are more tightly packed. (Recall that in other forms of cell injury, an early feature is cell swelling, not shrinkage.)

Chromatin condensation. This is the most characteristic feature of apoptosis. The chromatin aggregates peripherally, under the nuclear membrane, into dense masses of various shapes and sizes (Fig. 1–22B). The nucleus itself may break up, producing two or more fragments.

Formation of cytoplasmic blebs and apoptotic bodies. The apoptotic cell first shows extensive surface blebbing, then undergoes fragmentation into membrane-bound apoptotic bodies composed of cytoplasm and tightly packed organelles, with or without nuclear fragments (Fig. 1–22C).

Phagocytosis of apoptotic cells or cell bodies, usually by macrophages. The apoptotic bodies are rapidly ingested by phagocytes and degraded by the phagocyte's lysosomal enzymes.

Plasma membranes are thought to remain intact during apoptosis, until the last stages, when they become permeable to normally retained solutes. This classical description is accurate with respect to apop-

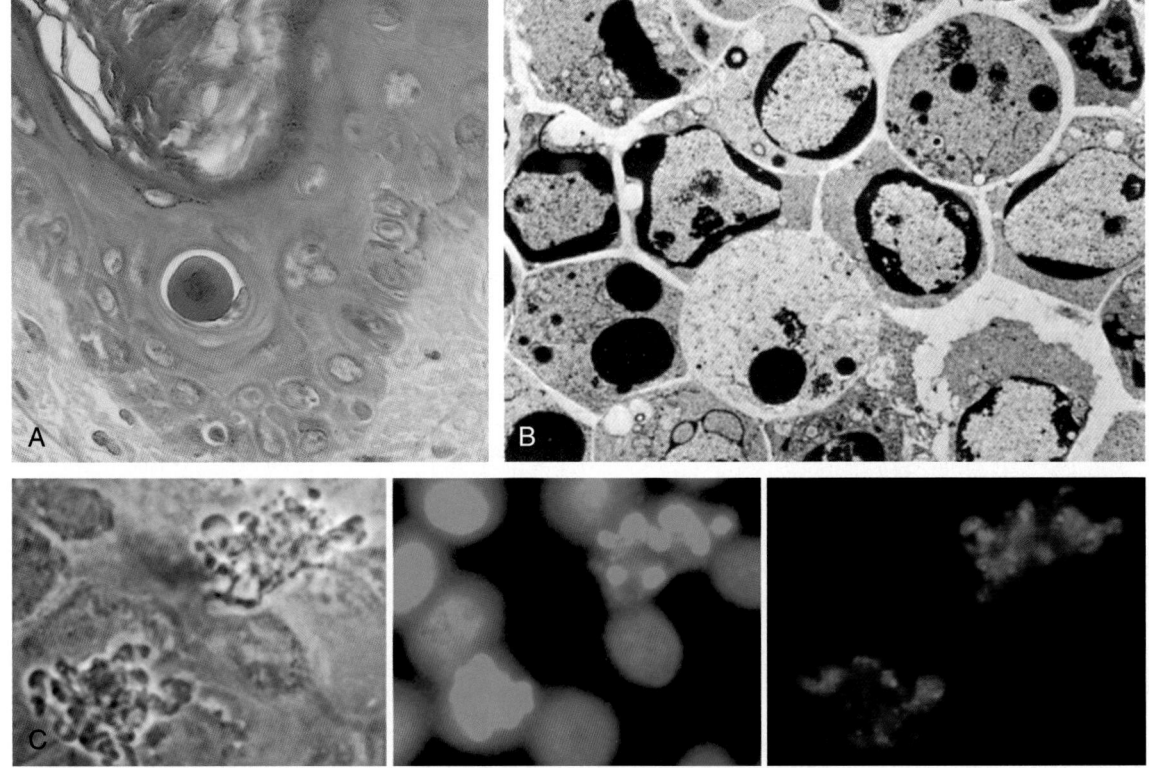

FIGURE 1–22 Morphologic features of apoptosis. **A,** Apoptosis of an epidermal cell in an immune reaction. The cell is reduced in size and contains brightly eosinophilic cytoplasm and a condensed nucleus. **B,** This electron micrograph of cultured cells undergoing apoptosis shows some nuclei with peripheral crescents of compacted chromatin, and others that are uniformly dense or fragmented. **C,** These images of cultured cells undergoing apoptosis show blebbing and formation of apoptotic bodies (*left panel*, phase contrast micrograph), a stain for DNA showing nuclear fragmentation (*middle panel*), and activation of caspase-3 (*right panel*, immunofluorescence stain with an antibody specific for the active form of caspase-3, revealed as red color). (**B,** From Kerr JFR, Harmon BV: Definition and incidence of apoptosis: a historical perspective. In Tomei LD, Cope FO (eds): Apoptosis: The Molecular Basis of Cell Death. Cold Spring Harbor, NY, Cold Spring Harbor Laboratory Press, 1991, pp 5–29; **C,** Courtesy of Dr. Zheng Dong, Medical College of Georgia, Augusta, GA.)

tosis during physiologic conditions such as embryogenesis and deletion of immune cells. However, forms of cell death with features of necrosis as well as of apoptosis are not uncommon after many injurious stimuli.[39] Under such conditions the severity rather than the nature of the stimulus determines the pathway of cell death, necrosis being the major pathway when there is advanced ATP depletion and membrane damage.

On histologic examination, in tissues stained with hematoxylin and eosin, the apoptotic cell appears as a round or oval mass of intensely eosinophilic cytoplasm with fragments of dense nuclear chromatin (Fig. 1–22A). Because the cell shrinkage and formation of apoptotic bodies are rapid and the pieces are quickly phagocytosed, considerable apoptosis may occur in tissues before it becomes apparent in histologic sections. In addition, apoptosis—in contrast to necrosis—does not elicit inflammation, making it more difficult to detect histologically.

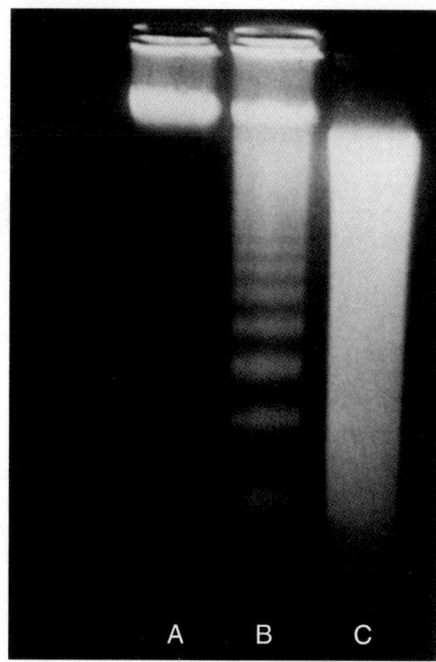

FIGURE 1–23 Agarose gel electrophoresis of DNA extracted from culture cells. Ethidium bromide stain; photographed under ultraviolet illumination. **Lane A**, Viable cells in culture. **Lane B**, Culture of cells exposed to heat showing extensive apoptosis; note ladder pattern of DNA fragments, which represent multiples of oligonucleosomes. **Lane C**, Culture showing cell necrosis; note diffuse smearing of DNA. (From Kerr JFR, Harmon BV: Definition and incidence of apoptosis: a historical perspective. In Tomei LD, Cope FO: Apoptosis: The Molecular Basis of Cell Death. Cold Spring Harbor, NY, Cold Spring Harbor Laboratory Press, 1991, p 13.)

Biochemical Features of Apoptosis

Apoptotic cells usually exhibit a distinctive constellation of biochemical alterations that underlie the structural changes described above.

Activation of Caspases. A specific feature of apoptosis is the activation of several members of a family of cysteine proteases named *caspases*.[40] The term *caspase* is based on two properties of this family of enzymes: the "c" refers to a cysteine protease (i.e., an enzyme with cysteine in its active site), and "aspase" refers to the unique ability of these enzymes to cleave after aspartic acid residues. The caspase family, now including more than 10 members, can be divided functionally into two groups—initiator and executioner—depending on the order in which they are activated during apoptosis. Initiator caspases include caspase-8 and caspase-9. Several other caspases, including caspase-3 and caspase-6, serve as executioners. Like many proteases, caspases exist as inactive pro-enzymes, or zymogens, and must undergo an enzymatic cleavage to become active. The presence of cleaved, active caspases is a marker for cells undergoing apoptosis (Fig. 1–22C). We will discuss the roles of these enzymes in apoptosis later in this section.

DNA and Protein Breakdown. Apoptotic cells exhibit a characteristic breakdown of DNA into large 50- to 300-kilobase pieces.[41] Subsequently, there is cleavage of DNA by Ca^{2+}- and Mg^{2+}-dependent endonucleases into fragments whose sizes are multiples of 180 to 200 base pairs, reflecting cleavage between nucleosomal subunits. The fragments may be visualized by electrophoresis as DNA "ladders" (Fig. 1–23). Endonuclease activity also forms the basis for detecting cell death by cytochemical techniques that recognize double-stranded breaks of DNA.[41] A "smeared" pattern of DNA fragmentation is thought to be indicative of necrosis, but this may be a late autolytic phenomenon, and typical DNA ladders are sometimes seen in necrotic cells as well.

Membrane Alterations and Recognition by Phagocytes. The plasma membrane of apoptotic cells changes in ways that promote the recognition of the dead cells by phagocytes. One of these changes is the movement of some phospholipids (notably phosphatidylserine) from the inner leaflet to the outer leaflet of the membrane, where they are recognized by a number of receptors on phagocytes. These lipids are also detectable by binding of a protein called annexin V; thus, annexin V staining is commonly used to identify apoptotic cells. The clearance of apoptotic cells by phagocytes is described later.

MECHANISMS OF APOPTOSIS

All cells contain intrinsic mechanisms that signal death or survival, and apoptosis results from an imbalance in these signals. Because too much or too little apoptosis is thought to underlie many diseases, such as degenerative diseases and cancer, there is great interest in elucidating the mechanisms of this form of cell death. One of the remarkable facts to emerge is that the basic mechanisms of apoptosis—the genes and proteins that control the process and the sequence of events—are conserved in all multicellular organisms.[38] In fact, some of the major breakthroughs came from observations made in the nematode *Caenorhabditis elegans*, whose development proceeds by a highly reproducible, programmed pattern of cell growth followed by cell death. Studies of mutant worms have allowed the identification of specific genes (called *ced* genes, for *cell death* abnormal) that initiate or inhibit apoptosis and for which there are defined mammalian homologues.[38]

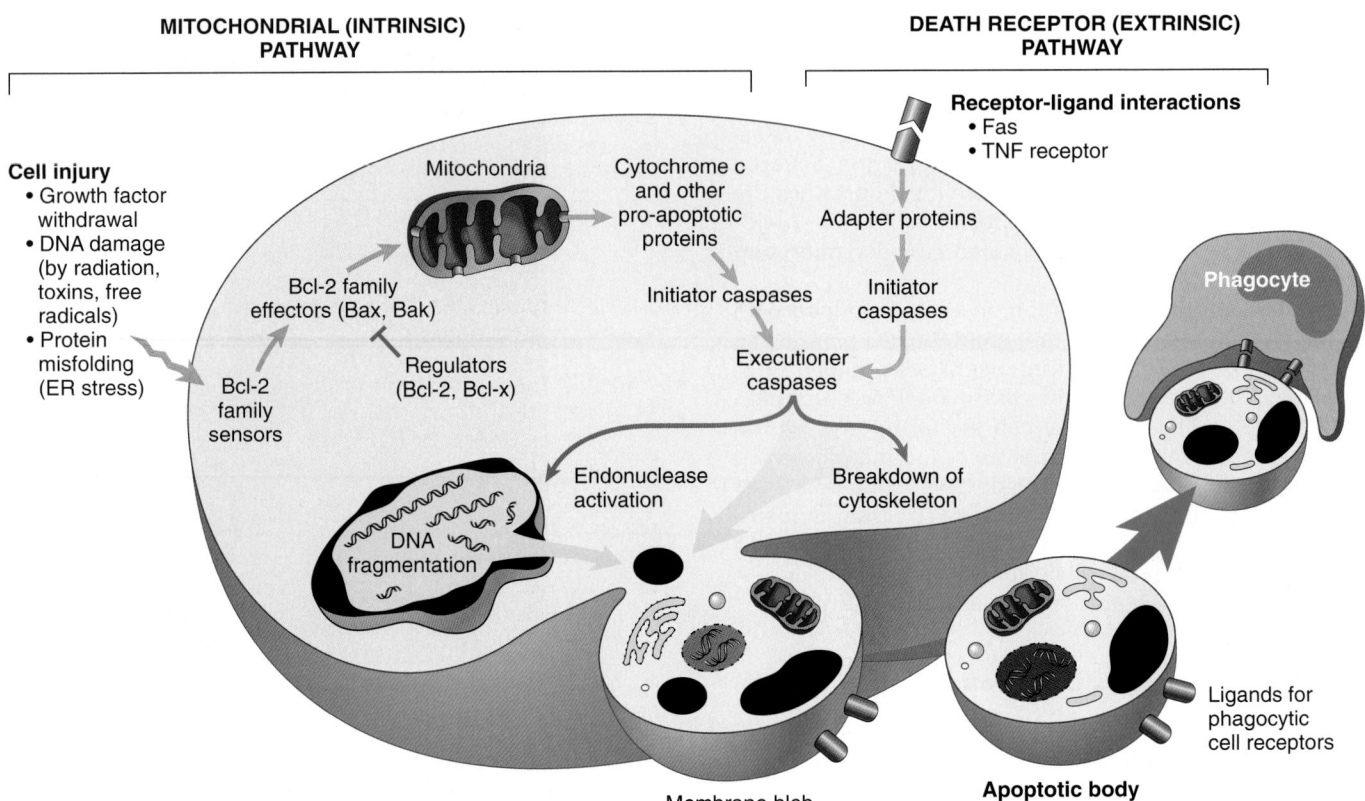

FIGURE 1–24 Mechanisms of apoptosis. The two pathways of apoptosis differ in their induction and regulation, and both culminate in the activation of "executioner" caspases. The induction of apoptosis by the mitochondrial pathway involves the action of sensors and effectors of the Bcl-2 family, which induce leakage of mitochondrial proteins. Also shown are some of the anti-apoptotic proteins ("regulators") that inhibit mitochondrial leakiness and cytochrome *c*–dependent caspase activation in the mitochondrial pathway. In the death receptor pathway engagement of death receptors leads directly to caspase activation. The regulators of death receptor–mediated caspase activation are not shown. ER, endoplasmic reticulum; TNF, tumor necrosis factor.

The process of apoptosis may be divided into an initiation phase, during which some caspases become catalytically active, and an execution phase, during which other caspases trigger the degradation of critical cellular components. *Initiation of apoptosis occurs principally by signals from two distinct pathways: the intrinsic, or mitochondrial, pathway, and the extrinsic, or death receptor–initiated, pathway* (Fig. 1–24).[42] These pathways are induced by distinct stimuli and involve different sets of proteins, although there is some cross-talk between them. Both pathways converge to activate caspases, which are the actual mediators of cell death.

The Intrinsic (Mitochondrial) Pathway of Apoptosis

The mitochondrial pathway is the major mechanism of apoptosis in all mammalian cells, and its role in a variety of physiologic and pathologic processes is well established. This pathway of apoptosis is the result of increased mitochondrial permeability and release of pro-apoptotic molecules (death inducers) into the cytoplasm (Fig. 1–25).[42] Mitochondria are remarkable organelles in that they contain proteins such as cytochrome *c* that are essential for life, but some of the same proteins, when released into the cytoplasm (an indication that the cell is not healthy), initiate the suicide program of apoptosis. The release of these mitochondrial proteins is controlled

by a finely orchestrated balance between pro- and anti-apoptotic members of the Bcl family of proteins.[43] This family is named after *Bcl-2*, which was identified as an oncogene in a B-cell lymphoma and is homologous to the *C. elegans* protein Ced-9. There are more than 20 members of the *Bcl* family, and most of them function to regulate apoptosis. Growth factors and other survival signals stimulate production of anti-apoptotic proteins, the main ones being Bcl-2, Bcl-x, and Mcl-1. These proteins normally reside in the cytoplasm and in mitochondrial membranes, where they control mitochondrial permeability and prevent leakage of mitochondrial proteins that have the ability to trigger cell death (Fig. 1–25A). When cells are deprived of survival signals or their DNA is damaged, or misfolded proteins induce ER stress, sensors of damage or stress are activated. These sensors are also members of the *Bcl* family, and they include proteins called Bim, Bid, and Bad that contain a single "Bcl-2 homology domain" (the third of the four such domains present in Bcl-2) and are called "BH3-only proteins." The sensors in turn activate two critical (pro-apoptotic) effectors, Bax and Bak, which form oligomers that insert into the mitochondrial membrane and create channels that allow proteins from the inner mitochondrial membrane to leak out into the cytoplasm. BH3-only proteins may also bind to and block the function of Bcl-2 and Bcl-x. At the same time, the synthesis of Bcl-2 and Bcl-x may decline. The net result of Bax-Bak activation coupled with loss of the protective

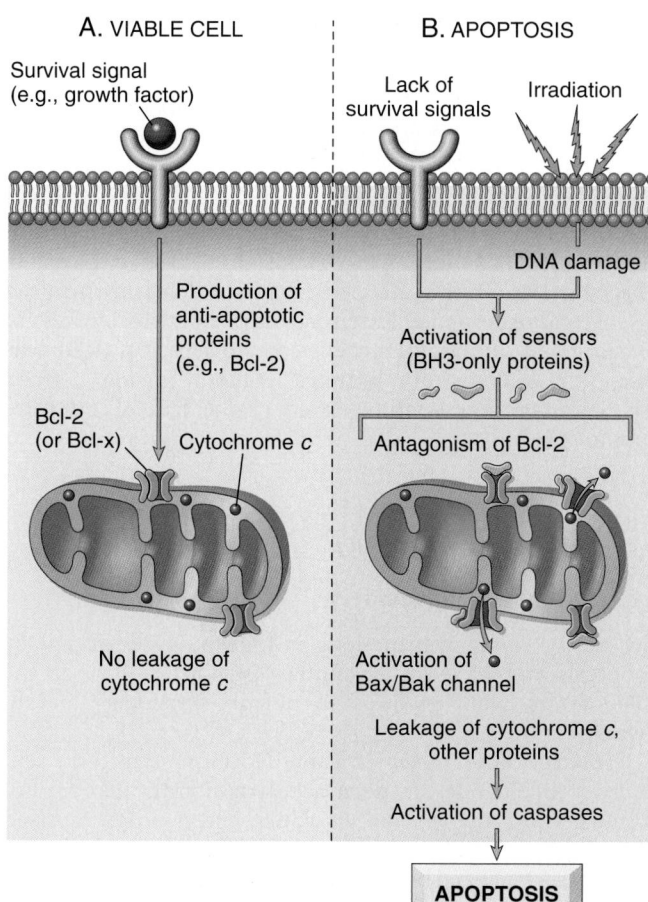

A. VIABLE CELL

Survival signal
(e.g., growth factor)

Production of
anti-apoptotic
proteins
(e.g., Bcl-2)

Bcl-2
(or Bcl-x)   Cytochrome *c*

No leakage of
cytochrome *c*

B. APOPTOSIS

Lack of
survival signals   Irradiation

DNA damage

Activation of sensors
(BH3-only proteins)

Antagonism of Bcl-2

Activation of
Bax/Bak channel

Leakage of cytochrome *c*,
other proteins

Activation of caspases

APOPTOSIS

FIGURE 1–25 The intrinsic (mitochondrial) pathway of apoptosis. **A,** Cell viability is maintained by the induction of anti-apoptotic proteins such as Bcl-2 by survival signals. These proteins maintain the integrity of mitochondrial membranes and prevent leakage of mitochondrial proteins. **B,** Loss of survival signals, DNA damage, and other insults activate sensors that antagonize the anti-apoptotic proteins and activate the pro-apoptotic proteins Bax and Bak, which form channels in the mitochondrial membrane. The subsequent leakage of cytochrome *c* (and other proteins, not shown) leads to caspase activation and apoptosis.

functions of the anti-apoptotic Bcl family members is the release into the cytoplasm of several mitochondrial proteins that can activate the caspase cascade (Fig. 1–25B). One of these proteins is *cytochrome c*, well known for its role in mitochondrial respiration. Once released into the cytosol, cytochrome *c* binds to a protein called Apaf-1 (apoptosis-activating factor-1, homologous to Ced-4 in *C. elegans*), which forms a wheel-like hexamer that has been called the *apoptosome*.[44] This complex is able to bind caspase-9, the critical initiator caspase of the mitochondrial pathway, and the enzyme cleaves adjacent caspase-9 molecules, thus setting up an auto-amplification process. Other mitochondrial proteins, with arcane names like Smac/DIABLO, enter the cytoplasm, where they bind to and neutralize cytoplasmic proteins that function as physiologic inhibitors of apoptosis (called IAPs). The normal function of the IAPs is to block the activation of caspases, including executioners like caspase-3, and keep cells alive.[45,46] Thus, the neutralization of these IAPs permits the initiation of a caspase cascade.

There is some evidence that the intrinsic pathway of apoptosis can be triggered without a role for mitochondria.[47] Apoptosis may be initiated by caspase activation upstream of mitochondria, and the subsequent increase in mitochondrial permeability and release of pro-apoptotic molecules serve to amplify the death signal. However, mechanisms of apoptosis involving mitochondria-independent initiation are not well defined.

The Extrinsic (Death Receptor–Initiated) Pathway of Apoptosis

This pathway is initiated by engagement of plasma membrane death receptors on a variety of cells.[48–50] Death receptors are members of the TNF receptor family that contain a cytoplasmic domain involved in protein-protein interactions that is called the *death domain* because it is essential for delivering apoptotic signals. (Some TNF receptor family members do not contain cytoplasmic death domains; their function is to activate inflammatory cascades [Chapter 2], and their role in triggering apoptosis is much less established.) The best-known death receptors are the type 1 TNF receptor (TNFR1) and a related protein called Fas (CD95), but several others have been described. The mechanism of apoptosis induced by these death receptors is well illustrated by Fas, a death receptor expressed on many cell types (Fig. 1–26). The ligand for Fas is called Fas ligand (FasL). FasL is expressed on T cells that recognize self antigens (and functions to eliminate

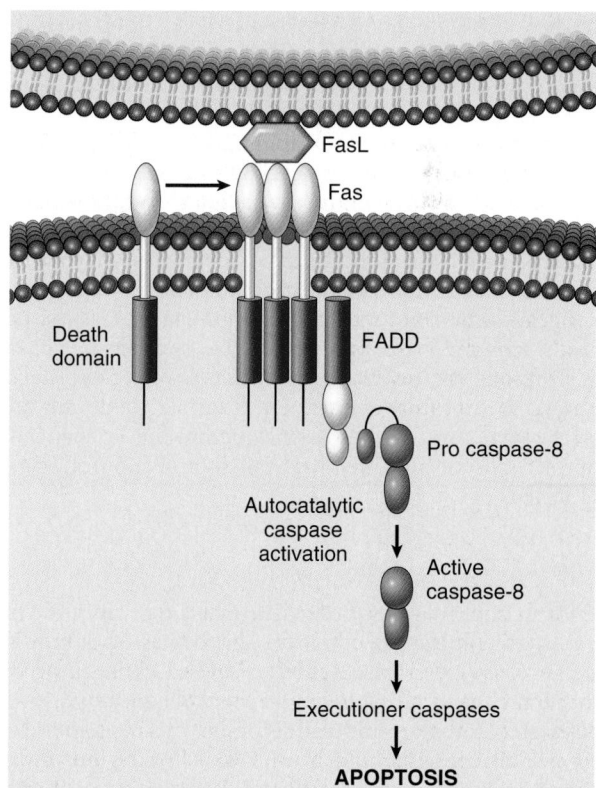

FasL

Fas

Death
domain   FADD

Pro caspase-8

Autocatalytic
caspase
activation   Active
caspase-8

Executioner caspases

APOPTOSIS

FIGURE 1–26 The extrinsic (death receptor–initiated) pathway of apoptosis, illustrated by the events following Fas engagement. FAAD, *Fas-*associated *death domain*; FasL, Fas ligand.

self-reactive lymphocytes), and on some cytotoxic T lympho-cytes (which kill virus-infected and tumor cells). When FasL binds to Fas, three or more molecules of Fas are brought together, and their cytoplasmic death domains form a binding site for an adapter protein that also contains a death domain and is called FADD (Fas-associated death domain). FADD that is attached to the death receptors in turn binds an inactive form of caspase-8 (and, in humans, caspase-10), again via a death domain. Multiple pro-caspase-8 molecules are thus brought into proximity, and they cleave one another to gener-ate active caspase-8. The enzyme then triggers a cascade of caspase activation by cleaving and thereby activating other pro-caspases, and the active enzymes mediate the execution phase of apoptosis (discussed below). This pathway of apop-tosis can be inhibited by a protein called FLIP, which binds to pro-caspase-8 but cannot cleave and activate the caspase because it lacks a protease domain.[51] Some viruses and normal cells produce FLIP and use this inhibitor to protect themselves from Fas-mediated apoptosis.

We have described the extrinsic and intrinsic pathways for initiating apoptosis as distinct because they involve funda-mentally different molecules for their initiation, but there may be interconnections between them. For instance, in hepato-cytes and several other cell types, Fas signaling activates a BH3-only protein called Bid, which then activates the mito-chondrial pathway.

The Execution Phase of Apoptosis

The two initiating pathways converge to a cascade of caspase activation, which mediates the final phase of apoptosis. As we have seen, the mitochondrial pathway leads to activation of the initiator caspase-9, and the death receptor pathway to the initiators caspase-8 and -10. After an initiator caspase is cleaved to generate its active form, the enzymatic death program is set in motion by rapid and sequential activation of the executioner caspases. Executioner caspases, such as caspase-3 and -6, act on many cellular components. For instance, these caspases, once activated, cleave an inhibitor of a cytoplasmic DNase and thus make the DNase enzymatically active; this enzyme induces the characteristic cleavage of DNA into nucleosome-sized pieces, described earlier. Caspases also degrade structural components of the nuclear matrix, and thus promote fragmentation of nuclei. Some of the steps in apoptosis are not fully defined. For instance, we do not know how the structure of the plasma membrane is changed in apoptotic cells, or how membrane blebs and apoptotic bodies are formed.

Removal of Dead Cells

The formation of apoptotic bodies breaks cells up into "bite-sized" fragments that are edible for phagocytes. Apoptotic cells and their fragments also undergo several changes in their membranes that actively promote their phagocytosis so they are cleared before they undergo secondary necrosis and release their cellular contents (which can result in injurious inflam-mation). In healthy cells phosphatidylserine is present on the inner leaflet of the plasma membrane, but in apoptotic cells this phospholipid "flips" out and is expressed on the outer layer of the membrane, where it is recognized by several mac-

rophage receptors. Cells that are dying by apoptosis secrete soluble factors that recruit phagocytes.[52] Some apoptotic bodies express thrombospondin, an adhesive glycoprotein that is recognized by phagocytes, and macrophages themselves may produce proteins that bind to apoptotic cells (but not to live cells) and thus target the dead cells for engulfment. Apop-totic bodies may also become coated with natural antibodies and proteins of the complement system, notably C1q, which are recognized by phagocytes.[53] Thus, numerous receptors on phagocytes and ligands induced on apoptotic cells are involved in the binding and engulfment of these cells. This process of phagocytosis of apoptotic cells is so efficient that dead cells disappear, often within minutes, without leaving a trace, and inflammation is absent even in the face of extensive apoptosis.

CLINICO-PATHOLOGIC CORRELATIONS: APOPTOSIS IN HEALTH AND DISEASE

Examples of Apoptosis

Cell death in many situations is known to be caused by apoptosis, and the selected examples listed below illustrate the role of this death pathway in normal physiology and in disease.[54]

Growth Factor Deprivation. Hormone-sensitive cells deprived of the relevant hormone, lymphocytes that are not stimulated by antigens and cytokines, and neurons deprived of nerve growth factor die by apoptosis. In all these situations, apoptosis is triggered by the intrinsic (mitochondrial) pathway and is attributable to decreased synthesis of Bcl-2 and Bcl-x and activation of Bim and other pro-apoptotic members of the Bcl family.

DNA Damage. Exposure of cells to radiation or chemo-therapeutic agents induces apoptosis by a mechanism that is initiated by DNA damage (genotoxic stress) and that involves the tumor-suppressor gene *p53*.[55] p53 protein accumulates in cells when DNA is damaged, and it arrests the cell cycle (at the G_1 phase) to allow time for repair (Chapter 7). However, if the damage is too great to be repaired successfully, p53 triggers apoptosis. When p53 is mutated or absent (as it is in certain cancers), it is incapable of inducing apoptosis, so that cells with damaged DNA are allowed to survive. In such cells the DNA damage may result in mutations or translocations that lead to neoplastic transformation (Chapter 7). Thus, p53 serves as a critical "life or death" switch following genotoxic stress. The mechanism by which p53 triggers the distal death effector machinery—the caspases—is complex but seems to involve its function in transcriptional activation. Among the proteins whose production is stimulated by p53 are several pro-apoptotic members of the Bcl family, notably Bax, Bak, and some BH3-only proteins, mentioned earlier.

Protein Misfolding. Chaperones in the ER control the proper folding of newly synthesized proteins, and misfolded polypeptides are ubiquitinated and targeted for proteolysis in proteasomes. If, however, unfolded or misfolded proteins accumulate in the ER, because of inherited mutations or stresses, they trigger a number of cellular responses, collec-tively called the *unfolded protein response*.[56,57] This unfolded protein response activates signaling pathways that increase the production of chaperones, enhance proteasomal degradation

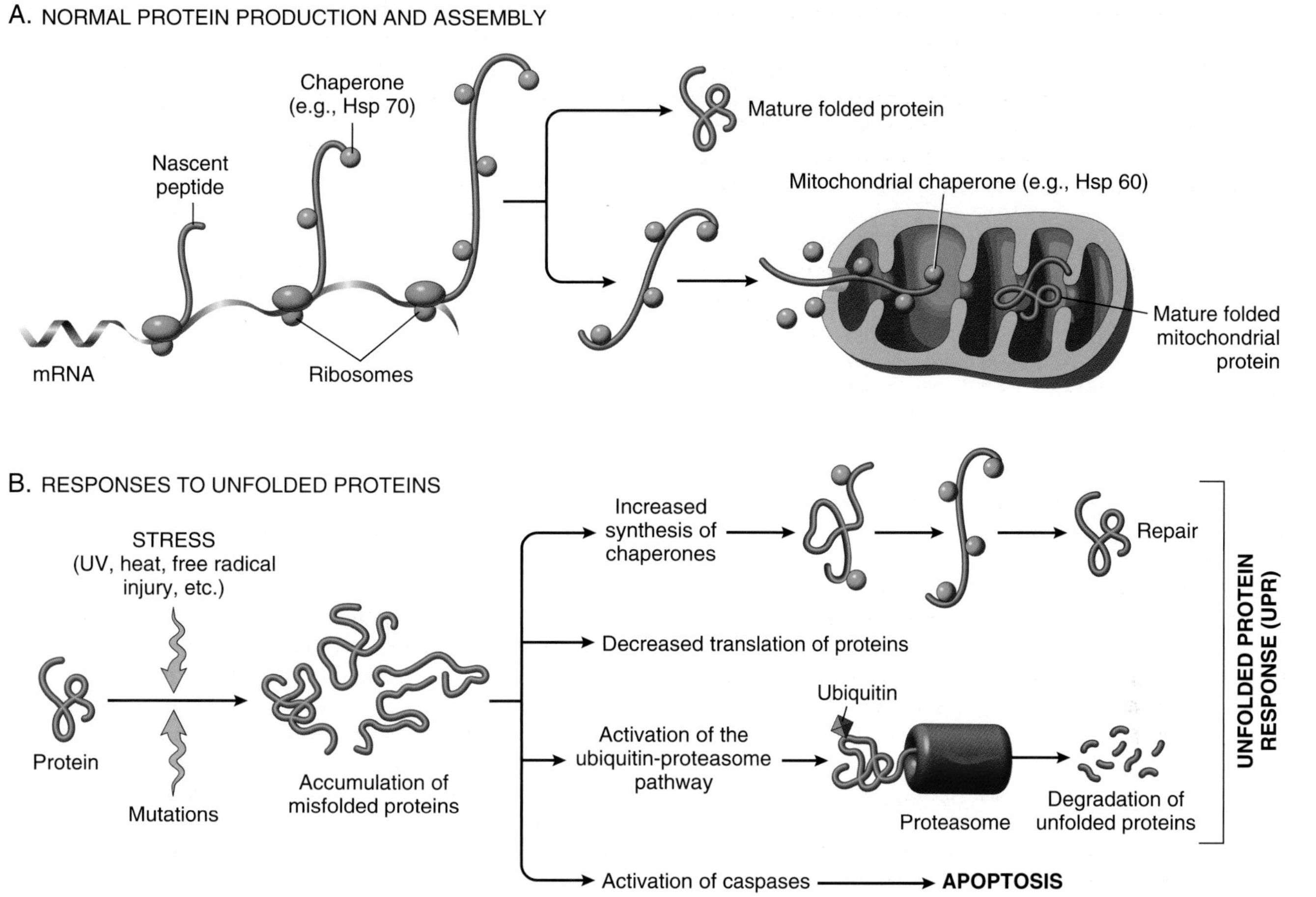

A. NORMAL PROTEIN PRODUCTION AND ASSEMBLY

B. RESPONSES TO UNFOLDED PROTEINS

FIGURE 1–27 Mechanisms of protein folding and the unfolded protein response. **A,** Chaperones, such as heat shock proteins (Hsp), protect unfolded or partially folded proteins from degradation and guide proteins into organelles. **B,** Misfolded proteins trigger a protective unfolded protein response (UPR). If this response is inadequate to cope with the level of misfolded proteins, it induces apoptosis.

of abnormal proteins, and slow protein translation, thus reducing the load of misfolded proteins in the cell (Fig. 1–27). However, if this cytoprotective response is unable to cope with the accumulation of misfolded proteins, the cell activates caspases and induces apoptosis.[58–60] This process is called *ER stress.* Intracellular accumulation of abnormally folded proteins, caused by genetic mutations, aging, or unknown environmental factors, is now recognized as a feature of a number of neurodegenerative diseases, including Alzheimer, Huntington, and Parkinson diseases (Chapter 28), and possibly type 2 diabetes.[61] Deprivation of glucose and oxygen, and stress such as heat, also result in protein misfolding, culminating in cell injury and death.

Apoptosis Induced By the TNF Receptor Family. FasL on T cells binds to Fas on the same or neighboring lymphocytes. This interaction plays a role in the elimination of lymphocytes that recognize self-antigens, and mutations affecting Fas or FasL result in autoimmune diseases in humans and mice (Chapter 6).[62] The cytokine TNF is an important mediator of the inflammatory reaction (Chapter 2), but it is also capable of inducing apoptosis. (The name "tumor necrosis factor" arose not because the cytokine kills tumor cells directly but because it induces thrombosis of tumor blood vessels, resulting in ischemic death of the

tumor.) TNF-mediated death is readily demonstrated in cell cultures, but its physiologic or pathologic significance in vivo is not known. In fact, the major physiologic functions of TNF are mediated not by inducing apoptosis but by activating the important transcription factor NF-κB (nuclear factor-κB), which promotes cell survival by stimulating synthesis of anti-apoptotic members of the Bcl-2 family and, as we shall see in Chapter 2, activates a number of inflammatory responses. Since TNF can induce cell death and promote cell survival, what determines this *yin* and *yang* of its action? The answer is unclear, but it probably depends on which signaling proteins attach to the TNF receptor after binding of the cytokine.

Cytotoxic T Lymphocyte–Mediated Apoptosis. Cytotoxic T lymphocytes (CTLs) recognize foreign antigens presented on the surface of infected host cells (Chapter 6). Upon activation, CTLs secrete *perforin,* a transmembrane pore-forming molecule, which promotes entry of the CTL granule serine proteases called *granzymes.* Granzymes have the ability to cleave proteins at aspartate residues and thus activate a variety of cellular caspases.[63] In this way the CTL kills target cells by directly inducing the effector phase of apoptosis. CTLs also express FasL on their surface and may kill target cells by ligation of Fas receptors.

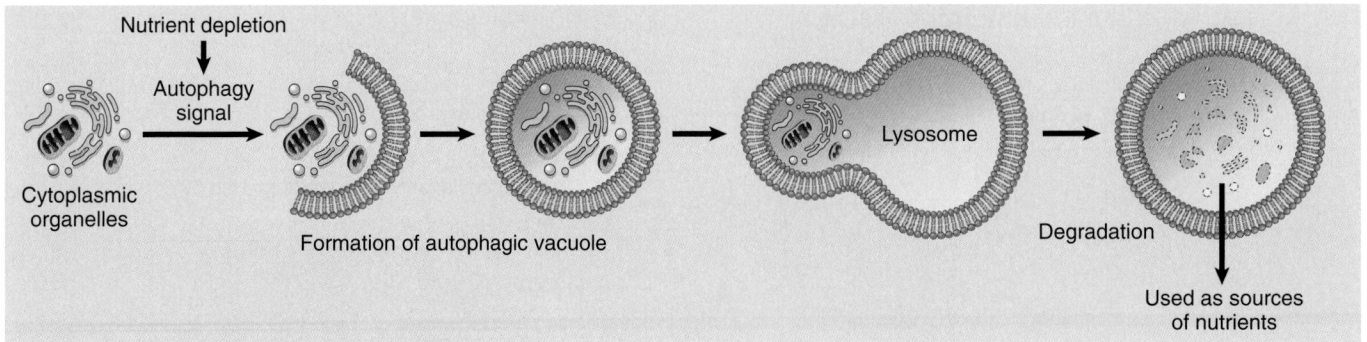

FIGURE 1–28   Autophagy. Cellular stresses, such as nutrient deprivation, activate autophagy genes that create vacuoles in which cellular organelles are sequestered and then degraded following fusion of the vesicles with lysosomes. The digested materials are recycled to provide nutrients for the cell.

Disorders Associated with Dysregulated Apoptosis

Dysregulated apoptosis ("too little or too much") has been postulated to explain aspects of a wide range of diseases.[56]

- *Disorders associated with defective apoptosis and increased cell survival.* An inappropriately low rate of apoptosis may permit the survival of abnormal cells, which may have a variety of consequences. For instance, if cells that carry mutations in *p53* are subjected to DNA damage, the cells not only fail to die but are susceptible to the accumulation of mutations because of defective DNA repair, and these abnormalities can give rise to *cancer*. The importance of apoptosis in preventing cancer development is emphasized by the fact that mutation of *p53* is the most common genetic abnormality found in human cancers (Chapter 7). In other situations defective apoptosis results in failure to eliminate potentially harmful cells, such as lymphocytes that can react against self-antigens, and failure to eliminate dead cells, a potential source of self-antigens. Thus, defective apoptosis may be the basis of *autoimmune disorders* (Chapter 6).
- *Disorders associated with increased apoptosis and excessive cell death.* These diseases are characterized by a loss of cells and include (1) *neurodegenerative diseases*, manifested by loss of specific sets of neurons, in which apoptosis is caused by mutations and misfolded proteins (Chapter 28); (2) *ischemic injury*, as in myocardial infarction (Chapter 12) and stroke (Chapter 28); and (3) *death of virus-infected cells*, in many viral infections (Chapter 8).

Autophagy

Autophagy is a process in which a cell eats its own contents. It is a survival mechanism in times of nutrient deprivation, when the starved cell lives by cannibalizing itself and recycling the digested contents. In this process intracellular organelles and portions of cytosol are first sequestered from the cytoplasm in an *autophagic vacuole*, which subsequently fuses with lysosomes to form an *autophagolysosome*, and the cellular components are digested by lysosomal enzymes (Fig. 1–28).[64,65]

Interest in autophagy has been spurred by the finding that it is regulated by a defined set of "autophagy genes" (called *Atgs*) in single-celled organisms and mammalian cells. The products of many of these genes function in the creation of the autophagic vacuole, but how they do so is unknown. It has also been suggested that autophagy triggers cell death that is distinct from necrosis and apoptosis.[66] However, the mechanism of this type of cell death is not known, nor is it clear that the cell death is caused by autophagy rather than by the stress that triggers autophagy. Nevertheless, autophagy has been invoked as a mechanism of cell loss in various diseases, including degenerative diseases of the nervous system and muscle; in many of these disorders, the damaged cells contain abundant autophagic vacuoles.[67]

Intracellular Accumulations

One of the manifestations of metabolic derangements in cells is the intracellular accumulation of abnormal amounts of various substances. The stockpiled substances fall into two categories: (1) a *normal cellular constituent*, such as water, lipids, proteins, and carbohydrates, that accumulates in excess; or (2) an *abnormal substance*, either exogenous, such as a mineral or products of infectious agents, or endogenous, such as a product of abnormal synthesis or metabolism. These substances may accumulate either transiently or permanently, and they may be harmless to the cells, but on occasion they are severely toxic. The substance may be located in either the cytoplasm (frequently within phagolysosomes) or the nucleus. In some instances the cell may be producing the abnormal substance, and in others it may be merely storing products of pathologic processes occurring elsewhere in the body.

Many processes result in abnormal intracellular accumulations, but most accumulations are attributable to four types of abnormalities (Fig. 1–29).

1. *A normal endogenous substance is produced at a normal or increased rate, but the rate of metabolism is inadequate to remove it.* Examples of this type of process are fatty change in the liver and reabsorption protein droplets in the tubules of the kidneys (see later).
2. An abnormal endogenous substance, typically the product of a mutated gene, accumulates because of defects in

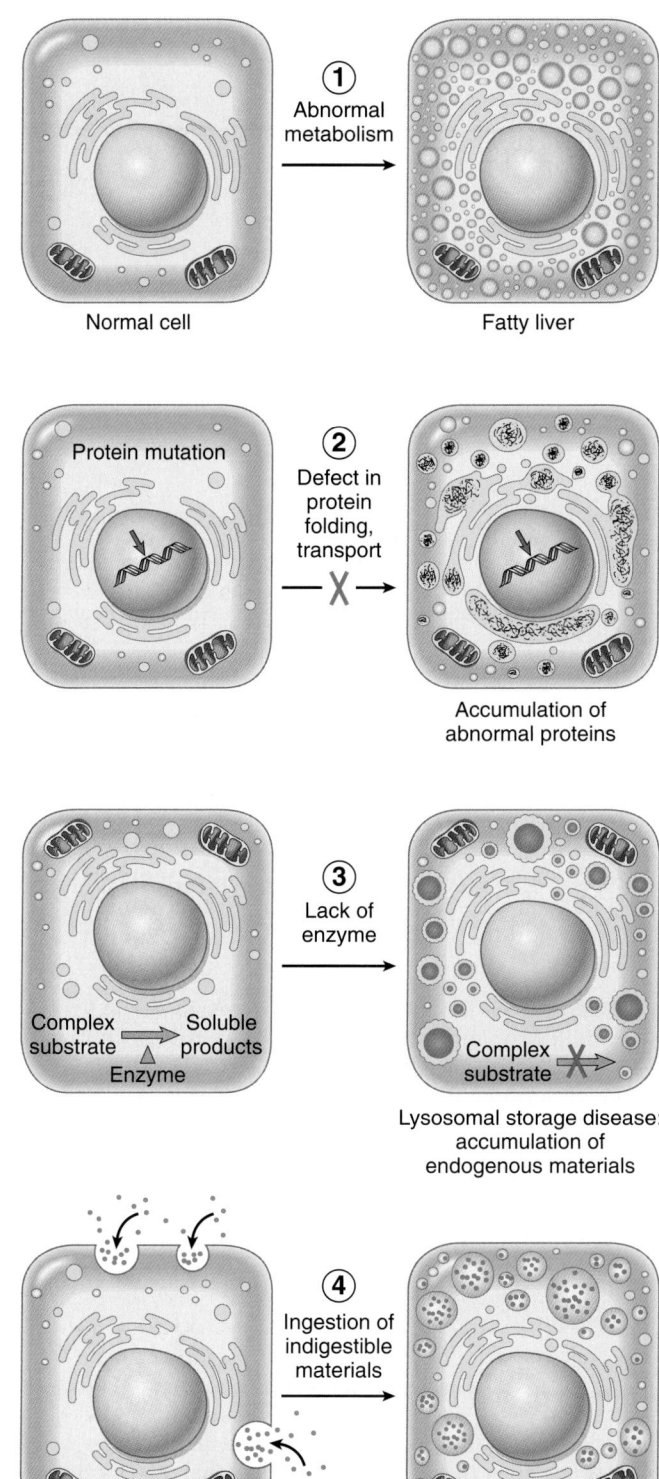

FIGURE 1–29 Mechanisms of intracellular accumulations discussed in the text.

protein folding and transport and an inability to degrade the abnormal protein efficiently. Examples include the accumulation of mutated α1-antitrypsin in liver cells (Chapter 18) and various mutated proteins in degenerative disorders of the central nervous system (Chapter 28).

3. A normal endogenous substance accumulates because of defects, usually inherited, in enzymes that are required for the metabolism of the substance. Examples include diseases caused by genetic defects in enzymes involved in the metabolism of lipid and carbohydrates, resulting in intracellular deposition of these substances, largely in lysosomes. These storage diseases are discussed in Chapter 5.

4. An abnormal exogenous substance is deposited and accumulates because the cell has neither the enzymatic machinery to degrade the substance nor the ability to transport it to other sites. Accumulations of carbon particles and nonmetabolizable chemicals such as silica are examples of this type of alteration.

In many cases, if the overload can be controlled or stopped, the accumulation is reversible. In inherited storage diseases accumulation is progressive, and the overload may cause cellular injury, leading in some instances to death of the tissue and the patient.

LIPIDS

All major classes of lipids can accumulate in cells: triglycerides, cholesterol/cholesterol esters, and phospholipids. Phospholipids are components of the myelin figures found in necrotic cells. In addition, abnormal complexes of lipids and carbohydrates accumulate in the lysosomal storage diseases (Chapter 5). Here we concentrate on triglyceride and cholesterol accumulations.

Steatosis (Fatty Change)

The terms *steatosis* and *fatty change* describe abnormal accumulations of triglycerides within parenchymal cells. Fatty change is often seen in the liver because it is the major organ involved in fat metabolism, but it also occurs in heart, muscle, and kidney. The causes of steatosis include toxins, protein malnutrition, diabetes mellitus, obesity, and anoxia. *In developed nations the most common causes of significant fatty change in the liver (fatty liver) are alcohol abuse and nonalcoholic fatty liver disease, which is often associated with diabetes and obesity* (Chapter 18).

Different mechanisms account for triglyceride accumulation in the liver. Free fatty acids from adipose tissue or ingested food are normally transported into hepatocytes. In the liver they are esterified to triglycerides, converted into cholesterol or phospholipids, or oxidized to ketone bodies. Some fatty acids are synthesized from acetate as well. Release of triglycerides from the hepatocytes requires association with apoproteins to form lipoproteins, which may then be transported from the blood into the tissues (Chapter 4). *Excess accumulation of triglycerides within the liver may result from excessive entry or defective metabolism and export of lipids* (Fig. 1–30A). Several such defects are induced by alcohol, a hepatotoxin that alters mitochondrial and microsomal functions, leading to increased synthesis and reduced breakdown of lipids (Chapter

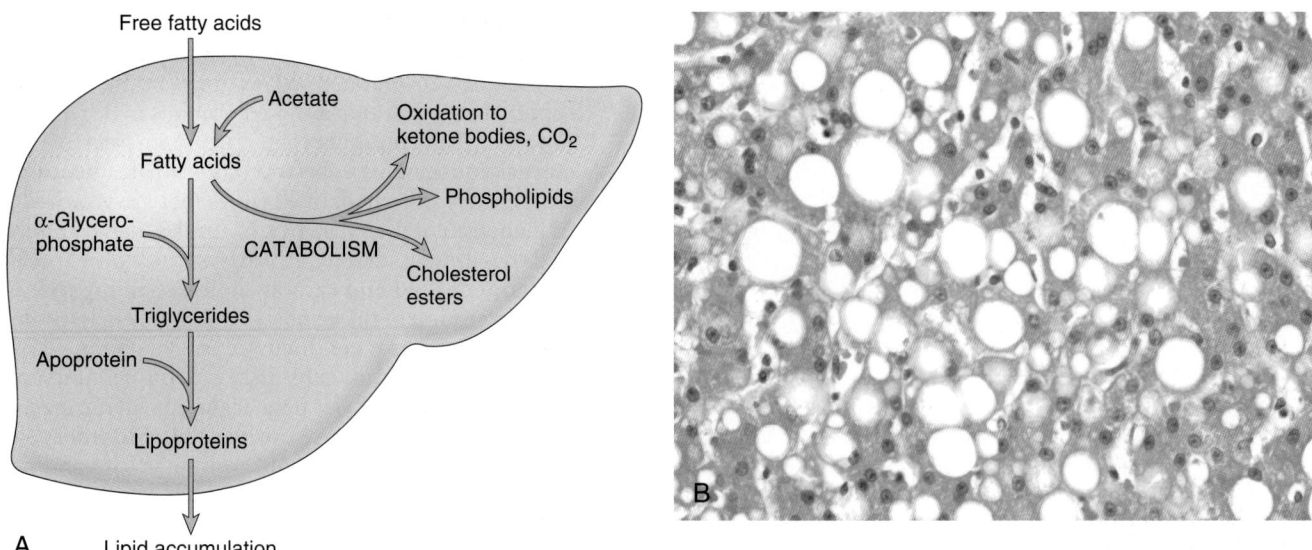

FIGURE 1–30   Fatty liver. **A,** Schematic diagram of the possible mechanisms leading to accumulation of triglycerides in fatty liver. Defects in any of the steps of uptake, catabolism, or secretion can result in lipid accumulation. **B,** High-power detail of fatty change of the liver. In most cells the well-preserved nucleus is squeezed into the displaced rim of cytoplasm about the fat vacuole. (**B,** Courtesy of Dr. James Crawford, Department of Pathology, University of Florida School of Medicine, Gainesville, FL.)

18). CCl_4 and protein malnutrition cause fatty change by reducing synthesis of apoproteins, hypoxia inhibits fatty acid oxidation, and starvation increases fatty acid mobilization from peripheral stores.

The significance of fatty change depends on the cause and severity of the accumulation. When mild it may have no effect on cellular function. More severe fatty change may impair cellular function and may be a harbinger of cell death.

Morphology. Fatty change is most often seen in the liver and heart. In all organs fatty change appears as clear vacuoles within parenchymal cells. Intracellular accumulations of water or polysaccharides (e.g., glycogen) may also produce clear vacuoles. The identification of lipids requires the avoidance of fat solvents commonly used in paraffin embedding for routine hematoxylin and eosin stains. To identify the fat, it is necessary to prepare frozen tissue sections of either fresh or aqueous formalin-fixed tissues. The sections may then be stained with Sudan IV or Oil Red-O, both of which impart an orange-red color to the contained lipids. The periodic acid-Schiff (PAS) reaction, coupled with digestion by the enzyme diastase, is used to identify glycogen, although it is not specific. When neither fat nor polysaccharide can be demonstrated within a clear vacuole, it is presumed to contain water or fluid with a low protein content.

Liver. In the liver, mild fatty change may not affect the gross appearance. With progressive accumulation, the organ enlarges and becomes increasingly yellow until, in extreme instances, the liver may weigh two to four times normal and be transformed into a bright yellow, soft, greasy organ.

Fatty change begins with the development of minute, membrane-bound inclusions (liposomes) closely applied to the ER. Accumulation of fat is first seen by light microscopy as small vacuoles in the cytoplasm around the nucleus. As the process progresses the vacuoles coalesce, creating cleared spaces that displace the nucleus to the periphery of the cell (Fig. 1–30B). Occasionally contiguous cells rupture and the enclosed fat globules coalesce, producing so-called fatty cysts.

Heart. Lipid is found in cardiac muscle in the form of small droplets, occurring in two patterns. In one, prolonged moderate hypoxia, such as that produced by profound anemia, causes intracellular deposits of fat, which create grossly apparent bands of yellowed myocardium alternating with bands of darker, red-brown, uninvolved myocardium (**tigered effect**). The other pattern of fatty change is produced by more profound hypoxia or by some forms of myocarditis (e.g., diphtheria infection) and shows more uniformly affected myocytes.

Cholesterol and Cholesterol Esters

The cellular metabolism of cholesterol (discussed in detail in Chapter 5) is tightly regulated such that most cells use cholesterol for the synthesis of cell membranes without intracellular accumulation of cholesterol or cholesterol esters. Accumulations manifested histologically by intracellular vacuoles are seen in several pathologic processes.

- *Atherosclerosis.* In atherosclerotic plaques, smooth muscle cells and macrophages within the intimal layer of the aorta and large arteries are filled with lipid vacuoles, most of which are made up of cholesterol and cholesterol esters. Such cells have a foamy appearance (foam cells), and aggregates of them in the intima produce the

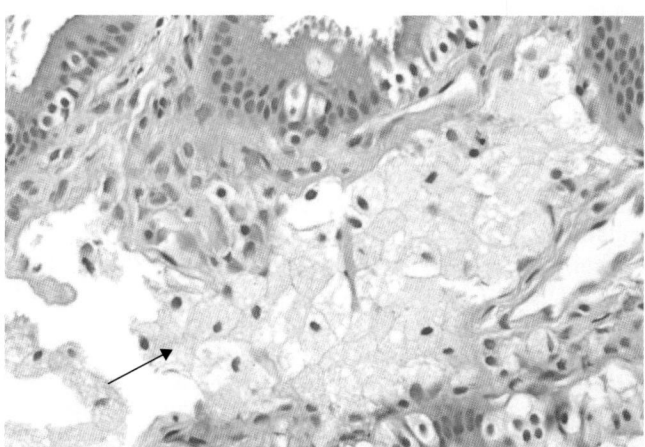

FIGURE 1–31   Cholesterolosis. Cholesterol-laden macrophages (foam cells, *arrow*) in a focus of gallbladder cholesterolosis. (Courtesy of Dr. Matthew Yeh, Department of Pathology, University of Washington, Seattle, WA.)

yellow cholesterol-laden atheromas characteristic of this serious disorder. Some of these fat-laden cells may rupture, releasing lipids into the extracellular space. The mechanisms of cholesterol accumulation in atherosclerosis are discussed in detail in Chapter 11. The extracellular cholesterol esters may crystallize in the shape of long needles, producing quite distinctive clefts in tissue sections.

- *Xanthomas.* Intracellular accumulation of cholesterol within macrophages is also characteristic of acquired and hereditary hyperlipidemic states. Clusters of foamy cells are found in the subepithelial connective tissue of the skin and in tendons, producing tumorous masses known as xanthomas.

- *Cholesterolosis.* This refers to the focal accumulations of cholesterol-laden macrophages in the lamina propria of the gallbladder (Fig. 1–31). The mechanism of accumulation is unknown.

- *Niemann-Pick disease, type C.* This lysosomal storage disease is caused by mutations affecting an enzyme involved in cholesterol trafficking, resulting in cholesterol accumulation in multiple organs (Chapter 5).

PROTEINS

Intracellular accumulations of proteins usually appear as rounded, eosinophilic droplets, vacuoles, or aggregates in the cytoplasm. By electron microscopy they can be amorphous, fibrillar, or crystalline in appearance. In some disorders, such as certain forms of amyloidosis, abnormal proteins deposit primarily in extracellular spaces (Chapter 6).

Excesses of proteins within the cells sufficient to cause morphologically visible accumulation have diverse causes.

- *Reabsorption droplets in proximal renal tubules* are seen in renal diseases associated with protein loss in the urine (proteinuria). In the kidney small amounts of protein filtered through the glomerulus are normally reabsorbed by pinocytosis in the proximal tubule. In disorders with heavy protein leakage across the glomerular filter there is increased reabsorption of the protein into vesicles, and the protein

appears as pink hyaline droplets within the cytoplasm of the tubular cell (Fig. 1–32). The process is reversible; if the proteinuria diminishes, the protein droplets are metabolized and disappear.

- The proteins that accumulate may be normal secreted proteins that are produced in excessive amounts, as occurs in certain plasma cells engaged in active synthesis of immunoglobulins. The ER becomes hugely distended, producing large, homogeneous eosinophilic inclusions called *Russell bodies*.

- *Defective intracellular transport and secretion of critical proteins.* In α_1-antitrypsin deficiency, mutations in the protein significantly slow folding, resulting in the buildup of partially folded intermediates, which aggregate in the ER of the liver and are not secreted. The resultant deficiency of the circulating enzyme causes emphysema (Chapter 15). In many of these diseases the pathology results not only from loss of protein function but also ER stress caused by the misfolded proteins, culminating in apoptotic death of cells (discussed above).

- *Accumulation of cytoskeletal proteins.* There are several types of cytoskeletal proteins, including microtubules (20–25 nm in diameter), thin actin filaments (6–8 nm), thick myosin filaments (15 nm) and intermediate filaments (10 nm). Intermediate filaments, which provide a flexible intracellular scaffold that organizes the cytoplasm and resists forces applied to the cell,[68] are divided into five classes – keratin filaments (characteristic of epithelial cells), neurofilaments (neurons), desmin filaments (muscle cells), vimentin filaments (connective tissue cells), and glial filaments (astrocytes). Accumulations of keratin filaments and neurofilaments are associated with certain types of cell injury. Alcoholic hyaline is an eosinophilic cytoplasmic inclusion in liver cells that is characteristic of alcoholic liver disease, and is composed predominantly of *keratin* intermediate filaments (Chapter 18). The *neurofibrillary tangle* found in the brain in Alzheimer disease contains neurofilaments and other proteins (Chapter 28).

- *Aggregation of abnormal proteins.* Abnormal or misfolded proteins may deposit in tissues and interfere with normal functions. The deposits can be intracellular, extracellular, or both, and the aggregates may either directly or indirectly

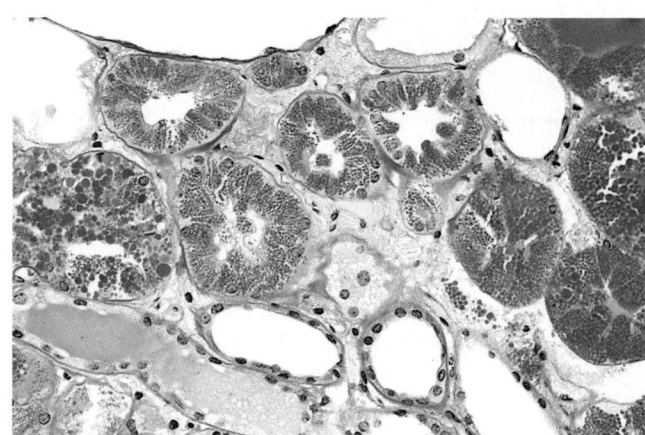

FIGURE 1–32   Protein reabsorption droplets in the renal tubular epithelium. (Courtesy of Dr. Helmut Rennke, Department of Pathology, Brigham and Women's Hospital, Boston, MA.)

cause the pathologic changes. Certain forms of *amyloidosis* (Chapter 6) fall in this category of diseases. These disorders are sometimes called *proteinopathies* or *protein-aggregation diseases*.

HYALINE CHANGE

The term *hyaline* usually refers to an alteration within cells or in the extracellular space that gives a homogeneous, glassy, pink appearance in routine histologic sections stained with hematoxylin and eosin. It is widely used as a descriptive histologic term rather than a specific marker for cell injury. This morphologic change is produced by a variety of alterations and does not represent a specific pattern of accumulation. Intracellular accumulations of protein, described earlier (reabsorption droplets, Russell bodies, alcoholic hyaline), are examples of intracellular hyaline deposits.

Extracellular hyaline has been more difficult to analyze. Collagenous fibrous tissue in old scars may appear hyalinized, but the biochemical basis of this change is not clear. In longstanding hypertension and diabetes mellitus, the walls of arterioles, especially in the kidney, become hyalinized, resulting from extravasated plasma protein and deposition of basement membrane material.

GLYCOGEN

Glycogen is a readily available energy source stored in the cytoplasm of healthy cells. Excessive intracellular deposits of glycogen are seen in patients with an abnormality in either glucose or glycogen metabolism. Whatever the clinical setting, the glycogen masses appear as clear vacuoles within the cytoplasm. Glycogen dissolves in aqueous fixatives; for its localization, tissues are best fixed in absolute alcohol. Staining with Best carmine or the PAS reaction imparts a rose-to-violet color to the glycogen, and diastase digestion of a parallel section before staining serves as a further control by hydrolyzing the glycogen.

Diabetes mellitus is the prime example of a disorder of glucose metabolism. In this disease glycogen is found in renal tubular epithelial cells, as well as within liver cells, β cells of the islets of Langerhans, and heart muscle cells.

Glycogen accumulates within the cells in a group of related genetic disorders that are collectively referred to as the *glycogen storage diseases*, or *glycogenoses* (Chapter 5). In these diseases enzymatic defects in the synthesis or breakdown of glycogen result in massive accumulation, causing cell injury and cell death.

PIGMENTS

Pigments are colored substances, some of which are normal constituents of cells (e.g., melanin), whereas others are abnormal and accumulate in cells only under special circumstances. Pigments can be exogenous, coming from outside the body, or endogenous, synthesized within the body itself.

Exogenous Pigments

The most common *exogenous pigment* is carbon (coal dust), a ubiquitous air pollutant of urban life. When inhaled it is picked up by macrophages within the alveoli and is then transported through lymphatic channels to the regional lymph nodes in the tracheobronchial region. Accumulations of this pigment blacken the tissues of the lungs *(anthracosis)* and the involved lymph nodes. In coal miners the aggregates of carbon dust may induce a fibroblastic reaction or even emphysema and thus cause a serious lung disease known as *coal worker's pneumoconiosis* (Chapter 15). *Tattooing* is a form of localized, exogenous pigmentation of the skin. The pigments inoculated are phagocytosed by dermal macrophages, in which they reside for the remainder of the life of the embellished (sometimes with embarrassing consequences for the bearer of the tattoo!). The pigments do not usually evoke any inflammatory response.

Endogenous Pigments

Lipofuscin is an insoluble pigment, also known as lipochrome or wear-and-tear pigment. Lipofuscin is composed of polymers of lipids and phospholipids in complex with protein, suggesting that it is derived through lipid peroxidation of polyunsaturated lipids of subcellular membranes. Lipofuscin is not injurious to the cell or its functions. Its importance lies in its being a telltale sign of free radical injury and lipid peroxidation. The term is derived from the Latin (*fuscus*, brown), referring to brown lipid. In tissue sections it appears as a yellow-brown, finely granular cytoplasmic, often perinuclear, pigment (Fig. 1–33). It is seen in cells undergoing slow, regressive changes and is particularly prominent in the liver and heart of aging patients or patients with severe malnutrition and cancer cachexia.

Melanin, derived from the Greek (*melas*, black), is an endogenous, non-hemoglobin-derived, brown-black pigment formed when the enzyme tyrosinase catalyzes the oxidation of tyrosine to dihydroxyphenylalanine in melanocytes. It is discussed further in Chapter 25. For practical purposes melanin is the *only endogenous brown-black pigment*. The only other that could be considered in this category is homogentisic acid, a black pigment that occurs in patients with *alkaptonuria*, a rare metabolic disease. Here the pigment is deposited in the skin, connective tissue, and cartilage, and the pigmentation is known as *ochronosis* (Chapter 5).

Hemosiderin is a hemoglobin-derived, golden yellow-to-brown, granular or crystalline pigment that serves as one of the major storage forms of iron. Iron metabolism and hemosiderin are considered in detail in Chapters 14 and 18. Iron is normally carried by specific transport proteins, transferrins. In cells, it is stored in association with a protein, apoferritin, to form ferritin micelles. Ferritin is a constituent of most cell types. *When there is a local or systemic excess of iron, ferritin forms hemosiderin granules*, which are easily seen with the light microscope (Fig. 1–34). Hemosiderin pigment represents aggregates of ferritin micelles. Under normal conditions small amounts of hemosiderin can be seen in the mononuclear phagocytes of the bone marrow, spleen, and liver, which are actively engaged in red cell breakdown.

Local or systemic excesses of iron cause hemosiderin to accumulate within cells. *Local excesses* result from hemorrhages in tissues. The best example of localized hemosiderosis is the common bruise. Extravasated red blood cells at the site of injury are phagocytosed over several days by macro-

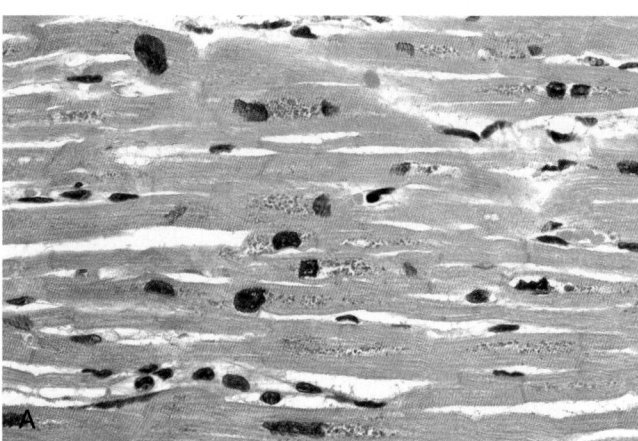
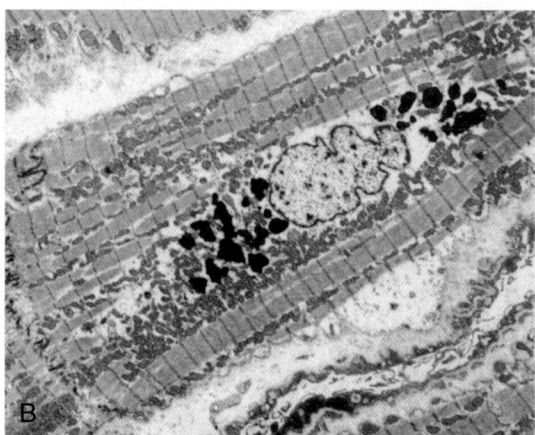

FIGURE 1–33 Lipofuscin granules in a cardiac myocyte shown by (**A**) light microscopy (deposits indicated by *arrows*), and (**B**) electron microscopy (note the perinuclear, intralysosomal location).

phages, which break down the hemoglobin and recover the iron. After removal of iron, the heme moiety is converted first to biliverdin ("green bile") and then to bilirubin ("red bile"). In parallel, the iron released from heme is incorporated into ferritin and eventually hemosiderin. These conversions account for the often dramatic play of colors seen in a healing bruise, which typically changes from red-blue to green-blue to golden-yellow before it is resolved.

When there is *systemic overload of iron* hemosiderin may be deposited in many organs and tissues, a condition called *hemosiderosis*. The main causes of hemosiderosis are (1) increased absorption of dietary iron, (2) hemolytic anemias, in which abnormal quantities of iron are released from erythrocytes, and (3) repeated blood transfusions because the transfused red cells constitute an exogenous load of iron. These conditions are discussed in Chapter 18.

Morphology. Iron pigment appears as a coarse, golden, granular pigment lying within the cell's cyto-

plasm (Fig. 1–34A). It can be visualized in tissues by the Prussian blue histochemical reaction, in which colorless potassium ferrocyanide is converted by iron to blue-black ferric ferrocyanide (Fig. 1–34B). When the underlying cause is the localized breakdown of red cells, the hemosiderin is found initially in the phagocytes in the area. In systemic hemosiderosis it is found at first in the mononuclear phagocytes of the liver, bone marrow, spleen, and lymph nodes and in scattered macrophages throughout other organs such as the skin, pancreas, and kidneys. With progressive accumulation, parenchymal cells throughout the body (principally in the liver, pancreas, heart, and endocrine organs) become pigmented.

In most instances of systemic hemosiderosis the pigment does not damage the parenchymal cells or impair organ function. The more extreme accumulation of iron, however, in an inherited disease called **hemochromatosis**, is associated with liver, heart, and

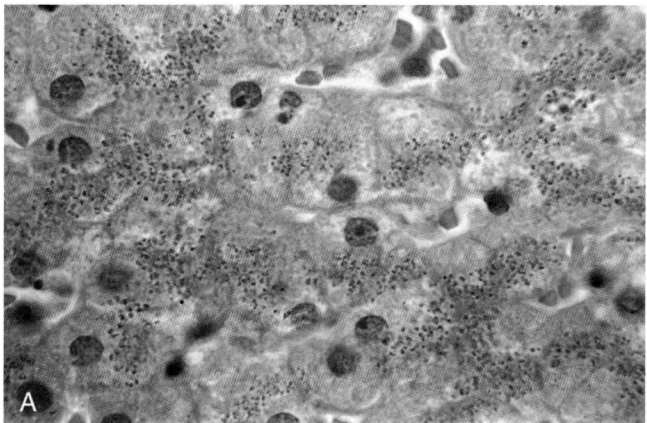
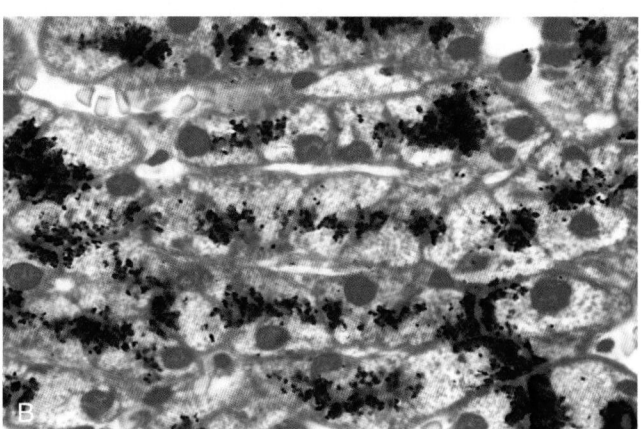

FIGURE 1–34 Hemosiderin granules in liver cells. **A,** H+E stain showing golden-brown, finely granular pigment. **B,** Prussian blue stain, specific for iron (seen as blue granules).

pancreatic damage, resulting in liver fibrosis, heart failure, and diabetes mellitus (Chapter 18).

Bilirubin is the normal major pigment found in bile. It is derived from hemoglobin but contains no iron. Its normal formation and excretion are vital to health, and jaundice is a common clinical disorder caused by excesses of this pigment within cells and tissues. Bilirubin metabolism and jaundice are discussed in Chapter 18.

Pathologic Calcification

Pathologic calcification is the abnormal tissue deposition of calcium salts, together with smaller amounts of iron, magnesium, and other mineral salts. There are two forms of pathologic calcification. When the deposition occurs locally in dying tissues it is known as *dystrophic calcification*; it occurs despite normal serum levels of calcium and in the absence of derangements in calcium metabolism. In contrast, the deposition of calcium salts in otherwise normal tissues is known as *metastatic calcification*, and it almost always results from hypercalcemia secondary to some disturbance in calcium metabolism.

DYSTROPHIC CALCIFICATION

Dystrophic calcification is encountered in areas of necrosis, whether they are of coagulative, caseous, or liquefactive type, and in foci of enzymatic necrosis of fat. Calcification is almost always present in the atheromas of advanced atherosclerosis. It also commonly develops in aging or damaged heart valves, further hampering their function (Fig. 1–35). Whatever the site of deposition, the calcium salts appear macroscopically as fine, white granules or clumps, often felt as gritty deposits. Sometimes a tuberculous lymph node is virtually converted to stone.

Morphology. Histologically, with the usual hematoxylin and eosin stain, calcium salts have a basophilic, amorphous granular, sometimes clumped appearance. They can be intracellular, extracellular, or in both locations. In the course of time, **heterotopic** bone may be formed in the focus of calcification. On occasion single necrotic cells may constitute seed crystals that become encrusted by the mineral deposits. The progressive acquisition of outer layers may create lamellated configurations, called **psammoma bodies** because of their resemblance to grains of sand. Some types of papillary cancers (e.g., thyroid) are apt to develop psammoma bodies. In asbestosis, calcium and iron salts gather about long slender spicules of asbestos in the lung, creating exotic, beaded dumbbell forms (Chapter 15).

Pathogenesis. In the pathogenesis of dystrophic calcification, the final common pathway is the formation of crystalline calcium phosphate mineral in the form of an apatite similar to the hydroxyapatite of bone. It is thought that calcium is

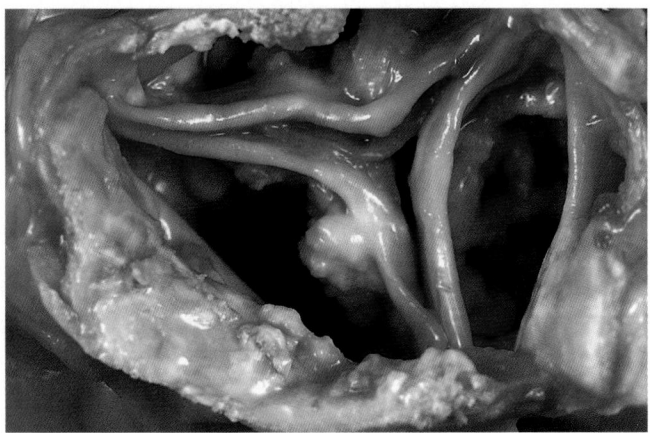

FIGURE 1–35 Dystrophic calcification of the aortic valve. View looking down onto the unopened aortic valve in a heart with calcific aortic stenosis. It is markedly narrowed (stenosis). The semilunar cusps are thickened and fibrotic, and behind each cusp are irregular masses of piled-up dystrophic calcification.

concentrated in membrane-bound vesicles in cells by a process that is initiated by membrane damage and has several steps: (1) calcium ion binds to the phospholipids present in the vesicle membrane; (2) phosphatases associated with the membrane generate phosphate groups, which bind to the calcium; (3) the cycle of calcium and phosphate binding is repeated, raising the local concentrations and producing a deposit near the membrane; and (4) a structural change occurs in the arrangement of calcium and phosphate groups, generating a microcrystal, which can then propagate and lead to more calcium deposition.

Although dystrophic calcification may simply be a telltale sign of previous cell injury, it is often a cause of organ dysfunction. Such is the case in calcific valvular disease and atherosclerosis, as will become clear in further discussion of these diseases.

METASTATIC CALCIFICATION

Metastatic calcification may occur in normal tissues whenever there is hypercalcemia. Hypercalcemia also accentuates dystrophic calcification. There are four principal causes of hypercalcemia: (1) increased secretion of parathyroid hormone (PTH) with subsequent bone resorption, as in *hyperparathyroidism* due to parathyroid tumors, and ectopic secretion of PTH-related protein by malignant tumors (Chapter 7); (2) *destruction of bone tissue*, secondary to primary tumors of bone marrow (e.g., multiple myeloma, leukemia) or diffuse skeletal metastasis (e.g., breast cancer), accelerated bone turnover (e.g., Paget disease), or immobilization; (3) *vitamin D–related disorders*, including vitamin D intoxication, sarcoidosis (in which macrophages activate a vitamin D precursor), and idiopathic hypercalcemia of infancy (Williams syndrome), characterized by abnormal sensitivity to vitamin D; and (4) *renal failure*, which causes retention of phosphate, leading to secondary hyperparathyroidism. Less common causes include aluminum intoxication, which occurs in patients on chronic renal dialysis, and milk-alkali syndrome, which is due to excessive ingestion of calcium and absorbable antacids such as milk or calcium carbonate.

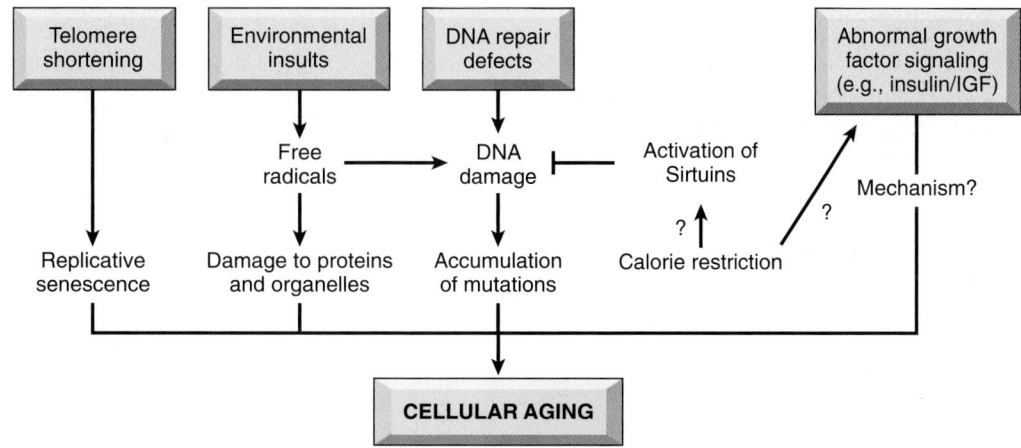

FIGURE 1–36   Mechanisms of cellular aging. Genetic factors and environmental insults combine to produce the cellular abnormalities characteristic of aging. How calorie restrictions prolong life span is net established. IGF, insulin-like growth factor.

Metastatic calcification may occur widely throughout the body but principally affects the interstitial tissues of the gastric mucosa, kidneys, lungs, systemic arteries, and pulmonary veins. Though quite different in location, all of these tissues excrete acid and therefore have an internal alkaline compartment that predisposes them to metastatic calcification. In all these sites the calcium salts morphologically resemble those described in dystrophic calcification. Thus, they may occur as noncrystalline amorphous deposits or, at other times, as hydroxyapatite crystals.

Usually the mineral salts cause no clinical dysfunction, but on occasion massive involvement of the lungs produces remarkable x-ray films and respiratory deficits. Massive deposits in the kidney (nephrocalcinosis) may in time cause renal damage (Chapter 20).

Cellular Aging

Shakespeare probably characterized aging best in his elegant description of the seven ages of man. It begins at the moment of conception, involves the differentiation and maturation of the organism and its cells, at some variable point in time leads to the progressive loss of functional capacity characteristic of senescence, and ends in death. With age there are physiologic and structural alterations in almost all organ systems. Aging in individuals is affected to a great extent by genetic factors, diet, social conditions, and occurrence of age-related diseases, such as atherosclerosis, diabetes, and osteoarthritis. In addition, there is good evidence that aging-induced alterations in cells are an important component of the aging of the organism. Here we discuss cellular aging because it could represent the progressive accumulation over the years of sublethal injury that may lead to cell death or to a diminished capacity of the cell to respond to injury.

Cellular aging is the result of a progressive decline in cellular function and viability caused by genetic abnormalities and the accumulation of cellular and molecular damage due to the effects of exposure to exogenous influences (Fig. 1–36). Studies in model systems have clearly established that aging is a regulated process that is influenced by a limited number of genes,[69] and

genetic anomalies underlie syndromes resembling premature aging in humans as well.[70] Such findings suggest that aging is associated with definable mechanistic alterations. The known changes that contribute to cellular aging include the following.

○ *Decreased cellular replication.* The concept that most normal cells have a limited capacity for replication was developed from a simple experimental model for aging. Normal human fibroblasts, when placed in tissue culture, have limited division potential.[71] After a fixed number of divisions all somatic cells become arrested in a terminally nondividing state, known as *senescence.* Cells from children undergo more rounds of replication than do cells from older people (Fig. 1–37). In contrast, cells from patients with *Werner syndrome,* a rare disease characterized by

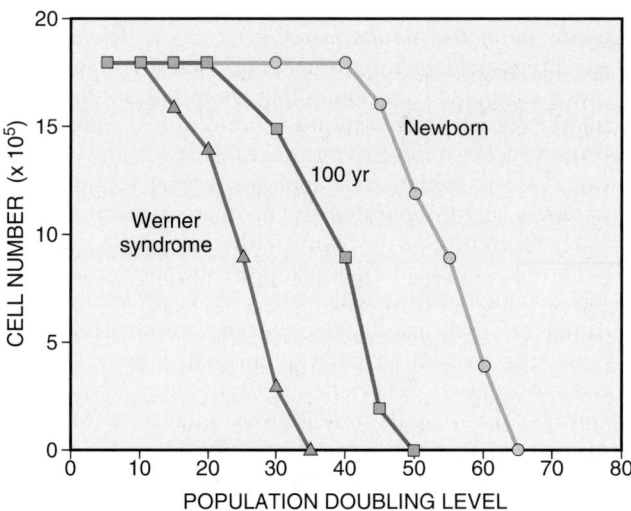

FIGURE 1–37   Finite population doublings of primary human fibroblasts derived from a newborn, a 100-year-old person, and a 20-year-old patient with Werner syndrome. The ability of cells to grow to a confluent monolayer decreases with increasing population-doubling levels. (From Dice JF: Cellular and molecular mechanisms of aging. Physiol Rev 73:150, 1993.)

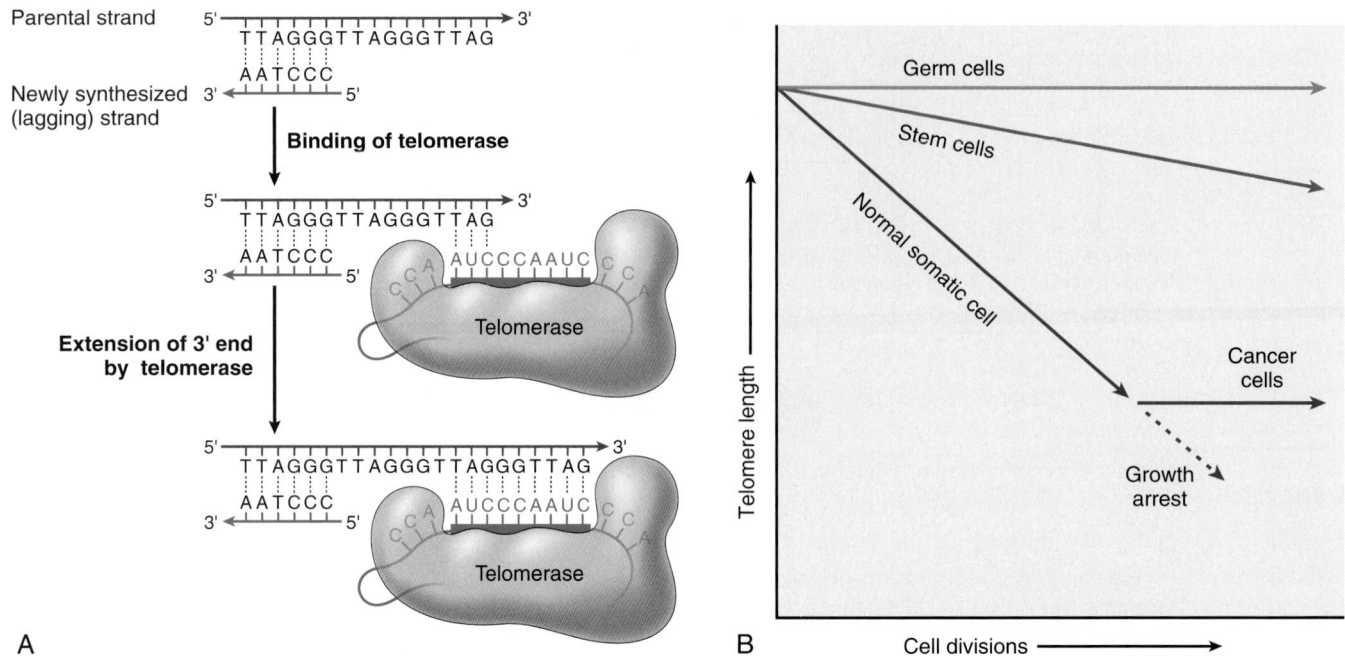

FIGURE 1–38 The role of telomeres and telomerase in replicative senescence of cells. **A,** Telomerase directs RNA template-dependent DNA synthesis, in which nucleotides are added to one strand at the end of a chromosome. The lagging strand is filled in by DNA polymerase. **B,** Telomere-telomerase hypothesis and proliferative capacity of cells. Telomere length is plotted against the number of cell divisions. Germ cells and stem cells both contain active telomerase, but only the germ cells have sufficient levels of the enzyme to stabilize telomere length completely. In normal somatic cells there is no telomerase activity, and telomeres progressively shorten with successive cell divisions until growth arrest, or senescence, occurs. Telomerase activation in cancer cells counteracts the telomere shortening that limits the proliferative capacity of normal somatic cells. (**A,** Data from Alberts BR, et al: Molecular Biology of the Cell. New York, Garland Science, 2002. **B,** Modified and redrawn with permission from Holt SE, et al: Refining the telomere-telomerase hypothesis of aging and cancer. Nat Biotechnol 14:836, 1996. Copyright 1996, Macmillan Magazines Limited.)

symptoms of premature aging, are defective in DNA replication and have a markedly reduced capacity to divide.

It is still not known why aging is associated with progressive senescence of cells.[72] One probable mechanism in human cells is that with each cell division there is *incomplete replication of chromosome ends (telomere shortening), which ultimately results in cell cycle arrest. Telomeres* are short repeated sequences of DNA (TTAGGG) present at the linear ends of chromosomes that are important for ensuring the complete replication of chromosomal ends and for protecting chromosomal termini from fusion and degradation.[73] When somatic cells replicate, a small section of the telomere is not duplicated and telomeres become progressively shortened. As the telomeres become shorter the ends of chromosomes cannot be protected and are seen as broken DNA, which activates the DNA damage response and signals cell cycle arrest. Telomere length is normally maintained by nucleotide addition mediated by an enzyme called *telomerase.* Telomerase is a specialized RNA-protein complex that uses its own RNA as a template for adding nucleotides to the ends of chromosomes (Fig. 1–38A). The activity of telomerase is repressed by regulatory proteins, which provide a mechanism for sensing telomere length and restrict unnecessary elongation. Telomerase activity is highest in germ cells and present at lower levels in stem cells, but it is usually undetectable in most somatic tissues (Fig. 1–38B). Therefore, as somatic cells divide, their telomeres become shorter, and they exit the cell cycle, resulting

in an inability to generate new cells to replace damaged ones. Thus, both accumulation of senescent cells and depletion of stem cell pools via senescence contribute to aging. Conversely, in immortal cancer cells telomerase is reactivated and telomeres are stable, suggesting that maintenance of telomere length might be an important—possibly essential—step in tumor formation (Chapter 7). Despite such alluring observations, however, the relationship of telomerase activity and telomeric length to aging and cancer still must be fully established.[74]

Replicative senescence can also be induced by increased expression of the cell cycle inhibitor p16INK4a and by DNA damage (discussed further below). How these factors contribute to normal aging is not known.[75]

● *Accumulation of metabolic and genetic damage.* Cellular life span is determined by a balance between damage resulting from *metabolic events* occurring within the cell and counteracting molecular responses that can repair the damage. One group of potentially toxic products of normal metabolism are *reactive oxygen species.* As we saw earlier, these by-products of oxidative phosphorylation cause covalent modifications of proteins, lipids, and nucleic acids. Increased oxidative damage could result from repeated environmental exposure to such influences as ionizing radiation, mitochondrial dysfunction, or reduction of antioxidant defense mechanisms with age (e.g., vitamin E, glutathione peroxidase). The amount of oxidative damage, which increases as an organism ages, may be an important cause of senescence.[76] Consistent with this proposal are the following observations: (1) variation in longevity among different species is inversely correlated with the rates of mitochondrial generation of O_2^- anion radical, and (2) overexpression of the antioxidative enzymes SOD and catalase extends life span in transgenic forms of *Drosophila*. Free radicals may have deleterious effects on DNA, leading to breaks and genome instability, thus affecting all cellular functions.[77]

Several protective responses counterbalance progressive damage in cells, and an important one is the recognition and repair of damaged DNA. Although most DNA damage is repaired by endogenous DNA repair enzymes, some persists and accumulates as cells age. Several lines of evidence point to the importance of DNA repair in the aging process. Patients with *Werner syndrome* show premature aging, and the defective gene product is a DNA helicase—a protein involved in DNA replication and repair and other functions requiring DNA unwinding.[78] A defect in this enzyme causes rapid accumulation of chromosomal damage that may mimic the injury that normally accumulates during cellular aging. Genetic instability in somatic cells is also characteristic of other disorders in which patients display some of the manifestations of aging at an increased rate, such as *ataxia-telangiectasia*, in which the mutated gene encodes a protein involved in repairing double-strand breaks in DNA (Chapter 7). Thus, the balance between cumulative metabolic damage and the response to that damage could determine the rate at which we age. In this scenario aging can be delayed by decreasing the accumulation of damage or by increasing the response to that damage.

Not only damaged DNA but damaged cellular organelles also accumulate as cells age. In part this may be the result of declining function of the proteasome, the proteolytic machine that serves to eliminate abnormal and unwanted intracellular proteins.[79]

Studies in model organisms, from yeast to mammals, have shown that the most effective way of prolonging life span is *calorie restriction*. How this works is still not established, but the effect of calorie restriction on longevity appears to be mediated by a family of proteins called *sirtuins*.[80] Sirtuins have histone deacetylase activity, and are thought to promote the expression of several genes whose products increase longevity. These products include proteins that increase metabolic activity, reduce apoptosis, stimulate protein folding, and inhibit the harmful effects of oxygen free radicals.[81] Sirtuins also increase insulin sensitivity and glucose metabolism, and may be targets for the treatment of diabetes. Not surprisingly, optimistic wine-lovers have been delighted to hear that a constituent of red wine may activate sirtuins and thus increase life span! Other studies have shown that growth factors, such as insulin-like growth factor, and intracellular signaling pathways triggered by these hormones also influence life span.[69] Transcription factors activated by insulin receptor signaling may induce genes that reduce longevity, and insulin receptor mutations are associated with increased life span. The relevance of these findings to aging in humans is an area of active investigation.

It should be apparent that the various forms of cellular derangements and adaptations described in this chapter cover a wide spectrum, ranging from adaptations in cell size, growth, and function; to the reversible and irreversible forms of acute cell injury; to the regulated type of cell death represented by apoptosis; to the pathologic alterations in cell organelles; and to the less ominous forms of intracellular accumulations, including pigmentations. Reference is made to all these alterations throughout this book, because all organ injury and ultimately all clinical disease arise from derangements in cell structure and function.

REFERENCES

1. Majno G: The Healing Hand: Man and Wound in the Ancient World. Cambridge, Harvard University Press, 1975, p 43.
2. Anversa P, Nadal-Ginard B: Myocyte renewal and ventricular remodeling. Nature 415:240, 2002.
3. Glass DJ: Signalling pathways that mediate skeletal muscle hypertrophy and atrophy. Nat Cell Biol 5:87, 2003.
4. Frey N, Olson EN: Cardiac hypertrophy: the good, the bad, and the ugly. Annu Rev Physiol 65:45, 2003.
5. Heineke J, Molkentin JD: Regulation of cardiac hypertrophy by intracellular signalling pathways. Nat Rev Mol Cell Biol 7:589, 2006.
6. Dorn GW: The fuzzy logic of physiological cardiac hypertrophy. Hypertension 49:962, 2007.
7. Roots I, et al. Genotype and phenotype relationship in drug metabolism. Ernst Schering Res Found Workshop 59:81, 2007.
8. Tanimizu N, Miyajima A: Molecular mechanism of liver development and regeneration. Int Rev Cytol 259:1, 2007.
9. Kandarian SC, Jackman RW: Intracellular signaling during skeletal muscle atrophy. Muscle Nerve 33:155, 2006.
10. Sacheck JM, et al.: Rapid disuse and denervation atrophy involve transcriptional changes similar to those of muscle wasting during systemic diseases. FASEB J 21:140, 2007.
11. Tosh D, Slack JM: How cells change their phenotype. Nat Rev Mol Cell Biol 3:187, 2002.
12. Slack JM: Metaplasia and transdifferentiation: from pure biology to the clinic. Nat Rev Mol Cell Biol 8:369, 2007.
13. Edinger AL, Thompson CB: Death by design: apoptosis, necrosis and autophagy. Curr Opin Cell Biol 16:663, 2004.
14. Kroemer G, et al.: Classification of cell death: recommendations of the Nomenclature Committee on Cell Death. Cell Death Differ 12 (Suppl 2):1463, 2005.
15. Golstein P, Kroemer G: Cell death by necrosis: towards a molecular definition. Trends Biochem Sci 32:37, 2007.
16. Vanlangenakker N et al.: Molecular mechanisms and pathophysiology of necrotic cell death. Curr Mol Med 8:207, 2008.
17. Newmeyer DD, Ferguson-Miller S: Mitochondria: releasing power for life and unleashing the machineries of death. Cell 112:481, 2003.
18. Bernardi P, et al.: The mitochondrial permeability transition from in vitro artifact to disease target. FEBS J 273:2077, 2006.
19. Deng Z, et al.: Calcium in cell injury and death. Annu Rev Pathol 1:405, 2006.
20. Orrenius S, et al.: Regulation of cell death: the calcium-apoptosis link. Nat Rev Mol Cell Biol 4:552, 2003.
21. Valko M, et al.: Free radicals and antioxidants in normal physiological functions and human disease. Int J Biochem Cell Biol 39:44, 2007.
22. Szabo C, et al.: Peroxynitrite: biochemistry, pathophysiology and development of therapeutics. Nat Rev Drug Discov 6:662, 2007.
23. Lambeth JD. NOX enzymes and the biology of reactive oxygen. Nat Rev Immunol 4:181, 2004.
24. Ryter SW, et al.: Mechanisms of cell death in oxidative stress. Antioxid Redox Signal 9:49, 2007.
25. D'Autreaux B, Toledano MB: ROS as signalling molecules: mechanisms that generate specificity in ROS homeostasis. Nat Rev Mol Cell Biol 8:813, 2007.
26. Afanas'ev IB: Signaling functions of free radicals superoxide and nitric oxide under physiological and pathological conditions. Mol Biotechnol 37:2, 2007.
27. Ke Q, Costa M: Hypoxia-inducible factor-1 (HIF-1). Mol Pharmacol 70:1469, 2006.
28. Rincon F, Mayer SA: Therapeutic hypothermia for brain injury after cardiac arrest. Semin Neurol 26:387, 2006.

29. de Groot H, Rauen U: Ischemia-reperfusion injury: processes in pathogenetic networks: a review. Transplant Proc 39:481, 2007.
30. Kaminski KA, et al.: Oxidative stress and neutrophil activation—the two keystones of ischemia/reperfusion injury. Int J Cardiol 86:41, 2002.
31. Zweier JL, Talukder MA: The role of oxidants and free radicals in reperfusion injury. Cardiovasc Res 70:181, 2006.
32. Frangogiannis NG, et al.: The inflammatory response in myocardial infarction. Cardiovasc Res 53:31, 2002.
33. Riedemann NC, Ward PA: Complement in ischemia reperfusion injury. Am J Pathol 162:363, 2003.
34. Zhang M, et al.: The role of natural IgM in myocardial ischemia-reperfusion injury. J Mol Cell Cardiol 41:62, 2006.
35. Bjornsson E: Drug-induced liver injury: Hy's rule revisited. Clin Pharmacol Ther 79:521, 2006.
36. Kaplowitz N: Biochemical and cellular mechanisms of toxic liver injury. Semin Liver Dis 22:137, 2002.
37. Kerr JF, et al.: Apoptosis: a basic biological phenomenon with wide-ranging implications in tissue kinetics. Br J Cancer 26:239, 1972.
38. Metzstein MM, et al.: Genetics of programmed cell death in *C. elegans*: past, present and future. Trends Genet 14:410, 1998.
39. Wyllie AH: Apoptosis: an overview. Br Med Bull 53:451, 1997.
40. Lavrik IN, et al.: Caspases: pharmacological manipulation of cell death. J Clin Invest 115:2665, 2005.
41. McCarthy NJ, Evan GI: Methods for detecting and quantifying apoptosis. Curr Top Dev Biol 36:259, 1998.
42. Danial NN, Korsmeyer SJ: Cell death: critical control points. Cell 116:205, 2004.
43. Cory S, Adams JM: The Bcl2 family: regulators of the cellular life-or-death switch. Nat Rev Cancer 2:647, 2002.
44. Riedl SJ, Salvesen GS: The apoptosome: signalling platform of cell death. Nat Rev Mol Cell Biol 8:405, 2007.
45. Vaux DL, Silke J: Mammalian mitochondrial IAP binding proteins. Biochem Biophys Res Commun 304:499, 2003.
46. Shiozaki EN, Shi Y: Caspases, IAPs and Smac/DIABLO: mechanisms from structural biology. Trends Biochem Sci 29:486, 2004.
47. Joza N, et al.: Genetic analysis of the mammalian cell death machinery. Trends Genet 18:142, 2002.
48. Wallach D, et al.: Tumor necrosis factor receptor and Fas signaling mechanisms. Annu Rev Immunol 17:331, 1999.
49. Nagata S: Fas ligand-induced apoptosis. Annu Rev Genet 33:29, 1999.
50. Peter ME, Krammer PH: The CD95(APO-1/Fas) DISC and beyond. Cell Death Differ 10:26, 2003.
51. Callus BA, Vaux DL: Caspase inhibitors: viral, cellular and chemical. Cell Death Differ 14:73, 2007.
52. Ravichandran KS: "Recruitment signals" from apoptotic cells: invitation to a quiet meal. Cell 113:817, 2003.
53. Ogden CA, Elkon KB: Role of complement and other innate immune mechanisms in the removal of apoptotic cells. Curr Dir Autoimmun 9:120, 2006.
54. Fadeel B, Orrenius S: Apoptosis: a basic biological phenomenon with wide-ranging implications in human disease. J Intern Med 258:479, 2005.
55. Roos WP, Kaina B: DNA damage-induced cell death by apoptosis. Trends Mol Med 12:440, 2006.
56. Patil C, Walter P: Intracellular signaling from the endoplasmic reticulum to the nucleus: the unfolded protein response in yeast and mammals. Curr Opin Cell Biol 13:349, 2001.
57. Schroder M, Kaufman RJ: The mammalian unfolded protein response. Annu Rev Biochem 74:739, 2005.
58. Xu C, et al.: Endoplasmic reticulum stress: cell life and death decisions. J Clin Invest 115:2656, 2005.
59. Macario AJ, Conway de Macario E: Sick chaperones, cellular stress, and disease. N Engl J Med 353:1489, 2005.
60. Marx J: Cell biology. A stressful situation. Science 313:1564, 2006.
61. Lin JH, et al.: Endoplasmic reticulum stress in disease pathogenesis. Annu Rev Pathol 3:399, 2008.
62. Rathmell JC, Thompson CB: Pathways of apoptosis in lymphocyte development, homeostasis, and disease. Cell 109 (Suppl):S97, 2002.
63. Russell JH, Ley TJ: Lymphocyte-mediated cytotoxicity. Annu Rev Immunol 20:323, 2002.
64. Levine B: Eating oneself and uninvited guests: autophagy-related pathways in cellular defense. Cell 120:159, 2005.
65. Kundu M, Thompson CB: Autophagy: basic principles and relevance to disease. Annu Rev Pathol 3:427, 2008.
66. Maiuri MC, et al.: Self-eating and self-killing: crosstalk between autophagy and apoptosis. Nat Rev Mol Cell Biol 8:741, 2007.
67. Huang J, Klionsky DJ: Autophagy and human disease. Cell Cycle 6:1837, 2007.
68. Omary MB, et al.: "Heads and tails" of intermediate filament phosphorylation: multiple sites and functional insights. Trends Biochem Sci 31:383, 2006.
69. Kenyon C: The plasticity of aging: insights from long-lived mutants. Cell 120:449, 2005.
70. Martin GM, Oshima J: Lessons from human progeroid syndromes. Nature 408:263, 2000.
71. Hayflick L, Moorhead PS: The serial cultivation of human diploid cell strains. Exp Cell Res 25:585, 1961.
72. Patil CK, et al.: The thorny path linking cellular senescence to organismal aging. Mech Ageing Dev 126:1040, 2005.
73. Blackburn EH: Switching and signaling at the telomere. Cell 106:661, 2001.
74. Stewart SA, Weinberg RA: Telomeres: cancer to human aging. Annu Rev Cell Dev Biol 22:531, 2006.
75. Collado M, Blasco MA, Serrano M: Cellular senescence in cancer and aging. Cell 130:223, 2007.
76. Balaban RS, et al.: Mitochondria, oxidants, and aging. Cell 120:483, 2005.
77. Lombard DB, et al.: DNA repair, genome stability, and aging. Cell 120:497, 2005.
78. Kyng KJ, Bohr VA: Gene expression and DNA repair in progeroid syndromes and human aging. Ageing Res Rev 4:579, 2005.
79. Carrard G, et al.: Impairment of proteasome structure and function in aging. Int J Biochem Cell Biol 34:1461, 2002.
80. Michan S, Sinclair D: Sirtuins in mammals: insights into their biological function. Biochem J 404:1, 2007.
81. Bordone L, Guarente L: Calorie restriction, SIRT1 and metabolism: understanding longevity. Nat Rev Mol Cell Biol 6:298, 2005.

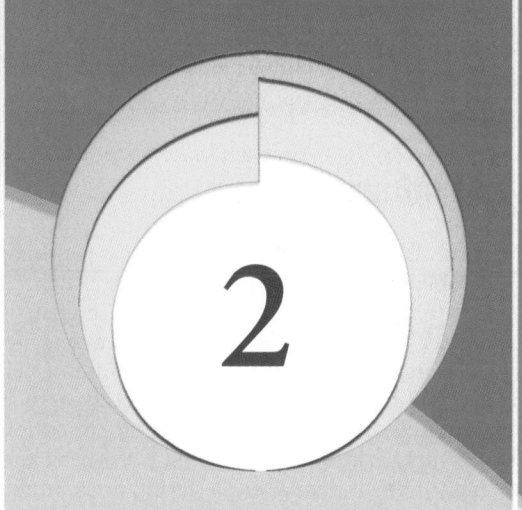

Acute and Chronic Inflammation

Overview of Inflammation

Historical Highlights

Acute Inflammation

  Stimuli for Acute Inflammation

  Reactions of Blood Vessels in Acute Inflammation
  Changes in Vascular Flow and Caliber
  Increased Vascular Permeability (Vascular Leakage)
  Responses of Lymphatic Vessels

  Reactions of Leukocytes in Inflammation
  Recruitment of Leukocytes to Sites of Infection and Injury
  Recognition of Microbes and Dead Tissues
  Removal of the Offending Agents
  Other Functional Responses of Activated Leukocytes
  Release of Leukocyte Products and Leukocyte-Mediated Tissue Injury
  Defects in Leukocyte Function

  Termination of the Acute Inflammatory Response

Mediators of Inflammation

  Cell-Derived Mediators
  Vasoactive Amines: Histamine and Serotonin
  Arachidonic Acid (AA) Metabolites: Prostaglandins, Leukotrienes, and Lipoxins
  Platelet-Activating Factor (PAF)

  Reactive Oxygen Species
  Nitric Oxide
  Cytokines and Chemokines
  Lysosomal Constituents of Leukocytes
  Neuropeptides

  Plasma Protein–Derived Mediators
  Complement System
  Coagulation and Kinin Systems

Outcomes of Acute Inflammation

Morphologic Patterns of Acute Inflammation

  Serous Inflammation

  Fibrinous Inflammation

  Suppurative or Purulent Inflammation; Abscess

  Ulcers

Summary of Acute Inflammation

Chronic Inflammation

  Causes of Chronic Inflammation

  Morphologic Features

  Role of Macrophages in Chronic Inflammation

  Other Cells in Chronic Inflammation

  Granulomatous Inflammation

Systemic Effects of Inflammation

Consequences of Defective or Excessive Inflammation

Overview of Inflammation

Essential to the survival of organisms is their ability to get rid of damaged or necrotic tissues and foreign invaders, such as microbes. The host response that accomplishes these goals is called *inflammation. This is fundamentally a protective response,* designed to rid the organism of both the initial cause of cell injury (e.g., microbes, toxins) and the consequences of such injury (e.g., necrotic cells and tissues). Without inflammation infections would go unchecked, wounds would never heal, and injured tissues might remain permanent festering sores. In the practice of medicine the importance of inflammation is that it can sometimes be inappropriately triggered or poorly controlled, and is thus the cause of tissue injury in many disorders.

Inflammation is a complex reaction in tissues that consists mainly of responses of blood vessels and leukocytes. The body's principal defenders against foreign invaders are plasma proteins and circulating leukocytes (white blood cells), as well as tissue phagocytes that are derived from circulating cells. The presence of proteins and leukocytes in the blood gives them the ability to home to any site where they may be needed. Because invaders such as microbes and necrotic cells are typically present in tissues, outside the circulation, it follows that the circulating cells and proteins have to be rapidly recruited to these extravascular sites. The inflammatory response coordinates the reactions of vessels, leukocytes, and plasma proteins to achieve this goal.

The vascular and cellular reactions of inflammation are triggered by soluble factors that are produced by various cells or derived from plasma proteins and are generated or activated in response to the inflammatory stimulus. Microbes, necrotic cells (whatever the cause of cell death) and even hypoxia can trigger the elaboration of inflammatory mediators, and thus elicit inflammation. Such mediators initiate and amplify the inflammatory response and determine its pattern, severity, and clinical and pathologic manifestations.

Inflammation may be acute or chronic, depending on the nature of the stimulus and the effectiveness of the initial reaction in eliminating the stimulus or the damaged tissues. *Acute inflammation* is rapid in onset (typically minutes) and is of short duration, lasting for hours or a few days; its main characteristics are the exudation of fluid and plasma proteins (edema) and the emigration of leukocytes, predominantly neutrophils (also called polymorphonuclear leukocytes). When acute inflammation is successful in eliminating the offenders the reaction subsides, but if the response fails to clear the invaders it can progress to a chronic phase. *Chronic inflammation* may follow acute inflammation or be insidious in onset. It is of longer duration and is associated with the presence of lymphocytes and macrophages, the proliferation of blood vessels, fibrosis, and tissue destruction.

Inflammation is terminated when the offending agent is eliminated. The reaction resolves rapidly, because the mediators are broken down and dissipated and the leukocytes have short life spans in tissues. In addition, anti-inflammatory mechanisms are activated that serve to control the response and prevent it from causing excessive damage to the host.

The inflammatory response is closely intertwined with the process of repair. At the same time as inflammation destroys, dilutes, and walls off the injurious agent, it sets into motion a series of events that try to heal the damaged tissue. Repair begins during inflammation but reaches completion usually after the injurious influence has been neutralized. In the process of repair the injured tissue is replaced through *regeneration* of native parenchymal cells, by filling of the defect with fibrous tissue *(scarring)* or, most commonly, by a combination of these two processes (Chapter 3).

Inflammation may be harmful in some situations. Mechanisms designed to destroy foreign invaders and necrotic tissues have an intrinsic ability to injure normal tissues. When inflammation is inappropriately directed against self tissues or is not adequately controlled, it becomes the cause of injury and disease. In fact, in clinical medicine, great attention is given to the damaging consequences of inflammation. Inflammatory reactions underlie common chronic diseases, such as rheumatoid arthritis, atherosclerosis, and lung fibrosis, as well as life-threatening hypersensitivity reactions to insect bites, drugs, and toxins. For this reason our pharmacies abound with anti-inflammatory drugs, which ideally would control the harmful sequelae of inflammation yet not interfere with its beneficial effects.

Inflammation may contribute to a variety of diseases that are not thought to be primarily due to abnormal host responses. For instance, chronic inflammation may play a role in atherosclerosis, type 2 diabetes, degenerative disorders like Alzheimer disease, and cancer. In recognition of the wide-ranging harmful consequences of inflammation, the lay press has rather melodramatically referred to it as "the silent killer."

This chapter describes the sequence of events and mediators of acute inflammation, and then its morphologic patterns. This is followed by a discussion of the major features of chronic inflammation. Inflammation has a rich history, and we first touch on some of the historical highlights in our consideration of this fascinating process.

Historical Highlights

Although clinical features of inflammation were described in an Egyptian papyrus dated around 3000 BC, Celsus, a Roman writer of the first century AD, first listed the four cardinal signs of inflammation: *rubor* (redness), *tumor* (swelling), *calor* (heat), and *dolor* (pain).[1] These signs are typically more prominent in acute inflammation than in chronic inflammation. A fifth clinical sign, loss of function *(functio laesa)*, was added by Rudolf Virchow in the 19th century. In 1793 the Scottish surgeon John Hunter noted what is now considered an obvious fact: that inflammation is not a disease but a nonspecific response that has a *salutary* effect on its host.[2] In the 1880s the Russian biologist Elie Metchnikoff discovered the process of *phagocytosis* by observing the ingestion of rose thorns by amebocytes of starfish larvae and of bacteria by mammalian leukocytes.[3] He concluded that the purpose of inflammation was to bring phagocytic cells to the injured area to engulf invading bacteria. This concept was elegantly satirized by George Bernard Shaw in his play "The Doctor's Dilemma," in which one physician's cure-all is to "stimulate the phagocytes"! Sir Thomas Lewis, studying the inflammatory response in skin, established the concept that *chemical substances, such as histamine (produced locally in response to injury), mediate the vascular changes of inflammation.* This fundamental concept underlies the important discoveries of chemical mediators of inflammation and the use of anti-inflammatory drugs in clinical medicine.

Acute Inflammation

Acute inflammation is a rapid host response that serves to deliver leukocytes and plasma proteins, such as antibodies, to sites of infection or tissue injury. Acute inflammation has three major components: (1) *alterations in vascular caliber that lead to an increase in blood flow*, (2) *structural changes in the microvasculature that permit plasma proteins and leukocytes to leave the circulation*, and (3) *emigration of the leukocytes* from the microcirculation, *their accumulation* in the focus of injury, and *their activation* to eliminate the offending agent (Fig. 2–1).

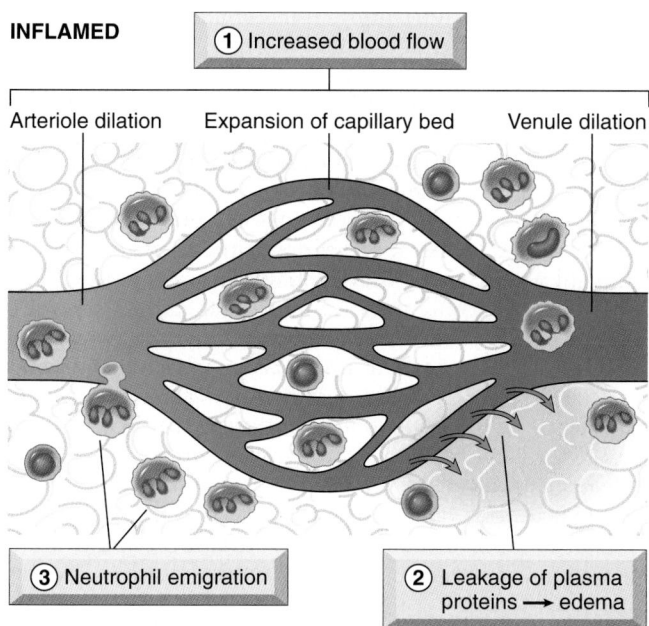

FIGURE 2–1 The major local manifestations of acute inflammation, compared to normal. (1) Vascular dilation and increased blood flow (causing erythema and warmth); (2) extravasation and extravascular deposition of plasma fluid and proteins (edema); (3) leukocyte emigration and accumulation in the site of injury.

STIMULI FOR ACUTE INFLAMMATION

Acute inflammatory reactions may be triggered by a variety of stimuli:

- *Infections* (bacterial, viral, fungal, parasitic) and microbial toxins are among the most common and medically important causes of inflammation. Mammals possess many mechanisms for sensing the presence of microbes. Among the most important receptors for microbial products are the family of Toll-like receptors (TLRs), named after the *Drosophila* protein Toll, and several cytoplasmic receptors, which can detect bacteria, viruses, and fungi (Chapter 6). Engagement of these receptors triggers signaling pathways that stimulate the production of various mediators.
- *Tissue necrosis* from any cause, including *ischemia* (as in a myocardial infarct), *trauma*, and *physical and chemical injury* (e.g., thermal injury, as in burns or frostbite; irradiation; exposure to some environmental chemicals). Several molecules released from necrotic cells are known to elicit inflammation; these include uric acid, a purine metabolite; adenosine triphosphate, the normal energy store; a DNA-binding protein of unknown function called HMGB-1; and even DNA when it is released into the cytoplasm and not sequestered in nuclei, as it should be normally.[4] *Hypoxia*, which often underlies cell injury, is also itself an inducer of the inflammatory response. This response is mediated largely by a protein called HIF-1α (hypoxia-induced factor-1α), which is produced by cells deprived of oxygen and activates the transcription of many genes involved in inflammation, including vascular endothelial growth factor (VEGF), which increases vascular permeability.[5]
- *Foreign bodies* (splinters, dirt, sutures) typically elicit inflammation because they cause traumatic tissue injury or carry microbes.
- *Immune reactions* (also called hypersensitivity reactions) are reactions in which the normally protective immune system damages the individual's own tissues. The injurious immune responses may be directed against self antigens, causing *autoimmune diseases*, or may be excessive reactions against environmental substances or microbes. Inflammation is a major cause of tissue injury in these diseases (Chapter 6). Because the stimuli for the inflammatory responses (i.e., self tissues) cannot be eliminated, autoimmune reactions tend to be persistent and difficult to cure, are associated with chronic inflammation, and are important causes of morbidity and mortality. The inflammation is induced by cytokines produced by T lymphocytes and other cells of the immune system (described later and in Chapter 6). The term *immune-mediated inflammatory disease* is often used to refer to this group of disorders.

All inflammatory reactions share the same basic features, although different stimuli may induce reactions with some distinctive characteristics. We first describe the typical sequence of events in acute inflammation, and then the chemical mediators responsible for inflammation and the morphologic appearance of these reactions.

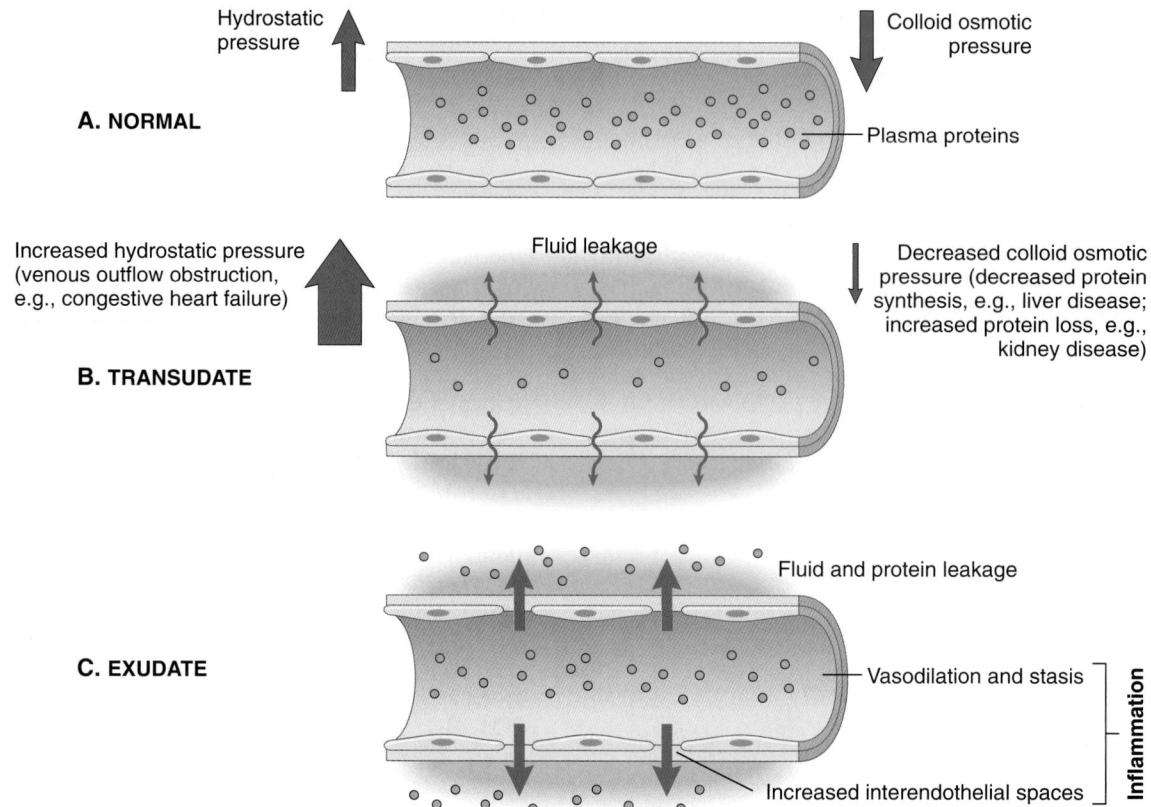

Hydrostatic pressure

Colloid osmotic pressure

A. NORMAL

Plasma proteins

Increased hydrostatic pressure (venous outflow obstruction, e.g., congestive heart failure)

Fluid leakage

Decreased colloid osmotic pressure (decreased protein synthesis, e.g., liver disease; increased protein loss, e.g., kidney disease)

B. TRANSUDATE

Fluid and protein leakage

C. EXUDATE

Vasodilation and stasis

Increased interendothelial spaces

Inflammation

FIGURE 2–2   Formation of transudates and exudates. **A,** Normal hydrostatic pressure *(blue arrows)* is about 32 mm Hg at the arterial end of a capillary bed and 12 mm Hg at the venous end; the mean colloid osmotic pressure of tissues is approximately 25 mm Hg *(green arrows)*, which is equal to the mean capillary pressure. Therefore, the net flow of fluid across the vascular bed is almost nil. **B,** A transudate is formed when fluid leaks out because of increased hydrostatic pressure or decreased osmotic pressure. **C,** An exudate is formed in inflammation, because vascular permeability increases as a result of increased interendothelial spaces.

REACTIONS OF BLOOD VESSELS IN ACUTE INFLAMMATION

In inflammation, blood vessels undergo a series of changes that are designed to maximize the movement of plasma proteins and circulating cells out of the circulation and into the site of infection or injury. The escape of fluid, proteins, and blood cells from the vascular system into the interstitial tissue or body cavities is known as *exudation*. An *exudate* is an extravascular fluid that has a high protein concentration, contains cellular debris, and has a high specific gravity. Its presence implies an increase in the normal permeability of small blood vessels in an area of injury and, therefore, an inflammatory reaction (Fig. 2–2). In contrast, a *transudate* is a fluid with low protein content (most of which is albumin), little or no cellular material, and low specific gravity. It is essentially an ultrafiltrate of blood plasma that results from osmotic or hydrostatic imbalance across the vessel wall without an increase in vascular permeability (Chapter 4). *Edema* denotes an excess of fluid in the interstitial tissue or serous cavities; it can be either an exudate or a transudate. *Pus*, a *purulent* exudate, is an inflammatory exudate rich in leukocytes (mostly neutrophils), the debris of dead cells and, in many cases, microbes.

The vascular reactions of acute inflammation consist of changes in the flow of blood and the permeability of vessels. Proliferation of blood vessels (angiogenesis) is prominent

during repair and in chronic inflammation; this process is discussed in Chapter 3.

Changes in Vascular Flow and Caliber

Changes in vascular flow and caliber begin early after injury and consist of the following.

- *Vasodilation* is one of the earliest manifestations of acute inflammation; sometimes it follows a transient constriction of arterioles, lasting a few seconds. Vasodilation first involves the arterioles and then leads to opening of new capillary beds in the area. The result is *increased blood flow*, which is the cause of heat and redness *(erythema)* at the site of inflammation. *Vasodilation is induced by the action of several mediators, notably histamine and nitric oxide (NO), on vascular smooth muscle.*
- Vasodilation is quickly followed by *increased permeability of the microvasculature*, with the outpouring of protein-rich fluid into the extravascular tissues; this process is described in detail below.
- The loss of fluid and increased vessel diameter lead to slower blood flow, concentration of red cells in small vessels, and increased viscosity of the blood. These changes result in dilation of small vessels that are packed with slowly moving red cells, a condition termed *stasis*, which is seen as

vascular congestion (producing localized redness) upon examination of the involved tissue.

- As stasis develops, blood leukocytes, principally neutrophils, accumulate along the vascular endothelium. At the same time endothelial cells are activated by mediators produced at sites of infection and tissue damage, and express increased levels of adhesion molecules. Leukocytes then adhere to the endothelium, and soon afterward they migrate through the vascular wall into the interstitial tissue, in a sequence that is described later.

Increased Vascular Permeability (Vascular Leakage)

A hallmark of acute inflammation is increased vascular permeability leading to the escape of a protein-rich exudate into the extravascular tissue, causing *edema*. Several mechanisms are responsible for the increased vascular permeability (Fig. 2–3):

- *Contraction of endothelial cells resulting in increased inter-endothelial spaces* is the most common mechanism of vascular leakage and is elicited by histamine, bradykinin, leukotrienes, the neuropeptide substance P, and many other chemical mediators.[6,7] It is called the *immediate transient response* because it occurs rapidly after exposure to the mediator and is usually short-lived (15–30 minutes). In some forms of mild injury (e.g. after burns, x-irradiation or ultraviolet radiation, and exposure to certain bacterial toxins), vascular leakage begins after a delay of 2 to 12 hours, and lasts for several hours or even days; this *delayed prolonged leakage* may be caused by contraction of endothelial cells or mild endothelial damage. Late-appearing sunburn is a good example of this type of leakage.

- *Endothelial injury, resulting in endothelial cell necrosis and detachment.*[8] Direct damage to the endothelium is encountered in severe injuries, for example, in burns, or by the actions of microbes that target endothelial cells.[9] Neutrophils that adhere to the endothelium during inflammation may also injure the endothelial cells and thus amplify the reaction. In most instances leakage starts immediately after injury and is sustained for several hours until the damaged vessels are thrombosed or repaired.

- Increased transport of fluids and proteins, called *transcytosis*, through the endothelial cell. This process may involve channels consisting of interconnected, uncoated vesicles and vacuoles called the *vesiculovacuolar organelle*, many of which are located close to intercellular junctions.[10] Certain factors, such as VEGF (Chapter 3), seem to promote vascular leakage in part by increasing the number and perhaps the size of these channels.

Although these mechanisms of increased vascular permeability are described separately, all probably contribute in varying degrees in responses to most stimuli. For example, at different stages of a thermal burn, leakage results from chemically mediated endothelial contraction and direct and leukocyte-dependent endothelial injury. The vascular leakage induced by all these mechanisms can cause life-threatening loss of fluid in severely burned patients.

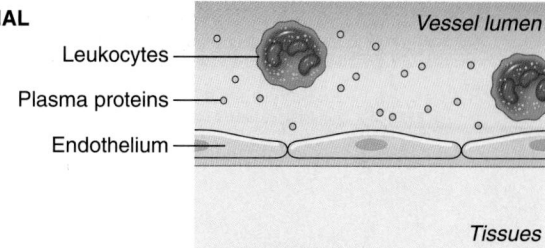

A. NORMAL

Leukocytes
Plasma proteins
Endothelium
Vessel lumen
Tissues

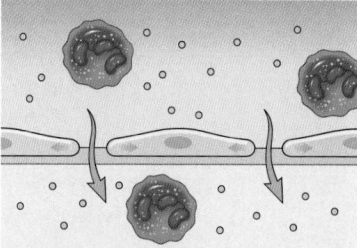

B. RETRACTION OF ENDOTHELIAL CELLS

- Occurs mainly in venules
- Induced by histamine, NO, other mediators
- Rapid and short-lived (minutes)

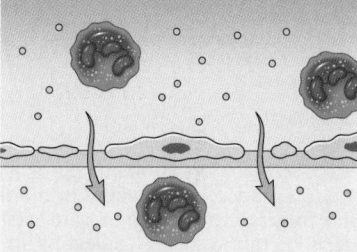

C. ENDOTHELIAL INJURY

- Occurs in arterioles, capillaries, venules
- Caused by burns, some microbial toxins
- Rapid; may be long-lived (hours to days)

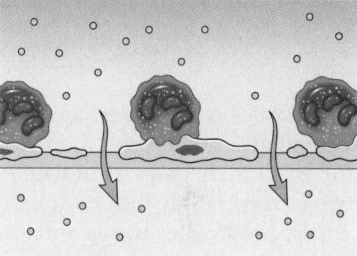

D. LEUKOCYTE-MEDIATED VASCULAR INJURY

- Occurs in venules, pulmonary capillaries
- Associated with late stages of inflammation
- Long-lived (hours)

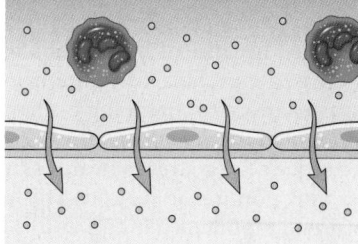

E. INCREASED TRANSCYTOSIS

- Occurs in venules
- Induced by VEGF

FIGURE 2–3   Principal mechanisms of increased vascular permeability in inflammation, and their features and underlying causes. NO, nitric oxide; VEGF, vascular endothelial growth factor.

Responses of Lymphatic Vessels

Although much of the emphasis in our discussion of inflammation is on the reactions of blood vessels, lymphatic vessels also participate in the response. The system of lymphatics and lymph nodes filters and polices the extravascular fluids. Recall that lymphatics normally drain the small amount of extravascular fluid that has seeped out of capillaries. In inflammation,

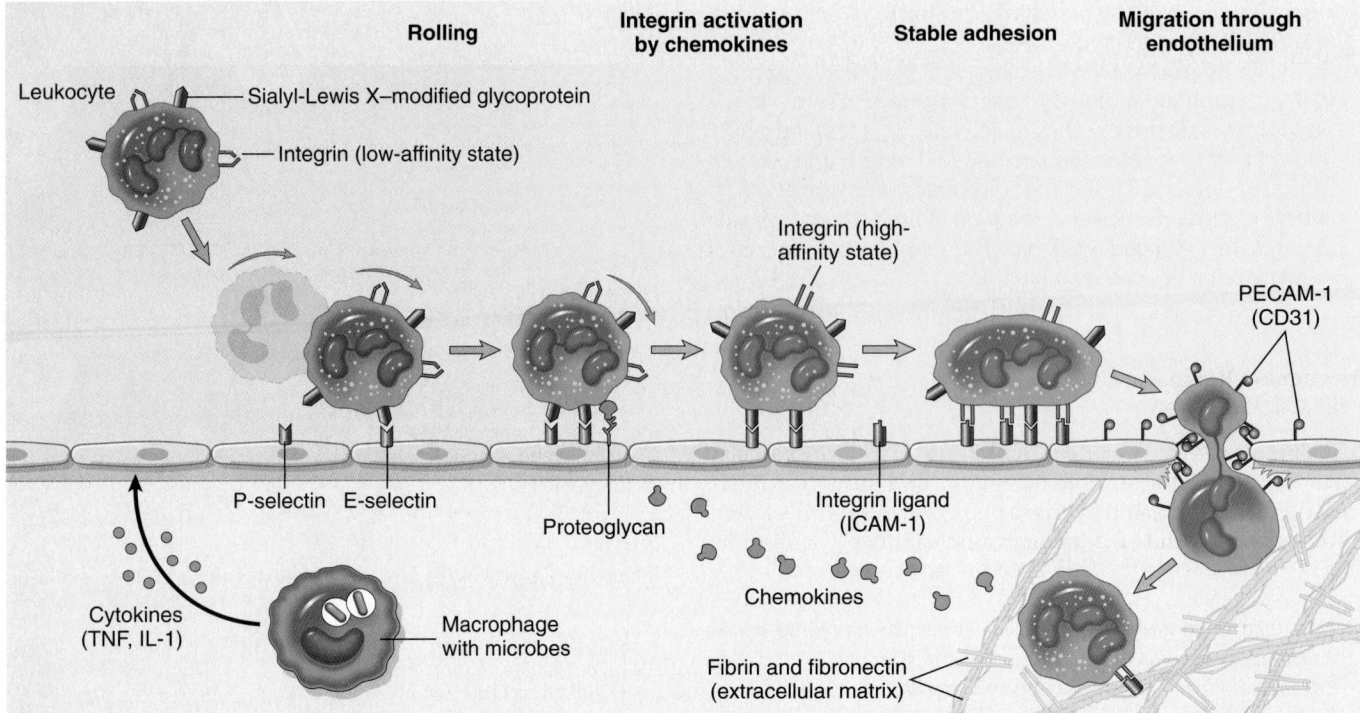

FIGURE 2–4   The multistep process of leukocyte migration through blood vessels, shown here for neutrophils. The leukocytes first roll, then become activated and adhere to endothelium, then transmigrate across the endothelium, pierce the basement membrane, and migrate toward chemoattractants emanating from the source of injury. Different molecules play predominant roles in different steps of this process—selectins in rolling; chemokines (usually displayed bound to proteoglycans) in activating the neutrophils to increase avidity of integrins; integrins in firm adhesion; and CD31 (PECAM-1) in transmigration. Neutrophils express low levels of L-selectin; they bind to endothelial cells predom in antly via P- and E-selectins. ICAM-1, intercellular adhesion molecule 1; TNF, tumor necrosis factor.

lymph flow is increased and helps drain edema fluid that accumulates due to increased vascular permeability. In addition to fluid, leukocytes and cell debris, as well as microbes, may find their way into lymph. Lymphatic vessels, like blood vessels, proliferate during inflammatory reactions to handle the increased load.[11,12] The lymphatics may become secondarily inflamed (*lymphangitis*), as may the draining lymph nodes (*lymphadenitis*). Inflamed lymph nodes are often enlarged because of hyperplasia of the lymphoid follicles and increased numbers of lymphocytes and macrophages. This constellation of pathologic changes is termed *reactive*, or *inflammatory, lymphadenitis* (Chapter 13). For clinicians the presence of red streaks near a skin wound is a telltale sign of an infection in the wound. This streaking follows the course of the lymphatic channels and is diagnostic of lymphangitis; it may be accompanied by painful enlargement of the draining lymph nodes, indicating lymphadenitis.

REACTIONS OF LEUKOCYTES IN INFLAMMATION

As mentioned earlier, a critical function of inflammation is to deliver leukocytes to the site of injury and to activate the leukocytes to eliminate the offending agents. The most important leukocytes in typical inflammatory reactions are the ones capable of phagocytosis, namely neutrophils and macrophages. These leukocytes ingest and kill bacteria and other microbes, and eliminate necrotic tissue and foreign substances. Leukocytes also produce growth factors that aid in repair. A price that is paid for

the defensive potency of leukocytes is that, when strongly activated, they may induce tissue damage and prolong inflammation, because the leukocyte products that destroy microbes and necrotic tissues can also injure normal host tissues.

The processes involving leukocytes in inflammation consist of: their recruitment from the blood into extravascular tissues, recognition of microbes and necrotic tissues, and removal of the offending agent.

Recruitment of Leukocytes to Sites of Infection and Injury

The journey of leukocytes from the vessel lumen to the interstitial tissue, called extravasation, can be divided into the following steps[13] (Fig. 2–4):

1. In the lumen: *margination, rolling, and adhesion to endothelium*. Vascular endothelium in its normal, unactivated state does not bind circulating cells or impede their passage. In inflammation the endothelium is activated and can bind leukocytes, as a prelude to their exit from the blood vessels.
2. Migration across the endothelium and vessel wall
3. Migration in the tissues toward a chemotactic stimulus

Leukocyte Adhesion to Endothelium.   In normally flowing blood in venules, red cells are confined to a central axial column, displacing the leukocytes toward the wall of the vessel. Because blood flow slows early in inflammation (stasis), hemodynamic

TABLE 2-1 Endothelial-Leukocyte Adhesion Molecules		
Endothelial Molecule	**Leukocyte Molecule**	**Major Role**
P-selectin	Sialyl-Lewis X–modified proteins	Rolling (neutrophils, monocytes, T lymphocytes)
E-selectin	Sialyl-Lewis X–modified proteins	Rolling and adhesion (neutrophils, monocytes, T lymphocytes)
GlyCam-1, CD34	L-selectin*	Rolling (neutrophils, monocytes)
ICAM-1 (immunoglobulin family)	CD11/CD18 (β_2) integrins (LFA-1, Mac-1)	Adhesion, arrest, transmigration (neutrophils, monocytes, lymphocytes)
VCAM-1 (immunoglobulin family)	VLA-4 (β_1) integrin	Adhesion (eosinophils, monocytes, lymphocytes)

*L-selectin is expressed weakly on neutrophils. It is involved in the binding of circulating T-lymphocytes to the high endothelial venules in lymph nodes and mucosal lymphoid tissues, and subsequent "homing" of lymphocytes to these tissues.

conditions change (wall shear stress decreases), and more white cells assume a peripheral position along the endothelial surface. This process of leukocyte redistribution is called *margination*. Subsequently, individual and then rows of leukocytes adhere transiently to the endothelium, detach and bind again, thus *rolling* on the vessel wall. The cells finally come to rest at some point where they *adhere* firmly (resembling pebbles over which a stream runs without disturbing them).

The adhesion of leukocytes to endothelial cells is mediated by complementary adhesion molecules on the two cell types whose expression is enhanced by secreted proteins called cytokines.[13,14] Cytokines are secreted by cells in tissues in response to microbes and other injurious agents, thus ensuring that leukocytes are recruited to the tissues where these stimuli are present. The initial rolling interactions are mediated by a family of proteins called *selectins*[15,16] (Table 2–1). There are three types of selectins: one expressed on leukocytes (L-selectin), one on endothelium (E-selectin), and one in platelets and on endothelium (P-selectin). The ligands for selectins are sialylated oligosaccharides bound to mucin-like glycoprotein backbones. The expression of selectins and their ligands is regulated by cytokines produced in response to infection and injury. Tissue macrophages, mast cells, and endothelial cells that encounter microbes and dead tissues respond by secreting several cytokines, including tumor necrosis factor (TNF),[17] interleukin-1 (IL-1),[18] and chemokines (chemoattractant cytokines).[19,20] (Cytokines are described in more detail below and in Chapter 6.) TNF and IL-1 act on the endothelial cells of post-capillary venules adjacent to the infection and induce the coordinate expression of numerous adhesion molecules (Fig. 2–5). Within 1 to 2 hours the endothelial cells begin to express E-selectin and the ligands for L-selectin. Other mediators such as histamine, thrombin, and platelet-activating factor (PAF), described later, stimulate the redistribution of P-selectin from its normal intracellular stores in endothelial cell granules (called Weibel-Palade bodies) to the cell surface. Leukocytes express L-selectin at the tips of their microvilli and also express ligands for E- and P-selectins, all of which bind to the complementary molecules on the endothelial cells. These are low-affinity interactions with a fast off-rate, and they are easily disrupted by the flowing blood. As a result, the bound leukocytes bind, detach, and bind again, and thus begin to roll along the endothelial surface.

These weak rolling interactions slow down the leukocytes and give them the opportunity to bind more firmly to the endothelium. Firm adhesion is mediated by a family of heterodimeric leukocyte surface proteins called *integrins*[21] (see Table 2–1). TNF and IL-1 induce endothelial expression of ligands for integrins, mainly vascular cell adhesion molecule 1 (VCAM-1, the ligand for the VLA-4 integrin) and intercellular adhesion molecule-1 (ICAM-1, the ligand for the LFA-1 and Mac-1 integrins). Leukocytes normally express integrins

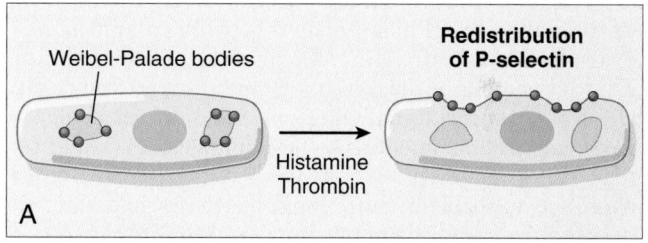

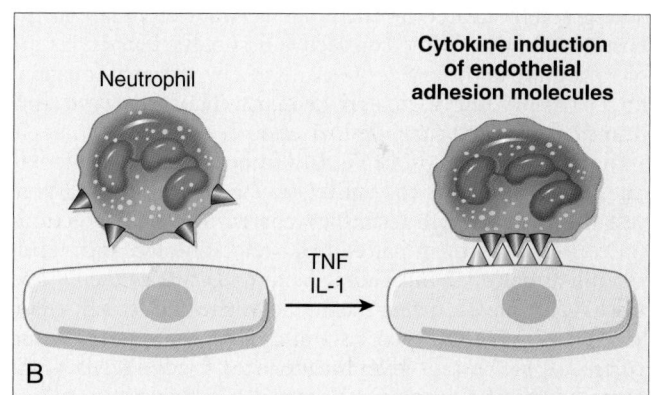

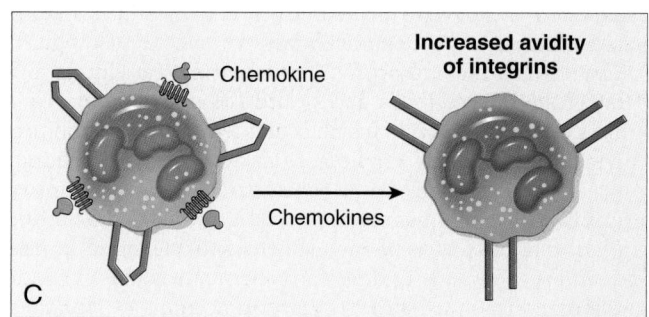

FIGURE 2–5 Regulation of expression of endothelial and leukocyte adhesion molecules. **A,** Redistribution of P-selectin from intracellular stores to the cell surface. **B,** Increased surface expression of selectins and ligands for integrins upon cytokine activation of endothelium. **C,** Increased binding avidity of integrins induced by chemokines. Clustering of integrins contributes to their increased binding avidity (not shown). IL-1, interleukin-1; TNF, tumor necrosis factor.

in a low-affinity state. Meanwhile, chemokines that were produced at the site of injury enter the blood vessel, bind to endothelial cell proteoglycans, and are displayed at high concentrations on the endothelial surface. These chemokines bind to and activate the rolling leukocytes. One of the consequences of activation is the conversion of VLA-4 and LFA-1 integrins on the leukocytes to a high-affinity state.[22] The combination of cytokine-induced expression of integrin ligands on the endothelium and activation of integrins on the leukocytes results in firm integrin-mediated binding of the leukocytes to the endothelium at the site of inflammation. The leukocytes stop rolling, their cytoskeleton is reorganized, and they spread out on the endothelial surface.

Leukocyte Migration through Endothelium. The next step in the process of leukocyte recruitment is *migration of the leukocytes through the endothelium,* called transmigration or *diapedesis.* Transmigration of leukocytes occurs mainly in post-capillary venules. Chemokines act on the adherent leukocytes and stimulate the cells to migrate through interendothelial spaces toward the chemical concentration gradient, that is, toward the site of injury or infection where the chemokines are being produced.[23] Several adhesion molecules present in the intercellular junctions between endothelial cells are involved in the migration of leukocytes. These molecules include a member of the immunoglobulin superfamily called PECAM-1 (platelet endothelial cell adhesion molecule) or CD31[24] and several junctional adhesion molecules.[25] After traversing the endothelium, leukocytes pierce the basement membrane, probably by secreting collagenases, and enter the extravascular tissue. The cells then migrate toward the chemotactic gradient created by chemokines and accumulate in the extravascular site. In the connective tissue, the leukocytes are able to adhere to the extracellular matrix by virtue of integrins and CD44 binding to matrix proteins. Thus, *leukocytes are retained at the site where they are needed.*

The most telling proof of the importance of leukocyte adhesion molecules is the existence of genetic deficiencies in these molecules, which result in recurrent bacterial infections as a consequence of impaired leukocyte adhesion and defective inflammation.[26] Individuals with *leukocyte adhesion deficiency type 1* have a defect in the biosynthesis of the β_2 chain shared by the LFA-1 and Mac-1 integrins. *Leukocyte adhesion deficiency type 2* is caused by the absence of sialyl-Lewis X, the fucose-containing ligand for E- and P-selectins, as a result of a defect in a fucosyl transferase, the enzyme that attaches fucose moieties to protein backbones.

Chemotaxis of Leukocytes. After exiting the circulation, leukocytes emigrate in tissues toward the site of injury by a process called *chemotaxis,* which is defined as locomotion oriented along a chemical gradient. Both exogenous and endogenous substances can act as chemoattractants. The most common exogenous agents are *bacterial products,* including peptides that possess an *N*-formylmethionine terminal amino acid, and some lipids. Endogenous chemoattractants include several chemical mediators (described later): (1) *cytokines,* particularly those of the chemokine family (e.g., IL-8); (2) *components of the complement system, particularly C5a;* and (3) *arachidonic acid (AA) metabolites, mainly leukotriene B_4 (LTB$_4$).* All these chemotactic agents bind to specific seven-transmembrane G protein–coupled receptors on the surface of leukocytes.[27] Signals initiated from these receptors result in activation

of second messengers that increase cytosolic calcium and activate small guanosine triphosphatases of the Rac/Rho/cdc42 family as well as numerous kinases. These signals induce polymerization of actin, resulting in increased amounts of polymerized actin at the leading edge of the cell and localization of myosin filaments at the back. The leukocyte moves by extending filopodia that pull the back of the cell in the direction of extension, much as an automobile with front-wheel drive is pulled by the wheels in front (Fig. 2–6). The net result is that leukocytes migrate toward the inflammatory stimulus in the direction of the gradient of locally produced chemoattractants.

The nature of the leukocyte infiltrate varies with the age of the inflammatory response and the type of stimulus. In most forms of acute inflammation *neutrophils predominate in the inflammatory infiltrate during the first 6 to 24 hours and are replaced by monocytes in 24 to 48 hours* (Fig. 2–7). Several reasons account for the early appearance of neutrophils: they are more numerous in the blood, they respond more rapidly to chemokines, and they may attach more firmly to the adhesion molecules that are rapidly induced on endothelial cells, such as P- and E-selectins. After entering tissues, neutrophils are short-lived; they undergo apoptosis and disappear after 24 to 48 hours. Monocytes not only survive longer but may proliferate in the tissues, and thus become the dominant population in chronic inflammatory reactions. There are, however, exceptions to this pattern of cellular infiltration. In certain infections—for example, those produced by *Pseudo-*

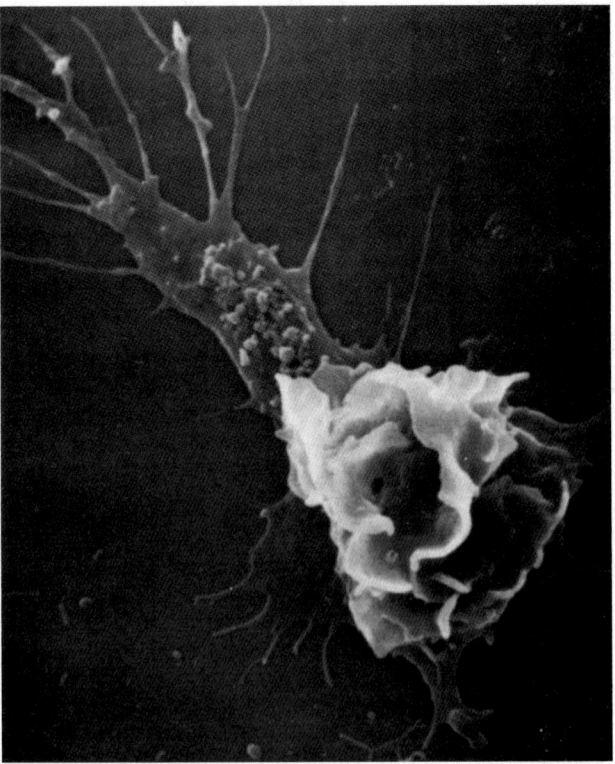

FIGURE 2–6 Scanning electron micrograph of a moving leukocyte in culture showing a filopodium *(upper left)* and a trailing tail. (Courtesy of Dr. Morris J. Karnovsky, Harvard Medical School, Boston, MA.)

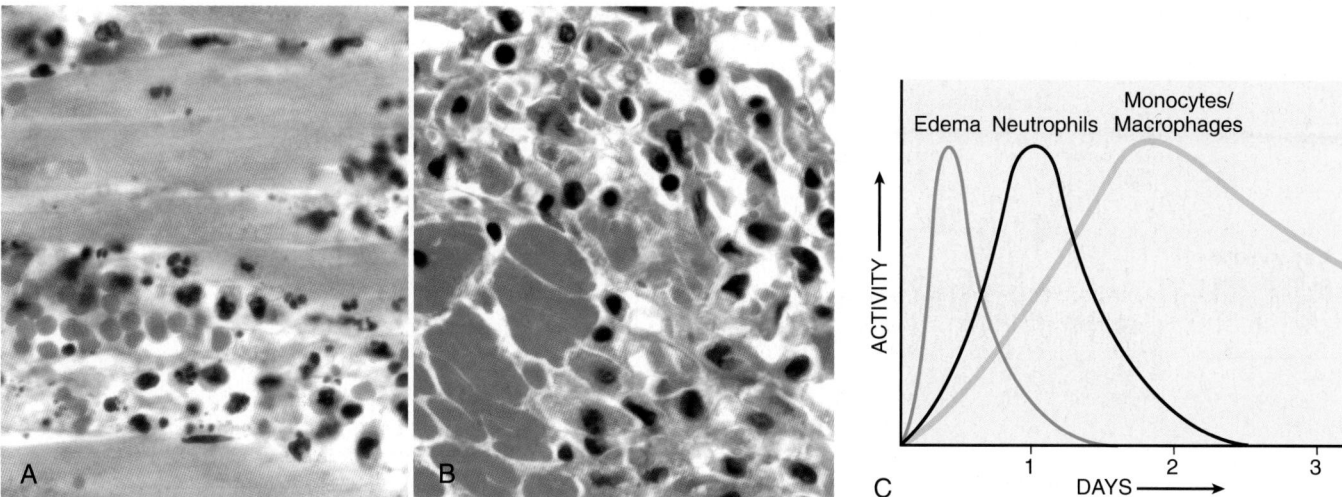

FIGURE 2–7   Nature of leukocyte infiltrates in inflammatory reactions. The photomicrographs are representative of the early (neutrophilic) (**A**) and later (mononuclear) cellular infiltrates (**B**) seen in an inflammatory reaction in the myocardium following ischemic necrosis (infarction). The kinetics of edema and cellular infiltration (**C**) are approximations.

monas bacteria—the cellular infiltrate is dominated by continuously recruited neutrophils for several days; in viral infections, lymphocytes may be the first cells to arrive; in some hypersensitivity reactions, eosinophils may be the main cell type.

The molecular understanding of leukocyte recruitment and migration has provided a large number of potential therapeutic targets for controlling harmful inflammation.[14] Agents that block TNF, one of the major cytokines in leukocyte recruitment, are among the most successful therapeutics ever developed for chronic inflammatory diseases, and antagonists of leukocyte integrins (e.g. VLA-4), selectins, and chemokines are approved for inflammatory diseases or in clinical trials. Predictably, these antagonists not only have the desired effect of controlling the inflammation but can compromise the ability of treated patients to defend themselves against microbes, which, of course, is the physiologic function of the inflammatory response.

Recognition of Microbes and Dead Tissues

Once leukocytes (neutrophils and monocytes) have been recruited to a site of infection or cell death, they must be activated to perform their functions. The responses of leukocytes consist of two sequential sets of events: (1) recognition of the offending agents, which deliver signals that (2) activate the leukocytes to ingest and destroy the offending agents and amplify the inflammatory reaction.

Leukocytes express several receptors that recognize external stimuli and deliver activating signals (Fig. 2–8).

○ *Receptors for microbial products: Toll-like receptors (TLRs)* recognize components of different types of microbes. Thus far 10 mammalian TLRs have been identified, and each seems to be required for responses to different classes of infectious pathogens.[28] Different TLRs play essential roles in cellular responses to bacterial lipopolysaccharide (LPS, or endotoxin), other bacterial proteoglycans and lipids, and

unmethylated CpG nucleotides, all of which are abundant in bacteria, as well as double-stranded RNA, which is produced by some viruses. TLRs are present on the cell surface and in the endosomal vesicles of leukocytes (and many other cell types), so they are able to sense products of extracellular and ingested microbes. These receptors function through receptor-associated kinases to stimulate the production of microbicidal substances and cytokines by the leukocytes. Various other cytoplasmic proteins in leukocytes recognize bacterial peptides and viral RNA.[29]

○ *G protein–coupled receptors* found on neutrophils, macrophages, and most other types of leukocytes recognize short bacterial peptides containing *N*-formylmethionyl residues. Because all bacterial proteins and few mammalian proteins (only those synthesized within mitochondria) are initiated by *N*-formylmethionine, this receptor enables neutrophils to detect and respond to bacterial proteins. Other G protein–coupled receptors recognize chemokines, breakdown products of complement such as C5a, and lipid mediators, including platelet activating factor, prostaglandins, and leukotrienes, all of which are produced in response to microbes and cell injury. Binding of ligands, such as microbial products and mediators, to the G protein–coupled receptors induces migration of the cells from the blood through the endothelium and production of microbicidal substances by activation of the respiratory burst.

○ *Receptors for opsonins*: Leukocytes express receptors for proteins that coat microbes. The process of coating a particle, such as a microbe, to target it for ingestion (phagocytosis) is called *opsonization*, and substances that do this are *opsonins*. These substances include antibodies, complement proteins, and lectins. One of the most efficient ways of enhancing the phagocytosis of particles is coating the particles with IgG antibodies specific for the particles, which are then recognized by the high-affinity Fcγ receptor of phagocytes, called FcγRI (Chapter 6). Components of the complement system, especially fragments of the complement

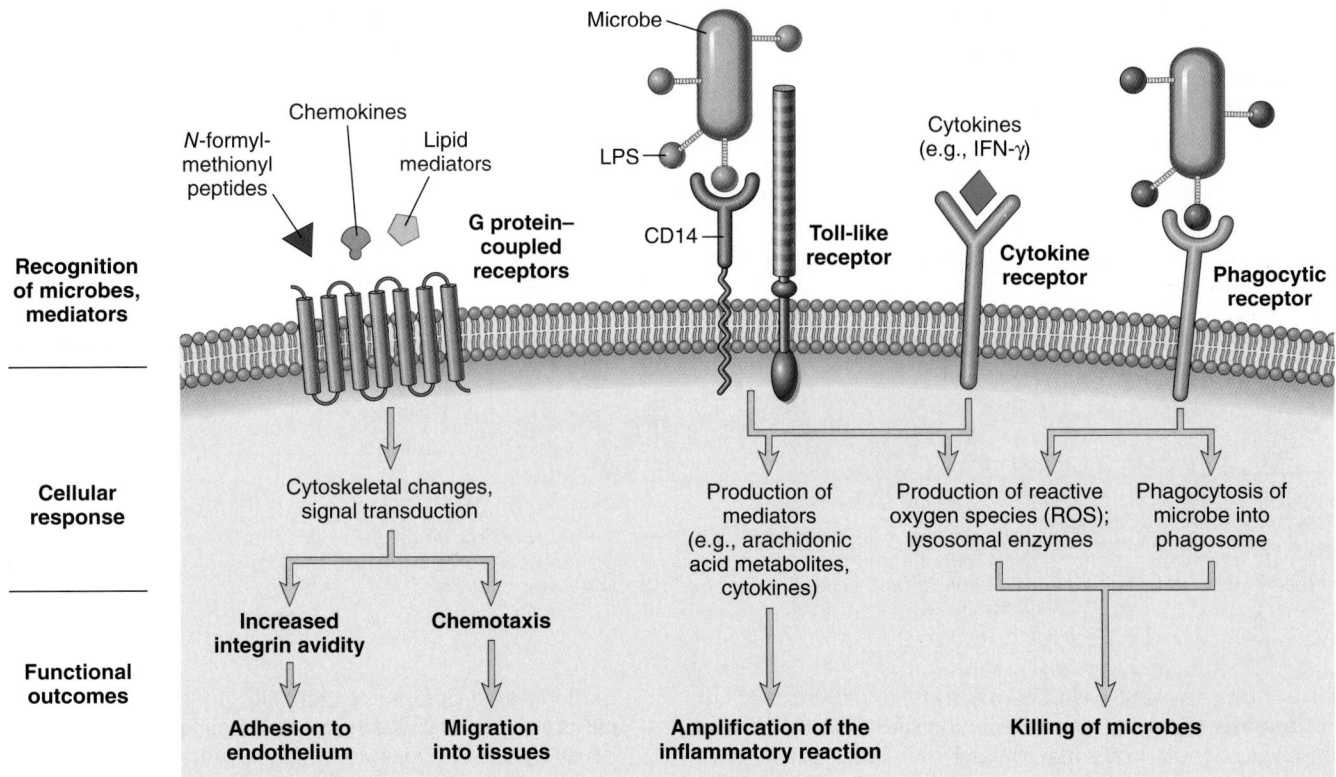

FIGURE 2–8 Leukocyte receptors and responses. Different classes of cell surface receptors of leukocytes recognize different stimuli. The receptors initiate responses that mediate the functions of the leukocytes. Only some receptors are depicted (see text for details). IFN-γ, interferon-γ; LPS, lipopolysaccharide(s).

protein C3, are also potent opsonins, because these fragments bind to microbes and phagocytes express a receptor, called the type 1 complement receptor (CR1), that recognizes breakdown products of C3 (discussed later). Plasma lectins, mainly mannan-binding lectin, also bind to bacteria and deliver them to leukocytes. The binding of opsonized particles to leukocyte Fc or C3 receptors promotes phagocytosis of the particles and activates the cells.

○ *Receptors for cytokines*: Leukocytes express receptors for cytokines that are produced in response to microbes. One of the most important of these cytokines is interferon-γ (IFN-γ), which is secreted by natural killer cells reacting to microbes and by antigen-activated T lymphocytes during adaptive immune responses (Chapter 6). IFN-γ is the major macrophage-activating cytokine.

Removal of the Offending Agents

Recognition of microbes or dead cells by the receptors described above induces several responses in leukocytes that are referred to under the rubric of *leukocyte activation* (see Fig. 2–8). Activation results from signaling pathways that are triggered in leukocytes, resulting in increases in cytosolic Ca^{2+} and activation of enzymes such as protein kinase C and phospholipase A_2. The functional responses that are most important for destruction of microbes and other offenders are phagocytosis and intracellular killing. Several other responses aid in

the defensive functions of inflammation and may contribute to its injurious consequences.

Phagocytosis. Phagocytosis involves three sequential steps (Fig. 2–9): (1) *recognition* and *attachment* of the particle to be ingested by the leukocyte; (2) its *engulfment*, with subsequent formation of a phagocytic vacuole; and (3) *killing* or *degradation* of the ingested material.[30]

Mannose receptors, scavenger receptors, and receptors for various opsonins all function to bind and ingest microbes. The macrophage mannose receptor is a lectin that binds terminal mannose and fucose residues of glycoproteins and glycolipids. These sugars are typically part of molecules found on microbial cell walls, whereas mammalian glycoproteins and glycolipids contain terminal sialic acid or N-acetylgalactosamine. Therefore, the mannose receptor recognizes microbes and not host cells. *Scavenger receptors* were originally defined as molecules that bind and mediate endocytosis of oxidized or acetylated low-density lipoprotein (LDL) particles that can no longer interact with the conventional LDL receptor. Macrophage scavenger receptors bind a variety of microbes in addition to modified LDL particles. Macrophage integrins, notably Mac-1 (CD11b/CD18), may also bind microbes for phagocytosis.

The efficiency of phagocytosis is greatly enhanced when microbes are opsonized by specific proteins (opsonins) for which the phagocytes express high-affinity receptors. As described above, the major opsonins are IgG antibodies, the C3b breakdown product of complement, and certain plasma lectins, notably mannan-binding lectin, all of which are recognized by specific receptors on leukocytes.

Engulfment. After a particle is bound to phagocyte receptors, extensions of the cytoplasm (pseudopods) flow around it, and the plasma membrane pinches off to form a vesicle (phagosome) that encloses the particle. The phagosome then fuses with a lysosomal granule, resulting in discharge of the granule's contents into the phagolysosome (see Fig. 2–9). During this process the phagocyte may also release granule contents into the extracellular space.

The process of phagocytosis is complex and involves the integration of many receptor-initiated signals to lead to membrane remodeling and cytoskeletal changes.[30] Phagocytosis is dependent on polymerization of actin filaments; it is, therefore, not surprising that the signals that trigger phagocytosis are many of the same that are involved in chemotaxis. (In contrast, fluid-phase pinocytosis and receptor-mediated endocytosis of small particles involve internalization into clathrin-coated pits and vesicles and are not dependent on the actin cytoskeleton.)

Killing and Degradation. The final step in the elimination of infectious agents and necrotic cells is their killing and degradation within neutrophils and macrophages, which occur most efficiently after activation of the phagocytes. *Microbial killing is accomplished largely by reactive oxygen species (ROS, also called reactive oxygen intermediates) and reactive nitrogen species,* mainly derived from NO (see Fig. 2–9).[31,32] The generation of ROS is due to the rapid assembly and activation of a multicomponent oxidase (NADPH oxidase, also called phagocyte oxidase), which oxidizes NADPH (reduced nicotinamide-adenine dinucleotide phosphate) and, in the process, reduces oxygen to superoxide anion ($O_2^{\overline{\cdot}}$). In neutrophils, this rapid oxidative reaction is triggered by activating signals and accompanies phagocytosis, and is called the *respiratory burst*. Phagocyte oxidase is an enzyme complex consisting of at least seven proteins.[33] In resting neutrophils, different components of the enzyme are located in the plasma membrane and the cytoplasm. In response to activating stimuli, the cytosolic protein components translocate to the phagosomal membrane, where they assemble and form the functional enzyme complex. Thus, the *ROS are produced within the lysosome* where the ingested substances are segregated, and the cell's own organelles are protected from the harmful effects of the ROS. $O_2^{\overline{\cdot}}$ is then converted into hydrogen peroxide (H_2O_2), mostly by spontaneous dismutation. H_2O_2 is not able to efficiently kill microbes by itself. However, the azurophilic granules of neutrophils contain the enzyme *myeloperoxidase* (MPO), which, in the presence of a halide such as Cl^-, converts H_2O_2 to hypochlorite ($OCl^{\cdot}$, the active ingredient in household bleach). The latter is a potent antimicrobial agent that destroys microbes by *halogenation* (in which the halide is bound covalently to cellular constituents) or by oxidation of proteins and lipids (lipid peroxidation). *The H_2O_2-MPO-halide system is the most efficient bactericidal system of neutrophils.* H_2O_2 is also converted to hydroxyl radical ($^{\cdot}OH$), another powerful destructive agent.

NO, produced from arginine by the action of nitric oxide synthase (NOS), also participates in microbial killing.[34] NO reacts with superoxide ($O_2^{\overline{\cdot}}$) to generate the highly reactive free radical peroxynitrite ($ONOO^{\cdot}$). These oxygen- and nitrogen-derived free radicals attack and damage the lipids,

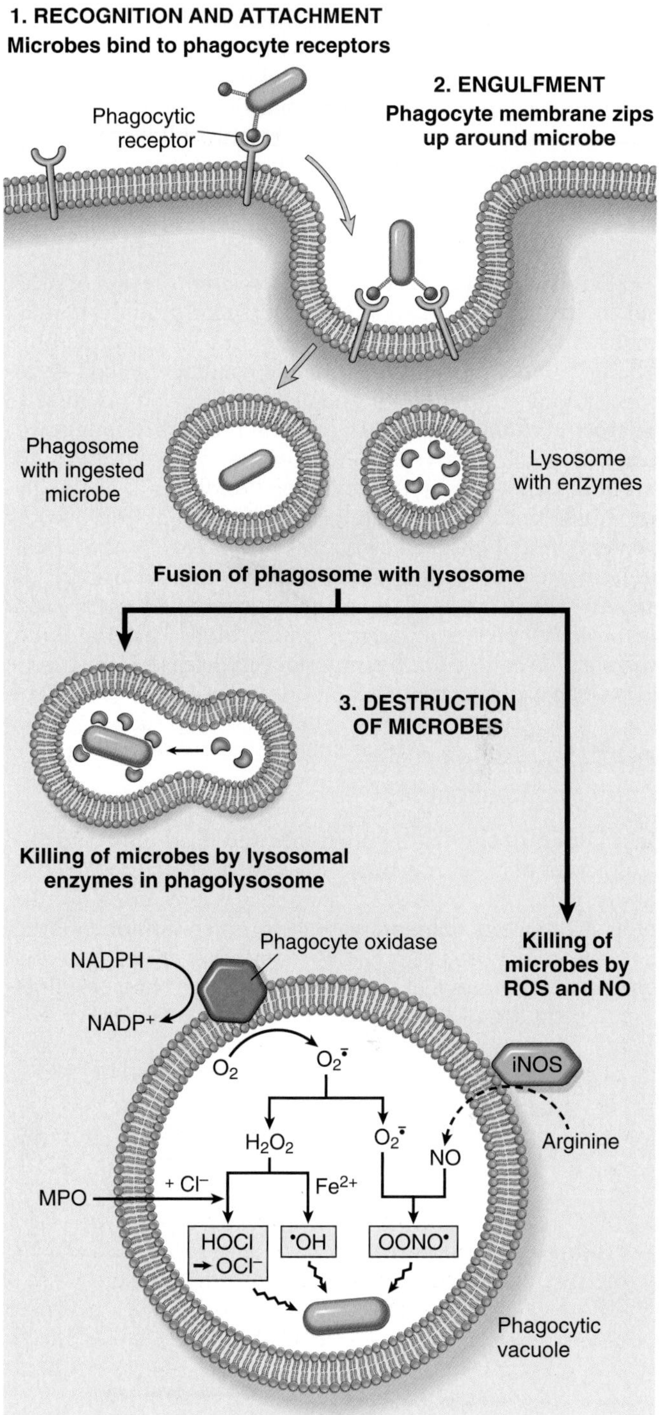

1. RECOGNITION AND ATTACHMENT
Microbes bind to phagocyte receptors

FIGURE 2–9 Phagocytosis and intracellular destruction of microbes. Phagocytosis of a particle (e.g., bacterium) involves binding to receptors on the leukocyte membrane, engulfment, and fusion of lysosomes with phagocytic vacuoles. This is followed by destruction of ingested particles within the phagolysosomes by lysosomal enzymes and by reactive oxygen and nitrogen species. The microbicidal products generated from superoxide ($O_2^{\overline{\cdot}}$) are hypochlorite ($HOCl^{\cdot}$) and hydroxyl radical ($^{\cdot}OH$), and from nitric oxide (NO) it is peroxynitrite ($OONO^{\cdot}$). During phagocytosis, granule contents may be released into extracellular tissues (not shown). MPO, myeloperoxidase; iNOS, inducible NO synthase.

proteins, and nucleic acids of microbes as they do with host macromolecules (Chapter 1). Reactive oxygen and nitrogen species have overlapping actions, as shown by the observation that knockout mice lacking either phagocyte oxidase or inducible nitric oxide synthase (iNOS) are only mildly susceptible to infections, but mice lacking both succumb rapidly to disseminated infections by normally harmless commensal bacteria. The roles of ROS and NO as mediators of inflammation are described later in the chapter.

Microbial killing can also occur through the action of other substances in leukocyte granules. Neutrophil granules contain many *enzymes*, such as elastase, that contribute to microbial killing.[35] Other microbicidal granule contents include *defensins*, cationic arginine-rich granule peptides that are toxic to microbes[36]; *cathelicidins*, antimicrobial proteins found in neutrophils and other cells[37]; *lysozyme*, which hydrolyzes the muramic acid–*N*-acetylglucosamine bond, found in the glycopeptide coat of all bacteria; *lactoferrin*, an iron-binding protein present in specific granules; *major basic protein*, a cationic protein of eosinophils, which has limited bactericidal activity but is cytotoxic to many parasites; and *bactericidal/permeability increasing protein*, which binds bacterial endotoxin and is believed to be important in defense against some gram-negative bacteria.

Other Functional Responses of Activated Leukocytes

In addition to eliminating microbes and dead cells, activated leukocytes play several other roles in host defense. Importantly, these cells, especially macrophages, produce a number of growth factors that stimulate the proliferation of endothelial cells and fibroblasts and the synthesis of collagen, and enzymes that remodel connective tissues. These products drive the process of repair after tissue injury (Chapter 3). An emerging concept is that macrophages can be activated to perform different functions—"classically activated" macrophages respond to microbial products and T-cell cytokines such as IFN-γ and have strong microbicidal activity, whereas "alternatively activated" macrophages respond to cytokines such as IL-4 and IL-13 (typically, the products of the T_H2 subset of T-cells, see Chapter 6) and are mainly involved in tissue repair and fibrosis (Fig. 2-10).[38] Different stimuli activate leukocytes to secrete mediators of inflammation as well as inhibitors of the inflammatory response, and thus serve to both amplify and control the reaction. This may be another distinction between classically and alternatively activated macrophages—the former trigger inflammation and the latter function to limit inflammatory reactions.

Release of Leukocyte Products and Leukocyte-Mediated Tissue Injury

Leukocytes are important causes of injury to normal cells and tissues under several circumstances:

- As part of a normal defense reaction against infectious microbes, when adjacent tissues suffer "collateral damage." In some infections that are difficult to eradicate, such as tuberculosis and certain viral diseases, the prolonged host response contributes more to the pathology than does the microbe itself.
- When the inflammatory response is inappropriately directed against host tissues, as in certain autoimmune diseases.
- When the host reacts excessively against usually harmless environmental substances, as in allergic diseases, including asthma.

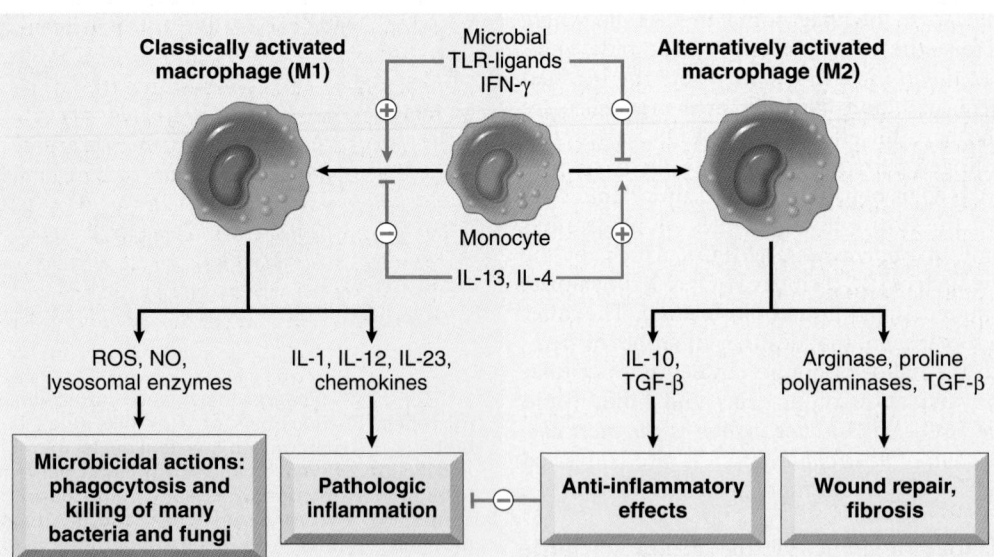

FIGURE 2-10 Subsets of activated macrophages. Different stimuli activate monocytes/macrophages to develop into functionally distinct populations. Classically activated macrophages are induced by microbial products and cytokines, particularly IFN-γ, and are microbicidal and involved in potentially harmful inflammation. Alternatively activated macrophages are induced by other cytokines and in response to helminths (not shown), and are important in tissue repair and the resolution of inflammation (and may play a role in defense against helminthic parasites, also not shown).

TABLE 2–2 Clinical Examples of Leukocyte-Induced Injury*	
Disorders	**Cells and Molecules Involved in Injury**
ACUTE	
Acute respiratory distress syndrome	Neutrophils
Acute transplant rejection	Lymphocytes; antibodies and complement
Asthma	Eosinophils; IgE antibodies
Glomerulonephritis	Neutrophils, monocytes; antibodies and complement
Septic shock	Cytokines
Lung abscess	Neutrophils (and bacteria)
CHRONIC	
Arthritis	Lymphocytes, macrophages; antibodies?
Asthma	Eosinophils; IgE antibodies
Atherosclerosis	Macrophages; lymphocytes?
Chronic transplant rejection	Lymphocytes; cytokines
Pulmonary fibrosis	Macrophages; fibroblasts

*Listed are selected examples of diseases in which the host response plays a significant role in tissue injury, and the principal cells and molecules that cause the injury. These diseases and their pathogenesis will be discussed in detail in relevant chapters.

In all these situations, the mechanisms by which leukocytes damage normal tissues are the same as the mechanisms involved in antimicrobial defense, because once the leukocytes are activated, their effector mechanisms do not distinguish between offender and host. During activation and phagocytosis, neutrophils and macrophages release microbicidal and other products not only within the phagolysosome but also into the extracellular space. The most important of these substances are *lysosomal enzymes*, present in the granules, and *reactive oxygen and nitrogen species*. These released substances are capable of damaging normal cells and vascular endothelium, and may thus amplify the effects of the initial injurious agent. In fact, if unchecked or inappropriately directed against host tissues, the leukocyte infiltrate itself becomes the offender,[39] and indeed leukocyte-dependent tissue injury underlies many acute and chronic human diseases (Table 2–2). This fact becomes evident in the discussion of specific disorders throughout the book.

The contents of lysosomal granules are secreted by leukocytes into the extracellular milieu by several mechanisms.[40] Controlled secretion of granule contents is a normal response of activated leukocytes. If phagocytes encounter materials that cannot be easily ingested, such as immune complexes deposited on immovable flat surfaces (e.g., glomerular basement membrane), the inability of the leukocytes to surround and ingest these substances (*frustrated phagocytosis*) triggers strong activation, and the release of large amounts of lysosomal enzymes into the extracellular environment. Phagocytosis of membrane-damaging substances, such as urate crystals, may injure the membrane of the phagolysosome and also lead to the release of lysosomal granule contents.

Defects in Leukocyte Function

Because leukocytes play a central role in host defense, defects in leukocyte function, both inherited and acquired, lead to increased vulnerability to infections (Table 2–3). Impairments of virtually every phase of leukocyte function have been identified—from adherence to vascular endothelium to microbicidal activity. These include the following:

- *Inherited defects in leukocyte adhesion.* We previously mentioned the genetic defects of integrins and selectin-ligands that cause leukocyte adhesion deficiencies types 1 and 2. The major clinical problem in both is recurrent bacterial infections.

- *Inherited defects in phagolysosome function.* One such disorder is *Chédiak-Higashi syndrome*, an autosomal recessive condition characterized by defective fusion of phagosomes and lysosomes in phagocytes (causing susceptibility to infections), and abnormalities in melanocytes (leading to albinism), cells of the nervous system (associated with nerve defects), and platelets (causing bleeding disorders).[41] The main leukocyte abnormalities are neutropenia (decreased numbers of neutrophils), defective degranulation, and delayed microbial killing. Leukocytes contain *giant granules*, which can be readily seen in peripheral blood smears and are thought to result from aberrant phagolysosome fusion. The gene associated with this disorder encodes a large cytosolic protein called LYST, which is believed to regulate lysosomal trafficking.

- *Inherited defects in microbicidal activity.* The importance of oxygen-dependent bactericidal mechanisms is shown by the existence of a group of congenital disorders called *chronic granulomatous disease*, which are characterized by defects in bacterial killing and render patients susceptible to recurrent bacterial infection. Chronic granulomatous disease results from *inherited defects in the genes encoding components of phagocyte oxidase*, which generates $O_2^{\bullet-}$. The most common variants are an X-linked defect in one of the membrane-bound components (gp91phox) and autosomal recessive defects in the genes encoding two of the cytoplasmic components (p47phox and p67phox).[42] The name of this disease comes from the macrophage-rich chronic inflammatory reaction that tries to control the infection when the initial neutrophil defense is inadequate. This often leads to collections of activated macrophages that wall off the microbes, forming aggregates called *granulomas* (described in more detail later in the chapter).

- *Acquired deficiencies.* Clinically, the most frequent cause of leukocyte defects is *bone marrow suppression*, leading to

TABLE 2–3 Defects in Leukocyte Functions	
Disease	**Defect**
GENETIC	
Leukocyte adhesion deficiency 1	Defective leukocyte adhesion because of mutations in β chain of CD11/CD18 integrins
Leukocyte adhesion deficiency 2	Defective leukocyte adhesion because of mutations in fucosyl transferase required for synthesis of sialylated oligosaccharide (ligand for selectins)
Chronic granulomatous disease	Decreased oxidative burst
X-linked	Phagocyte oxidase (membrane component)
Autosomal recessive	Phagocyte oxidase (cytoplasmic components)
MPO deficiency	Decreased microbial killing because of defective MPO— H_2O_2 system
Chédiak-Higashi syndrome	Decreased leukocyte functions because of mutations affecting protein involved in lysosomal membrane traffic
ACQUIRED	
Bone marrow suppression: tumors, radiation, and chemotherapy	Production of leukocytes
Diabetes, malignancy, sepsis, chronic dialysis	Adhesion and chemotaxis
Leukemia, anemia, sepsis, diabetes, malnutrition	Phagocytosis and microbicidal activity

MPO, myeloperoxidase.
Modified from Gallin JI: Disorders of phagocytic cells. In Gallin JI, et al (eds): Inflammation: Basic Principles and Clinical Correlates, 2nd ed. New York, Raven Press, 1992, pp 860, 861.

decreased production of leukocytes. This is seen following therapies for cancer (radiation and chemotherapy) and when the marrow space is compromised by tumors, which may arise in the marrow (e.g., leukemias) or be metastatic from other sites.

Although we have emphasized the role of leukocytes recruited from the circulation in the acute inflammatory response, *cells resident in tissues also serve important functions in initiating acute inflammation*. The two most important of these cell types are *mast cells* and tissue *macrophages*. These "sentinel" cells are stationed in tissues to rapidly recognize potentially injurious stimuli and initiate the host defense reaction. Mast cells react to physical trauma, breakdown products of complement, microbial products, and neuropeptides. These cells release histamine, leukotrienes, enzymes, and many cytokines (including TNF, IL-1, and chemokines), all of which contribute to inflammation. The functions of mast cells are discussed in more detail in Chapter 6. Macrophages recognize microbial products and secrete most of the cytokines important in acute inflammation. We will return to a discussion of the role of macrophages in inflammation later in the chapter.

TERMINATION OF THE ACUTE INFLAMMATORY RESPONSE

It is predictable that such a powerful system of host defense, with its inherent capacity to cause tissue damage, needs tight controls to minimize the damage. In part, inflammation declines simply because the mediators of inflammation are produced in rapid bursts, only as long as the stimulus persists, have short half-lives, and are degraded after their release. Neutrophils also have short half-lives in tissues and die by apoptosis within a few hours after leaving the blood. In addition,

as inflammation develops the process also triggers a variety of stop signals that serve to actively terminate the reaction.[43,44] These active termination mechanisms include a switch in the type of arachidonic acid metabolite produced, from pro-inflammatory leukotrienes to anti-inflammatory lipoxins (described below); the liberation of anti-inflammatory cytokines, including transforming growth factor-β (TGF-β) and IL-10, from macrophages and other cells; the production of anti-inflammatory lipid mediators, called resolvins and protectins, derived from polyunsaturated fatty acids[45]; and neural impulses (cholinergic discharge) that inhibit the production of TNF in macrophages.[46]

Mediators of Inflammation

Having described the sequence of events in acute inflammation, we can now turn to a discussion of the chemical mediators that are responsible for these reactions. Many mediators have been identified, and how they function in a coordinated manner is still not fully understood. The sources of the principal mediators and their roles in the inflammatory reaction are summarized in Table 2–4. We start our discussion of the mediators of inflammation by reviewing some of their shared properties and the general principles of their production and actions.

⊙ *Mediators are generated either from cells or from plasma proteins.* Cell-derived mediators are normally sequestered in intracellular granules and can be rapidly secreted by granule exocytosis (e.g., histamine in mast cell granules) or are synthesized de novo (e.g., prostaglandins, cytokines) in response to a stimulus. The major cell types that produce mediators of acute inflammation are platelets, neutrophils, monocytes/macrophages, and mast cells, but mesenchymal cells (endothelium, smooth muscle, fibroblasts) and most

TABLE 2–4 The Actions of the Principal Mediators of Inflammation

Mediator	Principal Sources	Actions
CELL-DERIVED		
Histamine	Mast cells, basophils, platelets	Vasodilation, increased vascular permeability, endothelial activation
Serotonin	Platelets	Vasodilation, increased vascular permeability
Prostaglandins	Mast cells, leukocytes	Vasodilation, pain, fever
Leukotrienes	Mast cells, leukocytes	Increased vascular permeability, chemotaxis, leukocyte adhesion and activation
Platelet-activating factor	Leukocytes, mast cells	Vasodilation, increased vascular permeability, leukocyte adhesion, chemotaxis, degranulation, oxidative burst
Reactive oxygen species	Leukocytes	Killing of microbes, tissue damage
Nitric oxide	Endothelium, macrophages	Vascular smooth muscle relaxation, killing of microbes
Cytokines (TNF, IL-1)	Macrophages, endothelial cells, mast cells	Local endothelial activation (expression of adhesion molecules), fever/pain/anorexia/hypotension, decreased vascular resistance (shock)
Chemokines	Leukocytes, activated macrophages	Chemotaxis, leukocyte activation
PLASMA PROTEIN–DERIVED		
Complement products (C5a, C3a, C4a)	Plasma (produced in liver)	Leukocyte chemotaxis and activation, vasodilation (mast cell stimulation)
Kinins	Plasma (produced in liver)	Increased vascular permeability, smooth muscle contraction, vasodilation, pain
Proteases activated during coagulation	Plasma (produced in liver)	Endothelial activation, leukocyte recruitment

IL-1, interleukin-1; MAC, membrane attack complex; TNF, tumor necrosis factor.

epithelia can also be induced to elaborate some of the mediators. Plasma-derived mediators (e.g., complement proteins, kinins) are produced mainly in the liver and present in the circulation as inactive precursors that must be activated, usually by a series of proteolytic cleavages, to acquire their biologic properties.

○ *Active mediators are produced in response to various stimuli.* These stimuli include microbial products, substances released from necrotic cells, and the proteins of the complement, kinin, and coagulation systems, which are themselves activated by microbes and damaged tissues. This requirement for microbes or dead tissues as the initiating stimulus ensures that inflammation is normally triggered only when and where it is needed.

○ *One mediator can stimulate the release of other mediators.* For instance, the cytokine TNF acts on endothelial cells to stimulate the production of another cytokine, IL-1, and many chemokines. The secondary mediators may have the same actions as the initial mediators but may also have different and even opposing activities. Such cascades provide mechanisms for amplifying—or, in certain instances, counteracting—the initial action of a mediator.

○ *Mediators vary in their range of cellular targets.* They can act on one or a few target cell types, can have diverse targets, or may even have differing effects on different types of cells.

○ *Once activated and released from the cell, most of these mediators are short-lived.* They quickly decay (e.g., arachidonic acid metabolites) or are inactivated by enzymes (e.g., kininase inactivates bradykinin), or they are otherwise scavenged (e.g., antioxidants scavenge toxic oxygen metabolites)

or inhibited (e.g., complement regulatory proteins break up and degrade activated complement components). There is thus a system of checks and balances that regulates mediator actions.

We now discuss some of the more important mediators of acute inflammation, starting with the cell-derived mediators and moving on to those derived from plasma proteins.

CELL-DERIVED MEDIATORS

Vasoactive Amines: Histamine and Serotonin

The two major vasoactive amines, so named because they have important actions on blood vessels, are histamine and serotonin. They are stored as preformed molecules in cells and are therefore among the first mediators to be released during inflammation. The richest sources of *histamine* are the mast cells that are normally present in the connective tissue adjacent to blood vessels. It is also found in blood basophils and platelets. Histamine is present in mast cell granules and is released by mast cell degranulation in response to a variety of stimuli, including (1) physical injury such as trauma, cold, or heat; (2) binding of antibodies to mast cells, which underlies allergic reactions (Chapter 6); (3) fragments of complement called *anaphylatoxins* (C3a and C5a); (4) histamine-releasing proteins derived from leukocytes; (5) neuropeptides (e.g., substance P); and (6) cytokines (IL-1, IL-8).

Histamine causes dilation of arterioles and increases the permeability of venules. It is considered to be the principal mediator of the immediate transient phase of increased

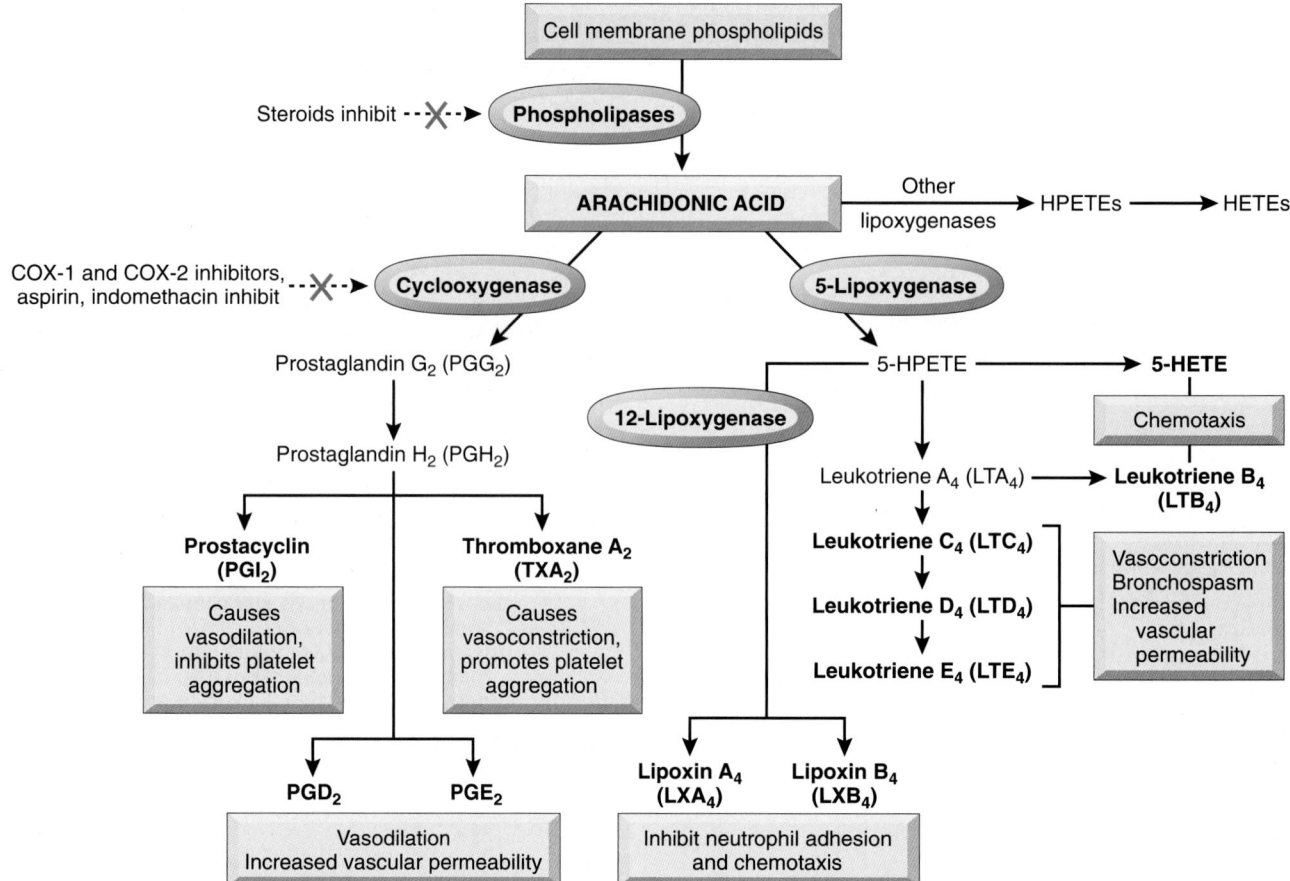

FIGURE 2–11 Generation of arachidonic acid metabolites and their roles in inflammation. The molecular targets of action of some anti-inflammatory drugs are indicated by a red X. Not shown are agents that inhibit leukotriene production by inhibition of 5-lipoxygenase (e.g., Zileuton) or block leukotriene receptors (e.g., Monteleukast). COX, cyclooxygenase; HETE, hydroxyeicosatetraenoic acid; HPETE, hydroperoxyeicosatetraenoic acid.

vascular permeability, producing interendothelial gaps in venules, as we have seen. Its vasoactive effects are mediated mainly via binding to H_1 receptors on microvascular endothelial cells.[47]

Serotonin (5-hydroxytryptamine) is a preformed vasoactive mediator with actions similar to those of histamine. It is present in platelets and certain neuroendocrine cells, e.g. in the gastrointestinal tract, and in mast cells in rodents but not humans. Release of serotonin (and histamine) from platelets is stimulated when platelets aggregate after contact with collagen, thrombin, adenosine diphosphate, and antigen-antibody complexes. Thus, the platelet release reaction, which is a key component of coagulation, also results in increased vascular permeability. This is one of several links between clotting and inflammation.

Arachidonic Acid (AA) Metabolites: Prostaglandins, Leukotrienes, and Lipoxins

When cells are activated by diverse stimuli, such as microbial products and various mediators of inflammation, membrane *AA* is rapidly converted by the actions of enzymes to produce *prostaglandins* and *leukotrienes*. These biologically active lipid mediators serve as intracellular or extracellular signals to affect a variety of biologic processes, including inflammation and hemostasis.[48–50]

AA is a 20-carbon polyunsaturated fatty acid (5,8,11,14-eicosatetraenoic acid) that is derived from dietary sources or by conversion from the essential fatty acid *linoleic acid*. It does not occur free in the cell but is normally esterified in membrane phospholipids. Mechanical, chemical, and physical stimuli or other mediators (e.g., C5a) release AA from membrane phospholipids through the action of cellular phospholipases, mainly phospholipase A_2. The biochemical signals involved in the activation of phospholipase A_2 include an increase in cytoplasmic Ca^{2+} and activation of various kinases in response to external stimuli.[51] AA-derived mediators, also called *eicosanoids*, are synthesized by two major classes of enzymes: cyclooxygenases (which generate prostaglandins) and lipoxygenases (which produce leukotrienes and lipoxins) (Fig. 2–11). Eicosanoids bind to G protein–coupled receptors on many cell types and can mediate virtually every step of inflammation (Table 2–5).

○ *Prostaglandins* (PGs) are produced by mast cells, macrophages, endothelial cells, and many other cell types, and are involved in the vascular and systemic reactions of inflam-

TABLE 2–5	Principal Inflammatory Actions of Arachidonic Acid Metabolites (Eicosanoids)
Action	**Eicosanoid**
Vasodilation	PGI$_2$ (prostacyclin), PGE$_1$, PGE$_2$, PGD$_2$
Vasoconstriction	Thromboxane A$_2$, leukotrienes C$_4$, D$_4$, E$_4$
Increased vascular permeability	Leukotrienes C$_4$, D$_4$, E$_4$
Chemotaxis, leukocyte adhesion	Leukotriene B$_4$, HETE

HETE, hydroxyeicosatetraenoic acid; PGI$_2$, etc., prostaglandin I$_2$, etc.

mation. They are produced by the actions of two *cyclooxygenases,* the constitutively expressed COX-1 and the inducible enzyme COX-2. Prostaglandins are divided into series based on structural features as coded by a letter (PGD, PGE, PGF, PGG, and PGH) and a subscript numeral (e.g., 1, 2), which indicates the number of double bonds in the compound. The most important ones in inflammation are PGE$_2$, PGD$_2$, PGF$_{2\alpha}$, PGI$_2$ (prostacyclin), and TxA$_2$ (thromboxane), each of which is derived by the action of a specific enzyme on an intermediate in the pathway. Some of these enzymes have restricted tissue distribution. For example, platelets contain the enzyme thromboxane synthetase, and hence TxA$_2$ is the major product in these cells. TxA$_2$, a potent platelet-aggregating agent and vasoconstrictor, is itself unstable and rapidly converted to its inactive form TxB$_2$. Vascular endothelium lacks thromboxane synthetase but possesses prostacyclin synthetase, which leads to the formation of prostacyclin (PGI$_2$) and its stable end product PGF$_{1\alpha}$. Prostacyclin is a vasodilator, a potent inhibitor of platelet aggregation, and also markedly potentiates the permeability-increasing and chemotactic effects of other mediators. A thromboxane-prostacyclin imbalance has been implicated as an early event in thrombus formation in coronary and cerebral blood vessels (Chapter 4). PGD$_2$ is the major prostaglandin made by mast cells; along with PGE$_2$ (which is more widely distributed), it causes vasodilation and increases the permeability of post-capillary venules, thus potentiating edema formation. PGF$_{2\alpha}$ stimulates the contraction of uterine and bronchial smooth muscle and small arterioles, and PGD$_2$ is a chemoattractant for neutrophils.

In addition to their local effects, the prostaglandins are involved in the pathogenesis of *pain* and *fever* in inflammation. PGE$_2$ is hyperalgesic and makes the skin hypersensitive to painful stimuli, such as intradermal injection of suboptimal concentrations of histamine and bradykinin. It is involved in cytokine-induced fever during infections (described later).

- The *lipoxygenase* enzymes are responsible for the production of *leukotrienes,* which are secreted mainly by leukocytes, are chemoattractants for leukocytes, and also have vascular effects. There are three different lipoxygenases, 5-lipoxygenase being the predominant one in neutrophils. This enzyme converts AA to 5-hydroxyeicosatetraenoic

acid, which is chemotactic for neutrophils, and is the precursor of the leukotrienes. *LTB$_4$* is a potent chemotactic agent and activator of neutrophils, causing aggregation and adhesion of the cells to venular endothelium, generation of ROS, and release of lysosomal enzymes. The cysteinyl-containing leukotrienes C$_4$, D$_4$, and E$_4$ *(LTC$_4$, LTD$_4$, LTE$_4$)* cause intense vasoconstriction, bronchospasm (important in asthma), and increased vascular permeability. The vascular leakage, as with histamine, is restricted to venules. Leukotrienes are much more potent than is histamine in increasing vascular permeability and causing bronchospasm.

- *Lipoxins* are also generated from AA by the lipoxygenase pathway, but unlike prostaglandins and leukotrienes, the *lipoxins are inhibitors of inflammation.*[45] They are also unusual in that two cell populations are required for the transcellular biosynthesis of these mediators. Leukocytes, particularly neutrophils, produce intermediates in lipoxin synthesis, and these are converted to lipoxins by platelets interacting with the leukocytes. *The principal actions of lipoxins are to inhibit leukocyte recruitment and the cellular components of inflammation.* They inhibit neutrophil chemotaxis and adhesion to endothelium. There is an inverse relationship between the production of lipoxin and leukotrienes, suggesting that the lipoxins may be endogenous negative regulators of leukotrienes and may thus play a role in the resolution of inflammation.

Many anti-inflammatory drugs work by inhibiting the synthesis of eicosanoids:

- *Cyclooxygenase inhibitors* include aspirin and other nonsteroidal anti-inflammatory drugs *(NSAIDs),* such as indomethacin. They inhibit both COX-1 and COX-2 and thus inhibit prostaglandin synthesis; aspirin does this by irreversibly acetylating and inactivating cyclooxygenases. Selective *COX-2 inhibitors* are a newer class of these drugs. There has been great interest in COX-2 as a therapeutic target because it is induced by a variety of inflammatory stimuli and is absent from most tissues under normal "resting" conditions.[52] COX-1, by contrast, is produced in response to inflammatory stimuli and is also constitutively expressed in most tissues. This difference has led to the notion that COX-1 is responsible for the production of prostaglandins that are involved in both inflammation and homeostatic functions (e.g., fluid and electrolyte balance in the kidneys, cytoprotection in the gastrointestinal tract), whereas COX-2 generates prostaglandins that are involved only in inflammatory reactions. If this idea is correct, the selective COX-2 inhibitors should be anti-inflammatory without having the toxicities of the nonselective inhibitors, such as gastric ulceration. However, these distinctions are not absolute, as COX-2 also seems to play a role in normal homeostasis. Recently, results from large clinical trials have raised concerns that selective COX-2 inhibitors may increase the risk of cardiovascular and cerebrovascular events, leading to the removal of several of these drugs from the market in the United States and elsewhere. A possible explanation for the increased risk of arterial thrombosis is that COX-2 inhibitors impair endothelial cell production of prostacyclin, a vasodilator and inhibitor of platelet aggregation, while leaving intact the COX-1–mediated production by platelets of TxA_2, an important inducer of platelet aggregation and vasoconstriction. Thus, according to this hypothesis, selective COX-2 inhibition tilts the balance toward thromboxane and promotes vascular thrombosis, especially in individuals with other factors that increase the risk of thrombosis.[50,53]

- *Lipoxygenase inhibitors.* 5-lipoxygenase is not affected by NSAIDs, and many new inhibitors of this enzyme pathway have been developed. Pharmacologic agents that inhibit leukotriene production (e.g. Zileuton) or block leukotriene receptors (e.g. Montelukast) are useful in the treatment of asthma.
- *Broad-spectrum inhibitors* include *corticosteroids.* These powerful anti-inflammatory agents may act by reducing the transcription of genes encoding COX-2, phospholipase A_2, pro-inflammatory cytokines (such as IL-1 and TNF), and iNOS.
- Another approach to manipulating inflammatory responses has been to modify the intake and content of dietary lipids by increasing the consumption of *fish oil.* The proposed explanation for the effectiveness of this approach is that the polyunsaturated fatty acids in fish oil serve as poor substrates for conversion to active metabolites by both the cyclooxygenase and lipoxygenase pathways but are excellent substrates for the production of anti-inflammatory lipid products called resolvins and protectins.[45]

Platelet-Activating Factor (PAF)

PAF is another phospholipid-derived mediator.[54] Its name comes from its discovery as a factor that causes platelet aggregation, but it is now known to have multiple inflammatory effects. A variety of cell types, including platelets themselves, basophils, mast cells, neutrophils, macrophages, and endothelial cells, can elaborate PAF, in both secreted and cell-bound forms. In addition to platelet aggregation, PAF causes vasoconstriction and bronchoconstriction, and at extremely low concentrations it induces vasodilation and increased venular permeability with a potency 100 to 10,000 times greater than that of histamine. PAF also causes increased leukocyte adhesion to endothelium (by enhancing integrin-mediated leukocyte binding), chemotaxis, degranulation, and the oxidative burst. Thus, PAF can elicit most of the vascular and cellular reactions of inflammation. PAF also boosts the synthesis of other mediators, particularly eicosanoids, by leukocytes and other cells. A role for PAF in vivo is supported by the ability of synthetic PAF receptor antagonists to inhibit inflammation in some experimental models.

Reactive Oxygen Species

Oxygen-derived free radicals may be released extracellularly from leukocytes after exposure to microbes, chemokines, and immune complexes, or following a phagocytic challenge.[55] Their production is dependent, as we have seen, on the activation of the NADPH oxidase system. Superoxide anion (O_2^-), hydrogen peroxide (H_2O_2), and hydroxyl radical ($^\bullet OH$) are the major species produced within cells, and O_2^- can combine with NO to form reactive nitrogen species. Extracellular

release of low levels of these potent mediators can increase the expression of chemokines (e.g., IL-8), cytokines, and endothelial leukocyte adhesion molecules, amplifying the inflammatory response. As mentioned earlier, the physiologic function of these ROS in leukocytes is to destroy phagocytosed microbes, but release of these potent mediators can be damaging to the host (Chapter 1). They are implicated in the following responses in inflammation:

- *Endothelial cell damage, with resultant increased vascular permeability.* Adherent neutrophils, when activated, not only produce their own toxic species but also stimulate production of ROS in the endothelial cells.
- *Injury to other cell types* (parenchymal cells, red blood cells).
- *Inactivation of antiproteases,* such as α_1-antitrypsin. This leads to unopposed protease activity, with increased destruction of extracellular matrix. In the lung, such inhibition of anti-proteases contributes to destruction of elastic tissues, as in emphysema (Chapter 15).

Serum, tissue fluids, and host cells possess *antioxidant mechanisms* that protect against these potentially harmful oxygen-derived radicals. These antioxidants were discussed in Chapter 1; they include (1) the enzyme *superoxide dismutase,* which is found in or can be activated in a variety of cell types; (2) the enzyme *catalase,* which detoxifies H_2O_2; (3) *glutathione peroxidase,* another powerful H_2O_2 detoxifier; (4) the copper-containing serum protein *ceruloplasmin*; and (5) the iron-free fraction of serum *transferrin.* Thus, the influence of oxygen-derived free radicals in any given inflammatory reaction depends on the balance between production and inactivation of these metabolites by cells and tissues.

Nitric Oxide (NO)

NO was discovered as a factor released from endothelial cells that caused vasodilation and was therefore called endothelium-derived relaxing factor. NO is a soluble gas that is produced not only by endothelial cells but also by macrophages and some neurons in the brain. It acts in a paracrine manner on target cells through induction of cyclic guanosine monophosphate, which, in turn, initiates a series of intracellular events leading to a response, such as the relaxation of vascular smooth muscle cells. Because the in vivo half-life of NO is only seconds, the gas acts only on cells in close proximity to where it is produced.

NO is synthesized from L-arginine by the enzyme nitric oxide synthase (NOS). There are three different types of NOS: endothelial (eNOS), neuronal (nNOS), and inducible (iNOS) (Fig. 2–12). eNOS and nNOS are constitutively expressed at low levels and can be activated rapidly by an increase in cytoplasmic Ca^{2+}. iNOS, in contrast, is induced when macrophages and other cells are activated by cytokines (e.g., TNF, IFN-γ) or microbial products.

NO has dual actions in inflammation: it relaxes vascular smooth muscle and promotes vasodilation, thus contributing to the vascular reaction, but it is also an inhibitor of the cellular component of inflammatory responses.[56,57] NO reduces platelet aggregation and adhesion (Chapter 4), inhibits several features of mast cell–induced inflammation, and

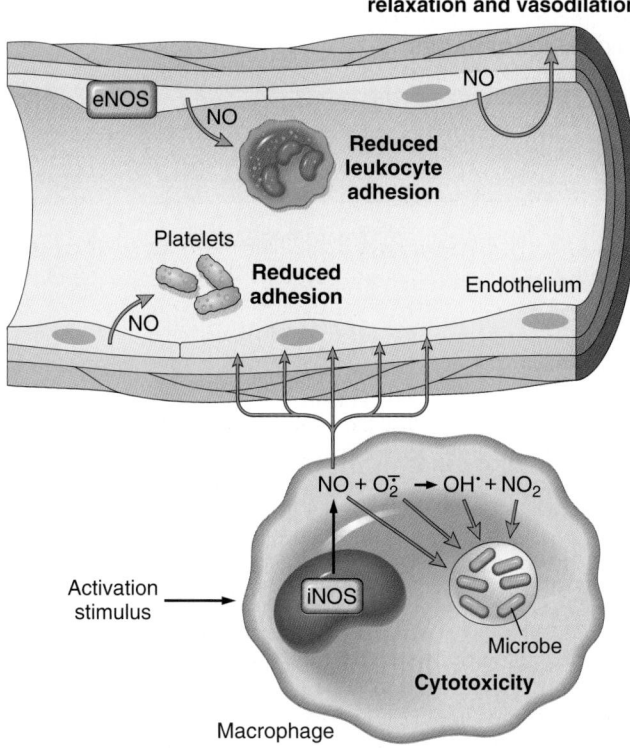

Vascular smooth muscle relaxation and vasodilation

FIGURE 2–12   Functions of nitric oxide (NO) in blood vessels and macrophages. NO is produced by two NO synthase (NOS) enzymes. It causes vasodilation, and NO-derived free radicals are toxic to microbial and mammalian cells.

inhibits leukocyte recruitment. *Because of these inhibitory actions, production of NO is thought to be an endogenous mechanism for controlling inflammatory responses.*

NO and its derivatives are microbicidal, and thus NO is a mediator of host defense against infection (discussed earlier). High levels of iNOS-induced NO are produced by leukocytes, mainly neutrophils and macrophages, in response to microbes.

Cytokines and Chemokines

Cytokines are proteins produced by many cell types (principally activated lymphocytes and macrophages, but also endothelial, epithelial, and connective tissue cells) that modulate the functions of other cell types. Long known to be involved in cellular immune responses, these products have additional effects that play important roles in both acute and chronic inflammation. Their general properties and functions are discussed in Chapter 6. Here we review the properties of cytokines that are involved in acute inflammation (Table 2–6).

Tumor Necrosis Factor and Interleukin-1. TNF and IL-1 are two of the major cytokines that mediate inflammation. They are produced mainly by activated macrophages. The secretion of TNF and IL-1 can be stimulated by endotoxin and other microbial products, immune complexes, physical injury, and a variety of inflammatory stimuli. Their most important actions in inflammation are their effects on endothelium, leukocytes, and fibroblasts, and induction of systemic acute-phase reactions (Fig. 2–13). In endothelium they induce a spectrum of changes referred to as *endothelial activation*.[58] In particular, they induce the expression of endothelial adhesion molecules; synthesis of chemical mediators, including other cytokines, chemokines, growth factors, eicosanoids, and NO; production of enzymes associated with matrix remodeling; and increases in the surface thrombogenicity of the endothelium.[59] TNF also augments responses of neutrophils to other stimuli such as bacterial endotoxin.

The production of IL-1 is controlled by a multi-protein cellular complex, sometimes called the "inflammasome," that responds to stimuli from microbes and dead cells. This complex activates proteases that are members of the caspase family, which function to cleave the newly synthesized inactive precursor of IL-1 into the biologically active cytokine. Mutations in genes encoding members of this protein complex are the cause of *inherited autoinflammatory syndromes,* the best known of which is familial Mediterranean fever.[60] The mutant proteins either constitutively activate the inflammatory caspases

TABLE 2–6 **Cytokines in Inflammation**		
Cytokine	**Principal Sources**	**Principal Actions in Inflammation**
IN ACUTE INFLAMMATION		
TNF	Macrophages, mast cells, T lymphocytes	Stimulates expression of endothelial adhesion molecules and secretion of other cytokines; systemic effects
IL-1	Macrophages, endothelial cells, some epithelial cells	Similar to TNF; greater role in fever
IL-6	Macrophages, other cells	Systemic effects (acute-phase response)
Chemokines	Macrophages, endothelial cells, T lymphocytes, mast cells, other cell types	Recruitment of leukocytes to sites of inflammation; migration of cells to normal tissues
IN CHRONIC INFLAMMATION		
IL-12	Dendritic cells, macrophages	Increased production of IFN-γ
IFN-γ	T lymphocytes, NK cells	Activation of macrophages (increased ability to kill microbes and tumor cells)
IL-17	T lymphocytes	Recruitment of neutrophils and monocytes

IFN-γ, interferon-γ; IL-1, interleukin-1; NK cells, natural killer cells; TNF, tumor necrosis factor.
The most important cytokines involved in inflammatory reactions are listed. Many other cytokines may play lesser roles in inflammation. There is also considerable overlap between the cytokines involved in acute and chronic inflammation. Specifically, all the cytokines listed under acute inflammation may also contribute to chronic inflammatory reactions.

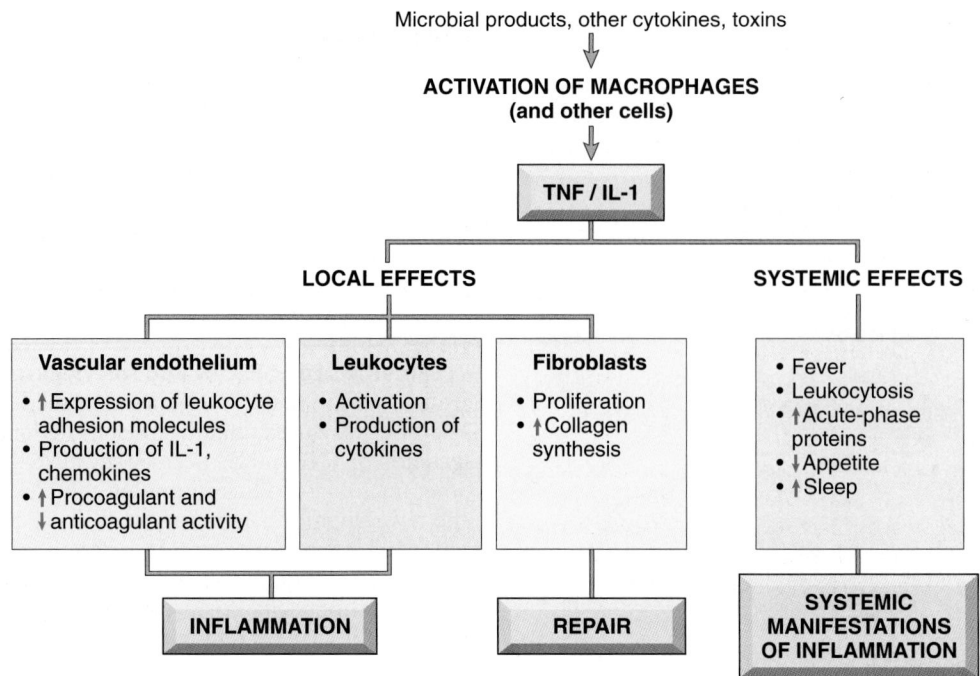

Microbial products, other cytokines, toxins

ACTIVATION OF MACROPHAGES
(and other cells)

TNF / IL-1

LOCAL EFFECTS

SYSTEMIC EFFECTS

Vascular endothelium
- ↑ Expression of leukocyte adhesion molecules
- Production of IL-1, chemokines
- ↑ Procoagulant and ↓ anticoagulant activity

Leukocytes
- Activation
- Production of cytokines

Fibroblasts
- Proliferation
- ↑ Collagen synthesis

- Fever
- Leukocytosis
- ↑ Acute-phase proteins
- ↓ Appetite
- ↑ Sleep

INFLAMMATION

REPAIR

SYSTEMIC MANIFESTATIONS OF INFLAMMATION

FIGURE 2–13   Principal local and systemic actions of tumor necrosis factor (TNF) and interleukin-1 (IL-1).

or interfere with the negative regulation of this enzymatic process. The net result is unregulated IL-1 production.[61,62] Affected patients present with fever and other systemic manifestations of inflammation without overt provocation. Over time, some of these patients also develop amyloidosis, a disease of extracellular protein deposition that is often the result of persistent inflammation (Chapter 6). IL-1 antagonists are effective for treating these disorders, an excellent example of molecularly targeted rational therapy. The same inflammasome complex may be activated by urate crystals in the disease called gout, and the inflammation in this disease also seems to be, at least partly, mediated by IL-1 (Chapter 26).

IL-1 and TNF (as well as IL-6) induce the systemic *acutephase responses* associated with infection or injury (described later in the chapter). TNF also regulates energy balance by promoting lipid and protein mobilization and by suppressing appetite. Therefore, sustained production of TNF contributes to *cachexia*, a pathologic state characterized by weight loss and anorexia that accompanies some chronic infections and neoplastic diseases (Chapter 9).

Chemokines. Chemokines are a family of small (8 to 10 kD) proteins that act primarily as chemoattractants for specific types of leukocytes.[63] About 40 different chemokines and 20 different receptors for chemokines have been identified. They are classified into four major groups, according to the arrangement of the conserved cysteine (C) residues in the mature proteins[64,65]:

○ *C-X-C chemokines* (also called α chemokines) have one amino acid residue separating the first two conserved cysteine residues. The C-X-C chemokines act primarily on neutrophils. *IL-8* is typical of this group. It is secreted by activated macrophages, endothelial cells, and other cell types, and causes activation and chemotaxis of neutrophils,

with limited activity on monocytes and eosinophils. Its most important inducers are microbial products and other cytokines, mainly IL-1 and TNF.

○ *C-C chemokines* (also called β chemokines) have the first two conserved cysteine residues adjacent. The C-C chemokines, which include *monocyte chemoattractant protein* (MCP-1), *eotaxin, macrophage inflammatory protein-1α* (MIP-1α), and *RANTES* (regulated and normal T-cell expressed and secreted), generally attract monocytes, eosinophils, basophils, and lymphocytes but not neutrophils. Although most of the chemokines in this class have overlapping actions, eotaxin selectively recruits eosinophils.

○ *C chemokines* (also called γ chemokines) lack two (the first and third) of the four conserved cysteines. The C chemokines (e.g., lymphotactin) are relatively specific for lymphocytes.

○ *CX3C chemokines* contain three amino acids between the two cysteines. The only known member of this class is called *fractalkine.* This chemokine exists in two forms: the cell surface-bound protein can be induced on endothelial cells by inflammatory cytokines and promotes strong adhesion of monocytes and T cells, and a soluble form, derived by proteolysis of the membrane-bound protein, has potent chemoattractant activity for the same cells.

Chemokines mediate their activities by binding to seventransmembrane G protein–coupled receptors. These receptors (called CXCR or CCR, for C-X-C or C-C chemokine receptors) usually exhibit overlapping ligand specificities, and leukocytes generally express more than one receptor type. As discussed in Chapter 6, certain chemokine receptors (CXCR-4, CCR-5) act as coreceptors for a viral envelope glycoprotein of human immunodeficiency virus 1 and are thus involved in binding and entry of the virus into cells.

Chemokines have two main functions: they stimulate leukocyte recruitment in inflammation and control the normal migration of cells through various tissues.[20,65] Some chemokines are produced transiently in response to inflammatory stimuli and promote the recruitment of leukocytes to the sites of inflammation. Other chemokines are produced constitutively in tissues and function to organize different cell types in different anatomic regions of the tissues. In both situations, chemokines may be displayed at high concentrations attached to proteoglycans on the surface of endothelial cells and in the extracellular matrix.

Other Cytokines in Acute Inflammation. The list of cytokines implicated in inflammation is huge and constantly growing.[66] Two that have received considerable recent interest are: IL-6, made by macrophages and other cells, which is involved in local and systemic reactions[67]; and IL-17, produced mainly by T lymphocytes, which promotes neutrophil recruitment.[68] Antagonists against both are in clinical trials for inflammatory diseases. Cytokines also play central roles in chronic inflammation; these are described later in the chapter.

Lysosomal Constituents of Leukocytes

Neutrophils and monocytes contain lysosomal granules, which, when released, may contribute to the inflammatory response. Neutrophils have two main types of granules. The smaller *specific* (or secondary) granules contain lysozyme, collagenase, gelatinase, lactoferrin, plasminogen activator, histaminase, and alkaline phosphatase. The larger *azurophil* (or primary) granules contain myeloperoxidase, bactericidal factors (lysozyme, defensins), acid hydrolases, and a variety of neutral proteases (elastase, cathepsin G, nonspecific collagenases, proteinase 3).[40] Both types of granules can fuse with phagocytic vacuoles containing engulfed material, or the granule contents can be released into the extracellular space.

Different granule enzymes serve different functions. *Acid proteases* degrade bacteria and debris *within the phagolysosomes,* in which an acid pH is readily reached. *Neutral proteases* are capable of degrading various *extracellular components,* such as collagen, basement membrane, fibrin, elastin, and cartilage, resulting in the tissue destruction that accompanies inflammatory processes. Neutral proteases can also cleave C3 and C5 complement proteins directly, releasing anaphylatoxins, and release a kinin-like peptide from kininogen. Neutrophil elastase has been shown to degrade virulence factors of bacteria and thus combat bacterial infections. *Monocytes* and *macrophages* also contain acid hydrolases, collagenase, elastase, phospholipase, and plasminogen activator. These may be particularly active in chronic inflammatory reactions.

Because of the destructive effects of lysosomal enzymes, the initial leukocytic infiltration, if unchecked, can potentiate further inflammation and tissue damage. These harmful proteases, however, are held in check by a system of *antiproteases* in the serum and tissue fluids. Foremost among these is α_1-antitrypsin, which is the major inhibitor of neutrophil elastase. A deficiency of these inhibitors may lead to sustained action of leukocyte proteases, as is the case in patients with α_1-antitrypsin deficiency (Chapter 15). α_2-Macroglobulin is another antiprotease found in serum and various secretions.

Neuropeptides

Neuropeptides are secreted by sensory nerves and various leukocytes, and play a role in the initiation and propagation of an inflammatory response. The small peptides, such as *substance P* and neurokinin A, belong to a family of tachykinin neuropeptides produced in the central and peripheral nervous systems.[69] Nerve fibers containing substance P are prominent in the lung and gastrointestinal tract. Substance P has many biologic functions, including the transmission of pain signals, regulation of blood pressure, stimulation of secretion by endocrine cells, and increasing vascular permeability. Sensory neurons can also produce other pro-inflammatory molecules, such as calcitonin-related gene product, which are thought to link the sensing of painful stimuli to the development of protective host responses.[70]

PLASMA PROTEIN–DERIVED MEDIATORS

A variety of phenomena in the inflammatory response are mediated by plasma proteins that belong to three interrelated systems: the complement, kinin, and clotting systems.

Complement System

The complement system consists of more than 20 proteins, some of which are numbered C1 through C9. This system functions in both innate and adaptive immunity for defense against microbial pathogens.[71-73] In the process of complement activation several cleavage products of complement proteins are elaborated that cause increased vascular permeability, chemotaxis, and opsonization. The activation and functions of the complement system are outlined in Figure 2–14.

Complement proteins are present in inactive forms in the plasma, and many of them are activated to become proteolytic enzymes that degrade other complement proteins, thus forming an enzymatic cascade capable of tremendous amplification. The critical step in complement activation is the proteolysis of the third (and most abundant) component, C3. Cleavage of C3 can occur by one of three pathways: the *classical pathway,* which is triggered by fixation of C1 to antibody (IgM or IgG) that has combined with antigen; the *alternative pathway,* which can be triggered by microbial surface molecules (e.g., endotoxin, or LPS), complex polysaccharides, cobra venom, and other substances, in the absence of antibody; and the *lectin pathway,* in which plasma mannose-binding lectin binds to carbohydrates on microbes and directly activates C1. Whichever pathway is involved in the early steps of complement activation, they all lead to the formation of an active enzyme called the *C3 convertase,* which splits C3 into two functionally distinct fragments, C3a and C3b. C3a is released, and C3b becomes covalently attached to the cell or molecule where complement is being activated. More C3b then binds to the previously generated fragments to form *C5 convertase,* which cleaves C5 to release C5a and leave C5b attached to the cell surface. C5b binds the late components (C6–C9), culminating in the formation of the membrane attack complex (MAC, composed of multiple C9 molecules).

The biologic functions of the complement system fall into three general categories (see Fig. 2–14):

COMPLEMENT ACTIVATION

EFFECTOR FUNCTIONS

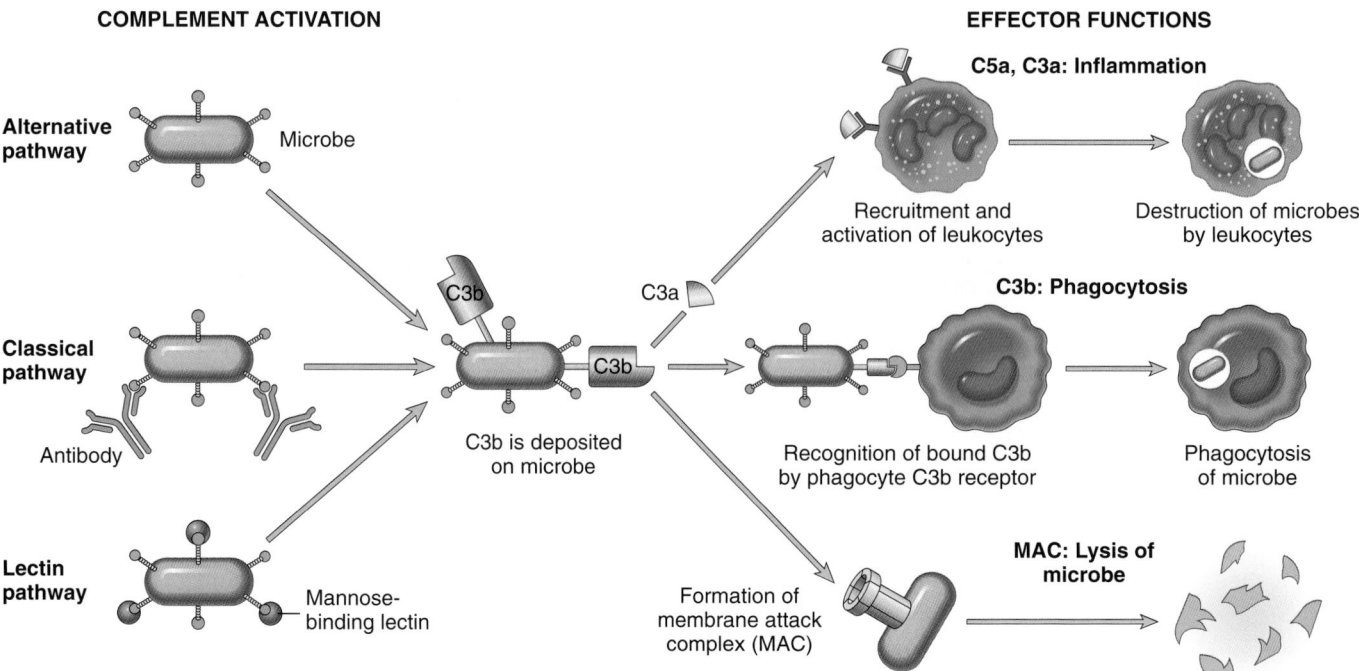

FIGURE 2–14 The activation and functions of the complement system. Activation of complement by different pathways leads to cleavage of C3. The functions of the complement system are mediated by breakdown products of C3 and other complement proteins, and by the membrane attack complex (MAC).

- *Inflammation. C3a, C5a,* and, to a lesser extent, *C4a* are cleavage products of the corresponding complement components that stimulate histamine release from mast cells and thereby increase vascular permeability and cause vasodilation. They are called *anaphylatoxins* because they have effects similar to those of mast cell mediators that are involved in the reaction called *anaphylaxis* (Chapter 6). C5a is also a powerful chemotactic agent for neutrophils, monocytes, eosinophils, and basophils. In addition, C5a activates the lipoxygenase pathway of AA metabolism in neutrophils and monocytes, causing further release of inflammatory mediators.
- *Phagocytosis. C3b* and its cleavage product *iC3b* (inactive C3b), when fixed to a microbial cell wall, act as opsonins and promote phagocytosis by neutrophils and macrophages, which bear cell surface receptors for the complement fragments.
- *Cell lysis.* The deposition of the MAC on cells makes these cells permeable to water and ions and results in death (lysis) of the cells.

Among the complement components, C3a and C5a are the most important inflammatory mediators. In addition to the mechanisms already discussed, *C3 and C5 can be cleaved by several proteolytic enzymes present within the inflammatory exudate.* These include plasmin and lysosomal enzymes released from neutrophils (discussed earlier). Thus, the chemotactic actions of complement and the complement-activating effects of neutrophils can initiate a self-perpetuating cycle of neutrophil recruitment.

The *activation of complement is tightly controlled by cell-associated and circulating regulatory proteins.* Different regulatory proteins inhibit the production of active complement

fragments or remove fragments that deposit on cells. These regulators are expressed on normal host cells and are thus designed to prevent healthy tissues from being injured at sites of complement activation. Regulatory proteins can be overwhelmed when large amounts of complement are deposited on host cells and tissues, as happens in autoimmune diseases, in which individuals produce complement-fixing antibodies against their own tissue antigens (Chapter 6).

Coagulation and Kinin Systems

Inflammation and blood clotting are often intertwined, with each promoting the other.[74] The clotting system is divided into two pathways that converge, culminating in the activation of thrombin and the formation of fibrin (Fig. 2–15) (Chapter 4). The intrinsic clotting pathway is a series of plasma proteins that can be activated by Hageman factor (factor XII), a protein synthesized by the liver that circulates in an inactive form. Factor XII is activated upon contact with negatively charged surfaces, for instance when vascular permeability increases and plasma proteins leak into the extravascular space and come into contact with collagen, or when it comes into contact with basement membranes exposed as a result of endothelial damage. Factor XII then undergoes a conformational change (becoming factor XIIa), exposing an active serine center that can subsequently cleave protein substrates and activate a variety of mediator systems (see later). Inflammation increases the production of several coagulation factors, makes the endothelial surface pro-thrombogenic, and inhibits anticoagulation mechanisms, thus promoting clotting. Conversely, thrombin, a product of clotting, promotes inflammation by engaging receptors that are called *protease-activated receptors* (PARs) because they bind multiple trypsin-like serine prote-

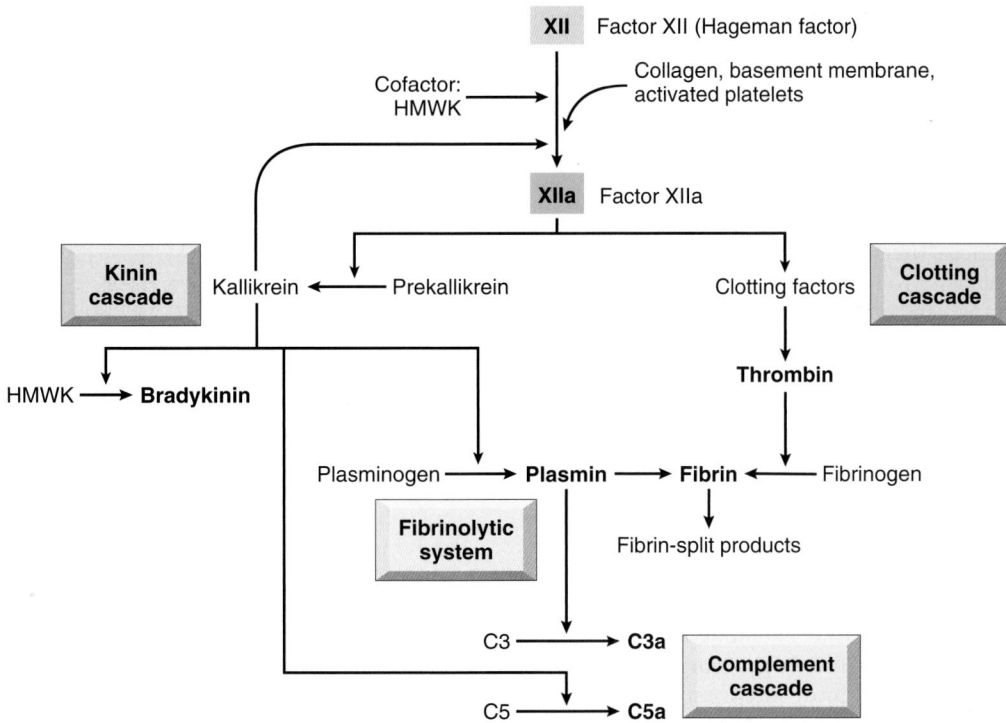

FIGURE 2–15 Interrelationships between the four plasma mediator systems triggered by activation of factor XII (Hageman factor). Note that thrombin induces inflammation by binding to protease-activated receptors (principally PAR-1) on platelets, endothelium, smooth muscle cells, and other cells. HMWK, high molecular weight kininogen.

ases in addition to thrombin.[75] These receptors are seven-transmembrane G protein–coupled receptors that are expressed on platelets, endothelial and smooth muscle cells, and many other cell types. Engagement of the so-called type 1 receptor (PAR-1) by proteases, particularly thrombin, triggers several responses that induce inflammation. They include mobilization of P-selectin; production of chemokines and other cytokines; expression of endothelial adhesion molecules for leukocyte integrins; induction of cyclooxygenase-2 and production of prostaglandins; production of PAF and NO; and changes in endothelial shape.[75] As we have seen, these responses promote the recruitment of leukocytes and many other reactions of inflammation. Because coagulation and inflammation can initiate a vicious cycle of amplification, interfering with clotting is a potential therapeutic strategy for the systemic inflammatory disease seen with severe, disseminated bacterial infections. This is the rationale for treating this disorder with the anticoagulant, activated protein C, which may benefit a subset of the patients (Chapter 4).[76]

Kinins are vasoactive peptides derived from plasma proteins, called kininogens, by the action of specific proteases called kallikreins. The kinin and coagulation systems are also intimately connected. The active form of factor XII, factor XIIa, converts plasma *prekallikrein* into an active proteolytic form, the enzyme *kallikrein*, which cleaves a plasma glycoprotein precursor, high-molecular-weight kininogen, to produce *bradykinin* (see Fig. 2–15).[77] *Bradykinin increases vascular permeability and causes contraction of smooth muscle, dilation of blood vessels, and pain when injected into the skin.* These effects are similar to those of histamine. The action of bradykinin is short-lived, because it is quickly inactivated by an enzyme called kininase. Any remaining kinin is inactivated during passage of plasma through the lung by angiotensin-converting enzyme. *Kallikrein itself is a potent activator of Hageman factor, allowing for autocatalytic amplification of the initial stimulus.* Kallikrein has chemotactic activity, and it also directly converts C5 to the chemoattractant product C5a.

At the same time that factor XIIa is inducing fibrin clot formation, it activates the *fibrinolytic system.* This cascade counterbalances clotting by cleaving fibrin, thereby solubilizing the clot. Kallikrein, as well as plasminogen activator (released from endothelium, leukocytes, and other tissues), cleaves plasminogen, a plasma protein that binds to the evolving fibrin clot to generate *plasmin*, a multifunctional protease. The fibrinolytic system contributes to the vascular phenomena of inflammation in several ways. Although the primary function of plasmin is to lyse fibrin clots, during inflammation it also cleaves the complement protein C3 to produce C3 fragments, and it degrades fibrin to form *fibrin split products*, which may have permeability-inducing properties. Plasmin can also activate Hageman factor, which can trigger multiple cascades (see Fig. 2–15), amplifying the response.

From this discussion of the plasma proteases activated by the complement, kinin, and clotting systems, a few general conclusions can be drawn:

- *Bradykinin, C3a, and C5a* (as mediators of increased vascular permeability); *C5a* (as the mediator of chemotaxis); and *thrombin* (which has effects on endothelial cells and many other cell types) are likely to be the most important in vivo.

- *C3a* and *C5a* can be generated by several types of reactions: (1) immunologic reactions, involving antibodies and complement (the classical pathway); (2) activation of the alternative and lectin complement pathways by microbes, in the absence of antibodies; and (3) agents not directly related to immune responses, such as plasmin, kallikrein, and some serine proteases found in normal tissue.
- *Activated Hageman factor (factor XIIa)* initiates four systems involved in the inflammatory response: (1) the *kinin system*, which produces vasoactive kinins; (2) the *clotting system*, which induces formation of thrombin, which has inflammatory properties; (3) the *fibrinolytic system*, which produces plasmin and degrades fibrin to produce fibrinopeptides, which induce inflammation; and (4) the *complement system*, which produces anaphylatoxins and other mediators. Some of the products of this initiation—particularly kallikrein—can, by feedback, activate Hageman factor, resulting in amplification of the reaction.

When Lewis discovered the role of histamine in inflammation, one mediator was thought to be enough. Now, we are wallowing in them! Yet, from this large compendium, it is likely that a few mediators are most important for the reactions of acute inflammation in vivo, and these are summarized in Table 2–7. The redundancy of the mediators and their actions ensures that this protective response remains robust and is not easy to perturb.

TABLE 2–7 Role of Mediators in Different Reactions of Inflammation

Role in Inflammation	Mediators
Vasodilation	Prostaglandins Nitric oxide Histamine
Increased vascular permeability	Histamine and serotonin C3a and C5a (by liberating vasoactive amines from mast cells, other cells) Bradykinin Leukotrienes C_4, D_4, E_4 PAF Substance P
Chemotaxis, leukocyte recruitment and activation	TNF, IL-1 Chemokines C3a, C5a Leukotriene B_4 (Bacterial products, e.g., *N*-formyl methyl peptides)
Fever	IL-1, TNF Prostaglandins
Pain	Prostaglandins Bradykinin
Tissue damage	Lysosomal enzymes of leukocytes Reactive oxygen species Nitric oxide

IL-1, interleukin-1; PAF, platelet-activating factor; TNF, tumor necrosis factor.

Outcomes of Acute Inflammation

Although, as might be expected, many variables may modify the basic process of inflammation, including the nature and intensity of the injury, the site and tissue affected, and the responsiveness of the host, *all acute inflammatory reactions may have one of three outcomes* (Fig. 2–16):

- *Complete resolution.* In a perfect world, all inflammatory reactions, once they have succeeded in neutralizing and eliminating the injurious stimulus, should end with restoration of the site of acute inflammation to normal. This is called *resolution* and is the usual outcome when the injury is limited or short-lived or when there has been little tissue destruction and the damaged parenchymal cells can regenerate. Resolution involves removal of cellular debris and microbes by macrophages, and resorption of edema fluid by lymphatics.
- *Healing by connective tissue replacement (fibrosis).* This occurs after substantial tissue destruction, when the inflammatory injury involves tissues that are incapable of regeneration, or when there is abundant fibrin exudation in tissue or serous cavities (pleura, peritoneum) that cannot be adequately cleared. In all these situations, connective tissue grows into the area of damage or exudate, converting it into a mass of fibrous tissue—a process also called *organization.*
- Progression of the response to *chronic inflammation* (discussed below). This may follow acute inflammation, or the response may be chronic from the onset. Acute to chronic transition occurs when the acute inflammatory response cannot be resolved, as a result of either the persistence of the injurious agent or some interference with the normal process of healing.[79] For example, bacterial infection of the lung may begin as a focus of acute inflammation (pneumonia), but its failure to resolve may lead to extensive tissue destruction and formation of a cavity in which the inflammation continues to smolder, leading eventually to a chronic lung abscess. Another example of chronic inflammation with a persisting stimulus is peptic ulcer of the duodenum or stomach. Peptic ulcers may persist for months or years and, as discussed below, are manifested by both acute and chronic inflammatory reactions.

Morphologic Patterns of Acute Inflammation

The morphologic hallmarks of all acute inflammatory reactions are dilation of small blood vessels, slowing of blood flow, and accumulation of leukocytes and fluid in the extravascular tissue (Fig. 2–17). However, special morphologic patterns are often superimposed on these general features, depending on the severity of the reaction, its specific cause, and the particular tissue and site involved. The importance of recognizing the gross and microscopic patterns is that they often provide valuable clues about the underlying cause.

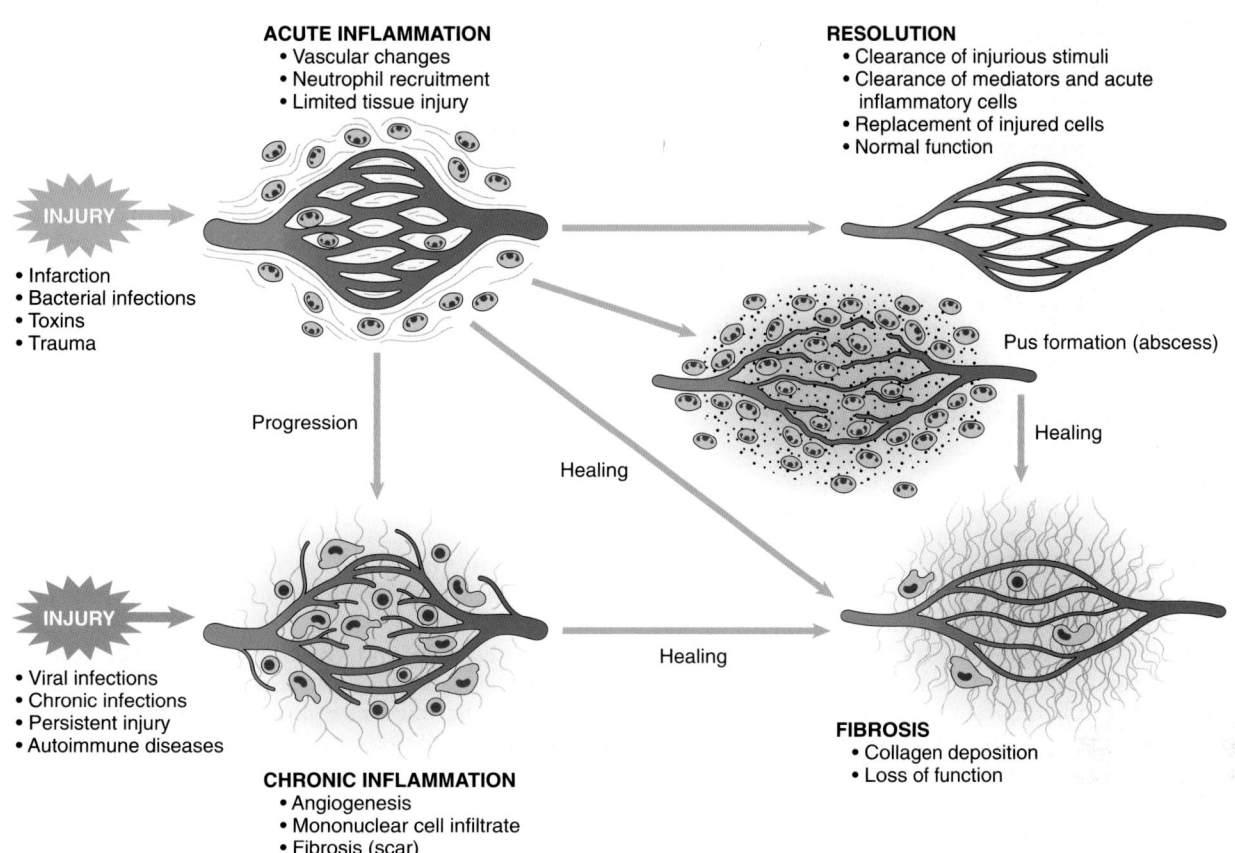

FIGURE 2–16 Outcomes of acute inflammation: resolution, healing by fibrosis, or chronic inflammation. The components of the various reactions and their functional outcomes are listed.

SEROUS INFLAMMATION

Serous inflammation is marked by the outpouring of a thin fluid that may be derived from the plasma or from the secretions of mesothelial cells lining the peritoneal, pleural, and pericardial cavities. Accumulation of fluid in these cavities is called an *effusion*. The skin blister resulting from a burn or viral infection represents a large accumulation of serous fluid, either within or immediately beneath the epidermis of the skin (Fig. 2–18).

FIBRINOUS INFLAMMATION

With greater increase in vascular permeability, large molecules such as fibrinogen pass the vascular barrier, and fibrin is formed

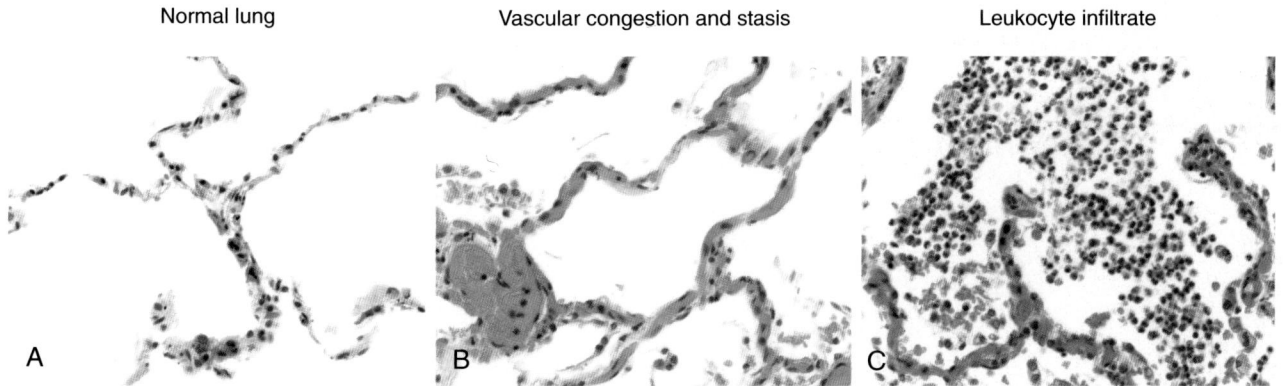

FIGURE 2–17 The characteristic histopathology of acute inflammation. **A,** Normal lung shows thin (virtually invisible) blood vessels in the alveolar walls and no cells in the alveoli. **B,** The vascular component of acute inflammation is manifested by congested blood vessels (packed with erythrocytes), resulting from stasis. **C,** The cellular component of the response is manifested by large numbers of leukocytes (neutrophils) in the alveoli.

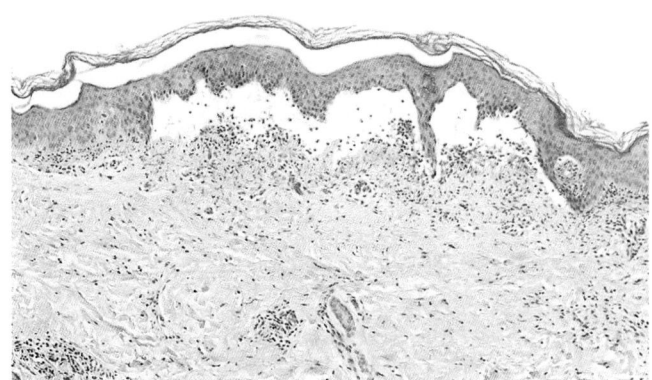

FIGURE 2–18 Serous inflammation. Low-power view of a cross-section of a skin blister showing the epidermis separated from the dermis by a focal collection of serous effusion.

and deposited in the extracellular space. A fibrinous exudate develops when the vascular leaks are large or there is a local procoagulant stimulus (e.g., cancer cells). A fibrinous exudate is characteristic of inflammation in the lining of body cavities, such as the meninges, pericardium (Fig. 2–19A) and pleura. Histologically, fibrin appears as an eosinophilic meshwork of threads or sometimes as an amorphous coagulum (Fig. 2–19B). Fibrinous exudates may be removed by fibrinolysis and clearing of other debris by macrophages. If the fibrin is not removed, over time it may stimulate the ingrowth of fibroblasts and blood vessels and thus lead to scarring. Conversion of the fibrinous exudate to scar tissue *(organization)* within the pericardial sac leads to opaque fibrous thickening of the pericardium and epicardium in the area of exudation and, if the fibrosis is extensive, obliteration of the pericardial space.

SUPPURATIVE OR PURULENT INFLAMMATION; ABSCESS

This type of inflammation is characterized by the production of large amounts of pus or purulent exudate consisting of neutrophils, liquefactive necrosis, and edema fluid. Certain bacteria (e.g., staphylococci) produce this localized suppuration and are therefore referred to as *pyogenic* (pus-producing) bacteria. A common example of an acute suppurative inflammation is acute appendicitis. *Abscesses are localized collections of purulent inflammatory tissue* caused by suppuration buried in a tissue, an organ, or a confined space. They are produced by deep seeding of pyogenic bacteria into a tissue (Fig. 2–20). Abscesses have a central region that appears as a mass of necrotic leukocytes and tissue cells. There is usually a zone of preserved neutrophils around this necrotic focus, and outside this region vascular dilation and parenchymal and fibroblastic proliferation occur, indicating chronic inflammation and repair. In time the abscess may become walled off and ultimately replaced by connective tissue.

ULCERS

An ulcer is a local defect, or excavation, of the surface of an organ or tissue that is produced by the sloughing (shedding) of inflamed necrotic tissue (Fig. 2–21). Ulceration can occur only when tissue necrosis and resultant inflammation exist on or near a surface. It is most commonly encountered in (1) the mucosa of the mouth, stomach, intestines, or genitourinary tract; and (2) the skin and subcutaneous tissue of the lower extremities in older persons who have circulatory disturbances that predispose to extensive ischemic necrosis.

Ulcerations are best exemplified by peptic ulcer of the stomach or duodenum, in which acute and chronic inflammation coexist. During the acute stage there is intense polymorphonuclear infiltration and vascular dilation in the margins of the defect. With chronicity, the margins and base of the ulcer develop fibroblastic proliferation, scarring, and the accumulation of lymphocytes, macrophages, and plasma cells.

Summary of Acute Inflammation

Now that we have described the components, mediators, and pathologic manifestations of acute inflammatory responses, it

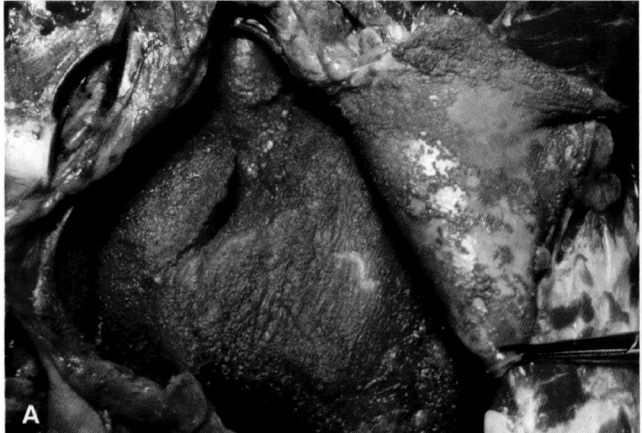
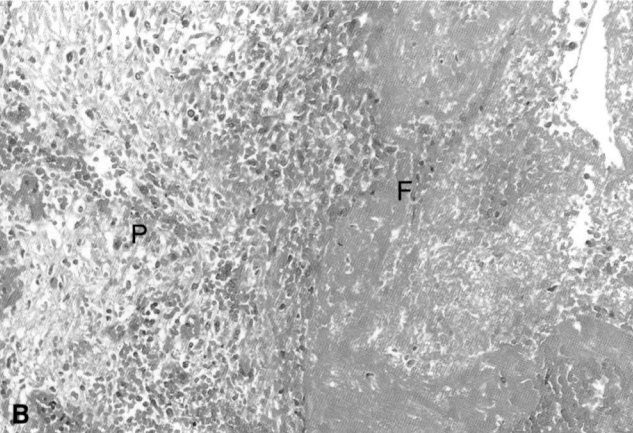

FIGURE 2–19 Fibrinous pericarditis. **A,** Deposits of fibrin on the pericardium. **B,** A pink meshwork of fibrin exudate (F) overlies the pericardial surface (P).

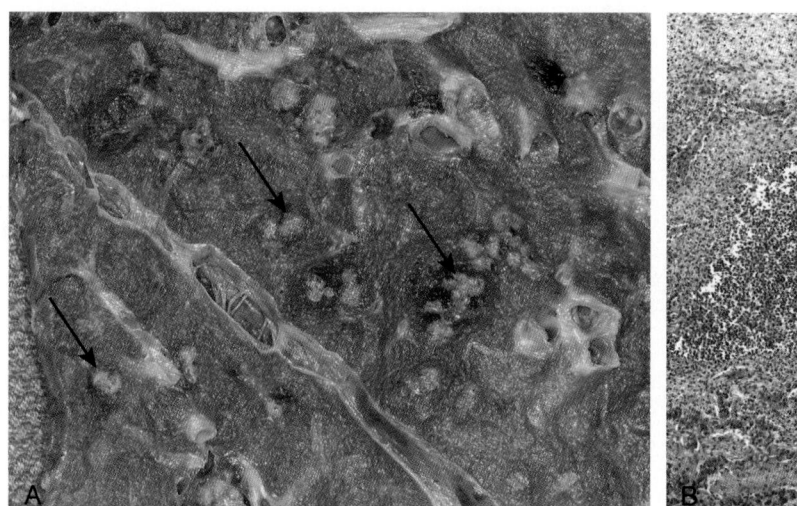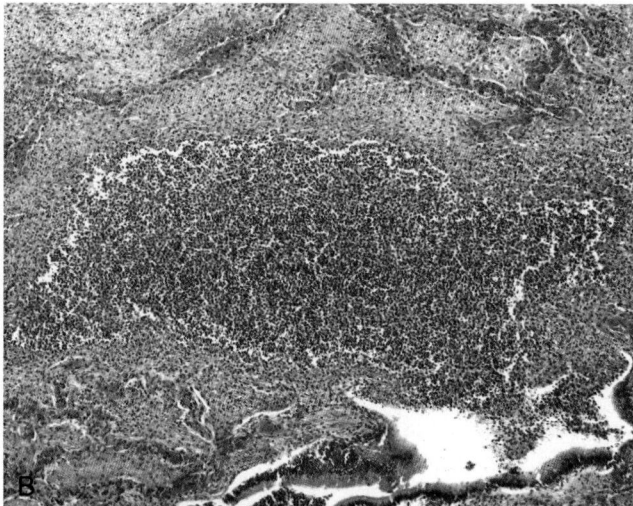

FIGURE 2–20   Purulent inflammation. **A,** Multiple bacterial abscesses in the lung, in a case of bronchopneumonia. **B,** The abscess contains neutrophils and cellular debris, and is surrounded by congested blood vessels.

is useful to summarize the sequence of events in a typical response of this type.[78] When a host encounters an injurious agent, such as an infectious microbe or dead cells, phagocytes that reside in all tissues try to eliminate these agents. At the same time phagocytes and other host cells react to the presence of the foreign or abnormal substance by liberating cytokines, lipid messengers, and other mediators of inflammation. Some of these mediators act on small blood vessels in the vicinity and promote the efflux of plasma and the recruitment of circulating leukocytes to the site where the offending agent is located. The recruited leukocytes are activated by the injurious agent and by locally produced mediators, and the activated leukocytes try to remove the offending agent by phagocytosis. As the injurious agent is eliminated and anti-inflammatory mechanisms become active, the process subsides and the host returns to a normal state of health. If the injurious agent cannot be quickly eliminated, the result may be chronic inflammation.

The clinical and pathologic manifestations of the inflammatory response are caused by several reactions. The vascular phenomena of acute inflammation are characterized by increased blood flow to the injured area, resulting mainly from arteriolar dilation and opening of capillary beds induced by mediators such as histamine. Increased vascular permeability results in the accumulation of protein-rich extravascular fluid, which forms the exudate. Plasma proteins leave the vessels, most commonly through widened interendothelial cell junctions of the venules. The redness *(rubor),* warmth *(calor),* and swelling *(tumor)* of acute inflammation are caused by the increased blood flow and edema. Circulating leukocytes, initially predominantly neutrophils, adhere to the endothelium via adhesion molecules, traverse the endothelium, and migrate to the site of injury under the influence of chemotactic agents. Leukocytes that are activated by the offending agent and by endogenous mediators may release toxic metabolites and proteases extracellularly, causing tissue damage. During the damage, and in part as a result of the liberation of prostaglandins, neuropeptides, and cytokines, one of the local symptoms is pain *(dolor).*

In clinical practice the underlying cause determines whether the therapeutic goal is to promote or reduce inflammation. In infections the treatment is intended to increase the host

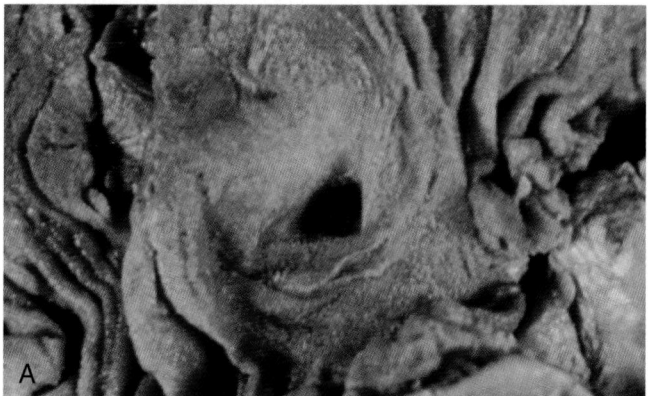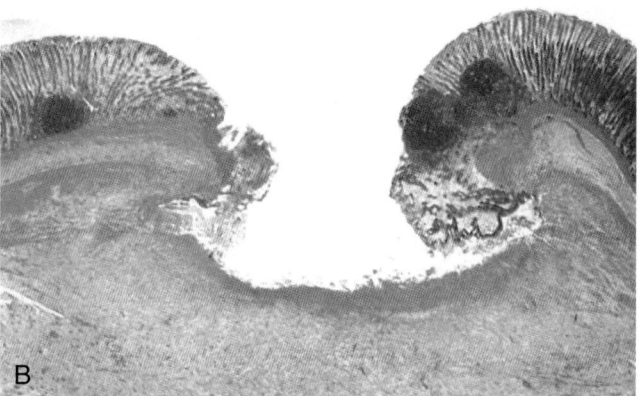

FIGURE 2–21   The morphology of an ulcer. **A,** A chronic duodenal ulcer. **B,** Low-power cross-section of a duodenal ulcer crater with an acute inflammatory exudate in the base.

response and eliminate the infection—hence the practice of warm compresses and gargles in case of pharyngitis (sore throat). On the other hand, in traumatic injuries and chronic inflammatory diseases, inflammation serves no useful purpose and the goal is to reduce it with application of cold (in trauma) and anti-inflammatory drugs. At certain locations, such as the cornea, it may be desirable to suppress even acute inflammation so that corneal transparency can be maintained.

Chronic Inflammation

Chronic inflammation is inflammation of prolonged duration (weeks or months) in which inflammation, tissue injury, and attempts at repair coexist, in varying combinations. It may follow acute inflammation, as described earlier, or chronic inflammation may begin insidiously, as a low-grade, smoldering response without any manifestations of an acute reaction. This latter type of chronic inflammation is the cause of tissue damage in some of the most common and disabling human diseases, such as rheumatoid arthritis, atherosclerosis, tuberculosis, and pulmonary fibrosis. It has also been implicated in the progression of cancer and in diseases once thought to be purely degenerative, such as Alzheimer disease.

CAUSES OF CHRONIC INFLAMMATION

Chronic inflammation arises in the following settings:

- *Persistent infections* by microorganisms that are difficult to eradicate, such as mycobacteria, and certain viruses, fungi, and parasites. These organisms often evoke an immune reaction called *delayed-type hypersensitivity* (Chapter 6). The inflammatory response sometimes takes a specific pattern called a *granulomatous reaction* (discussed later).
- *Immune-mediated inflammatory diseases.* Chronic inflammation plays an important role in a group of diseases that are caused by excessive and inappropriate activation of the immune system. Under certain conditions immune reactions develop against the individual's own tissues, leading to *autoimmune diseases* (Chapter 6). In these diseases, autoantigens evoke a self-perpetuating immune reaction that results in chronic tissue damage and inflammation; examples of such diseases are rheumatoid arthritis and multiple sclerosis. In other cases, chronic inflammation is the result of unregulated immune responses against microbes, as in inflammatory bowel disease. Immune responses against common environmental substances are the cause of *allergic diseases*, such as bronchial asthma (Chapter 6). Because these autoimmune and allergic reactions are inappropriately triggered against antigens that are normally harmless, the reactions serve no useful purpose and only cause disease. Such diseases may show morphologic patterns of mixed acute and chronic inflammation because they are characterized by repeated bouts of inflammation. Fibrosis may dominate the late stages.
- *Prolonged exposure to potentially toxic agents, either exogenous or endogenous.* An example of an exogenous agent is particulate silica, a nondegradable inanimate material that, when inhaled for prolonged periods, results in an inflammatory lung disease called *silicosis* (Chapter 15). *Atheroscle-*

rosis (Chapter 11) is thought to be a chronic inflammatory process of the arterial wall induced, at least in part, by endogenous toxic plasma lipid components.

MORPHOLOGIC FEATURES

In contrast to acute inflammation, which is manifested by vascular changes, edema, and predominantly neutrophilic infiltration, *chronic inflammation is characterized by:*

- *Infiltration with mononuclear cells,* which include macrophages, lymphocytes, and plasma cells (Fig. 2–22)
- *Tissue destruction,* induced by the persistent offending agent or by the inflammatory cells
- Attempts at *healing by connective tissue replacement of damaged tissue,* accomplished by proliferation of small blood vessels *(angiogenesis)* and, in particular, *fibrosis*[80]

Because angiogenesis and fibrosis are also components of wound healing and repair, they are discussed more fully in Chapter 3.

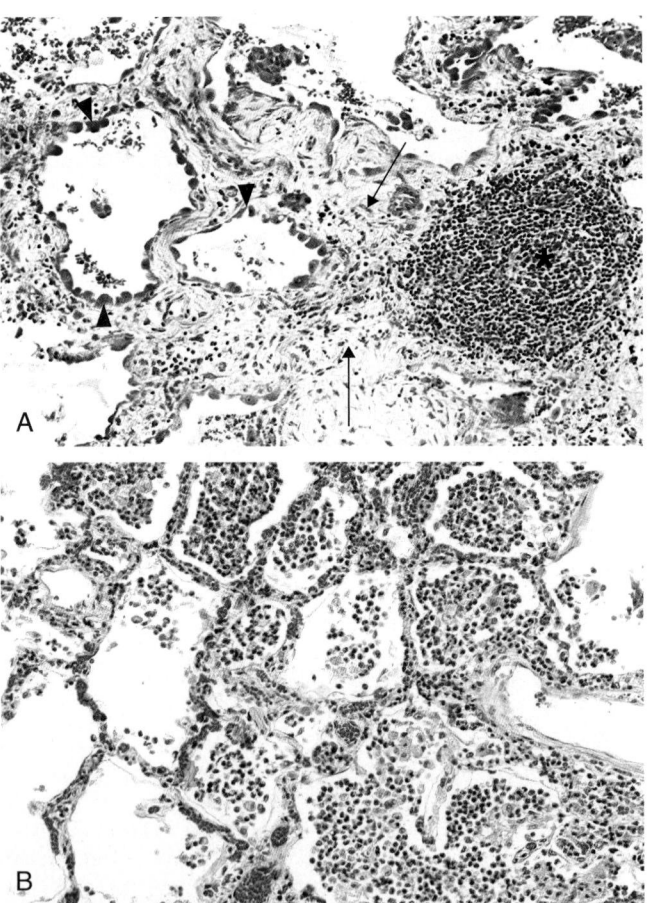

FIGURE 2–22   A, Chronic inflammation in the lung, showing all three characteristic histologic features: (1) collection of chronic inflammatory cells (*), (2) destruction of parenchyma (normal alveoli are replaced by spaces lined by cuboidal epithelium, *arrowheads*), and (3) replacement by connective tissue (fibrosis, *arrows*). **B,** By contrast, in acute inflammation of the lung (acute bronchopneumonia), neutrophils fill the alveolar spaces and blood vessels are congested.

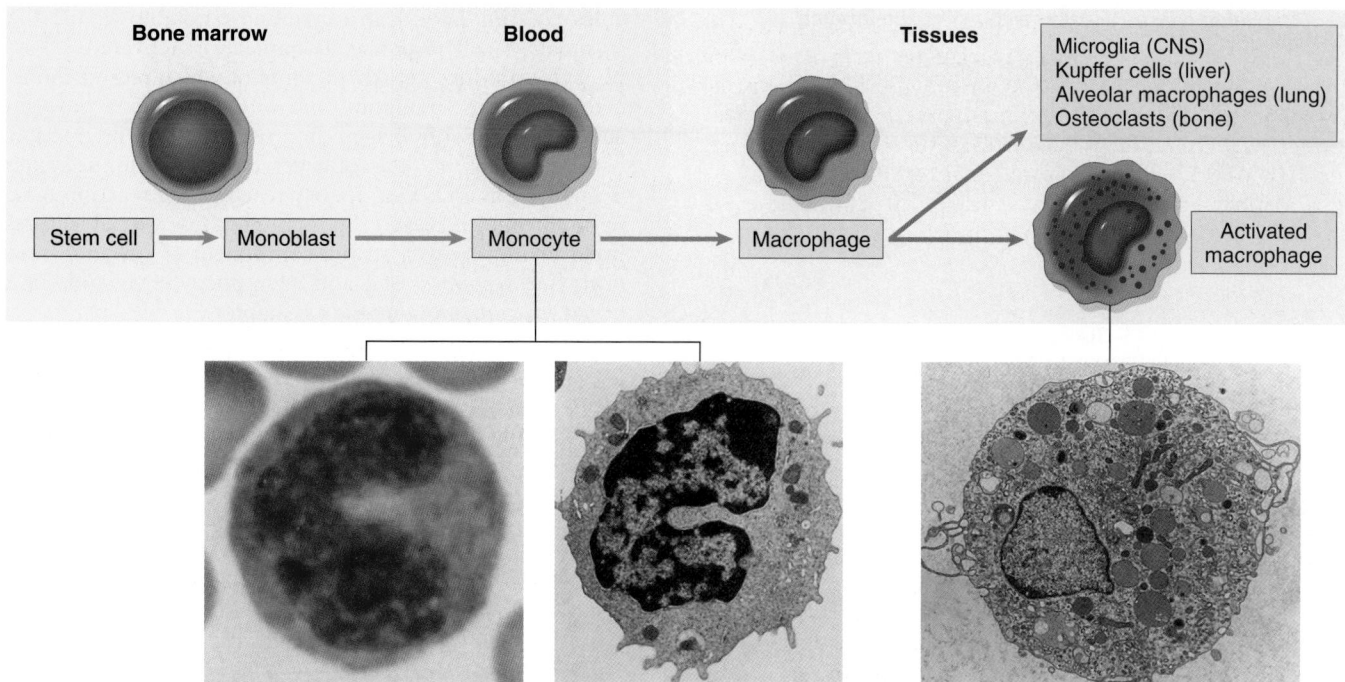

FIGURE 2–23   Maturation of mononuclear phagocytes. (From Abbas AK et al: Cellular and Molecular Immunology, 5th ed. Philadelphia, WB Saunders, 2003.)

ROLE OF MACROPHAGES IN CHRONIC INFLAMMATION

The *macrophage* is the dominant cellular player in chronic inflammation, and we begin our discussion with a brief review of its biology. *Macrophages* are one component of the *mononuclear phagocyte system* (Fig. 2–23). The mononuclear phagocyte system (sometimes called reticuloendothelial system) consists of closely related cells of bone marrow origin, including blood monocytes and tissue macrophages. The latter are diffusely scattered in the connective tissue or located in organs such as the liver (Kupffer cells), spleen and lymph nodes (sinus histiocytes), lungs (alveolar macrophages), and central nervous system (microglia). Mononuclear phagocytes arise from a common precursor in the bone marrow, which gives rise to blood monocytes. From the blood, monocytes migrate into various tissues and differentiate into macrophages. The half-life of blood monocytes is about 1 day, whereas the life span of tissue macrophages is several months or years. The journey from bone marrow stem cell to tissue macrophage is regulated by a variety of growth and differentiation factors, cytokines, adhesion molecules, and cellular interactions.

As discussed earlier, monocytes begin to emigrate into extravascular tissues quite early in acute inflammation, and within 48 hours they may constitute the predominant cell type. Extravasation of monocytes is governed by the same factors that are involved in neutrophil emigration, that is, adhesion molecules and chemical mediators with chemotactic and activating properties.[81] When a monocyte reaches the extravascular tissue, it undergoes transformation into a larger phagocytic cell, the *macrophage*. Macrophages may be *activated* by a variety of stimuli, including microbial products that engage TLRs and other cellular receptors, cytokines (e.g.,

IFN-γ) secreted by sensitized T lymphocytes and by natural killer cells, and other chemical mediators (Fig. 2–24).

The products of activated macrophages serve to eliminate injurious agents such as microbes and to initiate the process of repair, and are responsible for much of the tissue injury in chronic inflammation. Activation of macrophages results in increased levels of lysosomal enzymes and reactive oxygen and nitrogen species, and production of cytokines, growth factors, and other mediators of inflammation. Some of these products are toxic to microbes and host cells (e.g., reactive oxygen and nitrogen species) or to extracellular matrix (proteases); some cause influx of other cell types (e.g., cytokines, chemotactic factors); and still others cause fibroblast proliferation, collagen deposition, and angiogenesis (e.g., growth factors). As illustrated in Fig. 2–10, different macrophage populations may serve distinct functions—some may be important for microbial killing and inflammation, and others for repair.[38] Their impressive arsenal of mediators makes macrophages powerful allies in the body's defense against unwanted invaders, but the same weaponry can also induce considerable tissue destruction when macrophages are inappropriately activated. It is because of the activities of these macrophages that *tissue destruction is one of the hallmarks of chronic inflammation.* The ongoing tissue destruction can itself activate the inflammatory cascade, so that features of both acute and chronic inflammation may coexist in certain circumstances.

In short-lived inflammation, if the irritant is eliminated, macrophages eventually disappear (either dying off or making their way into the lymphatics and lymph nodes). In chronic inflammation, macrophage accumulation persists, as a result of continuous recruitment from the circulation and local proliferation at the site of inflammation.

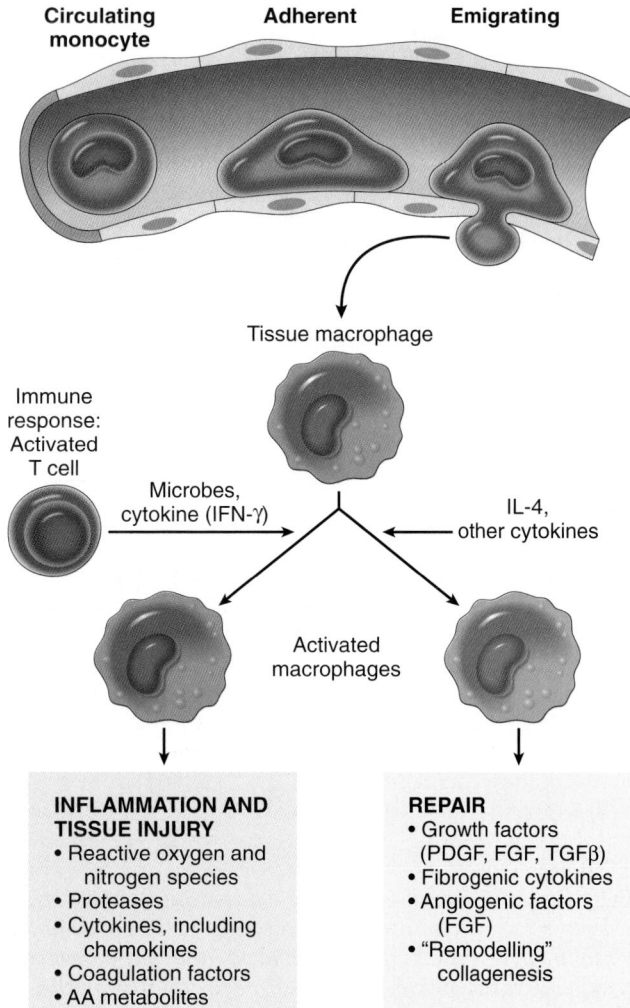

FIGURE 2-24 The roles of activated macrophages in chronic inflammation. Macrophages are activated by nonimmunologic stimuli such as endotoxin or by cytokines from immune-activated T cells (particularly IFN-γ). The products made by activated macrophages that cause tissue injury and fibrosis are indicated. AA, arachidonic acid; PDGF, platelet-derived growth factor; FGF, fibroblast growth factor; TGFβ, transforming growth factor β.

OTHER CELLS IN CHRONIC INFLAMMATION

Other cell types involved in chronic inflammation include lymphocytes, plasma cells, eosinophils, and mast cells:

○ *Lymphocytes* are mobilized in both antibody-mediated and cell-mediated immune reactions. Antigen-stimulated (effector and memory) lymphocytes of different types (T and B cells) use various adhesion molecule pairs (selectins, integrins and their ligands) and chemokines to migrate into inflammatory sites. Cytokines from activated macrophages, mainly TNF, IL-1, and chemokines, promote leukocyte recruitment, setting the stage for persistence of the inflammatory response. Lymphocytes and macrophages interact in a bidirectional way, and these reactions play an important role in chronic inflammation (Fig. 2–25). Macrophages display antigens to T cells and produce membrane mole-

cules (costimulators) and cytokines (notably IL-12) that stimulate T-cell responses (Chapter 6). Activated T lymphocytes produce cytokines, some of which recruit monocytes from the circulation and one, IFN-γ, is a powerful activator of macrophages. Because of these interactions between T cells and macrophages, once the immune system is involved in an inflammatory reaction the reaction tends to be chronic and severe. To highlight these special features, inflammation with a strong component of immune reactions (i.e., responses of T and B lymphocytes) is sometimes called *immune inflammation* (Chapter 6).

○ *Plasma cells* develop from activated B lymphocytes and produce antibodies directed either against persistent foreign or self antigens in the inflammatory site or against altered tissue components. In some strong chronic inflammatory reactions, the accumulation of lymphocytes, antigen-presenting cells, and plasma cells may assume the morphologic features of lymphoid organs, particularly lymph nodes, even containing well-formed germinal centers. These are called *tertiary lymphoid organs*; this type of *lymphoid organogenesis* is often seen in the synovium of patients with long-standing rheumatoid arthritis.[82]

○ *Eosinophils* are abundant in immune reactions mediated by IgE and in parasitic infections (Fig. 2–26). A chemokine that is especially important for eosinophil recruitment is eotaxin. Eosinophils have granules that contain *major basic protein*, a highly cationic protein that is toxic to parasites but also causes lysis of mammalian epithelial cells. This is why eosinophils are of benefit in controlling parasitic infections, but they contribute to tissue damage in immune reactions such as allergies (Chapter 6).[83]

○ *Mast cells* are widely distributed in connective tissues and participate in both acute and chronic inflammatory reactions. Mast cells express on their surface the receptor (FcεRI) that binds the Fc portion of IgE antibody. In immediate hypersensitivity reactions, IgE antibodies bound to the cells' Fc receptors specifically recognize antigen, and the cells degranulate and release mediators, such as histamine and prostaglandins (Chapter 6). This type of response occurs during allergic reactions to foods, insect venom, or drugs, sometimes with catastrophic results (e.g. anaphylactic shock). Mast cells are also present in chronic inflammatory reactions, and because they secrete a plethora of cytokines, they have the ability to both promote and limit inflammatory reactions in different situations.

Although *neutrophils* are characteristic of acute inflammation, many forms of chronic inflammation, lasting for months, continue to show large numbers of neutrophils, induced either by persistent microbes or by mediators produced by activated macrophages and T lymphocytes. In chronic bacterial infection of bone (osteomyelitis), a neutrophilic exudate can persist for many months. Neutrophils are also important in the chronic damage induced in lungs by smoking and other irritant stimuli (Chapter 15).

In addition to cellular infiltrates, growth of *blood vessels and lymphatic vessels* is often prominent in chronic inflammatory reactions. This growth of vessels is stimulated by growth factors, such as VEGF, produced by macrophages and endothelial cells (Chapter 3).

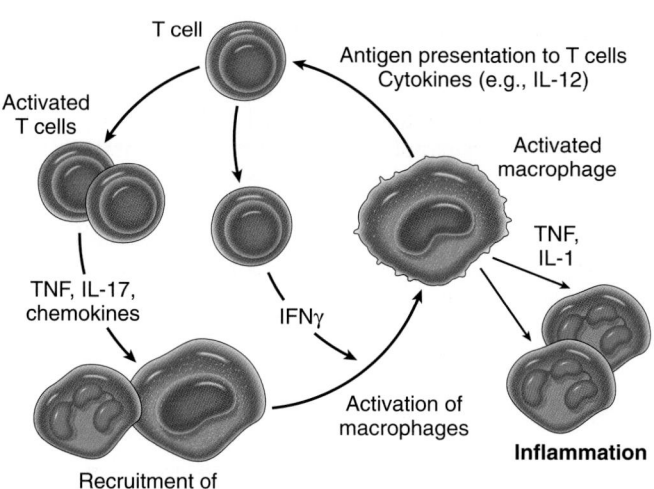

FIGURE 2–25 Macrophage-lymphocyte interactions in chronic inflammation. Activated T cells produce cytokines that recruit macrophages (TNF, IL-17, chemokines) and others that activate macrophages (IFNγ). Different subsets of T cells (called T$_H$1 and T$_H$17) may produce different sets of cytokines; these are described in Chapter 6. Activated macrophages in turn stimulate T cells by presenting antigens and via cytokines (such as IL-12).

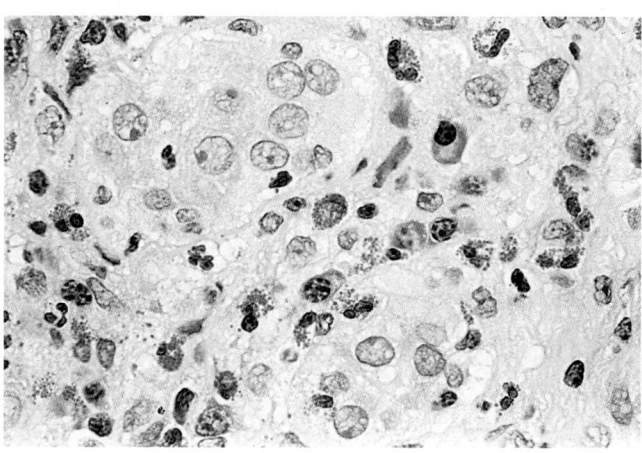

FIGURE 2–26 A focus of inflammation showing numerous eosinophils.

GRANULOMATOUS INFLAMMATION

Granulomatous inflammation is a distinctive pattern of chronic inflammation that is encountered in a limited number of infectious and some noninfectious conditions. Immune reactions are usually involved in the development of granulomas, and therefore this process is described in more detail in Chapter 6. Briefly, a granuloma is a cellular attempt to contain an offending agent that is difficult to eradicate. In this attempt there is often strong activation of T lymphocytes leading to macrophage activation, which can cause injury to normal tissues. Tuberculosis is the prototype of the granulomatous diseases, but sarcoidosis, cat-scratch disease, lymphogranuloma inguinale, leprosy, brucellosis, syphilis, some mycotic infections, berylliosis, reactions of irritant lipids, and some autoimmune diseases are also included (Table 2–8). Recognition of the granulomatous pattern in a biopsy specimen is important because of the limited number of possible conditions that cause it and the significance of the diagnoses associated with the lesions.

A granuloma is a focus of chronic inflammation consisting of a microscopic aggregation of macrophages that are transformed into epithelium-like cells, surrounded by a collar of mononuclear leukocytes, principally lymphocytes and occasionally plasma cells. In the usual hematoxylin and eosin–stained tissue sections, the epithelioid cells have a pale pink granular cytoplasm

TABLE 2–8 Examples of Diseases with Granulomatous Inflammation		
Disease	**Cause**	**Tissue Reaction**
Tuberculosis	*Mycobacterium tuberculosis*	Caseating granuloma (tubercle): focus of activated macrophages (epithelioid cells), rimmed by fibroblasts, lymphocytes, histiocytes, occasional Langhans giant cells; central necrosis with amorphous granular debris; acid-fast bacilli
Leprosy	*Mycobacterium leprae*	Acid-fast bacilli in macrophages; noncaseating granulomas
Syphilis	*Treponema pallidum*	Gumma: microscopic to grossly visible lesion, enclosing wall of histiocytes; plasma cell infiltrate; central cells necrotic without loss of cellular outline
Cat-scratch disease	Gram-negative bacillus	Rounded or stellate granuloma containing central granular debris and recognizable neutrophils; giant cells uncommon
Sarcoidosis	Unknown etiology	Noncaseating granulomas with abundant activated macrophages
Crohn disease (inflammatory bowel disease)	Immune reaction against intestinal bacteria, self-antigens	Occasional noncaseating granulomas in the wall of the intestine, with dense chronic inflammatory infiltrate

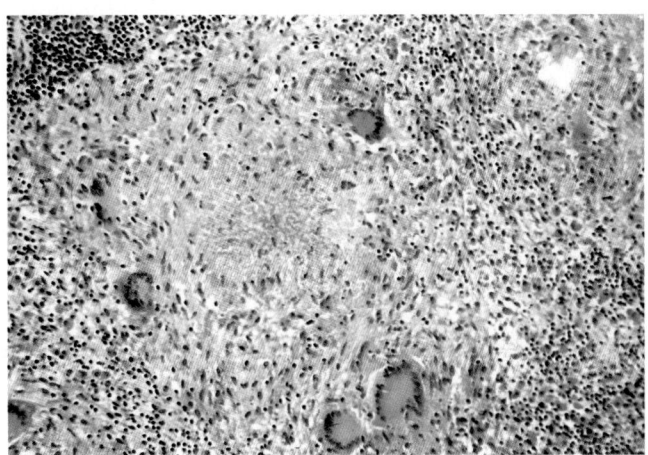

FIGURE 2–27 Typical tuberculous granuloma showing an area of central necrosis surrounded by multiple Langhans-type giant cells, epithelioid cells, and lymphocytes.

with indistinct cell boundaries, often appearing to merge into one another. The nucleus is less dense than that of a lymphocyte, is oval or elongate, and may show folding of the nuclear membrane. Older granulomas develop an enclosing rim of fibroblasts and connective tissue. Frequently, epithelioid cells fuse to form *giant cells* in the periphery or sometimes in the center of granulomas. These giant cells may attain diameters of 40 to 50 µm. They have a large mass of cytoplasm containing 20 or more small nuclei arranged either peripherally (Langhans-type giant cell) or haphazardly (foreign body–type giant cell) (Fig. 2–27). There is no known functional difference between these two types of giant cells, yet some pathologists persist in describing them—perhaps because they make nice exam questions!

There are two types of granulomas, which differ in their pathogenesis. *Foreign body granulomas* are incited by relatively inert foreign bodies. Typically, foreign body granulomas form around material such as talc (associated with intravenous drug abuse) (Chapter 9), sutures, or other fibers that are large enough to preclude phagocytosis by a single macrophage and do not incite any specific inflammatory or immune response. Epithelioid cells and giant cells are apposed to the surface of the foreign body. The foreign material can usually be identified in the center of the granuloma, particularly if viewed with polarized light, in which it appears refractile.

Immune granulomas are caused by a variety of agents that are capable of inducing a cell-mediated immune response (Chapter 6). This type of immune response produces granulomas usually when the inciting agent is poorly degradable or particulate. In such responses macrophages engulf foreign protein antigen, process it, and present peptides to antigen-specific T lymphocytes, causing their activation (Chapter 6). The responding T cells produce cytokines, such as IL-2, which activates other T cells, perpetuating the response, and IFN-γ, which is important in activating macrophages and transforming them into epithelioid cells and multinucleate giant cells.

The prototype of the immune granuloma is that caused by infection with *Mycobacterium tuberculosis*. In this disease the granuloma is referred to as a *tubercle. It is often characterized by the presence of central caseous necrosis* (see Fig. 2–27). In contrast, caseous necrosis is rare in other granulomatous diseases. The morphologic patterns in the various granulomatous diseases may be sufficiently different to allow reasonably accurate diagnosis by an experienced pathologist (see Table 2–8); however, there are so many atypical presentations that it is always necessary to identify the specific etiologic agent by special stains for organisms (e.g., acid-fast stains for tubercle bacilli), by culture methods (e.g., in tuberculosis and fungal diseases), by molecular techniques (e.g., the polymerase chain reaction in tuberculosis), and by serologic studies (e.g., in syphilis).

Systemic Effects of Inflammation

Anyone who has suffered a severe sore throat or a respiratory infection has experienced the systemic manifestations of acute inflammation. The systemic changes associated with acute inflammation are collectively called the *acute-phase response*, or the systemic inflammatory response syndrome. These changes are reactions to cytokines whose production is stimulated by bacterial products such as LPS and by other inflammatory stimuli. The acute-phase response consists of several clinical and pathologic changes:

- *Fever,* characterized by an elevation of body temperature, usually by 1° to 4°C, is one of the most prominent manifestations of the acute-phase response, especially when inflammation is associated with infection. Fever is produced in response to substances called *pyrogens* that act by stimulating prostaglandin synthesis in the vascular and perivascular cells of the hypothalamus. Bacterial products, such as LPS (called *exogenous pyrogens*), stimulate leukocytes to release cytokines such as IL-1 and TNF (called *endogenous pyrogens*) that increase the enzymes (cyclooxygenases) that convert AA into prostaglandins.[84] In the hypothalamus, the prostaglandins, especially PGE$_2$, stimulate the production of neurotransmitters such as cyclic adenosine monophosphate, which function to reset the temperature set point at a higher level. NSAIDs, including aspirin, reduce fever by inhibiting prostaglandin synthesis. An elevated body temperature has been shown to help amphibians ward off microbial infections, and it is assumed that fever does the same for mammals, although the mechanism is unknown. One hypothesis is that fever may induce heat shock proteins that enhance lymphocyte responses to microbial antigens.
- *Acute-phase proteins* are plasma proteins, mostly synthesized in the liver, whose plasma concentrations may increase several hundred-fold as part of the response to inflammatory stimuli.[85] Three of the best-known of these proteins are C-reactive protein (CRP), fibrinogen, and serum amyloid A (SAA) protein. Synthesis of these molecules by hepatocytes is up-regulated by cytokines, especially IL-6 (for CRP and fibrinogen) and IL-1 or TNF (for SAA). Many acute-phase proteins, such as CRP and SAA, bind to microbial cell walls, and they may act as opsonins and fix complement. They also bind chromatin, possibly aiding in the clearing of necrotic cell nuclei. During the acute-phase response SAA protein replaces apolipoprotein A, a component of high-density lipoprotein particles. This may alter

the targeting of high-density lipoproteins from liver cells to macrophages, which can use these particles as a source of energy-producing lipids. Fibrinogen binds to red cells and causes them to form stacks (rouleaux) that sediment more rapidly at unit gravity than do individual red cells. This is the basis for measuring the *erythrocyte sedimentation rate* as a simple test for the systemic inflammatory response, caused by any stimulus. Acute-phase proteins have beneficial effects during acute inflammation, but as we shall see in Chapter 6, prolonged production of these proteins (especially SAA) in states of chronic inflammation causes *secondary amyloidosis*. Elevated serum levels of CRP have been proposed as a marker for increased risk of myocardial infarction in patients with coronary artery disease.[86] It is postulated that inflammation involving atherosclerotic plaques in the coronary arteries may predispose to thrombosis and subsequent infarction, and CRP is produced during inflammation. Another peptide whose production is increased in the acute-phase response is the iron-regulating peptide *hepcidin*.[87] Chronically elevated plasma concentrations of hepcidin reduce the availability of iron and are responsible for the *anemia* associated with chronic inflammation (Chapter 14).

- *Leukocytosis* is a common feature of inflammatory reactions, especially those induced by bacterial infections. The leukocyte count usually climbs to 15,000 or 20,000 cells/μL, but sometimes it may reach extraordinarily high levels of 40,000 to 100,000 cells/μL. These extreme elevations are referred to as *leukemoid reactions*, because they are similar to the white cell counts observed in leukemia and have to be distinguished from leukemia. The leukocytosis occurs initially because of *accelerated release* of cells from the bone marrow postmitotic reserve pool (caused by cytokines, including TNF and IL-1) and is therefore associated with a rise in the number of more immature neutrophils in the blood *(shift to the left)*. Prolonged infection also induces proliferation of precursors in the bone marrow, caused by increased production of colony-stimulating factors. Thus, the bone marrow output of leukocytes is increased to compensate for the loss of these cells in the inflammatory reaction. (See also the discussion of leukocytosis in Chapter 13.) Most bacterial infections induce an increase in the blood neutrophil count, called *neutrophilia*. Viral infections, such as infectious mononucleosis, mumps, and German measles, cause an absolute increase in the number of lymphocytes *(lymphocytosis)*. In bronchial asthma, allergy, and parasitic infestations, there is an increase in the absolute number of eosinophils, creating an *eosinophilia*. Certain infections (typhoid fever and infections caused by some viruses, rickettsiae, and certain protozoa) are associated with a decreased number of circulating white cells *(leukopenia)*. Leukopenia is also encountered in infections that overwhelm patients debilitated by disseminated cancer, rampant tuberculosis, or severe alcoholism.

- Other manifestations of the acute-phase response include increased pulse and blood pressure; decreased sweating, mainly because of redirection of blood flow from cutaneous to deep vascular beds, to minimize heat loss through the skin; rigors (shivering), chills (search for warmth), anorexia, somnolence, and malaise, probably because of the actions of cytokines on brain cells.

- In severe bacterial infections *(sepsis)* the large amounts of organisms and LPS in the blood stimulate the production of enormous quantities of several cytokines, notably TNF and IL-1.[88,89] As a result, circulating levels of these cytokines increase and the nature of the host response changes. High levels of cytokines cause various clinical manifestations such as disseminated intravascular coagulation, cardiovascular failure, and metabolic disturbance, which are described as *septic shock*; it is discussed in more detail in Chapter 4.

Consequences of Defective or Excessive Inflammation

Now that we have described the process of inflammation and its outcomes, it is helpful to summarize the clinical and pathologic consequences of too much or too little inflammation.

- *Defective inflammation* typically results in increased susceptibility to infections, because the inflammatory response is a central component of the early defense mechanisms that immunologists call *innate immunity* (Chapter 6). It is also associated with delayed wound healing, because inflammation is essential for clearing damaged tissues and debris, and provides the necessary stimulus to get the repair process started.

- *Excessive inflammation* is the basis of many types of human disease. Allergies, in which individuals mount unregulated immune responses against commonly encountered environmental antigens, and autoimmune diseases, in which immune responses develop against normally tolerated self-antigens, are disorders in which the fundamental cause of tissue injury is inflammation (Chapter 6). In addition, as we mentioned at the outset, recent studies are pointing to an important role of inflammation in a wide variety of human diseases that are not primarily disorders of the immune system. These include atherosclerosis and ischemic heart disease, and some neurodegenerative diseases such as Alzheimer disease. Prolonged inflammation and the fibrosis that accompanies it are also responsible for much of the pathology in many infectious, metabolic, and other diseases. The specific diseases are discussed in relevant chapters later in the book.

Now that our discussion of the molecular and cellular events in acute and chronic inflammation is concluded, in Chapter 3 we consider the body's attempts to heal the damage, the process of *repair*. Repair begins almost as soon as the inflammatory reaction has started and involves several processes, including cell proliferation, angiogenesis, and collagen synthesis and deposition. Many aspects of repair were mentioned in this chapter, but the process is sufficiently complex and important to deserve its own chapter!

REFERENCES

1. Weissman G (ed): Inflammation: Historical Perspectives. New York, Raven Press, 1992.
2. Hunter J: A Treatise of the Blood, Inflammation, and Gunshot Wounds. London, J. Nicoli, 1794.

3. Heifets L: Centennial of Metchnikoff's discovery. J Reticuloendothel Soc 31:381, 1982.

4. Rock KL, Kono H: The inflammatory response to cell death. Annu Rev Pathol Mech Dis 3:99, 2008.

5. Hellwig-Burgel T et al: Review: hypoxia-inducible factor-1 (HIF-1): a novel transcription factor in immune reactions. J Interferon Cytokine Res 25:297, 2005.

6. Lampugnani MG, Dejana E: Interendothelial junctions: structure, signalling and functional roles. Curr Opin Cell Biol 9:674, 1997.

7. Mehta D, Malik AB: Signaling mechanisms regulating endothelial permeability. Physiol Rev 86:279, 2006.

8. Lentsch AB, Ward PA: Regulation of inflammatory vascular damage. J Pathol 190:343, 2000.

9. Valbuena G, Walker DH: Endothelium as a target of infections. Annu Rev Pathol Mech Dis 1:151, 2006.

10. Dvorak AM, Feng D: The vesiculo-vacuolar organelle (VVO). A new endothelial cell permeability organelle. J Histochem Cytochem 49:419, 2001.

11. Oliver G, Alitalo K: The lymphatic vasculature: recent progress and paradigms. Annu Rev Cell Dev Biol 21:457, 2005.

12. Adams RH, Alitalo K: Molecular regulation of angiogenesis and lymphangiogenesis. Nat Rev Mol Cell Biol 8:464, 2007.

13. Muller WA: Leukocyte-endothelial cell interactions in the inflammatory response. Lab Invest 82:521, 2002.

14. Luster AD et al: Immune cell migration in inflammation: present and future therapeutic targets. Nat Immunol 6:1182, 2005.

15. McEver RP: Selectins: lectins that initiate cell adhesion under flow. Curr Opin Cell Biol 14:581, 2002.

16. Sperandio M: Selectins and glycosyltransferases in leukocyte rolling in vivo. FEBS J 273:4377, 2006.

17. Hehlgans T, Pfeffer K: The intriguing biology of the tumour necrosis factor/tumour necrosis factor receptor superfamily: players, rules and the games. Immunology 115:1, 2005.

18. Dinarello CA. Interleukin-1β. Crit Care Med 33:S460, 2005.

19. Johnston B, Butcher EC: Chemokines in rapid leukocyte adhesion triggering and migration. Semin Immunol 14:83, 2002.

20. Sallusto F, Mackay CR: Chemoattractants and their receptors in homeostasis and inflammation. Curr Opin Immunol 16:724, 2004.

21. Hynes RO: Integrins: bidirectional, allosteric signaling machines. Cell 110:673, 2002.

22. Cook-Mills JM, Deem TL: Active participation of endothelial cells in inflammation. J Leukoc Biol 77:487, 2005.

23. Petri B, Bixel MG: Molecular events during leukocyte diapedesis. FEBS J 273:4399, 2006.

24. Muller WA: Leukocyte-endothelial-cell interactions in leukocyte transmigration and the inflammatory response. Trends Immunol 24:327, 2003.

25. Weber C et al: The role of junctional adhesion molecules in vascular inflammation. Nat Rev Immunol 7:467, 2007.

26. Bunting M et al: Leukocyte adhesion deficiency syndromes: adhesion and tethering defects involving beta 2 integrins and selectin ligands. Curr Opin Hematol 9:30, 2002.

27. Van Haastert PJ, Devreotes PN: Chemotaxis: signalling the way forward. Nat Rev Mol Cell Biol 5:626, 2004.

28. Akira S et al: Pathogen recognition and innate immunity. Cell 124:783, 2006.

29. Meylan E et al: Intracellular pattern recognition receptors in the host response. Nature 442:39, 2006.

30. Underhill DM, Ozinsky A: Phagocytosis of microbes: complexity in action. Annu Rev Immunol 20:825, 2002.

31. Segal AW: How neutrophils kill microbes. Annu Rev Immunol 23:197, 2005.

32. Fang FC: Antimicrobial reactive oxygen and nitrogen species: concepts and controversies. Nat Rev Microbiol 2:820, 2004.

33. Babior BM: NADPH oxidase. Curr Opin Immunol 16:42, 2004.

34. Nathan C, Shiloh MU: Reactive oxygen and nitrogen intermediates in the relationship between mammalian hosts and microbial pathogens. Proc Natl Acad Sci U S A 97:8841, 2000.

35. Belaaouaj A: Neutrophil elastase-mediated killing of bacteria: lessons from targeted mutagenesis. Microbes Infect 4:1259, 2002.

36. Selsted ME, Ouellette AJ: Mammalian defensins in the antimicrobial immune response. Nat Immunol 6:551, 2005.

37. Zanetti M: Cathelicidins, multifunctional peptides of the innate immunity. J Leukoc Biol 75:39, 2004.

38. Gordon S, Taylor PR: Monocyte and macrophage heterogeneity. Nat Rev Immunol 5:953, 2005.

39. Jaeschke H, Smith CW: Mechanisms of neutrophil-induced parenchymal cell injury. J Leukoc Biol 61:647, 1997.

40. Faurschou M, Borregaard N: Neutrophil granules and secretory vesicles in inflammation. Microbes Infect 5:1317, 2003.

41. Ward DM et al: Chediak-Higashi syndrome: a clinical and molecular view of a rare lysosomal storage disorder. Curr Mol Med 2:469, 2002.

42. Heyworth PG et al: Chronic granulomatous disease. Curr Opin Immunol 15:578, 2003.

43. Nathan C: Points of control in inflammation. Nature 420:846, 2002.

44. Serhan CN, Savill J: Resolution of inflammation: the beginning programs the end. Nat Immunol 6:1191, 2005.

45. Serhan CN, Chang N, van Dyke TE: Resolving inflammation: dual anti-inflammatory and pro-resolution lipid mediators. Nat Rev Immunol 8:349, 2008.

46. Tracey KJ: The inflammatory reflex. Nature 420:853, 2002.

47. Repka-Ramirez MS, Baraniuk JN: Histamine in health and disease. Clin Allergy Immunol 17:1, 2002.

48. Funk CD: Prostaglandins and leukotrienes: advances in eicosanoid biology. Science 294:1871, 2001.

49. Miller SB: Prostaglandins in health and disease: an overview. Semin Arthritis Rheum 36:37, 2006.

50. Khanapure SP et al: Eicosanoids in inflammation: biosynthesis, pharmacology, and therapeutic frontiers. Curr Top Med Chem 7:311, 2007.

51. Murakami M, Kudo I: Cellular arachidonate-releasing functions of various phospholipase A_2s. Adv Exp Med Biol 525:87, 2003.

52. Flower RJ: The development of COX2 inhibitors. Nat Rev Drug Discov 2:179, 2003.

53. Krotz F et al: Selective COX-2 inhibitors and risk of myocardial infarction. J Vasc Res 42:312, 2005.

54. Stafforini DM et al. Platelet-activating factor, a pleiotrophic mediator of physiological and pathological processes. Crit Rev Clin Lab Sci 40:643, 2003.

55. Salvemini D et al: Superoxide, peroxynitrite and oxidative/nitrative stress in inflammation. Biochem Soc Trans 34:965, 2006.

56. Laroux FS et al. Role of nitric oxide in inflammation. Acta Physiol Scand 173:113, 2001.

57. Cirino G et al: Nitric oxide and inflammation. Inflamm Allergy Drug Targets 5:115, 2006.

58. Mantovani A et al: Endothelial activation by cytokines. Ann N Y Acad Sci 832:93, 1997.

59. Madge LA, Pober JS: TNF signaling in vascular endothelial cells. Exp Mol Pathol 70:317, 2001.

60. Stojanov S, Kastner DL: Familial autoinflammatory diseases: genetics, pathogenesis and treatment. Curr Opin Rheumatol 17:586, 2005.

61. Ting JP et al: CATERPILLERs, pyrin and hereditary immunological disorders. Nat Rev Immunol 6:183, 2006.

62. Martinon F, Tschopp J: Inflammatory caspases and inflammasomes: master switches of inflammation. Cell Death Differ 14:10, 2007.

63. Charo IF, Ransohoff RM: The many roles of chemokines and chemokine receptors in inflammation. N Engl J Med 354:610, 2006.

64. Zlotnik A, Yoshie O: Chemokines: a new classification system and their role in immunity. Immunity 12:121, 2000.

65. Rot A, von Andrian UH: Chemokines in innate and adaptive host defense: basic chemokinese grammar for immune cells. Annu Rev Immunol 22:891, 2004.

66. Conti P et al: Modulation of autoimmunity by the latest interleukins (with special emphasis on IL-32). Autoimmun Rev 6:131, 2007.

67. Nishimoto N, Kishimoto T: Interleukin 6: from bench to bedside. Nat Clin Pract Rheumatol 2:619, 2006.

68. Kolls JK, Linden A: Interleukin-17 family members and inflammation. Immunity 21:467, 2004.

69. O'Connor TM et al: The role of substance P in inflammatory disease. J Cell Physiol 201:167, 2004.

70. Richardson JD, Vasko MR: Cellular mechanisms of neurogenic inflammation. J Pharmacol Exp Ther 302:839, 2002.

71. Walport MJ: Complement. First of two parts. N Engl J Med 344:1058, 2001.

72. Walport MJ: Complement. Second of two parts. N Engl J Med 344:1140, 2001.

73. Barrington R et al: The role of complement in inflammation and adaptive immunity. Immunol Rev 180:5, 2001.

74. Esmon CT: The interactions between inflammation and coagulation. Br J Haematol 131:417, 2005.

75. Coughlin SR, Camerer E: PARticipation in inflammation. J Clin Invest 111:25, 2003.

76. Esmon CT: Inflammation and the activated protein C anticoagulant pathway. Semin Thromb Hemost 32 (Suppl 1):49, 2006.

77. Joseph K, Kaplan AP: Formation of bradykinin: a major contributor to the innate inflammatory response. Adv Immunol 86:159, 2005.

78. Medzhitov R: Origin and physiological roles of inflammation. Nature 454:428, 2008.

79. Lawrence T, Gilroy DW: Chronic inflammation: a failure of resolution? Int J Exp Pathol 88:85, 2007.

80. Majno G: Chronic inflammation: links with angiogenesis and wound healing. Am J Pathol 153:1035, 1998.

81. Imhof BA, Aurrand-Lions M: Adhesion mechanisms regulating the migration of monocytes. Nat Rev Immunol 4:432, 2004.

82. Drayton DL et al: Lymphoid organ development: from ontogeny to neogenesis. Nat Immunol 7:344, 2006.

83. Rothenberg ME, Hogan SP: The eosinophil. Annu Rev Immunol 24:147, 2006.

84. Dinarello CA: Cytokines as endogenous pyrogens. J Infect Dis 179 (Suppl 2):S294, 1999.

85. Gabay C, Kushner I: Acute-phase proteins and other systemic responses to inflammation. N Engl J Med 340:448, 1999.

86. Ridker PM: C-reactive protein and the prediction of cardiovascular events among those at intermediate risk: moving an inflammatory hypothesis toward consensus. J Am Coll Cardiol 49:2129, 2007.

87. Ganz T: Molecular control of iron transport. J Am Soc Nephrol 18:394, 2007.

88. Hotchkiss RS, Karl IE: The pathophysiology and treatment of sepsis. N Engl J Med 348:138, 2003.

89. Munford RS: Severe sepsis and septic shock: the role of Gram-negative bacteremia. Annu Rev Pathology Mech Dis 1:467, 2006.

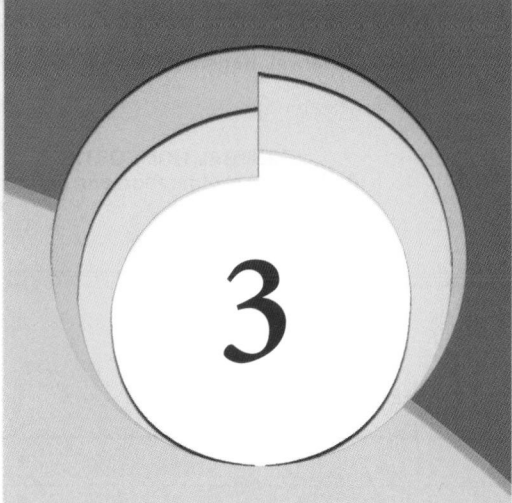

3

Tissue Renewal, Regeneration, and Repair

Control of Normal Cell Proliferation and Tissue Growth
   Tissue Proliferative Activity
   Stem Cells
      Embryonic Stem Cells
      Reprogramming of Differentiated Cells: Induced Pluripotent Stem Cells
      Adult (Somatic) Stem Cells
      Stem Cells in Tissue Homeostasis

Cell Cycle and the Regulation of Cell Replication
   Growth Factors
   Signaling Mechanisms in Cell Growth
      Receptors and Signal Transduction Pathways
      Transcription Factors

Mechanisms of Tissue and Organ Regeneration
   Liver Regeneration

Extracellular Matrix and Cell-Matrix Interactions
   Collagen
   Elastin, Fibrillin, and Elastic Fibers
   Cell Adhesion Proteins
   Glycosaminoglycans (GAGs) and Proteoglycans

Healing by Repair, Scar Formation, and Fibrosis
   Mechanisms of Angiogenesis
      Growth Factors and Receptors Involved in Angiogenesis
      ECM Proteins as Regulators of Angiogenesis
   Cutaneous Wound Healing
   Local and Systemic Factors That Influence Wound Healing
   Pathologic Aspects of Repair
      Fibrosis

Injury to cells and tissues sets in motion a series of events that contain the damage and initiate the healing process. This process can be broadly separated into *regeneration* and *repair* (Fig. 3–1). Regeneration results in the complete restitution of lost or damaged tissue; repair may restore some original structures but can cause structural derangements. In healthy tissues, healing, in the form of regeneration or repair, occurs after practically any insult that causes tissue destruction, and is essential for the survival of the organism.[1]

Regeneration refers to the proliferation of cells and tissues to replace lost structures, such as the growth of an amputated limb in amphibians. In mammals, whole organs and com-

plex tissues rarely regenerate after injury, and the term is usually applied to processes such as liver growth after partial resection or necrosis, but these processes consist of compensatory growth rather than true regeneration.[2] Regardless, the term *regeneration* is well established and is used throughout this book. Tissues with high proliferative capacity, such as the hematopoietic system and the epithelia of the skin and gastrointestinal (GI) tract, renew themselves continuously and can regenerate after injury, as long as the *stem cells* of these tissues are not destroyed.[3]

Repair most often consists of a combination of regeneration and scar formation by the deposition of collagen. The relative

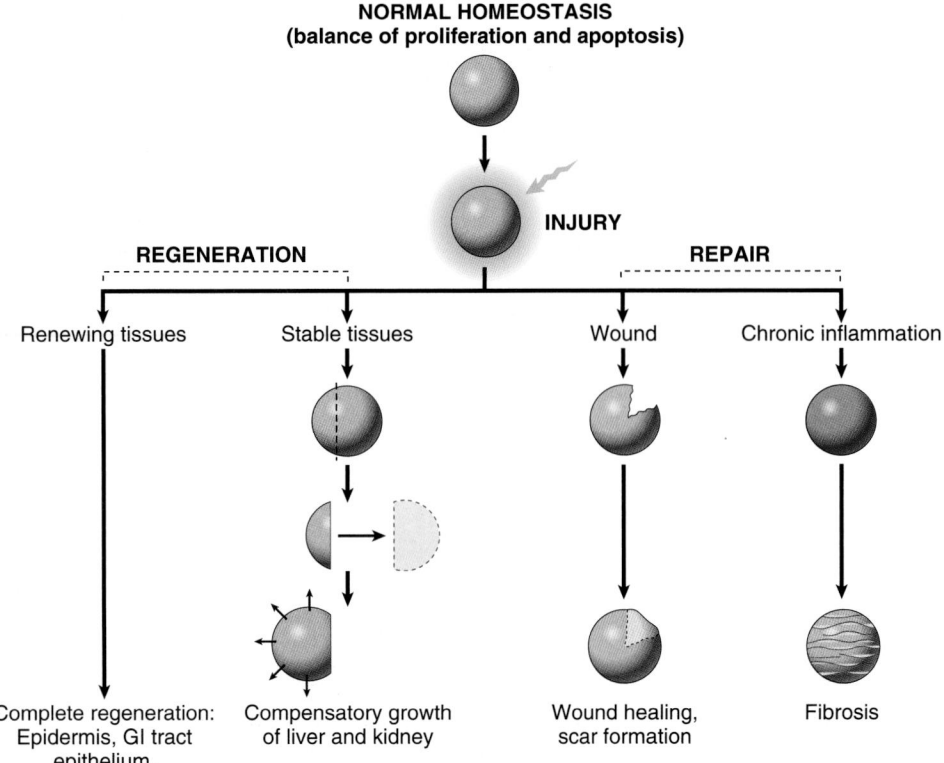

FIGURE 3–1 Overview of healing responses after injury. Healing after acute injury can occur by regeneration that restores normal tissue structure or by repair with scar formation. Healing in chronic injury involves scar formation and fibrosis (see text). GI, gastrointestinal.

contribution of regeneration and scarring in tissue repair depends on the ability of the tissue to regenerate and the extent of the injury. For instance, a superficial skin wound heals through the regeneration of the surface epithelium. However, as discussed later, scar formation is the predominant healing process that occurs when the extracellular matrix (ECM) framework is damaged by severe injury (Fig. 3–2). Chronic inflammation that accompanies persistent injury also stimulates scar formation because of local production of growth factors and cytokines that promote fibroblast proliferation and collagen synthesis. The term *fibrosis* is used to describe the extensive deposition of collagen that occurs under these situations. ECM components are essential for wound healing, because they provide the framework for cell migration, maintain the correct cell polarity for the re-assembly of multilayer structures,[4] and participate in the formation of new blood vessels (angiogenesis). Furthermore, cells in the ECM (fibroblasts, macrophages, and other cell types) produce growth factors, cytokines, and chemokines that are critical for regeneration and repair. Although repair is a healing process, it may itself cause tissue dysfunction, as, for instance, in the development of atherosclerosis (Chapter 11).

Understanding the mechanisms of regeneration and repair requires some knowledge of the control of cell proliferation and signal transduction pathways, and the many functions of ECM components.

In this chapter we first discuss the principles of cell proliferation, the proliferative capacity of tissues, and the role of stem cells in tissue homeostasis. This is followed by an overview of growth factors and cell signaling mechanisms relevant to healing processes. We then discuss regenerative processes

with emphasis on liver regeneration, and examine the properties of the ECM and its components. These sections lay the foundation for the consideration of the main features of wound healing and fibrosis.

Control of Normal Cell Proliferation and Tissue Growth

In adult tissues the size of cell populations is determined by the rates of cell proliferation, differentiation, and death by apoptosis (Fig. 3–3), and increased cell numbers may result from either increased proliferation or decreased cell death.[5] *Apoptosis* is a physiologic process required for tissue homeostasis, but it can also be induced by a variety of pathologic stimuli (see Chapter 1). Differentiated cells incapable of replication are referred to as *terminally differentiated* cells. The impact of *differentiation* depends on the tissue under which it occurs: in some tissues differentiated cells are not replaced, while in others they die but are continuously replaced by new cells generated from stem cells (discussed in the next section).

Cell proliferation can be stimulated by physiologic and pathologic conditions. The proliferation of endometrial cells under estrogen stimulation during the menstrual cycle and the thyroid-stimulating hormone–mediated replication of cells of the thyroid that enlarges the gland during pregnancy are examples of physiologic proliferation. Physiologic stimuli may become excessive, creating pathologic conditions such as nodular prostatic hyperplasia resulting from dihydrotestoster-

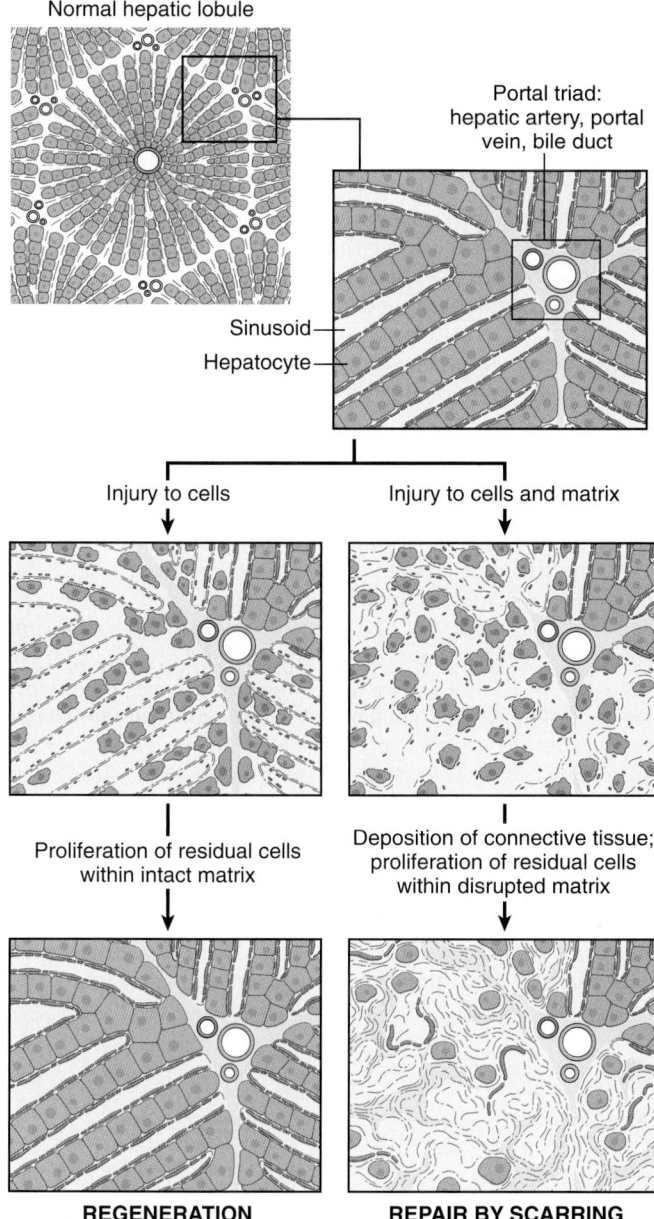

Normal hepatic lobule

Portal triad:
hepatic artery, portal
vein, bile duct

Sinusoid

Hepatocyte

Injury to cells

Injury to cells and matrix

Proliferation of residual cells
within intact matrix

Deposition of connective tissue;
proliferation of residual cells
within disrupted matrix

REGENERATION

REPAIR BY SCARRING

FIGURE 3–2 Role of the extracellular matrix in regeneration and repair. Liver regeneration with restoration of normal tissue after injury requires an intact cellular matrix. If the matrix is damaged the injury is repaired by fibrous tissue deposition and scar formation.

manent tissues). This time-honored classification should be interpreted in the light of recent findings on stem cells and the reprogramming of cell differentiation.

- In *continuously dividing tissues* cells proliferate throughout life, replacing those that are destroyed. These tissues include surface epithelia, such as stratified squamous epithelia of the skin, oral cavity, vagina, and cervix; the lining mucosa of all the excretory ducts of the glands of the body (e.g., salivary glands, pancreas, biliary tract); the columnar epithelium of the GI tract and uterus; the transitional epithelium of the urinary tract, and cells of the bone marrow and hematopoietic tissues. In most of these tissues mature cells are derived from adult *stem cells*, which have a tremendous capacity to proliferate and whose progeny may differentiate into several kinds of cells (discussed in more detail later).

- *Quiescent tissues* normally have a low level of replication; however, cells from these tissues can undergo rapid division in response to stimuli and are thus capable of reconstituting the tissue of origin. In this category are the parenchymal cells of liver, kidneys, and pancreas; mesenchymal cells such as fibroblasts and smooth muscle; vascular endothelial cells; and lymphocytes and other leukocytes. The regenerative capacity of stable cells is best exemplified by the ability of the liver to regenerate after partial hepatectomy and after acute chemical injury. Fibroblasts, endothelial cells, smooth muscle cells, chondrocytes, and osteocytes are quiescent in adult mammals but proliferate in response to injury. Fibroblasts in particular can proliferate extensively, as in healing processes and fibrosis, discussed later in this chapter.

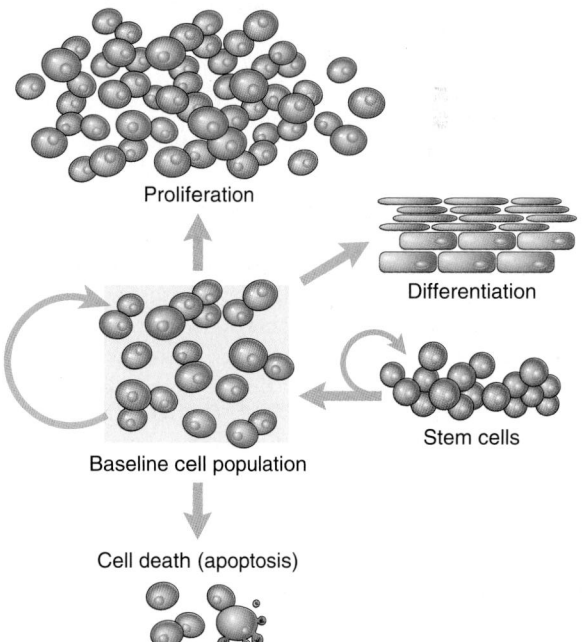

Proliferation

Differentiation

Baseline cell population

Stem cells

Cell death (apoptosis)

FIGURE 3–3 Mechanisms regulating cell populations. Cell numbers can be altered by increased or decreased rates of stem cell input, cell death due to apoptosis, or changes in the rates of proliferation or differentiation. (Modified from McCarthy NJ et al: Apoptosis in the development of the immune system: growth factors, clonal selection and bcl-2. Cancer Metastasis Rev 11:157, 1992.)

one stimulation (Chapter 21) and the development of nodular goiters in the thyroid as a consequence of increased serum levels of thyroid-stimulating hormone (Chapter 24). Cell proliferation is largely controlled by signals (soluble or contact-dependent) from the microenvironment that either stimulate or inhibit proliferation. An excess of stimulators or a deficiency of inhibitors leads to net growth and, in the case of cancer, uncontrolled growth.

TISSUE PROLIFERATIVE ACTIVITY

The tissues of the body are divided into three groups on the basis of the proliferative activity of their cells: continuously dividing (labile tissues), quiescent (stable tissues), and nondividing (per-

● *Nondividing tissues* contain cells that have left the cell cycle and cannot undergo mitotic division in postnatal life. To this group belong neurons and skeletal and cardiac muscle cells. If *neurons* in the central nervous system are destroyed, the tissue is generally replaced by the proliferation of the central nervous system–supportive elements, the glial cells. However, recent results demonstrate that limited neurogenesis from stem cells may occur in adult brains (discussed later). Although mature skeletal muscle cells do not divide, *skeletal muscle* does have regenerative capacity, through the differentiation of the *satellite cells* that are attached to the endomysial sheaths. *Cardiac muscle* has very limited, if any, regenerative capacity, and a large injury to the heart muscle, as may occur in myocardial infarction, is followed by scar formation.

STEM CELLS

Research on stem cells is at the forefront of modern-day biomedical investigation and stands at the core of a new field called *regenerative medicine*. The enthusiasm created by stem cell research derives from findings that challenge established views about cell differentiation, and from the hope that stem cells may one day be used to repair damaged human tissues, such as heart, brain, liver, and skeletal muscle.[3,6,7]

Stem cells are characterized by their self-renewal properties and by their capacity to generate differentiated cell lineages (Fig. 3–4). To give rise to these lineages, stem cells need to be maintained during the life of the organism. Such maintenance is achieved by two mechanisms[8]: (a) *obligatory asymmetric replication*, in which with each stem cell division, one of the daughter cells retains its self-renewing capacity while the other enters a differentiation pathway, and (b) *stochastic differentia-*

tion, in which a stem cell population is maintained by the balance between stem cell divisions that generate either two self-renewing stem cells or two cells that will differentiate. In early stages of embryonic development, stem cells, known as *embryonic stem cells* or *ES cells*, are *pluripotent*, that is, they can generate all tissues of the body (Fig. 3–4). Pluripotent stem cells give rise to multipotent stem cells, which have more restricted developmental potential, and eventually produce differentiated cells from the three embryonic layers. The term *transdifferentiation* (discussed later) indicates a change in the lineage commitment of a stem cell.

In adults, stem cells (often referred to as *adult stem cells* or *somatic stem cells*) with a more restricted capacity to generate different cell types have been identified in many tissues. They have been studied in detail in the skin, the lining of the gut, the cornea, and particularly in the hematopoietic tissue. An unexpected finding has been the discovery of stem cells and neurogenesis in areas of the central nervous system of adult animals and humans.[9] Somatic stem cells for the most part reside in special microenvironments called *niches* (Fig. 3–5), composed of mesenchymal, endothelial, and other cell types.[10,11] It is believed *that niche cells generate or transmit stimuli that regulate stem cell self-renewal and the generation of progeny cells.* Recent groundbreaking research has now demonstrated that *differentiated cells of rodents and humans can be reprogrammed into pluripotent cells, similar to ES cells, by the transduction of genes encoding ES cell transcription factors.*[12,13] These reprogrammed cells have been named *induced pluripotent stem cells (iPS cells).* Their discovery has opened open an exciting new era in stem cell research and its applications.

We start our discussion of stem cells with a brief consideration of ES cells and the newly identified iPS cells. This is followed by a presentation on adult stem cells from a few selected tissues and the role they play in regeneration and repair.

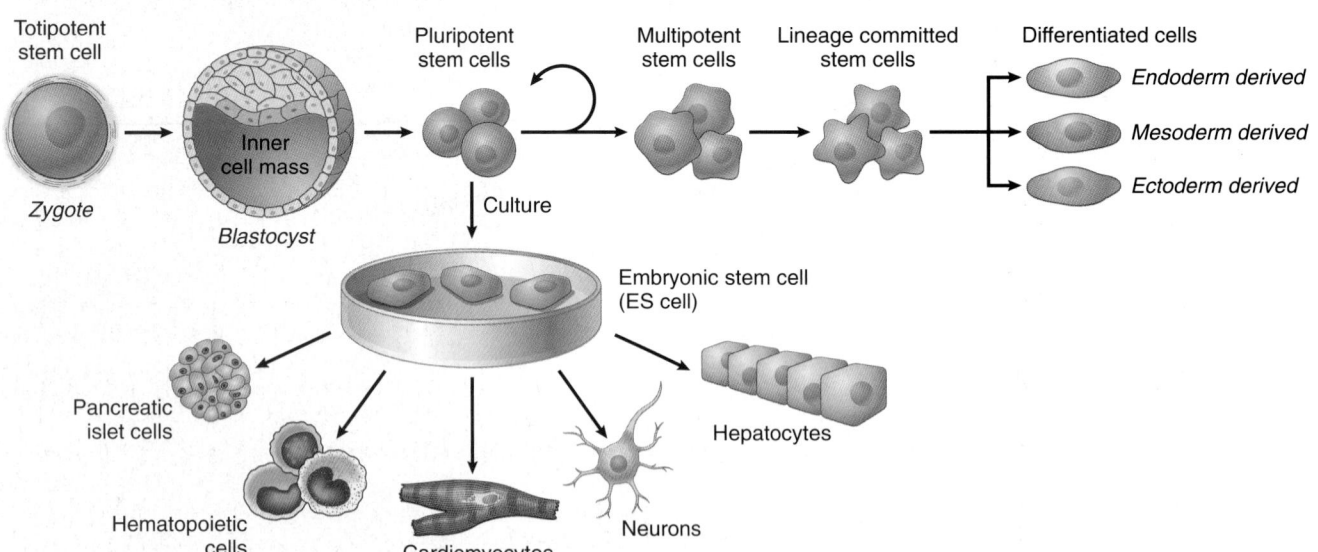

FIGURE 3–4 Stem cell generation and differentiation. The zygote, formed by the union of sperm and egg, divides to form blastocysts, and the inner cell mass of the blastocyst generates the embryo. The cells of the inner cell mass, known as embryonic stem (ES) cells, maintained in culture, can be induced to differentiate into cells of multiple lineages. In the embryo, pluripotent stem cells divide, but the pool of these cells is maintained (see text). As pluripotent cells differentiate, they give rise to cells with more restricted developmental capacity, and finally generate stem cells that are committed to specific lineages.

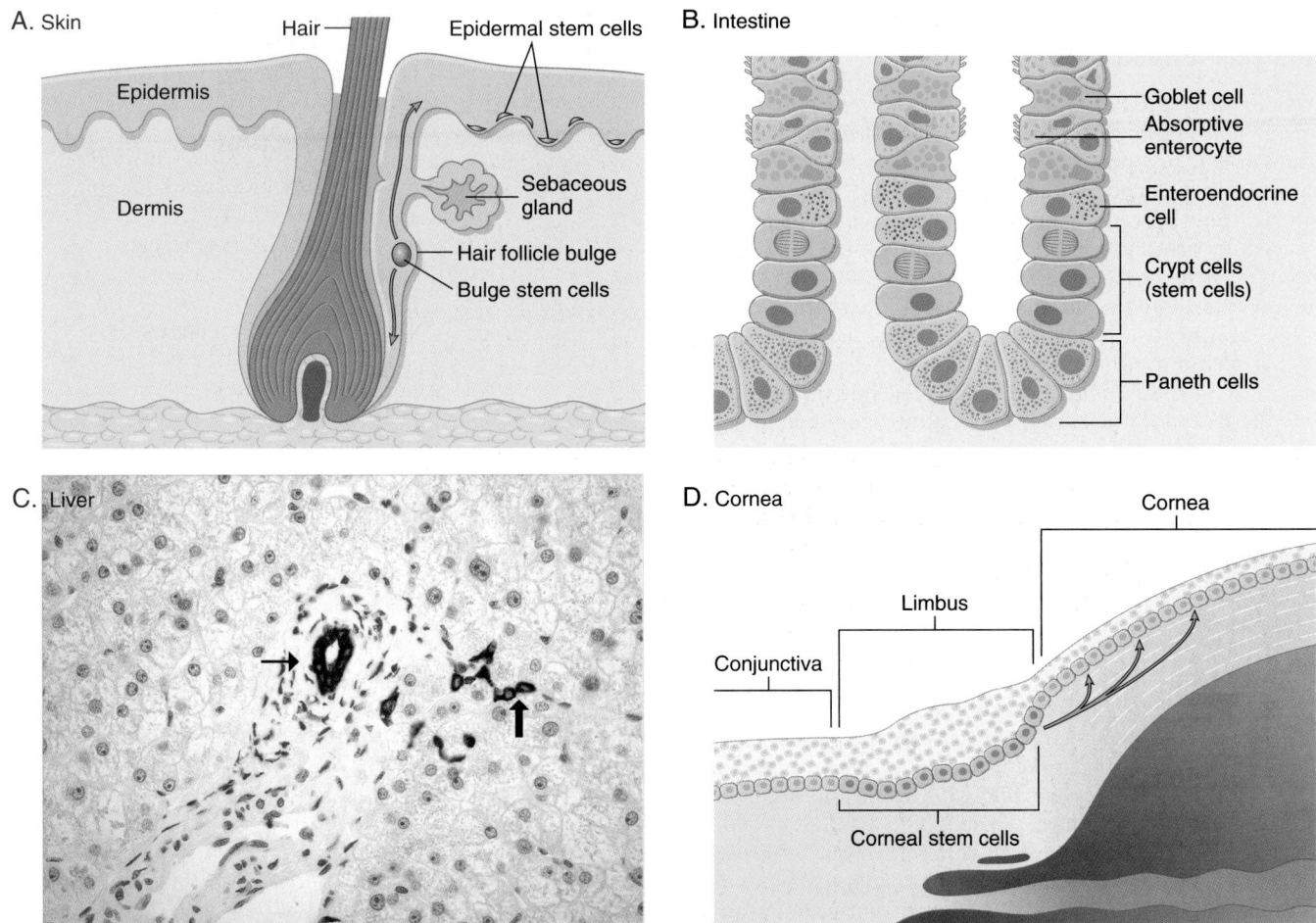

FIGURE 3–5 Stem cell niches in various tissues. **A,** Skin stem cells are located in the bulge area of the hair follicle, in sebaceous glands, and in the lower layer of the epidermis. **B,** Small intestine stem cells located near the base of a crypt, above Paneth cells (stem cells in the small intestine may also be located at the bottom of the crypt[25]). **C,** Liver stem (progenitor) cells, known as oval cells, are located in the canals of Hering *(thick arrow)*, structures that connect bile ductules *(thin arrow)* with parenchymal hepatocytes (bile duct and Hering canals are stained for cytokeratin 7). **D,** Corneal stem cells are located in the limbus region, between the conjunctiva and the cornea. (**C,** courtesy of Tania Roskams, MD, University of Leuven, Leuven, Belgium; **D,** Courtesy of T-T Sun, MD, New York University, New York, NY.)

Embryonic Stem Cells

The inner cell mass of blastocysts in early embryonic development contains pluripotent stem cells known as ES cells.[14] Cells isolated from blastocysts can be maintained in culture as undifferentiated cell lines or be induced to differentiate into specific lineages (see Fig. 3–4) such as heart and liver cells.[15]

The study of ES cells has had an enormous impact on biology and medicine:

○ ES cells have been used to study the specific signals and differentiation steps required for the development of many tissues.
○ *ES cells made possible the production of knockout mice, an essential tool to study the biology of particular genes and to develop models of human disease.* The first step in the production of knockout mice is the inactivation or deletion of a gene from cultured ES cells. The cells are then injected into blastocysts, which are implanted into the uterus of a surrogate mother. The genetically modified implanted blas-

tocysts develop into full embryos, as long as the gene defect does not cause embryonic lethality. Using similar techniques, "*knock-in*" mice have been developed, in which a mutated DNA sequence replaces the endogenous sequence.[16] Mice can also be produced with gene deficiencies that are specific for a single tissue or cell type, or to have "conditional gene deficiencies," that is, gene deficiencies that can be turned on and off in adult animals. Knockout mice have provided essential information about gene function in vivo. Thus far, more than 500 models of human diseases have been created using these animals.
○ *ES cells may in the future be used to repopulate damaged organs.* ES cells capable of differentiating into insulin-producing pancreatic cells, nerve cells, myocardial cells, or hepatocytes have been implanted in animals with experimentally produced diabetes, neurologic defects, myocardial infarction, and liver damage, respectively. The effectiveness of these procedures in animals is under intense study, and there is much debate about the ethical issues associated with the derivation of ES cells from human blastocytes.

Reprogramming of Differentiated Cells: Induced Pluripotent Stem Cells

Differentiated cells of adult tissues can be reprogrammed to become pluripotent by transferring their nucleus to an enucleated oocyte. The oocytes implanted into a surrogate mother can generate cloned embryos that develop into complete animals. This procedure, known as *reproductive cloning*, was successfully demonstrated in 1997 by the cloning of Dolly the sheep.[17] There has been great hope that the technique of nuclear transfer to oocytes may be used for *therapeutic cloning* in the treatment of human diseases (illustrated in Fig. 3–6). In this technique the nucleus of a skin fibroblast from a patient is introduced into an enucleated human oocyte to generate ES cells, which are kept in culture, and then induced to differentiate into various cell types. In principle, these cells can then be transplanted into the patient to repopulate damaged organs.[18] In addition to the ethical issues associated with this technique, therapeutic as well as reproductive cloning are inefficient and often inaccurate. One of the main reasons for the inaccuracy is the deficiency in histone methylation in reprogrammed ES cells, which results in improper gene expression.

Until recently there were no clues about the mechanisms that maintain pluripotency of ES cells. A series of landmark experiments have now demonstrated that the *pluripotency of mouse ES cells depends on the expression of four transcription factors, Oct3/4, Sox2, c-myc, and Klf4,* while the homeobox protein *Nanog* (named after Tir na n'Og, the Celtic land of the ever-young) acts to prevent differentiation.[19–22] *Human fibroblasts from adults and newborns have been reprogrammed into pluripotent cells by the transduction of four genes encoding transcription factors (Oct3/4, Sox2, c-myc and Kfl4 in one laboratory; Oct3/4, Sox2, Nanog, and Lin28 in experiments from another laboratory).*[12,13] The reprogrammed cells, known as *iPS cells*, are able to generate cells from endodermal, mesodermal, and ectodermal origin. They have also been used to rescue mice with a model of sickle cell anemia, proving that they function in vivo even after genetic manipulation and transplantation.[23] More recently, pluripotent iPS cells were generated by transfecting mouse hepatocytes, gastric cells, and terminally differentiated mature B lymphocytes with genes for the same four transcription factors.[24,25] Thus, *iPS cells may become a source of cells for patient-specific stem cell therapy, without the involvement of nuclear transfer into oocytes* (see Fig. 3–6). To make the dream of using iPS cells in human regenerative medicine a reality (iPS cells have been called ES cells without embryos), much additional work is required, including the development of new methods for gene delivery and the replacement of c-myc and Kfl4, which are oncogenes.[26] In any event, exciting new achievements can be expected in the near future from work on ES cells, iPS cells, and cell reprogramming.

Adult (Somatic) Stem Cells

In the adult organism, stem cells are present in tissues that continuously divide such as the bone marrow, the skin, and the lining of the GI tract. Stem cells may also be present in organs such as liver, pancreas, and adipose tissue, in which, under

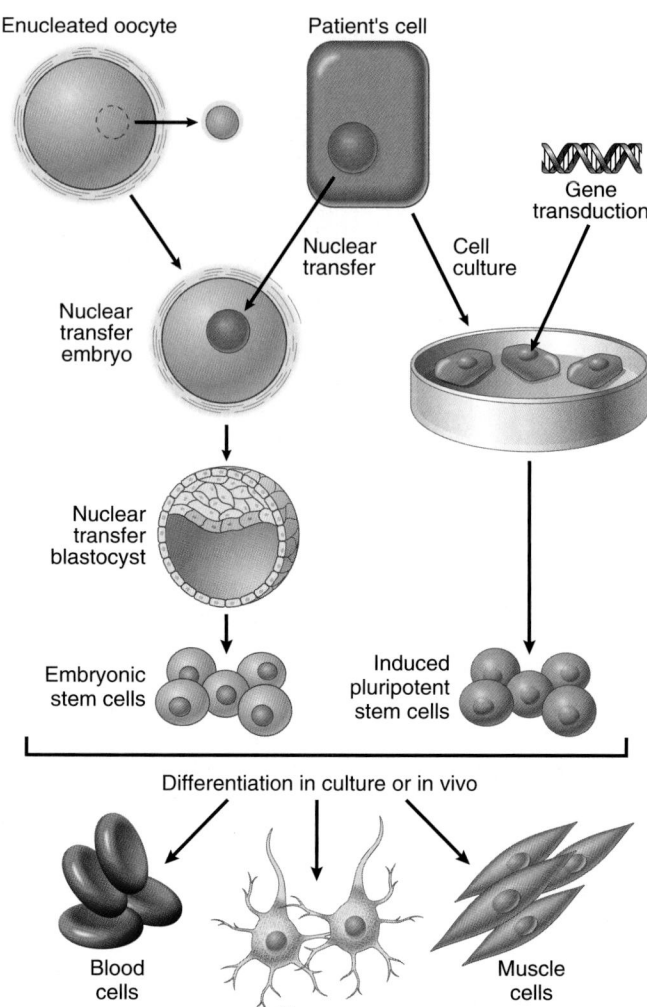

FIGURE 3–6   Steps involved in stem cell therapy, using embryonic stem (ES) cells or induced pluripotent stem (iPS) cells. *Left side,* Therapeutic cloning using ES cells. The diploid nucleus of an adult cell from a patient is introduced into an enucleated oocyte. The oocyte is activated, and the zygote divides to become a blastocyst that contains the donor DNA. The blastocyst is dissociated to obtain ES cells. *Right side,* Stem cell therapy using iPS cells. The cells of a patient are placed in culture and transduced with genes encoding transcription factors, to generate iPS cells. Both ES and iPS cells are capable of differentiating into various cell types. The goal of stem cell therapy is to repopulate damaged organs of a patient or to correct a genetic defect, using the cells of the same patient to avoid immunological rejection. (Modified from Hochedlinger K, Jaenisch R: Nuclear transplantation, embryonic stem cells, and the potential for cell therapy. N Engl J Med 349:275–286, 2003.)

normal conditions, they do not actively produce differentiated cell lineages. Stem cells divide very slowly in most tissues, but there is evidence that they may be continuously cycling in the small intestine epithelium.[27] Regardless of their proliferative activity, somatic stem cells generate rapidly dividing cells known as *transit amplifying cells.* These cells lose the capacity of self-perpetuation, and give rise to cells with restricted developmental potential known as *progenitor cells.* Regrettably, the terms *stem cell* and *progenitor cell* continue to be used interchangeably, despite the fact that cell lineage hierarchies have been well defined only for hemopoietic stem cells (HSC).

A change in the differentiation of a cell from one type to another is known as *transdifferentiation,* and the capacity of a cell to transdifferentiate into diverse lineages is referred to as *developmental plasticity.* HSCs maintained in culture have been shown to transdifferentiate into other cell types, such as hepatocytes and neurons. In addition, some studies indicated that when injected in appropriate sites, HSC could transdifferentiate in vivo into cells such as neurons, skeletal and cardiac myocytes, and hepatocytes. However, *many of the findings attributed to HSC transdifferentiation in vivo have been difficult to reproduce,* because cells assumed to be the product of transdifferentiation could not be detected or were present at a very low frequency.[28] Moreover, the reported generation of neurons, skeletal myocytes, and hepatocytes from injected HSCs seems to be caused primarily by *fusion of the hematopoietic cells or their progeny with differentiated or progenitor cells* of the appropriate tissues.[29,30] *Hence, so far, there is little conclusive evidence that transdifferentiation of HSCs contributes to tissue renewal in normal homeostasis or tissue regeneration and repair after injury.*[31] On the other hand, it is possible that HSCs may migrate to sites of inflammation and injury, where they generate innate immune cells, or release growth factors and cytokines that promote repair and cell replication through a paracrine effect.[32] The issue of transdifferentiation and developmental plasticity in tissue repopulation continues to be explored.

Stem Cells in Tissue Homeostasis

To illustrate the importance of stem cells in tissue maintenance and regeneration, we briefly discuss stem cells in the bone marrow, skin, gut, liver, brain, muscle, and cornea.

- *Bone marrow.* The bone marrow contains HSCs and stromal cells (also known as multipotent stromal cells, mesenchymal stem cells or MSCs).
  - *Hematopoietic Stem Cells.* HSCs generate all of the blood cell lineages (Chapter 13), can reconstitute the bone marrow after depletion caused by disease or irradiation, and are widely used for the treatment of hematologic diseases.[33] They can be collected directly from the bone marrow, from umbilical cord blood, and from the peripheral blood of individuals receiving cytokines such as granulocyte-macrophage colony-stimulating factor, which mobilize HSCs.[34] It is estimated that the human bone marrow produces approximately 1.5×10^6 blood cells per second, an astonishing rate of cell-generating activity!
  - *Marrow Stromal Cells.* MSCs are multipotent. *They have potentially important therapeutic applications, because they can generate chondrocytes, osteoblasts, adipocytes, myoblasts, and endothelial cell precursors depending on the tissue to which they migrate.* MSCs migrate to injured tissues and generate stromal cells or other cell lineages, but do not seem to participate in normal tissue homeostasis.[35,36]

- *Liver. The liver contains stem cells/progenitor cells in the canals of Hering* (see Fig. 3–5), the junction between the biliary ductular system and parenchymal hepatocytes (Chapter 18). Cells located in this niche can give rise to a population of precursor cells known as *oval cells,* which are bipotential progenitors, capable of differentiating into hepatocytes and biliary cells.[2,37] In contrast to stem cells in proliferating tissues, liver stem cells function as a secondary or reserve compartment activated only when hepatocyte proliferation is blocked. Oval cell proliferation and differentiation are prominent in the livers of patients recovering from fulminant hepatic failure, in liver tumorigenesis, and in some cases of chronic hepatitis and advanced liver cirrhosis.

- *Brain. Neurogenesis from neural stem cells (NSCs) occurs in the brain of adult rodents and humans.* Thus, the long-established dogma that no new neurons are generated in the brain of normal adult mammals is now known to be incorrect. NSCs (also known as *neural precursor cells*), capable of generating neurons, astrocytes, and oligodendrocytes, have been identified in two areas of adult brains, the subventricular zone (SVZ) and the dentate gyrus of the hippocampus.[38] It is not clear if newly generated neurons in the adult human brain are integrated into neural circuits under physiologic and pathologic conditions, and, more broadly, what might be the purpose of adult neurogenesis.[39] There is much hope that stem cell transplantation, or the induction of differentiation of endogenous NSCs, may be used in treatment of stroke, neurodegenerative disorders such as Parkinson and Alzheimer diseases, and spinal cord injury.[40]

- *Skin. Stem cells are located in three different areas of the epidermis: the hair follicle bulge, interfollicular areas of the surface epidermis, and sebaceous glands* (see Fig. 3–5).[41] The *bulge area of the hair follicle* constitutes a niche for stem cells that produce all of the cell lineages of the hair follicle.[42] *Interfollicular stem cells are scattered individually in the epidermis* and are not contained in niches. They divide infrequently but generate transit amplifying cells that generate the differentiated epidermis.[43] The human epidermis has a high turnover rate of about 4 weeks. Bulge stem cells have been characterized in mice and humans.[44] They contribute to the replenishment of surface epidermal cells after skin wounding but not during normal homeostasis. Their activation is regulated by stimulatory signals from the *Wnt pathway and inhibition of signaling from the bone morphogenetic protein (BMP) system.*

- *Intestinal epithelium. In the small intestine, crypts are monoclonal structures derived from single stem cells: the villus is a differentiated compartment that contains cells from multiple crypts* (see Fig. 3–5). Stem cells in small intestine crypts regenerate the crypt in 3 to 5 days.[45] As with skin stem cells, *the Wnt and BMP pathways are important in the regulation of proliferation and differentiation of intestinal stem cells.* Stem cells may be located immediately above Paneth cells in the small intestine, or at the base of the crypt, as is the case in the colon.[27,46]

- *Skeletal and cardiac muscle. Skeletal muscle myocytes do not divide, even after injury; growth and regeneration of injured skeletal muscle occur by replication of satellite cells.* These cells, located beneath the myocyte basal lamina, constitute a reserve pool of stem cells that can generate differentiated myocytes after injury.[47] Active Notch signaling, triggered by up-regulation of delta-like (Dll) ligands, stimulates the proliferation of satellite cells (Notch signaling is discussed later in "Mechanisms of Angiogenesis"). The presence of stem cells in the heart continues to be debated. It has been proposed that the heart may contain progenitor-like cells with the capacity to generate progeny after injury, but not during physiologic aging.[48,49]

○ *Cornea.* The transparency of the cornea depends on the integrity of the outermost corneal epithelium, which is maintained by *limbal stem cells (LSCs).* These cells are located at the junction between the epithelium of the cornea and the conjunctiva[50] (see Fig. 3–5). Hereditary or acquired conditions that result in LSC deficiency and corneal opacification can be treated by limbal transplantation or LSC grafting. Animal experiments indicate that it might also be possible to correct the loss of photoreceptors that occurs in *degenerative diseases of the retina* by transplanting retinal stem cells.[51]

Cell Cycle and the Regulation of Cell Replication

Cell proliferation is a tightly regulated process that involves a large number of molecules and interrelated pathways. To understand how cells proliferate during regeneration and repair, it is useful to summarize the key features of the normal cell cycle and its regulation. We discuss the details of the cell cycle and its abnormalities in Chapter 7, in the context of cancer. Here we summarize some salient features of the process of cellular proliferation.

The replication of cells is stimulated by growth factors or by signaling from ECM components through integrins. To achieve DNA replication and division, the cell goes through a tightly controlled sequence of events known as the *cell cycle. The cell cycle consists of G_1 (presynthetic), S (DNA synthesis), G_2 (premitotic), and M (mitotic) phases. Quiescent cells that have not entered the cell cycle are in the G_0 state* (Fig. 3–7). Each cell cycle phase is dependent on the proper activation and completion of the previous one, and the cycle stops at a place at which an essential gene function is deficient. Because of its central role in maintaining tissue homeostasis and regulating physiologic growth processes such as regeneration and repair, *the cell cycle has multiple controls and redundancies, particularly during the transition between the G_1 and S phases.* These controls include activators and inhibitors, as well as sensors that are responsible for checkpoints, described below.[52]

Cells can enter G_1 either from G_0 (quiescent cells) or after completing mitosis (continuously replicating cells). Quiescent cells first must go through the transition from G_0 to G_1, the first decision step, which functions as a gateway to the cell cycle. This transition involves the transcriptional activation of a large set of genes, including various proto-oncogenes and genes required for ribosome synthesis and protein translation. Cells in G_1 progress through the cycle and reach a critical stage at the G_1/S transition, known as a *restriction point*, a rate-limiting step for replication (see Fig. 3–7). Upon passing this restriction point, normal cells become irreversibly committed to DNA replication. *Progression through the cell cycle, particularly at the G_1/S transition, is tightly regulated by proteins called cyclins and associated enzymes called cyclin-dependent kinases*

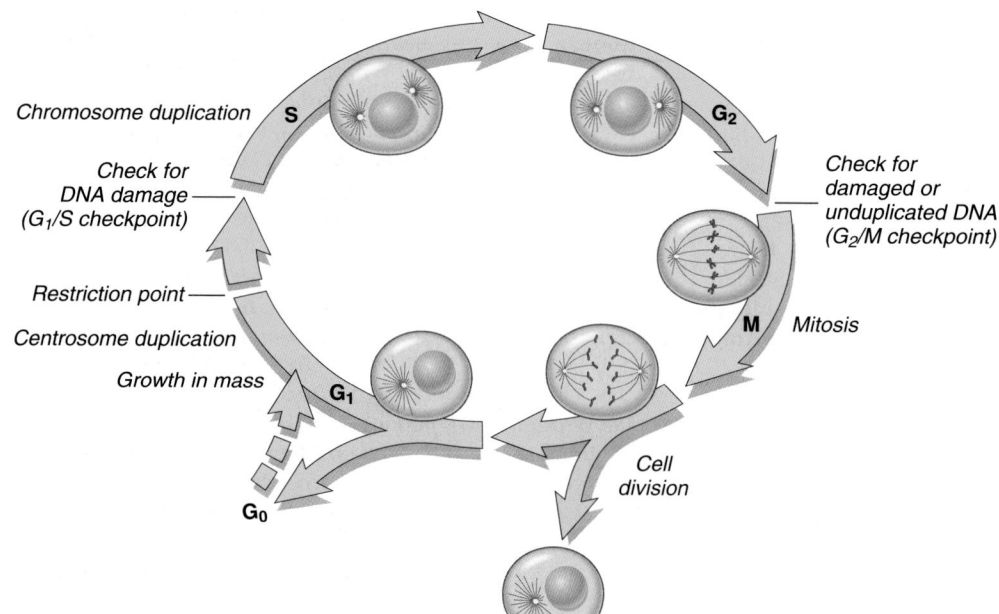

FIGURE 3–7 Cell cycle landmarks. The figure shows the cell cycle phases (G_0, G_1, G_2, S, and M), the location of the G_1 restriction point, and the G_1/S and G_2/M cell cycle checkpoints. Cells from labile tissues such as the epidermis and the GI tract may cycle continuously; stable cells such as hepatocytes are quiescent but can enter the cell cycle; permanent cells such as neurons and cardiac myocytes have lost the capacity to proliferate. (Modified from Pollard TD, Earnshaw WC: Cell Biology. Philadelphia, Saunders, 2002.)

(CDKs). CDKs acquire catalytic activity by binding to and forming complexes with the cyclins. Activated CDKs in these complexes drive the cell cycle by phosphorylating proteins that are critical for cell cycle transitions. One such protein is the retinoblastoma susceptibility (RB) protein, which normally prevents cells from replicating by forming a tight, inactive complex with the transcription factor E2F. Phosphorylation of RB causes its release, which activates E2F and allows it to stimulate transcription of genes whose products drive cells through the cycle. More details are provided in Chapter 7.

The activity of cyclin-CDK complexes is tightly regulated by *CDK inhibitors.* Some growth factors shut off production of these inhibitors. Embedded in the cell cycle are surveillance mechanisms that are geared primarily at sensing damage to DNA and chromosomes. These quality control checks are called *checkpoints;* they ensure that cells with damaged DNA or chromosomes do not complete replication.[53] The G_1/S checkpoint monitors the integrity of DNA before replication, whereas the G_2/M checkpoint checks DNA after replication and monitors whether the cell can safely enter mitosis. When cells sense DNA damage, checkpoint activation delays the cell cycle and triggers DNA repair mechanisms. If DNA damage is too severe to be repaired, the cells are eliminated by apoptosis, or enter a nonreplicative state called *senescence,* primarily through p53-dependent mechanisms. Checkpoint defects that allow cells with DNA strand breaks and chromosome abnormalities to divide produce mutations in daughter cells that may lead to neoplasia (Chapter 7).[54]

GROWTH FACTORS

The proliferation of many cell types is driven by polypeptides known as growth factors. These factors, which can have restricted or multiple cell targets, may also promote cell survival, locomotion, contractility, differentiation, and angiogenesis, activities that may be as important as their growth-promoting effects. All growth factors function as *ligands* that bind to specific *receptors,* which deliver signals to the target cells. These signals stimulate the transcription of genes that may be silent in resting cells, including genes that control *cell cycle entry and progression.* Table 3–1 lists some of

TABLE 3–1 Growth Factors and Cytokines Involved in Regeneration and Wound Healing			
Growth Factor	**Symbol**	**Source**	**Functions**
Epidermal growth α	EGF	Platelets, macrophages, saliva, urine, milk, plasma	Mitogenic for keratinocytes and fibroblasts; stimulates keratinocyte migration and granulation tissue formation
Transforming growth factor α	TGF-α	Macrophages, T lymphocytes, keratinocytes, and many tissues	Similar to EGF; stimulates replication of hepatocytes and most epithelial cells
Heparin-binding EGF	HB-EGF	Macrophages, mesenchymal cells	Keratinocyte replication
Hepatocyte growth factor/scatter factor	HGF	Mesenchymal cells	Enhances proliferation of hepatocytes, epithelial cells, and endothelial cells; increases cell motility, keratinocyte replication
Vascular endothelial cell growth factor (isoforms A, B, C, D)	VEGF	Many types of cells	Increases vascular permeability; mitogenic for endothelial cells (see Table 3–3); angiogenesis
Platelet-derived growth factor (isoforms A, B, C, D)	PDGF	Platelets, macrophages, endothelial cells, keratinocytes, smooth muscle cells	Chemotactic for PMNs, macrophages, fibroblasts, and smooth muscle cells; activates PMNs, macrophages, and fibroblasts; mitogenic for fibroblasts, endothelial cells, and smooth muscle cells; stimulates production of MMPs, fibronectin, and HA; stimulates angiogenesis and wound contraction
Fibroblast growth factor 1 (acidic), 2 (basic), and family	FGF	Macrophages, mast cells, T lymphocytes, endothelial cells, fibroblasts	Chemotactic for fibroblasts; mitogenic for fibroblasts and keratinocytes; stimulates keratinocyte migration, angiogenesis, wound contraction, and matrix deposition
Transforming growth factor β (isoforms 1, 2, 3); other members of the family are BMPs and activin	TGF-β	Platelets, T lymphocytes, macrophages, endothelial cells, keratinocytes, smooth muscle cells, fibroblasts	Chemotactic for PMNs, macrophages, lymphocytes, fibroblasts, and smooth muscle cells; stimulates TIMP synthesis, angiogenesis, and fibroplasia; inhibits production of MMPs and keratinocyte proliferation
Keratinocyte growth factor (also called FGF-7)	KGF	Fibroblasts	Stimulates keratinocyte migration, proliferation, and differentiation
Tumor necrosis factor	TNF	Macrophages, mast cells, T lymphocytes	Activates macrophages; regulates other cytokines; multiple functions

BMP, bone morphogenetic proteins; HA, hyaluronate; MMPs, matrix metalloproteinases; PMNs, polymorphonuclear leukocytes; TIMP, tissue inhibitor of MMP.
Modified from Schwartz SI: Principles of Surgery. New York, McGraw-Hill, 1999.

the most important growth factors involved in tissue regeneration and repair. Here we review only those that have major roles in these processes. Other growth factors are alluded to in various sections of the book.

Epidermal Growth Factor (EGF) and Transforming Growth Factor α (TGF-α). These two factors belong to the EGF family and share a common receptor (EGFR).[55] EGF is mitogenic for a variety of epithelial cells, hepatocytes, and fibroblasts, and is widely distributed in tissue secretions and fluids. In healing wounds of the skin, EGF is produced by keratinocytes, macrophages, and other inflammatory cells that migrate into the area. TGF-α was originally extracted from sarcoma virus–transformed cells and is involved in epithelial cell proliferation in embryos and adults, and in malignant transformation of normal cells to cancer. TGF-α has homology with EGF, binds to EGFR, and shares most of the biologic activities of EGF. The "EGF receptor" is actually a family of four membrane receptors with intrinsic tyrosine kinase activity. The best-characterized EGFR is referred to as EGFR1, ERB B1, or simply EGFR. It responds to EGF, TGF-α, and other ligands of the EGF family, such as *HB-EGF (heparin-binding EGF) and amphiregulin. EGFR1 mutations and amplification have been detected in cancers of the lung, head and neck, and breast, glioblastomas, and other cancers, leading to the development of new types of treatments for these conditions.* The *ERB B2 receptor* (also known as *HER-2* or HER2/Neu), whose main ligand has not been identified, has received great attention because it is overexpressed in a subset of breast cancers and is an important therapeutic target.

Hepatocyte Growth Factor (HGF). HGF was originally isolated from platelets and serum. Subsequent studies demonstrated that it is identical to a previously identified growth factor isolated from fibroblasts known as *scatter factor.*[56] The factor is often referred to as HGF/SF, but in this chapter we will use the simpler notation, HGF.

HGF has mitogenic effects on hepatocytes and most epithelial cells, including cells of the biliary epithelium, and epithelial cells of the lungs, kidney, mammary gland, and skin. HGF acts as a morphogen in embryonic development, promotes cell scattering and migration, and enhances survival of hepatocytes. It is produced by fibroblasts and most mesenchymal cells, endothelial cells, and liver nonparenchymal cells. It is produced as an inactive single-chain form (pro-HGF) that is activated by serine proteases released in damaged tissues. The receptor for HGF, c-MET, is often highly expressed or mutated in human tumors, especially in renal and thyroid papillary carcinomas. HGF signaling is required for survival during embryonic development, as demonstrated by defects in the development of muscles, kidney, liver, and brain, and the lethality of knockout mice that lack c-*met*. Several HGF and c-MET inhibitors are presently being evaluated in cancer therapy clinical trials.

Platelet-Derived Growth Factor (PDGF). PDGF is a family of several closely related proteins, each consisting of two chains. Three isoforms of PDGF (AA, AB, and BB) are secreted as biologically active molecules. The more recently identified isoforms PDGF-CC and PDGF-DD require extracellular proteolytic cleavage to release the active growth factor.[57] All PDGF isoforms exert their effects by binding to two cell surface receptors, designated PDGFR α and β, which have different ligand specificities. PDGF is stored in platelet granules and is released on platelet activation. It is produced by a variety of cells, including activated macrophages, endothelial cells, smooth muscle cells, and many tumor cells. PDGF causes migration and proliferation of fibroblasts, smooth muscle cells, and monocytes to areas of inflammation and healing skin wounds, as demonstrated by defects in these functions in mice deficient in either the A or the B chain of PDGF. PDGF-B and C participate in the activation of hepatic stellate cells in the initial steps of liver fibrosis (Chapter 18) and stimulate wound contraction.

Vascular Endothelial Growth Factor (VEGF). VEGFs are a family of homodimeric proteins that include *VEGF-A (referred throughout as VEGF), VEGF-B, VEGF-C, VEGF-D,* and *PIGF (placental growth factor).*[58] VEGF is a potent inducer of blood vessel formation in early development *(vasculogenesis)* and has a central role in the growth of new blood vessels *(angiogenesis)* in adults (see Table 3–3). *It promotes angiogenesis in chronic inflammation, healing of wounds, and in tumors* (discussed later in this chapter, in "Mechanisms of Angiogenesis"). Mice that lack a single VEGF allele (heterozygous VEGF knockout mice) die during embryonic development as a result of defective vasculogenesis and hematopoiesis. VEGF family members signal through three tyrosine kinase receptors: VEGFR-1, VEGFR-2, and VEGFR-3. VEGFR-2, located in endothelial cells and many other cell types, is the main receptor for the vasculogenic and angiogenic effects of VEGF. The role of VEGFR-1 is less well understood, but it may facilitate the mobilization of endothelial stem cells and has a role in inflammation. VEGF-C and VEGF-D bind to VEGFR-3 and act on lymphatic endothelial cells to induce the production of lymphatic vessels *(lymphangiogenesis)*.

Fibroblast Growth Factor (FGF). This is a family of growth factors containing more than 20 members, of which acidic FGF (aFGF, or FGF-1) and basic FGF (bFGF, or FGF-2) are the best characterized.[59] FGFs transduce signals through four tyrosine kinase receptors (FGFRs 1–4). FGF-1 binds to all receptors; FGF-7 is referred to as *keratinocyte growth factor* or *KGF*. Released FGFs associate with heparan sulfate in the ECM, which can serve as a reservoir for the storage of inactive factors. FGFs contribute to wound healing responses, hematopoiesis, angiogenesis, development, and other processes through several functions:

- *Wound repair:* FGF-2 and KGF (FGF-7) contribute to re-epithelialization of skin wounds.
- *New blood vessel formation (angiogenesis):* FGF-2, in particular, has the ability to induce new blood vessel formation (discussed later).
- *Hematopoiesis:* FGFs have been implicated in the differentiation of specific lineages of blood cells and development of bone marrow stroma.
- *Development:* FGFs play a role in skeletal and cardiac muscle development, lung maturation, and the specification of the liver from endodermal cells.

Transforming Growth Factor β (TGF-β) and Related Growth Factors. TGF-β belongs to a superfamily of about 30 members that includes three TGF-β isoforms (TGF-β1, TGF-β2, TGF-β3) and factors with wide-ranging functions, such as BMPs, activins, inhibins, and müllerian inhibiting substance.[60] TGF-β1 has the most widespread distribution in mammals and will be referred to as TGF-β. It is a homodimeric protein produced by a variety of different cell types, including platelets, endothelial cells, lymphocytes, and macrophages. Native TGF-β is synthesized as a precursor protein, which is secreted and then proteolytically cleaved to yield the biologically active growth factor and a second *latent* component. Active TGF-β binds to two cell surface receptors (types I and II) with serine/threonine kinase activity and triggers the phosphorylation of cytoplasmic transcription factors called *Smads* (of which there are several forms, e.g., Smad 1, 2, 3, 5, and 8). These phosphorylated Smads in turn form heterodimers with Smad 4, which enter the nucleus and associate with other DNA-binding proteins to activate or inhibit gene transcription. TGF-β has multiple and often opposing effects depending on the tissue and the type of injury. Agents that have multiple effects are called pleiotropic; because of the large diversity of TGF-β effects, it has been said that TGF-β is pleiotropic with a vengeance.

- *TGF-β is a growth inhibitor for most epithelial cells.* It blocks the cell cycle by increasing the expression of cell cycle inhibitors of the Cip/Kip and INK4/ARF families (see Chapter 7). The effects of TGF-β on mesenchymal cells depend on the tissue environment, but it can promote invasion and metastasis during tumor growth. Loss of TGF-β receptors frequently occurs in human tumors, providing a proliferative advantage to tumor cells. At the same time TGF-β expression may increase in the tumor microenvironment, creating stromal-epithelial interactions that enhance tumor growth and invasion.
- *TGF-β is a potent fibrogenic agent* that stimulates fibroblast chemotaxis and enhances the production of collagen, fibronectin, and proteoglycans. It inhibits collagen degradation by decreasing matrix proteases and increasing protease inhibitor activities. TGF-β is involved in the development of fibrosis in a variety of chronic inflammatory conditions particularly in the lungs, kidney, and liver. High TGF-β expression also occurs in hypertrophic scars (discussed later), systemic sclerosis (Chapter 6), and the Marfan syndrome (Chapter 5).
- *TGF-β has a strong anti-inflammatory effect but may enhance some immune functions.* Knockout mice lacking the *TGF-β1* gene in T cells have defects in regulatory T cells leading to widespread inflammation with abundant T-cell proliferation and CD4+ differentiation into T_H1 and T_H2 helper cells. However, TGF-β also enhances the development of interleukin-17 (IL-17)–producing T cells (T_H17) that may be involved in autoimmune tissue injury, and stimulates the production of IgA in the gut mucosa.

Cytokines. Cytokines have important functions as mediators of inflammation and immune responses (Chapter 6). Some of these proteins can also be considered as growth factors, because they have growth-promoting activities for a variety of cells. Cytokines are discussed in Chapters 2 and 6. Tumor necrosis factor (TNF) and IL-1 participate in wound healing reactions (see Table 3–1), and TNF and IL-6 are involved in the initiation of liver regeneration (discussed later).

SIGNALING MECHANISMS IN CELL GROWTH

In this section we review the process of *receptor-mediated signal transduction*, which is activated by the binding of ligands such as growth factors, and cytokines to specific receptors. Different classes of receptor molecules and pathways initiate a cascade of events by which receptor activation leads to expression of specific genes. Here we focus on the biochemical pathways and transcriptional regulation that mediate growth factor activity.

According to the source of the ligand and the location of its receptors (i.e., in the same, adjacent, or distant cells), three general modes of signaling, named autocrine, paracrine, and endocrine, can be distinguished (Fig. 3–8).

- *Autocrine signaling:* Cells respond to the signaling molecules that they themselves secrete, thus establishing an *autocrine loop*. Autocrine growth regulation plays a role in liver regeneration and the proliferation of antigen-stimulated lymphocytes. Tumors frequently overproduce growth factors and their receptors, thus stimulating their own proliferation through an autocrine loop.
- *Paracrine signaling:* One cell type produces the ligand, which then acts on adjacent target cells that express the appropriate receptor. The responding cells are in close proximity to the ligand-producing cell and are generally of a different type. Paracrine stimulation is common in connective tissue repair of healing wounds, in which a factor produced by one cell type (e.g., a macrophage) has a growth effect on adjacent cells (e.g., a fibroblast). It is also necessary for hepatocyte replication during liver regeneration (discussed later), and for Notch effects in embryonic development, wound healing, and renewing tissues.
- *Endocrine signaling:* Hormones synthesized by cells of endocrine organs act on target cells distant from their site of synthesis, being usually carried by the blood. Growth factors may also circulate and act at distant sites, as is the case for HGF. Several cytokines, such as those associated with the systemic aspects of inflammation discussed in Chapter 2, also act as endocrine agents.

Receptors and Signal Transduction Pathways

The binding of a ligand to its receptor triggers a series of events by which extracellular signals are transduced into the cell resulting in changes in gene expression. Although single receptor molecules can transduce some signals upon ligand binding, signaling typically involves clustering of two or more receptor molecules by the ligand. Receptors are generally located on the surface of the target cell but can also be found in the cytoplasm or nucleus.

It is useful at this point to summarize the properties of the major types of receptors and how they deliver signals to the cell interior (Fig. 3–9). This is pertinent to an understanding

AUTOCRINE SIGNALING

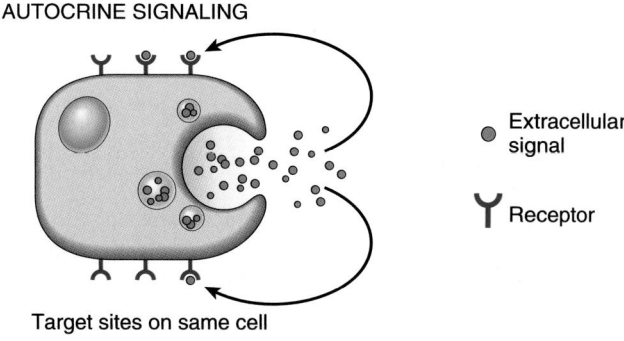

Target sites on same cell

PARACRINE SIGNALING

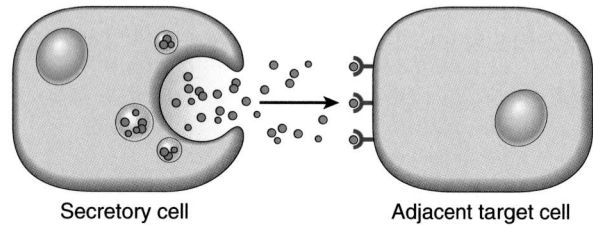

Secretory cell   Adjacent target cell

ENDOCRINE SIGNALING

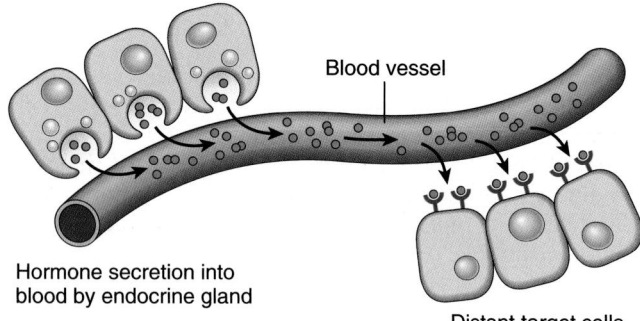

Hormone secretion into
blood by endocrine gland

Distant target cells

FIGURE 3–8   General patterns of intercellular signaling demonstrating autocrine, paracrine, and endocrine signaling (see text). (Modified from Lodish H et al [eds]: Molecular Cell Biology, 3rd ed. New York, WH Freeman, 1995, p 855. © 1995 by Scientific American Books. Used with permission of WH Freeman and Company.)

of normal and unregulated (neoplastic) cell growth (discussed in Chapter 7).

● *Receptors with intrinsic tyrosine kinase activity.* The ligands for receptors with tyrosine kinase activity include most growth factors such as EGF, TGF-α, HGF, PDGF, VEGF, FGF, c-KIT ligand, and insulin. Receptors belonging to this family have an extracellular ligand-binding domain, a transmembrane region, and a cytoplasmic tail that has intrinsic tyrosine kinase activity.[61] Binding of the ligand induces *dimerization of the receptor*, tyrosine phosphorylation, and activation of the receptor tyrosine kinase (Fig. 3–10). The active kinase then phosphorylates, and thereby activates, many downstream *effector molecules* (molecules that mediate the effects of receptor engagement with a ligand). Activation of effector molecules can be direct or through the involvement of *adapter proteins*. A prototypical

adapter protein is GRB-2, which binds a guanosine triphosphate–guanosine diphosphate (GTP-GDP) exchange factor called SOS. SOS acts on the GTP-binding (G) protein RAS and catalyzes the formation of RAS-GTP, which triggers the mitogen-activated protein kinase (MAP kinase) cascade (see Fig. 3–10). Active MAP kinases stimulate the synthesis and phosphorylation of transcription factors, such as FOS and JUN. The transcription factors activated by these various signaling cascades in turn stimulate the production of growth factors, receptors for growth factors, and proteins that directly control the entry of cells into the cell cycle. Other effector molecules activated by receptors with intrinsic tyrosine kinase activity include *phospholipase Cγ (PLCγ)* and *phosphatidyl inositol-3 kinase (PI3K)* (see Fig. 3–9). PLCγ catalyzes the breakdown of membrane inositol phospholipids into inositol 1,4,5-triphosphate (IP_3), which functions to increase concentrations of calcium, an important effector molecule, and diacylglycerol, which activates the serine-threonine kinase protein kinase C that in turn activates various transcription factors. PI3K phosphorylates a membrane phospholipid, generating products that activate the kinase Akt (also referred to as protein kinase B), which is involved in cell proliferation and cell survival through inhibition of apoptosis. Alterations in tyrosine kinase activity and receptor mutations have been detected in many forms of cancer and are important targets for therapy (Chapter 7).

● *Receptors lacking intrinsic tyrosine kinase activity that recruit kinases.* Ligands for these receptors include many cytokines, such as IL-2, IL-3, and other interleukins; interferons α, β, and γ; erythropoietin; granulocyte colony-stimulating factor; growth hormone; and prolactin. These receptors transmit extracellular signals to the nucleus by activating members of the JAK (Janus kinase) family of proteins (see Fig. 3–9). The JAKs link the receptors with and activate cytoplasmic transcription factors called STATs (signal transducers and activation of transcription), which directly shuttle into the nucleus and activate gene transcription.[62] Cytokine receptors can also activate other signaling pathways, such as the MAP kinase pathways already mentioned.

● *G protein–coupled receptors.* These receptors transmit signals into the cell through trimeric GTP-binding proteins *(G proteins)*. They contain *seven transmembrane α-helices* (see Fig. 3–9) and constitute the largest family of plasma membrane receptors, with nonodorant G protein–coupled receptors accounting for about 1% of the human genome. A large number of ligands signal through this type of receptor, including chemokines, vasopressin, serotonin, histamine, epinephrine and norepinephrine, calcitonin, glucagon, parathyroid hormone, corticotropin, and rhodopsin. An enormous number of common pharmaceutical drugs targets such receptors.[63] Binding of the ligand induces changes in the conformation of the receptors, causing their activation and allowing their interaction with many different G proteins. Activation of G proteins occurs by the exchange of GDP, present in the inactive protein, with GTP, which activates the protein. Among the many branches of this signal transduction pathway are those involving *calcium and 3′,5′-cyclic adenosine monophosphate (cAMP) as second messengers.* Activation of G protein–coupled receptors (as well as of tyrosine kinase receptors, discussed above) can

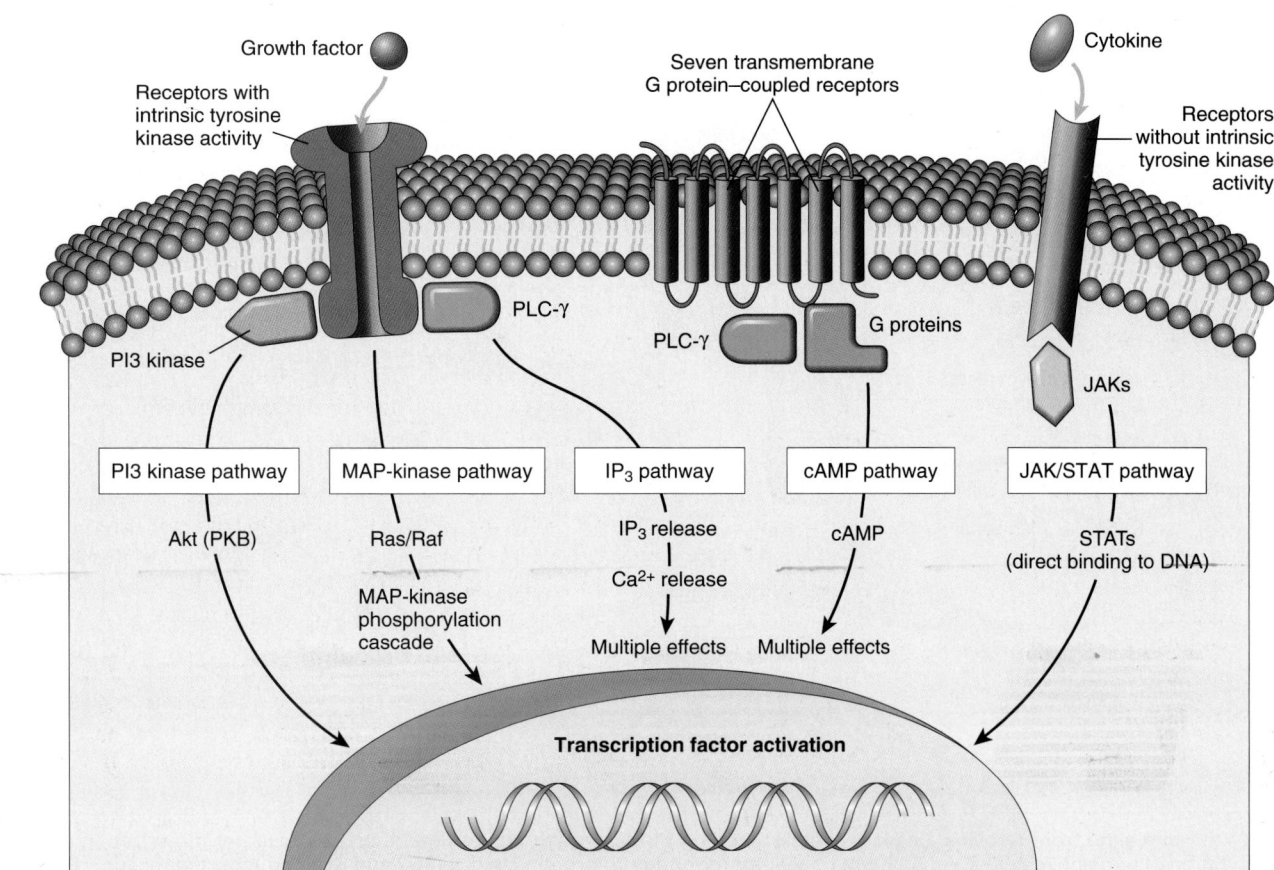

FIGURE 3–9 Overview of the main types of cell surface receptors and their principal signal transduction pathways (see text). Shown are receptors with intrinsic tyrosine kinase activity, seven transmembrane G protein–coupled receptors, and receptors without intrinsic tyrosine kinase activity. cAMP, cyclic adenosine monophosphate: IP_3, inositol triphosphate; JAK, Janus kinase; MAP kinase, mitogen-activated protein kinase; PI3 kinase, phosphatidylinositol 3-kinase; PKB, protein kinase B, also known as Akt; PLC-γ, phospholipase C gamma; STATs, signal transducers and activators of transcription.

produce inositol triphosphate (IP_3), which releases calcium from the endoplasmic reticulum. Calcium signals, which are generally oscillatory, have multiple targets, including cytoskeletal proteins, chloride- and potassium-activated ion pumps, enzymes such as calpain, and calcium-binding proteins such as calmodulin. cAMP activates a more restricted set of targets that include protein kinase A and cAMP-gated ion channels, important in vision and olfactory sensing. Inherited defects involving G protein–coupled receptor signal transduction are associated with retinitis pigmentosa, corticotropin deficiencies, and hyperparathyroidism.

○ *Steroid hormone receptors. These receptors are generally located in the nucleus and function as ligand-dependent transcription factors. The ligands diffuse through the cell membrane and bind the inactive receptors, causing their activation. The activated receptor then binds to specific DNA sequences known as hormone response elements within target genes, or they can bind to other transcription factors.* In addition to steroid hormones, other ligands that bind to members of this receptor family include thyroid hormone, vitamin D, and retinoids. A group of receptors belonging to this family are called *peroxisome proliferator-activated receptors.*[64] They are nuclear receptors that are involved in

a broad range of responses that include adipogenesis (Chapter 24), inflammation, and atherosclerosis.

Transcription Factors

Many of the signal transduction systems used by growth factors transfer information to the nucleus and modulate gene transcription through the activity of *transcription factors.* Among the transcription factors that regulate cell proliferation are products of several growth-promoting genes, such as c-*MYC* and c-*JUN*, and of cell cycle–inhibiting genes, such as *p53*. Transcription factors have a modular design and contain domains for DNA binding and for transcriptional regulation. The DNA-binding domain permits binding to short sequence motifs of DNA, which may be unique to a particular target gene or may be present in many genes. The transactivating domain stimulates transcription of the adjacent gene.

Growth factors induce the synthesis or activity of transcription factors. Cellular events requiring rapid responses do not rely on new synthesis of transcription factors but depend on post-translational modifications that lead to their activation. These modifications include (a) *heterodimerization*, as for instance, the dimerization of the products of the proto-

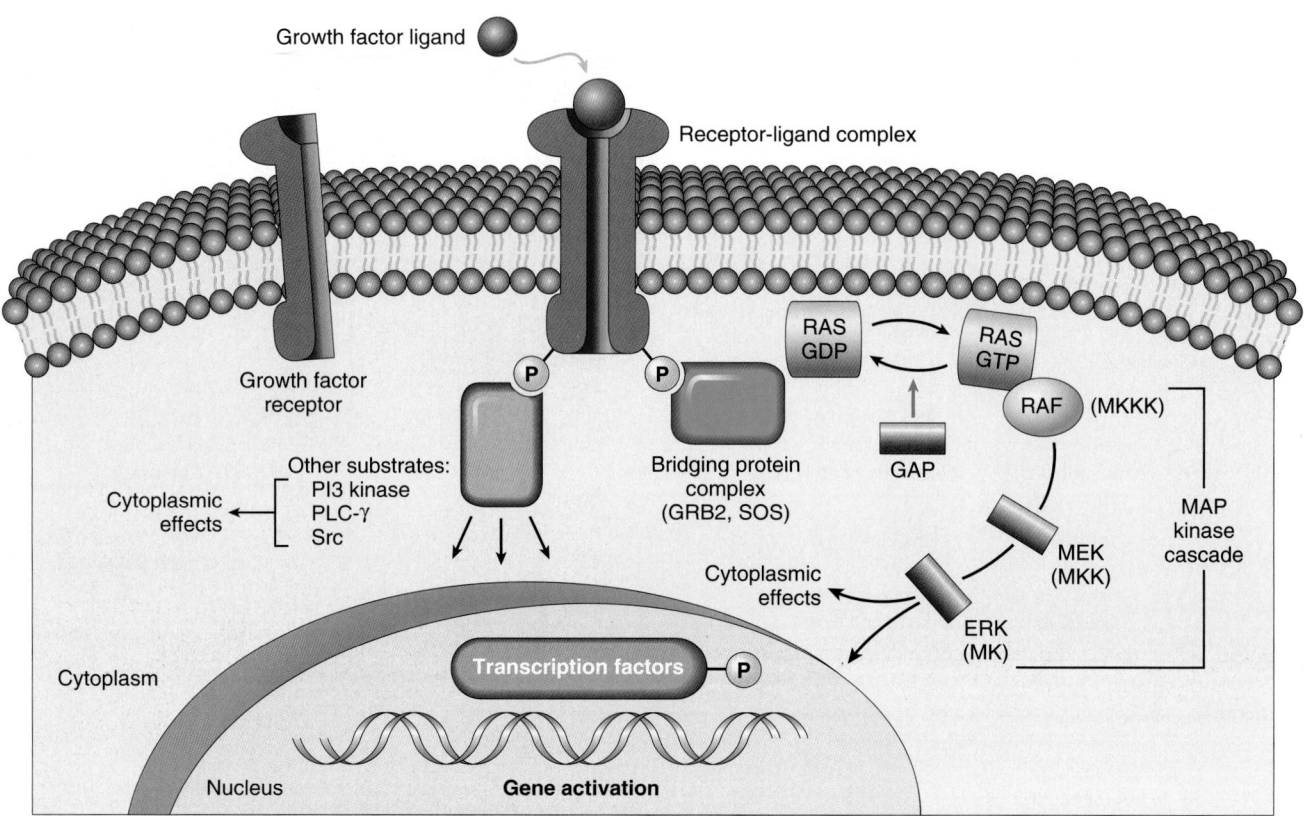

FIGURE 3–10 Signaling from tyrosine kinase receptors. Binding of the growth factor (ligand) causes receptor dimerization and auto-phosphorylation of tyrosine residues. Attachment of adapter (or bridging) proteins (e.g., GRB2 and SOS) couples the receptor to inactive RAS. Cycling of RAS between its inactive and active forms is regulated by GAP. Activated RAS interacts with and activates RAF (also known as MAP kinase kinase kinase). This kinase then phosphorylates a component of the MAP kinase signaling pathway, MEK (also known as MAP kinase kinase or MKK), which then phosphorylates ERK (MAP kinase or MK). Activated MAP kinase phosphorylates other cytoplasmic proteins and nuclear transcription factors, generating cellular responses. The phosphorylated tyrosine kinase receptor can also bind other components, such as phosphatidyl 3-kinase (PI3 kinase), which activates other signaling systems.

oncogenes c-*FOS* and c-*JUN* to form the transcription factor activator protein-1 (AP-1), which is activated by MAP kinase signaling pathways, (b) *phosphorylation*, as for STATs in the JAK/STAT pathway, (c) *release of inhibition* to permit migration into the nucleus, as for NF-κB, and (d) *release from membranes* by proteolytic cleavage, as for Notch receptors (see Fig. 3–16).

Mechanisms of Tissue and Organ Regeneration

Urodele amphibians such as the newt can regenerate their tails, limbs, lens, retina, jaws, and even a large portion of the heart, but *the capacity for regeneration of whole tissues and organs has been lost in mammals.*[1] The inadequacy of true regeneration in mammals has been attributed to the absence of *blastema* formation (the source of cells for regeneration) and to the rapid fibroproliferative response after wounding. *The Wnt/β-catenin is a highly conserved pathway* that participates in the regeneration of planaria flatworms, fin and heart regeneration in zebra fish, and blastema and patterning formation in limb regeneration in newts. In mammals, Wnt/β-catenin modulates stem cell functions in the intestinal epithelium, bone marrow, and muscle, participates in liver regeneration after partial hepatectomy, and stimulates oval cell proliferation after liver injury.[27,65,66]

In this section we have chosen the liver to illustrate the mechanisms of regeneration, because it has been studied in detail and has important biologic and clinical aspects. Even this process is not one of true regeneration, because the resection of tissue does not cause new growth of liver but instead triggers a process of compensatory hyperplasia in the remaining parts of the organ (discussed below). Other organs, including kidney, pancreas, adrenal glands, thyroid, and the lungs of very young animals, are also capable of compensatory growth, although they display it in less dramatic form than the liver. Because new nephrons cannot be generated in the adult kidney, the growth of the contralateral kidney after unilateral nephrectomy involves nephron hypertrophy and some replication of proximal tubule cells. The pancreas has a limited capacity to regenerate its exocrine components and islets. Regeneration of pancreatic beta cells may involve beta-cell replication, transdifferentiation of ductal cells, or differentiation of putative stem cells that express the transcription factors Oct4 and Sox2.[67] Recently, pancreatic exocrine cells have been reprogrammed into insulin-secreting β-cells.

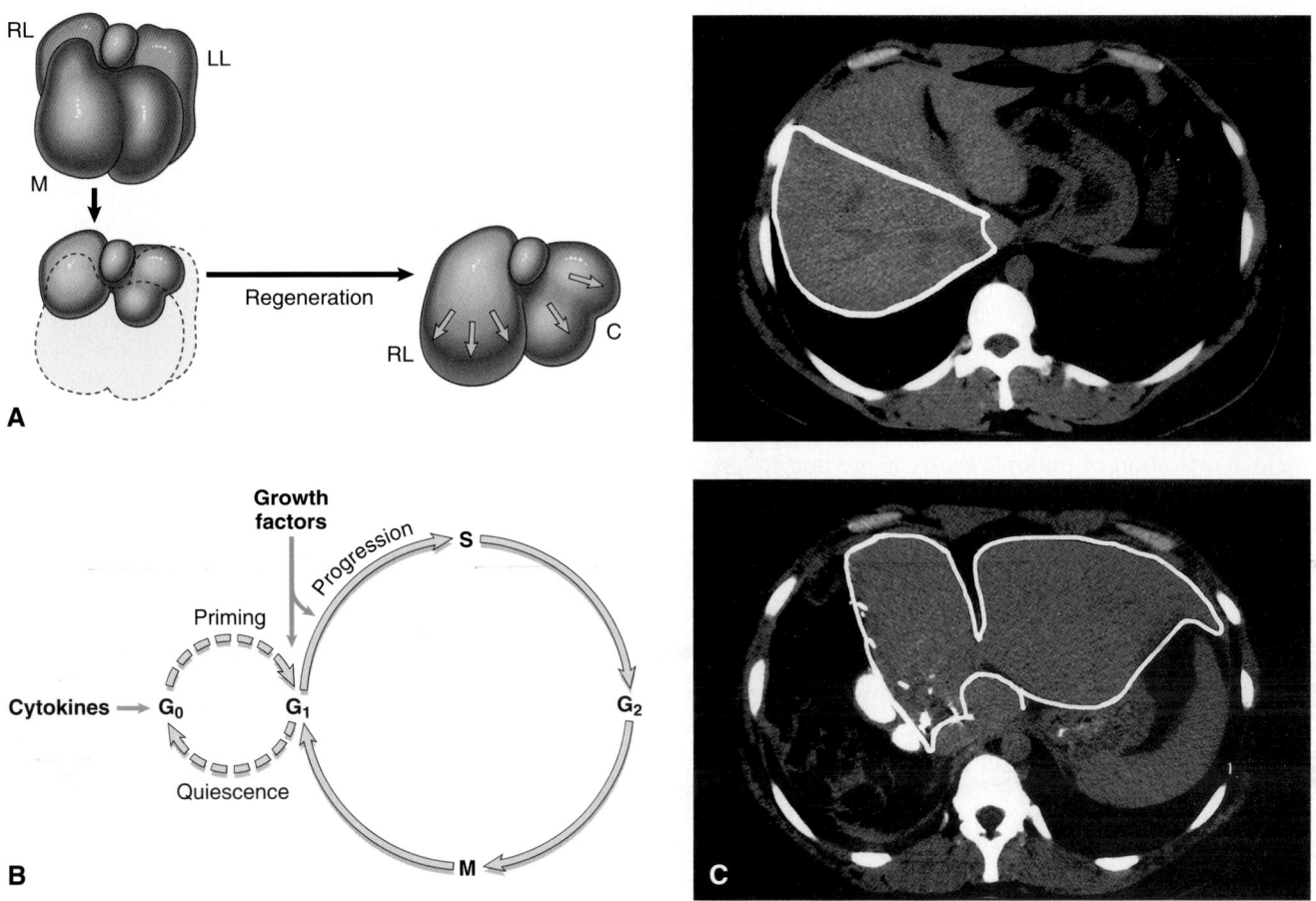

FIGURE 3–11 Liver regeneration after partial hepatectomy. **A,** The lobes of the liver of a rat (M, median; RL and LL, right and left lateral lobes; C, caudate lobe). Partial hepatectomy removes two thirds of the liver (median and left lateral lobes). After 3 weeks the right lateral and caudate lobes enlarge to reach a mass equivalent to that of the original liver without regrowth of the median and left lateral lobes. **B,** Entry and progression of hepatocytes in the cell cycle (see text for details). **C,** *Regeneration of the human liver in living-donor transplantation.* Computed tomography scans of the donor liver in living-donor hepatic transplantation. Upper panel is a scan of the liver of the donor before the operation. The right lobe, to be used as a transplant, is outlined. Lower panel is a scan of the liver 1 week after performance of partial hepatectomy. Note the great enlargement of the left lobe (outlined in the panel) without regrowth of the right lobe. (**A,** From Goss RJ: Regeneration versus repair. In Cohen IK et al [eds]: Wound Healing. Biochemical and Clinical Aspects. Philadelphia, WB Saunders, 1992, pp 20–39; **C,** courtesy of R. Troisi, MD, Ghent University, Ghent, Belgium; reproduced in part from Fausto N: Liver regeneration. In Arias I, et al: The Liver: Biology and Pathobiology, 4th ed. Philadelphia, Lippincott Williams & Wilkins, 2001.)

LIVER REGENERATION

The human liver has a remarkable capacity to regenerate, as demonstrated by its growth after partial hepatectomy, which may be performed for tumor resection or for living-donor hepatic transplantation (Fig. 3–11). The popular image of liver regeneration is the daily regrowth of the liver of Prometheus, which was eaten every day by an eagle sent by Zeus (Zeus was angry at Prometheus for stealing the secret of fire, but did he know that Prometheus's liver would regenerate?). The reality, although less dramatic, is still quite impressive. In humans, resection of approximately 60% of the liver in living donors results in the doubling of the liver remnant in about one month. The portions of the liver that remain after partial hepatectomy constitute an intact "mini-liver" that rapidly expands and reaches the mass of the original liver (see Fig. 3–11). *Restoration of liver mass is achieved without the regrowth of the lobes that were resected at the operation.* Instead, growth

occurs by enlargement of the lobes that remain after the operation, a process known as *compensatory growth or compensatory hyperplasia.* In both humans and rodents, the end point of liver regeneration after partial hepatectomy is the restitution of functional mass rather than the reconstitution of the original form.[69]

Almost all hepatocytes replicate during liver regeneration after partial hepatectomy. Because hepatocytes are quiescent cells, it takes them several hours to enter the cell cycle, progress through G_1, and reach the S phase of DNA replication. The wave of hepatocyte replication is synchronized and is followed by synchronous replication of nonparenchymal cells (Kupffer cells, endothelial cells, and stellate cells).

There is substantial evidence that *hepatocyte proliferation in the regenerating liver is triggered by the combined actions of cytokines and polypeptide growth factors.* With the exception of the autocrine activity of TGF-α, hepatocyte replication is strictly dependent on paracrine effects of growth factors and cytokines such as HGF and IL-6 produced by hepatic non-parenchymal cells. There are two major restriction points for hepatocyte replication: the G_0/G_1 transition that bring quiescent hepatocytes into the cell cycle, and the G_1/S transition needed for passage through the late G_1 restriction point. Gene expression in the regenerating liver proceeds in phases, starting with the immediate early gene response, which is a transient response that corresponds to the G_0/G_1 transition. More than 70 genes are activated during this response, including the proto-oncogenes c-*FOS* and c-*JUN*, whose products dimerize to form the transcription factor AP-1; c-*MYC*, which encodes a transcription factor that activates many different genes; and other transcription factors, such as NF-κB, STAT-3, and C/EBP.[70] The immediate early gene response sets the stage for the sequential activation of multiple genes, as hepatocytes progress into the G_1 phase. The G_1 to S transition occurs as previously described (see Fig. 3–7).

Quiescent hepatocytes become competent to enter the cell cycle through a priming phase that is mostly mediated by the cytokines TNF and IL-6, and components of the complement system. Priming signals activate several signal transduction pathways as a necessary prelude to cell proliferation. Under the stimulation of HGF, TGFα, and HB-EGF, primed hepatocytes enter the cell cycle and undergo DNA replication (Fig. 3–11). Norepinephrine, serotonin, insulin, thyroid and growth hormone, act as adjuvants for liver regeneration, facilitating the entry of hepatocytes into the cell cycle.

Individual hepatocytes replicate once or twice during regeneration and then return to quiescence in a strictly regulated sequence of events, but the mechanisms of growth cessation have not been established. Growth inhibitors, such as TGF-β and activins, may be involved in terminating hepatocyte replication, but there is no clear understanding of their mode of action. *Intrahepatic stem or progenitor cells do not play a role in the compensatory growth that occurs after partial hepatectomy,* and there is no evidence for hepatocyte generation from bone marrow–derived cells during this process.[28,37] However, endothelial cells and other nonparenchymal cells in the regenerating liver may originate from bone marrow precursors.

Extracellular Matrix and Cell-Matrix Interactions

Tissue repair and regeneration depend not only on the activity of soluble factors, but also on interactions between cells and the components of the *extracellular matrix (ECM)*. The ECM regulates the growth, proliferation, movement, and differentiation of the cells living within it. It is constantly remodeling, and its synthesis and degradation accompanies morphogenesis, regeneration, wound healing, chronic fibrotic processes, tumor invasion, and metastasis. The ECM sequesters water, providing turgor to soft tissues, and minerals that give rigidity to bone, but it does much more than just fill the spaces around cells to maintain tissue structure. Its various functions include:

- *Mechanical support* for cell anchorage and cell migration, and maintenance of cell polarity
- *Control of cell growth.* ECM components can regulate cell proliferation by signaling through cellular receptors of the integrin family.
- *Maintenance of cell differentiation.* The type of ECM proteins can affect the degree of differentiation of the cells in the tissue, also acting largely via cell surface integrins.
- *Scaffolding for tissue renewal.* The maintenance of normal tissue structure requires a basement membrane or stromal scaffold. The integrity of the basement membrane or the stroma of the parenchymal cells is critical for the organized regeneration of tissues. It is particularly noteworthy that although labile and stable cells are capable of regeneration, injury to these tissues results in restitution of the normal structure only if the ECM is not damaged. Disruption of these structures leads to collagen deposition and scar formation (see Fig. 3–2).
- *Establishment of tissue microenvironments.* Basement membrane acts as a boundary between epithelium and underlying connective tissue and also forms part of the filtration apparatus in the kidney.
- *Storage and presentation of regulatory molecules.* For example, growth factors like FGF and HGF are secreted and stored in the ECM in some tissues. This allows the rapid deployment of growth factors after local injury, or during regeneration.

The ECM is composed of three groups of macromolecules: *fibrous structural proteins,* such as collagens and elastins that provide tensile strength and recoil; *adhesive glycoproteins* that connect the matrix elements to one another and to cells; and *proteoglycans and hyaluronan* that provide resilience and lubrication. These molecules assemble to form two basic forms of ECM: *interstitial matrix and basement membranes.* The interstitial matrix is found in spaces between epithelial, endothelial, and smooth muscle cells, as well as in connective tissue. It consists mostly of fibrillar and nonfibrillar collagen, elastin, fibronectin, proteoglycans, and hyaluronan. Basement membranes are closely associated with cell surfaces, and consist of nonfibrillar collagen (mostly type IV), laminin, heparin sulfate, and proteoglycans.[71]

We will now consider the main components of the ECM.

COLLAGEN

Collagen is the most common protein in the animal world, providing the extracellular framework for all multicellular organisms. Without collagen, a human being would be reduced to a clump of cells, like the "Blob" (the "gelatinous horror from outer space" of 1950s movie fame), interconnected by a few neurons. Currently, 27 different types of collagens encoded by 41 genes dispersed on at least 14 chromosomes are known[72] (Table 3–2). Each *collagen* is composed of three chains that form a trimer in the shape of a triple helix. The polypeptide is characterized by a repeating sequence in which glycine is in every third position (Gly-X-Y, in which X and Y can be any amino acid other than cysteine or tryptophan), and it contains

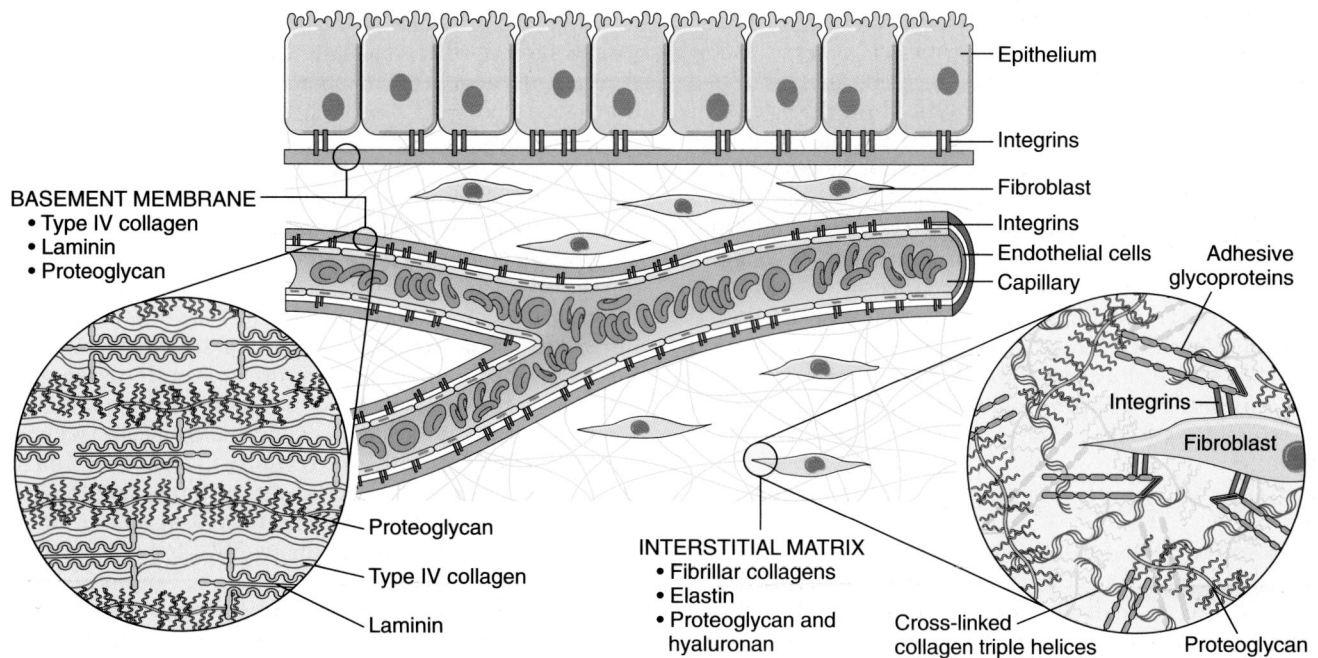

FIGURE 3–12 Main components of the extracellular matrix (ECM), including collagens, proteoglycans, and adhesive glycoproteins. Both epithelial and mesenchymal cells (e.g., fibroblasts) interact with ECM via integrins. Basement membranes and interstitial ECM have different architecture and general composition, although there is some overlap in their constituents. For the sake of simplification, many ECM components (e.g., elastin, fibrillin, hyaluronan, and syndecan) are not included.

the specialized amino acids 4-hydroxyproline and hydroxylysine. Prolyl residues in the Y-position are characteristically hydroxylated to produce hydroxyproline, which serves to stabilize the triple helix. Types I, II, III and V, and XI are the *fibrillar collagens*, in which the triple-helical domain is uninterrupted for more than 1000 residues; these proteins are found in extracellular fibrillar structures. *Type IV collagens have long but interrupted triple-helical domains and form sheets instead of fibrils; they are the main components of the basement*

membrane, together with laminin. Another collagen with a long interrupted triple-helical domain (type VII) forms the anchoring fibrils between some epithelial and mesenchymal structures, such as epidermis and dermis. Still other collagens are transmembrane and may also help to anchor epidermal and dermal structures.

The messenger RNAs transcribed from fibrillar collagen genes are translated into pre-pro-α chains that assemble in a type-specific manner into trimers. Hydroxylation of proline

TABLE 3–2 Main Types of Collagens, Tissue Distribution, and Genetic Disorders		
Collagen Type	**Tissue Distribution**	**Genetic Disorders**
FIBRILLAR COLLAGENS		
I	Ubiquitous in hard and soft tissues	Osteogenesis imperfecta; Ehlers-Danlos syndrome—arthrochalasias type I
II	Cartilage, intervertebral disk, vitreous	Achondrogenesis type II, spondyloepiphysea dysplasia syndrome
III	Hollow organs, soft tissues	Vascular Ehlers-Danlos syndrome
V	Soft tissues, blood vessels	Classical Ehlers-Danlos syndrome
IX	Cartilage, vitreous	Stickler syndrome
BASEMENT MEMBRANE COLLAGENS		
IV	Basement membranes	Alport syndrome
OTHER COLLAGENS		
VI	Ubiquitous in microfibrils	Bethlem myopathy
VII	Anchoring fibrils at dermal-epidermal junctions	Dystrophic epidermolysis bullosa
IX	Cartilage, intervertebral disks	Multiple epiphyseal dysplasias
XVII	Transmembrane collagen in epidermal cells	Benign atrophic generalized epidermolysis bullosa
XV and XVIII	Endostatin-forming collagens, endothelial cells	Knobloch syndrome (type XVIII collagen)

Courtesy of Dr. Peter H. Byers, Department of Pathology, University of Washington, Seattle, WA.

and lysine residues and lysine glycosylation occur during translation. Three chains of a particular collagen type assemble to form the triple helix (Fig. 3–15). Procollagen is secreted from the cell and cleaved by proteases to form the basic unit of the fibrils. Collagen fibril formation is associated with the oxidation of lysine and hydroxylysine residues by the extracellular enzyme *lysyl oxidase*. This results in *cross-linking* between the chains of adjacent molecules, which stabilizes the array, and is a major contributor to the tensile strength of collagen. *Vitamin C is required for the hydroxylation of procollagen*, a requirement that explains the inadequate wound healing in scurvy (Chapter 9). Genetic defects in collagen production (see Table 3–2) cause many inherited syndromes, including various forms of the Ehlers-Danlos syndrome and osteogenesis imperfecta[73] (Chapters 5 and 26).

ELASTIN, FIBRILLIN, AND ELASTIC FIBERS

Tissues such as blood vessels, skin, uterus, and lung require elasticity for their function. Proteins of the collagen family provide tensile strength, but the ability of these tissues to expand and recoil (compliance) depends on the elastic fibers. These fibers can stretch and then return to their original size after release of the tension. Morphologically, elastic fibers consist of a central core made of *elastin*, surrounded by a peripheral network of microfibrils. Substantial amounts of elastin are found in the walls of large blood vessels, such as the aorta, and in the uterus, skin, and ligaments. The peripheral microfibrillar network that surrounds the core consists largely of *fibrillin*, a 350-kD secreted glycoprotein, which associates either with itself or with other components of the ECM. The microfibrils serve, in part, as scaffolding for deposition of elastin and the assembly of elastic fibers. They also influence the availability of active TGFβ in the ECM. As already mentioned, inherited defects in fibrillin result in formation of abnormal elastic fibers in *Marfan syndrome*, manifested by changes in the cardiovascular system (aortic dissection) and the skeleton[74] (Chapter 5).

CELL ADHESION PROTEINS

Most adhesion proteins, also called CAMs (cell adhesion molecules), can be classified into four main families: immunoglobulin family CAMs, cadherins, integrins, and selectins. These proteins function as transmembrane receptors but are sometimes stored in the cytoplasm.[75] As receptors, CAMs can bind to similar or different molecules in other cells, providing for interaction between the same cells (homotypic interaction) or different cell types (heterotypic interaction). Selectins have been discussed in Chapter 2 in the context of leukocyte/endothelial interactions. Selected aspects of other cell adhesion proteins are described here. *Integrins* bind to ECM proteins such as fibronectin, laminin, and osteopontin providing a connection between cells and ECM, and also to adhesive proteins in other cells, establishing cell-to-cell contact. *Fibronectin* is a large protein that binds to many molecules, such as collagen, fibrin, proteoglycans, and cell surface receptors. It consists of two glycoprotein chains, held together by disulfide bonds. Fibronectin messenger RNA has two splice forms, giving rise to tissue fibronectin and plasma fibronectin. The plasma form binds to fibrin, helping to stabilize the blood clot that fills the gaps created by wounds, and serves as a substratum for ECM

deposition and formation of the provisional matrix during wound healing (discussed later). *Laminin* is the most abundant glycoprotein in the basement membrane and has binding domains for both ECM and cell surface receptors. In the basement membrane, polymers of laminin and collagen type IV form tightly bound networks. Laminin can also mediate the attachment of cells to connective tissue substrates.

Cadherins and integrins link the cell surface with the cytoskeleton through binding to actin and intermediate filaments. These linkages, particularly for the integrins, provide a mechanism for the transmission of mechanical force and the activation of intracellular signal transduction pathways that respond to these forces. Ligand binding to integrins causes clustering of the receptors in the cell membrane and formation of *focal adhesion* complexes. The cytoskeletal proteins that co-localize with integrins at the cell focal adhesion complex include talin, vinculin, and paxillin. The integrin-cytoskeleton complexes function as activated receptors and trigger a number of signal transduction pathways, including the MAP kinase, PKC, and PI3K pathways, which are also activated by growth factors. Not only is there a functional overlap between integrin and growth factor receptors, *but integrins and growth factor receptors interact ("crosstalk") to transmit environmental signals to the cell* that regulate proliferation, apoptosis, and differentiation (Fig. 3–13).

The name *cadherin* is derived from the term "calcium-dependent adherence protein." This family contains almost 90 members, which participate in interactions between cells of the same type. These interactions connect the plasma membrane of adjacent cells, forming two types of cell junctions called (1) *zonula adherens*, small, spotlike junctions located near the apical surface of epithelial cells, and (2) *desmosomes*, stronger and more extensive junctions, present in epithelial and muscle cells. Migration of keratinocytes in the re-epithelialization of skin wounds is dependent on the formation of dermosomal junctions. Linkage of cadherins with the cytoskeleton occurs through two classes of *catenins*. β-catenin links cadherins with α-catenin, which, in turn, connects to actin, thus completing the connection with the cytoskeleton. Cell-to-cell interactions mediated by cadherins and catenins play a major role in regulating cell motility, proliferation, and differentiation and account for the inhibition of cell proliferation that occurs when cultured normal cells contact each other ("contact inhibition"). Diminished function of E-cadherin contributes to certain forms of breast and gastric cancer. As already mentioned, free β-catenin acts independently of cadherins in the Wnt signaling pathway, which participates in stem cell homeostasis and regeneration. Mutation and altered expression of the Wnt/β-catenin pathway is implicated in cancer development, particularly in gastrointestinal and liver cancers (Chapter 7).

In addition to the main families of adhesive proteins described earlier, some other secreted adhesion molecules are mentioned because of their potential role in disease processes: (1) *SPARC* (secreted protein acidic and rich in cysteine), also known as *osteonectin*, contributes to tissue remodeling in response to injury and functions as an angiogenesis inhibitor; (2) the *thrombospondins*, a family of large multifunctional proteins, some of which, similar to SPARC, also inhibit angiogenesis; (3) *osteopontin (OPN)* is a glycoprotein that regulates calcification, is a mediator of leukocyte migration involved in inflammation, vascular remodeling, and fibrosis in various organs[76,77] (discussed later in this chapter); and (4) the

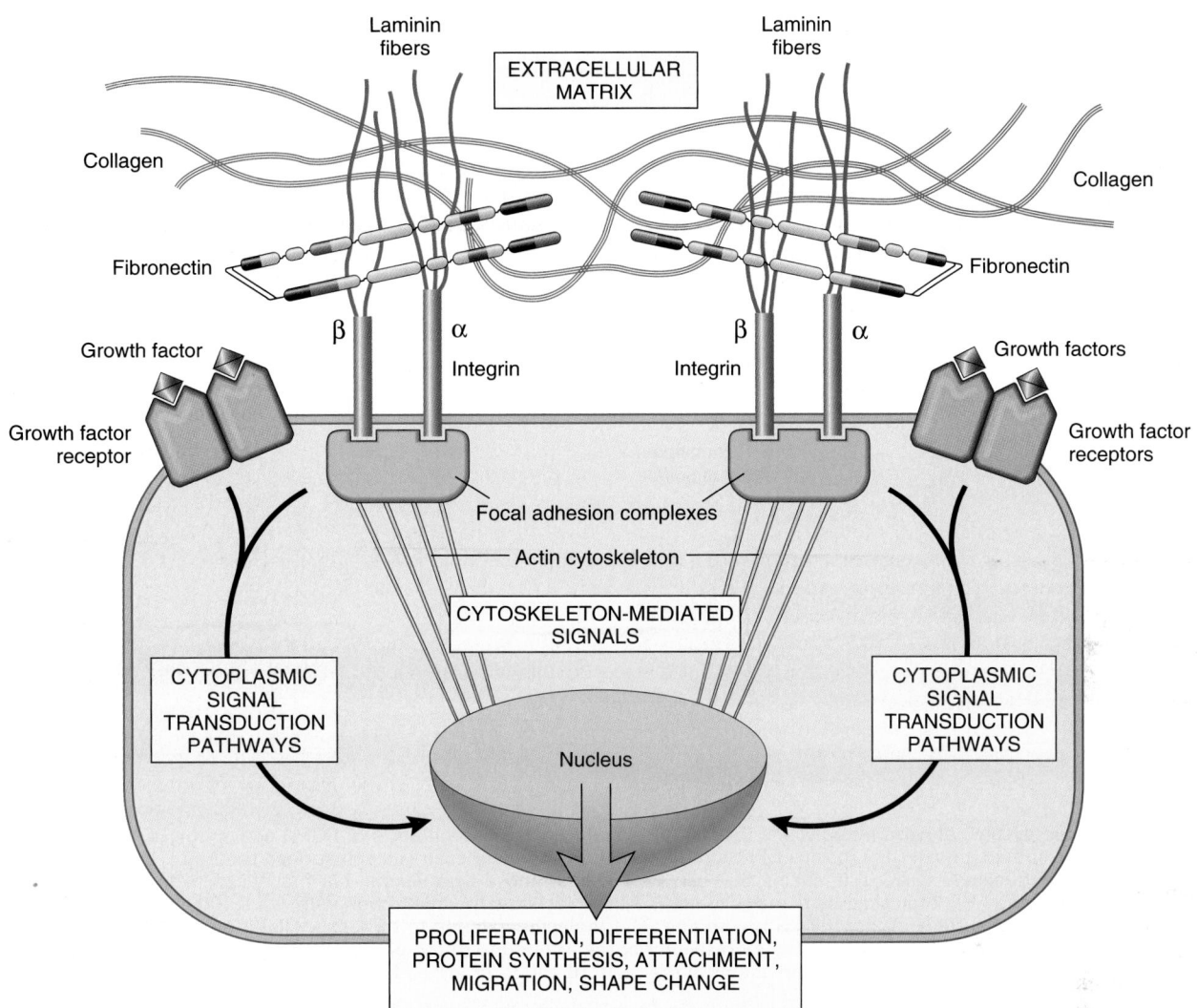

FIGURE 3–13 Mechanisms by which ECM components and growth factors interact and activate signaling pathways. Integrins bind ECM components and interact with the cytoskeleton at focal adhesion complexes (protein aggregates that include vinculin, α-actin, and talin). This can initiate the production of intracellular messengers or can directly mediate nuclear signals. Cell surface receptors for growth factors may activate signal transduction pathways that overlap with those activated by integrins. Signaling from ECM components and growth factors is integrated by the cell to produce various responses, including changes in cell proliferation, locomotion, and differentiation.

tenascin family, which consist of large multimeric proteins involved in morphogenesis and cell adhesion.

GLYCOSAMINOGLYCANS (GAGS) AND PROTEOGLYCANS

GAGs make up the third type of component in the ECM, besides the fibrous structural proteins and cell adhesion proteins. *GAGs consist of long repeating polymers of specific disaccharides.* With the exception of *hyaluronan* (discussed later), GAGs are linked to a core protein, forming molecules called *proteoglycans.*[78] Proteoglycans are remarkable in their diversity. At most sites, ECM may contain several different core proteins, each containing different GAGs. Proteoglycans were originally described as ground substances or *mucopolysaccharides*, whose main function was to organize the ECM, but it is now recognized that these molecules have diverse roles in regulating connective tissue structure and permeability (Fig. 3–14). Proteoglycans can be integral membrane proteins

and, through their binding to other proteins and the activation of growth factors and chemokines, act as modulators of inflammation, immune responses, and cell growth and differentiation.

There are four structurally distinct families of GAGs: *heparan sulfate, chondroitin/dermatan sulfate, keratan sulfate, and hyaluronan (HA).* The first three of these families are synthesized and assembled in the Golgi apparatus and rough endoplasmic reticulum as proteoglycans. By contrast, HA is produced at the plasma membrane by enzymes called hyaluronan synthases and is not linked to a protein backbone.

HA is a polysaccharide of the GAG family found in the ECM of many tissues and is abundant in heart valves, skin and skeletal tissues, synovial fluid, the vitreous of the eye, and the umbilical cord.[79] It is a huge molecule that consists of many repeats of a simple disaccharide stretched end-to-end. It binds a large amount of water (about 1000-fold its own weight), forming a viscous hydrated gel that gives connective tissue the ability to resist compression forces. HA helps provide

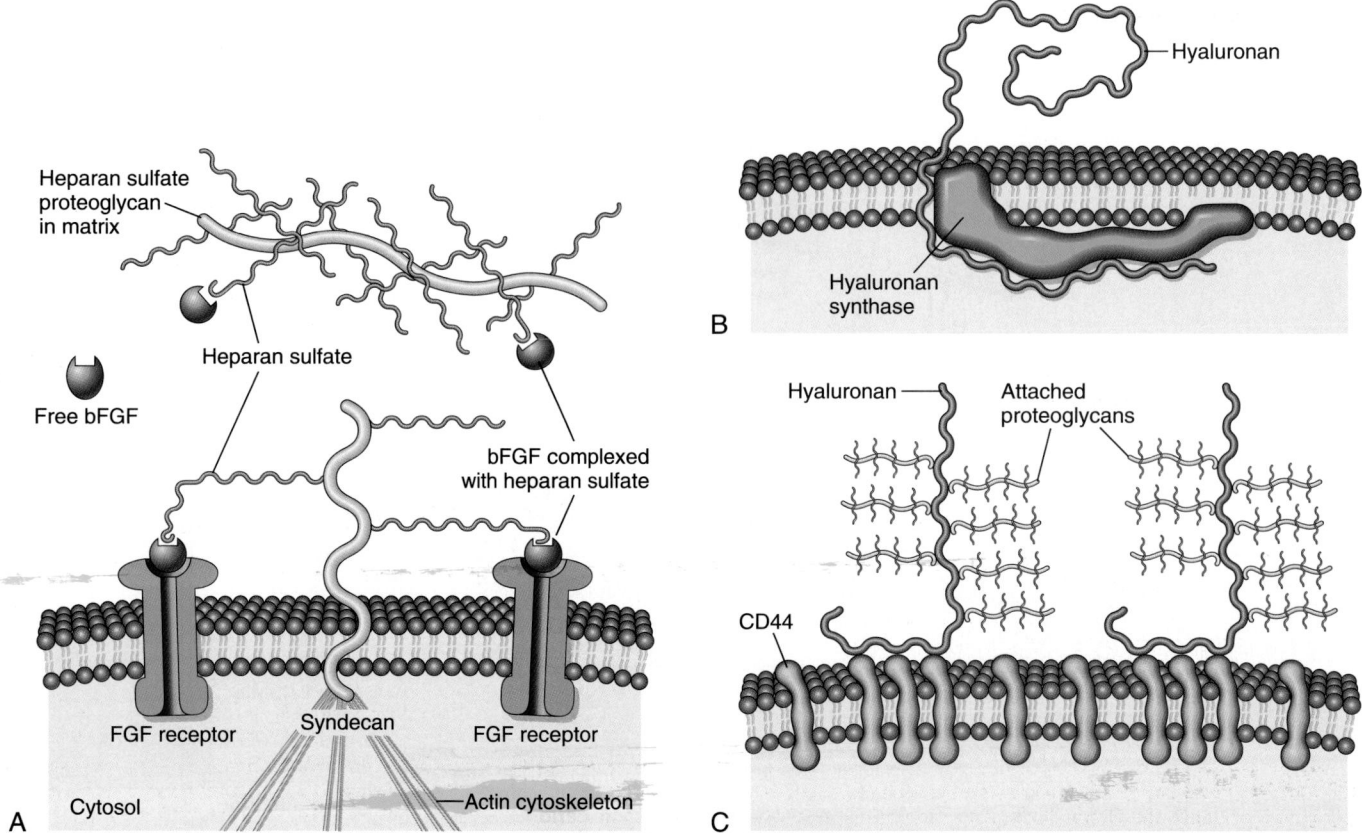

FIGURE 3–14   Proteoglycans, glycosaminoglycans (GAGs), and hyaluronan. **A,** Regulation of FGF-2 activity by ECM and cellular proteoglycans. Heparan sulfate binds FGF-2 (basic FGF) secreted into the ECM. Syndecan is a cell surface proteoglycan with a transmembrane core protein, extracellular GAG side chains that can bind FGF-2, and a cytoplasmic tail that binds to the actin cytoskeleton. Syndecan side chains bind FGF-2 released by damage to the ECM and facilitate the interaction with cell surface receptors. **B,** Synthesis of hyaluronan at the inner surface of the plasma membrane. The molecule extends to the extracellular space, while still attached to hyaluronan synthase. **C,** Hyaluronan chains in the extracellular space are bound to the plasma membrane through the CD44 receptor. Multiple proteoglycans may attach to hyaluronan chains in the ECM. (**B** and **C,** modified from Toole KR: Hyaluronan: from extracellular glue to pericellular cue. Nat Rev Cancer 4:528, 2004.)

resilience and lubrication to many types of connective tissue, notably for the cartilage in joints. Its concentration increases in inflammatory diseases such as rheumatoid arthritis, scleroderma, psoriasis, and osteoarthritis. Enzymes called hyaluronidases fragment HA into lower molecular weight molecules (LMW HA) that have different functions than the parent molecule. LMW HA produced by endothelial cells binds to the CD44 receptor on leukocytes, promoting the recruitment of leukocytes to the sites of inflammation. In addition, LMW HA molecules stimulate the production of inflammatory cytokines and chemokines by white cells recruited to the sites of injury. The leukocyte recruitment process and the production of pro-inflammatory molecules by LMW HA are strictly regulated processes; these activities are beneficial if short-lived, but their persistence may lead to prolonged inflammation.

Healing by Repair, Scar Formation and Fibrosis

If tissue injury is severe or chronic, and results in damage of both parenchymal cells and the stromal framework of the tissue, healing can not be accomplished by regeneration.

Under these conditions, the main healing process is *repair by deposition of collagen and other ECM components, causing the formation of a scar.* In contrast to regeneration which involves the restitution of tissue components, repair is a fibroproliferative response that "patches" rather than restores the tissue. The term scar is most often used in connection to *wound healing* in the skin, but is also used to describe the replacement of parenchymal cells in any tissue by collagen, as in the heart after myocardial infarction. Repair by connective tissue deposition includes the following basic features:

- *inflammation*
- *angiogenesis,*
- *migration and proliferation of fibroblasts,*
- *scar formation*
- *connective tissue remodeling.*

We will examine all of these events under the context of cutaneous wound healing, as a prototype repair process. Suffice to say here that regardless of site, the inflammatory reaction elicited by the injury contains the damage, removes injured tissue, and promotes the deposition of ECM components in the area of injury, at the same time that angiogenesis is stimulated. However, if the damage persists, inflammation

A. Angiogenesis from pre-existing vessels

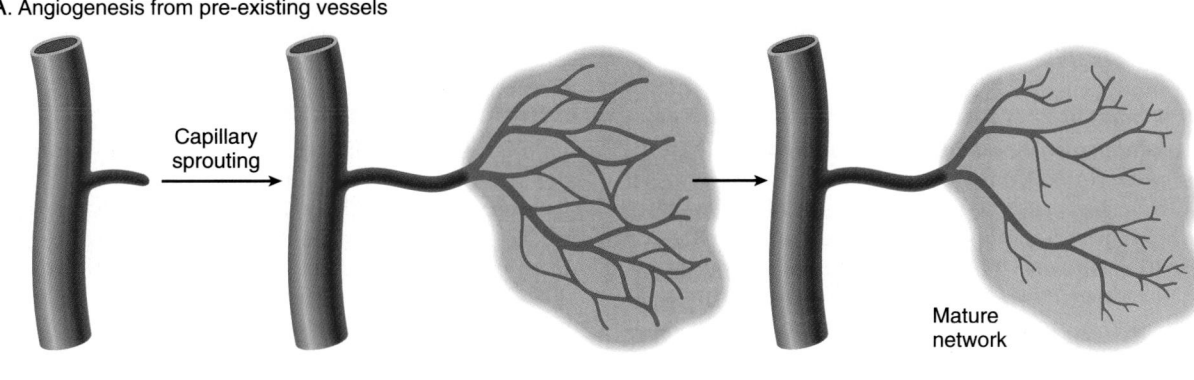

B. Angiogenesis by mobilization of EPCs from the bone marrow

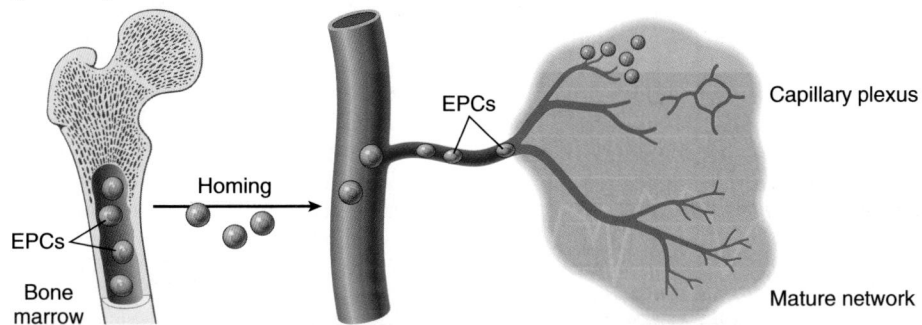

FIGURE 3–15 Angiogenesis by mobilization of endothelial precursor cells (EPCs) from the bone marrow and from preexisting vessels (capillary growth). **A,** In angiogenesis from preexisting vessels, endothelial cells from these vessels become motile and proliferate to form capillary sprouts. Regardless of the initiating mechanism, vessel maturation (stabilization) involves the recruitment of pericytes and smooth muscle cells to form the periendothelial layer. **B,** EPCs are mobilized from the bone marrow and may migrate to a site of injury or tumor growth. At these sites, EPCs differentiate and form a mature network by linking to existing vessels. (Modified from Conway EM et al: Molecular mechanisms of blood vessel growth. Cardiovasc Res 49:507, 2001.)

becomes chronic, leading to an excess deposition of connective tissue known as *fibrosis*. In most healing processes, a combination of repair and regeneration occurs. The relative contributions of repair and regeneration are influenced by: (1) the proliferative capacity of the cells of the tissue; (2) the integrity of the extracellular matrix; and (3) the resolution or chronicity of the injury and inflammation.

Because of the great importance of angiogenesis in processes other than wound healing, we start with a discussion of the mechanisms of angiogenesis before considering the steps of cutaneous wound healing.

MECHANISMS OF ANGIOGENESIS

Angiogenesis is a fundamental process that affects physiologic reactions (e.g. wound healing, regeneration, the vascularization of ischemic tissues, and menstruation), and pathologic processes, such as tumor development and metastasis, diabetic retinopathy, and chronic inflammation. Therefore great efforts have been made to understand the mechanisms of angiogenesis, and to develop agents that have pro- or anti-angiogenic activity.

Around 4000 BC, Egyptian physicians believed that there were "vessels for every part of the body, which are hollow, having a mouth which opens to absorb medications and eliminate waste".[80] Fortunately, our understanding of blood vessels

has clearly improved since then.[81,82] We know now that blood vessels are assembled during embryonic development by *vasculogenesis*, in which a primitive vascular network is established from endothelial cell precursors (*angioblasts*), or from dual hemopoietic/endothelial cell precursors called *hemangioblasts*. Blood vessel formation in adults, known as *angiogenesis* or *neovascularization*, involves the branching and extension of adjacent pre-existing vessels, but it can also occur by recruitment of endothelial progenitor cells (EPCs) from the bone marrow (Fig. 3–15).[81]

Angiogenesis from Preexisting Vessels. In this type of angiogenesis there is vasodilation and increased permeability of the existing vessels, degradation of ECM, and migration of endothelial cells. The major steps are listed below.

- ○ *Vasodilation* in response to nitric oxide, and VEGF-induced increased permeability of the preexisting vessel
- ○ Proteolytic *degradation of the basement membrane of* the parent vessel by matrix metalloproteinases (MMPs) and disruption of cell-to-cell contact between endothelial cells by plasminogen activator
- ○ *Migration of endothelial cells* toward the angiogenic stimulus
- ○ *Proliferation of endothelial cells*, just behind the leading front of migrating cells

○ *Maturation of endothelial cells*, which includes inhibition of growth and remodeling into capillary tubes
○ *Recruitment of periendothelial cells* (pericytes and vascular smooth muscle cells) to form the mature vessel

Angiogenesis from Endothelial Precursor Cells (EPCs).
EPCs can be recruited from the bone marrow into tissues to initiate angiogenesis (Fig. 3–15). The nature of the homing mechanism is uncertain. These cells express some markers of hematopoietic stem cells as well as VEGFR-2, and vascular endothelial–cadherin (VE-cadherin). EPCs may contribute to the re-endothelization of vascular implants and the neovascularization of ischemic organs, cutaneous wounds, and tumors. The number of circulating EPCs increases greatly in patients with ischemic conditions, suggesting that EPCs may influence vascular function and determine the risk of cardiovascular diseases.

Growth Factors and Receptors Involved in Angiogenesis

Despite the diversity of factors that participate in angiogenesis, VEGF is the most important growth factor in adult tissues undergoing physiologic angiogenesis (e.g., proliferating endometrium) as well as angiogenesis occurring in chronic inflammation, wound healing, tumors, and diabetic retinopathy.[81,82]

As mentioned earlier,[58] VEGF is secreted by many mesenchymal and stromal cells. Of the various receptors for VEGF, VEGFR-2, a tyrosine kinase receptor, is the most important in angiogenesis. It is expressed by endothelial cells and their precursors, by other cell types, and by many tumor cells. VEGF, or more specifically, its circulating isoforms $VEGF_{121}$ and $VEGF_{165}$, signal through VEGFR-2 (also known as KDR in humans and flk-1 in mice). VEGF induces the migration of EPCs in the bone marrow, and enhances the proliferation and differentiation of these cells at sites of angiogenesis. In angiogenesis originating from preexisting local vessels, VEGF signaling stimulates the survival of endothelial cells, their proliferation and their motility, initiating the sprouting of new capillaries. The main components of the VEGF/VEGFR system and their main actions are listed in Table 3–3. Endothelial cell proliferation, differentiation, and migration can also be stimulated by FGF-2.

Given the multiplicity of VEGF effects and the diverse mechanisms that regulate its expression, how do endothelial cells develop into a perfect pattern of vessels during angiogenesis? One recently identified mechanism for the modulation of vasculogenesis is the Notch pathway, which promotes the proper branching of new vessels and prevents excessive angiogenesis by decreasing the responsiveness to VEGF.[83–85] Notch ligands and receptors are membrane-bound molecules conserved between species. In mammals there are five Notch ligands (Jagged 1 and 2, and Delta-like ligand [Dll] 1, 3, and 4) and four transmembrane receptors (Notch 1–4). The receptors contain EGF-like repeats on their extracellular surface that serve as ligand-binding sites (Fig. 3–16). The Delta-like ligand 4 (Dll4) ligand is endothelial cell–specific and is expressed in arteries and capillaries but not in veins; the importance of this ligand is demonstrated by the embryonic lethality of mice that lack a single Delta-like ligand 4 allele. During angiogenesis the leading cell, known as a tip cell, undergoes proliferation and migration, but stalk cells maintain their connection with the existing vessel. VEGF induces Delta-like ligand 4 in tip cells, while Notch1 and Notch4 are expressed in stalk cells (see Fig. 3–16C). The interaction between Delta-like ligand 4 and Notch receptors in adjacent tip and stalk cells leads to a two-step proteolytic cleavage of the receptor, releasing the Notch intracellular domain, which translocates to the nucleus and activates genes that dampen responsiveness to VEGF. Blockade of Delta-like ligand 4 causes increased proliferation of endothelial cells and capillary sprouting; VEGF blockade has the opposite effects

TABLE 3–3 Vascular Endothelial Growth Factor (VEGF)	
Proteins	Family members: VEGF (VEGF-A), VEGF-B, VEGF-C, VEGF-D Dimeric glycoprotein with multiple isoforms Targeted mutations in VEGF result in defective vasculogenesis and angiogenesis.
Production	Expressed at low levels in a variety of adult tissues and at higher levels in a few sites, such as podocytes in the glomerulus and cardiac myocytes
Inducing agents	Hypoxia TGF-β PDGF TGF-α
Receptors	VEGFR-1 VEGFR-2 VEGFR-3 (lymphatic endothelial cells) Targeted mutations in the receptors result in lack of vasculogenesis
Functions	Promotes angiogenesis Increases vascular permeability Stimulates endothelial cell migration Stimulates endothelial cell proliferation VEGF-C selectively induces hyperplasia of lymphatic vasculature Up-regulates endothelial expression of plasminogen activator, plasminogen activator inhibitor 1, and collagenase

PDGF, platelet-derived growth factor; TGF-β, -α, transforming growth factor beta, alpha.

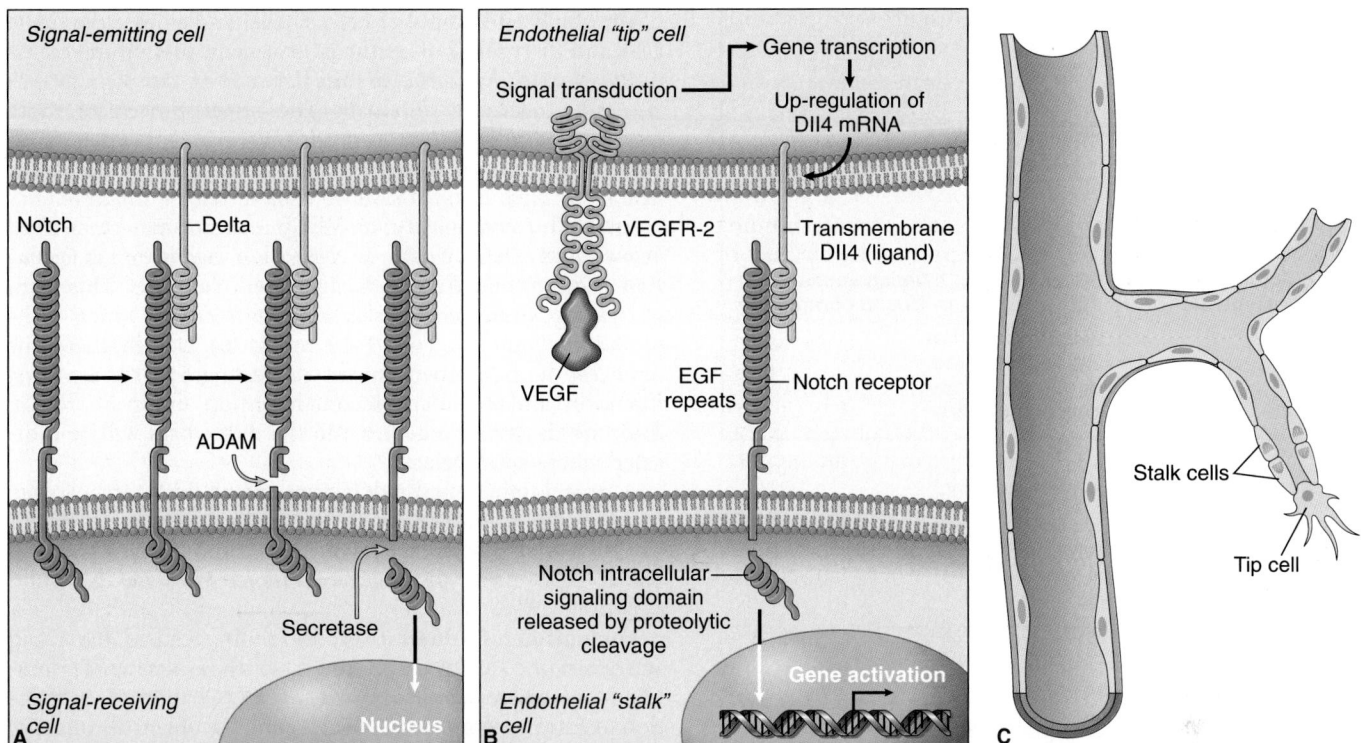

FIGURE 3–16 Notch signaling and angiogenesis. **A,** The Notch receptor binds a ligand (a delta-like ligand, Dll, is shown in the figure) located in an adjacent cell, and undergoes two proteolytic cleavages (the first cleavage by ADAM protease, the second by δ-secretase), releasing a C-terminal fragment known as Notch intracellular domain (Notch-ICD). **B,** Notch signaling in endothelial cells during angiogenesis, triggered by the binding of the Dll4 ligand in a tip cell to a Notch receptor in a stalk cell. Notch-ICD migrates into the nucleus and activates the transcription of target genes. **C,** Sprouting angiogenesis, showing a migrating tip cell and stalk cells connected to the endothelial cells of the main vessel. (**A,** modified from Weinberg RA: The Biology of Cancer. New York, Garland Science, 2007, Fig. 5.22; **B,** modified from Kerbel RS: Tumor angiogenesis. N Engl J Med 358:2039, 2008.)

and also decreases the survival of endothelial cells (Fig. 3–17).

Regardless of the process that leads to capillary formation, newly formed vessels are fragile and need to become "stabilized." Stabilization requires the recruitment of pericytes and smooth muscle cells (periendothelial cells) and the deposition of ECM proteins. *Angiopoietins 1 and 2 (Ang1 and Ang2)*, PDGF, and TGF-β participate in the stabilization process. Ang1 interacts with a receptor on endothelial cells called *Tie2* to recruit periendothelial cells. PDGF participates in the recruitment of

DLL4 blockade		VEGF blockade
Sprouting ↑	DLL4/Notch	Sprouting ↓
EC proliferation ↑		EC proliferation ↓
Vessel lumen size ↓		EC survival ↓
Vascular organization ↓	VEGF/VEGFR	Vascular organization ↑

FIGURE 3–17 Interactions between Notch and VEGF during angiogenesis. VEGF stimulates delta-like ligand 4 (Dll4)/Notch, which inhibits VEGFR signaling. Compared with unperturbed angiogenesis, Dll4 blockade causes an increase in capillary sprouting and endothelial cell (EC) proliferation, creating vessels that are disorganized and have a small lumen size. VEGF blockade decreases capillary sprouting, and the proliferation and survival of ECs. (Courtesy of Minhong Yan, Genentech, San Francisco, CA).

smooth muscle cells, while TGF-β stabilizes newly formed vessels by enhancing the production of ECM proteins.[58] The Ang1-Tie2 interaction mediates vessel maturation from simple endothelial tubes into more elaborate vascular structures and helps maintain endothelial quiescence. Ang2, in contrast, which also interacts with Tie2, has the opposite effect, making endothelial cells become either more responsive to stimulation by growth factors such as VEGF or, in the absence of VEGF, more responsive to inhibitors of angiogenesis. A telling proof of the importance of these molecules is the existence of a genetic disorder caused by mutations in *Tie2* that is characterized by venous malformations. Agents or conditions that stimulate VEGF expression, such as certain cytokines and growth factors (e.g., TGF-β, PDGF, TGF-α), and notably, *tissue hypoxia*, can influence physiologic and pathologic angiogenesis. *VEGF transcription is regulated by the transcription factor HIF, which is induced by hypoxia.*

ECM Proteins as Regulators of Angiogenesis

A key component of angiogenesis is the motility and directed migration of endothelial cells, required for the formation of new blood vessels. These processes are controlled by several classes of proteins, including (1) *integrins*, especially $\alpha_v\beta_3$, which is critical for the formation and maintenance of newly formed blood vessels, (2) *matricellular proteins*, including thrombospondin 1, SPARC, and tenascin C, which destabilize

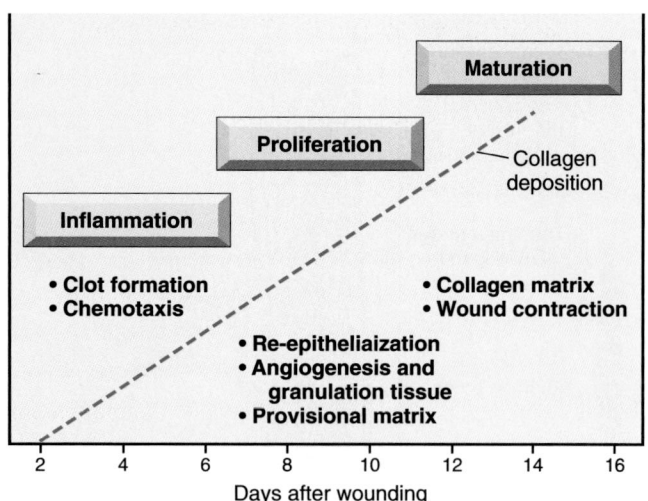

FIGURE 3-18 Phases of cutaneous wound healing: inflammation, proliferation, and maturation (see text for details). (Modified from Broughton G et al: The basic science of wound healing. Plast Reconstr Surg 117:12S–34S, 2006.)

cell-matrix interactions and therefore promote angiogenesis, and (3) *proteinases*, such as the plasminogen activators and MMPs, which are important in tissue remodeling during endothelial invasion. Additionally, these proteinases cleave extracellular proteins, releasing matrix-bound growth factors such as VEGF and FGF-2 that stimulate angiogenesis. Proteinases can also release inhibitors such as *endostatin*, a small fragment of collagen that inhibits endothelial proliferation and angiogenesis. $\alpha_V\beta_3$ Integrin expression in endothelial cells is stimulated by hypoxia and has multiple effects on angiogenesis: it interacts with a metalloproteinase (MMP-2, discussed below), it binds to and regulates the activity of VEGFR-2, and it mediates adhesion to ECM components such as fibronectin, thrombospondin, and OPN.[72]

The review of ECM components, cell-matrix interactions, and the mechanisms of angiogenesis sets the stage for the discussion of tissue healing that involves repair and scar formation, with special emphasis on the steps and main mechanisms of cutaneous wound healing.

CUTANEOUS WOUND HEALING

Cutaneous wound healing is divided into three phases: inflammation, proliferation, and maturation[86] (Fig. 3–18). These phases overlap, and their separation is somewhat arbitrary, but they help to understand the sequence of events that take place in the healing of skin wounds. The initial injury causes platelet adhesion and aggregation and the formation of a clot in the surface of the wound, leading to *inflammation*. In the *proliferative phase* there is formation of granulation tissue, proliferation and migration of connective tissue cells, and re-epithelialization of the wound surface. *Maturation* involves ECM deposition, tissue remodeling, and wound contraction.

The simplest type of cutaneous wound repair is the healing of a clean, uninfected surgical incision approximated by surgical sutures (Fig. 3–19). Such healing is referred to as *healing by primary union* or *by first intention*.[86–88] The incision causes

death of a limited number of epithelial and connective tissue cells and disruption of epithelial basement membrane continuity. *Re-epithelialization to close the wound occurs with formation of a relatively thin scar.* The repair process is more complicated in excisional wounds that create large defects on the skin surface, causing extensive loss of cells and tissue. *The healing of these wounds involves a more intense inflammatory reaction, the formation of abundant granulation tissue (described below), and extensive collagen deposition, leading to the formation of a substantial scar, which generally contracts.* This form of healing is referred to as *healing by secondary union* or *by second intention* (see Figs. 3–19 and 3–20). Despite these differences, the basic mechanisms of healing by primary (first intention) and secondary (second intention) union are similar. They are described together and the differences will be indicated where appropriate.

A large number of growth factors and cytokines are involved in cutaneous wound healing.[89] The main agents, and the steps at which they participate in the repair process, are listed in Table 3–4. We next discuss the sequence of events in wound healing.

Formation of Blood Clot. Wounding causes the rapid activation of coagulation pathways, which results in *the formation of a blood clot on the wound surface* (Chapter 4). In addition to entrapped red cells, the clot contains fibrin, fibronectin, and complement components. *The clot serves to stop bleeding and also as a scaffold for migrating cells, which are attracted by growth factors, cytokines and chemokines released into the area.*[89] Release of VEGF leads to increased vessel permeability and edema. However, dehydration occurs at the external surface of the clot, forming a scab that covers the wound. In wounds causing large tissue deficits, the fibrin clot is larger, and there is more exudate and necrotic debris in the wounded area. Within 24 hours, *neutrophils* appear at the margins of the incision, and use the scaffold provided by the fibrin clot to march in. They release proteolytic enzymes that clean out debris and invading bacteria.

Formation of Granulation Tissue. Fibroblasts and vascular endothelial cells proliferate in the first 24 to 72 hours of the repair process to form a specialized type of tissue called *granulation tissue*, which is a hallmark of tissue repair. The term derives from its pink, soft, granular appearance on the surface of wounds. Its characteristic histologic feature is *the presence of new small blood vessels (angiogenesis) and the proliferation of fibroblasts* (Fig. 3–21). These new vessels are leaky, allowing the passage of plasma proteins and fluid into the extravascular space. Thus, new granulation tissue is often edematous. Granulation tissue progressively invades the incision space; the amount of *granulation tissue that is formed depends on the size of the tissue deficit created by the wound and the intensity of inflammation.* Hence, it is much more prominent in healing by secondary union. By 5 to 7 days, granulation tissue fills the wound area and neovascularization is maximal. The mechanisms of angiogenesis in repair processes were discussed earlier in this chapter.

Cell Proliferation and Collagen Deposition. Neutrophils are largely replaced by *macrophages* by 48 to 96 hours. *Macrophages are key cellular constituents of tissue repair*, clearing extracellular debris, fibrin, and other foreign material at the site of repair, and promoting angiogenesis and ECM deposition (Fig. 3–22).

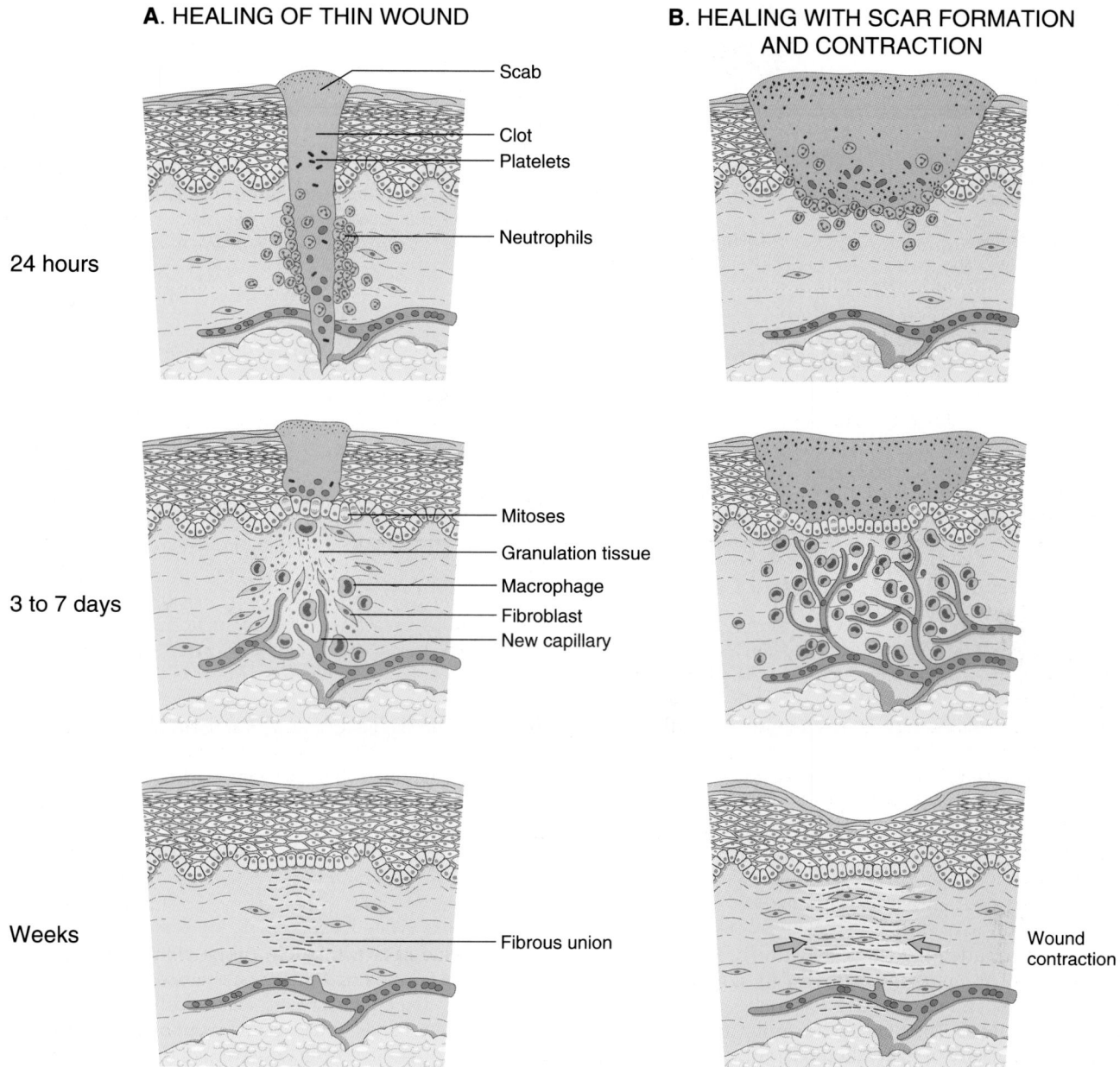

A. HEALING OF THIN WOUND

Scab
Clot
Platelets
Neutrophils

24 hours

Mitoses
Granulation tissue
Macrophage
Fibroblast
New capillary

3 to 7 days

Weeks

Fibrous union

B. HEALING WITH SCAR FORMATION
AND CONTRACTION

Wound
contraction

FIGURE 3–19 Wound healing and scar formation. **A,** Healing of wound that caused little loss of tissue: note the small amount of granulation tissue, and formation of a thin scar with minimal contraction. **B,** Healing of large wound: note large amounts of granulation tissue and scar tissue, and wound contraction.

Migration of fibroblasts to the site of injury is driven by chemokines, TNF, PDGF, TGF-β, and FGF. Their subsequent proliferation is triggered by multiple growth factors, including PDGF, EGF, TGF-β, FGF, and the cytokines IL-1 and TNF (see Table 3–4). Macrophages are the main source for these factors, although other inflammatory cells and platelets may also produce them. Collagen fibers are now present at the margins of the incision, but at first these are vertically oriented and do not bridge the incision. In 24 to 48 hours, *spurs of epithelial cells move from the wound edge (initially with little cell proliferation) along the cut margins of the dermis, depositing basement membrane components* as they move. They fuse in the midline beneath the surface scab, producing a thin, continuous epithelial layer that closes the wound. Full epithelialization of the wound surface is much slower in healing by secondary union because the gap to be

bridged is much greater. Subsequent epithelial cell proliferation thickens the epidermal layer. Macrophages stimulate fibroblasts to produce FGF-7 (keratinocyte growth factor) and IL-6, which enhance keratinocyte migration and proliferation. Other mediators of re-epithelialization are HGF and HB-EGF.[89] Signaling through the chemokine receptor CXCR 3 also promotes skin re-epithelialization.

Concurrently with epithelialization, collagen fibrils become more abundant and begin to bridge the incision. At first a provisional matrix containing fibrin, plasma fibronectin, and type III collagen is formed, but this is replaced by a matrix composed primarily of type I collagen. *TGF-β is the most important fibrogenic agent* (see Table 3–4). It is produced by most of the cells in granulation tissue and causes fibroblast migration and proliferation, increased synthesis of collagen

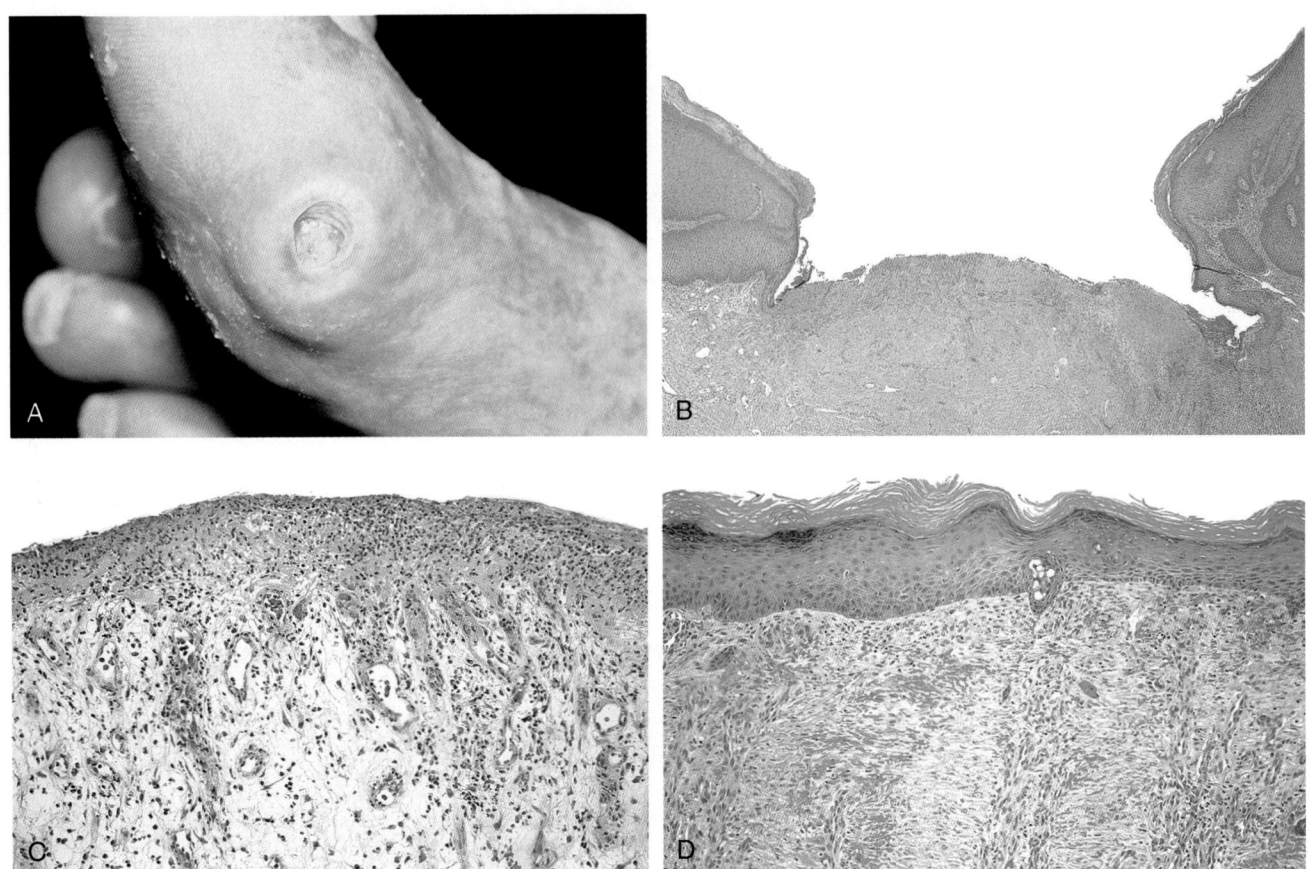

FIGURE 3–20 Healing of skin ulcers. **A,** Pressure ulcer of the skin, commonly found in diabetic patients. The histologic slides show: **B,** a skin ulcer with a large gap between the edges of the lesion; **C,** a thin layer of epidermal re-epithelialization and extensive granulation tissue formation in the dermis; and **D,** continuing re-epithelialization of the epidermis and wound contraction. (Courtesy of Z. Argenyi, MD, University of Washington, Seattle, WA.)

and fibronectin, and decreased degradation of ECM by metal-loproteinases. The epidermis recovers its normal thickness and architecture, and surface keratinization.

Scar Formation. The leukocytic infiltrate, edema, and increased vascularity largely disappear during the second week. Blanching begins, accomplished by the increased accumulation of collagen within the wound area and regression of

TABLE 3–4 Growth Factors and Cytokines Affecting Various Steps in Wound Healing

Monocyte chemotaxis	Chemokines, TNF, PDGF, FGF, TGF-β
Fibroblast migration/replication	PDGF, EGF, FGF, TGF-β, TNF, IL-1
Keratinocyte replication	HB-EGF, FGF-7, HGF
Angiogenesis	VEGF, angiopoietins, FGF
Collagen synthesis	TGF-β, PDGF
Collagenase secretion	PDGF, FGF, TNF; TGF-β inhibits

HB-EGF, heparin-binding EGF; IL-1, interleukin 1; TNF, tumor necrosis factor; other abbreviations as given in Table 3–1.

vascular channels. Ultimately, the original granulation tissue scaffolding is converted into a pale, avascular scar, composed of spindle-shaped fibroblasts, dense collagen, fragments of elastic tissue, and other ECM components. The dermal appendages that have been destroyed in the line of the incision are permanently lost, although in rats new hair follicles may develop in large healing wounds under Wnt stimulation.[90] This result suggests that, with appropriate treatment procedures, regrowth of skin appendages during wound healing might be achieved in humans. *By the end of the first month, the scar is made up of acellular connective tissue devoid of inflammatory infiltrate, covered by intact epidermis.*

Wound Contraction. *Wound contraction generally occurs in large surface wounds.* The contraction helps to close the wound by decreasing the gap between its dermal edges and by reducing the wound surface area. Hence, it is an important feature in healing by secondary union. The initial steps of wound contraction involve the formation, at the edge of the wound, of a network of *myofibroblasts* that express smooth muscle α-actin and vimentin. These cells have ultrastructural characteristics of smooth muscle cells, contract in the wound tissue, and may produce large amounts of ECM components (see discussion of hypertrophic scars in this chapter), such as type I collagen, tenascin-C, SPARC, and extra-domain fibro-

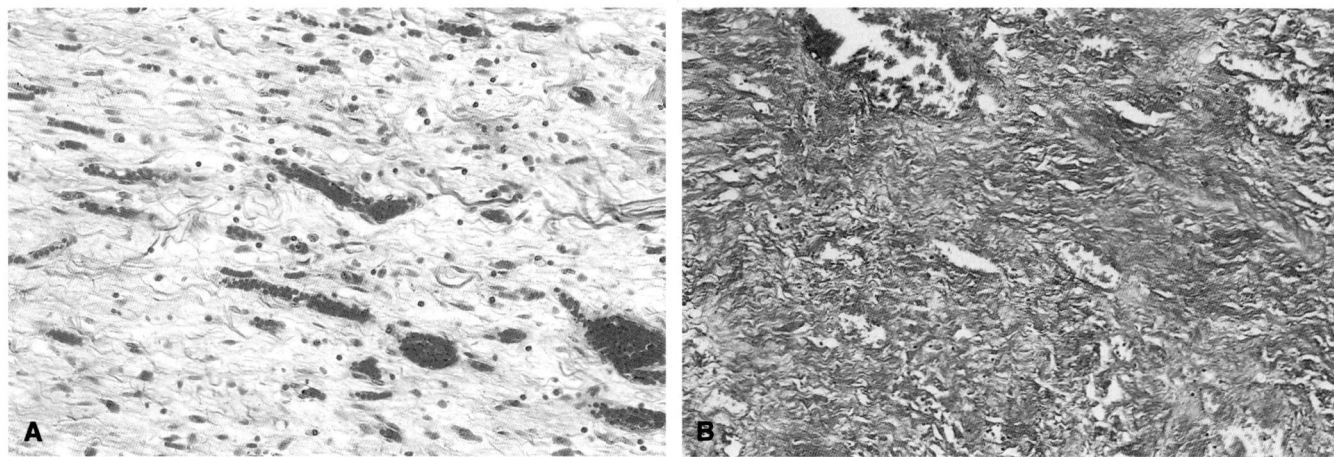

FIGURE 3–21 **A,** Granulation tissue showing numerous blood vessels, edema, and a loose ECM containing occasional inflammatory cells. Collagen is stained blue by the trichrome stain; minimal mature collagen can be seen at this point. **B,** Trichrome stain of mature scar, showing dense collagen, with only scattered vascular channels.

nectin.[91] Myofibroblasts are formed from tissue fibroblasts through the effects of PDGF, TGF-β, and FGF-2 released by macrophages at the wound site, but they can also originate from bone marrow precursors known as fibrocytes, or from epithelial cells, through the process of epithelial-to-mesenchymal transition.

Connective Tissue Remodeling. *The replacement of granulation tissue with a scar involves changes in the composition of the ECM. The balance between ECM synthesis and degradation results in remodeling of the connective tissue framework – an important feature of tissue repair.* Some of the growth factors that stimulate synthesis of collagen and other connective tissue molecules also modulate the synthesis and activation of metalloproteinases, enzymes that degrade these ECM components.

Degradation of collagen and other ECM proteins is achieved by matrix metalloproteinases (MMPs), a family of enzymes that includes more than 20 members that have in common a 180-residue zinc-protease domain (MMPs should be distinguished from neutrophil elastase, cathepsin G, kinins, plasmin, and other important proteolytic enzymes, which also degrade EMC components and which are *serine proteinases, not metalloenzymes*). Matrix metalloproteinases include *interstitial collagenases (MMP-1, -2, and -3),* which cleave the fibrillar collagen types I, II, and III; *gelatinases (MMP-2 and 9),* which degrade amorphous collagen as well as fibronectin; *stromelysins (MMP-3, 10, and 11),* which act on a variety of ECM components, including proteoglycans, laminin, fibronectin, and amorphous collagens; and the family of *membrane-bound MMPs* (ADAMs) described below. MMPs are produced by fibroblasts, macrophages, neutrophils, synovial cells, and some epithelial cells. Their secretion is induced by growth factors (PDGF, FGF), cytokines (IL-1, TNF), and phagocytosis in macrophages, and is inhibited by TGF-β and steroids. Collagenases cleave collagen under physiologic conditions. They are synthesized as a latent precursor (procollagenase) that is activated by chemicals, such as free radicals produced during the oxidative burst of leukocytes, and proteinases (plasmin). Once formed, activated collagenases are rapidly inhibited by a family of specific tissue *inhibitors of metalloproteinases,* which are produced by most mesenchymal cells, thus preventing uncontrolled action of these proteases. Collagenases and their inhibitors are essential in the debridement of injured sites and in the remodeling of connective tissue necessary to repair the defect.

A large and important family of enzymes related to MMPs is called ADAM (disintegrin and metalloproteinase-domain family). Most ADAMs are anchored by a single transmembrane domain to cell surface. ADAM-17 (also known as TACE, for TNF-converting enzyme) cleaves the membrane-bound precursor forms of TNF and TGF-α, releasing the active molecules. ADAM-17 deficiency in mice causes embryonic or neonatal lethality associated with pulmonary hypoplasia. Members of the ADAM family are also involved in the pathogenesis of bronchial asthma (Chapter 15), and thrombotic microangiopathies (Chapter 13).

Recovery of Tensile Strength. Fibrillar collagens (mostly type I collagen) form a major portion of the connective tissue in repair sites and are essential for the development of strength in healing wounds. *Net collagen accumulation, however, depends not only on increased collagen synthesis but also on decreased*

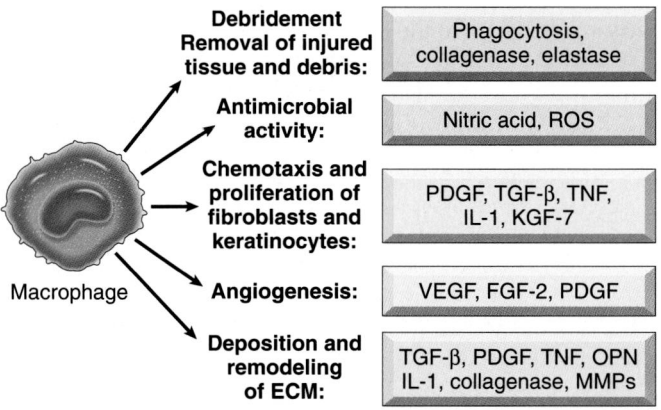

FIGURE 3–22 Multiple roles of macrophages in wound healing. Macrophages participate in wound debridement, have antimicrobial activity, stimulate chemotaxis and the activation of inflammatory cells and fibroblasts, promote angiogenesis, and stimulate matrix remodeling and synthesis. ROS, reactive oxygen species.

degradation. How long does it take for a skin wound to achieve its maximal strength? When sutures are removed from an incisional surgical wound, usually at the end of the first week, wound strength is approximately 10% that of unwounded skin. *Wound strength* increases rapidly over the next 4 weeks, slows down at approximately the third month after the original incision, and reaches a plateau at about 70% to 80% of the tensile strength of unwounded skin. Lower tensile strength in the healed wound area may persist for life. The recovery of tensile strength results from the excess of collagen synthesis over collagen degradation during the first 2 months of healing, and, at later times, from structural modifications of collagen fibers (cross-linking, increased fiber size) after collagen synthesis ceases.

LOCAL AND SYSTEMIC FACTORS THAT INFLUENCE WOUND HEALING

The adequacy of wound repair may be impaired by systemic and local host factors.

Systemic factors include those listed below:

- *Nutrition* has profound effects on wound healing. Protein deficiency, for example, and particularly vitamin C deficiency, inhibit collagen synthesis and retard healing.
- *Metabolic status* can change wound healing. Diabetes mellitus, for example, is associated with delayed healing, as a consequence of the microangiopathy that is a frequent feature of this disease (Chapter 24).
- *Circulatory status* can modulate wound healing. *Inadequate blood supply*, usually caused by arteriosclerosis or venous abnormalities (e.g., varicose veins) that retard venous drainage, also impairs healing.
- *Hormones* such as *glucocorticoids* have well-documented anti-inflammatory effects that influence various components of inflammation. These agents also inhibit collagen synthesis.

Local factors that influence healing include those listed here:

- *Infection* is the single most important cause of delay in healing, because it results in persistent tissue injury and inflammation.

- *Mechanical factors*, such as early motion of wounds, can delay healing, by compressing blood vessels and separating the edges of the wound.
- *Foreign bodies*, such as unnecessary sutures or fragments of steel, glass, or even bone, constitute impediments to healing.
- *Size, location, and type of wound.* Wounds in richly vascularized areas, such as the face, heal faster than those in poorly vascularized ones, such as the foot. As we have discussed, small incisional injuries heal faster and with less scar formation than large excisional wounds or wounds caused by blunt trauma.

PATHOLOGIC ASPECTS OF REPAIR

Complications in wound healing can arise from abnormalities in any of the basic components of the repair process. These aberrations can be grouped into three general categories: (1) *deficient scar formation*, (2) *excessive formation of the repair components*, and (3) *formation of contractures*.

- *Inadequate formation of granulation tissue or assembly of a scar* can lead to two types of complications: *wound dehiscence* and *ulceration*. Dehiscence or rupture of a wound is most common after abdominal surgery and is due to increased abdominal pressure. Vomiting, coughing, or ileus can generate mechanical stress on the abdominal wound. Wounds can ulcerate because of inadequate vascularization during healing. For example, lower extremity wounds in individuals with atherosclerotic peripheral vascular disease typically ulcerate (Chapter 11). Nonhealing wounds also form in areas devoid of sensation. These neuropathic ulcers are occasionally seen in patients with diabetic peripheral neuropathy (Chapters 24 and 27).
- *Excessive formation of the components of the repair process* can give rise to hypertrophic scars and keloids. The accumulation of excessive amounts of collagen may give rise to a raised scar known as a *hypertrophic scar*; if the scar tissue grows beyond the boundaries of the original wound and does not regress, it is called a *keloid* (Fig. 3–23). Keloid formation seems to be an individual predisposition, and for unknown reasons this aberration is somewhat more

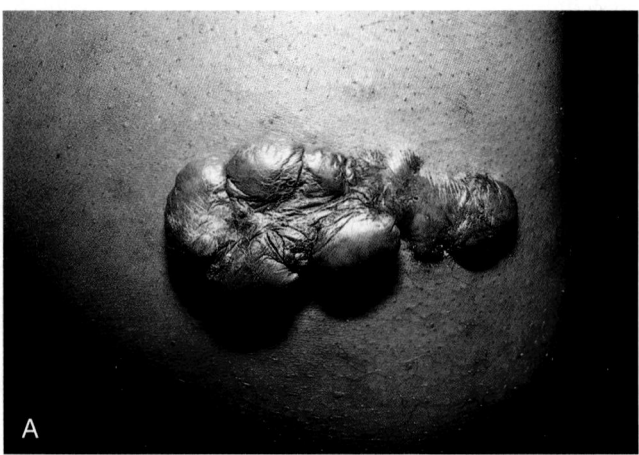
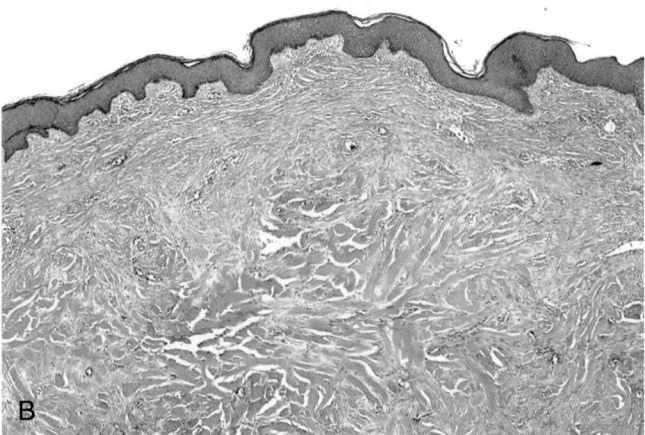

FIGURE 3–23   Keloid. **A,** Excess collagen deposition in the skin forming a raised scar known as keloid. **B,** Note the thick connective tissue deposition in the dermis. (**A,** from Murphy GF, Herzberg AJ: Atlas of Dermatopathology. Philadelphia, WB Saunders, 1996, p 219; **B,** courtesy of Z. Argenyi, MD, University of Washington, Seattle, WA.)

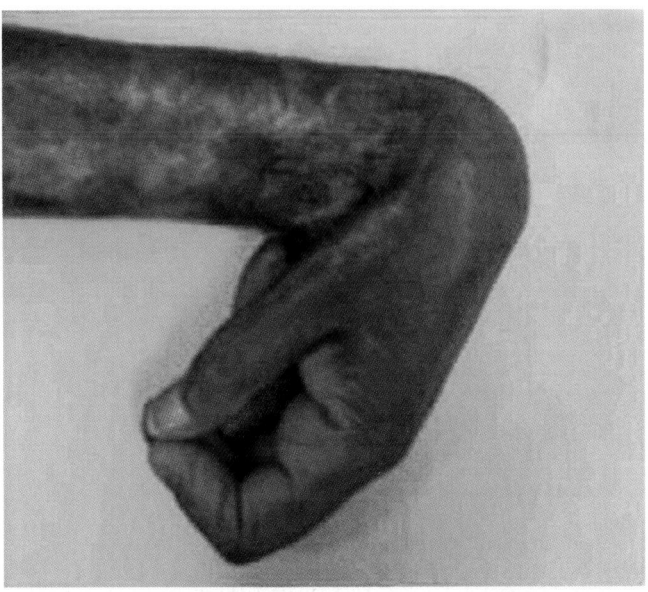

FIGURE 3-24 Wound contracture. Severe contracture of a wound after deep burn injury. (From Aarabi S et al: Hypertrophic scar formation following burns and trauma: new approaches to treatment. PLOS Med 4:e234, 2007.)

common in African Americans. Hyperthrophic scars generally develop after thermal or traumatic injury that involves the deep layers of the dermis. Collagen is produced by myofibroblasts, which persist in the lesion through the autocrine production of TGF-β, and the establishment of focal adhesions.[92]

Exuberant granulation is another deviation in wound healing consisting of the formation of excessive amounts of granulation tissue, which protrudes above the level of the surrounding skin and blocks re-epithelialization (this process has been called, with more literary fervor, *proud flesh*). Excessive granulation must be removed by cautery or surgical excision to permit restoration of the continuity of the epithelium. Finally (fortunately rarely), incisional scars or trau-

matic injuries may be followed by exuberant proliferation of fibroblasts and other connective tissue elements that may, in fact, recur after excision. Called *desmoids*, or *aggressive fibromatoses*, these lie in the interface between benign proliferations and malignant (though low-grade) tumors. The line between the benign hyperplasias characteristic of repair and neoplasia is frequently finely drawn (Chapter 7).

○ *Contraction* in the size of a wound is an important part of the normal healing process. An exaggeration of this process gives rise to *contracture* and results in deformities of the wound and the surrounding tissues. Contractures are particularly prone to develop on the palms, the soles, and the anterior aspect of the thorax. Contractures are commonly seen after serious burns and can compromise the movement of joints (Fig. 3-24).

Fibrosis

Deposition of collagen is part of normal wound healing. However, the term *fibrosis* is used more broadly to denote the excessive deposition of collagen and other ECM components in a tissue. As already mentioned, the terms *scar* and *fibrosis* are used interchangeably, but *fibrosis* most often indicates the deposition of collagen in chronic diseases. The basic mechanisms that occur in the development of fibrosis associated with chronic inflammatory diseases are generally similar to the mechanisms of skin wound healing that have been discussed in this chapter. However, in contrast to the short-lived stimulus that triggers the orderly steps of wound healing in the skin, the injurious stimulus caused by infections, autoimmune reactions, trauma, and other types of tissue injury persists in chronic diseases, causing organ dysfunction and often organ failure.

The persistence of injury leads to chronic inflammation, which is associated with the proliferation and activation of macrophages and lymphocytes, and the production of a plethora of inflammatory and fibrogenic growth factors and cytokines, mentioned earlier and summarized in Figure 3-25.

FIGURE 3-25 Development of fibrosis in chronic inflammation. The persistent stimulus of chronic inflammation activates macrophages and lymphocytes, leading to the production of growth factors and cytokines, which increase the synthesis of collagen. Deposition of collagen is enhanced by decreased activity of metalloproteinases.

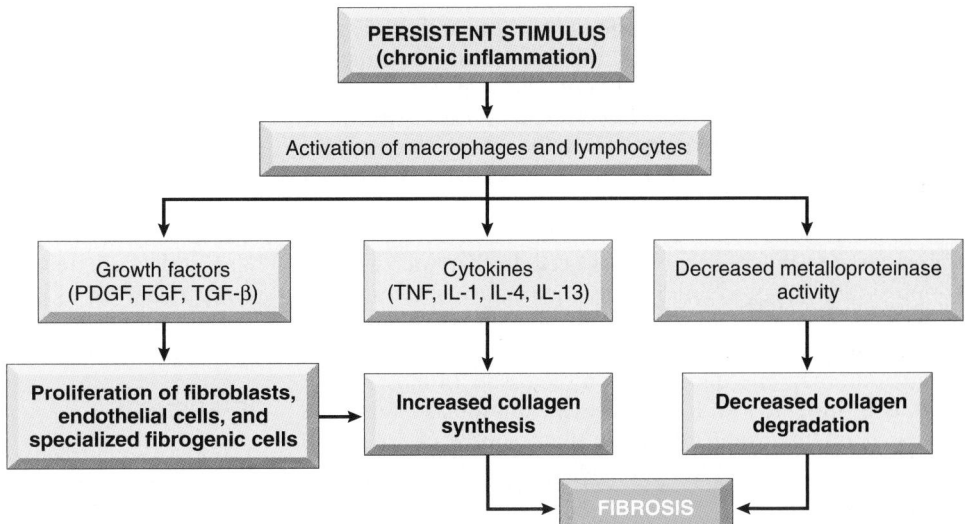

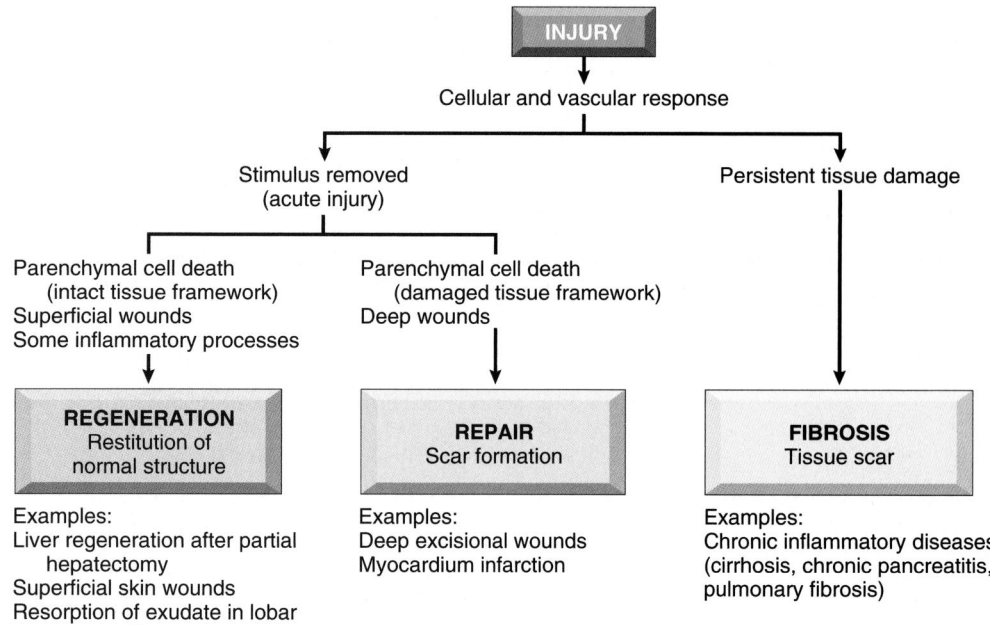

FIGURE 3–26 Repair, regeneration, and fibrosis after injury and inflammation.

The host response to harmful stimuli is orchestrated to first clear these stimuli and then heal the damage. As we discussed in Chapter 2 (see Fig. 2–10), the initial wave of the host response to external invaders and tissue injury generates "classically activated macrophages", which are effective in ingesting and destroying microbes and dead tissues. This is followed by the accumulation of "alternatively activated macrophages", which suppress the microbicidal activities and instead function to remodel tissues and promote angiogenesis and scar formation.[93] The cytokines that induce classical macrophage activation are those produced by T_H1 cells, notably IFN-γ and TNF, whereas alternative macrophage activation is best induced by IL-4 and IL-13, cytokines produced by T_H2 cells and other cells including mast cells and eosinophils. Alternatively activated macrophages produce TGF-β and other growth factors that are involved in the repair process.

TGF-β is practically always involved as an important fibrogenic agent (see Table 3–4) in these diseases, regardless of the original cause. It is produced by most of the cells in granulation tissue and causes fibroblast migration and proliferation, increased synthesis of collagen and fibronectin, and decreased degradation of ECM due to inhibition of metalloproteinases. The levels of TGF-β in tissues are not primarily regulated by the transcription of the gene but depend on the post-transcriptional activation of latent TGF-β, the rate of secretion of the active molecule, and factors in the ECM that enhance or diminish TGF-β activity.

The mechanisms that lead to the activation of TGF-β in fibrosis are not precisely known, but cell death by necrosis or apoptosis and the production of reactive oxygen species seem to be important triggers of the activation, regardless of the tissue. Similarly, the cells that produce collagen under TGF-β stimulation may vary depending on the tissue. In most cases, such as in lung and kidney fibrosis, myofibroblasts (already discussed in this chapter) are the main source of collagen, but stellate cells are the major collagen producers in liver cirrhosis.

Recent studies provide evidence for an important role for osteopontin (OPN) in would healing and fibrosis.[77] OPN is strongly expressed in fibrosis of the heart, lung, liver, kidney and some other tissues. In animal experiments, blockage of OPN expression during wound healing decreases the formation of granulation tissue and scarring.[94] Although the mechanisms by which OPN promotes fibrosis are not completely understood, recent data show that OPN is a mediator of the differentiation of myofibroblasts induced by TGF-β.

In marked contrast to wounds in adults, fetal cutaneous wounds heal without scar formation.[95,96] Several factors have been proposed to promote scarless healing, including the secretion of non-fibrogenic forms of TGF-β, the lack of osteopontin, and the absence of a T_H2 response, but no definitive results have been obtained. Given the serious organ dysfunction produced by fibrosis, there is a major effort to develop clinically useful antifibrotic agents. Among agents being tested are inhibitors of TGF-β binding or signaling, angiogenesis inhibitors, Toll-like receptors antagonists, and the decoy receptor IL-13Rα2 which blocks IL-13.

Fibrotic disorders include diverse diseases such as liver cirrhosis, systemic sclerosis, fibrosing diseases of the lung (*idiopathic pulmonary fibrosis, pneumoconioses, and drug-, radiation-induced pulmonay fibrosis), chronic pancreatitis, glomerulonephritis, and constrictive pericarditis*. These conditions are discussed in the appropriate chapters throughout the book.

This concludes the discussion, begun in Chapter 1, of cellular and tissue injury, the inflammatory reaction to such injury (Chapter 2), and tissue healing by regeneration and repair. An overview of the relationships between these processes is illustrated in Fig. 3–26.

REFERENCES

1. Goss RJ: Regeneration versus repair. In Cohen IK, Diegelman RF, Lindblad WJ (eds): Wound Healing: Biochemical and Clinical Aspects. Philadelphia: WB Saunders, 1992, p 20.

2. Fausto N, Campbell JS: The role of hepatocytes and oval cells in liver regeneration and repopulation. Mech Dev 120:117, 2003.

3. Mimeault M et al: Stem cells: a revolution in therapeutics—recent advances in stem cell biology and their therapeutic applications in regenerative medicine and cancer therapies. Clin Pharmacol Ther 82:252, 2007.

4. Ott HC et al: Perfusion-decellularized matrix: using nature's platform to engineer a bioartificial heart. Nat Med 14:213, 2008.

5. Pellettieri J, Alvarado AS: Cell turnover and adult tissue homeostasis: from humans to planarians. Annu Rev Genet 41:83, 2007.

6. Park IH et al.: Disease-specific induced pluripotent stem cells. Cell 134:877, 2008.

7. Gardner RL: Stem cells and regenerative medicine: principles, prospects and problems. C R Biol 330:465, 2007.

8. Schroeder M: Asymmetric cell division in normal and malignant hematopoietic precursor cells. Cell Stem Cell 1:479, 2007.

9. Conover JC, Notti RQ: The neural stem cell niche. Cell Tissue Res 331:211, 2008.

10. Moore KA, Lemischka IR: Stem cells and their niches. Science 311:1880, 2006.

11. Xie T, Li L: Stem cells and their niche: an inseparable relationship. Development 134:2001, 2007.

12. Takahashi K et al: Induction of pluripotent stem cells from adult human fibroblasts by defined factors. Cell 131:861, 2007.

13. Yu J et al: Induced pluripotent stem cell lines derived from human somatic cells. Science 318:1916, 2007.

14. Wu DC et al: Embryonic stem cell transplantation: potential applicability in cell replacement therapy and regenerative medicine. Front Biosci 12:4525, 2007.

15. Laflamme MA et al: Cardiomyocytes derived from human embryonic stem cells in pro-survival factors enhance function of infarcted rat hearts. Nat Biotechnol 25:1015, 2007.

16. Manis JP: Knock out, knock in, knock down—genetically manipulated mice and the Nobel Prize. N Engl J Med 357:2426, 2007.

17. Paterson L et al: Application of reproductive biotechnology in animals: implications and potentials. Applications of reproductive cloning. Anim Reprod Sci 79:137, 2003.

18. Han Z et al: Therapeutic cloning: status and prospects. Curr Opin Mol Ther 9:392, 2007.

19. Okita K et al: Generation of germline-competent induced pluripotent stem cells. Nature 448:313, 2007.

20. Lowry WE et al.: Generation of human induced pluripotent stem cells from dermal fibroblasts. Proc Natl Acad Sci USA 105:2883, 2008.

21. Chambers I et al: Nanog safeguards pluripotency and mediates germline development. Nature 450:1230, 2007.

22. Chen L, Daley GQ: Molecular basis of pluripotency. Hum Mol Genet 17: R23, 2008.

23. Hanna J et al: Treatment of sickle cell anemia mouse model with iPS cells generated from autologous skin. Science 318:1920, 2007.

24. Aoi T et al: Generation of pluripotent stem cells from adult mouse liver and stomach cells. Science 321:699, 2008.

25. Hanna J et al.: Direct reprogramming of terminally differentiated mature B lymphocytes to pluripotency. Cell 133:250, 2008.

26. Nakagawa M et al: Generation of induced pluripotent stem cells without Myc from mouse and human fibroblasts. Nat Biotechnol 26:101, 2008.

27. Barker N et al: Identification of stem cells in the small intestine and colon by marker gene *Lgr5*. Nature 449:1003, 2007.

28. Thorgeirsson SS, Grisham JW: Hematopoietic cells as hepatocyte stem cells: a critical review of the evidence. Hepatology 43:2, 2006.

29. Rizvi AZ et al: Bone marrow–derived cells fuse with normal and transformed intestinal stem cells. Proc Natl Acad Sci U S A 103:6321, 2006.

30. Camargo FD et al: Hematopoietic myelomonocytic cells are the major source of hepatocyte fusion partners. J Clin Invest 113:1266, 2004.

31. Vieyra DS et al: Plasticity and tissue regenerative potential of bone marrow–derived cells. Stem Cell Rev 1:65, 2005.

32. Massberg S et al: Immunosurveillance by hematopoietic progenitor cells trafficking through blood, lymph, and peripheral tissues. Cell 131:994, 2007.

33. Bryder D et al: Hematopoietic stem cells: the paradigmatic tissue-specific stem cell. Am J Pathol 169:338, 2006.

34. Levesque JP, Winkler IG: Mobilization of hematopoietic stem cells: state of the art. Curr Opin Organ Transplant 13:53, 2008.

35. Fox JM et al: Recent advances into the understanding of mesenchymal stem cell trafficking. Br J Haematol 137:491, 2007.

36. Caplan AI: Adult mesenchymal stem cells for tissue engineering versus regenerative medicine. J Cell Physiol 213:341, 2007.

37. Fausto N: Liver regeneration and repair: hepatocytes, progenitor cells, and stem cells. Hepatology 39:1477, 2004.

38. Taupin P: Adult neural stem cells, neurogenic niches, and cellular therapy. Stem Cell Rev 2:213, 2006.

39. Okano H et al: Regeneration of the central nervous system using endogenous repair mechanisms. J Neurochem 102:1459, 2007.

40. Sieber-Blum M, Hu Y: Epidermal neural crest stem cells (EPI-NCSC) and pluripotency. Stem Cell Rev, August 2008, Epub.

41. Fuchs E: Skin stem cells: rising to the surface. J Cell Biol 180:273, 2008.

42. Braun KM, Prowse DM: Distinct epidermal stem cell compartments are maintained by independent niche microenvironments. Stem Cell Rev 2:221, 2006.

43. Watt FM et al: Epidermal stem cells: an update. Curr Opin Genet Dev 16:518, 2006.

44. Ohyama M et al: Characterization and isolation of stem cell–enriched human hair follicle bulge cells. J Clin Invest 116:249, 2006.

45. Yen TH, Wright NA: The gastrointestinal tract stem cell niche. Stem Cell Rev 2:203, 2006.

46. Barker N et al.: The intestinal stem cell. Genes Dev 22:1856, 2008.

47. Shi X, Garry DJ: Muscle stem cells in development, regeneration, and disease. Genes Dev 20:1692, 2006.

48. Hsieh PCH et al: Evidence from a genetic fate-mapping study that stem cells refresh adult mammalian cardiomyocytes after injury. Nat Med 13:970, 2007.

49. Murry CE: Cardiac aid to the injured but not the elderly? Nat Med 13:901, 2007.

50. Daniels JT et al: Corneal epithelial stem cells in health and disease. Stem Cell Rev 2:247, 2006.

51. Djojosubroto MW, Arsenijevic Y: Retinal stem cells: promising candidates for retina transplantation. Cell Tissue Res 331:347, 2008.

52. Massague J: G1 cell-cycle control and cancer. Nature 432:298, 2004.

53. Bartek J, Lukas J: DNA damage checkpoints: from initiation to recovery or adaptation. Curr Opin Cell Biol 19:238, 2007.

54. Ashwell S, Zabludoff S: DNA damage detection and repair pathways—recent advances with inhibitors of checkpoint kinases in cancer therapy. ClinCancer Res 14:4032, 2008.

55. Zandi R et al: Mechanisms for oncogenic activation of the epidermal growth factor receptor. Cell Signal 19:2013, 2007.

56. Conway K et al: The molecular and clinical impact of hepatocyte growth factor, its receptor, activators, and inhibitors in wound healing. Wound Repair Regen 14:2, 2006.

57. Andrae J et al.: Role of platelet-derived growth factors in physiology and medicine. Genes Dev 22:1276, 2008.

58. Nagy JA et al: VEGF-A and the induction of pathological angiogenesis. Annu Rev Pathol 2:251, 2007.

59. Itoh N: The Fgf families in humans, mice, and zebrafish: their evolutional processes and roles in development, metabolism, and disease. Biol Pharm Bull 30:1819, 2007.

60. Bierie B, Moses HL: Tumour microenvironment: TGFbeta: the molecular Jekyll and Hyde of cancer. Nat Rev Cancer 6:506, 2006.

61. Johnson GL, Lapadat R: Mitogen-activated protein kinase pathways mediated by ERK, JNK, and p38 protein kinases. Science 298:1911, 2002.

62. Rawlings JS et al: The JAK/STAT signaling pathway. J Cell Sci 117:1281, 2004.

63. Deupi X, Kobilka B: Activation of G protein–coupled receptors. Adv Protein Chem 74:137, 2007.

64. Ahmed W et al: PPARs and their metabolic modulation: new mechanisms for transcriptional regulation? J Intern Med 262:184, 2007.

65. Thompson MD, Monga SP: WNT/beta-catenin signaling in liver health and disease. Hepatology 45:1298, 2007.

66. Stoick-Cooper CL et al: Advances in signaling in vertebrate regeneration as a prelude to regenerative medicine. Genes Dev 21:1292, 2007.

67. Zhao M et al: Evidence for the presence of stem cell-like progenitor cells in human adult pancreas. J Endocrinol 195:407, 2007.

68. Zhou Q et al.: In vivo reprogramming of adult pancreatic exocrine cells to beta-cells. Nature, Aug 2008, Epub.

69. Fausto N et al: Liver regeneration. Hepatology 43:S45, 2006.

70. Taub R: Liver regeneration: from myth to mechanism. Nat Rev Mol Cell Biol 5:836, 2004.

71. LeBleu VS et al: Structure and function of basement membranes. Exp Biol Med (Maywood) 232:112, 2007.

72. Myllyharju J, Kivirikko KI: Collagens, modifying enzymes and their mutations in humans, flies and worms. Trends Genet 20:33, 2004.

73. Byers PH et al: Genetic evaluation of suspected osteogenesis imperfecta (OI). Genet Med 8:383, 2006.

74. Robinson PN et al: The molecular genetics of Marfan syndrome and related disorders. J Med Genet 43:769, 2006.

75. Morgan MR et al: Synergistic control of cell adhesion by integrins and syndecans. Nat Rev Mol Cell Biol 8:957, 2007.

76. Scatena M et al: Osteopontin: a multifunctional molecule regulating chronic inflammation and vascular disease. Arterioscler Thromb Vasc Biol 27:2302, 2007.

77. Lenga Y et al.: Osteopontin expression is required for myofibroblast differentiation. Circ Res 102:319, 2008.

78. Taylor KR, Gallo RL: Glycosaminoglycans and their proteoglycans: host-associated molecular patterns for initiation and modulation of inflammation. FASEB J 20:9, 2006.

79. Toole BP: Hyaluronan: from extracellular glue to pericellular cue. Nat Rev Cancer 4:528, 2004.

80. Carmeliet P: Manipulating angiogenesis in medicine. J Intern Med 255:538, 2004.

81. Carmeliet P: Angiogenesis in life, disease and medicine. Nature 438:932, 2005.

82. Adams RH, Alitalo K: Molecular regulation of angiogenesis and lymphangiogenesis. Nat Rev Mol Cell Biol 8:464, 2007.

83. Kerbel RS: Tumor angiogenesis. N Engl J Med 358:2039, 2008.

84. Holderfield MT, Hughes CCW: Crosstalk between vascular endothelial growth factor, Notch and transforming growth factor-β in vascular morphogenesis. Circ Res 102:637, 2008.

85. Siekmann AF et al: Modulation of VEGF signaling output by the NOTCH pathway. BioEssays 30:303, 2008.

86. Broughton G et al: The basic science of wound healing. Plast Reconstr Surg 117:12S, 2006.

87. Gurtner GC et al: Wound repair and regeneration. Nature 453:314, 2008.

88. Diegelmann RF, Evans MC: Wound healing: an overview of acute, fibrotic and delayed healing. Front Biosci 9:283, 2004.

89. Werner S, Grose R: Regulation of wound healing by growth factors and cytokines. Physiol Rev 83:835, 2003.

90. Ito M et al: Wnt-dependent de novo hair follicle regeneration in adult mouse skin after wounding. Nature 447:316, 2007.

91. Darby IA, Hewitson TD: Fibroblast differentiation in wound healing and fibrosis. Int Rev Cytol 257:143, 2007.

92. Dabiri G et al: Hic-5 promotes the hypertrophic scar myofibroblast phenotype by regulating the TGF-β1 autocrine loop. J Invest Dermatol [serial on the internet], 10 April 2008 (doi: 10.1038/jid.2008.90).

93. Martinez FO et al.: Macrophage activation and polarization. Front Biosci 13:453, 2008.

94. Mori R et al: Molecular mechanisms linking wound inflammation and fibrosis: knockdown of osteopontin leads to rapid repair and reduced scarring. J Exp Med 205:43, 2008.

95. Ferguson MW, O'Kane S: Scar-free healing: from embryonic mechanisms to adult therapeutic intervention. Philos Trans R Soc Lond B Biol Sci 359:839, 2004.

96. Hantash BM et al.: Adult and fetal wound healing. Front Biosci 13:51, 2008.

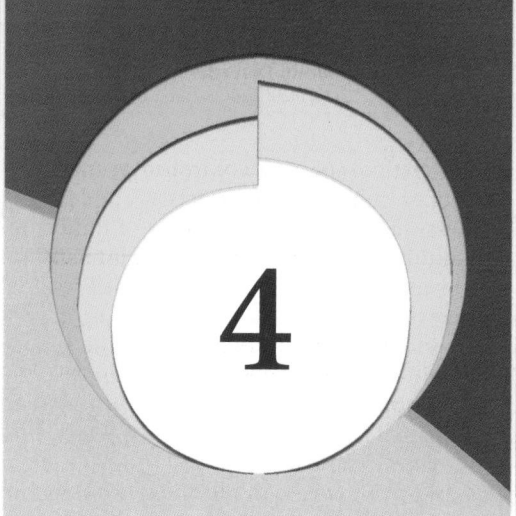

Hemodynamic Disorders, Thromboembolic Disease, and Shock

Richard N. Mitchell

Edema

Hyperemia and Congestion

Hemorrhage

Hemostasis and Thrombosis
    Normal Hemostasis
        Endothelium
        Platelets
        Coagulation Cascade
    Thrombosis
    Disseminated Intravascular Coagulation
    (DIC)

Embolism
    Pulmonary Embolism
    Systemic Thromboembolism
    Fat and Marrow Embolism
    Air Embolism
    Amniotic Fluid Embolism

Infarction

Shock
    Pathogenesis of Septic Shock
    Stages of Shock

As a group, cardiovascular diseases are the most important cause of morbidity and mortality in Western society. In the year 2005, it was estimated that 81 million people in the United States had one or more forms of cardiovascular disease, which were responsible for 35% to 40% of deaths. Included in this category are diseases that primarily affect one of the three major components of the cardiovascular system: the heart; the blood vessels; and the blood itself, which is composed of water, salts, a wide variety of proteins, elements that regulate clotting (the coagulation factors and platelets), and other formed elements (red cells and white cells). For the sake of simplicity we will consider disorders affecting each component of the cardiovascular system separately, recognizing that disturbances affecting one component often lead to adaptations and abnormalities involving others. Here, we focus on disorders of hemodynamics (edema, congestion, and shock) and hemostasis (hemorrhage and thrombosis), as well as various forms of embolism. Diseases that primarily affect the blood vessels and the heart will be discussed in Chapters 11 and 12, respectively.

Edema

Approximately 60% of lean body weight is water. Two thirds of the body's water is intracellular, and the remainder is in extracellular compartments, mostly the interstitium (or third space) that lies between cells; only about 5% of total body water is in blood plasma. The movement of water and low molecular weight solutes such as salts between the intravascular and interstitial spaces is controlled primarily by the opposing effect of vascular hydrostatic pressure and plasma colloid osmotic pressure. Normally the outflow of fluid from the arteriolar end of the microcirculation into the interstitium is nearly balanced by inflow at the venular end; a small residual amount of fluid may be left in the interstitium and is drained by the lymphatic vessels, ultimately returning to the bloodstream via the thoracic duct. *Either increased capillary pressure or diminished colloid osmotic pressure can result in increased interstitial fluid* (Fig. 4–1). If the movement of water into tissues (or body cavities) exceeds lymphatic drainage, fluid accumulates. An abnormal increase in interstitial fluid within tissues is called *edema*, while fluid collections in the different body cavities are variously designated *hydrothorax, hydropericardium, and hydroperitoneum* (the last is more commonly called *ascites*). *Anasarca* is a severe and generalized edema with widespread subcutaneous tissue swelling.

There are several pathophysiologic categories of edema (Table 4–1). Edema caused by increased hydrostatic pressure or reduced plasma protein is typically a protein-poor fluid called a *transudate*. Edema fluid of this type is seen in patients suffering from heart failure, renal failure, hepatic failure, and certain forms of malnutrition, as described below and outlined in Figure 4–2. In contrast, inflammatory edema is a protein-rich *exudate* that is a result of increased vascular per-

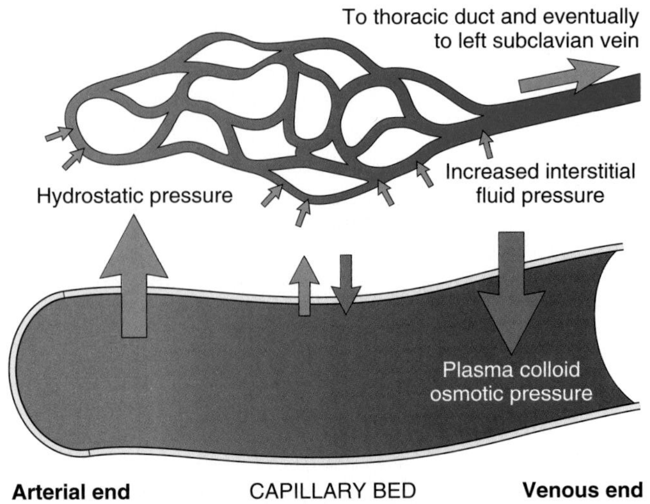

FIGURE 4–1 Factors influencing fluid transit across capillary walls. Capillary hydrostatic and osmotic forces are normally balanced so that there is no *net* loss or gain of fluid across the capillary bed. However, *increased* hydrostatic pressure or *diminished* plasma osmotic pressure will cause extravascular fluid to accumulate. Tissue lymphatics remove much of the excess volume, eventually returning it to the circulation via the thoracic duct; however, if the capacity for lymphatic drainage is exceeded, tissue *edema* results.

TABLE 4–1 Pathophysiologic Categories of Edema

INCREASED HYDROSTATIC PRESSURE

Impaired venous return
    Congestive heart failure
    Constrictive pericarditis
    Ascites (liver cirrhosis)
    Venous obstruction or compression
        Thrombosis
        External pressure (e.g., mass)
        Lower extremity inactivity with prolonged dependency
Arteriolar dilation
    Heat
    Neurohumoral dysregulation

REDUCED PLASMA OSMOTIC PRESSURE (HYPOPROTEINEMIA)

Protein-losing glomerulopathies (nephrotic syndrome)
Liver cirrhosis (ascites)
Malnutrition
Protein-losing gastroenteropathy

LYMPHATIC OBSTRUCTION

Inflammatory
Neoplastic
Postsurgical
Postirradiation

SODIUM RETENTION

Excessive salt intake with renal insufficiency
Increased tubular reabsorption of sodium
    Renal hypoperfusion
    Increased renin-angiotensin-aldosterone secretion

INFLAMMATION

Acute inflammation
Chronic inflammation
Angiogenesis

Modified from Leaf A, Cotran RS: Renal Pathophysiology, 3rd ed. New York, Oxford University Press, 1985, p 146.

meability. Edema in inflamed tissues is discussed in Chapter 2; *noninflammatory causes of edema* (see Fig. 4–2) are described below.

Increased Hydrostatic Pressure. *Regional increases* in hydrostatic pressure can result from a focal impairment in venous return. Thus, *deep venous thrombosis* in a lower extremity may cause localized edema in the affected leg. On the other hand, *generalized increases* in venous pressure, with resulting systemic edema, occur most commonly in *congestive heart failure* (Chapter 12), where compromised right ventricular function leads to pooling of blood on the venous side of the circulation.

Reduced Plasma Osmotic Pressure. Reduced plasma osmotic pressure occurs when albumin, the major plasma protein, is not synthesized in adequate amounts or is lost from the circulation. An important cause of albumin loss is the *nephrotic syndrome* (Chapter 20), in which glomerular capillaries become leaky; patients typically present with generalized edema. Reduced albumin synthesis occurs in the setting of severe liver diseases (e.g., cirrhosis, Chapter 18) or protein malnutrition (Chapter 9). In each case, reduced plasma osmotic pressure leads to a net movement of fluid into the interstitial tissues with subsequent plasma volume contraction. The reduced intravascular volume leads to decreased renal perfusion. This triggers increased production of renin, angiotensin, and aldosterone, but the resulting salt and water retention cannot correct the plasma volume deficit because the primary defect of low serum protein persists.

Sodium and Water Retention. Salt and water retention can also be a primary cause of edema. Increased salt retention—with obligate associated water—causes both increased hydrostatic pressure (due to intravascular fluid volume expansion) and diminished vascular colloid osmotic pressure (due to dilution). Salt retention occurs whenever renal function is

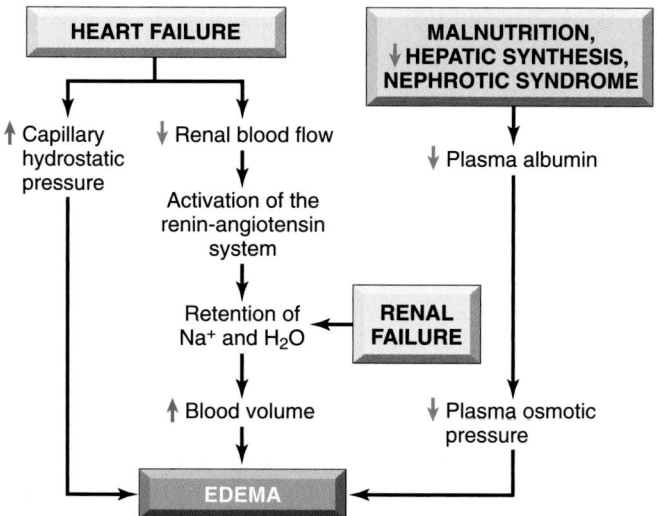

FIGURE 4–2   Pathways leading to systemic edema from primary heart failure, primary renal failure, or reduced plasma osmotic pressure (e.g., from malnutrition, diminished hepatic synthesis, or protein loss from nephrotic syndrome).

compromised, such as in primary disorders of the kidney and disorders that decrease renal perfusion. One of the most important causes of renal hypoperfusion is congestive heart failure, which (like hypoproteinemia) results in the activation of the renin-angiotensin-aldosterone axis. In early heart failure, this response tends to be beneficial, as the retention of sodium and water and other adaptations, including increased vascular tone and elevated levels of antidiuretic hormone (ADH), improve cardiac output and restore normal renal perfusion.[1,2] However, as heart failure worsens and cardiac output diminishes, the retained fluid merely increases the venous pressure, which (as already mentioned) is a major cause of edema in this disorder. Unless cardiac output is restored or renal sodium and water retention is reduced (e.g., by salt restriction, diuretics, or aldosterone antagonists), a downward spiral of fluid retention and worsening edema ensues. Salt restriction, diuretics, and aldosterone antagonists are also of value in managing generalized edema arising from other causes. Primary retention of water (and modest vasoconstriction) is produced by the release of ADH from the posterior pituitary, which normally occurs in the setting of reduced plasma volumes or increased plasma osmolarity.[2] Inappropriate increases in ADH are seen in association with certain malignancies and lung and pituitary disorders and can lead to hyponatremia and cerebral edema (but interestingly not to peripheral edema).

Lymphatic Obstruction. Impaired lymphatic drainage results in *lymphedema* that is typically localized; causes include chronic inflammation with fibrosis, invasive malignant tumors, physical disruption, radiation damage, and certain infectious agents. One dramatic example is seen in parasitic *filariasis*, in which lymphatic obstruction due to extensive inguinal lymphatic and lymph node fibrosis can result in edema of the external genitalia and lower limbs that is so massive as to earn the appellation *elephantiasis*. Severe edema of the upper extremity may also complicate surgical removal and/or irradiation of the breast and associated axillary lymph nodes in patients with breast cancer.

Morphology. Edema is easily recognized grossly; microscopically, it is appreciated as clearing and separation of the extracellular matrix and subtle cell swelling. Any organ or tissue can be involved, but edema is most commonly seen in subcutaneous tissues, the lungs, and the brain. **Subcutaneous edema** can be diffuse or more conspicuous in regions with high hydrostatic pressures. In most cases the distribution is influenced by gravity and is termed **dependent edema** (e.g., the legs when standing, the sacrum when recumbent). Finger pressure over substantially edematous subcutaneous tissue displaces the interstitial fluid and leaves a depression, a sign called **pitting edema**.

Edema as a result of **renal dysfunction** can **affect all parts of the body**. It often initially manifests in tissues with loose connective tissue matrix, such as the eyelids; **periorbital edema** is thus a characteristic finding in severe renal disease. With **pulmonary edema**, the lungs are often two to three times their normal weight, and sectioning yields frothy, blood-tinged fluid—a mixture of air, edema, and extravasated red cells. **Brain edema** can be localized or generalized depending on the nature and extent of the pathologic process or injury. With generalized edema the brain is grossly swollen with narrowed sulci; distended gyri show evidence of compression against the unyielding skull (Chapter 28).

Clinical Consequences. The consequences of edema range from merely annoying to rapidly fatal. Subcutaneous tissue edema is important primarily because it signals potential underlying cardiac or renal disease; however, when significant, it can also impair wound healing or the clearance of infection. Pulmonary edema is a common clinical problem that is most frequently seen in the setting of left ventricular failure; it can also occur with renal failure, acute respiratory distress syndrome (Chapter 15), and pulmonary inflammation or infection. Not only does fluid collect in the alveolar septa around capillaries and impede oxygen diffusion, but edema fluid in the alveolar spaces also creates a favorable environment for bacterial infection. Brain edema is life-threatening; if severe, brain substance can *herniate* (extrude) through the foramen magnum, or the brain stem vascular supply can be compressed. Either condition can injure the medullary centers and cause death (Chapter 28).

Hyperemia and Congestion

Hyperemia and congestion both stem from locally increased blood volumes. *Hyperemia* is an *active process* in which arteriolar dilation (e.g., at sites of inflammation or in skeletal muscle during exercise) leads to increased blood flow. Affected tissues turn red (*erythema*) because of the engorgement of vessels with oxygenated blood. *Congestion* is a *passive process* resulting from reduced outflow of blood from a tissue. It can be systemic, as in cardiac failure, or local, as in isolated venous obstruction. Congested tissues take on a dusky reddish-blue color (*cyanosis*) due to red cell stasis and the accumulation of deoxygenated hemoglobin.

As a result of the increased volumes and pressures, congestion commonly leads to edema. In long-standing *chronic passive congestion,* the lack of blood flow causes chronic hypoxia, potentially resulting in ischemic tissue injury and scarring. Capillary rupture in chronic congestion can also cause small hemorrhagic foci; subsequent catabolism of extravasated red cells can leave residual telltale clusters of hemosiderin-laden macrophages.

> **Morphology.** The cut surfaces of congested tissues are often discolored due to the presence of high levels of poorly oxygenated blood. Microscopically, **acute pulmonary congestion** exhibits engorged alveolar capillaries often with alveolar septal edema and focal intra-alveolar hemorrhage. In **chronic pulmonary congestion** the septa are thickened and fibrotic, and the alveoli often contain numerous hemosiderin-laden macrophages called **heart failure cells**. In **acute hepatic congestion**, the central vein and sinusoids are distended; centrilobular hepatocytes can be frankly ischemic while the periportal hepatocytes—better oxygenated because of proximity to hepatic arterioles—may only develop fatty change. In **chronic passive hepatic congestion** the centrilobular regions are grossly red-brown and slightly depressed (because of cell death) and are accentuated against the surrounding zones of uncongested tan liver **(nutmeg liver)** (Fig. 4–3A). Microscopically, there is centrilobular hemorrhage, hemosiderin-laden macrophages, and degeneration of hepatocytes (Fig. 4–3B). Because the centrilobular area is at the distal end of the blood supply to the liver, it is prone to undergo necrosis whenever the blood supply is compromised.

Hemorrhage

Hemorrhage is defined as the extravasation of blood into the extravascular space. As described above, capillary bleeding can occur under conditions of chronic congestion; an increased tendency to hemorrhage (usually with insignificant injury) also occurs in a variety of clinical disorders that are collectively called *hemorrhagic diatheses*. Rupture of a large artery or vein results in severe hemorrhage and is almost always due to vascular injury, including trauma, atherosclerosis, or inflammatory or neoplastic erosion of the vessel wall.

Tissue hemorrhage can occur in distinct patterns, each with its own clinical implications:

- Hemorrhage may be external or contained within a tissue; any accumulation is called a *hematoma*. Hematomas may be relatively insignificant or so massive that death ensues.
- Minute 1- to 2-mm hemorrhages into skin, mucous membranes, or serosal surfaces are called *petechiae* (Fig. 4–4A). These are most commonly associated with locally increased intravascular pressure, low platelet counts (*thrombocytopenia*), or defective platelet function (as in uremia).
- Slightly larger (≥3 mm) hemorrhages are called *purpura*. These may be associated with many of the same disorders that cause petechiae or can be secondary to trauma, vascular inflammation (*vasculitis*), or increased vascular fragility (e.g., in amyloidosis).
- Larger (>1 to 2 cm) subcutaneous hematomas (i.e., bruises) are called *ecchymoses*. The red cells in these lesions are degraded and phagocytized by macrophages; the hemoglobin (red-blue color) is then enzymatically converted into bilirubin (blue-green color) and eventually into hemosiderin (gold-brown color), accounting for the characteristic color changes in a bruise.
- Depending on the location, a large accumulation of blood in a body cavity is denoted as a *hemothorax, hemopericardium, hemoperitoneum,* or *hemarthrosis* (in joints). Patients with extensive bleeding can develop jaundice from the massive breakdown of red cells and hemoglobin.

The clinical significance of hemorrhage depends on the volume and rate of bleeding. Rapid loss of up to 20% of the blood volume or slow losses of even larger amounts may have little impact in healthy adults; greater losses, however, can cause *hemorrhagic (hypovolemic) shock* (discussed later). The site of hemorrhage is also important. For example,

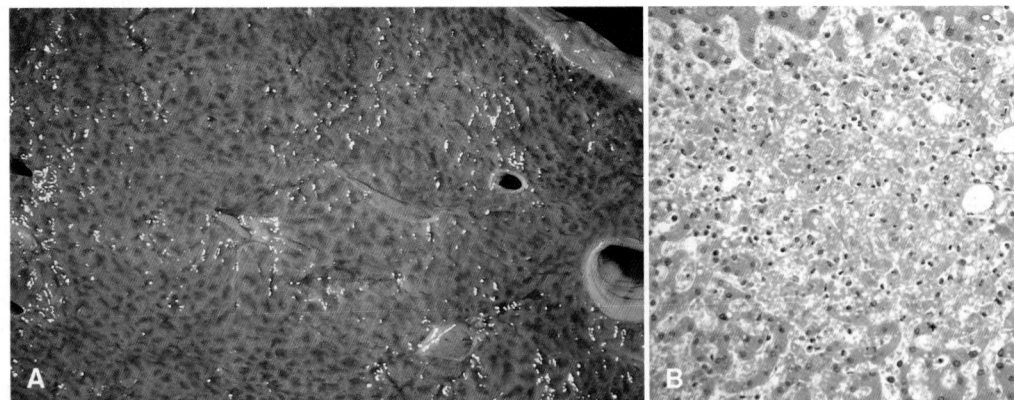

FIGURE 4–3 Liver with chronic passive congestion and hemorrhagic necrosis. **A,** Central areas are red and slightly depressed compared with the surrounding tan viable parenchyma, forming a "nutmeg liver" pattern (so-called because it resembles the cut surface of a nutmeg). **B,** Centrilobular necrosis with degenerating hepatocytes and hemorrhage. (Courtesy of Dr. James Crawford, Department of Pathology, University of Florida, Gainesville, FL.)

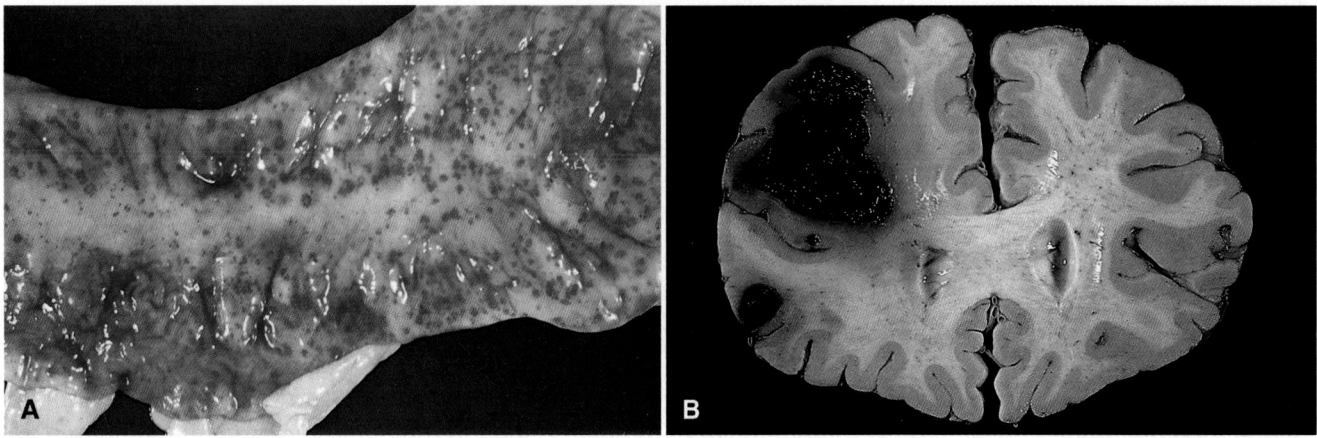

FIGURE 4–4 **A,** Punctate petechial hemorrhages of the colonic mucosa, a consequence of thrombocytopenia. **B,** Fatal intracerebral bleed.

bleeding that is trivial in the subcutaneous tissues can cause death if located in the brain (Fig. 4–4B); because the skull is unyielding, intracranial hemorrhage can result in an increase in pressure that is sufficient to compromise the blood supply or to cause the herniation of the brainstem (Chapter 28). Finally, chronic or recurrent external blood loss (e.g., peptic ulcer or menstrual bleeding) causes a net loss in iron and can lead to an iron deficiency anemia. In contrast, when red cells are retained (e.g., hemorrhage into body cavities or tissues), iron is recovered and recycled for use in the synthesis of hemoglobin.

Hemostasis and Thrombosis

Normal hemostasis is a consequence of tightly regulated processes that maintain blood in a fluid state in normal vessels, yet also permit the rapid formation of a *hemostatic clot* at the site of a vascular injury. The pathologic counterpart of hemostasis is *thrombosis*; it involves blood clot *(thrombus)* formation within intact vessels. Both hemostasis and thrombosis involve three components: the *vascular wall* (particularly the *endothelium*), *platelets*, and the *coagulation cascade*. We begin the discussion with the normal hemostatic pathway and how it is regulated.

NORMAL HEMOSTASIS

The general sequence of events in hemostasis at a site of vascular injury is shown in Figure 4–5.[3,4]

- After initial injury there is a brief period of *arteriolar vasoconstriction* mediated by reflex neurogenic mechanisms and augmented by the local secretion of factors such as *endothelin* (a potent endothelium-derived vasoconstrictor; Fig. 4–5A). The effect is transient, however, and bleeding would resume if not for activation of the platelet and coagulation systems.
- Endothelial injury exposes highly thrombogenic subendothelial extracellular matrix (ECM), facilitating *platelet adherence and activation.* Activation of platelets results in a dramatic shape change (from small rounded discs to flat

plates with markedly increased surface area), as well as the release of secretory granules. Within minutes the secreted products recruit additional platelets *(aggregation)* to form a *hemostatic plug*; this process is referred to as *primary hemostasis* (Fig. 4–5B).
- *Tissue factor* is also exposed at the site of injury. Also known as *factor III* and *thromboplastin*, tissue factor is a membrane-bound procoagulant glycoprotein synthesized by endothelial cells. It acts in conjunction with factor VII (see below) as the major in vivo initiator of the coagulation cascade, eventually culminating in *thrombin* generation. Thrombin cleaves circulating fibrinogen into insoluble *fibrin*, creating a fibrin meshwork, and also induces additional platelet recruitment and activation. This sequence, *secondary hemostasis*, consolidates the initial platelet plug (Fig. 4–5C).
- Polymerized fibrin and platelet aggregates form a solid, *permanent plug* to prevent any further hemorrhage. At this stage, counter-regulatory mechanisms (e.g., *tissue plasminogen activator, t-PA*) are set into motion to limit the hemostatic plug to the site of injury (Fig. 4–5D).

The following sections discuss the roles of the endothelium, platelets, and the coagulation cascade in greater detail.

Endothelium

Endothelial cells are key players in the regulation of homeostasis, as the balance between the anti- and prothrombotic activities of endothelium determines whether thrombus formation, propagation, or dissolution occurs.[5-7] Normally, endothelial cells exhibit antiplatelet, anticoagulant, and fibrinolytic properties; however, after injury or activation they acquire numerous *procoagulant* activities (Fig. 4–6). Besides trauma, endothelium can be activated by infectious agents, hemodynamic forces, plasma mediators, and cytokines.

Antithrombotic Properties

Under normal circumstances endothelial cells actively prevent thrombosis by producing factors that variously block platelet adhesion and aggregation, inhibit coagulation, and lyse clots.

A. VASOCONSTRICTION

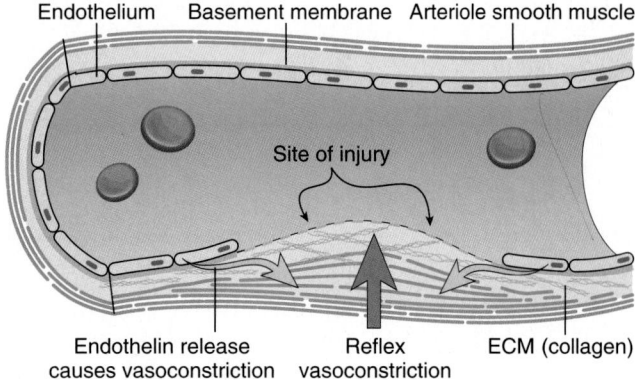

B. PRIMARY HEMOSTASIS

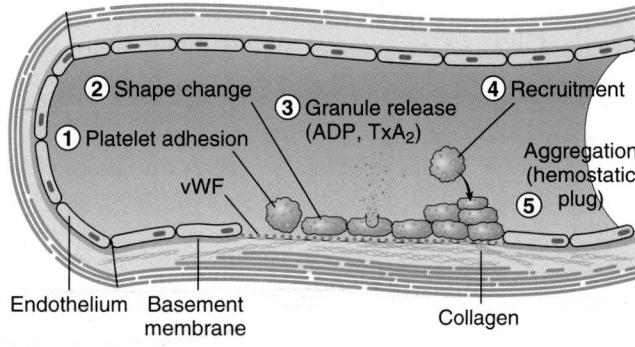

C. SECONDARY HEMOSTASIS

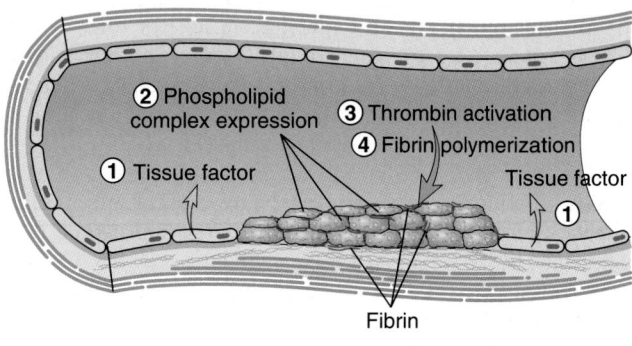

D. THROMBUS AND ANTITHROMBOTIC EVENTS

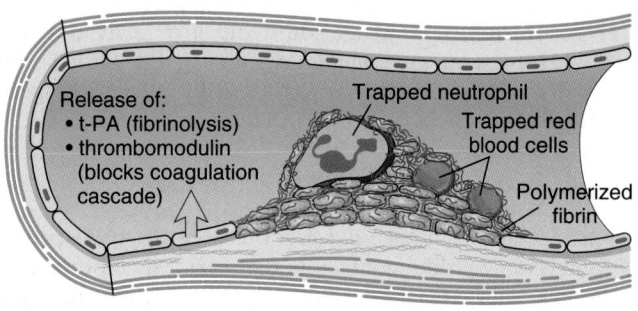

FIGURE 4–5 Normal hemostasis. **A,** After vascular injury local neurohumoral factors induce a transient vasoconstriction. **B,** Platelets bind via glycoprotein Ib (GpIb) receptors to von Willebrand factor (vWF) on exposed extracellular matrix (ECM) and are activated, undergoing a shape change and granule release. Released adenosine diphosphate (ADP) and thromboxane A_2 (TxA$_2$) induce additional platelet aggregation through platelet GpIIb-IIIa receptor binding to fibrinogen, and form the *primary* hemostatic plug. **C,** Local activation of the coagulation cascade (involving tissue factor and platelet phospholipids) results in fibrin polymerization, "cementing" the platelets into a definitive *secondary* hemostatic plug. **D,** Counter-regulatory mechanisms, mediated by tissue plasminogen activator (t-PA, a fibrinolytic product) and thrombomodulin, confine the hemostatic process to the site of injury.

- *Antiplatelet effects.* Intact endothelium prevents platelets (and plasma coagulation factors) from engaging the highly thrombogenic subendothelial ECM. Nonactivated platelets do not adhere to endothelial cells, and even if platelets are activated, prostacyclin (PGI_2) and nitric oxide produced by the endothelial cells impede platelet adhesion. Both of these mediators are potent vasodilators and inhibitors of platelet aggregation; their synthesis by the endothelium is stimulated by several factors produced during coagulation (e.g., thrombin and cytokines). Endothelial cells also elaborate adenosine diphosphatase, which degrades adenosine diphosphate (ADP) and further inhibits platelet aggregation (see below).

- *Anticoagulant effects.*[8] These effects are mediated by endothelial membrane-associated heparin-like molecules, thrombomodulin, and tissue factor pathway inhibitor (see Fig. 4–6). The *heparin-like molecules* act indirectly; they are cofactors that greatly enhance the inactivation of thrombin and several other coagulation factors by the plasma protein *antithrombin III* (see later). *Thrombomodulin* binds to thrombin and converts it from a procoagulant into an anticoagulant via its ability to activate protein C, which inhibits clotting by inactivating factors Va and VIIIa.[9] Endothelium also produces protein S, a co-factor for protein C, and *tissue factor pathway inhibitor (TFPI)*, a cell surface protein that directly inhibits tissue factor–factor VIIa and factor Xa activities.[10]

- *Fibrinolytic effects.* Endothelial cells synthesize tissue-type plasminogen activator (*t-PA*), a protease that cleaves plasminogen to form plasmin; plasmin, in turn, cleaves fibrin to degrade thrombi.[9]

Prothrombotic Properties

While normal endothelial cells limit clotting, trauma and inflammation of endothelial cells induce a prothrombotic state that alters the activities of platelets, coagulation proteins, and the fibrinolytic system.

- *Platelet effects.* Endothelial injury allows platelets to contact the underlying extracellular matrix; subsequent adhesion occurs through interactions with *von Willebrand factor (vWF)*, which is a product of normal endothelial cells and an essential cofactor for platelet binding to matrix elements (Fig. 4–7).[11]

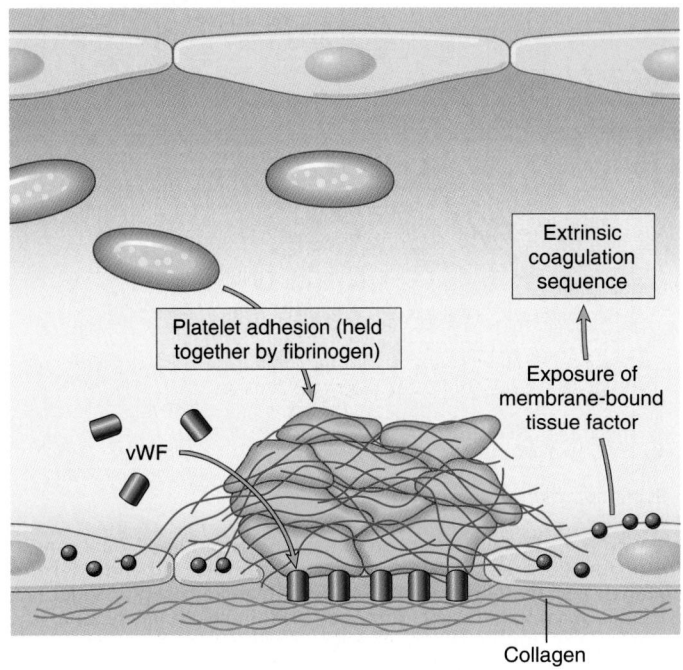

INHIBIT THROMBOSIS

FAVOR THROMBOSIS

Inactivates factors Xa and IXa

Proteolysis of factors Va and VIIIa

(requires protein S)

Active protein C ⟸ Protein C

Fibrinolytic cascade

Inactivates thrombin

Inactivates tissue factor-VIIa complexes

Inhibit platelet aggregation

Antithrombin III

Thrombin

PGI$_2$, NO, and adenosine diphosphatase

t-PA

Endothelial effects

Heparin-like molecule

Thrombin receptor

Tissue factor pathway inhibitor

Thrombomodulin

Platelet adhesion (held together by fibrinogen)

vWF

Extrinsic coagulation sequence

Exposure of membrane-bound tissue factor

Collagen

FIGURE 4–6 Anti- and procoagulant activities of endothelium. NO, nitric oxide; PGI$_2$, prostacyclin; t-PA, tissue plasminogen activator; vWF, von Willebrand factor. The thrombin receptor is also called a protease-activated receptor (PAR).

- *Procoagulant effects.* In response to cytokines (e.g., tumor necrosis factor [TNF] or interleukin-1 [IL-1]) or bacterial endotoxin, endothelial cells synthesize *tissue factor,* the major activator of the extrinsic clotting cascade.[10,12] In addition, activated endothelial cells augment the catalytic function of activated coagulation factors IXa and Xa.
- *Antifibrinolytic effects.* Endothelial cells secrete inhibitors of plasminogen activator (PAIs), which limit fibrinolysis and tend to favor thrombosis.

In summary, intact, nonactivated endothelial cells inhibit platelet adhesion and blood clotting. Endothelial injury or activation, however, results in a procoagulant phenotype that enhances thrombus formation.

Platelets

Platelets are disc-shaped, anucleate cell fragments that are shed from megakaryocytes in the bone marrow into the blood stream. They play a critical role in normal hemostasis,[13] by forming the hemostatic plug that initially seals vascular defects, and by providing a surface that recruits and concentrates activated coagulation factors. Their function depends on several glycoprotein receptors, a contractile cytoskeleton, and two types of cytoplasmic granules. *α-Granules* have the adhesion molecule P-selectin on their membranes (Chapter 2) and contain fibrinogen, fibronectin, factors V and VIII, platelet factor 4 (a heparin-binding chemokine), platelet-derived growth factor (PDGF), and transforming growth factor-β

(TGF-β). *Dense (or δ) granules* contain ADP and ATP, ionized calcium, histamine, serotonin, and epinephrine.

After vascular injury, platelets encounter ECM constituents such as collagen and the adhesive glycoprotein vWF. On contact with these proteins, platelets undergo: (1) adhesion and shape change, (2) secretion (release reaction), and (3) aggregation (see Fig. 4–5B).

- *Platelet adhesion* to ECM is mediated largely via interactions with vWF, which acts as a bridge between platelet surface receptors (e.g., glycoprotein Ib [GpIb]) and exposed collagen (Fig. 4–8). Although platelets can also adhere to other components of the ECM (e.g., fibronectin), vWF-GpIb associations are necessary to overcome the high shear forces of flowing blood. Reflecting the importance of these interactions, genetic deficiencies of vWF (von Willebrand disease; Chapter 14) or its receptor (Bernard-Soulier syndrome) result in bleeding disorders.
- *Secretion (release reaction)* of both granule types occurs soon after adhesion. Various agonists can bind platelet surface receptors and initiate an intracellular protein phosphorylation cascade ultimately leading to degranulation. Release of the contents of dense-bodies is especially important, since calcium is required in the coagulation cascade, and ADP is a potent activator of *platelet aggregation.* ADP also begets additional ADP release, amplifying the aggregation process. Finally, platelet activation leads to the appearance of *negatively charged phospholipids* (particularly phosphatidylserine) on their surfaces. These phospholipids

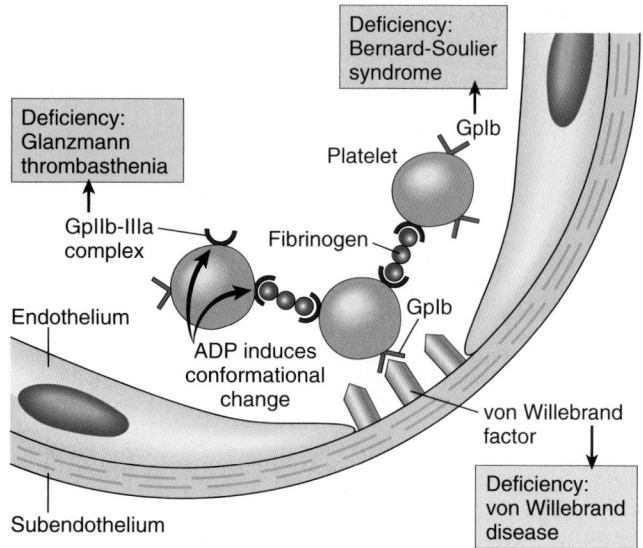

FIGURE 4–7 Platelet adhesion and aggregation. Von Willebrand factor functions as an adhesion bridge between subendothelial collagen and the glycoprotein Ib (GpIb) platelet receptor. Aggregation is accomplished by fibrinogen bridging GpIIb-IIIa receptors on different platelets. Congenital deficiencies in the various receptors or bridging molecules lead to the diseases indicated in the colored boxes. ADP, adenosine diphosphate.

bind calcium and serve as critical nucleation sites for the assembly of complexes containing the various coagulation factors.[14,15]

- *Platelet aggregation* follows adhesion and granule release. In addition to ADP, the vasoconstrictor thromboxane A_2 (TxA_2; Chapter 2) is an important platelet-derived stimulus that amplifies platelet aggregation, which leads to the formation of the primary hemostatic plug. Although this initial wave of aggregation is reversible, concurrent activation of the coagulation cascade generates thrombin, which stabilizes the platelet plug via two mechanisms. First, thrombin binds to a protease-activated receptor (PAR, see below) on the platelet membrane and in concert with ADP and TxA_2 causes further platelet aggregation. This is followed by *platelet contraction*, an event that is dependent on the platelet cytoskeleton that creates an irreversibly fused mass of platelets, which constitutes the definitive *secondary hemostatic plug*. Second, thrombin converts fibrinogen to *fibrin* in the vicinity of the platelet plug, functionally cementing the platelets in place.

Noncleaved *fibrinogen* is also an important component of platelet aggregation. Platelet activation by ADP triggers a conformational change in the platelet GpIIb-IIIa receptors that induces binding to fibrinogen, a large protein that forms bridging interactions between platelets that promote platelet aggregation (see Fig. 4–7). Predictably, inherited deficiency of GpIIb-IIIa results in a bleeding disorder *(Glanzmann thrombasthenia)*.[16] The recognition of the central role of the various receptors and mediators in platelet cross-linking has led to the development of therapeutic agents that block platelet aggregation—for example, by interfering with thrombin activity,[17] by blocking ADP binding (clopidogrel), or by binding to the GpIIb-IIIa

receptors (synthetic antagonists or monoclonal antibodies).[18] Antibodies against GpIb are on the horizon.

Red cells and leukocytes are also found in hemostatic plugs. Leukocytes adhere to platelets via P-selectin and to endothelium using several adhesion receptors (Chapter 2); they contribute to the inflammation that accompanies thrombosis. Thrombin also drives thrombus-associated inflammation by directly stimulating neutrophil and monocyte adhesion and by generating chemotactic *fibrin split products* during fibrinogen cleavage.

Platelet-Endothelial Cell Interactions. The interplay of platelets and endothelium has a profound impact on clot formation. The endothelial cell-derived prostaglandin PGI$_2$ (prostacyclin) inhibits platelet aggregation and is a potent vasodilator; conversely, the platelet-derived prostaglandin TxA_2 activates platelet aggregation and is a vasoconstrictor (Chapter 2). Effects mediated by PGI$_2$ and TxA_2 are exquisitely balanced to effectively modulate platelet and vascular wall function: at baseline, platelet aggregation is prevented, whereas endothelial injury promotes hemostatic plug formation. The clinical utility of aspirin (an irreversible cyclooxygenase inhibitor) in persons at risk for coronary thrombosis resides in its ability to permanently block platelet TxA_2 synthesis. Although endothelial PGI$_2$ production is also inhibited by aspirin, endothelial cells can resynthesize active cyclooxygenase and thereby overcome the blockade. In a manner similar to PGI$_2$, endothelial-derived nitric oxide also acts as a vasodilator and inhibitor of platelet aggregation (see Fig. 4–6).

Coagulation Cascade

The coagulation cascade is the third arm of the hemostatic process. The pathways are schematically presented in Figure 4–8; only general principles are discussed here.[4,19]

The coagulation cascade is essentially an amplifying series of enzymatic conversions; each step proteolytically cleaves an inactive proenzyme into an activated enzyme, culminating in *thrombin* formation. Thrombin is the most important coagulation factor, and indeed can act at numerous stages in the process (see blue boxes in Fig. 4–8).[20] At the conclusion of the proteolytic cascade, thrombin converts the soluble plasma protein *fibrinogen* into *fibrin* monomers that polymerize into an insoluble gel. The fibrin gel encases platelets and other circulating cells in the definitive secondary hemostatic plug, and the fibrin polymers are covalently cross-linked and stabilized by factor XIIIa (which itself is activated by thrombin).

Each reaction in the pathway results from the assembly of a complex composed of an *enzyme* (activated coagulation factor), a *substrate* (proenzyme form of coagulation factor), and a *cofactor* (reaction accelerator). These components are typically assembled on a *phospholipid surface* and held together by *calcium ions* (as an aside, the clotting of blood is prevented by the presence of calcium chelators). The requirement that coagulation factors be brought close together ensures that clotting is normally localized to the surface of activated platelets or endothelium;[4] as shown in Figure 4–9, it can be likened to a "dance" of complexes, in which coagulation factors are passed successfully from one partner to the next. Parantheti-

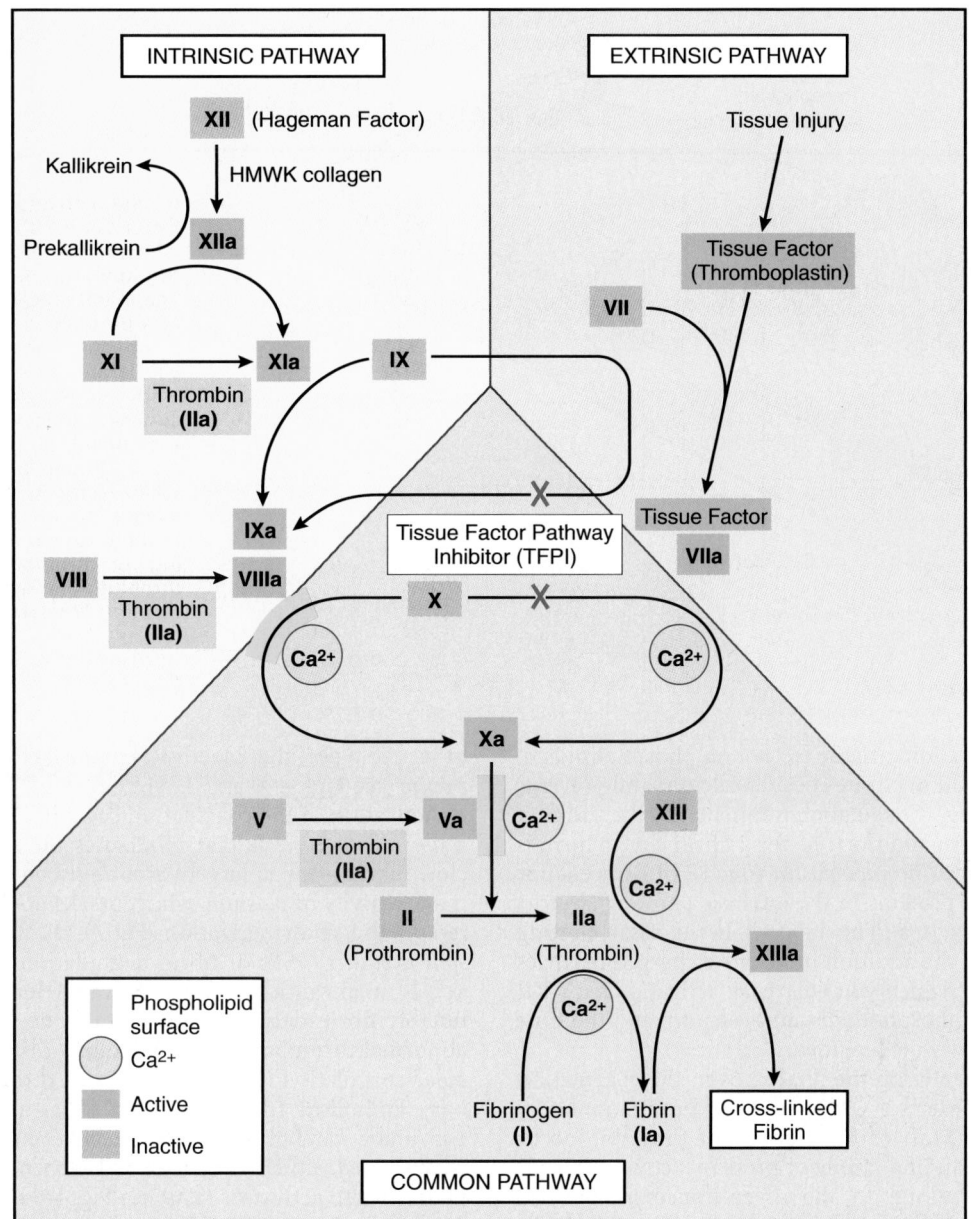

FIGURE 4–8 The coagulation cascade. Factor IX can be activated either by factor XIa or factor VIIa; in lab tests, activation is predominantly dependent on factor XIa of the intrinsic pathway. Factors in red boxes represent inactive molecules; activated factors are indicated with a lower case "a" and a green box. Note also the multiple points where thrombin (factor IIa; light blue boxes) contributes to coagulation through positive feedback loops. The red "X"s denote points of action of tissue factor pathway inhibitor (TFPI), which inhibits the activation of factors X and IX by factor VIIa. PL, phospholipid; HMWK, high-molecular-weight kininogen.

cally, the binding of coagulation factors II, XII, IX, and X to calcium depends on the addition of γ-carboxyl groups to certain glutamic acid residues on these proteins. This reaction uses vitamin K as a cofactor and is antagonized by drugs such as *coumadin*, which is a widely used anticoagulant.

Blood coagulation is traditionally classified into *extrinsic* and *intrinsic* pathways that converge on the activation of factor X (see Fig. 4–8). The extrinsic pathway was so designated because it required the addition of an exogenous trigger (originally provided by tissue extracts); the intrinsic pathway only required exposing factor XII (Hageman factor) to thrombogenic surfaces (even glass would suffice). However, such a

division is largely an artifact of in vitro testing; there are, in fact, several interconnections between the two pathways. Moreover, the extrinsic pathway is the most physiologically relevant pathway for coagulation occurring when vascular damage has occurred; it is activated by *tissue factor* (also known as *thromboplastin* or factor III), a membrane-bound lipoprotein expressed at sites of injury (see Fig. 4–8).[12]

Clinical laboratories assess the function of the two arms of the coagulation pathway through two standard assays: *prothrombin time* (PT) and *partial thromboplastin time* (PTT). The PT assay assesses the function of the proteins in the extrinsic pathway (factors VII, X, II, V, and fibrinogen). This

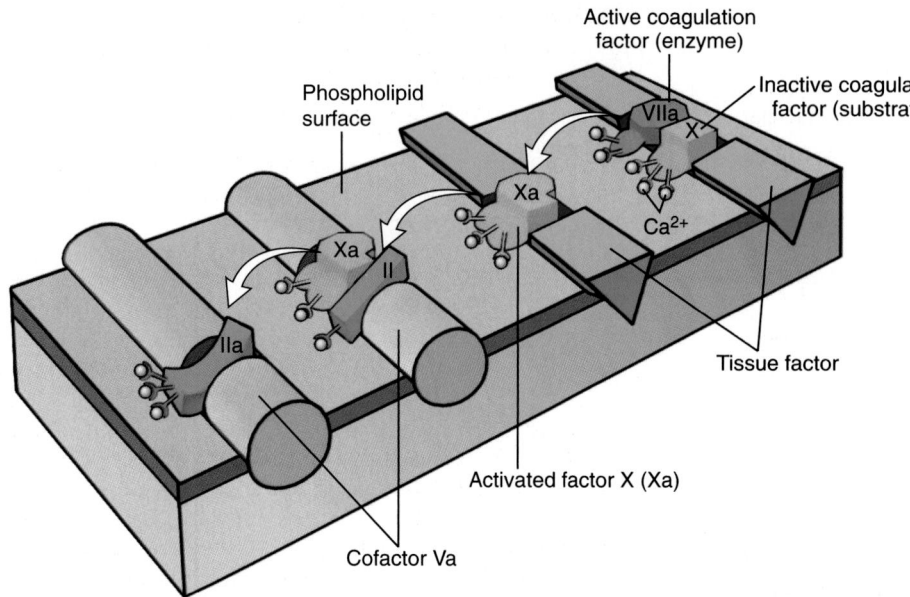

FIGURE 4–9 Schematic illustration of the conversion of factor X to factor Xa via the extrinsic pathway, which in turn converts factor II (prothrombin) to factor IIa (thrombin). The initial reaction complex consists of a proteolytic enzyme (factor VIIa), a substrate (factor X), and a reaction accelerator (tissue factor), all assembled on a platelet phospholipid surface. Calcium ions hold the assembled components together and are essential for the reaction. Activated factor Xa becomes the protease for the second adjacent complex in the coagulation cascade, converting prothrombin substrate (II) to thrombin (IIa) using factor Va as the reaction accelerator.

is accomplished by adding tissue factor and phospholipids to citrated plasma (sodium citrate chelates calcium and prevents spontaneous clotting). Coagulation is initiated by the addition of exogenous calcium and the time for a fibrin clot to form is recorded. The *partial thromboplastin time* (PTT) screens for the function of the proteins in the intrinsic pathway (factors XII, XI, IX, VIII, X, V, II, and fibrinogen). In this assay, clotting is initiated through the addition of negative charged particles (e.g., ground glass), which you will recall activates factor XII (Hageman factor), phospholipids, and calcium, and the time to fibrin clot formation is recorded.

In addition to catalyzing the final steps in the coagulation cascade, thrombin exerts a wide variety of proinflammatery effects (Fig. 4–10). Most of these effects of thrombin occur through its activation of a family of protease activated receptors (PARs) that belong to the seven-transmembrane G protein–coupled receptor family[21,22] (see also Fig. 4–6). PARs are expressed on endothelium, monocytes, dendritic cells, T lymphocytes, and other cell types. Receptor activation is initiated by cleavage of the extracellular end of the PAR; this generates a tethered peptide that binds to the "clipped" receptor, causing a conformational change that triggers signaling.

Once activated, the coagulation cascade must be restricted to the site of vascular injury to prevent runaway clotting of the entire vascular tree. Besides restricting factor activation to sites of exposed phospholipids, three categories of endogenous anticoagulants also control clotting. (1) *Antithrombins* (e.g., antithrombin III) inhibit the activity of thrombin and other serine proteases, including factors IXa, Xa, XIa, and XIIa. Antithrombin III is activated by binding to heparin-like molecules on endothelial cells; hence the clinical usefulness of administering heparin to minimize thrombosis (see Fig. 4–6). (2) *Proteins C and S* are vitamin K–dependent proteins that act in a complex that proteolytically inactivates factors Va and VIIIa. Protein C activation by thrombomodulin was described earlier. (3) *TFPI* is a protein produced by endothelium (and

other cell types) that inactivates tissue factor–factor VIIa complexes (see Figs. 4–6 and 4–8).[10]

Activation of the coagulation cascade also sets into motion a *fibrinolytic cascade* that moderates the size of the ultimate clot. Fibrinolysis is largely accomplished through the enzymatic activity of *plasmin*, which breaks down fibrin and interferes with its polymerization (Fig. 4–11).[23] The resulting *fibrin split products* (FSPs or fibrin degradation products) can also act as weak anticoagulants. Elevated levels of FSPs (most notably fibrin-derived *D-dimers*) can be used in diagnosing abnormal thrombotic states including disseminated intravascular coagulation (DIC), deep venous thrombosis, or pulmonary embolism (described later). Plasmin is generated by enzymatic catabolism of the inactive circulating precursor *plasminogen,* either by a factor XII–dependent pathway or by plasminogen activators (PAs; see Fig. 4–11). The most important of the PAs is t-PA; it is synthesized principally by endothelium and is most active when bound to fibrin. The affinity for fibrin makes t-PA a useful therapeutic agent, since it largely confines fibrinolytic activity to sites of recent thrombosis. *Urokinase-like PA (u-PA)* is another PA present in plasma and in various tissues; it can activate plasmin in the fluid phase. Finally, plasminogen can be cleaved to plasmin by the bacterial enzyme *streptokinase,* an activity that may be clinically significant in certain bacterial infections. As with any potent regulator, plasmin activity is tightly restricted. To prevent excess plasmin from lysing thrombi indiscriminately elsewhere in the body, free plasmin is rapidly inactivated by α_2-plasmin inhibitor (see Fig. 4–11).

Endothelial cells also fine-tune the coagulation/anticoagulation balance by releasing plasminogen activator inhibitor (PAI); it blocks fibrinolysis by inhibiting t-PA binding to fibrin and confers an overall procoagulant effect (see Fig. 4–11). PAI production is increased by thrombin as well as certain cytokines, and probably plays a role in the intravascular thrombosis accompanying severe inflammation.[24]

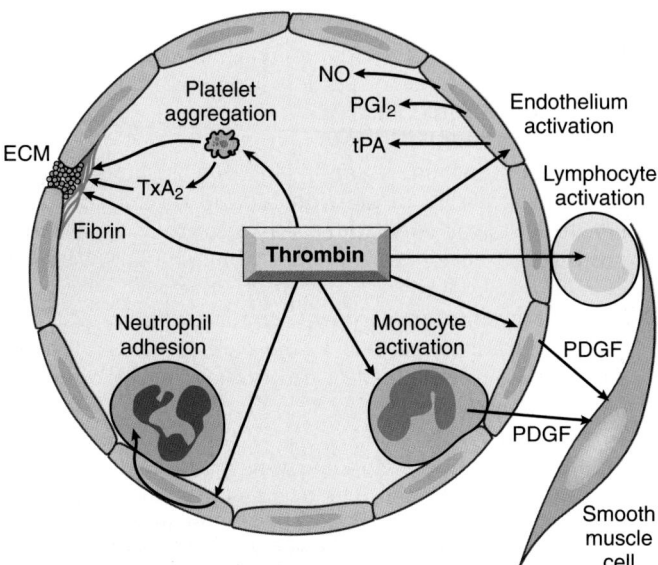

FIGURE 4–10 Role of thrombin in hemostasis and cellular activation. Thrombin plays a critical role in generating cross-linked fibrin (by cleaving fibrinogen to fibrin, and by activating factor XIII), as well as activating several other coagulation factors (see Fig. 4–8). Through protease-activated receptors (PARs, see text), thrombin also modulates several cellular activities. It directly induces platelet aggregation and TxA_2 production, and activates ECs to express adhesion molecules, and a variety of fibrinolytic (t-PA), vasoactive (NO, PGI_2), and cytokine mediators (e.g., PDGF). Thrombin also directly activates leukocytes. ECM, extracellular matrix; NO, nitric oxide; PDGF, platelet-derived growth factor; PGI_2, prostacyclin; TxA_2, thromboxane A_2; t-PA, tissue plasminogen activator. See Figure 4–7 for additional anticoagulant activities mediated by thrombin, including via thrombomodulin. (Courtesy of Shaun Coughlin, MD, PhD, Cardiovascular Research Institute, University of California at San Francisco; modified with permission.)

THROMBOSIS

Having discussed the components of normal hemostasis, we now turn our attention to the three primary *abnormalities that lead to thrombus formation (called Virchow's triad)*: (1) endothelial injury, (2) stasis or turbulent blood flow, and (3) hypercoagulability of the blood (Fig. 4–12).

Endothelial Injury. Endothelial injury is particularly important for thrombus formation in the heart or the arterial circulation, where the normally high flow rates might otherwise impede clotting by preventing platelet adhesion and washing out activated coagulation factors. Thus, thrombus formation within cardiac chambers (e.g., after endocardial injury due to myocardial infarction), over ulcerated plaques in atherosclerotic arteries, or at sites of traumatic or inflammatory vascular injury *(vasculitis)* is largely a consequence of endothelial cell injury. Clearly, physical loss of endothelium can lead to exposure of the subendothelial ECM, adhesion of platelets, release of tissue factor, and local depletion of PGI_2 and plasminogen activators. *However, it should be emphasized that endothelium need not be denuded or physically disrupted to contribute to the development of thrombosis; any perturbation in the dynamic balance of the prothombotic and antithrombotic activities of endothelium can influence local clotting events* (see Fig. 4–6). Thus, dysfunctional endothelial cells can produce more procoagulant factors (e.g., platelet adhesion molecules, tissue factor, PAIs) or may synthesize less anticoagulant effectors (e.g., thrombomodulin, PGI_2, t-PA). Endothelial dysfunction can be induced by a wide variety of insults, including hypertension, turbulent blood flow, bacterial endotoxins, radiation injury, metabolic abnormalities such as homocystinemia or hypercholesterolemia, and toxins absorbed from cigarette smoke.

Alterations in Normal Blood Flow. *Turbulence* contributes to arterial and cardiac thrombosis by causing endothelial injury or dysfunction, as well as by forming countercurrents and local pockets of stasis; *stasis* is a major contributor in the development of venous thrombi.[25] Normal blood flow is *laminar* such that the platelets (and other blood cellular elements) flow centrally in the vessel lumen, separated from endothelium by a slower moving layer of plasma. Stasis and turbulence therefore:

- Promote endothelial activation, enhancing procoagulant activity, leukocyte adhesion, etc., in part through flow-induced changes in endothelial cell gene expression.[21]
- Disrupt laminar flow and bring platelets into contact with the endothelium[26]

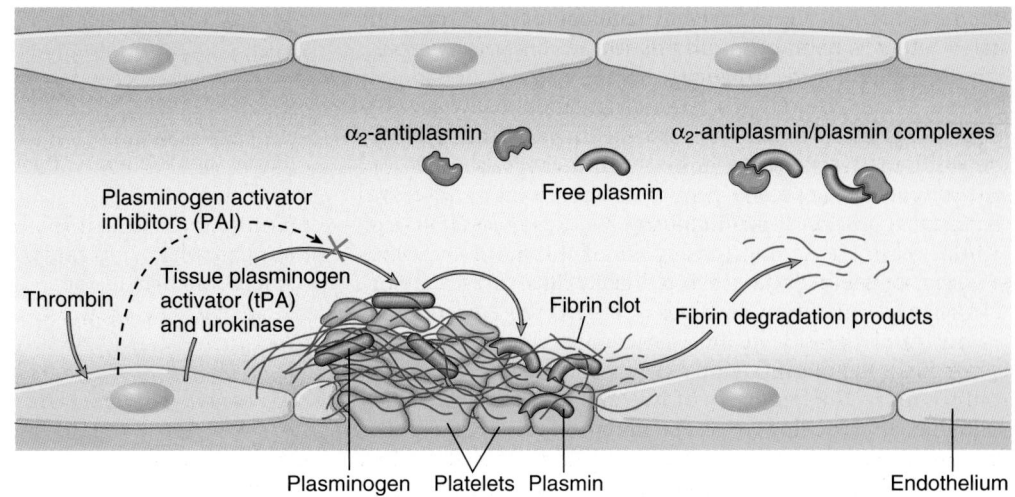

FIGURE 4–11 The fibrinolytic system, illustrating various plasminogen activators and inhibitors (see text).

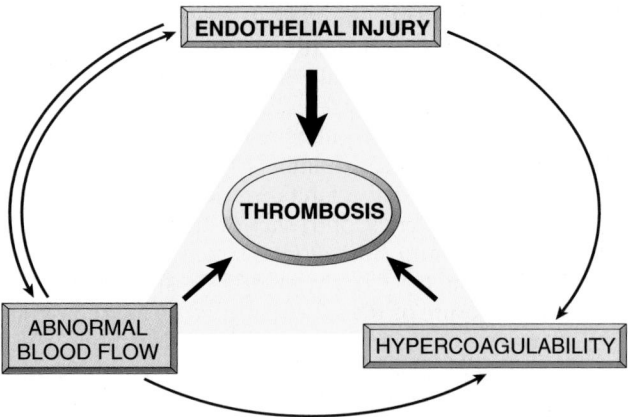

FIGURE 4–12 Virchow's triad in thrombosis. Endothelial integrity is the most important factor. Injury to endothelial cells can alter local blood flow and affect coagulability. Abnormal blood flow (stasis or turbulence), in turn, can cause endothelial injury. The factors promote thrombosis independently or in combination.

○ Prevent washout and dilution of activated clotting factors by fresh flowing blood and the inflow of clotting factor inhibitors

Turbulence and stasis contribute to thrombosis in several clinical settings. Ulcerated atherosclerotic plaques not only expose subendothelial ECM but also cause turbulence. Aortic and arterial dilations called *aneurysms* result in local stasis and are therefore fertile sites for thrombosis (Chapter 11). Acute myocardial infarctions result in areas of noncontractile myocardium and sometimes cardiac aneurysms; both are associated with stasis and flow abnormalities that promote the formation of cardiac mural thrombi (Chapter 12). Rheumatic mitral valve stenosis results in left atrial dilation; in conjunction with atrial fibrillation, a dilated atrium is a site of profound stasis and a prime location for developing thrombi (Chapter 12). *Hyperviscosity* (such as is seen with polycythemia vera; Chapter 13) increases resistance to flow and causes small vessel stasis; the deformed red cells in *sickle cell anemia* (Chapter 14) cause vascular occlusions, with the resulting stasis also predisposing to thrombosis.

Hypercoagulability. Hypercoagulability (also called *thrombophilia*) is a less frequent contributor to thrombotic states but is nevertheless an important component in the equation, and in some situations can predominate. It is loosely defined as any alteration of the coagulation pathways that predisposes to thrombosis; it can be divided into *primary* (genetic) and *secondary* (acquired) disorders (Table 4–2).[27–29] *Of the inherited causes of hypercoagulability, point mutations in the factor V gene and prothrombin gene are the most common.*

○ Approximately 2% to 15% of Caucasians carry a single-nucleotide mutation in factor V (called the *Leiden mutation*, after the city in the Netherlands where it was discovered). Among individuals with recurrent deep venous thrombosis the frequency of this mutation is considerably higher, approaching 60%. The mutation results in a glutamine to arginine substitution at position 506 that renders factor V resistant to cleavage by protein C. As a result, an

important antithrombotic counter-regulatory pathway is lost (see Fig. 4–6). Indeed, heterozygotes have a five-fold increased relative risk of venous thrombosis, and homozygotes have a 50-fold increase![30]

○ A single nucleotide change (G20210A) in the 3′-untranslated region of the *prothrombin gene* is another fairly common mutation in individuals with hypercoagulability (1% to 2% of the population); it is associated with elevated prothrombin levels and an almost threefold increased risk of venous thromboses.[28,31]

○ Elevated levels of *homocysteine* contribute to arterial and venous thrombosis, as well as the development of atherosclerosis (Chapter 11). The prothrombotic effects of homocysteine may be due to thioester linkages formed between homocysteine metabolites and a variety of proteins, including fibrinogen.[32] Marked elevations of homocysteine may be caused by an inherited deficiency of cystathione β-synthetase. Much more common is a variant form of the enzyme 5,10-methylenetetrahydrofolate reductase that causes mild homocysteinemia in 5% to 15% of Caucasian and eastern Asian populations; this possible etiology for hypercoagulability is therefore as common as factor V Leiden.[27] However, while folic acid, pyridoxine, and/or vitamin B_{12} supplements can reduce plasma homocysteine concentrations (by stimulating its metabolism), they fail to

TABLE 4–2   **Hypercoagulable States**
PRIMARY (GENETIC)
Common
Factor V mutation (G1691A mutation; factor V Leiden)
Prothrombin mutation (G20210A variant)
5,10-Methylenetetrahydrofolate reductase (homozygous C677T mutation)
Increased levels of factors VIII, IX, XI, or fibrinogen
Rare
Antithrombin III deficiency
Protein C deficiency
Protein S deficiency
Very Rare
Fibrinolysis defects
Homozygous homocystinuria (deficiency of cystathione β-synthetase)
SECONDARY (ACQUIRED)
High Risk for Thrombosis
Prolonged bedrest or immobilization
Myocardial infarction
Atrial fibrillation
Tissue injury (surgery, fracture, burn)
Cancer
Prosthetic cardiac valves
Disseminated intravascular coagulation
Heparin-induced thrombocytopenia
Antiphospholipid antibody syndrome
Lower Risk for Thrombosis
Cardiomyopathy
Nephrotic syndrome
Hyperestrogenic states (pregnancy and postpartum)
Oral contraceptive use
Sickle cell anemia
Smoking

lower the risk of thromboses, raising questions about the significance of modest homocysteinemia.[33]

⬤ Rare inherited causes of primary hypercoagulability include deficiencies of anticoagulants such as antithrombin III, protein C, or protein S; affected individuals typically present with venous thrombosis and recurrent thromboembolism beginning in adolescence or early adulthood.[27] Various polymorphisms in coagulant factor genes can result in increased synthesis and impart an elevated risk of venous thrombosis.[34]

The most common thrombophilic genotypes found in various populations (heterozygosity for factor V Leiden and heterozygosity for prothrombin) impart only a moderately increased risk of thrombosis; most individuals with these genotypes, when otherwise healthy, are free of thrombotic complications. However, mutations in factor V and prothrombin are frequent enough that homozygosity and compound heterozygosity are not rare, and such genotypes are associated with greater risk.[35] Moreover, individuals with such mutations have a significantly increased frequency of venous thrombosis in the setting of other acquired risk factors (e.g., pregnancy or prolonged bedrest). Thus, factor V Leiden heterozygosity (which by itself has only a modest effect) may trigger deep venous thrombosis when combined with enforced inactivity, such as during prolonged plane travel. Consequently, *inherited causes of hypercoagulability must be considered in patients under the age of 50 who present with thrombosis—even when acquired risk factors are present.*[36,37]

Unlike hereditary disorders, the pathogenesis of *acquired thrombophilia* is frequently multifactorial (see Table 4–2). In some cases (e.g., cardiac failure or trauma), stasis or vascular injury may be most important. Hypercoagulability due to oral contraceptive use or the hyperestrogenic state of pregnancy is probably caused by increased hepatic synthesis of coagulation factors and reduced anticoagulant synthesis.[38] In disseminated cancers, release of procoagulant tumor products predisposes to thrombosis.[39] The hypercoagulability seen with advancing age may be due to reduced endothelial PGI_2. Smoking and obesity promote hypercoagulability by unknown mechanisms.

Among the acquired thrombophilic states, two that are particularly important clinical problems deserve special mention.

Heparin-induced thrombocytopenia (HIT) syndrome. HIT occurs following the administration of *unfractionated heparin*, which may induce the appearance of antibodies that recognize complexes of heparin and platelet factor 4 on the surface of platelets (Chapter 14), as well as complexes of heparin-like molecules and platelet factor 4-like proteins on endothelial cells.[40–42] Binding of these antibodies to platelets results in their activation, aggregation, and consumption (hence the *thrombocytopenia* in the syndrome name). This effect on platelets and endothelial damage combine to produce a *prothrombotic state*, even in the face of heparin administration and low platelet counts. Newer low-molecular weight heparin preparations induce antibody formation less frequently, but still cause thrombosis if antibodies have already formed.[41] Other anticoagulants such as fondaparinux (a pentasaccharide inhibitor of factor X) also cause a HIT-like syndrome on rare occasions.[42]

Antiphospholipid antibody syndrome[43] (previously called the lupus anticoagulant syndrome). This syndrome has protean clinical manifestations, including recurrent thromboses, repeated miscarriages, cardiac valve vegetations, and thrombocytopenia. Depending on the vascular bed involved, the clinical presentations can include pulmonary embolism (following lower extremity venous thrombosis), pulmonary hypertension (from recurrent subclinical pulmonary emboli), stroke, bowel infarction, or renovascular hypertension. Fetal loss is attributable to antibody-mediated inhibition of t-PA activity necessary for trophoblastic invasion of the uterus. Antiphospholipid antibody syndrome is also a cause of renal microangiopathy, resulting in renal failure associated with multiple capillary and arterial thromboses (Chapter 20).

The name *antiphospholipid antibody syndrome* is a bit of a misnomer, as it is believed that the most important pathologic effects are mediated through binding of the antibodies to epitopes on plasma proteins (e.g., prothrombin) that are somehow induced or "unveiled" by phospholipids. In vivo, these autoantibodies induce a *hypercoagulable state* by causing endothelial injury, by activating platelets and complement directly, and through interaction with the catalytic domains of certain coagulation factors.[43] However, in vitro (in the absence of platelets and endothelial cells), the autoantibodies interfere with phospholipids and thus inhibit coagulation. The antibodies also frequently give a false-positive serologic test for syphilis because the antigen in the standard assay is embedded in cardiolipin.

Antiphospholipid antibody syndrome has primary and secondary forms. Individuals with a well-defined autoimmune disease, such as systemic lupus erythematosus (Chapter 6), are designated as having *secondary antiphospholipid syndrome* (hence the earlier term *lupus anticoagulant syndrome*). In *primary antiphospholipid syndrome*, patients exhibit only the manifestations of a hypercoagulable state and lack evidence of other autoimmune disorders; occasionally this happens in association with certain drugs or infections. A particularly aggressive form (*catastrophic antiphospholipid syndrome*) characterized by widespread small-vessel thrombi and multiorgan failure has a 50% mortality.[44] The antibodies also make surgical procedures more difficult; for example, nearly 90% of patients with anti-phospholipid antibodies undergoing cardiovascular surgery have complications related to the antibodies.[45] Therapy involves anticoagulation and immunosuppression. Although antiphospholipid antibodies are clearly associated with thrombotic diatheses, they have also been identified in 5% to 15% of apparently normal individuals, implying that they are necessary but not sufficient to cause the full-blown syndrome.

Morphology. Thrombi can develop anywhere in the cardiovascular system (e.g., in cardiac chambers, on valves, or in arteries, veins, or capillaries). The size and shape of thrombi depend on the site of origin and the cause. Arterial or cardiac thrombi usually begin at sites of turbulence or endothelial injury; venous thrombi characteristically occur at sites of stasis. Thrombi are focally attached to the underlying vascular surface; arterial thrombi tend to grow retrograde from the point of attachment, while venous thrombi extend in the direction of blood flow (thus both propagate toward the heart). The propagating

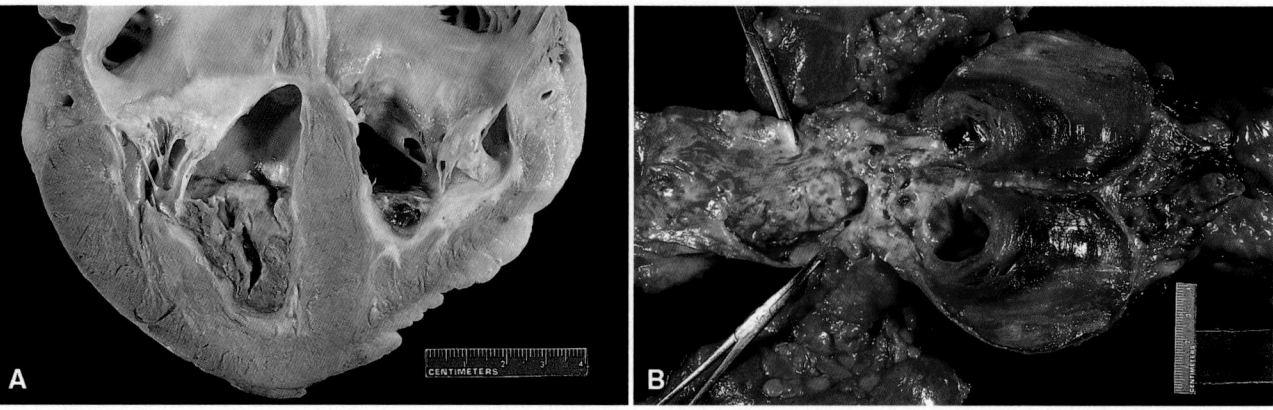

FIGURE 4–13   Mural thrombi. **A,** Thrombus in the left and right ventricular apices, overlying white fibrous scar. **B,** Laminated thrombus in a dilated abdominal aortic aneurysm. Numerous friable mural thrombi are also superimposed on advanced atherosclerotic lesions of the more proximal aorta *(left side of picture).*

portion of a thrombus is often poorly attached and therefore prone to fragmentation and embolization.

Thrombi often have grossly and microscopically apparent laminations called **lines of Zahn**; these represent pale platelet and fibrin deposits alternating with darker red cell–rich layers. Such laminations signify that a thrombus has formed in flowing blood; their presence can therefore distinguish antemortem thrombosis from the bland nonlaminated clots that occur postmortem (see below).

Thrombi occurring in heart chambers or in the aortic lumen are designated **mural thrombi**. Abnormal myocardial contraction (arrhythmias, dilated cardiomyopathy, or myocardial infarction) or endomyocardial injury (myocarditis or catheter trauma) promotes cardiac mural thrombi (Fig. 4–13A), while ulcerated atherosclerotic plaque and aneurysmal dilation are the precursors of aortic thrombus (Fig. 4–13B).

Arterial thrombi are frequently **occlusive**; the most common sites in decreasing order of frequency are the coronary, cerebral, and femoral arteries. They typically cosist of a friable meshwork of platelets, fibrin, red cells, and degenerating leukocytes. Although these are usually superimposed on a ruptured atherosclerotic plaque, other vascular injuries (vasculitis, trauma) may be the underlying cause.

Venous thrombosis (phlebothrombosis) is almost invariably occlusive, with the thrombus forming a long cast of the lumen. Because these thrombi form in the sluggish venous circulation, they tend to contain more enmeshed red cells (and relatively few platelets) and are therefore known as **red**, or **stasis**, **thrombi**. The veins of the lower extremities are most commonly involved (90% of cases); however, upper extremities, periprostatic plexus, or the ovarian and periuterine veins can also develop venous thrombi. Under special circumstances, they can also occur in the dural sinuses, portal vein, or hepatic vein.

Postmortem clots can sometimes be mistaken for antemortem venous thrombi. However, postmortem clots are gelatinous with a dark red dependent portion where red cells have settled by gravity and a yellow "chicken fat" upper portion; they are usually not attached to the underlying wall. In comparison, red thrombi are firmer and are focally attached, and sectioning typically reveals gross and/or microscopic lines of Zahn.

Thrombi on heart valves are called **vegetations**. Blood-borne bacteria or fungi can adhere to previously damaged valves (e.g., due to rheumatic heart disease) or can directly cause valve damage; in both cases, endothelial injury and disturbed blood flow can induce the formation of large thrombotic masses (**infective endocarditis**; Chapter 12). Sterile vegetations can also develop on noninfected valves in persons with hypercoagulable states, so-called **nonbacterial thrombotic endocarditis** (Chapter 12). Less commonly, sterile, verrucous endocarditis (**Libman-Sacks endocarditis**) can occur in the setting of systemic lupus erythematosus (Chapter 6).

Fate of the Thrombus. If a patient survives the initial thrombosis, in the ensuing days to weeks thrombi undergo some combination of the following four events:

- *Propagation.* Thrombi accumulate additional platelets and fibrin. This process was discussed earlier.
- *Embolization.* Thrombi dislodge and travel to other sites in the vasculature. This process is described below.
- *Dissolution.* Dissolution is the result of fibrinolysis, which can lead to the rapid shrinkage and total disappearance of recent thrombi. In contrast, the extensive fibrin deposition and crosslinking in older thrombi renders them more resistant to lysis. This distinction explains why therapeutic administration of fibrinolytic agents such as t-PA (e.g., in the setting of acute coronary thrombosis) is generally effective only when given in the first few hours of a thrombotic episode.
- *Organization and recanalization.* Older thrombi become organized by the ingrowth of endothelial cells, smooth

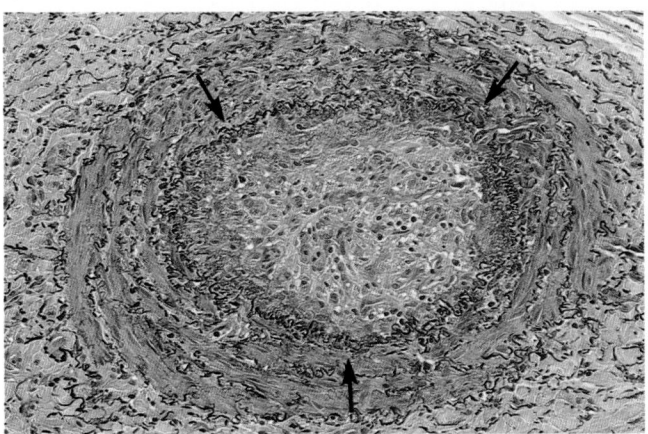

FIGURE 4–14 Low-power view of a thrombosed artery stained for elastic tissue. The original lumen is delineated by the internal elastic lamina *(arrows)* and is totally filled with organized thrombus, now punctuated by several recanalized endothelium-lined channels (white spaces).

muscle cells, and fibroblasts (Fig. 4–14). Capillary channels eventually form that re-establish the continuity of the original lumen, albeit to a variable degree.

Although the earliest capillary channels may not restore significant flow to obstructed vessels, continued recanalization may convert a thrombus into a smaller mass of connective tissue that becomes incorporated into the vessel wall. Eventually, with remodeling and contraction of the mesenchymal elements, only a fibrous lump may remain to mark the original thrombus. Occasionally the centers of thrombi undergo enzymatic digestion, presumably as a result of the release of lysosomal enzymes from trapped leukocytes and platelets. In the setting of bacteremia such thrombi may become infected, producing an inflammatory mass that erodes and weakens the vessel wall. If unchecked, this may result in a mycotic aneurysm (Chapter 11).

Clinical Consequences. Thrombi are significant because *they cause obstruction of arteries and veins,* and *are sources of emboli.* Which effect predominates depends on the site of the thrombosis. Venous thrombi can cause congestion and edema in vascular beds distal to an obstruction, but they are far more worrisome for their capacity to embolize to the lungs and cause death (see below). Conversely, although arterial thrombi can embolize and cause downstream infarctions, a thrombotic occlusion at a critical site (e.g., a coronary artery) can have more serious clinical consequences.

Venous Thrombosis (Phlebothrombosis). Most venous thrombi occur in the superficial or deep veins of the leg.[25] Superficial venous thrombi typically occur in the saphenous veins in the setting of varicosities. Although such thrombi can cause local congestion, swelling, pain, and tenderness, they rarely embolize. Nevertheless, the local edema and impaired venous drainage do predispose the overlying skin to infections from slight trauma and to the development of *varicose ulcers.* *Deep venous thrombosis (DVT) in the larger leg veins—at or above the knee* (e.g., popliteal, femoral, and iliac veins)—is more serious because such thrombi more often embolize to the lungs and give rise to pulmonary infarction (see below and Chapter 15). Although they can cause local pain and edema,

venous obstructions from DVTs can be rapidly offset by collateral channels. Consequently, DVTs are asymptomatic in approximately 50% of affected individuals and are recognized only in retrospect after embolization.

Lower extremity DVTs are associated with hypercoagulable states, as described earlier (see Table 4–2). Common predisposing factors include bed rest and immobilization (because they reduce the milking action of the leg muscles, resulting in reduced venous return), and congestive heart failure (also a cause of impaired venous return). Trauma, surgery, and burns not only immobilize a person but are also associated with vascular insults, procoagulant release from injured tissues, increased hepatic synthesis of coagulation factors, and altered t-PA production. Many elements contribute to the thrombotic diathesis of pregnancy; besides the potential for amniotic fluid infusion into the circulation at the time of delivery, late pregnancy and the postpartum period are also associated with systemic hypercoagulability. Tumor-associated inflammation and coagulation factors (tissue factor, factor VIII) and procoagulants (e.g., mucin) released from tumor cells all contribute to the increased risk of thromboembolism in disseminated cancers, so-called *migratory thrombophlebitis* or *Trousseau syndrome.*[39,46] Regardless of the specific clinical setting, advanced age also increases the risk of DVT.

Arterial and Cardiac Thrombosis. *Atherosclerosis* is a major cause of arterial thromboses, because it is associated with loss of endothelial integrity and with abnormal vascular flow (see Fig. 4–13B). Myocardial infarction can predispose to cardiac mural thrombi by causing dyskinetic myocardial contraction as well as damage to the adjacent endocardium (see Fig. 4–13A), and rheumatic heart disease may engender atrial mural thrombi as discussed above. Besides local obstructive consequences, cardiac and aortic mural thrombi can also embolize peripherally. Although any tissue can be affected, the brain, kidneys, and spleen are particularly likely targets because of their rich blood supply.

DISSEMINATED INTRAVASCULAR COAGULATION (DIC)

Disorders ranging from obstetric complications to advanced malignancy can be complicated by DIC, the sudden or insidious onset of widespread fibrin thrombi in the microcirculation. Although these thrombi are not grossly visible, they are readily apparent microscopically and can cause diffuse circulatory insufficiency, particularly in the brain, lungs, heart, and kidneys. To complicate matters, the widespread microvascular thrombosis results in platelet and coagulation protein consumption (hence the synonym *consumption coagulopathy*), and at the same time, fibrinolytic mechanisms are activated. Thus, an initially thrombotic disorder can evolve into a bleeding catastrophe. *It should be emphasized that DIC is not a primary disease but rather a potential complication of any condition associated with widespread activation of thrombin.*[47] It is discussed in greater detail along with other bleeding diatheses in Chapter 14.

Embolism

An embolus is a detached intravascular solid, liquid, or gaseous mass that is carried by the blood to a site distant from its point of origin. The term *embolus* was coined by Rudolf Virchow in 1848 to describe objects that lodge in blood vessels and obstruct the flow of blood. Almost all emboli represent some part of a dislodged thrombus, hence the term *thromboembolism.* Rare forms of emboli include fat droplets, nitrogen bubbles, atherosclerotic debris *(cholesterol emboli)*, tumor fragments, bone marrow, or even foreign bodies. However, unless otherwise specified, emboli should be considered thrombotic in origin. Inevitably, emboli lodge in vessels too small to permit further passage, causing partial or complete vascular occlusion; a major consequence is ischemic necrosis *(infarction)* of the downstream tissue. Depending on where they originate, emboli can lodge anywhere in the vascular tree; the clinical outcomes are best understood based on whether emboli lodge in the pulmonary or systemic circulations.

PULMONARY EMBOLISM

Pulmonary embolism (PE) has had a fairly stable incidence since the 1970s of roughly 2 to 4 per 1000 hospitalized patients in the United States, although the numbers vary depending on the mix of patient age and diagnosis (i.e., surgery, pregnancy, and malignancy all increase the risk).[48] While the rate of fatal PEs (as assessed at autopsy) has declined from 6% to 2% over the last quarter century, PE still causes about 200,000 deaths per year in the United States.[49] In more than 95% of cases, PEs originate from leg deep vein thromboses (DVTs), although it is important to realize that DVTs occur roughly two to three times more frequently than PEs.[48]

Fragmented thrombi from DVTs are carried through progressively larger channels and the right side of the heart before slamming into the pulmonary arterial vasculature. Depending on the size of the embolus, it can occlude the main pulmonary artery, straddle the pulmonary artery bifurcation *(saddle embolus)*, or pass out into the smaller, branching arteries (Fig. 4–15). Frequently there are multiple emboli, perhaps sequentially or as a shower of smaller emboli from a single large mass; in general, *the patient who has had one PE is at high risk of having more.* Rarely, an embolus can pass through an interatrial or interventricular defect and gain access to the systemic circulation *(paradoxical embolism).* A more complete discussion of PEs is presented in Chapter 15; an overview is offered here.[49-51]

- Most pulmonary emboli (60% to 80%) are clinically silent because they are small. With time they become organized and are incorporated into the vascular wall; in some cases organization of the thromboembolus leaves behind a delicate, bridging fibrous *web.*
- Sudden death, right heart failure *(cor pulmonale)*, or cardiovascular collapse occurs when emboli obstruct 60% or more of the pulmonary circulation.
- Embolic obstruction of medium-sized arteries with subsequent vascular rupture can result in pulmonary hemorrhage but usually does not cause pulmonary infarction. This is because the lung has a dual blood supply, and the intact bronchial circulation continues to perfuse the affected area. However, a similar embolus in the setting of left-sided cardiac failure (and compromised bronchial artery flow) can result in infarction.
- Embolic obstruction of small end-arteriolar pulmonary branches usually does result in hemorrhage or infarction.
- Multiple emboli over time may cause pulmonary hypertension and right ventricular failure.

SYSTEMIC THROMBOEMBOLISM

Systemic thromboembolism refers to emboli in the arterial circulation. Most (80%) arise from intracardiac mural thrombi, two thirds of which are associated with left ventricular wall infarcts and another quarter with left atrial dilation and fibrillation. The remainder originate from aortic aneurysms, thrombi on ulcerated atherosclerotic plaques, or fragmentation of a valvular vegetation, with a small fraction due to *paradoxical emboli*; 10% to 15% of systemic emboli are of unknown origin. In contrast to venous emboli, which tend to lodge primarily in one vascular bed (the lung), arterial emboli can travel to a wide variety of sites; the point of arrest depends on the source and the relative amount of blood flow that downstream tissues receive. Major sites for arteriolar embolization are the lower extremities (75%) and the brain (10%), with the intestines, kidneys, spleen, and upper extremities involved to a lesser extent. The consequences of embolization in a tissue depend on its vulnerability to ischemia, the caliber of the occluded vessel, and whether there is a collateral blood supply; in general, arterial emboli cause infarction of the affected tissues.

FAT AND MARROW EMBOLISM

Microscopic fat globules—with or without associated hematopoietic marrow elements—can be found in the circulation and impacted in the pulmonary vasculature after fractures of long bones (which have fatty marrow) or, rarely, in the setting of soft tissue trauma and burns. Fat and associated cells released by marrow or adipose tissue injury may enter the circulation after the rupture of the marrow vascular sinusoids or venules. Fat and marrow PEs are very common incidental findings after vigorous cardiopulmonary resuscitation and are probably of no clinical consequence. Indeed, fat embolism occurs in some 90% of individuals with severe skeletal injuries (Fig. 4–16), but less than 10% of such patients have any clinical findings.

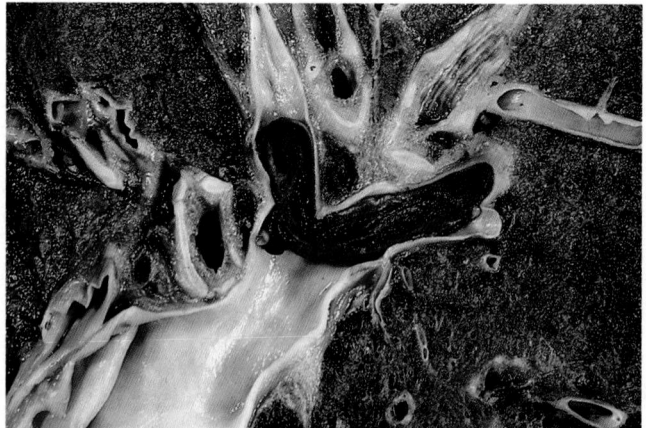

FIGURE 4–15 Embolus from a lower extremity deep venous thrombosis, now impacted in a pulmonary artery branch.

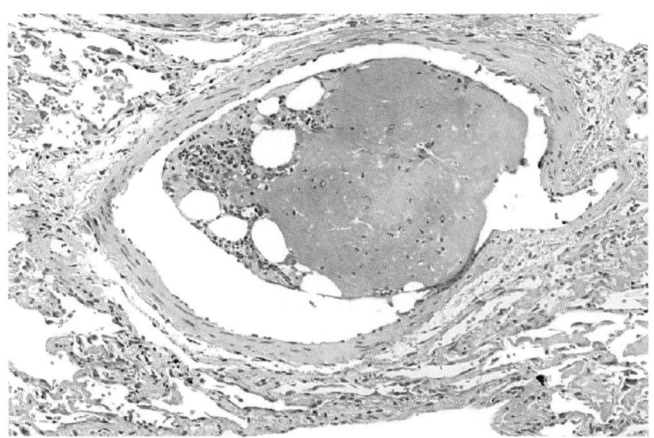

FIGURE 4–16 Bone marrow embolus in the pulmonary circulation. The cellular elements on the left side of the embolus are hematopoietic precursors, while the cleared vacuoles represent marrow fat. The relatively uniform red area on the right of the embolus is an early organizing thrombus.

Fat embolism syndrome is the term applied to the minority of patients who become symptomatic. It is characterized by pulmonary insufficiency, neurologic symptoms, anemia, and thrombocytopenia, and is fatal in about 5% to 15% of cases.[52,53] Typically, 1 to 3 days after injury there is a sudden onset of tachypnea, dyspnea, and tachycardia; irritability and restlessness can progress to delirium or coma. Thrombocytopenia is attributed to platelet adhesion to fat globules and subsequent aggregation or splenic sequestration; anemia can result from similar red cell aggregation and/or hemolysis. A diffuse petechial rash (seen in 20% to 50% of cases) is related to rapid onset of thrombocytopenia and can be a useful diagnostic feature.

The pathogenesis of fat emboli syndrome probably involves both mechanical obstruction and biochemical injury.[52] Fat microemboli and associated red cell and platelet aggregates can occlude the pulmonary and cerebral microvasculature. Release of free fatty acids from the fat globules exacerbates the situation by causing local toxic injury to endothelium, and platelet activation and granulocyte recruitment (with free radical, protease, and eicosanoid release) complete the vascular assault. Because lipids are dissolved out of tissue preparations by the solvents routinely used in paraffin embedding, the microscopic demonstration of fat microglobules (in the absence of accompanying marrow) typically requires specialized techniques, including frozen sections and stains for fat.

AIR EMBOLISM

Gas bubbles within the circulation can coalesce to form frothy masses that obstruct vascular flow (and cause distal ischemic injury). For example, a very small volume of air trapped in a coronary artery during bypass surgery, or introduced into the cerebral circulation by neurosurgery in the "sitting position," can occlude flow with dire consequences. Generally, more than 100 cc of air are required to have a clinical effect in the pulmonary circulation; however, this volume of air can be inadvertently introduced during obstetric or laparoscopic procedures, or as a consequence of chest wall injury.[54]

A particular form of gas embolism, called *decompression sickness*, occurs when individuals experience sudden decreases in atmospheric pressure.[55] Scuba and deep sea divers, underwater construction workers, and individuals in unpressurized aircraft in rapid ascent are all at risk. When air is breathed at high pressure (e.g., during a deep sea dive), increased amounts of gas (particularly nitrogen) are dissolved in the blood and tissues. If the diver then ascends (depressurizes) too rapidly, the nitrogen comes out of solution in the tissues and the blood.

The rapid formation of gas bubbles within skeletal muscles and supporting tissues in and about joints is responsible for the painful condition called *the bends*. In the lungs, gas bubbles in the vasculature cause edema, hemorrhage, and focal atelectasis or emphysema, leading to a form of respiratory distress called the *chokes*. A more chronic form of decompression sickness is called *caisson disease* (named for the pressurized vessels used in the bridge construction; workers in these vessels suffered both acute and chronic forms of decompression sickness). In caisson disease, persistence of gas emboli in the skeletal system leads to multiple foci of ischemic necrosis; the more common sites are the femoral heads, tibia, and humeri.

Acute decompression sickness is treated by placing the individual in a high pressure chamber, which serves to force the gas bubbles back into solution. Subsequent slow decompression theoretically permits gradual resorption and exhalation of the gases so that obstructive bubbles do not re-form.

AMNIOTIC FLUID EMBOLISM

Amniotic fluid embolism is an ominous complication of labor and the immediate postpartum period. Although the incidence is only approximately 1 in 40,000 deliveries, the mortality rate is up to 80%, making amniotic fluid embolism the fifth most common cause of maternal mortality worldwide; it accounts for roughly 10% of maternal deaths in the United States and results in permanent neurologic deficit in as many as 85% of survivors.[56] The onset is characterized by sudden severe dyspnea, cyanosis, and shock, followed by neurologic impairment ranging from headache to seizures and coma. If the patient survives the initial crisis, pulmonary edema typically develops, along with (in half the patients) DIC, as a result of release of thrombogenic substances from the amniotic fluid.[56]

The underlying cause is the infusion of amniotic fluid or fetal tissue into the maternal circulation via a tear in the placental membranes or rupture of uterine veins. Classic findings include the presence of squamous cells shed from fetal skin, lanugo hair, fat from vernix caseosa, and mucin derived from the fetal respiratory or gastrointestinal tract in the maternal pulmonary microvasculature (Fig. 4–17). Other findings include marked pulmonary edema, *diffuse alveolar damage* (Chapter 15), and the presence of fibrin thrombi in many vascular beds due to DIC.

Infarction

An infarct is an area of ischemic necrosis caused by occlusion of either the arterial supply or the venous drainage. Tissue

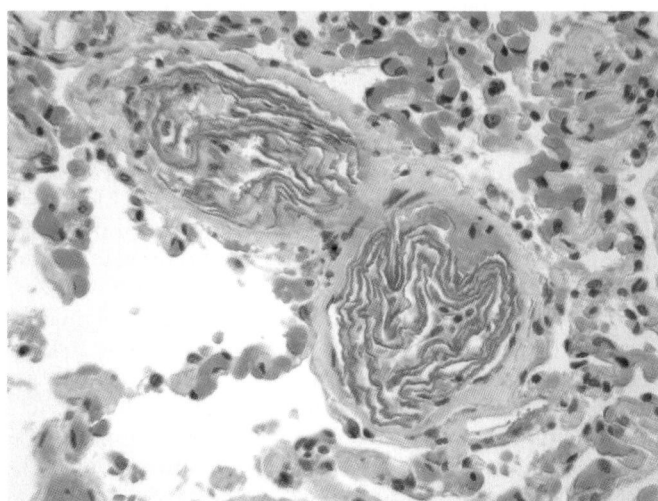

FIGURE 4–17   Amniotic fluid embolism. Two small pulmonary arterioles are packed with laminated swirls of fetal squamous cells. There is marked edema and congestion, and elsewhere in the lung were small organizing thrombi consistent with disseminated intravascular coagulation. (Courtesy of Dr. Beth Schwartz, Baltimore, MD.)

infarction is a common and extremely important cause of clinical illness. Roughly 40% of all deaths in the United States are caused by cardiovascular disease, and most of these are attributable to myocardial or cerebral infarction. Pulmonary infarction is also a common complication in many clinical settings, bowel infarction is frequently fatal, and ischemic necrosis of the extremities *(gangrene)* is a serious problem in the diabetic population.

Nearly all infarcts result from thrombotic or embolic arterial occlusions. Occasionally infarctions are caused by other mechanisms, including local vasospasm, hemorrhage into an atheromatous plaque, or extrinsic vessel compression (e.g., by tumor). Rarer causes include torsion of a vessel (e.g., in testicular torsion or bowel volvulus), traumatic rupture, or vascular compromise by edema (e.g., *anterior compartment syndrome*) or by entrapment in a hernia sac. Although venous thrombosis can cause infarction, the more common outcome is just congestion; in this setting, bypass channels rapidly open and permit vascular outflow, which then improves arterial inflow. Infarcts caused by venous thrombosis are thus more likely in organs with a single efferent vein (e.g., testis and ovary).

Morphology. Infarcts are classified according to color and the presence or absence of infection; they are either red (hemorrhagic) or white (anemic) and may be septic or bland.

- **Red infarcts** (Fig. 4–18A) occur (1) with venous occlusions (e.g., ovary), (2) in loose tissues (e.g., lung) where blood can collect in the infarcted zone, (3) in tissues with dual circulations (e.g., lung and small intestine) that allow blood flow from an unobstructed parallel supply into a necrotic zone, (4) in tissues previously congested by sluggish venous

outflow, and (5) when flow is re-established to a site of previous arterial occlusion and necrosis (e.g., following angioplasty of an arterial obstruction).
- **White infarcts** (Fig. 4–18B) occur with arterial occlusions in solid organs with end-arterial circulation (e.g., heart, spleen, and kidney), and where tissue density limits the seepage of blood from adjoining capillary beds into the necrotic area.

Infarcts tend to be wedge-shaped, with the occluded vessel at the apex and the periphery of the organ forming the base (see Fig. 4–18); when the base is a serosal surface there can be an overlying fibrinous exudate. Acute infarcts are poorly defined and slightly hemorrhagic. With time the margins tend to become better defined by a narrow rim of congestion attributable to inflammation.

Infarcts resulting from arterial occlusions in organs without a dual blood supply typically become progressively paler and more sharply defined with time (see Fig. 4–18B). By comparison, in the lung hemorrhagic infarcts are the rule (see Fig. 4–18A). Extravasated red cells in hemorrhagic infarcts are phagocytosed by macrophages, which convert heme iron into hemosiderin; small amounts do not grossly impart any appreciable color to the tissue, but extensive hemorrhage can leave a firm, brown residuum.

The dominant histologic characteristic of infarction is **ischemic coagulative necrosis** (Chapter 1). It is important to recall that if the vascular occlusion has occurred shortly (minutes to hours) before the death of the person, no demonstrable histologic changes may be evident; it takes 4 to 12 hours for the tissue to show frank necrosis. Acute inflammation is present along the margins of infarcts within a few hours and is usually well defined within 1 to 2 days. Eventually the inflammatory response is followed by a reparative response beginning in the preserved margins (Chapter 2). In stable or labile tissues, parenchymal

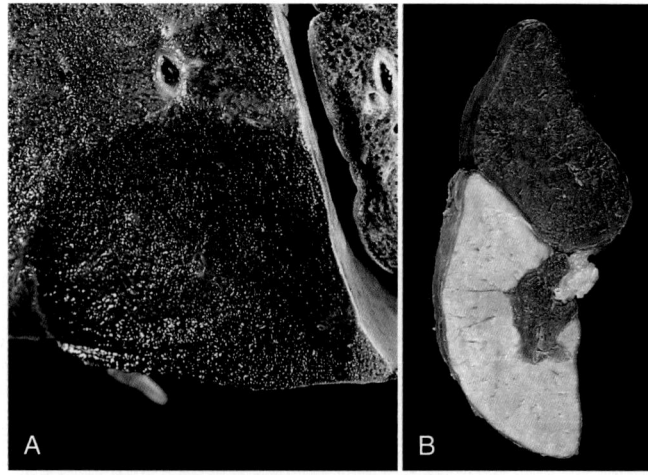

FIGURE 4–18   Red and white infarcts. **A,** Hemorrhagic, roughly wedge-shaped pulmonary *red infarct.* **B,** Sharply demarcated *white infarct* in the spleen.

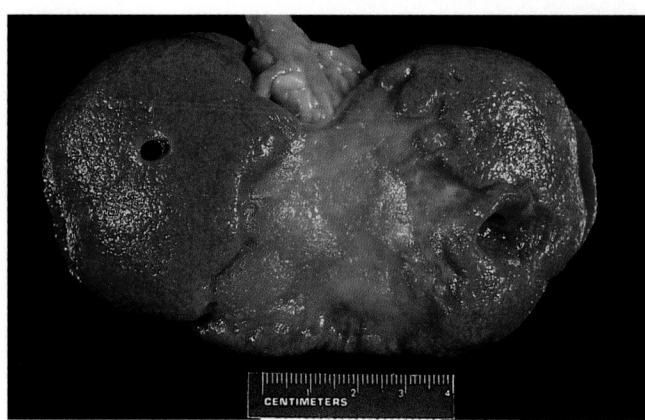

FIGURE 4–19 Remote kidney infarct, now replaced by a large fibrotic scar.

regeneration can occur at the periphery where underlying stromal architecture is preserved. However, most infarcts are ultimately replaced by **scar** (Fig. 4–19). The brain is an exception to these generalizations, as central nervous system infarction results in **liquefactive necrosis** (Chapter 1).

Septic infarctions occur when infected cardiac valve vegetations embolize or when microbes seed necrotic tissue. In these cases the infarct is converted into an **abscess**, with a correspondingly greater inflammatory response (Chapter 2). The eventual sequence of organization, however, follows the pattern already described.

Factors That Influence Development of an Infarct. The effects of vascular occlusion can range from no or minimal effect to causing the death of a tissue or person. *The major determinants of the eventual outcome are:* (1) *the nature of the vascular supply,* (2) *the rate at which an occlusion develops,* (3) *vulnerability to hypoxia,* and (4) *the oxygen content of the blood.*

○ *Nature of the vascular supply.* The availability of an alternative blood supply is the most important determinant of whether vessel occlusion will cause damage. As already mentioned, the lungs have a dual pulmonary and bronchial artery blood supply that provides protection from thromboembolism-induced infarction. Similarly, the liver, with its dual hepatic artery and portal vein circulation, and the hand and forearm, with their dual radial and ulnar arterial supply, are all relatively resistant to infarction. In contrast, renal and splenic circulations are end-arterial, and vascular obstruction generally causes tissue death.

○ *Rate of occlusion development.* Slowly developing occlusions are less likely to cause infarction, because they provide time to develop alternate perfusion pathways. For example, small interarteriolar anastomoses—normally with minimal functional flow—interconnect the three major coronary arteries in the heart. If one of the coronaries is only slowly occluded (i.e., by an encroaching atherosclerotic plaque), flow within this *collateral circulation* may increase sufficiently to prevent infarction, even though the larger coronary artery is eventually occluded.

○ *Vulnerability to hypoxia.* Neurons undergo irreversible damage when deprived of their blood supply for only 3 to 4 minutes. Myocardial cells, though hardier than neurons, are also quite sensitive and die after only 20 to 30 minutes of ischemia. In contrast, fibroblasts within myocardium remain viable even after many hours of ischemia (Chapter 12).

○ *Oxygen content of blood.* A partial obstruction of a small vessel that would be without effect in an otherwise normal individual might cause infarction in an anemic or cyanotic patient.

Shock

Shock is the final common pathway for several potentially lethal clinical events, including severe hemorrhage, extensive trauma or burns, large myocardial infarction, massive pulmonary embolism, and microbial sepsis. *Shock is characterized by systemic hypotension due either to reduced cardiac output or to reduced effective circulating blood volume.* The consequences are *impaired tissue perfusion and cellular hypoxia.* At the outset the cellular injury is reversible; however, prolonged shock eventually leads to irreversible tissue injury that often proves fatal.

The causes of shock fall into three general categories (Table 4–3):

○ *Cardiogenic shock* results from low cardiac output due to myocardial pump failure. This can be due to intrinsic myocardial damage (infarction), ventricular arrhythmias, extrinsic compression (cardiac tamponade; Chapter 12), or outflow obstruction (e.g., pulmonary embolism).

○ *Hypovolemic shock* results from low cardiac output due to the loss of blood or plasma volume, such as can occur with massive hemorrhage or fluid loss from severe burns.

○ *Septic shock* results from vasodilation and peripheral pooling of blood as part of a systemic immune reaction to bacterial or fungal infection. Its complex pathogenesis is discussed in further detail below.

Less commonly, shock can occur in the setting of anesthetic accident or a spinal cord injury *(neurogenic shock),* as a result of loss of vascular tone and peripheral pooling of blood. *Anaphylactic shock* denotes systemic vasodilation and increased vascular permeability caused by an IgE–mediated hypersensitivity reaction (Chapter 6). In these situations, acute widespread vasodilation results in tissue hypoperfusion and hypoxia.

PATHOGENESIS OF SEPTIC SHOCK

Septic shock is associated with severe hemodynamic and hemostatic derangements, and therefore merits more detailed consideration here. With a mortality rate near 20%, septic shock ranks first among the causes of death in intensive care units and accounts for over 200,000 lost lives each year in the United States.[57] Its incidence is rising, ironically due to improvements in life support for critically ill patients and the growing ranks of immunocompromised hosts (due to chemotherapy, immunosuppression, or HIV infection). Currently, septic shock is most frequently triggered by gram-positive

TABLE 4–3 **Three Major Types of Shock**

Type of Shock	Clinical Example	Principal Mechanisms
CARDIOGENIC		
	Myocardial infarction Ventricular rupture Arrhythmia Cardiac tamponade Pulmonary embolism	Failure of myocardial pump resulting from intrinsic myocardial damage, extrinsic pressure, or obstruction to outflow
HYPOVOLEMIC		
	Fluid loss (e.g., hemorrhage, vomiting, diarrhea, burns, or trauma)	Inadequate blood or plasma volume
SEPTIC		
	Overwhelming microbial infections (bacterial and fungal) Superantigens (e.g., toxic shock syndrome)	Peripheral vasodilation and pooling of blood; endothelial activation/injury; leukocyte-induced damage, disseminated intravascular coagulation; activation of cytokine cascades

bacterial infections, followed by gram-negative bacteria and fungi.[57] Hence, the older synonym of "endotoxic shock" is not appropriate.

In septic shock, systemic vasodilation and pooling of blood in the periphery leads to tissue hypoperfusion, even though cardiac output may be preserved or even increased early in the course. This is accompanied by widespread endothelial cell activation and injury, often leading to a hypercoagulable state that can manifest as DIC. In addition, septic shock is associated with changes in metabolism that directly suppress cellular function. The net effect of these abnormalities is hypoperfusion and dysfunction of multiple organs—culminating in the extraordinary morbidity and mortality associated with sepsis.

The ability of diverse microorganisms to cause septic shock (sometimes even when the infection is localized to one area of the body)[58] is consistent with the idea that several microbial constituents can initiate the process. As you will recall from Chapter 2, macrophages, neutrophils, and other cells of the innate immune system express a number of receptors that respond to a variety of substances derived from microorganisms. Once activated, these cells release inflammatory mediators, as well as a variety of immunosuppressive factors that modify the host response. In addition, microbial constituents also activate humoral elements of innate immunity, particularly the complement and coagulation pathways. These mediators combine with the direct effects of microbial constituents on endothelium in a complex, incompletely understood fashion to produce septic shock (Fig. 4-20).[59–61] The major factors contributing to its pathophysiology include the following:

○ *Inflammatory mediators.* Various microbial cell wall constituents engage receptors on neutrophils, mononuclear inflammatory cells, and endothelial cells, leading to cellular activation. Toll-like receptors (TLRs, Chapter 2) recognize microbial elements and trigger the responses that initiate sepsis. However, mice genetically deficient in TLRs still succumb to sepsis,[59,60] and it is believed that other pathways are probably also involved in the initiation of sepsis in humans (e.g., G-protein coupled receptors that detect bacterial peptides and nucleotide oligomerization domain

proteins 1 and 2 [NOD1, NOD2]).[62] Upon activation, inflammatory cells produce TNF, IL-1, IFN-γ, IL-12, and IL-18, as well as other inflammatory mediators such as high mobility group box 1 protein (HMGB1).[62] Reactive oxygen species and lipid mediators such as prostaglandins and platelet activating factor (PAF) are also elaborated. These effector molecules activate endothelial cells (and other cell types) resulting in adhesion molecule expression, a procoagulant phenotype, and secondary waves of cytokine production.[61] The *complement cascade* is also activated by microbial components, both directly and through the proteolytic activity of plasmin (Chapter 2), resulting in the production of anaphylotoxins (C3a, C5a), chemotactic fragments (C5a), and opsonins (C3b) that contribute to the pro-inflammatory state.[63] In addition, microbial components such as endotoxin can activate coagulation directly through factor XII and indirectly through altered endothelial function (discussed below). The systemic procoagulant state induced by sepsis not only leads to thrombosis, but also augments inflammation through effects mediated by protease-activated receptors (PARs) found on inflammatory cells.

○ *Endothelial cell activation and injury.* Endothelial cell activation by microbial constituents or inflammatory mediators produced by leukocytes has three major sequelae: (1) thrombosis; (2) increased vascular permeability; and (3) vasodilation. *The derangement in coagulation is sufficient to produce the fearsome complication of DIC in up to half of septic patients.*[60] Sepsis alters the expression of many factors so as to favor coagulation. Pro-inflammatory cytokines result in increased tissue factor production by endothelial cells (and monocytes as well), while at the same time reining in fibrinolysis by increasing PAI-1 expression (see Fig. 4-6*B* and Fig. 4-8). The production of other endothelial anticoagulant factors, such as tissue factor pathway inhibitor, thrombomodulin, and protein C (see Fig. 4-6 and Fig. 4-8), are diminished.[60,61,64] The procoagulant tendency is further exacerbated by decreased blood flow at the level of small vessels, producing stasis and diminishing the washout of activated coagulation factors. Acting in concert, these effects promote the deposition of fibrin-rich thrombi in small vessels, often throughout the body, which also contributes

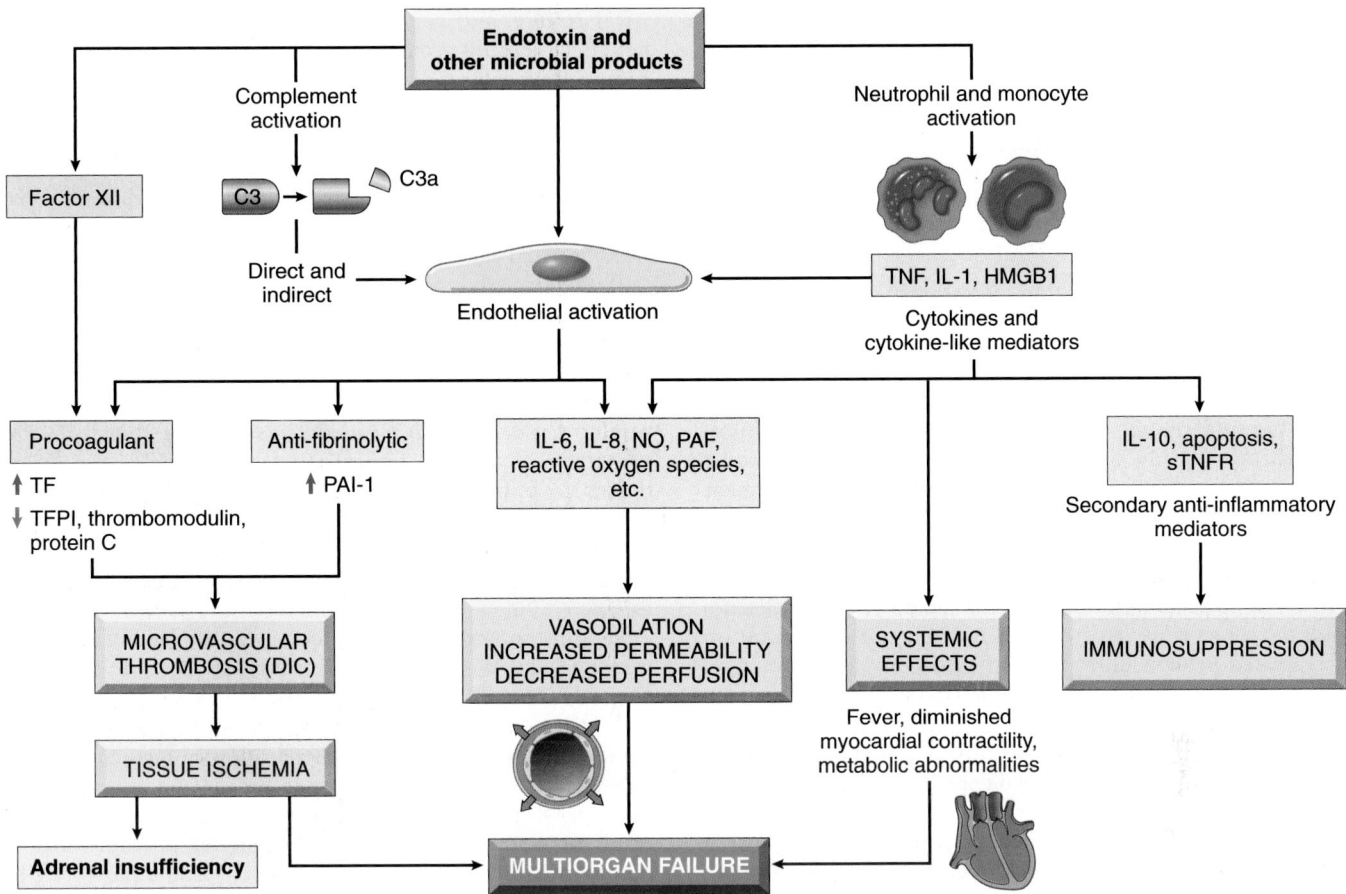

FIGURE 4–20   Major pathogenic pathways in septic shock. Microbial products activate endothelial cells and cellular and humoral elements of the innate immune system, initiating a cascade of events that lead to end-stage multiorgan failure. Additional details are given in the text. DIC, disseminated vascular coagulation; HMGB1, high mobility group box 1 protein; NO, nitric oxide; PAF, platelet activating factor; PAI-1, plasminogen activator inhibitor 1; STNFR, soluble TNF receptor; TF, tissue factor; TFPI, tissue factor pathway inhibitor.

to the hypoperfusion of tissues.[60] In full-blown DIC, the consumption of coagulation factors and platelets is so great that deficiencies of these factors appear, leading to concomitant bleeding and hemorrhage (Chapter 14). The increase in vascular permeability leads to exudation of fluid into the interstitium, causing edema and an increase in interstitial fluid pressure that may further impede blood flow into tissues, particularly following resuscitation of the patient with intravenous fluids. The endothelium also increases its expression of inducible nitric oxide synthetase and the production of nitric oxide (NO). These alterations, along with increases in vasoactive inflammatory mediators (e.g., C3a, C5a, and PAF), cause the systemic relaxation of vascular smooth muscle, leading to hypotension and diminished tissue perfusion.

- *Metabolic abnormalities.* Septic patients exhibit insulin resistance and hyperglycemia. Cytokines such as TNF and IL-1, stress-induced hormones (such as glucagon, growth hormone, and glucocorticoids), and catecholamines all drive gluconeogenesis. At the same time, the pro-inflammatory cytokines suppress insulin release while simultaneously promoting insulin resistance in the liver and other tissues, likely by impairing the surface expression of GLUT-4,[65] a glucose transporter. Hyperglycemia decreases

neutrophil function—thereby suppressing bactericidal activity—and causes increased adhesion molecule expression on endothelial cells.[65] Although sepsis is initially associated with an acute surge in glucocorticoid production, this phase is frequently followed by adrenal insufficiency and a functional deficit of glucocorticoids. This may stem from depression of the synthetic capacity of intact adrenal glands or frank adrenal necrosis due to DIC (*Waterhouse-Friderichsen syndrome*, Chapter 24).

- *Immune suppression.* The hyperinflammatory state initiated by sepsis can activate counter-regulatory immunosuppressive mechanisms, which may involve both innate and adaptive immunity.[59–61] Proposed mechanisms for the immune suppression include a shift from pro-inflammatory (T_H1) to anti-inflammatory (T_H2) cytokines (Chapter 6), production of anti-inflammatory mediators (e.g., soluble TNF receptor, IL-1 receptor antagonist, and IL-10), lymphocyte apoptosis, the immunosuppressive effects of apoptotic cells, and the induction of cellular anergy.[59–61] It is still debated whether immunosuppressive mediators are deleterious or protective in sepsis.[59]

- *Organ dysfunction.* Systemic hypotension, interstitial edema, and small vessel thrombosis all decrease the delivery of oxygen and nutrients to the tissues, which fail to properly utilize those nutrients that are delivered due to changes in cellular metabolism. High levels of cytokines and secondary mediators may diminish myocardial contractility and cardiac output, and increased vascular permeability and endothelial injury can lead to the *adult respiratory distress syndrome* (Chapter 15). Ultimately, these factors may conspire to cause the failure of multiple organs, particularly the kidneys, liver, lungs, and heart, culminating in death.

The severity and outcome of septic shock are likely dependent upon the extent and virulence of the infection; the immune status of the host; the presence of other co-morbid conditions; and the pattern and level of mediator production. The multiplicity of factors and the complexity of the interactions that underlie sepsis explain why most attempts to intervene therapeutically with antagonists of specific mediators have been of very modest benefit at best, and may even have had deleterious effects in some cases.[59] The standard of care remains treatment with appropriate antibiotics, intensive insulin therapy for hyperglycemia, fluid resuscitation to maintain systemic pressures, and "physiologic doses" of corticosteroids to correct relative adrenal insufficiency.[59] Administration of activated protein C (to prevent thrombin generation and thereby reduce coagulation and inflammation) may have some benefit in cases of severe sepsis, but this remains controversial. Suffice it to say, even in the best of clinical centers, septic shock remains an obstinate clinical challenge.[58]

It is worth mentioning here that an additional group of secreted bacterial proteins called *superantigens* also cause a syndrome similar to septic shock (e.g., *toxic shock syndrome*). Superantigens are polyclonal T-lymphocyte activators that induce the release of high levels of cytokines that result in a variety of clinical manifestations, ranging from a diffuse rash to vasodilation, hypotension, and death.[66]

STAGES OF SHOCK

Shock is a progressive disorder that, if uncorrected, leads to death. The exact mechanism(s) of death from sepsis are still unclear; aside from increased lymphocyte and enterocyte apoptosis there is only minimal cell death, and patients rarely have refractory hypotension.[61] For hypovolemic and cardiogenic shock, however, the pathways to death are reasonably well understood. Unless the insult is massive and rapidly lethal (e.g., a massive hemorrhage from a ruptured aortic aneurysm), shock in those settings tends to evolve through three general (albeit somewhat artificial) phases:

- An initial *nonprogressive phase* during which reflex compensatory mechanisms are activated and perfusion of vital organs is maintained
- A *progressive stage* characterized by tissue hypoperfusion and onset of worsening circulatory and metabolic imbalances, including acidosis
- An *irreversible stage* that sets in after the body has incurred cellular and tissue injury so severe that even if the hemodynamic defects are corrected, survival is not possible

In the early nonprogressive phase of shock, a variety of *neurohumoral mechanisms* help to maintain cardiac output and blood pressure. These include baroreceptor reflexes, catecholamine release, activation of the renin-angiotensin axis,

ADH release, and generalized sympathetic stimulation. The net effect is *tachycardia, peripheral vasoconstriction, and renal conservation of fluid*. Cutaneous vasoconstriction, for example, is responsible for the characteristic coolness and pallor of the skin in well-developed shock (although septic shock can initially cause cutaneous *vasodilation* and thus present with warm, flushed skin). Coronary and cerebral vessels are less sensitive to the sympathetic response and thus maintain relatively normal caliber, blood flow, and oxygen delivery.

If the underlying causes are not corrected, shock passes imperceptibly to the progressive phase, during which there is widespread tissue hypoxia. In the setting of persistent oxygen deficit, intracellular aerobic respiration is replaced by anaerobic glycolysis with excessive production of lactic acid. The resultant metabolic *lactic acidosis lowers the tissue pH and blunts the vasomotor response*; arterioles dilate, and blood begins to pool in the microcirculation. Peripheral pooling not only worsens the cardiac output, but also puts EC at risk for developing anoxic injury with subsequent DIC. With widespread tissue hypoxia, vital organs are affected and begin to fail.

Without intervention, the process eventually enters an irreversible stage. Widespread cell injury is reflected in lysosomal enzyme leakage, further aggravating the shock state. Myocardial contractile function worsens in part because of nitric oxide synthesis. If ischemic bowel allows intestinal flora to enter the circulation, bacteremic shock may be superimposed. At this point the patient has complete renal shutdown as a result of acute tubular necrosis (Chapter 20), and despite heroic measures the downward clinical spiral almost inevitably culminates in death.

Morphology. The cellular and tissue changes induced by cardiogenic or hypovolemic shock are essentially those of hypoxic injury (Chapter 1); changes can manifest in any tissue although they are particularly evident in brain, heart, lungs, kidneys, adrenals, and gastrointestinal tract. The **adrenal** changes in shock are those seen in all forms of stress; essentially there is cortical cell lipid depletion. This does not reflect adrenal exhaustion but rather conversion of the relatively inactive vacuolated cells to metabolically active cells that utilize stored lipids for the synthesis of steroids. The **kidneys** typically exhibit acute tubular necrosis (Chapter 20). The **lungs** are seldom affected in pure hypovolemic shock, because they are somewhat resistant to hypoxic injury. However, when shock is caused by bacterial sepsis or trauma, changes of **diffuse alveolar damage** (Chapter 15) may develop, the so-called shock lung. In septic shock, the development of DIC leads to widespread deposition of fibrin-rich microthrombi, particularly in the brain, heart, lungs, kidney, adrenal glands, and gastrointestinal tract. The consumption of platelets and coagulation factors also often leads to the appearance of petechial hemorrhages on serosal surface and the skin.

With the exception of neuronal and myocyte ischemic loss, virtually all of these tissues may revert to normal if the individual survives. Unfortunately, most patients with irreversible changes due to severe shock die before the tissues can recover.

Clinical Consequences. The clinical manifestations of shock depend on the precipitating insult. In hypovolemic and cardiogenic shock *the patient presents with hypotension; a weak, rapid pulse; tachypnea; and cool, clammy, cyanotic skin.* In septic shock *the skin may initially be warm and flushed because of peripheral vasodilation.* The initial threat to life stems from the underlying catastrophe that precipitated the shock (e.g., myocardial infarct, severe hemorrhage, or sepsis). Rapidly, however, the cardiac, cerebral, and pulmonary changes secondary to shock worsen the problem. Eventually, electrolyte disturbances and metabolic acidosis also exacerbate the situation. Individuals who survive the initial complications may enter *a second phase dominated by renal insufficiency* and marked by a progressive fall in urine output as well as severe fluid and electrolyte imbalances.

The prognosis varies with the origin of shock and its duration. Thus, greater than 90% of young, otherwise healthy patients with hypovolemic shock survive with appropriate management; in comparison, septic shock, or cardiogenic shock associated with extensive myocardial infarction, can have substantially worse mortality rates, even with optimal care.

REFERENCES

1. Schrier R, Abraham W: Hormones and hemodynamics in heart failure. N Engl J Med 341:57, 1999.
2. Chen H, Schrier R: Pathophysiology of volume overload in acute heart failure syndromes. Am J Med 119:S11, 2006.
3. Arnout J et al.: Haemostasis. Handb Exp Pharmacol 176 (Pt 2):1, 2006.
4. Hoffman M, Monroe D: Coagulation 2006: a modern view of hemostasis. Hematol Oncol Clin North Am 21:1, 2007.
5. Michiels C: Endothelial cell functions. J Cell Physiol 196:430, 2003.
6. Galley H, Webster N: Physiology of the endothelium. Br J Anaesth 93:105, 2004.
7. Pries A, Kuebler W: Normal endothelium. Handb Exp Pharmacol 176 (Pt 1):1, 2006.
8. Mackman N: Tissue-specific hemostasis in mice. Arterioscler Thromb Vasc Biol 25:2273, 2005.
9. Esmon C: Inflammation and the activated protein C anticoagulant pathway. Semin Thromb Hemost 32 (Suppl 1):49, 2006.
10. Crawley J, Lane D: The haemostatic role of tissue factor pathway inhibitor. Arterioscler Thromb Vasc Biol 2007.
11. Ruggeri Z: Von Willebrand factor: looking back and looking forward. Thromb Haemost 98:55, 2007.
12. Monroe D, Key N: The tissue factor–factor VIIa complex: procoagulant activity, regulation, and multitasking. J Thromb Haemost 5:1097, 2007.
13. Andrews R, Berndt M: Platelet physiology and thrombosis. Thromb Res 114:447, 2004.
14. Briedé J et al.: von Willebrand factor stimulates thrombin-induced exposure of procoagulant phospholipids on the surface of fibrin-adherent platelets. J Thromb Haemost 1:559, 2003.
15. Lentz B: Exposure of platelet membrane phosphatidylserine regulates blood coagulation. Prog Lipid Res 42:423, 2003.
16. Salles I et al.: Inherited traits affecting platelet function. Blood Rev 2008.
17. Husmann M, Barton M: Therapeutical potential of direct thrombin inhibitors for atherosclerotic vascular disease. Expert Opin Investig Drugs 16:563, 2007.
18. Schneider D, Aggarwal A: Development of glycoprotein IIb–IIIa antagonists: translation of pharmacodynamic effects into clinical benefit. Expert Rev Cardiovasc Ther 2:903, 2004.
19. Mackman N et al.: Role of the extrinsic pathway of blood coagulation in hemostasis and thrombosis. Arterioscler Thromb Vasc Biol 27:1687, 2007.
20. Crawley J et al.: The central role of thrombin in hemostasis. J Thromb Haemost 5 (Suppl 1):95, 2007.
21. Coughlin S: Protease-activated receptors in hemostasis, thrombosis and vascular biology. J Thromb Haemost 3:1800, 2005.
22. Landis R: Protease activated receptors: clinical relevance to hemostasis and inflammation. Hematol Oncol Clin North Am 21:103, 2007.
23. Cesarman-Maus G, Hajjar K: Molecular mechanisms of fibrinolysis. Br J Haematol 129:307, 2005.
24. Cale J, Lawrence D: Structure-function relationships of plasminogen activator inhibitor-1 and its potential as a therapeutic agent. Curr Drug Targets 8:971, 2007.
25. Cushman M: Epidemiology and risk factors for venous thrombosis. Semin Hematol 44:62, 2007.
26. Nesbitt W et al.: The impact of blood rheology on the molecular and cellular events underlying arterial thrombosis. J Mol Med 84:989, 2006.
27. Seligsohn U, Lubetsky A: Genetic susceptibility to venous thrombosis. N Engl J Med 344:1222, 2001.
28. Feero W: Genetic thrombophilia. Prim Care 31:685, 2004.
29. Middeldorp S, Levi M: Thrombophilia: an update. Semin Thromb Hemost 33:563, 2007.
30. Rosendorff A, Dorfman D: Activated protein C resistance and factor V Leiden. Arch Pathol Lab Med 131:866, 2007.
31. Danckwardt S et al.: 3′ end processing of the prothrombin mRNA in thrombophilia. Acta Haematol 115:192, 2006.
32. Jakubowski H: The molecular basis of homocysteine thiolactone-mediated vascular disease. Clin Chem Lab Med 45:1704, 2007.
33. Gatt A, Makris M: Hyperhomocysteinemia and venous thrombosis. Semin Hematol 44:70, 2007.
34. Kottke-Marchant K: Genetic polymorphisms associated with venous and arterial thrombosis: an overview. Arch Pathol Lab Med 126:295, 2002.
35. Emmerich J et al.: Combined effect of factor V Leiden and prothrombin 20210A on the risk of venous thromboembolism—pooled analysis of 8 case-control studies including 2310 cases and 3204 controls. Study Group for Pooled-Analysis in Venous Thromboembolism. Thromb Haemost 86:809, 2001.
36. Gallus A: Travel, venous thromboembolism, and thrombophilia. Semin Thromb Hemost 31:90, 2005.
37. Kuipers S et al.: Travel and venous thrombosis: a systematic review. J Intern Med 262:615, 2007.
38. Rosendaal F et al.: Estrogens, progestogens and thrombosis. J Thromb Haemost 1:1371, 2003.
39. Zwicker J et al.: Cancer-associated thrombosis. Crit Rev Oncol Hematol 62:126, 2007.
40. Castelli R et al.: Heparin induced thrombocytopenia: pathogenetic, clinical, diagnostic and therapeutic aspects. Cardiovasc Hematol Disord Drug Targets 7:153, 2007.
41. Warkentin T: Heparin-induced thrombocytopenia. Hematol Oncol Clin North Am 21:589, 2007.
42. Warkentin T et al.: Heparin-induced thrombocytopenia associated with fondaparinux. N Engl J Med 356:2653, 2007.
43. Pierangeli S et al.: Antiphospholipid antibodies and the antiphospholipid syndrome: an update on treatment and pathogenic mechanisms. Curr Opin Hematol 13:366, 2006.
44. Merrill J, Asherson R: Catastrophic antiphospholipid syndrome. Nat Clin Pract Rheumatol 2:81, 2006.
45. Hegde V et al.: Cardiovascular surgical outcomes in patients with the antiphospholipid syndrome—a case-series. Heart Lung Circ 16:4237, 2007.
46. Varki A: Trousseau's syndrome: multiple definitions and multiple mechanisms. Blood 110:1723, 2007.
47. Levi M: Disseminated intravascular coagulation. Crit Care Med 35:21915, 2007.
48. Stein P et al.: Trends in the incidence of pulmonary embolism and deep venous thrombosis in hospitalized patients. Am J Cardiol 95:1525, 2005.
49. Heit J: Venous thromboembolism epidemiology: implications for prevention and management. Semin Thromb Hemost 28 (Suppl 2):3, 2002.
50. Goldhaber S: Pulmonary embolism. Lancet 363:1295, 2004.
51. Rahimtoola A, Bergin J: Acute pulmonary embolism: an update on diagnosis and management. Curr Probl Cardiol 30:61, 2005.
52. Parisi D et al.: Fat embolism syndrome. Am J Orthop 31:507, 2002.
53. Habashi N et al.: Therapeutic aspects of fat embolism syndrome. Injury 37 (Suppl 4):S68, 2006.
54. Mirski M et al.: Diagnosis and treatment of vascular air embolism. Anesthesiology 106:164, 2007.

55. Tetzlaff K, Thorsen E: Breathing at depth: physiologic and clinical aspects of diving while breathing compressed gas. Clin Chest Med 26:355, 2005.

56. Moore J, Baldisseri M: Amniotic fluid embolism. Crit Care Med 33 (10 Suppl):S279, 2005.

57. Martin G et al.: The epidemiology of sepsis in the United States from 1979 through 2000. N Engl J Med 348:1546, 2003.

58. Munford R: Severe sepsis and septic shock: the role of gram-negative bacteremia. Annu Rev Pathol 1:467, 2006.

59. Hotchkiss R, Karl I: The pathophysiology and treatment of sepsis. N Engl J Med 348:138, 2003.

60. Remick D: Pathophysiology of sepsis. Am J Pathol 170:1435, 2007.

61. Cohen J: The immunopathogenesis of sepsis. Nature 420:885, 2002.

62. Fink M: Neuropetide modulators of high mobility group box 1 secretion as potential therapeutic agents for severe sepsis. Am J Pathol 172:1171, 2008.

63. Albrecht E, Ward P: Complement-induced impairment of the innate immune system during sepsis. Curr Infect Dis Rep 7:349, 2005.

64. vanAmersfoort E et al.: Receptors, mediators, and mechanisms involved in bacterial sepsis and septic shock. Clin Microbiol Rev 16:379, 2003.

65. Marik P, Raghaven M: Stress-hyperglycemia, insulin and immunomodulation in sepsis. Int Care Med 30:748, 2004.

66. Zamoyska R: Superantigens: supersignalers? Sci STKE 358:45, 2006.

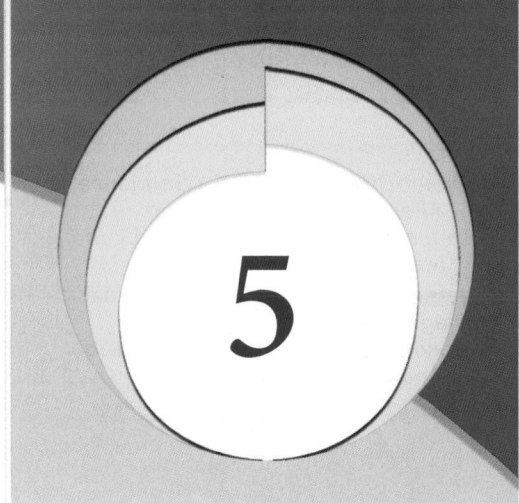

Genetic Disorders

Human Genetic Architecture

Genes and Human Diseases
  Mutations

Mendelian Disorders
  Transmission Patterns of Single-Gene
    Disorders
    Autosomal Dominant Disorders
    Autosomal Recessive Disorders
    X-Linked Disorders
  Biochemical and Molecular Basis of
    Single-Gene (Mendelian) Disorders
    *Enzyme Defects and Their
      Consequences*
    *Defects in Receptors and Transport
      Systems*
    *Alterations in Structure, Function, or
      Quantity of Nonenzyme Proteins*
    *Genetically Determined Adverse
      Reactions to Drugs*
  Disorders Associated with Defects in
    Structural Proteins
    Marfan Syndrome
    Ehlers-Danlos Syndromes (EDS)
  Disorders Associated with Defects in
    Receptor Proteins
    Familial Hypercholesterolemia
  Disorders Associated with Defects in
    Enzymes
    Lysosomal Storage Diseases
    *Glycogen Storage Diseases
      (Glycogenoses)*
    Alkaptonuria (Ochronosis)
  Disorders Associated with Defects in
    Proteins That Regulate Cell Growth

Complex Multigenic Disorders

Chromosomal Disorders
  Normal Karyotype
  Structural Abnormalities of Chromosomes
  Cytogenetic Disorders Involving
    Autosomes
    Trisomy 21 (Down Syndrome)
    Other Trisomies
    *Chromosome 22q11.2 Deletion
      Syndrome*
  Cytogenetic Disorders Involving Sex
    Chromosomes
    Klinefelter Syndrome
    Turner Syndrome
    *Hermaphroditism and
      Pseudohermaphroditism*

**Single-Gene Disorders with Nonclassic
  Inheritance**
  Diseases Caused by Trinucleotide-Repeat
    Mutations
    Fragile-X Syndrome
  Mutations in Mitochondrial Genes—Leber
    Hereditary Optic Neuropathy
  Genomic Imprinting
    *Prader-Willi Syndrome and Angelman
      Syndrome*
  Gonadal Mosaicism

**Molecular Diagnosis of Genetic
  Diseases***
  Indications for Analysis of Germ Line
    Genetic Alterations
  Indications for Analysis of Acquired
    Genetic Alterations
  PCR and Detection of DNA Sequence
    Alterations

*The assistance of Dr. A. John Iafrate (Massachusetts General Hospital, Boston, MA) in the revision of the section on molecular diagnosis is greatly appreciated.

Direct Detection of DNA Sequence
Alterations by Sequencing
Detection of DNA Mutations by Indirect
Methods
**Polymorphic Markers and Molecular
Diagnosis**
Polymorphisms and Genome-Wide
Analysis (GWAS)

**Molecular Analysis of Genomic
Alterations**
Southern Blotting
Fluorescence in Situ Hybridization
Array-Based Comparative Genomic
Hybridization (Array CGH)
Epigenetic Alterations
RNA Analysis

Human Genetic Architecture

The sequence of the human genome is complete, and much has been learned about the "genetic architecture" of humans.[1] Some of what has been revealed was quite unexpected. For example, we now know that less than 2% of the human genome encodes proteins, whereas more than one half represents blocks of repetitive DNA sequences whose functions remain mysterious. What was totally unexpected was that humans have a mere 20,000 to 25,000 genes that code for proteins rather than the 100,000 predicted. Quite remarkably, this figure is about the same as that of the mustard plant, with 26,000 genes! However, it is also known that by alternative splicing, the 25,000 human genes can give rise to greater than 100,000 proteins. Humans are not so poor, after all. With the completion of the Human Genome Project, a new term, *genomics*, has been added to the medical vocabulary. Whereas genetics is the study of single or a few genes and their phenotypic effects, genomics is the study of all the genes in the genome and their interactions.[2] DNA microarray analysis of tumors (Chapter 7) is an excellent example of genomics in current clinical use.

Another surprising revelation from the recent progress in genomics is that, on average, any two individuals share greater than 99.5% of their DNA sequences.[3] Thus, the remarkable diversity of humans is encoded in less than 0.5% of our DNA. The secrets to disease predisposition and response to environmental agents and drugs must therefore reside within these variations. Though small when compared to the total nucleotide sequences, this 0.5% represents about 15 million base pairs. The two most common forms of DNA variations in the human genome are *single-nucleotide polymorphisms (SNPs)* and *copy number variations (CNVs)*. SNPs represent variation at single isolated nucleotide positions and are almost always biallelic (i.e., one of only two choices exist at a given site within the population, such as A or T). Much effort has been devoted to making SNP maps of the human genome. These efforts have identified over 6 million SNPs in the human population, many of which show wide variation in frequency in different populations. SNPs may occur anywhere in the genome—within exons, introns, or intergenic regions, but less than 1% of SNPs occur in coding regions. These coding sequence variations are important, since they could of course alter the gene product and predispose to a phenotypic difference or to a disease. Much more commonly, however, the SNP is just a marker that is co-inherited with a disease-associated gene as

a result of physical proximity. Another way of expressing this is to say that the SNP and the causative genetic factor are in *linkage disequilibrium*. There is optimism that groups of SNPs could serve as reliable markers of risk for multigenic complex diseases such as type II diabetes and hypertension, and that by identifying such variants strategies for disease prevention could be developed (discussed later).

CNVs are a recently identified form of genetic variation consisting of different numbers of large contiguous stretches of DNA from 1000 base pairs to millions of base pairs.[4,5] In some instances these loci are, like SNPs, biallelic and simply duplicated or deleted in a subset of the population. In other instances there are complex rearrangements of genomic material, with multiple alleles in the human population. Current estimates are that CNVs are responsible for between 5 and 24 million base pairs of sequence difference between any two individuals.[6] Approximately 50% of CNVs involve gene-coding sequences; thus, CNVs may underlie a large portion of human phenotypic diversity. There is a significant over-representation of certain gene families in regions affected by CNVs; these include genes involved in the immune system and in the nervous system. It is assumed that copy number diversity in such gene families has been subject to strong evolutionary selection, since they would enhance human adaptation to changing environmental factors. We currently know much less about CNVs than SNPs, therefore their influence on disease susceptibility is less established, though predicted to be substantial.

It should be pointed out that despite all these advances in the understanding of human variations, it is clear that alterations in DNA sequence cannot by themselves explain the diversity of phenotypes in human populations. Nor can classic genetics explain how monozygotic twins can have differing phenotypes.[7] The answer must lie in *epigenetics*, which is defined as heritable changes in gene expression that are not caused by alterations in DNA sequence. Epigenetic changes are involved in tissue-specific expression of genes and genomic imprinting. The biochemical basis of epigenetic changes and its detection are discussed under "Molecular Diagnosis."

Just as genomics involves the study of all the DNA sequences, *proteomics* concerns itself with the measurement of all proteins expressed in a cell or tissue. To simultaneously analyze patterns of expression involving thousands of genes and proteins has required the parallel development of computer-based techniques that can manage vast collections of data. In response to this, an exciting new discipline called *bioinformatics* has sprouted.[8]

It is worth noting that until recently the major focus of gene hunting has been discovery of structural genes whose products encode proteins. Recent studies indicate, however, that a very large number of genes do not encode proteins. Instead, their products play important regulatory functions. The most recently discovered among this class of genes are those that encode small RNA molecules, so-called microRNAs (miRNAs). miRNAs, unlike other RNAs, do not encode proteins but instead inhibit gene expression. Silencing of gene expression by miRNA is preserved in all living forms from plants to humans and therefore must be a fundamental mechanism of gene regulation. Because of their profound influence on gene regulation, miRNAs are assuming central importance in understanding normal developmental pathways, as well as pathologic conditions, such as cancer.[9] Such is the importance of the discovery of gene silencing by miRNAs that Andrew Fire and Craig Mello were awarded the Nobel Prize in physiology or medicine in 2006, a mere 8 years after they published their initial work.

By current estimates there are approximately 1000 genes in humans that encode miRNAs, accounting for about 5% of the human genome. Transcription of miRNA genes produces primary miRNA transcripts, which is processed within the nucleus to form another structure, called pre-miRNA (Fig. 5–1). With the help of specific transporter proteins, pre-miRNA is exported to the cytoplasm. Additional "cutting" by an enzyme, appropriately called Dicer, generates mature miRNAs that are about 21 to 30 nucleotides in length (hence the name "micro"). At this stage the miRNA is still double-stranded. Next, the miRNA unwinds, and single strands of this duplex are incorporated into a multiprotein complex called RNA-induced silencing complex (RISC). Base-pairing between the miRNA strand and its target messenger RNA (mRNA) directs the RISC to either cause mRNA cleavage or repress its translation. In this way, the gene from which the target mRNA was derived is silenced (at a post-transcriptional level).[10] Given that the numbers of miRNA genes are far fewer than those that encode proteins, it follows that a given miRNA can silence many target genes. The precise mechanism by which the target specificity of miRNA is determined remains to be fully elucidated.

Another species of gene-silencing RNA, called *small interfering RNAs* (siRNAs), works in a manner quite similar to that of miRNA. Unlike miRNA, however, siRNA precursors are introduced by investigators into the cell. Their processing by Dicer and functioning via RISC are essentially similar to that described for miRNA. siRNAs are becoming powerful tools for studying gene function and may in the future be used therapeutically to silence specific genes, such as oncogenes, whose products are involved in neoplastic transformation.

Genes and Human Diseases

Genetic disorders are far more common than is widely appreciated. The lifetime frequency of genetic diseases is estimated to be 670 per 1000.[11] Furthermore, the genetic diseases encountered in medical practice represent only the tip of the iceberg, that is, those with less extreme genotypic errors permitting full embryonic development and live birth. It is estimated that 50% of spontaneous abortuses during the early months of gestation have a demonstrable chromosomal abnormality;

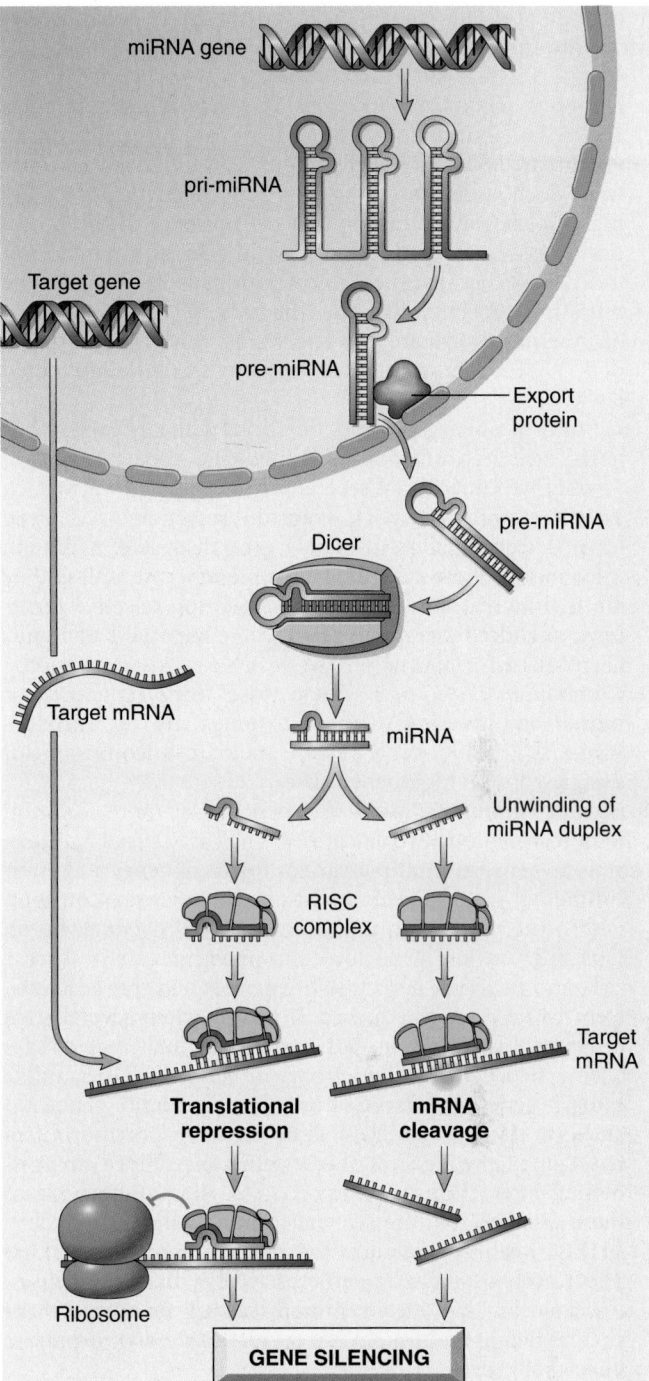

FIGURE 5–1 Generation of microRNAs and their mode of action in regulating gene function. Pri-miRNA, primary microRNA transcript; pre-miRNA, precursor microRNA; RISC, RNA-induced silencing complex.

there are, in addition, numerous smaller detectable errors and many others still beyond our range of identification. About 1% of all newborn infants possess a gross chromosomal abnormality, and approximately 5% of individuals under age 25 develop a serious disease with a significant genetic component. How many more mutations remain hidden?

Before discussing specific aberrations that may cause genetic diseases, it is useful to summarize the genetic contribution to human disease. Human genetic disorders can be broadly classified into three categories

- *Disorders related to mutations in single genes with large effects.* These mutations cause the disease or predispose to the disease and are typically not present in normal population. Such mutations and their associated disorders are highly penetrant, meaning that the presence of the mutation is associated with the disease in a large proportion of individuals. Because these diseases are caused by single gene mutations, they usually follow the classic Mendelian pattern of inheritance and are also referred to as Mendelian disorders. A few important exceptions to this rule are noted later.

  Study of single genes and mutations with large effects has been extremely informative in medicine since a great deal of what we know about several physiologic pathways (such as cholesterol transport, chloride secretion) has been learned from analysis of single gene disorders. Although informative, these disorders are generally rare unless they are maintained in a population by strong selective forces (e.g., sickle cell anemia in areas where malaria is endemic, Chapter 14).

- *Chromosomal disorders.* These arise from structural or numerical alteration in the autosomes and sex chromosomes. Like monogenic disease they are uncommon but associated with high penetrance.

- *Complex multigenic disorders.* These are far more common than the previous two categories. They are caused by interactions between multiple variant forms of genes and environmental factors. Such variations in genes are common within the population and are also called *polymorphisms.* Each such variant gene confers a small increase in disease risk, and no single susceptibility gene is necessary or sufficient to produce the disease. It is only when several such polymorphisms are present in an individual that disease occurs, hence the term *multigenic* or *polygenic.* Thus, unlike mutant genes with large effects that are highly penetrant and give rise to Mendelian disorders, each polymorphism has a small effect and is of low penetrance. Since environmental interactions are important in the pathogenesis of these diseases, they are also called multifactorial disorders. In this category are some of the most common diseases that afflict humans, including atherosclerosis, diabetes mellitus, hypertension, and autoimmune diseases. Even normal traits such as height and weight are governed by polymorphisms in several genes.

  Since complex traits do not follow a Mendelian pattern of inheritance, the genes and polymorphisms that contribute to such diseases have been very difficult to discern. However, recent progress in genomics and high throughput sequencing technology has made possible genome wide association studies (GWAS), a systematic method of identifying disease-associated polymorphisms that is beginning to unravel the molecular basis of complex disorders. We will discuss the principle of GWAS later in the chapter.

We begin our discussion with a description of mutations that affect single genes, since they underlie Mendelian disorders. We follow with transmission patterns and selected samples of single gene disorders.

MUTATIONS

A *mutation* is defined as a permanent change in the DNA. Mutations that affect germ cells are transmitted to the progeny and can give rise to inherited diseases. Mutations that arise in somatic cells understandably do not cause hereditary diseases but are important in the genesis of cancers and some congenital malformations.

Mutations may result in partial or complete deletion of a gene or, more often, affect a single base. For example, a single nucleotide base may be *substituted* by a different base, resulting in a *point mutation.* Less commonly, one or two base pairs may be *inserted* into or *deleted* from the DNA, leading to alterations in the reading frame of the DNA strand; hence these are referred to as *frameshift* mutations (Figs. 5–2 and 5–3). Next we briefly review some general principles relating to the effects of gene mutations.

- *Point mutations within coding sequences:* A point mutation may alter the code in a triplet of bases and lead to the replacement of one amino acid by another in the gene product. Because these mutations alter the meaning of the sequence of the encoded protein, they are often termed *missense mutations.* If the substituted amino acid causes little change in the function of the protein, the mutation is called a "conservative" missense mutation. On the other hand, a "nonconservative" missense mutation replaces the normal amino acid with a very different one. An excellent example of this type is the sickle mutation affecting the β-globin chain of hemoglobin (Chapter 14). Here the nucleotide triplet CTC (or GAG in mRNA), which encodes glutamic acid, is changed to CAC (or GUG in mRNA), which encodes valine. This single amino acid substitution alters the physicochemical properties of hemoglobin, giving rise to sickle cell anemia. Besides producing an amino acid substitution, a point mutation may change an amino acid codon to a chain terminator, or *stop codon (nonsense mutation).* Taking again the example of β-globin, a point mutation affecting the codon for glutamine (CAG) creates a stop codon (UAG) if U is substituted for C (Fig. 5–4). This change leads to premature termination of β-globin gene translation, and the short peptide that is produced is rapidly degraded. The resulting deficiency of β-globin chains can give rise to a severe form of anemia called β^0-thalassemia (Chapter 14).

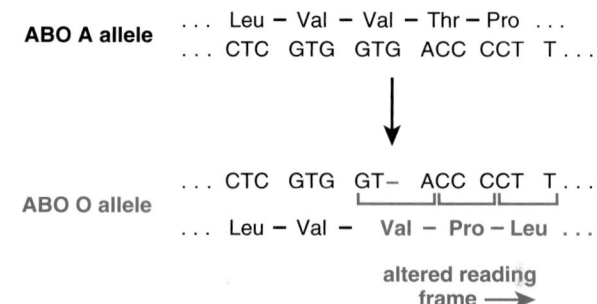

FIGURE 5–2   Single-base deletion at the ABO (glycosyltransferase) locus, leading to a frameshift mutation responsible for the O allele. (From Thompson MW et al.: Thompson and Thompson Genetics in Medicine, 5th ed. Philadelphia, WB Saunders, 1991, p 134.)

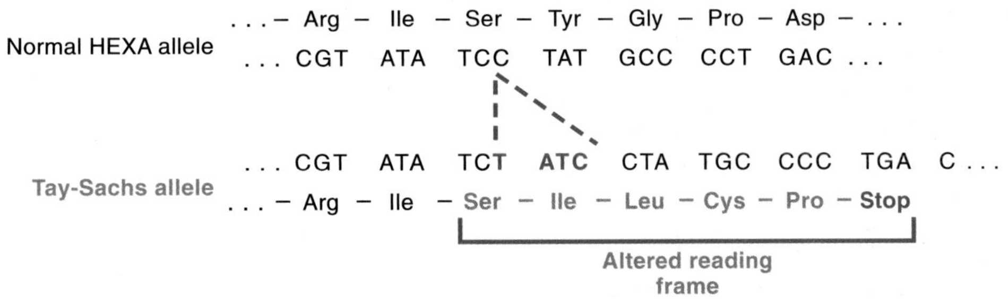

FIGURE 5–3 Four-base insertion in the hexosaminidase A gene, leading to a frameshift mutation. This mutation is the major cause of Tay-Sachs disease in Ashkenazi Jews. (From Nussbaum RL et al.: Thompson and Thompson Genetics in Medicine, 6th ed. Philadelphia, WB Saunders, 2001, p 212.)

- *Mutations within noncoding sequences:* Deleterious effects may also result from mutations that do not involve the exons. Recall that transcription of DNA is initiated and regulated by promoter and enhancer sequences. Point mutations or deletions involving these regulatory sequences may interfere with binding of transcription factors and thus lead to a marked reduction in or total lack of transcription. Such is the case in certain forms of hereditary anemias. In addition, point mutations within introns may lead to defective splicing of intervening sequences. This, in turn, interferes with normal processing of the initial mRNA transcripts and results in a failure to form mature mRNA. Therefore, translation cannot take place, and the gene product is not synthesized.

- *Deletions and insertions:* Small deletions or insertions involving the coding sequence lead to alterations in the reading frame of the DNA strand; hence, they are referred to as *frameshift mutations* (see Figs. 5–2 and 5–3). If the number of base pairs involved is three or a multiple of three, frameshift does not occur (Fig. 5–5); instead an abnormal protein lacking or gaining one or more amino acids is synthesized.

- *Trinucleotide-repeat mutations:* Trinucleotide-repeat mutations belong to a special category of genetic anomaly. These mutations are characterized by amplification of a sequence of three nucleotides. Although the specific nucleotide sequence that undergoes amplification differs in various disorders, almost all affected sequences share the nucleotides guanine (G) and cytosine (C). For example, in fragile-X syndrome, prototypical of this category of disorders, there are 250 to 4000 tandem repeats of the sequence CGG within a gene called familial mental retardation 1 (*FMR1*). In normal populations the number of repeats is small, averaging 29. Such expansions of the trinucleotide sequences prevent normal expression of the *FMR1* gene, thus giving rise to mental retardation. Another *distinguishing feature of trinucleotide-repeat mutations is that they are dynamic* (i.e., the degree of amplification increases during gametogenesis). These features, discussed in greater detail later, influence the pattern of inheritance and the phenotypic manifestations of the diseases caused by this class of mutation.

To summarize, mutations can interfere with protein synthesis at various levels. Transcription may be suppressed with gene deletions and point mutations involving promoter sequences. Abnormal mRNA processing may result from mutations affecting introns or splice junctions or both. Translation is affected if a stop codon (chain termination mutation) is created within an exon. Finally, some point mutations may lead to the formation of an abnormal protein without impairing any step in protein synthesis.

In closing, it should be noted that, uncommonly, mutations are beneficial. As will be discussed in Chapter 6, the human immunodeficiency virus (HIV) uses a chemokine receptor, CCR5, to enter cells; a deletion in the *CCR5* gene thus protects from HIV infection.

Against this background, we now turn our attention to the three major categories of genetic disorders: (1) disorders related to mutant genes of large effect, (2) diseases with multifactorial inheritance, and (3) chromosomal disorders. To

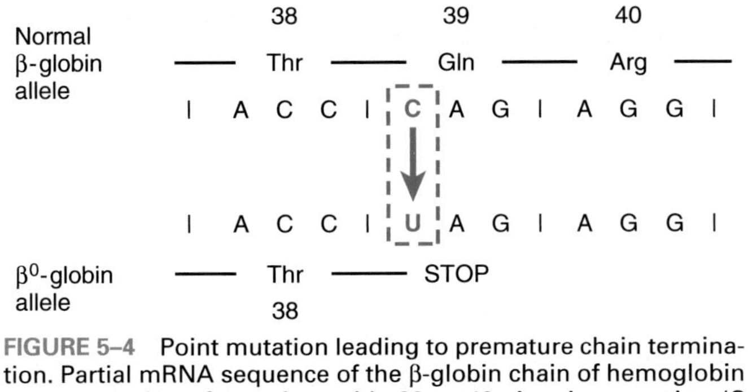

FIGURE 5–4 Point mutation leading to premature chain termination. Partial mRNA sequence of the β-globin chain of hemoglobin showing codons for amino acids 38 to 40. A point mutation (C → U) in codon 39 changes glutamine (Gln) codon to a stop codon, and hence protein synthesis stops at amino acid 38.

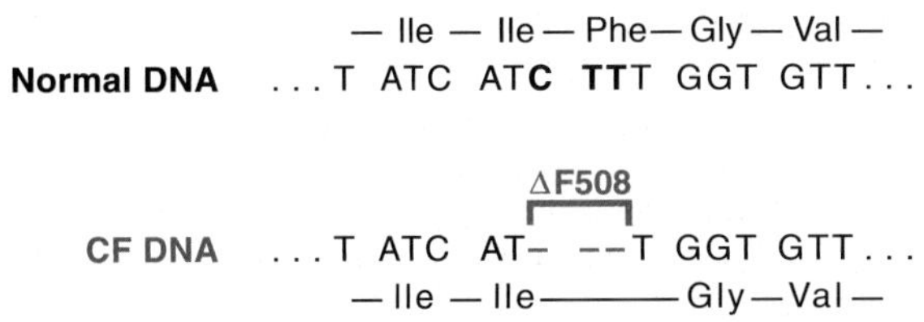

FIGURE 5–5 Three-base deletion in the common cystic fibrosis (CF) allele results in synthesis of a protein that lacks amino acid 508 (phenylalanine). Because the deletion is a multiple of three, this is not a frameshift mutation. (From Thompson MW et al.: Thompson and Thompson Genetics in Medicine, 5th ed. Philadelphia, WB Saunders, 1991, p 135.)

these three well-known categories must be added a heterogeneous group of *single-gene disorders with nonclassic patterns of inheritance.* This group includes disorders resulting from triplet-repeat mutations, those arising from mutations in mitochondrial DNA (mtDNA), and those in which the transmission is influenced by genomic imprinting or gonadal mosaicism. Diseases within this group are caused by mutations in single genes, but they do not follow the mendelian pattern of inheritance. These are discussed later in this chapter.

It is beyond the scope of this book to review normal human genetics. It is, however, important to clarify several commonly used terms—*hereditary, familial,* and *congenital.* Hereditary disorders, by definition, are derived from one's parents and are transmitted in the germ line through the generations and therefore are familial. The term *congenital* simply implies "born with." Some congenital diseases are not genetic; for example, congenital syphilis. Not all genetic diseases are congenital; individuals with Huntington disease, for example, begin to manifest their condition only after their 20s or 30s.

Mendelian Disorders

All mendelian disorders are the result of mutations in single genes that have large effects. It is not necessary to detail Mendel's laws here, since every student in biology, and possibly every garden pea, has learned about them at an early age. Only some comments of medical relevance are made.

It is estimated that every individual is a carrier of five to eight deleterious genes. Most of these are recessive and therefore do not have serious phenotypic effects. About 80% to 85% of these mutations are familial. The remainder represent new mutations acquired de novo by an affected individual.

Some autosomal mutations produce partial expression in the heterozygote and full expression in the homozygote. Sickle cell anemia is caused by substitution of normal hemoglobin (HbA) by hemoglobin S (HbS). When an individual is homozygous for the mutant gene, all the hemoglobin is of the abnormal, HbS, type, and even with normal saturation of oxygen the disorder is fully expressed (i.e., sickling deformity of all red cells and hemolytic anemia). In the heterozygote, only a proportion of the hemoglobin is HbS (the remainder being HbA), and therefore red cell sickling occurs only when there is exposure to lowered oxygen tension. This is referred to as the *sickle cell trait* to differentiate it from full-blown sickle cell anemia.

Although gene expression and mendelian traits are usually described as dominant or recessive, in some cases both of the alleles of a gene pair contribute to the phenotype—a condition called *codominance.* Histocompatibility and blood group antigens are good examples of codominant inheritance.

A single mutant gene may lead to many end effects, termed *pleiotropism;* conversely, mutations at several genetic loci may produce the same trait *(genetic heterogeneity).* Sickle cell anemia is an example of pleiotropism. In this hereditary disorder not only does the point mutation in the gene give rise to HbS, which predisposes the red cells to hemolysis, but also the abnormal red cells tend to cause a logjam in small vessels, inducing, for example, splenic fibrosis, organ infarcts, and

bone changes. The numerous differing end-organ derangements are all related to the primary defect in hemoglobin synthesis. On the other hand, profound childhood deafness, an apparently homogeneous clinical entity, results from many different types of autosomal recessive mutations. Recognition of genetic heterogeneity not only is important in genetic counseling but also is relevant in the understanding of the pathogenesis of some common disorders, such as diabetes mellitus.

TRANSMISSION PATTERNS OF SINGLE-GENE DISORDERS

Mutations involving single genes typically follow one of three patterns of inheritance: autosomal dominant, autosomal recessive, and X-linked. The general rules that govern the transmission of single-gene disorders are well known; only a few salient features are summarized.[12] Single-gene disorders with nonclassic patterns of inheritance are described later.

Autosomal Dominant Disorders

Autosomal dominant disorders are manifested in the heterozygous state, so at least one parent of an index case is usually affected; both males and females are affected, and both can transmit the condition. When an affected person marries an unaffected one, every child has one chance in two of having the disease. In addition to these basic rules, autosomal dominant conditions are characterized by the following:

- With every autosomal dominant disorder, some proportion of patients do not have affected parents. Such patients owe their disorder to new mutations involving either the egg or the sperm from which they were derived. Their siblings are neither affected nor at increased risk for developing the disease. The proportion of patients who develop the disease as a result of a new mutation is related to the effect of the disease on reproductive capability. If a disease markedly reduces reproductive fitness, most cases would be expected to result from new mutations. Many new mutations seem to occur in germ cells of relatively older fathers.
- Clinical features can be modified by variations in penetrance and expressivity. Some individuals inherit the mutant gene but are phenotypically normal. This is referred to as *incomplete penetrance.* Penetrance is expressed in mathematical terms. Thus, 50% penetrance indicates that 50% of those who carry the gene express the trait. In contrast to penetrance, if a trait is seen in all individuals carrying the mutant gene but is expressed differently among individuals, the phenomenon is called *variable expressivity.* For example, manifestations of neurofibromatosis type 1 range from brownish spots on the skin to multiple skin tumors and skeletal deformities. The mechanisms underlying incomplete penetrance and variable expressivity are not fully understood, but they most likely result from effects of other genes or environmental factors that modify the phenotypic expression of the mutant allele. For example, the phenotype of a patient with sickle cell anemia (resulting from mutation at the β-globin locus) is influenced by the genotype at the α-globin locus, because the latter influences the total amount of hemoglobin made (Chapter 14). The influence of environmental factors

is exemplified by familial hypercholesterolemia. The expression of the disease in the form of atherosclerosis is conditioned by the dietary intake of lipids.

○ In many conditions the age at onset is delayed: symptoms and signs may not appear until adulthood (as in Huntington disease).

The biochemical mechanisms of autosomal dominant disorders are best considered in the context of the nature of the mutation and the type of protein affected. Most mutations lead to the reduced production of a gene product or give rise to an inactive protein. The effect of such *loss-of-function* *mutations* depends on the nature of the protein affected. If the mutation affects an enzyme protein the heterozygotes are usually normal. Because up to 50% loss of enzyme activity can be compensated for, mutation in genes that encode enzymes do not manifest an autosomal dominant pattern of inheritance. By contrast, two major categories of nonenzyme proteins are affected in autosomal dominant disorders:

1. Those involved in regulation of complex metabolic pathways that are subject to feedback inhibition: Membrane receptors such as the low-density lipoprotein (LDL) receptor provide one such example; in familial hypercholesterolemia, discussed in detail later, a 50% loss of LDL receptors results in a secondary elevation of cholesterol that, in turn, predisposes to atherosclerosis in affected heterozygotes.
2. Key structural proteins, such as collagen and cytoskeletal elements of the red cell membrane (e.g., spectrin): The biochemical mechanisms by which a 50% reduction in the amounts of such proteins results in an abnormal phenotype are not fully understood. In some cases, especially when the gene encodes one subunit of a multimeric protein, the product of the mutant allele can interfere with the assembly of a functionally normal multimer. For example, the collagen molecule is a trimer in which the three collagen chains are arranged in a helical configuration. Each of the three collagen chains in the helix must be normal for the assembly and stability of the collagen molecule. Even with a single mutant collagen chain, normal collagen trimers cannot be formed, and hence there is a marked deficiency of collagen. In this instance the mutant allele is called *dominant negative*, because it impairs the function of a normal allele. This effect is illustrated by some forms of osteogenesis imperfecta, characterized by marked deficiency of collagen and severe skeletal abnormalities (Chapter 26).

Less common than loss-of-function mutations are *gain-of-function* mutations. As the name indicates, in this type of mutation the protein product of the mutant allele acquires new properties not normally associated with the wild-type protein. The transmission of disorders produced by gain-of-function mutations is almost always autosomal dominant, as illustrated by Huntington disease (Chapter 28). In this disease the trinucleotide-repeat mutation affecting the Huntington gene (see later) gives rise to an abnormal protein, called huntingtin, that is toxic to neurons, and hence even heterozygotes develop a neurologic deficit.

To summarize, two types of mutations and two categories of proteins are involved in the pathogenesis of autosomal

TABLE 5–1	Autosomal Dominant Disorders
System	**Disorder**
Nervous	Huntington disease Neurofibromatosis Myotonic dystrophy Tuberous sclerosis
Urinary	Polycystic kidney disease
Gastrointestinal	Familial polyposis coli
Hematopoietic	Hereditary spherocytosis von Willebrand disease
Skeletal	Marfan syndrome* Ehlers-Danlos syndrome (some variants)* Osteogenesis imperfecta Achondroplasia
Metabolic	Familial hypercholesterolemia* Acute intermittent porphyria

*Discussed in this chapter. Other disorders listed are discussed in appropriate chapters in the book.

dominant diseases. The more common loss-of-function mutations affect regulatory proteins and subunits of multimeric proteins, the latter acting through a dominant-negative effect. Gain-of-function mutations are less common; they often endow normal proteins with toxic properties, or more rarely increase a normal activity (e.g., activating mutation in the erythropoetin receptor associated with a pathologic increase in red cell production).

Table 5–1 lists common autosomal dominant disorders. Many are discussed more logically in other chapters. A few conditions not considered elsewhere are discussed later in this chapter to illustrate important principles.

Autosomal Recessive Disorders

Autosomal recessive traits make up the largest category of mendelian disorders. Because autosomal recessive disorders result only when both alleles at a given gene locus are mutated, such disorders are characterized by the following features: (1) The trait does not usually affect the parents of the affected individual, but siblings may show the disease; (2) siblings have one chance in four of having the trait (i.e., the recurrence risk is 25% for each birth); and (3) if the mutant gene occurs with a low frequency in the population, there is a strong likelihood that the affected individual (proband) is the product of a consanguineous marriage. The following features generally apply to most autosomal recessive disorders and distinguish them from autosomal dominant diseases:

○ The expression of the defect tends to be more uniform than in autosomal dominant disorders.
○ Complete penetrance is common.
○ Onset is frequently early in life.
○ Although new mutations associated with recessive disorders do occur, they are rarely detected clinically. Since the individual with a new mutation is an asymptomatic heterozygote, several generations may pass before the descendants of such a person mate with other heterozygotes and produce affected offspring.

TABLE 5–2	Autosomal Recessive Disorders
System	**Disorder**
Metabolic	Cystic fibrosis
	Phenylketonuria
	Galactosemia
	Homocystinuria
	Lysosomal storage diseases*
	α_1-Antitrypsin deficiency
	Wilson disease
	Hemochromatosis
	Glycogen storage diseases*
Hematopoietic	Sickle cell anemia
	Thalassemias
Endocrine	Congenital adrenal hyperplasia
Skeletal	Ehlers-Danlos syndrome (some variants)*
	Alkaptonuria*
Nervous	Neurogenic muscular atrophies
	Friedreich ataxia
	Spinal muscular atrophy

*Discussed in this chapter. Many others are discussed elsewhere in the text.

● Many of the mutated genes encode enzymes. In heterozygotes, equal amounts of normal and defective enzyme are synthesized. Usually the natural "margin of safety" ensures that cells with half the usual complement of the enzyme function normally.

Autosomal recessive disorders include almost all inborn errors of metabolism. The various consequences of enzyme deficiencies are discussed later. The more common of these conditions are listed in Table 5–2. Most are presented elsewhere; a few prototypes are discussed later in this chapter.

X-Linked Disorders

All sex-linked disorders are X-linked, and almost all are recessive. Several genes are located in the "male-specific region of Y"; all of these are related to spermatogenesis.[13] Males with mutations affecting the Y-linked genes are usually infertile, and hence there is no Y-linked inheritance. As discussed later, a few additional genes with homologues on the X chromosome have been mapped to the Y chromosome, but no disorders resulting from mutations in such genes have been described.

X-linked recessive inheritance accounts for a small number of well-defined clinical conditions. The Y chromosome, for the most part, is not homologous to the X, and so mutant genes on the X do not have corresponding alleles on the Y. Thus, the male is said to be *hemizygous* for X-linked mutant genes, so these disorders are expressed in the male. Other features that characterize these disorders are as follows:

● An affected male does not transmit the disorder to his sons, but all daughters are carriers. Sons of heterozygous women have, of course, one chance in two of receiving the mutant gene.
● The heterozygous female usually does not express the full phenotypic change because of the paired normal allele. Because of the random inactivation of one of the X chromosomes in the female, however, females have a variable proportion of cells in which the mutant X chromosome is active. Thus, it is remotely possible for the normal allele to be inactivated in most cells, permitting full expression of heterozygous X-linked conditions in the female. Much more commonly, the normal allele is inactivated in only some of the cells, and thus the heterozygous female expresses the disorder partially. An illustrative condition is *glucose-6-phosphate dehydrogenase (G6PD) deficiency.* Transmitted on the X chromosome, this enzyme deficiency, which predisposes to red cell hemolysis in patients receiving certain types of drugs (Chapter 14), is expressed principally in males. In the female, a proportion of the red cells may be derived from marrow cells with inactivation of the normal allele. Such red cells are at the same risk for undergoing hemolysis as are the red cells in the hemizygous male. Thus, the female is not only a carrier of this trait but also is susceptible to drug-induced hemolytic reactions. Because the proportion of defective red cells in heterozygous females depends on the random inactivation of one of the X chromosomes, however, the severity of the hemolytic reaction is almost always less in heterozygous women than in hemizygous men. Most of the X-linked conditions listed in Table 5–3 are covered elsewhere in the text.

There are only a few *X-linked dominant* conditions. They are caused by dominant disease-associated alleles on the X chromosome. These disorders are transmitted by an affected heterozygous female to half her sons and half her daughters and by an affected male parent to all his daughters but none of his sons, if the female parent is unaffected. Vitamin D–resistant rickets is an example of this type of inheritance.

BIOCHEMICAL AND MOLECULAR BASIS OF SINGLE-GENE (MENDELIAN) DISORDERS

Mendelian disorders result from alterations involving single genes. The genetic defect may lead to the formation of an abnormal protein or a reduction in the output of the gene product. Virtually any type of protein may be affected in

TABLE 5–3	X-Linked Recessive Disorders
System	**Disease**
Musculoskeletal	Duchenne muscular dystrophy
Blood	Hemophilia A and B
	Chronic granulomatous disease
	Glucose-6-phosphate dehydrogenase deficiency
Immune	Agammaglobulinemia
	Wiskott-Aldrich syndrome
Metabolic	Diabetes insipidus
	Lesch-Nyhan syndrome
Nervous	Fragile-X syndrome*

*Discussed in this chapter. Others are discussed in appropriate chapters in the text.

TABLE 5–4　Biochemical and Molecular Basis of Some Mendelian Disorders

Protein Type/Function	Example	Molecular Lesion	Disease
ENZYME	Phenylalanine hydroxylase	Splice-site mutation: reduced amount	Phenylketonuria
	Hexosaminidase	Splice-site mutation or frameshift mutation with stop codon: reduced amount	Tay-Sachs disease
	Adenosine deaminase	Point mutations: abnormal protein with reduced activity	Severe combined immunodeficiency
ENZYME INHIBITOR	α_1-Antitrypsin	Missense mutations: impaired secretion from liver to serum	Emphysema and liver disease
RECEPTOR	Low-density lipoprotein receptor	Deletions, point mutations: reduction of synthesis, transport to cell surface, or binding to low-density lipoprotein	Familial hypercholesterolemia
	Vitamin D receptor	Point mutations: failure of normal signaling	Vitamin D–resistant rickets
TRANSPORT			
Oxygen	Hemoglobin	Deletions: reduced amount	α-Thalassemia
		Defective mRNA processing: reduced amount	β-Thalassemia
		Point mutations: abnormal structure	Sickle cell anemia
Ions	Cystic fibrosis transmembrane conductance regulator	Deletions and other mutations: nonfunctional or misfolded proteins	Cystic fibrosis
STRUCTURAL			
Extracellular	Collagen	Deletions or point mutations cause reduced amount of normal collagen or normal amounts of defective collagen	Osteogenesis imperfecta; Ehlers-Danlos syndromes
	Fibrillin	Missense mutations	Marfan syndrome
Cell membrane	Dystrophin	Deletion with reduced synthesis	Duchenne/Becker muscular dystrophy
	Spectrin, ankyrin, or protein 4.1	Heterogeneous	Hereditary spherocytosis
HEMOSTASIS	Factor VIII	Deletions, insertions, nonsense mutations, and others: reduced synthesis or abnormal factor VIII	Hemophilia A
GROWTH REGULATION	Rb protein	Deletions	Hereditary retinoblastoma
	Neurofibromin	Heterogeneous	Neurofibromatosis type 1

single-gene disorders and by a variety of mechanisms (Table 5–4). To some extent the pattern of inheritance of the disease is related to the kind of protein affected by the mutation, as was discussed earlier and is reiterated subsequently. For the purposes of this discussion, the mechanisms involved in single-gene disorders can be classified into four categories: (1) *enzyme defects and their consequences*; (2) *defects in membrane receptors and transport systems*; (3) *alterations in the structure, function, or quantity of nonenzyme proteins*; and (4) *mutations resulting in unusual reactions to drugs*.

Enzyme Defects and Their Consequences

Mutations may result in the synthesis of a defective enzyme with reduced activity or in a reduced amount of a normal enzyme. In either case, the consequence is a metabolic block. Figure 5–6 provides an example of an enzyme reaction in which the substrate is converted by intracellular enzymes, denoted as 1, 2, and 3, into an end product through intermediates 1 and 2. In this model the final product exerts feedback control on enzyme 1. A minor pathway producing small quantities of M1 and M2 also exists. The biochemical consequences

of an enzyme defect in such a reaction may lead to three major consequences:

1. *Accumulation of the substrate*, depending on the site of block, may be accompanied by accumulation of one or both intermediates. Moreover, an increased concentration of intermediate 2 may stimulate the minor pathway and thus lead to an excess of M1 and M2. Under these conditions tissue injury may result if the precursor, the intermediates, or the products of alternative minor pathways are toxic in high concentrations. For example, in galactosemia, the deficiency of galactose-1-phosphate uridyltransferase (Chapter 10) leads to the accumulation of galactose and consequent tissue damage. Excessive accumulation of complex substrates within the lysosomes as a result of deficiency of degradative enzymes is responsible for a group of diseases generally referred to as *lysosomal storage diseases*.

2. *An enzyme defect can lead to a metabolic block and a decreased amount of end product* that may be necessary for normal function. For example, a deficiency of melanin may result from lack of tyrosinase, which is necessary for the biosynthesis of melanin from its precursor, tyrosine. This results

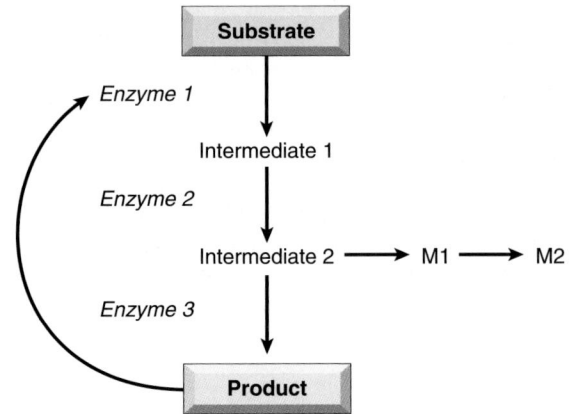

FIGURE 5-6 A possible metabolic pathway in which a substrate is converted to an end product by a series of enzyme reactions. M1, M2, products of a minor pathway.

in the clinical condition called *albinism*. If the end product is a feedback inhibitor of the enzymes involved in the early reactions (in Fig. 5–6 it is shown that the product inhibits enzyme 1), the deficiency of the end product may permit overproduction of intermediates and their catabolic products, some of which may be injurious at high concentrations. A prime example of a disease with such an underlying mechanism is the Lesch-Nyhan syndrome (Chapter 26).

3. *Failure to inactivate a tissue-damaging substrate* is best exemplified by α_1-antitrypsin deficiency. Individuals who have an inherited deficiency of serum α_1-antitrypsin are unable to inactivate neutrophil elastase in their lungs. Unchecked activity of this protease leads to destruction of elastin in the walls of lung alveoli, leading eventually to pulmonary emphysema (Chapter 15).

Defects in Receptors and Transport Systems

Many biologically active substances have to be actively transported across the cell membrane. This transport is generally achieved by one of two mechanisms—through receptor-mediated endocytosis or by a transport protein. A genetic defect in a receptor-mediated transport system is exemplified by familial hypercholesterolemia, in which reduced synthesis or function of LDL receptors leads to defective transport of LDL into the cells and secondarily to excessive cholesterol synthesis by complex intermediary mechanisms. In cystic fibrosis the transport system for chloride ions in exocrine glands, sweat ducts, lungs, and pancreas is defective. By mechanisms not fully understood, impaired chloride transport leads to serious injury to the lungs and pancreas (Chapter 10).

Alterations in Structure, Function, or Quantity of Nonenzyme Proteins

Genetic defects resulting in alterations of nonenzyme proteins often have widespread secondary effects, as exemplified by sickle cell disease. The hemoglobinopathies, sickle cell disease being one, all of which are characterized by defects in the structure of the globin molecule, best exemplify this category. In contrast to the hemoglobinopathies, the thalassemias result from mutations in globin genes that affect the amount of globin chains synthesized. Thalassemias are associated with reduced amounts of structurally normal α-globin or β-globin chains (Chapter 14). Other examples of genetically defective structural proteins include collagen, spectrin, and dystrophin, giving rise to osteogenesis imperfecta (Chapter 26), hereditary spherocytosis (Chapter 14), and muscular dystrophies (Chapter 27), respectively.

Genetically Determined Adverse Reactions to Drugs

Certain genetically determined enzyme deficiencies are unmasked only after exposure of the affected individual to certain drugs. This special area of genetics, called *pharmacogenetics*, is of considerable clinical importance.[14] The classic example of drug-induced injury in the genetically susceptible individual is associated with a deficiency of the enzyme G6PD. Under normal conditions glucose-6 phosphate-dehydrogenase (G6PD) deficiency does not result in disease, but on administration, for example, of the antimalarial drug primaquine, a severe hemolytic anemia results (Chapter 14). In recent years an increasing number of polymorphisms of genes encoding drug-metabolizing enzymes, transporters, and receptors are being identified. In some cases these genetic factors have major impact on drug sensitivity and adverse reactions. It is expected that advances in pharmacogenetics will lead to patient-tailored therapy, or "personalized medicine."

With this overview of the biochemical basis of single-gene disorders, we now consider selected examples grouped according to the underlying defect.

DISORDERS ASSOCIATED WITH DEFECTS IN STRUCTURAL PROTEINS

Several diseases caused by mutations in genes that encode structural proteins are listed in Table 5–4. Many are discussed elsewhere in the text. Only Marfan syndrome and Ehlers-Danlos syndromes (EDSs) are discussed here, because they affect connective tissue and hence involve multiple organ systems.

Marfan Syndrome

Marfan syndrome is a disorder of connective tissues, manifested principally by changes in the skeleton, eyes, and cardiovascular system.[15] Its prevalence is estimated to be 1 in 5000. Approximately 70% to 85% of cases are familial and transmitted by autosomal dominant inheritance. The remainder are sporadic and arise from new mutations.

Pathogenesis.   Marfan syndrome results from an inherited defect in an extracellular glycoprotein called *fibrillin-1*. As alluded to in Chapter 3, fibrillin is the major component of microfibrils found in the extracellular matrix. These fibrils provide a scaffolding on which tropoelastin is deposited to form elastic fibers. Although microfibrils are widely distributed in the body, they are particularly abundant in the aorta, ligaments, and the ciliary zonules that support the lens; these tissues are prominently affected in Marfan syndrome.

Fibrillin occurs in two homologous forms, fibrillin-1 and fibrillin-2, encoded by two separate genes, *FBN1* and

FBN2, mapped on chromosomes 15q21.1 and 5q23.31, respectively. Mutations of *FBN1* underlie Marfan syndrome; mutations of the related *FBN2* gene are less common, and they give rise to *congenital contractural arachnodactyly*, an autosomal dominant disorder characterized by skeletal abnormalities. Mutational analysis has revealed more than 600 distinct mutations of the *FBN1* gene in individuals with Marfan syndrome. Most of these are missense mutations that give rise to abnormal fibrillin-1. While many clinical manifestations of Marfan syndrome can be explained by changes in the mechanical properties of the extracellular matrix resulting from abnormalities of fibrillin, several others such as bone overgrowth cannot be attributed to changes in tissue elasticity. Recent studies indicate that loss of microfibrils gives rise to abnormal and excessive activation of transforming growth factor β (TGF-β), since normal microfibrils sequester TGF-β and thus control the bioavailability of this cytokine. Excessive TGF-β signaling has deleterious effects on vascular smooth muscle development and the integrity of extracellular matrix. This hypothesis is supported by two sets of observations. First, in a small number of individuals with clinical features of Marfan syndrome (MFS2) there are no mutations in *FBN1* but mutations in genes that encode TGF-β receptors. Second, in mouse models of Marfan syndrome generated by mutations in *Fbn1*, administration of antibodies to TGF-β prevents alterations in the aorta and mitral valves.[16] Human trials with a similar strategy seem to be promising.

Morphology. **Skeletal abnormalities** are the most striking feature of Marfan syndrome. Typically the patient is unusually tall with exceptionally long extremities and long, tapering fingers and toes. The joint ligaments in the hands and feet are lax, suggesting that the patient is double-jointed; typically the thumb can be hyperextended back to the wrist. The head is commonly dolichocephalic (long-headed) with bossing of the frontal eminences and prominent supraorbital ridges. A variety of spinal deformities may appear, including kyphosis, scoliosis, or rotation or slipping of the dorsal or lumbar vertebrae. The chest is classically deformed, presenting either pectus excavatum (deeply depressed sternum) or a pigeon-breast deformity.

The **ocular changes** take many forms. Most characteristic is bilateral subluxation or dislocation (usually outward and upward) of the lens, referred to as ectopia lentis. This abnormality is so uncommon in persons who do not have this genetic disease that the finding of bilateral ectopia lentis should raise the suspicion of Marfan syndrome.

Cardiovascular lesions are the most life-threatening features of this disorder. The two most common lesions are mitral valve prolapse and, of greater importance, dilation of the ascending aorta due to cystic medionecrosis. Histologically the changes in the media are virtually identical to those found in cystic medionecrosis not related to Marfan syndrome (see Chapter 12). Loss of medial support results in progressive dilation of the aortic valve ring and the root of the aorta, giving rise to severe aortic incom-

petence. In addition, excessive TGF-β signaling in the adventia also probably contributes to aortic dilation. Weakening of the media predisposes to an intimal tear, which may initiate an intramural hematoma that cleaves the layers of the media to produce aortic dissection. After cleaving the aortic layers for considerable distances, sometimes back to the root of the aorta or down to the iliac arteries, the hemorrhage often ruptures through the aortic wall. Such a calamity is the cause of death in 30% to 45% of these individuals.

Clinical Features. Although mitral valve lesions are more frequent, they are clinically less important than aortic lesions. Loss of connective tissue support in the mitral valve leaflets makes them soft and billowy, creating the so-called floppy valve (Chapter 12). Valvular lesions, along with lengthening of the chordae tendineae, frequently give rise to mitral regurgitation. Similar changes may affect the tricuspid and, rarely, the aortic valves. Echocardiography greatly enhances the ability to detect the cardiovascular abnormalities and is therefore extremely valuable in the diagnosis of Marfan syndrome. The great majority of deaths are caused by rupture of aortic dissections, followed in importance by cardiac failure.

While the lesions just described typify Marfan syndrome, it must be emphasized that there is great variation in the clinical expression of this genetic disorder. Patients with prominent eye or cardiovascular changes may have few skeletal abnormalities, whereas others with striking changes in body habitus have no eye changes. Although variability in clinical expression may be seen within a family, interfamilial variability is much more common and extensive. Because of such variations, the clinical diagnosis of Marfan syndrome must be based on major involvement of two of the four organ systems (skeletal, cardiovascular, ocular, and skin) and minor involvement of another organ.

To account for the variable expression of the Marfan defect, it has been hypothesized that Marfan syndrome is genetically heterogeneous. With one exception, however, all studies thus far point to mutations in the *FBN1* gene, on chromosome 15q21.1, as the cause of this disease.[15] Thus, variable expressivity is best explained on the basis of allelic mutations within the same locus. Because the *FBN1* gene is large and many different mutations have been identified, direct diagnosis by DNA sequencing is not currently feasible, but this may change in the near future as new technologies are being developed.

Ehlers-Danlos Syndromes (EDS)

EDSs comprise a clinically and genetically heterogeneous group of disorders that result from some defect in the synthesis or structure of fibrillar collagen. Other disorders resulting from mutations affecting collagen synthesis include osteogenesis imperfecta (Chapter 26), Alport syndrome (Chapter 20), and epidermolysis bullosa (Chapter 25).

Biosynthesis of collagen is a complex process that can be disturbed by genetic errors that may affect any one of the numerous structural collagen genes or enzymes necessary for post-transcriptional modifications of collagen. Hence, the

TABLE 5–5	Classification of Ehlers-Danlos Syndromes		
EDS Type*	**Clinical Findings**	**Inheritance**	**Gene Defects**
Classical (I/II)	Skin and joint hypermobility, atrophic scars, easy bruising	Autosomal dominant	*COL5A1, COL5A2*
Hypermobility (III)	Joint hypermobility, pain, dislocations	Autosomal dominant	Unknown
Vascular (IV)	Thin skin, arterial or uterine rupture, bruising, small joint hyperextensibility	Autosomal dominant	*COL3A1*
Kyphoscoliosis (VI)	Hypotonia, joint laxity, congenital scoliosis, ocular fragility	Autosomal recessive	Lysyl hydroxylase
Arthrochalasia (VIIa,b)	Severe joint hypermobility, skin changes (mild), scoliosis, bruising	Autosomal dominant	*COL1A1, COL1A2*
Dermatosparaxsis (VIIc)	Severe skin fragility, cutis laxa, bruising	Autosomal recessive	Procollagen *N*-peptidase

*EDS types were previously classified by Roman numerals. Parentheses show previous numerical equivalents.

mode of inheritance of EDS encompasses all three mendelian patterns. On the basis of clinical and molecular characteristics, six variants of EDS have been recognized.[17] These are listed in Table 5–5. It is beyond the scope of this book to discuss each variant individually; instead, we first summarize the important clinical features that are common to most variants and then correlate some of the clinical manifestations with the underlying molecular defects in collagen synthesis or structure.

As might be expected, tissues rich in collagen, such as skin, ligaments, and joints, are frequently involved in most variants of EDS. Because the abnormal collagen fibers lack adequate tensile strength, *skin is hyperextensible, and the joints are hypermobile.* These features permit grotesque contortions, such as bending the thumb backward to touch the forearm and bending the knee forward to create almost a right angle. It is believed that most contortionists have one of the EDSs. A predisposition to joint dislocation, however, is one of the prices paid for this virtuosity. *The skin is extraordinarily stretchable, extremely fragile, and vulnerable to trauma.* Minor injuries produce gaping defects, and surgical repair or intervention is accomplished with great difficulty because of the lack of normal tensile strength. *The basic defect in connective tissue may lead to serious internal complications.* These include rupture of the colon and large arteries (vascular EDS), ocular fragility with rupture of cornea and retinal detachment (kyphoscoliosis EDS), and diaphragmatic hernia (classical EDS).

The biochemical and molecular bases of these abnormalities are known in several forms of EDS. These are described briefly, because they offer some insights into the perplexing clinical heterogeneity of EDS. Perhaps the best characterized is the *kyphoscoliosis type, the most common autosomal recessive form of EDS.* It results from mutations in the gene encoding lysyl hydroxylase, an enzyme necessary for hydroxylation of lysine residues during collagen synthesis.[18] Affected patients have markedly reduced levels of this enzyme. Because hydroxylysine is essential for the cross-linking of collagen fibers, a deficiency of lysyl hydroxylase results in the synthesis of collagen that lacks normal structural stability.

The *vascular type of EDS results from abnormalities of type III collagen.*[19] This form is genetically heterogeneous, because at least three distinct types of mutations affecting the *COL3A1*

gene encoding collagen type III can give rise to this variant. Some affect the rate of synthesis of pro α1 (III) chains, others affect the secretion of type III procollagen, and still others lead to the synthesis of structurally abnormal type III collagen. Some mutant alleles behave as dominant negatives (see discussion under "Autosomal Dominant Disorders") and thus produce severe phenotypic effects. These molecular studies provide a rational basis for the pattern of transmission and clinical features that are characteristic of this variant. First, because vascular-type EDS results from mutations involving a structural protein (rather than an enzyme protein), an autosomal dominant pattern of inheritance would be expected. Second, because blood vessels and intestines are known to be rich in collagen type III, an abnormality of this collagen is consistent with severe defects (e.g., spontaneous rupture) in these organs.

In two forms of EDS—arthrochalasia type and dermatosparaxis type—the fundamental defect is in the conversion of type I procollagen to collagen. This step in collagen synthesis involves cleavage of noncollagen peptides at the N terminus and C terminus of the procollagen molecule. This is accomplished by N terminal–specific and C terminal–specific peptidases. *The defect in the conversion of procollagen to collagen in the arthrochalasia type has been traced to mutations that affect one of the two type I collagen genes, COL1A1 and COL1A2.* As a result, structurally abnormal pro α1 (I) or pro α2 (I) chains that resist cleavage of N-terminal peptides are formed. In patients with a single mutant allele, only 50% of the type I collagen chains are abnormal, but because these chains interfere with the formation of normal collagen helices, heterozygotes manifest the disease. By contrast, the related dermatosparaxis type is caused by mutations in the procollagen-N-peptidase genes, essential for the cleavage of collagens. In this case the enzyme deficiency leads to an autosomal recessive form of inheritance.

Finally, the *classical type of EDS* is worthy of brief mention, since molecular analysis of this variant suggests that genes other than collagen genes may be involved in the pathogenesis of EDS. In 30% to 50% of these cases, mutations in the genes for type V collagen (*COL5A1* and *COL5A2*) have been detected.[20] Surprisingly, despite a phenotype typical of EDS, no other collagen gene abnormalities have been found in the remaining cases.

To summarize, the common thread in EDS is some abnormality of collagen. These disorders, however, are extremely heterogeneous. At the molecular level, a variety of defects, varying from mutations involving structural genes for collagen to those involving enzymes that are responsible for post-transcriptional modifications of mRNA, have been detected. Such molecular heterogeneity results in the expression of EDS as a clinically variable disorder with several patterns of inheritance.

DISORDERS ASSOCIATED WITH DEFECTS IN RECEPTOR PROTEINS

Familial Hypercholesterolemia

Familial hypercholesterolemia is a "receptor disease" that is the consequence of *a mutation in the gene encoding the receptor for LDL, which is involved in the transport and metabolism of cholesterol.* As a consequence of receptor abnormalities there is a loss of feedback control and elevated levels of cholesterol that induce premature atherosclerosis, leading to a greatly increased risk of myocardial infarction.[21]

Familial hypercholesterolemia is one of the most frequently occurring mendelian disorders. Heterozygotes with one mutant gene, representing about 1 in 500 individuals, have from birth a two-fold to three-fold elevation of plasma cholesterol level, leading to tendinous xanthomas and premature atherosclerosis in adult life (Chapter 11). Homozygotes, having a double dose of the mutant gene, are much more severely affected, and may have five-fold to six-fold elevations in plasma cholesterol levels. These individuals develop skin xanthomas and coronary, cerebral, and peripheral vascular atherosclerosis at an early age. Myocardial infarction may develop before age 20. Large-scale studies have found that familial hypercholesterolemia is present in 3% to 6% of survivors of myocardial infarction.

An understanding of this disorder requires that we briefly review the normal process of cholesterol metabolism and transport. Approximately 7% of the body's cholesterol circulates in the plasma, predominantly in the form of LDL. As might be expected, the amount of plasma cholesterol is influenced by its synthesis and catabolism, and the liver plays a crucial role in both these processes (Fig. 5–7). The first step in this complex sequence is the secretion of very-low-density lipoproteins (VLDLs) by the liver into the bloodstream. VLDL particles are rich in triglycerides, but they contain lesser amounts of cholesteryl esters. When a VLDL particle reaches the capillaries of adipose tissue or muscle, it is cleaved by lipoprotein lipase, a process that extracts most of the triglycerides. The resulting molecule, called *intermediate-density lipoprotein (IDL)*, is reduced in triglyceride content and enriched in cholesteryl esters, but it retains two of the three apoproteins (B-100 and E) present in the parent VLDL particle (see Fig. 5–7). After release from the capillary endothelium, the IDL particles have one of two fates. Approximately 50% of newly formed IDL is rapidly taken up by the liver by receptor-mediated transport. The receptor responsible for the binding of IDL to the liver cell membrane recognizes both apoprotein B-100 and apoprotein E. It is called the *LDL receptor,* however, because it is also involved in the hepatic clearance of LDL, as described later. In the liver cells, IDL is recycled to generate VLDL. The IDL particles not taken up by the liver are

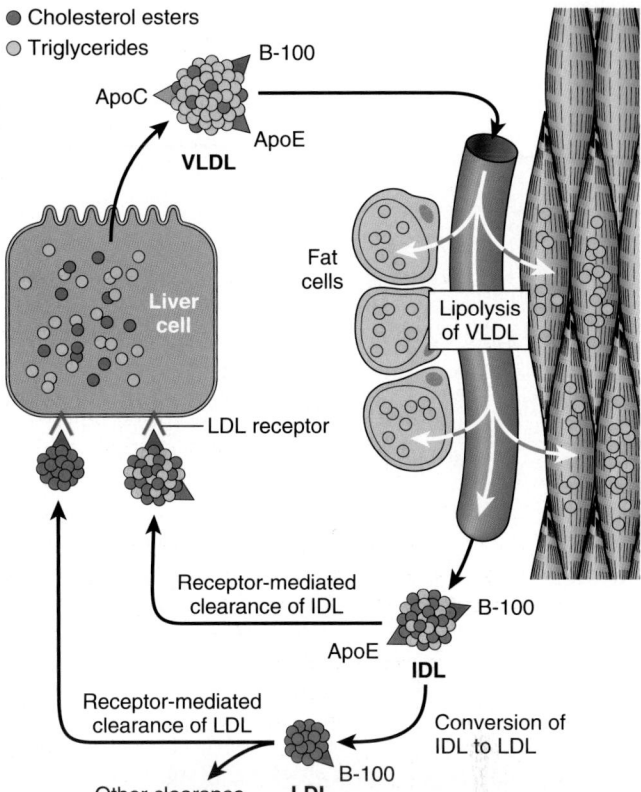

FIGURE 5–7   Low-density lipoprotein (LDL) metabolism and the role of the liver in its synthesis and clearance. Lipolysis of very-low-density lipoprotein (VLDL) by lipoprotein lipase in the capillaries releases triglycerides, which are then stored in fat cells and used as a source of energy in skeletal muscles. See text for explanation of abbreviations used.

subjected to further metabolic processing that removes most of the remaining triglycerides and apoprotein E, yielding cholesterol-rich LDL particles. *It should be emphasized that IDL is the immediate and major source of plasma LDL.* There seem to be two mechanisms for removal of LDL from plasma, one mediated by an LDL receptor and the other by a receptor for oxidized LDL (scavenger receptor), described later. Although many cell types, including fibroblasts, lymphocytes, smooth muscle cells, hepatocytes, and adrenocortical cells, possess high-affinity LDL receptors, approximately 70% of the plasma LDL seems to be cleared by the liver, using a quite sophisticated transport process (Fig. 5–8). The first step involves binding of LDL to cell surface receptors, which are clustered in specialized regions of the plasma membrane called *coated pits.* After binding, the coated pits containing the receptor-bound LDL are internalized by invagination to form coated vesicles, after which they migrate within the cell to fuse with the lysosomes. Here the LDL dissociates from the receptor, which is recycled to the surface. In the lysosomes the LDL molecule is enzymatically degraded; the apoprotein part is hydrolyzed to amino acids, whereas the cholesteryl esters are broken down to free cholesterol. This free cholesterol, in turn, crosses the lysosomal membrane to enter the cytoplasm, where it is used for membrane synthesis and as a regulator of cholesterol homeostasis. The exit of cholesterol from the lysosomes requires the action of two proteins called NPC1 and

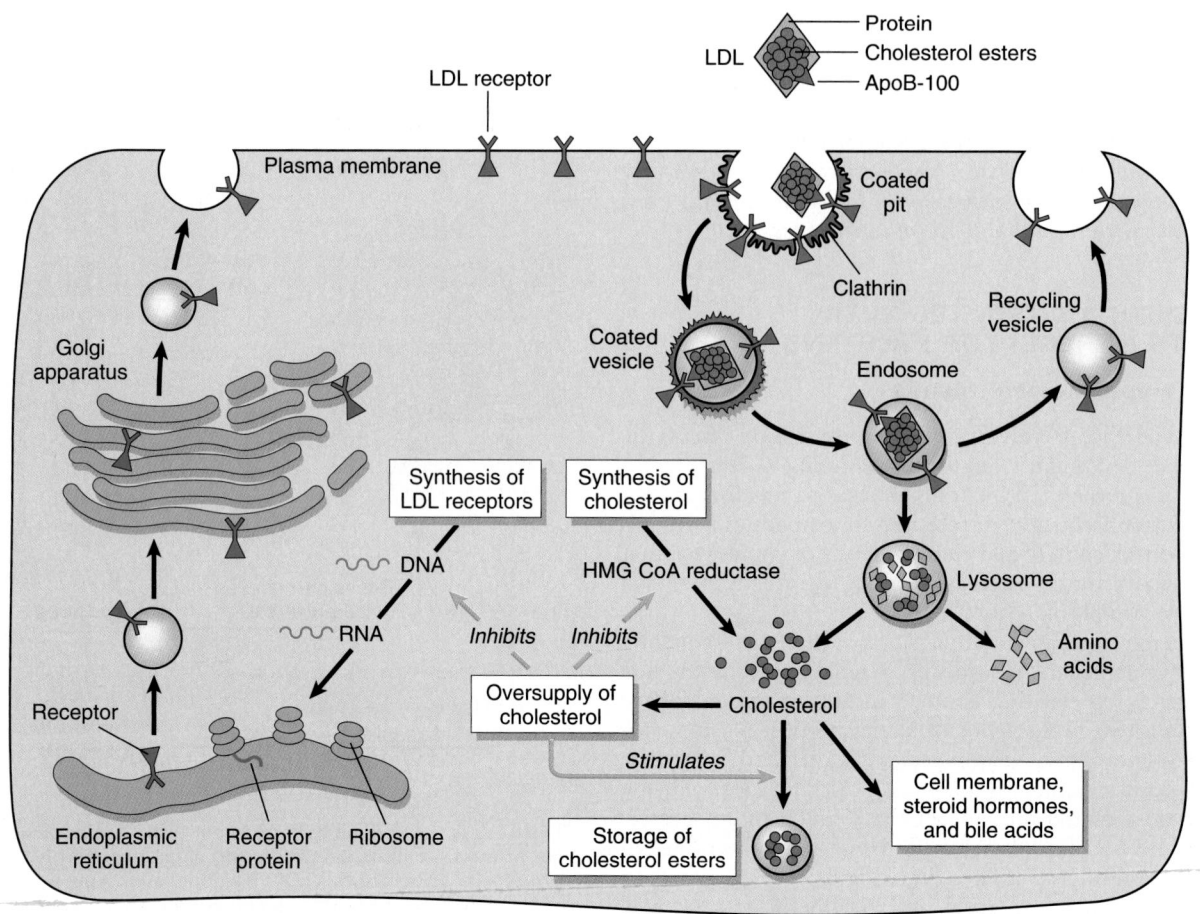

FIGURE 5–8   The LDL receptor pathway and regulation of cholesterol metabolism.

NPC2 (see "Niemann-Pick Disease, Type C"). Three separate processes are affected by the released intracellular cholesterol, as follows:

○ Cholesterol *suppresses* cholesterol synthesis within the cell by inhibiting the activity of the enzyme 3-hydroxy-3-methylglutaryl coenzyme A (HMG CoA) reductase, which is the rate-limiting enzyme in the synthetic pathway.

○ Cholesterol *activates* the enzyme acyl-coenzyme A : cholesterol acyltransferase, favoring esterification and storage of excess cholesterol.

○ Cholesterol *suppresses* the synthesis of LDL receptors, thus protecting the cells from excessive accumulation of cholesterol.

As mentioned earlier, familial hypercholesterolemia results from mutations in the gene specifying the receptor for LDL. Heterozygotes with familial hypercholesterolemia possess only 50% of the normal number of high-affinity LDL receptors, because they have only one normal gene. As a result of this defect in transport, the catabolism of LDL by the receptor-dependent pathways is impaired, and the plasma level of LDL increases approximately two-fold. Homozygotes have virtually no normal LDL receptors in their cells and have much higher levels of circulating LDL. In addition to defective LDL clearance, both the homozygotes and heterozygotes have increased

synthesis of LDL. The mechanism of increased synthesis that contributes to hypercholesterolemia also results from a lack of LDL receptors (see Fig. 5–7). Recall that IDL, the immediate precursor of plasma LDL, also uses hepatic LDL receptors (apoprotein B-100 and E receptors) for its transport into the liver. In familial hypercholesterolemia, impaired IDL transport into the liver secondarily diverts a greater proportion of plasma IDL into the precursor pool for plasma LDL.

The transport of LDL via the scavenger receptor seems to occur at least in part into the cells of the mononuclear phagocyte system. Monocytes and macrophages have receptors for chemically altered (e.g., acetylated or oxidized) LDL. Normally the amount of LDL transported along this scavenger receptor pathway is less than that mediated by the LDL receptor–dependent mechanisms. In the face of hypercholesterolemia, however, there is a marked increase in the scavenger receptor–mediated traffic of LDL cholesterol into the cells of the mononuclear phagocyte system and possibly the vascular walls (Chapter 11). This increase is responsible for the appearance of xanthomas and contributes to the pathogenesis of premature atherosclerosis.

The molecular genetics of familial hypercholesterolemia is extremely complex. More than 900 mutations, including insertions, deletions, and missense and nonsense mutations, involving the LDL receptor gene have been identified. These can be classified into five groups (Fig. 5–9): *Class I mutations*

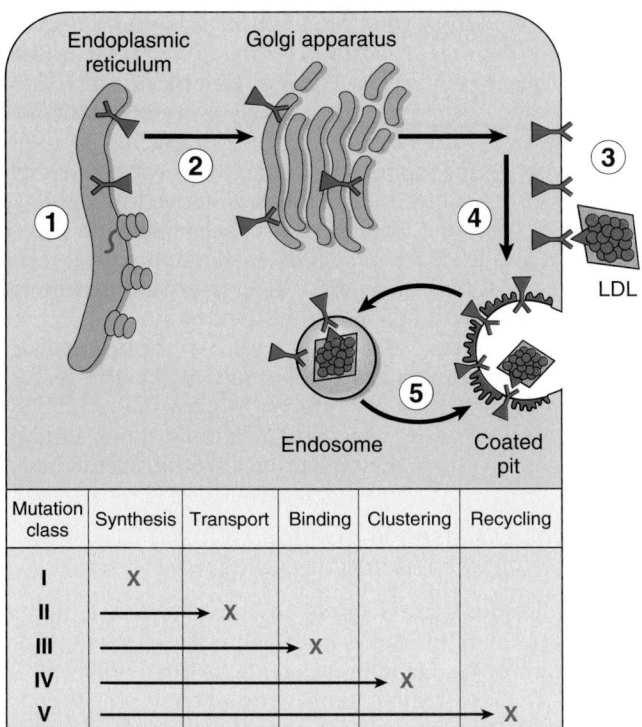

FIGURE 5–9   Classification of LDL receptor mutations based on abnormal function of the mutant protein. These mutations disrupt the receptor's synthesis in the endoplasmic reticulum, transport to the Golgi complex, binding of apoprotein ligands, clustering in coated pits, and recycling in endosomes. Each class is heterogeneous at the DNA level. (Modified with permission from Hobbs HH et al.: The LDL receptor locus in familial hypercholesterolemia: mutational analysis of a membrane protein. Annu Rev Genet 24:133–170, 1990. © 1990 by Annual Reviews.)

are relatively uncommon, and they lead to a complete failure of synthesis of the receptor protein (null allele). *Class II mutations* are fairly common; they encode receptor proteins that accumulate in the endoplasmic reticulum because their folding defects make it impossible for them to be transported to the Golgi complex. *Class III mutations* affect the LDL-binding domain of the receptor; the encoded proteins reach the cell surface but fail to bind LDL or do so poorly. *Class IV mutations* encode proteins that are synthesized and transported to the cell surface efficiently. They bind LDL normally, but they fail to localize in coated pits, and hence the bound LDL is not internalized. *Class V mutations* encode proteins that are expressed on the cell surface, can bind LDL, and can be internalized; however, the pH-dependent dissociation of the receptor and the bound LDL fails to occur. Such receptors are trapped in the endosome, where they are degraded, and hence they fail to recycle to the cell surface.

The discovery of the critical role of LDL receptors in cholesterol homeostasis has led to the rational design of drugs that lower plasma cholesterol by increasing the number of LDL receptors. One strategy is based on the ability of certain drugs (statins) to suppress intracellular cholesterol synthesis by inhibiting the enzyme HMG CoA reductase. This, in turn, allows greater synthesis of LDL receptors (see Fig. 5–8).

DISORDERS ASSOCIATED WITH DEFECTS IN ENZYMES

Lysosomal Storage Diseases

Lysosomes are key components of the "intracellular digestive tract." They contain a battery of hydrolytic enzymes, which have two special properties. First, they function in the acidic milieu of the lysosomes. Second, these enzymes constitute a special category of secretory proteins that are destined not for the extracellular fluids but for intracellular organelles. This latter characteristic requires special processing within the Golgi apparatus, which is reviewed briefly. Similar to all other secretory proteins, lysosomal enzymes (or acid hydrolases, as they are sometimes called) are synthesized in the endoplasmic reticulum and transported to the Golgi apparatus. Within the Golgi complex they undergo a variety of post-translational modifications, of which one is worthy of special note. This modification involves the attachment of terminal mannose-6-phosphate groups to some of the oligosaccharide side chains. The phosphorylated mannose residues serve as an "address label" that is recognized by specific receptors found on the inner surface of the Golgi membrane. Lysosomal enzymes bind these receptors and are thereby segregated from the numerous other secretory proteins within the Golgi. Subsequently, small transport vesicles containing the receptor-bound enzymes are pinched off from the Golgi and proceed to fuse with the lysosomes. Thus, the enzymes are targeted to their intracellular abode, and the vesicles are shuttled back to the Golgi (Fig. 5–10). As indicated later, genetically determined errors in this remarkable sorting mechanism may give rise to one form of lysosomal storage disease.[22]

The lysosomal acid hydrolases catalyze the breakdown of a variety of complex macromolecules. These large molecules may be derived from the metabolic turnover of intracellular organelles (autophagy), or they may be acquired from outside the cells by phagocytosis (heterophagy). With an inherited deficiency of a functional lysosomal enzyme, catabolism of its substrate remains incomplete, leading to the accumulation of the partially degraded insoluble metabolite within the lysosomes. Stuffed with incompletely digested macromolecules, these organelles become large and numerous enough to interfere with normal cell functions, giving rise to the so-called *lysosomal storage disorders* (Fig. 5–11). In addition to "missing enzymes," lysosomal storage diseases can result from lack of any protein essential for normal function of lysosomes. Examples are:

- Lack of an enzyme activator or protector protein.
- Lack of a substrate activator protein. In some instances, proteins that react with the substrate to facilitate its hydrolysis may be missing or defective.
- Lack of a transport protein required for egress of the digested material from the lysosomes.

There are three general approaches to the treatment of lysosomal storage diseases. The most obvious is enzyme replacement therapy, currently in use for several lysosomal storage diseases. Another approach, the "substrate reduction therapy," is based on the premise that if the substrate to be degraded by

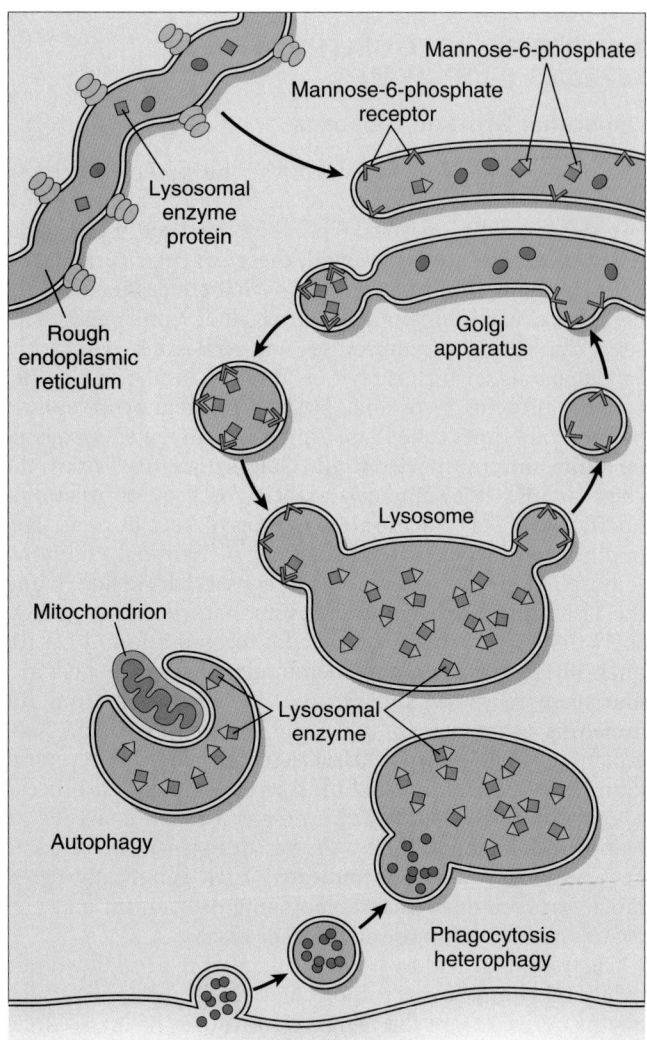

FIGURE 5–10   Synthesis and intracellular transport of lysosomal enzymes.

defective hydrolysis of gangliosides, as occurs in G_{M1} *and* G_{M2} *gangliosidoses, results primarily in accumulation within neurons and consequent neurologic symptoms.* Defects in degradation of mucopolysaccharides affect virtually every organ, because mucopolysaccharides are widely distributed in the body. Because cells of the mononuclear phagocyte system are especially rich in lysosomes and are involved in the degradation of a variety of substrates, organs rich in phagocytic cells, such as the spleen and liver, are frequently enlarged in several forms of lysosomal storage disorders. The ever-expanding number of lysosomal storage diseases can be divided into rational categories based on the biochemical nature of the accumulated metabolite, thus creating such subgroups as the *glycogenoses, sphingolipidoses (lipidoses), mucopolysaccharidoses (MPSs),* and *mucolipidoses* (see Table 5–6). Only the most common disorders among the remaining groups are considered here.

Tay-Sachs Disease (G_{M2} Gangliosidosis: Hexosaminidase α-Subunit Deficiency)

G_{M2} gangliosidoses are a group of three lysosomal storage diseases caused by an inability to catabolize G_{M2} gangliosides. Degradation of G_{M2} gangliosides requires three polypeptides encoded by three distinct genes. The phenotypic effects of mutations affecting these genes are fairly similar, because they result from accumulation of G_{M2} gangliosides.[24] The underlying enzyme defect, however, is different for each. Tay-Sachs

the lysosomal enzyme can be reduced, the residual enzyme activity may be sufficient to catabolize it and prevent accumulation. A more recent strategy is based on the understanding of the molecular basis of enzyme deficiency. In many disorders, exemplified by Gaucher disease, the enzyme activity is low because the mutant proteins are unstable and prone to misfolding, and hence degraded in the endoplasmic reticulum. In such diseases an exogenous competitive inhibitor of the enzyme can, paradoxically, bind to the mutant enzyme and act as the "folding template" that assists proper folding of the enzyme and thus prevents its degradation. Such *molecular chaperone therapy* is under active investigation.[23]

Several distinctive and separable conditions are included among the lysosomal storage diseases (Table 5–6). In general, the distribution of the stored material, and hence the organs affected, is determined by two interrelated factors: (1) the tissue where most of the material to be degraded is found and (2) the location where most of the degradation normally occurs. *For example, brain is rich in gangliosides, and hence*

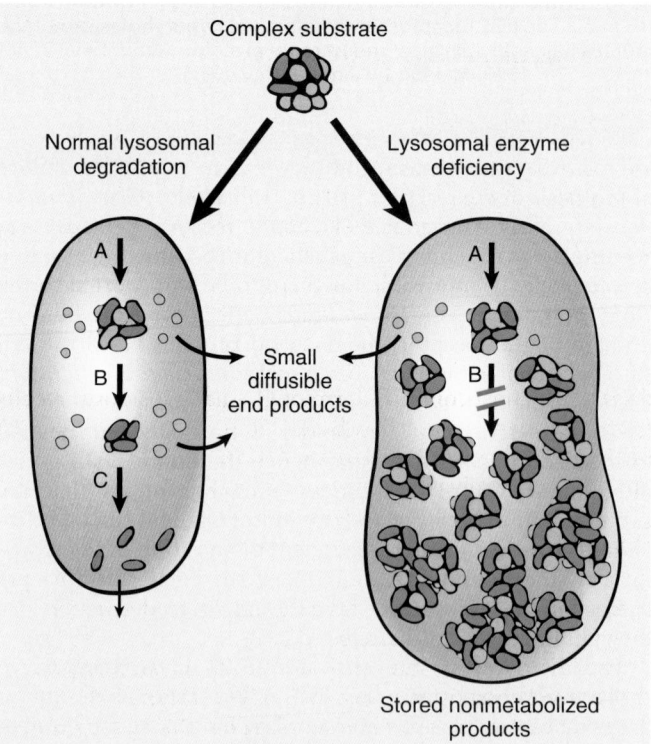

FIGURE 5–11   Pathogenesis of lysosomal storage diseases. In the example shown a complex substrate is normally degraded by a series of lysosomal enzymes (A, B, and C) into soluble end products. If there is a deficiency or malfunction of one of the enzymes (e.g., B), catabolism is incomplete and insoluble intermediates accumulate in the lysosomes.

TABLE 5–6 Lysosomal Storage Diseases		
Disease	**Enzyme Deficiency**	**Major Accumulating Metabolites**
GLYCOGENOSIS		
Type 2—Pompe disease	α-1,4-Glucosidase (lysosomal glucosidase)	Glycogen
SPHINGOLIPIDOSES		

G_{M1} gangliosidosis
    Type 1—infantile, generalized
    Type 2—juvenile
	G_{M1} ganglioside β-galactosidase	G_{M1} ganglioside, galactose-containing oligosaccharides

G_{M2} gangliosidosis
    Tay-Sachs disease
    Sandhoff disease
    G_{M2} gangliosidosis variant AB
	Hexosaminidase, α subunit
	Hexosaminidase, β subunit
	Ganglioside activator protein
		G_{M2} ganglioside
		G_{M2} ganglioside, globoside
		G_{M2} ganglioside

SULFATIDOSES		
Metachromatic leukodystrophy	Arylsulfatase A	Sulfatide
Multiple sulfatase deficiency	Arylsulfatase A, B, C; steroid sulfatase; iduronate sulfatase; heparan N-sulfatase	Sulfatide, steroid sulfate, heparan sulfate, dermatan sulfate
Krabbe disease	Galactosylceramidase	Galactocerebroside
Fabry disease	α-Galactosidase A	Ceramide trihexoside
Gaucher disease	Glucocerebrosidase	Glucocerebroside
Niemann-Pick disease: types A and B	Sphingomyelinase	Sphingomyelin
MUCOPOLYSACCHARIDOSES (MPSs)		
MPS I H (Hurler) MPS II (Hunter)	α-L-Iduronidase L-Iduronosulfate sulfatase	Dermatan sulfate, heparan sulfate
MUCOLIPIDOSES (MLs)		
I-cell disease (ML II) and pseudo-Hurler polydystrophy	Deficiency of phosphorylating enzymes essential for the formation of mannose-6-phosphate recognition marker; acid hydrolases lacking the recognition marker cannot be targeted to the lysosomes but are secreted extracellularly	Mucopolysaccharide, glycolipid
OTHER DISEASES OF COMPLEX CARBOHYDRATES		
Fucosidosis	α-Fucosidase	Fucose-containing sphingolipids and glycoprotein fragments
Mannosidosis	α-Mannosidase	Mannose-containing oligosaccharides
Aspartylglycosaminuria	Aspartylglycosamine amide hydrolase	Aspartyl-2-deoxy-2-acetamido-glycosylamine
OTHER LYSOSOMAL STORAGE DISEASES		
Wolman disease	Acid lipase	Cholesterol esters, triglycerides
Acid phosphate deficiency	Lysosomal acid phosphatase	Phosphate esters

disease, the most common form of G_{M2} gangliosidosis, results from mutations in the α-subunit locus on chromosome 15 that cause a severe deficiency of hexosaminidase A. This disease is especially prevalent among Jews, particularly among those of Eastern European (Ashkenazic) origin, in whom a carrier rate of 1 in 30 has been reported.

Morphology. The hexosaminidase A is absent from virtually all the tissues, so G_{M2} ganglioside accumulates in many tissues (e.g., heart, liver, spleen), but the **involvement of neurons in the central and autonomic nervous systems and retina dominates the clinical picture.** On histologic examination, the neurons are ballooned with cytoplasmic vacuoles, each representing a markedly distended lysosome filled with gangliosides (Fig. 5–12A). Stains for fat such as oil red O and Sudan black B are positive. With

the electron microscope, several types of cytoplasmic inclusions can be visualized, the most prominent being whorled configurations within lysosomes composed of onion-skin layers of membranes (Fig. 5–12B). In time there is progressive destruction of neurons, proliferation of microglia, and accumulation of complex lipids in phagocytes within the brain substance. A similar process occurs in the cerebellum as well as in neurons throughout the basal ganglia, brain stem, spinal cord, and dorsal root ganglia and in the neurons of the autonomic nervous system. The ganglion cells in the retina are similarly swollen with G_{M2} ganglioside, particularly at the margins of the macula. A **cherry-red spot** thus appears in the macula, representing accentuation of the normal color of the macular choroid contrasted with the pallor produced by the swollen ganglion cells in the remainder of the

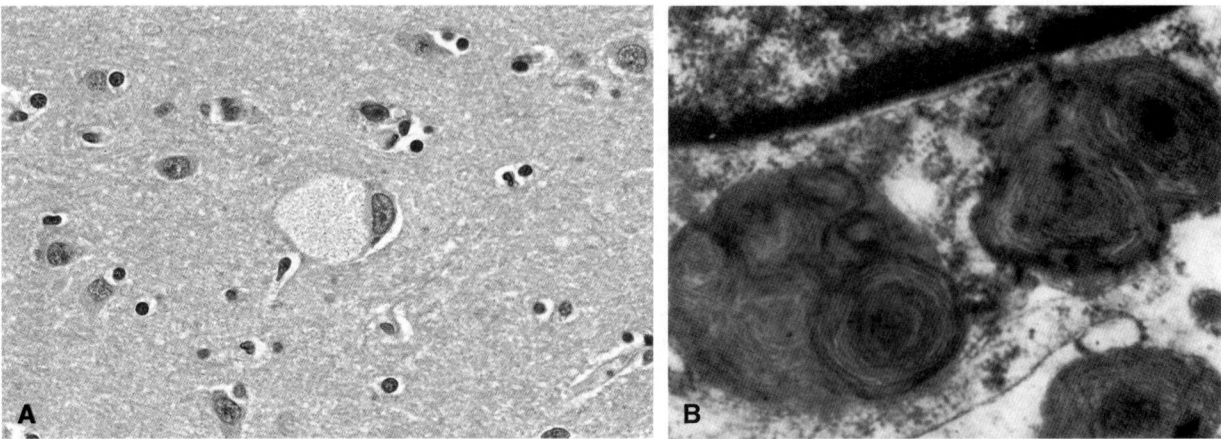

FIGURE 5–12   Ganglion cells in Tay-Sachs disease. **A,** Under the light microscope a large neuron has obvious lipid vacuolation. **B,** A portion of a neuron under the electron microscope shows prominent lysosomes with whorled configurations. Part of the nucleus is shown above. (**A,** courtesy of Dr. Arthur Weinberg, Department of Pathology, University of Texas Southwestern Medical Center, Dallas, TX; **B,** electron micrograph courtesy of Dr. Joe Rutledge, University of Texas Southwestern Medical Center, Dallas, TX.)

retina (Chapter 29). This finding is characteristic of Tay-Sachs disease and other storage disorders affecting the neurons.

Clinical Features. The affected infants appear normal at birth but begin to manifest signs and symptoms at about age 6 months. There is relentless motor and mental deterioration, beginning with motor incoordination, mental obtundation leading to muscular flaccidity, blindness, and increasing dementia. Sometime during the early course of the disease, the characteristic, but not pathognomonic, cherry-red spot appears in the macula of the eye in almost all patients. Over the span of 1 or 2 years a complete vegetative state is reached, followed by death at age 2 to 3 years. More than 100 mutations have been described in the α-subunit gene; most affect protein folding. Such misfolded proteins trigger the "unfolded protein" response (Chapter 1) leading to apoptosis. These findings have given rise to the possibility of chaperone therapy of Tay-Sachs disease.

Antenatal diagnosis and carrier detection are possible by enzyme assays and DNA-based analysis. The clinical features of the two other forms of G_{M2} gangliosidosis, Sandhoff disease, resulting from β-subunit defect, and G_{M2} activator deficiency, are similar to those of Tay-Sachs disease.

Niemann-Pick Disease, Types A and B

Niemann-Pick disease types A and B refers to two related disorders that are characterized by lysosomal accumulation of sphingomyelin due to an inherited deficiency of sphingomyelinase.[25] *Type A is a severe infantile form with extensive neurologic involvement, marked visceral accumulations of sphingomyelin, and progressive wasting and early death within the first 3 years of life.* In contrast, type B disease patients have organomegaly but generally no central nervous system involvement. They usually survive into adulthood. As with Tay-Sachs disease, Niemann-Pick disease types A and B are common in Ashkenazi Jews. The acid sphingomyelinase gene maps to chromosome 11p15.4 and is one of the imprinted genes that

is preferentially expressed from the maternal chromosome as a result of epigenetic silencing of the paternal gene (discussed later). More than 100 mutations have been found in the acid sphingomyelinase gene and there seems to be a correlation between the type of mutation, the severity of enzyme deficiency, and the phenotype.

Morphology. In the classic infantile type A variant, a missense mutation causes almost complete deficiency of sphingomyelinase. Sphingomyelin is a ubiquitous component of cellular (including organellar) membranes, and so the enzyme deficiency blocks degradation of the lipid, resulting in its progressive accumulation within lysosomes, particularly within cells of the mononuclear phagocyte system. Affected cells become enlarged, sometimes to 90 μm in diameter, due to the distention of lysosomes with sphingomyelin and cholesterol. Innumerable small vacuoles of relatively uniform size are created, imparting foaminess to the cytoplasm (Fig. 5–13). In frozen sections of fresh tissue, the vacuoles stain for fat. Electron microscopy confirms that the vacuoles are engorged secondary lysosomes that often contain membranous cytoplasmic bodies resembling concentric lamellated myelin figures, sometimes called "zebra" bodies.

The lipid-laden phagocytic foam cells are widely distributed in the spleen, liver, lymph nodes, bone marrow, tonsils, gastrointestinal tract, and lungs. **The involvement of the spleen generally produces massive enlargement**, sometimes to ten times its normal weight, but the hepatomegaly is usually not quite so striking. The lymph nodes are generally moderately to markedly enlarged throughout the body.

Involvement of the brain and eye deserves special mention. In the brain the gyri are shrunken and the sulci widened. The neuronal involvement is diffuse, affecting all parts of the nervous system.

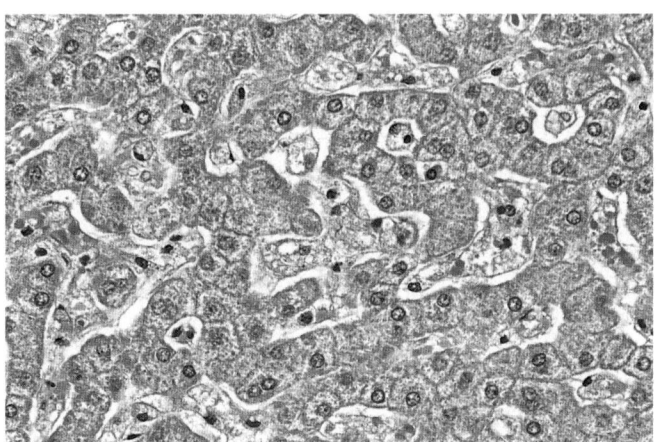

FIGURE 5–13 Niemann-Pick disease in liver. The hepatocytes and Kupffer cells have a foamy, vacuolated appearance due to deposition of lipids. (Courtesy of Dr. Arthur Weinberg, Department of Pathology, University of Texas Southwestern Medical Center, Dallas, TX.)

Vacuolation and ballooning of neurons constitute the dominant histologic change, which in time leads to cell death and loss of brain substance. A retinal cherry-red spot similar to that seen in Tay-Sachs disease is present in about one third to one half of affected individuals.

Clinical manifestations in type A disease may be present at birth and almost invariably become evident by age 6 months. Infants typically have a protuberant abdomen because of the hepatosplenomegaly. Once the manifestations appear, they are followed by progressive failure to thrive, vomiting, fever, and generalized lymphadenopathy as well as progressive deterioration of psychomotor function. Death comes, usually within the first or second year of life.

The diagnosis is established by biochemical assays for sphingomyelinase activity in liver or bone marrow biopsy. Individuals affected with types A and B as well as carriers can be detected by DNA analysis.

Niemann-Pick Disease, Type C (NPC)

Although previously considered to be related to types A and B, Niemann-Pick disease type C (NPC) is quite distinct at the biochemical and molecular levels and is more common than types A and B combined. Mutations in two related genes, *NPC1* and *NPC2*, can give rise to it, with *NPC1* being responsible for 95% of cases. Unlike most other lysosomal storage diseases, NPC is due to a primary defect in lipid transport. Affected cells accumulate cholesterol as well as gangliosides such as G_{M1} and G_{M2}. Both NPC1 and NPC2 are involved in the transport of free cholesterol from the lysosomes to the cytoplasm.[26] NPC is clinically heterogeneous. It may present as hydrops fetalis and stillbirth, as neonatal hepatitis, or as a chronic form characterized by progressive neurologic damage. The most common form presents in childhood and is marked by ataxia, vertical supranuclear gaze palsy, dystonia, dysarthria, and psychomotor regression.

Gaucher Disease

Gaucher disease refers to a cluster of autosomal recessive disorders resulting from mutations in the gene encoding glucocerebrosidase.[27] This disease is the most common lysosomal storage disorder. The affected gene encodes glucocerebrosidase, an enzyme that normally cleaves the glucose residue from ceramide. As a result of the enzyme defect, glucocerebroside accumulates principally in phagocytes but in some subtypes also in the central nervous system. Glucocerebrosides are continually formed from the catabolism of glycolipids derived mainly from the cell membranes of senescent leukocytes and erythrocytes. It is clear now that the pathologic changes in Gaucher disease are caused not just by the burden of storage material but also by activation of macrophages and the consequent secretion of cytokines such as IL-1, IL-6, and tumor necrosis factor (TNF). Three clinical subtypes of Gaucher disease have been distinguished. The most common, accounting for 99% of cases, is called *type I*, or the chronic non-neuronopathic form. In this type, *storage of glucocerebrosides is limited to the mononuclear phagocytes throughout the body without involving the brain. Splenic and skeletal involvements dominate this pattern of the disease.* It is found principally in Jews of European stock. Individuals with this disorder have reduced but detectable levels of glucocerebrosidase activity. Longevity is shortened but not markedly. *Type II*, or acute neuronopathic Gaucher disease, is the *infantile acute cerebral pattern. This form has no predilection for Jews. In these patients there is virtually no detectable glucocerebrosidase activity in the tissues.* Hepatosplenomegaly is also seen in this form of Gaucher disease, but the clinical picture is dominated by progressive central nervous system involvement, leading to death at an early age. A third pattern, type III, is intermediate between types I and II. These patients have the systemic involvement characteristic of type I but have progressive central nervous system disease that usually begins in adolescence or early adulthood.

Morphology. Glucocerebrosides accumulate in massive amounts within phagocytic cells throughout the body in all forms of Gaucher disease. The distended phagocytic cells, known as **Gaucher cells**, are found in the spleen, liver, bone marrow, lymph nodes, tonsils, thymus, and Peyer's patches. Similar cells may be found in both the alveolar septa and the air spaces in the lung. In contrast to other lipid storage diseases, Gaucher cells rarely appear vacuolated but instead have a fibrillary type of cytoplasm likened to crumpled tissue paper (Fig. 5–14). Gaucher cells are often enlarged, sometimes up to 100 μm in diameter, and have one or more dark, eccentrically placed nuclei. Periodic acid–Schiff staining is usually intensely positive. With the electron microscope the fibrillary cytoplasm can be resolved as elongated, distended lysosomes, containing the stored lipid in stacks of bilayers.

In type I disease, the spleen is enlarged, sometimes up to 10 kg. The lymphadenopathy is mild to moderate and is body-wide. The accumulation of Gaucher cells in the bone marrow occurs in 70% to 100% of

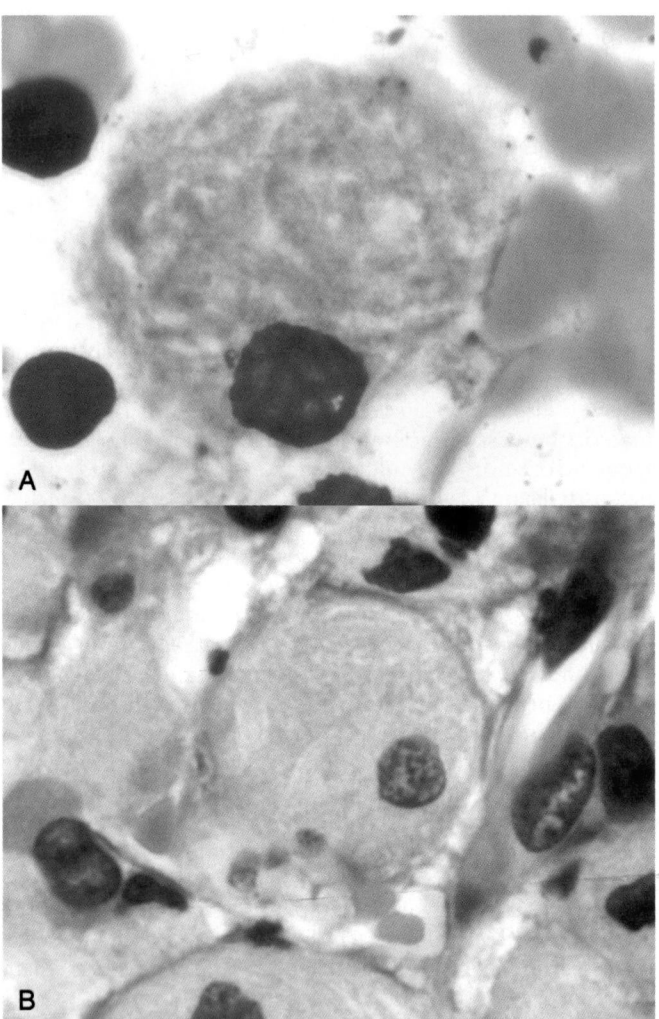

A

B

FIGURE 5–14 Gaucher disease involving the bone marrow. Gaucher cells (**A**, H&E; **B**, Wright stain) are plump macrophages that characteristically have the appearance in the cytoplasm of crumpled tissue paper (**B**), due to accumulation of glucocerebroside. (Courtesy of Dr. John Anastasi, Department of Pathology, University of Chicago, Chicago, IL.)

cases of type I Gaucher disease. It produces areas of bone erosion that are sometimes small but in other cases sufficiently large to give rise to pathologic fractures. Bone destruction occurs due to the secretion of cytokines by activated macrophages. In patients with cerebral involvement, Gaucher cells are seen in the Virchow-Robin spaces, and arterioles are surrounded by swollen adventitial cells. There is no storage of lipids in the neurons, yet neurons appear shriveled and are progressively destroyed. It is suspected that the lipids that accumulate in the phagocytic cells around blood vessels secrete cytokines that damage nearby neurons.

Clinical Features. The clinical course of Gaucher disease depends on the clinical subtype. In type I, symptoms and signs first appear in adult life and are related to splenomegaly or bone involvement. Most commonly there is pancytopenia or

thrombocytopenia secondary to hypersplenism. Pathologic fractures and bone pain occur if there has been extensive expansion of the marrow space. Although the disease is progressive in the adult, it is compatible with long life. In types II and III, central nervous system dysfunction, convulsions, and progressive mental deterioration dominate, although organs such as the liver, spleen, and lymph nodes are also affected.

The diagnosis of homozygotes can be made by measurement of glucocerebrosidase activity in peripheral blood leukocytes or in extracts of cultured skin fibroblasts. In principle, heterozygotes can be identified by detection of mutations. However, because more than 150 mutations in the glucocerebroside gene can cause Gaucher disease, it is not possible to use a single genetic test.

Replacement therapy with recombinant enzymes is the mainstay for treatment of Gaucher disease; it is effective, and those with type I disease can expect normal life expectancy with this form of treatment. However, such therapy is extremely expensive. Because the fundamental defect resides in mononuclear phagocytic cells originating from marrow stem cells, bone marrow transplantation has been attempted. Other work is directed toward correction of the enzyme defect by transfer of the normal glucocerebrosidase gene into the patient's bone marrow cells. Substrate reduction therapy with inhibitors of glucosylceramide synthetase is also being evaluated.

Mucopolysaccharidoses

The MPSs are a group of closely related syndromes that result from genetically determined deficiencies of lysosomal enzymes involved in the degradation of mucopolysaccharides (glycosaminoglycans). Chemically, mucopolysaccharides are long-chain complex carbohydrates that are linked with proteins to form proteoglycans. They are abundant in the ground substance of connective tissue. The glycosaminoglycans that accumulate in MPSs are dermatan sulfate, heparan sulfate, keratan sulfate, and chondroitin sulfate. The enzymes involved in the degradation of these molecules cleave terminal sugars from the polysaccharide chains disposed along a polypeptide or core protein. In the absence of enzymes, these chains accumulate within lysosomes in various tissues and organs of the body.

Several clinical variants of MPS, classified numerically from MPS I to MPS VII, have been described, each resulting from the deficiency of one specific enzyme. All the MPSs except one are inherited as autosomal recessive traits; the exception, called *Hunter syndrome*, is an X-linked recessive trait. Within a given group (e.g., MPS I, characterized by a deficiency of α-l-iduronidase), subgroups exist that result from different mutant alleles at the same genetic locus. Thus, the severity of enzyme deficiency and the clinical picture even within subgroups are often different.

In general, MPSs are progressive disorders, characterized by *coarse facial features*, *clouding of the cornea*, *joint stiffness*, and *mental retardation*. Urinary excretion of the accumulated mucopolysaccharides is often increased.

Morphology. The accumulated mucopolysaccharides are generally found in mononuclear phagocytic cells, endothelial cells, intimal smooth muscle cells, and fibroblasts throughout the body. Common sites of involvement are thus the spleen, liver, bone marrow, lymph nodes, blood vessels, and heart.

Microscopically, affected cells are distended and have apparent clearing of the cytoplasm to create so-called balloon cells. Under the electron microscope, the clear cytoplasm can be resolved as numerous minute vacuoles. These are swollen lysosomes containing a finely granular periodic acid–Schiff–positive material that can be identified biochemically as mucopolysaccharide. Similar lysosomal changes are found in the neurons of those syndromes characterized by central nervous system involvement. In addition, however, some of the lysosomes in neurons are replaced by lamellated zebra bodies similar to those seen in Niemann-Pick disease. **Hepatosplenomegaly, skeletal deformities, valvular lesions, and subendothelial arterial deposits, particularly in the coronary arteries, and lesions in the brain, are common threads that run through all of the MPSs.** In many of the more protracted syndromes, coronary subendothelial lesions lead to myocardial ischemia. Thus, myocardial infarction and cardiac decompensation are important causes of death.

Clinical Features. Of the seven recognized variants, only two well-characterized syndromes are described briefly here. *Hurler syndrome*, also called MPS I-H, results from a deficiency of α-l-iduronidase.[28] It is one of the most severe forms of MPS. Affected children appear normal at birth but develop hepatosplenomegaly by age 6 to 24 months. Their growth is retarded, and, as in other forms of MPS, they develop coarse facial features and skeletal deformities. Death occurs by age 6 to 10 years and is often due to cardiovascular complications. *Hunter syndrome*, also called MPS II, differs from Hurler syndrome in mode of inheritance (X-linked), absence of corneal clouding, and milder clinical course.[29]

Glycogen Storage Diseases (Glycogenoses)

The *glycogen storage diseases* result from a hereditary deficiency of one of the enzymes involved in the synthesis or sequential degradation of glycogen. Depending on the tissue or organ distribution of the specific enzyme in the normal state, *glycogen storage in these disorders may be limited to a few tissues, may be more widespread while not affecting all tissues, or may be systemic in distribution.*[30]

The significance of a specific enzyme deficiency is best understood from the perspective of the normal metabolism of glycogen (Fig. 5–15). Glycogen is a storage form of glucose. Glycogen synthesis begins with the conversion of glucose to glucose-6-phosphate by the action of a hexokinase (glucokinase). A phosphoglucomutase then transforms the glucose-6-phosphate to glucose-1-phosphate, which, in turn, is converted to uridine diphosphoglucose. A highly branched, large polymer is then built (molecular weight as high as 100 million), containing as many as 10,000 glucose molecules linked together by α-1,4-glucoside bonds. The glycogen chain and branches continue to be elongated by the addition of glucose molecules

mediated by glycogen synthetases. During degradation, distinct phosphorylases in the liver and muscle split glucose-1-phosphate from the glycogen until about four glucose residues remain on each branch, leaving a branched oligosaccharide called *limit dextrin*. This can be further degraded only by the debranching enzyme. In addition to these major pathways, glycogen is also degraded in the lysosomes by acid maltase. If the lysosomes are deficient in this enzyme, the glycogen contained within them is not accessible to degradation by cytoplasmic enzymes such as phosphorylases.

On the basis of specific enzyme deficiencies and the resultant clinical pictures, glycogenoses have traditionally been divided into a dozen or so syndromes designated by roman numerals, and the list continues to grow.[31] On the basis of pathophysiology glycogenoses can be divided into three major subgroups (Table 5–7).

- *Hepatic forms:* The liver is a key player in glycogen metabolism. It contains enzymes that synthesize glycogen for storage and ultimately break it down into free glucose, which is then released into the blood. An inherited deficiency of hepatic enzymes that are involved in glycogen degradation therefore leads not only to the storage of glycogen in the liver but also to a reduction in blood glucose concentrations (hypoglycemia) (Fig. 5–16). Deficiency of the enzyme glucose-6-phosphatase (von Gierke disease, or type I glycogenosis) is a prime example of the hepatic-hypoglycemic form of glycogen storage disease (see Table 5–7). Other examples include deficiencies of liver phosphorylase and debranching enzyme, both involved in the breakdown of glycogen (see Fig. 5–15). In all these disorders glycogen is stored in many organs, but *hepatic enlargement and hypoglycemia dominate the clinical picture.*[32]
- *Myopathic forms:* In the skeletal muscles, as opposed to the liver, glycogen is used predominantly as a source of energy during physical activity. ATP is generated by glycolysis, which leads ultimately to the formation of lactate (see Fig. 5–16). If the enzymes that fuel the glycolytic pathway are deficient, glycogen storage occurs in the muscles and is associated with muscular weakness due to impaired energy production. Examples in this category include deficiencies of muscle phosphorylase (McArdle disease, or type V glycogenosis), muscle phosphofructokinase (type VII glycogen storage disease), and several others. *Typically, individuals with the myopathic forms present with muscle cramps after exercise and lactate levels in the blood fail to rise after exercise due to a block in glycolysis.*[33]
- Glycogen storage diseases associated with (1) deficiency of α-glucosidase (acid maltase) and (2) lack of branching enzyme do not fit into the hepatic or myopathic categories. They are associated with glycogen storage in many organs and death early in life. Acid maltase is a lysosomal enzyme, and hence its deficiency leads to lysosomal storage of glycogen (type II glycogenosis, or Pompe disease) in all organs, but cardiomegaly is the most prominent feature[34] (Fig. 5–17).

Alkaptonuria (Ochronosis)

Alkaptonuria, the first human inborn error of metabolism to be discovered, is an autosomal recessive disorder in which

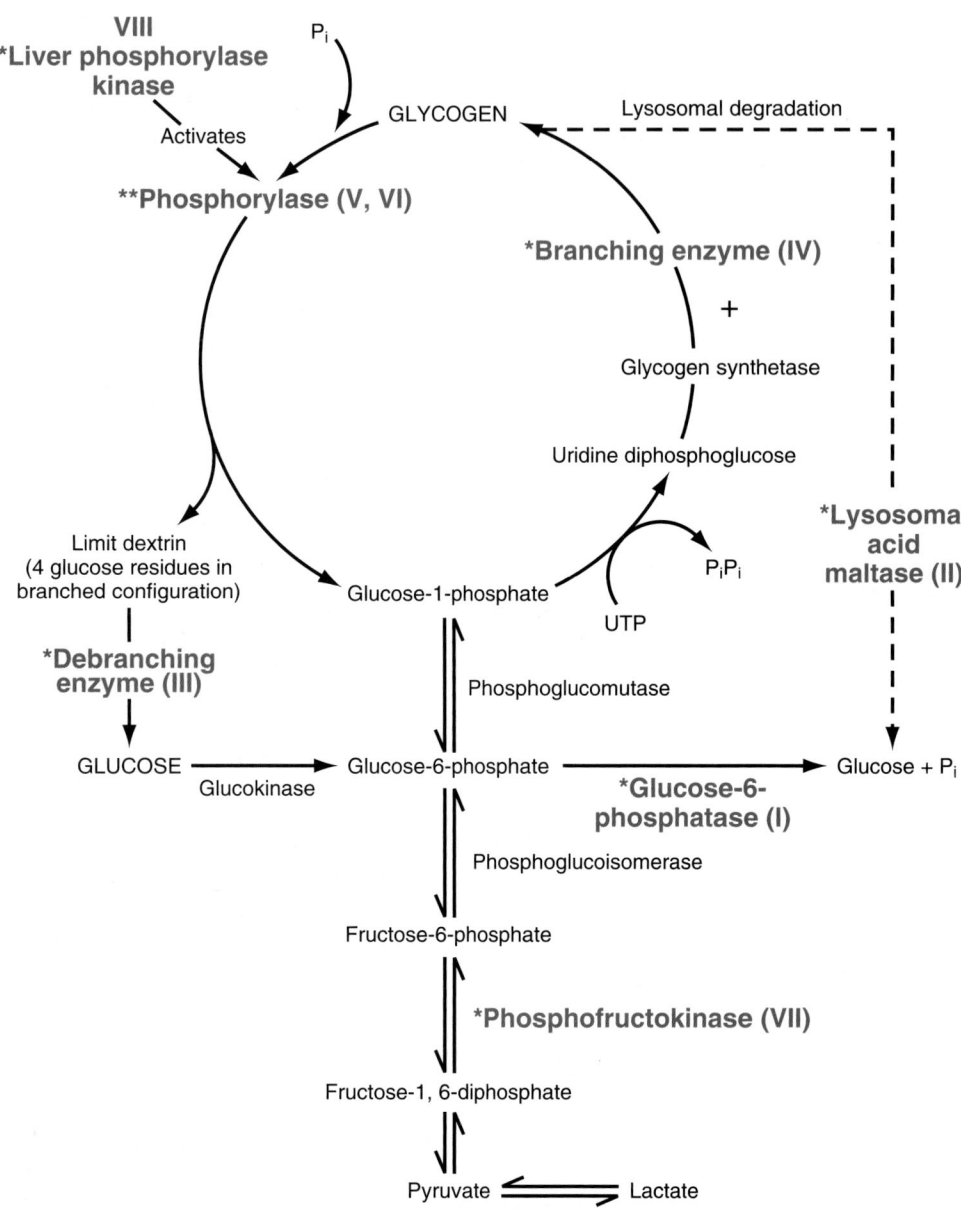

FIGURE 5–15 Pathways of glycogen metabolism. Asterisks mark the enzyme deficiencies associated with glycogen storage diseases. Roman numerals indicate the type of glycogen storage disease associated with the given enzyme deficiency. Types V and VI result from deficiencies of muscle and liver phosphorylases, respectively. (Modified from Hers H et al.: Glycogen storage diseases. In Scriver CR et al. [eds]: The Metabolic Basis of Inherited Disease, 6th ed. New York, McGraw-Hill, 1989, p 425.)

there is lack of homogentisic oxidase, an enzyme that converts homogentisic acid to methylacetoacetic acid in the tyrosine degradation pathway.[35] Thus, homogentisic acid accumulates in the body. A large amount is excreted, imparting a black color to the urine if allowed to stand and undergo oxidation.

> **Morphology.** The retained homogentisic acid binds to collagen in connective tissues, tendons, and cartilage, imparting to these tissues a blue-black pigmentation (**ochronosis**) most evident in the ears, nose, and cheeks. **The most serious consequences of ochronosis, however, stem from deposits of the pigment in the articular cartilages of the joints.** The pigment accumulation causes the cartilage to lose its normal resiliency and become brittle and fibrillated. Wear-and-tear erosion of this abnormal cartilage leads to denudation of the subchondral bone, and often tiny fragments of the fibrillated cartilage are driven into the underlying bone, worsening the damage. The vertebral column, particularly the intervertebral disc, is the prime site of attack, but later the knees, shoulders, and hips may be affected. The small joints of the hands and feet are usually spared.

Clinical Features. The metabolic defect is present from birth, but the degenerative arthropathy develops slowly and usually does not become clinically evident until the 30s. Although it is not life-threatening, it may be severely crippling. The arthropathy may be as extreme as that encountered in the severe forms of osteoarthritis (Chapter 26) of the elderly, but it occurs at a much earlier age.

	TABLE 5-7	Principal Subgroups of Glycogenoses		
Clinicopathologic Category	Specific Type	Enzyme Deficiency	Morphologic Changes	Clinical Features
Hepatic type	Hepatorenal—von Gierke disease (type I)	Glucose-6-phosphatase	Hepatomegaly—intracytoplasmic accumulations of glycogen and small amounts of lipid; intranuclear glycogen Renomegaly—intracytoplasmic accumulations of glycogen in cortical tubular epithelial cells	*In untreated patients:* Failure to thrive, stunted growth, hepatomegaly, and renomegaly Hypoglycemia due to failure of glucose mobilization, often leading to convulsions Hyperlipidemia and hyperuricemia resulting from deranged glucose metabolism; many patients develop gout and skin xanthomas Bleeding tendency due to platelet dysfunction *With treatment:* Most survive and develop late complications (e.g., hepatic adenomas)
Myopathic type	McArdle syndrome (type V)	Muscle phosphorylase	Skeletal muscle only—accumulations of glycogen predominant in subsarcolemmal location	Painful cramps associated with strenuous exercise; myoglobinuria occurs in 50% of cases; onset in adulthood (>20 years); muscular exercise fails to raise lactate level in venous blood; serum creatine kinase always elevated; compatible with normal longevity
Miscellaneous types	Generalized glycogenosis—Pompe disease (type II)	Lysosomal glucosidase (acid maltase)	Mild hepatomegaly—ballooning of lysosomes with glycogen, creating lacy cytoplasmic pattern Cardiomegaly—glycogen within sarcoplasm as well as membrane-bound Skeletal muscle—similar to changes in heart	Massive cardiomegaly, muscle hypotonia, and cardiorespiratory failure within 2 years; a milder adult form with only skeletal muscle involvement, presenting with chronic myopathy

DISORDERS ASSOCIATED WITH DEFECTS IN PROTEINS THAT REGULATE CELL GROWTH

Normal growth and differentiation of cells are regulated by two classes of genes; proto-oncogenes and tumor suppressor genes, whose products promote or restrain cell growth (Chapter 7). It is now well established that mutations in these two classes of genes are important in the pathogenesis of tumors. In the vast majority of cases, cancer-causing mutations affect somatic cells and hence are not passed in the germ line. In approximately 5% of all cancers, however, mutations transmitted through the germ line contribute to the development of cancer. Most familial cancers are inherited in an autosomal dominant fashion, but a few recessive disorders have also been described. This subject is discussed in Chapter 7. Specific forms of familial tumors are described in various chapters.

Complex Multigenic Disorders

As discussed previously, such disorders are caused by interactions between variant forms of genes and environmental factors.

A genetic variant that has at least two alleles and occurs in at least 1% of the population is called a polymorphism. According to the common disease/common variant hypothesis, complex genetic disorders occur when many polymorphisms, each with a modest effect and low penetrance, are inherited.[36] Two additional facts that have emerged from studies of common complex disorders, such as type I diabetes, are:

- While complex disorders result from the collective inheritance of many polymorphisms, different polymorphisms vary in significance. For example, of the 20–30 genes implicated in type I diabetes, 6–7 are most important, and a few HLA-alleles contribute >50% of the risk (Chapter 24).
- Some polymorphisms are common to multiple diseases of the same type, while others are disease specific. This is best illustrated in immune-mediated inflammatory diseases (Chapter 6).

Several normal phenotypic characteristics are governed by multifactorial inheritance, such as hair color, eye color, skin color, height, and intelligence. These characteristics show a continuous variation in population groups, producing the standard bell-shaped curve of distribution. Environmental

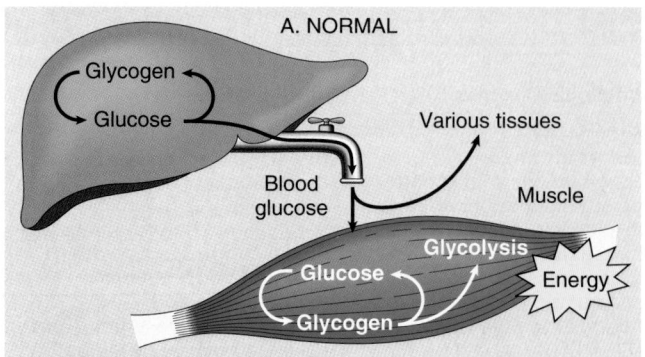

A. NORMAL

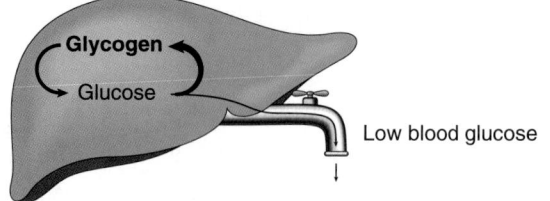

B. GLYCOGEN STORAGE DISEASE—HEPATIC TYPE

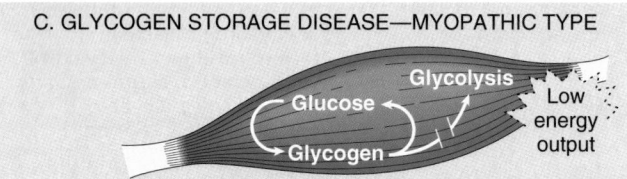

C. GLYCOGEN STORAGE DISEASE—MYOPATHIC TYPE

FIGURE 5–16 **A,** Normal glycogen metabolism in the liver and skeletal muscles. **B,** Effects of an inherited deficiency of hepatic enzymes involved in glycogen metabolism. **C,** Consequences of a genetic deficiency in the enzymes that metabolize glycogen in skeletal muscles.

influences, however, significantly modify the phenotypic expression of complex traits. For example, type II diabetes mellitus has many of the features of a multifactorial disorder. It is well recognized clinically that individuals often first manifest this disease after weight gain. Thus, obesity as well as other environmental influences unmasks the diabetic genetic trait. Nutritional influences may cause even monozygous twins to achieve different heights. The culturally deprived child cannot achieve his or her full intellectual capacity.

Assigning a disease to this mode of inheritance must be done with caution. It depends on many factors but first on familial clustering and the exclusion of mendelian and chromosomal modes of transmission. A range of levels of severity of a disease is suggestive of a complex multigenic disorder, but, as pointed out earlier, variable expressivity and reduced penetrance of single mutant genes may also account for this phenomenon. Because of these problems, sometimes it is difficult to distinguish between mendelian and multifactorial disease.

Chromosomal Disorders

NORMAL KARYOTYPE

As is well known, human somatic cells contain 46 chromosomes; these comprise 22 homologous pairs of autosomes and two sex chromosomes, XX in the female and XY in the male. The study of chromosomes—*karyotyping*—is the basic tool of the cytogeneticist. The usual procedure to examine chromosomes is to arrest dividing cells in metaphase with mitotic spindle inhibitors (e.g., *N*-deacetyl-*N*-methylcolchicine [Colcemid]) and then to stain the chromosomes. In a metaphase spread, the individual chromosomes take the form of two chromatids connected at the centromere. A karyotype is obtained by arranging each pair of autosomes according to length, followed by sex chromosomes.

A variety of staining methods have been developed that allow identification of individual chromosomes on the basis of a distinctive and reliable pattern of alternating light and dark bands. The one most commonly used involves a Giemsa stain and is hence called *G banding*. A normal male karyotype with G banding is illustrated in Figure 5–18. With standard G

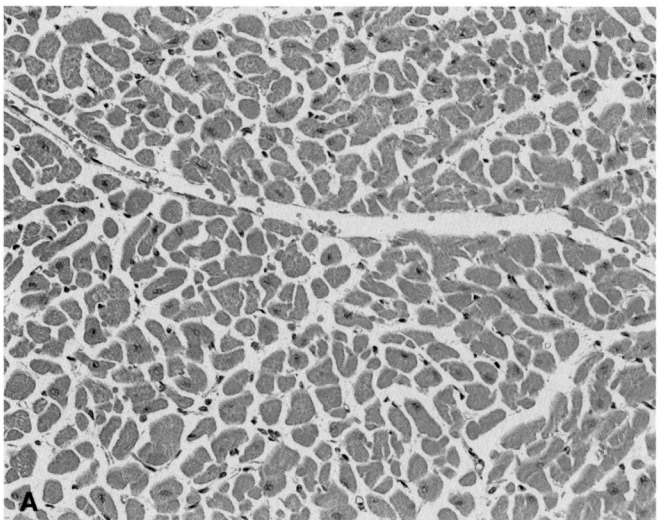
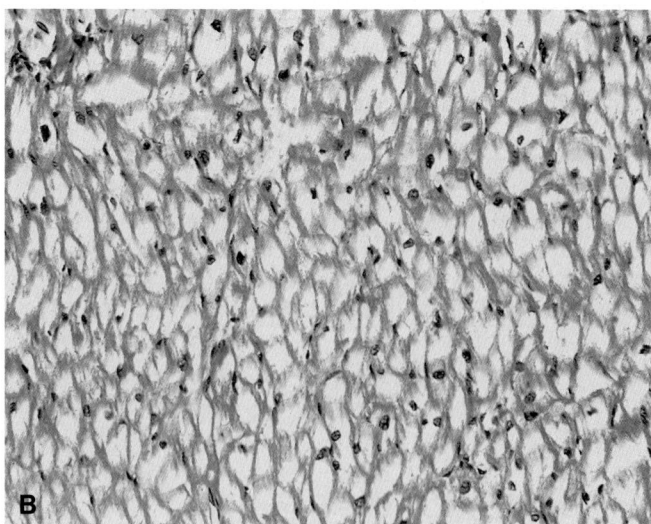

FIGURE 5–17 Pompe disease (glycogen storage disease type II). **A,** Normal myocardium with abundant eosinophilic cytoplasm. **B,** Patient with Pompe disease (same magnification) showing the myocardial fibers full of glycogen seen as clear spaces. (Courtesy of Dr. Trace Worrell, Department of Pathology, University of Texas Southwestern Medical Center, Dallas, TX.)

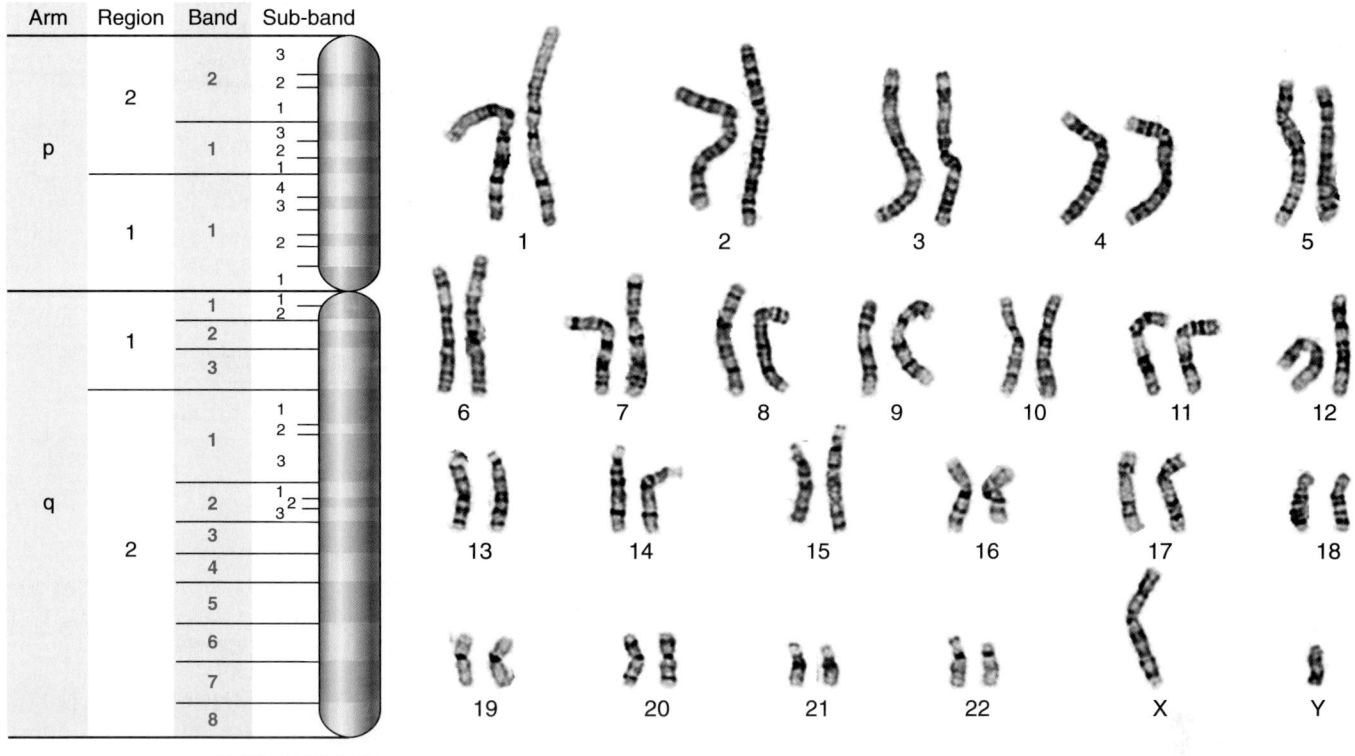

Arm	Region	Band	Sub-band

FIGURE 5–18 G-banded karyotype from a normal male (46,XY). (Courtesy of Dr. Stuart Schwartz, Department of Pathology, University of Chicago, Chicago, IL.) Also shown is the banding pattern of the X-chromosome with nomenclature of arms, regions, bands, and sub-bands.

banding, approximately 400 to 800 bands per haploid set can be detected. The resolution obtained by banding can be markedly improved by obtaining the cells in prophase. The individual chromosomes appear markedly elongated, and as many as 1500 bands per karyotype can be recognized. The use of these banding techniques permits certain identification of each chromosome and roughly delineates breakpoints and other gross alterations, to be described later.

Before this discussion of the normal karyotype is concluded, reference must be made to commonly used cytogenetic terminology. Karyotypes are usually described using a shorthand system of notations. The following order is used: Total number of chromosomes is given first, followed by the sex chromosome complement, and finally the description of abnormalities in ascending numerical order. For example, a male with trisomy 21 is designated *47,XY,+21*. Some of the notations denoting structural alterations of chromosomes are described along with the abnormalities in a later section. Here we should mention that the short arm of a chromosome is designated *p* (for petit), and the long arm is referred to as *q* (the next letter of the alphabet). In a banded karyotype, each arm of the chromosome is divided into two or more regions bordered by prominent bands. The regions are numbered (e.g., 1, 2, 3) from the centromere outward. Each region is further subdivided into bands and sub-bands, and these are ordered numerically as well (see Fig. 5–18). Thus, the notation *Xp21.2* refers to a chromosomal segment located on the short arm of the X chromosome, in region 2, band 1, and sub-band 2.

STRUCTURAL ABNORMALITIES OF CHROMOSOMES

The aberrations underlying cytogenetic disorders may take the form of an abnormal number of chromosomes or alterations in the structure of one or more chromosomes. The normal chromosome complement is expressed as 46,XX for the female and 46,XY for the male. Any exact multiple of the haploid number is called *euploid*. If an error occurs in meiosis or mitosis and a cell acquires a chromosome complement that is not an exact multiple of 23, it is referred to as *aneuploidy*. The usual causes for aneuploidy are *nondisjunction* and *anaphase lag*. When nondisjunction occurs during gametogenesis, the gametes formed have either an extra chromosome (n + 1) or one less chromosome (n − 1). Fertilization of such gametes by normal gametes results in two types of zygotes—trisomic (2n + 1) or monosomic (2n − 1). In anaphase lag, one homologous chromosome in meiosis or one chromatid in mitosis lags behind and is left out of the cell nucleus. The result is one normal cell and one cell with monosomy. As seen subsequently, monosomy or trisomy involving the sex chromosomes, or even more bizarre aberrations, are compatible with life and are usually associated with variable degrees of phenotypic abnormalities. *Monosomy involving an autosome generally causes loss of too much genetic information to permit live birth or even embryogenesis, but several autosomal trisomies do permit survival.* With the exception of trisomy 21, all yield severely handicapped infants who almost invariably die at an early age.

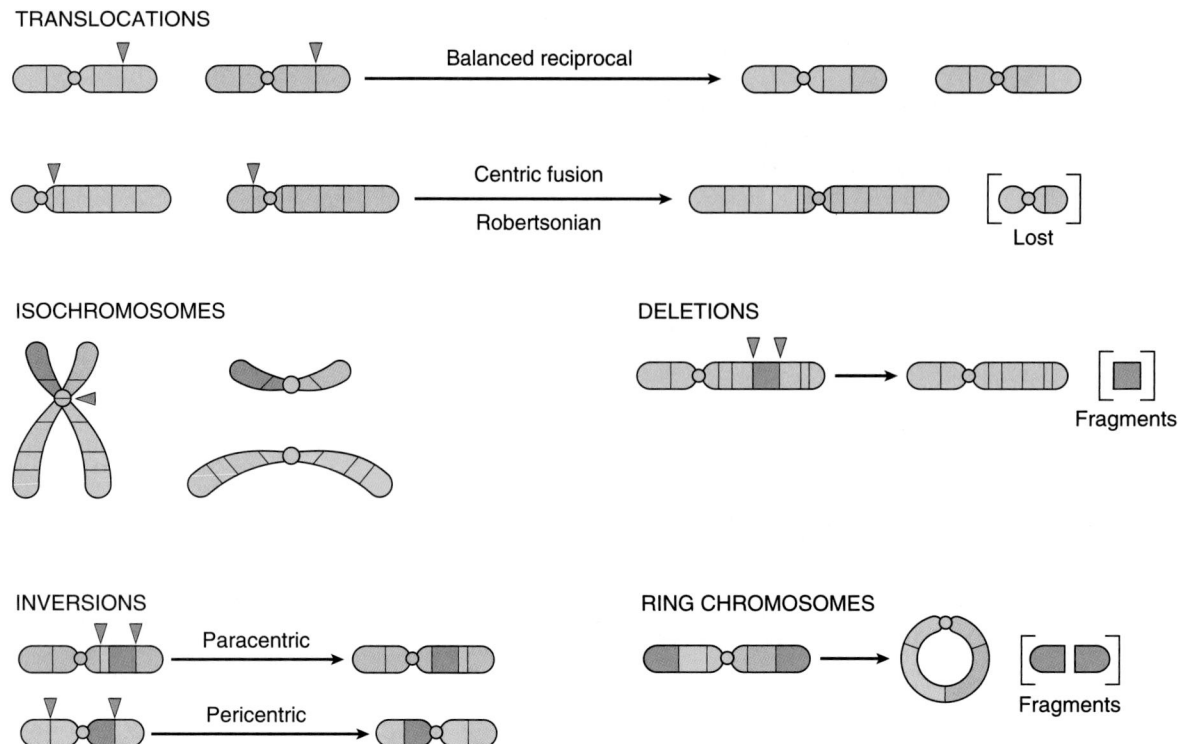

TRANSLOCATIONS

Balanced reciprocal

Centric fusion

Robertsonian

Lost

ISOCHROMOSOMES

DELETIONS

Fragments

INVERSIONS

Paracentric

Pericentric

RING CHROMOSOMES

Fragments

FIGURE 5–19 Types of chromosomal rearrangements.

Occasionally, *mitotic errors in early development give rise to two or more populations of cells with different chromosomal complement, in the same individual*, a condition referred to as *mosaicism*. Mosaicism can result from mitotic errors during the cleavage of the fertilized ovum or in somatic cells. Mosaicism affecting the sex chromosomes is relatively common. In the division of the fertilized ovum, an error may lead to one of the daughter cells receiving three sex chromosomes, whereas the other receives only one, yielding, for example, a 45,X/47,XXX mosaic. All descendent cells derived from each of these precursors thus have either a 47,XXX complement or a 45,X complement. Such a patient is a mosaic variant of Turner syndrome, with the extent of phenotypic expression dependent on the number and distribution of the 45,X cells.

Autosomal mosaicism seems to be much less common than that involving the sex chromosomes. An error in an early mitotic division affecting the autosomes usually leads to a nonviable mosaic due to autosomal monosomy. Rarely, the nonviable cell population is lost during embryogenesis, yielding a viable mosaic (e.g., 46,XY/47,XY,+21). Such a patient is a trisomy 21 mosaic with variable expression of Down syndrome, depending on the proportion of cells containing the trisomy.

A second category of chromosomal aberrations is associated with changes in the structure of chromosomes. To be visible by routine banding techniques, a fairly large amount of DNA (approximately 2–4 million base pairs), containing many genes, must be involved. The resolution is much higher with fluorescence in situ hybridization (FISH), which can detect changes as small as kilobases. Structural changes in chromosomes usually result from chromosome breakage followed by loss or rearrangement of material. Such alterations

occur spontaneously at a low rate that is increased by exposure to environmental mutagens, such as chemicals and ionizing radiation. In the next section we briefly review the more common forms of alterations in chromosome structure and the notations used to signify them.

Deletion refers to loss of a portion of a chromosome (Fig. 5–19). Most deletions are interstitial, but rarely terminal deletions may occur. Interstitial deletions occur when there are two breaks within a chromosome arm, followed by loss of the chromosomal material between the breaks and fusion of the broken ends. One can specify in which region(s) and at what bands the breaks have occurred. For example, *46,XY,del (16)(p11.2p13.1)* describes breakpoints in the short arm of chromosome 16 at 16p11.2 and 16p13.1 with loss of material between breaks. Terminal deletions result from a single break in a chromosome arm, producing a fragment with no centromere, which is then lost at the next cell division, and a chromosome bearing a deletion. The end of the chromosome is protected by acquiring telomeric sequences.

A *ring chromosome* is a special form of deletion. It is produced when a break occurs at both ends of a chromosome with fusion of the damaged ends (see Fig. 5–19). If significant genetic material is lost, phenotypic abnormalities result. This might be expressed as *46,XY,r(14)*. Ring chromosomes do not behave normally in meiosis or mitosis and usually result in serious consequences.

Inversion refers to a rearrangement that involves two breaks within a single chromosome with reincorporation of the inverted, intervening segment (see Fig. 5–19). An inversion involving only one arm of the chromosome is known as *paracentric*. If the breaks are on opposite sides of the centromere, it is known as *pericentric*. Inversions are often fully compatible with normal development.

Isochromosome formation results when one arm of a chromosome is lost and the remaining arm is duplicated, resulting in a chromosome consisting of two short arms only or of two long arms (see Fig. 5–19). An isochromosome has morphologically identical genetic information in both arms. The most common isochromosome present in live births involves the long arm of the X and is designated *i(X)(q10)*. The Xq isochromosome is associated with monosomy for genes on the short arm of X and with trisomy for genes on the long arm of X.

In a *translocation*, a segment of one chromosome is transferred to another (see Fig. 5–19). In one form, called *balanced reciprocal translocation*, there are single breaks in each of two chromosomes, with exchange of material. A balanced reciprocal translocation between the long arm of chromosome 2 and the short arm of chromosome 5 would be written *46,XX,t(2;5)(q31;p14)*. This individual has 46 chromosomes with altered morphology of one of the chromosomes 2 and one of the chromosomes 5. Because there has been no loss of genetic material, the individual is likely to be phenotypically normal. A balanced translocation carrier, however, is at increased risk for producing abnormal gametes. For example, in the case cited above, a gamete containing one normal chromosome 2 and a translocated chromosome 5 may be formed. Such a gamete would be unbalanced because it would not contain the normal complement of genetic material. Subsequent fertilization by a normal gamete would lead to the formation of an abnormal (unbalanced) zygote, resulting in spontaneous abortion or birth of a malformed child. The other important pattern of translocation is called a *robertsonian translocation* (or centric fusion), a translocation between two acrocentric chromosomes. Typically the breaks occur close to the centromeres of each chromosome. Transfer of the segments then leads to one very large chromosome and one extremely small one. Usually the small product is lost (see Fig. 5–19); however, because it carries only highly redundant genes (e.g., ribosomal RNA genes), this loss is compatible with a normal phenotype. Robertsonian translocation between two chromosomes is encountered in 1 in 1000 apparently normal individuals. The significance of this form of translocation also lies in the production of abnormal progeny, as discussed later with Down syndrome.

Many more numerical and structural chromosomal aberrations are described in specialized texts, and more and more abnormal karyotypes are being identified in disease. As pointed out earlier, the clinically detected chromosome disorders represent only the "tip of the iceberg." It is estimated that approximately 7.5% of all conceptions have a chromosomal abnormality, most of which are not compatible with survival or live birth. Even in live-born infants the frequency is approximately 0.5% to 1.0%. It is beyond the scope of this book to discuss most of the clinically recognizable chromosomal disorders. Hence, we focus attention on those few that are most common.

CYTOGENETIC DISORDERS INVOLVING AUTOSOMES

Trisomy 21 (Down Syndrome)

Down syndrome is the most common of the chromosomal disorders and is a *major cause of mental retardation*. In the United States the incidence in newborns is about 1 in 700.

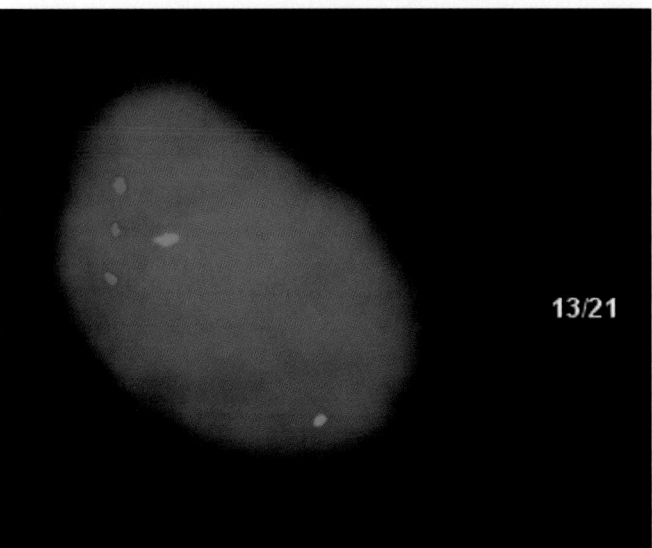

FIGURE 5–20 FISH analysis of an interphase nucleus, using locus-specific probes to chromosome 13 (green) and chromosome 21 (red), revealing three red signals consistent with trisomy 21. (Courtesy of Dr. Stuart Schwartz, Department of Pathology, University of Chicago, Chicago, IL.)

Approximately 95% of affected individuals have trisomy 21, so their chromosome count is 47. FISH with chromosome 21–specific probes reveals the extra copy of chromosome 21 in such cases (Fig. 5–20). Most others have normal chromosome numbers, but the extra chromosomal material is present as a translocation. As mentioned earlier, the most common cause of trisomy and therefore of Down syndrome is meiotic nondisjunction. The parents of such children have a normal karyotype and are normal in all respects.

Maternal age has a strong influence on the incidence of trisomy 21. It occurs once in 1550 live births in women under age 20, in contrast to 1 in 25 live births for mothers over age 45. The correlation with maternal age suggests that in most cases the meiotic nondisjunction of chromosome 21 occurs in the ovum. Studies in which DNA polymorphisms were used to trace the parental origin of chromosome 21 have revealed that in 95% of the cases with trisomy 21 the extra chromosome is of maternal origin. Although many hypotheses have been advanced, the reason for the increased susceptibility of the ovum to nondisjunction remains unknown.

In about 4% of cases of Down syndrome, the extra chromosomal material derives from the presence of a robertsonian translocation of the long arm of chromosome 21 to another acrocentric chromosome (e.g., 22 or 14). Because the fertilized ovum already possesses two normal autosomes 21, the translocated material provides the same triple gene dosage as in trisomy 21. Such cases are frequently (but not always) familial, and the translocated chromosome is inherited from one of the parents (usually the mother), who is a carrier of a robertsonian translocation, for example, a mother with karyotype 45,XX,der(14;21)(q10;q10).

Approximately 1% of Down syndrome patients are mosaics, usually having a mixture of cells with 46 and 47 chromosomes. This mosaicism results from mitotic nondisjunction of chromosome 21 during an early stage of embryogenesis.

Symptoms in such cases are variable and milder, depending on the proportion of abnormal cells. Clearly, *in cases of translocation or mosaic Down syndrome, maternal age is of no importance.*

The diagnostic clinical features of this condition—flat facial profile, oblique palpebral fissures, and epicanthic folds (Fig. 5–21)—are usually readily evident, even at birth.[37] Down syndrome is a leading cause of severe mental retardation; approximately 80% of those afflicted have an IQ of 25 to 50. Ironically, these severely disadvantaged children may have a gentle, shy manner and may be more easily directed than their more fortunate normal siblings. It should be pointed out that some mosaics with Down syndrome have mild phenotypic changes and often even have normal or near-normal intelligence. In addition to the phenotypic abnormalities and the mental retardation already noted, some other clinical features are worthy of note.

- Approximately 40% of the patients have congenital heart disease, most commonly defects of the endocardial cushion, including ostium primum, atrial septal defects, atrioventricular valve malformations, and ventricular septal defects. Cardiac problems are responsible for the majority of the deaths in infancy and early childhood. Several other congenital malformations, including atresias of the esophagus and small bowel, are also common.
- Children with trisomy 21 have a 10-fold to 20-fold increased risk of developing acute leukemia. Both acute lymphoblastic leukemias and acute myeloid leukemias occur. The latter, most commonly, is acute megakaryoblastic leukemia.[38]
- Virtually all patients with trisomy 21 older than age 40 develop neuropathologic changes characteristic of Alzheimer disease, a degenerative disorder of the brain.
- Patients with Down syndrome have abnormal immune responses that predispose them to serious infections, particularly of the lungs, and to thyroid autoimmunity. Although several abnormalities, affecting mainly T-cell functions, have been reported, the basis of immunological disturbances is not clear.

Despite all these problems, improved medical care has increased the longevity of individuals with trisomy 21. Currently the median age at death is 47 years (up from 25 years in 1983).

Although the karyotype and clinical features of trisomy 21 have been known for decades, little is known about the molecular basis of Down syndrome. Chromosome 21 contains approximately 430 genes. Interestingly, there are several gene clusters, each of which is predicted to participate in the same biologic pathway. For example, there are 16 genes that are involved in the mitochondrial energy pathway, several that are likely to influence central nervous system development, and a group that is involved in folate metabolism. It is not known how each of these groups of genes is related to Down syndrome. The gene dosage hypothesis assumes that the phenotypic features of the trisomy 21 are related to overexpression of genes. In reality only about 37% of the genes on chromosomes 21 are overexpressed by 150%, whereas others have variable degrees of changes in expression. Further complexity in defining the specific genes involved in the pathogenesis of Down syndrome is related to the presence of several miRNA genes on chromosome 21 that can shut down translation of genes that map elsewhere in the genome.[39] Thus, despite the availability of the gene map of chromosome 21, the progress in understanding the molecular basis of Down syndrome remains slow.[40]

Other Trisomies

A variety of other trisomies, involving chromosomes 8, 9, 13, 18, and 22, have been described. Only trisomy 18 (Edwards syndrome) and trisomy 13 (Patau syndrome) are common enough to merit brief mention here. As noted in Figure 5–21, they share several karyotypic and clinical features with trisomy 21. Thus, most cases result from meiotic nondisjunction and therefore carry a complete extra copy of chromosome 18 or 13. As in Down syndrome, an association with increased maternal age is also noted. In contrast to trisomy 21, however, the malformations are much more severe and wide-ranging. As a result, only rarely do these infants survive beyond the first year of life. Most succumb within a few weeks to months.

Chromosome 22q11.2 Deletion Syndrome

Chromosome 22q11.2 deletion syndrome encompasses a spectrum of disorders that result from a small deletion of band q11.2 on the long arm of chromosome 22.[41] The syndrome is fairly common, occurring in as many as 1 in 4000 births, but it is often missed because of variable clinical features. These include congenital heart defects, abnormalities of the palate, facial dysmorphism, developmental delay, and variable degrees of T-cell immunodeficiency and hypocalcemia. Previously, these clinical features were considered to represent two different disorders—*DiGeorge syndrome* and *velocardiofacial syndrome.* Patients with DiGeorge syndrome have thymic hypoplasia, with resultant T-cell immunodeficiency (Chapter 6), parathyroid hypoplasia giving rise to hypocalcemia, a variety of cardiac malformations affecting the outflow tract, and mild facial anomalies. The clinical features of the so-called velocardiofacial syndrome include facial dysmorphism (prominent nose, retrognathia), cleft palate, cardiovascular anomalies, and learning disabilities. Less frequently, these patients also have immunodeficiency. Until recently the overlapping clinical features of these two conditions (e.g., cardiac malformations, facial dysmorphology) were not appreciated; it was only after these two apparently unrelated syndromes were found to be associated with a similar cytogenetic abnormality that the clinical overlap came into focus. Recent studies indicate that in addition to the numerous structural malformations, individuals with the 22q11.2 deletion syndrome are at a particularly high risk for psychotic illnesses, such as schizophrenia and bipolar disorders.[42] In fact, it is estimated that approximately 25% of adults with this syndrome develop schizophrenia. Conversely, deletions of the region can be found in 2% to 3% of individuals with childhood-onset schizophrenia. In addition, attention deficit hyperactivity disorder is seen in 30% to 35% of affected children.

The diagnosis of this condition may be suspected on clinical grounds but can be established only by detection of the deletion by FISH (Fig. 5–22). By this test, approximately 90% of those previously diagnosed as having DiGeorge syndrome and

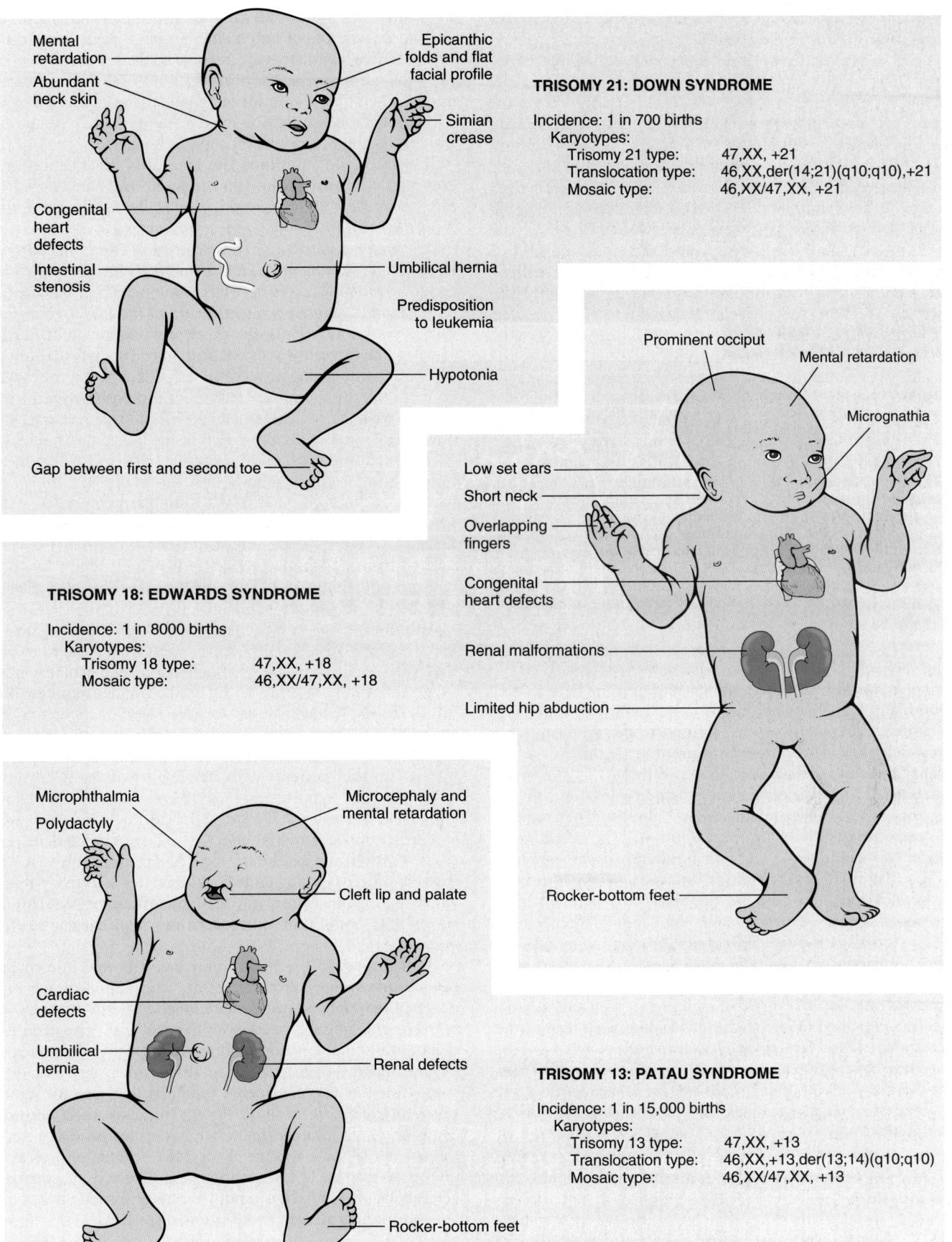

TRISOMY 21: DOWN SYNDROME

Incidence: 1 in 700 births
Karyotypes:
Trisomy 21 type: 47,XX, +21
Translocation type: 46,XX,der(14;21)(q10;q10),+21
Mosaic type: 46,XX/47,XX, +21

TRISOMY 18: EDWARDS SYNDROME

Incidence: 1 in 8000 births
Karyotypes:
Trisomy 18 type: 47,XX, +18
Mosaic type: 46,XX/47,XX, +18

TRISOMY 13: PATAU SYNDROME

Incidence: 1 in 15,000 births
Karyotypes:
Trisomy 13 type: 47,XX, +13
Translocation type: 46,XX,+13,der(13;14)(q10;q10)
Mosaic type: 46,XX/47,XX, +13

Labels for Down syndrome figure:
Mental retardation
Abundant neck skin
Epicanthic folds and flat facial profile
Simian crease
Congenital heart defects
Intestinal stenosis
Umbilical hernia
Predisposition to leukemia
Hypotonia
Gap between first and second toe

Labels for Patau syndrome figure:
Microphthalmia
Polydactyly
Microcephaly and mental retardation
Cleft lip and palate
Cardiac defects
Umbilical hernia
Renal defects
Rocker-bottom feet

Labels for Edwards syndrome figure:
Prominent occiput
Mental retardation
Micrognathia
Low set ears
Short neck
Overlapping fingers
Congenital heart defects
Renal malformations
Limited hip abduction
Rocker-bottom feet

FIGURE 5–21 Clinical features and karyotypes of selected autosomal trisomies.

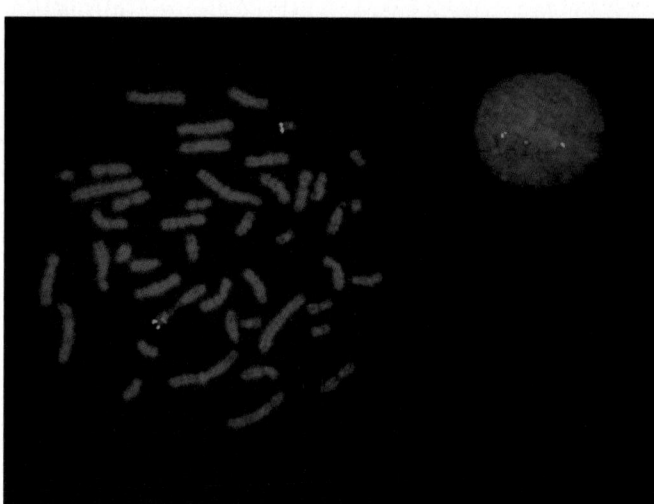

FIGURE 5–22 FISH on both metaphase chromosomes and an interphase cell from a patient with Di George syndrome demonstrating the deletion of the *TUPLE1* probe (official name *HIRA*) localized to chromosome 22q11.2. The *TUPLE1* probe is in red, and the control probe, localized to 22q, is in green. The metaphase spread shows one chromosome 22 with both a green signal (control probe) and a red signal (from the *TUPLE1* probe). The other chromosome 22 shows only hybridization with the control probe (green), but no red signal since there is a deletion on this chromosome. The interphase cell shows two areas of hybridization with the control probe (in green) but also only one area of hybridization with the *TUPLE1* probe (in red), illustrating a deletion of chromosome 22q11.2. (Courtesy of Dr. Stuart Schwartz, Department of Pathology, University of Chicago, Chicago, IL.)

80% of those with the velocardiofacial syndrome have a deletion of 22q11.2. Thirty percent of individuals with conotruncal cardiac defects but no other features of this syndrome also reveal deletions of the same chromosomal region.

The molecular basis of this syndrome is not fully understood. The deleted region is large (approximately 1.5 megabases) and includes many genes. The clinical heterogeneity, with predominant immunodeficiency in some cases (DiGeorge syndrome) and predominant dysmorphology and cardiac malformations in other cases, probably reflects the variable position and size of the deleted segment from this genetic region. Approximately 30 candidate genes have been mapped to the deleted region. Among these, *TBX1*, a T-box transcription factor is most closely associated with the phenotypic features of this syndrome.[41] This gene is expressed in the pharyngeal mesenchyme and endodermal pouch from which facial structures, thymus, and parathyroid are derived. The targets of *TBX1* include *PAX9*, a gene that controls the development of the palate, parathyroids, and thymus. Clearly there are other genes that contribute to the behavioral and psychiatric disorders that remain to be identified.

CYTOGENETIC DISORDERS INVOLVING SEX CHROMOSOMES

Genetic diseases associated with changes involving the sex chromosomes are far more common than those related to autosomal aberrations. Furthermore, imbalances (excess or loss) of sex chromosomes are much better tolerated than are similar imbalances of autosomes. In large part, this latitude relates to two factors that are peculiar to the sex chromosomes: (1) lyonization or inactivation of all but one X chromosome and (2) the modest amount of genetic material carried by the Y chromosome.[43] We discuss these features briefly to aid our understanding of sex chromosomal disorders.

In 1961, Lyon[44] outlined the idea of X-inactivation, now commonly known as the Lyon hypothesis. It states that (1) *only one of the X chromosomes is genetically active*, (2) *the other X of either maternal or paternal origin undergoes heteropyknosis and is rendered inactive*, (3) *inactivation of either the maternal or paternal X occurs at random among all the cells of the blastocyst on or about day 16 of embryonic life*, and (4) *inactivation of the same X chromosome persists in all the cells derived from each precursor cell*. Thus, the great preponderance of normal females are in reality mosaics and have two populations of cells, one with an inactivated maternal X and the other with an inactivated paternal X. Herein lies the explanation of why females have the same dosage of X-linked active genes as have males. The inactive X can be seen in the interphase nucleus as a darkly staining small mass in contact with the nuclear membrane known as the Barr body, or X chromatin. The molecular basis of X inactivation involves a unique gene called *XIST*, whose product is a noncoding RNA that is retained in the nucleus, where it "coats" the X chromosome that it is transcribed from and initiates a gene-silencing process by chromatin modification and DNA methylation. The *XIST* allele is switched off in the active X.[45]

Although it was initially thought that all the genes on the inactive X are "switched off," more recent studies have revealed that many genes escape X inactivation. Molecular studies suggest that 21% of genes on Xp, and a smaller number (3%) on Xq escape X inactivation. At least some of the genes that are expressed from both X chromosomes are important for normal growth and development.[46] This notion is supported by the fact that patients with monosomy of the X chromosome (Turner syndrome: 45,X) have severe somatic and gonadal abnormalities. If a single dose of X-linked genes were sufficient, no detrimental effect would be expected in such cases. Furthermore, although one X chromosome is inactivated in all cells during embryogenesis, it is selectively reactivated in oogonia before the first meiotic division. Thus, it seems that both X chromosomes are required for normal oogenesis.

With respect to the Y chromosome, it is well known that this chromosome is both necessary and sufficient for male development. *Regardless of the number of X chromosomes, the presence of a single Y determines the male sex.* The gene that dictates testicular development (*SRY*: sex-determining region Y gene) has been located on its distal short arm. For quite some time this was considered to be the only gene of significance on the Y chromosome. Recent studies of the Y chromosome, however, have yielded a rich harvest of gene families in the so-called "male-specific Y," or MSY region.[47] All of these are believed to be testes-specific genes involved in spermatogenesis. With this background, we review some features that are common to all sex chromosome disorders.

○ In general, they cause subtle, chronic problems relating to sexual development and fertility.

- They are often difficult to diagnose at birth, and many are first recognized at the time of puberty.
- In general, the higher the number of X chromosomes, in both male and female, the greater the likelihood of mental retardation.

The most important disorders arising in aberrations of sex chromosomes are described briefly here.

Klinefelter Syndrome

Klinefelter syndrome is best defined as male hypogonadism that occurs when there are two or more X chromosomes and one or more Y chromosomes.[48] It is one of the most frequent forms of genetic disease involving the sex chromosomes as well as one of the most common causes of hypogonadism in the male. The incidence of this condition is approximately 1 in 660 live male births.[49] It can rarely be diagnosed before puberty, particularly because the testicular abnormality does not develop before early puberty. Most patients have a distinctive body habitus with an increase in length between the soles and the pubic bone, which creates the appearance of an elongated body. Also characteristic are eunuchoid body habitus with abnormally long legs; small atrophic testes often associated with a small penis; and lack of such secondary male characteristics as deep voice, beard, and male distribution of pubic hair. Gynecomastia may be present. The mean IQ is somewhat lower than normal, but mental retardation is uncommon. There is increased incidence of type 2 diabetes and the metabolic syndrome; and curiously, mitral valve prolapse is seen in about 50% of adults with Klinefelter syndrome. It should be evident that the clinical features of this condition are variable, the only consistent finding being hypogonadism. Plasma gonadotropin concentrations, particularly follicle-stimulating hormone, are consistently elevated, whereas testosterone levels are variably reduced. Mean plasma estradiol levels are elevated by an as yet unknown mechanism. The ratio of estrogens and testosterone determines the degree of feminization in individual cases.

Klinefelter syndrome is an important genetic cause of reduced spermatogenesis and male infertility.[50] In some patients the testicular tubules are totally atrophied and replaced by pink, hyaline, collagenous ghosts. In others, apparently normal tubules are interspersed with atrophic tubules. In some patients all tubules are primitive and appear embryonic, consisting of cords of cells that never developed a lumen or progressed to mature spermatogenesis. Leydig cells appear prominent, as a result of the atrophy and crowding of tubules and elevation of gonadotropin concentrations.

Patients with Klinefelter syndrome have a higher risk for breast cancer (20 times more common than in normal males), extragonadal germ cell tumors, and autoimmune diseases such as systemic lupus erythematosus.

The classic pattern of Klinefelter syndrome is associated with a 47,XXY karyotype (90% of cases). This complement of chromosomes results from nondisjunction during the meiotic divisions in one of the parents. Maternal and paternal nondisjunction at the first meiotic division are roughly equally involved. There is no phenotypic difference between those who receive the extra X chromosome from their father and those who receive it from their mother. Maternal age is increased in the cases associated with errors in oogenesis. In addition to this classic karyotype, approximately 15% of patients with Klinefelter syndrome have been found to have a variety of mosaic patterns, most of them being 46,XY/47,XXY. Other patterns are 47,XXY/48,XXXY and variations on this theme. As is the case with normal females, all but one X undergoes inactivation in patients with Klinefelter syndrome. Why then, do the patients with this disorder have hypogonadism and associated features? The explanation of this lies in the pattern of X inactivation. The gene encoding the androgen receptor, through which testosterone mediates its effects, maps on the X chromosome. The androgen receptor gene contains highly polymorphic CAG (trinucleotide) repeats. The functional response to androgens is dictated, in part, by the number of CAG repeats. With shorter CAG repeats, the effect of androgens is more pronounced. In persons with Klinefelter syndrome the X chromosome, bearing androgen receptor with the shortest CAG repeat, is preferentially inactivated. Such nonrandom X inactivation leaves the allele with the longest CAG repeat active, thus accounting for hypogonadism.

Turner Syndrome

Turner syndrome results from complete or partial monosomy of the X chromosome and is characterized primarily by hypogonadism in phenotypic females.[51] It is the most common sex chromosome abnormality in females, affecting about 1 in 2000 live-born females.

With routine cytogenetic methods, three types of karyotypic abnormalities are seen in individuals with Turner syndrome. Approximately 57% are missing an entire X chromosome, resulting in a 45,X karyotype. Of the remaining 43%, approximately one third (approximately 14%) have structural abnormalities of the X chromosomes, and two thirds (approximately 29%) are mosaics. The common feature of the structural abnormalities is to produce partial monosomy of the X chromosome. In order of frequency, the structural abnormalities of the X chromosome include (1) an isochromosome of the long arm, 46,X,i(X)(q10) resulting in the loss of the short arm; (2) deletion of portions of both long and short arms, resulting in the formation of a ring chromosome, 46,X,r(X); and (3) deletion of portions of the short or long arm, 46X,del(Xq) or 46X,del(Xp). The mosaic patients have a 45,X cell population along with one or more karyotypically normal or abnormal cell types. Examples of karyotypes that mosaic Turner females may have are the following: (1) 45,X/46,XX; (2) 45,X/46,XY; (3) 45,X/47,XXX; or (4) 45,X/46,X,i(X)(q10). Studies suggest that the prevalence of mosaicism in Turner syndrome may be much higher than the 30% detected by conventional cytogenetic studies. With the use of more sensitive techniques, including FISH (discussed later) and polymerase chain reaction (PCR), and analysis of more than one cell type (e.g., peripheral blood and fibroblasts), the prevalence of mosaic Turner syndrome increases to 75%. Because 99% of 45,X conceptuses are nonviable, many authorities believe that there are no truly nonmosaic Turner syndrome patients. While this issue remains controversial, it is important to appreciate the karyotypic heterogeneity associated with Turner syndrome, because it is responsible for significant variations in phenotype. In patients who are truly 45,X, or in whom the proportion of 45,X cells is high, the phenotypic changes are more severe than in those who have readily

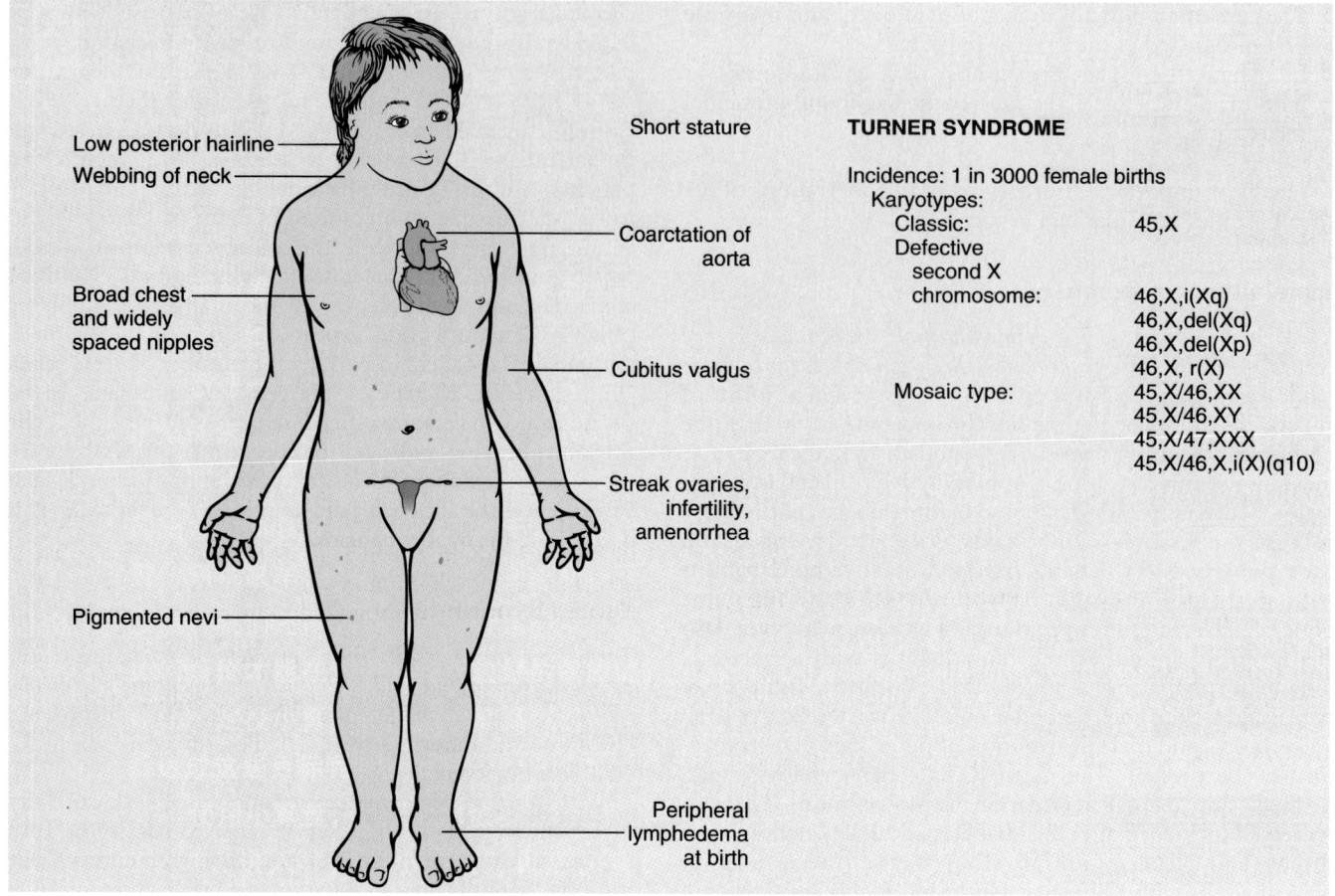

TURNER SYNDROME	
Incidence: 1 in 3000 female births	
Karyotypes:	
Classic:	45,X
Defective second X chromosome:	46,X,i(Xq)
	46,X,del(Xq)
	46,X,del(Xp)
	46,X, r(X)
Mosaic type:	45,X/46,XX
	45,X/46,XY
	45,X/47,XXX
	45,X/46,X,i(X)(q10)

Labels on figure: Low posterior hairline; Webbing of neck; Broad chest and widely spaced nipples; Pigmented nevi; Short stature; Coarctation of aorta; Cubitus valgus; Streak ovaries, infertility, amenorrhea; Peripheral lymphedema at birth

FIGURE 5–23   Clinical features and karyotypes of Turner syndrome.

detectable mosaicism. The latter may have an almost normal appearance and may present only with primary amenorrhea. Similarly, those with a Y chromosome–containing population (e.g., 45,X/46,XY karyotype) may be at risk of developing a gonadal tumor (gonadoblastoma).

The most severely affected patients generally present during infancy with edema of the dorsum of the hand and foot due to lymph stasis, and sometimes *swelling of the nape of the neck.* The latter is related to markedly distended lymphatic channels, producing a so-called cystic hygroma (Chapter 10). As these infants develop, the swellings subside but often leave bilateral *neck webbing* and persistent looseness of skin on the back of the neck. *Congenital heart disease* is also common, affecting 25% to 50% of patients. Left-sided cardiovascular abnormalities, particularly preductal coarctation of the aorta and bicuspid aortic valve, are seen most frequently. Cardiovascular abnormalities are the most important cause of increased mortality in children with Turner syndrome.[52]

The principal clinical features in the adolescent and adult are illustrated in Figure 5–23. At puberty there is *failure to develop normal secondary sex characteristics.* The genitalia remain infantile, breast development is inadequate, and there is little pubic hair. The mental status of these patients is usually normal, but subtle defects in nonverbal, visual-spatial information processing have been noted. Of particular importance in establishing the diagnosis in the adult is the shortness of stature (rarely exceeding 150 cm in height) and amenorrhea.

Turner syndrome is the single most important cause of primary amenorrhea, accounting for approximately one third of the cases. For reasons not quite clear, approximately 50% of patients develop autoantibodies that react with the thyroid gland, and up to half of these develop clinically manifest hypothyroidism. Equally mysterious is the presence of glucose intolerance, obesity, and insulin resistance in a minority of patients. The last mentioned is significant, because therapy with growth hormone, commonly used in these patients, worsens insulin resistance.

The molecular pathogenesis of Turner syndrome is not completely understood, but studies have begun to shed some light.[53] As mentioned earlier, both X chromosomes are active during oogenesis and are essential for normal development of the ovaries. During normal fetal development, ovaries contain as many as 7 million oocytes. The oocytes gradually disappear so that by menarche their numbers have dwindled to a mere 400,000, and when menopause occurs fewer than 10,000 remain. In Turner syndrome, fetal ovaries develop normally early in embryogenesis, but the absence of the second X chromosome leads to an accelerated loss of oocytes, which is complete by age 2 years. In a sense, therefore, "menopause occurs before menarche," and the ovaries are reduced to atrophic fibrous strands, devoid of ova and follicles *(streak ovaries).* Because patients with Turner syndrome also have other (nongonadal) abnormalities, it follows that some genes for normal growth and development of somatic tissues must also reside on the X chromosome. Among the genes involved in the Turner phenotype is the short stature homeobox (*SHOX*) gene at Xp22.33. This is one of several genes that remain active in both X chromosomes and has an active homologue on the short arm of the Y chromosome. Thus, both normal males and females have two copies of this gene. Haploinsufficiency of *SHOX* gives rise to short stature. Indeed, deletions of the *SHOX* gene are noted in 2% to 5% of otherwise normal children with short stature. In keeping with its role as a critical regulator of growth, the *SHOX* gene is expressed during fetal life in the growth plates of several long bones including the radius, ulna, tibia, and fibula. It is also expressed in the first and second pharyngeal arches. Just as the loss of *SHOX* is always associated with short stature, excess copies of this gene are associated with tall stature. Whereas haploinsufficiency of *SHOX* can explain growth deficit in Turner syndrome, it cannot explain other important clinical features such as cardiac malformations and endocrine abnormalities. Clearly several other genes located on the X chromosome are also involved.

Hermaphroditism and Pseudohermaphroditism

The problem of sexual ambiguity is exceedingly complex, and only limited observations are possible here; for more details, reference should be made to specialized sources.[54] It will be no surprise to medical students that the sex of an individual can be defined on several levels. *Genetic sex* is determined by the presence or absence of a Y chromosome. No matter how many X chromosomes are present, a single Y chromosome dictates testicular development and the genetic male gender. The initially indifferent gonads of both the male and the female embryos have an inherent tendency to feminize, unless influenced by Y chromosome–dependent masculinizing factors. *Gonadal sex* is based on the histologic characteristics of the gonads. *Ductal sex* depends on the presence of derivatives of the müllerian or wolffian ducts. *Phenotypic*, or *genital, sex* is based on the appearance of the external genitalia. Sexual ambiguity is present whenever there is disagreement among these various criteria for determining sex.

The term true hermaphrodite implies the presence of both ovarian and testicular tissue. In contrast, a pseudohermaphrodite represents a disagreement between the phenotypic and gonadal sex (i.e., a female pseudohermaphrodite has ovaries but male external genitalia; a male pseudohermaphrodite has testicular tissue but female-type genitalia).

True hermaphroditism, implying the presence of both ovarian and testicular tissue, is an extremely rare condition. In some cases there is a testis on one side and an ovary on the other, whereas in other cases there may be combined ovarian and testicular tissue, referred to as ovotestes. The karyotype is 46,XX in 50% of patients; of the remaining, most are mosaics with a 46,XX/46,XY karyotype. Only rarely is the chromosomal constitution 46,XY. The presence of testes implies that those with the 46,XX karyotype might possess Y-chromosomal material, in particular, the *SRY* gene, which dictates testicular differentiation. Indeed, molecular analysis has revealed *SRY* gene expression in the ovotestis of 46,XX true hermaphrodites, indicating either cryptic chimerism localized to the gonads or possibly a Y-to-autosome translocation.[55]

Female pseudohermaphroditism is much less complex. The genetic sex in all cases is XX, and the development of the gonads (ovaries) and internal genitalia is normal. Only the external genitalia are ambiguous or virilized. The basis of female pseudohermaphroditism is excessive and inappropriate exposure to androgenic steroids during the early part of gestation. Such steroids are most commonly derived from the fetal adrenal affected by congenital adrenal hyperplasia, which is transmitted as an autosomal recessive trait. Biosynthetic defects in the pathway of cortisol synthesis are present in these patients, which lead secondarily to excessive synthesis of androgenic steroids by the fetal adrenal cortex (Chapter 24).

Male pseudohermaphroditism represents the most complex of all disorders of sexual differentiation. These individuals possess a Y chromosome, and thus their gonads are exclusively testes, but the genital ducts or the external genitalia are incompletely differentiated along the male phenotype. Their external genitalia are either ambiguous or completely female. Male pseudohermaphroditism is extremely heterogeneous, with a multiplicity of causes. Common to all is defective virilization of the male embryo, which usually results from genetically determined defects in androgen synthesis or action or both. The most common form, called *complete androgen insensitivity syndrome (testicular feminization)*, results from mutations in the gene encoding the androgen receptor.[56] This gene is located at Xq12, and hence this disorder is inherited as an X-linked recessive.

Single-Gene Disorders with Nonclassic Inheritance

It has become increasingly evident that transmission of certain single-gene disorders does not follow classic mendelian principles. This group of disorders can be classified into four categories:

- Diseases caused by trinucleotide-repeat mutations
- Disorders caused by mutations in mitochondrial genes
- Disorders associated with genomic imprinting
- Disorders associated with gonadal mosaicism

Clinical and molecular features of some single-gene diseases that exemplify nonclassic patterns of inheritance are described next.

DISEASES CAUSED BY TRINUCLEOTIDE-REPEAT MUTATIONS

The discovery in 1991 of expanding trinucleotide repeats as a cause of fragile-X syndrome was a landmark in human genetics. Since then the origins of about 40 human diseases (Table 5–8) have been traced to unstable nucleotide repeats,[57] and the number continues to grow. Some general principles that apply to these diseases are as follows:

- The causative mutations are associated with the expansion of a stretch of trinucleotides that usually share the nucleotides G and C. In all cases the DNA is unstable, and an expansion of the repeats above a certain threshold impairs gene function in various ways, discussed below.

Disease	Gene	Locus	Protein	Repeat	No. of Repeats	
					Normal	**Disease**
EXPANSIONS AFFECTING NONCODING REGIONS						
Fragile-X syndrome	*FMRI (FRAXA)*	Xq27.3	FMR-1 protein (FMRP)	CGG	6–53	60–200 (pre); >230 (full)
Friedreich ataxia	*FXN*	9q21.1	Frataxin	GAA	7–34	34–80 (pre); >100 (full)
Myotonic dystrophy	*DMPK*	19q13.3	Myotonic dystrophy protein kinase (DMPK)	CTG	5–37	34–80 (pre); >100 (full)
EXPANSIONS AFFECTING CODING REGIONS						
Spinobulbar muscular atrophy (Kennedy disease)	*AR*	Xq12	Androgen receptor (AR)	CAG	9–36	38–62
Huntington disease	*HTT*	4p16.3	Huntingtin	CAG	6–35	36–121
Dentatorubral-pallidoluysian atrophy (Haw River syndrome)	*ATNL*	12p13.31	Atrophin-1	CAG	6–35	49–88
Spinocerebellar ataxia type 1	*ATXN1*	6p23	Ataxin-1	CAG	6–44	39–82
Spinocerebellar ataxia type 2	*ATXN2*	12q24.1	Ataxin-2	CAG	15–31	36–63
Spinocerebellar ataxia type 3 (Machado-Joseph disease)	*ATXN3*	14q21	Ataxin-3	CAG	12–40	55–84
Spinocerebellar ataxia type 6	*CACNA2A*	19p13.3	α_{1A}-Voltage-dependent calcium channel subunit	CAG	4–18	21–33
Spinocerebellar ataxia type 7	*ATXN7*	3p14.1	Ataxin-7	CAG	4–35	37–306

TABLE 5–8 **Examples of Trinucleotide-Repeat Disorders**

- The proclivity to expand depends strongly on the sex of the transmitting parent. In the fragile-X syndrome, expansions occur during oogenesis, whereas in Huntington disease they occur during spermatogenesis.
- From a mechanistic standpoint, the mutations can be divided into two groups. In the first group of disorders, exemplified by fragile-X syndrome and myotonic dystrophy, the repeat expansions occur in noncoding regions, whereas in other disorders, such as Huntington disease, expansions occur in the coding regions (Fig. 5–24).

The pathogenetic mechanisms underlying disorders caused by mutations that affect coding regions seem to be distinct from those in which the expansions affect noncoding regions.[58] The former usually involve CAG repeats coding for polyglutamine tracts in the corresponding proteins. Such "polyglutamine diseases" are characterized by progressive neurodegeneration, typically striking in midlife. Polyglutamine expansions lead to toxic gain of function, whereby the abnormal protein interferes with the function of the normal protein.[59] The precise mechanisms by which expanded polyglutamine proteins cause disease is not fully understood. However, some general features have emerged. In most cases the proteins are misfolded and tend to aggregate; the aggregates may suppress transcription of other genes, cause mitochondrial dysfunction, or trigger the unfolded-protein stress response and apoptosis (Chapter 1). A morphologic hallmark of these diseases is the accumulation of aggregated mutant proteins in large intranuclear inclusions. By contrast, when expansions affect noncoding regions the resulting mutations are loss-of-function type, since protein synthesis (e.g., FMRP) is suppressed. Typically, such disorders affect many systems. Finally, many noncoding repeat disorders are characterized by intermediate-size expansions, or premutations, that expand to full mutations in germ cells.

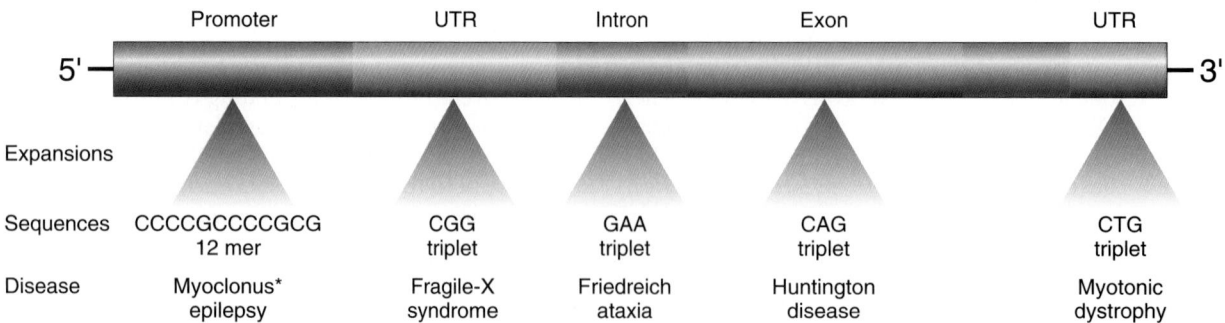

FIGURE 5–24 Sites of expansion and the affected sequence in selected diseases caused by nucleotide-repeat mutations. UTR, untranslated region.
*Though not strictly a trinucleotide-repeat disease, progressive myoclonus epilepsy is caused, like others in this group, by a heritable DNA expansion. The expanded segment is in the promoter region of the gene.

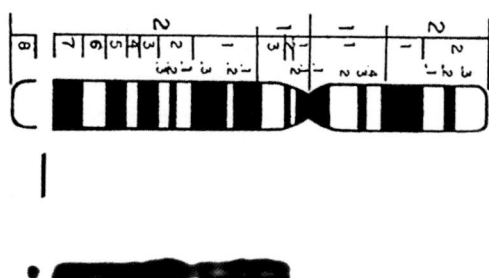

FIGURE 5–25 Fragile X, seen as discontinuity of staining. (Courtesy of Dr. Patricia Howard-Peebles, University of Texas Southwestern Medical Center, Dallas, TX.)

Fragile-X Syndrome

Fragile-X syndrome is the prototype of diseases in which the mutation is characterized by a long repeating sequence of three nucleotides. Although the specific nucleotide sequence that undergoes amplification differs in the 20 or so disorders included in this group, in most cases the affected sequences share the nucleotides guanine (G) and cytosine (C). In the ensuing discussion we consider the clinical features and inheritance pattern of the fragile-X syndrome, to be followed by the causative molecular lesion. The remaining disorders in this group are discussed later, in this chapter and elsewhere in the book.

With a frequency of 1 in 1550 for affected males and 1 in 8000 for affected females, *fragile-X syndrome is the second most common genetic cause of mental retardation, after Down syn-*

drome. It is an X-linked disorder characterized by an inducible cytogenetic abnormality in the X chromosome and an unusual mutation within the familial mental retardation-1 (*FMR1*) gene. The cytogenetic alteration is seen as a discontinuity of staining or as a constriction in the long arm of the X chromosome when cells are cultured in a folate-deficient medium. Because it appears that the chromosome is "broken" at this locale, it is referred to as a *fragile site* (Fig. 5–25). It should be noted that more than 100 "fragile sites" have been found in the human genome.[60] Many, like the one seen in fragile-X syndrome, are sensitive to lack of folate in the medium, whereas others require different culture conditions. The significance of most fragile sites is unknown, since many are present in normal individuals.

In fragile-X syndrome, the affected males are *mentally retarded*, with an IQ in the range of 20 to 60. They express a characteristic physical phenotype that includes a *long face with a large mandible, large everted ears*, and *large testicles (macro-orchidism)*. Hyperextensible joints, a high arched palate, and mitral valve prolapse noted in some patients mimic a connective tissue disorder. These and other physical abnormalities described in this condition, however, are not always present and, in some cases, are quite subtle. *The most distinctive feature is macro-orchidism, which is observed in at least 90% of postpubertal males.*

As with all X-linked diseases, fragile-X syndrome affects males. Analysis of several pedigrees, however, reveals some patterns of transmission not typically associated with other X-linked recessive disorders (Fig. 5–26). These include the following[61]:

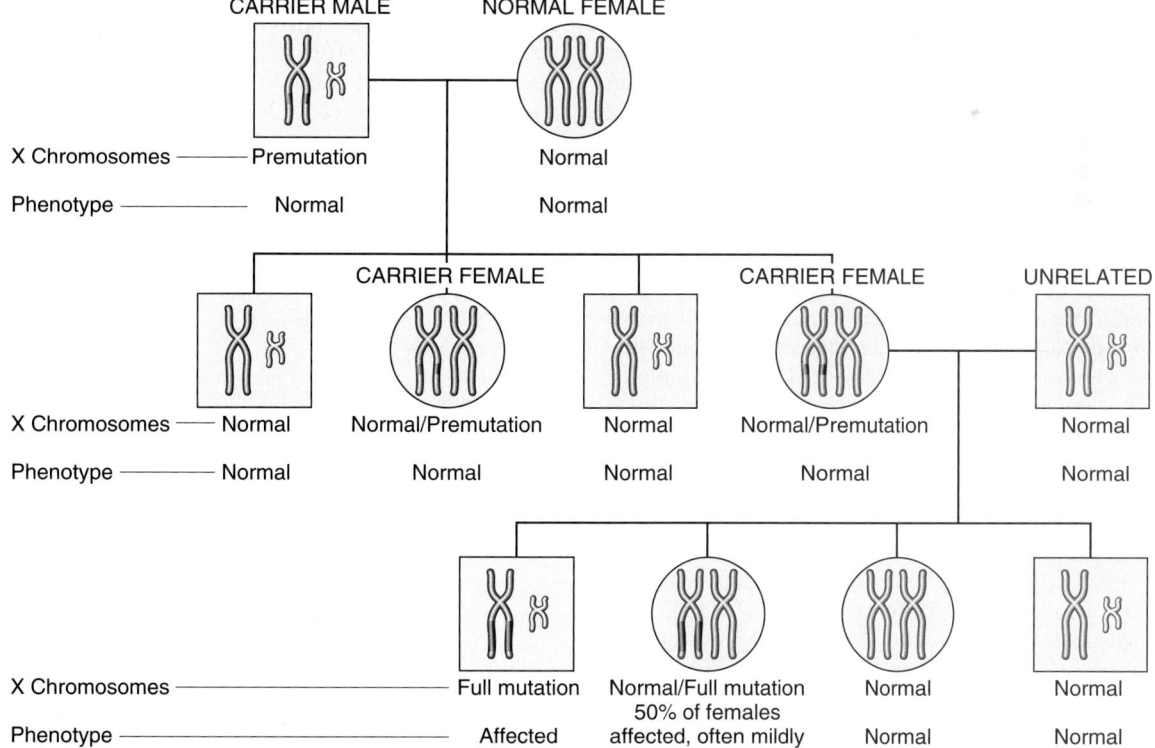

FIGURE 5–26 Fragile-X pedigree. Note that in the first generation all sons are normal and all females are carriers. During oogenesis in the carrier female, premutation expands to full mutation; hence, in the next generation all males who inherit the X with full mutation are affected. However, only 50% of females who inherit the full mutation are affected, and only mildly. (Courtesy of Dr. Nancy Schneider, Department of Pathology, University of Texas Southwestern Medical Center, Dallas, TX.)

- *Carrier males:* Approximately 20% of males who, by pedigree analysis and by molecular tests, are known to carry a fragile-X mutation are clinically and cytogenetically normal. Because carrier males transmit the trait through all their daughters (phenotypically normal) to affected grandchildren, they are called *normal transmitting males.*

- *Affected females:* 30% to 50% of carrier females are affected (i.e., mentally retarded), a number much higher than that in other X-linked recessive disorders.

- *Risk of phenotypic effects:* Risk depends on the position of the individual in the pedigree. For example, brothers of transmitting males are at a 9% risk of having mental retardation, whereas grandsons of transmitting males incur a 40% risk.

- *Anticipation:* This refers to the observation that clinical features of fragile-X syndrome worsen with each successive generation, as if the mutation becomes increasingly deleterious as it is transmitted from a man to his grandsons and great-grandsons.

These unusual patterns perplexed geneticists for years, but molecular studies have begun to unravel the complexities of this condition.[62,63] The first breakthrough came when linkage studies localized the mutation responsible for this disease to Xq27.3, within the cytogenetically abnormal region. Within this region lies the *FMR1* gene, characterized by multiple tandem repeats of the nucleotide sequence CGG in its 5′ untranslated region. In the normal population, the number of CGG repeats is small, ranging from 6 to 55 (average, 29). The presence of clinical symptoms and a cytogenetically detectable fragile site is related to the amplification of the CGG repeats. Thus, normal transmitting males and carrier females carry 55 to 200 CGG repeats. Expansions of this size are called *premutations.* In contrast, affected individuals have an extremely large expansion of the repeat region (200–4000 repeats, or *full mutations*). Full mutations are believed to arise by further amplification of the CGG repeats seen in premutations. How this process takes place is quite peculiar. Carrier males transmit the repeats to their progeny with small changes in repeat number. When the premutation is passed on by a carrier female, however, there is a high probability of a dramatic amplification of the CGG repeats, leading to mental retardation in most male offspring and 50% of female offspring. Thus, *it seems that during the process of oogenesis, but not spermatogenesis, premutations can be converted to mutations by triplet-repeat amplification.* This explains the unusual inheritance pattern; that is, the likelihood of mental retardation is much higher in grandsons than in brothers of transmitting males because grandsons incur the risk of inheriting a premutation from their grandfather that is amplified to a "full mutation" in their mothers' ova. By comparison, brothers of transmitting males, being "higher up" in the pedigree, are less likely to have a full mutation. These molecular details also provide a satisfactory explanation of anticipation—a phenomenon observed by clinical geneticists but not believed by molecular geneticists until triplet-repeat mutations were identified. Why only 50% of the females with the full mutation are clinically affected is not clear. Presumably in those that are clinically affected there is unfavorable lyonization (i.e., there is a higher frequency of cells in which the X chromosome carrying the mutation is active). Recent studies indicate that premutations are not so benign after all. *Approximately 30% of females carrying the premutation have premature ovarian failure (before the age of 40 years), and about one third of premutation-carrying males exhibit a progressive neurodegenerative syndrome starting in their sixth decade.* This syndrome, referred to as fragile X–associated tremor/ataxia, is characterized by intention tremors and cerebellar ataxia and may progress to parkinsonism. However, it is clear that the abnormalities in premutation carriers are milder and occur later in life.

The molecular basis of mental retardation and other somatic changes is related to a loss of function of the familial mental retardation protein (FMRP). As mentioned earlier, the normal *FMR1* gene contains up to 46 CGG repeats in its 5′ untranslated region. When the trinucleotide repeats in the *FMR1* gene exceed approximately 230, the DNA of the entire 5′ region of the gene becomes abnormally methylated. Methylation also extends upstream into the promoter region of the gene, resulting in transcriptional suppression of *FMR1.* The resulting absence of FMRP is believed to cause the phenotypic changes.

FMRP is a widely expressed cytoplasmic protein, most abundant in the brain and testis, the two organs most affected in this disease. The function of FMRP in the brain is beginning to be unraveled.[64] FMRP is an RNA-binding protein associated with polysomes. Unlike other cells, in neurons protein synthesis occurs both in the perinuclear cytoplasm and in dendritic spines. According to current understanding, FMRP is first transported from the cytoplasm to the nucleus, where it assembles into a complex containing specific mRNA transcripts. The assembled complex is then exported to the cytoplasm. From here the FMRP-mRNA complex is transported to the dendrites close to the synapse (Fig. 5–27). Not all species of mRNA are transported by FMRP to the dendrites. Only those that encode proteins that regulate synaptic function are so shuttled by FMRP. At the synaptic junctions, FMRP

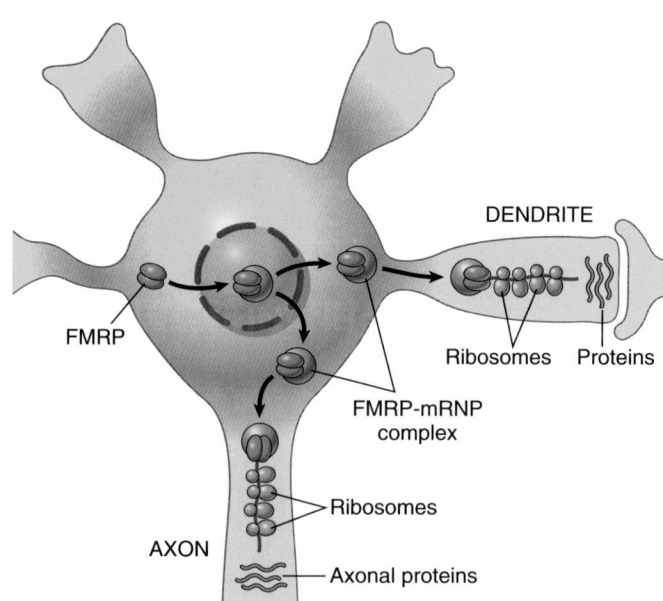

FIGURE 5–27 A model for the action of familial mental retardation protein (FMRP) in neurons. (Adapted from Hin P, Warren ST: New insights into fragile X syndrome: from molecules to neurobehavior. Trends Biochem Sci 28:152, 2003.)

suppresses protein synthesis from the bound mRNAs in response to signaling through group I metabotropic glutamate receptors (mGlu-R). In fragile-X syndrome a reduction in FMRP results in increased translation of the bound mRNAs at the synaptic junctions. Such imbalance in turn causes permanent changes in synaptic activity and ultimately mental retardation.

Although demonstration of an abnormal karyotype led to the identification of this disorder, PCR-based detection of the repeats is now the method of choice for diagnosis. With Southern blot analysis, distinction between premutations and mutations can be made prenatally as well as postnatally. Hence, this technique is valuable not only for establishing the diagnosis, but also for guiding genetic counseling. These techniques are described later.

MUTATIONS IN MITOCHONDRIAL GENES—LEBER HEREDITARY OPTIC NEUROPATHY

The vast majority of genes are located on chromosomes in the cell nucleus and are inherited in classical Mendelian fashion. There exist several mitochondrial genes, however, that are inherited in quite a different manner. *A feature unique to mtDNA is maternal inheritance.* This peculiarity exists because ova contain numerous mitochondria within their abundant cytoplasm, whereas spermatozoa contain few, if any. Hence, the mtDNA complement of the zygote is derived entirely from the ovum. Thus, mothers transmit mtDNA to all their offspring, male and female; however, daughters but not sons transmit the DNA further to their progeny (Fig. 5–28). Several other features apply to mitochondrial inheritance.[65,66] They are as follows:

- Human mtDNA contains 37 genes, of which 22 are transcribed into transfer RNAs and two into ribosomal RNAs. The remaining 13 genes encode subunits of the respiratory chain enzymes. Because mtDNA encodes enzymes involved in oxidative phosphorylation, mutations affecting these genes exert their deleterious effects primarily on the organs most dependent on oxidative phosphorylation such as the central nervous system, skeletal muscle, cardiac muscle, liver, and kidneys.
- Each mitochondrion contains thousands of copies of mtDNA, and, typically, deleterious mutations of mtDNA

affect some but not all of these copies. Thus, tissues and, indeed, whole individuals may harbor both wild-type and mutant mtDNA, a situation called *heteroplasmy*. It should be evident that a minimum number of mutant mtDNA must be present in a cell or tissue before oxidative dysfunction gives rise to disease. This is called the "threshold effect." Not surprisingly, the threshold is reached most easily in the metabolically active tissues listed earlier.[67]

- During cell division, mitochondria and their contained DNA are randomly distributed to the daughter cells. Thus, when a cell containing normal and mutant mtDNA divides, the proportion of the normal and mutant mtDNA in daughter cells is extremely variable. Therefore, the expression of disorders resulting from mutations in mtDNA is quite variable.

Diseases associated with mitochondrial inheritance are rare and, as mentioned earlier, many of them affect the neuromuscular system. *Leber hereditary optic neuropathy* is a prototype of this type of disorder. It is a neurodegenerative disease that manifests as a progressive bilateral loss of central vision. Visual impairment is first noted between ages 15 and 35, and it leads eventually to blindness. Cardiac conduction defects and minor neurologic manifestations have also been observed in some families.[68]

GENOMIC IMPRINTING

We all inherit two copies of each autosomal gene, carried on homologous maternal and paternal chromosomes. In the past, it had been assumed that there is no functional difference between the alleles derived from the mother or the father. Studies over the past two decades have provided definite evidence that, at least with respect to some genes, important functional differences exist between the paternal allele and the maternal allele. These differences result from an epigenetic process (discussed later), called *imprinting*. In most cases, *imprinting selectively inactivates either the maternal or paternal allele*. Thus, *maternal imprinting* refers to transcriptional silencing of the maternal allele, whereas *paternal imprinting* implies that the paternal allele is inactivated. Imprinting occurs in the ovum or the sperm, before fertilization, and then is stably transmitted to all somatic cells through mitosis.[69] As with other instances of epigenetic regulation, imprinting is

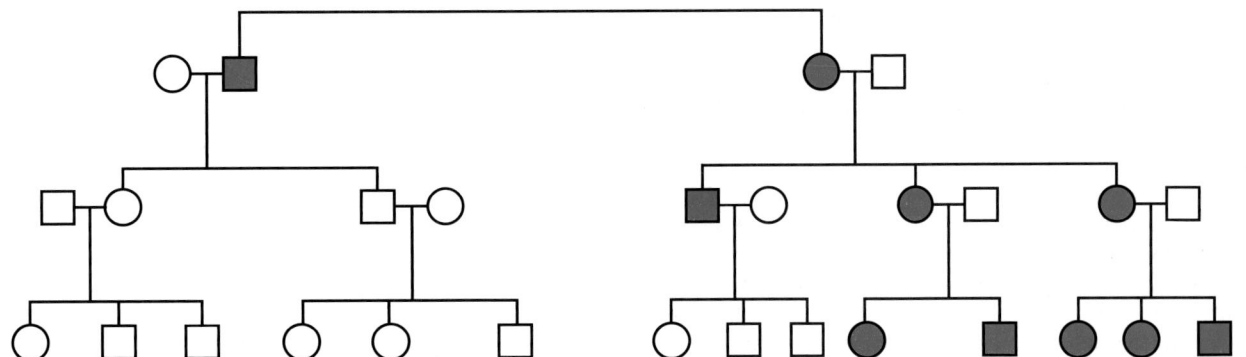

FIGURE 5–28 Pedigree of Leber hereditary optic neuropathy, a disorder caused by mutation in mitochondrial DNA. Note that all progeny of an affected male (shaded squares) are normal, but all children, male and female, of the affected female (shaded circles) manifest disease.

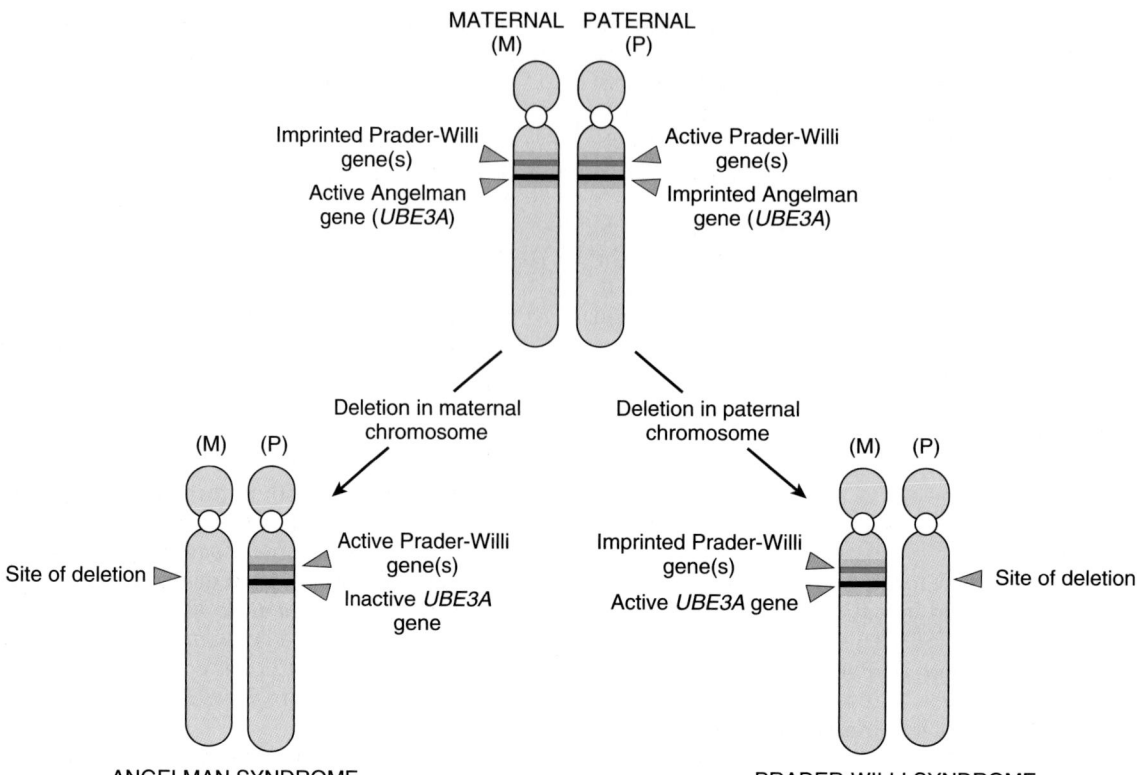

MATERNAL PATERNAL
(M)   (P)

Imprinted Prader-Willi
gene(s)

Active Angelman
gene (*UBE3A*)

Active Prader-Willi
gene(s)

Imprinted Angelman
gene (*UBE3A*)

Deletion in maternal
chromosome

Deletion in paternal
chromosome

(M)   (P)   (M)   (P)

Site of deletion

Active Prader-Willi
gene(s)

Inactive *UBE3A*
gene

Imprinted Prader-Willi
gene(s)

Active *UBE3A* gene

Site of deletion

ANGELMAN SYNDROME   PRADER-WILLI SYNDROME

FIGURE 5–29 Diagrammatic representation of Prader-Willi and Angelman syndromes.

associated with differential patterns of DNA methylation at CG nucleotides. Other mechanisms include histone H4 deacetylation and methylation. Regardless of the mechanism, it is believed that such marking of paternal and maternal chromosomes occurs during gametogenesis, and thus it seems that from the moment of conception some chromosomes remember where they came from. The exact number of imprinted genes is not known; estimates range from 200 to 600. Although imprinted genes may occur in isolation, more commonly they are found in groups that are regulated by common *cis*-acting elements called imprinting control regions. As is often the case in medicine, genomic imprinting is best illustrated by considering two uncommon genetic disorders: Prader-Willi syndrome and Angelman syndrome.

Prader-Willi Syndrome and Angelman Syndrome

Prader-Willi syndrome is characterized by mental retardation, short stature, hypotonia, profound hyperphagia, obesity, small hands and feet, and hypogonadism.[70] In 65% to 70% of cases, an interstitial deletion of band q12 in the long arm of chromosome 15, del(15)(q11.2q13), can be detected. In most cases the breakpoints are the same, causing a 5-Mb deletion. *It is striking that in all cases the deletion affects the paternally derived chromosome 15.* In contrast with the Prader-Willi syndrome, patients with the phenotypically distinct Angelman syndrome are *born with a deletion of the same chromosomal region derived from their mothers.* Patients with Angelman syndrome are also mentally retarded, but in addition they present with ataxic gait, seizures, and inappropriate laughter. Because of their laughter and ataxia they have been referred to as

"happy puppets."[71] A comparison of these two syndromes clearly demonstrates the *parent-of-origin* effects on gene function.

The molecular basis of these two syndromes lies in the genomic imprinting (Fig. 5–29). It is known that a gene or set of genes on maternal chromosome 15q12 is imprinted (and hence silenced), and thus the only functional allele(s) are provided by the paternal chromosome. When these are lost as a result of a deletion, the person develops Prader-Willi syndrome. Conversely, a distinct gene that also maps to the same region of chromosome 15 is imprinted on the paternal chromosome. Only the maternally derived allele of this gene is normally active. Deletion of this maternal gene on chromosome 15 gives rise to the Angelman syndrome. Molecular studies of cytogenetically normal patients with the Prader-Willi syndrome (i.e., those without the deletion) have revealed that they have two maternal copies of chromosome 15. Inheritance of both chromosomes of a pair from one parent is called *uniparental disomy.* The net effect is the same (i.e., the person does not have a functional set of genes from the [nonimprinted] paternal chromosomes 15). Angelman syndrome, as might be expected, can also result from uniparental disomy of paternal chromosome 15.

The genetic basis of these two imprinting disorders is now being unraveled. In the Angelman syndrome, the affected gene is a ubiquitin ligase that is involved in catalyzing the transfer of activated ubiquitin to target protein substrates. The gene, called *UBE3A,* maps within the 15q12 region, is imprinted on the paternal chromosome, and is expressed from the maternal allele primarily in specific regions of the brain.[72] The imprinting is tissue-specific in that *UBE3A* is expressed from both alleles in most tissues. In approximately 10% of cases, Angelman syndrome occurs not as a result of imprinting but of a point mutation in the maternal allele, thus establishing a firm link between the *UBE3A* gene and Angelman syndrome. In contrast to Angelman syndrome, no single gene has been implicated in Prader-Willi syndrome. Instead, a series of genes located in the 15q11.2–q13 interval (which are imprinted on the maternal chromosome and expressed from the paternal chromosome) are believed to be involved. These include a gene that encodes small nuclear riboprotein N, which controls gene splicing and is expressed highly in the brain and heart. Loss of small nuclear riboprotein N function is believed to contribute to Prader-Willi syndrome. Molecular diagnosis (see later) of these syndromes is based on assessment of methylation status of marker genes and FISH.

The importance of imprinting is not restricted to rare chromosomal disorders. Parent-of-origin effects have been identified in a variety of inherited diseases, such as Huntington disease and myotonic dystrophy and in tumorigenesis.

GONADAL MOSAICISM

It was mentioned earlier that with every autosomal dominant disorder some patients do not have affected parents. In such patients the disorder results from a new mutation in the egg or the sperm from which they were derived; as such, their siblings are neither affected nor at increased risk of developing the disease. This is not always the case, however. In some autosomal dominant disorders, exemplified by osteogenesis imperfecta, phenotypically normal parents have more than one affected child. This clearly violates the laws of mendelian inheritance. Studies indicate that gonadal mosaicism may be responsible for such unusual pedigrees.[73] Gonadal mosaicism results from a mutation that occurs postzygotically during early (embryonic) development. If the mutation affects only cells destined to form the gonads, the gametes carry the mutation, but the somatic cells of the individual are completely normal. Such an individual is said to exhibit *germ line* or *gonadal mosaicism*. A phenotypically normal parent who has germ line mosaicism can transmit the disease-causing mutation to the offspring through the mutant gamete. Because the progenitor cells of the gametes carry the mutation, there is a definite possibility that more than one child of such a parent would be affected. Obviously the likelihood of such an occurrence depends on the proportion of germ cells carrying the mutation.

Molecular Diagnosis of Genetic Diseases

Medical applications of recombinant DNA technology have come of age. With the completion of the Human Genome Project, DNA-based analysis has become a powerful tool for the diagnosis of human disease, both genetic and acquired. Molecular diagnostic techniques have found application in virtually all areas of medicine. In the era predating the ready availability of molecular diagnostic assays, assays for single-gene ("mendelian") disorders depended on the identification of abnormal gene products (e.g., mutant hemoglobin or abnormal metabolites) or their clinical effects, such as mental retardation (e.g., in phenylketonuria). Now, it is possible to identify mutations at the DNA level and offer diagnostic tests for an increasing number of genetic disorders. In addition, molecular tools have become extremely important in discovery of the genetic basis of common complex disorders such as diabetes mellitus, atherosclerosis, and cancer. The molecular diagnosis of inherited diseases at the nucleic acid level has distinct advantages over other surrogate techniques:

- Molecular assays are remarkably sensitive. For example, the use of PCR allows several million-fold amplification of DNA or RNA, making it possible to use as few as 1 or 100 cells for analysis. $0.1\mu l$ of blood or cells scraped from buccal mucosa can supply sufficient DNA for PCR amplification.
- DNA-based tests are not dependent on a gene product that may be produced only in certain specialized cells (e.g., brain) or expression of a gene that may occur late in life. Because the defective gene responsible for inherited genetic disorders is present in germ line samples, every postzygotic cell carries the mutation.

INDICATIONS FOR ANALYSIS OF GERM LINE GENETIC ALTERATIONS

While many techniques are available today for the diagnosis of genetic diseases, to judiciously use these methods it is important to ascertain which individuals require genetic testing. In general, testing for alterations inherited in the germ line can be divided into prenatal and postnatal analysis. It may involve conventional cytogenetics, fluorescent in situ hybridization (FISH), other molecular diagnostic assays, or a combination of these techniques.

Prenatal genetic analysis should be offered to all patients who are at risk of having cytogenetically abnormal progeny. It can be performed on cells obtained by amniocentesis, on chorionic villus biopsy material, or on umbilical cord blood. Some important indications are as follows[74]:

- A mother of advanced age (>35 years) because of greater risk of trisomies
- A parent who is a carrier of a balanced reciprocal translocation, robertsonian translocation, or inversion (in these cases the gametes may be unbalanced, and hence the progeny would be at risk for chromosomal disorders)
- A parent with a previous child with a chromosomal abnormality
- A fetus with ultrasound-detected abnormalities
- A parent who is a carrier of an X-linked genetic disorder (to determine fetal sex)
- Abnormal levels of AFP, βHCG, and estriol performed as the triple test.

Postnatal genetic analysis is usually performed on peripheral blood lymphocytes. Indications are as follows:

- Multiple congenital anomalies
- Unexplained mental retardation and/or developmental delay
- Suspected aneuploidy (e.g., features of Down syndrome)

- Suspected unbalanced autosome (e.g., Prader-Willi syndrome)
- Suspected sex chromosomal abnormality (e.g., Turner syndrome)
- Suspected fragile-X syndrome
- Infertility (to rule out sex chromosomal abnormality)
- Multiple spontaneous abortions (to rule out the parents as carriers of balanced translocation; both partners should be evaluated)

INDICATIONS FOR ANALYSIS OF ACQUIRED GENETIC ALTERATIONS

In this era of molecularly targeted therapies it is becoming increasingly important to identify specific molecular genetic signatures for acquired diseases (i.e., cancer and infectious disease), which were formerly diagnosed and managed with nonmolecular clinicopathologic data. The technical approaches are the same as those used for germ line mendelian disorders, and the common indications include:

Diagnosis and management of cancer (see also Chapter 7)
- Detection of tumor-specific acquired mutations and cytogenetic alterations that are the hallmarks of specific tumors (e.g., *BCR-ABL1* in chronic myeloid leukemia or CML)
- Determination of clonality as an indicator of a neoplastic (i.e., nonreactive) condition
- The identification of specific genetic alterations that can direct therapeutic choices (e.g., *HER2/Neu* [official name *ERBB2*] in breast cancer or *EGFR* mutations in lung cancer)
- Determination of treatment efficacy (e.g., minimal residual disease detection of BCR-ABL1 by PCR in CML)
- Detection of Gleevec-resistant forms of chronic myeloid leukemia and gastrointestinal stromal tumors

Diagnosis and management of infectious disease (see also Chapter 8)
- Detection of microorganism-specific genetic material for definitive diagnosis (e.g., HIV, mycobacteria, human papillomavirus, herpesvirus in central nervous system)
- The identification of specific genetic alterations in the genomes of microbes that are associated with drug resistance
- Determination of treatment efficacy (e.g., assessment of viral loads in HIV and hepatitis C virus infection)

PCR AND DETECTION OF DNA SEQUENCE ALTERATIONS

PCR analysis, which involves exponential amplification of DNA, has revolutionized molecular biology and is now widely used in the molecular diagnosis of human disease. By using appropriate DNA polymerases and thermal cycling, the target DNA is greatly amplified, producing millions of copies of the DNA sequence between the two primer sites. The subsequent identification of an abnormal sequence can then be performed using an ever-increasing number of assays. Direct sequence analysis of PCR products is currently the most straightforward method.

Direct Detection of DNA Sequence Alterations by DNA Sequencing

DNA can be sequenced to obtain a readout of the order of nucleotides, and by comparison with a normal (wild-type) sequence, mutations can be identified. The ready availability of Sanger di-deoxynucleotide sequencing and automated capillary electrophoresis allows thousands of base pairs of genomic DNA to be routinely sequenced in a matter of hours.[75] The genes mutated in hundreds of mendelian disorders have been identified, and definitive diagnosis is possible by direct sequencing in most of them. Some disorders, most with recessive inheritance, are associated with a limited number of recurrent mutations, such as cystic fibrosis. Many others, especially those with dominant inheritance, can have mutations throughout the gene-coding region. Challenges to sole use of gene sequencing for the diagnosis of such diseases include the difficulty and high cost of analyzing large genes. For example, the gene associated with Duchenne muscular dystrophy possesses 79 exons, and the *FBN1* gene mutated in Marfan syndrome possesses 65 exons; the sequencing of these genes in their entirety can be prohibitively expensive with current methodologies. Among other difficulties, it is not uncommon to detect sequence alterations of unknown significance, which cannot be definitively determined to be pathogenic in the absence of any functional data.

However, this picture is changing with remarkable speed. Rapidly advancing technology will make large-scale germ line sequencing applications feasible and may lead in the not distant future to the routine sequencing of entire individual human genomes. One high-throughput technology uses gene chips (microarrays) to sequence genes or portions of genes.[76] Short sequences of DNA (oligonucleotides) that are complementary to the wild-type sequence and to known mutations are "tiled" adjacent to each other on the gene chip, and the DNA sample to be tested is hybridized to the array (Fig. 5–30). Before hybridization the sample is labeled with fluorescent dyes. The hybridization (and consequently, the fluorescent signal emitted) will be strongest at the oligonucleotide that is complementary to wild-type sequence if no mutations are present, while the presence of a mutation will cause hybridization to occur at the complementary mutant oligonucleotide. Computerized algorithms can then rapidly "decode" the DNA sequence for hundreds of thousands of base pairs of sequence from the fluorescent hybridization pattern on the chip, and identify potential mutations. Perhaps the most exciting recent advance is technology termed "next-generation" sequencing, which involves PCR performed in an oil emulsion that allows over one million individual PCR reactions at once.[77] While at present very costly, over one billion nucleotides (one third of the human genome!) can be sequenced per run. Bioinformatics challenges of handling and interpreting such massive amounts of data are currently staggering, and much effort is devoted to such analysis.

Detection of DNA Mutations by Indirect Methods

There are a large number of molecular techniques that detect DNA mutations without direct sequencing.

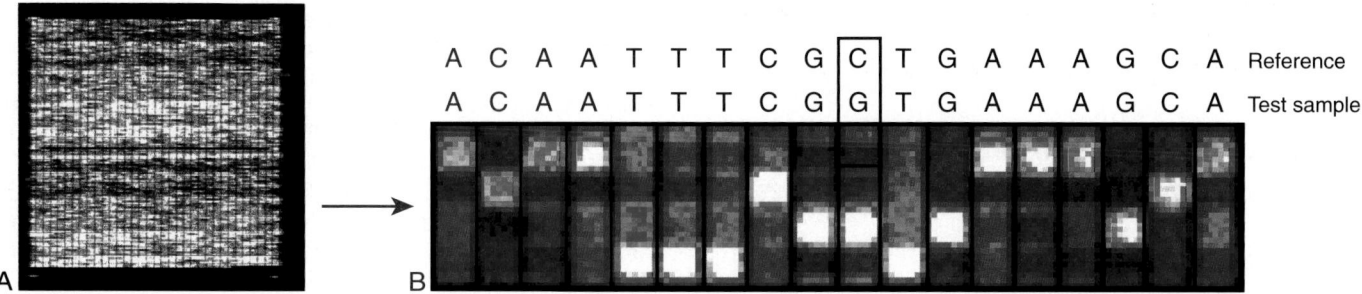

A C A A T T T C G [C] T G A A A G C A Reference
A C A A T T T C G [G] T G A A A G C A Test sample

FIGURE 5–30 Microarray-based DNA sequencing. **A,** A low-power digitized scan of a "gene chip" that is no larger than a nickel in size but is capable of sequencing thousands of base pairs of DNA. High-throughput microarrays have been used for sequencing whole organisms (such as viruses), organelles (such as mitochondria), and entire human chromosomes. **B,** A high-resolution view of the gene chip illustrates hybridization patterns corresponding to a stretch of DNA sequence. Typically, a computerized algorithm is available that can convert the individual hybridization patterns across the entire chip into actual sequence data within a matter of minutes ("conventional" sequencing technologies would require days to weeks for such analysis). Here, the upper sequence is the reference (wild-type) sequence, while the lower one corresponds to the test sample sequence. As shown, the computerized algorithm has identified a C→G mutation in the test sample. (Adapted from Maitra A et al.: The Human MitoChip: a high-throughput sequencing microarray for the mitochondrial mutation detection. Genome Res 14:812, 2004.)

Their development is driven by lower costs and higher throughput.

- One simple approach takes advantage of the digestion of DNA with enzymes known as restriction enzymes that recognize, and then cut, DNA at specific sequences. If the specific mutation is known to affect a restriction site, then the amplified DNA can be digested. Because the mutation affects a restriction site, the mutant and normal alleles give rise to PCR products of different sizes. These would appear as different bands on agarose gel electrophoresis. Needless to say, this approach is considerably less comprehensive than direct sequencing but remains useful for molecular diagnosis when the causal mutation always occurs at an invariant nucleotide position.
- Another approach for identifying mutations at a specific nucleotide position (say, a codon 12 mutation in the *KRAS* oncogene that converts glycine [GGT] to aspartic acid [GAT]) would be to add fluorescently labeled nucleotides C and T to the PCR mixture, which are complementary to either the wild-type (G) or mutant (A) sequence, respectively. Since these two nucleotides are labeled with different fluorophores, the fluorescence emitted by the resulting PCR product can be of one or another color, depending on whether a "C" or a "T" becomes incorporated in the process of primer extension (Fig. 5–31). The advantage of this "allele-specific extension" strategy is that it can detect the presence of mutant DNA even in heterogeneous mixtures of normal and abnormal cells (for example, in clinical specimens obtained from individuals with a suspected malignancy).
- A variety of PCR-based technologies that use fluorophore indicators can detect the presence or absence of mutations in "real time" (i.e., during the exponential phase of DNA amplification). This has significantly reduced the time required for mutation detection by removing the restriction digestion and electrophoresis steps used in conventional PCR assays.
- Mutations that affect the length of DNA (e.g., deletions or expansions) can also be detected by PCR analysis. As dis-

cussed earlier, several diseases, such as the fragile-X syndrome, are associated with trinucleotide repeats. Figure 5–32 reveals how PCR analysis can be used to detect this mutation. Two primers that flank the region affected by trinucleotide repeats at the 5′ end of the *FMR1* gene are used to amplify the intervening sequences. Because there are large differences in the number of repeats, the size of the PCR products obtained from the DNA of normal individuals, or those with premutation, is quite different. These size differences are revealed by differential migration of the

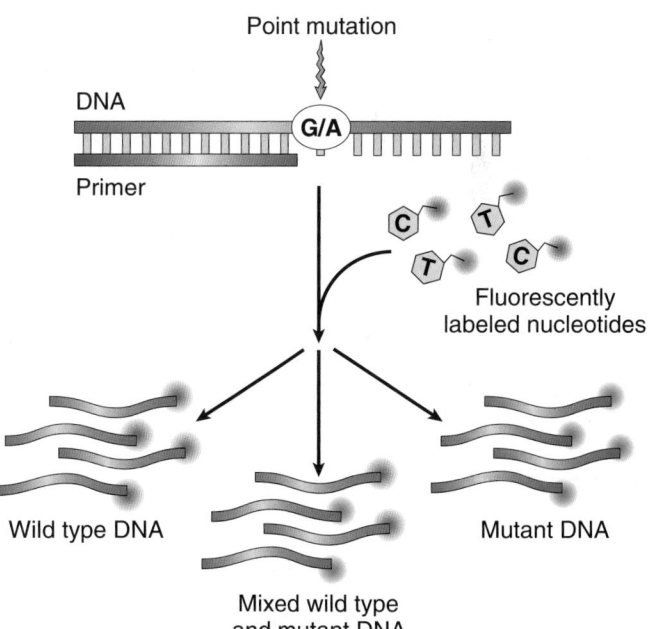

FIGURE 5–31 Allele-specific PCR for mutation detection in a heterogeneous sample containing an admixture of normal and mutant DNA. Nucleotides complementary to the mutant and wild-type nucleotides at the queried base position are labeled with different fluorophores, such that incorporation into the resulting PCR product yields fluorescent signals of varying intensity based on the ratio of mutant to wild-type DNA present.

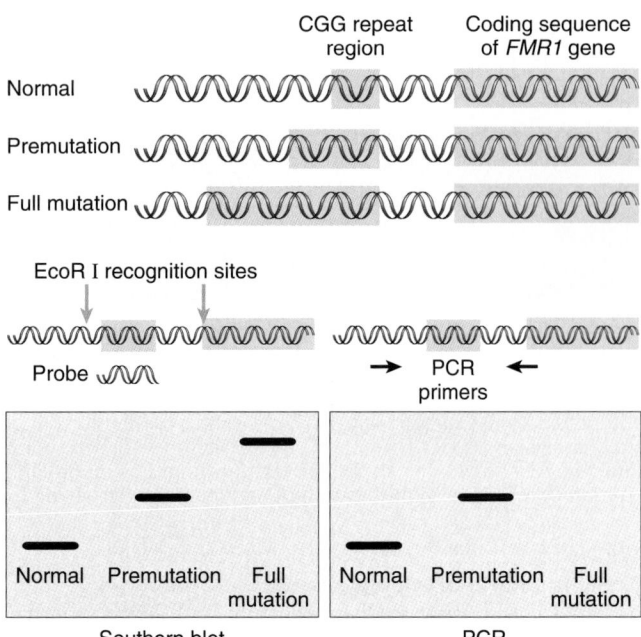

FIGURE 5–32 Diagnostic application of PCR and Southern blot analysis in fragile-X syndrome. With PCR the differences in the size of CGG repeats between normal and premutation give rise to products of different sizes and mobility. With a full mutation, the region between the primers is too large to be amplified by conventional PCR. In Southern blot analysis the DNA is cut by enzymes that flank the CGG repeat region, and is then probed with a complementary DNA that binds to the affected part of the gene. A single small band is seen in normal males, a band of higher molecular weight in males with premutation, and a very large (usually diffuse) band in those with the full mutation.

amplified DNA products on a gel. At this point the full mutation cannot be detected by PCR analysis, because the affected segment of DNA is too large for conventional PCR. In such cases, a Southern blot analysis of genomic DNA must be performed (see "Southern Blotting").

POLYMORPHIC MARKERS AND MOLECULAR DIAGNOSIS

Detection of mutations by the methods outlined above is possible only if the gene responsible for a genetic disorder is known and its sequence has been identified. In some diseases that have a genetic basis such approaches are not possible, either because the causal gene has not been identified or because the disease is multifactorial and no single gene is involved. In such cases, surrogate markers in the genome, also known as marker loci, can be used to localize the chromosomal regions of interest, on the basis of their linkage to one or more putative disease-causing genes. *Linkage analysis* deals with assessing these marker loci in family members having the disease or trait of interest, with the assumption that marker loci very close to the disease allele are transmitted through pedigrees (linkage disequilibrium). With time it becomes possible to define a "disease haplotype" based on a panel of marker loci, all of which co-segregate with the putative disease allele. Eventually, linkage analysis facilitates localization and cloning of the disease allele. The marker loci used in linkage studies

are naturally occurring variations in DNA sequences known as *polymorphisms*. Two types of genetic polymorphism are most useful for linkage analysis. They are SNPs (including small insertion-deletion polymorphisms) and repeat-length polymorphisms known as minisatellite and microsatellite repeats. Each of the two types is described next.

SNPs occur at a frequency of approximately one nucleotide in every stretch of approximately 1000 base pairs and are found throughout the genome (e.g., in exons and introns and in regulatory sequences). They serve both as a physical landmark within the genome and as a genetic marker whose transmission can be followed from parent to child. Because of their prevalence throughout the genome and relative stability, SNPs can be used in linkage analysis for identifying haplotypes associated with disease.

Human DNA contains short repetitive sequences of DNA giving rise to what are called *repeat-length polymorphisms*. These polymorphisms are often subdivided on the basis of their length into microsatellite repeats and minisatellite repeats. Microsatellites are usually less than 1 kilobase and are characterized by a repeat size of 2 to 6 base pairs. Minisatellite repeats, by comparison, are larger (1–3 kilobases), and the repeat motif is usually 15 to 70 base pairs. It is important to note that the number of repeats, both in microsatellites and minisatellites, is extremely variable within a given population, and hence these stretches of DNA can be used quite effectively to establish genetic identity for linkage analysis. Microsatellites and the smaller minisatellites can be readily distinguished by utilizing PCR primers that flank the repeat region (Fig. 5–33A). Note that in the example given in Figure 5–33, three different alleles generate PCR products of different lengths (hence the name "length polymorphism").

Linkage analysis can be been useful in the antenatal or presymptomatic diagnosis of disorders such as Huntington disease and autosomal dominant polycystic kidney disease, even though the disease-associated gene is known in each of these conditions. In general, when the disease-associated gene is known, detection of the causative mutation by direct sequencing is the method of choice. However, if the disease originates from several different mutations in a given gene (e.g., *fibrillin-1*; see earlier), and gene sequencing is either not practical or negative but there is very strong clinical suspicion, linkage analysis can be useful. Figure 5–33B illustrates how microsatellite polymorphisms can be used to track the inheritance of autosomal-dominant polycystic kidney disease. In this case allele C, which produces a larger PCR product than allele A or B, carries the disease-related gene. Hence all individuals who carry the C allele are affected.

Assays to detect genetic polymorphisms are also important in many other areas of medicine, including in the determination of relatedness and identity in transplantation, cancer genetics, paternity testing, and forensic medicine. Since microsatellite markers are scattered throughout the human genome and have such a high level of polymorphism, they are ideal for differentiating two individuals and to follow transmission of the marker from parent to child. Panels of microsatellite marker PCR assays have been extensively validated and are now routinely used for determining paternity and for criminal investigations. Since PCR can be performed even with highly degraded biologic samples, DNA technology is critical in forensic identifications. The same assays have been

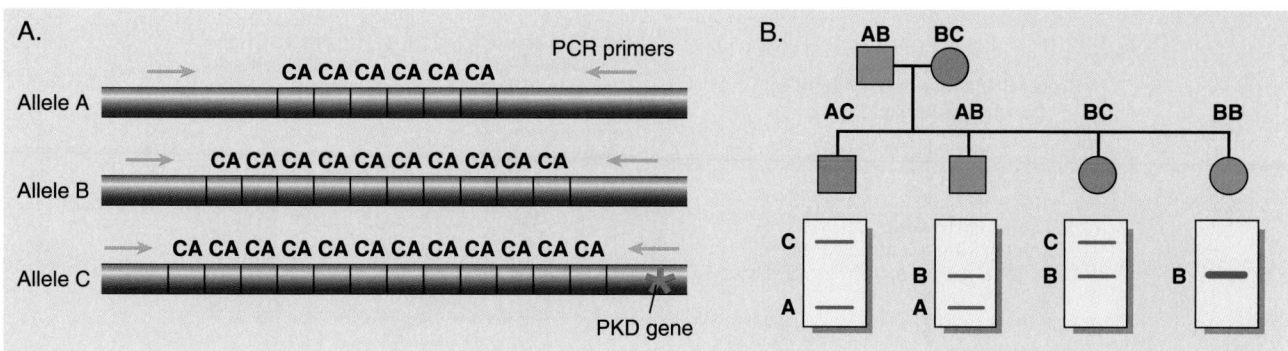

FIGURE 5-33 DNA polymorphisms resulting from a variable number of CA repeats. The three alleles produce PCR products of different sizes, thus identifying their origins from specific chromosomes. In the example depicted, allele C is linked to a mutation responsible for autosomal-dominant polycystic kidney disease (PKD). Application of this to detect progeny carrying the disease-related gene (red symbols) is illustrated in one hypothetical pedigree. Males (squares); females (circles).

applied to the detection and quantification of transplant chimerism in allogeneic bone marrow transplants.

Polymorphisms and Genome-Wide Analyses

As described earlier, linkage analysis utilizing DNA of affected families has been used to detect the presence of genes with large effects and high penetrance, the kind that give rise to Mendelian diseases. Similar analyses of complex (multifactorial) disorders, however, have been unsuccessful since conventional linkage studies lack the statistical power to detect variants with small effects and low penetrance, which are typical of the genes that contribute to complex disorders.

These limitations appear to have been overcome through genome-wide association studies (GWAS), a powerful method of identifying genetic variants that are associated with an increased risk of developing a particular disease.[78] Such variants may themselves be causative, or may be in *linkage disequilibrium* with other genetic variants that are responsible for the increased risk. In GWAS large cohorts of patients with and without a disease (rather than families) are examined across the entire genome for genetic variants or polymorphisms that are over-represented in patients with the disease. This identifies regions of the genome that contain a variant gene or genes that confer disease susceptibility. The causal variant within the region is then provisionally identified using a "candidate gene" approach, in which genes are selected based on how tightly they are associated with the disease and whether their biologic function seems likely to be involved in the disease under study. For example, a variant in a gene whose product regulates vascular smooth muscle tone (e.g., angiotensinogen) is a strong candidate to influence the risk of hypertension. As might be imagined, however, some linked genes would not have been expected to be associated with particular diseases based on prior knowledge; such surprises are one of the benefits of the unbiased, systematic nature of GWAS.

GWAS have been enabled by two major technological breakthroughs. First is the completion of the so-called "HapMap" project, which has provided more complete linkage disequilibrium patterns in three major ethno-racial groups, based on genome-wide single nucleotide polymorphism (SNP) mapping. The entire human genome can now be divided into blocks known as "haplotypes," which contain varying numbers of contiguous SNPs on the same chromosome that are in linkage disequilibrium and hence inherited together as a cluster. As a result, rather than querying every single SNP in the human genome, it is possible to glean comparable information about shared DNA by simply looking for shared haplotypes, using single or a small number of SNPs that "tag" or identify a specific haplotype. Second, it is now possible to simultaneously genotype hundreds of thousands to a million SNPs at one time, in a cost-effective way, using high-density SNP-chip technology. Figure 5-34 demonstrates how information from the publicly available "HapMap" is utilized to manufacture SNP chips that can query genome-wide haplotypes in an unbiased manner. Thereafter, DNA from a cohort of individuals with a defined trait (say, hypertension) is analyzed using SNP chips for haplotypes that are overrepresented compared to individuals without the trait (i.e., in controls). This is followed by the "candidate gene" approach described above to further localize the causal gene (and in some instances, the functional polymorphism within that gene), associated with the trait.

In addition to shedding light on some of the most frequent human ailments such as diabetes, hypertension, coronary artery disease, schizophrenia and other mental disorders, and asthma, GWAS have also led to the identification of genetic loci that modulate common quantitative traits in humans, such as height, body mass, hair and eye color, and bone density. An updated catalog of published GWAS is maintained by the National Human Genome Research Institute (www.genome.gov), with the list currently at >200 studies and growing. The power of GWAS is underscored by the fact that within a very short time, nearly a dozen genes that confer risk for type 2 diabetes have been identified, of which one in particular, *TCF7L2*, has emerged as a strong candidate gene (see Chapter 24 for a detailed discussion).

With the incrementally lowered costs for genotyping individual patients for SNPs that might render them "at-risk" for a variety of multifactorial disease over their lifetime, there is emerging concern in the biomedical community that such information would be utilized for discrimination in the workplace or by healthcare agencies. In the United States, a law was passed in 2008 that explicitly prohibits discrimination based on an individual's genetic makeup.

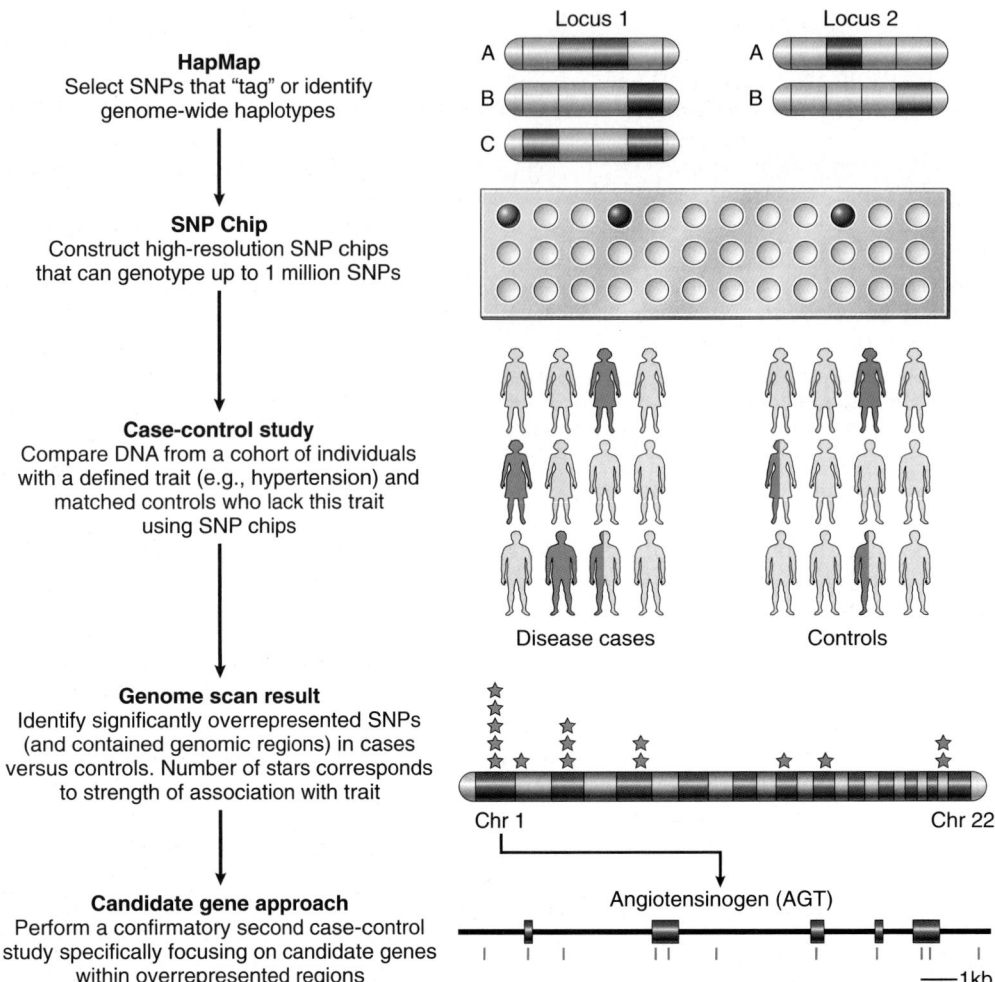

FIGURE 5–34 **General scheme for conducting a genome wide association study (GWAS).** Using the publicly available "HapMap" data, the human genome is divided into "haplotypes" or regions of contiguous DNA inherited as a block, each identified by one or a few "tag" SNPs that identify the haplotype. In the example shown, locus 1 contains three haplotypes defined by different combinations of SNPs, where white signifies the more common "normal" sequence and each color designates a different SNP; thus, these haplotypes can be distinguished by assaying for only the blue and purple "tag" SNPs. Thereafter, high density SNP chips are constructed that contain these "tag" SNPs, in order to enable an unbiased genome-wide assessment of shared haplotypes between disease and control populations. Of note, "disease" refers to any defined phenotype, and could pertain to an actual disease entity like hypertension, or simply a quantitative trait like hair or eye color. Next, DNA obtained from the two cohorts is analyzed for overrepresented SNPs in the disease population ("cases") *versus* the control samples—this is known as a case-control study. The most significant shared genomic regions of interest are then examined for candidate genes of interest—an example shown here in a search for loci associated with hypertension is *angiotensinogen*, a gene on chromosome 1 whose product regulates vascular smooth muscle tone. The final step is to perform a second case control study, this time using SNPs located within the gene of interest in order to confirm or refute the association with the trait, often in an independent population from the one in which the initial GWAS was conducted. In this example, individual SNPs within angiotensinogen gene are denoted as red vertical bars, and these SNPs will be tested in the second round of case-control study. (Modified from Mathew CG: New links to the pathogenesis of Crohn disease provided by genome-wide association scans. Nat Rev Genet 9(1):9–14, 2008.)

MOLECULAR ANALYSIS OF GENOMIC ALTERATIONS

A significant number of genetic lesions involve large deletions, duplications, or more complex rearrangements that are not easily assayed using PCR methods or sequence analysis. Such "genomic" alterations can be studied using a variety of hybridization-based techniques.

Southern Blotting

Changes in the structure of specific loci can be detected by Southern blotting, which involves hybridization of radiola- beled sequence-specific probes to genomic DNA that has been first digested with a restriction enzyme and separated by gel electrophoresis. The probe usually detects one germ line band in normal individuals. Importantly, a normal DNA sample is required to compare the pattern of the DNA in question. With the advent of FISH and microarray technology, Southern blotting is rarely used but remains useful in the detection of large-trinucleotide-expansion diseases including the fragile-X syndrome (see Fig. 5–32), and in detection of clonal immunoglobulin gene rearrangements in the diagnosis of lymphoma. The latter is being replaced by PCR-based methods.

Fluorescence in Situ Hybridization

FISH uses DNA probes that recognize sequences specific to particular chromosomal regions. As part of the Human Genome Project, large libraries of bacterial artificial chromosomes that span the entire human genome were created. The human DNA insert in these clones is on the order of 100,000–200,000 base pairs, which defines the limit of resolution of FISH for identifying chromosomal changes. These DNA clones are labeled with fluorescent dyes and applied to metaphase spreads or interphase nuclei. The probe hybridizes to its homologous genomic sequence and thus labels a specific chromosomal region that can be visualized under a fluorescent microscope. The ability of FISH to circumvent the need for dividing cells is invaluable when a rapid diagnosis is warranted (e.g., when deciding to treat a patient with acute myeloid leukemia with retinoic acid, which is only effective in a particular subtype with a chromosomal translocation involving the retinoic acid receptor gene [Chapter 14]). FISH can be performed on prenatal samples (e.g., cells obtained by amniocentesis, chorionic villus biopsy, or umbilical cord blood), peripheral blood lymphocytes, touch preparations from cancer biopsies, and even archival tissue sections. FISH has been used for detection of numeric abnormalities of chromosomes (aneuploidy) (see Fig. 5–20); for the demonstration of subtle microdeletions (see Fig. 5–22) or complex translocations not detectable by routine karyotyping; for analysis of gene amplification (e.g., *HER2/NEU* in breast cancer or *N-MYC* amplification in neuroblastomas); and for mapping newly isolated genes of interest to their chromosomal loci. Chromosome painting is an extension of FISH, whereby probes are prepared for entire chromosomes. The number of chromosomes that can be *detected simultaneously* by chromosome painting is limited by the availability of fluorescent dyes that emit different wavelengths of visible light. This limitation has been overcome by the introduction of spectral karyotyping (also called multicolor FISH). By using a combination of five fluorochromes and appropriate computer-generated signals, the entire human genome can be visualized (Fig. 5–35). So powerful is spectral karyotyping that it might well be called "spectacular karyotyping."

Array-Based Comparative Genomic Hybridization (Array CGH)

It is obvious from the preceding discussion that FISH requires prior knowledge of the one or few specific chromosomal regions suspected of being altered in the test sample. However, genomic abnormalities can also be detected without prior knowledge of what these aberrations may be, using a global strategy such as array CGH. In array CGH the test DNA and a reference (normal) DNA are labeled with two different fluorescent dyes (most commonly Cy5 and Cy3, which fluoresce red and green, respectively) (Fig. 5–36). The differentially

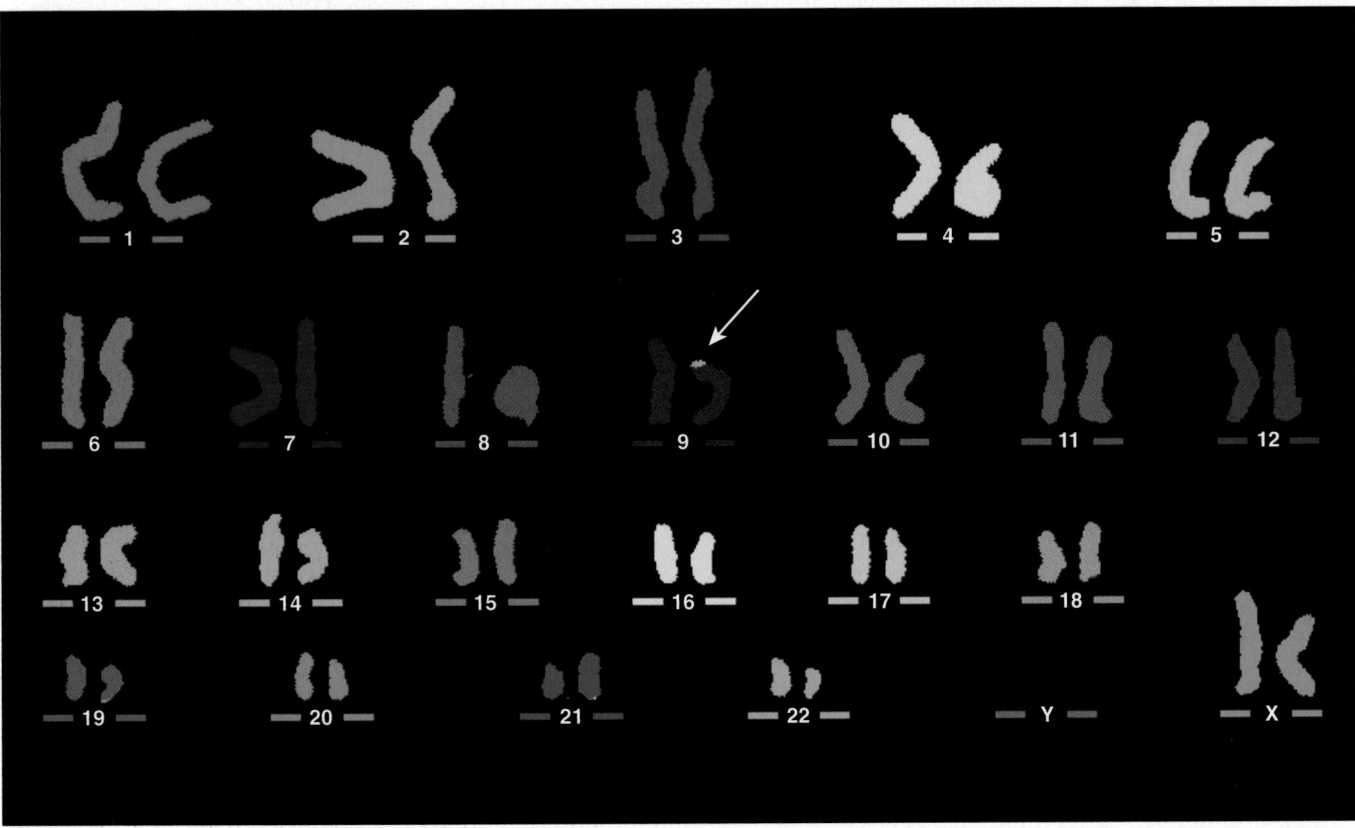

FIGURE 5–35 FISH studies using multicolor FISH in a child with an undetermined abnormality. This technique uses ratio-labeled probes labeled with 23 distinct mixtures of 5 fluorophores to create a unique "color" for each chromosome. This analysis revealed a derivative chromosome 9, with 9p containing additional material from 22q. (Courtesy of Dr. Stuart Schwartz, Department of Pathology, University of Chicago, Chicago, IL.)

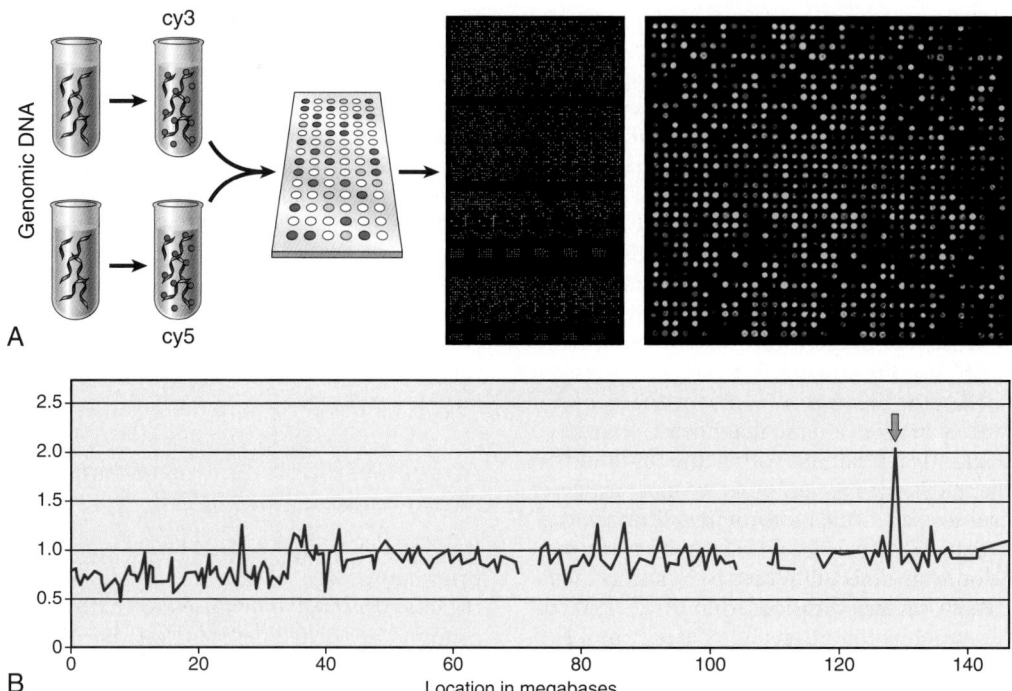

FIGURE 5–36 **A,** Array CGH is performed by hybridization of fluorescently labeled "test" DNA and "control" DNA on a slide that contains thousands of probes corresponding to defined chromosomal regions across the human genome. The resolution of most currently available array CGH assays is in the order of about 200 to 500 kilobases. Higher power view of the array demonstrates copy number aberrations in the "test" sample (Cy5, red), including regions of amplification (spots with excess of red signal) and deletion (spots with excess of green signal); yellow spots correspond to regions of normal (diploid) copy number. **B,** The hybridization signals are digitized, resulting in a virtual karyotype of the genome of the "test" sample. In the illustrated example, array CGH of a cancer cell line identifies an amplification on the distal long arm of chromosome 8, which corresponds to increased number of the oncogenic *MYC*. (**A,** From Snijders AM et al.: Assembly of microarrays for genome-wide measurement of DNA copy number. Nat Genet 29:263, 2001. Web Figure A, Copyright 2001. Reprinted by permission from Macmillan Publishers Ltd.)

labeled samples are then hybridized to a glass slide spotted with DNA probes that span the human genome at regularly spaced intervals, and usually cover all 22 autosomes and the X chromosome. If the contributions of both samples are equal for a given chromosomal region (i.e., the test sample is diploid), then all spots on the array will fluoresce yellow (the result of an equal admixture of green and red dyes). In contrast, if the test sample shows an excess of DNA at any given chromosomal region (such as resulting from an amplification), there will be a corresponding excess of signal from the dye with which this sample was labeled. The reverse will be true in the event of a deletion, with an excess of the signal used for labeling the reference sample. Amplifications and deletions in the test sample can now be significantly better localized, often down to a few thousand base pairs. Newer arrays provide even higher resolution with more than 100,000 probes per array, and are at present being used to uncover copy number abnormalities in a variety of diseases, from cancer to autism. Array CGH is regularly performed in cases of mental retardation–developmental delay of unknown etiology or in children with dysmorphic features with negative karyotypes.

As discussed earlier in the chapter, CNVs are a recently discovered source of genetic polymorphism, which was uncovered using array CGH technology. While intriguing in terms of understanding the marked differences between individual genomes, they can be problematic in the clinical interpretation of array CGH data.[79] There are usually many CNVs observed when comparing any two genomes encompassing millions of bases of DNA. Deciding whether a specific change is a benign polymorphism or a critical disease-causing duplication or deletion can be difficult. Databases of CNVs now exist that are very helpful guides in deciding on the relevance of questionable CNVs. Another limitation of existing array CGH platforms is that they cannot detect balanced translocations, since there is a rearrangement but no genetic material is gained or lost. Nonetheless, the vastly superior sensitivity of molecular approaches should make assays such as array CGH first-line genomic diagnostic tests that have the potential of replacing traditional karyotyping.

EPIGENETIC ALTERATIONS

Epigenetics is defined as the study of heritable chemical modification of DNA or chromatin that does not alter the DNA sequence itself. Examples of such modification include the methylation of DNA, and the methylation and acetylation of histones. Our understanding of these types of molecular alterations is rapidly growing, and it is clear that epigenetic modifications are critical for normal human development—including the regulation of tissue-specific gene expression, X chromosome inactivation, and imprinting, as well as for understanding of the cellular perturbations in the aging process and cancer.[80,81]

Gene expression frequently correlates with the level of methylation of DNA, usually of cytosines specifically in the

CG dinucleotide-rich promoter regions known as CpG islands. As discussed earlier in the section on genomic imprinting, increased methylation of these loci is associated with decreased gene expression and is accompanied by concomitant specific patterns of histone methylation and acetylation. An ever-increasing number of disease states warrant analysis of promoter methylation—for example, in the diagnosis of fragile-X syndrome, in which hypermethylation results in *FMR1* silencing. Methylation analysis is also essential in the diagnosis of Prader-Willi and Angelman syndromes.

Since traditional Sanger sequencing alone cannot detect DNA methylation, other techniques have been developed to uncover these chemical modifications. One common approach is to treat genomic DNA with sodium bisulfite, a chemical that converts unmethylated cytosines to uracil, while methylated cytosines are protected from modification. An assay termed methylation-specific PCR uses two PCR primer sets to analyze single DNA loci: one to detect a DNA sequence with unmethylated cytosines (which are converted to uracils after bisulfite treatment) and the other to detect DNA sequences with methylated cytosines (which remain cytosines after bisulfite treatment).[82] Additional techniques are evolving that provide a genome-wide snapshot of epigenetically altered DNA. These techniques are based on the ability to detect histone modifications such as methylation and acetylation (which, like DNA methylation, are important regulators of gene expression) by using antibodies against specifically modified histones. Such antibodies can be used to pull down bound DNA sequences, a method termed chromatin immunoprecipitation (ChIP). These pulled-down sequences can be amplified and analyzed by hybridizing to microarrays ("ChIP on Chip") or sequencing ("ChIP-Seq") to map epigenetically modified genes throughout the genome.[83,84]

RNA ANALYSIS

Changes in DNA lead to alterations in mRNA expression; hence in principle it should be possible to use mRNA expression analysis in the diagnosis of genetic diseases. From a practical standpoint, however, DNA-based diagnosis is much preferred, since DNA is much more stable. Nonetheless, RNA analysis is critical in several areas of molecular diagnostics. The most important application is the detection and quantification of RNA viruses such as HIV and hepatitis C virus. Furthermore, mRNA expression profiling (described in Chapters 7 and 23) is rapidly becoming an important tool for molecular stratification of tumors. In some instances cancer cells bearing particular chromosomal translocations are detected with greater sensitivity by analyzing mRNA (e.g., *BCR-ABL* fusion in CML). The principal reason for this is that most translocations occur in scattered locations within particular introns, which can be very large, beyond the capacity of conventional PCR amplification. Since introns are removed by splicing during the formation of mRNA, PCR analysis is possible if RNA is first converted to cDNA by reverse transcriptase. PCR performed on cDNA is the method of choice for detection of minimal residual disease in patients with chronic myeloid leukemia (Chapter 13).

In closing, it should be pointed out that the progress in unraveling the genetic basis of human disease promises to be breathtaking in the coming years. An entirely new field of personalized and genomic medicine is waiting to be developed.

REFERENCES

1. International Human Genome Sequencing Consortium: Finishing the euchromatic sequence of the human genome. Nature 431:931, 2004.
2. Plomin R, Schalkwyk LC: Microarrays. Dev Sci 10:19, 2007.
3. Gresham D et al.: Comparing whole genomes using DNA microarrays. Nat Rev Genet 9:291, 2008.
4. Iafrate AJ et al.: Detection of large-scale variation in the human genome. Nat Genet 36:949, 2004.
5. Sebat J et al.: Large-scale copy number polymorphism in the human genome. Science 305:525, 2004.
6. Redon R et al.: Global variation in copy number in the human genome. Nature 444:444, 2006.
7. Esteller M: Epigenetics and cancer. N Engl J Med 358:1148, 2008.
8. Bayat A: Science, medicine, and the future: bioinformatics. BMJ 324:1018, 2002.
9. Jay C et al.: miRNA profiling for diagnosis and prognosis of human cancer. DNA Cell Biol 26:293, 2007.
10. Eulalio A et al.: Getting to the root of miRNA-mediated gene silencing. Cell 132:9, 2008.
11. Rimoin DL et al.: Nature and frequency of genetic disease. In Rimoin DL, et al (eds): Emery and Rimoin's Principles and Practice of Medical Genetics, 3rd ed. New York, Churchill Livingstone, 1997, p 32.
12. Ensenauer RE et al.: Primer on medical genomics. Part VIII: essentials of medical genetics for the practicing physician. Mayo Clin Proc 78:846, 2003.
13. Willard HF: Tales of the Y chromosome. Nature 423:810, 2003.
14. Gomase VS et al.: Pharmacogenomics. Curr Drug Metab 9:207, 2008.
15. Ramirez F, Dietz HC: Marfan syndrome: from molecular pathogenesis to clinical treatment. Curr Opin Genet Dev 17:252, 2007.
16. Judge DP, Dietz HC: Therapy of Marfan syndrome. Ann Rev Med 59:43, 2008.
17. Mao JR, Bristow J: The Ehlers-Danlos syndrome: on beyond collagens. J Clin Invest 07:1063, 2001.
18. Yeowell HN, Walker LC: Mutations in the lysyl hydroxylase 1 gene that result in enzyme deficiency and the clinical phenotype of Ehlers-Danlos syndrome type VI. Mol Genet Metab 71:212, 2000.
19. Pepin MG, Byers PH: Ehler-Danlos syndrome, vascular type. Gene Rev. Available at <http://www.ncbi.nlm.nih.gov/bookshelf/br.fcgi?book=gene&part=eds4> (2006).
20. Wenstrup R, De Paepe A: Ehler-Danlos syndrome, classic type. Gene Rev. Available at <http://www.ncbi.nlm.nih.gov/bookshelf/br.fcgi?book=gene&part=eds> (2007).
21. Soutar AK, Naoumova RP: Mechanisms of disease: genetic causes of familial hypercholesterolemia. Nat Clin Pract Cardiovasc Med 4:214, 2007.
22. Vellodi A: Lysosomal storage disorders. Br J Hematol 128:413, 2004.
23. Fan JQ: A counterintuitive approach to treat enzyme deficiencies: use of enzyme inhibitors for restoring mutant enzyme activity. Biol Chem 389:1, 2008.
24. Kaback MM: Hexosaminidase A deficiency. Gene Rev. Available at <http://www.ncbi.nlm.nih.gov/bookshelf/br.fcgi?book=gene&part=tay-sachs> (2006).
25. Schuchman EH: The pathogenesis and treatment of acid sphingo-myelinase-deficient Niemann-Pick disease. J Inherit Metab Dis 30:654, 2007.
26. Liu B et al.: Receptor-mediated and bulk-phase endocytosis cause macrophage and cholesterol accumulation in Niemann-Pick C disease. J Lipid Res 48:1710, 2007.
27. Pastores GM, Hughes DA: Gaucher disease. Gene Rev. Available at <http://www.ncbi.nlm.nih.gov/bookshelf/br.fcgi?book=gene&part=gaucher> (2008).
28. Clarke LA: Mucopolysaccharidosis type I. Gene Rev. Available at <http://www.ncbi.nlm.nih.gov/bookshelf/br.fcgi?book=gene&part=mps1> (2007).
29. Martin RA: Mucopolysaccharidosis type II. Gene Rev. Available at <http://www.ncbi.nlm.nih.gov/bookshelf/br.fcgi?book=gene&part=hunter> (2007).
30. Ozen H: Glycogen storage diseases: new perspectives. World J Gastroenterol 13:2541, 2007.

31. Shin YS: Glycogen storage disease: clinical, biochemical, and molecular heterogeneity. Semin Pediatr Neurol 13:115, 2006.

32. Bali DS, Chen YT: Glycogen storage disease type I. Gene Rev. Available at <http://www.ncbi.nlm.nih.gov/bookshelf/br.fcgi?book=gene&part=gsd1> (2006).

33. Arenas J et al.: Glycogen storage disease type V. Gene Rev. Available at <http://www.ncbi.nlm.nih.gov/bookshelf/br.fcgi?book=gene&part=gsd5> (2007).

34. Tinkle BT, Leslie N: Glycogen storage disease type II (Pompe disease). Gene Rev. Available at <http://www.ncbi.nlm.nih.gov/bookshelf/br.fcgi?book=gene&part=gsd2> (2007).

35. Introne WJ et al.: Alkaptonuria. Gene Rev. Available at <http://www.ncbi.nlm.nih.gov/bookshelf/br.fcgi?book=gene&part=alkap> (2007).

36. Lango H, Weedon MN: What will whole genome searches for susceptibility genes for common complex disease offer to clinical practice? J Internal Med 263:16, 2007.

37. Roizen NJ, Patterson D: Down's syndrome. Lancet 361:1281, 2003.

38. Izraeli S et al.: Trisomy of chromosome 21 in leukemogenesis. Blood Cells Mol Dis 39:156, 2007.

39. Patterson D: Genetic mechanisms involved in the phenotype of Down syndrome. Ment Retard Dev Disabil Res Rev 13:199, 2007.

40. Antonarakis SE et al.: Chromosome 21 and Down syndrome: from genomics to pathophysiology. Nat Rev Genet 5:725, 2004.

41. Sullivan KE: Chromosome 22q11.2 deletion syndrome: DiGeorge syndrome/velocardiofacial syndrome. Immunol Allergy Clin N Am 28:353, 2008.

42. Arinami T: Analyses of the associations between the genes of 22q11 deletion syndrome and schizophrenia. J Hum Genet 51:1037, 2006.

43. Ross MT et al.: The sequences of the human sex chromosomes. Curr Opin Genet Dev 16:213, 2006.

44. Lyon MF: X-chromosome inactivation and human genetic disease. Acta Paediatr 91 (Suppl):107, 2002.

45. Salstrom JL: X-inactivation and the dynamic maintenance of gene silencing. Mol Genet Metab 92:56, 2007.

46. Heard E, Disteche M: Dosage compensation in mammals: fine-tuning the expression of the X chromosome. Genes Dev 20:1848, 2006.

47. Hawley RS: The human Y chromosome: rumors of its death have been greatly exaggerated. Cell 113:825, 2003.

48. Visootsak J, Graham JM Jr: Klinefelter syndrome and other sex chromosomal aneuploidies. Orphanet J Rare Dis 1:42, 2006.

49. Bojesen A, Gravholt CH: Klinefelter syndrome in clinical practice. Nat Clin Pract Urol 4:192, 2007.

50. Ferlin A et al.: Genetic causes of male infertility. Reprod Toxicol 22:133, 2006.

51. Hjerrild BE et al.: Turner syndrome and clinical treatment. Br Med Bull 86:77, 2008.

52. Bondy CA: Congenital cardiovascular disease in Turner syndrome. Congenit Heart Dis 3:2, 2008.

53. Marchini A et al.: SHOX at a glance: from gene to protein. Arch Physiol Biochem 113:116, 2007.

54. McLauglin DT, Donahoe PK: Sex determination and differentiation. N Engl J Med 350:367, 2004.

55. Ortenberg J et al.: *SRY* gene expression in the ovotestes of XX true hermaphrodites. J Urol 167:1828, 2002.

56. Brinkmann AO: Molecular basis of androgen insensitivity. Mol Cell Endocrinol 179:105, 2001.

57. Lutz RE: Trinucleotide repeat disorders. Semin Pediatr Neurol 14:26, 2007.

58. Orr HT, Zoghbi HY: Trinucleotide repeat disorders. Annu Rev Neurosci 30:575, 2007.

59. Shao J, Diamond MI: Polyglutamine diseases: emerging concepts in pathogenesis and therapy. Hum Mol Genet 16:R115, 2007.

60. Debacker K, Kooy RF: Fragile sites and human disease. Hum Mol Genet 16:R150, 2007.

61. Penagarikano O et al.: The pathophysiology of fragile X syndrome. Annu Rev Genomics Hum Genet 8:109, 2007.

62. Venkitaramani DV, Lombroso PJ: Molecular basis of genetic neuropsychiatric disorders. Child Adolesc Psychiatr Clin N Am 16:541, 2007.

63. Bear MF et al.: Fragile X: translation in action. Neuropsychopharmacology 33:84, 2008.

64. Garber KB et al.: Fragile X syndrome. Eur J Hum Genet 16:666, 2008.

65. Haas RH et al.: Mitochondrial disease: a practical approach for primary care physicians. Pediatrics 120:1326, 2007.

66. Schapira AH: Mitochondrial disease. Lancet 368:70, 2006.

67. Mancuso M et al.: Mitochondrial DNA-related disorders. Biosci Rep 27:31, 2007.

68. Man PY, Turnbull DM et al.: Leber hereditary optic neuropathy. J Med Genet 39:162, 2002.

69. Wood AJ, Oakey RJ: Genomic imprinting in mammals: emerging themes and established theories. PLoS Genet 2:e147, 2006.

70. Chen C et al.: Prader-Willi syndrome: an update and review for the primary pediatrician. Clin Pediatr 46:580, 2007.

71. Williams CA: Neurological aspects of the Angelman syndrome. Brain Dev 27: 88, 2005.

72. Lalande M, Calciano MA: Molecular epigenetics of Angelman syndrome. Cell Mol Life Sci 64:947, 2007.

73. Bernards A, Gusella JF: The importance of genetic mosaicism in human disease. N Engl J Med 331:1447, 1994.

74. American College of Obstetricians and Gynecologists: ACOG Practice Bulletin No. 88, December 2007. Invasive prenatal testing for aneuploidy. Obstet Gynecol 110:1459, 2007.

75. Metzker ML: Emerging technologies in DNA sequencing. Genome Res 15:1767, 2005.

76. Gresham D, Dunham MJ et al.: Comparing whole genomes using DNA microarrays. Nat Rev Genet 9:291, 2008.

77. Shendure J et al.: Accurate multiplex polony sequencing of an evolved bacterial genome. Science 309:1728, 2005.

78. Altshuler D, Daly MJ, Lander ES: Genetic mapping of human disease. Science 322:881, 2008.

79. Beaudet AL, Belmont JW: Array-based DNA diagnostics: let the revolution begin. Ann Rev Med 59:113, 2008.

80. Esteller M: Epigenetics in cancer. N Engl J Med 358:1148, 2008.

81. Gosden RG, Feinberg AP: Genetics and epigenetics—nature's pen-and-pencil set. N Engl J Med 356:731, 2007.

82. Herman JG et al.: Methylation-specific PCR: a novel PCR assay for methylation status of CpG islands. Proc Natl Acad Sci USA 93:9821, 1996.

83. Wu J et al.: ChIP—chip comes of age for genome-wide functional analysis. Cancer Res 66:6899, 2006.

84. Barski A et al.: High-resolution profiling of histone methylations in the human genome. Cell 129:823, 2007.

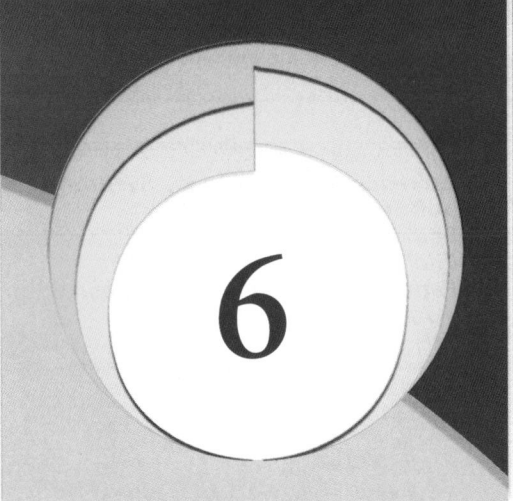

6

Diseases of the Immune System

The Normal Immune Response

Innate Immunity

Adaptive Immunity

Components of the Immune System:
Cells, Tissues, and Selected Molecules
Cells of the Immune System
Tissues of the Immune System
MHC Molecules: Peptide Display
System of Adaptive Immunity
Cytokines: Messenger Molecules of the
Immune System

Overview of Lymphocyte Activation
and Immune Responses
The Display and Recognition of
Antigens
Cell-Mediated Immunity: Activation of
T Lymphocytes and Elimination of
Intracellular Microbes
Humoral Immunity: Activation of B
Lymphocytes and Elimination of
Extracellular Microbes
Decline of Immune Responses and
Immunological Memory

Hypersensitivity and Autoimmune
Disorders

Mechanisms of Hypersensitivity
Reactions
Immediate (Type I) Hypersensitivity
Antibody-Mediated (Type II)
Hypersensitivity
Immune Complex–Mediated (Type III)
Hypersensitivity
T Cell–Mediated (Type IV)
Hypersensitivity

Autoimmune Diseases
Immunological Tolerance
Mechanisms of Autoimmunity: General
Principles

General Features of Autoimmune
Diseases

Systemic Lupus Erythematosus (SLE)
Spectrum of Autoantibodies in SLE
Etiology and Pathogenesis of SLE
Drug-Induced Lupus Erythematosus

Rheumatoid Arthritis

Sjögren Syndrome
Etiology and Pathogenesis

Systemic Sclerosis (Scleroderma)
Etiology and Pathogenesis

Inflammatory Myopathies

Mixed Connective Tissue Disease

Polyarteritis Nodosa and Other
Vasculitides

Rejection of Tissue Transplants
Mechanisms of Recognition and
Rejection of Allografts
Rejection of Kidney Grafts
Transplantation of Other Solid Organs
Transplantation of Hematopoietic Cells

Immunodeficiency Syndromes

Primary Immunodeficiencies
X-Linked Agammaglobulinemia
(Bruton's Agammaglobulinemia)
Common Variable Immunodeficieny
Isolated IgA Deficiency
Hyper-IgM Syndrome
DiGeorge Syndrome (Thymic
Hypoplasia)
Severe Combined Immunodeficiency
Immunodeficiency with
Thrombocytopenia and Eczema
(Wiskott-Aldrich Syndrome)
Genetic Deficiencies of the Complement
System

Secondary Immunodeficiencies

Acquired Immunodeficiency Syndrome (AIDS)
Epidemiology
Etiology: The Properties of HIV
Pathogenesis of HIV Infection and AIDS

Natural History of HIV Infection
Clinical Features of AIDS
Amyloidosis
    Properties of Amyloid Proteins
    Pathogenesis of Amyloidosis
    Classification of Amyloidosis

The immune system is vital for survival, because our environment is teeming with potentially deadly microbes and the immune system protects us from infectious pathogens. Predictably, immune deficiencies render individuals easy prey to infections. But the immune system is similar to the proverbial double-edged sword. Although it normally defends us against infections, a hyperactive immune system may cause diseases that can sometimes be fatal. Examples of disorders caused by immune responses include allergic reactions and reactions against an individual's own tissues and cells *(autoimmunity)*.

This chapter is devoted to diseases caused by too little immunity or too much immunologic reactivity. We also consider amyloidosis, a disease in which an abnormal protein, derived in some cases from fragments of immunoglobulins, is deposited in tissues. First, we review some of the important features of normal immune responses, to provide a foundation for understanding the abnormalities that give rise to immunological diseases.

The Normal Immune Response

The normal immune response is best understood in the context of defense against infectious pathogens, the classical definition of immunity. The mechanisms of protection against infections fall into two broad categories. *Innate immunity* (also called natural, or native, immunity) refers to defense mechanisms that are present even before infection and that have evolved to specifically recognize microbes and protect individuals against infections. *Adaptive immunity* (also called acquired, or specific, immunity) consists of mechanisms that are stimulated by ("adapt to") microbes and are capable of recognizing microbial and nonmicrobial substances. Innate immunity is the first line of defense, because it is always ready to prevent and eradicate infections. Adaptive immunity develops later, after exposure to microbes, and is even more powerful than innate immunity in combating infections. By convention, the term "immune response" refers to adaptive immunity.

INNATE IMMUNITY

The major components of innate immunity are epithelial barriers that block entry of microbes, phagocytic cells (mainly neutrophils and macrophages), dendritic cells, natural killer (NK) cells, and several plasma proteins, including the proteins of the complement system. The two most important cellular reactions of innate immunity are: *inflammation*, the process in which phagocytic leukocytes are recruited and activated to kill microbes, and *anti-viral defense*, mediated by dendritic cells and NK cells. Leukocytes and epithelial cells that participate in innate immunity are capable of recognizing components of microbes that are shared among related microbes and are often essential for the infectivity of these pathogens (and thus cannot be mutated to allow the microbes to evade the defense mechanisms). These microbial structures are called *pathogen-associated molecular patterns*. Leukocytes also recognize molecules released by injured and necrotic cells, which are sometimes called *danger-associated molecular patterns*. The cellular receptors that recognize these molecules are often called *pattern recognition receptors*. The best-defined pattern recognition receptors are a family of proteins called *Toll-like receptors (TLRs)*[1] that are homologous to the *Drosophila* protein Toll. Different TLRs are specific for components of different bacteria and viruses. TLRs are located on the cell surface and in endosomes, so they are able to recognize and initiate cellular responses to extracellular and ingested microbes. Other microbial sensors are located in the cytoplasm, where they recognize bacteria and viruses that may have colonized cells. Upon recognition of microbes, the TLRs and other sensors signal by a common pathway that leads to the activation of transcription factors, notably NF-κB (nuclear factor κB). NF-κB turns on the production of cytokines and proteins that stimulate the microbicidal activities of various cells, notably the phagocytes. Other cellular receptors bind microbes for phagocytosis; these include receptors for mannose residues, which are typical of microbial but not host glycoproteins, and receptors for opsonins such as antibodies and complement proteins that coat microbes.

Epithelia of the skin and gastrointestinal and respiratory tracts provide mechanical barriers to the entry of microbes from the external environment. Epithelial cells also produce anti-microbial molecules such as defensins, and lymphocytes located in the epithelia combat microbes at these sites. If microbes do breach epithelial boundaries, other defense mechanisms are called in.

Monocytes and *neutrophils* are phagocytes in the blood that can rapidly be recruited to any site of infection; monocytes that enter the tissues and mature are called *macrophages* (Chapter 2). *Dendritic cells* produce type I interferons, anti-viral cytokines that inhibit viral infection and replication; these cells are described below, in the context of antigen display to lymphocytes. *Natural killer cells* provide early protection against many viruses and intracellular bacteria; their properties and functions are also described below.

The proteins of the *complement system*, which were described in Chapter 2, are some of the most important plasma proteins

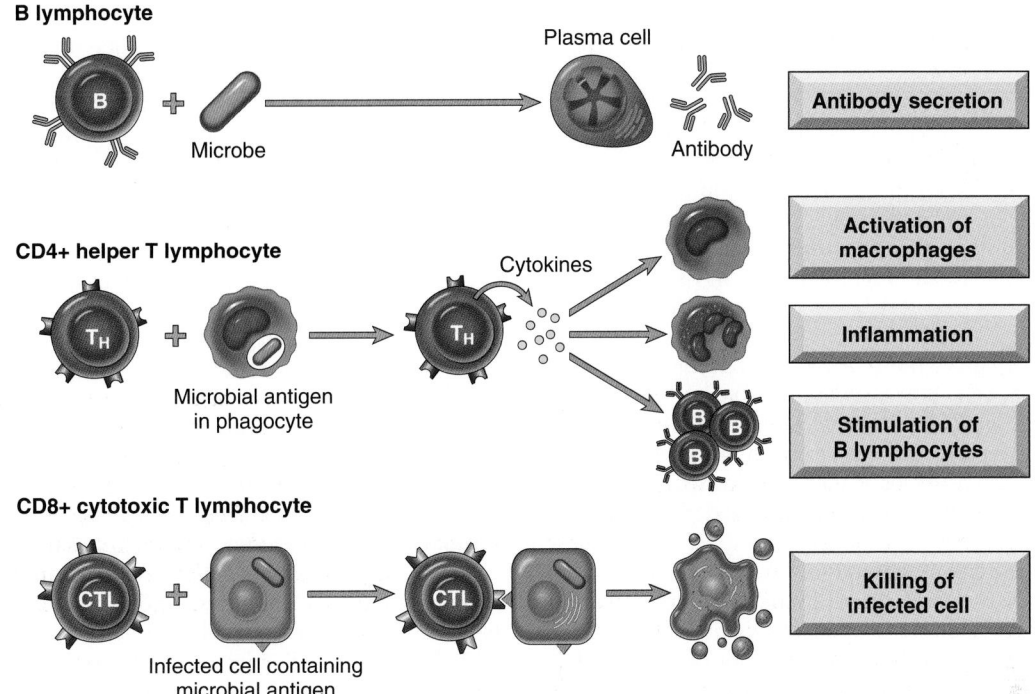

FIGURE 6–1 The principal classes of lymphocytes and their functions in adaptive immunity.

of the innate immune system. Recall that in innate immunity the complement system is activated by microbes using the alternative and lectin pathways; in adaptive immunity it is activated by antibodies using the classical pathway. Other circulating proteins of innate immunity are mannose-binding lectin and C-reactive protein, both of which coat microbes for phagocytosis. Lung surfactant is also a component of innate immunity, providing protection against inhaled microbes.

The early innate immune response not only provides the initial defense against infections but is also involved in triggering the subsequent, more powerful adaptive immune response.

ADAPTIVE IMMUNITY

The adaptive immune system consists of lymphocytes and their products, including antibodies. The receptors of lymphocytes are much more diverse than those of the innate immune system, but lymphocytes are not inherently specific for microbes, and they are capable of recognizing a vast array of foreign substances. In the remainder of this introductory section we focus on lymphocytes and the reactions of the adaptive immune system.

There are two types of adaptive immunity: humoral immunity, which protects against extracellular microbes and their toxins, and cell-mediated (or cellular) immunity, which is responsible for defense against intracellular microbes. Humoral immunity is mediated by B (bone marrow–derived) lymphocytes and their secreted products, antibodies (also called immunoglobulins, Ig), and cellular immunity is mediated by T (thymus-derived) lymphocytes. Both classes of lymphocytes express highly specific receptors for a wide variety of substances, called *antigens*.

COMPONENTS OF THE IMMUNE SYSTEM: CELLS, TISSUES, AND SELECTED MOLECULES

Before describing normal and pathologic immune responses, it is important to summarize the salient characteristics of some of the important participants in these responses.

Cells of the Immune System

Although lymphocytes appear morphologically unimpressive and similar to one another, they are actually remarkably heterogeneous and specialized in molecular properties and functions. The major classes of lymphocytes and their functions in adaptive immunity are illustrated in Figure 6–1. Lymphocytes and other cells involved in immune responses are not fixed in particular tissues (as are cells in most of the organs of the body) but are capable of migrating among lymphoid and other tissues and the vascular and lymphatic circulations. This feature permits lymphocytes to home to any site of infection. In lymphoid organs, different classes of lymphocytes are anatomically segregated in such a way that they interact with one another only when stimulated to do so by encounter with antigens and other stimuli. Mature lymphocytes that have not encountered the antigen for which they are specific are said to be *naive* (immunologically inexperienced). After they are activated by recognition of antigens and other signals described later, lymphocytes differentiate into *effector cells*, which perform the function of eliminating microbes, and *memory cells*, which live in a state of heightened awareness and are better able to combat the microbe in case it returns. The process of lymphocyte differentiation into effector and memory cells is summarized below.

T Lymphocytes

T lymphocytes develop from precursors in the thymus. Mature T cells are found in the blood, where they constitute 60% to 70% of lymphocytes, and in T-cell zones of peripheral lymphoid organs (described below). Each T cell recognizes a specific cell-bound antigen by means of an antigen-specific T-cell receptor (TCR).[2] In approximately 95% of T cells the TCR consists of a disulfide-linked heterodimer made up of an α and a β polypeptide chain (Fig. 6–2), each having a variable (antigen-binding) region and a constant region. *The αβ TCR recognizes peptide antigens that are displayed by major histocompatibility complex (MHC) molecules on the surfaces of antigen-presenting cells (APCs).* (The function of MHC proteins is described later.) By limiting the specificity of T cells for peptides displayed by cell surface MHC molecules, called MHC *restriction,* the immune system ensures that T cells see only cell-associated antigens (e.g., those derived from microbes in cells).

TCR diversity is generated by somatic rearrangement of the genes that encode the TCR α and β chains.[3] All cells of the body, including lymphocyte progenitors, contain TCR genes in the germ-line configuration, which cannot be expressed as TCR proteins. During T cell development in the thymus, the TCR genes rearrange to form many different combinations that can be transcribed and translated into functional antigen receptors. The enzyme in developing lymphocytes that mediates rearrangement of antigen receptor genes is the product of *RAG-1* and *RAG-2* (recombination activating genes); inherited defects in RAG proteins result in a failure to generate mature lymphocytes. Whereas each T cell expresses TCR molecules of one specificity, collectively, the full complement of T cells in an individual is capable of recognizing a very large number of antigens. It is important to note that unrearranged (germ-line) TCR genes are present in all non-T cells in the body, but only T cells contain rearranged TCR genes. Hence, the *presence of rearranged TCR genes, which can be demonstrated by molecular analysis, is a marker of T-lineage cells.* Furthermore, because each T cell and its clonal progeny have a unique DNA rearrangement (and hence a unique TCR), it is possible to distinguish polyclonal (non-neoplastic) T-cell proliferations from monoclonal (neoplastic) T-cell proliferations. Thus, *analysis of antigen receptor gene rearrangements is a valuable assay for detecting lymphoid tumors* (Chapter 13).

Each TCR is noncovalently linked to five polypeptide chains, which form the CD3 complex and the ζ chain dimer (see Fig. 6–2).[4] The CD3 and ζ proteins are invariant (i.e., identical) in all T cells. They are involved in the transduction of signals into the T cell after the TCR has bound the antigen. Together with the TCR, these proteins form the "TCR complex."

A small population of mature T cells expresses another type of TCR composed of γ and δ polypeptide chains.[5] The γδ TCR recognizes peptides, lipids, and small molecules, without a requirement for display by MHC proteins. γδ T cells tend to aggregate at epithelial surfaces, such as the skin and mucosa of the gastrointestinal and urogenital tracts, suggesting that these cells are sentinels that protect against microbes that try to enter through epithelia. However, the functions of γδ T cells are not known. Another small subset of T cells expresses markers that are found on NK cells; these cells are called NK-T cells.[6] NK-T cells express a very limited diversity of TCRs, and they recognize glycolipids that are displayed by the MHC-like molecule CD1. The functions of NK-T cells are also not well defined.

In addition to CD3 and ζ proteins, T cells express several other proteins that assist the TCR complex in functional responses. These include CD4, CD8, CD2, integrins, and CD28.[7] CD4 and CD8 are expressed on two mutually exclusive subsets of αβ T cells. CD4 is expressed on approximately 60% of mature CD3+ T cells, which function as cytokine-secreting helper cells that help macrophages and B lymphocytes to combat infections, whereas CD8 is expressed on about 30% of T cells, which function as cytotoxic (killer) T lymphocytes (CTLs) to destroy host cells harboring microbes. CD4 and CD8 serve as "coreceptors" in T-cell activation, so called because they work with the antigen receptor in responses to antigen. During antigen presentation, CD4 molecules bind to class II MHC molecules that are displaying antigen (see Fig. 6–2), and CD8 molecules bind to class I MHC molecules. When the antigen receptor of a T cell recognizes antigen, the CD4 or CD8 coreceptor initiates signals that are necessary for activation of the T cells. Because of this requirement for coreceptors, CD4+ helper T cells can recognize and respond to antigen displayed only by class II MHC molecules, whereas CD8+ cytotoxic T cells recognize cell-bound antigens only in association with class I MHC molecules; this segregation is described below.

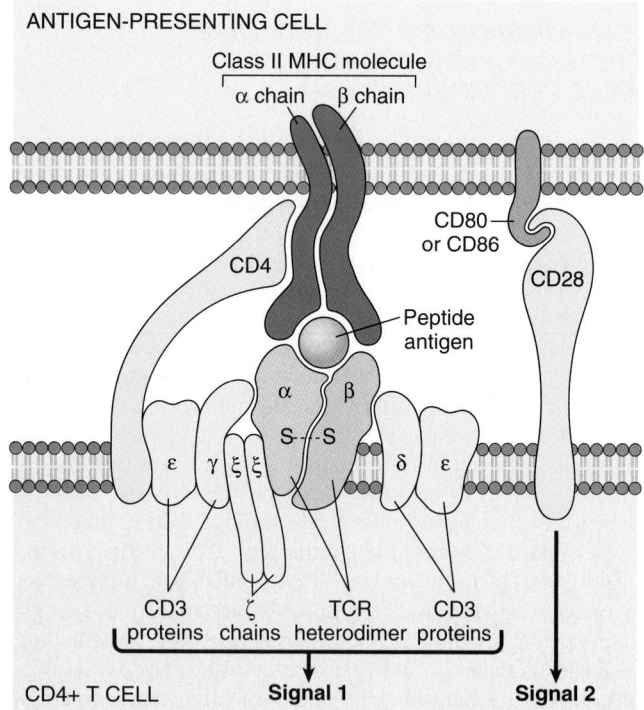

FIGURE 6–2 The T-cell receptor (TCR) complex and other molecules involved in T-cell activation. The TCR heterodimer, consisting of an α and a β chain, recognizes antigen (in the form of peptide-MHC complexes expressed on antigen-presenting cells, or APCs), and the linked CD3 complex and ζ chains initiate activating signals. CD4 and CD28 are also involved in T-cell activation. (Note that some T cells express CD8 and not CD4; these molecules serve analogous roles.) The sizes of the molecules are not drawn to scale. MHC, major histocompatibility complex.

To respond, T cells have to recognize not only antigen-MHC complexes but additional signals provided by APCs. We will describe these later, when we summarize the steps in cell-mediated immune responses.

B Lymphocytes

B lymphocytes develop from precursors in the bone marrow. Mature B cells constitute 10% to 20% of the circulating peripheral lymphocyte population and are also present in peripheral lymphoid tissues such as lymph nodes, spleen, and mucosa-associated lymphoid tissues. B cells recognize antigen via the B-cell antigen receptor complex. Membrane-bound antibodies called IgM and IgD, present on the surface of all mature, naive B cells, are the antigen-binding component of the B-cell receptor complex (Fig. 6–3). As with T cells, each B-cell receptor has a unique antigen specificity, derived from RAG-mediated

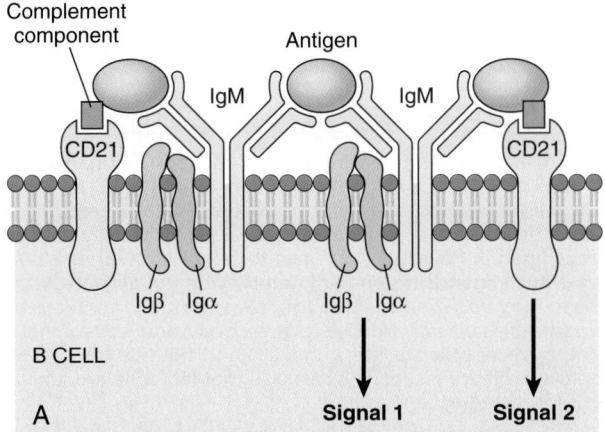

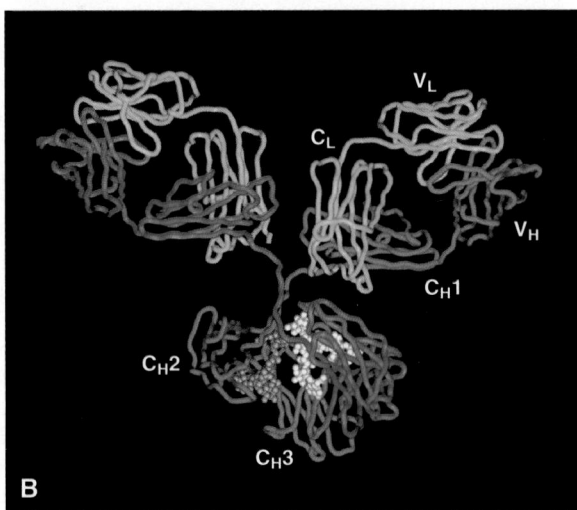

FIGURE 6–3   Structure of antibodies and the B-cell antigen receptor. **A,** The B-cell receptor complex is composed of membrane immunoglobulin M (IgM; or IgD, not shown), which recognize antigens, and the associated signaling proteins Igα and Igβ. CD21 is a receptor for a complement component that also promotes B-cell activation. **B,** Crystal structure of a secreted IgG molecule, showing the arrangement of the variable (V) and constant (C) regions of the heavy (H) and light (L) chains. (Courtesy of Dr. Alex McPherson, University of California, Irvine, CA.)

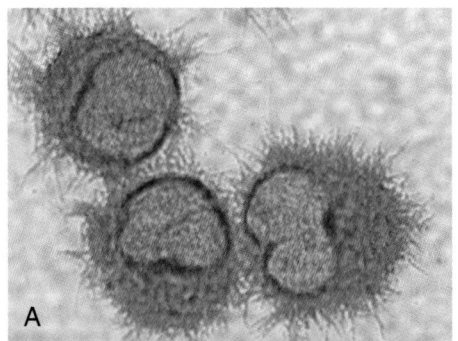

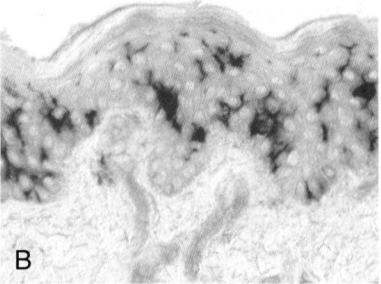

FIGURE 6–4   Dendritic cells. **A,** Cultured dendritic cells showing the prominent surface projections. **B,** The location of dendritic cells (Langerhans cells) in the epidermis (stained blue using an immunohistochemical method). (Courtesy of Dr. Y-J. Liu, M.D. Anderson Cancer Center, Houston, TX.)

rearrangements of Ig genes. Thus, as in T cells, *analysis of Ig gene rearrangements is useful for identifying monoclonal B-cell tumors.* After stimulation by antigen and other signals (described later), B cells develop into *plasma cells* that secrete antibodies, the mediators of humoral immunity. In addition to membrane Ig, the B-cell antigen receptor complex contains a heterodimer of two invariant proteins called Igα and Igβ. Similar to the CD3 and ζ proteins of the TCR complex, Igα and Igβ are essential for signal transduction through the antigen receptor. B cells also express several other molecules that are essential for their responses. These include complement receptors, Fc receptors, and CD40. The type 2 complement receptor (CR2, or CD21) is also the receptor for the Epstein-Barr virus (EBV), and hence EBV readily infects B cells.

Dendritic Cells

There are two types of cells with dendritic morphology that are functionally quite different. Both have numerous fine cytoplasmic processes that resemble dendrites, from which they derive their name. One type is called *interdigitating dendritic cells,* or just *dendritic cells* (Fig. 6–4).[8] These cells are the most important *antigen-presenting cells (APCs) for initiating primary T-cell responses against protein antigens* (described later). Several features of dendritic cells account for their key role in antigen presentation. First, these cells are located at the right place to capture antigens—under epithelia, the common site of entry of microbes and foreign antigens, and in the interstitia of all tissues, where antigens may be produced. Immature dendritic cells within the epidermis are called *Langerhans cells.* Second, dendritic cells express many receptors for capturing and responding to microbes (and other antigens), including TLRs and mannose receptors. Third, in response to microbes, dendritic cells are recruited to the T-cell zones of lymphoid organs, where they are ideally located to present antigens to T cells. Fourth, dendritic cells express high levels of the molecules needed for presenting antigens to and activating CD4+ T cells.

The other type of cell with dendritic morphology is present in the germinal centers of lymphoid follicles in the spleen and lymph nodes and is hence called *follicular dendritic cell*.[9] These cells bear Fc receptors for IgG and receptors for C3b and can trap antigen bound to antibodies or complement proteins. Such cells play a role in humoral immune responses by presenting antigens to B cells and selecting the B cells that have the highest affinity for the antigen, thus improving the quality of the antibody produced.

Macrophages

Macrophages are a part of the mononuclear phagocyte system; their origin, differentiation, and role in inflammation are discussed in Chapter 2. Here we need only to emphasize their important functions in the induction and effector phases of adaptive immune responses.

- Macrophages that have phagocytosed microbes and protein antigens process the antigens and present peptide fragments to T cells. Thus, macrophages function as APCs in T-cell activation.
- Macrophages are key effector cells in certain forms of cell-mediated immunity, the reaction that serves to eliminate intracellular microbes. In this type of response, T cells activate macrophages and enhance their ability to kill ingested microbes (discussed below).
- Macrophages also participate in the effector phase of humoral immunity. As discussed in Chapter 2, macrophages efficiently phagocytose and destroy microbes that are opsonized (coated) by IgG or C3b.

Natural Killer Cells

NK cells make up approximately 10% to 15% of peripheral blood lymphocytes. They do not express TCRs or Ig. Morphologically, NK cells are somewhat larger than small lymphocytes, and they contain abundant azurophilic granules; because of these characteristics, they are also called *large granular lymphocytes*. NK cells are endowed with the ability to kill a variety of infected and tumor cells, without prior exposure to or activation by these microbes or tumors. This ability makes NK cells an early line of defense against viral infections and, perhaps, some tumors. Two cell surface molecules, CD16 and CD56, are commonly used to identify NK cells. CD16 is an Fc receptor for IgG, and it confers on NK cells the ability to lyse IgG-coated target cells. This phenomenon is known as *antibody-dependent cell-mediated cytotoxicity (ADCC)*.

The functional activity of NK cells is regulated by a balance between signals from activating and inhibitory receptors[10] (Fig. 6–5). There are many types of activating receptors, of which the NKG2D family is the best characterized. The NKG2D receptors recognize surface molecules that are induced by various kinds of stress, such as infection and DNA damage.

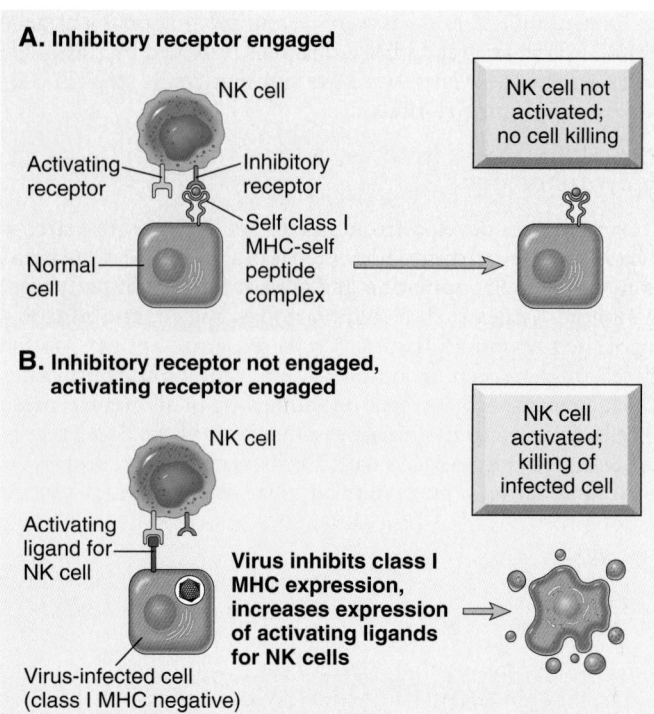

A. Inhibitory receptor engaged

NK cell

Activating receptor
Inhibitory receptor
Self class I MHC-self peptide complex
Normal cell

NK cell not activated; no cell killing

B. Inhibitory receptor not engaged, activating receptor engaged

NK cell

Activating ligand for NK cell

Virus inhibits class I MHC expression, increases expression of activating ligands for NK cells

Virus-infected cell (class I MHC negative)

NK cell activated; killing of infected cell

FIGURE 6–5 Activating and inhibitory receptors of natural killer (NK) cells. **A,** Healthy cells express self–class I MHC molecules, which are recognized by inhibitory receptors, thus ensuring that NK cells do not attack normal cells. Note that healthy cells may express ligands for activating receptors (not shown) or may not express such ligands (as shown), but they do not activate NK cells because they engage the inhibitory receptors. **B,** In infected and stressed cells, class I MHC expression is reduced so that the inhibitory receptors are not engaged, and ligands for activating receptors are expressed. The result is that NK cells are activated and the infected cells are killed.

NK cell inhibitory receptors recognize self–class I MHC molecules, which are expressed on all healthy cells. These receptors belong to two major families: killer cell Ig-like receptors and the CD94 family of lectins (carbohydrate-recognizing proteins). The inhibitory receptors prevent NK cells from killing normal cells. Virus infection or neoplastic transformation often induces expression of ligands for activating receptors and at the same time reduces the expression of class I MHC molecules. As a result the balance is tilted toward activation, and the infected or tumor cell is killed.

NK cells also secrete cytokines, such as interferon-γ (IFN-γ), which activates macrophages to destroy ingested microbes, and thus NK cells provide early defense against intracellular microbial infections. The activity of NK cells is regulated by many cytokines, including the interleukins IL-2, IL-15, and IL-12. IL-2 and IL-15 stimulate proliferation of NK cells, whereas IL-12 activates killing and secretion of IFN-γ.

Tissues of the Immune System

The tissues of the immune system consist of the generative (also called primary, or central) lymphoid organs, in which T and B lymphocytes mature and become competent to respond to antigens, and the peripheral (or secondary) lymphoid organs, in which adaptive immune responses to microbes are initiated.

Generative Lymphoid Organs

The principal generative lymphoid organs are the thymus, where T cells develop, and the bone marrow, the site of production of all blood cells and where B lymphocytes mature. These organs are described in Chapter 13.

Peripheral Lymphoid Organs

The peripheral lymphoid organs consist of the lymph nodes, spleen, and the mucosal and cutaneous lymphoid tissues. These tissues are organized to concentrate antigens, APCs, and lymphocytes in a way that optimizes interactions among these cells and the development of adaptive immune responses.

Lymph nodes are nodular aggregates of lymphoid tissues located along lymphatic channels throughout the body (Fig. 6–6). As lymph passes through lymph nodes, APCs in the nodes are able to sample the antigens of microbes that may enter through epithelia into tissues and are carried in the lymph. In addition, dendritic cells pick up and transport antigens of microbes from epithelia via the lymphatic vessels to the lymph nodes. Thus, the antigens of microbes that enter through epithelia or colonize tissues become concentrated in draining lymph nodes.

The *spleen* is an abdominal organ that serves the same role in immune responses to blood-borne antigen as that of lymph nodes in responses to lymph-borne antigens. Blood entering the spleen flows through a network of sinusoids. Blood-borne antigens are trapped by dendritic cells and macrophages in the spleen.

The cutaneous and mucosal lymphoid systems are located under the epithelia of the skin and the gastrointestinal and respiratory tracts, respectively. They respond to antigens that enter by breaches in the epithelium. Pharyngeal tonsils and Peyer's patches of the intestine are two anatomically defined mucosal lymphoid tissues. At any time, more than half the body's lymphocytes are in the mucosal tissues (reflecting the large size of these tissues), and many of these are memory cells.

Within the peripheral lymphoid organs, T lymphocytes and B lymphocytes are segregated into different regions (see Fig. 6–6). In lymph nodes the B cells are concentrated in discrete structures, called *follicles*, located around the periphery, or cortex, of each node. If the B cells in a follicle have recently responded to an antigen, this follicle may contain a central region called a *germinal center*. The T lymphocytes are concentrated in the paracortex, adjacent to the follicles. The follicles contain the follicular dendritic cells that are involved in the activation of B cells, and the paracortex contains the dendritic cells that present antigens to T lymphocytes. In the spleen, T lymphocytes are concentrated in periarteriolar lymphoid sheaths surrounding small arterioles, and B cells reside in the follicles.

The anatomic organization of peripheral lymphoid organs is tightly regulated to allow immune responses to develop.[11–13] The location of B cells and T cells in the lymphoid follicles and paracortical areas, respectively, is dictated by chemokines

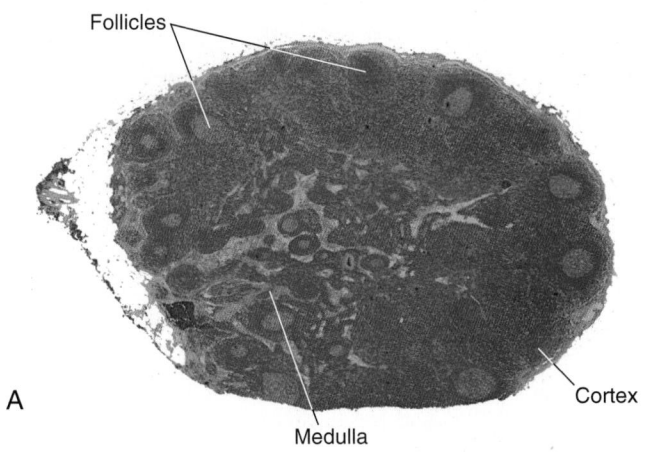

A

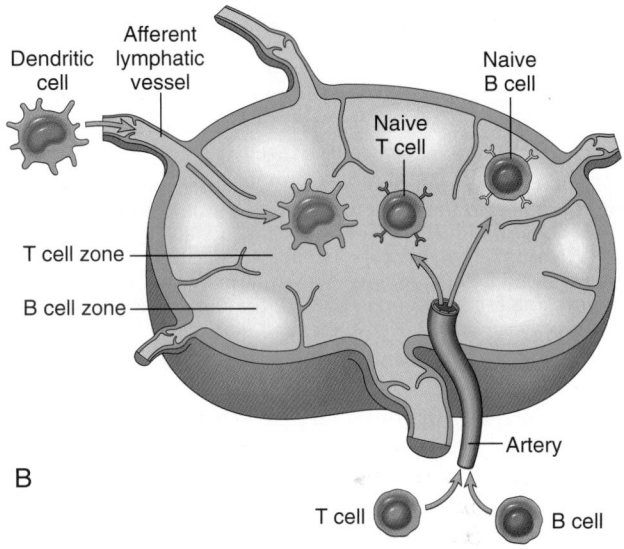

B

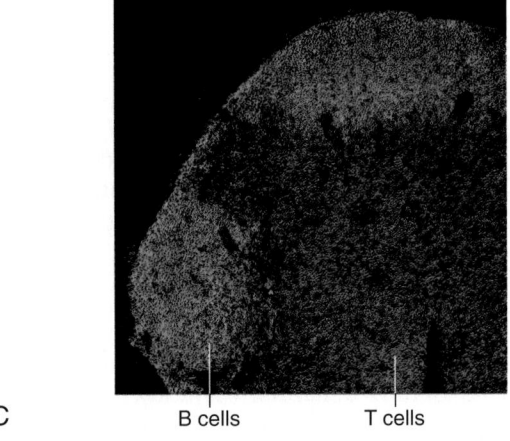

C

FIGURE 6–6 Morphology of a lymph node. **A,** The histology of a lymph node, with an outer cortex containing follicles and an inner medulla. **B,** The segregation of B cells and T cells in different regions of the lymph node, illustrated schematically. **C,** The location of B cells (stained green, using the immunofluorescence technique) and T cells (stained red) in a lymph node. (Courtesy of Drs. Kathryn Pape and Jennifer Walter, University of Minnesota School of Medicine, Minneapolis, MN.)

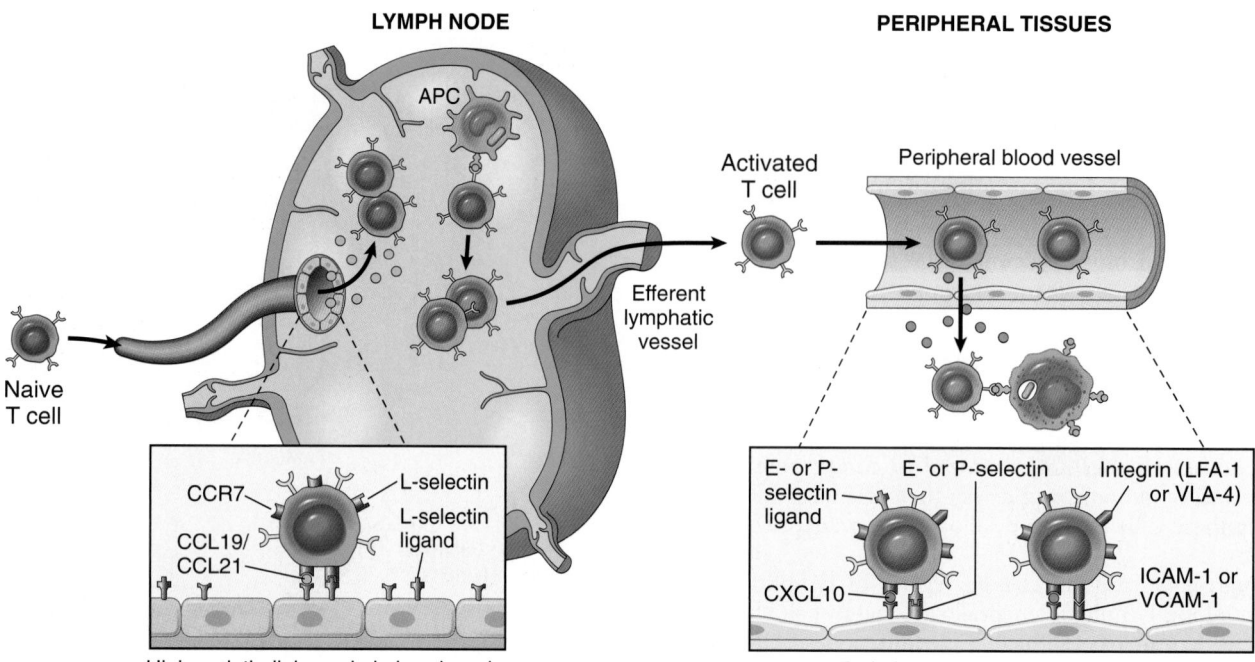

LYMPH NODE

PERIPHERAL TISSUES

High endothelial venule in lymph node

Endothelium at the site of infection

FIGURE 6–7 Migration of naive and effector T lymphocytes. Naive T lymphocytes home to lymph nodes as a result of L-selectin and integrin binding to their ligands on high endothelial venules (HEVs). Chemokines expressed in lymph nodes (called CCL19 and CCL21) bind to receptors (CCR7) on naive T cells, enhancing integrin-dependent adhesion and inducing migration of the cells through the HEV wall. Activated T lymphocytes, including effector and memory cells, home to sites of infection in peripheral tissues, and this migration is mediated by E-selectin and P-selectin, integrins, and chemokines secreted at inflammatory sites (e.g., CXCL10) that are recognized by chemokine receptors (e.g., CXCR3) that are expressed on activated T cells. APC, antigen-presenting cell; ICAM-1, intercellular adhesion molecule 1; VCAM-1, vascular cell adhesion molecule 1.

produced in these anatomic locales. When the lymphocytes are activated by antigens they alter their expression of chemokine receptors. As a result, the B cells and T cells leave their homes, migrate toward each other and meet at the edge of follicles, where helper T cells interact with and help B cells to differentiate into antibody-producing cells.

Lymphocyte Recirculation

Lymphocytes constantly recirculate between tissues and home to particular sites; naive lymphocytes traverse the peripheral lymphoid organs where immune responses are initiated, and effector lymphocytes migrate to sites of infection and inflammation[14] (Fig. 6–7). This process of lymphocyte recirculation is most relevant for T cells, because effector T cells have to locate and eliminate microbes at any site of infection. By contrast, plasma cells remain in lymphoid organs and do not need to migrate to sites of infection because they secrete antibodies that are carried to distant tissues. Therefore, we will limit our discussion of lymphocyte recirculation to T lymphocytes.

Naive T lymphocytes that have exited the thymus migrate to lymph nodes and enter the T-cell zones through specialized postcapillary venules, called *high endothelial venules (HEVs)* (see Fig. 6–7). In the lymph node, a naive T cell may encounter the antigen that it specifically recognizes on the surface of an APC and is activated. During this process, the cells alter their expression of adhesion molecules and chemokine receptors. Differentiated effector T cells ultimately leave the lymph nodes, enter the circulation, and migrate into the tissues that harbor the microbes.

Major Histocompatibility Complex (MHC) Molecules: Peptide Display System of Adaptive Immunity

Because MHC molecules are fundamental to the recognition of antigens by T cells and are linked to many autoimmune diseases, it is important to briefly review the structure and function of these molecules.[15] MHC molecules were discovered as products of genes that evoke rejection of transplanted organs, and their name derives from the recognition that they are responsible for tissue compatibility between individuals. *The physiologic function of MHC molecules is to display peptide fragments of proteins for recognition by antigen-specific T cells.*[16] In humans the genes encoding the major histocompatibility molecules are clustered on a small segment of chromosome 6, the *major histocompatibility complex,* or the *human leukocyte antigen* (HLA) complex (Fig. 6–8), so named because in humans MHC-encoded proteins were initially detected on leukocytes by the binding of antibodies. The HLA system is highly polymorphic, meaning that there are many alleles of each MHC gene in the population and each individual inherits one set of these alleles that is different from the alleles in most other individuals. This, as we see subsequently, constitutes a formidable barrier in organ transplantation.

On the basis of their structure, cellular distribution, and function, MHC gene products are classified into three groups.

○ *Class I MHC molecules* are expressed on all nucleated cells and platelets. They are encoded by three closely linked loci,

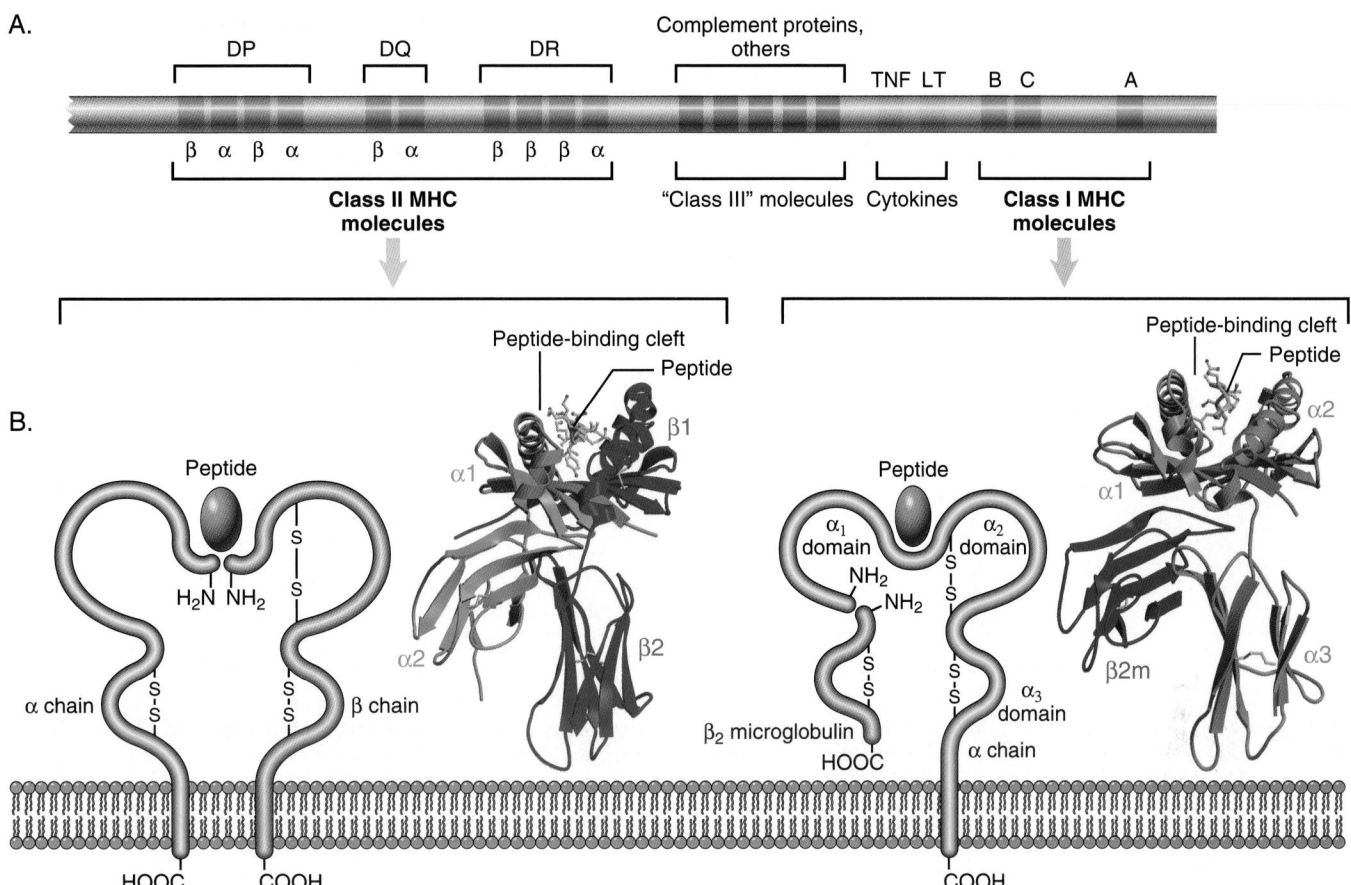

FIGURE 6–8 The human leukocyte antigen (HLA) complex and the structure of HLA molecules. **A,** The location of genes in the HLA complex. The relative locations, sizes, and distances between genes are not to scale. Genes that encode several proteins involved in antigen processing (the TAP transporter, components of the proteasome, and HLA-DM) are located in the class II region (not shown). **B,** Schematic diagrams and crystal structures of class I and class II HLA molecules. (Crystal structures are courtesy of Dr. P. Bjorkman, California Institute of Technology, Pasadena, CA.)

designated *HLA-A, HLA-B,* and *HLA-C* (see Fig. 6–9). Each class I MHC molecule is a heterodimer consisting of a polymorphic α, or heavy, chain (44-kD) linked noncovalently to a smaller (12-kD) nonpolymorphic peptide called β2-microglobulin, which is not encoded within the MHC. The extracellular region of the α chain is divided into three domains: α1, α2, and α3. Crystal structure of class I molecules has revealed that the α1 and α2 domains form a cleft, or groove, where peptides bind.[16] The polymorphic residues line the sides and the base of the peptide-binding groove; the variation in this region explains why different class I alleles bind different peptides.

Class I MHC molecules display peptides that are derived from proteins, such as viral antigens, that are located in the cytoplasm and usually produced in the cell, and class I–associated peptides are recognized by CD8+ T lymphocytes (Fig. 6–9A). Cytoplasmic proteins are degraded in proteasomes and peptides are transported into the endoplasmic reticulum (ER) where the peptides bind to newly synthesized class I molecules.[17] Peptide-loaded MHC molecules associate with β2-microglobulin to form a stable trimer that is transported to the cell surface. The nonpolymorphic α3 domain of class I MHC molecules has a binding site for CD8, and therefore the peptide–class I complexes are rec-

ognized by CD8+ T cells, which function as CTLs. In this interaction, the TCR recognizes the MHC-peptide complex, and the CD8 molecule, acting as a coreceptor, binds to the class I heavy chain. Thus, CD8+ cytotoxic T cells recognize peptides that are produced by cytoplasmic microbes (typically viruses) or in tumors and kill cells harboring these infections or the tumor cells. Since CD8+ T cells recognize peptides only if presented as a complex with self–class I MHC molecules, CD8+ T cells are said to be *class I MHC–restricted*. Because one of the important functions of CD8+ CTLs is to eliminate viruses, which may infect any nucleated cell, it makes good sense that all nucleated cells express class I HLA molecules and can be surveyed by CD8+ T cells.

○ *Class II MHC molecules* are encoded in a region called *HLA-D,* which has three subregions: *HLA-DP, HLA-DQ,* and *HLA-DR.* Each class II molecule is a heterodimer consisting of a noncovalently associated α chain and β chain, both of which are polymorphic. The extracellular portions of the α and β chains have two domains each: α1, α2 and β1, β2. Crystal structure of class II molecules has revealed that, similar to class I molecules, they have peptide-binding clefts facing outward[16] (see Fig. 6–8). This cleft is formed by an interaction of the α1 and β1 domains, and it

A. CLASS I MHC PATHWAY   **B. CLASS II MHC PATHWAY**

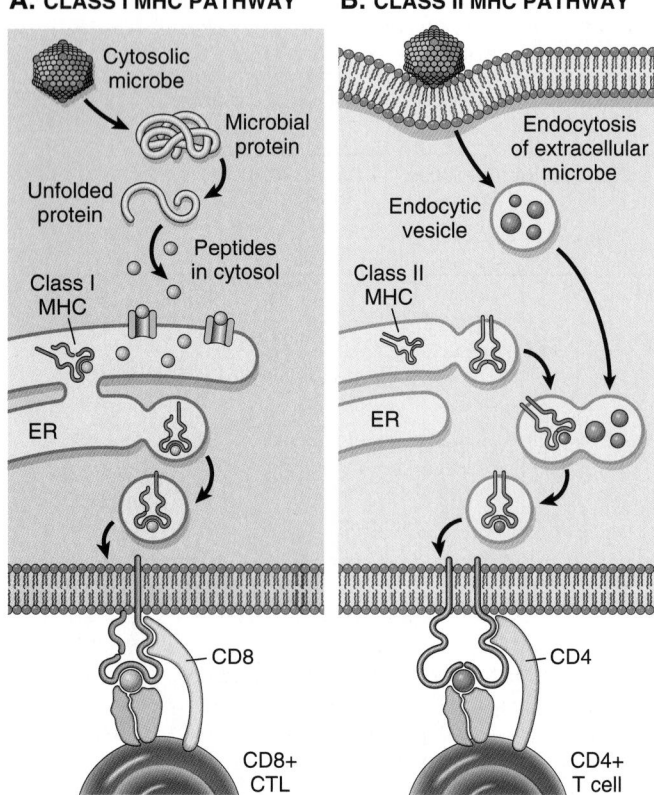

FIGURE 6–9   Antigen processing and display by major histocompatibility complex (MHC) molecules. **A,** In the class I MHC pathway, peptides are produced from proteins in the cytosol and transported to the endoplasmic reticulum (ER), where they bind to class I MHC molecules. The peptide-MHC complexes are transported to the cell surface and displayed for recognition by CD8+ T cells. **B,** In the class II MHC pathway, proteins are ingested into vesicles and degraded into peptides, which bind to class II MHC molecules being transported in the same vesicles. The class II–peptide complexes are expressed on the cell surface and recognized by CD4+ T cells.

is in this portion that most class II alleles differ. Thus, as with class I molecules, polymorphism of class II molecules is associated with differential binding of antigenic peptides.

Class II MHC molecules present antigens that are internalized into vesicles, and are typically derived from extracellular microbes and soluble proteins (Fig. 6–9B). The internalized proteins are proteolytically digested in endosomes or lysosomes. Peptides resulting from proteolytic cleavage then associate with class II heterodimers in the vesicles, and the stable peptide-MHC complexes are transported to the cell surface. The class II β2 domain has a binding site for CD4, and therefore, the class II–peptide complex is recognized by CD4+ T cells, which function as helper cells. In this interaction, the CD4 molecule acts as the co-receptor. Because CD4+ T cells can recognize antigens only in the context of self–class II molecules, they are referred to as *class II MHC–restricted.* In contrast to class I molecules, class II MHC molecules are mainly expressed on cells that present ingested antigens and respond to T-cell help (macrophages, B lymphocytes, and dendritic cells).

The MHC locus also contains genes that encode some complement components and the cytokines tumor necrosis factor (TNF) and lymphotoxin, as well as some proteins that have no apparent role in the immune system. The class II locus contains genes that encode many proteins involved in antigen processing and presentation, such as components of the proteasome, peptide transporter, and a class II–like molecule called DM that facilitates peptide binding to class II molecules.

The combination of HLA alleles in each individual is called the *HLA haplotype.* Any given individual inherits one set of HLA genes from each parent and thus typically expresses two different molecules for every locus. Because of the polymorphism of the HLA loci, virtually innumerable combinations of molecules exist in the population, and each individual expresses an MHC profile on his or her cell surface that is different from the haplotypes of most other individuals. It is believed that this polymorphism evolved to ensure that at least some individuals in a species would be able to display any microbial peptide and thus provide protection against any infection. The same polymorphism means that no two individuals (other than identical twins) are likely to express the same MHC molecules, and therefore grafts exchanged between these individuals are recognized as foreign and attacked by the immune system.

MHC molecules play key roles in regulating T cell–mediated immune responses in several ways. First, because different antigenic peptides bind to different MHC molecules, it follows that an individual mounts an immune response against a protein antigen only if he or she inherits the gene(s) for those MHC molecule(s) that can bind peptides derived from the antigen and present it to T cells. The consequences of inheriting a given MHC (e.g., class II) gene depend on the nature of the antigen bound by the class II molecule. For example, if the antigen is a peptide from ragweed pollen, the individual who expresses class II molecules capable of binding the antigen would be genetically prone to allergic reactions against pollen. In contrast, an inherited capacity to bind a bacterial peptide may provide resistance to the infection by evoking a protective antibody response. Second, by segregating cytoplasmic and internalized antigens, MHC molecules ensure that the correct immune response is mounted against different microbes—CTLs against cytoplasmic microbes, and antibodies and macrophages (both of which are activated by helper T cells) against extracellular microbes.

HLA and Disease Association

A variety of diseases are associated with the inheritance of certain HLA alleles (Table 6–1).[18] The most striking of these is the association between ankylosing spondylitis and *HLA-B27*; individuals who inherit this class I HLA allele have a 90-fold greater chance (relative risk) of developing the disease as compared with those who do not carry *HLA-B27*. The diseases that show association with the HLA locus can be broadly grouped into the following categories:

1. *Inflammatory diseases,* including ankylosing spondylitis and several postinfectious arthropathies, all associated with *HLA-B27*

TABLE 6–1   Association of HLA Alleles and Inflammatory Diseases

Disease	HLA Allele	Relative Risk (%)
Ankylosing spondylitis	B27	90–100
Postgonococcal arthritis	B27	14
Acute anterior uveitis	B27	14
Rheumatoid arthritis	DR4	4
Chronic active hepatitis	DR3	13
Primary Sjögren syndrome	DR3	9
Type 1 diabetes	DR3	5
	DR4	6
	DR3/DR4	20

2. *Autoimmune diseases*, including autoimmune endocrinopathies, associated mainly with alleles at the *DR* locus

3. *Inherited errors of metabolism*, such as 21-hydroxylase deficiency (*HLA-BW47*) and hereditary hemochromatosis (*HLA-A*)

The mechanisms underlying these associations are not fully understood. In the immunological and inflammatory diseases, the inheritance of particular HLA alleles likely influences the T-cell response, but it has proved difficult to define precisely how. In some cases (e.g., 21-hydroxylase deficiency), the linkage results because the relevant disease-associated gene, in this case the gene for 21-hydroxylase, maps within the HLA complex. Similarly, in hereditary hemochromatosis, a gene that is mutated, called *HFE*, maps within the HLA locus. The HFE protein resembles MHC molecules structurally, but its function is in the regulation of iron transport (Chapter 18).

Cytokines: Messenger Molecules of the Immune System

The induction and regulation of immune responses involve multiple interactions among lymphocytes, dendritic cells, macrophages, other inflammatory cells (e.g., neutrophils), and endothelial cells. Some of these interactions depend on cell-to-cell contact; however, many interactions and effector functions of leukocytes are mediated by short-acting secreted mediators called *cytokines*. Molecularly defined cytokines are called *interleukins*, because they mediate communications between leukocytes. Most cytokines have a wide spectrum of effects, and some are produced by several different cell types.

It is convenient to classify cytokines into distinct functional classes, although many belong to multiple categories.

- *Cytokines of innate immunity* are produced rapidly in response to microbes and other stimuli, are made principally by macrophages, dendritic cells, and NK cells, and mediate inflammation and anti-viral defense; these include TNF, IL-1, IL-12, type I IFNs, IFN-γ, and chemokines (Chapter 2).
- *Cytokines of adaptive immune responses* are made principally by CD4+ T lymphocytes in response to antigen and other signals, and function to promote lymphocyte proliferation and differentiation and to activate effector cells. The main ones in this group are IL-2, IL-4, IL-5, IL-17, and IFN-γ; their roles in immune responses are described below.

- Some cytokines stimulate hematopoiesis and are called *colony-stimulating factors* because they are assayed by their ability to stimulate formation of blood cell colonies from bone marrow progenitors (Chapter 13). Their functions are to increase leukocyte numbers during immune and inflammatory responses, and to replace leukocytes that are consumed during such responses.

The knowledge gained about cytokines has numerous practical therapeutic applications. Inhibiting cytokine production or actions is an approach for controlling the harmful effects of inflammation and tissue-damaging immune reactions. Patients with rheumatoid arthritis often show dramatic responses to TNF antagonists, an elegant example of rationally designed and molecularly targeted therapy. Conversely, recombinant cytokines can be administered to enhance immunity against cancer or microbial infections (immunotherapy).

OVERVIEW OF LYMPHOCYTE ACTIVATION AND IMMUNE RESPONSES

All adaptive immune responses develop in steps, consisting of: antigen recognition, activation of specific lymphocytes to proliferate and differentiate into effector and memory cells, elimination of the antigen, and decline of the response, with memory cells being the long-lived survivors. The major events in each step are summarized below; these general principles apply to protective responses against microbes as well as pathologic responses that injure the host.

The Display and Recognition of Antigens

Lymphocytes specific for a large number of antigens exist before exposure to the antigen, and when an antigen enters, it selects the specific cells and activates them. This fundamental concept is called the *clonal selection hypothesis*. According to this hypothesis, antigen-specific clones of lymphocytes develop before and independent of exposure to antigen. The cells constituting each clone have identical antigen receptors, which are different from the receptors on the cells of all other clones. It is estimated that there are about 10^7 to 10^9 different specificities in the total pool of about 10^{12} lymphocytes in an adult, and therefore, at least this many antigens can be recognized by the adaptive immune system. It follows that the number of lymphocytes specific for any one antigen is very small, probably less than 1 in 100,000 to 1 in 1 million cells. To permit a small number of lymphocytes to find antigen anywhere in the body, the immune system has specialized mechanisms for capturing antigens and displaying them to lymphocytes. Microbes and their protein antigens are captured by dendritic cells that are resident in epithelia and tissues. These cells carry their antigenic cargo to draining lymph nodes (Fig. 6–10).[19] Here the antigens are processed and displayed complexed with MHC molecules on the cell surface (see Fig. 6–9).

B lymphocytes use their antigen receptors (membrane-bound antibody molecules) to recognize antigens of many different chemical types, including proteins, polysaccharides, and lipids.

At the same time as the antigens of a microbe are recognized by T and B lymphocytes, the microbe elicits an innate immune response; in the case of immunization with a protein antigen,

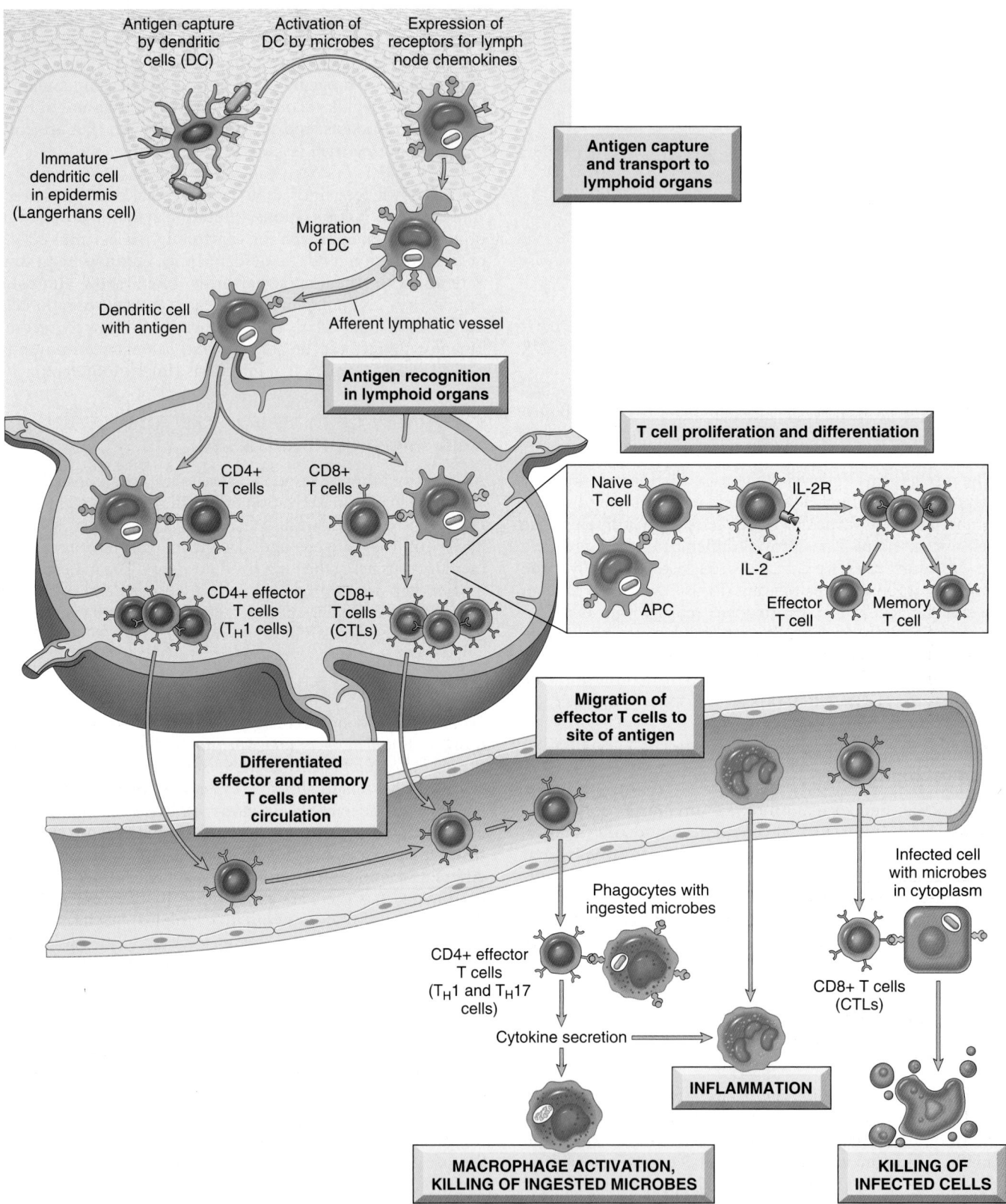

FIGURE 6–10 Cell-mediated immunity. Dendritic cells (DCs) capture microbial antigens from epithelia and tissues and transport the antigens to lymph nodes. During this process, the DCs mature, and express high levels of MHC molecules and costimulators. Naive T cells recognize MHC-associated peptide antigens displayed on DCs. The T cells are activated to proliferate and to differentiate into effector and memory cells, which migrate to sites of infection and serve various functions in cell-mediated immunity. CD4+ effector T cells of the T$_H$1 subset recognize the antigens of microbes ingested by phagocytes, and activate the phagocytes to kill the microbes. CD4+ T cells also induce inflammation. CD8+ cytotoxic T lymphocytes (CTLs) kill infected cells harboring microbes in the cytoplasm. Not shown are T$_H$2 cells, which are especially important in defense against helminthic infections. Some activated T cells differentiate into long-lived memory cells. APC, antigen-presenting cell.

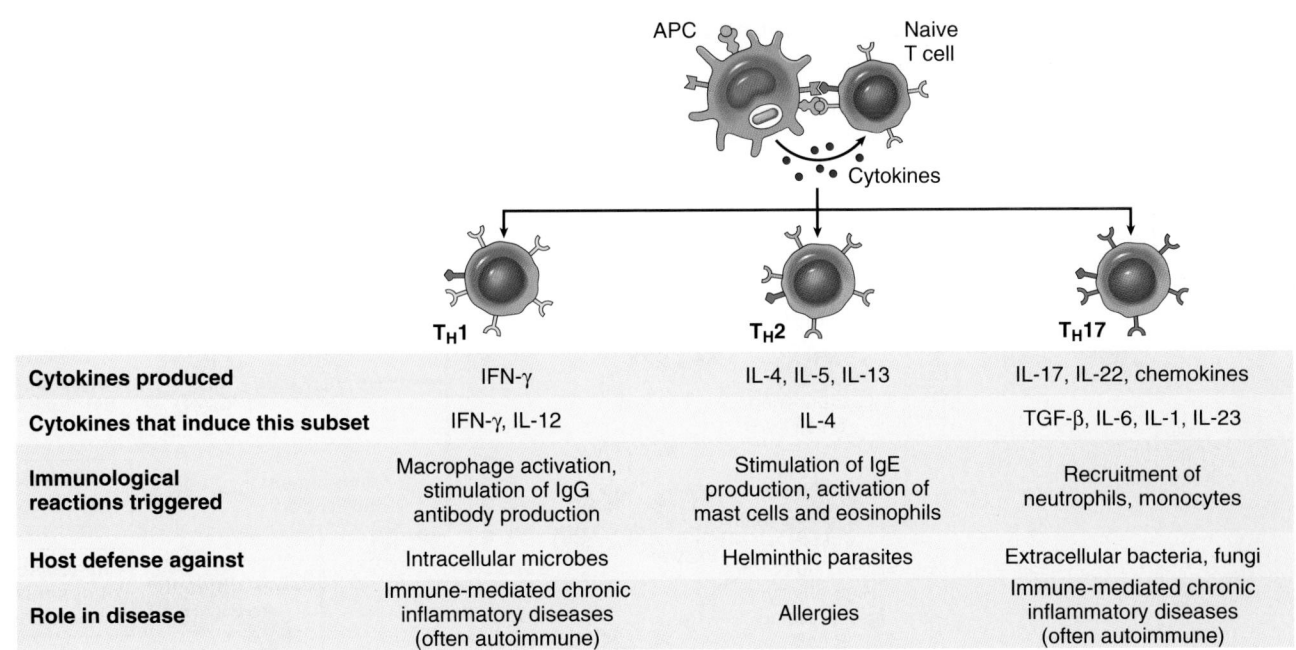

	TH1	TH2	TH17
Cytokines produced	IFN-γ	IL-4, IL-5, IL-13	IL-17, IL-22, chemokines
Cytokines that induce this subset	IFN-γ, IL-12	IL-4	TGF-β, IL-6, IL-1, IL-23
Immunological reactions triggered	Macrophage activation, stimulation of IgG antibody production	Stimulation of IgE production, activation of mast cells and eosinophils	Recruitment of neutrophils, monocytes
Host defense against	Intracellular microbes	Helminthic parasites	Extracellular bacteria, fungi
Role in disease	Immune-mediated chronic inflammatory diseases (often autoimmune)	Allergies	Immune-mediated chronic inflammatory diseases (often autoimmune)

FIGURE 6–11 Subsets of helper T (T$_H$) cells. In response to stimuli (mainly cytokines) present at the time of antigen recognition, naive CD4+ T$_H$ cells may differentiate into populations of effector cells that produce distinct sets of cytokines and perform different functions. The dominant immune reactions elicited by each subset, and its role in host defense and immunological diseases, are summarized.

the innate response is induced by the adjuvant given with the antigen. During this innate response the microbe activates APCs to express molecules called *costimulators* and to secrete cytokines that stimulate the proliferation and differentiation of T lymphocytes. The principal costimulators for T cells are the B7 proteins (CD80 and CD86) that are expressed on APCs and are recognized by the CD28 receptor on naive T cells.[20] Thus, antigen ("signal 1") and costimulatory molecules produced during innate immune responses to microbes ("signal 2") function cooperatively to activate antigen-specific lymphocytes (see Fig. 6–3). The requirement for microbe-triggered signal 2 ensures that the adaptive immune response is induced by microbes and not by harmless substances. In immune responses to tumors and transplants, "signal 2" may be provided by substances released from necrotic cells (the "danger-associated molecular patterns" mentioned earlier).

The reactions and functions of T and B lymphocytes differ in important ways and are best considered separately.

Cell-Mediated Immunity: Activation of T Lymphocytes and Elimination of Intracellular Microbes

Naive T lymphocytes are activated by antigen and costimulators in peripheral lymphoid organs, and proliferate and differentiate into effector cells that migrate to any site where the antigen (microbe) is present (see Fig. 6–10). One of the earliest responses of CD4+ helper T cells is secretion of the cytokine IL-2 and expression of high-affinity receptors for IL-2. IL-2 is a growth factor that acts on these T lymphocytes and stimulates their proliferation, leading to an increase in the number of antigen-specific lymphocytes. The functions of helper T cells are mediated by the combined actions of CD40-ligand (CD40L) and cytokines. When CD4+ helper T cells recognize antigens being displayed by macrophages or B lymphocytes, the T cells express

CD40L, which engages CD40 on the macrophages or B cells and activates these cells.

Some of the progeny of the expanded T cells differentiate into effector cells that can secrete different sets of cytokines, and thus perform different functions (Fig. 6–11).[21] The best defined subsets of differentiated CD4+ helper cells are the T$_H$1 and T$_H$2 subsets. Cells of the T$_H$1 subset secrete the cytokine IFN-γ, which is a potent macrophage activator. The combination of CD40- and IFN-γ–mediated activation results in the induction of microbicidal substances in macrophages, leading to the destruction of ingested microbes. T$_H$2 cells produce IL-4, which stimulates B cells to differentiate into IgE-secreting plasma cells, and IL-5, which activates eosinophils. Eosinophils and mast cells bind to IgE-coated microbes such as helminthic parasites, and function to eliminate helminths. A third subset of CD4+ T cells that has been discovered recently is called the T$_H$17 subset because the signature cytokine of these cells is IL-17.[22,23] T$_H$17 cells are powerful recruiters of neutrophils and monocytes, and thus play major roles in several inflammatory diseases. They may also be important for defense against some bacterial and fungal infections in which neutrophilic inflammation is a prominent feature. We will return to the generation and functions of these subsets when we discuss hypersensitivity reactions.

Activated CD8+ lymphocytes differentiate into CTLs that kill cells harboring microbes in the cytoplasm. By destroying the infected cells, CTLs eliminate the reservoirs of infection.

Humoral Immunity: Activation of B Lymphocytes and Elimination of Extracellular Microbes

Upon activation, B lymphocytes proliferate and then differentiate into plasma cells that secrete different classes of antibodies with distinct functions (Fig. 6–12). Many

B Lymphocyte activation

Effector functions of secreted antibodies

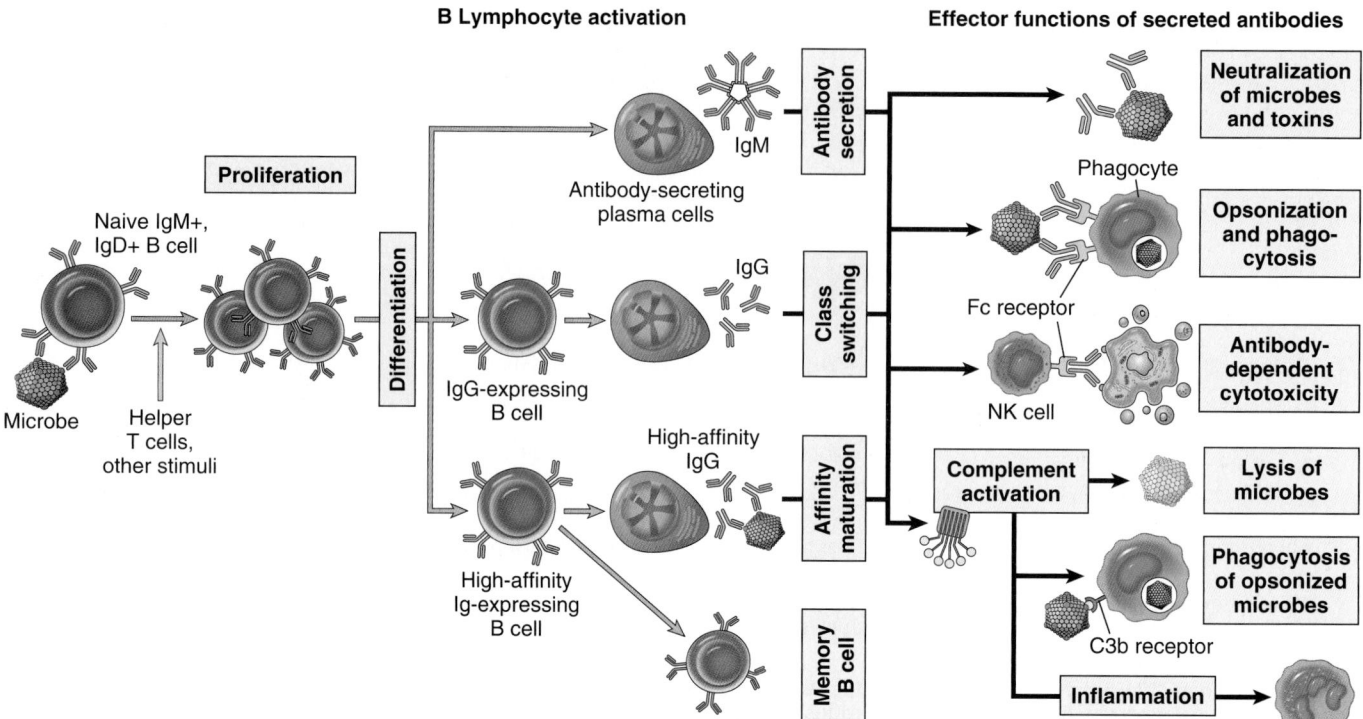

FIGURE 6–12 Humoral immunity. Naive B lymphocytes recognize antigens, and under the influence of T_H cells and other stimuli (not shown), the B cells are activated to proliferate and to differentiate into antibody-secreting plasma cells. Some of the activated B cells undergo heavy-chain class switching and affinity maturation, and some become long-lived memory cells. Antibodies of different heavy-chain classes (isotypes) perform different effector functions, shown on the right. See text for abbreviations.

polysaccharide and lipid antigens have multiple identical antigenic determinants (epitopes) that are able to engage many antigen receptor molecules on each B cell and initiate the process of B-cell activation. Typical globular protein antigens are not able to bind to many antigen receptors, and the full response of B cells to protein antigens requires help from CD4+ T cells.[24] B cells ingest protein antigens into vesicles, degrade them, and display peptides bound to MHC molecules for recognition by helper T cells. The helper T cells express CD40L and secrete cytokines, which work together to activate the B cells.

Each plasma cell secretes antibodies that have the same antigen binding site as the cell surface antibodies (B-cell receptors) that first recognized the antigen. Polysaccharides and lipids stimulate secretion mainly of IgM antibody. Protein antigens, by virtue of CD40L- and cytokine-mediated helper T-cell actions, induce the production of antibodies of different classes, or isotypes (IgG, IgA, IgE). Cytokines that induce isotype switching include IFN-γ and IL-4. Helper T cells also stimulate the production of antibodies with high affinities for the antigen. This process, called *affinity maturation*, improves the quality of the humoral immune response. Isotype switching and affinity maturation occur mainly in germinal centers, which are formed by proliferating B cells, especially in helper T cell-dependent responses to protein antigens.

The humoral immune response combats microbes in many ways (see Fig. 6–12). Antibodies bind to microbes and prevent them from infecting cells, thus "neutralizing" the microbes. IgG antibodies coat ("opsonize") microbes and target them for phagocytosis, since phagocytes (neutrophils and macro-

phages) express receptors for the Fc tails of IgG. IgG and IgM activate the complement system by the classical pathway, and complement products promote phagocytosis and destruction of microbes. The production of most opsonizing and complement-fixing IgG antibodies is stimulated by T_H1 helper cells, which respond to many bacteria and viruses; thus, the protective response to most bacteria and viruses is driven by T_H1 cells. Some antibodies serve special roles at particular anatomic sites. IgA is secreted from mucosal epithelia and neutralizes microbes in the lumens of the respiratory and gastrointestinal tracts (and other mucosal tissues). IgG is actively transported across the placenta and protects the newborn until the immune system becomes mature. IgE and eosinophils cooperate to kill parasites, mainly by release of eosinophil granule contents that are toxic to the worms. As mentioned above, T_H2 cells secrete cytokines that stimulate the production of IgE and activate eosinophils, and thus the response to helminths is orchestrated by T_H2 cells.

Most circulating IgG antibodies have half-lives of about 3 weeks. Some antibody-secreting plasma cells migrate to the bone marrow and live for years, continuing to produce low levels of antibodies.

Decline of Immune Responses and Immunological Memory

The majority of effector lymphocytes induced by an infectious pathogen die by apoptosis after the microbe is eliminated, thus returning the immune system to its basal resting state, called homeostasis. The initial activation of lymphocytes also generates long-lived *memory cells*, which may survive for years after the infection. Memory cells are an expanded pool of antigen-specific lymphocytes (more numerous than the naive cells specific for any antigen that are present before encounter with that antigen), and that respond faster and more effectively when re-exposed to the antigen than do naive cells.[25] This is why the generation of memory cells is an important goal of vaccination.

The brief outline of basic immunology presented above provides a foundation for considering the diseases of the immune system. Our subsequent discussion will be divided into disorders caused by an abnormally active immune system, called *hypersensitivity disorders*, and the rejection of transplants, followed by diseases caused by a defective immune system, called *immunodeficiency diseases*. We close with a consideration of amyloidosis, a disorder that is often associated with immune and inflammatory diseases.

Hypersensitivity and Autoimmune Disorders

Before discussing specific immunological diseases, we start with a summary of the general mechanisms of hypersensitivity.

MECHANISMS OF HYPERSENSITIVITY REACTIONS

Individuals who have been previously exposed to an antigen are said to be sensitized. Sometimes, repeat exposures to the same antigen trigger a pathologic reaction; such reactions are described as *hypersensitivity*, implying an excessive response to antigen. There are several important general features of hypersensitivity disorders.

- *Both exogenous and endogenous antigens may elicit hypersensitivity reactions.* Humans live in an environment teeming with substances capable of eliciting immune responses. Exogenous antigens include those in dust, pollens, foods, drugs, microbes, chemicals, and some blood products that are used in clinical practice. The immune responses against such exogenous antigens may take a variety of forms, ranging from annoying but trivial discomforts, such as itching of the skin, to potentially fatal diseases, such as bronchial asthma and anaphylaxis. Injurious immune reactions may also be evoked by endogenous tissue antigens. Immune responses against self, or autologous, antigens, cause the important group of *autoimmune diseases*.
- *The development of hypersensitivity diseases (both allergic and autoimmune disorders) is often associated with the inheritance of particular susceptibility genes.* HLA genes and many non-HLA genes have been implicated in different diseases; specific examples will be described in the context of the diseases.
- A general principle that has emerged is that *hypersensitivity reflects an imbalance between the effector mechanisms of immune responses and the control mechanisms that serve to normally limit such responses.* We will return to this concept when we consider autoimmunity.

Hypersensitivity diseases can be classified on the basis of the immunologic mechanism that mediates the disease (Table 6–2). This classification is of value in distinguishing the manner in which the immune response causes tissue injury

TABLE 6–2	Mechanisms of Immunologically Mediated Hypersensitivity Reactions		
Type of Reaction	**Prototypic Disorder**	**Immune Mechanisms**	**Pathologic Lesions**
Immediate (type I) hypersensitivity	Anaphylaxis; allergies; bronchial asthma (atopic forms)	Production of IgE antibody → immediate release of vasoactive amines and other mediators from mast cells; later recruitment of inflammatory cells	Vascular dilation, edema, smooth muscle contraction, mucus production, tissue injury, inflammation
Antibody-mediated (type II) hypersensitivity	Autoimmune hemolytic anemia; Goodpasture syndrome	Production of IgG, IgM → binds to antigen on target cell or tissue → phagocytosis or lysis of target cell by activated complement or Fc receptors; recruitment of leukocytes	Phagocytosis and lysis of cells; inflammation; in some diseases, functional derangements without cell or tissue injury
Immune complex–mediated (type III) hypersensitivity	Systemic lupus erythematosus; some forms of glomerulonephritis; serum sickness; Arthus reaction	Deposition of antigen-antibody complexes → complement activation → recruitment of leukocytes by complement products and Fc receptors → release of enzymes and other toxic molecules	Inflammation, necrotizing vasculitis (fibrinoid necrosis)
Cell-mediated (type IV) hypersensitivity	Contact dermatitis; multiple sclerosis; type I diabetes; rheumatoid arthritis; inflammatory bowel disease; tuberculosis	Activated T lymphocytes → (i) release of cytokines → inflammation and macrophage activation; (ii) T cell–mediated cytotoxicity	Perivascular cellular infiltrates; edema; granuloma formation; cell destruction

and disease, and the accompanying pathologic and clinical manifestations. However, it is now increasingly recognized that multiple mechanisms may be operative in any one hypersensitivity disease. The main types of hypersensitivity reactions are the following:

- In *immediate hypersensitivity (type I hypersensitivity)*, the immune response is mediated by T_H2 cells, IgE antibodies, and mast cells, and results in the release of mediators that act on vessels and smooth muscle and of pro-inflammatory cytokines that recruit inflammatory cells.
- In *antibody-mediated disorders (type II hypersensitivity)*, secreted IgG and IgM antibodies participate directly in injury to cells by promoting their phagocytosis or lysis and in injury to tissues by inducing inflammation. Antibodies may also interfere with cellular functions and cause disease without tissue injury.
- In *immune complex–mediated disorders (type III hypersensitivity)*, IgG and IgM antibodies bind antigens usually in the circulation, and the antigen-antibody complexes deposit in tissues and induce inflammation. The leukocytes that are recruited (neutrophils and monocytes) produce tissue damage by release of lysosomal enzymes and generation of toxic free radicals.
- In *cell-mediated immune disorders (type IV hypersensitivity)*, sensitized T lymphocytes (T_H1 and T_H17 cells and CTLs) are the cause of the cellular and tissue injury. T_H2 cells induce lesions that are part of immediate hypersensitivity reactions, and are not considered a form of type IV hypersensitivity.

Immediate (Type I) Hypersensitivity

Immediate, or type I, hypersensitivity is a rapid immunologic reaction occurring within minutes after the combination of an antigen with antibody bound to mast cells in individuals previously sensitized to the antigen.[26] These reactions are often called *allergy*, and the antigens that elicit them are allergens. Immediate hypersensitivity may occur as a systemic disorder or as a local reaction. The systemic reaction usually follows injection of an antigen into a sensitized individual. Sometimes, within minutes the patient goes into a state of shock, which may be fatal. Local reactions are diverse and vary depending on the portal of entry of the allergen. They may take the form of localized cutaneous swellings (skin allergy, hives), nasal and conjunctival discharge (allergic rhinitis and conjunctivitis), hay fever, bronchial asthma, or allergic gastroenteritis (food allergy). Many local type I hypersensitivity reactions have two well-defined phases (Fig. 6–13). The *immediate* or *initial reaction* is characterized by vasodilation, vascular leakage, and depending on the location, smooth muscle spasm or glandular secretions. These changes usually become evident within 5 to 30 minutes after exposure to an allergen and tend to subside in 60 minutes. In many instances (e.g., allergic rhinitis and bronchial asthma), a second, *late-phase reaction* sets in 2 to 24 hours later without additional exposure to antigen and may last for several days. This late-phase reaction is characterized by infiltration of tissues with eosinophils, neutrophils, basophils, monocytes, and CD4+ T cells as well as tissue destruction, typically in the form of mucosal epithelial cell damage.

Most immediate hypersensitivity reactions are mediated by IgE antibody–dependent activation of mast cells and other leukocytes (Fig. 6–14). Because mast cells are central to the development of immediate hypersensitivity, we first review some of their salient characteristics.[27] *Mast cells* are bone marrow–derived cells that are widely distributed in the tissues. They are abundant near blood vessels and nerves and in subepithelial tissues, which explains why local immediate hypersensitivity reactions often occur at these sites. Mast cells have cytoplasmic membrane-bound granules that contain a variety of biologically active mediators. The granules also contain acidic proteoglycans that bind basic dyes such as toluidine blue. As is

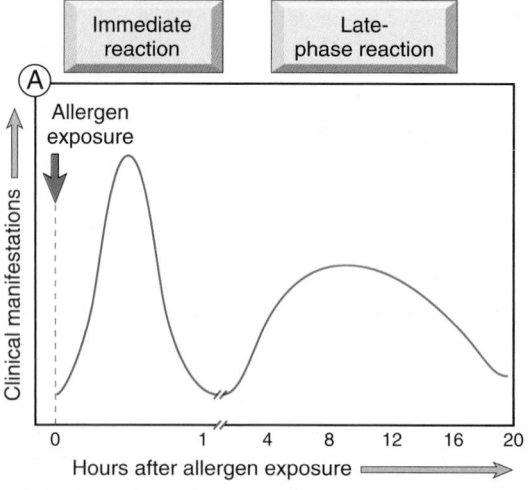
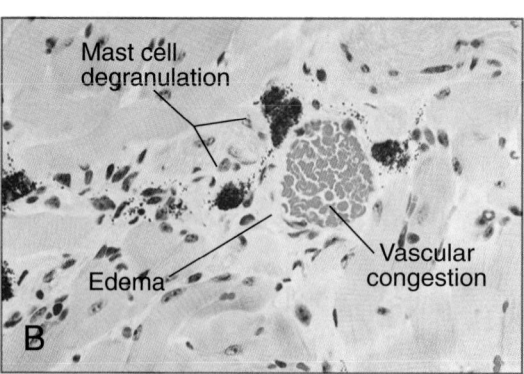
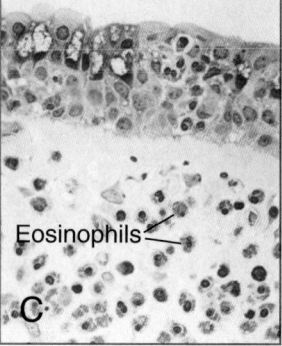

FIGURE 6–13   Immediate hypersensitivity. **A,** Kinetics of the immediate and late-phase reactions. The immediate vascular and smooth muscle reaction to allergen develops within minutes after challenge (allergen exposure in a previously sensitized individual), and the late-phase reaction develops 2 to 24 hours later. **B, C,** Morphology: The immediate reaction (**B**) is characterized by vasodilation, congestion, and edema, and the late-phase reaction (**C**) is characterized by an inflammatory infiltrate rich in eosinophils, neutrophils, and T cells. (Courtesy of Dr. Daniel Friend, Department of Pathology, Brigham and Women's Hospital, Boston, MA.)

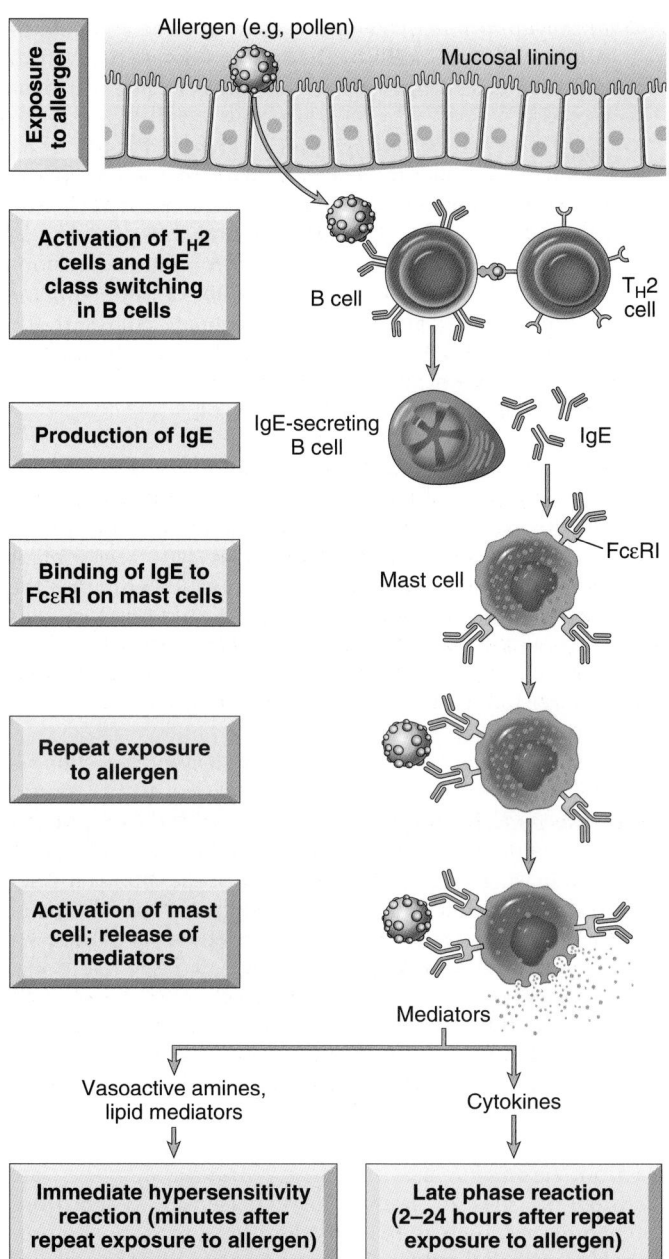

FIGURE 6–14 Sequence of events in immediate (type I) hypersensitivity. Immediate hypersensitivity reactions are initiated by the introduction of an allergen, which stimulates T_H2 responses and IgE production in genetically susceptible individuals. IgE binds to Fc receptors ($Fc\varepsilon RI$) on mast cells, and subsequent exposure to the allergen activates the mast cells to secrete the mediators that are responsible for the pathologic manifestations of immediate hypersensitivity. See text for abbreviations.

detailed next, mast cells (and basophils) are activated by the cross-linking of high-affinity IgE Fc receptors; in addition, mast cells may also be triggered by several other stimuli, such as complement components C5a and C3a (called *anaphyla-toxins* because they elicit reactions that mimic anaphylaxis), both of which act by binding to receptors on the mast cell membrane. Other mast cell secretagogues include some chemokines (e.g., IL-8), drugs such as codeine and morphine, adenosine, mellitin (present in bee venom), and physical

stimuli (e.g., heat, cold, sunlight). Basophils are similar to mast cells in many respects, including the presence of cell surface IgE Fc receptors as well as cytoplasmic granules. In contrast to mast cells, however, basophils are not normally present in tissues but rather circulate in the blood in extremely small numbers. (Most allergic reactions occur in tissues, and the role of basophils in these reactions is not as well established as that of mast cells.) Similar to other granulocytes, basophils can be recruited to inflammatory sites.

T_H2 cells play a central role in the initiation and propagation of immediate hypersensitivity reactions by stimulating IgE production and promoting inflammation.[28,29] The first step in the generation of T_H2 cells is the presentation of the antigen to naive CD4+ helper T cells, probably by dendritic cells that capture the antigen from its site of entry. In response to antigen and other stimuli, including cytokines such as IL-4 produced at the local site, the T cells differentiate into T_H2 cells. The newly minted T_H2 cells produce a number of cytokines upon subsequent encounter with the antigen; as we mentioned earlier, the signature cytokines of this subset are IL-4, IL-5, and IL-13. IL-4 acts on B cells to stimulate class switching to IgE, and promotes the development of additional T_H2 cells. IL-5 is involved in the development and activation of eosinophils, which, as we discuss subsequently, are important effectors of type I hypersensitivity. IL-13 enhances IgE production and acts on epithelial cells to stimulate mucus secretion. In addition, T_H2 cells (as well as mast cells and epithelial cells) produce chemokines that attract more T_H2 cells, as well as other leukocytes, to the reaction site.[28]

Mast cells and basophils express a high-affinity receptor, called $Fc\varepsilon RI$, that is specific for the Fc portion of IgE, and therefore avidly binds IgE antibodies. When a mast cell, armed with IgE antibodies, is exposed to the specific allergen, a series of reactions takes place, leading eventually to the release of an arsenal of powerful mediators responsible for the clinical expression of immediate hypersensitivity reactions. In the first step in this sequence, antigen (allergen) binds to the IgE antibodies previously attached to the mast cells. Multivalent antigens bind to and cross-link adjacent IgE antibodies and the underlying IgE Fc receptors. The bridging of the $Fc\varepsilon$ receptors activates signal transduction pathways from the cytoplasmic portion of the receptors. These signals lead to mast cell degranulation with the discharge of preformed (primary) mediators that are stored in the granules, and de novo synthesis and release of secondary mediators, including lipid products and cytokines (Fig. 6–15). These mediators are responsible for the initial, sometimes explosive, symptoms of immediate hypersensitivity, and they also set into motion the events that lead to the late-phase reaction.[26]

Preformed Mediators. Mediators contained within mast cell granules are the first to be released, and can be divided into three categories:

- *Vasoactive amines.* The most important mast cell–derived amine is *histamine*. Histamine causes intense smooth muscle contraction, increased vascular permeability, and increased mucus secretion by nasal, bronchial, and gastric glands.
- *Enzymes.* These are contained in the granule matrix and include neutral proteases (chymase, tryptase) and several acid hydrolases. The enzymes cause tissue damage and

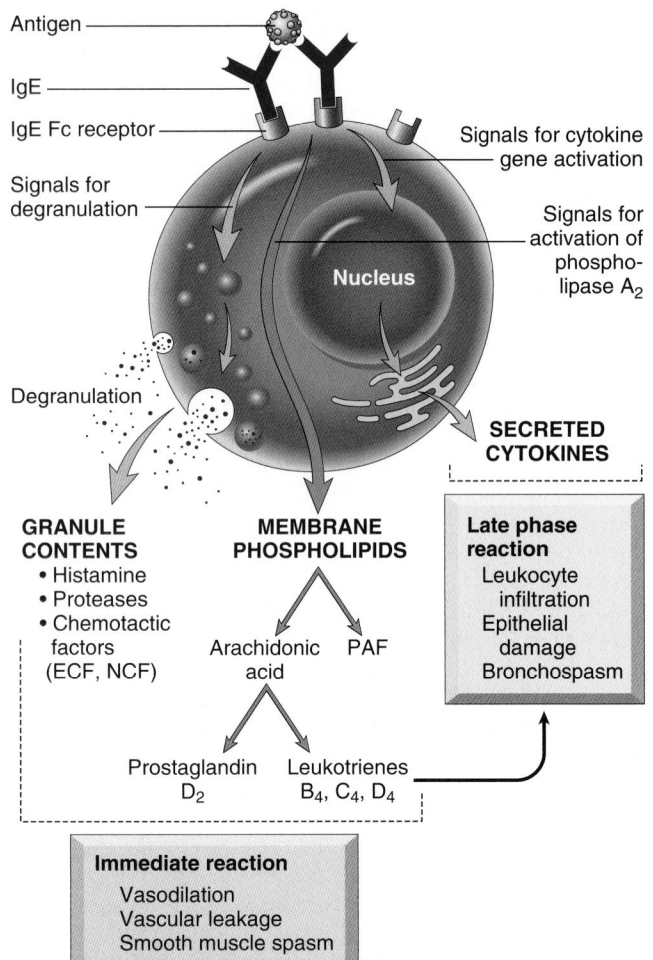

FIGURE 6–15   Mast cell mediators. Upon activation, mast cells release various classes of mediators that are responsible for the immediate and late-phase reactions. ECF, eosinophil chemotactic factor; NCF, neutrophil chemotactic factor (neither of these is biochemically defined); PAF, platelet-activating factor.

lead to the generation of kinins and activated components of complement (e.g., C3a) by acting on their precursor proteins.

○ *Proteoglycans.* These include heparin, a well-known anticoagulant, and chondroitin sulfate. The proteoglycans serve to package and store the amines in the granules.

Lipid Mediators.   The major *lipid mediators* are synthesized by sequential reactions in the mast cell membranes that lead to activation of phospholipase A_2, an enzyme that acts on membrane phospholipids to yield *arachidonic acid*. This is the parent compound from which leukotrienes and prostaglandins are derived by the 5-lipoxygenase and cyclooxygenase pathways (Chapter 2).

○ *Leukotrienes.* Leukotrienes C_4 and D_4 are the most potent vasoactive and spasmogenic agents known. On a molar basis, they are several thousand times more active than histamine in increasing vascular permeability and causing bronchial smooth muscle contraction. Leukotriene B_4 is highly chemotactic for neutrophils, eosinophils, and monocytes.

○ *Prostaglandin D_2.* This is the most abundant mediator produced in mast cells by the cyclooxygenase pathway. It causes intense bronchospasm as well as increased mucus secretion.

○ *Platelet-activating factor (PAF).* PAF (Chapter 2) is produced by some mast cell populations. It causes platelet aggregation, release of histamine, bronchospasm, increased vascular permeability, and vasodilation. In addition, it is chemotactic for neutrophils and eosinophils, and at high concentrations it activates the inflammatory cells, causing them to degranulate. Although the production of PAF is also triggered by the activation of phospholipase A_2, it is not a product of arachidonic acid metabolism.

Cytokines.   Mast cells are sources of many cytokines, which may play an important role at several stages of immediate hypersensitivity reactions. The cytokines include: TNF, IL-1, and chemokines, which promote leukocyte recruitment (typical of the late-phase reaction); IL-4, which amplifies the T_H2 response; and numerous others. The inflammatory cells that are recruited by mast cell–derived TNF and chemokines are additional sources of cytokines and of histamine-releasing factors that cause further mast cell degranulation.

The development of immediate hypersensitivity reactions is dependent on the coordinated actions of a variety of chemotactic, vasoactive, and spasmogenic compounds (Table 6–3). Some, such as histamine and leukotrienes, are released rapidly from sensitized mast cells and are responsible for the intense immediate reactions characterized by edema, mucus secretion, and smooth muscle spasm; others, exemplified by cytokines, set the stage for the late-phase response by recruiting additional leukocytes. Not only do these inflammatory cells release additional waves of mediators (including cytokines), but they also cause epithelial cell damage. Epithelial cells themselves are not passive bystanders in this reaction; they can also produce soluble mediators, such as chemokines.

Among the cells that are recruited in the late-phase reaction, *eosinophils* are particularly important.[30] They are recruited to sites of immediate hypersensitivity reactions by chemokines, such as eotaxin and others, that may be produced by epithelial cells, T_H2 cells, and mast cells. The survival of eosinophils in tissues is favored by IL-3, IL-5, and granulocyte-macrophage colony-stimulating factor (GM-CSF), and IL-5 is the most potent eosinophil-activating cytokine known. Eosinophils liberate proteolytic enzymes as well as two unique proteins called major basic protein and eosinophil cationic protein, which are toxic to epithelial cells. Activated eosinophils and other leukocytes also produce leukotriene C_4 and PAF and directly activate mast cells to release mediators. Thus, *the recruited cells amplify and sustain the inflammatory response without additional exposure to the triggering antigen.* It is now believed that this late-phase reaction is a major cause of symptoms in some type I hypersensitivity disorders, such as allergic asthma. Therefore, treatment of these diseases requires the use of broad-spectrum anti-inflammatory drugs, such as steroids.

Susceptibility to immediate hypersensitivity reactions is genetically determined. The term *atopy* refers to a predisposition to develop localized immediate hypersensitivity reactions to a

TABLE 6–3	Summary of the Action of Mast Cell Mediators in Immediate (Type I) Hypersensitivity
Action	**Mediators**
Vasodilation, increased vascular permeability	Histamine PAF Leukotrienes C_4, D_4, E_4 Neutral proteases that activate complement and kinins Prostaglandin D_2
Smooth muscle spasm	Leukotrienes C_4, D_4, E_4 Histamine Prostaglandins PAF
Cellular infiltration	Cytokines (e.g., chemokines, TNF) Leukotriene B_4 Eosinophil and neutrophil chemotactic factors (not defined biochemically)

PAF, platelet-activating factor; TNF, tumor necrosis factor.

variety of inhaled and ingested allergens. Atopic individuals tend to have higher serum IgE levels, and more IL-4–producing T_H2 cells, compared with the general population. A positive family history of allergy is found in 50% of atopic individuals. The basis of familial predisposition is not clear, but studies in patients with asthma reveal linkage to several gene loci.[31] Candidate genes have been mapped to 5q31, where genes encoding the cytokines IL-3, IL-4, IL-5, IL-9, IL-13, and GM-CSF are located. This locus has attracted great attention because of the known roles of many of these cytokines in the reaction, but how the disease-associated polymorphisms influence the biology of the cytokines is not known. Linkage has also been noted to 6p, close to the HLA complex, suggesting that the inheritance of certain HLA alleles permits reactivity to certain allergens.

A significant proportion of immediate hypersensitivity reactions are triggered by temperature extremes and exercise, and do not involve T_H2 cells or IgE; such reactions are sometimes called "non-atopic allergy." It is believed that in these cases mast cells are abnormally sensitive to activation by various non-immune stimuli.

A final point that should be mentioned in this general discussion of immediate hypersensitivity disorders is that the incidence of many of these diseases is increasing in developed countries, and seems to be related to a decrease in infections during early life. These observations have led to an idea, sometimes called the *hygiene hypothesis*, that reduced exposure to microbes resets the immune system in such a way that T_H2 responses develop more readily against common environmental antigens. This hypothesis, however, is controversial, and the underlying mechanisms are not defined.

To summarize, immediate (type I) hypersensitivity is a complex disorder resulting from an IgE-mediated triggering of mast cells and subsequent accumulation of inflammatory cells at sites of antigen deposition. These events are regulated mainly by the induction of T_H2 helper T cells that stimulate production of IgE (which promotes mast cell activation), cause accumulation of inflammatory cells (particularly eosinophils), and trigger secretion of mucus. The clinical features result from release of mast cell mediators as well as the eosinophil-rich inflammation.

With this consideration of the basic mechanisms of type I hypersensitivity, we turn to some conditions that are important examples of IgE-mediated disease.

Systemic Anaphylaxis

Systemic anaphylaxis is characterized by vascular shock, widespread edema, and difficulty in breathing. It may occur in sensitized individuals in hospital settings after administration of foreign proteins (e.g., antisera), hormones, enzymes, polysaccharides, and drugs (such as the antibiotic penicillin), or in the community setting following exposure to food allergens (e.g. peanuts, shellfish) or insect toxins (e.g. those in bee venom).[32] Extremely small doses of antigen may trigger anaphylaxis, for example, the tiny amounts used in skin testing for various forms of allergies. Because of the risk of severe allergic reactions to minute quantities of peanuts, the U.S. Congress is considering a bill to ban peanut snacks from the confined quarters of commercial airplanes. Within minutes after exposure, itching, hives, and skin erythema appear, followed shortly thereafter by a striking contraction of respiratory bronchioles and respiratory distress. Laryngeal edema results in hoarseness and further compromises breathing. Vomiting, abdominal cramps, diarrhea, and laryngeal obstruction follow, and the patient may go into shock and even die within the hour. The risk of anaphylaxis must be borne in mind when certain therapeutic agents are administered. Although patients at risk can generally be identified by a previous history of some form of allergy, the absence of such a history does not preclude the possibility of an anaphylactic reaction.

Local Immediate Hypersensitivity Reactions

About 10% to 20% of the population suffers from allergies involving localized reactions to common environmental allergens, such as pollen, animal dander, house dust, foods, and the like. Specific diseases include urticaria, angioedema, allergic rhinitis (hay fever), and bronchial asthma; these are discussed elsewhere in the book.

Antibody-Mediated (Type II) Hypersensitivity

This type of hypersensitivity is caused by antibodies that react with antigens present on cell surfaces or in the extracellular matrix. The antigenic determinants may be intrinsic to the cell membrane or matrix, or they may take the form of an exogenous antigen, such as a drug metabolite, that is adsorbed on a cell surface or matrix. In either case the hypersensitivity reaction results from the binding of antibodies to normal or altered cell surface antigens. The antibody-dependent mechanisms that cause tissue injury and disease are illustrated in Figure 6–16 and described next.

Opsonization and Phagocytosis

Phagocytosis is largely responsible for depletion of cells coated with antibodies. Cells opsonized by IgG antibodies are recognized by phagocyte Fc receptors, which are specific for the Fc portions of some IgG subclasses. In addition, when IgM or IgG antibodies are deposited on the surfaces of cells, they may activate the complement system by the classical pathway. Complement activation generates by-products, mainly C3b and C4b, which are deposited on the surfaces of the cells and recognized by phagocytes that express receptors for these proteins. The net result is phagocytosis of the opsonized cells and their destruction (Fig. 6–16A). Complement activation on cells also leads to the formation of the membrane attack complex, which disrupts membrane integrity by "drilling

holes" through the lipid bilayer, thereby causing osmotic lysis of the cells. This mechanism of depletion is probably effective only with cells that have thin cell walls, such as *Neisseria* bacteria.

Antibody-mediated destruction of cells may occur by another process called *antibody-dependent cellular cytotoxicity (ADCC)*. Cells that are coated with low concentrations of IgG antibody are killed by a variety of effector cells, which bind to the target by their receptors for the Fc fragment of IgG, and cell lysis proceeds without phagocytosis. ADCC may be mediated by monocytes, neutrophils, eosinophils, and NK cells. The role of ADCC in particular hypersensitivity diseases is uncertain.

Clinically, antibody-mediated cell destruction and phagocytosis occur in the following situations: (1) *transfusion reactions*, in which cells from an incompatible donor react with and are opsonized by preformed antibody in the host; (2) *hemolytic disease of the newborn (erythroblastosis fetalis)*, in which there is an antigenic difference between the mother and the fetus, and antibodies (of the IgG class) from the mother cross the placenta and cause destruction of fetal red cells; (3)

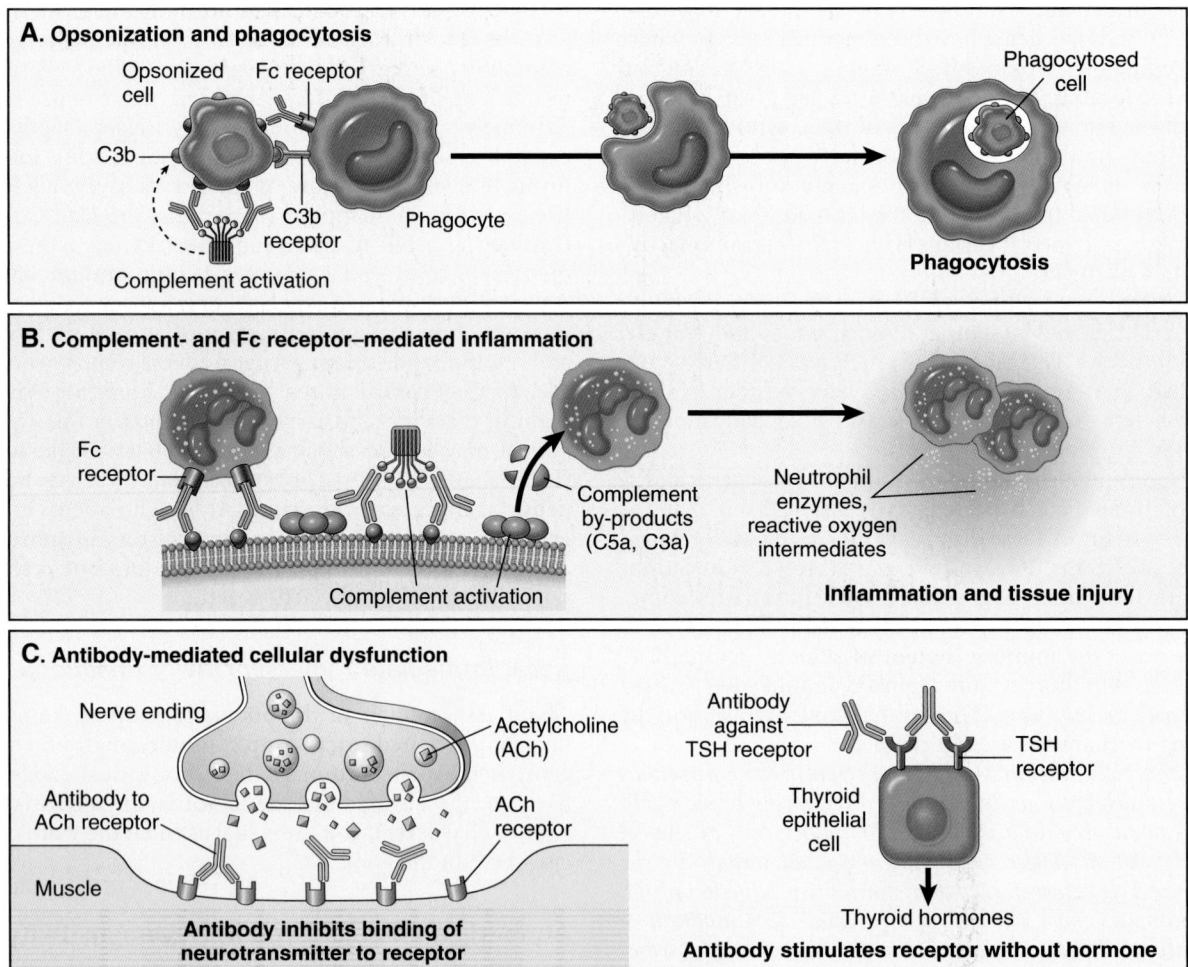

FIGURE 6–16 Mechanisms of antibody-mediated injury. **A,** Opsonization of cells by antibodies and complement components and ingestion by phagocytes. **B,** Inflammation induced by antibody binding to Fc receptors of leukocytes and by complement breakdown products. **C,** Anti-receptor antibodies disturb the normal function of receptors. In these examples, antibodies to the acetylcholine (ACh) receptor impair neuromuscular transmission in myasthenia gravis, and antibodies against the thyroid-stimulating hormone (TSH) receptor activate thyroid cells in Graves disease.

autoimmune hemolytic anemia, agranulocytosis, and *thrombocytopenia,* in which individuals produce antibodies to their own blood cells, which are then destroyed; and (4) *certain drug reactions,* in which a drug acts as a "hapten" by attaching to surface molecules of red cells and antibodies are produced against the drug–membrane protein complex.

Inflammation

When antibodies deposit in fixed tissues, such as basement membranes and extracellular matrix, the resultant injury is due to inflammation. The deposited antibodies activate complement, generating by-products, including chemotactic agents (mainly C5a), which direct the migration of polymorphonuclear leukocytes and monocytes, and anaphylatoxins (C3a and C5a), which increase vascular permeability (Fig. 6–16B). The leukocytes are activated by engagement of their C3b and Fc receptors. This results in the release or generation of a variety of pro-inflammatory substances, including prostaglandins, vasodilator peptides, and chemotactic substances. Leukocyte activation leads to the production of other substances that damage tissues, such as lysosomal enzymes, including proteases capable of digesting basement membrane,

collagen, elastin, and cartilage, and reactive oxygen species. It was once thought that complement was the major mediator of antibody-induced inflammation, but knockout mice lacking Fc receptors also show striking reduction in these reactions. It is now believed that inflammation in antibody-mediated (and immune complex–mediated) diseases is due to both complement- and Fc receptor–dependent reactions.[33]

Antibody-mediated inflammation is the mechanism responsible for tissue injury in some forms of *glomerulonephritis, vascular rejection* in organ grafts, and other disorders (Table 6–4).

Cellular Dysfunction

In some cases, antibodies directed against cell surface receptors impair or dysregulate function without causing cell injury or inflammation (Fig. 6–16C). For example, in *myasthenia gravis,* antibodies reactive with acetylcholine receptors in the motor end plates of skeletal muscles block neuromuscular transmission and therefore cause muscle weakness. The converse (i.e., antibody-mediated stimulation of cell function) is the basis of *Graves disease.* In this disorder, antibodies against the thyroid-stimulating hormone receptor

TABLE 6–4 Examples of Antibody-Mediated Diseases (Type II Hypersensitivity)

Disease	Target Antigen	Mechanisms of Disease	Clinicopathologic Manifestations
Autoimmune hemolytic anemia	Red cell membrane proteins (Rh blood group antigens, I antigen)	Opsonization and phagocytosis of red cells	Hemolysis, anemia
Autoimmune thrombocytopenic purpura	Platelet membrane proteins (GpIIb:IIIa integrin)	Opsonization and phagocytosis of platelets	Bleeding
Pemphigus vulgaris	Proteins in intercellular junctions of epidermal cells (epidermal cadherin)	Antibody-mediated activation of proteases, disruption of intercellular adhesions	Skin vesicles (bullae)
Vasculitis caused by ANCA	Neutrophil granule proteins, presumably released from activated neutrophils	Neutrophil degranulation and inflammation	Vasculitis
Goodpasture syndrome	Noncollagenous protein in basement membranes of kidney glomeruli and lung alveoli	Complement- and Fc receptor–mediated inflammation	Nephritis, lung hemorrhage
Acute rheumatic fever	Streptococcal cell wall antigen; antibody cross-reacts with myocardial antigen	Inflammation, macrophage activation	Myocarditis, arthritis
Myasthenia gravis	Acetylcholine receptor	Antibody inhibits acetylcholine binding, down-modulates receptors	Muscle weakness, paralysis
Graves disease (hyperthyroidism)	TSH receptor	Antibody-mediated stimulation of TSH receptors	Hyperthyroidism
Insulin-resistant diabetes	Insulin receptor	Antibody inhibits binding of insulin	Hyperglycemia, ketoacidosis
Pernicious anemia	Intrinsic factor of gastric parietal cells	Neutralization of intrinsic factor, decreased absorption of vitamin B_{12}	Abnormal erythropoiesis, anemia

ANCA, antineutrophil cytoplasmic antibodies; TSH, thyroid-stimulating hormone.

TABLE 6–5	Examples of Immune Complex–Mediated Diseases	
Disease	**Antigen Involved**	**Clinicopathologic Manifestations**
Systemic lupus erythematosus	Nuclear antigens	Nephritis, skin lesions, arthritis, others
Poststreptococcal glomerulonephritis	Streptococcal cell wall antigen(s); may be "planted" in glomerular basement membrane	Nephritis
Polyarteritis nodosa	Hepatitis B virus antigens in some cases	Systemic vasculitis
Reactive arthritis	Bacterial antigens (e.g., *Yersinia*)	Acute arthritis
Serum sickness	Various proteins, e.g., foreign serum protein (horse anti-thymocyte globulin)	Arthritis, vasculitis, nephritis
Arthus reaction (experimental)	Various foreign proteins	Cutaneous vasculitis

on thyroid epithelial cells stimulate the cells, resulting in hyperthyroidism.

Immune Complex–Mediated (Type III) Hypersensitivity

Antigen-antibody complexes produce tissue damage mainly by eliciting inflammation at the sites of deposition. The pathologic reaction is initiated when antigen combines with antibody within the circulation (circulating immune complexes), and these are deposited typically in vessel walls.[34] Sometimes the complexes are formed at extravascular sites where antigen may have been "planted" previously (called in situ immune complexes). The antigens that form immune complexes may be *exogenous*, such as a foreign protein that is injected or produced by an infectious microbe, or *endogenous*, if the individual produces antibody against self-components (autoimmunity). Examples of immune complex disorders and the antigens involved are listed in Table 6–5. Immune complex–mediated diseases can be *systemic*, if immune complexes are formed in the circulation and are deposited in many organs, or *localized* to particular organs, such as the kidney (glomerulonephritis), joints (arthritis), or the small blood vessels of the skin if the complexes are deposited or formed in these tissues.

Systemic Immune Complex Disease

Acute serum sickness is the prototype of a systemic immune complex disease; it was once a frequent sequela to the administration of large amounts of foreign serum (e.g., serum from immunized horses used for protection against diphtheria). In modern times the disease is infrequent, but it is an informative model that has taught us a great deal about systemic immune complex disorders.

The pathogenesis of systemic immune complex disease can be divided into three phases: (1) formation of antigen-antibody complexes in the circulation; (2) deposition of the immune complexes in various tissues, thus initiating (3) an inflammatory reaction at the sites of immune complex deposition (Fig. 6–17).

Formation of Immune Complexes. The introduction of a protein antigen triggers an immune response that results in the formation of antibodies, typically about a week after the injection of the protein. These antibodies are secreted into

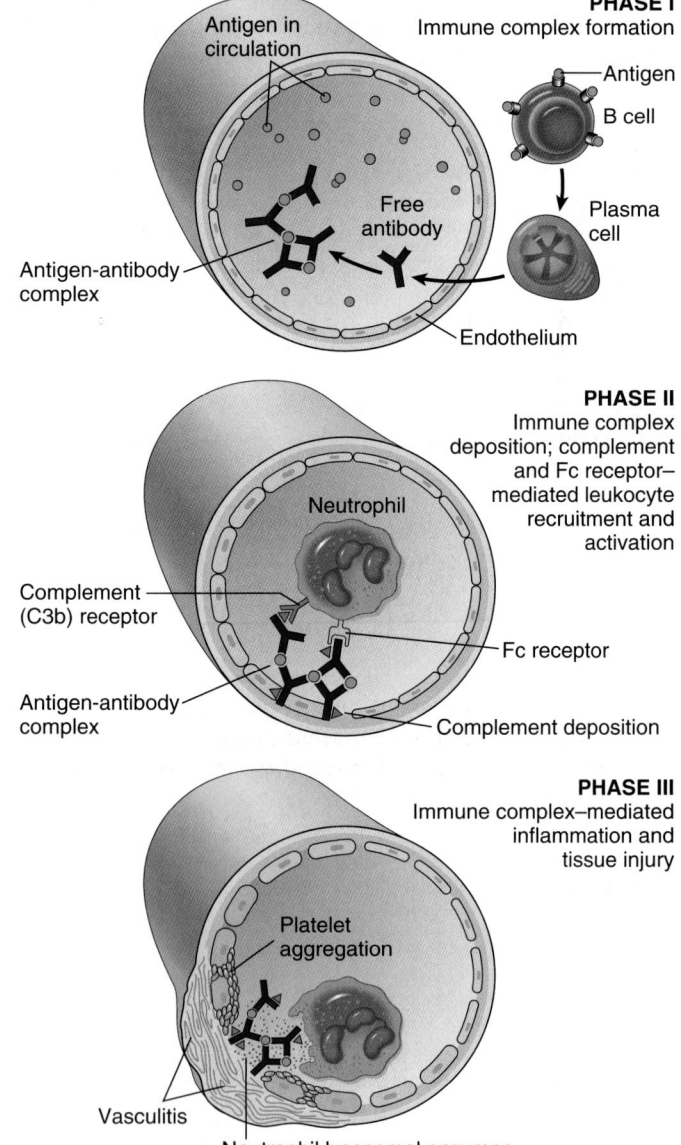

PHASE I
Immune complex formation

PHASE II
Immune complex deposition; complement and Fc receptor–mediated leukocyte recruitment and activation

PHASE III
Immune complex–mediated inflammation and tissue injury

FIGURE 6–17 Pathogenesis of systemic immune complex–mediated disease (type III hypersensitivity). The three sequential phases in the development of immune complex diseases are shown.

the blood, where they react with the antigen still present in the circulation and form antigen-antibody complexes.

Deposition of Immune Complexes. In the next phase the circulating antigen-antibody complexes are deposited in various tissues. The factors that determine whether immune complex formation will lead to tissue deposition and disease are not fully understood, but the major influences seem to be the characteristics of the complexes and local vascular alterations.

In general, complexes that are of medium size, formed in slight antigen excess, are the most pathogenic. Organs where blood is filtered at high pressure to form other fluids, like urine and synovial fluid, are favored; hence, immune complexes frequently deposit in glomeruli and joints.[35]

Tissue Injury Caused by Immune Complexes. Once complexes are deposited in the tissues, they initiate an acute inflammatory reaction (the third phase). During this phase (approximately 10 days after antigen administration), clinical features such as fever, urticaria, joint pains (arthralgias), lymph node enlargement, and proteinuria appear. Wherever complexes deposit the tissue damage is similar. The mechanisms of inflammation and injury were discussed above, in the discussion of antibody-mediated injury. The resultant inflammatory lesion is termed *vasculitis* if it occurs in blood vessels, *glomerulonephritis* if it occurs in renal glomeruli, *arthritis* if it occurs in the joints, and so on.

It is clear that complement-fixing antibodies (i.e., IgG and IgM) and antibodies that bind to leukocyte Fc receptors (some subclasses of IgG) induce the pathologic lesions of immune complex disorders. The important role of complement in the pathogenesis of the tissue injury is supported by the observations that during the active phase of the disease, consumption of complement leads to a decrease in serum levels of C3. In fact, serum C3 levels can, in some cases, be used to monitor disease activity.

> **Morphology.** The principal morphologic manifestation of immune complex injury is acute necrotizing vasculitis, with necrosis of the vessel wall and intense neutrophilic infiltration. The necrotic tissue and deposits of immune complexes, complement, and plasma protein produce a smudgy eosinophilic deposit that obscures the underlying cellular detail, an appearance termed **fibrinoid necrosis** (Fig. 6–18). When deposited in the kidney, the **complexes can be seen on immunofluorescence microscopy as granular lumpy deposits of immunoglobulin and complement** and on electron microscopy as electron-dense deposits along the glomerular basement membrane (see Figs. 6–30 and 6–31).

If the disease results from a single large exposure to antigen (e.g., acute serum sickness and perhaps acute post-streptococcal glomerulonephritis), the lesions tend to resolve, as a result of catabolism of the immune complexes. A *chronic form of serum sickness* results from repeated or prolonged exposure to an antigen. This occurs in several human diseases, such as systemic lupus erythematosus (SLE), which is associated with persistent antibody responses to autoantigens. In many diseases, however, the morphologic changes and other findings suggest immune complex deposition but the inciting antigens are unknown. Included in this category are membranous glomerulonephritis, many cases of polyarteritis nodosa, and several other vasculitides.

Local Immune Complex Disease (Arthus Reaction)

The *Arthus reaction* is a localized area of tissue necrosis resulting from acute immune complex vasculitis, usually elicited in the skin. The reaction can be produced experimentally by intracutaneous injection of antigen in a previously immunized animal that contains circulating antibodies against the antigen. As the antigen diffuses into the vascular wall, it binds the preformed antibody, and large immune complexes are formed locally. These complexes precipitate in the vessel walls and cause fibrinoid necrosis, and superimposed thrombosis worsens the ischemic injury.

T Cell–Mediated (Type IV) Hypersensitivity

The cell-mediated type of hypersensitivity is initiated by antigen-activated (sensitized) T lymphocytes, including CD4+ and CD8+ T cells (Fig. 6–19). CD4+ T cell–mediated hypersensitivity induced by environmental and self-antigens can be a cause of chronic inflammatory disease. Many autoimmune diseases are now known to be caused by inflammatory reactions driven by CD4+ T cells (Table 6–6). In some of these T cell–mediated autoimmune diseases, CD8+ cells may also be involved. In fact, in certain forms of T cell–mediated reactions, especially those that follow viral infections, CD8+ cells may be the dominant effector cells.

Reactions of CD4+ T Cells: Delayed-Type Hypersensitivity and Immune Inflammation

Inflammatory reactions caused by CD4+ T cells were initially characterized on the basis of *delayed-type hypersensitivity (DTH)* to exogenously administered antigens. The same

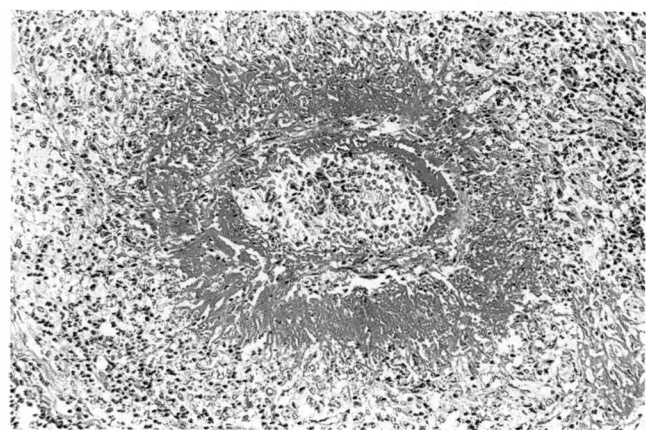

FIGURE 6–18 Immune complex vasculitis. The necrotic vessel wall is replaced by smudgy, pink "fibrinoid" material. (Courtesy of Dr. Trace Worrell, Department of Pathology, University of Texas Southwestern Medical School, Dallas, TX.)

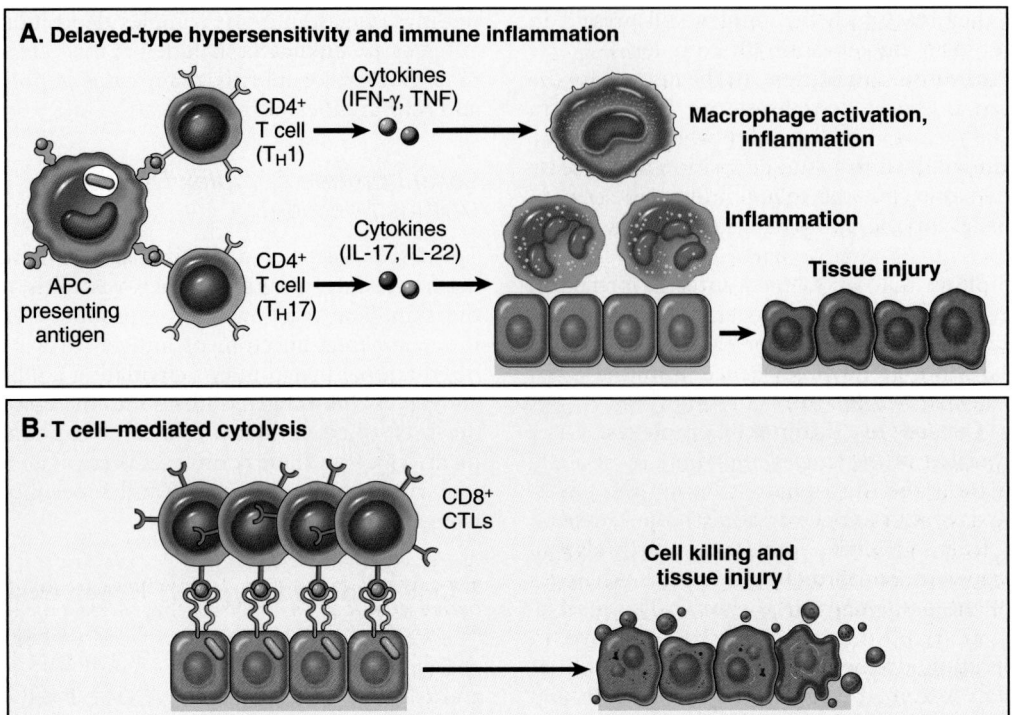

FIGURE 6–19 Mechanisms of T cell–mediated (type IV) hypersensitivity reactions. **A,** In delayed-type hypersensitivity reactions, CD4+ T$_H$1 cells (and sometimes CD8+ T cells, not shown) respond to tissue antigens by secreting cytokines that stimulate inflammation and activate phagocytes, leading to tissue injury. CD4+ T$_H$17 cells contribute to inflammation by recruiting neutrophils (and, to a lesser extent, monocytes). **B,** In some diseases, CD8+ cytotoxic T lymphocytes (CTLs) directly kill tissue cells. APC, antigen-presenting cell. See text for other abbreviations.

immunological events are responsible for chronic inflammatory reactions against self-tissues. Because of the central role of the adaptive immune system in such inflammation, it is sometimes referred to as *immune inflammation*. Both T$_H$1 and T$_H$17 cells contribute to organ-specific diseases in which inflammation is a prominent aspect of the pathology.[36] The inflammatory reaction associated with T$_H$1 cells is dominated by activated macrophages, and that triggered by T$_H$17 cells has a greater neutrophil component.

The cellular events in T cell–mediated hypersensitivity consist of a series of reactions in which cytokines play important roles. The reactions can be divided into the following stages.

Proliferation and Differentiation of CD4+ T Cells. Naive CD4+ T cells recognize peptides displayed by dendritic cells and secrete IL-2, which functions as an autocrine growth factor to stimulate proliferation of the antigen-responsive T cells. The subsequent differentiation of antigen-stimulated T cells to T$_H$1 or T$_H$17 cells is driven by the cytokines produced

TABLE 6–6 Examples of T Cell–Mediated (Type IV) Hypersensitivity

Disease	Specificity of Pathogenic T Cells	Clinicopathologic Manifestations
Type 1 diabetes mellitus	Antigens of pancreatic islet β cells (insulin, glutamic acid decarboxylase, others)	Insulitis (chronic inflammation in islets), destruction of β cells; diabetes
Multiple sclerosis	Protein antigens in CNS myelin (myelin basic protein, proteolipid protein)	Demyelination in CNS with perivascular inflammation; paralysis, ocular lesions
Rheumatoid arthritis	Unknown antigen in joint synovium (type II collagen?); role of antibodies?	Chronic arthritis with inflammation, destruction of articular cartilage and bone
Crohn disease	Unknown antigen; role for commensal bacteria	Chronic intestinal inflammation, obstruction
Peripheral neuropathy; Guillain-Barré syndrome?	Protein antigens of peripheral nerve myelin	Neuritis, paralysis
Contact sensitivity (dermatitis)	Various environmental antigens (e.g., poison ivy)	Skin inflammation with blisters

CNS, central nervous system.

by APCs at the time of T-cell activation (see Fig. 6–13).[36] In some situations the APCs (dendritic cells and macrophages) produce IL-12, which induces differentiation of CD4+ T cells to the T_H1 subset. IFN-γ produced by these effector cells promotes further T_H1 development, thus amplifying the reaction. If the APCs produce inflammatory cytokines such as IL-1, IL-6, and a close relative of IL-12 called IL-23, these work in collaboration with transforming growth factor-β (TGF-β) (made by many cell types) to stimulate differentiation of T cells to the T_H17 subset. Some of the differentiated effector cells enter the circulation and may remain in the memory pool of T cells for long periods, sometimes years.

Responses of Differentiated Effector T Cells. Upon repeat exposure to an antigen, previously activated T cells recognize the antigen displayed by APCs and respond. T_H1 cells secrete cytokines, mainly IFN-γ, which are responsible for many of the manifestations of delayed-type hypersensitivity. IFN-γ–activated macrophages are altered in several ways: their ability to phagocytose and kill microorganisms is markedly augmented; they express more class II MHC molecules on the surface, thus facilitating further antigen presentation; they secrete TNF, IL-1, and chemokines, which promote inflammation (Chapter 2); and they produce more IL-12, thereby amplifying the T_H1 response. Thus, activated macrophages serve to eliminate the offending antigen; if the activation is sustained, continued inflammation and tissue injury result.

T_H17 cells are activated by some microbial antigens and by self-antigens in autoimmune diseases. Activated T_H17 cells secrete IL-17, IL-22, chemokines, and several other cytokines. Collectively, these cytokines recruit neutrophils and monocytes to the reaction, thus promoting inflammation. T_H17 cells also produce IL-21, which amplifies the T_H17 response.

The classic example of DTH is the *tuberculin reaction*, which is produced by the intracutaneous injection of purified protein derivative (PPD, also called tuberculin), a protein-containing antigen of the tubercle bacillus. In a previously sensitized individual, reddening and induration of the site appear in 8 to 12 hours, reach a peak in 24 to 72 hours, and thereafter slowly subside. Morphologically, delayed-type hypersensitivity is characterized by the accumulation of mononuclear cells, mainly CD4+ T cells and macrophages, around venules, producing perivascular "cuffing" (Fig. 6–20). In fully developed lesions, the venules show marked endothelial hypertrophy, reflecting cytokine-mediated endothelial activation.

With certain persistent or nondegradable antigens, such as tubercle bacilli colonizing the lungs or other tissues, the perivascular infiltrate is dominated by macrophages over a period of 2 or 3 weeks. The activated macrophages often undergo a morphologic transformation into epithelium-like cells and are then referred to as *epithelioid cells*. A microscopic aggregation of epithelioid cells, usually surrounded by a collar of lymphocytes, is referred to as a *granuloma* (Fig. 6–21). This pattern of inflammation, called *granulomatous inflammation* (Chapter 2), is typically associated with strong T-cell activation with cytokine production (Fig. 6–22). It can also be caused by foreign bodies that activate macrophages without eliciting an adaptive immune response.

Contact dermatitis is a common example of tissue injury resulting from DTH reactions. It may be evoked by contact with urushiol, the antigenic component of poison ivy or poison oak, and presents as a vesicular dermatitis (Fig. 6–23).

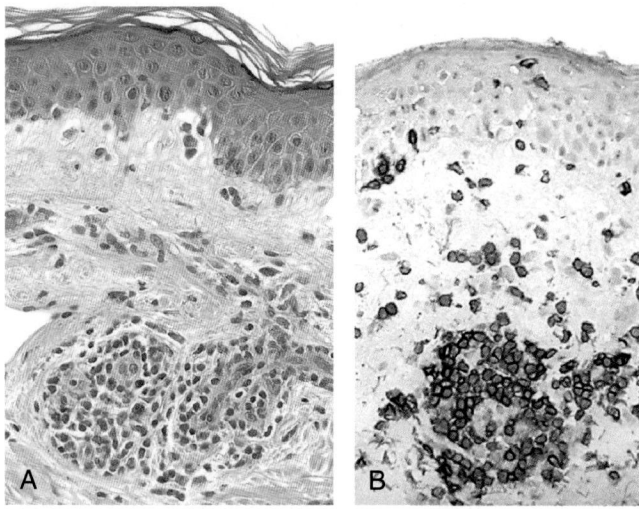

FIGURE 6–20 Delayed hypersensitivity reaction in the skin. **A,** Perivascular infiltration by T cells and mononuclear phagocytes. **B,** Immunoperoxidase staining reveals a predominantly perivascular cellular infiltrate that marks positively with antibodies specific to CD4. (Courtesy of Dr. Louis Picker, Department of Pathology, University of Texas Southwestern Medical School, Dallas, TX.)

Reactions of CD8+ T Cells: Cell-Mediated Cytotoxicity

In this type of T cell–mediated reaction, CD8+ CTLs kill antigen-bearing target cells. Tissue destruction by CTLs may be an important component of many T cell–mediated diseases, such as type 1 diabetes. CTLs directed against cell surface histocompatibility antigens play an important role in graft rejection, to be discussed later. They also play a role in reactions against viruses. In a virus-infected cell, viral peptides are displayed by class I MHC molecules and the complex is recognized by the TCR of CD8+ T lymphocytes. The killing of infected cells leads to the elimination of the infection, and is responsible for cell damage that accompanies the infection

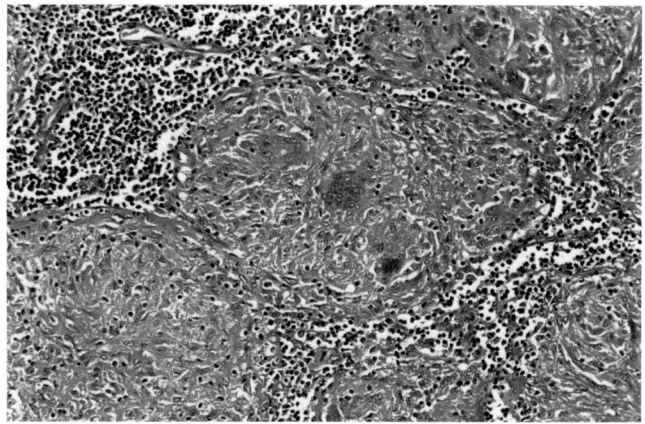

FIGURE 6–21 Granulomatous inflammation. A section of a lymph node shows several granulomas, each made up of an aggregate of epithelioid cells and surrounded by lymphocytes. The granuloma in the center shows several multinucleate giant cells. (Courtesy of Dr. Trace Worrell, Department of Pathology, University of Texas Southwestern Medical School, Dallas, TX.)

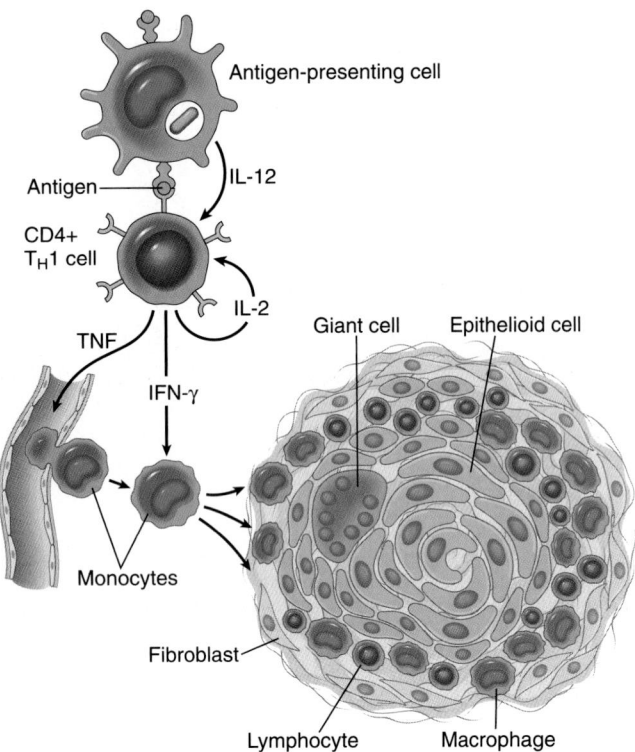

FIGURE 6–22 Mechanisms of granuloma formation. Schematic illustration of the events that give rise to the formation of granulomas in cell-mediated (type IV) hypersensitivity reactions. Note the role played by cytokines. See text for abbreviations.

(e.g., in viral hepatitis). Tumor-associated antigens are also presented on the cell surface, and CTLs are involved in tumor rejection (Chapter 7).

The principal mechanism of T cell–mediated killing of targets involves *perforins* and *granzymes*, preformed mediators contained in the lysosome-like granules of CTLs.[37] CTLs that recognize the target cells secrete a complex consisting of perforin, granzymes, and a protein called serglycin, which enters target cells by endocytosis. In the target cell cytoplasm, perfo-

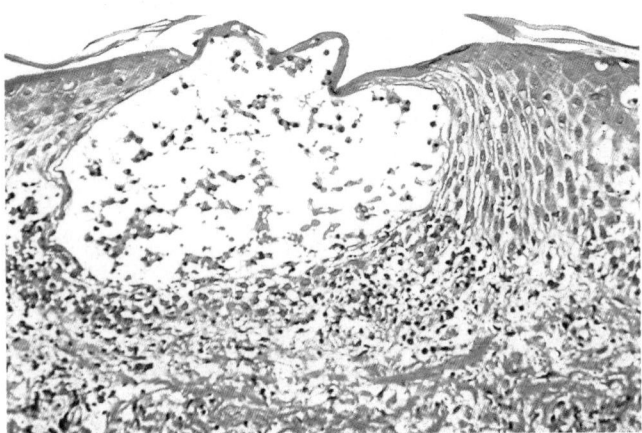

FIGURE 6–23 Contact dermatitis. The lesion shows an epidermal blister (vesicle) with dermal and epidermal mononuclear infiltrates. (Courtesy of Dr. Louis Picker, Department of Pathology, University of Texas Southwestern Medical School, Dallas, TX.)

rin facilitates the release of the granzymes from the complex. Granzymes are proteases that cleave and activate caspases, which induce apoptosis of the target cells (Chapter 1). Activated CTLs also express Fas ligand, a molecule with homology to TNF, which can bind to Fas expressed on target cells and trigger apoptosis.

CD8+ T cells also produce cytokines, notably IFN-γ, and are involved in inflammatory reactions resembling DTH, especially following virus infections and exposure to some contact sensitizing agents.

AUTOIMMUNE DISEASES

Immune reactions against self-antigens—*autoimmunity*—are an important cause of certain diseases in humans, estimated to affect at least 1% to 2% of the US population. A growing number of diseases have been attributed to autoimmunity (Table 6–7). Autoantibodies can be found in the serum of apparently normal individuals, particularly in older age groups. Furthermore, innocuous autoantibodies are also formed after damage to tissue and may serve a physiologic role in the removal of tissue breakdown products. How, then, does one define *pathologic autoimmunity*? Ideally, at least three requirements should be met before a disorder is categorized as truly due to autoimmunity: (1) the presence of an immune reaction specific for some self-antigen or self-tissue; (2) evidence that such a reaction is not secondary to tissue damage but is of primary pathogenic significance; and (3) the absence of another well-defined cause of the disease. Similarity with experimental models of proven autoimmunity is also often used to support this mechanism in human diseases. Because of the uncertainty about the target antigens and the contribution of "true" autoimmunity, these disorders are often grouped

TABLE 6–7   Immune-Mediated Inflammatory Diseases
DISEASES MEDIATED BY ANTIBODIES AND IMMUNE COMPLEXES
Organ-specific autoimmune diseases
Autoimmune hemolytic anemia
Autoimmune thrombocytopenia
Myasthenia gravis
Graves disease
Goodpasture syndrome
Systemic autoimmune diseases
Systemic lupus erythematosus (SLE)
Diseases caused by autoimmunity or by reactions to microbial antigens
Polyarteritis nodosa
DISEASES MEDIATED BY T CELLS
Organ-specific autoimmune diseases
Type 1 diabetes mellitus
Multiple sclerosis
Systemic autoimmune diseases
Rheumatoid arthritis*
Systemic sclerosis*
Sjogren syndrome*
Diseases caused by autoimmunity or by reactions to microbial antigens
Inflammatory bowel disease (Crohn disease, ulcerative colitis)
Inflammatory myopathies

*Antibodies may also play a role in these diseases.

under *immune-mediated inflammatory diseases.* This term also emphasizes the important contribution of chronic inflammation to the pathogenesis of these diseases.

The clinical manifestations of autoimmune disorders are extremely varied. On one end are conditions in which the immune responses are directed against a single organ or tissue, resulting in *organ-specific disease*, and on the other end are diseases in which the autoimmune reactions are against widespread antigens, resulting in *systemic* or *generalized disease*. Examples of organ-specific autoimmunity are type 1 diabetes mellitus, in which the autoreactive T cells and antibodies are specific for β cells of the pancreatic islets, and multiple sclerosis, in which autoreactive T cells react against central nervous system myelin. The best example of systemic autoimmune disease is SLE, in which a diversity of antibodies directed against DNA, platelets, red cells, and protein-phospholipid complexes result in widespread lesions throughout the body. In the middle of the spectrum falls Goodpasture's syndrome, in which antibodies to basement membranes of lung and kidney induce lesions in these organs.

It is obvious that autoimmunity results from the loss of self-tolerance, and the question arises as to how this happens. Before we look for answers to this question, we review the mechanisms of immunological tolerance to self-antigens.

Immunological Tolerance

Immunological tolerance is the phenomenon of unresponsiveness to an antigen as a result of exposure of lymphocytes to that antigen. Self-tolerance refers to lack of responsiveness to an individual's own antigens, and it underlies our ability to live in harmony with our cells and tissues. Lymphocytes with receptors capable of recognizing self-antigens are being generated constantly, and these cells have to be eliminated or inactivated as soon as they recognize the antigens, to prevent them from causing harm. The mechanisms of self-tolerance can be broadly classified into two groups: central tolerance and peripheral tolerance (Fig. 6–24).[38–40] Each of these is considered briefly.

Central Tolerance. In this process, immature self-reactive T- and B-lymphocyte clones that recognize self-antigens during their maturation in the central (or generative) lymphoid organs (the thymus for T cells and the bone marrow for B cells) are killed or rendered harmless.[41] The mechanisms of central tolerance in T and B cells show some similarities and differences.

- In developing T cells, random somatic gene rearrangements generate diverse TCRs. Such antigen-independent TCR generation produces many lymphocytes that express high-affinity receptors for self-antigens. When immature lymphocytes encounter the antigens in the thymus, the cells die by apoptosis. This process, called *negative selection* or *deletion*, is responsible for eliminating many self-reactive lymphocytes from the T-cell pool. A wide variety of autologous protein antigens, including antigens thought to be restricted to peripheral tissues, are processed and presented by thymic antigen-presenting cells in association with self-MHC molecules and can, therefore, be recognized by potentially self-reactive T cells. A protein called AIRE (autoimmune regulator) stimulates expression of some "peripheral tissue-

restricted" self-antigens in the thymus and is thus critical for deletion of immature T cells specific for these antigens.[42] Mutations in the *AIRE* gene are the cause of an autoimmune polyendocrinopathy (Chapter 24). In the CD4+ T-cell lineage, some of the cells that see self antigens in the thymus do not die but develop into regulatory T cells (described later).

- When developing B cells strongly recognize self-antigens in the bone marrow, many of them reactivate the machinery of antigen receptor gene rearrangement and begin to express new antigen receptors, not specific for self-antigens. This process is called *receptor editing*; it is estimated that a quarter to half of all B cells in the body may have undergone receptor editing during their maturation.[43] If receptor editing does not occur, the self-reactive cells undergo apoptosis, thus purging potentially dangerous lymphocytes from the mature pool.

Central tolerance, however, is far from perfect. Not all self-antigens may be present in the thymus, and hence T cells bearing receptors for such autoantigens escape into the periphery. There is similar "slippage" in the B-cell system. Self-reactive lymphocytes that escape negative selection can inflict tissue injury unless they are deleted or muzzled in the peripheral tissues.

Peripheral Tolerance. Several mechanisms silence potentially autoreactive T and B cells in peripheral tissues; these are best defined for T cells.[40] These mechanisms include the following:

- *Anergy:* This refers to prolonged or irreversible functional inactivation of lymphocytes, induced by encounter with antigens under certain conditions.[44] We discussed earlier that activation of antigen-specific T cells requires two signals: recognition of peptide antigen in association with self-MHC molecules on the surface of APCs and a set of costimulatory signals ("second signals") from APCs. These second signals are provided by certain T cell–associated molecules, such as CD28, that bind to their ligands (the costimulators B7-1 and B7-2) on APCs. If the antigen is presented by cells that do not bear the costimulators a negative signal is delivered, and the cell becomes anergic (see Fig. 6–24). Because costimulatory molecules are not expressed or are weakly expressed on resting dendritic cells in normal tissues, the encounter between autoreactive T cells and their specific self-antigens displayed by these dendritic cells may lead to anergy. Two mechanisms of T-cell anergy have been demonstrated in various experimental systems. First, the cells lose their ability to trigger biochemical signals from the TCR complex, in part because of activation of ubiquitin ligases and proteolytic degradation of receptor-associated signaling proteins.[45] Second, T cells that recognize self-antigens receive an inhibitory signal from receptors that are structurally homologous to CD28 but serve the opposite functions. Two of these inhibitory receptors are CTLA-4, which (like CD28) also binds to B7 molecules, and PD-1, which binds to two ligands that are expressed on a wide variety of cells.[46] How T cells choose to use CD28 to recognize B7 molecules and be activated, or CTLA-4 to recognize the same B7 molecules and become anergic, is an intriguing question to which there are no

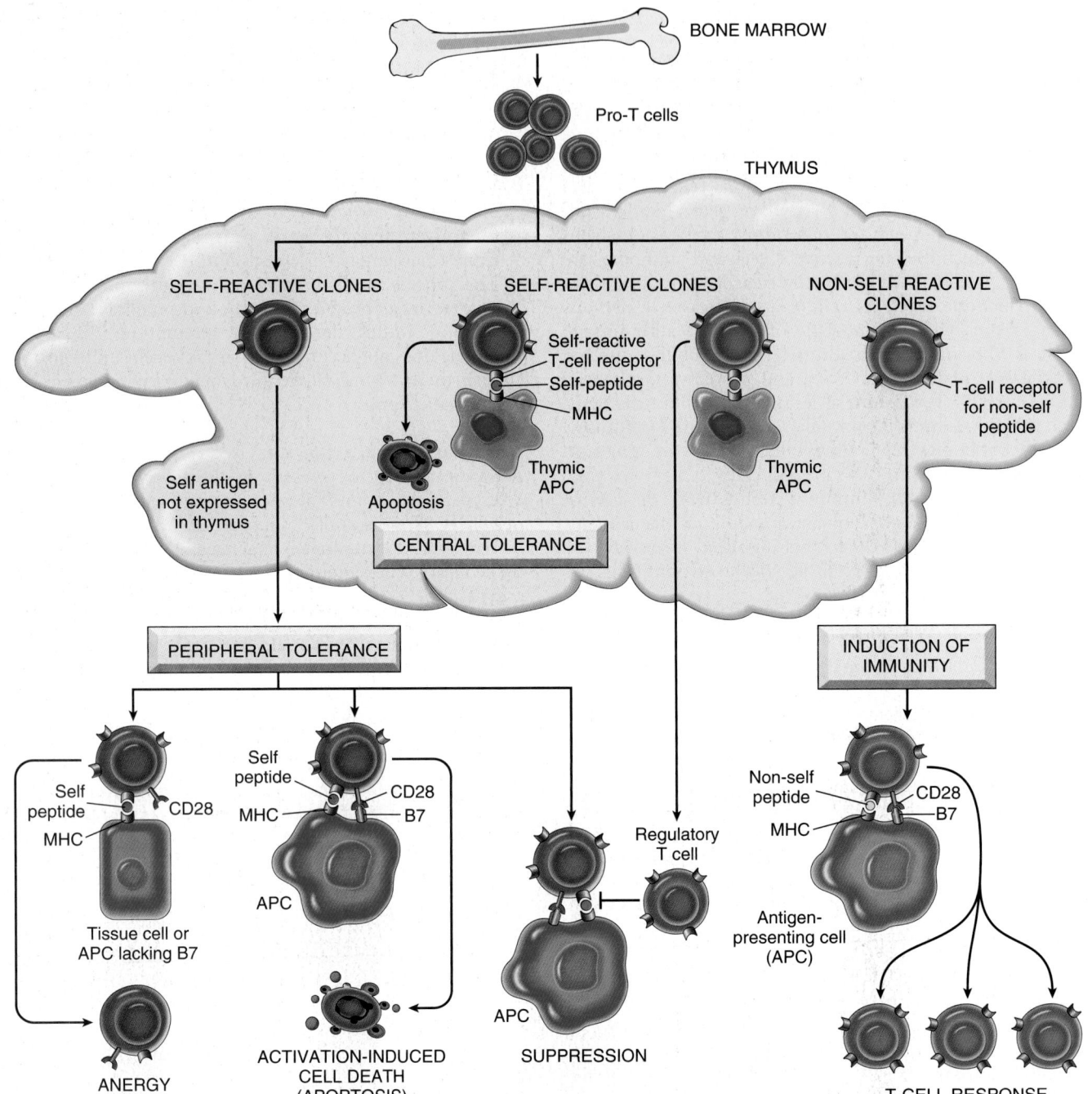

FIGURE 6–24 Mechanisms of immunological tolerance. Schematic illustration of the mechanisms of central and peripheral tolerance to self-antigens, shown for CD4+ T cells. APC, antigen-presenting cell. See text for other abbreviations.

clear answers. Nevertheless, the importance of these inhibitory mechanisms has been established by the finding that mice in which the gene encoding CTLA-4 or PD-1 is knocked out develop autoimmune diseases. Furthermore, polymorphisms in the *CTLA4* gene are associated with some autoimmune endocrine diseases in humans. Interestingly, some tumors and viruses may have evolved to use the same pathways of immune regulation to evade immune attack.

Anergy also affects mature B cells in peripheral tissues. It is believed that if B cells encounter self-antigen in periph-

eral tissues, especially in the absence of specific helper T cells, the B cells become unable to respond to subsequent antigenic stimulation and may be excluded from lymphoid follicles, resulting in their death.

○ *Suppression by regulatory T cells:* A population of T cells called *regulatory T cells* plays a major role in preventing immune reactions against self-antigens.[47] Regulatory T cells develop mainly in the thymus, as a result of recognition of self-antigens (see Fig. 6–24), but they may also be induced in peripheral lymphoid tissues. The best-defined regulatory T cells are CD4+ cells that constitutively express CD25, the α chain of the IL-2 receptor, and a transcription factor of the forkhead family, called Foxp3. Both IL-2 and Foxp3 are required for the development and maintenance of functional CD4+ regulatory T cells.[48] Mutations in *Foxp3* result in severe autoimmunity in humans and mice; in humans these mutations are the cause of a systemic autoimmune disease called IPEX (for immune dysregulation, polyendocrinopathy, enteropathy, X-linked). In mice knockout of the gene encoding IL-2 or the IL-2 receptor α or β chain also results in severe multi-organ autoimmunity, because IL-2 is essential for the maintenance of regulatory T cells. Recent genome-wide association studies have revealed that polymorphisms in the *CD25* gene are associated with multiple sclerosis and other autoimmune diseases, raising the possibility of a regulatory T-cell defect contributing to these diseases. The mechanisms by which regulatory T cells suppress immune responses are not fully defined. The inhibitory activity of these cells may be mediated by the secretion of immunosuppressive cytokines such as IL-10 and TGF-β, which inhibit lymphocyte activation and effector functions.

○ *Deletion by activation-induced cell death:* CD4+ T cells that recognize self-antigens may receive signals that promote their death by apoptosis. This process has been called activation-induced cell death, because it is a consequence of T-cell activation. Two mechanisms of activation-induced cell death have been proposed, based on studies in mice.[49] It is postulated that if T cells recognize self-antigens, they may express a pro-apoptotic member of the Bcl family, called Bim, without anti-apoptotic members of the family like Bcl-2 and Bcl-x (whose induction requires the full set of signals for lymphocyte activation). Unopposed Bim triggers apoptosis by the mitochondrial pathway (Chapter 1). A second mechanism of activation-induced death of CD4+ T cells and B cells involves the Fas-Fas ligand system. Lymphocytes as well as many other cells express Fas (CD95), a member of the TNF-receptor family. FasL, a membrane protein that is structurally homologous to the cytokine TNF, is expressed mainly on activated T lymphocytes. The engagement of Fas by FasL induces apoptosis of activated T cells by the death receptor pathway (Chapter 1). It is postulated that if self-antigens engage antigen receptors of self-antigen–specific T cells, Fas and FasL are co-expressed, leading to elimination of the cells via Fas-mediated apoptosis (see Fig. 6–24). Self-reactive B cells may also be deleted by FasL on T cells engaging Fas on the B cells. The importance of this mechanism in the peripheral deletion of autoreactive lymphocytes is highlighted by two strains of mice that are natural mutants of Fas or FasL. Both these strains of mice develop an autoimmune disease resembling human SLE, associated with generalized lymphoproliferation. In humans a similar disease is caused by mutations in the *FAS* gene; it is called the autoimmune lymphoproliferative syndrome.[50]

Some antigens are hidden (sequestered) from the immune system, because the tissues in which these antigens are located do not communicate with the blood and lymph. Thus, self-antigens in these tissues do not induce tolerance but fail to elicit immune responses and are essentially ignored by the immune system. This is believed to be the case for the testis,

eye, and brain, all of which are called *immune-privileged sites* because it is difficult to induce immune responses to antigens introduced into these sites. If the antigens of these tissues are released, for example, as a consequence of trauma or infection, the result may be an immune response that leads to prolonged tissue inflammation and injury. This is the postulated mechanism for post-traumatic orchitis and uveitis.

Mechanisms of Autoimmunity: General Principles

Autoimmunity arises from a combination of the inheritance of susceptibility genes, which may contribute to the breakdown of self-tolerance, and environmental triggers, such as infections and tissue damage, which promote the activation of self-reactive lymphocytes (Fig. 6–25).[51,52] In general, these genetic and environmental influences conspire to create an imbalance between control mechanisms that normally function to prevent self-reactivity and pathways that lead to the generation and

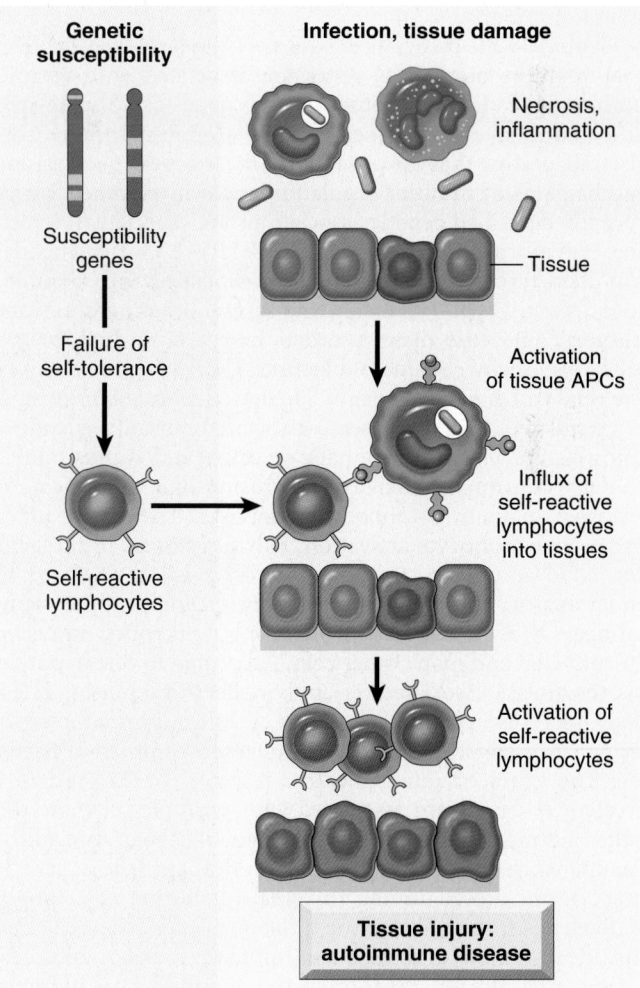

FIGURE 6–25 Pathogenesis of autoimmunity. Autoimmunity results from multiple factors, including susceptibility genes that may interfere with self-tolerance and environmental triggers (tissue injury, inflammation) that promote lymphocyte entry into tissues, activation of self-reactive lymphocytes, and tissue damage.

activation of pathogenic effector lymphocytes. In the following section we discuss how genetic and other factors contribute to the development of autoimmunity.

Role of Susceptibility Genes. It has been known for decades that autoimmunity has a genetic component. The incidence of the disease is greater in twins of affected individuals than in the general population, and greater in monozygotic than in dizygotic twins. *Most autoimmune diseases are complex multigenic disorders.*[53–55] Among the genes known to be associated with autoimmunity, the greatest contribution is that of HLA genes. The concept of HLA association with diseases was mentioned earlier (see Table 6–1). Although this association has been well established for many years, the underlying mechanisms remain obscure. It is postulated that the presence of particular MHC alleles affects the negative selection of T cells in the thymus or the development of regulatory T cells, but there is little proof for either possibility. It should be pointed out that many normal individuals inherit the MHC alleles that are disease-associated in patient populations, and normal MHC molecules are capable of presenting self-antigens. Therefore, the presence of particular MHC alleles is not, by itself, the cause of autoimmunity.

Genome-wide association studies (Chapter 5) have shown that multiple non-MHC genes are associated with various autoimmune diseases. Some of these genes are disease-specific, but many of the associations are seen in multiple disorders, suggesting that the products of these genes affect general mechanisms of immune regulation and self-tolerance. Three recently described genetic associations are especially interesting. Polymorphisms in a gene called *PTPN-22*, which encodes a protein tyrosine phosphatase, are associated with rheumatoid arthritis, type 1 diabetes, and several other autoimmune diseases.[56] Because these disorders have a fairly high prevalence (especially rheumatoid arthritis), *PTPN-22 is said to be the gene that is most frequently implicated in autoimmunity*. It is postulated that the disease-associated variants encode a phosphatase that is functionally defective and is thus unable to fully control the activity of tyrosine kinases, which are involved in many lymphocyte responses. The net result is excessive lymphocyte activation. Polymorphisms in the gene for *NOD-2* are associated with Crohn disease, a form of inflammatory bowel disease, especially in certain ethnic populations.[57] NOD-2 is a cytoplasmic sensor of microbes, expressed in epithelial and many other cells. According to one hypothesis, the disease-associated variant is ineffective at sensing intestinal microbes, resulting in entry of and chronic inflammatory responses against normally well-tolerated commensal bacteria. The genes encoding the *IL-2 receptor (CD25)* and *IL-7 receptor* α chains are associated with multiple sclerosis and other autoimmune diseases. These cytokines may control the maintenance of regulatory T cells. Although these genetic associations are beginning to reveal interesting clues about pathogenesis, the links between the genes, functions of their encoded proteins, and the diseases remain to be established.

We have already mentioned that in mice and humans, knockouts and natural mutations affecting several individual genes result in autoimmunity. These genes include *AIRE*, *CTLA4*, *PD1*, *Fas*, *FasL*, and *IL2* and its receptor *CD25*. In addition, B cells express an Fc receptor that recognizes IgG antibodies bound to antigens and switches off further antibody production (a normal negative-feedback mechanism). Knockout of this receptor results in autoimmunity, presumably because the B cells can no longer be controlled. These examples are very informative about pathways of self-tolerance and immune regulation, but the diseases caused by these single gene mutations are rare and not representative of the common autoimmune disorders.

Role of Infections. Many autoimmune diseases are associated with infections, and clinical flare-ups are often preceded by infectious prodromes. Two mechanisms have been postulated to explain the link between infections and autoimmunity (Fig. 6–26). First, infections may up-regulate the expression of costimulators on APCs. If these cells are presenting self-antigens, the result may be a breakdown of anergy and activation of T cells specific for the self-antigens. Second, some microbes may express antigens that have the same amino acid sequences as self-antigens. Immune responses against the microbial antigens may result in the activation of self-reactive lymphocytes. This phenomenon is called *molecular mimicry*. A clear example of such mimicry is rheumatic heart disease, in which antibodies against streptococcal proteins cross-react with myocardial proteins and cause myocarditis (Chapter 12). But more subtle molecular mimicry may be involved in classical autoimmune diseases as well.

Microbes may induce other abnormalities that promote autoimmune reactions. Some viruses, such as Epstein-Barr virus (EBV) and HIV, cause polyclonal B-cell activation, which may result in production of autoantibodies. The tissue injury that is common in infections may release self-antigens and structurally alter self-antigens so that they are able to activate T cells that are not tolerant to these new, modified antigens. Infections may induce the production of cytokines that recruit lymphocytes, including potentially self-reactive lymphocytes, to sites of self-antigens.

Although the role of infections in triggering autoimmunity has received a great deal of attention, recent epidemiologic studies suggest that the incidence of autoimmune diseases is increasing in developed countries as infections are better controlled. In some animal models (e.g., of type 1 diabetes) infections greatly reduce the incidence of disease. Thus, *paradoxically, infections may protect against some autoimmune diseases.*[58] The underlying mechanisms are unclear; an intriguing possibility is that infections promote low-level IL-2 production, and this is essential for maintaining regulatory T cells.

General Features of Autoimmune Diseases

Diseases caused by autoimmunity have some important general features.

- Once an autoimmune disease has been induced it tends to be progressive, sometimes with sporadic relapses and remissions, and the damage becomes inexorable. One reason for this is that the immune system contains many intrinsic amplification loops that allow small numbers of antigen-specific lymphocytes to accomplish their task of eradicating complex infections. When the response is inappropriately directed against self-tissues, the very same amplification mechanisms exacerbate injury. Another reason for the persistence and progression of autoimmune disease is the phenomenon of *epitope spreading*. Infections,

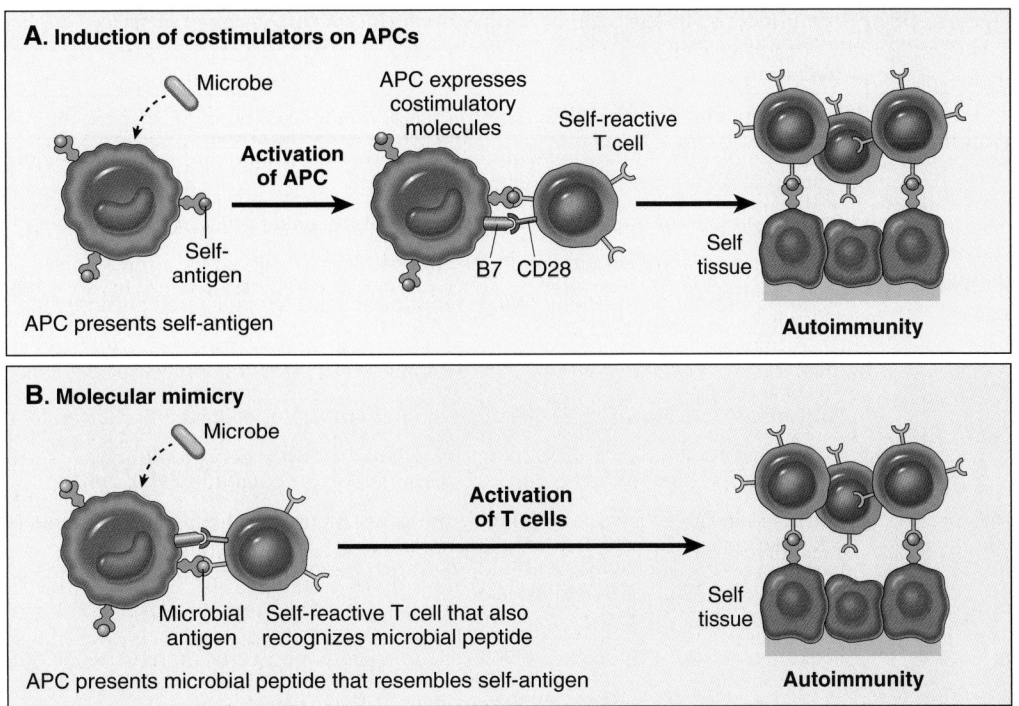

A. Induction of costimulators on APCs

Microbe

APC expresses
costimulatory
molecules

Self-reactive
T cell

**Activation
of APC**

Self-
antigen

B7 CD28

APC presents self-antigen

Self
tissue

Autoimmunity

B. Molecular mimicry

Microbe

**Activation
of T cells**

Microbial   Self-reactive T cell that also
antigen   recognizes microbial peptide

APC presents microbial peptide that resembles self-antigen

Self
tissue

Autoimmunity

FIGURE 6–26 Postulated role of infections in autoimmunity. Infections may promote activation of self-reactive lymphocytes by inducing the expression of costimulators (**A**), or microbial antigens may mimic self-antigens and activate self-reactive lymphocytes as a cross-reaction (**B**).

and even the initial autoimmune response, may damage tissues, release self-antigens and expose epitopes of the antigens that are normally concealed from the immune system. The result is continuing activation of lymphocytes that recognize these previously hidden epitopes; since these epitopes were not expressed normally, the lymphocytes did not become tolerant to them. The activation of such autoreactive T cells is referred to as epitope spreading because the immune response "spreads" to epitopes that were initially not recognized.[59]

● The clinical and pathologic manifestations of an autoimmune disease are determined by the nature of the underlying immune response. T_H1 responses are associated with destructive macrophage-rich inflammation and the production of antibodies that cause tissue damage by activating complement and binding to Fc receptors. T_H17 responses are believed to underlie inflammatory lesions dominated by neutrophils as well as monocytes.

● Different autoimmune diseases show substantial clinical, pathologic, and serologic overlaps. For this reason, precise phenotypic classification of these disorders is often a challenge.

With this background we can proceed to a discussion of specific autoimmune diseases. Table 6–7 lists both systemic and organ-specific autoimmune disorders. The systemic diseases tend to involve blood vessels and connective tissues, and therefore, they are often classified as *collagen vascular diseases.* Our focus here is on prototypic systemic autoimmune diseases; organ-specific disorders are covered elsewhere in the book.

SYSTEMIC LUPUS ERYTHEMATOSUS (SLE)

SLE is the prototype of a multisystem disease of autoimmune origin, characterized by a vast array of autoantibodies, particularly antinuclear antibodies (ANAs). *Acute or insidious in its onset, it is a chronic, remitting and relapsing, often febrile illness characterized principally by injury to the skin, joints, kidney, and serosal membranes.* Virtually every other organ in the body, however, may also be affected. The clinical presentation of SLE is so variable that the American College of Rheumatology has established a complex set of criteria for this disorder (Table 6–8). SLE is a fairly common disease, with a prevalence that may be as high as 1 in 2500 in certain populations.[60] Similar to many autoimmune diseases, SLE predominantly affects women, with a frequency of 1 in 700 among women of childbearing age and a female-to-male ratio of 9:1. By comparison, the female-to-male ratio is only 2:1 for disease developing during childhood or after the age of 65. The prevalence of the disease is 2–3 fold higher in blacks and Hispanics than in whites. Although SLE usually arises in the 20s and 30s, it may manifest at any age, even in early childhood.

Spectrum of Autoantibodies in SLE

The hallmark of the disease is the production of autoantibodies. Some antibodies recognize diverse nuclear and cytoplasmic components of the cell that are neither organ- nor species-specific, and others are directed against cell surface antigens of blood cells. Apart from their value in the diagnosis and management of patients with SLE, these antibodies are of major pathogenetic significance, as, for example, in the

TABLE 6–8	1997 Revised Criteria for Classification of Systemic Lupus Erythematosus*
Criterion	**Definition**
1. Malar rash	Fixed erythema, flat or raised, over the malar eminences, tending to spare the nasolabial folds
2. Discoid rash	Erythematous raised patches with adherent keratotic scaling and follicular plugging; atrophic scarring may occur in older lesions
3. Photosensitivity	Rash as a result of unusual reaction to sunlight, by patient history or physician observation
4. Oral ulcers	Oral or nasopharyngeal ulceration, usually painless, observed by a physician
5. Arthritis	Nonerosive arthritis involving two or more peripheral joints, characterized by tenderness, swelling, or effusion
6. Serositis	Pleuritis—convincing history of pleuritic pain or rub heard by a physician or evidence of pleural effusion, or Pericarditis—documented by electrocardiogram or rub or evidence of pericardial effusion
7. Renal disorder	Persistent proteinuria >0.5 gm/dL or >3 if quantitation not performed or Cellular casts—may be red blood cell, hemoglobin, granular, tubular, or mixed
8. Neurologic disorder	Seizures—in the absence of offending drugs or known metabolic derangements (e.g., uremia, ketoacidosis, or electrolyte imbalance), or Psychosis—in the absence of offending drugs or known metabolic derangements (e.g., uremia, ketoacidosis, or electrolyte imbalance)
9. Hematologic disorder	Hemolytic anemia—with reticulocytosis, or Leukopenia—<4.0×10^9 cells/L (4000 cells/mm³) total on two or more occasions, or Lymphopenia—<1.5×10^9 cells/L (1500 cells/mm³) on two or more occasions, or Thrombocytopenia—<100×10^9 cells/L (100×10^3 cells/mm³) in the absence of offending drugs
10. Immunological disorder	Anti-DNA antibody to native DNA in abnormal titer, or Anti-Sm—presence of antibody to Sm nuclear antigen, or Positive finding of antiphospholipid antibodies based on (1) an abnormal serum level of IgG or IgM anticardiolipin antibodies, (2) a positive test for lupus anticoagulant using a standard test, or (3) a false-positive serologic test for syphilis known to be positive for at least 6 months and confirmed by negative *Treponema pallidum* immobilization or fluorescent treponemal antibody absorption test
11. Antinuclear antibody	An abnormal titer of antinuclear antibody by immunofluorescence or an equivalent assay at any point in time and in the absence of drugs known to be associated with drug-induced lupus syndrome

*This classification, based on 11 criteria, was proposed for the purpose of identifying patients in clinical studies. A person is said to have systemic lupus erythematosus if any 4 or more of the 11 criteria are present, serially or simultaneously, during any period of observation.
From Tan EM et al: The revised criteria for the classification of systemic lupus erythematosus. Arthritis Rheum 25:1271, 1982; and Hochberg MC: Updating the American College of Rheumatology revised criteria for the classification of systemic lupus erythematosus. Arthritis Rheum 40:1725, 1997.

immune complex–mediated glomerulonephritis so typical of this disease.[61,62]

Antinuclear antibodies (ANAs) are directed against nuclear antigens and can be grouped into four categories[63]: (1) antibodies to DNA, (2) antibodies to histones, (3) antibodies to nonhistone proteins bound to RNA, and (4) antibodies to nucleolar antigens. Table 6–9 lists several ANAs and their association with SLE as well as with other autoimmune diseases to be discussed later. The most widely used method for detecting ANAs is indirect immunofluorescence, which can identify antibodies that bind to a variety of nuclear antigens, including DNA, RNA, and proteins (collectively called *generic ANAs*). The pattern of nuclear fluorescence suggests the type of antibody present in the patient's serum. Four basic patterns are recognized:

○ *Homogeneous or diffuse nuclear staining* usually reflects antibodies to chromatin, histones, and, occasionally, double-stranded DNA.
○ *Rim or peripheral staining* patterns are most often indicative of antibodies to double-stranded DNA.

○ *Speckled pattern* refers to the presence of uniform or variable-sized speckles. This is one of the most commonly observed patterns of fluorescence and therefore the least specific. It reflects the presence of antibodies to non-DNA nuclear constituents. Examples include Sm antigen, ribonucleoprotein, and SS-A and SS-B reactive antigens (see Table 6–9).
○ *Nucleolar pattern* refers to the presence of a few discrete spots of fluorescence within the nucleus and represents antibodies to RNA. This pattern is reported most often in patients with systemic sclerosis.

The fluorescence patterns are not absolutely specific for the type of antibody, and because many autoantibodies may be present, combinations of patterns are frequent. *The immunofluorescence test for ANAs is sensitive because it is positive in virtually every patient with SLE, but it is not specific because patients with other autoimmune diseases also frequently score positive* (see Table 6–9). Furthermore, approximately 5% to 15% of normal individuals have low titers of these antibodies, and the incidence increases with age. *Antibodies to double-*

TABLE 6–9 Antinuclear Antibodies in Various Autoimmune Diseases

Nature of Antigen	Antibody System	Disease, % Positive					
		SLE	Drug-Induced LE	Systemic Sclerosis—Diffuse	Limited Scleroderma—CREST	Sjögren Syndrome	Inflammatory Myopathies
Many nuclear antigens (DNA, RNA, proteins)	Generic ANA (indirect IF)	>95	>95	70–90	70–90	50–80	40–60
Native DNA	Anti–double-stranded DNA	40–60	<5	<5	<5	<5	<5
Histones	Antihistone	50–70	>95	<5	<5	<5	<5
Core proteins of small nuclear RNP particles (Smith antigen)	Anti-Sm	20–30	<5	<5	<5	<5	<5
RNP (U1RNP)	Nuclear RNP	30–40	<5	15	10	<5	<5
RNP	SS-A(Ro)	30–50	<5	<5	<5	70–95	10
RNP	SS-B(La)	10–15	<5	<5	<5	60–90	<5
DNA topoisomerase I	Scl-70	<5	<5	28–70	10–18	<5	<5
Centromeric proteins	Anticentromere	<5	<5	22–36	90	<5	<5
Histidyl-tRNA synthetase	Jo-1	<5	<5	<5	<5	<5	25

ANA, antinuclear antibodies; IF, immunofluorescence; LE, lupus erythematosus; RNP, ribonucleoprotein; SLE, systemic lupus erythematosus.

stranded DNA and the so-called Smith (Sm) antigen are virtually diagnostic of SLE.[64]

In addition to ANAs, lupus patients have a host of other autoantibodies. Some are directed against blood cells, such as red cells, platelets, and lymphocytes; others react with proteins in complex with phospholipids. In recent years there has been much interest in these so-called *antiphospholipid antibodies*. They are present in 40% to 50% of lupus patients. They are actually directed against epitopes of plasma proteins that are revealed when the proteins are in complex with phospholipids. Included among these proteins are prothrombin, annexin V, β_2-glycoprotein I, protein S, and protein C.[65] *Antibodies against the phospholipid–β_2-glycoprotein complex also bind to cardiolipin antigen, used in syphilis serology, and therefore lupus patients may have a false-positive test result for syphilis.* Some of these antibodies interfere with in vitro clotting tests, such as partial thromboplastin time. Therefore, these antibodies are sometimes referred to as *lupus anticoagulant*. Despite having a circulating anticoagulant that delays clotting in vitro, these patients have complications associated with a *hypercoagulable state*.[66] They have venous and arterial thromboses, which may be associated with recurrent spontaneous miscarriages and focal cerebral or ocular ischemia. This constellation of clinical features, in association with lupus, is referred to as the *secondary antiphospholipid antibody syndrome*. The pathogenesis of thrombosis in these patients is unknown; possible mechanisms are discussed in Chapter 4. Some patients develop these autoantibodies and the clinical syndrome without associated SLE. They are said to have the primary antiphospholipid syndrome (Chapter 4).

Etiology and Pathogenesis of SLE

The cause of SLE remains unknown, but the existence in these patients of a seemingly limitless number of antibodies against self-constituents indicates that the *fundamental defect in SLE is a failure of the mechanisms that maintain self-tolerance*. As is true of most autoimmune diseases, both genetic and environmental factors play a role in the pathogenesis of SLE.[67]

Genetic Factors. SLE is a genetically complex disease with contributions from MHC and multiple non-MHC genes. Many lines of evidence support a genetic predisposition.[68,69]

- Family members of patients have an increased risk of developing SLE. As many as 20% of clinically unaffected first-degree relatives of SLE patients reveal autoantibodies and other immunoregulatory abnormalities.
- There is a higher rate of concordance (>20%) in monozygotic twins when compared with dizygotic twins (1% to 3%).
- Studies of HLA associations support the concept that MHC genes regulate production of particular autoantibodies. Specific alleles of the *HLA-DQ* locus have been linked to the production of anti–double-stranded DNA, anti-Sm, and antiphospholipid antibodies, although the relative risk is small.
- Some lupus patients (~6%) have inherited deficiencies of early complement components, such as C2, C4, or C1q. Lack of complement may impair removal of circulating immune complexes by the mononuclear phagocyte system, thus favoring tissue deposition. Knockout mice lacking C4 or certain complement receptors are also prone to develop lupus-like autoimmunity. Various mechanisms have been invoked, including failure to clear immune complexes and loss of B-cell self-tolerance. It has also been proposed that deficiency of C1q results in defective phagocytic clearance of apoptotic cells.[70] Many cells normally undergo apoptosis, and if they are not cleared their nuclear components may elicit immune responses.
- In animal models of SLE, several non-MHC susceptibility loci have been identified. The best-known animal model is

the (NZB × NZW)F$_1$ mouse strain. In different versions of this strain, as many as 20 loci are believed to be associated with the disease.[71]

Immunological Factors. Recent studies in animal models and patients are revealing several immunological aberrations that collectively may result in the persistence and uncontrolled activation of self-reactive lymphocytes.

- Defective elimination of self-reactive B cells in the bone marrow or defects in peripheral tolerance mechanisms may lead to *failure of self-tolerance in B cells.*[72]
- In models of SLE and in some patients there is evidence that *CD4+ helper T cells* specific for nucleosomal antigens also *escape tolerance* and contribute to the production of high-affinity pathogenic autoantibodies.[73]
- Nuclear DNA and RNA contained in immune complexes may activate B lymphocytes by engaging *TLRs*, which function normally to sense microbial products, including nucleic acids. Thus, B cells specific for nuclear antigens may get second signals from TLRs and may be activated, resulting in increased production of anti-nuclear autoantibodies.[74]
- Recent analyses of patients have revealed a striking molecular signature in peripheral blood lymphocytes that suggests exposure to *type I interferons.*[75] These cytokines are antiviral cytokines that are normally produced during innate immune responses to viruses. It may be that nucleic acids engage TLRs on dendritic cells and stimulate the production of interferons. In other words, self–nucleic acids mimic their microbial counterparts. The role of interferons in SLE is also unclear; these cytokines may activate dendritic cells and B cells and promote T$_H$1 responses, all of which may contribute to the production of pathogenic autoantibodies.
- Other cytokines that may play a role in unregulated B-cell activation include the TNF family member, BAFF, which promotes survival of B cells. In some patients and animal models, increased production of BAFF has been reported, prompting attempts to block the cytokine or its receptor as therapy for autoimmune diseases.[76]

Environmental Factors. There are many indications that *environmental* or nongenetic factors must also be involved in the pathogenesis of SLE. Exposure to *ultraviolet (UV) light* exacerbates the disease in many individuals. UV irradiation may induce apoptosis in cells and may alter the DNA in such a way that it becomes immunogenic, perhaps because of enhanced recognition by TLRs.[77] In addition, UV light may modulate the immune response, for example, by stimulating keratinocytes to produce IL-1, a cytokine known to promote inflammation. *Sex hormones* seem to exert an important influence on the occurrence and manifestations of SLE. During the reproductive years the frequency of SLE is 10 times greater in women than in men in the age group of 17 through 55 years, and exacerbation has been noted during normal menses and pregnancy. *Drugs* such as hydralazine, procainamide, and D-penicillamine can induce an SLE-like response in humans.[78]

A Model for the Pathogenesis of SLE. It is clear from this discussion that the immunological abnormalities in SLE—

both documented and postulated—are as varied and complex as is the clinical presentation (discussed later). Nevertheless, an attempt can be made to synthesize the new results into a hypothetical model of the pathogenesis of SLE (Fig. 6–27). UV irradiation and other environmental insults lead to the apoptosis of cells. Inadequate clearance of the nuclei of these cells results in a large burden of nuclear antigens.[79] An underlying abnormality in B and T lymphocytes is responsible for defective tolerance, because of which self-reactive lymphocytes survive and remain functional. These lymphocytes are stimulated by self nuclear antigens, and antibodies are produced against the antigens. Complexes of the antigens and antibodies bind to Fc receptors on B cells and dendritic cells, and may be internalized. The nucleic acid components engage TLRs and stimulate B cells to produce autoantibodies and activate dendritic cells to produce interferons and other cytokines, which further enhance the immune response and cause more apop-

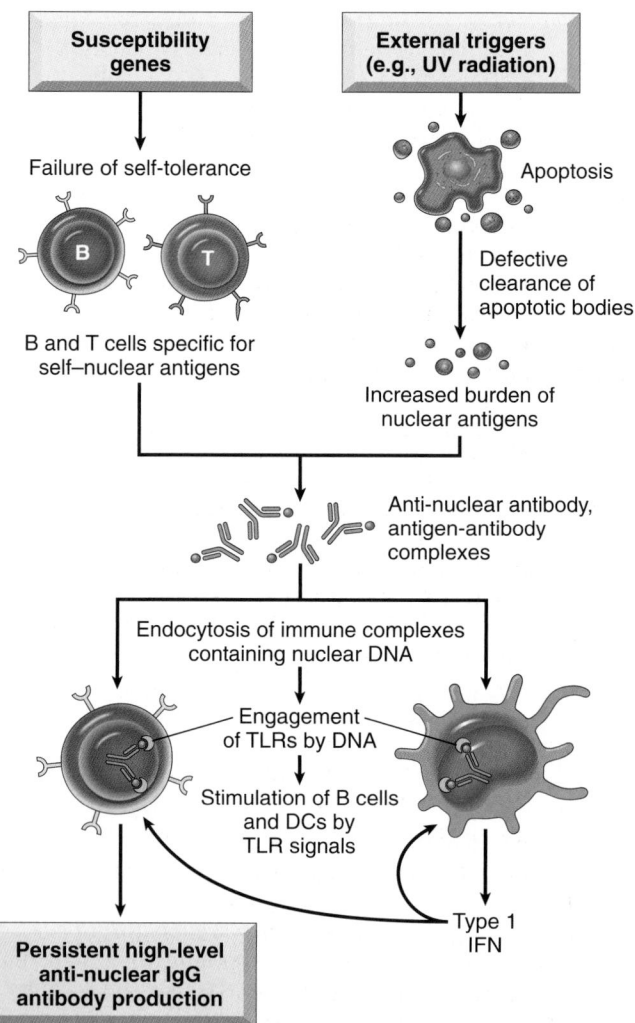

FIGURE 6–27 Model for the pathogenesis of systemic lupus erythematosus. In this hypothetical model, susceptibility genes interfere with the maintenance of self-tolerance and external triggers lead to persistence of nuclear antigens. The result is an antibody response against self–nuclear antigens, which is amplified by the action of nucleic acids on dendritic cells (DCs) and B cells, and the production of type 1 interferons. TLRs, Toll-like receptors.

tosis. The net result is a cycle of antigen release and immune activation resulting in the production of high-affinity autoantibodies.

Mechanisms of Tissue Injury. Regardless of the exact mechanisms by which autoantibodies are formed, they are clearly the mediators of tissue injury. *Most of the visceral lesions are caused by immune complexes (type III hypersensitivity).* DNA–anti-DNA complexes can be detected in the glomeruli and small blood vessels. Low levels of serum complement (secondary to consumption of complement proteins) and granular deposits of complement and immunoglobulins in the glomeruli further support the immune complex nature of the disease. *Autoantibodies specific for red cells, white cells, and platelets opsonize these cells and promote their phagocytosis and lysis.* There is no evidence that ANAs, which are involved in immune complex formation, can penetrate intact cells. If cell nuclei are exposed, however, the ANAs can bind to them. In tissues, nuclei of damaged cells react with ANAs, lose their chromatin pattern, and become homogeneous, to produce so-called LE bodies or hematoxylin bodies. Related to this phenomenon is the LE cell, which is readily seen when blood is agitated in vitro. The LE cell is any phagocytic leukocyte (blood neutrophil or macrophage) that has engulfed the denatured nucleus of an injured cell. The demonstration of LE cells in vitro was used in the past as a test for SLE. With new techniques for detection of ANAs, however, this test is now largely of historical interest. Sometimes, LE cells are found in pericardial or pleural effusions in patients.

To summarize, SLE is a complex disorder of multifactorial origin resulting from interactions among genetic, immunological, and environmental factors that act in concert to cause activation of helper T cells and B cells and result in the production of several species of pathogenic autoantibodies.

Morphology. The morphologic changes in SLE are extremely variable, as are the clinical manifestations and course of disease. The constellation of clinical, serologic, and morphologic changes is essential for diagnosis (see Table 6–8). The frequency of individual organ involvement is shown in Table 6–10. The most characteristic lesions result from immune complexes depositing in blood vessels, kidneys, connective tissue, and skin.

An acute necrotizing vasculitis involving capillaries, small arteries and arterioles may be present in any tissue.[80] The arteritis is characterized by fibrinoid deposits in the vessel walls. In chronic stages, vessels undergo fibrous thickening with luminal narrowing.

Kidney. Lupus nephritis affects up to 50% of SLE patients. The principal mechanism of injury is immune complex deposition in the glomeruli, tubular or peritubular capillary basement membranes, or larger blood vessels. Other injuries may include thrombi in glomerular capillaries, arterioles, or arteries, often associated with antiphospholipid antibodies.

All of the glomerular lesions described below are the result of deposition of immune complexes that are regularly present in the mesangium or along the entire basement membrane and sometimes through-

TABLE 6–10 Clinical and Pathologic Manifestations of Systemic Lupus Erythematosus

Clinical Manifestation	Prevalence in Patients (%)*
Hematologic	100
Arthritis	80–90
Skin	85
Fever	55–85
Fatigue	80–100
Weight loss	60
Renal	50–70
Neuropsychiatric	25–35
Pleuritis	45
Myalgia	35
Pericarditis	25
Gastrointestinal	20
Raynaud phenomenon	15–40
Ocular	15
Peripheral neuropathy	15

*The percentages are approximate and may vary with age, ethnicity, and other factors.

out the glomerulus. The immune complexes consist of DNA and anti-DNA antibodies, but other antigens such as histones have also been implicated. Both in situ formation and deposition of preformed circulating immune complexes may contribute to the injury, but the reason for the wide spectrum of histopathologic lesions (and clinical manifestations) in lupus nephritis patients remains uncertain.

A morphologic classification of lupus nephritis has proven to be clinically useful.[81] Five patterns are recognized: minimal mesangial (class I); mesangial proliferative (class II); focal proliferative (class III); diffuse proliferative (class IV); and membranous (class V). None of these patterns is specific for lupus.

Mesangial lupus glomerulonephritis is seen in 10% to 25% of patients and is characterized by mesangial cell proliferation and immune complex deposition without involvement of glomerular capillaries. There is no or slight (class I) to moderate (class II) increase in both mesangial matrix and number of mesangial cells. **Granular mesangial deposits of immunoglobulin and complement are always present.** Classes III to V nephritis, described below, are usually superimposed on some degree of mesangial changes.

Focal proliferative glomerulonephritis (class III) is seen in 20% to 35% of patients, and is defined by fewer than 50% involvement of all glomeruli. The lesions may be segmental (affecting only a portion of the glomerulus) or global (involving the entire glomerulus). Affected glomeruli may exhibit crescent formation, fibrinoid necrosis, proliferation of endothelial

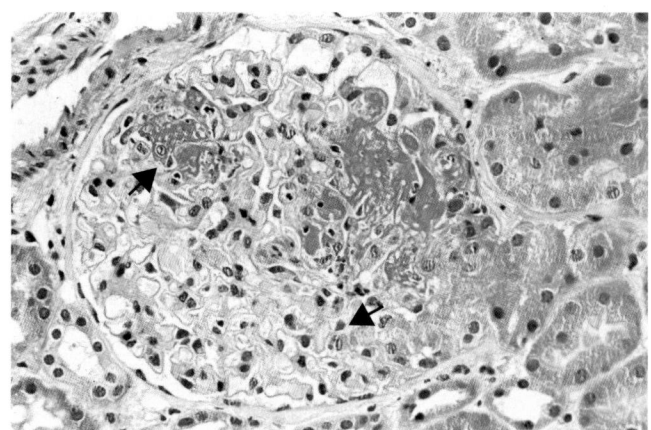

FIGURE 6–28 Lupus nephritis, focal proliferative type. There are two focal necrotizing lesions in the glomerulus *(arrows)*. (Courtesy of Dr. Helmut Rennke, Department of Pathology, Brigham and Women's Hospital, Boston, MA.)

and mesangial cells, infiltrating leukocytes, and eosinophilic deposits or intracapillary thrombi (Fig. 6–28), which often correlate with hematuria and proteinuria. Some patients may progress to diffuse proliferative glomerulonephritis. The active (or proliferative) inflammatory lesions can heal completely or lead to chronic global or segmental glomerular scarring.

Diffuse proliferative glomerulonephritis (class IV) is the most severe form of lupus nephritis, occurring in 35% to 60% of patients. Pathologic glomerular changes may be identical to focal (class III) lupus nephritis, including proliferation of endothelial, mesangial and, sometimes, epithelial cells (Fig. 6–29), with the latter producing cellular crescents that fill Bowman's space (Chapter 20). The entire glomerulus is frequently affected but segmental lesions also may occur. Both acutely injured and chronically scarred

glomeruli in focal or diffuse lupus nephritis are qualitatively indistinguishable from one another; the distinction is based solely on the percentage of glomerular involvement (<50% for class III vs >50% for class IV). Patients with diffuse glomerulonephritis are usually symptomatic, showing hematuria as well as proteinuria. Hypertension and mild to severe renal insufficiency are also common.

Membranous glomerulonephritis (class V) is characterized by diffuse thickening of the capillary walls, which is similar to idiopathic membranous glomerulonephritis, described in Chapter 20. This lesion is seen in 10% to 15% of lupus nephritis patients, is usually accompanied by severe proteinuria or nephrotic syndrome, and may occur concurrently with focal or diffuse lupus nephritis.

Granular deposits of antibody and complement can be detected by immunofluorescence (Fig. 6–30). Electron microscopy demonstrates electron-dense deposits that represent immune complexes in mesangial, intramembranous, subepithelial, or subendothelial locations. All classes show variable amounts of mesangial deposits. In membranous lupus nephritis, the deposits are predominantly subepithelial (between the basement membrane and visceral epithelial cells). Subendothelial deposits (between the endothelium and the basement membrane) are seen in the proliferative types (classes III and IV) but may be encountered rarely in class I, II, and V lupus nephritis (Fig. 6–31). When prominent, subendothelial deposits create a homogeneous thickening of the capillary wall, which are seen by light microscopy as a **"wire-loop"** lesion (Fig. 6–32). Such wire loops are often

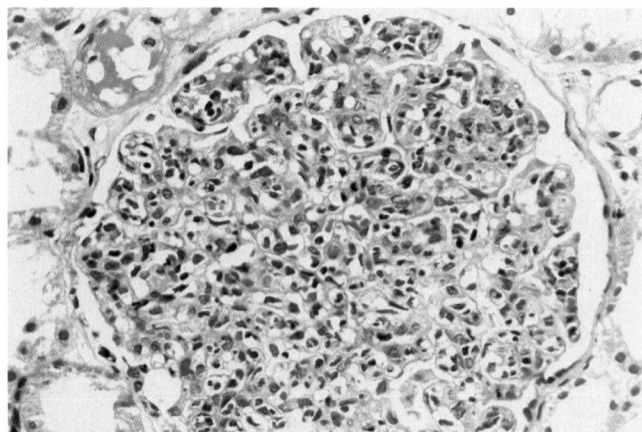

FIGURE 6–29 Lupus nephritis, diffuse proliferative type. Note the marked increase in cellularity throughout the glomerulus. (Courtesy of Dr. Helmut Rennke, Department of Pathology, Brigham and Women's Hospital, Boston, MA.)

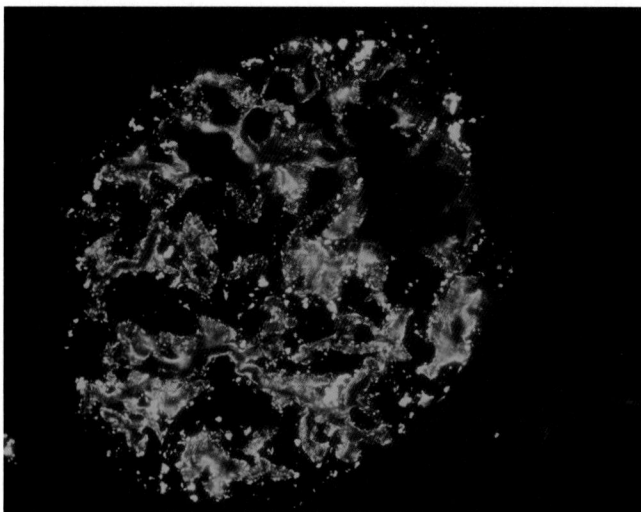

FIGURE 6–30 Immune complex deposition in systemic lupus erythematosus. Immunofluorescence micrograph of a glomerulus stained with fluorescent anti-IgG from a patient with diffuse proliferative lupus nephritis. Note the mesangial and capillary wall deposits of IgG. (Courtesy of Dr. Jean Olson, Department of Pathology, University of California San Francisco, San Francisco, CA.)

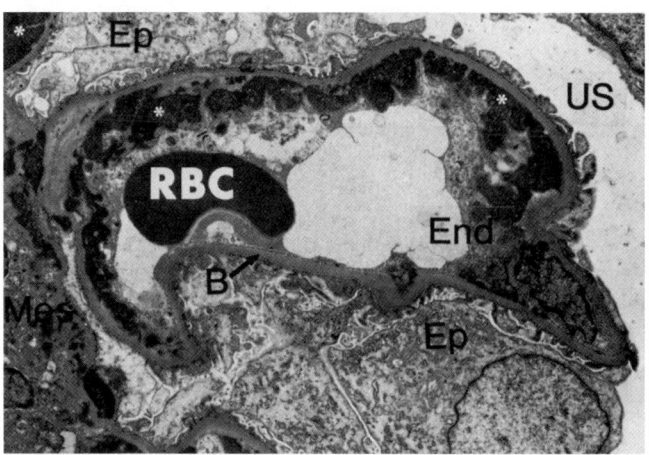

FIGURE 6–31 Immune complex deposition in systemic lupus erythematosus (SLE). Electron micrograph of a renal glomerular capillary loop from a patient with SLE nephritis shows subendothelial dense deposits corresponding to "wire loops" seen by light microscopy. Deposits are also present in the mesangium. B, basement membrane; End, endothelium; Ep, epithelium; RBC, red blood cell; US, urinary space (Courtesy of Dr. Edwin Eigenbrodt, Department of Pathology, University of Texas Southwestern Medical School, Dallas, TX.)

found in both focal and diffuse proliferative (class III or IV) lupus nephritis, which reflects active disease.

Changes in the **interstitium and tubules are frequently present** in lupus nephritis patients. Rarely, tubulointerstitial lesions may be the dominant abnormality. Discrete immune complexes similar to those in glomeruli are present in the tubular or peritubular capillary basement membranes in many lupus nephritis patients.

Skin. Characteristic erythema affects the facial butterfly (malar) area (bridge of the nose and cheeks) in approximately 50% of patients, but a similar rash may also be seen on the extremities and trunk. Urticaria, bullae, maculopapular lesions, and ulcerations also occur. **Exposure to sunlight incites or accentuates the erythema.** Histologically the involved areas show vacuolar degeneration of the basal layer of the epidermis (Fig. 6–33A). In the dermis, there is variable edema and perivascular inflammation. Vasculitis with fibrinoid necrosis may be prominent. Immunofluorescence microscopy shows deposition of immunoglobulin and complement along the dermoepidermal junction (Fig. 6–33B), which may also be present in uninvolved skin. This finding is not diagnostic of SLE and is sometimes seen in scleroderma or dermatomyositis.

Joints. Joint involvement is typically a nonerosive synovitis with little deformity, which contrasts with rheumatoid arthritis.

Central Nervous System. The pathologic basis of central nervous system symptoms is not entirely clear, but antibodies against a synaptic membrane protein have been implicated.[82,83] Neuropsychiatric symptoms of SLE have often been ascribed to acute

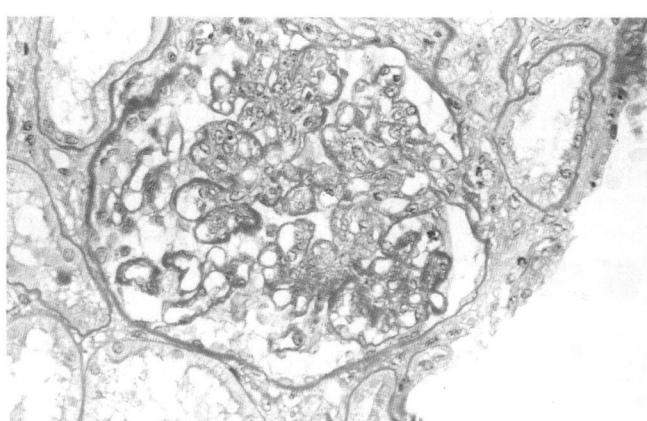

FIGURE 6–32 Lupus nephritis. A glomerulus with several "wire loop" lesions representing extensive subendothelial deposits of immune complexes is seen. (Periodic acid-Schiff [PAS] stain.) (Courtesy of Dr. Helmut Rennke, Department of Pathology, Brigham and Women's Hospital, Boston, MA.)

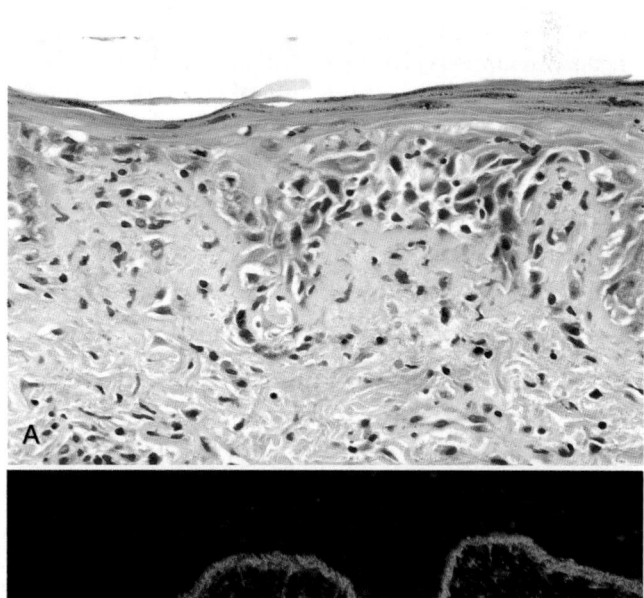

FIGURE 6–33 Systemic lupus erythematosus involving the skin. **A,** An H&E-stained section shows liquefactive degeneration of the basal layer of the epidermis and edema at the dermoepidermal junction. (Courtesy of Dr. Jag Bhawan, Boston University School of Medicine, Boston, MA.) **B,** An immunofluorescence micrograph stained for IgG reveals deposits of Ig along the dermoepidermal junction. (Courtesy of Dr. Richard Sontheimer, Department of Dermatology, University of Texas Southwestern Medical School, Dallas, TX.)

vasculitis, but in histologic studies of the nervous system in such patients significant vasculitis is rarely present. Instead, noninflammatory occlusion of small vessels by intimal proliferation is sometimes noted, which may be due to endothelial damage by antiphospholipid antibodies.

Pericarditis and Other Serosal Cavity Involvement. Inflammation of the serosal lining membranes may be acute, subacute, or chronic. During the acute phases, the mesothelial surfaces are sometimes covered with fibrinous exudate. Later they become thickened, opaque, and coated with a shaggy fibrous tissue that may lead to partial or total obliteration of the serosal cavity.

Cardiovascular system involvement may manifest as damage to any layer of the heart.[84] Symptomatic or asymptomatic pericardial involvement is present in up to 50% of patients. Myocarditis, or mononuclear cell infiltration, is less common and may cause resting tachycardia and electrocardiographic abnormalities. Valvular abnormalities primarily of the mitral and aortic valves manifest as diffuse leaflet thickening that may be associated with dysfunction (stenosis and/or regurgitation). Valvular (or so-called Libman-Sacks) endocarditis was more common prior to the widespread use of steroids. This **nonbacterial verrucous endocarditis** takes the form of single or multiple 1- to 3-mm warty deposits on any heart valve, distinctively on either surface of the leaflets (Fig. 6–34). By comparison, the vegetations in infective endocarditis are considerably larger, and those in rheumatic heart disease (Chapter 12) are smaller and confined to the lines of closure of the valve leaflets.

An increasing number of patients have clinical evidence of coronary artery disease (angina, myocardial infarction) owing to coronary atherosclerosis. This complication is noted particularly in young patients with long-standing disease and especially in those who have been treated with corticosteroids. The pathogenesis of accelerated coronary atherosclerosis is unclear but is probably multifactorial. The traditional risk factors, including hypertension, obesity, and hyperlipidemia, are more common in SLE patients than in control populations. In addition, immune complexes and antiphospholipid antibodies may cause endothelial damage and promote atherosclerosis.

Spleen. Splenomegaly, capsular thickening, and follicular hyperplasia are common features. Central penicilliary arteries may show concentric intimal and smooth muscle cell hyperplasia, producing so-called onion-skin lesions.

Lungs. Pleuritis and pleural effusions are the most common pulmonary manifestations, affecting almost 50% of patients. Alveolar injury with edema and hemorrhage is less common. In some cases, there is chronic interstitial fibrosis and secondary pulmonary hypertension. None of these changes is specific for SLE.

Other Organs and Tissues. LE, or hematoxylin, bodies in the bone marrow or other organs are strongly indicative of SLE. Lymph nodes may be enlarged with hyperplastic follicles or even demonstrate necrotizing lymphadenitis.

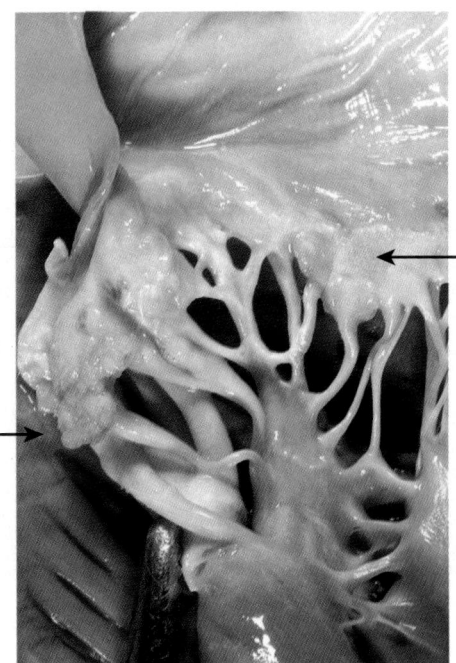

FIGURE 6–34 Libman-Sacks endocarditis of the mitral valve in lupus erythematosus. The vegetations attached to the margin of the thickened valve leaflet are indicated by *arrows*. (Courtesy of Dr. Fred Schoen, Department of Pathology, Brigham and Women's Hospital, Boston, MA.)

Clinical Features. SLE is a multisystem disease that is highly variable in its clinical presentation. Typically, the patient is a young woman with some, but not necessarily all, of the following features: a butterfly rash over the face, fever, pain but no deformity in one or more peripheral joints (feet, ankles, knees, hips, fingers, wrists, elbows, shoulders), pleuritic chest pain, and photosensitivity. In many patients, however, the presentation of SLE is subtle and puzzling, taking forms such as a febrile illness of unknown origin, abnormal urinary findings, or joint disease masquerading as rheumatoid arthritis or rheumatic fever. ANAs are found in virtually 100% of patients, but it must be remembered that ANAs are not specific (see Table 6–9). A variety of clinical findings may point toward renal involvement, including hematuria, red cell casts, proteinuria, and in some cases the classic nephrotic syndrome (Chapter 20). Laboratory evidence of some hematologic derangement is seen in virtually every case, but in some patients anemia or thrombocytopenia may be the presenting manifestation as well as the dominant clinical problem. In still others, mental aberrations, including psychosis or convulsions, or coronary artery disease may be prominent clinical problems. Patients with SLE are also prone to infections, presumably because of their underlying immune dysfunction and treatment with immunosuppressive drugs.

The course of the disease is variable and unpredictable. Rare acute cases result in death within weeks to months. More often, with appropriate therapy, the disease is characterized by flare-ups and remissions spanning a period of years or even decades. During acute flare-ups, increased formation of immune complexes and the accompanying complement activation often result in hypocomplementemia. Disease exacerbations are usually treated by corticosteroids or other immunosuppressive drugs. Even without therapy, in some patients the disease may run a benign course with skin manifestations and mild hematuria for years. The outcome has improved significantly, and an approximately 90% 5-year and 80% 10-year survival can be expected. *The most common causes of death are renal failure and intercurrent infections.* Coronary artery disease is also becoming an important cause of death. Patients treated with steroids and immunosuppressive drugs incur the usual risks associated with such therapy.

As mentioned earlier, involvement of skin along with multisystem disease is fairly common in SLE. The following sections describe two syndromes in which the cutaneous involvement is the exclusive or most prominent feature.

Chronic Discoid Lupus Erythematosus. Chronic discoid lupus erythematosus is a disease in which the skin manifestations may mimic SLE, but systemic manifestations are rare.[85] It is characterized by the presence of skin plaques showing varying degrees of edema, erythema, scaliness, follicular plugging, and skin atrophy surrounded by an elevated erythematous border. The face and scalp are usually affected, but widely disseminated lesions occasionally occur. The disease is usually confined to the skin, but 5% to 10% of patients with discoid lupus erythematosus develop multisystem manifestations after many years. Conversely, some patients with SLE may have prominent discoid lesions in the skin. Approximately 35% of patients show a positive ANA test, but *antibodies to double-stranded DNA are rarely present.* Immunofluorescence studies of skin biopsy specimens show deposition of immunoglobulin and C3 at the dermoepidermal junction similar to that in SLE.

Subacute Cutaneous Lupus Erythematosus. This condition also presents with predominant skin involvement and can be distinguished from chronic discoid lupus erythematosus by several criteria. The skin rash in this disease tends to be widespread, superficial, and nonscarring, although scarring lesions may occur in some patients. Most patients have mild systemic symptoms consistent with SLE. Furthermore, there is a strong association with antibodies to the SS-A antigen and with the *HLA-DR3* genotype. Thus, the term *subacute cutaneous lupus erythematosus* seems to define a group intermediate between SLE and lupus erythematosus localized only to skin.[85]

Drug-Induced Lupus Erythematosus

A lupus erythematosus–like syndrome may develop in patients receiving a variety of drugs, including hydralazine, procainamide, isoniazid, and D-penicillamine, to name only a few.[78] Many of these drugs are associated with the development of ANAs, but most patients do not have symptoms of lupus erythematosus. For example, 80% of patients receiving procain-

amide test positive for ANAs, but only one third of these manifest clinical symptoms, such as arthralgias, fever, and serositis. *Although multiple organs are affected, renal and central nervous system involvement is distinctly uncommon.* There are serologic and genetic differences from classical SLE, as well. Antibodies specific for double-stranded DNA are rare, but there is an *extremely high frequency of antibodies specific for histone.* Persons with the *HLA-DR4* allele are at a greater risk of developing lupus erythematosus after administration of hydralazine. The disease remits after withdrawal of the offending drug.

RHEUMATOID ARTHRITIS

Rheumatoid arthritis is a chronic inflammatory disease that affects primarily the joints but may involve extra-articular tissues such as the skin, blood vessels, lungs, and heart. Abundant evidence supports the autoimmune nature of the disease. Because the principal manifestations of the disease are in the joints, it is discussed in Chapter 26.

SJÖGREN SYNDROME

Sjögren syndrome is a chronic disease characterized by dry eyes (keratoconjunctivitis sicca) and dry mouth (xerostomia) resulting from immunologically mediated destruction of the lacrimal and salivary glands. It occurs as an isolated disorder (primary form), also known as the sicca syndrome, or more often in association with another autoimmune disease (secondary form). Among the associated disorders, rheumatoid arthritis is the most common, but some patients have SLE, polymyositis, scleroderma, vasculitis, mixed connective tissue disease, or thyroiditis.

Etiology and Pathogenesis

The characteristic decrease in tears and saliva (sicca syndrome) is the result of *lymphocytic infiltration* and fibrosis of the lacrimal and salivary glands.[86,87] The infiltrate contains predominantly activated CD4+ helper T cells and some B cells, including plasma cells. About 75% of patients have rheumatoid factor (an antibody reactive with self-IgG) whether or not coexisting rheumatoid arthritis is present. ANAs are detected in 50% to 80% of patients. A host of other organ-specific and non–organ-specific antibodies have also been identified. Most important, however, are antibodies directed against two ribonucleoprotein antigens, SS-A (Ro) and SS-B (La) (see Table 6–9), which can be detected in as many as 90% of patients by sensitive techniques. These antibodies are thus considered serologic markers of the disease. Patients with high titers of antibodies to SS-A are more likely to have early disease onset, longer disease duration, and extraglandular manifestations, such as cutaneous vasculitis and nephritis.[62] These autoantibodies are also present in a smaller percentage of patients with SLE and hence are not diagnostic of Sjögren syndrome.

As with other autoimmune diseases, Sjögren syndrome shows some association, albeit weak, with certain HLA alleles. Studies of whites and blacks suggest linkage of the primary form with *HLA-B8*, *HLA-DR3*, and *DRW52* as well as *HLA-DQA1* and *HLA-DQB1* loci; in patients with anti-SS-A or anti-SS-B antibodies, specific alleles of *HLA-DQA1* and

HLA-DQB1 are frequent. This suggests that, as in SLE, inheritance of certain class II molecules predisposes to the development of particular autoantibodies.

Although the pathogenesis of Sjögren syndrome remains obscure, aberrant T-cell and B-cell activation are both implicated. The initiating trigger may be a viral infection of the salivary glands, which causes local cell death and release of tissue self-antigens. In genetically susceptible individuals, CD4+ T cells and B cells specific for these self-antigens may have escaped tolerance and are able to react. The result is inflammation, tissue damage, and, eventually, fibrosis. The nature of the autoantigen(s) recognized by these lymphocytes is still mysterious. A cytoskeletal protein called α-fodrin is a candidate autoantigen, but its role in disease development has not been established yet.[88] The viruses that may serve as the initiating stimuli are also unknown but may include the perennial culprit in chronic inflammatory diseases, Epstein-Barr virus, and hepatitis C virus.[89] In addition, a small proportion of individuals infected with the human retrovirus human T-cell lymphotropic virus type 1 develop a clinical picture and pathologic changes virtually identical to those seen in Sjögren syndrome.

Morphology. As mentioned earlier, lacrimal and salivary glands are the major targets of the disease, although other exocrine glands, including those lining the respiratory and gastrointestinal tracts and the vagina, may also be involved. The earliest histologic finding in both the major and the minor salivary glands is **periductal and perivascular lymphocytic infiltration**. Eventually the lymphocytic infiltrate becomes extensive (Fig. 6–35), and in the larger salivary glands lymphoid follicles with germinal centers may be seen. The ductal lining epithelial cells may show hyperplasia, thus obstructing the ducts. Later there is atrophy of the acini, fibrosis, and hyalinization; still later in the course atrophy and replacement of parenchyma with fat are seen. In some cases the lymphoid infiltrate may be so intense as to give the

appearance of a lymphoma. Indeed, these patients are at high risk for development of B-cell lymphomas, and molecular assessments of clonality may be necessary to distinguish intense reactive chronic inflammation from early involvement by lymphoma.

The lack of tears leads to drying of the corneal epithelium, which becomes inflamed, eroded, and ulcerated; the oral mucosa may atrophy, with inflammatory fissuring and ulceration; and dryness and crusting of the nose may lead to ulcerations and even perforation of the nasal septum.

Clinical Features. Sjögren syndrome occurs most commonly in women between the ages of 50 and 60. As might be expected, symptoms result from inflammatory destruction of the exocrine glands. The keratoconjunctivitis produces blurring of vision, burning, and itching, and thick secretions accumulate in the conjunctival sac. The xerostomia results in difficulty in swallowing solid foods, a decrease in the ability to taste, cracks and fissures in the mouth, and dryness of the buccal mucosa. Parotid gland enlargement is present in half the patients; dryness of the nasal mucosa, epistaxis, recurrent bronchitis, and pneumonitis are other symptoms. Manifestations of extraglandular disease are seen in one third of patients and include synovitis, diffuse pulmonary fibrosis, and peripheral neuropathy. These are more common in patients with high titers of antibodies specific for SS-A. In contrast to SLE, glomerular lesions are extremely rare in Sjögren syndrome. Defects of tubular function, however, including renal tubular acidosis, uricosuria, and phosphaturia, are often seen and are associated histologically with tubulointerstitial nephritis (Chapter 20). About 60% of patients have another accompanying autoimmune disorder, such as rheumatoid arthritis, and these patients also have the symptoms and signs of that disorder.

The combination of lacrimal and salivary gland inflammatory involvement was once called *Mikulicz disease*. The name has now been replaced, however, by *Mikulicz syndrome*, broadened to include lacrimal and salivary gland enlargement from

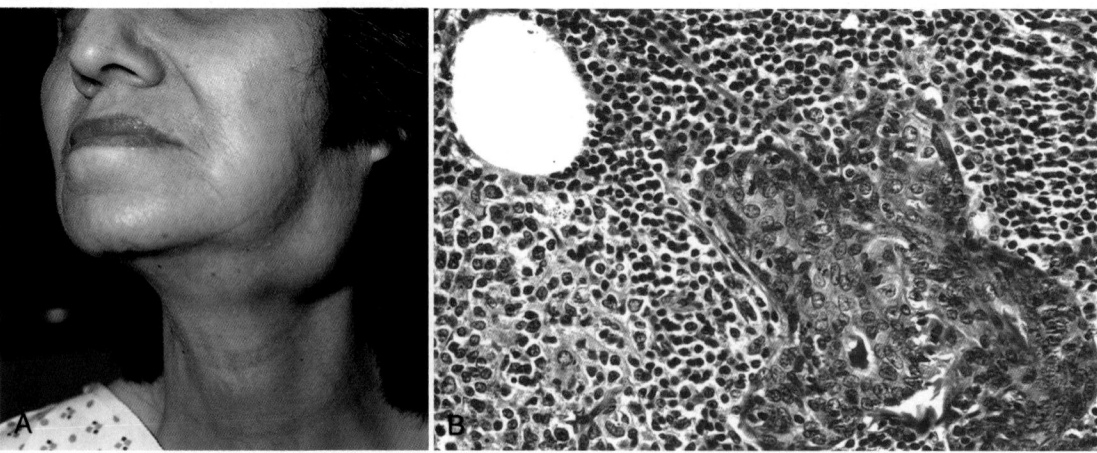

FIGURE 6–35 Sjögren syndrome. **A,** Enlargement of the salivary gland. (Courtesy of Dr. Richard Sontheimer, Department of Dermatology, University of Texas Southwestern Medical School, Dallas, TX.) **B,** Intense lymphocytic and plasma cell infiltration with ductal epithelial hyperplasia in a salivary gland. (Courtesy of Dr. Dennis Burns, Department of Pathology, University of Texas Southwestern Medical School, Dallas, TX.)

any cause, including sarcoidosis, leukemia, lymphoma, and other tumors. *Biopsy of the lip (to examine minor salivary glands) is essential for the diagnosis of Sjögren syndrome.*

The lymph nodes of patients with Sjögren syndrome are often hyperplastic, but the most intense lymphocytic response is seen in the tissues that are the focal point of the autoimmune response, particularly the salivary and lacrimal glands. In early stages of the disease, this immune infiltrate consists of a mixture of polyclonal T and B cells. However, if the reaction continues unabated there is a strong tendency over time for individual clones within the population of B cells to gain a growth advantage, presumably because of the acquisition of somatic mutations. Emergence of a dominant B cell clone is usually indicative of the development of a marginal zone lymphoma, a specific type of B cell malignancy that often arises in the setting of chronic lymphocytic inflammation. About 5% of Sjögren patients develop lymphoma, an incidence that is 40-fold greater than normal. Certain other autoimmune disorders (e.g., Hashimoto thyroiditis) are also associated with a high risk of marginal zone lymphoma (Chapter 13).

SYSTEMIC SCLEROSIS (SCLERODERMA)

Systemic sclerosis is a chronic disease characterized by: (1) chronic inflammation thought to be the result of autoimmunity, (2) widespread damage to small blood vessels, and (3) progressive interstitial and perivascular fibrosis in the skin and multiple organs.[90] Although the term *scleroderma* is ingrained in clinical medicine, this disease is better named systemic sclerosis because it is characterized by excessive fibrosis throughout the body. The skin is most commonly affected, but the gastrointestinal tract, kidneys, heart, muscles, and lungs also are frequently involved. In some patients the disease seems to remain confined to the skin for many years, but in the majority it progresses to visceral involvement with death from renal failure, cardiac failure, pulmonary insufficiency, or intestinal malabsorption. The clinical heterogeneity of systemic sclerosis has been recognized by classifying the disease into two major categories: *diffuse scleroderma*, characterized by widespread skin involvement at onset, with rapid progression and early visceral involvement; and *limited scleroderma*, in which the skin involvement is often confined to fingers, forearms, and face. Visceral involvement occurs late; hence, the clinical course is relatively benign. Some patents with the limited disease also develop a combination of calcinosis, Raynaud's phenomenon, esophageal dysmotility, sclerodactyly, and telangiectasia, called the *CREST syndrome*. Several other variants and related conditions, such as eosinophilic fasciitis, occur far less frequently and are not described here.

Etiology and Pathogenesis

The cause of systemic sclerosis is not known. *Autoimmune responses, vascular damage, and collagen deposition all contribute to the ultimate tissue injury* (Fig. 6–36).[90,91]

Abnormal Immune Responses. It is proposed that *CD4+ T cells responding to an as yet unidentified antigen accumulate in the skin and release cytokines that activate inflammatory cells and fibroblasts.*[92] Although inflammatory infiltrates are typically sparse in the skin of patients with systemic sclerosis, activated CD4+ T cells can be found in many patients, and

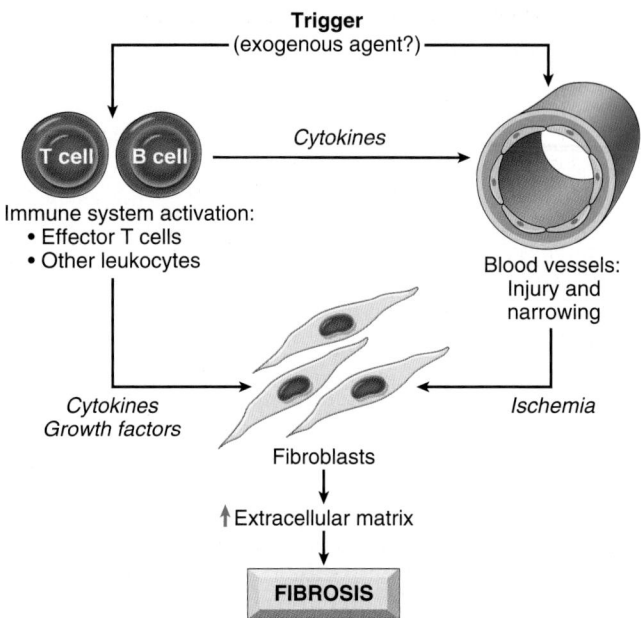

FIGURE 6–36 Possible mechanisms leading to systemic sclerosis.

T_H2 cells have been isolated from the skin. Several cytokines produced by these T cells, including TGF-β and IL-13, can stimulate transcription of genes that encode collagen and other extracellular matrix proteins (e.g., fibronectin) in fibroblasts. Other cytokines recruit leukocytes and propagate the chronic inflammation.

There is also evidence for inappropriate activation of humoral immunity, and the presence of various autoantibodies provides diagnostic and prognostic information.[93] Virtually all patients have ANAs that react with a variety of nuclear antigens. Two ANAs strongly associated with systemic sclerosis have been described. One of these, directed against *DNA topoisomerase* I (anti-Scl 70), is highly specific. Depending on the ethnic group and the assay, it is present in 10% to 20% of patients with diffuse systemic sclerosis. Patients who have this antibody are more likely to have pulmonary fibrosis and peripheral vascular disease. The other, an *anticentromere antibody*, is found in 20% to 30% of patients, who tend to have the CREST syndrome or limited cutaneous systemic sclerosis. Only rarely does the same patient have both antibodies. The role of these ANAs in the pathogenesis of the disease is unclear; it has been postulated that some of these antibodies may stimulate fibrosis, but the evidence in support of this idea is not convincing.

Vascular Damage. *Microvascular disease is consistently present early in the course of systemic sclerosis and may be the initial lesion.* Intimal proliferation is evident in 100% of digital arteries of patients with systemic sclerosis. Capillary dilation with leaking, as well as destruction, is also common. Nailfold capillary loops are distorted early in the course of disease, and later they disappear. Thus, there is unmistakable morphologic evidence of microvascular injury. Telltale signs of endothelial activation and injury (e.g., increased levels of von Willebrand factor) and increased platelet activation (increased percentage of circulating platelet aggregates) have also been noted.

However, what causes the vascular injury is not known; it could be the initiating event or the result of chronic inflammation, with mediators released by inflammatory cells inflicting damage on microvascular endothelium. Repeated cycles of endothelial injury followed by platelet aggregation lead to release of platelet and endothelial factors (e.g., PDGF, TGF-β) that trigger perivascular fibrosis. Activated or injured endothelial cells themselves may release PDGF and factors chemotactic for fibroblasts. Vascular smooth muscle cells also show abnormalities, such as increased expression of adrenergic receptors. Eventually, widespread narrowing of the microvasculature leads to ischemic injury and scarring. Whether endothelial injury can also be initiated by toxic effects of environmental triggers remains uncertain but cannot be definitively excluded.

Fibrosis. The progressive fibrosis characteristic of the disease may be the culmination of multiple abnormalities, including the actions of fibrogenic cytokines produced by infiltrating leukocytes, hyperresponsiveness of fibroblasts to these cytokines, and scarring following upon ischemic damage caused by the vascular lesions. There is also evidence for a primary abnormality in collagen production. Consistent with this notion is the finding that a polymorphism in the gene encoding connective tissue growth factor is associated with systemic sclerosis.[94] In mouse models of Marfan syndrome caused by mutations in the fibrillin-1 gene, some features of systemic sclerosis are also seen,[95] suggesting again that connective tissue abnormalities may contribute to this disease.

Morphology. Virtually all organs can be involved in systemic sclerosis. Prominent changes occur in the skin, alimentary tract, musculoskeletal system, and kidney, but lesions also are often present in the blood vessels, heart, lungs, and peripheral nerves.

Skin. A great majority of patients have diffuse, sclerotic atrophy of the skin, which usually begins in the fingers and distal regions of the upper extremities and extends proximally to involve the upper arms, shoulders, neck, and face. Histologically, there are edema and perivascular infiltrates containing CD4+ T cells, together with swelling and degeneration of collagen fibers, which become eosinophilic. Capillaries and small arteries (150 to 500 μm in diameter) may show thickening of the basal lamina, endothelial cell damage, and partial occlusion. With progression of the disease, there is increasing fibrosis of the dermis, which becomes tightly bound to the subcutaneous structures. There is marked increase of compact collagen in the dermis, usually with thinning of the epidermis, loss of rete pegs, atrophy of the dermal appendages, and hyaline thickening of the walls of dermal arterioles and capillaries (Fig. 6–37). Focal and sometimes diffuse subcutaneous calcifications may develop, especially in patients with the CREST syndrome. In advanced stages the fingers take on a tapered, clawlike appearance with limitation of motion in the joints, and the face becomes a drawn mask. Loss of blood supply may lead to cutaneous ulcerations and to atrophic changes in the terminal phalanges (Fig. 6–38). Sometimes the tips of the fingers undergo autoamputation.

Alimentary Tract. The alimentary tract is affected in approximately 90% of patients. Progressive atrophy and collagenous fibrous replacement of the muscularis may develop at any level of the gut but are most severe in the esophagus. The lower two thirds of the esophagus often develops a rubber-hose inflexibility.

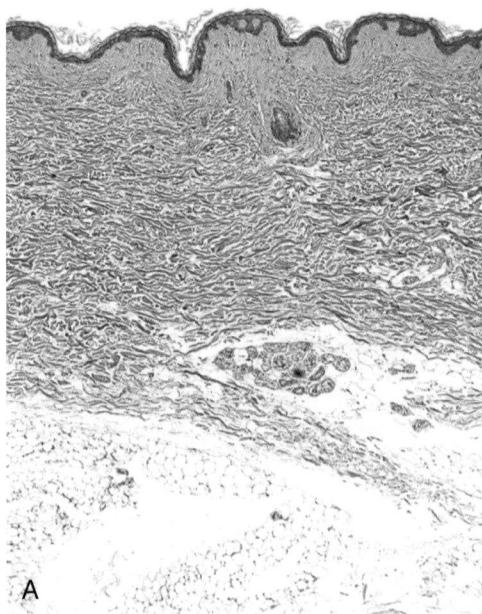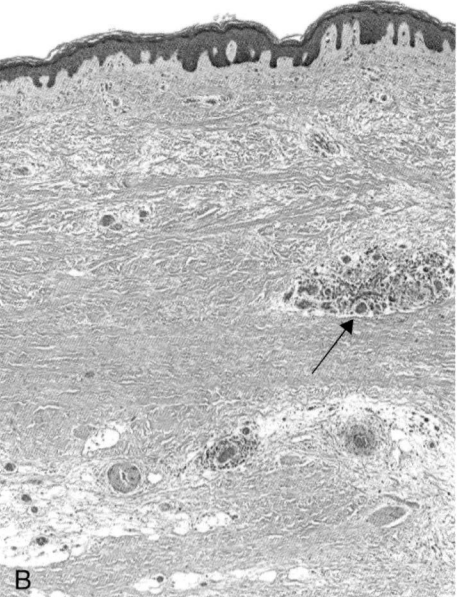

FIGURE 6–37 Systemic sclerosis. **A,** Normal skin. **B,** Skin biopsy from a patient with systemic sclerosis. Note the extensive deposition of dense collagen in the dermis with virtual absence of appendages (e.g., hair follicles) and foci of inflammation *(arrow).*

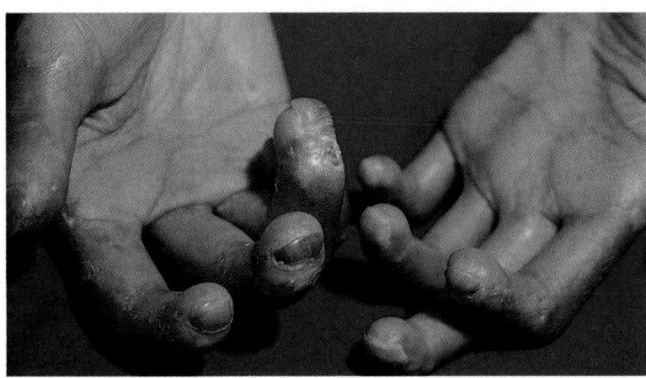

FIGURE 6–38 Advanced systemic sclerosis. The extensive subcutaneous fibrosis has virtually immobilized the fingers, creating a clawlike flexion deformity. Loss of blood supply has led to cutaneous ulcerations. (Courtesy of Dr. Richard Sontheimer, Department of Dermatology, University of Texas Southwestern Medical School, Dallas, TX.)

The associated dysfunction of the lower esophageal sphincter gives rise to gastroesophageal reflux and its complications, including Barrett metaplasia (Chapter 17) and strictures. The mucosa is thinned and may be ulcerated, and there is excessive collagenization of the lamina propria and submucosa. Loss of villi and microvilli in the small bowel is the anatomic basis for the malabsorption syndrome sometimes encountered.

Musculoskeletal System. Inflammation of the synovium, associated with hypertrophy and hyperplasia of the synovial soft tissues, is common in the early stages; fibrosis later ensues. These changes are reminiscent of rheumatoid arthritis, but joint destruction is not common in systemic sclerosis. In a small subset of patients (approximately 10%), inflammatory myositis indistinguishable from polymyositis may develop.

Kidneys. Renal abnormalities occur in two thirds of patients with systemic sclerosis. The most prominent are the vascular lesions. Interlobular arteries show intimal thickening as a result of deposition of mucinous or finely collagenous material, which stains histochemically for glycoprotein and acid mucopolysaccharides. There is also concentric proliferation of intimal cells. These changes may resemble those seen in malignant hypertension, but in scleroderma the alterations are restricted to vessels 150 to 500 μm in diameter and are not always associated with hypertension. Hypertension, however, does occur in 30% of patients with scleroderma, and in 20% it takes an ominously rapid, downhill course (malignant hypertension). In hypertensive patients, vascular alterations are more pronounced and are often associated with fibrinoid necrosis involving the arterioles together with thrombosis and infarction. Such patients often die of renal failure, which accounts for about 50% of deaths in persons with this disease. There are no specific glomerular changes.

Lungs. The lungs are involved in more than 50% of individuals with systemic sclerosis. This involvement may manifest as pulmonary hypertension and interstitial fibrosis. Pulmonary vasospasm, secondary to pulmonary vascular endothelial dysfunction, is considered important in the pathogenesis of pulmonary hypertension. Pulmonary fibrosis, when present, is indistinguishable from that seen in idiopathic pulmonary fibrosis (Chapter 15).

Heart. Pericarditis with effusion and myocardial fibrosis, along with thickening of intramyocardial arterioles, occurs in one third of the patients. Clinical myocardial involvement, however, is less common.

Clinical Features. Systemic sclerosis has a female-to-male ratio of 3:1, with a peak incidence in the 50- to 60-year age group. Although systemic sclerosis shares many features with SLE, rheumatoid arthritis (Chapter 26), and polymyositis (Chapter 27), *its distinctive features are the striking cutaneous changes*, notably skin thickening. *Raynaud's phenomenon*, manifested as episodic vasoconstriction of the arteries and arterioles of the extremities, is seen in virtually all patients and precedes other symptoms in 70% of cases. *Dysphagia* attributable to esophageal fibrosis and its resultant hypomotility are present in more than 50% of patients. Eventually, destruction of the esophageal wall leads to atony and dilation, especially at its lower end. Abdominal pain, intestinal obstruction, or malabsorption syndrome with weight loss and anemia reflect involvement of the small intestine. Respiratory difficulties caused by the pulmonary fibrosis may result in right-sided cardiac dysfunction, and myocardial fibrosis may cause either arrhythmias or cardiac failure. Mild proteinuria occurs in as many as 30% of patients, but rarely is the proteinuria severe enough to cause a nephrotic syndrome. The most ominous manifestation is malignant hypertension, with the subsequent development of fatal renal failure, but in its absence progression of the disease may be slow. The disease tends to be more severe in blacks, especially black women. As treatment of the renal crises has improved, pulmonary disease has become the major cause of death in systemic sclerosis.

As mentioned earlier, the CREST syndrome is seen in some patients with limited systemic sclerosis. It is characterized by calcinosis, Raynaud phenomenon, esophageal dysfunction, sclerodactyly, telangiectasia, and the presence of anticentromere antibodies. Patients with the CREST syndrome have relatively limited involvement of skin, often confined to fingers, forearms, and face, and calcification of the subcutaneous tissues. Involvement of the viscera, including esophageal lesions, pulmonary hypertension, and biliary cirrhosis, may not occur at all or occur late. In general the patients live longer than those with systemic sclerosis with diffuse visceral involvement at the outset.

INFLAMMATORY MYOPATHIES

Inflammatory myopathies comprise an uncommon, heterogeneous group of disorders characterized by injury and inflammation of mainly the skeletal muscles, which are probably immunologically mediated. Three distinct disorders, *dermatomyositis, polymyositis,* and *inclusion-body myositis,* are included in this category. These may occur alone or with other immune-mediated diseases, particularly systemic sclerosis. These diseases are described in Chapter 27.

MIXED CONNECTIVE TISSUE DISEASE

The term *mixed connective tissue disease* is used to describe a disease with clinical features that are a mixture of the features of SLE, systemic sclerosis, and polymyositis.[96] The disease is characterized *serologically by high titers of antibodies to ribonucleoprotein particle–containing U1 ribonucleoprotein.* Typically, mixed connective tissue disease shows modest renal involvement and a good response to corticosteroids, at least in the short term. Because the clinical features overlap with other diseases, it has been suggested that mixed connective tissue disease is not a distinct entity but that different patients represent subsets of SLE, systemic sclerosis, and polymyositis. The disease can also, over time, evolve into classical SLE or systemic sclerosis. Two of the more serious complications of mixed connective tissue disease are pulmonary hypertension and renal disease resembling that associated with systemic sclerosis.

POLYARTERITIS NODOSA AND OTHER VASCULITIDES

Polyarteritis nodosa belongs to a group of diseases characterized by necrotizing inflammation of the walls of blood vessels and showing strong evidence of an immunological pathogenetic mechanism.[97,98] The general term *noninfectious vasculitis* differentiates these conditions from those due to direct infection of the blood vessel wall (such as occurs in the wall of an abscess) and serves to emphasize that any type of vessel may be involved—arteries, arterioles, veins, or capillaries.

Noninfectious vasculitis is encountered in many clinical settings. A detailed classification and description of vasculitides is presented in Chapter 11 on blood vessels, where the immunological mechanisms are also discussed.

Rejection of Tissue Transplants

Transplant rejection is discussed here because it involves several of the immunological reactions that underlie immune-mediated inflammatory diseases. A major barrier to transplantation is the process of *rejection,* in which the recipient's immune system recognizes the graft as being foreign and attacks it.

Mechanisms of Recognition and Rejection of Allografts

Rejection is a complex process in which both cell-mediated immunity and circulating antibodies play a role[99]; moreover, the contributions of these two mechanisms are often reflected in the histologic features of the rejected organs.

T Cell–Mediated Reactions

The critical role of T cells in transplant rejection has been documented both in humans and in experimental animals. T

cell–mediated graft rejection is called *cellular rejection,* and it involves destruction of graft cells by CD8+ CTLs and delayed hypersensitivity reactions triggered by activated CD4+ helper cells. The major antigenic differences between a donor and recipient that result in rejection of transplants are differences in highly polymorphic HLA alleles. The recipient's T cells recognize donor antigens from the graft (the allogeneic antigens, or alloantigens) by two pathways, called *direct* and *indirect* (Fig. 6–39).[100]

○ In the *direct pathway,* T cells of the transplant recipient recognize allogeneic (donor) MHC molecules on the surface of APCs in the graft. It is believed that dendritic cells carried in the donor organs are the most important APCs for initiating the antigraft response, because they not only express high levels of class I and II MHC molecules but also are endowed with costimulatory molecules (e.g., B7-1 and B7-2). The T cells of the host encounter the donor dendritic cells either within the grafted organ or after the dendritic cells migrate to the draining lymph nodes. CD8+ T cells recognize class I MHC molecules and differentiate into active CTLs, which can kill the graft cells by mechanisms already discussed. CD4+ helper T cells recognize allogeneic class II molecules and proliferate and differentiate into T_H1 (and possibly T_H17) effector cells. Cytokines secreted by the activated CD4+ T cells trigger a delayed hypersensitivity reaction in the graft, resulting in increased vascular permeability and local accumulation of mononuclear cells (lymphocytes and macrophages), and graft injury caused by the activated macrophages. The direct recognition of allogeneic MHC molecules seems paradoxical to the rules of self-MHC restriction: If T cells normally are restricted to recognizing foreign peptides displayed by self-MHC molecules, why should these T cells recognize foreign MHC? The probable explanation is that allogeneic MHC molecules, with their bound peptides, resemble, or mimic, the self-MHC–foreign peptide complexes that are recognized by self-MHC–restricted T cells. Thus, recognition of allogeneic MHC molecules is a cross-reaction of T cells selected to recognize self-MHC plus foreign peptides.

○ In the *indirect pathway* of allorecognition, recipient T lymphocytes recognize MHC antigens of the graft donor after they are presented by the recipient's own APCs. This process involves the uptake and processing of MHC and other foreign molecules from the grafted organ by host APCs. The peptides derived from the donor tissue are presented by the host's own MHC molecules, like any other foreign peptide. Thus, the indirect pathway is similar to the physiologic processing and presentation of other foreign (e.g., microbial) antigens. The indirect pathway generates CD4+ T cells that enter the graft and recognize graft antigens being displayed by host APCs that have also entered the graft, and the result is a delayed hypersensitivity type of reaction. However, CD8+ CTLs that may be generated by the indirect pathway cannot directly recognize or kill graft cells, because these CTLs recognize graft antigens presented by the host's APCs. Therefore, when T cells react to a graft by the indirect pathway, the principal mechanism of cellular rejection may be T-cell cytokine production and delayed hypersensitivity. It is postulated that the direct pathway is the major pathway in acute cellular rejection, whereas the

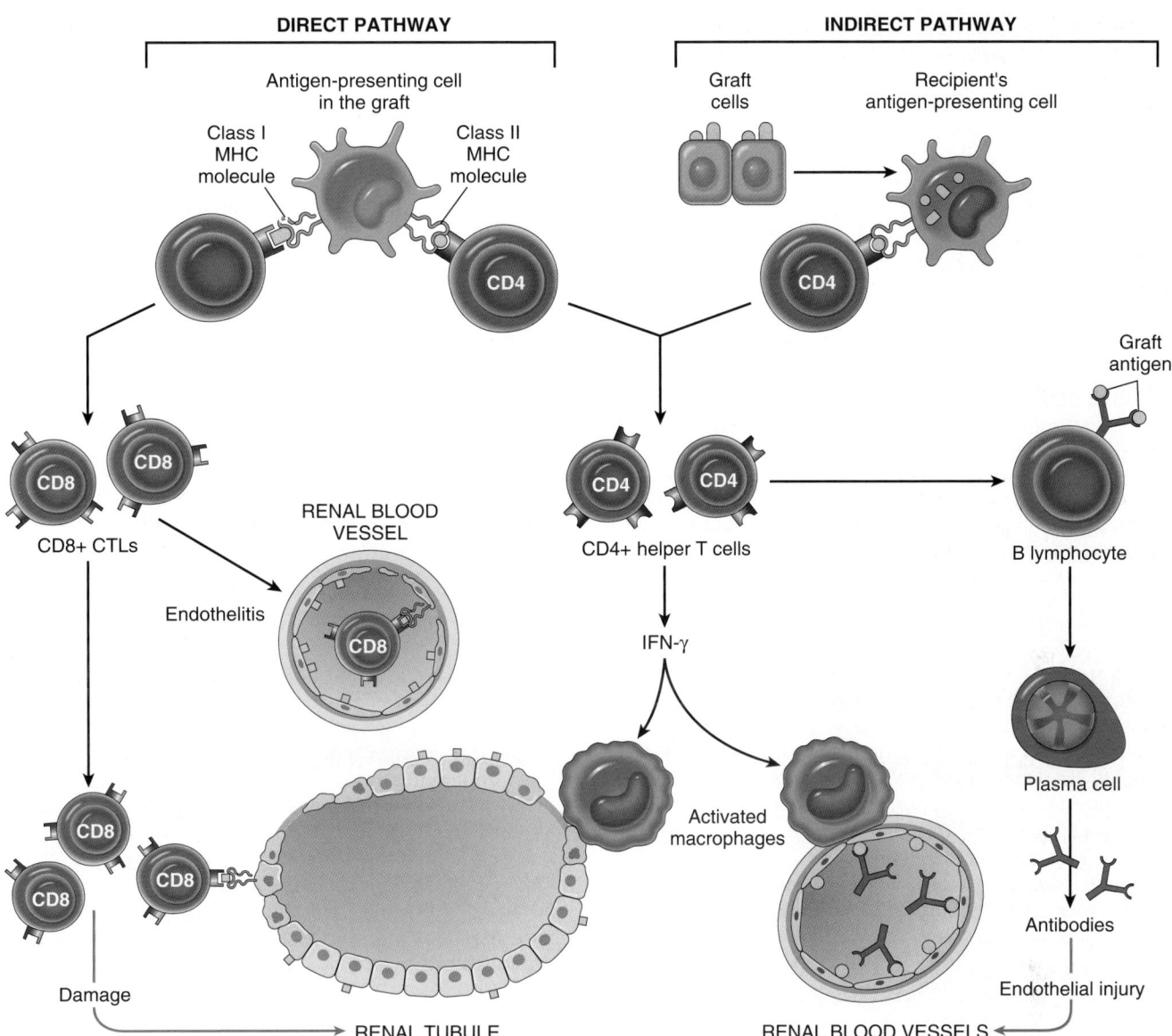

DIRECT PATHWAY

Antigen-presenting cell
in the graft

Class I
MHC
molecule

Class II
MHC
molecule

CD4

CD8

CD8

CD8+ CTLs

RENAL BLOOD
VESSEL

Endothelitis

CD8

CD8

CD8

CD8

Damage

RENAL TUBULE

INDIRECT PATHWAY

Graft
cells

Recipient's
antigen-presenting cell

CD4

CD4

CD4

CD4+ helper T cells

IFN-γ

Activated
macrophages

Graft
antigen

B lymphocyte

Plasma cell

Antibodies

Endothelial injury

RENAL BLOOD VESSELS

FIGURE 6–39 Recognition and rejection of organ allografts. In the direct pathway, donor class I and class II MHC antigens on antigen-presenting cells in the graft (along with costimulators, not shown) are recognized by host CD8+ cytotoxic T cells and CD4+ helper T cells, respectively. CD4+ cells proliferate and produce cytokines (e.g., IFN-γ), which induce tissue damage by a local delayed hypersensitivity reaction. CD8+ T cells responding to graft antigens differentiate into CTLs that kill graft cells. In the indirect pathway graft antigens are picked up, processed, and displayed by host APCs and activate CD4+ T cells, which damage the graft by a local delayed hypersensitivity reaction and stimulate B lymphocytes to produce antibodies.

indirect pathway is more important in chronic rejection. However, this separation is by no means absolute.

Antibody-Mediated Reactions

Although T cells are pivotal in the rejection of organ transplants, antibodies produced against alloantigens in the graft are also important mediators of rejection.[101] This process is called *humoral rejection*, and it can take two forms. *Hyperacute rejection occurs when preformed antidonor antibodies are present in the circulation of the recipient.* Such antibodies may be present in a recipient who has previously rejected a kidney transplant. Multiparous women who develop anti-HLA antibodies against paternal antigens shed from the fetus may

have preformed antibodies to grafts taken from their husbands or children, or even from unrelated individuals who share HLA alleles with the husbands. Prior blood transfusions can also lead to presensitization, because platelets and white blood cells are rich in HLA antigens and donors and recipients are usually not HLA-identical. With the current practice of cross-matching, that is, testing recipient's serum for antibodies against donor's cells, hyperacute rejection is no longer a significant clinical problem.

In recipients not previously sensitized to transplantation antigens, exposure to the class I and class II HLA antigens of the donor graft may evoke antibodies. The antibodies formed by the recipient may cause injury by several mechanisms, including complement-dependent cytotoxicity, inflammation, and antibody-dependent cell-mediated cytotoxicity. *The initial target of these antibodies in rejection seems to be the graft vasculature.* Thus, antibody-dependent *acute humoral rejection* is usually manifested by a vasculitis, sometimes referred to as *rejection vasculitis.*

Rejection of Kidney Grafts

Because kidneys were the first solid organs to be transplanted and more kidneys have been transplanted than any other organ, much of our understanding of the clinical and pathologic aspects of solid-organ transplantation is based on studies of renal allografts.

> **Morphology.** On the basis of the morphology and the underlying mechanism, **rejection reactions are classified as hyperacute, acute, and chronic.** The morphologic changes in these patterns are described below as they relate to renal transplants. Similar changes may occur in any other vascularized organ transplant and are discussed in relevant chapters.
>
> *Hyperacute Rejection.* This form of rejection occurs within minutes or hours after transplantation. A hyperacutely rejecting kidney rapidly becomes cyanotic, mottled, and flaccid, and may excrete a mere few drops of bloody urine. Immunoglobulin and complement are deposited in the vessel wall, causing endothelial injury and fibrin-platelet thrombi (Fig. 6–40A). Neutrophils rapidly accumulate within arterioles, glomeruli, and peritubular capillaries. As these changes become diffuse and intense, the glomeruli undergo thrombotic occlusion of the capillaries, and fibrinoid necrosis occurs in arterial walls. The kidney cortex then undergoes outright necrosis (infarction), and such nonfunctioning kidneys have to be removed.

> *Acute Rejection.* This may occur within days of transplantation in the untreated recipient or may appear suddenly months or even years later, after immunosuppression has been used and terminated. In any one patient, cellular or humoral immune mechanisms may predominate. Histologically, humoral rejection is associated with vasculitis, whereas cellular rejection is marked by an interstitial mononuclear cell infiltrate.
>
> **Acute cellular rejection** is most commonly seen within the initial months after transplantation and is heralded by clinical and biochemical signs of renal failure (Chapter 20). Histologically, there may be extensive interstitial mononuclear cell infiltration and edema as well as mild interstitial hemorrhage (Fig. 6–40B). As might be expected, immunohistochemical staining reveals both CD4+ and CD8+ T lymphocytes, which express markers of activated T cells, such as the α chain of the IL-2 receptor. Glomerular and peritubular capillaries contain large numbers of mononuclear cells that may also invade the tubules, causing focal tubular necrosis. In addition to causing tubular damage, CD8+ T cells may injure vascular endothelial cells, causing a so-called **endothelitis**. The affected vessels have swollen endothelial cells, and at places the lymphocytes can be seen between the endothelium and the vessel wall. The recognition of cellular rejection is important because, in the absence of an accompanying humoral rejection, patients respond well to immunosuppressive therapy. Cyclosporine, a widely used immunosuppressive drug, is also nephrotoxic, and hence the histologic changes resulting from cyclosporine may be superimposed.
>
> **Acute humoral rejection (rejection vasculitis)** is mediated by antidonor antibodies, and hence it is manifested mainly by damage to the blood vessels.

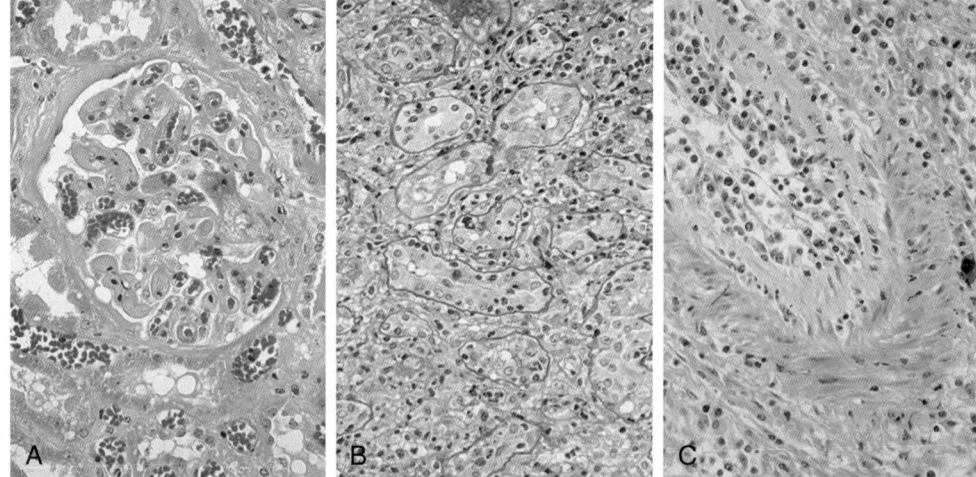

FIGURE 6–40 Morphology of hyperacute and acute graft rejection. **A,** Hyperacute rejection of a kidney allograft showing endothelial damage, platelet and thrombin thrombi, and early neutrophil infiltration in a glomerulus. **B,** Acute cellular rejection of a kidney allograft with inflammatory cells in the interstitium and between epithelial cells of the tubules. **C,** Acute humoral rejection of a kidney allograft (rejection vasculitis) with inflammatory cells and proliferating smooth muscle cells in the intima. (Courtesy of Dr. Helmut Rennke, Department of Pathology, Brigham and Women's Hospital and Harvard Medical School, Boston, MA.)

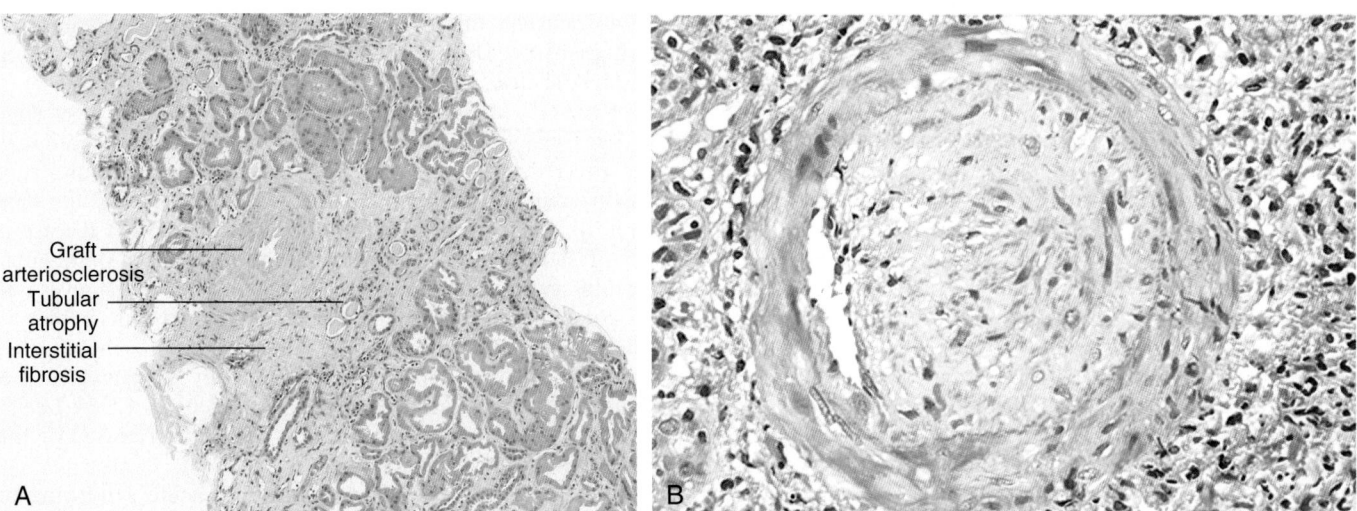

Graft arteriosclerosis
Tubular atrophy
Interstitial fibrosis

A

B

FIGURE 6–41 Chronic rejection of a kidney allograft. **A,** Changes in the kidney in chronic rejection. **B,** Graft arteriosclerosis. The vascular lumen is replaced by an accumulation of smooth muscle cells and connective tissue in the vessel intima. (Courtesy of Dr. Helmut Rennke, Department of Pathology, Brigham and Women's Hospital and Harvard Medical School, Boston, MA.)

This may take the form of necrotizing vasculitis with endothelial cell necrosis, neutrophilic infiltration, deposition of immunoglobulins, complement, and fibrin, and thrombosis. Such lesions are associated with extensive necrosis of the renal parenchyma. In many cases, the vasculitis is less acute and is characterized by marked thickening of the intima with proliferating fibroblasts, myocytes, and foamy macrophages (Fig. 6–40C). The resultant narrowing of the arterioles may cause infarction or renal cortical atrophy. The proliferative vascular lesions mimic arteriosclerotic thickening and are believed to be caused by cytokines that cause proliferation of vascular smooth muscle cells. Deposition of the complement breakdown product C4d in allografts is a strong indicator of humoral rejection, because C4d is produced during activation of the complement system by the antibody-dependent classical pathway.[101,102] The importance of making this diagnosis is that it provides a rationale for treating affected patients with B cell–depleting agents.

Chronic Rejection. In recent years acute rejection has been significantly controlled by immunosuppressive therapy, and chronic rejection has emerged as an important cause of graft failure.[103] Patients with chronic rejection present clinically with a progressive renal failure manifested by a rise in serum creatinine over a period of 4 to 6 months. Chronic rejection is dominated by vascular changes, interstitial fibrosis, and tubular atrophy with loss of renal parenchyma (Fig. 6–41). The **vascular changes** consist of dense, obliterative intimal fibrosis, principally in the cortical arteries. These vascular lesions result in renal ischemia, manifested by glomerular loss, interstitial fibrosis and tubular atrophy, and shrinkage of the renal parenchyma. The glomeruli may show scarring, with duplication of basement membranes; this appearance is sometimes called chronic transplant glomerulopathy. Chronically rejecting kidneys usually have interstitial mononuclear cell infiltrates of plasma cells and numerous eosinophils.

Methods of Increasing Graft Survival

The value of HLA matching between donor and recipient varies in different solid-organ transplants. In kidney transplants, there is substantial benefit if all the polymorphic HLA alleles are matched (both inherited alleles of *HLA-A, -B* and *DR*). However, HLA matching is usually not even done for transplants of liver, heart, and lungs, because other considerations, such as anatomic compatibility, severity of the underlying illness, and the need to minimize the time of organ storage, override the potential benefits of HLA matching.

Except in the case of identical twins, who obviously express the same histocompatibility antigens, *immunosuppressive therapy* is a practical necessity in all other donor-recipient combinations.[104] The mainstay of immunosuppression is the drug *cyclosporine.* Cyclosporine works by blocking activation of a transcription factor called nuclear factor of activated T cells (NFAT), which is required for transcription of cytokine genes, in particular, the gene that encodes IL-2. Additional drugs that are used to treat rejection include azathioprine (which inhibits leukocyte development from bone marrow precursors), steroids (which block inflammation), rapamycin and mycophenolate mofetil (both of which inhibit lymphocyte proliferation), and monoclonal anti–T-cell antibodies (e.g., monoclonal anti-CD3 and antibodies against the IL-2 receptor α chain [CD25], which opsonize and eliminate the cells and may also block T-cell activation). Another, more recent, strategy for reducing antigraft immune responses is to prevent host T cells from receiving costimulatory signals from dendritic cells during the initial phase of sensitization. This can be accomplished by interrupting the interaction between the B7 molecules on the dendritic cells of the graft donor with the CD28 receptors on host T cells, for example, by administration of proteins that bind to B7 costimulators.

Although immunosuppression prolongs graft survival, it carries its own risks. The price paid in the form of increased susceptibility to opportunistic infections is not small. These patients are also at increased risk for developing EBV-induced lymphomas, human papillomavirus–induced squamous cell carcinomas, and Kaposi sarcoma (Chapter 11), all probably the result of reactivation of latent viral infections because of diminished host defenses. To circumvent the untoward effects of immunosuppression, much effort is being devoted to induce donor-specific tolerance in graft recipients.[105] For instance, giving donor cells to graft recipients may prevent reactions to the graft, perhaps because the donor inoculum contains cells, such as immature dendritic cells, that induce tolerance to the donor alloantigens. This approach may result in long-term *mixed chimerism,* in which the recipient lives with the injected donor cells. Other strategies being tested include injecting regulatory T cells at the time of transplantation, and promoting the death of alloreactive T cells in the recipient.

Transplantation of Other Solid Organs

In addition to the kidney, a variety of organs, such as the liver (Chapter 18), heart (Chapter 12), lungs, and pancreas, are also transplanted. The rejection reaction against liver transplants is not as vigorous as might be expected from the degree of HLA disparity. The molecular basis of this "privilege" is not understood.

Transplantation of Hematopoietic Cells

Use of hematopoietic stem cell transplants for hematologic malignancies, certain nonhematologic cancers, aplastic anemias, thalassemias, and certain immunodeficiency states is increasing. Transplantation of genetically engineered hematopoietic stem cells may also be useful for somatic cell gene therapy, and is being evaluated in some immunodeficiencies. Hematopoietic stem cells are usually obtained from the bone marrow but may also be harvested from peripheral blood after they are mobilized from the bone marrow by administration of hematopoietic growth factors. In most of the conditions in which bone marrow transplantation is indicated, the recipient is irradiated to destroy the immune system (and sometimes, cancer cells) and to create a graft bed. Several features distinguish bone marrow transplants from solid-organ transplants. Two problems that are unique to bone marrow transplantation are graft-versus-host (GVH) disease and immunodeficiency.

GVH disease occurs in any situation in which immunologically competent cells or their precursors are transplanted into immunologically crippled recipients, and the transferred cells recognize alloantigens in the host.[106] It is seen most commonly in the setting of bone marrow transplantation but, rarely, may occur following transplantation of solid organs rich in lymphoid cells (e.g., the liver) or transfusion of unirradiated blood. When immune-compromised recipients receive normal bone marrow cells from allogeneic donors, the immunocompetent T cells present in the donor marrow recognize the recipient's HLA antigens as foreign and react against them. To try to minimize GVH disease, bone marrow transplants are

done between donor and recipient that are HLA-matched using sensitive DNA sequencing methods for molecular typing of HLA alleles.

Acute GVH disease occurs within days to weeks after allogeneic bone marrow transplantation. Although any organ may be affected, the major clinical manifestations result from involvement of the *immune system and epithelia of the skin, liver, and intestines.* Involvement of skin in GVH disease is manifested by a generalized rash that may lead to desquamation in severe cases. Destruction of small bile ducts gives rise to jaundice, and mucosal ulceration of the gut results in bloody diarrhea. Although tissue injury may be severe, the affected tissues are usually not heavily infiltrated by lymphocytes. It is believed that in addition to direct cytotoxicity by CD8+ T cells, considerable damage is inflicted by cytokines released by the sensitized donor T cells.

Chronic GVH disease may follow the acute syndrome or may occur insidiously. These patients have extensive cutaneous injury, with destruction of skin appendages and fibrosis of the dermis. The changes may resemble systemic sclerosis (discussed earlier). Chronic liver disease manifested by cholestatic jaundice is also frequent. Damage to the gastrointestinal tract may cause esophageal strictures. The immune system is devastated, with involution of the thymus and depletion of lymphocytes in the lymph nodes. Not surprisingly, the patients experience recurrent and life-threatening infections. Some patients develop manifestations of autoimmunity, postulated to result from the grafted CD4+ helper T cells reacting with host B cells and stimulating these cells, some of which may be capable of producing autoantibodies.

Because GVH disease is mediated by T lymphocytes contained in the donor bone marrow, depletion of donor T cells before transfusion virtually eliminates the disease. This protocol, however, has proved to be a mixed blessing: GVH disease is ameliorated, but the incidence of graft failures and EBV-related B-cell lymphoma and the recurrence of disease in leukemic patients increase. It seems that the multifaceted T cells not only mediate GVH disease but also are required for engraftment of the transplanted marrow stem cells, suppression of EBV-infected B-cell clones, and control of leukemic cells. The latter, called *graft-versus-leukemia* effect, can be quite dramatic. Deliberate induction of graft-versus-leukemia effect by infusion of allogeneic T cells is being used in the treatment of chronic myelogenous leukemia when patients relapse after bone marrow transplantation.

Immunodeficiency is a frequent complication of bone marrow transplantation. The immunodeficiency may be a result of prior treatment, myeloablative preparation for the graft, a delay in repopulation of the recipient's immune system, and attack on the host's immune cells by grafted lymphocytes. Affected individuals are profoundly immunosuppressed and are easy prey to infections. Although many different types of organisms may infect patients, infection with cytomegalovirus is particularly important. This usually results from activation of previously silent infection. Cytomegalovirus-induced pneumonitis can be a fatal complication.

Immunodeficiency Syndromes

Immunodeficiencies can be divided into the *primary immunodeficiency* disorders, which are almost always genetically

TABLE 6–11 Examples of Infections in Immunodeficiencies

Pathogen Type	T-Cell Defect	B-Cell Defect	Granulocyte Defect	Complement Defect
Bacteria	Bacterial sepsis	Streptococci, staphylococci, *Haemophilus*	Staphylococci, *Pseudomonas*	Neisserial infections, other pyogenic infections
Viruses	Cytomegalovirus, Epstein-Barr virus, severe varicella, chronic infections with respiratory and intestinal viruses	Enteroviral encephalitis		
Fungi and parasites	*Candida, Pneumocystis jiroveci*	Severe intestinal giardiasis	*Candida, Nocardia, Aspergillus*	
Special features	Aggressive disease with opportunistic pathogens, failure to clear infections	Recurrent sinopulmonary infections, sepsis, chronic meningitis		

determined, and *secondary immunodeficiency* states, which may arise as complications of cancers, infections, malnutrition, or side effects of immunosuppression, irradiation, or chemotherapy for cancer and other diseases. The primary immunodeficiency syndromes are accidents of nature that provide valuable insights into some of the critical molecules of the human immune system. Here we briefly discuss the more important primary immunodeficiencies, to be followed by a more detailed description of acquired immunodeficiency syndrome (AIDS), the most devastating example of secondary immunodeficiency.

PRIMARY IMMUNODEFICIENCIES

Most primary immunodeficiency diseases are genetically determined and affect the humoral and/or cellular arms of adaptive immunity (mediated by B and T lymphocytes, respectively) or the defense mechanisms of innate immunity (NK cells, phagocytes, or complement). Defects in adaptive immunity are often subclassified on the basis of the primary component involved (i.e., B cells or T cells or both). However, these distinctions are not clear-cut; for instance, T-cell defects almost always lead to impaired antibody synthesis, and hence isolated deficiencies of T cells are often indistinguishable clinically from combined deficiencies of T and B cells. Although these disorders were once thought to be quite rare, some form of mild genetic immune deficiency is, in fact, present in many individuals.[107] Most primary immunodeficiencies manifest themselves in infancy, between 6 months and 2 years of life, and they are detected because the affected infants are susceptible to recurrent infections. The nature of infecting organisms depends to some extent on the nature of the underlying defect, as summarized in Table 6–11. Defects of phagocytes were discussed in Chapter 2. Here we present selected examples of other immunodeficiencies. We begin with isolated defects in B cells, followed by a discussion of combined immunodeficiencies and defects in complement proteins. Finally, Wiskott-Aldrich syndrome, a complex disorder affecting lymphocytes as well as platelets, is presented. With advances in genetic analyses, the mutations responsible for many of the common primary immunodeficiencies have now been identified (Fig. 6–42).[108,109]

X-Linked Agammaglobulinemia (Bruton's Agammaglobulinemia)

X-linked agammaglobulinemia is one of the more common forms of primary immunodeficiency.[110] *It is characterized by the failure of B-cell precursors (pro-B cells and pre-B cells) to develop into mature B cells.* During normal B-cell maturation in the bone marrow, the Ig heavy-chain genes are rearranged first, in pre-B cells, and these are expressed on the cell surface in association with a "surrogate" light chain, where they deliver signals that induce rearrangement of the Ig light-chain genes and further maturation. This need for Ig-initiated signals is a quality control mechanism that ensures that maturation will proceed only if functional Ig proteins are expressed. X-linked agammaglobulinemia is caused by mutations in a cytoplasmic tyrosine kinase, called *Bruton tyrosine kinase (Btk)*; the gene that encodes it is located on the long arm of the X chromosome at Xq21.22.[95] Btk is a protein tyrosine kinase that is associated with the Ig receptor complex of pre-B and mature B cells and is needed to transduce signals from the receptor. When it is mutated, the pre-B cell receptor cannot deliver signals, and maturation stops at this stage. Because light chains are not produced, the complete antigen receptor molecule (which contains Ig heavy and light chains) cannot be assembled and transported to the cell membrane.

As an X-linked disease, this disorder is seen almost entirely in males, but sporadic cases have been described in females, possibly caused by mutations in some other gene that functions in the same pathway. *The disease usually does not become apparent until about 6 months of age, as maternal immunoglobulins are depleted.* In most cases, recurrent bacterial infections of the respiratory tract, such as acute and chronic pharyngitis, sinusitis, otitis media, bronchitis, and pneumonia, call attention to the underlying immune defect. Almost always the causative organisms are *Haemophilus influenzae*, *Streptococcus pneumoniae*, or *Staphylococcus aureus*. These organisms are normally opsonized by antibodies and cleared by phagocytosis. Because antibodies are important for neutralizing infectious viruses that are present in the bloodstream or mucosal secretions or being passed from cell to cell, individuals with this disease are also susceptible to certain viral infections, especially those caused by enteroviruses, such as

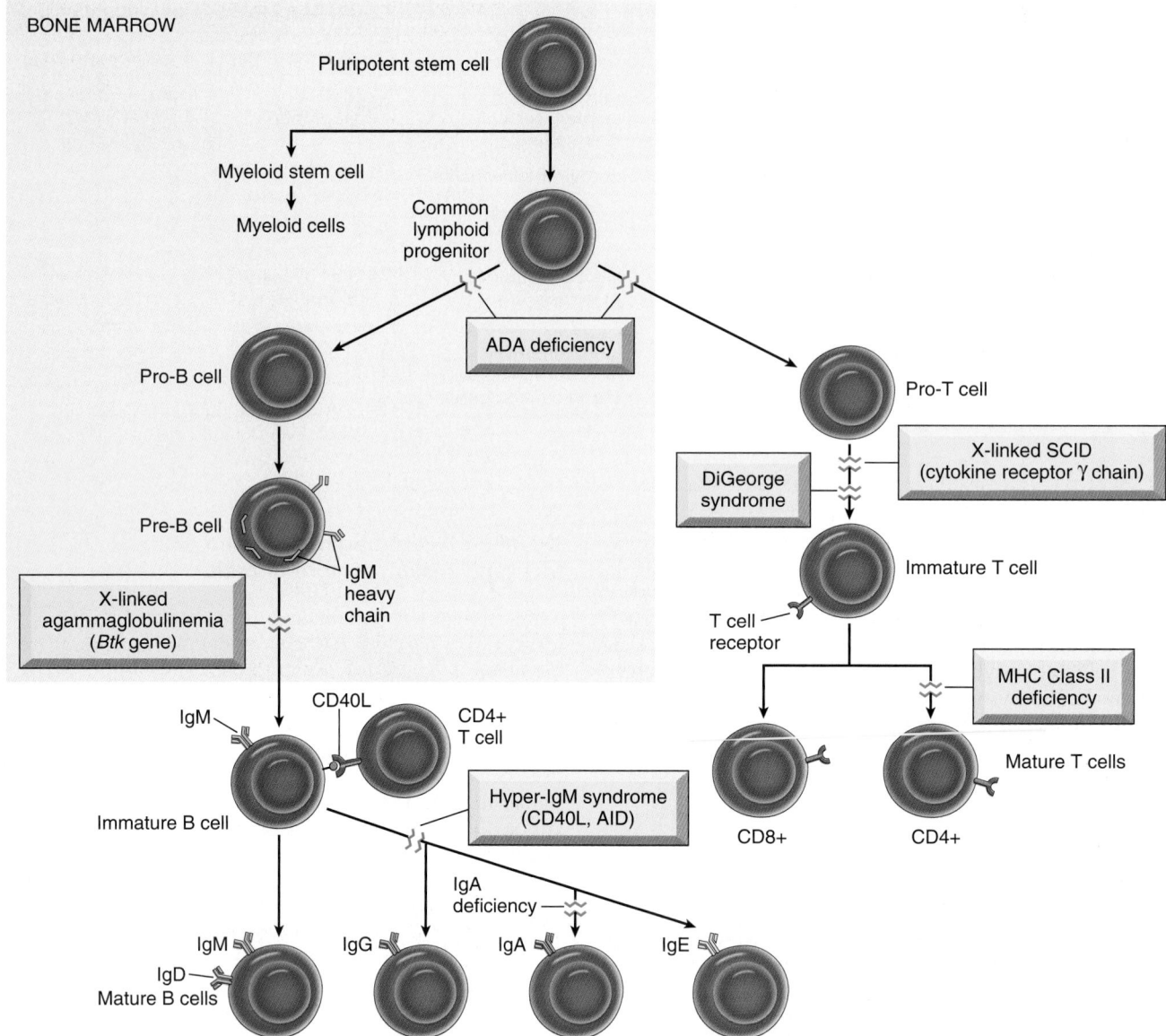

FIGURE 6–42 Simplified scheme of lymphocyte development and sites of block in some primary immunodeficiency diseases are shown. The affected genes are indicated in parentheses for some of the disorders. ADA, adenosine deaminase; AID, activation-induced deaminase; CD40L, CD40 ligand (also known as CD154); SCID, severe combined immune deficiency.

echovirus, poliovirus, and coxsackievirus. These viruses infect the gastrointestinal tract, and from here they can disseminate to the nervous system via the blood. Thus, immunization with live poliovirus carries the risk of paralytic poliomyelitis, and echovirus can cause fatal encephalitis. For similar reasons, *Giardia lamblia*, an intestinal protozoan that is normally resisted by secreted IgA, causes persistent infections in persons with this disorder. In general, however, most intracellular viral, fungal, and protozoal infections are handled quite well by the intact T cell–mediated immunity.

The classic form of this disease has the following characteristics:

● B cells are absent or markedly decreased in the circulation, and the serum levels of all classes of immunoglobulins are depressed. Pre-B cells, which express the B-lineage marker CD19 but not membrane Ig, are found in normal numbers in the bone marrow.
● Germinal centers of lymph nodes, Peyer's patches, the appendix, and tonsils are underdeveloped.
● Plasma cells are absent throughout the body.
● T cell–mediated reactions are normal.

Autoimmune diseases, such as arthritis and dermatomyositis, occur with increased frequency, in as many as 35% of individuals with this disease, which is paradoxical in the presence of an immune deficiency. It is likely that these autoimmune disorders are caused by a breakdown of self-tolerance resulting in autoimmunity, but chronic infections associated with the immune deficiency may play a role in inducing the inflammatory reactions. The treatment of X-linked agammaglobulinemia is replacement therapy with immunoglobulins.

In the past, most patients succumbed to infection in infancy or early childhood. Prophylactic intravenous Ig therapy allows most individuals to reach adulthood.

Common Variable Immunodeficiency

This relatively common but poorly defined entity represents a heterogeneous group of disorders.[111,112] The feature common to all patients is hypogammaglobulinemia, generally affecting all the antibody classes but sometimes only IgG. The diagnosis of common variable immunodeficiency is based on exclusion of other well-defined causes of decreased antibody production.

As might be expected in a heterogeneous group of disorders, both sporadic and inherited forms of the disease occur. In familial forms there is no single pattern of inheritance. Relatives of such patients have a high incidence of selective IgA deficiency (see later). These studies suggest that at least in some cases, selective IgA deficiency and common variable immunodeficiency may represent different expressions of a common genetic defect in antibody synthesis. In contrast to X-linked agammaglobulinemia, most individuals with common variable immunodeficiency have normal or near-normal numbers of B cells in the blood and lymphoid tissues. These B cells, however, are not able to differentiate into plasma cells.

Both intrinsic B-cell defects and abnormalities in T helper cell–mediated activation of B cells may account for the antibody deficiency in this disease. Families have been reported in which the underlying abnormality is in a receptor for a cytokine called BAFF that promotes the survival and differentiation of B cells, or in a molecule called ICOS (inducible costimulator) that is homologous to CD28 and is involved in T-cell activation and in interactions between T and B cells.[111] However, the known mutations account for a minority of cases.

The clinical manifestations of common variable immunodeficiency are caused by antibody deficiency, and hence they resemble those of X-linked agammaglobulinemia. The patients typically present with recurrent sinopulmonary pyogenic infections. In addition, about 20% of patients present with recurrent herpesvirus infections. Serious enterovirus infections causing meningoencephalitis may also occur. Individuals with this disorder are also prone to the development of persistent diarrhea caused by *G. lamblia*. In contrast to X-linked agammaglobulinemia, common variable immunodeficiency affects both sexes equally, and the onset of symptoms is later—in childhood or adolescence. Histologically the B-cell areas of the lymphoid tissues (i.e., lymphoid follicles in nodes, spleen, and gut) are hyperplastic. The enlargement of B-cell areas probably reflects defective regulation, that is, B cells can proliferate in response to antigen but do not produce antibodies, and therefore the normal feedback inhibition by IgG is absent.

As in X-linked agammaglobulinemia, these patients have a high frequency of autoimmune diseases (approximately 20%), including rheumatoid arthritis. The risk of lymphoid malignancy is also increased, and an increase in gastric cancer has been reported.

Isolated IgA Deficiency

Isolated IgA deficiency is a common immunodeficiency. In the United States it occurs in about 1 in 600 individuals of European descent.[113] It is far less common in blacks and Asians. Affected individuals have extremely *low levels of both serum and secretory IgA*. It may be familial, or acquired in association with toxoplasmosis, measles, or some other viral infection. The association of IgA deficiency with common variable immunodeficiency was mentioned earlier. Most individuals with this disease are asymptomatic. Because IgA is the major Ig in external secretions, mucosal defenses are weakened, and infections occur in the respiratory, gastrointestinal, and urogenital tracts. Symptomatic patients commonly present with recurrent sinopulmonary infections and diarrhea. Some individuals with IgA deficiency are also deficient in the IgG2 and IgG4 subclasses of IgG. This group of patients is particularly prone to developing infections. In addition, IgA-deficient patients have a high frequency of respiratory tract allergy and a variety of autoimmune diseases, particularly SLE and rheumatoid arthritis. The basis of the increased frequency of autoimmune and allergic diseases is not known. When transfused with blood containing normal IgA, some of these patients develop severe, even fatal, anaphylactic reactions, because the IgA behaves like a foreign antigen (since the patients do not produce it and are not tolerant to it).

The basic defect in IgA deficiency is impaired differentiation of naive B lymphocytes to IgA-producing cells. The molecular basis of this defect in most patients is still unknown. Defects in a receptor for the B cell–activating cytokine, BAFF, have been described in some patients.

Hyper-IgM Syndrome

In hyper-IgM syndrome the *affected patients make IgM antibodies but are deficient in their ability to produce IgG, IgA, and IgE antibodies*. It is now known that the defect in this disease affects the ability of helper T cells to deliver activating signals to B cells and macrophages. As discussed earlier in the chapter, many of the functions of CD4+ helper T cells require the engagement of CD40 on B cells, macrophages and dendritic cells by CD40L (also called CD154) expressed on antigen-activated T cells. This interaction triggers Ig class switching and affinity maturation in B cells, and stimulates the microbicidal functions of macrophages. Approximately 70% of individuals with hyper-IgM syndrome have the X-linked form of the disease, caused by mutations in the gene encoding CD40L located on Xq26.[114] In the remaining persons the disease is inherited in an autosomal recessive pattern. Most of these patients have mutations in the gene encoding CD40 or the enzyme called activation-induced deaminase, a DNA-editing cytosine deaminase that is required for class switching and affinity maturation.

The serum of persons with this syndrome contains normal or elevated levels of IgM but no IgA or IgE and extremely low levels of IgG. The number of B and T cells is normal. Many of the IgM antibodies react with elements of blood, giving rise to autoimmune hemolytic anemia, thrombocytopenia, and neutropenia. In older patients there may be uncontrolled proliferation of IgM-producing plasma cells with infiltrations of the gastrointestinal tract. Although the proliferating B cells are polyclonal, extensive infiltration may lead to death.

Clinically, individuals with the hyper-IgM syndrome present with recurrent pyogenic infections, because the level of opsonizing IgG antibodies is low. In addition, those with CD40L mutations are also susceptible to pneumonia caused by the intracellular organism *Pneumocystis jiroveci*, because of the defect in cell-mediated immunity.

DiGeorge Syndrome (Thymic Hypoplasia)

DiGeorge syndrome is a T-cell deficiency that results from failure of development of the third and fourth pharyngeal pouches. The latter give rise to the thymus, the parathyroids, some of the clear cells of the thyroid, and the ultimobranchial body. Thus, individuals with this syndrome have a variable loss of T cell–mediated immunity (resulting from hypoplasia or lack of the thymus), tetany (resulting from lack of the parathyroids), and congenital defects of the heart and great vessels. In addition, the appearance of the mouth, ears, and facies may be abnormal. Absence of cell-mediated immunity is caused by low numbers of T lymphocytes in the blood and lymphoid tissues and poor defense against certain fungal and viral infections. The T-cell zones of lymphoid organs—paracortical areas of the lymph nodes and the periarteriolar sheaths of the spleen—are depleted. Ig levels may be normal or reduced, depending on the severity of the T-cell deficiency.

DiGeorge syndrome is not a familial disorder. It results from the deletion of a gene that maps to chromosome 22q11.[115] This deletion is seen in 90% of patients, and DiGeorge syndrome is now considered a component of the *22q11 deletion syndrome*, discussed in Chapter 5. One mutation that has been associated with the DiGeorge syndrome affects a member of the T-box family of transcription factors, which may be involved in development of the branchial arch and the great vessels.

Severe Combined Immunodeficiency

Severe combined immunodeficiency (SCID) represents a constellation of genetically distinct syndromes, all having in common *defects in both humoral and cell-mediated immune responses.*[116] Affected infants present with prominent thrush (oral candidiasis), extensive diaper rash, and failure to thrive. Some patients develop a morbilliform rash shortly after birth because maternal T cells are transferred across the placenta and attack the fetus, causing GVH disease. Persons with SCID are extremely susceptible to recurrent, severe infections by a wide range of pathogens, including *Candida albicans*, *P. jiroveci*, *Pseudomonas*, cytomegalovirus, varicella, and a whole host of bacteria. Without bone marrow transplantation, death occurs within the first year of life. Despite the common clinical manifestations, the underlying defects are quite different in different forms of SCID, and in many cases the genetic lesion is not known. Often, the SCID defect resides in the T-cell compartment, with a secondary impairment of humoral immunity.

The most common form, accounting for 50% to 60% of cases, is X-linked, and hence SCID is more common in boys than in girls. The genetic defect in the X-linked form is a *mutation in the common γ-chain (γc) subunit of cytokine receptors.* This transmembrane protein is part of the signal-transducing components of the receptors for IL-2, IL-4, IL-7, IL-9, IL-11, IL-15, and IL-21. IL-7 is required for the survival and proliferation of lymphoid progenitors, particularly T-cell precursors. As a result of defective IL-7 receptor signaling, there is a profound defect in the earliest stages of lymphocyte development, especially T-cell development.[117] T-cell numbers are greatly reduced, and although B cells are normal in number, antibody synthesis is severely impaired because of lack of T-cell help. IL-15 is important for the maturation and proliferation of NK cells, and because the common γ chain is a component of the receptor for IL-15, these individuals often have a deficiency of NK cells as well.

The remaining cases of SCID are inherited as autosomal recessive. The most common cause of autosomal recessive SCID is a *deficiency of the enzyme adenosine deaminase (ADA).* Although the mechanisms by which ADA deficiency causes SCID are not entirely clear, it has been proposed that deficiency of ADA leads to accumulation of deoxyadenosine and its derivatives (e.g., deoxy-ATP), which are toxic to rapidly dividing immature lymphocytes, especially those of the T-cell lineage.[118] Hence there may be a greater reduction in the number of T lymphocytes than of B lymphocytes.

Several other less common causes of autosomal recessive SCID have been discovered:

- Mutations in recombinase-activating genes prevent the somatic gene rearrangements essential for the assembly of T-cell receptor and Ig genes.[119] This blocks the development of T and B cells.
- An intracellular kinase called Jak3 is essential for signal transduction through the common cytokine receptor γ chain (which is mutated in X-linked SCID, as discussed above). Mutations of Jak3 therefore have the same effects as mutations in the γc chain.[120]
- Several mutations have been described in signaling molecules, including kinases associated with the T-cell antigen receptor and components of calcium channels that are required for entry of calcium and activation of many signaling pathways.
- Mutations that impair the expression of class II MHC molecules prevent the development of CD4+ T cells.[121] CD4+ T cells are involved in cellular immunity and provide help to B cells, and hence class II MHC deficiency results in combined immunodeficiency. This disease, called the *bare lymphocyte syndrome*, is usually caused by mutations in transcription factors that are required for class II MHC gene expression.

The histologic findings in SCID depend on the underlying defect. In the two most common forms (ADA deficiency and γc mutation), the thymus is small and devoid of lymphoid cells. In SCID caused by ADA deficiency, remnants of Hassall's corpuscles can be found, whereas in X-linked SCID the thymus contains lobules of undifferentiated epithelial cells resembling fetal thymus. In either case other lymphoid tissues are hypoplastic as well, with marked depletion of T-cell areas and in some cases both T-cell and B-cell zones.

Currently, bone marrow transplantation is the mainstay of treatment, but X-linked SCID is the first human disease in which gene therapy has been successful.[122] For gene therapy a normal γc gene is expressed in bone marrow stem cells of patients using a retroviral vector, and the cells are transplanted back into the patients. The clinical experience is small, but some patients have shown reconstitution of their immune systems for over a year after therapy. Unfortunately, however, 20% of these patients have developed acute T-cell leukemias, which appear to have been triggered by the activation of oncogenes by the integrated retrovirus,[123] highlighting the dangers of this particular approach to gene therapy. Patients with ADA deficiency have also been treated with bone marrow transplantation and, more recently, with gene therapy to introduce a normal ADA gene into T-cell precursors.

Immunodeficiency with Thrombocytopenia and Eczema (Wiskott-Aldrich Syndrome)

Wiskott-Aldrich syndrome is an X-linked recessive disease characterized by thrombocytopenia, eczema, and a marked vulnerability to recurrent infection, ending in early death.[124] The thymus is morphologically normal, at least early in the course of the disease, but there is progressive secondary depletion of T lymphocytes in the peripheral blood and in the T-cell zones (paracortical areas) of the lymph nodes, with variable loss of cellular immunity. Patients do not make antibodies to polysaccharide antigens, and the response to protein antigens is poor. IgM levels in the serum are low, but levels of IgG are usually normal. Paradoxically the levels of IgA and IgE are often elevated. Patients are also prone to developing non-Hodgkin B-cell lymphomas. The Wiskott-Aldrich syndrome is caused by mutations in the gene encoding *Wiskott-Aldrich syndrome protein (WASP)*, which is located at Xp11.23. This protein belongs to a family of proteins that are believed to link membrane receptors, such as antigen receptors, to cytoskeletal elements. The WASP protein may be involved in cytoskeleton-dependent responses, including cell migration and signal transduction, but the essential functions of this protein in lymphocytes and platelets are unclear. The only treatment is bone marrow transplantation.

Genetic Deficiencies of the Complement System

The complement system plays critical roles in host defense and inflammation. Hereditary deficiencies have been described for virtually all components of the complement system and several of the regulators.[125] A deficiency of C2 is the most common of all. With a deficiency of C2 or the other early components of the classical pathway (i.e., C1 [C1q, r, or s] or C4), there is little or no increase in susceptibility to infections, but the dominant manifestation is an increased incidence of an SLE-like autoimmune disease, as discussed earlier. Presumably, the alternative complement pathway is adequate for the control of most infections. Deficiency of components of the alternative pathway (properdin and factor D) is rare. It is associated with recurrent pyogenic infections. The C3 component of complement is required for both the classical and alternative pathways, and hence a deficiency of this protein results in susceptibility to serious and recurrent pyogenic infections. There is also increased incidence of immune complex–mediated glomerulonephritis; in the absence of complement, immune complex–mediated inflammation is presumably caused by Fc receptor–dependent leukocyte activation. The terminal components of complement C5, 6, 7, 8, and 9 are required for the assembly of the membrane attack complex involved in the lysis of organisms. With a deficiency of these

late-acting components, there is increased susceptibility to recurrent neisserial (gonococcal and meningococcal) infections; *Neisseria* bacteria have thin cell walls and are especially susceptible to the lytic actions of complement. Some patients inherit a form of mannose-binding lectin, the plasma protein that initiates the lectin pathway of complement, that does not polymerize normally and is functionally defective. These individuals also show increased susceptibility to infections.

A deficiency of C1 inhibitor gives rise to *hereditary angioedema*.[126] This autosomal dominant disorder is more common than complement deficiency states. The C1 inhibitor is a protease inhibitor whose target enzymes are C1r and C1s of the complement cascade, factor XII of the coagulation pathway, and the kallikrein system. As discussed in Chapter 2, these pathways are closely linked, and their unregulated activation can give rise to vasoactive peptides such as bradykinin. Although the exact nature of the bioactive compound produced in hereditary angioedema is uncertain, these patients have episodes of edema affecting skin and mucosal surfaces such as the larynx and the gastrointestinal tract. This may result in life-threatening asphyxia or nausea, vomiting, and diarrhea after minor trauma or emotional stress. Acute attacks of hereditary angioedema can be treated with C1 inhibitor concentrates prepared from human plasma.

Deficiency of other complement-regulatory proteins is the cause of paroxysmal nocturnal hemoglobinuria. In this disease there are mutations in enzymes required for glycophosphatidyl inositol linkages, which are essential for the assembly of decay-accelerating factor and CD59, both of which regulate complement.[127] Uncontrolled complement activation on the surface of red cells is believed to be the basis of hemolysis (Chapter 14). Mutations in the complement-regulatory protein factor H underlie about 10% of cases of a renal disease called hemolytic uremic syndrome, which is characterized by microvascular thrombosis in the kidneys (Chapter 20).

SECONDARY IMMUNODEFICIENCIES

Secondary immune deficiencies may be encountered in individuals with cancer, diabetes and other metabolic diseases, malnutrition, chronic infection, and renal disease. They also occur in persons receiving chemotherapy or radiation therapy for cancer, or immunosuppressive drugs to prevent graft rejection or to treat autoimmune diseases. Some of these secondary immunodeficiency states can be caused by defective lymphocyte maturation (when the bone marrow is damaged by radiation or chemotherapy or involved by tumors, such as leukemias and metastatic cancers), loss of immunoglobulins (as in proteinuric renal diseases), inadequate Ig synthesis (as in malnutrition), or lymphocyte depletion (from drugs or severe infections). *As a group, the secondary immune deficiencies are more common than the disorders of primary genetic origin.* The most common secondary immunodeficiency is AIDS, and we will describe this in the next section.

ACQUIRED IMMUNODEFICIENCY SYNDROME (AIDS)

AIDS is a disease caused by the retrovirus human immunodeficiency virus (HIV) and characterized by profound immuno-

suppression that leads to opportunistic infections, secondary neoplasms, and neurologic manifestations. The magnitude of this modern plague is truly staggering. By the end of 2006, more than a million cases of AIDS had been reported in the United States, where AIDS is the second leading cause of death in men between ages 25 and 44, and the third leading cause of death in women in this age group. Though initially recognized in the United States, AIDS is a global problem. It has now been reported from more than 190 countries around the world, and the pool of HIV-infected persons in Africa and Asia is large and expanding. By the year 2006, HIV had infected 60 million people worldwide, and nearly 20 million adults and children have died of the disease. There are about 33 million people living with HIV, of whom 65% are in Africa and over 20% in Asia; the prevalence rate in adults in sub-Saharan Africa is over 8%. It is estimated that 2.5 million people were newly infected with HIV during 2006, and 2.1 million deaths were caused by AIDS in that year alone. In this dismal scenario, there may be some good news. Because of public health measures, the infection rate seems to be decreasing, and some authorities believe it may have peaked in the late 1990s. Furthermore, improved antiviral therapies have resulted in fewer people dying of the disease. This, however, raises its own tragic concern; because more people are living with HIV, the risk of spreading the infection will increase if vigilance is relaxed.

The enormous medical and social burden of the AIDS problem has led to an explosion of research aimed at understanding HIV and its remarkable ability to cripple host defenses. The literature on AIDS is vast and expanding. Here we summarize the currently available data on the epidemiology, pathogenesis, and clinical features of HIV infection.

Epidemiology

Epidemiologic studies in the United States have identified five groups of adults at risk for developing AIDS. The case distribution in these groups is as follows:

- *Homosexual or bisexual men* constitute the largest group, accounting for over 50% of the reported cases. This includes about 5% who were intravenous drug abusers as well. Transmission of AIDS in this category appears to be on the decline: in 2005 about 48% of new cases were attributed to male homosexual contacts.
- *Intravenous drug abusers* with no previous history of homosexuality are the next largest group, representing about 20% of infected individuals.
- *Hemophiliacs*, especially those who received large amounts of factor VIII or factor IX concentrates before 1985, make up about 0.5% of all cases.
- *Recipients of blood and blood components* who are not hemophiliacs but who received transfusions of HIV-infected whole blood or components (e.g., platelets, plasma) account for about 1% of patients. (Organs obtained from HIV-infected donors can also transmit AIDS.)
- *Heterosexual contacts* of members of other high-risk groups (chiefly intravenous drug abusers) constitute about 10% of the patient population. About 30% of new cases in 2005 were attributable to heterosexual contact. This is the most

rapidly growing group of infected individuals, particularly women; in sub-Saharan Africa, where the infection rate is estimated to be about 10,000 new cases every day, more than half the infected individuals are women.
- In approximately 5% of cases the risk factors cannot be determined.

The epidemiology of AIDS is quite different in children under age 13. Close to 2% of all AIDS cases occur in this pediatric population, and worldwide over 500,000 new cases and almost 400,000 deaths were reported in children in the year 2006. In this group the vast majority acquired the infection by transmission of the virus from mother to child (discussed later).

It should be apparent from the preceding discussion that transmission of HIV occurs under conditions that facilitate exchange of blood or body fluids containing the virus or virus-infected cells. The three major routes of transmission are *sexual contact, parenteral inoculation,* and *passage of the virus from infected mothers to their newborns.*

- *Sexual transmission* is clearly the predominant mode of infection worldwide, accounting for over 75% of all cases of HIV transmission. Because the majority of infected people in the United States are men who have sex with men, most sexual transmission has occurred among homosexual men. The virus is carried in the semen, and it enters the recipient's body through abrasions in rectal or oral mucosa or by direct contact with mucosal lining cells. Viral transmission occurs in two ways: (1) direct inoculation into the blood vessels breached by trauma, and (2) infection of dendritic cells or CD4+ cells within the mucosa. Heterosexual transmission, though initially of less numerical importance in the United States, is globally the most common mode by which HIV is spread. In the past few years, even in the United States, *the rate of increase of heterosexual transmission has outpaced transmission by other means.* Such spread is occurring most rapidly in female sex partners of male intravenous drug abusers. As such, the number of women with AIDS is rising rapidly. In contrast to the U.S. experience, heterosexual transmission has always been the dominant mode of HIV infection in Asia and Africa.

In addition to male-to-male and male-to-female transmission, there is evidence supporting female-to-male transmission. HIV is present in vaginal secretions and cervical cells of infected women. In the United States this form of heterosexual spread is approximately 20-fold less common than male-to-female transmission. By contrast, in Africa and parts of Asia, the risk of female-to-male transmission is much higher. This observation is believed to be attributable to the presence of concurrent sexually transmitted disease. All forms of sexual transmission of HIV are enhanced by coexisting sexually transmitted diseases, especially those associated with genital ulceration. In this regard, syphilis, chancroid, and herpes are particularly important. Other sexually transmitted diseases, including gonorrhea and chlamydia, are also cofactors for HIV transmission, perhaps because in these genital inflammatory states there is greater concentration of the virus and virus-containing cells in genital fluids, as a result of increased numbers of inflammatory cells in the semen.

○ *Parenteral transmission* of HIV has occurred in three groups of individuals: intravenous drug abusers, hemophiliacs who received factor VIII and factor IX concentrates, and random recipients of blood transfusion. Of these three, intravenous drug users constitute by far the largest group. Transmission occurs by sharing of needles, syringes, and other paraphernalia contaminated with HIV-containing blood.

Transmission of HIV by transfusion of blood or blood products, such as lyophilized factor VIII and factor IX concentrates, has been virtually eliminated. This fortunate outcome resulted from increasing use of recombinant clotting factors and from three public health measures: screening of donated blood and plasma for antibody to HIV, stringent purity criteria for factor VIII and factor IX preparations, and screening of donors on the basis of history. However, an extremely small risk of acquiring AIDS through transfusion of seronegative blood persists, because a recently infected individual may be antibody-negative. Currently, this risk is estimated to be 1 in more than 2 million units of blood transfused. Because it is now possible to detect HIV-associated p24 antigens in the blood before the development of humoral antibodies, this small risk is likely to decrease even further.

○ As alluded to earlier, *mother-to-infant transmission* is the major cause of pediatric AIDS. Infected mothers can transmit the infection to their offspring by three routes: (1) in utero by transplacental spread, (2) during delivery through an infected birth canal, and (3) after birth by ingestion of breast milk. Of these, transmission during birth (intrapartum) and in the immediate period thereafter (peripartum) is considered to be the most common mode in the United States. The reported transmission rates vary from 7% to 49% in different parts of the world. Higher risk of transmission is associated with high maternal viral load and low CD4+ T-cell counts as well as chorioamnionitis. Currently, with antiretroviral therapy given to infected pregnant women in the United States, the mother-to-child transmission has been virtually eliminated.

Much concern has arisen in the lay public and among health care workers about spread of HIV infection outside the high-risk groups. Extensive studies indicate that *HIV infection cannot be transmitted by casual personal contact in the household, workplace, or school.* Spread by insect bites is virtually impossible. Regarding transmission of HIV infection to health care workers, an extremely small but definite risk seems to be present. Seroconversion has been documented after accidental needle-stick injury or exposure of nonintact skin to infected blood in laboratory accidents. After needle-stick accidents, the risk of seroconversion is believed to be about 0.3%, and antiretroviral therapy given within 24 to 48 hours of a needle stick can reduce the risk of infection eightfold. By comparison, approximately 30% of those accidentally exposed to hepatitis B–infected blood become seropositive.

Etiology: The Properties of HIV

AIDS is caused by HIV, a nontransforming human retrovirus belonging to the lentivirus family. Included in this group are feline immunodeficiency virus, simian immunodeficiency virus, visna virus of sheep, bovine immunodeficiency virus, and the equine infectious anemia virus.

Two genetically different but related forms of HIV, called *HIV-1 and HIV-2,* have been isolated from patients with AIDS. HIV-1 is the most common type associated with AIDS in the United States, Europe, and Central Africa, whereas HIV-2 causes a similar disease principally in West Africa and India. Specific tests for HIV-2 are available, and blood collected for transfusion is routinely screened for both HIV-1 and HIV-2 seropositivity. The ensuing discussion relates primarily to HIV-1 and diseases caused by it, but the information is generally applicable to HIV-2 as well.

Structure of HIV

Similar to most retroviruses, the HIV-1 virion is spherical and contains an electron-dense, cone-shaped core surrounded by a lipid envelope derived from the host cell membrane (Fig. 6–43). The virus core contains (1) the major capsid protein p24; (2) nucleocapsid protein p7/p9; (3) two copies of genomic RNA; and (4) the three viral enzymes (protease, reverse transcriptase, and integrase). p24 is the most readily detected viral antigen and is the target for the antibodies that are used for the diagnosis of HIV infection in the widely used enzyme-linked immunosorbent assay. The viral core is surrounded by a matrix protein called p17, which lies underneath the virion envelope. Studding the viral envelope are two viral glycoproteins, gp120 and gp41, which are critical for HIV infection of cells.

The HIV-1 RNA genome contains the *gag, pol,* and *env* genes, which are typical of retroviruses (Fig. 6–44). The products of the *gag* and *pol* genes are translated initially into large precursor proteins that are cleaved by the viral protease to yield the mature proteins. The highly effective anti-HIV-1 protease inhibitor drugs prevent viral assembly by inhibiting

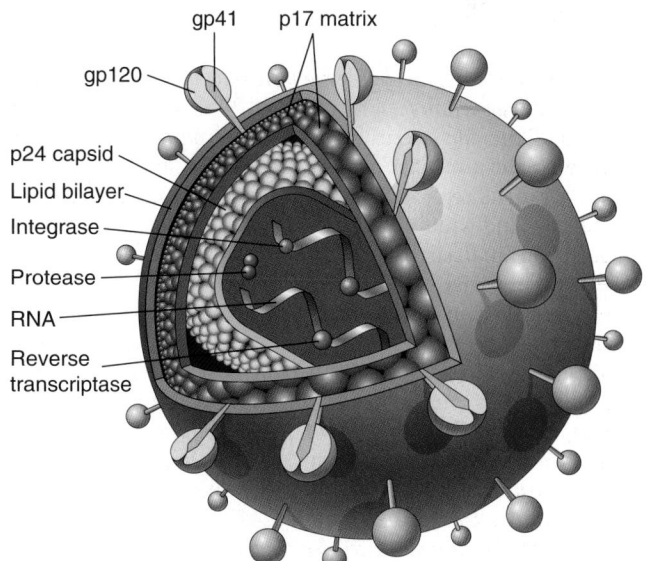

FIGURE 6–43 The structure of the human immune deficiency virus (HIV)–1 virion. The viral particle is covered by a lipid bilayer derived from the host cell and studded with viral glycoproteins gp41 and gp120.

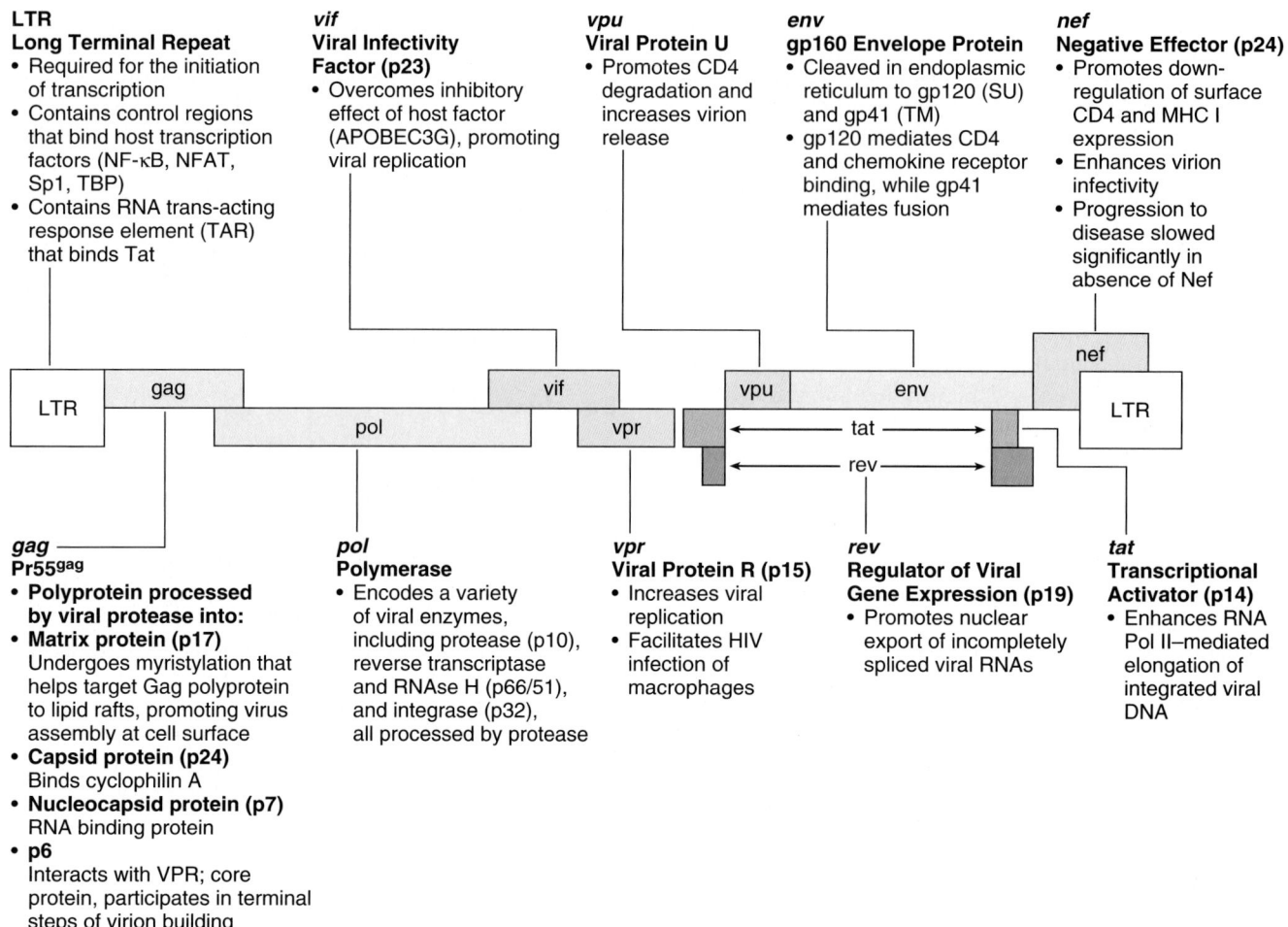

LTR
Long Terminal Repeat
- Required for the initiation of transcription
- Contains control regions that bind host transcription factors (NF-κB, NFAT, Sp1, TBP)
- Contains RNA trans-acting response element (TAR) that binds Tat

vif
Viral Infectivity Factor (p23)
- Overcomes inhibitory effect of host factor (APOBEC3G), promoting viral replication

vpu
Viral Protein U
- Promotes CD4 degradation and increases virion release

env
gp160 Envelope Protein
- Cleaved in endoplasmic reticulum to gp120 (SU) and gp41 (TM)
- gp120 mediates CD4 and chemokine receptor binding, while gp41 mediates fusion

nef
Negative Effector (p24)
- Promotes down-regulation of surface CD4 and MHC I expression
- Enhances virion infectivity
- Progression to disease slowed significantly in absence of Nef

gag
Pr55^{gag}
- **Polyprotein processed by viral protease into:**
- **Matrix protein (p17)**
  Undergoes myristylation that helps target Gag polyprotein to lipid rafts, promoting virus assembly at cell surface
- **Capsid protein (p24)**
  Binds cyclophilin A
- **Nucleocapsid protein (p7)**
  RNA binding protein
- **p6**
  Interacts with VPR; core protein, participates in terminal steps of virion building

pol
Polymerase
- Encodes a variety of viral enzymes, including protease (p10), reverse transcriptase and RNAse H (p66/51), and integrase (p32), all processed by protease

vpr
Viral Protein R (p15)
- Increases viral replication
- Facilitates HIV infection of macrophages

rev
Regulator of Viral Gene Expression (p19)
- Promotes nuclear export of incompletely spliced viral RNAs

tat
Transcriptional Activator (p14)
- Enhances RNA Pol II–mediated elongation of integrated viral DNA

FIGURE 6–44   The HIV genome. Several viral genes and the functions of the encoded proteins are illustrated. The genes outlined in red are unique to HIV; others are shared by all retroviruses.

the formation of mature viral proteins. In addition to these three standard retroviral genes, HIV contains several other accessory genes, including *tat, rev, vif, nef, vpr,* and *vpu,* that regulate the synthesis and assembly of infectious viral particles and the pathogenicity of the virus.[128–130] For example, the product of the *tat* (transactivator) gene causes a 1000-fold increase in the transcription of viral genes and is therefore critical for virus replication. The functions of other accessory proteins are indicated in Figure 6–44.

Molecular analysis of different HIV-1 isolates has revealed considerable variability in certain parts of their genome. Most variations are clustered in particular regions of the envelope glycoproteins. Because the humoral immune response against HIV-1 is targeted against its envelope, such variability poses problems for the development of a single antigen vaccine. On the basis of genetic analysis, HIV-1 can be divided into three subgroups, designated *M* (major), *O* (outlier), and *N* (neither *M* nor *O*). Group M viruses are the most common form worldwide, and they are further divided into several subtypes, or clades, designated A through K. Various subtypes differ in their geographic distribution; for example, subtype B is the most common form in western Europe and the United States, whereas subtype E is the most common clade in Thailand. Currently, clade C is the fastest-spreading clade worldwide, being present in India, Ethiopia, and Southern Africa.

Pathogenesis of HIV Infection and AIDS

While HIV can infect many tissues, *there are two major targets of HIV infection: the immune system and the central nervous system.* The effects of HIV infection on each of these two systems are discussed separately.

Profound immune deficiency, primarily affecting cell-mediated immunity, is the hallmark of AIDS. This results chiefly from infection of and a severe loss of CD4+ T cells as well as impairment in the function of surviving helper T cells.[131,132] As discussed later, macrophages and dendritic cells are also targets of HIV infection. HIV enters the body through mucosal tissues and blood and first infects T cells as well as dendritic cells and macrophages. The infection becomes established in lymphoid tissues, where the virus may remain latent for long periods. Active viral replication is associated with more infection of cells and progression to AIDS. We first describe the mechanisms involved in viral entry into T cells and macrophages and the replicative cycle of the virus within cells. This is followed by a more detailed review of the interaction between HIV and its cellular targets.

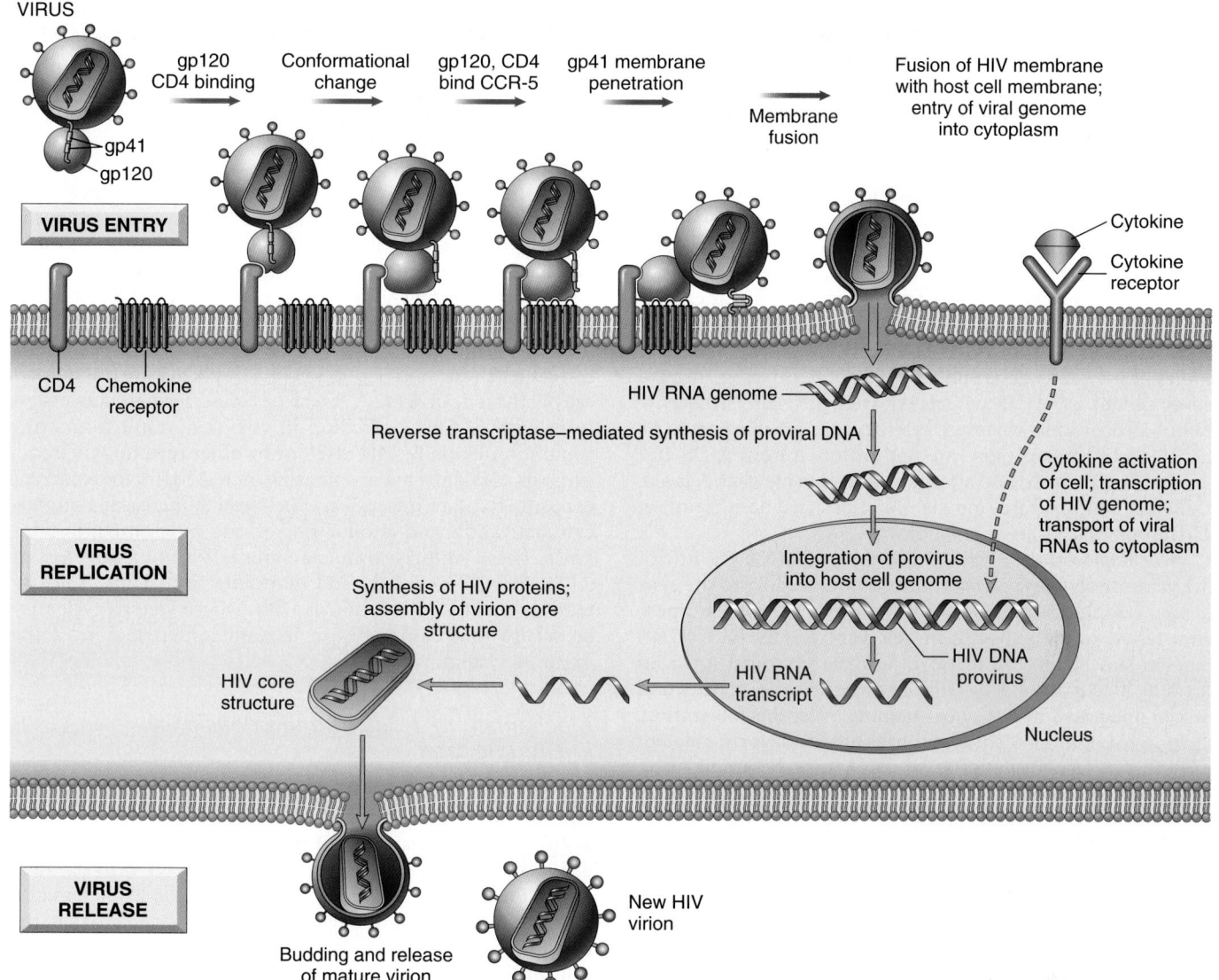

VIRUS

gp120
CD4 binding

Conformational
change

gp120, CD4
bind CCR-5

gp41 membrane
penetration

Membrane
fusion

Fusion of HIV membrane
with host cell membrane;
entry of viral genome
into cytoplasm

gp41
gp120

VIRUS ENTRY

Cytokine

Cytokine
receptor

CD4   Chemokine
receptor

HIV RNA genome

Reverse transcriptase–mediated synthesis of proviral DNA

Cytokine activation
of cell; transcription
of HIV genome;
transport of viral
RNAs to cytoplasm

**VIRUS
REPLICATION**

Synthesis of HIV proteins;
assembly of virion core
structure

Integration of provirus
into host cell genome

HIV core
structure

HIV RNA
transcript

HIV DNA
provirus

Nucleus

**VIRUS
RELEASE**

New HIV
virion

Budding and release
of mature virion

FIGURE 6–45   The life cycle of HIV, showing the steps from viral entry to production of infectious virions. (Adapted with permission from Wain-Hobson S: HIV. One on one meets two. Nature 384:117, 1996. Copyright 1996, Macmillan Magazines Limited.)

Life Cycle of HIV

The life cycle of HIV consists of infection of cells, integration of the provirus into the host cell genome, activation of viral replication, and production and release of infectious virus (Fig. 6–45).[133] The molecules and mechanisms of each of these steps are understood in considerable detail.

Infection of Cells by HIV.   *HIV infects cells by using the CD4 molecule as receptor and various chemokine receptors as coreceptors* (Fig. 6–45). The requirement for CD4 binding explains the selective tropism of the virus for CD4+ T cells and other CD4+ cells, particularly monocytes/macrophages and dendritic cells. Binding to CD4 is not sufficient for infection, however. HIV gp120 must also bind to other cell surface molecules (coreceptors) for entry into the cell. Chemokine receptors, particularly CCR5 and CXCR4, serve this role.[134] HIV isolates can be distinguished by their use of these receptors: R5 strains use CCR5, X4 strains use CXCR4, and some strains

(R5X4) are dual-tropic. In approximately 90% of cases, the R5 (M-tropic) type of HIV is the dominant virus found in the blood of acutely infected individuals and early in the course of infection. Over the course of infection, however, T-tropic viruses gradually accumulate; these are especially virulent because T-tropic viruses are capable of infecting many T cells and even thymic T-cell precursors and cause greater T-cell depletion and impairment.

Molecular details of the deadly handshake between HIV glycoproteins and their cell surface receptors have been uncovered by elegant studies and are important to understand because they may provide the basis of anti-HIV therapy. The HIV envelope contains two glycoproteins, surface gp120 noncovalently attached to a transmembrane protein, gp41. *The initial step in infection is the binding of the gp120 envelope glycoprotein to CD4 molecules.* This binding leads to a conformational change that results in the formation of a new recognition site on gp120 for the coreceptors CCR5 or CXCR4. Binding to the coreceptors induces conformational changes in gp41 that result in the exposure of a hydrophobic region called the fusion peptide at the tip of gp41. This peptide inserts into the cell membrane of the target cells (e.g., T cells or macrophages), leading to fusion of the virus with the host cell.[135] After fusion the virus core containing the HIV genome enters the cytoplasm of the cell. The requirement for HIV binding to coreceptors may have important implications for the pathogenesis of AIDS. Chemokines sterically hinder HIV infection of cells in culture by occupying their receptors, and therefore, the level of chemokines in the tissues may influence the efficiency of viral infection in vivo. Also, polymorphisms in the gene encoding CCR5 are associated with different susceptibility to HIV infection. About 1% of white Americans inherit two defective copies of the CCR5 gene and are resistant to infection and the development of AIDS associated with R5 HIV isolates.[125] About 20% of individuals are heterozygous for this protective CCR5 allele; these persons are not protected from AIDS, but the onset of their disease after infection is somewhat delayed. Only rare homozygotes for the mutation have been found in African or East Asian populations.

Viral Replication. Once internalized, the RNA genome of the virus undergoes reverse transcription, leading to the synthesis of double-stranded complementary DNA (cDNA; proviral DNA) (see Fig. 6–45). In quiescent T cells, HIV cDNA may remain in the cytoplasm in a linear episomal form. In dividing T cells, the cDNA circularizes, enters the nucleus, and is then integrated into the host genome. After this integration, the provirus may be silent for months or years, a form of latent infection. Alternatively, proviral DNA may be transcribed, with the formation of complete viral particles that bud from the cell membrane. Such productive infection, when associated with extensive viral budding, leads to death of infected cells.

In vivo, HIV infects memory and activated T cells but is inefficient at productively infecting naive (unactivated) T cells. Naive T cells contain an active form of an enzyme that introduces mutations in the HIV genome. This enzyme has been given the rather cumbersome name APOBEC3G (for "apolipoprotein B mRNA-editing enzyme catalytic polypeptide-like editing complex 3").[136] It is a cytidine deaminase that introduces cytosine-to-uracil mutations in the viral DNA that is produced by reverse transcription. These mutations inhibit further DNA replication by mechanisms that are not fully defined. Activation of T cells converts cellular APOBEC3G into an inactive, high-molecular-mass complex, which explains why the virus can replicate in previously activated (e.g., memory) T cells and T-cell lines. HIV has also evolved to counteract this cellular defense mechanism; the viral protein Vif binds to APOBEC3G and promotes its degradation by cellular proteases.

Completion of the viral life cycle in latently infected cells occurs only after cell activation, and in the case of most CD4+ T cells virus activation results in cell lysis. Activation of T cells by antigens or cytokines upregulates several transcription factors, including NF-κB, which stimulate transcription of genes encoding cytokines such as IL-2 and its receptor. In resting T cells, NF-κB is sequestered in the cytoplasm in a complex with members of the IκB (inhibitor of κB) protein. Cellular activation by antigen or cytokines induces cytoplasmic kinases that phosphorylate IκB and target it for enzymatic

degradation, thus releasing NF-κB and allowing it to translocate to the nucleus. In the nucleus, NF-κB binds to sequences within the promoter regions of several genes, including those of cytokines that are expressed in activated T cells. The long-terminal-repeat sequences that flank the HIV genome also contain NF-κB–binding sites that can be triggered by the same transcription factors.[137] Imagine now a latently infected CD4+ cell that encounters an environmental antigen. Induction of NF-κB in such a cell (a physiologic response) activates the transcription of HIV proviral DNA (a pathologic outcome) and leads ultimately to the production of virions and to cell lysis. Furthermore, TNF and other cytokines produced by activated macrophages also stimulate NF-κB activity and thus lead to production of HIV RNA. Thus, it seems that HIV thrives when the host T cells and macrophages are physiologically activated, an act that can be best described as "subversion from within." Such activation in vivo may result from antigenic stimulation by HIV itself or by other infecting microorganisms. HIV-infected people are at increased risk for recurrent exposure to other infections, which lead to increased lymphocyte activation and production of pro-inflammatory cytokines. These, in turn, stimulate more HIV production, loss of additional CD4+ T cells, and more infection. Thus, it is easy to visualize how in individuals with AIDS a vicious cycle may be set up that culminates in inexorable destruction of the immune system.

Mechanism of T-Cell Immunodeficiency in HIV Infection

Loss of CD4+ T cells is mainly because of infection of the cells and the direct cytopathic effects of the replicating virus (Fig. 6–46).[138] Approximately 100 billion new viral particles are produced every day, and 1 to 2 billion CD4+ T cells die each day.[139] Because the frequency of infected cells in the circulation is very low, for many years it was suspected that the immunodeficiency is out of proportion to the level of infection and cannot be attributed to death of infected cells. In fact, many infected cells may be in mucosal and other peripheral lymphoid organs, and death of these cells is a major cause of the relentless, and eventually profound, cell loss. Also, to a point the immune system can replace the dying T cells, and hence the rate of T cell loss may appear deceptively low, but as the disease progresses, renewal of CD4+ T cells cannot keep up with the loss of these cells. Possible mechanisms by which the virus directly kills infected cells include increased plasma membrane permeability associated with budding of virus particles from the infected cells, and virus replication interfering with protein synthesis.

In addition to direct killing of cells by the virus, other mechanisms may contribute to the loss of T cells (see Fig. 6–46).[140] These include:

- HIV colonizes the lymphoid organs (spleen, lymph nodes, tonsils) and may cause progressive destruction of the architecture and cellular composition of lymphoid tissues.
- Chronic activation of uninfected cells, responding to HIV itself or to infections that are common in individuals with AIDS, leads to apoptosis of these cells by the process of *activation-induced cell death*.[140,141] Thus, the numbers of CD4+ T cells that die are far greater than the numbers

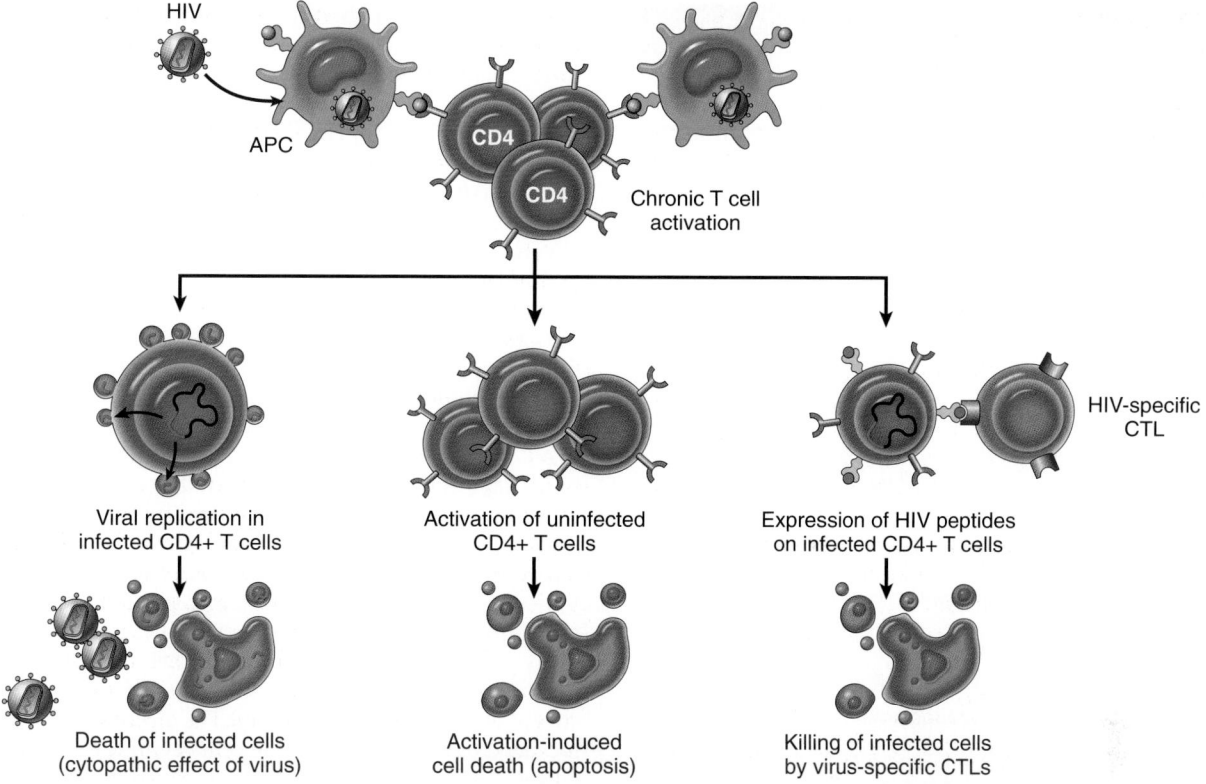

FIGURE 6–46 Mechanisms of CD4+ T-cell loss in HIV infection, showing some of the known and postulated mechanisms of T-cell depletion after HIV infection. APC, antigen-presenting cell; CTL, cytotoxic T lymphocyte.

of infected cells. The molecular mechanism of this type of cell death is not known.

○ Loss of immature precursors of CD4+ T cells can also occur, either by direct infection of thymic progenitor cells or by infection of accessory cells that secrete cytokines essential for CD4+ T-cell maturation.

○ Fusion of infected and uninfected cells with formation of syncytia (giant cells) can occur. In tissue culture the gp120 expressed on productively infected cells binds to CD4 molecules on uninfected T cells, followed by cell fusion. Fused cells develop ballooning and usually die within a few hours. This property of syncytia formation is generally confined to the T-tropic X4 type of HIV-1. For this reason, this type is often referred to as syncytia-inducing (SI) virus, in contrast to the R5 virus.

○ Apoptosis of uninfected CD4+ T cells by binding of soluble gp120 to the CD4 molecule, followed by activation through the T-cell receptor by antigens. It has been suggested that such cross-linking of CD4 molecules and T-cell activation lead to aberrant signaling and activation of death pathways. CD8+ CTLs may kill uninfected CD4+ T cells that are coated with gp120 released from infected cells.

Although marked reduction in CD4+ T cells, a hallmark of AIDS, can account for most of the immunodeficiency late in the course of HIV infection, there is compelling evidence for *qualitative defects in T cells that can be detected even in asymptomatic HIV-infected persons.* Reported defects include a reduction in antigen-induced T-cell proliferation, a decrease in T_H1-type responses relative to the T_H2 type, defects in intra-

cellular signaling, and many more. The loss of T_H1 responses results in profound deficiency in cell-mediated immunity, leading to increased susceptibility to infections by viruses and other intracellular microbes. There is also a selective loss of the memory subset of CD4+ helper T cells early in the course of disease, which explains poor recall responses to previously encountered antigens.

Low-level chronic or latent infection of T cells (and macrophages, discussed below) is an important feature of HIV infection. It is widely believed that integrated provirus, without virus expression (latent infection), can remain in the cells for months to years. Even with potent antiviral therapy, which practically sterilizes the peripheral blood, latent virus lurks within the CD4+ cells (both T cells and macrophages) in the lymph nodes. According to some estimates, 0.05% of resting CD4+ T cells in the lymph nodes are latently infected. Because these CD4+ T cells are memory T cells, they are long-lived, with a life span of months to years, and thus provide a persistent reservoir of virus.

CD4+ T cells play a pivotal role in regulating both cellular and humoral immune responses. Therefore, loss of this "master regulator" has ripple effects on virtually every other component of the immune system, as summarized in Table 6–12.

HIV Infection of Non-T Cells

In addition to infection and loss of CD4+ T cells, infection of macrophages[142] and dendritic cells[143] is also important in the pathogenesis of HIV infection. Similar to T cells, the majority

TABLE 6–12   Major Abnormalities of Immune Function in AIDS

LYMPHOPENIA

Predominantly caused by selective loss of the CD4+ helper T-cell subset

DECREASED T-CELL FUNCTION IN VIVO

Preferential loss of activated and memory T cells
Decreased delayed-type hypersensitivity
Susceptibility to opportunistic infections
Susceptibility to neoplasms

ALTERED T-CELL FUNCTION IN VITRO

Decreased proliferative response to mitogens, alloantigens, and soluble antigens
Decreased cytotoxicity
Decreased helper function for B-cell antibody production
Decreased IL-2 and IFN-γ production

POLYCLONAL B-CELL ACTIVATION

Hypergammaglobulinemia and circulating immune complexes
Inability to mount de novo antibody response to new antigens
Poor responses to normal B-cell activation signals in vitro

ALTERED MONOCYTE OR MACROPHAGE FUNCTIONS

Decreased chemotaxis and phagocytosis
Decreased class II HLA expression
Diminished capacity to present antigen to T cells

HLA, human leukocyte antigen; IFN-γ, interferon-γ; IL-1, etc., interleukin-1; TNF, tumor necrosis factor.

of the *macrophages* that are infected by HIV are found in the tissues and the number of blood monocytes infected by the virus may be low. In certain tissues, such as the lungs and brain, as many as 10% to 50% of macrophages are infected. Several aspects of HIV infection of macrophages should be emphasized:

- Although cell division is required for replication of most retroviruses, HIV-1 can infect and multiply in terminally differentiated nondividing macrophages. This property of HIV-1 is dependent on the HIV-1 *vpr* gene. The Vpr protein allows nuclear targeting of the HIV preintegration complex through the nuclear pore.
- Infected macrophages bud relatively small amounts of virus from the cell surface, but these cells contain large numbers of virus particles often located in intracellular vacuoles. Even though macrophages allow viral replication, they are quite resistant to the cytopathic effects of HIV, in contrast to CD4+ T cells. Thus, macrophages may be reservoirs of infection, whose output remains largely protected from host defenses. In late stages of HIV infection, when CD4+ T-cell numbers decline greatly, macrophages may be an important site of continued viral replication.[144]
- Macrophages, in all likelihood, act as gatekeepers of infection. Recall that in more than 90% of cases acute HIV infection is characterized by predominantly circulating M-tropic strains. This finding suggests that the initial infection of macrophages or dendritic cells may be important in the pathogenesis of HIV disease.

Even uninfected monocytes are reported to have unexplained functional defects that may have important consequences for host defense. These defects include impaired microbicidal activity, decreased chemotaxis, decreased secretion of IL-1, inappropriate secretion of TNF, and poor capacity to present antigens to T cells. Also, even the low number of infected blood monocytes may be vehicles for HIV to be transported to various parts of the body, including the nervous system.

Studies have documented that, in addition to macrophages, two types of *dendritic cells* are also important targets for the initiation and maintenance of HIV infection: mucosal and follicular dendritic cells. It is thought that *mucosal dendritic cells are infected by the virus and transport it to regional lymph nodes*, where the virus is transmitted to CD4+ T cells.[143] Dendritic cells also express a lectin-like receptor that specifically binds HIV and displays it in an intact, infectious form to T cells, thus promoting infection of the T cells.[145] *Follicular dendritic cells in the germinal centers of lymph nodes, similar to macrophages, are potential reservoirs of HIV.* Although some follicular dendritic cells may be susceptible to HIV infection, most virus particles are found on the surface of their dendritic processes. Follicular dendritic cells have receptors for the Fc portion of immunoglobulins, and hence they trap HIV virions coated with anti-HIV antibodies. The antibody-coated virions localized to follicular dendritic cells retain the ability to infect CD4+ T cells as they traverse the intricate meshwork formed by the dendritic processes of the follicular dendritic cells.

Although much attention has been focused on T cells, macrophages, and dendritic cells because they can be infected by HIV, individuals with AIDS also display profound abnormalities of B-cell function. Paradoxically, there is polyclonal activation of B cells, resulting in germinal center B-cell hyperplasia (particularly early in the disease course), bone marrow plasmacytosis, hypergammaglobulinemia, and formation of circulating immune complexes. This activation may result from multiple interacting factors: reactivation of or reinfection with cytomegalovirus and EBV, both of which are polyclonal B-cell activators, can occur; gp41 itself can promote B-cell growth and differentiation; and HIV-infected macrophages produce increased amounts of IL-6, which stimulates proliferation of B cells. *Despite the presence of spontaneously activated B cells, patients with AIDS are unable to mount antibody responses to newly encountered antigens.* This could be due, in part, to lack of T-cell help, but antibody responses against T-independent antigens are also suppressed, and hence there may be other intrinsic defects in B cells as well. Impaired humoral immunity renders these patients prey to disseminated infections caused by encapsulated bacteria, such as *S. pneumoniae* and *H. influenzae*, both of which require antibodies for effective opsonization and clearance.

Pathogenesis of Central Nervous System Involvement

The pathogenesis of neurologic manifestations deserves special mention because, in addition to the lymphoid system, the nervous system is a major target of HIV infection. Macrophages and microglia, cells in the central nervous system that belong to the macrophage lineage, are the predominant cell types in the brain that are infected with HIV.[146] It is believed that HIV is carried into the brain by infected monocytes. In keeping with this, the HIV isolates from the brain are almost exclusively M-tropic. The mechanism of HIV-induced damage of the brain, however, remains obscure. Because neurons are not infected by HIV, and the extent of neuropathologic changes is often less than might be expected from the severity of neurologic symptoms, most workers believe that the neurologic deficit is caused indirectly by viral products and by soluble factors produced by infected microglia. Included among the soluble factors are the usual culprits, such as IL-1, TNF, and IL-6. In addition, nitric oxide induced in neuronal cells by gp41 has been implicated. Direct damage of neurons by soluble HIV gp120 has also been postulated.

Natural History of HIV Infection

HIV disease begins with acute infection, which is only partly controlled by the adaptive immune response, and advances to chronic progressive infection of peripheral lymphoid tissues (Fig. 6–47). Virus typically enters through mucosal epithelia. The subsequent pathogenetic events and clinical manifestations of the infection can be divided into several phases: (1) an acute retroviral syndrome; (2) a middle, chronic phase, in which most individuals are asymptomatic; and (3) clinical AIDS (Figs. 6–47 and 6–48).[131,132]

Primary Infection, Virus Dissemination, and the Acute Retroviral Syndrome. *Acute (early) infection is characterized by infection of memory CD4+ T cells (which express CCR5) in mucosal lymphoid tissues, and death of many infected cells.* Because the mucosal tissues are the largest reservoir of T cells in the body, and a major site of residence of memory T cells, this local loss results in considerable depletion of lymphocytes.[147,148] Few infected cells are detectable in the blood and other tissues.

Mucosal infection is followed by dissemination of the virus and the development of host immune responses. Dendritic cells in epithelia at sites of virus entry capture the virus and then migrate into the lymph nodes. Once in lymphoid tissues, dendritic cells may pass HIV on to CD4+ T cells through direct cell-cell contact. Within days after the first exposure to HIV, viral replication can be detected in the lymph nodes. This replication leads to viremia, during which high numbers of HIV particles are present in the patient's blood. The virus disseminates throughout the body and infects helper T cells, macrophages, and dendritic cells in peripheral lymphoid tissues.

As the HIV infection spreads, the individual mounts antiviral humoral and cell-mediated immune responses.[149] These responses are evidenced by seroconversion (usually within 3 to 7 weeks of presumed exposure) and by the development of virus-specific CD8+ cytotoxic T cells. *HIV-specific CD8+ T cells are detected in the blood at about the time viral titers begin to fall and are most likely responsible for the initial containment of HIV infection.* These immune responses partially control the infection and viral production, and such control is reflected by a drop in viremia to low but detectable levels by about 12 weeks after the primary exposure.

The *acute retroviral syndrome* is the clinical presentation of the initial spread of the virus and the host response.[150] It is estimated that 40% to 90% of individuals who acquire

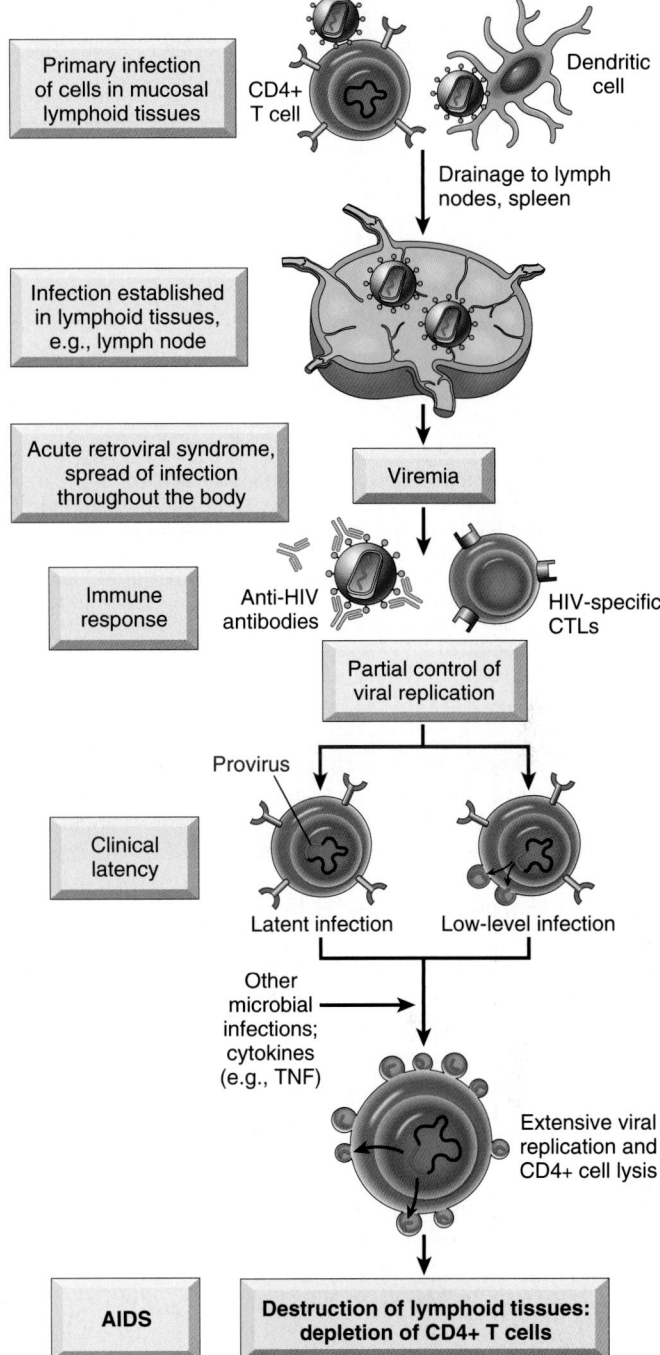

FIGURE 6–47 Pathogenesis of HIV-1 infection. The initial infection starts in mucosal tissues, involving mainly memory CD4+ T cells and dendritic cells, and spreads to lymph nodes. Viral replication leads to viremia and widespread seeding of lymphoid tissue. The viremia is controlled by the host immune response (not shown), and the patient then enters a phase of clinical latency. During this phase, viral replication in both T cells and macrophages continues unabated, but there is some immune containment of virus (not illustrated). There continues a gradual erosion of CD4+ cells and ultimately, CD4+ T-cell numbers decline, and the patient develops clinical symptoms of full-blown AIDS. CTL, cytotoxic T lymphocyte.

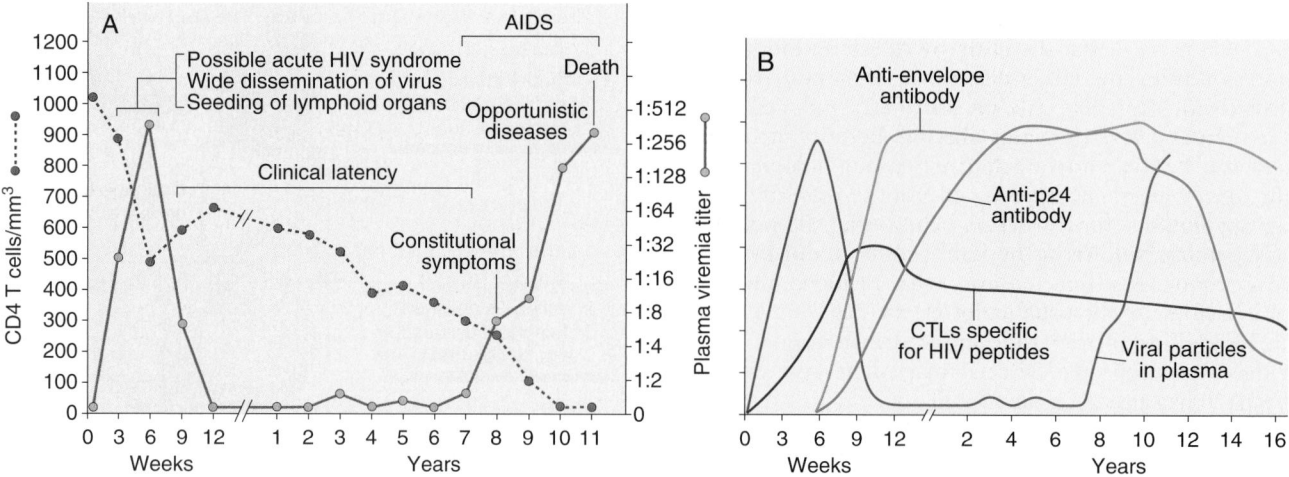

FIGURE 6–48 Clinical course of HIV infection. **A,** During the early period after primary infection there is dissemination of virus, development of an immune response to HIV, and often an acute viral syndrome. During the period of clinical latency, viral replication continues and the CD4+ T-cell count gradually decreases, until it reaches a critical level below which there is a substantial risk of AIDS-associated diseases. (Redrawn from Fauci AS, Lane HC: Human immunodeficiency virus disease: AIDS and related conditions. In Fauci AS, et al (eds): Harrison's Principles of Internal Medicine, 14th ed. New York, McGraw-Hill, 1997, p 1791.) **B,** Immune response to HIV infection. A cytotoxic T lymphocyte (CTL) response to HIV is detectable by 2 to 3 weeks after the initial infection, and it peaks by 9 to 12 weeks. Marked expansion of virus-specific CD8+ T-cell clones occurs during this time, and up to 10% of a patient's CTLs may be HIV specific at 12 weeks. The humoral immune response to HIV peaks at about 12 weeks.

a primary infection develop the viral syndrome. This typically occurs 3 to 6 weeks after infection, and resolves spontaneously in 2 to 4 weeks. Clinically, this phase is associated with a self-limited acute illness with nonspecific symptoms, including sore throat, myalgias, fever, weight loss, and fatigue, resembling a flulike syndrome. Other clinical features, such as rash, cervical adenopathy, diarrhea, and vomiting, may also occur.

The viral load at the end of the acute phase reflects the equilibrium reached between the virus and the host response, and in a given patient it may remain fairly stable for several years. This level of steady-state viremia, or the viral "set point," is a predictor of the rate of decline of CD4+ T cells, and, therefore, progression of HIV disease. In one study, only 8% of patients with a viral load of less than 4350 copies of viral mRNA per microliter of blood progressed to clinical AIDS in 5 years, whereas 62% of those with a viral load of greater than 36,270 copies had developed AIDS in the same period.[151] From a practical standpoint, therefore, *the extent of viremia, measured as HIV-1 RNA levels, is a useful surrogate marker of HIV disease progression and is of clinical value in the management of people with HIV infection.*

Because the loss of immune containment is associated with declining CD4+ T-cell counts, the Centers for Disease Control (CDC) classification of HIV infection stratifies patients into three categories on the basis of CD4+ cell counts: CD4+ cells greater than or equal to 500 cells/μL, 200 to 499 cells/μL, and fewer than 200 cells/μL (Table 6–13). For clinical management, blood CD4+ T-cell counts are perhaps the most reliable short-term indicator of disease progression. For this reason, CD4+ cell counts and not viral load are the primary clinical measurements used to determine when to start combination antiretroviral therapy.

Chronic Infection: Phase of Clinical Latency. *In the next, chronic phase of the disease, lymph nodes and the spleen are sites of continuous HIV replication and cell destruction* (see Fig. 6–47). During this period of the disease, few or no clinical manifestations of the HIV infection are present. Therefore, this phase of HIV disease is called the clinical latency period. Although the majority of peripheral blood T cells do not harbor the virus, destruction of CD4+ T cells within lymphoid tissues continues during this phase, and the number of circulating blood CD4+ T cells steadily declines. More than 90% of

Clinical Categories	CD4+ T-Cell Categories		
	1 ≥500 cells/μL	**2** 200–499 cells/μL	**3** <200 cells/μL
A. Asymptomatic, acute (primary) HIV, or persistent generalized lymphadenopathy	A1	A2	A3
B. Symptomatic, not A or C conditions	B1	B2	B3
C. AIDS indicator conditions: including constitutional disease, neurologic disease, or neoplasm			

TABLE 6–13 CDC Classification Categories of HIV Infection

Data from CDC. Centers for Disease Control and Prevention: 1993 revised classification system and expanded surveillance definition for AIDS among adolescents and adults. MMWR 41(RR-17):1, 1992.

the body's approximately 10^{12} T cells are normally found in lymphoid tissues, and it is estimated that HIV destroys up to 1×10^9 to 2×10^9 CD4+ T cells every day. Early in the course of the disease, the body may continue to make new CD4+ T cells, and therefore CD4+ T cells can be replaced almost as quickly as they are destroyed. At this stage, up to 10% of CD4+ T cells in lymphoid organs may be infected, but the frequency of circulating CD4+ T cells that are infected at any one time may be less than 0.1% of the total CD4+ T cells. Eventually, over a period of years, the continuous cycle of virus infection, T-cell death, and new infection leads to a steady decline in the number of CD4+ T cells in the lymphoid tissues and the circulation.

Concomitant with this loss of CD4+ T cells, host defenses begin to wane, and the proportion of the surviving CD4+ cells infected with HIV increases, as does the viral burden per CD4+ cell. Not unexpectedly, HIV RNA levels may begin to increase as the host begins to lose the battle with the virus. How HIV escapes immune control is not entirely clear, but several mechanisms have been proposed.[152,153] These include destruction of the CD4+ T cells that are critical for effective immunity, antigenic variation, and down-modulation of class I MHC molecules on infected cells so that viral antigens are not recognized by CD8+ CTLs. During this period the virus may evolve and switch from relying solely on CCR5 to enter its target cells to relying on either CXCR4 or both CCR5 and CXCR4. This coreceptor switch is associated with more rapid decline in CD4+ T-cell counts, presumably because of greater infection of T cells.

In this chronic phase of infection, patients are either asymptomatic or develop minor opportunistic infections, such as oral candidiasis (thrush), vaginal candidiasis, herpes zoster, and perhaps mycobacterial tuberculosis (the latter being particularly common in resource-poor regions such as sub-Saharan Africa). Autoimmune thrombocytopenia may also be noted (Chapter 14).

AIDS. The final phase is *progression to AIDS,* characterized by a breakdown of host defense, a dramatic increase in plasma virus, and severe, life-threatening clinical disease. Typically the patient presents with long-lasting fever (>1 month), fatigue, weight loss, and diarrhea. After a variable period, serious opportunistic infections, secondary neoplasms, or clinical neurologic disease (grouped under the rubric *AIDS indicator diseases,* discussed below) emerge, and the patient is said to have developed AIDS.

In the absence of treatment, most but not all patients with HIV infection progress to AIDS after a chronic phase lasting from 7 to 10 years. Exceptions to this typical course are exemplified by rapid progressors and long-term nonprogressors. In *rapid progressors* the middle, chronic phase is telescoped to 2 to 3 years after primary infection. About 5% to 15% of infected individuals are *long-term nonprogressors,* defined as untreated HIV-1–infected individuals who remain asymptomatic for 10 years or more, with stable CD4+ T-cell counts and low levels of plasma viremia (usually less than 500 viral RNA copies per milliliter).[154] Remarkably, about 1% of infected individuals have undetectable plasma virus (50–75 RNA copies/mL); these have been called *elite controllers.* Individuals with such an uncommon clinical course have attracted great attention in the hope that studying them may shed light on host and viral factors that influence disease progression. Studies thus far

indicate that this group is heterogeneous with respect to the variables that influence the course of the disease. In most cases, the viral isolates do not show qualitative abnormalities, suggesting that the course of the disease cannot be attributed to a "wimpy" virus. In all cases there is evidence of a vigorous anti-HIV immune response, but the immune correlates of protection are still unknown. Some of these individuals have high levels of HIV-specific CD4+ and CD8+ T-cell responses, and these levels are maintained over the course of infection. Further studies, it is hoped, will provide the answers to this and other questions critical to understanding disease progression.

Clinical Features of AIDS

The clinical manifestations of HIV infection can be readily surmised from the foregoing discussion. They range from a mild acute illness to severe disease. Because the salient clinical features of the acute early and chronic middle phases of HIV infection were described earlier, here we summarize the clinical manifestations of the terminal phase, AIDS. At the outset it should be pointed out that the clinical manifestations and opportunistic infections associated with HIV infection may differ in different parts of the world. Also, the course of the disease has been greatly modified by new antiretroviral therapies, and many complications that were once devastating are now infrequent.

In the United States, the typical adult patient with AIDS presents with fever, weight loss, diarrhea, generalized lymphadenopathy, multiple opportunistic infections, neurologic disease, and, in many cases, secondary neoplasms. The infections and neoplasms listed in Table 6–14 are included in the surveillance definition of AIDS.

TABLE 6–14 AIDS-Defining Opportunistic Infections and Neoplasms Found in Patients with HIV Infection
PROTOZOAL AND HELMINTHIC INFECTIONS
Cryptosporidiosis or isosporidiosis (enteritis)
Toxoplasmosis (pneumonia or CNS infection)
FUNGAL INFECTIONS
Pneumocystosis (pneumonia or disseminated infection)
Candidiasis (esophageal, tracheal, or pulmonary)
Cryptococcosis (CNS infection)
Coccidioidomycosis (disseminated)
Histoplasmosis (disseminated)
BACTERIAL INFECTIONS
Mycobacteriosis ("atypical," e.g., *Mycobacterium avium-intracellulare*, disseminated or extrapulmonary; *M. tuberculosis*, pulmonary or extrapulmonary)
Nocardiosis (pneumonia, meningitis, disseminated)
Salmonella infections, disseminated
VIRAL INFECTIONS
Cytomegalovirus (pulmonary, intestinal, retinitis, or CNS infections)
Herpes simplex virus (localized or disseminated)
Varicella-zoster virus (localized or disseminated)
Progressive multifocal leukoencephalopathy

CNS, central nervous system.

Opportunistic Infections

Opportunistic infections account for the majority of deaths in untreated patients with AIDS. Many of these infections represent reactivation of latent infections, which are normally kept in check by a robust immune system but are not completely eradicated because the infectious agents have evolved to coexist with their hosts. The actual frequency of infections varies in different regions of the world, and has been markedly reduced by the advent of highly active antiretroviral therapy (HAART).[155] A brief summary of selected opportunistic infections is provided here.

Approximately 15% to 30% of untreated HIV-infected people develop pneumonia at some time during the course of the disease, caused by the fungus *Pneumocystis jiroveci* (reactivation of a prior latent infection). Before the advent of HAART, this infection was the presenting feature in about 20% of cases, but the incidence is much less in patients who respond to HAART.

Many patients present with an opportunistic infection other than *P. jiroveci* pneumonia. Among the most common pathogens are *Candida*, cytomegalovirus, atypical and typical mycobacteria, *Cryptococcus neoformans, Toxoplasma gondii, Cryptosporidium,* herpes simplex virus, papovaviruses, and *Histoplasma capsulatum.*

Candidiasis is the most common fungal infection in patients with AIDS, and infection of the oral cavity, vagina, and esophagus are its most common clinical manifestations. In asymptomatic HIV-infected individuals oral candidiasis is a sign of immunological decompensation, and it often heralds the transition to AIDS. Invasive candidiasis is infrequent in patients with AIDS, and it usually occurs when there is drug-induced neutropenia or use of indwelling catheters.

Cytomegalovirus may cause disseminated disease, although, more commonly, it affects the eye and gastrointestinal tract. Chorioretinitis was seen in approximately 25% of patients before the advent of HAART, but this has decreased dramatically after the initiation of HAART. Cytomegalovirus retinitis occurs almost exclusively in patients with CD4+ T cell counts below 50 per microliter. Gastrointestinal disease, seen in 5% to 10% of cases, manifests as esophagitis and colitis, the latter associated with multiple mucosal ulcerations.

Disseminated bacterial infection with *atypical mycobacteria* (mainly *M. avium-intracellulare*) also occurs late, in the setting of severe immunosuppression. Coincident with the AIDS epidemic, the incidence of tuberculosis has risen dramatically. Worldwide, almost a third of all deaths in AIDS patients are attributable to tuberculosis, but this complication remains uncommon in the United States. Patients with AIDS have reactivation of latent pulmonary disease as well as outbreaks of primary infection. In contrast to infection with atypical mycobacteria, *M. tuberculosis* manifests itself early in the course of AIDS. As with tuberculosis in other settings, the infection may be confined to lungs or may involve multiple organs. The pattern of expression depends on the degree of immunosuppression; dissemination is more common in patients with very low CD4+ T-cell counts. Most worrisome are reports indicating that a growing number of isolates are resistant to multiple anti-mycobacterial drugs.

Cryptococcosis occurs in about 10% of AIDS patients. As in other settings with immunosuppression, meningitis is the major clinical manifestation of cryptococcosis. *Toxoplasma gondii,* another frequent invader of the central nervous system in AIDS, causes encephalitis and is responsible for 50% of all mass lesions in the central nervous system.

JC virus, a human papovavirus, is another important cause of central nervous system infections in HIV-infected patients. It causes progressive multifocal leukoencephalopathy (Chapter 28). *Herpes simplex virus infection* is manifested by mucocutaneous ulcerations involving the mouth, esophagus, external genitalia, and perianal region. *Persistent diarrhea,* which is common in untreated patients with advanced AIDS, is often caused by infections with protozoans such as *Cryptosporidium, Isospora belli,* or microsporidia. These patients have chronic, profuse, watery diarrhea with massive fluid loss. Diarrhea may also result from infection with enteric bacteria, such as *Salmonella* and *Shigella,* as well as *M. avium-intracellulare.*

Tumors

Patients with AIDS have a high incidence of certain tumors, especially *Kaposi sarcoma (KS),* non-Hodgkin B-cell lymphoma, cervical cancer in women, and anal cancer in men.[156] It is estimated that 25% to 40% of untreated HIV-infected individuals will eventually develop a malignancy. A common feature of these tumors is that they are all believed to be caused by oncogenic DNA viruses, that is, kaposi sarcoma herpesvirus (Kaposi sarcoma), EBV (B-cell lymphoma), and human papillomavirus (cervical and anal carcinoma). Even in healthy people, any of these viruses may establish latent infections that are kept in check by a competent immune system. The increased risk of malignancy in AIDS patients exists mainly because of failure to contain the infections and reactivation of the viruses, as well as decreased immunity against the tumors.

Kaposi Sarcoma. Kaposi sarcoma, a vascular tumor that is otherwise rare in the United States, is the most common neoplasm in patients with AIDS. The morphology of KS and its occurrence in patients not infected with HIV are discussed in Chapter 11. At the onset of the AIDS epidemic, up to 30% of infected homosexual or bisexual men had KS, but in recent years, with use of HAART there has been a marked decline in its incidence, from 15 cases per 1000 person years to less than 5 cases.[157]

The lesions of KS are characterized by the proliferation of spindle-shaped cells that express markers of both endothelial cells (vascular or lymphatic) and smooth muscle cells (Chapter 11). There is also a profusion of slitlike vascular spaces, suggesting that the lesions may arise from primitive mesenchymal precursors of vascular channels. In addition, KS lesions display chronic inflammatory cell infiltrates. Many of the features of KS suggest that it is not a malignant tumor (despite its ominous name).[158] For instance, spindle cells in many KS lesions are polyclonal or oligoclonal, although more advanced lesions occasionally show monoclonality. The spindle cells in many KS lesions are diploid and are dependent on growth factors for their proliferation. When these cells are implanted subcutaneously in immunodeficient mice they do not form tumors but transiently induce slitlike new blood vessels and inflammatory infiltrates in the surrounding tissue. These elements recall features of human KS but surprisingly are of murine origin, and when the human KS cells involute, these elements also regress. Based on these observations, the current model of KS pathogenesis is that the spindle cells produce

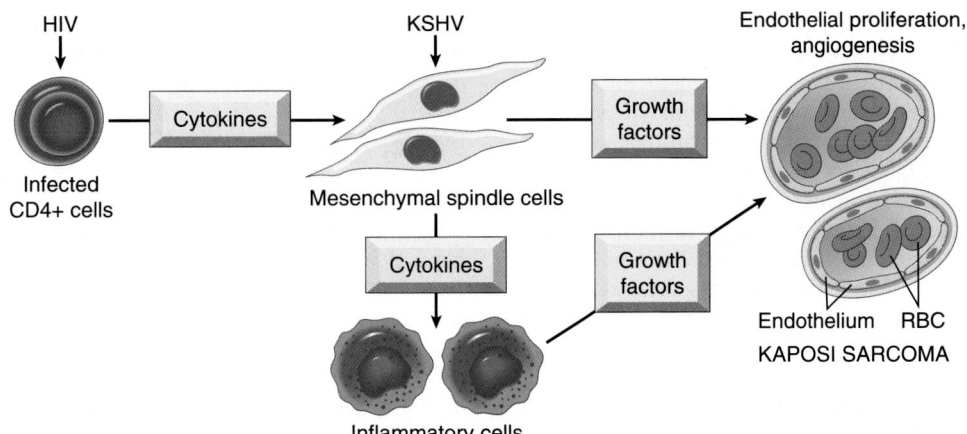

FIGURE 6–49 Postulated pathogenesis of Kaposi sarcoma (KS). Proposed roles of HIV, KS herpesvirus (KSHV; HHV8), and cytokines in the development of KS. Cytokines are produced by the mesenchymal cells infected by KSHV, or by HIV-infected CD4+ cells. B cells may also be infected by KSHV; they are the probable cells in body cavity lymphomas, also associated with KSHV infection, but their role in KS is unclear.

pro-inflammatory and angiogenic factors, which recruit the inflammatory and neovascular components of the lesion, and the latter components supply signals that aid in spindle cell survival or growth (Fig. 6–49).

But what initiates this cycle of events? There is compelling evidence that HIV itself is not the culprit, and that KS is caused by the *KS herpesvirus* (KSHV), also called *human herpesvirus 8* (HHV8).[159] Epidemiologic and molecular studies have established the link between KSHV and KS development. KSHV DNA is found in virtually all KS lesions, including those that occur in HIV-negative populations, and in the lesions, KSHV is strikingly localized to the spindle cells, which display predominantly latent infection. However, KSHV infection, while necessary for KS development, is not sufficient, and additional cofactors are needed. In the AIDS-related form, that cofactor is clearly HIV. (The relevant cofactors for HIV-negative KS remain unknown.) Debate continues over exactly how HIV contributes to KS development. The simplest model is that HIV-mediated immune suppression allows widespread dissemination of KSHV in the host, allowing it to access more spindle cells and set them on the path to uncontrolled growth. Another idea is that HIV-infected T cells produce cytokines or other proteins that promote spindle cell proliferation and survival. Clearly, these possibilities are not mutually exclusive.

Exactly how KSHV infection leads to KS is also still unclear.[158] Like other herpesviruses, KSHV establishes latent infection, during which several proteins are produced with potential roles in stimulating spindle cell proliferation and preventing apoptosis. These include a viral homologue of cyclin D and several inhibitors of p53. Such proteins could give latently infected cells a survival and growth advantage in vivo that would allow them to begin proliferating. But in addition to latent infection, a small subpopulation of cells in KS is undergoing lytic viral replication, with cell death and the release of viral progeny. The KSHV lytic cycle is remarkable for its production of numerous paracrine signaling molecules, including a viral homologue of the cytokine IL-6 and several chemokines. The latter probably play prominent roles in eliciting the inflammatory infiltrates that are an important feature of KS. The contribution of viral IL-6 is not yet clear. Another viral protein produced during lytic infection is a constitutively active G protein–coupled receptor. This protein has attracted attention because its expression activates the release of vascular endothelial growth factor (VEGF), which can promote angiogenesis in the surrounding tissue. Interestingly, expression of the viral G protein–coupled receptor in transgenic mice leads to the development of neovascular spaces vaguely reminiscent of those in KS. Thus, there is ample reason to believe that both latent and lytic KSHV infection contributes to KS pathogenesis.

KSHV infection is not restricted to endothelial cells. The virus is related phylogenetically to the lymphotropic subfamily of herpesviruses (γ-herpesvirus); in keeping with this, its genome is found in B cells of infected subjects. In fact, KSHV infection is also linked to rare B-cell lymphomas in AIDS patients (called *body cavity-based primary effusion lymphoma*) and to multicentric Castleman disease, a B-cell lymphoproliferative disorder.

Clinically, AIDS-associated KS is quite different from the sporadic form (Chapter 11). In HIV-infected individuals the tumor is usually widespread, affecting the skin, mucous membranes, gastrointestinal tract, lymph nodes, and lungs. These tumors also tend to be more aggressive than classic KS.

Lymphomas. AIDS-related lymphomas can be divided into three groups on the basis of their location: systemic, primary central nervous system, and body cavity–based lymphomas.[160] Systemic lymphomas involve lymph nodes as well as extranodal, visceral sites; they constitute 80% of all AIDS-related lymphomas. The central nervous system is the most common extranodal site affected, followed by the gastrointestinal tract and, less commonly, virtually any other location, including the orbit, salivary glands, and lungs. The vast majority of these lymphomas are aggressive B-cell tumors that present in an advanced stage (Chapter 13). In addition to being commonly involved by systemic non-Hodgkin lymphomas, the central nervous system is also the primary site of lymphomatous involvement in 20% of HIV-infected patients who develop lymphomas. Primary central nervous system lymphoma is 1000 times more common in patients with AIDS than in the general population. Body cavity lymphomas are rare, but they attract attention because of their unusual presentation as pleural, peritoneal, or pericardial effusions.

The pathogenesis of AIDS-associated B-cell lymphomas probably involves sustained polyclonal B-cell activation, followed by the emergence of monoclonal or oligoclonal B-cell populations. It is believed that during the frenzy of proliferation, some clones undergo mutations or chromosomal translocations involving oncogenes or tumor suppressor genes, and subsequent neoplastic transformation (Chapter 7). There is morphologic evidence of B-cell activation in lymph nodes, and it is believed that such triggering of B cells is multifactorial. Patients with AIDS have high levels of several cytokines, some of which, including IL-6, are growth factors for B cells. In addition, there seems to be a role for EBV, known to be a polyclonal mitogen for B cells. Half of the systemic B-cell lymphomas and virtually all lymphomas primary in the central nervous system are latently infected with EBV. Other evidence of EBV infection includes oral hairy leukoplakia (white projections on the tongue), resulting from EBV-driven squamous cell proliferation of the oral mucosa (Chapter 16). In cases in which molecular footprints of EBV infection cannot be detected, other viruses and microbes may initiate polyclonal B-cell proliferation. There is no evidence that HIV by itself is capable of causing neoplastic transformation. The rare body cavity–based primary effusion lymphomas are uniformly latently infected with KSHV, discussed earlier.

With prolonged survival, the number of AIDS patients who develop non-Hodgkin lymphoma has increased steadily. It is currently believed that approximately 6% of all patients with AIDS develop lymphoma during their lifetime. Thus, the risk of developing non-Hodgkin lymphoma is approximately 120-fold greater than in the general population. In contrast to KS, immunodeficiency is firmly implicated as the central predisposing factor. It seems that patients with CD4+ T-cell counts below 50 per microliter incur an extremely high risk.

Other Tumors. In addition to KS and lymphomas, patients with AIDS also have an increased occurrence of carcinoma of the uterine cervix and of anal cancer. This is most likely due to reactivation of latent human papillomavirus (HPV) infection as a result of immunosuppression.[161] This virus is believed to be intimately associated with squamous cell carcinoma of the cervix and its precursor lesions, cervical dysplasia and carcinoma in situ (Chapters 7 and 22). HPV-associated cervical dysplasia is 10 times more common in HIV-infected women as compared with uninfected women attending family planning clinics. Hence it is recommended that gynecologic examination be part of a routine work-up of HIV-infected women.

Central Nervous System Disease

Involvement of the central nervous system is a common and important manifestation of AIDS. Ninety percent of patients demonstrate some form of neurologic involvement at autopsy, and 40% to 60% have clinically manifest neurologic dysfunction. Importantly, in some patients, neurologic manifestations may be the sole or earliest presenting feature of HIV infection. In addition to opportunistic infections and neoplasms, several virally determined neuropathologic changes occur. These include a self-limited meningoencephalitis occurring at the time of seroconversion, aseptic meningitis, vacuolar myelopathy, peripheral neuropathies, and, most commonly, a progressive encephalopathy designated clinically as the AIDS-dementia complex (Chapter 28).

Effect of Antiretroviral Drug Therapy on the Clinical Course of HIV Infection

The advent of new antiretroviral drugs that target the viral reverse transcriptase, protease, and integrase has changed the clinical face of AIDS. These drugs are given in combination to reduce the emergence of mutants that develop resistance to any one; treatment regimens are commonly called *highly active antiretroviral therapy (HAART)* or *combination antiretroviral therapy*. Over 25 antiretroviral drugs from six distinct drug classes have been developed for the management of HIV infection. When a combination of at least three effective drugs is used in a motivated, adherent patient, HIV replication is invariably reduced to below the level of quantification (<50 copies RNA per milliliter) and remains there indefinitely (as long as the patient adheres to therapy). Even when a drug-resistant virus breaks through, there are several second- and third-line options to again suppress the virus. Once the virus is suppressed, the progressive loss of CD4+ T cells is halted. Over a period of several years the peripheral CD4+ T-cell count slowly increases and often returns to a normal level (although for unclear reasons, a significant proportion of patients with suppressed viremia fail to fully reconstitute a normal CD4+ T-cell count). With the use of these drugs, in the United States the annual death rate from AIDS has decreased from its peak of 16 to 18 per 100,000 people in 1995–1996 to about 4 per 100,000 in 2005. Many AIDS-associated disorders, such as opportunistic infections with *P. jiroveci* and KS, are very uncommon now. Because of the greatly reduced mortality, an increased number of people are living with HIV, but since they are not virus-free, there is increased risk of spreading the infection.

Despite these dramatic improvements, several complications associated with HIV infection and its treatment have emerged. Some patients with advanced disease who are given antiretroviral therapy develop a paradoxical clinical deterioration during the period of recovery of the immune system. This occurs despite increasing CD4+ T-cell counts and decreasing viral load. This disorder has been called the *immune reconstitution inflammatory syndrome*.[162] Its basis is not understood but is postulated to be a poorly regulated host response to the high antigenic burden of persistent microbes. Perhaps a more important complication of long-term HAART pertains to an evolving series of long-term toxicities. These include but are not limited to lipoatrophy (loss of facial fat), lipoaccumulation (excess fat deposition centrally), elevated lipids, insulin resistance, peripheral neuropathy, premature cardiovascular disease, kidney disease, and hepatic dysfunction. The mechanisms underlying these toxicities remain undefined. Finally, it is now well recognized that non-AIDS morbidity is far more common than classic AIDS-related morbidity in long-term HAART-treated patients. Major causes of morbidity are cancer (including those not believed to be HIV related), accelerated cardiovascular disease, kidney disease, and liver disease. Many of these complications are occurring at a younger age in HIV-infected persons than in persons not infected with HIV. The mechanism for these non-AIDS related complications is not known, but persistent inflammation and/or T-cell dysfunction may be playing a role.

Morphology. The anatomic changes in the tissues (with the exception of lesions in the brain) are neither specific nor diagnostic. In general, the pathologic features of AIDS include those of widespread opportunistic infections, KS, and lymphoid tumors. Most of these lesions are discussed elsewhere, because they also occur in individuals who do not have HIV infection. Lesions in the central nervous system are described in Chapter 28.

Biopsy specimens from enlarged lymph nodes in the early stages of HIV infection reveal a **marked follicular hyperplasia**. The mantle zones that surround the follicles are attenuated, and hence the germinal centers seem to merge with the interfollicular area. These changes, affecting primarily the B-cell areas of the node, are the morphologic reflections of the polyclonal B-cell activation and hypergammaglobulinemia seen in patients with AIDS. Under the electron microscope and by in situ hybridization, HIV particles can be detected within the germinal centers. Here they seem to be concentrated on the processes of follicular dendritic cells, presumably trapped in the form of immune complexes. During the early phase of HIV infection, viral DNA can be found within the nuclei of CD4+ T cells located predominantly in the parafollicular regions. The B cell hyperplasia is also reflected in the bone marrow, which typically contains increased numbers of plasma cells, and in peripheral blood smears, which often demonstrate rouleaux, the abnormal stacking of red cells that results from hypergammaglobulinemia.

With disease progression, the frenzy of B-cell proliferation subsides and gives way to a pattern of severe follicular involution. The follicles are depleted of cells, and the **organized network of follicular dendritic cells is disrupted**. The germinal centers may even become hyalinized. During this advanced stage viral burden in the nodes is reduced, in part because of the disruption of the follicular dendritic cells. These "burnt-out" lymph nodes are atrophic and small and may harbor numerous opportunistic pathogens. Because of profound immunosuppression, the inflammatory response to infections both in the lymph nodes and at extranodal sites may be sparse or atypical. For example, mycobacteria may not evoke granuloma formation because CD4+ cells are deficient. In the empty-looking lymph nodes and in other organs, the presence of infectious agents may not be readily apparent without special stains. As might be expected, lymphoid depletion is not confined to the nodes; in later stages of AIDS, the spleen and thymus also appear to be "wastelands."

Despite spectacular advances in our understanding of HIV infection, the prognosis of patients with AIDS remains dismal. Although with effective drug therapy the mortality rate has declined in the United States, the treated patients still carry viral DNA in their lymphoid tissues. In fact, there is compelling evidence that even treated patients who remain asymptomatic, with virtually undetectable plasma virus, for years, develop active infection if they stop the treatment. Can there be a cure with persistent virus? Although a considerable effort has been mounted to develop a vaccine, many hurdles remain to be crossed before vaccine-based prophylaxis becomes a reality.[163,164] Molecular analyses have revealed an alarming degree of polymorphism in viral isolates from different patients; this renders the task of producing a vaccine extremely difficult. This task is further complicated by the fact that the correlates of immune protection are not yet fully understood. At present, therefore, prevention, effective public health measures, and antiretroviral drugs remain the mainstays in the fight against AIDS.

Amyloidosis

Immunological mechanisms are suspected of contributing to a large number of diseases in addition to those already described in this chapter. Some of the entities are discussed in the chapters dealing with individual organs and systems. Amyloidosis is described here because it is a systemic disease that may involve components of the immune system, although the pathogenesis of the disease is probably related to abnormal protein folding and immunological abnormalities are associated with only some forms of amyloidosis.

Amyloid is a pathologic proteinaceous substance, deposited in the extracellular space in various tissues and organs of the body in a wide variety of clinical settings. Because amyloid deposition appears insidiously and sometimes mysteriously, its clinical recognition ultimately depends on morphologic identification of this distinctive substance in appropriate biopsy specimens. With the light microscope and hematoxylin and eosin stains, amyloid appears as an amorphous, eosinophilic, hyaline, extracellular substance that, with progressive accumulation, encroaches on and produces pressure atrophy of adjacent cells. To differentiate amyloid from other hyaline deposits (e.g., collagen, fibrin), a variety of histochemical techniques, described later, are used. Perhaps most widely used is the Congo red stain, which under ordinary light imparts a pink or red color to tissue deposits, but far more striking and specific is the green birefringence of the stained amyloid when observed by polarizing microscopy (Fig. 6–50).

Even though all deposits have a uniform appearance and staining characteristics, *amyloid is not a chemically distinct entity.*[165] There are three major and several minor biochemical forms. These are deposited by several different pathogenetic mechanisms, and therefore amyloidosis *should not be considered a single disease; rather it is a group of diseases having in common the deposition of similar-appearing proteins.* At the heart of the morphologic similarity is the remarkably uniform physical organization of amyloid protein, which we consider first.

Properties of Amyloid Proteins

Physical Nature of Amyloid

By electron microscopy amyloid is seen to be made up largely of continuous, nonbranching fibrils with a diameter of approximately 7.5 to 10 nm. This electron-microscopic

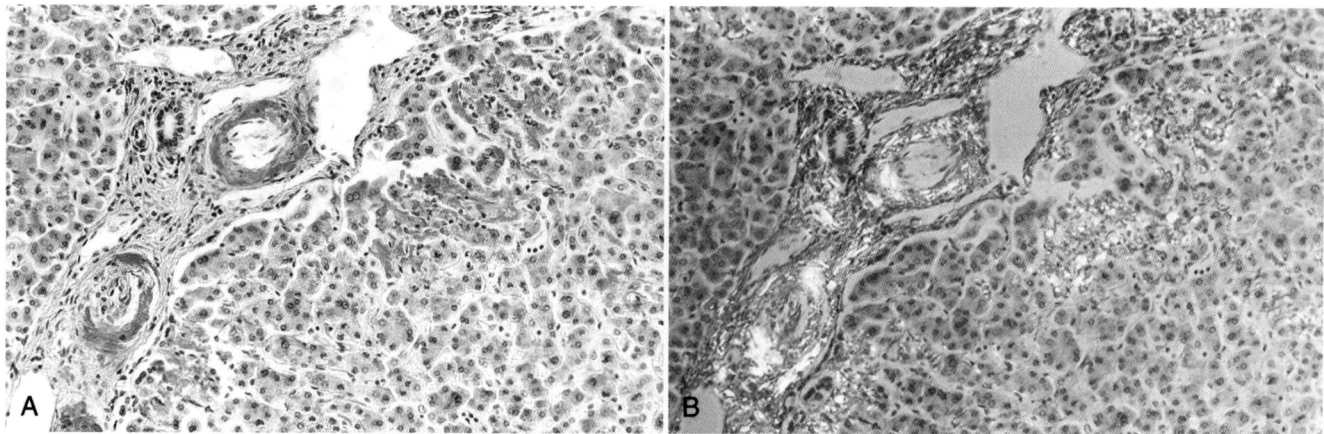

FIGURE 6–50   Amyloidosis. **A,** A section of the liver stained with Congo red reveals pink-red deposits of amyloid in the walls of blood vessels and along sinusoids. **B,** Note the yellow-green birefringence of the deposits when observed by polarizing microscope. (Courtesy of Dr. Trace Worrell and Sandy Hinton, Department of Pathology, University of Texas Southwestern Medical School, Dallas TX.)

structure is identical in all types of amyloidosis. X-ray crystallography and infrared spectroscopy demonstrate a characteristic cross-β-pleated sheet conformation (Fig. 6–51). This conformation is seen regardless of the clinical setting or chemical composition and is responsible for the distinctive Congo red staining and birefringence of amyloid.

Chemical Nature of Amyloid

Approximately 95% of the amyloid material consists of fibril proteins, the remaining 5% being the P component and other glycoproteins. *Of the more than 20 biochemically distinct forms of amyloid proteins that have been identified, three are most common:* (1) *AL (amyloid light chain)* is derived from Ig light chains produced in plasma cells; (2) *AA (amyloid-associated)* is derived from a unique non-Ig protein synthesized by the liver; and (3) *Aβ amyloid* is produced from β amyloid precursor protein and is found in the cerebral lesions of Alzheimer disease.

○ The AL protein is made up of complete immunoglobulin light chains, the amino-terminal fragments of light chains, or both. Most of the AL proteins analyzed are composed of λ light chains or their fragments, but in some cases κ chains have been identified. The amyloid fibril protein of the AL type is produced from free Ig light chains secreted by a monoclonal population of plasma cells, and its deposition is associated with certain forms of plasma cell tumors (Chapter 13).

○ The second major class of amyloid fibril protein (AA) does not have structural homology to immunoglobulins. It has a molecular weight of 8500 and consists of 76 amino acid residues. AA fibrils are derived by proteolysis from a larger (12,000 daltons) precursor in the serum called SAA (serum amyloid–associated) protein that is synthesized in the liver and circulates in association with high density lipoproteins. The production of SAA protein is increased in inflammatory states as part of the "acute phase response"; therefore, this form of amyloidosis is associated with chronic inflammation, and is often called *secondary amyloidosis.*

○ β-*amyloid protein* (Aβ) is a 4000-dalton peptide that constitutes the core of cerebral plaques found in Alzheimer disease as well as the amyloid deposited in walls of cerebral blood vessels in individuals with this disease. The Aβ protein is derived by proteolysis from a much larger trans-

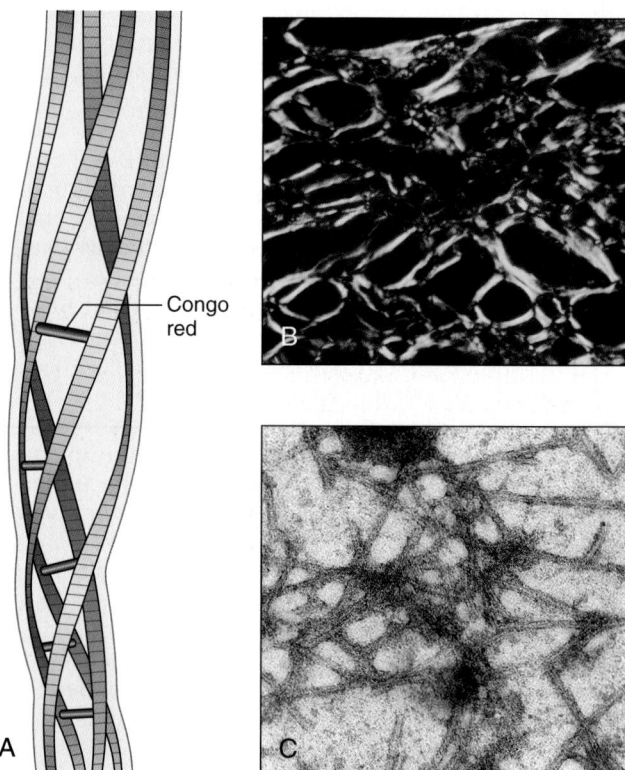

FIGURE 6–51   Structure of amyloid. **A,** An amyloid fiber schematically showing four fibrils (there can be as many as six in each fiber) wound around one another with regularly spaced binding of the Congo red dye. **B,** Congo red staining shows apple-green birefringence under polarized light, a diagnostic feature of amyloid. **C,** Electron micrograph of 7.5- to 10-nm amyloid fibrils. (Reproduced from Merlini G and Bellotti V. Molecular mechanisms of amyloidosis. N Engl J Med 349:583–596, 2003, with permission of the Massachusetts Medical Society.)

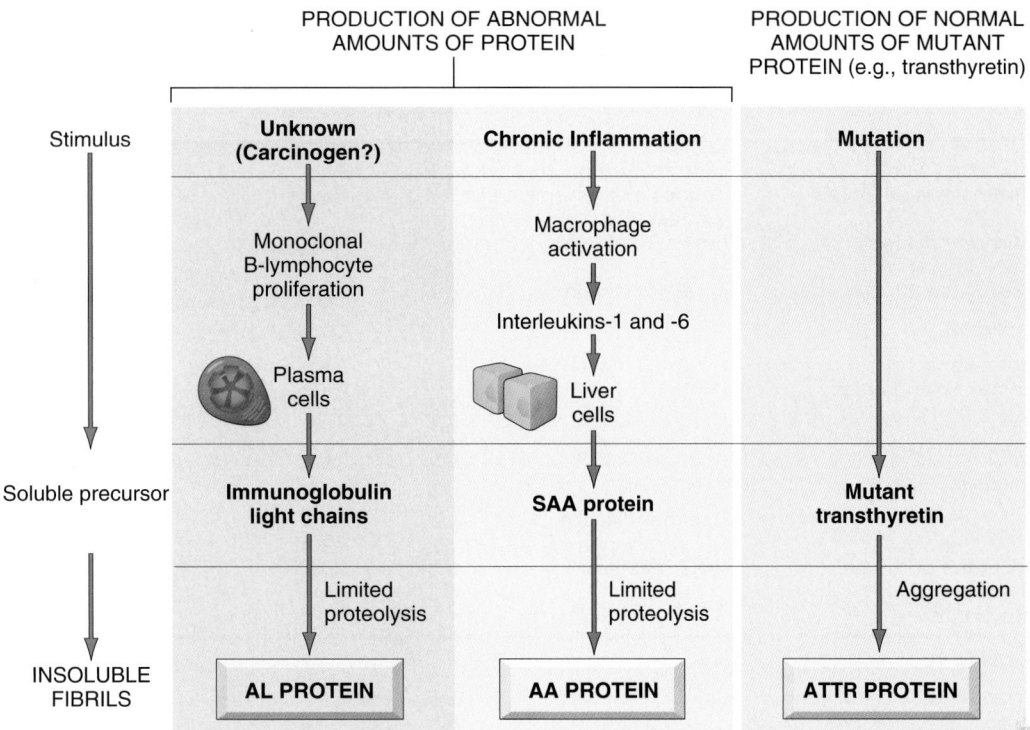

PRODUCTION OF ABNORMAL
AMOUNTS OF PROTEIN

PRODUCTION OF NORMAL
AMOUNTS OF MUTANT
PROTEIN (e.g., transthyretin)

Stimulus

**Unknown
(Carcinogen?)**

Chronic Inflammation

Mutation

Monoclonal
B-lymphocyte
proliferation

Macrophage
activation

Interleukins-1 and -6

Plasma
cells

Liver
cells

Soluble precursor

**Immunoglobulin
light chains**

SAA protein

**Mutant
transthyretin**

Limited
proteolysis

Limited
proteolysis

Aggregation

INSOLUBLE
FIBRILS

AL PROTEIN

AA PROTEIN

ATTR PROTEIN

FIGURE 6–52 Pathogenesis of amyloidosis, showing the proposed mechanisms underlying deposition of the major forms of amyloid fibrils. See text for abbreviations.

membrane glycoprotein, called *amyloid precursor protein.* This form of amyloid is discussed in Chapter 28.

Several other biochemically distinct proteins have been found in amyloid deposits in a variety of clinical settings. Some of the more common ones are the following:

- *Transthyretin (TTR)* is a normal serum protein that binds and transports thyroxine and retinol. A mutant form of TTR (and its fragments) is deposited in a group of genetically determined disorders referred to as familial amyloid polyneuropathies.[167] Several mutations have been identified in the TTR protein that contribute to its deposition in tissues in the form of amyloid. TTR is also deposited in the heart of aged individuals (senile systemic amyloidosis), but in such cases the amino acid sequence of the TTR molecule is normal.

- *β_2-microglobulin,* a component of MHC class I molecules and a normal serum protein, has been identified as the amyloid fibril subunit ($A\beta_2m$) in amyloidosis that complicates the course of patients on *long-term hemodialysis.*

- In a minority of cases of prion disease in the central nervous system, the misfolded *prion proteins* aggregate in the extracellular space and acquire the structural and staining characteristics of amyloid protein. Therefore, prion diseases are sometimes considered examples of local amyloidosis.

In addition, other minor components are always present in amyloid. These include serum amyloid P component, proteoglycans, and highly sulfated glycosaminoglycans. Serum amyloid P protein may contribute to amyloid deposition by stabilizing the fibrils and decreasing their clearance.

Pathogenesis of Amyloidosis

Amyloidosis results from abnormal folding of proteins, which are deposited as fibrils in extracellular tissues and disrupt normal function.[165,166] Misfolded proteins are often unstable and self-associate, ultimately leading to the formation of oligomers and fibrils that are deposited in tissues. The reason diverse conditions are associated with amyloidosis may be that each results in excessive production of proteins that are prone to misfolding (Fig. 6–52). The proteins that form amyloid fall into two general categories: (1) normal proteins that have an inherent tendency to fold improperly, associate and form fibrils, and do so when they are produced in increased amounts; and (2) mutant proteins that are prone to misfolding and subsequent aggregation.

Normally, misfolded proteins are degraded intracellularly in proteasomes, or extracellularly by macrophages. It seems that in amyloidosis these quality control mechanisms fail so that too much of a misfolded protein accumulates outside cells. This proposed mechanism may explain most forms of amyloidosis. For instance, SAA is synthesized by the liver cells under the influence of cytokines such as IL-6 and IL-1 that are produced during inflammation; thus, long-standing inflammation leads to elevated SAA levels. However, increased production of SAA by itself is not sufficient for the deposition of amyloid. There are two possible explanations for this. According to one view, SAA is normally degraded to soluble end products by the action of monocyte-derived enzymes. Conceivably, individuals who develop amyloidosis have an enzyme defect that results in incomplete breakdown of SAA, thus generating insoluble AA molecules. Alternatively, a genetically determined structural abnormality in the

TABLE 6–15 Classification of Amyloidosis

Clinicopathologic Category	Associated Diseases	Major Fibril Protein	Chemically Related Precursor Protein
SYSTEMIC (GENERALIZED) AMYLOIDOSIS			
Immunocyte dyscrasias with amyloidosis (primary amyloidosis)	Multiple myeloma and other monoclonal plasma cell proliferations	AL	Immunoglobulin light chains, chiefly λ type
Reactive systemic amyloidosis (secondary amyloidosis)	Chronic inflammatory conditions	AA	SAA
Hemodialysis-associated amyloidosis	Chronic renal failure	Aβ$_2$m	β$_2$-microglobulin
HEREDITARY AMYLOIDOSIS			
Familial Mediterranean fever		AA	SAA
Familial amyloidotic neuropathies (several types)		ATTR	Transthyretin
SYSTEMIC SENILE AMYLOIDOSIS		ATTR	Transthyretin
LOCALIZED AMYLOIDOSIS			
Senile cerebral	Alzheimer disease	A*b*	APP
Endocrine		A Cal	Calcitonin
Medullary carcinoma of thyroid	Type 2 diabetes	AIAPP	Islet amyloid peptide
Islets of Langerhans		AANF	Atrial natriuretic factor
Isolated atrial amyloidosis			

SAA molecule itself renders it resistant to degradation by macrophages.

In familial amyloidosis the deposition of TTRs as amyloid fibrils does not result from overproduction of TTRs. It has been proposed that genetically detemined alterations of structure render the TTRs prone to misfolding and aggregation, and resistant to proteolysis.

Classification of Amyloidosis

Because a given biochemical form of amyloid (e.g., AA) may be associated with amyloid deposition in diverse clinical settings, we follow a combined biochemical-clinical classification for our discussion (Table 6–15). Amyloid may be *systemic* (generalized), involving several organ systems, or it may be *localized*, when deposits are limited to a single organ, such as the heart.

On clinical grounds, the systemic, or generalized, pattern is subclassified into *primary amyloidosis*, when associated with some immunocyte disorder, or *secondary amyloidosis*, when it occurs as a complication of an underlying chronic inflammatory or tissue-destructive process.[167] *Hereditary* or *familial amyloidosis* constitutes a separate, albeit heterogeneous group, with several distinctive patterns of organ involvement.

Primary Amyloidosis: Immunocyte Dyscrasias with Amyloidosis

Amyloid in this category is usually systemic in distribution and is of the AL type. With approximately 1275 to 3200 new cases every year in the United States, this is the most common form of amyloidosis. In many of these cases, the patients have some form of plasma cell dyscrasia. Best defined is the occurrence of systemic amyloidosis in 5% to 15% of individuals with multiple myeloma, a plasma-cell tumor characterized by multiple osteolytic lesions throughout the skeletal system

(Chapter 13). The malignant B cells characteristically synthesize abnormal amounts of a single specific Ig (monoclonal gammopathy), producing an M (myeloma) protein spike on serum electrophoresis. In addition to the synthesis of whole Ig molecules, only the light chains (referred to as *Bence-Jones protein*) of either the κ or the λ variety may be elaborated and found in the serum. By virtue of the small molecular size of the Bence-Jones protein, it is frequently excreted in the urine. The amyloid deposits contain the same light chain protein. Almost all the individuals with myeloma who develop amyloidosis have Bence-Jones proteins in the serum or urine, or both, but the great majority of myeloma patients who have free light chains do not develop amyloidosis. Clearly, therefore, *the presence of Bence-Jones proteins, though necessary, is by itself not enough to produce amyloidosis.* Other factors, such as the type of light chain produced (*amyloidogenic potential*) and the susceptibility to degradation, may have a bearing on whether Bence-Jones proteins are deposited as amyloid.

The great majority of persons with AL amyloid do not have classic multiple myeloma or any other overt B-cell neoplasm; such cases have been traditionally classified as primary amyloidosis, because their clinical features derive from the effects of amyloid deposition without any other associated disease. In virtually all such cases, however, monoclonal immunoglobulins or free light chains, or both, can be found in the serum or urine. Most of these patients also have a modest increase in the number of plasma cells in the bone marrow, which presumably secrete the precursors of AL protein. Clearly, these patients have an underlying plasma cell dyscrasia in which production of an abnormal protein, rather than production of tumor masses, is the predominant manifestation.

Reactive Systemic Amyloidosis

The amyloid deposits in this pattern are systemic in distribution and are composed of AA protein. This category was previously referred to as *secondary amyloidosis* because it is secondary to an associated inflammatory condition. At one time, tuberculosis, bronchiectasis, and chronic osteomyelitis were the most important underlying conditions, but with the advent of effective antimicrobial chemotherapy the importance of these conditions has diminished. More commonly now, reactive systemic amyloidosis complicates rheumatoid arthritis, other connective tissue disorders such as ankylosing spondylitis, and inflammatory bowel disease, particularly Crohn disease and ulcerative colitis. Among these the most frequent associated condition is rheumatoid arthritis. Amyloidosis is reported to occur in approximately 3% of patients with rheumatoid arthritis and is clinically significant in one half of those affected. Heroin abusers who inject the drug subcutaneously also have a high occurrence rate of generalized AA amyloidosis. The chronic skin infections associated with "skin-popping" of narcotics seem to be responsible for the amyloidosis. Reactive systemic amyloidosis may also occur in association with non-immunocyte–derived tumors, the two most common being renal cell carcinoma and Hodgkin lymphoma.

Hemodialysis-Associated Amyloidosis

Patients on long-term hemodialysis for renal failure develop amyloidosis as a result of deposition of β_2-microglobulin. This protein is present in high concentrations in the serum of persons with renal disease and is retained in the circulation because it cannot be filtered through dialysis membranes. Patients often present with carpal tunnel syndrome because of β_2-microglobulin deposition. In some series, over half the patients on long-term dialysis (>20 years) developed amyloid deposits in the synovium, joints, or tendon sheaths.

Heredofamilial Amyloidosis

A variety of familial forms of amyloidosis have been described. Most of them are rare and occur in limited geographic areas. The most common and best studied is an autosomal recessive condition called *familial Mediterranean fever*.[168] This is an "autoinflammatory" syndrome associated with abnormally high production of the cytokine IL-1, and characterized clinically by attacks of fever accompanied by inflammation of serosal surfaces, including peritoneum, pleura, and synovial membrane. The gene for familial Mediterranean fever encodes a protein called *pyrin* (for its relation to fever), which is one of a complex of proteins that regulate inflammatory reactions via the production of pro-inflammatory cytokines (Chapter 2).[169,170] This disorder is encountered largely in individuals of Armenian, Sephardic Jewish, and Arabic origins. It is sometimes associated with widespread amyloidosis. The amyloid fibril proteins are made up of AA proteins, suggesting that this form of amyloidosis is related to the recurrent bouts of inflammation.

In contrast to familial Mediterranean fever, a group of autosomal dominant familial disorders is characterized by deposition of amyloid predominantly in peripheral and autonomic nerves. These familial amyloidotic polyneuropathies have been described in different parts of the world. As mentioned before, in all of these genetic disorders, the fibrils are made up of mutant TTRs.

Localized Amyloidosis

Sometimes, amyloid deposits are limited to a single organ or tissue without involvement of any other site in the body. The deposits may produce grossly detectable nodular masses or be evident only on microscopic examination. Nodular deposits of amyloid are most often encountered in the lung, larynx, skin, urinary bladder, tongue, and the region about the eye. Frequently, there are infiltrates of lymphocytes and plasma cells in the periphery of these amyloid masses. At least in some cases, the amyloid consists of AL protein and may therefore represent a localized form of immunocyte-derived amyloid.

Endocrine Amyloid

Microscopic deposits of localized amyloid may be found in certain endocrine tumors, such as medullary carcinoma of the thyroid gland, islet tumors of the pancreas, pheochromocytomas, and undifferentiated carcinomas of the stomach, and in the islets of Langerhans in individuals with type II diabetes mellitus. In these settings the amyloidogenic proteins seem to be derived either from polypeptide hormones (e.g., medullary carcinoma) or from unique proteins (e.g., islet amyloid polypeptide).

Amyloid of Aging

Several well-documented forms of amyloid deposition occur with aging. *Senile systemic amyloidosis* refers to the systemic deposition of amyloid in elderly patients (usually in their 70s and 80s). Because of the dominant involvement and related dysfunction of the heart, this form was previously called *senile cardiac amyloidosis*. Those who are symptomatic present with a restrictive cardiomyopathy and arrhythmias (Chapter 12). The amyloid in this form is composed of the normal TTR molecule. In addition to the sporadic senile systemic amyloidosis, another form, affecting predominantly the heart, that results from the deposition of a mutant form of TTR has also been recognized. Approximately 4% of the black population in the United States is a carrier of the mutant allele, and cardiomyopathy has been identified in both homozygous and heterozygous patients. The precise prevalence of patients with this muta-tion who develop clinically manifest cardiac disease is not known.

Morphology. There are no consistent or distinctive patterns of organ or tissue distribution of amyloid deposits in any of the categories cited. Kidneys, liver, spleen, lymph nodes, adrenals, and thyroid as well as many other tissues are classically involved. Macroscopically the affected organs are often enlarged and firm and have a waxy appearance. If the deposits are sufficiently large, painting the cut surface with iodine imparts a yellow color that is transformed to blue violet after application of sulfuric acid.

As noted earlier, the histologic diagnosis of amyloid is based on its staining characteristics. The most commonly used staining technique uses the dye **Congo red**, which under ordinary light imparts a pink or red color to amyloid deposits. Under polarized light, the Congo red–stained amyloid shows a green birefringence (see Fig. 6–50B). This reaction is shared by all forms of amyloid and is due to the cross-β-pleated configuration of amyloid fibrils. Confirmation can be obtained by electron microscopy. AA, AL, and TTR amyloid can be distinguished in histologic sections by specific immunohistochemical staining. Because the pattern of organ involvement in different clinical forms of amyloidosis is variable, each of the major organ involvements is described separately.

Kidney. Amyloidosis of the kidney is the most common and potentially the most serious form of organ involvement. Grossly, the kidneys may be of normal size and color, or, in advanced cases, they may be shrunken because of ischemia caused by vascular narrowing induced by the deposition of amyloid within arterial and arteriolar walls.

Histologically, the amyloid is deposited primarily in the glomeruli, but the interstitial peritubular tissue, arteries, and arterioles are also affected. The glomerular deposits first appear as subtle thickenings of the mesangial matrix, accompanied usually by uneven widening of the basement membranes of the glomerular capillaries. In time the mesangial depositions and the deposits along the basement membranes cause capillary narrowing and distortion of the glomerular vascular tuft. With progression of the glomerular amyloidosis, the capillary lumens are obliterated, and the obsolescent glomerulus is flooded by confluent masses or interlacing broad ribbons of amyloid (Fig. 6–53).

Spleen. Amyloidosis of the spleen may be inapparent grossly or may cause moderate to marked splenomegaly (up to 800 gm). For completely mysterious reasons, one of two patterns of deposition is seen. In one, the deposits are largely limited to the splenic follicles, producing tapioca-like granules on gross inspection, designated **sago spleen**. In the other pattern, the amyloid involves the walls of the splenic sinuses and connective tissue framework in the red pulp. Fusion of the early deposits gives rise to large, maplike areas of amyloidosis, creating what has been designated **lardaceous spleen**.

Liver. The deposits may be inapparent grossly or may cause moderate to marked hepatomegaly. Amyloid appears first in the space of Disse and then progressively encroaches on adjacent hepatic parenchymal cells and sinusoids (see Fig. 6–50). In time, deformity, pressure atrophy, and disappearance of hepatocytes occur, causing total replacement of large areas of liver parenchyma. Vascular involvement and deposits in Kupffer cells are frequent. Normal liver function is usually preserved despite sometimes quite severe involvement of the liver.

Heart. Amyloidosis of the heart (Chapter 12) may occur in any form of systemic amyloidosis. It is also the major organ involved in senile systemic amyloidosis. The heart may be enlarged and firm, but more often it shows no significant changes on gross inspection. Histologically the deposits begin as focal subendocardial accumulations and within the myocardium between the muscle fibers. Expansion of these myocardial deposits eventually causes pressure atrophy of myocardial fibers. When the amyloid deposits are subendocardial, the conduction system may be damaged, accounting for the electrocardiographic abnormalities noted in some patients.

Other Organs. Amyloidosis of other organs is generally encountered in systemic disease. The adrenals, thyroid, and pituitary are common sites of involvement. The gastrointestinal tract may be involved at any level, from the oral cavity (gingiva, tongue) to the anus. The early lesions mainly affect blood vessels but eventually extend to involve the adjacent areas of the submucosa, muscularis, and subserosa.

Nodular depositions in the tongue may cause macroglossia, giving rise to the designation **tumor-forming amyloid of the tongue**. The respiratory tract may be involved focally or diffusely from the larynx down to the smallest bronchioles. It involves so-called plaques as well as blood vessels (Chapter 28). Amyloidosis of peripheral and autonomic nerves is a feature of several familial amyloidotic neuropathies. Depositions of amyloid in patients on long-term hemodialysis are most prominent in the carpal ligament of the wrist, resulting in compression of the median nerve (carpal tunnel syndrome). These patients may also have extensive amyloid deposition in the joints.

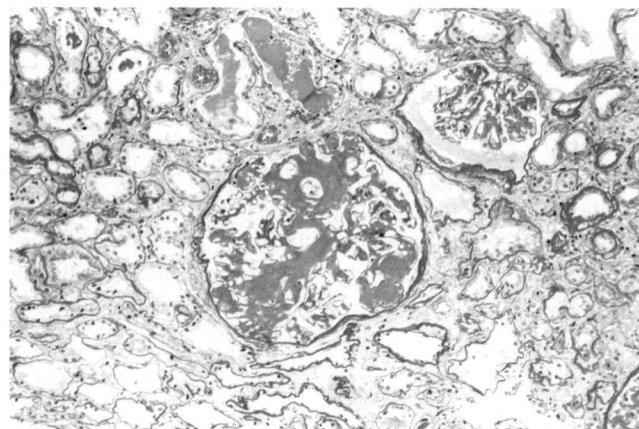

FIGURE 6–53 Amyloidosis of the kidney. The glomerular architecture is almost totally obliterated by the massive accumulation of amyloid.

Clinical Features. Amyloidosis may be found as an unsuspected anatomic change, having produced no clinical manifestations, or it may cause death. The symptoms depend on the magnitude of the deposits and on the particular sites or organs affected. Clinical manifestations at first are often entirely nonspecific, such as weakness, weight loss, light-headedness, or syncope. Somewhat more specific findings appear later and most often relate to renal, cardiac, and gastrointestinal involvement.

Renal involvement gives rise to proteinuria that may be severe enough to cause the nephrotic syndrome (Chapter 20). Progressive obliteration of glomeruli in advanced cases ultimately leads to renal failure and uremia. Renal failure is a common cause of death. *Cardiac amyloidosis* may present as an insidious congestive heart failure. The most serious aspects of cardiac amyloidosis are conduction disturbances and arrhythmias, which may prove fatal. Occasionally, cardiac amyloidosis produces a restrictive pattern of cardiomyopathy and masquerades as chronic constrictive pericarditis (Chapter 12). *Gastrointestinal amyloidosis* may be entirely asymptomatic, or it may present in a variety of ways. Amyloidosis of the tongue may cause sufficient enlargement and inelasticity to hamper speech and swallowing. Depositions in the stomach and intestine may lead to malabsorption, diarrhea, and disturbances in digestion.

The diagnosis of amyloidosis depends on the histologic demonstration of amyloid deposits in tissues. The most common sites biopsied are the kidney, when renal manifestations are present, or rectal or gingival tissues in patients suspected of having systemic amyloidosis. Examination of abdominal fat aspirates stained with Congo red can also be used for the diagnosis of systemic amyloidosis. The test is quite specific, but its sensitivity is low. In suspected cases of immunocyte-associated amyloidosis, serum and urine protein electrophoresis and immunoelectrophoresis should be performed. Bone marrow aspirates in such cases often show monoclonal plasmacytosis, even in the absence of overt multiple myeloma. Scintigraphy with radiolabeled serum amyloid P (SAP) component is a rapid and specific test, since SAP binds to the amyloid deposits and reveals their presence. It also gives a measure of the extent of amyloidosis and can be used to follow patients undergoing treatment.

The prognosis for individuals with generalized amyloidosis is poor. Those with immunocyte-derived amyloidosis (not including multiple myeloma) have a median survival of 2 years after diagnosis. Persons with myeloma-associated amyloidosis have a poorer prognosis. The outlook for individuals with reactive systemic amyloidosis is somewhat better and depends to some extent on the control of the underlying condition. Resorption of amyloid after treatment of the associated condition has been reported, but this is a rare occurrence. New therapeutic strategies aimed at correcting protein misfolding and inhibiting fibrillogenesis are being developed.

REFERENCES

1. Akira S et al: Pathogen recognition and innate immunity. Cell 124:783, 2006.
2. Krogsgaard M, Davis MM: How T cells "see" antigen. Nat Immunol 6:239, 2005.
3. Jung D, Alt FW: Unraveling V(D)J recombination; insights into gene regulation. Cell 116:299, 2004.
4. Kuhns MS et al: Deconstructing the form and function of the TCR/CD3 complex. Immunity 24:133, 2006.
5. Carding SR, Egan PJ: Gammadelta T cells: functional plasticity and heterogeneity. Nat Rev Immunol 2:336, 2002.
6. Bendelac A et al: The biology of NKT cells. Annu Rev Immunol 25:297, 2007.
7. Davis SJ et al: The nature of molecular recognition by T cells. Nat Immunol 4:217, 2003.
8. Steinman RM, Banchereau J: Taking dendritic cells into medicine. Nature 449:419, 2007.
9. Allen CD et al: Germinal-center organization and cellular dynamics. Immunity 27:190, 2007.
10. Lanier LL: NK cell recognition. Annu Rev Immunol 23:225, 2005.
11. Cyster JG: Chemokines and cell migration in secondary lymphoid organs. Science 286:2098, 1999.
12. von Andrian UH, Mempel TR: Homing and cellular traffic in lymph nodes. Nat Rev Immunol 3:867, 2003.
13. Bajenoff M et al: Highways, byways and breadcrumbs: directing lymphocyte traffic in the lymph node. Trends Immunol 28:346, 2007.
14. von Andrian UH, Mackay CR: T-cell function and migration. Two sides of the same coin. N Engl J Med 343:1020, 2000.
15. Klein J, Sato A: The HLA system. N Engl J Med 343:702; 782, 2000.
16. Hennecke J, Wiley DC: T cell receptor–MHC interactions up close. Cell 104:1, 2001.
17. Trombetta ES, Mellman I: Cell biology of antigen processing in vitro and in vivo. Annu Rev Immunol 23:975, 2005.
18. Thorsby E, Lie BA: HLA associated genetic predisposition to autoimmune diseases: genes involved and possible mechanisms. Transpl Immunol 14:175, 2005.
19. Germain RN, Jenkins MK: In vivo antigen presentation. Curr Opin Immunol 16:120, 2004.
20. Greenwald RJ et al: The B7 family revisited. Annu Rev Immunol 23:515, 2005.
21. Reiner SL: Development in motion: helper T cells at work. Cell 129:33, 2007.
22. Bettelli E et al: T(H)-17 cells in the circle of immunity and autoimmunity. Nat Immunol 8:345, 2007.
23. Steinman L: A brief history of T(H)17, the first major revision in the T(H)1/T(II)2 hypothesis of T cell-mediated tissue damage. Nat Med 13:139, 2007.
24. McHeyzer-Williams LJ et al: Helper T cell–regulated B cell immunity. Curr Top Microbiol Immunol 311:59, 2006.
25. Sallusto F et al: Central memory and effector memory T cell subsets: function, generation, and maintenance. Annu Rev Immunol 22:745, 2004.
26. Kay AB: Allergy and allergic diseases. N Engl J Med 344:30, 2001.
27. Galli SJ et al: The development of allergic inflammation. Nature 454:445, 2008.
28. Romagnani S: Cytokines and chemoattractants in allergic inflammation. Mol Immunol 38:881, 2002.
29. Stetson DB et al: Th2 cells: orchestrating barrier immunity. Adv Immunol 83:163, 2004.
30. Rothenberg ME, Hogan SP: The eosinophil. Annu Rev Immunol 24:147, 2006.
31. Wills-Karp M, Ewart SL: Time to draw breath: asthma-susceptibility genes are identified. Nat Rev Genet 5:376, 2004.
32. Golden DB: What is anaphylaxis? Curr Opin Allergy Clin Immunol 7:331, 2007.
33. Baumann U, Schmidt RE: The role of Fc receptors and complement in autoimmunity. Adv Exp Med Biol 495:219, 2001.
34. Jancar S, Sanchez Crespo M: Immune complex–mediated tissue injury: a multistep paradigm. Trends Immunol 26:48, 2005.
35. Nigrovic PA, Lee DM: Synovial mast cells: role in acute and chronic arthritis. Immunol Rev 217:19, 2007.
36. Gutcher I, Becher B: APC-derived cytokines and T cell polarization in autoimmune inflammation. J Clin Invest 117:1119, 2007.
37. Russell JH, Ley TJ: Lymphocyte-mediated cytotoxicity. Annu Rev Immunol 20:323, 2002.
38. Goodnow CC et al: Cellular and genetic mechanisms of self tolerance and autoimmunity. Nature 435:590, 2005.
39. Singh NJ, Schwartz RH: Primer: mechanisms of immunologic tolerance. Nat Clin Pract Rheumatol 2:44, 2006.
40. Walker LS, Abbas AK: The enemy within: keeping self-reactive T cells at bay in the periphery. Nat Rev Immunol 2:11, 2002.
41. Mathis D, Benoist C: Back to central tolerance. Immunity 20:509, 2004.
42. Mathis D, Benoist C: A decade of AIRE. Nat Rev Immunol 7:645, 2007.

43. Nemazee D: Receptor editing in lymphocyte development and central tolerance. Nat Rev Immunol 6:728, 2006.

44. Schwartz RH: T cell anergy. Annu Rev Immunol 21:305, 2003.

45. Mueller DL: E3 ubiquitin ligases as T cell anergy factors. Nat Immunol 5:883, 2004.

46. Riley JL, June CH: The CD28 family: a T-cell rheostat for therapeutic control of T-cell activation. Blood 105:13, 2005.

47. Sakaguchi S, Powrie F: Emerging challenges in regulatory T cell function and biology. Science 317:627, 2007.

48. Zheng Y, Rudensky AY: Foxp3 in control of the regulatory T cell lineage. Nat Immunol 8:457, 2007.

49. Bidere N et al: Genetic disorders of programmed cell death in the immune system. Annu Rev Immunol 24:321, 2006.

50. Rieux-Laucat F: Inherited and acquired death receptor defects in human autoimmune lymphoproliferative syndrome. Curr Dir Autoimmun 9:18, 2006.

51. Goodnow CC: Multistep pathogenesis of autoimmune disease. Cell 130:25, 2007.

52. Davidson A, Diamond B: Autoimmune diseases. N Engl J Med 345:340, 2001.

53. Gregersen PK, Behrens TW: Genetics of autoimmune diseases—disorders of immune homeostasis. Nat Rev Genet 7:917, 2006.

54. Rioux JD, Abbas AK: Paths to understanding the genetic basis of autoimmune disease. Nature 435:584, 2005.

55. Xavier RJ, Rioux JD: Genome-wide association studies: a new window into immune-mediated diseases. Nat Rev Immunol 8:631, 2008.

56. Gregersen PK et al: PTPN22: setting thresholds for autoimmunity. Semin Immunol 18:214, 2006.

57. Cho JH, Abraham C: Inflammatory bowel disease genetics: Nod2. Annu Rev Med 58:401, 2007.

58. Bach JF: Infections and autoimmune diseases. J Autoimmun 25 (Suppl):74, 2005.

59. Vanderlugt CL, Miller SD: Epitope spreading in immune-mediated diseases: implications for immunotherapy. Nat Rev Immunol 2:85, 2002.

60. D'Cruz DP et al: Systemic lupus erythematosus. Lancet 369:587, 2007.

61. Riemekasten G, Hahn BH: Key autoantigens in SLE. Rheumatology (Oxford) 44:975, 2005.

62. Migliorini P et al: Anti-Sm and anti-RNP antibodies. Autoimmunity 38:47, 2005.

63. Hahn BH: Antibodies to DNA. N Engl J Med 338:1359, 1998.

64. Keren DF: Antinuclear antibody testing. Clin Lab Med 22:447, 2002.

65. Koike T et al: Antiphospholipid antibodies: lessons from the bench. J Autoimmun 28:129, 2007.

66. Fischer MJ et al: The antiphospholipid syndrome. Semin Nephrol 27:35, 2007.

67. Kyttaris VC et al: Systems biology in systemic lupus erythematosus: integrating genes, biology and immune function. Autoimmunity 39:705, 2006.

68. Morel L: Genetics of human lupus nephritis. Semin Nephrol 27:2, 2007.

69. Harley JB et al: Unraveling the genetics of systemic lupus erythematosus. Springer Semin Immunopathol 28:119, 2006.

70. Manderson AP et al: The role of complement in the development of systemic lupus erythematosus. Annu Rev Immunol 22:431, 2004.

71. Fairhurst AM et al: Systemic lupus erythematosus: multiple immunological phenotypes in a complex genetic disease. Adv Immunol 92:1, 2006.

72. Yurasov S et al: B-cell tolerance checkpoints in healthy humans and patients with systemic lupus erythematosus. Ann N Y Acad Sci 1062:165, 2005.

73. Hoffman RW: T cells in the pathogenesis of systemic lupus erythematosus. Clin Immunol 113:4, 2004.

74. Rahman AH, Eisenberg RA: The role of toll-like receptors in systemic lupus erythematosus. Springer Semin Immunopathol 28:131, 2006.

75. Banchereau J, Pascual V: Type I interferon in systemic lupus erythematosus and other autoimmune diseases. Immunity 25:383, 2006.

76. Mackay F et al: B cells and the BAFF/APRIL axis: fast-forward on autoimmunity and signaling. Curr Opin Immunol 19:327, 2007.

77. White S, Rosen A: Apoptosis in systemic lupus erythematosus. Curr Opin Rheumatol 15:557, 2003.

78. Borchers AT et al: Drug-induced lupus. Ann N Y Acad Sci 1108:166, 2007.

79. Sigal LH: Basic science for the clinician 42: handling the corpses: apoptosis, necrosis, nucleosomes and (quite possibly) the immunopathogenesis of SLE. J Clin Rheumatol 13:44, 2007.

80. Calamia KT, Balabanova M: Vasculitis in systemic lupus erythematosis. Clin Dermatol 22:148, 2004.

81. Schwartz MM: The pathology of lupus nephritis. Semin Nephrol 27:22, 2007.

82. Stojanovich L et al: Psychiatric manifestations in systemic lupus erythematosus. Autoimmun Rev 6:421, 2007.

83. Hanly JG: Neuropsychiatric lupus. Rheum Dis Clin North Am 31:273, 2005.

84. Tincani A et al: Heart involvement in systemic lupus erythematosus, anti-phospholipid syndrome and neonatal lupus. Rheumatology (Oxford) 45 (Suppl 4):iv8, 2006.

85. Patel P, Werth V: Cutaneous lupus erythematosus: a review. Dermatol Clin 20:373, 2002.

86. Garcia-Carrasco M et al: Pathophysiology of Sjögren's syndrome. Arch Med Res 37:921, 2006.

87. Jonsson R et al: Sjögren's syndrome—a plethora of clinical and immunological phenotypes with a complex genetic background. Ann N Y Acad Sci 1108:433, 2007.

88. Witte T: Antifodrin antibodies in Sjögren's syndrome: a review. Ann N Y Acad Sci 1051:235, 2005.

89. James JA et al: Role of viruses in systemic lupus erythematosus and Sjögren syndrome. Curr Opin Rheumatol 13:370, 2001.

90. Varga J, Abraham D: Systemic sclerosis: a prototypic multisystem fibrotic disorder. J Clin Invest 117:557, 2007.

91. Boin F, Rosen A: Autoimmunity in systemic sclerosis: current concepts. Curr Rheumatol Rep 9:165, 2007.

92. Sakkas LI et al: Mechanisms of disease: the role of immune cells in the pathogenesis of systemic sclerosis. Nat Clin Pract Rheumatol 2:679, 2006.

93. Cepeda EJ, Reveille JD: Autoantibodies in systemic sclerosis and fibrosing syndromes: clinical indications and relevance. Curr Opin Rheumatol 16:723, 2004.

94. Fonseca C et al: A polymorphism in the *CTGF* promoter region associated with systemic sclerosis. N Engl J Med 357:1210, 2007.

95. Lemaire R et al: Fibrillin in Marfan syndrome and tight skin mice provides new insights into transforming growth factor-beta regulation and systemic sclerosis. Curr Opin Rheumatol 18:582, 2006.

96. Venables PJ: Mixed connective tissue disease. Lupus 15:132, 2006.

97. Jennette JC, Falk RJ: Nosology of primary vasculitis. Curr Opin Rheumatol 19:10, 2007.

98. Guillevin L, Dorner T: Vasculitis: mechanisms involved and clinical manifestations. Arthritis Res Ther 9 (Suppl 2):S9, 2007.

99. Rocha PN et al: Effector mechanisms in transplant rejection. Immunol Rev 196:51, 2003.

100. Heeger PS: T-cell allorecognition and transplant rejection: a summary and update. Am J Transplant 3:525, 2003.

101. Colvin RB: Antibody-mediated renal allograft rejection: diagnosis and pathogenesis. J Am Soc Nephrol 18:1046, 2007.

102. Truong LD et al: Acute antibody-mediated rejection of renal transplant: pathogenetic and diagnostic considerations. Arch Pathol Lab Med 131:1200, 2007.

103. Mitchell RN: Graft vascular disease: immune response meets the vessel wall. Annu Rev Pathol 4:19, 2009.

104. Tang IY et al: Immunosuppressive strategies to improve outcomes of kidney transplantation. Semin Nephrol 27:377, 2007.

105. Girlanda R, Kirk AD: Frontiers in nephrology: immune tolerance to allografts in humans. J Am Soc Nephrol 18:2242, 2007.

106. Shlomchik WD: Graft-versus-host disease. Nat Rev Immunol 7:340, 2007.

107. Casanova JL, Abel L: Primary immunodeficiencies: a field in its infancy. Science 317:617, 2007.

108. Cunningham-Rundles C, Ponda PP: Molecular defects in T- and B-cell primary immunodeficiency diseases. Nat Rev Immunol 5:880, 2005.

109. Notarangelo L et al: Primary immunodeficiency diseases: an update from the International Union of Immunological Societies Primary Immunodeficiency Diseases Classification Committee Meeting in Budapest, 2005. J Allergy Clin Immunol 117:883, 2006.

110. Conley ME et al: Genetic analysis of patients with defects in early B-cell development. Immunol Rev 203:216, 2005.

111. Schaffer AA et al: Deconstructing common variable immunodeficiency by genetic analysis. Curr Opin Genet Dev 17:201, 2007.

112. Castigli E, Geha RS: Molecular basis of common variable immunodeficiency. J Allergy Clin Immunol 117:740, 2006.

113. Latiff AH, Kerr MA: The clinical significance of immunoglobulin A deficiency. Ann Clin Biochem 44:131, 2007.
114. Durandy A et al: Pathophysiology of B-cell intrinsic immunoglobulin class switch recombination deficiencies. Adv Immunol 94:275, 2007.
115. Sullivan KE: DiGeorge syndrome/velocardiofacial syndrome: the chromosome 22q11.2 deletion syndrome. Adv Exp Med Biol 601:37, 2007.
116. Buckley RH: Molecular defects in human severe combined immunodeficiency and approaches to immune reconstitution. Annu Rev Immunol 22:625, 2004.
117. Kovanen PE, Leonard WJ: Cytokines and immunodeficiency diseases: critical roles of the gamma(c)-dependent cytokines interleukins 2, 4, 7, 9, 15, and 21, and their signaling pathways. Immunol Rev 202:67, 2004.
118. Blackburn MR, Kellems RE: Adenosine deaminase deficiency: metabolic basis of immune deficiency and pulmonary inflammation. Adv Immunol 86:1, 2005.
119. Sobacchi C et al: RAG-dependent primary immunodeficiencies. Hum Mutat 27:1174, 2006.
120. O'Shea JJ et al: Jak3 and the pathogenesis of severe combined immunodeficiency. Mol Immunol 41:727, 2004.
121. Reith W, Mach B: The bare lymphocyte syndrome and the regulation of MHC expression. Annu Rev Immunol 19:331, 2001.
122. Cavazzana-Calvo M et al: Gene therapy for severe combined immunodeficiency. Annu Rev Med 56:585, 2005.
123. Pike-Overzet K et al: New insights and unresolved issues regarding insertional mutagenesis in X-linked SCID gene therapy. Mol Ther 15:1910, 2007.
124. Ochs HD, Thrasher AJ: The Wiskott-Aldrich syndrome. J Allergy Clin Immunol 117:725, 2006.
125. Sjoholm AG et al: Complement deficiency and disease: an update. Mol Immunol 43:78, 2006.
126. Cicardi M et al: C1 inhibitor: molecular and clinical aspects. Springer Semin Immunopathol 27:286, 2005.
127. Smith LJ: Paroxysmal nocturnal hemoglobinuria. Clin Lab Sci 17:172, 2004.
128. Frankel AD, Young JA: HIV-1: fifteen proteins and an RNA. Annu Rev Biochem 67:1, 1998.
129. Li L et al: Roles of HIV-1 auxiliary proteins in viral pathogenesis and host-pathogen interactions. Cell Res 15:923, 2005.
130. Rohr O et al: Regulation of HIV-1 gene transcription: from lymphocytes to microglial cells. J Leukoc Biol 74:736, 2003.
131. Stevenson M: HIV-1 pathogenesis. Nat Med 9:853, 2003.
132. Letvin NL, Walker BD: Immunopathogenesis and immunotherapy in AIDS virus infections. Nat Med 9:861, 2003.
133. Sierra S et al: Basics of the virology of HIV-1 and its replication. J Clin Virol 34:233, 2005.
134. Lusso P: HIV and the chemokine system: 10 years later. EMBO J 25:447, 2006.
135. Arenzana-Seisdedos F, Parmentier M: Genetics of resistance to HIV infection: role of co-receptors and co-receptor ligands. Semin Immunol 18:387, 2006.
136. Harris RS, Liddament MT: Retroviral restriction by APOBEC proteins. Nat Rev Immunol 4:868, 2004.
137. Greene WC, Peterlin BM: Charting HIV's remarkable voyage through the cell: basic science as a passport to future therapy. Nat Med 8:673, 2002.
138. Hazenberg MD et al: T cell depletion in HIV-1 infection: how CD4+ T cells go out of stock. Nat Immunol 1:285, 2000.
139. Simon V, Ho DD: HIV-1 dynamics in vivo: implications for therapy. Nat Rev Microbiol 1:181, 2003.
140. Grossman Z et al: CD4+ T-cell depletion in HIV infection: are we closer to understanding the cause? Nat Med 8:319, 2002.
141. McCune JM: The dynamics of CD4+ T-cell depletion in HIV disease. Nature 410:974, 2001.
142. Verani A et al: Macrophages and HIV-1: dangerous liaisons. Mol Immunol 42:195, 2005.
143. Larsson M: HIV-1 and the hijacking of dendritic cells: a tug of war. Springer Semin Immunopathol 26:309, 2005.
144. Blankson JN et al: The challenge of viral reservoirs in HIV-1 infection. Annu Rev Med 53:557, 2002.
145. Wu L, KewalRamani VN: Dendritic-cell interactions with HIV: infection and viral dissemination. Nat Rev Immunol 6:859, 2006.
146. Gonzalez-Scarano F, Martin-Garcia J: The neuropathogenesis of AIDS. Nat Rev Immunol 5:69, 2005.
147. Haase AT: Perils at mucosal front lines for HIV and SIV and their hosts. Nat Rev Immunol 5:783, 2005.
148. Brenchley JM et al: HIV disease: fallout from a mucosal catastrophe? Nat Immunol 7:235, 2006.
149. Gandhi RT, Walker BD: Immunologic control of HIV-1. Annu Rev Med 53:149, 2002.
150. Picker LJ: Immunopathogenesis of acute AIDS virus infection. Curr Opin Immunol 18:399, 2006.
151. Mellors JW et al: Prognosis in HIV-1 infection predicted by the quantity of virus in plasma. Science 272:1167, 1996.
152. Peterlin BM, Trono D: Hide, shield and strike back: how HIV-infected cells avoid immune eradication. Nat Rev Immunol 3:97, 2003.
153. Johnson WE, Desrosiers RC: Viral persistance: HIV's strategies of immune system evasion. Annu Rev Med 53:499, 2002.
154. Deeks SG, Walker BD: Human immunodeficiency virus controllers: mechanisms of durable virus control in the absence of antiretroviral therapy. Immunity 27:406, 2007.
155. Kaplan JE et al: Epidemiology of human immunodeficiency virus–associated opportunistic infections in the United States in the era of highly active antiretroviral therapy. Clin Infect Dis 30 (Suppl 1):S5, 2000.
156. Scadden DT: AIDS-related malignancies. Annu Rev Med 54:285, 2003.
157. Yarchoan R et al: Therapy insight: AIDS-related malignancies—the influence of antiviral therapy on pathogenesis and management. Nat Clin Pract Oncol 2:406, 2005.
158. Ganem D: KSHV infection and the pathogenesis of Kaposi's sarcoma. Annu Rev Pathol Mech Dis 1:273, 2006.
159. Moore PS, Chang Y: Molecular virology of Kaposi's sarcoma-associated herpesvirus. Philos Trans R Soc Lond B Biol Sci 356:499, 2001.
160. Carbone A, Gloghini A: AIDS-related lymphomas: from pathogenesis to pathology. Br J Haematol 130:662, 2005.
161. Einstein MH, Kadish AS: Anogenital neoplasia in AIDS. Curr Opin Oncol 16:455, 2004.
162. Murdoch DM et al: Immune reconstitution inflammatory syndrome (IRIS): review of common infectious manifestations and treatment options. AIDS Res Ther 4:9, 2007.
163. McMichael AJ: HIV vaccines. Annu Rev Immunol 24:227, 2006.
164. Letvin NL: Correlates of immune protection and the development of a human immunodeficiency virus vaccine. Immunity 27:366, 2007.
165. Merlini G, Bellotti V: Molecular mechanisms of amyloidosis. N Engl J Med 349:583, 2003.
166. Pepys MB: Amyloidosis. Annu Rev Med 57:223, 2006.
167. Obici L et al: Clinical aspects of systemic amyloid diseases. Biochim Biophys Acta 1753:11, 2005.
168. van der Hilst JC et al: Hereditary periodic fever and reactive amyloidosis. Clin Exp Med 5:87, 2005.
169. Stojanov S, Kastner DL: Familial autoinflammatory diseases: genetics, pathogenesis and treatment. Curr Opin Rheumatol 17:586, 2005.
170. Ting JP et al: CATERPILLERs, pyrin and hereditary immunological disorders. Nat Rev Immunol 6:183, 2006.

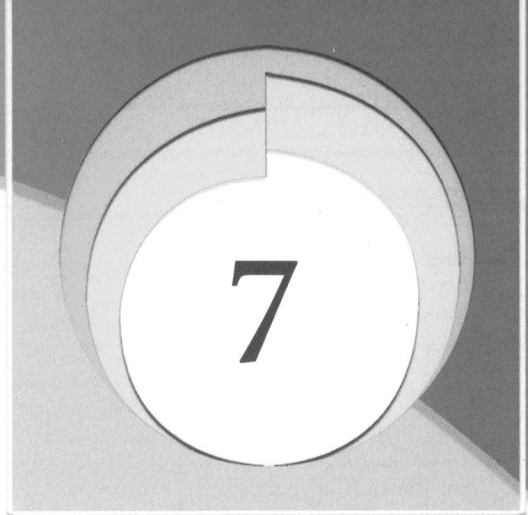

Neoplasia

THOMAS P. STRICKER · VINAY KUMAR

Nomenclature

Characteristics of Benign and Malignant Neoplasms
Differentiation and Anaplasia
Rates of Growth
Cancer Stem Cells and Cancer Cell Lineages
Local Invasion
Metastasis
Pathways of Spread

Epidemiology
Cancer Incidence
Geographic and Environmental Factors
Age
Genetic Predisposition to Cancer
Nonhereditary Predisposing Conditions

Molecular Basis of Cancer
Essential Alterations for Malignant Transformation
Self-Sufficiency in Growth Signals: Oncogenes
Proto-oncogenes, Oncogenes, and Oncoproteins
Alterations in Nonreceptor Tyrosine Kinases
Insensitivity to Growth Inhibition and Escape from Senescence: Tumor Suppressor Genes
Evasion of Apoptosis
Limitless Replicative Potential: Telomerase
Angiogenesis
Invasion and Metastasis
Invasion of Extracellular Matrix

Vascular Dissemination and Homing of Tumor Cells
Molecular Genetics of Metastasis Development
Genomic Instability—Enabler of Malignancy
Stromal Microenvironment and Carcinogenesis
Metabolic Alterations: The Warburg Effect
Dysregulation of Cancer-Associated Genes
Chromosomal Changes
Gene Amplification
Epigenetic Changes
miRNAs and Cancer

Molecular Basis of Multistep Carcinogenesis

Carcinogenic Agents and Their Cellular Interactions
Steps Involved in Chemical Carcinogenesis
Direct-Acting Agents
Indirect-Acting Agents
Initiation and Promotion of Chemical Carcinogenesis
Radiation Carcinogenesis
Ultraviolet Rays
Ionizing Radiation
Microbial Carcinogenesis
Oncogenic RNA Viruses
Oncogenic DNA Viruses
Helicobacter pylori

Host Defense against Tumors—Tumor Immunity
Tumor Antigens
Antitumor Effector Mechanisms

Immune Surveillance and Escape

Clinical Aspects of Neoplasia
Local and Hormonal Effects
Cancer Cachexia

Paraneoplastic Syndromes
Grading and Staging of Tumors
Laboratory Diagnosis of Cancer
Molecular Profiles of Tumors
Tumor Markers

Cancer is the second leading cause of death in the United States; only cardiovascular diseases exact a higher toll. Even more agonizing than the mortality rate is the emotional and physical suffering inflicted by neoplasms. Patients and the public often ask, "When will there be a cure for cancer?" The answer to this simple question is difficult, because cancer is not one disease but many disorders that share a profound growth dysregulation. Some cancers, such as Hodgkin lymphoma, are curable, whereas others, such as pancreatic adenocarcinoma, have a high mortality. The only hope for controlling cancer lies in learning more about its cause and pathogenesis, and great strides have been made in understanding its molecular basis. Indeed, some good news has emerged: cancer mortality for both men and women in the United States declined during the last decade of the twentieth century and has continued its downward course in the 21st.[1] The discussion that follows deals with both benign and malignant tumors, focusing on the basic morphologic and biologic properties of tumors and the molecular basis of carcinogenesis. We also discuss the interactions of the tumor with the host and the host response to tumors.

Nomenclature

Neoplasia means "new growth," and a new growth is called a *neoplasm.* *Tumor* originally applied to the swelling caused by inflammation, but the non-neoplastic usage of *tumor* has almost vanished; thus, the term is now equated with neoplasm. *Oncology* (Greek *oncos* = tumor) is the study of tumors or neoplasms.

Although all physicians know what they mean when they use the term *neoplasm*, it has been surprisingly difficult to develop an accurate definition. The eminent British oncologist Willis[2] has come closest: "A neoplasm is an abnormal mass of tissue, the growth of which exceeds and is uncoordinated with that of the normal tissues and persists in the same excessive manner after cessation of the stimuli which evoked the change." We know that the persistence of tumors, even after the inciting stimulus is gone, results from *genetic alterations that are passed down to the progeny of the tumor cells. These genetic changes allow excessive and unregulated proliferation that becomes autonomous (independent of physiologic growth stimuli)*, although tumors generally remain dependent on the host for their nutrition and blood supply. As we shall discuss later, the entire population of neoplastic cells within an individual tumor arises from a single cell that has incurred genetic change, and hence tumors are said to be *clonal.*

A tumor is said to be *benign* when its microscopic and gross characteristics are considered relatively innocent, implying that it will remain localized, it cannot spread to other sites, and it is generally amenable to local surgical removal; the patient generally survives. It should be noted, however, that benign tumors can produce more than localized lumps, and sometimes they are responsible for serious disease.

Malignant tumors are collectively referred to as *cancers,* derived from the Latin word for *crab,* because they adhere to any part that they seize on in an obstinate manner, similar to a crab. *Malignant,* as applied to a neoplasm, implies that the lesion can invade and destroy adjacent structures and spread to distant sites (metastasize) to cause death. Not all cancers pursue so deadly a course. Some are discovered early and are treated successfully, but the designation *malignant* always raises a red flag.

All tumors, benign and malignant, have two basic components: (1) clonal neoplastic cells that constitute their *parenchyma* and (2) reactive *stroma* made up of connective tissue, blood vessels, and variable numbers of macrophages and lymphocytes. Although the neoplastic cells largely determine a tumor's behavior and pathologic consequences, their growth and evolution is critically dependent on their stroma. An adequate stromal blood supply is requisite for the tumor cells to live and divide, and the stromal connective tissue provides the structural framework essential for the growing cells. In addition, there is cross-talk between tumor cells and stromal cells that directly influences the growth of tumors. In some tumors, the stromal support is scant and so the neoplasm is soft and fleshy. In other cases the parenchymal cells stimulate the formation of an abundant collagenous stroma, referred to as *desmoplasia.* Some demoplastic tumors—for example, some cancers of the female breast—are stony hard or *scirrhous.* The nomenclature of tumors and their biologic behavior are based primarily on the parenchymal component.

Benign Tumors. In general, benign tumors are designated by attaching the suffix *-oma* to the cell of origin. Tumors of mesenchymal cells generally follow this rule. For example, a benign tumor arising in fibrous tisssue is called a *fibroma,* whereas a benign cartilaginous tumor is a *chondroma.* In contrast, the nomenclature of benign epithelial tumors is more complex. These are variously classified, some based on their cells of origin, others on microscopic pattern, and still others on their macroscopic architecture.

Adenoma is applied to a benign epithelial neoplasm derived from glands, although they may or may not form glandular structures. On this basis, a benign epithelial neoplasm that arises from renal tubular cells growing in the form of numerous tightly clustered small glands would be termed an *adenoma,* as would a heterogeneous mass of adrenal cortical cells growing as a solid sheet. Benign epithelial neoplasms producing microscopically or macroscopically visible finger-like or warty projections from epithelial surfaces are referred to as *papillomas.* Those that form large cystic masses, as in the ovary, are referred to as *cystadenomas.* Some tumors produce papillary patterns that protrude into cystic

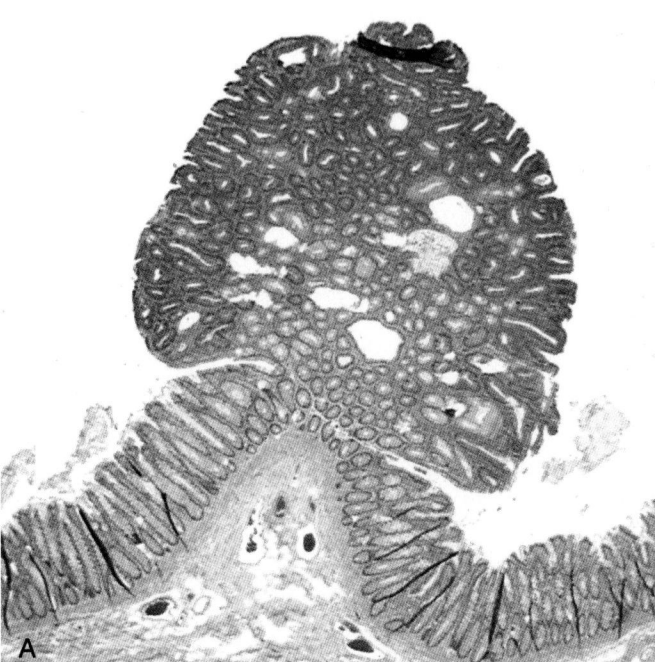
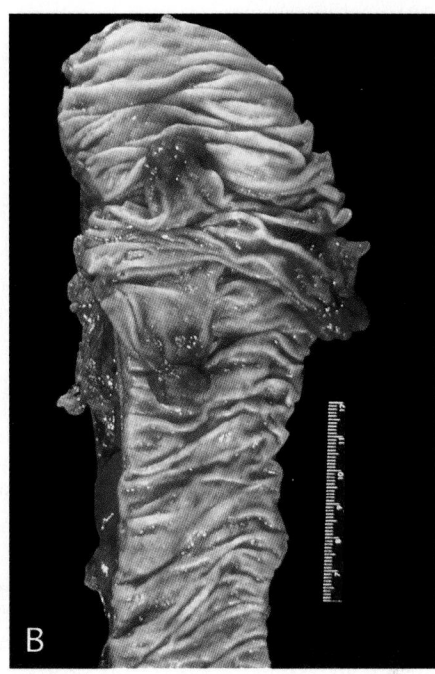

FIGURE 7–1   Colonic polyp. **A,** This benign glandular tumor (adenoma) is projecting into the colonic lumen and is attached to the mucosa by a distinct stalk. **B,** Gross appearance of several colonic polyps.

spaces and are called *papillary cystadenomas.* When a neoplasm, benign or malignant, produces a macroscopically visible projection above a mucosal surface and projects, for example, into the gastric or colonic lumen, it is termed a *polyp* (Fig. 7–1).

Malignant Tumors. The nomenclature of malignant tumors essentially follows the same schema used for benign neoplasms, with certain additions. *Malignant tumors arising in mesenchymal tissue are usually called sarcomas* (Greek *sar* = fleshy), because they have little connective tissue stroma and so are fleshy (e.g., fibrosarcoma, chondrosarcoma, leiomyosarcoma, and rhabdomyosarcoma). Malignant neoplasms of epithelial cell origin, derived from any of the three germ layers, are called *carcinomas.* Thus, cancer arising in the epidermis of ectodermal origin is a carcinoma, as is a cancer arising in the mesodermally derived cells of the renal tubules and the endodermally derived cells of the lining of the gastrointestinal tract. Carcinomas may be further qualified. *Squamous cell carcinoma* would denote a cancer in which the tumor cells resemble stratified squamous epithelium, and *adenocarcinoma* denotes a lesion in which the neoplastic epithelial cells grow in glandular patterns. Sometimes the tissue or organ of origin can be identified, as in the designation of renal cell adenocarcinoma or bronchogenic squamous cell carcinoma. Not infrequently, however, a cancer is composed of undifferentiated cells of unknown tissue origin, and must be designated merely as an undifferentiated malignant tumor.

In many benign and malignant neoplasms, the parenchymal cells bear a close resemblance to each other, as though all were derived from a single cell. Indeed, neoplasms are of monoclonal origin, as is documented later. Infrequently, divergent differentiation of a single neoplastic clone along two lineages creates what are called *mixed tumors.* The best example of this is the *mixed tumor of salivary gland origin.* These tumors contain epithelial components scattered within a myxoid stroma that sometimes contains islands of cartilage or bone (Fig. 7–2). All these elements, it is believed, arise from a single clone capable of giving rise to epithelial and myoepithelial cells; thus, the preferred designation of these neoplasms is *pleomorphic adenoma.* The great majority of neoplasms, even mixed tumors, are composed of cells representative of a single germ layer. The multifaceted mixed tumors should not be confused with a *teratoma,* which contains recognizable mature or immature cells or tissues representative of more than one germ cell layer and sometimes all three. Teratomas originate from totipotential cells such as those normally present in the ovary and testis and sometimes abnormally present in

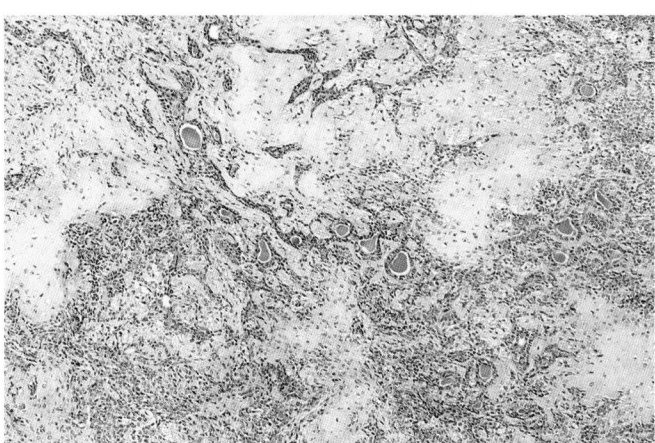

FIGURE 7–2   This mixed tumor of the parotid gland contains epithelial cells forming ducts and myxoid stroma that resembles cartilage. (Courtesy of Dr. Trace Worrell, University of Texas Southwestern Medical School, Dallas, TX.)

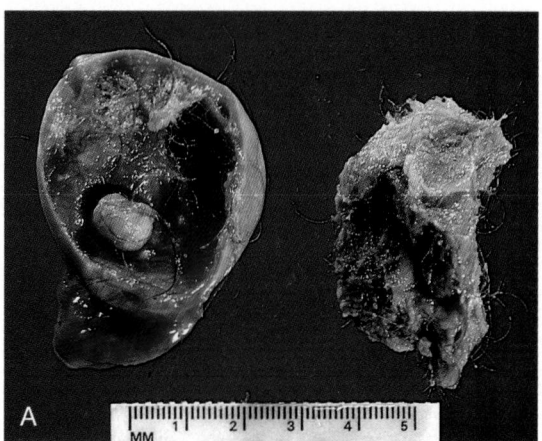 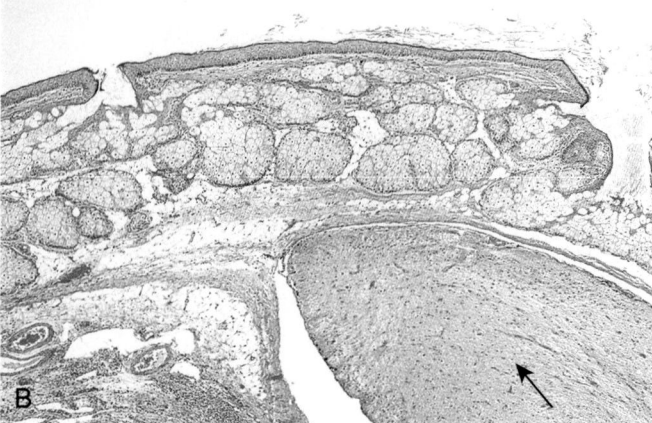

FIGURE 7–3   **A,** Gross appearance of an opened cystic teratoma of the ovary. Note the presence of hair, sebaceous material, and tooth. **B,** A microscopic view of a similar tumor shows skin, sebaceous glands, fat cells, and a tract of neural tissue *(arrow).*

sequestered midline embryonic rests. Such cells have the capacity to differentiate into any of the cell types found in the adult body and so, not surprisingly, may give rise to neoplasms that mimic, in a helter-skelter fashion, bits of bone, epithelium, muscle, fat, nerve, and other tissues. When all the component parts are well differentiated, it is a *benign (mature) teratoma*; when less well differentiated, it is an immature, potentially or overtly, *malignant teratoma.* A particularly common pattern is seen in the ovarian *cystic teratoma* (dermoid cyst), which differentiates principally along ectodermal lines to create a cystic tumor lined by skin replete with hair, sebaceous glands, and tooth structures (Fig. 7–3).

The nomenclature of the more common forms of neoplasia is presented in Table 7–1. It is evident from this compilation that there are some inappropriate but deeply entrenched usages. For generations, benign-sounding designations such as lymphoma, melanoma, mesothelioma, and seminoma have been used for certain malignant neoplasms. The converse is also true; ominous terms may be applied to trivial lesions. *Hamartomas* present as disorganized but benign-appearing masses composed of cells indigenous to the particular site. They were once thought to be a developmental malformation, unworthy of the -oma designation. For example, pulmonary chondroid harmatoma contains islands of disorganized, but histologically normal cartilage, bronchi, and vessels. However, many hamartomas, including pulmonary chondroid hamartoma, have clonal, recurrent translocations involving genes encoding certain chromatin proteins.[3] Thus, through molecular biology they have finally earned their -oma designation. Another misnomer is the term *choristoma.* This congenital anomaly is better described as a *heterotopic rest* of cells. For example, a small nodule of well-developed and normally organized pancreatic substance may be found in the submucosa of the stomach, duodenum, or small intestine. This heterotopic rest may be replete with islets of Langerhans and exocrine glands. The term *choristoma,* connoting a neoplasm, imparts to the heterotopic rest a gravity far beyond its usual trivial significance. Although regrettably the terminology of neoplasms is not simple, it is important because it is the language by which the nature and significance of tumors are categorized.

Characteristics of Benign and Malignant Neoplasms

Nothing is more important to the individual with a tumor than being told "It is benign," and so the differentiation between benign and malignant tumors is one of the most important distinctions a pathologist can make. In the great majority of instances, a benign tumor may be distinguished from a malignant tumor with considerable confidence on the basis of morphology. Occasionally, despite the pathologist's best efforts, a neoplasm defies categorization. Certain anatomic features may suggest innocence, whereas others point toward cancerous potential. In a few instances there is not perfect concordance between the appearance of a neoplasm and its biologic behavior. In these cases molecular profiling (see below) or other molecular ancillary tests may provide useful information. Although an innocent face may mask an ugly nature, in general, benign and malignant tumors can be distinguished on the basis of differentiation and anaplasia, rate of growth, local invasion, and metastasis.

DIFFERENTIATION AND ANAPLASIA

Differentiation refers to the extent to which neoplastic parenchymal cells resemble the corresponding normal parenchymal cells, both morphologically and functionally; lack of differentiation is called anaplasia. In general, benign tumors are well differentiated (Figs. 7–4 and 7–5). The neoplastic cell in a benign adipocyte tumor—a lipoma—so closely resembles the normal cell that it may be impossible to recognize it as a tumor by microscopic examination of individual cells. Only the growth of these cells into a discrete mass discloses the neoplastic nature of the lesion. One may get so close to the tree that one loses sight of the forest. In well-differentiated benign tumors, mitoses are extremely scant in number and are of normal configuration.

Malignant neoplasms are characterized by a wide range of parenchymal cell differentiation, from surprisingly well differentiated (Fig. 7–6) to completely undifferentiated. Certain well-differentiated adenocarcinomas of the thyroid, for

TABLE 7–1	Nomenclature of Tumors	
Tissue of Origin	**Benign**	**Malignant**
COMPOSED OF ONE PARENCHYMAL CELL TYPE		
Tumors of Mesenchymal Origin		
Connective tissue and derivatives	Fibroma Lipoma Chondroma Osteoma	Fibrosarcoma Liposarcoma Chondrosarcoma Osteogenic sarcoma
Endothelial and Related Tissues		
Blood vessels	Hemangioma	Angiosarcoma
Lymph vessels	Lymphangioma	Lymphangiosarcoma
Synovium		Synovial sarcoma
Mesothelium		Mesothelioma
Brain coverings	Meningioma	Invasive meningioma
Blood Cells and Related Cells		
Hematopoietic cells		Leukemias
Lymphoid tissue		Lymphomas
Muscle		
Smooth	Leiomyoma	Leiomyosarcoma
Striated	Rhabdomyoma	Rhabdomyosarcoma
Tumors of Epithelial Origin		
Stratified squamous	Squamous cell papilloma	Squamous cell carcinoma
Basal cells of skin or adnexa		Basal cell carcinoma
Epithelial lining of glands or ducts	Adenoma Papilloma Cystadenoma	Adenocarcinoma Papillary carcinomas Cystadenocarcinoma
Respiratory passages	Bronchial adenoma	Bronchogenic carcinoma
Renal epithelium	Renal tubular adenoma	Renal cell carcinoma
Liver cells	Liver cell adenoma	Hepatocellular carcinoma
Urinary tract epithelium (transitional)	Transitional-cell papilloma	Transitional-cell carcinoma
Placental epithelium	Hydatidiform mole	Choriocarcinoma
Testicular epithelium (germ cells)		Seminoma Embryonal carcinoma
Tumors of Melanocytes	Nevus	Malignant melanoma
MORE THAN ONE NEOPLASTIC CELL TYPE—MIXED TUMORS, USUALLY DERIVED FROM ONE GERM CELL LAYER		
Salivary glands	Pleomorphic adenoma (mixed tumor of salivary origin)	Malignant mixed tumor of salivary gland origin
Renal anlage		Wilms tumor
MORE THAN ONE NEOPLASTIC CELL TYPE DERIVED FROM MORE THAN ONE GERM CELL LAYER—TERATOGENOUS		
Totipotential cells in gonads or in embryonic rests	Mature teratoma, dermoid cyst	Immature teratoma, teratocarcinoma

example, may form normal-appearing follicles, and some squamous cell carcinomas contain cells that do not differ cytologically from normal squamous epithelial cells (Fig. 7–7). Thus, the morphologic diagnosis of malignancy in well-differentiated tumors may sometimes be quite difficult. In between the two extremes lie tumors that are loosely referred to as *moderately well differentiated.*

Malignant neoplasms that are composed of poorly differentiated cells are said to be *anaplastic.* Lack of differentiation, or anaplasia, is considered a hallmark of malignancy. The term *anaplasia* literally means "to form backward," implying a reversal of differentiation to a more primitive level. It is believed, however, that most cancers do not represent "reverse differentiation" of mature normal cells but, in fact, arise from less mature cells with "stem-cell-like" properties, such as tissue

stem cells (Chapter 3). In well-differentiated tumors (Fig. 7–7), daughter cells derived from these "cancer stem cells" retain the capacity for differentiation, whereas in poorly differentiated tumors that capacity is lost.

Lack of differentiation, or anaplasia, is often associated with many other morphologic changes.

- *Pleomorphism.* Both the cells and the nuclei characteristically display *pleomorphism*—variation in size and shape (Fig. 7–8). Thus, cells within the same tumor are not uniform, but range from large cells, many times larger than their neighbors, to extremely small and primitive appearing.
- *Abnormal nuclear morphology.* Characteristically the nuclei contain abundant chromatin and are dark staining *(hyperchromatic).* The nuclei are disproportionately large

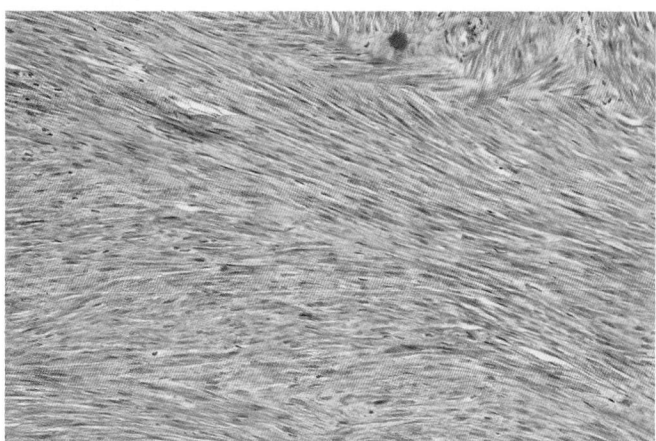

FIGURE 7–4   Leiomyoma of the uterus. This benign, well-differentiated tumor contains interlacing bundles of neoplastic smooth muscle cells that are virtually identical in appearance to normal smooth muscle cells in the myometrium.

for the cell, and the nuclear-to-cytoplasm ratio may approach 1 : 1 instead of the normal 1 : 4 or 1 : 6. The nuclear shape is variable and often irregular, and the chromatin is often coarsely clumped and distributed along the nuclear membrane. Large nucleoli are usually present in these nuclei.

○ *Mitoses.* As compared with benign tumors and some well-differentiated malignant neoplasms, undifferentiated tumors usually possess large numbers of mitoses, reflecting the higher proliferative activity of the parenchymal cells. *The presence of mitoses, however, does not necessarily indicate that a tumor is malignant or that the tissue is neoplastic.* Many normal tissues exhibiting rapid turnover, such as bone marrow, have numerous mitoses, and non-neoplastic proliferations such as hyperplasias contain many cells in mitosis. More important as a morphologic feature of malignancy are atypical, bizarre mitotic figures, sometimes producing tripolar, quadripolar, or multipolar spindles (Fig. 7–9).

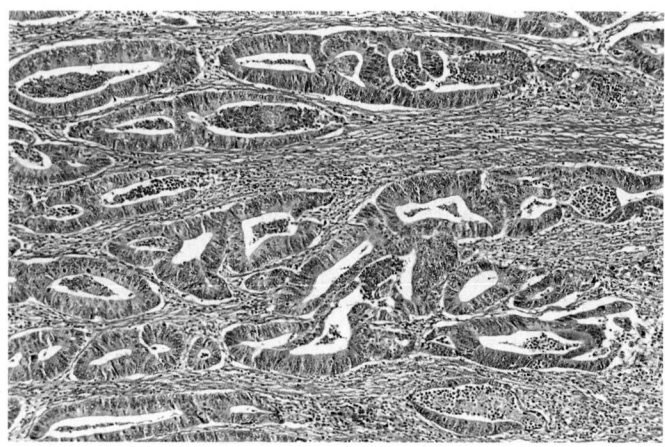

FIGURE 7–6   Malignant tumor (adenocarcinoma) of the colon. Note that compared with the well-formed and normal-looking glands characteristic of a benign tumor (see Fig. 7–5), the cancerous glands are irregular in shape and size and do not resemble the normal colonic glands. This tumor is considered differentiated because gland formation can be seen. The malignant glands have invaded the muscular layer of the colon. (Courtesy of Dr. Trace Worrell, University of Texas Southwestern Medical School, Dallas, TX.)

○ *Loss of polarity.* In addition to the cytologic abnormalities, the *orientation of anaplastic cells is markedly disturbed (i.e., they lose normal polarity).* Sheets or large masses of tumor cells grow in an anarchic, disorganized fashion.

○ *Other changes.* Another feature of anaplasia is the formation of *tumor giant cells,* some possessing only a single huge polymorphic nucleus and others having two or more large, hyperchromatic nuclei (Fig. 7–8). These giant cells are not to be confused with inflammatory Langhans or foreign body giant cells, which are derived from macrophages and contain many small, normal-appearing nuclei. Although growing tumor cells obviously require a blood supply, often the vascular stroma is scant, and in many anaplastic tumors, large central areas undergo ischemic *necrosis.*

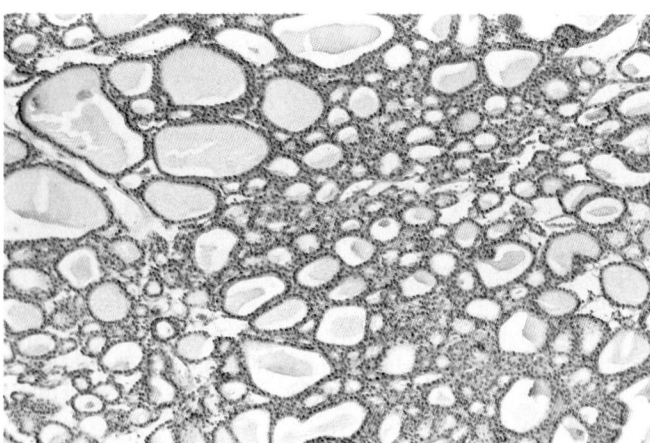

FIGURE 7–5   Benign tumor (adenoma) of the thyroid. Note the normal-looking (well-differentiated), colloid-filled thyroid follicles. (Courtesy of Dr. Trace Worrell, University of Texas Southwestern Medical School, Dallas, TX.)

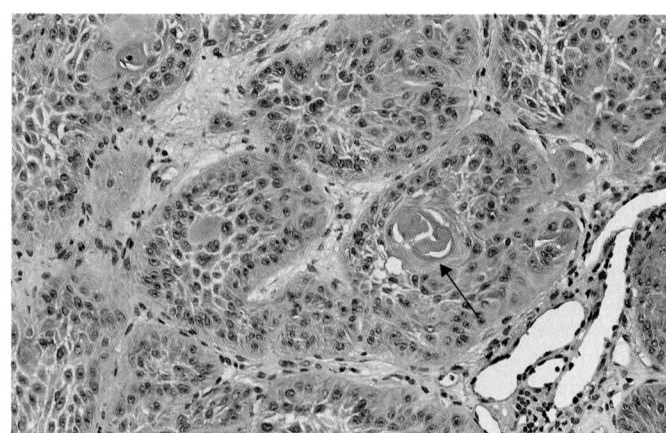

FIGURE 7–7   Well-differentiated squamous cell carcinoma of the skin. The tumor cells are strikingly similar to normal squamous epithelial cells, with intercellular bridges and nests of keratin pearls *(arrow).* (Courtesy of Dr. Trace Worrell, University of Texas Southwestern Medical School, Dallas, TX.)

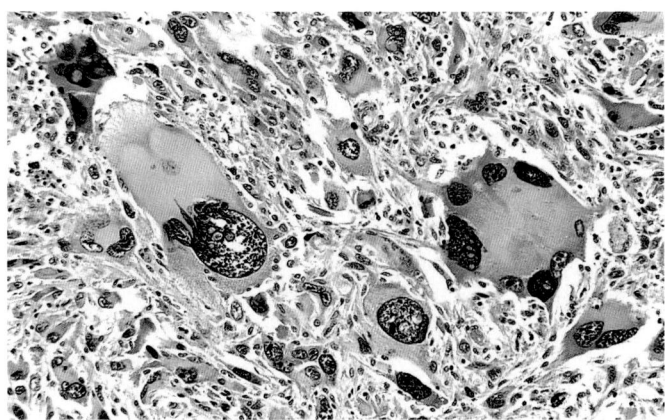

FIGURE 7-8 Anaplastic tumor of the skeletal muscle (rhabdo-myosarcoma). Note the marked cellular and nuclear pleomorphism, hyperchromatic nuclei, and tumor giant cells. (Courtesy of Dr. Trace Worrell, University of Texas Southwestern Medical School, Dallas, TX.)

Before we leave the subject of differentiation and anaplasia, we should discuss metaplasia and dysplasia. *Metaplasia is defined as the replacement of one type of cell with another type.* Metaplasia is nearly always found in association with tissue damage, repair, and regeneration. Often the replacing cell type is more suited to a change in environment. For example, gastroesophageal reflux damages the squamous epithelium of the esophagus, leading to its replacement by glandular (gastric or intestinal) epithelium, more suited to the acidic environment. *Dysplasia* is a term that literally means disordered growth. Dysplasia often occurs in metaplastic epithelium, but not all metaplastic epithelium is also dysplastic. Dysplasia is encountered principally in epithelia, and it is characterized by a constellation of changes that *include a loss in the uniformity of the individual cells as well as a loss in their architectural orientation.* Dysplastic cells exhibit considerable pleomorphism and often contain large hyperchromatic nuclei with a high nuclear-to-cytoplasmic ratio. The architecture of the tissue may be disorderly. For example, in squamous epithelium the usual progressive maturation of tall cells in the basal layer to flat-

tened squames on the surface may be lost and replaced by a scrambling of dark basal-appearing cells throughout the epithelium. Mitotic figures are more abundant than usual, although almost invariably they have a normal configuration. Frequently, however, the mitoses appear in abnormal locations within the epithelium. For example, in dysplastic stratified squamous epithelium, mitoses are not confined to the basal layers but instead may appear at all levels, including surface cells. When dysplastic changes are marked and involve the entire thickness of the epithelium but the lesion remains confined by the basement membrane, it is considered a preinvasive neoplasm and is referred to as *carcinoma in situ* (Fig. 7-10). Once the tumor cells breach the basement membrane, the tumor is said to be *invasive.* Dysplastic changes are often found adjacent to foci of invasive carcinoma, and in some situations, such as in long-term cigarette smokers and persons with Barrett esophagus, severe epithelial dysplasia frequently antedates the appearance of cancer. However, *dysplasia does not necessarily progress to cancer.* Mild to moderate changes that do not involve the entire thickness of epithelium may be reversible, and with removal of the inciting causes the epithelium may revert to normal. Even carcinoma in situ may take years to become invasive.

As you might presume, the better the differentiation of the transformed cell, the more completely it retains the functional capabilities found in its normal counterparts. Thus, benign neoplasms and well-differentiated carcinomas of endocrine glands frequently elaborate the hormones characteristic of their origin. Increased levels of these hormones in the blood are used clinically to detect and follow such tumors. Well-differentiated squamous cell carcinomas of the epidermis elaborate keratin, just as well-differentiated hepatocellular carcinomas elaborate bile. Highly anaplastic undifferentiated cells, whatever their tissue of origin, lose their resemblance to the normal cells from which they have arisen. In some instances, new and unanticipated functions emerge. Some tumors may elaborate fetal proteins not produced by comparable cells in the adult. Carcinomas of nonendocrine origin may produce a variety of hormones. For example, bronchogenic carcinomas may produce corticotropin, parathyroid-like hormone, insulin, and glucagon, as well as others. *Despite exceptions, the more rapidly growing and the more anaplastic a tumor, the less likely it will have specialized functional activity. The cells in benign tumors are almost always well differentiated and resemble their normal cells of origin; the cells in cancer are more or less differentiated, but some derangement of differentiation is always present.*

RATES OF GROWTH

A fundamental issue in tumor biology is to understand the factors that affect the growth rates of tumors and their influence on clinical outcome and therapeutic responses. One can begin the consideration of tumor cell kinetics by asking the question: How long does it take to produce a clinically overt tumor mass? It is a reasonable estimate the original transformed cell (approximately 10 μm in diameter) must undergo at least 30 population doublings to produce 10^9 cells (weighing approximately 1 gm), which is the smallest clinically detectable mass. In contrast, only 10 additional doubling cycles are required to produce a tumor containing 10^{12} cells (weighing ~1 kg), which is usually

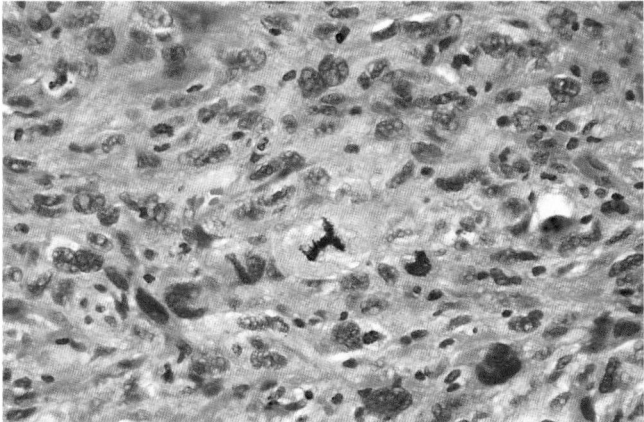

FIGURE 7-9 Anaplastic tumor showing cellular and nuclear variation in size and shape. The prominent cell in the center field has an abnormal tripolar spindle.

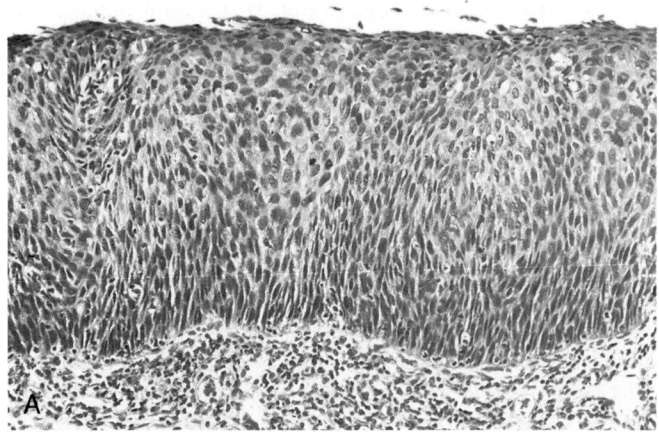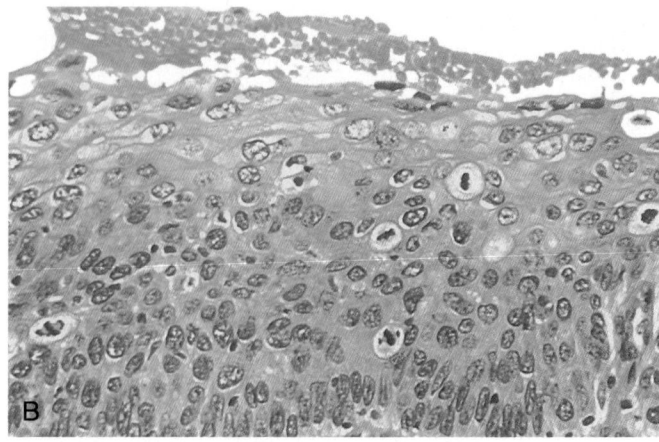

FIGURE 7–10 **A,** Carcinoma in situ. This low-power view shows that the entire thickness of the epithelium is replaced by atypical dysplastic cells. There is no orderly differentiation of squamous cells. The basement membrane is intact, and there is no tumor in the subepithelial stroma. **B,** A high-power view of another region shows failure of normal differentiation, marked nuclear and cellular pleomorphism, and numerous mitotic figures extending toward the surface. The basement membrane is not seen in this section.

the maximal size compatible with life. These are minimal estimates, based on the assumption that all descendants of the transformed cell retain the ability to divide and that there is no loss of cells from the replicative pool. This concept of tumor as a "pathologic dynamo" is not entirely correct, as we discuss subsequently. Nevertheless, this calculation highlights an extremely important concept about tumor growth: *By the time a solid tumor is clinically detected, it has already completed a major portion of its life span.* This is a major impediment in the treatment of cancer and underscores the need to develop diagnostic markers to detect early cancers.

The rate of growth of a tumor is determined by three main factors: the doubling time of tumor cells, the fraction of tumor cells that are in the replicative pool, and the rate at which cells are shed or die. Because cell cycle controls are deranged in most tumors, tumor cells can be triggered to cycle without the usual restraints. The dividing cells, however, do not necessarily complete the cell cycle more rapidly than do normal cells. In reality, total cell cycle time for many tumors is equal to or longer than that of corresponding normal cells. Thus, it can be safely concluded that growth of tumors is not commonly associated with a shortening of cell cycle time.

The proportion of cells within the tumor population that are in the proliferative pool is referred to as the *growth fraction.* Clinical and experimental studies suggest that during the early, submicroscopic phase of tumor growth, the vast majority of transformed cells are in the proliferative pool (Fig. 7–11). As tumors continue to grow, cells leave the proliferative pool in ever-increasing numbers as a result of shedding, lack of nutrients, necrosis, apoptosis, differentiation, and reversion to the nonproliferative phase of the cell cycle (G_0). Thus, by the time a tumor is clinically detectable, most cells are not in the replicative pool. Even in some rapidly growing tumors, the growth fraction is only about 20% or less.

Ultimately the progressive growth of tumors and the rate at which they grow are determined by an *excess of cell production over cell loss.* In some tumors, especially those with a relatively high growth fraction, the imbalance is large, resulting in more rapid growth than in those in which cell production exceeds cell loss by only a small margin. Some leukemias and lymphomas and certain lung cancers (i.e., small-cell carcinoma) have

a relatively high growth fraction, and their clinical course is rapid. By comparison, many common tumors, such as cancers of the colon and breast, have low growth fractions, and cell production exceeds cell loss by only about 10%; they tend to grow at a much slower pace.

Several important conceptual and practical lessons can be learned from studies of tumor cell kinetics:

● Fast-growing tumors may have a high *cell turnover,* implying that rates of both proliferation and apoptosis are high. Obviously if the tumor is to grow, the rate of proliferation must exceed that of cell death.

● The growth fraction of tumor cells has a profound effect on their susceptibility to cancer chemotherapy. Because most anticancer agents act on cells that are in cycle, it is not difficult to imagine that a tumor that contains 5% of all cells in the replicative pool will be slow growing but relatively refractory to treatment with drugs that kill dividing cells. One strategy used in the treatment of tumors with low growth fraction (e.g., cancer of colon and breast) is first to shift tumor cells from G_0 into the cell cycle. This can be

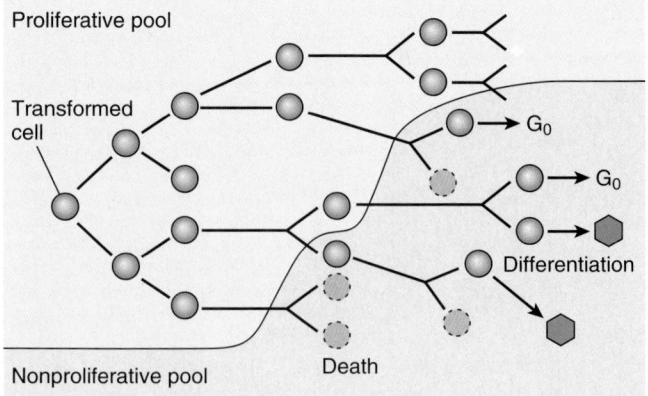

FIGURE 7–11 Schematic representation of tumor growth. As the cell population expands, a progressively higher percentage of tumor cells leaves the replicative pool by reversion to G_0, differentiation, and death.

accomplished by debulking the tumor with surgery or radiation. The surviving tumor cells tend to enter the cell cycle and thus become susceptible to drug therapy. Such considerations form the basis of combined-modality treatment. Some aggressive tumors (such as certain lymphomas and leukemias) that contain a large pool of dividing cells literally melt away with chemotherapy and may even be cured.

We can now return to the question posed earlier: How long does it take for one transformed cell to produce a clinically detectable tumor containing 10^9 cells? If every one of the daughter cells remained in cell cycle and no cells were shed or lost, we could anticipate the answer to be 90 days (30 population doublings, with a cell cycle time of 3 days). In reality, *the latent period before which a tumor becomes clinically detectable is unpredictable but typically much longer than 90 days, as long as many years for most solid tumors, emphasizing once again that human cancers are diagnosed only after they are fairly advanced in their life cycle.* After they become clinically detectable, the average volume-doubling time for such common killers as cancer of the lung and colon is about 2 to 3 months. As might be anticipated from the discussion of the variables that affect growth rate, however, the range of doubling time values is extremely broad, varying from less than 1 month for some childhood cancers to more than 1 year for certain salivary gland tumors. Cancer is indeed an unpredictable group of disorders.

In general, *the growth rate of tumors correlates with their level of differentiation, and thus most malignant tumors grow more rapidly than do benign lesions.* There are, however, many exceptions to such an oversimplification. Some benign tumors have a higher growth rate than malignant tumors. Moreover, the rate of growth of benign as well as malignant neoplasms may not be constant over time. Factors such as hormonal stimulation, adequacy of blood supply, and unknown influences may affect their growth. For example, the growth of uterine leiomyomas (benign smooth muscle tumors) may change over time because of hormonal variations. Not infrequently, repeated clinical examination of women bearing such neoplasms over the span of decades discloses no significant increase in size. After menopause the neoplasms may atrophy and may be replaced largely by collagenous, sometimes calcified, tissue. During pregnancy leiomyomas frequently enter a growth spurt. Such changes reflect the responsiveness of the tumor cells to circulating levels of steroid hormones, particularly estrogens. Cancers show a wide range of growth. Some malignant tumors grow slowly for years and then suddenly increase in size, explosively disseminating to cause death within a few months of discovery. It is possible that such behavior results from the emergence of an aggressive subclone of transformed cells. At the other extreme are malignant neoplasms that grow more slowly than do benign tumors and may even enter periods of dormancy lasting for years. On occasion, cancers decrease in size and even spontaneously disappear, but such "miracles" are rare enough that they remain intriguing curiosities.

CANCER STEM CELLS AND CANCER CELL LINEAGES

The continued growth and maintenance of many tissues that contain short-lived cells, such as the formed elements of the blood and the epithelial cells of the gastrointestinal tract and skin, require a resident population of tissue stem cells that are long-lived and capable of self-renewal. Tissue stem cells are rare and exist in a niche created by support cells, which produce paracrine factors that sustain the stem cell.[4] Recall from Chapter 3 that tissue stem cells divide asymmetrically to produce two types of daughter cells—those with limited proliferative potential, which undergo terminal differentiation and die, and those that retain stem cell potential.

Cancers are immortal and have limitless proliferative capacity, indicating that like normal tissues, they also must contain cells with "stemlike" properties.[5,6] The concept of cancer stem cells has several important implications. Most notably, if cancer stem cells are essential for tumor persistence, it follows that these cells must be eliminated to cure the affected patient. It is hypothesized that like normal stem cells, cancer stem cells have a high intrinsic resistance to conventional therapies, because of their low rate of cell division and the expression of factors, such as multiple drug resistance-1 (MDR1), that counteract the effects of chemotherapeutic drugs.[5,6] Thus, the limited success of current therapies may in part be explained by their failure to kill the malignant stem cells that lie at the root of cancer. Cancer stem cells could arise from normal tissue stem cells or from more differentiated cells that, as part of the transformation process, acquire the property of self-renewal. Studies of certain leukemias (Chapter 13) support both of these possibilities. For example, chronic myelogenous leukemia (CML) originates from the malignant counterpart of a normal hematopoietic stem cell, whereas certain acute myeloid leukemias (AMLs) are derived from more differentiated myeloid precursors that acquire an abnormal capacity for self-renewal. The identification of "leukemia stem cells" has spurred the search for cancer stem cells in solid tumors. Most such studies have focused on the identification of tumor-initiating cells (T-ICs), which are defined as cells that allow a human tumor to grow and maintain itself indefinitely when transplanted into an immunodeficient mouse. T-ICs have been identified in several human tumors, including breast carcinoma, glioblastoma multiforme, colon cancer, and AML,[5–8] in which they constitute 0.1% to 2% of the total cellularity.

More recent studies have shown that in some cancers, T-ICs are very common, representing 25% of the total cellularity.[9] Thus some tumors may have a small number of T-ICs that then "differentiate" to form the bulk of the tumor, while other tumors may be primarily composed of T-ICs. In the future, it will be important to identify the tumorigenic population in each tumor to direct therapy against tumor stem cells. An emerging theme is that the genes and pathways that maintain cancer stem cells are the same as those that regulate normal tissue stem cell homeostasis. Examples include BMI1, a component of the polycomb chromatin-remodeling complex that promotes "stem-ness" in both normal hematopoietic and leukemic stem cells; and the WNT pathway, a key regulator of normal colonic crypt stem cells that has been implicated in the maintenance of colonic adenocarcinoma "stem cells."[9,10] Important remaining questions revolve around whether T-ICs are an accurate measure of cancer stem cells, if cancer stem cells remain dependent on the "niche" that supports normal stem cells, and if it will be possible to selectively target cancer cell "stem-ness" factors.

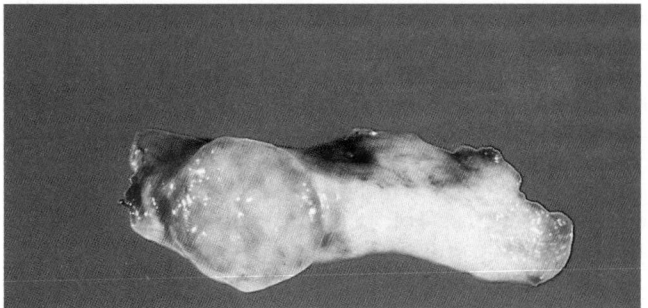

FIGURE 7–12 Fibroadenoma of the breast. The tan-colored, encapsulated small tumor is sharply demarcated from the whiter breast tissue.

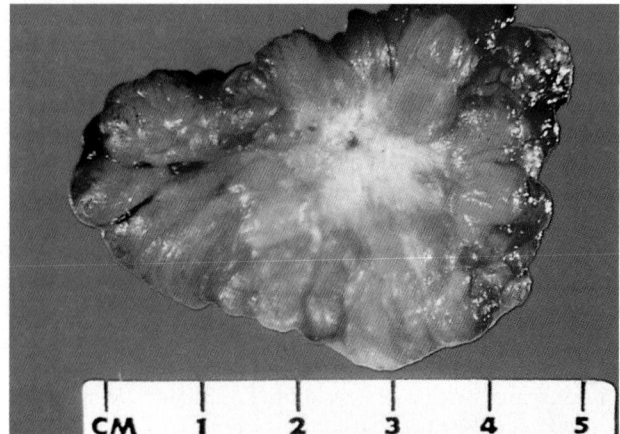

FIGURE 7–14 Cut section of an invasive ductal carcinoma of the breast. The lesion is retracted, infiltrating the surrounding breast substance, and would be stony hard on palpation.

LOCAL INVASION

Nearly all benign tumors grow as cohesive expansile masses that remain localized to their site of origin and do not have the capacity to infiltrate, invade, or metastasize to distant sites, as do malignant tumors. Because they grow and expand slowly, they usually develop a rim of compressed connective tissue, sometimes called a fibrous *capsule,* which separates them from the host tissue. This capsule is derived largely from the extracellular matrix of the native tissue due to atrophy of normal parenchymal cells under the pressure of an expanding tumor. Such encapsulation does not prevent tumor growth, but it keeps the benign neoplasm as a discrete, readily palpable, and easily movable mass that can be surgically enucleated (Figs. 7–12 and 7–13). Although a well-defined cleavage plane exists around most benign tumors, in some it is lacking. For example, hemangiomas (neoplasms composed of tangled blood vessels) are often unencapsulated and may appear to permeate the site in which they arise (commonly the dermis of the skin).

The growth of cancers is accompanied by progressive infiltration, invasion, and destruction of the surrounding tissue. In general, malignant tumors are poorly demarcated from the surrounding normal tissue, and a well-defined cleavage plane is lacking (Figs. 7–14 and 7–15). Slowly expanding malignant tumors, however, may develop an apparently enclosing fibrous capsule and may push along a broad front into adjacent normal structures. Histologic examination of such pseudo-encapsulated masses almost always shows rows of cells penetrating the margin and infiltrating the adjacent structures, a crablike pattern of growth that constitutes the popular image of cancer.

Most malignant tumors are obviously invasive and can be expected to penetrate the wall of the colon or uterus, for example, or fungate through the surface of the skin. They recognize no normal anatomic boundaries. Such invasiveness makes their surgical resection difficult or impossible, and even if the tumor appears well circumscribed it is necessary to remove a considerable margin of apparently normal tissues adjacent to the infiltrative neoplasm. *Next to the development*

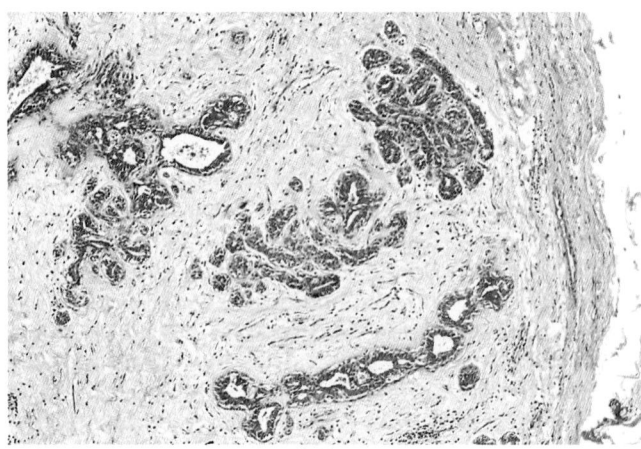

FIGURE 7–13 Microscopic view of fibroadenoma of the breast seen in Figure 7–12. The fibrous capsule *(right)* delimits the tumor from the surrounding tissue. (Courtesy of Dr. Trace Worrell, University of Texas Southwestern Medical School, Dallas, TX.)

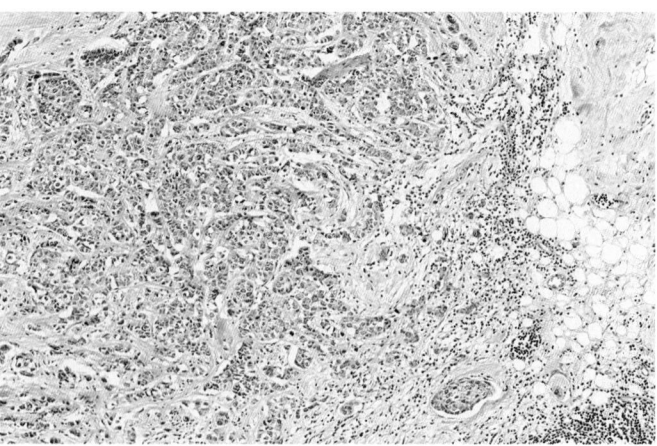

FIGURE 7–15 The microscopic view of the breast carcinoma seen in Figure 7–14 illustrates the invasion of breast stroma and fat by nests and cords of tumor cells (compare with fibroadenoma shown in Fig. 7–13). The absence of a well-defined capsule should be noted. (Courtesy of Dr. Trace Worrell, University of Texas Southwestern Medical School, Dallas, TX.)

of metastases, invasiveness is the most reliable feature that differentiates malignant from benign tumors. We noted earlier that some cancers seem to evolve from a preinvasive stage referred to as *carcinoma in situ*. This commonly occurs in carcinomas of the skin, breast, and certain other sites and is best illustrated by carcinoma of the uterine cervix (Chapter 22). *In situ epithelial cancers display the cytologic features of malignancy without invasion of the basement membrane.* They may be considered one step removed from invasive cancer; with time, most penetrate the basement membrane and invade the subepithelial stroma.

METASTASIS

Metastases are tumor implants discontinuous with the primary tumor. *Metastasis unequivocally marks a tumor as malignant because benign neoplasms do not metastasize.* The invasiveness of cancers permits them to penetrate into blood vessels, lymphatics, and body cavities, providing the opportunity for spread. *With few exceptions, all malignant tumors can metastasize.* The major exceptions are most malignant neoplasms of the glial cells in the central nervous system, called *gliomas*, and basal cell carcinomas of the skin. Both are locally invasive forms of cancer, but they rarely metastasize. It is evident then that the properties of invasion and metastasis are separable.

In general, the more aggressive, the more rapidly growing, and the larger the primary neoplasm, the greater the likelihood that it will metastasize or already has metastasized. There are innumerable exceptions, however. Small, well-differentiated, slowly growing lesions sometimes metastasize widely; conversely, some rapidly growing, large lesions remain localized for years. Many factors relating to both invader and host are involved.

Approximately 30% of newly diagnosed individuals with solid tumors (excluding skin cancers other than melanomas) present with metastases. Metastatic spread strongly reduces the possibility of cure; hence, short of prevention of cancer, no achievement would be of greater benefit to patients than methods to block metastases.

Pathways of Spread

Dissemination of cancers may occur through one of three pathways: (1) direct seeding of body cavities or surfaces, (2) lymphatic spread, and (3) hematogenous spread. Although direct transplantation of tumor cells, as for example on surgical instruments, may theoretically occur, it is rare and we do not discuss this artificial mode of dissemination further. Each of the three major pathways is described separately.

Seeding of Body Cavities and Surfaces. Seeding of body cavities and surfaces may occur whenever a malignant neoplasm penetrates into a natural "open field." Most often involved is the peritoneal cavity (Fig. 7–16), but any other cavity—pleural, pericardial, subarachnoid, and joint space—may be affected. Such seeding is particularly characteristic of carcinomas arising in the ovaries, when, not infrequently, all peritoneal surfaces become coated with a heavy layer of cancerous glaze. Remarkably, the tumor cells may remain confined to the surface of the coated abdominal viscera without penetrating into the substance. Sometimes mucus-secreting appendiceal carcinomas fill the peritoneal cavity

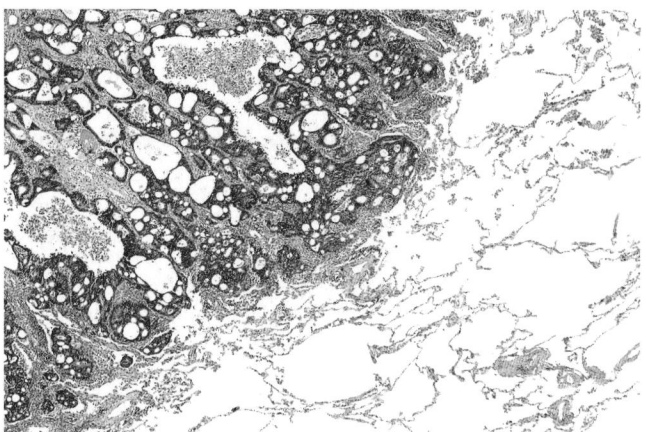

FIGURE 7–16 Colon carcinoma invading pericolonic adipose tissue. (Courtesy of Dr. Melissa Upton, University of Washington, Seattle, WA.)

with a gelatinous neoplastic mass referred to as *pseudomyxoma peritonei*.

Lymphatic Spread. Transport through lymphatics is the most common pathway for the initial dissemination of carcinomas (Fig. 7–17), and sarcomas may also use this route. Tumors do not contain functional lymphatics, but lymphatic vessels located at the tumor margins are apparently sufficient for the lymphatic spread of tumor cells.[11] The emphasis on lymphatic spread for carcinomas and hematogenous spread for sarcomas is misleading, because ultimately there are numerous interconnections between the vascular and the lymphatic systems. *The pattern of lymph node involvement follows the natural routes of lymphatic drainage.* Because carcinomas of the breast usually arise in the upper outer quadrants, they generally disseminate first to the axillary lymph nodes. Cancers of the inner quadrants drain to the nodes along the internal mammary arteries. Thereafter the infraclavicular and supraclavicular nodes may become involved. Carcinomas of the lung arising in the major respiratory passages metastasize first to the perihilar tracheobronchial and mediastinal

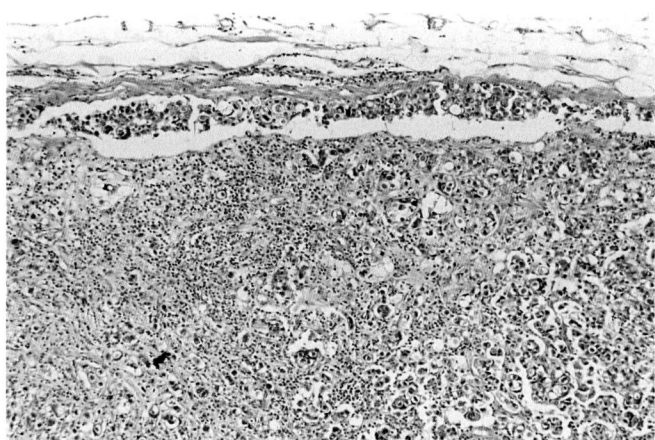

FIGURE 7–17 Axillary lymph node with metastatic breast carcinoma. The subcapsular sinus *(top)* is distended with tumor cells. Nests of tumor cells have also invaded the subcapsular cortex. (Courtesy of Dr. Trace Worrell, University of Texas Southwestern Medical School, Dallas, TX.)

nodes. Local lymph nodes, however, may be bypassed—so-called "skip metastasis"—because of venous-lymphatic anastomoses or because inflammation or radiation has obliterated lymphatic channels.

In breast cancer, determining the involvement of axillary lymph nodes is very important for assessing the future course of the disease and for selecting suitable therapeutic strategies. To avoid the considerable surgical morbidity associated with a full axillary lymph node dissection, *biopsy of sentinel nodes* is often used to assess the presence or absence of metastatic lesions in the lymph nodes. A sentinel lymph node is defined as "the first node in a regional lymphatic basin that receives lymph flow from the primary tumor."[12] Sentinel node mapping can be done by injection of radiolabeled tracers and blue dyes, and the use of frozen section upon the sentinel lymph node at the time of surgery can guide the surgeon to the appropriate therapy. Sentinel node biopsy has also been used for detecting the spread of melanomas, colon cancers, and other tumors.[12,13]

In many cases the regional nodes serve as effective barriers to further dissemination of the tumor, at least for a while. Conceivably the cells, after arrest within the node, may be destroyed by a tumor-specific immune response. Drainage of tumor cell debris or tumor antigens, or both, also induces reactive changes within nodes. Thus, enlargement of nodes may be caused by (1) the spread and growth of cancer cells or (2) reactive hyperplasia (Chapter 13). Therefore, *nodal enlargement in proximity to a cancer, while it must arouse suspicion, does not necessarily mean dissemination of the primary lesion.*

Hematogenous Spread. Hematogenous spread is typical of sarcomas but is also seen with carcinomas. Arteries, with their thicker walls, are less readily penetrated than are veins. Arterial spread may occur, however, when tumor cells pass through the pulmonary capillary beds or pulmonary arteriovenous shunts or when pulmonary metastases themselves give rise to additional tumor emboli. In such vascular spread, several factors influence the patterns of distribution of the metastases. With venous invasion the blood-borne cells follow the venous flow draining the site of the neoplasm, and the tumor cells often come to rest in the first capillary bed they encounter. Understandably the liver and lungs are most frequently involved in such hematogenous dissemination (Figs. 7–18 and 7–19), because all portal area drainage flows to the liver and all caval blood flows to the lungs. Cancers arising in close proximity to the vertebral column often embolize through the paravertebral plexus, and this pathway is involved in the frequent vertebral metastases of carcinomas of the thyroid and prostate.

Certain cancers have a propensity for invasion of veins. Renal cell carcinoma often invades the branches of the renal vein and then the renal vein itself to grow in a snakelike fashion up the inferior vena cava, sometimes reaching the right side of the heart. Hepatocellular carcinomas often penetrate portal and hepatic radicles to grow within them into the main venous channels. Remarkably, such intravenous growth may not be accompanied by widespread dissemination. Histologic evidence of penetration of small vessels at the site of the primary neoplasm is obviously an ominous feature. Such changes, however, must be viewed guardedly because, for reasons discussed later, they do not indicate the inevitable development of metastases.

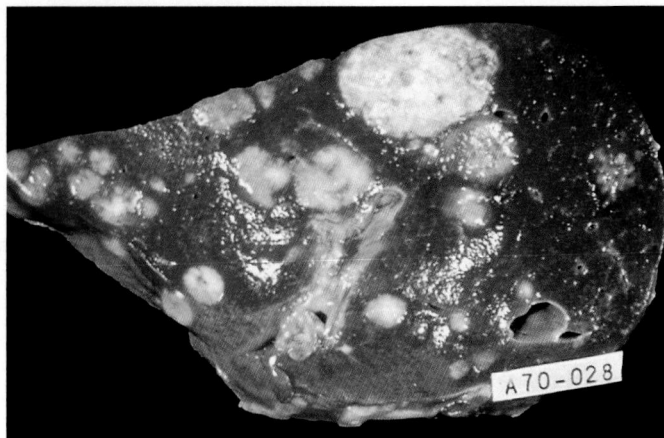

FIGURE 7–18   A liver studded with metastatic cancer.

Many observations suggest that mere anatomic localization of the neoplasm and natural pathways of venous drainage do not wholly explain the systemic distributions of metastases. For example, breast carcinoma preferentially spreads to bone, bronchogenic carcinomas tend to involve the adrenals and the brain, and neuroblastomas spread to the liver and bones. Conversely, skeletal muscles and the spleen, despite the large percentage of blood flow they receive and the enormous vascular beds present, are rarely the site of secondary deposits. The probable basis of such tissue-specific homing of tumor cells is discussed later.

The distinguishing features of benign and malignant tumors discussed in this overview are summarized in Table 7–2 and Figure 7–20. With this background on the structure and behavior of neoplasms, we now discuss the origin of tumors, starting with insights gained from the epidemiology of cancer and followed by the molecular basis of carcinogenesis.

Epidemiology

Because cancer is a disorder of cell growth and behavior, its ultimate cause has to be defined at the cellular and subcellular levels. Study of cancer patterns in populations, however, can

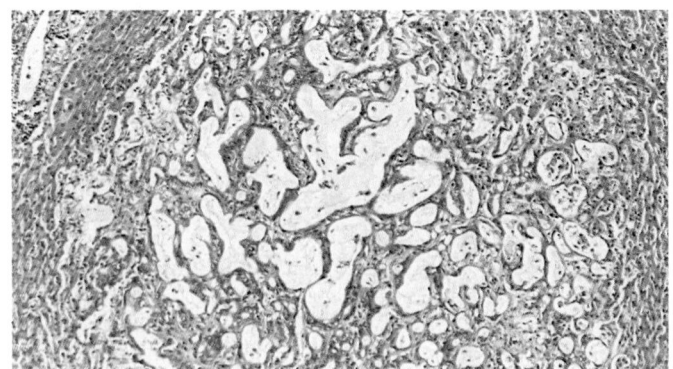

FIGURE 7–19   Microscopic view of liver metastasis. A pancreatic adenocarcinoma has formed a metastatic nodule in the liver. (Courtesy of Dr. Trace Worrell, University of Texas Southwestern Medical School, Dallax, TX.)

TABLE 7–2 **Comparisons between Benign and Malignant Tumors**

Characteristics	Benign	Malignant
Differentiation/anaplasia	Well differentiated; structure sometimes typical of tissue of origin	Some lack of differentiation with anaplasia; structure often atypical
Rate of growth	Usually progressive and slow; may come to a standstill or regress; mitotic figures rare and normal	Erratic and may be slow to rapid; mitotic figures may be numerous and abnormal
Local invasion	Usually cohesive expansile well-demarcated masses that do not invade or infiltrate surrounding normal tissues	Locally invasive, infiltrating surrounding tissue; sometimes may be seemingly cohesive and expansile
Metastasis	Absent	Frequently present; the larger and more undifferentiated the primary, the more likely are metastases

contribute substantially to knowledge about the origins of cancer. Epidemiologic studies have established the causative link between smoking and lung cancer, and comparison of diet and cancer rates in the Western world and Africa has implicated high dietary fat and low fiber in the development of colon cancer. Major insights into the causes of cancer can be obtained by epidemiologic studies that relate particular environmental, racial (possibly hereditary), and cultural influences to the occurrence of specific neoplasms. Certain diseases associated with an increased risk of developing cancer (preneoplastic disorders) also provide clues to the pathogenesis of cancer. In the following discussion we first summarize the overall incidence of cancer to gain an insight into the magnitude of the cancer problem, then we review some factors relating to the patient and environment that influence the predisposition to cancer.

CANCER INCIDENCE

In some measure, an individual's likelihood of developing a cancer is expressed by national incidence and mortality rates. For example, residents of the United States have about a one in five chance of dying of cancer. There were, it is estimated, about 1,437,180 new cancer cases and 565,650 deaths from cancer in 2008, representing 23% of all mortality,[1] a frequency surpassed only by deaths caused by cardiovascular diseases. These data do not include an additional 1 million, for the most part readily curable, non-melanoma cancers of the skin and

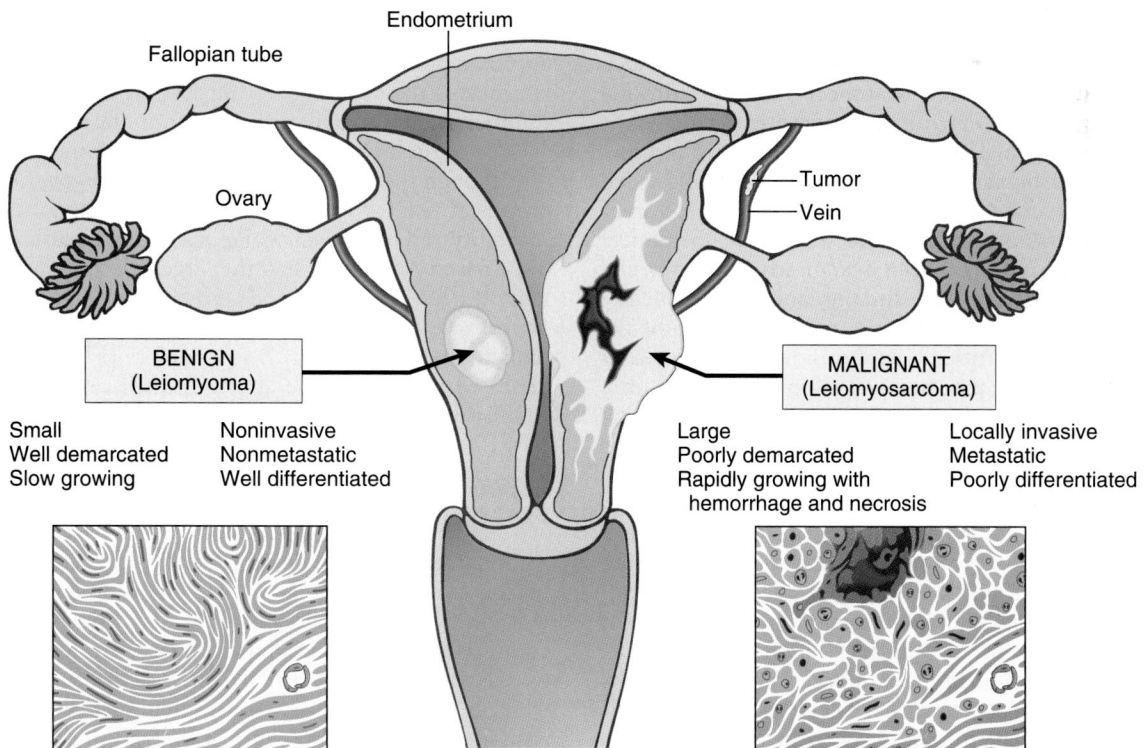

FIGURE 7–20 Comparison between a benign tumor of the myometrium (leiomyoma) and a malignant tumor of the same origin (leiomyosarcoma).

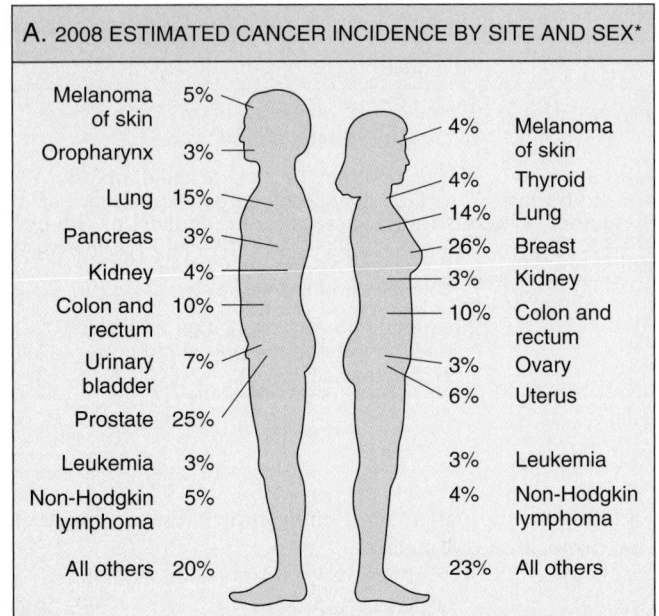

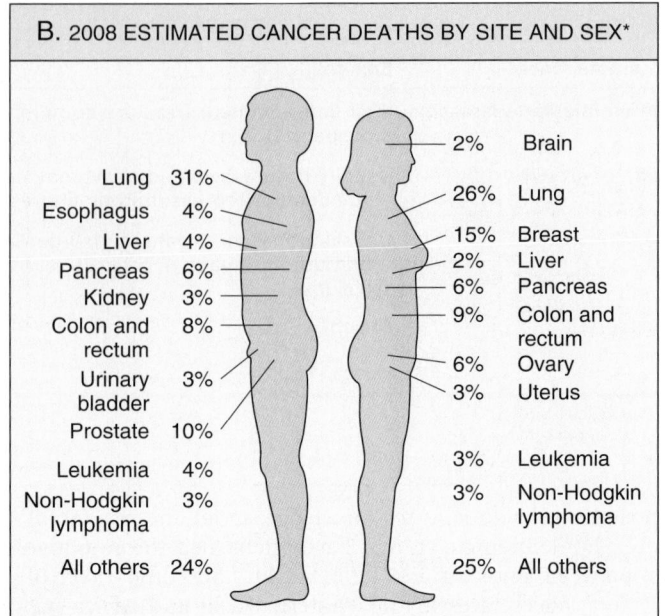

FIGURE 7–21   Cancer incidence and mortality by site and sex. Excludes basal cell and squamous cell skin cancers and in situ carcinomas, except urinary bladder. (Adapted from Jemal A et al.: Cancer statistics, 2008. CA Cancer J Clin 58:2, 2008.)

122,000 cases of carcinoma in situ, largely of the female breast and melanomas.[1] The major organ sites affected and the estimated frequency of cancer deaths are shown in Figure 7–21. The most common tumors in men arise in the prostate, lung, and colorectum. In women, cancers of the breast, lung, and colon and rectum are the most frequent. Cancers of the lung, female breast, prostate, and colon/rectum constitute more than 50% of cancer diagnoses and cancer deaths in the U.S. population.[1]

The age-adjusted death rates (number of deaths per 100,000 population) for many forms of cancer have significantly changed over the years. Many of the long-term comparisons are noteworthy. Over the last 50 years of the twentieth century, the overall age-adjusted cancer death rate significantly increased in both men and women. However, since 1995 the cancer incidence rate in men has stabilized and since 1990 the cancer death rate in men has decreased 18.4%.[1] In women the cancer incidence rate stabilized in 1995, and the cancer death rate has decreased 10.4% since 1991.[1] Among men nearly 80% of the total decrease in cancer death rates is accounted for by decreases in death rates from lung, prostate, and colorectal cancers since 1990.[1] Among women nearly 60% of the decrease in cancer death rates is due to reductions in death rates from breast and colorectal cancers.[1] Nearly 40% of the sex-specific decreases in cancer death rates is accounted for by a reduction in lung cancer deaths in men and breast cancer deaths in women.[1] Decreased use of tobacco products is responsible for the reduction in lung cancer deaths, while improved detection and treatment are responsible for the decrease in death rates for colorectal, female breast, and prostate cancer.[1] The last half century has seen a decline in the number of deaths caused by cervical cancer that relates to earlier diagnosis made possible by the Papanicolaou (Pap) smear. The downward trend in deaths from stomach cancer has been attributed to a decrease in some dietary carcinogens, as a consequence of better food

preservation or changes in dietary habits. Unfortunately, between 1990–1991 and 2004, lung cancer death rates in women, and liver and intrahepatic bile duct cancer death rates in men, increased substantially, offsetting some of the improvement in survival from other cancers.[1] Indeed, although in women carcinomas of the breast occur about 2.5 times more frequently than those of the lung, lung cancer has become the leading cause of cancer deaths in women. Deaths from primary liver cancers, which declined between 1930 and 1970, have approximately doubled during the past 30 years. This number is expected to increase over the coming decades, as the large number of individuals infected with the hepatitis C virus (HCV) begin to develop hepatocellular carcinoma.

Although race is not a strict biologic category, it can define groups at risk for certain cancers.[14,15] The disparity in cancer mortality rates between white and black Americans persists, but African Americans had the largest decline in cancer mortality during the past decade. Hispanics living in the United States have a lower frequency of the most common tumors than the white non-Hispanic population but a higher incidence of tumors of the stomach, liver, uterine cervix, and gallbladder, as well as certain childhood leukemias.

GEOGRAPHIC AND ENVIRONMENTAL FACTORS

Although genetics and environmental triggers both play a role in the pathogenesis of cancer, environmental factors are thought to be the more significant contributors in most common sporadic cancers. In one large study the proportion of risk from environmental causes was found to be 65%, whereas heritable factors contributed 26% to 42% of cancer risk. Remarkable differences found in the incidence and death rates of specific forms of cancer around the world also suggest a role for environmental factors.[16,17] For example, the

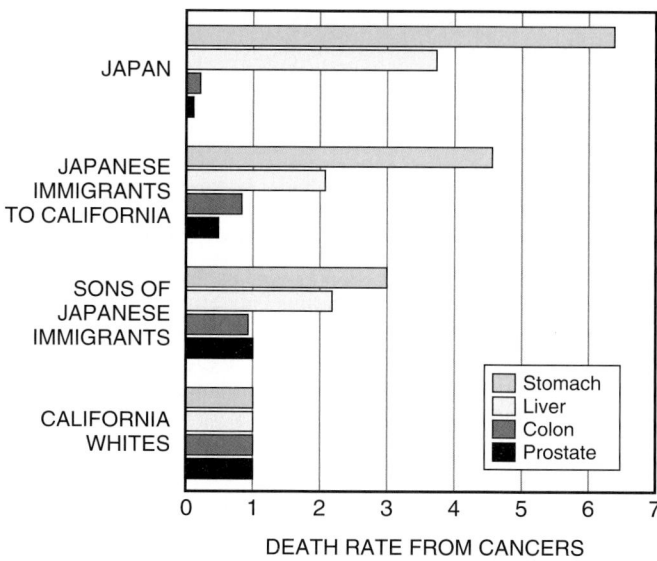

DEATH RATE FROM CANCERS
(Compared with rate for California whites)

FIGURE 7–22 The change in incidence of various cancers with migration from Japan to the United States provides evidence that the occurrence of cancers is related to components of the environment that differ in the two countries. The incidence of each kind of cancer is expressed as the ratio of the death rate in the population being considered to that in a hypothetical population of California whites with the same age distribution; the death rates for whites are thus defined as 1. The death rates among immigrants and immigrants' sons tend consistently toward California norms. (From Cairns J: The cancer problem. In Readings from Scientific American—Cancer Biology. New York, WH Freeman, 1986, p 13.)

death rate for stomach carcinoma in both men and women is seven to eight times higher in Japan than in the United States. In contrast, the death rate from carcinoma of the lung is slightly more than twice as great in the United States as in Japan. Although racial predispositions cannot be ruled out, it is generally believed that most of these geographic differences are the consequence of environmental influences. Indeed, comparing mortality rates for Japanese immigrants to the United States and Japanese born in the United States of immigrant parents (Nisei) with those of long-term residents of both countries shows that cancer mortality rates for first-generation Japanese immigrants are intermediate between those of natives of Japan and natives of California, and the two rates come closer with each passing generation (Fig. 7–22). This points strongly to environmental and cultural factors rather than genetic predisposition.

There is no paucity of carcinogenic environmental factors: they lurk in the ambient environment, in the workplace, in food, and in personal practices. Individuals may be exposed to carcinogenic factors when they go outside (ultraviolet [UV] rays, smog), in their medication (methotrexate), at work (asbestos, vinyl chloride; Table 7–3), or at home (high-fat diet, alcohol). Overall, mortality data indicate that the most overweight individuals in the U.S. population have a 52% (men) and 62% (women) higher death rate from cancer than do their slimmer counterparts. Indeed, obesity is associated with approximately 14% of cancer deaths in men and 20% in women.[18] Alcohol abuse alone increases the risk of carcinomas of the oropharynx (excluding lip), larynx, and esophagus and,

by the development of alcoholic cirrhosis, hepatocellular carcinoma. Smoking, particularly of cigarettes, has been implicated in cancer of the mouth, pharynx, larynx, esophagus, pancreas, bladder, and most significantly, about 90% of lung cancer deaths (Chapter 9). Cigarette smoking has been called the single most important environmental factor contributing to premature death in the United States. Alcohol and tobacco together synergistically increase the danger of incurring cancers in the upper aerodigestive tract. The risk of cervical cancer is linked to age at first intercourse and the number of sex partners, and it is now known that infection by venereally transmitted human papillomavirus (HPV) contributes to cervical dysplasia and cancer. It appears that almost everything one does to gain a livelihood or for pleasure is fattening, immoral, illegal, or, even worse, oncogenic.

AGE

Age has an important influence on the likelihood of being afflicted with cancer. Most carcinomas occur in the later years of life (>55 years). Cancer is the main cause of death among women aged 40 to 79 and among men aged 60 to 79; the decline in deaths after age 80 is due to the lower number of individuals who reach this age. The rising incidence with age may be explained by the accumulation of somatic mutations associated with the emergence of malignant neoplasms (discussed later). The decline in immune competence that accompanies aging may also be a factor.

However, children are not spared; cancer accounts for slightly more than 10% of all deaths in children under age 15 in the United States, second only to accidents. However, the types of cancers that predominate in children are significantly different from those seen in adults. Carcinomas, the most common general category of tumor in adults, are extraordinarily rare among children. Instead, acute leukemia and primitive neoplasms of the central nervous system are responsible for approximately 60% of childhood cancer deaths. The common neoplasms of infancy and childhood include the so-called small round blue cell tumors such as neuroblastoma, Wilms tumor, retinoblastoma, acute leukemias, and rhabdomyosarcomas. These are discussed in Chapter 10 and elsewhere in the text.

GENETIC PREDISPOSITION TO CANCER

One frequently asked question is: "My mother and father both died of cancer. Does that mean I am doomed to get it?" Based on current knowledge, the answer must be carefully qualified.[19,20] Evidence now indicates that for a large number of cancer types, including the most common forms, there exist not only environmental influences but also hereditary predispositions. For example, lung cancer is in most instances clearly related to cigarette smoking, yet mortality from lung cancer has been shown to be four times greater among nonsmoking relatives (parents and siblings) of lung cancer patients than among nonsmoking relatives of controls (the effects of secondhand smoke may confound some of these results). Less than 10% of cancer patients have inherited mutations that predispose to cancer, and the frequency is even lower (around 0.1%) for certain types of tumors. Despite the low frequency, the

TABLE 7–3   Occupational Cancers

Agents or Groups of Agents	Human Cancer Site for Which Reasonable Evidence Is Available	Typical Use or Occurrence
Arsenic and arsenic compounds	Lung, skin, hemangiosarcoma	Byproduct of metal smelting; component of alloys, electrical and semiconductor devices, medications and herbicides, fungicides, and animal dips
Asbestos	Lung, mesothelioma; gastrointestinal tract (esophagus, stomach, large intestine)	Formerly used for many applications because of fire, heat, and friction resistance; still found in existing construction as well as fire-resistant textiles, friction materials (i.e., brake linings), underlayment and roofing papers, and floor tiles
Benzene	Leukemia, Hodgkin lymphoma	Principal component of light oil; despite known risk, many applications exist in printing and lithography, paint, rubber, dry cleaning, adhesives and coatings, and detergents; formerly widely used as solvent and fumigant
Beryllium and beryllium compounds	Lung	Missile fuel and space vehicles; hardener for lightweight metal alloys, particularly in aerospace applications and nuclear reactors
Cadmium and cadmium compounds	Prostate	Uses include yellow pigments and phosphors; found in solders; used in batteries and as alloy and in metal platings and coatings
Chromium compounds	Lung	Component of metal alloys, paints, pigments, and preservatives
Nickel compounds	Nose, lung	Nickel plating; component of ferrous alloys, ceramics, and batteries; by-product of stainless-steel arc welding
Radon and its decay products	Lung	From decay of minerals containing uranium; potentially serious hazard in quarries and underground mines
Vinyl chloride	Angiosarcoma, liver	Refrigerant; monomer for vinyl polymers; adhesive for plastics; formerly inert aerosol propellant in pressurized containers

Modified from Stellman JM, Stellman SD: Cancer and workplace. CA Cancer J Clin 46:70, 1996.

recognition of inherited predisposition to cancer has had a major impact on the understanding of cancer pathogenesis. Moreover, genes that are causally associated with cancers that have a strong hereditary component are generally also involved in the much more common sporadic forms of the same tumor. Genetic predisposition to cancer can be divided into three categories (Table 7–4).

Autosomal Dominant Inherited Cancer Syndromes. Inherited cancer syndromes include several well-defined cancers in which inheritance of a single autosomal dominant mutant gene greatly increases the risk of developing a tumor. The inherited mutation is usually a point mutation occurring in a single allele of a tumor suppressor gene. The silencing of the second allele occurs in somatic cells, generally as a consequence of deletion or recombination. Childhood *retinoblastoma* is the most striking example in this category. Approximately 40% of retinoblastomas are inherited. Carriers of a mutant of the *RB tumor suppressor gene* have a 10,000-fold increased risk of developing retinoblastoma, usually bilateral. They also have a greatly increased risk of developing a second cancer, particularly osteosarcoma. Familial adenomatous polyposis is an autosomal dominant hereditary disorder caused by mutation of the adenomatous polyposis coli (*APC*) tumor suppressor gene. Other autosomal dominant cancer syn-

dromes include Li-Fraumeni syndrome resulting from germline mutations of the *p53* gene; multiple endocrine neoplasia types 1 and 2 (MEN-1 and MEN-2) caused by mutation in the genes that encode the menin transcription factor and the RET tyrosine kinase, respectively; hereditary nonpolyposis colon cancer (HNPCC), a condition caused by inactivation of a DNA mismatch repair gene (also listed below among repair defects); and several others listed in Table 7–4.

There are several features that characterize inherited cancer syndromes:

○ In each syndrome, tumors tend to arise in specific sites and tissues, although they may involve more than one site. There is no increase in predisposition to cancers in general. For example, in MEN-2, thyroid, parathyroid, and adrenals are involved, while in MEN-1, the pituitary, parathyroid, and pancreas are involved. Patients with familial adenomatous polyposis develop innumerable polypoid adenomas of the colon, and virtually 100% of those affected develop a colonic adenocarcinoma by age 50. The one exception to this tumor specific tissue involvement is Li-Fraumeni syndrome.

○ Tumors within this group are often associated with a specific marker phenotype. For example, there may be multiple

TABLE 7–4 Examples of Inherited Predisposition to Cancer	
INHERITED CANCER SYNDROMES (AUTOSOMAL DOMINANT)	
Gene	*Inherited Predisposition*
RB	Retinoblastoma
p53	Li-Fraumeni syndrome (various tumors)
p16/INK4A	Melanoma
APC	Familial adenomatous polyposis/colon cancer
NF1, NF2	Neurofibromatosis 1 and 2
BRCA1, BRCA2	Breast and ovarian tumors
MEN1, RET	Multiple endocrine neoplasia 1 and 2
MSH2, MLH1, MSH6	Hereditary nonpolyposis colon cancer
PTCH	Nevoid basal cell carcinoma syndrome
PTEN	Cowden syndrome (epithelial cancers)
LKB1	Peutz-Jegher syndrome (epithelial cancers)
VHL	Renal cell carcinomas
INHERITED AUTOSOMAL RECESSIVE SYNDROMES OF DEFECTIVE DNA REPAIR	
Xeroderma pigmentosum	
Ataxia-telangiectasia	
Bloom syndrome	
Fanconi anemia	
FAMILIAL CANCERS	
Familial clustering of cases, but role of inherited predisposition not clear for each individual	
Breast cancer	
Ovarian cancer	
Pancreatic cancer	

benign tumors in the affected tissue, as occurs in familial polyposis of the colon and in MEN. Sometimes, there are abnormalities in tissue that are not the target of transformation (e.g., Lisch nodules and café-au-lait spots in neurofibromatosis type 1; see Chapter 27).

As in other autosomal dominant conditions, both incomplete penetrance and variable expressivity occur.

Defective DNA-Repair Syndromes. Besides the dominantly inherited precancerous conditions, a group of cancer-predisposing conditions is collectively characterized by defects in DNA repair and resultant DNA instability. These conditions generally have an autosomal recessive pattern of inheritance. Included in this group are xeroderma pigmentosum, ataxia-telangiectasia, and Bloom syndrome, all rare diseases characterized by genetic instability resulting from defects in DNA-repair genes. Also included here is HNPCC, an autosomal dominant condition caused by inactivation of a DNA mismatch repair gene.[21] HNPCC is the most common cancer predisposition syndrome, increasing the susceptibility of cancer of the colon, the small intestine, endometrium, and ovary (Chapter 17).

Familial Cancers. Besides the inherited syndromes of cancer susceptibility, cancer may occur at higher frequency in certain families without a clearly defined pattern of transmission. Virtually all the common types of cancers that occur sporadically have also been reported to occur in familial forms. Examples include carcinomas of colon, breast, ovary, and brain, as well as melanomas and lymphomas. *Features that characterize familial cancers include early age at onset, tumors arising in two or more close relatives of the index case, and sometimes, multiple or bilateral tumors.* Familial cancers are not associated with specific marker phenotypes. For example,

in contrast to the familial adenomatous polyp syndrome, familial colonic cancers do not arise in preexisting benign polyps. The transmission pattern of familial cancers is not clear. In general, siblings have a risk between two and three times greater than unrelated individuals. Segregation analyses of large families usually show that predisposition to the tumors is dominant, but multifactorial inheritance cannot be easily ruled out. It is likely that familial susceptibility to cancer may depend on multiple low-penetrance alleles, each contributing to only a small increase in the risk of tumor development. Genome-wide association studies show great promise in identifying such alleles (Chapter 5).[22] It has been estimated that 10% to 20% of patients with breast or ovarian cancer have a first- or second-degree relative with one of these tumors. Although two breast cancer susceptibility genes, named *BRCA1* and *BRCA2*, have been identified, mutation of these genes occurs in no more than 3% of breast cancers.[20] A similar situation occurs in familial melanomas, in which a mutation of the *p16* tumor suppressor gene has been identified. However, mutation in this gene accounts for only about 20% of familial melanoma kindreds, suggesting that other factors are involved in the familial predisposition.[23]

Interactions between Genetic and Nongenetic Factors. What can be said about the influence of heredity on the majority of malignant neoplasms? It could be argued that they are largely of environmental origin, but lack of family history does not preclude an inherited component. It is generally difficult to sort out the hereditary and acquired basis of a tumor, because these factors often interact closely. The interaction between genetic and nongenetic factors is particularly complex when tumor development depends on the action of multiple contributory genes. Even in tumors with a well-defined inherited component, the risk of developing the tumor can be greatly influenced by nongenetic factors. For instance, breast cancer risk in female carriers of *BRCA1* or *BRCA2* mutations is almost threefold higher for women born after 1940, as compared with the risks for women born before that year.[20] Furthermore, the genotype can significantly influence the likelihood of developing environmentally induced cancers. Inherited variations (polymorphisms) of enzymes that metabolize procarcinogens to their active carcinogenic forms (see "Initiation of Carcinogenesis") can influence the susceptibility to cancer. Of interest in this regard are genes that encode the cytochrome P-450 enzymes. As discussed later under "Chemical Carcinogenesis," polymorphism at one of the P-450 loci confers inherited susceptibility to lung cancers in cigarette smokers. More such associations are likely to be found.

NONHEREDITARY PREDISPOSING CONDITIONS

The only certain way of avoiding cancer is not to be born; to live is to incur the risk. Certain predisposing influences, such as environment, behaviors, and clinical conditions, can increase that risk, however. For example, regenerative, metaplastic, hyperplastic, and dysplastic proliferations are fertile soil for the origin of a malignant tumor, because cell replication is involved in neoplastic transformation. Indeed, proliferation may be required for neoplastic transformation in some settings, since it is proliferating cells that accumulate the genetic lesions required for carcinogenesis.

Chronic Inflammation and Cancer. In 1863 Virchow proposed that *cancer develops at sites of chronic inflammation*, and the potential relationships between cancer and inflammation have been studied since then.[24] This is exemplified by the increased risk of cancer in individuals affected by a variety of chronic inflammatory diseases of the gastrointestinal tract (Table 7–5). These include ulcerative colitis, *Helicobacter pylori* gastritis, viral hepatitis, and chronic pancreatitis. Although the precise mechanisms that link inflammation and cancer development have not been established, recent work has demonstrated that in the setting of unresolved chronic inflammation, as occurs in viral hepatitis or chronic gastritis, the immune response may become maladaptive, promoting tumorigenesis.[24] As with any cause of tissue injury, there is a compensatory proliferation of cells so as to repair the damage. This regenerative process is aided and abetted by a plethora of growth factors, cytokines, chemokines, and other bioactive substances produced by activated immune cells that promote cell survival, tissue remodeling, and angiogenesis. In some cases, chronic inflammation may increase the pool of tissue stem cells, which become subject to the effect of mutagens. These mediators also cause genomic stress and mutations; additionally the activated immune cells produce reactive oxygen species that are directly genotoxic. To add insult to injury, many of these mediators promote cell survival, even in the face of genomic damage. In the short term this can be adaptive; the organism must survive, and the damaged cells can be repaired or eliminated later. However, in chronic inflammation such behavior is maladaptive, since it allows the creation and fixation of such mutations, eventually leading to cancer. Whatever the precise mechanism, the link between chronic inflammation and cancer has practical implications. For instance, expression of the enzyme *cyclooxygenase-2*

(COX-2), which brings about the conversion of arachidonic acid into prostaglandins (Chapter 2), is induced by inflammatory stimuli and is increased in colon cancers and other tumors.[25] The development of COX-2 inhibitors for cancer treatment is an active area of research.[26]

Precancerous Conditions. Certain non-neoplastic disorders—*the chronic atrophic gastritis of pernicious anemia, solar keratosis of the skin, chronic ulcerative colitis, and leukoplakia of the oral cavity, vulva, and penis*—have such a well-defined association with cancer that they have been termed *precancerous conditions*. This designation is somewhat unfortunate, because in the great majority of these lesions no malignant neoplasm emerges. Nonetheless, the term persists because it calls attention to the increased risk. Certain forms of benign neoplasia also constitute precancerous conditions. The villous adenoma of the colon, as it increases in size, becomes malignant in up to 50% of cases. It might be asked: Is there not a risk with all benign neoplasms? Although some risk may be inherent, a large cumulative experience indicates that most benign neoplasms do not become cancerous. Nonetheless, numerous examples could be offered of cancers arising, albeit rarely, in benign tumors—for example, a leiomyosarcoma beginning in a leiomyoma, and carcinoma appearing in long-standing pleomorphic adenomas. Generalization is impossible, because each type of benign neoplasm is associated with a particular level of risk ranging from virtually never to frequently. Only follow-up studies of large series of each neoplasm can establish the level of risk, and always the question remains: Did the cancer arise from a nonmalignant cell in the benign tumor, or did the benign tumor contain, from the outset, a silent or indolent malignant focus?

Molecular Basis of Cancer

The literature on the molecular basis of cancer continues to proliferate at such a rapid pace that it is easy to get lost in the growing forest of information. We list some fundamental principles before delving into the details of the molecular basis of cancer.

- *Nonlethal genetic damage lies at the heart of carcinogenesis.* Such genetic damage (or mutation) may be acquired by the action of environmental agents, such as chemicals, radiation, or viruses, or it may be inherited in the germ line.[26] The term *environmental*, used in this context, involves any acquired defect caused by exogenous agents or endogenous products of cell metabolism. Not all mutations, however, are "environmentally" induced. Some may be spontaneous and stochastic, falling into the category of bad luck.

- *A tumor is formed by the clonal expansion of a single precursor cell that has incurred genetic damage (i.e., tumors are monoclonal).* Clonality of tumors can be assessed in women who are heterozygous for polymorphic X-linked markers, such as the androgen receptor. The principle underlying such an analysis is illustrated in Figure 7–23. The most commonly used method to determine tumor clonality involves the analysis of methylation patterns adjacent to the highly polymorphic locus of the human androgen receptor gene, *AR*.[27] The frequency of such polymorphisms in the general population is more than 90%, so it is easy to estab-

TABLE 7-5 Chronic Inflammatory States and Cancer		
Pathologic Condition	**Associated Neoplasm(s)**	**Etiologic Agent**
Asbestosis, silicosis	Mesothelioma, lung carcinoma	Asbestos fibers, silica particles
Bronchitis	Lung carcinoma	Silica, asbestos, smoking (nitrosamines, peroxides)
Cystitis, bladder inflammation	Bladder carcinoma	Chronic indwelling urinary catheters
Gingivitis, lichen planus	Oral squamous cell carcinoma	
Inflammatory bowel disease	Colorectal carcinoma	
Lichen sclerosis	Vulvar squamous cell carcinoma	
Chronic pancreatitis	Pancreatic carcinoma	Alcoholism
Hereditary pancreatitis	Pancreatic carcinoma	Mutation in trypsinogen gene
Reflux esophagitis, Barrett esophagus	Esophageal carcinoma	Gastric acids
Sialadenitis	Salivary gland carcinoma	
Sjögren syndrome, Hashimoto thyroiditis	MALT lymphoma	
CANCERS ASSOCIATED WITH INFECTIOUS AGENTS		
Opisthorchis, cholangitis	Cholangiosarcoma, colon carcinoma	Liver flukes (*Opisthorchis viverrini*) Bile acids
Chronic cholecystitis	Gallbladder cancer	Bacteria, gallbladder stones
Gastritis/ulcers	Gastric adenocarcinoma, MALT	*Helicobacter pylori*
Hepatitis	Hepatocellular carcinoma	Hepatitis B and/or C virus
Mononucleosis	B-cell non-Hodgkin lymphoma and Hodgkin lymphoma	Epstein-Barr virus
AIDS	Non-Hodgkin lymphoma, squamous cell carcinoma, Kaposi sarcoma	Human immunodeficiency virus, human herpesvirus type 8
Osteomyelitis	Carcinoma in draining sinuses	Bacterial infection
Pelvic inflammatory disease, chronic cervicitis	Ovrian carcinoma, cervical/anal carcinoma	Gonorrhea, chlamydia, human papillomavirus
Chronic cystitis	Bladder, liver, rectal carcinoma	Schistosomiasis

Adapted from TIsty TD, Coussens LM: Tumor stroma and regulation of cancer development. Ann Rev Pathol Mech Dis 1:119, 2006.

lish clonality by showing that all the cells in a tumor express the same allele. For tumors with acquired cytogenetic aberrations of any type (e.g., a translocation) their presence can be taken as evidence that the proliferation is clonal. Immunoglobulin receptor and T-cell receptor gene rearrangements serve as markers of clonality in B- and T-cell lymphomas, respectively.

● *Four classes of normal regulatory genes—the growth-promoting proto-oncogenes, the growth-inhibiting tumor suppressor genes, genes that regulate programmed cell death (apoptosis), and genes involved in DNA repair—are the principal targets of genetic damage.* Mutant alleles of proto-oncogenes are considered dominant, because they transform cells despite the presence of a normal counterpart. In contrast, typically, both normal alleles of the tumor suppressor genes must be damaged before transformation can occur. However, there are exceptions to this rule; sometimes, loss of a single allele of a tumor suppressor gene reduces levels or activity of the protein enough that the brakes on cell proliferation and survival are released. Loss of gene function caused by damage to a single allele is called *haploinsufficiency.* Such a finding indicates that dosage of the gene is important, and that two copies are required for normal function.[28] Genes that regulate apoptosis may behave as proto-oncogenes or tumor suppressor genes. Mutations of DNA repair genes do not directly transform cells by affecting proliferation or apoptosis. Instead, DNA-repair genes affect cell proliferation or survival indirectly by influencing the ability of the organism to repair nonlethal damage in other genes, including proto-oncogenes, tumor suppressor genes, and genes that regulate apoptosis. A disability in the DNA-repair

genes can predispose cells to widespread mutations in the genome and thus to neoplastic transformation. Cells with mutations in DNA repair genes are said to have developed a *mutator phenotype.*[29] Interestingly, a new class of regulatory molecules, called microRNAs (miRNAs), has recently been discovered (Chapter 5). Even though they do not encode proteins, different families of miRNAs have been shown to act as either oncogenes or tumor suppressors.[29,30] They do so by affecting the translation of other genes as will be discussed later.

● *Carcinogenesis is a multistep process at both the phenotypic and the genetic levels, resulting from the accumulation of multiple mutations.*[31] As discussed earlier, malignant neoplasms have several phenotypic attributes, such as excessive growth, local invasiveness, and the ability to form distant metastases. Furthermore, it is well established that over a period of time many tumors become more aggressive and acquire greater malignant potential. This phenomenon is referred to as tumor progression and is not simply a function of an increase in tumor size. Careful clinical and experimental studies reveal that increasing malignancy is often acquired in an incremental fashion. At the molecular level, tumor progression and associated heterogeneity most likely result from multiple mutations that accumulate independently in different cells, generating subclones with varying abilities to grow, invade, metastasize, and resist (or respond to) therapy (Fig. 7–24). Some of the mutations may be lethal; others may spur cell growth by affecting additional proto-oncogenes or tumor suppressor genes. *Even though most malignant tumors are monoclonal in origin, by the time they become clinically evident their constituent cells are*

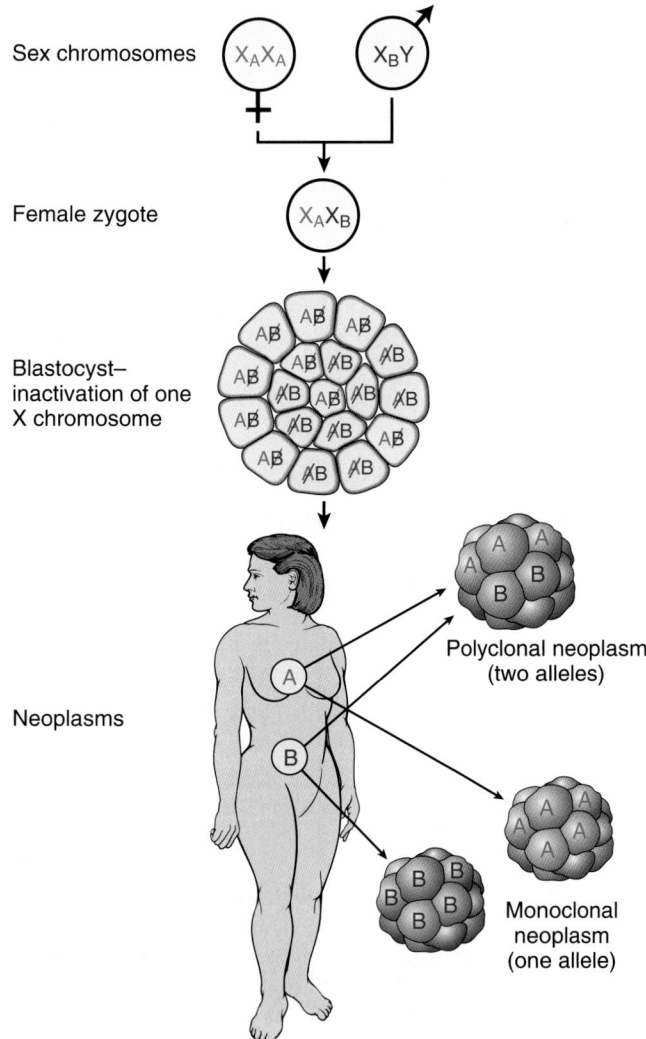

Sex chromosomes

Female zygote

Blastocyst–
inactivation of one
X chromosome

Neoplasms

Polyclonal neoplasm
(two alleles)

Monoclonal
neoplasm
(one allele)

FIGURE 7–23 The use of X-linked markers as evidence of the monoclonality of neoplasms. Because of random X inactivation, all females are mosaics with two cell populations (with different alleles for the androgen receptor labeled A and B in this case). When neoplasms that arise in women who are heterozygous for X-linked markers are analyzed, they are made up of cells that contain the active maternal (X_A) or the paternal (X_B) X chromosome but not both.

decades, hundreds of cancer-associated genes have been discovered. Some, such as *p53*, are mutated in many different cancers; others, such as *ABL1*, are affected only in one or few. Each of the cancer-associated genes has a specific function, the dysregulation of which contributes to the origin or progression of malignancy. It is traditional to describe cancer-associated genes on the basis of their presumed function. It is beneficial, however, to consider cancer-related genes in the context of *seven fundamental changes in cell physiology that together determine malignant phenotype.*[32] (Another important change for tumor development is *escape from immune attack*. This property is discussed later in this chapter.) The seven key changes are the following:

- *Self-sufficiency in growth signals*: Tumors have the capacity to proliferate without external stimuli, usually as a consequence of oncogene activation.
- *Insensitivity to growth-inhibitory signals*: Tumors may not respond to molecules that are inhibitory to the proliferation of normal cells such as transforming growth factor β (TGF-β) and direct inhibitors of cyclin-dependent kinases (CDKIs).
- *Evasion of apoptosis*: Tumors may be resistant to programmed cell death, as a consequence of inactivation of *p53* or activation of anti-apoptotic genes.
- *Limitless replicative potential*: Tumor cells have unrestricted proliferative capacity, avoiding cellular senescence and mitotic catastrophe.
- *Sustained angiogenesis*: Tumor cells, like normal cells, are not able to grow without formation of a vascular supply to bring nutrients and oxygen and remove waste products. Hence, tumors must induce angiogenesis.
- *Ability to invade and metastasize*: Tumor metastases are the cause of the vast majority of cancer deaths and depend on processes that are intrinsic to the cell or are initiated by signals from the tissue environment.
- *Defects in DNA repair*: Tumors may fail to repair DNA damage caused by carcinogens or incurred during unregulated cellular proliferation, leading to genomic instability and mutations in proto-oncogenes and tumor suppressor genes.

Mutations in one or more genes that regulate these cellular traits are seen in every cancer. However, the precise genetic pathways that give rise to these attributes differ between individual cancers, even within the same organ. It is widely believed that the occurrence of mutations in cancer-related genes is conditioned by the robustness of the DNA-repair machinery, as well as protective mechanisms such as apoptosis and senescence that prevent the proliferation of cells with damaged DNA. Indeed, recent studies in a variety of human tumors, such as melanoma and prostate adenocarcinoma, have shown that oncogene-induced senescence, wherein mutation of a proto-oncogene drives cells into senescence rather than proliferation, is an important barrier to carcinogenesis.[33] Some limits to neoplastic growth are even physical. If a tumor is to grow larger than 1 to 2 mm, mechanisms that allow the delivery of nutrients and the elimination of waste products must

extremely heterogeneous. During progression, tumor cells are subjected to immune and nonimmune selection pressures. For example, cells that are highly antigenic are destroyed by host defenses, whereas those with reduced growth factor requirements are positively selected. A growing tumor therefore tends to be enriched for subclones that "beat the odds" and are adept at survival, growth, invasion, and metastasis.

ESSENTIAL ALTERATIONS FOR MALIGNANT TRANSFORMATION

With this overview we can now address in some detail the molecular pathogenesis of cancer and then discuss the carcinogenic agents that inflict genetic damage. Over the past two

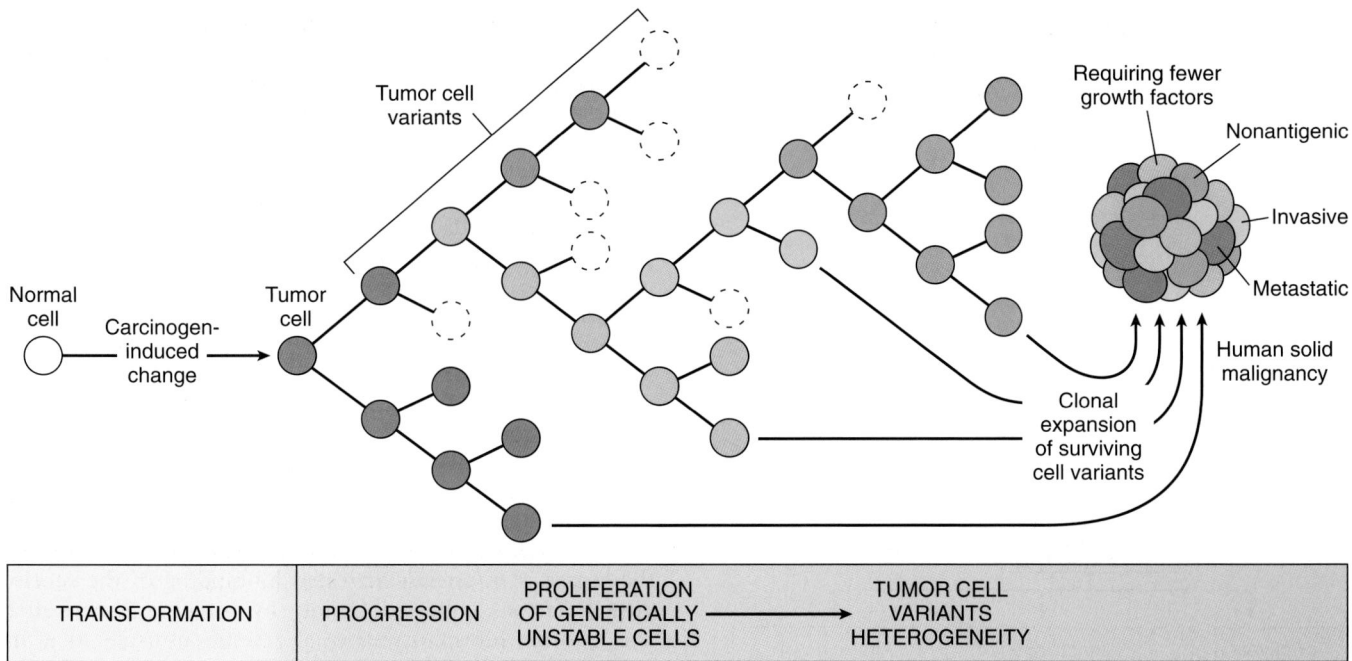

FIGURE 7–24 Tumor progression and generation of heterogeneity. New subclones arise from the descendants of the original transformed cell by multiple mutations. With progression the tumor mass becomes enriched for variants that are more adept at evading host defenses and are likely to be more aggressive.

be provided (angiogenesis). Furthermore, epithelia are separated from the interstitial matrix by a basement membrane, composed of extracellular matrix molecules, that must be broken down by invasive carcinoma cells. These protective barriers, both intrinsic and extrinsic to the cell, must be breached, and feedback loops that normally prevent uncontrolled cell division must be disabled by mutations before a fully malignant tumor can emerge. The main principles of the molecular basis of cancer are summarized in a simplified form in Figure 7–25.

In the following sections we discuss the nature of the genes involved in each of the seven biologic alterations listed earlier. We end with a discussion of epigenetic changes and chromosomal abnormalities in cancer.

SELF-SUFFICIENCY IN GROWTH SIGNALS: ONCOGENES

Genes that promote autonomous cell growth in cancer cells are called *oncogenes*, and their unmutated cellular counterparts are called *proto-oncogenes*. Oncogenes are created by mutations in proto-oncogenes and are characterized by the ability to promote cell growth in the absence of normal growth-promoting signals. Their products, called *oncoproteins*, resemble the normal products of proto-oncogenes except that oncoproteins are often devoid of important internal regulatory elements, and their production in the transformed cells does not depend on growth factors or other external signals. In this way cell growth becomes autonomous, freed from checkpoints and dependence upon external signals. To aid in the understanding of the nature and functions of oncoproteins and their role in cancer, it is necessary to briefly mention the sequential steps that characterize normal cell proliferation.

Under physiologic conditions cell proliferation can be readily resolved into the following steps:

- The binding of a growth factor to its specific receptor
- Transient and limited activation of the growth factor receptor, which, in turn, activates several signal-transducing proteins on the inner leaflet of the plasma membrane
- Transmission of the transduced signal across the cytosol to the nucleus via second messengers or by a cascade of signal transduction molecules
- Induction and activation of nuclear regulatory factors that initiate DNA transcription
- Entry and progression of the cell into the cell cycle, ultimately resulting in cell division

With this background we can readily identify the strategies used by cancer cells to acquire self-sufficiency in growth signals. They can be grouped on the basis of their role in growth factor–mediated signal transduction cascades and cell cycle regulation.

Proto-oncogenes, Oncogenes, and Oncoproteins

Proto-oncogenes have multiple roles, participating in cellular functions related to growth and proliferation. Proteins encoded by proto-oncogenes may function as growth factors or their receptors, signal transducers, transcription factors, or cell cycle components. Oncoproteins encoded by oncogenes generally serve functions similar to their normal counterparts (Table 7–6). However, *mutations convert proto-oncogenes into constitutively active cellular oncogenes that are involved in tumor development because the oncoproteins they encode endow the cell with self-sufficiency in growth.*[34]

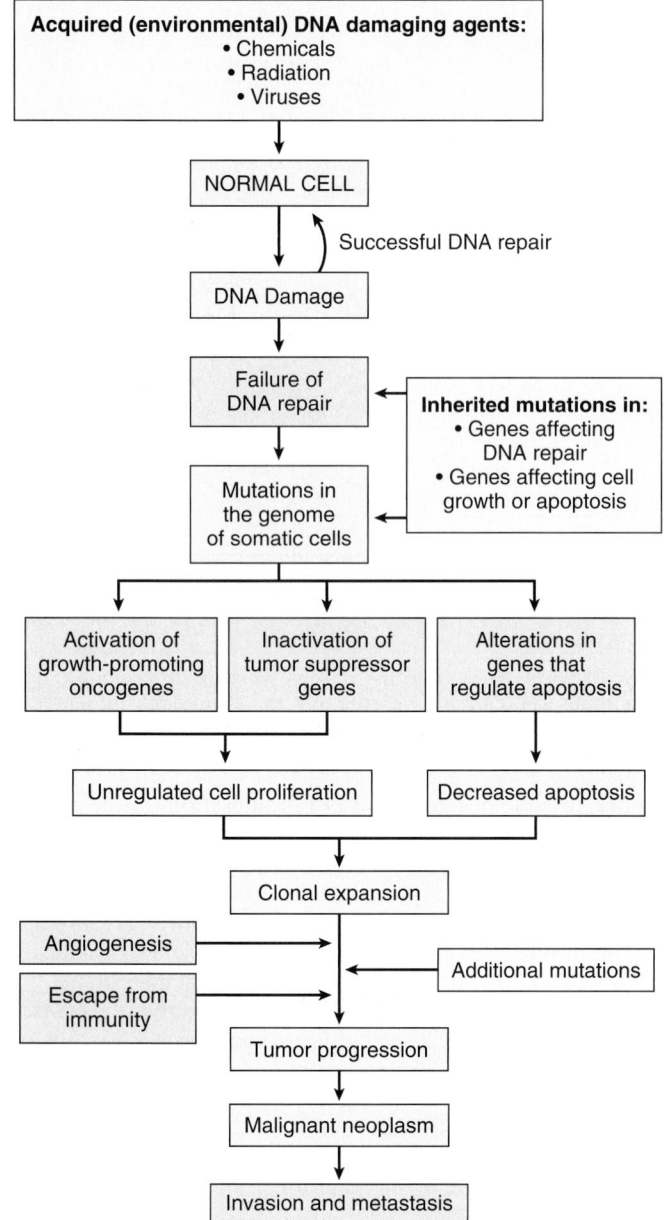

FIGURE 7–25 Flowchart depicting a simplified scheme of the molecular basis of cancer.

Two questions follow: (1) What are the functions of oncogene products, the oncoproteins? (2) How do the normally "civilized" proto-oncogenes turn into "enemies within"? These issues are discussed below.

Growth Factors. Normal cells require stimulation by growth factors to undergo proliferation. Most soluble growth factors are made by one cell type and act on a neighboring cell to stimulate proliferation (paracrine action). Many cancer cells, however, acquire the ability to synthesize the same growth factors to which they are responsive, generating an autocrine loop. For example, many glioblastomas secrete platelet-derived growth factor (PDGF) and express the PDGF receptor, and many sarcomas make both transforming growth factor α (TGF-α) and its receptor. Although an auto-

crine loop is considered to be an important element in the pathogenesis of several tumors, in most instances the growth factor gene itself is not altered or mutated. More commonly, products of other oncogenes that lie along many signal transduction pathways, such as *RAS,* cause overexpression of growth factor genes, thus forcing the cells to secrete large amounts of growth factors, such as TGF-α. Nevertheless, increased growth factor production is not sufficient for neoplastic transformation. In all likelihood growth factor driven proliferation contributes to the malignant phenotype by increasing the risk of spontaneous or induced mutations in the proliferating cell population.

Growth Factor Receptors. Several oncogenes that encode growth factor receptors have been found. To understand how mutations affect the function of these receptors, it should be recalled that one important class of growth factor receptors are transmembrane proteins with an external ligand-binding domain and a cytoplasmic tyrosine kinase domain (Chapter 3). In the normal forms of these receptors, the kinase is *transiently* activated by binding of the specific growth factors, followed rapidly by receptor dimerization and tyrosine phosphorylation of several substrates that are a part of the signaling cascade. *The oncogenic versions of these receptors are associated with constitutive dimerization and activation without binding to the growth factor.* Hence, the mutant receptors deliver continuous mitogenic signals to the cell, even in the absence of growth factor in the environment.

Growth factor receptors can be constitutively activated in tumors by multiple different mechanisms, including mutations, gene rearrangements, and overexpression. The *RET* proto-oncogene, a receptor tyrosine kinase, exemplifies oncogenic conversion via mutations and gene rearrangements.[33] The RET protein is a receptor for the glial cell line–derived neurotrophic factor and structurally related proteins that promote cell survival during neural development. RET is normally expressed in neuroendocrine cells, such as parafollicular C cells of the thyroid, adrenal medulla, and parathyroid cell precursors. Point mutations in the *RET* proto-oncogene are associated with dominantly inherited MEN types 2A and 2B and familial medullary thyroid carcinoma (Chapter 24). In MEN-2A, point mutations in the *RET* extracellular domain cause constitutive dimerization and activation, leading to medullary thyroid carcinomas and adrenal and parathyroid tumors. In MEN-2B, point mutations in the *RET* cytoplasmic catalytic domain alter the substrate specificity of the tyrosine kinase and lead to thyroid and adrenal tumors without involvement of the parathyroid. In all these familial conditions, the affected individuals inherit the *RET* mutation in the germline. Sporadic medullary carcinomas of the thyroid are associated with somatic rearrangements of the *RET* gene, generally similar to those found in MEN-2B.[35,36]

Oncogenic conversions by mutations and rearrangements have been found in other growth factor receptor genes. Point mutations in *FLT3*, the gene encoding the FMS-like tyrosine kinase 3 receptor, that lead to constitutive signaling have been detected in myeloid leukemias. In certain chronic myelomonocytic leukemias with the (5;12) translocation, the entire cytoplasmic domain of the PDGF receptor is fused with a segment of an ETS family transcription factor, resulting in permanent dimerization of the PDGF receptor. Greater than

TABLE 7–6 Selected Oncogenes, Their Mode of Activation, and Associated Human Tumors			
Category	**Proto-oncogene**	**Mode of Activation**	**Associated Human Tumor**
GROWTH FACTORS			
PDGF-β chain	*SIS* (official name *PBGFB*)	Overexpression	Astrocytoma Osteosarcoma
Fibroblast growth factors	*HST1* *INT2* (official name *FGF3*)	Overexpression Amplification	Stomach cancer Bladder cancer Breast cancer Melanoma
TGF-α	*TGFA*	Overexpression	Astrocytomas Hepatocellular carcinomas
HGF	*HGF*	Overexpression	Thyroid cancer
GROWTH FACTOR RECEPTORS			
EGF-receptor family	*ERBB1* (*EGFR*), *ERRB2*	Overexpression	Squamous cell carcinoma of lung, gliomas
FMS-like tyrosine kinase 3	*FLT3*	Amplification	Breast and ovarian cancers

Receptor for neurotrophic
  factors
	RET	Point mutation
		Point mutation
			Leukemia
			Multiple endocrine neoplasia 2A
			  and B, familial medullary thyroid
			  carcinomas

PDGF receptor	*PDGFRB*	Overexpression, translocation	Gliomas, leukemias

Receptor for stem cell
  (steel) factor
	KIT	Point mutation	Gastrointestinal stromal tumors,
			  seminomas, leukemias

PROTEINS INVOLVED IN SIGNAL TRANSDUCTION			
GTP-binding	*KRAS* *HRAS* *NRAS*	Point mutation Point mutation Point mutation	Colon, lung, and pancreatic tumors Bladder and kidney tumors Melanomas, hematologic malignancies
Nonreceptor tyrosine kinase	*ABL*	Translocation	Chronic myeloid leukemia Acute lymphoblastic leukemia
RAS signal transduction	*BRAF*	Point mutation	Melanomas
WNT signal transduction	β-catenin	Point mutation Overexpression	Hepatoblastomas, hepatocellular carcinoma
NUCLEAR-REGULATORY PROTEINS			
Transcriptional activators	C-*MYC* N-*MYC* L-*MYC*	Translocation Amplification Amplification	Burkitt lymphoma Neuroblastoma, small-cell carcinoma of lung Small-cell carcinoma of lung
CELL CYCLE REGULATORS			
Cyclins	Cyclin D Cyclin E	Translocation Amplification Overexpression	Mantle cell lymphoma Breast and esophageal cancers Breast cancer
Cyclin-dependent kinase	*CDK4*	Amplification or point mutation	Glioblastoma, melanoma, sarcoma

90% of gastrointestinal stromal tumors have a constitutively activating mutation in the receptor tyrosine kinase c-KIT or PDGFR, which are the receptors for stem cell factor and PDGF, respectively. These mutations are amenable to specific inhibition by the tyrosine kinase inhibitor imatinib mesylate. This type of therapy, directed to a specific alteration in the cancer cell, is called *targeted therapy*.[37]

Far more common than mutations of these proto-oncogenes is overexpression of normal forms of growth factor receptors. In some tumors increased receptor expression results from gene amplification, but in many cases the molecular basis of increased receptor expression is not fully known. Two members of the epidermal growth factor (EGF) receptor family are the best described. The normal form of *ERBB1*, the EGF receptor gene, is overexpressed in up to 80% of squamous cell carcinomas of the lung, in 50% or more of *glioblastomas*

(Chapter 28), and in 80% to 100% of head and neck tumors.[38,39] Likewise, the *ERBB2* gene (also called *HER-2/NEU*), the second member of the EGF receptor family, is amplified in approximately 25% of breast cancers and in human adenocarcinomas arising within the ovary, lung, stomach, and salivary glands.[36] Because the molecular alteration in *ERBB2* is specific for the cancer cells, new therapeutic agents consisting of monoclonal antibodies specific to *ERBB2* have been developed and are currently in use clinically, providing yet another example of targeted therapy.[38,39]

Signal-Transducing Proteins. Several examples of oncoproteins that mimic the function of normal cytoplasmic signal-transducing proteins have been found. Most such proteins are strategically located on the inner leaflet of the plasma membrane, where they receive signals from outside the cell (e.g., by activation of growth factor receptors) and transmit them to the cell's nucleus. Biochemically, the signal-transducing proteins are heterogeneous. *The most well-studied example of a signal-transducing oncoprotein is the RAS family of guanine triphosphate (GTP)-binding proteins (G proteins).*

The RAS Oncogene. The *RAS* genes, of which there are three in the human genome (*HRAS, KRAS, NRAS*), were discovered initially in transforming retroviruses. *Point mutation of RAS family genes is the single most common abnormality of proto-oncogenes in human tumors.* Approximately 15% to 20% of all human tumors contain mutated versions of RAS proteins.[40] The frequency of such mutations varies with different tumors, but in some types of cancers it is very high. For example, 90% of pancreatic adenocarcinomas and cholangiocarcinomas contain a *RAS* point mutation, as do about 50% of colon, endometrial, and thyroid cancers and 30% of lung adenocarcinomas and myeloid leukemias.[41,42] In general, carcinomas (particularly from colon and pancreas) have mutations of *KRAS*, bladder tumors have *HRAS* mutations, and hematopoietic tumors bear *NRAS* mutations. *RAS* mutations are infrequent in certain other cancers, such as those arising in the uterine cervix or breast.

RAS plays an important role in signaling cascades downstream of growth factor receptors, resulting in mitogenesis. For example, abrogation of RAS function blocks the prolifera-tive response to EGF, PDGF, and CSF-1. Normal RAS proteins are tethered to the cytoplasmic aspect of the plasma membrane, as well as the endoplasmic reticulum and Golgi membranes. They can be activated by growth factor binding to receptors at the plasma membrane.[40] RAS is a member of a family of small G proteins that bind guanosine nucleotides (guanosine triphosphate, GTP and guanosine diphosphate, GDP), similar to the larger trimolecular G proteins. Normally RAS proteins flip back and forth between an excited signal-transmitting state and a quiescent state. In the inactive state, RAS proteins bind GDP. Stimulation of cells by growth factors leads to exchange of GDP for GTP and subsequent conformational changes that generates active RAS (Fig. 7–26). The activated RAS stimulates downstream regulators of proliferation, such as the *mitogen-activated protein (MAP) kinase cascade*, which floods the nucleus with signals for cell proliferation.

The orderly cycling of the RAS protein depends on two reactions: (1) nucleotide exchange (GDP by GTP), which activates RAS protein, and (2) GTP hydrolysis, which converts the GTP-bound, active RAS to the GDP-bound, inactive form. Both these processes are extrinsically regulated by other proteins. The removal of GDP and its replacement by GTP during RAS activation are catalyzed by a family of guanine nucleo-

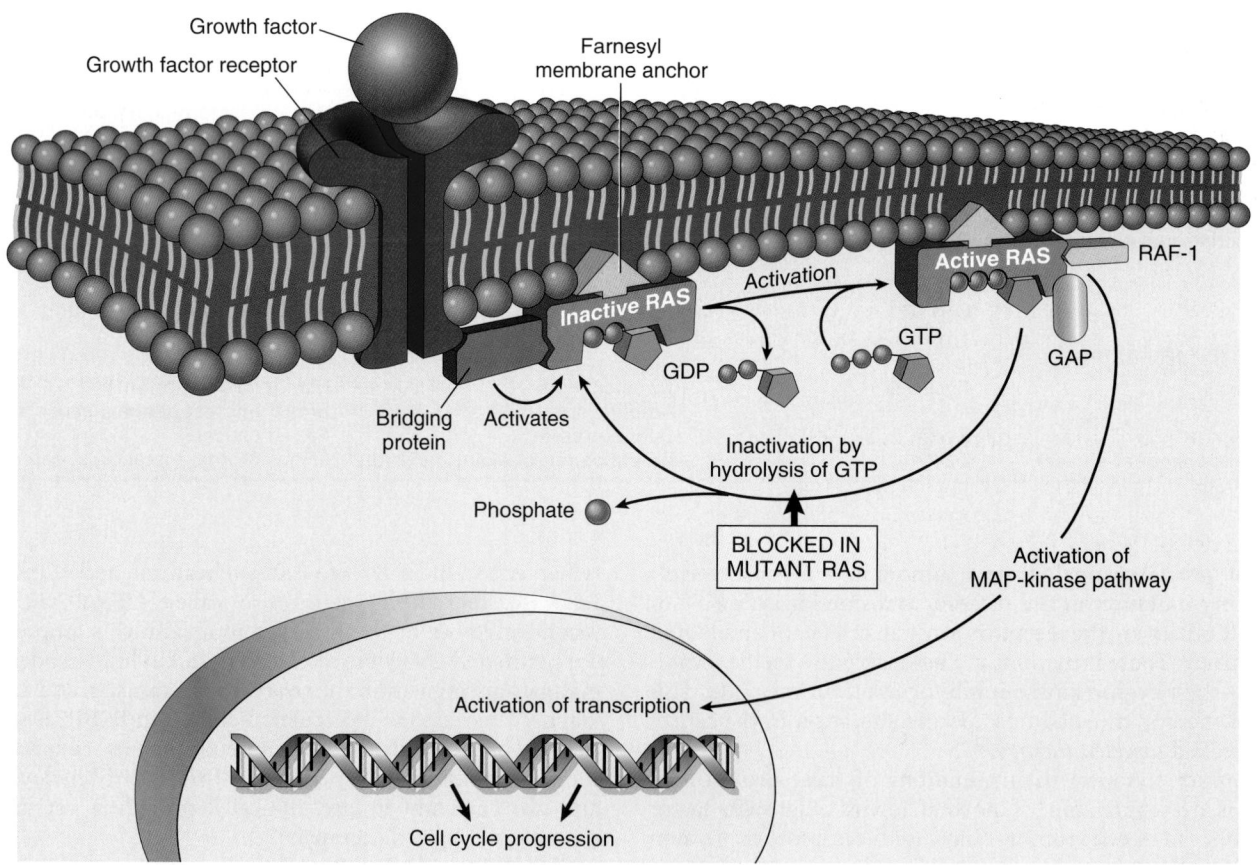

FIGURE 7–26   Model for action of *RAS* genes. When a normal cell is stimulated through a growth factor receptor, inactive (GDP-bound) RAS is activated to a GTP-bound state. Activated RAS recruits RAF and stimulates the MAP-kinase pathway to transmit growth-promoting signals to the nucleus. The mutated RAS protein is permanently activated because of inability to hydrolyze GTP, leading to continuous stimulation of cells without any external trigger. The anchoring of RAS to the cell membrane by the farnesyl moiety is essential for its action. See text for explanation of abbreviations.

tide–releasing proteins. Conversely, the GTPase activity intrinsic to normal RAS proteins is dramatically accelerated by *GTPase-activating proteins (GAPs)*. These widely distributed proteins bind to the active RAS and augment its GTPase activity by more than 1000-fold, leading to termination of signal transduction. Thus, GAPs function as "brakes" that prevent uncontrolled RAS activity.

Several distinct point mutations of *RAS* have been identified in cancer cells. The affected residues lie within either the GTP-binding pocket or the enzymatic region essential for GTP hydrolysis, and thus markedly reduce the GTPase activity of the RAS protein. Mutated RAS is trapped in its activated GTP-bound form, and the cell is forced into a continuously proliferating state. It follows from this scenario that the consequences of mutations in RAS protein would be mimicked by mutations in the GAPs that fail to activate the GTPase activity and thus restrain normal RAS proteins. Indeed, disabling mutation of neurofibromin 1, a GAP, is associated with the inherited cancer syndrome familial neurofibromatosis type 1 (Chapter 27).

In addition to RAS, downstream members of the RAS signaling cascade (RAS/RAF/MAP kinase) may also be altered in cancer cells, resulting in a similar phenotype. Thus, mutations in *BRAF*, one of the members of the *RAF* family, have been detected in more than 60% of melanomas and in more than 80% of benign nevi.[44,45] This suggests that dysregulation of the RAS/RAF/MAP kinase pathway may be one of the initiating events in the development of melanomas, although it is not sufficient by itself to cause tumorigenesis. Indeed, *BRAF* mutations alone lead to oncogene-induced senescence giving rise to benign nevi rather than malignant melanoma. Thus, oncogene-induced senescence is a barrier to carcinogenesis that must be overcome by mutation and disabling of key protective mechanisms, such as those provided by the *p53* gene (discussed later).[33]

Because *RAS* is so frequently mutated in human cancers, much effort has been spent to develop anti-RAS modalities of targeted therapy. Unfortunately, none of these strategies has so far proven to be successful for clinical use.

Alterations in Nonreceptor Tyrosine Kinases

Mutations that unleash latent oncogenic activity occur in several non-receptor-associated tyrosine kinases, which normally function in signal transduction pathways that regulate cell growth (Chapter 3). As with receptor tyrosine kinases, in some instances the mutations take the form of chromosomal translocations or rearrangements that create fusion genes encoding constitutively active tyrosine kinases. An important example of this oncogenic mechanism involves the c-ABL tyrosine kinase. In CML and some acute lymphoblastic leukemias, the *ABL* gene is translocated from its normal abode on chromosome 9 to chromosome 22 (Fig. 7–27), where it fuses with the *BCR* gene (see discussion of chromosomal translocations, later in this chapter). The resultant chimeric gene encodes a constitutively active, oncogenic BCR-ABL tyrosine kinase. Several structural features of the BCR-ABL fusion protein contribute to the increased kinase activity, but the most important is that the BCR moiety promotes the self-association of BCR-ABL. This is a common theme, since many

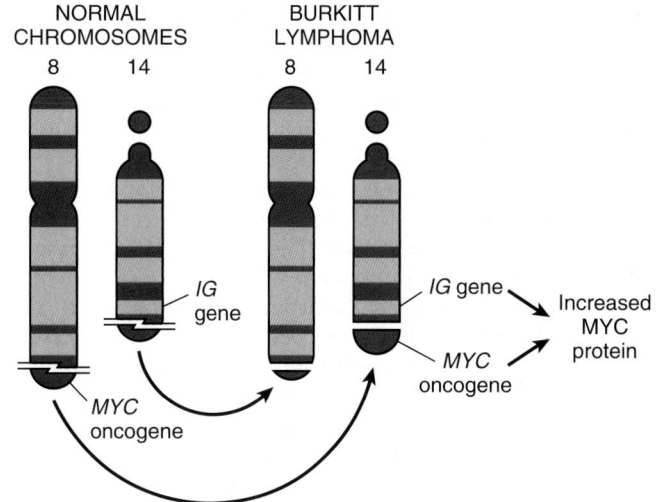

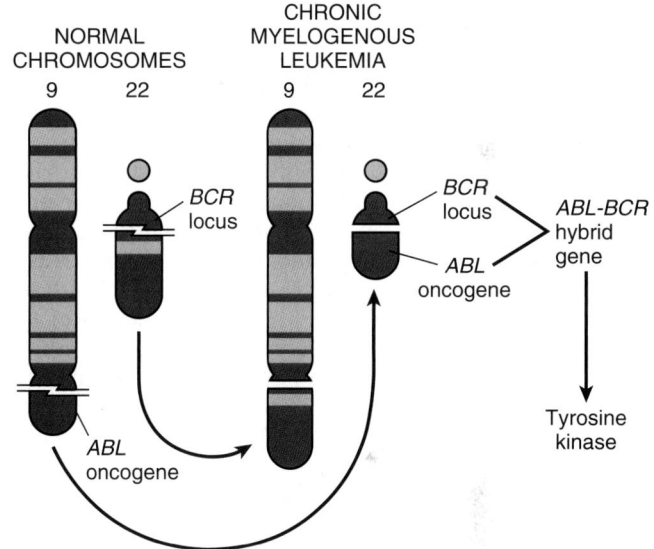

FIGURE 7–27 The chromosomal translocation and associated oncogenes in Burkitt lymphoma and chronic myelogenous leukemia.

different oncogenic tyrosine kinases consist of fusion proteins in which the non–tyrosine kinase partner drives self-association.[46] Treatment of CML has been revolutionized by the development of imatinib mesylate, a "designer" drug with low toxicity and high therapeutic efficacy that inhibits the BCR-ABL kinase.[47–49] This is another example of rational drug design emerging from an understanding of the molecular basis of cancer. It is also an example of the concept of oncogene addiction.[50] Despite accumulation of numerous mutations throughout the genome, signaling through the BCR-ABL gene is required for the tumor to persist, hence inhibition of its activity is effective therapy. BCR-ABL translocation is an early, perhaps initiating event, during leukemogenesis. The remaining mutations are selected for, and built around, the constant signaling through BCR-ABL. BCR-ABL signaling can be seen as the central lodgepole around which the structure is built. Remove the lodgepole by inhibition of the BCR-ABL kinase, and the structure collapses.

In other instances, nonreceptor tyrosine kinases are activated by point mutations that abrogate the function of negative regulatory domains that normally hold enzyme activity in check. For example, several myeloproliferative disorders, particularly polycythemia vera and primary myelofibrosis, are highly associated with activating point mutations in the tyrosine kinase JAK2 (Chapter 13).[51] The aberrant JAK2 kinase in turn activates transcription factors of the STAT family, which promote the growth factor–independent proliferation and survival of the tumor cells. Recognition of this molecular lesion has led to trials of JAK2 inhibitors in myeloproliferative disorders, and stimulated searches for activating mutations in other nonreceptor tyrosine kinases in a wide variety of human cancers.

Transcription Factors. Just as all roads lead to Rome, all signal transduction pathways converge to the nucleus, where a large bank of responder genes that orchestrate the cell's orderly advance through the mitotic cycle are activated. Indeed, the ultimate consequence of signaling through oncogenes like *RAS* or *ABL* is inappropriate and continuous stimulation of nuclear transcription factors that drive growth-promoting genes. Transcription factors contain specific amino acid sequences or motifs that allow them to bind DNA or to dimerize for DNA binding. Binding of these proteins to specific sequences in the genomic DNA activates transcription of genes. Growth autonomy may thus occur as a consequence of mutations affecting genes that regulate transcription. A host of oncoproteins, including products of the *MYC*, *MYB*, *JUN*, *FOS*, and *REL* oncogenes, are transcription factors that regulate the expression of growth-promoting genes, such as cyclins. *Of these, MYC is most commonly involved in human tumors*, and hence a brief overview of its function is warranted.

The MYC Oncogene. The *MYC* proto-oncogene is expressed in virtually all eukaryotic cells and belongs to the immediate early response genes, which are rapidly induced when quiescent cells receive a signal to divide (see discussion of liver regeneration in Chapter 3). After a transient increase of *MYC* messenger RNA, the expression declines to a basal level. The molecular basis of MYC function in cell replication is not entirely clear. As with many transcription factors, it is thought that MYC is involved in carcinogenesis by activating genes that are involved in proliferation. Indeed, some of its target genes, such as ornithine decarboxylase and cyclin D2, are known to be associated with cell proliferation. However, the range of activities modulated by MYC is very broad and includes histone acetylation, reduced cell adhesion, increased cell motility, increased telomerase activity, increased protein synthesis, decreased proteinase activity, and other changes in cellular matbolism that enable a high rate of cell division.[52] Genomic mapping of MYC binding sites has identified thousands of different sites and an equivalent number of genes that might be regulated.[53] However, there is little overlap in the MYC target genes in different cancers, preventing identification of a canonical MYC carcinogenesis program. Interestingly, it has been recently suggested that MYC interacts with components of the DNA-replication machinery, and plays a role in the selection of origins of replication.[54] Thus, overexpression of MYC may drive activation of more origins than needed for normal cell division, or bypass checkpoints involved in replication, leading to genomic damage and accumulation of mutations. Finally, MYC is one of a handful of transcription factors that can act in concert to reprogram somatic cells into pluripotent stem cells (Chapter 3); MYC may also enhance self-renewal, block differentiation, or both.

While on one hand *MYC* activation is linked to proliferation, on the other hand, cells in culture undergo apoptosis if *MYC* activation occurs in the absence of survival signals (growth factors).[55] The *MYC* proto-oncogene contains separate domains that encode the growth-promoting and apoptotic activities, but it is not clear whether MYC-induced apoptosis occurs in vivo.

In contrast to the regulated expression of *MYC* during normal cell proliferation, persistent expression, and in some cases overexpression, of the MYC protein are commonly found in tumors. Dysregulation of *MYC* expression resulting from translocation of the gene occurs in Burkitt lymphoma, a B-cell tumor (see Fig. 7–27). *MYC* is amplified in some cases of breast, colon, lung, and many other carcinomas. The related N-*MYC* and L-*MYC* genes are amplified in neuroblastomas (Fig. 7–28) and small-cell cancers of the lung, respectively.

Cyclins and Cyclin-Dependent Kinases. The ultimate outcome of all growth-promoting stimuli is the entry of quiescent cells into the cell cycle. Cancers may grow autonomously if the genes that drive the cell cycle become dysregulated by mutations or amplification. As described in Chapter 3, the

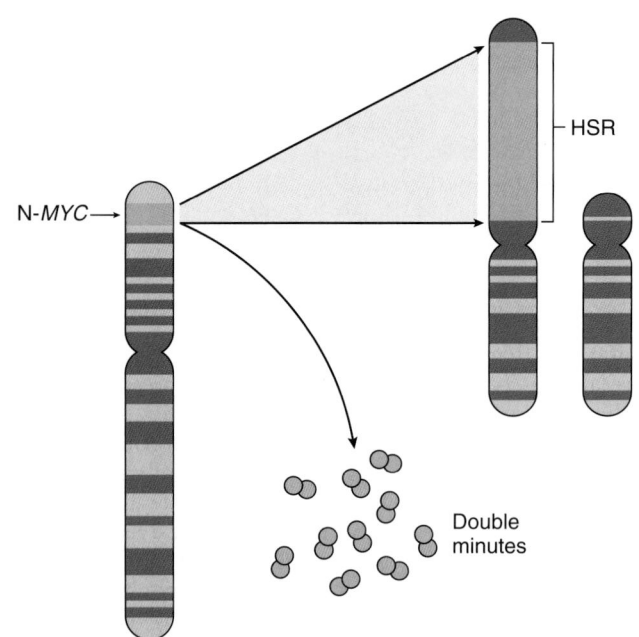

FIGURE 7–28 Amplification of the N-*MYC* gene in human neuroblastomas. The N-*MYC* gene, normally present on chromosome 2p, becomes amplified and is seen either as extra chromosomal double minutes or as a chromosomally integrated, homogeneous staining region (HSR). The integration involves other autosomes, such as 4, 9, or 13. (Modified from Brodeur GM: Molecular correlates of cytogenetic abnormalities in human cancer cells: implications for oncogene activation. In Brown EB (ed): Progress in Hematology, Vol 14. Orlando, FL, Grune & Stratton, 1986, p 229–256.)

orderly progression of cells through the various phases of the cell cycle is orchestrated by cyclin-dependent kinases (CDKs), which are activated by binding to *cyclins*, so called because of the cyclic nature of their production and degradation. The CDK-cyclin complexes phosphorylate crucial target proteins that drive the cell through the cell cycle. On completion of this task, cyclin levels decline rapidly. More than 15 cyclins have been identified; cyclins D, E, A, and B appear sequentially during the cell cycle and bind to one or more CDK. The cell cycle may thus be seen as a relay race in which each lap is regulated by a distinct set of cyclins, and as one set of cyclins leaves the track, the next set takes over (Fig. 7–29 and Table 7–7).

With this background it is easy to appreciate that mutations that dysregulate the activity of cyclins and CDKs favor cell proliferation. Mishaps affecting the expression of cyclin D or CDK4 seem to be a common event in neoplastic transformation. The cyclin D genes are overexpressed in many cancers,

including those affecting the breast, esophagus, liver, and a subset of lymphomas. Amplification of the *CDK4* gene occurs in melanomas, sarcomas, and glioblastomas. Mutations affecting cyclin B and cyclin E and other CDKs also occur, but they are much less frequent.

While cyclins arouse the CDKs, their inhibitors (CDKIs), of which there are many, silence the CDKs and exert negative control over the cell cycle. The CIP/WAF family of CDKIs, composed of three proteins, called p21 (CDKN1A), p27 (CDKN1B), and p57 (CDKN1C), inhibits the CDKs broadly, whereas the INK4 family of CDK1s, made up of p15 (CDKN2B), p16 (CDKN2A), p18 (CDKN2C), and p19 (CDKN2D), has selective effects on cyclin D/CDK4 and cyclin D/CDK6. Expression of these inhibitors is down-regulated by mitogenic signaling pathways, thus promoting the progression of the cell cycle. For example, p27 (CDKN1B), a CDKI that inhibits cyclin E, is expressed throughout G_1. Mitogenic signals dampen the activity of p27 in a variety of ways, relieving

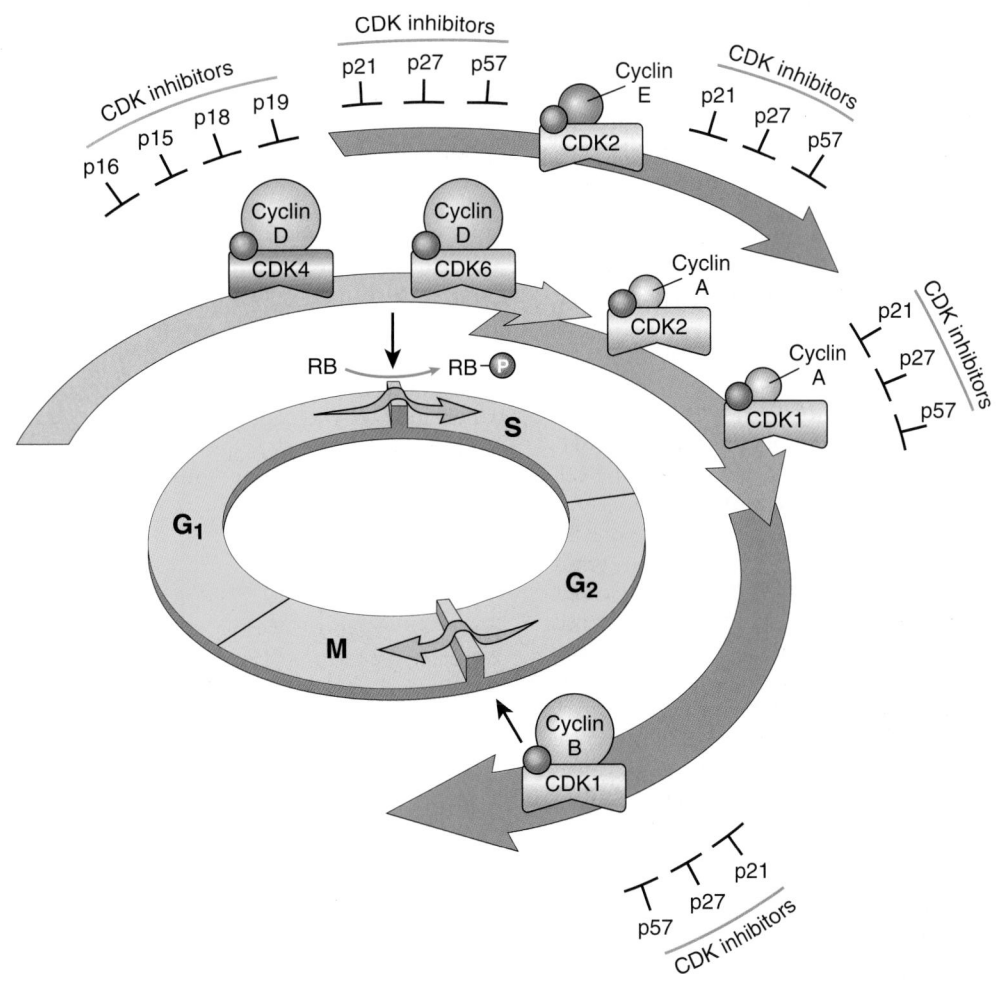

FIGURE 7–29 Schematic illustration of the role of cyclins, CDKs, and CDK inhibitors (CDKIs) in regulating the cell cycle. The shaded arrows represent the phases of the cell cycle during which specific cyclin-CDK complexes are active. As illustrated, cyclin D–CDK4, cyclin D–CDK6, and cyclin E–CDK2 regulate the G_1-to-S transition by phosphorylation of the RB protein (pRB). Cyclin A–CDK2 and cyclin A–CDK1 are active in the S phase. Cyclin B–CDK1 is essential for the G_2-to-M transition. Two families of CDKIs can block activity of CDKs and progression through the cell cycle. The so-called INK4 inhibitors, composed of p16, p15, p18, and p19, act on cyclin D–CDK4 and cyclin D–CDK6. The other family of three inhibitors, p21, p27, and p57, can inhibit all CDKs.

TABLE 7–7   Main Cell Cycle Components and Their Inhibitors

Cell Cycle Component	Main Function
CYCLIN-DEPENDENT KINASES	
CDK4	Forms a complex with cyclin D that phosphorylates RB, allowing the cell to progress through the G_1 restriction point.
CDK2	Forms a complex with cyclin E in late G_1, which is involved in G_1/S transition. Forms a complex with cyclin A at the S phase that facilitates G_2/M transition.
CDK1	Forms a complex with cyclin B that facilitates G_2/M transition.
INHIBITORS	
CIP/KIP family: p21, p27 (CDKN2A-C)	Block the cell cycle by binding to cyclin-CDK complexes; p21 is induced by the tumor suppressor p53; p27 responds to growth suppressors such as TGF-β.
INK4/ARF family (CDKN1A-D)	p16/INK4a binds to cyclin D–CDK4 and promotes the inhibitory effects of RB; p14/ARF increases p53 levels by inhibiting MDM2 activity.
CHECKPOINT COMPONENTS	
p53	Tumor suppressor gene altered in the majority of cancers; causes cell cycle arrest and apoptosis. Acts mainly through p21 to cause cell cycle arrest. Causes apoptosis by inducing the transcription of pro-apoptotic genes such as *BAX*. Levels of p53 are negatively regulated by MDM2 through a feedback loop. p53 is required for the G_1/S checkpoint and is a main component of the G_2/M checkpoint.
Ataxia-telangiectasia mutated	Activated by mechanisms that sense double-stranded DNA breaks. Transmits signals to arrest the cell cycle after DNA damage. Acts through p53 in the G_1/S checkpoint. At the G_2/M checkpoint, it acts both through p53-dependent mechanisms and through the inactivation of CDC25 phosphatase, which disrupts the cyclin B–CDK1 complex. Component of a network of genes that include *BRCA1* and *BRCA2*, which link DNA damage with cell cycle arrest and apoptosis.

inhibition of cyclin E-CDK2 and thus allowing the cell cycle to proceed.[56] The CDKIs are frequently mutated or otherwise silenced in many human malignancies. Germline mutations of *p16* (*CDKN2A*) are associated with 25% of melanoma-prone kindreds.[23] Somatically acquired deletion or inactivation of *p16* is seen in 75% of pancreatic carcinomas, 40% to 70% of glioblastomas, 50% of esophageal cancers, 20% to 70% of acute lymphoblastic leukemias, and 20% of non-small-cell lung carcinomas, soft-tissue sarcomas, and bladder cancers.[57]

Before closing this discussion of the cell cycle and its regulation, we should briefly discuss the internal controls of the cell cycle called *checkpoints*, since later discussion of tumor suppressor genes will illustrate the importance of cell cycle checkpoints in maintaining genomic integrity. There are two main cell cycle checkpoints, one at the G_1/S transition and the other at G_2/M. The S phase is the point of no return in the cell cycle. Before a cell makes the final commitment to replicate, the G_1/S checkpoint checks for DNA damage; if damage is present, the DNA-repair machinery and mechanisms that arrest the cell cycle are put in motion. The delay in cell cycle progression provides the time needed for DNA repair; if the damage is not repairable, apoptotic pathways are activated to kill the cell. Thus, the G_1/S checkpoint prevents the replication of cells that have defects in DNA, which would be perpetuated as mutations or chromosomal breaks in the progeny of the cell. DNA damaged after its replication can still be repaired as long as the chromatids have not separated. The G_2/M checkpoint monitors the completion of DNA replication and checks whether the cell can safely initiate mitosis and separate sister chromatids. This checkpoint is particularly important in cells exposed to ionizing radiation. Cells damaged by ionizing radiation activate the G_2/M checkpoint and arrest in G_2; defects in this checkpoint give rise to chromosomal

abnormalities. To function properly, cell cycle checkpoints require sensors of DNA damage, signal transducers, and effector molecules.[58] The sensors and transducers of DNA damage seem to be similar for the G_1/S and G_2/M checkpoints. They include, as sensors, proteins of the RAD family and ataxia telangiectasia mutated (ATM) and as transducers, the CHK kinase families.[59] The checkpoint effector molecules differ, depending on the cell cycle stage at which they act. In the G_1/S checkpoint, cell cycle arrest is mostly mediated through p53, which induces the cell cycle inhibitor p21. Arrest of the cell cycle by the G_2/M checkpoint involves both p53-dependent and p53-independent mechanisms. *Defects in cell cycle checkpoint components are a major cause of genetic instability in cancer cells.*

INSENSITIVITY TO GROWTH INHIBITION AND ESCAPE FROM SENESCENCE: TUMOR SUPPRESSOR GENES

Failure of growth inhibition is one of the fundamental alterations in the process of carcinogenesis. Whereas oncogenes drive the proliferation of cells, the products of *tumor suppressor genes apply brakes to cell proliferation* (Table 7–8). It has become apparent that the tumor suppressor proteins form a network of checkpoints that prevent uncontrolled growth. Many tumor suppressors, such as RB and p53, are part of a regulatory network that recognizes genotoxic stress from any source, and responds by shutting down proliferation. Indeed, expression of an oncogene in an otherwise completely normal cell leads to quiescence, or to permanent cell cycle arrest (oncogene-induced senescence), rather than uncontrolled proliferation. Ultimately, the growth-inhibitory pathways may prod the cells into apoptosis. Another set of tumor suppressors seem to be involved in cell differentiation, causing cells

TABLE 7–8 Selected Tumor Suppressor Genes Involved in Human Neoplasms

Subcellular Locations	Gene	Function	Tumors Associated with Somatic Mutations	Tumors Assocated with Inherited Mutations
Cell surface	TGF-β receptor E-cadherin	Growth inhibition Cell adhesion	Carcinomas of colon Carcinoma of stomach	Unknown Familial gastric cancer
Inner aspect of plasma membrane	NF1	Inhibition of RAS signal transduction and of p21 cell cycle inhibitor	Neuroblastomas	Neurofibromatosis type 1 and sarcomas
Cytoskeleton	NF2	Cytoskeletal stability	Schwannomas and meningiomas	Neurofibromastosis type 2, acoustic schwannomas, and meningiomas
Cytosol	APC/β-catenin	Inhibition of signal transduction	Carcinomas of stomach, colon, pancreas; melanoma	Familial adenomatous polyposis coli/colon cancer
	PTEN	PI3 kinase signal transduction	Endometrial and prostate cancers	Cowden syndrome
	SMAD2 and SMAD4	TGF-β signal transduction	Colon, pancreas tumors	Unknown
Nucleus	RB1	Regulation of cell cycle	Retinoblastoma; osteosarcoma carcinomas of breast, colon, lung	Retinoblastomas, osteosarcoma
	p53	Cell cycle arrest and apoptosis in response to DNA damage	Most human cancers	Li-Fraumeni syndrome; multiple carcinomas and sarcomas
	WT1	Nuclear transcription	Wilms' tumor	Wilms' tumor
	P16/INK4a	Regulation of cell cycle by inhibition of cyclin-dependent kinases	Pancreatic, breast, and esophageal cancers	Malignant melanoma
	BRCA1 and BRCA2	DNA repair	Unknown	Carcinomas of female breast and ovary; carcinomas of male breast

PI3 kinase, phosphatidylinositol 3-kinase.

to enter a postmitotic, differentiated pool without replicative potential. Similar to mitogenic signals, growth-inhibitory, pro-differentiation signals originate outside the cell and use receptors, signal transducers, and nuclear transcription regulators to accomplish their effects; tumor suppressors form a portion of these networks.

In this section we describe tumor suppressor genes, their products, and possible mechanisms by which loss of their function contributes to unregulated cell growth. The protein products of tumor suppressor genes may function as transcription factors, cell cycle inhibitors, signal transduction molecules, cell surface receptors, and regulators of cellular responses to DNA damage. In the following section we discuss the functions of the most important tumor suppressor genes, and how their defects contribute to carcinogenesis.

We begin our discussion with *RB*, the first, and prototypic, tumor suppressor gene discovered. Like many discoveries in medicine, *RB* was discovered by studying a rare disease, in this case retinoblastoma. Approximately 60% of retinoblastomas are sporadic, and the remaining are familial, with the predisposition to develop the tumor being transmitted as an autosomal dominant trait. Patients with familial retinoblastoma are also at greatly increased risk of developing osteosarcoma and other soft-tissue sarcomas. To explain the inherited and sporadic occurrence of an apparently identical tumor, Knudson proposed his now canonical *"two-hit"* hypothesis of oncogene-

sis.[19,60] In molecular terms, Knudson's hypothesis can be stated as follows (Fig. 7–30):

○ Two mutations (hits), involving both alleles of *RB* at chromosome locus 13q14, are required to produce retinoblastoma. In some cases, the genetic damage is large enough to be visible in the form of a deletion of 13q14.

○ In familial cases, children inherit one defective copy of the *RB* gene in the germ line (one hit); the other copy is normal (Fig. 7–30). Retinoblastoma develops when the normal *RB* allele is mutated in retinoblasts as a result of spontaneous somatic mutation (second hit). Because only a single somatic mutation is required for loss of RB function in retinoblastoma families, familial retinoblastoma is inherited as an autosomal dominant trait.

○ In sporadic cases both normal *RB* alleles must undergo somatic mutation in the same retinoblast (two hits). The end result is the same: a retinal cell that has completely lost *RB* function becomes cancerous.

At this point we should clarify some terminology. A child carrying an inherited mutant *RB* allele in all somatic cells is perfectly normal (except for the increased risk of developing cancer). Because such a child is heterozygous at the *RB* locus, this implies that heterozygosity for the *RB* gene does not affect cell behavior. *Cancer develops when the cell becomes*

PATHOGENESIS OF RETINOBLASTOMA

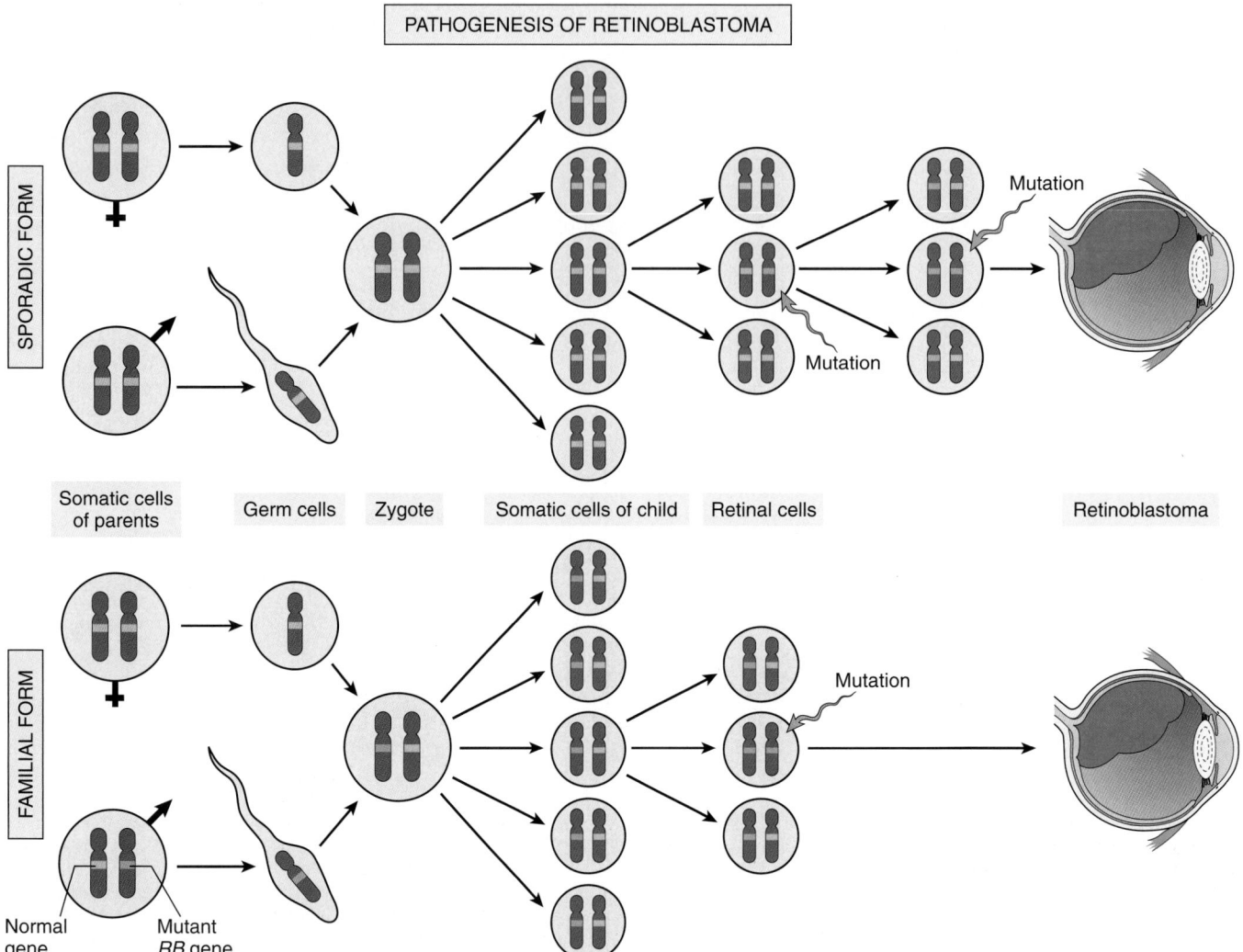

FIGURE 7–30 Pathogenesis of retinoblastoma. Two mutations of the *RB* locus on chromosome 13q14 lead to neoplastic proliferation of the retinal cells. In the sporadic form both mutations at the *RB* locus are acquired by the retinal cells after birth. In the familial form, all somatic cells inherit one mutant *RB* gene from a carrier parent. The second mutation affects the *RB* locus in one of the retinal cells after birth.

homozygous for the mutant allele or, put another way, when the cell loses heterozygosity for the normal RB gene (a condition known as LOH, for loss of heterozygosity). The RB gene stands as a paradigm for several other genes that act similarly. For example, one or more genes on the short arm of chromosome 11 play a role in the formation of Wilms' tumor, hepatoblastoma, and rhabdomyosarcoma. The von Hippel-Lindau (*VHL*) gene is a tumor suppressor gene that causes familial clear cell renal carcinomas and is also involved in sporadic forms of the same tumor.[61] *Consistent and nonrandom LOH has provided important clues to the location of several tumor suppressor genes.*

RB. RB protein, the product of the *RB* gene, is a ubiquitously expressed nuclear phosphoprotein that plays a key role in regulating the cell cycle. RB exists in an active hypophosphorylated state in quiescent cells and an inactive hyperphosphorylated state in the G_1/S cell cycle transition (Fig. 7–31). The importance of RB lies in its enforcement of G_1, or the gap between mitosis (M) and DNA replication (S). In embryos, cell divisions proceed at an amazing clip, with DNA replica-

tion beginning immediately after mitosis ends. However, as development proceeds, two gaps are incorporated into the cell cycle: Gap 1 (G_1) between mitosis (M) and DNA replication (S), and Gap 2 (G_2) between DNA replication (S) and mitosis (M) (see Fig. 7–29). Although each phase of the cell cycle circuitry is monitored carefully, the transition from G_1 to S is believed to be an extremely important checkpoint in the cell cycle clock. Once cells cross the G_1 checkpoint they can pause the cell cycle for a time, but they are obligated to complete mitosis. In G_1, however, cells can exit the cell cycle, either temporarily, called quiescence, or permanently, called senescence. In G_1, therefore, diverse signals are integrated to determine whether the cell should enter the cell cycle, exit the cell cycle and differentiate, or die. RB is a key node in this decision process. To understand why RB is such a crucial player, we must review the mechanisms that police the G_1 phase.[62]

The initiation of DNA replication requires the activity of cyclin E–CDK2 complexes, and expression of cyclin E is dependent on the E2F family of transcription factors. Early in

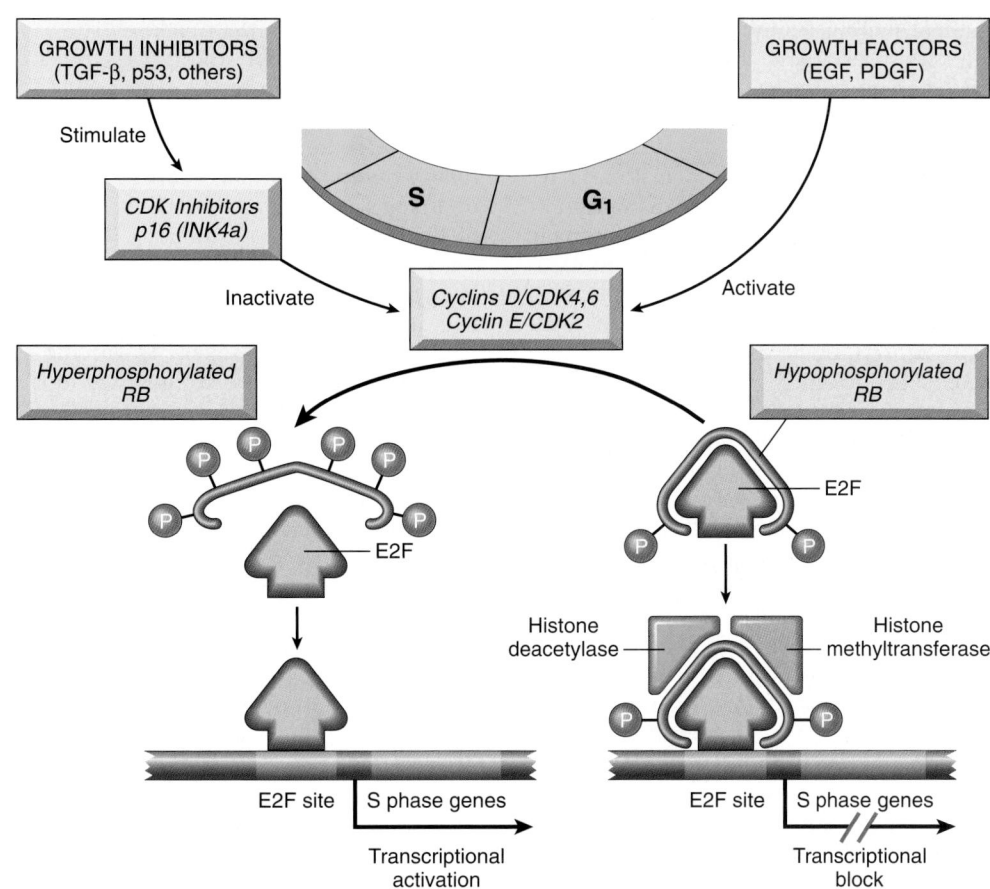

FIGURE 7–31 The role of RB in regulating the G_1-S checkpoint of the cell cycle. Hypophosphorylated RB in complex with the E2F transcription factors binds to DNA, recruits chromatin-remodeling factors (histone deacetylases and histone methyltransferases), and inhibits transcription of genes whose products are required for the S phase of the cell cycle. When RB is phosphorylated by the cyclin D–CDK4, cyclin D–CDK6, and cyclin E–CDK2 complexes, it releases E2F. The latter then activates transcription of S-phase genes. The phosphorylation of RB is inhibited by CDKIs, because they inactivate cyclin-CDK complexes. Virtually all cancer cells show dysregulation of the G_1-S checkpoint as a result of mutation in one of four genes that regulate the phosphorylation of RB; these genes are *RB1*, *CDK4*, the genes encoding cyclin D proteins, and *CDKN2A* (p16). EGF, epidermal growth factor; PDGF, platelet-derived growth factor; TGF-β, transforming growth factor-beta.

G_1, RB is in its hypophosphorylated active form, and it binds to and inhibits the E2F family of transcription factors, preventing transcription of cyclin E. Hypophosphorylated RB blocks E2F-mediated transcription in at least two ways (see Fig. 7–31). First, it sequesters E2F, preventing it from interacting with other transcriptional activators. Second, RB recruits chromatin-remodeling proteins, such as histone deacetylases and histone methyltransferases, which bind to the promoters of E2F-responsive genes such as cyclin E. These enzymes modify chromatin so as to make promoters insensitive to transcription factors. Mitogenic signaling leads to cyclin D expression and activation of cyclin D–CDK4/6 complexes. These complexes phosphorylate RB, inactivating the protein and releasing E2F to induce target genes such as cyclin E. Expression of cyclin E then stimulates DNA replication and progression through the cell cycle. When the cells enter S phase, they are committed to divide without additional growth factor stimulation. During the ensuing M phase the phosphate groups are removed from RB by cellular phosphatases, regenerating the hypophosphorylated form of RB. E2Fs are not the sole effectors of Rb-mediated G_1 arrest. Rb also controls the stability of the cell cycle inhibitor p27.[63,64]

If RB is absent (as a result of gene mutations) or its ability to regulate E2F transcription factors is derailed, the molecular brakes on the cell cycle are released, and the cells move through the cell cycle. The mutations of *RB* genes found in tumors are localized to a region of the RB protein, called the "RB pocket," that is involved in binding to E2F. However, the versatile RB protein has also been shown to bind to a variety of other transcription factors that regulate cell differentiation.[65] For example, RB stimulates myocyte-, adipocyte-, melanocyte-, and macrophage-specific transcription factors. Thus, the RB pathway couples control of cell cycle progression at G_1 with differentiation, which may explain how differentiation is associated with exit from the cell cycle. In addition to these dual activities, RB can also induce senescence, discussed below.

It was mentioned previously that germline loss or mutations of the *RB* gene predispose to occurrence of retinoblastomas and to a lesser extent osteosarcomas. Furthermore, somatically acquired RB mutations have been described in glioblastomas, small-cell carcinomas of lung, breast cancers, and bladder carcinomas. Given the presence of RB in every cell and its importance in cell cycle control, two questions arise: (1) Why do patients with germline mutation of the *RB* locus develop mainly retinoblastomas? (2) Why are inactivating mutations of *RB* not much more common in human cancers? The reason for the occurrence of tumors restricted to the retina in persons who inherit one defective allele of *RB* is not fully understood, but some possible explanations have emerged from the study of mice with targeted disruption of the *rb* locus. For instance, RB family members may partially complement its function in cell types other than retinoblasts. Indeed, RB is a member of a small family of proteins, so-called pocket proteins, which also include p107 and p130.[66] All three proteins bind to E2F transcription factors. The complexity grows; there are seven E2F proteins (named E2F1 through E2F7), which function as either transcriptional activators or repressors. The pocket proteins are all thought to regulate progression through the cell cycle as well as differentiation in a manner similar to that described for RB above. However, each member of this protein family binds a different set of E2F proteins and is also expressed at different times in the cell cycle. Thus, although there is some redundancy in the network, their functions are not completely overlapping. The complexity of the pocket protein–E2F network is just now being unraveled. For example, in a mouse model of retinoblastoma, it has been shown that mutation of different members of the network in various combinations generates retinoblastomas not just from retinoblasts, but also from differentiated cells in the retina, such as horizontal interneurons.[67]

With respect to the second question (i.e., why the loss of *RB* is not more common in human tumors), the answer is much simpler: Mutations in other genes that control RB phosphorylation can mimic the effect of *RB* loss, and such genes are mutated in many cancers that may have normal *RB* genes. Thus, for example, mutational activation of cyclin D or CDK4 would favor cell proliferation by facilitating RB phosphorylation. As previously discussed, cyclin D is overexpressed in many tumors because of gene amplification or translocation. Mutational inactivation of CDKIs would also drive the cell cycle by unregulated activation of cyclins and CDKs. Thus, *the emerging paradigm is that loss of normal cell cycle control is central to malignant transformation and that at least one of four key regulators of the cell cycle* (p16/INK4a, cyclin D, CDK4, RB) *is dysregulated in the vast majority of human cancers.*[68] In cells that harbor mutations in any one of these other genes, the function of RB is disrupted even if the *RB* gene itself is not mutated.[34]

The transforming proteins of several oncogenic animal and human DNA viruses seem to act, in part, by neutralizing the growth-inhibitory activities of RB. In these cases, RB protein is functionally inactivated by the binding of a viral protein and no longer acts as a cell cycle inhibitor. Simian virus 40 and polyomavirus large T antigens, adenoviruses EIA protein, and HPV E7 protein all bind to the hypophosphorylated form of RB. The binding occurs in the same RB pocket that normally sequesters E2F transcription factors; in the case of HPV the binding is particularly strong for viral types, such as HPV type 16, that confer high risk for the development of cervical carcinomas. Thus, the RB protein, unable to bind the E2F transcription factors, is functionally inactivated, and the transcription factors are free to cause cell cycle progression.

Several other pathways of cell growth regulation, some to be discussed in more detail later, also converge on RB (see Fig. 7–31):

p53: Guardian of the Genome. The *p53* gene is located on chromosome 17p13.1, and it is the most common target for genetic alteration in human tumors.[69] (The official name of the gene is *TP53* and the protein is p53; for the sake of simplicity, we refer to both as "p53".) *A little over 50% of human tumors contain mutations in this gene.* Homozygous loss of *p53* occurs in virtually every type of cancer, including carcinomas of the lung, colon, and breast—the three leading causes of cancer death. In most cases, the inactivating mutations affect both *p53* alleles and are acquired in somatic cells (not inherited in the germ line). Less commonly, some individuals inherit one mutant *p53* allele. As with the *RB* gene, inheritance of one mutant allele predisposes individuals to develop malignant tumors because only one additional "hit" is needed to inactivate the second, normal allele. Such individuals, said to have the *Li-Fraumeni syndrome*, have a 25-fold greater chance of developing a malignant tumor by age 50 than the general population.[70] In contrast to individuals who inherit a mutant *RB* allele, the spectrum of tumors that develop in persons with the Li-Fraumeni syndrome is quite varied; the most common types of tumors are sarcomas, breast cancer, leukemia, brain tumors, and carcinomas of the adrenal cortex. As compared with sporadic tumors, those that afflict patients with the Li-Fraumeni syndrome occur at a younger age, and a given individual may develop multiple primary tumors.[71]

The fact that *p53* mutations are common in a variety of human tumors suggests that the p53 protein functions as a critical gatekeeper against the formation of cancer. Indeed, it is evident that p53 acts as a "*molecular policeman*" that prevents the propagation of genetically damaged cells. p53 is a transcription factor that is at the center of a large network of signals that sense cellular stress, such as DNA damage, shortened telomeres, and hypoxia. Many activities of the p53 protein are related to its function as a transcription factor. Several hundred genes have been shown to be regulated by p53 in numerous different contexts, but which genes are the key for the p53 response is not yet clear. Approximately 80% of the *p53* point mutations present in human cancers are located in the DNA-binding domain of the protein. However, the effects of different point mutations vary considerably; in some cases there is complete abrogation of transcriptional capabilities, whereas other mutants retain the ability to bind to and activate a subset of genes. In addition to somatic and inherited mutations, p53 functions can be inactivated by other mechanisms. As with RB, the transforming proteins of several DNA viruses, including the E6 protein of HPV, can bind to and promote the degradation of p53. Also, analogous to RB, it is thought that in the majority of tumors without a *p53* mutation, the function of the p53 pathway is blocked by mutation in another gene that regulates p53 function. For example, MDM2 and MDMX stimulate the degradation of p53; these proteins are frequently overexpressed in malignancies in which the gene encoding p53 is not mutated. Indeed, MDM2 is amplified in 33% of human sarcomas, thereby causing functional loss of p53 in these tumors.[72,73]

p53 thwarts neoplastic transformation by three interlocking mechanisms: activation of temporary cell cycle arrest (quiescence), induction of permanent cell cycle arrest (senescence), or triggering of programmed cell death (apoptosis).

In nonstressed, healthy cells, p53 has a short half-life (20 minutes), because of its association with MDM2, a protein that targets it for destruction. When the cell is stressed, for example by an assault on its DNA, p53 undergoes post-transcriptional modifications that release it from MDM2 and increase its half-life. Unshackled from MDM2, p53 also becomes activated as a transcription factor. Hundreds of genes whose transcription is triggered by p53 have been found.[74,75] They can be grouped into two broad categories: those that cause cell cycle arrest and those that cause apoptosis. If DNA damage can be repaired during cell cycle arrest, the cell reverts to a normal state; if the repair fails, p53 induces apoptosis or senescence. Recently, however, the plot has thickened. It has been known that repression of a subset of pro-proliferative and anti-apoptotic genes is key to the p53 response, but it was not clear how p53 achieved repression, since in most assays it seemed to be an activator of transcription. At this point enter the recently famous miRNAs, the small guys with big clubs. It

has been shown that p53 activates transcription of the mir34 family of miRNAs (mir34a–mir34c).[76] miRNAs, as discussed in Chapter 5, bind to cognate sequences in the 3′ untranslated region of mRNAs, preventing translation (Fig. 7–32B). Interestingly, blocking mir34 severely hampered the p53 response in cells, while ectopic expression of mir34 without p53 activation is sufficient to induce growth arrest and apoptosis. Thus, mir34 microRNAs are able to recapitulate many of the functions of p53 and are necessary for these functions, demonstrating the importance of mir34 to the p53 response. Targets of mir34s include pro-proliferative genes such as cyclins, and anti-apoptotic genes such as *BCL2*. p53 regulation of mir34 explains, at least in part, how p53 is able to repress gene expression, and it seems that regulation of this miRNA is crucial for the p53 response.

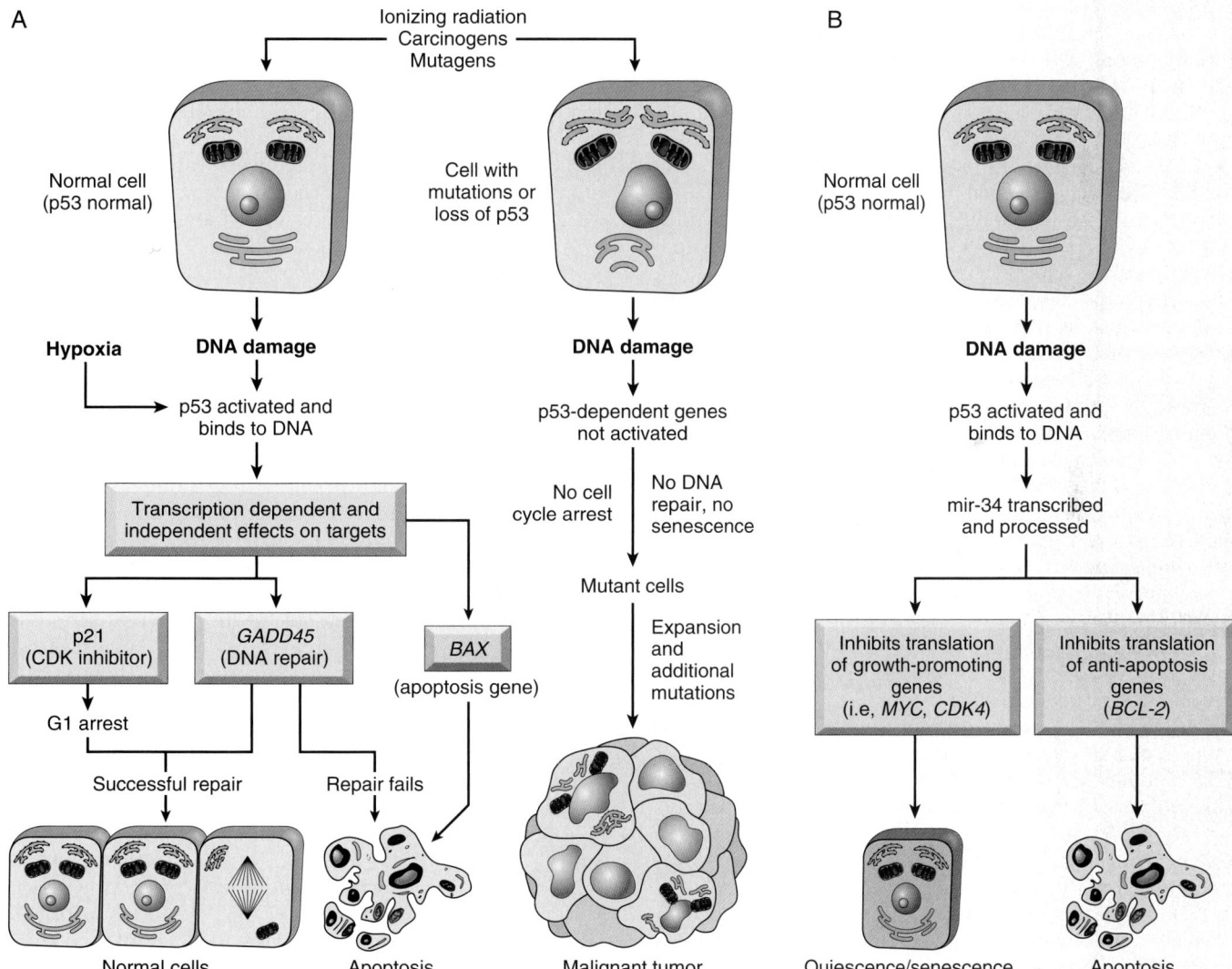

FIGURE 7–32 **A,** The role of *p53* in maintaining the integrity of the genome. Activation of normal *p53* by DNA-damaging agents or by hypoxia leads to cell cycle arrest in G₁ and induction of DNA repair, by transcriptional up-regulation of the cyclin-dependent kinase inhibitor *CDKN1A* (p21) and the *GADD45* genes. Successful repair of DNA allows cells to proceed with the cell cycle; if DNA repair fails, *p53* triggers either apoptosis or senescence. In cells with loss or mutations of *p53*, DNA damage does not induce cell cycle arrest or DNA repair, and genetically damaged cells proliferate, giving rise eventually to malignant neoplasms. **B,** p53 mediates gene repression by activating transcription of miRNAs. p53 activates transcription of the mir34 family of miRNAs. mir34s repress translation of both proliferative genes, such as cyclins, and anti-apoptotic genes, such as *BCL2*. Repression of these genes can promote either quiescence or senescence as well as apoptosis.

The manner in which p53 senses DNA damage and determines the adequacy of DNA repair is beginning to be understood. The key initiators of the DNA-damage pathway are two related protein kinases: *ataxia-telangiectasia mutated (ATM)* and *ataxia-telangiectasia and Rad3 related (ATR).*[77,78] As the name implies, the *ATM* gene was originally identified as the germ-line mutation in individuals with ataxia-telangiectasia. Persons with this disease, which is characterized by an inability to repair certain kinds of DNA damage, suffer from an increased incidence of cancer. The types of damage sensed by ATM and ATR are different, but the downstream pathways they activate are similar. Once triggered, both ATM and ATR phosphorylate a variety of targets, including p53 and DNA-repair proteins. Phosphorylation of these two targets leads to a pause in the cell cycle and stimulation of DNA-repair pathways, respectively.

p53-*mediated cell cycle arrest may be considered the primordial response to DNA damage* (Fig. 7–32). It occurs late in the G_1 phase and is caused mainly by p53-dependent transcription of the CDK inhibitor *CDKN1A (p21)*. As discussed, p21 inhibits cyclin-CDK complexes and phosphorylation of RB, thereby preventing cells from entering G_1 phase. Such a pause in cell cycling is welcome, because it gives the cells "breathing time" to repair DNA damage. p53 also helps the process by inducing certain proteins, such as GADD45 (growth arrest and DNA damage), that help in DNA repair.[75] p53 can stimulate DNA-repair pathways by transcription-independent mechanisms as well. If DNA damage is repaired successfully, p53 up-regulates transcription of MDM2, leading to its own destruction and thus releasing the cell cycle block. If the damage cannot be repaired, the cell may enter p53-induced senescence or undergo p53-directed apoptosis.

p53-*induced senescence is a permanent cell cycle arrest* characterized by specific changes in morphology and gene expression that differentiate it from quiescence or reversible cell cycle arrest. Senescence requires activation of p53 and/or RB and expression of their mediators, such as the CDK inhibitors, and is generally irreversible, although it may require the continued expression of p53. The mechanisms of senescence are unclear but involve epigenetic changes that result in the formation of heterochromatin at different loci throughout the genome.[80] These senescence-associated heterochromatin foci include pro-proliferative genes regulated by E2F; this drastically and permanently alters expression of these E2F targets. Like all p53 responses, senescence may be stimulated in response to a variety of stresses, such as unopposed oncogene signaling, hypoxia, and shortened telomeres.

p53-*induced apoptosis of cells with irreversible DNA damage* is the ultimate protective mechanism against neoplastic transformation. p53 directs the transcription of several pro-apoptotic genes such as *BAX* and *PUMA* (approved name *BBC3*; described later). Exactly how a cell decides whether to repair its DNA or to enter apoptosis is unclear. It appears that the affinity of p53 for the promoters and enhancers of DNA-repair genes is stronger than its affinity for pro-apoptotic genes.[80] Thus, the DNA-repair pathway is stimulated first, while p53 continues to accumulate. Eventually, if the DNA damage is not repaired, enough p53 accumulates to stimulate transcription of the pro-apoptotic genes and the cell dies. While this scheme is generally correct, there seem to be important cell type–specific responses as well, with some cell types succumbing to apoptosis early, while others opt for senes-

cence.[80] Such differential responses may be related to the functions of other p53 family members expressed in different cell types (see below).

To summarize, p53 links cell damage with DNA repair, cell cycle arrest, and apoptosis. In response to DNA damage, p53 is phosphorylated by genes that sense the damage and are involved in DNA repair. p53 assists in DNA repair by causing G_1 arrest and inducing DNA-repair genes. A cell with damaged DNA that cannot be repaired is directed by p53 to undergo apoptosis (see Fig. 7–32). In view of these activities, p53 has been rightfully called a "guardian of the genome." With loss of function of p53, DNA damage goes unrepaired, mutations accumulate in dividing cells, and the cell marches along a one-way street leading to malignant transformation.

The ability of p53 to control apoptosis in response to DNA damage has important practical therapeutic implications. Irradiation and chemotherapy, the two common modalities of cancer treatment, mediate their effects by inducing DNA damage and subsequent apoptosis. Tumors that retain normal p53 are more likely to respond to such therapy than tumors that carry mutated alleles of the gene. Such is the case with testicular teratocarcinomas and childhood acute lymphoblastic leukemias. By contrast, tumors such as lung cancers and colorectal cancers, which frequently carry *p53* mutations, are relatively resistant to chemotherapy and irradiation. Various therapeutic modalities aimed at increasing normal p53 activity in tumor cells that retain this type of activity or selectively killing cells with defective p53 function are being investigated.

The discovery of p53 family members p63 and p73 has revealed that p53 has collaborators. Indeed, p53, p63, and p73 are players in a complex network with significant cross-talk that is only beginning to be unraveled.[81,82] p53 is ubiquitously expressed, while p63 and p73 show more tissue specificity. For example, p63 is essential for the differentiation of stratified squamous epithelia, while p73 has strong pro-apoptotic effects after DNA damage induced by chemotheraputic agents. Furthermore, both p63 and p73, and probably p53 as well, are expressed as different isoforms, some of which act as transcriptional activators and others that function as dominant negatives. An illustrative example of the concerted actions of these three musketeers is seen in the so-called basal subset of breast cancers, which have a poor prognosis. These tumors have been shown to have mutations in *p53* and additionally express a dominant-negative version of p63 that antagonizes the apoptotic activity of p73. This perturbation of the p53-p63-p73 network contributes to the chemoresistance and poor prognosis of these tumors.[83]

APC/β-Catenin Pathway. Adenomatous polyposis coli genes (APC) represents a class of tumor suppressors whose main function is to down-regulate growth-promoting signals. Germ-line mutations at the *APC* (5q21) loci are associated with familial adenomatous polyposis, in which all individuals born with one mutant allele develop thousands of adenomatous polyps in the colon during their teens or 20s (familial adenomatous polyposis; Chapter 17). Almost invariably, one or more of these polyps undergoes malignant transformation, giving rise to colon cancer. As with other tumor suppressor genes, both copies of the *APC* gene must be lost for a tumor to arise. This conclusion is supported by the development of colon adenomas in mice with targeted disruption of *apc* genes

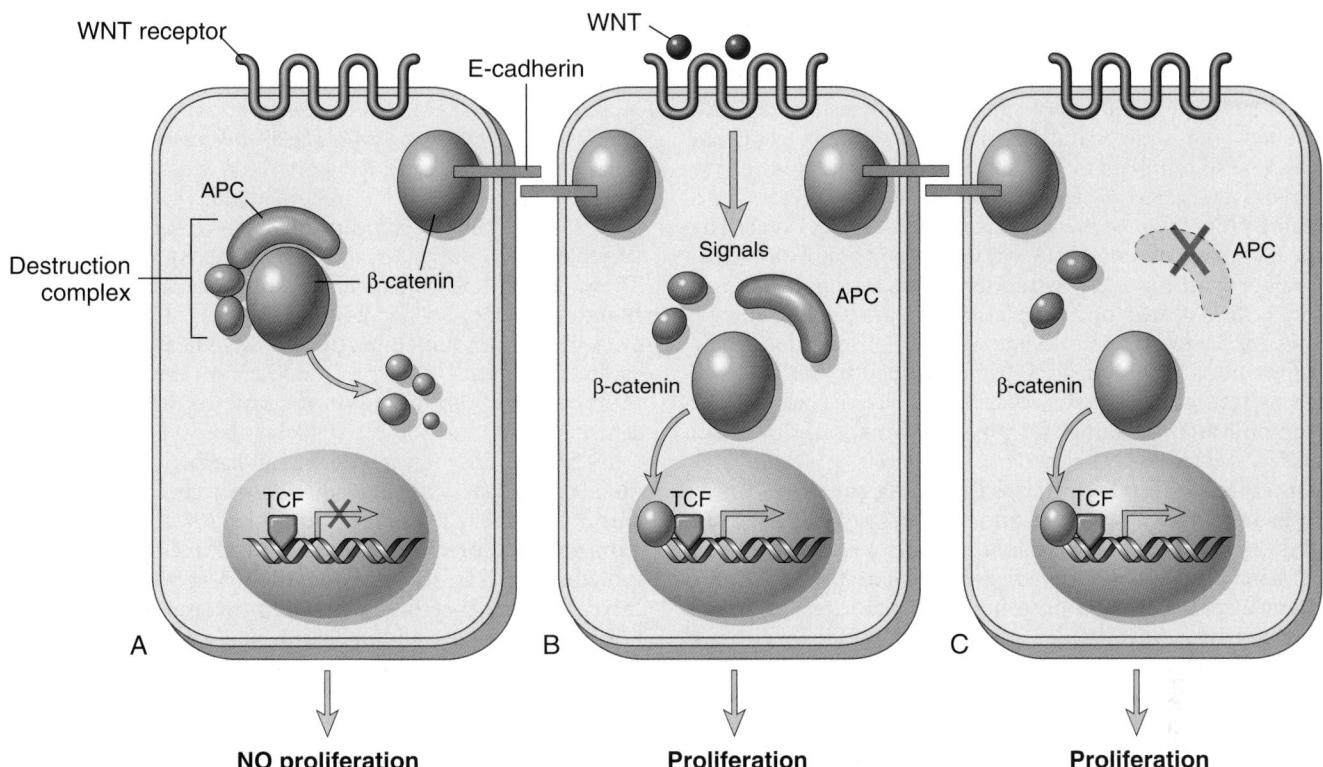

NO proliferation   **Proliferation**   **Proliferation**

FIGURE 7–33 **A,** The role of APC in regulating the stability and function of β-catenin. APC and β-catenin are components of the WNT signaling pathway. In resting cells (not exposed to WNT), β-catenin forms a macromolecular complex containing the APC protein. This complex leads to the destruction of β-catenin, and intracellular levels of β-catenin are low. **B,** When cells are stimulated by WNT molecules, the *destruction complex* is deactivated, β-catenin degradation does not occur, and cytoplasmic levels increase. β-catenin translocates to the nucleus, where it binds to TCF, a transcription factor that activates genes involved in cell cycle progression. **C,** When *APC* is mutated or absent, the destruction of β-catenin cannot occur. β-catenin translocates to the nucleus and coactivates genes that promote entry into the cell cycle, and cells behave as if they are under constant stimulation by the WNT pathway.

in the colonic mucosa.[84] As discussed later, several additional mutations must occur if cancers are to develop in the adenomas. In addition to these tumors, which have a strong hereditary predisposition, 70% to 80% of nonfamilial colorectal carcinomas and sporadic adenomas also show homozygous loss of the *APC* gene, thus firmly implicating *APC* loss in the pathogenesis of colonic tumors.[85]

APC is a component of the WNT signaling pathway, which has a major role in controlling cell fate, adhesion, and cell polarity during embryonic development (Fig. 7–33). WNT signaling is also required for self-renewal of hematopoietic stem cells. WNT signals through a family of cell surface receptors called frizzled (FRZ), and stimulates several pathways, the central one involving β-catenin and APC.

An important function of the APC protein is to down-regulate β-catenin. In the absence of WNT signaling APC causes degradation of β-catenin, preventing its accumulation in the cytoplasm.[85] It does so by forming a macromolecular complex with β-catenin, axin, and GSK3β, which leads to the phosphorylation and eventually ubiquitination of β-catenin and destruction by the proteasome. Signaling by WNT blocks the APC-AXIN-GSK3β destruction complex, allowing β-catenin to translocate from the cytoplasm to the nucleus. In the cell nucleus, β-catenin forms a complex with TCF, a transcription factor that up-regulates cellular proliferation by increasing the transcription of c-*MYC*, *cyclin D1*, and other genes. Since inactivation

of the *APC* gene disrupts the destruction complex, β-catenin survives and translocates to the nucleus, where it can activate transcription in cooperation with TCF.[85] Thus, cells with loss of APC behave as if they are under continuous WNT signaling. The importance of the APC/β-catenin signaling pathway in tumorigenesis is attested to by the fact that colon tumors that have normal *APC* genes harbor mutations in β-catenin that prevent its destruction by APC, allowing the mutant protein to accumulate in the nucleus. Dysregulation of the APC/β-catenin pathway is not restricted to colon cancers; mutations in the β-catenin gene are present in more than 50% of hepatoblastomas and in approximately 20% of hepatocellular carcinomas.[86] As mentioned in Chapter 3, β-catenin binds to the cytoplasmic tail of E-cadherin, a cell surface protein that maintains intercellular adhesiveness. Loss of cell-cell contact, such as in a wound or injury to the epithelium, disrupts the interaction between E-cadherin and β-catenin, and allows β-catenin to travel to the nucleus and stimulate proliferation; this is an appropriate response to injury that can help repair the wound. Re-establishment of these E-cadherin contacts as the wound heals leads to β-catenin again being sequestered at the membrane and reduction in the proliferative signal; these cells are said to be "contact-inhibited." Loss of contact inhibition, by mutation of the E-cadherin/β-catenin axis, or by other methods, is a key characteristic of carcinomas. Furthermore, loss of cadherins can favor the malignant phenotype by allowing easy disaggregation of cells, which can then invade locally or metastasize. Reduced cell surface expression of E-cadherin has been noted in many types of cancers, including those that arise in the esophagus, colon, breast, ovary, and prostate.[87] Germline mutations of the E-cadherin gene can predispose to familial gastric carcinoma, and mutation of the gene and decreased E-cadherin expression are present in a variable proportion of gastric cancers of the diffuse type. The molecular basis of reduced E-cadherin expression is varied. In a small proportion of cases, there are mutations in the E-cadherin gene (located on 16q); in other cancers, E-cadherin expression is reduced as a secondary effect of mutations in β-catenin genes. Additionally, E-cadherin may be down-regulated by transcription repressors, such as SNAIL, which have been implicated in epithelial-to-mesenchymal transition and metastasis[88] (discussed below).

Other Genes That Function as Tumor Suppressors. There is little doubt that many more tumor suppressor genes remain to be discovered. Often, their location is suspected by the detection of consistent sites of *chromosomal deletions* or by analysis of *LOH*. Some of the tumor suppressor genes that are associated with well-defined clinical syndromes are briefly described below (see Table 7–8):

INK4a/ARF. Also called the *CDKN2A* gene locus, the *INK4a/ARF* locus encodes two protein products; the p16/INK4a CDKI, which blocks cyclin D/CDK2-mediated phosphorylation of RB, keeping the RB checkpoint in place. The second gene product, p14/ARF, activates the p53 pathway by inhibiting MDM2 and preventing destruction of p53. Both protein products function as tumor suppressors, and thus mutation or silencing of this locus impacts both the RB and p53 pathways. p16 in particular is crucial for the induction of senescence. Mutations at this locus have been detected in bladder, head and neck tumors, acute lymphoblastic leukemias, and cholangiocarcinomas. In some tumors, such as cervical cancer, p16/INK4a is frequently silenced by hypermethylation of the gene, without the presence of a mutation (see discussion of epigenetic changes). The other CDKIs also function as tumor suppressors and are frequently mutated or otherwise silenced in many human malignancies, including 20% of familial melanomas, 50% of sporadic pancreatic adenocarcinomas, and squamous cell carcinomas of the esophagus.

The TGF-β Pathway. In most normal epithelial, endothelial, and hematopoietic cells, TGF-β is a potent inhibitor of proliferation. It regulates cellular processes by binding to a serine-threonine kinase complex composed of TGF-β receptors I and II. Dimerization of the receptor upon ligand binding leads to activation of the kinase and phosphorylation of receptor SMADs (R-SMADs). Upon phosphorylation, R-SMADs can enter the nucleus, bind to SMAD-4, and activate transcription of genes, including the CDKIs p21 and p15/INK4b. In addition, TGF-β signaling leads to repression of c-MYC, CDK2, CDK4, and cyclins A and E. As can be inferred from our earlier discussion, these changes result in decreased phosphorylation of RB and cell cycle arrest.

In many forms of cancer the growth-inhibiting effects of TGF-β pathways are impaired by mutations in the TGF-β signaling pathway. These mutations may affect the type II TGF-β receptor or interfere with SMAD molecules that serve to transduce antiproliferative signals from the receptor to the nucleus. Mutations affecting the type II receptor are seen in cancers of the colon, stomach, and endometrium. Mutational inactivation of SMAD4 is common in pancreatic cancers. *In 100% of pancreatic cancers and 83% of colon cancers, at least one component of the TGF-β pathway is mutated.* However, in many cancers, loss of TGF-β-mediated growth inhibition occurs at a level downstream of the core signaling pathway, for example, loss of p21 and/or persistent expression of c-Myc. These tumor cells can then use other elements of the TGF-β–induced program, including immune system suppression/evasion or promotion of angiogenesis, to facilitate tumor progression.[89] Thus TGF-β can function to prevent or promote tumor growth, depending on the state of other genes in the cell.

PTEN. PTEN (Phosphatase and *ten*sin homologue) is a membrane-associated phosphatase encoded by a gene on chromosome 10q23 that is mutated in Cowden syndrome, an autosomal dominant disorder marked by frequent benign growths, such as tumors of the skin appendages, and an increased incidence of epithelial cancers, particularly of the breast (Chapter 23), endometrium, and thyroid. PTEN acts as a tumor suppressor by serving as a brake on the pro-survival/pro-growth PI3K/AKT pathway.[90,91] As you will recall from Chapter 3, this pathway is normally stimulated (along with the RAS and JAK/STAT pathways) when ligands bind to receptor tyrosine kinases and involves a cascade of phosphorylation events. First, PI3K (phosphoinositide 3-kinase) phosphorylates the lipid inositide-3-phosphate to give rise to inositide-3,4,5-triphosphate, which binds and activates the kinase PDK1. PDK1 and other factors in turn phosphorylate and activate the serine/threonine kinase AKT, which is a major node in the pathway with several important functions. By phosphorylating a number of substrates, including BAD and MDM2, AKT enhances cell survival. AKT also inactivates the TSC1/TSC2 complex. TSC1 and TSC2 are the products of two tumor suppressor genes that are mutated in tuberous sclerosis (Chapter 28), an autosomal dominant disorder associated with developmental malformations and unusual benign neoplasms such as cardiac rhabdomyomas (Chapter 12), renal angiomyolipomas, and giant cell astrocytomas. Inactivation of TSC1/TSC2 unleashes the activity of yet another kinase called mTOR (mammalian target of rapamycin, a potent immunosuppressive drug), which stimulates the uptake of nutrients such as glucose and amino acids that are needed for growth and augments the activity of several factors that are required for protein synthesis. Although acquired loss of PTEN function is one of the most common ways that PI3K/AKT signaling is upregulated in various cancers, many other components of the pathway, including PI3K itself, may also be mutated so as to increase signaling. Considering all of these molecular lesions collectively, it is said that this may be the most commonly mutated pathway in human cancer. As a result there is great interest in targeting the PI3K/AKT pathway with inhibitors of mTOR, AKT, and other kinases in the pathway.

NF1. Individuals who inherit one mutant allele of the *NF1* gene develop numerous benign neurofibromas and optic nerve gliomas as a result of inactivation of the second copy of the gene.[92] This condition is called *neurofibromatosis type 1*

(Chapter 27). Some of the neurofibromas later develop into malignant peripheral nerve sheath tumors. *Neurofibromin*, the protein product of the *NF1* gene, contains a GTPase-activating domain, which regulates signal transduction through RAS proteins. Recall that RAS transmits growth-promoting signals and flips back and forth between GDP-binding (inactive) and GTP-binding (active) states. Neurofibromin facilitates conversion of RAS from an active to an inactive state. With loss of neurofibromin function, RAS is trapped in an active, signal-emitting state.

NF2. Germline mutations in the *NF2* gene predispose to the development of *neurofibromatosis type 2*.[93] As discussed in Chapter 27, individuals with mutations in *NF2* develop benign bilateral schwannomas of the acoustic nerve. In addition, somatic mutations affecting both alleles of *NF2* have also been found in sporadic meningiomas and ependymomas. The product of the *NF2* gene, called *neurofibromin 2* or *merlin*, shows a great deal of homology with the red cell membrane cytoskeletal protein 4.1 (Chapter 14), and is related to the ERM (ezrin, radixin, and moesin) family of membrane cytoskeleton-associated proteins. Although the mechanism by which *merlin* deficiency leads to carcinogenesis is not known, cells lacking this protein are not capable of establishing stable cell-to-cell junctions and are insensitive to normal growth arrest signals generated by cell-to-cell contact. Merlin is a key member of the Salvador-Warts-Hippo (SWH) tumor suppressor pathway, originally described in *Drosophila*. The signaling pathway controls organ size by modulating cell growth, proliferation, and apoptosis. Many human homologues of genes in the SWH pathway have been implicated in human cancers.[94]

VHL. Germline mutations of the von Hippel-Lindau (*VHL*) gene on chromosome 3p are associated with hereditary renal cell cancers, pheochromocytomas, hemangioblastomas of the central nervous system, retinal angiomas, and renal cysts.[60] Mutations of the *VHL* gene have also been noted in sporadic renal cell cancers (Chapter 20). The VHL protein is part of a ubiquitin ligase complex. A critical substrate for this activity is HIF1α (hypoxia-inducible transcription factor 1α). In the presence of oxygen, HIF1α is hydroxylated and binds to the VHL protein, leading to ubiquitination and proteasomal degradation. This hydroxylation reaction requires oxygen; in hypoxic environments the reaction cannot occur, and HIF1α escapes recognition by VHL and subsequent degradation. HIF1α can then translocate to the nucleus and turn on many genes, such as the growth/angiogenic factors vascular endothelial growth factor (VEGF) and PDGF. Lack of VHL activity prevents ubiquitination and degradation of HIF1α and is associated with increased levels of angiogenic growth factors.

WT1. The *WT1* gene, located on chromosome 11p13, is associated with the development of Wilms' tumor, a pediatric kidney cancer.[95] Both inherited and sporadic forms of Wilms' tumor occur, and mutational inactivation of the *WT1* locus has been seen in both forms. The WT1 protein is a transcriptional activator of genes involved in renal and gonadal differentiation. It regulates the mesenchymal-to-epithelial transition that occurs in kidney development. Though not precisely known, it is likely that the tumorigenic effect of WT1 deficiency is intimately connected with the role of the gene in the differentiation of genitourinary tissues. Interestingly, although WT1 is a tumor suppressor in Wilms' tumor, a variety of adult cancers, including leukemias and breast carcinomas, have also been shown to overexpress WT1. Since these tissues do not normally express WT1 at all, it has been suggested that WT1 may function as an oncogene in these cancers. Another Wilms' gene, *WT2*, located on 11p15, is associated with the Beckwith-Wiedemann syndrome (Chapter 10).

Patched (PTCH). *PTCH1* and *PTCH2* are tumor suppressor genes that encode a cell membrane protein (PATCHED), which functions as a receptor for a family of proteins called *Hedgehog*.[96] The Hedgehog/PATCHED pathway regulates several genes, including *TGF-β* and *PDGFRA* and *PDGFRB*. Mutations in *PTCH* are related to Gorlin syndrome, an inherited condition also known as nevoid basal cell carcinoma syndrome (see Chapter 26). *PTCH* mutations are present in 20% to 50% of sporadic cases of basal cell carcinoma. About one half of such mutations are of the type caused by UV exposure.

EVASION OF APOPTOSIS

Accumulation of neoplastic cells may result not only from activation of growth-promoting oncogenes or inactivation of growth-suppressing tumor suppressor genes, but also from mutations in the genes that regulate apoptosis.[97–99] Thus, apoptosis represents a barrier that must be surmounted for cancer to occur. In the adult, cell death by apoptosis is a physiologic response to several pathologic conditions that might contribute to malignancy if the cells remained viable. A cell with genomic injury can be induced to die, preventing the accumulation of cells with mutations. A variety of signals, ranging from DNA damage to loss of adhesion to the basement membrane (termed *anoikis*), can trigger apoptosis. A large family of genes that regulate apoptosis has been identified. Before we can understand how tumor cells evade apoptosis, it is essential to review briefly the biochemical pathways to apoptosis.

As discussed in Chapter 1, there are two distinct programs that activate apoptosis, the extrinsic and intrinsic pathways. Figure 7–34 shows, in simplified form, the sequence of events that lead to apoptosis by signaling through the death receptor CD95/Fas (extrinsic pathway) and by DNA damage (intrinsic pathway). The extrinsic pathway is initiated when CD95/Fas binds to its ligand, CD95L/FasL, leading to trimerization of the receptor and its cytoplasmic *death domains*, which attract the intracellular adaptor protein FADD. This protein recruits procaspase 8 to form the death-inducing signaling complex. Procaspase 8 is activated by cleavage into smaller subunits, generating caspase 8. Caspase 8 then activates downstream caspases such as caspase 3, a typical *executioner caspase* that cleaves DNA and other substrates to cause cell death. Additionally, caspase 8 can cleave and activate the BH3-only protein BID, activating the intrinsic pathway as well. The intrinsic pathway of apoptosis is triggered by a variety of stimuli, including withdrawal of survival factors, stress, and injury. Activation of this pathway leads to permeabilization of the mitochondrial outer membrane, with resultant release of molecules, such as cytochrome *c*, that initiate apoptosis. The integrity of the mitochondrial outer membrane is regulated by pro-apoptotic and anti-apoptotic members of the BCL2 family of proteins.[100] The pro-apoptotic proteins BAX and BAK are required for apoptosis and directly promote mitochondrial permeabilization. Their action is inhibited by the

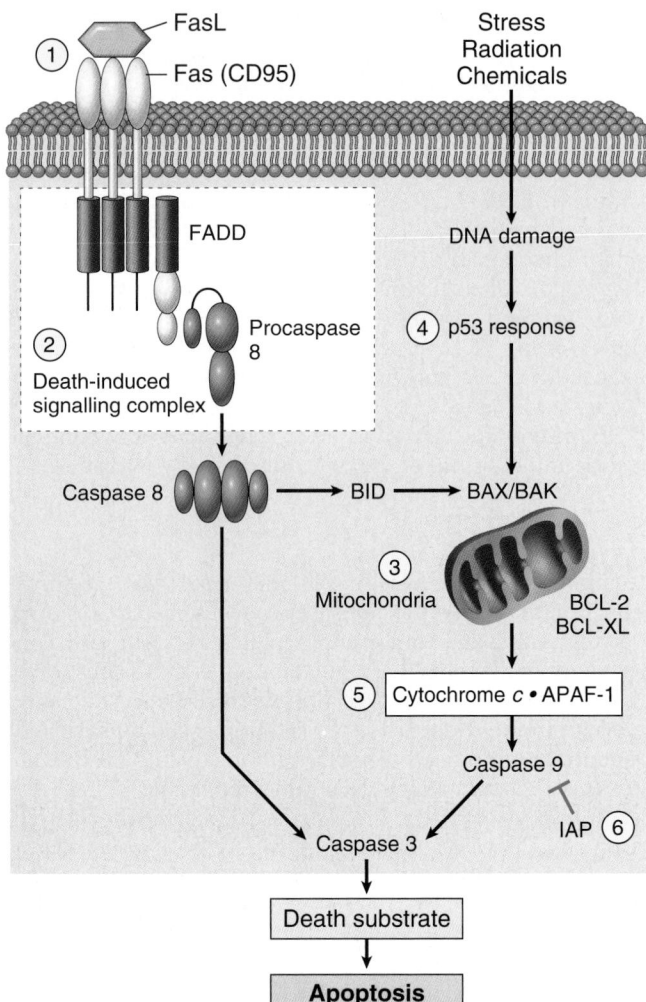

FIGURE 7–34 CD95 receptor–induced and DNA damage–triggered pathways of apoptosis and mechanisms used by tumor cells to evade cell death. (1) Reduced CD95 level. (2) Inactivation of death-induced signaling complex by FLICE protein (caspase 8; apoptosis-related cysteine peptidase). (3) Reduced egress of cytochrome *c* from mitochondrion as a result of up-regulation of BCL2. (4) Reduced levels of pro-apoptotic BAX resulting from loss of p53. (5) Loss of apoptotic peptidase activating factor 1 (APAF1). (6) Up-regulation of inhibitors of apoptosis (IAP). FADD, Fas-associated via death domain.

anti-apoptotic members of this family exemplified by BCL2 and BCL-XL. A third set of proteins (so-called BH3-only proteins), including BAD, BID, and PUMA, regulate the balance between the pro- and anti-apoptotic members of the BCL2 family. The BH3-only proteins sense death-inducing stimuli and promote apoptosis by neutralizing the actions of anti-apoptotic proteins like BCL2 and BCL-XL. When the sum total of all BH3 proteins expressed "overwhelms" the anti-apoptotic BCL2/BCL-XL protein barrier, BAX and BAK are activated and form pores in the mitochondrial membrane. Cytochrome *c* leaks into the cytosol, where it binds to APAF1, activating caspase 9. Like caspase 8 of the extrinsic pathway, caspase 9 can cleave and activate the executioner caspases. The caspases can be inhibited by a family of proteins called Inhibitors of Apoptosis Proteins (IAPs). Some tumors avoid apop-

tosis by upregulating these proteins, and there is interest in developing drugs that can block the interaction between IAPs and caspases. Because of the pro-apoptotic effect of BH3-only proteins, efforts are underway to develop BH3 mimetic drugs.

Within this framework it is possible to illustrate the multiple sites at which apoptosis is frustrated by cancer cells[101] (see Fig. 7–34). Starting from the surface, reduced levels of CD95/Fas may render the tumor cells less susceptible to apoptosis by CD95L/FasL. Some tumors have high levels of FLIP, a protein that can bind death-inducing signaling complex and prevent activation of caspase 8. Of all these genes, perhaps *best established is the role of BCL2 in protecting tumor cells from apoptosis.* As discussed later, approximately 85% of B-cell lymphomas of the follicular type (Chapter 13) carry a characteristic t(14;18)(q32;q21) translocation. Recall that 14q32, the site where immunoglobulin heavy-chain (IgH) genes are found, is also involved in the pathogenesis of Burkitt lymphoma. Juxtaposition of this transcriptionally active locus with *BCL2* (located at 18q21) causes overexpression of the BCL2 protein. This in turn increases the BCL2/BCL-XL buffer, protecting lymphocytes from apoptosis and allowing them to survive for long periods; there is therefore a steady accumulation of B lymphocytes, resulting in lymphadenopathy and marrow infiltration. Because BCL2-overexpressing lymphomas arise in large part from reduced cell death rather than explosive cell proliferation, they tend to be indolent (slow growing) compared with many other lymphomas.

As mentioned before, *p53 is an important pro-apoptotic gene that induces apoptosis in cells that are unable to repair DNA damage.* The actions of p53 are mediated in part by transcriptional activation of BAX, but there are other connections as well between p53 and the apoptotic machinery. Thus, the apoptotic machinery in cancer may be thwarted by mutations affecting the component proteins directly, as well as by loss of sensors of genomic integrity such as p53.

LIMITLESS REPLICATIVE POTENTIAL: TELOMERASE

As was discussed in the section on cellular aging (Chapter 1), most normal human cells have a capacity of 60 to 70 doublings. After this, the cells lose their ability to divide and become senescent. This phenomenon has been ascribed to progressive shortening of *telomeres* at the ends of chromosomes. Indeed, short telomeres seem to be recognized by the DNA-repair machinery as double-stranded DNA breaks, and this leads to cell cycle arrest mediated by p53 and RB.[102] In cells in which the checkpoints are disabled by *p53* or *RB1* mutations, the nonhomologous end-joining pathway is activated as a last-ditch effort to save the cell, joining the shortened ends of two chromosomes.[103] This inappropriately activated repair system results in dicentric chromosomes that are pulled apart at anaphase, resulting in new double-stranded DNA breaks. The resulting genomic instability from the repeated bridge-fusion-breakage cycles eventually produces mitotic catastrophe, characterized by massive cell death. *It follows that for tumors to grow indefinitely, as they often do, loss of growth restraints is not enough. Tumor cells must also develop ways to avoid both cellular senescence and mitotic catastrophe* (Fig. 7–35). If during crisis a cell manages to reactivate telom-

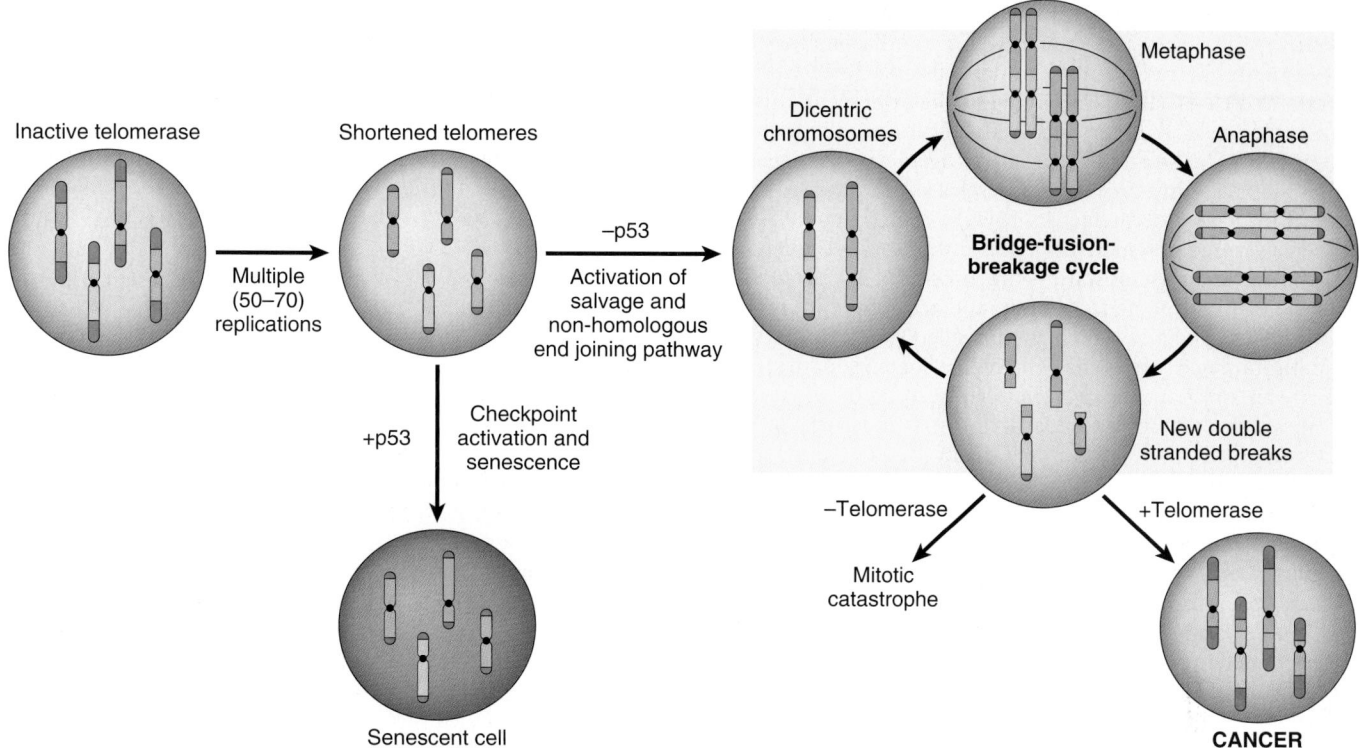

FIGURE 7–35 Sequence of events in the development of limitless replicative potential. Replication of somatic cells, which do not express telomerase, leads to shortened telomeres. In the presence of competent checkpoints, cells undergo arrest and enter nonreplicative senescence. In the absence of checkpoints, DNA-repair pathways are inappropriately activated, leading to the formation of dicentric chromosomes. At mitosis the dicentric chromosomes are pulled apart, generating random double-stranded breaks, which then activate DNA-repair pathways, leading to the random association of double-stranded ends and the formation, again, of dicentric chromosomes. Cells undergo numerous rounds of this bridge-fusion-breakage cycle, which generates massive chromosomal instability and numerous mutations. If cells fail to re-express telomerase, they eventually undergo mitotic catastrophe and death. Re-expression of telomerase allows the cells to escape the bridge-fusion-breakage cycle, thus promoting their survival and tumorigenesis.

erase, the bridge-fusion-breakage cycles cease and the cell is able to avoid death. However, during the period of genomic instability that precedes telomerase activation, numerous mutations could accumulate, helping the cell march toward malignancy. Passage through a period of genomic instability may explain the complex karyotypes frequently seen in human carcinomas. Telomerase, active in normal stem cells, is normally absent, or expressed at very low levels in most somatic cells. By contrast, telomere maintenance is seen in virtually all types of cancers. In 85% to 95% of cancers, this is due to up-regulation of the enzyme telomerase. A few tumors use other mechanisms, termed *alternative lengthening of telomeres*, which probably depend on DNA recombination. Interestingly, in the progression from colonic adenoma to colonic adenocarcinoma, early lesions had a high degree of genomic instability with low telomerase expression, whereas malignant lesions had complex karyotypes with high levels of telomerase activity, consistent with a model of telomere-driven tumorigenesis in human cancer. Several other mechanisms of genomic instability are discussed later.

ANGIOGENESIS

Even with all the genetic abnormalities discussed above, solid tumors cannot enlarge beyond 1 to 2 mm in diameter unless they are vascularized. Like normal tissues, tumors require

delivery of oxygen and nutrients and removal of waste products; presumably the 1- to 2-mm zone represents the maximal distance across which oxygen, nutrients, and waste can diffuse from blood vessels. Cancer cells can stimulate neoangiogenesis, during which new vessels sprout from previously existing capillaries, or, in some cases, vasculogenesis, in which endothelial cells are recruited from the bone marrow (Chapter 3). Tumor vasculature is abnormal, however. The vessels are leaky and dilated, and have a haphazard pattern of connection. Neovascularization has a dual effect on tumor growth: perfusion supplies needed nutrients and oxygen, and newly formed endothelial cells stimulate the growth of adjacent tumor cells by secreting growth factors, such as insulin-like growth factors (IGFs), PDGF, and granulocyte-macrophage colony-stimulating factor. Angiogenesis is required not only for continued tumor growth but also for access to the vasculature and hence for metastasis. *Angiogenesis is thus a necessary biologic correlate of malignancy.*[104]

How do growing tumors develop a blood supply? The emerging paradigm is that tumor angiogenesis is controlled by the balance between angiogenesis promoters and inhibitors. Early in their growth, most human tumors do not induce angiogenesis. They remain small or in situ, possibly for years, until the *angiogenic switch* terminates this stage of vascular quiescence.[105] The molecular basis of the angiogenic switch involves increased production of angiogenic factors and/or loss of angiogenic inhibitors. These factors may be produced directly by the tumor cells themselves or by inflammatory cells (e.g., macrophages) or other stromal cells associated with the tumors. Proteases, either elaborated by the tumor cells directly or from stromal cells in response to the tumor, are also involved in regulating the balance between angiogenic and anti-angiogenic factors. Many proteases can release the proangiogenic basic fibroblast growth factors (bFGF) stored in the ECM; conversely, three potent angiogenesis inhibitors—angiostatin, endostatin, and vasculostatin—are produced by proteolytic cleavage of plasminogen, collagen, and transthyretin, respectively. The angiogenic switch is controlled by several physiologic stimuli, such as hypoxia. Relative lack of oxygen stimulates HIF1α, an oxygen-sensitive transcription factor mentioned above, which then activates transcription of a variety of pro-angiogenic cytokines, such as VEGF and bFGF. These factors create an angiogenic gradient that stimulates the proliferation of endothelial cells and guides the growth of new vessels toward the tumor. VEGF also increases the expression of ligands that activate the Notch signaling pathway, which plays a crucial role in regulating the branching and density of the new vessels (Chapter 3). Both pro- and anti-angiogenic factors are regulated by many other genes frequently mutated in cancer. For example, in normal cells, p53 can stimulate expression of anti-angiogenic molecules such as thrombospondin-1, and repress expression of pro-angiogenic molecules such as VEGF. Thus, loss of p53 in tumor cells not only removes the cell cycle checkpoints listed above but also provides a more permissive environment for angiogenesis. The transcription of VEGF is also influenced by signals from the RAS-MAP kinase pathway, and mutations of *RAS* or *MYC* up-regulate the production of VEGF. The mechanisms whereby bFGF, VEGF, and the Notch pathway work together to coordinate angiogenesis were discussed in Chapter 3. bFGF and VEGF are commonly expressed in a wide variety of tumor cells, and elevated levels can be detected in the serum and urine of a significant fraction of cancer patients. Indeed, an anti-VEGF monoclonal antibody, bevacizumab, has recently been approved for use in the treatment of multiple cancers.[106] Another emerging strategy involves the use of antibodies that inhibit Notch activation. These antibodies cause new vessels to be so malformed that they cannot deliver blood to the tumor effectively.[107,108]

INVASION AND METASTASIS

Invasion and metastasis are biologic hallmarks of malignant tumors. They are the major cause of cancer-related morbidity and mortality and hence are the subjects of intense scrutiny. Studies in mice and humans reveal that although millions of cells are released into the circulation each day from a primary tumor, only a few metastases are produced. Indeed, tumor cells can be frequently detected in the blood and marrow of patients with breast cancer who have not, and do not ever, develop gross metastatic disease. Why is the metastatic process so inefficient? Each step in the process is subject to a multitude of controls; hence, at any point in the sequence the breakaway cell may not survive.[109] For tumor cells to break loose from a primary mass, enter blood vessels or lymphatics, and produce a secondary growth at a distant site, they must go through a series of steps (summarized in Fig. 7–36). For the purpose of this discussion, the metastatic cascade will be divided into two

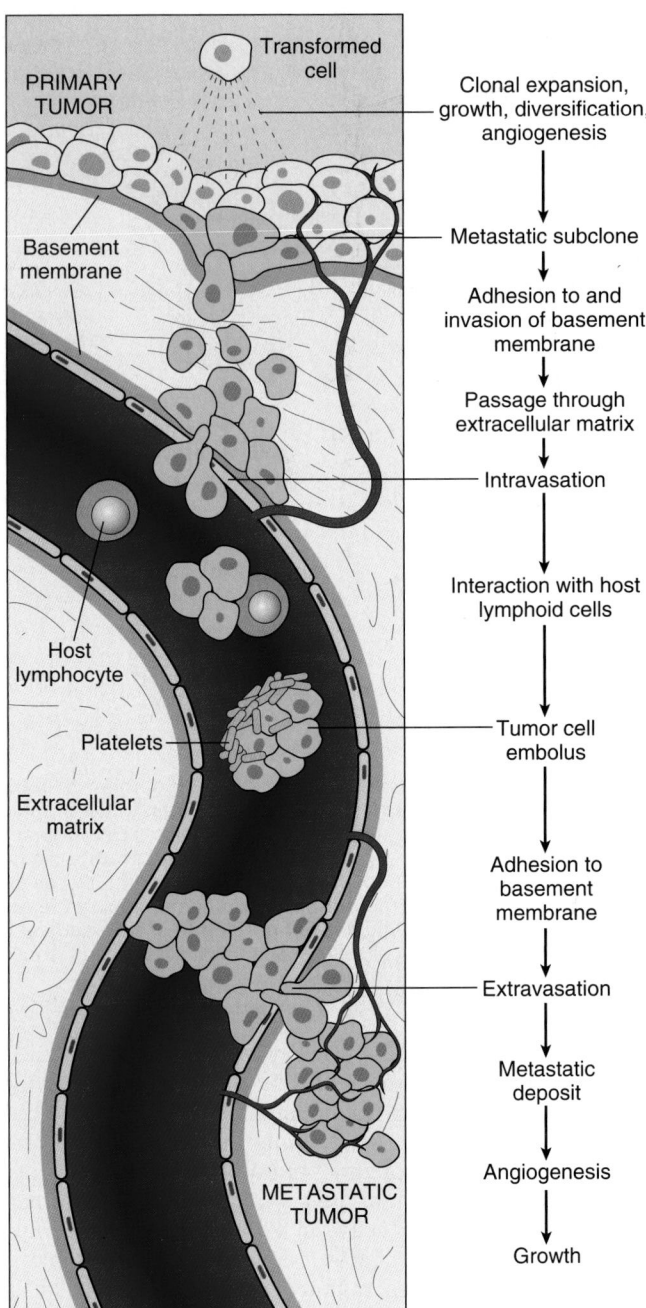

FIGURE 7–36 The metastatic cascade. Sequential steps involved in the hematogenous spread of a tumor.

phases: (1) invasion of the extracellular matrix (ECM); (2) vascular dissemination, homing of tumor cells, and colonization. Subsequently, the molecular genetics of the metastatic cascade, as currently understood, will be presented.

Invasion of Extracellular Matrix

The structural organization and function of normal tissues is to a great extent determined by interactions between cells and the ECM.[110] As we discussed in Chapter 3, tissues are organized into compartments separated from each other by two types of ECM: basement membrane and interstitial connec-

FIGURE 7–37 **A–D,** Sequence of events in the invasion of epithelial basement membranes by tumor cells. Tumor cells detach from each other because of reduced adhesiveness, then secrete proteolytic enzymes, degrading the basement membrane. Binding to proteolytically generated binding sites and tumor cell migration follow.

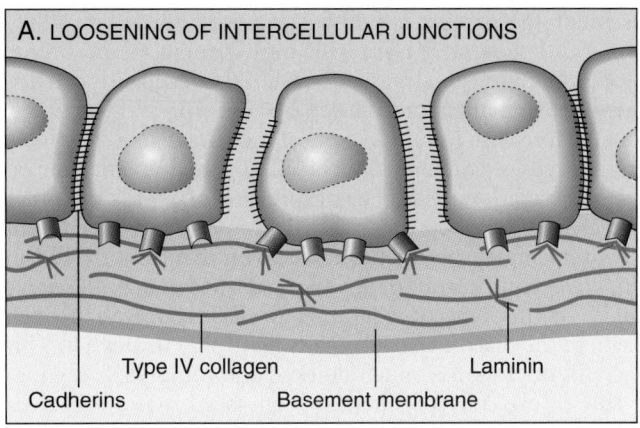

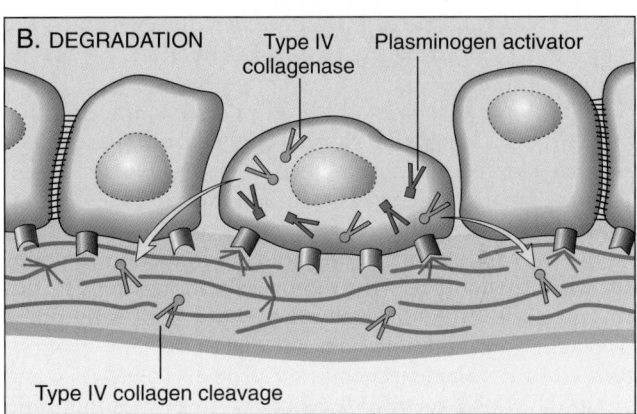

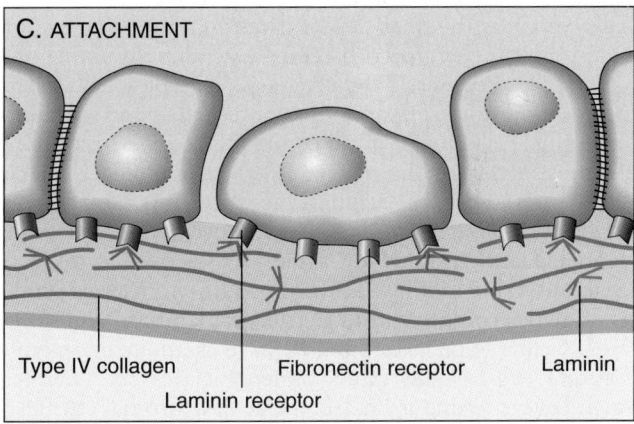

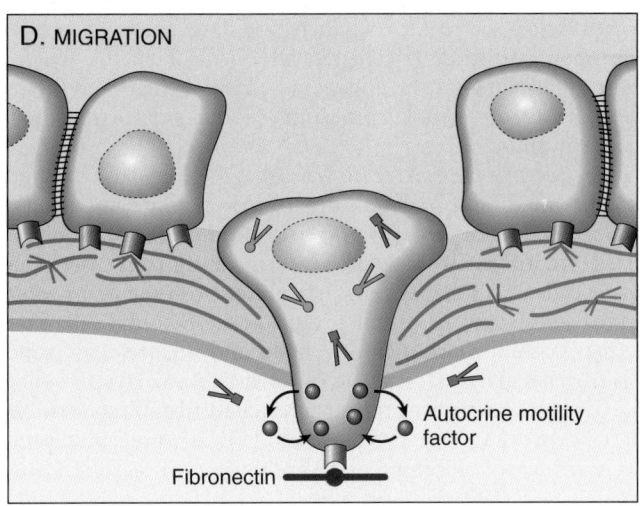

tive tissue. Though organized differently, each of these components of ECM is made up of collagens, glycoproteins, and proteoglycans. As shown in Figure 7–36, tumor cells must interact with the ECM at several stages in the metastatic cascade. A carcinoma must first breach the underlying basement membrane, then traverse the interstitial connective tissue, and ultimately gain access to the circulation by penetrating the vascular basement membrane. This process is repeated in reverse when tumor cell emboli extravasate at a distant site. Invasion of the ECM initiates the metastatic cascade and *is an active process that can be resolved into several steps* (Fig. 7–37):

- Changes ("loosening up") of tumor cell-cell interactions
- Degradation of ECM
- Attachment to novel ECM components
- Migration of tumor cells

Dissociation of cells from one another is often the result of alterations in intercellular adhesion molecules. Normal cells are neatly glued to each other and their surroundings by a variety of adhesion molecules.[111] Cell-cell interactions are mediated by the cadherin family of transmembrane glycoproteins. E-cadherins mediate homotypic adhesions in epithelial tissue, thus serving to keep the epithelial cells together and to relay signals between the cells; intracellularly the E-cadherins are connected to β-catenin and the actin cytoskeleton. In several epithelial tumors, including adenocarcinomas of the colon and breast, there is a down-regulation of E-cadherin expression. Presumably, this down-regulation reduces the ability of cells to adhere to each other and facilitates their detachment from the primary tumor and their advance into the surrounding tissues. E-cadherins are linked to the cytoskeleton by the *catenins*, proteins that lie under the plasma membrane (see Fig. 7–33). The normal function of E-cadherin is dependent on its linkage to catenins. In some tumors E-cadherin is normal, but its expression is reduced because of mutations in the gene for α catenin.

The second step in invasion is local *degradation of the basement membrane and interstitial connective tissue.* Tumor cells may either secrete proteolytic enzymes themselves or induce stromal cells (e.g., fibroblasts and inflammatory cells) to elaborate proteases. Many different families of proteases, such as matrix metalloproteinases (MMPs), cathepsin D, and urokinase plasminogen activator, have been implicated in tumor cell invasion. MMPs regulate tumor invasion not only by remodeling insoluble components of the basement membrane and interstitial matrix but also by releasing ECM-sequestered growth factors. Indeed, cleavage products of collagen and proteoglycans also have chemotactic, angiogenic, and growth-promoting effects.[112] For example, MMP9 is a gelatinase that cleaves type IV collagen of the epithelial and vascular basement membrane and also stimulates release of VEGF from ECM-sequestered pools. Benign tumors of the breast, colon, and stomach show little type IV collagenase activity, whereas their malignant counterparts overexpress this enzyme. Concurrently, the concentrations of metalloproteinase inhibitors are reduced so that the balance is tilted greatly toward tissue degradation. Indeed, overexpression of MMPs and other proteases has been reported for many tumors. However, recent in vivo imaging experiments have shown that tumor cells can adopt a second mode of invasion, termed *ameboid migration*.[113] In this type of migration the cell squeezes through spaces in the matrix instead of cutting its way through it. This ameboid migration is much quicker, and tumor cells seem to be able to use collagen fibers as high-speed railways in their travels. Tumor cells, in vitro at least, seem to be able to switch between the two forms of migration, perhaps explaining the disappointing performance of MMP inhibitors in clinical trials.

The third step in invasion involves *changes in attachment of tumor cells to ECM proteins*. Normal epithelial cells have receptors, such as integrins, for basement membrane laminin and collagens that are polarized at their basal surface; these receptors help to maintain the cells in a resting, differentiated state. Loss of adhesion in normal cells leads to induction of apoptosis, while, not surprisingly, tumor cells are resistant to this form of cell death. Additionally, the matrix itself is modified in ways that promote invasion and metastasis. For example, cleavage of the basement membrane proteins collagen IV and laminin by MMP2 or MMP9 generates novel sites that bind to receptors on tumor cells and stimulate migration.

Locomotion is the final step of invasion, propelling tumor cells through the degraded basement membranes and zones of matrix proteolysis. Migration is a complex, multistep process that involves many families of receptors and signaling proteins that eventually impinge on the actin cytoskeleton. Cells must attach to the matrix at the leading edge, detach from the matrix at the trailing edge, and contract the actin cytoskeleton to ratchet forward. Such movement seems to be potentiated and directed by tumor cell–derived cytokines, such as autocrine motility factors. In addition, cleavage products of matrix components (e.g., collagen, laminin) and some growth factors (e.g., IGFs I and II) have chemotactic activity for tumor cells. Furthermore, proteolytic cleavage liberates growth factors bound to matrix molecules. Stromal cells also produce paracrine effectors of cell motility, such as hepatocyte growth factor–scatter factor, which bind to receptors on tumor cells. Concentrations of hepatocyte growth factor–scatter factor are elevated at the advancing edges of the highly invasive brain tumor glioblastoma multiforme, supporting their role in motility.

It has become clear in recent years that the ECM and stromal cells surrounding tumor cells do not merely represent a static barrier for tumor cells to traverse but instead represent a varied environment in which reciprocal signaling between tumor cells and stromal cells may either promote or prevent tumorigenesis and/or tumor progression.[24] Stromal cells that interact with tumors include innate and adaptive immune cells (discussed later), as well as fibroblasts. A variety of studies have demonstrated that tumor-associated fibroblasts exhibit altered expression of genes that encode ECM molecules, proteases, protease inhibitors, and various growth factors. Thus,

tumor cells live in a complex and ever-changing milieu composed of ECM, growth factors, fibroblasts, and immune cells, with significant cross-talk among all the components. The most successful tumors may be those that can co-opt and adapt this environment to their own nefarious ends.

Vascular Dissemination and Homing of Tumor Cells

Once in the circulation, tumor cells are vulnerable to destruction by a variety of mechanisms, including mechanical shear stress, apoptosis stimulated by loss of adhesion, (which has been termed *anoikis*), and innate and adaptive immune defenses. The details of tumor immunity are considered later.

Within the circulation, tumor cells tend to aggregate in clumps. This is favored by homotypic adhesions among tumor cells as well as heterotypic adhesion between tumor cells and blood cells, particularly platelets (see Fig. 7–36). Formation of platelet-tumor aggregates may enhance tumor cell survival and implantability. Tumor cells may also bind and activate coagulation factors, resulting in the formation of emboli. Arrest and extravasation of tumor emboli at distant sites involves adhesion to the endothelium, followed by egress through the basement membrane. Involved in these processes are adhesion molecules (integrins, laminin receptors) and proteolytic enzymes, discussed earlier. Of particular interest is the CD44 adhesion molecule, which is expressed on normal T lymphocytes and is used by these cells to migrate to selective sites in the lymphoid tissue. Such migration is accomplished by the binding of CD44 to hyaluronate on high endothelial venules, and overexpression of CD44 may favor metastatic spread. At the new site, tumor cells must proliferate, develop a vascular supply, and evade the host defenses.[109]

The site at which circulating tumor cells leave the capillaries to form secondary deposits is related, in part, to the anatomic location of the primary tumor, with most metastases occurring in the first capillary bed available to the tumor. Many observations, however, suggest that natural pathways of drainage do not wholly explain the distribution of metastases. For example, prostatic carcinoma preferentially spreads to bone, bronchogenic carcinomas tend to involve the adrenals and the brain, and neuroblastomas spread to the liver and bones. Such organ tropism may be related to the following mechanisms:

- Because the first step in extravasation is adhesion to the endothelium, tumor cells may have adhesion molecules whose ligands are expressed preferentially on the endothelial cells of the target organ. Indeed, it has been shown that the endothelial cells of the vascular beds of various tissues differ in their expression of ligands for adhesion molecules.
- Chemokines have an important role in determining the target tissues for metastasis. For instance, some breast cancer cells express the chemokine receptors CXCR4 and CCR7.[114] The chemokines that bind to these receptors are highly expressed in tissues to which breast cancers commonly metastasize. Blockage of the interaction between CXCR4 and its receptor decreases breast cancer metastasis to lymph nodes and lungs. Some target organs may liberate chemoattractants that recruit tumor cells to the site. Examples include IGFs I and II.

● In some cases, the target tissue may be a nonpermissive environment—unfavorable soil, so to speak, for the growth of tumor seedlings. For example, though well vascularized, skeletal muscles are rarely the site of metastases.

Despite their "cleverness" in escaping their sites of origin, tumor cells are quite inefficient in colonizing distant organs. Millions of tumors cells are shed daily from even small tumors. These cells can be detected in the bloodstream and in small foci in the bone marrow, even in patients that never develop gross metastatic lesions. Indeed, the concept of dormancy, referring to the prolonged survival of micrometastases without progression, is well described in melanoma and in breast and prostate cancer. Although the molecular mechanisms of colonization are just beginning to be unraveled in mouse models, a constant pattern seems to be that tumor cells secrete cytokines, growth factors, and ECM molecules that act on the resident stromal cells, which in turn make the metastatic site habitable for the cancer cell.[115] For example, breast cancer metastases to bone are osteolytic because of the activation of osteoclasts in the metastatic site. Breast cancer cells secrete parathyroid hormone–related protein (PTHRP), which stimulates osteoblasts to make RANK ligand (RANKL). RANKL then activates osteoclasts, which degrade the bone matrix and release growth factors embedded within it, like IGF and TGF-β. With a better molecular understanding of the mechanisms of metastasis our ability to target them therapeutically will be greatly enhanced.

Molecular Genetics of Metastasis Development

Why do only some tumors metastasize? What are the genetic changes that allow metastases? Why is the metastatic process so inefficient? Several competing theories have been proposed to explain how the metastatic phenotype arises. The clonal evolution model suggest that, as mutations accumulate in genetically unstable cancer cells and the tumor become heterogeneous (Fig. 7–38A), a subset of tumor cell subclones develop the right combination of gene products to complete all the steps involved in metastasis. Thus, metastatic subclones result from clonal evolution, and it is only the rare cell that acquires all the necessary genetic alterations and can complete all the steps. However, recent experiments, in which gene expression profiles of primary tumors and metastatic deposits have been compared, challenge this hypothesis. For example, a subset of breast cancers has a gene expression signature similar to that found in metastases, although no clinical evidence for metastasis is apparent. In these tumors it seems that most if not all cells develop a predilection for metastatic spread during early stages of carcinogenesis. Metastases, according to this view, are not dependent on the stochastic generation of metastatic subclones postulated above. The alternative hypothesis suggested by these data is that metastasis is the result of multiple abnormalities that occur in many, perhaps most, cells of a primary tumor, and perhaps early in the development of the tumor (Fig. 7–38B and C). Such abnormalities give most cells within the tumor a general predisposition for metastasis, often called the "metastasis signature."[116] This signature may involve not only properties intrinsic to the cancer cells but also the characteristics of their

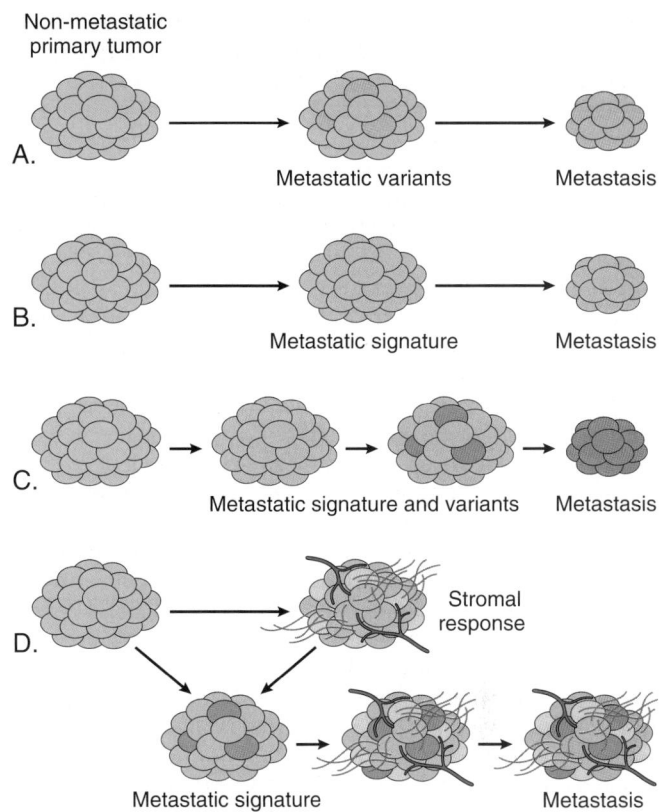

FIGURE 7–38 Mechanisms of metastasis development within a primary tumor. A nonmetastatic primary tumor is shown (light blue) on the left side of all diagrams. Four models are presented: **A,** Metastasis is caused by rare variant clones that develop in the primary tumor; **B,** Metastasis is caused by the gene expression pattern of most cells of the primary tumor, referred to as a metastatic signature; **C,** A combination of **A** and **B**, in which metastatic variants appear in a tumor with a metastatic gene signature; **D,** Metastasis development is greatly influenced by the tumor stroma, which may regulate angiogenesis, local invasiveness, and resistance to immune elimination, allowing cells of the primary tumor, as in **C,** to become metastatic.

microenvironment, such as the components of the stroma, the presence of infiltrating immune cells, and angiogenesis (Fig. 7–38D). It should be noted, however, that gene expression analyses like those described above would not detect a small subset of metastatic subclones within a large tumor. Perhaps both mechanisms are operative, with aggressive tumors acquiring a metastases-permissive gene expression pattern early in tumorigenesis that requires some additional random mutations to complete the metastatic phenotype. A third hypothesis suggests that background genetic variation, and the resulting variation in gene expression, in the human population contributes to the generation of metastases. In mouse models, cancers induced with the same oncogenic mutations can have very different metastatic outcomes depending on the strain (i.e., background genetics) of the mouse used. Even very strong oncogenes can be significantly affected by background genetics. The fourth hypothesis is a corollary of the tumor stem cell hypothesis, which suggests that if tumors derive from rare tumor stem cells, metastases require the spread of the tumor stem cells themselves.

One open question in the field is, are there genes whose principal or sole contribution to tumorigenesis is to control metastasis? This question is of more than academic interest, because if altered forms of certain genes promote or suppress the metastatic phenotype, their detection in a primary tumor would have both prognostic and therapeutic implications. Since metastasis is a complex phenomenon involving a variety of steps and pathways described above, it is thought that, unlike transformation, in which a subset of proteins like p53 and RB seem to play a key role, genes that function as "metastasis oncogenes" or "metastatic suppressors" are rare. A metastasis suppressor gene is defined as a gene whose loss promotes the development of metastasis without an effect on the primary tumor. Accordingly, expression of a metastasis oncogene favors the development of metastasis without effect upon the primary tumor. At least a dozen genes lost in metastatic lesions have been confirmed to function as "metastasis suppressors".[117,118] Their molecular functions are varied and not yet completely clear; however, most appear to affect various signaling pathways. Interestingly, recent work has suggested that two miRNAs, mir335 and mir126, suppress the metastasis of breast cancer, while a second set (mir10b) promotes metastasis.[119,120]

Among candidates for metastasis oncogenes are SNAIL and TWIST, which encode transcription factors whose primary function is to promote a process called epithelial-to-mesenchymal transition (EMT).[88] In EMT, carcinoma cells down-regulate certain epithelial markers (e.g., E-cadherin) and up-regulate certain mesenchymal markers (e.g., vimentin and smooth muscle actin). These changes are believed to favor the development of a promigratory phenotype that is essential for metastasis. Loss of E-cadherin expression seems to be a key event in EMT, and SNAIL and TWIST are transcriptional repressors that down-regulate E-cadherin expression.[121] EMT has been documented mainly in breast cancers; whether this is a general phenomenon remains to be established.

GENOMIC INSTABILITY—ENABLER OF MALIGNANCY

Although humans literally swim in environmental agents that are mutagenic (e.g., chemicals, radiation, sunlight), cancers are relatively rare outcomes of these encounters. This state of affairs results from the ability of normal cells to repair DNA damage, the death of cells with unrepairable damage[122] (see "Evasion of Apoptosis" above), and other mechanisms, such as oncogene-induced senescence and immune surveillance (discussed later). The importance of DNA repair in maintaining the integrity of the genome is highlighted by several inherited disorders in which genes that encode proteins involved in DNA repair are defective. *Individuals born with such inherited defects in DNA-repair proteins are at a greatly increased risk of developing cancer.* Moreover, defects in repair mechanisms are present in sporadic human cancers. *DNA-repair genes themselves are not oncogenic, but their abnormalities allow mutations in other genes during the process of normal cell division.* Typically, genomic instability occurs when both copies of the DNA repair gene are lost; however, recent work has suggested that at least a subset of these genes may promote cancer in a haploinsufficient manner. Defects in three types of DNA-repair systems—mismatch repair, nucleotide excision repair, and recombination repair—contribute to different types of cancers.

Hereditary Nonpolyposis Colon Cancer Syndrome. HNPCC syndrome, characterized by familial carcinomas of the colon affecting predominantly the cecum and proximal colon (Chapter 17), results from defects in genes involved in DNA mismatch repair.[123] When a strand of DNA is being replicated, these genes act as "spell checkers." For example, if there is an erroneous pairing of G with T rather than the normal A with T, the mismatch-repair genes correct the defect. Without these "proofreaders," errors gradually accumulate randomly in the genome, and some of these errors may involve proto-oncogenes and tumor suppressor genes. One of the hallmarks of patients with mismatch-repair defects is microsatellite instability.[21] Microsatellites are tandem repeats of one to six nucleotides found throughout the genome. In normal people the length of these microsatellites remains constant. However, in people with HNPCC, these satellites are unstable and increase or decrease in length in tumor cells, creating alleles not found in normal cells of the same patient. Of the various DNA mismatch-repair genes, at least four are involved in the pathogenesis of HNPCC, but germline mutations in the *MSH2* (2p16) and *MLH1* (3p21) genes each account for approximately 30% of cases. The remaining cases have mutations in other mismatch repair genes. Each affected individual inherits one defective copy of a DNA mismatch-repair gene and acquires the second hit in colonic epithelial cells. Thus, DNA-repair genes behave like tumor suppressor genes in their mode of inheritance, but in contrast to tumor suppressor genes (and oncogenes), they affect cell growth only indirectly—by allowing mutations in other genes during the process of normal cell division. Although HNPCC accounts only for 2% to 4% of all colonic cancers, microsatellite instability can be detected in about 15% of sporadic colon cancers. The growth-regulating genes that are mutated in HNPCC tumors have not yet been fully characterized but include the genes encoding TGF-β receptor II, the TCF component of the β-catenin pathway, *BAX*, and other oncogenes and tumor suppressor genes.[124]

Xeroderma Pigmentosum. Individuals with another inherited disorder of defective DNA repair, xeroderma pigmentosum, are at increased risk for the development of cancers of the skin particularly following exposure to the UV light contained in sun rays.[125] UV radiation causes cross-linking of pyrimidine residues, preventing normal DNA replication. Such DNA damage is repaired by the nucleotide excision repair system. Several proteins are involved in nucleotide excision repair, and an inherited loss of any one can give rise to xeroderma pigmentosum.

Diseases with Defects in DNA Repair by Homologous Recombination. A group of autosomal recessive disorders comprising Bloom syndrome, ataxia-telangiectasia, and Fanconi anemia is characterized by hypersensitivity to other DNA-damaging agents, such as ionizing radiation (Bloom syndrome and ataxia-telangiectasia), or DNA cross-linking agents, such as many chemotherapeutic agents (Fanconi anemia).[126,127] Their phenotype is complex and includes, in addition to predisposition to cancer, features such as neural symptoms (ataxia-telangiectasia), bone marrow aplasia (Fanconi anemia), and developmental defects (Bloom syndrome). As mentioned earlier, the gene mutated in ataxia-telangiectasia, *ATM*, is important in recognizing and responding to DNA damage caused by ionizing radiation. Persons with Bloom syndrome have a predisposition to a very broad spectrum of tumors. The defective gene is located on chromosome 15 and encodes a helicase that participates in DNA repair by homologous recombination. There are 13 genes that make up the Fanconi anemia complex; mutation of any one of these genes can result in the phenotype.[126,128] Interestingly, *BRCA2*, which is mutated in some individuals with familial breast cancer, is also mutated in a subset of persons with Fanconi anemia. Evidence for the role of DNA-repair genes in the origin of cancer also comes from the study of hereditary breast cancer. Mutations in two genes, *BRCA1* (chromosome 17q21) and *BRCA2* (chromosome 13q12–13), account for 25% of cases of familial breast cancer. In addition to breast cancer, women with *BRCA1* mutations have a substantially higher risk of epithelial ovarian cancers, and men have a slightly higher risk of prostate cancer. Likewise, mutations in the *BRCA2* gene increase the risk of breast cancer in both men and women as well as cancer of the ovary, prostate, pancreas, bile ducts, stomach, and melanocytes. Although the functions of these genes have not been elucidated fully, cells that lack these genes develop chromosomal breaks and severe aneuploidy. Indeed, both *BRCA1* and *BRCA2* have been shown to associate with a variety of proteins involved in the homologous recombination repair pathway. The Fanconi anemia proteins and the BRCA proteins form a DNA-damage response network whose purpose is to resolve and repair intrastrand and interstrand DNA cross-links induced by chemical cross-linking agents. Failure to resolve these cross-links before separation of the two strands would lead to chromosome breakage and exposed chromosome ends. Generation of such ends would, as with short telomeres (see above), lead to the activation of the salvage nonhomologous end joining pathway, formation of dicentric chromosomes, bridge-fusion-breakage cycles, and massive aneuploidy. Similar to other tumor suppressor genes, both copies of *BRCA1* and *BRCA2* must be inactivated for cancer to develop. Although linkage of *BRCA1* and *BRCA2* to familial breast cancers is established, these genes are rarely inactivated in sporadic cases of breast cancer. In this regard, *BRCA1* and *BRCA2* are different from other tumor suppressor genes, such as *APC* and *p53*, which are inactivated in both familial and sporadic cancers.

STROMAL MICROENVIRONMENT AND CARCINOGENESIS

Although we have mostly focused on the neoplastic parenchymal cells in our discussion, tumors are not composed of a single cell type. Indeed, tumors are comprised of a complex mixture of cells of numerous lineages, including the tumor cells themselves, innate and adaptive immune cells, fibroblasts, endothelial cells, and others. Additionally, numerous examples of cross-talk between the ECM and tumor cells have been described. For example, cleavage of matrix components such as type IV collagen releases angiogenic factors (VEGF), and enzymatic degradation of laminin-5 by MMP2 reveals a cryptic proteolytic fragment that favors cancer cell motility.[112] The ECM also stores growth factors in inactive forms, which are released by active matrix proteases. Such factors include PDGF, TGF-β, and bFGF, which in turn affect the growth of tumor cells in a paracrine manner. Successful tumor cells must co-opt these and other interactions and use them to promote their growth and invasion. More interesting is whether tumor cells are dependent upon these interactions for proliferation, survival, or metastases. If so, these interactions, and the stromal cells themselves, become potential therapeutic targets.

Both the inflammatory cells and fibroblasts within the tumor have been shown to have a complex relationship to the cancer cells and to each other. The role of chronic inflammation in the development of cancer has already been described (see above). Various mechanisms, such as the expression of pro-survival and pro-proliferation cytokines by immune cells, not only promote the development of cancer, but also promote survival and progression of tumor cells. Additionally, it has been suggested that macrophages infiltrating the tumor can be induced by the tumor cells to secrete factors that promote metastasis.[129] In a mouse model of breast cancer, genetic deletion of macrophages prevented metastases. Furthermore, in vivo imaging of tumors in animal models has shown that macrophages surrounding blood vessels secrete EGF, resulting in chemotactic migration of tumor cells toward the vasculature.[113] Fibroblasts play an important role in tumors as well. Fibroblasts secrete the matrix that results in the desmoplastic response to tumors. Interestingly, in vitro experiments that altered the stiffness of the matrix alone could change the aggressiveness of a cancer cell line. Thus, the desmoplastic response to cancer may be stimulated by the cancer cells and may promote their growth. On the other hand, in a prostate cancer model, injection of immortalized, but nontumorigenic cells, together with fibroblasts derived from a tumor (cancer-associated fibroblasts) led to the development of poorly differentiated tumors in athymic mice.[130] These carcinomas had multiple genetic abnormalities that were not present in the parent cell line, suggesting that the stroma can drive genetic changes that promote carcinogenesis. Indeed, some of the predictions of tumor behavior based on gene expression profiling are turning out to be based on genes highly expressed in stromal cells, rather than tumor cells. How such changes come about remains mysterious, as does their relevance to carcinogenesis in vivo. However, the results are sufficiently intriguing to merit attention, since they suggest a novel form of cancer therapy that could be targeted to stromal cells. The role of stromal cells in tumor growth and progression is highlighted by recent studies in which gene expression profiles of stroma cells predicted clinical outcome in human breast cancer.[131]

METABOLIC ALTERATIONS: THE WARBURG EFFECT

Even in the presence of ample oxygen, cancer cells shift their glucose metabolism away from the oxygen hungry, but efficient, mitochondria to glycolysis.[132–134] This phenomenon, called the Warburg effect and also known as aerobic glycolysis, has been recognized for many years (indeed, Otto Warburg received the Nobel Prize for discovery of the effect that bears his name in 1931), but was largely neglected until recently. This metabolic alteration is so common to tumors that some would call it the eighth hallmark of cancer. Indeed, clinically, the "glucose-hunger" of tumors is used to visualize tumors via positron emission tomography (PET) scanning, in which patients are injected with 18F-fluorodeoxyglucose, a non-metabolizable derivative of glucose that is preferentially taken up into tumor cells (as well as normal, actively dividing tissues such as the bone marrow). Most tumors are PET-positive, and rapidly growing ones are markedly so. However, the causal relationship between aerobic glycolysis and tumor progression is not entirely clear, nor is the initial insult that drives these metabolic changes.

Indeed, as is well known, glycolysis generates 2 ATP molecules per molecule of glucose, while oxidative phosphorylation in the mitochondria generates more than 20. How does a switch to the less efficient glycolysis lead to a growth advantage for a tumor? Several mutually non-exclusive hypotheses have been offered. One attractive hypothesis to explain the Warburg effect is that altered metabolism confers a growth advantage in the hypoxic tumor microenvironment.[133–134] Although angiogenesis generates increased vasculature, the vessels are poorly formed, and tumors are still relatively hypoxic compared to normal tissues. Indeed, the activation of HIF1α by hypoxia not only stimulates angiogenesis, but also increases the expression of numerous metabolic enzymes in the glycolytic pathway as well as downregulates genes involved in oxidative phosphorylation. So the simplest explanation is basic economics: supply and demand. Decreased demand by individual tumor cells increases the oxygen supply, thus increasing the number of tumor cells that can be supported by the vasculature and increasing the size of the tumor.

However, the Warburg effect refers to aerobic glycolysis; glycolysis that occurs in the face of adequate oxygen for oxidative phosphorylation. Thus, the changes that promote the switch in metabolism during hypoxia must become fixed in the tumor cell. It may be that continuous rounds of hypoxia followed by normoxia, as is frequently seen in tumors, select for tumor cells that constitutively upregulate glycolysis. Additionally, or perhaps alternatively, mutations in oncogenes and tumor suppressors that favor growth, such as *RAS*, *p53* and *PTEN*, also stimulate metabolic changes in the cell. Which brings us to the second part of the supply and demand equation that may help explain why tumor cells opt for a less efficient energy production pipeline.

In addition to doubling its DNA content prior to division, an actively dividing cell (whether normal or transformed) must also double all of its other components, including membranes, proteins, and organelles. This task requires increased uptake of nutrients, particularly glucose (which produces the energy needed for biosynthesis of these components) and amino acids (which provide the building blocks used for protein synthesis) as well as increased synthesis of the necessary building blocks. Halting the breakdown of glucose at pyruvate allows these carbons to be shunted to anabolic pathways, such as lipid and nucleotide production; additionally, tumor cells are able to shunt glutamine into both the glycolytic as well as anabolic pathways.[134–135] Thus, the metabolic changes that tumor cells undergo increase their ability to synthesize the building blocks they need for cell division. Indeed, alterations in signaling pathways involved in cancer also stimulate the uptake of glucose and other nutrients, favor glycolysis over oxidative phosphorylation, and increase anabolic pathways in the cell. Normally, growth factors stimulate glucose and amino acid uptake through the PI3K/AKT/mTOR pathway, which is downstream of receptor tyrosine kinases and other growth factor receptors; in tumors, these signals are cell autonomous. Thus, mutation of tumor suppressors and oncogenes not only leads to constitutive activation of pathways that favor survival and proliferation, but they also make glycolysis and anabolic biosynthesis a permanent fixture of the tumor cell.[135–136]

Now that the Warburg effect has been "rediscovered," other fascinating connections between metabolism and neoplasia are emerging that involve both tumor suppressors and onco-

proteins. One example of the former involves *LKB1*, a tumor suppressor gene encoding a threonine kinase that is mutated in Peutz-Jegher syndrome (Chapter 17), which is associated with benign and malignant epithelial proliferations of the gastrointestinal tract. At least one aspect of LKB1's tumor suppressive activity is mediated through its ability to activate AMP-dependent protein kinase (AMPK), a conserved sensor of cellular energy status that is an important negative regulator of mTOR. Thus LKB1 suppresses tumor formation, at least in part, by putting the brakes on anabolic metabolism. Of note, two other tumor suppressors that are mutated in tuberous sclerosis, TSC1 and TSC2 (Chapter 28), also negatively regulate mTOR. On the other side of the ledger, it has been claimed that the transforming effects of many oncoproteins, including mutated receptor tyrosine kinases and the notorious oncogenic transcription factor c-MYC, are mediated in part through induction of the "Warburg effect." These kinds of insights have spurred many recent attempts to target signaling pathways that drive anabolic metabolism in cancer cells, such as the PI3K/AKT/mTOR pathway.

As we have discussed earlier, cells have many regulatory barriers to prevent inappropriate growth. One adaptive response of normal cells to oxygen and glucose deprivation is *autophagy*, a state in which cells arrest their growth and cannibalize their own organelles, proteins, and membranes as carbon sources for energy production (Chapter 1). If this adaptation fails, the cells die. Tumor cells often seem to be able to grow under marginal environmental conditions without triggering autophagy, suggesting that the pathways that induce autophagy are deranged. In keeping with this, several genes that promote autophagy are tumor suppressors, most notable PTEN (a negative regulator of the PI3K/AKT pathway), which is mutated or epigenetically silenced in a wide variety of human cancers. Whether autophagy is always bad from the vantage point of the tumor, however, is a matter of active investigation and debate. For example, under conditions of severe nutrient deprivation tumor cells may use autophagy to become "dormant," a state of metabolic hibernation that allows cells to survive hard times for long periods. Such cells are believed to be resistant to therapies that kill actively dividing cells, and could therefore be responsible for therapeutic failures. Thus, autophagy may be a tumor's friend or foe depending on how the signaling pathways that regulate it are "wired" in a given tumor.

DYSREGULATION OF CANCER-ASSOCIATED GENES

The genetic damage that activates oncogenes or inactivates tumor suppressor genes may be subtle (e.g., point mutations) or may involve segments of chromosomes large enough to be detected in a routine karyotype. Activation of oncogenes and loss of function of tumor suppressor genes by mutations were discussed earlier in this chapter. Here we discuss chromosomal abnormalities. We end this section by discussing the epigenetic changes that contribute to carcinogenesis.

Chromosomal Changes

In certain neoplasms, karyotypic abnormalities are nonrandom and common. Specific chromosomal abnormalities have been identified in most leukemias and lymphomas, many sar-

TABLE 7–9 Selected Examples of Oncogenes Activated by Translocation

Malignancy	Translocation	Affected Genes*	
Chronic myeloid leukemia	(9;22)(q34;q11)	ABL	9q34
		BCR	22q11
Acute leukemias (AML and ALL)	(8;21)(q22;q22)	AML	8q22
		ETO	21q22
	(15;17)(q22;q21)	PML	15q22
		RARA	17q21
Burkitt lymphoma	(8;14)(q24;q32)	c-MYC	8q24
		IGH	14q32
Mantle cell lymphoma	(11;14)(q13;q32)	CCND1	11q13
		IGH	14q32
Follicular lymphoma	(14;18)(q32;q21)	IGH	14q32
		BCL2	18q21
T-cell ALL	(10;14)(q24;q11)	HOX 11	10q24
		TCRA	14q11
Ewing sarcoma	(11;22)(q24;q12)	FLI1	11q24
		EWSR1	22q12
Prostatic adenocarcinoma	(21;21)(q22;q22)	TMPRSS2 (21q22.3)	
	(7;21)(p22;q22)	ERG (21q22.2)	
	(17;21)(p21;q22)	ETV1 (7p21.2)	
		ETV4 (17q21)	

*Genes in boldface are involved in multiple translocations.
AML, acute myeloid leukemia; ALL, acute lymphoblastic leukemia.

comas, and an increasing number of carcinomas. In addition, whole chromosomes may be gained or lost. Although changes in chromosome number (aneuploidy) and structure are generally considered to be late phenomena in cancer progression, it has been suggested that aneuploidy and chromosomal instability may be the initiating events in tumor growth.

The study of chromosomal changes in tumor cells is important on two accounts. First, molecular cloning of genes in the vicinity of chromosomal breakpoints or deletions has been extremely useful in identification of oncogenes (e.g., BCL2, ABL) and tumor suppressor genes (e.g., APC, RB). Second, certain karyotypic abnormalities are specific enough to be of diagnostic value, and in some cases they are predictive of clinical course. The translocations associated with the ABL oncogene in CML and with c-MYC in Burkitt lymphoma have been mentioned earlier, in the context of molecular defects in cancer cells (see Fig. 7–27). Several other karyotype alterations in cancer cells are presented in the discussion of specific tumors in later chapters.

Two types of chromosomal rearrangements can activate proto-oncogenes—translocations and inversions. Chromosomal translocations are much more common (Table 7–9) and are discussed here. Translocations can activate proto-oncogenes in two ways:

- In lymphoid tumors specific translocations result in overexpression of proto-oncogenes by swapping their regulatory elements with those of another gene.
- In many hematopoietic tumors, sarcomas, and certain carcinomas, the translocations allow normally unrelated sequences from two different chromosomes to recombine and form hybrid fusion genes that encode chimeric pro-

teins that variously promote growth and survival, or enhance self-renewal and block differentiation.

Overexpression of a proto-oncogene caused by translocation is best exemplified by Burkitt lymphoma. All such tumors carry one of three translocations, each involving chromosome 8q24, where the MYC gene has been mapped, as well as one of the three immunoglobulin gene–carrying chromosomes. At its normal locus, MYC is tightly controlled, and is most highly expressed in actively dividing cells. In Burkitt lymphoma the most common form of translocation results in the movement of the MYC-containing segment of chromosome 8 to chromosome 14q32 (see Fig. 7–27), placing it close to the IGH gene. The genetic notation for the translocation is t(8:14)(q24;q32). The molecular mechanisms of the translocation-associated activation of MYC are variable, as are the precise breakpoints within the gene. In most cases the translocation causes mutation or loss of the regulatory sequences of the MYC gene, replacing them with the control regions of the IGH locus, which is highly expressed in B-cell precursors. As the coding sequences remain intact, the gene is constitutively expressed at high levels. The invariable presence of the translocated MYC gene in Burkitt lymphomas attests to the importance of MYC overactivity in the pathogenesis of this tumor.

There are other examples of oncogenes translocated to antigen receptor loci in lymphoid tumors. As mentioned earlier, in mantle cell lymphoma the cyclin D1 gene (CCND1) on chromosome 11q13 is overexpressed by juxtaposition to the IGH locus on 14q32. In follicular lymphomas, a t(14;18)(q32;q21) translocation, the most common translocation in lymphoid malignancies, causes activation of the BCL2 gene. Not unexpectedly, all these tumors in which the immunoglobulin gene is involved are of B-cell origin. In an analogous situation, overexpression of several proto-oncogenes in T-cell tumors results from translocations of oncogenes into the T-cell antigen receptor locus. The affected oncogenes are diverse, but in most cases, as with MYC, they encode nuclear transcription factors.

The Philadelphia chromosome, characteristic of CML and a subset of acute lymphoblastic leukemias, provides the prototypic example of an oncogene formed by *fusion of two separate genes*. In these cases, a reciprocal translocation between chromosomes 9 and 22 relocates a truncated portion of the proto-oncogene c-ABL (from chromosome 9) to the BCR (breakpoint cluster region) on chromosome 22 (see Fig. 7–27). The hybrid fusion gene BCR-ABL encodes a chimeric protein that has constitutive tyrosine kinase activity. As mentioned, BCR-ABL tyrosine kinase has served as a target for leukemia therapy, with remarkable success so far. Although the translocations are cytogenetically identical in CML and acute lymphoblastic leukemias, they usually differ at the molecular level. In most cases of CML the chimeric protein has a molecular weight of 210 kD, whereas in the more aggressive acute leukemias a 190-kD BCR-ABL fusion protein is typically formed.[48,49]

Transcription factors are often the partners in gene fusions occurring in cancer cells. For instance, the MLL (myeloid, lymphoid leukemia) gene on 11q23, which itself is a component of a chromatin-remodeling complex, is known to be involved in 50 different translocations with several different partner genes, some of which encode transcription factors (see

Table 7–9). Ewing sarcoma/primitive neuroectodermal tumor (PNET) is defined by translocation of the Ewing sarcoma (*EWSR1*) gene at 22q12, which is involved in numerous translocations, and all of its partner genes analyzed so far also encode a transcription factor. In Ewing sarcoma/PNET, for example, the *EWSR1* gene fuses with the *FLI1* gene, also a member of the ETS transcription factor family; the resultant chimeric EWS-FLI1 protein has transforming ability. One might ask, why are particular translocations so strongly associated with specific tumors? This is incompletely understood, but one recurrent theme is that at least one of the affected genes often encodes a transcription factor that is required for the development and differentiation of normal cells of the same lineage as the tumor. For example, in acute leukemias many genes involved by recurrent translocations (such as *MLL*) play essential roles in regulating the self-renewal of hematopoietic stem cells and the normal differentiation of lymphoid and myeloid cells. The fusion proteins resulting from translocations most often inhibit, but occasionally increase, transcriptional function. Until recently, most known translocations were discovered in leukemias/lymphomas and sarcomas; few common translocations had been identified in carcinomas, even though carcinomas are more common. The complex karyotypes of most carcinomas have made identifying translocations difficult. Recently, however, a translocation involving an androgen-regulated gene, *TMPRSS2* (21q22), and one of three ETS family transcription factors (*ERG* [21q22], *ETV1* [7p22.2], or *ETV4* [17q21]) was found to be present in 50% or more prostate adenocarcinomas.[137,138] Development of this translocation seems to occur early in carcinogenesis, in that it is also present in high-grade prostatic intraepithelial neoplasia, a precursor lesion. Although the mechanism by which this translocation causes cancer is not completely understood, it removes the ETS family gene from its normal control region and fuses it to the androgen-regulated *TMPRSS2*. Thus, the ETS family transcription factor is inappropriately expressed in prostate cells, and as noted above with Ewing sarcoma, when ETS proteins are inappropriately expressed they have transforming ability. There is significant interest in identifying additional fusion genes in other carcinomas. Many fusion genes are thought to be initiators in carcinogenesis, and it is postulated that many cancers may be "addicted" to their properties, similar to the oncogene addiction seen in CML with the BCR-ABL fusion. Thus, inhibition of these genes may provide an avenue for targeted therapy.

Deletions. Chromosomal deletions are the second most prevalent structural abnormality in tumor cells. *Compared with translocations, deletions are more common in nonhematopoietic solid tumors.* Deletion of specific regions of chromosomes is associated with the loss of particular tumor suppressor genes. As discussed, deletions involving chromosome 13q14, the site of the *RB* gene, are associated with retinoblastoma. Deletions of 17p, 5q, and 18q have all been noted in colorectal cancers; these regions harbor three tumor suppressor genes. Deletion of 3p, noted in several tumors, is extremely common in small-cell lung carcinomas, and the hunt is on for one or more cancer suppressor genes at this locale.

Gene Amplification

Activation of proto-oncogenes associated with overexpression of their products may result from reduplication and *amplification* of their DNA sequences.[139] Such amplification may produce several hundred copies of the proto-oncogene in the tumor cell. The amplified genes can be readily detected by molecular hybridization with appropriate DNA probes. In some cases the amplified genes produce chromosomal changes that can be identified microscopically. Two mutually exclusive patterns are seen: multiple small, centric structures called *double minutes* and *homogeneous staining regions.* The latter derive from the insertion of the amplified genes into new chromosomal locations, which may be distant from the normal location of the involved genes; because regions containing amplified genes lack a normal banding pattern, they appear homogeneous in a G-banded karyotype (see Fig. 7–28). The most interesting cases of amplification involve N-*MYC* in neuroblastoma and *ERBB2* in breast cancers. N-*MYC* is amplified in 25% to 30% of neuroblastomas, and the amplification is associated with poor prognosis. In neuroblastomas with N-*MYC* amplification, the gene is present both in double minutes and homogeneous staining regions. *ERBB2* amplification occurs in about 20% of breast cancers, and antibody therapy directed against this receptor has proven effective in this subset of tumors. Amplification of C-*MYC*, L-*MYC*, or N-*MYC* correlates with disease progression in small-cell cancer of the lung.

Epigenetic Changes

Epigenetics refers to reversible, heritable changes in gene expression that occur without mutation. Such changes involve post-translational modifications of histones and DNA methylation, both of which affect gene expression. In normal, differentiated cells, the majority of the genome is not expressed. Some portions of the genome are silenced by DNA methylation and histone modifications that lead to the compaction of DNA into heterochromatin. On the other hand, cancer cells are characterized by a global DNA hypomethylation and selective promoter-localized hypermethylation.[140] Indeed, it has become evident during the past few years that tumor suppressor genes are sometimes silenced by hypermethylation of promoter sequences rather than mutation. One example is CDKN2A, a complex locus that encodes two tumor suppressors, p14/ARF and p16/INK4a from two different reading frames; p14/ARF is epigenetically silenced in colon and gastric cancers, while p16/INK4a is silenced in a wide variety of cancers. Since this locus produces two tumor suppressors which affect the p53 and Rb pathways, silencing this locus has the pleasing effect (from the cancer's point of view) of removing two checkpoints with a single alteration. Other tumor suppressor genes subject to silencing by methylation include *BRCA1* in breast cancer, *VHL* in renal cell carcinomas, and the *MLH1* mismatch-repair gene in colorectal cancer.[140] You will recall from Chapter 5 that methylation also participates in the phenomenon called *genomic imprinting*, in which the maternal or paternal allele of a gene or chromosome is modified by methylation and is inactivated. The reverse phenomenon—that is, demethylation of an imprinted gene leading to its biallelic expression (loss of imprinting)—can also occur in tumor cells.[141] There has been great interest in developing potential therapeutic agents that act to demethylate DNA sequences in tumor suppressor genes. Recent data demonstrating that genomic hypomethylation causes chromosomal instability and induces tumors in mice greatly strengthen the notion that epigenetic changes may directly contribute to tumor development.[141]

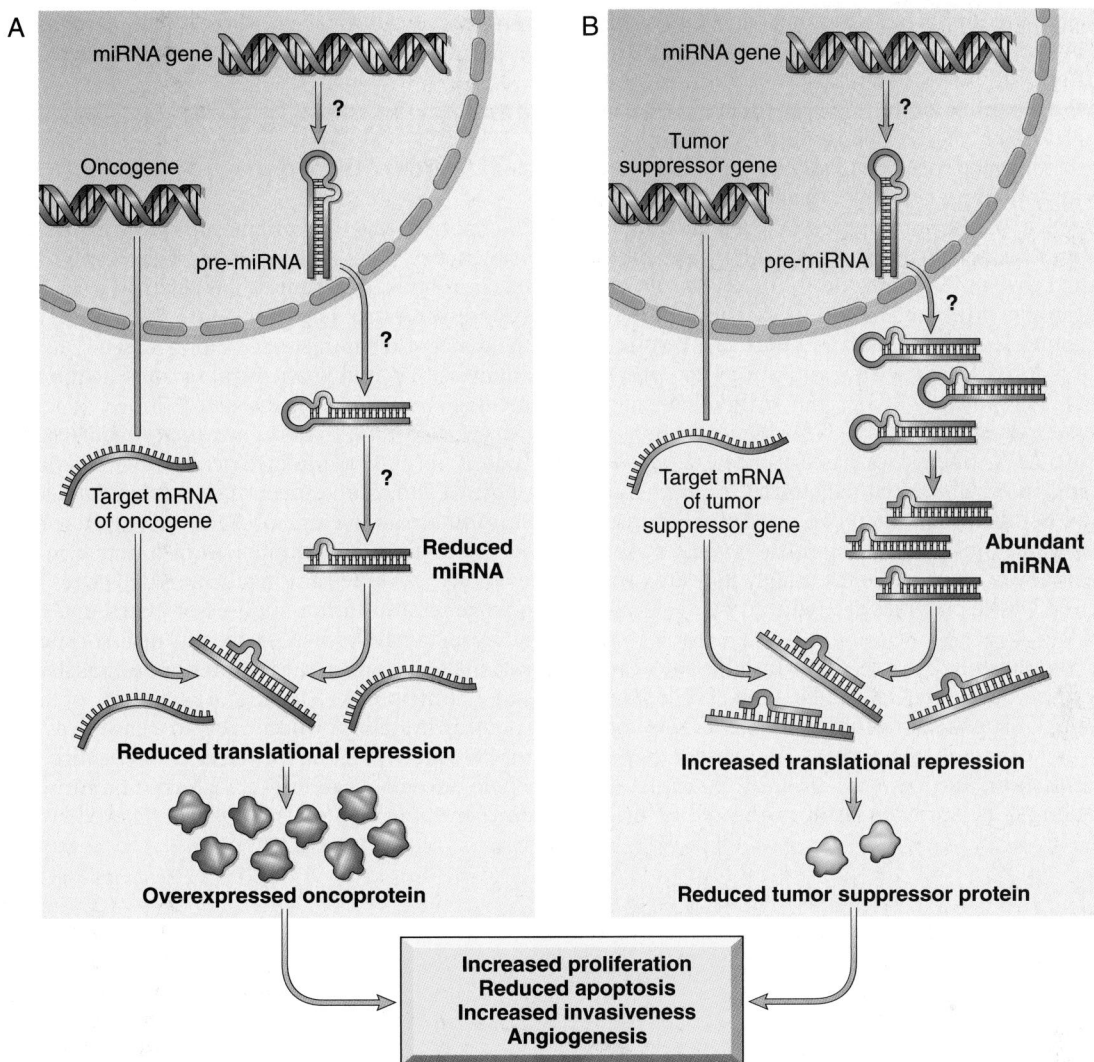

FIGURE 7–39 Role of miRNAs in tumorigenesis. **A,** Reduced activity of a miRNA that inhibits translation of an oncogene gives rise to an excess of oncoproteins. **B,** Overactivity of a miRNA that targets a tumor suppression gene reduces the production of the tumor suppressor protein. Question marks in **A** and **B** indicate that the mechanisms by which changes in the level or activity of miRNA are not entirely known.

The chromatin changes that contribute to carcinogenesis are less well understood. The current paradigm is that there is a histone code in which various modifications to the tails of histones, such as acetylation and methylation, lead to activation or repression of transcription. Several chromatin-modifying enzymes, such as EZH2, have been shown to be overexpressed in breast and prostate carcinomas.[141] EZH2 is the enzymatic component of the multiprotein polycomb repressive complex 2, which places repressive chromatin marks at the promoter of genes. Although its targets in cancer in vivo have not yet been defined, in cell lines overexpression of EZH2 leads to the repression of tumor suppressors, such as p21. Interestingly, in flies and mammals the polycomb repressive complexes are required for the maintenance of stem cells, as well as to silence lineage-specific transcription factors until the proper cues signal differentiation. Inappropriate repression or expression of such genes could give cancer cells a stem cell–like, undifferentiated quality. There is, of course, significant cross-talk between the chromatin-remodeling enzymes and the DNA-methylation

machinery. For example, the placement of repressive chromatin marks by enzymes like EZH2 in cancer cells results in the recruitment of DNA methylases, methylation of promoters, and durable repression of gene expression.

miRNAs and Cancer

As discussed in Chapter 5, miRNAs are small noncoding, single-stranded RNAs, approximately 22 nucleotides in length, that are incorporated into the RNA-induced silencing complex. The miRNAs mediate sequence-specific recognition of mRNAs and, through the action of the RNA-induced silencing complex, mediate post-transcriptional gene silencing. Given that miRNAs control cell growth, differentiation, and cell survival, it is not surprising that they play a role in carcinogenesis.[142] miRNAs have been shown to undergo changes in expression in cancer cells, and frequent amplifications and deletions of miRNA loci have been identified in many cancers. As illustrated in Figure 7–39, miRNAs can participate in neoplastic transformation either by increasing the expression of oncogenes or by reducing the expression of tumor suppressor genes. If a miRNA inhibits the translation of an oncogene, a reduction in the quantity or function of that miRNA will lead to overproduction of the oncogene product; thus, the miRNA acts as a tumor suppressor. Conversely, if the target of a miRNA is a tumor suppressor gene, then overactivity of the miRNA can reduce the tumor suppressor protein; thus, the miRNA acts as an oncogene. Such relationships have already been established by miRNA profiling of several human tumors. For example, down-regulation or deletion of certain miRNAs in some leukemias and lymphomas results in increased expression of BCL2, the anti-apoptotic protein. Thus, by negatively regulating BCL2, such miRNAs behave as tumor suppressor genes. Similar miRNA-mediated upregulation of *RAS* and *MYC* oncogenes has also been detected in lung tumors and in certain B-cell leukemias, respectively. In some brain and breast tumors there is 5- to 100-fold greater expression of certain miRNAs. Although the targets of these miRNAs have not been identified, presumably they are tumor suppressor genes, whose activities are reduced by the overexpressed miRNA.

These findings not only provide novel insights into carcinogenesis, they also have practical implications. For instance, drugs that inhibit or augment the functions of miRNAs could be useful in chemotherapy. Since miRNAs regulate normal cellular differentiation, the patterns of miRNA expression ("miRNA profiling") can provide clues to the cell of origin and classification of tumors. Much remains to be learned about these oncogenic miRNAs, or so called "oncomirs."

Molecular Basis of Multistep Carcinogenesis

The notion that malignant tumors arise from a protracted sequence of events is supported by epidemiologic, experimental, and molecular studies. The study of oncogenes and tumor suppressor genes has provided a firm molecular footing for the concept of multistep carcinogenesis.[143]

Given that malignant tumors must acquire several fundamental abnormalities, discussed above, it follows that *each cancer must result from the accumulation of multiple mutations.* Indeed, recently completed genome-wide sequencing analysis of breast and colon cancers has revealed that individual tumors accumulate an average of 90 mutant genes. A much smaller subset of these (11/tumor) were mutated at significant frequency.[144] Included among the mutated genes are some known oncogenes and tumor suppressor genes, and others that were not previously known to be tumor-associated. It is not yet established which of these mutations establish the transformed state, contribute to tumor progression, or are "passengers" (neutral mutations) occurring in genomically unstable cells that are merely "along for the ride". More directly, however, no single oncogene can fully transform nonimmortalized cells in vitro, but *cells can generally be transformed by combinations of*

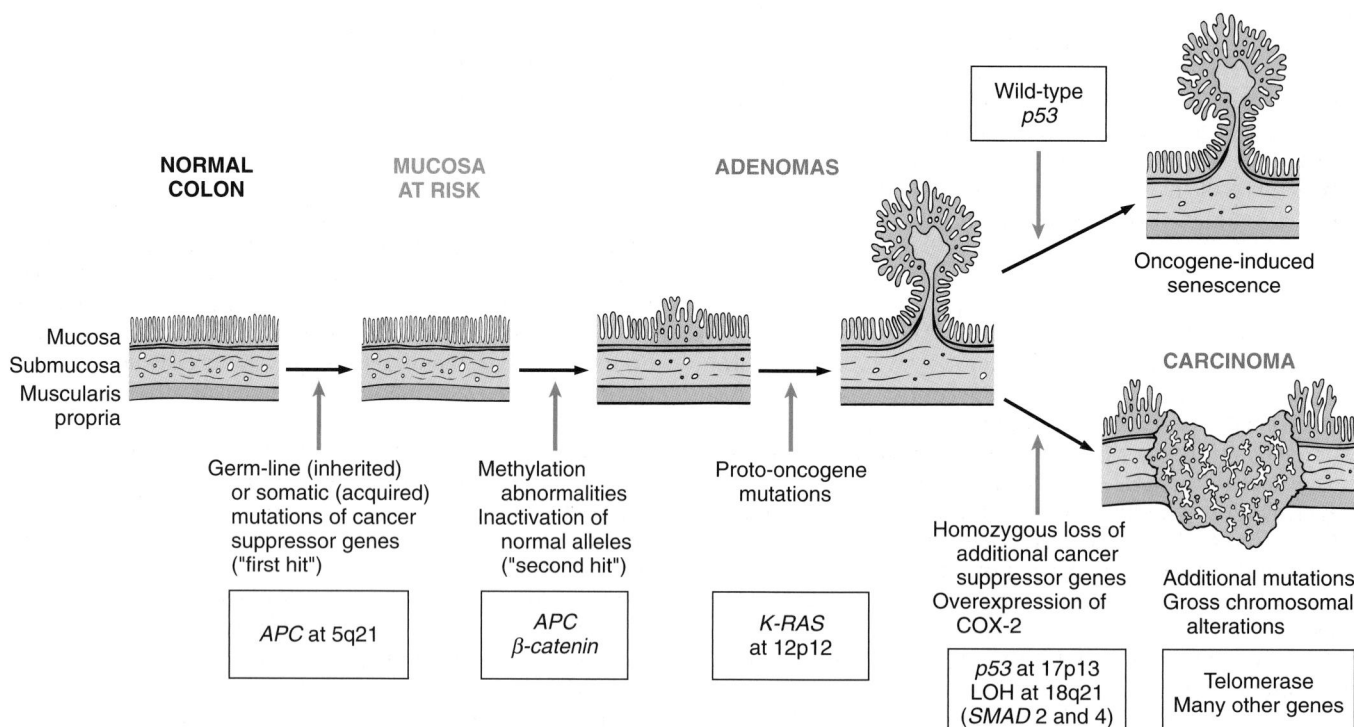

FIGURE 7–40 Molecular model for the evolution of colorectal cancers through the adenoma-carcinoma sequence. Although *APC* mutation is an early event and loss of *p53* occurs late in the process of tumorigenesis, the timing for the other changes may be variable. Note also that individual tumors may not have all of the changes listed. *Top right,* cells that gain oncogene signaling without loss of p53 eventually enter oncogene-induced senescence.

oncogenes. Such cooperation is required because each onco-gene is specialized to induce part of the phenotype necessary for full transformation. For instance, the *RAS* oncogene induces cells to secrete growth factors and permits them to grow without anchorage to a normal substrate (anchorage independence), whereas the *MYC* oncogene renders cells more sensitive to growth factors and immortalizes cells. These two genes, acting in conjunction, can cause neoplastic transforma-tion of mouse fibroblasts in culture.

Furthermore, it seems that evolution has installed a variety of "intrinsic tumor-suppressive mechanisms" such as apopto-sis and senescence that thwart the actions of growth-promot-ing mutations. Indeed, in cells with competent checkpoints, oncogenic signaling through proteins like RAS leads not to transformation but to senescence or apoptosis.[33] Thus, emer-gence of malignant tumors requires mutational loss of many genes, including those that regulate apoptosis and senes-cence.[145] A classic example of incremental acquisition of the malignant phenotype is documented by the study of colon carcinoma. Many of these cancers are believed to evolve through a series of morphologically identifiable stages: colon epithelial hyperplasia followed by formation of adenomas that progressively enlarge and ultimately undergo malignant trans-formation (Chapter 17). The proposed molecular correlates of this adenoma-carcinoma sequence are illustrated in Figure 7–40. According to this scheme, inactivation of the *APC* tumor suppressor gene occurs first, followed by activation of *RAS* and, ultimately, loss of a tumor suppressor gene on 18q and loss of *p53.* Also depicted is the senescence pathway if *p53* loss does not occur. Indeed, it has been shown that most cells in most adenomas are senescent. It is thought that mutation of a proto-oncogene such as *RAS* drives a cell into senescence instead of proliferation[33] by activating the DNA-damage checkpoint, as discussed previously. The loss of p53 in adeno-mas prevents oncogene-induced senescence, allowing the adenomatous cells to continue to proliferate, generating a car-cinoma. While multiple mutations, including gain of onco-genes and loss of tumor suppressors, are required for carcinogenesis, the precise temporal sequence of mutations may be different in each organ and tumor type.

Carcinogenic Agents and Their Cellular Interactions

More than 200 years ago the London surgeon Sir Percival Pott correctly attributed scrotal skin cancer in chimney sweeps to chronic exposure to soot. Based on this observation, the Danish Chimney Sweeps Guild ruled that its members must bathe daily. No public health measure since that time has achieved so much in the control of a form of cancer. Subse-quently, hundreds of chemicals have been shown to be carci-nogenic in animals.

Some of the major agents are presented in Table 7–10. A few comments are offered on a handful of these.

Steps Involved in Chemical Carcinogenesis

As discussed earlier, carcinogenesis is a multistep process. This is most readily demonstrated in experimental models of

TABLE 7–10 Major Chemical Carcinogens

DIRECT-ACTING CARCINOGENS

Alkylating Agents

β-Propiolactone
Dimethyl sulfate
Diepoxybutane
Anticancer drugs (cyclophosphamide, chlorambucil, nitrosoureas, and others)

Acylating Agents

1-Acetyl-imidazole
Dimethylcarbamyl chloride

PROCARCINOGENS THAT REQUIRE METABOLIC ACTIVATION

Polycyclic and Heterocyclic Aromatic Hydrocarbons

Benz[*a*]anthracene
Benzo[*a*]pyrene
Dibenz[*a,h*]anthracene
3-Methylcholanthrene
7,12-Dimethylbenz[*a*]anthracene

Aromatic Amines, Amides, Azo Dyes

2-Naphthylamine (β-naphthylamine)
Benzidine
2-Acetylaminofluorene
Dimethylaminoazobenzene (butter yellow)

Natural Plant and Microbial Products

Aflatoxin B_1
Griseofulvin
Cycasin
Safrole
Betel nuts

Others

Nitrosamine and amides
Vinyl chloride, nickel, chromium
Insecticides, fungicides
Polychlorinated biphenyls

chemical carcinogenesis, in which the stages of initiation and progression during cancer development were first described.[146] The classic experiments that allowed the distinction between initiation and promotion were performed on mouse skin and are outlined in Figure 7–41. The following concepts relating to the initiation-promotion sequence have emerged from these experiments:

- *Initiation* results from exposure of cells to a sufficient dose of a carcinogenic agent (initiator); an initiated cell is altered, making it potentially capable of giving rise to a tumor (groups 2 and 3). *Initiation alone, however, is not sufficient for tumor formation* (group 1).
- *Initiation causes permanent DNA damage (mutations). It is therefore rapid and irreversible and has "memory."* This is illustrated by group 3, in which tumors were produced even if the application of the promoting agent was delayed for several months after a single application of the initiator.
- *Promoters can induce tumors in initiated cells, but they are nontumorigenic by themselves* (group 5). Furthermore, tumors do not result when the promoting agent is applied

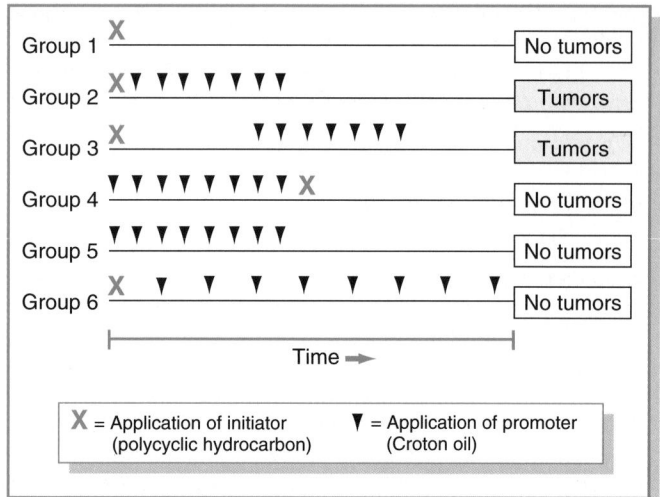

FIGURE 7–41 Experiments demonstrating the initiation and promotion phases of carcinogenesis in mice. Group 2: application of promoter repeated at twice-weekly intervals for several months. Group 3: application of promoter delayed for several months and then applied twice weekly. Group 6: promoter applied at monthly intervals.

controlled, or delayed recurrence of certain types of cancer (e.g., leukemia, lymphoma, and ovarian carcinoma), only to evoke later a second form of cancer, usually acute myeloid leukemia. The risk of induced cancer is low, but its existence dictates judicious use of such agents.

Indirect-Acting Agents

The designation *indirect-acting agent* refers to chemicals that require metabolic conversion to an *ultimate carcinogen* before they become active. Some of the most potent indirect chemical carcinogens—the polycyclic hydrocarbons—are present in fossil fuels. Others, for example, benzo[*a*]pyrene and other carcinogens, are formed in the high-temperature combustion of tobacco in cigarette smoking. *These products are implicated in the causation of lung cancer in cigarette smokers.* Polycyclic hydrocarbons may also be produced from animal fats during the process of broiling meats and are present in smoked meats and fish. The principal active products in many hydrocarbons are epoxides, which form covalent adducts (addition products) with molecules in the cell, principally DNA, but also with RNA and proteins.

before, rather than after, the initiating agent (group 4). This indicates that, *in contrast to the effects of initiators, the cellular changes resulting from the application of promoters do not affect DNA directly and are reversible.* As discussed later, promoters enhance the proliferation of initiated cells, an effect that may contribute to the development of additional mutations in these cells. That the effects of promoters are reversible is further documented in group 6, in which tumors failed to develop in initiated cells if the time between multiple applications of the promoter was sufficiently extended.

Although the concepts of initiation and promotion have been derived largely from experiments involving induction of skin cancer in mice, these stages are also discernible in the development of cancers of the liver, urinary bladder, breast, colon, and respiratory tract. With this brief overview of two major steps in carcinogenesis, we can examine initiation and promotion in more detail (Fig. 7–42). All initiating chemical carcinogens are highly reactive electrophiles (have electron-deficient atoms) that can react with nucleophilic (electron-rich) sites in the cell. Their targets are DNA, RNA, and proteins, and in some cases these interactions cause cell death. Initiation, obviously, inflicts nonlethal damage on the DNA that cannot be repaired. The mutated cell then passes on the DNA lesions to its daughter cells. Chemicals that can cause initiation of carcinogenesis can be classified into two categories: direct acting and indirect acting.

Direct-Acting Agents

Direct-acting agents require no metabolic conversion to become carcinogenic. Most of them are weak carcinogens but are important because some are cancer chemotherapeutic drugs (e.g., alkylating agents) that have successfully cured,

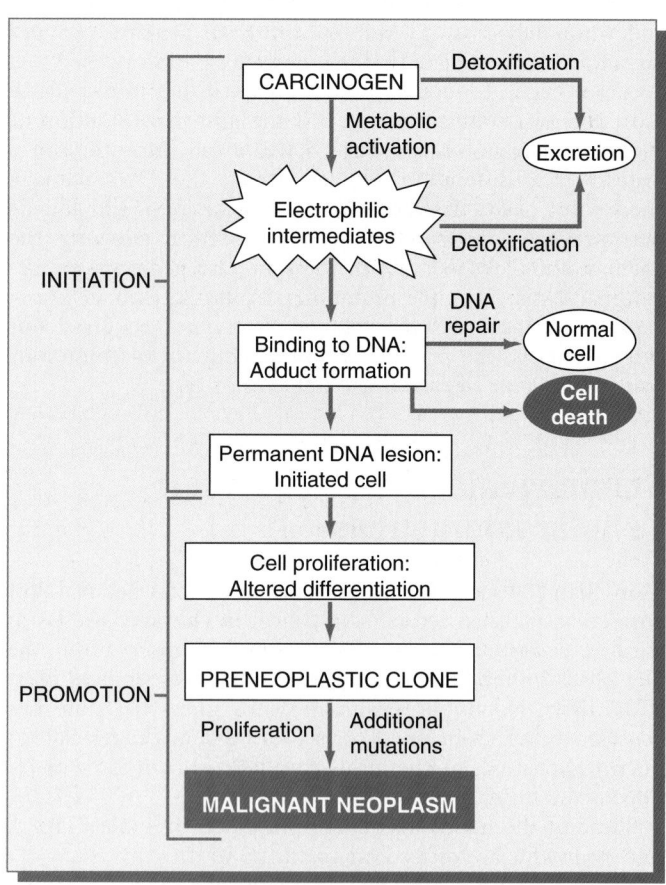

FIGURE 7–42 General schema of events in chemical carcinogenesis. Note that promoters cause clonal expansion of the initiated cell, thus producing a preneoplastic clone. Further proliferation induced by the promoter or other factors causes accumulation of additional mutations and emergence of a malignant tumor.

The aromatic amines and azo dyes are another class of indirect-acting carcinogens that were widely used in the past in the aniline dye and rubber industries.[147] Many other occupational carcinogens are listed in Table 7–3.

Most chemical carcinogens require metabolic activation for conversion into ultimate carcinogens (see Fig. 7–42). Other metabolic pathways may lead to the inactivation (detoxification) of the procarcinogen or its derivatives. Thus, *the carcinogenic potency of a chemical is determined not only by the inherent reactivity of its electrophilic derivative but also by the balance between metabolic activation and inactivation reactions.*

Most of the known carcinogens are metabolized by cytochrome P-450–dependent mono-oxygenases. The genes that encode these enzymes are quite polymorphic, and the activity and inducibility of these enzymes have been shown to vary among different individuals. Because these enzymes are essential for the activation of procarcinogens, the susceptibility to carcinogenesis is regulated in part by polymorphisms in the genes that encode these enzymes. Thus, it may be possible to assess cancer risk in a given individual by genetic analysis of such enzyme polymorphisms.[147]

The metabolism of polycyclic aromatic hydrocarbons, such as benzo[a]pyrene by the product of the P-450 gene, *CYP1A1*, provides an instructive example. Approximately 10% of the white population has a highly inducible form of this enzyme that is associated with an increased risk of lung cancer in smokers.[148,149] Light smokers with the susceptible genotype *CYP1A1* have a sevenfold higher risk of developing lung cancer, compared with smokers without the permissive genotype. Not all variations in the activation or detoxification of carcinogens are genetically determined. Age, sex, and nutritional status also determine the internal dose of toxicants produced and hence influence the risk of cancer development in a particular individual.[150]

Molecular Targets of Chemical Carcinogens. Because malignant transformation results from mutations, it comes as no surprise that the majority of initiating chemicals are mutagenic. Thus, DNA is the primary target for chemical carcinogens, but there is no single or unique alteration associated with initiation of chemical carcinogenesis. Although any gene may be the target of chemical carcinogens, the commonly mutated oncogenes and tumor suppressors, such as *RAS* and *p53*, are particularly important targets. An illustrative example of a chemical carcinogenesis is aflatoxin B₁, a naturally occurring agent produced by some strains of *Aspergillus*, a mold that grows on improperly stored grains and nuts. There is a *strong correlation between the dietary level of this food contaminant and the incidence of hepatocellular carcinoma in parts of Africa and the Far East.* Interestingly, aflatoxin B₁ produces mutations in the *p53* gene; 90% or more of these mutations are a characteristic G:C→T:A transversion in codon 249 (called *249(ser) p53* mutation).[151] By contrast, *p53* mutations are much less frequent in liver tumors from areas where aflatoxin contamination of food is not a risk factor, and the *249(ser)* mutation is uncommon. Thus, the detection of the "*signature mutation*" within the *p53* gene establishes aflatoxin as the causative agent. These associations are proving to be useful tools in epidemiologic studies of chemical carcinogenesis.

Additionally, vinyl chloride, arsenic, nickel, chromium, insecticides, fungicides, and polychlorinated biphenyls are potential carcinogens in the workplace and at home. Finally, nitrites used as food preservatives have caused concern, since they cause nitrosylation of amines contained in the food. The nitrosoamines so formed are suspected to be carcinogenic.

Initiation and Promotion of Chemical Carcinogenesis

Unrepaired alterations in the DNA are essential first steps in the process of initiation. *For the change to be heritable, the damaged DNA template must be replicated. Thus, for initiation to occur, carcinogen-altered cells must undergo at least one cycle of proliferation so that the change in DNA becomes fixed.* In the liver, many chemicals are activated to reactive electrophiles, yet most of them do not produce cancers unless the liver cells proliferate within a few days of the formation of DNA adducts. In tissues that are normally quiescent, the mitogenic stimulus may be provided by the carcinogen itself, because many cells die as a result of toxic effects of the carcinogenic chemical, thereby stimulating regeneration in the surviving cells. Alternatively, cell proliferation may be induced by concurrent exposure to biologic agents such as viruses and parasites, dietary factors, or hormonal influences. Agents that do not cause mutation but instead stimulate the division of mutated cells are known as *promoters.*

The carcinogenicity of some initiators is augmented by subsequent administration of *promoters* (such as phorbol esters, hormones, phenols, and drugs) that by themselves are nontumorigenic. Application of promoters leads to proliferation and clonal expansion of initiated (mutated) cells. Such cells have reduced growth factor requirements and may also be less responsive to growth-inhibitory signals in their extracellular milieu. Driven to proliferate, the initiated clone of cells suffers additional mutations, developing eventually into a malignant tumor. Thus, the process of tumor promotion includes multiple steps: proliferation of preneoplastic cells, malignant conversion, and eventually tumor progression, which depends on changes in tumor cells and the tumor stroma—the process of multistep carcinogenesis highlighted above.

RADIATION CARCINOGENESIS

Radiant energy, whether in the form of the UV rays of sunlight or as ionizing electromagnetic and particulate radiation, is a well-established carcinogen. UV light is clearly implicated in the causation of skin cancers, and ionizing radiation exposure from medical or occupational exposure, nuclear plant accidents, and atomic bomb detonations has produced a variety of cancers. Although the contribution of radiation to the total human burden of cancer is probably small, the well-known latency of damage caused by radiant energy and its cumulative effect require extremely long periods of observation and make it difficult to ascertain its full significance. An increased incidence of breast cancer has become apparent decades later among women exposed during childhood to atomic bomb tests. The incidence peaked during 1988–1992 and then declined.[152] Moreover, radiation's possible additive or synergistic effects with other potential carcinogenic influences add another dimension to the picture.

Ultraviolet Rays

There is ample evidence from epidemiologic studies that *UV rays* derived from the sun cause an increased incidence of squamous cell carcinoma, basal cell carcinoma, and possibly melanoma of the skin.[153] The degree of risk depends on the type of UV rays, the intensity of exposure, and the quantity of the light-absorbing "protective mantle" of melanin in the skin. Persons of European origin who have fair skin that repeatedly becomes sunburned but stalwartly refuses to tan and who live in locales receiving a great deal of sunlight (e.g., Queensland, Australia, close to the equator) have among the highest incidence of skin cancers (melanomas, squamous cell carcinomas, and basal cell carcinomas) in the world. Nonmelanoma skin cancers are associated with total cumulative exposure to UV radiation, whereas melanomas are associated with intense intermittent exposure—as occurs with sunbathing. The UV portion of the solar spectrum can be divided into three wavelength ranges: UVA (320–400 nm), UVB (280–320 nm), and UVC (200–280 nm). Of these, UVB is believed to be responsible for the induction of cutaneous cancers. UVC, although a potent mutagen, is not considered significant because it is filtered out by the ozone shield around the earth (hence the concern about ozone depletion).

The carcinogenicity of UVB light is attributed to its formation of pyrimidine dimers in DNA. This type of DNA damage is repaired by the nucleotide excision repair pathway. There are five steps in nucleotide excision repair, and in mammalian cells the process may involve 30 or more proteins. It is postulated that with excessive sun exposure, the capacity of the nucleotide excision repair pathway is overwhelmed, and error-prone nontemplated DNA-repair mechanisms become operative that provide for the survival of the cell at the cost of genomic mutations that in some instances, lead to cancer. The importance of the nucleotide excision repair pathway of DNA repair is most graphically illustrated by the high frequency of cancers in individuals with the hereditary disorder *xeroderma pigmentosum* (discussed previously).[126]

Ionizing Radiation

Electromagnetic (x-rays, γ rays) and particulate (α particles, β particles, protons, neutrons) radiations are all carcinogenic. The evidence is so voluminous that a few examples suffice.[152,154] Many individuals pioneering the use of x-rays developed skin cancers. Miners of radioactive elements in central Europe and the Rocky Mountain region of the United States have a tenfold increased incidence of lung cancers compared to the rest of the population. Most telling is the follow-up of survivors of the atomic bombs dropped on Hiroshima and Nagasaki. Initially there was a marked increase in the incidence of leukemias—principally acute and chronic myelogenous leukemia—after an average latent period of about 7 years. Subsequently the incidence of many solid tumors with longer latent periods (e.g., breast, colon, thyroid, and lung) increased.

In humans there is a hierarchy of vulnerability of different tissues to radiation-induced cancers. Most frequent are the acute and chronic myeloid leukemia. Cancer of the thyroid follows closely but only in the young. In the intermediate category are cancers of the breast, lungs, and salivary glands. In contrast, skin, bone, and the gastrointestinal tract are relatively resistant to radiation-induced neoplasia, even though the gastrointestinal epithelial cells are vulnerable to the acute cell-killing effects of radiation, and the skin is in the pathway of all external radiation. Nonetheless, the physician dare not forget: practically *any* cell can be transformed into a cancer cell by sufficient exposure to radiant energy.

MICROBIAL CARCINOGENESIS

Many RNA and DNA viruses have proved to be oncogenic in animals as disparate as frogs and primates. Despite intense scrutiny, however, only a few viruses have been linked with human cancer. Our discussion focuses on human oncogenic viruses as well as the emerging role of the bacterium *Helicobacter pylori* in gastric cancer.

Oncogenic RNA Viruses

Human T-Cell Leukemia Virus Type 1. Although the study of animal retroviruses has provided spectacular insights into the molecular basis of cancer, only one human retrovirus, human T-cell leukemia virus type 1 (HTLV-1), is firmly implicated in the causation of cancer in humans.

HTLV-1 causes a form of T-cell leukemia/lymphoma that is endemic in certain parts of Japan and the Caribbean basin but is found sporadically elsewhere, including the United States.[155] Similar to the human immunodeficiency virus, which causes acquired immunodeficiency syndrome (AIDS), HTLV-1 has tropism for CD4+ T cells, and hence this subset of T cells is the major target for neoplastic transformation. Human infection requires transmission of infected T cells via sexual intercourse, blood products, or breastfeeding. Leukemia develops in only 3% to 5% of the infected individuals after a long latent period of 40 to 60 years.

There is little doubt that HTLV-1 infection of T lymphocytes is necessary for leukemogenesis, but the molecular mechanisms of transformation are not entirely clear. In contrast to several murine retroviruses, HTLV-1 does not contain an oncogene, and no consistent integration next to a proto-oncogene has been discovered. In leukemic cells, however, viral integration shows a clonal pattern. In other words, although the site of viral integration in host chromosomes is random (the viral DNA is found at different locations in different cancers), the site of integration is identical within all cells of a given cancer. This would not occur if HTLV-1 were merely a passenger that infects cells after transformation. The HTLV-1 genome contains the *gag, pol, env,* and long-terminal-repeat regions typical of other retroviruses, but, in contrast to other leukemia viruses, it contains another region, referred to as *tax.* It seems that the secrets of its transforming activity are locked in the *tax* gene.[156] The product of this gene is essential for viral replication, because it stimulates transcription of viral mRNA by acting on the 5′ long terminal repeat. It is now established that the Tax protein can also activate the transcription of several host cell genes involved in proliferation and differentiation of T cells. These include the immediate early gene *FOS,* genes encoding interleukin-2 (IL-2) and its receptor, and the gene for the myeloid growth factor granulocyte-macrophage colony-stimulating factor. In addition, Tax protein inactivates the cell cycle inhibitor p16/INK4a and enhances cyclin D activation, thus dysregulating the cell cycle. Tax also activates NF-κb, a transcription factor that regulates a host of genes, including pro-survival/anti-apoptotic genes. Another mechanism by which Tax may contribute to malignant transformation is through genomic instability. Recent data show that Tax interferes with DNA-repair functions and inhibits ATM-mediated cell cycle checkpoints activated by DNA damage.[156]

The main steps that lead to the development of adult T-cell leukemia/lymphoma may be summarized as follows. Infection by HTLV-1 causes the expansion of a nonmalignant polyclonal cell population through stimulatory effects of Tax on cell proliferation. The proliferating T cells are at increased risk of mutations and genomic instability induced by Tax. This instability allows the accumulation of mutations and chromosomal abnormalities, and eventually a monoclonal neoplastic T-cell population emerges. The malignant cells replicate independently of IL-2 and contain molecular and chromosomal abnormalities.

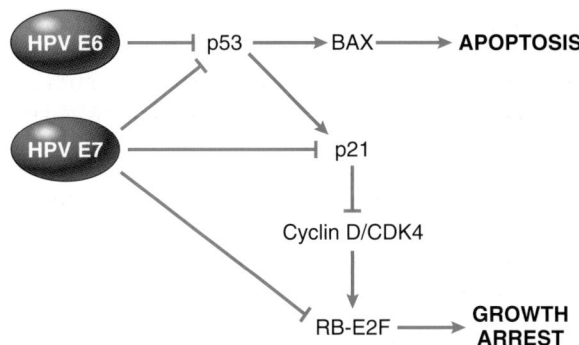

FIGURE 7–43 Effect of HPV proteins E6 and E7 on the cell cycle. E6 and E7 enhance p53 degradation, causing a block in apoptosis and decreased activity of the p21 cell cycle inhibitor. E7 associates with p21 and prevents its inhibition of the cyclin-CDK4 complex; E7 can bind to RB, removing cell cycle restriction. The net effect of HPV E6 and E7 proteins is to block apoptosis and remove the restraints to cell proliferation (see Fig. 7–29). (Modified from Münger K, Howley PM: Human papillomavirus immortalization and transformation functions. Virus Res 89:213–228, 2002.)

Oncogenic DNA Viruses

As with RNA viruses, several oncogenic DNA viruses that cause tumors in animals have been identified. Of the various human DNA viruses, four—HPV, Epstein-Barr virus (EBV), hepatitis B virus (HBV), and Kaposi sarcoma herpesvirus, also called human herpesvirus 8—have been implicated in the causation of human cancer. A fifth virus, Merkel cell polyomavirus, has been identified in Merkel cell carcinomas and may soon join the rogue's gallery; it is described in Chapter 25. Kaposi sarcoma herpesvirus is discussed in Chapters 6 and 11. Though not a DNA virus, HCV is also associated with cancer and is discussed briefly here.[157]

Human Papillomavirus. At least 70 genetically distinct types of HPV have been identified. Some types (e.g., 1, 2, 4, and 7) cause benign squamous papillomas (warts) in humans (Chapters 19 and 22). By contrast, high-risk HPVs (e.g., types 16 and 18) have been implicated in the genesis of several cancers, particularly squamous cell carcinoma of the cervix and anogenital region.[158,159] Thus, cervical cancer is a sexually transmitted disease, caused by transmission of HPV. In addition, at least 20% of oropharyngeal cancers are associated with HPV. In contrast to cervical cancers, genital warts have low malignant potential and are associated with low-risk HPVs, predominantly HPV-6 and HPV-11. Interestingly, in benign warts the HPV genome is maintained in a nonintegrated episomal form, while in cancers the HPV genome is integrated into the host genome, suggesting that integration of viral DNA is important for malignant transformation. As with HTLV-1, the site of viral integration in host chromosomes is random, but the pattern of integration is clonal. Cells in which the viral genome has integrated show significantly more genomic instability. Furthermore, since the integration site is random there is no consistent association with a host proto-oncogene. Rather, integration interrupts the viral DNA within the E1/E2 open reading frame, leading to loss of the E2 viral repressor and overexpression of the oncoproteins E6 and E7.

Indeed, the oncogenic potential of HPV can be related to the products of two viral genes, E6 and E7. Together, they interact with a variety of growth-regulating proteins encoded by proto-oncogenes and tumor suppressor genes (Fig. 7–43). The E7 protein binds to the RB protein and displaces the E2F transcription factors that are normally sequestered by RB, promoting progression through the cell cycle. Of note, E7 protein from high-risk HPV types has a higher affinity for RB than does E7 from low-risk HPV types. E7 also inactivates the CDKIs p21 and p27. E7 proteins from high-risk HPV types (types 16, 18, and 31) also bind and presumably activate cyclins E and A. The E6 protein has complementary effects. It binds to and mediates the degradation of p53 and BAX, a pro-apoptotic member of the BCL2 family, and it activates telomerase. Like E7, E6 from high-risk HPV types has a higher affinity for p53 than E6 from low-risk HPV types. Interestingly the E6-p53 interaction may offer some clues regarding polymorphisms and risk factors for development of cervical cancer. Human *p53* is polymorphic at amino acid 72, encoding either a proline or arginine residue at that position. The p53 Arg72 variant is much more susceptible to degradation by E6. Not surprisingly, infected individuals with the Arg72 polymorphism are more likely to develop cervical carcinomas.[160]

To summarize, *high-risk HPV types express oncogenic proteins that inactivate tumor suppressors, activate cyclins, inhibit apoptosis, and combat cellular senescence.* Thus, it is evident that many of the hallmarks of cancer discussed earlier are driven by HPV proteins. The primacy of HPV infection in the causation of cervical cancer is confirmed by the effectiveness of anti-HPV vaccines in preventing cervical cancer. However, infection with HPV itself is not sufficient for carcinogenesis. For example, when human keratinocytes are transfected with DNA from HPV types 16, 18, or 31 in vitro, they are immortalized but do not form tumors in experimental animals. Cotransfection with a mutated *RAS* gene results in full malignant transformation. In addition to such genetic co-factors, HPV in all likelihood also acts in concert with environmental factors (Chapter 22). These include cigarette smoking, coexisting microbial infections, dietary deficiencies, and hormonal changes, all of which have been implicated in the pathogenesis of cervical cancers. A high proportion of women infected with

HPV clear the infection by immunological mechanisms, but some do not for unknown reasons.

Epstein-Barr Virus. EBV, a member of the herpes family, has been implicated in the pathogenesis of several human tumors: the African form of Burkitt lymphoma; B-cell lymphomas in immunosuppressed individuals (particularly in those with HIV infection or undergoing immunosuppressive therapy after organ transplantation); a subset of Hodgkin lymphoma; nasopharyngeal and some gastric carcinomas and rare forms of T cell lymphomas and natural killer (NK) cell lymphomas.[161] Except for nasopharyngeal carcinoma, all others are B-cell tumors. These neoplasms are reviewed elsewhere in this book; therefore, only their association with EBV is discussed here.

EBV infects B lymphocytes and possibly epithelial cells of the oropharynx. EBV uses the complement receptor CD21 to attach to and infect B cells. The infection of B cells is latent; that is, there is no viral replication and the cells are not killed, but the B cells latently infected with EBV are immortalized and acquire the ability to propagate indefinitely in vitro. The molecular basis of B-cell proliferations induced by EBV is complex, but as with other viruses it involves the "hijacking" of several normal signaling pathways.[162] One EBV gene, latent membrane protein-1 (*LMP-1*), acts as an oncogene, in that its expression in transgenic mice induces B-cell lymphomas. LMP-1 behaves like a constitutively active CD40 receptor, a key recipient of helper T-cell signals that stimulate B-cell growth (Chapter 6). LMP-1 activates the NF-κB and JAK/STAT signaling pathways and promotes B-cell survival and proliferation, all of which occur autonomously (i.e., without T cells or other outside signals) in EBV-infected B cells. Concurrently, LMP-1 prevents apoptosis by activating BCL2. Thus, the virus "borrows" a normal B-cell activation pathway to expand the pool of latently infected cells. Another EBV gene, *EBNA-2*, encodes a nuclear protein that mimics a constitutively active Notch receptor. EBNA-2 transactivates several host genes, including cyclin D and the *src* family of proto-oncogenes. In addition, the EBV genome contains a viral cytokine, vIL-10, that was hijacked from the host genome. This viral cytokine can prevent macrophages and monocytes from activating T cells and is required for EBV-dependent transformation of B cells. In immunologically normal individuals EBV-driven polyclonal B-cell proliferation in vivo is readily controlled, and the individual either remains asymptomatic or develops a self-limited episode of infectious mononucleosis (Chapter 8). Evasion of the immune system seems to be a key step in EBV-related oncogenesis.

Burkitt lymphoma is a neoplasm of B lymphocytes that is the most common childhood tumor in central Africa and New Guinea. A morphologically identical lymphoma occurs sporadically throughout the world. The association between endemic Burkitt lymphoma and EBV is quite strong (Fig. 7–44):

- More than 90% of African tumors carry the EBV genome.
- One hundred percent of the patients have elevated antibody titers against viral capsid antigens.
- Serum antibody titers against viral capsid antigens are correlated with the risk of developing the tumor.

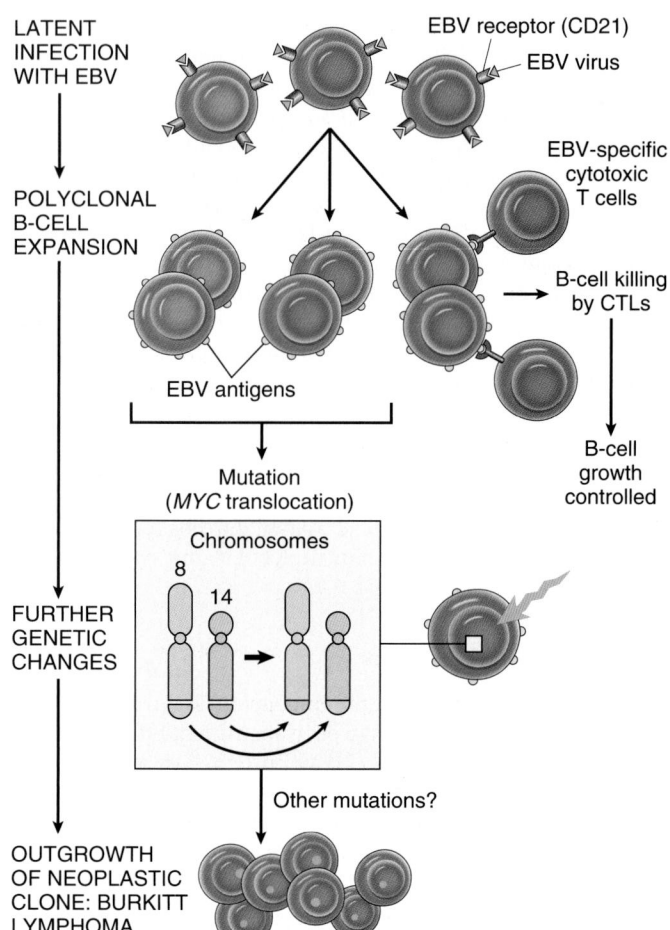

FIGURE 7–44 Possible evolution of EBV-induced Burkitt lymphoma.

Although EBV is intimately involved in the causation of Burkitt lymphoma, several observations suggest that additional factors must also be involved.[163,164] (1) EBV infection is not limited to the geographic locales where Burkitt lymphoma is found, but it is a ubiquitous virus that asymptomatically infects almost all humans worldwide. (2) The EBV genome is found in only 15% to 20% of sufferers of Burkitt lymphoma outside Africa. (3) There are significant differences in the patterns of viral gene expression in EBV-transformed (but not tumorigenic) B-cell lines and Burkitt lymphoma cells. Most notably, Burkitt lymphoma cells do not express LMP-1, EBNA2, and other EBV proteins that drive B-cell growth and immortalization.

Given these observations, how then does EBV contribute to the genesis of endemic Burkitt lymphoma? A plausible scenario is shown in Figure 7–44. In regions of the world where Burkitt lymphoma is endemic, concomitant infections such as malaria impair immune competence, allowing sustained B-cell proliferation. Eventually, however, T-cell immunity directed against EBV antigens such as EBNA2 and LMP-1 eliminates most of the EBV-infected B cells, but a small number of cells downregulate expression of these immunogenic antigens. These cells persist indefinitely, even in the face of normal immunity. Lymphoma cells may emerge from this population only with the acquisition of specific mutations, most notably translocations that activate the c-*MYC* oncogene. It should be noted that in nonendemic areas 80% of tumors do not harbor the EBV genome, but all tumors possess the t(8;14) or other translocations that dysregulate c-*MYC*. This observation suggests that, although non-African Burkitt lymphomas are triggered by mechanisms other than EBV, they develop through very similar oncogenic pathways.

In summary, in the case of Burkitt lymphoma, it seems that EBV is not directly oncogenic, but by acting as a polyclonal B-cell mitogen, it sets the stage for the acquisition of the t(8;14) translocation and other mutations, which ultimately release the cells from normal growth regulation. In normal individuals, EBV infection is readily controlled by effective immune responses directed against viral antigens expressed on the cell membranes. Hence, the vast majority of infected individuals remain asymptomatic or develop self-limited infectious mononucleosis. In regions of Africa where Burkitt lymphoma is endemic, poorly understood cofactors (e.g., chronic malaria) may favor the acquisition of genetic events (e.g., the t(8;14) translocation) that lead to transformation.

The role played by EBV is more direct in B-cell lymphomas in immunosuppressed patients. Some persons with AIDS and those who receive long-term immunosuppressive therapy for preventing allograft rejection present with multifocal B-cell tumors within lymphoid tissue or in the central nervous system. These tumors are polyclonal at the outset but can develop into monoclonal neoplasms. In contrast to Burkitt lymphoma, the tumors in immunosuppressed patients uniformly express LMP-1 and EBNA2, that are recognized by cytotoxic T cells. These potentially lethal proliferations can be subdued if the immunological status of the host improves, as may occur with withdrawal of immunosuppressive drugs in transplant recipients.

Nasopharyngeal carcinoma is also associated with EBV infection. This tumor is endemic in southern China, in some parts of Africa, and in the Inuit population of the Arctic. In contrast to Burkitt lymphoma, 100% of nasopharyngeal carcinomas obtained from all parts of the world contain EBV DNA.[165] The viral integration in the host cells is clonal, thus ruling out the possibility that EBV infection occurred after tumor development. Antibody titers to viral capsid antigens are greatly elevated, and in endemic areas patients develop IgA antibodies before the appearance of the tumor. The 100% correlation between EBV and nasopharyngeal carcinoma suggests that EBV[110] plays a role in the genesis of this tumor, but (as with Burkitt tumor) the restricted geographic distribution indicates that genetic or environmental cofactors, or both, also contribute to tumor development. LMP-1 is expressed in epithelial cells as well. In these cells, as in B cells, *LMP-1* activates the NF-κB pathway. Furthermore, *LMP-1* induces the expression of pro-angiogenic factors such as VEGF, FGF-2, MMP9, and COX2, which may contribute to oncogenesis. The relationship of EBV to the pathogenesis of Hodgkin lymphoma is discussed in Chapter 13.

Hepatitis B and C Viruses. Epidemiologic studies strongly suggest a close association between HBV infection and the occurrence of liver cancer (Chapter 18). It is estimated that 70% to 85% of hepatocellular carcinomas worldwide are due to infection with HBV or HCV.[111,166–168] HBV is endemic in countries of the Far East and Africa; correspondingly, these areas have the highest incidence of hepatocellular carcinoma. Despite compelling epidemiologic and experimental evidence, the mode of action of these viruses in liver tumorigenesis is not fully elucidated. The HBV and HCV genomes do not encode any viral oncoproteins, and although the HBV DNA is integrated within the human genome, there is no consistent pattern of integration in liver cells. Indeed, the oncogenic effects of HBV and HCV are multifactorial, but the dominant effect seems to be immunologically mediated chronic inflammation with hepatocyte death leading to regeneration and genomic damage. Although the immune system is generally thought to be protective, recent work has demonstrated that in the setting of unresolved chronic inflammation, as occurs in viral hepatitis or chronic gastritis caused by *H. pylori* (see below), the immune response may become maladaptive, promoting tumorigenesis.

As with any cause of hepatocellular injury, chronic viral infection leads to the compensatory proliferation of hepatocytes. This regenerative process is aided and abetted by a plethora of growth factors, cytokines, chemokines, and other bioactive substances that are produced by activated immune cells and promote cell survival, tissue remodeling, and angiogenesis (Chapter 3). The activated immune cells also produce other mediators, such as reactive oxygen species, that are genotoxic and mutagenic. One key molecular step seems to be activation of the NF-κB pathway in hepatocytes in response to mediators derived from the activated immune cells. Activation of the NF-κB pathway within hepatocytes blocks apoptosis, allowing the dividing hepatocytes to incur genotoxic stress and to accumulate mutations. Although this seems to be the dominant mechanism in the pathogenesis of viral-induced hepatocellular carcinoma, both HBV and HCV also contain proteins within their genomes that may more directly promote the development of cancer. The HBV genome contains a gene known as *HBx* that can directly or indirectly activate a variety of transcription factors and several signal transduction pathways. In addition, viral integration can cause secondary rearrangements of chromosomes, including multiple deletions that may harbor unknown tumor suppressor genes.

Though not a DNA virus, HCV is also strongly linked to the pathogenesis of liver cancer. The molecular mechanisms used by HCV are less well defined than are those of HBV. In addition to chronic liver cell injury and compensatory regeneration, components of the HCV genome, such as the HCV core protein, may have a direct effect on tumorigenesis, possibly by activating a variety of growth-promoting signal transduction pathways.

Helicobacter pylori

First incriminated as a cause of peptic ulcers, *H. pylori* now has acquired the dubious distinction of being the first bacterium classified as a carcinogen. Indeed, *H. pylori* infection is implicated in the genesis of both gastric adenocarcinomas and gastric lymphomas.[169]

The scenario for the development of gastric adenocarcinoma is similar to that of HBV- and HCV-induced liver cancer. It involves increased epithelial cell proliferation in a background of chronic inflammation. As in viral hepatitis, the inflammatory milieu contains numerous genotoxic agents, such as reactive oxygen species. There is an initial development of chronic gastritis, followed by gastric atrophy, intestinal metaplasia of the lining cells, dysplasia, and cancer. This sequence takes decades to complete and occurs in only 3% of infected patients. Like HBV and HCV, the *H. pylori* genome also contains genes directly implicated in oncogenesis. Strains associated with gastric adenocarcinoma have been shown to contain a "pathogenicity island" that contains cytotoxin-associated A (*CagA*) gene. Although *H. pylori* is noninvasive, *CagA* penetrates into gastric epithelial cells, where it has a variety of effects, including the initiation of a signaling cascade that mimics unregulated growth factor stimulation.

As mentioned above, *H. pylori* is associated with an increased risk for the development of gastric lymphomas as well. The gastric lymphomas are of B-cell origin, and because the tumors recapitulate some of the features of normal Peyer's patches, they are often called lymphomas of mucosa-associated lymphoid tissue, or MALTomas (also discussed in Chapters 13 and 17). Their molecular pathogenesis is incompletely understood but seems to involve strain-specific *H. pylori* factors, as well as host genetic factors, such as polymorphisms in the promoters of inflammatory cytokines such as IL-1β and tumor necrosis factor (TNF). It is thought that *H. pylori* infection leads to the appearance of *H. pylori*–reactive T cells, which in turn stimulate a polyclonal B-cell proliferation. In chronic infections, currently unknown mutations may be acquired that give individual cells a growth advantage. These cells grow out into a monoclonal "MALToma" that nevertheless remains dependent on T-cell stimulation of B-cell pathways that activate the transcription factor NF-κB. At this stage, eradication of *H. pylori* by antibiotic therapy "cures" the lymphoma by removing the antigenic stimulus for T cells. At later stages, however, additional mutations may be acquired, such as an (11;18) translocation, that cause NF-κB to be activated constitutively. At this point, the MALToma no longer requires the antigenic stimulus of the bacterium for growth and survival and develops the capacity to spread beyond the stomach to other tissues.

Host Defense against Tumors— Tumor Immunity

The idea that tumors are not entirely self and may be recognized by the immune system was conceived by Paul Ehrlich, who proposed that immune recognition of autologous tumor cells may be capable of eliminating tumors. Subsequently, Lewis Thomas and Macfarlane Burnet formalized this concept by coining the term *immune surveillance,* which implies that a normal function of the immune system is to survey the body for emerging malignant cells and destroy them.[170,171] This idea has been supported by many observations—the occurrence of lymphocytic infiltrates around tumors and in lymph nodes draining sites of cancer; experimental results, mostly with transplanted tumors; the increased incidence of some cancers in immunodeficient individuals; and the direct demonstration of tumor-specific T cells and antibodies in patients. The fact that cancers occur in immunocompetent individuals suggests that immune surveillance is imperfect; however, that some tumors escape such policing does not preclude the possibility

that others may have been aborted.[172] The concept of tumor immune surveillance has recently been expanded to encompass not only the protective role of the immune system in tumor development but also the effect of the immune system in selecting for tumor variants.[173,174] These variants have reduced immunogenicity and can more easily escape immunological detection and rejection. The term *cancer immunoediting* is now being used to describe the effects of the immune system in preventing tumor formation and also in "sculpting" the immunogenic properties of tumors to select tumor cells that escape immune elimination.[175]

In the following section we explore some of the important questions about tumor immunity: What is the nature of tumor antigens? What host effector systems may recognize tumor cells? Is antitumor immunity effective against spontaneous neoplasms? Can immune reactions against tumors be exploited for immunotherapy?

TUMOR ANTIGENS

Antigens that elicit an immune response have been demonstrated in many experimentally induced tumors and in some human cancers.[176] Initially, they were broadly classified into two categories based on their patterns of expression: *tumor-specific antigens,* which are present only on tumor cells and not on any normal cells, and *tumor-associated antigens,* which are present on tumor cells and also on some normal cells. This classification, however, is imperfect because many antigens thought to be tumor-specific turned out to be expressed by some normal cells as well. The modern classification of tumor antigens is based on their molecular structure and source.

The early attempts to purify and characterize tumor antigens relied on producing monoclonal antibodies specific for tumor cells and defining the antigens that these antibodies recognized. An important advance in the field was the development of techniques for identifying tumor antigens that were recognized by cytotoxic T lymphocytes (CTLs), because CTLs are the major immune defense mechanism against tumors. Recall that CTLs recognize peptides derived from cytoplasmic proteins that are displayed bound to class I major histocompatibility complex (MHC) molecules (Chapter 6). Below we describe the main classes of tumor antigens (Fig. 7–45).

Products of Mutated Genes. Neoplastic transformation, as we have discussed, results from genetic alterations in proto-oncogenes and tumor suppressor genes; these mutated proteins represent antigens that have never been seen by the immune system and thus can be recognized as non-self.[177,178] Additionally, because of the genetic instability of tumor cells, many different genes may be mutated in these cells, including genes whose products are not related to the transformed phenotype and have no known function. Products of these mutated genes can also be potential tumor antigens. The products of altered proto-oncogenes, tumor suppressor genes, or other mutated genes not associated with transformation are synthesized in the cytoplasm of tumor cells, and like any cytoplasmic protein, they may enter the class I MHC antigen-processing pathway and be recognized by CD8+ T cells. In addition, these proteins may enter the class II antigen-processing pathway in antigen-presenting cells that have phagocy-

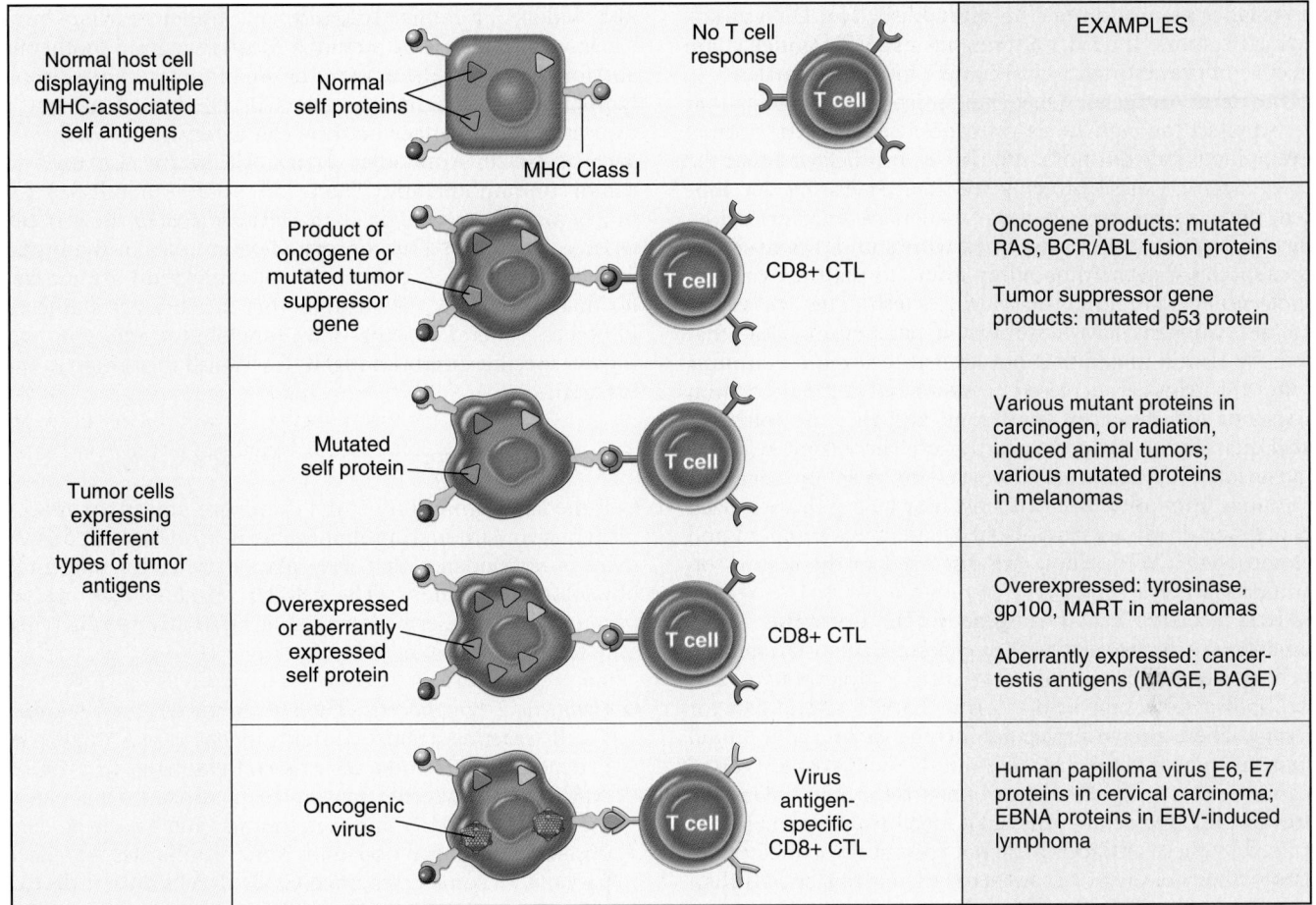

Normal host cell displaying multiple MHC-associated self antigens	Normal self proteins — MHC Class I	No T cell response — T cell	EXAMPLES
Tumor cells expressing different types of tumor antigens	Product of oncogene or mutated tumor suppressor gene	T cell — CD8+ CTL	Oncogene products: mutated RAS, BCR/ABL fusion proteins Tumor suppressor gene products: mutated p53 protein
	Mutated self protein	T cell	Various mutant proteins in carcinogen, or radiation, induced animal tumors; various mutated proteins in melanomas
	Overexpressed or aberrantly expressed self protein	T cell — CD8+ CTL	Overexpressed: tyrosinase, gp100, MART in melanomas Aberrantly expressed: cancer-testis antigens (MAGE, BAGE)
	Oncogenic virus	T cell — Virus antigen-specific CD8+ CTL	Human papilloma virus E6, E7 proteins in cervical carcinoma; EBNA proteins in EBV-induced lymphoma

FIGURE 7–45 Tumor antigens recognized by CD8+ T cells. (Modified from Abbas AK, Lichtman AH: Cellular and Molecular Immunology, 5th ed. Philadelphia, WB Saunders, 2003.)

tosed dead tumor cells, and thus be recognized by CD4+ T cells also. Because these altered proteins are not present in normal cells, they do not induce self-tolerance. Some cancer patients have circulating CD4+ and CD8+ T cells that can respond to the products of mutated oncogenes such as RAS, p53, and BCR-ABL proteins. In animals, immunization with mutated RAS or p53 proteins induces CTLs and rejection responses against tumors expressing these mutants. However, these oncoproteins do not seem to be major targets of tumor-specific CTLs in most patients.

Overexpressed or Aberrantly Expressed Cellular Proteins. Tumor antigens may be normal cellular proteins that are abnormally expressed in tumor cells and elicit immune responses. In a subset of human melanomas some tumor antigens are structurally normal proteins that are produced at low levels in normal cells and overexpressed in tumor cells. One such antigen is tyrosinase, an enzyme involved in melanin biosynthesis that is expressed only in normal melanocytes and melanomas.[179] T cells from melanoma patients recognize peptides derived from tyrosinase, raising the possibility that tyrosinase vaccines may stimulate such responses to melanomas; clinical trials with these vaccines are ongoing. It may be surprising that these patients are able to respond to a normal self-antigen. The probable explanation is that tyrosinase is normally produced in such small amounts and in so few cells

that it is not recognized by the immune system and fails to induce tolerance.

Another group, the "cancer-testis" antigens, are encoded by genes that are silent in all adult tissues except the testis—hence their name. Although the protein is present in the testis it is not expressed on the cell surface in an antigenic form, because sperm do not express MHC class I antigens. Thus, for all practical purposes these antigens are tumor specific. Prototypic of this group is the melanoma antigen gene (MAGE) family. Although originally described in melanomas, MAGE antigens are expressed by a variety of tumor types. For example, MAGE-1 is expressed on 37% of melanomas and a variable number of lung, liver, stomach, and esophageal carcinomas.[180] Similar antigens called GAGE, BAGE, and RAGE have been detected in other tumors.

Tumor Antigens Produced by Oncogenic Viruses. As we have discussed, several viruses are associated with cancers. Not surprisingly, these viruses produce proteins that are recognized as foreign by the immune system. The most potent of these antigens are proteins produced by latent DNA viruses; examples in humans include HPV and EBV. There is abundant evidence that CTLs recognize antigens of these viruses and that a competent immune system plays a role in surveillance against virus-induced tumors because of its ability to recognize and kill virus-infected cells. In fact, the concept of immune surveillance against tumors is best established for DNA virus–induced tumors. Indeed, vaccines against HPV antigens are effective in preventing cervical cancers in young females.

Oncofetal Antigens. Oncofetal antigens are proteins that are expressed at high levels on cancer cells and in normal developing (fetal) but not adult tissues. It is believed that the genes encoding these proteins are silenced during development and are derepressed upon malignant transformation. Oncofetal antigens were identified with antibodies raised in other species, and their main importance is that they provide markers that aid in tumor diagnosis. As techniques for detecting these antigens have improved, it has become clear that their expression in adults is not limited to tumors. Amounts of these proteins are increased in tissues and in the circulation in various inflammatory conditions, and they are found in small quantities even in normal tissues. There is no evidence that oncofetal antigens are important inducers or targets of antitumor immunity. The two most thoroughly characterized oncofetal antigens are carcinoembryonic antigen (CEA) and α-fetoprotein (AFP). These are discussed in the section on "Tumor Markers".

Altered Cell Surface Glycolipids and Glycoproteins. Most human and experimental tumors express higher than normal levels and/or abnormal forms of surface glycoproteins and glycolipids, which may be diagnostic markers and targets for therapy. These altered molecules include gangliosides, blood group antigens, and mucins. Many antibodies have been raised in animals that recognize the carbohydrate groups or peptide cores of these molecules. Although most of the epitopes recognized by these antibodies are not specifically expressed on tumors, they are present at higher levels on cancer cells than on normal cells. This class of antigens is a target for cancer therapy with specific antibodies.

Among the glycolipids expressed at high levels in melanomas are the gangliosides GM_2, GD_2, and GD_3. Clinical trials of anti-GM_2 and anti-GD_3 antibodies and immunization with vaccines containing GM_2 are underway in melanoma patients. Mucins are high-molecular-weight glycoproteins containing numerous O-linked carbohydrate side chains on a core polypeptide. Tumors often have dysregulated expression of the enzymes that synthesize these carbohydrate side chains, which leads to the appearance of tumor-specific epitopes on the carbohydrate side chains or on the abnormally exposed polypeptide core. Several mucins have been the focus of diagnostic and therapeutic studies, including CA-125 and CA-19-9, expressed on ovarian carcinomas, and MUC-1, expressed on breast carcinomas. Unlike many mucins, MUC-1 is an integral membrane protein that is normally expressed only on the apical surface of breast ductal epithelium, a site that is relatively sequestered from the immune system. In ductal carcinomas of the breast, however, the molecule is expressed in an unpolarized fashion and contains new, tumor-specific carbohydrate and peptide epitopes detectable by mouse monoclonal antibodies. The peptide epitopes induce both antibody and T-cell responses in cancer patients and are therefore being considered as candidates for tumor vaccines.

Cell Type–Specific Differentiation Antigens. Tumors express molecules that are normally present on the cells of origin. These antigens are called *differentiation antigens* because they are specific for particular lineages or differentiation stages of various cell types. Such differentiation antigens are typically normal self-antigens, and therefore they do not induce immune response in tumor-bearing hosts. Their importance is as potential targets for immunotherapy and for identifying the tissue of origin of tumors. For example, lymphomas may be diagnosed as B cell–derived tumors by the detection of surface markers characteristic of this lineage, such as CD20. Antibodies against CD20 are also used for tumor immunotherapy. These kill normal B cells as well but because hemopoietic stem cells are spared, new B cells emerge eventually. The idiotypic determinants of the surface immunoglobulin of a clonal B-cell population are markers for that B-cell clone, because all other B cells express different idiotypes. Therefore, the immunoglobulin idiotype is a highly specific tumor antigen for B-cell lymphomas and leukemias.

ANTITUMOR EFFECTOR MECHANISMS

Cell-mediated immunity is the dominant antitumor mechanism in vivo. Although antibodies can be made against tumors, there is no evidence that they play a protective role under physiologic conditions. The cellular effectors that mediate immunity were described in Chapter 6, so it is necessary here only to characterize them briefly.

- *Cytotoxic T lymphocytes:* The antitumor effect of cytotoxic T cells reacting against tumor antigens is well established in experimentally induced tumors. In humans, CD8+ CTLs play a protective role against virus-associated neoplasms (e.g., EBV- and HPV-induced tumors) and have been demonstrated in the blood and tumor infiltrates of cancer patients. In some cases, such CD8+ T cells do not develop spontaneously in vivo but can be generated by immunization with tumor antigen–pulsed dendritic cells.

- *Natural killer cells:* NK cells are lymphocytes that are capable of destroying tumor cells without prior sensitization and thus may provide the first line of defense against tumor cells.[181] After activation with IL-2 and IL-15, NK cells can lyse a wide range of human tumors, including many that seem to be nonimmunogenic for T cells. T cells and NK cells seem to provide complementary antitumor mechanisms. Tumors that fail to express MHC class I antigens cannot be recognized by T cells, but these tumors may trigger NK cells because the latter are inhibited by recognition of normal autologous class I molecules (Chapter 6). The triggering receptors on NK cells are extremely diverse and belong to several gene families. NKG2D proteins expressed on NK cells and some T cells are important activating receptors. They recognize stress-induced antigens that are expressed on tumor cells and cells that have incurred DNA damage and are at risk for neoplastic transformation.

- *Macrophages:* Activated macrophages exhibit cytotoxicity against tumor cells in vitro. T cells, NK cells, and macrophages may collaborate in antitumor reactivity, because interferon-γ, a cytokine secreted by T cells and NK cells, is a potent activator of macrophages. Activated macrophages may kill tumors by mechanisms similar to those used to kill microbes (e.g., production of reactive oxygen metabolites; Chapter 2) or by secretion of TNF.

- *Antibodies:* Although there is no evidence for the protective effects of antitumor antibodies against spontaneous tumors, administration of monoclonal antibodies against tumor cells can be therapeutically effective. A monoclonal anti-

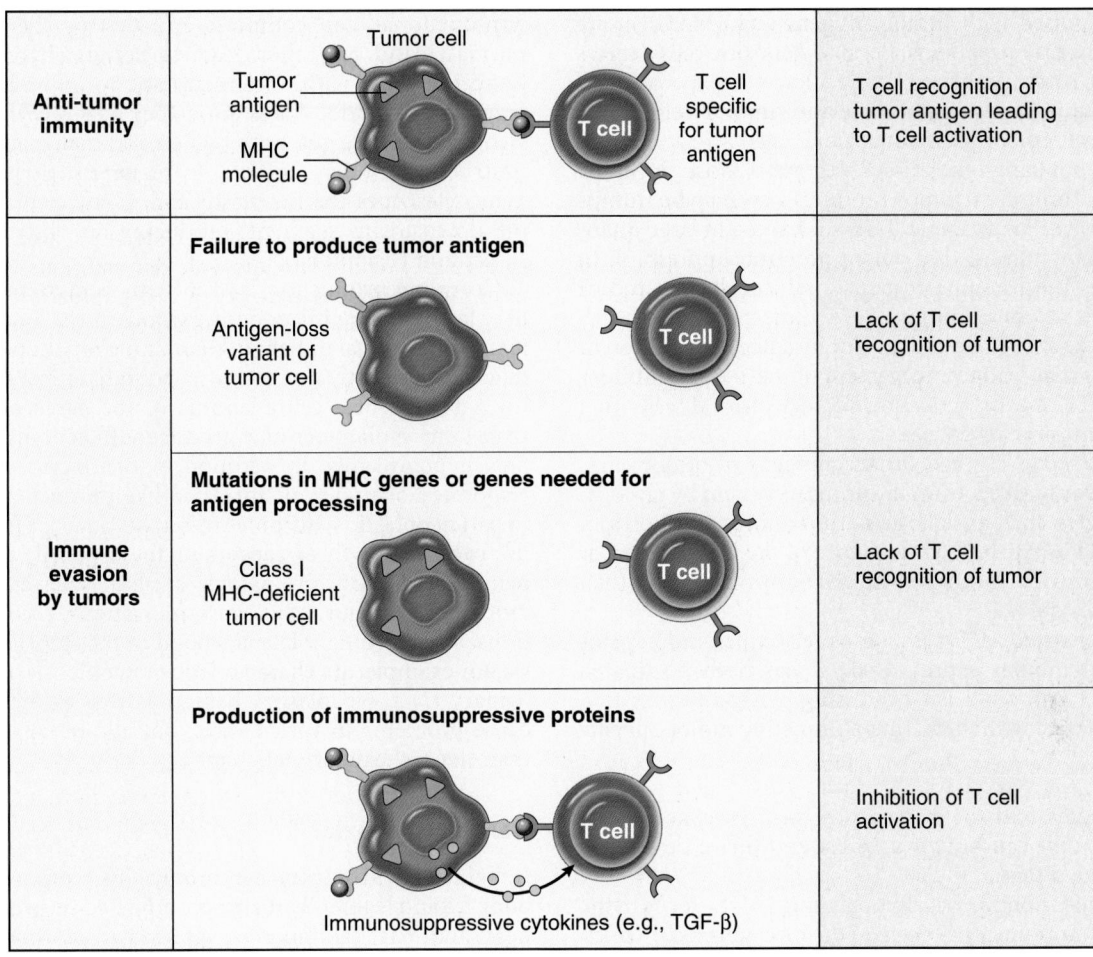

	Tumor cell / T cell specific for tumor antigen	
Anti-tumor immunity	Tumor antigen / MHC molecule / T cell	T cell recognition of tumor antigen leading to T cell activation
Immune evasion by tumors	**Failure to produce tumor antigen** Antigen-loss variant of tumor cell / T cell	Lack of T cell recognition of tumor
	Mutations in MHC genes or genes needed for antigen processing Class I MHC-deficient tumor cell / T cell	Lack of T cell recognition of tumor
	Production of immunosuppressive proteins T cell Immunosuppressive cytokines (e.g., TGF-β)	Inhibition of T cell activation

FIGURE 7–46 Mechanisms by which tumors evade the immune system. (Reprinted from Abbas AK, Lichtman AH: Cellular and Molecular Immunology, 5th ed. Philadelphia, WB Saunders, 2003)

body against CD20, a B-cell surface antigen, is widely used for treatment of lymphomas.

IMMUNE SURVEILLANCE AND ESCAPE

Given the many potential antitumor mechanisms, is there any evidence that they operate in vivo to prevent emergence of neoplasms? The strongest argument for the existence of immune surveillance is the increased frequency of cancers in immunodeficient hosts. About 5% of persons with congenital immunodeficiencies develop cancers, about 200 times the rate in immunocompetent individuals. Immunosuppressed transplant recipients and persons with AIDS also have an increased incidence of malignancies. Most (but not all) of these neoplasms are lymphomas, often diffuse large B-cell lymphomas. Particularly illustrative is the rare X-linked recessive immunodeficiency disorder termed *XLP (X-linked lymphoproliferative syndrome)*, caused by mutations in the gene encoding an adapter protein *(SAP)*, which participates in lymphocyte signaling pathways.[182] When affected boys develop an EBV infection, such infection does not take the usual self-limited form of infectious mononucleosis but instead evolves into a chronic or sometimes fatal form of infectious mononucleosis or, even worse, B-cell lymphoma.

Most cancers occur in persons who do not suffer from any overt immunodeficiency. It is evident, then, that *tumor cells must develop mechanisms to escape or evade the immune system in immunocompetent hosts.* Several such mechanisms may be operative (Fig. 7–46).

- *Selective outgrowth of antigen-negative variants:* During tumor progression, strongly immunogenic subclones may be eliminated.
- *Loss or reduced expression of MHC molecules:* Tumor cells may fail to express normal levels of HLA class I molecules, thereby escaping attack by cytotoxic T cells. Such cells, however, may trigger NK cells.
- *Lack of costimulation:* It may be recalled that sensitization of T cells requires two signals, one by a foreign peptide presented by MHC molecules and the other by costimulatory molecules (Chapter 6); although tumor cells may express peptide antigens with class I molecules, they often do not express costimulatory molecules. This not only prevents sensitization but also may render T cells anergic or, worse, cause them to undergo apoptosis. To bypass this problem, attempts are being made to immunize patients with autologous tumor cells that have been transfected with the gene for the costimulatory molecule B7-1 (CD 80). In another approach, autologous dendritic cells expanded in

vitro and pulsed with tumor antigens (e.g., MAGE1) are infused into cancer patients. Because dendritic cells express high levels of costimulatory molecules, it is expected that such immunization will stimulate antitumor T cells.

- *Immunosuppression:* Many oncogenic agents (e.g., chemicals and ionizing radiation) suppress host immune responses. Tumors or tumor products also may be immunosuppressive. For example, TGF-β, secreted in large quantities by many tumors, is a potent immunosuppressant. In some cases the immune response induced by the tumor may inhibit tumor immunity. Several mechanisms of such inhibition have been described. For instance, recognition of tumor cells may lead to engagement of the T-cell inhibitory receptor, CTLA4, or activation of regulatory T cells that suppress immune responses.
- *Antigen masking:* The cell surface antigens of tumors may be hidden, or masked, from the immune system by glycocalyx molecules, such as sialic acid–containing mucopolysaccharides. This may be a consequence of the fact that tumor cells often express more of these glycocalyx molecules than normal cells do.
- *Apoptosis of cytotoxic T cells:* Some melanomas and hepatocellular carcinomas express FasL. It has been postulated that these tumors kill Fas-expressing T lymphocytes that come in contact with them, thus eliminating tumor-specific T cells.[183]

Thus, it seems that there is no dearth of mechanisms by which tumor cells can outwit the host and thrive despite an intact immune system.

It is worth mentioning that although much of the focus in the field of tumor immunity has been on the mechanisms by which the host immune system defends against tumors, there is some recent evidence that, paradoxically, the immune system may promote the growth of tumors.[184] It is possible that activated lymphocytes and macrophages produce growth factors for tumor cells, and regulatory T-cells and certain subtypes of macrophages may suppress the host response to tumors. Enzymes, such as MMPs, that enhance tumor invasion, may also be produced. Harnessing the protective actions of the immune system and abolishing its ability to increase tumor growth are obviously important goals of immunologists and oncologists.

Clinical Aspects of Neoplasia

Ultimately the importance of neoplasms lies in their effects on patients. Although malignant tumors are of course more threatening than benign tumors, any tumor, even a benign one, may cause morbidity and mortality. Indeed, both malignant and benign tumors may cause problems because of (1) location and impingement on adjacent structures, (2) functional activity such as hormone synthesis or the development of paraneoplastic syndromes, (3) bleeding and infections when the tumor ulcerates through adjacent surfaces, (4) symptoms that result from rupture or infarction, and (5) cachexia or wasting.

Local and Hormonal Effects

Location is crucial in both benign and malignant tumors. A small (1-cm) pituitary adenoma, though benign and possibly nonfunctional, can compress and destroy the surrounding normal gland and thus lead to serious hypopituatarism. Cancers arising within or metastatic to an endocrine gland may cause an endocrine insufficiency by destroying the gland. Neoplasms in the gut, both benign and malignant, may cause obstruction as they enlarge. Infrequently, peristaltic movement telescopes the neoplasm and its affected segment into the downstream segment, producing an obstructing intussusception (Chapter 17).

Hormone production is seen with benign and malignant neoplasms arising in endocrine glands. Such functional activity is more typical of benign than of malignant tumors, which may be sufficiently undifferentiated to have lost such capability. A benign beta-cell adenoma of the pancreatic islets less than 1 cm in diameter may produce sufficient insulin to cause fatal hypoglycemia. In addition, nonendocrine tumors may elaborate hormones or hormone-like products and give rise to paraneoplastic syndromes (discussed later). The erosive and destructive growth of cancers or the expansile pressure of a benign tumor on any natural surface, such as the skin or mucosa of the gut, may cause ulcerations, secondary infections, and bleeding. Melena (blood in the stool) and hematuria, for example, are characteristic of neoplasms of the gut and urinary tract. Neoplasms, benign as well as malignant, may cause problems in varied ways, but all are far less common than the cachexia of malignancy.

Cancer Cachexia

Individuals with cancer commonly suffer progressive loss of body fat and lean body mass accompanied by profound weakness, anorexia, and anemia, referred to as *cachexia*. Unlike starvation, the weight loss seen in cachexia results equally from loss of fat and lean muscle. There is some correlation between the tumor burden and the severity of the cachexia. However, cachexia is not caused by the nutritional demands of the tumor. In persons with cancer, the basal metabolic rate is increased, despite reduced food intake. This is in contrast to the lower metabolic rate that occurs as an adaptational response in starvation. Although patients with cancer are often anorexic, cachexia probably results from the action of soluble factors such as cytokines produced by the tumor and the host rather than reduced food intake. The basis of these metabolic abnormalities is not fully understood. It is suspected that TNF produced by macrophages in response to tumor cells or by the tumor cells themselves mediates cachexia. TNF at high concentrations may mobilize fats from tissue stores and suppress appetite; both activities would contribute to cachexia. Other cytokines, such as IL-1, interferon-γ, and leukemia inhibitory factor, synergize with TNF. Additionally, other soluble factors produced by tumors, such as proteolysis-inducing factor and a lipid-mobilizing factor, increase the catabolism of muscle and adipose tissue.[185] These factors reduce protein synthesis by decreasing m-RNA translation and by stimulating protein catabolism through the activation of the ATP-dependent ubiquitin-proteasome pathway. It is now thought that there is a balance between factors that regulate muscle hypertrophy, such as IGF, and factors that regulate muscle catabolism. In cachexia these homeostatic mechanisms are disrupted, tilting the scales toward cachectic factors. There is currently no satisfactory treatment for cancer cachexia other than removal of the underlying cause, the tumor. However, cachexia clearly hampers effective chemotherapy, by reducing the dosages that can be given. Furthermore, it has been estimated that a third of deaths of cancer are attributable to cachexia, rather than directly due to the tumor burden itself. Identification of the molecular mechanisms involved in cancer cachexia may allow treatment of cachexia itself.

Paraneoplastic Syndromes

Symptom complexes in cancer-bearing individuals that cannot readily be explained, either by the local or distant spread of the tumor or by the elaboration of hormones indigenous to the tissue from which the tumor arose, are known as *paraneoplastic syndromes*.[186] These occur in about 10% of persons with malignant disease. Despite their relative infrequency, paraneo-

plastic syndromes are important to recognize, for several reasons:

- They may represent the earliest manifestation of an occult neoplasm.
- In affected patients they may represent significant clinical problems and may even be lethal.
- They may mimic metastatic disease and therefore confound treatment.

A classification of paraneoplastic syndromes and their presumed origins is presented in Table 7–11. A few comments on some of the more common and interesting syndromes follow.

The *endocrinopathies* are frequently encountered paraneoplastic syndromes.[187] Because the cancer cells are not of

TABLE 7–11 Paraneoplastic Syndromes

Clinical Syndromes	Major Forms of Underlying Cancer	Causal Mechanism
ENDOCRINOPATHIES		
Cushing syndrome	Small-cell carcinoma of lung Pancreatic carcinoma Neural tumors	ACTH or ACTH-like substance
Syndrome of inappropriate antidiuretic hormone secretion	Small-cell carcinoma of lung; intracranial neoplasms	Antidiuretic hormone or atrial natriuretic hormones
Hypercalcemia	Squamous cell carcinoma of lung Breast carcinoma Renal carcinoma Adult T-cell leukemia/lymphoma	Parathyroid hormone–related protein (PTHRP), TGF-α, TNF, IL-1
Hypoglycemia	Ovarian carcinoma Fibrosarcoma Other mesenchymal sarcomas	Insulin or insulin-like substance
Carcinoid syndrome	Hepatocellular carcinoma Bronchial adenoma (carcinoid) Pancreatic carcinoma Gastric carcinoma	Serotonin, bradykinin
Polycythemia	Renal carcinoma Cerebellar hemangioma Hepatocellular carcinoma	Erythropoietin
NERVE AND MUSCLE SYNDROMES		
Myasthenia Disorders of the central and peripheral nervous system	Bronchogenic carcinoma Breast carcinoma	Immunological
DERMATOLOGIC DISORDERS		
Acanthosis nigricans	Gastric carcinoma Lung carcinoma Uterine carcinoma	Immunological; secretion of epidermal growth factor
Dermatomyositis	Bronchogenic, breast carcinoma	Immunological
OSSEOUS, ARTICULAR, AND SOFT-TISSUE CHANGES		
Hypertrophic osteoarthropathy and clubbing of the fingers	Bronchogenic carcinoma	Unknown
VASCULAR AND HEMATOLOGIC CHANGES		
Venous thrombosis (Trousseau phenomenon)	Pancreatic carcinoma Bronchogenic carcinoma Other cancers	Tumor products (mucins that activate clotting)
Nonbacterial thrombotic endocarditis	Advanced cancers	Hypercoagulability
Red cell aplasia	Thymic neoplasms	Unknown
OTHERS		
Nephrotic syndrome	Various cancers	Tumor antigens, immune complexes

ACTH, adrenocorticotropic hormone; IL, interleukin; TGF, transforming growth factor; TNF, tumor necrosis factor.

endocrine origin, the functional activity is referred to as *ectopic hormone production.* Cushing syndrome is the most common endocrinopathy. Approximately 50% of individuals with this endocrinopathy have carcinoma of the lung, chiefly the small-cell type. It is caused by excessive production of corticotropin or corticotropin-like peptides. The precursor of corticotropin is a large molecule known as pro-opiomelanocortin. Lung cancer patients with Cushing syndrome have elevated serum levels of pro-opiomelanocortin and of corticotropin. The former is not found in serum of patients with excess corticotropin produced by the pituitary.

Hypercalcemia is probably the most common paraneoplastic syndrome; overtly symptomatic hypercalcemia is most often related to some form of cancer rather than to hyperparathyroidism. Two general processes are involved in cancer-associated hypercalcemia: (1) osteolysis induced by cancer, whether primary in bone, such as multiple myeloma, or metastatic to bone from any primary lesion, and (2) the production of calcemic humoral substances by extraosseous neoplasms. *Hypercalcemia due to skeletal metastases is not a paraneoplastic syndrome.*

Several humoral factors have been associated with paraneoplastic hypercalcemia of malignancy. The most important, parathyroid hormone–related protein (PTHRP), is a molecule related to, but distinct from, parathyroid hormone (PTH). PTHRP resembles the native hormone only in its N terminus.[188] It has some biologic actions similar to those of PTH, and both hormones share a G protein–coupled receptor, known as PTH/PTHRP receptor (often referred to as PTH-R or PTHRP-R). In contrast to PTH, PTHRP is produced in small amounts by many normal tissues, including keratinocytes, muscles, bone, and ovary. It regulates calcium transport in the lactating breast and across the placenta, and seems to regulate development and remodeling in the lung. Tumors most often associated with paraneoplastic hypercalcemia are carcinomas of the breast, lung, kidney, and ovary. In breast cancers, PTHRP production is associated with osteolytic bone disease, bone metastasis, and humoral hypercalcemia. The most common lung neoplasm associated with hypercalcemia is squamous cell bronchogenic carcinoma. In addition to PTHRP, several other factors, such as IL-1, TGF-α, TNF, and dihydroxyvitamin D, have also been implicated in causing the hypercalcemia of malignancy.

The *neuromyopathic paraneoplastic syndromes* take diverse forms, such as peripheral neuropathies, cortical cerebellar degeneration, a polymyopathy resembling polymyositis, and a myasthenic syndrome similar to *myasthenia gravis* (Chapter 27). The cause of these syndromes is poorly understood. In some cases, antibodies, presumably induced against tumor cell antigens (Chapter 28) that cross-react with neuronal cell antigens, have been detected. It is postulated that some neural antigens are ectopically expressed by visceral cancers. For some unknown reason, the immune system recognizes these antigens as foreign and mounts an immune response.

Acanthosis nigricans is characterized by gray-black patches of verrucous hyperkeratosis on the skin. This disorder occurs rarely as a genetically determined disease in juveniles or adults (Chapter 25). In addition, in about 50% of the cases, particularly in those over age 40, the appearance of such lesions is associated with some form of cancer. Sometimes the skin changes appear before discovery of the cancer.

Hypertrophic osteoarthropathy is encountered in 1% to 10% of patients with bronchogenic carcinomas. Rarely, other forms of cancer are involved. This disorder is characterized by (1) periosteal new bone formation, primarily at the distal ends of long bones, metatarsals, metacarpals, and proximal phalanges; (2) arthritis of the adjacent joints; and (3) clubbing of the digits. Although the osteoarthropathy is seldom seen in non-cancer patients, clubbing of the fingertips may be encountered in liver diseases, diffuse lung disease, congenital cyanotic heart disease, ulcerative colitis, and other disorders. The cause of hypertrophic osteoarthropathy is unknown.

Several *vascular and hematologic manifestations* may appear in association with a variety of forms of cancer. As mentioned in the discussion of thrombosis (Chapter 4), *migratory thrombophlebitis* (Trousseau syndrome) may be encountered in association with deep-seated cancers, most often carcinomas of the pancreas or lung. Disseminated intravascular coagulation may complicate a diversity of clinical disorders (Chapter 14). Acute disseminated intravascular coagulation is most commonly associated with acute promyelocytic leukemia and prostatic adenocarcinoma. Bland, small, nonbacterial fibrinous vegetations sometimes form on the cardiac valve leaflets (more often on left-sided valves), particularly in individuals with advanced mucin-secreting adenocarcinomas. These lesions, called *nonbacterial thrombotic endocarditis*, are described further in Chapter 12. The vegetations are potential sources of emboli that can further complicate the course of cancer.

GRADING AND STAGING OF TUMORS

Methods to quantify the probable clinical aggressiveness of a given neoplasm and its apparent extent and spread in the individual patient are necessary for making an accurate prognosis and for comparing end results of various treatment protocols. For instance, the results of treating well-differentiated thyroid adenocarcinoma that is localized to the thyroid gland will be different from those obtained from treating highly anaplastic thyroid cancers that have invaded the neck organs. Systems have been developed to express, at least in semiquantitative terms, the level of differentiation, or *grade*, and extent of spread of a cancer within the patient, or *stage*, as parameters of the clinical gravity of the disease.

Grading of a cancer is based on the degree of differentiation of the tumor cells and, in some cancers, the number of mitoses or architectural features. Grading schemes have evolved for each type of malignancy, and generally range from two categories (low grade and high grade) to four categories. Criteria for the individual grades vary with each form of neoplasia and so are not detailed here, but all attempt, in essence, to judge the extent to which the tumor cells resemble or fail to resemble their normal counterparts. Although histologic grading is useful, the correlation between histologic appearance and biologic behavior is less than perfect. In recognition of this problem and to avoid spurious quantification, it is common practice to characterize a particular neoplasm in descriptive terms, for example, well-differentiated, mucin-secreting adenocarcinoma of the stomach, or poorly differentiated pancreatic adenocarcinoma. In general, with a few exceptions, such as soft-tissue sarcomas, grading of cancers has proved of less clinical value than has staging.

The staging of cancers is based on the size of the primary lesion, its extent of spread to regional lymph nodes, and the presence or absence of blood-borne metastases. The major staging system currently in use is the American Joint Committee on Cancer Staging. This system uses a classification called the *TNM system*—T for primary tumor, N for regional lymph node involvement, and M for metastases. The TNM staging varies for each specific form of cancer, but there are general principles. With increasing size the primary lesion is characterized as T1 to T4. T0 is used to indicate an in situ lesion. N0 would mean no nodal involvement, whereas N1 to N3 would denote involvement of an increasing number and range of nodes. M0 signifies no distant metastases, whereas M1 or sometimes M2 indicates the presence of metastases and some judgment as to their number.

LABORATORY DIAGNOSIS OF CANCER

Every year the approach to laboratory diagnosis of cancer becomes more complex, more sophisticated, and more specialized. For virtually every neoplasm mentioned in this text, the experts have characterized several subcategories; we must walk, however, before we can run. Each of the following sections attempts to present the state of the art, avoiding details of method.

Histologic and Cytologic Methods. The laboratory diagnosis of cancer is, in most instances, not difficult. The two ends of the benign-malignant spectrum pose no problems; however, in the middle lies a gray zone that the novices dread and where experts tread cautiously. The focus here is on the roles of the clinician (often a surgeon) and the pathologist in facilitating the correct diagnosis.

Clinical data are invaluable for optimal pathologic diagnosis, but often clinicians underestimate its value. Radiation changes in the skin or mucosa can be similar to those associated with cancer. Sections taken from a healing fracture can mimic an osteosarcoma. Moreover, the laboratory evaluation of a lesion can be only as good as the specimen made available

for examination. It must be adequate, representative, and properly preserved. Several sampling approaches are available: (1) excision or biopsy, (2) needle aspiration, and (3) cytologic smears. When excision of a small lesion is not possible, selection of an appropriate site for biopsy of a large mass requires awareness that the periphery may not be representative and the center largely necrotic. Appropriate preservation of the specimen is obvious, yet it involves such actions as prompt immersion in a usual fixative (commonly formalin solution, but other fluids can be used), preservation of a portion in a special fixative (e.g., glutaraldehyde) for electron microscopy, or prompt refrigeration to permit optimal hormone, receptor, or other types of molecular analysis. Requesting "quick-frozen section" diagnosis is sometimes desirable, for example, in determining the nature of a mass lesion or in evaluating the margins of an excised cancer to ascertain that the entire neoplasm has been removed. This method permits histologic evaluation within minutes. In experienced, competent hands, frozen-section diagnosis is highly accurate, but there are particular instances in which the better histologic detail provided by the more time-consuming routine methods is needed—for example, when extremely radical surgery, such as the amputation of an extremity, may be indicated. Better to wait a day or two despite the drawbacks, than to perform inadequate or unnecessary surgery.

Fine-needle aspiration of tumors is another approach that is widely used. The procedure involves aspirating cells and attendant fluid with a small-bore needle, followed by cytologic examination of the stained smear. This method is used most commonly for the assessment of readily palpable lesions in sites such as the breast, thyroid, and lymph nodes. Modern imaging techniques permit extension of the method to lesions in deep-seated structures, such as pelvic lymph nodes and pancreas. Fine-needle aspiration is less invasive and more rapidly performed than are needle biopsies. It obviates surgery and its attendant risks. Although it entails some difficulties, such as small sample size and sampling errors, in experienced hands it is extremely reliable, rapid, and useful.

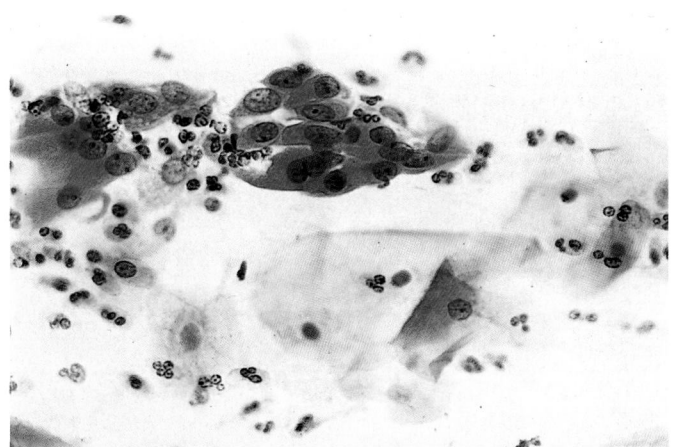

FIGURE 7–47 A normal cervicovaginal smear shows large, flattened squamous cells and groups of metaplastic cells; interspersed are some neutrophils. There are no malignant cells. (Courtesy of Dr. P.K. Gupta, University of Pennsylvania, Philadelphia, PA.)

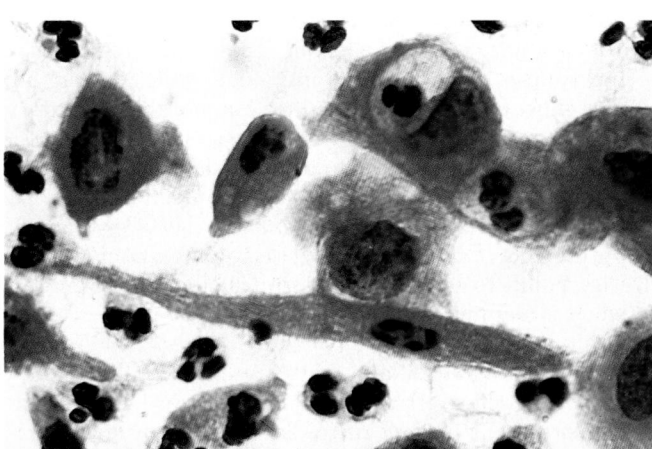

FIGURE 7–48 An abnormal cervicovaginal smear shows numerous malignant cells that have pleomorphic, hyperchromatic nuclei; interspersed are some normal polymorphonuclear leukocytes. (Courtesy of Dr. P.K. Gupta, University of Pennsylvania, Philadelphia, PA.)

Cytologic (Pap) smears provide yet another method for the detection of cancer (Chapter 22). This approach is widely used to screen for carcinoma of the cervix, often at an in situ stage, but it is also used with many other forms of suspected malignancy, such as endometrial carcinoma, bronchogenic carcinoma, bladder and prostatic tumors, and gastric carcinomas; for the identification of tumor cells in abdominal, pleural, joint, and cerebrospinal fluids; and, less commonly, with other forms of neoplasia.

As pointed out earlier, cancer cells have lowered cohesiveness and exhibit a range of morphologic changes encompassed by the term *anaplasia*. Thus, shed cells can be evaluated for the features of anaplasia indicative of their origin from a tumor (Figs. 7–47 and 7–48). In contrast to the histologist's task, judgment here must be rendered based on the features of individual cells or, at most, a clump of cells, without the supporting evidence of loss of orientation of one cell to another, and (most importantly) evidence of invasion. This method permits differentiation among normal, dysplastic, and malignant cells and, in addition, permits the recognition of cellular changes characteristic of carcinoma in situ. The gratifying control of cervical cancer is the best testament to the value of the cytologic method.

Although histology and exfoliative cytology remain the most commonly used methods in the diagnosis of cancer, new techniques are being constantly added to the tools of the surgical pathologist. Some, such as immunohistochemistry, are already well established and widely used; others, including molecular methods, are rapidly finding their way into the "routine" category. Only some highlights of these diagnostic modalities are presented.

Immunohistochemistry. The availability of specific antibodies has greatly facilitated the identification of cell products or surface markers. Some examples of the utility of immunohistochemistry in the diagnosis or management of malignant neoplasms follow.

- *Categorization of undifferentiated malignant tumors:* In many cases malignant tumors of diverse origin resemble each other because of limited differentiation. These tumors are often quite difficult to distinguish on the basis of routine hematoxylin and eosin (H&E)–stained tissue sections. For example, certain anaplastic carcinomas, lymphomas, melanomas, and sarcomas may look quite similar, but they must be accurately identified because their treatment and prognosis are different. Antibodies specific to intermediate filaments have proved to be of particular value in such cases, because solid tumor cells often contain intermediate filaments characteristic of their cell of origin. For example, the presence of cytokeratins, detected by immunohistochemistry, points to an epithelial origin (carcinoma) (Fig. 7–49), whereas desmin is specific for neoplasms of muscle cell origin.

- *Determination of site of origin of metastatic tumors:* Many cancer patients present with metastases. In some the primary site is obvious or readily detected on the basis of clinical or radiologic features. In cases in which the origin of the tumor is obscure, immunohistochemical detection of tissue-specific or organ-specific antigens in a biopsy specimen of the metastatic deposit can lead to the identification of the tumor source. For example, prostate-specific

antigen (PSA) and thyroglobulin are markers of carcinomas of the prostate and thyroid, respectively.

- *Detection of molecules that have prognostic or therapeutic significance:* Immunohistochemical detection of hormone (estrogen/progesterone) receptors in breast cancer cells is of prognostic and therapeutic value because these cancers are susceptible to anti-estrogen therapy (Chapter 23). In general, receptor-positive breast cancers have a better prognosis. Protein products of oncogenes such as *ERBB2* in breast cancers can also be detected by immunostaining. Breast cancers with overexpression of ERBB2 protein generally have a poor prognosis. In general practice, the overexpression of ERBB2 is confirmed by fluorescent in situ hybridization (FISH) to confirm amplification of the genomic region containing the *ERBB2* gene.

Flow Cytometry. Flow cytometry can rapidly and quantitatively measure several individual cell characteristics, such as membrane antigens and the DNA content of tumor cells. *Flow cytometry* has also proved useful in the identification and classification of tumors arising from T and B lymphocytes and from mononuclear-phagocytic cells. Monoclonal antibodies directed against various lymphohematopoietic cells are listed in Chapter 13.

Molecular Diagnosis. Several molecular techniques—some established, others emerging—have been used for diagnosis and, in some cases, for predicting behavior of tumors.

- *Diagnosis of malignant neoplasms:* Although molecular methods are not the primary modality of cancer diagnosis, they are of considerable value in selected cases. Molecular techniques are useful in differentiating benign (polyclonal) proliferations of T or B cells from malignant (monoclonal) proliferations. Because each T and B cell has unique rearrangements of its antigen receptor genes (Chapter 6), PCR–based detection of T-cell receptor or immunoglobulin genes allows distinction between monoclonal (neoplastic) and polyclonal (reactive) proliferations. Many hematopoietic neoplasms (leukemias and lymphomas) are associated with specific translocations that activate oncogenes. Detection of such translocations, usually by routine cytogenetic analysis or by FISH technique (Chapter 5), is often extremely

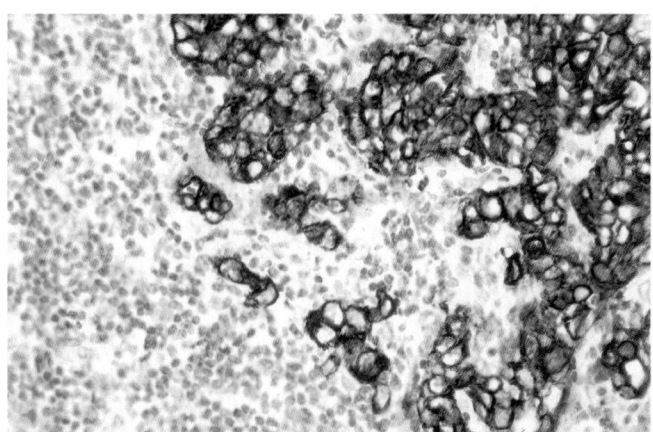

FIGURE 7–49 Anti-cytokeratin immunoperoxidase stain of a tumor of epithelial origin (carcinoma). (Courtesy of Dr. Melissa Upton, University of Washington, Seattle, WA.)

helpful in diagnosis.[189] In some cases, molecular techniques, such as PCR, can detect residual disease in cases that appear negative by conventional analysis. Diagnosis of sarcomas (Chapter 26) with characteristic translocations is also aided by molecular techniques, because chromosome preparations are often difficult to obtain from solid tumors. For example, many sarcomas of childhood, so-called round blue cell tumors (Chapter 10), can be difficult to distinguish from each other on the basis of morphology. However, the presence of the characteristic [t(11;22)(q24;q12)] translocation, established by PCR, in one of these tumors confirms the diagnosis of Ewing sarcoma.[190] A molecular cytogenetic technique called *spectral karyotyping* has great sensitivity and allows the examination of all chromosomes in a single experiment.[191] This technique, which is based on 24-color chromosomal painting with a mixture of fluorochromes, can detect all types of chromosomal rearrangements in tumor cells, even small, cryptic translocations and insertions (Chapter 5; see Fig. 5–35). It can also detect the origin of unidentified chromosomes, called *marker chromosomes*, seen in many hematopoietic malignancies. Another available technique is *comparative genomic hybridization, now more conveniently converted to microarray format,* which allows the analysis of chromosomal gains and losses in tumor cells. The use of DNA microarrays (discussed later), either tiling arrays, which cover the entire human genome, or single-nucleotide polymorphism arrays (SNP chips), also allows analysis of genomic amplifications and deletions at very high resolution.

- *Prognosis of malignant neoplasms:* Certain genetic alterations are associated with poor prognosis, and hence their detection allows stratification of patients for therapy. For example, amplification of the N-*MYC* gene and deletions of 1p bode poorly for patients with neuroblastoma, while amplification of *HER-2/NEU* in breast cancer is an indication that therapy with antibodies against the ERBB2 receptor may be effective. These can be detected by routine cytogenetics and also by FISH or PCR assays. Oligodendrogliomas in which the only genomic abnormality is the loss of chromosomes 1p and 19q respond well to therapy and are associated with long-term survival when compared to tumors with intact 1p and 19q but with EGF receptor amplification.[192]

- *Detection of minimal residual disease:* After treatment of patients with leukemia or lymphoma, the presence of minimal disease or the onset of relapse can be monitored by PCR-based amplification of nucleic acid sequences unique to the malignant clone. For example, detection of *BCR-ABL* transcripts by PCR gives a measure of the residual leukemia cells in treated patients with CML. Similarly, detection of specific *KRAS* mutations in stool samples of persons previously treated for colon cancer can alert the clinician to the possible recurrence of the tumor. The prognostic importance of minimal disease has been established in acute lymphoblastic leukemia, and is being evaluated in other neoplasms.

- *Diagnosis of hereditary predisposition to cancer:* As was discussed earlier, germ-line mutations in several tumor suppressor genes, including *BRCA1*, *BRCA2*, and the *RET* proto-oncogene, are associated with a high risk of developing specific cancers. Thus, detection of these mutated alleles may allow the patient and physician to devise an aggressive screening program, consider the option of prophylactic surgery, and counseling of relatives at risk. Such analysis usually requires detection of a specific mutation (e.g., *RET* gene) or sequencing of the entire gene. The latter is necessitated when several different cancer-associated mutations are known to exist. Although the detection of mutations in such cases is relatively straightforward, the ethical issues surrounding such presymptomatic diagnosis are complex.

Molecular Profiles of Tumors

Until recently, studies of gene expression in tumors involved the analysis of individual genes. These studies have been revolutionized by the introduction of methods that can measure the expression of essentially all the genes in the genome simultaneously.[193,194] The most common method for large-scale analysis of gene expression in use today is based on DNA microarray technology. There are essentially two methods for expression analysis. Either PCR products from cloned genes or oligonucleotides homologous to genes of interest are spotted onto a glass slide. Each method has its advantages and disadvantages. Chips can be purchased from commercial suppliers or produced on the premises, and high-density oligonucleotide arrays can contain more than 2 million elements. The gene chip is then hybridized to "probes" prepared from tumor and control samples (the probes are usually complementary DNA copies of RNAs extracted from tumor and uninvolved tissues) that have been labeled with a fluorochrome. After hybridization the chip is read using a laser scanner (Fig. 7–50); sophisticated software has been developed to measure the intensity of the fluorescence for each spot. A variety of analyses can then be performed with these data; one of the most useful for cancer research has been hierarchical clustering, which can be used in many ways to understand the molecular heterogeneity and biologic behavior of cancer. One can determine the expression profiles of many different individual tumors that have different outcomes, for example, breast cancers that relapsed and those that did not. Using a hierarchical clustering, a (hopefully) short list of genes that are differentially expressed in these two groups can be generated. This "signature" may then be used to predict the behavior of tumors. In this way it is hoped that gene expression profiles will improve our ability to stratify patients' risk and guide treatment beyond the limits of histology and pathologic staging. Indeed, analysis of phenotypically identical large B-cell lymphomas (Chapter 13) from different individuals shows that these tumors are heterogeneous with respect to their gene expression profiles. Importantly, gene expression signatures have been identified that allow segregation of morphologically similar lymphomas into distinct subcategories with markedly different survival rates.[195]

A major problem in the analysis of gene expression in tumors is the heterogeneity of the tissue. In addition to the heterogeneity of the tumor cells, samples may contain variable amounts of stromal connective tissue, inflammatory infiltrates, and normal tissue cells. One way to overcome this problem is to obtain nearly pure tumor cells or small tumors free from associated stroma using *laser capture microdissection*. In this technique, the dissection of tumor cells is made under a microscope through a focused laser. The dissected material

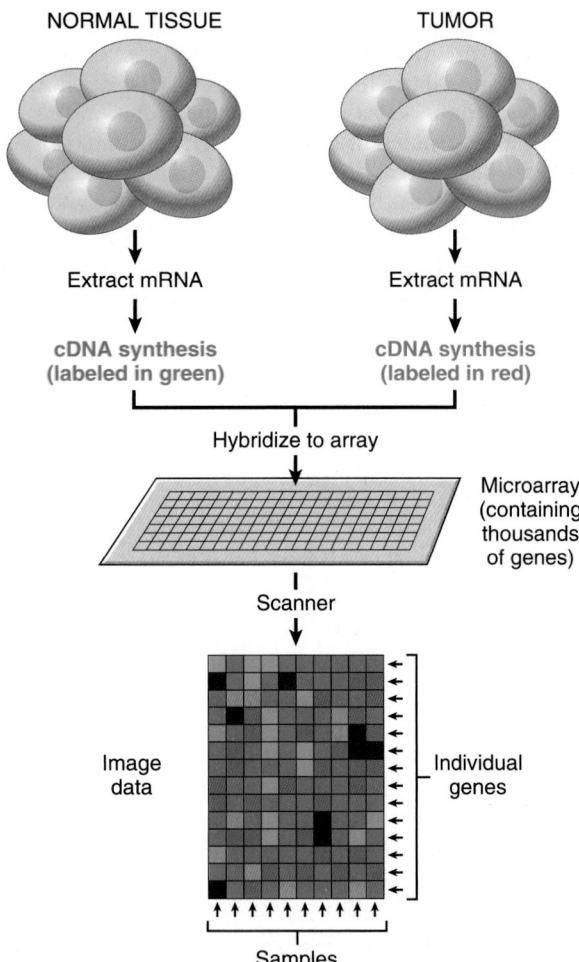

NORMAL TISSUE   TUMOR

Extract mRNA   Extract mRNA

cDNA synthesis   cDNA synthesis
(labeled in green)   (labeled in red)

Hybridize to array

Microarray
(containing
thousands
of genes)

Scanner

Image
data

Individual
genes

Samples

FIGURE 7–50 Steps required for the analysis of global gene expression by DNA microarray. RNA is extracted from tumor and normal tissue. Complementary DNA (cDNA) synthesized from each preparation is labeled with fluorescent dyes (in the example shown, normal tissue cDNA is labeled with a green dye; tumor cDNA is labeled with a red dye). The array consists of a solid support in which DNA fragments from many thousands of genes are spotted. The labeled cDNAs from tumor and normal tissue are combined and hybridized to the genes contained in the array. Hybridization signals are detected using a confocal laser scanner and downloaded to a computer for analysis (*red squares*, expression of the gene is higher in tumor; *green squares*, expression of the gene is higher in normal tissue; *black squares*, no difference in the expression of the gene between tumor and normal tissue). In the display the horizontal rows correspond to each gene contained in the array; each vertical row corresponds to single samples.

is then captured or "catapulted" into a small cap and processed for RNA and DNA isolation.

The applications of molecular profiling technology keep expanding and being refined, but much has already been accomplished. The work that has received the most publicity involves gene expression profiling of breast cancers. In addition to identifying new subtypes of breast cancers, a 70-gene prognosis signature has been established.[196] It has been reported that the signature is a powerful predictor of disease prognosis for young patients and is particularly accurate for predicting metastasis during the first 5 years after diagnosis.

Prognosis determined by gene expression profile correlates highly with histologic grade and estrogen receptor status but not with lymphatic spread of the tumor. A smaller panel of 21 genes is currently being used to assess the risk or recurrence and likely benefit of chemotherapy in a subset of breast cancer patients.[197]

The development of new microarray platforms and new technologies, such as high-throughput sequencing, make the methodical categorization of all the genomic changes present in a cancer cell a realistic possibility. Array-based comparative genomic hybridization can be used to look for alterations in genomic structure, such as amplifications and deletions. These changes can then be correlated to changes in gene expression. So-called single nucleotide polymorphism (SNP) chips, which include SNPs that span the entire genome, have been used in genome-wide linkage analysis (Chapter 5) and association studies to identify genes associated with increased risk of cancer.[198–200] Arrays tiled across the entire genome can be used to look for novel transcripts, novel promoters, and novel splice variants. These tiling arrays can also be used to identify epigenetic events, such as DNA methylation, and, when combined with a technique called chromatin immunoprecipitation, can map the genomic site of chromatin marks, as well as genomic binding sites of transcription factors. High-throughput resequencing methods, which can generate hundreds of millions to billions of base pairs in a single run, may allow identification of unknown fusion gene products, as well as efficient resequencing of entire cancer genomes.[201]

Next on the horizon of molecular techniques for the global analysis of cancers is *proteomics*, a technique used to obtain profiles of proteins contained in tissues, serum, or other body fluids. Indeed, with the realization that mRNA levels are regulated post-transcriptionally, it is not clear how closely the levels of proteins, the molecules that execute cellular processes, actually correlate with mRNA levels. Technologies to achieve global protein measurements, such as mass spectroscopy and antibody arrays, are currently being developed.

The excitement created by the development of new techniques for the global molecular analysis of tumors has led some scientists to predict that the end of histopathology is in sight, and to consider existing approaches to tumor diagnosis as the equivalent of magical methods of divination. Indeed, it is hard to escape the excitement generated by the development of entirely new and powerful methods of molecular analysis. However, what lies ahead is not the replacement of one set of techniques by another. On the contrary, the most accurate diagnosis and prognosis of cancer will be arrived at by a combination of morphologic and molecular techniques.

Tumor Markers

Biochemical assays for tumor-associated enzymes, hormones, and other tumor markers in the blood cannot be used for definitive diagnosis of cancer; however, they contribute to the detection of cancer and in some instances are useful in determining the effectiveness of therapy or the appearance of a recurrence.

A host of tumor markers have been described, and new ones are identified every year. Only a few have stood the test of time and proved to have clinical usefulness.

TABLE 7–12	**Selected Tumor Markers**
HORMONES	
Human chorionic gonadotropin	Trophoblastic tumors, nonseminomatous testicular tumors
Calcitonin	Medullary carcinoma of thyroid
Catecholamine and metabolites	Pheochromocytoma and related tumors
Ectopic hormones	See "Paraneoplastic Syndromes" (Table 7–11)
ONCOFETAL ANTIGENS	
α-Fetoprotein	Liver cell cancer, nonseminomatous germ cell tumors of testis
Carcinoembryonic antigen	Carcinomas of the colon, pancreas, lung, stomach, and heart
ISOENZYMES	
Prostatic acid phosphatase	Prostate cancer
Neuron-specific enolase	Small-cell cancer of lung, neuroblastoma
SPECIFIC PROTEINS	
Immunoglobulins	Multiple myeloma and other gammopathies
Prostate-specific antigen and prostate-specific membrane antigen	Prostate cancer
MUCINS AND OTHER GLYCOPROTEINS	
CA-125	Ovarian cancer
CA-19-9	Colon cancer, pancreatic cancer
CA-15-3	Breast cancer
NEW MOLECULAR MARKERS	
p53, APC, RAS mutants in stool and serum	Colon cancer
p53 and RAS mutants in stool and serum	Pancreatic cancer
p53 and RAS mutants in sputum and serum	Lung cancer
p53 mutants in urine	Bladder cancer

The application of several markers, listed in Table 7–12, is considered in the discussion of specific forms of neoplasia in other chapters, so only a few widely used examples suffice here. PSA, used to screen for prostatic adenocarcinoma, may be one of the most used, and most successful, tumor markers in clinical practice.[202] Prostatic carcinoma can be suspected when elevated levels of PSA are found in the blood. However, PSA screening also highlights problems encountered with virtually every tumor marker. Although PSA levels are often elevated in cancer, PSA levels also may be elevated in benign prostatic hyperplasia (Chapter 18). Furthermore, there is no PSA level that ensures that a person does not have prostate cancer. *Thus, the PSA test suffers from both low sensitivity and low specificity.* Other tumor markers occasionally used in clinical practice include CEA, which is elaborated by carcinomas of the colon, pancreas, stomach, and breast, and AFP, which is produced by hepatocellular carcinomas, yolk sac remnants in the gonads, and occasionally teratocarcinomas and embryonal cell carcinomas. Unfortunately, like PSA, both of these markers can be produced by a variety of non-neoplastic conditions as well. Thus, as with PSA levels, CEA and AFP assays lack both specificity and sensitivity required for the early detection of cancers. They are still useful in the detection of recurrences after excision. With successful resection of the tumor, these markers disappear from the serum; their reappearance almost always signifies the beginning of the end.

Other widely used markers include human chorionic gonadotropin for testicular tumors, CA-125 for ovarian tumors, and immunoglobulins in multiple myeloma and other secretory plasma cell tumors. The development of tests to detect cancer markers in blood and body fluids is an active area of research. Some of the markers being evaluated include the detection of mutated *APC, p53,* and *RAS* in the stool of individuals with colorectal carcinomas; the presence of mutated *p53* and of hypermethylated genes in the sputum of persons with lung cancer and in the saliva of persons with head and neck cancers; and the detection of mutated *p53* in the urine of patients with bladder cancer.

REFERENCES

1. Jemal A et al.: Cancer Statistics, 2008. CA Cancer J Clin 58:71, 2008.
2. Willis R: The Spread of Tumors in the Human Body. London, Butterworth, 1952.
3. Fusco A, Fedele M: Roles of HMGA proteins in cancer. Nat Rev Cancer 7:899, 2007.
4. Morrison SJ, Spradling C: Stem cells and niches: mechanisms that promote stem cell maintenance throughout life. Cell 132:598, 2008.
5. Jordan C, Guzman M, Noble M: Cancer stem cells. N Engl J Med 355:1253, 2006.
6. Ward R, Dirks P: Cancer stem cells: at the headwaters of tumor development. Annu Rev Pathol 2:175, 2007.
7. Al-Hajj M et al.: Prospective identification of tumorigenic breast cancer cells. Proc Natl Acad Sci U S A 100:3983, 2003.
8. O'Brien CA et al.: A human colon cancer cell capable of initiating tumour growth in immunodeficient mice. Nature 445:106, 2007.
9. Quintana E et al.: Efficient tumor formation by single human melanoma cells. Nature 456:593, 2008.
10. Park IK et al.: Bmi-1 is required for maintenance of adult self-renewing haematopoietic stem cells. Nature 423:302, 2003.
11. Padera T et al.: Lymphatic metastasis in the absence of functional intratumor lymphatics. Science 296:1883, 2002.
12. Choi S-H et al.: Clinicopathologic analysis of sentinel lymph node mapping in early breast cancer. Breast J 9:153, 2003.

13. Covens A: Sentinel lymph nodes. Cancer 97:2945, 2003.
14. Ghafoor A et al.: Cancer statistics for African Americans. CA Cancer J Clin 52:326, 2002.
15. O'Brien K et al.: Cancer statistics for Hispanics, 2003. CA Cancer J Clin 53:208, 2003.
16. Parkin DM: Global cancer statistics in the year 2000. Lancet Oncol 2:533, 2001.
17. Parkin DM et al.: Global cancer statistics, 2002. CA Cancer J Clin 55:74, 2005.
18. Calle E, Kaaks R: Overweight, obesity and cancer: epidemiological evidence and proposed mechanisms. Nat Rev Cancer 4:579, 2004.
19. Knudson AG: Cancer genetics. Am J Med Genet 111:96, 2002.
20. Narod S: Modifiers of risk of hereditary breast cancer. Oncogene 25:5832, 2005.
21. Rustgi A: The genetics of hereditary colon cancer. Genes Dev 21:2525, 2007.
22. Easton D et al.: Genome-wide association study identifies novel breast cancer susceptibility loci. Nature 447:1087, 2007.
23. Pho LG et al.: Melanoma genetics: a review of genetic factors and clinical phenotypes in familial melanoma. Curr Opin Oncol 18:173, 2006.
24. Tlsty TD, Coussens LM: Tumor stroma and regulation of cancer development. Annu Rev Pathol 1:119, 2006.
25. Sinicrope FA: Targeting cyclooxygenase-2 for prevention and therapy of colorectal cancer. Mol Carcinog 45:447, 2006.
26. Howe LR, Dannenberg AJ: A role for cyclooxygenase-2 inhibitors in the prevention and treatment of cancer. Semin Oncol 29:111, 2002.
27. Gale RE: Evaluation of clonality in myeloid stem-cell disorders. Semin Hematol 36:361, 1999.
28. Santarosa M, Ashworth A: Haploinsufficiency for tumour suppressor genes: when you don't need to go all the way. Biochim Biophys Acta 1654:105, 2004.
29. Zhang W et al.: MicroRNAs in tumorigenesis: a primer. Am J Pathol 171:728, 2007.
30. Rana TM: Illuminating the silence: understanding the structure and function of small RNAs. Nat Rev Mol Cell Biol 8:23, 2007.
31. Loeb LA et al.: Multiple mutations and cancer. Proc Natl Acad Sci U S A 100:776, 2003.
32. Weinberg RA, Hanahan D: The hallmarks of cancer. Cell 100:57, 2000.
33. Halazonetis TD et al.: An oncogene-induced DNA damage model for cancer development. Science 319:1352, 2008.
34. Kern SE: Progressive genetic abnormalities in human neoplasia. In Mendelsohn J, Howley PM, Israel MA, et al (eds): The Molecular Basis of Cancer, 2nd ed. Philadelphia, WB Saunders, 2001, p 41.
35. Plaza-Menacho I et al.: Current concepts in RET-related genetics, signaling and therapeutics. Trends Genet 22:627, 2006.
36. Lakhani VT et al.: The multiple endocrine neoplasia syndromes. Annu Rev Med 58:253, 2007.
37. Badalamenti G et al.: Gastrointestinal stromal tumors (GISTs): focus on histopathological diagnosis and biomolecular features. Ann Oncol 18 (Suppl 6):vi36, 2007.
38. Rowinsky EK: The erbB family: targets for therapeutic development against cancer and therapeutic strategies using monoclonal antibodies and tyrosine kinase inhibitors. Annu Rev Med 55:433, 2004.
39. Hudis C: Trastuzumab—mechanism of action and use in clinical practice. N Engl J Med 357:39, 2007.
40. Malumbres M, Barbacid M: *RAS* oncogenes: the first 30 years. Nat Rev Cancer 3:459, 2003.
41. Jaffee EM et al.: Focus on pancreas cancer. Cancer Cell 2:25, 2002.
42. Minna JD et al.: Focus on lung cancer. Cancer Cell 1:49, 2002.
43. Hingorani SR, Tuveson DA: Ras redux: rethinking how and where Ras acts. Curr Opin Genet Dev 13:6, 2003.
44. Michaloglou C et al.: BRAFE600 in benign and malignant human tumours. Oncogene 27:877, 2007.
45. Pollock P et al.: High frequency of BRAF mutations in nevi. Nat Genet 33:19, 2003.
46. Krause DS, Van Eetten RA: Tyrosine kinases as targets for cancer therapy. N Engl J Med 353:172, 2005.
47. Goldman JM, Melo JV: Chronic myeloid leukemia—advances in biology and new approaches to treatment. N Engl J Med 349:1451, 2003.
48. Kurzrock R et al.: Philadelphia chromosome-positive leukemias: from basic mechanisms to molecular therapeutics. Ann Intern Med 138:819, 2003.
49. Sattler M, Griffin JD: Molecular mechanisms of transformation by the *BCR-ABL* oncogene. Semin Hematol 40:4, 2003.
50. Sharma SV and Settleman J: Oncogene addiction: setting the stage for molecularly targeted cancer therapy. Genes and Development 21:3214, 2007.
51. Campbell PJ, Green AR: The myeloproliferative disorders. N Engl J Med 355:2452, 2006.
52. Patel JH et al.: Analysis of genomic targets reveals complex functions of MYC. Nat Rev Cancer 4:562, 2004.
53. Adhikary S, Eilers M: Transcriptional regulation and transformation by Myc proteins. Nat Rev Mol Cell Biol 6:635, 2005.
54. Dominguez-Sola D et al.: Non-transcriptional control of DNA replication by c-Myc. Nature 448:445, 2007.
55. Meyer N et al.: The Oscar-worthy role of Myc in apoptosis. Semin Cancer Biol 16:275, 2006.
56. Chu I et al.: The Cdk inhibitor p27 in human cancer: prognostic potential and relevance to anticancer therapy. Nat Rev Cancer 8:253, 2008.
57. Kim WY, Sharpless NE: The regulation of INK4/ARF in cancer and aging. Cell 127:265, 2006.
58. Bartek J, Lukas J: Mammalian G_1- and S-phase checkpoints in response to DNA damage. Curr Opin Cell Biol 13:738, 2001.
59. Kastan MB, Bartek J: Cell cycle checkpoints and cancer. Nature 432:316, 2004.
60. Knudson A: Two genetic hits (more or less) to cancer. Nat Rev Cancer 1:157, 2001.
61. Kaelin WG: von Hippel-Lindau disease. Annu Rev Pathol 2:145, 2007.
62. Massague J: G_1 cell-cycle control and cancer. Nature 432:298, 2004.
63. Ji P et al.: An Rb–Skp2–p27 pathway mediates acute cell cycle inhibition by Rb and is retained in a partial-penetrance Rb mutant. Mol Cell 16:47, 2004.
64. Binne UK et al.: Retinoblastoma protein and anaphase-promoting complex physically interact and functionally cooperate during cell-cycle exit. Nature Cell Biol 9:225, 2007.
65. Skapek SX et al.: Regulation of cell lineage specification by the retinoblastoma tumor suppressor. Oncogene 25:5268, 2006.
66. Macaluso M et al.: Rb family proteins as modulators of gene expression and new aspects regarding the interaction with chromatin remodeling enzymes. Oncogene 25:5263, 2006.
67. Ajioka I et al.: Differentiated horizontal interneurons clonally expand to form metastatic retinoblastoma in mice. Cell 131:378, 2007.
68. Sherr CJ, McCormick F: The RB and p53 pathways in cancer. Cancer Cell 2:103, 2002.
69. Vousden K, Lane D: p53 in health and disease. Nat Rev Mol Cell Biol 8:275, 2007.
70. Frebourg T et al.: Germ-line p53 mutations in 15 families with Li-Fraumeni syndrome. Am J Hum Genet 56:608, 1995.
71. Nichols KE et al.: Germ-line p53 mutations predispose to a wide spectrum of early-onset cancers. Cancer Epidemiol Biomarkers Prev 10:83, 2001.
72. Onel K, Cordon-Cardo C: MDM2 and prognosis. Mol Cancer Res 2:1, 2004.
73. Shmueli A, Oren M: Regulation of p53 by Mdm2: fate is in the numbers. Mol Cell 13:4, 2004.
74. Wei CL et al.: A global map of p53 transcription-factor binding sites in the human genome. Cell 124: 207, 2006.
75. Riley T et al.: Transcriptional control of human p53-regulated genes. Nature Rev Mol Cell Biol 402:402, 2008.
76. He L et al.: microRNAs join the p53 network—another piece in the tumour-suppression puzzle. Nat Rev Cancer 7:819, 2007.
77. Shiloh Y: The ATM-mediated DNA-damage response: taking shape. Trends Biochem Sci 31:402, 2006.
78. Cimprich KA, Cortez D: ATR: an essential regulator of genome integrity. Nature Rev Med 9:616, 2008.
79. Di Micco R et al.: Breaking news: high-speed race ends in arrest—how oncogenes induce senescence. Trends Cell Biol 17:529, 2007.
80. Murray-Zmijewski et al.: A complex barcode underlies the heterogenous response of p53 to stress. Nature Rev Med 9:702, 2008.
81. Deyoung M, Ellisen L: p63 and p73 in human cancer: defining the network. Oncogene 26:5169, 2007.
82. Ratovitski E et al.: p63 and p73: teammates or adversaries? Cancer Cell 9:1, 2006.
83. Leong C et al.: The p63/p73 network mediates chemosensitivity to cisplatin in a biologically defined subset of primary breast cancers. J Clin Invest 117:1370, 2007.
84. Shibata H et al.: Rapid colorectal adenoma formation initiated by conditional targeting of the *Apc* gene. Science 278:120, 1997.

85. Polakis P: The many ways of Wnt in cancer. Curr Opin Genet Dev 17:45, 2007.

86. Wei Y et al.: Activation of β-catenin in epithelial and mesenchymal hepatoblastomas. Oncogene 19:498, 2000.

87. Hirohashi S, Kanai Y: Cell adhesion system and human cancer morphogenesis. Cancer Sci 94:575, 2003.

88. Thiery J, Sleeman J: Complex networks orchestrate epithelial-mesenchymal transitions. Nat Rev Mol Cell Biol 7:131, 2006.

89. Bierie B, Moses H: Tumour microenvironment: TGFβ: the molecular Jekyll and Hyde of cancer. Nat Rev Cancer 6:506, 2006.

90. Jiang B-H, Liu L-Z: PI3K/PTEN signaling in tumorigenesis and angiogenesis. Biochim Biophys Acta 1784:150, 2008.

91. Chaloub N, Baker SJ: PTEN and PI3-kinase pathway in cancer. Ann Rev Path Mech Dis 4:97, 2009.

92. Gutmann D, Collins F (eds): Neurofibromatosis 1, 2nd ed. In Vogelstein B, Kinzler K (eds): The Genetic Basis of Human Cancer. New York, McGraw-Hill, 2002, p 417–437.

93. MacCollin M, Gusella J (eds): Neurofibromatosis 2. In Vogelstein B, Kinzler K (eds): The Genetic Basis of Human Cancer. New York, McGraw-Hill, 2002, p 439.

94. Harvey K, Tapon N: The Salvador-Warts-Hippo pathway—an emerging tumour-suppressor network. Nat Rev Cancer 7:182, 2007.

95. Haber D (ed): Wilms tumor. In Vogelstein B, Kinzler K (eds): The Genetic Basis of Human Cancer. New York, McGraw-Hill, 2002, p 403.

96. Beachy PA et al.: Tissue repair and stem cell renewal in carcinogenesis. Nature 432:324, 2004.

97. Evan GI, Vousden KH: Proliferation, cell cycle and apoptosis in cancer. Nature 411:342, 2001.

98. Korsmeyer SJ: Programmed cell death and the regulation of homeostasis. Harvey Lect 95:21, 1999.

99. Igney FH, Krammer PH: Death and anti-death: tumour resistance to apoptosis. Nat Rev Cancer 2:277, 2002.

100. Green D, Kroemer G: The pathophysiology of mitochondrial cell death. Science 305:626, 2004.

101. Danial NN, Korsmeyer SJ: Cell death: critical control points. Cell 116:205, 2004.

102. Deng Y et al.: Telomere dysfunction and tumor suppression: the senescence connection. Nature Rev. Cancer 8:450, 2008.

103. Sharpless N, DePinho R: Telomeres, stem cells, senescence, and cancer. J Clin Invest 113:160, 2004.

104. Nagy J et al.: VEGF-A and the induction of pathological angiogenesis. Annu Rev Pathol 2:251, 2007.

105. Bergers G, Benjamin L: Tumorigenesis and the angiogenic switch. Nat Rev Cancer 3:401, 2003.

106. Sonpavde G et al.: Bevacizumab in colorectal cancer. N Engl J Med 351:1690, 2004.

107. Noguera-Troise I et al.: Blockade of Dll4 inhibits tumour growth by promoting non-productive angiogenesis. Nature 444:1032, 2006.

108. Ridgway J et al.: Inhibition of Dll4 signalling inhibits tumour growth by deregulating angiogenesis. Nature 444:1083, 2006.

109. Fidler IJ: The pathogenesis of cancer metastasis: the "seed and soil" hypothesis revisited. Nat Rev Cancer 3:453, 2003.

110. Bissell MJ, Radisky D: Putting tumours in context. Nat Rev Cancer 1:46, 2001.

111. Radisky D, Muschler J, Bissell MJ: Order and disorder: the role of extracellular matrix in epithelial cancer. Cancer Invest 20:139, 2002.

112. Overall CM, Kleifeld O: Validating matrix metalloproteinases as drug targets and anti-targets for cancer therapy. Nature Rev Cancer 6:227, 2006.

113. Sahai E: Illuminating the metastatic cascade. Nature Rev Cancer 7:737, 2007.

114. Epstein RJ: The CXCL12-CXCR4 chemotactic pathway as a target of adjuvant breast cancer therapies. Nat Rev Cancer 4:901, 2004.

115. Steeg P: Tumor metastasis: mechanistic insights and clinical challenges. Nat Med 12:895, 2006.

116. Ramaswamy S et al.: A molecular signature of metastasis in primary solid tumors. Nat Genet 33:49, 2003.

117. Nguyen D, Massague J: Genetic determinants of cancer metastasis. Nat Rev Genet 8:341, 2007.

118. Steeg PZ: Metastasis suppressors alter the signal transduction of cancer cells. Nat Rev Cancer 3:55, 2003.

119. Tavazoie SF et al.: Endogenous human microRNAs that suppress breast cancer metastases. Nature 451:157, 2008.

120. Ma L et al.: Tumor invasions and metastases initiated by microRNA-10b in breast cancer. Nature 449:682, 2008.

121. Peindao H et al.: Snail, ZEB and bHLH factors in tumour progression; an alliance against the epithelial phenotype? Nature Rev Cancer 7:415, 2007.

122. Hoeijmakers JH: Genome maintenance mechanisms for preventing cancer. Nature 411:366, 2001.

123. Lynch HT, de la Chapelle A: Hereditary colorectal cancer. N Engl J Med 348:919, 2003.

124. Jiricny J, Marra G: DNA repair defects in colon cancer. Curr Opin Genet Dev 13:61, 2003.

125. Friedberg EC: How nucleotide excision repair protects against cancer. Nat Rev Cancer 1:22, 2001.

126. Wang W: Emergence of a DNA-damage response network consisting of Fanconi anaemia and BRCA proteins. Nat Rev Genet 8:735, 2007.

127. Hickson ID et al.: Role of the Bloom's syndrome helicase in maintenance of genome stability. Biochem Soc Trans 29:201, 2001.

128. Venkatiraman AR: Linking the cellular functions of *BRCA* gene to cancer pathogenesis and treatment. Ann Rev Path Mech Dis 4:435, 2009.

129. Condeelis J, Pollard JW: Macrophages: obligate partners for tumor cell migration, invasion, and metastasis. Cell 124:263, 2006.

130. Cunha GR et al.: Role of stromal microenvironment in carcinogenesis of prostate. Int J Cancer 107:1, 2003.

131. Finak G et al.: Stromal gene expression predicts clinical outcome in breast cancer. Nat Med 14:518, 2008.

132. Yeung SJ et al.: Roles of p53, Myc, and HIF1 in regulating glycolysis—the seventh hallmark of cancer. Cell Mol Life Sci 2008. Advance Online Publication.

133. DeBerardinis RJ et al.: Brick by brick: metabolism and tumor cell growth. Curr Opin Gen Devel 18:54, 2008.

134. Hsu PP, Sabatini DM: Cancer cell metabolism: warburg and beyond. Cell 134:703, 2008.

135. Dang CV et al.: The interplay between MYC and HIF in cancer. Nature Rev Cancer 8:51, 2008.

136. Denko NC: Hypoxia, HIF1 and glucose metabolism in the solid tumor. Nature Rev Cancer 8:705, 2008.

137. Tomlins SA et al.: Recurrent fusion of TMPRSS2 and ETS transcription factor genes in prostate cancer. Science 310:644, 2005.

138. Kumar-Sinha C et al.: Recurrent gene fusions in prostate cancer. Nature Rev Cancer 8:497, 2008.

139. Hogarty MD, Brodeur GM: Gene amplification in human cancers: biological and clinical significance. In Vogelstein B, Kinzler KW (eds): The Genetic Basis of Human Cancer, 2nd ed. New York, McGraw-Hill, 2002, pp 115–128.

140. Ting A et al.: The cancer epigenome—components and functional correlates. Genes Dev 20:3215, 2006.

141. Esteller M: Epigenetics in cancer. N Engl J Med 358:1148, 2008.

142. Dutta A, Lee YS: MicroRNA in cancer. Ann Rev Path Mech Dis 4:175, 2009.

143. Hahn W, Weinberg R: Rules for making human tumor cells. N Engl J Med 347:1593, 2002.

144. Wood LD et al.: The genomic landscapes of human breast and colorectal cancers. Science. 318(5853):1108, 2007.

145. Cichowski K, Hahn WC: Unexpected pieces of the senescence puzzle. Cell 133:958, 2008.

146. Tennant R: Chemical carcinogenesis. In Franks LM, Teich NM (eds): An Introduction to the Cellular and Molecular Biology of Cancer, 3rd ed. Oxford, Oxford University Press, 1997, pp 106–125.

147. Perera F: Environment and cancer: who are susceptible? Science 278:1068, 1997.

148. Vineis P et al.: CYP1A1 T3801 C polymorphism and lung cancer: a pooled analysis of 2,451 cases and 3,358 controls. Int J Cancer 104:650, 2003.

149. Hecht SS: Cigarette smoking and lung cancer: chemical mechanisms and approaches to prevention. Lancet Oncol 3:461, 2002.

150. Palli D et al.: Biomarkers of dietary intake of micronutrients modulate DNA adduct levels in healthy adults. Carcinogenesis 24:739, 2003.

151. Hussain S et al.: *TP53* mutations and hepatocellular carcinoma: insights into the etiology and pathogenesis of liver cancer. Oncogene 26:2166, 2007.

152. Preston DL et al.: Radiation effects on breast cancer risk: a pooled analysis of eight cohorts. Radiat Res 158:220, 2002.

153. Cleaver JE, Crowley E: UV damage, DNA repair and skin carcinogenesis. Front Biosci 7:1024, 2002.

154. Neronova E et al.: Chromosome alterations in cleanup workers sampled years after the Chernobyl accident. Radiat Res 160:46, 2003.

155. Matsuoka M, Jeang K.-T: Human T-cell leukaemia virus type 1 (HTLV-1) infectivity and cellular transformation. Nat Rev Cancer 7:270, 2007.

156. Grassmann R et al.: Molecular mechanisms of cellular transformation by HTLV-1 Tax. Oncogene 24:5976, 2005.

157. McLaughlin-Drubin ME, Munger K: Viruses associated with human cancer. Biochim Biophys Acta 1782:127, 2008.

158. Woodman C et al.: The natural history of cervical HPV infection: unresolved issues. Nat Rev Cancer 7:11, 2007.

159. zur Hausen H: Papillomaviruses and cancer: from basic studies to clinical application. Nat Rev Cancer 2:342, 2002.

160. Zehbe I et al.: Codon 72 polymorphism of and its association with cervical cancer. The Lancet 354:218, 1999.

161. Kutok J, Wang F: Spectrum of Epstein-Barr virus–associated diseases. Annu Rev Pathol 1:375, 2006.

162. Thorley-Lawson D: Epstein-Barr virus: exploiting the immune system. Nat Rev Immunol 1:75, 2001.

163. Thorley-Lawson DA, Gross A: Mechanism of disease: persistence of Epstein-Barr virus and the origins of associated lymphomas. N Engl J Med 350:1328, 2004.

164. Lindstrom MS, Wiman KG: Role of genetic and epigenetic changes in Burkitt lymphoma. Semin Cancer Biol 12:381, 2002.

165. Raab-Traub N: Epstein-Barr virus in the pathogenesis of NPC. Semin Cancer Biol 12:431, 2002.

166. Tang H et al.: Molecular functions and biological roles of hepatitis B virus x protein. Cancer Sci 97:977, 2006.

167. Kremsdorf D et al.: Hepatitis B virus–related hepatocellular carcinoma: paradigms for viral-related human carcinogenesis. Oncogene 25:3823, 2006.

168. Levrero M: Viral hepatitis and liver cancer: the case of hepatitis C. Oncogene 25:3834, 2006.

169. Peek RM Jr, Crabtree JE: *Helicobacter* infection and gastric neoplasia. J Pathol 208:233, 2006.

170. Burnet FM: The concept of immunological surveillance. Prog Exper Tumor Res 13:1, 1970.

171. Dunn GP et al.: Cancer immunoediting: from immunosurveillance to tumor escape. Nat Immunol 3:991, 2002.

172. Aptsiauri N et al.: MHC class I antigens and immune surveillance in transformed cells. Int Rev Cytol 256:139, 2007.

173. Zitvogel L et al.: Cancer despite immunosurveillance: immunoselection and immunosubversion. Nat Rev Immunol 6:715, 2006.

174. Kim R et al.: Cancer immunoediting from immune surveillance to immune escape. Immunology 121:1, 2007.

175. Dunn GP et al.: Interferons, immunity and cancer immunoediting. Nat Rev Immunol 6(11):836, 2006.

176. Coulie PG, Hanagiri T, Takenoyama M: From tumor antigens to immunotherapy. Int J Clin Oncol 6:163, 2001.

177. Pardoll D: Does the immune system see tumors as foreign or self? Annu Rev Immunol 21:807, 2003.

178. Boon T, Van den Eynde B: Tumour immunology. Curr Opin Immunol 15:129, 2003.

179. Castelli C et al.: T-cell recognition of melanoma-associated antigens. J Cell Physiol 182:323, 2000.

180. Barker PA, Salehi A: The MAGE proteins: emerging roles in cell cycle progression, apoptosis, and neurogenetic disease. J Neurosci Res 67:705, 2002.

181. Cerwenka A, Lanier LL: Natural killer cells, viruses and cancer. Nat Rev Immunol 1:41, 2001.

182. Latour S, Veillette A: Molecular and immunological basis of X-linked lymphoproliferative disease. Immunol Rev 192:212, 2003.

183. Strand S, Galle PR: Immune evasion by tumours: involvement of the CD95 (APO-1/Fas) system and its clinical implications. Mol Med Today 4:63, 1998.

184. Hanahan D, Lanzavecchia A, Mihich E: The novel dichotomy of immune interactions with tumors. Cancer Res 63:3005, 2003.

185. Acharyya S, Guttridge D: Cancer cachexia signaling pathways continue to emerge yet much still points to the proteasome. Clin Cancer Res 13:1356, 2007.

186. Darnell R, Posner J: Paraneoplastic syndromes involving the nervous system. N Engl J Med 349:1543, 2003.

187. Mazzone PJ, Arroliga AC: Endocrine paraneoplastic syndromes in lung cancer. Curr Opin Pulm Med 9:313, 2003.

188. Hoey RP et al.: The parathyroid hormone-related protein receptor is expressed in breast cancer bone metastases and promotes autocrine proliferation in breast carcinoma cells. Br J Cancer 88:567, 2003.

189. Swansbury J: Some difficult choices in cytogenetics. Methods Mol Biol 220:245, 2003.

190. Rowland JM: Molecular genetic diagnosis of pediatric cancer: current and emerging methods. Pediatr Clin North Am 49:1415, 2002.

191. Bayani J, Squire JA: Advances in the detection of chromosomal aberrations using spectral karyotyping. Clin Genet 59:65, 2001.

192. Louis DN, Pomeroy SL, Cairncross JG: Focus on central nervous system neoplasia. Cancer Cell 1:125, 2002.

193. Lakhani SR, Ashworth A: Microarray and histopathological analysis of tumours: the future and the past? Nat Rev Cancer 1:151, 2001.

194. Riggins GJ, Morin PJ: Gene expression profiling in cancer. In Vogelstein B, Kinzler KW (eds): The Genetic Basis of Human Cancers, 2nd ed. New York, McGraw-Hill, 2002, pp 131–141.

195. Rosenwald A et al.: The use of molecular profiling to predict survival after chemotherapy for diffuse large-B-cell lymphoma. New Engl J Med 346:1937, 2002.

196. van de Vijver MJ et al.: A gene-expression signature as a predictor of survival in breast cancer. N Engl J Med 347:1999, 2002.

197. Paik S et al.: A Multigene assay to predict recurrence of tamoxifen-treated, node-negative breast cancer. N Engl J Med 351(27):2817, 2004.

198. Eeles RA et al.: Multiple newly identified loci associated with prostate cancer susceptibility. Nat Genet 40(3):316, 2008.

199. Thomas G et al.: Multiple loci identified in a genome-wide association study of prostate cancer. Nat Genet 40(3):310, 2008.

200. Hunter DJ et al.: A genome-wide association study identifies alleles in FGFR2 associated with risk of sporadic postmenopausal breast cancer. Nat Genet 39(7):870, 2007.

201. Campbell PJ et al.: Identification of somatically acquired rearrangements in cancer using genome-wide massively parallel paired-end sequencing. Nat Genet 40(6):722, 2008.

202. Lilja H et al.: Prostate-specific antigen and prostate cancer: prediction, detection and monitoring. Nature Rev Cancer 8(4):268, 2008.

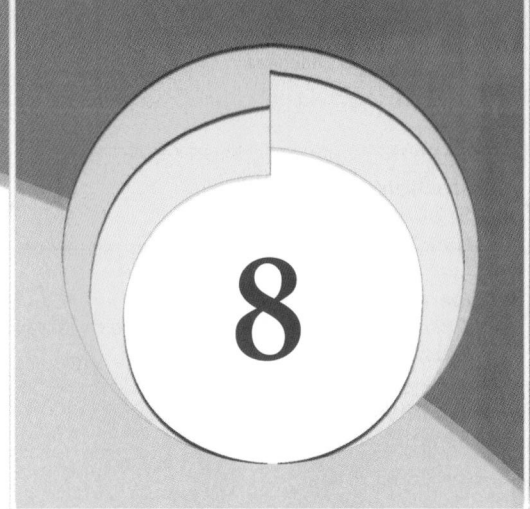

Infectious Diseases

ALEXANDER J. McADAM · ARLENE H. SHARPE

General Principles of Microbial Pathogenesis
  Categories of Infectious Agents
    Prions
    Viruses
    Bacteria
    Fungi
    Protozoa
    Helminths
    Ectoparasites
  Special Techniques for Diagnosing Infectious Agents
  New and Emerging Infectious Diseases
  Agents of Bioterrorism
  Transmission and Dissemination of Microbes
    Routes of Entry of Microbes
    Spread and Dissemination of Microbes
    Release of Microbes from the Body
    Sexually Transmitted Infections
    Healthcare-Associated Infections
    Host Defenses Against Infections
  How Microorganisms Cause Disease
    Mechanisms of Viral Injury
    Mechanisms of Bacterial Injury
    Injurious Effects of Host Immunity
  Immune Evasion by Microbes
  Infections in Immunosuppressed Hosts
  Spectrum of Inflammatory Responses to Infection
    Suppurative (Purulent) Inflammation
    Mononuclear and Granulomatous Inflammation
    Cytopathic-Cytoproliferative Reaction
    Tissue Necrosis
    Chronic Inflammation and Scarring

Viral Infections
  Acute (Transient) Infections
    Measles
    Mumps
    Poliovirus Infection
    West Nile Virus
    Viral Hemorrhagic Fevers
  Chronic Latent Infections (Herpesvirus Infections)
    Herpes Simplex Virus (HSV)
    Varicella-Zoster Virus (VZV)
    Cytomegalovirus (CMV)
  Chronic Productive Infections
    Hepatitis B Virus
  Transforming Infections
    Epstein-Barr Virus (EBV)

Bacterial Infections
  Gram-Positive Bacterial Infections
    Staphylococcal Infections
    Streptococcal and Enterococcal Infections
    Diphtheria
    Listeriosis
    Anthrax
    Nocardia
  Gram-Negative Bacterial Infections
    Neisserial Infections
    Whooping Cough
    Pseudomonas Infection
    Plague
    Chancroid (Soft Chancre)
    Granuloma Inguinale
  Mycobacteria
    Tuberculosis
    Mycobacterium avium-intracellulare Complex
    Leprosy

Spirochetes
   Syphilis
   Relapsing Fever
   Lyme Disease
Anaerobic Bacteria
   Abscesses Caused by Anaerobes
   Clostridial Infections
Obligate Intracellular Bacteria
   Chlamydial Infections
   Rickettsial Infections
Fungal Infections
   Candidiasis
   Cryptococcosis
   Aspergillosis
   Zygomycosis (Mucormycosis)

Parasitic Infections
Protozoa
   Malaria
   Babesiosis
   Leishmaniasis
   African Trypanosomiasis
   Chagas Disease
Metazoa
   Strongyloidiasis
   Tapeworms (Cestodes): Cysticercosis
      and Hydatid Disease
   Trichinosis
   Schistosomiasis
   Lymphatic Filariasis
   Onchocerciasis

General Principles of Microbial Pathogenesis

Despite the availability and use of effective vaccines and antibiotics, infectious diseases remain an important health problem in the United States and worldwide. In the United States, 2 of the top 10 leading causes of death are infectious diseases (pneumonia and influenza, and septicemia).[1] Infectious diseases are particularly important causes of death among the elderly, people with acquired immunodeficiency syndrome (AIDS), those with chronic diseases, and those receiving immunosuppressive drugs. In developing countries, unsanitary living conditions and malnutrition contribute to a massive burden of infectious diseases that kills more than 10 million people each year. Most of these deaths are among children, especially from respiratory and diarrheal infections.[2]

CATEGORIES OF INFECTIOUS AGENTS

Infectious agents belong to a wide range of classes and vary in size from the approximately 27-kD nucleic acid–free prion to 20-nm poliovirus to 10-m tapeworms (Table 8–1).

Prions

Prions are composed of abnormal forms of a host protein, termed *prion protein* (PrP).[3] These agents cause transmissible spongiform encephalopathies, including kuru (associated with human cannibalism), Creutzfeldt-Jakob disease (CJD), bovine spongiform encephalopathy (BSE; better known as mad cow disease), and variant Creutzfeldt-Jakob disease (vCJD; probably transmitted to humans from BSE-infected cattle).[4] PrP is normally found in neurons. Diseases occur when the PrP undergoes a conformational change that confers resistance to proteases. The protease-resistant PrP promotes conversion of the normal protease-sensitive PrP to the abnor-

mal form, explaining the infectious nature of these diseases. Accumulation of abnormal PrP leads to neuronal damage and distinctive spongiform pathologic changes in the brain. Spontaneous or inherited mutations in PrP, which make PrP resistant to proteases, have been observed in the sporadic and familial forms of CJD, respectively. CJD can be transmitted from person to person iatrogenically, by surgery, organ transplant, or blood transfusion. These diseases are discussed in detail in Chapter 28.

Viruses

Viruses are obligate intracellular parasites that depend on the host cell's metabolic machinery for their replication. They consist of a nucleic acid genome surrounded by a protein coat (called a capsid) that is sometimes encased in a lipid membrane. Viruses are classified by their nucleic acid genome (DNA or RNA but not both), the shape of the capsid (icosahedral or helical), the presence or absence of a lipid envelope, their mode of replication, the preferred cell type for replication (called tropism), or the type of pathology. Because viruses are only 20 to 300 nm in size, they are best visualized with the electron microscope (Fig. 8–1). However, some viral particles aggregate within the cells they infect and form characteristic inclusion bodies, which may be seen with the light microscope and are useful for diagnosis. For example, cytomegalovirus (CMV)-infected cells are enlarged and show a large eosinophilic nuclear inclusion and smaller basophilic cytoplasmic inclusions; herpesviruses form a large nuclear inclusion surrounded by a clear halo; and both smallpox and rabies viruses form characteristic cytoplasmic inclusions. Many viruses do not produce inclusions (e.g., Epstein-Barr virus [EBV]).

Viruses account for a large share of human infections. Many viruses cause transient illnesses (e.g., colds, influenza). Other viruses are not eliminated from the body and persist within cells of the host for years, either continuing to multiply (e.g., chronic infection with hepatitis B virus [HBV]) or surviving

TABLE 8–1 Classes of Human Pathogens and Their Lifestyles

Taxonomic	Size	Site of Propagation	Examples	Disease
Prions	30–50 kD	Intracellular	Prion protein	Creutzfeld-Jacob disease
Viruses	20–300 nm	Obligate intracellular	Poliovirus	Poliomyelitis
Bacteria	0.2–15 μm	Obligate intracellular Extracellular Facultative intracellular	*Chlamydia trachomatis* *Streptococcus pneumoniae* *Mycobacterium tuberculosis*	Trachoma, urethritis Pneumonia Tuberculosis
Fungi	2–200 μm	Extracellular Facultative intracellular	*Candida albicans* *Histoplasma capsulatum*	Thrush Histoplasmosis
Protozoa	1–50 μm	Extracellular Facultative intracellular Obligate intracellular	*Trypanosoma gambiense* *Trypanosoma cruzi* *Leishmania donovani*	Sleeping sickness Chagas disease Kala-azar
Helminths	3 mm–10 m	Extracellular Intracellular	*Wuchereria bancrofti* *Trichinella spiralis*	Filariasis Trichinosis

in some nonreplicating form (termed *latent infection*) with the potential to be reactivated later. For example, herpes zoster virus, the cause of chickenpox, can enter dorsal root ganglia and establish latency there and later be periodically activated to cause shingles, a painful skin condition. Some viruses are involved in transformation of a host cell into a benign or malignant tumor (e.g., human papillomavirus [HPV]-induced benign warts and cervical carcinoma). Different species of viruses can produce the same clinical picture (e.g., upper respiratory infection); conversely, a single virus can cause different clinical manifestations depending on host age or immune status (e.g., CMV).

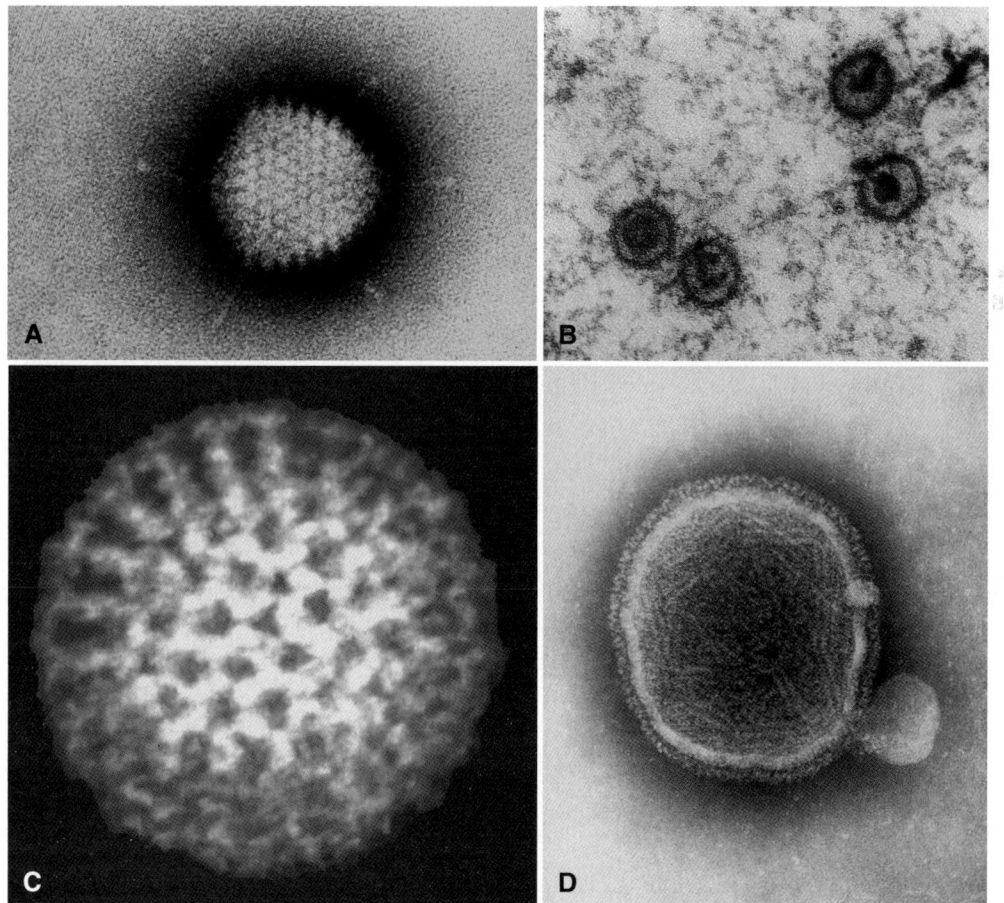

FIGURE 8–1 The variety of viral structures, as seen by electron microscopy. **A,** Adenovirus, an icosahedral nonenveloped DNA virus with fibers. **B,** Epstein-Barr virus, an icosahedral enveloped DNA virus. **C,** Rotavirus, a nonenveloped, wheel-like, RNA virus. **D,** Paramyxovirus, a spherical enveloped RNA virus. RNA is seen spilling out of the disrupted virus. (Photos courtesy of Science Source; © Photo Researchers, Inc., New York, NY.)

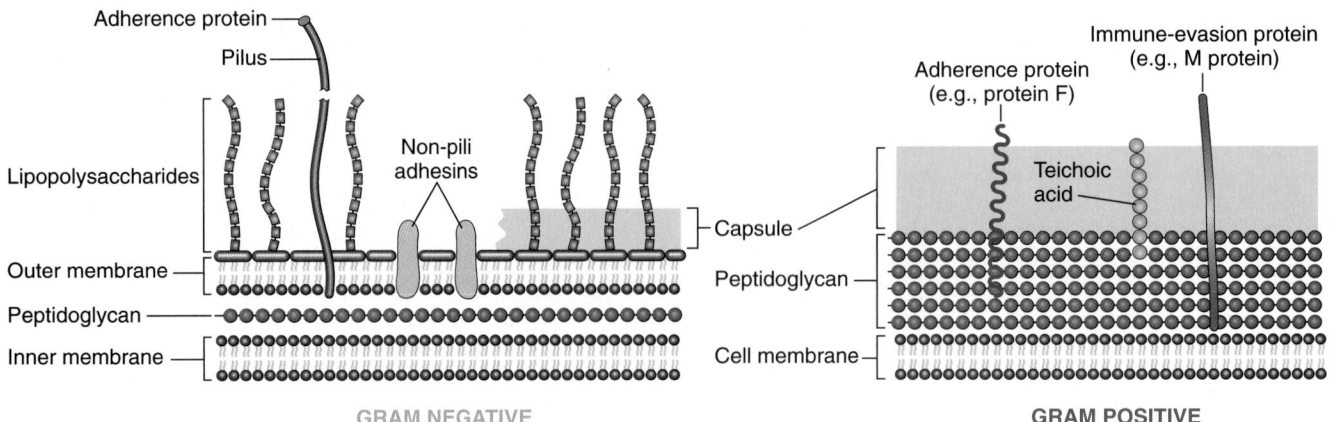

FIGURE 8–2   Molecules on the surface of gram-negative and gram-positive bacteria involved in pathogenesis. Not shown is the type 3 secretory apparatus of gram-negative bacteria (see text).

Bacteria

Bacteria are prokaryotes, meaning that they have a cell membrane but lack membrane-bound nuclei and other membrane-enclosed organelles. Most bacteria are bound by a cell wall consisting of peptidoglycan, a polymer of long sugar chains linked by peptide bridges. There are two forms of cell wall structures: a thick wall surrounding the cell membrane that retains crystal-violet stain (gram-positive bacteria) or a thin cell wall sandwiched between two phospholipid bilayer membranes (gram-negative bacteria) (Fig. 8–2). Bacteria are classified by Gram staining (positive or negative), shape (spherical ones are cocci; rod-shaped ones are bacilli) (Fig. 8–3), and need for oxygen (aerobic or anaerobic). Many bacteria have flagella, long helical filaments extending from the cell surface that enable bacteria to move. Some bacteria possess pili, another kind of surface projection that can attach bacteria to host cells or extracellular matrix. Most bacteria

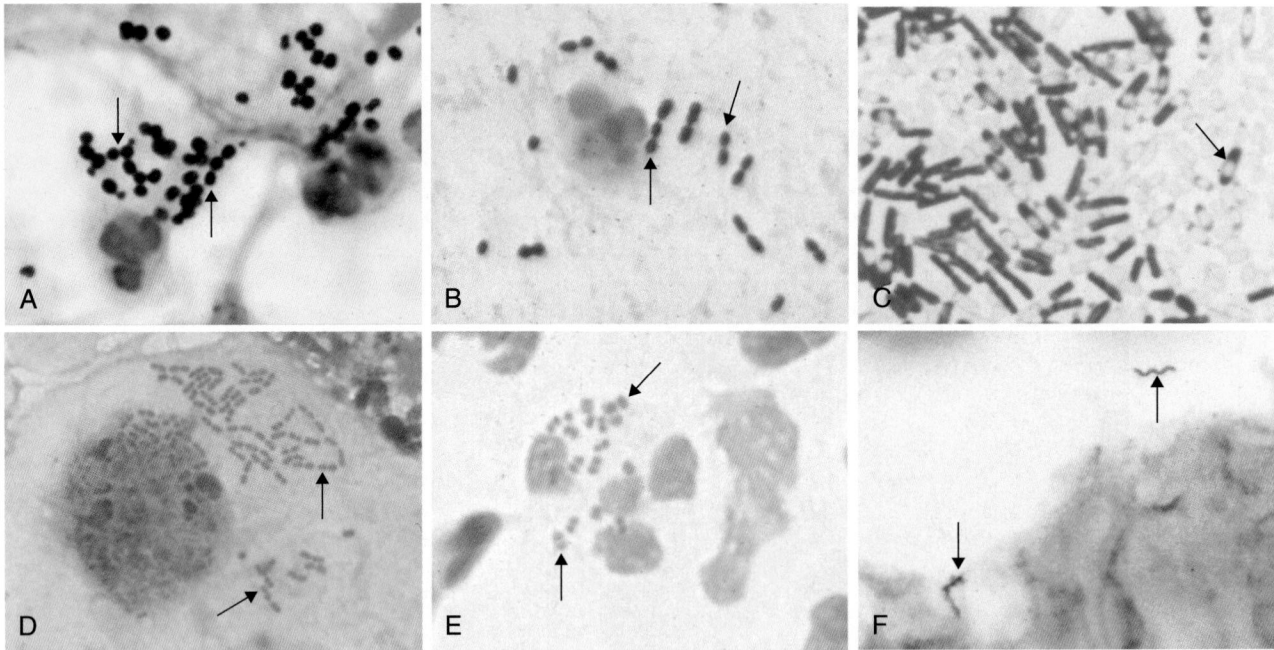

FIGURE 8–3   The variety of bacterial morphology. The bacteria are indicated by arrows in each panel. **A,** Gram stain of sputum from a patient with pneumonia. There are gram-positive cocci in clusters *(Staphylococcus aureus)* with degenerating neutrophils. **B,** Gram stain of sputum from a patient with pneumonia. Gram-positive, elongated cocci in pairs and short chains *(Streptococcus pneumoniae)* and a neutrophil are seen. **C,** Gram stain of *Clostridium sordellii* grown in culture. A mixture of gram-positive and gram-negative rods, many of which have subterminal spores (clear areas), are present. *Clostridia* species often stain as both gram-positive and gram-negative, although they are true gram-positive bacteria. **D,** Gram stain of a bronchoalveolar lavage specimen showing gram-negative intracellular rods typical of Enterobacteriaceae such as *Klebsiella pneumoniae* or *Escherichia coli.* **E,** Gram stain of urethral discharge from a patient with gonorrhea. Many gram-negative diplococci *(Neisseria gonorrhoeae)* are present within a neutrophil. **F,** Silver stain of brain tissue from a patient with Lyme disease meningoencephalitis. Two helical spirochetes *(Borrelia burgdorferi)* are indicated by arrows. The panels are at different magnifications. **(D,** Courtesy of Dr. Karen Krisher, Clinical Microbiology Institute, Wilsonville, OR. Other panels courtesy of Dr. Kenneth Van Horn, Focus Diagnostics.)

synthesize their own DNA, RNA, and proteins, but they depend on the host for favorable growth conditions.

Normal healthy people can be colonized by as many as 10^{12} bacteria on the skin, 10^{10} bacteria in the mouth, and 10^{14} bacteria in the gastrointestinal tract. Bacteria colonizing the skin include *Staphylococcus epidermidis* and *Propionibacterium acnes*, the cause of acne. Aerobic and anaerobic bacteria in the mouth, particularly *Streptococcus mutans*, contribute to dental plaque, a major cause of tooth decay. High-throughput sequencing methods have recently allowed detailed analysis of the diversity of intestinal bacterial flora. There are at least 395 species of bacteria in the normal intestinal flora, but only a small subset, mainly anaerobes, account for the great majority. In-depth analysis of the collective genome (called the "microbiome") of the intestinal flora may yield insights into the evolutionary pressures that have selected the organisms that have succeeded in making humans their home, as well as disturbances in this symbiotic relationship, as in inflammatory bowel diseases.[5] Many bacteria remain extracellular when they invade the body, while others can survive and replicate either outside or inside of host cells (*facultative intracellular* bacteria) and some grow only inside host cells (*obligate intracellular* bacteria).

Obligate intracellular bacteria include *Chlamydia* and *Rickettsia*, which replicate inside membrane-bound vacuoles in epithelial and endothelial cells, respectively. These bacteria get most or all of their energy source, ATP, from the host cell. *Chlamydia trachomatis* is the most frequent infectious cause of female sterility (by scarring and narrowing of the fallopian tubes) and blindness (by chronic inflammation of the conjunctiva that eventually causes scarring and opacification of the cornea). Rickettsiae injure the endothelial cells in which they grow, and so cause a hemorrhagic vasculitis, often visible as a rash, but they may also injure the central nervous system (CNS) and cause death (Rocky Mountain spotted fever [RMSF] and epidemic typhus). Rickettsiae are transmitted by arthropod vectors, including lice (epidemic typhus), ticks (RMSF and ehrlichiosis), and mites (scrub typhus).[6]

Mycoplasma organisms and those belonging to the related genus *Ureaplasma* are unique among extracellular bacterial pathogens, because they do not have a cell wall. These are the tiniest free-living organisms known (125–300 nm).

Fungi

Fungi are eukaryotes that possess thick chitin-containing cell walls and ergosterol-containing cell membranes. Fungi can grow either as rounded yeast cells or as slender filamentous hyphae. Hyphae may be septate (with cell walls separating individual cells) or aseptate, which is an important distinguishing characteristic in clinical material. Some of the most important pathogenic fungi exhibit thermal dimorphism; that is, they grow as hyphal forms at room temperature but as yeast forms at body temperature. Fungi may produce sexual spores or, more commonly, asexual spores referred to as *conidia*. The latter are produced on specialized structures or fruiting bodies arising along the hyphal filament. Fungi may cause superficial or deep infections. Superficial infections involve the skin, hair, and nails. Fungal species that are confined to superficial layers of the human skin are known as dermatophytes. These infec-

tions are commonly referred to by the term "tinea" followed by the area of the body affected (e.g., tinea pedis, "athlete's foot"; tinea capitis, "ringworm of the scalp"). Certain fungal species invade the subcutaneous tissue, causing abscesses or granulomas (e.g., sporotrichosis and tropical mycoses).

Deep fungal infections can spread systemically and invade tissues, destroying vital organs in immunocompromised hosts, but usually heal or remain latent in otherwise normal hosts. Some deep fungal species are limited to a particular geographic region (e.g., *Coccidioides* in the southwestern United States and *Histoplasma* in the Ohio River Valley). Opportunistic fungi (e.g., *Candida*, *Aspergillus*, *Mucor*, and *Cryptococcus*), by contrast, are ubiquitous organisms that either colonize individuals or are encountered from environmental sources. In immunodeficient individuals, opportunistic fungi give rise to life-threatening infections characterized by tissue necrosis, hemorrhage, and vascular occlusion, with little or no inflammatory response. AIDS patients are often infected by the opportunistic fungus *Pneumocystis jiroveci* (previously called *Pneumocystis carinii*).

Protozoa

Parasitic protozoa are single-celled eukaryotes that are major causes of disease and death in developing countries. Protozoa can replicate intracellularly within a variety of cells (e.g., *Plasmodium* in red blood cells, *Leishmania* in macrophages) or extracellularly in the urogenital system, intestine, or blood. *Trichomonas vaginalis* are flagellated protozoal parasites that are sexually transmitted and can colonize the vagina and male urethra. The most prevalent intestinal protozoans, *Entamoeba histolytica* and *Giardia lamblia*, have two forms: (1) motile trophozoites that attach to the intestinal epithelial wall and may invade, and (2) immobile cysts that are resistant to stomach acids and are infectious when ingested. Blood-borne protozoa (e.g., *Plasmodium*, *Trypanosoma*, and *Leishmania*) are transmitted by insect vectors, in which they replicate before being passed to new human hosts. Intestinal protozoa are acquired by ingestion of cysts from contaminated food or water. *Toxoplasma gondii* is acquired either by contact with oocyst-shedding kittens or by eating cyst-ridden, undercooked meat.

Helminths

Parasitic worms are highly differentiated multicellular organisms. Their life cycles are complex; most alternate between sexual reproduction in the definitive host and asexual multiplication in an intermediary host or vector. Thus, depending on parasite species, humans could harbor adult worms (e.g., *Ascaris lumbricoides*) or immature stages (e.g., *Toxocara canis*) or asexual larval forms (e.g., *Echinococcus* species). Once adult worms take up residence in humans, they do not multiply but they produce eggs or larvae that are usually passed out in stool. Often, the severity of disease is in proportion to the number of organisms that have infected the individual (e.g., 10 hookworms cause little disease, whereas 1000 hookworms cause severe anemia by consuming 100 mL of blood per day). In some helminthic infections, disease is caused by inflammatory responses to the eggs or larvae rather than to the adults (e.g., schistosomiasis).

Ectoparasites

Ectoparasites are insects (lice, bedbugs, fleas) or arachnids (mites, ticks, spiders) that attach to and live on or in the skin. Arthropods may produce disease directly by damaging the human host or indirectly by serving as the vectors for transmission of an infectious agent into a human host. Some arthropods cause itching and excoriations (e.g., pediculosis caused by lice attached to hair shafts, or scabies caused by mites burrowing into the stratum corneum). At the site of the bite, mouth parts may be found associated with a mixed infiltrate of lymphocytes, macrophages, and eosinophils. In addition, attached arthropods can be vectors for other pathogens. For example, deer ticks transmit the Lyme disease spirochete *Borrelia burgdorferi*.

SPECIAL TECHNIQUES FOR DIAGNOSING INFECTIOUS AGENTS

Some infectious agents or their products can be directly observed in hematoxylin and eosin–stained sections (e.g., the inclusion bodies formed by CMV and herpes simplex virus (HSV); bacterial clumps, which usually stain blue; *Candida* and *Mucor* among the fungi; most protozoans; and all helminths). Many infectious agents, however, are best visualized by special stains that identify organisms on the basis of particular characteristics of their cell wall or coat—Gram, acid-fast, silver, mucicarmine, and Giemsa stains—or after labeling with specific antibody probes (Table 8–2). Regardless of the staining technique, organisms are usually best visualized at the advancing edge of a lesion rather than at its center, particularly if there is necrosis.

Acute infections can be diagnosed serologically by detecting pathogen-specific antibodies in the serum. The presence of specific IgM antibody shortly after the onset of symptoms is often diagnostic. Alternatively, specific antibody titers can be measured early ("acute") and 4–6 weeks ("convalescent") after infection; a four-fold rise in titer is usually considered diagnostic.

Nucleic acid–based tests, collectively called *molecular diagnostics*, have become routine methods for detecting and quantifying several pathogens. For instance, in people infected with the human immunodeficiency virus (HIV), quantification of HIV RNA is an important guide to antiretroviral therapy.[7] The management of HBV and HCV infections is similarly guided by nucleic acid–based viral quantification or typing to predict resistance to antiviral drugs.

Nucleic acid amplification tests, such as polymerase chain reaction (PCR) and transcription-mediated amplification, have become routine for diagnosis of gonorrhea, chlamydial infection, tuberculosis, and herpes encephalitis. In some cases, molecular assays are much more sensitive than conventional testing.[8,9] PCR testing of cerebrospinal fluid (CSF) for herpes simplex virus (HSV) encephalitis has a sensitivity of about 80%, while viral culture of CSF has a sensitivity of less than 10%. Similarly, nucleic acid tests for genital chlamydia detect 10% to 30% more infections than does conventional chlamydia culture. In other cases, such as gonorrhea, the sensitivity of nucleic acid testing is similar to that of culture.

NEW AND EMERGING INFECTIOUS DISEASES

Although infectious diseases such as leprosy have been known since biblical times, and parasitic schistosomes and mycobacteria have been demonstrated in Egyptian mummies, a surprising number of new infectious agents continue to be discovered (Table 8–3). The infectious causes of some diseases with significant morbidity and mortality were previously unrecognized, because some of the infectious agents are difficult to culture; examples include *Helicobacter pylori* gastritis, HBV and HCV, and Legionnaires pneumonia. Some infectious agents are genuinely new to humans, e.g., HIV, which causes AIDS, and *B. burgdorferi*, which causes Lyme disease. Other infections have become much more common because of immunosuppression caused by AIDS or therapy for transplant rejection and some cancers (e.g., CMV, Kaposi sarcoma herpesvirus, *Mycobacterium avium-intracellulare*, *P. jiroveci*, and *Cryptosporidium parvum*).[10,11] Finally, infectious diseases that are common in one area may be introduced into a new area. For example, West Nile virus has been common in Europe, Asia, and Africa for years but was first described in the United States in 1999.

Human demographics and behavior are among the many variables that contribute to the emergence of infectious diseases. AIDS was first recognized in the United States as predominantly a disease of homosexuals and drug abusers, but heterosexual transmission is now common. In sub-Saharan Africa, the area of the world with the highest number of AIDS cases, it is predominantly a heterosexual disease.[12] Changes in the environment occasionally drive rates of infectious diseases. Reforestation of the eastern United States has led to massive increases in the populations of deer and mice, which carry the ticks that transmit Lyme disease, babesiosis, and ehrlichiosis.[13] Failure of DDT to control the mosquitoes that transmit malaria and the development of drug-resistant parasites have dramatically increased the morbidity and mortality of *Plasmodium falciparum* in Asia, Africa, and Latin America. Microbial adaptation to widespread antibiotic use contributed to the emergence of drug resistance in many species of bacteria, including *Mycobacterium tuberculosis*, *Neisseria gonorrhoeae*, *Staphylococcus aureus*, and *Enterococcus faecium*.

TABLE 8–2	Special Techniques for Diagnosing Infectious Agents
Techniques	**Infectious Agents**
Gram stain	Most bacteria
Acid-fast stain	Mycobacteria, nocardiae (modified)
Silver stains	Fungi, legionellae, pneumocystis
Periodic acid–Schiff	Fungi, amebae
Mucicarmine	Cryptococci
Giemsa	Campylobacteria, leishmaniae, malaria parasites
Antibody probes	All classes
Culture	All classes
DNA probes	All classes

TABLE 8–3	Some Recently Recognized Infectious Agents and Manifestations	
Date Recognized	**Infectious Agent**	**Manifestations**
1977	Ebola virus	Epidemic Ebola hemorrhagic fever
	Hantaan virus	Hemorrhagic fever with renal syndrome
	Legionella pneumophila	Legionnaires disease
	Campylobacter jejuni	Enteritis
1980	HTLV-I	T-cell lymphoma or leukemia, HTLV-associated myelopathy
1981	*Staphylococcus aureus*	Toxic shock syndrome
1982	*Escherichia coli* O157:H7	Hemorrhagic colitis, hemolytic-uremic syndrome
	Borrelia burgdorferi	Lyme disease
1983	HIV	AIDS
	Helicobacter pylori	Gastric ulcers
1988	Hepatitis E	Enterically transmitted hepatitis
1989	Hepatitis C	Hepatitis C
1992	*Vibrio cholerae* O139	New epidemic cholera strain
	Bartonella henselae	Cat-scratch disease
1995	KSHV (HHV-8)	Kaposi sarcoma in AIDS
1999	West Nile virus	West Nile fever, neuroinvasive disease
2003	SARS coronavirus	Severe acute respiratory syndrome

Infections with antibiotic-resistant bacteria are becoming a serious problem, such as methicillin-resistant staphylococcus (discussed later).

AGENTS OF BIOTERRORISM

Sadly, the anthrax attacks in the United States in 2001 transformed the theoretical threat of bioterrorism into reality. The Centers for Disease Control and Prevention (CDC) have evaluated the microorganisms that pose the greatest danger as weapons on the basis of the efficiency with which disease can be transmitted, how difficult the microorganisms are to produce and distribute, what can be done to defend against them, and the extent to which they are likely to alarm the public and produce widespread fear. The CDC has ranked bioweapons into three categories, A, B, and C, based on these criteria (Table 8–4).[14]

Category A agents pose the highest risk and can be readily disseminated or transmitted from person to person, can cause high mortality with potential for major public health impact, might cause public panic and social disruption, and might require special action for public health preparedness. For example, smallpox is a category A agent because of its high transmissibility in any climate or season, case mortality rate of 30% or greater, and lack of effective antiviral therapy. This agent can be easily disseminated because of the stability of the virus in aerosol form and the very small dose needed for infection. Smallpox naturally spreads from person to person mainly by direct contact with virus in skin lesions or contaminated clothing or bedding. Symptoms appear after 7 to 17 days. Initially there is high fever, headache, and backache, followed by the appearance of the rash, which first appears on the mucosa of the mouth and pharynx, face, and forearms and later spreads to the trunk and legs and becomes vesicular and later pustular. Because people can be contagious during the incuba-

tion period, this virus has the potential to continue to spread throughout an unprotected population. Since vaccination ended in the United States in 1972 and vaccination immunity has waned, the population is highly susceptible to smallpox. Recent concern that smallpox could be used for bioterrorism

TABLE 8–4   Potential Agents of Bioterrorism
Category A Diseases/Agents
Anthrax *(Bacillus anthracis)*
Botulism *(Clostridium botulinum* toxin*)*
Plague *(Yersinia pestis)*
Smallpox *(Variola major virus)*
Tularemia *(Francisella tularensis)*
Viral hemorrhagic fevers (filoviruses [e.g., Ebola, Marburg] and arenaviruses [e.g., Lassa, Machupo])
Category B Diseases/Agents
Brucellosis *(Brucella* sp.*)*
Epsilon toxin of *Clostridium perfringens*
Food safety threats (e.g., *Salmonella* sp., *Escherichia coli* O157:H7, *Shigella*)
Glanders *(Burkholderia mallei)*
Melioidosis *(Burkholderia pseudomallei)*
Psittacosis *(Chlamydia psittaci)*
Q fever *(Coxiella burnetti)*
Ricin toxin from *Ricinus communis* (castor beans)
Staphylococcal enterotoxin B
Typhus fever *(Rickettsia prowazekii)*
Viral encephalitis (alphaviruses [e.g., Venezuelan equine encephalitis, eastern equine encephalitis, western equine encephalitis])
Water safety threats (e.g., *Vibrio cholerae, Cryptosporidium parvum*)
Category C Diseases/Agents
Emerging infectious disease threats such as Nipah virus and Hantavirus

Adapted from Centers for Disease Control Information.

has led to a return of vaccination for selected groups in the United States and Israel.

Category B agents are moderately easy to disseminate, produce moderate morbidity but low mortality, and require specific diagnostic and disease surveillance. Many of these agents are food-borne or water-borne. Category C agents include emerging pathogens that could be engineered for mass dissemination because of availability, ease of production and dissemination, potential for high morbidity and mortality, and great impact on health.

TRANSMISSION AND DISSEMINATION OF MICROBES

Routes of Entry of Microbes

Microbes can enter the host by inhalation, ingestion, sexual transmission, insect or animal bites, or injection. The first defenses against infection are intact skin and mucosal surfaces, which provide physical barriers and produce antimicrobial substances. In general, respiratory, gastrointestinal, or genito-urinary tract infections that occur in healthy persons are caused by relatively virulent microorganisms that are capable of damaging or penetrating intact epithelial barriers. In contrast, most skin infections in healthy persons are caused by less virulent organisms entering the skin through damaged sites (cuts and burns).

Skin. The dense, keratinized outer layer of skin is a natural barrier to infection, and the low pH of the skin (~5.5) and the presence of fatty acids inhibit growth of microorganisms other than residents of the normal flora. Human skin is normally inhabited by a variety of bacterial and fungal species, including some potential opportunists, such as *S. epidermidis* and *Candida albicans*. Although skin is usually an effective barrier, certain types of fungi (dermatophytes) can infect the stratum corneum, hair, and nails, and a few microorganisms are able to traverse the unbroken skin. For example, *Schistosoma* larvae released from freshwater snails penetrate swimmers' skin by releasing collagenase, elastase, and other enzymes that dissolve the extracellular matrix. *Most microorganisms, however, penetrate through breaks in the skin*, including superficial pricks (fungal infections), wounds (staphylococci), burns *(Pseudomonas aeruginosa)*, and diabetic and pressure-related foot sores (multibacterial infections). Intravenous catheters in hospitalized patients can produce local or systemic infection (bacteremia). Needle sticks can expose the recipient to potentially infected blood and may transmit HBV, hepatitis C virus (HCV), or HIV. Some pathogens penetrate the skin via an insect or animal bite. For instance, bites by fleas, ticks, mosquitoes, mites, and lice break the skin and transmit arboviruses (causes of yellow fever and encephalitis), rickettsiae (Rocky Mountain spotted fever [RMSF]), bacteria (plague, Lyme disease), protozoa (malaria, leishmaniasis), and helminths (filariasis). Animal bites can lead to infections with bacteria or certain viruses such as rabies.

Gastrointestinal Tract. Most gastrointestinal pathogens are transmitted by food or drink contaminated with fecal material. Where hygiene fails, diarrheal disease becomes rampant.

Acidic gastric secretions are important defenses within the gastrointestinal tract and are lethal for many gastrointestinal pathogens.[14] Healthy volunteers do not become infected by *Vibrio cholerae* unless they are fed 10^{11} organisms, whereas volunteers given *V. cholerae* and sodium bicarbonate have a 10,000-fold increase in susceptibility to cholera. In contrast, some ingested agents, such as *Shigella* and *Giardia* cysts, are relatively resistant to gastric acid; hence, as few as 100 organisms of each are sufficient to cause illness.

Other normal defenses within the gastrointestinal tract include (1) the layer of viscous mucus covering the intestinal epithelium, (2) lytic pancreatic enzymes and bile detergents, (3) mucosal antimicrobial peptides called defensins, (4) normal flora, and (5) secreted IgA antibodies. IgA antibodies are made by plasma cells located in mucosa-associated lymphoid tissues (MALT). These lymphoid aggregates are covered by a single layer of specialized epithelial cells called M cells. M cells are important for transport of antigens to mucosa-associated lymphoid tissues and for binding and uptake of numerous gut pathogens, including poliovirus, enteropathic *Escherichia coli*, *V. cholerae*, *Salmonella typhi*, and *Shigella flexneri*.[15]

Infections via the gastrointestinal tract occur when local defenses are weakened or the organisms develop strategies to overcome these defenses. Host defenses are weakened by low gastric acidity, by antibiotics that alter the normal bacterial flora (e.g., in pseudomembranous colitis), or when there is stalled peristalsis or mechanical obstruction (e.g., in blind-loop syndrome). Most enveloped viruses are inactivated by bile and digestive enzymes, but nonenveloped viruses may be resistant (e.g., the hepatitis A virus, rotaviruses, reoviruses, and norovirus).

Enteropathogenic bacteria elicit gastrointestinal disease by a variety of mechanisms:

- While growing on contaminated food, certain staphylococcal strains release powerful enterotoxins that cause food poisoning without any bacterial multiplication in the gut.
- *V. cholerae* and toxigenic *E. coli* multiply inside the mucous layer overlying the gut epithelium and release exotoxins that cause the gut epithelium to secrete large volumes of fluid, resulting in watery diarrhea.
- *Shigella*, *Salmonella*, and *Campylobacter* invade and damage the intestinal mucosa and lamina propria and so cause ulceration, inflammation, and hemorrhage that is clinically manifested as dysentery.
- *Salmonella typhi* passes from the damaged mucosa through Peyer patches and mesenteric lymph nodes and into the bloodstream, resulting in a systemic infection.

Fungal infection of the gastrointestinal tract occurs mainly in immunologically compromised people. *Candida*, part of the normal gastrointestinal flora, shows a predilection for stratified squamous epithelium, causing oral thrush or membranous esophagitis, but may also spread to the stomach, lower gastrointestinal tract, and systemic organs.

The cyst forms of *intestinal protozoa* are essential for their transmission, because cysts resist stomach acid. In the gut, cysts convert to motile trophozoites and attach to sugars on the intestinal epithelia through surface lectins. What happens next differs among pathogens. *Giardia lamblia* attaches to the epithelial brush border, whereas cryptosporidia are taken up by enterocytes, in which they form gametes and spores. *E. histolytica* causes contact-mediated cytolysis through a channel-forming pore protein and thereby ulcerates and invades the colonic mucosa. Intestinal helminths, as a rule, cause disease only when they are present in large numbers or in ectopic sites, for example, by obstructing the gut or invading and damaging the bile ducts *(Ascaris lumbricoides)*. Hookworms may cause iron deficiency anemia by chronic loss of blood sucked from intestinal villi; the fish tapeworm *Diphyllobothrium latum* can deplete its host of vitamin B_{12}, giving rise to an illness resembling pernicious anemia. Finally, the larvae of several helminths pass through the gut briefly on their way to another organ; for example, *Trichinella spiralis* larvae preferentially encyst in muscle, *Echinococcus* species larvae in the liver or lung.

Respiratory Tract. A large number of microorganisms, including viruses, bacteria, and fungi, are inhaled daily by every city inhabitant. In many cases, the microbes are inhaled in dust or aerosol particles. The distance these particles travel into the respiratory system is inversely proportional to their size. Large particles are trapped in the mucociliary blanket that lines the nose and the upper respiratory tract. Inhaled microorganisms are trapped in the mucus secreted by goblet cells and are then transported by ciliary action to the back of the throat, where they are swallowed and cleared. Particles smaller than 5 μm travel directly to the alveoli, where they are phagocytosed by alveolar macrophages or by neutrophils recruited to the lung by cytokines.

Microorganisms that invade the normal healthy respiratory tract have developed specific mechanisms to overcome the mucociliary defenses or to avoid destruction by alveolar macrophages. Some successful respiratory pathogens evade these defenses by attaching to epithelial cells in the lower respiratory tract and pharynx. For example, influenza viruses possess hemagglutinin proteins that project from the surface of the virus and bind to sialic acid on the surface of epithelial cells. This attachment induces the host cell to engulf the virus, leading to viral entry and replication within the host cell. However, sialic acid also interferes with shedding of newly synthesized viruses from the host cell. Influenza viruses have another cell surface protein, neuraminidase, which cleaves sialic acid and allows virus to release from the host cell. Neuraminidase also lowers the viscosity of mucus and facilitates viral transit within the respiratory tract. Interestingly, some anti-influenza drugs are sialic acid analogues that inhibit neuraminidase and prevent viral release from host cells.

Certain bacterial respiratory pathogens can impair ciliary activity. For instance, *Haemophilus influenzae* and *Bordetella pertussis* elaborate toxins that paralyze mucosal cilia; *P. aeruginosa*, a cause of severe respiratory infection in persons with cystic fibrosis, and *M. pneumoniae* produce ciliostatic substances. Some bacteria such as *Streptococcus pneumoniae* or *Staphylococcus* species lack specific adherence factors and often gain access after viral infection causes loss of ciliated epithelium, making individuals with a viral respiratory infection more susceptible to these secondary bacterial superinfections. Chronic damage to mucociliary defense mechanisms occurs in smokers and people with cystic fibrosis, while acute injury occurs in intubated patients and in those who aspirate gastric acid.

Some respiratory pathogens avoid phagocytosis or destruction after phagocytosis. M. tuberculosis, for example, gains its foothold in normal alveoli because it is able to escape killing within the phagolysosomes of macrophages. Opportunistic fungi infect the lungs when cellular immunity is depressed or when leukocytes are reduced in number (e.g., *P. jiroveci* in AIDS patients and *Aspergillus* species following chemotherapy).

Urogenital Tract. *The urinary tract is almost always invaded from the exterior via the urethra.* The regular flushing of the urinary tract with urine serves as a defense against invading microorganisms. Urine in the bladder is normally sterile, and successful pathogens (e.g., *N. gonorrhoeae, E. coli*) adhere to the urinary epithelium. Anatomy plays an important role in infection. Women have more than 10 times as many urinary tract infections as men, because the distance between the urinary bladder and skin (i.e., the length of the urethra) is 5 cm in women, in contrast to 20 cm in men. Obstruction of urinary flow and/or reflux can compromise normal defenses and increase susceptibility to urinary tract infections. Urinary tract infections can spread retrogradely from the bladder to the kidney and cause acute and chronic pyelonephritis, which is the major preventable cause of renal failure.

From puberty until menopause the vagina is protected from pathogens by a low pH resulting from catabolism of glycogen in the normal epithelium by lactobacilli. Antibiotics can kill the lactobacilli and make the vagina susceptible to infection. Sexually transmitted pathogens have developed specific mechanisms for attaching to the vaginal or cervical mucosa, or they enter via local breaks in the mucosa during sexual intercourse (HIV, HPV, *Treponema pallidum*).

Spread and Dissemination of Microbes

Some microorganisms proliferate locally, at the site of infection, whereas others penetrate the epithelial barrier and spread to distant sites via the lymphatics, the blood, or nerves (Fig. 8–4). Pathogens that cause superficial infections stay confined to the lumen of hollow viscera (e.g., *Vibrio cholera*), or adhere to or proliferate exclusively in or on epithelial cells (e.g., papillomaviruses, dermatophytes). A variety of pathogenic bacteria, fungi, and helminths are invasive by virtue of their motility or ability to secrete lytic enzymes (e.g., streptococci and staphylococci secrete hyaluronidase, which degrades the extracellular matrix between host cells). Microbial spread initially follows tissue planes of least resistance and to sites drained by regional lymphatics. For example, staphylococcal infections may progress from a localized abscess or furuncle to regional lymph nodes. This can sometimes leads to bacteremia and colonization of distant organs (heart, liver, brain, kidney, bone). Within the blood, microorganisms may be transported free or within host cells. Some viruses (e.g., poliovirus and HBV), most bacteria and fungi, some protozoa (e.g., African trypanosomes), and all helminths are transported free in the plasma. Leukocytes can carry herpesviruses, HIV, mycobacteria, and *Leishmania* and *Toxoplasma* organisms. Certain viruses (e.g., Colorado tick fever virus) and parasites (*Plasmodium* and *Babesia*) are carried by red blood cells. Most viruses spread from cell to cell by replication and release of infectious virions, but others may propagate from cell to cell by fusion or transport within nerves (e.g., rabies virus). Infectious foci seeded by blood are called secondary foci. They can be single and large (a solitary abscess or tuberculoma) or multiple and tiny

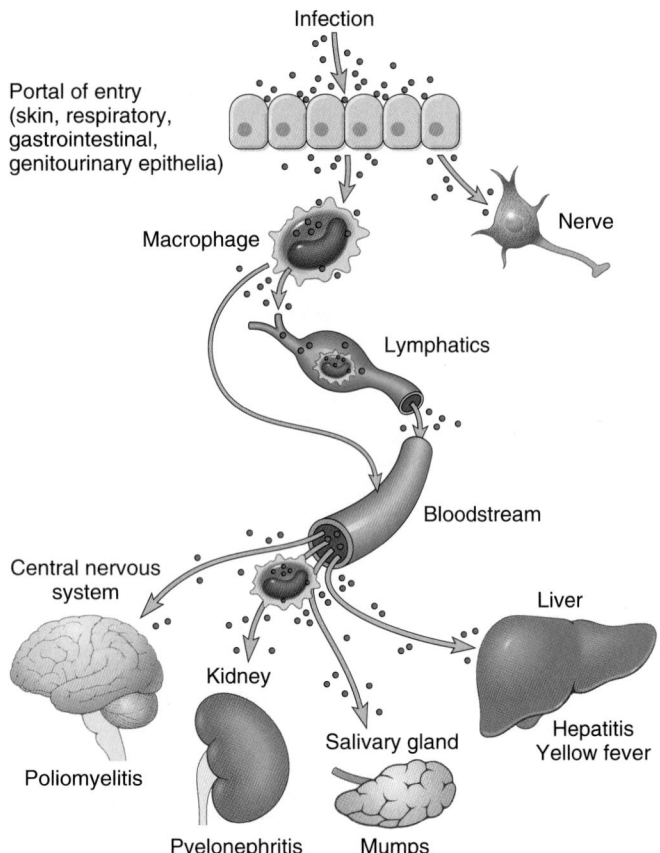

FIGURE 8–4 Routes of entry and dissemination of microbes. To enter the body microbes penetrate the epithelial or mucosal barriers. Infection may remain localized at the site of entry or spread to other sites in the body. Most common microbes (selected examples are shown) spread through the lymphatics or bloodstream (either freely or within inflammatory cells). However, certain viruses and bacterial toxins may also travel through nerves. (Adapted from Mims CA: The Pathogenesis of Infectious Disease, 4th ed. San Diego, Academic Press, 1996.)

(e.g., miliary tuberculosis or *Candida* microabscesses in many tissues). Sporadic bloodstream invasion by low-virulence or nonvirulent microbes (e.g., during brushing of teeth) is common but is quickly controlled by normal host defenses. By contrast, disseminated viremia, bacteremia, fungemia, or parasitemia by virulent pathogens is a serious insult and manifests itself by fever, low blood pressure, and multiple other systemic signs and symptoms of sepsis. Massive bloodstream invasion by bacteria or their endotoxins can rapidly become fatal, even for previously healthy individuals.

The major manifestations of infectious disease may appear at sites distant from the point of microbe entry. For example, chickenpox and measles viruses enter through the airways but cause rashes in the skin; poliovirus enters through the intestine but kills motor neurons. *Schistosoma mansoni* parasites penetrate the skin but eventually localize in blood vessels of the portal system and mesentery, damaging the liver and intestine. *Schistosoma hematobium*, on the other hand, localizes to the urinary bladder and causes cystitis. The rabies virus travels to the brain in a retrograde fashion within nerves, while the varicella zoster virus (VZV) hides in dorsal root ganglia, and on reactivation, travels along nerves to cause shingles.

The placental-fetal route is an important mode of transmission (Chapter 10). When infectious organisms reach the pregnant uterus through the cervical orifice or the bloodstream and are able to traverse the placenta, severe damage to the fetus can result. Bacterial or mycoplasmal placentitis can cause premature delivery or stillbirth. Viral infections can cause maldevelopment of the fetus, with infection early in pregnancy resulting in the most severe disease. Rubella infection during the first trimester can cause congenital heart disease, mental retardation, cataracts, or deafness in the infant, while little damage is caused by rubella infection during the third trimester. Transmission of treponemes leads to congenital syphilis only when *T. pallidum* infects the mother late in the second trimester but then causes severe fetal osteochondritis and periostitis that leads to multiple bony lesions. Infection also can occur during passage through the birth canal (e.g., gonococcal or chlamydial conjunctivitis) or through maternal milk (e.g., CMV, HBV, human T-cell leukemia virus-1 [HTLV-1]). Maternal transmission of HIV is the major cause of AIDS in children. Maternal transmission of HBV can later cause chronic hepatitis or liver cancer.

Release of Microbes from the Body

For transmission of disease, the mode of exit of a microorganism from the host's body is as important as entry into it. Depending on the location of infection, release may be accomplished by skin shedding, coughing, sneezing, voiding of urine or feces, during sexual contact, or through insect vectors. Some microbes are hardy and can survive for extended periods in dust, food, or water. Bacterial spores, protozoan cysts, and thick-shelled helminth eggs can survive in a cool and dry environment. Some enteric pathogens are shed for long periods by asymptomatic carrier hosts (e.g., *S. typhi*). Less hardy microorganisms must be quickly passed from person to person, often by direct contact.

Transmission from person to person can occur by respiratory, fecal-oral, or sexual routes (discussed below). Viruses and bacteria transmitted by the respiratory route (e.g., *M. tuberculosis*) are infectious only when lesions are open to the airways. Many pathogens, ranging from viruses to helminths, can be transmitted by the fecal-oral route, that is, by ingestion of stool-contaminated food or water. Water-borne viruses involved in epidemic outbreaks include hepatitis A and E viruses, poliovirus, and rotavirus. Some parasitic helminths (e.g., hookworms, schistosomes) shed eggs in stool that gain access to new hosts by larval penetration of the skin rather than by oral intake. Protozoa and helminths have evolved complex transmission cycles involving a chain of intermediate and vector hosts bearing successive developmental stages of the parasites. Viruses infecting the oropharynx (e.g., EBV, CMV, mumps viruses) are transmitted principally through saliva. Other pathogens are spread mainly by prolonged intimate or mucosal contact (as occurs during sexual transmission) including viruses (HPV, HSV, HBV, HIV), bacteria (*T. pallidum, N. gonorrhoeae, Chlamydia trachomatis*), fungi (*Candida* species), protozoa (*Trichomonas* species), and arthropods (*Phthirus pubis*, or crab lice). Transmission of HBV, HCV, and HIV infections through blood and blood products may be caused by human behavior, e.g., needle sharing by drug abusers, cuts, and needle sticks.

TABLE 8–5 Classification of Important Sexually Transmitted Diseases

Pathogens	Disease or Syndrome and Population Principally Affected		
	Males	*Females*	*Both*
VIRUSES			
Herpes simplex virus			Primary and recurrent herpes, neonatal herpes
Hepatitis B virus			Hepatitis
Human papillomavirus	Cancer of penis (some cases)	Cervical dysplasia and cancer, vulvar cancer	Condyloma acuminatum
Human immunodeficiency virus			Acquired immunodeficiency syndrome
CHLAMYDIAE			
Chlamydia trachomatis	Urethritis, epididymitis, proctitis	Urethral syndrome, cervicitis, bartholinitis, salpingitis and sequelae	Lymphogranuloma venereum
MYCOPLASMAS			
Ureaplasma urealyticum	Urethritis		
BACTERIA			
Neisseria gonorrhoeae	Epididymitis, prostatitis, urethral stricture	Cervicitis, endometritis, bartholinitis, salpingitis, and sequelae (infertility, ectopic pregnancy, recurrent salpingitis)	Urethritis, proctitis, pharyngitis, disseminated gonococcal infection
Treponema pallidum			Syphilis
Haemophilus ducreyi			Chancroid
Klebsiella granulomatis			Granuloma inguinale (donovanosis)
PROTOZOA			
Trichomonas vaginalis	Urethritis, balanitis	Vaginitis	

Microbes can be transmitted from animal to human (termed *zoonotic infections*), either by direct contact or consumption of animal products or indirectly via an invertebrate vector. Invertebrate vectors (insects, ticks, mites) can spread infection passively in some cases or serve as necessary hosts for replication and development of the pathogen.

Sexually Transmitted Infections

A number of organisms can be transmitted through sexual contact (Table 8–5). Some, such as *C. trachomatis* and *N. gonorrhoeae*, are usually spread by sexual intercourse, while others, such as *Shigella* species and *E. histolytica*, are typically spread by other means but are also occasionally spread by oral-anal sex. Groups that are at greater risk for some sexually transmitted infections (STIs) include adolescents, men who have sex with men, and people who use illegal drugs. While the increased risk among these groups is partially due to unsafe sexual practices, limited access to health care is also often a contributing factor. The presence of an STI in young children, unless acquired during birth, strongly suggests sexual abuse.

The initial site of an STI may be the urethra, vagina, cervix, rectum, or oral pharynx. The organisms that cause these infections tend to be short-lived outside of the host, so they usually depend on direct person-to-person spread. Most of these agents can be infectious in the absence of symptoms, so transmission often occurs from people who do not realize that they have an infection. To reduce the spread of STIs, these infections are often reported to public health authorities so that people who have had intimate contact with the person may be tested and treated.

Although the various pathogens that cause STIs differ in many ways, some general features should be noted.

- *Infection with one STI-associated organism increases the risk for additional STIs.* This is mainly because the risk factors are the same for all STIs, which probably explains the association between two common STIs in the United States: chlamydia and gonorrhea. Infection with both of these bacteria is so common that the diagnosis of either should lead to treatment for both. In addition, the epithelial injury caused by *N. gonorrhoeae* or *C. trachomatis* can increase the chance of co-infection with the other, as well as the risk of HIV infection with concomitant exposure.

- *The microbes that cause STIs can be spread from a pregnant woman to the fetus and cause severe damage to the fetus or child.* Perinatally acquired *C. trachomatis* causes conjunctivitis, and neonatal HSV infection is much more likely to cause visceral and CNS disease than is infection acquired later in life. Syphilis frequently causes miscarriage. HIV infection may be fatal to children infected with the virus prenatally or perinatally. Diagnosis of STIs in pregnant women is critical, because intrauterine or neonatal STI transmission can often be prevented by treatment of the mother or newborn. Bacterial infections such as gonorrhea, syphilis, and chlamydia can be easily cured with antibiotics. Antiretroviral treatment of pregnant women with HIV infection and treatment of the newborn can reduce transmission of HIV to children from 25% to less than 2%.

Syphilis is discussed later in this chapter, and other STIs are described in Chapters 21 and 22.

Healthcare-Associated Infections

An increasingly important source of infections is the healthcare setting. "Nosocomial" infections are those acquired in the hospital. It is estimated that about 1.7 million patients each year get nosocomial infections in the United States.[15] These infections can be transmitted in many ways (e.g. blood transfusion or organ transplant), but perhaps the most common, and readily preventable, means of transmission include spread from the hands of healthcare workers or from contaminated surfaces such as bedrails. Proper attention to hygiene and cleansing (e.g., hand washing) can greatly reduce the transmission of important pathogens such as methicillin-resistant *S. aureus* and vancomycin-resistant enterococci.

Host Defenses Against Infections

The outcome of infection is determined by the ability of the microbe to infect, colonize, and damage host tissues and the ability of host defense mechanisms to eradicate the infection. *Host barriers to infection prevent microbes from entering the body and consist of innate and adaptive immune defenses.* Innate immune defense mechanisms exist before infection and respond rapidly to microbes. These mechanisms include physical barriers to infection, phagocytic cells, natural killer (NK) cells, and plasma proteins, including the complement system proteins and other mediators of inflammatory responses (cytokines, collectins, acute-phase reactants). Adaptive immune responses are stimulated by exposure to microbes and increase in magnitude, speed, and effectiveness with successive exposures to microbes. Adaptive immunity is mediated by T and B lymphocytes and their products (Chapter 6).

Microbes and the immune system have been engaged in an evolutionary battle, in which each tries to outwit the other. The immune system is capable of effectively combating many infections, but different microbes have developed ways of evading host defenses (discussed later). In some infections, a balance is reached between the microbe and the host such that the infection persists in a state of latency but does not cause significant pathology. In such situations, decline of immune responses can result in rapid reactivation of the infection and severe pathologic manifestations. Such reactivation is seen in latent viral infections (e.g., EBV) and some bacterial infections (e.g., tuberculosis).

HOW MICROORGANISMS CAUSE DISEASE

Infectious agents establish infection and damage tissues by three mechanisms:

- They can contact or enter host cells and directly cause cell death.

- They may release toxins that kill cells at a distance, release enzymes that degrade tissue components, or damage blood vessels and cause ischemic necrosis.
- They can induce host immune responses that, though directed against the invader, cause additional tissue damage. Thus, as we discussed in Chapters 2 and 6, the defensive responses of the host constitute a double-edged sword: They are necessary to overcome the infection but at the same time may directly contribute to tissue damage.

Here we describe some of the mechanisms whereby viruses and bacteria damage host tissues.

Mechanisms of Viral Injury

Viruses can directly damage host cells by entering them and replicating at the host's expense. The predilection for viruses to infect certain cells and not others is called *tropism* and is determined by several factors, including (1) expression of host cell receptors for the virus, (2) presence of cellular transcription factors that recognize viral enhancer and promoter sequences, (3) anatomic barriers, and (4) local temperature, pH, and host defenses.[17] Each of these is described briefly.

A major determinant of tissue tropism is the presence of viral receptors on host cells. Viruses possess specific cell-surface proteins that bind to particular host cell-surface proteins. Many viruses use normal cellular receptors of the host to enter cells. For example, HIV glycoprotein gp120 binds to CD4 on T cells and to the chemokine receptors CXCR4 (mainly on T cells) and CCR5 (mainly on macrophages) (Chapter 6). EBV envelope glycoprotein gp350 binds to complement receptor 2 (CR2/CD21) on B cells. In some cases, host proteases are needed to enable binding of virus to host cells; for instance, a host protease cleaves and activates the influenza virus hemagglutinin. Another determinant of viral tropism is the ability of the virus to replicate inside some cells but not in others, and this is related to the presence of cell type–specific transcription factors. For example, the JC virus, which causes leukoencephalopathy (Chapter 28), is restricted to oligodendroglia in the CNS, because the promoter and enhancer DNA sequences upstream from the viral genes are active in glial cells but not in neurons or endothelial cells. Physical barriers also can contribute to tissue tropism. For example, enteroviruses replicate in the intestine in part because they can resist inactivation by acids, bile, and digestive enzymes. Rhinoviruses infect only within the upper respiratory tract because they replicate optimally at the lower temperature of the upper respiratory tract.

Once viruses are inside host cells, they can damage or kill the cells by a number of mechanisms (Fig. 8–5):

- *Direct cytopathic effects.* Some viruses kill cells by preventing synthesis of host macromolecules (e.g., host cell DNA, RNA, or proteins), by producing degradative enzymes and toxic proteins, or by inducing apoptosis. For example, poliovirus inactivates cap-binding protein, which is essential for translation of host cell mRNAs but leaves translation of poliovirus mRNAs unaffected. HSV produces proteins that inhibit synthesis of cellular DNA and mRNA and other proteins that degrade host DNA. Some viruses can stimulate apoptosis by production of proteins that are pro-apoptotic (e.g., HIV vpr protein). Viral replication also can trigger apoptosis of host cells by cell-intrinsic mecha-

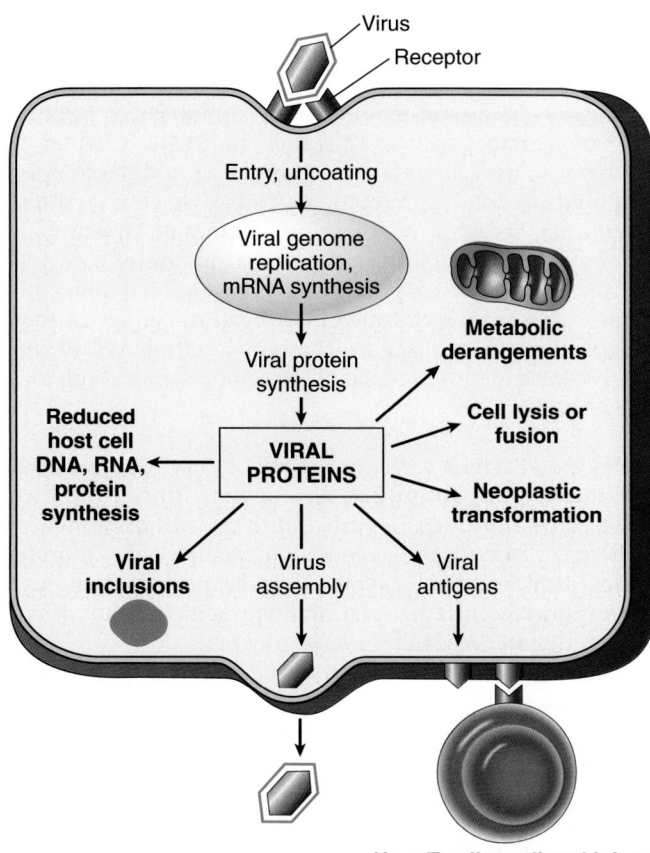

FIGURE 8–5 Mechanisms by which viruses cause injury to cells.

nisms, such as perturbations of the endoplasmic reticulum during virus assembly, which can activate proteases that mediate apoptosis (caspases).

○ *Antiviral immune responses.* Viral proteins on the surface of the host cells may be recognized by the immune system, and the host lymphocytes may attack virus-infected cells. Cytotoxic T lymphocytes (CTLs) are important for defense against viral infections, but CTLs also can be responsible for tissue injury. Lymphocytic choriomeningitis virus infection in mice is an experimental model in which disease is caused by the host immune response. Acute liver failure during hepatitis B infection may be accelerated by CTL-mediated destruction of infected hepatocytes (a normal response to clear the infection).

○ *Transformation of infected cells* into benign or malignant tumor cells. Different oncogenic viruses can stimulate cell growth and survival by a variety of mechanisms, including expression of virus-encoded oncogenes, anti-apoptotic strategies, or insertional mutagenesis (in which the function of host genes is altered by viral genes inserted into the host genome). The mechanisms of viral transformation are numerous and are discussed in Chapter 7.

Mechanisms of Bacterial Injury

Bacterial Virulence. *Bacterial damage to host tissues depends on the ability of the bacteria to adhere to host cells, invade cells and tissues, or deliver toxins.* Pathogenic bacteria have virulence genes that encode proteins that confer these properties. Virulence genes are frequently found grouped together in clusters called *pathogenicity islands*. All of the *Salmonella* strains that infect humans are closely related enough to form a single species, meaning that they share many "housekeeping" genes.[16] Differences in a relatively small number of pathogenicity genes determine whether an isolate of *Salmonella* can cause life-threatening typhoid fever or self-limited enteritis.

Plasmids and bacteriophages (viruses) are mobile genetic elements that spread between bacteria and can encode virulence factors (e.g., toxins, or enzymes that confer antibiotic resistance). Bacteriophages or plasmids can convert otherwise nonpathogenic bacteria into virulent ones. Exchange of these elements between bacteria can endow the recipient with a survival advantage, with the capacity to cause disease, or both. Plasmids or transposons encoding antibiotic resistance can convert an antibiotic-susceptible bacterium into a resistant one, making therapy difficult (e.g., vancomycin-resistant enterococci and methicillin-resistant staphylococci are endemic in many hospitals).

Many bacteria coordinately regulate gene expression within a large population of organisms by *quorum sensing.* For example, bacteria can induce expression of virulence factors as their concentration in the tissues increases. This may allow bacteria growing in discrete host sites, such as an abscess or consolidated pneumonia, to overcome host defenses. *S. aureus* coordinately regulates virulence factors by secreting *autoinducer peptides.*[17] As the bacteria grow to increasing concentrations, the level of the autoinducer peptide increases, stimulating toxin production. Within the population, some bacteria produce the autoinducer peptide and others respond to it by secreting toxins. Thus, because of quorum sensing, unicellular bacteria acquire some of the more complex properties of multicellular organisms, in which different cells perform different functions.

Communities of bacteria can form *biofilms* in which the organisms live within a viscous layer of extracellular polysaccharides that adhere to host tissues or devices such as intravascular catheters and artificial joints. In addition to enhancing adherence to host tissues, biofilms increase the virulence of bacteria by making them inaccessible to immune effector mechanisms and increasing their resistance to antimicrobial drugs. Biofilm formation seems to be important in the persistence and relapse of infections such as bacterial endocarditis, artificial joint infections, and respiratory infections in people with cystic fibrosis.

Bacterial Adherence to Host Cells. *Adhesins* are bacterial surface molecules that bind to host cells or extracellular matrix. Bacterial adhesins that bind bacteria to host cells are limited in structural type but have a broad range of host cell specificity. *Streptococcus pyogenes* is a gram-positive bacterium that adheres to host tissues by virtue of protein F and teichoic acid projecting from the bacterial cell wall and binding to fibronectin on the surface of host cells and in the extracellular matrix.

Pili are filamentous proteins on the surface of bacteria. The stalks of pili are composed of conserved repeating subunits, while the variable amino acids on the tips of the pili determine the binding specificity of the bacteria. Strains of *E. coli* that cause urinary tract infections uniquely express a specific P pilus, which binds to a gal(α1–4)gal moiety expressed on uroepithelial cells.[18] Pili on *N. gonorrhoeae* bacteria mediate adherence of the bacteria to host cells and also are targets of the antibody response against *N. gonorrhoeae*. Variation in the type of pili expressed is an important mechanism by which *N. gonorrhoeae* escapes the immune response.[19]

Virulence of Intracellular Bacteria. Facultative intracellular bacteria infect either epithelial cells (*Shigella* and enteroinvasive *E. coli*), macrophages (*M. tuberculosis, M. leprae*), or both (*S. typhi*). The growth of bacteria in cells may allow the bacteria to escape from certain effector mechanisms of the immune response (e.g., antibodies), or it may facilitate spread of the bacteria, as migration of macrophages carries *M. tuberculosis* bacteria from the lung to other sites.

Bacteria have a number of mechanisms for entering host cells. Some bacteria use the host immune response to gain entry into macrophages. Coating of bacteria with antibodies or the complement protein C3b (opsonization) normally results in phagocytosis of bacteria by macrophages. Like many bacteria, *M. tuberculosis* activates the alternative complement pathway, resulting in opsonization with C3b. Once coated with C3b, *M. tuberculosis* binds to the CR3 complement receptor on macrophages and is endocytosed into the cell.[20] Gram-negative bacteria use a complex secretion system to enter epithelial cells.[21] This system consists of needle-like structures projecting from the bacterial surface that bind to host cells, form pores in the host cell membrane, and then inject proteins that mediate rearrangement of the cell cytoskeleton, facilitating bacterial entry. Bacteria such as *Listeria monocytogenes* can manipulate the cell cytoskeleton to spread directly from cell to cell, perhaps allowing the bacteria to evade immune effector mechanisms.[22]

Once in the cytoplasm, bacteria have different strategies for interacting with the host cell. *Shigella* and *E. coli* inhibit host protein synthesis, replicate rapidly, and lyse the host cell within 6 hours. Within macrophages, most bacteria are killed when the phagosome fuses with an acidic lysosome to form a phagolysosome, but certain bacteria elude this host defense. For example, *M. tuberculosis* blocks fusion of the lysosome with the phagosome,[23] allowing it to proliferate unchecked within the macrophage. Other bacteria avoid destruction in macrophages by escaping from the phagosome. *L. monocytogenes* produces a pore-forming protein called listeriolysin O and two phospholipases that degrade the phagosome membrane, allowing the bacteria to escape into the cytoplasm.[22]

Bacterial Toxins. Any bacterial substance that contributes to illness can be considered a toxin. Toxins are classified as endotoxins, which are components of the bacterial cell, and exotoxins, which are proteins that are secreted by the bacterium.

Bacterial endotoxin is a lipopolysaccharide (LPS) that is a large component of the outer membrane of gram-negative bacteria. LPS is composed of a long-chain fatty acid anchor (lipid A) connected to a core sugar chain, both of which are very similar in all gram-negative bacteria. Attached to the core sugar is a variable carbohydrate chain (O antigen), which is used diagnostically to serotype and discriminate between different strains of bacteria. The response to bacterial LPS can be both beneficial and harmful to the host. The response is beneficial in that LPS activates protective immunity in several ways, including induction of important cytokines and chemoattractants (chemokines) of the immune system as well as increased expression of costimulatory molecules, which

enhance T-lymphocyte activation. However, high levels of LPS are thought to play an important role in septic shock, disseminated intravascular coagulation (DIC), and adult respiratory distress syndrome, mainly through induction of excessive levels of cytokines such as TNF, IL-1, and IL-12 (Chapter 4). LPS binds to the cell-surface receptor CD14, and the complex then binds to Toll-like receptor 4 (TLR4), which is a pattern recognition receptor of the innate immune system and transmits signals that lead to the cellular response.[24]

Exotoxins are secreted proteins that cause cellular injury and disease. They can be classified into broad categories by their site and mechanism of action. These are briefly described next and discussed in more detail in the specific sections about each type of bacteria.

- *Enzymes.* Bacteria secrete a variety of enzymes (proteases, hyaluronidases, coagulases, fibrinolysins) that act on their respective substrates in vitro, but the role of only a few of these in disease is understood. For example, certain proteases produced by *S. aureus* degrade proteins that hold keratinocytes together, causing the epidermis to detach from the deeper skin.[25]
- *Toxins that alter intracellular signaling or regulatory pathways.* Most of these toxins have an active (A) subunit with enzymatic activity and a binding (B) subunit that binds receptors on the cell surface and delivers the A subunit into the cell cytoplasm. The effect of these toxins depends on the binding specificity of the B domain and the cellular pathways affected by the A domain. A-B toxins are made by many bacteria including *Bacillus anthracis, V. cholerae,* and some strains of *E. coli.*
- *Neurotoxins* produced by *Clostridium botulinum* and *Clostridium tetani* inhibit release of neurotransmitters, resulting in paralysis.[26] These toxins do not kill neurons; instead, the A domains interact specifically with proteins involved in secretion of neurotransmitters at the synaptic junction. Both tetanus and botulism can result in death from respiratory failure due to paralysis of the chest and diaphragm muscles.
- *Superantigens* are bacterial toxins that stimulate very large number of T lymphocytes by binding to conserved portions of the T-cell receptor, leading to massive T-lymphocyte proliferation and cytokine release. The high levels of cytokines can lead to capillary leak and shock.[27] Superantigens made by *S. aureus* and *S. pyogenes* cause toxic shock syndrome (TSS).

Injurious Effects of Host Immunity

As was mentioned earlier, the host immune response to microbes can sometimes be the cause of tissue injury. The granulomatous inflammatory reaction to *M. tuberculosis* is a delayed hypersensitivity response that sequesters the bacilli and prevents spread but also can produce tissue damage and fibrosis. Similarly, the liver damage following HBV and HCV infection of hepatocytes is mainly due to the immune response to the infected liver cells and not to cytopathic effects of the virus. The humoral immune response to microbes also can have pathologic consequences. For example, following infection with *S. pyogenes,* antibodies produced against the streptococcal M protein can cross-react with cardiac proteins and damage the heart, leading to rheumatic heart disease. Post-streptococcal glomerulonephritis, which also can develop following infection with *S. pyogenes*, is caused by antistreptococcal antibodies that bind to streptococcal antigens and form immune complexes, which deposit in renal glomeruli and produce nephritis. Thus, antimicrobial immune responses can have beneficial and pathologic consequences.

The examples provided above are relatively infrequent situations in which specific immune responses to microbes have been identified as causative agents of various diseases. Recent clinical, epidemiologic, and experimental studies suggest that infections may be associated with a wide variety of chronic inflammatory disorders as well as cancer.[28] In some chronic inflammatory diseases, such as inflammatory bowel disease (Chapter 17), an important early event may be compromise of the intestinal epithelial barrier, which enables the entry of both pathogenic and commensal microbes and their interactions with local immune cells, resulting in inflammation. The cycle of inflammation and epithelial injury may be the basis of the disease, with microbes playing the central role. Viruses (HBV, HCV) and bacteria (*H. pylori*) that are not known to carry or activate oncogenes are associated with cancers, presumably because these microbes trigger chronic inflammation, which provides fertile ground for the development of cancer (Chapter 7).

IMMUNE EVASION BY MICROBES

Humoral and cellular immune responses that protect the host from most infections were discussed in Chapter 6. Not surprisingly, microorganisms have developed many means to resist and evade the immune system (Fig. 8–6).[29] These mechanisms are important determinants of microbial viru-lence and pathogenicity. They include (1) growth in niches that are inaccessible to the host immune system, (2) antigenic variation, (3) resistance to innate immune defenses, and (4) impairment of effective T-cell antimicrobial responses by specific or nonspecific immunosuppression.

Some microorganisms replicate in sites that are inaccessible to the host immune response. Microbes that propagate in the lumen of the intestine (e.g., toxin-producing *Clostridium difficile*) or gallbladder (e.g., *S. typhi*) are concealed from cell-mediated immune defenses. Some organisms establish infections by rapidly invading host cells before the host humoral response becomes effective (e.g., malaria sporozoites entering liver cells, *Trichinella* and *Trypanosoma cruzi* entering skeletal or cardiac muscle cells). Some larger parasites (e.g., the larvae of tapeworms) form cysts in host tissues that are covered by a dense capsule and are thus inaccessible to host immune cells and antibodies. Viral latency is the ultimate strategy for hiding antigens from the immune system. During the latent state, many viral genes are not expressed.

Some microbes can evade immune responses by varying the antigens they express. Neutralizing antibodies block the ability of microbes to infect cells and recruit effector mechanisms to kill pathogens. To escape recognition, microbes use many strategies that involve genetic mechanisms for generating antigenic variation. The low fidelity of viral RNA polymerases (in HIV and many respiratory viruses including influenza virus) and reassortment of viral genomes (influenza viruses) create viral antigenic variation (Table 8–6). The spirochete *Borrelia recurrentis* repeatedly switches its surface antigens, and the Lyme disease *Borrelia* organisms use similar mechanisms to vary their outer membrane proteins.[30] *Trypanosoma* species have many genes for their major surface antigen, VSG, and can vary the expression of this surface protein. There are

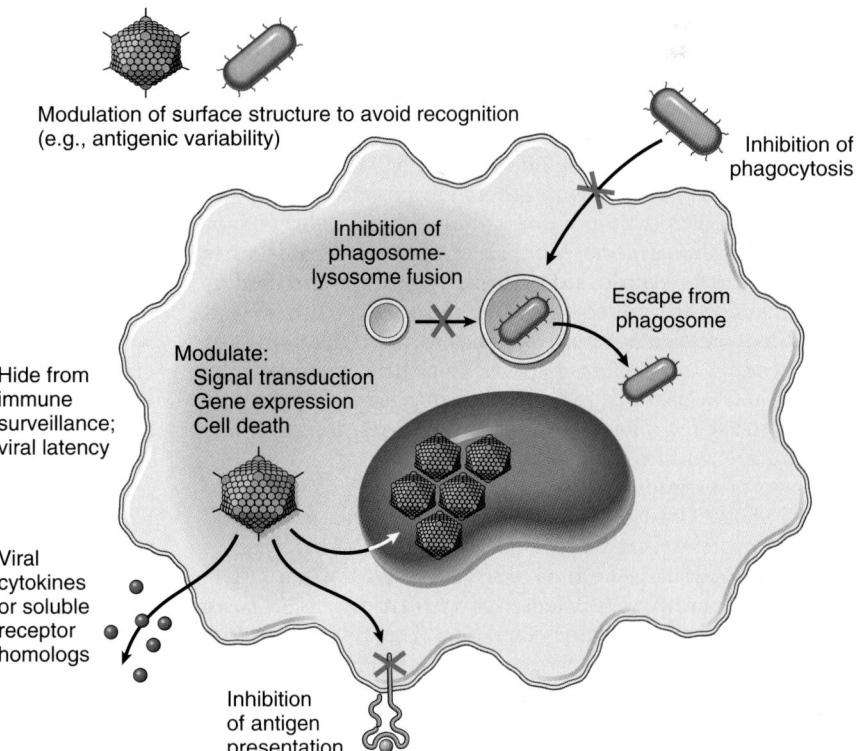

FIGURE 8–6 An overview of mechanisms used by viral and bacterial pathogens to evade innate and adaptive immunity. (Modified with permission from Finlay B, McFadden G: Anti-immunology: evasion of the host immune system by bacterial and viral pathogens. Cell 124:767–782, 2006.)

TABLE 8–6 Mechanisms of Antigenic Variation		
Type	**Example**	**Disease**
High mutation rate	HIV Influenza virus	AIDS Influenza
Genetic reassortment	Influenza virus Rotavirus	Influenza Diarrhea
Genetic rearrangement (e.g., gene recombination, gene conversion, site-specific inversion)	*Borrelia burgdorferi* *Neisseria gonorrhoeae* *Trypanosoma* sp. *Plasmodium* sp.	Lyme disease Gonorrhea African sleeping sickness Malaria
Large diversity of serotypes	Rhinoviruses *Streptococcus pneumoniae*	Colds Pneumonia Meningitis

at least 80 different serotypes of *S. pneumoniae*, each with different capsular polysaccharides.

Some microbes have devised methods for evading innate immune defenses, such as escaping killing by phagocytic cells and complement.[31] Cationic antimicrobial peptides, including defensins, cathelicidins, and thrombocidins, provide important initial defense against invading microbes. Resistance to these antimicrobial peptides is key to the virulence of a number of bacterial pathogens, enabling them to avoid killing by neutrophils and macrophages.[32] The carbohydrate capsule on the surface of all the major bacteria that cause pneumonia or meningitis (pneumococcus, meningococcus, *H. influenzae*) makes them more virulent by shielding bacterial antigens and by preventing phagocytosis of the organisms by neutrophils. For example, *E. coli* with the sialic acid–containing K1 capsule causes meningitis in newborns. Sialic acid will not bind C3b, which is critical for activation of the alternative complement pathway, so the bacteria escape from complement-mediated lysis and opsonization-directed phagocytosis. Many bacteria make toxic proteins that kill phagocytes, prevent their migration, or diminish their oxidative burst. Bacteria also can circumvent immune defenses by covering themselves with host proteins. Some bacterial pathogens including *Salmonella* can modify the lipid moiety of LPS to reduce Toll-like receptor (TLR) activation. *S. aureus* are covered by protein A molecules that bind the Fc portion of antibodies and so inhibit phagocytosis. *Neisseria*, *Haemophilus*, and *Streptococcus* all secrete proteases that degrade antibodies. As already mentioned, another successful strategy for circumventing defense mechanisms is to replicate within phagocytic cells. A number of viruses, some intracellular bacteria (including mycobacteria, *Listeria*, and *Legionella*), fungi (e.g., *Cryptococcus neoformans*), and protozoa (e.g., leishmania, trypanosomes, toxoplasmas) can multiply within phagocytes.

Viruses can produce molecules that inhibit innate immunity.[29,33] Some viruses (e.g., herpesviruses and poxviruses) produce proteins that block complement activation. Viruses have developed a large number of strategies to combat interferons (IFNs), an early host defense against viruses. Some viruses produce soluble homologues of IFN-α/β or IFN-γ receptors that bind to and inhibit actions of secreted IFNs, or produce proteins that inhibit intracellular JAK/STAT signaling downstream of IFN receptors. They may also inactivate or inhibit double-stranded RNA–dependent protein kinase (PKR), a key mediator of the antiviral effects of IFN. Some viruses encode within their genomes homologues of other cytokines and chemokines, or their receptors, which act in various ways to inhibit immune responses. Many viruses have developed strategies to block apoptosis in the host cell, which may give the viruses time to complete replication, assembly, and exit, promote viral persistence, and contribute to cell transformation.

Some microbes produce factors that decrease recognition of infected cells by CD4+ helper T cells and CD8+ cytotoxic T cells. For example, several DNA viruses (e.g., herpesviruses, including HSV, CMV, and EBV) can bind to or alter localization of major histocompatibility complex (MHC) class I proteins, impairing peptide presentation to CD8+ T cells.[34,35] Downregulation of MHC class I molecules might make it likely that virus-infected cells would be targets for NK cells. However, herpesviruses also express MHC class I homologues that act as effective inhibitors of NK cells by engaging killer inhibitory receptors (Chapter 6). Herpesviruses can target MHC class II molecules for degradation, impairing antigen presentation to CD4+ T helper cells. Viruses also can infect leukocytes and directly compromise their function. HIV infects CD4+ T cells, macrophages, and dendritic cells, and EBV infects B lymphocytes.

INFECTIONS IN IMMUNOSUPPRESSED HOSTS

Inherited or acquired defects in immunity (Chapter 6) often impair only part of the immune system, rendering the affected individual susceptible to specific types of infections. Patients with antibody deficiency, as in X-linked agammaglobulinemia, contract severe bacterial infections by organisms including *S. pneumoniae*, *H. influenzae*, and *S. aureus*, as well as a few viral infections (rotavirus and enteroviruses). Patients with T-cell defects are especially susceptible to infections with intracellular pathogens, notably viruses and some parasites. Patients with deficiencies in complement proteins are particularly susceptible to infections by *S. pneumoniae*, *H. influenzae*, and *N. meningitidis*. Some children have deficiencies in neutrophil function, leading to increased infections with *S. aureus* as well as some gram-negative bacteria and fungi.

Acquired immunodeficiencies have a variety of causes, the most important being infection with HIV, which causes AIDS. HIV infects and eventually kills CD4+ helper T lymphocytes. As discussed in Chapter 6, this leads to profound immunosuppression and a multitude of infections. While most organisms that infect people with AIDS were common pathogens before the era of HIV, others were uncommon (cryptococcus, pneumocystis), and one, Kaposi sarcoma herpesvirus (KSHV), also called human herpesvirus-8 (HHV-8), was discovered as a result of research in AIDS patients.[36]

Diseases that impair production of leukocytes, such as leukemia, which fills the bone marrow with cancerous cells, make patients vulnerable to opportunistic infections. Iatrogenic causes of immunosuppression include immunosuppressive drugs used to treat patients with autoimmune diseases and organ transplant recipients, as well as drugs used to treat cancer. Therapy to prevent rejection of organ transplants leads to severe immunosuppression, making transplant recipients very susceptible to infectious diseases. Patients receiving bone marrow transplants have profound defects in innate and adaptive immunity during the long time that it takes for the donated bone marrow to engraft, and become susceptible to infection with almost any organism, including opportunistic organisms that seldom cause disease in healthy people (e.g., *Aspergillus* species and *Pseudomonas* species).

Diseases of organ systems other than the immune system can also make patients susceptible to specific microorganisms. People with cystic fibrosis commonly get respiratory infections with *P. aeruginosa, S. aureus,* and *Burkholdaria cepacia.*[37] The lack of splenic function in individuals with sickle cell disease makes them susceptible to infection with encapsulated bacteria such as *S. pneumoniae,* which are normally opsonized and phagocytosed by splenic macrophages. Burns destroy skin, removing this barrier to microbes, allowing infection with pathogens such as *P. aeruginosa.* Finally, malnutrition may impair the host defenses.

SPECTRUM OF INFLAMMATORY RESPONSES TO INFECTION

In contrast to the vast molecular diversity of microbes, the morphologic patterns of tissue responses to microbes are limited, as are the mechanisms directing these responses. Therefore, many pathogens produce similar reaction patterns, and few features are unique or pathognomonic for a particular microorganism. Moreover, it is the interaction between the microorganism and the host that determines the histologic features of the inflammatory response. Thus, pyogenic bacteria, which normally evoke vigorous leukocyte responses, may cause rapid tissue necrosis with little leukocyte exudation in a profoundly neutropenic host. Similarly, in a normal patient, *M. tuberculosis* causes well-formed granulomas with few mycobacteria present, whereas in an AIDS patient the same mycobacteria multiply profusely in macrophages, which fail to coalesce into granulomas.

There are five major histologic patterns of tissue reaction in infections.

Suppurative (Purulent) Inflammation

This pattern is the reaction to acute tissue damage, described in Chapter 2, characterized by increased vascular permeability and leukocytic infiltration, predominantly of neutrophils (Fig. 8–7). The neutrophils are attracted to the site of infection by

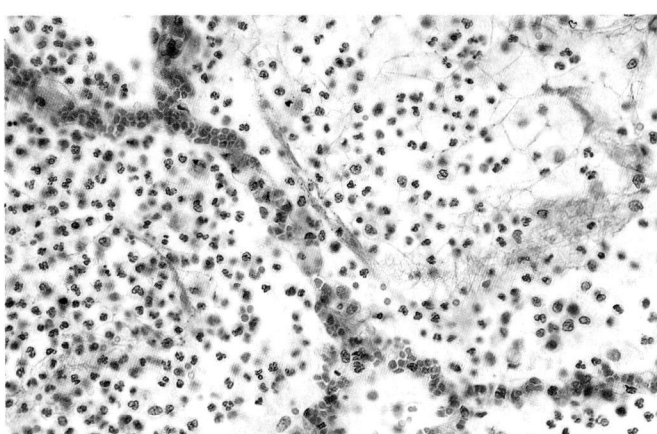

FIGURE 8–7 Pneumococcal pneumonia. Note the intra-alveolar polymorphonuclear exudate and intact alveolar septa.

release of chemoattractants from the "pyogenic" (pus-forming) bacteria that evoke this response, mostly extracellular gram-positive cocci and gram-negative rods. Massing of neutrophils and liquefactive necrosis of the tissue form pus. The sizes of exudative lesions range from tiny microabscesses formed in multiple organs during bacterial sepsis secondary to a colonized heart valve to diffuse involvement of entire lobes of the lung in pneumonia. How destructive the lesions are depends on their location and the organism involved. For example, pneumococci usually spare alveolar walls and cause lobar pneumonia that resolves completely, whereas staphylococci and *Klebsiella* species destroy alveolar walls and form abscesses that heal with scar formation. Bacterial pharyngitis resolves without sequelae, whereas untreated acute bacterial inflammation of a joint can destroy it in a few days.

Mononuclear and Granulomatous Inflammation

Diffuse, predominantly mononuclear, interstitial infiltrates are a common feature of all chronic inflammatory processes, but when they develop acutely, they often are a response to viruses, intracellular bacteria, or intracellular parasites. In addition, spirochetes and helminths provoke chronic inflammatory responses. Which mononuclear cell predominates within the inflammatory lesion depends on the host immune response to the organism. For example, plasma cells are abundant in the primary and secondary lesions of syphilis (Fig. 8–8), whereas lymphocytes predominate in HBV infection or viral infections of the brain. The presence of these lymphocytes reflects cell-mediated immune responses against the pathogen or pathogen-infected cells. At the other extreme, macrophages may become filled with organisms, as occurs in *M. avium-intracellulare* infections in AIDS patients, who cannot mount an effective immune response to the organisms. *Granulomatous inflammation* is a distinctive form of mononuclear inflammation usually evoked by infectious agents that resist eradication and are capable of stimulating strong T cell–mediated immunity (e.g., *M. tuberculosis, Histoplasma capsulatum,* schistosome eggs). Granulomatous inflammation is characterized by accumulation of activated macrophages

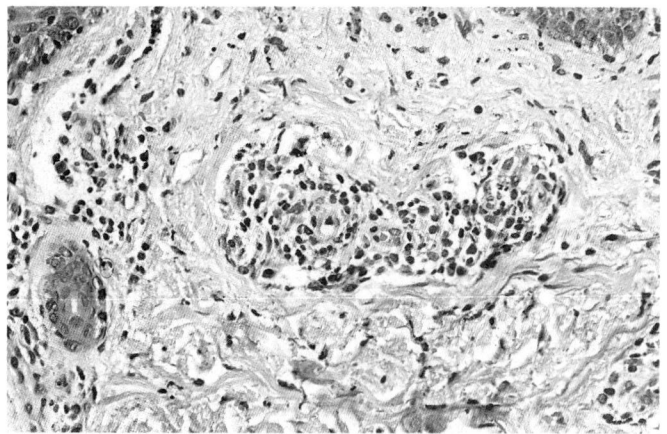

FIGURE 8–8 Secondary syphilis in the dermis with perivascular lymphoplasmacytic infiltrate and endothelial proliferation.

called "epithelioid" cells, which may fuse to form giant cells. In some cases there is a central area of caseous necrosis (see Chapter 2 and "Tuberculosis" in this chapter).

Cytopathic-Cytoproliferative Reaction

These reactions are usually produced by viruses. The lesions are characterized by cell necrosis or cellular proliferation, usually with sparse inflammatory cells. Some viruses replicate within cells and make viral aggregates that are visible as inclusion bodies (e.g., herpesviruses or adenovirus) or induce cells to fuse and form multinucleated cells called polykaryons (e.g., measles virus or herpesviruses). Focal cell damage in the skin may cause epithelial cells to become detached, forming blisters (Fig. 8–9). Some viruses can cause epithelial cells to proliferate (e.g., venereal warts caused by HPV or the umbilicated papules of molluscum contagiosum caused by poxviruses). Finally, viruses can contribute to the development of malignant neoplasms (Chapter 7).

Tissue Necrosis

Clostridium perfringens and other organisms that secrete powerful toxins can cause such rapid and severe necrosis

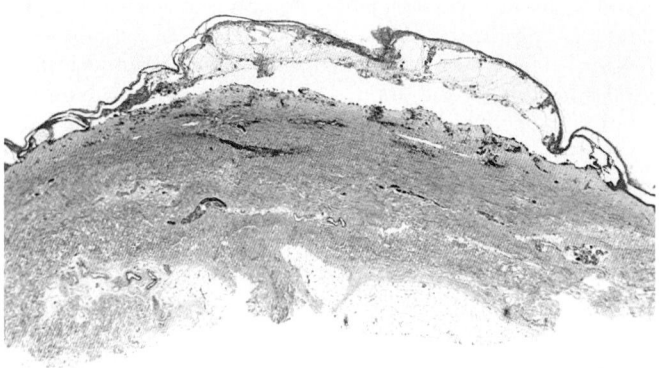

FIGURE 8–9 Herpesvirus blister in mucosa. See Figure 8–12 for viral inclusions.

(gangrenous necrosis) that tissue damage is the dominant feature. Because few inflammatory cells are present, these lesions resemble infarcts with disruption or loss of basophilic nuclear staining and preservation of cellular outlines. Clostridia are often opportunistic pathogens that are introduced into muscle tissue by penetrating trauma or infection of the bowel in a neutropenic host. Similarly, the parasite *E. histolytica* causes colonic ulcers and liver abscesses characterized by extensive tissue destruction with liquefactive necrosis and without a prominent inflammatory infiltrate. By entirely different mechanisms, viruses can cause widespread and severe necrosis of host cells associated with inflammation, as exemplified by total destruction of the temporal lobes of the brain by herpesvirus or the liver by HBV.

Chronic Inflammation and Scarring

Many infections elicit chronic inflammation, which can lead either to complete healing or to extensive scarring. For example, chronic HBV infection may cause cirrhosis of the liver, in which dense fibrous septae surround nodules of regenerating hepatocytes. Sometimes the exuberant scarring response is the major cause of dysfunction (e.g., the "pipestem" fibrosis of the liver or fibrosis of the bladder wall caused by schistosomal eggs [Fig. 8–10] or the constrictive fibrous pericarditis in tuberculosis).

These patterns of tissue reaction are useful guidelines for analyzing microscopic features of infectious processes, but they rarely appear in pure form because different types of host reactions often occur at the same time. For example, the lung of an AIDS patient may be infected with CMV, which causes cytolytic changes, and at the same time by *Pneumocystis*, which causes interstitial inflammation. Similar patterns of inflammation also can be seen in tissue responses to physical or chemical agents and in inflammatory diseases of unknown cause (Chapter 2).

This concludes our discussion of the general principles of the pathogenesis and pathology of infectious disease. We now turn to descriptions of specific infections caused by viruses, bacteria, fungi, and parasites. In this discussion we emphasize *pathogenic mechanisms* and *pathologic changes*, rather than details of clinical features, which are available in clinical textbooks. Infections that typically involve a specific organ are discussed in other chapters.

Viral Infections

Viruses are the cause of many clinically important acute and chronic infections affecting virtually every organ system (Table 8–7).

ACUTE (TRANSIENT) INFECTIONS

The viruses that cause transient infections are structurally heterogeneous, but each elicits an effective immune response that eliminates the organism and may or may not confer lifelong protection. The mumps virus, for example, has only one serotype and infects people only once, whereas other transient viruses, such as influenza viruses, can repeatedly infect the

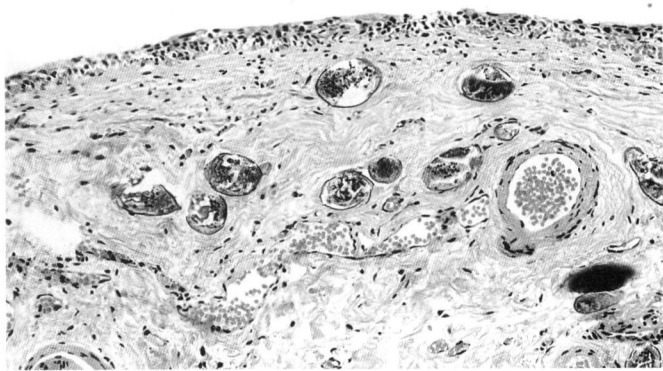

FIGURE 8–10 *Schistosoma haematobium* infection of the bladder with numerous calcified eggs and extensive scarring.

same individual because of antigenic variation. The immune response to some transient viruses wanes with time, allowing even the same serotype of virus to infect repeatedly (e.g., respiratory syncytial virus).

Measles

Measles (rubeola) virus is a leading cause of vaccine-preventable death and illness worldwide. More than 20 million people are affected by measles each year. In 2005, there were an estimated 345,000 deaths globally, the majority of them in children in developing countries. Because of poor nutrition, children in developing countries are 10 to 1000 times more likely to die of measles pneumonia than are children in devel-

oped countries.[38] Epidemics of measles occur among unvaccinated individuals. Measles can produce severe disease in people with defects in cellular immunity (such as HIV-infected people or people with hematologic malignancy). In the United States the incidence of measles has decreased dramatically since 1963, when a measles vaccine was licensed. The diagnosis is usually made clinically, or by serology or detection of viral antigen in nasal exudate or urinary sediment.

Pathogenesis. Measles virus is a single-stranded RNA virus of the paramyxovirus family that includes mumps, respiratory syncytial virus (the major cause of lower respiratory infections in infants), parainfluenza virus (a cause of croup), and human metapneumovirus. There is only one serotype of measles virus. Two cell-surface receptors have been identified for the virus: CD46, a complement-regulatory protein that inactivates C3 convertases, and signaling lymphocytic activation molecule (SLAM), a molecule involved in T-cell activation.[39] CD46 is expressed on all nucleated cells, while SLAM is expressed on cells of the immune system. Both these receptors bind the viral hemagglutinin protein. Measles virus is transmitted by respiratory droplets. The virus initially multiplies within upper respiratory epithelial cells and then spreads to local lymphoid tissue. Measles can replicate in epithelial cells, endothelial cells, monocytes, macrophages, dendritic cells, and lymphocytes. Replication of the virus in lymphatic tissue is followed by viremia and systemic dissemination of the virus to many tissues, including the conjunctiva, respiratory tract, urinary tract, small blood vessels, lymphatic system, and CNS. Measles may cause croup, pneumonia, diarrhea with protein-losing enteropathy, keratitis with scarring and blindness, encephalitis, and hemorrhagic rashes ("black measles")

TABLE 8–7	Selected Human Viruses and Viral Diseases	
Organ System	**Species**	**Disease**
Respiratory	Adenovirus	Upper and lower respiratory tract infections, conjunctivitis, diarrhea
	Rhinovirus	Upper respiratory tract infection
	Influenza viruses A, B	Influenza
	Respiratory syncytial virus	Bronchiolitis, pneumonia
Digestive	Mumps virus	Mumps, pancreatitis, orchitis
	Rotavirus	Childhood gastroenteritis
	Norovirus	Gastroenteritis
	Hepatitis A virus	Acute viral hepatitis
	Hepatitis B virus	Acute or chronic hepatitis
	Hepatitis D virus	With HBV, acute or chronic hepatitis
	Hepatitis C virus	Acute or chronic hepatitis
	Hepatitis E virus	Enterically transmitted hepatitis
Systemic with Skin Eruptions	Measles virus	Measles (rubeola)
	Rubella virus	German measles (rubella)
	Varicella-zoster virus	Chickenpox, shingles
	Herpes simplex virus 1	Oral herpes ("cold sore")
	Herpes simplex virus 2	Genital herpes
Systemic with Hematopoietic Disorders	Cytomegalovirus	Cytomegalic inclusion disease
	Epstein-Barr virus	Infectious mononucleosis
	HIV-1 and HIV-2	AIDS
Arboviral and Hemorrhagic Fevers	Dengue virus 1–4	Dengue hemorrhagic fever
	Yellow fever virus	Yellow fever
Skin/Genital Warts	Papillomavirus	Condyloma; cervical carcinoma
Central Nervous System	Poliovirus	Poliomyelitis
	JC virus	Progressive multifocal leukoencephalopathy (opportunistic)

in malnourished children with poor medical care. Most children develop T cell–mediated immunity to measles virus that controls the viral infection and produces the measles rash, a hypersensitivity reaction to measles-infected cells in the skin. The rash is less frequent in people with deficiencies in cell-mediated immunity but does occur in agammaglobulinemic people. Antibody-mediated immunity to measles virus protects against reinfection. Measles also can cause transient but profound immunosuppression, resulting in secondary bacterial and viral infection, which are responsible for much of measles-related morbidity and mortality. Alterations of both innate and adaptive immune responses occur following measles infection, including defects in dendritic cell and lymphocyte function.[40] Subacute sclerosing panencephalitis (described in Chapter 28) and measles inclusion body encephalitis (in immunocompromised individuals) are rare late complications of measles. The pathogenesis of subacute sclerosing panencephalitis is not well understood, but a replication-defective variant of measles may be involved in this persistent viral infection.[41]

Morphology. The blotchy, reddish brown rash of measles virus infection on the face, trunk, and proximal extremities is produced by dilated skin vessels, edema, and a moderate, nonspecific, mononuclear perivascular infiltrate. Ulcerated mucosal lesions in the oral cavity near the opening of Stensen ducts (the pathognomonic Koplik spots) are marked by necrosis, neutrophilic exudate, and neovascularization. The lymphoid organs typically have marked follicular hyperplasia, large germinal centers, and randomly distributed multinucleate giant cells, called Warthin-Finkeldey cells, which have eosinophilic nuclear and cytoplasmic inclusion bodies. These are pathognomonic of measles and are also found in the lung and sputum (Fig. 8–11). The milder forms of measles pneumonia show the same peribronchial and interstitial mononuclear cell infiltration that is seen in other nonlethal viral infections. In severe or neglected cases, bacterial superinfection may be a cause of death.

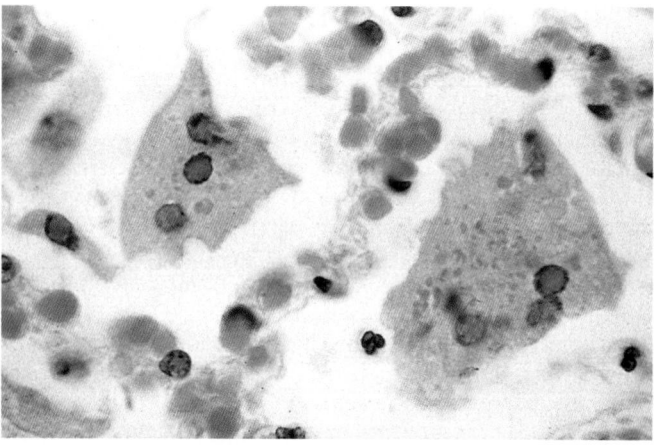

FIGURE 8–11 Measles giant cells in the lung. Note the glassy eosinophilic intranuclear inclusions.

Mumps

Like measles virus, mumps virus is a member of the paramyxovirus family. Mumps virus has two types of surface glycoproteins, one with hemagglutinin and neuraminidase activities and the other with cell fusion and cytolytic activities. Mumps viruses enter the upper respiratory tract through inhalation of respiratory droplets, spread to draining lymph nodes where they replicate in lymphocytes (preferentially in activated T cells), and then spread through the blood to the salivary and other glands. Mumps virus infects salivary gland ductal epithelial cells, resulting in desquamation of involved cells, edema, and inflammation that leads to the classic salivary gland pain and swelling of mumps. Mumps virus also can spread to other sites, including the CNS, testis and ovary, and pancreas. Aseptic meningitis is the most common extrasalivary gland complication of mumps infection, occurring in about 10% of cases. The mumps vaccine has reduced the incidence of mumps by 99% in the United States. The diagnosis is usually made clinically, but serology or viral culture can be used for definitive diagnosis.

Morphology. In **mumps parotitis**, which is bilateral in 70% of cases, affected glands are enlarged, have a doughy consistency, and are moist, glistening, and reddish brown on cross-section. On microscopic examination the gland interstitium is edematous and diffusely infiltrated by macrophages, lymphocytes, and plasma cells, which compress acini and ducts. Neutrophils and necrotic debris may fill the ductal lumen and cause focal damage to the ductal epithelium.

In **mumps orchitis** testicular swelling may be marked, caused by edema, mononuclear cell infiltration, and focal hemorrhages. Because the testis is tightly contained within the tunica albuginea, parenchymal swelling may compromise the blood supply and cause areas of infarction. Sterility, when it occurs, is caused by scars and atrophy of the testis after resolution of viral infection.

In the enzyme-rich **pancreas**, lesions may be destructive, causing parenchymal and fat necrosis and neutrophil-rich inflammation. **Mumps encephalitis** causes perivenous demyelination and perivascular mononuclear cuffing.

Poliovirus Infection

Poliovirus is a spherical, unencapsulated RNA virus of the enterovirus genus. Other enteroviruses cause childhood diarrhea as well as rashes (coxsackievirus A), conjunctivitis (enterovirus 70), viral meningitis (coxsackieviruses and echovirus), and myopericarditis (coxsackievirus B). There are three major strains of poliovirus, each of which is included in the Salk formalin-fixed (killed) vaccine and the Sabin oral, attenuated (live) vaccine.[42] These vaccines have nearly eliminated poliovirus from the Western hemisphere, because the poliovirus, like smallpox virus, infects people but not other animals, is only briefly shed, does not undergo antigenic variation, and is effectively prevented by immunization.[43] Poliovirus still persists in parts of Africa.

Poliovirus, like other enteroviruses, is transmitted by the fecal-oral route. It first infects tissues in the oropharynx, then is secreted into the saliva and swallowed, and subsequently multiplies in the intestinal mucosa and lymph nodes, causing a transient viremia and fever. The virus infects only humans because it uses human CD155 to gain entry into cells but does not bind to cells in other species.[44] Although most polio infections are asymptomatic, in about 1 of 100 infected persons poliovirus invades the CNS and replicates in motor neurons of the spinal cord (spinal poliomyelitis) or brain stem (bulbar poliomyelitis). Antiviral antibodies control the disease in most cases, and it is not known why they fail to contain the virus in some individuals. Viral spread to the nervous system may be secondary to viremia or occur by retrograde transport of the virus along axons of motor neurons.[45] Rare cases of poliomyelitis that occur after vaccination are caused by mutations of the attenuated viruses to wild-type forms. The diagnosis can be made by viral culture of throat secretions or stool, or by serology. The neurologic features and neuropathology of poliovirus infection are described in Chapter 28.

West Nile Virus

West Nile virus is an arthropod-borne virus (arbovirus) of the flavivirus group, which also includes viruses that cause dengue fever and yellow fever. West Nile virus has a broad geographic distribution in the Old World, with outbreaks in Africa, the Middle East, Europe, Southeast Asia, and Australia. This virus was first detected in the United States in 1999 during an outbreak in New York City.[46] West Nile virus is transmitted by mosquitoes to birds and to mammals. Wild birds develop prolonged viremia and are the major reservoir for the virus. Humans are usually incidental hosts. However, West Nile virus has been transmitted by blood transfusion, transplanted organs, breast milk, and transplacentally.[47]

After inoculation by a mosquito, West Nile virus replicates in skin dendritic cells, which then migrate to lymph nodes, where virus replicates further, enters the bloodstream, and, in some individuals, crosses the blood-brain barrier. In the CNS the virus infects neurons. Chemokines have essential roles in directing leukocytes to the CNS for viral clearance. In humans and in mice, the chemokine receptor CCR5 functions as an essential host factor to resist neuroinvasive infection. The CCR5Δ32 allele, which contains a 32–base pair deletion in the coding sequence and results in a complete loss of function in a homozygous individual, is associated with symptomatic and lethal West Nile virus infection. Thus, the loss of CCR5 receptor increases the risk of fatal West Nile virus infection but is protective against HIV-1 infection because HIV uses the receptor to infect host cells (Chapter 6).[48]

West Nile virus infection is usually asymptomatic, but in 20% of infected individuals it gives rise to a mild, short-lived febrile illness associated with headache and myalgia. A maculopapular rash is seen in approximately half the cases. CNS complications (meningitis, encephalitis, meningoencephalitis) are not frequent, occurring in about 1 in 150 clinically apparent infections. There is a mortality of about 10% in people with meningoencephalitis and long-term cognitive and neurologic impairment in many survivors. Perivascular and leptomeningeal chronic inflammation, microglial nodules (Chapter 28), and neuronophagia predominantly involving the temporal lobes and brain stem have been observed in the brains of patients who died of West Nile virus infection. Immunosuppressed persons and the elderly appear to be at the greatest risk for severe disease. Rare complications include hepatitis, myocarditis, and pancreatitis. The diagnosis is usually made by serology, but viral culture and PCR-based tests are also used.

Viral Hemorrhagic Fevers

Viral hemorrhagic fevers (VHFs) are systemic infections. They are caused by enveloped RNA viruses in four different families: arenaviruses, filoviruses, bunyaviruses, and flaviviruses. Although structurally distinct, these viruses all depend on an animal or insect host for survival and transmission. VHF viruses are restricted geographically to areas in which their hosts reside. Humans are infected when they come into contact with infected hosts or insect vectors, but humans are not the natural reservoir for any of these viruses. Some viruses that cause hemorrhagic fever (Ebola, Marburg, Lassa) also can spread from person to person. VHF viruses produce a spectrum of illnesses, ranging from relatively mild acute disease characterized by fever, headache, myalgia, rash, neutropenia, and thrombocytopenia to severe, life-threatening disease in which there is sudden hemodynamic deterioration and shock. These viruses are potential biologic weapons because of their infectious properties, morbidity and mortality, and the absence of therapy and vaccines.

The pathogenesis of viral hemorrhagic fevers is not well understood. The hemorrhagic manifestations are due to thrombocytopenia or severe platelet or endothelial dysfunction. Typically there is increased vascular permeability. There may be necrosis and hemorrhage in many organs, particularly the liver. Although the viruses that cause hemorrhagic fever can replicate in endothelial cells and direct cytopathic effects may contribute to disease, most disease manifestations are related to activation of innate immune responses.[49] Viral infection of macrophages and dendritic cells leads to release of mediators that modify vascular function and have procoagulant activity.

CHRONIC LATENT INFECTIONS (HERPESVIRUS INFECTIONS)

Herpesviruses are large encapsulated viruses that have a double-stranded DNA genome that encodes approximately 70 proteins. Herpesviruses cause acute infection followed by latent infection in which the viruses persist in a noninfectious form with periodic reactivation and shedding of infectious virus. Latency is operationally defined as the inability to recover infectious particles from cells that harbor the virus. There are eight types of human herpesviruses, belonging to three subgroups defined by the type of cell most frequently infected and the site of latency: α-*group viruses*, including HSV-1, HSV-2, and VZV, which infect epithelial cells and produce latent infection in neurons; lymphotropic β-*group viruses*, including CMV, human herpesvirus-6 (which causes exanthem subitum, also known as roseola infantum and sixth disease, a benign rash of infants), and human herpesvirus-7 (a virus without a known disease association), which infect and produce latent infection in a variety of cell types; and the γ-*group viruses* EBV and KSHV/HHV-8, the cause of Kaposi sarcoma,[58] which produce latent infection mainly in lymphoid cells. In addition, herpesvirus simiae is an Old World monkey virus that resembles HSV-1 and can cause fatal neurologic disease in animal handlers, usually resulting from an animal bite.

Herpes Simplex Virus (HSV)

HSV-1 and HSV-2 differ serologically but are genetically similar and cause a similar set of primary and recurrent infections.[50] These viruses produce acute and latent infections. Both viruses replicate in the skin and the mucous membranes at the site of entrance of the virus (usually oropharynx or genitals), where they produce infectious virions and cause vesicular lesions of the epidermis. The viruses spread to sensory neurons that innervate these primary sites of replication. Viral nucleocapsids are transported along axons to the neuronal cell bodies, where the viruses establish latent infection. In immunocompetent hosts, primary HSV infection resolves in a few weeks, although the virus remains latent in nerve cells. During latency the viral DNA remains within the nucleus of the neuron, and only latency-associated viral RNA transcripts (LATs) are synthesized.[51] In this state, no viral proteins appear to be produced. Recent data suggest that some LATs may be microRNAs that confer resistance to apoptosis and thus contribute to virus persistence in sensory neurons.[52] Reactivation of HSV-1 and HSV-2 may occur repeatedly with or without symptoms, and results in the spread of virus from the neurons to the skin or to mucous membranes. Reactivation occurs in the presence of host immunity, because herpesviruses have developed ways to avoid immune recognition. For example, HSVs can evade antiviral CTLs by inhibiting the MHC class I recognition pathway, and elude humoral immune defenses by producing receptors for the Fc domain of immunoglobulin and inhibitors of complement.[34,35]

In addition to causing cutaneous lesions, HSV-1 is the major infectious cause of corneal blindness in the United States; corneal epithelial disease is thought to be due to direct viral damage, while corneal stromal disease appears to be immune mediated. HSV-1 is also the major cause of fatal sporadic encephalitis in the United States, when the virus spreads to the brain, particularly the temporal lobes and orbital gyri of the frontal lobes. In addition, neonates and individuals with compromised cellular immunity (e.g., secondary to HIV infection or chemotherapy) may suffer disseminated herpesvirus infections.

Morphology. HSV-infected cells contain large, pink to purple intranuclear inclusions (Cowdry type A) that consist of intact and disrupted virions with the stained host cell chromatin pushed to the edges of the nucleus (Fig. 8–12). Due to cell fusion, HSV also produces inclusion-bearing multinucleated syncytia.

HSV-1 and HSV-2 cause lesions ranging from self-limited cold sores and gingivostomatitis to life-threatening disseminated visceral infections and encephalitis. **Fever blisters or cold sores** favor the facial skin around mucosal orifices (lips, nose), where their distribution is frequently bilateral and independent of skin dermatomes. Intraepithelial vesicles (blisters), which are formed by intracellular edema

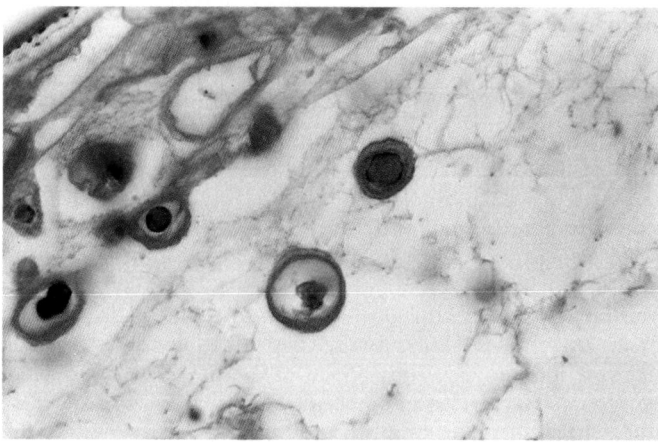

FIGURE 8–12 High-power view of cells from the blister in Figure 8–9 showing glassy intranuclear herpes simplex inclusion bodies.

and ballooning degeneration of epidermal cells, frequently burst and crust over, but some may result in superficial ulcerations.

Gingivostomatitis, which is usually encountered in children, is caused by HSV-1. It is a vesicular eruption extending from the tongue to the retropharynx and causing cervical lymphadenopathy. Swollen, erythematous HSV lesions of the fingers or palm (herpetic whitlow) occur in infants and, occasionally, in health care workers.

Genital herpes is more often caused by HSV-2 than by HSV-1. It is characterized by vesicles on the genital mucous membranes as well as on the external genitalia that are rapidly converted into superficial ulcerations, rimmed by an inflammatory infiltrate (Chapter 22). Herpesvirus (usually HSV-2) can be transmitted to neonates during passage through the birth canal of infected mothers. Although HSV-2 infection in the neonate may be mild, more commonly it is fulminating with generalized lymphadenopathy, splenomegaly, and necrotic foci throughout the lungs, liver, adrenals, and CNS.

Two forms of **corneal lesions** are caused by HSV (Chapter 29). **Herpes epithelial keratitis** shows typical virus-induced cytolysis of the superficial epithelium. In contrast, **herpes stromal keratitis** is characterized by infiltrates of mononuclear cells around keratinocytes and endothelial cells, leading to neovascularization, scarring, opacification of the cornea, and eventual blindness. This is an immunological reaction to the HSV infection.

Herpes simplex encephalitis is described in Chapter 28.

Disseminated skin and visceral herpes infections are usually encountered in hospitalized patients with some form of underlying cancer or immunosuppression. **Kaposi varicelliform eruption** is a generalized vesiculating involvement of the skin, whereas **eczema herpeticum** is characterized by confluent, pustular, or hemorrhagic blisters, often with bacterial superinfection and viral dissemination to internal viscera. **Herpes esophagitis** is frequently complicated by superinfection with bacteria or fungi. **Herpes bronchopneumonia**, which may be introduced by intubation of a patient with active oral lesions, is often necrotizing, and **herpes hepatitis** may cause liver failure.

Varicella-Zoster Virus (VZV)

Two conditions—*chickenpox* and *shingles*—are caused by VZV. Acute infection with VZV causes chickenpox; reactivation of latent VZV causes shingles (also called herpes zoster). Chickenpox is mild in children but more severe in adults and in immunocompromised people. Shingles is a source of morbidity in elderly and immunosuppressed persons.[53] Like HSV, VZV infects mucous membranes, skin, and neurons and causes a self-limited primary infection in immunocompetent individuals. Also like HSV, VZV evades immune responses and establishes a latent infection in sensory ganglia.[51] In contrast to HSV, VZV is transmitted in epidemic fashion by aerosols, disseminates hematogenously, and causes widespread vesicular skin lesions. VZV infects neurons and/or satellite cells around neurons in the dorsal root ganglia and may recur many years after the primary infection, causing shingles. Localized recurrence of VZV is most frequent and painful in dermatomes innervated by the trigeminal ganglia, where it is most likely to exist in a state of latency. In contrast to numerous recurrences of HSV, most people do not have a recurrence of VZV. VZV usually recurs only once in immunocompetent individuals, but immunosuppressed or elderly persons can have multiple recurrences of VZV. VZV infection is diagnosed by viral culture or detection of viral antigens in cells scraped from superficial lesions.

> **Morphology.** The **chickenpox** rash occurs approximately 2 weeks after respiratory infection. Lesions appear in multiple waves centrifugally from the torso to the head and extremities. Each lesion progresses rapidly from a macule to a vesicle, which resembles a dewdrop on a rose petal. On histologic examination, chickenpox vesicles contain intranuclear inclusions in the epithelial cells like those of HSV-1 (Fig. 8–13). After a few days most chickenpox vesicles rupture, crust over, and heal by regeneration, leaving no scars. However, bacterial superinfection of vesicles that are ruptured by trauma may lead to destruction of the basal epidermal layer and residual scarring.
> **Shingles** occurs when VZV that has long remained latent in the dorsal root ganglia after a previous chickenpox infection is reactivated and infects sensory nerves that carry it to one or more dermatomes. There, the virus infects keratinocytes and causes vesicular lesions, which, unlike chickenpox, are often associated with intense itching, burning, or sharp pain because of the simultaneous radiculoneuritis. This pain is especially severe when the trigeminal nerves are involved; rarely, the geniculate nucleus is involved, causing facial paralysis (Ramsay Hunt syn-

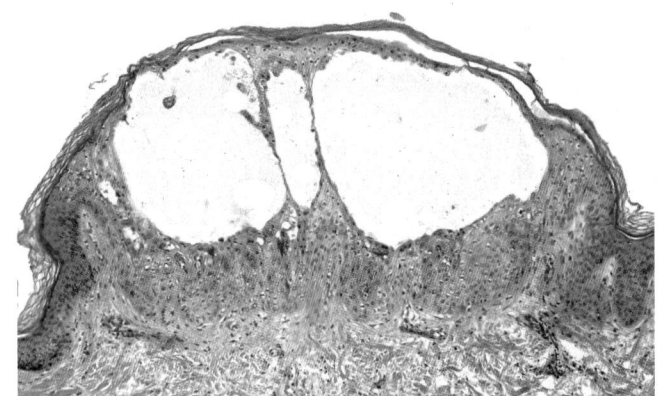

FIGURE 8–13 Skin lesion of chickenpox (varicella zoster virus) with intraepithelial vesicle.

> drome). The sensory ganglia contain a dense, predominantly mononuclear infiltrate, with herpetic intranuclear inclusions within neurons and their supporting cells (Fig. 8–14). VZV can also cause interstitial pneumonia, encephalitis, transverse myelitis, and necrotizing visceral lesions, particularly in immunosuppressed people.

Cytomegalovirus (CMV)

Cytomegalovirus (CMV), a β-group herpesvirus, can produce a variety of disease manifestations, depending on the age of the host, and, more important, on the host's immune status. CMV latently infects monocytes and their bone marrow progenitors and can be reactivated when cellular immunity is depressed. CMV causes an asymptomatic or mononucleosis-like infection in healthy individuals but devastating systemic infections in neonates and in immunocompromised people. As its name implies, CMV-infected cells exhibit gigantism of both the entire cell and its nucleus. Within the nucleus is a large inclusion surrounded by a clear halo (owl's eye).

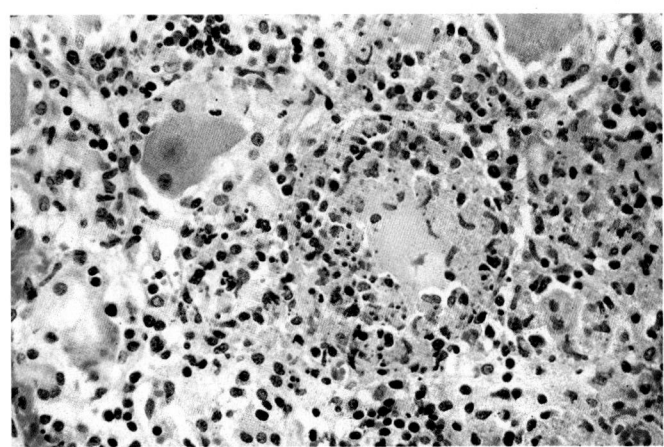

FIGURE 8–14 Dorsal root ganglion with varicella zoster virus infection. Note the ganglion cell necrosis and associated inflammation. (Courtesy of Dr. James Morris, Radcliffe Infirmary, Oxford, England.)

Transmission of CMV can occur by several mechanisms, depending on the age group affected.[54,55] These include the following:

- Transplacental transmission can occur from a newly acquired or primary infection in a mother who does not have protective antibodies ("congenital CMV").
- Neonatal transmission can occur through cervical or vaginal secretions at birth or, later, through breast milk from a mother who has active infection ("perinatal CMV").
- Transmission can occur through saliva during preschool years, especially in day care centers. Toddlers so infected readily transmit the virus to their parents.
- Transmission by the venereal route is the dominant mode after about 15 years of age, but spread may also occur via respiratory secretions and the fecal-oral route.
- Iatrogenic transmission can occur at any age through organ transplants or blood transfusions.

Acute CMV infection induces transient but severe immunosuppression. CMV can infect dendritic cells and impair their maturation and ability to stimulate T cells.[55] Similar to other herpesviruses, CMV can elude immune responses by downmodulating MHC class I and II molecules and producing homologues of TNF receptor, IL-10, and MHC class I molecules.[29,34,35] Interestingly, CMV can both activate and evade NK cells by inducing ligands for activating receptors and class I–like proteins that engage inhibitory receptors. Thus, CMV can both hide from immune defenses and actively suppress immune responses.

Morphology. The characteristic enlargement of infected cells can be appreciated histologically. Prominent **intranuclear basophilic inclusions** spanning half the nuclear diameter are usually set off from the nuclear membrane by a clear halo (Fig. 8–15). Within the cytoplasm of these cells, smaller basophilic inclusions can also be seen. In the glandular organs, the parenchymal epithelial cells are affected; in the brain, the neurons; in the lungs, the alveolar macrophages and epithelial and endothelial cells; and in the kidneys, the tubular epithelial and glomerular endothelial cells. Affected cells are strikingly enlarged, often to a diameter of 40 μm, and they show cellular and nuclear pleomorphism. Disseminated CMV causes focal necrosis with minimal inflammation in virtually any organ.

Congenital Infections. Infection acquired in utero may take many forms. In approximately 95% of cases it is asymptomatic. However, sometimes when the virus is acquired from a mother with primary infection (who does not have protective antibodies), classic *cytomegalic inclusion disease* develops. Cytomegalic inclusion disease resembles erythroblastosis fetalis. Affected infants may suffer intrauterine growth retardation, be profoundly ill, and manifest jaundice, hepatosplenomegaly, anemia, bleeding due to thrombocytopenia, and encephalitis. In fatal cases the brain is often smaller than

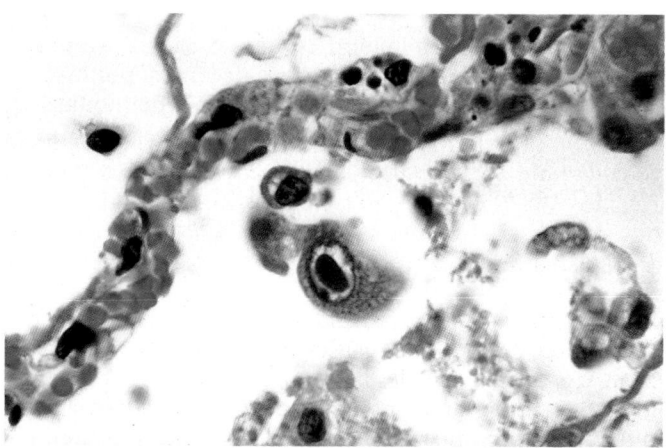

FIGURE 8–15 Cytomegalovirus: distinct nuclear and ill-defined cytoplasmic inclusions in the lung.

normal (microcephaly) and may show foci of calcification. Diagnosis of neonatal CMV is made by shell-virus culture of urine or oral secretions.

The infants who survive usually have permanent deficits, including mental retardation, hearing loss, and other neurologic impairments. The congenital infection is not always devastating, however, and may take the form of interstitial pneumonitis, hepatitis, or a hematologic disorder. Most infants with this milder form of cytomegalic inclusion disease recover, although a few develop mental retardation later. Uncommonly, a totally asymptomatic infection may be followed months to years later by neurologic sequelae, including delayed-onset mental retardation and deafneas.

Perinatal Infections. Infection acquired during passage through the birth canal or from breast milk is asymptomatic in the vast majority of cases, although, uncommonly, infants may develop an interstitial pneumonitis, failure to thrive, skin rash, or hepatitis. These children have acquired maternal antibodies against CMV, which reduce the severity of disease. Despite the lack of symptoms, many of these people continue to excrete CMV in their urine or saliva for months to years. Subtle effects on hearing and intelligence later in life have been reported in some studies.

Cytomegalovirus Mononucleosis. In healthy young children and adults the disease is nearly always asymptomatic. In surveys around the world, 50% to 100% of adults demonstrate antibodies to CMV in the serum, indicating previous exposure. *The most common clinical manifestation of CMV infection in immunocompetent hosts beyond the neonatal period is an infectious mononucleosis–like illness, with fever, atypical lymphocytosis, lymphadenopathy, and hepatomegaly accompanied by abnormal liver function test results, suggesting mild hepatitis.* The diagnosis is made by serology. Most people recover without any sequelae, although excretion of the virus may occur in body fluids for months to years.

Irrespective of the presence or absence of symptoms, once infected a person becomes seropositive for life. The virus remains latent within leukocytes.

CMV in Immunosuppressed Individuals. Immunocompromised individuals (e.g., transplant recipients, HIV-infected individuals) are susceptible to severe CMV infection. This can be either primary infection or reactivation of latent CMV.

CMV is the most common opportunistic viral pathogen in AIDS. Recipients of solid-organ transplants (heart, liver, kidney) also may contract CMV from the donor organ.

In all these settings, serious, life-threatening disseminated CMV infections primarily affect the lungs (pneumonitis) and gastrointestinal tract (colitis). In the pulmonary infection an interstitial mononuclear infiltrate with foci of necrosis develops, accompanied by the typical enlarged cells with inclusions. The pneumonitis can progress to full-blown acute respiratory distress syndrome. Intestinal necrosis and ulceration can develop and be extensive, leading to the formation of pseudo-membranes and debilitating diarrhea. Diagnosis of CMV infections is made by demonstration of characteristic morphologic alterations in tissue sections, viral culture, rising antiviral antibody titer, detection of CMV antigens, and PCR-based detection of CMV DNA. The antigen- and PCR-based methods have revolutionized the approach to monitoring CMV infection in people after transplantation.

CHRONIC PRODUCTIVE INFECTIONS

In some infections the immune system is unable to eliminate the virus, and continued viral replication leads to persistent viremia. The high mutation rate of viruses such as HIV and HBV may allow them to escape control by the immune system.

Hepatitis B Virus

HBV is a significant cause of acute and chronic liver disease worldwide. Here we will briefly discuss HBV as an example of a chronic productive viral infection; viral hepatitis is discussed in detail in Chapter 18. HBV, a member of the hepadnavirus family, is a DNA virus that can be transmitted percutaneously (e.g., intravenous drug use or blood transfusion), perinatally, and sexually. HBV infects hepatocytes, and cellular injury occurs mainly from the immune response to infected liver cells and not to cytopathic effects of the virus.[56] The effectiveness of the cytotoxic T-lymphocyte (CTL) response is a major determinant of whether a person clears the virus or becomes a chronic carrier. When infected hepatocytes are destroyed by CTLs, replicating virus is also eliminated and the infection is cleared. However, if the rate of infection of hepatocytes outpaces the ability of CTLs to eliminate infected cells, a chronic infection is established. This may happen in about 5% of adults and up to 90% of children infected perinatally. In this setting the liver develops a chronic hepatitis, with lymphocytic inflammation, apoptotic hepatocytes resulting from CTL-mediated killing, and progressive destruction of the liver parenchyma. Long-term viral replication and recurrent immune-mediated liver injury can lead to cirrhosis of the liver and an increased risk for hepatocellular carcinoma. The morphology and pathogenesis of hepatocellular carcinoma and the role of HBV are discussed in Chapter 18. In some infected individuals, hepatocytes are infected but the CTL response is dormant, resulting in the establishment of a "carrier" state, without progressive liver damage.

TRANSFORMING INFECTIONS

This group includes several viruses that have been implicated in the causation of human cancer: EBV, HPV, HBV, and HTLV-1. EBV is discussed here; others are discussed in later chapters.

Epstein-Barr Virus (EBV)

EBV causes *infectious mononucleosis*, a benign, self-limited lymphoproliferative disorder, and is associated with the development of a number of neoplasms, most notably certain lymphomas and nasopharyngeal carcinoma.[57] Infectious mononucleosis is characterized by fever, generalized lymphadenopathy, splenomegaly, sore throat, and the appearance in the blood of atypical activated T lymphocytes (mononucleosis cells). Some people develop hepatitis, meningoencephalitis, and pneumonitis. Infectious mononucleosis occurs principally in late adolescents or young adults among upper socioeconomic classes in developed nations. In the rest of the world, primary infection with EBV occurs in childhood and is usually asymptomatic.

Pathogenesis. EBV is transmitted by close human contact, frequently with the saliva during kissing. An EBV envelope glycoprotein binds to CD21 (CR2), the receptor for the C3d component of complement (Chapter 2), present on B cells.[58] The viral infection begins in nasopharyngeal and oropharyngeal lymphoid tissues, particularly the tonsils (Fig. 8–16). Either through transient infection of epithelium or transcytosis into the submucosa, EBV gains access to submucosal lymphoid tissues. Here, infection of B cells may take one of two forms. In a minority of B cells there is productive infection with lysis of infected cells and release of virions, which may infect other B cells. In most B cells, EBV establishes latent infection. Of note, people with X-linked agammaglobulinemia, who lack B cells, do not become latently infected with EBV or shed virus, suggesting B cells are the main reservoir of latent infection. During latent infection, a small number of EBV genes are expressed and they are involved in the establishment of latency. The gene products include EBNA1, which binds the EBV genome to chromosomes, mediating episomal persistence and maintenance, and EBNA2 and latent membrane protein 1 (LMP1), which drive B-cell activation and proliferation.[59] LMP1 appears to act by binding to TNF receptor–associated factors, and activates signaling pathways that mimic B-cell activation by CD40, which is involved in normal B-cell responses (Chapter 6). EBNA2 stimulates transcription of many host cell genes, including genes that drive cell cycle entry. The activated B cells then disseminate in the circulation and secrete antibodies with several specificities, including the heterophile anti–sheep red blood cell antibodies used for the diagnosis of infectious mononucleosis. Heterophile antibodies bind to antigens that differ from the antigens that induced them. Thus, people with mononucleosis make antibodies that agglutinate sheep or horse red blood cells in the laboratory, but these antibodies do not react with EBV.

The symptoms of infectious mononucleosis appear upon initiation of the host immune response. Cellular immunity mediated by CD8+ cytotoxic T cells and NK cells is the most important component of this response. The *atypical lymphocytes* seen in the blood, so characteristic of this disease, are mainly EBV-specific CD8+ cytotoxic T cells, but also include CD16+ NK cells. The reactive proliferation of T cells is largely centered in lymphoid tissues, which accounts for the lymphadenopathy and splenomegaly. Early in the course of

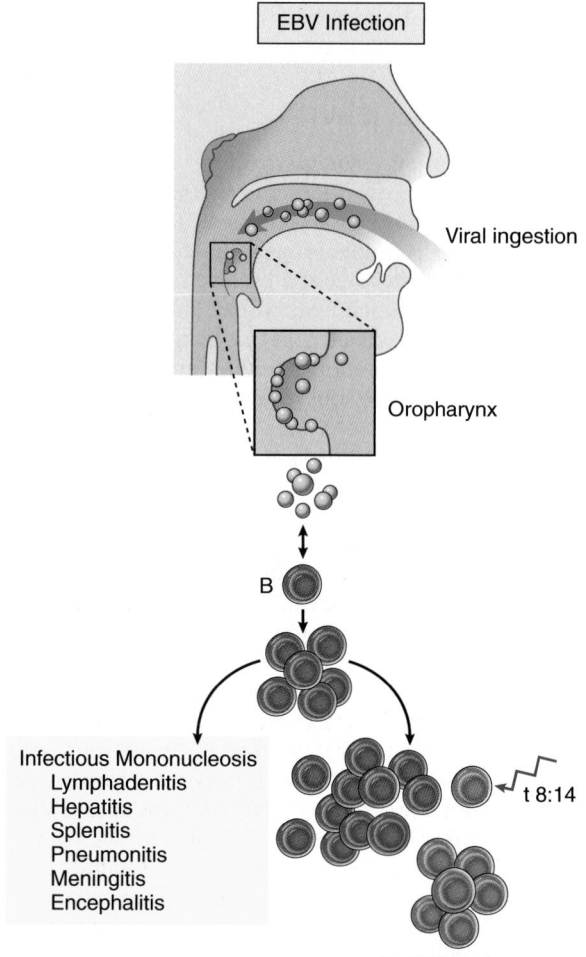

EBV Infection

Viral ingestion

Oropharynx

B

Infectious Mononucleosis
Lymphadenitis
Hepatitis
Splenitis
Pneumonitis
Meningitis
Encephalitis

t 8:14

Burkitt lymphoma

FIGURE 8–16 Outcome of Epstein-Barr virus (EBV) infection. In an individual with normal immune function, infection is usually either asymptomatic or leads to mononucleosis. In the setting of cellular immunodeficiency, the proliferation of infected B cells may be uncontrolled, leading to the development of B-cell neoplasms. In other instances, persons without overt evidence of immunodeficiency develop EBV-positive tumors, which are usually (but not always) also derived from B cells. One secondary genetic event that collaborates with EBV to cause B-cell transformation is a balanced 8;14 chromosomal translocation, which is seen in Burkitt lymphoma. EBV is also implicated in the pathogenesis of nasopharyngeal carcinoma, Hodgkin lymphoma, and certain other rare non-Hodgkin lymphomas.

phoma (Chapter 13), in which a chromosomal translocation (most commonly an 8:14 translocation) involving the c-*myc* oncogene is the critical oncogenic event (see Fig. 8–16).

Morphology. The major alterations involve the blood, lymph nodes, spleen, liver, CNS, and, occasionally, other organs. The **peripheral blood** shows absolute lymphocytosis; more than 60% of white blood cells are lymphocytes. Between 5% and 80% of these are large, **atypical lymphocytes**, 12 to 16 µm in diameter, characterized by an abundant cytoplasm containing multiple clear vacuolations, an oval, indented, or folded nucleus, and scattered cytoplasmic azurophilic granules (Fig. 8–17). These atypical lymphocytes, most of which express CD8, are sufficiently distinctive to strongly suggest the diagnosis.

The **lymph nodes** are typically discrete and enlarged throughout the body, principally in the posterior cervical, axillary, and groin regions. On histologic examination the most striking feature is the expansion of paracortical areas by activated T cells (immunoblasts). A minor population of EBV-infected B cells expressing *EBNA2*, *LMP1*, and other latency-specific genes can also be detected in the paracortex using specific antibodies. Occasionally, EBV-infected B cells resembling Reed-Sternberg cells (the malignant cells of Hodgkin lymphoma, Chapter 13) may be found. B-cell areas (follicles) may also be hyperplastic, but this is usually mild. The T-cell proliferation is sometimes so exuberant that it is difficult to distinguish the nodal morphology from that seen in malignant lymphomas. Similar changes commonly occur in the tonsils and lymphoid tissue of the oropharynx.

The **spleen** is enlarged in most cases, weighing between 300 and 500 gm. It is usually soft and fleshy, with a hyperemic cut surface. The histologic changes are analogous to those of the lymph nodes, showing an expansion of white pulp follicles and red pulp sinusoids due to the presence of numerous activated T cells. These spleens are especially vulnerable to rupture, possibly in part because the rapid increase in size produces a tense, fragile splenic capsule.

the infection, IgM antibodies are formed against viral capsid antigens; later, IgG antibodies are formed that persist for life. In otherwise healthy persons, the fully developed humoral and cellular responses to EBV act as brakes on viral shedding, resulting in the elimination of B cells expressing the full complement of EBV latency–associated genes. However, EBV persists throughout life in a small population of resting B cells in which expression of EBV genes is limited to *EBNA1* and *LMP2*. Cells within this pool are thought to occasionally reactivate expression of the other latency-associated genes, such as *EBNA2* and *LMP1*, causing them to proliferate. In hosts with acquired defects in cellular immunity (e.g., AIDS, organ transplantation), this proliferation can progress through a multistep process to EBV-associated B-cell lymphomas. EBV also contributes to the development of some cases of Burkitt lym-

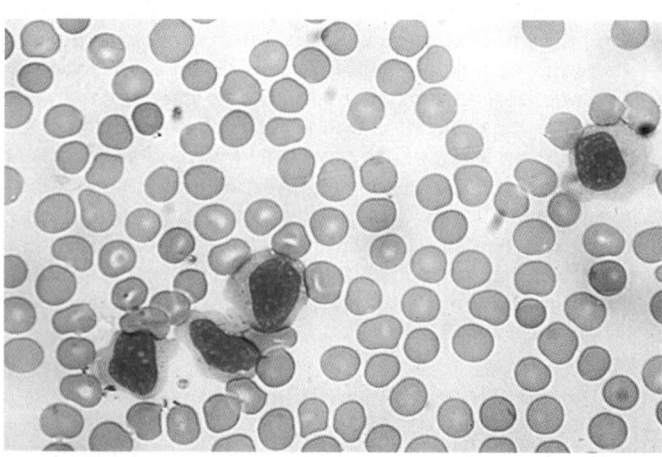

FIGURE 8–17 Atypical lymphocytes in infectious mononucleosis.

The **liver** is usually involved to some degree, although hepatomegaly is at most moderate. On histologic examination, atypical lymphocytes are seen in the portal areas and sinusoids, and scattered, isolated cells or foci of parenchymal necrosis may be present. This histologic picture is similar to that of other forms of viral hepatitis.

Clinical Features. Infectious mononucleosis classically presents with fever, sore throat, lymphadenitis, and the other features mentioned earlier. However, atypical presentations are common, and include malaise, fatigue, and lymphadenopathy, raising the specter of leukemia or lymphoma; a fever of unknown origin without significant lymphadenopathy or other localized findings; hepatitis resembling one of the hepatotropic viral syndromes; or a febrile rash resembling rubella. The diagnosis depends on the following findings (in increasing order of specificity): (1) lymphocytosis with the characteristic atypical lymphocytes in the peripheral blood, (2) a positive heterophile antibody reaction (monospot test), and (3) specific antibodies for EBV antigens (viral capsid antigens, early antigens, or Epstein-Barr nuclear antigen). In most patients, infectious mononucleosis resolves within 4 to 6 weeks, but sometimes the fatigue lasts longer. One or more complications occasionally supervene. Perhaps most common is marked hepatic dysfunction with jaundice, elevated hepatic enzyme levels, disturbed appetite, and rarely even liver failure. Other complications involve the nervous system, kidneys, bone marrow, lungs, eyes, heart, and spleen. Splenic rupture can occur even with minor trauma, leading to hemorrhage that may be fatal. A more serious complication in those suffering from some form of immunodeficiency, such as AIDS, or receiving immunosuppressive therapy (e.g., bone marrow or solid-organ transplant recipients) is B-cell lymphomas. As detailed in Chapter 13, EBV also causes another distinctive form of lymphoma, called *Burkitt lymphoma*, particularly in certain geographic locales.

Unfortunate consequences also occur in individuals suffering from the X-linked lymphoproliferation syndrome (also known as Duncan disease), a disorder caused by a defect in a gene, *SH2D1A*, that is expressed primarily in cytotoxic T cells and NK cells.[60] SH2D1A (also called SAP) participates in a signaling pathway critical for an effective cellular response to EBV-infected B cells. Patients are often normal until they are acutely infected with EBV, often during adolescence. The failure to control EBV infection variously leads to chronic infectious mononucleosis, agammaglobulinemia, and B-cell lymphoma, each of which proves fatal in about a third of patients.

Bacterial Infections

Different classes of bacteria are responsible for diverse infections (Table 8–8).

GRAM-POSITIVE BACTERIAL INFECTIONS

Common gram-positive pathogens include *Staphylococcus*, *Streptococcus*, and *Enterococcus*, each of which causes many types of infections. Four less common diseases caused by gram-positive rod-shaped organisms are also discussed here:

diphtheria, listeriosis, anthrax, and nocardiosis. *Clostridia*, which are gram-positive, are discussed with the anaerobes. All these infections are diagnosed by culture and some special tests mentioned below.

Staphylococcal Infections

Staphylococcus aureus are pyogenic gram-positive cocci that form clusters like bunches of grapes. *These bacteria cause a myriad of skin lesions (boils, carbuncles, impetigo, and scalded-skin syndrome) as well as abscesses, sepsis, osteomyelitis, pneumonia, endocarditis, food poisoning, and toxic shock syndrome (TSS)* (Fig. 8–18). Here we review the general characteristics of *S. aureus* infection. Specific organ infections are described in other chapters. *S. epidermidis*, a species that is related to *S. aureus*, causes opportunistic infections in catheterized patients, patients with prosthetic cardiac valves, and drug addicts. *S. saprophyticus* is a common cause of urinary tract infections in young women.

Pathogenesis. *S. aureus* possess a multitude of virulence factors, which include surface proteins involved in adherence, secreted enzymes that degrade proteins, and secreted toxins that damage host cells.

S. aureus expresses surface receptors for fibrinogen (called clumping factor), fibronectin, and vitronectin, and uses these molecules as a bridge to bind to host endothelial cells.[61] Staphylococci infecting prosthetic valves and catheters have a polysaccharide capsule that allows them to attach to the artificial materials and to resist host cell phagocytosis. The lipase of *S. aureus* degrades lipids on the skin surface, and its expression is correlated with the ability of the bacteria to produce skin abscesses. Staphylococci also have protein A on their surface, which binds the Fc portion of immunoglobulins, allowing the organism to escape antibody-mediated killing.

S. aureus produces multiple membrane-damaging (hemolytic) toxins, including α-toxin, a pore-forming protein that intercalates into the plasma membrane of host cells and depolarizes them[62]; β-toxin, a sphingomyelinase; and δ-toxin, which is a detergent-like peptide. Staphylococcal γ-toxin and leukocidin lyse erythrocytes and phagocytic cells, respectively.

The exfoliative A and B toxins produced by *S. aureus* are serine proteases that cleave the protein desmoglein 1, which is part of the desmosomes that hold epidermal cells tightly together.[25] This causes keratinocytes to detach from one another and the underlying skin, resulting in a loss of barrier function that often leads to secondary skin infections. Exfoliation can occur locally at the site of infection (bullous impetigo) or can be widespread, when secreted toxin causes disseminated loss of the superficial epidermis (staphylococcal scalded-skin syndrome).

Superantigens produced by *S. aureus* cause food poisoning and TSS. TSS came to public attention because of its association with the use of hyperabsorbent tampons, which became colonized with *S. aureus* during use. It is now clear that TSS can be caused by growth of *S. aureus* at many sites, most commonly the vagina and infected surgical sites. TSS is characterized by hypotension (shock), renal failure, coagulopathy, liver disease, respiratory distress, a generalized erythematous rash, and soft tissue necrosis at the site of infection. If not promptly treated, TSS can be fatal. TSS can also be caused by *Streptococcus pyogenes*. As mentioned earlier, bacterial superantigens

TABLE 8–8 Selected Human Bacterial Diseases and Their Pathogens

Clinical or Microbiologic Category	Species	Frequent Disease Presentations
Infections by pyogenic cocci	*Staphylococcus aureus, S. epidermidis* *Streptococcus pyogenes* *Streptococcus pneumoniae* (pneumococcus) *Neisseria meningitidis* (meningococcus) *Neisseria gonorrhoea* (gonococcus)	Abscess, cellulitis, pneumonia, sepsis Pharyngitis, erysipelas, scarlet fever Lobar pneumonia, meningitis Meningitis Gonorrhea

Gram-negative infections	*Escherichia coli,* Klebsiella pneumoniae**
	Enterobacter (Aerobacter) aerogenes*
	Proteus spp. *(P. mirabilis, P. morgagni)**
	Serratia marcescens,* Pseudomonas spp.
	  (P. aeruginosa)*
	Bacteroides spp. *(B. fragilis)*
	Legionella spp. *(L. pneumophila)*
		Urinary tract infection, wound infection,
		  abscess, pneumonia, sepsis, shock,
		  endocarditis
		
		Anaerobic infection
		Legionnaires disease

Contagious childhood bacterial diseases	*Haemophilus influenzae* *Bordetella pertussis* *Corynebacterium diphtheriae*	Meningitis, upper and lower respiratory tract infections Whooping cough Diphtheria
Enteric infections	Enteropathogenic *E. coli, Shigella* spp. *Vibrio cholerae,* *Campylobacter jejuni, C. coli* *Yersinia enterocolitica,* *Salmonella* spp. (1000 strains) *Salmonella typhi*	Invasive or noninvasive gastroenterocolitis Typhoid fever
Clostridial infections	*Clostridium tetani* *Clostridium botulinum* *Clostridium perfringens, C. septicum* *Clostridium difficile**	Tetanus (lockjaw) Botulism (paralytic food poisoning) Gas gangrene, necrotizing cellulitis Pseudomembranous colitis
Zoonotic bacterial infections	*Bacillus anthracis* *Yersinia pestis* *Francisella tularensis* *Brucella melitensis, B. suis, B. abortus* *Borrelia recurrentis* *Borrelia burgdorferi*	Anthrax Bubonic plague Tularemia Brucellosis (undulant fever) Relapsing fever Lyme disease
Human treponemal infections	*Treponema pallidum*	Syphilis
Mycobacterial infections	*Mycobacterium tuberculosis,* M. bovis* *M. leprae* *M. kansasii,* M. avium, M. intracellulare*	Tuberculosis Leprosy Atypical mycobacterial infections
Actinomycetaceae	*Nocardia asteroides** *Actinomyces israelii*	Nocardiosis Actinomycosis

*Important opportunistic infections.

bind to conserved portions of MHC molecules and to relatively conserved portions of T-cell receptor β chains. In this manner superantigens may stimulate up to 20% of T lymphocytes, leading to release of large amounts of cytokines such as TNF and IL-1, which can produce a condition resembling septic shock (Chapter 4). Superantigens produced by *S. aureus* also cause vomiting, presumably by affecting the CNS or the enteric nervous system.[63]

Morphology. Whether the lesion is located in the skin, lungs, bones, or heart valves, *S. aureus* causes pyogenic inflammation that is distinctive for its local destructiveness.

Excluding impetigo, which is a staphylococcal or streptococcal infection restricted to the superficial epidermis, staphylococcal skin infections are centered around the hair follicles. A **furuncle**, or **boil**, is a focal suppurative inflammation of the skin and subcutaneous tissue, either solitary or multiple or recurrent in successive crops. Furuncles are most frequent in moist, hairy areas, such as the face, axillae, groin, legs, and submammary folds. Beginning in a single hair follicle, a boil develops into a growing and deepening abscess that eventually "comes to a head" by thinning and rupturing the overlying skin. A **carbuncle** is a deeper suppurative infection that spreads laterally beneath the deep subcutaneous fascia and then burrows superficially to erupt in multiple adjacent skin sinuses. Carbuncles typically appear beneath the skin of the upper back and posterior neck, where fascial planes favor their spread. **Hidradenitis** is a chronic suppurative infection of apocrine glands,

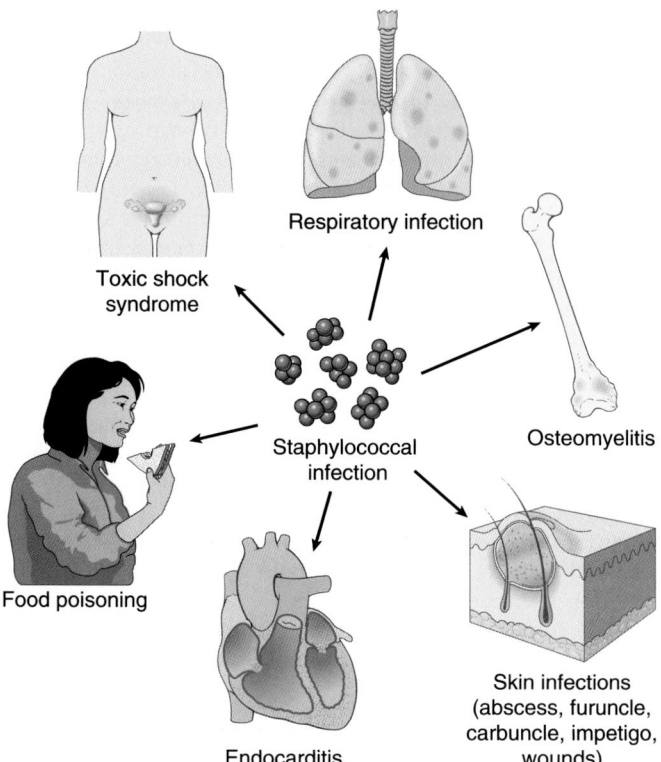

FIGURE 8–18 The many consequences of staphylococcal infection.

care-associated infections, but community-acquired MRSA infections have now become common in many areas.[64] As a result, empiric treatment of staphylococcal infections with beta-lactam antibiotics has become less effective. Community-acquired MRSA commonly produce a potent membrane damaging toxin, which kills leukocytes and may make these strains of *S. aureus* particularly virulent.

Streptococcal and Enterococcal Infections

Streptococci are gram-positive cocci that grow in pairs or chains and cause a myriad of suppurative infections of the skin, oropharynx, lungs, and heart valves. They are also responsible for a number of post-infectious syndromes, including rheumatic fever (Chapter 12), immune complex glomerulonephritis (Chapter 20), and erythema nodosum (Chapter 25). β-hemolytic streptococci are typed according to their surface carbohydrate (Lancefield) antigens. *S. pyogenes* (group A) causes pharyngitis, scarlet fever, erysipelas, impetigo, rheumatic fever, TSS, and glomerulonephritis. *S. agalactiae* (group B) colonizes the female genital tract and causes sepsis and meningitis in neonates and chorioamnionitis in pregnancy. *S. pneumoniae*, the most important α-hemolytic streptococcus, is a common cause of community-acquired pneumonia and meningitis in adults. The viridans group streptococci include several species of α-hemolytic and non-hemolytic streptococci that are normal oral flora and are also a common cause of endocarditis. Finally, *S. mutans* is the major cause of dental caries. Streptococcal infections are diagnosed by culture, and the rapid antigen test for pharyngitis.

Enterococci are also gram-positive cocci that grow in chains. Enterococci are often resistant to commonly used antibiotics and are a significant cause of endocarditis and urinary tract infections.

Pathogenesis. The different species of streptococci produce many virulence factors and toxins. *S. pyogenes*, *S. agalactiae*, and *S. pneumoniae* have capsules that resist phagocytosis. *S. pyogenes* also expresses M protein, a surface protein that prevents bacteria from being phagocytosed, and a complement C5a peptidase, which degrades this chemotactic peptide.[64] *S. pyogenes* secrete a phage-encoded pyrogenic

most often in the axilla. Infections of the nail bed **(paronychia)** or on the palmar side of the fingertips **(felons)** are exquisitely painful. They may follow trauma or embedded splinters and, if deep enough, destroy the bone of the terminal phalanx or detach the fingernail.

Staphylococcal lung infections (Fig. 8–19) have a polymorphonuclear infiltrate similar to that of pneumococcus (Fig. 8–7) but cause much more tissue destruction. *S. aureus* lung infections usually occur in people with a hematogenous source, such as an infected thrombus, or a predisposing condition such as influenza.

Staphylococcal scalded-skin syndrome, also called **Ritter disease**, most frequently occurs in children with staphylococcal infections of the nasopharynx or skin. There is a sunburn-like rash that spreads over the entire body and evolves into fragile bullae that lead to partial or total skin loss. The desquamation of the epidermis in staphylococcal scalded-skin syndrome occurs at the level of the granulosa layer, distinguishing it from toxic epidermal necrolysis, or Lyell's disease, which is secondary to drug hypersensitivity and causes desquamation at the level of the epidermal-dermal junction (Chapter 25).

Antibiotic resistance is a growing problem in treatment of *S. aureus* infections. Methicillin-resistant *S. aureus* (MRSA) are resistant to all currently available beta-lactam cell-wall synthesis inhibitors (which include the penicillins and cephalosporins). Until recently, MRSA was mainly found in health-

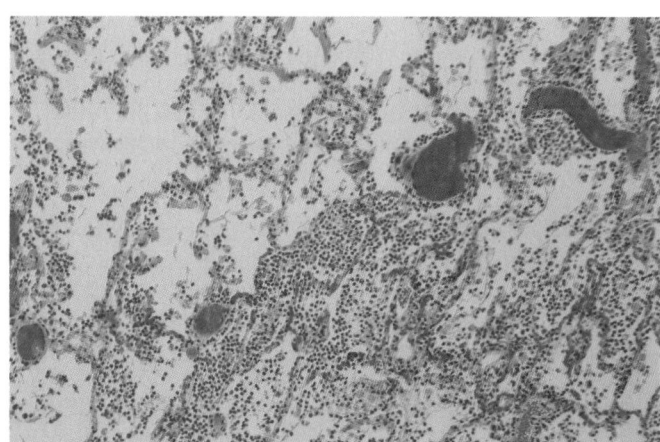

FIGURE 8–19 Staphylococcal abscess of the lung with extensive neutrophilic infiltrate and destruction of the alveoli (contrast with Fig. 8–7).

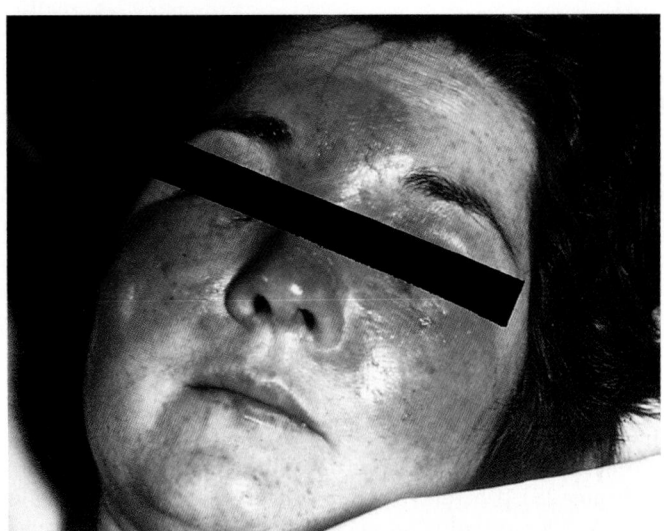

FIGURE 8–20 Streptococcal erysipelas.

exotoxin that causes fever and rash in scarlet fever. Poststreptococcal acute rheumatic fever is probably caused by antistreptococcal M protein antibodies and T cells that cross-react with cardiac proteins.[66] Virulent *S. pyogenes* have been referred to as flesh-eating bacteria because they cause a rapidly progressive necrotizing fasciitis. Pneumolysin is a cytosolic bacterial protein released on disruption of *S. pneumoniae.*[67] Pneumolysin inserts into host cell membranes and lyses them, greatly increasing tissue damage. This toxin also activates the classical pathway of complement, reducing complement available for opsonization of bacteria. *S. mutans* produces caries by metabolizing sucrose to lactic acid (which causes demineralization of tooth enamel) and by secreting high-molecular-weight glucans that promote aggregation of bacteria and plaque formation.

Enterococci have an antiphagocytic capsule and produce enzymes that cleave host tissues, but they are relatively low-virulence bacteria. The emergence of enterococci as pathogens is primarily due to their resistance to antibiotics, including the broad-spectrum antibiotic vancomycin.

Morphology. Streptococcal infections are characterized by diffuse interstitial neutrophilic infiltrates with minimal destruction of host tissues. The skin lesions caused by streptococci (furuncles, carbuncles, and impetigo) resemble those of staphylococci, although streptococci are less likely to cause the formation of discrete abscesses.

Erysipelas is most common among middle-aged persons in warm climates and is caused by exotoxins from superficial infection with *S. pyogenes.* It is characterized by rapidly spreading erythematous cutaneous swelling that may begin on the face or, less frequently, on the body or an extremity. The rash has a sharp, well-demarcated, serpiginous border and may form a "butterfly" distribution on the face (Fig. 8–20). On histologic examination there is a diffuse, edematous, neutrophilic inflammatory reaction in the dermis and epidermis extending into the subcutane-

---

ous tissues. Microabscesses may be formed, but tissue necrosis is usually minor.

Streptococcal pharyngitis, which is the major antecedent of poststreptococcal glomerulonephritis (Chapter 20), is marked by edema, epiglottic swelling, and punctate abscesses of the tonsillar crypts, sometimes accompanied by cervical lymphadenopathy. Swelling associated with severe pharyngeal infection may encroach on the airways, especially if there is peritonsillar or retropharyngeal abscess formation.

Scarlet fever, associated with pharyngitis caused by *S. pyogenes*, is most common between the ages of 3 and 15 years. It is manifested by a punctate erythematous rash that is most prominent over the trunk and inner aspects of the arms and legs. The face is also involved, but usually a small area about the mouth remains relatively unaffected to produce a circumoral pallor. The inflammation of the skin usually leads to hyperkeratosis and scaling during defervescence.

S. pneumoniae is an important cause of lobar pneumonia (described in Chapter 15 and pictured in Fig. 8–7).

Diphtheria

Diphtheria is caused by *Corynebacterium diphtheriae*, a slender gram-positive rod with clubbed ends, that is passed from person to person through aerosols or skin exudate. *C. diphtheriae* may be carried asymptomatically or cause illnesses ranging from skin lesions in neglected wounds of combat troops in the tropics, and a life-threatening syndrome that includes formation of a tough pharyngeal membrane and toxin-mediated damage to the heart, nerves, and other organs. *C. diphtheriae* produces only one toxin, which is a phage-encoded A-B toxin that blocks host cell protein synthesis.[68] The A fragment does this by catalyzing the covalent transfer of adenosine diphosphate (ADP)-ribose to elongation factor-2 (EF-2). This inhibits EF-2 function, which is essential for the translation of mRNA into protein. A single molecule of diphtheria toxin can kill a cell by ADP-ribosylating, and thus inactivating, more than a million EF-2 molecules. Immunization with diphtheria toxoid (formalin-fixed toxin) does not prevent colonization with *C. diphtheriae* but protects immunized people from the lethal effects of the toxin.

Morphology. Inhaled *C. diphtheriae* proliferate at the site of attachment on the mucosa of the nasopharynx, oropharynx, larynx, or trachea but also form satellite lesions in the esophagus or lower airways. Release of exotoxin causes necrosis of the epithelium, accompanied by an outpouring of a dense fibrinosuppurative exudate. The coagulation of this exudate on the ulcerated necrotic surface creates a tough, dirty gray to black, superficial membrane (Fig. 8–21). Neutrophilic infiltration in the underlying tissues is intense and is accompanied by marked vascular congestion, interstitial edema, and fibrin exudation. When the membrane sloughs off its inflamed and vascularized

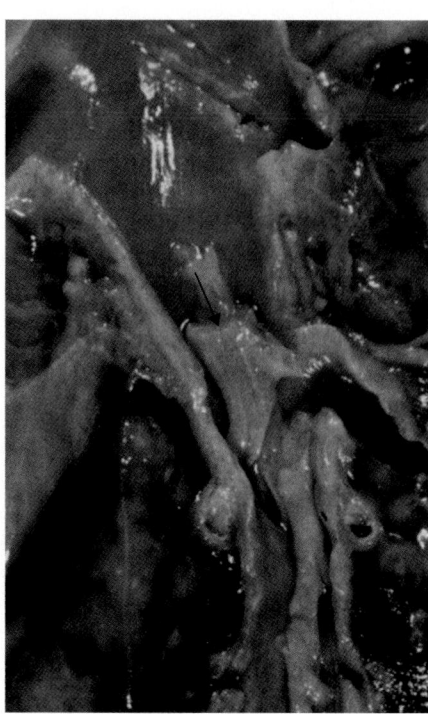

FIGURE 8–21 Membrane of diphtheria *(arrow)* lying within a transverse bronchus.

bed, bleeding and asphyxiation may occur. With control of the infection, the membrane is coughed up or removed by enzymatic digestion, and the inflammatory reaction subsides.

Although the bacterial invasion remains localized, generalized hyperplasia of the spleen and lymph nodes ensues as a result of the entry of soluble exotoxin into the blood. The exotoxin may cause fatty change in the myocardium with isolated myofiber necrosis, polyneuritis with degeneration of the myelin sheaths and axis cylinders, and (less commonly) fatty change and focal necroses of parenchymal cells in the liver, kidneys, and adrenals.

Listeriosis

Listeria monocytogenes is a gram-positive, facultative intracellular bacillus that causes severe food-borne infections. Miniepidemics of *L. monocytogenes* infection have been linked to dairy products, chicken, and hot dogs. Pregnant women, their neonates, the elderly, and immunosuppressed persons (e.g., transplant recipients or AIDS patients) are particularly susceptible to severe *L. monocytogenes* infection. In pregnant women (and pregnant sheep and cattle), *L. monocytogenes* causes an amnionitis that may result in abortion, stillbirth, or neonatal sepsis. In neonates, *L. monocytogenes* may cause disseminated disease (granulomatosis infantiseptica) and an exudative meningitis, both of which are also seen in immunosuppressed adults.

Listeria monocytogenes has leucine-rich proteins on its surface called *internalins*, which bind to E-cadherin on host epithelial cells and induce internalization of the bacterium.[69] Inside the cell, the bacteria escape from the membrane-bound

phagolysosome by the action of a pore-forming protein, listeriolysin O, and two phospholipases.[22] In the host cell cytoplasm, ACTA, a bacterial surface protein, binds to host cell cytoskeletal proteins and induces actin polymerization, which propels the bacteria into adjacent, uninfected host cells. Resting macrophages, which internalize *L. monocytogenes* through C3 activated on the bacterial surface, fail to kill the bacteria. In contrast, macrophages that are activated by IFN-γ phagocytose and kill the bacteria. Hence protection against *L. monocytogenes* is mediated largely by IFN-γ produced by NK cells and T cells.

Morphology. In acute human infections, *L. monocytogenes* evokes an exudative pattern of inflammation with numerous neutrophils. The meningitis it causes is macroscopically and microscopically indistinguishable from that caused by other pyogenic bacteria (Chapter 28). The finding of gram-positive, mostly intracellular, bacilli in the CSF is virtually diagnostic. More varied lesions may be encountered in neonates and immunosuppressed adults. Focal abscesses alternate with grayish or yellow nodules representing necrotic amorphous basophilic tissue debris. These can occur in any organ, including the lung, liver, spleen, and lymph nodes. In infections of longer duration, macrophages appear in large numbers, but granulomas are rare. Infants born with *L. monocytogenes* sepsis often have a papular red rash over the extremities, and listerial abscesses can be seen in the placenta. A smear of the meconium will disclose the gram-positive organisms.

Anthrax

Bacillus anthracis is a large, spore-forming gram-positive rod-shaped bacterium. These bacteria are common pathogens in farm and wild animals that have contact with soil contaminated with *B. anthracis* spores. Anthrax spores can be ground to a fine powder, making a potent biologic weapon. There are between 20,000 and 100,000 cases of anthrax each year, and recent use of the microbe as an agent of bioterrorism has heightened concern about this organism. In 1979, accidental release of *B. anthracis* spores at a military research institute in Russia killed 66 people. In 2001, 22 people in the United States were infected with *B. anthracis*, mostly through spores delivered in the mail.

B. anthracis is typically acquired through exposure to animals or animal products such as wool or hides.[70] There are three major anthrax syndromes.

- *Cutaneous anthrax*, which makes up 95% of naturally occurring infections, begins as a painless, pruritic papule that develops into a vesicle within 2 days. As the vesicle enlarges, striking edema may form around it, and regional lymphadenopathy develops. After the vesicle ruptures, the remaining ulcer becomes covered with a characteristic black eschar, which dries and falls off as the person recovers. Bacteremia is rare with cutaneous anthrax.
- *Inhalational anthrax* occurs when spores are inhaled. The organism is carried by phagocytes to lymph nodes where

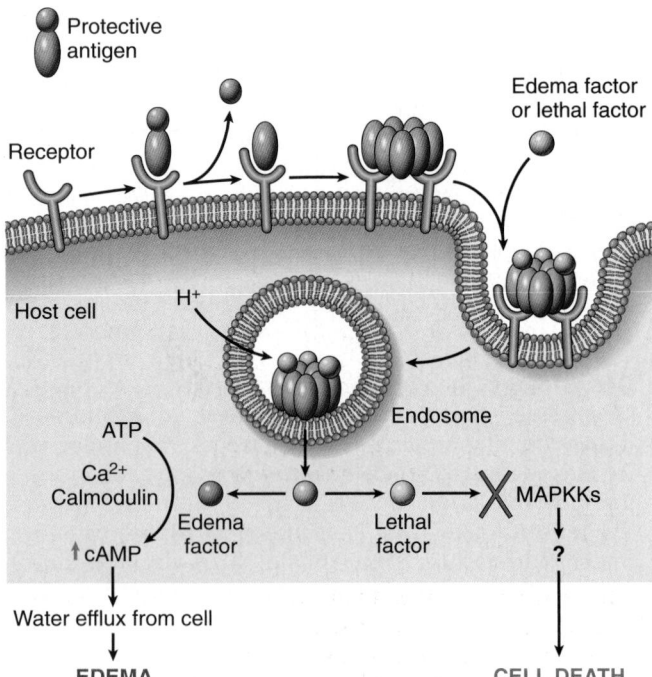

FIGURE 8–22 Mechanism of action of anthrax toxins. (Adapted from Mourez M et al.: 2001: a year of major advances in anthrax toxin research. Trends Microbiol 10:287, 2002.)

the spores germinate, and the release of toxins causes hemorrhagic mediastinitis. After a prodromal illness of 1 to 6 days characterized by fever, cough, and chest or abdominal pain, there is abrupt onset of increased fever, hypoxia, and sweating. Frequently, anthrax meningitis develops from bacteremia. Inhalational anthrax rapidly leads to shock and frequently death within 1 to 2 days.

○ *Gastrointestinal anthrax* is an uncommon form of this infection that is usually contracted by eating undercooked meat contaminated with *B. anthracis*. Initially, the person has nausea, abdominal pain, and vomiting, followed by severe, bloody diarrhea. Mortality is over 50%.

Pathogenesis. *Bacillus anthracis* produces potent toxins and a polyglutamyl capsule that is antiphagocytic. The mode of action of anthrax toxin is well understood[85] (Fig. 8–22). It has A and B subunits. The B subunit is also referred to as the *protective antigen*, because antibodies against this protein protect animals against the toxin. The protective antigen binds to a cell-surface protein, and then a host protease clips off a 20-kD fragment of the B subunit. The remaining 63-kD fragment self-associates to form a heptamer. Anthrax toxin has two alternate A subunits: edema factor (EF) and lethal factor (LF), each named for the effect of the toxin in experimental animals. Three A subunits bind to the B heptamer, and this complex is endocytosed into the host cell. The low pH of the endosome causes a conformational change in the B heptamer, which then forms a selective channel in the endosome membrane through which EF and LF move into the cytoplasm. In the cytoplasm, EF binds to calcium and calmodulin to form an adenylate cyclase. The active EF converts ATP to cyclic adenosine monophosphate (cAMP), an important signaling molecule that stimulates efflux of water from the cell, leading

to interstitial edema. LF has a different mechanism of action. LF is a protease that destroys mitogen-activated protein kinase kinases (MAPKKs). These kinases regulate the activity of MAPKs, which are important regulators of cell growth and differentiation (Chapter 3). The mechanism of cell death due to dysregulation of MAPKs is not understood.

Morphology. Anthrax lesions at any site are typified by necrosis and exudative inflammation with infiltration of neutrophils and macrophages. The presence of large, boxcar-shaped gram-positive extracellular bacteria in chains, seen histopathologically or recovered in culture, should suggest the diagnosis.

Inhalational anthrax causes numerous foci of hemorrhage in the mediastinum with hemorrhagic, enlarged hilar and peribronchial lymph nodes.[72] Microscopic examination of the lungs typically shows a perihilar interstitial pneumonia with infiltration of macrophages and neutrophils and pulmonary vasculitis. Hemorrhagic lesions associated with vasculitis are also present in about half of cases. Mediastinal lymph nodes show lymphocytosis, macrophages with phagocytosed apoptotic lymphocytes, and a fibrin-rich edema (Fig. 8–23). *B. anthracis* is present predominantly in the alveolar capillaries and venules and, to a lesser degree, within the alveolar space. In fatal cases, *B. anthracis* is evident in multiple organs (spleen, liver, intestines, kidneys, adrenal glands, and meninges).

Nocardia

Nocardia are aerobic gram-positive bacteria that grow in distinctive branched chains. In culture, *Nocardia* form thin aerial filaments resembling hyphae. Despite this morphologic similarity to molds, *Nocardia* are true bacteria.

Nocardia are found in soil and cause opportunistic infections in immunocompromised people.[73] *Nocardia asteroides* causes respiratory infections, while other species, mainly *Nocardia brasiliensis*, infect the skin. A fifth of *N. asteroides*

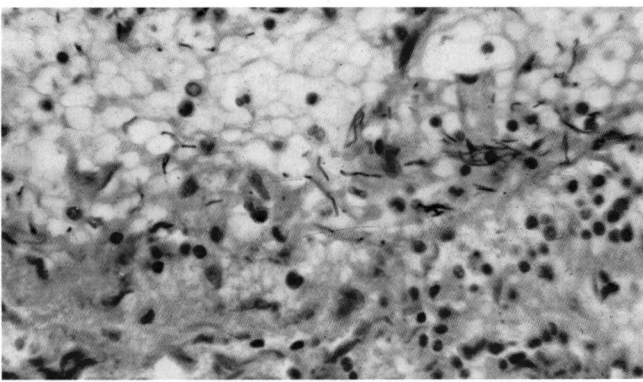

FIGURE 8–23 *Bacillus anthracis* in the subcapsular sinus of a hilar lymph node of a patient who died of inhalational anthrax. (Courtesy of Dr. Lev Grinberg, Department of Pathology, Hospital 40, Ekaterinburg, Russia and Dr. David Walker, UTMB Center for Biodefense and Emerging Infectious Diseases, Galveston, TX.)

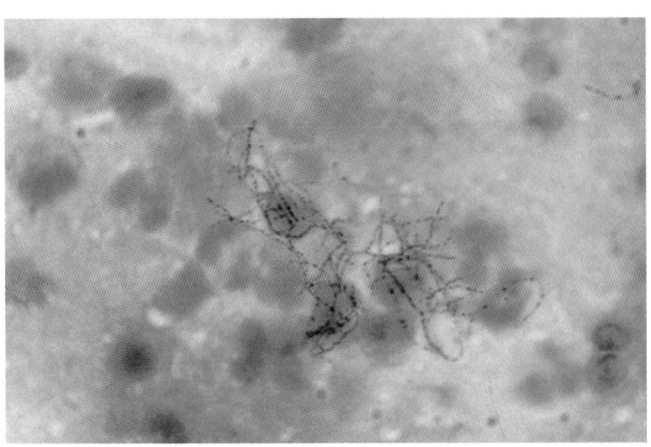

FIGURE 8–24 *Nocardia asteroides* in a Gram-stained sputum sample. Note the beaded, branched gram-positive organisms and leukocytes. (Courtesy of Dr. Ellen Jo Baron, Stanford University Medical Center, Stanford, CA.)

infections involve the CNS, presumably after dissemination from the lungs. Most patients with *N. asteroides* have defects in T cell–mediated immunity, often due to prolonged steroid use or HIV infection, or diabetes mellitus. Respiratory infection with *N. asteroides* causes an indolent illness with fever, weight loss, and cough, which may be mistaken for tuberculosis or malignancy. CNS infections with *N. asteroides* are also indolent and cause varying neurologic deficits depending on the site of the infection. Skin infections have a range of manifestations, from rapidly progressive infections resembling those of *Staphylococcus* or *Streptococcus* to slowly progressive lesions.

> **Morphology.** *Nocardia* appear in tissue as slender gram-positive organisms arranged in branching filaments (Fig. 8–24). Irregular staining gives the filaments a beaded appearance. *Nocardia* stain with modified acid-fast stains (Fite-Faraco stain), unlike *Actinomyces*, which may appear similar on Gram stain of tissue. At any site of infection, *Nocardia* elicit a suppurative response with central liquefaction and surrounding granulation and fibrosis. Granulomas do not form.

GRAM-NEGATIVE BACTERIAL INFECTIONS

Only a few gram-negative bacteria are considered in this section. A number of important gram-negative pathogens are discussed in the appropriate chapters of organ systems, including bacterial causes of gastrointestinal infections and urinary tract infections. Anaerobic gram-negative organisms are considered later in this chapter. Gram-negative bacterial infections are usually diagnosed by culture.

Neisserial Infections

Neisseria are gram-negative diplococci that are flattened on the adjoining sides, giving the pair the shape of a coffee bean (see Fig. 8–3E). These aerobic bacteria have stringent nutritional requirements and grow best on enriched media such as lysed sheep's blood agar ("chocolate" agar). The two clinically significant *Neisseria* are *N. meningitidis* and *N. gonorrhoeae*.

N. meningitidis is a significant cause of bacterial meningitis, particularly among children younger than 2 years of age. The organism is a common colonizer of the oropharynx and is spread by the respiratory route. Approximately 10% of the population is colonized at any one time, and each episode of colonization lasts, on average, for several months. An immune response leads to elimination of the organism in most people, and this response is protective against subsequent disease with the same serotype of bacteria. There are at least 13 serotypes of *N. meningitidis*. Invasive disease mainly occurs when people encounter new strains to which they are not immune, as may happen to young children or young adults living in crowded quarters such as military barracks or college dormitories. *N. meningitidis* disease is endemic in the United States, but epidemics occur periodically in sub-Saharan Africa and cause thousands of deaths.[74]

Even in the absence of pre-existing immunity, only a small fraction of people infected with *N. meningitidis* develop meningitis. The bacteria must invade respiratory epithelial cells and travel to the basolateral side of the cells to enter the blood.[75] In the blood, the capsule of the bacteria inhibits opsonization and destruction of the bacteria by complement proteins. Despite this, the importance of complement as a first-line defense against *N. meningitidis* is shown by the increased rates of serious infection among people who have inherited defects in the complement proteins (C5 to C9) that form the membrane attack complex. If *N. meningitidis* escapes the host response, the consequences can be severe. Although antibiotic treatment of meningitis has greatly reduced mortality of *N. meningitidis* infection, the death rate is still about 10%. The pathology of pyogenic meningitides is discussed in Chapter 28.

N. gonorrhoeae is an important cause of sexually transmitted disease (STD), infecting about 700,000 people each year in the United States. It is second only to *C. trachomatis* as a bacterial causative agent of STDs. Infection in men causes urethritis. In women, *N. gonorrhoeae* infection is often asymptomatic and so may go unnoticed. Untreated infection can lead to pelvic inflammatory disease, which can cause infertility or ectopic pregnancy (Chapter 22). Infection is diagnosed by PCR tests, in addition to culture.

Although *N. gonorrhoeae* infection usually manifests locally in the genital or cervical mucosa, pharynx, or anorectum, disseminated infections may occur. Like *N. meningitidis*, *N. gonorrhoeae* is much more likely to become disseminated in people who lack the complement proteins that form the membrane attack complex. Disseminated infection of adults and adolescents usually causes septic arthritis accompanied by a rash of hemorrhagic papules and pustules. Neonatal *N. gonorrhoeae* infection causes blindness and, rarely, sepsis. The eye infection, which is preventable by instillation of silver nitrate or antibiotics in the newborn's eyes, remains an important cause of blindness in some developing nations.

Pathogenesis. *Neisseria* use antigenic variation as a strategy to escape the immune response. The existence of multiple serotypes of *N. meningitidis* results in meningitis in some people on exposure to a new strain, as discussed above. In addition, *Neisseria* species also generate antigenic variation by special genetic mechanisms, which permit a single bacterial clone to change its expressed antigens (see below) and escape immune defenses.[19] *Neisseria* organisms adhere to and invade nonciliated epithelial cells at the site of entry (nasopharynx, urethra, or cervix). Two surface proteins of *Neisseria*, both of which bind the bacteria to host cells, undergo antigenic variation through different mechanisms. Although both *N. meningitidis* and *N. gonorrhoeae* use these mechanisms, they seem to be more important in *N. gonorrhoeae*.

○ Pili proteins are altered by *genetic recombination*. Adherence of *N. gonorrhoeae* to epithelial cells is initially mediated by long pili, which bind to CD46, a complement-regulatory protein expressed on all human nucleated cells. The pili are composed of polypeptides encoded by the pili gene, which consists of a promoter and coding sequences for 10–15 pili protein variants. At any point in time, only one of these coding sequences is juxtaposed to the promoter, allowing it to be expressed. Periodically, homologous recombination shuttles one of the other coding sequences next to the promoter, resulting in expression of a different pili variant. Sometimes, only part of the second coding sequence is swapped, creating an entirely new chimeric variant.

○ *N. gonorrhoeae* has three or four genes for OPA proteins, and *N. meningitidis* has up to 12. OPA proteins (so named because they make bacterial colonies opaque) are located in the outer membrane of the bacteria. They increase binding of *Neisseria* organisms to epithelial cells and promote entry of bacteria into cells. Each *OPA* gene has several repeats of a five-nucleotide sequence, which are frequently deleted or duplicated. These changes shift the reading frame of the gene so that it encodes new sequences. Stop codons are also introduced by the additions and deletions, which determine whether each *OPA* gene is expressed or silent. This allows *N. gonorrhoeae* to express none, one, or several *OPA* genes at a time.

Whooping Cough

Whooping cough, caused by the gram-negative coccobacillus *Bordetella pertussis*, is an acute, highly communicable illness characterized by paroxysms of violent coughing followed by a loud inspiratory "whoop." *B. pertussis* vaccination, whether with killed bacteria or the newer acellular vaccine, has been effective in preventing whooping cough. Since the 1980s, however, rates of pertussis have been increasing in the United States particularly in adolescents and adults, despite continued high rates of vaccination.[76] The cause of this increase is not known, but antigenic divergence of clinical strains from vaccine strains and waning immunity in young adults may play a role. In parts of the developing world, where vaccination is not widely practiced, pertussis kills hundreds of thousands of children each year. The diagnosis is best made by PCR, because culture is less sensitive.

Pathogenesis. *Bordetella pertussis* colonizes the brush border of the bronchial epithelium and also invades macrophages. Coordinated expression of virulence factors is regulated by the *Bordetella* virulence gene locus *(bvg)*.[77] BVGS is a transmembrane protein that "senses" signals that induce expression of virulence factors. On activation, BVGS phosphorylates the protein BVGA, which regulates transcription of mRNA for adhesins and toxins. The filamentous hemagglu-

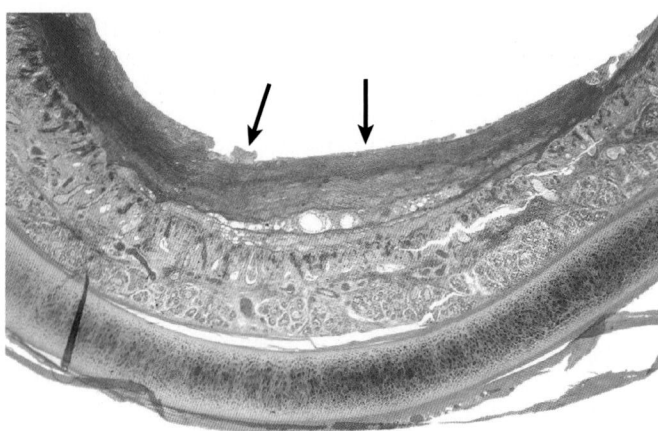

FIGURE 8–25 Whooping cough showing a haze of bacilli *(arrows)* entangled with the cilia of bronchial epithelial cells.

nin adhesin binds to carbohydrates on the surface of respiratory epithelial cells, as well as to CR3 (Mac-1) integrins on macrophages. Pertussis toxin is an exotoxin composed of five distinct proteins, including a catalytic peptide S1 that shows homology with the catalytic peptides of cholera toxin and *E. coli* heat-labile toxin.[78] Like cholera toxin, pertussis toxin ADP-ribosylates and inactivates guanine nucleotide–binding proteins, so these G proteins no longer transduce signals from host plasma membrane receptors. The toxin produced by *B. pertussis* paralyzes the cilia, thus impairing an important pulmonary defense.

> **Morphology.** *Bordetella* bacteria cause a laryngotracheobronchitis that in severe cases features bronchial mucosal erosion, hyperemia, and copious mucopurulent exudate (Fig. 8–25). Unless superinfected, the lung alveoli remain open and intact. In parallel with a striking peripheral lymphocytosis (up to 90%), there is hypercellularity and enlargement of the mucosal lymph follicles and peribronchial lymph nodes.

Pseudomonas Infection

Pseudomonas aeruginosa is an opportunistic aerobic gram-negative bacillus that is a frequent, deadly pathogen of people with cystic fibrosis, severe burns, or neutropenia.[93] Many people with cystic fibrosis die of pulmonary failure secondary to chronic infection with *P. aeruginosa*. *P. aeruginosa* can be very resistant to antibiotics, making these infections difficult to treat. *P. aeruginosa* often infects extensive skin burns, which can be a source of sepsis. *P. aeruginosa* is a common cause of hospital-acquired infections; it has been cultured from washbasins, respirator tubing, nursery cribs, and even antiseptic-containing bottles. *P. aeruginosa* also causes corneal keratitis in wearers of contact lenses, endocarditis and osteomyelitis in intravenous drug abusers, external otitis (swimmer's ear) in healthy individuals, and severe external otitis in diabetics.

Pathogenesis. *P. aeruginosa* has pili and adherence proteins that bind to epithelial cells and lung mucin, and expresses an endotoxin that causes the symptoms and signs of gram-negative sepsis. *Pseudomonas* also has a number of distinctive virulence factors. In the lungs of people with cystic fibrosis, these bacteria secrete a mucoid exopolysaccharide called *alginate*, forming a slimy biofilm that protects bacteria from antibodies, complement, phagocytes, and antibiotics. The organisms also secrete an exotoxin and several other virulence factors. Exotoxin A, like diphtheria toxin, inhibits protein synthesis by ADP-ribosylating the ribosomal protein EF-2.[80] *P. aeruginosa* also releases exoenzyme S, which ADP-ribosylates RAS and other G proteins that regulate cell growth and metabolism. The organisms also secrete a phospholipase C that lyses red cells and degrades pulmonary surfactant, and an elastase that degrades IgGs and extracellular matrix proteins. These enzymes may be important in tissue invasion and destruction of the cornea in keratitis. Finally, *P. aeruginosa* produces iron-containing compounds that are extremely toxic to endothelial cells and so may cause the vascular lesions that are characteristic of this infection.[81]

> **Morphology.** *Pseudomonas* causes a **necrotizing pneumonia** that is distributed through the terminal airways in a fleur-de-lis pattern, with striking pale necrotic centers and red, hemorrhagic peripheral areas. On microscopic examination, masses of organisms cloud the tissue with a bluish haze, concentrating in the walls of blood vessels, where host cells undergo coagulative necrosis (Fig. 8–26). This picture of gram-negative vasculitis accompanied by thrombosis and hemorrhage, although not pathognomonic, is highly suggestive of *P. aeruginosa* infection.
>
> Bronchial obstruction caused by mucus plugging and subsequent *P. aeruginosa* infection are frequent complications of cystic fibrosis. Despite antibiotic treatment and the host immune response, chronic *P. aeruginosa* infection may result in bronchiectasis and pulmonary fibrosis (Chapter 15).
>
> In skin burns, *P. aeruginosa* proliferates widely, penetrating deeply into the veins and spreading hematogenously. Well-demarcated necrotic and hemorrhagic oval skin lesions, called **ecthyma gangreno-sum**, often appear. Disseminated intravascular coagulation (DIC) is a frequent complication of bacteremia.

Plague

Yersinia pestis is a gram-negative facultative intracellular bacterium that is transmitted from rodents to humans by fleabites or, less often, from one human to another by aerosols. It causes an invasive, frequently fatal infection called *plague*. Plague, also named Black Death, caused three great pandemics that killed an estimated 100 million people in Egypt and Byzantium in the sixth century; one quarter of Europe's population in the fourteenth and fifteenth centuries; and tens of millions in India, Myanmar, and China at the beginning of the twentieth century. Currently, 1000 to 3000 cases of plague occur each year worldwide. Wild rodents in the rural western United States are infected with *Y. pestis*, and 10 to 15 human cases occur per year. *Y. enterocolitica* and *Y. pseudotuberculosis* are genetically similar to *Y. pestis*; these bacteria cause fecal-orally transmitted ileitis and mesenteric lymphadenitis.

Pathogenic *Yersinia* proliferate within lymphoid tissue. These organisms have a complex of genes, called the Yop virulon, which enable the bacteria to kill host phagocytes.[82] The Yop virulon encodes proteins that assemble into a type III secretion system, which is a hollow syringe-like structure that projects from the bacterial surface, binds to host cells, and injects bacterial toxins, called Yops (Yersinia outercoat proteins), into the cell. YopE, YopH, and YopT block phagocytosis by inactivating molecules that regulate actin polymerization. YopJ inhibits the signaling pathways that are activated by LPS, blocking the production of inflammatory cytokines. *Y. pestis* ensures its own spread by forming a biofilm that obstructs the gut of the infected flea. The flea must regurgitate before it feeds, and thus infects the rodent or human that it is biting.

> **Morphology.** *Yersinia pestis* causes lymph node enlargement (buboes), pneumonia, or sepsis with a striking neutrophilia. The distinctive histologic features include (1) massive proliferation of the organisms, (2) early appearance of protein-rich and polysaccharide-rich effusions with few inflammatory cells but with marked tissue swelling, (3) necrosis of tissues and blood vessels with hemorrhage and thrombosis, and (4) neutrophilic infiltrates that accumulate adjacent to necrotic areas as healing begins.
>
> In **bubonic plague** the infected fleabite is usually on the legs and is marked by a small pustule or ulcer. The draining lymph nodes enlarge dramatically within a few days and become soft, pulpy, and plum colored, and may infarct or rupture through the skin. In **pneumonic plague** there is a severe, confluent, hemorrhagic and necrotizing bronchopneumonia, often with fibrinous pleuritis. In **septicemic plague** lymph nodes throughout the body as well as organs rich in mononuclear phagocytes develop foci of necrosis. Fulminant bacteremias also induce DIC with widespread hemorrhages and thrombi.

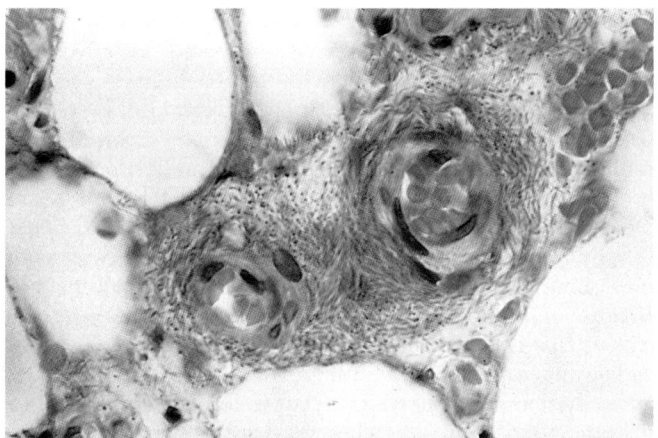

FIGURE 8–26 *Pseudomonas* vasculitis in which masses of organisms form a perivascular blue haze.

Chancroid (Soft Chancre)

Chancroid is an acute, sexually transmitted, ulcerative infection caused by *Hemophilus ducreyi*.[83] The disease is most common in tropical and subtropical areas among lower socio-economic groups and men who have regular contact with prostitutes. *Chancroid is one of the most common causes of genital ulcers in Africa and Southeast Asia*, where it probably serves as an important cofactor in the transmission of HIV infection. Chancroid is uncommon in the United States, with 20 to 50 cases per year reported to the CDC in the past several years. The organism must be cultured in special conditions and PCR-based tests are not widely available, so chancroid may be underdiagnosed.

Morphology. Four to seven days after inoculation the person develops a tender, erythematous papule involving the external genitalia. In males the primary lesion is usually on the penis; in females most lesions occur in the vagina or the periurethral area. Over the course of several days the surface of the primary lesion erodes to produce an irregular ulcer, which is more apt to be painful in males than in females. In contrast to the primary chancre of syphilis, the ulcer of chancroid is not indurated, and multiple lesions may be present. The base of the ulcer is covered by shaggy, yellow-gray exudate. The regional lymph nodes, particularly in the inguinal region, become enlarged and tender in about 50% of cases within 1 to 2 weeks of the primary inoculation. In untreated cases the inflamed and enlarged nodes (buboes) may erode the overlying skin to produce chronic, draining ulcers.

Microscopically, the ulcer of chancroid contains a superficial zone of neutrophilic debris and fibrin, with an underlying zone of granulation tissue containing areas of necrosis and thrombosed vessels. A dense, lymphoplasmacytic inflammatory infiltrate is present beneath the layer of granulation tissue. Coccobacilli are sometimes demonstrable in Gram or silver stains, but they are often obscured by other bacteria that colonize the ulcer base.

Granuloma Inguinale

Granuloma inguinale, or donovanosis, is a chronic inflammatory disease caused by *Klebsiella granulomatis* (formerly called *Calymmatobacterium donovani*), a minute, encapsulated, coccobacillus. The organism is sexually transmitted. Granuloma inguinale is uncommon in the United States and western Europe but is endemic in rural areas in certain tropical and subtropical regions. Untreated cases are characterized by the development of extensive scarring, often associated with lymphatic obstruction and lymphedema (elephantiasis) of the external genitalia. Culture of the organism is difficult, and PCR assays are still in development, so the diagnosis is made by microscopic examination of smears or biopsy samples of the ulcer.

Morphology. Granuloma inguinale begins as a raised, papular lesion on the moist, stratified squamous epithelium of the genitalia or, rarely, the oral mucosa or pharynx. The lesion eventually ulcerates and develops abundant granulation tissue, which is manifested grossly as a protuberant, soft, painless mass. As the lesion enlarges, its borders become raised and indurated. Disfiguring scars may develop in untreated cases and are sometimes associated with urethral, vulvar, or anal strictures. Regional lymph nodes typically are spared or show only nonspecific reactive changes, in contrast to chancroid.

Microscopic examination of active lesions reveals marked epithelial hyperplasia at the borders of the ulcer, sometimes mimicking carcinoma **(pseudoepitheliomatous hyperplasia)**. A mixture of neutrophils and mononuclear inflammatory cells is present at the base of the ulcer and beneath the surrounding epithelium. The organisms are demonstrable in Giemsa-stained smears of the exudate as minute, encapsulated coccobacilli (Donovan bodies) in macrophages. Silver stains (e.g., the Warthin-Starry stain) may also be used to demonstrate the organism.

MYCOBACTERIA

Bacteria in the genus *Mycobacterium* are slender, aerobic rods that grow in straight or branching chains. Mycobacteria have a unique waxy cell wall composed of mycolic acid, which makes them *acid fast*, meaning they will retain stains even on treatment with a mixture of acid and alcohol. Mycobacteria are weakly Gram positive.

Tuberculosis

Mycobacterium tuberculosis is responsible for most cases of tuberculosis; the reservoir of infection is humans with active tuberculosis. Oropharyngeal and intestinal tuberculosis contracted by drinking milk contaminated with *M. bovis* is rare in countries where milk is routinely pasteurized, but it is still seen in countries that have tuberculous dairy cows and unpasteurized milk.

Epidemiology. Tuberculosis is estimated to affect 1.7 billion individuals worldwide, with 8 to 10 million new cases and 1.6 million deaths each year, a toll second only to HIV disease. Infection with HIV makes people susceptible to rapidly progressive tuberculosis; over 10 million people are infected with both HIV and *M. tuberculosis*. From 1985 to 1992, the number of tuberculosis cases in the United States rose by 20% because of increase in the disease in people with HIV, immigrants, and those in jail or homeless shelters. Because of public health efforts, the number of cases of tuberculosis has declined since 1993. Currently, there are about 14,000 new cases of active tuberculosis in the United States annually, about half of which occur in foreign-born people.

Tuberculosis flourishes wherever there is poverty, crowding, and chronic debilitating illness. In the United States tuberculosis is mainly a disease of the elderly, the urban poor, and people with AIDS. *Certain disease states also increase the risk*: diabetes mellitus, Hodgkin lymphoma, chronic lung disease (particularly silicosis), chronic renal failure, malnutrition, alcoholism, and immunosuppression.

It is important that *infection* with *M. tuberculosis* be differentiated from *disease*. Infection is the presence of organisms, which may or may not cause clinically significant disease. Most infections are acquired by person-to-person transmission of airborne organisms from an active case to a susceptible host. In most people primary tuberculosis is asymptomatic, although it may cause fever and pleural effusion. Generally, the only evidence of infection, if any remains, is a tiny, fibrocalcific nodule at the site of the infection. Viable organisms may remain dormant in such lesions for decades. If immune defenses are lowered, the infection may reactivate to produce communicable and potentially life-threatening disease.

Infection typically leads to the development of delayed hypersensitivity to *M. tuberculosis* antigens, which can be detected by the tuberculin (Mantoux) skin test. About 2 to 4 weeks after infection, intracutaneous injection of purified protein derivative of *M. tuberculosis* induces a visible and palpable induration that peaks in 48 to 72 hours. *A positive tuberculin test result signifies T cell–mediated immunity to mycobacterial antigens.* It does not differentiate between infection and disease. False-negative reactions may occur in the setting of certain viral infections, sarcoidosis, malnutrition, Hodgkin lymphoma, immunosuppression, and (notably) overwhelming active tuberculous disease. False-positive reactions may result from infection by atypical mycobacteria or prior vaccination with BCG (*Bacillus Calmette-Guerin*), an attenuated strain of *M. bovis* that is used as a vaccine in some countries.

Pathogenesis. The pathogenesis of tuberculosis in a previously unexposed, immunocompetent person depends on the development of anti-mycobacterial cell-mediated immunity, which confers resistance to the bacteria and also results in development of hypersensitivity to mycobacterial antigens. The pathologic manifestations of tuberculosis, such as caseating granulomas and cavitation, are the result of the hypersensitivity that develops in concert with the protective host immune response. Because the effector cells that mediate immune protection also mediate hypersensitivity and tissue destruction, the appearance of hypersensitivity also signals the acquisition of immunity to the organism. A summary of the pathogenesis of tuberculosis is shown in Figure 8–27.

A. PRIMARY PULMONARY TUBERCULOSIS (0–3 weeks)

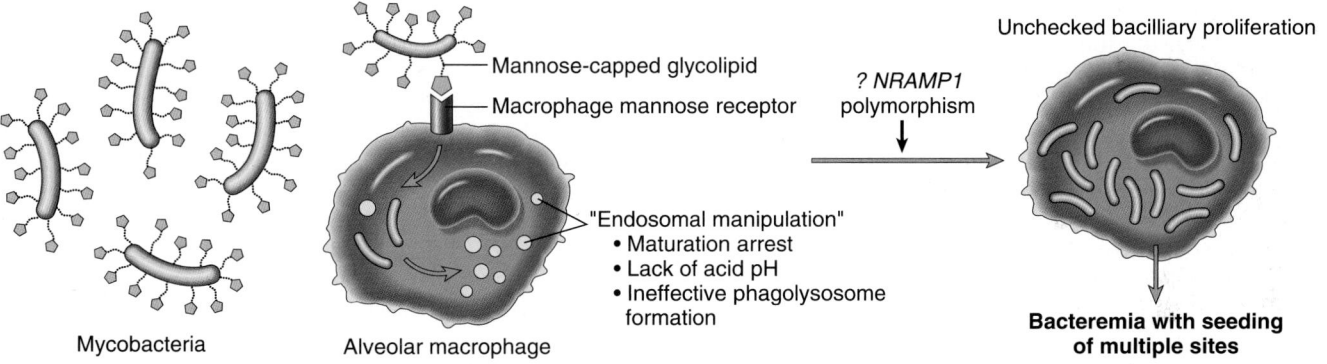

B. PRIMARY PULMONARY TUBERCULOSIS (>3 weeks)

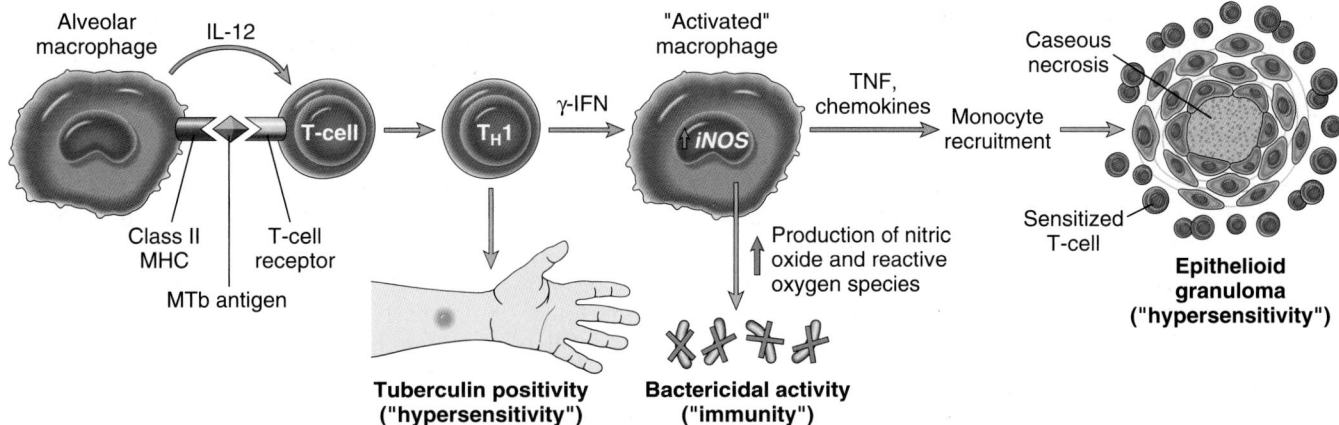

FIGURE 8–27 The sequence of events in primary pulmonary tuberculosis, commencing with inhalation of virulent *Mycobacterium tuberculosis* organisms and culminating with the development of cell-mediated immunity to the organism. **A,** Events occurring in the first 3 weeks after exposure. **B,** Events thereafter. The development of resistance to the organism is accompanied by the appearance of a positive tuberculin test. γ-IFN, interferon-γ; iNOS, inducible nitric oxide synthase; MHC, major histocompatibility complex; MTB, *M. tuberculosis*; NRAMP1, natural resistance–associated macrophage protein; TNF, tumor necrosis factor.

Macrophages are the primary cells infected by *M. tuberculosis*. Early in infection, tuberculosis bacilli replicate essentially unchecked, while later in infection, the cell response stimulates macrophages to contain the proliferation of the bacteria.

- *M. tuberculosis* enters macrophages by endocytosis mediated by several macrophage receptors: mannose receptors bind lipoarabinomannan, a glycolipid in the bacterial cell wall, and complement receptors (already discussed) bind opsonized mycobacteria.[23]
- Once inside the macrophage, *M. tuberculosis* organisms replicate within the phagosome by blocking fusion of the phagosome and lysosome. *M. tuberculosis* blocks phagolysosome formation by inhbiting Ca^{2+} signals and the recruitment and assembly of the proteins that mediate phagosome-lysosome fusion.[84] Thus, during the earliest stage of primary tuberculosis (<3 weeks) in the nonsensitized individual, bacteria proliferate in the pulmonary alveolar macrophages and airspaces, resulting in bacteremia and seeding of multiple sites. *Despite the bacteremia, most people at this stage are asymptomatic or have a mild flulike illness.*
- The genetic makeup of the host may influence the course of the disease. In some people with polymorphisms in the *NRAMP1* gene, the disease may progress due to the absence of an effective immune response. NRAMP1 is a transmembrane protein found in endosomes and lysosomes that pumps divalent cations (e.g. Fe^{2+}) out of the lysosome. NRAMP1 may inhibit microbial growth by limiting availability of ions needed by the bacteria.[85]
- About 3 weeks after infection, a T-helper 1 (T_H1) response is mounted that activates macrophages to become bactericidal.[86] The response is initiated by mycobacterial antigens that enter draining lymph nodes and are displayed to T cells. Differentiation of T_H1 cells depends on IL-12, which is produced by antigen-presenting cells that have encountered the mycobacteria. *M. tuberculosis* makes several molecules that are ligands for TLR2, and stimulation of TLR2 by these ligands promotes production of IL-12 by dendritic cells.
- Mature T_H1 cells, both in lymph nodes and in the lung, produce IFN-γ. *INF-γ is the critical mediator that enables macrophages to contain the M. tuberculosis infection.* IFN-γ stimulates formation of the phagolysosome in infected macrophages, exposing the bacteria to an inhospitable acidic environment. IFN-γ also stimulates expression of inducible nitric oxide synthase, which produces nitric oxide, capable of destroying several mycobacterial constituents, from cell wall to DNA.
- In addition to stimulating macrophages to kill mycobacteria, the T_H1 response orchestrates the formation of granulomas and caseous necrosis. Macrophages activated by IFN-γ differentiate into the "epithelioid histiocytes" that characterize the granulomatous response, and may fuse to form giant cells. In many people this response halts the infection before significant tissue destruction or illness. In other people the infection progresses due to advanced age or immunosuppression, and the ongoing immune response results in tissue destruction due to caseation and cavitation. Activated macrophages also secrete TNF, which promotes recruitment of more monocytes. The importance of TNF is underscored by the fact that patients with rheumatoid arthritis who are treated with a TNF antagonist have an increased risk of tuberculosis reactivation.
- In addition to the T_H1 response, NK-T cells that recognize mycobacterial lipid antigens bound to CD1 on antigen-presenting cells, or T cells that express a γδ T-cell receptor, also make IFN-γ. However, it is clear that T_H1 cells have a central role in this process, since defects in any of the steps in generating a T_H1 response result in absence of resistance and disease progression.

In summary, immunity to *M. tuberculosis* is primarily mediated by T_H1 cells, which stimulate macrophages to kill the bacteria. This immune response, while largely effective, comes at the cost of hypersensitivity and accompanying tissue destruction. Reactivation of the infection or re-exposure to the bacilli in a previously sensitized host results in rapid mobilization of a defensive reaction but also increased tissue necrosis. Just as hypersensitivity and resistance are correlated, so, too, the loss of hypersensitivity (indicated by tuberculin negativity in a previously tuberculin-positive individual) may be an ominous sign that resistance to the organism has faded.

Clinical Features of Tuberculosis. The many clinicalpathologic patterns of tuberculosis are shown in Figure 8–28. *Primary tuberculosis is the form of disease that develops in a previously unexposed, and therefore unsensitized, person.* About 5% of newly infected people develop clinically significant disease. The elderly and profoundly immunosuppressed persons may lose their immunity to *M. tuberculosis* and so may develop primary tuberculosis more than once. With primary tuberculosis the source of the organism is exogenous.

In most people, the primary infection is contained, but in others, primary tuberculosis is progressive. The diagnosis of progressive primary tuberculosis in adults can be difficult. In contrast to secondary tuberculosis (apical disease with cavitation; see below), progressive primary tuberculosis more often resembles an acute bacterial pneumonia, with lower and middle lobe consolidation, hilar adenopathy, and pleural effusion; cavitation is rare, especially in people with severe immunosuppression. Lymphohematogenous dissemination may result in the development of *tuberculous meningitis* and *miliary tuberculosis* (discussed below).

Secondary tuberculosis is the pattern of disease that arises in a previously sensitized host. It may follow shortly after primary tuberculosis, but more commonly it appears many years after the initial infection, usually when host resistance is weakened. It most commonly stems from reactivation of a latent infection, but may also result from exogenous reinfection in the face of waning host immunity or when a large inoculum of virulent bacilli overwhelms the host immune system. Reactivation is more common in low-prevalence areas, while reinfection plays an important role in regions of high contagion.

Secondary pulmonary tuberculosis classically involves the apex of the upper lobes of one or both lungs. Because of the pre-existence of hypersensitivity, the bacilli elicit a prompt and marked tissue response that tends to wall off the focus of infection. As a result, the regional lymph nodes are less prominently involved early in secondary disease than they are in primary tuberculosis. On the other hand, cavitation occurs readily in the secondary form. Indeed, cavitation is almost inevitable in neglected secondary tuberculosis, and erosion of

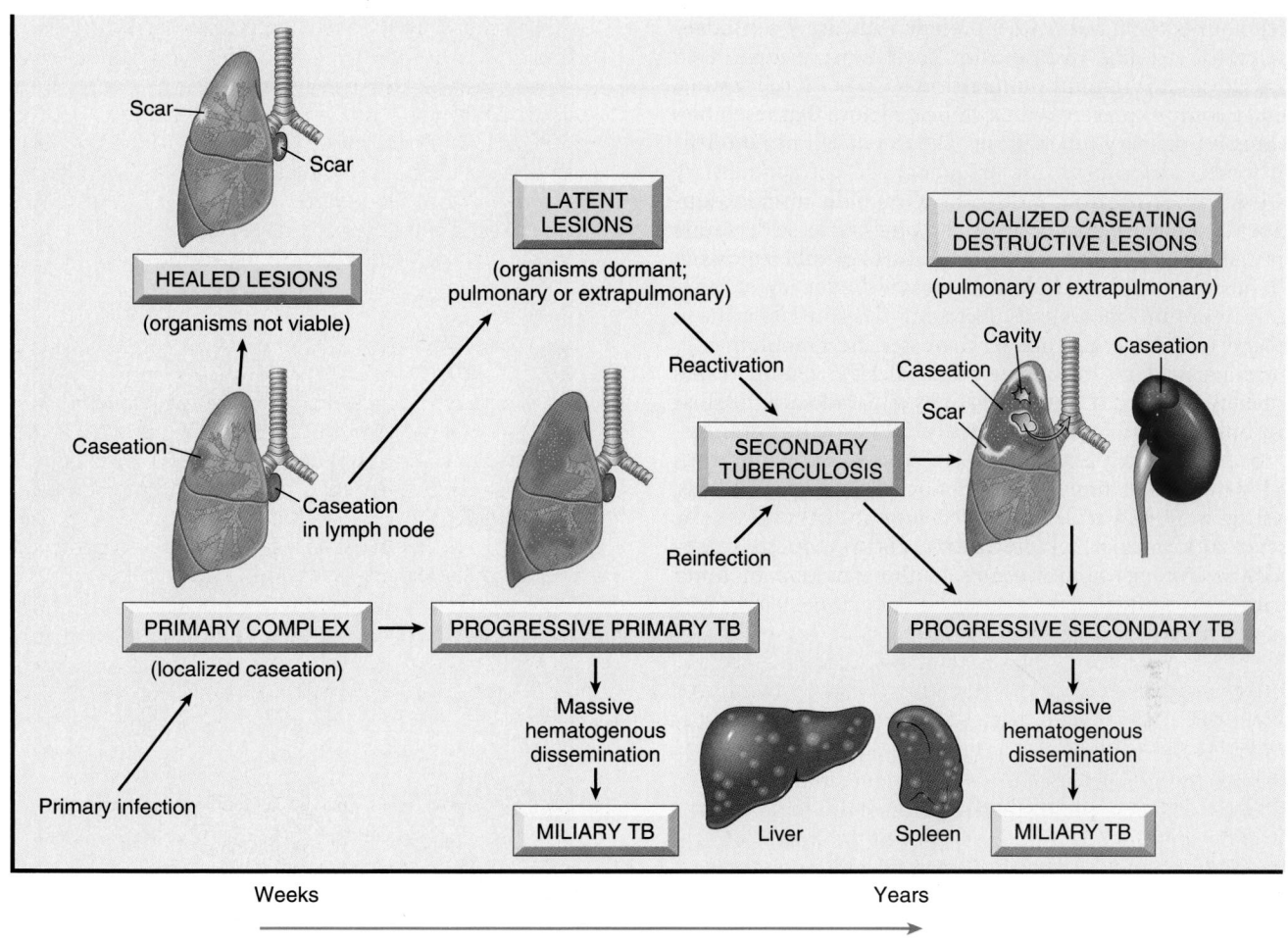

FIGURE 8–28 The natural history and spectrum of tuberculosis. (Adapted from a sketch provided by Professor R.K. Kumar, The University of New South Wales, School of Pathology, Sydney, Australia.)

the cavities into an airway is an important source of infection because the person now coughs sputum that contains bacteria.

Localized secondary tuberculosis may be asymptomatic. When manifestations appear, they are usually *insidious* in onset. Systemic symptoms, probably related to cytokines released by activated macrophages (e.g., TNF and IL-1), often appear early in the course and include malaise, anorexia, weight loss, and fever. Commonly, the *fever is low grade* and remittent (appearing late each afternoon and then subsiding), and *night sweats* occur. With progressive pulmonary involvement, increasing amounts of sputum, at first mucoid and later purulent, appear. Some degree of *hemoptysis* is present in about half of all cases of pulmonary tuberculosis. *Pleuritic pain* may result from extension of the infection to the pleural surfaces. Extrapulmonary manifestations of tuberculosis are legion and depend on the organ system involved.

The diagnosis of pulmonary disease is based in part on the history and on physical and radiographic findings of consolidation or cavitation in the apices of *the lungs*. Ultimately, however, *tubercle bacilli must be identified*. Acid-fast smears and cultures of the sputum of patients suspected of having tuberculosis should be performed. Conventional cultures require up to 10 weeks, but culture in liquid media can provide

an answer within 2 weeks. PCR amplification of *M. tuberculosis* DNA allows for even more rapid diagnosis. PCR assays can detect as few as 10 organisms in clinical specimens, compared with more than 10,000 organisms required for smear positivity. However, culture remains the gold standard because it also allows testing of drug susceptibility. Multidrug resistance is now seen more commonly than it was in past years; hence, all newly diagnosed cases in the United States are assumed to be resistant and are treated with multiple drugs. The prognosis is generally good if infections are localized to the lungs, except when they are caused by drug-resistant strains or occur in aged, debilitated, or immunosuppressed individuals, who are at high risk for developing miliary tuberculosis (see below).

All stages of HIV infection are associated with an increased risk of tuberculosis. The use of highly active antiretroviral therapy (HAART) reduces the risk of tuberculosis in people with HIV infection, but even with HAART, people infected with HIV are more likely to get tuberculosis than the uninfected. A low CD4 count before starting HAART is an important risk factor for development of tuberculosis, which underscores the role of the immune response in keeping reactivation of *M. tuberculosis* in check. The manifestations of tuberculosis differ depending on the degree of immunosuppression. People with less severe immunosuppression (CD4+

T-cell counts >300 cells/mm³) present with usual secondary tuberculosis (apical disease with cavitation). People with more advanced immunosuppression (CD4+ T-cell counts <200 cells/mm³) present with a clinical picture that resembles progressive primary tuberculosis. The extent of immunodeficiency also determines the frequency of extrapulmonary involvement, rising from 10% to 15% in mildly immunosuppressed people to greater than 50% in those with severe immune deficiency. Other atypical features of tuberculosis in HIV-positive people include an increased frequency of false-negative sputum smears and tuberculin tests (the latter due to "anergy"), and the absence of characteristic granulomas in tissues, particularly in the late stages of HIV. The increased frequency of sputum smear-negativity is paradoxical because these immunosuppressed patients typically have higher bacterial loads. The likely explanation is that cavitation and bronchial damage are more in immunocompetent individuals, resulting in more bacilli in expelled sputum. In contrast, the absence of bronchial wall destruction due to reduced T-cell–mediated hypersensitivity results in the excretion of fewer bacilli in the sputum.

Morphology.

Primary Tuberculosis. In countries where infected milk has been eliminated, primary tuberculosis almost always begins in the lungs. Typically, the inhaled bacilli implant in the distal airspaces of the lower part of the upper lobe or the upper part of the lower lobe, usually close to the pleura. As sensitization develops, a 1- to 1.5-cm area of gray-white inflammation with consolidation emerges, known as the Ghon focus. In most cases, the center of this focus undergoes caseous necrosis. Tubercle bacilli, either free or within phagocytes, drain to the regional nodes, which also often caseate. This combination of parenchymal lung lesion and nodal involvement is referred to as the Ghon complex (Fig. 8–29). During the first few weeks there is also lymphatic and hematogenous dissemination to other parts of the body. In approximately 95% of cases, development of cell-mediated immunity controls the infection. Hence, the Ghon complex undergoes progressive fibrosis, often followed by radiologically detectable calcification (Ranke complex), and despite seeding of other organs, no lesions develop.

Histologically, sites of active involvement are marked by a characteristic granulomatous inflammatory reaction that forms both caseating and noncaseating tubercles (Fig. 8–30A to C). Individual tubercles are microscopic; it is only when multiple granulomas coalesce that they become macroscopically visible. The granulomas are usually enclosed within a fibroblastic rim punctuated by lymphocytes. Multinucleate giant cells are present in the granulomas. Immunocompromised people do not form the characteristic granulomas (Fig. 8–30D).

Secondary Tuberculosis. The initial lesion is usually a small focus of consolidation, less than 2 cm in diameter, within 1 to 2 cm of the apical pleura. Such

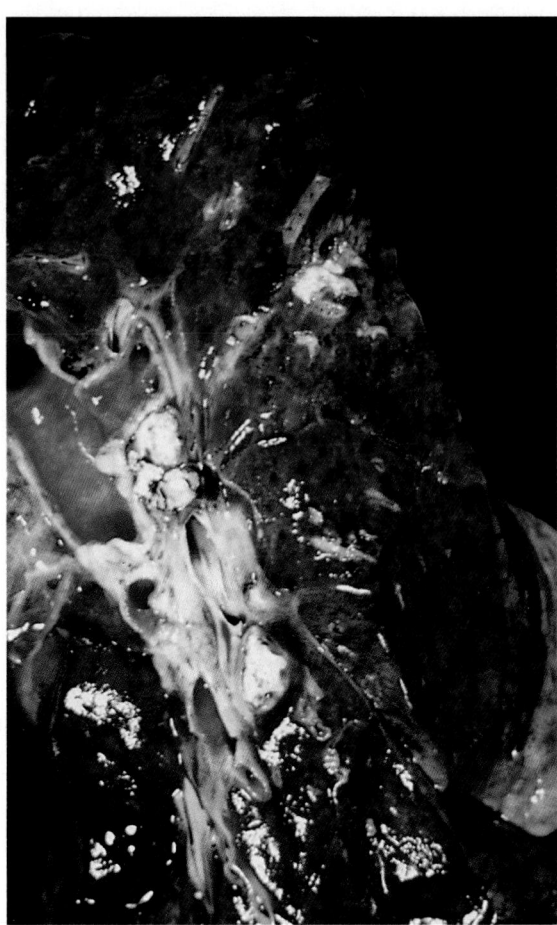

FIGURE 8–29   Primary pulmonary tuberculosis, Ghon complex. The gray-white parenchymal focus is under the pleura in the lower part of the upper lobe. Hilar lymph nodes with caseation are seen on the left.

foci are sharply circumscribed, firm, gray-white to yellow areas that have a variable amount of central caseation and peripheral fibrosis (Fig. 8–31). In immunocompetent individuals, the initial parenchymal focus undergoes progressive fibrous encapsulation, leaving only fibrocalcific scars. Histologically, the active lesions show characteristic coalescent tubercles with central caseation. Tubercle bacilli can often be identified with acid-fast stains in early exudative and caseous phases of granuloma formation but are usually too few to be found in the late, fibrocalcific stages. Localized, apical, secondary pulmonary tuberculosis may heal with fibrosis either spontaneously or after therapy, or the disease may progress and extend along several different pathways.

Progressive pulmonary tuberculosis may ensue in the elderly and immunosuppressed. The apical lesion expands into adjacent lung and eventually erodes into bronchi and vessels. This evacuates the caseous center, creating a ragged, irregular cavity that is poorly walled off by fibrous tissue. Erosion of blood vessels results in hemoptysis. With adequate treatment the process may be arrested, although healing

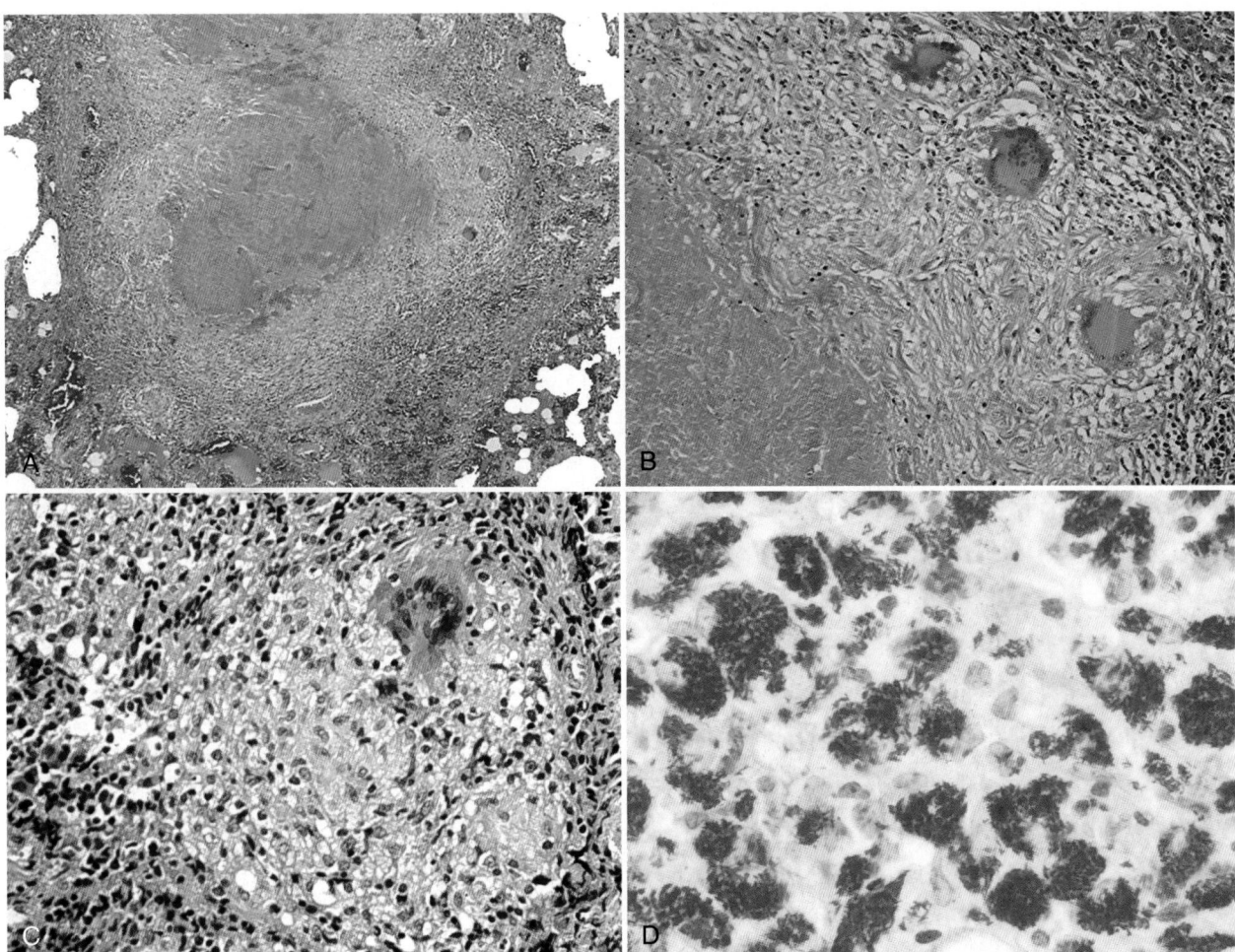

FIGURE 8–30   The morphologic spectrum of tuberculosis. A characteristic tubercle at low magnification (**A**) and in detail (**B**) illustrates central caseation surrounded by epithelioid and multinucleated giant cells. This is the usual response seen in patients who have cell-mediated immunity to the organism. Not all tubercular granulomas might show central caseation (**C**); hence, irrespective of the presence or absence of caseous necrosis, special stains for acid-fast organisms must be performed when granulomas are present. In immuno-suppressed individuals without cellular immunity sheets of foamy macrophages are seen that are packed with mycobacteria (demonstrable with acid-fast stains) (**D**). (**D**, Courtesy of Dr. Dominick Cavuoti, Department of Pathology, University of Texas Southwestern Medical School, Dallas, TX.)

by fibrosis often distorts the pulmonary architecture. The cavities, now free of inflammation, may persist or become fibrotic. If the treatment is inadequate or if host defenses are impaired, the infection may spread via airways, lymphatic channels, or the vascular system. **Miliary pulmonary disease** occurs when organisms draining through lymphatics enter the venous blood and circulate back to the lung. Individual lesions are either microscopic or small, visible (2-mm) foci of yellow-white consolidation scattered through the lung parenchyma (the adjective "miliary" is derived from the resemblance of these foci to millet seeds). Miliary lesions may expand and coalesce, resulting in consolidation of large regions or even whole lobes of the lung. With progressive pulmonary tuberculosis, the pleural cavity is invariably involved, and serous **pleural effusions**, **tuberculous empyema**, or **obliterative fibrous pleuritis** may develop.

Endobronchial, **endotracheal**, and **laryngeal tuberculosis** may develop by spread through lymphatic channels or from expectorated infectious material. The mucosal lining may be studded with minute granulomatous lesions that may only be apparent microscopically.

Systemic miliary tuberculosis occurs when bacteria disseminate through the systemic arterial system. Miliary tuberculosis is most prominent in the liver, bone marrow, spleen, adrenals, meninges, kidneys, fallopian tubes, and epididymis, but could involve any organ (Fig. 8–32).

Isolated tuberculosis may appear in any of the organs or tissues seeded hematogenously and may be the presenting manifestation. Organs that are commonly involved include the meninges (tuberculous meningitis), kidneys (renal tuberculosis), adrenals (formerly an important cause of Addison disease),

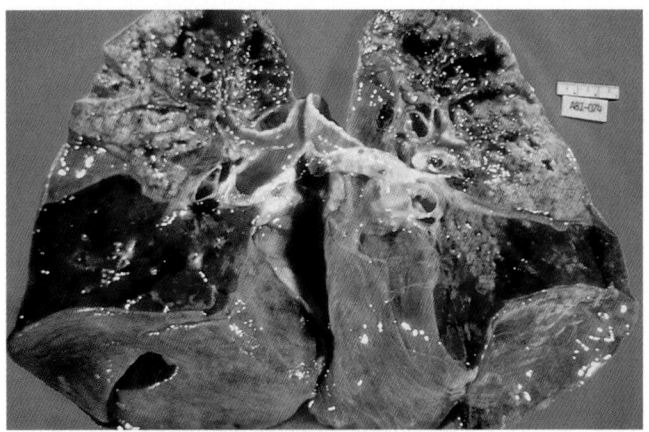

FIGURE 8–31 Secondary pulmonary tuberculosis. The upper parts of both lungs are riddled with gray-white areas of caseation and multiple areas of softening and cavitation.

bones (osteomyelitis), and fallopian tubes (salpingitis). When the vertebrae are affected, the disease is referred to as **Pott disease**. Paraspinal "cold" abscesses in these patients may track along tissue planes and present as an abdominal or pelvic mass.

Lymphadenitis is the most frequent presentation of extrapulmonary tuberculosis, usually occurring in the cervical region ("scrofula"). In HIV-negative individuals, lymphadenitis tends to be unifocal and localized. HIV-positive people, on the other hand, almost always have multifocal disease, systemic symptoms, and either pulmonary or other organ involvement by active tuberculosis.

In years past, **intestinal tuberculosis** contracted by the drinking of contaminated milk was a fairly common primary focus of disease. In countries where milk is pasteurized, intestinal tuberculosis is more often caused by the swallowing of coughed-up infective material in patients with advanced pulmonary disease. Typically the organisms are seed to mucosal lymphoid aggregates of the small and large bowel, which then undergo granulomatous inflammation that can lead to ulceration of the overlying mucosa, particularly in the ileum.

Mycobacterium avium-intracellulare Complex

Mycobacterium avium and *M. intracellulare* are separate species, but the infections they cause are so similar that they are simply referred to as *M. avium-intracellulare* complex, or MAC. MAC is common in soil, water, dust, and domestic animals. Clinically significant infection with MAC is uncommon except among people with AIDS and low numbers of CD4+ lymphocytes (<60 cells/mm^3).

In AIDS patients MAC causes widely disseminated infections, and organisms proliferate abundantly in many organs, including the lungs and gastrointestinal system. Unchecked by the immune response, the organisms reach very high levels: up to 10^4 organisms/mL of blood and 10^6 organisms/gm in tissue. Patients are feverish, with drenching night sweats and

weight loss. In the rare case of MAC in a person without HIV, the organisms primarily infect the lung, causing a productive cough and sometimes fever and weight loss.

> **Morphology. The hallmark of MAC infections in patients with HIV is abundant acid-fast bacilli within macrophages** (Fig. 8–33). Depending on the severity of immune deficiency, MAC infections can be widely disseminated throughout the mononuclear phagocyte system, causing enlargement of involved lymph nodes, liver, and spleen, or localized to the lungs. There may be a yellowish pigmentation to these organs secondary to the large number of organisms present in swollen macrophages. Granulomas, lymphocytes, and tissue destruction are rare.

Leprosy

Leprosy, or Hansen's disease, is a slowly progressive infection caused by *Mycobacterium leprae* that mainly affects the skin and peripheral nerves and results in disabling deformities. *M. leprae* is likely to be transmitted from person to person through aerosols from asymptomatic lesions in the upper respiratory tract. Inhaled *M. leprae*, like *M. tuberculosis*, is taken up by alveolar macrophages and disseminates through the blood, but replicates only in relatively cool tissues of the skin and extremities. Despite its low communicability, leprosy remains endemic among an estimated 10 to 15 million people living in poor tropical countries.

Pathogenesis. *M. leprae* is an acid-fast obligate intracellular organism that grows very poorly in culture but can be propagated in the armadillo. It proliferates best at 32° to 34°C, the temperature of the human skin and the core temperature of armadillos. Like *M. tuberculosis*, *M. leprae* secretes no toxins, and its virulence is based on properties of its cell wall. The cell wall is similar enough to that of *M. tuberculosis* that immunization with BCG confers some protection against *M. leprae* infection. Cell-mediated immunity is reflected by delayed-type hypersensitivity reactions to dermal injections of a bacterial extract called *lepromin*.

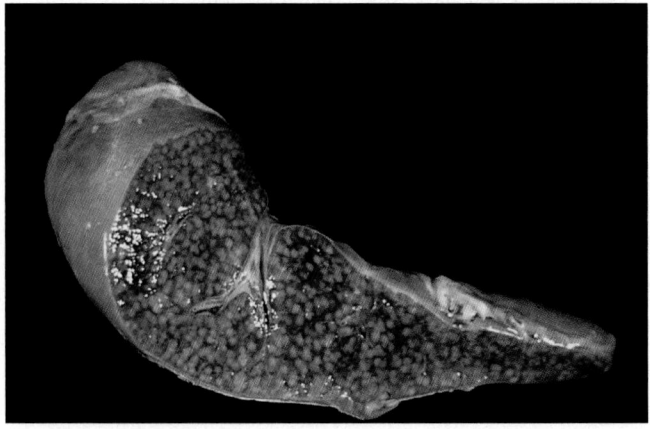

FIGURE 8–32 Miliary tuberculosis of the spleen. The cut surface shows numerous gray-white tubercles.

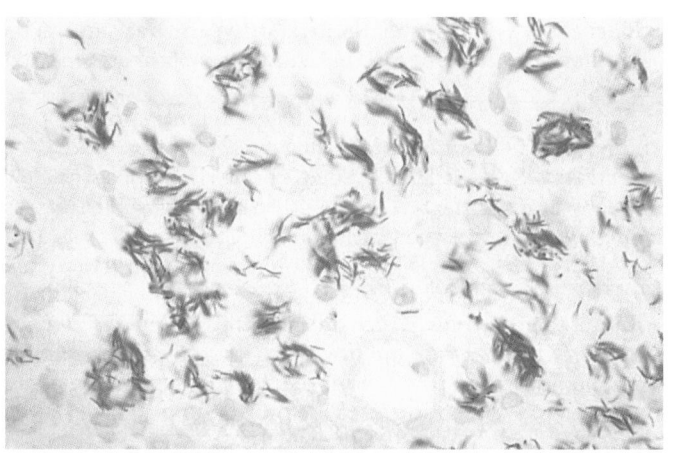

FIGURE 8–33 *Mycobacterium avium* infection in a patient with AIDS, showing massive infection with acid-fast organisms.

M. leprae causes *two strikingly different patterns of disease*. People with the less severe form, *tuberculoid leprosy*, have dry, scaly skin lesions that lack sensation. They often have asymmetric involvement of large peripheral nerves. The more severe form, *lepromatous leprosy*, includes symmetric skin thickening and nodules. This is also called *anergic leprosy*, because of the unresponsiveness (anergy) of the host immune system. Cooler areas of skin, including the earlobes and feet, are more severely affected than warmer areas, such as the axilla and groin. In lepromatous leprosy, widespread invasion of the mycobacteria into Schwann cells and into endoneural and perineural macrophages damages the peripheral nervous system. In advanced cases of lepromatous leprosy, *M. leprae* is present in sputum and blood. People can also have intermediate forms of disease, called *borderline leprosy*.

The T-helper lymphocyte response to *M. leprae* determines whether an individual has tuberculoid or lepromatous leprosy.[88] People with tuberculoid leprosy have a T_H1 response associated with production of IL-2 and IFN-γ. As with *M. tuberculosis*, IFN-γ is critical to mobilizing an effective host macrophage response. Lepromatous leprosy is associated with a weak T_H1 response and, in some cases, a relative increase in the T_H2 response. The net result is weak cell-mediated immunity and an inability to control the bacteria. Occasionally, most often in the lepromatous form, antibodies are produced against *M. leprae* antigens. Paradoxically, these antibodies are usually not protective, but they may form immune complexes with free antigens that can lead to erythema nodosum, vasculitis, and glomerulonephritis.

Morphology. Tuberculoid leprosy begins with localized flat, red skin lesions that enlarge and develop irregular shapes with indurated, elevated, hyperpigmented margins and depressed pale centers (central healing). Neuronal involvement dominates tuberculoid leprosy. Nerves become enclosed within granulomatous inflammatory reactions and, if small (e.g., the peripheral twigs), are destroyed (Fig. 8–34). Nerve degeneration causes skin anesthesias and skin and muscle atrophy that render the person liable to trauma of the affected parts, leading to the develop-

ment of chronic skin ulcers. Contractures, paralyses, and autoamputation of fingers or toes may ensue. Facial nerve involvement can lead to paralysis of the eyelids, with keratitis and corneal ulcerations. On microscopic examination, all sites of involvement have granulomatous lesions closely resembling those found in tuberculosis, and bacilli are almost never found, hence the name "paucibacillary" leprosy. The presence of granulomas and absence of bacteria reflect strong T-cell immunity. Because leprosy pursues an extremely slow course, spanning decades, most patients die with leprosy rather than of it.

Lepromatous leprosy involves the skin, peripheral nerves, anterior chamber of the eye, upper airways (down to the larynx), testes, hands, and feet. The vital organs and CNS are rarely affected, presumably because the core temperature is too high for growth of *M. leprae*. Lepromatous lesions contain large aggregates of lipid-laden macrophages (lepra cells), often filled with masses ("globi") of acid-fast bacilli (Fig. 8–35). Because of the abundant bacteria, lepromatous leprosy is referred to as **"multibacillary"**. Macular, papular, or nodular lesions form on the face, ears, wrists, elbows, and knees. With progression, the nodular lesions coalesce to yield a distinctive leonine facies. Most skin lesions are hypoesthetic or anesthetic. Lesions in the nose may cause persistent inflammation and bacilli-laden discharge. The peripheral nerves, particularly the ulnar and peroneal nerves

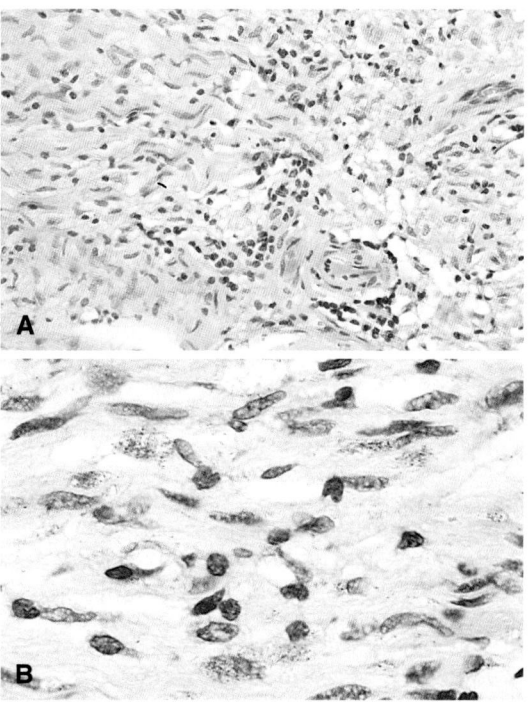

FIGURE 8–34 Leprosy. **A,** Peripheral nerve. Note the inflammatory cell infiltrates in the endoneural and epineural compartments. **B,** Cells within the endoneurium contain acid-fast positive lepra bacilli. (Courtesy of E.P. Richardson, Jr., and U. De Girolami, Harvard Medical School.)

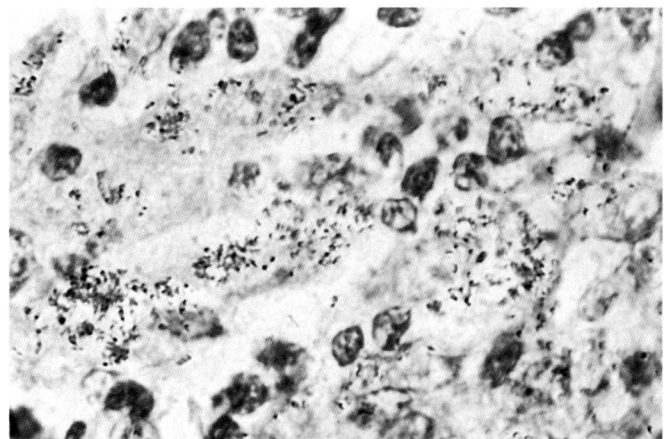

FIGURE 8–35 Lepromatous leprosy. Acid-fast bacilli ("red snappers") within macrophages.

where they approach the skin surface, are symmetrically invaded with mycobacteria, with minimal inflammation. Loss of sensation and trophic changes in the hands and feet follow the nerve lesions. Lymph nodes contain aggregates of bacteria-filled foamy macrophages in the paracortical (T-cell) areas and reactive germinal centers. In advanced disease, aggregates of macrophages are also present in the splenic red pulp and the liver. The testes are usually extensively involved, leading to destruction of the seminiferous tubules and consequent sterility.

SPIROCHETES

Spirochetes are gram-negative, slender corkscrew-shaped bacteria with axial periplasmic flagella wound around a helical protoplasm. The bacteria are covered in a membrane called an outer sheath, which may mask bacterial antigens from the host immune response. *Treponema pallidum* subsp. *pallidum* is the microaerophilic spirochete that causes syphilis, a chronic venereal disease with multiple clinical presentations. Other closely related treponemes cause yaws (*Treponema pallidum* subsp. *pertenue*) and pinta (*Treponema pallidum* subsp. *carateum*).

Syphilis

Syphilis is a chronic venereal disease with multiple presentations. The causative spirochete, *T. pallidum* subsp. *pallidum*, hereafter referred to simply as *T. pallidum*, is too slender to be seen in Gram stain, but it can be visualized by silver stains, dark-field examination, and immunofluorescence techniques (Fig. 8–36). Sexual contact is the usual mode of spread. Transplacental transmission of *T. pallidum* occurs readily, and active disease during pregnancy results in congenital syphilis. *T. pallidum* cannot be grown in culture.

Public health programs and penicillin treatment reduced the number of cases of syphilis in the United States from the late 1940s until the 1970s. Cases of syphilis surged upward in the mid-1980s, reaching a total of 50,000 cases in 1990. Renewed public health efforts led to a sharp drop in the

incidence of syphilis over the next 10 years, but since 2000 there has been a steady rise in the number of cases reported annually, to ~10,000 in 2006.

Syphilis is divided into three stages, with distinct clinical and pathologic manifestations (Fig. 8–37).

Primary Syphilis. This stage, occurring approximately 3 weeks after contact with an infected individual, features a single firm, nontender, raised, red lesion (chancre) located at the site of treponemal invasion on the penis, cervix, vaginal wall, or anus. The chancre heals in 3 to 6 weeks with or without therapy. *Spirochetes are plentiful within the chancre and can be seen by immunofluorescent stains of serous exudate.* Treponemes spread throughout the body by hematologic and lymphatic dissemination even before the appearance of the chancre.

Secondary Syphilis. This stage usually occurs 2 to 10 weeks after the primary chancre and is due to spread and proliferation of the spirochetes within the skin and mucocutaneous tissues. Secondary syphilis occurs in approximately 75% of untreated people. *The skin lesions, which frequently occur on the palms or soles of the feet, may be maculopapular, scaly, or pustular.* Moist areas of the skin, such as the anogenital region, inner thighs, and axillae, may have *condylomata lata*, which are broad-based, elevated plaques. Silvery-gray superficial erosions may form on any of the mucous membranes but are particularly common in the mouth, pharynx, and external genitalia. All these painless superficial lesions contain spirochetes and so are infectious. Lymphadenopathy, mild fever, malaise, and weight loss are also common in secondary syphilis. The symptoms of secondary syphilis last several weeks, after which the person enters the latent phase of the disease. Superficial lesions may recur during the early latent phase, although they are milder.

Tertiary Syphilis. This stage is rare where adequate medical care is available, but it occurs in approximately one third of untreated patients, usually after a latent period of 5 years or more. Tertiary syphilis has three main manifestations: cardiovascular syphilis, neurosyphilis, and so-called benign tertiary syphilis. These may occur alone or in combination.

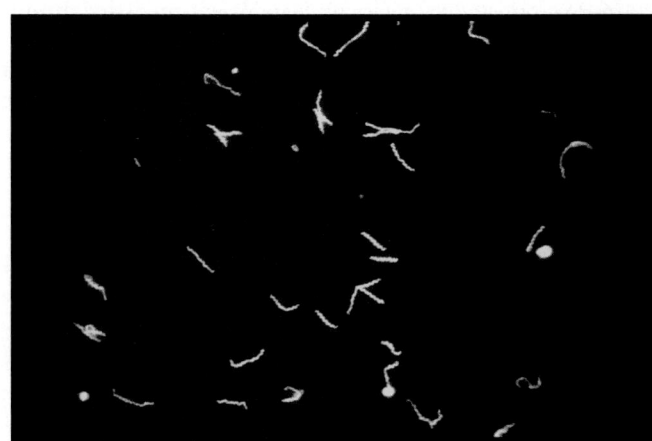

FIGURE 8–36 *Treponema pallidum* (dark-field microscopy) showing several spirochetes in scrapings from the base of a chancre. (Courtesy of Dr. Paul Southern, Department of Pathology, University of Texas Southwestern Medical School, Dallas, TX.)

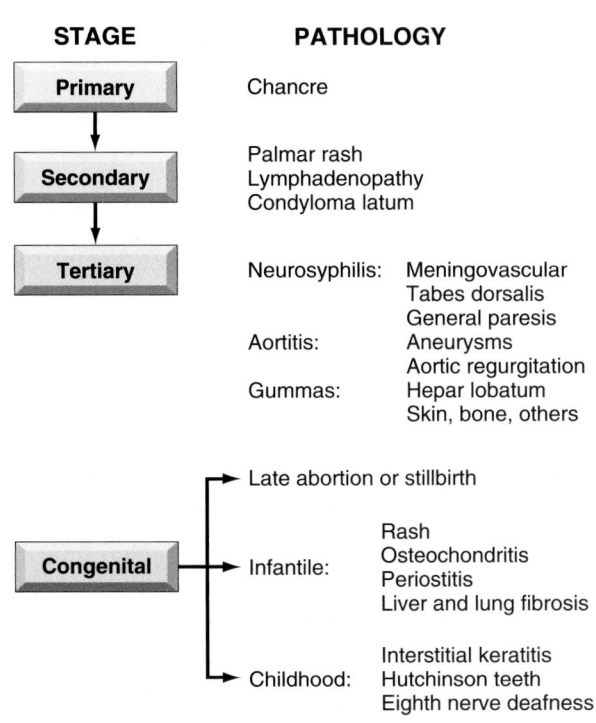

STAGE	PATHOLOGY	
Primary	Chancre	
Secondary	Palmar rash Lymphadenopathy Condyloma latum	
Tertiary	Neurosyphilis:	Meningovascular Tabes dorsalis General paresis
	Aortitis:	Aneurysms Aortic regurgitation
	Gummas:	Hepar lobatum Skin, bone, others
Congenital	Late abortion or stillbirth	
	Infantile:	Rash Osteochondritis Periostitis Liver and lung fibrosis
	Childhood:	Interstitial keratitis Hutchinson teeth Eighth nerve deafness

FIGURE 8–37 Protean manifestations of syphilis.

Cardiovascular syphilis, in the form of syphilitic aortitis, accounts for more than 80% of cases of tertiary disease. The aortitis leads to slowly progressive dilation of the aortic root and arch, which causes aortic valve insufficiency and aneurysms of the proximal aorta (see Chapter 11).

Neurosyphilis may be symptomatic or asymptomatic. Symptomatic disease manifests in several ways, including chronic meningovascular disease, tabes dorsalis, and a generalized brain parenchymal disease called *general paresis*. These are discussed in Chapter 28. Asymptomatic neurosyphilis, which accounts for about one third of neurosyphilis cases, is detected when a patient's CSF exhibits abnormalities such as pleocytosis (increased numbers of inflammatory cells), elevated protein levels, or decreased glucose. Antibodies stimulated by the spirochetes, discussed below, can also be detected in the CSF, and this is the most specific test for neurosyphilis. Antibiotics are given for a longer time if the spirochetes have spread to the CNS, and so patients with tertiary syphilis should be tested for neurosyphilis even if they do not have neurologic symptoms.

So-called *benign tertiary syphilis* is characterized by the formation of gummas in various sites. Gummas are nodular lesions probably related to the development of delayed hypersensitivity to the bacteria. They occur most commonly in bone, skin, and the mucous membranes of the upper airway and mouth, although any organ may be affected. Skeletal involvement characteristically causes local pain, tenderness, swelling, and sometimes pathologic fractures. Involvement of skin and mucous membranes may produce nodular lesions or, rarely, destructive, ulcerative lesions that mimic malignant neoplasms. Gummas are now very rare because of the use of effective antibiotics and are seen mainly in individuals with AIDS.

Congenital Syphilis. Congenital syphilis occurs when *T. pallidum* crosses the placenta from an infected mother to the fetus. Maternal transmission happens most frequently during primary or secondary syphilis, when the spirochetes are most numerous. Because the manifestations of maternal syphilis may be subtle, routine serologic testing for syphilis is mandatory in all pregnancies. Intrauterine death and perinatal death each occurs in approximately 25% of cases of untreated congenital syphilis.

Manifestations of congenital disease are divided into early (infantile) and late (tardive) syphilis, depending on whether they occur in the first 2 years of life or later. Early congenital syphilis is often manifested by nasal discharge and congestion (snuffles) in the first few months of life. A desquamating or bullous rash can lead to sloughing of the skin, particularly of the hands and feet and around the mouth and anus. Hepatomegaly and skeletal abnormalities are also common.

Nearly half of untreated children with neonatal syphilis will develop late manifestations, which are discussed below.

Serologic Tests for Syphilis. Serology remains the mainstay of diagnosis, although microscopy and PCR are also useful. Serologic tests include nontreponemal antibody tests and antitreponemal antibody tests. Nontreponemal tests measure antibody to cardiolipin, a phospholipid present in both host tissues and *T. pallidum*. These antibodies are detected in the rapid plasma reagin and Venereal Disease Research Laboratory (VDRL) tests. Nontreponemal tests typically become positive 4 to 6 weeks after infection, and so immunofluorescence of exudate from the chancre is important for diagnosis early in infection. The nontreponemal tests are nearly always positive in secondary syphilis, but they usually become negative in tertiary syphilis. The VDRL and rapid plasma reagin tests are used as screening tests for syphilis and to monitor response to therapy, since these tests become negative after successful treatment of infection. False-positive VDRL test results are not uncommon and are associated with certain acute infections, collagen vascular diseases (e.g., systemic lupus erythematosus), drug addiction, pregnancy, hypergammaglobulinemia of any cause, and lepromatous leprosy.

Treponemal antibody tests measure antibodies that specifically react with *T. pallidum*. These include the fluorescent treponemal antibody absorption test and the microhemagglutination assay for *T. pallidum* antibodies. These tests also become positive 4 to 6 weeks after infection, but unlike nontreponemal antibody tests, they remain positive indefinitely, even after successful treatment. They are not recommended as primary screening tests because they are significantly more expensive than nontreponemal tests. While more specific than the nontreponemal tests, false-positive treponemal antibody tests can also occur.

Serologic response may be delayed, absent, or exaggerated (false-positive results) in people co-infected with syphilis and HIV. However, in most cases, these tests remain useful in the diagnosis and management of syphilis even in people infected with HIV.

Morphology. In **primary syphilis** a chancre occurs on the penis or scrotum of 70% of men and on the vulva or cervix of 50% of women. The chancre is a slightly elevated, firm, reddened papule, up to several centimeters in diameter, that erodes to create a clean-based shallow ulcer. The contiguous induration

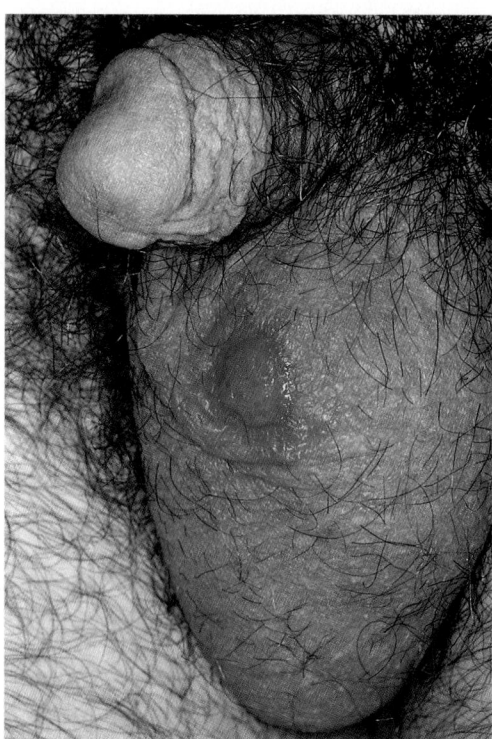

FIGURE 8–38   Syphilitic chancre in the scrotum (see Figure 8–8 for the histopathology of syphilis). (Courtesy of Dr. Richard Johnson, Beth Israel–Deaconess Hospital, Boston, MA.)

creates a button-like mass directly adjacent to the eroded skin, providing the basis for the designation hard chancre (Fig. 8–38). On histologic examination, treponemes are visible at the surface of the ulcer with silver stains (e.g., Warthin-Starry stain) or immunofluorescence techniques. The chancre contains an intense infiltrate of plasma cells, with scattered macrophages and lymphocytes and a proliferative endarteritis (see Fig. 8–8). The endarteritis, which is seen in all stages of syphilis, starts with endothelial cell activation and proliferation and progresses to intimal fibrosis. The regional nodes are usually enlarged due to nonspecific acute or chronic lymphadenitis, plasma cell–rich infiltrates, or granulomas.

In **secondary syphilis** widespread mucocutaneous lesions involve the oral cavity, palms of the hands, and soles of the feet. The rash frequently consists of discrete red-brown macules less than 5 mm in diameter, but it may be follicular, pustular, annular, or scaling. Red lesions in the mouth or vagina contain the most organisms and are the most infectious. Histologically, the mucocutaneous lesions of secondary syphilis show the same plasma cell infiltrate and obliterative endarteritis as the primary chancre, although the inflammation is often less intense.

Tertiary syphilis most frequently involves the aorta; the CNS; and the liver, bones, and testes. The aortitis is caused by endarteritis of the vasa vasorum of the proximal aorta. Occlusion of the vasa vasorum results in scarring of the media of the proximal aortic wall, causing a loss of elasticity. There may be narrowing of the coronary artery ostia caused by subintimal scarring with resulting myocardial ischemia. The morphologic and clinical features of syphilitic aortitis are discussed in greater detail with diseases of the blood vessels (Chapter 11). **Neurosyphilis** takes one of several forms, designated meningovascular syphilis, tabes dorsalis, and general paresis (Chapter 28). **Syphilitic gummas** are white-gray and rubbery, occur singly or multiply, and vary in size from microscopic lesions resembling tubercles to large tumor-like masses. They occur in most organs but particularly in skin, subcutaneous tissue, bone, and joints. In the liver, scarring as a result of gummas may cause a distinctive hepatic lesion known as hepar lobatum (Fig. 8–39). On histologic examination, the gummas have centers of coagulated, necrotic material and margins composed of plump, palisading macrophages and fibroblasts surrounded by large numbers of mononuclear leukocytes, chiefly plasma cells. Treponemes are scant in gummas and are difficult to demonstrate.

The rash of **congenital syphilis** is more severe than that of adult secondary syphilis. It is a bullous eruption of the palms and soles of the feet associated with epidermal sloughing. **Syphilitic osteochondritis and periostitis** affect all bones, but lesions of the nose and lower legs are most distinctive. Destruction of the vomer causes collapse of the bridge of the nose and, later on, the characteristic saddle nose deformity. Periostitis of the tibia leads to excessive new bone growth on the anterior surfaces and anterior bowing, or saber shin. There is also widespread disturbance in endochondral bone formation. The epiphyses become widened as the cartilage overgrows, and cartilage is found in displaced islands within the metaphysis.

The **liver** is often severely affected in congenital syphilis. Diffuse fibrosis permeates lobules to isolate hepatic cells into small nests, accompanied by the

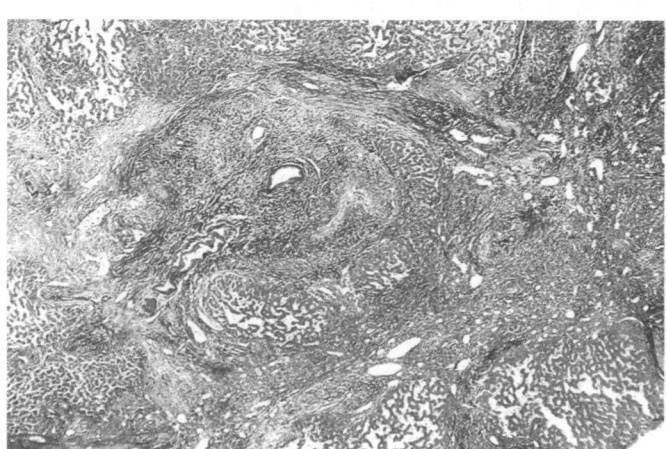

FIGURE 8–39   Trichrome stain of liver shows a gumma (scar), stained blue, caused by tertiary syphilis (the hepatic lesion is also known as hepar lobatum).

characteristic lymphoplasmacytic infiltrate and vascular changes. Gummas are occasionally found in the liver, even in early cases. The **lungs** may be affected by a diffuse interstitial fibrosis. In the syphilitic stillborn, the lungs appear pale and airless (pneumonia alba). The generalized spirochetemia may lead to diffuse interstitial inflammatory reactions in virtually any other organ (e.g., the pancreas, kidneys, heart, spleen, thymus, endocrine organs, and CNS).

The late manifestations of congenital syphilis include a distinctive **triad of interstitial keratitis, Hutchinson teeth, and eighth-nerve deafness**. In addition to interstitial keratitis, the ocular changes include choroiditis and abnormal retinal pigmentation. Hutchinson teeth are small incisors shaped like a screwdriver or a peg, often with notches in the enamel. Eighth-nerve deafness and optic nerve atrophy develop secondary to meningovascular syphilis.

Pathogenesis. There are no good animal models of syphilis, and *T. pallidum* has never been grown in culture (it lacks genes for making nucleotides, fatty acids, and most amino acids). As a result, our scant knowledge of *T. pallidum* pathogenesis comes mainly from observations of the disease in humans.

Proliferative endarteritis occurs in all stages of syphilis. The pathophysiology of the endarteritis is not known, although the scarcity of treponemes and the intense inflammatory infiltrate suggest that the immune response plays a role in the development of these lesions. Regardless of the mechanism, much of the pathology of the disease, such as syphilitic aortitis, can be ascribed to the vascular abnormalities.

The immune response to *T. pallidum* reduces the burden of bacteria, but it may also have a central role in the pathogenesis of the disease. The T cells that infiltrate the chancre are T_H1 cells, suggesting that activation of macrophages to kill bacteria may cause resolution of the local infection.[89] Although there are many plasma cells in the syphilitic lesions and treponeme-specific antibodies are readily detectable, the antibody response does not eliminate the infection. The outer membrane of *T. pallidum* seems to protect the bacteria from antibody binding. The mechanism of this effect is not well understood, but either the paucity of bacterial proteins in the membrane or absorption (coating) of the membrane by host proteins may play a role.[90] The immune response is ultimately inadequate, since the spirochetes disseminate, persist, and cause secondary and tertiary syphilis.

In passing, it should be noted that antibiotic treatment of syphilis, in patients with a high bacterial load, can cause a massive release of endotoxins, resulting in a cytokine storm that manifests with high fever, rigors, hypotension, and leukopenia. This syndrome, called the Jarisch-Herxheimer reaction, is seen not only in syphilis but in other spirochetal diseases, such as Lyme disease, and can be mistaken for drug allergy.

Relapsing Fever

Relapsing fever is an insect-transmitted disease characterized by recurrent fevers with spirochetemia. *Epidemic relapsing fever* is caused by body louse-transmitted *Borrelia recurrentis*, which infects only humans. *B. recurrentis*, which is associated with overcrowding due to poverty or war, caused multiple large epidemics in Africa, Eastern Europe, and Russia in the first half of the twentieth century, infecting 15 million people and killing 5 million, and is still a problem in some developing countries. *Endemic relapsing fever* is caused by several *Borrelia* species, which are transmitted from small animals to humans by *Ornithodorus* (soft-bodied) ticks.

In both louse- and tick-transmitted borreliosis, there is a 1- to 2-week incubation period after the bite as the spirochetes multiply in the blood. Clinical infection is heralded by shaking chills, fever, headache, and fatigue, followed by DIC and multiorgan failure. Spirochetes are temporarily cleared from the blood by anti-*Borrelia* antibodies, which target a single major surface protein called the variable major protein.[91] After a few days, bacteria bearing a different surface antigen emerge and reach high densities in the blood, and symptoms return until a second set of host antibodies clears these organisms. The lessening severity of successive attacks of relapsing fever and its spontaneous cure in many untreated patients have been attributed to the limited genetic repertoire of *Borrelia*, enabling the host to build up cross-reactive as well as clone-specific antibodies.

Morphology. The diagnosis can be made by identification of spirochetes in blood smears obtained during febrile periods. In fatal louse-borne disease, the spleen is moderately enlarged (300–400 gm) and contains focal necrosis and miliary collections of leukocytes, including neutrophils, and numerous borreliae. There is congestion and hypercellularity of the red pulp, which contains macrophages with phagocytosed red cells (erythrophagocytosis). The liver may also be enlarged and congested, with prominent Kupffer cells and septic foci. Scattered hemorrhages resulting from DIC may be found in serosal and mucosal surfaces, skin, and viscera. Pulmonary bacterial superinfection is a frequent complication.

Lyme Disease

Lyme disease is named for the Connecticut town where there was an epidemic of arthritis associated with skin erythema in the mid-1970s. It is caused by several subspecies of the spirochete *Borrelia burgdorferi*, which is transmitted from rodents to people by *Ixodes* deer ticks.[92,93] Lyme disease is a common arthropod-borne disease in the United States, Europe, and Japan. In the United States the incidence of Lyme disease has risen, with approximately 23,000 cases in 2005. Most cases occur in the Northeastern states and in some parts of Midwestern states. In endemic areas, as many as 50% of ticks are infected with *B. burgdorferi*, and ticks may also be infected with *Ehrlichia* and *Babesia* (discussed later). Serology is the main method of diagnosis, but PCR can be done on infected tissue.

Lyme disease involves multiple organ systems and is divided into three stages (Fig. 8–40). In *stage 1*, spirochetes multiply and spread in the dermis at the site of a tick bite, causing an expanding area of redness, often with a pale center. This skin

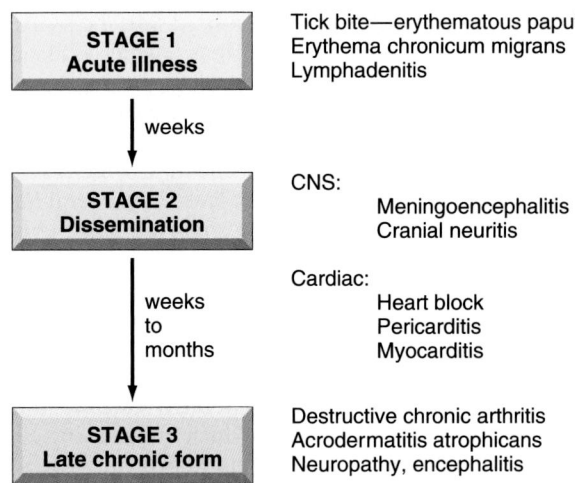

FIGURE 8–40 Clinical stages of Lyme disease.

lesion, called *erythema chronicum migrans*, may be accompanied by fever and lymphadenopathy but usually disappears in 4 to 12 weeks. In *stage 2, the early disseminated stage*, spirochetes spread hematogenously throughout the body and cause secondary skin lesions, lymphadenopathy, migratory joint and muscle pain, cardiac arrhythmias, and meningitis often associated with cranial nerve involvement. In *stage 3, the late disseminated stage*, 2 or 3 years after the initial bite, Lyme borreliae cause a chronic arthritis sometimes with severe damage to large joints and a polyneuropathy and encephalitis that vary from mild to debilitating.

Pathogenesis. *Borrelia burgdorferi* does not produce LPS or exotoxins that damage the host. *Much of the pathology associated with B. burgdorferi is thought to be secondary to the immune response against the bacteria and the inflammation that accompanies it.* The initial immune response is stimulated by binding of bacterial lipoproteins to TLR2 expressed by macrophages. In response, these cells release proinflammatory cytokines (IL-6 and TNF) and generate bactericidal nitric oxide, reducing but usually not eliminating the infection.

The adaptive immune response to Lyme disease is mediated by CD4+ helper T cells and B cells. *Borrelia*-specific antibodies, made 2 to 4 weeks after infection, drive complement-mediated killing of the bacteria; however, *B. burgdorferi* escapes the antibody response through antigenic variation. Similar to *Borrelia hermsii*, a cause of endemic relapsing fever, *B. burgdorferi* has a plasmid with a single promoter sequence and multiple coding sequences for an antigenic surface protein, VlsE, each of which can shuttle into position next to the promoter and be expressed. Thus, as the antibody response to one VlsE protein is mounted, bacteria expressing an alternate VlsE protein can escape immune recognition. Chronic manifestations of Lyme disease, such as the late arthritis, are probably caused by the immune response against persistent bacteria.

Morphology. Skin lesions caused by *B. burgdorferi* are characterized by edema and a lymphocytic–plasma cell infiltrate. In early Lyme arthritis, the synovium resembles early rheumatoid arthritis, with villous hypertrophy, lining-cell hyperplasia, and abundant lymphocytes and plasma cells in the subsy-

novium. A distinctive feature of Lyme arthritis is an arteritis, which produces onionskin-like lesions resembling those seen in lupus (Chapter 6). In late Lyme disease there may be extensive erosion of the cartilage in large joints. In Lyme meningitis the CSF is hypercellular, due to a marked lymphoplasmacytic infiltrate, and contains anti-spirochete IgGs.

ANAEROBIC BACTERIA

Many anaerobic bacteria are normal flora in sites of the body that have low oxygen levels. The anaerobic flora cause disease (abscesses or peritonitis) when they are introduced into normally sterile sites or when the balance of organisms is upset and pathogenic anaerobes overgrow (e.g., *Clostridium difficile* colitis with antibiotic treatment). Environmental anaerobes also cause disease (tetanus, botulism, and gas gangrene).

Abscesses Caused by Anaerobes

Abscesses are usually caused by mixed anaerobic and facultative aerobic bacteria (able to grow with or without oxygen). On average, abscesses have 2.5 species of bacteria, 1.6 of which are anaerobes and 0.9 of which are aerobic or facultative bacteria.[94] *Commensal bacteria from adjacent sites (oropharynx, intestine, and female genital tract) are the usual cause of abscesses, so the species found in the abscess reflect the normal flora.* Since most anaerobes that cause abscesses are part of the normal flora, it is not surprising that these organisms do not produce significant toxins.

The bacteria found in head and neck abscesses reflect oral and pharyngeal flora. Common anaerobes at this site include the gram-negative bacilli *Prevotella* and *Porphyromonas* species, often mixed with the facultative *S. aureus* and *S. pyogenes*. *Fusobacterium necrophorum*, an oral commensal, causes Lemierre syndrome, characterized by infection of the lateral pharyngeal space and septic jugular vein thrombosis. Abdominal abscesses are caused by the anaerobes of the gastrointestinal tract, including gram-positive *Peptostreptococcus* and *Clostridium* species, as well as the gram-negative *Bacteriodes fragilis* and *E. coli*. Genital tract infections in women are caused by anaerobic gram-negative bacilli, including *Prevotella* species that are found in Bartholin cyst abscesses and tubo-ovarian abscesses, often mixed with *E. coli* or *Streptococcus agalactiae*.

Morphology. Abscesses caused by anaerobes contain discolored and foul-smelling pus that is often poorly walled off. Otherwise, these lesions pathologically resemble those of the common pyogenic infections. Gram stain reveals mixed infection with gram-positive and gram-negative rods and gram-positive cocci mixed with neutrophils.

Clostridial Infections

Clostridium species are gram-positive bacilli that grow under anaerobic conditions and produce spores that are present in the soil. Four types of disease are caused by *Clostridium*:

- *C. perfringens, C. septicum,* and other species cause cellulitis and myonecrosis of traumatic and surgical wounds *(gas gangrene)*, uterine myonecrosis often associated with illegal abortions, mild food poisoning, and infection of the small bowel associated with ischemia or neutropenia that often leads to severe sepsis.
- *C. tetani*, the cause of *tetanus*, proliferates in puncture wounds and in the umbilical stump of newborn infants and releases a potent neurotoxin, called tetanospasmin, that causes convulsive contractions of skeletal muscles (lockjaw). Tetanus toxoid (formalin-fixed neurotoxin) is part of the DPT (diphtheria, pertussis, and tetanus) immunization, which has greatly decreased the incidence of tetanus worldwide.
- *C. botulinum* grows in inadequately sterilized canned foods and releases a potent neurotoxin that blocks synaptic release of acetylcholine and causes a severe paralysis of respiratory and skeletal muscles *(botulism)*.
- *C. difficile* overgrows other intestinal flora in antibiotic-treated people, releases toxins, and causes *pseudomembranous colitis* (Chapter 17).

Clostridial infections can be diagnosed by culture (cellulitis, myonecrosis), toxin assays (pseudomembranous colitis), or both (botulism).

Pathogenesis. *Clostridium perfringens* does not grow in the presence of oxygen, so tissue death is essential for growth of the bacteria in the host. These bacteria release collagenase and hyaluronidase that degrade extracellular matrix proteins and contribute to bacterial invasiveness, but their most powerful virulence factors are the many toxins they produce. *C. perfringens* secretes 14 toxins, the most important of which is α-toxin.[95] This toxin has multiple actions. It is a phospholipase C that degrades lecithin, a major component of cell membranes, and so destroys red cells, platelets, and muscle cells, causing myonecrosis. It also has a sphingomyelinase activity that contributes to nerve sheath damage.

Ingestion of food contaminated with *C. perfringens* causes a brief diarrhea. Spores, usually in contaminated meat, survive cooking, and the organism proliferates in cooling food. *C. perfringens* enterotoxin forms pores in the epithelial cell membranes, lysing the cells and disrupting tight junctions between epithelial cells.[96]

The neurotoxins produced by *C. botulinum* and *C. tetani* both inhibit release of neurotransmitters, resulting in paralysis.[26] Botulism toxin, eaten in contaminated foods or absorbed from wounds infected with *C. botulinum*, binds gangliosides on motor neurons and is transported into the cell. In the cytoplasm, the A fragment of botulism toxin cleaves a protein, called synaptobrevin, that mediates fusion of neurotransmitter-containing vesicles with the neuron membrane. By blocking vesicle fusion, botulism toxin prevents the release of acetylcholine at the neuromuscular junction, resulting in flaccid paralysis. If the respiratory muscles are affected, botulism can lead to death. Indeed, the widespread use of botulism toxin (Botox) in cosmetic surgery is based on its ability to cause paralysis of strategically chosen muscles on the face. The mechanism of tetanus toxin is similar to that of botulism toxin, but tetanus toxin causes a violent spastic paralysis by blocking release of γ-aminobutyric acid, a neurotransmitter that inhibits motor neurons.

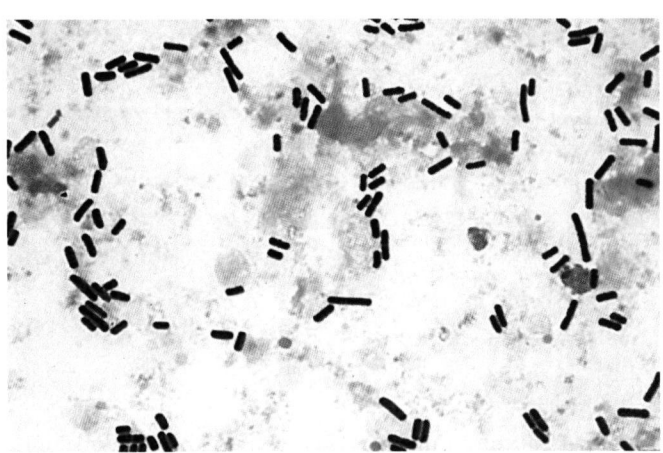

FIGURE 8–41   Boxcar-shaped gram-positive *Clostridium perfringens* in gangrenous tissue.

Clostridium difficile produces toxin A, an enterotoxin that stimulates chemokine production and thus attracts leukocytes, and toxin B, a cytotoxin, which causes distinctive cytopathic effects in cultured cells. Both toxins are glucosyl transferases and are part of a pathogenicity island that is absent from the chromosomes of nonpathogenic strains of *C. difficile*.[97]

Morphology. Clostridial cellulitis, which originates in wounds, can be differentiated from infection caused by pyogenic cocci by its foul odor, its thin, discolored exudate, and the relatively quick and wide tissue destruction. On microscopic examination, the amount of tissue necrosis is disproportionate to the number of neutrophils and gram-positive bacteria present (Fig. 8–41). Clostridial cellulitis, which often has granulation tissue at its borders, is treatable by debridement and antibiotics.

In contrast, **clostridial gas gangrene** is life-threatening and is characterized by marked edema and enzymatic necrosis of involved muscle cells 1 to 3 days after injury. An extensive fluid exudate, which is lacking in inflammatory cells, causes swelling of the affected region and the overlying skin, forming large, bullous vesicles that rupture. Gas bubbles caused by bacterial fermentation appear within the gangrenous tissues. As the infection progresses, the inflamed muscles become soft, blue-black, friable, and semifluid as a result of the massive proteolytic action of the released bacterial enzymes. On microscopic examination there is severe **myonecrosis**, extensive hemolysis, and marked vascular injury, with thrombosis. *C. perfringens* is also associated with dusk-colored, wedge-shaped infarcts in the small bowel, particularly in neutropenic people. Regardless of the site of entry, when *C. perfringens* disseminates hematogenously there is widespread formation of gas bubbles.

Despite the severe neurologic damage caused by botulinum and tetanus toxins, the neuropathologic changes are subtle and nonspecific.

OBLIGATE INTRACELLULAR BACTERIA

Obligate intracellular bacteria proliferate only within host cells, although some may survive outside of cells. These organisms are well adapted to the intracellular environment, with membrane pumps to capture amino acids and ATP for energy. Some are unable to synthesize ATP at all (e.g., *Chlamydia*), while others synthesize at least some of their own ATP (e.g., the rickettsiae).

Chlamydial Infections

Chlamydia trachomatis is a small gram-negative bacterium that is an obligate intracellular parasite. *C. trachomatis* exists in two forms during its unique life cycle. The infectious form, called the elementary body (EB), is a metabolically inactive, sporelike structure. The EB is taken up by host cells by receptor-mediated endocytosis. The bacteria prevent fusion of the endosome and lysosome by an unknown mechanism. Inside the endosome the elementary body differentiates into a metabolically active form, called the reticulate body. Using energy sources and amino acids from the host cell, the reticulate body replicates and ultimately forms new elementary bodies that are capable of infecting additional cells.

The various diseases caused by *C. trachomatis* infection are associated with different serotypes of the bacteria: urogenital infections and inclusion conjunctivitis (serotypes D through K), lymphogranuloma venereum (serotypes L1, L2, and L3), and an ocular infection of children, trachoma (serotypes A, B, and C). The venereal infections caused by *C. trachomatis* will be discussed here.

Genital infection by *C. trachomatis is the most common sexually transmitted bacterial disease in the world.*[98] In 2006 approximately a million cases of genital chlamydia were reported to the CDC; this is more than twice the number of cases of gonorrhea. Before the identification of *C. trachomatis*, people infected with this organism were diagnosed with nongonococcal urethritis (NGU). Indeed, *C. trachomatis* is the cause of over half the cases of NGU. Current CDC recommendations call for treatment of both *N. gonorrhoeae* and *C. trachomatis* in patients who are diagnosed with either infection, because co-infection with both is common.

Genital *C. trachomatis* infections (other than lymphogranuloma venereum, discussed below) are associated with clinical features that are similar to those caused by *N. gonorrhoeae*. Patients may develop epididymitis, prostatitis, pelvic inflammatory disease, pharyngitis, conjunctivitis, perihepatic inflammation, and proctitis. Unlike *N. gonorrhoeae* urethritis, *C. trachomatis* urethritis in men may be asymptomatic and so may go untreated. Both *N. gonorrhoeae* and *C. trachomatis* frequently cause asymptomatic infections in women. *C. trachomatis* urethritis can be diagnosed by culture of the bacteria in human cell lines, but amplified nucleic acid tests performed on genital swabs or urine specimens are more sensitive and have supplanted cultures.

Genital infection with the L serotypes of *C. trachomatis* causes *lymphogranuloma venereum*, a chronic, ulcerative disease. Lymphogranuloma venereum is a sporadic disease in the United States and Western Europe, but it is endemic in parts of Asia, Africa, the Caribbean region, and South America. The infection initially manifests as a small, often unnoticed, papule on the genital mucosa or nearby skin. Two to six weeks later, growth of the organism and the host response in draining lymph nodes produce swollen, tender lymph nodes, which may coalesce and rupture. If not treated, the infection can subsequently cause fibrosis and strictures in the anogenital tract. Rectal strictures are particularly common in women.

> **Morphology.** The morphologic features of *C. trachomatis* **urethritis** are virtually identical to those of gonorrhea. The primary infection is characterized by a mucopurulent discharge containing a predominance of neutrophils. Organisms are not visible in Gram-stained smears or sections.
>
> The lesions of **lymphogranuloma venereum** contain a mixed granulomatous and neutrophilic inflammatory response. Variable numbers of chlamydial inclusions are seen in the cytoplasm of epithelial cells or inflammatory cells. Regional lymphadenopathy is common, usually occurring within 30 days of infection. Lymph node involvement is characterized by a granulomatous inflammatory reaction associated with irregularly shaped foci of necrosis and neutrophilic infiltration (stellate abscesses). With time, the inflammatory reaction is dominated by nonspecific chronic inflammatory infiltrates and extensive fibrosis. The latter, in turn, may cause local lymphatic obstruction, lymphedema, and strictures. In active lesions, the diagnosis of lymphogranuloma venereum may be made by demonstration of the organism in biopsy sections or smears of exudate. In more chronic cases, the diagnosis rests with the demonstration of antibodies to the appropriate chlamydial serotypes in the patient's serum.

Rickettsial Infections

Members of the order *Rickettsiales* are vector-borne obligate intracellular bacteria that cause epidemic typhus (*Rickettsia prowazekii*), scrub typhus (*Orienta tsutsugamushi*), and spotted fevers (*Rickettsia rickettsii* and others).[6] These organisms have the structure of gram-negative, rod-shaped bacteria, although they stain poorly with Gram stain. Epidemic typhus, which is transmitted from person to person by body lice, is associated with wars and human deprivation, when individuals are forced to live in close contact without changing clothes. Scrub typhus, transmitted by chiggers, was a major problem for US soldiers in the Pacific in World War II and in Vietnam. Rocky Mountain spotted fever (RMSF), transmitted to humans by dog ticks, is most common in the southeastern and south-central United States. Rickettsiae of RMSF are transmitted after several hours of the tick feeding or, less commonly, when the tick is crushed during removal from the skin.

Ehrlichiosis is a recently discovered, tick-transmitted disease caused by *Rickettsiales*. The bacteria predominantly infect neutrophils (*Anaplasma phagocytophilum* and *Ehrlichia ewingii*) or macrophages (*Ehrlichia chaffeensis*). Characteristic cytoplasmic inclusions (morulae), occasionally shaped like mulberries and composed of masses of bacteria, can be seen in leukocytes (Fig. 8–42). Ehrlichiosis is characterized by abrupt onset of fever, headache, and malaise, and may pro-

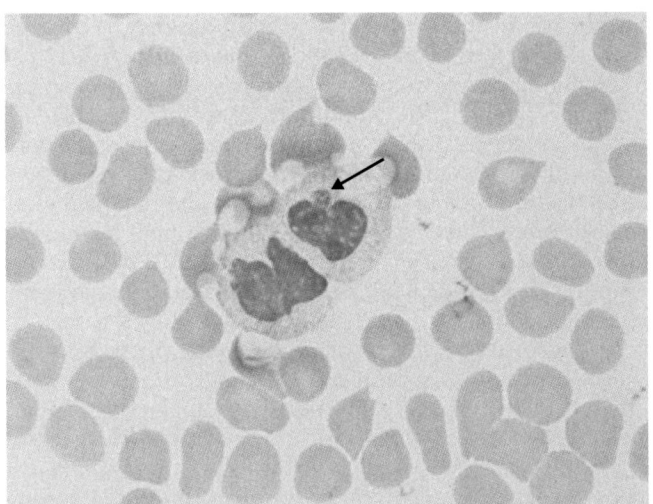

FIGURE 8–42 Peripheral blood granulocyte (band neutrophil) containing an *Ehrlichia* inclusion *(arrow)*. (Courtesy of Dr. Stephen Dumler, Johns Hopkins Medical Institution, Baltimore, MD.)

gress to respiratory insufficiency, renal failure, and shock. Rash occurs in approximately 40% of people with *E. chaffeensis* infections.

Rickettsial diseases are usually diagnosed clinically and confirmed by serology.

Pathogenesis. Rickettsiae do not produce significant toxins. The rickettsiae that cause typhus and spotted fevers predominantly infect vascular endothelial cells, especially those in the lungs and brain. The bacteria enter the endothelial cells by endocytosis, but they escape from the endosome into the cytoplasm before formation of the acidic phagolysosome. The organisms proliferate in the endothelial cell cytoplasm and then either lyse the cell (typhus group) or spread from cell to cell through actin-mobilized motion (spotted fever group). *The severe manifestations of rickettsial infection are primarily due to vascular leakage secondary to endothelial cell damage.*[6] This causes hypovolemic shock with peripheral edema, as well as pulmonary edema, renal failure, and a variety of CNS manifestations that can include coma.

The innate immune response to rickettsial infection is mounted by NK cells, which produce IFN-γ, reducing bacterial proliferation. Subsequent CTL responses are critical for elimination of rickettsial infections. IFN-γ and TNF, from activated NK cells and T cells, stimulate the production of bactericidal nitric oxide. CTLs lyse infected cells, reducing bacterial proliferation. Rickettsial infections are diagnosed by immunostaining of organisms or by detection of antirickettsial antibodies in the serum.

Morphology

Typhus Fever. In mild cases the gross changes are limited to a rash and small hemorrhages due to the vascular lesions. In more severe cases, there may be areas of necrosis of the skin and gangrene of the tips of the fingers, nose, earlobes, scrotum, penis, and vulva. In such cases, irregular ecchymotic hemorrhages may be found internally, principally in the brain, heart muscle, testes, serosal membrane, lungs, and kidneys.

The most prominent microscopic changes are small-vessel lesions and focal areas of hemorrhage and inflammation in various organs and tissues. Endothelial swelling in the capillaries, arterioles, and venules may narrow the lumens of these vessels. A cuff of mononuclear inflammatory cells usually surrounds the affected vessel. The vascular lumens are sometimes thrombosed. Necrosis of the vessel wall is unusual in typhus (as compared to RMSF). Vascular thromboses lead to gangrenous necrosis of the skin and other structures in a minority of cases. In the brain, characteristic typhus nodules are composed of focal microglial proliferations with an infiltrate of mixed T lymphocytes and macrophages (Fig. 8–43).

Scrub typhus, or mite-borne infection, is usually a milder version of typhus fever. The rash is usually transitory or might not appear. Vascular necrosis or thrombosis is rare, but there may be a prominent inflammatory lymphadenopathy.

Rocky Mountain Spotted Fever. A hemorrhagic rash that extends over the entire body, including the palms of the hands and soles of the feet, is the hallmark of RMSF. An eschar at the site of the tick bite is uncommon with RMSF but is common with *R. akari,* *R. africae,* and *R. conorii* infection. The vascular lesions that underlie the rash often lead to acute necrosis, fibrin extravasation, and occasionally thrombosis of the small blood vessels, including arterioles (Fig. 8–44). In severe RMSF, foci of necrotic skin appear, particularly on the fingers, toes, elbows, ears, and scrotum. The perivascular inflammatory response, similar to that of typhus, is seen in the brain, skeletal muscle, lungs, kidneys, testes, and heart muscle. The vascular lesions in the brain may involve larger vessels and produce microinfarcts. A noncardiogenic pulmonary edema causing adult respiratory distress syndrome is the major cause of death in patients with RMSF.

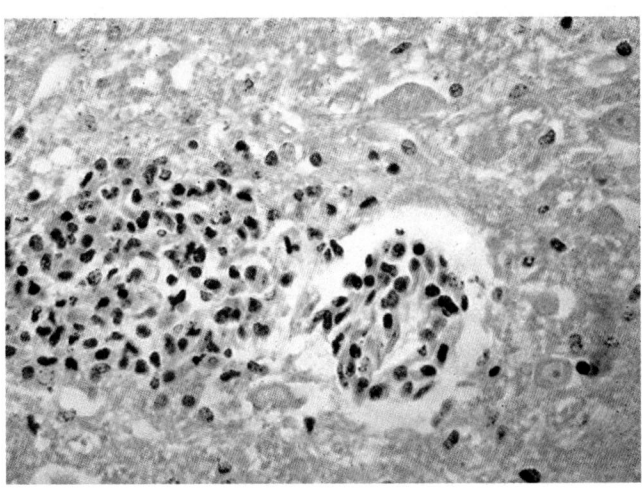

FIGURE 8–43 Typhus nodule in the brain.

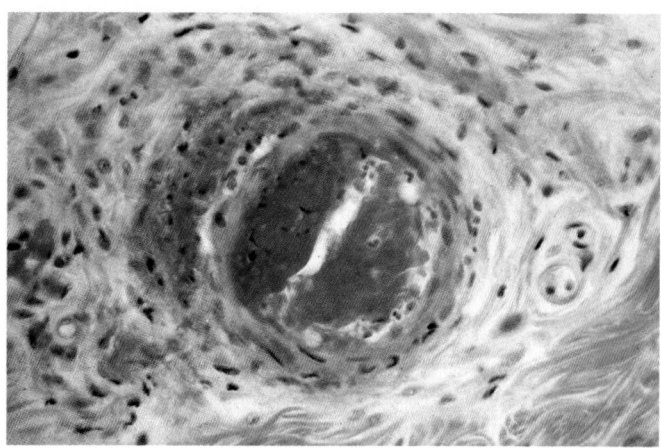

FIGURE 8–44   Rocky Mountain spotted fever with a thrombosed vessel and vasculitis.

Fungal Infections

Fungi are eukaryotes with cell walls that give them their shape. Fungal cells can grow as multicellular filaments called molds or as single cells or chains of cells called yeast. Most yeasts reproduce by budding. Some yeasts, such as *Candida albicans*, can produce buds that fail to detach and become elongated, producing a chain of elongated yeast cells called pseudohyphae. Molds consist of threadlike filaments (hyphae) that grow and divide at their tips. They can produce round cells, called conidia, that easily become airborne, disseminating the fungus. Many medically important fungi are dimorphic, existing as yeast or molds, depending on environmental conditions (yeast form at human body temperature and a mold form at room temperature).[99] Fungal infections can be diagnosed by histologic examination, although definitive identification of some species requires culture.

Fungal infections, also called *mycoses*, are of four major types: (1) superficial and cutaneous mycoses, which are common and limited to the very superficial or keratinized layers of skin, hair, and nails; (2) subcutaneous mycoses, which involve the skin, subcutaneous tissues, and lymphatics and rarely disseminate systemically; (3) endemic mycoses, which are caused by dimorphic fungi that can produce serious systemic illness in healthy individuals; and (4) opportunistic mycoses, which can cause life-threatening systemic diseases in individuals who are immunosuppressed or who carry implanted prosthetic devices or vascular catheters. Some of the fungi that cause opportunistic mycoses are discussed below; those involving specific organs are discussed in other chapters.

Candidiasis

Residing normally in the skin, mouth, gastrointestinal tract, and vagina, *Candida* species usually live as benign commensals and seldom produce disease in healthy people. However, *Candida* species, most often *C. albicans*, are the most frequent cause of human fungal infections. Most types of *Candida* infections originate when the normal commensal flora breach the skin or mucosal barriers. These infections may be confined to the skin or mucous membranes or disseminate widely.[99] In otherwise healthy people *Candida* organisms cause vaginitis and diaper rash. Diabetics and burn patients are particularly susceptible to superficial candidiasis. In individuals with indwelling intravenous lines or catheters, or undergoing peritoneal dialysis, *Candida* organisms can spread into the bloodstream. Severe disseminated candidiasis most commonly occurs in patients who are neutropenic due to leukemia, chemotherapy, or bone marrow transplantation, and may cause shock and DIC.

Pathogenesis. A single strain of *Candida* can be successful as a commensal or a pathogen. *Candida* can shift between different phenotypes in a reversible and apparently random fashion. Phenotypic switching involves coordinated regulation of phase-specific genes and provides a way for *Candida* to adapt to changes in the host environment (produced by antibiotic therapy, the immune response, or altered host physiology). These variants can exhibit altered colony morphology, cell shape, antigenicity, and virulence.[100]

Candida produce a large number of functionally distinct adhesins that mediate adherence to host cells, some of which also function in *Candida* morphogenesis or signaling.[101] These adhesins include (1) an integrin-like protein, which binds arginine-glycine-aspartic acid (RGD) groups on fibrinogen, fibronectin, and laminin; (2) a protein that resembles transglutaminase substrates and binds to epithelial cells; and (3) several agglutinins that bind to endothelial cells or fibronectin. Adhesion is an important determinant of virulence, since strains with reduced adherence to cells in vitro are avirulent in experimental models in vivo. Differential expression of adhesins by yeast and filamentous forms leads to recognition of distinct receptors on host cells.

Candida produce a number of enzymes that contribute to invasiveness, including at least nine secreted aspartyl proteinases, which may promote tissue invasion by degrading extracellular matrix proteins, and catalases, which may enable the organism to resist oxidative killing by phagocytic cells.[101,102] *Candida* also secrete adenosine, which blocks neutrophil oxygen radical production and degranulation.

The ability of *C. albicans* to grow as biofilms also contributes to its capacity to cause disease.[103] *Candida* biofilms are microbial communities consisting of mixtures of yeast, filamentous forms, and fungal-derived extracellular matrix. *C. albicans* can form biofilms on implanted medical devices that reduce susceptibility of the organism to immune responses and antifungal drug therapy.

The immune response to *Candida* is complex. Innate immunity and T-cell responses are important for protection against *Candida* infection.[104] Neutrophils and macrophages phagocytose *Candida*, and oxidative killing by these phagocytes is a first line of host defense. The important role of neutrophils and macrophages is illustrated by the increased risk of *Candida* infections in individuals with neutropenia or defects in NADPH oxidase or myeloperoxidase. Filamentous forms, but not yeast, can escape from phagosomes and enter the cytoplasm and proliferate. *Candida* yeast activate dendritic cells to produce IL-12 more than do the filamentous forms of the fungi. As a result, the yeast forms elicit a protective antifungal T_H1 response, while filamentous forms tend to stimulate a nonprotective T_H2 response. Like other fungi, *Candida*

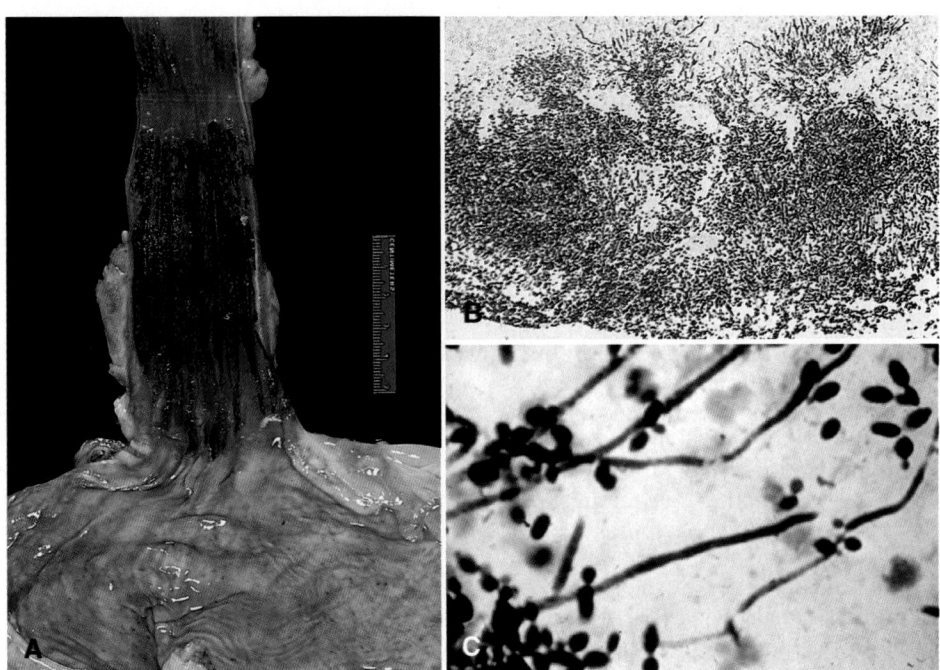

FIGURE 8–45 The morphology of *Candida* infections. **A,** Severe candidiasis of the distal esophagus. **B,** Silver stain of esophageal candidiasis reveals the dense mat of *Candida*. **C,** Characteristic pseudohyphae and blastoconidia (budding yeast) of *Candida*. (**C,** Courtesy of Dr. Dominick Cuvuoti, Department of Pathology, University of Texas Southwestern Medical School, Dallas, TX.)

also elicit T_H17 responses, which are responsible for recruiting neutrophils and monocytes (Chapter 6). *Candida* T-cell responses are particularly important for protection against mucosal and cutaneous *Candida* infection, as shown by recurrent mucocutaneous *Candida* infections in individuals with HIV infection and low T-cell counts.

Morphology. In tissue sections, *C. albicans* can appear as yeastlike forms (blastoconidia), pseudohyphae, and, less commonly, true hyphae, defined by the presence of septae (Fig. 8–45). Pseudohyphae, an important diagnostic clue, represent budding yeast cells joined end to end at constrictions. All forms may be present together in the same tissue. The organisms may be visible with routine hematoxylin and eosin stains, but a variety of special "fungal" stains (Gomori methenamine–silver, periodic acid–Schiff) are commonly used to better visualize them.

Most commonly candidiasis takes the form of a superficial infection on mucosal surfaces of the oral cavity **(thrush)**. Florid proliferation of the fungi creates gray-white, dirty-looking pseudomembranes composed of matted organisms and inflammatory debris. Deep to the surface, there is mucosal hyperemia and inflammation. This form of candidiasis is seen in newborns, debilitated people, children receiving oral steroids for asthma, and following a course of broad-spectrum antibiotics that destroy competing normal bacterial flora. The other major risk group includes HIV-positive patients; people with oral thrush for no obvious reason should be evaluated for HIV infection.

Candida esophagitis is commonly seen in AIDS patients and in those with hematolymphoid malignancies. These patients present with dysphagia (painful swallowing) and retrosternal pain; endoscopy demonstrates white plaques and pseudomembranes resembling oral thrush on the esophageal mucosa (see Fig. 8–45).

Candida vaginitis is a common form of vaginal infection in women, especially those who are diabetic, pregnant, or on oral contraceptive pills. It is usually associated with intense itching and a thick, curdlike discharge.

Cutaneous candidiasis can present in many different forms, including infection of the nail proper ("onychomycosis"), nail folds ("paronychia"), hair follicles ("folliculitis"), moist, intertriginous skin such as armpits or webs of the fingers and toes ("intertrigo"), and penile skin ("balanitis"). "Diaper rash" is a cutaneous candidial infection seen in the perineum of infants, in the region of contact with wet diapers.

Invasive candidiasis is caused by blood-borne dissemination of organisms to various tissues or organs. Common patterns include (1) renal abscesses, (2) myocardial abscesses and endocarditis, (3) brain microabscesses and meningitis, (4) endophthalmitis (virtually any eye structure can be involved), and (5) hepatic abscesses. In any of these locations, depending on the immune status of the infected person, the fungus may evoke little inflammatory reaction, cause the usual suppurative response, or occasionally produce granulomas. People with acute leukemias who are profoundly neutropenic after chemotherapy are particularly prone to developing systemic disease. *Candida* endocarditis is the most common fungal endocarditis, usually occurring in the setting of prosthetic heart valves or in intravenous drug abusers.

Cryptococcosis

Cryptococcus neoformans grows as an encapsulated yeast that causes meningoencephalitis in otherwise healthy individuals but more frequently presents as an opportunistic infection in people with AIDS, leukemia, lymphoma, systemic lupus erythematosus, or sarcoidosis, as well as in transplant recipients. Many of these patients receive high-dose corticosteroids, a major risk factor for *Cryptococcus* infection.

Pathogenesis. *Cryptococcus neoformans* is present in the soil and in bird (particularly pigeon) droppings and infects people when it is inhaled. Several virulence factors enable it to evade host defenses, including (1) a polysaccharide capsule, (2) melanin production, and (3) enzymes.[105] These mechanisms are not very effective when *C. neoformans* infects hosts with intact immune defenses, but they can lead to disseminated disease in immunosuppressed individuals.

Glucuronoxylomannin, the principal capsular polysaccharide of *C. neoformans*, is a major virulence factor that inhibits phagocytosis by alveolar macrophages, leukocyte migration, and recruitment of inflammatory cells. *C. neoformans* can undergo phenotypic switching, which leads to changes in the structure and size of the capsule polysaccharide, providing a means to evade immune responses.[106]

Cryptococcus neoformans makes laccase, which catalyzes the formation of a melanin-like pigment.[105] Laccase mutants of *C. neoformans* have reduced virulence in animal models. The effects of melanin may be related to its antioxidant properties. These fungi also make a number of other enzymes, including a serine proteinase that cleaves fibronectin and other basement membrane proteins, which may aid tissue invasion.[107] *C. neoformans* can establish latent infections accompanied by granuloma formation that can reactivate in immunosuppressed hosts.[108]

Morphology. Cryptococcus has yeast but not pseudohyphal or hyphal forms. The 5- to 10-μm cryptococcal yeast has a highly characteristic thick gelatinous capsule. Capsular polysaccharide stains intense red with periodic acid–Schiff and mucicarmine in tissues and can be detected with antibody-coated beads in an agglutination assay. India ink preparations create a negative image, visualizing the thick capsule as a clear halo within a dark background. Although the lung is the primary site of infection, pulmonary involvement is usually mild and asymptomatic, even while the fungus is spreading to the CNS. *C. neoformans*, however, may form a solitary pulmonary granuloma similar to the circumscribed (coin) lesions caused by *Histoplasma*. The major lesions caused by *C. neoformans* are in the CNS, involving the meninges, cortical gray matter, and basal nuclei. The host

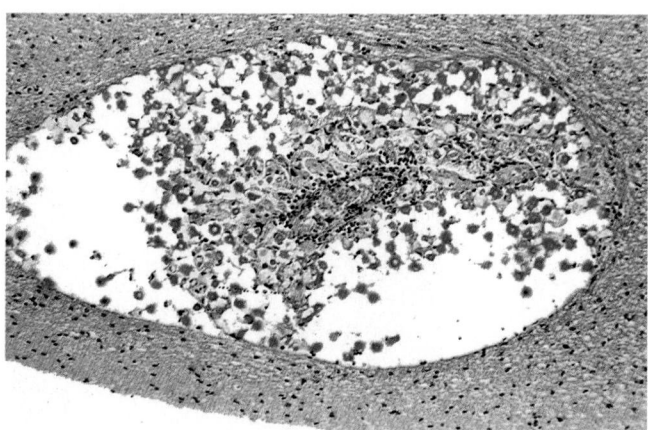

FIGURE 8–46 Mucicarmine stain of cryptococci (staining red) in a Virchow-Robin perivascular space of the brain (soap-bubble lesion).

response to cryptococci is extremely variable. In immunosuppressed people, organisms may evoke virtually no inflammatory reaction, so gelatinous masses of fungi grow in the meninges or expand the perivascular Virchow-Robin spaces within the gray matter, producing the so-called soap-bubble lesions (Fig. 8–46). In severely immunosuppressed persons, *C. neoformans* may disseminate widely to the skin, liver, spleen, adrenals, and bones. In nonimmunosuppressed people or in those with protracted disease, the fungi induce a chronic granulomatous reaction composed of macrophages, lymphocytes, and foreign body–type giant cells. Suppuration also may occur, as well as a rare granulomatous arteritis of the circle of Willis.

Aspergillosis

Aspergillus is a ubiquitous mold that causes allergies (allergic bronchopulmonary aspergillosis) in otherwise healthy people and serious *sinusitis, pneumonia,* and invasive disease in immunocompromised individuals. The major conditions that predispose to *Aspergillus* infection are neutropenia and corticosteroids. *Aspergillus fumigatus* is the most common species to cause disease, and it produces severe invasive infections in immunocompromised individuals.

Pathogenesis. *Aspergillus* species are transmitted by airborne conidia, and the lung is the major portal of entry. The small size of *A. fumigatus* spores, approximately 2 to 3 μm, enables them to reach alveoli. Conidia germinate into hyphae, which then invade tissues. Neutrophils and macrophages are the major host defenses against *Aspergillus*. Alveolar macrophages ingest and kill the conidia, while neutrophils produce reactive oxygen intermediates that kill hyphae. Invasive aspergillosis is highly associated with neutropenia and impaired neutrophil defenses.

Aspergillus produces several virulence factors, including adhesins, antioxidants, enzymes, and toxins.[108] Conidia can bind to fibrinogen, laminin, complement, fibronectin, colla-

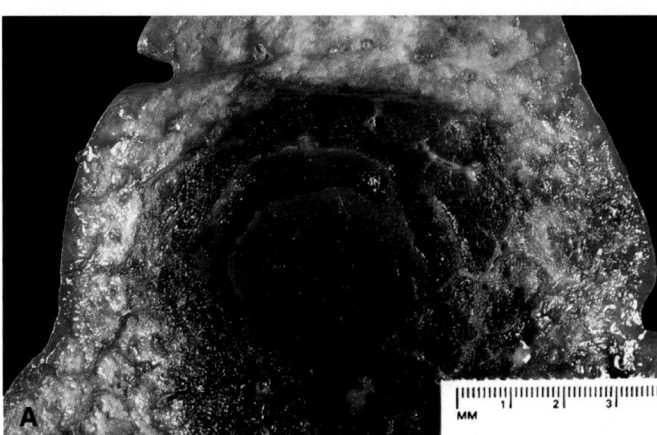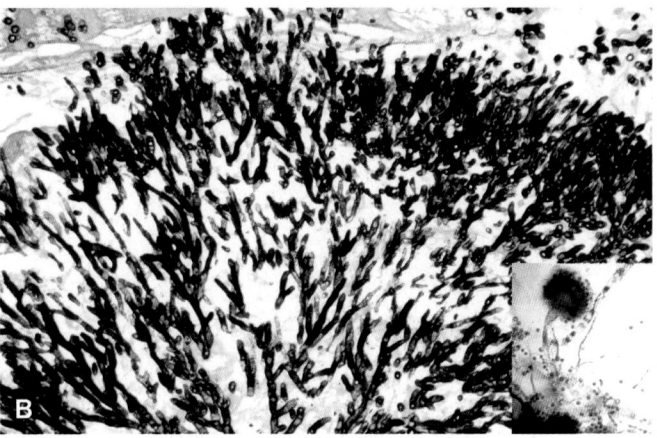

FIGURE 8–47 *Aspergillus* morphology. **A,** Invasive aspergillosis of the lung in a bone marrow transplant patient. **B,** Histologic sections from this case, stained with Gomori methenamine-silver stain, show septate hyphae with acute-angle branching, features consistent with *Aspergillus*. Occasionally, *Aspergillus* may demonstrate fruiting bodies *(inset)* when it grows in areas that are well aerated (such as the upper respiratory tract).

gen, albumin, and surfactant proteins, but receptor-ligand interactions are not well defined. *Aspergillus* produces several antioxidant defenses, including melanin pigment, mannitol, catalases, and superoxide dismutases. This fungus also produces phospholipases, proteases, and toxins, but their roles in pathogenicity are not yet clear. *Restrictocin* and *mitogillin* are ribotoxins that inhibit host-cell protein synthesis by degrading mRNAs. The carcinogen *aflatoxin* is made by *Aspergillus* species growing on the surface of peanuts and may be a cause of liver cancer in Africa.[109] Sensitization to *Aspergillus* spores produces an allergic alveolitis[110] (Chapter 15). *Allergic bronchopulmonary aspergillosis*, associated with hypersensitivity arising from superficial colonization of the bronchial mucosa, often occurs in asthmatic people.

> **Morphology. Colonizing aspergillosis (aspergilloma)** usually implies growth of the fungus in pulmonary cavities with minimal or no invasion of the tissues (the nose also is often colonized). The cavities are usually the result of prior tuberculosis, bronchiectasis, old infarcts, or abscesses. Proliferating masses of hyphae form brownish "fungal balls" lying free within the cavities. The surrounding inflammatory reaction may be sparse, or there may be chronic inflammation and fibrosis. People with aspergillomas usually have recurrent hemoptysis.
>
> **Invasive aspergillosis** is an opportunistic infection that is confined to immunosuppressed hosts. The primary lesions are usually in the lung, but widespread hematogenous dissemination with involvement of the heart valves and brain is common. The pulmonary lesions take the form of necrotizing pneumonia with sharply delineated, rounded, gray foci and hemorrhagic borders; they are often referred to as **target lesions** (Fig. 8–47A). *Aspergillus* forms fruiting bodies (usually in lung cavities) and septate filaments, 5 to 10 μm thick, branching at acute angles (40

> degrees) (Fig. 8–47B). *Aspergillus* hyphae cannot be distinguished from *Pseudallescheria boydii* and *Fusarium* species by morphology alone. *Aspergillus* has a tendency to invade blood vessels; therefore, areas of hemorrhage and infarction are usually superimposed on the necrotizing, inflammatory tissue reactions. Rhinocerebral *Aspergillus* infection in immunosuppressed individuals resembles that caused by Zygomycetes (e.g., mucormycosis).

Zygomycosis (Mucormycosis)

Zygomycosis (mucormycosis, phycomycosis) is an opportunistic infection caused by "bread mold fungi," including *Mucor, Rhizopus, Absidia,* and *Cunninghamella,* which belong to the class Zygomycetes.[111] These fungi are widely distributed in nature and cause no harm to immunocompetent individuals, but they infect immunosuppressed people, albeit somewhat less frequently than do *Candida* and *Aspergillus.* Major predisposing factors are neutropenia, corticosteroid use, diabetes mellitus, iron overload, and breakdown of the cutaneous barrier (e.g., as a result of burns, surgical wounds, or trauma).

Pathogenesis. Similar to *Aspergillus*, zygomycetes fungi are transmitted by airborne asexual spores. Most commonly, inhaled spores produce infection in the sinuses and the lungs, but percutaneous exposure or ingestion can also lead to infection. The thermotolerance of the spores of some species of zygomycetes might contribute to their spread. Macrophages provide the initial defenses by phagocytosis and oxidative killing of germinating spores.[111] Neutrophils have a key role in killing fungi during established infection.

> **Morphology.** Zygomycetes form nonseptate, irregularly wide (6 to 50 μm) fungal hyphae with frequent

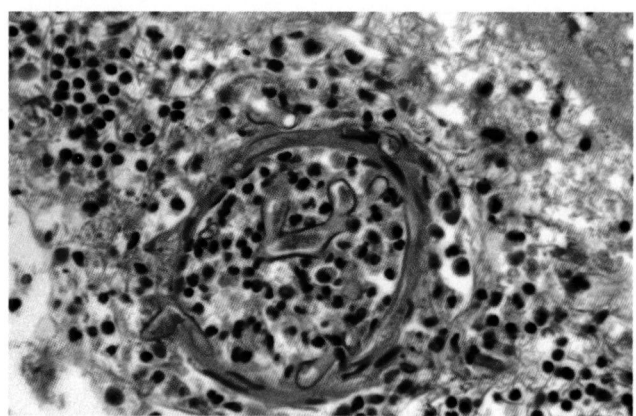

FIGURE 8–48 Meningeal blood vessels with angioinvasive *Mucor* species. Note the irregular width and near right-angle branching of the hyphae. (Courtesy of Dr. Dan Milner, Department of Pathology, Brigham and Women's Hospital, Boston, MA.)

right-angle branching, which are readily demonstrated in necrotic tissues by hematoxylin and eosin or special fungal stains (Fig. 8–48). The three primary sites of invasion are the nasal sinuses, lungs, and gastrointestinal tract, depending on whether the spores (which are widespread in dust and air) are inhaled or ingested. Most commonly in diabetics, the fungus may spread from nasal sinuses to the orbit and brain, giving rise to **rhinocerebral mucormycosis**. The zygomycetes cause local tissue necrosis, invade arterial walls, and penetrate the periorbital tissues and cranial vault. Meningoencephalitis follows, sometimes complicated by cerebral infarctions when fungi invade arteries and induce thrombosis.

Lung involvement with zygomycetes may be secondary to rhinocerebral disease, or it may be primary in people with severe immunodeficiency. The lung lesions combine areas of hemorrhagic pneumonia with vascular thrombi and distal infarctions.

Parasitic Infections

PROTOZOA

Protozoa are unicellular, eukaryotic organisms. The parasitic protozoa are transmitted by insects or by the fecal-oral route and, in humans, mainly reside in the blood or intestine (Table 8–9). Most of these infections are diagnosed by microscopic examination of blood smears or lesions.

Malaria

Malaria, caused by the intracellular parasite *Plasmodium*, is a worldwide infection that affects 500 million and kills more than 1 million people each year. According to the World Health Organization, 90% of deaths from malaria occur in sub-Saharan Africa, where malaria is the leading cause of death in children younger than 5 years old. *Plasmodium falciparum*, which causes severe malaria, and the three other malaria parasites that infect humans (*P. vivax, P. ovale,* and *P. malariae*) are transmitted by female *Anopheles* mosquitoes that are widely distributed throughout Africa, Asia, and Latin America. Nearly all of the approximately 1500 new cases of malaria each year in the United States occur in travelers or immigrants, although rare cases transmitted by *Anopheles* mosquitoes or blood transfusion do occur. Worldwide public health efforts to control malaria in the 1950s through 1980s failed, leaving mosquitoes resistant to DDT and malathion and *Plasmodium* resistant to chloroquine and pyrimethamine.

Life Cycle and Pathogenesis. *Plasmodium vivax, P. ovale,* and *P. malariae* cause low levels of parasitemia, mild anemia, and, in rare instances, splenic rupture and nephrotic syndrome. *P. falciparum* causes high levels of parasitemia, severe anemia, cerebral symptoms, renal failure, pulmonary edema, and death. The life cycles of the *Plasmodium* species are similar, although *P. falciparum* differs in ways that contribute to its greater virulence.

The infectious stage of malaria, the *sporozoite,* is found in the salivary glands of female mosquitoes. When the mosquito takes a blood meal, sporozoites are released into the human's

TABLE 8–9 Selected Human Protozoal Diseases		
Location	**Species**	**Disease**
Luminal or Epithelial	*Entamoeba histolytica*	Amebic dysentery; liver abscess
	Balantidium coli	Colitis
	Giardia lamblia	Diarrheal disease, malabsorption
	Isospora belli	Chronic enterocolitis or malabsorption or both
	Cryptosporidium sp.	
	Trichomonas vaginalis	Urethritis, vaginitis
Central Nervous System	*Naegleria fowleri*	Meningoencephalitis
	Acanthamoeba sp.	Meningoencephalitis or ophthalmitis
Bloodstream	*Plasmodium* sp.	Malaria
	Babesia microti, B. bovis	Babesiosis
	Trypanosoma sp.	African sleeping sickness
Intracellular	*Trypanosoma cruzi*	Chagas disease
	Leishmania donovani	Kala-azar
	Leishmania sp.	Cutaneous and mucocutaneous leishmaniasis
	Toxoplasma gondii	Toxoplasmosis

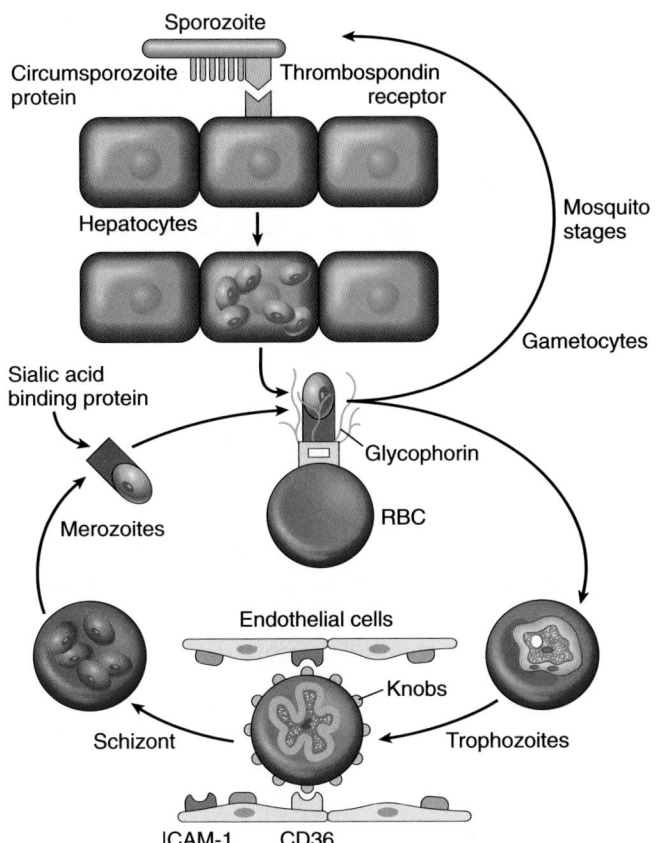

FIGURE 8–49 Life cycle of *Plasmodium falciparum*. ICAM-1, intercellular adhesion molecule 1; RBC, red blood cell. (Drawn by Dr. Jeffrey Joseph, Beth Israel–Deaconess Hospital, Boston, MA.)

blood and within minutes attach to and invade liver cells by binding to the hepatocyte receptor for the serum proteins thrombospondin and properdin[112] (Fig. 8–49). Within liver cells, malaria parasites multiply rapidly, releasing as many as 30,000 *merozoites* (asexual, haploid forms) when each infected hepatocyte ruptures. *P. vivax* and *P. ovale* form latent *hypnozoites* in hepatocytes, which cause relapses of malaria long after initial infection.

Once released from the liver, *Plasmodium* merozoites bind by a parasite lectin-like molecule to sialic acid residues on glycophorin molecules on the surface of red cells. Within the red cells the parasites grow in a membrane-bound digestive vacuole, hydrolyzing hemoglobin through secreted enzymes. The *trophozoite* is the first stage of the parasite in the red cell and is defined by the presence of a single chromatin mass. The next stage, the *schizont*, has multiple chromatin masses, each of which develops into a merozoite. On lysis of the red cell, the new merozoites infect additional red cells. Although most malaria parasites within the red cells develop into merozoites, some parasites develop into sexual forms called *gametocytes* that infect the mosquito when it takes its blood meal.

Plasmodium falciparum causes more severe disease than the other *Plasmodium* species do. Several features of *P. falciparum* account for its greater pathogenicity:

- *P. falciparum* is able to infect red blood cells of any age, leading to high parasite burdens and profound anemia. The other species infect only young or old red cells, which are a smaller fraction of the red cell pool.

- *P. falciparum* causes infected red cells to clump together (rosette) and to stick to endothelial cells lining small blood vessels (sequestration), which blocks blood flow. Several proteins, including *P. falciparum* erythrocyte membrane protein 1 (PfEMP1), form knobs on the surface of red cells (Fig. 8–49).[113] PfEMP1 binds to ligands on endothelial cells, including CD36, thrombospondin, VCAM-1, ICAM-1, and E-selectin. *Ischemia due to poor perfusion causes the manifestations of cerebral malaria, which is the main cause of death due to malaria in children.*

- *P. falciparum* stimulates production of high levels of cytokines, including TNF, IFN-γ, and IL-1. GPI-linked proteins, including merozoite surface antigens, are released from infected red cells and induce cytokine production by host cells by a mechanism that is not yet understood. These cytokines suppress production of red blood cells, increase fever, stimulate nitric oxide production (leading to tissue damage), and induce expression of endothelial receptors for PfEMP1 (increasing sequestration).

Host Resistance to *Plasmodium*. There are two general mechanisms of host resistance to *Plasmodium*. First, inherited alterations in red cells make people resistant to *Plasmodium*. Second, repeated or prolonged exposure to *Plasmodium* species stimulates an immune response that reduces the severity of the illness caused by malaria.

Several common mutations in hemoglobin genes confer resistance to malaria. People who are heterozygous for the sickle cell trait (HbS) become infected with *P. falciparum*, but they are less likely to die from infection. The HbS trait causes the parasites to grow poorly or die because of the low oxygen concentrations. The geographic distribution of the HbS trait is similar to that of *P. falciparum*, suggesting evolutionary selection of the HbS trait in people by the parasite. HbC, another common hemoglobin mutation, also protects against severe malaria by reducing parasite proliferation. People can also be resistant to malaria due to the absence of proteins to which the parasites bind. *P. vivax* enters red cells by binding to the Duffy blood group antigen. Many Africans, including most Gambians, are not susceptible to infection by *P. vivax* because they do not have the Duffy antigen.

Individuals living where *Plasmodium* is endemic often gain partial immune-mediated resistance to malaria, evidenced by reduced illness despite infection. Antibodies and T lymphocytes specific for *Plasmodium* reduce disease manifestations, although the parasite has developed strategies to evade the host immune response. *P. falciparum* uses antigenic variation to escape from antibody responses to PfEMP1. Each haploid *P. falciparum* genome has about 50 *var* genes, each encoding a variant of PfEMP1. The mechanism of *var* regulation is not known, but at least 2% of the parasites switch PfEMP1 genes each generation. CTLs may also be important in resistance to *P. falciparum*. Despite enormous efforts, there has been little progress in developing a vaccine for malaria.

Morphology. *Plasmodium falciparum* infection initially causes congestion and enlargement of the spleen, which may eventually exceed 1000 gm in

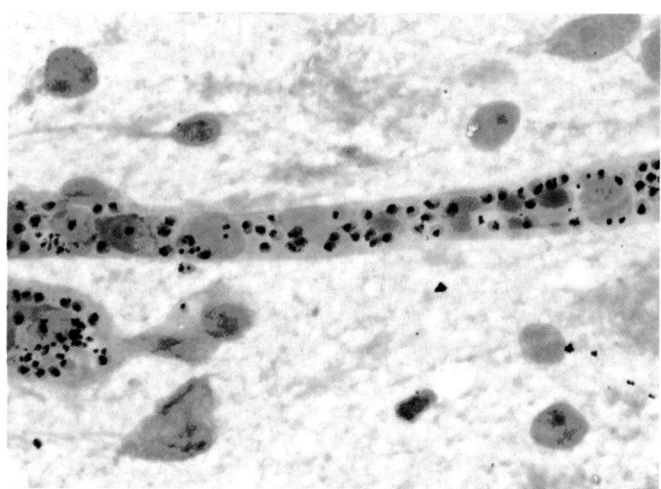

FIGURE 8–50 Field's stain of *Plasmodium falciparum*–infected red cells marginating within a capillary in cerebral malaria. (Courtesy of Dr. Dan Milner, Department of Pathology, Brigham and Women's Hospital, Boston, MA.)

weight. Parasites are present within red cells, which is the basis of the diagnostic test, and there is increased phagocytic activity of the macrophages in the spleen. In chronic malaria infection, the spleen becomes increasingly fibrotic and brittle, with a thick capsule and fibrous trabeculae. The parenchyma is gray or black because of phagocytic cells containing granular, brown-black, faintly birefringent hemozoin pigment. In addition, macrophages with engulfed parasites, red blood cells, and debris are numerous.

With progression of malaria, the liver becomes progressively enlarged and pigmented. Kupffer cells are heavily laden with malarial pigment, parasites, and cellular debris, while some pigment is also present in the parenchymal cells. Pigmented phagocytic cells may be found dispersed throughout the bone marrow, lymph nodes, subcutaneous tissues, and lungs. The kidneys are often enlarged and congested with a dusting of pigment in the glomeruli and hemoglobin casts in the tubules.

In **malignant cerebral malaria** caused by *P. falciparum*, brain vessels are plugged with parasitized red cells (Fig. 8–50). Around the vessels there are ring hemorrhages that are probably related to local hypoxia incident to the vascular stasis and small focal inflammatory reactions (called **malarial** or **Dürck granulomas**). With more severe hypoxia, there is degeneration of neurons, focal ischemic softening, and occasionally scant inflammatory infiltrates in the meninges.

Nonspecific focal hypoxic lesions in the heart may be induced by the progressive anemia and circulatory stasis in chronically infected people. In some, the myocardium shows focal interstitial infiltrates. Finally, in the nonimmune patient, pulmonary edema or shock with DIC may cause death, sometimes in the absence of other characteristic lesions.

Babesiosis

Babesia microti and *Babesia divergens* are malaria-like protozoans transmitted by the same deer ticks that carry Lyme disease and granulocytic ehrlichiosis.[114] The white-footed mouse is the reservoir for *B. microti*, and in some areas, nearly all mice have a persistent low-level parasitemia. *B. microti* survives well in refrigerated blood, and several cases of transfusion-acquired babesiosis have been reported. Babesiae parasitize red blood cells and cause fever and hemolytic anemia. The symptoms are mild except in debilitated or splenectomized individuals, who develop severe and fatal parasitemias.

Morphology. In blood smears, *Babesia* organisms resemble *P. falciparum* ring stages, although they lack hemozoin pigment and are more pleomorphic. They form characteristic tetrads (Maltese cross), which are diagnostic if found (Fig. 8–51). The level of *B. microti* parasitemia is a good indication of the severity of infection (about 1% in mild cases and up to 30% in splenectomized persons). In fatal cases the anatomic findings are related to shock and hypoxia, and include jaundice, hepatic necrosis, acute renal tubular necrosis, adult respiratory distress syndrome, erythrophagocytosis, and visceral hemorrhages.

Leishmaniasis

Leishmaniasis is a chronic inflammatory disease of the skin, mucous membranes, or viscera caused by obligate intracellular, kinetoplast-containing (kinetoplastid) protozoan parasites transmitted through the bite of infected sandflies. Leishmaniasis is endemic throughout the Middle East, South Asia, Africa, and Latin America. It may also be epidemic, as is tragically the case in Sudan, India, Bangladesh, and Brazil, where tens of thousands of people have died of visceral leishmaniasis. Leishmanial infection, like other intracellular organisms (mycobacteria, *Histoplasma*, *Toxoplasma*, and trypanosomes), is exacerbated by conditions that interfere with T-cell function, such as AIDS.[115] Culture or histologic examination is used to diagnose the infection.

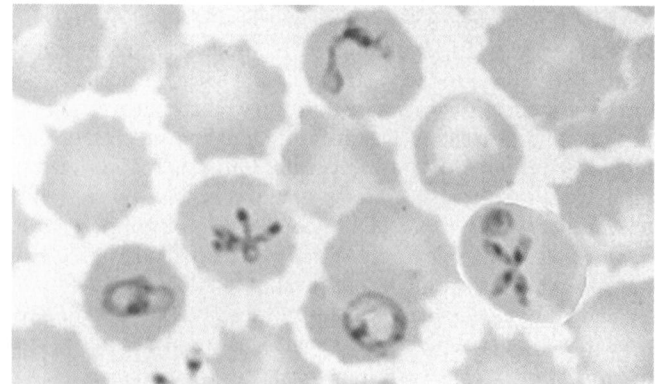

FIGURE 8–51 Erythrocytes with *Babesia*, including the distinctive Maltese cross form. (Courtesy of Lynne Garcia, LSG and Associates, Santa Monica, CA.)

Pathogenesis. The life cycle of *Leishmania* involves two forms: the promastigote, which develops and lives extracellularly in the sandfly vector, and the amastigote, which multiplies intracellularly in host macrophages. Mammals, including rodents, dogs, and foxes, are reservoirs of *Leishmania*. When sandflies bite infected humans or animals, macrophages harboring amastigotes are ingested. The amastigotes differentiate into promastigotes, multiply within the digestive tract of the sandfly and migrate to the salivary gland, where they are poised for transmission by the fly bite. When the infected fly bites a person, the slender, flagellated infectious promastigotes are released into the host dermis along with the sandfly saliva, which potentiates parasite infectivity.[116] The promastigotes are phagocytosed by macrophages, and the acidity within the phagolysosome induces them to transform into round amastigotes that lack flagella but contain a single mitochondrion with its DNA massed into a unique sub-organelle, the kinetoplast.[117] Amastigotes proliferate within macrophages, and dying macrophages release progeny amastigotes that can infect additional macrophages.

How far the amastigotes spread throughout the body depends on the *Leishmania* species and host. Cutaneous disease is caused primarily by *Leishmania major* and *Leishmania tropica* in the Old World and *Leishmania mexicana* and *Leishmania braziliensis* in the New World; mucocutaneous disease (also called espundia) is caused by *L. braziliensis* in the New World; and visceral disease involving the liver, spleen, and bone marrow is caused by *Leishmania donovani* and *Leishmania infantum* in the Old World and *Leishmania chagasi* in the New World. Tropism of *Leishmania* species seems to be linked in part to the optimal temperature for their growth. Parasites that cause visceral disease grow better at 37°C in vitro, whereas parasites that cause mucocutaneous disease grow better at lower temperatures. However, "cutaneous" *Leishmania* species often are viscerotropic in HIV patients.

Leishmania manipulate innate host defenses to facilitate their entry and survival in host macrophages.[118] Promastigotes produce two abundant surface glycoconjugates, which seem to be important for their virulence. The first, *lipophosphoglycan*, forms a dense glycocalyx that both activates complement (leading to C3b deposition on the parasite surface) and inhibits complement action (by preventing membrane attack complex insertion into the parasite membrane). Thus, the parasite becomes coated with C3b but avoids destruction by the membrane attack complex. Instead, the C3b on the surface of the parasite binds to Mac-1 and CR1 on macrophages, targeting the promastigote for phagocytosis. Once inside the cell, lipophosphoglycan protects the parasites within the phagolysosomes by scavenging oxygen radicals and by inhibiting lysosomal enzymes. The second surface glycoprotein, *gp63*, is a zinc-dependent proteinase that cleaves complement and some lysosomal antimicrobial enzymes. Gp63 also binds to fibronectin receptors on macrophages and promotes promastigote adhesion to macrophages. *Leishmania* amastigotes also produce molecules that facilitate their survival and replication within macrophages. Amastigotes reproduce in macrophage phagolysosomes, which normally have a pH of 4.5. However, the amastigotes protect themselves from this hostile environment by expressing a proton-transporting ATPase, which maintains the intracellular parasite pH at 6.5.

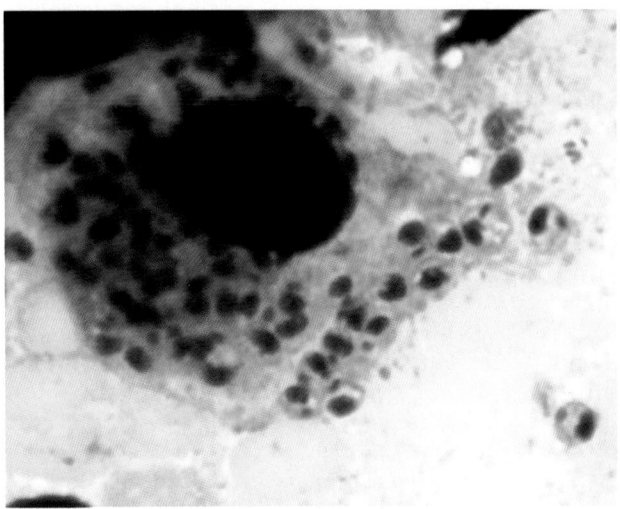

FIGURE 8–52 Giemsa stain of a tissue macrophage with *Leishmania donovani* parasites. (Courtesy of Dr. Dan Milner, Department of Pathology, Brigham and Women's Hospital, Boston, MA.)

Much of our knowledge of mechanisms of resistance and susceptibility to *Leishmania* comes from experimental mouse models.[118] Parasite-specific CD4+ helper T lymphocytes of the T_H1 subset are needed to control *Leishmania* in mice and humans. *Leishmania* evade host immunity by altering macrophage gene expression and impairing the development of the T_H1 response. In animal models, mice that are resistant to *Leishmania* infection produce high levels of T_H1-derived IFN-γ, which activates macrophages to kill the parasites through reactive oxygen species. In contrast, in mouse strains that are susceptible to leishmaniasis, there is a dominant T_H2 response, and T_H2 cytokines such as IL-4, IL-13, and IL-10 prevent effective killing of *Leishmania* by inhibiting the microbicidal activity of macrophages.

Morphology. *Leishmania* species produce four different types of lesions in humans: visceral, cutaneous, mucocutaneous, and diffuse cutaneous. In **visceral leishmaniasis**, *L. donovani* or *L. chagasi* parasites invade macrophages throughout the mononuclear phagocyte system (Figure 8–52), and cause severe systemic disease marked by hepatosplenomegaly, lymphadenopathy, pancytopenia, fever, and weight loss. The spleen may weigh as much as 3 kg, and the lymph nodes may measure 5 cm in diameter. Phagocytic cells are enlarged and filled with *Leishmania*, many plasma cells are present, and the normal architecture of the spleen is obscured. In the late stages the liver becomes increasingly fibrotic. Phagocytic cells crowd the bone marrow and also may be found in the lungs, gastrointestinal tract, kidneys, pancreas, and testes. Often there is hyperpigmentation of the skin in individuals of South Asian ancestry, which is why the disease is called kala-azar or "black fever" in Urdu (the language spoken in India and Pakistan). In the kidneys there may be an immune complex–mediated mesangioproliferative glomerulonephritis, and in advanced cases there may be amyloid deposition. The overloading of phagocytic cells with parasites predisposes the patients to secondary bacterial infections, the usual cause of death. Hemorrhages related to thrombocytopenia may also be fatal.

Cutaneous leishmaniasis, caused by *L. major, L. mexicana*, and *L. braziliensis*, is a relatively mild, localized disease consisting of ulcer(s) on exposed skin. The lesion begins as a papule surrounded by induration, changes into a shallow and slowly expanding ulcer, often with heaped-up borders, and usually heals by involution within 6 to 18 months without treatment. On microscopic examination, the lesion is granulomatous, usually with many giant cells and few parasites.

Mucocutaneous leishmaniasis, caused by *L. braziliensis*, is found only in the New World. Moist, ulcerating or nonulcerating lesions, which may be disfiguring, develop in the nasopharyngeal areas. Lesions may be progressive and highly destructive. Microscopic examination reveals a mixed inflammatory infiltrate composed of parasite-containing macrophages with lymphocytes and plasma cells. Later the tissue inflammatory response becomes granulomatous, and the number of parasites declines. Eventually, the lesions remit and scar, although reactivation may occur after long intervals by mechanisms that are not currently understood.

Diffuse cutaneous leishmaniasis is a rare form of dermal infection, thus far found in Ethiopia and adjacent East Africa and in Central and South America. Diffuse cutaneous leishmaniasis begins as a single skin nodule, which continues spreading until the entire body is covered by nodular lesions. Microscopically, they contain aggregates of foamy macrophages stuffed with leishmania.

African Trypanosomiasis

African trypanosomes are kinetoplastid parasites that proliferate as extracellular forms in the blood and cause sustained or intermittent fevers, lymphadenopathy, splenomegaly, progressive brain dysfunction (sleeping sickness), cachexia, and death. *Trypanosoma brucei rhodesiense* infections, which occur in East Africa, are often acute and virulent. *Trypanosoma brucei gambiense* infection tends to be chronic and occurs most frequently in the West African bush. Tsetse flies (genus *Glossina*) transmit African *Trypanosoma* to humans either from the reservoir of parasites found in wild and domestic animals (*T. brucei rhodesiense*) or from other humans (*T. brucei gambiense*). Within the fly, the parasites multiply in the stomach and then in the salivary glands before developing into nondividing trypomastigotes, which are transmitted to humans and animals.

Pathogenesis. African trypanosomes are covered by a single, abundant, glycolipid-anchored protein called the *variant surface glycoprotein (VSG)*.[119] As parasites proliferate in the bloodstream, the host produces antibodies to the VSG, which, in association with phagocytes, kill most of the organisms, causing a spike of fever. A small number of parasites,

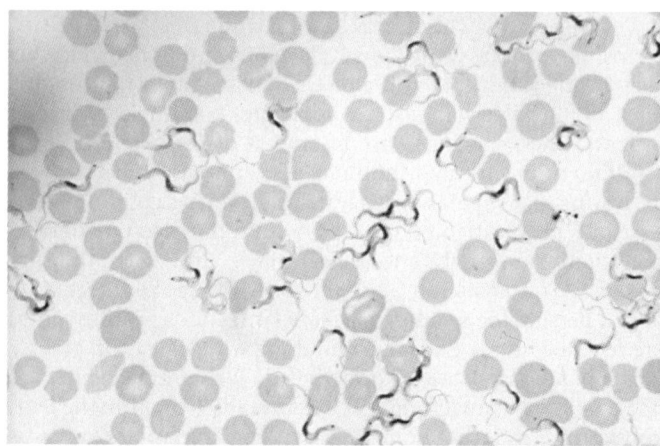

FIGURE 8–53 Slender bloodstream parasites of African trypanosomiasis.

however, undergo a genetic rearrangement and produce a different VSG on their surface and so escape the host immune response. These successor trypanosomes multiply until the host mounts an antibody response against their VSG and kills most of them, and another clone with a new VSG takes over. In this way, African trypanosomes escape the immune response to cause waves of fever before they finally invade the CNS.

Trypanosomes have many VSG genes, only one of which is expressed at a time. The parasite uses an elegant mechanism to turn VSG genes on and off.[119] Although VSG genes are scattered throughout the trypanosome genome, only VSG genes found within chromosomal regions called *bloodstream expression sites*, located in telomeres (the ends of chromosomes), are expressed. New VSG genes are moved into the bloodstream expression sites mainly by homologous recombination. A poorly understood transcription apparatus, which includes the RNA polymerase that transcribes VSG genes, associates with a single bloodstream expression site to limit expression to one VSG gene at a time.

Morphology. A large, red, rubbery chancre forms at the site of the insect bite, where large numbers of parasites are surrounded by a dense, predominantly mononuclear, inflammatory infiltrate. With chronicity, the lymph nodes and spleen enlarge due to infiltration by lymphocytes, plasma cells, and macrophages, which are filled with dead parasites. Trypanosomes, which are small and difficult to visualize (Fig. 8–53), concentrate in capillary loops, such as the choroid plexus and glomeruli. When parasites breach the blood-brain barrier and invade the CNS, a leptomeningitis develops that extends into the perivascular Virchow-Robin spaces, and eventually a demyelinating panencephalitis occurs. Plasma cells containing cytoplasmic globules filled with immunoglobulins are frequent and are referred to as **Mott cells**. Chronic disease leads to progressive cachexia, and patients, devoid of energy and normal mentation, waste away.

Chagas Disease

Trypanosoma cruzi is a kinetoplastid, intracellular protozoan parasite that causes American trypanosomiasis, or Chagas disease. Chagas disease occurs rarely in the United States and Mexico but is more common in South America, particularly Brazil. *T. cruzi* parasites infect many animals, including cats, dogs, and rodents. The parasites are transmitted between animals and to humans by "kissing bugs" (triatomids), which hide in the cracks of loosely constructed houses, feed on the sleeping inhabitants, and pass the parasites in the feces; the infectious parasites enter the host through damaged skin or through mucous membranes. At the site of skin entry there may be a transient, erythematous nodule called a *chagoma*.

Pathogenesis. While most intracellular pathogens avoid the toxic contents of lysosomes, *T. cruzi* actually requires brief exposure to the acidic phagolysosome to stimulate development of amastigotes, the intracellular stage of the parasite.[120] To gain exposure to lysosomes, *T. cruzi* trypomastigotes stimulate an increase in the concentration of cytoplasmic calcium in host cells, which promotes fusion of the phagosome and lysosome. In addition to stimulating amastigote development, the low pH of the lysosome activates pore-forming proteins that disrupt the lysosomal membrane, releasing the parasite into the cell cytoplasm. Parasites reproduce as rounded amastigotes in the cytoplasm of host cells and then develop flagella, lyse host cells, enter the bloodstream, and penetrate smooth, skeletal, and heart muscles.

In *acute Chagas disease*, which is mild in most individuals, cardiac damage results from direct invasion of myocardial cells by the organisms and the subsequent inflammation. Rarely, acute Chagas disease presents with high parasitemia, fever, or progressive cardiac dilation and failure, often with generalized lymphadenopathy or splenomegaly. In *chronic Chagas disease*, which occurs in 20% of people 5 to 15 years after initial infection, the mechanism of cardiac and digestive tract damage is controversial; it probably results from an immune response induced by *T. cruzi* parasites, which are still present in small numbers. A striking inflammatory infiltration of the myocardium may be induced by the scant organisms.[121] Alternatively, parasites may induce an autoimmune response, such that antibodies and T cells that recognize parasite proteins cross-react with host myocardial cells, nerve cells, and extracellular proteins such as laminin. Damage to myocardial cells and to conductance pathways causes a dilated cardiomyopathy and cardiac arrhythmias, whereas damage to the myenteric plexus causes dilation of the colon (megacolon) and esophagus.

> **Morphology.** In lethal **acute myocarditis**, the changes are diffusely distributed throughout the heart. Clusters of amastigotes cause swelling of individual myocardial fibers and create intracellular pseudocysts. There is focal myocardial cell necrosis accompanied by extensive, dense, acute interstitial inflammatory infiltration throughout the myocardium, often associated with four-chamber cardiac dilation (Chapter 12).
>
> In **chronic Chagas disease** the heart is typically dilated, rounded, and increased in size and weight.

Often, there are mural thrombi that, in about half of autopsy cases, have given rise to pulmonary or systemic emboli or infarctions. On histologic examination, there are interstitial and perivascular inflammatory infiltrates composed of lymphocytes, plasma cells, and monocytes. There are scattered foci of myocardial cell necrosis and interstitial fibrosis, especially toward the apex of the left ventricle, which may undergo aneurysmal dilation and thinning. In the Brazilian endemic foci, as many as half of the patients with lethal carditis also have dilation of the esophagus or colon, related to damage to the intrinsic innervation of these organs. At the late stages, however, when such changes appear, parasites cannot be found within these ganglia. Chronic Chagas cardiomyopathy is often treated by cardiac transplantation.

METAZOA

Metazoa are multicellular, eukaryotic organisms. The parasitic metazoa are contracted by consuming the parasite, often in undercooked meat, or by direct invasion of the host through the skin or via insect bites. Metazoa dwell in many sites of the body, including the intestine, skin, lung, liver, muscle, blood vessels, and lymphatics. The infections are diagnosed by microscopic identification of larvae or ova in excretions or tissues, and by serology.

Strongyloidiasis

Strongyloides stercoralis infects tens of million people worldwide. It is endemic in the southeastern United States, South America, sub-Saharan Africa, and Southeast Asia. The worms live in the soil and infect humans when larvae penetrate the skin, travel in the circulation to the lungs, and then travel up the trachea to be swallowed. Female worms reside in the mucosa of the small intestine, where they produce eggs by asexual reproduction (parthenogenesis). Most of the larvae are passed in the stool and then may contaminate soil to continue the cycle of infection.

In immunocompetent hosts, *S. stercoralis* may cause diarrhea, bloating, and occasionally malabsorption. Unlike other parasitic worms, *S. stercoralis* larvae hatched in the gut can invade the colon mucosa and reinitiate infection (autoinfection). *Immunocompromised hosts, particularly people on prolonged corticosteroid therapy, can have very high worm burdens due to uncontrolled autoinfection.* This hyperinfection can be complicated by sepsis caused by bacteria from the intestine, which are carried into the host's blood by the invading larvae.

> **Morphology.** In mild strongyloidiasis, worms, mainly larvae, are present in the duodenal crypts but are not seen in the underlying tissue. There is an eosinophil-rich infiltrate in the lamina propria with mucosal edema. Hyperinfection with *S. stercoralis* results in invasion of larvae into the colonic submucosa, lymphatics, and blood vessels, with an associated

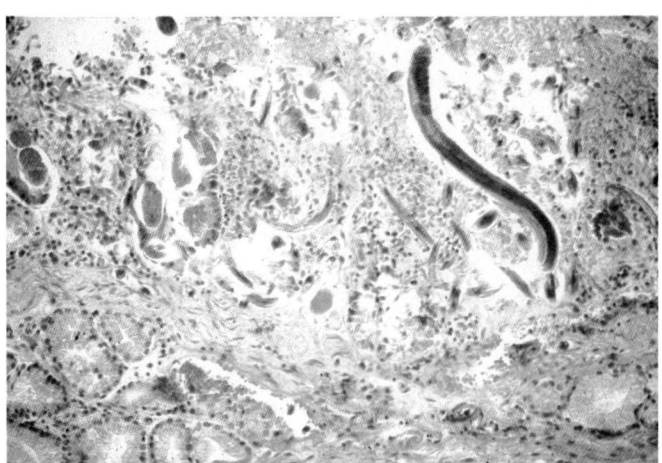

FIGURE 8–54 *Strongyloides* hyperinfection in a patient treated with high-dose cortisone. A female, her eggs, and rhabditoid larvae are in the duodenal crypts; filariform larvae are entering the blood vessels and muscularis mucosa. (Courtesy of Dr. Franz C. Von Lichtenberg, Brigham and Women's Hospital, Boston, MA.)

mononuclear infiltrate. There are many adult worms, larvae, and eggs in the crypts of the duodenum and ileum (Fig. 8–54). Worms of all stages may be found in other organs, including skin and lungs, and may even be found in large numbers in sputum.

Tapeworms (Cestodes): Cysticercosis and Hydatid Disease

Taenia solium and *Echinococcus granulosus* are cestode parasites (tapeworms) that cause cysticercosis and hydatid infections, respectively.[122,123] Both diseases are caused by larvae that develop after ingestion of tapeworm eggs. These tapeworms have a complex life cycle requiring two mammalian hosts: a definitive host, in which the worm reaches sexual maturity, and an intermediate host, in which the worm does not reach sexual maturity.

Taenia solium tapeworms consist of a head (scolex) that has suckers and hooklets that attach to the intestinal wall, a neck, and many flat segments called proglottids that contain both male and female reproductive organs. New proglottids develop behind the scolex. The most distal proglottids are mature and contain many eggs, and they can detach and be shed in the feces. *T. solium* can be transmitted to humans in two ways, with distinct outcomes. (1) Ingestion of undercooked pork containing larval cysts, called cysticerci, leads to development of adult tapeworms in the intestine. Ingested cysticerci attach to the intestinal wall and develop into mature adult tapeworms, which can grow to many meters in length and can produce mild abdominal symptoms. (2) When intermediate hosts (pigs or humans) ingest eggs in food or water contaminated with human feces, the larvae hatch, penetrate the gut wall, disseminate hematogenously, and encyst in many organs. Convulsions, increased intracranial pressure, and neurologic disturbances are caused by *T. solium* cysts in brain tissue.[124] Adult tapeworms are not produced with this mode of infection. Viable *T. solium* cysts often do not produce symptoms

and can evade host immune defenses by producing taeniaestatin and paramyosin, which seem to inhibit complement activation.[125] When the cysticerci die and degenerate, an inflammatory response develops. *Taenia saginata*, the beef tapeworm, and *Diphyllobothrium latum*, the fish tapeworm, are acquired by eating undercooked meat or fish. In humans these parasites live only in the gut, and they do not form cysticerci.

Hydatid disease is caused by ingestion of eggs of echinococcal species.[123] For *Echinococcus granulosus* the definitive hosts are dogs, and sheep are the usual intermediate hosts. For *Echinoccus multilocularis* foxes are the most important definitive host, and rodents are intermediate hosts. Humans are accidental intermediate hosts, infected by ingestion of food contaminated with eggs shed by dogs or foxes. Eggs hatch in the duodenum and invade the liver, lungs, or bones.

Morphology. Cysticerci may be found in any organ, but the more common locations include the brain, muscles, skin, and heart. Cerebral symptoms depend on the precise location of the cysts, which may be intraparenchymal, attached to the arachnoid, or freely floating in the ventricular system. The cysts are ovoid and white to opalescent, often grape-sized, and contain an invaginated scolex with hooklets that are bathed in clear cyst fluid (Fig. 8–55). The cyst wall is more than 100 µm thick, is rich in glycoproteins, and evokes little host reaction when it is intact. When cysts degenerate, however, there is inflammation, followed by focal scarring, and calcifications, which may be visible by radiography.

About two thirds of human *E. granulosus* cysts are found in the liver, 5% to 15% in the lung, and the rest in bones and brain or other organs. In the various organs the larvae lodge within the capillaries and first incite an inflammatory reaction composed principally of mononuclear leukocytes and eosinophils. Many such larvae are destroyed, but others encyst. The cysts begin at microscopic levels and progressively increase in size, so that in 5 years or more they may

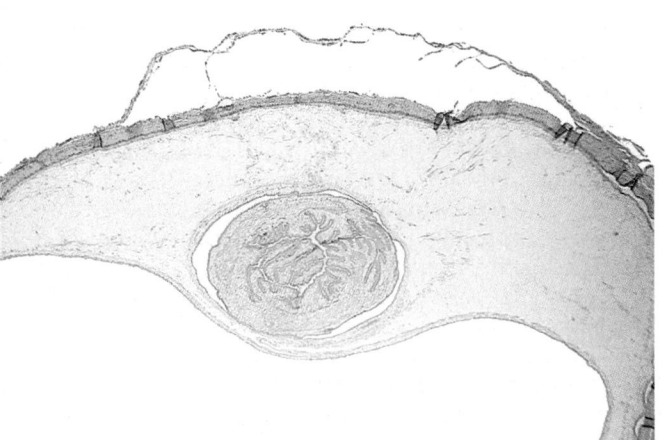

FIGURE 8–55 Portion of a cysticercus cyst in the skin.

have achieved dimensions of more than 10 cm in diameter. Enclosing an opalescent fluid is an inner, nucleated, germinative layer and an outer, opaque, non-nucleated layer. The outer non-nucleated layer is distinctive and has innumerable delicate laminations. Outside this opaque layer, there is a host inflammatory reaction that produces a zone of fibroblasts, giant cells, and mononuclear and eosinophilic cells. In time a dense fibrous capsule forms. Daughter cysts often develop within the large mother cyst. These appear first as minute projections of the germinative layer that develop central vesicles and thus form tiny brood capsules. Degenerating scolices of the worm produce a fine, sandlike sediment within the hydatid fluid ("hydatid sand").

Trichinosis

Trichinella spiralis is a nematode parasite that is acquired by ingestion of larvae in undercooked meat from infected animals (usually pigs, boars, or horses) that have themselves been infected by eating *T. spiralis*–infected rats or meat products. In the United States the number of *T. spiralis*–infected pigs has been greatly reduced by laws requiring cooking of food or garbage fed to hogs, and this has reduced the number of reported human infections in the United States to about 100 each year. Still, trichinosis is widespread where undercooked meat is eaten.

In the human gut, *T. spiralis* larvae develop into adults that mate and release new larvae, which penetrate into the tissues. Larvae disseminate hematogenously and penetrate muscle cells, causing fever, myalgias, marked eosinophilia, and periorbital edema. Much less commonly, patients develop dyspnea, encephalitis, and cardiac failure. In striated skeletal muscle, *T. spiralis* larvae become intracellular parasites, increase dramatically in size, and modify the host muscle cell (referred to as the nurse cell) so that it loses its striations, gains a collagenous capsule, and develops a plexus of new blood vessels around itself.[126] The nurse cell–parasite complex is largely asymptomatic, and the worm may persist for years before it dies and calcifies. Antibodies to larval antigens, which include an immunodominant carbohydrate epitope called tyvelose, may reduce reinfection and are useful for serodiagnosis of the disease.[127]

Trichinella spiralis and other invasive nematodes stimulate a T_H2 response, with production of IL-4, IL-5, IL-10, and IL-13. The cytokines produced by T_H2 cells activate eosinophils and mast cells, both of which are associated with the inflammatory response to these parasites. In animal models of *T. spiralis* infection, the T_H2 response is associated with increased contractility of the intestine, which expels adult worms from the gut and subsequently reduces the number of larvae in the muscles.[128] The mechanism by which the T_H2 response increases intestinal motility is unclear, although IL-4, IL-13, and mast cell degranulation have each been implicated. While the T_H2 response indirectly reduces the number of larvae in muscle by eliminating adults from the intestine, it is not clear whether the intramuscular inflammatory response, which is composed of mononuclear cells and eosinophils, is effective against the larvae.

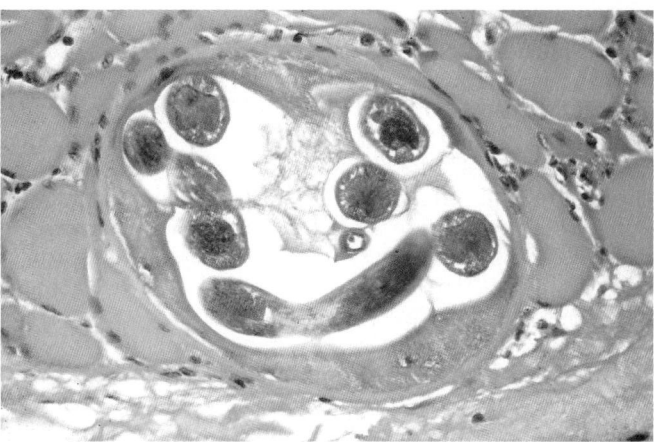

FIGURE 8–56 Coiled *Trichinella spiralis* larva within a skeletal muscle cell.

Morphology. During the invasive phase of trichinosis, cell destruction can be widespread during heavy infections and may be lethal. In the heart there is a patchy interstitial myocarditis characterized by many eosinophils and scattered giant cells. The myocarditis can lead to scarring. Larvae in the heart do not encyst and are difficult to identify, because they die and disappear. In the lungs, trapped larvae cause focal edema and hemorrhages, sometimes with an allergic eosinophilic infiltrate. In the CNS, larvae cause a diffuse lymphocytic and eosinophilic infiltrate, with focal gliosis in and about small capillaries of the brain.

Trichinella spiralis preferentially encysts in striated skeletal muscles with the richest blood supply, including the diaphragm and the extraocular, laryngeal, deltoid, gastrocnemius, and intercostal muscles (Fig. 8–56). Coiled larvae are approximately 1 mm long and are surrounded by membrane-bound vacuoles within nurse cells, which in turn are surrounded by new blood vessels and an eosinophil-rich mononuclear cell infiltrate. This infiltrate is greatest around dying parasites, which eventually calcify and leave behind characteristic scars, which are useful for retrospective diagnosis of trichinosis.

Schistosomiasis

Schistosomiasis infects approximately 200 million persons and kills over 100,000 individuals annually. Most of the mortality comes from hepatic cirrhosis, caused by *Schistosoma mansoni* in Latin America, Africa, and the Middle East and *Schistosoma japonicum* and *Schistosoma mekongi* in East Asia.[129] In addition, *Schistosoma haematobium*, found in Africa, causes hematuria and granulomatous disease of the bladder, resulting in chronic obstructive uropathy.

Pathogenesis. Schistosomiasis is transmitted by freshwater snails that live in the slow-moving water of tropical rivers, lakes, and irrigation ditches, ironically linking agricultural development with spread of the disease. Infectious schistosome larvae (cercariae) swim through fresh water and penetrate human skin with the aid of powerful proteolytic enzymes that degrade the keratinized layer. Schistosomes migrate into the peripheral vasculature, travel to the lung, and mature and mate in hepatic vessels, then migrate out as male-female worm pairs and settle in the portal or pelvic venous system. Females produce hundreds of eggs per day, around which granulomas and fibrosis form. Schistosome eggs produce proteases and elicit prominent inflammatory reactions. This inflammatory response is necessary for passive transfer of eggs across the intestine and bladder walls, allowing the eggs to be shed in stool or urine, respectively. Infection of freshwater snails completes the life cycle.

Eggs that are carried by the portal circulation into the hepatic parenchyma cause prominent inflammatory reactions. This immune response to *S. mansoni* and *S. japonicum* eggs in the liver causes the severe pathology of schistosomiasis.[130] While the immune response does provide some protection in animal models, the price of this response is granuloma formation and hepatic fibrosis. Acute schistosomiasis in humans can be a severe febrile illness that peaks about 2 months after infection. The helper T-cell response in this early stage is dominated by T_H1 cells that produce IFN-γ, which stimulates macrophages to secrete high levels of the cytokines TNF, IL-1, and IL-6 that cause fever. Chronic schistosomiasis is associated with a dominant T_H2 response, although T_H1 cells persist. Stimulation of T_H2 cells may be due to proteins in the parasite egg that cause mast cells to produce IL-4, which induces further T_H2 differentiation and amplifies the response. Both types of helper T cells contribute to the formation of granulomas surrounding eggs in the liver. Severe hepatic fibrosis is a serious manifestation of chronic schistosomiasis. In animal models, IL-13, produced by T_H2 cells, increases fibrosis by stimulating the synthesis of collagen.

Morphology. In mild *S. mansoni* or *S. japonicum* infections, white, pinhead-sized granulomas are scattered throughout the gut and liver. At the center of the granuloma is the schistosome egg, which contains a miracidium; this degenerates over time and calcifies. The granulomas are composed of macrophages, lymphocytes, neutrophils, and eosinophils; eosinophils are distinctive for helminth infections (Fig. 8–57). The liver is darkened by regurgitated heme-derived pigments from the schistosome gut, which, like malaria pigments, are iron-free and accumulate in Kupffer cells and splenic macrophages.

In severe *S. mansoni* or *S. japonicum* infections, inflammatory patches or pseudopolyps may form in the colon. The surface of the liver is bumpy, and cut surfaces reveal granulomas and widespread fibrosis and portal enlargement without intervening regenerative nodules. Because these fibrous triads resemble the stem of a clay pipe, the lesion is named **pipe-stem fibrosis** (Fig. 8–58). The fibrosis often obliterates the portal veins, leading to portal hypertension, severe congestive splenomegaly, esophageal varices, and ascites. Schistosome eggs, diverted to the lung through portal collaterals, may produce granulomatous pulmonary arteritis with intimal hyperplasia, progressive arterial obstruction, and ultimately heart

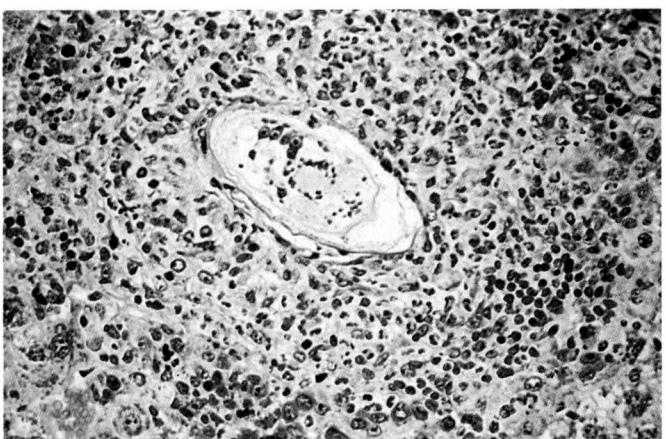

FIGURE 8–57   *Schistosoma mansoni* granuloma with a miracidium-containing egg *(center)* and numerous adjacent, scattered eosinophils.

failure (cor pulmonale). On histologic examination, arteries in the lungs show disruption of the elastic layer by granulomas and scars, luminal organizing thrombi, and angiomatoid lesions similar to those of idiopathic pulmonary hypertension (Chapter 15). Patients with hepatosplenic schistosomiasis also have an increased frequency of mesangioproliferative or membranous glomerulopathy (Chapter 20), in which glomeruli contain deposits of immunoglobulin and complement but rarely schistosome antigen.

In *S. haematobium* infection, inflammatory cystitis due to massive egg deposition and granulomas appear early, leading to mucosal erosions and hematuria (see Fig. 8–10). Later, the granulomas calcify and develop a "sandy" appearance, which, if severe, may line the wall of the bladder and cause a dense concentric rim (calcified bladder) on radiographic films. The most frequent complication of *S. haematobium* infec-

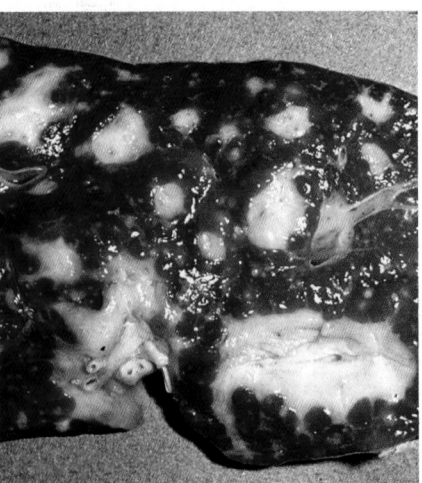

FIGURE 8–58   Pipe-stem fibrosis of the liver due to chronic *Schistosoma japonicum* infection.

tion is inflammation and fibrosis of the ureteral walls, leading to obstruction, hydronephrosis, and chronic pyelonephritis. There is also an association between urinary schistosomiasis and squamous cell carcinoma of the bladder (Chapter 21).

Lymphatic Filariasis

Lymphatic filariasis is transmitted by mosquitoes and is caused by closely related nematodes, *Wuchereria bancrofti* and *Brugia* species (*B. malayi* or *B. timori*), which are responsible for 90% and 10%, respectively, of the 90 million infections worldwide. In endemic areas, which include parts of Latin America, sub-Saharan Africa, and Southeast Asia, filariasis causes a spectrum of diseases, including (1) asymptomatic microfilaremia, (2) recurrent lymphadenitis, (3) chronic lymphadenitis with swelling of the dependent limb or scrotum (elephantiasis), and (4) tropical pulmonary eosinophilia. As is the case with leprosy and leishmanial infections, some of the different disease manifestations caused by lymphatic filariae are likely related to variations in host T-cell responses to the parasites.[131]

Pathogenesis. Infective larvae released by mosquitoes into the tissues during a blood meal develop within lymphatic channels into adult males and females, which mate and release microfilariae that enter into the bloodstream. When mosquitoes bite infected individuals they can take up the microfilariae and transmit the disease. The filarial genome project has led to the identification of a number of filarial molecules that enable the organism to evade or inhibit immune defenses. *Brugia malayi* produces (1) several surface glycoproteins with antioxidant function, which may protect from superoxide and free oxygen radicals; (2) homologues of cystatins, cysteine protease inhibitors, which can impair the MHC class II antigen-processing pathway; (3) serpins, serine protease inhibitors, which can inhibit neutrophil proteases, critical inflammatory mediators; and (4) homologues of TGF-β, which can bind to mammalian TGF-β receptors and may downregulate inflammatory responses.[132,133] In addition, endosymbiotic rickettsia-like *Wolbachia* bacteria infect filarial nematodes and contribute to pathogenesis of disease.[134] *Wolbachia* seem to be needed for nematode development and reproduction, since antibiotics that eradicate *Wolbachia* impair nematode survival and fertility. It has been hypothesized that LPS from *Wolbachia* also stimulates inflammatory responses.

In chronic lymphatic filariasis, damage to the lymphatics is caused directly by the adult parasites and by a T_H1-mediated immune response, which stimulates the formation of granulomas around the adult parasites. Microfilariae are most often absent from the bloodstream.

Finally, there may be an *IgE-mediated hypersensitivity* to microfilariae in *tropical pulmonary eosinophilia*. IgE and eosinophils may be stimulated by IL-4 and IL-5, respectively, secreted by filaria-specific T_H2 helper T cells. Tropical pulmonary eosinophilia is seen most commonly in individuals of Southern Asian descent or in northern Latin America, suggesting that host factors contribute to this disorder (Chapter 15).

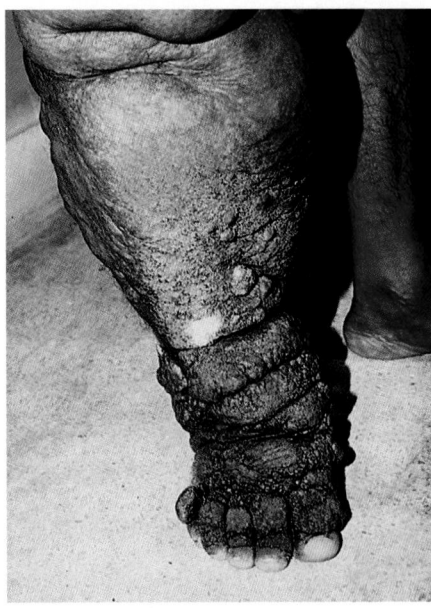

FIGURE 8–59 Massive edema and elephantiasis caused by filariasis of the leg. (Courtesy of Dr. Willy Piessens, Harvard School of Public Health, Boston, MA.)

Morphology. Chronic filariasis is characterized by persistent lymphedema of the extremities, scrotum, penis, or vulva (Fig. 8–59). Frequently there is hydrocele and lymph node enlargement. In severe and long-lasting infections, chylous weeping of the enlarged scrotum may ensue, or a chronically swollen leg may develop tough subcutaneous fibrosis and epithelial hyperkeratosis, termed **elephantiasis**. Elephantoid skin shows dilation of the dermal lymphatics, widespread lymphocytic infiltrates and focal cholesterol deposits; the epidermis is thickened and hyperkeratotic. Adult filarial worms—live, dead, or calcified—are present in the draining lymphatics or nodes, surrounded by (1) mild or no inflammation, (2) an intense eosinophilia with hemorrhage and fibrin (recurrent filarial funiculoepididymitis), or (3) granulomas. Over time, the dilated lymphatics develop polypoid infoldings. In the testis, hydrocele fluid, which often contains cholesterol crystals, red cells, and hemosiderin, induces thickening and calcification of the tunica vaginalis.

Lung involvement by microfilariae is marked by eosinophilia caused by T_H2 responses and cytokine production (tropical eosinophilia) or by dead microfilariae surrounded by stellate, hyaline, eosinophilic precipitates embedded in small epithelioid granulomas (Meyers-Kouvenaar bodies). Typically, these patients lack other manifestations of filarial disease.

Onchocerciasis

Onchocerca volvulus, a filarial nematode transmitted by black flies, affects millions of people in Africa, South America, and Yemen.[135] An aggressive campaign of ivermectin treatment has dramatically reduced the incidence of *Onchocerca* infection in

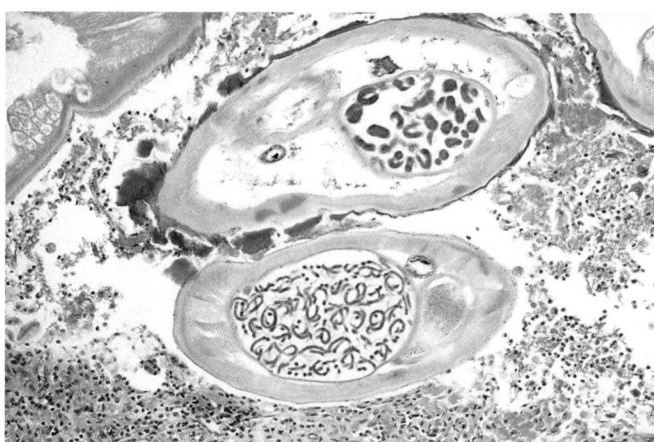

FIGURE 8–60 Microfilaria-laden gravid female of *Onchocerca volvulus* in a subcutaneous fibrous nodule.

West Africa; however, *O. volvulus* remains the second most common preventable cause of blindness in sub-Saharan Africa (called "river blindness" because of its prevalence near some rivers). It is estimated that there are half a million people who are blind due to onchocerciasis.

Adult *O. volvulus* parasites mate in the dermis, where they are surrounded by a mixed infiltrate of host cells that produces a characteristic subcutaneous nodule *(onchocercoma)*. The major pathologic process is caused by large numbers of microfilariae, released by females, that accumulate in the skin and in the eye chambers. *Punctate keratitis* is caused by inflammation around a degenerating microfilaria. Unfortunately, it is sometimes accentuated by treatment with antifilarial drugs (Mazzotti reaction). Ivermectin kills only immature worms, not adult worms, so parasites repopulate the host a few months after treatment. Doxycycline treatment blocks reproduction of *O. volvus* for up to 24 months. Doxycycline kills *Wolbachia*, symbiotic bacteria that live inside adult *O. volvulus* and are required for the fertility of the worm.[136]

Morphology. *Onchocerca volvulus* causes chronic, itchy dermatitis with focal darkening or loss of pigment and scaling, referred to as leopard, lizard, or elephant skin. Foci of epidermal atrophy and elastic fiber breakdown may alternate with areas of hyperkeratosis, hyperpigmentation with pigment incontinence, dermal atrophy, and fibrosis. The subcutaneous onchocercoma is composed of a fibrous capsule surrounding adult worms and a mixed chronic inflammatory infiltrate that includes fibrin, neutrophils, eosinophils, lymphocytes, and giant cells (Fig. 8–60). The progressive eye lesions begin with punctate keratitis along with small, fluffy opacities of the cornea caused by degenerating microfilariae, which evoke an eosinophilic infiltrate. This is followed by a sclerosing keratitis that opacifies the cornea, beginning at the scleral limbus. Microfilariae in the anterior chamber cause iridocyclitis and glaucoma, whereas involvement of the choroid and retina results in atrophy and loss of vision.

REFERENCES

1. Minino AM et al.: Deaths: final data for 2004. Natl Vital Stat Rep 55:1, 2007.
2. Lopez AD et al.: Global and regional burden of disease and risk factors, 2001: systematic analysis of population health data. Lancet 367:1747, 2006.
3. Caughey B, Baron GS: Prions and their partners in crime. Nature 443:803, 2006.
4. Aguzzi A et al.: Molecular mechanisms of prion pathogenesis. Annu Rev Pathol 3:1, 2008.
5. Ley RE, Peterson DA, Gordon JI: Ecological and evolutionary forces shaping microbial diversity in the human intestine. Cell 124:837, 2006.
6. Walker DH: Rickettsiae and rickettsial infections: the current state of knowledge. Clin Infect Dis 45 (Suppl 1):S39, 2007.
7. Clarke JR: Molecular diagnosis of HIV. Expert Rev Mol Diagn 2:233, 2002.
8. Cinque P et al.: Molecular analysis of cerebrospinal fluid in viral diseases of the central nervous system. J Clin Virol 26:1, 2003.
9. Watson EJ et al.: The accuracy and efficacy of screening tests for *Chlamydia trachomatis*: a systematic review. J Med Microbiol 51:1021, 2002.
10. Hui EK: Reasons for the increase in emerging and re-emerging viral infectious diseases. Microbes Infect 8:905, 2006.
11. Gillim-Ross L, Subbarao K: Emerging respiratory viruses: challenges and vaccine strategies. Clin Microbiol Rev 19:614, 2006.
12. Quinn TC: Circumcision and HIV transmission. Curr Opin Infect Dis 20:33, 2007.
13. Harrus S, Baneth G: Drivers for the emergence and re-emergence of vector-borne protozoal and bacterial diseases. Int J Parasitol 35:1309, 2005.
14. Centers for Disease Control and Prevention: Biological and chemical terrorism: strategic plan for preparedness and response. Recommendation of the CDC Strategic Planning Workgroup. MMWR Morb Mortal Wkly Rep 49:1, 2000.
15. Curtis LT: Prevention of hospital-acquired infections: review of non-pharmacological interventions. J Hosp Infect 69:204, 2008.
16. Edwards RA et al.: Comparative genomics of closely related salmonellae. Trends Microbiol 10:94, 2002.
17. Irie Y, Parsek MR: Quorum sensing and microbial biofilms. Curr Top Microbiol Immunol 322:67, 2008.
18. Mulvey MA: Adhesion and entry of uropathogenic *Escherichia coli*. Cell Microbiol 4:257, 2002.
19. Criss AK et al.: The frequency and rate of pilin antigenic variation in *Neisseria gonorrhoeae*. Mol Microbiol 58:510, 2005.
20. Velasco-Velazquez MA et al.: Macrophage–*Mycobacterium tuberculosis* interactions: role of complement receptor 3. Microb Pathog 35:125, 2003.
21. Coburn B et al.: Type III secretion systems and disease. Clin Microbiol Rev 20:535, 2007.
22. Portnoy DA et al.: The cell biology of *Listeria monocytogenes* infection: the intersection of bacterial pathogenesis and cell-mediated immunity. J Cell Biol 158:409, 2002.
23. Pieters J, Gatfield J: Hijacking the host: survival of pathogenic mycobacteria inside macrophages. Trends Microbiol 10:142, 2002.
24. Dobrovolskaia MA, Vogel SN: Toll receptors, CD14, and macrophage activation and deactivation by LPS. Microbes Infect 4:903, 2002.
25. Amagai M et al.: Toxin in bullous impetigo and staphylococcal scalded-skin syndrome targets desmoglein 1. Nat Med 6:1275, 2000.
26. Turton K et al.: Botulinum and tetanus neurotoxins: structure, function and therapeutic utility. Trends Biochem Sci 27:552, 2002.
27. Papageorgiou AC, Acharya KR: Microbial superantigens: from structure to function. Trends Microbiol 8:369, 2000.
28. Karin M, Lawrence T, Nizet V: Innate immunity gone awry: Linking microbial infections to chronic inflammation and cancer. Cell 124:823, 2006.
29. Finlay BB, McFadden G: Anti-immunology: evasion of the host immune system by bacterial and viral pathogens. Cell 124:767, 2006.
30. Fikrig E, Narasimhan S: *Borrelia burgdorferi*—traveling incognito? Microbes Infect 8:1390, 2006.
31. Hornef MW et al.: Bacterial strategies for overcoming host innate and adaptive immune responses. Nat Immunol 3:1033, 2002.
32. Brown KL, Hancock RE: Cationic host defense (antimicrobial) peptides. Curr Opin Immunol 18:24, 2006.

33. Lodoen MB, Lanier LL: Viral modulation of NK cell immunity. Nat Rev Microbiol 3:59, 2005.

34. Yewdell JW, Hill AB: Viral interference with antigen presentation. Nat Immunol 3:1019, 2002.

35. Lilley BN, Ploegh HL: Viral modulation of antigen presentation: manipulation of cellular targets in the ER and beyond. Immunol Rev 207:126, 2005.

36. Ganem D: KSHV infection and the pathogenesis of Kaposi's sarcoma. Annu Rev Pathol 1:273, 2006.

37. Lyczak JB et al.: Lung infections associated with cystic fibrosis. Clin Microbiol Rev 15:194, 2002.

38. Moss WJ, Griffin DE: Global measles elimination. Nat Rev Microbiol 4:900, 2006.

39. Yanagi Y et al.: Measles virus: cellular receptors, tropism and pathogenesis. J Gen Virol 87:2767, 2006.

40. Trifilo MJ et al.: Dendritic cell inhibition: memoirs from immunosuppressive viruses. J Infect Dis 194 (Suppl 1):S3, 2006.

41. Rima BK, Duprex WP: Molecular mechanisms of measles virus persistence. Virus Res 111:132, 2005.

42. De Jesus NH: Epidemics to eradication: the modern history of poliomyelitis. Virol J 4:70, 2007.

43. Chumakov K et al.: Vaccination against polio should not be stopped. Nat Rev Microbiol 5:952, 2007.

44. Racaniello VR: One hundred years of poliovirus pathogenesis. Virology 344:9, 2006.

45. Blondel B et al.: Poliovirus, pathogenesis of poliomyelitis, and apoptosis. Curr Top Microbiol Immunol 289:25, 2005.

46. Hayes EB, Gubler DJ: West Nile virus: epidemiology and clinical features of an emerging epidemic in the United States. Annu Rev Med 57:181, 2006.

47. Samuel MA, Diamond MS: Pathogenesis of West Nile Virus infection: a balance between virulence, innate and adaptive immunity, and viral evasion. J Virol 80:9349, 2006.

48. Diamond MS, Klein RS: A genetic basis for human susceptibility to West Nile virus. Trends Microbiol 14:287, 2006.

49. Bray M. Pathogenesis of viral hemorrhagic fever. Curr Opin Immunol 17:399, 2005.

50. Taylor TJ et al.: Herpes simplex virus. Front Biosci 7:d752, 2002.

51. Jones C: Herpes simplex virus type 1 and bovine herpesvirus 1 latency. Clin Microbiol Rev 16:79, 2003.

52. Gupta A et al.: Anti-apoptotic function of a microRNA encoded by the HSV-1 latency-associated transcript. Nature 442:82, 2006.

53. Quinlivan M, Breuer J: Molecular studies of Varicella zoster virus. Rev Med Virol 16:225, 2006.

54. Fishman JA et al.: Cytomegalovirus in transplantation—challenging the status quo. Clin Transplant 21:149, 2007.

55. Lehner PJ, Wilkinson GW: Cytomegalovirus: from evasion to suppression? Nat Immunol 2:993, 2001.

56. Guidotti LG, Chisari FV: Immunobiology and pathogenesis of viral hepatitis. Annu Rev Pathol 1:23, 2006.

57. Kutok JL, Wang F: Spectrum of Epstein-Barr virus–associated diseases. Annu Rev Pathol 1:375, 2006.

58. Szakonyi G et al.: Structure of the Epstein-Barr virus major envelope glycoprotein. Nat Struct Mol Biol 13:996, 2006.

59. Soni V et al.: LMP1 TRAFficking activates growth and survival pathways. Adv Exp Med Biol 597:173, 2007.

60. Morra M et al.: X-linked lymphoproliferative disease: a progressive immunodeficiency. Annu Rev Immunol 19:657, 2001.

61. Clarke SR, Foster SJ: Surface adhesins of Staphylococcus aureus. Adv Microb Physiol 51:187, 2006.

62. Menestrina G et al.: Ion channels and bacterial infection: the case of beta-barrel pore-forming protein toxins of Staphylococcus aureus. FEBS Lett 552:54, 2003.

63. Proft T, Fraser JD: Bacterial superantigens. Clin Exp Immunol 133:299, 2003.

64. Daum RS: Skin and soft-tissue infections caused by methicillin-resistant Staphyloccocus aureus. N Eng J Med 357:380, 2007.

65. Bisno AL et al.: Molecular basis of group A streptococcal virulence. Lancet Infect Dis 3:191, 2003.

66. Guilherme L et al.: Molecular mimicry in the autoimmune pathogenesis of rheumatic heart disease. Autoimmunity 39:31, 2006.

67. Jedrzejas MJ: Unveiling molecular mechanisms of bacterial surface proteins: Streptococcus pneumoniae as a model organism for structural studies. Cell Mol Life Sci 2007.

68. Hadfield TL et al.: The pathology of diphtheria. J Infect Dis 181 (Suppl 1):S116, 2000.

69. Seveau S et al.: Molecular mechanisms exploited by Listeria monocytogenes during host cell invasion. Microbes Infect 9:1167, 2007.

70. Swartz MN: Recognition and management of anthrax—an update. N Engl J Med 345:1621, 2001.

71. Young JA, Collier RJ: Anthrax toxin: receptor binding, internalization, pore formation, and translocation. Annu Rev Biochem 76:243, 2007.

72. Grinberg LM et al.: Quantitative pathology of inhalational anthrax I: quantitative microscopic findings. Mod Pathol 14:482, 2001.

73. Torres HA et al.: Nocardiosis in cancer patients. Medicine (Baltimore) 81:388, 2002.

74. Stephens DS et al.: Epidemic meningitis, meningococcaemia, and Neisseria meningitidis. Lancet 369:2196, 2007.

75. Pathan N et al.: Pathophysiology of meningococcal meningitis and septicaemia. Arch Dis Child 88:601, 2003.

76. Mooi FR et al.: Adaptation of Bordetella pertussis to vaccination: a cause for its reemergence? Emerg Infect Dis 7:526, 2001.

77. Locht C et al.: Bordetella pertussis, molecular pathogenesis under multiple aspects. Curr Opin Microbiol 4:82, 2001.

78. Ahuja N et al.: The adenylate cyclase toxins. Crit Rev Microbiol 30:187, 2004.

79. Driscoll JA et al.: The epidemiology, pathogenesis and treatment of Pseudomonas aeruginosa infections. Drugs 67:351, 2007.

80. Yates SP et al.: Stealth and mimicry by deadly bacterial toxins. Trends Biochem Sci 31:123, 2006.

81. DeWitte JJ et al.: Assessment of structural features of the pseudomonas siderophore pyochelin required for its ability to promote oxidant-mediated endothelial cell injury. Arch Biochem Biophys 393:236, 2001.

82. Prentice MB, Rahalison L: Plague. Lancet 369:1196, 2007.

83. Lewis DA: Chancroid: clinical manifestations, diagnosis, and management. Sex Transm Infect 79:68, 2003.

84. Fratti RA et al.: Role of phosphatidylinositol 3-kinase and Rab5 effectors in phagosomal biogenesis and mycobacterial phagosome maturation arrest. J Cell Biol 154:631, 2001.

85. Cellier MF et al.: NRAMP1 phagocyte intracellular metal withdrawal defense. Microbes Infect 9:1662, 2007.

86. Flynn JL, Chan J: Immunology of tuberculosis. Annu Rev Immunol 19:93, 2001.

87. Kaufmann SHE: Tuberculosis: back on the immunologists' agenda. Immunity 24:351, 2006.

88. Ottenhoff TH et al.: Control of human host immunity to mycobacteria. Tuberculosis (Edinb) 85:53, 2005.

89. Leader BT et al.: CD4+ lymphocytes and gamma interferon predominate in local immune responses in early experimental syphilis. Infect Immun 75:3021, 2007.

90. Lafond RE, Lukehart SA: Biological basis for syphilis. Clin Microbiol Rev 19:29, 2006.

91. Palmer GH, Brayton KA: Gene conversion is a convergent strategy for pathogen antigenic variation. Trends Parasitol 23:408, 2007.

92. Hengge UR et al.: Lyme borreliosis. Lancet Infect Dis 3:489, 2003.

93. Hoppa E, Bachur R: Lyme disease update. Curr Opin Pediatr 19:275, 2007.

94. Brook I: Microbiology of polymicrobial abscesses and implications for therapy. J Antimicrob Chemother 50:805, 2002.

95. Sakurai J et al.: Clostridium perfringens alpha-toxin: characterization and mode of action. J Biochem (Tokyo) 136:569, 2004.

96. McClane BA: Clostridium perfringens enterotoxin and intestinal tight junctions. Trends Microbiol 8:145, 2000.

97. Cloud J, Kelly CP: Update on Clostridium difficile associated disease. Curr Opin Gastroenterol 23:4, 2007.

98. Coonrod DV: Chlamydial infections. Curr Womens Health Rep 2:266, 2002.

99. Latge JP, Calderone R: Host-microbe interactions: fungi invasive human fungal opportunistic infections. Curr Opin Microbiol 5:355, 2002.

100. Whiteway M, Oberholzer U: Candida morphogenesis and host-pathogen interactions. Curr Opin Microbiol 7:350, 2004.

101. Calderone RA, Fonzi WA: Virulence factors of Candida albicans. Trends Microbiol 9:327, 2001.

102. Filler SG: Candida–host cell receptor–ligand interactions. Curr Opin Microbiol 9:333, 2006.

103. Nett J, Andes D: Candida albicans biofilm development, modeling a host-pathogen interaction. Curr Opin Microbiol 9:340, 2006.

104. Romani L: Immunity to fungal infections. Nat Rev Immunol 4:1, 2004.
105. Gomez BL, Nosanchuk JD: Melanin and fungi. Curr Opin Infect Dis 16:91, 2003.
106. Fries BC et al.: Phenotypic switching in *Cryptococcus neoformans*. Microbes Infect 4:1345, 2002.
107. Rodrigues ML et al.: Cleavage of human fibronectin and other basement membrane–associated proteins by a *Cryptococcus neoformans* serine proteinase. Microb Pathog 34:65, 2003.
108. Eisenman HC et al.: New Insights on the pathogenesis of invasive *Cryptococcus neoformans* infection. Curr Infect Dis Rep 9:457, 2007.
109. Groopman JD et al.: Protective interventions to prevent aflatoxin-induced carcinogenesis in developing countries. Annu Rev Public Health 29:187, 2008.
110. Kauffman HF: Immunopathogenesis of allergic bronchopulmonary aspergillosis and airway remodeling. Front Biosci 8:e190, 2003.
111. Greenberg RN et al.: Zygomycosis (mucormycosis): emerging clinical importance and new treatments. Curr Opin Infect Dis 17:517, 2004.
112. Mikolajczak SA, Kappe SH: A clash to conquer: the malaria parasite liver infection. Mol Microbiol 62:1499, 2006.
113. Haldar K, et al.: Malaria: mechanisms of erythrocytic infection and pathological correlates of severe disease. Annu Rev Pathol 2:217, 2007.
114. Krause PJ: Babesiosis diagnosis and treatment. Vector Borne Zoonotic Dis 3:45, 2003.
115. Banuls AL et al.: *Leishmania* and the leishmaniases: a parasite genetic update and advances in taxonomy, epidemiology and pathogenicity in humans. Adv Parasitol 64:1, 2007.
116. Rogers ME, Bates PA: *Leishmania* manipulation of sand fly feeding behavior results in enhanced transmission. PLoS Pathog 3:e91, 2007.
117. Liu B et al.: Fellowship of the rings: the replication of kinetoplast DNA. Trends Parasitol 21:363, 2005.
118. Sacks D, Noben-Trauth N: The immunology of susceptibility and resistance to *Leishmania major* in mice. Nat Rev Immunol 2:845, 2002.
119. Pays E: Regulation of antigen gene expression in *Trypanosoma brucei*. Trends Parasitol 21:517, 2005.
120. Andrews NW: Lysosomes and the plasma membrane: trypanosomes reveal a secret relationship. J Cell Biol 158:389, 2002.
121. Viotti R, Vigliano C: Etiological treatment of chronic Chagas disease: neglected "evidence" by evidence-based medicine. Expert Rev Anti Infect Ther 5:717, 2007.
122. Hoberg EP: *Taenia* tapeworms: their biology, evolution and socioeconomic significance. Microbes Infect 4:859, 2002.
123. Zhang W, Li Jet al.: Concepts in immunology and diagnosis of hydatid disease. Clin Microbiol Rev 16:18, 2003.
124. Kristensson K et al.: Parasites and the brain: neuroinvasion, immunopathogenesis and neuronal dysfunctions. Curr Top Microbiol Immunol 265:227, 2002.
125. White AJ: Neurocysticercosis: updates on epidemiology, pathogenesis, diagnosis, and management. Annu Rev Med 51:187, 2000.
126. Pozio E, Darwin Murrell K: Systematics and epidemiology of trichinella. Adv Parasitol 63:367, 2006.
127. Pozio E et al.: Clinical aspects, diagnosis and treatment of trichinellosis. Expert Rev Anti Infect Ther 1:471, 2003.
128. Finkelman FD et al.: Interleukin-4- and interleukin-13–mediated host protection against intestinal nematode parasites. Immunol Rev 201:139, 2004.
129. Ross AG et al.: Schistosomiasis. N Engl J Med 346:1212, 2002.
130. Pearce EJ, MacDonald AS: The immunobiology of schistosomiasis. Nat Rev Immunol 2:499, 2002.
131. King CL: Transmission intensity and human immune responses to lymphatic filariasis. Parasite Immunol 23:227, 2002.
132. Lawrence RA, Devaney E: Lymphatic filariasis: parallels between the immunology of infection in humans and mice. Parasite Immunol 23:353, 2001.
133. Maizels RM et al.: Helminth parasites—masters of regulation. Immunol Rev 201:89, 2004.
134. Taylor MJ et al.: *Wolbachia* bacterial endosymbionts of filarial nematodes. Adv Parasitol 60:245, 2005.
135. Hoerauf A et al.: Onchocerciasis. BMJ 326:207, 2003.
136. Hoerauf A et al.: Depletion of *Wolbachia* endobacteria in *Onchocerca volvulus* by doxycycline and microfilaridermia after ivermectin treatment. Lancet 357:1415, 2001.

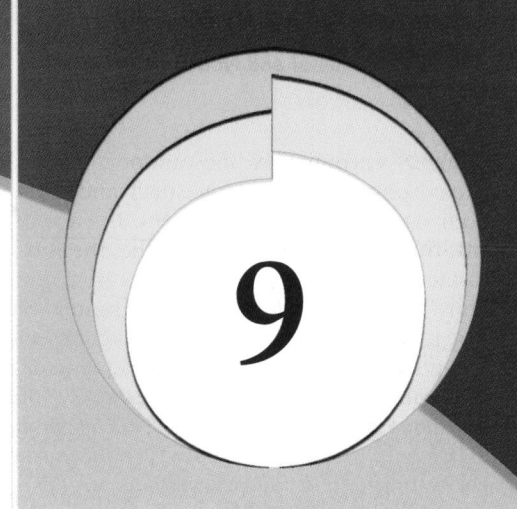

9

Environmental and Nutritional Diseases

The Global Burden of Disease

Health Effects of Climate Change

Toxicity of Chemical and Physical Agents

Environmental Pollution
  Air Pollution
    Outdoor Air Pollution
    Indoor Air Pollution
  Metals as Environmental Pollutants
    Lead
    Mercury
    Arsenic
    Cadmium

Occupational Health Risks: Industrial and Agricultural Exposures

Effects of Tobacco

Effects of Alcohol

Injury by Therapeutic Drugs and Drugs of Abuse
  Injury by Therapeutic Drugs (Adverse Drug Reactions)
    Hormonal Replacement Therapy (HRT)
    Oral Contraceptives (OCs)
    Anabolic Steroids
    Acetaminophen
    Aspirin (Acetylsalicylic Acid)

Injury by Nontherapeutic Agents (Drug Abuse)
  Cocaine
  Heroin
  Amphetamines
  Marijuana
  Other Drugs

Injury by Physical Agents
  Mechanical Trauma
  Thermal Injury
    Thermal Burns
    Hyperthermia
    Hypothermia
  Electrical Injury
  Injury Produced by Ionizing Radiation

Nutritional Diseases
  Dietary Insufficiency
  Protein-Energy Malnutrition (PEM)
  Anorexia Nervosa and Bulimia
  Vitamin Deficiencies
    Vitamin A
    Vitamin D
    Vitamin C (Ascorbic Acid)
  Obesity
    General Consequences of Obesity
    Obesity and Cancer
  Diets, Cancer, and Atherosclerosis
    Diet and Cancer
    Diet and Atherosclerosis

The term "environment" encompasses the outdoor, indoor, and occupational environments shared by small and large populations, and our own personal environment. In each of these environments, the air we collectively breathe, the food and water we consume, and exposure to toxic agents are major determinants of our health. Our personal environment is greatly influenced by tobacco use, alcohol ingestion, therapeutic and nontherapeutic drug consumption, and diet. Factors in the personal environment may have a larger effect on human health than the ambient environment. *The term environmental diseases refers to conditions caused by exposure to chemical or physical agents in the ambient, workplace, and personal environment, including diseases of nutritional origin.* Environmental diseases mostly come to the public's attention after major disasters, such as the methyl mercury contamination of Minamata Bay in Japan in the 1960s, the exposure to dioxin in Seveso, Italy, in 1976, the leakage of methyl isocyanate gas in Bhopal, India, in 1984, the Chernobyl nuclear accident in 1986, and the contamination of Tokyo subways by the organophosphate pesticide sarin. Fortunately, these are unusual and infrequent occurrences, but environmental diseases caused by chronic exposure to relatively low levels of contaminants, occupational injuries, and nutritional deficiencies are widespread. The International Labor Organization has estimated that work-related injuries and illnesses kill approximately 2 million people per year globally (more deaths than are caused by road accidents and wars combined). A comprehensive report from the Disease Control Priorities Project (http://www.dcp2.org) estimated that there are 130 million undernourished children worldwide, and that malnutrition alone is responsible for 2.67 million deaths per year. Estimating the burden of disease in the general population caused by nonoccupational exposures to toxic agents is complicated by the diversity of agents and difficulties in determining the extent and duration of exposures. Whatever the precise numbers, environmental (including nutritional) diseases are major causes of disability and suffering, and constitute a heavy financial burden, particularly in developing countries. During the last few years new concerns have been raised about air and water quality, and the potential health effects of climate change.

In this chapter, we first consider two key issues in global health: the global burden of disease, and the emerging problem of the health effects of climate change. We then discuss the mechanisms of toxicity of chemical and physical agents, and address specific environmental disorders, including those of nutritional origin.

The Global Burden of Disease

Until about 1990 global health data were fragmented and lacked a uniform standard of measurement.[1] Since then, a project entitled The Global Burden of Disease (GBD) has set the standard for reporting health information. The GBD approach is now applied to the measurement of the burden imposed by environmental disease, including those caused by communicable and nutritional diseases. In addition, a unit of measurement ("metric") called DALY (disability-adjusted life year, a time based measure that adds the years of life lost to premature mortality with the years lived with illness and disability), has been used to assess both premature mortality and disease morbidity. DALY reporting provides a high degree of uniformity for health information gathered about acute and chronic diseases in different parts of the world and at multiple locations in a single country. The new methodology has revealed important trends in the worldwide morbidity and mortality of disease.

- *Undernutrition is the single leading global cause of health loss (defined as morbidity and premature death).* It is estimated that about one third of the disease burden in developing countries is, directly or indirectly, due to poor general nutrition or deficiencies in specific nutrients that increase the risk of infections.
- *Ischemic heart disease and cerebrovascular disease are the leading causes of death in developed countries.* In these countries the main risk factors associated with loss of healthy life are smoking, high blood pressure, obesity, high cholesterol, and alcohol abuse.
- *In developing countries, infectious diseases constitute 5 of the 10 leading causes of death:* respiratory infections, human immunodeficiency virus/acquired immunodeficiency syndrome (HIV/AIDS), diarrheal diseases, tuberculosis, and malaria.[2] HIV/AIDS contributes 18% to the loss of healthy life in sub-Saharan Africa and 13% in South Asia.
- *About 70% of all child deaths are attributed to only five conditions, all of them preventable:* pneumonia, diarrheal diseases, malaria, measles, and perinatal/neonatal problems (mostly prematurity and neonatal infections).
- *Worldwide mortality of children under 5 years of age has declined* from 110 deaths per 1000 in 1980 to 72 per 1000 in 2005. Though impressive, the 27% decline in mortality under 5 years of age, expected to occur between 1990 and 2015, falls short of the United Nations Millennium Development Goal of achieving a 67% decline. To be noted is that under-5 mortality in Central and West Africa (about 210/1000) is almost 50 times higher than that in Western Europe[3] (Fig. 9–1) and has shown no significant decline.
- *Emerging infectious diseases (EIDs) constitute one of the most important components of the global burden of disease.* EIDs are correlated with environmental, and socioeconomic conditions, and include (1) *diseases caused by newly evolved strains or organisms,* such as rifampin/isoniazid-resistant and multidrug-resistant (XDR) tuberculosis, chloroquine-resistant malaria, and methicillin-resistant *Staphylococcus aureus*; (2) *diseases caused by pathogens endemic in other species (e.g., wild mammals and birds) that recently entered human populations,* such as HIV and severe acute respiratory syndrome (SARS); (3) *diseases caused by pathogens that have been present in human populations but show a recent increase in incidence,* such as dengue fever.
- Bacteria and rickettsia caused approximately 54% of worldwide emerging infectious diseases during the last 60 years (viruses represented ~25%). Drug-resistant bacteria were the most important group of pathogens. Their appearance relates to therapeutic use of antibiotics, and in agriculture as well as urban living in densely populated areas. During the last decade, vector-borne diseases constituted approximately 29% of emerging infectious disease, an increase that may be related to environmental changes such as global warming.[4]

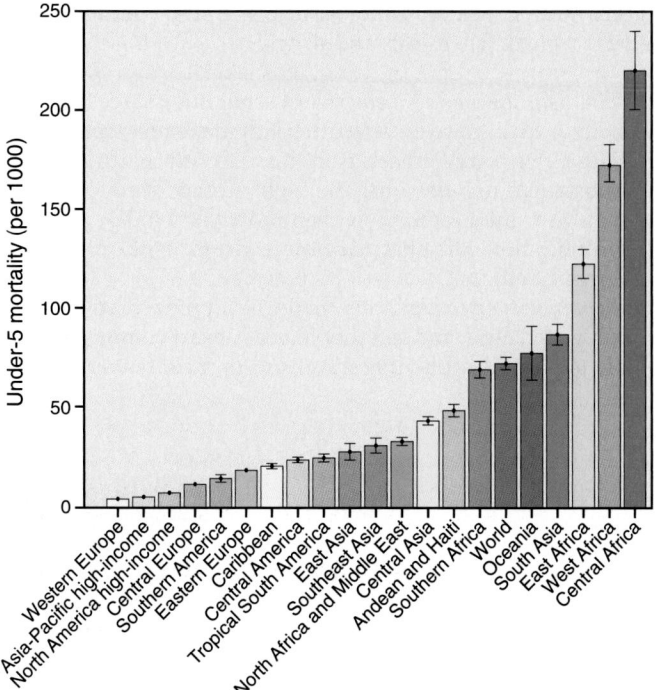

FIGURE 9–1 Worldwide mortality of children under 5 years of age. Note the more than 50-fold difference between areas with the lowest and highest mortality. Malnutrition and infections are major causes of the high mortality in East, Central, and West Africa.

Health Effects of Climate Change

There is general agreement that the earth has been warming at an accelerating pace during the last 40 years, and that the rate of warming is more rapid than at any other period in perhaps 1000 years.[5] Since 1960 the global average surface temperature increased by 0.6°C; the increase is not uniform, being greatest at latitudes between 40° N and 70° N.[6] Glacier melting has accelerated, and in polar regions, snow cover and ice thickness have diminished. At the same time, the sea level

has risen 1 to 2 mm/year as a result of thermal expansion.[6] The importance of climate change was highlighted by the awarding of the 2007 Nobel Peace Prize to individuals and organizations concerned with the impact of these changes on human health.

The causes of global climate change are the subject of debate, but human activity is a major contributor, through increases of *carbon dioxide* (CO_2), *methane*, and *ozone* (discussed later), the main agents of the *greenhouse effect*. These gases (along with water vapor) act like a blanket by absorbing energy radiated from the earth's surface that would otherwise be lost into space. Recent increases in levels of greenhouse gases, particularly CO_2 and ozone produced by the combustion of hydrocarbons in automobiles and energy plants, are strongly correlated with warming of the earth (Fig. 9–2). The present concentration of atmospheric CO_2, estimated to be 370 ppm (highest in about 1 million years), is expected to increase to 500 to 1200 ppm at the end of this century. Also contributing to the increase in atmospheric CO_2 is large-scale deforestation (present estimates are that the Amazon forest will lose 50% of the original area by 2050), which decreases carbon sequestration by trees. Beyond certain levels of warming of the land and seas, it is predicted that positive-feedback loops will amplify the process further. Examples include increases in heat absorption due to the loss of reflective snow and ice; increases in water vapor in the atmosphere due to greater evaporation from bodies of water and transpiration from trees; large releases of stored CO_2 and methane from thawing arctic tundra; and decreased sequestration of CO_2 in the oceans, due to diminished growth of diatoms, which serve as an important CO_2 sink. Depending on the model used, these changes are predicted to cause the global temperature to rise 2° to 5°C by the year 2100 (see Fig. 9–2).

The future impact of global warming on health will depend on the extent and rapidity of climate change, the severity of the ensuing consequences, and humankind's ability to adapt to or otherwise mitigate the damaging effects. Even in the best-case scenario, however, it is expected that climate change will seriously impact human health by increasing the incidence of several diseases.[7]

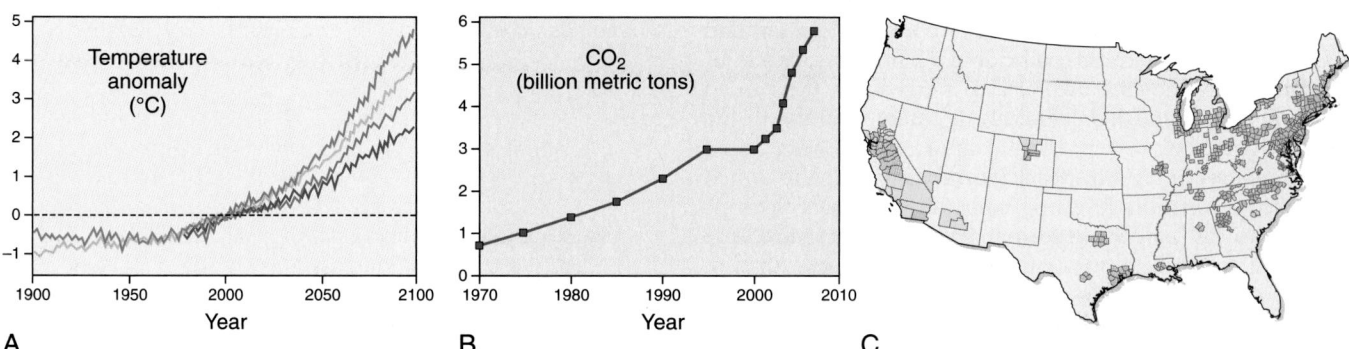

FIGURE 9–2 Sources and consequences of increased greenhouse gases. **A,** Predicted temperature increases during the twenty-first century. Different computer models plot anticipated rises in temperature of 2° to 5°C by the year 2100. **B,** Release of carbon dioxide (CO_2) from combustion sources in China, 1970 to 2005. China has now surpassed the United States as the world's largest producer of CO_2. **C,** Regions of the United States in which ozone levels are above existing accepted standards (80 ppb during an 8-hour period). These areas include about 500 counties located predominantly in the East Coast corridor, the Los Angeles basin, and areas with large coal-burning plants.

- *Cardiovascular, cerebrovascular, and respiratory diseases*, caused by heat waves and air pollution (e.g., the European summer of 2003, the warmest in 500 years, resulted in more than 25,000 heat- and pollution-related deaths)
- *Gastroenteritis and infectious disease epidemics*, caused by water and food contamination as a consequence of floods, and disruption of clean water supplies and sewage treatment, after heavy rains and other environmental disasters
- *Vector-borne infectious diseases*, such as dengue fever, malaria, West Nile virus infection, and hantavirus pulmonary syndrome, as a consequence of changes in vector number and geographic distribution caused by increased temperatures, crop failures, and more frequent El Nino climate cycles
- *Malnutrition*, caused by disruption of crops, mostly in tropical locations in which average temperatures are near or above crop tolerance levels; it is estimated that by 2080 agricultural productivity may decline by 10% to 25% in some developing countries as a consequence of warming, while it may decrease or even increase by up to 6% in developed countries with more moderate climates

Despite recognition of these dangers, climate change is just one of multiple factors that contribute to the incidence of a disease at a particular geographic location, making it difficult to establish precise risk estimates for effects which are specifically caused by global warming.[8]

Both developed and developing countries will suffer the consequences of climate change, but the burden will be heaviest in developing nations. Wealthy countries are the main producers of the emissions that cause global warming, but rapidly developing countries such as China and India are using increasingly large amounts of energy to sustain their growth. The urgent challenge ahead is to develop new methods of energy production that do not harm the environment and do not contribute to global warming.

Toxicity of Chemical and Physical Agents

Toxicology is defined as the science of poisons. It studies the distribution, effects, and mechanisms of action of toxic agents. More broadly, it also includes the study of the effects of physical agents such as radiation and heat. Approximately 4 billion pounds of toxic chemicals, including 72 million pounds of recognized carcinogens, are released per year in the United States. Of about 100,000 chemicals in commercial use in the United States, only a very small proportion has been tested experimentally for health effects. Several agencies in the United States set permissible levels of exposure to known environmental hazards (e.g., the maximum level of carbon monoxide in air that is noninjurious or the tolerable levels of radiation that are harmless or "safe"). But factors such as the complex interaction between various pollutants, and the age, genetic predisposition, and the different tissue sensitivities of exposed persons, create wide variations in individual sensitivity to toxic agents, limiting the value of establishing rigid "safe levels" for entire populations. Nevertheless, such levels are useful for comparative studies of the effects of harmful agents between specific populations, and for estimating risk of disease in heavily exposed individuals.

We now consider some basic principles relevant to the effects of toxic chemicals and drugs.

- The *definition of a poison* is not straightforward. It is basically a quantitative concept strictly dependent on *dosage*. The quote from Paracelsus in the sixteenth century that "all substances are poisons; the right dosage differentiates a poison from a remedy" is even more valid today, given the proliferation of pharmaceutical drugs with potentially harmful effects.
- *Xenobiotics* are exogenous chemicals in the environment in air, water, food, and soil that may be absorbed into the body through inhalation, ingestion, and skin contact (Fig. 9–3).

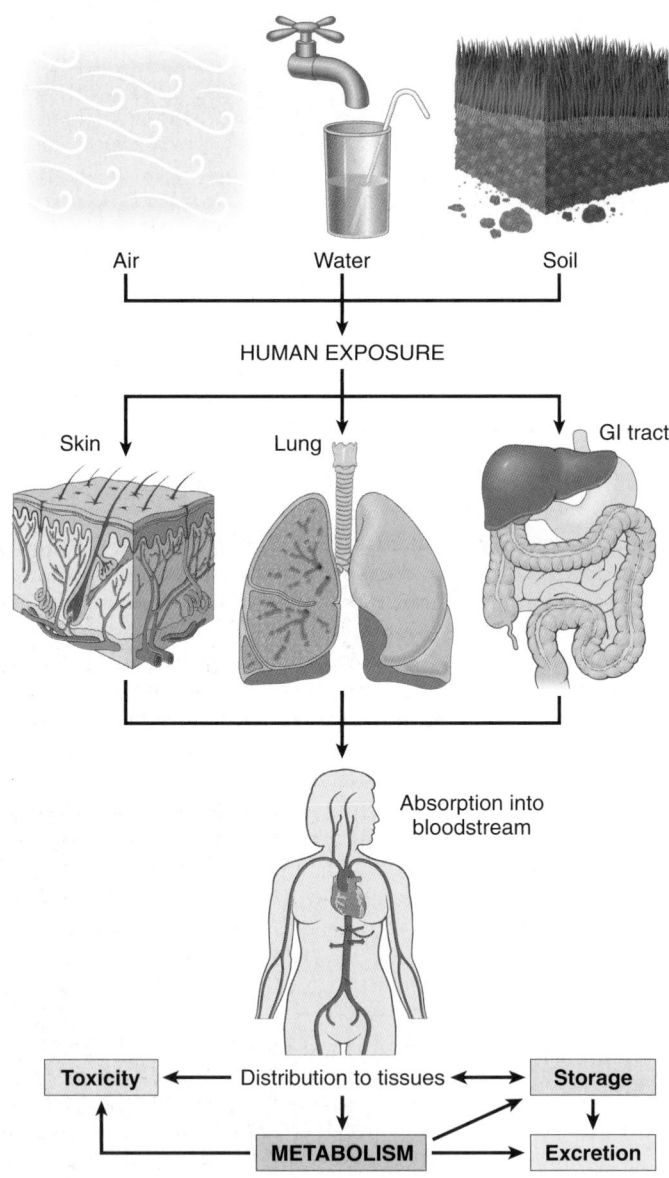

FIGURE 9–3 Human exposure to pollutants. Pollutants contained in air, water, and soil are absorbed through the lungs, gastrointestinal tract, and skin. In the body they may act at the site of absorption but are generally transported through the bloodstream to various organs where they may be stored or metabolized. Metabolism of xenobiotics may result in the formation of water-soluble compounds that are excreted, or in activation of the agent, creating a toxic metabolite.

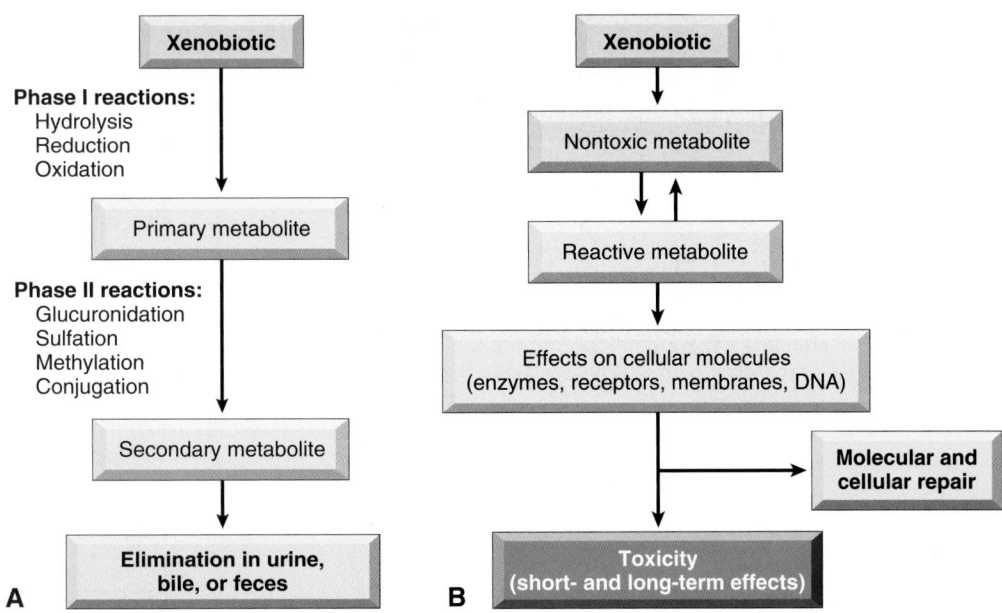

FIGURE 9–4 Xenobiotic metabolism. **A,** Xenobiotics can be metabolized to nontoxic metabolites and eliminated from the body (detoxification). **B,** Xenobiotic metabolism may also result in the formation of a reactive metabolite that is toxic to cellular components. If repair is not effective, short- and long-term effects develop. (Based on Hodgson E: A Textbook of Modern Toxicology, 3rd ed. Hoboken, NJ, Wiley, 2004.)

- Chemicals may be excreted in urine, feces, or eliminated in expired air, or may accumulate in bone, fat, brain, or other tissues.
- Chemicals may act at the site of entry or at other sites following transport through the blood.
- *Most solvents and drugs are lipophilic,* which facilitates their transport in the blood by lipoproteins and their penetration through the plasma membrane into cells.
- Some agents are not modified after entry in the body, but most solvents, drugs, and xenobiotics are metabolized to form inactive water-soluble products *(detoxification),* or are *activated to form toxic metabolites.* The reactions that metabolize xenobiotics into nontoxic products, or activate xenobiotics to generate toxic compounds (Figs. 9–3 and 9–4), occur in two phases. In *phase I* reactions, chemicals undergo hydrolysis, oxidation, or reduction. Products of phase I reactions are often metabolized into water-soluble compounds through *phase II* reactions, which include glucuronidation, sulfation, methylation, and conjugation with glutathione. Water-soluble compounds are readily excreted. Enzymes that catalyze the biotransformation of xenobiotics and drugs are known as *drug-metabolizing enzymes.*
- The most important catalyst of phase I reactions is the *cytochrome P-450 enzyme system (abbreviated as CYP)* located primarily in the endoplasmic reticulum of the liver but also present in skin, lungs, and gastrointestinal mucosa, and practically every organ.[9] CYPs are a large family of heme-containing enzymes with preferential affinity toward different substrates. The system catalyzes reactions that either *detoxify xenobiotics or activate xenobiotics into active compounds that cause cellular injury.* Both types of reactions may produce, as a byproduct, *reactive oxygen species (ROS),* which can cause cellular damage (Chapter 1). Examples of metabolic activation of chemicals through CYPs are the production of the toxic trichloromethyl free radical from carbon tetrachloride in the liver, and the generation of a DNA-binding metabolite from benzo[*a*]pyrene, a carcinogen present in cigarette smoke. CYPs participate in the metabolism of a large number of common therapeutic drugs such as acetaminophen, barbiturates, and anticonvulsants, and also in alcohol metabolism (discussed later in this chapter).

There is great variation in the activity of CYPs among individuals. The variation may be a consequence of *genetic polymorphisms in specific CYPs,* but more commonly it is due to exposure to drugs or chemicals that induce or diminish CYP activity. Known CYP inducers include environmental chemicals, drugs, smoking, alcohol, and hormones. In contrast, fasting or starvation can decrease CYP activity.

Inducers of CYP do so by binding to nuclear receptors, which then heterodimerize with the retinoic X receptor (RXR) to form a transcriptional activation complex that associates with promoter elements located in the 5′-flanking region of CYP genes.[10] Nuclear receptors participating in CYP induction responses include the *aryl hydrocarbon receptor,* the *peroxisome proliferator–activated receptors (PPAR),* and two orphan nuclear receptors, constitutive androstane receptor (CAR), and pregnane X receptor (PXR).

This brief overview of the general mechanisms of toxicity provides the background for the discussion of environmental diseases presented in this chapter.

Environmental Pollution

AIR POLLUTION

Precious as air is—especially to those deprived of it—it is often loaded with many potential causes of disease. Airborne microorganisms contaminating food and water have long

TABLE 9–1 Health Effects of Outdoor Air Pollutants		
Pollutant	**Populations at Risk**	**Effects**
Ozone	Healthy adults and children	Decreased lung function
		Increased airway reactivity
		Lung inflammation
	Athletes, outdoor workers	Decreased exercise capacity
	Asthmatics	Increased hospitalizations
Nitrogen dioxide	Healthy adults	Increased airway reactivity
	Asthmatics	Decreased lung function
	Children	Increased respiratory infections
Sulfur dioxide	Healthy adults	Increased respiratory symptoms
	Individuals with chronic lung disease	Increased mortality
	Asthmatics	Increased hospitalization
		Decreased lung function
Acid aerosols	Healthy adults	Altered mucociliary clearance
	Children	Increased respiratory infections
	Asthmatics	Decreased lung function
		Increased hospitalizations
Particulates	Children	Increased respiratory infections
	Individuals with chronic lung or heart disease	Decreased lung function
	Asthmatics	Excess mortality
		Increased attacks

Data from Bascom R, et al.: Health effects of outdoor air pollution. Am J Respir Crit Care Med 153:477, 1996.

been major causes of morbidity and mortality, especially in developing countries. More widespread are the chemical and particulate pollutants found in the air, especially in industrialized nations. Here, we consider these hazards in outdoor and indoor air.

Outdoor Air Pollution

The ambient air in industrialized nations is contaminated with an unsavory mixture of gaseous and particulate pollutants, more heavily in cities and in proximity to heavy industry. In the United States the Environmental Protection Agency monitors and sets allowable upper limits for six pollutants: sulfur dioxide, carbon monoxide, ozone, nitrogen dioxide, lead, and particulate matter. Collectively, these agents produce the well-known *smog* (smoke and fog) that sometimes stifles large cities such as Beijing, Los Angeles, Houston, Cairo, New Delhi, Mexico City, and São Paulo. It may seem that air pollution is a modern phenomenon. This is not so, since John Evelyn wrote in 1661 that inhabitants of London suffered from "Catharrs, Phthisicks and Consumptions" (bronchitis, pneumonia, and tuberculosis) and breathed "nothing but an impure and thick mist, accompanied by a fuliginous and filthy vapour, which renders them obnoxious to a thousand inconveniences, corrupting the lungs, and disordering the entire habit of their bodies." The first environmental control law, proclaimed by Edward I in 1306, was straightforward in its simplicity: "whoever should be found guilty of burning coal shall suffer the loss of his head." Thus, what has changed in modern times is the nature and sources of air pollutants, and the types of regulations that control their emission.

Although the lungs bear the brunt of the adverse consequences, air pollutants can affect many organ systems (see, for instance, the discussion of lead poisoning and carbon monoxide effects in this chapter). Except for some comments on

smoking, pollutant-caused lung diseases are discussed in Chapter 15. Major health effects of outdoor pollutants are described in Table 9–1. Here we discuss ozone, sulfur dioxide, particulates, and carbon monoxide.

Ozone. The interaction of ultraviolet (UV) radiation and oxygen (O_2) in the stratosphere leads to the formation of *ozone* (O_3), which accumulates in the so-called ozone layer 10 to 30 miles above the earth's surface. This layer protects life on earth by absorbing the most dangerous UV radiation emitted by the sun. During the last 30 years, the stratospheric ozone layer decreased in both thickness and extent due to the widespread use of aerosols, which drift up into the upper atmosphere and participate in chemical reactions that destroy ozone. The resulting depletion has been most profound over polar regions, particularly Antarctica, during the winter months. Recognition of the problem led to the ban of chlorofluorocarbons as aerosol propellants and their replacement by hydrofluoroalkanes, resulting in a decrease in the extent of stratospheric ozone "holes."

In contrast to the "good" ozone in the stratosphere, *ozone that accumulates in the lower atmosphere (ground-level ozone) is one of the most pernicious air pollutants* (see Fig. 9–2). Ground-level ozone is a gas formed by the reaction of nitrogen oxides and volatile organic compounds in the presence of sunlight. These chemicals are released by industrial emissions and motor vehicle exhaust. Ozone toxicity is in large part mediated by the production of free radicals, which injure epithelial cells along the respiratory tract and type I alveolar cells, and cause the release of inflammatory mediators. Healthy individuals exposed to ozone experience upper respiratory tract inflammation and mild symptoms (decreased lung function and chest discomfort), but exposure is much more dangerous for people with asthma or emphysema. Ozone-induced asthma is associated with airway hyper-reactivity and neutrophilia.[11]

Even low levels of ozone may be detrimental to the lung function of normal individuals when combined with other air pollutants. Unfortunately, air pollutants often combine to create a veritable "witches' brew" of ozone and other agents such as *sulfur dioxide* and particulates. Sulfur dioxide is produced by power plants burning coal and oil, from copper smelting, and as a byproduct of paper mills. Released into the air, it may be converted into sulfuric acid and sulfuric trioxide, which cause a burning sensation in the nose and throat, difficulty in breathing, and asthma attacks in susceptible individuals.

Particulate matter (known as "soot") is emitted by coal- and oil-fired power plants, by industrial processes burning these fuels, and by diesel exhaust. Exposure to particulates was the main cause of morbidity and mortality in the air pollution episodes that occurred in London in 1952 and 1962. Although the particles have not been well characterized chemically or physically, *fine or ultrafine particles that are less than 10 μm in diameter are the most harmful.* They are readily inhaled into the alveoli, where they are phagocytosed by macrophages and neutrophils, which release inflammatory mediators such as macrophage inflammatory protein 1α and endothelin. Acute exposure to diesel exhaust that contains fine particles may cause irritation to the eyes, throat, and lungs, induce asthma attacks,[12] and promote myocardial ischemia.[13] In contrast, exposure to particles that are greater than 10 μm in diameter is of lesser consequence, because these particles are generally removed in the nose, or trapped by the mucociliary epithelium of the airways.

Carbon monoxide (CO). CO is a nonirritating, colorless, tasteless, odorless gas produced by the incomplete oxidation of carbonaceous materials. Its sources include automotive engines, industrial processes using fossil fuels, wood and charcoal burning with an inadequate supply of oxygen, and cigarette smoke. The low levels often found in ambient air may contribute to impaired respiratory function, but of themselves they are not life-threatening. However, chronic poisoning can occur in individuals working in confined environments with high exposure to fumes, such as tunnels, underground garages, and in highway toll workers. *CO is included here as an air pollutant, but it is also an important cause of accidental and suicidal death.* In a small, closed garage, the average car exhaust can induce lethal coma within 5 minutes. CO is a systemic asphyxiant that kills by inducing central nervous system (CNS) depression, which appears so insidiously that victims are often unaware of their plight and fail to help themselves. Hemoglobin has 200-fold greater affinity for CO than for oxygen, and the resultant carboxyhemoglobin does not carry oxygen. Systemic hypoxia develops when the hemoglobin is 20% to 30% saturated with CO; unconsciousness and death are likely with 60% to 70% saturation.

Morphology. Chronic poisoning by CO develops because carboxyhemoglobin, once formed, is remarkably stable. Even with low-level, but persistent, exposure to CO, carboxyhemoglobin may rise to life-threatening levels in the blood. The slowly developing hypoxia can insidiously evoke widespread ischemic changes in the central nervous system; these are particularly marked in the basal ganglia and lenticular nuclei. With cessation of exposure to CO, the patient usually recovers, but often there are permanent neurologic sequelae such as impairment of memory, vision, hearing, and speech. The diagnosis is made by measuring carboxyhemoglobin levels in the blood.

Acute poisoning by CO is generally a consequence of accidental exposure or suicide attempt. In light-skinned individuals, **acute poisoning is marked by a characteristic generalized cherry-red color of the skin** and mucous membranes, which result from high levels of carboxyhemoglobin. If death occurs rapidly morphologic changes may not be present; with longer survival the brain may be slightly edematous, with punctate hemorrhages and hypoxia-induced neuronal changes. The morphologic changes are not specific and stem from systemic hypoxia.

Indoor Air Pollution

As we increasingly "button up" our homes to exclude the environment, the potential for pollution of the indoor air increases. The commonest pollutant is *tobacco smoke* (discussed later), but additional offenders are CO, nitrogen dioxide (both already mentioned as outdoor pollutants), and asbestos (discussed in Chapter 15). Volatile substances containing polycyclic aromatic hydrocarbons generated by cooking oils and coal burning are important indoor pollutants in some regions of China. Only a few comments about other agents will be made here.

Wood smoke, containing various oxides of nitrogen and carbon particulates, may not only be an irritant but also predisposes to lung infections and may contain the far more dangerous carcinogenic polycyclic hydrocarbons. *Bioaerosols* range from microbiologic agents capable of causing infectious diseases such as Legionnaires' disease, viral pneumonia, and the common cold, to less threatening but nonetheless distressing allergens derived from pet dander, dust mites, and fungi and molds responsible for rhinitis, eye irritation, and asthma. *Radon*, a radioactive gas derived from uranium widely present in soil and in homes, can cause lung cancer in uranium miners. However, it does not seem that low-level chronic exposures in the home increase lung cancer risk, at least for nonsmokers. Exposure to *formaldehyde*, used in the manufacture of building materials (cabinetry, furniture, adhesives, etc.) has become a common health problem in refugees from environmental disasters living in poorly ventilated trailers. Many of these cases occurred in trailers occupied by families displaced from their homes after Hurricane Katrina, which hit the southeastern United States in 2005. At concentrations of 0.1 ppm or higher, it causes breathing difficulties and a burning sensation in the eyes and throat, and can trigger asthma attacks. Formaldehyde is classified as a carcinogen for humans and animals. Finally, the so-called *sick building syndrome* remains an elusive problem, since it may be a consequence of exposure to one or more of the indoor pollutants already mentioned or be caused by poor ventilation.

METALS AS ENVIRONMENTAL POLLUTANTS

Lead, mercury, arsenic, and cadmium are the heavy metals most commonly associated with harmful effects in humans.

Lead

Lead exposure occurs through contaminated air and food and water. For most of the twentieth century the major sources of lead in the environment were lead-containing house paints and gasoline. Although limits have been set for the amounts of lead contained in residential paints, and leaded gasoline has practically disappeared in the United States, lead contamination remains an important health hazard, particularly for children. The large-scale recall of toys containing lead in 2007 alerted the general public to the dangers of lead exposures. There are many sources of lead in the environment, such as from mining, foundries, batteries, and spray painting, which constitute occupational hazards. However, *flaking lead paint* in older houses and soil contamination pose major hazards to youngsters, and ingestion of up to 200 mg/day can occur. During the last 30 years the median blood level of lead in preschool children in the United States decreased from 15 μg/dL to the present level of less than 2 μg/dL. However, lead blood levels in children living in older homes containing lead-based paint or lead-contaminated dust, often exceed the maximal allowed level of 10 μg/dL. *Subclinical lead poisoning* may occur in children exposed to levels of lead below 10 μg/dL, causing low intellectual capacity, behavioral problems such as hyperactivity, and poor organizational skills.[14,15] Lead poisoning, although less common in adults, occurs mainly as an occupational hazard in those involved in the manufacturing of batteries, pigments, car radiators, and tin cans. The main clinical features of lead poisoning in children and adults are shown in Figures 9–5 and 9–6.

Most of the absorbed lead (80% to 85%) is incorporated into bone and developing teeth, where it competes with calcium; its half-life in bone is 20 to 30 years. *High levels of lead cause disturbances in the CNS in adults and children,* but peripheral neuropathies predominate in adults. Children absorb more than 50% of ingested lead (as compared with ≤15% in adults); the higher intestinal absorption and the more permeable blood-brain barrier of children create a high susceptibility to brain damage. The neurotoxic effects of lead are attributed to the inhibition of neurotransmitters caused by the disruption of calcium homeostasis. Other effects of lead exposure are listed below.

○ *Lead interferes with the normal remodeling of cartilage* and primary bone trabeculae in the epiphyses in children. This causes increased bone density detected as radiodense "lead lines" (Fig. 9–7; another type of lead line appears in the gums as a result of hyperpigmentation). Lead *inhibits the healing of fractures* by increasing chondrogenesis and delaying cartilage mineralization.

○ Lead inhibits the activity of two enzymes involved in heme synthesis, δ-aminolevulinic acid dehydratase and ferrochelatase. Ferrochelatase catalyzes the incorporation of iron into protoporphyrin, and its inhibition causes a rise in protoporphyrin levels. The resulting heme deficiency causes various abnormalities, but the most obvious is a *microcytic,*

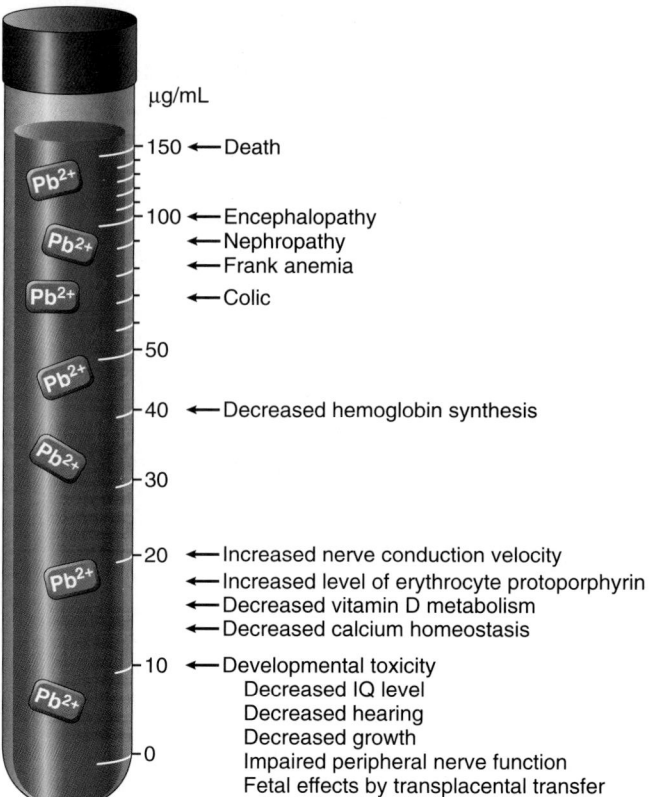

FIGURE 9–5 Effects of lead poisoning in children related to blood levels. (Modified from Bellinger DC, Bellinger AM: Childhood lead poisoning: the tortuous path from science to policy. J Clin Invest 116:853, 2006.)

hypochromic anemia stemming from the suppression of hemoglobin synthesis.

The diagnosis of lead poisoning requires constant awareness of its prevalence. In children it may be suspected on the basis of neurologic and behavioral changes, or by unexplained anemia with basophilic stippling in red cells. Definitive diagnosis requires the detection of elevated blood levels of lead and free (or zinc-bound) red cell protoporphyrin.

Morphology. The major anatomic targets of lead toxicity are the bone marrow and blood, nervous system, gastrointestinal tract, and kidneys (see Fig. 9–6).

Blood and marrow changes occur fairly early and are characteristic. The inhibition of ferrochelatase by lead results in the appearance of scattered **ringed sideroblasts,** red cell precursors with iron-laden mitochondria that are detected with a Prussian blue stain. In the peripheral blood the defect in hemoglobin synthesis appears as a **microcytic, hypochromic anemia** that is often accompanied by mild **hemolysis.** Even more distinctive is a **punctate basophilic stippling of the red cells.**

Brain damage is prone to occur in children. It can be very subtle, producing mild dysfunction, or it can be massive and lethal. In young children, sensory, motor, intellectual, and psychologic impairments

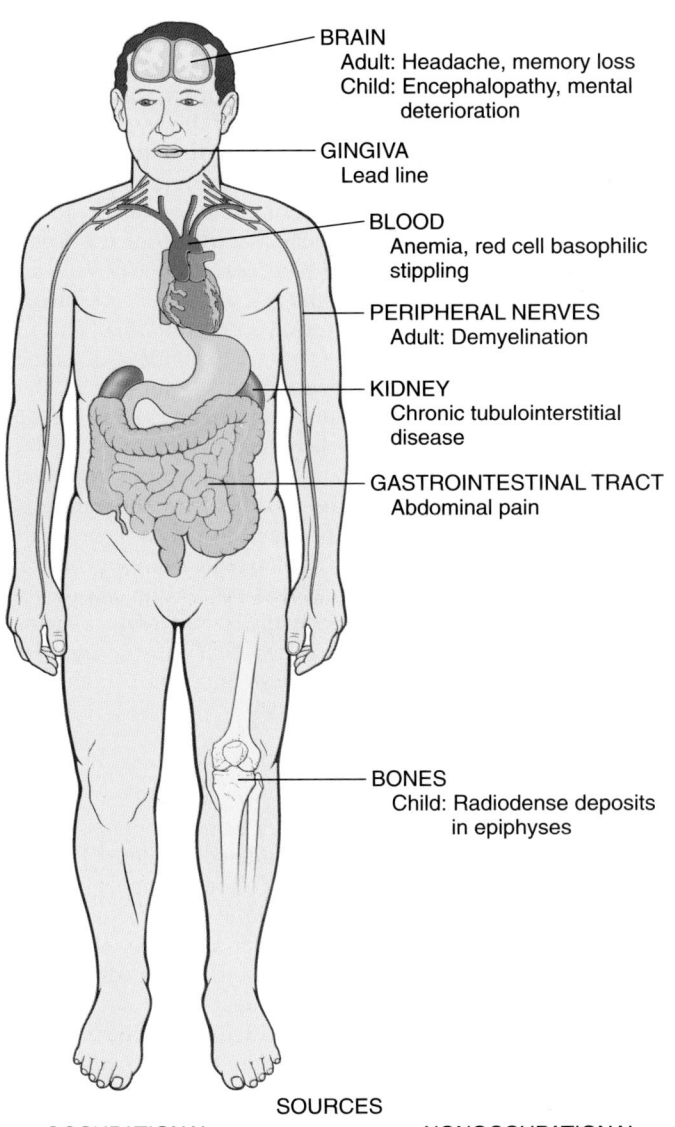

BRAIN
  Adult: Headache, memory loss
  Child: Encephalopathy, mental
    deterioration

GINGIVA
  Lead line

BLOOD
  Anemia, red cell basophilic
    stippling

PERIPHERAL NERVES
  Adult: Demyelination

KIDNEY
  Chronic tubulointerstitial
    disease

GASTROINTESTINAL TRACT
  Abdominal pain

BONES
  Child: Radiodense deposits
    in epiphyses

SOURCES

OCCUPATIONAL
  Spray painting
  Foundry work
  Mining and extracting lead
  Battery burning

NONOCCUPATIONAL
  Water supply
  Paint dust and flakes
  Automotive exhaust
  Urban soil

FIGURE 9–6 Pathologic features of lead poisoning in adults.

monly used muscles. Thus, the extensor muscles of the wrist and fingers are often the first to be affected (causing wristdrop), followed by paralysis of the peroneal muscles (causing footdrop).

The **gastrointestinal tract** is also a major source of clinical manifestations. Lead "colic" is characterized by extremely severe, poorly localized abdominal pain.

Kidneys may develop proximal tubular damage with intranuclear lead inclusions. Chronic renal damage leads eventually to interstitial fibrosis and possibly renal failure. Decreases in uric acid excretion can lead to gout ("saturnine gout").

Mercury

Mercury has had many uses throughout history such as a pigment in cave paintings, a cosmetic, a remedy for syphilis, and a component of diuretics. Alchemists tried (without much success) to produce gold from mercury. Poisoning from inhalation of mercury vapors has long been recognized and is associated with tremor, gingivitis, and bizarre behavior, such as that displayed by the Mad Hatter in *Alice in Wonderland*. There are three forms of mercury: metallic mercury (also referred to as elemental mercury), inorganic mercury compounds (mostly mercuric chloride), and organic mercury (mostly methyl mercury). Today, the main sources of exposure to mercury are contaminated fish (methyl mercury) and mercury vapors released from metallic mercury in dental amalgams, a possible occupational hazard for dental workers.

have been described, including reduced IQ, learning disabilities, retarded psychomotor development, blindness, and, in more severe cases, psychoses, seizures, and coma (see Fig. 9–5). Lead toxicity in the mother may impair brain development in the prenatal infant. The anatomic changes underlying the more subtle functional deficits are ill-defined, but there is concern that some of the defects may be permanent. At the more severe end of the spectrum are marked brain edema, demyelination of the cerebral and cerebellar white matter, and necrosis of cortical neurons accompanied by diffuse astrocytic proliferation. In adults the CNS is less often affected, but frequently **a peripheral demyelinating neuropathy** appears, typically involving the motor nerves of the most com-

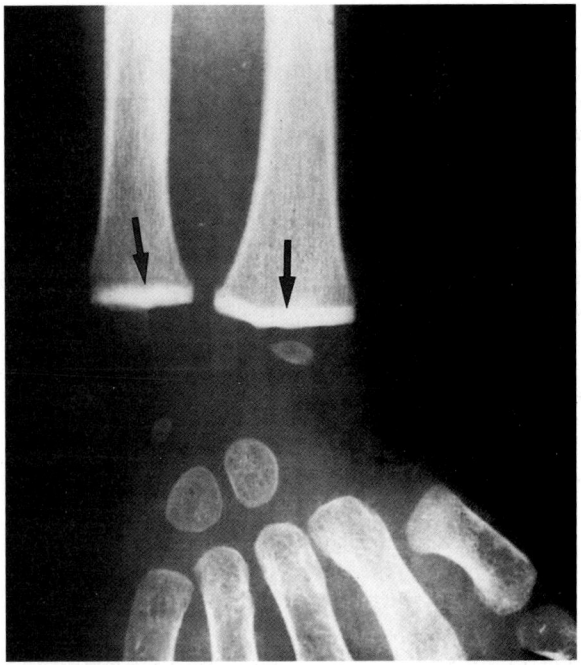

FIGURE 9–7 Lead poisoning. Impaired remodeling of calcified cartilage in the epiphyses *(arrows)* of the wrist has caused a marked increase in their radiodensity, so that they are as radiopaque as the cortical bone. (Courtesy of Dr. G.W. Dietz, Department of Radiology, University of Texas Southwestern Medical School, Dallas, TX.)

In some areas of the world, mercury used in gold mining has contaminated rivers and streams.

Inorganic mercury from the natural degassing of the earth's crust or from industrial contamination is converted to organic compounds such as methyl mercury by bacteria. Methyl mercury enters the food chain, and in carnivorous fish such as swordfish, shark, and bluefish, mercury may be concentrated to levels a million-fold higher than in the surrounding water. Disasters caused by the consumption of fish contaminated by the release of methyl mercury from industrial sources in Minamata Bay and the Agano River in Japan caused widespread mortality and morbidity. Acute exposure through consumption of bread made from grain treated with a methyl mercury–based fungicide in Iraq in 1971 resulted in hundreds of deaths and thousands of hospitalizations. The medical disorders associated with the Minamata episode became known as *"Minamata disease"* and include cerebral palsy, deafness, blindness, mental retardation, and major CNS defects in children exposed in utero. For unclear reasons, *the developing brain is extremely sensitive to methyl mercury.* The lipid solubility of methyl mercury and metallic mercury facilitate their accumulation in the brain, disturbing neuromotor, cognitive, and behavioral functions.[16] Mercury binds with high affinity to thiol groups, a property that contributes to its toxicity. *Intracellular glutathione, acting as thiol donor, is the main protective mechanism against mercury-induced CNS and kidney damage.*

Mercury continues to be released into the environment by power plants and other industrial sources, and there are serious concerns about the effects of chronic low-level exposure to methyl mercury in the food supply. To protect against potential fetal brain damage, the Centers for Disease Control and Prevention has recommended that pregnant women reduce their consumption of fish known to contain mercury to a minimum. There has been much publicity about a possible relationship between thimerosal (a compound that contains ethyl mercury, used until recently as a preservative in some vaccines) and the development of autism, but multiple studies have failed to find evidence of a causal relationship.[17]

Arsenic

Arsenic was the poison of choice in Renaissance Italy, with members of the Borgia and Medici families being highly skilled practitioners of the art. Because of its favored use as a murder weapon among royal families, arsenic has been called "the poison of kings and the king of poisons."[18] Deliberate poisoning by arsenic is exceedingly rare today, but exposure to arsenic is an important health problem in many areas of the world. Arsenic is found naturally in soils and water and is used in products such as wood preservers, as well as herbicides and other agricultural products. It may be released into the environment from mines and smelting industries. Arsenic is present in Chinese and Indian herbal medicine, and arsenic trioxide is used in the treatment of relapsing acute promyelocytic leukemia. Large concentrations of inorganic arsenic are present in ground water used for drinking in countries such as Bangladesh, Chile, and China. Between 35 and 77 million people in Bangladesh drink water contaminated by arsenic, constituting the highest environmental cancer risk ever found.

The most toxic forms of arsenic are the trivalent compounds arsenic trioxide, sodium arsenite, and arsenic trichloride.[19] If ingested in large quantities, arsenic causes acute toxic effects consisting of severe disturbances of the *gastrointestinal, cardiovascular, and central nervous systems* that are often fatal. These effects may be attributed to interference with mitochondrial oxidative phosphorylation, since trivalent arsenic can replace the phosphates in adenosine triphosphate. *Neurologic effects* usually occur 2 to 8 weeks after exposure and consist of a sensorimotor neuropathy that causes paresthesias, numbness, and pain. The most serious consequence of chronic exposure is the *increased risk for the development of cancers* in almost all tissues, but particularly in the lungs and skin. Chronic exposure to arsenic causes *skin changes* consisting of hyperpigmentation and hyperkeratosis, which may be followed by the development of basal and squamous cell carcinomas. Arsenic-induced skin tumors differ from those induced by sunlight; they are often multiple and usually appear on the palms and soles. The mechanisms of arsenic carcinogenesis in skin and lung have not been elucidated but may involve defects in nucleotide excision repair mechanisms that protect against DNA damage.[18] Recent studies suggest that chronic exposure to arsenic in drinking water can also cause non-malignant respiratory disease.[20]

Cadmium

In contrast to the other metals discussed in this section, cadmium toxicity is a relatively modern problem. It is an occupational and environmental pollutant generated by mining, electroplating, and production of nickel-cadmium batteries, which are usually disposed of as household waste. Cadmium can contaminate the soil and plants directly or through fertilizers and irrigation water. Food is the most important source of cadmium exposure for the general population. *The toxic effects of excess cadmium consist of obstructive lung disease caused by necrosis of alveolar macrophages, and kidney damage, initially consisting of tubular damage that may progress to end-stage renal disease.* Cadmium exposure can also cause skeletal abnormalities associated with calcium loss. Cadmium-containing water used to irrigate rice fields in Japan caused a disease in postmenopausal women known as "Itai-Itai" (ouch-ouch), a combination of osteoporosis and osteomalacia associated with renal disease. Cadmium exposure is also associated with elevated risk of lung cancer, which has been demonstrated in workers exposed occupationally and in populations living near zinc smelters.[21] Cadmium is not directly genotoxic and most likely produces DNA damage through the generation of reactive oxygen species (see Chapter 1). A recent survey showed that 5% of the US population age 20 years and older have urinary cadmium levels that may produce subtle kidney injury and calcium loss.

Occupational Health Risks: Industrial and Agricultural Exposures

More than 10 million injuries and about 100,000 deaths occur yearly in the United States as a consequence of work-related accidents and illnesses. Work-related accidents are the biggest

TABLE 9–2	Human Diseases Associated with Occupational Exposures	
Organ/System	Effect	Toxicant
Cardiovascular system	Heart disease	Carbon monoxide, lead, solvents, cobalt, cadmium
Respiratory system	Nasal cancer Lung cancer Chronic obstructive lung disease Hypersensitivity Irritation Fibrosis	Isopropyl alcohol, wood dust Radon, asbestos, silica, bis(chloromethyl)ether, nickel, arsenic, chromium, mustard gas, uranium Grain dust, coal dust, cadmium Beryllium, isocyanates Ammonia, sulfur oxides, formaldehyde Silica, asbestos, cobalt
Nervous system	Peripheral neuropathies Ataxic gait Central nervous system depression Cataracts	Solvents, acrylamide, methyl chloride, mercury, lead, arsenic, DDT Chlordane, toluene, acrylamide, mercury Alcohols, ketones, aldehydes, solvents Ultraviolet radiation
Urinary system	Toxicity Bladder cancer	Mercury, lead, glycol ethers, solvents Naphthylamines, 4-aminobiphenyl, benzidine, rubber products
Reproductive system	Male infertility Female infertility/stillbirths Teratogenesis	Lead, phthalate plasticizers, cadmium Lead, mercury Mercury, polychlorinated biphenyls
Hematopoietic system	Leukemia	Benzene
Skin	Folliculitis and acneiform dermatosis Cancer	Polychlorinated biphenyls, dioxins, herbicides Ultraviolet radiation
Gastrointestinal tract	Liver angiosarcoma	Vinyl chloride

Data from Leigh JP, et al.: Occupational injury and illness in the United States. Estimates of costs, morbidity, and mortality, Arch Intern Med 157:1557, 1997; Mitchell FL: Hazardous waste. In Rom WN (ed): Environmental and Occupational Medicine, 2nd ed. Boston, Little, Brown, 1992, p 1275; and Levi PE: Classes of toxic chemicals. In Hodgson E, Levi PE (eds): A Textbook of Modern Toxicology. Stamford, CT, Appleton & Lange, 1997, p 229.

problem in developing countries, while work-related diseases are more frequent in industrialized countries. The fraction of global disease attributed to occupational exposures includes 13% of all cases of chronic obstructive pulmonary disease, 9% of lung cancers, and 2 % of leukemias. Industrial exposures to toxic agents are as varied as the industries themselves. They range from mere irritation of the respiratory mucosa by formaldehyde or ammonia fumes; to lung cancer induced by exposure to asbestos, arsenic, or uranium mining; to leukemia caused by chronic exposure to benzene. Human diseases associated with occupational exposures are listed in Table 9–2. Here we provide a few examples of important agents that contribute to occupational diseases. Toxicity caused by metals has already been discussed in this chapter.

- *Organic solvents* are widely used in huge quantities worldwide. Some, such as *chloroform and carbon tetrachloride*, are found in degreasing and dry cleaning agents and paint removers. Acute exposure to high levels of vapors from these agents can cause dizziness and confusion, leading to central nervous system depression and even coma. Lower levels are toxic for the liver and kidneys. Occupational exposure of rubber workers to *benzene* and *1,3-butadiene* increases the risk of leukemia. Benzene is oxidized by hepatic CYP2E1 to toxic metabolites that disrupt the differentiation of hematopoietic cells in the bone marrow, leading to dose-dependent marrow aplasia and an increased risk of acute myeloid leukemia.
- *Polycyclic hydrocarbons* may be released during the combustion of fossil fuels, particularly when coal and gas are

burned at high temperatures (such as in steel foundries), and are also present in tar and soot (Pott identified soot as the cause of scrotal cancers in chimney sweeps in 1775, as mentioned in Chapter 7). Polycyclic hydrocarbons are among the most potent carcinogens, and industrial exposures have been implicated in the development of lung and bladder cancer.

- *Organochlorines.* Organochlorines (and halogenated organic compounds in general) are synthetic lipophilic products that resist degradation. Important organochlorines used as pesticides include *DDT (dichlorodiphenyltrichloroethane)*, Lindane, Aldrin, and Dieldrin. Nonpesticide organochlorines include *polychlorinated biphenyls (PCBs) and dioxin* (TCDD; 2,3,7,8-tetrachlorodibenzo-p-dioxin). DDT was banned in the United States in 1973, but more than half of the U.S. population has detectable levels of *p, p'*-DDE, a long-lasting DDT metabolite. This substance was even found in 12- to 19-year-olds born after the ban on DDT. PCB (another banned substance), dioxin, and PBDEs (polybrominated diphenyl ethers used as flame retardants) are also detectable in a large proportion of the U.S. population. *Most organochlorines are endocrine disruptors* with anti-estrogenic or anti-androgenic activity.
- *Dioxins and PCBs* can cause skin disorders such as folliculitis and a dermatosis known as *chloracne* that is characterized by acne, cyst formation, hyperpigmentation, and hyperkeratosis, generally around the face and behind the ears. These toxins can also cause abnormalities in the liver and central nervous system. Because PCBs induce CYPs,

workers exposed to these substances may show abnormal drug metabolism. Environmental disasters in Japan and China in the late 1960s caused by the consumption of rice oil contaminated by PCBs during its production, poisoned about 2000 people in each episode. The primary manifestation of the disease (Yusho in Japan; Yu-Cheng in China) was chloracne and hyperpigmentation of the skin and nails. A bizarre case of intentional dioxin poisoning, which made international headlines and was a front-page illustration of chloracne, involved a future president of Ukraine. This individual developed extensive chloracne and systemic symptoms, as a consequence of eating a meal spiked with dioxin that was offered by one of his political "friends."

● *Inhalation of mineral dusts causes chronic, non-neoplastic lung diseases known as pneumoconioses.* This term also includes diseases induced by organic and inorganic particulates, and chemical fume- and vapor-induced non-neoplastic lung diseases. The most common pneumoconioses are caused by exposures to *coal dust* (from mining of hard coal), *silica* (sandblasting, stone cutting, etc.), *asbestos* (mining, fabrication, insulation work), and *beryllium* (mining, fabrication). Exposure to these agents nearly always occurs in the workplace. However, the increased risk of cancer as a result of asbestos exposure extends to the family members of asbestos workers and to other individuals exposed outside the workplace. Pneumoconioses and their pathogenesis are discussed in Chapter 15.

● Exposure to *vinyl chloride* used in the synthesis of polyvinyl resins leads to the development of angiosarcoma of the liver, an uncommon type of hepatic tumor.

● Exposure to *phthalates* in laboratory animals causes endocrine disruption and a testicular dysgenesis syndrome involving hypospadias, cryptorchidism, and testicular cell abnormalities that are similar to conditions of generally unknown origin found in humans. Phthalates are widely used plasticizers found in flexible plastics (as in food wraps) and in medical containers, such as blood and serum bags. A matter of concern is that critically ill infants may receive large doses of phthalates from bags holding intravenous fluids, although the toxicity in humans has not been firmly established.

Effects of Tobacco

Tobacco is the most common exogenous cause of human cancers, being responsible for 90% of lung cancers. *The main culprit is cigarette smoking, but smokeless tobacco (snuff, chewing tobacco, etc.) is also harmful to health and an important cause of oral cancer.* The use of tobacco products not only creates personal risks, but passive tobacco inhalation from the environment *("second-hand smoke")* can cause lung cancer in nonsmokers.[22] Cigarette smoking causes, worldwide, more than 5 million deaths annually, mostly from cardiovascular disease, various types of cancers, and chronic respiratory problems, that result in a total of more than 35 million years of life lost. These figures are expected to rise to 8 million tobacco-related deaths by 2020, the major increase occurring in developing countries. It has been estimated that of people alive today, approximately 500 million will die from tobacco-related illnesses. In the United States alone, tobacco is responsible for

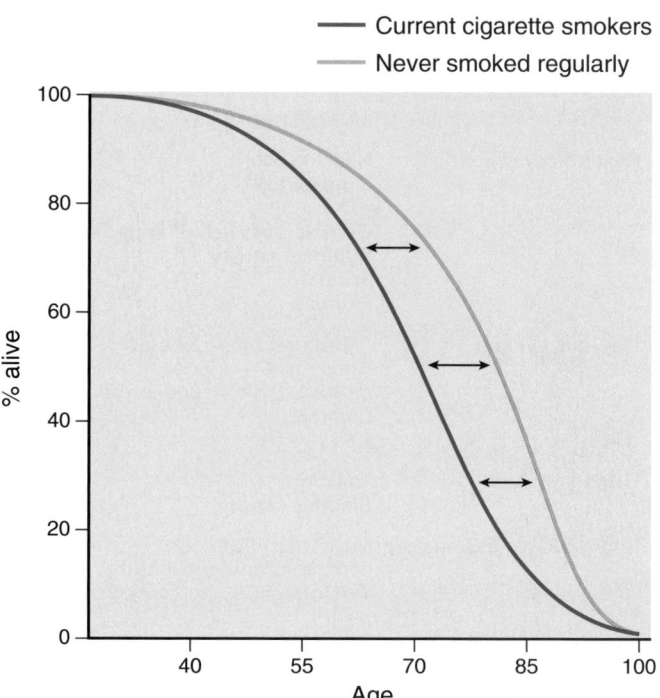

FIGURE 9–8 The effects of smoking on survival. The study compared age-specific death rates for current cigarette smokers with that of individuals who never smoked regularly (British Doctors Study). Measured at age 75, the difference in survival between smokers and nonsmokers is 7.5 years. (Modified from Stewart BW, Kleihues P (eds): World Cancer Report. Lyon, IARC Press, 2003.)

over 400,000 deaths annually, one third of these attributable to lung cancer. Two thirds of smokers live in 10 countries, led by China, which accounts for nearly 30%, and India with about 10%, followed by Indonesia, Russia, the United States, Japan, Brazil, Bangladesh, Germany, and Turkey.

Smoking is the most preventable cause of human death. It reduces overall survival through dose-dependent effects. For instance, while 80% of a population of nonsmokers is alive at age 70, only about 50% of smokers survive to that age (Fig. 9–8). The prevalence of smoking has decreased in US teenagers, a hopeful trend. However, recent surveys estimate that 7%, 14%, and 22% of students in grades 8, 10, and 12, respectively, had used tobacco products during the month before the survey. Delaying the age at which smoking is initiated reduces the future risk of lung and other types of cancers, but, unfortunately, initiation seems to be occurring at younger ages. *Cessation of smoking greatly reduces, within 5 years, the overall mortality and the risk of death from cardiovascular diseases. Lung cancer mortality decreases by 21% within 5 years, but the excess risk lasts for 30 years.*[22]

The number of potentially noxious chemicals in tobacco smoke is extraordinary. Tobacco contains between 2000 and 4000 substances, more than 60 of which have been identified as carcinogens. Table 9–3 provides only a partial list and includes various types of injuries produced by these agents. *Nicotine,* an alkaloid present in tobacco leaves, is not a direct cause of tobacco-related diseases, but is addictive. Without it, it would be easy for smokers to stop the habit. Nicotine binds to receptors in the brain, and through the release of catecholamines,

TABLE 9–3 Effects of Selected Tobacco Smoke Constituents

Substance	Effect
Tar	Carcinogenesis
Polycyclic aromatic hydrocarbons	Carcinogenesis
Nicotine	Ganglionic stimulation and depression; tumor promotion
Phenol	Tumor promotion; mucosal irritation
Benzopyrene	Carcinogenesis
Carbon monoxide	Impaired oxygen transport and utilization
Formaldehyde	Toxicity to cilia; mucosal irritation
Oxides of nitrogen	Toxicity to cilia; mucosal irritation
Nitrosamine	Carcinogenesis

is responsible for the acute effects of smoking, such as the increase in heart rate and blood pressure, and the elevation in cardiac contractility and output. The *most common diseases caused by cigarette smoking involve the lung and include emphysema, chronic bronchitis, chronic obstructive pulmonary disease, and lung cancer*, conditions that are discussed in Chapter 15. *Cigarette smoking is also strongly associated with the development of atherosclerosis, myocardial infarcts, and cancers of the lip, mouth, pharynx, esophagus, pancreas, bladder, kidney, and cervix*. Adverse effects of smoking in various organs systems are shown in Figure 9–9.

Smoking and Lung Cancer. Agents in smoke have a direct irritant effect on the tracheobronchial mucosa, producing *inflammation and increased mucus production (bronchitis)*. Cigarette smoke also causes the recruitment of leukocytes to the lung, with increased local elastase production and subsequent injury to lung tissue, leading to *emphysema. Components of cigarette smoke, particularly polycyclic hydrocarbons and nitrosamines* (Table 9–4), *are potent carcinogens in animals and likely to be directly involved in the development of lung cancer in humans* (see Chapter 15). CYPs (cytochrome P-450 phase I enzymes) and phase II enzymes increase the water solubility of the carcinogens, facilitating their excretion. However, some intermediates produced by CYPs are electrophilic and form DNA adducts. If such adducts persist, they can cause mutations in oncogenes and tumor suppressors such as *K-Ras* and *p53*,[23] respectively. The risk of developing lung cancer is related to the intensity of exposure, frequently expressed in terms of "pack years" (e.g., one pack smoked daily for 20 years equals 20 pack years) or in cigarettes smoked per day (Fig. 9–10). Moreover, *smoking multiplies the risk of other carcinogenic influences*. Witness the ten-fold higher incidence of lung carcinomas in asbestos workers and uranium miners who smoke over those who do not smoke, and the interaction between tobacco consumption and alcohol in the development of oral cancers (mentioned below).

Smoking and Other Diseases. In addition to lung cancers, *tobacco contributes to the development of cancers of the oral cavity, esophagus, pancreas, and bladder*. Smoke and smokeless tobacco interact with alcohol in the development of laryngeal

cancer. The combination of these agents has a multiplicative effect on the risk of developing this tumor (Fig. 9–11).

Cigarette smoking is strongly linked to the development of atherosclerosis and its major complication, myocardial infarction. The causal mechanisms probably relate to several factors, including increased platelet aggregation, decreased myocardial oxygen supply (because of significant lung disease coupled with the hypoxia related to the CO content of cigarette smoke) accompanied by an increased oxygen demand, and a decreased threshold for ventricular fibrillation. Smoking has a multiplicative effect on the incidence of myocardial infarction when combined with hypertension and hypercholesterolemia.

Maternal smoking increases the risk of spontaneous abortions and preterm births and results in intrauterine growth retardation (Chapter 10). Birth weights of infants born to mothers who stopped smoking before pregnancy are, however, normal.

Exposure to *environmental tobacco smoke (passive smoke inhalation)* is also associated with some of the same detrimental effects that result from active smoking. It is estimated that the relative risk of lung cancer in nonsmokers exposed to environmental smoke is about 1.3 times higher than that of nonsmokers who are not exposed to smoke. In the United States, approximately 3000 lung cancer deaths in nonsmokers over the age of 35 years can be attributed each year to envi-

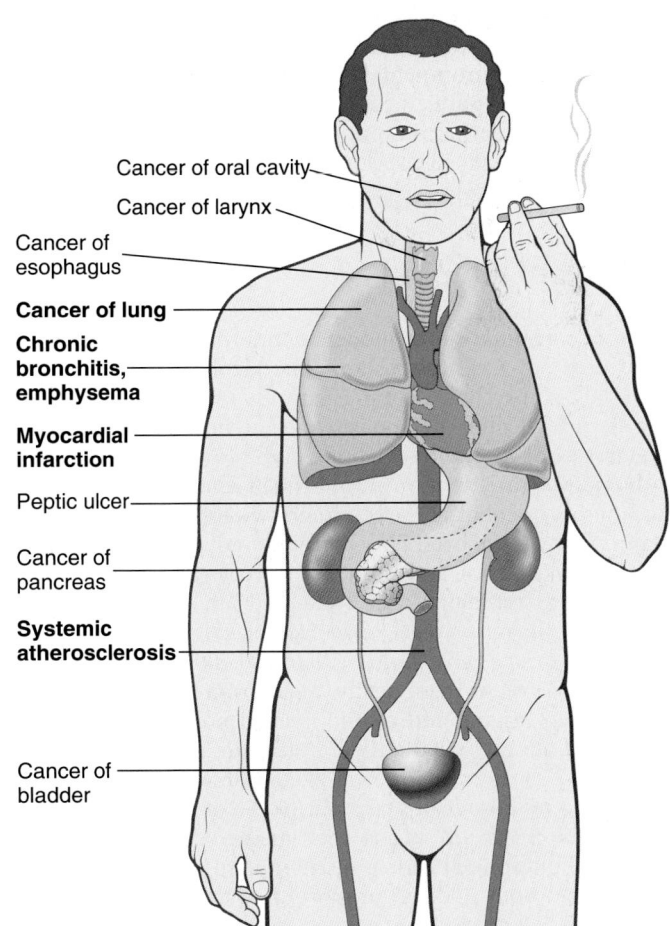

FIGURE 9–9 Adverse effects of smoking: those that are more common are in boldface.

TABLE 9–4	Organ-Specific Carcinogens in Tobacco Smoke
Organ	**Carcinogen**
Lung, larynx	Polycyclic aromatic hydrocarbons 4-(Methylnitrosoamino)-1-(3-pyridyl)-1-buta-none (NNK), polonium 210
Esophagus	N'-Nitrosonornicotine (NNN)
Pancreas	NNK (?)
Bladder	4-Aminobiphenyl, 2-naphthylamine
Oral cavity (smoking)	Polycyclic aromatic hydrocarbons, NNK, NNN
Oral cavity (snuff)	NNK, NNN, polonium 210

Data from Szczesny LB, Holbrook JH: Cigarette smoking. In Rom WH (ed): Environmental and Occupational Medicine, 2nd ed. Boston, Little, Brown, 1992, p 1211.

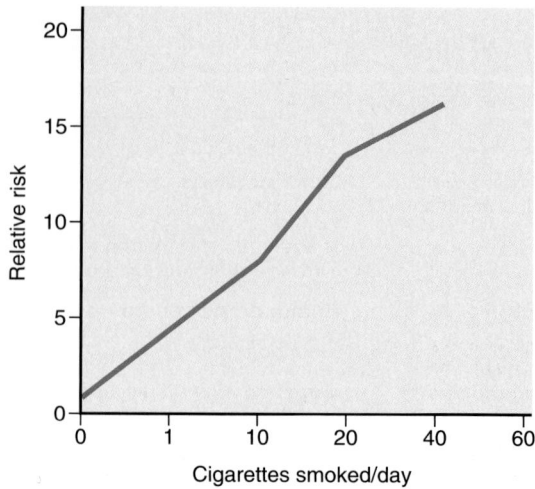

FIGURE 9–10 The risk of lung cancer is determined by the number of cigarettes smoked. (Modified from Stewart BW, Kleihues P (eds): World Cancer Report. Lyon, IARC Press, 2003.)

ronmental tobacco smoke. Even more striking is the increased risk of coronary atherosclerosis and fatal myocardial infarction. Studies report that every year 30,000 to 60,000 cardiac deaths in the United States are associated with exposure to passive smoke. Passive smoke inhalation in nonsmokers can be estimated by measuring the blood levels of *cotinine*, a metabolite of nicotine. Median cotinine levels in nonsmokers have decreased by more than 60% during the last 10 years, but exposure to environmental tobacco smoke in the home remains a major public health concern, particularly for children who may develop respiratory illnesses and asthma. It is clear that the transient pleasure a puff may give comes with a heavy long-term price.

Effects of Alcohol

Ethanol consumption in moderate amounts is generally not injurious, but in excessive amounts alcohol causes serious physical and psychologic damage. In this section we describe the steps of alcohol metabolism and the major health consequences associated with alcohol abuse.

Despite all the attention given to illicit drugs such as cocaine and heroin, alcohol abuse is a more widespread hazard and claims many more lives. Fifty percent of adults in the Western world drink alcohol, and about 5% to 10% have chronic alcoholism. It is estimated that *there are more than 10 million chronic alcoholics in the United States and that alcohol consumption is responsible for more than 100,000 deaths annually.* More than 50% of these deaths result from accidents caused by drunken driving and alcohol-related homicides and suicides, and about 15,000 annual deaths are a consequence of cirrhosis of the liver. Worldwide, alcohol accounts for approximately 1.8 million deaths per year (3.2% of all deaths). After consumption, ethanol is absorbed unaltered in the stomach and small intestine. It is then distributed to all the tissues and fluids of the body in direct proportion to the blood level. Less than 10% is excreted unchanged in the urine, sweat, and breath. The amount exhaled is proportional to the blood level and forms the basis of the breath test used by law enforcement

agencies. A concentration of 80 mg/dL in the blood constitutes the legal definition of drunk driving in the United States. For an average individual, this alcohol concentration may be reached after consumption of three standard drinks, contained in about 3 (12 ounce) bottles of beer, 15 ounces of wine, or 4–5 ounces of 80 proof distilled spirits. Drowsiness occurs at 200 mg/dL, stupor at 300 mg/dL, and coma, with possible respiratory arrest, at higher levels. The rate of metabolism affects the blood alcohol level. Chronic alcoholics can tolerate

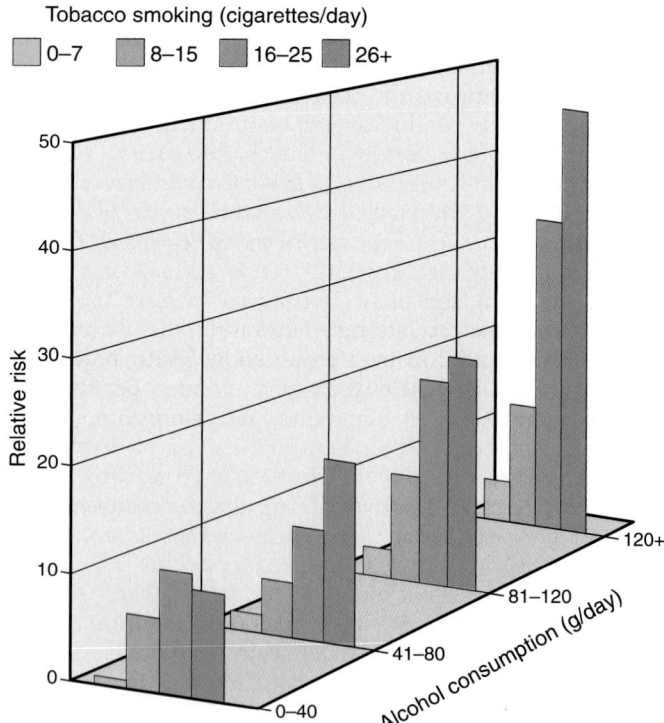

FIGURE 9–11 Multiplicative increase in the risk of laryngeal cancer from the interaction between cigarette smoking and alcohol consumption. (Modified from Stewart BW, Kleihues P (eds): World Cancer Report. Lyon, IARC Press, 2003.)

FIGURE 9–12 Metabolism of ethanol: oxidation of ethanol to acetaldehyde by three different routes, and the generation of acetic acid. Note that oxidation by ADH (alcohol dehydrogenase) takes place in the cytosol; the cytochrome P-450 system and its CYP2E1 isoform are located in the endoplasmic reticulum (microsomes), and catalase is located in peroxisomes. Oxidation of acetaldehyde by ALDH (aldehyde dehydrogenase) occurs in mitochondria. ADH oxidation is the most important route; catalase is involved in only 5% of ethanol metabolism. Oxidation through CYPs may also generate reactive oxygen species (not shown). (From Parkinson A: Biotransformation of xenobiotics. In Klassen CD [ed]: Casarett and Doull's Toxicology: The Basic Science of Poisons, 6th ed. New York, McGraw-Hill, 2001, p 133.)

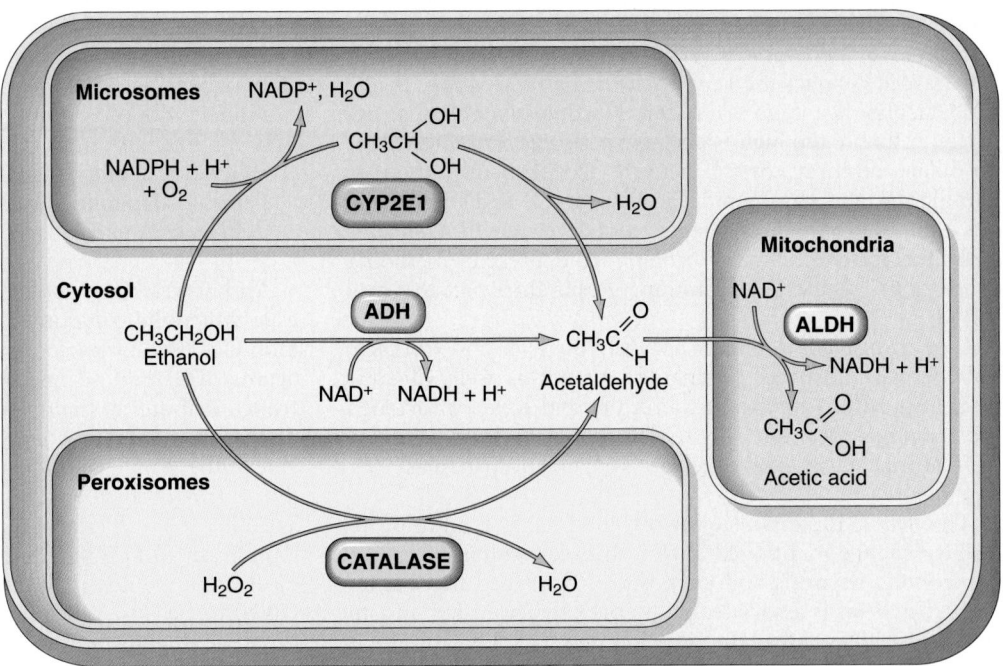

levels of up to 700 mg/dL, a situation that is partially explained by accelerated ethanol metabolism caused by a five- to tenfold induction of liver CYPs discussed below. The effects of alcohol also vary by age, sex, and body fat.

Most of the alcohol in the blood is biotransformed to acetaldehyde in the liver by three enzyme systems consisting of alcohol dehydrogenase (ADH), the microsomal ethanol-oxidizing system (MEOS), and catalase (Fig. 9–12). The *main enzyme system involved in alcohol metabolism is ADH,* located in the cytosol of hepatocytes. At high blood alcohol levels, the *microsomal ethanol-oxidizing system participates in its metabolism.* Catalase, which uses hydrogen peroxide as substrate, is of minor importance, since it metabolizes no more than 5% of ethanol in the liver. Acetaldehyde produced by alcohol metabolism through ADH or MEOS is converted to *acetate* by acetaldehyde dehydrogenase (ALDH), which is then utilized in the mitochondrial respiratory chain.

The microsomal oxidation system involves CYPs, particularly CYP2E1 located in the smooth endoplasmic reticulum. Induction of CYPs by alcohol explains the increased susceptibility of alcoholics to other compounds metabolized by the same enzyme system, which include drugs, anesthetics, carcinogens, and industrial solvents. Note, however, that when alcohol is present in the blood at high concentrations, it competes with other CYP2E1 substrates and delays drug catabolism, potentiating the depressant effects of narcotic, sedative, and psychoactive drugs in the central nervous system. The oxidation of ethanol produces toxic agents and disrupts metabolic pathways. Here we mention only the most important of these changes.

○ *Acetaldehyde* has many toxic effects and is responsible for some of the acute effects of alcohol and for the development of oral cancers. The efficiency of alcohol metabolism varies between populations, depending on the expression

levels of ADH and ALDH isozymes, and the presence of genetic variants that alter enzyme activity. About 50% of Asians have very low ALDH activity, due to the substitution of lysine for glutamine at residue 487 (the normal allele is termed ALDH2*1 and the inactive variant is designated as ALDH2*2). The ALDH2*2 protein has dominant-negative activity, such that even one copy of the ALDH2*2 allele reduces ALDH activity significantly. *Individuals homozygous for the ALDH2*2 allele are completely unable to oxidize acetaldehyde and cannot tolerate alcohol,* experiencing nausea, flushing, tachycardia, and hyperventilation after its ingestion.[24]

○ Alcohol oxidation by ADH causes the reduction of nicotinamide adenine dinucleotide (NAD) to NADH, with a consequent decrease in NAD and increase in NADH. NAD is required for fatty acid oxidation in the liver and for the conversion of lactate into pyruvate. Its deficiency is a main cause of the accumulation of fat in the liver of alcoholics. The increase in the NADH/NAD ratio in alcoholics also causes lactic acidosis.

○ *Metabolism of ethanol in the liver by CYP2E1 produces reactive oxygen species and causes lipid peroxidation of cell membranes.* However, the precise mechanisms that account for alcohol-induced cellular injury in the liver have not been well defined. Alcohol also causes the release of endotoxin (lipopolysaccharide) from gram-negative bacteria in the intestinal flora, which stimulates the production of TNF (tumor necrosis factor) and other cytokines from macrophages and Kupffer cells, leading to hepatic injury.

The adverse effects of ethanol can be classified as acute or chronic.

Acute alcoholism exerts its effects mainly on the CNS, but it may induce hepatic and gastric changes that are reversible if alcohol consumption is discontinued. Even with moderate intake of alcohol, multiple fat droplets accumulate in the cytoplasm of hepatocytes (fatty change or hepatic steatosis). The gastric changes are acute gastritis and ulceration. In the CNS, alcohol is a depressant, first affecting subcortical structures (probably the high brain stem reticular formation) that modulate cerebral cortical activity. Consequently, there is stimulation and disordered cortical, motor, and intellectual behavior. At progressively higher blood levels, cortical neurons and then lower medullary centers are depressed, including those that regulate respiration. Respiratory arrest may follow.

Chronic alcoholism affects not only the liver and stomach, but virtually all other organs and tissues as well. Chronic alcoholics suffer significant morbidity and have a shortened life span, related principally to damage to the liver, gastrointestinal tract, CNS, cardiovascular system, and pancreas.

- The liver is the main site of chronic injury. In addition to fatty change mentioned above, chronic alcoholism causes alcoholic hepatitis and cirrhosis, as described in Chapter 18. Cirrhosis is associated with portal hypertension and an increased risk for the development of hepatocellular carcinoma.

- In the gastrointestinal tract, chronic alcoholism can cause massive bleeding from gastritis, gastric ulcer, or esophageal varices (associated with cirrhosis), which may prove fatal.

- Thiamine (vitamin B_1) deficiency is common in chronic alcoholics. The principal lesions resulting from this deficiency are peripheral neuropathies and the Wernicke-Korsakoff syndrome (see Table 9–9 in this chapter, and Chapter 28); cerebral atrophy, cerebellar degeneration, and optic neuropathy may also occur.

- Alcohol has diverse effects on the cardiovascular system. Injury to the myocardium may produce dilated congestive cardiomyopathy (alcoholic cardiomyopathy, discussed in Chapter 12). Chronic alcoholism is also associated with an increased incidence of hypertension. Moderate amounts of alcohol (about 20–30 gm of daily intake, corresponding to approximately 250 mL of wine) have been reported to increase high-density lipoprotein (HDL) levels and inhibit platelet aggregation, thus protecting against coronary heart disease. However, heavy alcohol consumption, with attendant liver injury, results in decreased levels of HDL, increasing the likelihood of coronary heart disease.

- Excessive alcohol intake increases the risk of acute and chronic pancreatitis (Chapter 19).

- The use of ethanol during pregnancy—reportedly in very low amounts—can cause fetal alcohol syndrome.[25] It consists of microcephaly, growth retardation, and facial abnormalities in the newborn, and reduction in mental functions as the child grows older. It is difficult to establish the minimal amount of alcohol consumption that can cause fetal alcohol syndrome, but consumption during the first trimester of pregnancy is particularly harmful. It has been estimated that the prevalence of frequent and binge drinking among pregnant women is approximately 6% and that fetal alcohol syndrome affects 1 to 4.8 per 1000 children born in the United States.

- Chronic alcohol consumption is associated with an increased incidence of cancer of the oral cavity, esophagus, liver, and, possibly, breast in females. Acetaldehyde is considered to be the main agent associated with alcohol-induced laryngeal and esophageal cancer, in that acetaldehyde-DNA adducts have been detected in some tumors from these tissues. Individuals with one copy of the ALDH2*2 allele who drink are at a higher risk of developing cancer of the esophagus.

- Ethanol is a substantial source of energy (empty calories). Chronic alcoholism leads to malnutrition and nutritional deficiencies, particularly of the B vitamins.

And now, a bit of good news: red wine contains resveratrol, a polyphenolic compound that increases life span in worms and flies, promotes longevity in mice, and protects mice against diet-induced obesity and insulin resistance. Resveratrol contributes to the protective effect against cardiovascular disease in moderate wine drinkers and possibly provides the clue to the "French paradox," a wine- and food-loving population with a low incidence of obesity and cardiovascular disease. The effects of resveratrol on longevity have been attributed to its activation of protein deacetylases of the Sir2 (sirtuin) family of enzymes, which include histone deacetylases (Chapter 1). However, because resveratrol also interacts with various other proteins, ongoing studies seek to identify the precise mechanisms of its protective effects.[26,27]

Injury by Therapeutic Drugs and Drugs of Abuse

INJURY BY THERAPEUTIC DRUGS (ADVERSE DRUG REACTIONS)

Adverse drug reactions (ADRs) refer to untoward effects of drugs that are given in conventional therapeutic settings. These reactions are extremely common in the practice of medicine (Fig. 9–13) and affect almost 10% of patients admitted to a hospital. It is estimated that in about 10% of these patients, ADRs are fatal. Table 9–5 lists common pathologic findings in ADRs and the drugs most frequently involved. As can be seen in the table, many of the drugs that produce ADRs, such as antineoplastic agents, are highly potent, and the adverse reactions are expected risks of the treatment. In this section, we examine the adverse reactions to some commonly used drugs. We first discuss the adverse effects of hormonal replacement therapy (HRT), oral contraceptives (OCs), and anabolic steroids. This is followed by a discussion of the effects of the drugs acetaminophen and aspirin, because all of these are used very commonly.

Hormonal Replacement Therapy (HRT)

The most common type of HRT consists of the administration of estrogens together with progesterone. Because of the risk of uterine cancer, estrogen therapy alone is used only in hysterectomized women. Once prescribed primarily for distressing menopausal symptoms (e.g., hot flashes), HRT had been widely used in postmenopausal women to prevent or slow the progression of osteoporosis (Chapter 26) and to reduce the likelihood of myocardial infarction. However, the results of the Women's Health Initiative published in 2002, stunned the scientific community by failing to find support for some of the presumed beneficial effects of the therapy. This large epi-

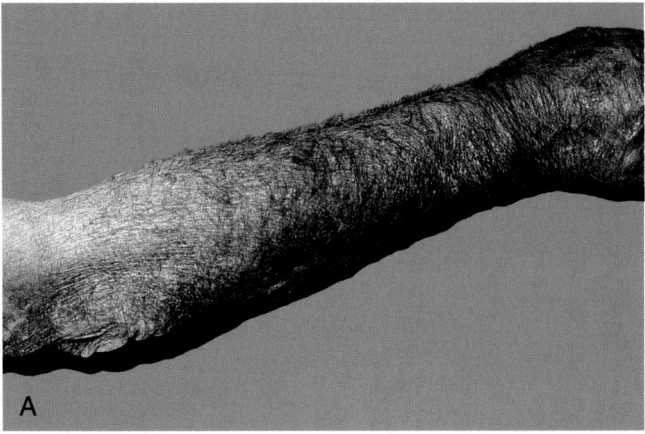

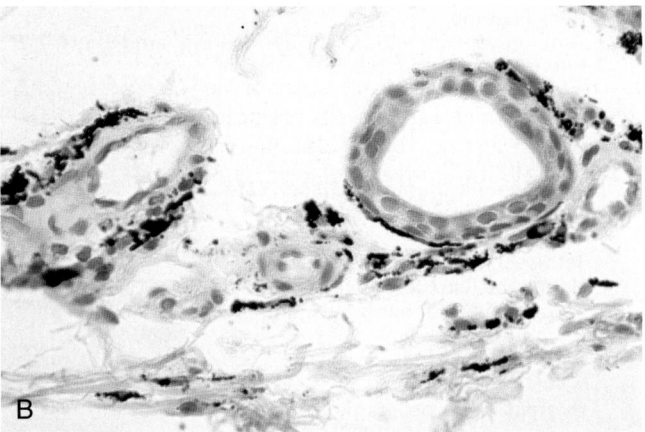

FIGURE 9–13 Adverse drug reaction. Skin pigmentation caused by minocycline, a long-acting tetracycline derivative. **A,** Diffuse blue-gray pigmentation of the forearm; **B,** Deposition of drug metabolite/iron/melanin pigment particles in the dermis. (Courtesy of Dr. Zsolt Argenyi, Department of Pathology, University of Washington, Seattle, WA.)

demiologic study involved approximately 17,000 women who were taking a combination of estrogen (equine estrogen) and progesterone (medroxyprogesterone acetate). Although the study found that HRT caused a reduction in the number of fractures, it also reported that after 5 years of treatment, HRT increased the risk of breast cancer (as discussed in Chapter 23) and thromboembolism, and had no effect on preventing cardiovascular disease. The wide dissemination of these findings led to a drastic decrease in the use of HRT, from 16 million prescriptions in 2001 to 6 million in 2006, which was accompanied by an apparent drop in the incidence of newly diagnosed breast cancers. During the last few years there has been a reappraisal of the risks and benefits of HRT.[28] The new analyses showed that HRT effects depend on the type of estrogen/progesterone used, the mode of drug administration, the age of the person at the start of treatment, the duration of the treatment, and the presence of associated diseases.

- *HRT increases the risk of breast cancer after a median time of 5 to 8 years.* The risk is highest and the latency times shorter for the development of lobular carcinomas and ductal-lobular cancer.[29]
- *HRT has a protective effect on the development of atherosclerosis and coronary disease in women under age 60, but*

there is no protection in women who started HRT at an older age.[30] These data support the notion that there is a critical therapeutic window for HRT effects on the cardiovascular system. Protective effects in younger women depend in part on the response of estrogen receptors that regulate calcium homeostasis in blood vessels.

- *HRT increases the risk of venous thromboembolism,* including deep vein thrombosis, pulmonary embolism, and stroke. The increase is more pronounced during the first 2 years of treatment and in women who have other risk factors such as immobilization, and hypercoagulable states caused by prothrombin or factor V Leiden mutations (Chapter 4).

Oral Contraceptives (OCs)

Worldwide, more than 100 million women use hormonal contraception. OCs nearly always contain a synthetic estradiol and a variable amount of a progestin, but some preparations contain only progestins. They act by inhibiting ovulation or preventing implantation. Currently prescribed OCs contain a much smaller amount of estrogens (as little as 20 µg of ethinyl estradiol) than the earliest formulations approved for use in the United States in 1960, and are associated with fewer side effects. Transdermal and implantable formulations have also become available. Hence, the results of epidemiologic studies should be interpreted in the context of the dosage and the delivery system. Nevertheless, there is good evidence that the use of OCs is associated with the following conditions[31]:

Thromboembolism. Most studies indicate that OC use results in an approximately three-fold increased risk of venous thrombosis and pulmonary thromboembolism. This risk is increased further in carriers of prothrombin and factor V Leiden mutations. The increased thrombotic risk seems to be a consequence of the generation of an acute-phase response, with increases in C-reactive protein and coagulation factors (factors VII, IX, X, XII, and XIII), and reduction in anticoagulants (protein S and anti-thrombin III).

Cardiovascular disease. OCs increase the risk of myocardial infarction in smoking women at all ages and in nonsmoking women over age 35. In women over 35 years of age, the effect is more than ten-fold higher in smokers than nonsmokers.

Cancers. OCs reduce the incidence of endometrial and ovarian cancers. They do not increase the lifetime risk for development of breast cancers, although a small increase in incidence has been detected during the first 5 years of use.

Hepatic adenoma. There is a well-defined association between the use of OCs and this hepatic tumor (Chapter 18), particularly in older women who have used OCs for prolonged periods of time. The tumor appears as a large, solitary, and well-encapsulated mass.

Anabolic Steroids

The use of steroids to increase performance by baseball players, track-and-field athletes, and wrestlers has received wide publicity during the last few years. Anabolic steroids are synthetic versions of testosterone, and for performance enhancement they are used at doses that are about 10 to 100 times higher

TABLE 9–5 Some Common Adverse Drug Reactions and Their Agents	
Reaction	**Major Offenders**
BONE MARROW AND BLOOD CELLS*	
Granulocytopenia, aplastic anemia, pancytopenia	Antineoplastic agents, immunosuppressives, and chloramphenicol
Hemolytic anemia, thrombocytopenia	Penicillin, methyldopa, quinidine, heparin
CUTANEOUS	
Urticaria, macules, papules, vesicles, petechiae, exfoliative dermatitis, fixed drug eruptions, abnormal pigmentation	Antineoplastic agents, sulfonamides, hydantoins, some antibiotics, and many other agents
CARDIAC	
Arrhythmias	Theophylline, hydantoins, digoxin
Cardiomyopathy	Doxorubicin, daunorubicin
RENAL	
Glomerulonephritis	Penicillamine
Acute tubular necrosis	Aminoglycoside antibiotics, cyclosporin, amphotericin B
Tubulointerstitial disease with papillary necrosis	Phenacetin, salicylates
PULMONARY	
Asthma	Salicylates
Acute pneumonitis	Nitrofurantoin
Interstitial fibrosis	Busulfan, nitrofurantoin, bleomycin
HEPATIC	
Fatty change	Tetracycline
Diffuse hepatocellular damage	Halothane, isoniazid, acetominophen
Cholestasis	Chlorpromazine, estrogens, contraceptive agents
SYSTEMIC	
Anaphylaxis	Penicillin
Lupus erythematosus syndrome (drug-induced lupus)	Hydralazine, procainamide
CENTRAL NERVOUS SYSTEM	
Tinnitus and dizziness	Salicylates
Acute dystonic reactions and parkinsonian syndrome	Phenothiazine antipsychotics
Respiratory depression	Sedatives

*Affected in almost half of all drug-related deaths.

than therapeutic indications. The high concentration of testosterone and its derivatives inhibits production and release of luteinizing hormone and follicle-stimulating hormone by a feedback mechanism, and increases the amount of estrogens, which are produced from anabolic steroids. Anabolic steroids have multiple adverse effects including stunted growth in adolescents, acne, gynecomastia and testicular atrophy in males, and growth of facial hair and menstrual changes in women. Other effects include psychiatric problems and premature heart attacks. Hepatic cholestasis may develop in individuals receiving orally administered anabolic steroids.

Acetaminophen

Acetaminophen is the most commonly used analgesic in the United States. It is present in over 300 products, alone or in combination with other agents. Hence, acetaminophen toxicity is common, being responsible for more than 50,000 emergency room visits per year. In the United States, it is the cause of about 50% of cases of acute liver failure, with 30% mortality. Intentional overdosage (suicide attempts) is the most common cause of acetaminophen toxicity in Great Britain, but unintentional overdosage is the most frequent cause in the United States, representing almost 50% of the total intoxication cases.

At therapeutic doses about 95% of acetaminophen undergoes detoxification in the liver by phase II enzymes and is excreted in the urine as glucuronate or sulfate conjugates (Fig. 9–14). About 5% or less is metabolized through the activity of CYPs (primarily CYP2E) to NAPQI (N-acetyl-p-benzoquinoneimine), a highly reactive metabolite.[32,33] NAPQI is normally conjugated with glutathione (GSH), but when taken in larger doses unconjugated *NAPQI accumulates and causes hepatocellular injury leading to centrilobular necrosis and liver failure.* The injury produced by NAPQI involves two mechanisms: (1) covalent binding to hepatic proteins, which causes damage to cellular membranes and mitochondrial dysfunction, and (2) depletion of GSH, making hepatocytes more susceptible to reactive oxygen species–induced injury. It should be noted that because alcohol induces CYP2E in the liver, toxicity can occur at lower doses in chronic alcoholics.

The window between the usual dose (0.5 gm) and the toxic dose (15 to 25 gm) is large, and the drug is ordinarily very safe. Toxicity begins with nausea, vomiting, diarrhea, and sometimes shock, followed in a few days by evidence of jaundice. Overdoses of acetaminophen can be treated at its early stages (within 12 hours) by administration of *N-acetylcysteine, which restores GSH.* In serious overdose liver failure ensues, starting with centrilobular necrosis that may extend to entire lobules,

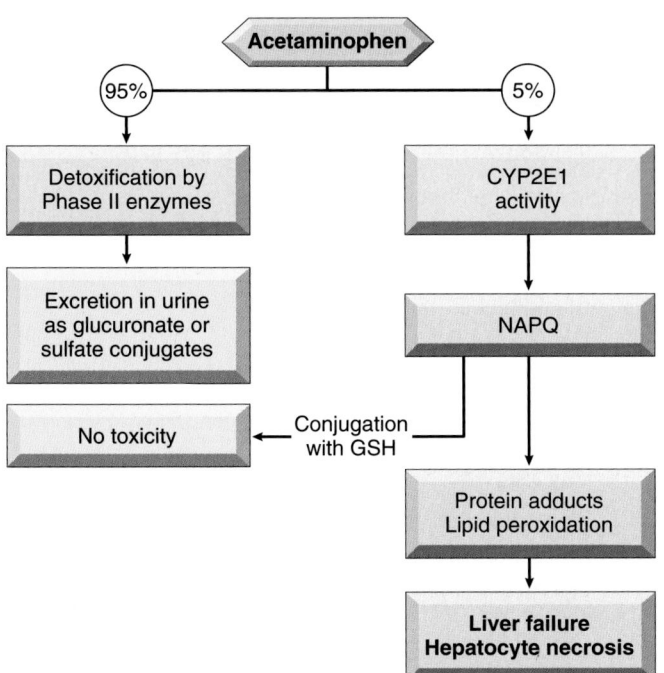

FIGURE 9–14 Acetaminophen metabolism and toxicity. (See text for details.) (Courtesy of Dr. Xavier Vaquero, Department of Pathology, University of Washington, Seattle, WA.)

requiring liver transplantation for survival. Some patients show evidence of concurrent renal damage.

Aspirin (Acetylsalicylic Acid)

Overdose may result from accidental ingestion of a large number of tablets by young children; in adults overdose is frequently suicidal. A source of salicylate poisoning is the excessive use of ointments containing oil of wintergreen (methyl salicylate). Acute salicylate overdose causes alkalosis as a consequence of the stimulation of the respiratory center in the medulla. This is followed by metabolic acidosis and accumulation of pyruvate and lactate, caused by uncoupling of oxidative phosphorylation and inhibition of the Krebs cycle. Metabolic acidosis enhances the formation of nonionized forms of salicylates, which diffuse into the brain and produce effects from nausea to coma. Ingestion of 2 to 4 gm by children or 10 to 30 gm by adults may be fatal, but survival has been reported after ingestion of doses five times larger.

Chronic aspirin toxicity (salicylism) may develop in persons who take 3 gm or more daily for long periods of time for treatment of chronic pain or inflammatory conditions. Chronic salicylism is manifested by headaches, dizziness, ringing in the ears (tinnitus), hearing impairment, mental confusion, drowsiness, nausea, vomiting, and diarrhea. The CNS changes may progress to convulsions and coma. The morphologic consequences of chronic salicylism are varied. Most often there is an acute erosive gastritis (Chapter 17), which may produce overt or covert gastrointestinal bleeding and lead to gastric ulceration. A bleeding tendency may appear concurrently with chronic toxicity, because aspirin acetylates platelet cyclooxygenase and irreversibly blocks the production of thromboxane A$_2$, an activator of platelet aggregation. Pete-

chial hemorrhages may appear in the skin and internal viscera, and bleeding from gastric ulcerations may be exaggerated. With the recognition of gastric ulceration and bleeding as an important complication of ingestion of large doses of aspirin, its chronic toxicity is now quite uncommon.

Proprietary analgesic mixtures of aspirin and phenacetin or its active metabolite, acetaminophen, when taken over several years, can cause tubulointerstitial nephritis with renal papillary necrosis, referred to as *analgesic nephropathy* (Chapter 20).

INJURY BY NONTHERAPEUTIC AGENTS (DRUG ABUSE)

Drug abuse generally involves the use of mind-altering substances, beyond therapeutic or social norms. Drug addiction and overdose are serious public health problems. Common drugs of abuse are listed in Table 9–6. Here we consider cocaine, heroin, amphetamines, and marijuana, and briefly mention a few others.

Cocaine

The use of cocaine and crack continues to increase. According to a 2006 survey, approximately 35.3 million Americans aged 12 or older have tried cocaine, with 6.1 million having used cocaine in the past year. Cocaine is extracted from the leaves of the coca plant, and is usually prepared as a water-soluble powder, cocaine hydrochloride. Sold on the street, it is liberally diluted with talcum powder, lactose, or other look-alikes. Cocaine can be snorted or dissolved in water and injected subcutaneously or intravenously. Crystallization of the pure alkaloid yields nuggets of *crack*, so called because of the cracking or popping sound it makes when heated to produce vapors that are inhaled. The pharmacologic actions of cocaine and crack are identical, but crack is far more potent.

Cocaine produces an intense euphoria and stimulation, making it one of the most addictive drugs. Experimental animals will press a lever more than 1000 times and forgo food and drink to obtain it. In the cocaine user, although physical dependence generally does not occur, the psychologic withdrawal is profound and can be extremely difficult to treat. Intense cravings are particularly severe in the first several months after abstinence and can recur for years. Acute overdose can produce seizures, cardiac arrhythmias, and respiratory arrest.

- *Cardiovascular effects.* The most serious physical effects of cocaine relate to its acute action on the cardiovascular system, where it behaves as a sympathomimetic (Fig. 9–15). It facilitates neurotransmission both in the CNS, where it blocks the reuptake of dopamine, and at adrenergic nerve endings, where it blocks the reuptake of both epinephrine and norepinephrine while stimulating the presynaptic release of norepinephrine. The net effect is the accumulation of these two neurotransmitters in synapses, resulting in excess stimulation, manifested by *tachycardia, hypertension*, and *peripheral vasoconstriction*. Cocaine also induces *myocardial ischemia*, by causing *coronary artery vasoconstriction*, and enhancing platelet aggregation and thrombus formation. Cigarette smoking potentiates cocaine-induced coronary vasospasm. Thus, the dual effect of cocaine, causing increased myocardial oxygen demand by its

TABLE 9–6	Common Drugs of Abuse	
Class	**Molecular Target**	**Example**
Opioid narcotics	Mu opioid receptor (agonist)	Heroin, hydromorphone (Dilaudid) Oxycodone (Percodan, Percocet, Oxycontin) Methadone (Dolophine) Meperidine (Demerol)
Sedative-hypnotics	GABA$_A$ receptor (agonist)	Barbiturates Ethanol Methaqualone (Quaalude) Glutethimide (Doriden) Ethchlorvynol (Placidyl)
Psychomotor stimulants	Dopamine transporter (antagonist) Serotonin receptors (toxicity)	Cocaine Amphetamines 3,4-methylenedioxymethamphetamine (MDMA, ecstasy)
Phencyclidine-like drugs	NMDA glutamate receptor channel (antagonist)	Phencyclidine (PCP, angel dust) Ketamine
Cannabinoids	CBI cannabinoid receptors (agonist)	Marijuana Hashish
Hallucinogens	Serotonin 5-HT$_2$ receptors (agonist)	Lysergic acid diethylamide (LSD) Mescaline Psilocybin

GABA, γ-aminobutyric acid; 5-HT$_2$, 5-hydroxytryptamine; NMDA, N-methyl D-aspartate.
Data from Hyman SE: A 28-year-old man addicted to cocaine. JAMA 286:2586, 2001.

sympathomimetic action, and, at the same time, decreasing coronary blood flow, sets the stage for myocardial ischemia that may lead to myocardial infarction. Cocaine can also precipitate *lethal arrhythmias* by enhanced sympathetic activity as well as by disrupting normal ion (K^+, Ca^{2+}, Na^+) transport in the myocardium. These toxic effects are not necessarily dose-related, and a fatal event may occur in a first-time user with what is a typical mood-altering dose.

- *CNS.* The most common CNS effects are hyperpyrexia (thought to be caused by aberrations of the dopaminergic pathways that control body temperature) and seizures.
- *Effects on pregnancy.* In pregnant women, cocaine may cause decreased blood flow to the placenta, resulting in fetal hypoxia and spontaneous abortion. Neurologic development may be impaired in the fetus of pregnant women who are chronic drug users.
- *Other effects.* Chronic cocaine use may cause (1) perforation of the nasal septum in snorters, (2) decreased lung diffusing capacity in those who inhale the smoke, and (3) the development of dilated cardiomyopathy.

Heroin

Heroin is an addictive opioid derived from the poppy plant that is closely related to morphine. Its use is even more harmful than that of cocaine. As sold on the street, it is cut (diluted) with an agent (often talc or quinine); thus, the size of the dose is not only variable but also usually unknown to the buyer. Heroin, along with any contaminating substances, is usually self-administered intravenously or subcutaneously. Effects are varied and include euphoria, hallucinations, somnolence, and sedation. Heroin has a wide range of adverse physical effects related to (1) the pharmacologic action of the agent, (2) reactions to the cutting agents or contaminants, (3) hypersensitivity reactions to the drug or its adulterants (quinine itself has

neurologic, renal, and auditory toxicity), and (4) diseases contracted incident to the use of infected needles. Some of the most important adverse effects of heroin are the following:

- *Sudden death.* Sudden death, usually related to overdose, is an ever-present risk, because drug purity is generally unknown (it may range from 2% to 90%). The yearly mortality among heroin users in the United States is estimated to be between 1% and 3%. Sudden death can also occur if heroin is taken after tolerance for the drug, built up over time, is lost (as during a period of incarceration). The mechanisms of death include profound respiratory depression, arrhythmia and cardiac arrest, and severe pulmonary edema.
- *Pulmonary injury.* Pulmonary complications include moderate to severe edema, septic embolism from endocarditis lung abscess, opportunistic infections, and foreign-body granulomas from talc and other adulterants. Although granulomas occur principally in the lung, they are sometimes found in the mononuclear phagocyte system, particularly in the spleen, liver, and lymph nodes that drain the upper extremities. Examination under polarized light often highlights trapped talc crystals, sometimes enclosed within foreign-body giant cells.
- *Infections.* Infectious complications are common. The four sites most commonly affected are the skin and subcutaneous tissue, heart valves, liver, and lungs. In a series of addicted patients admitted to the hospital, more than 10% had endocarditis, which often takes a distinctive form involving right-sided heart valves, particularly the tricuspid. Most cases are caused by *S. aureus*, but fungi and a multitude of other organisms have also been implicated. Viral hepatitis is the most common infection among addicted persons and is acquired by the sharing of dirty needles. In the United States, this practice has also led to a

CENTRAL NERVOUS SYSTEM SYNAPSE

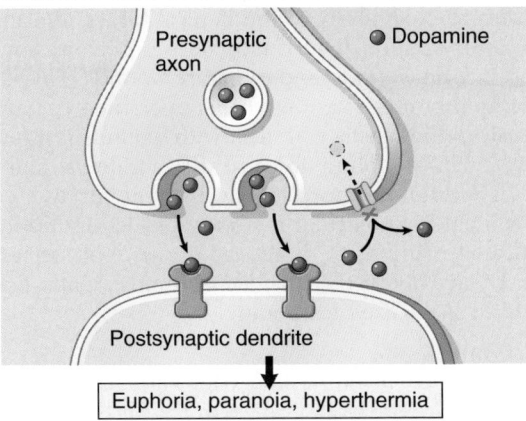

Euphoria, paranoia, hyperthermia

SYMPATHETIC NEURON–TARGET CELL INTERFACE

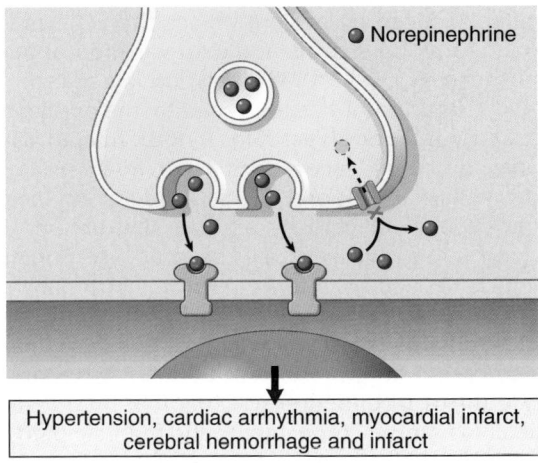

Hypertension, cardiac arrhythmia, myocardial infarct, cerebral hemorrhage and infarct

FIGURE 9–15 The effect of cocaine on neurotransmission. The drug inhibits reuptake of the neurotransmitters dopamine and norepinephrine in the central and peripheral nervous systems.

very high incidence of AIDS in intravenous drug abusers.
- *Skin.* Cutaneous lesions are probably the most frequent telltale sign of heroin addiction. Acute changes include abscesses, cellulitis, and ulcerations due to subcutaneous injections. Scarring at injection sites, hyperpigmentation over commonly used veins, and thrombosed veins are the usual sequelae of repeated intravenous inoculations.
- *Renal problems.* Kidney disease is a relatively common hazard. The two forms most frequently encountered are amyloidosis (generally secondary to skin infections) and focal glomerulosclerosis; both induce heavy proteinuria and the nephrotic syndrome.

Methadone, originally used in the treatment of heroin addiction, is increasingly being prescribed as a painkiller. Unfortunately, its careless use has contributed to more than 800 deaths per year in the United States.

Amphetamines

Methamphetamine. This addictive drug, known as *"speed"* or *"meth,"* is closely related to amphetamine but has stronger effects in the CNS. It is estimated that there are approximately 500,000 current users in the United States. Approximately 2.5% of youths in grade 8 and 6.5% in grade 12 have tried methamphetamine at least once. It acts by releasing dopamine in the brain, which inhibits presynaptic neurotransmission at corticostriatal synapses, slowing glutamate release.[34] Metamphetamine produces a feeling of euphoria, which is followed by a "crash." Long-term use leads to violent behaviors, confusion, and psychotic features that include paranoia and hallucinations.

MDMA. MDMA (3,4 methylenedioxymethamphetamine) is popularly known as *ecstasy*. MDMA is generally taken orally. Its effects, which include euphoria and hallucinogen-like feelings that last for 4 to 6 hours, are mainly due to an increase in serotonin release in the CNS. This is coupled with interference in serotonin synthesis, causing a reduction in serotonin that is only slowly replenished. MDMA use also reduces the number of serotonergic axon terminals in the striatum and the cortex, and it may increase the peripheral effects of dopamine and adrenergic agents. MDMA tablets may be spiked with other drugs, including methamphetamine and cocaine, which greatly enhance the effects on the CNS.

Marijuana

Marijuana, or "pot," is made from the leaves of the *Cannabis sativa* plant, which contain the psychoactive substance Δ^9-tetrahydrocannabinol (THC). About 5% to 10% of THC is absorbed when it is smoked in a hand-rolled cigarette ("joint"). Despite numerous studies, the central question of whether the drug has persistent adverse physical and functional effects remains unresolved.[35] Some of the untoward anecdotal effects may be allergic or idiosyncratic reactions or possibly related to contaminants in the preparations rather than to the pharmacologic effects of marijuana. Among the beneficial effects of marijuana is its potential use to treat nausea secondary to cancer chemotherapy, and as an agent capable of decreasing pain in some chronic conditions that are otherwise difficult to treat. The functional and organic CNS consequences of marijuana smoking have received most scrutiny. Its use distorts sensory perception and impairs motor coordination, but these acute effects generally clear in 4 to 5 hours. With continued use these changes may progress to cognitive and psychomotor impairments, such as inability to judge time, speed, and distance, a frequent cause of automobile accidents. Marijuana increases the heart rate and sometimes blood pressure, and it may cause angina in a person with coronary artery disease.

The respiratory system is also affected by chronic marijuana smoking; laryngitis, pharyngitis, bronchitis, cough and hoarseness, and asthma-like symptoms have all been described, along with mild but significant airway obstruction. Marijuana cigarettes contain a large number of carcinogens that are also present in tobacco. Smoking a marijuana cigarette, compared with a tobacco cigarette, is associated with a three-fold increase in the amount of tar inhaled and retained in the lungs, presumably because of the larger puff volume, deeper inhalation, and longer breath holding.

Regardless of the use of THC as a recreational drug, a large number of studies have characterized the *endogenous cannabinoid system*, which consists of the *cannabinoid receptors CB1 and CB2*, and the endogenous lipid ligands known as *endocannabinoids*.[36] This system participates in the regulation of the hypothalamic-pituitary-adrenal axis, and modulates the control of appetite, food intake, and energy balance, as well as fertility and sexual behavior.[37]

Other Drugs

The variety of drugs that have been tried by those seeking "new experiences" (e.g., "highs," "lows," "out-of-the-body experiences") defies belief. Overall, there has been a decrease in the use of most illegal drugs, but large increases have occurred in prescription and nonprescription drug abuse, and in the inhalation of potentially toxic household products. These drugs include various stimulants, depressants, analgesics, and hallucinogens (see Table 9–6). Among these are PCP (phenylcyclidine, an anesthetic agent), analgesics such as oxycontin and vicodin, and ketamine, an anesthetic agent used in animal surgery. Chronic inhalation of vapors of spray paints, paint thinners, and some glues that contain toluene ("glue sniffing") can cause cognitive abnormalities and magnetic resonance imaging–detectable brain damage that ranges from mild to severe dementia. Because they are used haphazardly and in various combinations, not much is known about the long-time deleterious effects of most of these agents. However, their acute effects are clear: they cause bizarre and often aggressive behavior that leads to violence, or depressed mood and suicidal ideation.

Injury by Physical Agents

Injury induced by physical agents is divided into the following categories: mechanical trauma, thermal injury, electrical injury, and injury produced by ionizing radiation. Each type is considered separately.

MECHANICAL TRAUMA

Mechanical forces may inflict a variety of forms of damage. *The type of injury depends on the shape of the colliding object, the amount of energy discharged at impact, and the tissues or organs that bear the impact.* Bone and head injuries result in

unique damage and are discussed elsewhere (Chapter 28). All soft tissues react similarly to mechanical forces, and the patterns of injury can be divided into abrasions, contusions, lacerations, incised wounds, and puncture wounds. This is just a small sampling of the various forms of trauma encountered by forensic pathologists, who deal with wounds produced by shooting, stabbing, blunt force, traffic accidents, and other causes. In addition to morphologic analyses, forensic pathology now includes molecular methods for identity testing and sophisticated methods to detect the presence of foreign substances. Details about the practice of forensic pathology can be found in specialized textbooks.

Morphology. An **abrasion** is a wound produced by scraping or rubbing, resulting in removal of the superficial layer. Skin abrasions may remove only the epidermal layer. A **contusion,** or bruise, is an injury usually produced by a blunt object characterized by damage to blood vessels and extravasation of blood into tissues (Fig. 9–16A). A **laceration** is a tear or disruptive stretching of tissue caused by the application of force by a blunt object (Fig. 9–16B). In contrast to an incision, most lacerations have intact bridging blood vessels and jagged, irregular edges. An **incised wound** is one inflicted by a sharp instrument. The bridging blood vessels are severed. A **puncture wound** is caused by a long, narrow instrument and is termed **penetrating** when the instrument pierces the tissue and **perforating** when it traverses a tissue to also create an exit wound. Gunshot wounds are special forms of puncture wounds that demonstrate distinctive features important to the forensic pathologist. For example, a wound from a bullet fired at close range leaves powder burns, whereas one fired from more than 4 or 5 feet away does not.

One of the most common causes of mechanical injury is vehicular accident. The typical injuries result from (1) hitting a part of the interior of the vehicle or being hit by an object that enters the passenger compartment during the crash, such as the motor; (2)

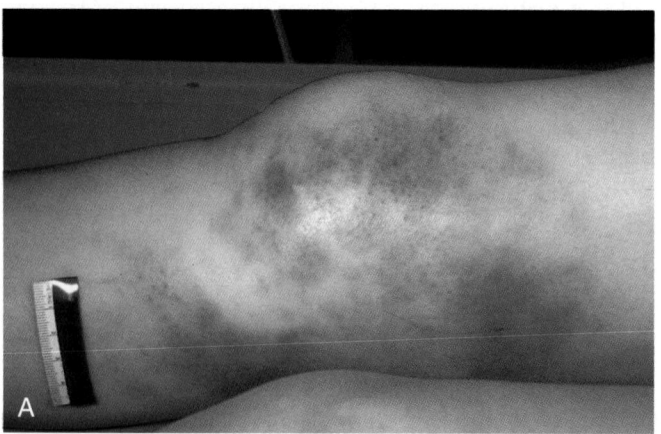

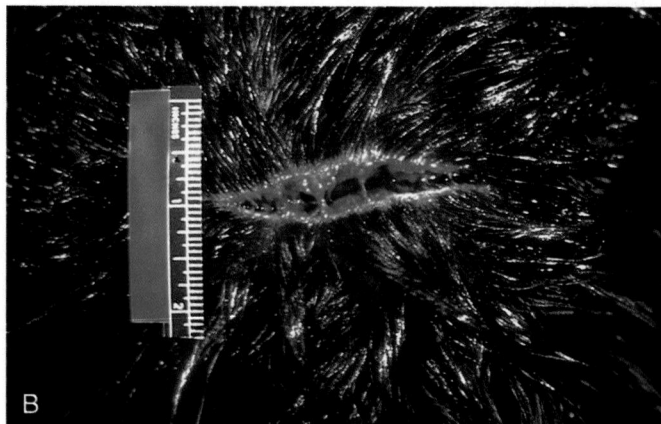

FIGURE 9–16 **A,** Contusion resulting from blunt trauma. The skin is intact, but there is hemorrhage of subcutaneous vessels, producing extensive discoloration. **B,** Laceration of the scalp; the bridging strands of fibrous tissues are evident. (From the Department of Pathology, Southwestern Medical School, Dallas, TX.)

being thrown from the vehicle; or (3) being trapped in a burning vehicle. The pattern of injury relates to whether one or all three of these mechanisms are operative. For example, in a head-on collision, a common pattern of injury sustained by a driver who is not wearing a seat belt includes trauma to the head (windshield impact), chest (steering column impact), and knees (dashboard impact). Under these conditions, common chest injuries include sternal and rib fractures, heart contusions, aortic lacerations, and (less commonly) lacerations of the spleen and liver. Thus, in caring for an automobile injury victim, it is essential to remember that internal wounds often accompany superficial abrasions, contusions, and lacerations. Indeed, in many cases external evidence of serious internal damage is completely absent.

THERMAL INJURY

Both excessive heat and excessive cold are important causes of injury. Burns are the most common cause of thermal injury and are discussed first; a brief discussion of hyperthermia and hypothermia follows.

Thermal Burns

In the United States, approximately 500,000 persons per year receive medical treatment for burn injuries. It is estimated that approximately 4000 persons per year die as a consequence of injuries caused by fire and smoke inhalation, mostly originating in homes. Fortunately, since the 1970s, marked decreases have been seen in both mortality rates and the length of hospitalizations of burn patients. In 2007 there were 40,000 hospitalizations in specialized burn centers, with a 90% survival. Eighty percent of the burns were caused by fire or scalding, the latter being a major cause of injury in children. Improvements in burn treatment have been achieved by a better understanding of the systemic effects of massive burns, the prevention of wound infection, and improvements in treatments that promote the healing of skin surfaces.

The clinical significance of a burn injury depends on the following factors:

- Depth of the burns
- Percentage of body surface involved
- Internal injuries caused by the inhalation of hot and toxic fumes
- Promptness and efficacy of therapy, especially fluid and electrolyte management and prevention or control of wound infections

Burns used to be classified as first to fourth degree, according to the depth of the injury (first-degree burns being the most superficial). This classification has been replaced by the terms *superficial, partial thickness, and full-thickness burns.*

- *Superficial burns* (formerly known as first-degree burns) are confined to the *epidermis.*

- *Partial thickness burns* (formerly known as second-degree burns) involve *injury to the dermis.*
- *Full-thickness burns* (formerly known as third-degree burns) extend to the *subcutaneous tissue.* Full-thickness burns may also involve *damage to muscle tissue* underneath the subcutaneous tissue (these were known formerly as fourth-degree burns).

Shock, sepsis, and respiratory insufficiency are the greatest threats to life in burn patients. Particularly in burns of more than 20% of the body surface, there is a rapid (within hours) shift of body fluids into the interstitial compartments, both at the burn site and systemically, which can result in *hypovolemic shock* (Chapter 4). Because protein from the blood is lost into interstitial tissue, generalized edema, including pulmonary edema, can be severe. An important pathophysiologic effect of burns is the development of a *hypermetabolic state* associated with excess heat loss and an increased need for nutritional support. It is estimated that when more than 40% of the body surface is burned, the resting metabolic rate may double.

The burn site is ideal for the growth of microorganisms; the serum and debris provide nutrients, and the burn injury compromises blood flow, blocking effective inflammatory responses. The most common offender is the opportunist *Pseudomonas aeruginosa,* but antibiotic-resistant strains of other common hospital-acquired bacteria, such as *S. aureus,* and fungi, particularly *Candida* species, may also be involved. Furthermore, cellular and humoral defenses against infections are compromised, and both lymphocyte and phagocyte functions are impaired. Direct bacteremic spread and release of toxic substances such as endotoxin from the local site have dire consequences. Pneumonia or septic shock with renal failure and/or the acute respiratory distress syndrome (Chapter 15) are the most common serious sequelae.

Organ system failure resulting from burn sepsis has greatly diminished during the last 30 years, because of the introduction of techniques for early excision and grafting of the burn wound. Removal of the burn wound decreases infection and reduces the need for reconstructive surgery.[38] Grafting is done with split-thickness skin grafts; dermal substitutes, which serve as a bed for cell repopulation, may be used in large full-thickness burns.

Injury to the airways and lungs may develop within 24 to 48 hours after the burn and may result from the direct effect of heat on the mouth, nose, and upper airways or from the inhalation of heated air and noxious gases in the smoke. Water-soluble gases, such as chlorine, sulfur oxides, and ammonia, may react with water to form acids or alkalis, particularly in the upper airways, producing inflammation and swelling, which may lead to partial or complete airway obstruction. Lipid-soluble gases, such as nitrous oxide and products of burning plastics, are more likely to reach deeper airways, producing pneumonitis.

In burn survivors the development of hypertrophic scars, both at the site of the original burn and at donor graft sites, and itching may become long-term, difficult-to-treat problems. Hypertrophic scars after burn injury may be a consequence of continuous angiogenesis in the wound caused by excess neuropeptides, such as substance P, released from injured nerve endings.[39]

Morphology. Grossly, full-thickness burns are white or charred, dry, and anesthetic (because of destruction of nerve endings), whereas, depending on the depth, partial-thickness burns are pink or mottled with blisters and are painful. Histologically, devitalized tissue reveals coagulative necrosis, adjacent to vital tissue that quickly accumulates inflammatory cells and marked exudation.

Hyperthermia

Prolonged exposure to elevated ambient temperatures can result in heat cramps, heat exhaustion, and heat stroke.

- *Heat cramps* result from loss of electrolytes via sweating. Cramping of voluntary muscles, usually in association with vigorous exercise, is the hallmark. Heat-dissipating mechanisms are able to maintain normal core body temperature.
- *Heat exhaustion* is probably the most common hyperthermic syndrome. Its onset is sudden, with prostration and collapse, and it results from a failure of the cardiovascular system to compensate for hypovolemia, secondary to water depletion. After a period of collapse, which is usually brief, equilibrium is spontaneously re-established.
- *Heat stroke* is associated with high ambient temperatures, high humidity, and exertion. Thermoregulatory mechanisms fail, sweating ceases, and the core body temperature rises to more than 40°C, leading to multi-organ dysfunction that can be rapidly fatal. The underlying mechanism is marked generalized vasodilation, with peripheral pooling of blood and a decreased effective circulating blood volume. Hyperkalemia, tachycardia, arrhythmias, and other systemic effects are common. *Necrosis of the muscles (rhabdomyolysis) and myocardium may occur as a consequence of the nitrosylation of the ryanodine receptor type 1 (RYR1) in skeletal muscle.*[40] RYR1 is located in the sarcoplasmic reticulum and regulates the release of calcium into the cytoplasm. Inherited mutations in *RYR1* occur in the condition called *malignant hyperthermia*, characterized by a rise in core body temperature and muscle contractures in response to exposure to common anesthetics. *RYR1* mutations may also increase the susceptibility to heat stroke. Elderly persons, individuals undergoing intense physical stress (including young athletes and military recruits), and persons with cardiovascular disease are potential candidates for heat stroke.

Hypothermia

Prolonged exposure to low ambient temperature leads to hypothermia, a condition seen all too frequently in homeless persons. High humidity, wet clothing, and dilation of superficial blood vessels resulting from the ingestion of alcohol hasten the lowering of body temperature. At a body temperature of about 90°F, loss of consciousness occurs, followed by bradycardia and atrial fibrillation at lower core temperatures.

Hypothermia causes injury by two mechanisms:

- *Direct effects* are probably mediated by physical disruptions within cells by high salt concentrations caused by the crystallization of intra- and extracellular water.
- *Indirect effects* resulting from circulatory changes, which vary depending on the rate and duration of the temperature drop. Slowly developing chilling may induce vasoconstriction and increased vascular permeability, leading to edema and hypoxia. Such changes are typical of "trench foot." This condition developed in soldiers who spent long periods of time in water-logged trenches during the First World War (1914–1918), frequently causing gangrene that necessitated amputation (the only protection was to cover the feet with whale-oil grease as insulation). With sudden, persistent chilling, the vasoconstriction and increased viscosity of the blood in the local area may cause ischemic injury and degenerative changes in peripheral nerves. In this situation, the vascular injury and increased permeability with exudation become evident only after the temperature begins to return to normal. However, during the period of ischemia, hypoxic changes and infarction of the affected tissues may develop (e.g., gangrene of toes or feet).

ELECTRICAL INJURY

Electrical injuries, which are often fatal, can arise from contact with low-voltage currents (i.e., in the home and workplace) or high-voltage currents carried by high-power lines or lightning. Injuries are of two types: (1) burns and (2) ventricular fibrillation or cardiac and respiratory center failure, resulting from disruption of normal electrical impulses. The type of injury and the severity and extent of burns depend on the strength (amperage), duration, and path of the electric current within the body.

Voltage in the household and workplace (120 or 220 V) is high enough that with low resistance at the site of contact (as when the skin is wet), sufficient current can pass through the body to cause serious injury, including *ventricular fibrillation*. If current flow continues long enough, it generates enough heat to produce burns at the site of entry and exit as well as in internal organs. An important characteristic of alternating current, the type available in most homes, is that it induces tetanic muscle spasm, so that when a live wire or switch is grasped, irreversible clutching is likely to occur, prolonging the period of current flow. This results in a greater likelihood of developing extensive electrical burns and, in some cases, spasm of the chest wall muscles, producing death from asphyxia. Currents generated from high-voltage sources cause similar damage; however, because of the large current flows generated, these are more likely to produce paralysis of medullary centers and extensive burns. Lightning is a classic cause of high-voltage electrical injury.

Earlier studies had linked exposure to high-voltage magnetic fields to an increased risk of cancer, mainly leukemias, among workers on electric high-power lines and children living near power transmission lines. However, further analyses have failed to find a consistent association between these exposures and cancer development. Electric and magnetic fields and microwave radiation, when sufficiently intense, may produce burns, usually of the skin and subjacent connective tissue, and both forms of radiation can interfere with cardiac pacemakers.

INJURY PRODUCED BY IONIZING RADIATION

Radiation is energy that travels in the form of waves or high-speed particles. Radiation has a wide range of energies that span the electromagnetic spectrum; it can be divided into non-ionizing and ionizing radiation. The energy of non-ionizing radiation such as UV and infrared light, microwave, and sound waves, can move atoms in a molecule or cause them to vibrate, but is not sufficient to displace bound electrons from atoms. By contrast, *ionizing radiation has sufficient energy to remove tightly bound electrons.* Collision of electrons with other molecules releases electrons in a reaction cascade, referred to as ionization. The main sources of ionizing radiation are *x-rays and gamma rays* (electromagnetic waves of very high frequencies), *high-energy neutrons, alpha particles* (composed of two protons and two neutrons), and *beta particles,* which are essentially electrons. At equivalent amounts of energy, alpha particles induce heavy damage in a restricted area, whereas x-rays and gamma rays dissipate energy over a longer, deeper course, and produce considerably less damage per unit of tissue. About 25% of the total dose of ionizing radiation received by the US population is human-made, mostly originated in medical devices and radioisotopes.

Ionizing radiation is a double-edged sword. It is indispensable in medical practice, being used in the treatment of cancer, in diagnostic imaging, and in therapeutic or diagnostic radioisotopes, but it also produces adverse short- and long-term effects such as *fibrosis, mutagenesis, carcinogenesis, and teratogenesis.*[41]

Radiation Units. Several somewhat confusing terms are used to describe the radiation doses. This is because radiation is measured in three different ways. These are, the amount of radiation emitted by a source, the radiation dose absorbed by a person, and the biologic effect of the radiation. These are described below:

- *Curie* (Ci) represents the disintegrations per second of a radionuclide (radioisotope). One Ci is equal to 3.7×10^{10} disintegrations per second. This is an expression of the amount of radiation emitted by a source.
- *Gray* (Gy) is a unit that expresses the energy absorbed by the target tissue per unit mass. It corresponds to the absorption of 10^4 erg/gm of tissue. The centigray (cGy), which is the absorption of 100 erg/gm of tissue, is equivalent to the exposure of tissue to 100 Rads (radiation absorbed dose), abbreviated as R. The cGy terminology has now replaced R.
- *Sievert* (Sv) is a unit of equivalent dose that depends on the biologic rather than the physical effects of radiation (it replaced a unit called "rem"). For the same absorbed dose, various types of radiation differ in the extent of damage they produce. The equivalent dose controls for this variation and thereby provides a uniform measure of biologic dose. *The equivalent dose (expressed in Sieverts) corresponds to the absorbed dose (expressed in Grays) multiplied by the relative biologic effectiveness of the radiation.* The relative biologic effectiveness depends on the type of radiation, the type and volume of the exposed tissue, the duration of the exposure, and some other biologic

factors (discussed below). The effective dose of x-rays in radiographs and computed tomography is commonly expressed in millisieverts (mSv). For x-radiation, 1 mSv = 1 mGy.

Main Determinants of the Biologic Effects of Ionizing Radiation. In addition to the physical properties of the radiation, its biologic effects depend heavily on the following factors.

- *Rate of delivery.* The rate of delivery significantly modifies the biologic effect. Although the effect of radiant energy is cumulative, divided doses may allow cells to repair some of the damage between exposures. Thus, fractionated doses of radiant energy have a cumulative effect only to the extent that repair during the "recovery" intervals is incomplete. Radiation therapy of tumors exploits the general capability of normal cells to repair themselves and recover more rapidly than tumor cells, and thus not sustain as much cumulative radiation damage.
- *Field size.* The size of the field exposed to radiation has a great influence on its consequences. The body can sustain relatively high doses of radiation when delivered to small, carefully shielded fields, whereas smaller doses delivered to larger fields may be lethal.
- *Cell proliferation.* Because ionizing radiation damages DNA, rapidly dividing cells are more vulnerable to injury than are quiescent cells (Fig. 9–17). Except at extremely high doses that impair DNA transcription, DNA damage is compatible with survival in nondividing cells, such as brain and myocardium. However, in dividing cells, certain types of mutations and chromosomal abnormalities are recognized by

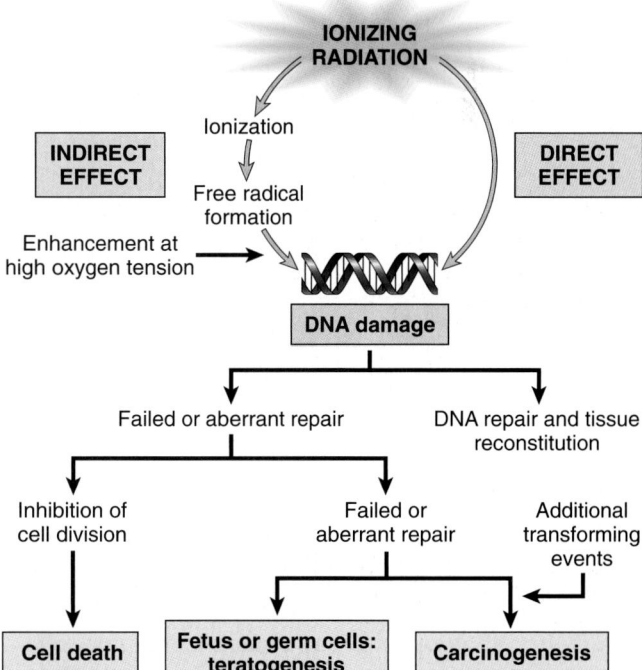

FIGURE 9–17 Effects of ionizing radiation on DNA and its consequences. The effects on DNA can be direct, or most importantly, indirect, through free radical formation.

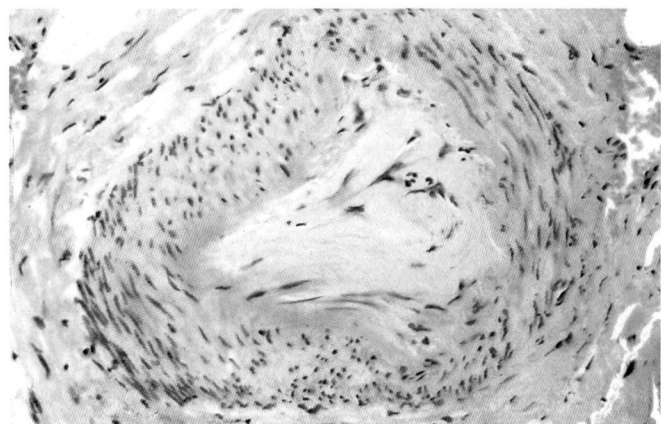

FIGURE 9–18 Chronic vascular injury with subintimal fibrosis occluding the lumen. (American Registry of Pathology © 1990.)

or more than one nucleus may appear and persist for years after exposure. At extremely high doses of radiant energy, markers of cell death, such as nuclear pyknosis, and lysis appear quickly.

In addition to affecting DNA and nuclei, radiant energy may induce a variety of **cytoplasmic changes**, including cytoplasmic swelling, mitochondrial distortion, and degeneration of the endoplasmic reticulum. Plasma membrane breaks and focal defects may be

cell cycle checkpoints, which initiate events that lead to growth arrest and apoptosis. Understandably, therefore, *tissues with a high rate of cell division, such as gonads, bone marrow, lymphoid tissue, and the mucosa of the gastrointestinal tract, are extremely vulnerable to radiation*, and the injury is manifested early after exposure.

● *Oxygen effects and hypoxia.* The production of reactive oxygen species from the radiolysis of water is the most important mechanism of DNA damage by ionizing radiation. Poorly vascularized tissues with low oxygenation, such as the center of rapidly growing tumors, are generally less sensitive to radiation therapy than nonhypoxic tissues.

● *Vascular damage.* Damage to endothelial cells, which are moderately sensitive to radiation, may cause narrowing or occlusion of the blood vessel leading to impaired healing, fibrosis, and chronic ischemic atrophy. These changes may appear months or years after exposure (Fig. 9–18). Late effects in tissues with a low rate of cell proliferation such as brain, kidney, liver, muscle, and subcutaneous tissue, may include diverse lesions such as cell death, atrophy, and fibrosis. These effects are associated with vascular damage and the release of pro-inflammatory cytokines in irradiated areas.

Figure 9–19 shows the overall consequences of radiation exposure. These consequences may vary according to the dose of radiation and the type of exposure. Table 9–7 lists the estimated threshold doses for acute effects of radiation aimed at specific organs; Table 9–8 shows the syndromes caused by exposure to various doses of total-body radiation.

Morphology. Cells surviving radiant energy damage show a wide range of structural changes in chromosomes, including deletions, breaks, translocations, and fragmentation. The mitotic spindle often becomes disorderly, and polyploidy and aneuploidy may be encountered. Nuclear swelling and condensation and clumping of chromatin may appear; sometimes the nuclear membrane breaks down. Apoptosis may occur. All forms of abnormal nuclear morphology may be seen. Giant cells with pleomorphic nuclei

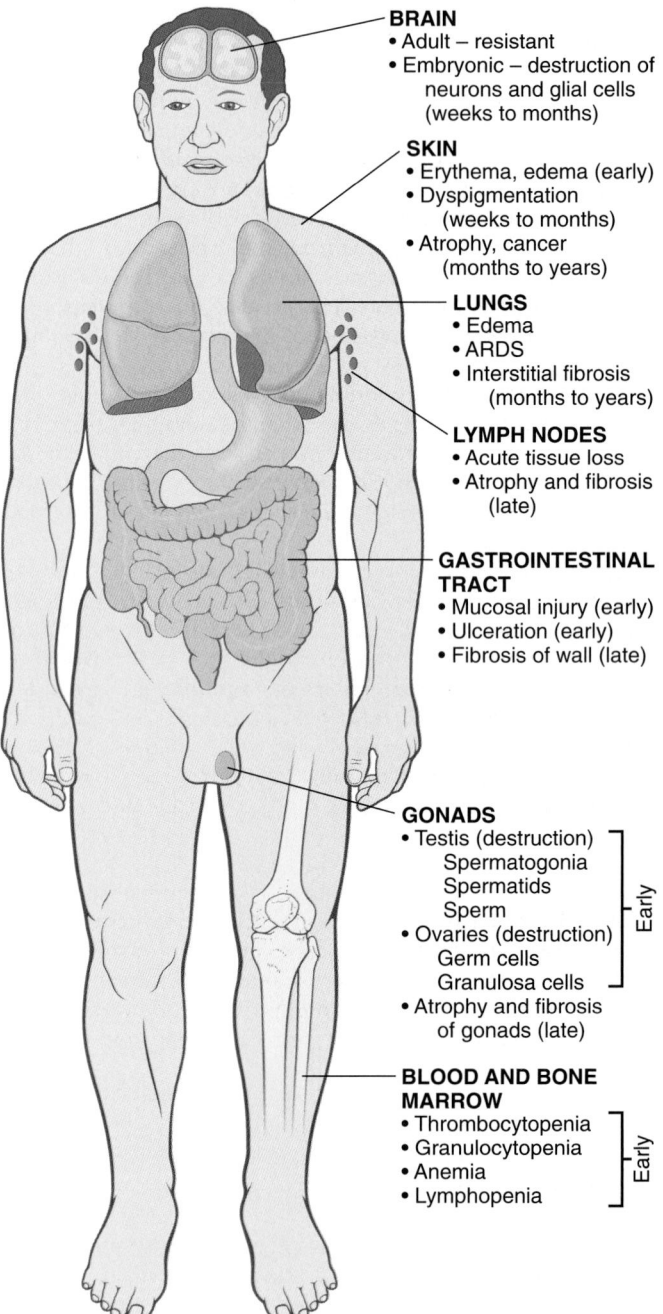

FIGURE 9–19 Overview of the major morphologic consequences of radiation injury. Early changes occur in hours to weeks; late changes occur in months to years. ARDS, acute respiratory distress syndrome.

TABLE 9–7 Estimated Threshold Doses for Acute Radiation Effects on Specific Organs

Health Effect	Organ	Dose (Sv)
Temporary sterility	Testes	0.15
Depression of hematopoiesis	Bone marrow	0.50
Reversible skin effects (e.g., erythema)	Skin	1.0–2.0
Permanent sterility	Ovaries	2.5–6.0
Temporary hair loss	Skin	3.0–5.0
Permanent sterility	Testis	3.5
Cataract	Lens of eye	5.0

seen. The histologic constellation of cellular pleomorphism, giant-cell formation, conformational changes in nuclei, and abnormal mitotic figures creates a more than passing similarity between radiation-injured cells and cancer cells, a problem that plagues the pathologist when evaluating post-irradiation tissues for the possible persistence of tumor cells.

At the light microscopic level, vascular changes and interstitial fibrosis are prominent in irradiated tissues (Fig. 9–20). During the immediate post-irradiation period, vessels may show only dilation. With time, or with higher doses, a variety of degenerative changes appear, including endothelial cell swelling and vacuolation, or even dissolution with total necrosis of the walls of small vessels such as capillaries and venules. Affected vessels may rupture or thrombose. Still later, endothelial cell proliferation and collagenous hyalinization with thickening of the media are seen in irradiated vessels, resulting in marked narrowing or even obliteration of the vascular lumens. At this time, an increase in interstitial collagen in the irradiated field usually becomes evident, leading to scarring and contractions.

Total-Body Irradiation. Exposure of large areas of the body to even very small doses of radiation may have devastating effects. Dosages below 1 Sv produce minimal or no symptoms. However, higher levels of exposure cause health effects known as acute radiation syndromes, which at progressively

higher doses involve the hematopoietic, gastrointestinal, and central nervous systems. The syndromes associated with total-body exposure to ionizing radiation are presented in Table 9–8.

Acute Effects on Hematopoietic and Lymphoid Systems. *The hematopoietic and lymphoid systems are extremely susceptible to radiation injury and deserve special mention.* With high dose levels and large exposure fields, severe lymphopenia may appear within hours of irradiation, along with shrinkage of the lymph nodes and spleen. Radiation directly destroys lymphocytes, both in the circulating blood and in tissues (nodes, spleen, thymus, gut). With sublethal doses of radiation, regeneration from viable precursors is prompt, leading to restoration of a normal lymphocyte count in the blood within weeks to months. *Hematopoietic precursors in the bone marrow* are also quite sensitive to radiant energy, which produces a dose-dependent marrow aplasia. Very high doses of radiation kill marrow stem cells and induce permanent aplasia (aplastic anemia), whereas with lower doses the aplasia is transient. The circulating *granulocyte count* may first rise but begins to fall toward the end of the first week. Levels near zero may be reached during the second week. If the patient survives, recovery of the normal granulocyte count may require 2 to 3 months. *Platelets* are similarly affected, with the nadir of the count occurring somewhat later than that of granulocytes; recovery is similarly delayed. Red cell counts fall and anemia appears after 2 to 3 weeks and may persist for months.

Fibrosis. A common consequence of radiation therapy for cancer is the development of fibrosis in the tissues included in the irradiated field (see Fig. 9–20). Fibrosis may occur weeks or months after irradiation as a consequence of the replacement of dead parenchymal cells by connective tissue, leading to the formation of scars and adhesions (see Chapter 3). Vascular damage, the killing of tissue stem cells, and the release of cytokines and chemokines that promote an inflammatory reaction and fibroblast activation are the main contributors to the development of radiation-induced fibrosis (Figs. 9–21 and 9–22). Common sites of fibrosis after radiation treatment are the lungs, the salivary glands after radiation therapy for head and neck cancers, and colorectal and pelvic areas after treatment for prostate cancer.

DNA Damage and Carcinogenesis. Ionizing radiation can cause multiple types of damage in DNA, including single-base damage, single- and double-stranded breaks, and DNA-protein cross-links. In surviving cells, simple defects may be repaired by various enzyme systems present in most mammalian cells (see Chapter 7). However, *the most serious damage*

TABLE 9–8 Effects of Total-Body Ionizing Radiation

	0–1 Sv	1–2 Sv	2–10 Sv	10–20 Sv	>50 Sv
Main site of injury	None	Lymphocytes	Bone marrow	Small bowel	Brain
Main signs and symptoms	None	Moderate granulocytopenia Lymphopenia	Leukopenia, hemorrhage, hair loss, vomiting	Diarrhea, fever, electrolyte imbalance, vomiting	Ataxia, coma, convulsions, vomiting
Time of development	–	1 day to 1 week	2–6 weeks	5–14 days	1–4 hours
Lethality	None	None	Variable (0% to 80%)	100%	100%

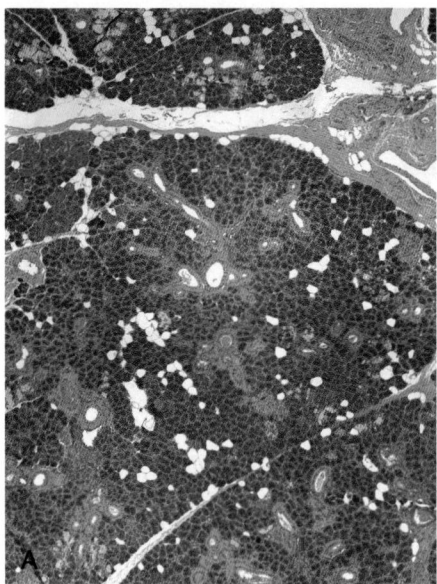
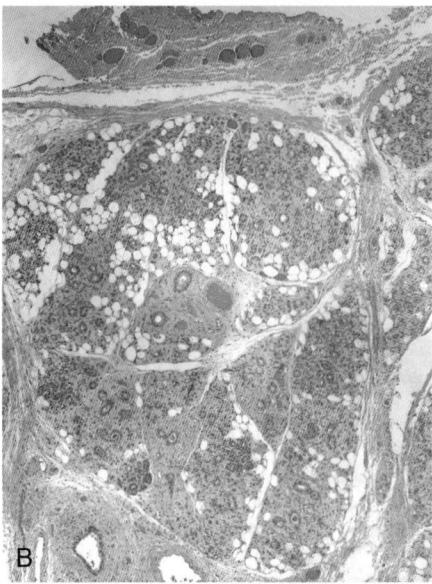
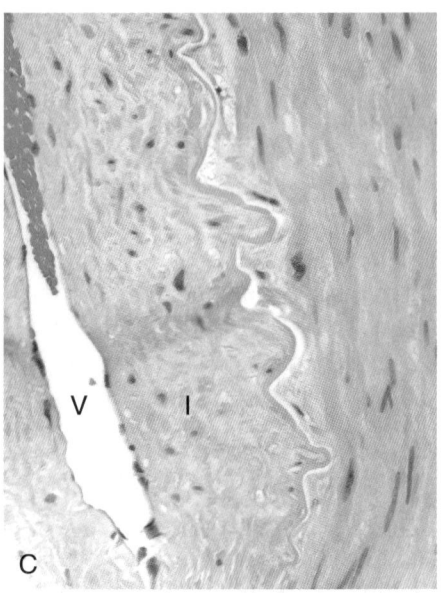

FIGURE 9–20 Fibrosis and vascular changes in salivary glands produced by radiation therapy of the neck region. **A,** Normal salivary gland; **B,** fibrosis caused by radiation; **C,** fibrosis and vascular changes consisting of fibrointimal thickening and arteriolar sclerosis. V, vessel lumen; I, thickened intima. (Courtesy of Dr. Melissa Upton, Department of Pathology, University of Washington, Seattle, WA.)

to DNA is caused by double-stranded breaks (DSBs). Two types of mechanisms can repair DSBs in mammalian cells: *homologous recombination and nonhomologous end joining (NHEJ)*, with NHEJ being the most common repair pathway. DNA repair through NHEJ often produces mutations, including short deletions or duplications, or gross chromosomal aberrations such as translocations and inversions. If the replication of cells containing DSBs is not stopped by cell cycle checkpoint controls (Chapter 3), cells with chromosomal damage persist and may initiate carcinogenesis many years later. More recently it has been recognized that these abnormal cells may also have a "bystander effect," that is, they may promote growth of non-irradiated surrounding cells through the production of growth factors and cytokines.[42,43] Bystander effects are referred to as non-target effects of radiation.

Cancer Risks from Exposures to Low-level Radiation. Any cell capable of division that has sustained a mutation has the potential to become cancerous. Thus, an increased incidence of neoplasms may occur in any organ after exposure to ionizing radiation. The level of radiation required to increase the risk of cancer development is difficult to determine, but there is little doubt that acute or prolonged exposures that result in doses of greater than 100 mSv cause serious consequences including cancer.[44] This is documented by the increased incidence of leukemias and tumors at various sites (such as thyroid, breast, and lungs) in survivors of the atomic bombings of Hiroshima and Nagasaki; the high number of thyroid cancers in survivors of the Chernobyl accident; the high incidence of thyroid tumors, and the elevated frequency of leukemias and birth defects in inhabitants of the Marshall Islands

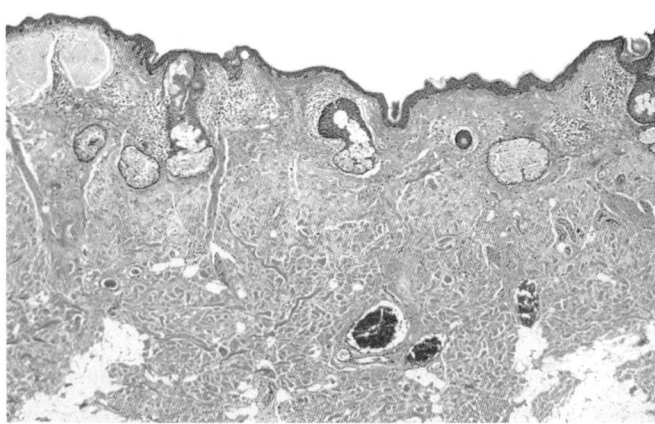

FIGURE 9–21 Chronic radiation dermatitis with atrophy of epidermis, dermal fibrosis, and telangiectasia of the subcutaneous blood vessels. (American Registry of Pathology © 1990.)

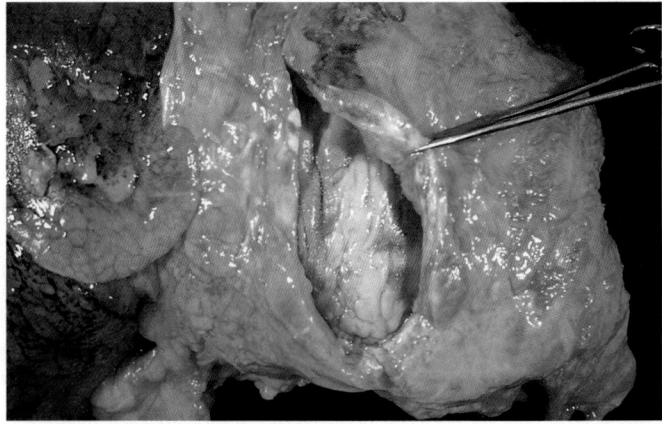

FIGURE 9–22 Extensive mediastinal fibrosis after radiotherapy for carcinoma of the lung. Note the markedly thickened cardium. (From the teaching collection of the Department Pathology, Southwestern Medical School, Dallas, TX.)

exposed to nuclear fallout; and the development of "second cancers," such as acute myeloid leukemia, myelodysplastic syndrome, Hodgkin lymphoma and solid tumors, in individuals who received radiation therapy for childhood cancers. The long-term cancer risks caused by radiation exposures in the range of 5 to 100 mSv are much more difficult to establish, because accurate measurements of risks require large population groups ranging from 50,000 to 5 million people.

Estimation of cancer risks at low levels of exposure to ionizing radiation relies in part on models that extrapolate from higher doses. Nevertheless, for x-rays and gamma rays there is good evidence for a statistically significant increase in the risk of cancer at acute doses of greater than 50 mSv and "reasonable" evidence for acute doses of greater than 5 mSv. For protracted exposures, the approximate values suggested are greater than 100 mSv (good evidence for a statistically significant increase of risk) and 50 mSv (reasonable evidence for increased risk). As a comparison, a single posterior-anterior chest radiograph, a lateral chest film chest radiograph, and a computed tomography of the chest deliver effective dosages to the lungs of 0.01, 0.15, and 10 mSv, respectively.[45]

Increased risk of cancer development may also be associated with occupational exposures. Radon gas is a ubiquitous product of the spontaneous decay of uranium. Its carcinogenic effects are largely attributable to two decay products, *polonium 214 and 218* (or "radon daughters"), which emit alpha particles. Polonium 214 and 218 produced from inhaled radon tend to deposit in the lung, and chronic exposure in uranium miners may give rise to lung carcinomas. Risks are also present in homes in which the levels of radon are very high, comparable to those found in mines. However, there is little or no evidence to suggest that radon contributes to the risk of lung cancer in the average household. Among other polonium isotopes, *polonium 210* came to the public attention in November 2006 with the highly publicized use of this isotope to kill an individual in England. For historical reasons, we also mention here the development of osteogenic sarcomas after radium exposure in radium dial painters, chemists, radiologists, and patients exposed to radium as a treatment for various ailments, during the first part of the twentieth century.

Nutritional Diseases

Malnutrition, also referred to as *protein energy malnutrition or PEM,* is a consequence of inadequate intake of proteins and calories, or deficiencies in the digestion or absorption of proteins, resulting in the loss of fat and muscle tissue, weight loss, lethargy, and generalized weakness. Millions of people in developing nations are malnourished and starving, or living on the cruel edge of starvation. In the industrial world and, more recently, also in developing countries, *obesity* has become a major public health problem, associated with the development of diseases such as diabetes and atherosclerosis.

The sections that follow barely skim the surface of nutritional disorders. Particular attention is devoted to PEM, anorexia nervosa and bulimia, deficiencies of vitamins and trace minerals, obesity, and a brief overview of the relationships of diet to atherosclerosis and cancer. Other nutrients and nutritional issues are discussed in the context of specific diseases.

DIETARY INSUFFICIENCY

An appropriate diet should provide (1) sufficient energy, in the form of carbohydrates, fats, and proteins, for the body's daily metabolic needs; (2) amino acids and fatty acids to be used as building blocks for synthesis of structural and functional proteins and lipids; and (3) vitamins and minerals, which function as coenzymes or hormones in vital metabolic pathways or, as in the case of calcium and phosphate, as important structural components. In *primary malnutrition,* one or all of these components are missing from the diet. By contrast, in *secondary malnutrition,* the supply of nutrients is adequate, but malnutrition results from insufficient intake, malabsorption, impaired utilization or storage, excess loss, or increased need for nutrients.

There are several conditions that may lead to dietary insufficiencies.

- *Poverty.* Homeless persons, aged individuals, and children of the poor often suffer from PEM as well as trace nutrient deficiencies. In poor countries, poverty, crop failures, livestock deaths, and drought, often in times of war and political upheaval, create the setting for the malnourishment of children and adults.

- *Infections.* PEM increases the susceptibility to many common infectious diseases. Conversely, infections have a negative effect on nutrition,[46] thus establishing a vicious cycle.

- *Acute and chronic illnesses.* The basal metabolic rate becomes accelerated in many illnesses resulting in increased daily requirements for all nutrients. Failure to recognize these nutritional needs may delay recovery. *PEM is often present in patients with wasting diseases such as advanced cancers and AIDS* (discussed later).

- *Chronic alcoholism.* Alcoholic persons may sometimes suffer PEM but more frequently have deficiency of several vitamins, especially thiamine, pyridoxine, folate, and vitamin A, as a result of dietary deficiency, defective gastrointestinal absorption, abnormal nutrient utilization and storage, increased metabolic needs, and an increased rate of loss. A failure to recognize the likelihood of thiamine deficiency in persons with chronic alcoholism may result in irreversible brain damage (e.g., Wernicke encephalopathy, discussed in Chapter 28).

- *Ignorance and failure of diet supplementation.* Even the affluent may fail to recognize that infants, adolescents, and pregnant women have increased nutritional needs. Ignorance about the nutritional content of various foods is also a contributing factor. Some examples are: iron deficiency in infants fed exclusively artificial milk diets; polished rice used as the mainstay of a diet may lack adequate amounts of thiamine; lack of iodine from food and water in regions removed from the oceans, unless supplementation is provided.

- *Self-imposed dietary restriction.* Anorexia nervosa, bulimia, and less overt eating disorders affect many individuals who are concerned about body image and are obsessed with body weight (anorexia and bulimia are discussed later).

- *Other causes.* Additional causes of malnutrition include gastrointestinal diseases and malabsorption syndromes, genetic diseases, specific drug therapies (which block uptake or utilization of particular nutrients), and total parenteral nutrition.

PROTEIN-ENERGY MALNUTRITION (PEM)

Severe PEM is a serious, often lethal disease affecting children. It is common in low-income countries, where up to 25% of children may be affected, and where it is a major factor in the high death rates among children younger than 5 years. In the West Africa country of Niger, which suffered a severe famine in 2005, United Nations reports estimate that there were, respectively, 150,000 and 650,000 children with severe and moderate malnutrition. In that country, malnutrition was a direct or indirect cause of mortality in 60% of children under age 5. Decreased food intake can also occur due to sharp increases in prices, as was seen in the first half of 2008. In developed countries, PEM occurs in elderly and debilitated patients in nursing homes and hospitals.

Malnutrition is determined according to the body mass index (BMI, weight in kilograms divided by height in meters squared). *A BMI less than 16 kg/m² is considered malnutrition* (normal range 18.5 to 25 kg/m²). In more practical ways, a child whose weight falls to less than 80% of normal (provided in standard tables) is considered malnourished. However, loss of weight may be masked by generalized edema, as discussed later. Other helpful parameters are the evaluation of fat stores (thickness of skin folds), muscle mass (reduced circumference of mid-arm), and serum proteins (albumin and transferrin measurements provide a measure of the adequacy of the visceral protein compartment).

Marasmus and Kwashiorkor. In malnourished children, PEM presents as a range of clinical syndromes, all characterized by a dietary intake of protein and calories inadequate to meet the body's needs. The two ends of the spectrum of PEM syndromes are known as *marasmus* and *kwashiorkor.* From a functional standpoint, there are two differentially regulated protein compartments in the body: the somatic compartment, represented by proteins in skeletal muscles, and the visceral compartment, represented by protein stores in the visceral organs, primarily the liver. As we shall see, the somatic compartment is affected more severely in marasmus, and the visceral compartment is depleted more severely in kwashiorkor.

A child is considered to have *marasmus* when weight falls to 60% of normal for sex, height, and age. A *marasmic child suffers growth retardation and loss of muscle,* the latter resulting from catabolism and depletion of the somatic protein compartment. This seems to be an adaptive response that provides the body with amino acids as a source of energy. The visceral protein compartment, which is presumably more precious and critical for survival, is only marginally depleted, and hence *serum albumin levels are either normal or only slightly reduced.* In addition to muscle proteins, subcutaneous fat is also mobilized and used as fuel. The production of leptin (discussed in "Obesity") is low, which may stimulate the hypothalamic-pituitary-adrenal axis to produce high levels of cortisol that contribute to lipolysis. With such losses of muscle and subcutaneous fat, the *extremities are emaciated;* by comparison, the head appears too large for the body (Fig. 9–23A). Anemia and manifestations of multiple vitamin deficiencies are present, and there is evidence of *immune deficiency,* particularly T

cell–mediated immunity. Hence, concurrent infections are usually present, which impose additional nutritional demands. Unfortunately, images of children dead or near death with marasmus, have become almost commonplace in television and newspaper reports of famine and disasters in various areas of the world.

Kwashiorkor occurs when protein deprivation is relatively greater than the reduction in total calories (Fig. 9–23B). This is the most common form of PEM seen in African children who have been weaned too early and subsequently fed, almost exclusively, a carbohydrate diet (the name kwashiorkor is from the Ga language in Ghana describing a disease of a baby due to the arrival of another child). The prevalence of kwashiorkor is also high in impoverished countries of Southeast Asia. Less severe forms may occur worldwide in persons with chronic diarrheal states in which protein is not absorbed or in those with chronic protein loss due to conditions such as protein-losing enteropathies, the nephrotic syndrome, or after extensive burns. Cases of kwashiorkor resulting from fad diets or replacement of milk by rice-based beverages have been reported in the United States.

In kwashiorkor, marked protein deprivation is associated with severe loss of the visceral protein compartment, and the resultant hypoalbuminemia gives rise to *generalized or dependent edema* (Fig. 9–23B). The loss of weight in these patients is masked by the increased fluid retention. In further contrast to marasmus, there is relative sparing of subcutaneous fat and muscle mass. Children with kwashiorkor have characteristic *skin lesions,* with alternating zones of hyperpigmentation, areas of desquamation, and hypopigmentation, giving a "flaky paint" appearance. *Hair changes* include overall loss of color or alternating bands of pale and darker hair. Other features that differentiate kwashiorkor from marasmus include an enlarged, *fatty liver* (resulting from reduced synthesis of the carrier protein component of lipoproteins), and the development of apathy, listlessness, and loss of appetite. Vitamin deficiencies are likely to be present, as are *defects in immunity* and *secondary infections. As already stated, marasmus and kwashiorkor are two ends of a spectrum, and considerable overlap exists between these conditions.*

Secondary PEM often develops in chronically ill, elderly, and bedridden patients. An 18-item questionnaire known as the Mininutritional Assessment (MNA) is often used to measure the nutritional status of elderly persons. It is estimated that more than 50% of elderly residents in nursing homes in the United States are malnourished. Weight loss of more than 5% associated with PEM increases the risk of mortality in nursing home patients by almost five-fold. The most obvious signs of secondary PEM include: (1) depletion of subcutaneous fat in the arms, chest wall, shoulders, or metacarpal regions; (2) wasting of the quadriceps femoris and deltoid muscles; and (3) ankle or sacral edema. Bedridden or hospitalized malnourished patients have an increased risk of infection, sepsis, impaired wound healing, and death after surgery.

> **Morphology.** The central anatomic changes in PEM are (1) growth failure, (2) peripheral edema in kwashiorkor, and (3) loss of body fat and atrophy of muscle, more marked in marasmus.

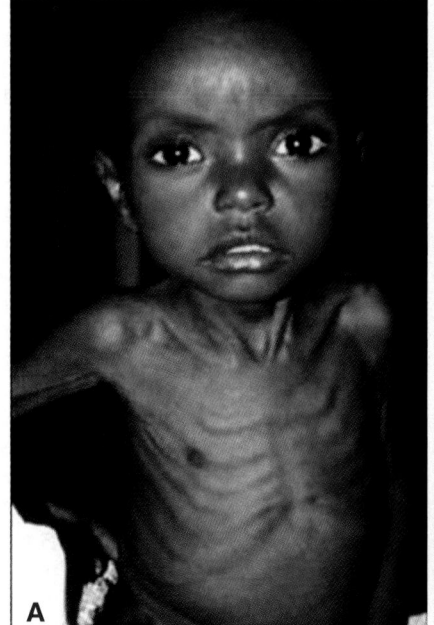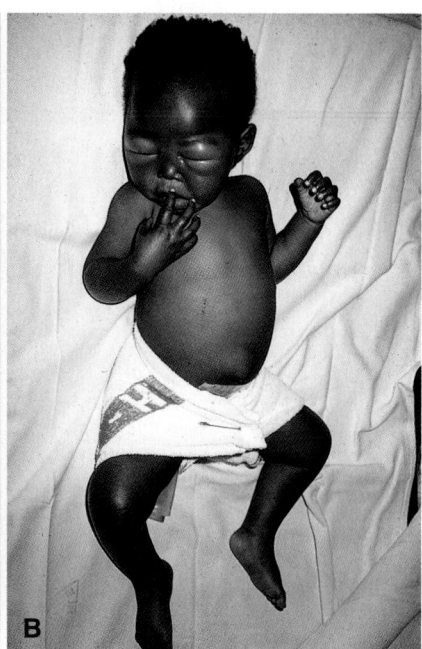

FIGURE 9–23 Childhood malnutrition. **A,** Marasmus. Note the loss of muscle mass and subcutaneous fat; the head appears to be too large for the emaciated body. **B,** Kwashiorkor. The infant shows generalized edema, seen as ascites and puffiness of the face, hands, and legs. (**A,** From Clinic Barak, Reisebericht Kenya.)

The **liver** in kwashiorkor, but not in marasmus, is enlarged and fatty; superimposed cirrhosis is rare.

In kwashiorkor (rarely in marasmus) the **small bowel** shows a decrease in the mitotic index in the crypts of the glands, associated with mucosal atrophy and loss of villi and microvilli. In such cases concurrent loss of small intestinal enzymes occurs, most often manifested as disaccharidase deficiency. Hence, infants with kwashiorkor initially may not respond well to full-strength, milk-based diets. With treatment, the mucosal changes are reversible.

The **bone marrow** in both kwashiorkor and marasmus may be hypoplastic, mainly as a result of decreased numbers of red cell precursors. The peripheral blood commonly reveals mild to moderate anemia, which often has a multifactorial origin; nutritional deficiencies of iron, folate, and protein, as well as the suppressive effects of infection (anemia of chronic disease) may all contribute. Depending on the predominant factor, the red cells may be microcytic, normocytic, or macrocytic.

The **brain** in infants who are born to malnourished mothers and who suffer PEM during the first 1 or 2 years of life has been reported by some to show cerebral atrophy, a reduced number of neurons, and impaired myelinization of white matter.

Many **other changes** may be present, including (1) thymic and lymphoid atrophy (more marked in kwashiorkor than in marasmus), (2) anatomic alterations induced by intercurrent infections, particularly with all manner of endemic worms and other parasites, and (3) deficiencies of other required nutrients such as iodine and vitamins.

Cachexia. *PEM is a common complication in patients with AIDS or advanced cancers, and in these settings it is known as cachexia.* Cachexia occurs in about 50% of cancer patients, most commonly in individuals with gastrointestinal, pancreatic, and lung cancers, and is responsible for about 30% of cancer deaths. It is a highly debilitating condition characterized by extreme weight loss, fatigue, muscle atrophy, anemia, anorexia, and edema. Mortality is generally the consequence of atrophy of the diaphragm and other respiratory muscles. The precise causes of cachexia are not known, but it is clear that agents secreted by tumors and host responses contribute to its development (Fig. 9–24). Cachetic agents produced by tumors include:

- *PIF (proteolysis-inducing factor)*, which is a glycosylated polypeptide excreted in the urine of weight-losing patients with pancreatic, breast, colon, and other cancers
- *LMF (lipid-mobilizing factor)*, which increases fatty acid oxidation, and pro-inflammatory cytokines such as TNF (originally known as cachetin), interleukin-2 (IL-2), and IL-6. TNF and IL-6 trigger an acute-phase response from the host, increasing the secretion of C-reactive protein and fibrinogen, and decreasing plasma concentrations of albumin.

Proteolysis-inducing factor (PIF) and pro-inflammatory cytokines cause skeletal muscle breakdown through the NF-κB-induced activation of the ubiquitin proteasome pathway, leading to the degradation of myosin heavy chain.[47] The induction of the ubiquitin proteasome pathway involves the production of two muscle-specific ubiquitin ligases, MuRF1 (muscle RING finger-1) and MAFBx (muscle atrophy F-box, or atroglin-1). More recent data also implicate alterations in the myofibrillar membrane of skeletal muscle with *loss of dystrophin caused by alterations in the dystrophin-glycoprotein complex* (Fig. 9–24) as contributors to muscle atrophy, through a mechanism similar to that which occurs in some muscular dystrophies.[48]

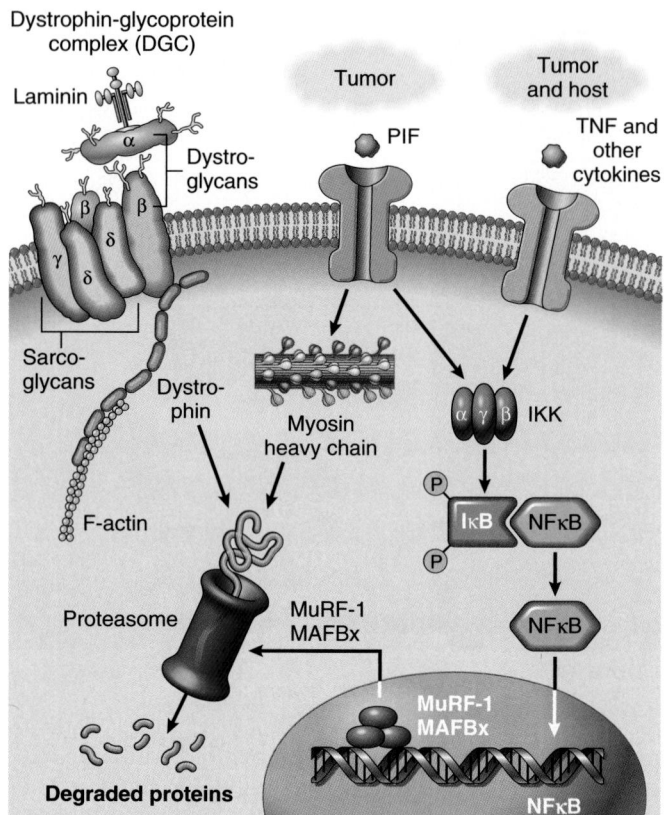

FIGURE 9–24 Mechanisms of cancer cachexia. The figure illustrates three mechanisms that cause muscle atrophy and muscle degradation leading to cachexia. (1) Proteolysis-inducing factor (PIF) produced by tumors degrades myosin heavy chain through the proteasome, causing muscle atrophy; (2) TNF and other cytokines produced by tumors and the host activate NF-κB and initiate the transcription of the ubiquitin ligases MAFBx and MuRF1, contributing to protein breakdown; (3) alterations in the dystrophin-glycoprotein complex leading to dystrophin-degradation by the proteasome also participate in the muscle atrophy of cachexia.

ANOREXIA NERVOSA AND BULIMIA

Anorexia nervosa is self-induced starvation, resulting in marked weight loss; *bulimia* is a condition in which the patient binges on food and then induces vomiting. Anorexia nervosa has the highest death rate of any psychiatric disorder. Bulimia is more common than anorexia nervosa, and generally has a better prognosis; it is estimated to occur in 1% to 2% of women and 0.1% of men, with an average onset at 20 years of age. These eating disorders occur primarily in previously healthy young women who have developed an obsession with body image and thinness. The neurobiologic underpinnings of these diseases are unknown, but it has been suggested that altered serotonin metabolism may be an important component.[49]

The clinical findings in anorexia nervosa are generally similar to those in severe PEM. In addition, effects on the endocrine system are prominent. *Amenorrhea*, resulting from decreased secretion of gonadotropin-releasing hormone, and subsequent decreased secretion of luteinizing hormone and follicle-stimulating hormone, is so common that its presence is a diagnostic feature for the disorder. Other common findings, related to decreased thyroid hormone release, include cold intolerance, bradycardia, constipation, and changes in the skin and hair. In addition, dehydration and electrolyte abnormalities are frequently present. The skin becomes dry and scaly. Bone density is decreased, most likely because of low estrogen levels, which mimics the postmenopausal acceleration of osteoporosis. Anemia, lymphopenia, and hypoalbuminemia may be present. A major complication of anorexia nervosa (and also bulimia) is an increased susceptibility to cardiac arrhythmia and sudden death, resulting from hypokalemia.

In bulimia, binge eating is the norm. Large amounts of food, principally carbohydrates, are ingested, only to be followed by induced vomiting. Although menstrual irregularities are common, amenorrhea occurs in less than 50% of bulimic patients, probably because weight and gonadotropin levels are maintained near normal. The major medical complications relate to continual induced vomiting, and the chronic use of laxatives and diuretics. They include (1) electrolyte imbalances (hypokalemia), which predispose the patient to cardiac arrhythmias; (2) pulmonary aspiration of gastric contents; and (3) esophageal and gastric cardiac rupture. Nevertheless, there are no signs and symptoms that are specific for bulimia; the diagnosis must rely on a comprehensive psychologic assessment of the person. A recent trend in bulimic patients has been the combination of binge eating with high ingestion of alcohol. Needless to say, the combined effects of bulimia and alcoholism are devastating.

VITAMIN DEFICIENCIES

Thirteen vitamins are necessary for health; vitamins A, D, E, and K are fat-soluble, and all others are water-soluble. The distinction between fat- and water-soluble vitamins is important. Fat-soluble vitamins are more readily stored in the body, but they may be poorly absorbed in fat malabsorption disorders, caused by disturbances of digestive functions (discussed in Chapter 17). Certain vitamins can be synthesized endogenously—vitamin D from precursor steroids, vitamin K and biotin by the intestinal microflora, and niacin from tryptophan, an essential amino acid. Notwithstanding this endogenous synthesis, a dietary supply of all vitamins is essential for health.

A deficiency of vitamins may be primary (dietary in origin) or secondary because of disturbances in intestinal absorption, transport in the blood, tissue storage, or metabolic conversion. In the following sections, vitamins A, D, and C are presented in some detail because of their wide-ranging activities and the morphologic changes of deficient states. This is followed by presentation in tabular form of the main consequences of deficiencies of the remaining vitamins (E, K, and the B complex) and some essential minerals. However, it should be emphasized that deficiency of a single vitamin is uncommon, and that single or multiple vitamin deficiencies may be associated with PEM.

Vitamin A

Vitamin A is the name given to a group of related compounds that include *retinol* (vitamin A alcohol), *retinal* (vitamin A aldehyde), *and retinoic acid* (vitamin A acid), which have similar biologic activities. Retinol is the chemical name given to vitamin A. It is the transport form and, as retinol ester, also the storage form. The generic term *retinoids* encompasses vitamin A in its various forms and both natural and synthetic chemicals that are structurally related to vitamin A, but may not necessarily have vitamin A–like biologic activity.[50] Animal-derived foods such as liver, fish, eggs, milk, and butter are important dietary sources of preformed vitamin A. Yellow and leafy green vegetables such as carrots, squash, and spinach supply large amounts of carotenoids, which are provitamins that can be metabolized to active vitamin A in the body. Carotenoids contribute approximately 30% of the vitamin A in human diets; the most important of these is β-carotene, which is efficiently converted to vitamin A. The Recommended Dietary Allowance for vitamin A is expressed in retinol equivalents, to take into account both preformed vitamin A and β-carotene.

Vitamin A is a fat-soluble vitamin, and its absorption requires bile, pancreatic enzymes, and some level of antioxidant activity in the food. Retinol (generally ingested as retinol ester) and β-carotene are absorbed in the intestine, where β-carotene is converted to retinol (Fig. 9–25). Retinol is then transported in chylomicrons to the liver for esterification and storage. Uptake in liver cells takes place through the apolipoprotein E receptor. More than 90% of the body's vitamin A reserves are stored in the liver, predominantly in the perisinusoidal stellate (Ito) cells. In healthy persons who consume an adequate diet, these reserves are sufficient to meet the body's demands for at least 6 months. Retinol esters stored in the liver can be mobilized; before release, retinol binds to a specific retinol-binding protein (RBP), synthesized in the liver. The uptake of retinol/RBP in peripheral tissues is dependent on cell surface receptors specific for RBP.[51] After uptake, retinol binds to a cellular RBP, and the RBP is released back into the blood. Retinol may be stored in peripheral tissues as retinol ester or be oxidized to form retinoic acid. Retinoic acid has important effects in epithelial differentiation and growth.

Function. In humans the main functions of vitamin A are the following:

○ *Maintenance of normal vision.* The *visual process* involves four forms of vitamin A–containing pigments: rhodopsin in the rods, the most light-sensitive pigment and therefore important in reduced light, and three iodopsins in cone cells, each responsive to specific colors in bright light. The synthesis of rhodopsin from retinol involves (1) oxidation to all-*trans*-retinal, (2) isomerization to 11-*cis*-retinal, and (3) covalent association with the 7-transmembrane rod protein opsin to form rhodopsin. A photon of light causes the isomerization of 11-*cis*-retinal to all-*trans*-retinal, which dissociates from rhodopsin. This induces a conformational change in opsin that triggers a series of downstream events and generates a nerve impulse, which is transmitted via neurons from the retina to the brain. During dark adaptation, some of the all-*trans*-retinal is reconverted to 11-*cis*-retinal, but most is reduced to retinol and lost to the retina, dictating the need for continuous supply.

○ *Cell growth and differentiation.* Vitamin A and retinoids play an important role in the orderly differentiation of mucus-secreting epithelium; *when a deficiency state exists, the epithelium undergoes squamous metaplasia, differentiat-*

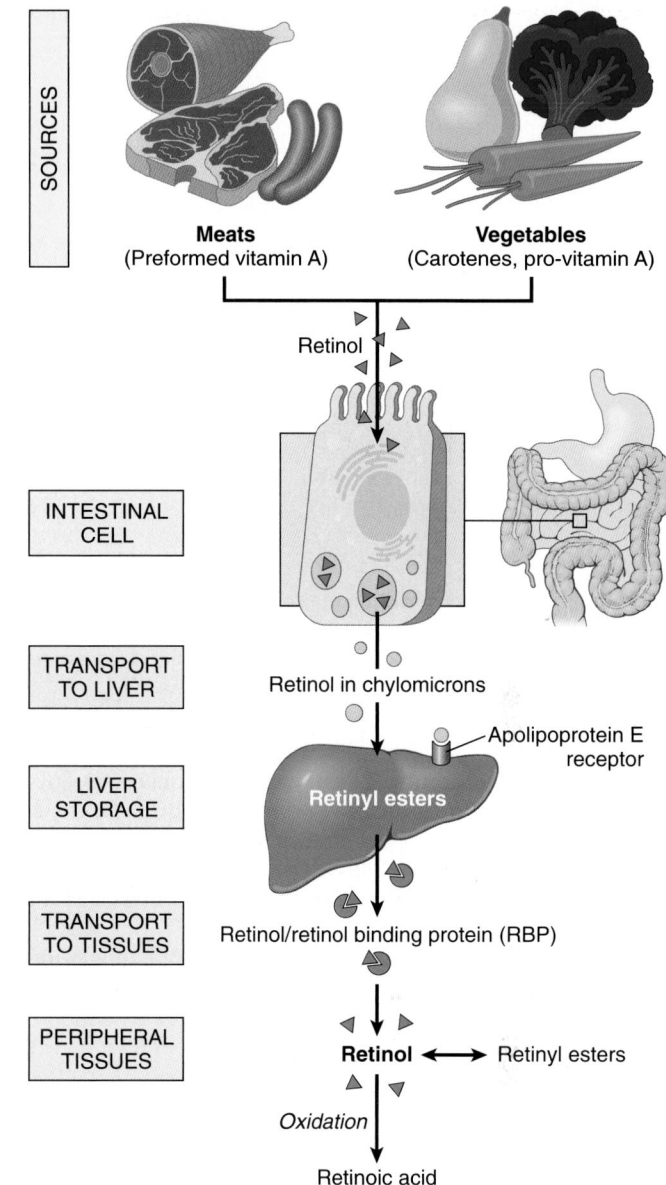

FIGURE 9–25 Vitamin A metabolism.

ing into a keratinizing epithelium. Activation of retinoic acid receptors (RARs) by their ligands causes the release of corepressors and the obligatory formation of heterodimers with another retinoid receptor, known as the retinoic X receptor (RXR). Both RAR and RXR have three isoforms, α, β, and γ. The RAR/RXR heterodimers bind to retinoic acid response elements located in the promoter region of genes that encode receptors for growth factors, tumor suppressor genes, and secreted proteins. Through these effects, retinoids participate in cell growth and differentiation, cell cycle control, and other biologic responses. *All-trans-retinoic acid*, a potent acid derivative of vitamin A, has the highest affinity for RARs compared with other retinoids.[51]

○ *Metabolic effects of retinoids.* The retinoic X receptor (RXR), believed to be activated by 9-*cis* retinoic acid, can form heterodimers with other nuclear receptors, such as (as we have seen) nuclear receptors involved in drug metabolism,

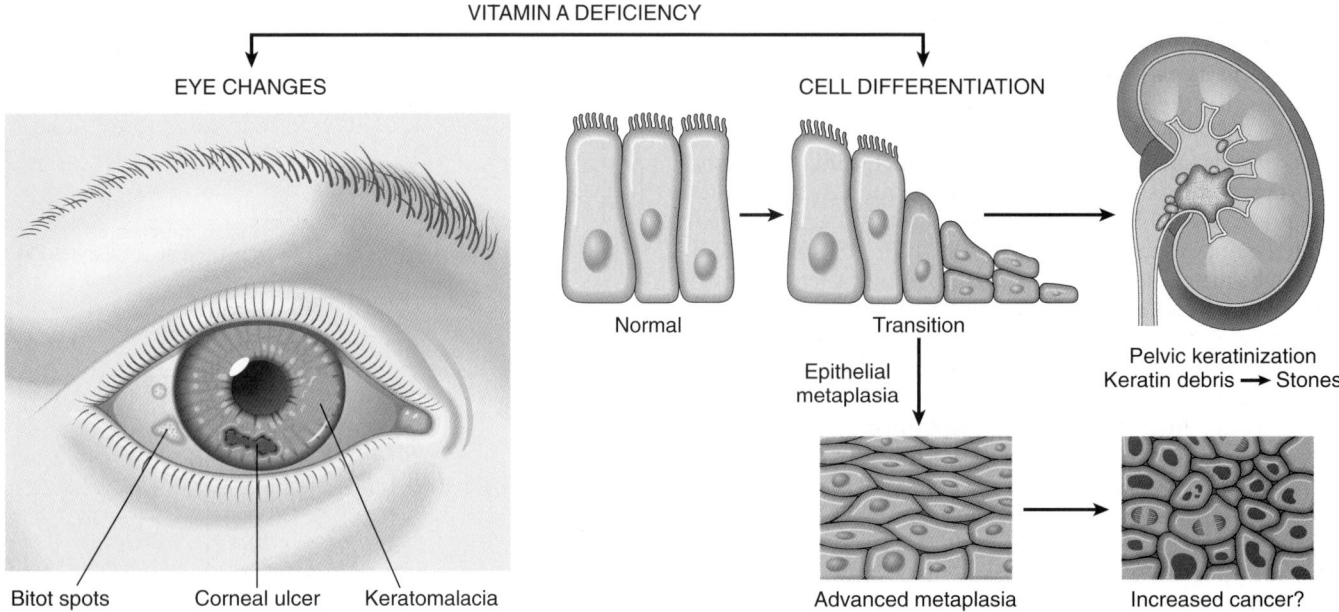

FIGURE 9–26 Vitamin A deficiency: its major consequences in the eye and in the production of keratinizing metaplasia of specialized epithelial surfaces, and its possible role in epithelial metaplasia. Not depicted are night blindness and immune deficiency.

the peroxisome proliferator-activated receptors (PPARs), and vitamin D receptors. PPARs are key regulators of fatty acid metabolism, including fatty acid oxidation in fat tissue and muscle, adipogenesis, and lipoprotein metabolism. The association between RXR and PPARγ provides an explanation for the metabolic effects of retinoids on adipogenesis and obesity.[52]

○ *Host resistance to infections.* Vitamin A supplementation can reduce morbidity and mortality from some forms of diarrhea, and in preschool children with measles, supplementation can quickly improve the clinical outcome. The beneficial effect of vitamin A in diarrheal diseases may be related to the maintenance and restoration of the integrity of the epithelium of the gut. The effects of vitamin A on infections also derive in part from its ability to stimulate the immune system, although the mechanisms are not entirely clear. Infections may reduce the bioavailability of vitamin A by inhibiting retinol binding protein synthesis in the liver through the acute-phase response associated with many infections. The drop in hepatic retinol binding protein causes a decrease in circulating retinol, which reduces the tissue availability of vitamin A.

In addition, the retinoids, β-carotene, and some related carotenoids can function as photoprotective and antioxidant agents.

Retinoids are used clinically for the treatment of skin disorders such as severe acne and certain forms of psoriasis, and also in the treatment of acute promyelocytic leukemia. In this leukemia, a (15:17) translocation (Chapter 13) results in the fusion of a truncated *RARα* gene on chromosome 17 with the *PML* gene on chromosome 15. The fusion gene encodes an abnormal RAR that blocks myeloid cell differentiation. Pharmacologic doses of all-*trans* retinoic acid overcome the block, causing leukemia cells to differentiate into neutrophils, which subsequently die by apoptosis. This "differentiation therapy"

induces remission in most individuals with acute promyelocytic leukemia and in combination with other chemotherapeutic agents can be curative. A different isomer, 13-*cis* retinoic acid, has been used with some success in the treatment of neuroblastomas in children.

Vitamin A Deficiency. Vitamin A deficiency occurs worldwide either as a consequence of general undernutrition or as a secondary deficiency in individuals with conditions that cause malabsorption of fats. In children, stores of vitamin A are depleted by infections, and the absorption of the vitamin is poor in newborn infants. Adult patients with malaborption syndromes, such as celiac disease, Crohn's disease, and colitis, may develop vitamin A deficiency, in conjunction with depletion of other fat-soluble vitamins. Bariatric surgery and, in elderly persons, continuous use of mineral oil as a laxative may lead to deficiency. The pathologic effects of vitamin A deficiency are summarized in Figure 9–26.

As already discussed, vitamin A is a component of rhodopsin and other visual pigments. Not surprisingly, one of the earliest manifestations of vitamin A deficiency is impaired vision, particularly in reduced light (*night blindness*). Other effects of deficiency are related to the role of vitamin A in maintaining the differentiation of epithelial cells. Persistent deficiency gives rise to a series of changes involving epithelial metaplasia and keratinization. The most devastating changes occur in the eyes and are referred to as *xerophthalmia* (dry eye). First, there is dryness of the conjunctiva (xerosis conjunctivae) as the normal lacrimal and mucus-secreting epithelium is replaced by keratinized epithelium. This is followed by buildup of keratin debris in small opaque plaques (*Bitot spots*) and, eventually, erosion of the roughened corneal surface with softening and destruction of the cornea (*keratomalacia*) and total blindness.

In addition to the ocular epithelium, the epithelium lining the upper respiratory passage and urinary tract is replaced by keratinizing squamous cells (*squamous metaplasia*). Loss of the mucociliary epithelium of the airways predisposes to secondary pulmonary infections, and desquamation of keratin debris in the urinary tract predisposes to renal and urinary bladder stones. Hyperplasia and *hyperkeratinization of the epidermis* with plugging of the ducts of the adnexal glands may produce follicular or papular dermatosis. Another very serious consequence is immune deficiency, which is responsible for higher mortality rates from common infections such as measles, pneumonia, and infectious diarrhea. In parts of the world where a deficiency of vitamin A is prevalent, dietary supplements reduce mortality by 20% to 30%.

Vitamin A Toxicity. Both short- and long-term excesses of vitamin A may produce toxic manifestations, a point of concern because of the megadoses touted by certain sellers of supplements. The consequences of acute hypervitaminosis A were first described by Gerrit de Veer in 1597, a ship's carpenter stranded in the Arctic, who recounted in his diary the serious symptoms that he and other members of the crew developed after eating polar bear liver. With this cautionary tale in mind, the adventurous eater should be aware that acute vitamin A toxicity has also been described in individuals who ingested the livers of whales, sharks, and even tuna! The symptoms of acute vitamin A toxicity include headache, dizziness, vomiting, stupor, and blurred vision, symptoms that may be confused with those of a brain tumor (pseudotumor cerebri). Chronic toxicity is associated with weight loss, anorexia, nausea, vomiting, and bone and joint pain. Retinoic acid stimulates osteoclast production and activity, which lead to increased bone resorption and high risk of fractures. Although synthetic retinoids used for the treatment of acne are not associated with these types of conditions, their use in pregnancy should be avoided because of the well-established teratogenic effects of retinoids.

Vitamin D

The major function of the fat-soluble vitamin D is the maintenance of adequate plasma levels of calcium and phosphorus to support metabolic functions, bone mineralization, and neuromuscular transmission.[53] Vitamin D is required for the prevention of bone diseases known as *rickets* (in children whose epiphyses have not already closed), *osteomalacia* (in adults), and hypocalcemic tetany. This latter condition is a convulsive state caused by an insufficient extracellular concentration of ionized calcium, which is required for normal neural excitation and the relaxation of muscles. Rickets was nearly endemic in large European cities and poor areas of New York and Boston at the end of the nineteenth century. Although cod liver oil was recognized for its anti-rachitic properties in the early part of that century, it took almost 100 years for it to be accepted by the medical profession as an effective preventive agent (it did not help that cod liver oil consumed in fishing villages in Northern Europe, Scandinavia, and Iceland was a dark, foul-smelling liquid).[54] In addition to its effects on calcium and phosphorus homeostasis, vitamin D has effects in non-skeletal tissues (so called "nonclassical" effects).

Metabolism of Vitamin D. The major source of vitamin D for humans is its endogenous synthesis in the skin by photochemical conversion of a precursor, 7-dehydrocholesterol, via the energy of solar or artificial UV light in the range of 290 to 315 nm (UVB radiation). Irradiation of 7-dehydrocho-

lesterol forms *cholecalciferol, known as vitamin D₃*. For the sake of simplicity we will use the term vitamin D to refer to this compound. Under usual conditions of sun exposure, about 90% of the vitamin D requirement is endogenously derived from 7-dehydrocholesterol present in the skin. However, individuals with dark skin generally have a lower level of vitamin D production because of melanin pigmentation. Dietary sources, such as deep-sea fish, plants, and grains, contribute about 10% of required vitamin D and depend on adequate intestinal fat absorption. In plants, vitamin D is present in its precursor form (ergosterol), which is converted to vitamin D in the body.

The main steps of vitamin D metabolism are summarized below[53] and shown in Figure 9–27.

1. Photochemical synthesis of vitamin D from 7-dehydrocholesterol in the skin and absorption of vitamin D from foods and supplements in the gut
2. Binding of vitamin D from both of these sources to plasma α1-globulin *(D-binding protein or DBP)* and transport into the liver
3. Conversion of vitamin D into 25-hydroxycholecalciferol (25-OH-D) in the liver, through the effect of 25-OHases (25-hydroxylases that include CYP27A1 and other CYPs)
4. Conversion of 25-OH-D *into 1,25-dihydroxyvitamin D, [1α,25(OH)₂D₃]* in the kidney, the most active form of vitamin D, through the activity of α1-hydroxylase

The production of 1,25-dihydroxyvitamin D in the kidney is regulated by three main mechanisms (Fig. 9–27): (a) *hypocalcemia stimulates secretion of parathyroid hormone (PTH)*, which in turn augments the conversion of 25-OH-D into 1,25-dihydroxyvitamin D by activating 1α-hydroxylase; (b) *hypophosphatemia directly activates α1-hydroxylase*, increasing the production of 1,25-dihydroxyvitamin D; (c) *through a feedback mechanism*, increased levels of 1,25-dihydroxyvitamin D down-regulate its own synthesis through inhibition of 1α-hydroxylase activity.

Mechanisms of Action. 1,25-dihydroxyvitamin D, the biologically active form of vitamin D, is best regarded as a steroid hormone. It binds to *the high-affinity vitamin D receptor (VDR)*, which associates with the already mentioned RXR. This heterodimeric complex binds to vitamin D response elements located in the promoter of vitamin D target genes. The receptors for 1,25-dihydroxyvitamin D are present in most cells of the body and transduce signals that regulate plasma levels of calcium and phosphorus, through action on the small intestine, bones, and kidneys. Beyond its role on skeletal homeostasis, vitamin D also has immunomodulatory and antiproliferative effects. More recently it has been proposed that 1,25-dihydroxyvitamin D may also act through nongenomic mechanisms, which do not require the transcription of target genes. Nongenomic mechanisms may involve the binding of 1,25-dihydroxyvitamin D to a membrane vitamin D receptor, leading to the activation of protein kinase C and opening of calcium channels.[55]

Effects of Vitamin D on Calcium and Phosphorus Homeostasis. The main functions of 1,25-dihydroxyvitamin D on calcium and phosphorus homeostasis are the following:

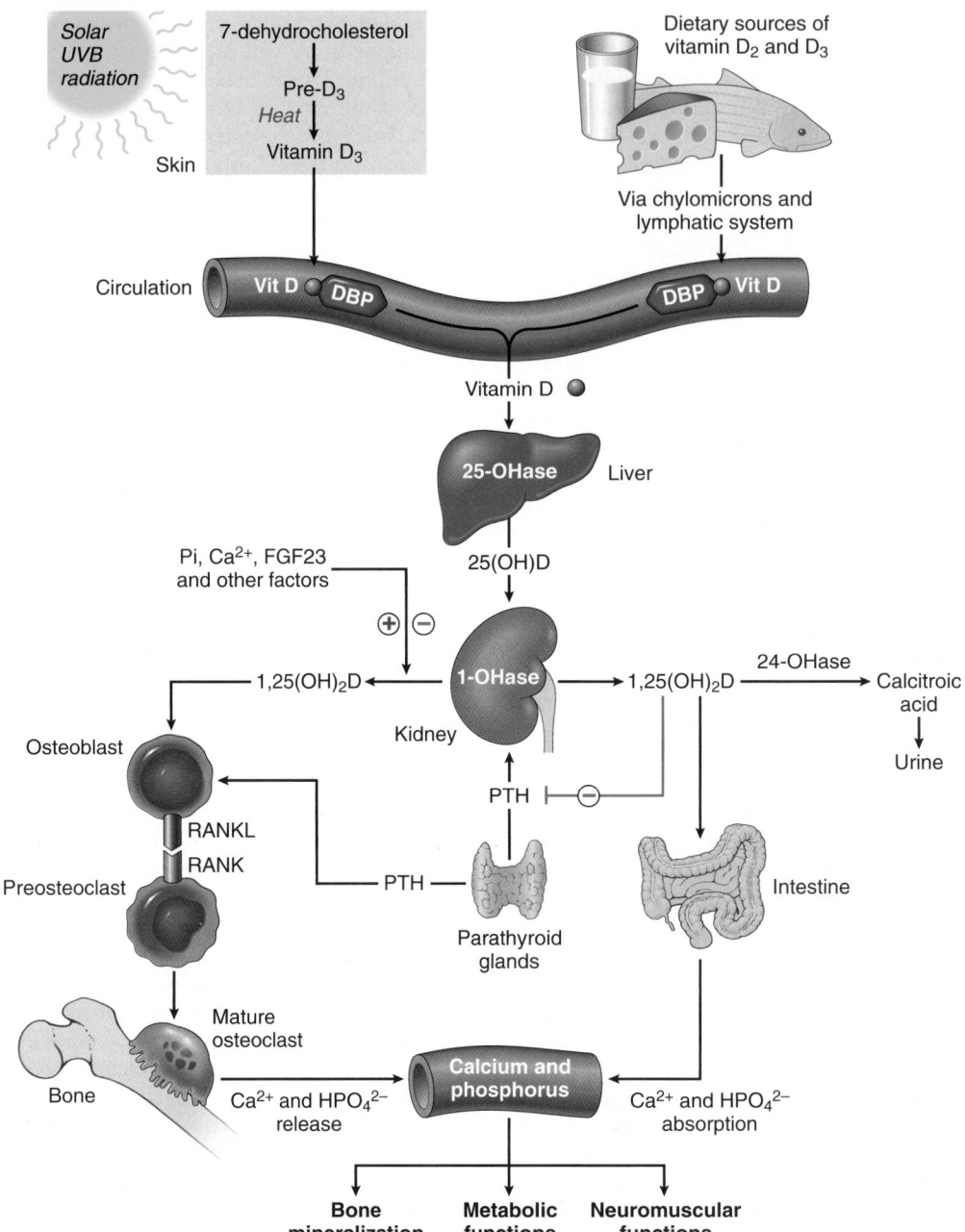

FIGURE 9–27 Vitamin D metabolism. Vitamin D is produced from 7-dehydrocholesterol in the skin or is ingested in the diet. It is converted in the liver into 25(OH)D, and in kidney into 1,25(OH)$_2$D (1,25-dihydroxyvitamin D), the active form of the vitamin. 1,25(OH)$_2$D stimulates the expression of RANKL, an important regulator of osteoclast maturation and function, on osteoblasts, and enhances the intestinal absorption of calcium and phosphorus in the intestine. See text for further details. DBP, vitamin D-binding protein (α1-globulin).

- *Stimulation of intestinal calcium absorption.* 1,25-dihydroxyvitamin D stimulates intestinal absorption of calcium in the duodenum through the *interaction of 1,25-dihydroxyvitamin D with nuclear vitamin D receptor and the formation of a complex with RXR.* The complex binds to vitamin D response elements and activates the transcription of TRPV6 (a member of the transient receptor potential vanilloid family), which encodes a critical calcium transport channel.
- *Stimulation of calcium reabsorption in the kidney.* 1,25-dihydroxyvitamin D increases calcium influx in distal tubules

of the kidney through the increased expression of TRPV5, another member of the transient receptor potential vanilloid family. TRPV5 expression is also regulated by PTH in response to hypocalcemia.[56]
- *Interaction with parathyroid hormone (PTH) in the regulation of blood calcium.* Vitamin D maintains calcium and phosphorus at supersaturated levels in the plasma. The parathyroid glands have a key role in the regulation of extracellular calcium concentrations. These glands have a calcium receptor that senses even small changes in blood calcium concentrations.[57] In addition to their effects on calcium absorption in the intes-

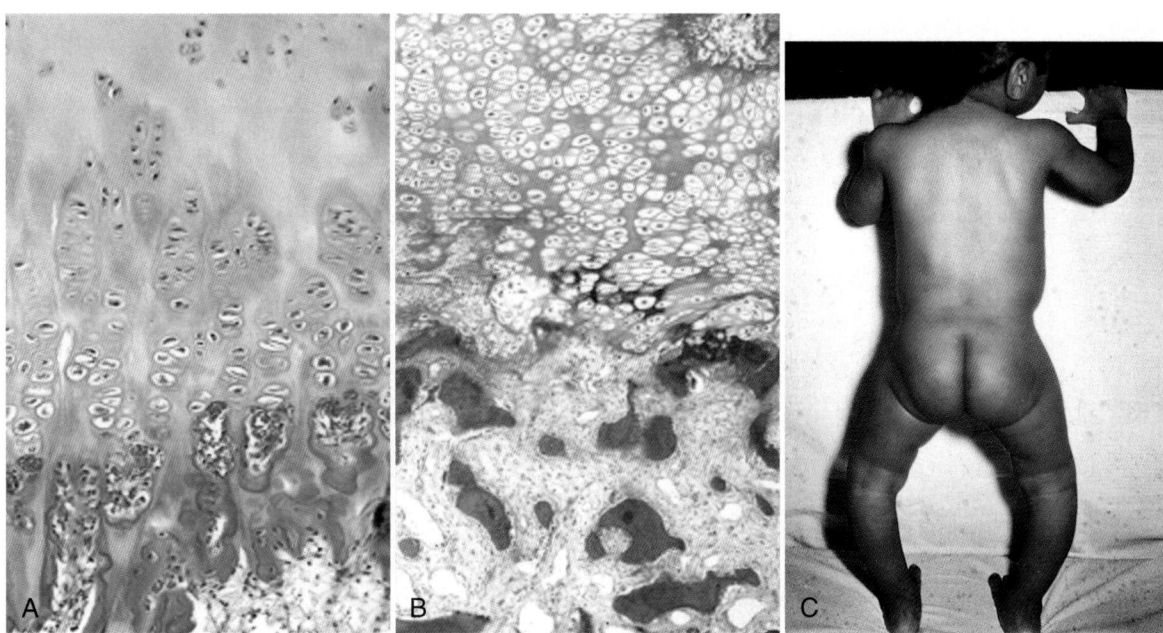

FIGURE 9–28   Rickets. **A,** Normal costochondral junction of a young child, illustrating formation of cartilage palisades and orderly transition from cartilage to new bone. **B,** Detail of a rachitic costochondral junction in which the palisades of cartilage is lost. Darker trabeculae are well-formed bone; paler trabeculae consist of uncalcified osteoid. **C,** Rickets, note bowing of legs due to formation of poorly mineralized bones. (**B,** Courtesy of Dr. Andrew E. Rosenberg, Massachusetts General Hospital, Boston, MA.)

tine and kidneys already described, both 1,25-dihydroxyvita-min D and parathyroid hormone enhance the expression of RANKL (receptor activator of NF-κB ligand) on osteoblasts. RANKL binds to its receptor (RANK) located in preosteo-clasts, inducing the differentiation of these cells into mature osteoclasts (Chapter 26). Through the secretion of hydro-chloric acid and activation of proteases such as cathepsin K, osteoclasts dissolve bone and release calcium and phosphorus into the circulation.

○ *Mineralization of bone.* Vitamin D contributes to the min-eralization of osteoid matrix and epiphyseal cartilage in the formation of both flat and long bones in the skeleton. It stimulates osteoblasts to synthesize the calcium-binding protein osteocalcin, involved in the deposition of calcium during bone development. Flat bones develop by intra-membranous bone formation, in which mesenchymal cells differentiate directly into osteoblasts, and synthesize the collagenous osteoid matrix on which calcium is deposited. Long bones develop by endochondral ossification, through which growing cartilage at the epiphyseal plates is provi-sionally mineralized and then progressively resorbed and replaced by osteoid matrix that is mineralized to create bone (Fig. 9–28A).

When *hypocalcemia* occurs in vitamin D deficiency (Fig. 9–29), PTH production is elevated, causing (1) activation of renal 1α-hydroxylase, increasing the amount of active vitamin D and calcium absorption; (2) increased resorption of calcium from bone by osteoclasts; (3) decreased renal calcium excre-tion; and (4) increased renal excretion of phosphate. Fibro-blast growth factor 23, which is produced by bone, is one of a group of agents known as *phosphatonins*, which block the absorption of phosphate in the intestine, and phosphate reab-sorption in the kidney, causing increased urinary excretion of

phosphate. Although a normal serum level of calcium may be restored, hypophosphatemia persists, impairing the mineral-ization of bone. Increased production of fibroblast growth factor 23 may be responsible for tumor-induced osteomalacia and some forms of hypophosphatemic rickets.[58]

Deficiency States. The normal reference range for circu-lating 25-(OH)-D is 20 to 100 ng/mL; concentrations of less than 20 ng/mL constitute vitamin D deficiency.

Rickets in growing children (see Fig. 9–28C) and osteoma-lacia in adults are skeletal diseases with worldwide distribu-tion. They may result from diets deficient in calcium and vitamin D, but an equally important cause of vitamin D deficiency is limited exposure to sunlight. This most often affects inhabitants of northern latitudes, but can even be a problem in tropical countries, in heavily veiled women, and in children born to mothers who have frequent pregnancies followed by lactation. In all of these situations, vitamin D deficiency can be prevented by a diet high in fish oils. Other, less common causes of rickets and osteomalacia include renal disorders causing decreased synthesis of 1,25-dihydroxyvitamin D, phosphate depletion, malabsorption dis-orders, and some rare inherited disorders.[53] Although rickets and osteomalacia rarely occur outside high-risk groups, milder forms of vitamin D deficiency (also called vitamin D insuffi-ciency), leading to an increase risk of bone loss and hip frac-tures, are quite common in the elderly in the United States and Europe.[59] Some genetically determined variants of the vitamin D receptors are associated with an accelerated loss of bone minerals with aging and in certain familial forms of osteoporosis (Chapter 26).

Morphology. The basic derangement in both rickets and osteomalacia is an excess of unmineral-

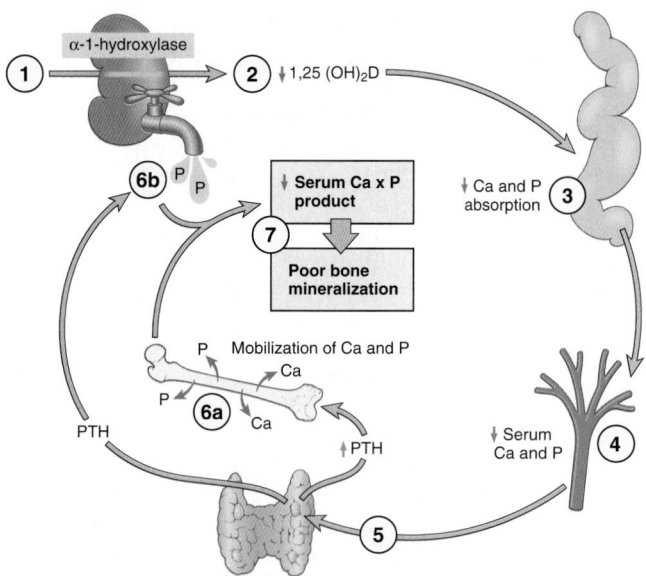

FIGURE 9–29 Vitamin D deficiency. There is inadequate substrate for the renal 1α-hydroxylase (1), yielding a deficiency of 1,25(OH)$_2$D (2), and deficient absorption of calcium and phosphorus from the gut (3), with consequently depressed serum levels of both (4). The hypocalcemia activates the parathyroid glands (5), causing mobilization of calcium and phosphorus from bone (6a). Simultaneously, the parathyroid hormone (PTH) induces wasting of phosphate in the urine (6b) and calcium retention. As a result, the serum levels of calcium are normal or nearly normal, but phosphate levels are low; hence, mineralization is impaired (7).

ized matrix. The following sequence ensues in rickets:

- Overgrowth of epiphyseal cartilage due to inadequate provisional calcification and failure of the cartilage cells to mature and disintegrate
- Persistence of distorted, irregular masses of cartilage, which project into the marrow cavity
- Deposition of osteoid matrix on inadequately mineralized cartilaginous remnants
- Disruption of the orderly replacement of cartilage by osteoid matrix, with enlargement and lateral expansion of the osteochondral junction (see Fig. 9–28B)
- Abnormal overgrowth of capillaries and fibroblasts in the disorganized zone resulting from microfractures and stresses on the inadequately mineralized, weak, poorly formed bone
- Deformation of the skeleton due to the loss of structural rigidity of the developing bones

Rickets is most common during the first year of life. The gross skeletal changes depend on the severity and duration of the process and, in particular, the stresses to which individual bones are subjected. During the nonambulatory stage of infancy, the head and chest sustain the greatest stresses. The softened occipital bones may become flattened, and the parietal bones can be buckled inward by pressure; with the release of the pressure, elastic recoil snaps the bones back into their original positions **(craniotabes)**. An excess of osteoid produces **frontal bossing** and a **squared appearance to the head**. Deformation of the chest results from overgrowth of cartilage or osteoid tissue at the costochondral junction, producing the **"rachitic rosary."** The weakened metaphyseal areas of the ribs are subject to the pull of the respiratory muscles and thus bend inward, creating anterior protrusion of the sternum **(pigeon breast deformity)**. When an ambulating child develops rickets, deformities are likely to affect the spine, pelvis, and tibia, causing **lumbar lordosis** and **bowing of the legs** (see Fig. 9–28C).

In adults, the lack of vitamin D deranges the normal bone remodeling that occurs throughout life. The newly formed osteoid matrix laid down by osteoblasts is inadequately mineralized, thus producing the excess of persistent osteoid that is characteristic of **osteomalacia**. Although the contours of the bone are not affected, the bone is weak and vulnerable to gross fractures or microfractures, which are most likely to affect vertebral bodies and femoral necks.

Histologically, the unmineralized osteoid can be visualized as a thickened layer of matrix (which stains pink in hematoxylin and eosin preparations) arranged about the more basophilic, normally mineralized trabeculae.

Non-Skeletal Effects of Vitamin D. It was mentioned earlier that the vitamin D receptor is present in various cells and tissues that do not participate in calcium and phophorus homeostasis. Macrophages, keratinocytes, and tissues such as breast, prostate, and colon can produce 1,25-dihydroxyvitamin D.[60] Within macrophages, synthesis of 1,25-dihydroxyvitamin D occurs through the activity of CYP27B located in the mitochondria. It has been proposed that pathogen-induced activation of Toll-like receptors in macrophages causes a transcription-induced increase in vitamin D receptor and CYP27B (Fig. 9–30). The resultant production of 1,25-dihydroxyvitamin D then stimulates the synthesis of *cathelicidin*, an antimicrobial peptide from the *defensin* family, which is effective against infection by *Mycobacterium tuberculosis*. Other effects of vitamin D in the innate and adaptive immune system have been reported,[61] but the data are often contradictory. Vitamin D regulates the expression of more than 200 genes, including genes that participate in cell proliferation, differentiation, apoptosis, and angiogenesis. It has been reported that levels of 1,25-dihydroxyvitamin D below 20 ng/mL are associated with a 30% to 50% increase in the incidence of colon, prostate, and breast cancers.

Vitamin D Toxicity. Prolonged exposure to normal sunlight does not produce an excess of vitamin D, but megadoses of orally administered vitamin can lead to hypervitaminosis. In children, hypervitaminosis D may take the form of metastatic calcifications of soft tissues such as the kidney; in adults it causes bone pain and hypercalcemia. In passing, we might point out that the toxic potential of this vitamin is so great that in sufficiently large doses it is a potent rodenticide!

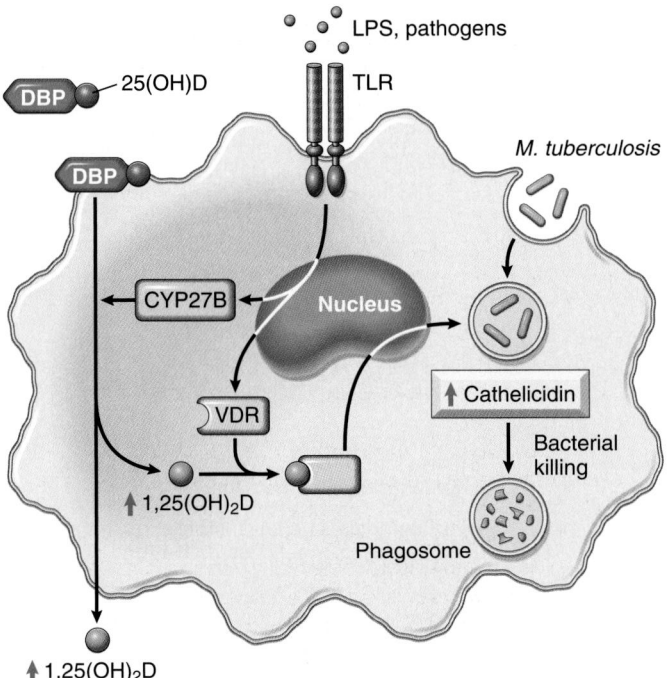

FIGURE 9–30 Anti-microbial effect of vitamin D. Pathogens and lipopolysaccharides (LPS) stimulate Toll-like receptors (TLRs) in macrophages, causing the transcription of vitamin D receptor (VDR) and an increase in CYP27B activity in mitochondria. This causes the production of 1,25(OH)$_2$D (1,25-dihydroxyvitamin D), which stimulates the synthesis of cathelicidin, an antimicrobial peptide that is particularly active against *Mycobacterium tuberculosis*.

Vitamin C (Ascorbic Acid)

A deficiency of water-soluble vitamin C leads to the development of *scurvy*, characterized principally by bone disease in growing children and by hemorrhages and healing defects in both children and adults. Sailors of the British Royal Navy were nicknamed "limeys," because at the end of the eighteenth century the Navy began to provide lime and lemon juice (rich sources of vitamin C) to sailors to prevent scurvy during their long sojourn at sea. It was not until 1932 that ascorbic acid was identified and synthesized. Ascorbic acid is not synthesized endogenously in humans; therefore, we are entirely dependent on the diet for this nutrient. Vitamin C is present in milk and some animal products (liver, fish) and is abundant in a variety of fruits and vegetables. All but the most restricted diets provide adequate amounts of vitamin C.

Function. Ascorbic acid functions in a variety of biosynthetic pathways by accelerating hydroxylation and amidation reactions. *The best-established function of vitamin C is the activation of prolyl and lysyl hydroxylases from inactive precursors, providing for hydroxylation of procollagen.* Inadequately hydroxylated procollagen cannot acquire a stable helical configuration or be adequately cross-linked, so it is poorly secreted from the fibroblast. Those molecules that are secreted lack tensile strength and are more soluble and vulnerable to enzymatic degradation. Collagen, which normally has the highest content, of hydroxyproline, of any polypeptide is most affected, particularly in blood vessels, accounting for the predisposition to hemorrhages in scurvy. In addition, a deficiency of vitamin C suppresses the rate of synthesis of procollagen, independent of an effect on proline hydroxylation.

While the role of vitamin C in collagen synthesis has been known for many decades, it is only in relatively recent years that its *antioxidant properties* have been recognized. Vitamin C can scavenge free radicals directly and can act indirectly by regenerating the antioxidant form of vitamin E.

Deficiency States. Consequences of vitamin C deficiency (scurvy) are illustrated in Figure 9–31. Fortunately, because of the abundance of ascorbic acid in many foods, scurvy has ceased to be a global problem. It is sometimes encountered even in affluent populations as a secondary deficiency, particularly among elderly individuals, persons who live alone, and chronic alcoholics, groups that often have erratic and inadequate eating patterns. Occasionally, scurvy appears in patients undergoing peritoneal dialysis and hemodialysis and among food faddists. Tragically, the condition sometimes appears in

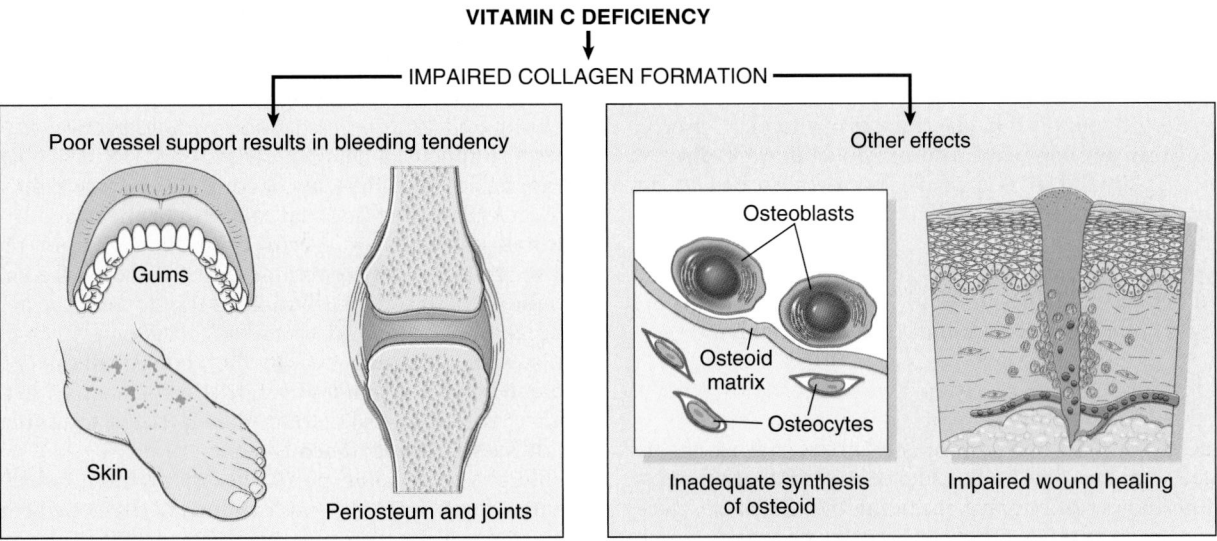

FIGURE 9–31 Major consequences of vitamin C deficiency caused by impaired formation of collagen.

TABLE 9–9	Vitamins: Major Functions and Deficiency Syndromes	
Vitamin	**Functions**	**Deficiency Syndromes**
FAT-SOLUBLE		
Vitamin A	A component of visual pigment Maintenance of specialized epithelia Maintenance of resistance to infection	Night blindness, xerophthalmia, blindness Squamous metaplasia Vulnerability to infection, particularly measles
Vitamin D	Facilitates intestinal absorption of calcium and phosphorus and mineralization of bone	Riskets in children Osteomalacia in adults
Vitamin E	Major antioxidant; scavenges free radicals	Spinocerebellar degeneration
Vitamin K	Cofactor in hepatic carboxylation of procoagulants— factors II (prothrombin), VII, IX, and X; and protein C and protein S	Bleeding diathesis (Chapter 14)
WATER-SOLUBLE		
Vitamin B_1 (thiamine)	As pyrophosphate, is coenzyme in decarboxylation reactions	Dry and wet beriberi, Wernicke syndrome, Korsakoff syndrome (Chapter 28)
Vitamin B_2 (riboflavin)	Converted to coenzymes flavin mononucleotide and flavin adenine dinucleotide, cofactors for many enzymes in intermediary metabolism	Ariboflavinosis, cheilosis, stomatitis, glossitis, dermatitis, corneal vascularization
Niacin	Incorporated into nicotinamide adenine dinucleotide (NAD) and NAD phosphate, involved in a variety of redox reactions	Pellagra—"three Ds": dementia, dermatitis, diarrhea
Vitamin B_6 (pyridoxine)	Derivatives serve as coenzymes in many intermediary reactions	Cheilosis, glossitis, dermatitis, peripheral neuropathy (Chapter 28)
Vitamin B_{12}	Required for normal folate metabolism and DNA synthesis Maintenance of myelinization of spinal cord tracts	Megaloblastic pernicious anemia and degeneration of posterolateral spinal cord tracts (Chapter 14)
Vitamin C	Serves in many oxidation-reduction (redox) reactions and hydroxylation of collagen	Scurvy
Folate	Essential for transfer and use of one-carbon units in DNA synthesis	Megaloblastic anemia, neural tube defects (Chapter 14)
Pantothenic acid	Incorporated in coenzyme A	No nonexperimental syndrome recognized
Biotin	Cofactor in carboxylation reactions	No clearly defined clinical syndrome

infants who are maintained on formulas of evaporated milk without supplementation of vitamin C.

Vitamin C Toxicity. The popular notion that megadoses of vitamin C protect against the common cold, or at least allay the symptoms, has not been borne out by controlled clinical studies. Such slight relief as may be experienced is probably due to the mild antihistamine action of ascorbic acid. Similarly there is little support that large doses of vitamin C protect against cancer development. The physiologic availability of vitamin C is limited. It is unstable, poorly absorbed in the intestine, and promptly excreted in the urine.

Other vitamins and some essential minerals are listed and briefly described in Tables 9–9 and 9–10. Some vitamins are discussed in other chapters, as indicated in the tables.

OBESITY

Excess adiposity (known as *obesity*) and *excess body weight* are associated with the increased incidence of several of the most important diseases of humans, including type 2 diabetes, dyslipidemias, cardiovascular disease, hypertension, and cancer. Obesity is defined as an accumulation of adipose tissue that is of sufficient magnitude to impair health. As with weight loss, excess weight is best assessed by *the body mass index or BMI*. For practical reasons, *body weight*, which generally correlates well with BMI, is often used as a surrogate for BMI measurements. *The normal BMI range is 18.5 to 25 kg/m², although the range may differ for different countries. Individuals with BMI above 30 kg/m² are classified as obese; those with BMI between 25 kg/m² and 30 kg/m² are considered to be overweight.* For the sake of simplicity, unless otherwise noted, the term obesity will be applied to both the truly obese and the overweight.

Accumulation of body fat may also be measured by triceps skinfold thickness, mid-arm circumference, and the ratio between waist and hip circumferences. Not only the total body weight but also the distribution of the stored fat is of importance in obesity. *Central, or visceral, obesity, in which fat accumulates in the trunk and in the abdominal cavity (in the mesentery and around viscera), is associated with a much higher risk for several diseases than is excess accumulation of fat diffusely in subcutaneous tissue.*

Obesity is a major public health problem, which, until about a dozen years ago, was confined to developed countries. Since then, it has also become an important health problem in developing nations, and in certain countries obesity coex-

	TABLE 9–10 Selected Trace Elements and Deficiency Syndromes		
Element	Function	Basis of Deficiency	Clinical Features
Zinc	Component of enzymes, principally oxidases	Inadequate supplementation in artificial diets Interference with absorption by other dietary constituents Inborn error of metabolism	Rash around eyes, mouth, nose, and anus called acrodermatitis enteropathica Anorexia and diarrhea Growth retardation in children Depressed mental function Depressed wound healing and immune response Impaired night vision Infertility
Iron	Essential component of hemoglobin as well as several iron-containing metalloenzymes	Inadequate diet Chronic blood loss	Hypochromic microcytic anemia (Chapter 14)
Iodine	Component of thyroid hormone	Inadequate supply in food and water	Goiter and hypothyroidism (Chapter 24)
Copper	Component of cytochrome *c* oxidase, dopamine β-hydroxylase, tyrosinase, lysyl oxidase, and unknown enzymes involved in cross-linking collagen	Inadequate supplementation in artificial diet Interference with absorption	Muscle weakness Neurologic defects Abnormal collagen cross-linking
Fluoride	Mechanism unknown	Inadequate supply in soil and water Inadequate supplementation	Dental caries (Chapter 16)
Selenium	Component of glutathione peroxidase Antioxidant with vitamin E	Inadequate amounts in soil and water	Myopathy Cardiomyopathy (Keshan disease)

ists with malnutrition in individual families. In the United States obesity has reached epidemic proportions. The prevalence of obesity increased from 13% to 32% between 1960 and 2004; currently 66% of adults in the United States are overweight or obese, and 16% of children are overweight. If current trends continue, it is projected that by the year 2015, 41% of adults will be obese.[62] The increase in obesity in the United States has been associated with the higher caloric content of the diet, mostly caused by increased consumption of refined sugars, sweetened beverages, and vegetable oils.

At its simplest level, obesity is a disease of caloric imbalance that results from an excess intake of calories above their consumption by the body. However, the pathogenesis of obesity is exceedingly complex and not yet completely understood. Ongoing research has identified complex humoral and neural mechanisms that control appetite and satiety. These neurohumoral mechanisms respond to genetic, nutritional, environmental, and psychologic signals, and trigger a metabolic response through the stimulation of centers located in the hypothalamus. There is little doubt that genetic influences play an important role in weight control, but obesity is a disease that depends on the interaction between multiple factors. After all, regardless of genetic makeup, obesity would not occur without intake of food!

In a simplified way the neurohumoral mechanisms that regulate energy balance can be subdivided into three components (illustrated in Figs. 9–29 and 9–30):

- *The peripheral or afferent system* generates signals from various sites. Its main components are *leptin and adiponectin* produced by fat cells, *ghrelin* from the stomach, *peptide YY (PYY)* from the ileum and colon, and *insulin* from the pancreas.

- *The arcuate nucleus in the hypothalamus* processes and integrates neurohumoral peripheral signals and generates efferent signals. It contains two subsets of first-order neurons: (1) *POMC* (pro-opiomelanocortin) and *CART* (cocaine and amphetamine-regulated transcripts) neurons, and (2) neurons containing *NPY* (neuropeptide Y) and *AgRP* (agouti-related peptide). These first order neurons communicate with second order neurons.

- *The efferent system* that carries the signals generated in the second order neurons of the hypothalamus to control food intake and energy expenditure. The hypothalamic system also communicates with forebrain and midbrain centers that control the autonomic nervous system.[63]

POMC/CART neurons enhance energy expenditure and weight loss through the production of the anorexigenic α-melanocyte-stimulating hormone (MSH), and the activation of the melanocortin receptors 3 and 4 (MC3/4R) in second-order neurons. NPY/AgRP neurons promote food intake (orexigenic effect) and weight gain, through the activation of Y1/5 receptors in secondary neurons.

We will now discuss three important components of the afferent system that regulates appetite and satiety: leptin, adiponectin, and gut hormones.

Leptin. The name leptin is derived from the Greek term *leptos*, meaning "thin." Leptin, a *16-kD hormone synthesized by fat cells*, is the product of the *ob* gene. The leptin receptor (OB-R) is the product of the diabetes (*db*) gene and belongs to the type I cytokine receptor superfamily that includes the gp130, granulocyte-colony-stimulating factor, IL-2, and IL-6 receptors. Mice genetically deficient in leptin (*ob/ob mice*) or leptin receptors (*db/db mice*) fail to sense the adequacy of fat stores, overeat, and gain weight, behaving as if they are undernourished. Thus, the obesity of these animals is a consequence

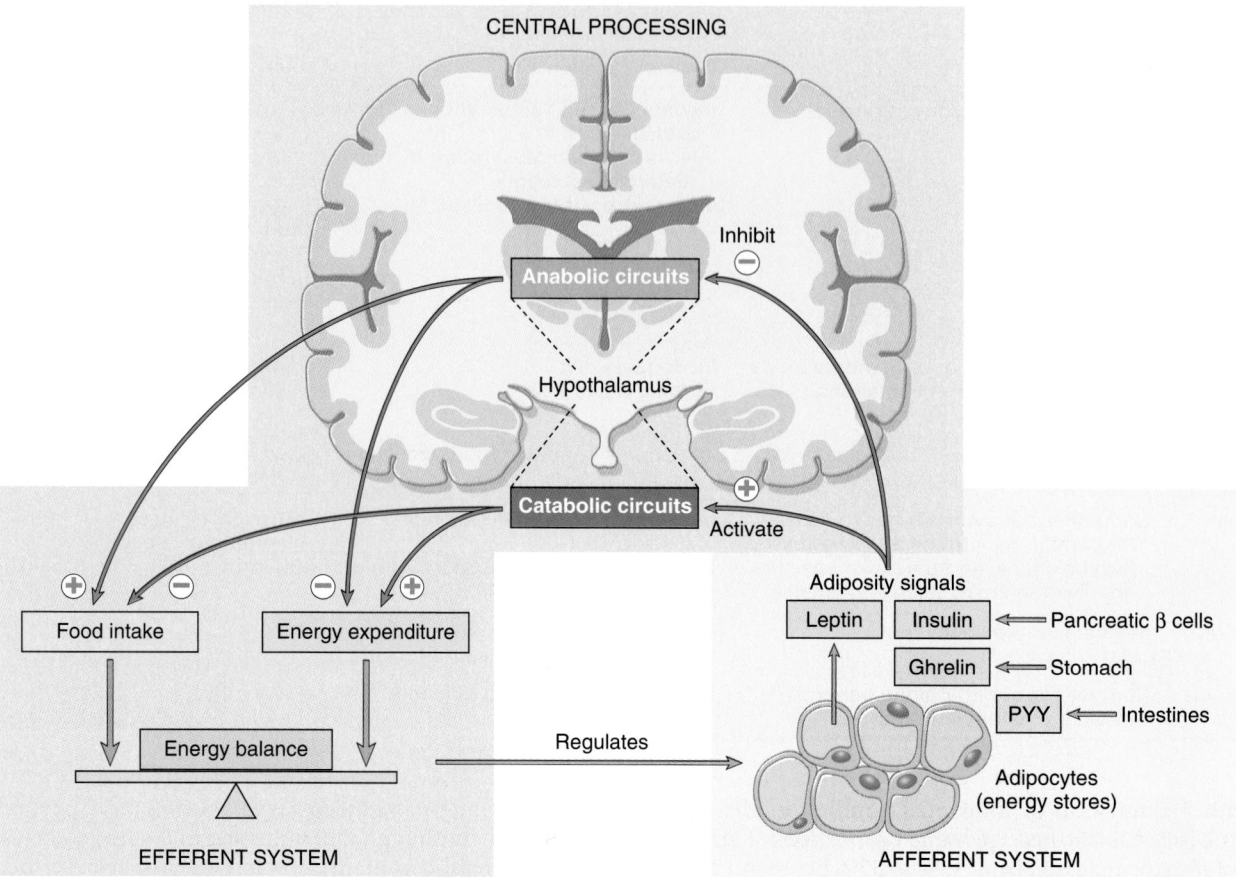

FIGURE 9–32 Regulation of energy balance. Adipose tissues generate afferent signals that influence the activity of the hypothalamus, which is the central regulator of appetite and satiety. These signals decrease food intake by inhibiting anabolic circuits, and enhance energy expenditure through the activation of catabolic circuits. PYY, peptide YY. See text for details.

of the lack of the signal for energy sufficiency that is normally provided by leptin.[63]

Although in a general sense leptin levels are regulated by the adequacy of fat stores, the precise mechanisms that regulate the output of leptin from adipose tissue have not been completely defined, but it has been established that leptin secretion is stimulated when fat stores are abundant. It is believed that insulin-stimulated glucose metabolism is an important factor in the regulation of leptin levels. *Leptin levels are regulated by multiple post-transcriptional mechanisms that affect its synthesis, secretion, and turnover. In the hypothalamus, leptin stimulates POMC/CART neurons that produce anorexigenic neuropeptides (primarily melanocyte-stimulating hormone) and inhibits NPY/AgRP neurons that produce feeding-inducing (orexigenic) neuropeptides* (see Figs. 9–32 and 9–33). In individuals with stable weight, the activities of the opposing POMC/CART and NPY/AgRP pathways are properly balanced. However, when there are inadequate stores of body fat, leptin secretion is diminished and food intake is increased.

Humans with loss-of-function mutations in the leptin system develop early-onset severe obesity, but this is a rare condition. Mutations of melanocortin receptor 4 (MC4R) and its downstream pathways are more frequent, being responsible for about 5% of massive obesity. In these individuals, sensing of satiety (anorexigenic signal) is not generated, and hence they behave as if they are undernourished. It has recently been

reported[64] that haplo-insufficiency of brain-derived neurotrophic factor (BDNF), an important component of MC4R downstream signaling in the hypothalamus, is associated with obesity in patients with the WAGR syndrome (this is a very rare condition that includes Wilms tumor, aniria, genitourinary defects, and mental retardation in addition to obesity Chapter 10). Although the defects in leptin and MC4R detected so far are uncommon, they underscore the importance of these systems in the control of energy balance and body weight. Perhaps other defects in these pathways may have pathogenic effects in more common forms of obesity. For instance, it has been proposed that leptin resistance rather than leptin deficiency may be prevalent in humans.

Leptin regulates not only food intake but also energy expenditure, through a distinct set of pathways. Thus, an abundance of leptin stimulates physical activity, heat production, and energy expenditure. The neurohumoral mediators of leptin-induced energy expenditure are less well defined. *Thermogenesis,* an important catabolic effect mediated by leptin, is controlled in part by hypothalamic signals that increase the release of norepinephrine from sympathetic nerve endings in adipose tissue. In addition to these effects, leptin can function as a pro-inflammatory cytokine and participates in the regulation of hematopoiesis and lymphopoiesis.[65] The OB-R receptor is highly similar structurally to the IL-6 receptor and activates the JAK/STAT pathway.

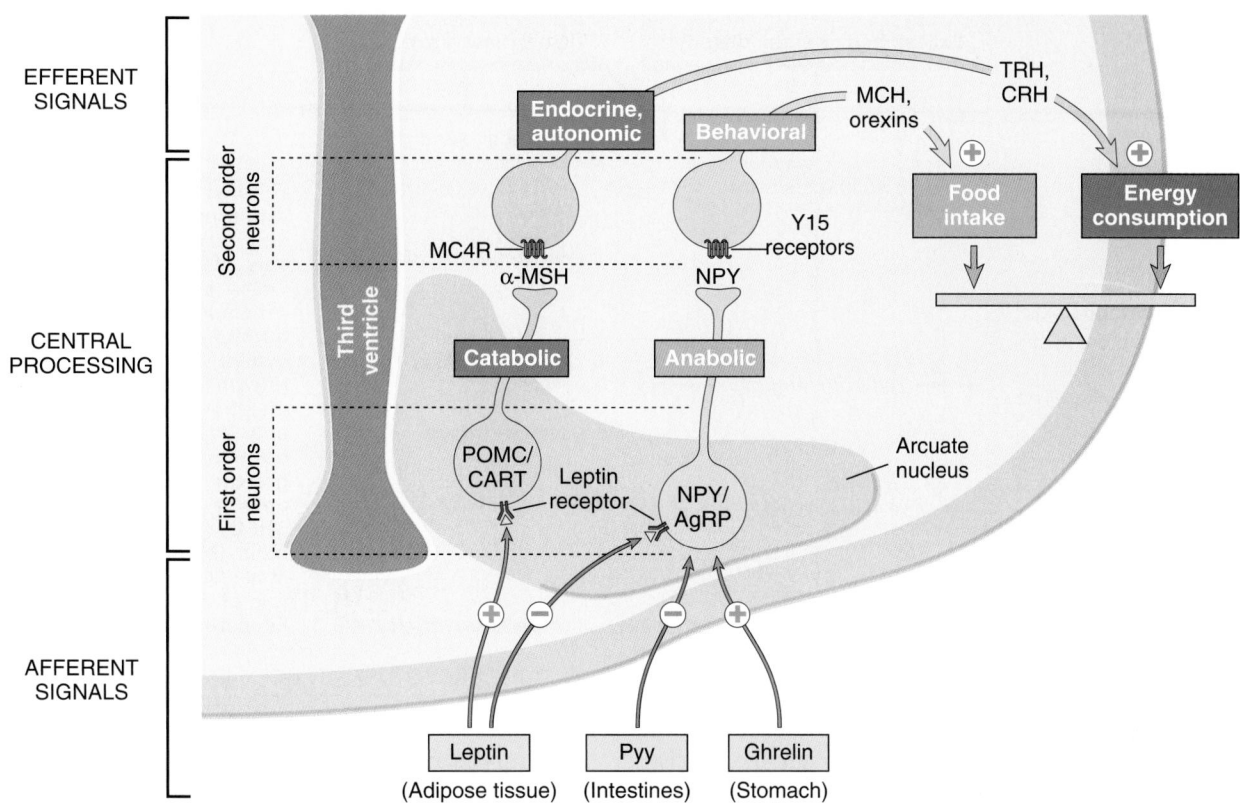

FIGURE 9–33 Neurohumoral circuits in the hypothalamus that regulate energy balance. Shown are POMC/CART anorexigenic neurons and NPY/AgRP orexigenic neurons in the arcuate nucleus of the hypothalamus, and their pathways. See text for details.

Adiponectin. *Injections of adiponectin in mice stimulate fatty acid oxidation in muscle, causing a decrease in fat mass.* This hormone is produced mainly by adipocytes. Its levels in the blood are very high, about 1000 times higher than those of other polypeptide hormones, and are lower in obese than in lean individuals.[66] Adiponectin, which has been called a "fat-burning molecule" and the "guardian angel against obesity," directs fatty acids to muscle for their oxidation. It decreases the influx of fatty acids to the liver and the total hepatic triglyceride content, and also decreases the glucose production in the liver, causing an increase in insulin sensitivity and a protection against the metabolic syndrome (described later).[67] Adiponectin circulates as a complex of three, six, or even more aggregates of the monomeric form, and binds to two receptors, AdipoR1 and AdipoR2. These receptors are found in many tissues, including the brain, but AdipoR1 and AdipoR2 are most highly expressed in skeletal muscle and liver, respectively. Binding of adiponectin to its receptors triggers signals that activate cyclic adenosine monophosphate–activated protein kinase, which in turn phosphorylates and inactivates acetyl coenzyme A carboxylase, a key enzyme required for fatty acid synthesis.

Adipose Tissue. *In addition to leptin and adiponectin, adipose tissue produces cytokines such as TNF, IL-6, IL-1, and IL-18, chemokines, and steroid hormones.* The increased production of cytokines and chemokines by adipose tissue in obese patients creates a chronic sub-clinical (asymptomatic) inflammatory state that includes high levels of circulating C-reactive protein. Through its multiple activities, adipose tissue participates in the control of energy balance and energy metabolism, functioning as a link between lipid metabolism, nutrition, and inflammatory responses. Thus, the adipocyte that was relegated to an obscure and passive role as the "Cinderella of cells of metabolism," is now "the Belle of the Ball" at the forefront of metabolic research.[68]

The total number of adipocytes is established during childhood and adolescence, and it is higher in obese than in lean individuals.[69] In adults the number of adipocytes remains constant, even after losses or weight gains, but there is a continuous turnover of the cell population. It is estimated that approximately 10% of adipocytes are renewed annually, regardless of the level of the individual's body mass. Thus, although the fat mass in an adult person can increase through the enlargement of existing adipocytes, their number is tightly controlled, and is predetermined in childhood and adolescence. In individuals who lose weight after dietary regimens, the well-known difficulties in maintaining weight losses are, in part, a consequence of the lack of a decrease in the number of adipocytes, and the enhanced appetite caused by leptin deficiency.

Gut Hormones. Gut peptides act as short-term meal initiators and terminators. They include ghrelin, PYY, pancreatic polypeptide, insulin, and amylin among others.[70] *Ghrelin* is produced in the stomach and in the arcuate nucleus of the hypothalamus. *It is the only known gut hormone that increases food intake (orexigenic effect).* Its injection in rodents elicits voracious feeding, even after repeated administration. Long-term injections cause weight gain, by increasing caloric intake and reducing energy utilization. Ghrelin acts by binding the growth hormone secretagogue receptor, which is abundant in

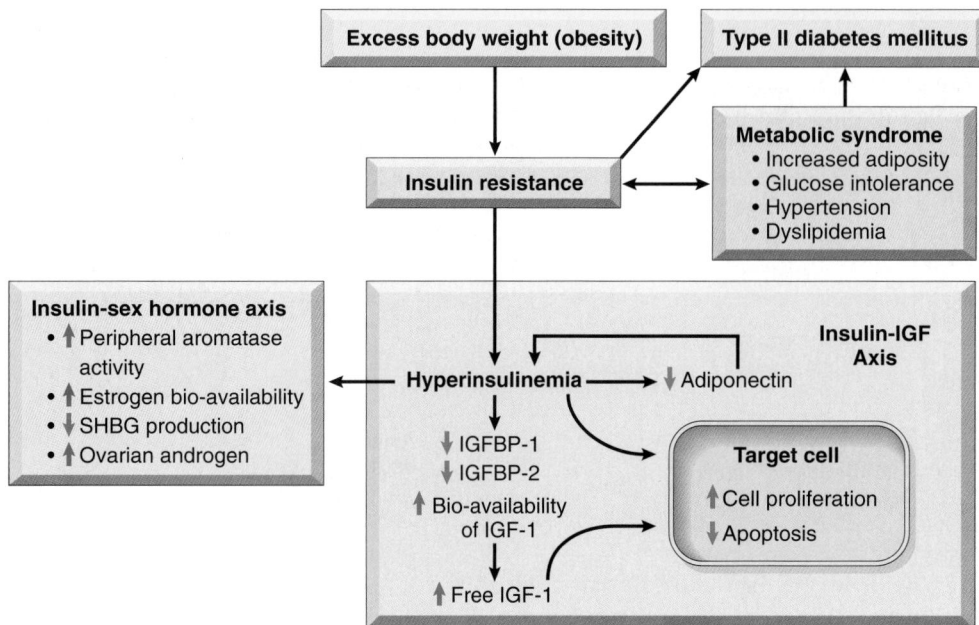

FIGURE 9–34 Obesity, metabolic syndrome, and cancer. Obesity and excessive weight are precursors of the metabolic syndrome, which is associated with insulin resistance, type 2 diabetes, and hormonal changes. Increases in insulin and IGF-1 (insulin-like growth factor-1) stimulate cell proliferation and inhibit apoptosis and may contribute to tumor development. IGF, insulin-like growth factor; IGFBP, insulin-like growth factor–binding protein; SHBG, sex hormone–binding globulin. (Modified from Renehan AG et al.: Obesity and cancer risk: the role of the insulin-I6F axis. Trends Endocrinol Metab 17:328, 2006.)

the hypothalamus and the pituitary. Although the precise mechanisms of ghrelin action have not been identified, it most likely stimulates NPY/AgRP neurons to increase food intake. Ghrelin levels rise before meals and fall between 1 and 2 hours after eating. However, in obese individuals the postprandial suppression of ghrelin is attenuated, leading to maintenance of the obesity.

PYY is secreted from endocrine cells in the ileum and colon. Plasma levels of PYY are low during fasting and increase shortly after food intake. Intravenous administration of PYY reduces energy intake, and its levels generally increase after gastric bypass surgery. By contrast, levels of PYY generally decrease in individuals with the *Prader-Willi syndrome* (caused by loss of imprinted genes on chromosome 15q11–q13),[71] and may contribute to the development of *hyperphagia and obesity* in these persons. These observations have led to ongoing work to produce PYYs for the treatment of obesity. *Amylin*, a peptide secreted with insulin from pancreatic β-cells that reduces food intake and weight gain, is also being evaluated for the treatment of obesity and diabetes. Both PYY and amylin act centrally by stimulating POMC/CART neurons in the hypothalamus, causing a decrease in food intake.

General Consequences of Obesity

Obesity, *particularly central obesity, increases the risk for a number of conditions, including type 2 diabetes and cardiovascular disease* (Fig. 9–34). Obesity is the main driver of a cluster of alterations known as the *metabolic syndrome* characterized by visceral or intra-abdominal adiposity, insulin resistance, hyperinsulinemia, glucose intolerance, hypertension, hypertriglyceridemia, and low HDL cholesterol (Chapter 11).

- Obesity is associated with *insulin resistance* and *hyperinsulinemia*, important features of type 2 diabetes, and weight loss is associated with improvement (Chapter 24). It has

been speculated that excess insulin, in turn, may play a role in the retention of sodium, expansion of blood volume, production of excess norepinephrine, and smooth muscle proliferation that are the hallmarks of hypertension. Regardless of the nature of the pathogenic mechanisms, *the risk of developing hypertension among previously normotensive persons increases proportionately with weight.*

- Obese persons generally have hypertriglyceridemia and low HDL, and these may increase the risk of *coronary artery disease* in the very obese. It should be emphasized that the association between obesity and heart disease is not straightforward, and such linkage as there may be relates more to the associated diabetes and hypertension than to weight.

- Obesity is associated with *non-alcoholic fatty liver disease* (Chapter 18). This condition occurs most often in diabetic patients and can progress to fibrosis and cirrhosis. *Cholelithiasis (gallstones)* is six times more common in obese than in lean subjects. An increase in total body cholesterol, increased cholesterol turnover, and augmented biliary excretion of cholesterol all act to predispose to the formation of cholesterol-rich gallstones (Chapter 18).

- *Obesity is associated with hypoventilation and hypersomnolence. Hypoventilation syndrome* is a constellation of respiratory abnormalities in very obese persons. It has been called the *pickwickian syndrome*, after the fat lad who was constantly falling asleep in Charles Dickens' *Pickwick Papers*. Hypersomnolence, both at night and during the day, is characteristic and is often associated with apneic pauses during sleep, polycythemia, and eventual right-sided heart failure.

- Marked adiposity predisposes to the development of degenerative joint disease (*osteoarthritis*). This form of arthritis, which typically appears in older persons, is attributed in large part to the cumulative effects of increased load on weight-bearing joints.

Obesity and Cancer

Approximately 4% of cancers in men and 7% in women are associated with obesity.[72] Data on the relationships between obesity and cancer have been obtained from the Million Women Study that examined the relationship between BMI and cancer in women aged 50 to 64 years in the United Kingdom, and from a systematic analysis of published data sets involving more than 280,000 cases of cancer in men and women.[73,74]

1. In men, a BMI greater than 25 kg/m^2 correlated strongly with an increased incidence of adenocarcinoma of the esophagus, and cancers of the thyroid, colon, and kidney.
2. In women, a BMI greater than 25 kg/m^2 correlated strongly with an increased incidence of adenocarcinoma of the esophagus, and of endometrial, gallbladder, and kidney cancers.

The mechanisms by which obesity is associated with these specific types of cancers are unknown, but a proposed hypothesis is that *the increased cancer risk in obese individuals is a consequence of hyperinsulinemia and insulin resistance* (Fig. 9–34). Insulin at high concentrations has multiple effects on cell growth, including the activation of phosphatidylinositol 3-kinase, extracellular-signal-regulated kinases 1 and 2, β-catenin, and Ras. All of these are important components of pathways that are dysregulated during cancer development. *Hyperinsulinemia also causes an increase in insulin-like growth factor-1 (IGF-1) concentrations, because insulin inhibits the production of the IGF-binding proteins IGFBP-1 and IGFBP-2.* IGF-1 is a mitogenic and anti-apoptotic agent that is highly expressed in many human cancers.[75] It binds with high affinity to the IGF-1R receptor, and with low affinity to the insulin receptor. IGF-1 activates many of the cell growth pathways that are also activated by insulin, and increases the production of vascular endothelial growth factor, by inducing the expression of hypoxia-inducible factor 1.

In addition to the obesity-associated effects of insulin and IGF-1 in cell growth pathways, obesity and hyperinsulimia have an effect on steroid hormones that regulate cell growth and differentiation in the breast, uterus, and other tissues: (1) obesity increases the synthesis of estrogen from androgen precursors through an effect of adipose tissue aromatases; (2) insulin increases androgen synthesis in ovaries and adrenals, and enhances estrogen availability in obese persons by inhibiting the production of sex-hormone-binding globulin (SHBG) in the liver (see Fig. 9–34).

As already discussed in this chapter, adiponectin, secreted mostly from adipose tissue, is an abundant hormone that is inversely correlated with obesity and acts as an insulin-sensitizing agent. Thus, *the decreased levels of adiponectin in obese persons contribute to hyperinsulinemia and the impairment of insulin sensitivity.*

DIETS, CANCER, AND ATHEROSCLEROSIS

Diet and Cancer

The incidence of specific cancers varies widely throughout the world. The frequency of some tumors varies as much as 100-fold in different geographic areas. It is also well known that differences in incidence of various cancers is not fixed and can be modified by nongenetic factors, including changes in diet. For instance, the incidence of colon cancer in Japanese men and women 55 to 60 years of age was negligible about 50 years ago, but it is now higher than that in men of the same age in the United Kingdom.[76] Studies have also shown a progressive increase in colon cancers in Japanese populations as they moved from Japan to Hawaii and from there to the continental United States. Nevertheless, despite the very large amount of experimental and epidemiologic research, relatively few mechanisms that link diets and specific types of cancer have been established.

With respect to carcinogenesis, three aspects of the diet are of major concern: (1) the content of exogenous carcinogens, (2) the endogenous synthesis of carcinogens from dietary components, and (3) the lack of protective factors.

- Regarding *exogenous* substances, *aflatoxin* is involved in the development of hepatocellular carcinomas in parts of Asia and Africa, generally in cooperation with hepatitis B virus. Exposure to aflatoxin causes a specific mutation in codon 249 of the *p53* gene; when found in hepatocellular carcinomas, this mutation serves as a molecular signature for aflatoxin exposure. Debate continues about the carcinogenicity of food additives, artificial sweeteners, and contaminating pesticides. Some artificial sweeteners (cyclamates and saccharin) have been implicated in bladder cancers, but convincing evidence is lacking.

- The concern about *endogenous* synthesis of carcinogens or enhancers of carcinogenicity from components of the diet relates principally to gastric carcinomas. *Nitrosamines and nitrosamides* are implicated in the generation of these tumors in humans, because they have been clearly shown to induce gastric cancer in animals. These compounds can be formed in the body from nitrites and amines or amides derived from digested proteins. Sources of nitrites include sodium nitrite added to foods as a preservative, and nitrates, present in common vegetables, which are reduced in the gut by bacterial flora. There is, then, the potential for endogenous production of carcinogenic agents from dietary components, which might well have an effect on the stomach.

- *High animal fat intake combined with low fiber intake has been implicated in the causation of colon cancer.* It has been estimated that doubling the average level of total fiber consumption to about 40 gm/day per person in most populations may decrease the risk of colon cancer by 50%.[75] The most convincing explanation of this association is that high fat intake increases the level of bile acids in the gut, which in turn modifies intestinal flora, favoring the growth of microaerophilic bacteria. Bile acid metabolites produced by these bacteria may function as carcinogens. The *protective effect of a high-fiber diet* might relate to (1) increased stool bulk and decreased transit time, which decreases the exposure of mucosa to putative offenders, and (2) the capacity of certain fibers to bind carcinogens and thereby protect the mucosa. However, attempts to document these theories in clinical and experimental studies have not generated consistent results.

- Although epidemiologic data from large populations show a strong positive correlation between total dietary fat intake and breast cancer, *it is still unclear whether increased fat consumption has a causal relationship to breast cancer development.*
- Vitamins C and E, β-carotenes, and selenium have been assumed to have anticarcinogenic effects because of their antioxidant properties. However, thus far there is no convincing evidence that these antioxidants act as chemopreventive agents. As discussed earlier in this chapter, retinoids are effective agents in the therapy of acute promyelocytic leukemia, and associations between low levels of vitamin D and cancer of the colon, prostate, and breast have been reported.

Thus, we must conclude that despite many tantalizing trends and proclamations by "diet gurus," thus far there is no definitive proof that a particular diet can cause or prevent cancer. On the other hand, given the relationships between obesity and cancer development, prevention of obesity through the consumption of a healthy diet is a commonsense measure that goes a long way in preserving good health. Concern persists that carcinogens lurk in things as pleasurable as a juicy steak, a rich ice cream, and in nuts contaminated with aflatoxin.

Diet and Atherosclerosis

A most important and controversial issue is the contribution of diet to atherogenesis. The central question is "can dietary modification—specifically, reduction in the consumption of cholesterol and saturated animal fats (e.g., eggs, butter, beef)—reduce serum cholesterol levels and prevent or retard the development of atherosclerosis (most importantly, coronary heart disease)?" The average adult in the United States consumes a large amount of fat and cholesterol daily, with a ratio of saturated fatty acids to polyunsaturated fatty acids of about 3 : 1. Lowering this ratio to 1 : 1 causes a 10% to 15% reduction in the serum cholesterol level within a few weeks. Vegetable oils (e.g., corn and safflower oils) and fish oil contain polyunsaturated fatty acids and are good sources of such cholesterol-lowering lipids. Fish oil fatty acids belonging to the omega-3 family have more double bonds than do the omega-6 fatty acids present in vegetable oils. A study of Dutch men whose usual daily diet contained 30 g of fish revealed a substantially lower frequency of death from coronary heart disease than that among comparable controls.

There is much talk about the role that caloric restriction and special diets may play in the control of body weight and prevention of cardiovascular disease. We offer just a few general observations on these topics.

- Caloric restriction has been convincingly demonstrated to decrease the incidence of some diseases, and to increase life span in experimental animals. The basis of this striking observation is not entirely clear but seems to depend on activation of sirtuins and on the lowering of insulin and IGF-1 levels (Chapter 1).[74] In calorie-restricted animals there is a more modest age-related decline in immunological functions, less oxidative damage, and greater resistance to carcinogenesis.

- Not surprisingly, there are a large number of commercial diets that are reported by its proponents to decrease the risk of heart disease. Among those are the low-carbohydrate diets (such as the Atkins Diet, the Zone, Sugar Busters, Protein Power), and others such as The Miami Diet/Hollywood 48-Hour Miracle Diet, and the South Beach Diet. The actual effect of these diets on heart disease is highly controversial.
- Most diets dictate what you cannot eat (of course, your favorite foods!). A better strategy is to simply focus on eating an enjoyable and healthy diet rich in fish, vegetables, whole grains, fruits, olive and peanut oils (to replace saturated and *trans* fats), complex carbohydrates (instead of simple carbohydrates contained in sweets and soft drinks), and low in salt (to control hypertension).
- Even lowly garlic has been touted to protect against heart disease (and also against, devils, werewolves, vampires, and, alas, kisses), although research has yet to prove this effect unequivocally. Of these, the effect on kisses is the best established!

REFERENCES

1. Stein C et al.: The global burden of disease assessments—WHO is responsible? PLoS Negl Trop Dis 1:e161, 2007.
2. Mathers CD et al.: Measuring the burden of neglected tropical diseases: the global burden of disease framework. PLoS Negl Trop Dis 1:e114, 2007.
3. Murray CJ et al.: Can we achieve Millennium Development Goal 4? New analysis of country trends and forecasts of under-5 mortality to 2015. Lancet 370:1040, 2007.
4. Jones KE et al.: Global trends in emerging infectious diseases. Nature 451:990, 2008.
5. Patz JA et al.: Impact of regional climate change on human health. Nature 438:310, 2005.
6. Shea KM: Global climate change and children's health. Pediatrics 120:e1359, 2007.
7. Patz JA, Kovats RS: Hotspots in climate change and human health. BMJ 325:1094, 2002.
8. McMichael AJ et al.: Climate change and human health: present and future risks. Lancet 367:859, 2006.
9. Iyanagi T: Molecular mechanism of phase I and phase II drug-metabolizing enzymes: implications for detoxification. Int Rev Cytol 260:35, 2007.
10. Tompkins LM, Wallace AD: Mechanisms of cytochrome P450 induction. J Biochem Mol Toxicol 21:176, 2007.
11. Pichavant M et al.: Ozone exposure in a mouse model induces airway hyperreactivity that requires the presence of natural killer T cells and IL-17. J Exp Med 205:385, 2008.
12. McCreanor J et al.: Respiratory effects of exposure to diesel traffic in persons with asthma. N Engl J Med 357:2348, 2007.
13. Mills NL et al.: Ischemic and thrombotic effects of dilute diesel-exhaust inhalation in men with coronary heart disease. N Engl J Med 357:1075, 2007.
14. Bellinger DC, Bellinger AM: Childhood lead poisoning: the torturous path from science to policy. J Clin Invest 116:853, 2006.
15. Bellinger DC: Very low lead exposures and children's neurodevelopment. Curr Opin Pediatr 20:172, 2008.
16. Guzzi G, La Porta CA: Molecular mechanisms triggered by mercury. Toxicology 244:1, 2008.
17. Thompson WW et al.: Early thimerosal exposure and neuropsychological outcomes at 7 to 10 years. N Engl J Med 357:1281, 2007.
18. Vahidnia A et al.: Arsenic neurotoxicity—a review. Hum Exp Toxicol 26:823, 2007.
19. Ratnaike RN: Acute and chronic arsenic toxicity. Postgrad Med J 79:391, 2003.
20. Parvez F et al.: Non-malignant respiratory effects of chronic arsenic exposure from drinking water in never-smokers in Bangladesh. Environ Health Perspect 116:190, 2008.

21. Nawrot T et al.: Environmental exposure to cadmium and risk of cancer: a prospective population-based study. Lancet Oncol 7:119, 2006.

22. Kenfield SA et al.: Smoking and smoking cessation in relation to mortality in women. JAMA 299:2037, 2008.

23. Sun S et al.: Lung cancer in never smokers—a different disease. Nat Rev Cancer 7:778, 2007.

24. Seitz HK, Stickel F: Molecular mechanisms of alcohol-mediated carcinogenesis. Nat Rev Cancer 7:599, 2007.

25. Bailey BA, Sokol RJ: Pregnancy and alcohol use: evidence and recommendations for prenatal care. Clin Obst Gyn 51:436, 2008.

26. Baur JA et al:. Resveratrol improves health and survival of mice on a high-calorie diet. Nature 444:337, 2006.

27. Lagouge M et al.: Resveratrol improves mitochondrial function and protects against metabolic disease by activating SIRT1 and PGC-1alpha. Cell 127:1109, 2006.

28. MacLennan AH. HRT: a reappraisal of the risks and benefits. Med J Aust 186:643, 2007.

29. Li CI et al.: Relationship between menopausal hormone therapy and risk of ductal, lobular, and ductal-lobular breast carcinomas. Cancer Epidemiol Biomarkers Prev 17:43, 2008.

30. Mendelsohn ME, Karas RH: HRT and the young at heart. N Engl J Med 356:2639, 2007.

31. American Society for Reproductive Medicine: Hormonal contraception: recent advances and controversies. Fertil Steril 86:S229, 2006.

32. Bessems JG, Vermeulen NP: Paracetamol (acetaminophen)-induced toxicity: molecular and biochemical mechanisms, analogues and protective approaches. Crit Rev Toxicol 31:55, 2001.

33. Liu ZX, Kaplowitz N: Role of innate immunity in acetaminophen-induced hepatotoxicity. Expert Opin Drug Metab Toxicol 2:493, 2006.

34. Bamford NS et al.: Repeated exposure to methamphetamine causes long-lasting presynaptic corticostriatal depression that is renormalized with drug readministration. Neuron 58:89, 2008.

35. Wilkins MR: Cannabis and cannabis-based medicines: potential benefits and risks to health. Clin Med 6:16, 2006.

36. Pagotto U et al.: The emerging role of the endocannabinoid system in endocrine regulation and energy balance. Endocr Rev 27:73, 2006.

37. Kunos G, Osei-Hyiaman D: Endocannabinoid involvement in obesity and hepatic steatosis. Am J Physiol Gastrointest Liver Physiol 294:G1101, 2008.

38. Gibran NS et al.: Cutaneous wound healing. J Burn Care Res 28:577, 2007.

39. Scott JR et al.: Making sense of hypertrophic scar: a role for nerves. Wound Repair Regen 15 (Suppl 1):S27, 2007.

40. Durham WJ et al.: RyR1 S-nitrosylation underlies environmental heat stroke and sudden death in Y522S RyR1 knockin mice. Cell 133:53, 2008.

41. Stone HB et al.: Effects of radiation on normal tissue: consequences and mechanisms. Lancet Oncol 4:529, 2003.

42. Wright EG, Coates PJ: Untargeted effects of ionizing radiation: implications for radiation pathology. Mutat Res 597:119, 2006.

43. Hagelstrom RT et al.: DNA-PKcs and ATM influence the generation of ionizing radiation-induced bystander effects. Oncogene Epub, 2008.

44. Brenner DJ et al.: Cancer risks attributable to low doses of ionizing radiation: assessing what we really know. Proc Natl Acad Sci U S A 100:13761, 2003.

45. Brenner DJ, Hall EJ: Computed tomography—an increasing source of radiation exposure. N Engl J Med 357:2277, 2007.

46. Schaible UE, Kaufmann SH: Malnutrition and infection: complex mechanisms and global impacts. PLoS Med 4:e115, 2007.

47. Acharyya S, Guttridge DC: Cancer cachexia signaling pathways continue to emerge yet much still points to the proteasome. Clin Cancer Res 13:1356, 2007.

48. Acharyya S et al.: Dystrophin glycoprotein complex dysfunction: a regulatory link between muscular dystrophy and cancer cachexia. Cancer Cell 8:421, 2005.

49. Kaye W: Neurobiology of anorexia and bulimia nervosa. Physiol Behav 94:121, 2008.

50. Ziouzenkova O, Plutzky J: Retinoid metabolism and nuclear receptor responses: new insights into coordinated regulation of the PPAR-RXR complex. FEBS Lett 582:32, 2008.

51. Germain P et al.: International Union of Pharmacology. LX. Retinoic acid receptors. Pharmacol Rev 58:712, 2006.

52. Ziouzenkova O, Plutsky J: Retinoid metabolism and nuclear receptor responses: new insights into coordinated regulation of the PPAR-RXR complex. FEBS Lett 9:582, 2008.

53. Holick MF: Resurrection of vitamin D deficiency and rickets. J Clin Invest 116:2062, 2006.

54. Rajakumar K et al.: Solar ultraviolet radiation and vitamin D: a historical perspective. Am J Public Health 97:1746, 2007.

55. Deeb KK et al.: Vitamin D signalling pathways in cancer: potential for anticancer therapeutics. Nat Rev Cancer 7:684, 2007.

56. Mensenkamp AR et al.: TRPV5, the gateway to Ca^{2+} homeostasis. Handb Exp Pharmacol 179:207, 2007.

57. Hoenderop JG et al.: Calcium absorption across epithelia. Physiol Rev 85:373, 2005.

58. Berndt T, Kumar R: Phosphatonins and the regulation of phosphate homeostasis. Annu Rev Physiol 69:341, 2007.

59. Holick MF: Vitamin D deficiency. N Engl J Med 357:266, 2007.

60. Schauber J et al.: Histone acetylation in keratinocytes enables control of the expression of cathelicidin and CD14 by 1,25-dihydroxyvitamin D3. J Invest Dermatol 128:816, 2008.

61. Adams JS, Hewison M: Unexpected actions of vitamin D: new perspectives on the regulation of innate and adaptive immunity. Nat Clin Pract Endocrinol Metab 4:80, 2008.

62. Wang Y, Beydoun MA: The obesity epidemic in the United States—gender, age, socioeconomic, racial/ethnic, and geographic characteristics: a systematic review and meta-regression analysis. Epidemiol Rev 29:6, 2007.

63. Badman MK, Flier JS: The adipocyte as an active participant in energy balance and metabolism. Gastroenterology 132:2103, 2007.

64. Froguel P, Blakemore AIF: The power of the extreme in elucidating obesity. N Engl J Med 359:891, 2008.

65. Lam QL, Lu L: Role of leptin in immunity. Cell Mol Immunol 4:1, 2007.

66. Guerre-Millo M: Adiponectin: an update. Diabetes Metab 34:12, 2008.

67. Garaulet M et al.: Adiponectin, the controversial hormone. Public Health Nutr 10:1145, 2007.

68. O'Rahilly S: Human obesity and insulin resistance: lessons from experiments of nature. Novartis Found Symp 286:13, 2007.

69. Spalding KL et al.: Dynamics of fat cell turnover in humans. Nature 453:783, 2008.

70. Huda MS et al.: Gut peptides and the regulation of appetite. Obes Rev 7:163, 2006.

71. Davies W et al.: Imprinted genes and neuroendocrine function. Front Neuroendocrinol 29:413, 2007.

72. Polednak AP: Estimating the number of U.S. incidence cancers attributable to obesity and the impact on temporal trends in incidence rates for obesity-related cancers. Cancer Detect Prev Epub, 2008.

73. Reeves GK et al.: Cancer incidence and mortality in relation to body mass index in the Million Women Study: cohort study. BMJ 335:1134, 2007.

74. Renehan AG et al.: Body-mass index and incidence of cancer: a systematic review and meta-analysis of prospective observational studies. Lancet 371:569, 2008.

75. Renehan AG et al.: Obesity and cancer risk: the role of the insulin-IGF axis. Trends Endocrinol Metab 17:328, 2006.

76. Bingham S, Riboli E: Diet and cancer—the European Prospective Investigation into Cancer and Nutrition. Nat Rev Cancer 4:206, 2004.

10

Diseases of Infancy and Childhood

ANIRBAN MAITRA

Congenital Anomalies
  Definitions
  Causes of Anomalies
    Genetic Causes
    Environmental Causes
    Multifactorial Causes
  Pathogenesis of Congenital Anomalies
Disorders of Prematurity
  **Causes of Prematurity and Fetal Growth
    Restriction**
  Neonatal Respiratory Distress Syndrome
  Necrotizing Enterocolitis
Perinatal Infections
  Transcervical (Ascending) Infections
  Transplacental (Hematologic) Infections
  Sepsis

Fetal Hydrops
  Immune Hydrops
  Nonimmune Hydrops
**Inborn Errors of Metabolism and Other
  Genetic Disorders**
  Phenylketonuria (PKU)
  Galactosemia
  Cystic Fibrosis (Mucoviscidosis)
Sudden Infant Death Syndrome (SIDS)
**Tumors and Tumor-like Lesions of
  Infancy and Childhood**
  Benign Tumors and Tumor-like Lesions
  Malignant Tumors
    Incidence and Types
    The Neuroblastic Tumors
    Wilms Tumor

Children are not merely little adults, and their diseases are not merely variants of adult diseases. Many childhood conditions are unique to, or at least take distinctive forms in, this stage of life and so are discussed separately in this chapter. Diseases originating in the perinatal period are important in that they account for significant morbidity and mortality. As would be expected, the chances for survival of live-born infants improve with each passing week. This progress represents, at least in part, a triumph of improved medical care. Better prenatal care, more effective methods of monitoring the condition of the fetus, and judicious resort to cesarean section before term when there is evidence of fetal distress,

have all contributed toward bringing into this "mortal coil" live-born infants who in past years might have been stillborn. These infants represent an increased number of *high-risk* infants. Nonetheless, the infant mortality rate in the United States has shown a decline from a level of 20.0 deaths per 1000 live births in 1970 to about 6.8 deaths in 2004, the latest year for which these data are systematically available.[1] Although the death rate has continued to decline for all infants, African Americans continue to have an infant mortality rate more than twice (13.6 deaths per 1000 live births) that of American whites (5.6 deaths). Worldwide, infant mortality rates vary widely, from as low as 2.3 deaths per 1000

447

live births in Singapore, to as high as 180 deaths in the African subcontinent.

Each stage of development of the infant and child is prey to a somewhat different group of disorders. The data available permit a survey of four time spans: (1) the neonatal period (the first 4 weeks of life), (2) infancy (the first year of life), (3) age 1 to 4 years, and (4) age 5 to 14 years.

The major causes of death in infancy and childhood are listed in Table 10–1. Congenital anomalies, disorders relating to short gestation (prematurity) and low birth weight, and sudden infant death syndrome (SIDS) represent the leading causes of death in the first 12 months of life. Once the infant survives the first year of life, the outlook brightens measurably. In the next two age groups—1 to 4 years and 5 to 14 years— injuries resulting from accidents have become the leading cause of death. Among the natural diseases, in order of importance, congenital anomalies and malignant neoplasms assume major significance. It would appear then that, in a sense, life is an obstacle course. For the great majority, the obstacles are surmounted or, even better, bypassed.

We now take a closer look at the specific conditions encountered during the various stages of infant and child development.

Congenital Anomalies

Congenital anomalies are morphologic defects that are present at birth, but some, such as cardiac defects and renal anomalies, may not become clinically apparent until years later. The term *congenital* means "born with," but it does not imply or exclude a genetic basis for the birth defect. It is estimated that about 120,000 (1 in 33) babies are born with a birth defect each year in the United States. They are the most common cause of mortality in the first year and contribute significantly to morbidity and mortality throughout the early years of life. In a sense, anomalies found in live-born infants represent the less serious developmental failures in embryogenesis that are compatible with live birth. Perhaps 20% of fertilized ova are so anomalous that they are blighted from the outset. Others may be compatible with early fetal development, only to lead to spontaneous abortion. Less severe anomalies allow more prolonged intrauterine survival, with some disorders terminating in stillbirth and those still less significant permitting live birth despite the handicaps imposed.

DEFINITIONS

Before proceeding, we define some of the terms used for various kinds of errors in morphogenesis—*malformations, disruptions, deformations, sequences,* and *syndromes.*

- *Malformations* represent primary errors of morphogenesis, in which there is an *intrinsically abnormal developmental process* (Fig. 10–1). They are usually associated with multiple genetic loci (multifactorial) and not the result of a single-gene or chromosomal defect. Malformations may present in several patterns. Some, such as congenital heart defects and anencephaly (absence of brain), involve single body systems, whereas in other cases multiple malformations involving many organs may coexist.

TABLE 10–1 Cause of Death Related with Age	
Causes*	**Rate†**
UNDER 1 YEAR	**685.2**
Congenital malformations, deformations, and chromosomal anomalies	
Disorders related to short gestation and low birth weight	
Sudden infant death syndrome (SIDS)	
Newborn affected by maternal complications of pregnancy	
Newborn affected by complications of placenta, cord, and membranes	
Respiratory distress of newborn	
Accidents (unintentional injuries)	
Bacterial sepsis of newborn	
Intrauterine hypoxia and birth asphyxia	
Diseases of the circulatory system	
1–4 YEARS	**29.9**
Accidents and adverse effects	
Congenital malformations, deformations, and chromosomal abnormalities	
Malignant neoplasms	
Homicide and legal intervention	
Diseases of the heart‡	
Influenza and pneumonia	
5–14 YEARS	**16.8**
Accidents and adverse effects	
Malignant neoplasms	
Homicide and legal intervention	
Congenital malformations, deformations, and chromosomal abnormalities	
Suicide	
Diseases of the heart	
15–24 YEARS	**80.1**
Accidents and adverse effects	
Homicide	
Suicide	
Malignant neoplasms	
Diseases of the heart	

*Causes are listed in decreasing order of frequency. All causes and rates are final 2004 statistics.
†Rates are expressed per 100,000 population from all causes within each age group.
‡Excludes congenital heart disease.
From Minino AM et al.: Deaths: final data for 2004. National Vital Statistics Rep 55:19, 2007.

- *Disruptions* result from secondary destruction of an organ or body region that was previously normal in development; thus, in contrast to malformations, disruptions arise from an *extrinsic disturbance in morphogenesis.* Amniotic bands, denoting rupture of amnion with resultant formation of "bands" that encircle, compress, or attach to parts of the developing fetus, are the classic example of a disruption (Fig. 10–2). A variety of environmental agents may cause disruptions (see below). Understandably, disruptions are not heritable and hence are not associated with risk of recurrence in subsequent pregnancies.
- *Deformations*, like disruptions, also represent an *extrinsic disturbance of development* rather than an intrinsic error of morphogenesis. Deformations are common problems, affecting approximately 2% of newborn infants to varying degrees. Fundamental to the pathogenesis of deformations

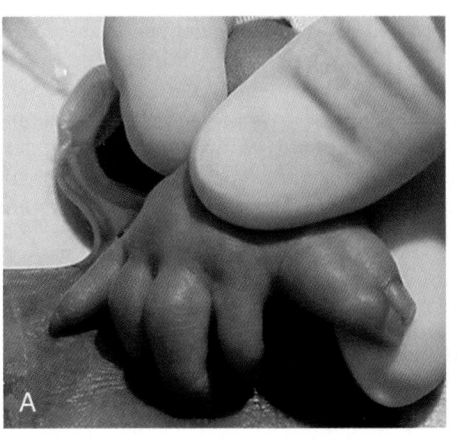
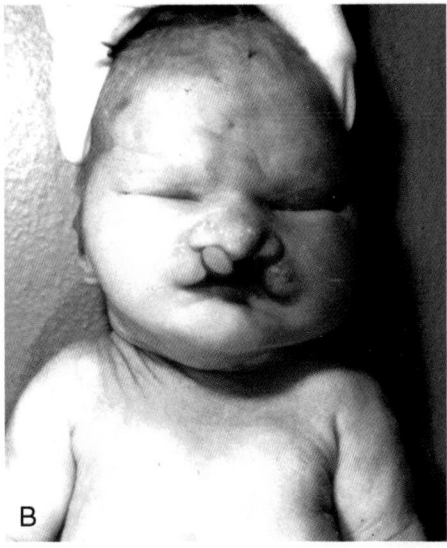
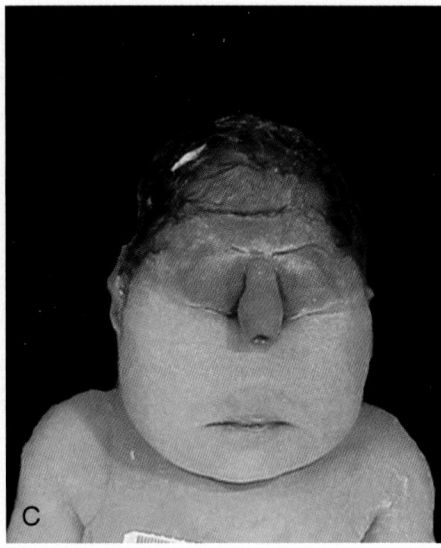

FIGURE 10–1 Examples of malformations. *Polydactyly* (one or more extra digits) and *syndactyly* (fusion of digits), both of which are illustrated in **A**, have little functional consequence when they occur in isolation. Similarly, *cleft lip* (**B**), with or without associated *cleft palate*, is compatible with life when it occurs as an isolated anomaly; in the present case, however, this neonate had an underlying *malformation syndrome* (trisomy 13) and expired because of severe cardiac defects. **C,** The stillbirth illustrated represents a severe and essentially lethal malformation, wherein the midface structures are fused or ill-formed; in almost all cases, this degree of external dysmorphogenesis is associated with severe internal anomalies such as maldevelopment of the brain and cardiac defects. (**A** and **C**, courtesy of Dr. Reade Quinton; and **B**, courtesy of Dr. Beverly Rogers, Department of Pathology, University of Texas Southwestern Medical Center, Dallas, TX.)

is localized or generalized compression of the growing fetus by *abnormal biomechanical forces*, leading eventually to a variety of structural abnormalities. The most common underlying factor responsible for deformations is *uterine constraint*. Between the thirty-fifth and thirty-eighth weeks of gestation, rapid increase in the size of the fetus outpaces the growth of the uterus, and the relative amount of amniotic fluid (which normally acts as a cushion) also decreases. Thus, even the normal fetus is subjected to some form of uterine constraint. Several factors increase the likelihood of

excessive compression of the fetus resulting in deformations. *Maternal factors* include first pregnancy, small uterus, malformed (bicornuate) uterus, and leiomyomas. *Fetal or placental factors* include oligohydramnios, multiple fetuses, and abnormal fetal presentation. An example of a deformation is clubfeet, often a component of Potter sequence, described later.

○ A *sequence* is a cascade of anomalies triggered by one initiating aberration. Approximately half the time, congenital anomalies occur singly; in the remaining cases, multiple congenital anomalies are recognized. In some instances the constellation of anomalies may be explained by a single, localized aberration in organogenesis (malformation, disruption, or deformation) that sets into motion secondary effects in other organs. A good example is the *oligohydramnios* (or *Potter*) *sequence* (Fig. 10–3). Oligohydramnios (decreased amniotic fluid) may be caused by a variety of

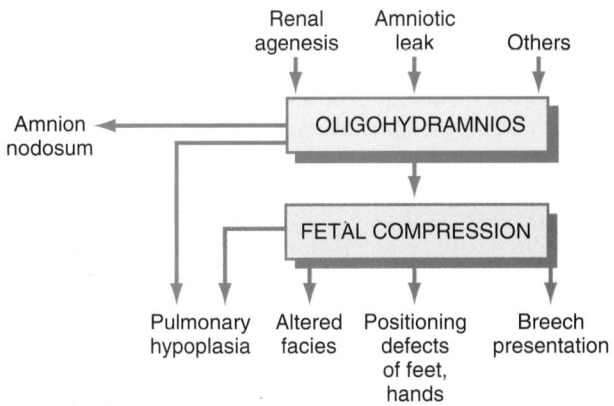

FIGURE 10–3 Schematic diagram of the pathogenesis of the oligohydramnios sequence.

FIGURE 10–2 Disruption of morphogenesis by an amniotic band. Note the placenta at the right of the diagram and the band of amnion extending from the top portion of the amniotic sac to encircle the leg of the fetus. (Courtesy of Dr. Theonia Boyd, Children's Hospital of Boston, Boston, MA.)

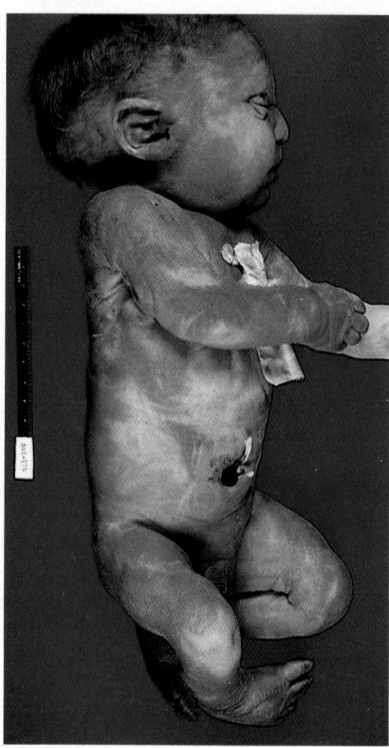

FIGURE 10–4 Infant with oligohydramnios sequence. Note the flattened facial features and deformed right foot (talipes equinovarus).

unrelated maternal, placental, or fetal abnormalities. Causes of oligohydramnios include chronic leakage of amniotic fluid because of rupture of the amnion, uteroplacental insufficiency resulting from maternal hypertension or severe toxemia, and renal agenesis in the fetus (because fetal urine is a major constituent of amniotic fluid). The fetal compression associated with significant oligohydramnios, in turn, results in a classic phenotype in the newborn infant, including flattened facies and positional abnormalities of the hands and feet (Fig. 10–4). The hips may be dislocated. Growth of the chest wall and the contained lungs is also compromised so that the lungs are frequently hypoplastic, occasionally to the degree that they are the cause of fetal demise. Nodules in the amnion (*amnion nodosum*) are frequently present.

- A *syndrome* is a constellation of congenital anomalies, believed to be pathologically related, that, in contrast to a sequence, *cannot* be explained on the basis of a single, localized, initiating defect. Syndromes are most often caused by a single etiologic agent, such as a viral infection or specific chromosomal abnormality, which simultaneously affects several tissues.

In addition to the aforementioned general definitions, a few organ-specific terms should be defined. *Agenesis* refers to the complete absence of an organ and its associated primordium. A closely related term, *aplasia*, refers also to the absence of an organ but one due to failure of development of the primordium. *Atresia* describes the absence of an opening, usually of a hollow visceral organ, such as the trachea and intestine. *Hypoplasia* refers to incomplete development or decreased size

of an organ with decreased numbers of cells, whereas *hyperplasia* refers to the converse, that is, the enlargement of an organ due to increased numbers of cells. An abnormality in an organ or a tissue as a result of an increase or a decrease in the size (rather than the number) of individual cells defines *hypertrophy* or *hypotrophy*, respectively. Finally, *dysplasia*, in the context of malformations (versus *neoplasia*) describes an abnormal organization of cells.

CAUSES OF ANOMALIES

At one time, it was believed that the presence of a visible, external anomaly was divine punishment for wickedness, a belief that occasionally jeopardized the mother's life. Although we are learning a great deal about some of the molecular bases of congenital anomalies, *the exact cause remains unknown in at least half to three quarters of the cases.* The common *known* causes of congenital anomalies can be grouped into three major categories: genetic, environmental, and multifactorial (Table 10–2).

Genetic Causes

Anomalies that are known to be genetic in origin can be divided into two groups:

- Those associated with chromosomal aberrations
- Those arising from single-gene mutations ("mendelian disorders")

TABLE 10–2 Causes of Congenital Anomalies in Humans

Cause	Frequency (%)
GENETIC	
Chromosomal aberrations	10–15
Mendelian inheritance	2–10
ENVIRONMENTAL	
Maternal/placental infections	2–3
Rubella	
Toxoplasmosis	
Syphilis	
Cytomegalovirus	
Human immunodeficiency virus	
Maternal disease states	6–8
Diabetes	
Phenylketonuria	
Endocrinopathies	
Drugs and chemicals	1
Alcohol	
Folic acid antagonists	
Androgens	
Phenytoin	
Thalidomide	
Warfarin	
13-*cis*-retinoic acid	
Others	
Irradiations	1
MULTIFACTORIAL	**20–25**
UNKNOWN	**40–60**

Adapted from Stevenson RE et al (eds): Human Malformations and related Anomalies. New York, Oxford University Press, 1993, p 115.

TABLE 10–3 National Prevalence Estimates for the Most Common Birth Defects in the United States, 1999–2001

Birth Defect	Estimated National Prevalence (per 10,000 live births)
CHROMOSOMAL DEFECTS	
Down syndrome (Trisomy 21)	12.8
Trisomy 13	1.3
Trisomy 18	2.3
OROFACIAL DEFECTS	
Cleft palate	6.4
Cleft lip with and without cleft palate	10.5
CARDIOVASCULAR DEFECTS	
Atrioventricular septal defect (endocardial cushion defect)	4.4
Transposition of great arteries	4.7
Tetrology of Fallot	3.9
CENTRAL NERVOUS SYSTEM DEFECTS	
Spina bifida without anencephalus	3.7
Anencephalus	2.5
GASTROINTESTINAL DEFECTS	
Rectal and large intestinal atresia/stenosis	4.8
Esophageal atresia/tracheoesophageal fistula	2.4
MUSCULOSKELETAL DEFECTS	
Gastroschisis	3.7
Diaphragmatic hernia	2.9
Omphalocele	2.1

Adapted from Canfield MA et al.: National estimates and race/ethnic-specific variation of selected birth defects in the United States, 1999–2001. Birth Defects Res A 76:747–756, 2006. The data have been adjusted for maternal race and ethnicity.

A third group is suspected of resulting from *multifactorial inheritance*, a term that implies the interaction of two or more genes of small effect with environmental factors, and is discussed separately.

Karyotypic abnormalities are present in approximately 10% to 15% of live-born infants with congenital anomalies, but trisomy 21 (Down syndrome) is the only one that approaches a birth frequency of greater than 10 in 10,000 total births. Next in order of frequency are trisomies 13 and 18 (Table 10–3). The remaining chromosomal syndromes associated with malformations are far rarer. *The great preponderance of these cytogenetic aberrations arises as defects in gametogenesis and so are not familial.* There are, however, several transmissible chromosomal abnormalities, for example, the form of Down syndrome associated with a robertsonian translocation in the parent, which is passed from one generation to the next, thus constituting a familial pattern of structural abnormalities (see Chapter 5). It should come as a sobering thought that *80% to 90% of fetuses with aneuploidy and other abnormalities of chromosome number die in utero, the majority in the earliest stages of gestation.*

Single-gene mutations of large effect may underlie major congenital anomalies, which, as expected, follow mendelian patterns of inheritance. Of these, approximately 90% are inherited in an autosomal dominant or recessive pattern, while the remainder segregates in an X-linked pattern. Not surprisingly, many of the mutations that give rise to birth defects involve loss of function of genes involved in normal organogenesis and development. For example, holoprosencephaly is the most common developmental defect of the forebrain and midface in humans (see Chapter 28); the Hedgehog signaling pathway plays a critical role in the morphogenesis of these structures, and loss-of-function mutations of individual components within this pathway are reported in families with a history of recurrent holoprosencephaly.[2] Similarly, achondroplasia, which is the most common form of short-limb dwarfism, is caused by gain-of-function mutations in *fibroblast growth factor receptor 3 (FGFR3)*.[3] The FGFR3 protein is a negative regulator of bone growth, and the activating FGFR3 mutations in achondroplasia are thought to exaggerate this physiologic inhibition, resulting in dwarfism.

Environmental Causes

Environmental influences, such as viral infections, drugs, and irradiation to which the mother was exposed during pregnancy, may cause fetal malformations (the appellation of "malformation" is loosely used in this context, since technically these anomalies represent *disruptions*).

Viruses. Many viruses have been implicated in causing malformations, including the agents responsible for rubella, cytomegalic inclusion disease, herpes simplex, varicella-zoster infection, influenza, mumps, human immunodeficiency virus (HIV), and enterovirus infections. Among these, the rubella virus and cytomegalovirus are the most extensively investigated agents. With all viruses, the gestational age at which the infection occurs in the mother is critically important. *The at-risk period for rubella infection extends from shortly before conception to the sixteenth week of gestation*, the hazard being greater in the first 8 weeks than in the second 8 weeks. The incidence of malformations is reduced from 50% to 20% to 7% if infection occurs in the first, second, or third month of gestation. The fetal defects are varied, but the major tetrad comprises cataracts, heart defects (persistent ductus arteriosus, pulmonary artery hypoplasia or stenosis, ventricular septal defect, tetralogy of Fallot), deafness, and mental retardation, referred to as *congenital rubella syndrome.*

Intrauterine infection with cytomegalovirus, mostly asymptomatic, is the most common fetal viral infection. This viral disease is considered in detail in Chapter 8; *the highest at-risk period is the second trimester of pregnancy.* Because organogenesis is largely completed by the end of the first trimester, congenital malformations occur less frequently than in rubella; nevertheless, the effects of virus-induced injury on the formed organs are often severe. Involvement of the central nervous system is a major feature, and the most prominent clinical changes are mental retardation, microcephaly, deafness, and hepatosplenomegaly.

Drugs and Other Chemicals. A variety of drugs and chemicals have been suspected to be teratogenic, but perhaps less than 1% of congenital malformations are caused by these agents. The list includes thalidomide, folate antagonists, androgenic hormones, alcohol, anticonvulsants, warfarin (oral anticoagulant), and 13-*cis*-retinoic acid used in the treatment of severe acne (see below). In many instances experimental studies in lower organisms (chick, zebrafish, etc.) have been instrumental in elucidating which developmental pathway(s) is affected by a given teratogen. For example, *thalidomide*, once used as a tranquilizer in Europe, caused an extremely high frequency (50% to 80%) of limb abnormalities in exposed fetuses. The mechanism of thalidomide teratogenicity involves downregulation of the developmentally important wingless (WNT) signaling pathway through upregulation of endogenous WNT repressors.[4] Thalidomide and related drugs have staged a remarkable comeback as antineoplastic agents, with potent immunomodulatory and anti-angiogenic properties. Much caution must be taken when these drugs are given to cancer patients who are of reproductive age. *Alcohol* is probably the most widely used teratogen. Alcohol is responsible for several structural anomalies, as well as more subtle cognitive and behavioral defects in the fetus, collectively termed *fetal alcohol spectrum disorders* (FASDs). The most severely affected infants with FASDs have growth retardation, microcephaly, atrial septal defect, short palpebral fissures, and maxillary hypoplasia, and this classic teratogenic phenotype is labeled as *fetal alcohol syndrome.* Experiments performed in animals suggest that prenatal exposure to alcohol disrupts at least two seminal developmental signaling pathways—retinoic acid and Hedgehog—with critical roles during development.[5,6] While cigarette smoke–derived nicotine has not been convincingly demonstrated to be a teratogen, there is a high incidence of spontaneous abortions, premature labor, and placental abnormalities in pregnant smokers; babies born to smoking mothers often have a low birth weight and may be prone to SIDS (see later). *In light of these findings, it is best to avoid nicotine exposure altogether during pregnancy.*

Radiation. In addition to being mutagenic and carcinogenic, radiation is teratogenic. Exposure to heavy doses of radiation during the period of organogenesis leads to malformations, such as microcephaly, blindness, skull defects, spina bifida, and other deformities. Such exposure occurred in the past when radiation was used to treat cervical cancer during pregnancy.

Maternal Diabetes. Diabetes mellitus is a common entity, and despite advances in antenatal obstetric monitoring and glucose control, the incidence of major malformations in infants of diabetic mothers stands between 6% and 10% in most series. Maternal hyperglycemia-induced fetal hyperinsulinemia results in increased body fat, muscle mass, and organomegaly *(fetal macrosomia)*; cardiac anomalies, neural tube defects, and other central nervous system malformations are some of the major anomalies seen in *diabetic embryopathy.*

Multifactorial Causes

In contrast to monogenic disorders like achondroplasia, which are caused by functional perturbation of a single gene, congenital anomalies with a multifactorial basis arise as a result of inheritance of multiple genetic polymorphisms that confer a "susceptibility phenotype." The interaction of this underlying phenotype with the environment is then required before the disorder becomes manifest. In the case of congenital dislocation of the hip, for example, a shallow acetabular socket and laxity of the supporting ligaments are believed to be genetically determined, whereas frank breech position in utero, with hips flexed and knees extended is a key environmental factor. Such complex gene-environment interactions might explain why the monozygotic concordance rate for some common congenital anomalies like cleft lip or cleft palate is only in the range of 25% to 50%. The importance of environmental contribution to multifactorial inheritance is further underscored by a marked reduction in the incidence of neural tube defects by periconceptional intake of folic acid in the diet.[7]

The estimated frequency of some common birth defects in the United States is presented in Table 10–3.

PATHOGENESIS OF CONGENITAL ANOMALIES

The pathogenesis of congenital anomalies is complex and still poorly understood, but two general principles of developmental pathology are relevant regardless of the etiologic agent.

1. *The timing of the prenatal teratogenic insult has an important impact on the occurrence and the type of anomaly produced* (Fig. 10–5). The intrauterine development of humans can be divided into two phases: (1) the embryonic period occupying the first 9 weeks of pregnancy and (2) the fetal period terminating at birth.
   - In the *early embryonic period* (first 3 weeks after fertilization), an injurious agent damages either enough cells to cause death and abortion or only a few cells, presumably allowing the embryo to recover without developing defects. *Between the third and the ninth weeks, the embryo is extremely susceptible to teratogenesis,* and the peak sensitivity during this period occurs between the fourth and the fifth weeks. During this period organs are being crafted out of the germ cell layers.
   - The *fetal period* that follows organogenesis is marked chiefly by the further growth and maturation of the organs, with greatly reduced susceptibility to teratogenic agents. Instead, the fetus is susceptible to growth retardation or injury to already formed organs. It is therefore

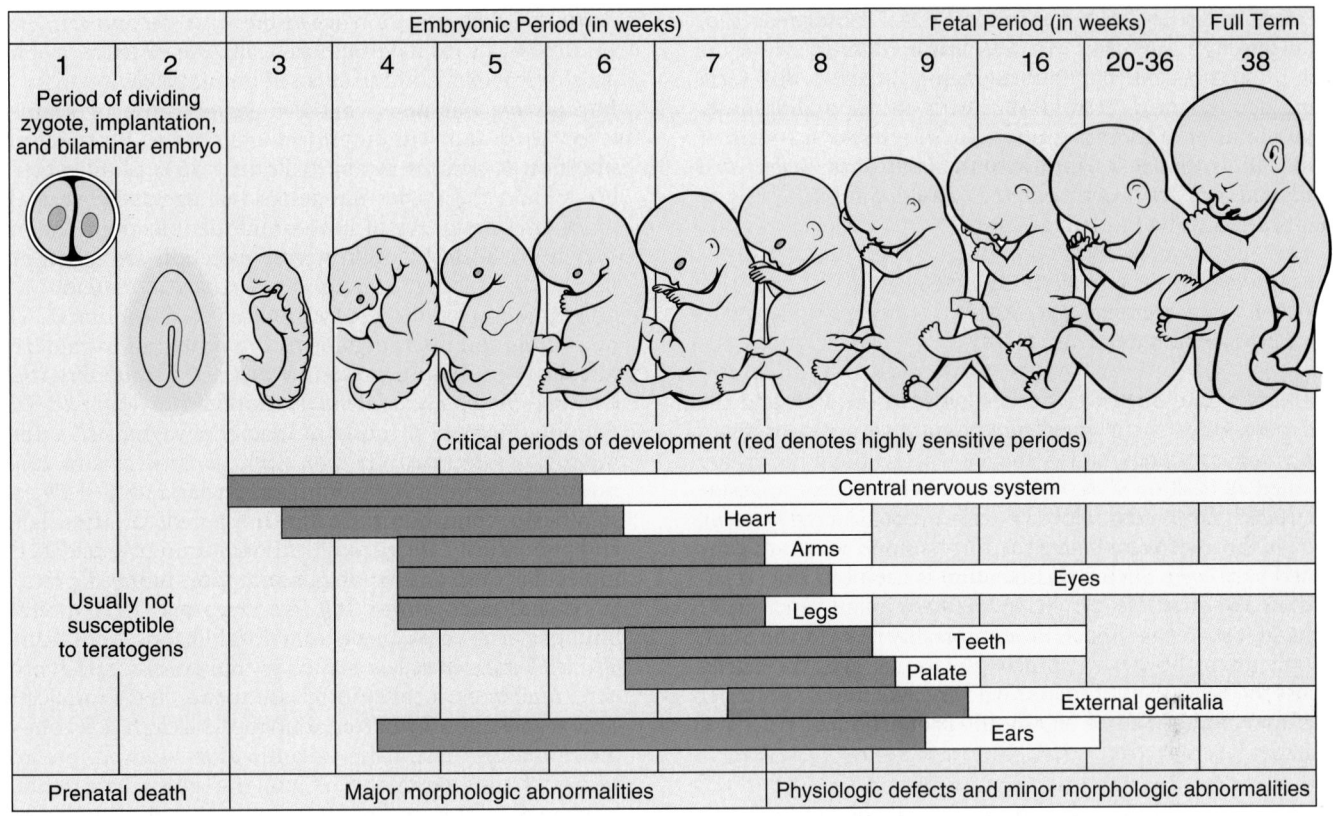

FIGURE 10–5 Critical periods of development for various organ systems and the resultant malformations. (Modified and redrawn from Moore KL: The Developing Human, 5th ed. Philadelphia, WB Saunders, 1993, p 156.)

possible for a given agent to produce different anomalies if exposure occurs at different times of gestation.

2. The complex interplay between environmental teratogens and intrinsic genetic defects is underscored by the fact that features of dysmorphogenesis caused by environmental insults can often be recapitulated by genetic defects in the pathways targeted by these teratogens. This is illustrated by the following representative examples.

- *Cyclopamine* is a teratogen derived from the roots of the plant *Veratrum californicum* (California lily). Pregnant ewes who feed on this plant give birth to lambs that have severe craniofacial abnormalities including holoprosencephaly and "cyclopia" (single fused eye, hence the origin of the moniker cyclopamine). This compound is a potent inhibitor of Hedgehog signaling in the embryo, and as stated above, mutations of Hedgehog genes are present in subsets of patients with holoprosencephaly.

- *Valproic acid* is an anti-epileptic and a recognized teratogen during pregnancy. Valproic acid disrupts expression of a family of highly conserved developmentally critical transcription factors known as *homeobox* (*HOX*) proteins.[8] The genes encoding HOX proteins have a 180-nucleotide motif, dubbed the homeobox, which binds DNA in a sequence-specific fashion. In vertebrates, HOX proteins have been implicated in the patterning of limbs, vertebrae, and craniofacial structures. Not surprisingly, mutations in HOX family genes are responsible for congenital anomalies that mimic features observed in *valproic acid embryopathy*.

- The vitamin A (retinol) derivative *all-trans-retinoic acid* is essential for normal development and differentiation, and its *absence* during embryogenesis results in a constellation of malformations affecting multiple organ systems, including the eyes, genitourinary system, cardiovascular system, diaphragm, and lungs (see Chapter 9 for vitamin A deficiency in the postnatal period). Conversely, *excessive exposure to retinoic acid is also teratogenic.* Infants born to mothers treated with retinoic acid for severe acne have a predictable phenotype (*retinoic acid embryopathy*), including central nervous system, cardiac, and craniofacial defects, such as *cleft lip and cleft palate.* The latter may stem from retinoic acid–mediated deregulation of components of the transforming growth factor-β (TGF-β) signaling pathway, which is involved in palatogenesis. Mice with knockout of the *Tgfb3* gene uniformly develop cleft palate,[9] once again underscoring the functional relationship between teratogenic exposure and signaling pathways in the causation of congenital anomalies.

Disorders of Prematurity

Infants born before completion of the normal gestation period or who have failed to grow normally during gestation have higher morbidity and mortality rates than full-term infants. For example, an infant weighing 2300 gm and born at 34 weeks of gestation is likely to be physiologically immature and therefore at greater risk for suffering the consequences of organ system immaturity (e.g., respiratory distress syndrome [RDS] or transient hyperbilirubinemia) than a full-term infant also weighing 2300 gm but with corresponding functional maturity of most organ systems. Therefore, a system of classification that takes into account *both birth weight and gestational age* has been adopted. Based on birth weight, infants are classified as being

- *Appropriate for gestational age (AGA)*
- *Small for gestational age (SGA)*
- *Large for gestational age (LGA)*

Infants whose birth weight falls between the 10th and the 90th percentiles for a given gestational age are considered AGA, whereas those who fall above or below these norms are classified as LGA or SGA, respectively. With respect to gestational age, infants born before 37 weeks are considered *preterm*, whereas those delivered after the forty-second week are considered *post-term*. Such a classification is useful in risk stratification. For example, an AGA 1500-gm infant born at 32 weeks' gestation has a much lower mortality risk than an SGA, 700-gm infant born at a similar gestational age. We briefly discuss the subgroups of infants who are SGA and/or preterm, since they account for a significant proportion of perinatal mortality.

CAUSES OF PREMATURITY AND FETAL GROWTH RESTRICTION

Prematurity, defined by a gestational age less than 37 weeks, is the second most common cause of neonatal mortality, behind only congenital anomalies. The American College of Obstetrics and Gynecology (ACOG) estimates that 12% of all births in the United States are preterm deliveries, and despite extensive research into this area, this rate has increased over the last two decades.[10] The major risk factors for prematurity include:

- *Preterm premature rupture of placental membranes (PPROM):* PPROM complicates about 3% of all pregnancies and is responsible for as many as a third of all preterm deliveries. Rupture of membranes (ROM) before the onset of labor can be spontaneous or induced. PPROM refers to spontaneous ROM occurring *before* 37 weeks' gestation (hence the annotation "preterm"). In contrast, PROM refers to spontaneous ROM occurring *after* 37 weeks' gestation. This distinction is important because after 37 weeks the associated risk to the fetus is considerably decreased. Several clinical risk factors have been identified for PPROM, including a prior history of preterm delivery, preterm labor and/or vaginal bleeding during the current pregnancy, maternal smoking, low socioeconomic status, and poor maternal nutrition. Polymorphisms in genes associated with immune regulation (e.g., tumor necrosis factor [TNF]) or collagen breakdown (e.g., matrix metalloproteinases 1, 8, and 9) have been identified as possible risk factors for PPROM association.[11] These findings are not unexpected, because the pathophysiology of PPROM typically includes inflammation of placental membranes and enhanced collagen degradation by matrix metalloproteinases. The fetal and maternal outcome after PPROM

depends on the gestation age of the fetus (second-trimester PPROM has a dismal prognosis), and the effective prophylaxis of infections in the exposed amniotic cavity.

- *Intrauterine infection:* This is a major cause of preterm labor with and without intact membranes. Intrauterine infection is present in approximately 25% of all preterm births, and the earlier the gestational age at delivery, the higher the frequency of intra-amniotic infection. The histologic correlates of intrauterine infection are inflammation of the placental membranes *(chorioamnionitis)* and inflammation of the fetal umbilical cord *(funisitis)*. The most common microorganisms implicated in intrauterine infections leading to preterm labor are *Ureaplasma urealyticum*, *Mycoplasma hominis*, *Gardnerella vaginalis* (the dominant organism found in "bacterial vaginosis," a polymicrobial infection), *Trichomonas*, *gonorrhea*, and *Chlamydia*. In developing countries, malaria and HIV are significant contributors to the burden of preterm labor and prematurity. Recent studies have begun to elucidate the molecular mechanisms of inflammation-induced preterm labor, and endogenous Toll-like receptors (TLRs), which bind bacterial components as natural ligands (see Chapter 6), have emerged as key players in this process. Specifically, experiments performed in mouse models have implicated TLR-4 activation by bacterial lipopolysaccharide as one of the initiating events in inflammation-induced preterm labor.[12] TLR-4 expression is also upregulated in preterm human placentas complicated by chorioamnionitis. It is postulated that signals produced by TLR-4 deregulate prostaglandin expression, which in turn induces uterine smooth muscle contractions.
- *Uterine, cervical, and placental structural abnormalities:* Uterine distortion (e.g., uterine fibroids), compromised structural support of the cervix ("cervical incompetence"), *placenta previa*, and *abruptio placentae* (Chapter 22) are associated with an increased risk of prematurity.
- *Multiple gestation* (twin pregnancy).

The hazards of prematurity are manifold for the newborn and include one or more of the entities listed below:

- Hyaline membrane disease (Neonatal respiratory distress syndrome)
- Necrotizing enterocolitis
- Sepsis
- Intraventricular hemorrhage
- Long-term complications, including developmental delay.

Although preterm infants have low birth weights, it is often appropriate once adjusted for their gestational age. In contrast, at least one third of infants who weigh less than 2500 gm are born at term and therefore are undergrown rather than immature. Hence, fetal growth restriction (FGR) commonly underlies SGA. FGR has also been called intrauterine growth retardation; however, the term *FGR* probably better reflects the pathophysiology of this disorder.[13] FGR can be detected before delivery by ultrasonographic measurement of various fetal dimensions, such as biparietal diameter, head circumference, abdominal circumference, femur length (as an indicator of fetal length), head-to-abdominal circumference ratio, femur length–to–abdominal circumference ratio, and total intrauterine volume. Influences known to result in FGR can be divided into three main groups: fetal, placental, and maternal.

Fetal. Fetal influences are those that intrinsically reduce growth potential of the fetus despite an adequate supply of nutrients from the mother. Prominent among such fetal conditions are *chromosomal disorders, congenital anomalies, and congenital infections.* Chromosomal abnormalities may be detected in up to 17% of fetuses sampled for FGR and in up to 66% of fetuses with documented ultrasonographic malformations. Among the first group, the abnormalities include triploidy (7%), trisomy 18 (6%), trisomy 21 (1%), trisomy 13 (1%), and a variety of deletions and translocations (2%). *Fetal infection* should be considered in all infants with FGR. Those most commonly responsible for FGR are the TORCH group of infections (toxoplasmosis, rubella, cytomegalovirus, herpesvirus, and other viruses and bacteria, such as syphilis). Infants who are SGA because of fetal factors are usually characterized by symmetric growth restriction (also referred to as *proportionate FGR*), meaning that all organ systems are similarly affected.

Placental. During the third trimester of pregnancy, vigorous fetal growth places particularly heavy demands on the uteroplacental supply line. Therefore, the adequacy of placental growth in the preceding midtrimester is extremely important, and *uteroplacental insufficiency is an important cause of growth restriction.* This insufficiency may result from *umbilical-placental vascular anomalies* (such as single umbilical artery, abnormal cord insertion, placental hemangioma), *placental abruption, placenta previa, placental thrombosis and infarction, placental infection,* or *multiple gestations*

(Chapter 22). In some cases the placenta may be small without any detectable underlying cause. Placental causes of FGR tend to result in *asymmetric* (or disproportionate) growth retardation of the fetus with relative sparing of the brain. Physiologically, this general type of FGR is viewed as a down-regulation of growth in the latter half of gestation because of limited availability of nutrients or oxygen.

Genetic mosaicism confined to the placenta (confined placental mosaicism) is a more recently discovered cause of FGR and has been documented in up to 15% of pregnancies with FGR.[14] Chromosomal mosaicism, in general, results from viable genetic mutations occurring after zygote formation. Depending on the developmental timing and cell of origin of the mutation, different forms of chromosomal mosaicism result. For example, genetic mutations occurring at the time of the first or second postzygotic division result in generalized constitutional mosaicism of the fetus and placenta. Conversely, if the mutation occurs later and within dividing trophoblast or extraembryonic progenitor cells of the inner cell mass (approximately 90% of the time), a genetic abnormality limited to the placenta results—confined placental mosaicism (Fig. 10–6). The phenotypic consequences of such placental mosaicism depend on both the specific cytogenetic abnormality and the percentage of cells involved. Chromosomal trisomies, in particular trisomy 7, are the abnormality most frequently documented.

Maternal. By far the most common factors associated with SGA infants are maternal conditions that result in decreased placental blood flow. Vascular diseases, such as *preeclampsia (toxemia of pregnancy)* and *chronic hypertension,* are often the underlying cause. Another class of maternal diseases

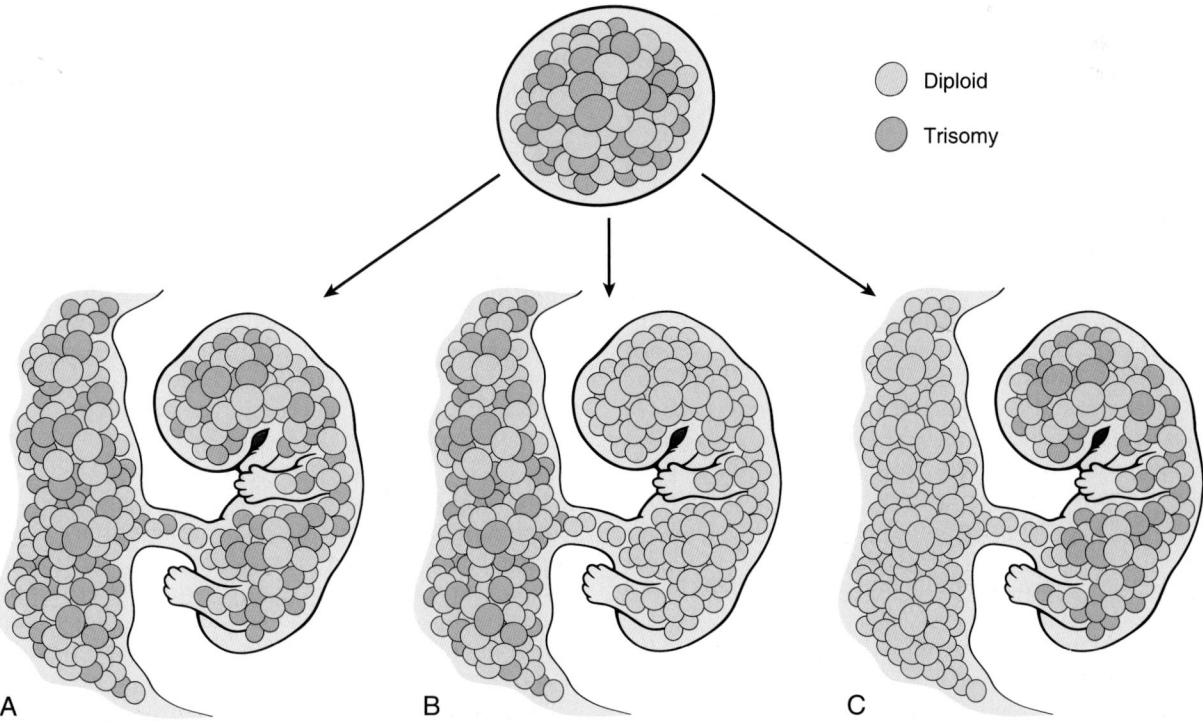

FIGURE 10–6 Diagrammatic representation of constitutional chromosomal mosaicism. **A,** Generalized. **B,** Confined to the placenta. **C,** Confined to the embryo. See text for details. See text for details. (Modified and redrawn from Kalousek DK: Confined placental mosaicism and intrauterine development. Pediatr Pathol 10:69, 1990.)

increasingly being recognized in the setting of FGR is *inherited thrombophilias,* such as the factor V Leiden mutation (Chapter 4).[15] Inherited diseases of hypercoagulability are also associated with recurrent early pregnancy losses. The list of other maternal conditions associated with SGA infants is long, but some of the avoidable factors worth mentioning are maternal *narcotic abuse, alcohol intake,* and *heavy cigarette smoking. Drugs* causing FGR include both classic teratogens, such as antimetabolites, and some commonly administered therapeutic agents, such as phenytoin (Dilantin). *Maternal malnutrition* (in particular, prolonged hypoglycemia) may also affect fetal growth, but the association between SGA infants and the nutritional status of the mother is complex.

The SGA infant faces a difficult course, not only during the struggle for survival in the perinatal period, but also in childhood and adult life. Depending on the underlying cause of FGR and, to a lesser extent, the degree of prematurity, there is a significant risk of morbidity in the form of a major handicap, cerebral dysfunction, learning disability, or hearing and visual impairment.

Neonatal Respiratory Distress Syndrome (RDS)

There are many causes of respiratory distress in the newborn, including excessive sedation of the mother, fetal head injury during delivery, aspiration of blood or amniotic fluid, and intrauterine hypoxia brought about by coiling of the umbilical cord about the neck. The most common cause, however, is RDS, also known as *hyaline membrane disease* because of the deposition of a layer of hyaline proteinaceous material in the peripheral airspaces of infants who succumb to this condition. An estimated 24,000 cases of RDS are reported annually in the United States, and improvements in management of this condition have sharply decreased deaths due to respiratory insufficiency from as many as 5000 per year a decade earlier to less than 900 cases.[16]

In untreated infants (not receiving surfactant), RDS generally presents in a stereotyped fashion, with characteristic clinical findings. The infant is almost always *preterm* and AGA, and there are strong, but not invariable, associations with *male gender, maternal diabetes,* and *delivery by cesarean section.* Resuscitation may be necessary at birth, but usually within a few minutes rhythmic breathing and normal color are reestablished. Soon afterward, often within 30 minutes, breathing becomes more difficult, and within a few hours cyanosis becomes evident. Fine rales can now be heard over both lung fields. A chest x-ray film at this time usually reveals uniform minute reticulogranular densities, producing a so-called *ground-glass picture.* In the full-blown condition the respiratory distress persists, cyanosis increases, and even the administration of 80% oxygen by a variety of ventilatory methods fails to improve the situation. If therapy staves off death for the first 3 or 4 days, however, the infant has an excellent chance of recovery.

Etiology and Pathogenesis. *Immaturity of the lungs is the most important substrate on which this condition develops.* It may be encountered in full-term infants but is much less frequent than in those "born before their time into this breathing world." The incidence of RDS is inversely proportional to gestational age. It occurs in about 60% of infants born at less

than 28 weeks of gestation, 30% of those born between 28 to 34 weeks' gestation, and less than 5% of those born after 34 weeks' gestation.

The *fundamental defect in RDS is a deficiency of pulmonary surfactant.* As described in Chapter 15, surfactant consists predominantly of dipalmitoyl phosphatidylcholine (lecithin), smaller amounts of phosphatidylglycerol, and two groups of surfactant-associated proteins. The first group is composed of hydrophilic glycoproteins SP-A and SP-D, which play a role in pulmonary host defense (innate immunity). The second group consists of hydrophobic surfactant proteins SP-B and SP-C, which, in concert with the surfactant lipids, are involved in the reduction of surface tension at the air-liquid barrier in the alveoli of the lung. With reduced surface tension in the alveoli, less pressure is required to keep them patent and hence aerated. The importance of surfactant proteins in normal lung function can be gauged by the occurrence of severe respiratory failure in neonates with congenital deficiency of surfactant caused by mutations in the *SFTPB* or *SFTBC* genes.[17]

Surfactant production by type II alveolar cells is accelerated after the thirty-fifth week of gestation in the fetus. At birth, the first breath of life requires high inspiratory pressures to expand the lungs. With normal levels of surfactant, the lungs retain up to 40% of the residual air volume after the first breath; thus, subsequent breaths require far lower inspiratory pressures. With a deficiency of surfactant, the lungs collapse with each successive breath, and so infants must work as hard with each successive breath as they did with the first. The problem of *stiff* atelectatic lungs is compounded by the *soft* thoracic wall that is pulled in as the diaphragm descends. Progressive atelectasis and reduced lung compliance then lead to a train of events as depicted in Figure 10–7, resulting in a protein-rich, fibrin-rich exudation into the alveolar spaces with the formation of hyaline membranes. The fibrin-hyaline membranes constitute barriers to gas exchange, leading to carbon dioxide retention and hypoxemia. The hypoxemia itself further impairs surfactant synthesis, and a vicious cycle ensues.

Surfactant synthesis is modulated by a variety of hormones and growth factors, including cortisol, insulin, prolactin, thyroxine, and TGF-β. *The role of glucocorticoids is particularly important.* Conditions associated with intrauterine stress and FGR that increase corticosteroid release lower the risk of developing RDS. Surfactant synthesis can be suppressed by the compensatory high blood levels of insulin in infants of diabetic mothers, which counteracts the effects of steroids. This may explain, in part, why infants of diabetic mothers have a higher risk of developing RDS. Labor is known to increase surfactant synthesis; hence, cesarean section before the onset of labor may increase the risk of RDS.

Morphology. The lungs are distinctive on gross examination. Though of normal size, they are solid, airless, and reddish purple, similar to the color of the liver, and they usually sink in water. Microscopically, alveoli are poorly developed, and those that are present are collapsed (Fig. 10–8). When the infant dies early in the course of the disease, necrotic cellular debris can be seen in the terminal bronchioles and alveolar ducts. The necrotic material becomes incorporated within eosinophilic hyaline membranes lining

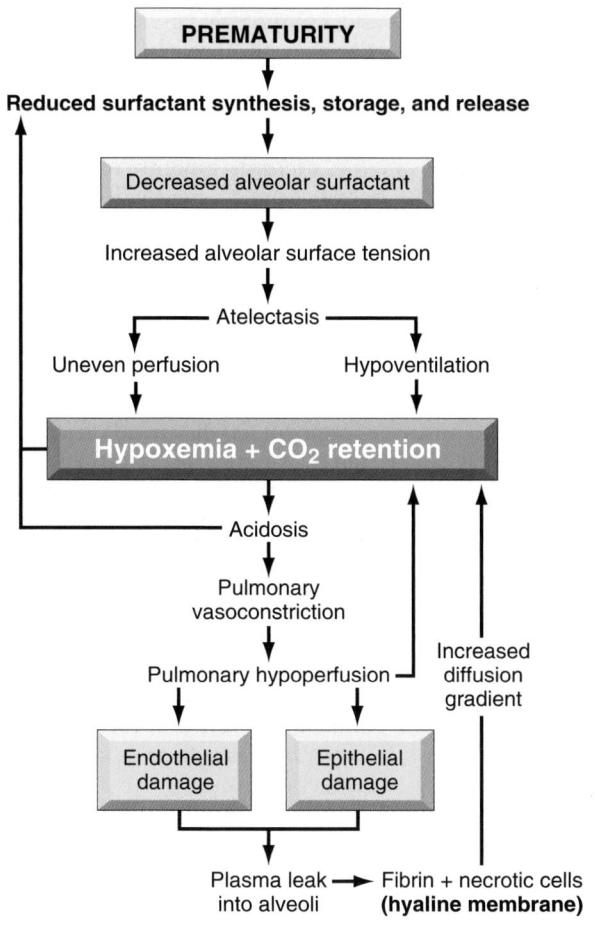

FIGURE 10–7 Schematic outline of the pathophysiology of respiratory distress syndrome (see text).

the respiratory bronchioles, alveolar ducts, and random alveoli. The membranes are largely made up of fibrin admixed with cell debris derived chiefly from necrotic type II pneumocytes. The sequence of events that leads to the formation of hyaline membranes is depicted in Figure 10–7. There is a remarkable paucity of neutrophilic inflammatory reaction associated with these membranes. The lesions of hyaline membrane disease are never seen in stillborn infants.

In infants who survive more than 48 hours, reparative changes occur in the lungs. The alveolar epithelium proliferates under the surface of the membrane, which may be desquamated into the airspace, where it may undergo partial digestion or phagocytosis by macrophages.

Clinical Course. Although a classic clinical presentation before the era of treatment with exogenous surfactant was described earlier, the actual clinical course and prognosis for neonatal RDS vary, dependent on the maturity and birth weight of the infant and the promptness of institution of therapy. A major thrust in the control of RDS focuses on prevention, either by delaying labor until the fetal lung reaches maturity or by inducing maturation of the lung in the fetus at risk. Critical to these objectives is the ability to assess fetal

lung maturity accurately. Because pulmonary secretions are discharged into the amniotic fluid, analysis of amniotic fluid phospholipids provides a good estimate of the level of surfactant in the alveolar lining. Prophylactic administration of exogenous surfactant at birth to extremely premature infants (gestational age ~26 to 28 weeks) and administration of surfactant to older premature infants who are symptomatic have been shown to be extremely beneficial, such that it is now uncommon for infants to die of acute RDS. In addition, antenatal corticosteroids decrease neonatal morbidity and mortality when administered to mothers with threatened premature delivery at 24 to 34 weeks' gestation. Once the infant is born, the cornerstone of treatment is the delivery of surfactant replacement therapy and oxygen, usually accomplished by a variety of ventilatory assistance methods, including high-frequency ventilation.

In uncomplicated cases, recovery begins to occur within 3 or 4 days. Therapy, however, carries with it the now well-recognized hazard of *oxygen toxicity*, caused by oxygen-derived free radicals. High concentrations of oxygen administered for prolonged periods cause two well-known complications: *retrolental fibroplasia* (also called *retinopathy of prematurity*) *in the eyes* (Chapter 29) and *bronchopulmonary dysplasia*. The retinopathy has been ascribed to changes in expression of vascular endothelial growth factor (VEGF), which is strongly induced by hypoxia, and also serves as a survival factor for endothelial cells and promotes angiogenesis (Chapter 3).[18] During the initial *hyperoxic* phase of RDS therapy (phase I), VEGF is markedly decreased, causing endothelial cell apoptosis; VEGF increases after return to relatively hypoxic room air ventilation, inducing the retinal vessel proliferation *(neovascularization)* characteristic of the lesions in the retina (phase II).

Bronchopulmonary dysplasia (BPD), originally described in 1967, is now infrequent in infants of more than 1200 gm birth weight or with gestations exceeding 30 weeks. Gentler ventilation techniques, antenatal glucocorticoid therapy, and surfactant treatments have minimized severe lung injury in larger and more mature infants. The definition of BPD has evolved in recent years to reflect these trends, and at least 28 days of oxygen therapy in an infant who is beyond 36 weeks'

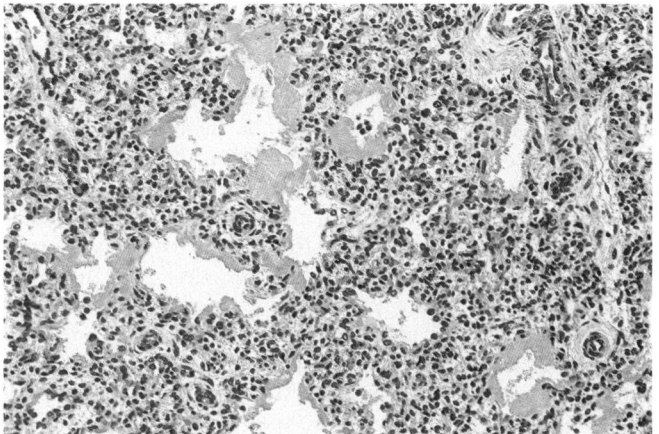

FIGURE 10–8 Hyaline membrane disease. There is alternating atelectasis and dilation of the alveoli. Note the eosinophilic thick hyaline membranes lining the dilated alveoli.

post-menstrual age is required to render a diagnosis of BPD.[19] The original histopathologic descriptions of BPD reported airway epithelial hyperplasia and squamous metaplasia, alveolar wall thickening, and peribronchial as well as interstitial fibrosis. The major abnormalities in "new" BPD are a striking decrease in alveolar septation (manifested as large, simplified alveolar structures) and a dysmorphic capillary configuration. Thus, the current view is that BPD is caused by a potentially reversible impairment in the development of alveolar septation at the saccular stage.

Multiple factors—hyperoxemia, hyperventilation, prematurity, inflammatory cytokines, and vascular maldevelopment—contribute to BPD and probably act additively or synergistically to promote injury.[20] Oxygen alone can arrest septation of lungs that are in the saccular stage of development, with infants receiving higher levels of supplemental oxygen having more persistent lung disease. Mechanical ventilation of preterm animals without simultaneous exposure to high levels of supplemental oxygen also results in the pathologic lesion of BPD. The levels of a variety of pro-inflammatory cytokines (TNF, interleukin-1β [IL-1β], IL-6, and IL-8) are increased in the alveoli of infants who develop BPD, and their deregulation in animal models can impair alveolar septation, suggesting a role for these cytokines in arresting pulmonary development.[21] Recent studies in experimental models of lung development have also elucidated the requirement of appropriate vascularization within the pulmonary mesenchyme for allowing branching morphogenesis of the epithelium. In corroboration, infants who succumb to BPD often demonstrate dysmorphic capillaries and reduced levels of the angiogenic growth factor, VEGF.[22]

If oxygen toxicity is avoided, as is usually the case, and the infant can be kept alive for about 3 or 4 days, recovery of infants of 31 weeks' gestation or more can be anticipated without permanent sequelae. Infants who recover from RDS are at increased risk for developing a variety of other complications associated with preterm birth; most important among these are *patent ductus arteriosus, intraventricular hemorrhage,* and *necrotizing enterocolitis.* Thus, although current high technology saves many infants with RDS, it also brings to the surface the exquisite fragility of the immature neonate.

NECROTIZING ENTEROCOLITIS

Necrotizing enterocolitis (NEC) is most common in premature infants, with the incidence of the disease being inversely proportional to the gestational age. It occurs in approximately 1 out of 10 very low birth weight infants (<1500 gm). Approximately 2500 cases occur annually in the United States.

The pathogenesis of NEC is uncertain, but is in all likelihood multifactorial. In addition to *prematurity,* most cases are associated with *enteral feeding,* suggesting that some postnatal insult (such as introduction of bacteria) sets in motion the cascade culminating in tissue destruction. While *infectious agents* likely play a role in NEC pathogenesis, no single bacterial pathogen has been linked to the disease. A large number of *inflammatory mediators* have been associated with NEC, and their discussion is beyond the scope of this book. One particular mediator, platelet activating factor (PAF), has been implicated in increasing mucosal permeability by promoting

enterocyte apoptosis and compromising intercellular tight junctions, thus adding "fuel to the fire."[23] Stool and serum samples of infants with NEC demonstrate higher PAF levels than age-matched controls. Ultimately, breakdown of mucosal barrier functions permits transluminal migration of gut bacteria, leading to a vicious cycle of inflammation, mucosal necrosis, and further bacterial entry, eventually culminating in sepsis and shock (Chapter 4).

The clinical course is fairly typical, with the onset of bloody stools, abdominal distention, and development of circulatory collapse. Abdominal radiographs often demonstrate gas within the intestinal wall *(pneumatosis intestinalis).* NEC typically involves the terminal ileum, cecum, and right colon, although any part of the small or large intestines may be involved. The involved segment is distended, friable, and congested, or it can be frankly gangrenous; intestinal perforation with accompanying peritonitis may be seen. Microscopically, mucosal or transmural coagulative necrosis, ulceration, bacterial colonization, and submucosal gas bubbles may be seen (Fig. 10–9). Reparative changes, such as the formation of granulation tissue and fibrosis, may begin shortly after the acute episode. When detected early on, NEC can be often managed conservatively, but many cases (20% to 60%) require resection of the necrotic segments of bowel. NEC is associated with high perinatal mortality; those who survive often develop *post-NEC strictures* from fibrosis caused by the healing process.

Perinatal Infections

Infections of the embryo, fetus, and neonate are manifested in a variety of ways and are mentioned as etiologic factors in numerous other sections within this chapter. In general, fetal and perinatal infections are acquired through one of two primary routes—*transcervically* (also referred to as *ascending*) or *transplacentally (hematologic).* Occasionally, infections occur by a combination of the two routes in that an ascending microorganism infects the endometrium and then the fetal bloodstream via the chorionic villi.

TRANSCERVICAL (ASCENDING) INFECTIONS

Most bacterial and a few viral (e.g., herpes simplex II) infections are acquired by the cervicovaginal route. Such infections may be acquired in utero or around the time of birth. In general the fetus acquires the infection either by inhaling infected amniotic fluid into the lungs shortly before birth or by passing through an infected birth canal during delivery. As stated before, preterm birth is often an unfortunate consequence and may be related either to damage and rupture of the amniotic sac as a direct consequence of the inflammation or to the induction of labor associated with a release of prostaglandins by the infiltrating neutrophils. Inflammation of the placental membranes and cord are usually demonstrable, although the presence or absence and severity of chorioamnionitis do not necessarily correlate with the severity of the fetal infection. In the fetus infected by inhalation of amniotic fluid, pneumonia, sepsis, and meningitis are the most common sequelae.

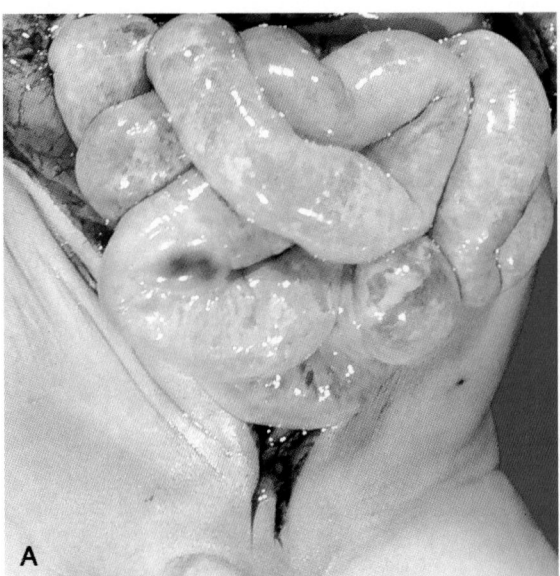
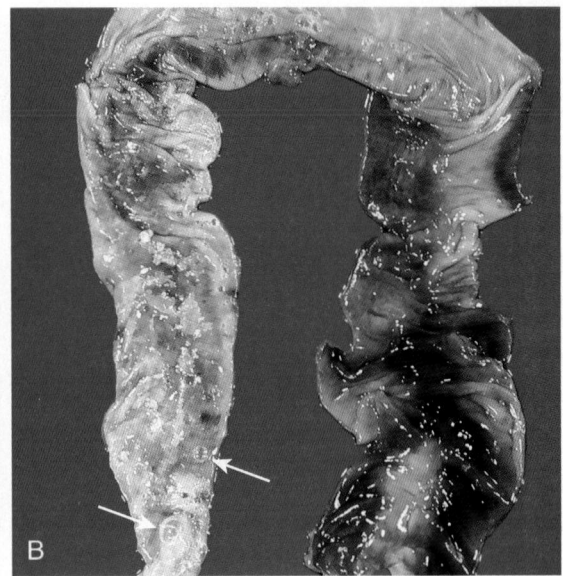

FIGURE 10–9 Necrotizing enterocolitis (NEC). **A,** Postmortem examination in a severe case of NEC shows the entire small bowel is markedly distended with a perilously thin wall (usually this implies impending perforation). **B,** The congested portion of the ileum corresponds to areas of hemorrhagic infarction and transmural necrosis microscopically. Submucosal gas bubbles *(pneumatosis intestinalis)* can be seen in several areas *(arrows).*

TRANSPLACENTAL (HEMATOLOGIC) INFECTIONS

Most parasitic (e.g., toxoplasma, malaria) and viral infections and a few bacterial infections (i.e., *Listeria*, *Treponema*) gain access to the fetal bloodstream transplacentally via the chorionic villi. This hematogenous transmission may occur at any time during gestation or occasionally, as may be the case with hepatitis B and HIV, at the time of delivery via maternal-to-fetal transfusion. The clinical manifestations of these infections are highly variable, depending largely on the gestational timing and microorganism involved.

Parvovirus B19, which causes *erythema infectiosum* or "fifth disease of childhood" in immunocompetent older children, can infect 1% to 5% of pregnant women, and the vast majority

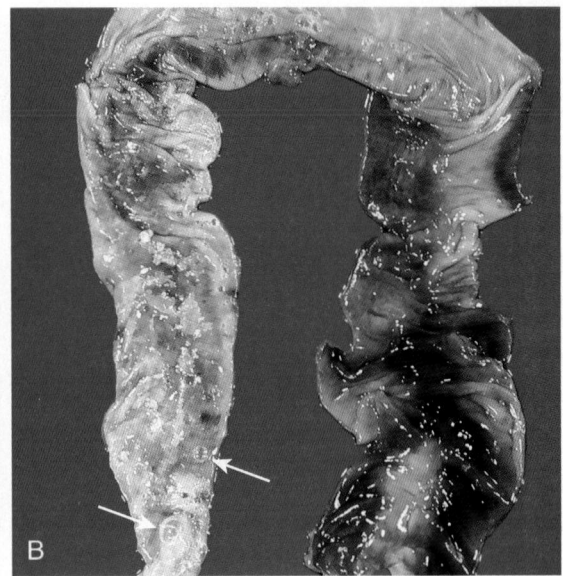

FIGURE 10–10 Bone marrow from an infant infected with parvovirus B19. The *arrows* indicate two erythroid precursors with large homogeneous intranuclear inclusions and a surrounding peripheral rim of residual chromatin.

have a normal pregnancy outcome. Adverse pregnancy outcomes in a minority of intrauterine infections include spontaneous abortion (particularly in the second trimester), stillbirth, hydrops fetalis (see below), and congenital anemia. Parvovirus B19 has a particular tropism for erythroid cells, and diagnostic viral inclusions can be seen in early erythroid progenitor cells in infected infants (Fig. 10–10).

The *TORCH group of infections* (see above) are grouped together because they may evoke similar clinical and pathologic manifestations, including *fever, encephalitis, chorioretinitis, hepatosplenomegaly, pneumonitis, myocarditis, hemolytic anemia, and vesicular or hemorrhagic skin lesions.* Such infections occurring early in gestation may also cause chronic sequelae in the child, including growth and mental retardation, cataracts, congenital cardiac anomalies, and bone defects.

SEPSIS

Perinatal sepsis can also be grouped clinically based on *early onset* (within the first 7 days of life) versus *late onset* (from 7 days to 3 months). Most cases of early-onset sepsis are acquired at or shortly before birth and tend to result in clinical signs and symptoms of pneumonia, sepsis, and occasionally meningitis within 4 or 5 days of life. Group B streptococcus is the most common organism isolated in early-onset sepsis and is also the most common cause of bacterial meningitis. Infections with *Listeria* and *Candida* follow a latent period between the time of microorganism inoculation and the appearance of clinical symptoms and present as late-onset sepsis.

Fetal Hydrops

Fetal hydrops refers to the accumulation of edema fluid in the fetus during intrauterine growth. Until recently, hemolytic anemia caused by Rh blood group incompatibility between mother and fetus *(immune hydrops)* was the most common cause, but with the successful prophylaxis of this disorder during pregnancy, causes of *nonimmune hydrops* have emerged as the principal culprits (Table 10–4). The intrauterine fluid accumulation can be quite variable, from progressive, generalized edema of the fetus *(hydrops fetalis)*, a usually lethal condition, to more localized degrees of edema, such as isolated pleural and peritoneal effusions, or postnuchal fluid accumulation *(cystic hygroma*, see later) that are compatible with life.

IMMUNE HYDROPS

Immune hydrops is a hemolytic disease caused by blood group incompatibility between mother and fetus. When the fetus inherits red cell antigenic determinants from the father that are foreign to the mother, a maternal immune reaction may occur, leading to hemolytic disease (*in utero*). The major antigens known to induce clinically significant immunological disease are certain of the Rh antigens the ABO and blood groups. The incidence of immune hydrops in urban populations has declined remarkably, mostly as a result of the current methods of preventing Rh immunization in at-risk women. Successful prophylaxis of this disorder has resulted from an understanding of its pathogenesis.

Etiology and Pathogenesis. The underlying basis of immune hydrops is the immunization of the mother by blood group antigens on fetal red cells and the free passage of antibodies from the mother through the placenta to the fetus (Fig. 10–11). Fetal red cells may reach the maternal circulation during the last trimester of pregnancy, when the cytotrophoblast is no longer present as a barrier, or during childbirth itself. The mother thus becomes sensitized to the foreign antigen.

Of the numerous antigens included in the Rh system, only the D antigen is a major cause of Rh incompatibility. Several factors influence the immune response to Rh-positive fetal red cells that reach the maternal circulation.

- Concurrent ABO incompatibility protects the mother against Rh immunization, because the fetal red cells are promptly coated and removed from the maternal circulation by anti-A or anti-B IgM antibodies that do not cross the placenta.
- The antibody response depends on the dose of immunizing antigen; hence, hemolytic disease develops only when the mother has experienced a significant transplacental bleed (more than 1 mL of Rh-positive fetal red cells).
- The initial exposure to Rh antigen evokes the formation of IgM antibodies, so Rh disease is uncommon with the first pregnancy. Exposure during a subsequent pregnancy generally leads to a brisk IgG antibody response and the risk of immune hydrops.

The incidence of maternal Rh isoimmunization has decreased significantly since the use of Rhesus immune globulin (RhIg) containing anti-D antibodies. Administration of RhIg at 28 weeks and within 72 hours of delivery to Rh-negative mothers significantly decreases the risk for hemolytic disease in Rh-positive neonates and in subsequent pregnancies; RhIg is also administered following abortions, as these

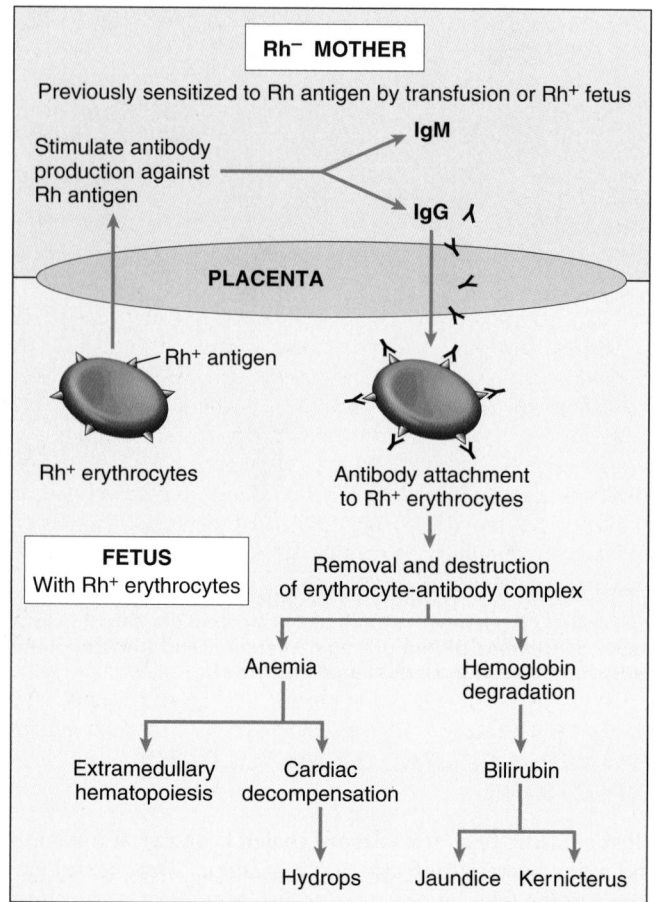

FIGURE 10–11 Pathogenesis of immune hydrops fetalis (see text).

too can lead to immunization. Antenatal identification and management of the at-risk fetus have been greatly facilitated by amniocentesis and the advent of chorionic villus and fetal blood sampling. In addition, cloning of the *RHD* gene has resulted in efforts to determine fetal Rh status using maternal blood. When identified, cases of severe intrauterine hemolysis may be treated by fetal intravascular transfusions via the umbilical cord and early delivery.

The pathogenesis of fetal hemolysis caused by maternal-fetal ABO incompatibility is slightly different from that caused by differences in the Rh antigens. ABO incompatibility occurs in approximately 20% to 25% of pregnancies, but laboratory evidence of hemolytic disease occurs in only 1 in 10 of such infants, and the hemolytic disease is severe enough to require treatment in only 1 in 200 cases. Several factors account for this. First, as mentioned, most anti-A and anti-B antibodies are of the IgM type and hence do not cross the placenta. Second, neonatal red cells express blood group antigens A and B poorly. Third, many cells other than red cells express A and B antigens and thus absorb some of the transferred antibody. ABO hemolytic disease occurs almost exclusively in infants of group A or B who are born of group O mothers. For reasons unknown, certain group O women possess IgG antibodies directed against group A or B antigens (or both) even without prior sensitization. Therefore, the firstborn may be affected.

Fortunately, even with transplacentally acquired antibodies, lysis of the infant's red cells is minimal. There is no effective protection against ABO reactions.

There are two consequences of excessive destruction of red cells in the neonate (see Fig. 10–11). The severity of these changes varies considerably, depending on the degree of hemolysis and the maturity of the infant.

- *Anemia* is a direct result of red cell loss. If hemolysis is mild, extramedullary hematopoeisis in the spleen and liver may suffice to maintain normal levels of red cells. However, with more severe hemolysis, progressive anemia develops, and may result in hypoxic injury to the heart and liver. Because of liver injury, plasma protein synthesis decreases, and levels of these proteins may drop to as low as 2 to 2.5 mg/dL. Cardiac hypoxia may lead to cardiac decompensation and failure. *The combination of reduced plasma oncotic pressure and increased hydrostatic pressure in the circulation (secondary to cardiac failure) results in generalized edema and anasarca, culminating in hydrops fetalis.*
- *Jaundice* develops because hemolysis produces unconjugated bilirubin (Chapter 18). Bilirubin also passes through the infant's poorly developed blood-brain barrier. Being water insoluble, it blinds to lipids in the brain, resulting in demage to the central nervous system, termed *kernicterus* (Fig. 10–14).

NONIMMUNE HYDROPS

The three major causes of nonimmune hydrops include *cardiovascular defects, chromosomal anomalies,* and *fetal anemia* (Table 10–4).[24] Both structural and functional cardiovascular defects, such as congenital cardiac defects and arrhythmias, may result in intrauterine cardiac failure and hydrops. Among the chromosomal anomalies, 45,X karyotype (Turner syndrome) and the trisomies 21 and 18 are associated with fetal hydrops. Most often, underlying structural cardiac anomalies associated with the chromosomal aberrations form the basis of fetal hydrops. In the Turner phenotype, however, abnormalities of lymphatic drainage from the neck may lead to postnuchal fluid accumulation *(cystic hygromas).* Fetal anemia, not caused by Rh- or ABO-associated antibodies, also results in hydrops. In fact, in some parts of the world (e.g., Southeast Asia), severe fetal anemia due to homozygous α-thalassemia is probably the most common cause of nonimmune hydrops. Transplacental infection by parvovirus B19 is rapidly emerging as an important cause of hydrops (see above). The virus gains preferential entry into erythroid precursors (normoblasts), where it replicates, leading to apoptosis of red cell progenitors and isolated red cell aplasia. Parvoviral intranuclear inclusions can be seen within circulating and marrow erythroid precursors (see Fig. 10–10). Approximately 10% of cases of nonimmune hydrops are related to monozygous twin pregnancies and twin-to-twin transfusion occurring through anastomoses between the two circulations.

Morphology of Hydrops Fetalis. The anatomic findings in fetuses with intrauterine fluid accumulation vary with both the severity of the disease and the underlying etiology. As previously noted, hydrops

TABLE 10–4 Selected Causes of Non-Immune Fetal Hydrops

CARDIOVASCULAR
Malformations
Tachyarrhythmia
High-output failure

CHROMOSOMAL
Turner syndrome
Trisomy 21, trisomy 18

THORACIC CAUSES
Cystic adenomatoid malformation
Diaphragmatic hernia

FETAL ANEMIA
Homozygous α-thalassemia
Parvovirus B19
Immune hydrops (Rh and ABO)

TWIN GESTATION
Twin-to-twin transfusion

INFECTION (EXCLUDING PARVOVIRUS)
Cytomegalovirus
Syphilis
Toxoplasmosis

GENITOURINARY TRACT MALFORMATIONS

TUMORS

GENETIC/METABOLIC DISORDERS

Note: The cause of fetal hydrops may be undetermined ("idiopathic") in up to 20% of cases.
Data from Machin GA: Hydrops, cystic hygroma, hydrothorax, pericardial effusions, and fetal ascites. In Gilbert-Barness E, et al (eds): Potter's Pathology of the Fetus, Infant, and Child. St. Louis, Mosby, 2007, p 33.

fetalis represents the most severe and generalized manifestation (Fig. 10–12), and lesser degrees of edema such as isolated pleural, peritoneal, or post-nuchal fluid collections can occur. Accordingly, infants may be stillborn, die within the first few days, or recover completely. The presence of dysmorphic features suggests a chromosomal abnormality; postmortem examination may reveal an underlying cardiac anomaly.

In hydrops associated with fetal anemia, both fetus and placenta are characteristically pale; in most cases the liver and spleen are enlarged from cardiac failure and congestion. Additionally, the bone marrow demonstrates compensatory hyperplasia of erythroid precursors (parvovirus-associated red cell aplasia being a notable exception), and extramedullary hematopoiesis is present in the liver, spleen, and lymph nodes, and possibly other tissues such as the kidneys, lungs, and even the heart. The increased hematopoietic activity accounts for the presence in the peripheral circulation of large numbers of immature red cells, including reticulocytes, normoblasts, and erythroblasts **(erythroblastosis fetalis)** (Fig. 10–13).

The most serious threat in fetal hydrops is central nervous system damage known as **"kernicterus"**

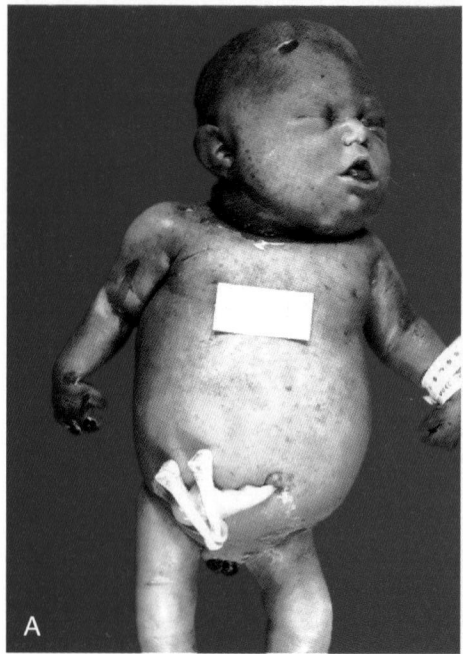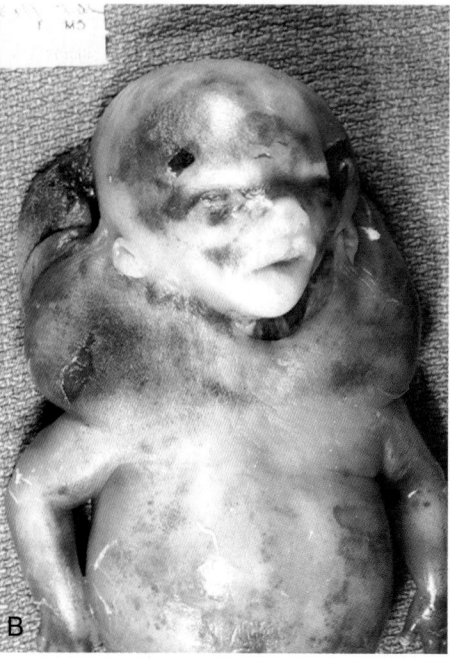

FIGURE 10–12 Hydrops fetalis. **A,** There is generalized accumulation of fluid in the fetus. **B,** Fluid accumulation is particularly prominent in the soft tissues of the neck, and this condition has been termed *cystic hygroma.* Cystic hygromas are characteristically seen, but not limited to, constitutional chromosomal anomalies such as 45,X0 karyotypes. (Courtesy of Dr. Beverly Rogers, Department of Pathology, University of Texas Southwestern Medical Center, Dallas, TX.)

(Fig. 10–14). The affected brain is enlarged and edematous and, when sectioned, has a bright yellow color, particularly the basal ganglia, thalamus, cerebellum, cerebral gray matter, and spinal cord. The precise level of bilirubin that induces kernicterus is unpredictable, but neural damage usually requires a blood bilirubin level greater than 20 mg/dL in term infants; in premature infants this threshold may be considerably lower.

Clinical Features. The clinical manifestations of fetal hydrops vary with the severity of the disease and can be inferred from the preceding discussion. Minimally affected infants display pallor, possibly accompanied by hepatosplenomegaly (to which may be added jaundice with more severe hemolytic reactions), whereas the most gravely ill neonates present with intense jaundice, generalized edema, and signs of neurologic involvement. These infants may be supported by a variety of measures, including phototherapy (visual light oxidizes toxic unconjugated bilirubin to harmless, readily excreted, water-soluble dipyrroles) and, in severe cases, total exchange transfusion of the infant.

Inborn Errors of Metabolism and Other Genetic Disorders

Sir Archibald Garrod coined the term *inborn errors of metabolism* in 1908; since that time the number of well-characterized

FIGURE 10–13 Numerous islands of extramedullary hematopoiesis (small blue cells) are scattered among mature hepatocytes in this infant with nonimmune hydrops fetalis.

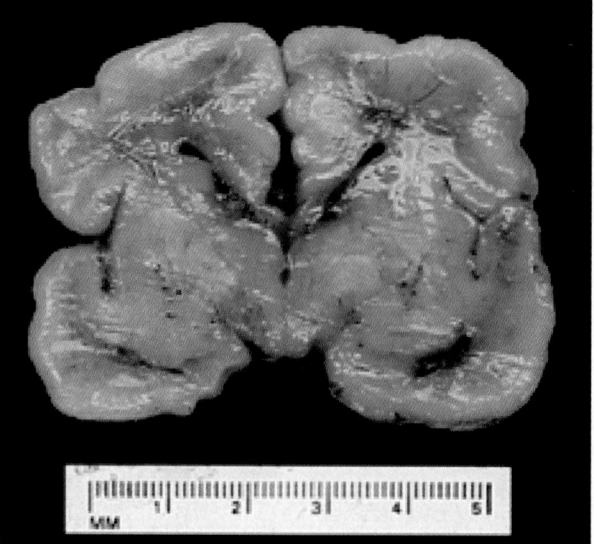

FIGURE 10–14 Kernicterus. Note the yellow discoloration of the brain parenchyma due to bilirubin accumulation, which is most prominent in the basal ganglia deep to the ventricles.

TABLE 10–5 Abnormalities Suggesting Inborn Errors of Metabolism

GENERAL

Dysmorphic features
Deafness
Self-mutilation
Abnormal hair
Abnormal body or urine odor ("sweaty feet"; "mousy or musty"; "maple syrup")
Hepatosplenomegaly; cardiomegaly
Hydrops

NEUROLOGIC

Hypotonia or hypertonia
Coma
Persistent lethargy
Seizures

GASTROINTESTINAL

Poor feeding
Recurrent vomiting
Jaundice

EYES

Cataract
Cherry red macula
Dislocated lens
Glaucoma

MUSCLE, JOINTS

Myopathy
Abnormal mobility

Adapted from Barness LA, Gilbert-Barness E: Metabolic diseases. In Gilbert-Barness E, et al (eds): Potter's Pathology of the Fetus, Infant, and Child. St. Louis, Mosby, 2007.

genetic disorders giving rise to congenital metabolic abnormalities has increased exponentially and is beyond the scope of this chapter. *Most inborn errors of metabolism are rare, and some were discussed in Chapter 5. They are inherited, most commonly, as autosomal recessive or X-linked diseases*; a few are inherited as dominant traits. Mitochondrial disorders (Chapter 5) form a distinct entity by themselves. Some of the clinical features that suggest an underlying metabolic disorder in a neonate are tabulated in Table 10–5. Three metabolic genetic defects, phenylketonuria (PKU), galactosemia, and cystic fibrosis, are selected for discussion here. PKU and galactosemia are reviewed because their early diagnosis (via neonatal screening programs) is particularly important, since appropriate dietary regimens can prevent early death or mental retardation. Cystic fibrosis is included because it is one of the most common, potentially lethal diseases occurring in individuals of Caucasian descent. Neonatal screening for cystic fibrosis remains a controversial topic, with the benefits and risks much less clear than in the other two diseases.

PHENYLKETONURIA (PKU)

PKU is characterized by abnormalities of phenylalanine metabolism, resulting in hyperphenylalaninemia. PKU is an autosomal recessive condition, and the vast majority of PKU is caused by bi-allelic mutations of the gene encoding the enzyme phenylalanine hydroxylase (PAH). Nevertheless, the great diversity in clinical presentation underscores the genetic complexities that underlie even classic "mendelian" diseases like PKU.[25] At the molecular level, more than 500 disease-associated alleles of the *PAH* gene have been identified in populations worldwide. Each mutation induces a particular alteration in the enzyme resulting in a corresponding quantitative effect on residual enzyme activity ranging from complete absence to 50% of normal values. The degree of hyperphenylalaninemia and clinical phenotype is inversely related to the amount of residual enzyme activity. Infants with mutations resulting in a lack of PAH activity present with the classic features of PKU, while those with up to 6% residual activity present with milder disease. Moreover, some mutations result in only modest elevations of blood phenylalanine levels without associated neurologic damage. This latter condition, referred to as *benign hyperphenylalaninemia*, is important to recognize, because the individuals may well have positive screening tests but do not develop the stigmata of classic PKU. Measurement of serum phenylalanine differentiates benign hyperphenylalaninemia and classic PKU, with the concentrations being typically above 600 μM in PKU (normal phenylalanine concentrations, by contrast, are less than 120 μM).

The biochemical abnormality in PKU is an inability to convert phenylalanine into tyrosine. In normal children, less than 50% of the dietary intake of phenylalanine is necessary for protein synthesis. The rest is irreversibly converted to tyrosine by PAH in the liver as part of a complex metabolic pathway, the *hepatic PAH system* (Fig. 10–15), which, in addition to the enzyme PAH, has two other components: the cofactor *tetrahydrobiopterin (BH_4)* and the enzyme *dihydropteridine reductase*, which regenerates BH_4. Although neonatal hyperphenylalaninemia can be caused by deficiencies in any of these components, about 98% of cases are attributable to abnormalities in PAH and the remaining 2% to abnormalities in synthesis or recycling of BH_4. BH_4 is not only an essential cofactor for PAH but is also required for tyrosine and tryptophan hydroxylation. Concomitant defects in BH_4 recycling disturb the synthesis of neurotransmitters. As a result, in patients with BH_4 recycling defects neurologic damage is not arrested despite normalization of phenylalanine levels. Although they account for a small minority of patients with hyperphenylalaninemia, *it is important to recognize these PKU variants because the ongoing neurologic disturbances cannot be treated by dietary control of phenylalanine levels alone.*

Individuals with "classic" PKU have a severe deficiency of PAH, leading to hyperphenylalaninemia and its pathologic consequences. With a block in phenylalanine metabolism due to lack of PAH, minor shunt pathways come into play, yielding phenylpyruvic acid, phenyllactic acid, phenylacetic acid, and o-hydroxyphenylacetic acid, which are excreted in large

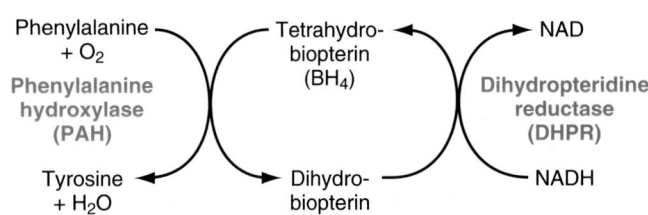

FIGURE 10–15 The phenylalanine hydroxylase system.

amounts in the urine in PKU. Some of these abnormal metabolites are excreted in the sweat, and phenylacetic acid in particular imparts a strong musty or mousy odor to affected infants. It is believed that excess phenylalanine or its metabolites contribute to the brain damage in PKU. Affected infants are normal at birth but within a few weeks develop a rising plasma phenylalanine level, which in some way impairs brain development. Usually by 6 months of life *severe mental retardation* becomes evident; fewer than 4% of untreated PKU children have intelligence quotient values greater than 50 or 60. About one third of these children are never able to walk, and two thirds cannot talk. Seizures, other neurologic abnormalities, decreased pigmentation of hair and skin, and eczema often accompany the mental retardation in untreated children. Hyperphenylalaninemia and the resultant mental retardation can be avoided by restriction of phenylalanine intake early in life. Hence, several screening procedures are routinely used for detection of PKU in the immediate postnatal period.

Many clinically normal female PKU patients who are treated with dietary control early in life reach childbearing age. If such individuals were to discontinue dietary treatment, the result would be marked hyperphenylalaninemia. Between 75% and 90% of children born to such women are mentally retarded and microcephalic, and 15% have congenital heart disease, even though the infants themselves are heterozygotes. This syndrome, termed *maternal PKU*, results from the teratogenic effects of phenylalanine or its metabolites that cross the placenta and affect specific fetal organs during development. The presence and severity of the fetal anomalies directly correlate with the maternal phenylalanine level, so *it is imperative that maternal dietary restriction of phenylalanine be initiated before conception and continue throughout pregnancy.*

Although dietary restriction of phenylalanine is usually successful in reducing or preventing the mental retardation associated with PKU, there are problems with long-term compliance (resulting in a decline in mental or behavioral status) and nutritional imbalances involving trace minerals, fatty acids, and lipids. A subset of patients with *PAH* missense mutations are responsive to pharmacologic dosages of BH$_4$; some recent analyses have predicted that as many as half of prevalent PAH mutations in some populations may be "BH$_4$ responsive."[26]

Since there are no primary abnormalities of BH$_4$ in these patients, it is believed that this cofactor acts as a "molecular chaperone," preventing the degradation of misfolded PAH protein. Permanent restitution of PAH activity through gene therapy remains the ultimate goal; recent studies in animal models of PKU have produced encouraging results.[27]

GALACTOSEMIA

Galactosemia is an autosomal recessive disorder of galactose metabolism. Normally, lactose, the major carbohydrate of mammalian milk, is split into glucose and galactose in the intestinal microvilli by lactase. Galactose is then converted to glucose in three steps (Fig. 10–16). *Two variants of galactosemia have been identified. In the more common variant there is a total lack of galactose-1-phosphate uridyl transferase (also known as GALT) involved in reaction 2. The rare variant arises from a deficiency of galactokinase, involved in reaction 1.* Because galactokinase deficiency leads to a milder form of the disease not associated with mental retardation, it is not considered in this discussion. As a result of the transferase lack, *galactose-1-phosphate* accumulates in many locations, including the liver, spleen, lens of the eye, kidneys, heart muscle, cerebral cortex, and erythrocytes. Alternative metabolic pathways are activated, leading to the production of *galactitol* (a polyol metabolite of galactose) and *galactonate*, an oxidized by-product of excess galactose, both of which also accumulate in the tissues. Long-term toxicity in galactosemics has been variously imputed to these metabolic intermediates.[28] Heterozygotes may have a mild deficiency but are spared the clinical and pathologic consequences of the homozygous state.

The clinical picture is variable, probably reflecting the heterogeneity of mutations in the galactose-1-phosphate uridyl transferase gene leading to galactosemia. The liver, eyes, and brain bear the brunt of the damage. The early-to-develop *hepatomegaly* is due largely to fatty change, but in time widespread scarring that closely resembles the cirrhosis of alcohol abuse may supervene (Fig. 10–17). *Opacification of the lens (cataract)* develops, probably because the lens absorbs water and swells as galactitol, produced by alternative metabolic

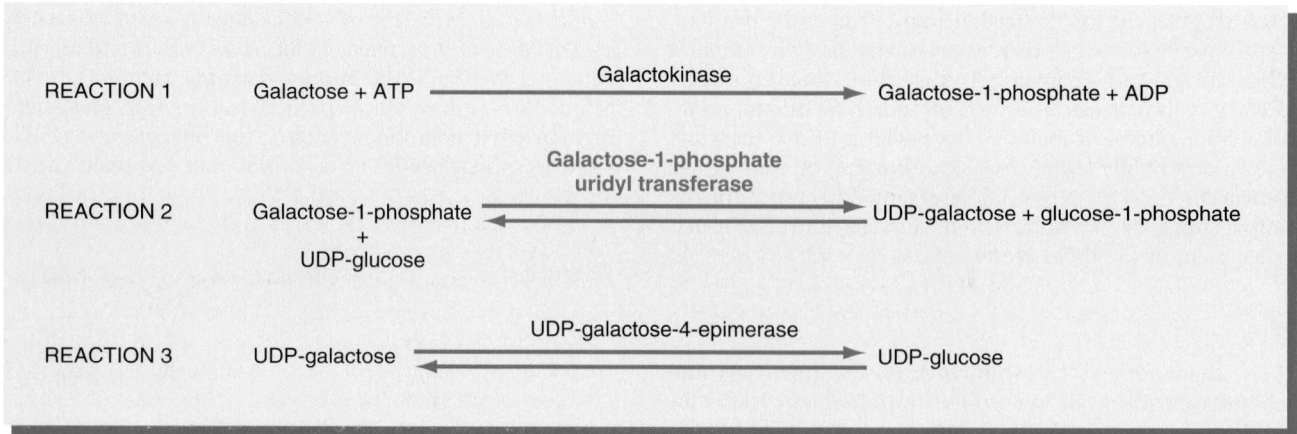

FIGURE 10–16 Pathways of galactose metabolism. ADP, adenosine diphosphate; ATP, adenosine triphosphate; UDP, uridine diphosphate.

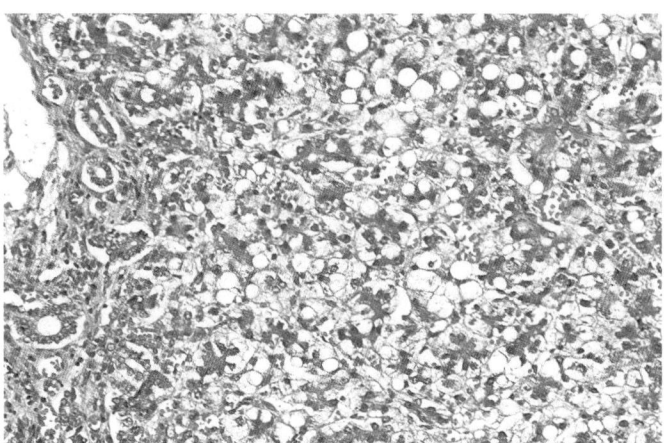

FIGURE 10–17 Galactosemia. The liver shows extensive fatty change and a delicate fibrosis. (Courtesy of Dr. Wesley Tyson, The Children's Hospital, Denver, CO.)

pathways, accumulates and increases its tonicity. *Nonspecific alterations appear in the central nervous system*, including loss of nerve cells, gliosis, and edema, particularly in the dentate nuclei of the cerebellum and the olivary nuclei of the medulla. Similar changes may occur in the cerebral cortex and white matter.

These infants *fail to thrive* almost from birth. *Vomiting* and *diarrhea* appear within a few days of milk ingestion. *Jaundice* and *hepatomegaly* usually become evident during the first week of life and may seem to be a continuation of the physiologic jaundice of the newborn. The *cataracts* develop within a few weeks, and within the first 6 to 12 months of life *mental retardation* may be detected. Even in untreated infants, however, the mental deficit is usually not as severe as that seen in PKU. Accumulation of galactose and galactose-1-phosphate in the kidney impairs amino acid transport, resulting in *aminoaciduria*. There is an increased frequency of fulminant *Escherichia coli septicemia*, possibly arising from depressed neutrophil bactericidal activity. *Hemolysis* and *coagulopathy* in the newborn period can occur as well.

The diagnosis of galactosemia can be suspected by the demonstration in the urine of a reducing sugar other than glucose, but tests that directly identify the deficiency of the transferase in leukocytes and erythrocytes are more reliable. Antenatal diagnosis is possible by the assay of GALT activity in cultured amniotic fluid cells or determination of galactitol level in amniotic fluid supernatant. More than 140 mutations have been documented in *GALT*; among these, a glutamine-to-arginine substitution at codon 188 *(Gln188Arg)* is the most prevalent mutation in non-Hispanic whites, while a serine-to-leucine substitution at codon 135 *(Ser135Leu)* is the most common mutation in African Americans.

Many of the clinical and morphologic changes of galactosemia can be prevented or ameliorated by early removal of galactose from the diet for at least the first 2 years of life. Control instituted soon after birth prevents the cataracts and liver damage and permits almost normal development. Even with dietary restrictions, however, it is now established that older patients are frequently affected by a speech disorder and gonadal failure (especially premature ovarian failure) and, less commonly, by an ataxic condition.

CYSTIC FIBROSIS (MUCOVISCIDOSIS)

Cystic fibrosis is a *disorder of ion transport in epithelial cells that affects fluid secretion in exocrine glands and the epithelial lining of the respiratory, gastrointestinal, and reproductive tracts.* In many infants this disorder leads to abnormally viscous secretions, which obstruct organ passages, resulting in most of the clinical features of this disorder, such as *chronic lung disease secondary to recurrent infections, pancreatic insufficiency, steatorrhea, malnutrition, hepatic cirrhosis, intestinal obstruction, and male infertility.* These manifestations may appear at any point in life from before birth to much later in childhood or even in adolescence.

With an incidence of 1 in 2500 live births, *cystic fibrosis is the most common lethal genetic disease that affects Caucasian populations.* The carrier frequency in the United States is 1 in 20 among Caucasians but significantly lower in African Americans, Asians, and Hispanics. Although cystic fibrosis follows an *autosomal recessive* transmission, recent data suggest that *even heterozygote carriers have a higher incidence of respiratory and pancreatic diseases* as compared with the general population.[29,30] In addition, despite the classification of cystic fibrosis as a "mendelian" disorder, there is a wide degree of phenotypic variation that results from diverse mutations in the gene associated with cystic fibrosis, the tissue-specific effects of this gene, and the influence of newly recognized disease modifiers.[31]

The Cystic Fibrosis–Associated Gene: Normal Structure and Function. In normal duct epithelia, chloride is transported by plasma membrane channels *(chloride channels). The primary defect in cystic fibrosis results from abnormal function of an epithelial chloride channel protein encoded by the cystic fibrosis transmembrane conductance regulator (CFTR) gene on chromosome 7q31.2.* The 1480–amino acid polypeptide encoded by *CFTR* has two transmembrane domains (each containing six α-helices), two cytoplasmic nucleotide-binding domains (NBDs), and a regulatory domain (R domain) that contains protein kinase A and C phosphorylation sites (Fig. 10–18). The two transmembrane domains form a channel through which chloride passes. Activation of the CFTR channel is mediated by agonist-induced increases in cyclic adenosine monophosphate (cAMP), followed by activation of a protein kinase A that phosphorylates the R domain. Adenosine triphosphate (ATP) binding and hydrolysis occurs at the NBD and is essential for the opening and closing of the channel pore in response to cAMP-mediated signaling. Several important facets of CFTR function have emerged in recent years:

○ *CFTR regulates multiple additional ion channels and cellular processes.* Although initially characterized as a chloride-conductance channel, it is now recognized that CFTR can regulate multiple ion channels and cellular processes, primarily through interactions involving its NBD. These include so-called outwardly rectified chloride channels, inwardly rectified potassium channels (Kir6.1), the epithelial sodium channel (ENaC), gap junction channels, and cellular processes involved in ATP transport and mucus secretion. Of these, the interaction of CFTR with the ENaC has possibly the most pathophysiologic relevance in cystic fibrosis. The ENaC is situated on the apical surface of exocrine epithelial cells and is responsible for sodium uptake

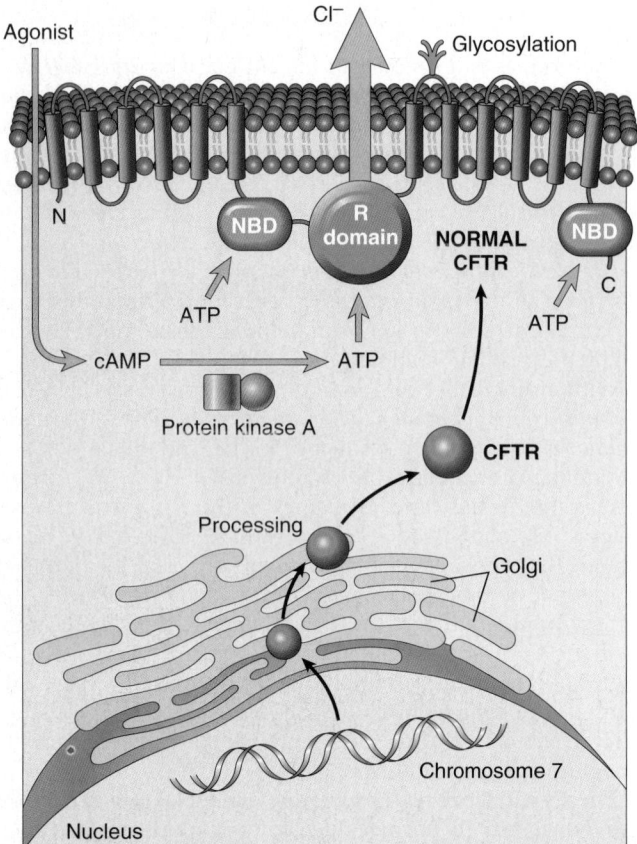

FIGURE 10–18   *Top*, Normal cystic fibrosis transmembrane conductance regulator (CFTR) structure and activation. CFTR consists of two transmembrane domains, two nucleotide-binding domains (NBDs), and a regulatory R domain. Agonists (e.g., acetylcholine) bind to epithelial cells and increase cyclic adenosine monophosphate (cAMP), which activates protein kinase A, the latter phosphorylating the CFTR at the R domain, resulting in opening of the chloride channel. *Bottom*, CFTR from gene to protein. The most common mutation in the *CFTR* gene results in defective protein folding in the Golgi/endoplasmic reticulum and degradation of CFTR before it reaches the cell surface. Other mutations affect synthesis of CFTR, NBDs and R domains, as well as membrane-spanning domains. (See text for details.)

from the luminal fluid, rendering it (the luminal fluid) hypotonic. The ENaC is *inhibited* by normally functioning CFTR; hence, *in cystic fibrosis, ENaC activity increases, markedly augmenting sodium uptake across the apical membrane.* The importance of this phenomenon is discussed below in the context of pulmonary and gastrointestinal pathology in cystic fibrosis. The one exception to this rule happens to be the human sweat ducts, where ENaC activity *decreases* as a result of *CFTR* mutations; therefore, a hypertonic luminal fluid containing both high sweat chloride (the sine qua non of classic cystic fibrosis) and high sodium content is formed. This is the basis for the "salty" sweat that mothers can often detect in their affected infants.

○ *The functions of* CFTR *are tissue-specific; therefore, the impact of a mutation in* CFTR *is also tissue-specific.* The major function of CFTR in the *sweat gland ducts* is to reabsorb luminal chloride ions and augment sodium reabsorption via the ENaC (see above). Therefore, in the sweat ducts,

loss of CFTR function leads to decreased reabsorption of sodium chloride and production of hypertonic sweat (Fig. 10–19). However, in the *respiratory and intestinal epithelium*, the CFTR is one of the most important avenues for *active luminal secretion of chloride*. At these sites, *CFTR* mutations result in loss or reduction of chloride secretion into the lumen (see Fig. 10–18). Active luminal sodium absorption is also increased (due to loss of inhibition of ENaC activity), and both of these ion changes increase passive water reabsorption from the lumen, *lowering the water content of the surface fluid layer coating mucosal cells.* Thus, unlike the sweat ducts, there is no difference in the salt concentration of the surface fluid layer coating the respiratory and intestinal mucosal cells in normal individuals versus those with cystic fibrosis. Instead, *the pathogenesis of respiratory and intestinal complications in cystic fibrosis seems to stem from an isotonic but low-volume surface fluid layer.* In the lungs, this dehydration leads to defective mucociliary action and the accumulation of hyperconcentrated, viscid secretions that obstruct the air passages and predispose to recurrent pulmonary infections.[32]

○ CFTR *mediates transport of bicarbonate ions.* The bicarbonate transport function of CFTR is mediated by reciprocal interactions with a family of anion exchangers called SLC26, which are co-expressed on the apical surface with CFTR.[33] It has been demonstrated in some *CFTR* mutant variants that chloride transport is completely or substantially preserved, while *bicarbonate transport is markedly abnormal.* Alkaline fluids are secreted by normal tissues, while acidic fluids (due to absence of bicarbonate ions) are secreted by epithelia harboring these mutant *CFTR* alleles. The decreased luminal pH can lead to a variety of adverse effects such as increased mucin precipitation and plugging of ducts, and increased binding of bacteria to plugged mucins. Pancreatic insufficiency, a feature of classic cystic fibrosis, is virtually always present when there are *CFTR* mutations with abnormal bicarbonate conductance.

The Cystic Fibrosis Gene: Mutational Spectra and Genotype-Phenotype Correlation. Since the *CFTR* gene was cloned in 1989, more than 1300 disease-associated mutations have been identified. Various mutations can be grouped into six "classes" based on their effect on the CFTR protein:

○ Class I: *Defective protein synthesis.* These mutations are associated with complete lack of CFTR protein at the apical surface of epithelial cells.

○ Class II: *Abnormal protein folding, processing, and trafficking.* These mutations result in defective processing of the protein from the endoplasmic reticulum to the Golgi apparatus; the protein does not become fully folded and glycosylated and is instead degraded before it reaches the cell surface. The most common class II mutation is a deletion of three nucleotides coding for phenylalanine at amino acid position 508 (ΔF508). Worldwide, this mutation can be found in approximately 70% of cystic fibrosis patients. Class II mutations are also associated with complete lack of CFTR protein at the apical surface of epithelial cells.

○ Class III: *Defective regulation.* Mutations in this class prevent activation of CFTR by preventing ATP binding and hydrolysis, an essential prerequisite for ion transport (see above).

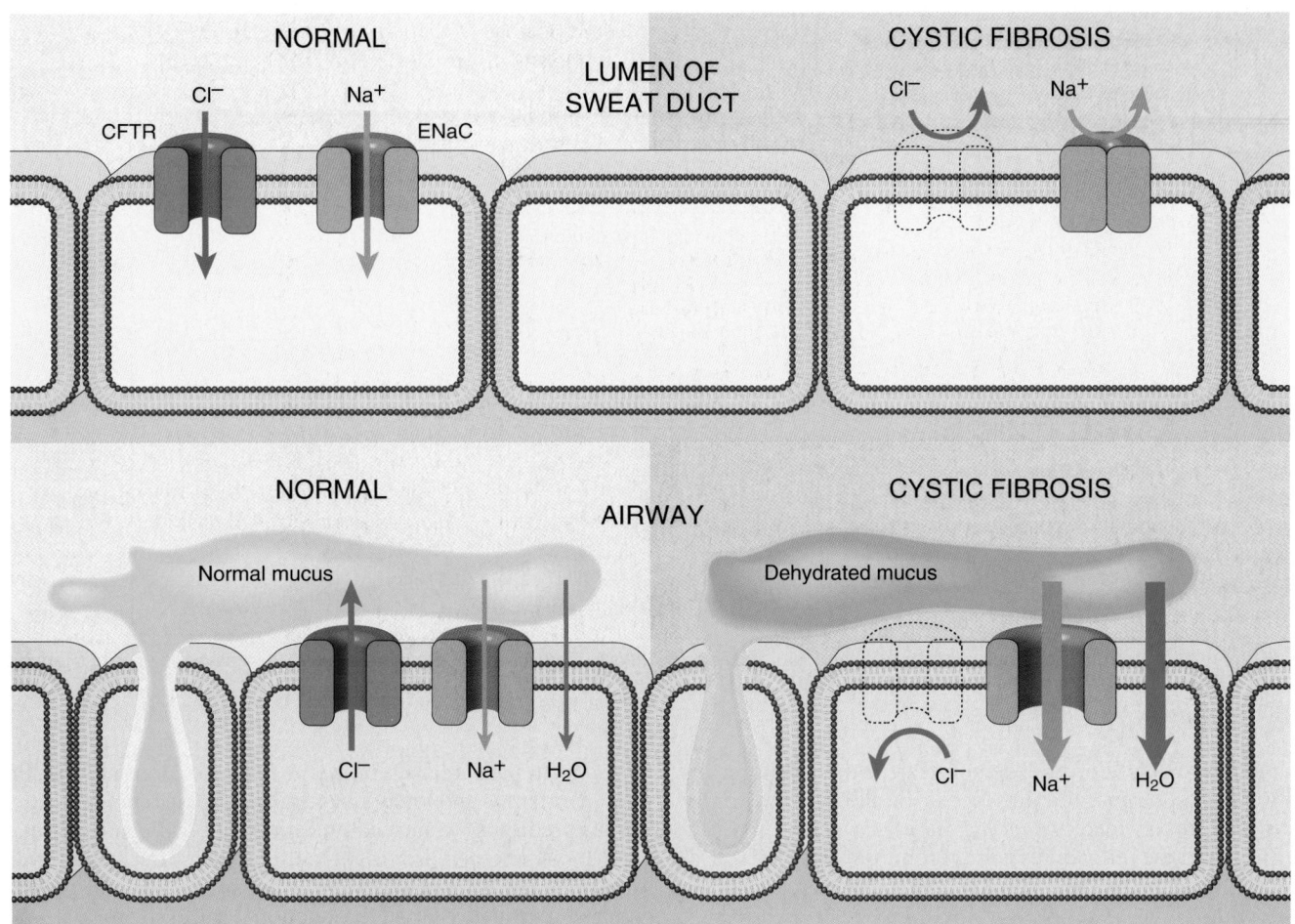

FIGURE 10–19 Chloride channel defect in the sweat duct *(top)* causes increased chloride and sodium concentration in sweat. In the airway *(bottom)*, cystic fibrosis patients have decreased chloride secretion and increased sodium and water reabsorption leading to dehydration of the mucus layer coating epithelial cells, defective mucociliary action, and mucus plugging of airways. CFTR, Cystic fibrosis transmembrane conductance regulator; ENaC, epithelial sodium channel.

Thus, there is a normal amount of CFTR on the apical surface, but it is nonfunctional.

- Class IV: *Decreased conductance.* These mutations typically occur in the transmembrane domain of *CFTR*, which forms the ionic pore for chloride transport. There is a normal amount of CFTR at the apical membrane, but with reduced function. This class is usually associated with a milder phenotype.
- Class V: *Reduced abundance.* These mutations typically affect intronic splice sites or the *CFTR* promoter, such that there is a reduced amount of normal protein. As discussed subsequently, class V mutations are also associated with a milder phenotype.
- Class VI: *Altered regulation of separate ion channels.* As previously described, CFTR is involved in the regulation of multiple distinct cellular ion channels. Mutations in this class affect the regulatory role of CFTR. In some cases, a given mutation affects the conductance by CFTR as well as regulation of other ion channels. For example, the ΔF508 mutation is both a class II and class VI mutation.

Since cystic fibrosis is an autosomal recessive disease, affected individuals harbor mutations on both alleles. However, the combination of mutations on the two alleles can have a remarkable effect on the overall phenotype, as well as on organ-specific manifestations (Fig. 10–20). Thus, two "severe" (class I, II, and III) mutations that produce virtual absence of membrane CFTR are associated with the *classic* cystic fibrosis phenotype (pancreatic insufficiency, sinopulmonary infections, and gastrointestinal symptoms), while the presence of a "mild" (class IV or V) mutation on one or both alleles results in a less severe phenotype. This general dictum of genotype-phenotype correlation is most consistent for pancreatic disease, wherein the presence of a "mild" mutation in one allele can revert to the pancreatic insufficiency phenotype conferred by homozygosity for "severe" mutations. By contrast, genotype-phenotype correlations are far less consistent in pulmonary disease, reflecting an effect of secondary modifiers (see below). As genetic testing for *CFTR* mutations has expanded, *it has become increasingly evident that patients who present with a variety of apparently unrelated clinical phenotypes may also harbor* CFTR *mutations.* These include individuals with *idiopathic chronic pancreatitis, late-onset chronic pulmonary disease, idiopathic bronchiectasis,* and *obstructive azoospermia* caused by bilateral absence of the vas deferens (see detailed discussion of individual phenotypes later). Most

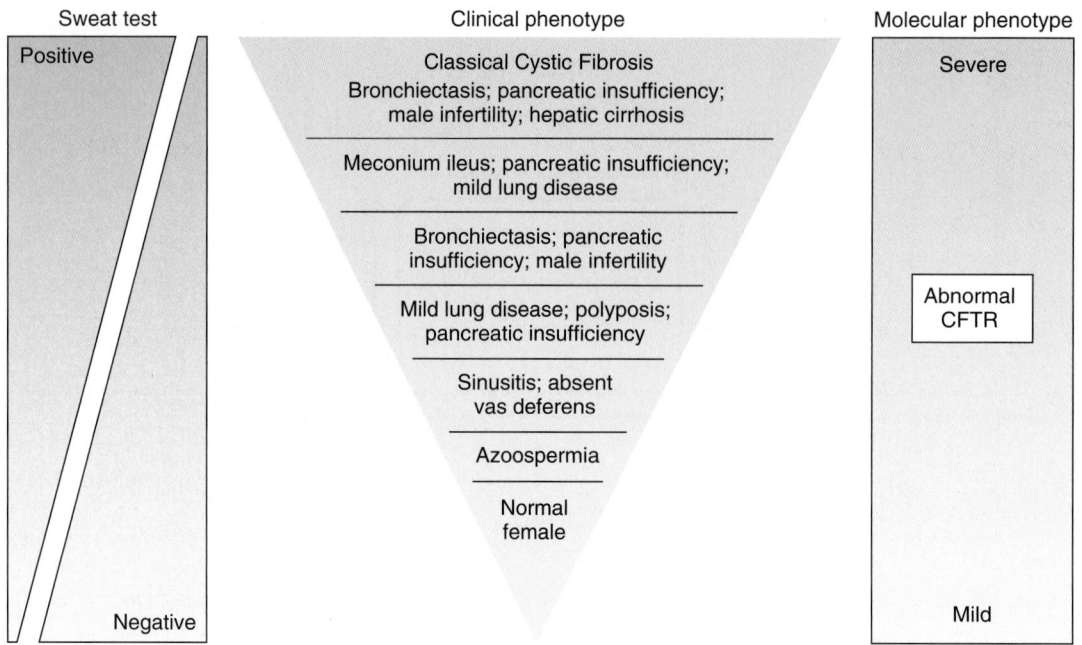

FIGURE 10–20 The many clinical manifestations of mutations in the cystic fibrosis gene, from most severe to asymptomatic. (Redrawn from Wallis C: Diagnosing cystic fibrosis: blood, sweat, and tears. Arch Dis Child 76:85, 1997.)

of these patients do not demonstrate other features of cystic fibrosis, despite the presence of bi-allelic *CFTR* mutations, and are classified as *nonclassic or atypical cystic fibrosis.*[34] Identifying these individuals is important not only for subsequent management, but also for the purposes of genetic counseling.

Genetic and Environmental Modifiers. Although cystic fibrosis remains one of the best-known examples of the "one gene, one disease" axiom, there is increasing evidence that genes other than *CFTR* modify the frequency and severity of organ-specific manifestations.[35] The severity of pulmonary manifestations in cystic fibrosis is associated with polymorphic variants at several genes, the best known examples of which are *mannose-binding lectin* 2 (*MBL2*) and *transforming growth factor β1* (*TGFB1*). MBL is a key effector of innate immunity involved in opsonization and phagocytosis of microorganisms, and polymorphisms in the *MBL2* gene that are associated with lower circulating levels of the protein confer a threefold higher risk of end-stage lung disease. TGFβ is a direct inhibitor of CFTR function.[36,37] A large multicenter study of patients homozygous for the ΔF508 *CFTR* mutation found two specific polymorphisms in the 5′ end of the *TGFB1* gene to be associated with severe pulmonary phenotypes.[38] Similarly, several putative genetic modifiers have been identified that influence the incidence of meconium ileus in cystic fibrosis, although the precise genes associated with the linked chromosomal regions have not yet been identified.[39]

Environmental modifiers may also cause significant phenotypic differences between individuals who share the same *CFTR* genotype. This is best exemplified in pulmonary disease, where *CFTR* genotype and phenotype correlations can be perplexing. As stated above, defective mucociliary action because of deficient hydration of the mucus results in an inability to clear bacteria from the airways. *Pseudomonas aeruginosa*

species, in particular, colonize the lower respiratory tract, first intermittently and then chronically. Concurrent viral infections predispose to such colonization. The static mucus creates a hypoxic microenvironment in the airway surface fluid, which in turn favors the production of *alginate*, a mucoid polysaccharide capsule. Alginate production permits the formation of a biofilm that protects the bacteria from antibodies and antibiotics, allowing them to evade host defenses, and produce a chronic destructive lung disease. Antibody- and cell-mediated immune reactions induced by the organisms result in further pulmonary destruction, but are ineffective against the organism. It is evident, therefore, that in addition to genetic factors (e.g., class of mutation), a plethora of environmental modifiers (e.g., virulence of organisms, efficacy of therapy, intercurrent and concurrent infections by other organisms, exposure to smoking and allergens) can influence the severity and progression of lung disease in cystic fibrosis.

Morphology. The anatomic changes are highly variable in distribution and severity. In individuals with nonclassic cystic fibrosis, the disease is quite mild and does not seriously disturb their growth and development. In others, the pancreatic involvement is severe and impairs intestinal absorption because of the pancreatic achylia, and so malabsorption stunts development and post-natal growth. In others, the mucus secretion defect leads to defective mucociliary action, obstruction of bronchi and bronchioles, and crippling fatal pulmonary infections (Fig. 10–21). In all variants, the sweat glands are morphologically unaffected.

Pancreatic abnormalities are present in approximately 85% to 90% of patients with cystic fibrosis. In the milder cases, there may be only accumulations of

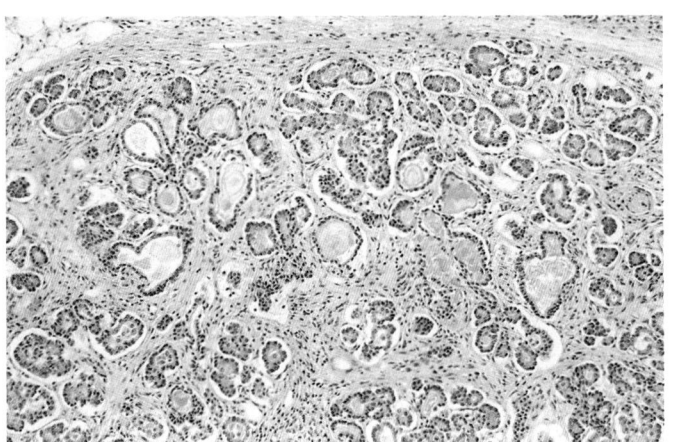

FIGURE 10–21 Mild to moderate cystic fibrosis changes in the pancreas. The ducts are dilated and plugged with eosinophilic mucin, and the parenchymal glands are atrophic and replaced by fibrous tissue.

mucus in the small ducts with some dilation of the exocrine glands. In more severe cases, usually seen in older children or adolescents, the ducts are completely plugged, causing atrophy of the exocrine glands and progressive fibrosis (Fig. 10–21). Atrophy of the exocrine portion of the pancreas may occur, leaving only the islets within a fibrofatty stroma. The loss of pancreatic exocrine secretion impairs fat absorption, and the associated avitaminosis A may contribute to squamous metaplasia of the lining epithelium of the ducts in the pancreas, which are already injured by the inspissated mucus secretions. Thick viscid plugs of mucus may also be found in the small intestine of infants. Sometimes these cause small-bowel obstruction, known as **meconium ileus**.

The **liver involvement** follows the same basic pattern. Bile canaliculi are plugged by mucinous material, accompanied by ductular proliferation and portal inflammation. Hepatic **steatosis** is not an uncommon finding in liver biopsies. Over time, **focal biliary cirrhosis** develops in approximately a third of patients (Chapter 18), which can eventually involve the entire liver, resulting in diffuse hepatic nodularity. Such severe hepatic involvement is encountered in less than 10% of patients.

The **salivary glands** frequently show histologic changes similar to those described in the pancreas: progressive dilation of ducts, squamous metaplasia of the lining epithelium, and glandular atrophy followed by fibrosis.

The **pulmonary changes** are the most serious complications of this disease (Fig. 10–22). These stem from the viscous mucus secretions of the submucosal glands of the respiratory tree leading to secondary obstruction and infection of the air passages. The bronchioles are often distended with thick mucus associated with marked hyperplasia and hypertrophy of the mucus-secreting cells. Superimposed infections give rise to severe chronic bronchitis and bron-

chiectasis (Chapter 15). In many instances, lung abscesses develop. *Staphylococcus aureus*, *Hemophilus influenzae*, and *Pseudomonas aeruginosa* are the three most common organisms responsible for lung infections. As mentioned above, a mucoid form of *P. aeruginosa* (alginate-producing) is particularly frequent and causes chronic inflammation. Even more sinister is the increasing frequency of infection with another group of pseudomonads, the *Burkholderia cepacia* complex, which includes at least nine different species; of these, infections with *B. cenocepacia* are the most common in cystic fibrosis patients. This opportunistic bacterium is particularly hardy, and infection with this organism has been associated with fulminant illness ("cepacia syndrome"), longer hospital stays, and increased mortality.[40] Other opportunistic bacterial pathogens include *Stenotrophomonas maltophila* and *nontuberculous mycobacteria*; *allergic bronchopulmonary aspergillosis* also occurs with increased frequency in cystic fibrosis.

Azoospermia and infertility are found in 95% of the males who survive to adulthood; **congenital bilateral absence of the vas deferens** is a frequent finding in these patients. In some males, bilateral absence of the vas deferens may be the only feature suggesting an underlying *CFTR* mutation.

Clinical Features. Few childhood diseases are as protean as cystic fibrosis in clinical manifestations (Table 10–6). The symptoms are extremely varied and may appear at birth to

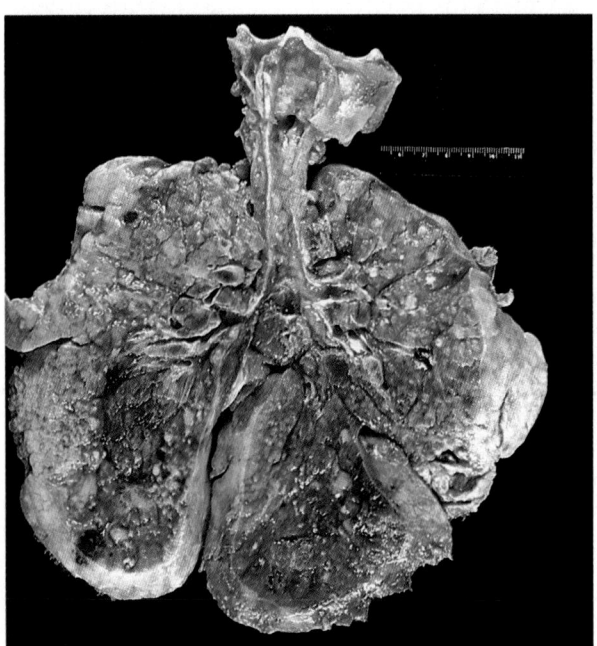

FIGURE 10–22 Lungs of a patient dying of cystic fibrosis. There is extensive mucus plugging and dilation of the tracheobronchial tree. The pulmonary parenchyma is consolidated by a combination of both secretions and pneumonia—the green color associated with *Pseudomonas* infections. (Courtesy of Dr. Eduardo Yunis, Children's Hospital of Pittsburgh, Pittsburgh, PA.)

TABLE 10–6 Clinical Features and Diagnostic Criteria for Cystic Fibrosis

CLINICAL FEATURES OF CYSTIC FIBROSIS

1. *Chronic sinopulmonary disease manifested by*
   a. Persistent colonization/infection with typical cystic fibrosis pathogens, including *Staphylococcus aureus*, nontypeable *Haemopilus influenzae*, mucoid and nonmucoid *Pseudomonas aeruginosa, Burkholderia cepacia*
   b. Chronic cough and sputum production
   c. Persistent chest radiograph abnormalities (e.g., brochiectasis, atelectasis, infiltrates, hyperinflation)
   d. Airway obstruction manifested by wheezing and air trapping
   e. Nasal polyps; radiographic or computed tomographic abnormalities of paranasal sinuses
   f. Digital clubbing
2. *Gastrointestinal and nutritional abnormalities, including*
   a. Intestinal: meconium ileus, distal intestinal obstruction syndrome, rectal prolapse
   b. Pancreatic: pancreatic insufficiency, recurrent acute pancreatitis, chronic pancreatitis
   c. Hepatic: chronic hepatic disease manifested by clinical or histologic evidence of focal biliary cirrhosis, or multilobular cirrhosis, prolonged neonatal jaundice
   d. Nutritional: failure to thrive (protein–calorie malnutrition), hypoproteinemia, edema, complications secondary to fat-soluble vitamin deficiency
3. *Salt-loss syndromes: acute salt depletion, chronic metabolic alkalosis*
4. *Male urogenital abnormalities resulting in obstructive azoospermia (congenital bilateral absence of vas deferens)*

CRITERIA FOR DIAGNOSIS OF CYSTIC FIBROSIS

One or more characteristic phenotypic features,
  OR a history of cystic fibrosis in a sibling,
  OR a positive newborn screening test result
AND
An increased sweat chloride concentration on two or more occasions
  OR identification of two cystic fibrosis mutations,
  OR demonstration of abnormal epithelial nasal ion transport

Adapted with permission from Rosenstein BJ, Cutting GR: The diagnosis of cystic fibrosis: a consensus statement. J Pediatr 132:589, 1998.

---

years later, and involve one organ system or many. Approximately 5% to 10% of the cases come to clinical attention at birth or soon after because of *meconium ileus*. Distal intestinal obstruction can also occur in older individuals, manifesting as recurrent episodes of right lower quadrant pain sometimes associated with a palpable mass in the right iliac fossa.

Exocrine pancreatic insufficiency occurs in the majority (85% to 90%) of patients with cystic fibrosis and is associated with "severe" *CFTR* mutations on *both* alleles (e.g., ΔF508/ΔF508), whereas 10% to 15% of patients with one "severe" and one "mild" *CFTR* mutation (ΔF508/R117H) or two "mild" *CFTR* mutations retain enough pancreatic exocrine function so as not to require enzyme supplementation (*pancreas-sufficient* phenotype). Pancreatic insufficiency is associated with protein and fat malabsorption and increased fecal loss. Manifestations of malabsorption (e.g., large, foul-smelling stools, abdominal distention, and poor weight gain) appear during the first year of life. The faulty fat absorption may induce deficiency of the fat-soluble vitamins, resulting in manifestations of avitaminosis A, D, or K. Hypoproteinemia may be severe enough to cause generalized edema. Persistent diarrhea may result in rectal prolapse in up to 10% of children with cystic fibrosis. The *pancreas-sufficient* phenotype is usually not associated with other gastrointestinal complications, and in general, these individuals demonstrate excellent growth and development. *"Idiopathic" chronic pancreatitis* occurs in a subset of patients with pancreas-sufficient cystic fibrosis and is associated with recurrent abdominal pain with life-threatening complications. These patients have other features of cystic fibrosis, such as pulmonary disease. By contrast, "idiopathic" chronic pancreatitis can also occur as an isolated late-onset finding in the absence of other stigmata of cystic fibrosis (Chapter 19); bi-allelic *CFTR* mutations (usually one "mild," one "severe") are demonstrable in the majority of these individuals who have *nonclassic or atypical cystic fibrosis. Endocrine pancreatic insufficiency* (i.e., diabetes) is uncommon in cystic fibrosis and is usually accompanied by substantial destruction of pancreatic parenchyma.

Cardiorespiratory complications, such as persistent lung infections, obstructive pulmonary disease, and *cor pulmonale,* are the most common cause of death (~80%) in patients in the United States. By age 18, 80% of patients with classic cystic fibrosis harbor *P. aeruginosa*. With the indiscriminate use of antibiotic prophylaxis against *Staphylococcus*, there has been an unfortunate resurgence of resistant strains of *Pseudomonas* in many patients. Individuals who carry one "severe" and one "mild" *CFTR* mutation may develop late-onset mild pulmonary disease, another example of nonclassic or atypical cystic fibrosis. Patients with mild pulmonary disease usually have little or no pancreatic disease. Adult-onset *"idiopathic" bronchiectasis,* has been linked to *CFTR* mutations in a subset of cases. *Recurrent sinonasal polyps* can occur in up to 25% of individuals with cystic fibrosis; hence, children who present with this finding should be tested for cystic fibrosis.

Significant *liver disease* occurs late in the natural history of cystic fibrosis and is gaining in clinical importance as life expectancies increase. In fact, after cardiopulmonary and transplantation-related complications, liver disease is the most common cause of death in cystic fibrosis. Most studies suggest that symptomatic or biochemical liver disease has its onset at or around puberty, with a prevalence of approximately 13% to 17%. However, *asymptomatic hepatomegaly* may be present in up to a third of individuals. Obstruction of the common bile duct may occur due to stones or sludge; it presents with abdominal pain and the acute onset of jaundice. As previously noted, *diffuse biliary cirrhosis* develops in less than 10% of individuals with cystic fibrosis.

Approximately 95% of males with cystic fibrosis are *infertile,* as a result of obstructive azoospermia. As mentioned earlier, this is most commonly due to congenital bilateral absence of the vas deferens, which is caused in 80% of cases by bi-allelic *CFTR* mutations.

In most cases, the diagnosis of cystic fibrosis is based on persistently elevated sweat electrolyte concentrations (often the mother makes the diagnosis by recognizing her infant's abnormally salty sweat), characteristic clinical findings (sinopulmonary disease and gastrointestinal manifestations), an abnormal newborn screening test, or a family history. A minority of patients with cystic fibrosis, especially those with at least one "mild" *CFTR* mutation, may have a normal or near-normal sweat test (<60 mM/L). Measurement of nasal transepithelial potential difference in vivo can be a useful adjunct test under these circumstances; individuals with cystic fibrosis demonstrate a significantly more negative baseline nasal potential difference than controls. Sequencing the *CFTR* gene is, of course, the "gold standard" for diagnosis of cystic fibrosis. Therefore, in patients with suggestive clinical findings or family history (or both), genetic analysis may be warranted.

There have been major improvements in the management of acute and chronic complications for cystic fibrosis, including more potent antimicrobial therapies, pancreatic enzyme replacement, and bilateral lung transplantation. Newer modalities for restituting endogenous CFTR function have also emerged in recent years. In principle, cystic fibrosis, like other single-gene disorders, should be amenable to gene therapy, and several adenoviral gene therapy vectors are currently undergoing early-phase clinical trials. Improvement in management of cystic fibrosis has resulted in enhancement of median life expectancy to above 36 years as of 2006,[41] and increasingly, a lethal disease of childhood is changing into a chronic disease of adults.

Sudden Infant Death Syndrome (SIDS)

The National Institute of Child Health and Human Development defines SIDS as "the sudden death of an infant under 1 year of age which remains unexplained after a thorough case investigation, *including performance of a complete autopsy, examination of the death scene, and review of the clinical history.*"[42] Thus, SIDS is a disease of unknown cause. It is important to emphasize that many cases of sudden death in infancy may have an unexpected anatomic or biochemical basis discernible at autopsy (Table 10–7), and these should *not* be labeled as SIDS. Furthermore, instances of sudden death during infancy wherein evidence for excluding alternative diagnoses is equivocal, or a postmortem diagnosis cannot be performed, are best labeled as *unclassified sudden infant death*, in line with the current rigorous definition of SIDS.[43] An aspect of SIDS that is not stressed in the definition is that the infant usually dies while asleep, mostly in the prone or side position, hence the pseudonyms of *crib death* or *cot death*.

Epidemiology. As infantile deaths due to nutritional problems and infections have come under control in developed countries, SIDS has assumed greater importance in these countries, including the United States. SIDS is the leading cause of death between age 1 month and 1 year in this country and the third leading cause of death overall in infancy, after congenital anomalies and diseases of prematurity and low birth weight. Mostly because of nationwide SIDS awareness campaigns by organizations such as the American Academy of Pediatrics, there has been a significant drop in SIDS-related mortality in the past decade, from an estimated 120 deaths per 100,000 live births in 1992 to 57 per 100,000 in 2002. Worldwide, in countries where unexpected infant deaths are diagnosed as SIDS only after postmortem examination, the death rates from SIDS range from 10 per 100,000 live births in the Netherlands to 80 per 100,000 in New Zealand.[44]

Approximately 90% of all SIDS deaths occur during the first 6 months of life, most between ages 2 and 4 months. This

TABLE 10–7 Risk Factors and Postmortem Findings Associated with Sudden Infant Death Syndrome
PARENTAL
Young maternal age (age <20 years)
Maternal smoking during pregnancy
Drug abuse in *either* parent, specifically paternal marijuana and maternal opiate, cocaine use
Short intergestational intervals
Late or no prenatal care
Low socioeconomic group
African-American and American Indian ethnicity (? socioeconomic factors)
INFANT
Brain stem abnormalities, associated with delayed development of arousal and cardiorespiratory control
Prematurity and/or low birth weight
Male sex
Product of a multiple birth
SIDS in a prior sibling
Antecedent respiratory infections
Germline polymorphisms in autonomic nervous system genes
ENVIRONMENT
Prone or side sleep position
Sleeping on a soft surface
Hyperthermia
Co-sleeping in first 3 months of life
POSTMORTEM ABNORMALITIES DETECTED IN CASES OF SUDDEN UNEXPECTED INFANT DEATH*
Infections
• Viral myocarditis
• Bronchopneumonia
Unsuspected congenital anomaly
• Congenital aortic stenosis
• Anomalous origin of the left coronary artery from the pulmonary artery
Traumatic child abuse
• Intentional suffocation (filicide)
Genetic and metabolic defects
• Long QT syndrome (*SCN5A* and *KCNQ1* mutations)
• Fatty acid oxidation disorders (*MCAD, LCHAD, SCHAD* mutations)
• Histiocytoid cardiomyopathy (*MTCYB* mutations)
• Abnormal inflammatory responsiveness (partial deletions in *C4a* and *C4b*)

*SIDS is not the only cause of sudden unexpected death in infancy but rather is a *diagnosis of exclusion*. Therefore, performance of an autopsy may often reveal findings that would explain the cause of sudden unexpected death. These cases should *not*, strictly speaking, be labeled as "SIDS." SCN5A, sodium channel, voltage-gated, type V, alpha polypeptide; KCNQ1, potassium voltage-gated channel, KQT-like subfamily, member 1; MCAD, medium-chain acyl coenzyme A dehydrogenase; LCHAD, long-chain 3-hydroxyacyl coenzyme A dehydrogenase; SCHAD, short-chain 3-hydroxyacyl coenzyme A dehydrogenase; MTCYB, mitochondrial cytochrome *b*; C4, complement component 4.

narrow window of peak susceptibility is a unique characteristic that is independent of other risk factors (to be described) and the geographic locale. Most infants who die of SIDS die at home, usually during the night after a period of sleep. For many years, prolonged apnea was considered to be a risk factor for SIDS. Infants who developed a so-called *"apparent life-threatening event"* (ALTE), characterized by some combination of apnea, marked change in color or muscle tone, choking or gagging, were considered at risk for subsequent SIDS.

However, epidemiologic studies have demonstrated that these "life-threatening events" and SIDS have different risk factors and ages of onset, and are probably unrelated entities. Children experiencing ALTEs are often premature or have a mechanical basis for respiratory compromise. This distinction might explain why home apnea monitors, which have proliferated among American families for "SIDS prevention," have had minimal impact on reducing the risk of SIDS.[45]

Morphology. In infants who have died of suspected SIDS, a variety of findings have been reported at postmortem examination. They are usually subtle and of uncertain significance and are not present in all cases. **Multiple petechiae** are the most common finding (~80% of cases); these are usually present on the thymus, visceral and parietal pleura, and epicardium. Grossly, the lungs are usually congested, and **vascular engorgement** with or without **pulmonary edema** is demonstrable microscopically in the majority of cases. These changes possibly represent agonal events, since they are found with comparable frequencies in *explained* sudden deaths in infancy. Within the upper respiratory system (larynx and trachea), there may be some histologic evidence of recent infection (correlating with the clinical symptoms), although the changes are not sufficiently severe to account for death and should not detract from the diagnosis of SIDS. The central nervous system demonstrates **astrogliosis** of the brain stem and cerebellum. Sophisticated morphometric studies have revealed quantitative brain-stem abnormalities such as **hypoplasia of the arcuate nucleus** or a decrease in brain-stem neuronal populations in several cases; these observations are not uniform, however. Nonspecific findings include frequent persistence of hepatic **extramedullary hematopoiesis** and **periadrenal brown fat**; it is tempting to speculate that these latter findings relate to chronic hypoxemia, retardation of normal development, and chronic stress. Thus, autopsy usually fails to provide a clear cause of death, and this may well be related to the etiologic heterogeneity of SIDS. The importance of a postmortem examination rests in identifying other causes of sudden unexpected death in infancy, such as unsuspected infection, congenital anomaly, or a genetic disorder (see Table 10–7), the presence of any of which would *exclude* a diagnosis of SIDS; and in ruling out the unfortunate possibility of traumatic child abuse.

Pathogenesis. The circumstances surrounding SIDS have been explored in great detail, and it is generally accepted that it is a *multifactorial condition,* with a variable mixture of contributing factors. A "triple-risk" model of SIDS has been proposed, which postulates the intersection of three overlapping factors: (1) *a vulnerable infant,* (2) *a critical developmental period in homeostatic control,* and (3) *an exogenous stressor(s).*[46] According to this model, several factors make the infant vulnerable to sudden death during the critical developmental period (i.e., the first 6 months of life). These vulnerability factors may be attributable to the parents or the infant, while the exogenous stressor(s) is attributable to the environment (see Table 10–7).

While numerous factors have been proposed to account for a vulnerable infant, *the most compelling hypothesis is that SIDS reflects a delayed development of "arousal" and cardiorespiratory control.* The brain stem, and in particular the medulla oblongata, plays a critical role in the body's "arousal" response to noxious stimuli such as episodic hypercarbia, hypoxia, and thermal stress encountered during sleep. The serotonergic (5-HT) system of the medulla is implicated in these "arousal" responses, as well as regulation of other critical homeostatic functions such as respiratory drive, blood pressure, and upper airway reflexes. Abnormalities in serotonin-dependent signaling in the brainstem may be the underlying basis for SIDS in some infants.[47] A recently developed mouse model of disrupted somatostatin signaling in the medulla recapitulates many of the features likely to contribute to sudden death in SIDS infants, including lack of an appropriate "arousal" response to environmental stressors.[48]

Epidemiologic and genetic studies have identified additional vulnerability factors for SIDS in the "triple-risk" model. Infants who are born before term or who are low birth weight are at increased risk, and risk increases with decreasing gestational age or birth weight. As stated, male sex is associated with a slightly greater incidence of SIDS. SIDS in a prior sibling is associated with a fivefold relative risk of recurrence, underscoring the importance of a genetic predisposition (see below); *traumatic child abuse must be carefully excluded under these circumstances.* Most SIDS babies have an immediate prior history of a mild respiratory tract infection, but no single causative organism has been isolated. These infections may predispose an already vulnerable infant to even greater impairment of cardiorespiratory control and delayed arousal. In this context, *laryngeal chemoreceptors* have emerged as a putative "missing link" between upper respiratory tract infections, the prone position (see below), and SIDS. When stimulated, these laryngeal chemoreceptors typically elicit an inhibitory cardiorespiratory reflex. Stimulation of the chemoreceptors is augmented by respiratory tract infections, which increase the volume of secretions, and by the prone position, which impairs swallowing and clearing of the airways even in healthy infants. In a previously vulnerable infant with impaired arousal, the resulting inhibitory cardiorespiratory reflex may prove fatal. Genetic vulnerability factors in the infant include polymorphic variants in genes that may confer an increased risk of SIDS. These genes include those related to serotonergic signaling and autonomic innervation, underscoring the importance of these processes in the pathophysiology of SIDS.[49]

In addition to infant vulnerability factors, several maternal risk factors have also been identified. Maternal smoking during pregnancy has consistently emerged as a risk factor in epidemiologic studies of SIDS, with children exposed to in utero nicotine having more than double the risk of SIDS as compared with children born to nonsmokers.[50] Young maternal age, frequent childbirths, and inadequate prenatal care are all risk factors associated with increased incidence of SIDS in the offspring.

Among the potential "environmental stressors," prone or side sleeping positions, sleeping with parents in the first 3 months, sleeping on soft surfaces, and thermal stress are possibly the most important modifiable risk factors for SIDS.[42,44] The prone or side positions predispose an infant to one or more recognized noxious stimuli (hypoxia, hypercarbia, and thermal stress) during sleep. The side position was considered a reliable alternative to the prone sleeping position, but a number of studies have established a substantial risk for both positions vis-à-vis SIDS. *The American Academy of Pediatrics now recognizes the supine sleeping position as the only safe position that reduces the risk of SIDS.* This "Back to Sleep" campaign has resulted in substantial reductions in SIDS-related deaths since its inception in 1994.

As has been stated, SIDS is not the only cause of sudden unexpected deaths in infancy. In fact, SIDS is a diagnosis of exclusion, requiring careful examination of the death scene and a complete postmortem examination. The latter can reveal an unsuspected cause of sudden death in as many as 20% or more of "SIDS" babies. Infections (e.g., viral myocarditis or bronchopneumonia) are the most common causes of sudden "unexpected" death, followed by unsuspected congenital anomalies. In part as a result of advancements in molecular diagnostics and knowledge of the human genome, several genetic causes of sudden "unexpected" infant death have emerged. For example, fatty acid oxidation disorders, characterized by defects in mitochondrial fatty acid oxidative enzymes, may be responsible for as many as 5% of sudden deaths in infancy. Other newly emerging genetic causes of *explained* sudden death are listed in Table 10–7.

Tumors and Tumor-like Lesions of Infancy and Childhood

Only 2% of all malignant tumors occur in infancy and childhood; nonetheless, cancer (including leukemia) accounts for about 9% of deaths in the United States in children over age 4 and up to age 14, and only accidents cause significantly more deaths. Benign tumors are even more common than cancers. Most benign tumors are of little concern, but on occasion they cause serious complications by virtue of their location or rapid increase in size.

It is sometimes difficult to separate, on morphologic grounds, true tumors or neoplasms from tumor-like lesions in the infant and child. In this context, two special categories of tumor-like lesions should be distinguished from true tumors.

The term *heterotopia* (or *choristoma*) is applied to microscopically normal cells or tissues that are present in abnormal locations. Examples of heterotopias include a rest of pancreatic tissue found in the wall of the stomach or small intestine, or a small mass of adrenal cells found in the kidney, lungs, ovaries, or elsewhere. These heterotopic rests are usually of little significance, but they can be confused clinically with neoplasms. Rarely, they are sites of origin of true neoplasms, producing paradoxes such as an adrenal carcinoma arising in the ovary.

The term *hamartoma* refers to an excessive, focal overgrowth of cells and tissues native to the organ in which it occurs. Although the cellular elements are mature and identical to those found in the remainder of the organ, they do not reproduce the normal architecture of the surrounding tissue. The line of demarcation between a hamartoma and a benign neoplasm is often unclear, as both lesions can be clonal. Hemangiomas, lymphangiomas, rhabdomyomas of the heart, adenomas of the liver, and developmental cysts within the kidneys, lungs, or pancreas are interpreted by some as hamartomas and by others as true neoplasms. The frequency of these lesions in infancy and childhood and their clinical behavior give credence to the belief that many are developmental aberrations. Their unequivocally benign histology, however, does not preclude bothersome and rarely life-threatening clinical problems in some cases.

BENIGN TUMORS AND TUMOR-LIKE LESIONS

Virtually any tumor may be encountered in children, but within this wide array hemangiomas, lymphangiomas, fibrous lesions, and teratomas deserve special mention. You will notice that the most common neoplasms of childhood are so-called soft-tissue tumors of mesenchymal derivation. This contrasts with adults, in whom the most common tumors, benign or malignant, have an epithelial origin. Benign tumors of various tissues are described in greater detail in appropriate chapters; here a few comments are made about their special features in childhood.

Hemangioma. Hemangiomas (Chapter 11) are the most common tumors of infancy. Architecturally, they do not differ from those occurring in adults. Both cavernous and capillary hemangiomas may be encountered, although the latter are often more cellular than in adults, a feature that is deceptively worrisome. In children, most are located in the skin, particularly on the face and scalp, where they produce flat to elevated, irregular, red-blue masses; some of the flat, larger lesions (considered by some to represent vascular ectasias) are referred to as *port-wine stains*. Hemangiomas may enlarge along with the growth of the child, but in many instances they spontaneously regress (Fig. 10–23). In addition to their cosmetic significance, they can represent one facet of the hereditary disorder von Hippel-Lindau disease (Chapter 20). A subset of central nervous system cavernous hemangiomas can occur in the familial setting; these families harbor mutations in one of three cerebral cavernous malformation (CCM) genes.

Lymphatic Tumors. A wide variety of lesions are of lymphatic origin. Some of them—*lymphangiomas*—are hamartomatous or neoplastic, whereas others seem to represent abnormal dilations of preexisting lymph channels known as *lymphangiectasis*. The *lymphangiomas* are usually characterized by cystic and cavernous spaces. Lesions of this nature may occur in the skin but are more often encountered in the deeper regions of the neck, axilla, mediastinum, retroperitoneal tissue, and elsewhere. Although histologically benign, they tend to increase in size after birth, owing to the accumulation of fluid and the budding of preexisting spaces. In this manner they may encroach on vital structures, such as those in the mediastinum or nerve trunks in the axilla, and give rise to clinical problems. *Lymphangiectasis*, in contrast, usually presents as a diffuse swelling of part or all of an extremity; considerable distortion and deformation may occur as a consequence of the spongy, dilated subcutaneous and deeper lymphatics. The lesion is not progressive, however, and does not extend beyond its original location. Nonetheless, it creates cosmetic problems that are often difficult to correct surgically.

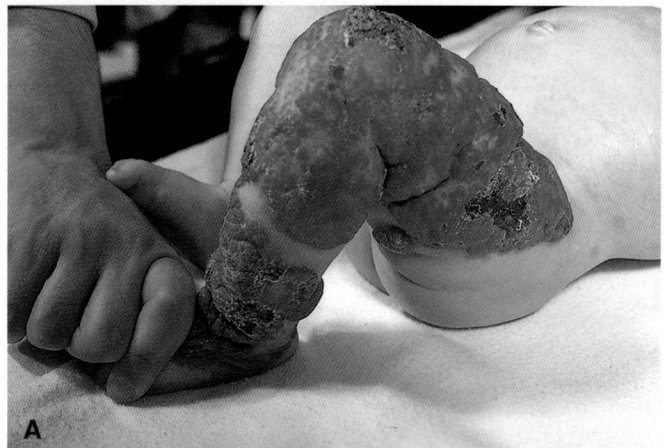

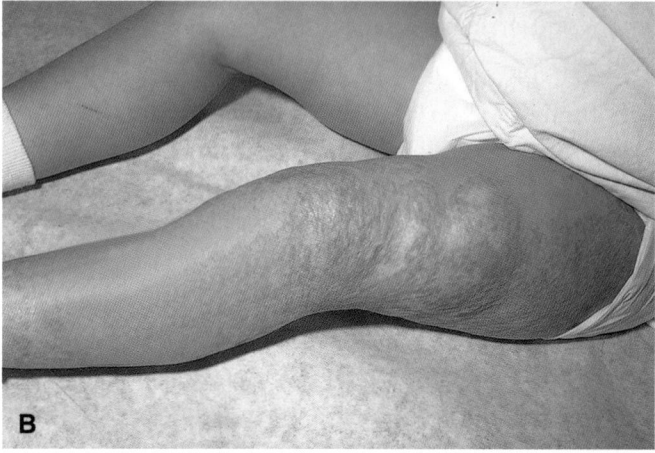

FIGURE 10–23 Congenital capillary hemangioma at birth (**A**) and at age 2 years (**B**) after spontaneous regression. (Courtesy of Dr. Eduardo Yunis, Children's Hospital of Pittsburgh, Pittsburgh, PA.)

Fibrous Tumors. Fibrous tumors occurring in infants and children range from sparsely cellular proliferations of spindle-shaped cells (designated as *fibromatosis*) to richly cellular lesions indistinguishable from fibrosarcomas occurring in adults (designated as *congenital-infantile fibrosarcomas*). Biologic behavior cannot be predicted based on histology alone, however, in that despite their histologic similarities with adult fibrosarcomas, the congenital-infantile variants have an excellent prognosis. Recently, a characteristic chromosomal translocation, t(12;15)(p13;q25), has been described in congenital-infantile fibrosarcomas, which results in generation of an *ETV6-NTRK3* fusion transcript.[51] The normal *ETV6* gene product is a transcription factor, while the *NTRK3* gene product (also known as TRKC, see below) is a tyrosine kinase. Like other tyrosine kinase fusion proteins found in human neoplasms, ETV6-TRKC is constitutively active and stimulates signaling through the oncogenic RAS and PI-3K/AKT pathways (Chapter 4). Among soft-tissue tumors, the ETV6-NTRK3 fusion transcript is unique to infantile fibrosarcomas, making it a useful diagnostic marker.

Teratomas. Teratomas illustrate the relationship of histologic maturity to biologic behavior. They may occur as benign, well-differentiated cystic lesions (mature teratomas), as lesions of indeterminate potential (immature teratomas), or as

unequivocally malignant teratomas (usually admixed with another germ cell tumor component such as endodermal sinus tumor) (Chapter 21). They exhibit two peaks in incidence: the first at approximately 2 years of age and the second in late adolescence or early adulthood. The first peak are congenital neoplasms; the later occurring lesions may also be of prenatal origin but are more slowly growing. *Sacrococcygeal teratomas* are the most common teratomas of childhood, accounting for 40% or more of cases (Fig. 10–24). They occur with a frequency of 1 in 20,000 to 40,000 live births, and are four times more common in girls than boys. In view of the overlap in the mechanisms underlying teratogenesis and oncogenesis, it is interesting that approximately 10% of sacrococcygeal teratomas are associated with congenital anomalies, primarily defects of the hindgut and cloacal region and other midline defects (e.g., meningocele, spina bifida) not believed to result from local effects of the tumor. Approximately 75% of these tumors are mature teratomas, and about 12% are unequivocally malignant and lethal. The remainder is immature teratomas; their malignant potential correlates with the amount of immature tissue, usually immature neuroepithelial elements, present. Most of the benign teratomas are encountered in younger infants (<4 months), whereas children with malignant lesions tend to be somewhat older. Other sites for teratomas in childhood include the testis (Chapter 21), ovaries (Chapter 22), and various midline locations, such as the mediastinum, retroperitoneum, and head and neck.

MALIGNANT TUMORS

Cancers of infancy and childhood differ biologically and histologically from their counterparts occurring later in life. The main differences, some of which have already been alluded to, include the following:

- Incidence and type of tumor
- Relatively frequent demonstration of a close relationship between abnormal development (teratogenesis) and tumor induction (oncogenesis)

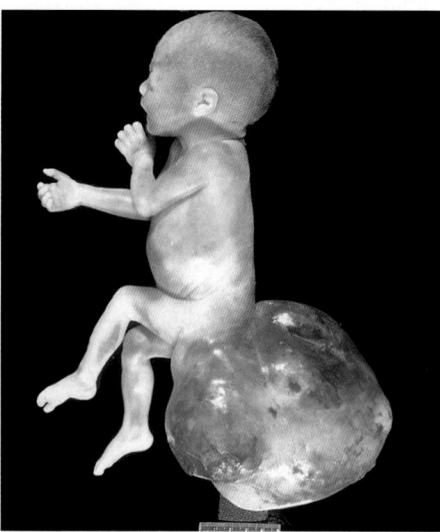

FIGURE 10–24 Sacrococcygeal teratoma. Note the size of the lesion compared with that of the stillbirth.

TABLE 10–8	Common Malignant Neoplasms of Infancy and Childhood	
0 to 4 Years	**5 to 9 Years**	**10 to 14 Years**
Leukemia	Leukemia	
Retinoblastoma	Retinoblastoma	
Neuroblastoma	Neuroblastoma	
Wilms tumor		
Hepatoblastoma	Hepatocellular carcinoma	Hepatocellular carcinoma
Soft-tissue sarcoma (especially rhabdomyosarcoma)	Soft-tissue sarcoma	Soft-tissue sarcoma
Teratomas		
Central nervous system tumors	Central nervous system tumors Ewing sarcoma Lymphoma	Osteogenic sarcoma Thyroid carcinoma Hodgkin disease

- Prevalence of underlying familial or genetic aberrations
- Tendency of fetal and neonatal malignancies to regress spontaneously or cytodifferentiate
- Improved survival or cure of many childhood tumors, so that more attention is now being devoted to minimizing the adverse delayed effects of chemotherapy and radiation therapy in survivors, including the development of second malignancies

Incidence and Types

The most frequent childhood cancers arise in the hematopoietic system, nervous tissue (including the central and sympathetic nervous system, adrenal medulla, and retina), soft tissues, bone, and kidney. This is in sharp contrast to adults, in whom the skin, lung, breast, prostate, and colon are the most common sites of tumors.

Neoplasms that exhibit sharp peaks in incidence in children younger than age 10 years include (1) leukemia (principally acute lymphoblastic leukemia), (2) neuroblastoma, (3) Wilms tumor, (4) hepatoblastoma, (5) retinoblastoma, (6) rhabdomyosarcoma, (7) teratoma, (8) Ewing sarcoma, and finally, posterior fossa neoplasms—principally (9) juvenile astrocytoma, (10) medulloblastoma, and (11) ependymoma. Other forms of cancer are also common in childhood but do not have the same striking early peak. The approximate age distribution of these cancers is indicated in Table 10–8. Within this large array, leukemia alone accounts for more deaths in children younger than age 15 years than all of the other tumors combined.

Histologically, many of the malignant non-hematopoietic pediatric neoplasms are unique. In general, they tend to have a more primitive *(embryonal)* rather than pleomorphic-anaplastic microscopic appearance, are often characterized by sheets of cells with small, round nuclei, and frequently show features of organogenesis specific to the site of tumor origin. Because of this latter characteristic, these tumors are frequently designated by the suffix *-blastoma*, for example, nephroblastoma (Wilms tumor), hepatoblastoma, and neuroblastoma. Because of their primitive histologic appearance, many childhood tumors have been collectively referred to as *small round blue cell tumors*. The differential diagnosis of such tumors includes neuroblastoma, Wilms tumor, lymphoma

(Chapter 14), rhabdomyosarcoma (Chapter 26), Ewing sarcoma/primitive neuroectodermal tumor (Chapter 26), medulloblastoma (Chapter 28), and retinoblastoma (Chapter 29). If the anatomic site of origin is known, diagnosis is usually possible on histologic grounds alone. Occasionally, a combination of chromosome analysis, immunoperoxidase stains, or electron microscopy is required. Two of these tumors are particularly illustrative and are discussed here: the neuroblastic tumors, specifically neuroblastoma, and Wilms tumor. The remaining tumors are discussed in their respective organ-specific chapters.

The Neuroblastic Tumors

The term *neuroblastic tumor* includes tumors of the sympathetic ganglia and adrenal medulla that are derived from primordial neural crest cells populating these sites. As a family, neuroblastic tumors demonstrate certain characteristic features including *spontaneous or therapy-induced differentiation of primitive neuroblasts into mature elements, spontaneous tumor regression*, and a *wide range of clinical behavior and prognosis*, which often mirror the extent of histologic differentiation. Neuroblastoma is the most important member of this family. It is the most common extracranial solid tumor of childhood, and the most frequently diagnosed tumor of infancy. The prevalence is about one case in 7000 live births, and there are approximately 700 cases diagnosed each year in the United States. The median age at diagnosis is 18 months; approximately 40% of cases are diagnosed in infancy. Most neuroblastomas occur sporadically, but 1% to 2% are familial, and in such cases the neoplasms may involve both of the adrenals or multiple primary autonomic sites. Germline mutations in the *anaplastic lymphoma kinase (ALK)* gene (Chapter 14) have recently been identified as a major cause of familial predisposition to neuroblastoma.[52] Somatic gain-of-function *ALK* mutations are also observed in a subset of sporadic neuroblastomas. It is envisioned that tumors harboring *ALK* mutations in either the germline or somatic setting will be amenable to treatment using drugs that target the activity of this kinase.

Despite the remarkable progress made in the therapy of this disease, long-term prognosis for the high-risk subsets remains modest, with a 5-year survival in the range of 40%. As will be

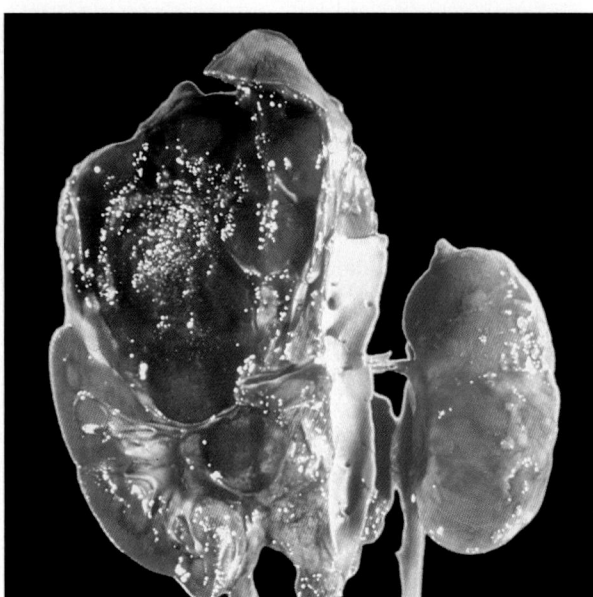

FIGURE 10–25 Adrenal neuroblastoma in a 6-month-old child. The hemorrhagic, partially encapsulated tumor has displaced the opened left kidney and is impinging on the aorta and left renal artery. (Courtesy of Dr. Arthur Weinberg, University of Texas Southwestern Medical School, Dallas, TX.)

evident later, age and stage have a remarkable effect on prognosis, and, in general, children younger than 18 months of age tend to have a significantly better prognosis than older individuals at comparable disease burdens.

Morphology. In childhood about 40% of neuroblastomas arise in the adrenal medulla. The remainder occur anywhere along the sympathetic chain, with the most common locations being the paravertebral region of the abdomen (25%) and posterior mediastinum (15%). Tumors may arise in numerous other sites, including the pelvis, the neck, and within the brain (cerebral neuroblastomas).

Neuroblastomas range in size from minute nodules (so-called **in situ lesions**) to large masses more than 1 kg in weight (Fig. 10–25). In situ neuroblastomas are reported to occur 40 times more frequently than clinically overt tumors. The great majority of these silent lesions spontaneously regress, leaving only a focus of fibrosis or calcification in the adult; this has led some to question the neoplastic connotation for the in situ lesions, arguing instead in favor of labeling them as developmental anomalies ("rests"). Some neuroblastomas are often sharply demarcated by a fibrous pseudo-capsule, but others are far more infiltrative and invade surrounding structures, including the kidneys, renal vein, and vena cava, and envelop the aorta. On transection, they are composed of soft, gray-tan, tissue. Larger tumors have areas of necrosis, cystic softening, and hemorrhage. Occasionally, foci of punctate intra-tumoral calcification can be palpated.

Histologically, classic neuroblastomas are composed of small, primitive-appearing cells with dark

nuclei, scant cytoplasm, and poorly defined cell borders growing in solid sheets. Such tumors may be difficult to differentiate morphologically from other small round blue cell tumors. Mitotic activity, nuclear breakdown ("karyorrhexis"), and pleomorphism may be prominent. The background often demonstrates a faintly eosinophilic fibrillary material (**neuropil**) that corresponds to neuritic processes of the primitive neuroblasts. Typically, rosettes (**Homer-Wright pseudorosettes**) can be found in which the tumor cells are concentrically arranged about a central space filled with neuropil (Fig. 10–26). Other helpful features include positive immunochemical reactions for neuron-specific enolase and ultrastructural demonstration of small, membrane-bound, cytoplasmic catecholamine-containing secretory granules; the latter contain characteristic central dense cores surrounded by a peripheral halo (dense core granules). Some neoplasms show signs of maturation that can be spontaneous or therapy-induced. Larger cells having more abundant cytoplasm, large vesicular nuclei, and a prominent nucleolus, representing *ganglion cells* in various stages of maturation, may be found in tumors admixed with primitive neuroblasts (**ganglioneuroblastoma**). Even better differentiated lesions contain many more large cells resembling mature ganglion cells with few if any residual neuroblasts; such neoplasms merit the designation **ganglioneuroma** (Fig. 10–27). Maturation of neuroblasts into ganglion cells is usually accompanied by the appearance of **Schwann cells**. In fact, the presence of a so-called schwannian stroma composed of organized fascicles of neuritic processes, mature Schwann cells, and fibroblasts is a histologic prerequisite for the designation of ganglioneuroblastoma and ganglioneuroma; ganglion cells in and of themselves do not fulfill the criteria for maturation. The origin of Schwann cells in neuroblastoma remains an issue of contention; some investigators believe they represent a reactive population recruited by the tumor cells. However, studies using

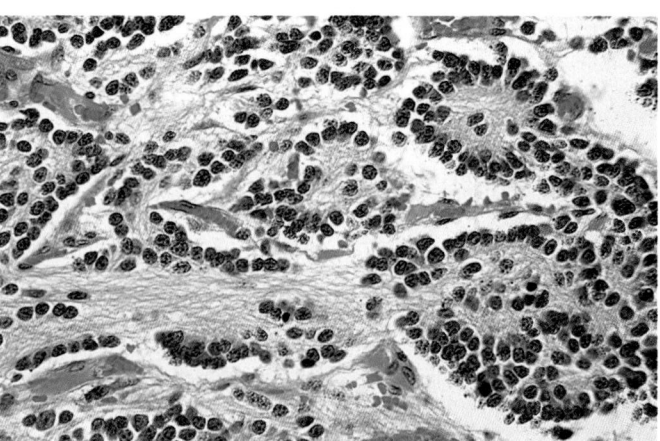

FIGURE 10–26 Adrenal neuroblastoma. This tumor is composed of small cells embedded in a finely fibrillar matrix.

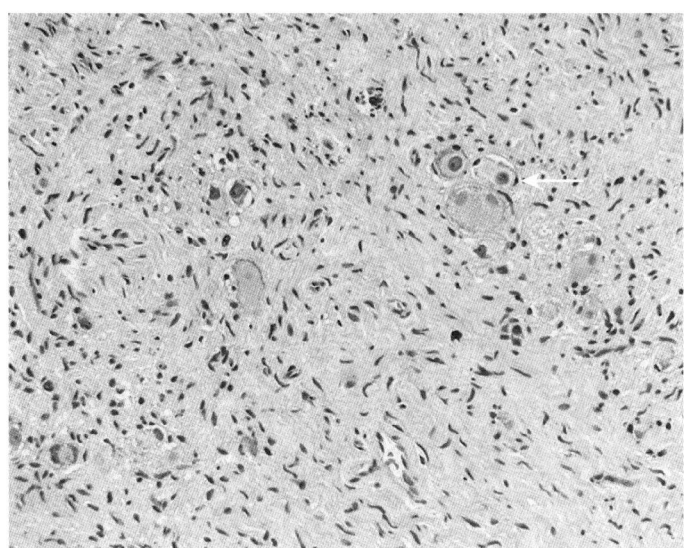

FIGURE 10–27 Ganglioneuromas, arising from spontaneous or therapy-induced maturation of neuroblastomas, are characterized by clusters of large cells with vesicular nuclei and abundant eosinophilic cytoplasm, representing neoplastic ganglion cells *(arrow)*. Spindle-shaped Schwann cells are present in the background stroma.

microdissection techniques have demonstrated that the Schwann cells harbor at least a subset of the same genetic alterations found in neuroblasts, and therefore are a component of the malignant clone.[53] Irrespective of histogenesis, documenting the presence of schwannian stroma is essential, since its presence is associated with a **favorable outcome** (Table 10–9).

Metastases, when they develop, appear early and widely. In addition to local infiltration and lymph node spread, there is a pronounced tendency to spread through the bloodstream to involve the liver, lungs, bone marrow, and bones.

Staging. The International Neuroblastoma Staging System, which is the most widely used staging scheme worldwide, is detailed below:

- **Stage 1:** Localized tumor with complete gross excision, with or without microscopic residual disease; representative ipsilateral nonadherent lymph nodes negative for tumor (nodes adherent to the primary tumor may be positive for tumor).
- **Stage 2A:** Localized tumor with incomplete gross resection; representative ipsilateral nonadherent lymph nodes negative for tumor microscopically.
- **Stage 2B:** Localized tumor with or without complete gross excision; ipsilateral nonadherent lymph nodes positive for tumor; enlarged contralateral lymph nodes, which are negative for tumor microscopically.
- **Stage 3:** Unresectable unilateral tumor infiltrating across the midline with or without regional lymph node involvement; or localized unilateral tumor with contralateral regional lymph node involvement.
- **Stage 4:** Any primary tumor with dissemination to distant lymph nodes, bone, bone marrow, liver, skin, and/or other organs *(except as defined for stage 4S)*.
- **Stage 4S** ("S" = special): Localized primary tumor (as defined for stages 1, 2A, or 2B) with dissemination limited to skin, liver, and/or bone marrow; *stage 4S is limited to infants younger than 1 year.*

TABLE 10–9 Prognostic Factors in Neuroblastomas		
Variable	**Favorable**	**Unfavorable**
Stage*	Stage 1, 2A, 2B, 4S	Stage 3, 4
Age*	<18 months	>18 months

Histology*
  Evidence of schwannian stroma and gangliocytic differentiation†
  Mitosis-karyorrhexis index‡
	Present
	<200/5000 cells
		Absent
		>200/5000 cells

DNA ploidy*	Hyperdiploid or near-triploid	Near-diploid
N-MYC*	Not amplified	Amplified
Chromosome 17q gain	Absent	Present
Chromosome 1p loss	Absent	Present
Chromosome 11q loss	Absent	Present
TRKA expression	Present	Absent
TRKB expression	Absent	Present
Telomerase expression	Low or absent	Highly expressed

*Corresponds to the most commonly used parameters in clinical practice for assessment of prognosis and risk stratification.
†It is not only the presence but also the amount of schwannian stroma that confers the designation of a favorable histology. At least *50% or more schwannian stroma* is required before a neoplasm can be classified as ganglioneuroblastoma or ganglioneuroma.
‡Mitotic karyorrhexis index (MKI) is defined as the number of mitotic or karyorrhectic cells per 5000 tumor cells in random foci.

Unfortunately, most (60% to 80%) children present with stage 3 or 4 tumors, and only 20% to 40% present with stage 1, 2A, 2B, or 4S neuroblastomas. The staging system is of paramount importance in determining prognosis.

Clinical Course and Prognostic Features. In young children, under age 2 years, neuroblastomas generally present with large abdominal masses, fever, and possibly weight loss. In older children, they may not come to attention until metastases produce manifestations, such as bone pain, respiratory symptoms, or gastrointestinal complaints. Neuroblastomas may metastasize widely through the hematogenous and lymphatic systems, particularly to liver, lungs, bones, and bone marrow. Proptosis and ecchymosis may also be present, because the periorbital region is a common metastatic site. Bladder and bowel dysfunction may be caused by paraspinal neuroblastomas that impinge on nerves. In neonates, disseminated neuroblastomas may present with multiple cutaneous metastases that cause deep blue discoloration of the skin (earning the unfortunate designation of "*blueberry muffin baby*"). *About 90% of neuroblastomas, regardless of location, produce catecholamines* (similar to the catecholamines associated with pheochromocytomas), which are an important diagnostic feature (i.e., elevated blood levels of catecholamines and elevated urine levels of the metabolites vanillylmandelic acid [VMA] and homovanillic acid [HVA]). Despite the elaboration of catecholamines, hypertension is much less frequent with these neoplasms than with pheochromocytomas (Chapter 24). Ganglioneuromas, unlike their malignant counterparts, tend to produce either asymptomatic mass lesions or symptoms related to compression.

The course of neuroblastomas is extremely variable. Several clinical, histopathologic, molecular, and biochemical factors have been identified that have a bearing on prognosis (see Table 10–9)[54]; based on the collection of prognostic factors present in a given patient, they are classified as either "low," "intermediate," or "high" risk. With improvements in therapy, the first two categories result in long-term survival of 80% to 90% of patients, while less than 40% of patients in the high-risk category are long-term survivors. The most pertinent prognostic factors in neuroblastomas include the following:

○ *Age and stage are the most important determinants of outcome.* Neuroblastomas at stages 1, 2A, or 2B tend to have an excellent prognosis, irrespective of age ("low" or "intermediate" risk); the one notable exception to this rule are tumors exhibiting amplification of the *N-MYC* oncogene (see below). Infants with localized primary tumors and widespread metastases to the liver, bone marrow, and skin (stage 4S) represent a special subtype, wherein it is not uncommon for the disease to regress spontaneously. The biologic basis of this welcome behavior is not clear. *The age of 18 months has emerged as a critical point of dichotomy in terms of prognosis.*[55] Children younger than 18 months of age, and especially those in the first year of life, have an excellent prognosis regardless of the stage of the neoplasm. Children older than 18 months fall into at least the "intermediate" risk category, while those with higher stage tumors or with confounding unfavorable prognostic variables like

N-MYC amplification in the neoplastic cells are considered "high" risk.

○ *Morphology* is an independent prognostic variable in neuroblastic tumors. An age-linked morphologic classification of neuroblastic tumors has recently been proposed that divides them into *favorable* and *unfavorable* histologic subtypes. The specific morphologic features that bear on prognosis are listed in Table 10–9.

○ *Amplification of the N-MYC oncogene in neuroblastomas is a molecular event that has possibly the most profound impact on prognosis*, particularly when it occurs in tumors that would otherwise portend a good outcome.[56] The presence of *N-MYC* amplification "bumps" the tumor into a "high"-risk category, irrespective of age, stage, or histology. *N-MYC* is located on the distal short arm of chromosome 2 (2p23–p24). Amplification of *N-MYC* does not karyotypically manifest at the resident 2p23–p24 site, but rather as extrachromosomal double minute chromatin bodies or homogeneously staining regions on other chromosomes (Fig. 10–28). *N-MYC* amplification is present in about 20% to 30% of primary tumors, most presenting as advanced-stage disease and the degree of amplification correlates with worse prognosis. *N-MYC* amplification is currently the most important genetic abnormality used in risk stratification of neuroblastic tumors (see below).

○ *Ploidy* of the tumor cells correlates with outcome in children less than 2 years of age but loses its independent prognostic significance in older children. Broadly, neuroblastomas can be divided into two categories: *near-diploid* and *hyper-diploid* (often near-triploid), with the latter being associated with a better prognosis. It is postulated that neuroblastomas with hyper-diploidy have an underlying defect in the mitotic machinery, leading to chromosomal nondisjunction and near-triploidy, but otherwise relatively banal karyotypes. On the contrary, the more aggressive near-diploid tumors harbor generalized genomic instability, with multiple unbalanced translocations and chromosomal rearrangements, which retains overall ploidy but results in a complex karyotype with adverse prognostic implications.

While *age, stage, N-MYC status, histology*, and *DNA ploidy* are currently the "core" criteria used for the purposes of formal risk stratification and therapeutic decision, several additional molecular variables have been described with prognostic implications. The most pertinent ones include the following:

○ *Hemizygous deletion of the distal short arm of chromosome 1 in the region of band p36* has been demonstrated in 25% to 35% of primary tumors. Loss of 1p36 in neuroblastomas has a strong correlation with *N-MYC* amplification, as well as advanced disease stage, and is associated with an increased risk of disease relapse in localized tumors.[57] *Hemizygous loss of chromosome 11q* genetic material is another adverse prognostic factor, and some recent high-resolution microarray studies suggest this abnormality may be the most common deletion event in neuroblastomas.[58]

○ *Partial gain of the distal long arm of chromosome 17 is present in up to 50% of tumors,* and associated with an adverse outcome, particularly with the risk of relapse in localized tumors without *N-MYC* amplification.[59]

Although discussion of the treatment modalities for neuroblastoma is beyond the scope of this book, we will mention in passing two promising experimental approaches that are being evaluated. The first involves the use of retinoids as an adjunct therapy for inducing the differentiation of neuroblastoma. Recall that the retinoic acid pathway plays a critical role in cellular differentiation during embryogenesis. Another emerging "targeted" therapy involves disrupting oncogenic TRKB signaling in neuroblastomas, by using small-molecule inhibitors of its tyrosine kinase activity. Finally, we should mention the current status of screening programs for neuroblastoma. Since the vast majority of neuroblastomas release catecholamines into the circulation, detection of catecholamine metabolites (VMA and HVA) in urine could, in principle, form the basis for screening for asymptomatic tumors in children. However, two large studies in Europe and North America have failed to demonstrate improved mortality rates with such population screening, because most tumors detected had favorable biologic characteristics, and the costs of screening failed to outweigh the benefits.[60,61] Therefore, community-based screening programs for neuroblastomas are not currently advocated.

Wilms Tumor

Wilms tumor afflicts approximately 1 in every 10,000 children in the United States, and it is the most common primary renal tumor of childhood and the fourth most common pediatric malignancy in the United States. The peak incidence for Wilms tumor is between 2 and 5 years of age, and 95% of tumors occur before the age of 10 years. Approximately 5% to 10% of Wilms tumors involve both kidneys, either simultaneously (*synchronous*) or one after the other (*metachronous*). Bilateral Wilms tumors have a median age of onset approximately 10 months earlier than tumors restricted to one kidney, and these patients are presumed to harbor a germline mutation in one of the Wilms tumor–predisposing genes (see below). The biology of this tumor illustrates several important aspects of childhood neoplasms, such as the relationship between *malformations* and *neoplasia*, the histologic similarities between *organogenesis* and *oncogenesis*, the *two-hit theory* of recessive tumor suppressor genes (Chapter 7), the role of *premalignant lesions*, and perhaps most importantly, the potential for *judicious treatment modalities* to dramatically affect prognosis and outcome.[62] Improvements in the cure rates for Wilms tumor (from as low as 30% a few decades ago, to 85% currently) represent one of the greatest successes of pediatric oncology.

Pathogenesis and Genetics. The risk of Wilms tumor is increased in association with at least four recognizable groups of congenital malformations associated with distinct chromosomal loci. Although Wilms tumors arising in this setting account for no more than 10% of cases, these *syndromic tumors* have provided important insight into the biology of this neoplasm.

The first group of patients has the *WAGR syndrome*, characterized by aniridia, genital anomalies, and mental retardation and a 33% chance of developing Wilms tumor. Individuals with WAGR syndrome carry constitutional (germline) deletions of 11p13. Studies on these patients led to the identification of the first Wilms tumor–associated gene, *WT1*, and a contiguously deleted autosomal dominant gene for aniridia,

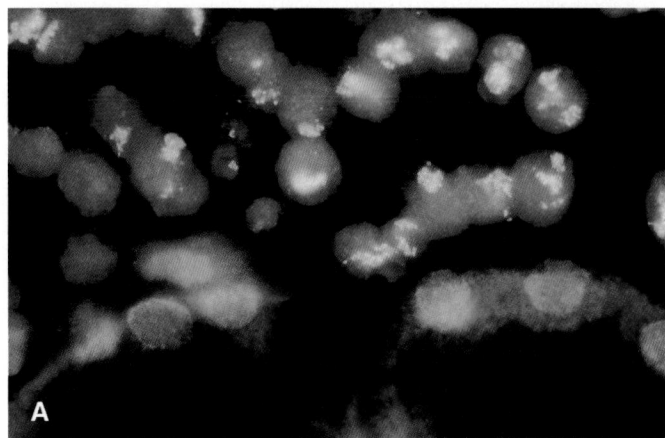

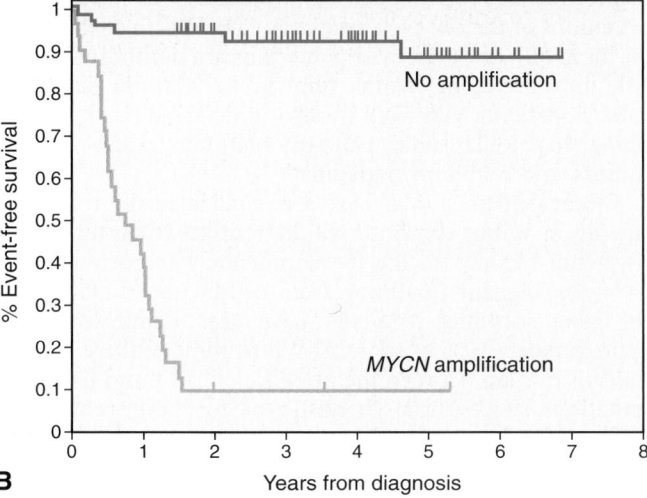

FIGURE 10–28 **A,** Fluorescence in situ hybridization using a fluorescein-labeled cosmid probe for *N-myc* on a tissue section. Note the neuroblastoma cells on the upper half of the photo with large areas of staining (*yellow-green*); this corresponds to amplified *N-MYC* in the form of homogeneously staining regions. Renal tubular epithelial cells in the lower half of the photograph show no nuclear staining and background (*green*) cytoplasmic staining. (Courtesy of Dr. Timothy Triche, Children's Hospital, Los Angeles, CA.) **B,** A Kaplan–Meier survival curve of infants younger than 1 year of age with metastatic neuroblastoma. The 3-year event-free survival (EFS) of infants whose tumors lacked *MYCN* amplification was 93%, whereas those with tumors that had *MYCN* amplification had only a 10% EFS. (Reproduced with permission from Brodeur GM: Neuroblastoma: biological insights into a clinical enigma. Nat Rev Cancer 3:203–216; 2003).

• *The expression of specific neurotrophin receptors* is also a prognostic marker for neuroblastoma. The neurotrophin receptors are a family of tyrosine kinase receptors, notably TrkA, TrkB, and TrkC (also known as NTRK3, see above), which regulate the growth, survival, and differentiation of neural cells. High TrkA expression is a favorable prognostic factor in neuroblastomas, generally associated with low-stage tumors lacking *N-MYC* amplification that occur in younger patients. In contrast, elevated TrkB expression is associated with unfavorable biological characteristics, including *N-MYC* amplification and a higher disease stage.

PAX6, both located on chromosome 11p13. Patients with deletions restricted to *PAX6*, with normal *WT1* function, develop sporadic aniridia, but they are *not* at increased risk for Wilms tumors. The presence of germline *WT1* deletions in WAGR syndrome represents the "first hit"; the development of Wilms tumor in these patients frequently correlates with the occurrence of a nonsense or frameshift mutation in the second *WT1* allele ("second hit").

A second group of patients at a much higher risk for Wilms tumor (~90%) have the *Denys-Drash syndrome*, which is characterized by *gonadal dysgenesis* (male pseudohermaphroditism) and *early-onset nephropathy* leading to renal failure. The characteristic glomerular lesion in these patients is a *diffuse mesangial sclerosis* (Chapter 20). As in patients with WAGR, these patients also demonstrate germline abnormalities in *WT1*. In patients with the Denys-Drash syndrome, however, the genetic abnormality is a *dominant-negative missense mutation* in the zinc-finger region of the *WT1* gene that affects its DNA-binding properties. This mutation interferes with the function of the remaining wild-type allele, yet strangely, it is sufficient only in causing genitourinary abnormalities, but not tumorigenesis; Wilms tumors arising in Denys-Drash syndrome demonstrate bi-allelic inactivation of *WT1*. In addition to Wilms tumors, these individuals are also at increased risk for developing germ cell tumors called *gonadoblastomas* (Chapter 21), almost certainly a consequence of disruption in normal gonadal development.

WT1 encodes a DNA-binding transcription factor that is expressed within several tissues, including the kidney and gonads, during embryogenesis. The WT1 protein is critical for normal renal and gonadal development. WT1 has multiple binding partners, and the choice of this partner can affect whether WT1 functions as a transcriptional activator or repressor in a given cellular context.[63] Numerous transcriptional targets of WT1 have been identified, including glomerular podocyte-specific proteins, and genes associated with inducing differentiation. Despite the importance of *WT1* in nephrogenesis and its unequivocal role as a tumor suppressor gene, only about 10% of patients with *sporadic* (nonsyndromic) Wilms tumors demonstrate *WT1* mutations, suggesting that the majority of these tumors arise by genetically distinct pathways.

Clinically distinct from these previous two groups of patients but also having an increased risk of developing Wilms tumor are children with *Beckwith-Wiedemann syndrome* (BWS), characterized by enlargement of body organs (organomegaly), macroglossia, hemihypertrophy, omphalocele, and abnormal large cells in the adrenal cortex (adrenal cytomegaly). BWS has served as a model for a nonclassical mechanism of tumorigenesis in humans—*genomic imprinting* (Chapter 5).[64] The chromosomal region implicated in BWS has been localized to band 11p15.5 ("WT2"), distal to the *WT1* locus. This region contains multiple genes that are normally expressed from only *one* of the two parental alleles, with transcriptional silencing (i.e., imprinting) of the other parental homologue by methylation of the promoter region. Unlike WAGR or Denys-Drash syndromes, the genetic basis for BWS is considerably more heterogeneous in that no single 11p15.5 gene is involved in all cases. Moreover, the phenotype of BWS, including the predisposition to tumorigenesis, is influenced by the specific "WT2" imprinting abnormalities present.

One of the genes in this region—insulin-like growth factor-2 (*IGF2*)—is normally expressed solely from the *paternal allele*, while the maternal allele is silenced by imprinting. In some Wilms tumors, *loss of imprinting* (i.e., re-expression of the maternal *IGF2* allele) can be demonstrated, leading to overexpression of the IGF-2 protein. In other instances there is a selective deletion of the imprinted maternal allele, combined with duplication of the transcriptionally active paternal allele in the tumor (*uniparental paternal disomy*), which has an identical functional effect in terms of overexpression of IGF-2. Since the IGF-2 protein is an embryonal growth factor, it could conceivably explain the features of overgrowth associated with BWS, as well as the increased risk for Wilms tumors in these patients. Of all the "WT2" genes, imprinting abnormalties of *IGF2* have the strongest relationship to tumor predisposition in BWS.[65] A subset of patients with BWS harbor mutations of the cell cycle regulator *CDKN1C* (also known as *p57* or *KIP2*); however, these patients have a significantly lower risk for developing Wilms tumors. In addition to Wilms tumors, patients with BWS are also at increased risk for developing hepatoblastoma, pancreatoblastoma, adrenocortical tumors, and rhabdomyosarcomas.

Recent genetic studies have also elucidated the role of β-catenin in Wilms tumor. It will be recalled (Chapter 7) that β-catenin belongs to the developmentally important *WNT* (*wingless*) signaling pathway. Gain-of-function mutations of the gene encoding β-catenin have been demonstrated in approximately 10% of sporadic Wilms tumors; there is a significant overlap between the presence of *WT1* and β-catenin mutations, suggesting a synergistic role for these events in the genesis of Wilms tumors.[66]

Nephrogenic Rests

Nephrogenic rests are putative precursor lesions of Wilms tumors and are seen in the renal parenchyma adjacent to approximately 25% to 40% of unilateral tumors; this frequency rises to nearly 100% in cases of bilateral Wilms tumors. In many instances the nephrogenic rests share genetic alterations with the adjacent Wilms tumor, underscoring their preneoplastic status. The appearance of nephrogenic rests varies from expansile masses that resemble Wilms tumors (hyperplastic rests) to sclerotic rests consisting predominantly of fibrous tissue and occasional admixed immature tubules or glomeruli. It is important to document the presence of nephrogenic rests in the resected specimen, since these patients are at an increased risk of developing Wilms tumors in the *contralateral* kidney and require frequent and regular surveillance for many years.

Morphology. Grossly, Wilms tumor tends to present as a large, solitary, well-circumscribed mass, although 10% are either bilateral or multicentric at the time of diagnosis. On cut section, the tumor is soft, homogeneous, and tan to gray with occasional foci of hemorrhage, cyst formation, and necrosis (Fig. 10–29).

Microscopically, Wilms tumors are characterized by recognizable attempts to recapitulate different stages of nephrogenesis. The classic triphasic combination of blastemal, stromal, and epithelial cell types

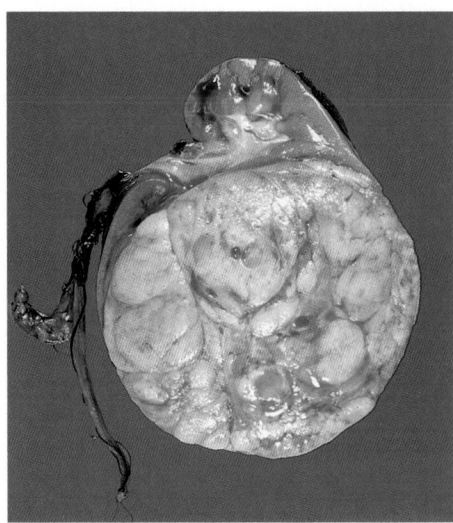

FIGURE 10–29 Wilms' tumor in the lower pole of the kidney with the characteristic tan-to-gray color and well-circumscribed margins.

pleomorphic nuclei and abnormal mitoses. The presence of anaplasia correlates with the presence of *p53* mutations and the emergence of resistance to chemotherapy.[67] Recall that p53 elicits pro-apoptotic signals in response to DNA damage (Chapter 1). The loss of p53 function might explain the relative unresponsiveness of anaplastic cells to cytotoxic chemotherapy.

Clinical Features. Most children with Wilms tumors present with a large abdominal mass that may be unilateral or, when very large, may extend across the midline and down into the pelvis. Hematuria, pain in the abdomen after some traumatic incident, intestinal obstruction, and appearance of hypertension are other patterns of presentation. In a considerable number of these patients, pulmonary metastases are present at the time of primary diagnosis.

As stated, most patients with Wilms tumor can expect to be cured of their malignancy. Anaplastic histology remains a critical determinant of adverse prognosis. Even anaplasia restricted to the kidney (i.e., without extra-renal spread) confers an increased risk of recurrence and death, underscoring the need for correctly identifying this histologic feature. Molecular parameters that correlate with adverse prognosis include loss of genetic material on chromosomes 11q and 16q, and gain of chromosome 1q in the tumor cells. Along with the increased survival of individuals with Wilms tumor have come reports of an increased relative risk of developing second primary tumors, including bone and soft-tissue sarcomas, leukemia and lymphomas, and breast cancers. While some of these neoplasms represent the presence of a germline mutation in a cancer predisposition gene, others are a consequence of therapy, most commonly radiation administered to the cancer field.[68] This tragic, albeit uncommon, outcome has mandated that radiation therapy be used judiciously in the treatment of this and other childhood cancers.

is observed in the vast majority of lesions, although the percentage of each component is variable (Fig. 10–30). Sheets of small blue cells with few distinctive features characterize the blastemal component. Epithelial differentiation is usually in the form of abortive tubules or glomeruli. Stromal cells are usually fibrocytic or myxoid in nature, although skeletal muscle differentiation is not uncommon. Rarely, other heterologous elements are identified, including squamous or mucinous epithelium, smooth muscle, adipose tissue, cartilage, and osteoid and neurogenic tissue. Approximately 5% of tumors reveal **anaplasia**, defined as the presence of cells with large, hyperchromatic,

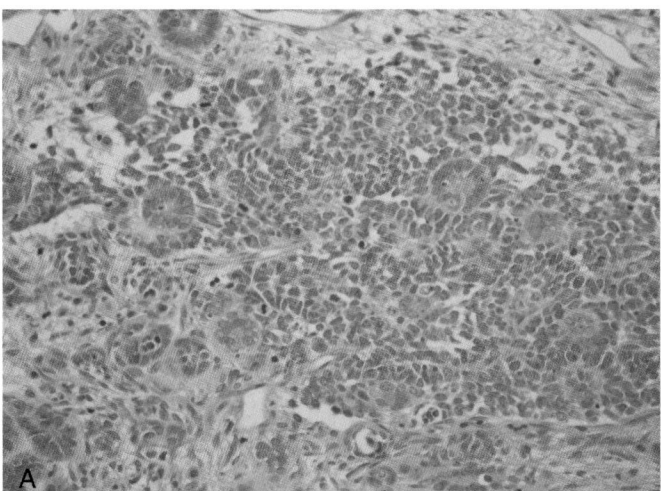
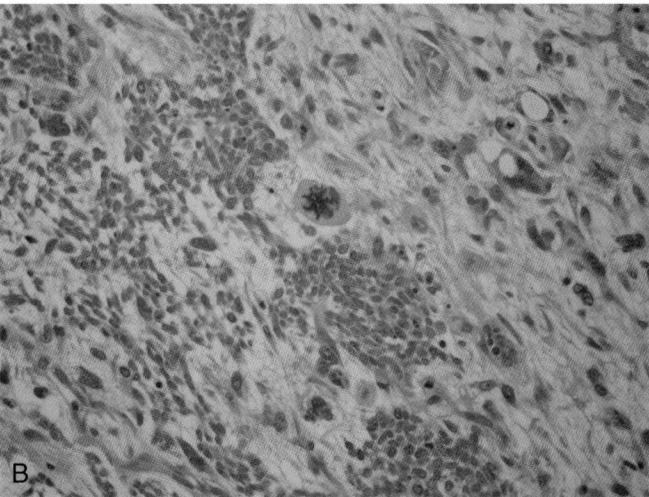

FIGURE 10–30 **A,** Wilms tumor with tightly packed blue cells consistent with the blastemal component and interspersed primitive tubules, representing the epithelial component. Although multiple mitotic figures are seen, none are atypical in this field. **B,** Focal anaplasia was present in this Wilms' tumor in other areas, characterized by cells with hyperchromatic, pleomorphic nuclei and abnormal mitoses.

REFERENCES

1. Minino AM, Heron MP, Murphy SL, Kochanek KD: Deaths: final data for 2004. Natl Vital Stat Rep 55:1, 2007.
2. Roessler E, Muenke M: How a Hedgehog might see holoprosencephaly. Hum Mol Genet 12 Spec No 1:R15, 2003.
3. Horton WA, Hall JG, Hecht JT: Achondroplasia. Lancet 370:162, 2007.
4. Knobloch J, Shaughnessy JD, Jr., Ruther U: Thalidomide induces limb deformities by perturbing the Bmp/Dkk1/Wnt signaling pathway. Faseb J 21:1410, 2007.
5. Yelin R, Schyr RB, Kot H et al: Ethanol exposure affects gene expression in the embryonic organizer and reduces retinoic acid levels. Dev Biol 279:193, 2005.
6. Li YX, Yang HT, Zdanowicz M et al: Fetal alcohol exposure impairs Hedgehog cholesterol modification and signaling. Lab Invest 87:231, 2007.
7. Blom HJ, Shaw GM, den Heijer M, Finnell RH: Neural tube defects and folate: case far from closed. Nat Rev Neurosci 7:724, 2006.
8. Faiella A, Wernig M, Consalez GG et al: A mouse model for valproate teratogenicity: parental effects, homeotic transformations, and altered HOX expression. Hum Mol Genet 9:227, 2000.
9. Koo SH, Cunningham MC, Arabshahi B, Gruss JS, Grant JH, 3rd: The transforming growth factor-beta 3 knock-out mouse: an animal model for cleft palate. Plast Reconstr Surg 108:938, 2001.
10. ACOG Practice Bulletin No. 80: premature rupture of membranes. Clinical management guidelines for obstetrician-gynecologists. Obstet Gynecol 109:1007, 2007.
11. Nesin M: Genetic basis of preterm birth. Front Biosci 12:115, 2007.
12. Elovitz MA, Wang Z, Chien EK, Rychlik DF, Phillippe M: A new model for inflammation-induced preterm birth: the role of platelet-activating factor and Toll-like receptor-4. Am J Pathol 163:2103, 2003.
13. Kinzler WL, Kaminsky L: Fetal growth restriction and subsequent pregnancy risks. Semin Perinatol 31:126, 2007.
14. Miura K, Yoshiura K, Miura S et al: Clinical outcome of infants with confined placental mosaicism and intrauterine growth restriction of unknown cause. Am J Med Genet A 140:1827, 2006.
15. Robertson L, Wu O, Langhorne P et al: Thrombophilia in pregnancy: a systematic review. Br J Haematol 132:171, 2006.
16. Hermansen CL, Lorah KN: Respiratory distress in the newborn. Am Fam Physician 76:987, 2007.
17. Hamvas A: Inherited surfactant protein-B deficiency and surfactant protein-C associated disease: clinical features and evaluation. Semin Perinatol 30:316, 2006.
18. Chen J, Smith LE: Retinopathy of prematurity. Angiogenesis 10:133, 2007.
19. Bancalari E, Claure N: Definitions and diagnostic criteria for bronchopulmonary dysplasia. Semin Perinatol 30:164, 2006.
20. Chess PR, D'Angio CT, Pryhuber GS, Maniscalco WM: Pathogenesis of bronchopulmonary dysplasia. Semin Perinatol 30:171, 2006.
21. Speer CP: Inflammation and bronchopulmonary dysplasia: a continuing story. Semin Fetal Neonatal Med 11:354, 2006.
22. Thebaud B: Angiogenesis in lung development, injury and repair: implications for chronic lung disease of prematurity. Neonatology 91:291, 2007.
23. Caplan MS, Simon D, Jilling T: The role of PAF, TLR, and the inflammatory response in neonatal necrotizing enterocolitis. Semin Pediatr Surg 14:145, 2005.
24. Abrams ME, Meredith KS, Kinnard P, Clark RH: Hydrops fetalis: a retrospective review of cases reported to a large national database and identification of risk factors associated with death. Pediatrics 120:84, 2007.
25. Scriver CR: The PAH gene, phenylketonuria, and a paradigm shift. Hum Mutat 28:831, 2007.
26. Zurfluh MR, Zschocke J, Lindner M et al: Molecular genetics of tetrahydrobiopterin-responsive phenylalanine hydroxylase deficiency. Hum Mutat 2008.
27. Harding CO, Gillingham MB, Hamman K et al: Complete correction of hyperphenylalaninemia following liver-directed, recombinant AAV2/8 vector-mediated gene therapy in murine phenylketonuria. Gene Ther 13:457, 2006.
28. Fridovich-Keil JL: Galactosemia: the good, the bad, and the unknown. J Cell Physiol 209:701, 2006.
29. Wang X, Kim J, McWilliams R, Cutting GR: Increased prevalence of chronic rhinosinusitis in carriers of a cystic fibrosis mutation. Arch Otolaryngol Head Neck Surg 131:237, 2005.
30. Cohn JA, Neoptolemos JP, Feng J et al: Increased risk of idiopathic chronic pancreatitis in cystic fibrosis carriers. Hum Mutat 26:303, 2005.
31. Castellani C, Cuppens H, Macek M Jr et al: Consensus on the use and interpretation of cystic fibrosis mutation analysis in clinical practice. J Cyst Fibros 7:179, 2008.
32. Boucher RC: Cystic fibrosis: a disease of vulnerability to airway surface dehydration. Trends in molecular medicine 13:231, 2007.
33. Shcheynikov N, Ko SB, Zeng W et al: Regulatory interaction between CFTR and the SLC26 transporters. Novartis Found Symp 273:177, 2006.
34. Farrell PM, Rosenstein BJ, White TB et al: Guidelines for diagnosis of cystic fibrosis in newborns through older adults: Cystic Fibrosis Foundation consensus report. The Journal of pediatrics 153:S4, 2008.
35. Cutting GR: Modifier genetics: cystic fibrosis. Annu Rev Genomics Hum Genet 6:237, 2005.
36. Howe KL, Wang A, Hunter MM, Stanton BA, McKay DM: TGFbeta downregulation of the CFTR: a means to limit epithelial chloride secretion. Exp Cell Res 298:473, 2004.
37. Pruliere-Escabasse V, Fanen P, Dazy AC et al: TGF-beta 1 downregulates CFTR expression and function in nasal polyps of non-CF patients. Am J Physiol Lung Cell Mol Physiol 288:L77, 2005.
38. Drumm ML, Konstan MW, Schluchter MD et al: Genetic modifiers of lung disease in cystic fibrosis. N Engl J Med 353:1443, 2005.
39. Blackman SM, Deering-Brose R, McWilliams R et al: Relative contribution of genetic and nongenetic modifiers to intestinal obstruction in cystic fibrosis. Gastroenterology 131:1030, 2006.
40. Mahenthiralingam E, Urban TA, Goldberg JB: The multifarious, multireplicon Burkholderia cepacia complex. Nat Rev Microbiol 3:144, 2005.
41. Boyle MP: Adult cystic fibrosis. JAMA 298:1787, 2007.
42. American Academy of Pediatrics Task Force on Sudden Infant Death Syndrome. The changing concept of sudden infant death syndrome: diagnostic coding shifts, controversies regarding the sleeping environment, and new variables to consider in reducing risk. Pediatrics 116:1245, 2005.
43. Krous HF, Beckwith JB, Byard RW et al: Sudden infant death syndrome and unclassified sudden infant deaths: a definitional and diagnostic approach. Pediatrics 114:234, 2004.
44. Moon RY, Horne RS, Hauck FR: Sudden infant death syndrome. Lancet 370:1578, 2007.
45. American Academy of Pediatrics, Committee on Fetus and Newborn. Apnea, sudden infant death syndrome, and home monitoring. Pediatrics 111:914, 2003.
46. Guntheroth WG, Spiers PS: The triple risk hypotheses in sudden infant death syndrome. Pediatrics 110:e64, 2002.
47. Paterson DS, Trachtenberg FL, Thompson EG et al: Multiple serotonergic brainstem abnormalities in sudden infant death syndrome. JAMA 296:2124, 2006.
48. Audero E, Coppi E, Mlinar B et al: Sporadic autonomic dysregulation and death associated with excessive serotonin autoinhibition. Science, New York, NY 321:130, 2008.
49. Weese-Mayer DE, Ackerman MJ, Marazita ML, Berry-Kravis EM: Sudden Infant Death Syndrome: review of implicated genetic factors. Am J Med Genet A 143:771, 2007.
50. Adgent MA: Environmental tobacco smoke and sudden infant death syndrome: a review. Birth Defects Res B Dev Reprod Toxicol 77:69, 2006.
51. Lannon CL, Sorensen PH: ETV6-NTRK3: a chimeric protein tyrosine kinase with transformation activity in multiple cell lineages. Semin Cancer Biol 15:215, 2005.
52. Mosse YP, Laudenslager M, Longo L et al: Identification of ALK as a major familial neuroblastoma predisposition gene. Nature 455:950, 2008.
53. Mora J, Cheung NK, Juan G et al: Neuroblastic and Schwannian stromal cells of neuroblastoma are derived from a tumoral progenitor cell. Cancer research 61:6892, 2001.
54. Maris JM, Hogarty MD, Bagatell R, Cohn SL: Neuroblastoma. Lancet 369:2106, 2007.
55. London WB, Castleberry RP, Matthay KK et al: Evidence for an age cutoff greater than 365 days for neuroblastoma risk group stratification in the Children's Oncology Group. J Clin Oncol 23:6459, 2005.
56. Brodeur GM, Maris JM: Neuroblastoma. In: Pizzo PA, Poplack DG, eds. Principles and Practice of Pediatric Oncology. Philadelphia: JB Lippincott; 2006:933.
57. Attiyeh EF, London WB, Mosse YP et al: Chromosome 1p and 11q deletions and outcome in neuroblastoma. N Engl J Med 353:2243, 2005.

58. George RE, Attiyeh EF, Li S et al: Genome-wide analysis of neuroblastomas using high-density single nucleotide polymorphism arrays. PLoS ONE 2:e255, 2007.
59. Schleiermacher G, Michon J, Huon I et al: Chromosomal CGH identifies patients with a higher risk of relapse in neuroblastoma without MYCN amplification. Br J Cancer 97:238, 2007.
60. Woods WG, Gao RN, Shuster JJ et al: Screening of infants and mortality due to neuroblastoma. N Engl J Med 346:1041, 2002.
61. Schilling FH, Spix C, Berthold F et al: Neuroblastoma screening at one year of age. N Engl J Med 346:1047, 2002.
62. Rivera MN, Haber DA: Wilms' tumour: connecting tumorigenesis and organ development in the kidney. Nat Rev Cancer 5:699, 2005.
63. Hohenstein P, Hastie ND: The many facets of the Wilms' tumour gene, WT1. Hum Mol Genet 15 Spec No 2:R196, 2006.
64. Feinberg AP: The epigenetics of cancer etiology. Semin Cancer Biol 14:427, 2004.
65. Bjornsson HT, Brown LJ, Fallin MD et al: Epigenetic specificity of loss of imprinting of the IGF2 gene in Wilms tumors. J Natl Cancer Inst 99:1270, 2007.
66. Tycko B, Li CM, Buttyan R: The Wnt/beta-catenin pathway in Wilms tumors and prostate cancers. Curr Mol Med 7:479, 2007.
67. Dome JS, Cotton CA, Perlman EJ et al: Treatment of anaplastic histology Wilms' tumor: results from the fifth National Wilms' Tumor Study. J Clin Oncol 24:2352, 2006.
68. Robison LL, Green DM, Hudson M et al: Long-term outcomes of adult survivors of childhood cancer. Cancer 104:2557, 2005.

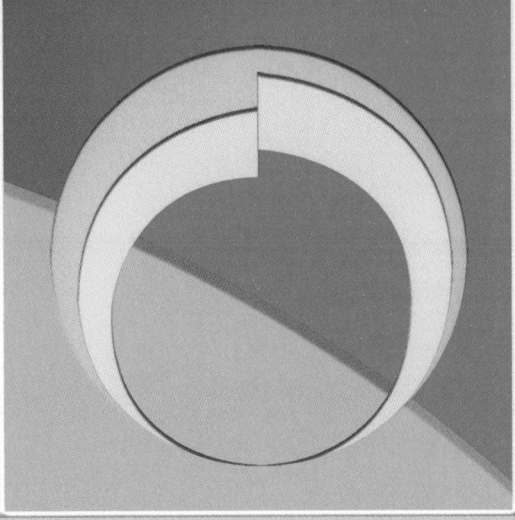

Systemic Pathology: Diseases of Organ Systems

11

Blood Vessels

RICHARD N. MITCHELL · FREDERICK J. SCHOEN

The Structure and Function of Blood Vessels

Vessel Development, Growth, and Remodeling

Congenital Anomalies

Vascular Wall Cells and Their Response to Injury

Hypertensive Vascular Disease
  Vascular Pathology in Hypertension

Arteriosclerosis

Atherosclerosis
  Epidemiology
  Pathogenesis of Atherosclerosis
    Endothelial Injury
    Smooth Muscle Proliferation
    Overview
  Consequences of Atherosclerotic Disease

Aneurysms and Dissection
  Abdominal Aortic Aneurysm (AAA)
  Thoracic Aortic Aneurysms
  Aortic Dissection

Vasculitis
  Noninfectious Vasculitis
  Giant-Cell (Temporal) Arteritis
  Takayasu Arteritis
  Polyarteritis Nodosa
  Kawasaki Disease
  Microscopic Polyangiitis

Churg-Strauss Syndrome
Wegener Granulomatosis
Thromboangiitis Obliterans (Buerger Disease)
Vasculitis Associated with Other Disorders
Infectious Vasculitis

Raynaud Phenomenon

Veins and Lymphatics
  Varicose Veins
  Thrombophlebitis and Phlebothrombosis
  Superior and Inferior Vena Caval Syndromes
  Lymphangitis and Lymphedema

Tumors
  Benign Tumors and Tumor-Like Conditions
    Hemangioma
    Lymphangiomas
    Glomus Tumor (Glomangioma)
    Vascular Ectasias
    Bacillary Angiomatosis
  Intermediate-Grade (Borderline) Tumors
    Kaposi Sarcoma
    Hemangioendothelioma
  Malignant Tumors
    Angiosarcoma
    Hemangiopericytoma

Pathology of Vascular Interventions
  Angioplasty and Endovascular Stents
  Vascular Replacement

Vascular disorders—and their downstream sequelae—are responsible for more morbidity and mortality than any other category of human disease. Although the most clinically significant lesions typically involve arteries, venous diseases also occur. Vascular pathology results in disease via two principal mechanisms: (1) *Narrowing (stenosis)* or *complete obstruction* of vessel lumens, either progressively (e.g., by atherosclerosis) or precipitously (e.g., by thrombosis or embolism); and (2) *weakening* of vessel walls, leading to dilation or rupture.

We will first describe the important structural and functional characteristics of blood vessels to better appreciate how pathologic changes can result in disease states.

The Structure and Function of Blood Vessels

The general architecture and cellular composition of blood vessels are the same throughout the cardiovascular system. However, certain features of the vasculature vary with and reflect distinct functional requirements at different locations (Fig. 11–1). To withstand the pulsatile flow and higher blood pressures in arteries, arterial walls are generally thicker than the walls of veins. Arterial wall thickness gradually diminishes as the vessels become smaller, but the ratio of wall thickness to lumen diameter becomes greater.

The basic constituents of the walls of blood vessels are endothelial cells and smooth muscle cells, and extracellular matrix (ECM), including elastin, collagen, and glycosoaminoglycans. The three concentric layers—*intima, media,* and *adventitia*—are most clearly defined in the larger vessels, particularly arteries. In normal arteries, the intima consists of a single layer of endothelial cells with minimal underlying subendothelial connective tissue. It is separated from the media by a dense elastic membrane called the *internal elastic lamina.* The smooth muscle cell layers of the media near the vessel lumen receive oxygen and nutrients by direct diffusion from the vessel lumen, facilitated by holes in the internal elastic membrane. However, diffusion from the lumen is inadequate for the outer portions of the media in large and medium-sized vessels, therefore these areas are nourished by small arterioles arising from outside the vessel (called *vasa vasorum,* literally "vessels of the vessels") coursing into the outer one half to two thirds of the media. The outer limit of the media of most arteries is a well-defined *external elastic lamina.* External to the media is the adventitia, consisting of connective tissue with nerve fibers and the vasa vasorum.

Based on their size and structural features, *arteries* are divided into three types: (1) large or *elastic arteries,* including

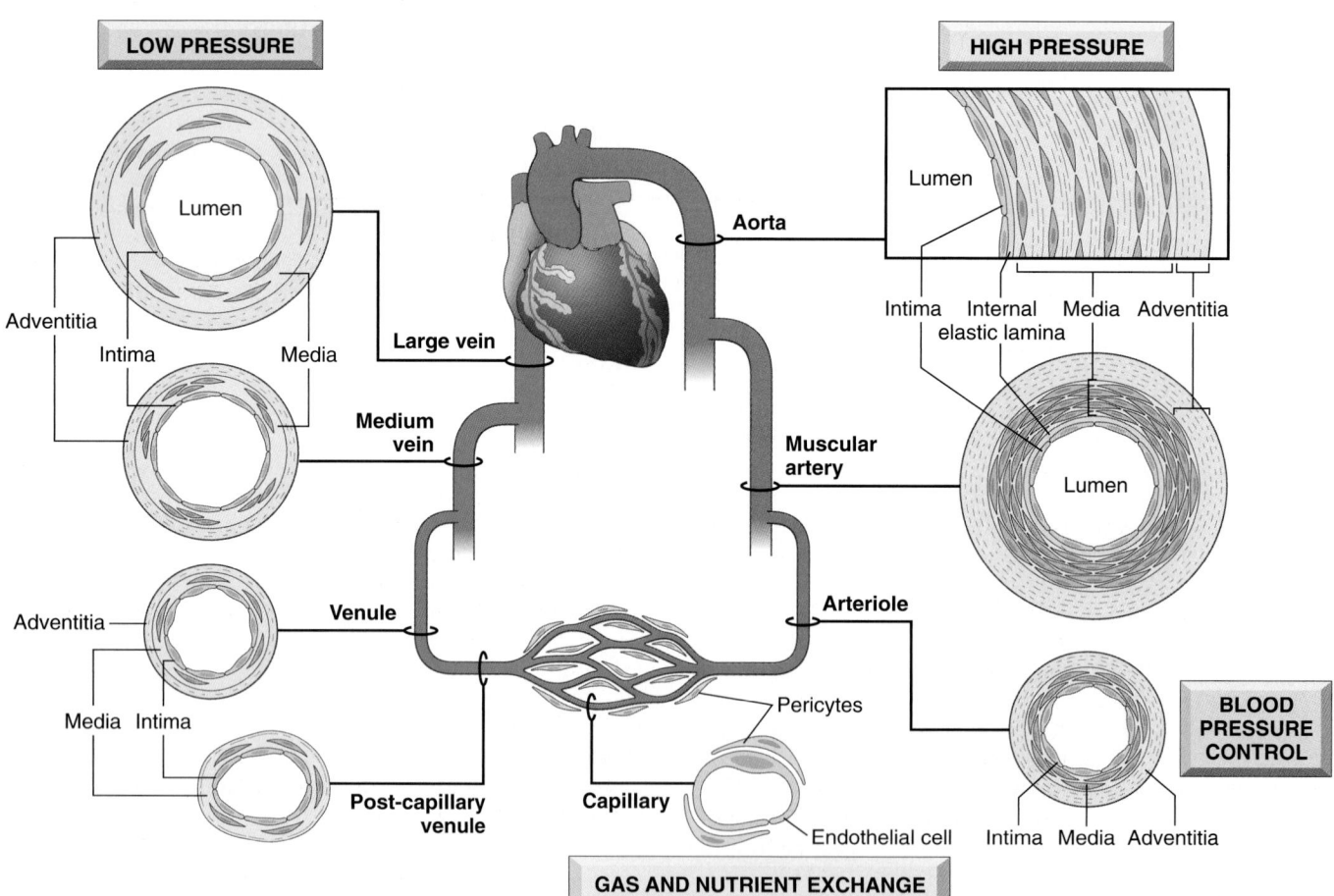

FIGURE 11–1   Regional specializations of the vasculature. Although the basic organization of the vasculature is constant, the thickness and composition of the various layers differ according to hemodynamic forces and tissue requirements.

the aorta, its large branches (particularly the innominate, sub-clavian, common carotid, and iliac), and pulmonary arteries; (2) medium-sized or *muscular arteries*, comprising other branches of the aorta (e.g., coronary and renal arteries); and (3) small arteries (less than approximately 2 mm in diameter) and *arterioles* (20 to 100 μm in diameter), within the substance of tissues and organs.

The relative amount and configuration of the basic constituents differ along the arterial system owing to local adaptations to mechanical or metabolic needs. These structural variations, from location to location, are principally in the media and in the ECM. In the elastic arteries the media is rich in elastic fibers. This allows vessels such as the aorta to expand during systole and recoil during diastole, thus propelling blood through the peripheral vascular system. With aging, the aorta loses elasticity, and large vessels expand less readily, particularly when blood pressure is increased. Thus, the arteries of older in-dividuals often become progressively tortuous and dilated *(ectatic)*. In *muscular arteries* the media is composed predominantly of circularly or spirally arranged smooth muscle cells. In the muscular arteries and arterioles (see below), regional blood flow and blood pressure are regulated by changes in lumen size through smooth muscle cell contraction *(vasoconstriction)* or relaxation *(vasodilation)*, controlled in part by the autonomic nervous system and in part by local metabolic factors and cellular interactions. Since the resistance of a tube to fluid flow is inversely proportional to the fourth power of the diameter (i.e., halving the diameter increases resistance 16-fold), small changes in the lumen size of small arteries caused by structural change or vasoconstriction can have a profound effect. Thus, *arterioles are the principal points of physiologic resistance to blood flow.*

Capillaries, approximately the diameter of a red blood cell (7 to 8 μm), have an endothelial cell lining but no media. Collectively, capillaries have a very large total cross-sectional area; within the capillaries, the flow rate slows dramatically. With thin walls only and slow flow, capillaries are ideally suited to the rapid exchange of diffusible substances between blood and tissues. As normal tissue function depends on an adequate supply of oxygen through blood vessels, and since diffusion of oxygen in solid tissues is inefficient over distances of greater than approximately 100 μm,[1] the capillary network of most tissues is very rich. Metabolically highly active tissues, such as the myocardium, have the highest density of capillaries.

Blood from capillary beds flows initially into the *postcapillary venules* and then sequentially through collecting venules and small, medium, and large veins. *In many types of inflammation, vascular leakage and leukocyte exudation occur preferentially in postcapillary venules* (Chapter 2).

Relative to arteries, veins have larger diameters, larger lumens, and thinner and less well organized walls (see Fig. 11-1). Thus, because of their poor support, *veins are predisposed to irregular dilation, compression, and easy penetration by tumors and inflammatory processes.* The venous system collectively has a large capacity; approximately two thirds of all the blood is in veins. Reverse flow is prevented by venous valves in the extremities, where blood flows against gravity.

Lymphatics are thin-walled, endothelium-lined channels that serve as a drainage system for returning interstitial tissue fluid and inflammatory cells to the blood. *Lymphatics consti-* *tute an important pathway for disease dissemination through transport of bacteria and tumor cells to distant sites.*

As will be discussed in detail in this chapter, pathologic lesions involve vessels of a characteristic size, range, and/or type. Atherosclerosis, for example, affects elastic and muscular arteries, hypertension affects small muscular arteries and arterioles, and specific types of vasculitis involve different vascular segments.

Vessel Development, Growth, and Remodeling

Three major processes characterize blood vessel formation and remodeling (covered in detail in Chapter 3): *vasculogenesis*, *angiogenesis*, and *arteriogenesis*.[1]

- *Vasculogenesis* is the de novo formation of blood vessels during embryogenesis. Hemangioblast angiogenic precursors develop and migrate to the sites of vascularization. These differentiate into endothelial cells that associate to form a primitive vascular plexus; with time and the influence of local genetic, metabolic, and hemodynamic factors, this network of cells remodels (through pruning and/or vessel enlargement) into the definitive vascular system.[2,3] The various isoforms of vascular endothelial growth factor (VEGF) are the primary growth factors involved in this process. Subsequent stabilization of the endothelial tubes during development (and induction of endothelial cell quiescence) also critically requires the recruitment of pericytes and smooth muscle cells, a process that involves *angiopoietin 1* binding to endothelial cell *Tie2 receptors*.
- *Angiogenesis* (or *neovascularization*) constitutes the process of new vessel formation in the mature organism.
- *Arteriogenesis* refers to the remodeling of existing arteries in response to chronic changes in pressure or flow, and results from an interplay of endothelial cell– and smooth muscle cell–derived factors.[4]

Congenital Anomalies

Though rarely symptomatic, variants of the usual anatomic pattern of vascular supply can become important during surgery when a vessel in an unexpected location is injured. Variations in the normal coronary artery anatomy are also extremely important to the cardiac surgeon or interventional cardiologist.[5,6] Among the other congenital vascular anomalies, three are particularly significant, though not necessarily common:

- *Developmental* or *berry aneurysms* occur in cerebral vessels; when ruptured these can be causes of fatal intracerebral hemorrhage. They are discussed in Chapter 28.
- *Arteriovenous fistulas* are abnormal, typically small, direct connections between arteries and veins that bypass the intervening capillaries. They occur most commonly as developmental defects but can also result from rupture of an arterial aneurysm into an adjacent vein, from penetrating injuries that pierce arteries and veins, or from

inflammatory necrosis of adjacent vessels; intentionally created arteriovenous fistulas are used to provide vascular access for chronic hemodialysis. Like berry aneurysms, ruptured arteriovenous fistulas can be an important cause of intracerebral hemorrhage.[7] Large or extensive arteriovenous fistulas become clinically significant by shunting blood from the arterial to the venous circulations and forcing the heart to pump additional volume; high-output cardiac failure can ensue.

○ *Fibromuscular dysplasia* is a focal irregular thickening of the walls of medium and large muscular arteries, including renal, carotid, splanchnic, and vertebral vessels. The cause is unknown but is probably developmental; first-degree relatives of affected individuals have an increased incidence. Segments of the vessel wall are focally thickened by a combination of irregular medial and intimal hyperplasia and fibrosis; this results in luminal stenosis, and in the renal arteries may be a cause of renovascular hypertension (Chapter 20). Vascular outpouchings *(aneurysms)* may develop in the vessel segments with attenuated media and in some cases can rupture. Fibromuscular dysplasia can manifest at any age, although it is seen most frequently in young women; there is no association with use of oral contraceptives or abnormalities of sex hormone expression.[8]

Vascular Wall Cells and Their Response to Injury

As the main cellular components of the blood vessels, endothelial cells and smooth muscle cells play central roles in vascular biology and pathology. Therefore, we will describe their functions and dysfunctions briefly before we discuss specific vascular disorders.

Endothelial Cells. Endothelium is critical for maintaining vessel wall homeostasis and circulatory function. Endothelial cells contain *Weibel-Palade bodies,* intracellular membrane-bound storage organelles for von Willebrand's factor (Chapter 4). Antibodies to von Willebrand's factor and/or platelet-endothelial cell adhesion molecule-1 (PECAM-1 or CD31, a protein localized to interendothelial junctions) can be used to identify endothelial cells immunohistochemically.

Vascular endothelium is a multifunctional tissue with a wealth of synthetic and metabolic properties; at baseline it has several constitutive activities critical for normal vessel homeostasis (Table 11–1). Thus, endothelial cells maintain a nonthrombogenic blood-tissue interface (until clotting is necessitated by local injury, Chapter 4), modulate vascular resistance, metabolize hormones, regulate inflammation, and affect the growth of other cell types, particularly smooth muscle cells. In most regions the interendothelial junctions are substantially impermeable. However, tight endothelial cell junctions can loosen under the influence of hemodynamic factors (e.g., high blood pressure) and/or vasoactive agents (e.g., histamine in inflammation), resulting in the flooding of adjacent tissues by electrolytes and protein; in inflammatory states, even leukocytes can slip between adjacent endothelial cells (Chapter 2).

Although endothelial cells share many general attributes, endothelial cell populations that line different portions of the

TABLE 11–1	Endothelial Cell Properties and Functions

MAINTENANCE OF PERMEABILITY BARRIER

ELABORATION OF ANTICOAGULANT, ANTITHROMBOTIC, FIBRINOLYTIC REGULATORS

Prostacyclin
Thrombomodulin
Heparin-like molecules
Plasminogen activator

ELABORATION OF PROTHROMBOTIC MOLECULES

Von Willebrand's factor
Tissue factor
Plasminogen activator inhibitor

EXTRACELLULAR MATRIX PRODUCTION (COLLAGEN, PROTEOGLYCANS)

MODULATION OF BLOOD FLOW AND VASCULAR REACTIVITY

Vasoconstrictors: endothelin, ACE
Vasodilators: NO, prostacyclin

REGULATION OF INFLAMMATION AND IMMUNITY

IL-1, IL-6, chemokines
Adhesion molecules: VCAM-1, ICAM, E-selectin, P-selectin
Histocompatibility antigens

REGULATION OF CELL GROWTH

Growth stimulators: PDGF, CSF, FGF
Growth inhibitors: heparin, TGF-β

OXIDATION OF LDL

ACE, angiotensin-converting enzyme; CSF, colony-stimulating factor; FGF, fibroblast growth factor; IL, interleukin; LDL, low-density lipoprotein; NO, nitric oxide; PDGF, platelet-derived growth factor; TGF-β, transforming growth factor-β.

vascular tree (large vessels vs. capillaries, arterial vs. venous) have distinct transcriptional repertoires and behavior.[9] There is also substantial phenotypic variability depending on specific anatomic site. Thus, endothelial cells in liver sinusoids or in renal glomeruli are fenestrated (they have *holes,* presumably to facilitate filtration), while the endothelial cells of the central nervous system (with the associated perivascular cells) create an impermeable blood-brain barrier.

Structurally intact endothelial cells can respond to various pathophysiologic stimuli by adjusting their usual (constitutive) functions and by expressing newly acquired (inducible) properties—a process termed *endothelial activation* (Fig. 11–2).[10,11] Inducers of endothelial activation include cytokines and bacterial products, which cause inflammation and septic shock (Chapter 2); hemodynamic stresses and lipid products, critical to the pathogenesis of atherosclerosis (see later); advanced glycosylation end products (important in diabetes, Chapter 24); as well as viruses, complement components, and hypoxia. Activated endothelial cells, in turn, express adhesion molecules (Chapter 2), and produce cytokines and chemokines, growth factors, vasoactive molecules that result either in vasoconstriction or in vasodilation, major histocompatibility complex molecules, procoagulant and anticoagulant moieties, and a variety of other biologically active products. Endothelial cells influence the vasoreactivity of the underlying smooth muscle cells through the production of both relaxing factors (e.g., nitric oxide [NO]) and contracting factors (e.g.,

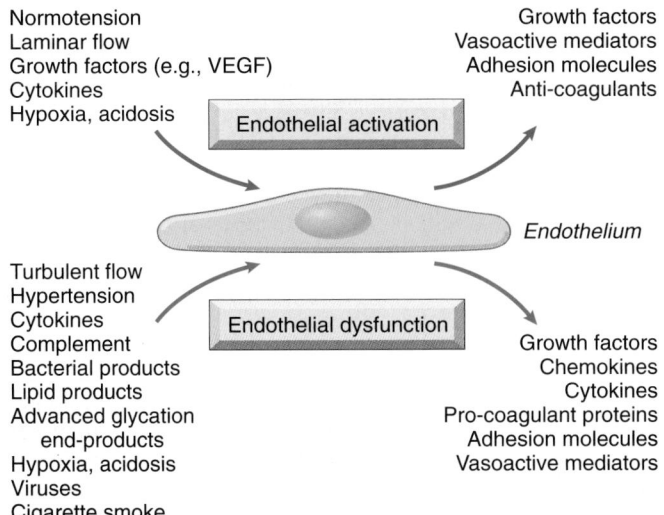

Normotension
Laminar flow
Growth factors (e.g., VEGF)
Cytokines
Hypoxia, acidosis

Growth factors
Vasoactive mediators
Adhesion molecules
Anti-coagulants

Endothelial activation

Endothelium

Turbulent flow
Hypertension
Cytokines
Complement
Bacterial products
Lipid products
Advanced glycation
  end-products
Hypoxia, acidosis
Viruses
Cigarette smoke

Endothelial dysfunction

Growth factors
Chemokines
Cytokines
Pro-coagulant proteins
Adhesion molecules
Vasoactive mediators

FIGURE 11–2 Endothelial cell responses to environmental stimuli. Certain cues (e.g., laminar flow and constant growth factor levels) lead to stable endothelial cell activation that maintains a nonthrombotic interface with appropriate smooth muscle cell tone. Pathologic mediators or excessive stimulation by normal physiologic pathways (e.g., increased inflammatory cytokines) can result in endothelial cell dysfunction. VEGF, vascular endothelial growth factor.

endothelin).[12] Normal endothelial function is characterized by a balance of these responses.

Endothelial dysfunction is defined as an altered phenotype that impairs vasoreactivity or induces a surface that is thrombogenic or abnormally adhesive to inflammatory cells. It is responsible, at least in part, for the initiation of thrombus formation, atherosclerosis, and the vascular lesions of hypertension and other disorders. Certain forms of endothelial cell dysfunction are rapid in onset (within minutes), reversible, and independent of new protein synthesis (e.g., endothelial cell contraction induced by histamine and other vasoactive mediators that cause gaps in venular endothelium, Chapter 2).

Other changes involve alterations in gene expression and protein synthesis and may require hours or even days to develop.

Vascular Smooth Muscle Cells. As the predominant cellular element of the vascular media, smooth muscle cells play important roles in normal vascular repair and pathologic processes such as atherosclerosis. Smooth muscle cells have the capacity to proliferate when appropriately stimulated; they can also synthesize ECM collagen, elastin, and proteoglycans and elaborate growth factors and cytokines. Smooth muscle cells are also responsible for the vasoconstriction or dilation that occurs in response to physiologic or pharmacologic stimuli.

The migratory and proliferative activities of smooth muscle cells are regulated by growth promoters and inhibitors. Promoters include PDGF, as well as endothelin-1, thrombin, fibroblast growth factor (FGF), interferon-γ (IFN-γ), and interleukin-1(IL-1). Inhibitors include heparan sulfates, nitric oxide, and TGF-β. Other regulators include the renin-angiotensin system (e.g., angiotensin II), catecholamines, the estrogen receptor, and osteopontin, a component of the ECM.[13]

Intimal Thickening—a Stereotypic Response To Vascular Injury. *Vascular injury—with endothelial cell loss or even just dysfunction—stimulates smooth muscle cell growth and associated matrix synthesis that thickens the intima. Healing of injured vessels is analogous to the healing process that occurs in other damaged tissues (Chapter 3); in vessels, it results in the formation of a neointima.* During the healing process, endothelial cells that fill areas of denudation may migrate from adjacent uninjured areas or may be derived from circulating precursors.[14] Medial smooth muscle cells or smooth muscle precursor cells also migrate into the intima, proliferate, and synthesize ECM in much the same way that fibroblasts fill in a wound (Fig. 11–3). The resulting neointima is typically completely covered by endothelial cells. This neointimal response occurs with any form of vascular damage or dysfunction, regardless of cause. *Thus, intimal thickening is the stereotypical response of the vessel wall to any insult.*

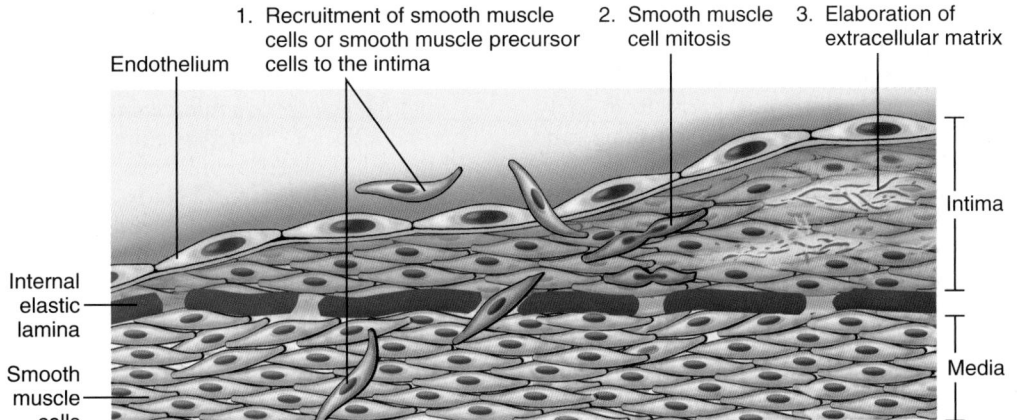

1. Recruitment of smooth muscle cells or smooth muscle precursor cells to the intima

2. Smooth muscle cell mitosis

3. Elaboration of extracellular matrix

Endothelium

Internal elastic lamina

Smooth muscle cells

Intima

Media

FIGURE 11–3 Schematic of intimal thickening, emphasizing smooth muscle cell migration and proliferation within the intima, with associated ECM synthesis. Intimal smooth muscle cells may derive from the underlying media or may be recruited from circulating precursors; they are shown in a different color from the medial cells to emphasize that they have a proliferative, synthetic, and non-contractile phenotype distinct from medial smooth muscle cells. (Modified and redrawn from Schoen FJ: Interventional and Surgical Cardiovascular Pathology: Clinical Correlations and Basic Principles. Philadelphia, WB Saunders, 1989, p 254.)

It should be emphasized that the phenotype of neointimal smooth muscle cells is distinct from that of medial smooth muscle cells; neointimal smooth muscle cells do not contract like medial smooth muscle cells but have the capacity to divide. Although these neointimal cells have long been thought to be derived from de-differentiation of smooth muscle cells migrating from the underlying media, there is increasing evidence that the intimal smooth muscle cells are at least in part derived from circulating precursor cells.[14–17] The migratory, proliferative, and synthetic activities of the intimal smooth muscle cells are physiologically regulated by products derived from platelets, endothelial cells, and macrophages, as well as by activated coagulation and complement factors. PDGF, endothelin-1, thrombin, FGF, IFN-γ, and IL-1 stimulate neointimal smooth muscle cells, while heparan sulfates, nitric oxide, and TGF-β antagonize their growth.

With time and restoration and/or normalization of the endothelial layer, the intimal smooth muscle cells can return to a nonproliferative state. However, the healing response results in permanent intimal thickening. With persistent or recurrent insults, excessive thickening can cause narrowing or stenosis of small and medium-sized blood vessels (e.g., atherosclerosis, see below), impeding downstream tissue perfusion. As a final note, it is important to remember that intimal thickening also occurs in otherwise normal arteries as a result of maturation and aging. In adult coronaries, for example, the intima and the media are frequently of approximately equal thickness. Such age-related intimal change is typically of no consequence, in part because a compensatory outward remodeling of the vessel results in little net change in the luminal diameter[18]; it also suggests that not all intimal thickening is a harbinger of disease.

Hypertensive Vascular Disease

Systemic and local tissue blood pressures must be maintained within a narrow range to prevent untoward consequences. Low pressures *(hypotension)* result in inadequate organ perfusion and can lead to dysfunction or tissue death. Conversely, high pressures *(hypertension)* can cause vessel and end-organ damage.

Like height and weight, blood pressure is a continuously distributed variable, and detrimental effects of blood pressure increase continuously as the pressure rises; no rigidly defined threshold level of blood pressure distinguishes risk from safety. Nevertheless, according to the National Heart, Lung, and Blood Institute of the U.S.A., a sustained diastolic pressure greater than 89 mm Hg, or a sustained systolic pressure in excess of 139 mm Hg, are associated with a measurably increased risk of atherosclerosis, and are therefore felt to represent clinically significant hypertension. Both the systolic and diastolic blood pressure are important in determining cardiovascular risk.[19] By either criterion, some 25% of individuals in the general population are hypertensive. However, it must be emphasized that these cut-offs are somewhat arbitrary, and in patients with other risk factors for vascular disease such as diabetes, lower thresholds are applicable.

Although we have an improved understanding of the molecular pathways that regulate normal blood pressure,[20,21] the mechanisms that result in hypertension remain largely unknown in most individuals. Typically, for individuals with such "essential hypertension," the best we can say is that the disorder is multifactorial, resulting from the combined effects of multiple genetic polymorphisms and interacting environmental factors.[22,23]

The prevalence and vulnerability to complications of hypertension increase with age; they are also higher in African Americans. As we will see below, hypertension is one of the major risk factors for atherosclerosis and underlies numerous other diseases. It can cause—among other things—cardiac hypertrophy and heart failure (*hypertensive heart disease*, Chapter 12), multi-infarct dementia (Chapter 28), aortic dissection, and renal failure. Unfortunately, hypertension typically remains asymptomatic until late in its course and even severely elevated pressures can be clinically silent for years. Left untreated, roughly half of hypertensive patients die of ischemic heart disease (IHD) or congestive heart failure, and another third die of stroke. Prophylactic blood pressure reduction dramatically reduces the incidence and death rates from all forms of hypertension-related pathology.

Table 11–2 lists the major causes of hypertension. A small number of patients (approximately 5%) have underlying renal or adrenal disease (such as primary aldosteronism, Cushing syndrome, pheochromocytoma), narrowing of the renal artery, usually by an atheromatous plaque (renovascular hypertension) or other identifiable cause (secondary hypertension). *However, about 95% of hypertension is idiopathic (called essential hypertension). This form of hypertension generally does not cause short-term problems.* When controlled, it is compatible with long life and is asymptomatic, unless a myocardial infarction, cerebrovascular accident, or other complication supervenes.

A small percentage, perhaps 5%, of hypertensive persons show a rapidly rising blood pressure that, if untreated, leads to death within a year or two. Called *accelerated* or *malignant hypertension*, this clinical syndrome is characterized by severe hypertension (i.e., systolic pressure over 200 mm Hg, diastolic pressure over 120 mm Hg), renal failure, and retinal hemorrhages and exudates, with or without papilledema. It may develop in previously normotensive persons but more often is superimposed on pre-existing benign hypertension, either essential or secondary.[24,25]

Regulation of Normal Blood Pressure. *Blood pressure is a function of cardiac output and peripheral vascular resistance* (Fig. 11–4A), *two hemodynamic variables that are influenced by multiple genetic, environmental, and demographic factors.* The major factors that determine blood pressure variation within and between populations include age, gender, body mass index, and diet, particularly sodium intake.

Cardiac output is highly dependent on blood volume, itself greatly influenced by the sodium homeostasis. Peripheral vascular resistance is determined mainly at the level of the arterioles and is affected by neural and hormonal factors. Normal vascular tone reflects the balance between humoral vasoconstricting influences (including angiotensin II, catecholamines, and endothelin) and vasodilators (including kinins, prostaglandins, and NO). Resistance vessels also exhibit *autoregulation*, whereby increased blood flow induces vasoconstriction to protect against tissue hyperperfusion. Other local factors such as pH and hypoxia, and the α- and β-adrenergic systems, which influence heart rate, cardiac contraction, and vascular

TABLE 11–2 Types and Causes of Hypertension (Systolic and Diastolic)

ESSENTIAL HYPERTENSION (90% TO 95% OF CASES)

SECONDARY HYPERTENSION

Renal

Acute glomerulonephritis
Chronic renal disease
Polycystic disease
Renal artery stenosis
Renal vasculitis
Renin-producing tumors

Endocrine

Adrenocortical hyperfunction (Cushing syndrome, primary aldosteronism, congenital adrenal hyperplasia, licorice ingestion)
Exogenous hormones (glucocorticoids, estrogen [including pregnancy-induced and oral contraceptives], sympathomimetics and tyramine-containing foods, monoamine oxidase inhibitors)
Pheochromocytoma
Acromegaly
Hypothyroidism (myxedema)
Hyperthyroidism (thyrotoxicosis)
Pregnancy-induced

Cardiovascular

Coarctation of aorta
Polyarteritis nodosa
Increased intravascular volume
Increased cardiac output
Rigidity of the aorta

Neurologic

Psychogenic
Increased intracranial pressure
Sleep apnea
Acute stress, including surgery

tone, may also be important in regulating blood pressure. The integrated function of these systems ensures adequate perfusion of all tissues, despite regional differences in demand.

The kidneys play an important role in blood pressure regulation as follows (Fig. 11–4B):

- Through the renin-angiotensin system, the kidney influences both peripheral resistance and sodium homeostasis. Renin is secreted by the juxtaglomerular cells of the kidney in response to fall in blood pressure. It converts *plasma angiotensinogen* to *angiotensin I*, which is then converted to *angiotensin II* by angiotensin-converting enzyme. Angiotensin II raises blood pressure by increasing both peripheral resistance (direct action on vascular smooth muscle cells) and blood volume (stimulation of aldosterone secretion, and increase in distal tubular reabsorption of sodium).
- The kidney also produces a variety of vascular relaxing, or antihypertensive, substances (including prostaglandins and NO), which presumably counterbalance the vasopressor effects of angiotensin.
- When blood volume is reduced, the *glomerular filtration rate* falls, leading to increased reabsorption of sodium by proximal tubules, thereby conserving sodium and expanding blood volume.

- *Natriuretic factors*, including the natriuretic peptides secreted by atrial and ventricular myocardium in response to volume expansion, inhibit sodium reabsorption in distal tubules and thereby cause sodium excretion and diuresis. Natriuretic peptides also induce vasodilation and may be considered to represent endogenous inhibitors of the renin-angiotensin system.

Mechanisms of Essential Hypertension. *Genetic factors* play a definite role in determining blood pressure levels, as shown by studies comparing blood pressure in monozygotic and dizygotic twins, and other types of family studies, including comparisons of genetically related and adopted family members. Moreover, several single-gene disorders cause relatively rare forms of hypertension (and hypotension) by altering net sodium reabsorption in the kidney. The importance of sodium balance is emphasized by considering that the kidneys filter 170 liters of plasma containing 23 moles of salt daily; on a typical 100-mEq sodium diet, this means that 99.5% of the filtered salt must be reabsorbed. About 98% of the filtered sodium is reabsorbed by a number of ion channels, exchangers, and transporters that are constitutively active and not subject to regulation. Absorption of the remaining 2% of sodium occurs via the epithelial Na^+ channel (ENaC), which is tightly regulated by the renin-angiotensin system in the cortical collecting tubule; it is this resorption pathway that determines net sodium balance.[26]

Single-gene disorders cause severe but rare forms of hypertension through several mechanisms. These include:

- Gene defects affecting enzymes involved in aldosterone metabolism (e.g., aldosterone synthase, 11β-hydroxylase, 17α-hydroxylase). These lead to an increase in secretion of aldosterone, increased salt and water resorption, plasma volume expansion and, ultimately, hypertension.
- Mutations affecting proteins that influence sodium reabsorption. For example, the moderately severe form of salt-sensitive hypertension, called *Liddle syndrome*, is caused by mutations in an epithelial Na^+ channel protein that lead to increased distal tubular reabsorption of sodium induced by aldosterone.

Inherited variations in blood pressure may also depend on the cumulative effects of polymorphisms in several genes that affect blood pressure. For example, predisposition to essential hypertension has been associated with variations in the genes encoding components of the renin-angiotensin system: there is an association of hypertension with polymorphisms in both the angiotensinogen locus and the angiotensin receptor locus. Genetic variants in the renin-angiotensin system may contribute to the known racial differences in blood pressure regulation.

Reduced renal sodium excretion in the presence of normal arterial pressure may be a key initiating event in essential hypertension and, indeed, a final common pathway for the pathogenesis of hypertension. Decreased sodium excretion may lead sequentially to an increase in fluid volume, increased cardiac output, and peripheral vasoconstriction, thereby elevating blood pressure. At the higher setting of blood pressure, enough additional sodium would be excreted by the kidneys to equal intake and prevent further fluid retention. Thus, an

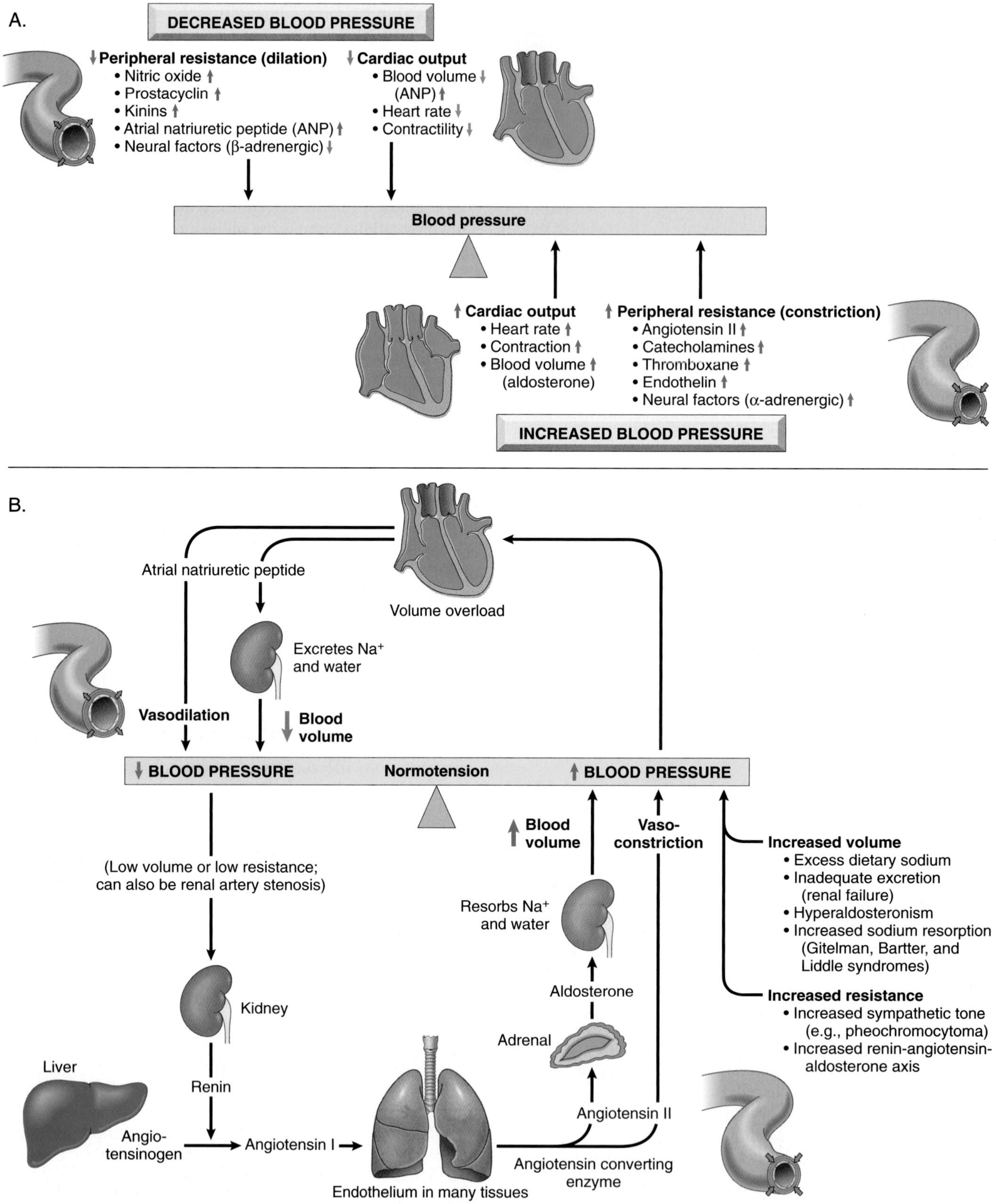

FIGURE 11–4 Blood pressure regulation. **A,** The critical roles played by cardiac output and peripheral resistance in modulating blood pressure. **B,** Interplay of renin-angiotensin-aldosterone and atrial natriuretic peptide in maintaining blood pressure homeostasis.

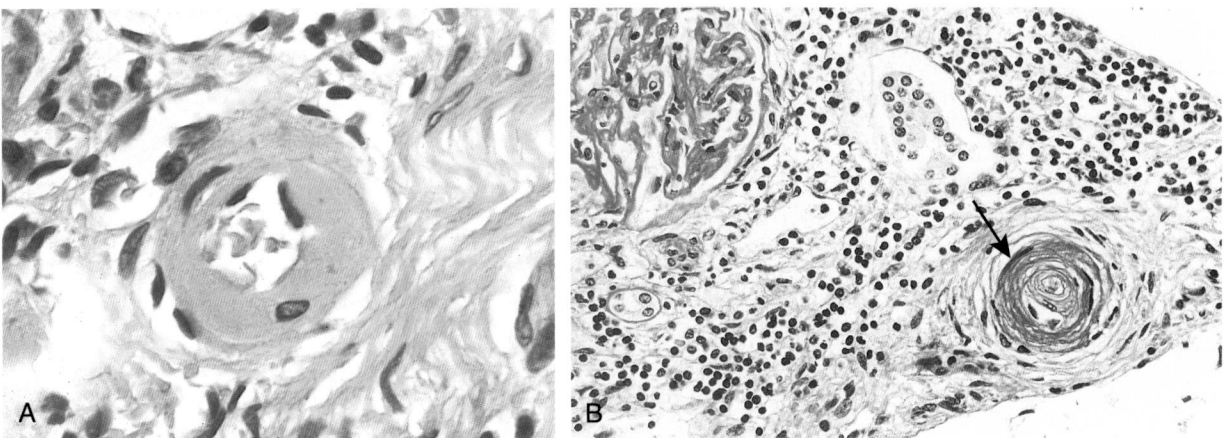

FIGURE 11–5   Vascular pathology in hypertension. **A,** Hyaline arteriolosclerosis. The arteriolar wall is thickened with increased protein deposition (hyalinized), and the lumen is markedly narrowed. **B,** Hyperplastic arteriolosclerosis (onion-skinning; *arrow*) causing lumenal obliteration (*arrow*; periodic acid–Schiff stain). (Courtesy of Helmut Rennke, M.D., Brigham and Women's Hospital, Boston, MA.)

altered but steady state of sodium excretion would be achieved ("resetting of pressure natriuresis"), but at the expense of an increase in blood pressure.

Vasoconstrictive influences, such as factors that induce vasoconstriction or stimuli that cause structural changes in the vessel wall, can lead to an increase in peripheral resistance and may also play a role in primary hypertension. Moreover, chronic or repeated vasoconstrictive influences could cause thickening and rigidity of the involved vessels.

Environmental factors can modify the impact of genetic determinants. Stress, obesity, smoking, physical inactivity, and heavy consumption of salt have all been implicated as exogenous factors in hypertension. Indeed, evidence linking the level of dietary sodium intake with the prevalence of hypertension in different population groups is particularly impressive. Moreover, in both essential and secondary hypertension, heavy sodium intake augments the condition.

To summarize, essential hypertension is a complex, multifactorial disorder. Although single gene disorders can be responsible for hypertension in rare cases, it is unlikely that such mutations are a major cause of essential hypertension. It is more likely that essential hypertension results from interactions of mutations or polymorphisms at several loci that influence blood pressure, with a variety of environmental factors (e.g., stress, salt intake). Mendelian forms of hypertension and hypotension are rare but yield insights into pathways and mechanisms of blood pressure regulation, and they may help define rational targets for therapeutic intervention. Sustained hypertension requires participation of the kidney, which normally responds to hypertension by eliminating salt and water. Susceptibility genes for essential hypertension in the larger population are currently unknown but may well include genes that govern responses to an increased renal sodium load, levels of pressor substances, reactivity of vascular smooth muscle cells to vasoconstrictive agents, or smooth muscle cell growth. In established hypertension, both increased blood volume and increased peripheral resistance contribute to the increased pressure.

Pathogenesis of Secondary Hypertension. For many of the secondary forms of hypertension, the underlying pathways are reasonably well understood. For example, in *renovascular*

hypertension, renal artery stenosis causes decreased glomerular flow and pressure in the afferent arteriole of the glomerulus. This (1) induces renin secretion, initiating angiotensin II–mediated vasoconstriction and increased peripheral resistance, and (2) increases sodium reabsorption and therefore blood volume through the aldosterone mechanism. Primary hyperaldosteronism is one of the most common causes of secondary hypertension (Chapter 24).

VASCULAR PATHOLOGY IN HYPERTENSION

Hypertension not only accelerates atherogenesis (see below) but also causes degenerative changes in the walls of large and medium arteries that can lead to aortic dissection and cerebrovascular hemorrhage.

Morphology

Hypertension is associated with two forms of small blood vessel disease: hyaline arteriolosclerosis and hyperplastic arteriolosclerosis.

Hyaline Arteriolosclerosis. Arterioles show homogeneous, pink hyaline thickening with associated luminal narrowing (Fig. 11–5A). These changes stem from plasma protein leakage across injured endothelial cells, and increased smooth muscle cell matrix synthesis in response to chronic hemodynamic stress. Although the vessels of elderly persons (either normo- or hypertensive) also frequently show hyaline arteriosclerosis, it is more generalized and severe in individuals with hypertension. The same lesions are also a common feature of diabetic microangiography; in that case the underlying etiology is hyperglycemia-induced endothelial cell dysfunction (Chapter 24). In **nephrosclerosis** due to chronic hypertension, the arteriolar narrowing of hyaline arteriosclerosis causes diffuse impairment of renal blood supply and causes glomerular scarring (Chapter 20).

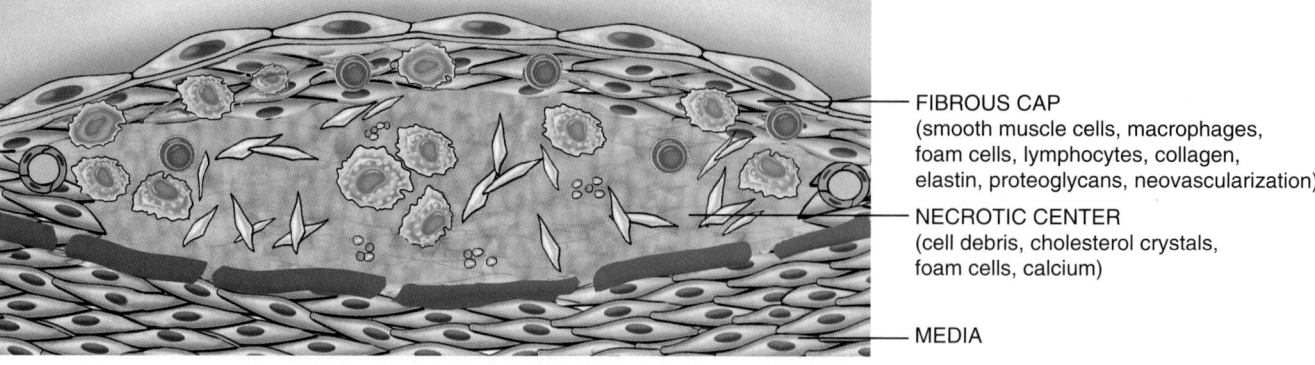

FIBROUS CAP
(smooth muscle cells, macrophages,
foam cells, lymphocytes, collagen,
elastin, proteoglycans, neovascularization)

NECROTIC CENTER
(cell debris, cholesterol crystals,
foam cells, calcium)

MEDIA

FIGURE 11–6 The major components of a well-developed intimal atheromatous plaque overlying an intact media.

Hyperplastic Arteriolosclerosis. This lesion occurs in severe (malignant) hypertension; vessels exhibit "onion-skin lesions," characterized by concentric, laminated thickening of the walls and luminal narrowing (Fig. 11–5B). The laminations consist of smooth muscle cells with thickened, reduplicated basement membranes; in malignant hypertension they are accompanied by fibrinoid deposits and vessel wall necrosis **(necrotizing arteriolitis)**, particularly in the kidney.

Arteriosclerosis

Arteriosclerosis literally means "hardening of the arteries"; it is a generic term reflecting arterial wall thickening and loss of elasticity. There are three general patterns, with differing clinical and pathologic consequences:

○ *Arteriolosclerosis* affects small arteries and arterioles, and may cause downstream ischemic injury. The anatomic variants, hyaline and hyperplastic, were discussed above in relation to hypertension.
○ *Mönckeberg medial sclerosis* is characterized by calcific deposits in muscular arteries in persons typically older than age 50. The deposits may undergo metaplastic change into bone. Nevertheless, the lesions do not encroach on the vessel lumen and are usually not clinically significant.
○ *Atherosclerosis*, from Greek root words for "gruel" and "hardening," is the most frequent and clinically important pattern and will now be discussed in detail.

Atherosclerosis

Atherosclerosis is characterized by intimal lesions called *atheromas* (also called *atheromatous* or *atherosclerotic plaques*) that protrude into vessel lumens. An atheromatous plaque consists of a raised lesion with a soft, yellow, grumous core of lipid (mainly cholesterol and cholesterol esters) covered by a white fibrous cap (Fig. 11–6). Besides mechanically obstructing blood flow, atherosclerotic plaques can rupture, leading to catastrophic vessel thrombosis; plaques also weaken the underlying media and thereby lead to aneurysm formation.

Atherosclerosis causes far more morbidity and mortality (roughly half of all deaths) in the Western world than any other disorder. Because coronary artery disease is an important manifestation of the disease, epidemiologic data related to atherosclerosis mortality typically reflect deaths caused by heart disease (Chapter 12); indeed, myocardial infarction is responsible for almost a quarter of all deaths in the United States. Significant morbidity and mortality are also caused by aortic and carotid atherosclerotic disease and stroke.

EPIDEMIOLOGY

Virtually ubiquitous among most developed nations, atherosclerosis is much less prevalent in Central and South America, Africa, and parts of Asia. The mortality rate for ischemic heart disease (IHD) in the United States is among the highest in the world and is approximately five times higher than that in Japan. Nevertheless, IHD has been increasing in Japan and is now the second leading cause of death there. Moreover, Japanese immigrants who adopt American life styles and dietary customs acquire the same predisposition to atherosclerosis as the indigenous population.

The prevalence and severity of atherosclerosis and IHD among individuals and groups are related to several risk factors, some constitutional (and therefore less controllable), others acquired or related to behaviors that are potentially amenable to intervention (Table 11–3). Risk factors have been identified through several prospective studies in well-defined populations, most notably the Framingham Heart Study and Atherosclerosis Risk in Communities Study (Fig. 11–7).[27,28] *Risk factors have a multiplicative effect*; two risk factors increase the risk approximately fourfold. When three risk factors are present (e.g., hyperlipidemia, hypertension, and smoking), the rate of myocardial infarction is increased seven times.

Constitutional risk factors in IHD. *These include age, gender, and genetics.*

○ *Age* is a dominant influence. Although atherosclerosis is typically progressive, it usually does not become clinically manifest until middle age or later (see below). Between ages 40 and 60 the incidence of myocardial infarction increases fivefold. Death rates from IHD rise with each decade even into advanced age.
○ *Gender.* Other factors being equal, premenopausal women are relatively protected against atherosclerosis and its

TABLE 11–3 Major Risk Factors for Atherosclerosis	
NONMODIFIABLE	
Increasing age	Family history
Male gender	Genetic abnormalities
MODIFIABLE	
Hyperlipidemia	Diabetes
Hypertension	C-reactive protein
Cigarette smoking	

consequences compared to age-matched men. Thus, myocardial infarction and other complications of atherosclerosis are uncommon in premenopausal women in the absence of risk factors such as diabetes, hyperlipidemia, or severe hypertension. After menopause, however, the incidence of atherosclerosis-related diseases increases and at older ages actually exceeds that of men. Although a favorable influence of estrogen has long been proposed to explain the protective effect, some clinical trials have failed to demonstrate any utility of hormonal therapy for vascular disease prevention. As discussed in greater detail in Chapter 9, the atheroprotective effect of estrogens is related to the age at which the therapy is initiated. In younger postmenopausal women, there is a reduction in coronary atherosclerosis with estrogen therapy. The effect is unclear in older women. In addition to atherosclerosis, gender also affects a number of parameters that can influence outcomes of IHD; thus, women show differences in hemostasis, infarct healing, and myocardial remodeling.[29]

○ *Genetics.* Family history is the most significant independent risk factor for atherosclerosis. Many mendelian disorders associated with atherosclerosis, such as familial hypercholesterolemia (Chapter 5), have been characterized. Nevertheless, these genetic diseases account for only a small percentage of cases. The well-established familial predisposition to atherosclerosis and IHD is usually multifactorial, relating to inheritance of various genetic polymorphisms, and familial clustering of other established risk factors, such as hypertension or diabetes.[30]

Modifiable risk factors in IHD. *These include hyperlipidemia, hypertension, cigarette smoking, and diabetes.*

○ *Hyperlipidemia*—and more specifically *hypercholesterolemia*—is a major risk factor for atherosclerosis; even in the absence of other factors, hypercholesterolemia is sufficient to stimulate lesion development.[28] The major component of serum cholesterol associated with increased risk is low-density lipoprotein (LDL) cholesterol ("bad cholesterol"); LDL cholesterol is the form of cholesterol that is delivered to peripheral tissues. In contrast, high-density lipoprotein (HDL, "good cholesterol") mobilizes cholesterol from tissue and transports it to the liver for excretion in the bile. Consequently, higher levels of HDL correlate with reduced risk.

Understandably, dietary and pharmacologic approaches that lower LDL or total serum cholesterol, and/or raise serum HDL, are of considerable interest. High dietary intake of cholesterol and saturated fats (present in egg yolks, animal fats, and butter, for example) raises plasma cholesterol levels. Conversely, diets low in cholesterol and/or with higher ratios of polyunsaturated fats lower plasma cholesterol levels. Omega-3 fatty acids (abundant in fish oils) are beneficial, whereas *trans*-unsaturated fats produced by artificial hydrogenation of polyunsaturated oils (used in baked goods and margarine) adversely affect cholesterol profiles. Exercise and moderate consumption of ethanol raise HDL levels, whereas obesity and smoking lower it.[28] *Statins* are a class of drugs that lower circulating cholesterol levels by inhibiting hydroxymethylglutaryl coenzyme A (HMG-CoA) reductase, the rate-limiting enzyme in hepatic cholesterol biosynthesis.[31]

○ *Hypertension* (see above) is another major risk factor for atherosclerosis; both systolic and diastolic levels are important. On its own, hypertension increases the risk of IHD by approximately 60% (see Fig. 11–7). Hypertension is the

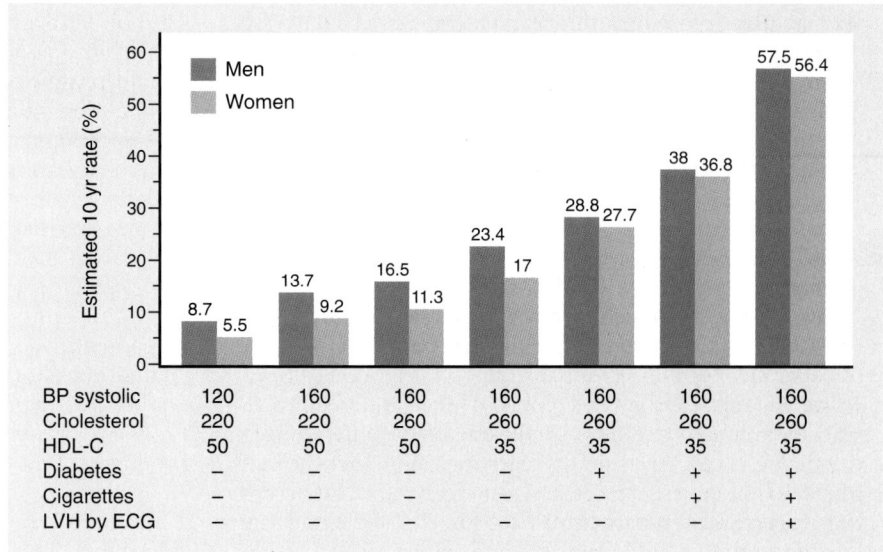

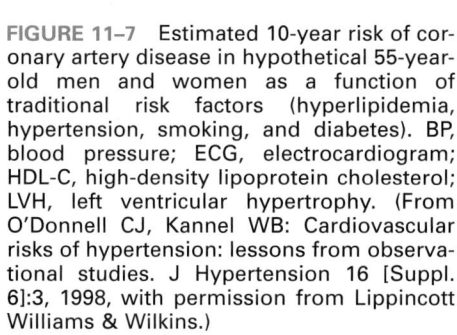

FIGURE 11–7   Estimated 10-year risk of coronary artery disease in hypothetical 55-year-old men and women as a function of traditional risk factors (hyperlipidemia, hypertension, smoking, and diabetes). BP, blood pressure; ECG, electrocardiogram; HDL-C, high-density lipoprotein cholesterol; LVH, left ventricular hypertrophy. (From O'Donnell CJ, Kannel WB: Cardiovascular risks of hypertension: lessons from observational studies. J Hypertension 16 [Suppl. 6]:3, 1998, with permission from Lippincott Williams & Wilkins.)

BP systolic	120	160	160	160	160	160	160
Cholesterol	220	220	260	260	260	260	260
HDL-C	50	50	50	35	35	35	35
Diabetes	–	–	–	–	+	+	+
Cigarettes	–	–	–	–	–	+	+
LVH by ECG	–	–	–	–	–	–	+

most important cause of left ventricular hypertrophy and hence the latter is also related to IHD.

○ *Cigarette smoking* is a well-established risk factor in men and probably accounts for the increasing incidence and severity of atherosclerosis in women. Prolonged (years) smoking of one pack of cigarettes or more daily doubles the death rate from IHD. Smoking cessation reduces the risk substantially.

○ *Diabetes mellitus* induces hypercholesterolemia (Chapter 24) and markedly increases the risk of atherosclerosis. Other factors being equal, the incidence of myocardial infarction is twice as high in diabetics as in nondiabetics. There is also an increased risk of strokes and a 100-fold increased risk of atherosclerosis-induced gangrene of the lower extremities.

Additional risk factors. As many as 20% of all cardiovascular events occur in the absence of hypertension, hyperlipidemia, smoking, or diabetes. Indeed, more than 75% of cardiovascular events in previously healthy women occurred with LDL cholesterol levels below 160 mg/dL (a cutoff generally considered to connote low risk).[32] Clearly, other factors contribute to risk; the assessment of some of these has entered clinical practice.

○ *Inflammation.* Inflammation is present during all stages of atherogenesis and is intimately linked with atherosclerotic plaque formation and rupture (see below). With increasing recognition that inflammation plays a significant causal role in IHD, assessment of systemic inflammation has become important in overall risk stratification. While a number of circulating markers of inflammation correlate with IHD risk, *C-reactive protein (CRP)* has emerged as one of the simplest and most sensitive.[33]

CRP is an acute-phase reactant synthesized primarily by the liver. It is downstream of a number of inflammatory triggers and plays a role in the innate immune response by opsonizing bacteria and activating complement. When CRP is secreted from cells within the atherosclerotic intima, it can activate local endothelial cells and induce a prothrombotic state and also increase the adhesiveness of endothelium for leukocytes. Most importantly, it strongly and independently predicts the risk of myocardial infarction, stroke, peripheral arterial disease, and sudden cardiac death, even among apparently healthy individuals (Fig. 11–8). Indeed, CRP levels have recently been incorporated into risk stratification algorithms.[34] Interestingly, although there is as yet no direct evidence that lowering CRP directly reduces cardiovascular risk, smoking cessation, weight loss, and exercise all reduce CRP; moreover, statins reduce CRP levels largely independent of their effects on LDL cholesterol.

○ *Hyperhomocystinemia.* Clinical and epidemiologic studies show a strong relationship between total serum homocysteine levels and coronary artery disease, peripheral vascular disease, stroke, and venous thrombosis.[35] Elevated homocysteine levels can be caused by low folate and vitamin B_{12} intake, although the jury is still out on whether supplemental folate and vitamin B_{12} ingestion can reduce the incidence of cardiovascular disease. *Homocystinuria*, due to rare inborn errors of metabolism, results in elevated circulating homocysteine (>100 µmol/L) and premature vascular disease.

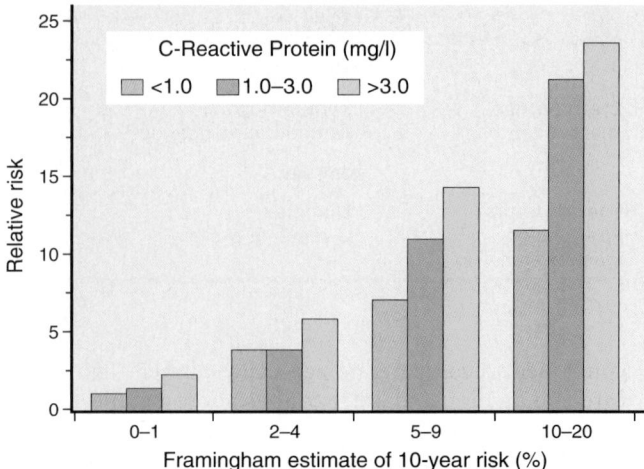

FIGURE 11–8 C-reactive protein (CRP) adds prognostic information at all levels of traditional risk identified from the Framingham Heart Study. Relative risk (*y*-axis) refers to the risk of a cardiovascular event (e.g., myocardial infarction). The *x*-axis is the 10-year risk of a cardiovascular event derived from the traditional risk factors identified in the Framingham Study. In each group of Framingham "risk", CRP values further stratify the patients. (Adapted from Ridker PM et al: Comparison of C-reactive protein and low-density lipoprotein cholesterol levels in the prediction of first cardiovascular events. N Engl J Med 347:1557, 2002.)

○ *Metabolic syndrome.* The metabolic syndrome is characterized by a number of abnormalities that are associated with insulin resistance.[36] Besides glucose intolerance, patients exhibit hypertension and central obesity; indeed, abnormal adipose tissue signaling has been proposed to drive the syndrome. Dyslipidemia leads to endothelial cell dysfunction secondary to increased oxidative stress; there is also a systemic proinflammatory state that further predisposes to vascular thrombosis. Regardless of the etiology, metabolic syndrome clearly plays into many of the known risk factors for atherosclerosis.

○ *Lipoprotein (a)* is an altered form of LDL that contains the apolipoprotein B-100 portion of LDL linked to apolipoprotein A. Lipoprotein (a) levels are associated with coronary and cerebrovascular disease risk, independent of total cholesterol or LDL levels.[37]

○ *Factors affecting hemostasis.* Several markers of hemostatic and/or fibrinolytic function (e.g., elevated plasminogen activator inhibitor 1) are predictors of risk for major atherosclerotic events, including myocardial infarction and stroke. Thrombin, through both its procoagulant and proinflammatory effects, as well as platelet-derived factors both are increasingly recognized as major contributors to local vascular pathology.[38,39]

○ *Other factors.* Factors associated with a less pronounced and/or difficult-to-quantitate risk include lack of exercise; competitive, stressful life style ("type A" personality); and obesity (which is often associated with hypertension, diabetes, hypertriglyceridemia, and decreased HDL).

PATHOGENESIS OF ATHEROSCLEROSIS

The clinical importance of atherosclerosis has stimulated enormous interest in understanding the mechanisms that underlie this disease and its complications. Historically, there

FIGURE 11–9 Evolution of arterial wall changes in the response to injury hypothesis. *1,* Normal. *2,* Endothelial injury with adhesion of monocytes and platelets (the latter to sites where endothelium has been lost). *3,* Migration of monocytes and smooth muscle cells into the intima. *4,* Smooth muscle cell proliferation in the intima with ECM production. *5,* Well-developed plaque.

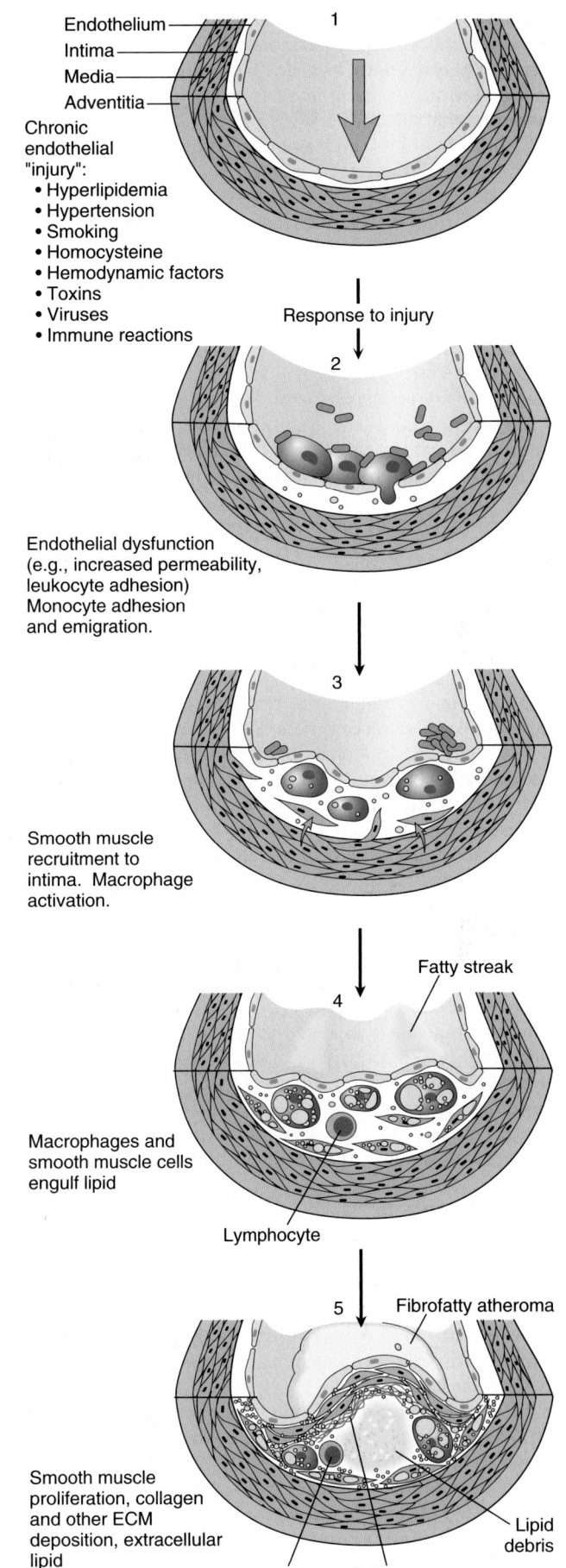

have been two dominant hypotheses: one emphasizes intimal cellular proliferation, while the other focuses on the repetitive formation and organization of thrombi. The contemporary view of atherogenesis incorporates elements of both theories and also integrates the risk factors previously discussed.[40,41] Called the *response-to-injury hypothesis,*[42] the model views *atherosclerosis as a chronic inflammatory and healing response of the arterial wall to endothelial injury. Lesion progression occurs through the interaction of modified lipoproteins, monocyte-derived macrophages, and T lymphocytes with the normal cellular constituents of the arterial wall* (Fig. 11–9). According to this model, atherosclerosis is produced by the following pathogenic events:

- *Endothelial injury,* which causes (among other things) increased vascular permeability, leukocyte adhesion, and thrombosis
- *Accumulation of lipoproteins* (mainly LDL and its oxidized forms) in the vessel wall
- *Monocyte adhesion to the endothelium,* followed by migration into the intima and transformation into *macrophages* and *foam cells*
- *Platelet adhesion*
- *Factor release* from activated platelets, macrophages, and vascular wall cells, inducing *smooth muscle cell recruitment,* either from the media or from circulating precursors
- *Smooth muscle cell proliferation and ECM production*
- *Lipid accumulation* both extracellularly and within cells (macrophages and smooth muscle cells)

The major mechanisms of atherogenesis will now be considered in detail.

Endothelial Injury

Endothelial cell injury is the cornerstone of the response-to-injury hypothesis. Endothelial loss due to *any* kind of injury—induced experimentally by mechanical denudation, hemodynamic forces, immune complex deposition, irradiation, or chemicals—results in intimal thickening; in the presence of high-lipid diets, typical atheromas ensue. However, early human lesions begin at sites of morphologically *intact endothelium.* Thus, *endothelial dysfunction* underlies human atherosclerosis; in this setting, dysfunctional endothelial cells show increased endothelial permeability, enhanced leukocyte adhesion, and altered gene expression.

The specific pathways and factors contributing to endothelial cell dysfunction in early atherosclerosis are not completely understood; etiologic culprits include hypertension, hyperlipidemia, toxins from cigarette smoke, homocysteine, and even infectious agents. Inflammatory cytokines (e.g., tumor necrosis factor [TNF]) can also stimulate pro-atherogenic patterns of endothelial cell gene expression. However, the two most important causes of endothelial dysfunction are hemodynamic disturbances and hypercholesterolemia.

Hemodynamic Disturbances. The importance of hemodynamic turbulence in atherogenesis is illustrated by the observation that plaques tend to occur at ostia of exiting vessels, branch points, and along the posterior wall of the abdominal aorta, where there are disturbed flow patterns.[43] In vitro studies further demonstrate that nonturbulent laminar flow in the normal vasculature leads to the induction of endothelial genes whose products (e.g., the antioxidant superoxide dismutase) *protect* against atherosclerosis. Such "atheroprotective" genes could explain the nonrandom localization of early atherosclerotic lesions.[11]

Lipids. Lipids are typically transported in the bloodstream bound to specific apoproteins (forming lipoprotein complexes). *Dyslipoproteinemias* can result from mutations that alter the apoproteins or the lipoprotein receptors on cells,[44] or from other disorders that affect the circulating levels of lipids (e.g., nephrotic syndrome, alcoholism, hypothyroidism, or diabetes mellitus).[45] Common lipoprotein abnormalities in the general population (indeed, present in many myocardial infarction survivors) include (1) increased LDL cholesterol levels, (2) decreased HDL cholesterol levels, and (3) increased levels of the abnormal lipoprotein (a) (see above).

The evidence implicating hypercholesterolemia in atherogenesis includes the following observations:

- The dominant lipids in atheromatous plaques are cholesterol and cholesterol esters.
- Genetic defects in lipoprotein uptake and metabolism that cause hyperlipoproteinemia are associated with accelerated atherosclerosis. Thus, homozygous familial hypercholesterolemia, caused by defective LDL receptors and inadequate hepatic LDL uptake (Chapter 5) can lead to myocardial infarction before age 20 years. Similarly, accelerated atherosclerosis occurs in animal models with engineered deficiencies in apolipoproteins or LDL receptors.
- Other genetic or acquired disorders (e.g., diabetes mellitus, hypothyroidism) that cause hypercholesterolemia lead to premature atherosclerosis.
- Epidemiologic analyses demonstrate a significant correlation between the severity of atherosclerosis and the levels of total plasma cholesterol or LDL.
- Lowering serum cholesterol by diet or drugs slows the rate of progression of atherosclerosis, causes regression of some plaques, and reduces the risk of cardiovascular events.

The mechanisms by which hyperlipidemia contributes to atherogenesis include the following:[44]

- Chronic hyperlipidemia, particularly hypercholesterolemia, can directly impair endothelial cell function by increasing local oxygen free radical production; oxygen free radicals can injure tissues and accelerate nitric oxide decay, reducing its vasodilator activity.
- With chronic hyperlipidemia, lipoproteins accumulate within the intima. These lipids are *oxidized* through the action of oxygen free radicals locally generated by macrophages or endothelial cells. Oxidized LDL is ingested by macrophages through a *scavenger receptor*, distinct from the LDL receptor, and accumulates in phagocytes, which are

then called *foam cells*. In addition, oxidized LDL stimulates the release of growth factors, cytokines, and chemokines by endothelial cells and macrophages that increase monocyte recruitment into lesions. Finally, oxidized LDL is cytotoxic to endothelial cells and smooth muscle cells and can induce endothelial cell dysfunction. The importance of oxidized LDL in atherogenesis is suggested by the fact that it accumulates within macrophages in all stages of plaque formation.

Inflammation. Inflammatory cells and pathways contribute to the initiation, progression, and complications of atherosclerotic lesions.[41,46] Although normal vessels do not bind inflammatory cells, early in atherogenesis, dysfunctional arterial endothelial cells express adhesion molecules that encourage leukocyte adhesion; vascular cell adhesion molecule 1 (VCAM-1), in particular, binds monocytes and T cells. After these cells adhere to the endothelium, they migrate into the intima under the influence of locally produced chemokines.

- Monocytes transform into macrophages and avidly engulf lipoproteins including oxidized LDL. Monocyte recruitment and differentiation into macrophages (and ultimately into foam cells) is theoretically protective, because these cells remove potentially harmful lipid particles. However, the oxidized LDL augments macrophage activation and cytokine production (e.g., TNF). This further increases leukocyte adhesion and production of chemokines (e.g., monocyte chemotactic protein 1), creating a stimulus for recruitment of additional mononuclear inflammatory cells. Activated macrophages also produce reactive oxygen species that aggravate LDL oxidation and elaborate growth factors that drive smooth muscle cell proliferation.
- T lymphocytes recruited to the intima interact with the macrophages and can generate a chronic inflammatory state. It is not clear whether the T cells are responding to specific antigens (e.g., bacterial or viral antigens, heat-shock proteins [see below], or modified arterial wall constituents and lipoproteins) or are nonspecifically activated by the local inflammatory milieu. Nevertheless, activated T cells in the growing intimal lesions elaborate inflammatory cytokines, (e.g., IFN-γ), which can stimulate macrophages as well as endothelial cells and smooth muscle cells.
- As a consequence of the chronic inflammatory state, activated leukocytes and vascular wall cells release growth factors that promote smooth muscle cell proliferation and ECM synthesis.

Infection. Although there is tantalizing evidence that infections may drive the local inflammatory process that underlies atherosclerosis, this hypothesis has yet to be conclusively proven. Herpesvirus, cytomegalovirus, and *Chlamydia pneumoniae* have all been detected in atherosclerotic plaques but not in normal arteries, and seroepidemiologic studies find increased antibody titers to *C. pneumoniae* in patients with more severe atherosclerosis. Of course, some of these observations are confounded by the fact that *C. pneumoniae* bronchitis is also associated with smoking, a well-established IHD risk factor. Moreover, infections with these organisms are exceedingly common (as is atherosclerosis), so that distinguishing

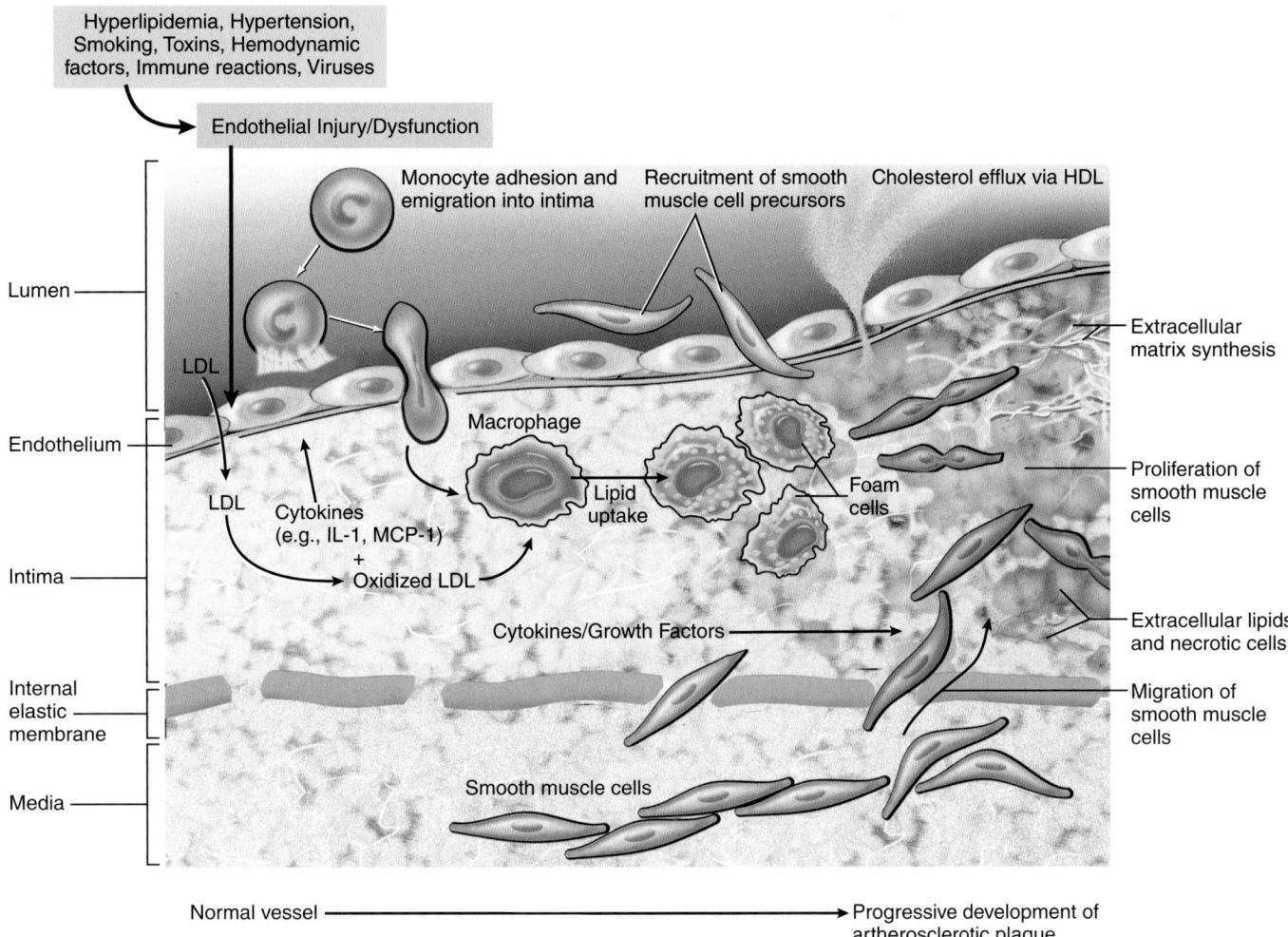

FIGURE 11–10 Hypothetical sequence of cellular interactions in atherosclerosis. Hyperlipidemia and other risk factors are thought to cause endothelial injury, resulting in adhesion of platelets and monocytes and release of growth factors, including platelet-derived growth factor (PDGF), which lead to smooth muscle cell migration and proliferation. Foam cells of atheromatous plaques are derived from both macrophages and smooth muscle cells—from macrophages via the very-low-density lipoprotein (VLDL) receptor and low-density lipoprotein (LDL) modifications recognized by scavenger receptors (e.g., oxidized LDL), and from smooth muscle cells by less certain mechanisms. Extracellular lipid is derived from insudation from the vessel lumen, particularly in the presence of hypercholesterolemia, and also from degenerating foam cells. Cholesterol accumulation in the plaque reflects an imbalance between influx and efflux, and high-density lipoprotein (HDL) probably helps clear cholesterol from these accumulations. Smooth muscle cells migrate to the intima, proliferate, and produce ECM, including collagen and proteoglycans. IL-1, interleukin-1; MCP-1, monocyte chemoattractant protein 1.

coincidence from causality is difficult. Nevertheless, it is certainly possible that such organisms could infect sites of early atheroma formation; their foreign antigens could potentiate atherogenesis by driving local immune responses, or infectious agents could contribute to the local prothrombotic state.[47]

Smooth Muscle Proliferation

Intimal smooth muscle cell proliferation and ECM deposition convert a *fatty streak*, the earliest lesion, into a mature atheroma and contribute to the progressive growth of atherosclerotic lesions (see Fig. 11–9, steps 4 and 5). (Recall that the intimal smooth muscle cells may be recruited from circulating precursors and they have a proliferative and synthetic phenotype distinct from the underlying medial smooth muscle cells.)

Several growth factors are implicated in smooth muscle cell proliferation and ECM synthesis, including PDGF (released by locally adherent platelets, as well as macrophages, endothelial cells, and smooth muscle cells), FGF, and TGF-α. The recruited smooth muscle cells synthesize ECM (notably collagen) that stabilizes atherosclerotic plaques. However, activated inflammatory cells in atheromas can cause intimal smooth muscle cell apoptosis, and also increase ECM catabolism resulting in unstable plaques (see below).

Overview

Figure 11–10 highlights the concept of atherosclerosis as a chronic inflammatory response—and ultimately an attempt at vascular "healing"—driven by a variety of insults, including endothelial cell injury, lipid accumulation and oxidation, and

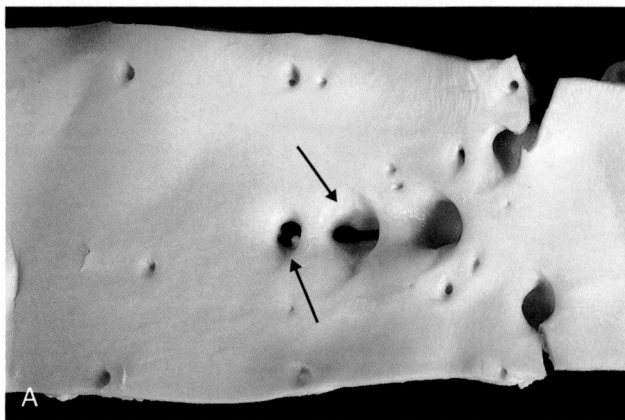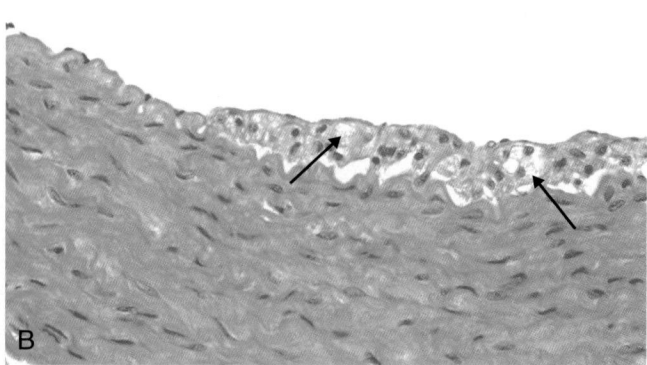

FIGURE 11–11 Fatty streak, a collection of foamy macrophages in the intima. **A,** Aorta with fatty streaks *(arrows)*, associated largely with the ostia of branch vessels. **B,** Photomicrograph of fatty streak in an experimental hypercholesterolemic rabbit, demonstrating intimal, macrophage-derived foam cells *(arrows)*. (**B,** Courtesy of Myron I. Cybulsky, M.D., University of Toronto, Toronto, ON, Canada.)

thrombosis. Atheromas are dynamic lesions consisting of dysfunctional endothelial cells, recruited and proliferating smooth muscle cells, and admixed lymphocytes and macrophages. All four cell types are capable of liberating mediators that can influence atherogenesis. Thus, at early stages, intimal plaques are little more than smooth muscle cell and macrophage foam cell aggregates. With progression, the atheroma is modified by ECM synthesized by smooth muscle cells; connective tissue is particularly prominent in the intima, where it forms a fibrous cap, although lesions also typically retain a central core of lipid-laden cells and fatty debris that can become calcified. The intimal plaque may progressively encroach on the vessel lumen, or compress and cause degeneration of the underlying media; disruption of the fibrous cap can lead to thrombosis and acute vascular occlusion.

With this overview of pathogenesis, we will now discuss the morphologic features and evolution of atherosclerosis.

Morphology

Fatty Streaks. Fatty streaks are the earliest lesions in atherosclerosis. They are composed of lipid-filled foamy macrophages. Beginning as multiple minute flat yellow spots, they eventually coalesce into elongated streaks 1 cm or more in length. These lesions are not significantly raised and do not cause any flow disturbance (Fig. 11–11). Aortas of infants less than 1 year old can exhibit fatty streaks, and such lesions are seen in virtually all children older than 10 years, regardless of geography, race, sex, or environment. The relationship of fatty streaks to atherosclerotic plaques is uncertain; although they may evolve into precursors of plaques, not all fatty streaks are destined to become advanced lesions. Nevertheless, coronary fatty streaks begin to form in adolescence, at the same anatomic sites that later tend to develop plaques.

Atherosclerotic Plaque. The key processes in atherosclerosis are intimal thickening and lipid accumulation (see Fig. 11–10). Atheromatous plaques impinge

on the lumen of the artery and grossly appear white to yellow; superimposed thrombus over ulcerated plaques is red-brown. Plaques vary from 0.3 to 1.5 cm in diameter but can coalesce to form larger masses (Fig. 11–12).

Atherosclerotic lesions are patchy, usually involving only a portion of any given arterial wall, and are rarely circumferential; on cross-section, the lesions therefore appear "eccentric" (Fig. 11–13A). The focality of atherosclerotic lesions—despite the uniform exposure of vessel walls to such factors as cigarette smoke toxins, elevated LDL, hyperglycemia, etc.—is attributable to the vagaries of vascular hemodynamics. Local flow disturbances (e.g., turbulence at branch points) leads to increased susceptibility of certain portions of a vessel wall to plaque formation. Though focal and sparsely distributed at first, atherosclerotic lesions can become more numerous and more diffuse with time.

In humans, the abdominal aorta is typically involved to a much greater degree than the thoracic aorta. In descending order, the most extensively involved vessels are the lower abdominal aorta, the coronary arteries, the popliteal arteries, the internal carotid arteries, and the vessels of the circle of Willis. Vessels of the upper extremities are usually spared, as are the mesenteric and renal arteries, except at their ostia. Nevertheless, in an individual case, the severity of atherosclerosis in one artery does not predict its severity in another. Moreover, in any given vessel, lesions at various stages often coexist.

Atherosclerotic plaques have three principal components: (1) cells, including smooth muscle cells, macrophages, and T cells; (2) ECM, including collagen, elastic fibers, and proteoglycans; and (3) intracellular and extracellular lipid (Fig. 11–13). These components occur in varying proportions and configurations in different lesions. Typically, there is a superficial fibrous cap composed of smooth muscle

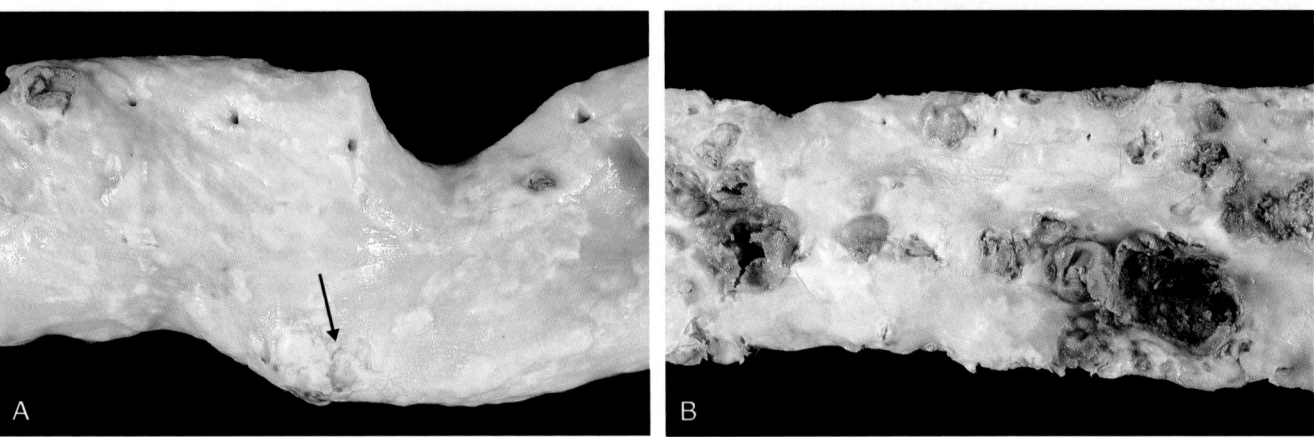

FIGURE 11–12   Gross views of atherosclerosis in the aorta. **A,** Mild atherosclerosis composed of fibrous plaques, one of which is denoted by the *arrow*. **B,** Severe disease with diffuse and complicated lesions (with plaque rupture and superimposed thrombosis), some of which have coalesced.

cells and relatively dense collagen. Beneath and to the side of the cap (the "shoulder") is a more cellular area containing macrophages, T cells, and smooth muscle cells. Deep to the fibrous cap is a necrotic core, containing lipid (primarily cholesterol and cholesterol esters), debris from dead cells, foam cells (lipid-laden macrophages and smooth muscle cells), fibrin, variably organized thrombus, and other plasma proteins; the cholesterol is frequently present as crystalline aggregates that are washed out during routine tissue processing and leave behind only empty "clefts." The periphery of the lesions show neovascularization (proliferating small blood vessels; Fig. 11–13C). Typical atheromas contain abundant lipid, but some plaques ("fibrous plaques") are composed

almost exclusively of smooth muscle cells and fibrous tissue.

Plaques generally continue to change and progressively enlarge due to cell death and degeneration, synthesis and degradation (remodeling) of ECM, and organization of thrombus. Moreover, atheromas often undergo **calcification** (see Fig. 11–13C).

Atherosclerotic plaques are susceptible to the following clinically important changes (see also subsequent discussion):

• **Rupture, ulceration, or erosion** of the intimal surface of atheromatous plaques exposes the blood to highly thrombogenic substances and induces **thrombosis**. Such thrombosis can partially or

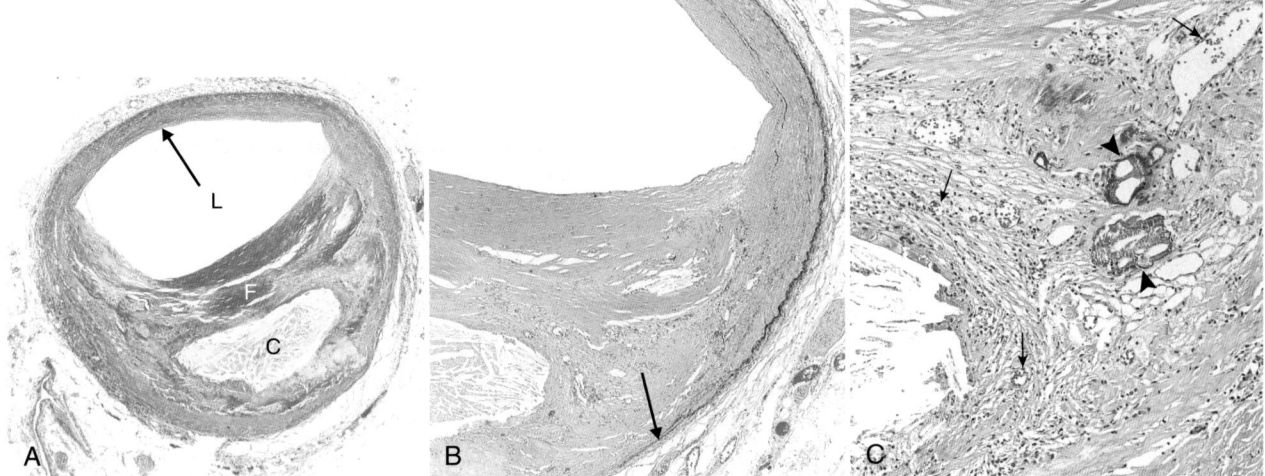

FIGURE 11–13   Histologic features of atheromatous plaque in the coronary artery. **A,** Overall architecture demonstrating fibrous cap (F) and a central necrotic (largely lipid) core (C). The lumen (L) has been moderately compromised. Note that a segment of the wall is free of plaque *(arrow)*; the lesion is therefore "eccentric". In this section, collagen has been stained blue (Masson's trichrome stain). **B,** Higher power photograph of a section of the plaque shown in **A,** stained for elastin (black), demonstrating that the internal and external elastic membranes are attenuated and the media of the artery is thinned under the most advanced plaque *(arrow)*. **C,** Higher magnification photomicrograph at the junction of the fibrous cap and core, showing scattered inflammatory cells, calcification *(arrowhead)* and neovascularization *(small arrows)*.

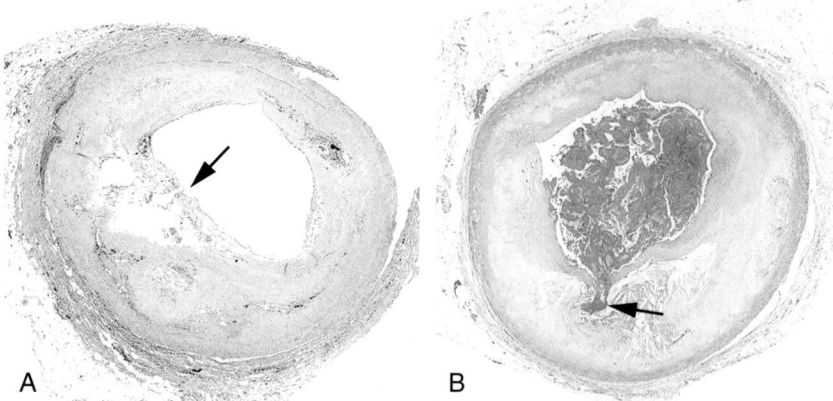

FIGURE 11–14 Atherosclerotic plaque rupture. **A,** Plaque rupture without superimposed thrombus, in a patient who died suddenly. **B,** Acute coronary thrombosis superimposed on an atherosclerotic plaque with focal disruption of the fibrous cap, triggering fatal myocardial infarction. In both **A** and **B,** an *arrow* points to the site of plaque rupture. (**B,** Reproduced from Schoen FJ: Interventional and Surgical Cardiovascular pathology: Clinical Correlations and Basic Principles. Philadelphia, WB Saunders, 1989, p 61.)

completely occlude the lumen and lead to downstream ischemia (Chapter 12) (Fig. 11–14). If the patient survives the initial thrombotic occlusion, the clot may become organized and incorporated into the growing plaque.

- **Hemorrhage into a plaque.** Rupture of the overlying fibrous cap, or of the thin-walled vessels in the areas of neovascularization, can cause intra-plaque hemorrhage; a contained hematoma may expand the plaque or induce plaque rupture.
- **Atheroembolism.** Plaque rupture can discharge atherosclerotic debris into the bloodstream, producing microemboli.
- **Aneurysm formation.** Atherosclerosis-induced pressure or ischemic atrophy of the underlying media, with loss of elastic tissue, causes weakness resulting in aneurysmal dilation and potential rupture (see below).

CONSEQUENCES OF ATHEROSCLEROTIC DISEASE

Large elastic arteries (e.g., the aorta, carotid, and iliac arteries) and large and medium-sized muscular arteries (e.g., coronary and popliteal arteries) are the major targets of atherosclerosis. Symptomatic atherosclerotic disease most often involves the arteries supplying the heart, brain, kidneys, and lower extremities. *Myocardial infarction (heart attack), cerebral infarction (stroke), aortic aneurysms, and peripheral vascular disease (gangrene of the legs) are the major consequences of atherosclerosis.* The natural history, principal morphologic features, and main pathogenic events are schematized in Figure 11–15. The principal outcomes depend on the size of the involved vessels, the relative stability of the plaque itself, and the degree of degeneration of the underlying arterial wall:

- Smaller vessels can become occluded, compromising distal tissue perfusion.
- Ruptured plaque can embolize atherosclerotic debris and cause distal vessel obstruction, or can lead to acute (and frequently catastrophic) vascular thrombosis.

- Destruction of the underlying vessel wall can lead to aneurysm formation, with secondary rupture and/or thrombosis.

Chronic stenosis and plaque rupture will be covered next, followed by a discussion of aneurysms.

Atherosclerotic Stenosis. In small arteries, atherosclerotic plaques can gradually occlude vessel lumens, compromising blood flow and causing ischemic injury. At early stages of stenosis, outward remodeling of the vessel media tends to preserve luminal diameter as the total circumference expands.[18] However, there are limits on this outward remodeling, and eventually the expanding atheroma impinges on blood flow. *Critical stenosis* is the Rubicon at which chronic occlusion significantly limits flow, and demand begins exceeding supply. In the coronary (and other) circulations, this typically occurs at approximately 70% fixed occlusion (i.e., loss of area through which blood can flow); at this degree of stenosis, patients classically develop chest pain *(angina)* on exertion (so-called *stable angina;* see Chapter 12). Although acute plaque rupture (below) is the most dangerous complication, atherosclerosis also takes a toll through chronically diminished arterial perfusion: *mesenteric occlusion and bowel ischemia, chronic IHD, ischemic encephalopathy,* and *intermittent claudication* (diminished extremity perfusion) are all consequences of flow-limiting stenoses. The effects of vascular occlusion ultimately depend on arterial supply and the metabolic demand of the affected tissue.

Acute Plaque Change. *Plaque erosion or rupture is typically promptly followed by partial or complete vascular thrombosis* (see Fig. 11–14), *resulting in acute tissue infarction (e.g., myocardial or cerebral infarction).*[40,48] Plaque changes fall into three general categories:

- *Rupture/fissuring,* exposing highly thrombogenic plaque constituents
- *Erosion/ulceration,* exposing the thrombogenic subendothelial basement membrane to blood
- *Hemorrhage into the atheroma,* expanding its volume

It is now recognized that the precipitating lesion in patients who develop myocardial infarction and other acute coronary syndromes is not necessarily a severely stenotic and

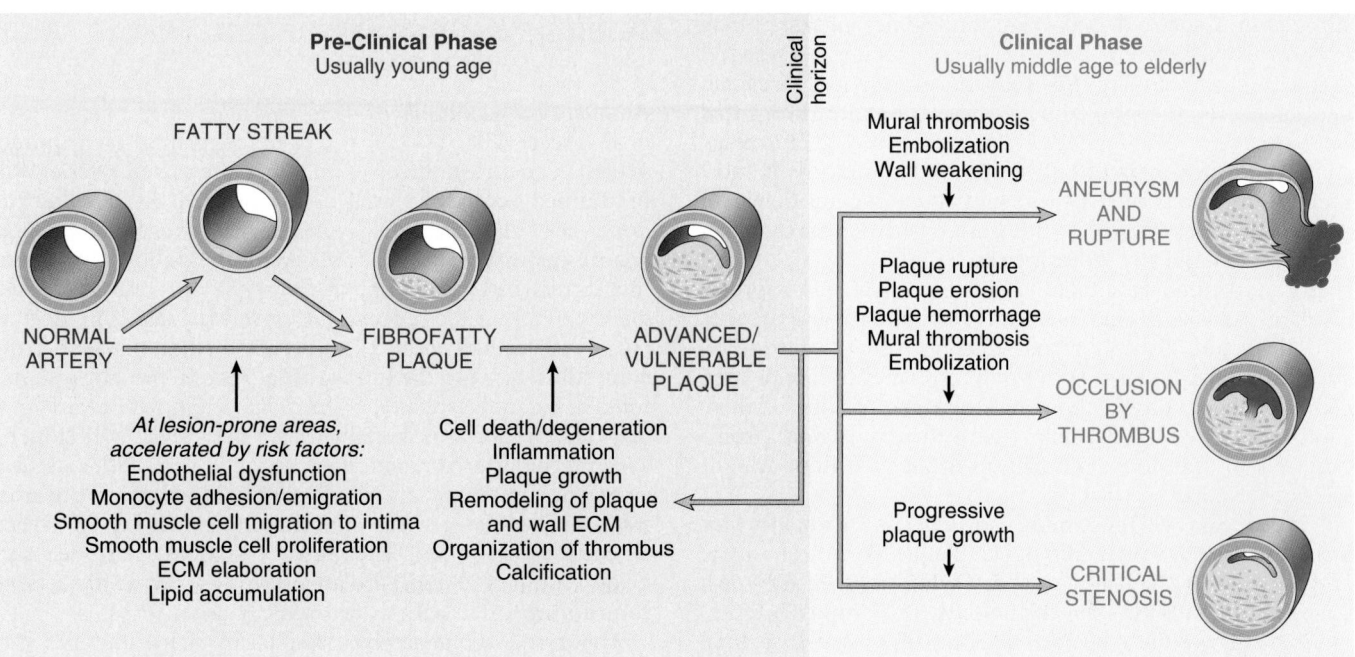

FIGURE 11–15 The natural history, morphologic features, main pathogenic events, and clinical complications of atherosclerosis.

hemodynamically significant lesion before its acute change. Pathologic and clinical studies show that the majority of plaques that undergo abrupt disruption and coronary occlusion previously showed only mild to moderate luminal stenosis.[49] The worrisome conclusion is that a rather large number of now asymptomatic adults may well have a real but unpredictable risk of a catastrophic coronary event. Regrettably, it is presently impossible to reliably detect individuals who will have plaque disruption or subsequent thrombosis.

The events that trigger abrupt changes in plaque configuration and superimposed thrombosis are complex and include both intrinsic factors (e.g., plaque structure and composition) and extrinsic factors (e.g., blood pressure, platelet reactivity)[40,50]; rupture of a plaque indicates that it was unable to withstand the mechanical stresses of vascular shear forces. We next discuss the intrinsic and extrinsic factors that influence the risk of plaque rupture.

It is important to remember that the composition of plaques is dynamic and can materially contribute to risk of rupture. Thus, plaques that contain large areas of foam cells and extracellular lipid, and those in which the fibrous caps are thin or contain few smooth muscle cells or have clusters of inflammatory cells, are more likely to rupture, and are therefore called "vulnerable plaques"[48] (Fig. 11–16).

It is also established that the fibrous cap undergoes continuous remodeling that may make the plaque susceptible to acute alterations. Collagen represents the major structural component of the fibrous cap, and accounts for its mechanical strength and stability. Thus, the balance of collagen synthesis versus degradation affects cap stability. Collagen in atherosclerotic plaque is produced primarily by smooth muscle cells, so that loss of these cellular elements results in a weaker cap. Moreover, collagen turnover is controlled by matrix metalloproteinases (MMPs), enzymes elaborated largely by macrophages within the atheromatous plaque; conversely, tissue inhibitors of metalloproteinases (TIMPs), produced by endothelial cells, smooth muscle cells, and macrophages, modulate MMP activity. In general, plaque inflammation results in a net increase in collagen degradation and reduces collagen synthesis, thereby destabilizing the mechanical integrity of the fibrous cap (see below). Interestingly, statins may have a beneficial therapeutic effect not only by reducing circulating cholesterol levels but also by stabilizing plaques through a reduction in plaque inflammation.[51]

Influences extrinsic to plaques are also important. Thus, adrenergic stimulation can increase systemic blood pressure or induce local vasoconstriction, thereby increasing the physical stresses on a given plaque. Indeed, the adrenergic

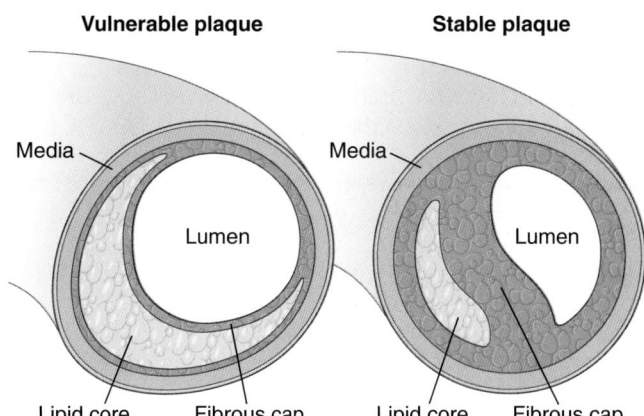

FIGURE 11–16 Schematic comparing vulnerable and stable atherosclerotic plaque. Whereas stable plaques have densely collagenous and thickened fibrous caps with minimal inflammation and negligible underlying atheromatous core, vulnerable plaques (prone to rupture) are characterized by thin fibrous caps, large lipid cores, and increased inflammation. (Adapted from Libby P: Circulation 91:2844, 1995.)

stimulation associated with waking and rising can cause blood pressure spikes (followed by heightened platelet reactivity) that have been causally linked to the pronounced circadian periodicity for the peak time of onset of acute myocardial infarction (between 6 AM and 12 noon).[52] Intense emotional stress can also contribute to plaque disruption; this is most dramatically illustrated by the uptick in the incidence of sudden death associated with disasters such as earthquakes and the September 11, 2001 attacks.[53]

It is also important to note that not all plaque ruptures result in occlusive thromboses with catastrophic consequences. Indeed, plaque disruption and ensuing platelet aggregation and thrombosis are probably common, repetitive, and often clinically silent complications of atheroma. Healing of these subclinical plaque disruptions—with their overlying thromboses—is an important mechanism in the growth of atherosclerotic lesions.

Thrombosis. As mentioned above, partial or total thrombosis associated with a disrupted plaque is critical to the pathogenesis of the acute coronary syndromes. In the most serious form, thrombus superimposed on a disrupted but previously only partially stenotic plaque converts it to a total occlusion. In contrast, in other coronary syndromes (Chapter 12), luminal obstruction by thrombosis is usually incomplete, and can even wax and wane with time.

Mural thrombus in a coronary artery can also embolize. Indeed, small fragments of thrombotic material in the distal intra-myocardial circulation or microinfarcts can be found at autopsy in patients after sudden death or in rapidly accelerating anginal syndromes. Finally, thrombus is a potent activator of multiple growth-related signals in smooth muscle cells, which can contribute to the growth of atherosclerotic lesions.

Vasoconstriction. Vasoconstriction compromises lumen size, and, by increasing the local mechanical forces can potentiate plaque disruption. Vasoconstriction at sites of atheroma is stimulated by (1) circulating adrenergic agonists, (2) locally released platelet contents, (3) impaired secretion of endothelial cell relaxing factors (nitric oxide) relative to contracting factors (endothelin) as a result of endothelial cell dysfunction, and possibly (4) mediators released from perivascular inflammatory cells.

Aneurysms and Dissection

An *aneurysm* is a *localized abnormal dilation of a blood vessel or the heart* (Fig. 11–17); it can be congenital or acquired. When an aneurysm involves an intact attenuated arterial wall or thinned ventricular wall of the heart, it is called a *true aneurysm.* Atherosclerotic, syphilitic, and congenital vascular aneurysms, and ventricular aneurysms that follow transmural myocardial infarctions are of this type. In contrast, a *false aneurysm* (also called *pseudo-aneurysm*) is a defect in the vascular wall leading to an extravascular hematoma that freely communicates with the intravascular space ("pulsating hematoma"). Examples include a ventricular rupture after myocardial infarction that is contained by a pericardial adhesion, or a leak at the sutured junction of a vascular graft with a natural artery. An arterial *dissection* arises when blood enters the arterial wall itself, as a hematoma dissecting between its layers. Dissections are often but not always aneurysmal (see also below). Both true and false aneurysms as well as dissections can rupture, often with catastrophic consequences.

Aneurysms are generally classified by shape and size (see Fig. 11–17). *Saccular* aneurysms are spherical outpouchings (involving only a portion of the vessel wall); they vary from 5 to 20 cm in diameter and often contain thrombus. *Fusiform* aneurysms involve diffuse, circumferential dilation of a long vascular segment; they vary in diameter (up to 20 cm) and in length, and can involve extensive portions of the aortic arch, abdominal aorta, or even the iliac arteries. These types are not specific for any disease or clinical manifestations.

Pathogenesis of Aneurysms. Arteries are dynamically remodeling tissues that maintain their integrity by constantly synthesizing, degrading, and repairing damage to their ECM constituents. Aneurysms can occur when the structure or function of the connective tissue within the vascular wall is compromised. Although we cite here examples of inherited defects in connective tissues, weakening of vessel walls is important in the common, sporadic forms of aneurysms as well.

○ *The intrinsic quality of the vascular wall connective tissue is poor.* In *Marfan syndrome,* for example (Chapter 5), defec-

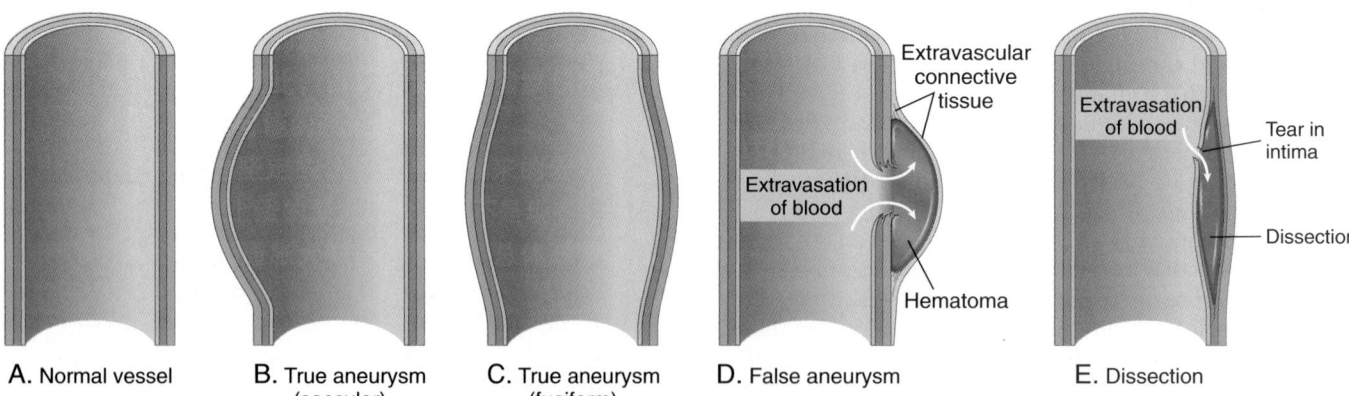

A. Normal vessel   B. True aneurysm (saccular)   C. True aneurysm (fusiform)   D. False aneurysm   E. Dissection

FIGURE 11–17   Aneurysms. **A,** Normal vessel. **B,** True aneurysm, saccular type. The wall focally bulges outward and may be attenuated but is otherwise intact. **C,** True aneurysm, fusiform type. There is circumferential dilation of the vessel, without rupture. **D,** False aneurysm. The wall is ruptured, and there is a collection of blood (hematoma) that is bounded externally by adherent extravascular tissues. **E,** Dissection. Blood has entered *(dissected)* the wall of the vessel and separated the layers. Although this is shown as occurring through a tear in the lumen, dissections can also occur by rupture of the vessels of the vaso vasorum within the media.

tive synthesis of the scaffolding protein *fibrillin* leads to aberrant TGF-β activity and progressive weakening of elastic tissue; in the aorta, the consequence is progressive dilation due to remodeling of the inelastic media.[54] *Loeys-Dietz syndrome* is another recently recognized cause of aneurysms; in this disorder, mutations in TGF-β receptors lead to abnormalities in elastin and collagen I and III. Aneurysms in such individuals can rupture fairly easily (even at small size).[55] Weak vessel walls due to defective type III collagen synthesis are also a hallmark of the vascular forms of *Ehlers-Danlos syndrome* (Chapter 5), and altered collagen cross-linking associated with vitamin C (ascorbate) deficiency is an example of a nutritional basis for aneurysm formation.

- *The balance of collagen degradation and synthesis is altered by local inflammatory infiltrates and the destructive proteolytic enzymes they produce.* In particular, increased MMP production, especially by macrophages in atherosclerotic plaque or in vasculitis, probably contributes to aneurysm development[56]; these enzymes have the capacity to degrade virtually all components of the ECM in the arterial wall (collagens, elastin, proteoglycans, laminin, fibronectin). Concurrently, decreased tissue inhibitor of metalloproteinase (TIMP) expression can also contribute to the overall ECM degradation. Genetic predisposition to aneurysm formation in the setting of inflammatory lesions (such as atherosclerosis) may be related to polymorphisms of MMP and/or TIMP genes, or to the nature of the local inflammatory response that results in increased production of MMP.[57]

- *The vascular wall is weakened through loss of smooth muscle cells or the inappropriate synthesis of noncollagenous or non-elastic ECM.* Ischemia of the inner media occurs when there is atherosclerotic thickening of the intima, which increases the distance that oxygen and nutrients must diffuse. Systemic hypertension can also cause significant narrowing of arterioles of the vasa vasorum (e.g., in the aorta), which can cause outer medial ischemia. Ischemia is reflected in "degenerative changes" of the aorta, whereby smooth muscle cell loss—or change in synthetic phenotype—leads to scarring (and loss of elastic fibers), inadequate ECM synthesis, and production of increasing amounts of amorphous ground substance (glycosaminoglycan). Histologically these changes are collectively called *cystic medial degeneration* (Fig. 11–18). These changes are nonspecific and can be seen in a variety of settings, including Marfan disease and scurvy.

The two most important disorders that predispose to aortic aneurysms are atherosclerosis and hypertension; atherosclerosis is a greater factor in abdominal aortic aneurysms, while hypertension is the most common condition associated with aneurysms of the ascending aorta.[58] Other conditions that weaken vessel walls and lead to aneurysms include trauma, vasculitis (see below), congenital defects (e.g., *berry aneurysms* typically in the circle of Willis; Chapter 28), and infections (*mycotic aneurysms*). Mycotic aneurysms can originate (1) from embolization of a septic embolus, usually as a complication of infective endocarditis; (2) as an extension of an adjacent suppurative process; or (3) by circulating organisms directly infecting the arterial wall. Tertiary syphilis is now a rare cause of aortic

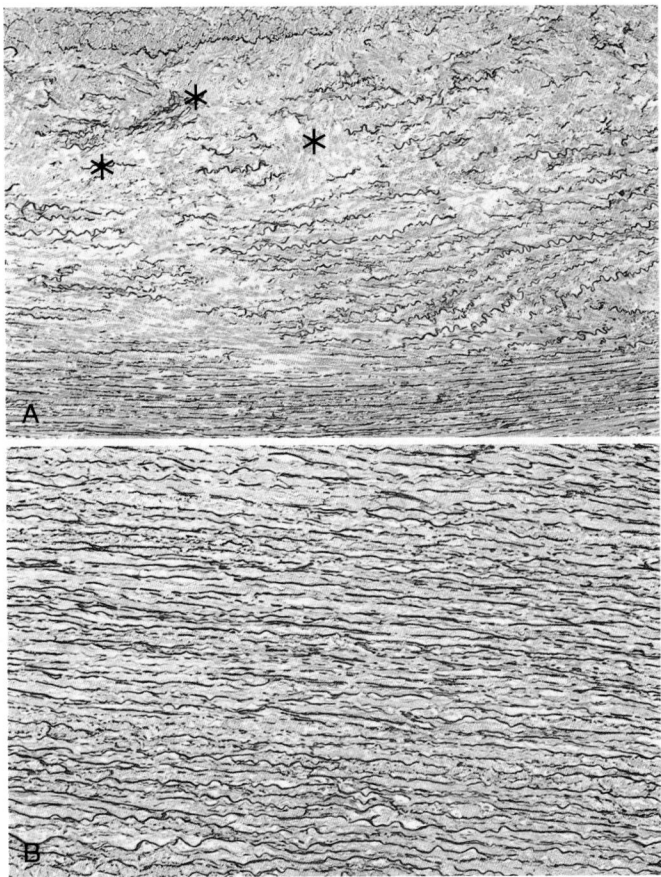

FIGURE 11–18 Cystic medial degeneration. **A,** Cross-section of aortic media from a patient with Marfan syndrome, showing marked elastin fragmentation and formation of areas devoid of elastin that resemble cystic spaces *(asterisks)*. **B,** Normal media for comparison, showing the regular layered pattern of elastic tissue. In both **A** and **B,** elastin is stained black.

aneurysms. The obliterative endarteritis characteristic of late-stage syphilis shows a predilection for small vessels, including those of the vasa vasorum of the thoracic aorta. This leads to ischemic injury of the aortic media and aneurysmal dilation, which sometimes involves the aortic valve annulus.[59]

ABDOMINAL AORTIC ANEURYSM (AAA)

Aneurysms associated with atherosclerosis occur most commonly in the abdominal aorta. Atherosclerotic plaque in the intima compresses the underlying media and compromises nutrient and waste diffusion from the vascular lumen into the arterial wall. The media therefore undergoes degeneration and necrosis that results in arterial wall weakness and consequent thinning. Nevertheless, as described above, the major influence that leads to aneurysm formation is the production of MMP by inflammatory cell infiltrates.[56]

Abdominal aortic aneurysms occur more frequently in men and in smokers, and rarely develop before age 50. Atherosclerosis is a major cause of AAAs, but other factors clearly contribute since the incidence is less than 5% in men older than 60 years of age, despite almost universal abdominal aortic atherosclerosis in that population.

Morphology. Usually positioned below the renal arteries and above the bifurcation of the aorta, AAAs can be saccular or fusiform, up to 15 cm in diameter, and up to 25 cm in length (Fig. 11–19). Typically the intimal surface of the aneurysm shows severe complicated atherosclerosis with destruction and thinning of the underlying aortic media; the aneurysm frequently contains a bland, laminated, poorly organized mural thrombus that may fill some or all of the dilated segment. Occasionally the aneurysm can affect the renal and superior or inferior mesenteric arteries, either by producing direct pressure or by narrowing or occluding vessel ostia with mural thrombi. Not infrequently, AAAs are accompanied by smaller aneurysms of the iliac arteries.

Two AAA variants merit special mention:

- **Inflammatory AAAs** are characterized by dense periaortic fibrosis containing abundant lymphoplasmacytic inflammation with many macrophages and often giant cells. Their cause is uncertain.
- **Mycotic AAAs** are lesions that have become infected by the lodging of circulating microorganisms in the wall, particularly in bacteremia from a primary *Salmonella* gastroenteritis. In such cases suppuration further destroys the media, potentiating rapid dilation and rupture.

Clinical Features. The clinical consequences of AAA include

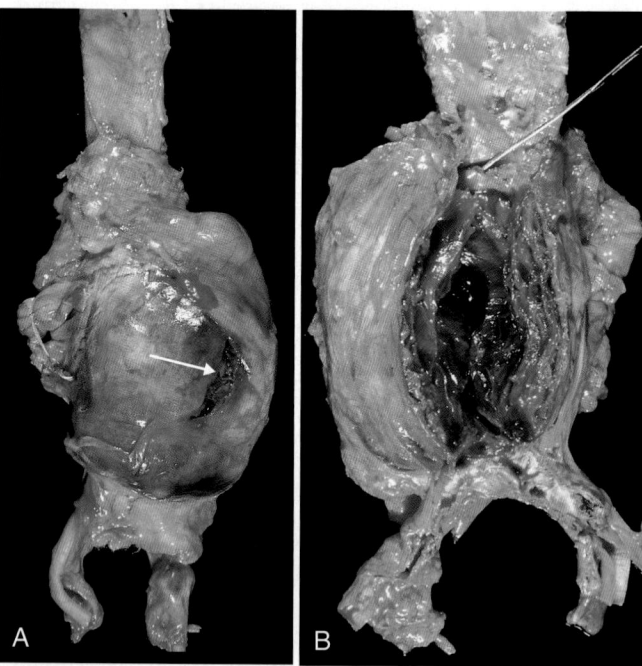

FIGURE 11–19 Abdominal aortic aneurysm. **A,** External view, gross photograph of a large aortic aneurysm that ruptured; the rupture site is indicated by the *arrow*. **B,** Opened view, with the location of the rupture tract indicated by a probe. The wall of the aneurysm is exceedingly thin, and the lumen is filled by a large quantity of layered but largely unorganized thrombus.

- Rupture into the peritoneal cavity or retroperitoneal tissues with massive, potentially fatal hemorrhage
- Obstruction of a branch vessel resulting in ischemic injury of downstream tissues, for example, iliac (leg), renal (kidney), mesenteric (gastrointestinal tract), or vertebral (spinal cord) arteries
- Embolism from atheroma or mural thrombus
- Impingement on an adjacent structure, e.g., compression of a ureter or erosion of vertebrae
- Presentation as an abdominal mass (often palpably pulsating) that simulates a tumor

The risk of rupture is directly related to the size of the aneurysm,[60] varying from nil for AAAs of 4 cm or less in diameter, to 1% per year for AAAs between 4 and 5 cm, to 11% per year for AAAs between 5 and 6 cm, and 25% per year for aneurysms greater than 6 cm in diameter. Most aneurysms expand at a rate of 0.2 to 0.3 cm/yr, but 20% expand more rapidly. In general, aneurysms of 5 cm and larger are managed aggressively, usually by surgical bypass involving prosthetic grafts. Currently, aneurysm treatment is evolving toward endoluminal approaches using stent grafts (expandable wire frames covered by a cloth sleeve) in selected patients.[61] Timely surgery is critical; operative mortality for unruptured aneurysms is approximately 5%, whereas emergency surgery after rupture carries a mortality rate of more than 50%. It is worth reiterating that because atherosclerosis is a systemic disease, a person with AAA is also very likely to have atherosclerosis in other vascular beds and is at a significantly increased risk of IHD and stroke.

THORACIC AORTIC ANEURYSMS

Thoracic aortic aneurysms are most commonly associated with hypertension, although other causes such as Marfan and Loeys-Dietz syndromes are increasingly recognized.[58] Regardless of etiology, these give rise to signs and symptoms referable to (1) encroachment on mediastinal structures, (2) respiratory difficulties due to encroachment on the lungs and airways, (3) difficulty in swallowing due to compression of the esophagus, (4) persistent cough due to irritation of or pressure on the recurrent laryngeal nerves, (5) pain caused by erosion of bone (i.e., ribs and vertebral bodies), (6) cardiac disease as the aortic aneurysm leads to aortic valve dilation with valvular insufficiency or narrowing of the coronary ostia causing myocardial ischemia, and (7) rupture. Most patients with syphilitic aneurysms die of heart failure induced by aortic valvular incompetence.

AORTIC DISSECTION

Aortic dissection occurs when blood splays apart the laminar planes of the media to form a blood-filled channel within the aortic wall (Fig. 11–20); this can be catastrophic if the dissection then ruptures through the adventitia and hemorrhages into adjacent spaces.[62] In contrast to atherosclerotic and syphilitic aneurysms, aortic dissection may or may not be associated with aortic dilation. Consequently, the older term "dissecting aneurysm" should be avoided.

Aortic dissection occurs principally in two groups: (1) men aged 40 to 60, with antecedent hypertension (more than 90% of cases of dissection); and (2) younger patients with systemic or localized abnormalities of connective tissue affecting the

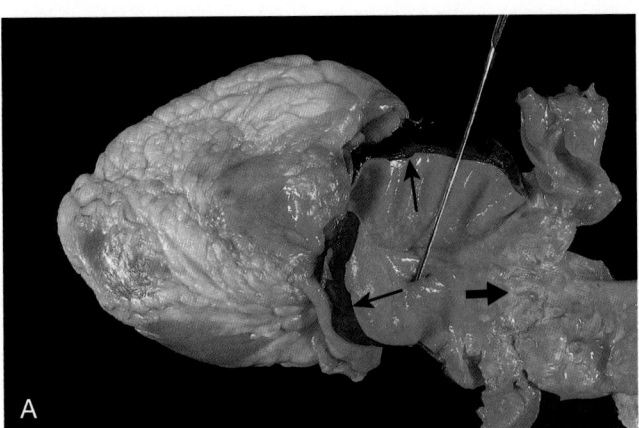 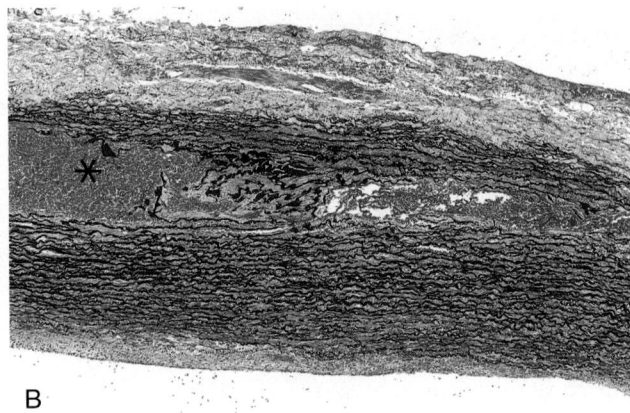

FIGURE 11–20 Aortic dissection. **A,** An opened aorta with proximal dissection originating from a small, oblique intimal tear *(identified by the probe)*, allowing blood to enter the media and creating an intramural hematoma *(narrow arrows)*. Note that the intimal tear has occurred in a region largely free of atherosclerotic plaque and that propagation of the intramural hematoma is arrested at a site more distally where atherosclerosis begins *(broad arrow)*. **B,** Histologic view of the dissection demonstrating an aortic intramural hematoma *(asterisk)*. Aortic elastic layers are black and blood is red in this section, stained with the Movat stain.

aorta (e.g., Marfan syndrome). Dissections can also be iatrogenic (e.g., complicating arterial cannulations during diagnostic catheterization or cardiopulmonary bypass). Rarely, for unknown reasons, dissection of the aorta or other branches, including the coronary arteries, occurs during or after pregnancy. Dissection is unusual in the presence of substantial atherosclerosis or other cause of medial scarring such as syphilis, presumably because the medial fibrosis inhibits propagation of the dissecting hematoma.

Pathogenesis. Hypertension is the major risk factor in aortic dissection. Aortas of hypertensive patients have medial hypertrophy of the vasa vasorum associated with degenerative changes in the aortic media and variable loss of medial smooth muscle cells, suggesting that pressure-related mechanical injury and/or ischemic injury (due to diminished flow through the vasa vasorum) is contributory. A considerably smaller number of dissections are related to inherited or acquired connective tissue disorders causing abnormal vascular ECM (e.g., Marfan syndrome, Ehlers-Danlos syndrome, vitamin C deficiency, copper metabolic defects). However, recognizable medial damage seems to be neither a prerequisite for dissection nor a guarantee that dissection is imminent. Regardless of the underlying etiology causing medial weakness, the trigger for the intimal tear and initial intramural aortic hemorrhage is not known in most cases. Nevertheless, once the tear has occurred, blood flow under systemic pressure dissects through the media, fostering progression of the medial hematoma. Accordingly, aggressive pressure-reducing therapy may be effective in limiting an evolving dissection. In some cases disruption of penetrating vessels of the vasa vasorum can give rise to an intramural hematoma *without* an intimal tear.

> **Morphology.** In most cases, no specific underlying causal pathology is identified in the aortic wall. The most frequent preexisting histologically detectable lesion is **cystic medial degeneration** (see Fig. 11–18); inflammation is characteristically absent. However, dissections can occur in the setting of rather trivial medial degeneration, and the relationship of the

> structural changes to the pathogenesis of dissection is uncertain.
>
> An aortic dissection usually initiates with an intimal tear. In the vast majority of spontaneous dissections, the tear is found in the ascending aorta, usually within 10 cm of the aortic valve (Fig. 11–20A). Such tears are typically transverse or oblique and 1 to 5 cm in length, with sharp, jagged edges. The dissection can extend along the aorta retrograde toward the heart as well as distally, sometimes into the iliac and femoral arteries. The dissecting hematoma spreads characteristically along the laminar planes of the aorta, usually between the middle and outer thirds (Fig. 11–20B). It often ruptures out through the adventitia causing massive hemorrhage (e.g., in the thoracic or abdominal cavities) or cardiac tamponade (hemorrhage into the pericardial sac).[62] In some (lucky) instances, the dissecting hematoma reenters the lumen of the aorta through a second distal intimal tear, creating a new vascular channel and forming a "double-barreled aorta" with a false channel.[62] This averts a fatal extra-aortic hemorrhage. In the course of time, false channels may be endothelialized and become chronic dissections.

Clinical Features. The risk and nature of complications of aorta dissection depend strongly on the region(s) affected; the most serious complications occur with dissections that involve the aorta from the aortic valve to the arch. Thus, aortic dissections are generally classified into two types (Fig. 11–21). They are named after Dr. Michael DeBakey, a pioneer in vascular surgery.

- More common (and dangerous) *proximal* lesions (called *type A dissections*), involving either both the ascending and descending aorta or just the ascending aorta (types I and II of the DeBakey classification)
- *Distal lesions not involving the ascending part* and usually beginning distal to the subclavian artery (called *type B dissections* or DeBakey type III)

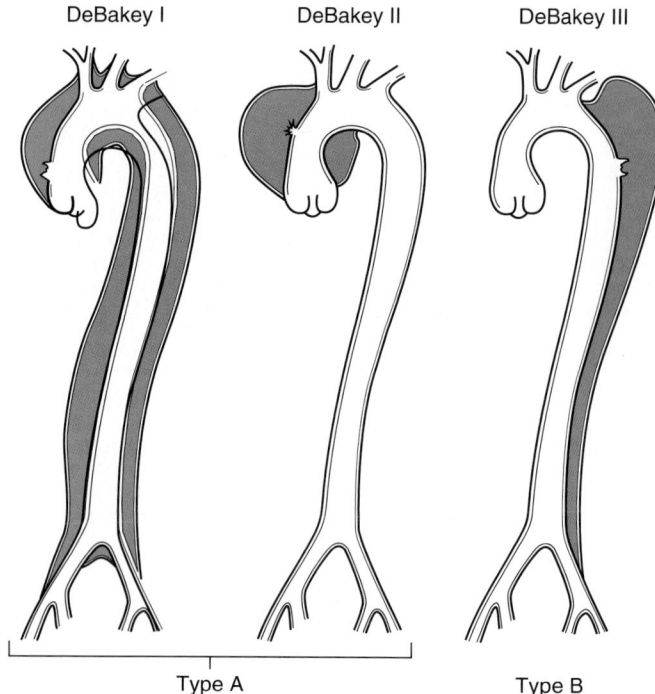

FIGURE 11–21 Classification of dissections. Type A (proximal) involves the ascending aorta, either as part of a more extensive dissection (DeBakey I) or in isolation (DeBakey II). Type B (distal or DeBakey III) dissections arise beyond the takeoff of the great vessels. The serious complications predominantly occur in type A dissections.

The classic clinical symptoms of aortic dissection are the sudden onset of excruciating pain, usually beginning in the anterior chest, radiating to the back between the scapulae, and moving downward as the dissection progresses; the pain can be confused with that of myocardial infarction.

The most common cause of death is rupture of the dissection outward into the pericardial, pleural, or peritoneal cavities. Retrograde dissection into the aortic root can cause disruption of the aortic valvular apparatus. Thus, common clinical manifestations include cardiac tamponade, aortic insufficiency, and myocardial infarction or extension of the dissection into the great arteries of the neck or into the coronary, renal, mesenteric, or iliac arteries, causing critical vascular obstruction and associated ischemic consequences; compression of spinal arteries may cause transverse myelitis.

In the past aortic dissection was typically fatal, but the prognosis has markedly improved. Rapid diagnosis and institution of intensive antihypertensive therapy, coupled with surgical procedures involving plication of the aortic wall, permit 65% to 75% of stricken individuals to be saved.

Vasculitis

Vasculitis is a general term for vessel wall inflammation. The clinical features of the various vasculitides are diverse and largely depend on the vascular bed affected (e.g., central nervous system vs. heart vs. small bowel). Besides the findings referable to the specific tissue(s) involved, the clinical mani-festations typically include constitutional signs and symptoms such as fever, myalgias, arthralgias, and malaise.

Vessels of any type in virtually any organ can be affected; most vasculitides involve small vessels, from arterioles to capillaries to venules.[63] Several of the vasculitides tend to affect only vessels of a particular size or particular vessel beds. There are vasculitic entities that primarily affect the aorta and medium-sized arteries, while others principally affect only smaller arterioles. Some 20 primary forms of vasculitis are recognized, and classification schemes attempt (with variable success) to group them according to vessel size, role of immune complexes, presence of specific autoantibodies, granuloma formation, organ specificity, and even population demographics! Though a subject of ongoing evolution,[64] the so-called Chapel Hill nomenclature remains the most widely accepted approach to organizing this diverse group of entities[65] (Table 11–4 and Fig. 11–22). As we will see, there is considerable clinical and pathologic overlap among many of them.

The two most common pathogenic mechanisms of vasculitis are immune-mediated inflammation and direct invasion of vascular walls by infectious pathogens. Predictably, *infections can also indirectly induce a noninfectious vasculitis,* for example, by generating immune complexes or triggering cross-reactivity. In any given patient, it is critical to distinguish between infectious and immunological mechanisms, because immunosuppressive therapy is appropriate for immune-mediated vasculitis but could very well worsen infectious vasculitis. Physical and chemical injury, such as from irradiation, mechanical trauma, and toxins, can also cause vasculitis.

NONINFECTIOUS VASCULITIS

The main immunological mechanisms that initiate noninfectious vasculitis are (1) immune complex deposition, (2) antineutrophil cytoplasmic antibodies, and (3) anti–endothelial cell antibodies.

Immune Complex–Associated Vasculitis. The lesions resemble those found in experimental immune complex–mediated conditions such as the Arthus reaction and serum sickness (Chapter 6). Many systemic immunological diseases, such as systemic lupus erythematosus (SLE) and polyarteritis nodosa, manifest as immune complex-mediated vasculitis. Antibody and complement are typically detected in vasculitic lesions, although the nature of the antigens responsible for their deposition cannot usually be determined. Circulating antigen-antibody complexes may also be seen (e.g., DNA–anti-DNA complexes in SLE–associated vasculitis [Chapter 6]), but the sensitivity and specificity of circulating immune complex assays in such diseases are low. In addition, immune complexes are implicated in the following vasculitides:

○ Immune complex deposition underlies the vasculitis associated with *drug hypersensitivity.* In some cases (e.g., penicillin) the drugs bind to serum proteins; other agents, like streptokinase, are themselves foreign proteins. In either case, antibodies directed against the drug-modified proteins or foreign molecules lead to the formation of immune complexes. Manifestations vary widely but are most frequently seen in the skin (see below); they can be mild and self-limiting, or severe and even fatal. It is important to

TABLE 11–4 **Classification and Characteristics of Selected Immune-Mediated Vasculitides**

Vasculitis Type*	Examples	Description
LARGE-VESSEL VASCULITIS *Aorta and large branches to extremities, head, and neck*	Giant-cell (temporal) arteritis	Granulomatous inflammation; frequently involves the temporal artery. Usually occurs in patients older than age 50 and is associated with polymyalgia rheumatica.
	Takayasu arteritis	Granulomatous inflammation usually occurring in patients younger than age 50
MEDIUM-VESSEL VASCULITIS *Main visceral arteries and their branches*	Polyarteritis nodosa	Necrotizing inflammation typically involving renal arteries but sparing pulmonary vessels
	Kawasaki disease	Arteritis with mucocutaneous lymph node syndrome; usually occurs in children. Coronary arteries can be involved with aneurysm formation and/or thrombosis.
SMALL-VESSEL VASCULITIS *Arterioles, venules, capillaries, and occasionally small arteries*	Wegener granulomatosis	Granulomatous inflammation involving the respiratory tract and necrotizing vasculitis affecting small vessels, including glomerular vessels. Associated with PR3-ANCAs.
	Churg-Strauss syndrome	Eosinophil-rich granulomatous inflammation involving the respiratory tract and necrotizing vasculitis affecting small vessels. Associated with asthma and blood eosinophilia. Associated with MPO-ANCAs.
	Microscopic polyangiitis	Necrotizing small-vessel vasculitis with few or no immune deposits; necrotizing arteritis of small and medium-sized arteries can occur. Necrotizing glomerulonephritis and pulmonary capillaritis are common. Associated with MPO-ANCAs.

MPO-ANCAs, antineutrophil cytoplasmic antibodies, directed against myeloperoxidase (p-ANCA); PR3-ANCAs, antineutrophil cytoplasmic antibodies, directed against proteinase 3 (c-ANCA).
*Note that some small- and large-vessel vasculitides may involve medium-sized arteries, but large- and medium-sized vessel vasculitides do not involve vessels smaller than arteries.
Modified from Jennette JC, et al. Nomenclature of systemic vasculitides: The proposal of an international consensus conference. Arthritis Rheum 37:187, 1994.

identify vasculitis due to drug hypersensitivities, since discontinuation of the offending agent will typically lead to resolution.
- In vasculitis secondary to *viral infections*, antibody to viral proteins forms immune complexes that can be found in the serum and the vascular lesions. Thus, as many as 30% of patients with polyarteritis nodosa (see below) have an underlying hepatitis B infection that produces a vasculitis attributable to complexes of hepatitis B surface antigen (HBsAg) and anti-HbsAg antibody.

In many cases of immune complex vasculitis, it is not clear whether the antigen-antibody complexes form elsewhere and then deposit in a particular vascular bed, or if they form in situ from the seeding of antigen in a vessel wall followed by antibody binding (Chapter 6). Moreover, in many cases of presumed immune complex vasculitis, antigen-antibody deposits are scarce. Either the immune complexes have been largely cleared at the time that the tissue diagnosis is made, or else other mechanisms may apply in such "pauci-immune" cases.

Antineutrophil Cytoplasmic Antibodies. Many patients with vasculitis have circulating antibodies that react with neutrophil cytoplasmic antigens, so-called *antineutrophil cytoplasmic antibodies (ANCAs)*. ANCAs are a heterogeneous group of autoantibodies directed against constituents (mainly enzymes) of neutrophil primary granules, monocyte lysosomes, and endothelial cells. These were previously classified according to their intracellular distribution, either cytoplasmic (c-ANCA) or perinuclear (p-ANCA). More commonly now, they are discriminated based on their target antigens:

- Anti-myeloperoxidase (MPO-ANCA): MPO is a lysosomal granule constituent normally involved in generating oxygen free radicals (Chapter 2). MPO-ANCAs can be induced by a variety of therapeutic agents, in particular propylthiouracil. These have been called p-ANCA.
- Anti-proteinase-3 (PR3-ANCA): PR3 is also a neutrophil azurophilic granule constituent. That it shares homology with numerous microbial peptides may explain how PR3-ANCAs develop.[66] These have been called c-ANCA.

Although not entirely specific, PR3-ANCAs are typical of Wegener granulomatosis and MPO-ANCAs are characteristic of microscopic polyangiitis and Churg-Strauss syndrome (see below); racial and geographic variables also influence the association of particular ANCAs and disease entities.

ANCAs serve as useful diagnostic markers for the ANCA-associated vasculitides, and their titers may reflect the degree of inflammatory activity. ANCA titers also rise with recurrent disease and are therefore useful in clinical management. The close association between ANCA titers and disease activity suggests a pathogenic role. Although the precise mechanisms are unknown, ANCA can directly activate neutrophils and may thereby stimulate neutrophils to release reactive oxygen species and proteolytic enzymes; within the vasculature, this also leads to endothelial cell-neutrophil interactions and subsequent endothelial cell damage.[67] Moreover, the antigenic targets of ANCAs are primarily intracellular and therefore might not be expected to be accessible to circulating antibodies, but there is now abundant evidence that ANCA antigens (in particular PR3) are either constitutively present at low levels on the plasma membrane or are

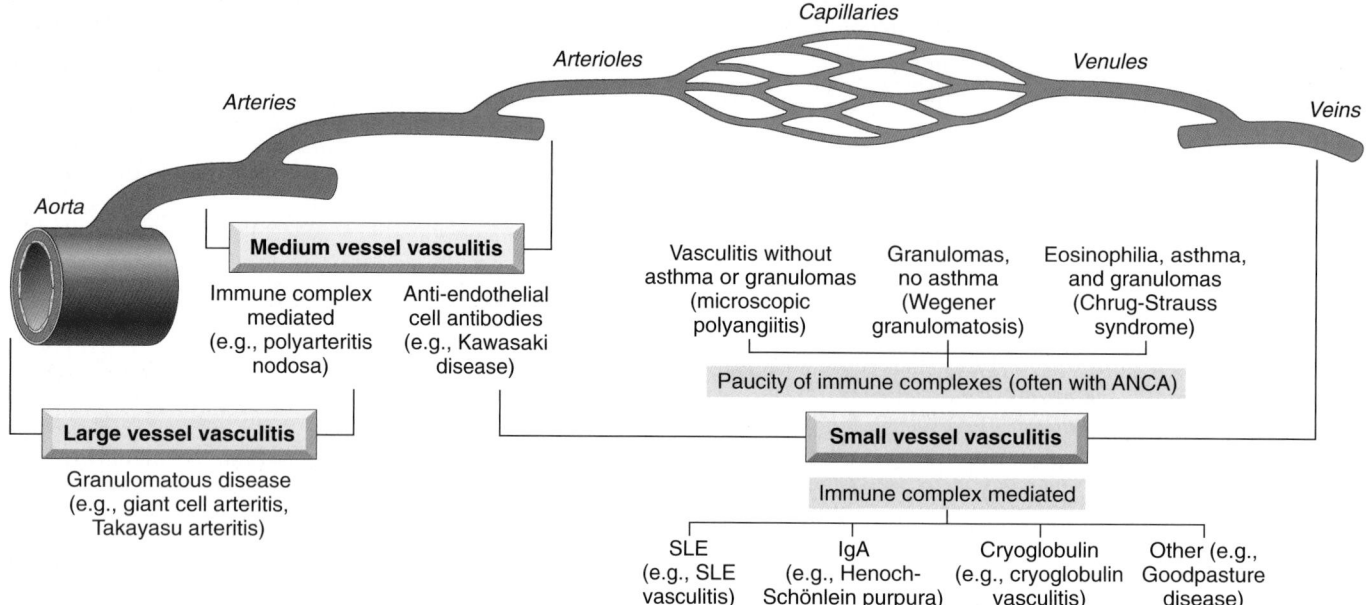

FIGURE 11–22 Diagrammatic representation of the typical vascular sites involved with the more common forms of vasculitis, as well as the presumptive etiologies. Note that there is a substantial overlap in distributions. ANCA, antineutrophil cytoplasmic antibody; SLE, systemic lupus erythematosus. (Modified from Jennette JC, Falk RJ: Nosology of primary vasculitis. Curr Opin Rheumatol 19:10, 2007.)

translocated to the cell surface in activated and apoptotic neutrophils.[66,68]

A plausible mechanism for ANCA vasculitis is the following[66,68]:

○ Drugs or cross-reactive microbial antigens induce ANCAs; alternatively, neutrophil surface expression or release of PR3 and MPO (e.g., in the setting of infections) incites ANCA formation in a susceptible host.
○ Subsequent infection, endotoxin exposure, or other inflammatory stimuli elicit cytokines such as TNF that cause surface expression of PR3 and MPO on neutrophils and other cell types.
○ ANCAs react with these cytokine-activated cells and either cause direct injury (e.g., to endothelial cells) or induce further activation (e.g., in neutrophils).
○ ANCA-activated neutrophils degranulate and also cause injury by releasing reactive oxygen species, engendering endothelial cell toxicity and other indirect tissue injury.

Interestingly, ANCAs directed against constituents other than PR3 and MPO are also found in some patients with inflammatory disorders that do not involve vasculitis (e.g., inflammatory bowel disease, primary sclerosing cholangitis, rheumatoid arthritis).

Anti-Endothelial Cell Antibodies. Antibodies to endothelial cells may predispose to certain vasculitides, for example, Kawasaki disease[69,70] (see below).

We will now briefly present several of the best-characterized vasculitides, again emphasizing that there is substantial overlap among the different entities. Moreover, it should be kept in mind that some patients with vasculitis do not have a classic constellation of findings that allows them to be neatly pigeonholed into one specific diagnosis.

GIANT-CELL (TEMPORAL) ARTERITIS

Giant-cell (temporal) arteritis is the most common form of vasculitis among elderly individuals in the United States and Europe. It is a chronic, typically granulomatous inflammation of large to small-sized arteries that affects principally the arteries in the head—especially the temporal arteries—but also the vertebral and ophthalmic arteries.[71] Ophthalmic arterial involvement can lead to permanent blindness; consequently, giant-cell arteritis is a medical emergency requiring prompt recognition and treatment. Lesions also occur in other arteries, including the aorta (giant-cell aortitis).

Pathogenesis. The cause of giant-cell arteritis remains elusive, although most evidence supports an initial T cell–mediated immune response against an unknown, possibly vessel wall, antigen. Pro-inflammatory cytokines (in particular TNF), and anti–endothelial cell humoral immune responses also probably contribute.[72] An immune etiology is supported by the characteristic granulomatous reaction, a correlation with certain HLA class II haplotypes, and a therapeutic response to steroids. The extraordinary predilection for a single vascular site (temporal artery) remains unexplained.

Morphology. Involved arterial segments develop **nodular intimal thickening** (with occasional thromboses) **that reduces the lumenal diameter**. Classic lesions exhibit medial **granulomatous inflammation** that leads to **elastic lamina fragmentation**; there is an infiltrate of T cells (CD4+ > CD8+) and macrophages. Multinucleated giant cells are found in upwards of 75% of adequately biopsied specimens (Fig. 11–23). Occasionally, granulomas and giant cells are rare or absent, and lesions show only a nonspecific panarteri-

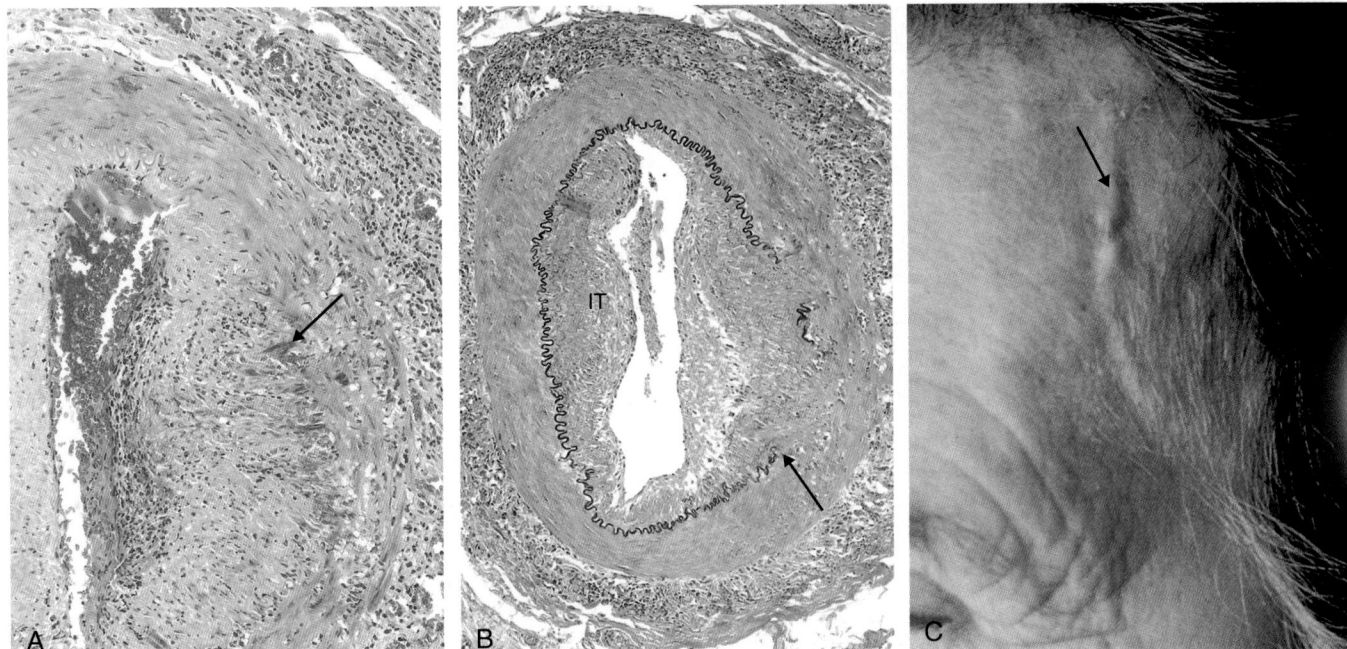

FIGURE 11–23 Giant-cell (temporal) arteritis. **A,** H&E stain of section of temporal artery showing giant cells at the degenerated internal elastic lamina in active arteritis *(arrow).* **B,** Elastic tissue stain demonstrating focal destruction of internal elastic lamina *(arrow)* and intimal thickening (IT) characteristic of long-standing or healed arteritis. **C,** Examination of the temporal artery of a patient with giant-cell arteritis shows a thickened, nodular, and tender segment of a vessel on the surface of head *(arrow).* (**C** from Salvarani C et al.: Polymyalgia rheumatica and giant-cell arteritis. N Engl J Med 347:261, 2002.)

tis composed predominantly of lymphocytes and macrophages. Inflammatory lesions are not continuous along the vessel, and long segments of relatively normal artery may be interposed. The healed stage is marked by medial scarring and intimal thickening, typically with residual elastic tissue fragmentation.

Clinical Features. Temporal arteritis is rare before the age of 50. Symptoms may be vague and constitutional—fever, fatigue, weight loss—or include facial pain or headache that is most intense along the course of the superficial temporal artery, which can be painful to palpation. Ocular symptoms (associated with involvement of the ophthalmic artery) appear abruptly in about 50% of patients; these range from diplopia to complete vision loss. Diagnosis depends on biopsy and histologic confirmation. However, because giant-cell arteritis is extremely segmental, adequate biopsy requires at least a 2- to 3-cm length of artery; even then, a negative biopsy result does not exclude the diagnosis. Treatment with corticosteroids is generally effective, with anti-TNF therapy showing promise in refractory cases.[71]

TAKAYASU ARTERITIS

This is a *granulomatous vasculitis* of medium and larger arteries characterized principally by ocular disturbances and marked weakening of the pulses in the upper extremities (hence, its other name, *pulseless disease*). Takayasu arteritis manifests with transmural fibrous thickening of the aorta—particularly the aortic arch and great vessels—and severe luminal narrowing of the major branch vessels (Fig. 11–24).

Aortic lesions share many attributes with giant-cell aortitis, including clinical features and histology; indeed, the distinction is typically made only on the basis of the age of the patient. Those over 50 years of age are designated as having giant-cell aortitis, while those under 50 have Takayasu aortitis.[64] Though traditionally associated with the Japanese population and a subset of HLA haplotypes, Takayasu aortitis has a global distribution. The cause and pathogenesis are unknown, although immune mechanisms are suspected.[71,72]

Morphology. Takayasu arteritis classically involves the aortic arch. In a third of patients it also affects the remainder of the aorta and its branches. The pulmonary artery is involved in half of cases; coronary and renal arteries may be similarly affected. There is irregular thickening of the vessel wall with intimal hyperplasia; when the aortic arch is involved the great vessel lumens can be markedly narrowed or even obliterated (Fig. 11–24A and B). Such narrowing explains the weakness of the peripheral pulses. Histological changes range from adventitial mononuclear infiltrates with perivascular cuffing of the vasa vasorum, to intense mononuclear inflammation in the media, to granulomatous inflammation, replete with giant cells and patchy medial necrosis. The histologic appearance (Fig. 11–24C) is indistinguishable from that of giant-cell (temporal) arteritis. As the disease progresses, collagenous scarring, with admixed chronic inflammatory infiltrates, occurs in all three layers of the vessel wall. Occasionally, aortic root involvement causes aortic insufficiency.

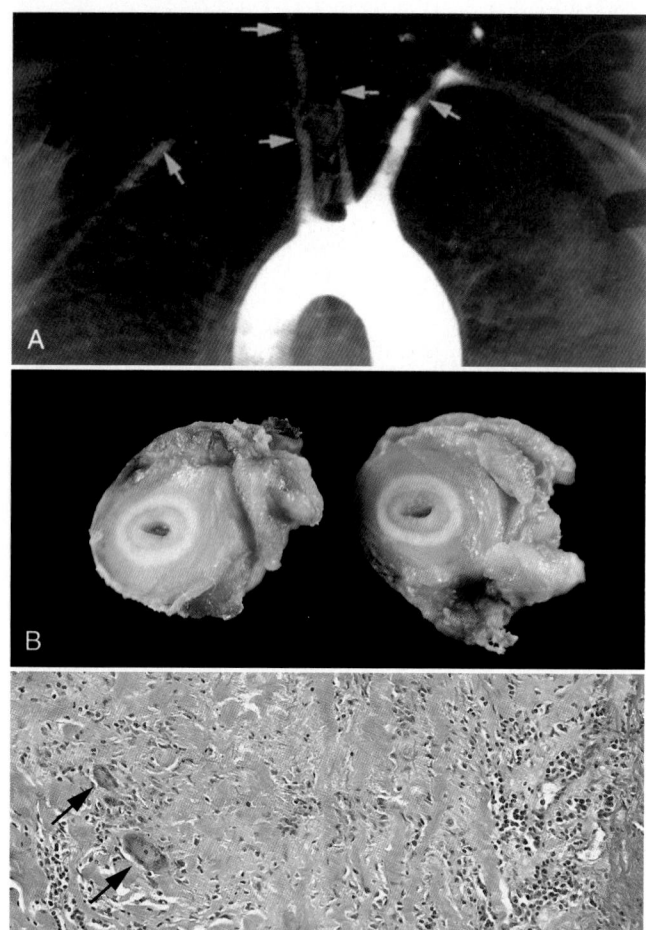

FIGURE 11–24 Takayasu arteritis. **A,** Aortic arch angiogram showing narrowing of brachiocephalic, carotid, and subclavian arteries *(arrows)*. **B,** Gross photograph of two cross-sections of the right carotid artery taken at autopsy of the patient shown in **A,** demonstrating marked intimal thickening with minimal residual lumen. **C,** Histologic view of active Takayasu aortitis, illustrating destruction of the arterial media by mononuclear inflammation with giant cells *(arrows)*.

Clinical Features. Initial symptoms are usually nonspecific, including fatigue, weight loss, and fever. With progression, vascular symptoms appear and dominate the clinical picture, including reduced blood pressure and weaker pulses in the upper extremities; ocular disturbances, including visual defects, retinal hemorrhages, and total blindness; and neurologic deficits. Involvement of the more distal aorta may lead to claudication of the legs; pulmonary artery involvement may cause pulmonary hypertension. Narrowing of the coronary ostia may lead to myocardial infarction, and involvement of the renal arteries leads to systemic hypertension in roughly half of patients. The course of the disease is variable. In some there is rapid progression, while others enter a quiescent stage at 1 to 2 years, permitting long-term survival, albeit sometimes with visual or neurologic deficits.

POLYARTERITIS NODOSA

Polyarteritis nodosa (PAN) is a systemic vasculitis of small or medium-sized muscular arteries (but not arterioles, capillaries, or venules), typically involving renal and visceral vessels but sparing the pulmonary circulation. There is no association with ANCAs, but about 30% of patients with PAN have chronic hepatitis B with HBsAg-HbsAb complexes in affected vessels, indicating an immune complex–mediated etiology (see Chapter 6) in that subset. Nevertheless, the cause remains unknown in the majority of cases; there may be etiologic and important clinical distinctions between classic idiopathic PAN, the cutaneous forms of PAN, and the PAN associated with chronic hepatitis.[73,74] Clinical manifestations result from ischemia and infarction of affected tissues and organs.[73]

Morphology. Classic PAN is characterized by **segmental transmural necrotizing inflammation of small to medium-sized arteries**. Vessels of the kidneys, heart, liver, and gastrointestinal tract are involved in descending order of frequency. Lesions usually affect only part of the vessel circumference and show a predilection for branch points. The inflammatory process **weakens the arterial wall** and can lead to aneurysms or even rupture. **Impaired perfusion** resulting in ulcerations, infarcts, ischemic atrophy, or hemorrhages in the distribution of affected vessels may be the first sign of disease.

During the acute phase there is **transmural inflammation** of the arterial wall with a mixed infiltrate of neutrophils, eosinophils, and mononuclear cells, frequently accompanied by **fibrinoid necrosis** (Fig. 11–25). Luminal thrombosis can occur. Later, the acute inflammatory infiltrate is replaced by **fibrous** (occasionally nodular) **thickening of the vessel wall** that can extend into the adventitia. **Characteristically,**

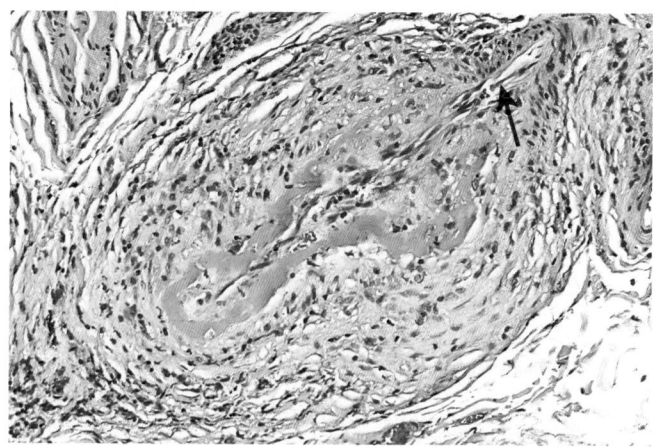

FIGURE 11–25 Polyarteritis nodosa. There is segmental fibrinoid necrosis and thrombotic occlusion of the lumen of this small artery. Note that part of the vessel wall at the upper right *(arrow)* is uninvolved. (Courtesy of Sidney Murphree, M.D., Department of Pathology, University of Texas Southwestern Medical School, Dallas, TX.)

all stages of activity (from early to late) **coexist in different vessels or even within the same vessel, suggesting ongoing and recurrent insults.**

Clinical Features. Though typically a disease of young adults, PAN can also occur in pediatric and geriatric populations. The course may be acute, subacute, or chronic, and is frequently remitting and episodic, with long symptom-free intervals. Because the vascular involvement is widely scattered, the clinical signs and symptoms of PAN may be varied, puzzling, and not always referable to a vascular source. The most common manifestations are malaise, fever, and weight loss; hypertension, usually developing rapidly due to renal involvement; abdominal pain and melena (bloody stool) due to vascular lesions in the gastrointestinal tract; diffuse muscular aches and pains; and peripheral neuritis. Renal arterial involvement is often prominent and a major cause of death. Untreated, the disease is fatal in most cases, either during an acute fulminant attack or following a protracted course. However, therapy with corticosteroids and cyclophosphamide results in remissions or cures in 90% of cases.

KAWASAKI DISEASE

The leading cause of acquired heart disease in children, *Kawasaki disease*, is an acute febrile, usually self-limited illness of infancy and childhood (80% are younger than 4 years) associated with an *arteritis affecting large to medium-sized, and even small, vessels.* Its clinical significance stems primarily from a predilection for coronary artery involvement; such coronary arteritis can cause aneurysms that rupture or thrombose, resulting in acute myocardial infarctions. Originally described in Japan, the disease is now increasingly reported in the United States and other countries. The etiology is uncertain, but the vasculitis is thought to result from a delayed-type hypersensitivity reaction of T cells to an as yet uncharacterized antigen. This leads to cytokine production and macrophage activation, and is accompanied by polyclonal B-cell activation. This results in formation of autoantibodies to endothelial cells and smooth muscle cells, which precipitate the acute vasculitis. It is currently speculated that a variety of infectious agents (most likely viral) can trigger the disease in genetically susceptible persons.[69,70]

Morphology. As with polyarteritis nodosa, lesions exhibit pronounced inflammation affecting the entire thickness of the vessel wall; however, fibrinoid necrosis is usually less prominent. Although the acute vasculitis subsides spontaneously or in response to treatment, aneurysm formation with thrombosis can supervene. As with other causes of arteritis, healed lesions may have obstructive intimal thickening. Pathologic changes outside the cardiovascular system are rarely significant.

Clinical Features. Kawasaki disease is also known as mucocutaneous lymph node syndrome, because it presents with conjunctival and oral erythema and erosion, edema of the hands and feet, erythema of the palms and soles, a desquamative rash, and cervical lymph node enlargement. Approximately 20% of untreated patients develop cardiovascular sequelae, ranging from asymptomatic coronary arteritis, to coronary artery ectasia and aneurysm formation, to giant coronary artery aneurysms (7–8 mm) with rupture or thrombosis, myocardial infarction, and sudden death. With intravenous immunoglobulin therapy and aspirin, the rate of coronary artery disease is reduced to about 4%.[69,70]

MICROSCOPIC POLYANGIITIS

This is *a necrotizing vasculitis that generally affects capillaries, as well as arterioles and venules* of a size smaller than those involved in polyarteritis nodosa; rarely, larger arteries may be involved. It is also called *hypersensitivity vasculitis* or *leukocytoclastic vasculitis.* Unlike polyarteritis nodosa, *all lesions of microscopic polyangiitis tend to be of the same age in any given patient.* The skin, mucous membranes, lungs, brain, heart, gastrointestinal tract, kidneys, and muscle can all be involved; *necrotizing glomerulonephritis (90% of patients) and pulmonary capillaritis are particularly common.* Disseminated vascular lesions of hypersensitivity angiitis can also occur as a presentation of other disorders (e.g., Henoch-Schönlein purpura, essential mixed cryoglobulinemia, and vasculitis associated with connective tissue disorders).[66,75]

Pathogenesis. In some cases, an antibody response to antigens such as drugs (e.g., penicillin), microorganisms (e.g., streptococci), heterologous proteins, or tumor proteins has been implicated; this can either result in immune complex deposition or may trigger secondary immune responses (e.g., the development of p-ANCAs) that are ultimately pathogenic. However, most lesions are pauci-immune (devoid of immune complexes), and increasingly, MPO-ANCAs are causally implicated.[68] Recruitment and activation of neutrophils within a particular vascular bed may be responsible for the disease manifestations.

Morphology. Microscopic polyangiitis is characterized by segmental fibrinoid necrosis of the media with focal transmural necrotizing lesions; granulomatous inflammation is absent. These lesions morphologically resemble polyarteritis nodosa but typically spare medium-sized and larger arteries; consequently, macroscopic infarcts are uncommon. In some areas (typically post-capillary venules), only infiltrating and fragmenting neutrophils are seen, giving rise to the term **leukocytoclastic vasculitis** (Fig. 11–26A). Although immunoglobulins and complement components can be demonstrated in early skin lesions, little or no immunoglobulin can be seen in most lesions (so-called **pauci-immune injury**).

Clinical Features. Depending on the vascular bed involved, major clinical features include hemoptysis; hematuria, and proteinuria; bowel pain or bleeding; muscle pain or weakness; and palpable cutaneous purpura. With the exception of those who develop widespread renal or brain involvement, cyclophosphamide and steroid immunosuppression induces remission and markedly improves long-term survival.[76]

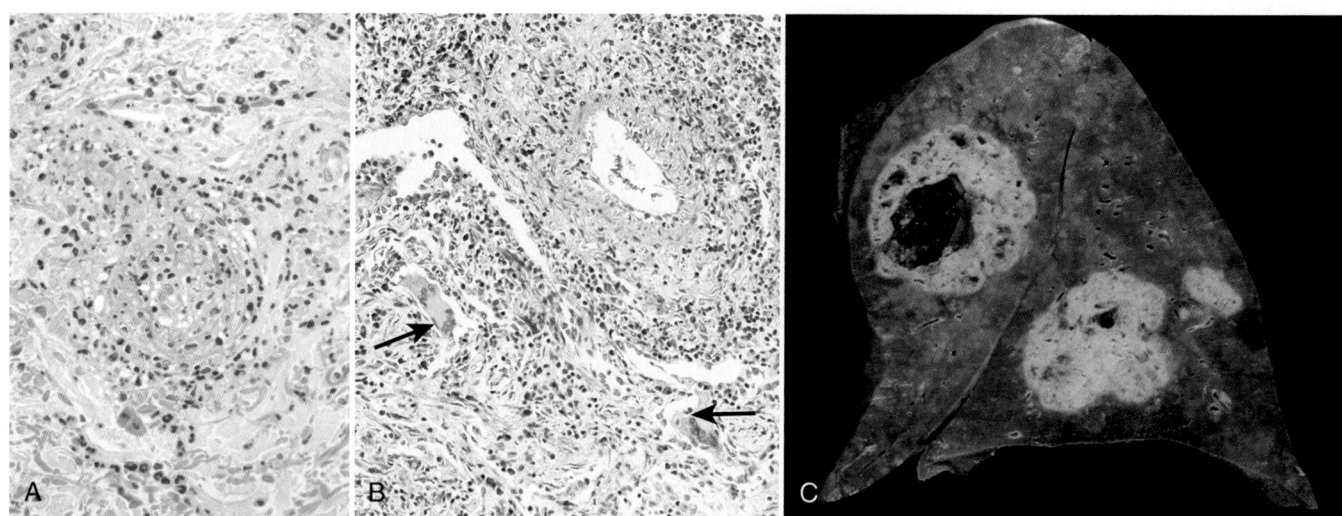

FIGURE 11–26 Representative forms of ANCA-associated small-vessel vasculitis. **A,** Leukocytoclastic vasculitis (microscopic polyangiitis) with fragmentation of neutrophils in and around blood vessel walls. **B** and **C,** Wegener granulomatosis. **B,** Vasculitis of a small artery with adjacent granulomatous inflammation including epithelioid cells and giant cells *(arrows)*. **C,** Gross photo from the lung of a patient with fatal Wegener granulomatosis, demonstrating large nodular centrally cavitating lesions. (**A,** Courtesy of Scott Granter, M.D., Brigham and Women's Hospital, Boston, MA; **C,** courtesy of Sidney Murphree, M.D., Department of Pathology, University of Texas Southwestern Medical School, Dallas, TX.)

CHURG-STRAUSS SYNDROME

Churg-Strauss syndrome (also called *allergic granulomatosis and angiitis*) is a relatively rare (roughly one in a million people) *small-vessel necrotizing vasculitis classically associated with asthma, allergic rhinitis, lung infiltrates, peripheral hypereosinophilia, and extravascular necrotizing granulomas.* Vascular lesions can be histologically similar to polyarteritis nodosa or microscopic polyangiitis but are also characteristically accompanied by granulomas and eosinophils.[77] ANCAs (mostly MPO-ANCAs) are present in less than half the cases and raise the possibility that there are distinct subsets of patients with the syndrome. Nevertheless, when present, the ANCAs are probably responsible for the vascular manifestations of the disease. Cutaneous involvement (palpable purpura), gastrointestinal tract bleeding, and renal disease (primarily as focal and segmental glomerulosclerosis) are the major associations. Myocardial infiltrates of eosinophils and cytotoxicity caused by them are implicated in the cardiomyopathy seen in Churg-Strauss syndrome; the heart is involved in 60% of patients, and accounts for almost half of the deaths in the syndrome.[77] The etiology remains obscure, but has been suggested to result from hyper-responsiveness to an allergic stimulus; in asthmatics, leukotriene receptor antagonists are reported as a trigger.[78]

WEGENER GRANULOMATOSIS

Wegener granulomatosis is a necrotizing vasculitis characterized by a triad of

- *Acute necrotizing granulomas* of the upper respiratory tract (ear, nose, sinuses, throat) or the lower respiratory tract (lung) or both
- *Necrotizing or granulomatous vasculitis* affecting *small to medium-sized vessels* (e.g., capillaries, venules, arterioles,

and arteries), most prominent in the lungs and upper airways but affecting other sites as well
- Renal disease in the form of *focal necrotizing, often crescentic, glomerulonephritis*

"Limited" forms of Wegener granulomatosis may be restricted to the respiratory tract. Conversely, a widespread form of the disease can affect eyes, skin, and other organs, notably the heart; clinically, this resembles polyarteritis nodosa except that there is also respiratory involvement.

Pathogenesis. Wegener granulomatosis probably represents a form of T cell–mediated hypersensitivity reaction, possibly to an inhaled infectious or other environmental agent; such a pathogenesis is supported by the presence of granulomas and a dramatic response to immunosuppressive therapy. PR3-ANCAs are present in up to 95% of cases; they are a useful marker of disease activity and may participate in disease pathogenesis. After immunosuppressive treatment, a rising PR3-ANCA titer suggests a relapse; most patients in remission have a negative test or falling titers.[79]

Morphology. Upper respiratory tract lesions range from inflammatory sinusitis with mucosal granulomas to ulcerative lesions of the nose, palate, or pharynx, rimmed by **granulomas with geographic patterns of central necrosis and accompanying vasculitis** (Fig. 11-26B). The necrotizing granulomas are surrounded by a zone of fibroblastic proliferation with giant cells and leukocyte infiltrate, reminiscent of mycobacterial or fungal infections. Multiple granulomas can coalesce to produce radiographically visible nodules that can also cavitate; late-stage disease may be marked by extensive necrotizing granulomatous involvement of the parenchyma (Fig. 11-26C); alveolar hemorrhage may be prominent. Lesions may ultimately undergo progressive fibrosis and organization.

A spectrum of **renal lesions** may be seen (Chapter 20). In early stages, glomeruli exhibit only focal necrosis with thrombosis of isolated glomerular capillary loops (focal and segmental necrotizing glomerulonephritis); there is minimal parietal cell proliferation in Bowman's capsule. More advanced glomerular lesions are characterized by diffuse necrosis and parietal cell proliferation to form crescents (crescentic glomerulonephritis).

Clinical Features. Males are affected more often than females, at an average age of about 40 years. Classic features include persistent pneumonitis with bilateral nodular and cavitary infiltrates (95%), chronic sinusitis (90%), mucosal ulcerations of the nasopharynx (75%), and evidence of renal disease (80%). Other features include rashes, muscle pains, articular involvement, mononeuritis or polyneuritis, and fever. Left untreated, the disease is usually rapidly fatal; 80% of patients die within 1 year. Treatment with steroids, cyclophosphamide, and more recently TNF-antagonists, have turned Wegener granulomatosis into a chronic remitting and relapsing disease.[80]

THROMBOANGIITIS OBLITERANS (BUERGER DISEASE)

Thromboangiitis obliterans (Buerger disease) is a distinctive disease that often leads to vascular insufficiency; it is characterized by *segmental, thrombosing, acute and chronic inflammation of medium-sized and small arteries*, principally the tibial and radial arteries, with occasional secondary extension into the veins and nerves of the extremities. Buerger disease is a condition that occurs almost exclusively in heavy cigarette smokers, usually before the age of 35.

Pathogenesis. The strong relationship to cigarette smoking is thought to be due to direct endothelial cell toxicity by some component of tobacco, or an idiosyncratic immune response to the same agents. Most patients have hypersensitivity to intradermally injected tobacco extracts, and their vessels exhibit impaired endothelium-dependent vasodilation when challenged with acetylcholine. Genetic influences are suggested by an increased prevalence in certain ethnic groups (Israeli, Indian subcontinent, Japanese) and an association with certain HLA haplotypes.[81]

Morphology. Thromboangiitis obliterans is characterized by a **sharply segmental acute and chronic vasculitis of medium-sized and small arteries**, predominantly of the extremities. Microscopically, there is acute and chronic inflammation, accompanied by luminal thrombosis. Typically, the thrombus contains small **microabscesses** composed of neutrophils surrounded by granulomatous inflammation (Fig. 11–27); the thrombus may eventually organize and recanalize. The inflammatory process extends into contiguous veins and nerves (rare with other forms of

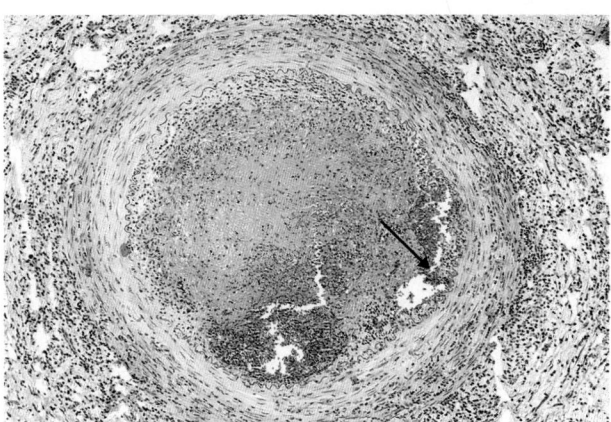

FIGURE 11–27 Thromboangiitis obliterans (Buerger disease). The lumen is occluded by a thrombus containing abscesses *(arrow)*, and the vessel wall is infiltrated with leukocytes.

vasculitis), and in time all three structures become encased in fibrous tissue.

Clinical Features. The early manifestations are a superficial nodular phlebitis, cold sensitivity of the Raynaud type (see below) in the hands, and pain in the instep of the foot induced by exercise (so-called *instep claudication*). In contrast to the insufficiency caused by atherosclerosis, in Buerger disease there tends to be severe pain, even at rest, related undoubtedly to the neural involvement. Chronic ulcerations of the toes, feet, or fingers may appear, which can be followed in time by frank gangrene. Abstinence from cigarette smoking in the early stages of the disease often brings dramatic relief from further attacks.

VASCULITIS ASSOCIATED WITH OTHER DISORDERS

Vasculitis resembling hypersensitivity angiitis or classic polyarteritis nodosa may sometimes be associated with other disorders, such as rheumatoid arthritis, SLE, cancer, or systemic illnesses such as mixed cryoglobulinemia, antiphospholipid antibody syndrome, and Henoch-Schönlein purpura. *Rheumatoid vasculitis* occurs predominantly after longstanding, severe rheumatoid arthritis and usually affects small and medium-sized arteries. It can lead to visceral infarction and sometimes causes a clinically significant aortitis. Identifying the underlying pathology may be therapeutically important. For example, although classic immune complex *lupus vasculitis* and antiphospholipid antibody syndrome are morphologically similar, anti-inflammatory therapy is required in the former while anticoagulant therapy is indicated in the latter.

INFECTIOUS VASCULITIS

Localized arteritis may be caused by the direct invasion of infectious agents, usually bacteria or fungi, and in particular *Aspergillus* and *Mucor* species. Vascular invasion can be part of a localized tissue infection (e.g., bacterial pneumonia or

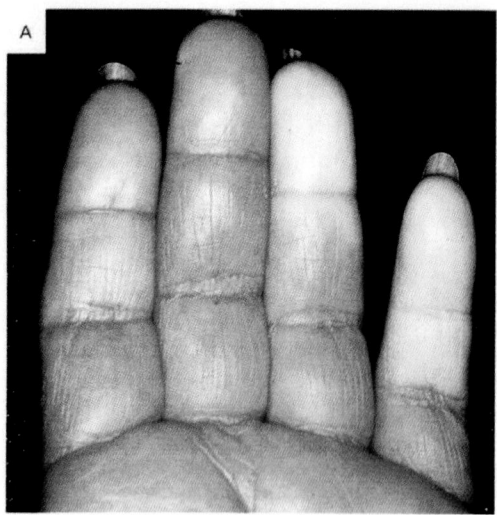
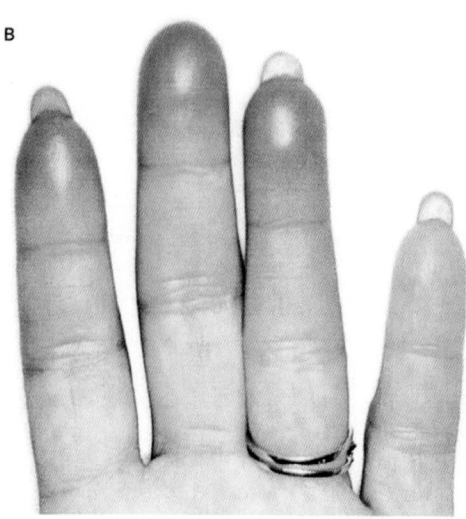

FIGURE 11–28 Raynaud's phenomenon. **A,** Sharply demarcated pallor of the distal fingers resulting from the closure of digital arteries. **B,** Cyanosis of the fingertips. (Reproduced from Salvarani C, et al.: Polymyalgia rheumatica and giant-cell arteritis. N Engl J Med 347:261, 2002.)

adjacent to abscesses), or—less commonly—it can arise from hematogenous seeding of bacteria during septicemia or embolization from sepsis of infective endocarditis.

Vascular infections can weaken arterial walls and culminate in *mycotic aneurysms* (see earlier), or can induce thrombosis and infarction. Thus, inflammation-induced thrombosis of meningeal vessels in bacterial meningitis can cause infarction of the underlying brain.

Raynaud Phenomenon

Raynaud phenomenon results from an exaggerated vasoconstriction of digital arteries and arterioles. These vascular changes induce paroxysmal pallor or cyanosis of the digits of the hands or feet; infrequently, the nose, earlobes, or lips can also be involved. Characteristically, the involved digits show red, white, and blue color changes from most proximal to most distal, correlating with proximal vasodilation, central vasoconstriction, and more distal cyanosis (Fig. 11–28). Raynaud phenomenon may be a primary disease entity or be secondary to a variety of conditions.[82]

Primary Raynaud phenomenon (previously called Raynaud disease) reflects an exaggeration of central and local vasomotor responses to cold or emotional stresses. It affects 3% to 5% of the general population and shows a predilection for young women. Structural changes in the arterial walls are absent except late in the course, when intimal thickening can appear. The course of Raynaud phenomenon is usually benign, but when long-standing can result in atrophy of the skin, subcutaneous tissues, and muscles. Ulceration and ischemic gangrene are rare.[83]

In contrast, *secondary Raynaud phenomenon* refers to vascular insufficiency of the extremities secondary to arterial disease caused by other entities including SLE, scleroderma, Buerger disease, or even atherosclerosis. Since Raynaud phenomenon may be the first manifestation of such conditions, any patient with new symptoms should be evaluated. Of these individuals, some 10% will eventually manifest an underlying disease.

Veins and Lymphatics

Varicose veins and phlebothrombosis/thrombophlebitis together account for at least 90% of clinical venous disease.

VARICOSE VEINS

Varicose veins are abnormally dilated, tortuous veins produced by prolonged, increased intraluminal pressure and loss of vessel wall support. The *superficial veins* of the upper and lower leg are typically involved (Fig. 11–29). When legs are dependent for prolonged periods, venous pressures in these sites can be markedly elevated (up to 10 times normal) and can lead to venous stasis and pedal edema, even in essentially normal veins *(simple orthostatic edema)*. Some 10% to 20% of adult males and 25% to 33% of adult females develop lower extremity varicose veins; obesity increases risk, and the higher incidence in women is a reflection of the elevated venous pressure in lower legs caused by pregnancy. A *familial tendency* toward premature varicosities has been noted.

Clinical Features. Varicose dilation renders the venous valves incompetent and leads to stasis, congestion, edema, pain, and thrombosis. The most disabling sequelae include persistent edema in the extremity and ischemic skin changes, including *stasis dermatitis* and ulcerations; poor wound healing and superimposed infections can lead to chronic *varicose ulcers. Notably, embolism from these superficial veins is very rare. This is in sharp contrast to the relatively frequent thromboembolism that arises from thrombosed deep veins* (see below and Chapter 4).

Varicosities that occur in two other sites deserve special mention:

● *Esophageal varices.* Liver cirrhosis (less frequently, portal vein obstruction or hepatic vein thrombosis) causes portal vein hypertension (Chapter 18). Portal hypertension leads to the opening of porto-systemic shunts that increase the blood flow into veins at the gastro-esophageal junction (forming *esophageal varices*), the rectum (forming *hemor-*

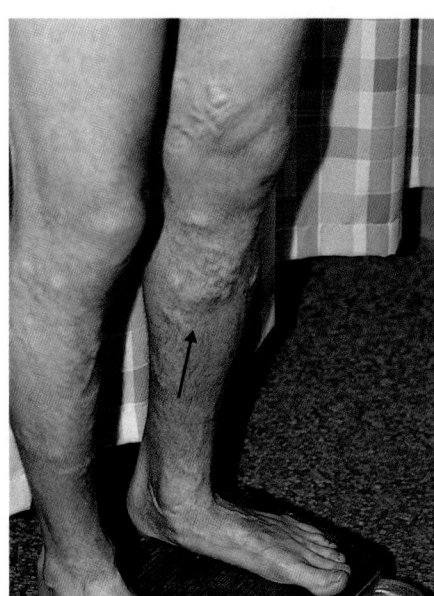

FIGURE 11–29 Varicose veins of the leg *(arrow)*. (Courtesy of Magruder C. Donaldson, M.D., Brigham and Women's Hospital, Boston, MA.)

rhoids), and periumbilical veins of the abdominal wall (forming a *caput medusa*). Esophageal varices are the most important, since their rupture can lead to massive (even fatal) upper gastrointestinal hemorrhage.

○ *Hemorrhoids* can also result from primary varicose dilation of the venous plexus at the anorectal junction (e.g., through prolonged pelvic vascular congestion due to pregnancy or chronic constipation). Hemorrhoids are uncomfortable and may be a source of bleeding; they can also thrombose and get inflamed, and are prone to painful ulceration.

THROMBOPHLEBITIS AND PHLEBOTHROMBOSIS

Deep leg veins are the site of more than 90% of cases of thrombophlebitis and *phlebothrombosis*; the two terms are largely interchangeable designations for venous thrombosis and inflammation. The periprostatic venous plexus in males and the pelvic venous plexus in females are additional sites, as are the large veins in the skull and the dural sinuses (especially in the setting of infection or inflammation). Peritoneal infections, including peritonitis, appendicitis, salpingitis, and pelvic abscesses, as well as certain thrombophilic conditions associated with platelet hyperactivity (e.g., polycythemia vera, Chapter 13), can lead to portal vein thrombosis. For deep venous thrombosis (DVT) of the legs, *prolonged immobilization resulting in decreased blood flow through the veins is the most important predisposing condition.* This can occur with extended bed rest or from just sitting during extended travel in an airplane or automobile; the postoperative state is another independent risk factor in DVT formation. Clearly, other mechanical factors that slow venous return also promote the development of DVT; these include congestive heart failure, pregnancy, and obesity.

Systemic hypercoagulability (Chapter 4) *often predisposes to thrombophlebitis.* In patients with cancer, particularly adenocarcinomas, hypercoagulability occurs as a paraneoplastic syndrome related to elaboration of pro-coagulant factors by the tumor cells (Chapter 7). In this setting, venous thromboses classically appear in one site, disappear, and then reoccur in other veins; this is referred to as *migratory thrombophlebitis (Trousseau sign).*

Thrombi in the legs tend to produce few, if any, reliable signs or symptoms. Indeed, local manifestations, including distal edema, cyanosis, superficial vein dilation, heat, tenderness, redness, swelling, and pain may be entirely absent, especially in bedridden patients. In some cases pain can be elicited by pressure over affected veins, squeezing the calf muscles, or forced dorsiflexion of the foot *(Homan sign)*; *absence of these findings does not exclude a diagnosis of DVT.*

Pulmonary embolism is a serious complication of DVT (Chapter 4), resulting from fragmentation or detachment of the whole venous thrombus. In many cases *the first manifestation of thrombophlebitis is a pulmonary embolus.* Depending on the size and number of emboli, the outcome can range from no symptoms to death.

SUPERIOR AND INFERIOR VENA CAVAL SYNDROMES

The *superior vena caval syndrome* is usually caused by neoplasms that compress or invade the superior vena cava, such as bronchogenic carcinoma or mediastinal lymphoma. The resulting obstruction produces a characteristic clinical complex that includes marked dilation of the veins of the head, neck, and arms and cyanosis. Pulmonary vessels can also be compressed, causing respiratory distress.

The *inferior vena caval syndrome* can be caused by neoplasms that compress or invade the inferior vena cava (IVC) or by a thrombus from the hepatic, renal, or lower extremity veins that propagates upward. Certain neoplasms—particularly hepatocellular carcinoma and renal cell carcinoma—show a striking tendency to grow within veins, and these may ultimately occlude the IVC. IVC obstruction induces marked lower extremity edema, distention of the superficial collateral veins of the lower abdomen, and—with renal vein involvement—massive proteinuria.

LYMPHANGITIS AND LYMPHEDEMA

Primary disorders of lymphatic vessels are extremely uncommon; secondary processes are much more frequent and develop in association with inflammation or malignancies.

Lymphangitis is the acute inflammation elicited when bacterial infections spread into lymphatics; the most common agents are group A β-hemolytic streptococci, although any microbe may be associated. The affected lymphatics are dilated and filled with an exudate of neutrophils and monocytes; these infiltrates can extend through the vessel wall into the perilymphatic tissues and, in severe cases, produce cellulitis or focal abscesses. Clinically, lymphangitis is recognized by red, painful subcutaneous streaks (the inflamed lymphatics), and painful enlargement of draining lymph nodes *(acute lymphadenitis)*. If bacteria are not successfully contained within the lymph nodes, subsequent passage into the venous circulation can result in bacteremia or sepsis.

Primary lymphedema can occur due to an isolated congenital defect (simple congenital lymphedema) or as the familial

Milroy disease (heredofamilial congenital lymphedema), which causes lymphatic agenesis or hypoplasia. *Secondary* or *obstructive lymphedema* stems from blockage of a previously normal lymphatic; such obstruction can result from

- Malignant tumors obstructing either the lymphatic channels or the regional lymph nodes
- Surgical procedures that remove regional groups of lymph nodes (e.g., axillary lymph nodes in radical mastectomy)
- Post-irradiation fibrosis
- Filariasis
- Post-inflammatory thrombosis and scarring

Regardless of the cause, lymphedema increases the hydrostatic pressure in the lymphatics distal to the obstruction and causes increased interstitial fluid accumulation. Persistence of this edema leads to increased deposition of interstitial connective tissue, *brawny induration* or *peau d'orange* (orange peel) appearance of the overlying skin, and eventually ulcers due to inadequate tissue perfusion. Milky accumulations of lymph in various spaces are designated *chylous ascites* (abdomen), *chylothorax,* and *chylopericardium;* these are caused by rupture of dilated lymphatics, typically obstructed secondary to an infiltrating tumor mass.

Tumors

Tumors of blood vessels and lymphatics range from benign hemangiomas to lesions that are locally aggressive but infrequently metastasize, to relatively rare, highly malignant angiosarcomas (Table 11–5). Primary tumors of large vessels (aorta, pulmonary artery, and vena cava) are extremely rare and are mostly connective tissue sarcomas. Congenital or developmental malformations and reactive vascular proliferations (e.g., *bacillary angiomatosis*) can also present as tumor-like lesions.

TABLE 11–5 **Classification of Vascular Tumors and Tumor-like Conditions**

BENIGN NEOPLASMS, DEVELOPMENTAL AND ACQUIRED CONDITIONS

Hemangioma
  Capillary hemangioma
  Cavernous hemangioma
  Pyogenic granuloma
Lymphangioma
  Simple (capillary) lymphangioma
  Cavernous lymphangioma (cystic hygroma)
Glomus tumor
Vascular ectasias
  Nevus flammeus
  Spider telangiectasia (arterial spider)
  Hereditary hemorrhagic telangiectasis (Osler-Weber-Rendu disease)
Reactive vascular proliferations
  Bacillary angiomatosis

INTERMEDIATE-GRADE NEOPLASMS

Kaposi sarcoma
Hemangioendothelioma

MALIGNANT NEOPLASMS

Angiosarcoma
Hemangiopericytoma

Vascular neoplasms can be endothelium-derived (e.g., hemangioma, lymphangioma, angiosarcoma) or arise from cells that support and/or surround blood vessels (e.g., glomus tumor, hemangiopericytoma). Although a benign, well-differentiated hemangioma can usually be readily discriminated from an anaplastic high-grade angiosarcoma, the distinction between benign and malignant can occasionally be difficult. Two general rules of thumb are as follows:

- Benign tumors usually produce obvious vascular channels filled with blood cells or lymph, lined by a layer of normal-appearing endothelial cells.
- Malignant tumors are more cellular, show cytologic atypia, and are proliferative, including mitotic figures; they usually do not form well-organized vessels. The endothelial derivation of neoplasms that do not form distinct vascular lumens can usually be confirmed by immunohistochemical demonstration of endothelial cell–specific markers such as CD31 or von Willebrand's factor.

Because vascular tumors result from dysregulated vascular proliferation, the possibility of controlling such growth by inhibitors of blood vessel formation (anti-angiogenic factors) is being explored.

BENIGN TUMORS AND TUMOR-LIKE CONDITIONS

Hemangioma

Hemangiomas are very common tumors characterized by increased numbers of normal or abnormal vessels filled with blood (Fig. 11–30); they may be difficult to distinguish from vascular malformations. These lesions constitute 7% of all benign tumors of infancy and childhood; most are present from birth and expand along with the growth of the child. Nevertheless, many of the capillary lesions eventually regress spontaneously. Although some hemangiomas can involve large portions of the body (*angiomatosis*), most are localized. The majority are superficial lesions, often of the head or neck, but they can occur internally, with nearly one third being found in the liver. Malignant transformation occurs rarely, if ever. There are several histologic and clinical variants:

Capillary Hemangioma. The most common variant, *capillary hemangiomas,* occur in the skin, subcutaneous tissues, and mucous membranes of the oral cavities and lips, as well as in the liver, spleen, and kidneys. The "strawberry type" or *juvenile hemangioma* of the skin of newborns is extremely common (1 in 200 births) and may be multiple. It grows rapidly in the first few months but then fades at 1 to 3 years of age and completely regresses by age 7 in 75% to 90% of cases.

Morphology. Capillary hemangiomas are bright red to blue and vary from a few millimeters to several centimeters in diameter; hemangiomas can be level with the surface of the skin or slightly elevated, and have an intact overlying epithelium (Fig. 11–30A). Histologically, these are unencapsulated aggregates of **closely packed, thin-walled capillaries**, usually blood-filled and lined by flattened endothelium; vessels are separated by scant connective tissue stroma (Fig. 11–30B). The lumens may be partially or completely thrombosed and organized. Vessel rupture accounts for hemosiderin pigment in these lesions as well as focal scarring.

Cavernous Hemangioma. These exhibit large, dilated vascular channels; compared with capillary hemangiomas, *cavernous hemangiomas* are less well circumscribed and more frequently involve deep structures. Since they may be locally destructive and show no spontaneous tendency to regress, some may require surgery. In most cases, the tumors are of little clinical significance; however, they can be a cosmetic disturbance and are vulnerable to traumatic ulceration and bleeding. Moreover, visceral hemangiomas detected by imaging studies may have to be distinguished from more ominous (e.g., malignant) lesions. Brain hemangiomas are most problematic, because they can cause pressure symptoms or rupture. Cavernous hemangiomas are a component of *von Hippel-Lindau disease* (Chapter 28), occurring within the cerebellum, brain stem, or retina, along with similar angiomatous lesions or cystic neoplasms in the pancreas and liver; von Hippel-Lindau disease is also associated with renal neoplasms.

Morphology. Cavernous hemangiomas are red-blue, soft, spongy masses 1 to 2 cm in diameter; rare giant forms can affect large subcutaneous areas of the face, extremities, or other body regions. Histologically, the mass is sharply defined but not encapsulated, and composed of **large, cavernous blood-filled vascular spaces**, separated by a modest connective tissue stroma (Fig. 11–30C). Intravascular thrombosis with associated dystrophic calcification is common.

Pyogenic Granuloma. This form of capillary hemangioma is a rapidly growing pedunculated red nodule on the skin, or gingival or oral mucosa; it bleeds easily and is often ulcerated (Fig. 11–30D). Roughly a third of the lesions develop after trauma, reaching a size of 1 to 2 cm within a few weeks. The proliferating capillaries are often accompanied by extensive edema and an acute and chronic inflammatory infiltrate, strikingly similar to exuberant granulation tissue. *Pregnancy tumor (granuloma gravidarum)* is a pyogenic granuloma that occurs infrequently (1% of patients) in the gingiva of pregnant women. These lesions can spontaneously regress (e.g., after pregnancy) or undergo fibrosis; in some cases surgical excision is required. Recurrence is rare.

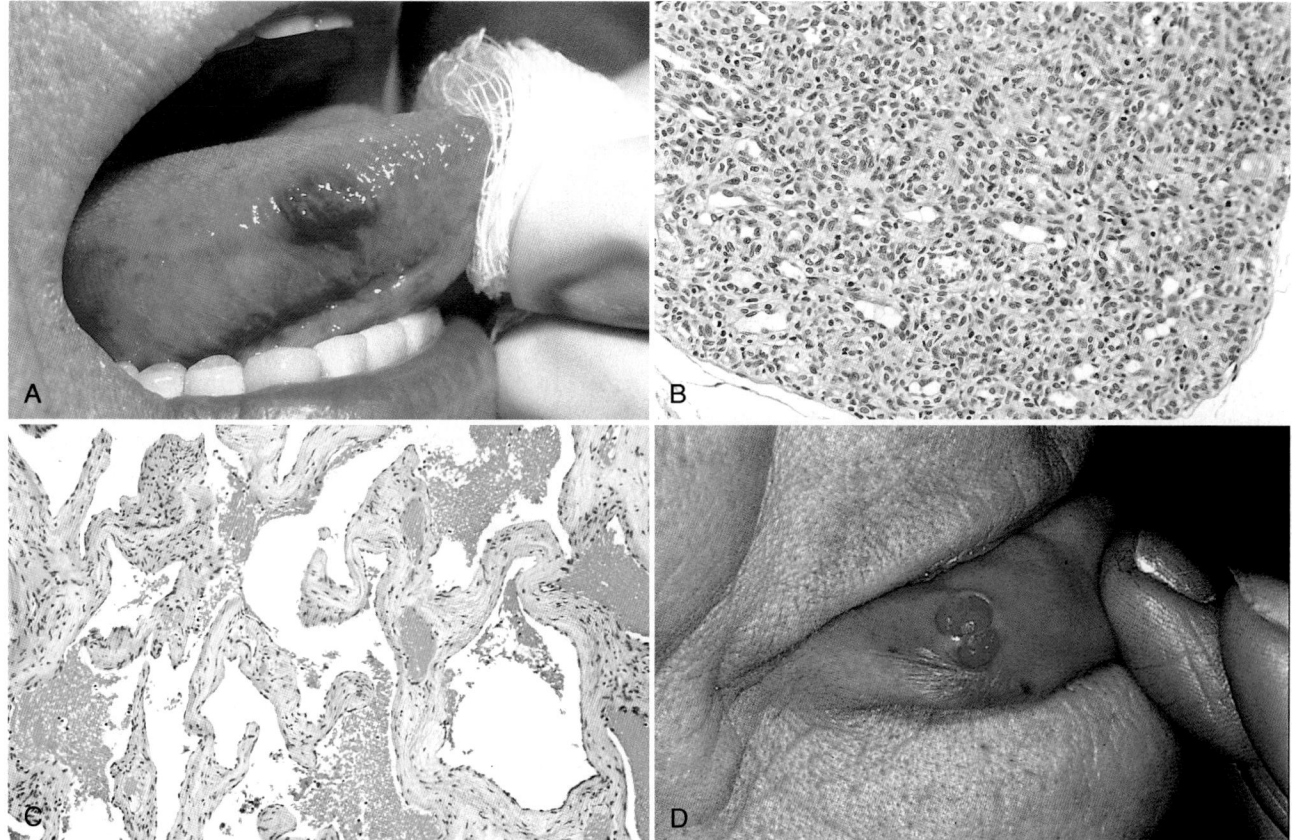

FIGURE 11–30 Hemangiomas. **A,** Hemangioma of the tongue. **B** and **C,** Histologic appearance of (**B**) juvenile capillary hemangioma and (**C**) cavernous hemangioma. **D,** Pyogenic granuloma of the lip. (**A** and **D,** Courtesy of John Sexton, M.D., Beth Israel Hospital, Boston, MA; **B,** courtesy of Christopher D.M. Fletcher, M.D., Brigham and Women's Hospital, Boston; **C,** courtesy of Thomas Rogers, M.D., University of Texas Southwestern Medical School, Dallas, TX.)

Lymphangiomas

Lymphangiomas are the benign lymphatic analogues of blood vessel hemangiomas.

Simple (Capillary) Lymphangioma. These are composed of small lymphatic channels predominantly occurring in the head, neck, and axillary subcutaneous tissues. They are slightly elevated or sometimes pedunculated lesions up to 1 to 2 cm in diameter. Histologically, lymphangiomas exhibit networks of endothelium-lined spaces that can be *distinguished from capillary channels only by the absence of erythrocytes.*

Cavernous Lymphangioma (Cystic Hygroma). These lesions are typically found in the neck or axilla of children, and rarely occur in the retroperitoneum; cavernous lymphangiomas of the neck are common in Turner syndrome (Chapter 10). Cavernous lymphangiomas can occasionally be enormous (up to 15 cm in diameter) and may fill the axilla or produce gross deformities about the neck. Tumors are composed of massively dilated lymphatic spaces lined by endothelial cells and separated by intervening connective tissue stroma containing lymphoid aggregates. The tumor margins are not discrete and the lesions are not encapsulated, making definitive resection difficult.

Glomus Tumor (Glomangioma)

Glomus tumors are benign, exquisitely painful tumors *arising from modified smooth muscle cells of the glomus body*, a specialized arteriovenous structure involved in thermoregulation. Although they can resemble cavernous hemangiomas, glomus tumors constitute a distinct entity by virtue of their constituent cells. They are most commonly found in the distal portion of the digits, especially under the fingernails. Excision is curative.

> **Morphology.** Glomus tumor lesions are round, slightly elevated, red-blue, firm nodules (usually <1 cm in diameter) that initially resemble a minute focus of hemorrhage. Histologically, these are **aggregates, nests, and masses of specialized glomus cells** intimately associated with branching vascular channels, all within a connective tissue stroma. Individual tumor cells are small, uniform, and round or cuboidal, with scant cytoplasm and ultrastructural features akin to smooth muscle cells.

Vascular Ectasias

Vascular ectasias are common lesions characterized by local dilation of preexisting vessels; *they are not true neoplasms. Telangiectasia* is a term used for a congenital anomaly or acquired exaggeration of preformed vessels—usually in the skin or mucous membranes—composed of capillaries, venules, and arterioles that creates a discrete red lesion.

Nevus Flammeus. This lesion is the ordinary "birthmark" and is the most common form of ectasia; it is characteristically a flat lesion on the head or neck, ranging in color from light pink to deep purple. Histologically, there is only vascular dilation; most ultimately regress.

The so-called *port wine stain* is a special form of nevus flammeus; these lesions tend to grow with a child, thicken the skin surface, and demonstrate no tendency to fade. Such lesions in a trigeminal nerve distribution are occasionally associated with the *Sturge-Weber syndrome* (also called *encephalotrigeminal angiomatosis*). Sturge-Weber syndrome is a rare congenital disorder associated with venous angiomatous masses in the cortical leptomeninges and ipsilateral facial port wine nevi; mental retardation, seizures, hemiplegia, and skull radioopacities also occur. Thus, *a large facial vascular malformation in a child with mental deficiency may indicate the presence of more extensive vascular malformations.*[84]

Spider Telangiectasia. This non-neoplastic vascular lesion grossly resembles a spider; there is a radial, often pulsatile array of dilated subcutaneous arteries or arterioles (resembling legs) about a central core (resembling a body) that blanches when pressure is applied to its center. It is commonly seen on the face, neck, or upper chest and is most frequently associated with hyper-estrogenic states such as pregnancy or patients with cirrhosis; how elevated estrogen levels contribute to "spider" formation is not known.

Hereditary Hemorrhagic Telangiectasia (Osler-Weber-Rendu Disease). In this autosomal dominant disorder the telangiectasias are malformations composed of dilated capillaries and veins. Present from birth, they are widely distributed over the skin and oral mucous membranes, as well as in the respiratory, gastrointestinal, and urinary tracts. Occasionally, these lesions rupture, causing serious epistaxis (nosebleeds), GI bleeding, or hematuria.

Bacillary Angiomatosis

Bacillary angiomatosis is a vascular proliferation resulting from an opportunistic infection in immunocompromised individuals; lesions can involve skin, bone, brain, and other organs. First described in patients with acquired immunodeficiency syndrome (AIDS), bacillary angiomatosis is caused by infection with gram-negative bacilli of the *Bartonella* family. Two species are implicated: *Bartonella henselae*, the organism responsible for cat-scratch disease (the domestic cat is the principal reservoir), and *B. quintana*, the cause of "trench fever" in World War I (the organism is transmitted by human body lice).[85]

> **Morphology.** Skin lesions are red papules and nodules, or rounded subcutaneous masses; histologically, there is capillary proliferation with prominent epithelioid endothelial cells exhibiting nuclear atypia and mitoses (Fig. 11–31). Lesions contain neutrophils, nuclear dust, and the causal bacteria.
>
> Though difficult to cultivate in the laboratory, the bacteria can be unequivocally demonstrated using molecular methods such as polymerase chain reaction with species-specific primers. The vascular proliferation results from induction of host HIF-1α by the bacteria; HIF-1α in turn drives VEGF production.[86] The infections (and lesions) are cleared by macrolide antibiotics (including erythromycin).

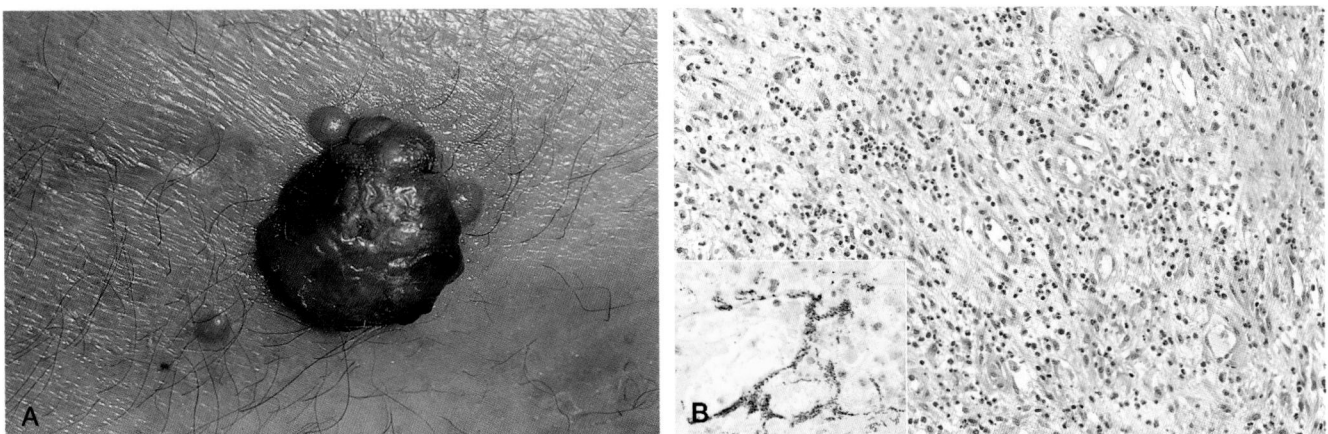

FIGURE 11–31 Bacillary angiomatosis. **A,** Photograph of a cutaneous lesion. **B,** Histologic appearance with acute neutrophilic inflammation and vascular (capillary) proliferation. *(Inset)* Demonstration by modified silver (Warthin-Starry) stain of clusters of tangled bacilli (black). (**A,** Courtesy of Richard Johnson, M.D., Beth Israel Deaconess Medical Center, Boston, MA; **B** and inset, courtesy of Scott Granter, M.D., Brigham and Women's Hospital, Boston.)

INTERMEDIATE-GRADE (BORDERLINE) TUMORS

Kaposi Sarcoma

Though rare in other populations, Kaposi sarcoma (KS) is common in patients with AIDS; indeed, its presence is used as a criterion for diagnosing AIDS (Chapter 6). Four forms of the disease are recognized (based primarily on population demographics and risks), although all share the same underlying viral pathogenesis[87] (see below):

- *Chronic KS* (also called *classic* or *European KS*) was first described by Kaposi in 1872; it characteristically occurs in older men of Eastern European (especially Ashkenazi Jews) or Mediterranean descent and is uncommon in the United States. While chronic KS can be associated with an underlying second malignancy or altered immunity, it is not associated with human immunodeficiency virus (HIV). Chronic KS presents with multiple red to purple skin plaques or nodules, usually in the distal lower extremities; these slowly increase in size and number and spread more proximally. Although locally persistent, the tumors are typically asymptomatic and remain localized to the skin and subcutaneous tissue.
- *Lymphadenopathic KS* (also called *African* or *endemic KS*) has the same general geographic distribution as Burkitt lymphoma and is particularly prevalent among South African Bantu children; it is also not associated with HIV. Skin lesions are sparse, and patients present instead with lymphadenopathy due to KS involvement; the tumor occasionally involves the viscera and is extremely aggressive. In combination with AIDS-associated KS (see below), KS is now the most common tumor in central Africa (50% of all tumors in men in some countries).
- *Transplant-associated KS* occurs in the setting of solid-organ transplantation with its attendant long-term immunosuppression. It tends to be aggressive (even fatal) with nodal, mucosal, and visceral involvement; cutaneous lesions may be absent. Lesions occasionally regress when immuno-

suppressive therapy is attenuated, but at the risk of organ rejection.

- *AIDS-associated (epidemic) KS* was originally found in a third of AIDS patients, particularly male homosexuals (Chapter 6). However, with current regimens of antiretroviral therapy, KS incidence is now less than 1% (although it is still the most prevalent malignancy in AIDS patients in the United States). AIDS-associated KS can involve lymph nodes or viscera and disseminates widely early in the course of the disease. Most patients eventually die of opportunistic infections rather than from KS.

Pathogenesis. In 1994, a previously unrecognized herpesvirus—*human herpesvirus-8 (HHV-8)* or *KS-associated herpesvirus (KSHV)*—was identified in a cutaneous KS lesion in an AIDS patient (Chapter 6). Indeed, regardless of the clinical subtype (described above), 95% of KS lesions have subsequently been shown to be KSHV-infected.[88] Like Epstein-Barr virus, KSHV is a member of the γ-herpesvirus subfamily; it is transmitted sexually and by poorly understood nonsexual routes—perhaps including saliva.

KSHV is accepted as a necessary requirement for KS development, but tumor progression also requires a cofactor; HIV clearly can provide this, but the identity of the cofactor in non-HIV-associated KS is controversial. KSHV induces a lytic as well as a latent infection in endothelial cells, both of which are probably important in KS pathogenesis. Cytokines derived from HIV-infected T cells, or inflammatory cells recruited in response to the lytic infection, create a local proliferative milieu; a virally encoded G protein also induces local VEGF production. In latently infected cells, KSHV proteins disrupt normal cellular proliferation controls and prevent apoptosis by viral production of p53 inhibitors and a viral homologue of cyclin D. Thus, latently infected cells have a growth advantage; the local environment also favors cellular proliferation. The increasing recognition of the various viral gene products has nevertheless opened a number of new avenues for therapeutic interventions against affected intracellular kinase pathways and downstream targets. In its early stages, only a few

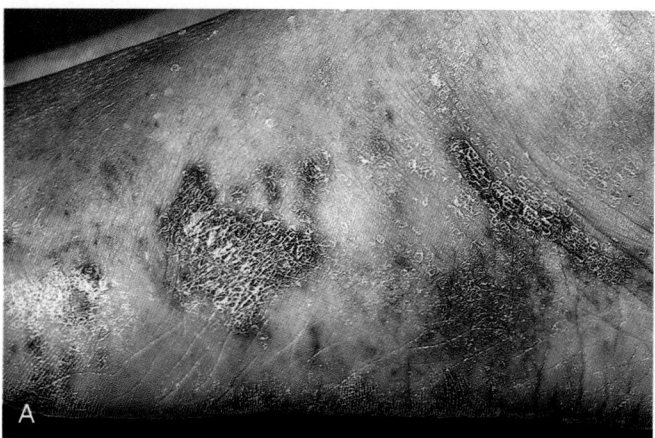
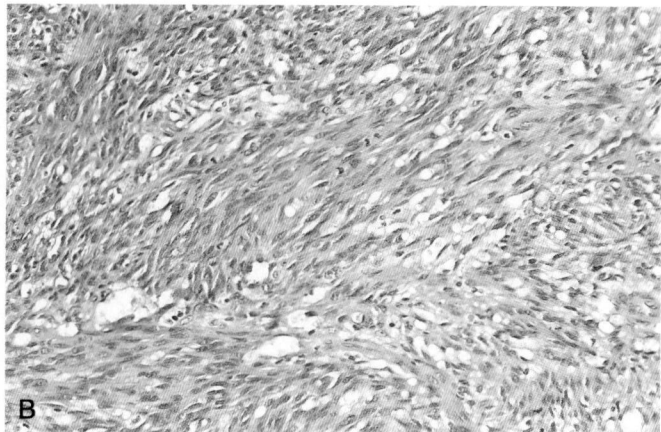

FIGURE 11–32 Kaposi sarcoma. **A,** Gross photograph, illustrating coalescent red-purple macules and plaques of the skin. **B,** Histologic appearance of nodular form, demonstrating sheets of plump, proliferating spindle cells. (**B,** Courtesy of Christopher D.M. Fletcher, M.D., Brigham and Women's Hospital, Boston, MA.)

cells are infected; with time virtually all spindle cells of late-stage lesions carry KSHV; these spindle cells express both endothelial cell and smooth muscle cell markers.

Morphology. In the indolent, classic disease of older men (and sometimes in other variants), three stages are recognized: patch, plaque, and nodule.

- **Patches** are red to purple macules typically confined to the distal lower extremities (Fig. 11–32A). Histology shows only dilated irregular endothelial cell–lined vascular spaces with interspersed lymphocytes, plasma cells, and macrophages (sometimes containing hemosiderin). The lesions can be difficult to distinguish from granulation tissue.
- With time, lesions spread proximally and become larger, violaceous, **raised plaques** (see Fig. 11–32A) composed of dermal accumulations of dilated, jagged vascular channels lined and surrounded by plump spindle cells. Scattered between the vascular channels are extravasated red cells, hemosiderin-laden macrophages, and other mononuclear inflammatory cells.
- Eventually, lesions become **nodular** and more distinctly neoplastic. These lesions are composed of sheets of plump, proliferating spindle cells, mostly in the dermis or subcutaneous tissues (Fig. 11–32B), encompassing small vessels and slitlike spaces containing red cells. More marked hemorrhage, hemosiderin pigment, and mononuclear inflammation is present; mitotic figures are common, as are round, pink, cytoplasmic globules of uncertain nature. The nodular stage often heralds nodal and visceral involvement, particularly in the African and AIDS-associated variants.

Clinical Features. The course of KS varies widely and is significantly affected by the clinical setting. Most primary KSHV infections are asymptomatic. Classic KS is—at least initially—largely restricted to the surface of the body, and surgical resection is usually adequate for an excellent prognosis. Radiation can be used for multiple lesions in a restricted area, and chemotherapy yields satisfactory results for more disseminated disease. Lymphadenopathic KS can also be treated with chemotherapy or radiation therapy with good results. In immunosuppression-associated KS, withdrawal of immunosuppression (perhaps with adjunct chemotherapy or radiation therapy) is often effective. For AIDS-associated KS, antiretroviral therapy for HIV is usually helpful, with or without therapy targeted to the KS lesions. IFN-α and angiogenesis inhibitors are variably effective, while newer strategies aimed at specific intracellular kinase pathways or the downstream mammalian target of rapamycin are showing promise.[89,90]

Hemangioendothelioma

Hemangioendothelioma denotes a wide spectrum of vascular neoplasms with clinical behaviors *intermediate between benign, well-differentiated hemangiomas and highly malignant angiosarcomas*, described below.

Epithelioid hemangioendothelioma is an example; it is a vascular tumor of adults occurring around medium-sized and large veins. The tumor cells are plump and often cuboidal (resembling epithelial cells); well-defined vascular channels are inconspicuous. Clinical behavior is variable; most are cured by excision, but up to 40% recur, 20% to 30% eventually metastasize, and perhaps 15% of patients die of the tumors.

MALIGNANT TUMORS

Angiosarcoma

Angiosarcomas are malignant endothelial neoplasms (Fig. 11–33) with histology varying from well-differentiated tumors that resemble hemangiomas (*hemangiosarcoma*) to anaplastic lesions difficult to distinguish from carcinomas or melanomas. Older adults are more commonly affected, with equal gender predilections; they occur at any site but most often involve skin, soft tissue, breast, and liver.

Hepatic angiosarcomas are associated with carcinogen exposures, including arsenic (arsenical pesticides), Thorotrast

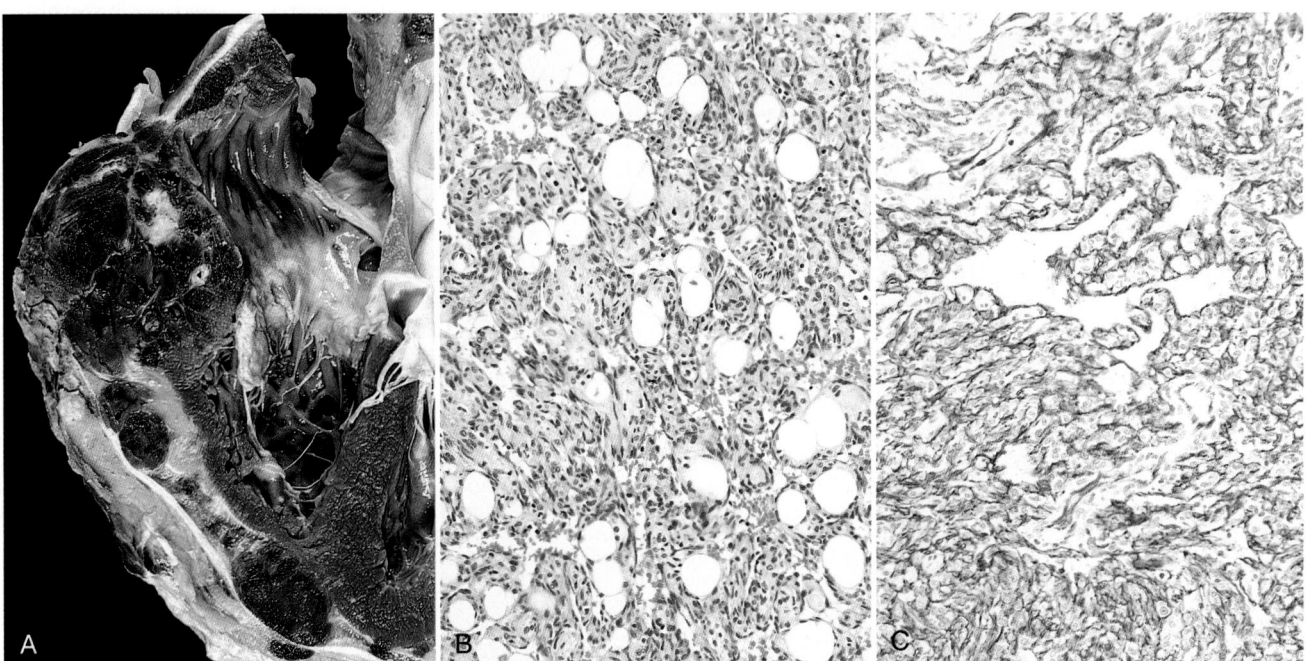

FIGURE 11–33 Angiosarcoma. **A,** Gross photograph of angiosarcoma of the heart (right ventricle). **B,** Photomicrograph of moderately well-differentiated angiosarcoma with dense clumps of irregular, moderate anaplastic cells and distinct vascular lumens. **C,** Immunohistochemical staining for the endothelial cell marker CD31, demonstrating the endothelial nature of the tumor cells.

(a radioactive contrast agent formerly used for radiologic imaging), and polyvinyl chloride (a widely used plastic). All of these agents have long latent periods between initial exposure and eventual tumor development. The increased frequency of angiosarcomas among polyvinyl chloride workers is one of the well-documented instances of human chemical carcinogenesis.

Angiosarcomas can also arise in the setting of lymphedema, classically in the ipsilateral upper extremity several years after radical mastectomy (i.e., with lymph node resection) for breast cancer; the tumor presumably arises from lymphatic vessels (lymphangiosarcoma). Angiosarcomas have also been induced by radiation and are rarely associated with foreign material introduced into the body either iatrogenically or accidentally.

> **Morphology.** Cutaneous angiosarcomas can begin as deceptively small, sharply demarcated, asymptomatic, often multiple red nodules; most eventually become large, fleshy masses of red-tan to gray-white tissue (Fig. 11–33A). The margins blend imperceptibly with surrounding structures. Central areas of necrosis and hemorrhage are frequent.
>
> Microscopically, **all degrees of differentiation can be seen,** from plump, anaplastic but recognizable endothelial cells producing vascular channels (Fig. 11–33B) to wildly undifferentiated tumors with a solid spindle cell appearance and without definite blood vessels. The endothelial cell origin of these tumors can be demonstrated by staining for CD31 or von Willebrand factor (Fig. 11–33C).

Clinically, angiosarcomas are locally invasive and can metastasize readily. Angiosarcomas are aggressive tumors with current 5-year survival rates approaching 30%.

Hemangiopericytoma

Hemangiopericytomas are rare tumors derived from pericytes—myofibroblast-like cells that are normally arranged around capillaries and venules. Hemangiopericytomas can occur as slowly enlarging, painless masses at any anatomic site, but are most common on the lower extremities (especially the thigh) and in the retroperitoneum. They consist of numerous branching capillary channels and gaping sinusoidal spaces enclosed within nests of spindle-shaped to round cells. Special stains confirm that these cells are outside the endothelial cell basement membrane and are therefore pericytes. The tumors may recur after excision, and roughly half will metastasize, usually hematogenously to lungs, bone, or liver.

Pathology of Vascular Interventions

The morphologic changes that occur in vessels after therapeutic intervention—balloon angioplasty, stenting, or bypass surgery—typically recapitulate many of the changes that occur in the setting of any vascular insult. Local endothelial cell trauma (e.g., due to a stent), vascular thrombosis (after angioplasty), or abnormal mechanical forces (e.g., a saphenous vein inserted into the arterial circulation as a coronary artery bypass graft), all induce similar responses characteristic of vessel wall healing. Thus, in the same way that various injuries can induce an intimal hyperplastic response that we recognize as atherosclerosis (see above), the trauma caused by

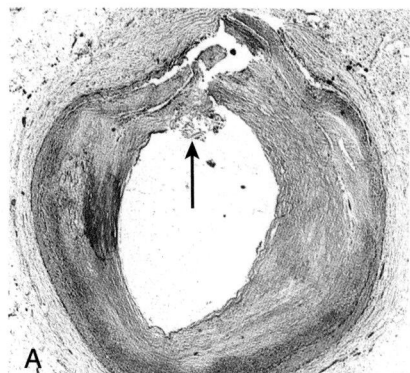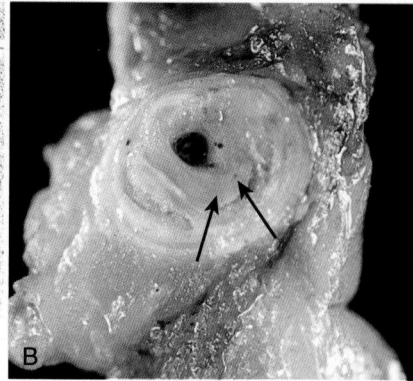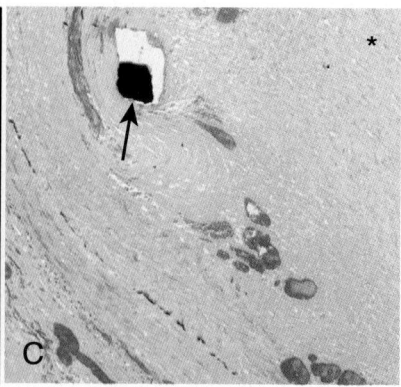

FIGURE 11–34 Balloon angioplasty and endovascular stents. **A,** Coronary artery after balloon angioplasty, showing the dissection encompassing the intima and media *(arrow).* **B,** Gross photograph of restenosis following balloon angioplasty, demonstrating residual atherosclerotic plaque *(left arrow)* and a new, glistening proliferative lesion *(right arrow).* **C,** Coronary arterial stent implanted long term, demonstrating thickened neointima separating the stent wires (black spot shown by *arrow*) from the lumen *(asterisk).* (**C,** Reproduced from Schoen FJ, Edwards WD: Pathology of cardiovascular interventions, including endovascular therapies, revascularization, vascular replacement, cardiac assist/replacement, arrhythmia control, and repaired congenital heart disease. In Silver MD et al. (eds): Cardiovascular Pathology, 3rd ed. Philadelphia, Churchill Livingstone, 2001.)

vascular interventions tends to induce a concentric intimal thickening composed of recruited smooth muscle cells and their associated matrix deposition.

ANGIOPLASTY AND ENDOVASCULAR STENTS

Balloon angioplasty (dilation of a stenotic artery by inserting an intravascular catheter), with or without endovascular stenting, is used extensively to restore flow at sites of focal vascular stenosis—especially in the coronary circulation *(percutaneous transluminal coronary angioplasty).* The morphologic outcomes of angioplasty, as well as the now more commonly used *endovascular stents,* are demonstrated in Figure 11–34.

Simple balloon dilation (without stenting) of an atherosclerotic vessel induces medial stretching and causes plaque fracture, often with accompanying localized hemorrhagic dissection of the adjacent arterial wall (Fig. 11–34A); in this manner vascular flow is restored, albeit with the attendant risks of more extensive dissection and luminal thrombosis (to prevent the latter, anticoagulation is required for a period of time after the procedure). Most patients improve symptomatically, at least in the short term. *Abrupt reclosure* may occur as a result of compression of the lumen by an extensive circumferential or longitudinal dissection or by thrombosis. The long-term success of angioplasty is primarily limited by the development of *proliferative restenosis,* due to intimal thickening; this occurs in approximately 30% to 50% of patients within the first 4 to 6 months after the procedure (Fig. 11–34B). The conditions causing restenosis are undoubtedly the same as those that occur in response to vascular damage of any type (e.g., atherosclerosis); in this case the injury is mechanical and is also compounded by the resolution of any associated thrombosis. The end result is an occlusive, progressive fibrous lesion that contains abundant smooth muscle cells and extracellular matrix.

Coronary stents are expandable tubes of metallic mesh that are inserted to preserve lumenal patency during angioplasty; they are now used in over 90% of angioplasty procedures.

Stents provide a larger and more regular lumen, "tack down" the intimal flaps and dissections that occur during angioplasty, and mechanically limit vascular spasm. Nevertheless, by also causing focal plaque erosion and/or endothelial cell disruption, stents can cause acute thrombosis, and a successful procedure also requires at least transient anticoagulation with potent anti-thrombotic agents (platelet antagonists).[91] A *late complication* of bare metal stents involves proliferative intimal thickening leading to proliferative restenosis much like that seen with percutaneous transluminal coronary angioplasty alone (Fig. 11–34C). The newest generation of stents are coated with anti-proliferative drugs (e.g., paclitaxel or rapamycin) that limit smooth muscle cell hyperplasia; this results in markedly diminished intimal thickening, although there is evidence that the anti-proliferative agents also slow the process of re-endothelialization of the coated stents and prolong the required period of anticoagulation therapy.[92]

VASCULAR REPLACEMENT

Synthetic or autologous vascular grafts are increasingly used to replace damaged vessels or bypass diseased arteries. With synthetic grafts (usually expanded polytetrafluoroethylene, a spongy Teflon fabric), large-bore (12- to 18-mm) conduits function well in high-flow locations such as the aorta; unfortunately, small-diameter artificial grafts (≤8 mm in diameter) generally fail because of early thrombosis or late intimal hyperplasia, primarily at the junction of the graft with the native vasculature (Fig. 11–35).

Consequently, where small-bore vessels are needed (e.g., for coronary artery bypass surgery performed in more than 400,000 U.S. patients per year), grafts are most commonly composed of either reversed autologous saphenous vein (taken from the patient's own leg) or left internal mammary artery (because of its proximity to the heart). The long-term patency of saphenous vein grafts is only 50% at 10 years; grafts occlude because of thrombosis (typically early), intimal thickening (months to years postoperatively), and vein graft atherosclerosis—sometimes with superimposed plaque rupture,

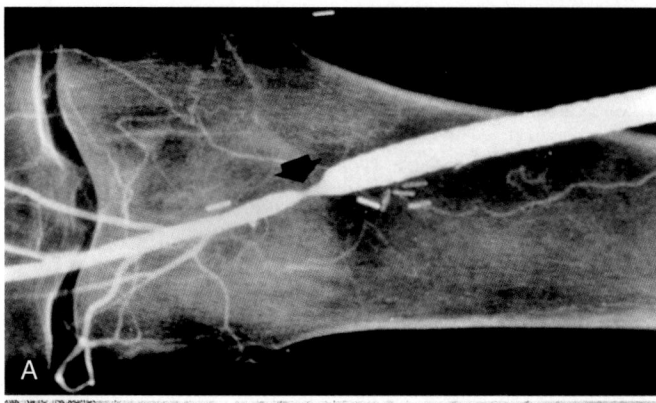

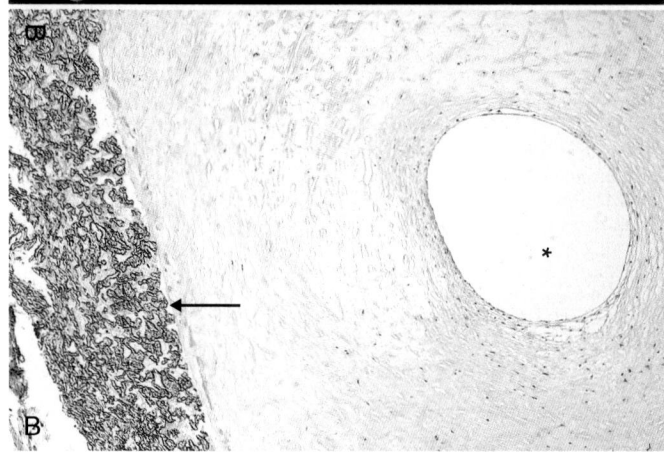

FIGURE 11–35 Anastomotic hyperplasia at the distal anastomosis of synthetic femoropopliteal graft. **A,** Angiogram demonstrating constriction *(arrow).* **B,** Photomicrograph demonstrating Gore-Tex graft *(arrow)* with prominent intimal proliferation and very small residual lumen *(asterisk).* (A, Courtesy of Anthony D. Whittemore, M.D., Brigham and Women's Hospital, Boston, MA.)

thrombi, or aneurysms (usually >2–3 years). In contrast, greater than 90% of internal mammary artery grafts are patent at 10 years.[93]

REFERENCES

1. Carmeliet P: Angiogenesis in life, disease and medicine. Nature 438:932, 2005.
2. Carmeliet P: Manipulating angiogenesis in medicine. J Intern Med 255:538, 2004.
3. Semenza G: Vasculogenesis, angiogenesis, and arteriogenesis: mechanisms of blood vessel formation and remodeling. J Cell Biochem 102:840, 2007.
4. Heil M et al.: Arteriogenesis versus angiogenesis: similarities and differences. J Cell Mol Med 10:45, 2006.
5. Angelini P et al.: Coronary anomalies: incidence, pathophysiology, and clinical relevance. Circulation 105:2449, 2002.
6. Angelini P: Coronary artery anomalies: an entity in search of an identity. Circulation 115:1296, 2007.
7. Friedlander R: Clinical practice. Arteriovenous malformations of the brain. N Engl J Med 356:2704, 2007.
8. Slovut D, Olin J: Fibromuscular dysplasia. N Engl J Med 350:1862, 2004.
9. Shin D et al.: Expression of ephrinB2 identifies a stable genetic difference between arterial and venous vascular smooth muscle as well as endothelial cells, and marks subsets of microvessels at sites of adult neovascularization. Dev Biol 230:139, 2001.
10. Garcia-Cardena G, Gimbrone M: Biomechanical modulation of endothelial phenotype: implications for health and disease. Handb Exp Pharmacol 176:79, 2006.
11. Pober JS, Min W, Bradley JR: Mechanisms of endothelial dysfunction, injury, and death. Annu Rev Pathol Mech Dis 4:71, 2009.
12. Stevens T et al.: NHLBI workshop report: endothelial cell phenotypes in heart, lung, and blood diseases. Am J Physiol Cell Physiol 281:C1422, 2001.
13. Berk B: Vascular smooth muscle growth: autocrine growth mechanisms. Physiol Rev 81:999, 2001.
14. Sata M: Role of circulating vascular progenitors in angiogenesis, vascular healing, and pulmonary hypertension: lessons from animal models. Arterioscler Thromb Vasc Biol 26:1008, 2006.
15. Shimizu K, Mitchell R: Stem cell origins of intimal cells in graft arterial disease. Curr Athero Rep 5:230, 2003.
16. Hillebrands J et al.: Origin of vascular smooth muscle cells and the role of circulating stem cells in transplant arteriosclerosis. Arterioscler Thromb Vasc Biol 23:380, 2003.
17. Caplice N, Doyle B: Vascular progenitor cells: origin and mechanisms of mobilization, differentiation, integration, and vasculogenesis. Stem Cells Dev 14:122, 2005.
18. Korshunov V et al.: Vascular remodeling: hemodynamic and biochemical mechanisms underlying Glagov's phenomenon. Arterioscler Thromb Vasc Biol 27:1722, 2007.
19. Kannel W et al.: Concept and usefulness of cardiovascular risk profiles. Am Heart J 148:16, 2004.
20. Kaplan N: Systemic hypertension: mechanisms and diagnosis. In Zipes D et al. (eds): Braunwald's Heart Disease, 7th ed. Philadelphia, Elsevier Saunders, 2005, p 959.
21. Lifton R et al.: Molecular mechanisms of human hypertension. Cell 104:545, 2001.
22. Puddu P et al.: The genetic basis of essential hypertension. Acta Cardiol 62:281, 2007.
23. Messerli F et al.: Essential hypertension. Lancet 370:591, 2007.
24. Scarpelli P et al.: Continuing follow-up of malignant hypertension. J Nephrol 15:431, 2002.
25. Aggarwal M, Khan I: Hypertensive crisis: hypertensive emergencies and urgencies. Cardiol Clin 24:135, 2006.
26. Rodriguez-Iturbe B et al.: Pathophysiological mechanisms of salt-dependent hypertension. Am J Kidney Dis 50:655, 2007.
27. Chambless L et al.: Coronary heart disease risk prediction in the Atherosclerosis Risk in Communities (ARIC) study. J Clin Epidemiol 56:880, 2003.
28. Ridker P, Libby P: Risk factors for atherothrombotic disease. In Zipes D et al. (eds): Braunwald's Heart Disease, 7th ed. Philadelphia, Elsevier Saunders, 2005, p 939.
29. Sweitzer N, Douglas P: Cardiovascular disease in women. In Zipes D et al. (eds): Braunwald's Heart Disease, 7th ed. Philadelphia, Elsevier Saunders, 2005, p 1951.
30. Miller D et al.: Atherosclerosis: the path from genomics to therapeutics. J Am Coll Cardiol 49:1589, 2007.
31. Glassberg H, Rader D: Management of lipids in the prevention of cardiovascular events. Annu Rev Med 59:79–94, 2008.
32. Ridker P et al.: Comparison of C-reactive protein and low-density lipoprotein cholesterol levels in the prediction of first cardiovascular events. N Engl J Med 347:1557, 2002.
33. Ridker P: C-reactive protein and the prediction of cardiovascular events among those at intermediate risk: moving an inflammatory hypothesis toward consensus. J Am Coll Cardiol 49:2129, 2007.
34. Ridker P et al.: Development and validation of improved algorithms for the assessment of global cardiovascular risk in women: the Reynolds Risk Score. JAMA 297:611, 2007.
35. Guthikonda S, Haynes W: Homocysteine: role and implications in atherosclerosis. Curr Atheroscler Rep 8:100, 2006.
36. Meerarani P et al.: Metabolic syndrome and diabetic atherothrombosis: implications in vascular complications. Curr Mol Med 6:501, 2006.
37. Anuurad E et al.: Lipoprotein(a): a unique risk factor for cardiovascular disease. Clin Lab Med 26:751, 2006.
38. Croce K, Libby P: Intertwining of thrombosis and inflammation in atherosclerosis. Curr Opin Hematol 14:55, 2007.
39. Meadows T, Bhatt D: Clinical aspects of platelet inhibitors and thrombus formation. Circ Res 100:1261, 2007.
40. Libby P: The vascular biology of atherosclerosis. In Zipes D et al. (eds): Braunwald's Heart Disease, 7th ed. Philadelphia, Elsevier Saunders, 2005, p 921.

41. Hansson G et al.: Inflammation and atherosclerosis. Annu Rev Pathol 1:297, 2006.

42. Ross R: Atherosclerosis—an inflammatory disease. N Engl J Med 340:115, 1999.

43. Chatzizisis Y et al.: Role of endothelial shear stress in the natural history of coronary atherosclerosis and vascular remodeling: molecular, cellular, and vascular behavior. J Am Coll Cardiol 49:2379, 2007.

44. Gau G, Wright R: Pathophysiology, diagnosis, and management of dyslipidemia. Curr Probl Cardiol 31:445, 2006.

45. Schiffrin E et al.: Chronic kidney disease: effects on the cardiovascular system. Circulation 116:85, 2007.

46. Hansson G: Inflammation, atherosclerosis, and coronary artery disease. N Engl J Med 352:1685, 2005.

47. Mussa F et al.: *Chlamydia pneumoniae* and vascular disease: an update. J Vasc Surg 43:1301, 2006.

48. Libby P: Atherosclerosis: disease biology affecting the coronary vasculature. Am J Cardiol 98:3Q, 2006.

49. Davies M: A macro and micro view of coronary vascular insult in ischemic heart disease. Circulation 82 (3 Suppl):II38, 1990.

50. Libby P, Theroux P: Pathophysiology of coronary artery disease. Circulation 111:3481, 2005.

51. Libby P, Sasiela W: Plaque stabilization: can we turn theory into evidence? Am J Cardiol 98 (11A):26P, 2006.

52. Curtis A, Fitzgerald G: Central and peripheral clocks in cardiovascular and metabolic function. Ann Med 38:552, 2006.

53. Brotman D et al.: The cardiovascular toll of stress. Lancet 370:1089, 2007.

54. Ramirez F, Dietz H: Marfan syndrome: from molecular pathogenesis to clinical treatment. Curr Opin Genet Dev 17:252, 2007.

55. Loeys B et al.: Aneurysm syndromes caused by mutations in the TGF-beta receptor. N Engl J Med 355:788, 2006.

56. Hobeika M et al.: Matrix metalloproteinases in peripheral vascular disease. J Vasc Surg 45:849, 2007.

57. Shimizu K et al. Inflammation and cellular immune responses in abdominal aortic aneurysms. Arterioscler Thromb Vasc Biol 26:987, 2006.

58. Homme J et al.: Surgical pathology of the ascending aorta: a clinicopathologic study of 513 cases. Am J Surg Pathol 30:1159, 2006.

59. Pagnoux C et al.: Vasculitides secondary to infections. Clin Exp Rheumatol 24 (2 Suppl 41):S71, 2006.

60. Fillinger M: Who should we operate on and how do we decide: predicting rupture and survival in patients with aortic aneurysm. Semin Vasc Surg 20:121, 2007.

61. Eliason J, Clouse W: Current management of infrarenal abdominal aortic aneurysms. Surg Clin North Am 87:1017, 2007.

62. Kamalakannan D et al.: Acute aortic dissection. Crit Care Clin 23:779, 2007.

63. Iglesias-Gamarra A et al.: Small-vessel vasculitis. Curr Rheumatol Rep 9:304, 2007.

64. Jennette J, Falk R: Nosology of primary vasculitis. Curr Opin Rheumatol 19:10, 2007.

65. Jennette J et al.: Nomenclature of systemic vasculitides. Proposal of an international consensus conference. Arthritis Rheum 37:187, 1994.

66. Kallenberg C: Antineutrophil cytoplasmic antibody–associated small-vessel vasculitis. Curr Opin Rheumatol 19:17, 2007.

67. Heeringa P et al.: Anti-neutrophil cytoplasmic autoantibodies and leukocyte-endothelial interactions: a sticky connection? Trends Immunol 26:561, 2005.

68. Jennette J et al.: Pathogenesis of vascular inflammation by antineutrophil cytoplasmic antibodies. J Am Soc Nephrol 17:1235, 2006.

69. Falcini F: Kawasaki disease. Curr Opin Rheumatol 18:33, 2006.

70. Gedalia A: Kawasaki disease: 40 years after the original report. Curr Rheumatol Rep 9:336, 2007.

71. Seko Y: Giant cell and Takayasu arteritis. Curr Opin Rheumatol 19:39, 2007.

72. Arnaud L et al.: Takayasu's arteritis: an update on physiopathology. Eur J Intern Med 17:241, 2006.

73. Colmegna I, Maldonado-Cocco J: Polyarteritis nodosa revisited. Curr Rheumatol Rep 7:288, 2007.

74. Segelmark M, Selga D: The challenge of managing patients with polyarteritis nodosa. Curr Opin Rheumatol 19:33, 2007.

75. Kallenberg C et al.: Mechanisms of disease: pathogenesis and treatment of ANCA-associated vasculitides. Nat Clin Pract Rheumatol 2:661, 2006.

76. Langford C: Small-vessel vasculitis: therapeutic management. Curr Rheumatol Rep 9:328, 2007.

77. Pagnoux C et al.: Churg-Strauss syndrome. Curr Opin Rheumatol 19:25, 2007.

78. Cuchacovich R et al.: Churg-Strauss syndrome associated with leukotriene receptor antagonists (LTRA). Clin Rheumatol 26:1769, 2007.

79. Sarraf P, Sneller M: Pathogenesis of Wegener's granulomatosis: current concepts. Expert Rev Mol Med 7:1, 2005.

80. Erickson V, Hwang P: Wegener's granulomatosis: current trends in diagnosis and management. Curr Opin Otolaryngol Head Neck Surg 15:170, 2007.

81. Olin J, Shih A: Thromboangiitis obliterans (Buerger's disease). Curr Opin Rheumatol 18:18, 2006.

82. Cooke J, Marshall J: Mechanisms of Raynaud's disease. Vasc Med 10:293, 2005.

83. Boin F, Wigley F: Understanding, assessing and treating Raynaud's phenomenon. Curr Opin Rheumatol 17:752, 2005.

84. Garzon M et al.: Vascular malformations. Part II: associated syndromes. J Am Acad Dermatol 56:541, 2007.

85. Chian C et al.: Skin manifestations of Bartonella infections. Int J Dermatol 41:461, 2002.

86. Kempf V et al.: Activation of hypoxia-inducible factor-1 in bacillary angiomatosis: evidence for a role of hypoxia-inducible factor-1 in bacterial infections. Circulation 111:1054, 2005.

87. Geraminejad P et al.: Kaposi's sarcoma and other manifestations of human herpesvirus 8. J Am Acad Dermatol 47:641, 2002.

88. Ganem D: KSHV infection and pathogenesis of Kaposi's sarcoma. Annu Rev Pathol 1:273, 2006.

89. Dittmer D, Krown S: Targeted therapy for Kaposi's sarcoma and Kaposi's sarcoma-associated herpesvirus. Curr Opin Oncol 19:452, 2007.

90. Lambert P et al.: Targeting the PI3K and MAPK pathways to treat Kaposi's-sarcoma-associated herpes virus infection and pathogenesis. Expert Opin Ther Targets 11:589, 2007.

91. Jaffe R, Strauss B: Late and very late thrombosis of drug-eluting stents: evolving concepts and perspectives. J Am Coll Cardiol 50:119, 2007.

92. VanBelle E et al.: Drug-eluting stents: trading restenosis for thrombosis? J Thromb Haemost 5 (Suppl 1):238, 2007.

93. Wallitt E et al.: Therapeutics of vein graft intimal hyperplasia: 100 years on. Ann Thorac Surg 84:317, 2007.

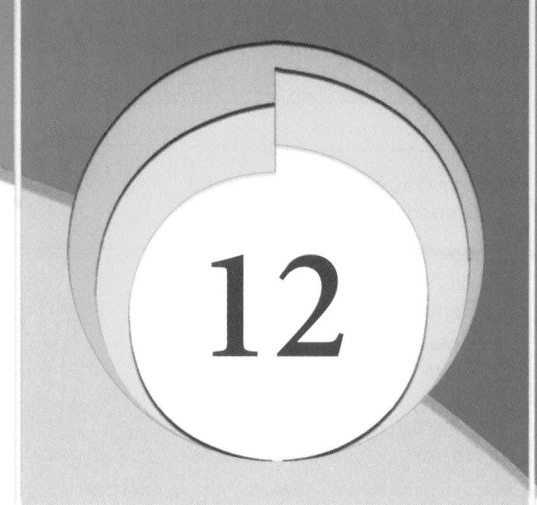

The Heart

FREDERICK J. SCHOEN · RICHARD N. MITCHELL

Cardiac Structure and Specializations
Myocardium
Valves
Conduction System
Blood Supply

Effects of Aging on the Heart

Heart Disease: Overview of Pathophysiology

Heart Failure
Cardiac Hypertrophy: Pathophysiology and Progression to Failure
Left-Sided Heart Failure
Right-Sided Heart Failure

Congenital Heart Disease
Left-to-Right Shunts
Atrial Septal Defect
Patent Foramen Ovale
Ventricular Septal Defect
Patent Ductus Arteriosus
Atrioventricular Septal Defect
Right-to-Left Shunts
Tetralogy of Fallot
Transposition of the Great Arteries
Persistent Truncus Arteriosus
Tricuspid Atresia
Total Anomalous Pulmonary Venous Connection
Obstructive Congenital Anomalies
Coarctation of the Aorta
Pulmonary Stenosis and Atresia
Aortic Stenosis and Atresia

Ischemic Heart Disease
Angina Pectoris

Myocardial Infarction
Chronic Ischemic Heart Disease
Sudden Cardiac Death

Hypertensive Heart Disease
Systemic (Left-Sided) Hypertensive Heart Disease
Pulmonary (Right-Sided) Hypertensive Heart Disease (Cor Pulmonale)

Valvular Heart Disease
Calcific Valvular Degeneration
Calcific Aortic Stenosis
Calcific Stenosis of Congenitally Bicuspid Aortic Valve
Mitral Annular Calcification
Mitral Valve Prolapse (Myxomatous Degeneration of the Mitral Valve)
Rheumatic Fever and Rheumatic Heart Disease
Infective Endocarditis
Noninfected Vegetations
Nonbacterial Thrombotic Endocarditis
Endocarditis of Systemic Lupus Erythematosus (Libman-Sacks Disease)
Carcinoid Heart Disease
Complications of Artificial Valves

Cardiomyopathies
Dilated Cardiomyopathy
Arrhythmogenic Right Ventricular Cardiomyopathy
Hypertrophic Cardiomyopathy
Restrictive Cardiomyopathy
Myocarditis

Other Causes of Myocardial Disease

Pericardial Disease
Pericardial Effusion and Hemopericardium
Pericarditis
Acute Pericarditis
Chronic or Healed Pericarditis
Heart Disease Associated with Rheumatologic Disorders

Tumors of the Heart
Primary Cardiac Tumors
Myxoma
Lipoma
Papillary Fibroelastoma
Rhabdomyoma
Sarcoma
Cardiac Effects of Noncardiac Neoplasms

Cardiac Transplantation

The human heart is a remarkably efficient, durable, and reliable pump that propels over 6000 liters of blood through the body daily and beats more than 40 million times a year, thereby providing the tissues with a steady supply of vital nutrients and facilitating the excretion of waste products. As might be anticipated, cardiac dysfunction can be associated with devastating physiologic consequences. Cardiovascular disease is the number one cause of death worldwide, with about 80% of the burden occurring in developing countries.[1,2] In the United States, heart disease accounts for nearly 40% of all postnatal deaths, totaling about 750,000 individuals annually; this is nearly 1.5 times the number of deaths caused by all forms of cancer combined. It is estimated that one third of Americans have one or more types of cardiovascular disease. Moreover, 32% of heart disease deaths are "premature," occurring in individuals younger than age 75.[3] If all major forms of cardiovascular disease were eliminated, life expectancy would increase by 7 years. The yearly economic burden of ischemic heart disease, the most prevalent subgroup, is estimated to be in excess of $100 billion in the United States.

The major categories of cardiac diseases considered in this chapter include congenital heart abnormalities, ischemic heart disease, heart disease caused by systemic hypertension, heart disease caused by pulmonary diseases (cor pulmonale), diseases of the cardiac valves, and primary myocardial diseases. A few comments about pericardial diseases and cardiac neoplasms as well as cardiac transplantation are also offered. Before considering details of specific conditions, we will briefly review the anatomy of the normal heart, because many diseases cause changes in the size and appearance of one or more of its components. We will also discuss the principles of cardiac hypertrophy and failure, the common end points of many different types of heart disease; these are essential for later discussion of disease processes.

Cardiac Structure and Specializations

Heart weight varies with body height and weight; it normally averages approximately 250 to 300 gm in females and 300 to 350 gm in males, or roughly 0.4% to 0.5% of body weight. The usual thickness of the free wall of the right ventricle is 0.3 to 0.5 cm, and that of the left ventricle 1.3 to 1.5 cm. Increases in cardiac size and weight accompany many forms of heart disease. Greater heart weight or ventricular thickness indicates

hypertrophy, and an enlarged chamber size implies *dilation*. An increase in cardiac weight or size or both (resulting from hypertrophy and/or dilation) is termed *cardiomegaly*.

The efficient pumping of blood by the heart to the entire body requires the normal function of each of its key components, the myocardium, valves, conduction system, and coronary arterial circulation.

MYOCARDIUM

The pumping function of the heart is accomplished by the cardiac muscle, the *myocardium*, composed primarily of a collection of specialized muscle cells called *cardiac myocytes*. Ventricular myocytes are arranged circumferentially in a spiral orientation and contract during systole and relax during diastole. The contractile unit is the *sarcomere*, an orderly arrangement of thick filaments composed principally of *myosin*, thin filaments containing *actin*, and regulatory proteins such as troponin and tropomyosin. Cardiac muscle cells contain strings of sarcomeres in series, which are responsible for the striated appearance of these cells. Contraction depends on a coordinated ratcheting mechanism whereby each myosin filament pulls the neighboring actin filaments toward the center of the sarcomere, leading to the shortening of the myocyte. The amount of force generated is determined by the distance each sarcomere shortens. Moderate ventricular dilation during diastole increases the extent of sarcomere shortening and the force of contraction during systole. With further dilation, however, there is a point at which effective overlap of the actin and myosin filaments is reduced and the force of contraction decreases sharply, as occurs in heart failure.

Atrial myocytes are generally smaller and arranged more haphazardly than their ventricular counterparts. Some atrial cells have distinctive electron-dense granules in the cytoplasm called *specific atrial granules*; these are the storage sites of *atrial natriuretic peptide*. Atrial natriuretic peptide can produce a variety of physiologic effects, including vasodilation, natriuresis, and diuresis, actions beneficial in pathologic states such as hypertension and congestive heart failure.[4]

Functional integration of cardiac myocytes is mediated by structures called *intercalated discs*, which link individual cells and contain specialized intercellular junctions that permit both mechanical and electrical (ionic) coupling. Within the intercalated discs, *gap junctions* facilitate synchronous myocyte contraction through electrical coupling by permitting relatively unrestricted passage of ions across the membranes of adjoining cells. Abnormalities in the spatial distribution of gap junctions and their respective proteins in ischemic and myocardial heart disease may contribute to electromechanical dysfunction (*arrhythmia*) and heart failure.[5]

VALVES

The four cardiac valves (tricuspid, pulmonary, mitral, and aortic) maintain unidirectional blood flow through the heart. Their function depends on the mobility, pliability, and structural integrity of their delicate flaps, called leaflets (in the tricuspid and mitral valves) or cusps (in the aortic and pulmonary valves, also known as the semilunar valves). All four valves have a similar, layered architecture: a dense collagenous core (fibrosa) close to the outflow surface and continuous with valvular supporting structures, a central core of loose connective tissue (spongiosa), a layer rich in elastin (ventricularis or atrialis depending on which chamber it faces) below the inflow surface, and an endothelial covering. The collagen is responsible for the mechanical integrity of a valve. The valve is populated throughout by interstitial cells, which produce and continuously repair the extracellular matrix (especially collagen), allowing the valve to respond and adapt to changing mechanical conditions.[6,7]

The function of the semilunar valves depends on the integrity and coordinated movements of the cuspal attachments. Thus, dilation of the aortic root can hinder coaptation of the aortic valve cusps during closure, yielding regurgitation. In contrast, the competence of the atrioventricular valves depends on not only the leaflets and their attachments, but also on tendinous connections to the papillary muscles of the ventricular wall. Left ventricular dilation, a ruptured tendon, or papillary muscle dysfunction can all interfere with mitral valve closure, leading to regurgitation.

Because they are thin enough to be nourished by diffusion from the heart's blood, normal leaflets and cusps have only scant blood vessels limited to the proximal portion. Pathologic changes of valves are largely of three types: damage to collagen that weakens the leaflets, exemplified by mitral valve prolapse; nodular calcification beginning in interstitial cells, as in calcific aortic stenosis; and fibrotic thickening, the key feature in rheumatic heart disease (see later).

CONDUCTION SYSTEM

Coordinated contraction of the cardiac muscle depends on propagation of electrical impulses, which is accomplished by specialized excitatory and conducting myocytes within the cardiac conduction system that regulate heart rate and rhythm. Key components of the conduction system include (1) the sinoatrial (SA) pacemaker of the heart, the *SA node*, located near the junction of the right atrial appendage and the superior vena cava; (2) the *AV node*, located in the right atrium along the atrial septum; (3) the *bundle of His*, which courses from the right atrium to the summit of the ventricular septum; and its major divisions (4) the *right and left bundle branches*, which further arborize in the respective ventricles through the anterior-superior and posterior-inferior divisions of the left

bundle and the Purkinje network. The cells of the specialized cardiac conduction system depolarize spontaneously, enabling them to function as cardiac pacemakers. Because the normal rate of spontaneous depolarization in the SA node (60 to 100 beats/minute) is faster than the other components, it normally sets the pace. The AV node serves as a kind of "gatekeeper"; by delaying the transmission of signals from the atria to the ventricles, it ensures that atria contraction precedes ventricular contraction.

The *autonomic nervous system* (the same part of the nervous system involved in blood pressure control) controls the rate of firing of the SA node to trigger the start of the cardiac cycle. Autonomic inputs can increase the heart rate to twice normal within only 3 to 5 seconds, and are important in cardiac responses to exercise or other states associated with increased oxygen demand.

BLOOD SUPPLY

To meet their energy needs, cardiac myocytes rely almost exclusively on oxidative phosphorylation, which is manifest by the abundant mitochondria that are found in these cells.[5] Oxydative phosphorylation requires oxygen, making cardiac myocytes extremely vulnerable to ischemia. A constant supply of oxygenated blood is thus essential for cardiac function. Most of the myocardium depends on nutrients and oxygen delivered via the the coronary arteries, which arise immediately distal to the aortic valve, initially running along the external surface of the heart (*epicardial coronary arteries*) and then penetrating the myocardium (*intramural arteries*). These small penetrating arteries yield arterioles and, ultimately, provide a rich network of capillaries enveloping individual cardiac muscle cells.

The three major epicardial coronary arteries are (1) the left anterior descending (LAD) and (2) the left circumflex (LCX) arteries, both arising from branches of the left (main) coronary artery, and (3) the right coronary artery. Branches of the LAD are called "diagonal" and "septal perforators," and those of the LCX are "obtuse marginals." Most coronary arterial blood flow to the myocardium occurs during ventricular diastole, when the microcirculation is not compressed by cardiac contraction.

There are a number of normal variations on the anatomy of the coronary arteries, which determine the areas of myocardium that are "at risk" in coronary artery disease and are of great practical importance to the heart surgeon and the invasive cardiologist; these are discussed later.

Effects of Aging on the Heart

The number of individuals aged 65 years and older will approximately double from 2000 to 2050 (from 35 million to 79 million in the United States). Considering this, one can see that knowledge of changes that occur in the cardiovascular system with aging will become increasingly important. Changes associated with aging can affect the pericardium, cardiac chambers, valves, coronary arteries, conduction system, myocardium, and aorta (Table 12–1).

TABLE 12–1   Changes in the Aging Heart
CHAMBERS
Increased left atrial cavity size
Decreased left ventricular cavity size
Sigmoid-shaped ventricular septum
VALVES
Aortic valve calcific deposits
Mitral valve annular calcific deposits
Fibrous thickening of leaflets
Buckling of mitral leaflets toward the left atrium
Lambl excrescences
EPICARDIAL CORONARY ARTERIES
Tortuosity
Increased cross-sectional luminal area
Calcific deposits
Atherosclerotic plaque
MYOCARDIUM
Increased mass
Increased subepicardial fat
Brown atrophy
Lipofuscin deposition
Basophilic degeneration
Amyloid deposits
AORTA
Dilated ascending aorta with rightward shift
Elongated (tortuous) thoracic aorta
Sinotubular junction calcific deposits
Elastic fragmentation and collagen accumulation
Atherosclerotic plaque

With advancing age, the amount of epicardial fat increases, particularly over the anterior surface of the right ventricle and in the atrial septum. A reduction in the size of the left ventricular cavity, particularly in the base-to-apex dimension, occurs with aging and may be exacerbated by systemic hypertension and sometimes by bulging of the basal ventricular septum into the left ventricular outflow tract (termed *sigmoid septum*). These changes in the left ventricular cavity can produce a functional outflow obstruction similar to that seen in hypertrophic cardiomyopathy, discussed later in this chapter.

Valvular aging changes include calcification of the mitral annulus and aortic valve, the latter frequently leading to aortic stenosis. In addition, the valves can develop fibrous thickening, and the mitral leaflets tend to buckle back toward the left atrium during ventricular systole, simulating a prolapsing (myxomatous) mitral valve. Moreover, many older persons develop small filiform processes *(Lambl excrescences)* on the closure lines of aortic and mitral valves, probably resulting from the organization of small thrombi.

Compared with younger myocardium, "elderly" myocardium has fewer myocytes, increased collagenized connective tissue and, in some individuals, deposition of amyloid. Lipofuscin deposits (Chapter 1) and *basophilic degeneration*, an accumulation within cardiac myocytes of a gray-blue byproduct of glycogen metabolism, may also be present. Extensive lipofuscin deposition in a small, atrophied heart is called

brown atrophy; this change often accompanies cachexia, as seen in terminal cancer.

Heart Disease: Overview of Pathophysiology

Although many diseases can involve the heart and blood vessels,[8,9] cardiovascular dysfunction results from one or more of six principal mechanisms, most with detectable morphologic manifestations:

- *Failure of the pump.* In the most common circumstance, the cardiac muscle contracts weakly, and the chambers cannot empty properly. In some conditions, the muscle cannot relax sufficiently to permit ventricular filling.
- *Obstruction to flow.* Lesions can obstruct blood flow through a vessel (e.g., atherosclerotic plaque) or prevent valve opening or otherwise cause increased ventricular chamber pressure (e.g., aortic valvular stenosis, systemic hypertension, or aortic coarctation). In the case of a valvular blockage, the increased pressure overworks the chamber that pumps against the obstruction.
- *Regurgitant flow.* In this situation, at least part of the output from each contraction flows backward, adding a volume workload to each of the chambers (e.g., left ventricle in aortic regurgitation; left atrium and left ventricle in mitral regurgitation).
- *Shunted flow.* Blood can be diverted from one part of the heart to another (e.g., from the left ventricle to the right ventricle), through defects that may be congenital or acquired (such as following myocardial infarction). Shunted flow can also occur between blood vessels, as in patent ductus arteriosus.
- *Disorders of cardiac conduction.* Conduction defects or arrhythmias due to uncoordinated generation of impulses (e.g., atrial or ventricular fibrillation) lead to nonuniform and inefficient contractions of the muscular walls.
- *Rupture of the heart or a major vessel.* In such circumstances (e.g., a gunshot wound through the thoracic aorta), there is massive bleeding into body cavities or externally.

Most cardiovascular disease results from a complex interplay of genetics and environmental factors that disrupt networks of genes and signaling pathways that control morphogenesis, myocyte survival and response to injury, biomechanical stress responses, contractility, or electrical conduction.[10] For example, the pathogenesis of many congenital heart defects involves an underlying genetic abnormality whose expression is modified by environmental or maternal factors (see later). Moreover, genes that control the development of the heart may also regulate the response of the heart to aging or to various types of injuries and stresses. As we will discuss, certain types of adult-onset heart disease have a predominantly genetic basis, and it is suspected that genetic polymorphisms in the same genes (or other genes in the same pathways) are likely to modify the risk of many forms of heart disease. These genetic discoveries are providing new insights into the molecular causes of heart disease and are likely to increasingly become part of its diagnosis and classification.

Heart Failure

Heart failure, often called congestive heart failure (CHF), is a common, usually progressive condition with a poor prognosis. Each year in the United States, CHF affects nearly 5 million individuals (approximately 2% of the population), necessitates over 1 million hospitalizations, and is the primary or contributing cause of death of an estimated 300,000 people. It is the leading discharge diagnosis in patients over 65 years of age in the United States and has an associated annual cost of $18 billion.

CHF occurs when the heart is unable to pump blood at a rate sufficient to meet the metabolic demands of the tissues or can do so only at an elevated filling pressure. It can appear during the end stage of many forms of chronic heart disease. In this setting, it most often develops insidiously due to the cumulative effects of chronic work overload (such as in valve disease or hypertension) or ischemic heart disease (e.g., following myocardial infarction with extensive heart damage). However, acute hemodynamic stresses, such as fluid overload, acute valvular dysfunction, or a large myocardial infarction, can cause CHF to appear suddenly.

When cardiac function is impaired or the work load increases, several physiologic mechanisms maintain arterial pressure and perfusion of vital organs. The most important of these are the following:

- *The Frank-Starling mechanism*, in which increased filling volumes dilate the heart and thereby increase functional cross-bridge formation within the sarcomeres, enhancing contractility.
- *Myocardial adaptations, including hypertrophy with or without cardiac chamber dilation.* The collective molecular, cellular, and structural changes that occur as a response to injury or changes in loading conditions are called *ventricular remodeling.*[11] Often adaptive, especially in early stages, these changes can culminate in impaired cardiac function. In many pathologic states, heart failure is preceded by cardiac hypertrophy, the compensatory response of the myocardium to increased mechanical work.
- *Activation of neurohumoral systems*, especially (1) release of norepinephrine by adrenergic cardiac nerves of the autonomic nervous system (which increases heart rate and augments myocardial contractility and vascular resistance); (2) activation of the renin-angiotensin-aldosterone system; and (3) release of atrial natriuretic peptide. The latter two factors act to adjust filling volumes and pressures.

These adaptive mechanisms may be adequate to maintain normal cardiac output in the face of heart disease, but their capacity to do so may ultimately be overwhelmed. Moreover, superimposed pathologic changes, such as myocyte apoptosis, cytoskeletal alterations, and the deposition of extracellular matrix may cause further structural and functional disturbances. Most frequently, heart failure results from progressive deterioration of myocardial contractile function *(systolic dysfunction)*; this may be attributable to ischemic injury, pressure or volume overload due to valvular disease or hypertension,

or dilated cardiomyopathy. Sometimes, however, failure results from an inability of the heart chamber to expand and fill sufficiently during diastole *(diastolic dysfunction)*, as can occur with massive left ventricular hypertrophy, myocardial fibrosis, deposition of amyloid, or constrictive pericarditis (see below).[12]

CARDIAC HYPERTROPHY: PATHOPHYSIOLOGY AND PROGRESSION TO FAILURE

Increased mechanical work due to pressure or volume overload (e.g., systemic hypertension or aortic stenosis), or trophic signals (e.g., those mediated through the activation of β-adrenergic receptors) causes myocytes to increase in size *(hypertrophy)*; cumulatively, this causes an increase in the size and weight of the heart (Fig. 12–1). Hypertrophy is dependent upon increased protein synthesis, which enables the assembly of additional sarcomeres. Hypertrophic myocytes also contain increased numbers of mitochondria and have enlarged nuclei. The latter alteration appears to be due to increases in DNA ploidy, which result from DNA replication in the absence of cell division. The pattern of hypertrophy reflects the nature of the stimulus. In response to increases in pressure (e.g., hypertension or aortic stenosis), ventricles develop *pressure-overload hypertrophy*, which usually causes a concentric increase in wall thickness. In pressure overload, new sarcomeres are predominantly assembled in parallel to the long axes of cells, expanding the cross-sectional area of myocytes. In contrast, *volume-overload hypertrophy* is characterized by ventricular dilation. This is because the new sarcomeres assembled in response to volume overload are largely positioned in series with existing sarcomeres. As a result, in dilation due to volume overload the wall thickness may be increased, normal, or less than normal; thus, heart weight, rather than wall thickness, is the best measure of hypertrophy in volume overloaded hearts.

Cardiac hypertrophy can be substantial in clinical heart disease. Heart weights of two to three times normal are common in patients with systemic hypertension, ischemic heart disease, aortic stenosis, mitral regurgitation, or dilated cardiomyopathy, and heart weights can be threefold to fourfold greater than normal in those with aortic regurgitation or hypertrophic cardiomyopathy.

Important changes at the tissue and cell level occur with cardiac hypertrophy. The increase in myocyte size is not accompanied by a proportional increase in capillary numbers. As a result, the supply of oxygen and nutrients to the hypertrophied heart, particularly one undergoing pressure overload hypertrophy, is more tenuous than in the normal heart. At the same time, oxygen consumption by the hypertrophied heart is elevated due to the increased workload that drives the process. Hypertrophy is also often accompanied by deposition of fibrous tissue. Molecular changes include the expression of immediate-early genes (e.g., *c-fos, c-myc, c-jun,* and *EGR1*) (Chapter 1).[13] With prolonged hemodynamic overload, there may be a shift to a gene expression pattern resembling that seen during fetal cardiac development (including selective expression of embryonic/fetal forms of β-myosin heavy chain, natriuretic peptides, and collagen).

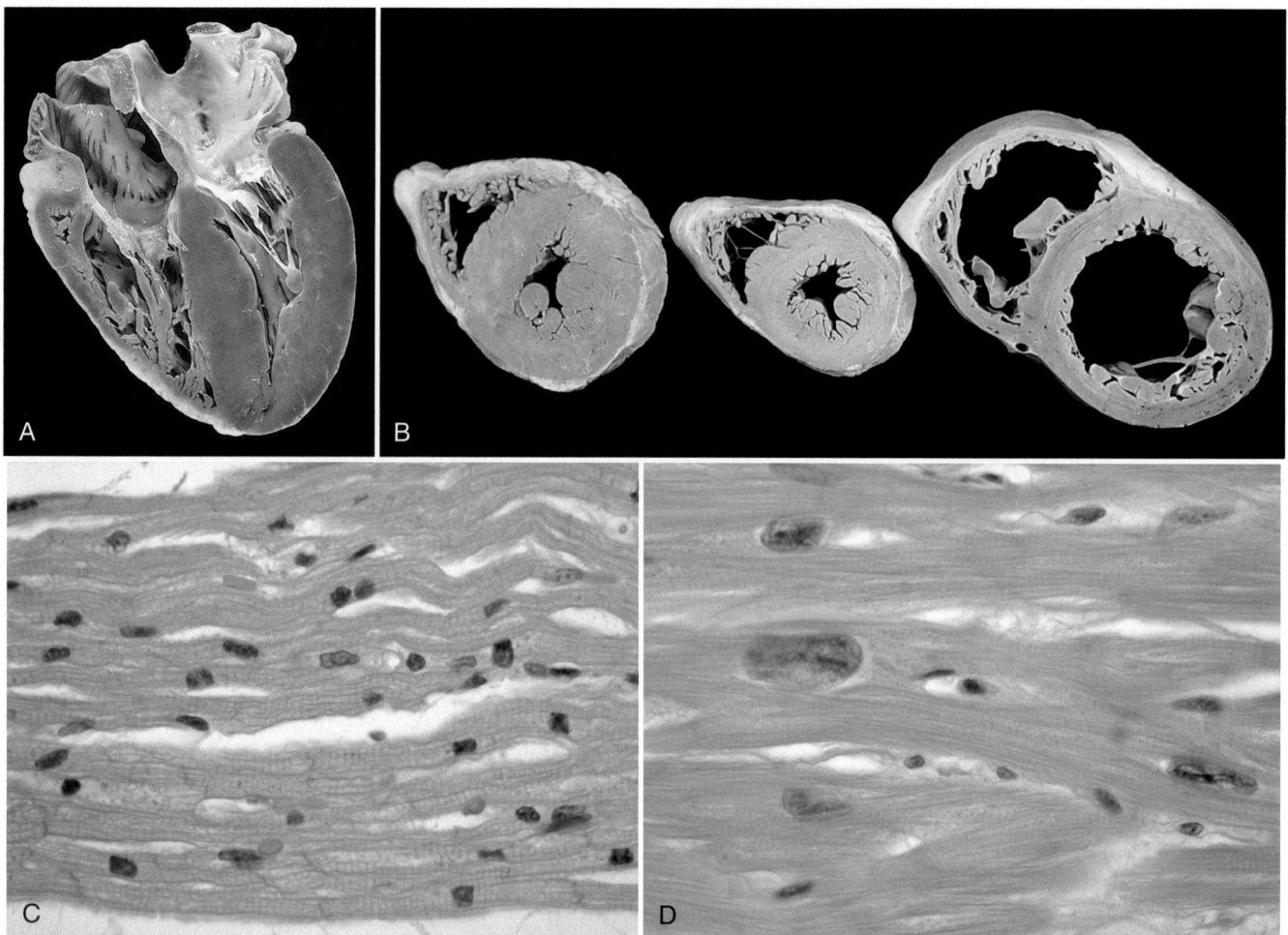

FIGURE 12-1 Left ventricular hypertrophy. **A,** Pressure hypertrophy due to left ventricular outflow obstruction. The left ventricle is on the lower right in this apical four-chamber view of the heart. **B,** Left ventricular hypertrophy with and without dilation, viewed in transverse heart sections. Compared with a normal heart *(center)*, the pressure-hypertrophied hearts *(left* and in **A)** have increased mass and a thick left ventricular wall, while the hypertrophied, dilated heart *(right)* has increased mass and a normal wall thickness. **C,** Normal myocardium. **D,** Hypertrophied myocardium. Note the increases in both cell size and nuclear size in the hypertrophied myocytes. (A,B, Reproduced by permission from Edwards WD: Cardiac anatomy and examination of cardiac specimens. In Emmanouilides GC et al. (eds): Moss and Adams Heart Disease in Infants, Children, and Adolescents: Including the Fetus and Young Adults, 5th ed. Philadelphia, Williams & Wilkins, 1995, p 86.)

At a functional level, cardiac hypertrophy is associated with heightened metabolic demands due to increases in wall tension, heart rate, and contractility (inotropic state, or force of contraction), all of which increase cardiac oxygen consumption. *As a result of these changes, the hypertrophied heart is vulnerable to decompensation,* which can evolve to cardiac failure and eventually lead to death.[14] The proposed sequence of initially beneficial, and later harmful, events in response to increased cardiac work is summarized in Figure 12–2. *The molecular and cellular changes in hypertrophied hearts that initially mediate enhanced function may themselves contribute to the development of heart failure.* This can occur through (1) abnormal myocardial metabolism,[15,16] (2) alterations of intracellular handling of calcium ions, (3) apoptosis of myocytes, and (4) reprogramming of gene expression.[17,18] The latter appears to occur in part through changes in expression of miRNAs, small noncoding RNAs that inhibit the expression of proteins at the level of mRNA stability or translation (Chapter 5). Cardiac hypertrophy is

associated with down-regulation of miR-208 and upregulation of miR-195; of interest, enforced over-expression of miR-195 can produce cardiac hypertrophy and dilation in the mouse, whereas over-expression of miR-208 is protective even in the setting of pressure overload, suggesting a cause and effect relationship.

The degree of structural abnormality of the heart in CHF does not always reflect the level of dysfunction, and the structural, biochemical, and molecular basis for myocardial contractile failure can be obscure. Indeed, it may be impossible from morphologic examination to distinguish a damaged but functional heart from one that has failed. At autopsy, the hearts of patients with CHF are generally heavy, dilated, and thin-walled and exhibit microscopic evidence of hypertrophy, but the extent of these changes is extremely variable. In myocardial infarction, loss of pumping capacity due to myocyte death leads to work-related hypertrophy of the surrounding viable myocardium. In valvular heart disease, the increased pressure or volume overloads the myocardium globally.

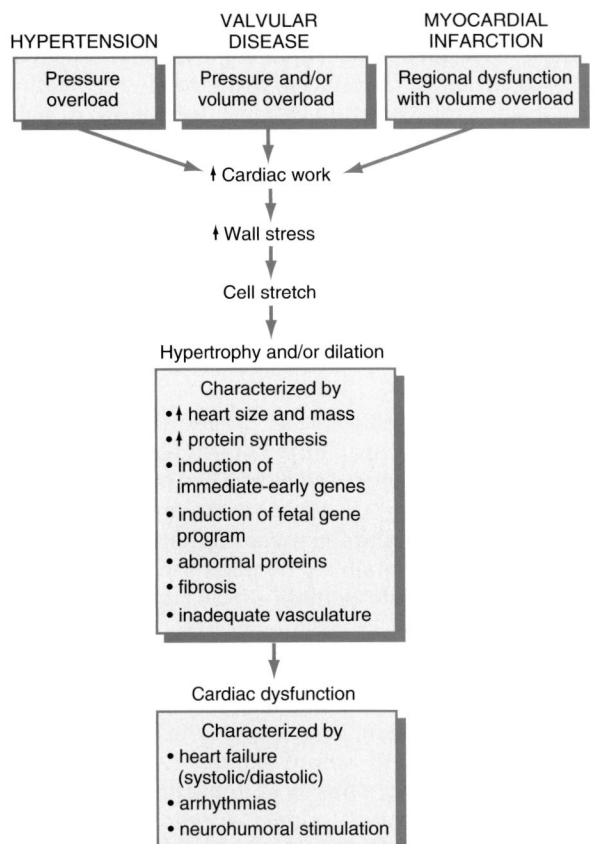

HYPERTENSION — Pressure overload

VALVULAR DISEASE — Pressure and/or volume overload

MYOCARDIAL INFARCTION — Regional dysfunction with volume overload

↑ Cardiac work

↑ Wall stress

Cell stretch

Hypertrophy and/or dilation

Characterized by
• ↑ heart size and mass
• ↑ protein synthesis
• induction of immediate-early genes
• induction of fetal gene program
• abnormal proteins
• fibrosis
• inadequate vasculature

Cardiac dysfunction

Characterized by
• heart failure (systolic/diastolic)
• arrhythmias
• neurohumoral stimulation

FIGURE 12–2 Schematic representation of the causes and consequences of cardiac hypertrophy.

Increased heart mass is correlated with excess cardiac mortality and morbidity; indeed, cardiomegaly is an independent risk factor for sudden death.[19] In contrast to pathologic hypertrophy (which is often associated with contractile impairment), hypertrophy induced by regular strenuous exercise has varied effects on the heart depending on the type of exercise. Aerobic exercise (e.g., long distance running) tends to be associated with volume-load hypertrophy that may be accompanied by increases in capillary density (unlike other forms of hypertrophy) and decreases in resting heart rate and blood pressure, effects that are all beneficial. These changes are sometimes referred to as *physiologic hypertrophy*. Static exercise (e.g., weight lifting) is associated with pressure hypertrophy and appears more likely to be associated with deleterious changes.

Whatever its basis, CHF is characterized by variable degrees of decreased cardiac output and tissue perfusion (sometimes called forward failure), as well as pooling of blood in the venous system (backward failure); the latter may cause pulmonary edema, peripheral edema, or both. Thus, many of the significant clinical features and morphologic changes noted in CHF are secondary to injuries induced by hypoxia and congestion in tissues distant from the heart.

The cardiovascular system is a closed circuit. Thus, although left-sided and right-sided failure can occur independently, failure of one side (particularly the left) often produces excessive strain on the other, terminating in global heart failure.

Despite this interdependency, it is easiest to understand the pathology of heart failure by considering right- and left-sided heart failure separately.

LEFT-SIDED HEART FAILURE

Left-sided heart failure is most often caused by (1) ischemic heart disease, (2) hypertension, (3) aortic and mitral valvular diseases, and (4) myocardial diseases. The morphologic and clinical effects of left-sided CHF primarily result from congestion of the pulmonary circulation, stasis of blood in the left-sided chambers, and hypoperfusion of tissues leading to organ dysfunction.

Morphology.

Heart. The findings in the heart vary depending on the disease process; gross structural abnormalities such as myocardial infarcts or a deformed, stenotic, or regurgitant valve may be present. Except for failure caused by mitral valve stenosis or unusual restrictive cardiomyopathies (described later), the left ventricle is usually hypertrophied and often dilated, sometimes massively. The microscopic changes are non-specific, consisting mainly of myocyte hypertrophy and variable degrees of interstitial fibrosis. The impaired left ventricular function usually causes dilation of the left atrium and increases the risk of atrial fibrillation. This in turn results in stasis, particularly in the atrial appendage, which is a common site of thrombus formation.

Lungs. Pulmonary congestion and **edema** produce heavy, wet lungs, as described elsewhere (Chapters 4 and 15). Pulmonary changes include, in sequence from mildest to most severe, the following: (1) perivascular and interstitial edema, particularly in the interlobular septa, which is responsible for the characteristic Kerley B lines noted on chest roentgenogram; (2) progressive edematous widening of alveolar septa; and (3) accumulation of edema fluid in the alveolar spaces. Some red cells extravasate into the edema fluid within the alveolar spaces, where they are phagocytosed and digested by macrophages, which store the iron recovered from hemoglobin in the form of hemosiderin. These hemosiderin-laden macrophages are telltale signs of previous episodes of pulmonary edema and are often referred to as **heart failure cells**.

Clinically, in early left-sided heart failure symptoms may be quite subtle and are often related to pulmonary congestion and edema. Cough and *dyspnea* (breathlessness), initially with exertion and later at rest, are two of the earliest complaints. As failure progresses, worsening pulmonary edema may lead to *orthopnea* (dyspnea when lying down that is relieved by standing), requiring the patient to sleep in an upright position; or *paroxysmal nocturnal dyspnea*, a form of dyspnea usually occurring at night that is so severe that it induces a feeling of suffocation. Particularly in the setting of *atrial fibrillation*, an arrhythmia characterized by uncoordinated, chaotic contraction of the atrium, stasis greatly increases the risk of thrombosis and thomboembolic stroke.[20]

Decreased cardiac output causes a reduction in renal perfusion, which leads to the activation of the renin-angiotensin-aldosterone system. This in turn induces the retention of salt and water and the expansion of the interstitial and intravascular fluid volumes (Chapters 4 and 11), compensatory effects that can contribute to or exacerbate pulmonary edema. If the hypoperfusion of the kidney becomes sufficiently severe, impaired excretion of nitrogenous products may cause azotemia (called *prerenal azotemia* because of its vascular origin; Chapter 20). In far-advanced CHF, cerebral hypoxia can give rise to *hypoxic encephalopathy* (Chapter 28), with irritability, loss of attention span, and restlessness. In end-stage CHF, this can even progress to stupor and coma.

Left-sided heart failure can be divided on clinical grounds into systolic and diastolic failure. Systolic failure is defined by insufficient cardiac output (pump failure), and can thus be caused by any of the many disorders that damage or derange the contractile function of the left ventricle. In diastolic failure, cardiac output is relatively preserved at rest, but the left ventricle is abnormally stiff or otherwise restricted in its ability to relax during diastole. As a result, the heart is unable to increase its output in response to increases in the metabolic demands of peripheral tissues (e.g., during exercise). Moreover, because the left ventricle cannot expand normally, any increase in filling pressure is immediately referred back to the pulmonary circulation, producing rapid onset pulmonary edema (sometimes referred to as *flash pulmonary edema*), which may be severe. Diastolic failure predominantly occurs in patients over the age of 65 and for unclear reasons is more common in women. Hypertension is the most common underlying etiology. Other risk factors include diabetes mellitus, obesity, and bilateral renal artery stenosis. The reduction in the ability of the left ventricle to relax and fill may stem from myocardial fibrosis (such as occurs in cardiomyopathies and ischemic heart disease), infiltrative disorders associated with restrictive cardiomyopathies (e.g., cardiac amyloidosis), and restrictive pericarditis. Diastolic failure may also appear in elderly patients without any known predisposing factors, possibly as an exaggeration of the normal stiffening of the heart with age, as discussed previously.

RIGHT-SIDED HEART FAILURE

Most commonly, right-sided heart failure is caused by left-sided heart failure, as any increase in pressure in the pulmonary circulation incidental to left-sided failure inevitably burdens the right side of the heart. The causes of right-sided heart failure must then include all of those that induce left-sided heart failure. Pure right-sided heart failure is infrequent and usually occurs in patients with any one of a variety of disorders affecting the lungs; hence, it is often referred to as *cor pulmonale*. Cor pulmonale is most commonly associated with parenchymal diseases of the lung, but can also arise secondary to disorders that affect the pulmonary vasculature (e.g., primary pulmonary hypertension (Chapter 15), recurrent pulmonary thromboembolism (Chapter 4)), or that merely produce hypoxia (e.g., chronic sleep apnea, altitude sickness),

with its associated pulmonary vasoconstriction. *The common feature of these diverse disorders is pulmonary hypertension* (discussed later), which results in hypertrophy and dilation of the right side of the heart. In extreme cases, leftward bulging of the ventricular septum can cause left ventricular dysfunction. The major morphologic and clinical effects of right-sided heart failure differ from those of left-sided heart failure in that pulmonary congestion is minimal, whereas engorgement of the systemic and portal venous systems may be pronounced.

Morphology.

Heart. As in left-heart failure, the morphology varies with cause. Rarely, structural defects such as valvular abnormalities or endocardial fibrosis (as in carcinoid heart disease) may be present. However, since isolated right heart failure is most often caused by lung disease, in a vast majority of cases the only findings are hypertrophy and dilation of the right atrium and ventricle.

Liver and Portal System. Congestion of the hepatic and portal vessels may produce pathologic changes in the liver, the spleen, and the gut. The liver is usually increased in size and weight (**congestive hepatomegaly**) due to prominent **passive congestion** (Chapter 4). Congestion is most prominent around central veins within hepatic lobules, which show red-brown centrilobular discoloration and paler, sometimes fatty, peripheral regions; this combination produces a characteristic appearance that is referred to as "nutmeg liver" (Chapter 4). In some instances, especially when left-sided heart failure is also present, severe central hypoxia produces **centrilobular necrosis**. With long-standing severe right-sided heart failure, the central areas can become fibrotic, creating so-called **cardiac sclerosis** and, in extreme case, **cardiac cirrhosis** (Chapter 18). Portal hypertension produces enlargement of the spleen (**congestive splenomegaly**), which often weighs from 300 to 500 gm (normal, <150 gm); it can also contribute to chronic congestion and edema of the bowel wall, which may be so severe as to interfere with the absorption of nutrients.

Pleural, Pericardial, and Peritoneal Spaces. Systemic venous congestion can lead to accumulation of fluid in the pleural, pericardial, or peritoneal spaces (effusions). Thus, pulmonary edema and pleural effusions are associated with left-sided heart failure. Large pleural effusions (over 1 liter) can cause portions of the corresponding lung to be poorly inflated (atelectasis). In addition, transudation of fluid into the peritoneal cavity may give rise to **ascites**.

Subcutaneous Tissues. Edema of the peripheral and dependent portions of the body, especially ankle (pedal) and pretibial edema, is a hallmark of right-sided heart filure. In chronically bedridden patients presacral edema may predominate. Generalized massive edema (anasarca) may also occur.

The clinical features of isolated right-sided heart failure are those related to systemic (and portal) venous congestion, and include hepatosplenomegaly, peripheral edema, pleural effusions, and ascites. Organs that are prominently affected in right-sided heart failure include the kidney and the brain. Congestion of the kidneys is more marked with right-sided than left-sided heart failure, leading to greater fluid retention and peripheral edema, and more pronounced azotemia. Venous congestion and hypoxia of the central nervous system can produce deficits of mental function that are essentially identical to those described in left-sided heart failure.

Although we have discussed right and left heart failure separately, it is again worth emphasizing that *in many cases of chronic cardiac decompensation, the patient presents in biventricular CHF with symptoms that encompass the clinical syndromes of both right-sided and left-sided heart failure.* Standard therapy for CHF relies mainly on pharmacologic approaches. Drugs that relieve fluid overload (e.g., diuretics), that block the renin-angiotensin-aldosterone axis (e.g., angiotensin converting enzyme inhibitors), and that lower adrenergic tone (e.g., β_1-adrenergic blockers) are particularly useful. The efficacy of the latter two classes of drugs supports the idea that the neurohumoral changes that are seen in CHF (including elevated circulating levels of norepinephrine and renin) are maladaptive and contribute to heart failure. Newer approaches to improving cardiac function include devices that provide the heart with a mechanical assist, and resynchronization of electrical impulses to maximize cardiac efficiency. Because of the prevalence and severity of CHF, there is considerable interest in novel therapies, including cell-based approaches.[21] Of note in this regard, a growing body of evidence indicates that the adult heart may have limited capacity for stem cell–mediated self-renewal. Whether and to what extent this potential can be harnessed to therapeutic advantage is not yet known.[22]

Congenital Heart Disease

Congenital heart disease is a general term used to describe abnormalities of the heart or great vessels that are present from birth. Most such disorders arise from faulty embryogenesis during gestational weeks 3 through 8, when major cardiovascular structures form and begin to function. The most severe anomalies are incompatible with intrauterine survival. Congenital heart defects compatible with embryologic maturation and birth generally affect individual chambers or discrete regions of the heart, with the remainder of the heart developing relatively normally. Examples are infants born with a defect in septation ("hole in the heart"), such as an atrial septal defect (ASD) or a ventricular septal defect (VSD), stenotic valvular lesions, or with abnormalities in the coronary arteries.[23] Some forms of congenital heart disease produce clinically important manifestations soon after birth, which are frequently brought on by the change from fetal to postnatal circulatory patterns (with reliance on the lungs for oxygenation birth, rather than the placenta as in intrauterine life). Approximately half of congenital cardiovascular malformations are diagnosed in the first year of life, but some mild forms may not become evident until adulthood (e.g., ASD).

TABLE 12–2 Frequencies of Congenital Cardiac Malformations*

Malformation	Incidence per Million Live Births	%
Ventricular septal defect	4482	42
Atrial septal defect	1043	10
Pulmonary stenosis	836	8
Patent ductus arteriosus	781	7
Tetralogy of Fallot	577	5
Coarctation of the aorta	492	5
Atrioventricular septal defect	396	4
Aortic stenosis	388	4
Transposition of the great arteries	388	4
Truncus arteriosus	136	1
Total anomalous pulmonary venous connection	120	1
Tricuspid atresia	118	1
TOTAL	9757	

*Presented as upper quartile of 44 published studies. Percentages do not add up to 100% because of rounding.
Source: Hoffman JIE, Kaplan S: The incidence of congenital heart disease. J Am Coll Cardiol 39:1890, 2002.

Incidence. With an incidence of approximately 1% (estimates range from 4 to 50 per 1000 live births), congenital cardiovascular defects are among the most prevalent malformations and are the most common type of heart disease among children.[24] The incidence is higher in premature infants and in stillborns. Twelve disorders account for about 85% of cases; their frequencies are presented in Table 12–2.

The number of individuals who have survived with congenital heart disease into adulthood is increasing rapidly and is presently estimated at nearly 1 million individuals in the United States.[25] Many of those with congenital heart disease have benefited greatly from rapid advances in the surgical and interventional repair of various structural heart defects. Nevertheless, such repairs may not restore the heart to normal; in such instances, patients may suffer from arrhythmias or ventricular dysfunction, and require additional surgery.[26] Other factors that impact the long-term outcome include risks associated with the use of prosthetic materials and devices,[27] such as substitute valves or myocardial patches, and maternal risks associated with childbearing.[28]

Cardiac Development. The diverse malformations seen in congenital heart disease are caused by errors that occur during cardiac development; thus, a brief review how the heart normally forms is in order before discussing the specific defects (Fig. 12–3). The fine details of this complex process are beyond our scope here. Suffice it to say that the earliest cardiac precursors originate in lateral mesoderm and move to the mid-line in two migratory waves to create a crescent of cells consisting of the first and second heart fields by about day 15 of development.[29,30] Each heart field is marked by the expression of different sets of genes; for example, the first heart field expresses the transcription factors TBX5 and Hand1, whereas the

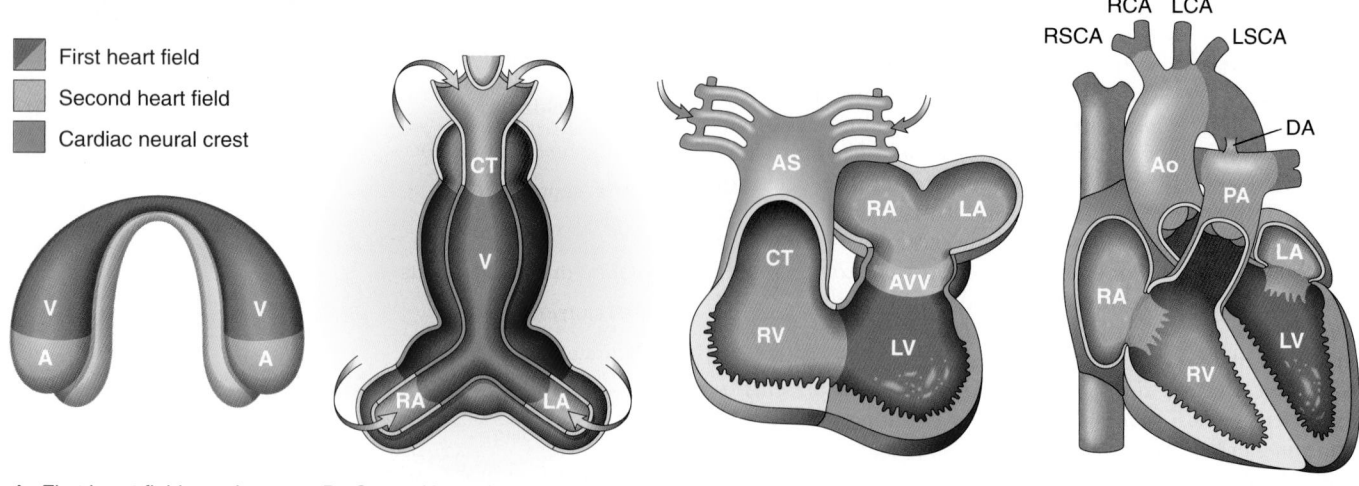

A First heart field template   B Second heart field migration   C   Neural crest migration   D Completed formation of
                                                                                                                four-chambered heart

FIGURE 12–3   Human cardiac development, emphasizing the three sources of cells. **A,** Day 15. First heart field (FHF) cells (shown in red) form a crescent shape in the anterior embryo with second heart field (SHF) cells (shown in yellow) near the FHF. **B,** Day 21. SHF cells lie dorsal to the straight heart tube and begin to migrate *(arrows)* into the anterior and posterior ends of the tube to form the right ventricle (RV), conotruncus (CT), and part of the atria (A). **C,** Day 28. Following rightward looping of the heart tube, cardiac neural crest cells (shown in blue) also migrate *(arrow)* into the outflow tract from the neural folds to septate the outflow tract and pattern the bilaterally symmetric aortic arch arteries (III, IV, and VI). **D,** Day 50. Septation of the ventricles, atria, and atrioventricular valves (AVV) results in the appropriately configured four-chambered heart. Ao, aorta; AS, aortic sac; DA, ductus arteriosus; LA, left atrium; LCA, left carotid artery; LSCA, left subclavian artery; LV, left ventricle; PA, pulmonary artery; RA, right atrium; RCA, right carotid artery; RSCA, right subclavian artery; V, ventricle. (Modified by permission from Srivastava D: Making or breaking the heart: from lineage determination to morphogenesis. Cell 126:1037, 2006.)

second heart field expresses the transcription factor Hand2 and fibroblast growth factor-10. Both fields contain multipotent progenitor cells that can produce all of the major cell types of the heart; endocardium, myocardium, and smooth muscle cells. As an aside, there is considerable interest in the therapeutic potential of such early cardiac progenitors, which could conceivably be used to regenerate portions of the adult heart that are damaged or otherwise dysfunctional.

Even at this very early stage of development, each heart field is destined to give rise to particular portions of the heart. Cells derived from the first heart field mainly give rise to the left ventricle, whereas cells derived from the second heart field give rise to the outflow tract, right ventricle, and most of the atria. By day 20, the initial cell crescent develops into a beating tube, which loops to the right and begins to form the heart chambers by day 28. Around this time, two other critical events occur: (1) cells derived from the neural crest migrate into the outflow tract, where they participate in the septation of the outflow tract and the formation of the aortic arches; and (2) the extracellular matrix (ECM) underlying the future atrioventricular canal and outflow tract enlarges to produce swellings known as endocardial cushions. This process depends on the delamination of a subset of endocardial cells, which invade the ECM and subsequently proliferate and differentiate into the mesenchymal cells that are responsible for valve development. By day 50, further septation of the ventricles, atria, and atrioventricular valves produces the four-chambered heart.

Proper orchestration of these remarkable transformations depends on a network of transcription factors that are regulated by a number of signaling pathways, particularly the Wnt, VEGF, bone morphogenetic factor, TGF-β, fibroblast growth

factor, and Notch pathways. It should also be remembered that the heart is a mechanical organ that is exposed to flowing blood from its earliest stages of development. It is likely that hemodynamic forces play an important role in cardiac development, just as they influence adaptations in the adult heart such as hypertrophy and dilation. In addition, specific micro-RNAs play critical roles in cardiac development by coordinating patterns and levels of transcription factor expression.[18]

Many of the genetic defects that affect heart development are autosomal dominant mutations that cause partial loss of function in one or another required factor, which are often transcription factors (discussed below). Thus, even relatively minor changes in the activity of one of the many factors necessary for normal development can lead to defects in the final product, the fully developed heart. It can be imagined (but is unproved) that transient environmental stresses during the first trimester of pregnancy that alter the activity of these same genes might give rise to defects resembling those produced by inherited mutations.

Etiology and Pathogenesis. *The main known causes of congenital heart disease consist of sporadic genetic abnormalities*, which can take the form of single gene mutations, small chromosomal deletions, and additions or deletions of whole chromosomes (trisomies and monosomies). In the case of single gene mutations, the affected genes encode proteins belonging to several different functional classes, examples of which are provided in Table 12–3. Many of these mutations affect genes encoding transcription factors that are required for normal heart development. Since the affected patients are heterozygous for these mutations, it follows that a 50% reduction in the activity of these factors is probably sufficient to derange cardiac development. Some of the affected transcription

TABLE 12–3	Selected Examples of Genetic Causes of Congenital Heart Disease		
Affected Gene(s)	**Normal Function**	**Syndrome Name**	**Congenital Cardiac Disease**
Non-syndromic			
NKX2–5	Transcription factor	—	ASD, VSD, conduction defects
GATA-4*	Transcription factor	—	ASD, VSD
TBX20*	Transcription factor	—	ASD, VSD, valve abnormalities
Syndromic			
TBX5	Transcription factor	Holt-Oram	ASD, VSD, Conduction defects
TBX1	Transcription factor	DiGeorge	Cardiac outflow tract defects
JAG1, NOTCH2	Notch signaling	Alagille	Pulmonary artery stenosis, Tetralogy of Fallot
Fibrillin	Structural protein TGFβ signaling	Marfan	Aortic aneurysm Valve abnormalities

*Associated with adult-onset cardiomyopathy. ASD, atrial septal defect; VSD, ventricular septal defect (Modified by permission from Srivastava D: Making or breaking the heart: from lineage determination to morphogenesis. Cell 126:1037, 2006.)

factors appear to work together in large protein complexes, providing an explanation for why mutations in any one of several genes produce similar defects. For example, GATA4, TBX5, and NKX2-5, three transcription factors that are mutated in some patients with atrial and ventricular septal defects, all bind to one another and co-regulate the expression of target genes that are required for the proper development of the heart. Of further interest, GATA4 and TBX20 are also mutated in rare forms of adult-onset cardiomyopathy (discussed later), indicating that they are not only important developmentally but are also needed to maintain the function of the postnatal heart.

Other single gene mutations associated with congenital heart disease affect proteins within signaling pathways or that have structural roles. Mutations in genes encoding various components of the Notch pathway, such as JAGGED1, NOTCH1, and NOTCH2, are associated with a number of different congenital heart defects, including bicuspid aortic valve (NOTCH1, discussed later) and Tetralogy of Fallot (JAGGED1 and NOTCH2).[29,30] As you will recall from Chapter 11, fibrillin mutations underlie Marfan syndrome, which is associated with valvular defects and aortic aneurysms. Although fibrillin was initially described as a structural protein, it is also an important negative regulator of TGFβ signaling, and hyperactive TGFβ signaling is at least partially responsible for the cardiovascular abnormalities in Marfan syndrome.

A notable example of a small chromosomal lesion that causes congenital heart disease is deletion of chromosome 22q11.2, which is found in up to 50% of patients with DiGeorge syndrome. In this syndrome the fourth branchial arch and the derivatives of the third and fourth pharyngeal pouches, which contribute to the formation of the thymus, parathyroids, and heart, develop abnormally. One candidate gene in the deleted region is TBX1, which encodes a transcription factor that regulates the expansion of cardiac progenitors in the second heart field. Other important genetic causes of congenital heart disease include chromosomal aneuploidies, particularly Turner syndrome (monosomy X) and trisomies 13, 18, and 21.[31] Indeed, *the most common genetic cause of congenital heart*

disease is trisomy 21 (Down syndrome),[32] in which about 40% of patients have one or more heart defects, most often affecting structures derived from the endocardial cushions (e.g., the atrioventricular septae and valves). The mechanisms by which aneuploidy leads to congenital heart defects remain largely unknown, but are likely to involve the dysregulated expression of multiple genes.

Beyond these known associations, more subtle forms of genetic variation probably also contribute to congenital heart disease. This assertion is based in part on the recognition that first-degree relatives of affected patients are at increased risk for congenital heart defects compared to the general population. For example, a child of a father with a VSD has a risk of 2%; if the VSD occurred in the mother, the risk to her offspring is 6% to 10%.

Despite these genetic clues, it must be acknowledged that our understanding of the mechanisms that lead to heart defects remains rudimentary. Most affected patients have no identifiable genetic risk factor, and even in those that do, the nature and severity of the defect are highly variable. As a result, it is thought that *environmental factors*, alone or in combination with genetic factors, also contribute to congenital heart disease and in some cases may be the primary cause. Examples of known exposures that are associated with heart defects include congenital rubella infection, gestational diabetes, and exposure to teratogens (including some therapeutic drugs).[33] There is also great interest in identifying nutritional factors that may modify risk. For instance, intake of multivitamin supplements containing folate may reduce the risk of congenital heart defects.[34]

Clinical Features. The varied structural anomalies in congenital heart disease fall primarily into three major categories:

- Malformations causing a *left-to-right shunt*
- Malformations causing a *right-to-left shunt*
- Malformations causing an *obstruction*.

A *shunt* is an abnormal communication between chambers or blood vessels. Abnormal channels permit the flow of blood down pressure gradients from the left (systemic) side to the right (pulmonary) side of the circulation or vice versa. When blood from the right side of the circulation flows directly into the left side *(right-to-left shunt)*, hypoxemia and *cyanosis* (a dusky blueness of the skin and mucous membranes) result because of the admixture of poorly oxygenated venous blood with systemic arterial blood (called *cyanotic congenital heart disease*). The most important congenital causes of right-to-left shunts are tetralogy of Fallot, transposition of the great arteries, persistent truncus arteriosus, tricuspid atresia, and total anomalous pulmonary venous connection. Moreover, with right-to-left shunts, emboli arising in peripheral veins can bypass the lungs and directly enter the systemic circulation *(paradoxical embolism)*; brain infarction and abscess are potential consequences. Severe, long-standing cyanosis also causes *clubbing of the tips of the fingers and toes* (called hypertrophic osteoarthropathy) and polycythemia.

In contrast, *left-to-right shunts* (such as ASD, VSD, and patent ductus arteriosus) increase pulmonary blood flow and are not initially associated with cyanosis. However, left-to-right shunts raise both flow volumes and pressures in the normally low-pressure, low-resistance pulmonary circulation, which can lead to right ventricular hypertrophy and atherosclerosis of the pulmonary vasculature. The muscular pulmonary arteries (<1 mm diameter) first respond to increased pressure and flow by undergoing medial hypertrophy and vasoconstriction, which maintains relatively normal distal pulmonary capillary and venous pressures, and prevents pulmonary edema. Prolonged pulmonary arterial vasoconstriction, however, stimulates the proliferation of the vascular wall cells and the consequent development of irreversible obstructive intimal lesions analogous to the arteriolar changes seen in systemic hypertension (Chapter 11). Eventually, pulmonary vascular resistance approaches systemic levels, thereby producing a new right-to-left shunt that introduces unoxygenated blood into the systemic circulation *(late cyanotic congenital heart disease, or Eisenmenger syndrome)*.

Once irreversible pulmonary hypertension develops, the structural defects of congenital heart disease are considered irreparable. The secondary pulmonary vascular changes can eventually lead to the patient's death. This provides the rationale for early intervention, either surgical or nonsurgical, in those with left-to-right shunts.

Some developmental anomalies of the heart (e.g., coarctation of the aorta, aortic valvular stenosis, and pulmonary valvular stenosis) produce abnormal narrowing of chambers, valves, or blood vessels and therefore are called *obstructive congenital heart disease*. A complete obstruction is called an *atresia*. In some disorders (e.g., Tetralogy of Fallot), an obstruction (pulmonary stenosis) and a shunt (right-to-left through a VSD) are both present.

The altered hemodynamics of congenital heart disease usually cause cardiac dilation or hypertrophy (or both). However, some defects induce a decrease in the volume and muscle mass of a cardiac chamber; this is called *hypoplasia* if it occurs before birth and *atrophy* if it develops postnatally.

LEFT-TO-RIGHT SHUNTS

The most commonly encountered left-to-right shunts include ASDs, VSDs, patent ductus arteriosus, and atrioventricular septal defects, and are shown in Figure 12–4.

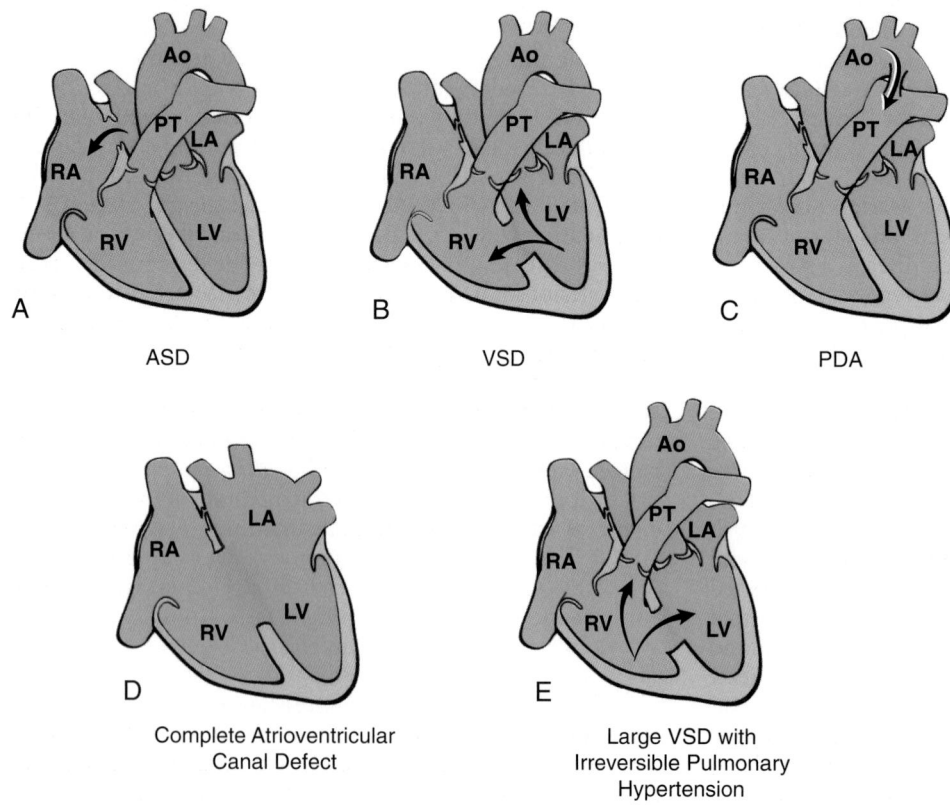

FIGURE 12–4 Schematic of congenital left-to-right shunts. *Arrows* indicate the direction of blood flow. **A,** Atrial septal defect (ASD). **B,** Ventricular septal defect (VSD). With VSD the shunt is left-to-right, and the pressures are the same in both ventricles. Pressure hypertrophy of the right ventricle and volume hypertrophy of the left ventricle are generally present. **C,** Patent ductus arteriosus (PDA). **D,** Atrioventricular septal defect (AVSD). **E,** Large VSD with irreversible pulmonary hypertension. The shunt is right-to-left (shunt reversal). Volume hypertrophy and pressure hypertrophy of the right ventricle are present. The right ventricular pressure is now sufficient to yield a right-to-left shunt. Ao, aorta; LA, left atrium; LV, left ventricle; PT, pulmonary trunk; RA, right atrium; RV, right ventricle.

A   ASD

B   VSD

C   PDA

D   Complete Atrioventricular Canal Defect

E   Large VSD with Irreversible Pulmonary Hypertension

Atrial Septal Defect

An atrial septal defect (ASD) is an abnormal, fixed opening in the atrial septum caused by incomplete tissue formation that allows communication of blood between the left and right atria (not to be confused with patent foramen ovale, see below). ASDs are usually asymptomatic until adulthood (Fig. 12–4A).[35]

> **Morphology.** The three major types of ASDs are classified according to their location as secundum, primum, and sinus venosus. **Secundum ASDs** (90% of all ASDs) result from a deficient or fenestrated oval fossa near the center of the atrial septum. These are usually not associated with other anomalies, and may be of any size, be single or multiple, or be fenestrated. **Primum** anomalies (5% of ASDs) occur adjacent to the AV valves. **Sinus venosus** defects (5%) are located near the entrance of the superior vena cava and may be associated with anomalous pulmonary venous return to the right atrium.

Clinical Features. ASDs result in a left-to-right shunt, largely because pulmonary vascular resistance is considerably less than systemic vascular resistance and because the compliance (distensibility) of the right ventricle is much greater than that of the left. Pulmonary blood flow may be two to four times normal. A murmur is often present as a result of excessive flow through the pulmonary valve. Despite the right-sided volume overload, ASDs are generally well tolerated and usually do not become symptomatic before age 30; irreversible pulmonary hypertension is unusual. Surgical or catheter-based closure of an ASD reverses the hemodynamic abnormalities and prevents complications, including heart failure, paradoxical embolization, and irreversible pulmonary vascular disease.[36] Mortality is low, and long-term survival is comparable to that of a normal population.

Patent Foramen Ovale

A patent foramen ovale is a small hole created by an open flap of tissue in the atrial septum at the oval fossa.[37] In the fetus, the foramen ovale is an important functional right-to-left shunt that allows oxygen-rich blood from the placenta to bypass the not yet inflated lungs by traveling directly from the right to left atrium. The hole is forced shut at birth as a result of increased blood pressure on the left side of the heart, and the tissue flap closes permanently in approximately 80% of people. In the remaining 20% of people, the unsealed flap can open when there is more pressure on the right side of the heart. Thus, sustained pulmonary hypertension or even transient increases in right-sided pressures, such as occurs during a bowel movement, coughing, or sneezing, can produce brief periods of right-to-left shunting, with the possibility of paradoxical embolism.[38]

Ventricular Septal Defect

Incomplete closure of the ventricular septum, allowing free communication of blood between the left to right ventricles, is the most common form of congenital cardiac anomaly (Fig.

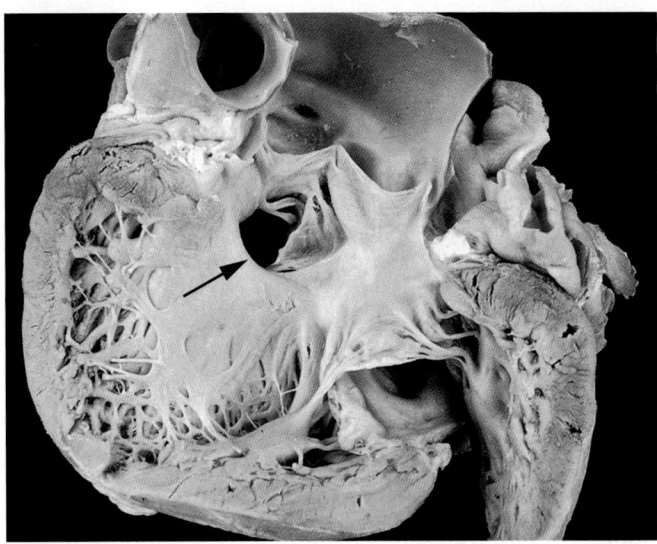

FIGURE 12–5 A ventricular septal defect (membranous type), denoted by the *arrow*. (Courtesy of William D. Edwards, MD, Mayo Clinic, Rochester, MN.)

12–4B). Most ventricular septal defects (VSDs) are associated with other congenital cardiac anomalies such as tetralogy of Fallot; only 20% to 30% are isolated.

> **Morphology.** VSDs are classified according to their size and location. Most are about the size of the aortic valve orifice. About 90% involve the region of the membranous interventricular septum (membranous VSD) (Fig. 12–5). The remainder lie below the pulmonary valve (infundibular VSD) or within the muscular septum. Although most VSDs are single, those in the muscular septum may be multiple (so-called "Swisscheese" septum).

Clinical Features. The functional consequences of a VSD depend on the size of the defect and whether there are associated with right-sided malformations. Large VSDs cause difficulties virtually from birth; smaller lesions are generally well tolerated for years, and may not be recognized until much later in life. Approximately 50% of small muscular VSDs close spontaneously.[39] Large defects are usually membranous or infundibular, and they generally cause significant left-to-right shunting, leading to right ventricular hypertrophy and pulmonary hypertension virtually from birth. Over time, irreversible pulmonary vascular disease develops in essentially all persons with large unclosed VSDs, ultimately resulting in shunt reversal, cyanosis, and death. Surgical or catheter-based closure of asymptomatic VSDs is generally delayed beyond infancy, in hope of spontaneous closure. Early correction, however, must be performed in babies with large defects to prevent the development of irreversible obstructive pulmonary vascular disease.

Patent Ductus Arteriosus

Patent (also called persistent) ductus arteriosus (PDA) results when the ductus arteriosus, an essential fetal structure that normally spontaneously closes, remains open after birth (see

Fig. 12–4C). In the fetal circulation the ductus arteriosus shunts blood from the pulmonary artery to the aorta, which (like the patent foramen ovale) serves to bypass the lungs. About 90% of PDAs occur as an isolated anomaly. The remainder are most often associated with VSD, coarctation of the aorta, or pulmonary or aortic valve stenosis.

PDA produces a characteristic continuous harsh murmur, described as "machinery-like". The clinical impact of a PDA depends on its diameter and the cardiovascular status of the individual.[40] PDA is usually asymptomatic at birth, and a narrow PDA may have no effect on the child's growth and development. Because the shunt is at first left-to-right, there is no cyanosis, but eventually the additional volume and pressure overload produce obstructive changes in small pulmonary arteries, leading to reversal of flow and its associated consequences.

There is general agreement that an isolated PDA should be closed as early in life as is feasible. Conversely, preservation of ductal patency (by administering prostaglandin E) assumes great importance in the survival of infants with various congenital malformations that obstruct the pulmonary or systemic outflow tracts. For example, in aortic valve atresia a PDA provides the bulk of the systemic blood flow. Depending on the context, therefore, a PDA may be either life-threatening or lifesaving.

Atrioventricular Septal Defect

Atrioventricular septal defect (AVSD, also called complete atrioventricular canal defect) results from the embryologic failure of the superior and inferior endocardial cushions of the AV canal to fuse adequately. The consequence is incomplete closure of the AV septum and malformation of the tricuspid and mitral valves (see Fig. 12–4D). The two most common forms are *partial* AVSD (consisting of a primum ASD and a cleft anterior mitral leaflet, causing mitral insufficiency) and *complete* AVSD (consisting of a large combined AV septal defect and a large common AV valve—essentially a hole in the center of the heart). In the complete form, all four cardiac chambers freely communicate, inducing volume hypertrophy of each. More than one third of all patients with a complete AVSD have Down syndrome. Surgical repair is possible.

RIGHT-TO-LEFT SHUNTS

The diseases in this group cause cyanosis early in postnatal life (*cyanotic* congenital heart disease). Tetralogy of Fallot, the most common in this group, and transposition of the great arteries are illustrated schematically in Figure 12–6. The others include persistent truncus arteriosus, tricuspid atresia, and total anomalous pulmonary venous connection.

Tetralogy of Fallot

The four cardinal features of the tetralogy of Fallot (TOF) are (1) VSD, (2) obstruction of the right ventricular outflow tract (subpulmonary stenosis), (3) an aorta that overrides the VSD, and (4) right ventricular hypertrophy (Fig. 12–6A). All of the features result embryologically from anterosuperior displacement of the infundibular septum.

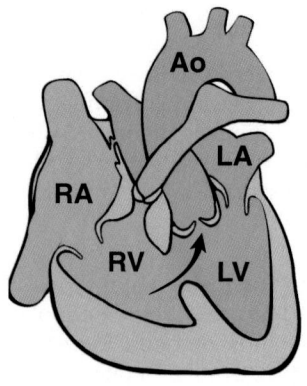

A   Classic Tetralogy of Fallot

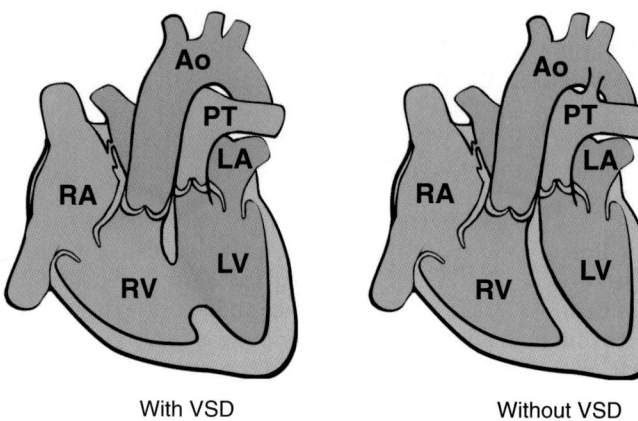

With VSD   Without VSD

B   Complete Transposition

FIGURE 12–6 Schematic of the most important right-to-left shunts *(cyanotic congenital heart disease).* **A,** Classic tetralogy of Fallot. The direction of shunting across the ventricular septal defect (VSD) depends on the degree of the subpulmonary stenosis; when severe, a right-to-left shunt results *(arrow).* **B,** Transposition of the great arteries with and without VSD. Ao, aorta; LA, left atrium; LV, left ventricle; PT, pulmonary trunk; RA, right atrium; RV, right ventricle. (Courtesy of William D. Edwards, MD, Mayo Clinic, Rochester, MN.)

Morphology. The heart is often enlarged and may be "boot-shaped" as a result of marked right ventricular hypertrophy, particularly of the apical region. The VSD is usually large. The aortic valve forms the superior border of the VSD, thereby overriding the defect and both ventricular chambers. The obstruction to right ventricular outflow is most often due to narrowing of the infundibulum (subpulmonic stenosis) but can be accompanied by pulmonary valvular stenosis. Sometimes there is complete atresia of the pulmonary valve and variable portions of the pulmonary arteries, such that blood flow through a patent ductus arteriosus, dilated bronchial arteries, or both, is necessary for survival. Aortic valve insufficiency or an ASD may also be present; a right aortic arch is present in about 25% of cases.

Clinical Features. Even untreated, some patients with TOF survive into adult life (in reports of untreated patients with this condition, 10% were alive at 20 years and 3% at 40 years).[49] The clinical consequences depend primarily on the severity of the subpulmonary stenosis, as this determines the direction of blood flow. If the subpulmonary stenosis is mild, the abnormality resembles an isolated VSD, and the shunt may be left-to-right, without cyanosis (so-called pink tetralogy). As the obstruction increases in severity, there is commensurately greater resistance to right ventricular outflow. *As right-sided pressures approach or exceed left-sided pressures, right-to-left shunting develops, producing cyanosis (classic TOF).* With increasingly severe subpulmonic stenosis, the pulmonary arteries become progressively smaller and thinner walled (hypoplastic), and the aorta grows progressively larger in diameter. As the child grows and the heart increases in size, the pulmonic orifice does not expand proportionally, making the obstruction progressively worse. Most infants with TOF are cyanotic from birth or soon thereafter. The subpulmonary stenosis, however, protects the pulmonary vasculature from pressure overload, and right ventricular failure is rare because the right ventricle is decompressed by the shunting of blood into the left ventricle and aorta. Complete surgical repair is possible for classic TOF but is more complicated for persons with pulmonary atresia and dilated bronchial arteries.

Transposition of the Great Arteries

Transposition of the great arteries (TGA) produces ventriculoarterial discordance: the aorta arises from the right ventricle, and lies anterior and to the right of the pulmonary artery, which emanates from the left ventricle (Fig. 12–7; see also Fig. 12–5B). The AV connections are normal (concordant), with the right atrium joining the right ventricle and the left atrium emptying into the left ventricle. The embryologic defect in complete TGA stems from abnormal formation of the truncal and aortopulmonary septa. The result is separation of the systemic and pulmonary circulations, a condition incompatible with postnatal life unless a shunt exists for adequate mixing of blood.

The outlook for infants with TGA depends on the degree of "mixing" of the blood, the magnitude of the tissue hypoxia, and the ability of the right ventricle to maintain the systemic circulation. Patients with TGA and a VSD (~35%) may have a stable shunt. Those with only a patent foramen ovale or ductus arteriosus (~65%), however, have unstable shunts that tend to close and therefore require immediate intervention to create a new shunt (such as balloon atrial septostomy) within the first few days of life. Right ventricular hypertrophy becomes prominent, because this chamber functions as the systemic ventricle. Concurrently, the left ventricle becomes thin-walled (atrophic) as it supports the low-resistance pulmonary circulation. Without surgery, most patients die during the first few months of life. However, as a result of considerable improvements in surgical repair over the past several decades, many persons with TGA now survive to adulthood.[41]

Persistent Truncus Arteriosus

Persistent truncus arteriosus (PTA) arises from a developmental failure of separation of the embryologic truncus arteriosus into the aorta and pulmonary artery. This results in a single great artery that receives blood from both ventricles and gives rise to the systemic, pulmonary, and coronary circulations.

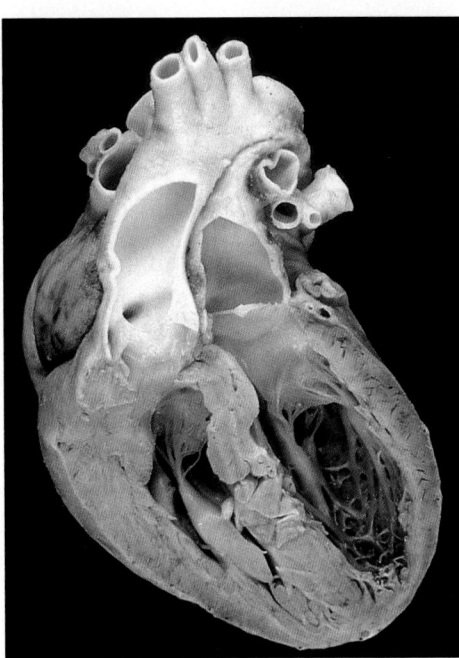

FIGURE 12–7   Transposition of the great arteries. (Courtesy of William D. Edwards, MD, Mayo Clinic, Rochester, MN.)

Because there is an associated VSD and mixing of blood from the right and left ventricles, PTA produces systemic cyanosis as well as increased pulmonary blood flow, with the danger of irreversible pulmonary hypertension.

Tricuspid Atresia

Complete occlusion of the tricuspid valve orifice is known as *tricuspid atresia.* It results embryologically from unequal division of the AV canal; thus, the mitral valve is larger than normal, and there is almost always underdevelopment (hypoplasia) of the right ventricle. The circulation is maintained to some degree by a right-to-left shunt through an interatrial communication (ASD or patent foramen ovale) and a VSD, which affords communication between the left ventricle and the pulmonary artery that arises from the hypoplastic right ventricle. Cyanosis is present virtually from birth, and there is a high mortality in the first weeks or months of life.

Total Anomalous Pulmonary Venous Connection

Total anomalous pulmonary venous connection (TAPVC), in which the pulmonary veins fail to directly join the left atrium, results embryologically when the common pulmonary vein fails to develop or becomes atretic. Fetal development is made possible by primitive systemic venous channels that usually drain from the lung into the left innominate vein or to the coronary sinus. Either a patent foramen ovale or an ASD is always present, allowing pulmonary venous blood to enter the left atrium. Consequences of TAPVC include volume and pressure hypertrophy and dilation of the right side of the heart, and dilation of the pulmonary trunk. The left atrium is hypoplastic, but the left ventricle is usually normal in size. Cyanosis may be present as a result of mixing of

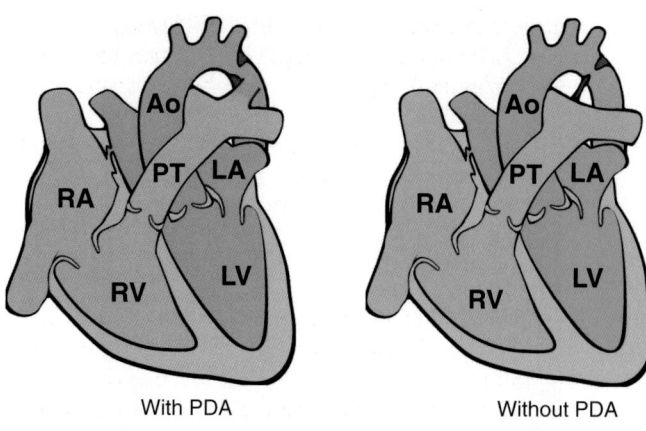

With PDA   Without PDA

Coarctation of Aorta

FIGURE 12–8   Diagram showing coarctation of the aorta with and without patent ductus arteriosus (PDA). Ao, aorta; LA, left atrium; LV, left ventricle; PT, pulmonary trunk; RA, right atrium; RV, right ventricle; PDA, patent ductus arteriosus. (Courtesy of William D. Edwards, MD, Mayo Clinic, Rochester, MN.)

well-oxygenated and poorly oxygenated blood at the site of the anomalous pulmonary venous connection and large right-to-left shunting through an ASD.

OBSTRUCTIVE CONGENITAL ANOMALIES

Congenital obstruction to blood flow may occur at the level of the heart valves or within a great vessel.[42] Relatively common examples include stenosis or atresia of the aortic or pulmonary valves, and coarctation of the aorta. Obstruction can also occur within a chamber, as with subpulmonary stenosis in TOF.

Coarctation of the Aorta

Coarctation (narrowing, constriction) of the aorta ranks high in frequency among the common structural anomalies. Males are affected twice as often as females, although females with Turner syndrome frequently have a coarctation (Chapter 5). Two classic forms have been described: (1) an "infantile" form with tubular hypoplasia of the aortic arch proximal to a patent ductus arteriosus that is often symptomatic in early childhood, and (2) an "adult" form in which there is a discrete ridgelike infolding of the aorta, just opposite the closed ductus arteriosus *(ligamentum arteriosum)* distal to the arch vessels (Fig. 12–8). Encroachment on the aortic lumen is of variable severity, sometimes leaving only a small channel and at other times producing only minimal narrowing. Although coarctation of the aorta may occur as a solitary defect, it is accompanied by a bicuspid aortic valve in 50% of cases and may also be associated with congenital aortic stenosis, ASD, VSD, mitral regurgitation, or berry aneurysms of the circle of Willis in the brain.

Clinical manifestations depend on the severity of the narrowing and the patency of the ductus arteriosus. *Coarctation of the aorta with a patent ductus arteriosus* usually leads to manifestations early in life; indeed, it may cause signs and symptoms immediately after birth. Many infants with this anomaly do not survive the neonatal period without surgical

or catheter-based intervention. In such cases, the delivery of unsaturated blood through the patent ductus arteriosus produces cyanosis localized to the lower half of the body.

The outlook is different with *coarctation of the aorta without a patent ductus arteriosus,* unless it is very severe. Most children are asymptomatic, and the disease may go unrecognized until well into adult life. Typically there is hypertension in the upper extremities; in contrast, there are weak pulses and hypotension in the lower extremities, associated with manifestations of arterial insufficiency (i.e., claudication and coldness). Particularly characteristic in adults is the development of collateral circulation between the precoarctation arterial branches and the postcoarctation arteries through enlarged intercostal and internal mammary arteries, which produce radiographically visible erosions ("notching") of the undersurfaces of the ribs.

With significant coarctations, murmurs are present throughout systole; sometimes a thrill may be present. There is cardiomegaly due to left ventricular pressure-overload hypertrophy. With uncomplicated coarctation of the aorta, surgical resection and end-to-end anastomosis or replacement of the affected aortic segment by a prosthetic graft yields excellent results.

Pulmonary Stenosis and Atresia

This relatively frequent malformation constitutes an obstruction at the pulmonary valve, which may be mild to severe; the lesion can be isolated or part of a more complex anomaly—either tetralogy of Fallot or transposition of the great arteries. Right ventricular hypertrophy often develops, and there is sometimes poststenotic dilation of the pulmonary artery due to injury of the wall by "jetting" blood. With coexistent subpulmonary stenosis (as in tetralogy of Fallot), the high ventricular pressure is not transmitted to the valve, and the pulmonary trunk is not dilated and may in fact be hypoplastic. When the valve is entirely atretic, there is no communication between the right ventricle and lungs. In such cases the anomaly is associated with a hypoplastic right ventricle and an ASD; blood reaches the lungs through a patent ductus arteriosus. Mild stenosis may be asymptomatic and compatible with long life, whereas symptomatic cases require surgical correction.

Aortic Stenosis and Atresia

Congenital narrowing and obstruction of the aortic valve can occur at three locations: valvular, subvalvular, and supravalvular. With *valvular aortic stenosis* the cusps may be hypoplastic (small), dysplastic (thickened, nodular), or abnormal in number (usually acommissural or unicommissural). In severe congenital aortic stenosis or atresia, obstruction of the left ventricular outflow tract leads to underdevelopment (hypoplasia) of the left ventricle and ascending aorta, sometimes accompanied by dense, porcelain-like left ventricular endocardial fibroelastosis. The ductus must be open to allow blood flow to the aorta and coronary arteries. This constellation of findings, called the *hypoplastic left heart syndrome,* is nearly always fatal in the first week of life, when the ductus closes, unless a palliative procedure is done. Less severe degrees of congenital aortic stenosis may be compatible with long survival. Congenital aortic stenosis is an isolated lesion in 80% of cases.

Subaortic stenosis can be caused by a thickened ring (discrete type) or collar (tunnel type) of dense endocardial fibrous tissue below the level of the cusps. *Supravalvular aortic stenosis* is an inherited form of aortic dysplasia in which the ascending aortic wall is greatly thickened, causing luminal constriction. In some cases it is a component of a multiorgan developmental disorder resulting from deletions on chromosome 7 that include the gene for elastin. Other features of the syndrome include hypercalcemia, cognitive abnormalities, and hallmark facial anomalies (Williams-Beuren syndrome).[43] Mutations in the elastin gene probably cause supravalvular aortic stenosis by disrupting elastin–smooth muscle cell interactions during arterial morphogenesis.

Subaortic stenosis is usually associated with a prominent systolic murmur and sometimes a thrill. Pressure hypertrophy of the left ventricle develops as a consequence of the obstruction to blood flow, but congenital stenoses are well tolerated unless very severe. Mild stenoses can be managed conservatively with antibiotic prophylaxis (to prevent endocarditis) and avoidance of strenuous activity, but owing to left ventricular hypertrophy the threat of sudden death with exertion always looms.

Ischemic Heart Disease

Ischemic heart disease (IHD) is the leading cause of death worldwide for both men and women (7 million total per year). IHD is the generic designation for a group of pathophysiologically related syndromes resulting from *myocardial ischemia*—an imbalance between the supply (perfusion) and demand of the heart for oxygenated blood. Ischemia brings not only an insufficiency of oxygen, but also reduces the availability of nutrients and the removal of metabolites (Chapter 1). For this reason, ischemia is generally less well tolerated by the heart than pure hypoxia, such as may be seen with severe anemia, cyanotic heart disease, or advanced lung disease.

In more than 90% of cases, the cause of myocardial ischemia is reduced blood flow due to obstructive atherosclerotic lesions in the coronary arteries. Thus, IHD is often termed coronary artery disease (CAD) or coronary heart disease. In most cases there is a long period (up to decades) of silent, slow progression of coronary lesions before symptoms appear. Thus, *the syndromes of IHD are only the late manifestations of coronary atherosclerosis that may have started during childhood or adolescence* (Chapter 11).

IHD usually presents as one or more of the following clinical syndromes:

○ *Myocardial infarction*, the most important form of IHD, in which ischemia causes the death of heart muscle.
○ *Angina pectoris*, in which the ischemia is of insufficient severity to cause infarction, but may be a harbinger of MI.
○ *Chronic IHD with heart failure*.
○ *Sudden cardiac death*.

In addition to coronary atherosclerosis, myocardial ischemia may be caused by coronary emboli, blockage of small myocardial blood vessels, and lowered systemic blood pressure (e.g., shock). Moreover, in the setting of coronary arterial obstruction, ischemia can be aggravated by an increase in cardiac energy demand (e.g., as occurs with myocardial hypertrophy or increased heart rate [*tachycardia*]), by diminished availability of blood or oxygen due to shock, or by hypoxemia. Some conditions have several deleterious effects; for example, tachycardia increases oxygen demand (because of more contractions per unit time) and decreases supply (by decreasing the relative time spent in diastole, when cardiac perfusion occurs).

Epidemiology. IHD in its various forms is the leading cause of death for both males and females in the United States and other industrialized nations. Each year nearly 500,000 Americans die of IHD. As troublesome as these numbers may be, they represent an improvement over those that prevailed 2 to 3 decades ago. Since its peak in 1963, the overall death rate from IHD has fallen in the United States by approximately 50%. This remarkable improvement has resulted primarily from (1) *prevention*, achieved by modification of important risk factors, such as smoking, elevated blood cholesterol, and hypertension, and (2) *diagnostic and therapeutic advances*, allowing earlier, more effective, and safer treatments. The latter include new medications, coronary care units, thrombolysis for MI, percutaneous transluminal coronary angioplasty, endovascular stents, coronary artery bypass graft (CABG) surgery, and improved control of heart failure and arrhythmias. Additional risk reduction may potentially be achieved by maintenance of normal blood glucose levels in diabetic patients, control of obesity, and prophylactic anticoagulation of middle-aged men with aspirin. Nevertheless, continuing this encouraging trend in the 21st century will be challenging, in view of the predicted doubling of the number of individuals over age 65 by 2050 and the increased longevity of "baby boomers," the "obesity epidemic," and other factors. Interestingly, the genetic determinants of coronary atherosclerosis and IHD may not be identical, since MI occurs in only a small fraction of individuals with coronary disease. For example, the risk of MI but not coronary atherosclerosis is associated with genetic variants that modify leukotriene B4 metabolism.[44]

Pathogenesis. *The dominant cause of the IHD syndromes is insufficient coronary perfusion relative to myocardial demand, due to chronic, progressive atherosclerotic narrowing of the epicardial coronary arteries, and variable degrees of superimposed acute plaque change, thrombosis, and vasospasm.* The individual elements and their interactions are discussed below.

Chronic Atherosclerosis. More than 90% of patients with IHD have atherosclerosis of one or more of the epicardial coronary arteries. The clinical manifestations of coronary atherosclerosis are generally due to progressive narrowing of the lumen leading to stenosis ("fixed" obstructions) or to acute plaque disruption with thrombosis, both of which compromise blood flow. A fixed lesion obstructing 75% or greater of the lumen is generally required to cause symptomatic ischemia precipitated by exercise (most often manifested as chest pain, known as angina); with this degree of obstruction, compensatory coronary arterial vasodilation is no longer sufficient to meet even moderate increases in myocardial demand. Obstruction of 90% of the lumen can lead to inadequate coronary blood flow even at rest. The progressive myocardial ischemia induced by slowly developing occlusions may stimulate the formation of collateral vessels over time, which can protect against myocardial ischemia and infarction and mitigate the effects of high-grade stenoses.[45]

Although only a single major coronary epicardial trunk may be affected, two or all three—the left anterior descending (LAD), the left circumflex (LCX), and the right coronary artery (RCA)—are often involved by atherosclerosis. Clinically significant stenosing plaques may be located anywhere within these vessels but tend to predominate within the first several centimeters of the LAD and LCX and along the entire length of the RCA. Sometimes the major secondary epicardial branches are also involved (i.e., diagonal branches of the LAD, obtuse marginal branches of the LCX, or posterior descending branch of the RCA), but atherosclerosis of the intramural (penetrating) branches is rare.

Acute Plaque Change. The risk of an individual developing clinically important IHD depends in part on the number, distribution, structure, and degree of obstruction of atheromatous plaques. However, the varied clinical manifestations of IHD cannot be explained by the anatomic disease burden alone. This is particularly true for the so-called acute coronary syndromes, unstable angina, acute MI, and sudden death. The acute coronary syndromes are typically initiated by an unpredictable and abrupt conversion of a stable atherosclerotic plaque to an unstable and potentially life-threatening atherothrombotic lesion through rupture, superficial erosion, ulceration, fissuring, or deep hemorrhage (Chapter 11). In most instances, the plaque change causes the formation of a superimposed thrombus that partially or completely occludes the affected artery.[46, 47] These acute events are often associated with intralesional inflammation, which you will remember mediates the initiation, progression, and acute complications of atherosclerosis (discussed in Chapter 11). For purposes of simplicity, the spectrum of acute alterations in atherosclerotic lesions will be termed either plaque disruption or plaque change.

Consequences of Myocardial Ischemia. In each syndrome the critical consequence is downstream myocardial ischemia. *Stable angina* results from increases in myocardial oxygen demand that outstrip the ability of stenosed coronary arteries to increase oxygen delivery; it is usually not associated with plaque disruption. *Unstable angina* is caused by plaque rupture complicated by partially occlusive thrombosis and vasoconstriction, which lead to severe but transient reductions in coronary blood flow. In some cases, microinfarcts can occur distal to disrupted plaques due to thromboemboli. In *MI*, acute plaque change induces total thrombotic occlusion and the subsequent death of heart muscle. Finally, *sudden cardiac death* frequently involves an atherosclerotic lesion in which a disrupted plaque causes regional myocardial ischemia that induces a fatal ventricular arrhythmia. Each of these important syndromes is discussed in detail below, followed by an examination of the important myocardial consequences.

ANGINA PECTORIS

Angina pectoris (literally, chest pain) is characterized by paroxysmal and usually recurrent attacks of substernal or precordial chest discomfort (variously described as constricting, squeezing, choking, or knifelike) caused by transient (15 seconds to 15 minutes) myocardial ischemia that falls short of inducing

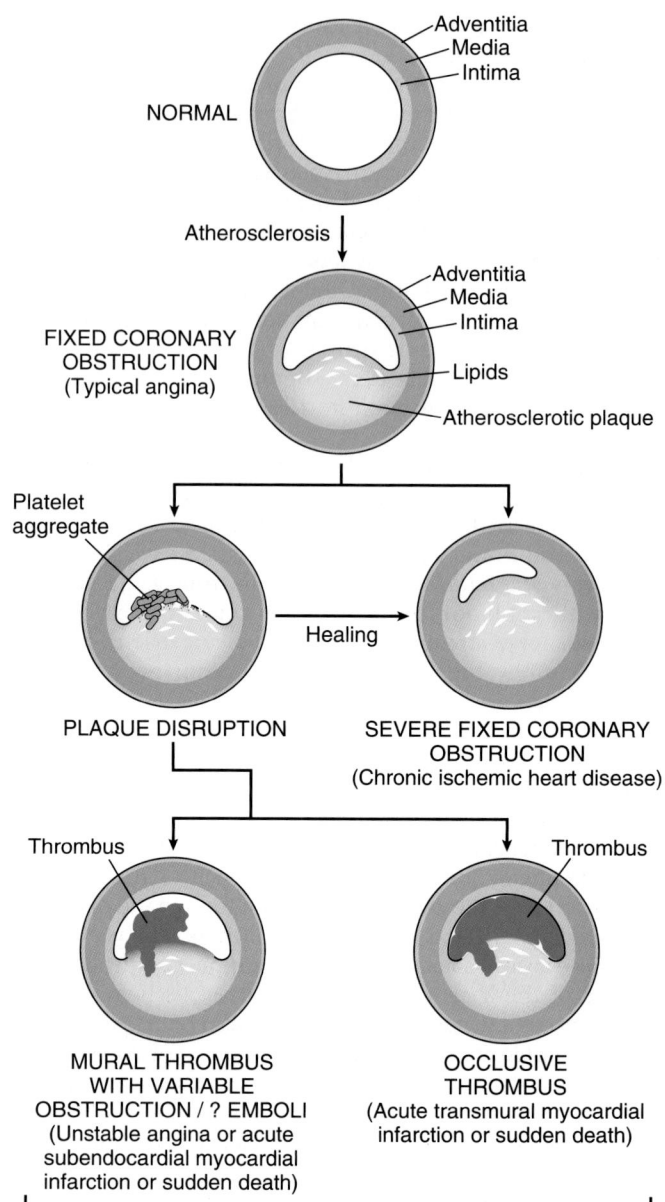

FIGURE 12–9 Schematic of sequential progression of coronary artery lesions and their association with various acute coronary syndromes. (Modified and redrawn from Schoen FJ: Interventional and Surgical Cardiovascular Pathology: Clinical Correlations and Basic Principles. Philadelphia, WB Saunders, 1989, p 63.)

myocyte necrosis. The three overlapping patterns of angina pectoris—(1) stable or typical angina, (2) Prinzmetal variant angina, and (3) unstable or crescendo angina—are caused by varying combinations of increased myocardial demand, decreased myocardial perfusion, and coronary arterial pathology. Moreover, not all ischemic events are perceived by patients (silent ischemia).[48]

Stable angina, the most common form, is also called *typical angina pectoris. It is caused by an imbalance in coronary perfusion (due to chronic stenosing coronary atherosclerosis) relative to myocardial demand,* such as that produced by physical activity, emotional excitement, or any other cause of increased cardiac workload. Typical angina pectoris is usually relieved by rest (which decreases demand) or administering nitroglycerin, a strong vasodilator (which increases perfusion).

Prinzmetal variant angina is an uncommon from of episodic myocardial ischemia that is caused by coronary artery spasm. Although individuals with Prinzmetal variant angina may well have significant coronary atherosclerosis, the anginal attacks are unrelated to physical activity, heart rate, or blood pressure. Prinzmetal angina generally responds promptly to vasodilators, such as nitroglycerin and calcium channel blockers.

Unstable or crescendo angina refers to *a pattern of increasingly frequent pain, often of prolonged duration, that is precipitated by progressively lower levels of physical activity or that even occurs at rest.* In most patients, unstable angina is caused by the disruption of an atherosclerotic plaque with superimposed partial (mural) thrombosis and possibly embolization or vasospasm (or both). Unstable angina thus serves as a warning that an acute MI may be imminent; indeed, this syndrome is sometimes referred to as *preinfarction angina.*

MYOCARDIAL INFARCTION (MI)

MI, also known as "heart attack," is the death of cardiac muscle due to prolonged severe ischemia. It is by far the most important form of IHD. About 1.5 million individuals in the United States suffer an MI annually.

Incidence and Risk Factors. MI can occur at virtually any age, but its frequency rises progressively with increasing age and when predispositions to atherosclerosis are present. Nearly 10% of myocardial infarcts occur in people under age 40, and 45% occur in people under age 65. Blacks and whites are equally affected. Throughout life, men are at significantly greater risk than women.[49] Indeed, except for those having some predisposing atherogenic condition, women are protected against MI and other heart diseases during the reproductive years. However, the decrease of estrogen following menopause is associated with rapid development of CAD, and IHD is the most common cause of death in elderly women. Postmenopausal hormonal replacement therapy is not currently felt to protect against atherosclerosis and IHD (Chapter 11).[50]

Pathogenesis. We now consider the basis for and consequences of myocardial ischemia.

Coronary Arterial Occlusion. In the typical case of MI, the following sequence of events is considered most likely (see Chapter 11 for more detail):

- The initial event is a sudden change in an atheromatous plaque, which may consist of intraplaque hemorrhage, erosion or ulceration, or rupture or fissuring.
- When exposed to subendothelial collagen and necrotic plaque contents, platelets adhere, become activated, release their granule contents, and aggregate to form microthrombi.
- Vasospasm is stimulated by mediators released from platelets.
- Tissue factor activates the coagulation pathway, adding to the bulk of the thrombus.

- Frequently within minutes, the thrombus evolves to completely occlude the lumen of the vessel.

Compelling evidence for this sequence has been obtained from (1) autopsy studies of patients dying of acute MI, (2) angiographic studies demonstrating a high frequency of thrombotic occlusion early after MI, (3) the high success rate of coronary revascularization (i.e., thrombolysis, angioplasty, stent placement, and surgery) following MI, and (4) the demonstration of residual disrupted atherosclerotic lesions by angiography after thrombolysis. Coronary angiography performed within 4 hours of the onset of an MI shows a thrombosed coronary artery in almost 90% of cases. However, when angiography is delayed until 12 to 24 hours after onset, occlusion is seen only about 60% of the time, suggesting that some occlusions resolve due to fibrinolysis, relaxation of spasm, or both.

In approximately 10% of cases, transmural MI occurs in the absence of the typical coronary vascular pathology. In such situations, other mechanisms may be responsible for the reduced coronary blood flow, including:

- *Vasospasm* with or without coronary atherosclerosis, perhaps in association with platelet aggregation or due to cocaine abuse
- *Emboli* from the left atrium in association with atrial fibrillation, a left-sided mural thrombus, vegetations of infective endocarditis, intracardiac prosthetic material; or *paradoxical emboli* from the right side of the heart or the peripheral veins, which travel through a patent foramen ovale to the coronary arteries
- *Ischemia without detectable coronary atherosclerosis and thrombosis* may be caused by disorders of small intramural coronary vessels, such as vasculitis, hematologic abnormalities such as sickle cell disease, amyloid deposition in vascular walls, and vascular dissection; lowered systemic blood pressure (shock); or inadequate myocardial "protection" during cardiac surgery

Myocardial Response. Coronary arterial obstruction compromises the blood supply to a region of myocardium (Fig. 12–10), *causing ischemia,* myocardial dysfunction, and potentially myocyte death. The anatomic region supplied by that artery is referred to as the *area at risk.* The outcome depends predominantly on the severity and duration of flow deprivation (Fig. 12–11).

The early biochemical consequence of myocardial ischemia is the cessation of aerobic metabolism within seconds, leading to inadequate production of high-energy phosphates (e.g., creatine phosphate and adenosine triphosphate) and accumulation of potentially noxious metabolites (such as lactic acid) (Fig. 12–11A). Because of the exquisite dependence of myocardial function on oxygen, severe ischemia induces loss of contractility within 60 seconds. This cessation of function can precipitate acute heart failure long before myocardial cell death. As detailed in Chapter 1, ultrastructural changes (including myofibrillar relaxation, glycogen depletion, cell and mitochondrial swelling) also develop within a few minutes of the onset of ischemia. *Nevertheless, these early changes are potentially reversible. As demonstrated both experimentally and in clinical studies, only severe ischemia lasting 20 to 30 minutes*

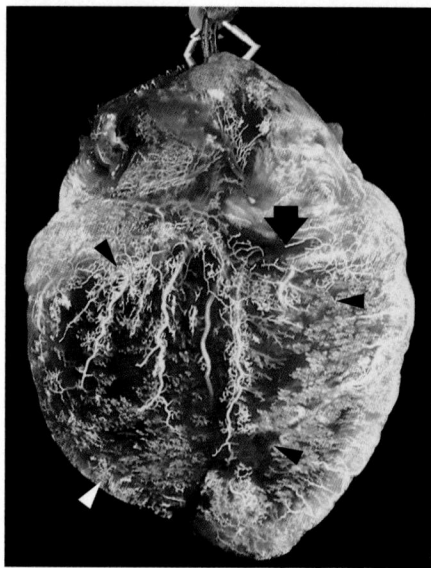

FIGURE 12–10 Postmortem angiogram showing the posterior aspect of the heart of a patient who died during the evolution of acute myocardial infarction, demonstrating total occlusion of the distal right coronary artery by an acute thrombus *(arrow)* and a large zone of myocardial hypoperfusion involving the posterior left and right ventricles, as indicated by *arrowheads,* and having almost absent filling of capillaries. The heart has been fixed by coronary arterial perfusion with glutaraldehyde and cleared with methyl salicylate, followed by intracoronary injection of silicone polymer (yellow). Photograph courtesy of Lewis L. Lainey. (Reproduced by permission from Schoen FJ: Interventional and Surgical Cardiovascular Pathology: Clinical Correlations and Basic Principles. Philadelphia, WB Saunders, 1989, p. 60.)

TABLE 12–4 Approximate Time of Onset of Key Events in Ischemic Cardiac Myocytes	
Feature	**Time**
Onset of ATP depletion	Seconds
Loss of contractility	<2 min

ATP reduced
    to 50% of normal
    to 10% of normal
	10 min
	40 min

Irreversible cell injury	20–40 min
Microvascular injury	>1 hr

ATP, adenosine triphosphate.

A key feature that marks the early phases of myocyte necrosis is the disruption of the integrity of the sarcolemmal membrane, which allows intracellular macromolecules to leak out of cells into the cardiac interstitium and ultimately into the microvasculature and lymphatics in the region of the infarct. Tests that measure the levels of myocardial proteins in the blood are important in the diagnosis and management of MI (see later). With prolonged severe ischemia, injury to the microvasculature then follows. The temporal progression of these events is summarized in Table 12–4.

In most cases of acute MI, permanent damage to the heart occurs when the perfusion of the myocardium is severely reduced for an extended interval (usually at least 2 to 4 hours), (Fig. 12–11B). *This delay in the onset of permanent myocardial injury provides the rationale for rapid diagnosis in acute MI—to permit early coronary intervention, the purpose of which is to establish reperfusion and salvage as much "at risk" myocardium as possible.*

The progression of ischemic necrosis in the myocardium is summarized in Figure 12–12. Ischemia is most pronounced in the subendocardium; thus, irreversible injury of ischemic myocytes occurs first in the subendocardial zone. With more extended ischemia, a *wavefront* of cell death moves through

or longer leads to irreversible damage (necrosis) of cardiac myocytes. Ultrastructural evidence of *irreversible* myocyte injury (primary structural defects in the sarcolemmal membrane) develops only after prolonged, severe myocardial ischemia (such as occurs when blood flow is 10% or less of normal).

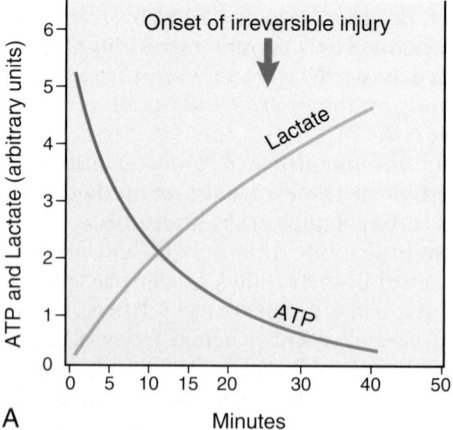

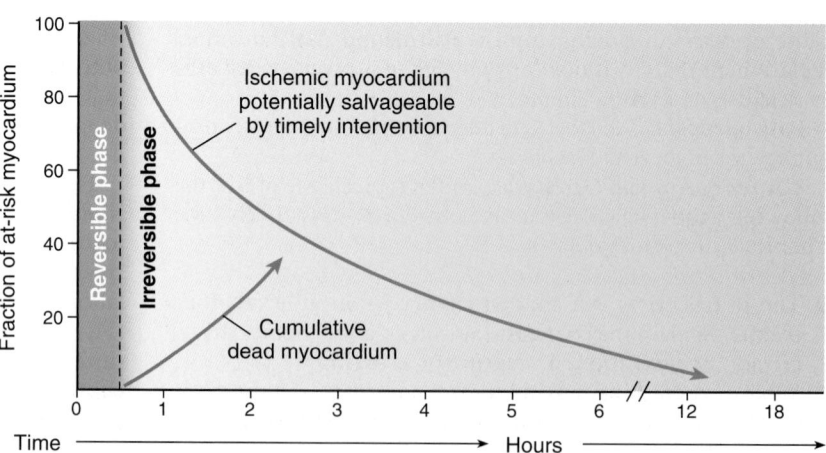

FIGURE 12–11 Temporal sequence of early biochemical findings and progression of necrosis after onset of severe myocardial ischemia. **A,** Early changes include loss of adenosine triphosphate (ATP) and accumulation of lactate. **B,** For approximately 30 minutes after the onset of even the most severe ischemia, myocardial injury is potentially reversible. Thereafter, progressive loss of viability occurs that is complete by 6 to 12 hours. The benefits of reperfusion are greatest when it is achieved early, and are progressively lost when reperfusion is delayed. (Modified with permission from Antman E: Acute myocardial infarction. In Braunwald E et al. (eds): Heart Disease: A Textbook of Cardiovascular Medicine, 6th ed. Philadelphia, WB Saunders, 2001, pp 1114–1231.)

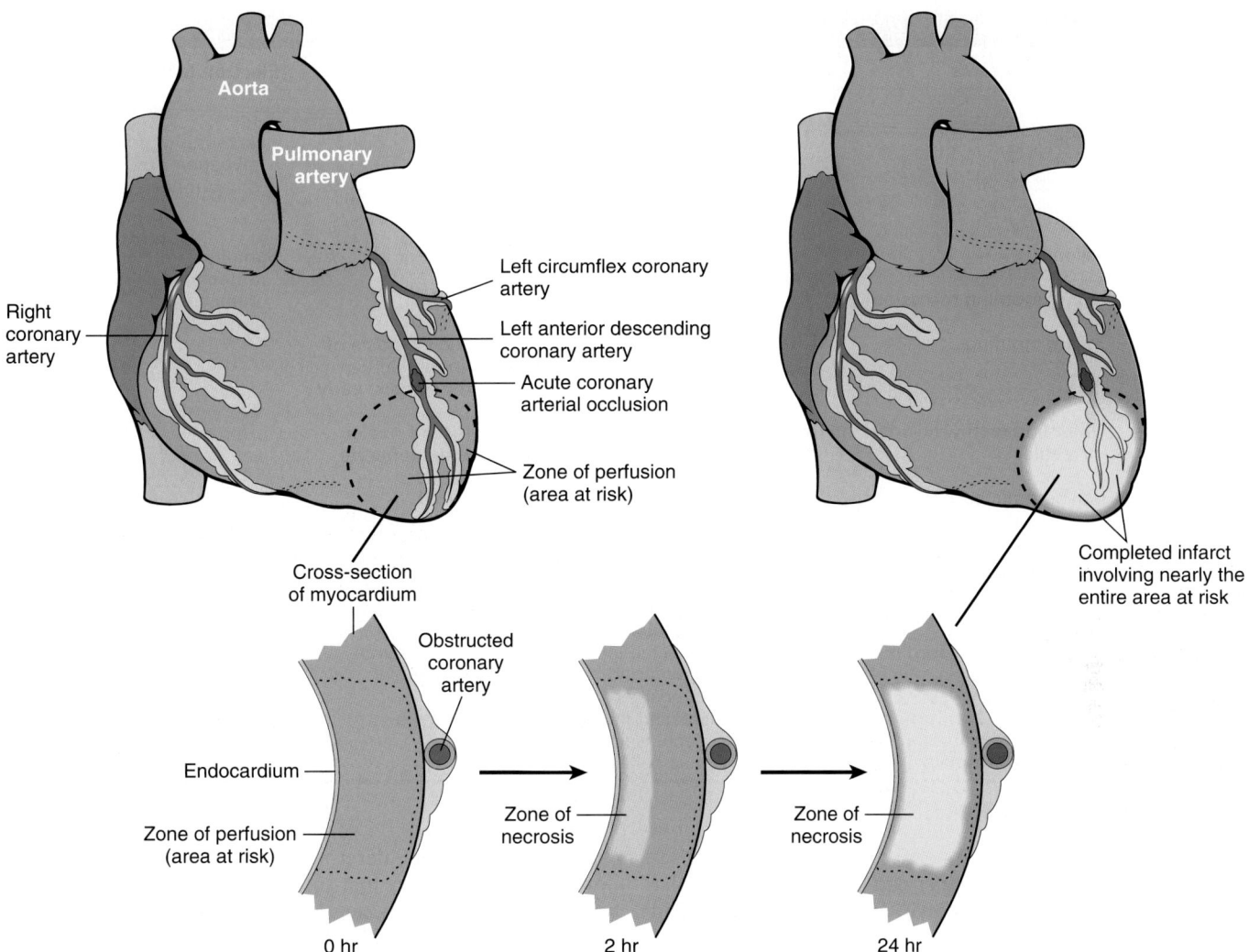

FIGURE 12–12 Progression of myocardial necrosis after coronary artery occlusion. Necrosis begins in a small zone of the myocardium beneath the endocardial surface in the center of the ischemic zone. The area that depends on the occluded vessel for perfusion is the "at risk" myocardium (*shaded*). Note that a very narrow zone of myocardium immediately beneath the endocardium is spared from necrosis because it can be oxygenated by diffusion from the ventricle.

the myocardium to involve progressively more of the transmural thickness and breadth of the ischemic zone. The precise location, size, and specific morphologic features of an acute MI depend on:

○ The location, severity, and rate of development of coronary obstructions due to atherosclerosis and thromboses
○ The size of the vascular bed perfused by the obstructed vessels
○ The duration of the occlusion
○ The metabolic/oxygen needs of the myocardium at risk
○ The extent of collateral blood vessels
○ The presence, site, and severity of coronary arterial spasm
○ Other factors, such as heart rate, cardiac rhythm, and blood oxygenation

Necrosis is usually complete within 6 hours of the onset of severe myocardial ischemia. However, in instances where the

coronary arterial collateral system, stimulated by chronic ischemia, is better developed and thereby more effective, the progression of necrosis may follow a more protracted course (possibly over 12 hours or longer).

Knowledge of the areas of myocardium perfused by the three major coronary arteries helps correlate sites of vascular obstruction with regions of myocardial infarction. Typically, the left anterior descending branch of the left coronary artery (LAD) supplies most of the apex of the heart (distal end of the ventricles), the anterior wall of the left ventricle, and the anterior two thirds of the ventricular septum. By convention, the coronary artery (either the right coronary artery [RCA] or the left circumflex artery [LCX]) that perfuses the posterior third of the septum is called "dominant" (even though the LAD and LCX collectively perfuse the majority of the left ventricular myocardium). In a right dominant circulation, present in approximately four fifths of individuals, the LCX generally perfuses only the lateral wall of the left ventricle, and the RCA supplies the entire right ventricular free wall, the posterobasal wall of the left ventricle, and the posterior third

TABLE 12–5	Evolution of Morphologic Changes in Myocardial Infarction		
Time	**Gross Features**	**Light Microscope**	**Electron Microscope**
REVERSIBLE INJURY			
0–½ hr	None	None	Ralaxation of myofibrils; glycogen loss; mitochondrial swelling
IRREVERSIBLE INJURY			
½–4 hr	None	Usually none; variable waviness of fibers at border	Sarcolemmal disruption; mitochondrial amorphous densities
4–12 hr	Dark mottling (occasional)	Early coagulation necrosis; edema; hemorrhage	
12–24 hr	Dark mottling	Ongoing coagulation necrosis; pyknosis of nuclei; myocyte hypereosinophilia; marginal contraction band necrosis; early neutrophilic infiltrate	
1–3 days	Mottling with yellow-tan infarct center	Coagulation necrosis, with loss of nuclei and striations; brisk interstitial infiltrate of neutrophils	
3–7 days	Hyperemic border; central yellow-tan softening	Beginning disintegration of dead myofibers, with dying neutrophils; early phagocytosis of dead cells by macrophages at infarct border	
7–10 days	Maximally yellow-tan and soft, with depressed red-tan margins	Well-developed phagocytosis of dead cells; early formation of fibrovascular granulation tissue at margins	
10–14 days	Red-gray depressed infarct borders	Well-established granulation tissue with new blood vessels and collagen deposition	
2–8 wk	Gray-white scar, progressive from border toward core of infarct	Increased collagen deposition, with decreased cellularity	
>2 mo	Scarring complete	Dense collagenous scar	

of the ventricular septum. Thus, occlusions of the RCA (as well as the left coronary artery) can cause left ventricular damage. The right and left coronary arteries function as end arteries, although anatomically most hearts have numerous intercoronary anastomoses (connections called the collateral circulation). Little blood courses through the collateral circulation in the normal heart. However, when one artery is severely narrowed, blood flows via collaterals from the high- to the low-pressure system, and causes the channels to enlarge. Thus, progressive dilation and growth of collaterals, stimulated by ischemia, may play a role in providing blood flow to areas of the myocardium otherwise deprived of adequate perfusion.

Transmural Versus Subendocardial Infarction. The distribution of myocardial necrosis correlates with the location and cause of the decreased perfusion (Fig. 12–16). Most myocardial infarcts are *transmural*, in which the ischemic necrosis involves the full or nearly full thickness of the ventricular wall in the distribution of a single coronary artery. This pattern of infarction is usually associated with a combination of chronic coronary atherosclerosis, acute plaque change, and superimposed thrombosis (as discussed previously). In contrast, a *subendocardial (nontransmural) infarct* constitutes an area of ischemic necrosis limited to the inner one third to one half of the ventricular wall. As the subendocardial zone is normally the least perfused region of myocardium, this area is most vulnerable to any reduction in coronary flow. A subendocardial infarct can occur as a result of a plaque disruption followed by a coronary thrombus that becomes lysed before myocardial necrosis extends across the full thickness of the

wall; in this case the infarct will be limited to the distribution of the coronary artery that suffered plaque change. However, subendocardial infarcts can also result from prolonged, severe reduction in systemic blood pressure, as in shock superimposed on chronic, otherwise noncritical, coronary stenoses. In the subendocardial infarcts that occur as a result of global hypotension, myocardial damage is usually circumferential, rather than being limited to the distribution of a single major coronary artery. Owing to the characteristic electrocardiographic changes resulting from myocardial ischemia/necrosis in various distributions, transmural infarcts are often referred to as "ST elevation infarcts" and subendocardial infarcts are known as "non-ST elevation infarcts."

Morphology. The temporal evolution of the morphologic changes in acute MI and subsequent healing are summarized in Table 12–5.

Nearly all transmural infarcts involve at least a portion of the left ventricle (comprising the free wall and ventricular septum) and encompass nearly the entire perfusion zone of the occluded coronary artery save for a narrow rim (~0.1 mm) of preserved subendocardial myocardium that is sustained by the diffusion of oxygen and nutrients from the ventricular lumen.

Of MIs caused by a right coronary obstruction, 15% to 30% extend from the posterior free wall of the septal portion of the left ventricle into the adjacent right ventricular wall. Isolated infarction of the right

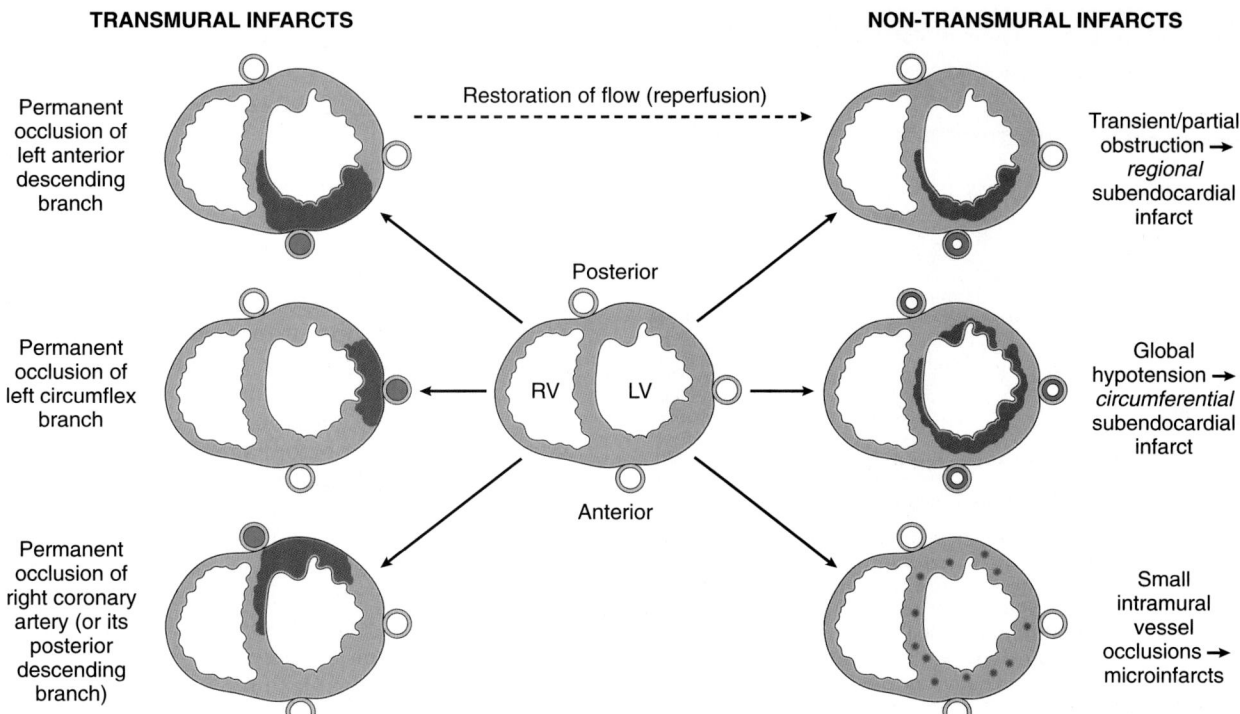

TRANSMURAL INFARCTS

Permanent occlusion of left anterior descending branch

Permanent occlusion of left circumflex branch

Permanent occlusion of right coronary artery (or its posterior descending branch)

Restoration of flow (reperfusion)

Posterior

RV   LV

Anterior

NON-TRANSMURAL INFARCTS

Transient/partial obstruction → *regional* subendocardial infarct

Global hypotension → *circumferential* subendocardial infarct

Small intramural vessel occlusions → microinfarcts

FIGURE 12–13 Distribution of myocardial ischemic necrosis correlated with the location and nature of decreased perfusion. Left, The positions of transmural acute infarcts resulting from occlusions of the major coronary arteries; *top to bottom,* left anterior descending, left circumflex, and right coronary arteries. Right, The types of infarcts that result from a partial or transient occlusion, global hypotension, or intramural small vessel occlusions.

ventricle is unusual (1% to 3% of cases), as is infarction of the atria.

The frequencies of involvement of each of the three main arterial trunks and the corresponding sites of myocardial lesions resulting in infarction (in the typical right dominant heart) are as follows (Fig. 12–13A):

- Left anterior descending coronary artery (40% to 50%): infarcts involving the anterior wall of left ventricle near the apex; the anterior portion of ventricular septum; and the apex circumferentially
- Right coronary artery (30% to 40%): infarcts involving the inferior/posterior wall of left ventricle; posterior portion of ventricular septum; and the inferior/posterior right ventricular free wall in some cases
- Left circumflex coronary artery (15% to 20%): infarcts involving the lateral wall of left ventricle except at the apex

Other locations of critical coronary arterial lesions causing infarcts are sometimes encountered, such as the left main coronary artery, the secondary branches of the left anterior descending coronary artery, or the marginal branches of the left circumflex coronary artery.

The gross and microscopic appearance of an infarct depends on the duration of survival of the patient following the MI. Areas of damage undergo a progressive sequence of morphologic changes that consist of typical ischemic coagulative necrosis (the predominant mechanism of cell death in MI, although apoptosis may also occur), followed by inflammation and repair that closely parallels tissue responses to injury at other sites.

Early recognition of acute MI can be difficult, particularly when death has occurred within a few hours after the onset of symptoms. MIs less than 12 hours old are usually not apparent on gross examination. If the patient died at least 2 to 3 hours after the infarct, however, it is possible to highlight the area of necrosis by immersion of tissue slices in a solution of **triphenyltetrazolium chloride**. This histochemical stain imparts a brick-red color to intact, noninfarcted myocardium where dehydrogenase (e.g., lactate dehydrogenase) activity is preserved. Because dehydrogenases leak out through the damaged membranes of dead cell, an infarct appears as an unstained pale zone (Fig. 12–14). By 12 to 24 hours an infarct can be identified grossly in transverse slices as a reddish-blue area of discoloration caused by stagnated, trapped blood. Thereafter, the infarct becomes progressively more sharply defined, yellow-tan, and soft. By 10 days to 2 weeks, it is rimmed by a hyperemic zone of highly vascularized granulation tissue. Over the succeeding weeks, the injured region evolves to a fibrous scar.

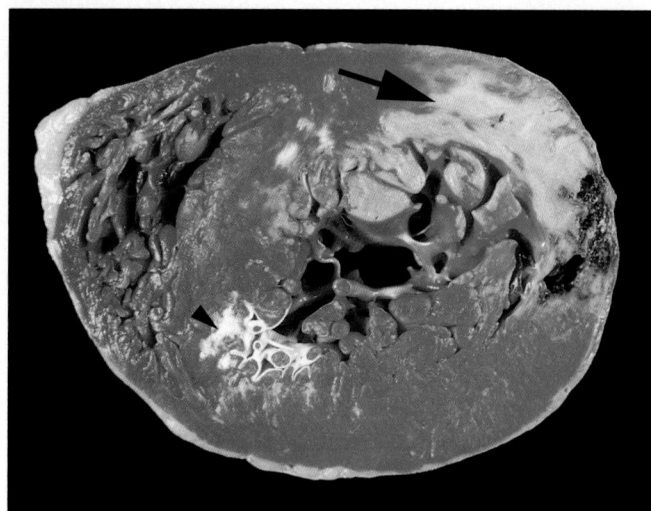

FIGURE 12–14 Acute myocardial infarct, predominantly of the posterolateral left ventricle, demonstrated histochemically by a lack of staining by triphenyltetrazolium chloride in areas of necrosis *(arrow)*. The staining defect is due to the enzyme leakage that follows cell death. Note the myocardial hemorrhage at one edge of the infarct that was associated with cardiac rupture, and the anterior scar *(arrowhead),* indicative of old infarct. Specimen is oriented with the posterior wall at the top.

The histopathologic changes also proceed in a fairly predictable sequence (summarized in Fig. 12–15). The typical changes of coagulative necrosis become detectable in the first 6 to 12 hours. "Wavy fibers" may be present at the periphery of the infarct; these changes probably result from the forceful systolic tugs of the viable fibers on immediately adjacent, noncontractile dead fibers, which stretches and folds them. An additional sublethal ischemic change may be seen in the margins of infarcts: so-called vacuolar degeneration or **myocytolysis**, which takes the form of large vacuolar spaces within cells that probably contain water. The necrotic muscle elicits acute inflammation (most prominent between 1 and 3 days). Thereafter macrophages remove the necrotic myocytes (most pronounced at 3 to 7 days), and the damaged zone is progressively replaced by the ingrowth of highly vascularized granulation tissue (most prominent at 1 to 2 weeks); as healing progresses, this is replaced by fibrous tissue. In most instances, scarring is well advanced by the end of the sixth week, but the efficiency of repair depends on the size of the original lesion.

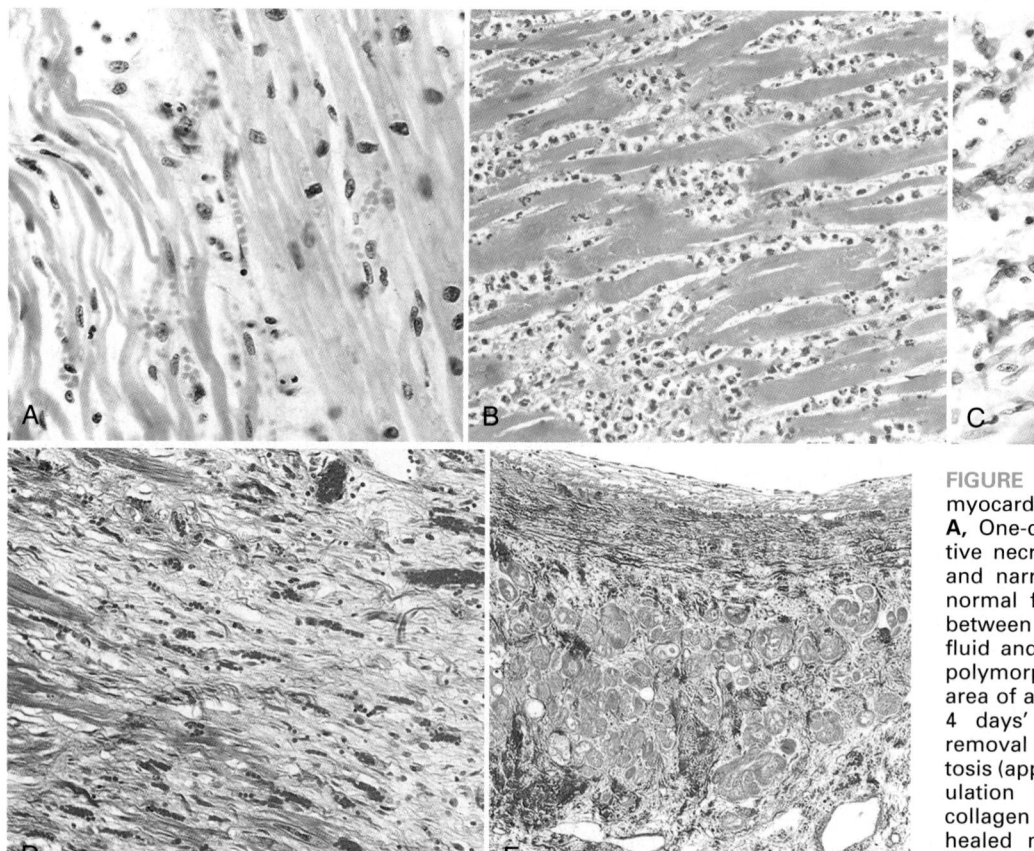

FIGURE 12–15 Microscopic features of myocardial infarction and its repair. **A,** One-day-old infarct showing coagulative necrosis and wavy fibers (elongated and narrow, as compared with adjacent normal fibers *at right*). Widened spaces between the dead fibers contain edema fluid and scattered neutrophils. **B,** Dense polymorphonuclear leukocytic infiltrate in area of acute myocardial infarction of 3 to 4 days' duration. **C,** Nearly complete removal of necrotic myocytes by phagocytosis (approximately 7 to 10 days). **D,** Granulation tissue characterized by loose collagen and abundant capillaries. **E,** Well-healed myocardial infarct with replacement of the necrotic fibers by dense collagenous scar. A few residual cardiac muscle cells are present.

Since healing requires the participation of inflammatory cells that migrate to the region of damage through intact blood vessels, which often survive only at the infarct margins, the infarct heals from its margins toward its center. Thus, a large infarct may not heal as quickly or as completely as a small one. A healing infarct may appear nonuniform, with the most advanced healing at the periphery. Once a lesion is completely healed, it is impossible to determine its age (i.e., the dense fibrous scar of 8-week-old and 10-year-old infarcts may look identical).

Infarcts may expand beyond their original borders over a period of days to weeks via a process of repetitive necrosis of adjacent regions **(extension)**. In such cases, there is a central zone in which healing is more advanced than the periphery of the infarct. This contrasts with the appearance of a simple infarct described above, in which the most advanced repair is peripheral. Infarct extension may occur because of retrograde propagation of a thrombus, proximal vasospasm, progressively impaired cardiac contractility that renders flow through moderate stenoses insufficient, the deposition of platelet-fibrin microemboli, or an arrhythmia that impairs cardiac function.

We now consider interventions that seek to limit infarct size by salvaging myocardium that is not yet necrotic.

Infarct Modification by Reperfusion. The most effective way to "rescue" ischemic myocardium threatened by infarction is to restore myocardial blood flow as rapidly as possible, a process referred to as *reperfusion*.[51] Although this can often be accomplished, reperfusion may also trigger deleterious complications, including arrhythmias, myocardial hemorrhage with contraction bands, irreversible cell damage superimposed on the original ischemic injury *(reperfusion injury)*, microvascular injury, and prolonged ischemic dysfunction *(myocardial stunning)*; these are discussed below and summarized in Figures 12–16 and 12–17. Coronary intervention (i.e., thrombolysis, angioplasty, stent placement, or coronary artery bypass graft [CABG] surgery) is often used in an attempt to dissolve, mechanically alter, or bypass the lesion that initiated the acute MI. The purpose of these treatments is to restore blood flow to the area at risk for infarction and rescue the ischemic (but not yet necrotic) heart muscle. Because loss of myocardial viability in infarction is progressive, occurring over a period of at least several hours (see Fig. 12–11B and Fig. 12–17A), early reperfusion can salvage myocardium and thereby limit infarct size, with consequent improvement in both short- and long-term function and survival. The potential benefit of reperfusion is related to (1) the rapidity with which the coronary obstruction is alleviated (the first 3 to 4 hours following onset are critical) and (2) the extent of correction of the vascular occlusion and the underlying causal lesion. For example, thrombolysis can remove a thrombus occluding a coronary artery, but does not alter the underlying atherosclerotic plaque that initiated it. In contrast, percutaneous transluminal coronary angioplasty (PTCA) with stent placement not only eliminates a thrombotic occlusion but also can relieve some of the original obstruction and insta-

bility caused by the underlying disrupted plaque. CABG provides flow around a blocked vessel.

Recall that (1) severe ischemia does not cause immediate cell death even in the most severely affected regions of myocardium, and (2) not all regions of myocardium are equally ischemic. Therefore, the outcome following the restoration of blood flow may vary from region to region. As indicated in Figure 12–16A, reperfusion of myocardium within 20 minutes of the onset of ischemia may completely prevent necrosis. Reperfusion after a longer interval may not prevent all necrosis but can salvage at least some myocytes that would have otherwise died.

The typical appearance of reperfused myocardium is illustrated in Figure 12–16B and C. A reperfused infarct is usually hemorrhagic because the vasculature is injured during the period of ischemia and leaks when flow is restored. Microscopic examination reveals that myocytes that were irreversibly injured at the time of reperfusion often contain *contraction bands*, intensely eosinophilic intracellular "stripes" composed of closely packed sarcomeres. These result from the exaggerated contraction of myofibrils when perfusion is reestablished, at which time the interior of dead cells with damaged plasma membranes are exposed to a high concentration of calcium ions from the plasma. Thus, *reperfusion not only salvages reversibly injured cells but also alters the morphology of lethally injured cells*.

In addition to its benefits, reperfusion may also have some deleterious effects on the vulnerable ischemic myocardium *(reperfusion injury;* see Fig. 12–17B).[52] The clinical significance of myocardial reperfusion injury is uncertain. As discussed in Chapter 1, reperfusion injury may be mediated by oxidative stress, calcium overload, and potentially inflammation initiated during reperfusion. Reperfusion-induced microvascular injury causes not only hemorrhage but also endothelial swelling that occludes capillaries and may limit the reperfusion of critically injured myocardium (called *no-reflow*).

Biochemical abnormalities may also persist for a period of days to several weeks in myocytes that are rescued from ischemia by reperfusion. These are thought to underlie a phenomenon referred to as *stunned myocardium,* a state of reversible cardiac failure that usually recovers after several days.[53] Reperfusion also frequently induces arrhythmias. Myocardium that is subjected to chronic, sublethal ischemia may also enter into a state of lowered metabolism and function that is referred to as *hibernation*.[54] The function of hibernating myocardium may be restored by revascularization (e.g., by CABG surgery, angioplasty, or stenting). Paradoxically, repetitive short-lived transient severe ischemia may protect the myocardium against infarction (a phenomenon known as *preconditioning*) by mechanisms that are not understood.[55]

Clinical Features. MI is diagnosed by clinical symptoms, laboratory tests for the presence of myocardial proteins in the plasma, and characteristic electrocardiographic changes. Patients with MI often present with a rapid, weak pulse and profuse sweating (diaphoresis). Dyspnea due to impaired contractility of the ischemic myocardium and the resultant pulmonary congestion and edema is common. However, in about 10% to 15% of patients the onset is entirely asymptomatic and the disease is discovered only by electrocardiographic changes or laboratory tests that show evidence of myocardial damage

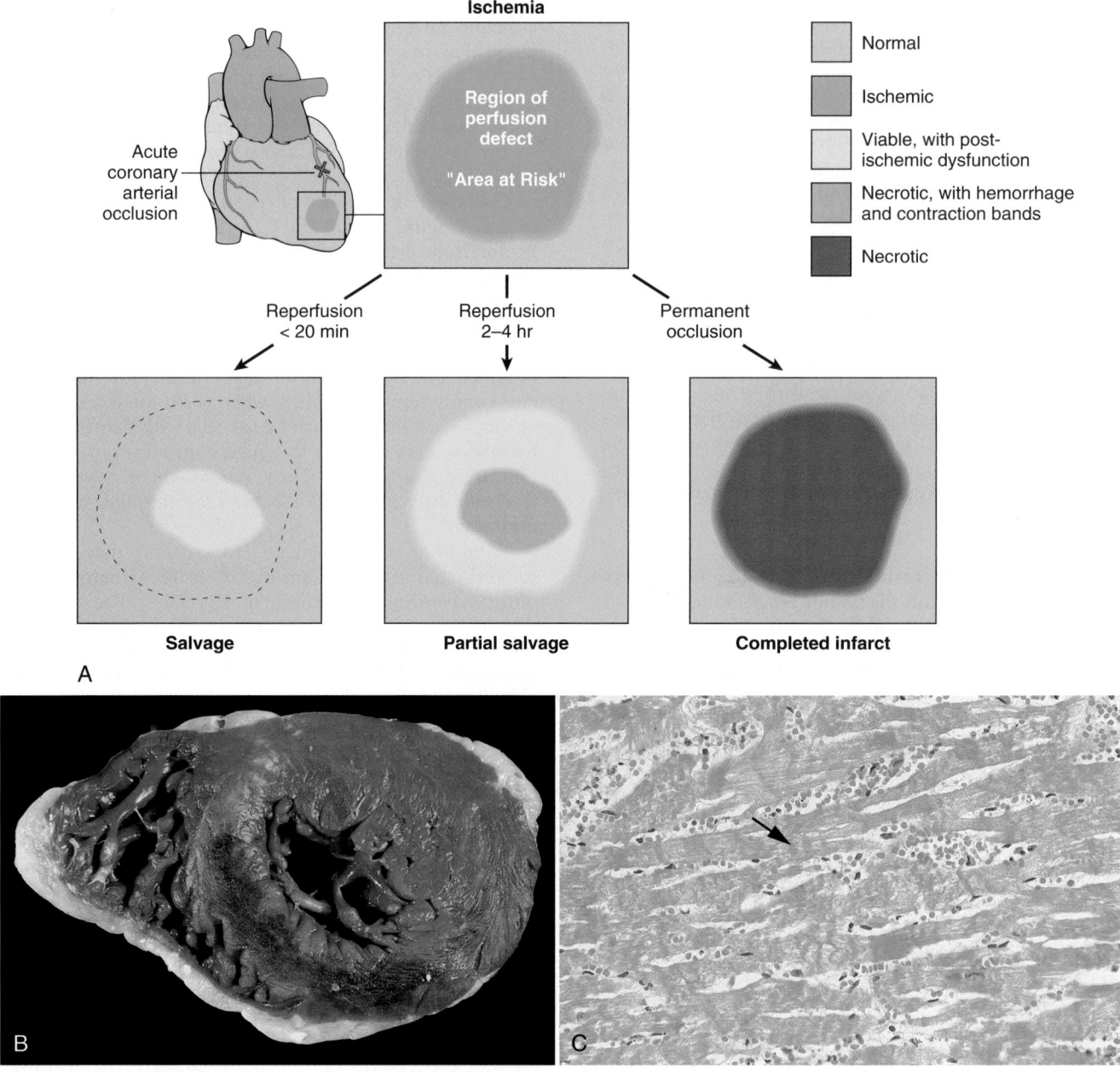

FIGURE 12–16 Consequences of myocardial ischemia followed by reperfusion. **A,** Schematic illustration of the progression of myocardial ischemic injury and its modification by restoration of flow (reperfusion). Hearts suffering brief periods of ischemia of longer than 20 minutes followed by reperfusion do not develop necrosis (reversible injury). Brief ischemia followed by reperfusion results in stunning. If coronary occlusion is extended beyond 20 minutes' duration, a wavefront of necrosis progresses from subendocardium to subepicardium over time. Reperfusion before 3 to 6 hours of ischemia salvages ischemic but viable tissue. This salvaged tissue may also demonstrate stunning. Reperfusion beyond 6 hours does not appreciably reduce myocardial infarct size. **B,** Gross and **C,** microscopic appearance of myocardium modified by reperfusion. **B,** Large, densely hemorrhagic, anterior wall acute myocardial infarction in a patient with left anterior descending artery thrombus treated with streptokinase, a fibrinolytic agent (triphenyl tetrazolium chloride–stained heart slice). Specimen oriented with posterior wall at top. **C,** Myocardial necrosis with hemorrhage and contraction bands, visible as dark bands spanning some myofibers *(arrow)*. This is the characteristic appearance of markedly ischemic myocardium that has been reperfused.

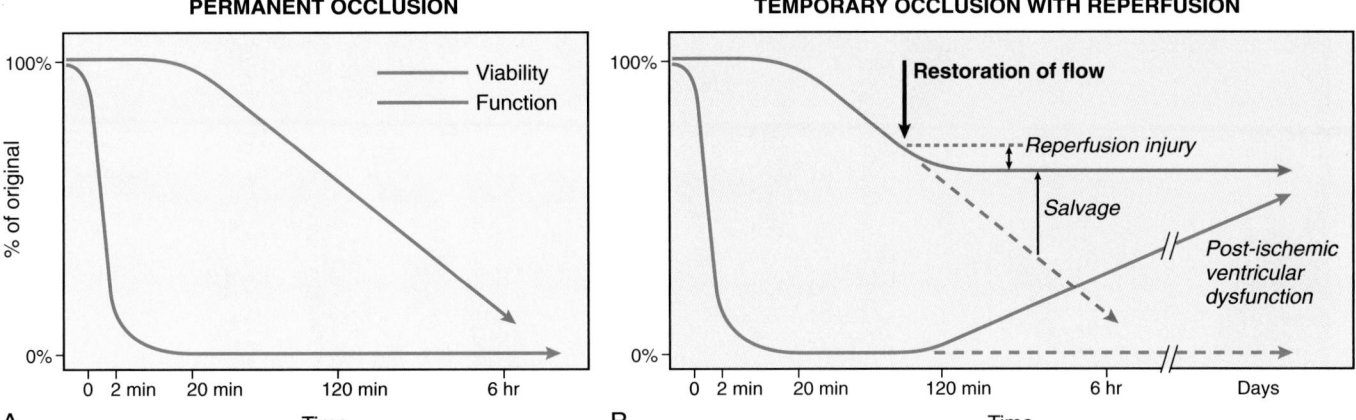

FIGURE 12–17 Effects of reperfusion on myocardial viability and function. Following coronary occlusion, contractile function is lost within 2 minutes and viability begins to diminish after approximately 20 minutes. If perfusion is not restored (**A**), then nearly all myocardium in the affected region will die. **B,** If flow is restored, then some necrosis is prevented, myocardium is salvaged, and at least some function will return. The earlier reperfusion occurs, the greater the degree of salvage. However, the process of reperfusion itself may induce some damage *(reperfusion injury)*, and return of function of salvaged myocardium may be delayed for hours to days *(post-ischemic ventricular dysfunction).*

(see below). Such "silent" MIs are particularly common in elderly patients and in the setting of diabetes mellitus.

The laboratory evaluation of MI is based on measuring the blood levels of proteins that leak out of fatally injured myocytes; these molecules include myoglobin, cardiac troponins T and I, the MB fraction of creatine kinase (CK-MB), lactate dehydrogenase, and many others (Fig. 12–18).[56] The diagnosis of myocardial injury is established when blood levels of these cardiac biomarkers are increased in the clinical setting of acute ischemia. The rate of appearance of these markers in the peripheral circulation depends on several factors, including their intracellular location and molecular weight, the blood flow and lymphatic drainage in the area of the infarct, and the rate of elimination of the marker from the blood.

The most sensitive and specific biomarkers of myocardial damage are cardiac-specific proteins, particularly Troponins I and T (proteins that regulate calcium-mediated contraction of cardiac and skeletal muscle). Troponins I and T are not normally detectable in the circulation. Following an MI, levels of both begin to rise at 2 to 4 hours and peak at 48 hours. Formerly the "gold standard," cardiac creatine kinase remains useful. Creatine kinase, an enzyme that is present in brain, myocardium, and skeletal muscle, is a dimer composed of two isoforms designated "M" and "B." MM homodimers are found predominantly in cardiac and skeletal muscle; BB homodimers in brain, lung, and many other tissues; and MB heterodimers principally in cardiac muscle, with lesser amounts also being found in skeletal muscle. As a result, the MB form of

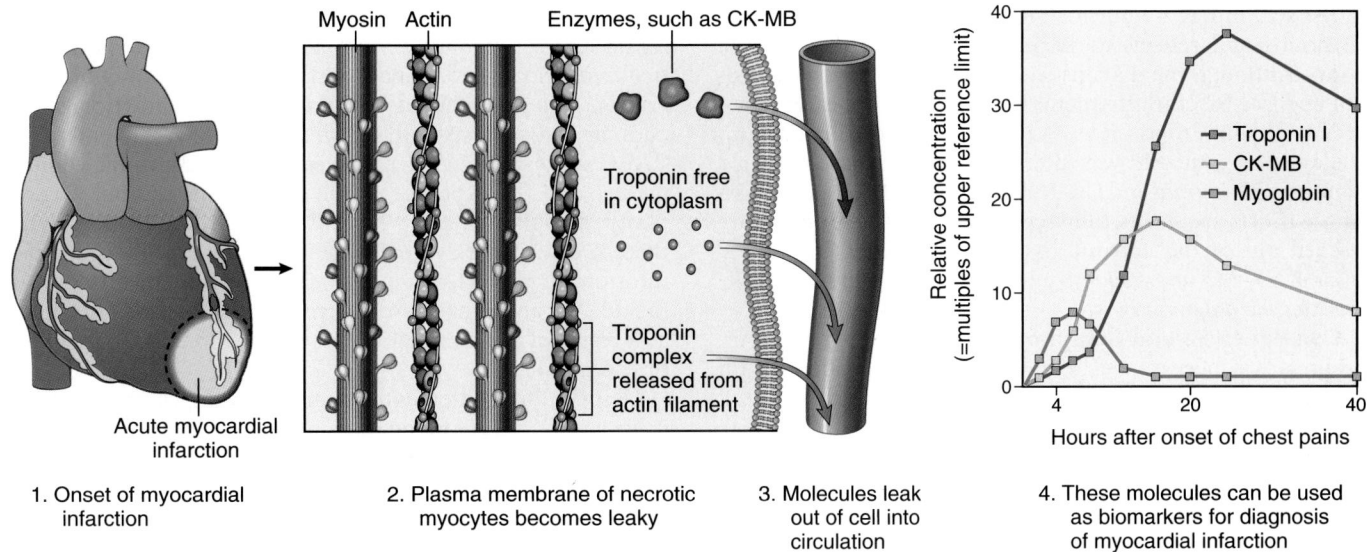

FIGURE 12–18 Release of myocyte proteins in myocardial infarction. Some of these proteins (e.g., troponin I, C, or T and creatine phosphokinase, MB fraction [CK-MB]) are used as diagnostic biomarkers.

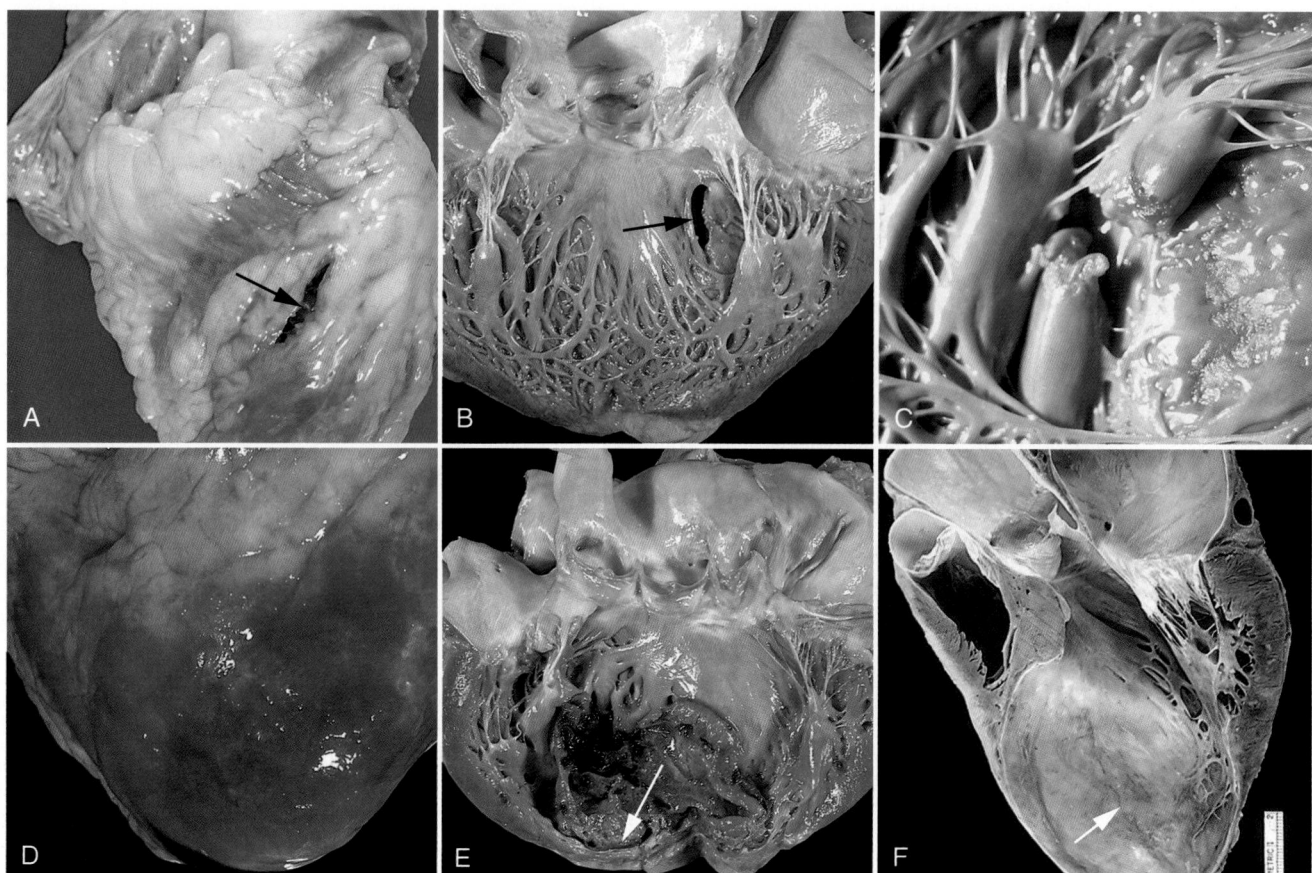

FIGURE 12–19 Complications of myocardial infarction. Cardiac rupture syndromes (**A–C**). **A,** Anterior myocardial rupture in an acute infarct *(arrow).* **B,** Rupture of the ventricular septum *(arrow).* **C,** Complete rupture of a necrotic papillary muscle. **D,** Fibrinous pericarditis, showing a dark, roughened epicardial surface overlying an acute infarct. **E,** Early expansion of anteroapical infarct with wall thinning *(arrow)* and mural thrombus. **F,** Large apical left ventricular aneurysm. The left ventricle is on the *right* in this apical four-chamber view of the heart. (**A–E,** Reproduced by permission from Schoen FJ: Interventional and Surgical Cardiovascular Pathology: Clinical Correlations and Basic Principles. Philadelphia, WB Saunders, 1989; **F,** Courtesy of William D. Edwards, MD, Mayo Clinic, Rochester, MN.)

creatine kinase (CK-MB) is sensitive but not specific, since it is also elevated when skeletal muscle is injured. CK-MB begins to rise within 2 to 4 hours of the onset of MI, peaks at about 24 hours, and returns to normal within approximately 72 hours. Although the diagnostic sensitivities of cardiac troponin and CK-MB measurements are similar in the early stages of MI, elevated troponin levels persist for approximately 7 to 10 days after acute MI, well after CK-MB levels have returned to normal. Troponin and CK-MB levels peak earlier in patients whose hearts are successfully reperfused, because proteins are washed out of the necrotic tissue more rapidly. *Unchanged levels of CK-MB and troponin over a period of 2 days essentially excludes the diagnosis of MI.*

Consequences and Complications of MI. Extraordinary progress has been made in the treatment of patients with acute MI. Concurrent with the decrease in the overall mortality of IHD since the 1960s, the in-hospital death rate has declined from around 30% to approximately 7% in patients receiving timely therapy. Half of the deaths associated with acute MI occur within 1 hour of onset; most of these individuals never reach the hospital. Therapies given routinely in the setting of acute MI include aspirin and heparin (to prevent further thrombosis); oxygen (to minimize ischemia);

nitrates (to induce vasodilation and reverse vasospasm); beta-adrenergic inhibitors (beta-blockers, to diminish cardiac oxygen demand and decrease the risk of arrythmias); angiotensinogen converting enzyme (ACE) inhibitors (to limit ventricular dilation); and maneuvers that aim to open up blocked vessels, including the administration of fibrinolytic agents, coronary angioplasty with or without stenting, and emergent CABG surgery. The choice of therapy depends on the clinical picture and the expertise of the treating institution. Angioplasty is highly effective in skilled hands, while fibinolytic therapy can be given with almost equivalent efficacy by simple infusion. In general, factors associated with a poor prognosis include advanced age, female gender, diabetes mellitus, and, as a result of the cumulative loss of functional myocardium, previous MI.

Despite these interventions, many patients have one or more complications following acute MI, including the following (some of which are illustrated in Fig. 12–19):

- *Contractile dysfunction. Myocardial infarcts produce abnormalities in left ventricular function roughly proportional to their size.* There is usually some degree of left ventricular failure with hypotension, pulmonary vascular congestion, and interstitial pulmonary transudates, which may progress to frank pulmonary edema and respiratory impairment. Severe "pump failure" *(cardiogenic shock)* occurs in 10% to 15% of patients following acute MI, generally those with a large infarct (>40% of the left ventricle). Cardiogenic shock has a nearly 70% mortality rate and accounts for two thirds of in-hospital deaths.

- *Arrhythmias.* Many patients have *myocardial irritability* and/or conduction disturbances following MI that lead to potentially fatal arrhythmias. MI-associated arrhythmias include sinus bradycardia, heart block (asystole), tachycardia, ventricular premature contractions or ventricular tachycardia, and ventricular fibrillation. Because of the location of portions of the atrioventricular conduction system (bundle of His) in the inferoseptal myocardium, infarcts of this region may also be associated with heart block.

- *Myocardial rupture.* The *cardiac rupture syndromes* result from softening and weakening of the necrotic and subsequently inflamed myocardium. They include (1) rupture of the ventricular free wall (most common), with hemopericardium and cardiac tamponade (Fig. 12–19A); (2) rupture of the ventricular septum (less common), leading to an *acute VSD* and left-to-right shunting (Fig. 12–19B); and (3) papillary muscle rupture (least common), resulting in the acute onset of severe mitral regurgitation (Fig. 12–19C). Free-wall rupture is most frequent 3 to 7 days after MI, when coagulative necrosis, neutrophilic infiltration, and lysis of the myocardial connective tissue have appreciably weakened the infarcted myocardium (mean, 4 to 5 days; range, 1 to 10 days). The anterolateral wall at the midventricular level is the most common site for postinfarction free-wall rupture. Risk factors for free-wall rupture include age over 60, female gender, and preexisting hypertension. This complication occurs less frequently in patients without prior MI because associated fibrotic scarring tends to inhibit myocardial tearing. Acute free-wall ruptures are usually rapidly fatal. However, a fortuitously located pericardial adhesion that partially aborts a rupture may result in a *false aneurysm* (localized hematoma communicating with the ventricular cavity). The wall of a false aneurysm consists only of epicardium and adherent parietal pericardium and thus many still ultimately rupture.

- *Pericarditis.* A fibrinous or fibrinohemorrhagic pericarditis (Dressler syndrome) usually develops about the second or third day following a transmural infarct as a result of underlying myocardial inflammation (Fig. 12–19D).

- *Right ventricular infarction.* Isolated infarction of the right ventricle is unusual, but infarction of some right ventricular myocardium often accompanies ischemic injury of the adjacent posterior left ventricle and ventricular septum. Right ventricular infarcts of either type cause acute right-sided heart failure associated with pooling of blood in the venous circulation and systemic hypotension.

- Infarct *extension.* New necrosis may occur adjacent to an existing infarct.

- Infarct *expansion.* As a result of the weakening of necrotic muscle, there may be disproportionate stretching, thinning, and dilation of the infarct region (especially with anteroseptal infarcts), which is often associated with mural thrombus (Fig. 12–19E).

- *Mural thrombus.* With any infarct, the combination of a local abnormality in contractility (causing stasis) and endocardial damage (creating a thrombogenic surface) can foster *mural thrombosis* (Chapter 4) and potentially *thromboembolism.*

- *Ventricular aneurysm.* In contrast to the *false aneurysms* mentioned above, *true* aneurysms of the ventricular wall are bounded by myocardium that has become scarred. Aneurysms of the ventricular wall are a late complication of large transmural infarcts that experience early expansion. The thin scar tissue wall of an aneurysm paradoxically bulges during systole (Fig. 12–19F). Complications of ventricular aneurysms include mural thrombus, arrhythmias, and heart failure; rupture of the tough fibrotic wall is not a concern.

- *Papillary muscle dysfunction.* As mentioned above, rupture of a papillary muscle may occur following an MI. More frequently, postinfarct mitral regurgitation results from ischemic dysfunction of a papillary muscle and underlying myocardium and later from papillary muscle fibrosis and shortening, or from ventricular dilation (see below).

- *Progressive late heart failure* (chronic IHD is discussed below).

The risk of specific postinfarct complications and the prognosis depend primarily on the infarct size, location, and thickness (subendocardial or transmural). Large transmural infarcts yield a higher probability of cardiogenic shock, arrhythmias, and late CHF. Patients with anterior transmural infarcts are at greatest risk for free-wall rupture, expansion, mural thrombi, and aneurysm. In contrast, posterior transmural infarcts are more likely to be complicated by conduction blocks, right ventricular involvement, or both; when acute VSDs occur in this area they are more difficult to manage. Overall, however, patients with anterior infarcts have a worse clinical course than those with inferior (posterior) infarcts. With subendocardial infarcts, only rarely do pericarditis, rupture, and aneurysms occur.

In addition to the sequence of repair in the infarcted tissues described above, the noninfarcted segments of the ventricle undergo hypertrophy and dilation; collectively, these changes are termed *ventricular remodeling.* The compensatory hypertrophy of noninfarcted myocardium is initially hemodynamically beneficial. However, this adaptive effect may be overwhelmed by ventricular dilation (with or without ventricular aneurysm) and increased oxygen demand, which can exacerbate ischemia and depress cardiac function. There may also be changes in ventricular shape and stiffening of the ventricle due to scar formation and hypertrophy that further diminish cardiac output. Some of these deleterious effects appear to be reduced by ACE inhibitors, which lessen the ventricular dilation that occurs after MI.

Long-term prognosis after MI depends on many factors, the most important of which are the quality of residual left ventricular function and the extent of vascular obstructions in vessels that perfuse the viable myocardium. The overall total mortality within the first year is about 30%. Thereafter there is a 3% to 4% mortality among survivors with each passing year. Infarct prevention through control of risk factors in individuals who have never experienced MI *(primary prevention)* and prevention of reinfarction in those who have recovered from an acute MI *(secondary prevention)* are important

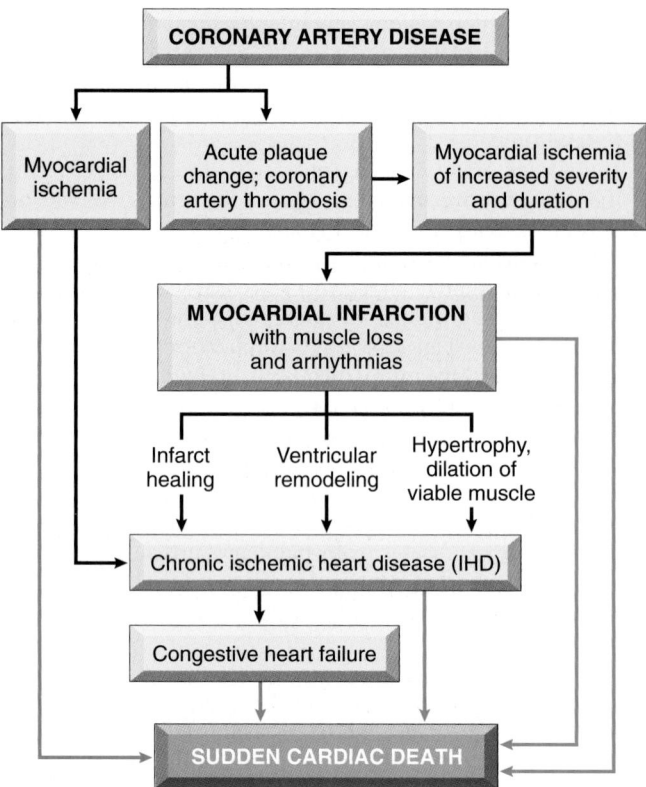

FIGURE 12–20 Schematic of the various pathways in the progression of ischemic heart disease (IHD), showing the interrelationships among coronary artery disease, acute plaque change, myocardial ischemia, myocardial infarction, chronic IHD, congestive heart failure, and sudden cardiac death.

strategies that have received much attention and achieved considerable success.

The relationship of the causes, pathophysiology, and consequences of MI are summarized in Figure 12–20, including the possible outcomes of chronic IHD and sudden death, to be discussed next.

CHRONIC IHD

The designation chronic IHD is used here to describe progressive heart failure as a consequence of ischemic myocardial damage. The term *ischemic cardiomyopathy* is often used by clinicians to describe chronic IHD. In most instances there has been prior MI and sometimes previous coronary arterial interventions and/or bypass surgery. Chronic IHD usually appears postinfarction due to the functional decompensation of hypertrophied noninfarcted myocardium (see earlier discussion of cardiac hypertrophy). However, in other cases severe obstructive coronary artery disease may present as chronic IHD in the absence of prior infarction.

Morphology. Hearts from patients with chronic IHD are usually enlarged and heavy, due to left ventricular hypertrophy and dilation. Invariably there is some degree of obstructive coronary atherosclerosis. Discrete scars representing healed infarcts are usually

present. The mural endocardium may have patchy, fibrous thickenings, and mural thrombi may be present. Microscopic findings include myocardial hypertrophy, diffuse subendocardial vacuolization, and fibrosis.

Clinically, progressive CHF may occur in patients who have had past episodes of MI or anginal attacks. In some individuals, however, progressive myocardial damage is silent, and heart failure is the first indication of IHD. The diagnosis rests largely on the exclusion of other cardiac diseases. Patients with chronic IHD account for nearly half of cardiac transplant recipients.

SUDDEN CARDIAC DEATH

Sudden cardiac death (SCD) strikes down about 300,000 to 400,000 individuals annually in the United States. It is defined as unexpected death from cardiac causes in individuals without symptomatic heart disease or early after symptom onset (usually within 1 hour). *SCD is usually the consequence of a lethal arrhythmia (e.g., asystole, ventricular fibrillation).* It most frequently occurs in the setting of IHD; in some cases, SCD is the first clinical manifestation of IHD.

Acute myocardial ischemia is the most common trigger for fatal arrhythmias.[57] Although ischemic injury can affect the conduction system and create electromechanical cardiac instability, fatal arrhythmias usually result from acute ischemia-induced electrical instability of myocardium that is distant from the conduction system. Arrythmogenic foci are often located adjacent to scars left by old MIs.

Nonatherosclerotic conditions associated with SCD include

- Congenital structural or coronary arterial abnormalities
- Aortic valve stenosis
- Mitral valve prolapse
- Myocarditis
- Dilated or hypertrophic cardiomyopathy
- Pulmonary hypertension
- Hereditary or acquired cardiac arrhythmias
- Cardiac hypertrophy of any cause (e.g., hypertension)
- Other miscellaneous causes, such as systemic metabolic and hemodynamic alterations, catecholamines, and drugs of abuse, particularly cocaine and methamphetamine.

Morphology. Marked coronary atherosclerosis with a critical (>75%) stenosis involving one or more of the three major vessels is present in 80% to 90% of SCD victims; only 10% to 20% of cases are of nonatherosclerotic origin. Usually there are high-grade stenoses (>90%); in approximately one half, acute plaque disruption is observed, and in approximately 25% diagnostic changes of acute MI are seen.[58] This suggests that many patients who die suddenly are suffering an MI, but the short interval from onset to death precludes the development of diagnostic myocardial changes. However, in one study of those who had been successfully resuscitated from a sudden cardiac arrest, a new MI occurred in only 39% of the patients.[59] Thus, most SCD is not associated with acute MI; most of these deaths are thought to result from myocardial ischemia–induced irritability that initiates malignant ventricular arrhythmias. Scars of previous infarcts and subendocardial myocyte vacuolization indicative of severe chronic ischemia are common in such patients.

Heritable conditions associated with SCD are of importance, since they may provide a basis for intervention in surviving family members.[60] Some of these disorders are associated with recognizable anatomic abnormalities (e.g., congenital anomalies, hypertrophic cardiomyopathy, mitral valve prolapse). However, other heritable arrhythmias can precipitate sudden death in the absence of structural cardiac pathology (so-called primary electrical disorders). These syndromes can only be diagnosed definitively by genetic testing, which is performed in those with a positive family history or an unexplained nonlethal arrhythmia.

The primary electrical abnormalities of the heart that predispose to SCD include long QT syndrome, Brugada syndrome, short QT syndrome, catecholaminergic polymorphic ventricular tachycardia, Wolff-Parkinson-White syndrome, congenital sick sinus syndrome, and isolated cardiac conduction disease.[61] The most important of these disorders are the so-called *channelopathies*, which are caused by mutations in genes that are required for normal ion channel function.[62] These disorders (mostly with autosomal-dominant inheritance) either involve genes that encode the ion channels (including Na[+], K[+], and Ca[+]), or accessory proteins that are essential for the normal function of the same channels, which are responsible for conducting the electrical currents that mediate contraction of the heart. The prototype is the *long QT syndrome*, characterized by prolongation of the QT segment in electrocardiograms and susceptibility to malignant ventricular arrhythmias. Mutations in seven different genes account for the majority of cases of long QT syndrome. The most frequent mutations are in the gene encoding KCNQ1 and result in decreased potassium currents. Ion channels are needed for the normal function of many tissues, and certain channelopathies are also associated with skeletal muscle disorders and diabetes; however, the most common cardiac channelopathies are isolated disorders of the heart.

The prognosis of many patients vulnerable to SCD, including those with chronic IHD, is markedly improved by implantation of a pacemaker or an automatic cardioverter defibrillator, which senses and electrically counteracts an episode of ventricular fibrillation.[63]

Hypertensive Heart Disease

Hypertensive heart disease (HHD) stems from the increased demands placed on the heart by hypertension, which causes pressure overload and ventricular hypertrophy. Although most commonly seen in the left heart as the result of systemic hypertension, pulmonary hypertension can cause right-sided HHD, or *cor pulmonale.*

SYSTEMIC (LEFT-SIDED) HYPERTENSIVE HEART DISEASE

In hypertension, hypertrophy of the heart is an adaptive response to pressure overload that can lead to myocardial dysfunction, cardiac dilation, CHF, and in some cases sudden death. *The minimal criteria for the diagnosis of systemic HHD are the following: (1) left ventricular hypertrophy (usually concentric) in the absence of other cardiovascular pathology and (2) a history or pathologic evidence of hypertension.* The Framingham Study established unequivocally that even mild hypertension (levels only slightly above 140/90 mm Hg), if sufficiently prolonged, induces left ventricular hypertrophy. Approximately 25% of the population of the United States suffers from hypertension of at least this degree. The pathogenesis of hypertension is discussed in Chapter 11.

Morphology. Hypertension induces left ventricular pressure overload hypertrophy, initially without ventricular dilation. As a result, the left ventricular wall thickening increases the weight of the heart disproportionately to the increase in overall cardiac size (Fig. 12–21A). The thickness of the left ventricular wall may exceed 2.0 cm, and the heart weight may exceed 500 gm. In time the increased thickness of the left ventricular wall imparts a stiffness that impairs diastolic filling, often inducing left atrial enlargement.

Microscopically, the earliest change of systemic HHD is an increase in the transverse diameter of myocytes, which may be difficult to appreciate on routine microscopy. At a more advanced stage variable degrees of cellular and nuclear enlargement become apparent, often accompanied by interstitial fibrosis. The biochemical, molecular, and morphologic changes that occur in hypertensive hypertrophy are similar to those noted in other conditions associated with myocardial pressure overload.

Compensated systemic HHD may be asymptomatic, producing only electrocardiographic or echocardiographic evidence of left ventricular enlargement. In many patients, systemic HHD comes to attention due to new atrial fibrillation induced by left atrial enlargement or CHF. Depending on the severity, duration, and underlying basis of the hypertension, and on the adequacy of therapeutic control, the patient may (1) enjoy normal longevity and die of unrelated causes, (2) develop IHD due to the potentiating effects of hypertension on coronary atherosclerosis, (3) suffer renal damage or cerebrovascular stroke as direct effects of hypertension, or (4) experience progressive heart failure or SCD. Effective control of hypertension can prevent or lead to regression of cardiac hypertrophy and its associated risks.

PULMONARY (RIGHT-SIDED) HYPERTENSIVE HEART DISEASE (COR PULMONALE)

Normally, because the pulmonary vasculature is the low pressure side of the circulation, the right ventricle has a thinner and more compliant wall than the left ventricle.[64] *Cor*

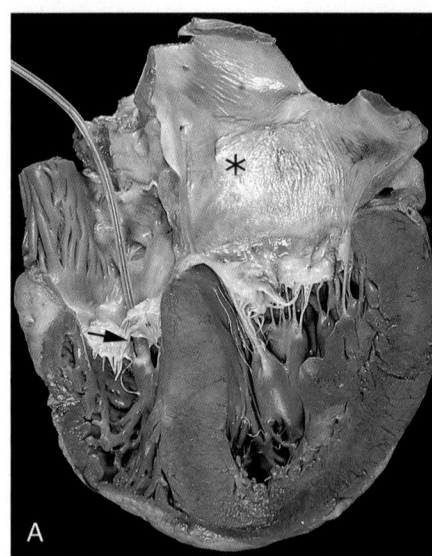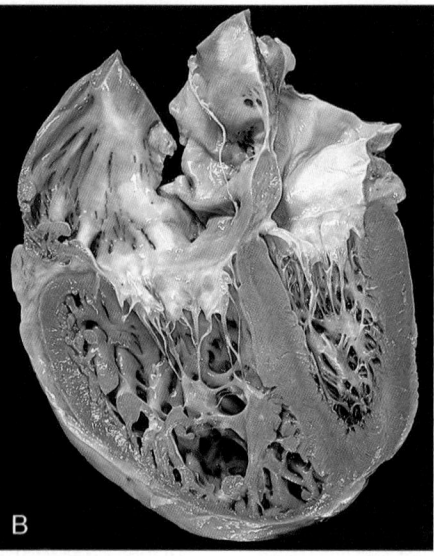

FIGURE 12–21 Hypertensive heart disease, systemic and pulmonary. **A,** Systemic (left-sided) hypertensive heart disease. There is marked concentric thickening of the left ventricular wall causing reduction in lumen size. The left ventricle and left atrium (*asterisk*) is on the *right* in this apical four-chamber view of the heart. A pacemaker is present in the right ventricle *(arrow)*. **B,** Pulmonary (right-sided) hypertensive heart disease (cor pulmonale). The right ventricle is markedly dilated and has a thickened free wall and hypertrophied trabeculae (apical four-chamber view of heart, right ventricle on *left*). The shape of the left ventricle (to the *right*) has been distorted by the enlarged right ventricle.

pulmonale, as isolated pulmonary HHD is frequently called, stems from pressure overload of the right ventricle,[65] and is characterized by right ventricular hypertrophy, dilation, and potentially failure secondary to pulmonary hypertension. The most frequent causes are disorders of the lungs, especially chronic respiratory diseases such as emphysema, or primary pulmonary hypertension (Table 12–6). It should be remembered, however, that pulmonary venous hypertension most commonly occurs as a complication of left-sided heart diseases of various etiologies.

Cor pulmonale may be acute or chronic. *Acute cor pulmonale* can follow massive pulmonary embolism. *Chronic cor*

pulmonale results from right ventricular hypertrophy (and dilation) secondary to prolonged pressure overload, such as can occur with chronic lung diseases and a variety of other conditions, many of which are discussed in more detail in Chapter 15.

> **Morphology.** In acute cor pulmonale there is marked dilation of the right ventricle without hypertrophy. On cross-section the normal crescent shape of the right ventricle is transformed to a dilated ovoid. In chronic cor pulmonale the right ventricular wall thickens, sometimes up to 1.0 cm or more (Fig. 12–21B). More subtle right ventricular hypertrophy may take the form of thickening of the muscle bundles in the outflow tract, immediately below the pulmonary valve, or thickening of the moderator band, the muscle bundle that connects the ventricular septum to the anterior right ventricular papillary muscle. Sometimes, the hypertrophied right ventricle compresses the left ventricular chamber, or leads to regurgitation and fibrous thickening of the tricuspid valve. Normally, the myocytes of the right ventricle are haphazardly arranged and the wall contains transmural fat; in right ventricular hypertrophy, fat in the wall disappears and the myocytes align themselves circumferentially.

Valvular Heart Disease

Valvular disease can come to clinical attention due to stenosis, insufficiency (regurgitation or incompetence), or both. *Stenosis is the failure of a valve to open completely, which impedes forward flow. Insufficiency, in contrast, results from failure of a valve to close completely, thereby allowing reversed flow.* These abnormalities can be present alone or coexist, and may involve only a single valve (*isolated disease*) or more than one valve (*combined disease*). *Functional regurgitation* is used to describe the incompetence of a valve stemming from an abnormality in one of its support structures. For example, dilation of the

TABLE 12–6 Disorders Predisposing to Cor Pulmonale
DISEASES OF THE PULMONARY PARENCHYMA
Chronic obstructive pulmonary disease
Diffuse pulmonary interstitial fibrosis
Pneumoconioses
Cystic fibrosis
Bronchiectasis
DISEASES OF THE PULMONARY VESSELS
Recurrent pulmonary thromboembolism
Primary pulmonary hypertension
Extensive pulmonary arteritis (e.g., Wegener granulomatosis)
Drug-, toxin-, or radiation-induced vascular obstruction
Extensive pulmonary tumor microembolism
DISORDERS AFFECTING CHEST MOVEMENT
Kyphoscoliosis
Marked obesity (sleep apnea, pickwickian syndrome)
Neuromuscular diseases
DISORDERS INDUCING PULMONARY ARTERIAL CONSTRICTION
Metabolic acidosis
Hypoxemia
Chronic altitude sickness
Obstruction of major airways
Idiopathic alveolar hypoventilation

TABLE 12–7 Major Etilogies of Acquired Heart Valve Disease	
Mitral Valve Disease	**Aortic Valve Disease**
MITRAL STENOSIS	**AORTIC STENOSIS**
Postinflammatory scarring (rheumatic heart disease)	Postinflammatory scarring (rheumatic heart disease) Senile calcific aortic stenosis Calcification of congenitally deformed valve
MITRAL REGURGITATION	**AORTIC REGURGITATION**
Abnormalities of Leaflets and Commissures Postinflammatory scarring Infective endocarditis Mitral valve prolapse Drugs (e.g., fen-phen) **Abnormalities of Tensor Apparatus** Rupture of papillary muscle Papillary muscle dysfunction (fibrosis) Rupture of chordae tendineae	Postinflammatory scarring (rheumatic heart disease) Infective endocarditis Marfan syndrome **Aortic Disease** Degenerative aortic dilation Syphilitic aortitis Ankylosing spondylitis Rheumatoid arthritis Marfan syndrome
Abnormalities of Left Ventricular Cavity and/or Annulus LV enlargement (myocarditis, dilated cardiomyopathy) Calcification of mitral ring	

LV, Left ventricular.
Modified from Schoen FJ: Surgical pathology of removed natural and prosthetic valves. Hum Pathol 18:558, 1987.

right or left ventricle can pull the ventricular papillary muscles down and outward, thereby preventing proper closure of otherwise normal mitral or tricuspid leaflets. Similarly, dilation of the aortic or pulmonary artery may pull the valve commissures apart and prevent full closure of the aortic or pulmonary valve cusps. Functional mitral valve regurgitation is particularly common in IHD (*ischemic mitral regurgitation*).[66]

The clinical consequences of valve dysfunction vary depending on the valve involved, the degree of impairment, how fast it develops, and the rate and quality of compensatory mechanisms. For example, sudden destruction of an aortic valve cusp by infection (infective endocarditis; see later) can cause acute, massive regurgitation that can be rapidly fatal. In contrast, rheumatic mitral stenosis usually develops indolently over years, and its clinical effects are often remarkably well tolerated. Certain conditions can complicate valvular heart disease by increasing the demands on the heart; for example, pregnancy can exacerbate valve disease and lead to an unfavorable maternal or fetal outcome.[67] Valvular stenosis or insufficiency often produces secondary changes, both proximal and distal to the affected valve. Generally, valvular stenosis leads to pressure overload of the heart, whereas valvular insufficiency leads to volume overload of the heart. In addition, the ejection of blood through narrowed stenotic valves can produce high speed "jets" of blood that injure the endocardium where they impact.

Valvular abnormalities may be congenital (discussed earlier) or acquired. *Acquired stenoses of the aortic and mitral valves account for approximately two thirds of all cases of valve disease.* Valvular stenosis is almost always due to a chronic abnormality of the valve cusp that becomes clinically evident after many years. Relatively few disorders produce valvular stenosis. In contrast, valvular insufficiency can result from intrinsic disease of the valve cusps or damage to or distortion of the supporting structures (e.g., the aorta, mitral annulus, tendinous cords,

papillary muscles, ventricular free wall). Valvular insufficiency has many causes and may appear acutely, as with rupture of the cords, or chronically in disorders associated with leaflet scarring and retraction.

The causes of acquired heart valve diseases are summarized in Table 12–7 and discussed in the following sections. The most frequent causes of the major functional valvular lesions are:

- Aortic stenosis: calcification of anatomically normal and congenitally bicuspid aortic valves
- Aortic insufficiency: dilation of the ascending aorta, usually related to hypertension and aging
- Mitral stenosis: rheumatic heart disease
- Mitral insufficiency: myxomatous degeneration (mitral valve prolapse)

VALVULAR DEGENERATION ASSOCIATED WITH CALCIFICATION

Heart valves are subjected to high levels of repetitive mechanical stress, particularly at the hinge points of the cusps and leaflets, as a result of (1) 40 million or more cardiac contractions per year, (2) substantial tissue deformations during each contraction, and (3) transvalvular pressure gradients in the closed phase of each contraction of approximately 120 mm Hg for the mitral and 80 mm Hg for the aortic valve. It is therefore not surprising that these delicate structures can suffer cumulative damage and dystrophic calcification (deposits of calcium phosphate salts) that lead to clinically important dysfunction.[68]

Calcific Aortic Stenosis

The most common of all valvular abnormalities, acquired aortic stenosis, is usually the consequence of age-associated

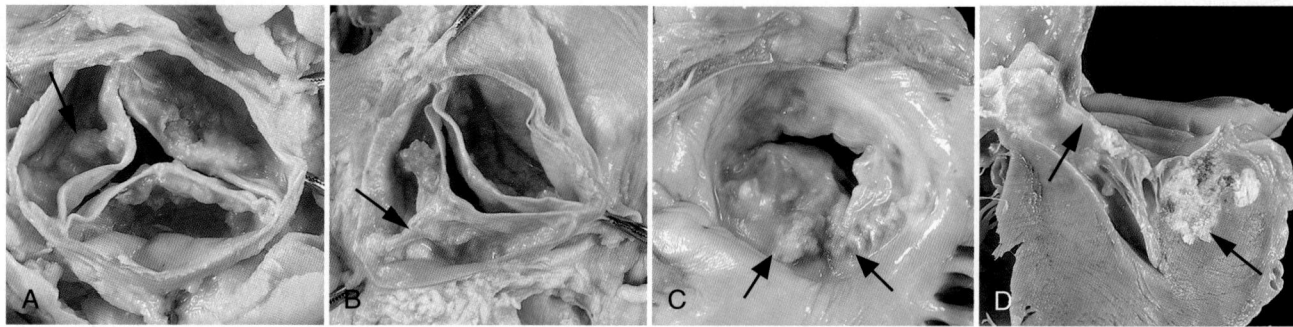

FIGURE 12–22 Calcific valvular degeneration. **A,** Calcific aortic stenosis of a previously normal valve (viewed from aortic aspect). Nodular masses of calcium are heaped up within the sinuses of Valsalva *(arrow).* Note that the commissures are not fused, as in postrheumatic aortic valve stenosis (see Fig. 12–27E). **B,** Calcific aortic stenosis of a congenitally bicuspid valve. One cusp has a partial fusion at its center, called a *raphe (arrow).* **C** and **D,** Mitral annular calcification, with calcific nodules at the base (attachment margin) of the anterior mitral leaflet *(arrows).* **C,** Left atrial view. **D,** Cut section of myocardium.

"wear and tear" of either anatomically normal valves or congenitally bicuspid valves (~1% of the population).[69] The prevalence of aortic stenosis, estimated at 2%, is increasing with the rising average age of the population. Aortic stenosis of previously normal valves (termed senile calcific aortic stenosis) usually comes to clinical attention in the seventh to ninth decades of life, whereas stenotic bicuspid valves tend to present in patients 50 to 70 years of age.

Prior work attributed aortic valve calcification to wear and tear degeneration and dystrophic and passive accumulation of hydroxyapatite, the same calcium salt that is found in bone.[70] More recent studies suggest that chronic injury due to hyperlipidemia, hypertension, inflammation, and other factors implicated in atherosclerosis may have a role and perhaps even precede the calcification. It is clear, however, that the valve injury of calcific aortic stenosis differs in some respects from atherosclerosis. Most notably, instead of accumulating smooth muscle cells, the abnormal valves contain cells resembling osteoblasts that synthesize bone matrix proteins and promote the deposition of calcium salts. Bicuspid valves incur greater mechanical stress than normal tricuspid valves, which may explain why they become stenotic more rapidly.

Morphology. The morphologic hallmark of nonrheumatic, calcific aortic stenosis (with either tricuspid or bicuspid valves) is heaped-up calcified masses within the aortic cusps that ultimately protrude through the outflow surfaces into the sinuses of Valsalva, preventing the opening of the cusps. The free edges of the cusps are usually not involved (Fig. 12–22A). The calcific process begins in the valvular fibrosa, at the points of maximal cusp flexion (near the margins of attachment). Microscopically, the layered architecture of the valve is largely preserved. An earlier, hemodynamically inconsequential stage of the calcification process is called **aortic valve sclerosis.** In aortic stenosis the functional valve area is decreased sufficiently by large nodular calcific deposits to cause measurable obstruction to outflow; this subjects the left ventricular myocardium to progressively increasing pressure overload.

In contrast to rheumatic (and congenital) aortic stenosis (see Fig. 12–24E), commissural fusion is not usually seen. The mitral valve is generally normal, although some patients may have direct extension of aortic valve calcific deposits onto the anterior mitral leaflet. In contrast, virtually all patients with rheumatic aortic stenosis also have concomitant and characteristic structural abnormalities of the mitral valve (see later).

Clinical Features. In calcific aortic stenosis (superimposed on a previously normal or bicuspid aortic valve), the obstruction to left ventricular outflow leads to gradual narrowing of the valve orifice (valve area approximately 0.5 to 1 cm^2 in severe aortic stenosis; normal, ~4 cm^2) and an increasing pressure gradient across the calcified valve, reaching 75 to 100 mm Hg in severe cases. Left ventricular pressures rise to 200 mm Hg or more in such instances, producing concentric left ventricular (pressure overload) hypertrophy. The hypertrophied myocardium tends to be ischemic (as a result of diminished microcirculatory perfusion, often complicated by coronary atherosclerosis), and angina pectoris may appear. Both systolic and diastolic myocardial function may be impaired; eventually, cardiac decompensation and CHF may ensue. The onset of symptoms (angina, CHF, or syncope, for which the pathophysiologic basis is poorly understood) in aortic stenosis heralds cardiac decompensation and carries a poor prognosis; ~50% with angina will die within 5 years, and 50% with CHF will die within 2 years, if the obstruction is not alleviated by surgical valve replacement. Medical therapy is ineffective in severe symptomatic aortic stenosis. In contrast, asymptomatic patients with aortic stenosis generally have an excellent prognosis.

Calcific Stenosis of Congenitally Bicuspid Aortic Valve

With a prevalence of approximately 1%, bicuspid aortic valve (BAV) is the most frequent congenital cardiovascular malformation in humans.[71] Although BAV is usually uncomplicated early in life, late complications of BAV include aortic stenosis or regurgitation, infective endocarditis, and aortic dilation and/or dissection. BAVs are predisposed to progressive degenerative calcification, similar to that occurring in aortic valves with initially normal anatomy (see Fig. 12–22B). Bicuspid aortic valves are responsible for approximately 50% of cases of aortic stenosis in adults.[72] Structural abnormalities of the aortic wall commonly accompany BAV, even when the valve is hemodynamically normal, and this may potentiate aortic dilation or aortic dissection (see later). Recent studies have confirmed previous reports of familial clustering of BAV and left ventricular outflow tract obstruction malformations, and their association with other cardiovascular malformations.[73]

In a congenitally bicuspid aortic valve, there are only two functional cusps, usually of unequal size, with the larger cusp having a midline *raphe*, resulting from incomplete commissural separation during development; less frequently the cusps are of equal size and the raphe is absent. The raphe is frequently a major site of calcific deposits. Once stenosis is present, the clinical course is similar to that described above for calcific aortic stenosis. Valves that become bicuspid because of an acquired deformity (e.g., rheumatic valve disease) have a fused commissure that produces a conjoined cusp that is generally twice the size of the nonconjoined cusp. BAVs may also become incompetent as a result of aortic dilation, cusp prolapse, or infective endocarditis. The mitral valve is generally normal in patients with a congenitally bicuspid aortic valve.

Mitral Annular Calcification

Degenerative calcific deposits can develop in the peripheral fibrous ring *(annulus)* of the mitral valve. Grossly, these appear as irregular, stony hard, occasionally ulcerated nodules (2–5 mm in thickness) that lie behind the leaflets (see Fig. 12–22C and D). The process generally does not affect valvular function or otherwise become clinically important. In unusual cases, however, mitral annular calcification may lead to (1) regurgitation by interfering with physiologic contraction of the valve ring, (2) stenosis by impairing opening of the mitral leaflets, or (3) arrhythmias and occasionally sudden death by penetration of calcium deposits to a depth sufficient to impinge on the atrioventricular conduction system. Because calcific nodules may also provide a site for thrombi that can embolize, patients with mitral annular calcification have an increased risk of stroke, and the calcific nodules can also be the nidus for infective endocarditis. Heavy calcific deposits are sometimes visualized on echocardiography or seen as a distinctive, ringlike opacity on chest radiographs. Mitral annular calcification is most common in women over age 60 and individuals with mitral valve prolapse (see below) or elevated left ventricular pressure (as in systemic hypertension, aortic stenosis, or hypertrophic cardiomyopathy).

MITRAL VALVE PROLAPSE (MYXOMATOUS DEGENERATION OF THE MITRAL VALVE)

In mitral valve prolapse (MVP), one or both mitral valve leaflets are "floppy" and *prolapse*, or balloon back, into the left atrium during systole.[74] The key histologic change in the tissue is called *myxomatous degeneration*. MVP affects approximately

3% of adults in the United States; it is most often an incidental finding on physical examination (particularly in young women), but in a small minority of affected individuals may lead to serious complications.

> **Morphology.** The characteristic anatomic change in MVP is interchordal ballooning (hooding) of the mitral leaflets or portions thereof (Fig. 12–23A–C). The affected leaflets are often enlarged, redundant, thick, and rubbery. The associated tendinous cords may be elongated, thinned, or even ruptured, and the annulus may be dilated. The tricuspid, aortic, or pulmonary valves may also be affected. Histologically, there is attenuation of the collagenous fibrosa layer of the valve, on which the structural integrity of the leaflet depends, accompanied by marked thickening of the spongiosa layer with deposition of mucoid (myxomatous) material (Fig. 12–23E). Secondary changes reflect the stresses and injury incident to the billowing leaflets: (1) fibrous thickening of the valve leaflets, particularly where they rub against each other; (2) linear fibrous thickening of the left ventricular endocardial surface where the abnormally long cords snap or rub against it; (3) thickening of the mural endocardium of the left ventricle or atrium as a consequence of friction-induced injury induced by the prolapsing, hyper-mobile leaflets; (4) thrombi on the atrial surfaces of the leaflets or the atrial walls; and (5) focal calcifications at the base of the posterior mitral leaflet. Mild myxomatous degeneration can also occur in mitral valves secondary to regurgitation of other etiologies (e.g., ischemic dysfunction).

Pathogenesis. The basis for the changes that weaken the valve leaflets and associated structures is unknown in most cases. Uncommonly, MVP is associated with heritable disorders of connective tissue including Marfan syndrome, which is usually caused by mutations in fibrillin-1 (FBN-1) (Chapter 5). As you will recall, defects in FBN-1 alter cell-matrix interactions and also dysregulate TGF-β signaling.[75] Of interest, mice engineered to express mutated FBN-1 develop a form of mitral valve prolapse that can be prevented by inhibitors of TGF-β,[76] indicating that excess TGF-β can cause the characteristic structural laxity and myxomatous change. Whether similar mechanisms contribute to sporadic MVP is unknown. Studies utilizing genetic linkage analysis have also mapped autosomal-dominant forms of MVP to several other genetic loci that may be involved in remodeling of the valvular extracellular matrix.[77]

Clinical Features. Most individuals diagnosed with MVP are asymptomatic, and the condition is discovered incidentally by detection of a midsystolic click on physical examination. The diagnosis can be confirmed by echocardiography. Those cases with mitral regurgitation are also associated with a systolic murmur. A minority of patients have chest pain mimicking angina, dyspnea, and fatigue. Although the great majority of persons with MVP have no untoward effects, approximately 3% develop one of four serious complications: (1) infective endocarditis; (2) mitral insufficiency, sometimes with chordal rupture; (3) stroke or other systemic

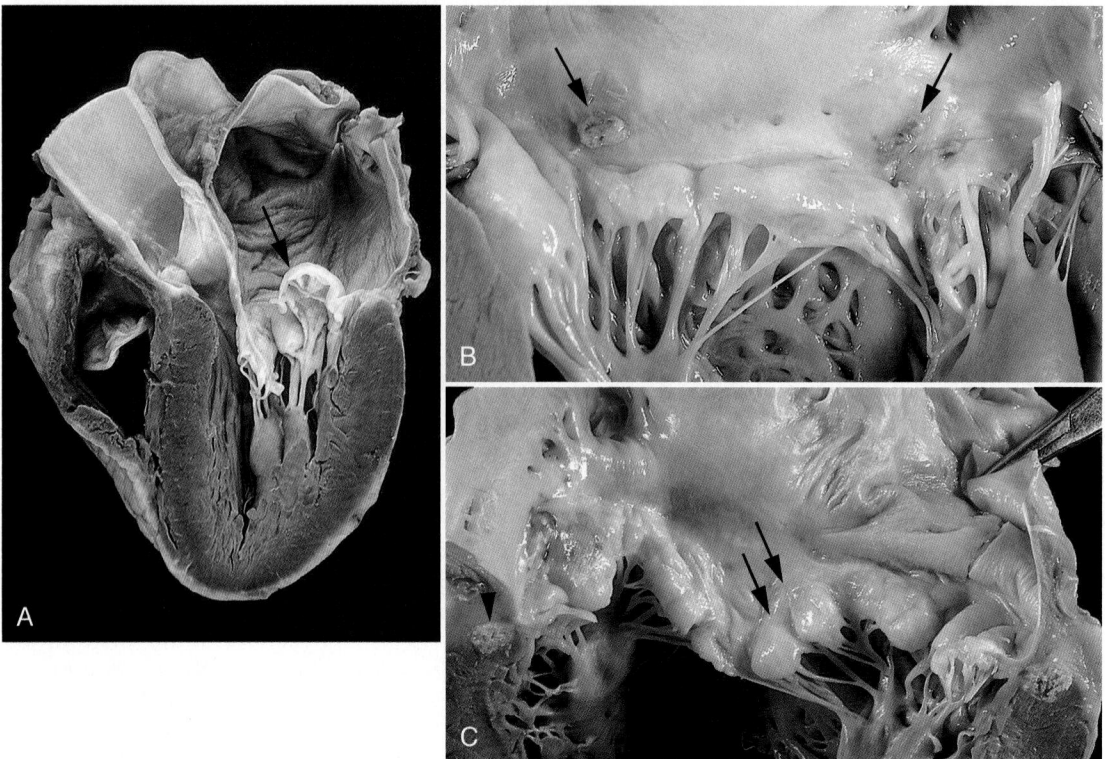

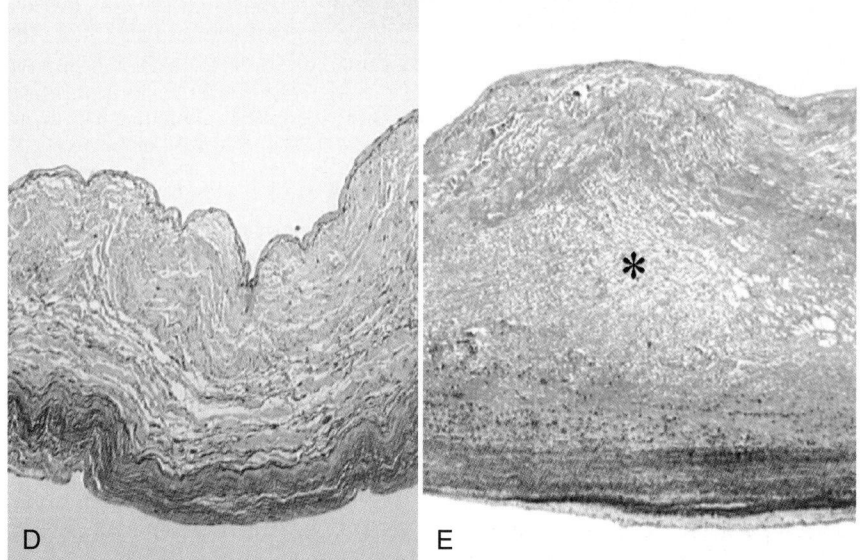

FIGURE 12–23 Myxomatous degeneration of the mitral valve. **A,** Long axis of left ventricle demonstrating hooding with prolapse of the posterior mitral leaflet into the left atrium *(arrow).* The left ventricle is on right in this apical four-chamber view. **B,** Opened valve, showing pronounced hooding of the posterior mitral leaflet with thrombotic plaques at sites of leaflet–left atrium contact *(arrows).* **C,** Opened valve with pronounced hooding from patient who died suddenly *(double arrows).* Note also mitral annular calcification *(arrowhead).* Normal heart valve **(D)** and myxomatous mitral valve **(E)** (Movat pentachrome stain, in which collagen is yellow, elastin is black, and proteoglycans are blue). In myxomatous valves, collagen in the fibrosa is loose and disorganized, proteolgycans *(asterisk)* are deposited in the spongiosa, and elastin in the atrialis is disorganized. (**A,** Courtesy of William D. Edwards, MD, Mayo Clinic, Rochester, MN; **D,E,** From Rabkin E, et al: Activated interstitial myofibroblasts express catabolic enzymes and mediate matrix remodeling in myxomatous heart valves. Circulation 104:2525–2532, 2001.)

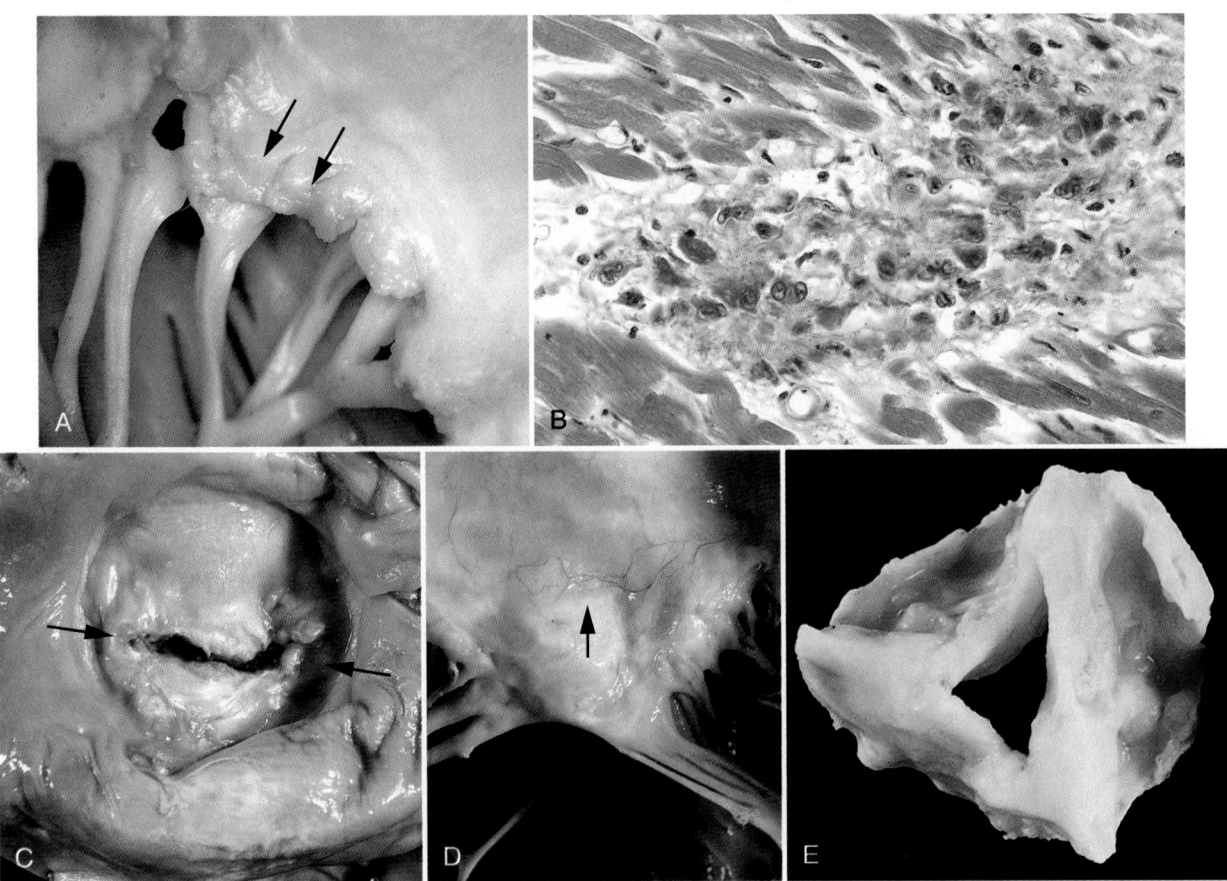

FIGURE 12–24 Acute and chronic rheumatic heart disease. **A,** Acute rheumatic mitral valvulitis superimposed on chronic rheumatic heart disease. Small vegetations (verrucae) are visible along the line of closure of the mitral valve leaflet *(arrows)*. Previous episodes of rheumatic valvulitis have caused fibrous thickening and fusion of the chordae tendineae. **B,** Microscopic appearance of Aschoff body in a patient with acute rheumatic carditis. The myocardial interstitium has a circumscribed collection of mononuclear inflammatory cells, including some large macrophages with prominent nucleoli and a binuclear macrophage, associated with necrosis. **C** and **D,** Mitral stenosis with diffuse fibrous thickening and distortion of the valve leaflets and commissural fusion *(arrows,* C), and thickening of the chordae tendineae (**D**). Note neovascularization of anterior mitral leaflet *(arrow,* D). **E,** Rheumatic aortic stenosis, demonstrating thickening and distortion of the cusps with commissural fusion. (**E,** Reproduced from Schoen FJ, St. John-Sutton M: Contemporary issues in the pathology of valvular heart disease. Hum Pathol 18:568, 1967.)

infarct, resulting from embolism of leaflet thrombi; or (4) arrhythmias, both ventricular and atrial.

The risk of complications is very low when MVP is discovered incidentally in young asymptomatic patients, and higher in men, older patients, and those with arrhythmias or mitral regurgitation. For patients with symptoms or at high risk for serious complications, valve surgery is often done; indeed, MVP is presently the most common cause for surgical repair or replacement of the mitral valve.

RHEUMATIC FEVER AND RHEUMATIC HEART DISEASE

Rheumatic fever (RF) is an acute, immunologically mediated, multisystem inflammatory disease that occurs a few weeks after an episode of group A streptococcal pharyngitis.[78] Acute rheumatic carditis is a frequent manifestation during the active phase of RF and may progress over time to chronic rheumatic heart disease (RHD), of which valvular abnormalities are key manifestations.

RHD is characterized principally by deforming fibrotic valvular disease, particularly mitral stenosis, of which it is virtually the only cause. The incidence and mortality rate of RF and RHD have declined remarkably in many parts of the world over the past century, as a result of improved socioeconomic conditions and rapid diagnosis and treatment of streptococcal pharyngitis. Nevertheless, in developing countries, and in many crowded, economically depressed urban areas in the Western world, RHD remains an important public health problem, affecting an estimated 15 million people. Rheumatic fever only rarely follows infections by streptococci at other sites, such as the skin.

Morphology. Key pathologic features of acute RF and chronic RHD are shown in Figure 12–24. During acute RF, focal inflammatory lesions are found in various tissues. Distinctive lesions occur in the heart, called **Aschoff bodies**, which consist of foci of lymphocytes (primarily T cells), occasional plasma cells, and plump activated macrophages called Anitschkow cells (pathognomonic for RF). These macrophages have abundant cytoplasm and central round-to-ovoid nuclei in which the chromatin is disposed in a central, slender, wavy ribbon (hence the designation **"caterpillar cells"**), and may become multinucleated.

During acute RF, diffuse inflammation and Aschoff bodies may be found in any of the three layers of the heart, causing pericarditis, myocarditis, or endocarditis (**pancarditis**).

Inflammation of the endocardium and the left-sided valves typically results in fibrinoid necrosis within the cusps or along the tendinous cords. Overlying these necrotic foci are small (1- to 2-mm) vegetations, called **verrucae**, along the lines of closure. These vegetations place RHD within a small group of disorders that are associated with vegetative valve disease, each with its own characteristic morphologic features (Fig. 12–25). Subendocardial lesions, perhaps exacerbated by regurgitant jets, may induce irregular thickenings called **MacCallum plaques**, usually in the left atrium.

The cardinal anatomic changes of the mitral valve in chronic RHD are **leaflet thickening, commissural fusion and shortening, and thickening and fusion of the tendinous cords** (Fig. 12–24D). In chronic disease the mitral valve is virtually always involved. The mitral valve is affected alone in 65% to 70% of cases, and along with the aortic valve in another 25% of cases. Tricuspid valve involvement is infrequent, and the pulmonary valve is only rarely affected. Because of the increase in calcific aortic stenosis (see earlier) and the reduced frequency of RHD, rheumatic aortic stenosis now accounts for less than 10% of cases of acquired aortic stenosis. Fibrous bridging across the valvular commissures and calcification create "fish mouth" or "buttonhole" stenoses. With tight mitral stenosis, the left atrium progressively dilates and may harbor mural thrombi in the appendage or along the wall, either of which can embolize. Long-standing congestive changes in the lungs may induce pulmonary vascular and parenchymal changes and in time lead to right ventricular hypertrophy. The left ventricle is largely unaffected by isolated pure mitral stenosis. Microscopically, in the mitral leaflets there is organization of the acute inflammation and subsequent diffuse fibrosis and neovascularization that obliterate the originally layered and avascular leaflet architecture. Aschoff bodies are rarely seen in surgical specimens or autopsy tissue from patients with chronic RHD, as a result of the long times between the initial insult and the development of the chronic deformity.

Pathogenesis. *Acute rheumatic fever results from immune responses to group A streptococci*, which happen to cross-react with host tissues. Antibodies directed against the M proteins of streptococci have been shown to cross-react with self antigens in the heart. In addition, CD4+ T cells specific for streptococcal peptides also react with self proteins in the heart, and produce cytokines that activate macrophages (such as those found in Aschoff bodies). Damage to heart tissue may thus be caused by a combination of antibody- and T cell–mediated reactions (Chapter 6).

Clinical Features. *RF is characterized by a constellation of findings that includes as major manifestations: (1) migratory polyarthritis of the large joints, (2) pancarditis, (3) subcutaneous nodules, (4) erythema marginatum of the skin, and (5) Sydenham chorea, a neurologic disorder with involuntary rapid, purposeless movements.* The diagnosis is established by the so-called Jones criteria: evidence of a preceding group A streptococcal infection, with the presence of two of the major manifestations listed above or one major and two minor manifestations (nonspecific signs and symptoms that include fever, arthralgia, or elevated blood levels of acute-phase reactants).[80]

Acute RF typically appears 10 days to 6 weeks after an episode of pharyngitis caused by group A streptococci in about 3% of infected patients. It occurs most often in children between ages 5 and 15, but first attacks can occur in middle to later life. Although pharyngeal cultures for streptococci are negative by the time the illness begins, antibodies to one or more streptococcal enzymes, such as streptolysin O and DNase B, can be detected in the sera of most patients with RF. The predominant clinical manifestations are carditis and arthritis, the latter more common in adults than in children. Clinical features related to *acute carditis* include pericardial friction rubs, weak heart sounds, tachycardia, and arrhythmias. Myocarditis may cause cardiac dilation that can evolve to functional mitral valve insufficiency or even heart failure. Approximately 1% of patients die from fulminant RF. *Arthritis* typically begins with migratory polyarthritis (accompanied by fever) in which one large joint after another becomes painful and swollen for a period of days and then subsides spontaneously, leaving no residual disability.

After an initial attack there is increased vulnerability to reactivation of the disease with subsequent pharyngeal infections, and the same manifestations are likely to appear with each recurrent attack. Damage to the valves is cumulative. Turbulence induced by ongoing valvular deformities begets additional fibrosis. Clinical manifestations appear years or even decades after the initial episode of RF and depend on which cardiac valves are involved. In addition to various cardiac murmurs, cardiac hypertrophy and dilation, and heart failure, individuals with chronic RHD may suffer from arrhythmias (particularly atrial fibrillation in the setting of mitral stenosis), thromboembolic complications, and infective endocarditis (see below). The long-term prognosis is highly variable. Surgical repair or prosthetic replacement of diseased valves has greatly improved the outlook for persons with RHD.

INFECTIVE ENDOCARDITIS

Infective endocarditis (IE) is a serious infection characterized by colonization or invasion of the heart valves or the mural endocardium by a microbe.[81] This leads to the formation of *vegetations* composed of thrombotic debris and organisms, often associated with destruction of the underlying cardiac tissues. The aorta, aneurysmal sacs, other blood vessels, and prosthetic devices can also become infected. Although fungi and other classes of microorganisms can be responsible, most cases are caused by bacterial infections *(bacterial endo-*

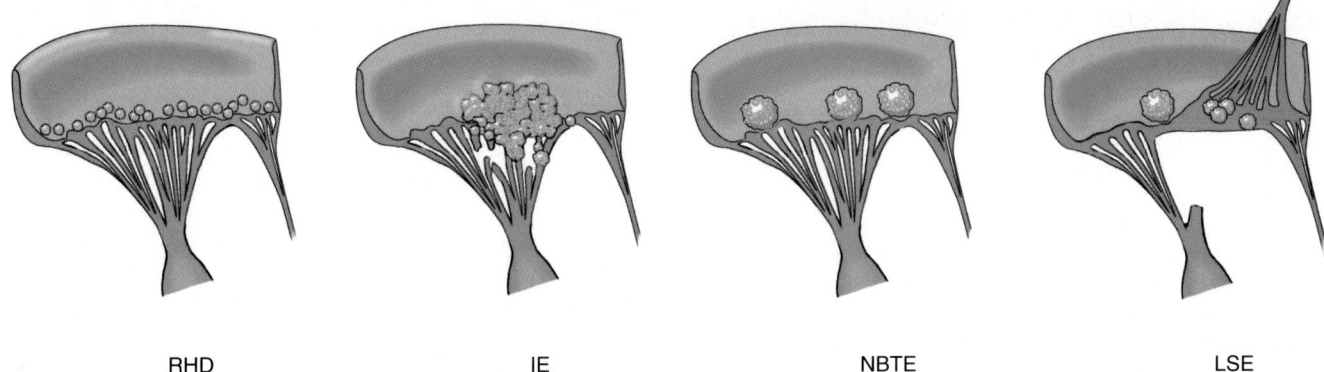

RHD   IE   NBTE   LSE

FIGURE 12–25 Comparison of the four major forms of vegetative endocarditis. The rheumatic fever phase of rheumatic heart disease (RHD) is marked by small, warty vegetations along the lines of closure of the valve leaflets. Infective endocarditis (IE) is characterized by large, irregular masses on the valve cusps that can extend onto the chordae (see Fig. 12–25). Nonbacterial thrombotic endocarditis (NBTE) typically exhibits small, bland vegetations, usually attached at the line of closure. One or many may be present (see Fig. 12–27). Libman-Sacks endocarditis (LSE) has small or medium-sized vegetations on either or both sides of the valve leaflets.

carditis). Prompt diagnosis and effective treatment of IE is important.

Traditionally, IE has been classified on clinical grounds into acute and subacute forms. This subdivision reflects the range of the disease severity and tempo, which are determined in large part by the virulence of the infecting microorganism and whether underlying cardiac disease is present. *Acute infective endocarditis* is typically caused by infection of a previously normal heart valve by a highly virulent organism that produces necrotizing, ulcerative, destructive lesions. These infections are difficult to cure with antibiotics and usually require surgery. Death within days to weeks ensues in many patients with acute IE, despite treatment. In contrast, in *subacute IE*, the organisms are of lower virulence. These organisms cause insidious infections of deformed valves that are less destructive. In such cases the disease may pursue a protracted course of weeks to months, and cures are often produced with antibiotics.

Etiology and Pathogenesis. As mentioned above, IE can develop on previously normal valves, especially with highly virulent organisms, but a variety of cardiac and vascular abnormalities predispose to this form of infection. In years past, rheumatic heart disease was the major antecedent disorder, but more common now are mitral valve prolapse, degenerative calcific valvular stenosis, bicuspid aortic valve (whether calcified or not), artificial (prosthetic) valves, and unrepaired and repaired congenital defects.[82] The causative organisms differ somewhat in the major high-risk groups. Endocarditis of native but previously damaged or otherwise abnormal valves is caused most commonly (50% to 60% of cases) by *Streptococcus viridans*, which is part of the normal flora of the oral cavity. In contrast, more virulent *S. aureus* organisms commonly found on the skin can infect either healthy or deformed valves and are responsible for 10% to 20% of cases overall; *S. aureus* is the major offender in intravenous drug abusers with IE. The roster of the remaining bacteria includes enterococci and the so-called HACEK group (*Haemophilus, Actinobacillus, Cardiobacterium, Eikenella*, and *Kingella*), all commensals in the oral cavity. Prosthetic valve endocarditis is caused most commonly by coagulase-negative staphylococci

(e.g., *S. epidermidis*). Other agents causing endocarditis include gram-negative bacilli and fungi. In about 10% to 15% of all cases of endocarditis, no organism can be isolated from the blood ("culture-negative" endocarditis).

Foremost among the factors predisposing to the development of endocarditis are those that lead to bacteremia. The source of the organism may be an obvious infection elsewhere, a dental or surgical procedure, a contaminated needle shared by intravenous drug users, or seemingly trivial breaks in the epithelial barriers of the gut, oral cavity, or skin. The risk can be lowered in those with predisposing factors (e.g., valve abnormalities, conditions causing bacteremia) by prophylaxis with antibiotics.

Morphology. The hallmark of IE is the presence of friable, bulky, potentially destructive **vegetations** containing fibrin, inflammatory cells, and bacteria or other organisms on the heart valves (Figs. 12–25B and 12–26). The aortic and mitral valves are the most common sites of infection, although the valves of the right heart may also be involved, particularly in intravenous drug abusers. The vegetations may be single or multiple and may involve more than one valve. Vegetations sometimes erode into the underlying myocardium and produce an abscess (**ring abscess**). **Emboli** may be shed from the vegetations at any time; because the embolic fragments may contain large numbers of virulent organisms, abscesses often develop at the sites where the emboli lodge, leading to sequelae such as **septic infarcts** or mycotic aneurysms.

The vegetations of **subacute endocarditis** are associated with less valvular destruction than those of acute endocarditis, although the distinction between the two forms may blur. Microscopically, the vegetations of typical subacute IE often have granulation tissue indicative of healing at their bases. With time, fibrosis, calcification, and a chronic inflammatory infiltrate can develop.

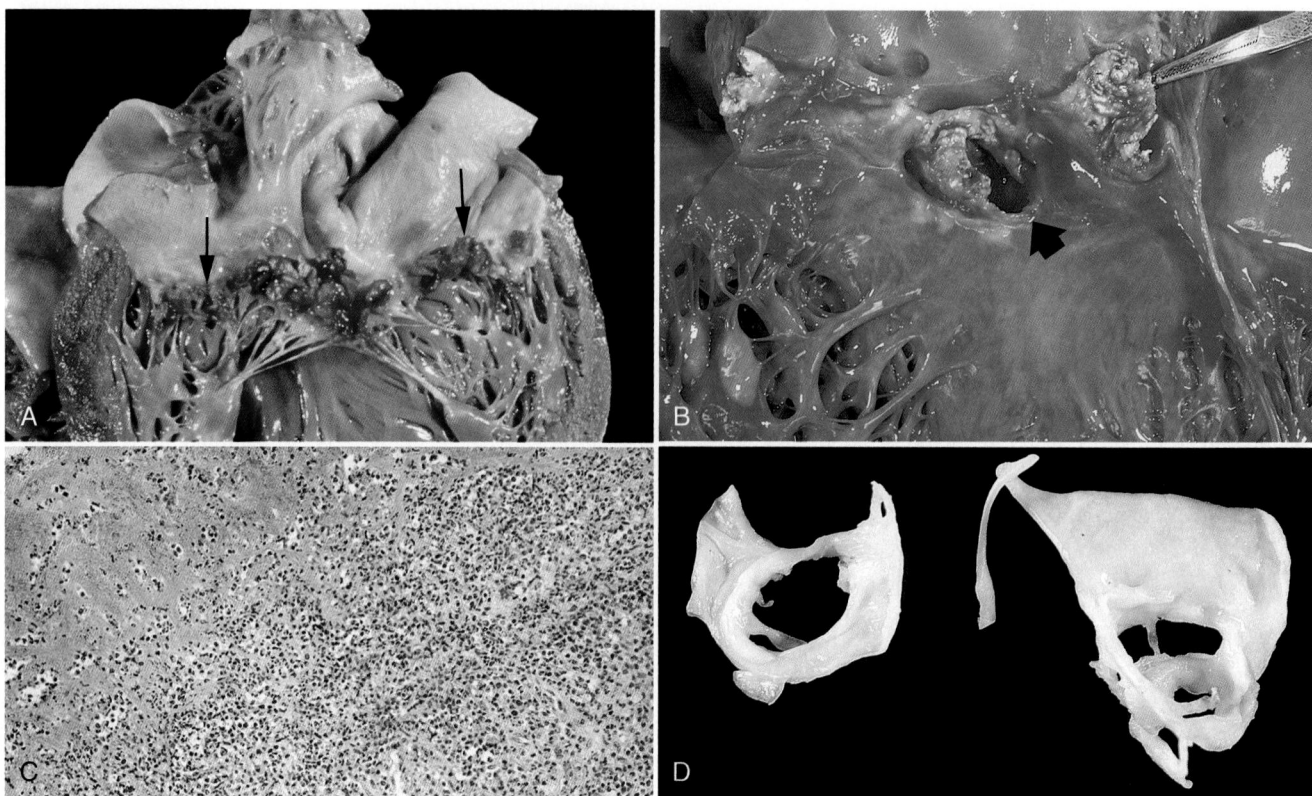

FIGURE 12–26 Infective (bacterial) endocarditis. **A,** Endocarditis of mitral valve (subacute, caused by *Streptococcus viridans*). The large, friable vegetations are denoted by *arrows*. **B,** Acute endocarditis of congenitally bicuspid aortic valve (caused by *Staphylococcus aureus)* with extensive cuspal destruction and ring abscess *(arrow)*. **C,** Histologic appearance of vegetation of endocarditis with extensive acute inflammatory cells and fibrin. Bacterial organisms were demonstrated by tissue Gram stain. **D,** Healed endocarditis, demonstrating mitral valvular destruction but no active vegetations. (**C,** Reproduced from Schoen FJ: Surgical pathology of removed natural and prosthetic heart valves. Hum Pathol 18:558, 1987.)

Clinical Features. Fever is the most consistent sign of IE. Acute endocarditis has a stormy onset with rapidly developing fever, chills, weakness, and lassitude. However, fever may be slight or absent, particularly in the elderly, and the only manifestations may be nonspecific fatigue, loss of weight, and a flu-like syndrome. Complications of IE generally begin within the first few weeks of onset. They may be immunologically mediated, as exemplified by glomerulonephritis caused by the deposition of antigen-antibody complexes (Chapter 20). Murmurs are present in 90% of patients with left-sided IE and may stem from a new valvular defect or represent a preexisting abnormality. The so-called Duke criteria (Table 12–8) provide a standardized assessment of individuals with suspected IE that takes into account predisposing factors, physical findings, blood culture results, echocardiographic findings, and laboratory information.[83] Earlier diagnosis and effective treatment has nearly eliminated some previously common clinical manifestations of long-standing IE—for example, microthromboemboli (manifest as splinter or subungual hemorrhages), erythematous or hemorrhagic nontender lesions on the palms or soles (Janeway lesions), subcutaneous nodules in the pulp of the digits (Osler nodes), and retinal hemorrhages in the eyes (Roth spots).

NONINFECTED VEGETATIONS

Noninfected (sterile) vegetations are caused by nonbacterial thrombotic endocarditis and the endocarditis of systemic lupus erythematosus (SLE), called Libman-Sacks endocarditis (see below).

Nonbacterial Thrombotic Endocarditis (NBTE)

NBTE is characterized by the deposition of small sterile thrombi on the leaflets of the cardiac valves (Figs. 12–25C and 12–27). The lesions are 1 mm to 5 mm in size, and occur singly or multiply along the line of closure of the leaflets or cusps. Histologically they are composed of bland thrombi that are loosely attached to the underlying valve. The vegetations are not invasive and do not elicit any inflammatory reaction. Thus, the local effect of the vegetations is usually unimportant, but they may be the source of systemic emboli that produce infarcts in the brain, heart, or elsewhere.

NBTE is often encountered in debilitated patients, such as those with cancer or sepsis—hence the previously used term *marantic endocarditis*. It frequently occurs concomitantly with deep venous thromboses, pulmonary emboli, or other findings consistent with an underlying systemic hypercoagulable state (Chapter 4). Indeed, there is a striking association with mucinous adenocarcinomas, which may relate to the procoagulant effects of tumor-derived mucin or tissue factor, and NBTE can be a part of the Trousseau syndrome of migratory thrombophlebitis (Chapter 7). Endocardial trauma, as from an indwelling catheter, is another well-recognized predisposing condition, and right-sided valvular and endocar-

TABLE 12–8 Diagnostic Criteria for Infective Endocarditis*

PATHOLOGIC CRITERIA

Microorganisms, demonstrated by culture or histologic examination, in a vegetation, embolus from a vegetation, or intracardiac abscess

Histologic confirmation of active endocarditis in vegetation or intracardiac abscess

CLINICAL CRITERIA

Major

Blood culture(s) positive for a characteristic organism or persistently positive for an unusual organism

Echocardiographic identification of a valve-related or implant-related mass or abscess, or partial separation of artificial valve

New valvular regurgitaion

Minor

Predisposing heart lesion or intravenous drug use

Fever

Vascular lesions, including arterial petechiae, subungual/splinter hemorrhages, emboli, septic infarcts, mycotic aneurysm, intracranial hemorrhage, Janeway lesions[†]

Immunological phenomena, including glomerulonephritis, Osler nodes,[‡] Roth spots,[§] rheumatoid factor

Microbiologic evidence, including a single culture positive for an unusual organism

Echocardiographic findings consistent with but not diagnostic of endocarditis, including worsening or changing of a preexistent murmur

---

*Diagnosis by these guidelines, often called the Duke Criteria, requires either pathologic or clinical criteria; if clinical criteria are used, 2 major, 1 major + 3 minor, or 5 minor criteria are required for diagnosis.

[†]Janeway lesions are small erythematous or hemorrhagic, macular, nontender lesions on the palms and soles and are the consequence of septic embolic events.

[‡]Osler nodes are small, tender subcutaneous nodules that develop in the pulp of the digits or occasionally more proximally in the fingers and persist for hours to several days.

[§]Roth spots are oval retinal hemorrhages with pale centers.

Modified from Durack DT et al: Am J Med, 96:200, 1994 and Karchmer AW: In Braunwald E, Zipes DP, Libby P (eds): Heart Disease. A Textbook of Cardiovascular Medicine, 6th ed. Philadelphia, WB Saunders, 2001, p 1723.

dial thrombotic lesions frequently track along the course of Swan-Ganz pulmonary artery catheters.

Endocarditis of Systemic Lupus Erythematosus (Libman-Sacks Disease)

Mitral and tricuspid valvulitis with small, sterile vegetations, called *Libman-Sacks endocarditis*, is occasionally encountered in SLE. The lesions are small (1–4 mm in diameter) single or multiple, sterile, pink vegetations that often have a warty (verrucous) appearance. They may be located on the undersurfaces of the atrioventricular valves, on the valvular endocardium, on the chords, or on the mural endocardium of atria or ventricles. Histologically the vegetations consist of a finely granular, fibrinous eosinophilic material that may contain hematoxylin bodies, homogeneous remnants of nuclei damaged by anti-nuclear antigen bodies (see Chapter 6). An intense valvulitis may be present, characterized by fibrinoid necrosis of the valve substance that is often contiguous with the vegetation. Active leaflet vegetations can be difficult to distinguish from those of infective endocarditis (see Fig. 12–25); fibrosis and serious deformities can result that resemble chronic rheumatoid heart disease and require surgery.

Thrombotic heart valve lesions with sterile vegetations or rarely fibrous thickening commonly occur with the antiphospholipid syndrome (discussed in Chapter 4), which you will recall can also lead to a hypercoagulable state.[84] The mitral valve is more frequently involved than the aortic valve; regurgitation is the usual functional abnormality.

CARCINOID HEART DISEASE

Carcinoid heart disease is the cardiac manifestation of the systemic syndrome caused by carcinoid tumors. It generally involves the endocardium and valves of the right heart. Cardiac lesions are present in one half of patients with the *carcinoid syndrome*, which is characterized by *episodic flushing of the skin, cramps, nausea, vomiting, and diarrhea* (see Chapter 17).

Morphology. The cardiovascular lesions associated with the carcinoid syndrome are distinctive, consisting of firm plaquelike endocardial fibrous thickenings on the inside surfaces of the cardiac chambers and the tricuspid and pulmonary valves; occasionally they involve the major blood vessels of the right side, the inferior vena cava and the pulmonary artery (Fig. 12–28). The plaquelike thickenings are composed predominantly of smooth muscle cells and sparse collagen fibers embedded in an acid mucopolysaccharide-rich matrix material. Elastic fibers are not present in the plaques. Structures underlying the plaques are intact.

Although the mechanisms of the fibrosis are not understood, it appears that the clinical and pathologic findings relate to the elaboration by carcinoid tumors of a variety of bioactive products, such as serotonin (5-hydroxytryptamine), kallikrein, bradykinin, histamine, prostaglandins, and tachykinins. Plasma levels of serotonin and urinary excretion of the serotonin metabolite 5-hydroxyindoleacetic acid correlate with the severity of the right heart lesions.

The key bioactive mediators released into the portal circulation by gut carcinoid tumors are readily metabolized by the liver and do not reach the heart in high concentration. Thus, gastrointestinal carcinoids (with venous drainage via the portal system) do not usually induce carcinoid heart disease, unless there are extensive hepatic metastases that release the relevant mediators directly into the interior vena cava. Restriction of the cardiac changes to the right side of the heart is explained by inactivation of both serotonin and bradykinin during passage through the lungs by monoamine oxidase present in the pulmonary vascular endothelium. In contrast, primary carcinoid tumors in organs outside of the portal system of venous drainage that empty directly into the inferior vena cava (e.g., ovary and lung) can induce the syndrome in the absence of hepatic metastases.

The most common cardiac manifestation is tricuspid insufficiency, followed by pulmonary valve insufficiency, which usually occurs in combination with tricuspid disease. Stenoses of the right-sided valves may also develop, whereas left-sided

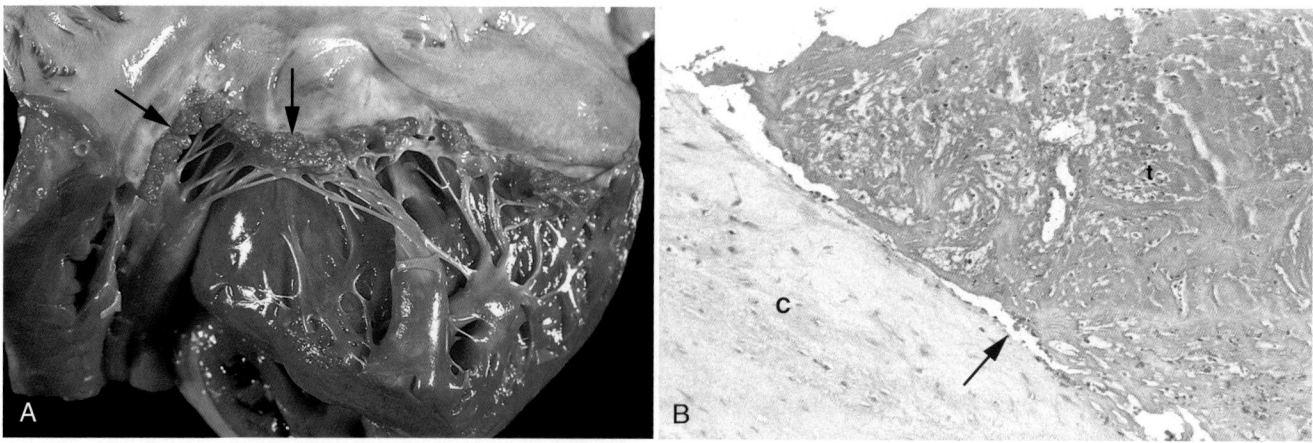

FIGURE 12–27 Nonbacterial thrombotic endocarditis (NBTE). **A,** Nearly complete row of thrombotic vegetations along the line of closure of the mitral valve leaflets *(arrows)*. **B,** Photomicrograph of NBTE, showing bland thrombus, with virtually no inflammation in the valve cusp (c) or the thrombotic deposit (t). The thrombus is only loosely attached to the cusp *(arrow)*.

valvular disease is only seen under unusual circumstances, such as when there is patent foramen ovale with right to left shunting or primary or metastatic carcinoid tumor involving the lung. Left-sided valvular abnormalities with pathologic features similar to those seen in the carcinoid syndrome have been reported to complicate the use of drugs that have serotonergic activity. These include fenfluramine (part of the "fen-phen" combination of appetite suppressants), some antiparkinsonian drugs, and methysergide or ergotamine, used to treat migraine headaches.[85]

COMPLICATIONS OF ARTIFICIAL VALVES

Replacement of damaged cardiac valves with prostheses is a common and often lifesaving mode of therapy.[86] Artificial valves are primarily of two types: (1) *mechanical prostheses,* consisting of different kinds of rigid mechanical valves, such as caged balls, tilting disks, or hinged semicircular flaps that are composed of nonphysiologic material; and (2) *tissue valves,* usually *bioprostheses,* consisting of chemically treated animal

tissue, especially porcine aortic valve tissue, which has been preserved in a dilute glutaraldehyde solution and subsequently mounted on a prosthetic frame. Tissue valves are flexible and function similarly to natural semilunar valves.

Approximately 60% of substitute valve recipients develop a serious prosthesis-related problem within 10 years postoperatively. The *nature* of these complications differs among types (Table 12–9 and Fig. 12–29).[87]

- *Thromboembolic complications,* either local obstruction of the prosthesis by thrombus or distant thromboemboli, are the major problem with mechanical valves (Fig. 12–29A). This complication necessitates long-term anticoagulation in all individuals with mechanical valves, with its attendant risk of hemorrhagic stroke or other forms of serious bleeding.
- *Infective endocarditis* is a potentially serious complication of valve replacement. The vegetations of prosthetic valve endocarditis are usually located at the prosthesis-tissue interface, and often cause the formation of a ring abscess,

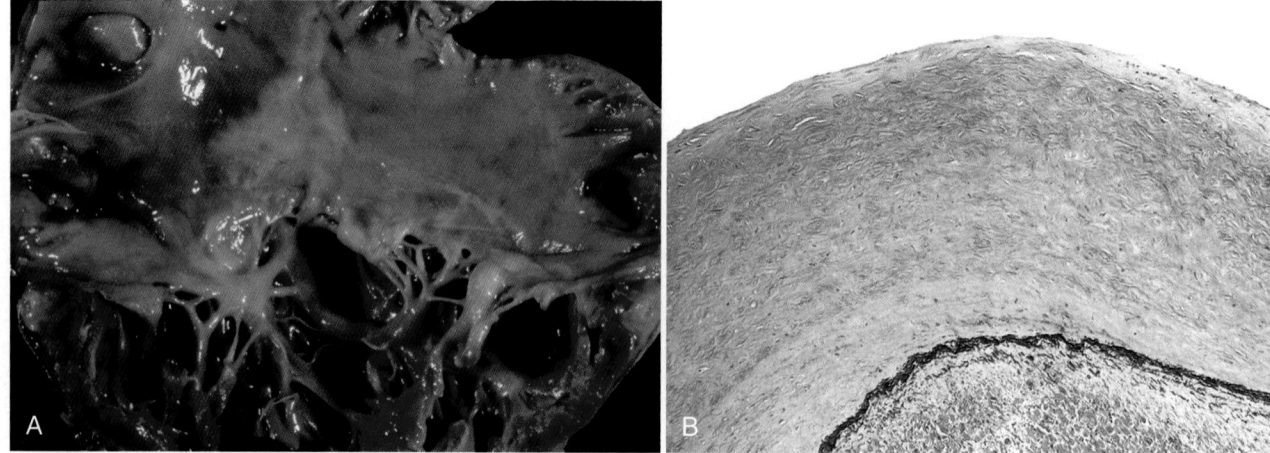

FIGURE 12–28 Carcinoid heart disease. **A,** Characteristic endocardial fibrotic lesion involving the right ventricle and tricuspid valve. **B,** Microscopic appearance of carcinoid heart disease with intimal thickening. Movat stain shows myocardial elastic tissue (black) underlying the acid mucopolysaccharide-rich lesion (blue-green).

TABLE 12–9	Complications of Cardiac Valve Prostheses
Thrombosis/thromboembolism
Anticoagulant-related hemorrhage
Prosthetic valve endocarditis
Structural deterioration (intrinsic)   Wear, fracture, poppet failure in ball valves, cuspal tear, calcification
Other forms of dysfunction   Inadequate healing (paravalvular leak), exuberant healing (obstruction), disproportion, hemolysis, noise

which can eventually lead to a paravalvular regurgitant blood leak if the prosthetic valve-tissue junction is disrupted. In addition, vegetations may directly involve the tissue of bioprosthetic valvular cusps. The major organisms causing such infections are staphylococcal skin contaminants (e.g., *S. epidermidis*), *S. aureus*, streptococci, and fungi.

- *Structural deterioration* rarely causes failure of contemporary mechanical valves. However, bioprostheses often eventually become incompetent due to calcification and/or tearing (Fig. 12–29B).[88]
- Other complications include intravascular hemolysis due to high shear forces, paravalvular leak due to inadequate healing, or obstruction due to overgrowth of fibrous tissue during the healing process.

Cardiomyopathies

The term *cardiomyopathy* (literally, heart muscle disease) is used to describe *heart disease resulting from an abnormality in the myocardium.*[89,90] Diseases of the myocardium usually produce abnormalities in cardiac wall thickness and chamber size, and mechanical and/or electrical dysfunction, and are associated with significant morbidity and mortality. Although chronic myocardial dysfunction secondary to ischemia, valvular abnormalities, or hypertension can cause ventricular dysfunction (see previous sections of this chapter), these conditions are not considered to be cardiomyopathies.

Clinical manifestations associated with the cardiomyopathies are either confined to the heart or can be a part of a generalized systemic disorder; in either situation, cardiac dysfunction is a key problem. *Primary* cardiomyopathies are diseases predominantly confined to the heart muscle, whereas *secondary* cardiomyopathies have myocardial involvement as a component of a systemic or multiorgan disorder. In most cases the mechanism by which the noncardiac problem affects the heart is well understood. In other disorders such as diabetes, the pathogenesis of the cardiac dysfunction is less obvious.[91] A major advance in our understanding of cardiomyopathies is the increasing appreciation that many cases have underlying genetic causes,[91,92] which we will discuss as we review the major categories of cardiomyopathy.

Cardiomyopathies of diverse etiology may have a similar morphologic appearance, and a clinician encountering a person with myocardial disease is usually unaware of the underlying cause. Hence the clinical approach is largely determined by which one of three clinical, functional, and pathologic patterns is present (Fig. 12–30 and Table 12–10): (1) dilated cardiomyopathy (DCM), (2) hypertrophic cardiomyopathy (HCM), or (3) restrictive cardiomyopathy. Another rare form of cardiomyopathy, left ventricular noncompaction, is characterized by a distinctive "spongy" appearance of the left ventricular myocardium. This congenital disorder is frequently associated with heart failure or arrhythmias and other clinical symptomatology; it may be diagnosed in children or adults as either an isolated finding or associated with other congenital heart anomalies, such as complex cyanotic congenital heart disease.[93] Gene mutations affecting myocardial

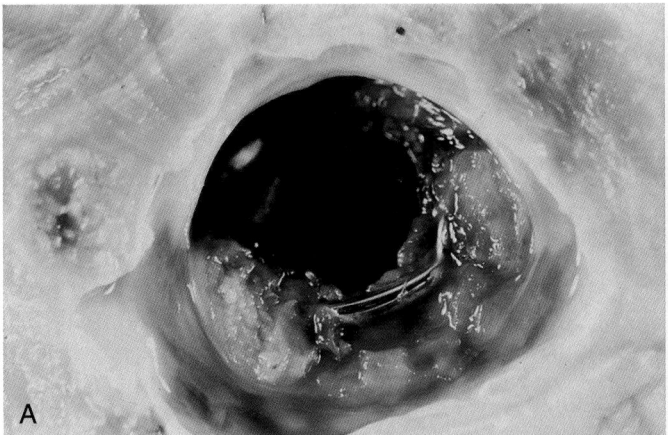
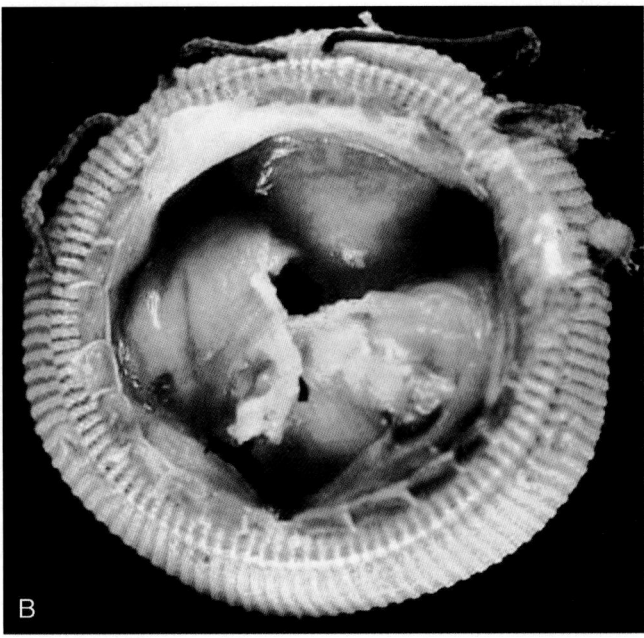

FIGURE 12–29 Complications of artificial heart valves. **A,** Thrombosis of a mechanical prosthetic valve. **B,** Calcification with secondary tearing of a porcine bioprosthetic heart valve, viewed from the inflow aspect.

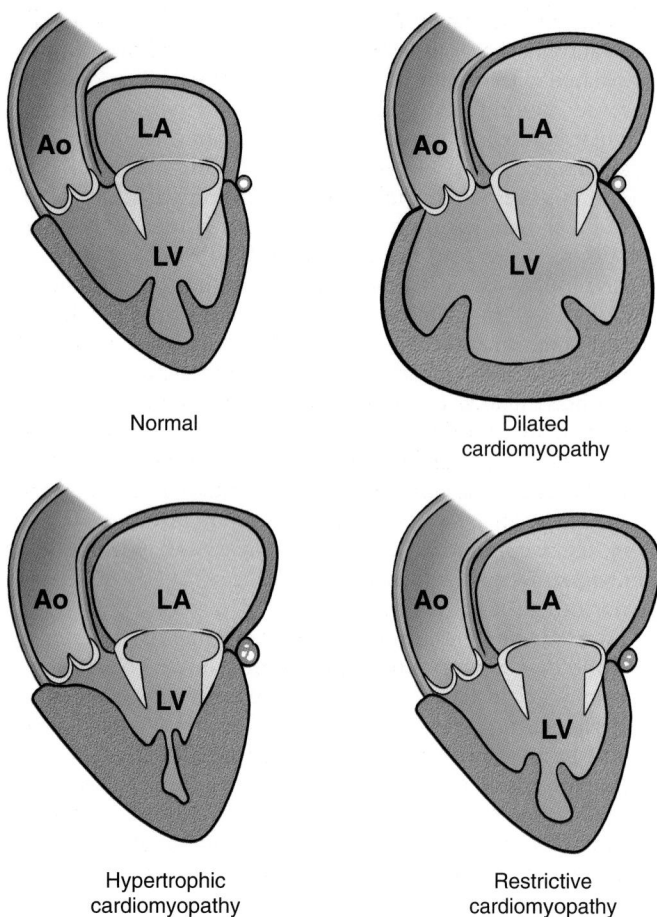

Normal

Dilated
cardiomyopathy

Hypertrophic
cardiomyopathy

Restrictive
cardiomyopathy

FIGURE 12–30 Representations of the three distinctive forms of myocardial disease. Ao, aorta; LA, left atrium; LV, left ventricle.

Within the hemodynamic patterns of myocardial dysfunction, there is a spectrum of clinical severity, and overlap of clinical features often occurs between groups. Moreover, each of these patterns can be either idiopathic or due to one of numerous specific identifiable causes (Table 12–11).

Endomyocardial biopsies are used in the diagnosis and management of individuals with myocardial disease and in cardiac transplant recipients.[94,95] Endomyocardial biopsy involves inserting a device (called a *bioptome*) transvenously into the right side of the heart and using its jaws to snip a small piece of septal myocardium, which is then analyzed by a pathologist.

DILATED CARDIOMYOPATHY

The term *dilated cardiomyopathy* (DCM) is applied to a form of cardiomyopathy characterized by *progressive cardiac dilation and contractile (systolic) dysfunction*, usually with concomitant hypertrophy. It is sometimes called congestive cardiomyopathy.

> **Morphology.** In DCM the heart is usually enlarged, heavy (often weighing two to three times normal), and flabby, due to dilation of all chambers (Fig. 12–31). Mural thrombi are common and may be a source of thromboemboli. There are no primary valvular alterations, and mitral (or tricuspid) regurgitation, when present, results from left (or right) ventricular chamber dilation (functional regurgitation). Either the coronary arteries are free of significant narrowing or the obstructions present are insufficient to explain the degree of cardiac dysfunction.
>
> The histologic abnormalities in DCM are nonspecific and usually do not point to a specific etiologic agent. Moreover, the severity of morphologic changes may not reflect either the degree of dysfunction or the patient's prognosis. Most muscle cells are hypertrophied with enlarged nuclei, but some are attenuated, stretched, and irregular. Interstitial and endocardial fibrosis of variable degree is present, and small subendocardial scars may replace individual cells or groups of cells, probably reflecting healing

ion channel function have also been included in recent classifications of primary cardiomyopathy (this group of disorders has been discussed in the context of sudden cardiac death). For the purposes of this discussion, arrhythmogenic right ventricular cardiomyopathy (arrhythmogenic right ventricular dysplasia), discussed below, is considered a variant of DCM.

TABLE 12–10	Cardiomyopathy and Indirect Myocardial Dysfunction: Functional Patterns and Causes			
Functional Pattern	**Left Ventricular Ejection Fraction***	**Mechanisms of Heart Failure**	**Causes of Phenotype**	**Indirect Myocardial Dysfunction (Mimicking Cardiomyopathy)**
Dilated	<40%	Impairment of contractility (systolic dysfunction)	Genetic; alcohol; peripartum; myocarditis; hemochromatosis; chronic anemia; doxorubicin (Adriamycin); sarcoidosis; idiopathic	Ischemic heart disease; valvular heart disease; hypertensive heart disease; congenital heart disease
Hypertrophic	50% to 80%	Impairment of compliance (diastolic dysfunction)	Genetic; Friedreich ataxia; storage diseases; infants of diabetic mother	Hypertensive heart disease; aortic stenosis
Restrictive	45% to 90%	Impairment of compliance (diastolic dysfunction)	Amyloidosis; radiation-induced fibrosis; idiopathic	Pericardial constriction

*Normal, approximately 50% to 65%.

TABLE 12–11   Conditions Associated with Heart Muscle Diseases

CARDIAC INFECTIONS

Viruses
Chlamydia
Rickettsia
Bacteria
Fungi
Protozoa

TOXINS

Alcohol
Cobalt
Catecholamines
Carbon monoxide
Lithium
Hydrocarbons
Arsenic
Cyclophosphamide
Doxorubicin (Adriamycin) and daunorubicin

METABOLIC

Hyperthroidism
Hypothyroidism
Hyperkalemia
Hypokalemia
Nutritional deficiency (protein, thiamine, other avitaminoses)
Hemochromatosis

NEUROMUSCULAR DISEASE

Friedreich ataxia
Muscular dystrophy
Congenital atrophies

STORAGE DISORDERS AND OTHER DEPOSITIONS

Hunter-Hurler syndrome
Glycogen storage disease
Fabry disease
Amyloidosis

INFILTRATIVE

Leukemia
Carcinomatosis
Sarcoidosis
Radiation-induced fibrosis

IMMUNOLOGICAL

Myocarditis (several forms)
Post-transplant rejection

of previous ischemic necrosis of myocytes caused by hypertrophy-induced imbalance between perfusion and demand.

Pathogenesis. Although many individuals with DCM have a familial (genetic) form, DCM can also result from various acquired myocardial insults or interactions of genetics and the environment that ultimately may yield a similar clinicopathologic pattern.[96] These include (1) myocarditis (an inflammatory disorder that precedes the development of cardiomyopathy in at least some cases, and is sometimes caused by viral infections), (2) toxicities (including adverse effects of chemotherapeutic agents and chronic alcoholism, a history of which can be elicited in 10% to 20% of patients), and (3) childbirth. Each of these subgroups are summarized in Figure 12–32 and described below.

- *Genetic influences.* In 20% to 50% of cases, DCM is familial and caused by inherited genetic abnormalities.[97] In the genetic forms of DCM, autosomal-dominant inheritance is the predominant pattern; X-linked, autosomal-recessive, and mitochondrial inheritance are less common. The genetic abnormalities identified as causes of familial DCM in humans most commonly affect genes that encode cytoskeletal proteins expressed by myocytes (Fig. 12–33).[98] In some families there are deletions in mitochondrial genes that result in defects in oxidative phosphorylation; in others there are mutations in genes encoding enzymes involved in beta-oxidation of fatty acids.[99] The mitochondrial defects most frequently cause dilated cardiomyopathy in children. X-linked dilated cardiomyopathy typically presents in the teenage years or in the early 20s and is usually rapidly progressive. X-linked cardiomyopathy is associated with mutations in the gene that encodes dystrophin, a cell membrane–associated cytoskeletal protein that plays a critical role in couping the internal cytoskeleton to the extracellular matrix; recall that dystrophin is mutated in the most common skeletal myopathies (i.e., Duchenne and Becker muscular dystrophies, see Chapter 27). Some patients and families with dystrophin gene mutations have DCM as the primary clinical feature. Other forms of DCM are associated with mutations in genes encoding cardiac α-actin (which links the sarcomere with dystrophin), desmin, and the nuclear lamina proteins, lamin A and lamin C. Interestingly, and probably resulting from the common developmental origin of contractile myocytes and conduction elements, congenital abnormalities of conduction may also be associated with DCM.[100]
- *Myocarditis.* Clinical studies using sequential endomyocardial biopsies have demonstrated progression from myocarditis to DCM; in other studies, *viral nucleic acids* from coxsackievirus B and other enteroviruses have been detected in the myocardium of patients with DCM. This suggests that, in at least some cases, DCM is a consequence of myocarditis. Myocarditis is discussed in more detail below.
- *Alcohol and other toxins. Alcohol abuse* is strongly associated with the development of DCM, raising the possibility that ethanol toxicity (Chapter 9) or a secondary nutritional disturbance may be the cause of the myocardial injury.[101] Alcohol or its metabolites (especially acetaldehyde) have a direct toxic effect on the myocardium; however, no morphologic features serve to distinguish *alcoholic cardiomyopathy* from DCM of other etiologies. Moreover, chronic alcoholism may be associated with thiamine deficiency, which can lead to beriberi heart disease (also indistinguishable from DCM) (see Chapter 9). In yet other cases a nonalcoholic *toxic insult* is the cause of the myocardial failure. Particularly important in this last group is myocardial injury caused by certain chemotherapeutic agents, including doxorubicin (Adriamycin), discussed later. In the past, cobalt has also caused DCM.
- *Childbirth.* A special form of DCM, termed *peripartum cardiomyopathy*, can occur late in pregnancy or several weeks to months postpartum. The cause of peripartum cardiomyopathy is poorly understood but is probably multifactorial.[102] Pregnancy-associated hypertension, volume overload, nutritional deficiency, other metabolic derangements, or an

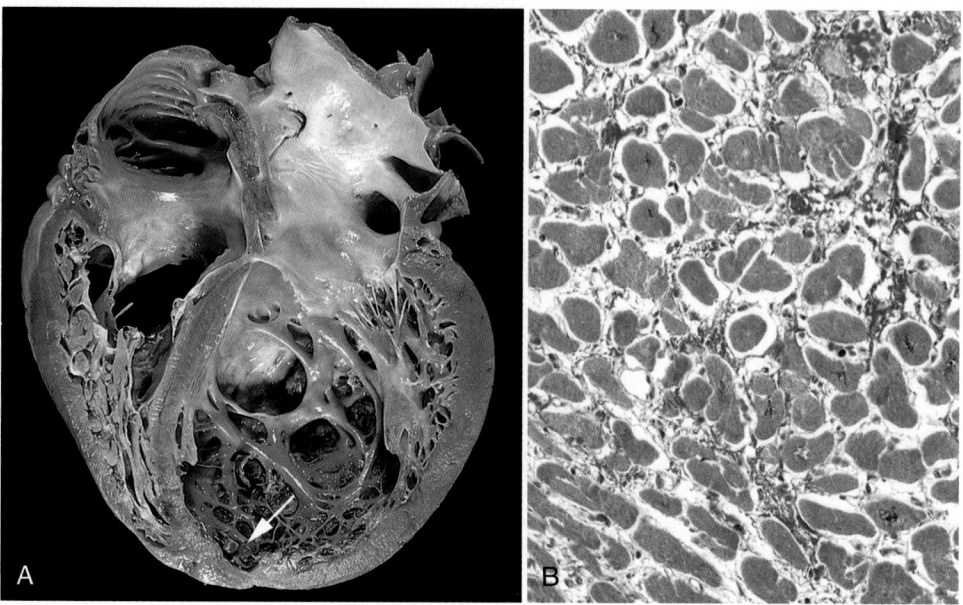

FIGURE 12–31 Dilated cardiomyopathy. **A,** Four-chamber dilatation and hypertrophy are evident. There is granular mural thrombus (*arrow*) at the apex of the left ventricle (on the *right* in this apical four-chamber view). The coronary arteries were patent. **B,** Histologic section demonstrating variable myocyte hypertrophy and interstitial fibrosis (collagen is highlighted as blue in this Masson trichrome stain).

as yet poorly characterized immunological reaction have been proposed as causes. Recent work suggests a relationship between elevated levels of an anti-angiogenic cleavage product of the hormone prolactin (which rises late in pregnancy) and peripartum cardiomyopathy.[103] Blocking prolactin secretion by bromocriptine in mouse models prevents peripartum cardiomyopathy, suggesting a potential novel therapeutic strategy.

Clinical Features. DCM may occur at any age, including in childhood, but it most commonly affects individuals between the ages of 20 and 50. It presents with slowly progressive signs and symptoms of CHF such as shortness of breath, easy fatigability, and poor exertional capacity. In the end stage, patients often have ejection fractions of less than 25% (normal, ~50% to 65%). Fifty percent of patients die within 2 years, and only 25% survive longer than 5 years, but some severely

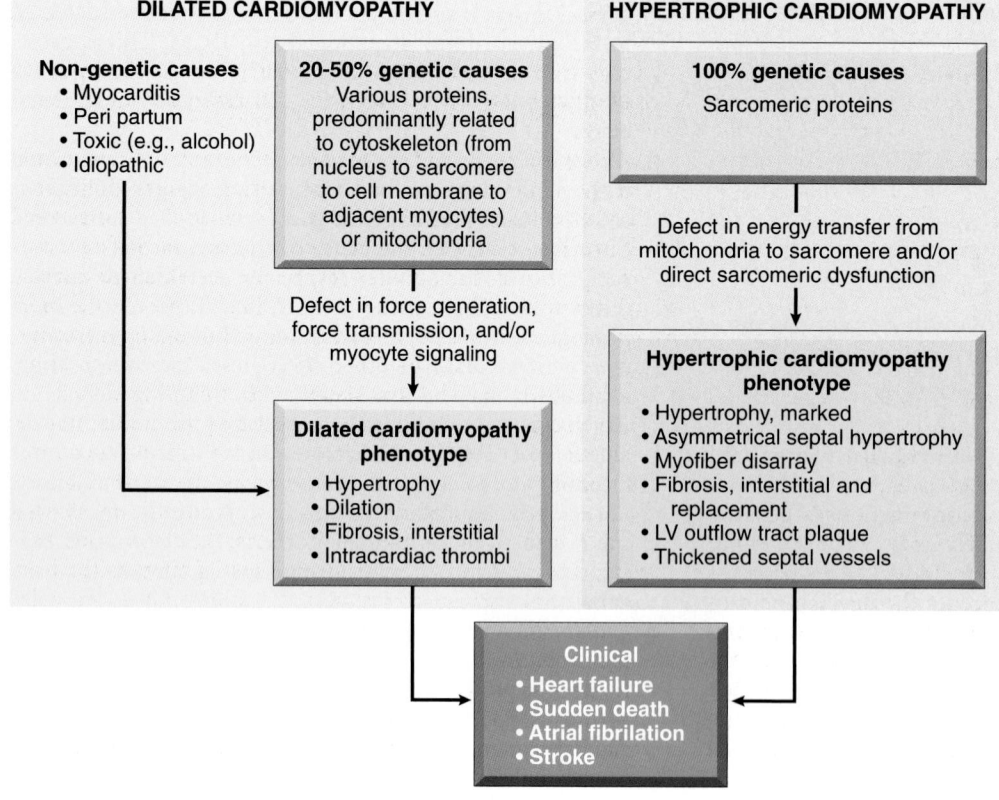

FIGURE 12–32 Causes and consequences of dilated and hypertrophic cardiomyopathy. Some dilated cardiomyopathies and virtually all hypertrophic cardiomyopathies are genetic in origin. The genetic causes of dilated cardiomyopathy involve mutations in any of a wide variety of proteins, predominantly of the cytoskeleton, but also the sarcomere, mitochondria, and nuclear envelope. In contrast, the mutated genes that cause hypertrophic cardiomyopathy encode proteins of the sarcomere. Although these two forms of cardiomyopathy differ greatly in subcellular basis and morphologic phenotypes, they share a common set of clinical complications. LV, left ventricle.

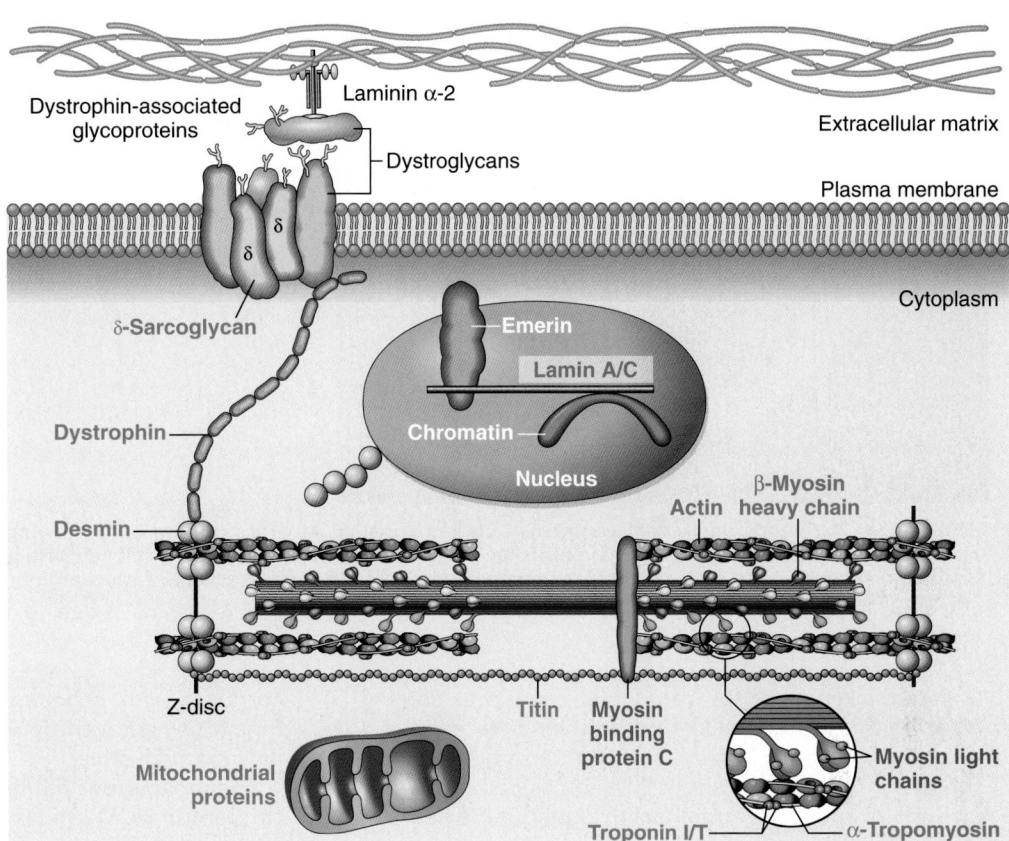

FIGURE 12–33 Schematic of a myocyte, showing key proteins mutated in dilated cardiomyopathy (red), hypertrophic cardiomyopathy (blue), or both (green).

affected patients may unexpectedly improve on therapy. Secondary mitral regurgitation and abnormal cardiac rhythms are common. Death is usually attributable to progressive cardiac failure or arrhythmia and can occur suddenly. Embolism from dislodgment of an intracardiac thrombus can occur. Cardiac transplantation is frequently done, and long-term ventricular assist may be beneficial in some patients. Interestingly, mechanical cardiac assist may induce lasting regression of cardiac dysfunction in some patients.[104]

Arrhythmogenic Right Ventricular Cardiomyopathy (Arrhythmogenic Right Ventricular Dysplasia)

Arrhythmogenic right ventricular cardiomyopathy (ARVC), or *arrhythmogenic right ventricular dysplasia*, is an inherited disease of the cardiac muscle that causes right ventricular failure and various rhythm disturbances, particularly ventricular tachycardia or fibrillation that can lead to sudden death, primarily in young people.[105] Left-sided involvement with left-sided heart failure may also occur. Morphologically, the right ventricular wall is severely thinned because of loss of myocytes, with extensive fatty infiltration and fibrosis (Fig. 12–34). The condition appears to have autosomal-dominant inheritance and variable penetrance. The disease seems to be related to defective cell adhesion proteins in the desmosomes that link adjacent cardiac myocytes. *Naxos syndrome* is a disorder characterized by arrhythmogenic right ventricular cardiomyopathy and hyperkeratosis of plantar palmar skin surfaces

that is associated with mutations in the gene encoding plakoglobin.[106]

HYPERTROPHIC CARDIOMYOPATHY

Hypertrophic cardiomyopathy (HCM) is characterized by *myocardial hypertrophy*, poorly compliant left ventricular myocardium *leading to abnormal diastolic filling*, and in about one third of cases, *intermittent ventricular outflow obstruction*. It is the leading cause of left ventricular hypertrophy unexplained by other clinical or pathologic causes.[107] As discussed below, HCM is caused by mutations in genes encoding sarcomeric proteins. Since the incidence of unexplained cardiac hypertrophy is approximately 1 in 500, HCM may be the most common cardiovascular disorder caused by single gene mutations. The heart is thick-walled, heavy, and *hyper*contracting, in striking contrast to the flabby, *hypo*contracting heart of DCM. HCM causes primarily diastolic dysfunction; systolic function is usually preserved. The two most common diseases that must be distinguished clinically from HCM are deposition diseases of the heart (e.g., amyloidosis, Fabry's disease) and hypertensive heart disease coupled with age-related subaortic septal hypertrophy (see "Hypertensive Heart Disease"). Occasionally, valvular or congenital subvalvular aortic stenosis can also mimic HCM.

Morphology. The essential feature of HCM is massive myocardial hypertrophy, usually without ventricular dilation (Fig. 12–35). The classic pattern is dispropor-

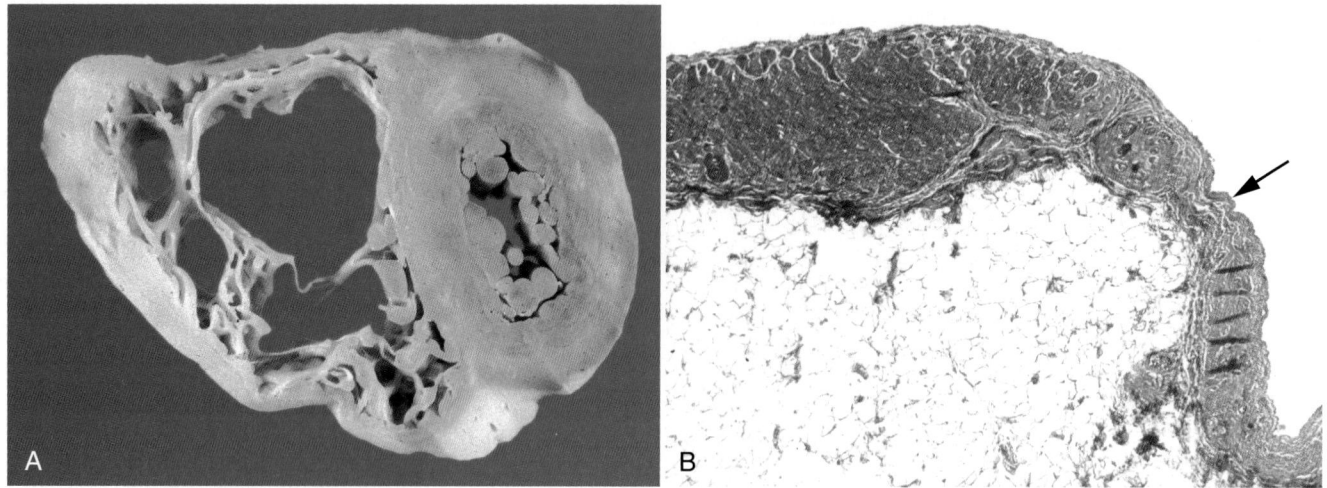

FIGURE 12–34 Arrhythmogenic right ventricular cardiomyopathy. **A,** Gross photograph, showing dilation of the right ventricle and near-transmural replacement of the right ventricular free-wall by fat and fibrosis. The left ventricle has a virtually normal configuration. **B,** Histologic section of the right ventricular free wall, demonstrating replacement of myocardium (red) by fibrosis (blue, *arrow*) and fat (Masson trichrome stain).

tionate thickening of the ventricular septum as compared with the free wall of the left ventricle (with a ratio greater than 1:3), frequently termed asymmetric septal hypertrophy. In about 10% of cases, however, the hypertrophy is symmetrical throughout the heart. On cross-section, the ventricular cavity loses its usual round-to-ovoid shape and may be compressed into a "banana-like" configuration by bulging of the ventricular septum into the lumen (Fig. 12–35A). Although marked hypertrophy can involve the entire septum, it is usually most prominent in the subaortic region. Often present are endocardial thickening or mural plaque formation in the left ventricular outflow tract and thickening of the anterior mitral leaflet. Both findings are a result of contact of the anterior mitral leaflet with the septum during ventricular systole, and they correlate with echocardiographically demonstrated functional left ventricular outflow tract obstruction during midsystole.

The most important histologic features of the myocardium in HCM are (1) extensive myocyte hypertrophy to a degree unusual in other conditions, with transverse myocyte diameters frequently greater than 40 μm (normal, ~15 μm); (2) haphazard disarray of bundles of myocytes, individual myocytes, and contractile elements in sarcomeres within cells (termed **myofiber disarray**); and (3) interstitial and replacement fibrosis (Fig. 12–35B).

Pathogenesis. HCM is caused by mutations in any one of several genes that encode sarcomeric proteins.[108] In most cases

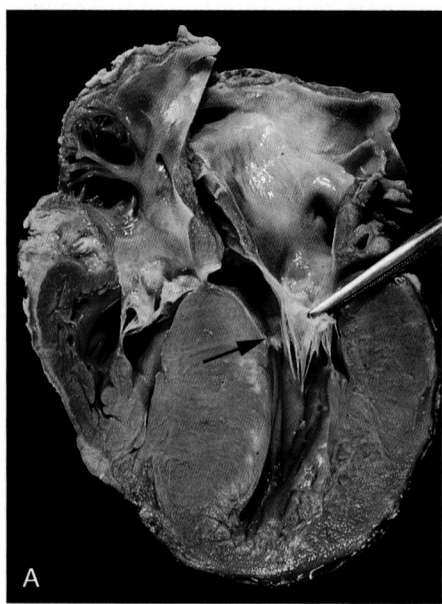
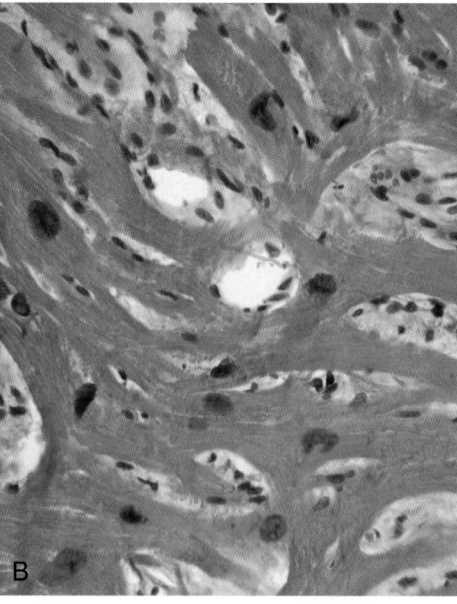

FIGURE 12–35 Hypertrophic cardiomyopathy with asymmetric septal hypertrophy. **A,** The septal muscle bulges into the left ventricular outflow tract, and the left atrium is enlarged. The anterior mitral leaflet has been moved away from the septum to reveal a fibrous endocardial plaque *(arrow)* (see text). **B,** Histologic appearance demonstrating disarray, extreme hypertrophy, and branching of myocytes as well as the characteristic interstitial fibrosis (collagen is blue in this Masson trichrome stain).

the pattern of transmission is autosomal dominant with variable penetrance. Remaining cases seem to be sporadic. More than 400 different mutations have been found in nine different genes in HCM, most being missense mutations. Mutations causing HCM are found most commonly in the gene encoding β-myosin heavy chain (β-MHC), with the genes for cardiac TnT, α-tropomyosin, and myosin-binding protein C (MYBP-C) being the next most frequently mutated. Mutations in β-MHC, MYBP-C, and TnT account for 70% to 80% of all cases of HCM. Different affected families may have distinct mutations involving the same protein. For example, approximately 50 different mutations of β-MHC are known to cause HCM. The prognosis of HCM varies widely and correlates strongly with specific mutations. Although it is clear that these genetic defects are critical to the etiology of HCM, the sequence of events leading from mutations to disease is still poorly understood. To make matters even more complicated, changes in certain genes, depicted in Figure 12–33, can give rise to both HCM and DCM.

Clinical Features. The basic physiologic abnormality in HCM is reduced stroke volume due to *impaired diastolic filling, which results from the reduced chamber size and compliance of the massively hypertrophied left ventricle.* In addition, approximately 25% of patients with HCM have dynamic obstruction to the left ventricular outflow. The limitation of cardiac output and a secondary increase in pulmonary venous pressure cause exertional dyspnea. Auscultation discloses a *harsh systolic ejection murmur,* caused by ventricular outflow obstruction as the anterior mitral leaflet moves toward the ventricular septum during systole. Because of the massive hypertrophy, high left ventricular chamber pressure, and frequently abnormal intramural arteries, focal myocardial ischemia commonly results, even in the absence of concomitant coronary artery disease; thus, anginal pain is frequent. The major clinical problems in HCM are atrial fibrillation, mural thrombus formation leading to embolization and possible stroke, intractable cardiac failure, ventricular arrhythmias, and, not infrequently, sudden death, especially in some affected families. Indeed, HCM is one of the most common causes of sudden, otherwise unexplained death in young athletes.[109]

The natural history of HCM is highly variable. Most patients can be helped by treatment with drugs that decrease heart rate and contractility, such as β-adrenergic blockers. Some benefit may also be gained from reduction of the mass of the septum, which relieves the outflow tract obstruction. This can be achieved either by surgical excision of muscle or carefully controlled septal infarction, which is induced by infusion of alcohol through a catheter.

As discussed above, HCM is a disease caused by mutations in proteins of the sarcomere, and DCM is mostly associated with abnormalities of cytoskeletal proteins (Fig. 12–33). DCM seems to be a disease of abnormal force generation, force transmission, or myocyte signaling. In the past, HCM has been considered a disorder of sarcomeres that impairs cardiac function and induces a compensatory hypertrophic response. However, recent evidence suggests that HCM may stem from a defect in energy transfer from its source of generation (mitochondria) to its site of use (sarcomeres), leading to subcellular energy deficiency. Despite these etiologic differences, there are some common mechanistic and clinicopathologic threads between HCM and the genetic and acquired forms of DCM, as summarized in Figure 12–32.

RESTRICTIVE CARDIOMYOPATHY

Restrictive cardiomyopathy is a disorder characterized by a *primary decrease in ventricular compliance, resulting in impaired ventricular filling during diastole.* Because the contractile (systolic) function of the left ventricle is usually unaffected, the functional abnormality can be confused with that of constrictive pericarditis or HCM.[110] Restrictive cardiomyopathy may be idiopathic or associated with distinct diseases or processes that affect the myocardium, principally radiation fibrosis, amyloidosis, sarcoidosis, metastatic tumors, or the deposition of metabolites that accumulate due to inborn errors of metabolism.

> **Morphology.** The ventricles are of approximately normal size or slightly enlarged, the cavities are not dilated, and the myocardium is firm and noncompliant. Biatrial dilation is commonly observed. Microscopically, there may be only patchy or diffuse interstitial fibrosis, which can vary from minimal to extensive. However, endomyocardial biopsy will often reveal a specific etiology. An important specific subgroup is amyloidosis (described later).

Several other restrictive conditions require brief mention. *Endomyocardial fibrosis* is principally a disease of children and young adults in Africa and other tropical areas, characterized by fibrosis of the ventricular endocardium and subendocardium that extends from the apex upward, often involving the tricuspid and mitral valves. The fibrous tissue markedly diminishes the volume and compliance of affected chambers and so induces a restrictive functional defect. Ventricular mural thrombi sometimes develop, and indeed there is a suggestion that the fibrous tissue results from the organization of mural thrombi. The etiology is unknown.

Loeffler endomyocarditis also results in endomyocardial fibrosis, typically with large mural thrombi. It is similar in morphology to the tropical disease, but in addition to the cardiac changes, there is often a peripheral eosinophilia (i.e., elevated blood eosinophils) and eosinophilic infiltrates in other organs. The release of toxic products of eosinophils, especially major basic protein, is postulated to initiate endomyocardial necrosis, followed by scarring of the necrotic area, layering of the endocardium by thrombus, and finally organization of the thrombus. It is now recognized that some patients with Loeffler endomyocarditis have a myeloproliferative disorder associated with chromosomal rearrangements involving either the PDGFRα or PDGFRβ genes (Chapter 13). These rearrangements produce fusion genes that encode constitutively active PDGFR tyrosine kinases. Treatment of such patients with the tyrosine kinase inhibitor imatinib has resulted in hematologic remissions associated with reversal of the endomyocarditis, which otherwise is often rapidly fatal.

Endocardial fibroelastosis is an uncommon heart disease of obscure etiology characterized by focal or diffuse fibroelastic thickening usually involving the mural left ventricular endocardium. It is most common in the first 2 years of life, and is accompanied by aortic valve obstruction or other congenital cardiac anomalies in about one third of cases. Diffuse involvement may be responsible for rapid and progressive cardiac decompensation and death.

MYOCARDITIS

Under the designation myocarditis are a diverse group of pathologic entities in which infectious microorganisms and/or an inflammatory process cause myocardial injury.[111] These disorders must be distinguished from conditions, such as ischemic heart disease, in which injuries caused by other mechanisms lead to inflammation secondarily.

Etiology and Pathogenesis. In the United States, *viral infections* are the most common cause of myocarditis. *Coxsackieviruses A and B* and other enteroviruses probably account for most of the cases. Other less common etiologic agents include cytomegalovirus, HIV, and a host of other agents (listed in Table 12–12). The responsible virus can sometimes be identified by serologic studies or, more recently, identification of viral nucleic acids (DNA or RNA) in myocardial biopsies. Whether viruses cause the myocardial injury directly or initiate a destructive immune response is unclear.

Nonviral agents are also important causes of infectious myocarditis, particularly the protozoa *Trypanosoma cruzi*, the agent of Chagas disease.[112] Chagas disease is endemic in some regions of South America; myocardial involvement is present in most infected individuals. About 10% of patients die during an acute attack; others develop a chronic immune-mediated myocarditis that may progress to cardiac insufficiency 10 to 20 years later. Trichinosis is the most common helminthic disease associated with myocarditis. Parasitic diseases, including toxoplasmosis, and bacterial infections, including Lyme disease and diphtheria, can also cause myocarditis. In the case of diphtheritic myocarditis, toxins released by *Corynebacterium diphtheriae* seem to be responsible for the myocardial injury. Myocarditis occurs in approximately 5% of patients with Lyme disease, a systemic illness caused by the bacterial spirochete *Borrelia burgdorferi* (Chapter 8). Lyme myocarditis manifests primarily as a self-limited conduction system disorder that frequently requires a temporary pacemaker. Myocarditis occurs in many patients with AIDS. Two types

have been identified: (1) inflammation and myocyte damage without a clear etiologic agent and (2) myocarditis caused by HIV directly or by an opportunistic pathogen.

There are also noninfectious causes of myocarditis. Myocarditis can be caused by hypersensitivity reactions *(hypersensitivity myocarditis)*, often to drugs such as antibiotics, diuretics, or antihypertensive agents. Myocarditis can also be associated with systemic diseases of immune origin, such as rheumatic fever, systemic lupus erythematosus, and polymyositis. Cardiac sarcoidosis and rejection of a transplanted heart (see Figure 12–40) are also considered forms of myocarditis.

Morphology. During the active phase of myocarditis the heart may appear normal or dilated; some hypertrophy may be present depending on disease duration. In advanced stages the ventricular myocardium is flabby and often mottled by either pale foci or minute hemorrhagic lesions. Mural thrombi may be present in any chamber.

During active disease, myocarditis is most frequently characterized by an interstitial inflammatory infiltrate associated with focal myocyte necrosis (Fig. 12–36). A diffuse, mononuclear, predominantly lymphocytic infiltrate is most common (Fig. 12–36A). Although endomyocardial biopsies are diagnostic in some cases, they can be spuriously negative because inflammatory involvement of the myocardium may be focal or patchy. If the patient survives the acute phase of myocarditis, the inflammatory lesions either resolve, leaving no residual changes, or heal by progressive fibrosis.

Hypersensitivity myocarditis has interstitial infiltrates, principally perivascular, composed of lymphocytes, macrophages, and a high proportion of eosinophils (Fig. 12–36B). A morphologically distinctive form of myocarditis of uncertain cause, called **giant-cell myocarditis**, is characterized by a widespread inflammatory cellular infiltrate containing multinucleate giant cells interspersed with lymphocytes, eosinophils, plasma cells, and macrophages. Focal to frequently extensive necrosis is present (see Fig. 12–36C). This variant carries a poor prognosis.

The myocarditis of **Chagas disease** is rendered distinctive by parasitization of scattered myofibers by trypanosomes accompanied by an inflammatory infiltrate of neutrophils, lymphocytes, macrophages, and occasional eosinophils (see Fig. 12–36D).

TABLE 12–12   **Major Causes of Myocarditis**
INFECTIONS
Viruses (e.g., coxsackievirus, ECHO, influenza, HIV, cytomegalovirus)
Chlamydiae (e.g., *C. psittaci*)
Rickettsiae (e.g., *R. typhi*, typhus fever)
Bacteria (e.g., *Corynebacterium diphtheriae*, *Neisseria meningococcus*, *Borrelia* (Lyme disease)
Fungi (e.g., *Candida*)
Protozoa (e.g., *Trypanosoma cruzi* [Chagas disease], toxoplasmosis)
Helminths (e.g. trichinosis)
IMMUNE-MEDIATED REACTIONS
Postviral
Poststreptococcal (rheumatic fever)
Systemic lupus erythematosus
Drug hypersensitivity (e.g., methyldopa, sulfonamides)
Transplant rejection
UNKNOWN
Sarcoidosis
Giant cell myocarditis

HIV, human immunodeficiency virus.

Clinical Features. The clinical spectrum of myocarditis is broad. At one end the disease is entirely asymptomatic, and such patients recover completely without sequelae; at the other extreme is the precipitous onset of heart failure or arrhythmias, occasionally with sudden death. Between these extremes are the many levels of involvement associated with symptoms such as fatigue, dyspnea, palpitations, precordial discomfort, and fever. The clinical features of myocarditis can mimic those of acute MI. Occasionally, patients develop dilated cardiomyopathy as a late complication of myocarditis.

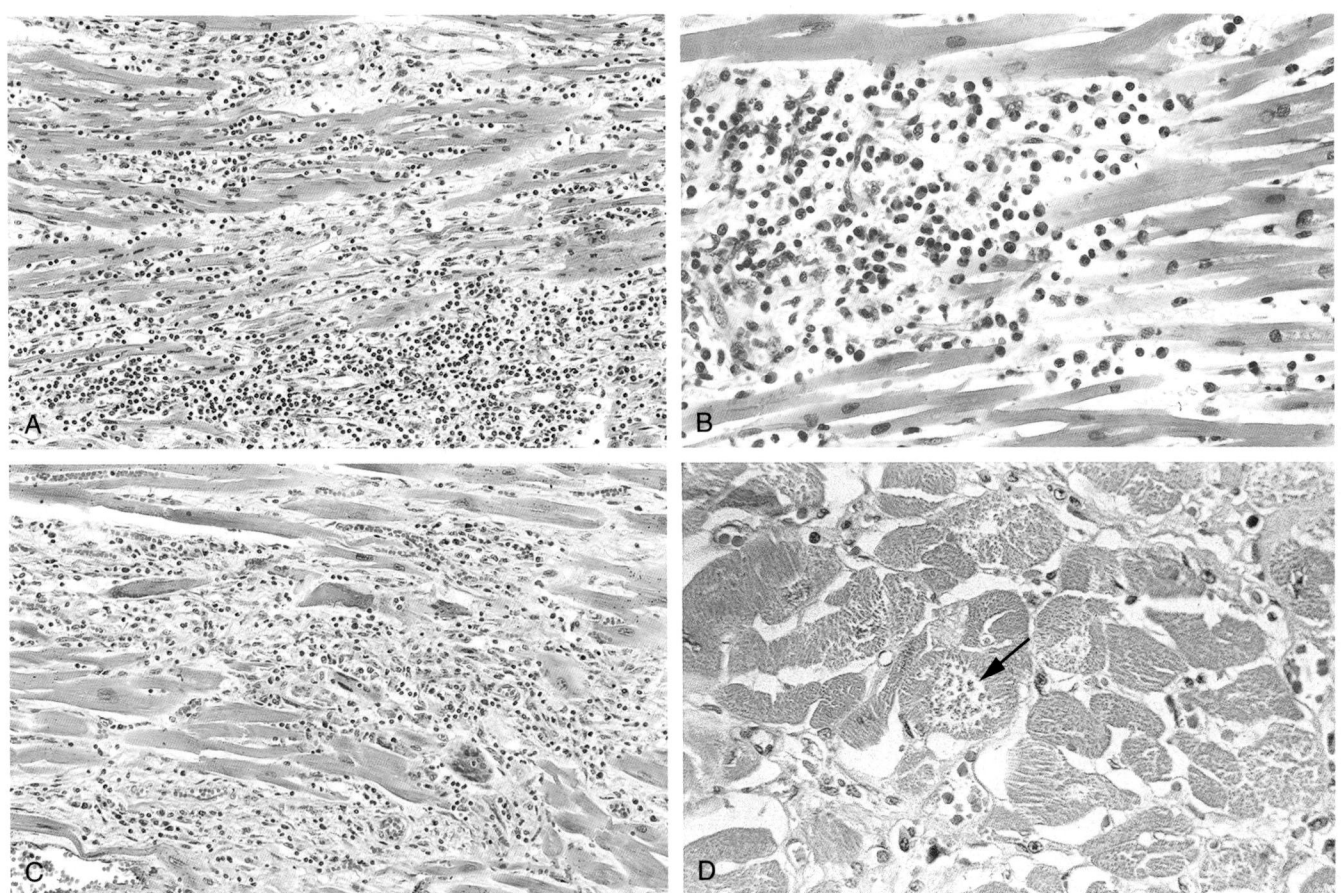

FIGURE 12–36 Myocarditis. **A,** Lymphocytic myocarditis, associated with myocyte injury. **B,** Hypersensitivity myocarditis, characterized by interstitial inflammatory infiltrate composed largely of eosinophils and mononuclear inflammatory cells, predominantly localized to perivascular and expanded interstitial spaces. **C,** Giant-cell myocarditis, with mononuclear inflammatory infiltrate containing lymphocytes and macrophages, extensive loss of muscle, and multinucleated giant cells. **D,** The myocarditis of Chagas disease. A myofiber distended with trypanosomes *(arrow)* is present along with inflammation and necrosis of individual myofibers.

OTHER CAUSES OF MYOCARDIAL DISEASE

Cardiotoxic Drugs. Cardiac complications of cancer therapy are an important clinical problem.[113] Cardiotoxicity can be associated with conventional chemotherapeutic agents, targeted drugs such as tyrosine kinase inhibitors, and certain forms of immunotherapy.[114,115] The anthracyclines doxorubicin and daunorubicin are the chemotherapeutic agents that are most often associated with toxic myocardial injury, which often leads to a dilated cardiomyopathy and heart failure. Anthracycline toxicity is dose-dependent (cardiotoxicity becomes progressively more frequent above a total dose of 500 mg/m^2) and is attributed primarily to peroxidation of lipids in myocyte membranes.

Many other pharmaceuticals and other agents, such as lithium, phenothiazines, chloroquine, and cocaine, have been implicated in myocardial injury and sometimes sudden death. Common findings in hearts injured by many of these chemicals and drugs (including diphtheria exotoxin and doxorubicin) are myofiber swelling, cytoplasmic vacuolization, and fatty change. With discontinuance of the toxic agent these changes may resolve completely, leaving no apparent sequelae. Sometimes, however, more extensive damage produces myocyte necrosis, which can evolve to a dilated cardiomyopathy.

Catecholamines. Foci of myocardial necrosis with contraction bands, often associated with a sparse mononuclear inflammatory infiltrate consisting mostly of macrophages, can occur in individuals with a pheochromocytoma, a tumor that elaborates catecholamines (Chapter 24). This is considered to be a manifestation of the general problem of "catecholamine effect," also seen in association with intense autonomic stimulation (secondary to intracranial lesions or stress), or the exogenous administration of large doses of vasopressor agents such as dopamine.[116] Sudden, intense emotional or physical stress can also induce acute left ventricular dysfunction due to myocardial stunning, a phenomenon known as Takotsubo cardiomyopathy.[117] Cocaine also causes similar catecholamine-mediated damage. The mechanism of catecholamine cardiotoxicity is uncertain, but it seems to relate either to direct toxicity of catecholamines to cardiac myocytes via calcium overload or to focal vasoconstriction in the coronary arterial macro- or microcirculation in the face of an increased heart rate. The mononuclear cell infiltrate is probably a secondary reaction to the foci of myocyte cell death. Similar changes may be encountered in individuals who have recovered from hypotensive episodes or have been resuscitated from a cardiac arrest; in such cases the damage is a result of ischemia-reperfusion (see earlier) with subsequent inflammation.

Amyloidosis. Amyloidosis is a prototypical myocardial disorder caused by deposition of an abnormal substance in the heart. Amyloidosis (Chapter 6) is caused by insoluble extracellular fibrillar deposits of protein fragments that are prone to forming β-pleated sheets.[118] Cardiac amyloidosis may appear along with systemic amyloidosis or be restricted to the heart, particularly in the aged (senile cardiac amyloidosis).[119] In senile cardiac amyloidosis, the amyloid deposits generally occur in the ventricles and atria. Senile cardiac amyloidosis occurs in older individuals and is caused by the deposition of transthyretin, a normal serum protein synthesized in the liver that is responsible for transporting thyroxine and retinol-binding protein. Senile cardiac amyloidosis[120] has a far better prognosis than systemic amyloidosis. Mutant forms of transthyretin can accelerate cardiac (and associated systemic) amyloidosis. For example, the risk of isolated cardiac amyloidosis is four times greater in African Americans than in Caucasians after 60 years of age because 4% of African Americans have a transthyretin mutation leading to the substitution of isoleucine for valine at position 122. This substitution produces an amyloidogenic form of transthyretin (responsible for autosomal-dominant familial transthyretin amyloidosis). Isolated atrial amyloidosis can also occur secondary to deposition of atrial natriuretic peptide, but its clinical significance is uncertain.

Cardiac amyloidosis most frequently produces a restrictive cardiomyopathy, but it can also be asymptomatic or manifest as dilation, arrhythmias, or symptoms mimicking those of ischemic or valvular disease. These varied presentations depend on the predominant location of the deposits, which can be found in the interstitium, conduction system, vasculature, or valves.

Morphology. The heart varies in consistency from normal to firm and rubbery. Usually the chambers are of normal size, but in some cases they are dilated and have thickened walls. Numerous small, semitranslucent nodules resembling drips of wax may be seen at the atrial endocardial surface, particularly on the left. Eosinophilic deposits of amyloid may be found in the interstitium, conduction tissue, valves, endocardium, pericardium, and small intramural coronary arteries; they can be distinguished from other hyaline deposits by special stains such as Congo red, which produces classic apple-green birefringence when viewed under polarized light (Fig. 12–37). Amyloid deposits often form rings around cardiac myocytes and capillaries. Intramural arteries and arterioles may have sufficient amyloid in their walls to compress and occlude their lumens, inducing myocardial ischemia ("small-vessel disease").

Iron Overload. *Iron overload* can result from either hereditary hemochromatosis (Chapter 18) or multiple blood transfusions (hemosiderosis). The heart in each is usually dilated. Iron deposition is more prominent in ventricles than atria and in the myocardium than in the conduction system. It is thought that iron causes systolic dysfunction by interfering with metal-dependent enzyme systems or by inducing oxygen free-radical injury.

Morphology. Grossly, the myocardium of the iron-overloaded heart is rust-brown in color but is usually otherwise indistinguishable from that of idiopathic dilated cardiomyopathy. Microscopically, there is marked accumulation of hemosiderin within cardiac myocytes, particularly in the perinuclear region, demonstrable with a Prussian blue stain. This is associated with varying degrees of cellular degeneration and fibrosis. Ultrastructurally, the cardiac myocytes contain abundant perinuclear siderosomes (iron-containing lysosomes).

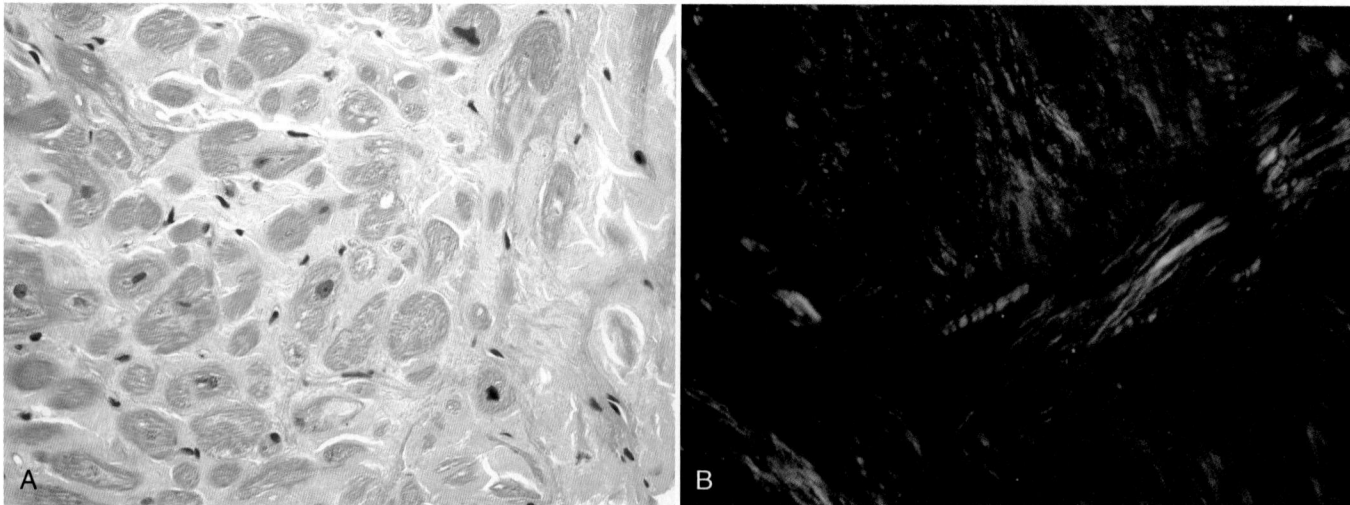

FIGURE 12–37 Cardiac amyloidosis. **A,** Hematoxylin and eosin stain, showing amyloid appearing as amorphous pink material around myocytes. **B,** Congo red stain viewed under polarized light, in which amyloid shows characteristic apple-green birefringence (compared with collagen, which appears white).

Hyperthyroidism and Hypothyroidism. Cardiac manifestations are among the earliest, most consistent features of hyperthyroidism and hypothyroidism, and they reflect direct and indirect effects of thyroid hormones on the cells of the heart.[121] In *hyperthyroidism* (Chapter 24), tachycardia, palpitations, and cardiomegaly are common; supraventricular arrhythmias occasionally appear. Cardiac failure is uncommon; when it occurs in this setting, it is usually superimposed on other cardiac diseases. In *hypothyroidism* (Chapter 24), cardiac output is decreased, due to reductions in stroke volume and heart rate. Increased peripheral vascular resistance and decreased blood volume result in narrowing of the pulse pressure, prolongation of circulation time, and decreased flow to peripheral tissues.

> **Morphology.** In hyperthyroidism the gross and histologic features are those of nonspecific hypertrophy and can also include ischemic foci. In well-advanced hypothyroidism (myxedema) the heart is flabby, enlarged, and dilated. Histologic features of hypothyroidism include myofiber swelling with loss of striations and basophilic degeneration, accompanied by interstitial mucopolysaccharide-rich edema fluid. A similar fluid sometimes accumulates within the pericardial sac. The term **myxedema heart** has been applied to these changes.

Pericardial Disease

The most important pericardial disorders cause fluid accumulation, inflammation, fibrous constriction, or some combination of these processes, usually in association with disease elsewhere in the heart or a systemic disease; isolated pericardial disease is unusual.[122]

PERICARDIAL EFFUSION AND HEMOPERICARDIUM

Normally, there are about 30 to 50 mL of thin, clear, straw-colored fluid in the pericardial sac. Under various circumstances the parietal pericardium may be distended by serous fluid *(pericardial effusion)*, blood (hemopericardium), or pus (purulent pericarditis). With long-standing pressure or volume overload, the pericardium dilates. This permits a slowly accumulating pericardial effusion to become quite large without interfering with cardiac function. Thus, with chronic effusions of less than 500 mL in volume, the only clinical significance is a characteristic globular enlargement of the heart shadow on chest radiographs. In contrast, rapidly developing fluid collections of as little as 200 to 300 mL—for example, due to hemopericardium caused by a ruptured MI or aortic dissection—may produce compression of the thin-walled atria and venae cavae, or the ventricles themselves. As a consequence, cardiac filling is restricted, producing potentially fatal *cardiac tamponade*.

PERICARDITIS

Pericardial inflammation may occur secondary to a variety of cardiac diseases, thoracic or systemic disorders, metastases

TABLE 12–13 Causes of Pericarditis
INFECTIOUS AGENTS
Viruses
Pyogenic becteria
Tuberculosis
Fungi
Other parasites
PRESUMABLY IMMUNOLOGICALLY MEDIATED
Rheumatic fever
Systemic lupus erythematosus
Scleroderma
Postcardiotomy
Postmyocardial infarction (Dressler) syndrome
Drug hypersensitivity reaction
MISCELLANEOUS
Myocardial infarction
Uremia
Following cardiac surgery
Neoplasia
Trauma
Radiation

from neoplasms arising in remote sites, or a surgical procedure on the heart. Primary pericarditis is unusual and almost always of viral origin. The major causes of pericarditis are listed in Table 12–13. Most evoke an acute pericarditis, but a few, such as tuberculosis and fungi, produce chronic reactions.

Acute Pericarditis

Serous Pericarditis. This is characteristically produced by noninfectious inflammatory diseases, such as rheumatic fever, SLE, and scleroderma, tumors, and uremia. An infection in the tissues contiguous to the pericardium—for example, a bacterial pleuritis—may incite sufficient irritation of the parietal pericardial serosa to cause a sterile serous effusion that may progress to serofibrinous pericarditis and ultimately to a frank suppurative reaction. In some instances a well-defined viral infection elsewhere—upper respiratory tract infection, pneumonia, parotitis—antedates the pericarditis and serves as the primary focus of infection. Infrequently, usually in young adults, a viral pericarditis occurs as an apparent primary infection that may be accompanied by myocarditis *(myopericarditis)*. Histologically, there is a mild inflammatory infiltrate in the epipericardial fat consisting predominantly of lymphocytes. Organization into fibrous adhesions rarely occurs.

Fibrinous and Serofibrinous Pericarditis. These two anatomic forms are *the most frequent type of pericarditis* and are composed of serous fluid mixed with a fibrinous exudate. Common causes include acute MI (recall Fig. 12–19D), the postinfarction (Dressler) syndrome (probably an autoimmune condition appearing several weeks after an MI), uremia, chest radiation, rheumatic fever, SLE, and trauma. A fibrinous reaction also follows routine cardiac surgery.

> **Morphology.** In fibrinous pericarditis the surface is dry, with a fine granular roughening. In serofibrinous pericarditis a more intense inflammatory process

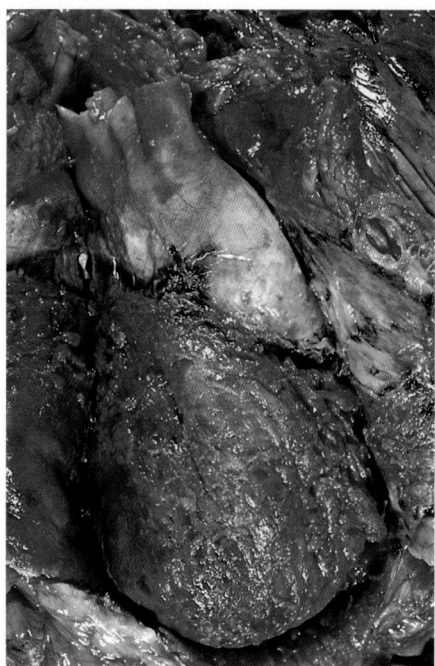

FIGURE 12-38 Acute suppurative pericarditis arising from direct extension of a pneumonia. Extensive purulent exudate is evident.

induces the accumulation of larger amounts of yellow to browen turbid fluid, which is made brown and cloudy by the presence of leukocytes and red cells (which may give the fluid a visibly bloody appearance), and often fibrin. As with all inflammatory exudates, fibrin may be lysed with resolution of the exudate, or it may become organized (see Chapter 3).

From the clinical standpoint *the development of a loud pericardial friction rub is the most striking characteristic of fibrinous pericarditis*, and pain, systemic febrile reactions, and signs suggestive of cardiac failure may be present. However, the collection of serous fluid may sometimes prevent rubbing by separating the two layers of the pericardium.

Purulent or Suppurative Pericarditis. This form of pericarditis is caused by invasion of the pericardial space by microbes, which may reach the pericardial cavity by several routes: (1) direct extension from neighboring infections, such as an empyema of the pleural cavity, lobar pneumonia, mediastinal infections, or extension of a ring abscess through the myocardium or aortic root; (2) seeding from the blood; (3) lymphatic extension; or (4) direct introduction during cardiotomy. Immunosuppression predisposes to infection by all of these pathways. The exudate ranges from a thin cloudy fluid to frank pus up to 400 to 500 mL in volume. The serosal surfaces are reddened, granular, and coated with the exudate (Fig. 12-38). Microscopically there is an acute inflammatory reaction, which sometimes extends into surrounding structures to induce *mediastinopericarditis*. Complete resolution is infrequent, and organization by scarring is the usual outcome. The intense inflammatory response and the subsequent scarring

frequently produce *constrictive pericarditis*, a serious consequence (see later).

The clinical findings in the active phase are essentially the same as those present in fibrinous pericarditis, but signs of systemic infection are usually marked: for example, spiking temperatures, chills, and fever.

Hemorrhagic Pericarditis. In this type of pericarditis the exudate is composed of blood mixed with a fibrinous or suppurative effusion; it is most commonly caused by the spread of a malignant neoplasm to the pericardial space. In such cases, cytologic examination of fluid removed through a pericardial tap often reveals the presence of neoplastic cells. Hemorrhagic pericarditis can also be found in bacterial infections, in persons with an underlying bleeding diathesis, and in tuberculosis. Hemorrhagic pericarditis often follows cardiac surgery and is occasionally responsible for significant blood loss or even tamponade, requiring a "second-look" operation. The clinical significance is similar to that of fibrinous or suppurative pericarditis.

Caseous Pericarditis. This rare type of pericarditis is, until proved otherwise, tuberculous in origin; infrequently, fungal infections evoke a similar reaction. Pericardial involvement occurs by direct spread from tuberculous foci within the tracheobronchial nodes. Caseous pericarditis is a frequent antecedent of disabling, fibrocalcific, chronic constrictive pericarditis.

Chronic or Healed Pericarditis

In some cases organization merely produces plaquelike fibrous thickenings of the serosal membranes ("soldier's plaque") or thin, delicate adhesions of obscure origin that are observed fairly frequently at autopsy and rarely cause impairment of cardiac function. In other cases, fibrosis in the form of delicate, stringy adhesions completely obliterates the pericardial sac. In most instances, this *adhesive pericarditis* has no effect on cardiac function.

Adhesive mediastinopericarditis may follow infectious pericarditis, previous cardiac surgery, or irradiation to the mediastinum. The pericardial sac is obliterated, and adherence of the external aspect of the parietal layer to surrounding structures produces a great strain on cardiac function. With each systolic contraction, the heart pulls not only against the parietal pericardium but also against the attached surrounding structures. Systolic retraction of the rib cage and diaphragm, pulsus paradoxus, and a variety of other characteristic clinical findings may be observed. The increased workload causes cardiac hypertrophy and dilation, which may be substantial in severe cases.

In *constrictive pericarditis* the heart is encased in a dense, fibrous or fibrocalcific scar that limits diastolic expansion and cardiac output, features that mimic a restrictive cardiomyopathy. A prior history of pericarditis may or may not be present. The scar, often 0.5 to 1.0 cm thick, obliterates the pericardial space and sometimes calcifies; in extreme cases it can resemble a plaster mold (*concretio cordis*). Because of the dense enclosing scar, cardiac hypertrophy and dilation cannot occur. Cardiac output may be reduced at rest, but more importantly the heart has little if any capacity to increase its output in response to increased peripheral needs. Heart sounds are understandably distant or muffled. Treatment consists of surgical removal of the shell of constricting fibrous tissue (pericardiectomy).

HEART DISEASE ASSOCIATED WITH RHEUMATOLOGIC DISORDERS

Paradoxically, the prevalence and importance of cardiovascular manifestations of rheumatologic diseases (including rheumatoid arthritis, SLE, systemic sclerosis, ankylosing spondylitis, and psoriatic arthritis) has increased as a result of the longer life expectancy of persons with these disorders and enhanced detection of milder cases.[123] Inflammatory mechanisms may cause vascular, myocardial, valvular, and pericardial manifestations. In addition, ischemic heart disease seems to be accelerated in individuals with inflammatory rheumatic conditions.

Rheumatoid arthritis is mainly a disorder of the joints, but it is also associated with many extra-articular features (e.g., subcutaneous rheumatoid nodules, acute vasculitis, and Felty syndrome; see Chapter 26). The heart is also involved in 20% to 40% of cases of severe prolonged rheumatoid arthritis. The most common finding is a *fibrinous pericarditis* that may progress to fibrous thickening of the visceral and parietal pericardium and dense adhesions. Granulomatous rheumatoid nodules resembling those that occur subcutaneously may also be identifiable in the myocardium. Much less frequently, rheumatoid nodules involve the endocardium, valves of the heart, and root of the aorta. *Rheumatoid valvulitis* can lead to marked fibrous thickening and secondary calcification of the aortic valve cusps, producing changes resembling those of chronic rheumatic valvular disease. The valvular lesions associated with SLE were discussed previously under "Valvular Heart Disease."

Tumors of the Heart

Primary tumors of the heart are rare; in contrast, metastatic tumors to the heart occur in about 5% of persons dying of cancer. The most common primary cardiac tumors, in descending order of frequency (overall, including adults and children), are myxomas, fibromas, lipomas, papillary fibroelastomas, rhabdomyomas, angiosarcomas, and other sarcomas. The five most common tumors are all benign and collectively account for 80% to 90% of primary tumors of the heart.

PRIMARY CARDIAC TUMORS

Myxoma

Myxomas are the most common primary tumor of the heart in adults (Fig. 12–39). They are benign neoplasms often associated with clonal abnormalities of chromosomes 12 and 17 that are thought to arise from primitive multipotent mesenchymal cells. Although they may arise in any of the four chambers or, rarely, on the heart valves, about 90% are located in the atria *(atrial myxomas)*, with a left-to-right ratio of approximately 4 : 1.

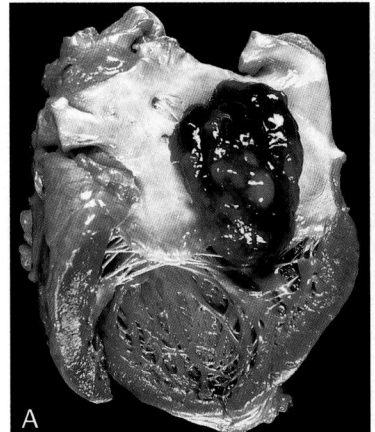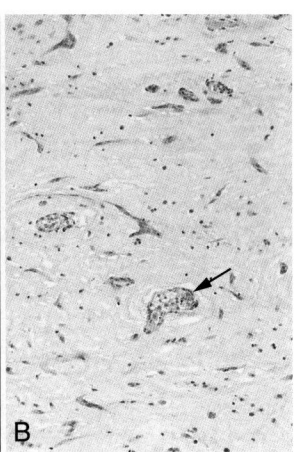

FIGURE 12–39 Left atrial myxoma. **A,** Gross photograph showing large pedunculated lesion arising from the region of the fossa ovalis and extending into the mitral valve orifice. **B,** Microscopic appearance, with abundant amorphous extracellular matrix in which there are scattered collections of myxoma cells in various groupings, including abnormal vessel-like formations *(arrow)*.

> **Morphology.** The tumors are usually single, but rarely several occur simultaneously. The region of the fossa ovalis in the atrial septum is the favored site of origin. Myxomas range in size from small (<1 cm) to large (≥10 cm). They are sessile or pedunculated lesions (Fig. 12–39A) that vary from globular hard masses mottled with hemorrhage to soft, translucent, papillary, or villous lesions having a gelatinous appearance. The pedunculated form is often sufficiently mobile to move into or even through the AV valves during systole, causing intermittent obstruction that may be position-dependent. Sometimes mobile tumors exert a "wrecking-ball" effect, causing damage to the valve leaflets.
>
> Histologically, myxomas are composed of stellate or globular myxoma cells embedded within an abundant acid mucopolysaccharide ground substance (Fig. 12–39B). Peculiar vessel-like or gland-like structures are characteristic. Hemorrhage and mononuclear inflammation are usually present.

The major clinical manifestations are due to valvular "ball-valve" obstruction, embolization, or a syndrome of constitutional symptoms, such as fever and malaise. Sometimes fragmentation and systemic embolization calls attention to these lesions. Constitutional symptoms are probably due to the elaboration by some myxomas of the cytokine IL-6, a major mediator of the acute-phase response. Echocardiography provides the opportunity to identify these masses noninvasively. Surgical removal is usually curative; rarely, the neoplasm recurs months to years later.

Approximately 10% of individuals with myxoma have a familial syndrome (known as *Carney complex*) characterized by autosomal-dominant transmission, multiple cardiac and often extracardiac (e.g., skin) myxomas, pigmented skin lesions, and endocrine overactivity. A careful history and physical examination in persons with cardiac myxoma is important to identify the extra-cardiac signs of the Carney complex, since this diagnosis carries implications for family members of the patient. The gene *PRKAR1* on chromosome 17 (encoding a regulatory subunit of cyclic adenosine monophosphate–dependent protein kinase A, possibly a tumor suppressor gene) is mutated in most Carney complex kindreds; other kindreds have abnormalities in a locus at chromosome 2p16.[124]

Lipoma

Lipomas are localized, well-circumscribed, benign tumors composed of mature fat cells that may occur in the subendocardium, subepicardium, or myocardium. They may be asymptomatic, or produce ball-valve obstructions or arrhythmias. Lipomas are most often located in the left ventricle, right atrium, or atrial septum and are not necessarily neoplastic. In the atrial septum, non-neoplastic depositions of fat sometimes occur that are called "lipomatous hypertrophy."

Papillary Fibroelastoma

Papillary fibroelastomas are curious, usually incidental, sea-anemone-like lesions, most often identified at autopsy. They may embolize and thereby become clinically important. Clonal cytogenetic abnormalities have been reported, suggesting that fibroelastomas are unusual benign neoplasms. They resemble the much smaller, usually trivial, *Lambl excrescences* that are frequently found on the aortic valves of older individuals.

Morphology. Papillary fibroelastomas are generally located on valves, particularly the ventricular surfaces of semilunar valves and the atrial surfaces of atrioventricular valves. They consist of a distinctive cluster of hairlike projections up to 1 cm in length, and several centimeters in diameter. Histologically, the projections are composed of a core of myxoid connective tissue containing abundant mucopolysaccharide matrix and elastic fibers that is covered by a surface endothelium.

Rhabdomyoma

Rhabdomyomas are the most frequent primary tumor of the heart in infants and children and are frequently discovered in the first years of life because of obstruction of a valvular orifice or cardiac chamber. Cardiac rhabdomyomas are often associated with tuberous sclerosis (see Chapter 28), which is caused by defects in the TSC1 or TSC2 tumor suppressor genes. The TSC1 and TSC2 proteins work together in a complex that inhibits the activity of the mammalian target of rapamycin (mTOR), a kinase that stimulates cell growth and regulates cell size. TSC1 or TSC2 expression is often completely lost in rhabdomyomas that occur in the setting of tuberous sclerosis, providing a mechanism for the myocyte overgrowth. Because they often regress spontaneously, rhabdomyomas are

considered by some to be hamartomas rather than true neoplasms.

Morphology. Rhabdomyomas are generally small, gray-white myocardial masses up to several centimeters in diameter. They are usually multiple in number and involve the ventricles preferentially, often protruding into the chambers. Histologically they are composed of bizarre, markedly enlarged myocytes. In sections the abundant myocyte cytoplasm is often reduced to thin webs or strands that extend to cell membranes, an appearance referred to as **spider cells**.

Sarcoma

Cardiac *angiosarcomas* and other sarcomas are not clinically or morphologically distinctive from their counterparts in other locations (see Fig. 11–35 and Chapter 26) and so require no further comment here.

CARDIAC EFFECTS OF NONCARDIAC NEOPLASMS

With enhanced patient survival due to diagnostic and therapeutic advances, significant cardiovascular effects of noncardiac neoplasms and their therapy are now commonly encountered (Table 12–14). Pathology derives from infiltration by tumor, circulating mediators, and complications of therapy.

The most frequent metastatic tumors involving the heart are carcinomas of the lung and breast, melanomas, leukemias, and lymphomas. Metastases can reach the heart and pericardium by retrograde lymphatic extension (most carcinomas), by hematogenous seeding (many tumors), by direct contiguous extension (primary carcinoma of the lung, breast, or esophagus), or by venous extension (tumors of the kidney or liver). Clinical symptoms are most often associated with pericardial spread, which can cause symptomatic pericardial effu-

TABLE 12–14 Cardiovascular Effects of Noncardiac Neoplasms

DIRECT CONSEQUENCES OF TUMOR

Pericardial and myocardial metastases
Large vessel obstruction
Pulmonary tumor emboli

INDIRECT CONSEQUENCES OF TUMOR (COMPLICATIONS OF CIRCULATING MEDIATORS)

Nonbacterial thrombotic endocarditis
Carcinoid heart disease
Pheochromocytoma-associated heart disease
Myeloma-associated amyloidosis

EFFECTS OF TUMOR THERAPY

Chemotherapy
Radiation therapy

Modified from Schoen FJ, et al: Cardiac effects of non-cardiac neoplasms. Cardiol Clin 2:657, 1984.

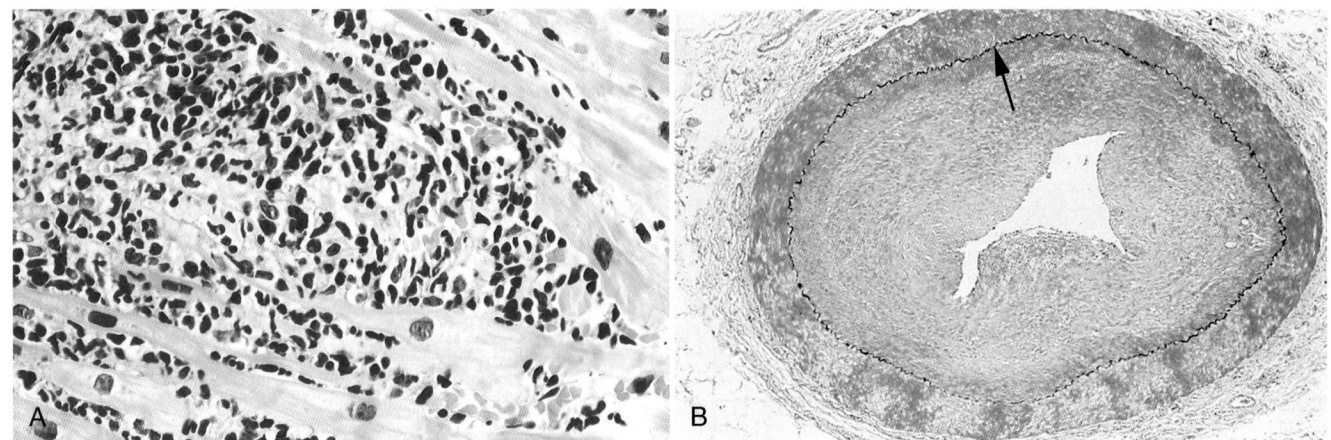

FIGURE 12–40 Complications of heart transplantation. **A,** Cardiac allograft rejection typified by lymphocytic infiltrate, with associated damage to cardiac myocytes. **B,** Graft coronary arteriosclerosis, demonstrating severe diffuse concentric intimal thickening producing critical stenosis. The internal elastic lamina *(arrow)* and media are intact (Movat pentachrome stain, elastin black). **(B,** Reproduced by permission from Salomon RN et al.: Human coronary transplantation-associated arteriosclerosis. Evidence for chronic immune reaction to activated graft endothelial cells. Am J Pathol 138:791, 1991.)

sions or a mass-effect that is sufficient to restrict cardiac filling. Myocardial metastases are usually clinically silent or have nonspecific features, such as a generalized defect in ventricular contractility or compliance. Bronchogenic carcinoma or malignant lymphoma may infiltrate the mediastinum extensively, causing encasement, compression, or invasion of the superior vena cava with resultant obstruction to blood coming from the head and upper extremities *(superior vena cava syndrome)*. Renal cell carcinoma often invades the renal vein, and may grow as a frond of tissue up the inferior vena cava and into the right atrium, blocking venous return to the heart.

Noncardiac tumors may also affect cardiac function indirectly, sometimes via circulating tumor-derived substances (e.g., nonbacterial thrombotic endocarditis, carcinoid heart disease, pheochromocytoma-associated myocardial damage, multiple myeloma–associated AL amyloidosis; all described earlier).

Complications of chemotherapy were discussed earlier in this chapter. Radiation used to treat breast, lung, or mediastinal neoplasms can cause pericarditis, pericardial effusion, myocardial fibrosis, and chronic pericardial disorders. Other cardiac effects of radiation therapy include accelerated coronary artery disease and mural and valvular endocardial fibrosis.

Cardiac Transplantation

Transplantation of cardiac allografts is now frequently performed (~3000 per year worldwide) for severe, intractable heart failure of diverse causes, the two most common being dilated cardiomyopathy and ischemic heart disease. Three major factors have contributed to the improved outcome of cardiac transplantation since the first human to human transplant in 1967: (1) more effective immunosuppressive therapy (including the use of cyclosporin A, glucocorticoids, and other agents), (2) careful selection of candidates, and (3) early histopathologic diagnosis of acute allograft rejection by endomyocardial biopsy.[125]

Of the major complications, allograft rejection is the primary problem requiring surveillance; scheduled endomyocardial biopsy is the only reliable means of diagnosing acute cardiac rejection before substantial myocardial damage has occurred and at a stage that is reversible in the majority of instances. Rejection is characterized by interstitial lymphocytic inflammation that, in its more advanced stages, damages adjacent myocytes; the histology resembles myocarditis (Fig. 12–40A). When myocardial injury is not extensive, the "rejection episode" is usually either self-limited or successfully reversed by increased immunosuppressive therapy. Advanced rejection may be irreversible and fatal if it is not promptly treated.

The major current limitation to the long-term success of cardiac transplantation is diffuse stenosing intimal proliferation of the coronary arteries, which may involve intramural vessels extensively *(graft arteriopathy)* (Fig. 12–40B). Because the transplanted heart is often denervated, patients with this disorder may not experience ischemic chest pain, and this vexing problem may lead to silent MI; in severe graft arteriopathy, CHF or sudden death is the usual outcome. The pathogenesis of these arterial lesions is uncertain. Low-level, chronic rejection reactions may induce inflammatory cells and vascular wall cells to secrete growth factors that promote the recruitment and proliferation of intimal smooth muscle cells and the synthesis of extracellular matrix, thereby expanding the intima (Chapter 6). Other postoperative problems include infection and malignancies, particularly Epstein-Barr virus-associated B cell lymphomas that arise in the setting of T-cell immunosuppression. Despite these problems, the overall outlook is good; the 1-year survival is 70% to 80% and 5-year survival is greater than 60%.

REFERENCES

1. Gaziano TA: Cardiovascular disease in the developing world and its cost-effective management. Circulation 112:3547, 2005.
2. Beaglehole R et al.: Poverty and human development. The global implications of cardiovascular disease. Circulation 116:1871, 2007.
3. Heart Association Statistics Committee and Stroke Statistics Subcommittee; Heart Disease and Stroke Statistics—2007 Update: a report from

the American Heart Association Statistics Committee and Stroke Statistics Subcommittee. Circulation 106:69, 2007.

4. Lee CY, Burnett JC Jr: Natriuretic peptides and therapeutic applications. Heart Fail Rev 12:131, 2007.

5. Saffitz JE: Adhesion molecules: why they are important to the electrophysiologist. J Cardiovasc Electrophysiol 17:225, 2006.

6. Liu AC et al.: The emerging role of valve interstitial cell phenotypes in regulating heart valve pathobiology. Am J Pathol 171:1407, 2007.

7. Aikawa E et al: Human semilunar cardiac valve remodeling by activated cells from fetus to adult: implications for postnatal adaptation, pathology, and tissue engineering. Circulation 113:1344, 2006.

8. Braunwald E et al. (eds): Braunwald's Heart Disease: A Textbook of Cardiovascular Medicine. Philadelphia, WB Saunders, 2008.

9. Silver MD et al. (eds): Cardiovascular Pathology, 3rd ed. New York, Churchill Livingstone, 2001, p 808.

10. Chien KR, Karsenty G: Longevity and lineages: toward the integrative biology of degenerative diseases in heart, muscle, and bone. Cell 120:533, 2005.

11. Opie LH et al.: Controversies in ventricular remodeling. Lancet 367:356, 2006.

12. Chinnaiyan KM et al.: Integrated diagnosis and management of diastolic heart failure. Am Heart J 153:189, 2007.

13. Oka T et al.: Re-employment of developmental transcription factors in adult heart disease. Semin Cell Develop Biol 18:117, 2007.

14. Diwan A, Dorn GW: Decompensation of cardiac hypertrophy: cellular mechanisms and novel therapeutic targets. Physiology 22:56, 2007.

15. Neubauer S: The failing heart—an engine out of fuel. N Engl J Med 356:1140, 2007.

16. Ashrafian H et al.: Metabolic mechanisms in heart failure. Circulation 116:434, 2007.

17. Thum T et al: MicroRNAs in the human heart. A clue to fetal gene reprogramming in heart failure. Circulation 116:258, 2007.

18. Van Rooij E: MicroRNAs: powerful new regulators of heart disease and provocative therapeutic targets. J Clin Invest 117:2369, 2007.

19. Rosanio S et al: Sudden death prophylaxis in heart failure. Int J Cardiol 119:291, 2007.

20. Lip GY, Tse HF: Management of atrial fibrillation. Lancet 370:604, 2007.

21. deGoma EM et al.: Emerging therapies for the management of decompensated heart failure. J Am Coll Cardiol 48:2397, 2006.

22. Anversa P et al.: Cardiac regeneration. J Am Coll Cardiol 47:1769, 2006.

23. Angelini P: Coronary artery anomalies. An entity in search of an identity. Circulation 115:1296, 2007.

24. Hoffman JIE, Kaplan S: The incidence of congenital heart disease. J Am Coll Cardiol 39:1890, 2002.

25. Williams RG et al: Report of the National Heart, Lung, and Blood Institute Working Group on Research in Adult Congenital Disease. J Am Coll Cardiol 47:701, 2006.

26. Warnes CA: The adult with congenital heart disease: born to be bad? J Am Coll Cardiol 46:1, 2005.

27. Schoen FJ, Edwards WD: Pathology of cardiovascular interventions, including endovascular therapies, revascularization, vascular replacement, cardiac assist/replacement, arrhythmia control and repaired congenital heart disease. In Silva MD et al. (eds): Cardiovascular Pathology, 3rd ed. Philadelphia, WB Saunders, 2001, p 678.

28. Drenthen W et al.: Outcome of pregnancy in women with congenital heart disease: a literature review. J Am Coll Cardiol 49:2303, 2007.

29. Srivastava D: Making or breaking the heart: from lineage determination to morphogenesis. Cell 126:1037, 2006.

30. Bruneau BG: The developmental genetics of congenital heart disease. Nature 451:943, 2008.

31. Pierpont ME et al.: Genetic basis for congenital heart defects: current knowledge. A scientific statement from the American Heart Association Council on Cardiovascular Disease in the Young. Circulation 115:3015, 2007.

32. Marino B: Congenital heart disease in patients with Down's syndrome: anatomic and genetic aspects. Biomed Pharmacother 47:197, 1993.

33. Jenkins KJ et al.: Noninherited risk factors and congenital cardiovascular defects: current knowledge. A scientific statement from the American Heart Association Council on Cardiovascular Disease in the Young. Circulation 115:2995, 2007.

34. Huhta JC, Hernandez-Robles JA: Homocysteine, folate, and congenital heart defects. Fetal Pediatr Pathol 24:71, 2005.

35. Webb G, Gatzoulis MA: Atrial septal defects in the adult. Recent progress and overview. Circulation 114:1645, 2006.

36. Hein R et al.: Atrial and ventricular septal defects can safely be closed by percutaneous intervention. J Interv Cardiol 18:515, 2005.

37. Hara H et al.: Patent foramen ovale: current pathology, pathophysiology, and clinical status. J Am Coll Cardiol 46:1768, 2005.

38. Homma S, Sacco RL: Patent foramen ovale and stroke. Circulation 112:1063, 2005.

39. Minette MS, Sahn DJ: Ventricular septal defects. Circulation 114:2190, 2006.

40. Schneider DJ, Moore JW: Patent ductus arteriosus. Circulation 114:1873, 2006.

41. Warnes CA: Transposition of the great arteries. Circulation 114:2699, 2006.

42. Aboulhosn J, Child JS: Left ventricular outflow obstruction. Subaortic stenosis, bicuspid aortic valve, supravalvar aortic stenosis, and coarctation of the aorta. Circulation 114:2412, 2006.

43. Lashkari A et al.: Williams-Beuren syndrome: an update and review for the primary physician. Clin Pediatr 38:189, 1999.

44. Topol EJ et al.: Genetic susceptibility to myocardial infarction and coronary artery disease. Hum Mol Gen 15:R117, 2006.

45. Regieli JJ et al.: Coronary collaterals—insights in molecular determinants and prognostic relevance. Int J Cardiol 116:139, 2007.

46. Fuster V et al.: Atherothrombosis and high-risk plaque: Part I: evolving concepts. J Am Coll Cardiol 46:937, 2005.

47. Falk E et al.: Coronary plaque disruption. Circulation 92:657, 1995.

48. Cohn PF: Silent myocardial ischemia: recent developments. Curr Atheroscler Rep 7:155, 2005.

49. Mendelsohn ME, Karas RH: Molecular and cellular basis of cardiovascular gender differences. Science 308:1583, 2005.

50. Wenger NK: Menopausal hormone therapy: is there evidence for cardiac protection? Int Urol Nephrol 36:617, 2004.

51. Boden WE et al.: Reperfusion strategies in acute ST-segment elevation myocardial infarction. J Am Coll Cardiol 50:917, 2007.

52. Yellon DM, Hausenloy DJ: Myocardial reperfusion injury. N Engl J Med 357:1121, 2007.

53. Kloner RA, Jennings RB: Consequences of brief ischemia: stunning, preconditioning, and their clinical implications: Part 1 and Part 2. Circulation 104:2981; 3158, 2001.

54. Heusch G et al.: Myocardial hibernation: a delicate balance. Am J Physiol Heart Circ Physiol 288:H984, 2005.

55. Eisen A et al.: Ischemic preconditioning: nearly two decades of research. A comprehensive review. Atherosclerosis 172:201, 2004.

56. Jaffe AS et al.: Biomarkers in acute cardiac disease: the present and the future. J Am Coll Cardiol 48:1, 2006.

57. Huikuri HV et al.: Sudden death due to cardiac arrhythmias. N Engl J Med 345:1473, 2001.

58. Farb A et al.: Sudden cardiac death. Frequency of active coronary lesions, inactive coronary lesions, and myocardial infarction. Circulation 92:1701, 1995.

59. Liberthson RR et al.: Prehospital ventricular defibrillation. Prognosis and followup course. N Engl J Med 291:317, 1974.

60. Roberts R: Genomics and cardiac arrhythmias. J Am Coll Cardiol 47:9, 2006.

61. Sarkozy A, Brugada P: Sudden cardiac death and inherited arrhythmia syndromes. J Cardiovasc Electrophysiol 16:S8, 2005.

62. Lehnart SE et al.: Inherited arrhythmias. A National Heart, Lung, and Blood Institute and Office of Rare Diseases Workshop consensus report about the diagnosis, phenotyping, molecular mechanisms, and therapeutic approaches for primary cardiomyopathies of gene mutations affecting ion channel function. Circulation 116:2325, 2007.

63. Passman R, Kadish A: Sudden death prevention with implantable devices. Circulation 16:561, 2007.

64. Voelkel NF et al.: Right ventricular function and failure. Report of a National Heart, Lung, and Blood Institute Working Group on Cellular and Molecular Mechanisms of Right Heart Failure. Circulation 114:1883, 2006.

65. Weitzenblum E: Chronic cor pulmonale. Heart 89:225, 2003.

66. Levine RA, Schwammenthal E: Ischemic mitral regurgitation on the threshold of a solution. From paradoxes to unifying concepts. Circulation 112:745, 2005.

67. Elkayam U, Bitar F: Valvular heart disease and pregnancy. Part I: Native valves. J Am Coll Cardiol 46:223, 2005.

68. Goldbarg SH et al.: Insights into degenerative aortic valve disease. J Am Coll Cardiol 50:1205, 2007.
69. Freeman RV, Otto CM: Spectrum of calcific aortic disease. Pathogenesis, disease progression, and treatment strategies. Circulation 111:3316, 2005.
70. Schoen FJ: Cardiac valves and valvular pathology. Update on function, disease, repair, and replacement. Cardiovasc Pathol 14:189, 2005.
71. Braverman AC et al.: The bicuspid aortic valve. Curr Probl Cardiol 30:470, 2005.
72. Roberts WC, Ko JM: Frequency by decades of unicuspid, bicuspid, and tricuspid aortic valves in adults having isolated aortic valve replacement for aortic stenosis, with or without associated aortic regurgitation. Circulation 111:920, 2005.
73. Cripe L et al.: Bicuspid aortic valve is heritable. J Am Coll Cardiol 44:138, 2004.
74. Hayek E et al.: Mitral valve prolapse. Lancet 365:507, 2005.
75. Robinson PN et al.: The molecular genetics of Marfan syndrome and related disorders. J Med Genet 43:769, 2006.
76. Ng CM et al.: TGF-β-dependent pathogenesis of mitral valve prolapse in a mouse model of Marfan syndrome. J Clin Invest 114:1586, 2004.
77. Roberts R: Another chromosomal locus for mitral valve prolapse. Close but no cigar. Circulation 112:1924, 2005.
78. Guilherme L, Kalil J: Rheumatic fever: from innate to acquired immune response. Ann NY Acad Sci 1107:426, 2007.
79. Carapetis JR et al.: Acute rheumatic fever. Lancet 366:155, 2005.
80. Ferrieri P: Proceedings of the Jones Criteria Workshop. Circulation 106:2521, 2002.
81. Beynon RP et al.: Infective endocarditis. BMJ 333:334, 2006.
82. Mylonakis E, Calderwood SB: Infective endocarditis in adults. N Engl J Med 345:1318, 2001.
83. Haldar SM, O'Gara PT: Infective endocarditis: diagnosis and management. Nat Clin Pract Cardiovasc Med 3:310; 2006.
84. Cervera R: Coronary and valvular syndromes and antiphospholipid antibodies. Thromb Res 114:501, 2004.
85. Roth BL: Drugs and valvular heart diseae. N Engl J Med 356:6, 2007.
86. Lifton RP: Lasker Award to heart valve pioneers. Cell 130:971, 2007.
87. Schoen FJ: Pathology of heart valve substitution with mechanical and tissue bioprostheses. In Silver MD et al. (eds): Cardiovascular Pathology, 3rd ed. Philadelphia, WB Saunders, 2001, p 629.
88. Schoen FJ, Levy RJ: Calcification of tissue heart valve substitutes: progress toward understanding and prevention. Ann Thorac Surg 79:1072, 2005.
89. Richardson P et al.: Report of the 1995 World Health Organization/International Society and Federation of Cardiology Task Force on the Definition and Classification of Cardiomyopathies. Circulation 93:841, 1996.
90. Maron BJ et al.: Contemporary definitions and classification of the cardiomyopathies. Circulation 113:1807, 2006.
91. Boudina S, Abel ED: Diabetic cardiomyopathy revisited. Circulation 115:3213, 2007.
92. Ahmad F et al.: The genetic basis for cardiac remodeling. Annu Rev Genomics Hum Genet 6:185, 2005.
93. Burke A et al.: Left ventricular noncompaction: a pathological study of 14 cases. Hum Pathol 36:403, 2005.
94. Cooper LT et al.: The role of endomyocardial biopsy in the management of cardiovascular disease. Circulation 116:2216, 2007.
95. Stewart S et al.: Revision of the 1990 working formulation for the standardization of nomenclature in the diagnosis of heart rejection. J Heart Lung Transplant 24:1710, 2005.
96. Poller W et al.: Genome-environment interactions in the molecular pathogenesis of dilated cardiomyopathy. J Mol Med 83:579, 2005.
97. Burkett EL, Hershberger RE: Clinical and genetic issues in familial dilated cardiomyopathy. J Am Coll Cardiol 45:969, 2005.
98. Towbin JA, Bowles NE: Dilated cardiomyopathy: a tale of cytoskeletal proteins and beyond. J Cardiovasc Electrophysiol 17:919, 2006.
99. Gilbert-Arness E: Metabolic cardiomyopathy and conduction system defects in children. Ann Clin Lab Sci 34:15, 2004.
100. Benson DW: Genetics of atrioventricular conduction disease in humans. Anat Rec 280:934, 2004.
101. Kloner RA, Rezkalla SH: To drink or not to drink: that is the question. Circulation 116:1306, 2007.
102. Sliwa K et al.: Peripartum cardiomyopathy. Lancet 368:687, 2006.
103. Hilfiker-Kleiner D et al.: A cathepsin D-cleaved 16 kDa form of prolactin mediates postpartum cardiomyopathy. Cell 128:589, 2007.
104. Birks EJ et al.: Left ventricular assist device and drug therapy for reversal of heart failure. N Engl J Med 355:1873, 2006.
105. Frances RJ: Arrhythmogenic right ventricular dysplasia/cardiomyopathy. A review and update. Int J Cardiol 110:279, 2006.
106. Corrado D, Thiene G: Arrhythmogenic right ventricular cardiomyopathy/dysplasia. Clinical impact of molecular genetic studies. Circulation 113:1634, 2006.
107. Ho CY, Seidman CE: A contemporary approach to hypertrophic cardiomyopathy. Circulation 113:e858, 2006.
108. Seidman JG, Seidman C: The genetic basis for cardiomyopathy: from mutation identification to mechanistic paradigms. Cell 104:557, 2001.
109. Maron BJ: Sudden death in young athletes. N Engl J Med 349:1064, 2003.
110. Hancock EW: Differential diagnosis of restrictive cardiomyopathy and constrictive pericarditis. Heart 86:343, 2001.
111. Magnani JW, Dec GW: Myocarditis. Current trends in diagnosis and treatment. Circulation 113:876, 2006.
112. Marin-Neto JA et al.: Pathogenesis of chronic Chagas heart disease. Circulation 115:1109, 2007.
113. Yeh ETH et al.: Cardiovascular complications of cancer therapy. Diagnosis, pathogenesis and management. Circulation 109:3122, 2004.
114. Floyd JD et al.: Cardiotoxicity of cancer therapy. J Clin Oncol 23:7685, 2005.
115. Force T et al.: Molecular mechanisms of cardiotoxicity of tyrosine kinase inhibition. Nature 7:332, 2007.
116. Samuels MA: The brain-heart connection. Circulation 116:77, 2007.
117. Lyon AR et al.: Stress (Takotsubo) cardiomyopathy—a novel pathophysiological hypothesis to explain catecholamine-induced myocardial stunning. Nat Rev Clin Pract Cardiovasc Med 5:2, 2008.
118. Merlini G, Bellotti V: Molecular mechanisms of amyloidosis. N Engl J Med 349:583, 2003.
119. Hassan W et al.: Amyloid heart disease. New frontiers and insights in pathophysiology, diagnosis and management. Tex Heart Inst J 32:178, 2005.
120. Shah KB et al.: Amyloidosis and the heart. Arch Intern Med 166:1805, 2006.
121. Klein I, Danzi S: Thyroid disease and the heart. Circulation 116:1725, 2007.
122. Little WC, Freeman GL: Pericardial disease. Circulation 113:1622, 2006.
123. Roman MJ, Salmon JE: Cardiovascular manifestations of rheumatologic diseases. Circulation 116:2346, 2007.
124. Wilkes D et al.: Inherited disposition to cardiac myxoma development. Nat Rev Cancer 6:157, 2006.
125. Tan CD et al.: Update on cardiac transplantation pathology. Arch Pathol Lab Med 131:1169, 2007.

Diseases of White Blood Cells, Lymph Nodes, Spleen, and Thymus

Development and Maintenance of Hematopoietic Tissues

▪ DISORDERS OF WHITE CELLS

Leukopenia
  Neutropenia, Agranulocytosis

Reactive (Inflammatory) Proliferations of White Cells and Lymph Nodes
  Leukocytosis
  Lymphadenitis
    Acute Nonspecific Lymphadenitis
    Chronic Nonspecific Lymphadenitis

Neoplastic Proliferations of White Cells
  Etiologic and Pathogenetic Factors in White Cell Neoplasia: Overview
  Lymphoid Neoplasms
    Definitions and Classifications
    Precursor B- and T-Cell Neoplasms
    Peripheral B-Cell Neoplasms
    Peripheral T-Cell and NK-Cell Neoplasms

Hodgkin Lymphoma
Myeloid Neoplasms
  Acute Myeloid Leukemia
  Myelodysplastic Syndromes
  Myeloproliferative Disorders
Langerhans Cell Histiocytosis

▪ SPLEEN

Splenomegaly
  Nonspecific Acute Splenitis
  Congestive Splenomegaly
  Splenic Infarcts

Neoplasms

Congenital Anomalies

Rupture

▪ THYMUS

Developmental Disorders

Thymic Hyperplasia

Thymomas

The components of the hematopoietic system have been traditionally divided into the *myeloid tissues,* which include the bone marrow and the cells derived from it (e.g., red cells, platelets, granulocytes, and monocytes), and the *lymphoid tissues,* consisting of the thymus, lymph nodes, and spleen. It is important to recognize, however, that this subdivision is artificial with respect to both the normal physiology of hema-

topoietic cells and the diseases affecting them. For example, although bone marrow contains relatively few lymphocytes, it is the source of all lymphoid progenitors. Similarly, neoplastic disorders of myeloid progenitor cells (myeloid leukemias) originate in the bone marrow but secondarily involve the spleen and (to a lesser degree) the lymph nodes. Some red cell disorders (such as immunohemolytic anemia, discussed in Chapter 14) result from the formation of autoantibodies, signifying a primary disorder of lymphocytes. Thus, it is not possible to draw neat lines between diseases involving the myeloid and lymphoid tissues. Recognizing this difficulty, we somewhat arbitrarily divide diseases of the hematopoietic tissues into two chapters. In this chapter we discuss white cell diseases and disorders affecting the spleen and thymus. In Chapter 14 we consider diseases of red cells and those affecting hemostasis. Before delving into specific diseases, we will briefly discuss the origins of hematopoietic cells, since many disorders of white cells and red cells involve disturbances of their normal development and maturation.

Development and Maintenance of Hematopoietic Tissues

Blood cell progenitors first appear during the third week of embryonic development in the yolk sac, but definitive *hematopoietic stem cells* (HSCs) are believed to arise several weeks later in the mesoderm of the intraembryonic aorta/gonad/mesonephros region.[1] During the third month of embryogenesis, HSCs migrate to the liver, which becomes the chief site of blood cell formation until shortly before birth. By the fourth month of development, HSCs begin to shift in location yet again, this time to the bone marrow. By birth, marrow throughout the skeleton is hematopoietically active and hepatic hematopoiesis dwindles to a trickle, persisting only in widely scattered foci that become inactive soon after birth. Until puberty, hematopoietically active marrow is found throughout the skeleton, but soon thereafter it becomes restricted to the axial skeleton. Thus, in normal adults, only about half of the marrow space is hematopoietically active.

The formed elements of blood—red cells, granulocytes, monocytes, platelets, and lymphocytes—have a common origin from HSCs, pluripotent cells that sit at the apex of a hierarchy of bone marrow progenitors (Fig. 13–1). Most evidence supporting this scheme comes from studies in mice, but human hematopoiesis is believed to proceed in a similar way. HSCs give rise to two kinds of multipotent cells, the common lymphoid and common myeloid progenitors. The common lymphoid progenitor is the source of T-cell, B-cell, and natural killer (NK) cell precursors. We will return to the origins of lymphoid cells when we discuss tumors derived from these cells. From the common myeloid progenitors arise various kinds of committed progenitors restricted to differentiation along particular lineages. These cells are referred to as colony-forming units (CFUs) (see Fig. 13–1), because they give rise to colonies composed of specific kinds of mature cells when grown in culture. From the various committed progenitors are derived the morphologically recognizable precursors, such as myeloblasts, proerythroblasts, and megakaryoblasts, which in turn give rise to mature granulocytes, red cells, and platelets.

HSCs have two essential properties that are required for the maintenance of hematopoiesis: pluripotency and the capacity for self-renewal. Pluripotency refers to the ability of a single HSC to generate all mature hematopoietic cells. When an HSC divides at least one daughter cell must self-renew to avoid stem cell depletion. Self-renewing divisions are believed to occur within a specialized marrow niche, in which stromal cells and secreted factors nurture and somehow maintain the HSCs.[2] As you may have already surmised from their ability to migrate during embryonic development, HSCs are not sessile. Particularly under conditions of marked stress, such as severe anemia, HSCs are mobilized from the bone marrow and appear in the peripheral blood. In such circumstances, additional HSC niches are sometimes induced or "unveiled" in other tissues, such as the spleen and liver, which can then become sites of extramedullary hematopoiesis.

The marrow response to short-term physiologic needs is regulated by hematopoietic growth factors through effects on the committed progenitors. Since mature blood elements are terminally differentiated cells with finite life spans, their numbers must be constantly replenished. In at least some divisions of HSCs, a single daughter cell begins to differentiate. Once past this threshold, these newly committed cells lose the capacity for self-renewal and commence an inexorable journey down a road that leads to terminal differentiation and death. However, as these progenitors differentiate they also begin to express receptors for lineage-specific growth factors, which stimulate their short-term growth and survival. Some growth factors, such as stem cell factor (also called *c-KIT ligand*) and FLT3-ligand, act on very early committed progenitors. Others, such as erythropoietin, granulocyte-macrophage colony-stimulating factor (GM-CSF), granulocyte colony-stimulating factor (G-CSF), and thrombopoietin, act on committed progenitors with more restricted potentials. Feedback loops that are mediated through growth factors tune the marrow output, allowing the numbers of formed blood elements (red cells, white cells, and platelets) to be maintained within appropriate ranges (given in Table 13–1).

Many diseases alter the production of blood cells. The marrow is the ultimate source of all cells of the innate and adaptive immune system and responds to infectious or inflammatory challenges by increasing its output of granulocytes under the direction of specific growth factors and cytokines. Conversely, other disorders are associated with defects in hematopoiesis that lead to deficiencies of one or more type of blood cell. Primary tumors of hematopoietic cells are among the most important diseases that interfere with marrow function, but specific genetic diseases, infections, toxins, and nutritional deficiencies, as well as chronic inflammation of any cause, can also decrease the production of blood cells by the marrow.

Tumors of hematopoietic origin are often associated with mutations that block progenitor cell maturation or abrogate their growth factor dependence. The net effect of such derangements is an unregulated clonal expansion of hematopoietic elements, which replace normal marrow progenitors and often spread to other hematopoietic tissues. In some instances, these tumors originate from transformed HSCs that retain the ability to differentiate along multiple lineages, whereas in other instances the origin is a more differentiated progenitor that has acquired an abnormal capacity for self-renewal. Whether this latter situation merely reflects a block in differentiation, or derives instead from the reactivation of a program of gene expression that supports the self-renewal of normal stem cells, is an area of current investigation.

Morphology. The bone marrow is a unique microenvironment that supports the orderly proliferation,

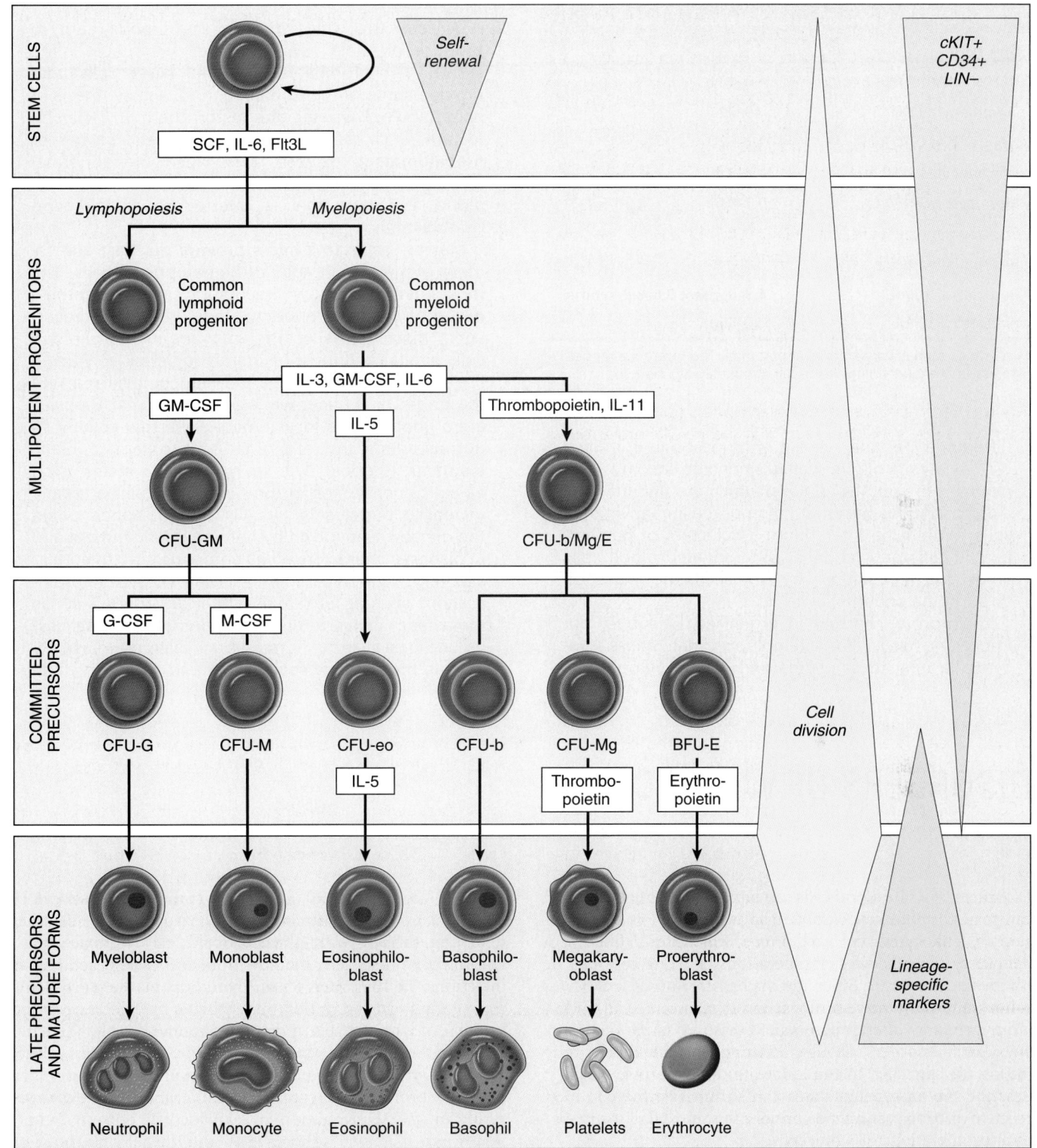

FIGURE 13–1 Differentiation of blood cells. CFU, colony forming unit; SCF, stem cell factor; Flt3L, Flt3 ligand; G-CSF, granulocyte colony-stimulating factor; GM-CSF, granulocyte-macrophage colony-stimulating factor; LIN–, negative for lineage-specific markers; M-CSF, macrophage colony-stimulating factor.

TABLE 13–1 Adult Reference Ranges for Blood Cells*	
Cell Type	
White cells (×10³/μL)	4.8–10.8
Granulocytes (%)	40–70
Neutrophils (×10³/μL)	1.4–6.5
Lymphocytes (×10³/μL)	1.2–3.4
Monocytes (×10³/μL)	0.1–0.6
Eosinophils (×10³/μL)	0–0.5
Basophils (×10³/μL)	0–0.2
Red cells (×10³/μL)	4.3–5, men; 3.5–5.0, women
Platelets (×10³/μL)	150–450

*Reference ranges vary among laboratories. The reference ranges for the laboratory providing the result should always be used.

differentiation, and release of blood cells. It is filled with a network of thin-walled sinusoids lined by a single layer of endothelial cells, which are underlaid by a discontinuous basement membrane and adventitial cells. Within the interstitium lie clusters of hematopoietic cells and fat cells. Differentiated blood cells enter the circulation by transcellular migration through the endothelial cells.

The normal marrow is organized in subtle, but important, ways. For example, normal megakaryocytes lie next to sinusoids and extend cytoplasmic processes that bud off into the bloodstream to produce platelets, while red cell precursors often surround macrophages (so-called **nurse cells**) that provide some of the iron needed for the synthesis of hemoglobin. Diseases that distort the marrow architecture, such as deposits of metastatic cancer or granulomatous disease, can cause the abnormal release of immature precursors into the peripheral blood, a finding that is referred to as **leukoerythroblastosis**.

Marrow aspirate smears provide the best assessment of the morphology of hematopoietic cells. The most mature marrow precursors can be identified based on their morphology alone. Immature precursors ("blast" forms) of different types are morphologically similar and must be identified definitively using lineage-specific antibodies and histochemical markers (described later under white cell neoplasms). Biopsies are a good means for estimating marrow activity. In normal adults, the ratio of fat cells to hematopoietic elements is about 1:1. In hypoplastic states (e.g., aplastic anemia) the proportion of fat cells is greatly increased; conversely, fat cells often disappear when the marrow is involved by hematopoietic tumors and in diseases characterized by compensatory hyperplasias (e.g., hemolytic anemias), and neoplastic proliferations such as leukemias. Other disorders (such as metastatic cancers and granulomatous diseases) induce local marrow fibrosis. Such lesions are usually inaspirable and best seen in biopsies.

DISORDERS OF WHITE CELLS

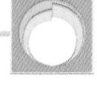

Disorders of white blood cells can be classified into two broad categories: *proliferative disorders*, in which there is an expansion of leukocytes, and *leukopenias*, which are defined as a deficiency of leukocytes. Proliferations of white cells can be *reactive* or *neoplastic*. Since the major function of leukocytes is host defense, reactive proliferation in response to an underlying primary, often microbial, disease is fairly common. Neoplastic disorders, though less frequent, are much more important clinically. In the following discussion we will first describe the leukopenic states and summarize the common reactive disorders, and then consider in some detail the malignant proliferations of white cells.

Leukopenia

The number of circulating white cells may be markedly decreased in a variety of disorders. An abnormally low white cell count *(leukopenia)* usually results from reduced numbers of neutrophils *(neutropenia, granulocytopenia)*. *Lymphopenia* is less common; in addition to congenital immunodeficiency diseases (see Chapter 6), it is most commonly observed in advanced human immunodeficiency virus (HIV) infection, following therapy with glucocorticoids or cytotoxic drugs, autoimmune disorders, malnutrition, and certain acute viral infections. In the latter setting lymphopenia actually stems from lymphocyte activation rather than a true decrease in the number of lymphocytes in the body. You will recall that acute viral infections induce production of type I interferons, which activate T lymphocytes and change the expression of a number of surface proteins that regulate T cell migration. These changes result in the sequestration of activated T cells in lymph nodes and increased adherence to endothelial cells, both of which contribute to lymphopenia. Granulocytopenia is more common and is often associated with significantly decreased granulocyte function, and thus merits further discussion.

NEUTROPENIA, AGRANULOCYTOSIS

Neutropenia, a reduction in the number of neutrophils in the blood, occurs in a wide variety of circumstances. *Agranulocytosis*, a clinically significant reduction in neutrophils, has the serious consequence of making individuals susceptible to bacterial and fungal infections.

Pathogenesis. A reduction in circulating granulocytes occurs if there is (1) inadequate or ineffective granulopoiesis, or (2) accelerated removal of neutrophils from the blood. *Inadequate or ineffective granulopoiesis* is observed in the setting of

- *Suppression of hematopoietic stem cells*, as occurs in aplastic anemia (see Chapter 14) and a variety of infiltrative marrow disorders (tumors, granulomatous disease, etc.); in these conditions granulocytopenia is accompanied by anemia and thrombocytopenia
- *Suppression of committed granulocytic precursors* by exposure to certain drugs (discussed below)
- Disease states associated with *ineffective hematopoiesis*, such as megaloblastic anemias (Chapter 14) and myelodysplastic syndromes, where defective precursors die in the marrow
- Rare *congenital conditions* (such as Kostmann syndrome) in which inherited defects in specific genes impair granulocytic differentiation

Accelerated removal or destruction of neutrophils occurs with

- *Immunologically mediated injury* to neutrophils, which can be idiopathic, associated with a well-defined immunological disorder (e.g., systemic lupus erythematosus), or caused by exposure to drugs
- *Splenomegaly*, in which splenic sequestration of neutrophils leads to excessive destruction, usually associated with increased destruction of red cells and platelets as well
- *Increased peripheral utilization*, which can occur in overwhelming bacterial, fungal, or rickettsial infections

The most common cause of agranulocytosis is drug toxicity. Certain drugs, such as alkylating agents and antimetabolites used in cancer treatment, produce agranulocytosis in a predictable, dose-related fashion. Because such drugs cause a generalized suppression of the bone marrow, production of red cells and platelets is also affected. Agranulocytosis can also occur as an idiosyncratic reaction to a large variety of agents. The roster of implicated drugs includes aminopyrine, chloramphenicol, sulfonamides, chlorpromazine, thiouracil, and phenylbutazone. The neutropenia induced by chlorpromazine and related phenothiazines results from a toxic effect on granulocytic precursors in the bone marrow. In contrast, agranulocytosis following administration of aminopyrine, thiouracil, and certain sulfonamides probably stems from antibody-mediated destruction of mature neutrophils through mechanisms similar to those involved in drug-induced immunohemolytic anemias (Chapter 14).

In some patients with acquired idiopathic neutropenia, autoantibodies directed against neutrophil-specific antigens are detected. Severe neutropenia can also occur in association with monoclonal proliferations of large granular lymphocytes (so-called LGL leukemia).[3] The mechanism of this neutropenia is not clear; suppression of marrow granulocytic progenitors by products of the neoplastic cell (usually a CD8+ cytotoxic T cell) is considered most likely.

Morphology. The alterations in the bone marrow vary with cause. With excessive destruction of neutrophils in the periphery, the marrow is usually hypercellular due to a compensatory increase in granulocytic precursors. Hypercellularity is also the rule with neutropenias caused by ineffective granulopoiesis, as occurs in megaloblastic anemias and myelodysplastic syndromes. Agranulocytosis caused by agents that suppress or destroy granulocytic precursors is understandably associated with marrow hypocellularity.

Infections are a common consequence of agranulocytosis. Ulcerating necrotizing lesions of the gingiva, floor of the mouth, buccal mucosa, pharynx, or elsewhere in the oral cavity (agranulocytic angina) are quite characteristic. These are typically deep, undermined, and covered by gray to green-black necrotic membranes from which numerous bacteria or fungi can be isolated. Less frequently, similar ulcerative lesions occur in the skin, vagina, anus, or gastrointestinal tract. Severe life-threatening invasive bacterial or fungal infections may occur in the lungs, urinary tract, and kidneys. The neutropenic patient is at particularly high risk for deep fungal infections caused by *Candida* and *Aspergillus*. Sites of infection often show a massive growth of organisms with little leukocytic response. In the most dramatic instances, bacteria grow in colonies (botryomycosis) resembling those seen on agar plates.

Clinical Features. The symptoms and signs of neutropenia are related to infection, and include malaise, chills, and fever, often followed by marked weakness and fatigability. With agranulocytosis, infections are often overwhelming and may cause death within hours to days.

Serious infections are most likely when the neutrophil count falls below 500 per mm³. Because infections are often fulminant, broad-spectrum antibiotics must be given expeditiously whenever signs or symptoms appear. In some instances, such as following myelosuppressive chemotherapy, neutropenia is treated with G-CSF, a growth factor that stimulates the production of granulocytes from marrow precursors.

Reactive (Inflammatory) Proliferations of White Cells and Lymph Nodes

LEUKOCYTOSIS

Leukocytosis refers to an increase in the number of white cells in the blood. It is a common reaction to a variety of inflammatory states.

Pathogenesis. The peripheral blood leukocyte count is influenced by several factors, including

- The size of the myeloid and lymphoid precursor and storage cell pools in the bone marrow, thymus, circulation, and peripheral tissues
- The rate of release of cells from the storage pools into the circulation

TABLE 13–2	Mechanisms and Causes of Leukocytosis

INCREASED PRODUCTION IN THE MARROW

Chronic infection or inflammation (growth factor-dependent)
Paraneoplastic (e.g., Hodgkin lymphoma; growth factor-dependent)
Myeloproliferative disorders (e.g., chronic myeloid leukemia; growth factor-independent)

INCREASED RELEASE FROM MARROW STORES

Endotoxemia
Infection
Hypoxia

DECREASED MARGINATION

Exercise
Catecholamines

DECREASED EXTRAVASATION INTO TISSUES

Glucocorticoids

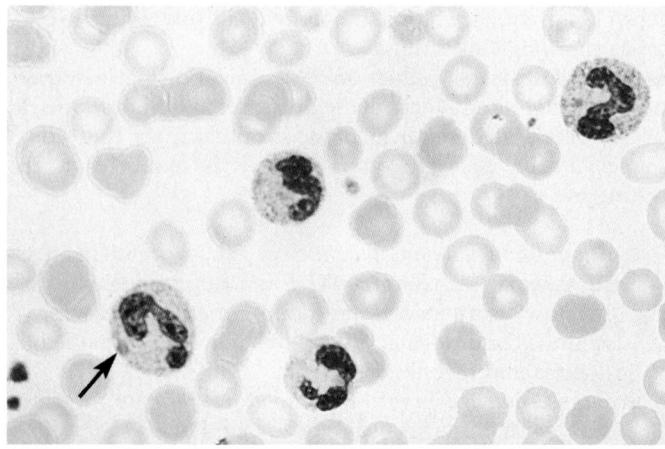

FIGURE 13–2   Reactive changes in neutrophils. Neutrophils containing coarse purple cytoplasmic granules (toxic granulations) and blue cytoplasmic patches of dilated endoplasmic reticulum (Döhle bodies, *arrow*) are observed in this peripheral blood smear prepared from a patient with bacterial sepsis.

○ The proportion of cells that are adherent to blood vessel walls at any time (the marginal pool)
○ The rate of extravasation of cells from the blood into tissues

As was discussed in Chapter 2, leukocyte homeostasis is maintained by cytokines, growth factors, and adhesion molecules through their effects on the commitment, proliferation, differentiation, and extravasation of leukocytes and their progenitors. Table 13–2 summarizes the major mechanisms of neutrophilic leukocytosis and its causes, the most important of which is infection. In acute infection there is a rapid increase in the egress of mature granulocytes from the bone marrow pool. If the infection is prolonged, the release of interleukin-1 (IL-1), tumor necrosis factor (TNF), and other inflammatory cytokines stimulates bone marrow stromal cells and T cells to produce increased amounts of hematopoietic growth factors, which enhance the proliferation and differentiation of committed granulocytic progenitors and, over several days, cause a sustained increase in neutrophil production.

Some growth factors preferentially stimulate the production of a single type of leukocyte. For example, IL-5 mainly stimulates eosinophil production, while G-CSF induces neutrophilia. Such factors are differentially produced in response to various pathogenic stimuli and, as a result, the five principal types of leukocytosis (neutrophilia, eosinophilia, basophilia, monocytosis, and lymphocytosis) tend to be observed in different clinical settings (summarized in Table 13–3).

In sepsis or severe inflammatory disorders (such as Kawasaki disease), leukocytosis is often accompanied by morphologic changes in the neutrophils, such as toxic granulations, Döhle bodies, and cytoplasmic vacuoles (Fig. 13–2). *Toxic granules*, which are coarser and darker than the normal neutrophilic granules, represent abnormal azurophilic (primary) granules. *Döhle bodies* are patches of dilated endoplasmic reticulum that appear as sky-blue cytoplasmic "puddles."

In most instances it is not difficult to distinguish reactive and neoplastic leukocytoses, but uncertainties may arise in two settings. Acute viral infections, particularly in children, can cause the appearance of large numbers of activated lym-

TABLE 13–3	Causes of Leukocytosis
Type of Leukocytosis	**Causes**
Neutrophilic leukocytosis	Acute bacterial infections, especially those caused by pyogenic organisms; sterile inflammation caused by, for example, tissue necrosis (myocardial infarction, burns)
Eosinophilic leukocytosis (eosinophilia)	Allergic disorders such as asthma, hay fever; certain skin diseases (e.g., pemphigus, dermatitis herpetiformis); parasitic infestations; drug reactions; certain malignancies (e.g., Hodgkin and some non-Hodgkin lymphomas); collagen vascular disorders and some vasculitides; atheroembolic disease (transient)
Basophilic leukocytosis (basophilia)	Rare, often indicative of a myeloproliferative disease (e.g., chronic myeloid leukemia)
Monocytosis	Chronic infections (e.g., tuberculosis), bacterial endocarditis, rickettsiosis, and malaria; collagen vascular diseases (e.g., systemic lupus erythematosus); inflammatory bowel diseases (e.g., ulcerative colitis)
Lymphocytosis	Accompanies monocytosis in many disorders associated with chronic immunological stimulation (e.g., tuberculosis, brucellosis); viral infections (e.g., hepatitis A, cytomegalovirus, Epstein-Barr virus); *Bordetella pertussis* infection

phocytes that resemble neoplastic lymphoid cells. At other times, particularly in severe infections, many immature granulocytes appear in the blood, simulating a myeloid leukemia (*leukemoid reaction*). Special laboratory studies (discussed later) are helpful in distinguishing reactive and neoplastic leukocytoses.

LYMPHADENITIS

Following their initial development from precursors in the bone marrow (B cells) and the thymus (T cells), lymphocytes circulate through the blood and, under the influence of specific cytokines and chemokines, home to lymph nodes, spleen, tonsils, adenoids, and Peyer's patches, which constitute the peripheral lymphoid tissues. Lymph nodes, the most widely distributed and easily accessible lymphoid tissue, are frequently examined for diagnostic purposes. They are discrete encapsulated structures that contain well-organized B-cell and T-cell zones, which are richly invested with phagocytes and antigen-presenting cells (Fig. 6–6, Chapter 6).

The activation of resident immune cells leads to morphologic changes in lymph nodes. Within several days of antigenic stimulation, the primary follicles enlarge and are transformed into pale-staining *germinal centers*, highly dynamic structures in which B cells acquire the capacity to make high-affinity antibodies against specific antigens. Paracortical T-cell zones may also undergo hyperplasia. The degree and pattern of the morphologic changes are dependent on the inciting stimulus and the intensity of the response. Trivial injuries and infections induce subtle changes, while more significant infections inevitably produce nodal enlargement and sometimes leave residual scarring. For this reason, lymph nodes in adults are almost never "normal" or "resting," and it is often necessary to distinguish morphologic changes secondary to past experience from those related to present disease. Infections and inflammatory stimuli often elicit regional or systemic immune reactions within lymph nodes. Some that produce distinctive morphologic patterns are described in other chapters. Most, however, cause stereotypical patterns of lymph node reaction designated acute and chronic nonspecific lymphadenitis.

Acute Nonspecific Lymphadenitis

Acute lymphadenitis in the cervical region is most often due to microbial drainage from infections of the teeth or tonsils, while in the axillary or inguinal regions it is most often caused by infections in the extremities. Acute lymphadenitis also occurs in mesenteric lymph nodes draining acute appendicitis. Unfortunately, other self-limited infections may also cause acute mesenteric adenitis and induce symptoms mimicking acute appendicitis, a differential diagnosis that plagues the surgeon. Systemic viral infections (particularly in children) and bacteremia often produce acute generalized lymphadenopathy.

> **Morphology.** Grossly, the nodes are swollen, gray-red, and engorged. Microscopically, there is prominence of large reactive germinal centers containing numerous mitotic figures. Macrophages often contain particulate debris derived from dead bacteria or necrotic cells. When pyogenic organisms are the cause, the centers of the follicles may undergo necrosis; sometimes the entire node is converted into a bag of pus. With less severe reactions, scattered neutrophils infiltrate about the follicles and accumulate within the lymphoid sinuses. The endothelial cells lining the sinuses undergo hyperplasia.

Nodes involved by acute lymphadenitis are enlarged and painful. When abscess formation is extensive the nodes become fluctuant. The overlying skin is red. Sometimes, suppurative infections penetrate through the capsule of the node and track to the skin to produce draining sinuses. Healing of such lesions is associated with scarring.

Chronic Nonspecific Lymphadenitis

Chronic immunological stimuli produce several different patterns of lymph node reaction.

> **Morphology.** **Follicular hyperplasia** is caused by stimuli that activate humoral immune responses. It is defined by the presence of large oblong germinal centers (secondary follicles), which are surrounded by a collar of small resting naive B cells (the mantle zone) (Fig. 13–3). Germinal centers are normally polarized into two distinct regions: (1) a dark zone containing proliferating blastlike B cells (centroblasts) and (2) a light zone composed of B cells with irregular or cleaved nuclear contours (centrocytes). Interspersed between the germinal B centers is an inconspicuous network of antigen-presenting follicular dendritic cells and macrophages (often referred to as **tingible-body macrophages**) containing the nuclear debris of B cells, which undergo apoptosis if they fail to produce an antibody with a high affinity for antigen.
>
> Causes of follicular hyperplasia include rheumatoid arthritis, toxoplasmosis, and early stages of infection with HIV. This form of hyperplasia is morphologically similar to follicular lymphoma (discussed later). Features favoring a reactive (non-neoplastic) hyperplasia include (1) preservation of the lymph node architecture, including the interfollicular T-cell zones and the sinusoids; (2) marked variation in the shape and size of the follicles; and (3) the presence of frequent mitotic figures, phagocytic macrophages, and recognizable light and dark zones, all of which tend to be absent from neoplastic follicles.
>
> **Paracortical hyperplasia** is caused by stimuli that trigger T cell–mediated immune responses, such as acute viral infections (e.g., infectious mononucleosis). The T-cell regions typically contain immunoblasts, activated T cells three to four times the size of resting lymphocytes that have round nuclei, open chromatin, several prominent nucleoli, and moderate amounts of pale cytoplasm. The expanded T-cell zones encroach on and, in particularly exuberant reactions, efface the B-cell follicles. In such cases

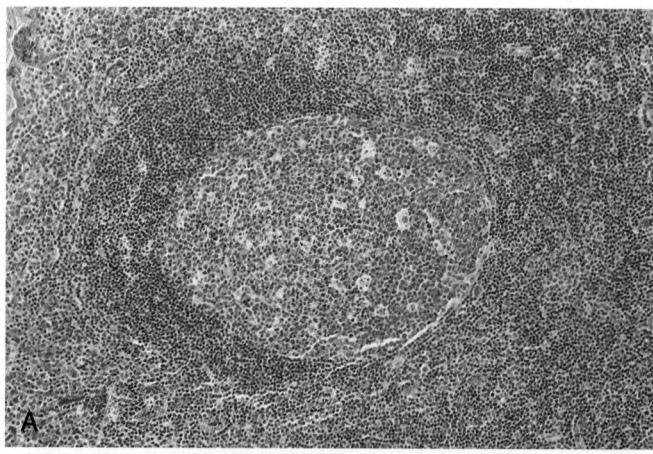

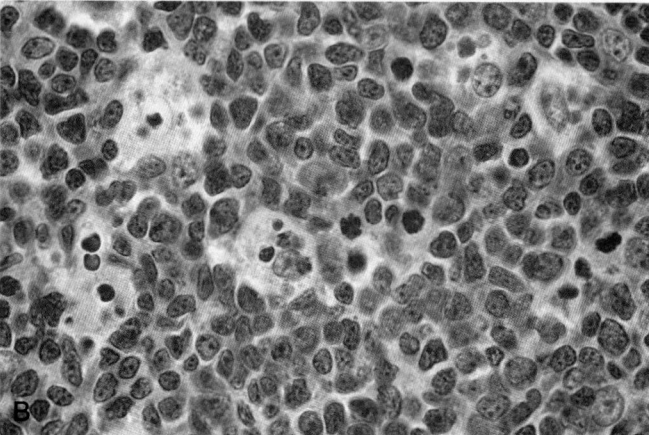

FIGURE 13–3 Follicular hyperplasia. **A,** Low-power view showing a reactive follicle and surrounding mantle zone. The dark-staining mantle zone is more prominent adjacent to the germinal-center light zone in the left half of the follicle. The right half of the follicle consists of the dark zone. **B,** High-power view of the dark zone shows several mitotic figures and numerous macrophages containing phagocytosed apoptotic cells (tingible bodies).

immunoblasts may be so numerous that special studies are needed to exclude a lymphoid neoplasm. In addition, there is often a hypertrophy of sinusoidal and vascular endothelial cells, sometimes accompanied by infiltrating macrophages and eosinophils.

Sinus histiocytosis (also called reticular hyperplasia) refers to an increase in the number and size of the cells that line lymphatic sinusoids. Although nonspecific, this form of hyperplasia may be particularly prominent in lymph nodes draining cancers such as carcinoma of the breast. The lining lymphatic endothelial cells are markedly hypertrophied and macrophages are greatly increased in numbers, resulting in the expansion and distension of the sinuses.

Characteristically, lymph nodes in chronic reactions are nontender, because nodal enlargement occurs slowly over time. Chronic lymphadenitis is particularly common in inguinal and axillary nodes, which drain relatively large areas of the body and are challenged frequently.

Before leaving the reactive disorders of lymphocytes, it is worth pointing out that chronic immune reactions can promote the appearance of organized collections of immune cells in nonlymphoid tissues. A classic example is seen in chronic gastritis caused by *Helicobacter pylori*, in which aggregates of mucosal lymphocytes are seen that simulate the appearance of Peyer's patches. A similar phenomenon occurs in rheumatoid athritis, in which B-cell follicles often appear in the inflamed synovium. Lymphotoxin, a cytokine required for the formation of normal Peyer's patches, is probably involved in the establishment of these "extranodal" inflammation-induced collections of lymphoid cells.[4]

Neoplastic Proliferations of White Cells

Malignancies are clinically the most important disorders of white cells. These diseases fall into several broad categories:

○ *Lymphoid neoplasms* include a diverse group of tumors of B-cell, T-cell, and NK-cell origin. In many instances the phenotype of the neoplastic cell closely resembles that of a particular stage of normal lymphocyte differentiation, a feature that is used in the diagnosis and classification of these disorders.
○ *Myeloid neoplasms* arise from early hematopoietic progenitors. Three categories of myeloid neoplasia are recognized: *acute myeloid leukemias*, in which immature progenitor cells accumulate in the bone marrow; *myelodysplastic syndromes*, which are associated with ineffective hematopoiesis and resultant peripheral blood cytopenias; and *chronic myeloproliferative disorders*, in which increased production of one or more terminally differentiated myeloid elements (e.g., granulocytes) usually leads to elevated peripheral blood counts.
○ The *histiocytoses* are uncommon proliferative lesions of macrophages and dendritic cells. Although "histiocyte" (literally, "tissue cell") is an archaic morphologic term, it is still often used. A special type of immature dendritic cell, the Langerhans cell, gives rise to a spectrum of neoplastic disorders referred to as the *Langerhans cell histiocytoses*.

ETIOLOGIC AND PATHOGENETIC FACTORS IN WHITE CELL NEOPLASIA: OVERVIEW

As we will see in the following sections, the neoplastic disorders of white cells are extremely varied. Before we delve into this complexity, it is worth considering a few themes of general relevance to their etiology and pathogenesis.

Chromosomal Translocations and Other Acquired Mutations. *Nonrandom chromosomal abnormalities, most commonly translocations, are present in the majority of white cell neoplasms.* As was discussed briefly in Chapter 7, many specific rearrangements are associated with particular neoplasms, suggesting a critical role in their genesis.

○ *The genes that are mutated or otherwise altered often play crucial roles in the development, growth, or survival of the normal counterpart of the malignant cell.* In some instances, the result of the aberration is to produce a "dominant-negative" protein that interferes with a normal function (a loss of function); in others the result is an inappropriate increase in some normal activity (a gain of function). In certain tumors, different aberrations have the same functional consequence as a result of their convergence on a common critical signaling pathway or transcription factor. An example of this is seen in so-called "MALTomas" (see also Chapter 17), B-cell lymphomas occurring in extranodal mucosal sites, which are often associated with translocations involving either the *MALT1* or the *BCL10* gene. The MALT1 and BCL10 proteins bind one another in a protein complex that regulates NF-κB, a transcription factor with important pro-survival functions in normal lymphocytes. The net effect of translocations involving either *MALT1* and *BCL10* is the same—a dysregulation of the MALT1/BCL10 complex that causes the constitutive activation of NF-κB,[5] which (as we will see) plays a role in the pathogenesis of many lymphoid malignancies.[6]

- *Oncoproteins created by genomic aberrations often block normal maturation.* Many oncoproteins cause an arrest in differentiation, often at a stage when cells are proliferating rapidly. The importance of this block in maturation is most evident in the acute leukemias, in which dominant-negative mutations involving transcription factors that interfere with early stages of lymphoid or myeloid cell differentiation often collaborate with activating mutations in tyrosine kinases that increase cell survival and proliferation (Fig. 13–4). However, this theme also applies to more mature lymphoid tumors. For example, *BCL6* encodes a transcription factor that is expressed in germinal center B cells. Without *BCL6*, germinal center B cells cannot form; however, *BCL6* must be turned off for germinal cell B cells to mature into memory B cells or plasma cells. As we will discuss, aberrations that up-regulate *BCL6* expression and prevent its down-regulation are very common in certain types of lymphomas derived from germinal center B cells.[7]

- *Proto-oncogenes are often activated in lymphoid cells by errors that occur during antigen receptor gene rearrangement and diversification.* Among lymphoid cells, *potentially oncogenic mutations occur most frequently in germinal center B cells during attempted antibody diversification.* After antigen stimulation, B cells enter germinal centers and upregulate the expression of activation-induced cytosine deaminase (AID), a specialized DNA-modifying enzyme that is essential for two types of Ig gene modifications: class switching, an intragenic recombination event in which the IgM heavy-chain constant gene segment is replaced with a different constant segment (e.g., IgG₃), thus allowing an isotype switch of antibody class; and somatic hypermutation, which creates point mutations within Ig genes that may by chance increase antibody affinity for antigen (Chapter 6). Certain proto-oncogenes, such as *c-MYC*, are activated in germinal center B-cell lymphomas by chromosomal translocations involving class switch regions. Remarkably, AID expression is sufficient to induce *c-MYC/ Ig* translocations in normal germinal center B cells,[8,9] apparently because it creates lesions in DNA that lead to chromosomal breaks. Parenthetically, it follows that even activation of a strong oncogene like *c-MYC* is not sufficient to cause transformation, emphasizing that (like other cancers) lymphomas arise due to a combination of multiple genetic lesions. Other proto-oncogenes, such as *BCL6*, are more commonly activated in germinal center B-cell lymphomas by point mutations,[10] which also seem to stem from "mistargeting" of AID. Undoubtedly, the selective advantage offered by antibody diversification against infection far outweighs the price that is paid in terms of potentially oncogenic mutations, but this is of little solace to individuals afflicted with tumors of germinal center B-cell origin, which include the most common and clinically important lymphoid neoplasms. A different type of regulated genomic instability is unique to precursor B and T cells, which express a V(D)J recombinase that cuts DNA at specific sites within the immunoglobulin (Ig) and T-cell receptor loci, respectively. This process is essential for the assembly of productive antigen receptor genes, but sometimes goes awry, leading to the joining of portions of other genes to antigen receptor gene regulatory elements. Particularly in tumors of precursor T cells, proto-oncogenes are often deregulated by their involvement in such aberrant recombination events.

Inherited Genetic Factors. As was discussed in Chapter 7, individuals with genetic diseases that promote genomic instability, such as Bloom syndrome, Fanconi anemia, and ataxia telangiectasia, are at increased risk of acute leukemia. In addition, both Down syndrome (trisomy 21) and type I neurofibromatosis are associated with an increased incidence of childhood leukemia.

Viruses. Three lymphotropic viruses—human T-cell leukemia virus-1 (HTLV-1), Epstein-Barr virus (EBV), and Kaposi sarcoma herpesvirus/human herpesvirus-8 (KSHV/ HHV-8)—have been implicated as causative agents in particular lymphomas. The possible mechanisms of transformation by viruses were discussed in Chapter 7. HTLV-1 is associated with adult T-cell leukemia/lymphoma. EBV is found in a subset of Burkitt lymphoma, 30% to 40% of Hodgkin lymphoma (HL), many B-cell lymphomas arising in the setting of T-cell immunodeficiency, and rare NK-cell lymphomas. In addition to Kaposi sarcoma, KSHV is uniquely associated with an unusual B-cell lymphoma that presents as a malignant effusion, often in the pleural cavity.

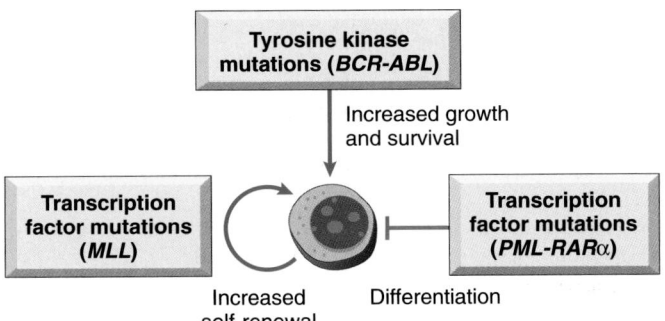

FIGURE 13–4 Molecular pathogenesis of acute leukemia. Acute leukemias arise from complementary mutations that block differentiation at early stages of white cell development, enhance self-renewal, and increase growth and survival. Important examples of each type of mutation are listed. BCR-ABL, breakpoint chromosomal region–Abelson kinase fusion gene; MLL, mixed-lineage leukemia gene; PML-RARα, promyelocytic leukemia–retinoic acid receptor α fusion gene.

Chronic Immune Stimulation. Several environmental agents that cause localized chronic immune stimulation predispose to lymphoid neoplasia, which almost always arises within the inflamed tissue. Examples include the associations between *H. pylori* infection and gastric B-cell lymphomas (Chapter 17), and gluten-sensitive enteropathy and intestinal T-cell lymphomas. This can be contrasted with HIV infection, which is associated with an increased risk of B-cell lymphomas that may arise within virtually any organ. Early in the course, T-cell dysregulation by HIV infection causes a systemic hyperplasia of germinal center B cells that is associated with an increased incidence of germinal center B-cell lymphomas. In advanced infection (acquired immunodeficiency syndrome), severe T-cell immunodeficiency further elevates the risk for B-cell lymphomas, particularly those associated with EBV and KSHV/HHV-8.

Iatrogenic Factors. Ironically, radiation therapy and certain forms of chemotherapy used to treat cancer increase the risk of subsequent myeloid and lymphoid neoplasms. This association stems from the mutagenic effects of ionizing radiation and chemotherapeutic drugs on hematolymphoid progenitor cells.

Smoking. The incidence of acute myeloid leukemia is increased 1.3- to 2-fold in smokers, presumably because of exposure to carcinogens, such as benzene, in tobacco smoke.

LYMPHOID NEOPLASMS

Definitions and Classifications

One confusing aspect of the lymphoid neoplasms concerns the use of the terms *lymphocytic leukemia* and *lymphoma*. *Leukemia* is used for neoplasms that present with widespread involvement of the bone marrow and (usually, but not always) the peripheral blood. *Lymphoma* is used for proliferations that arise as discrete tissue masses. Originally these terms were attached to what were considered distinct entities, but with time and increased understanding these divisons have blurred. Many entities called "lymphoma" occasionally have leukemic presentations, and evolution to "leukemia" is not unusual during the progression of incurable "lymphomas." Conversely, tumors identical to "leukemias" sometimes arise as soft-tissue masses unaccompanied by bone marrow disease. Hence, when applied to particular neoplasms, the terms *leukemia* and *lymphoma* merely reflect the usual tissue distribution of each disease at presentation.

Within the large group of lymphomas, *Hodgkin lymphoma* is segregated from all other forms, which constitute the *non-Hodgkin lymphomas (NHLs)*. As will be seen, Hodgkin lymphoma has distinctive pathologic features and is treated in a unique fashion. The other important group of lymphoid tumors is the *plasma cell neoplasms*. These most often arise in the bone marrow and only infrequently involve lymph nodes or the peripheral blood. Taken together, the diverse lymphoid neoplasms constitute a complex, clinically important group of cancers, with about 100,000 new cases being diagnosed each year in the United States.

The clinical presentation of the various lymphoid neoplasms is most often determined by the anatomic distribution of disease. Two thirds of NHLs and virtually all Hodgkin lymphomas present as enlarged nontender lymph nodes (often >2 cm).

The remaining one third of NHLs present with symptoms related to the involvement of extranodal sites (e.g., skin, stomach, or brain). The lymphocytic leukemias most often come to attention because of signs and symptoms related to the suppression of normal hematopoiesis by tumor cells in the bone marrow. Finally, the most common plasma cell neoplasm, multiple myeloma, causes bony destruction of the skeleton and often presents with pain due to pathologic fractures. However, it should also be kept in mind that *certain lymphoid tumors cause symptoms through the secretion of circulating factors*. Specific examples include the plasma cell tumors, in which much of the pathophysiology is related to the secretion of whole antibodies or Ig fragments; and Hodgkin lymphoma, which is often associated with fever related to the release of inflammatory cytokines.

Historically, few areas of pathology evoked as much controversy as the classification of lymphoid neoplasms, but this situation has improved greatly because of advances in the use of objective molecular diagnostic tools. The current World Health Organization (WHO) classification scheme (Table 13–4) uses morphologic, immunophenotypic, genotypic, and clinical fea-

---

TABLE 13–4   The WHO Classification of the Lymphoid Neoplasms

I. PRECURSOR B-CELL NEOPLASMS

B-cell acute lymphoblastic leukemia/lymphoma (B-ALL)

II. PERIPHERAL B-CELL NEOPLASMS

Chronic lymphocytic leukemia/small lymphocytic lymphoma
B-cell prolymphocytic leukemia
Lymphoplasmacytic lymphoma
Splenic and nodal marginal zone lymphomas
Extranodal marginal zone lymphoma
Mantle cell lymphoma
Follicular lymphoma
Marginal zone lymphoma
Hairy cell leukemia
Plasmacytoma/plasma cell myeloma
Diffuse large B-cell lymphoma
Burkitt lymphoma

III. PRECURSOR T-CELL NEOPLASMS

T-cell acute lymphoblastic leukemia/lymphoma (T-ALL)

IV. PERIPHERAL T-CELL AND NK-CELL NEOPLASMS

T-cell prolymphocytic leukemia
Large granular lymphocytic leukemia
Mycosis fungoides/Sézary syndrome
Peripheral T-cell lymphoma, unspecified
Anaplastic large-cell lymphoma
Angioimmunoblastic T-cell lymphoma
Enteropathy-associated T-cell lymphoma
Panniculitis-like T-cell lymphoma
Hepatosplenic γδ T-cell lymphoma
Adult T-cell leukemia/lymphoma
Extranodal NK/T-cell lymphoma
NK-cell leukemia

V. HODGKIN LYMPHOMA

Classical subtypes
   Nodular sclerosis
   Mixed cellularity
   Lymphocyte-rich
   Lymphocyte depletion
Lymphocyte predominance

NK, natural killer.

tures to sort the lymphoid neoplasms into five broad categories,[11] which are separated according to the cell of origin:

1. Precursor B-cell neoplasms (neoplasms of immature B cells)
2. Peripheral B-cell neoplasms (neoplasms of mature B cells)
3. Precursor T-cell neoplasms (neoplasms of immature T cells)
4. Peripheral T-cell and NK-cell neoplasms (neoplasms of mature T cells and NK cells)
5. Hodgkin lymphoma (neoplasms of Reed-Sternberg cells and variants)

Before we discuss the specific entities of the WHO classification, some important principles relevant to the lymphoid neoplasms should be emphasized.

○ Lymphoid neoplasia can be suspected from the clinical features, but *histologic examination of lymph nodes or other involved tissues is required for diagnosis.*

○ *In most lymphoid neoplasms, antigen receptor gene rearrangement precedes transformation; hence, all of the daughter cells derived from the malignant progenitor share the same antigen receptor gene configuration and sequence, and synthesize identical antigen receptor proteins* (either Igs or T-cell receptors). In contrast, normal immune responses comprise polyclonal populations of lymphocytes that express many different antigen receptors. Thus, analyses of antigen receptor genes and their protein products can be used to distinguish reactive (polyclonal) and malignant (monoclonal) lymphoid proliferations. In addition, each antigen receptor gene rearrangement produces a unique DNA sequence that constitutes a highly specific clonal marker, which can be used to detect small numbers of residual malignant lymphoid cells after therapy.[12,13]

○ *The vast majority (85% to 90%) of lymphoid neoplasms are of B-cell origin, with most of the remainder being T-cell tumors; only rarely are tumors of NK cell origin encountered.* Most lymphoid neoplasms resemble some recognizable stage of B- or T-cell differentiation (Fig. 13–5), a feature that is used in their classification. Markers recognized by

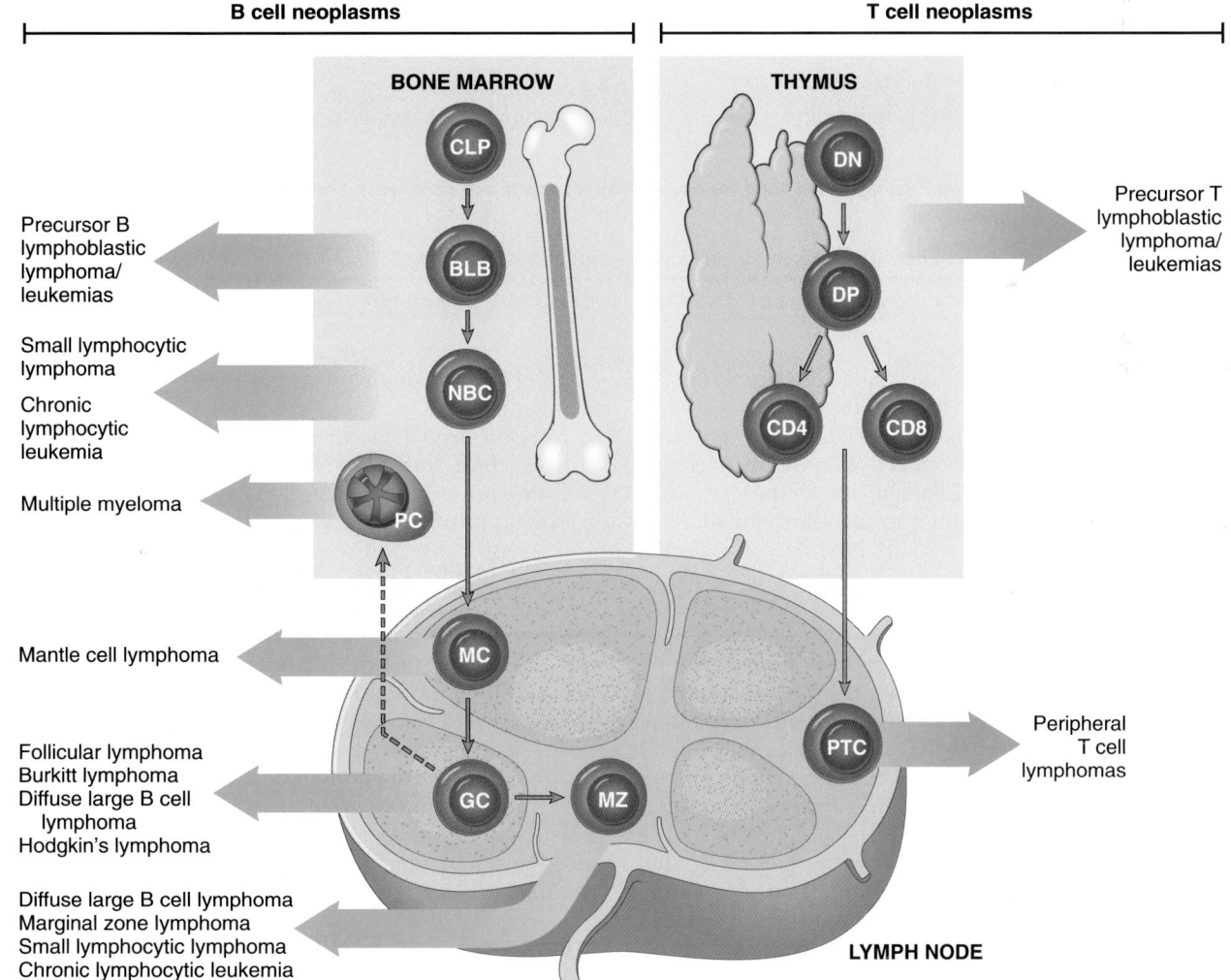

FIGURE 13–5 Origin of lymphoid neoplasms. Stages of B- and T-cell differentiation from which specific lymphoid tumors emerge are shown. CLP, common lymphoid precursor; BLB, pre-B lymphoblast; DN, CD4/CD8 double-negative pro-T cell; DP, CD4/CD8 double-positive pre-T cell; GC, germinal-center B cell; MC, mantle B cell; MZ, marginal zone B cell; NBC, naive B cell; PTC, peripheral T cell.

TABLE 13–5 Some Immune Cell Antigens Detected by Monoclonal Antibodies	
Antigen Designation	**Normal Cellular Distribution**
PRIMARILY T-CELL ASSOCIATED	
CD1	Thymocytes and Langerhans cells
CD3	Thymocytes, mature T cells
CD4	Helper T cells, subset of thymocytes
CD5	T cells and a small subset of B cells
CD8	Cytotoxic T cells, subset of thymocytes, and some NK cells
PRIMARILY B-CELL ASSOCIATED	
CD10	Pre-B cells and germinal-center B cells; also called CALLA
CD19	Pre-B cells and mature B cells but not plasma cells
CD20	Pre-B cells after CD19 and mature B cells but not plasma cells
CD21	EBV receptor; mature B cells and follicular dendritic cells
CD23	Activated mature B cells
CD79a	Marrow pre-B cells and mature B cells
PRIMARILY MONOCYTE- OR MACROPHAGE-ASSOCIATED	
CD11c	Granulocytes, monocytes, and macrophages; also expressed by hairy cell leukemias
CD13	Immature and mature monocytes and granulocytes
CD14	Monocytes
CD15	Granulocytes; Reed-Sternberg cells and variants
CD33	Myeloid progenitors and monocytes
CD64	Mature myeloid cells
PRIMARILY NK-CELL ASSOCIATED	
CD16	NK cells and granulocytes
CD56	NK cells and a subset of T cells
PRIMARILY STEM CELL– AND PROGENITOR CELL–ASSOCIATED	
CD34	Pluripotent hematopoietic stem cells and progenitor cells of many lineages
ACTIVATION MARKERS	
CD30	Activated B cells, T cells, and monocytes; Reed-Sternberg cells and variants
PRESENT ON ALL LEUKOCYTES	
CD45	All leukocytes; also known as leukocyte common antigen (LCA)

CALLA, common acute lymphoblastic leukemia antigen; CD, cluster designation; EBV, Epstein-Barr virus; NK, natural killer.

antibodies that are helpful in the characterization of lymphomas and leukemias are listed in Table 13–5.

○ *Lymphoid neoplasms are often associated with immune abnormalities.* Both a loss of protective immunity (susceptibility to infection) and a breakdown of tolerance (autoimmunity) can be seen, sometimes in the same patient. In a further ironic twist, individuals with inherited or acquired immunodeficiency are themselves at high risk of developing certain lymphoid neoplasms, particularly those caused by oncogenic viruses (e.g., EBV).

○ *Neoplastic B and T cells tend to recapitulate the behavior of their normal counterparts.* Like normal lymphocytes, neoplastic B and T cells home to certain tissue sites, leading to characteristic patterns of involvement. For example, follicular lymphomas home to germinal centers in lymph nodes, whereas cutaneous T-cell lymphomas home to the skin. Like their normal counterparts, particular adhesion molecules and chemokine receptors govern the homing of the neoplastic lymphoid cells. Variable numbers of neoplastic B and T lymphoid cells also recirculate through the lymphatics and peripheral blood to distant sites; as a result most lymphoid tumors are widely disseminated at the time of diagnosis. Notable exceptions to this rule include Hodgkin lymphomas, which are sometimes restricted to one group of lymph nodes, and marginal zone B-cell lymphomas, which are often restricted to sites of chronic inflammation.

○ *Hodgkin lymphoma spreads in an orderly fashion.* In contrast, most forms of NHL spread widely early in their course in a less predictable fashion. Hence, while lymphoma staging provides generally useful prognostic information, it is of most utility in guiding therapy in Hodgkin lymphoma.

We now turn to the specific entities of the WHO classification. We will begin with neoplasms of immature lymphoid cells and then move on to neoplasms of B cells, plasma cells, T cells, and NK cells. Some of the most salient molecular and clinical features of the group of neoplasms, which includes the lymphoid leukemias, non-Hodgkin lymphomas, and plasma cell tumors, are summarized in Table 13–6. We will then finish with a discussion of Hodgkin lymphoma. Throughout, the most common (and thus most important) entities will be emphasized.

Precursor B- and T-Cell Neoplasms

Acute Lymphoblastic Leukemia/Lymphoma

Acute lymphoblastic leukemia/lymphomas (ALLs) are neoplasms composed of immature B (pre-B) or T (pre-T)

TABLE 13–6   Summary of Major Types of Lymphoid Leukemias and Non-Hodgkin Lymphomas

Diagnosis	Cell of Origin	Genotype	Salient Clinical Features
NEOPLASMS OF IMMATURE B AND T CELLS			
B-cell acute lymphoblastic leukemia/lymphoma	Bone marrow precursor B cell	Diverse chromosomal translocations; t(12;21) involving *CBFα* and *ETV6* present in 25%	Predominantly children; symptoms relating to marrow replacement and pancytopenia; aggressive
T-cell acute lymphoblastic leukemia/lymphoma	Precursor T cell (often of thymic origin)	Diverse chromosomal translocations, *NOTCH1* mutations (50% to 70%)	Predominantly adolescent males; thymic masses and variable bone marrow involvement; aggressive
NEOPLASMS OF MATURE B CELLS			
Burkitt lymphoma	Germinal-center B cell	Translocations involving c-*MYC* and Ig loci, usually t(8;14); subset EBV-associated	Adolescents or young adults with extranodal masses; uncommonly presents as "leukemia"; aggressive
Diffuse large B-cell lymphoma	Germinal-center or post–germinal-center B cell	Diverse chromosomal rearrangements, most often of *BCL6* (30%), *BCL2* (10%), or c-*MYC* (5%)	All ages, but most common in adults; often appears as a rapidly growing mass; 30% extranodal; aggressive
Extranodal marginal zone lymphoma	Memory B cell	t(11;18), t(1;14), and t(14;18) creating *MALT1-IAP2*, *BCL10-IgH*, and *MALT1-IgH* fusion genes, respectively	Arises at extranodal sites in adults with chronic inflammatory diseases; may remain localized; indolent
Follicular lymphoma	Germinal-center B cell	t(14;18) creating *BCL2-IgH* fusion gene	Older adults with generalized lymphadenopathy and marrow involvement; indolent
Hairy cell leukemia	Memory B cell	No specific chromosomal abnormality	Older males with pancytopenia and splenomegaly; indolent
Mantle cell lymphoma	Naive B cell	t(11;14) creating *CyclinD1-IgH* fusion gene	Older males with disseminated disease; moderately aggressive
Multiple myeloma/solitary plasmacytoma	Post–germinal-center bone marrow homing plasma cell	Diverse rearrangements involving *IgH*; 13q deletions	Myeloma: older adults with lytic bone lesions, pathologic fractures, hypercalcemia, and renal failure; moderately aggressive Plasmacytoma: isolated plasma cell masses in bone or soft tissue; indolent
Small lymphocytic lymphoma/chronic lymphocytic leukemia	Naive B cell or memory B cell	Trisomy 12, deletions of 11q, 13q, and 17p	Older adults with bone marrow, lymph node, spleen, and liver disease; autoimmune hemolysis and thrombocytopenia in a minority; indolent
NEOPLASMS OF MATURE T CELLS OR NK CELLS			
Adult T-cell leukemia/lymphoma	Helper T cell	HTLV-1 provirus present in tumor cells	Adults with cutaneous lesions, marrow involvement, and hypercalcemia; occurs mainly in Japan, West Africa, and the Caribbean; aggressive
Peripheral T-cell lymphoma, unspecified	Helper or cytotoxic T cell	No specific chromosomal abnormality	Mainly older adults; usually presents with lymphadenopathy; aggressive
Anaplastic large-cell lymphoma	Cytotoxic T cell	Rearrangements of *ALK*	Children and young adults, usually with lymph node and soft-tissue disease; aggressive
Extranodal NK/T-cell lymphoma	NK-cell (common) or cytotoxic T cell (rare)	EBV-associated; no specific chromosomal abnormality	Adults with destructive extranodal masses, most commonly sinonasal; aggressive
Mycosis fungoides/Sézary syndrome	Helper T cell	No specific chromosomal abnormality	Adult patients with cutaneous patches, plaques, nodules, or generalized erythema; indolent
Large granular lymphocytic leukemia	Two types: cytotoxic T cell and NK cell	No specific chromosomal abnormality	Adult patients with splenomegaly, neutropenia, and anemia, sometimes accompanied by autoimmune disease

EBV, Epstein-Barr virus; HIV, human immunodeficiency virus; Ig, immunoglobulin; NK, natural killer.

cells, which are referred to as lymphoblasts. *About 85% are B-ALLs, which typically manifest as childhood acute "leukemias."* The less common *T-ALLs tend to present in adolescent males as thymic "lymphomas."* There is, however, considerable overlap in the clinical behavior of B- and T-ALL; for example, B-ALL uncommonly presents as a mass in the skin or a bone, and many T-ALLs present with or evolve to a leukemic picture. Because of their morphologic and clinical similarities, the various forms of ALL will be considered here together.

ALL is the most common cancer of children. Approximately 2500 new cases are diagnosed each year in the United States, most occurring in individuals under 15 years of age. ALL is almost three times as common in whites as in blacks, and slightly more frequent in boys than in girls. Hispanics have the highest incidence of any ethnic group. B-ALL peaks in incidence at about the age of 3, perhaps because the number of normal bone marrow pre-B cells (the cell of origin) is greatest very early in life. Similarly the peak incidence of T-ALL is in adolescence, the age when the thymus reaches its maximal size. B- and T-ALL also occur less frequently in adults of all ages.

> **Morphology.** In leukemic presentations, the marrow is hypercellular and packed with lymphoblasts, which replace the normal marrow elements. Mediastinal thymic masses occur in 50% to 70% of T-ALLs, which are also more likely to be associated with lymphadenopathy and splenomegaly. In both B- and T-ALL, the tumor cells have scant basophilic cytoplasm and nuclei somewhat larger than those of small lymphocytes (Fig. 13–6A). The nuclear chromatin is delicate and finely stippled, and nucleoli are either absent or inconspicuous. In many cases the nuclear membrane is deeply subdivided, imparting a convoluted appearance. In keeping with the aggressive clinical behavior, the mitotic rate is high. As with other rapidly growing lymphoid tumors, interspersed macrophages ingesting apoptotic tumor cells may impart a "starry sky" appearance (shown in Fig. 13–15).
>
> Because of differing responses to chemotherapy, ALL must be distinguished from acute myeloid leukemia (AML), a neoplasm of immature myeloid cells that can cause identical signs and symptoms. Compared with myeloblasts, lymphoblasts have more condensed chromatin, less conspicuous nucleoli, and smaller amounts of cytoplasm that usually lacks granules. However, these morphologic distinctions are not absolute and definitive diagnosis relies on stains performed with antibodies specific for B- and T-cell antigens (Fig. 13–6B and C). Histochemical stains are also helpful, in that (in contrast to myeloblasts) lymphoblasts are myeloperoxidase-negative and often contain periodic acid–Schiff-positive cytoplasmic material.

Immunophenotype. Immunostaining for terminal deoxynucleotidyl-transferase (TdT), a specialized DNA polymerase that is expressed only in pre-B and pre-T lymphoblasts, is positive in more than 95% of cases (Fig. 13–6B). B- and T-

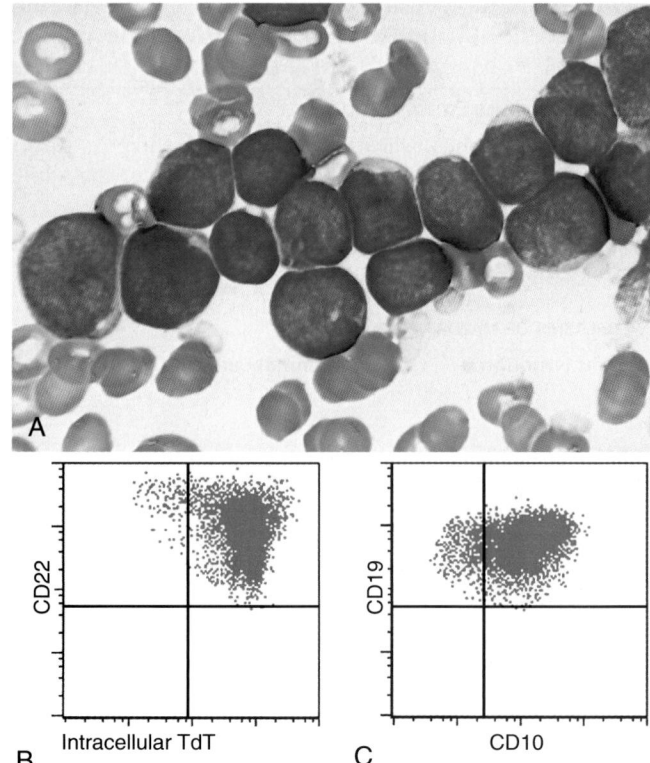

FIGURE 13–6   A, Acute lymphoblastic leukemia/lymphoma. Lymphoblasts with condensed nuclear chromatin, small nucleoli, and scant agranular cytoplasm. **B** and **C** represent the phenotype of the ALL shown in **A**, analyzed by flow cytometry. **B,** Note that the lymphoblasts represented by the red dots express terminal deoxynucleotidyl-transferase (TdT) and the B-cell marker CD22. **C,** The same cells are positive for two other markers, CD10 and CD19, commonly expressed on pre-B lymphoblasts. Thus, this is a B-ALL. (**A,** Courtesy of Dr. Robert W. McKenna; Department of Pathology, University of Texas Southwestern Medical School, Dallas, TX; **B** and **C,** courtesy of Dr. Louis Picker, Oregon Health Science Center, Portland, OR.)

ALLs are distinguished with stains for B- and T-cell–specific markers (summarized below).

B-ALLs are arrested at various stages of pre-B cell development. The lymphoblasts usually express the pan B-cell marker CD19 and the transcription factor PAX5, as well as CD10. In very immature B-ALLs, CD10 is negative. Alternatively, more mature "late pre-B" ALLs express CD10, CD19, CD20, and cytoplasmic IgM heavy chain (μ chain).

Similarly, T-ALLs are arrested at various stages of pre-T cell development. In most cases the cells are positive for CD1, CD2, CD5, and CD7. The more immature tumors are usually negative for surface CD3, CD4, and CD8, whereas "late" pre-T cell tumors are positive for these markers.

Molecular Pathogenesis. *Approximately 90% of ALLs have numerical or structural chromosomal changes.* Most common is hyperploidy (>50 chromosomes), but hypoploidy and a variety of balanced chromosomal translocations are also seen. These alterations frequently correlate with immunophenotype and sometimes prognosis. For example, hyperdiploidy and hypodiploidy are seen only in B-ALL. In addition, B- and T-ALL are associated with completely different sets of translocations, indicating that they are pathogenetically distinct.

RNA profiling using "gene chips" has also shown that certain chromosomal translocations correlate with unique patterns of gene expression.

Many of the chromosomal aberrations seen in ALL dysregulate the expression and function of transcription factors that are required for normal B- and T-cell development. Up to 70% of T-ALLs have gain-of-function mutations in *NOTCH1*, a gene that is essential for T-cell development.[14] On the other hand, a high fraction of B-ALLs have loss-of-function mutations in genes that are required for B-cell development, such as *PAX5*, *E2A*, and *EBF*,[15] or a balanced t(12;21) involving the genes *TEL* and *AML1*, two genes that are needed in very early hematopoietic precursors. All of these varied mutations seem to disturb the differentiation of lymphoid precursors and promote maturation arrest. As we will see, similar themes are relevant in the genesis of AML.

In keeping with the multistep origin of cancer (Chapter 7), *single mutations are not sufficient to produce ALL.* This conclusion stems in part from studies of identical twins with concordant B-ALL.[16] In these rare cases, the ALLs in both twins share a common chromosomal aberration and are derived from a single clone transmitted from one twin to the other by transfusion in utero. Despite the presence of the leukemogenic aberration at birth, ALL most often makes its clinical appearance in such patients between 4 and 12 years of age. This lengthy prodrome is most consistent with the existence of a "pre-leukemic" clone that must acquire additional mutations before ALL can develop. The identity of these complementary mutations is incomplete, but aberrations that increase growth and survival, such as activating mutations in tyrosine kinases, are commonly present.

Clinical Features. It should be emphasized that although ALL and AML are genetically and immunophenotypically distinct, they are clinically very similar. In both, the accumulation of neoplastic "blasts" in the bone marrow suppresses normal hematopoiesis by physical crowding, competition for growth factors, and other poorly understood mechanisms. The common features and those more characteristic of ALL are the following:

- *Abrupt stormy onset* within days to a few weeks of the first symptoms
- *Symptoms related to depression of marrow function*, including fatigue due to anemia; fever, reflecting infections secondary to neutropenia; and bleeding due to thrombocytopenia
- *Mass effects caused by neoplastic infiltration* (which are more common in ALL), including bone pain resulting from marrow expansion and infiltration of the subperiosteum; generalized lymphadenopathy, splenomegaly, and hepatomegaly; testicular enlargement; and in T-ALL, complications related to compression of large vessels and airways in the mediastinum
- *Central nervous system manifestations* such as headache, vomiting, and nerve palsies resulting from meningeal spread, all of which are also more common in ALL

Prognosis. Pediatric ALL is one of the great success stories of oncology. With aggressive chemotherapy about 95% of children with ALL obtain a complete remission, and 75% to 85% are cured. Despite these achievements, however, ALL

remains the leading cause of cancer deaths in children, and only 35% to 40% of adults are cured. *Several factors have been consistently associated with a worse prognosis: (1) age under 2,* largely because of the strong association of infantile ALL with translocations involving the *MLL* gene; *(2) presentation in adolescence or adulthood; (3) peripheral blood blast counts greater than 100,000,* which probably reflects a high tumor burden; and *(4) the presence of particular cytogenetic aberrations such as the t(9;22) (the Philadelphia chromosome).*[17] The t(9;22) is present in only 3% of childhood ALL, but up to 25% of adult cases, which partially explains the poor outcome in adults. Favorable prognostic markers include (1) an age of 2 to 10 years, (2) a low white cell count, (3) hyperploidy, (4) trisomy of chromosomes 4, 7, and 10, and (5) the presence of a t(12;21).[17] Notably, the molecular detection of residual disease after therapy is predictive of a worse outcome in both B- and T-ALL and is being used to guide new clinical trials.[12]

Although most chromosomal aberrations in ALL alter the function of transcription factors, the t(9;22) instead creates a fusion gene that encodes a constitutively active BCR-ABL tyrosine kinase (described in more detail under chronic myeloid leukemia). In B-ALL, the BCR-ABL protein is usually 190 kDa in size and has stronger tyrosine kinase activity than the form of BCR-ABL that is found in chronic myeloid leukemia, in which a BCR-ABL protein of 210 kDa in size is usually seen. Treatment of t(9;22)-positive ALLs with BCR-ABL kinase inhibitors leads to clinical responses, but patients relapse quickly because of acquired mutations in BCR-ABL that render the tumor cells drug-resistant.[18] BCR-ABL-positive B-ALL generates mutations at a high rate, a phenomenon referred to as genomic instability that contributes to the clinical progression and therapeutic resistance of many aggressive malignant tumors.

Peripheral B-Cell Neoplasms

Chronic Lymphocytic Leukemia (CLL)/Small Lymphocytic Lymphoma (SLL)

These two disorders differ only in the degree of peripheral blood lymphocytosis. Most affected patients have sufficient lymphocytosis to fulfill the diagnostic requirement for CLL (absolute lymphocyte count >4000 per mm³). CLL is the most common leukemia of adults in the Western world. There are about 15,000 new cases of CLL each year in the United States. The median age at diagnosis is 60 years, and there is a 2:1 male predominance. In contrast, SLL constitutes only 4% of NHLs. CLL/SLL is much less common in Japan and other Asian countries than in the West.

Morphology. Lymph nodes are diffusely effaced by an infiltrate of predominantly small lymphocytes 6 to 12 μm in diameter with round to slightly irregular nuclei, condensed chromatin, and scant cytoplasm (Fig. 13–7). Admixed are variable numbers of larger activated lymphocytes that often gather in loose aggregates referred to as **proliferation centers**, which contain mitotically active cells. When present, **proliferation centers are pathognomonic for CLL/ SLL**. The blood contains large numbers of small

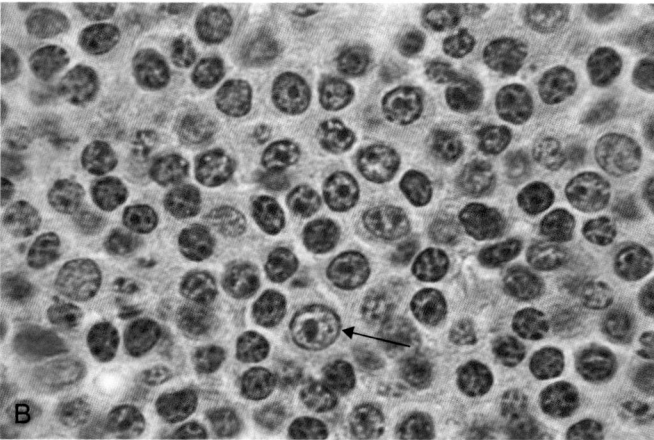

FIGURE 13–7 Small lymphocytic lymphoma/chronic lymphocytic leukemia (lymph node). **A,** Low-power view shows diffuse efface-ment of nodal architecture. **B,** At high power the majority of the tumor cells are small round lymphocytes. A "prolymphocyte," a larger cell with a centrally placed nucleolus, is also present in this field *(arrow)*. (**A,** Courtesy of Dr. José Hernandez, Department of Pathology, University of Texas Southwestern Medical School, Dallas, TX.)

round lymphocytes with scant cytoplasm (Fig. 13–8). Some of these cells are usually disrupted in the process of making smears, producing so-called **smudge cells.** The bone marrow is almost always involved by interstitial infiltrates or aggregates of tumor cells. Infiltrates are also virtually always seen in the splenic white and red pulp and the hepatic portal tracts (Fig. 13–9).

Immunophenotype. CLL/SLL has a distinctive immuno-phenotype. The tumor cells express the pan-B cell markers CD19 and CD20, as well as CD23 and CD5, the latter a marker that is found on a small subset of normal B cells. Low-level

expression of surface Ig (usually IgM or IgM and IgD) is also typical.

Molecular Pathogenesis. Unlike most other lymphoid malignancies, chromosomal translocations are rare in CLL/SLL. The most common findings are deletions of 13q14.3, 11q, and 17p, and trisomy 12q. Molecular character-ization of the region deleted on chromosome 13 has impli-cated two microRNAs, miR-15a and miR-16-1, as possible tumor suppressor genes.[19] DNA sequencing has revealed that the Ig genes of some CLL/SLL are somatically hypermutated, whereas others are not, suggesting that the cell of origin may be either a postgerminal center memory B cell or a naive B cell. For unclear reasons, tumors with unmutated Ig segments (those putatively of naive B-cell origin) pursue a more aggres-sive course.[20]

The growth of CLL/SLL cells is largely confined to prolifera-tion centers, where tumor cells must receive critical cues from the microenvironment. Stromal cells in proliferation centers seem to express a variety of factors that stimulate the activity

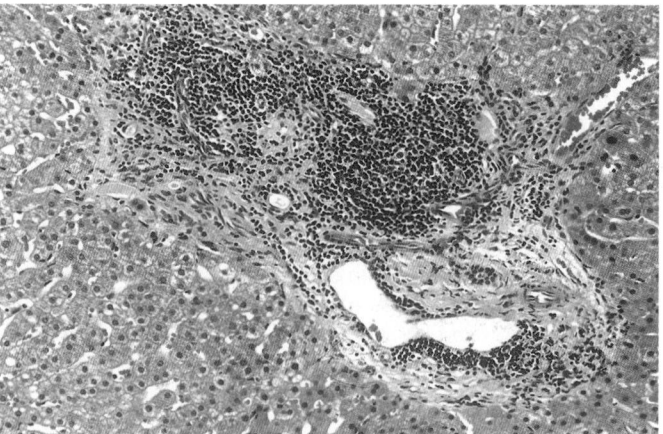

FIGURE 13–9 Small lymphocytic lymphoma/chronic lympho-cytic leukemia involving the liver. Low-power view of a typical periportal lymphocytic infiltrate. (Courtesy of Dr. Mark Fleming, Department of Pathology, Children's Hospital, Boston, MA.)

FIGURE 13–8 Chronic lymphocytic leukemia. This peripheral blood smear is flooded with small lymphocytes with condensed chromatin and scant cytoplasm. A characteristic finding is the pres-ence of disrupted tumor cells (smudge cells). A coexistent autoim-mune hemolytic anemia (Chapter 14) explains the presence of spherocytes (hyperchromatic, round erythrocytes). A nucleated erythroid cell is present in the lower left-hand corner of the field. In this setting, circulating nucleated red cells could stem from prema-ture release of progenitors in the face of severe anemia, marrow infiltration by tumor (leukoerythroblastosis), or both.

of the transcription factor NF-κB,[21] which promotes cell growth and survival.

Clinical Features. Patients are often asymptomatic at diagnosis. When symptoms appear, they are nonspecific and include easy fatigability, weight loss, and anorexia. Generalized lymphadenopathy and hepatosplenomegaly are present in 50% to 60% of symptomatic patients. The leukocyte count is highly variable; leukopenia can be seen in individuals with SLL and marrow involvement, while counts in excess of 200,000 per mm³ are sometimes seen in CLL patients with heavy tumor burdens. At the other end of the spectrum are asymptomatic patients that have in their peripheral blood monoclonal CD5+ B cells in numbers that are too few to merit the diagnosis of CLL. These abnormal B cells often have some of the same chromosomal aberrations that are seen in CLL, such as 13q deletions and trisomy 12, yet only about 1% of such patients progress to symptomatic CLL per year, presumably due to acquisition of additional genetic lesions that have yet to be identified. A small monoclonal Ig "spike" is present in the blood of some patients.

CLL/SLL disrupts normal immune function through uncertain mechanisms. Hypogammaglobulinemia is common and contributes to an increased susceptibility to infections, particularly those caused by bacteria. Conversely, 10% to 15% of patients develop hemolytic anemia or thrombocytopenia due to autoantibodies made by non-neoplastic B cells.

The course and prognosis are extremely variable and depend primarily on the clinical stage. Overall median survival is 4 to 6 years, but over 10 years in individuals with minimal tumor burdens at diagnosis. Other variables that correlate with a worse outcome include (1) the presence of deletions of 11q and 17p, (2) a lack of somatic hypermutation, and (3) the expression of ZAP-70, a protein that augments signals produced by the Ig receptor.[19] Patients are generally treated with "gentle" chemotherapy to control symptoms. Immunotherapy with antibodies against proteins found on the surface of CLL/SLL cells, such as CD20 and CD52, is finding increasing use.[22] Bone marrow transplantation is being offered to the relatively young.

An additional factor in patient survival is the tendency of CLL/SLL to transform to more aggressive tumors. Most commonly this takes the form of a prolymphocytic transformation (15% to 30% of patients) or a transformation to diffuse large B-cell lymphoma, so-called *Richter syndrome* (~5% to 10% of patients). Prolymphocytic transformation is marked by worsening cytopenias, increasing splenomegaly, and the appearance of increased numbers of "prolymphocytes" (large cells with a single prominent, centrally placed nucleolus) in the peripheral blood. Transformation to diffuse large B-cell lymphoma is often heralded by the development of a rapidly enlarging mass within a lymph node or the spleen. These transformations probably stem from the acquisition of additional, still unknown mutations that increase growth. Both prolymphocytic and large-cell transformation are ominous events, with most patients surviving less than 1 year.[23]

Follicular Lymphoma

Follicular lymphoma is the most common form of indolent NHL in the United States, affecting 15,000 to 20,000 individuals per year. It usually presents in middle age and afflicts males

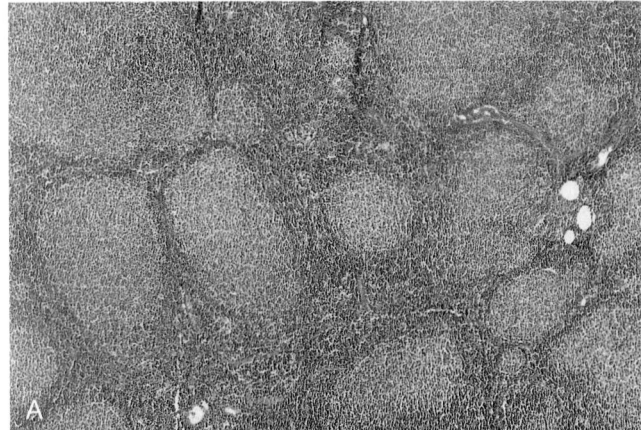
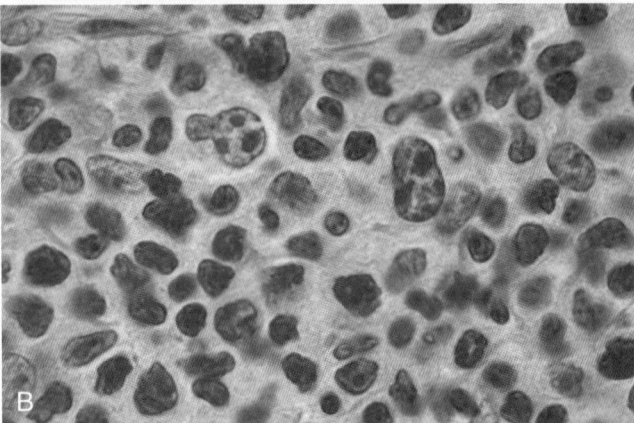

FIGURE 13–10   Follicular lymphoma (lymph node). **A,** Nodular aggregates of lymphoma cells are present throughout lymph node. **B,** At high magnification, small lymphoid cells with condensed chromatin and irregular or cleaved nuclear outlines (centrocytes) are mixed with a population of larger cells with nucleoli (centroblasts). (**A,** Courtesy of Dr. Robert W. McKenna, Department of Pathology, University of Texas Southwestern Medical School, Dallas, TX.)

and females equally. It is less common in Europe and rare in Asian populations. *The tumor likely arises from germinal center B cells and is strongly associated with chromosomal translocations involving BCL2.*

Morphology. In most cases, at low magnification, a predominantly nodular or nodular and diffuse growth pattern is observed in involved lymph nodes (Fig. 13–10A). **Two principal cell types are present in varying proportions: (1) small cells with irregular or cleaved nuclear contours and scant cytoplasm, referred to as centrocytes (small cleaved cells); and (2) larger cells with open nuclear chromatin, several nucleoli, and modest amounts of cytoplasm, referred to as centroblasts (Fig. 13–10B). In most follicular lymphomas, small cleaved cells are in the majority.** Peripheral blood involvement sufficient to produce lymphocytosis (usually under 20,000 cells per mm³) is seen in about 10% of cases. Bone marrow involvement occurs in 85% of cases and characteristically takes the form of paratrabecular lymphoid aggre-

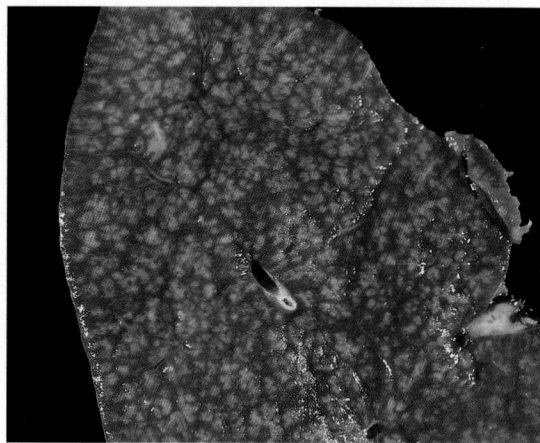

FIGURE 13–11 Follicular lymphoma (spleen). Prominent nodules represent white pulp follicles expanded by follicular lymphoma cells. Other indolent B-cell lymphomas (small lymphocytic lymphoma, mantle cell lymphoma, marginal zone lymphoma) can produce an identical pattern of involvement. (Courtesy of Dr. Jeffrey Jorgenson, Department of Hematopathology, M.D. Anderson Cancer Center, Houston, TX.)

gates. The splenic white pulp (Fig. 13–11) and hepatic portal triads are also frequently involved.

Immunophenotype. The neoplastic cells closely resemble normal germinal center B cells, expressing CD19, CD20, CD10, surface Ig, and BCL6. Unlike CLL/SLL and mantle cell lymphoma, CD5 is not expressed. BCL2 is expressed in more than 90% of cases, in distinction to normal follicular center B cells, which are BCL2-negative (Fig. 13–12).

Molecular Pathogenesis. *The hallmark of follicular lymphoma is a (14;18) translocation that juxtaposes the IgH locus on chromosome 14 and the BCL2 locus on chromosome 18.* The t(14;18) is seen in up to 90% of follicular lymphomas, and leads to overexpression of BCL2 (see Fig. 13–12). BCL2 antagonizes apoptosis (Chapter 7) and promotes the survival of follicular lymphoma cells. Notably, while normal germinal centers contain numerous B cells undergoing apoptosis, follicular lymphoma is characteristically devoid of apoptotic cells.

Particularly early in the disease, follicular lymphoma cells growing in lymph nodes are found within a network of reactive follicular dendritic cells admixed with macrophages and T cells. Expression profiling studies have shown that differences in the genes expressed by these reactive cells are predictive of outcome, implying that the response of follicular lymphoma cells to therapy is somehow influenced by the surrounding microenvironment.[24,25]

Clinical Features. Follicular lymphoma tends to present with painless, generalized lymphadenopathy. Involvement of extranodal sites, such as the gastrointestinal tract, central nervous system, or testis, is relatively uncommon. Although incurable, it usually follows an indolent waxing and waning course. Survival (median, 7–9 years) is not improved by aggressive therapy; hence, the usual approach is to palliate patients with low-dose chemotherapy or immunotherapy (such as anti-CD20 antibody) when they become symptomatic.

Histologic transformation occurs in 30% to 50% of follicular lymphomas, most commonly to diffuse large B-cell lymphoma. Less commonly, tumors resembling Burkitt lymphoma emerge that are associated with chromosomal translocations involving *c-MYC*. Like normal germinal center B cells, follicular lymphomas have ongoing somatic hypermutation, which may promote transformation by causing point mutations or chromosomal aberrations. The median survival is less than 1 year after transformation.

Diffuse Large B-Cell Lymphoma

Diffuse large B-cell lymphoma (DLBCL) is the most common form of NHL. Each year in the United States there are about 25,000 new cases. There is a slight male predominance. The median patient age is about 60 years, but DLBCL also occurs in young adults and children.

Morphology. The common features are a relatively large cell size (usually four to five times the diameter of a small lymphocyte) and a diffuse pattern of growth (Fig. 13–13). In other respects, substantial morphologic variation is seen. Most commonly, the tumor cells have a round or oval nucleus that appears vesicular due to margination of chromatin to the nuclear membrane, but large multilobated or cleaved nuclei are prominent in some cases. Nucleoli may be two to three in number and located adjacent to the nuclear membrane, or single and centrally placed. The cytoplasm is usually moderately abundant and may be pale or basophilic. More anaplastic tumors may even contain multinucleated cells with large inclusion-like nucleoli that resemble Reed-Sternberg cells (the malignant cell of Hodgkin lymphoma).

Immunophenotype. These mature B-cell tumors express CD19 and CD20 and show variable expression of germinal

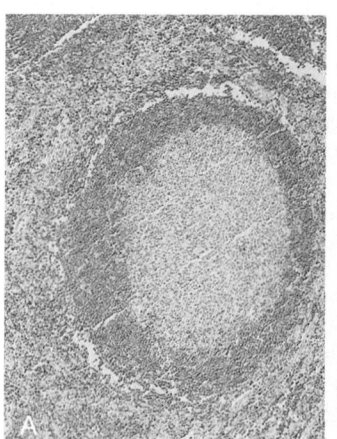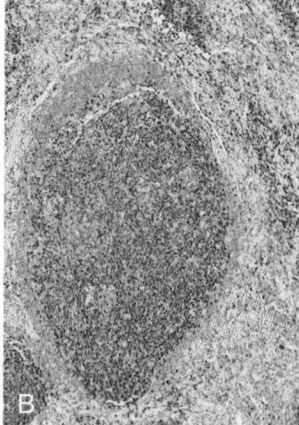

FIGURE 13–12 BCL2 expression in reactive and neoplastic follicles. BCL2 protein was detected by using an immunohistochemical technique that produces a brown stain. In reactive follicles (**A**), BCL2 is present in mantle zone cells but not follicular-center B cells, whereas follicular lymphoma cells (**B**) show strong BCL2 staining. (Courtesy of Dr. Jeffrey Jorgenson, Department of Hematopathology, M.D. Anderson Cancer Center, Houston, TX.)

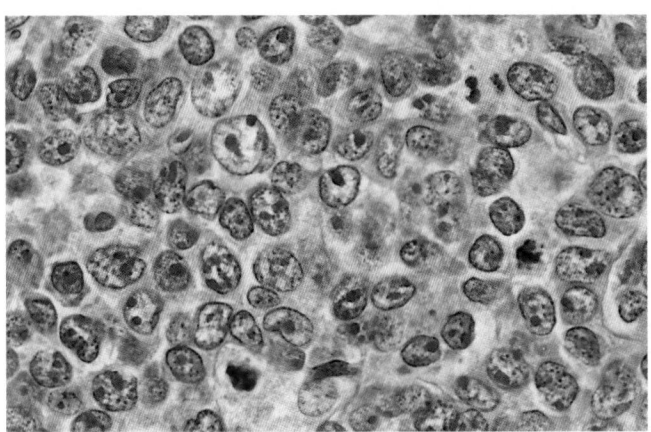

FIGURE 13–13 Diffuse large B-cell lymphoma. Tumor cells have large nuclei, open chromatin, and prominent nucleoli. (Courtesy of Dr. Robert W. McKenna, Department of Pathology, University of Texas Southwestern Medical School, Dallas, TX.)

center B-cell markers such as CD10 and BCL6. Most have surface Ig.

Molecular Pathogenesis. Cytogenetic, gene expression profiling, and immunohistochemical studies indicate that DLBCL is heterogeneous.[26,27] One frequent pathogenic event is dysregulation of BCL6, a DNA-binding zinc-finger transcriptional repressor that is required for the formation of normal germinal centers. About 30% of DLBCLs contain various translocations that have in common a breakpoint in *BCL6* at chromosome 3q27. Acquired mutations in *BCL6* promoter sequences that abrogate *BCL6* autoregulation (an important negative-regulatory mechanism) are seen even more frequently. It is hypothesized that both types of lesions are inadvertent byproducts of somatic hypermutation that result in overexpression of *BCL6*, which has several important consequences. BCL6 represses the expression of factors that promote germinal center B-cell differentiation and growth arrest, and thereby holds cells in a relatively undifferentiated, proliferative state.[28,29] BCL6 can also silence the expression of p53, the "guardian of the genome" (Chapter 7).[30] This "anti-p53" activity may serve to prevent the activation of DNA repair mechanisms in germinal center B cells undergoing somatic hypermutation and class switch recombination. Each of these activities is believed to contribute to the development of DLBCL. Mutations similar to those found in *BCL6* are also seen in multiple other oncogenes, including *c-MYC*,[10] suggesting that somatic hypermutation in DLBCL cells is "mistargeted" to a wide variety of loci.

Another 10% to 20% of tumors are associated with the t(14;18), which (as discussed under follicular lymphoma) leads to the overexpression of the anti-apoptotic protein BCL2. Tumors with *BCL2* rearrangements almost always lack *BCL6* rearrangements, suggesting that these rearrangements define two distinct molecular classes of DLBCL. Some tumors with *BCL2* rearrangements may arise from unrecognized underlying follicular lymphomas, which (as discussed already) frequently transform to DLBCL.

Special Subtypes Associated with Oncogenic Herpesviruses. Several other subtypes of DLBCL are sufficiently distinctive to merit brief discussion.

- *Immunodeficiency-associated large B-cell lymphoma* occurs in the setting of severe T-cell immunodeficiency (e.g., advanced HIV infection and allogeneic bone marrow transplantation). *The neoplastic B cells are usually infected with EBV, which plays a critical pathogenic role.* Restoration of T-cell immunity may lead to regression of these proliferations.
- *Primary effusion lymphoma* presents as a malignant pleural or ascitic effusion, mostly in patients with advanced HIV infection or the elderly. The tumor cells are often anaplastic in appearance and typically fail to express surface B- or T-cell markers, but have clonal IgH gene rearrangements. *In all cases the tumor cells are infected with KSHV/HHV-8, which appears to have a causal role.*

Clinical Features. *DLBCL typically presents as a rapidly enlarging mass at a nodal or extranodal site.* It can arise virtually anywhere in the body. Waldeyer ring, the oropharyngeal lymphoid tissue that includes the tonsils and adenoids, is involved commonly. Primary or secondary involvement of the liver and spleen may take the form of large destructive masses (Fig. 13–14). Extranodal sites include the gastrointestinal tract, skin, bone, brain, and other tissues. Bone marrow involvement is relatively uncommon and usually occurs late in the course. Rarely, a leukemic picture emerges.

DLBCLs are aggressive tumors that are rapidly fatal without treatment. With intensive combination chemotherapy, 60% to 80% of patients achieve a complete remission, and 40% to 50% are cured. Immunotherapy with anti-CD20 antibody seems to improve both the initial response and the overall outcome, particularly in the elderly. Individuals with limited disease fare better than those with widespread disease or bulky tumor masses. Expression profiling has identified distinct molecular subtypes with differing clinical outcomes and led to new targeted therapeutic approaches directed at components of the NF-κB and B cell receptor signaling pathways.[26,27]

Burkitt Lymphoma

Within this category fall (1) African (endemic) Burkitt lymphoma, (2) sporadic (nonendemic) Burkitt lymphoma, and

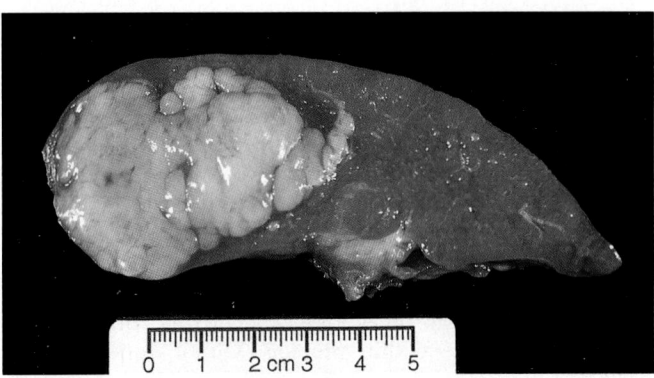

FIGURE 13–14 Diffuse large B-cell lymphoma involving the spleen. The isolated large mass is typical. In contrast, indolent B-cell lymphomas usually produce multifocal expansion of white pulp (see Fig. 13–11). (Courtesy of Dr. Mark Fleming, Department of Pathology, Children's Hospital, Boston, MA.)

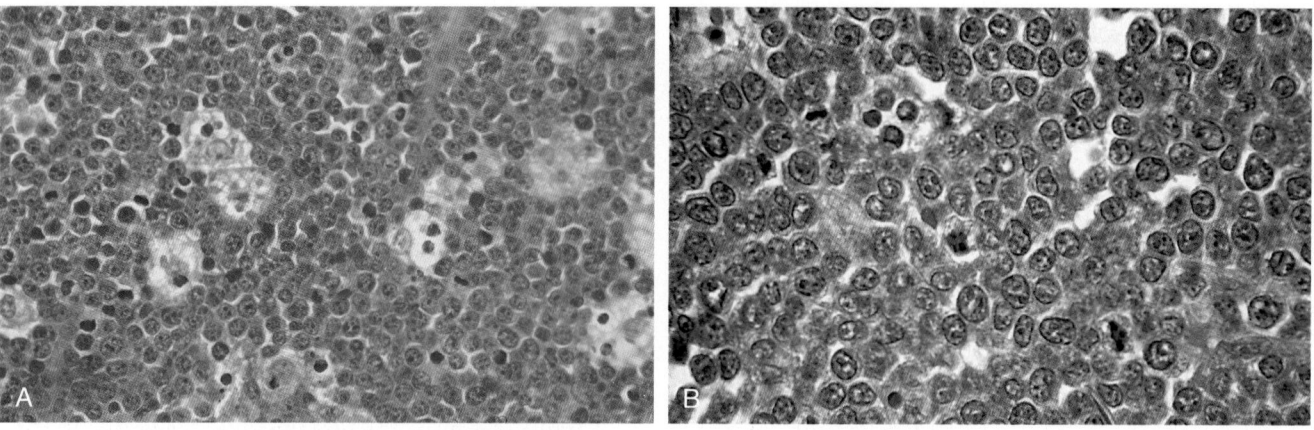

FIGURE 13–15 Burkitt lymphoma. **A,** At low power, numerous pale tingible body macrophages are evident, producing a "starry sky" appearance. **B,** At high power, tumor cells have multiple small nucleoli and high mitotic index. The lack of significant variation in nuclear shape and size lends a monotonous appearance. (**B,** Courtesy of Dr. José Hernandez, Department of Pathology, University of Texas Southwestern Medical School, Dallas, TX.)

(3) a subset of aggressive lymphomas occurring in individuals infected with HIV. Burkitt lymphomas occurring in each of these settings are histologically identical but differ in some clinical, genotypic, and virologic characteristics.

> **Morphology.** Involved tissues are effaced by a diffuse infiltrate of intermediate-sized lymphoid cells 10 to 25 μm in diameter with round or oval nuclei, coarse chromatin, several nucleoli, and a moderate amount of cytoplasm (Fig. 13–15). **The tumor exhibits a high mitotic index and contains numerous apoptotic cells**, the nuclear remnants of which are phagocytosed by interspersed benign macrophages. These phagocytes have abundant clear cytoplasm, creating a characteristic **"starry sky" pattern**. When the bone marrow is involved, aspirates reveal tumor cells with slightly clumped nuclear chromatin, two to five distinct nucleoli, and royal blue cytoplasm containing clear cytoplasmic vacuoles.

Immunophenotype. These are tumors of mature B cells that express surface IgM, CD19, CD20, CD10, and BCL6, a phenotype consistent with a germinal center B-cell origin. Unlike other tumors of germinal center origin, Burkitt lymphoma almost always fails to express the anti-apoptotic protein BCL2.

Molecular Pathogenesis. *All forms of Burkitt lymphoma are associated with translocations of the c-MYC gene on chromosome 8.* The translocation partner is usually the IgH locus [t(8;14)] but may also be the Ig κ [t(2;8)] or λ [t(8;22)] light-chain loci. The breakpoints in the IgH locus in sporadic Burkitt lymphoma are usually found in the class switch regions, whereas the breakpoints in endemic Burkitt lymphoma tend to lie within more 5′ V(D)J sequences. The basis for this subtle molecular distinction is not known, but both types of translocations can be induced in germinal center B cells by AID,[8,9] which you will recall is a specialized DNA-modifying enzyme that is required for both Ig class switching and somatic hypermutation. The net effect of these

translocations is similar; the *c-MYC* coding sequence is repositioned adjacent to strong Ig promoter and enhancer elements, which drive increased *c-MYC* expression. In addition, the translocated *c-MYC* allele often harbors point mutations that further increase its activity.[31] Burkitt lymphomas also commonly have mutations that inactivate p53, an event that increases the frequency of *c-MYC* translocations in germinal center B cells.[9] Hence, it is possible that pre-existent defects in p53 set the stage for the acquisition of *c-MYC* translocations.

Essentially all endemic tumors are latently infected with EBV, which is also present in about 25% of HIV-associated tumors and 15% to 20% of sporadic cases. The configuration of the EBV DNA is identical in all tumor cells within individual cases, indicating that infection precedes transformation. Although this places EBV at the "scene of the crime," its precise role in the genesis of Burkitt lymphoma remains poorly understood.

About 5% of DLBCLs have *c-MYC* translocations, and in such instances DLBCL may be difficult to distinguish from Burkitt lymphoma by conventional diagnostic tests. This distinction can be important, since DLBCL and Burkitt lymphoma are often treated with different chemotherapeutic regimens. Gene expression profiling may provide a more accurate assay for differentiating between these two tumors in difficult cases.[32]

Clinical Features. Both endemic and sporadic Burkitt lymphomas are found mainly in children or young adults; overall, it accounts for about 30% of childhood NHLs in the United States. *Most tumors manifest at extranodal sites.* Endemic Burkitt lymphoma often presents as a mass involving the mandible and shows an unusual predilection for involvement of abdominal viscera, particularly the kidneys, ovaries, and adrenal glands. In contrast, sporadic Burkitt lymphoma most often appears as a mass involving the ileocecum and peritoneum. Involvement of the bone marrow and peripheral blood is uncommon, especially in endemic cases. Burkitt lymphoma is very aggressive but responds well to intensive chemotherapy. Most children and young adults can be cured. The outcome is more guarded in older adults.

Plasma Cell Neoplasms and Related Disorders

These B-cell proliferations contain neoplastic plasma cells that virtually always secrete a monoclonal Ig or Ig fragment. Collectively, the plasma cell neoplasms (often referred to as dyscrasias) account for about 15% of the deaths caused by lymphoid neoplasms. The most common and deadly of these neoplasms is multiple myeloma, of which there are about 15,000 new cases per year in the United States.

A monoclonal Ig identified in the blood is referred to as an M component, in reference to myeloma. Since complete M components have molecular weights of 160,000 or higher, they are restricted to the plasma and extracellular fluid and excluded from the urine in the absence of glomerular damage. However, unlike normal plasma cells, in which the production and coupling of heavy and light chains are tightly balanced, *neoplastic plasma cells often synthesize excess light or heavy chains along with complete Igs.* Occasionally only light chains or heavy chains are produced. The free light chains are small enough to be excreted in the urine, where they are called *Bence-Jones proteins.* Free light chains can be detected and measured in the urine or the blood, the latter with new, highly sensitive tests that are in the process of being evaluated.

Terms used to describe the abnormal Igs include monoclonal gammopathy, dysproteinemia, and paraproteinemia. The following clinicopathologic entities are associated with monoclonal gammopathies.

○ *Multiple myeloma (plasma cell myeloma)*, the most important monoclonal gammopathy, usually presents as tumorous masses scattered throughout the skeletal system. *Solitary myeloma (plasmacytoma)* is an infrequent variant that presents as a single mass in bone or soft tissue. *Smoldering myeloma* refers to another uncommon variant defined by a lack of symptoms and a high plasma M component.
○ *Waldenström macroglobulinemia* is a syndrome in which high levels of IgM lead to symptoms related to hyperviscosity of the blood. It occurs in older adults, most commonly in association with lymphoplasmacytic lymphoma.
○ *Heavy-chain disease* is a rare monoclonal gammopathy that is seen in association with a diverse group of disorders, including lymphoplasmacytic lymphoma and an unusual small bowel marginal zone lymphoma that occurs in malnourished populations (so-called Mediterranean lymphoma). The common feature is the synthesis and secretion of free heavy-chain fragments.
○ *Primary or immunocyte-associated amyloidosis* results from a monoclonal proliferation of plasma cells secreting light chains (usually of λ isotype) that are deposited as amyloid. Some patients have overt multiple myeloma, but others have only a minor clonal population of plasma cells in the marrow.
○ *Monoclonal gammopathy of undetermined significance (MGUS)* is applied to patients without signs or symptoms who have small to moderately large M components in their blood. MGUS is very common in the elderly and has a low but constant rate of transformation to symptomatic monoclonal gammopathies, most often multiple myeloma.

With this background, we now turn to some of the specific clinicopathologic entities. Primary amyloidosis was discussed along with other disorders of the immune system in Chapter 6.

Multiple Myeloma. *Multiple myeloma is a plasma cell neoplasm characterized by multifocal involvement of the skeleton.* Although bony disease dominates, it can spread late in its course to lymph nodes and extranodal sites such as the skin. Multiple myeloma causes 1% of all cancer deaths in Western countries. Its incidence is higher in men and people of African descent. It is chiefly a disease of the elderly, with a peak age of incidence of 65 to 70 years.

Molecular Pathogenesis. The Ig genes in myeloma cells always show evidence of somatic hypermutation. On this basis, the cell of origin is considered to be a post-germinal center B cell that homes to the bone marrow and has differentiated into a plasma cell. Of interest, some studies suggest that the tumor originates in and is maintained by stem-like cells resembling small B lymphocytes that rely on signals generated by the "hedgehog" pathway for self-renewal.[33,34]

The proliferation and survival of myeloma cells are dependent on several cytokines, most notably IL-6. IL-6 is an important growth factor for plasma cells that is produced by the tumor cells themselves and resident marrow stromal cells. High serum levels of IL-6 are seen in patients with active disease and are associated with a poor prognosis. Myeloma cell growth and survival are also augmented by direct physical interactions with bone marrow stromal cells, which is a focus of new therapeutic approaches.[35]

Factors produced by neoplastic plasma cells mediate bone destruction, the major pathologic feature of multiple myeloma. Of particular importance, myeloma-derived MIP1α upregulates the expression of the receptor activator of NF-κB ligand (RANKL) by bone marrow stromal cells, which in turn activates osteoclasts.[36] Other factors released from tumor cells, such as modulators of the Wnt pathway, are potent inhibitors of osteoblast function. The net effect is a marked increase in bone resorption, which leads to hypercalcemia and pathologic fractures.[37]

Many myelomas have rearrangements involving the Ig heavy-chain gene on chromosome 14q32.[38,39] Common translocation partners include *FGFR3* (fibroblast growth factor receptor 3) on chromosome 4p16, a gene encoding a tyrosine kinase receptor implicated in the control of cellular proliferation; the cell cycle–regulatory genes cyclin D1 on chromosome 11q13 and cyclin D3 on chromosome 6p21; the gene for the transcription factor *c-MAF* on chromosome 16q23; and the gene encoding the transcription factor *MUM1/IRF4* on chromosome 6p25. As may be gathered from the involvement of two different D cyclin genes, dysregulation of D cyclins is a common feature.[38] The other most frequent karyotypic abnormalities are deletions of 13q. Consistent with the diversity of chromosomal aberrations, gene expression profiling studies suggest that myeloma is molecularly quite heterogeneous.[40]

Morphology. Multiple myeloma usually presents as destructive plasma cell tumors (plasmacytomas) involving the axial skeleton. The bones most commonly affected (in descending order of frequency) are the vertebral column, ribs, skull, pelvis, femur, clavicle, and scapula. Lesions begin in the medullary cavity, erode cancellous bone, and progressively

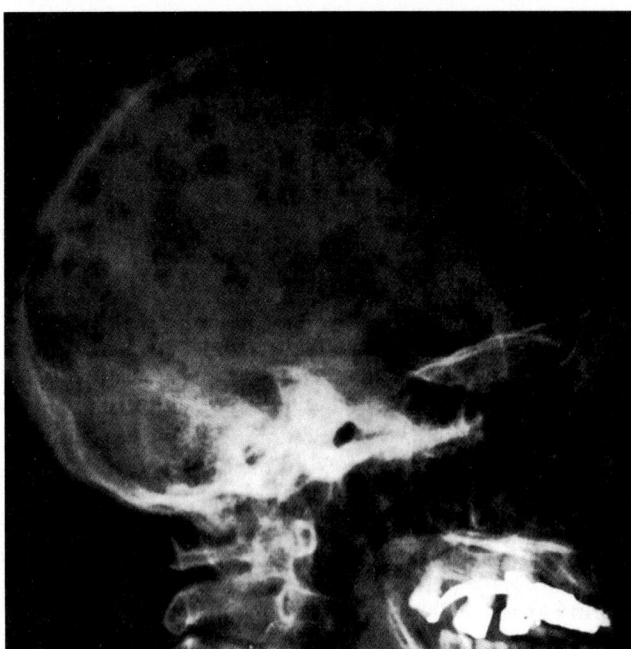

FIGURE 13–16 Multiple myeloma of the skull (radiograph, lateral view). The sharply punched-out bone lesions are most obvious in the calvarium.

destroy the bony cortex, often leading to pathologic fractures; these are most common in the vertebral column, but may occur in any affected bone. **The bone lesions appear radiographically as punched-out defects, usually 1 to 4 cm in diameter** (Fig. 13–16), and grossly consist of soft, gelatinous, red tumor masses. Less commonly, widespread myelomatous bone disease produces diffuse demineralization (osteopenia) rather than focal defects.

Even away from overt tumor masses, the marrow contains an increased number of plasma cells, which usually constitute more than 30% of the cellularity. The plasma cells may infiltrate the interstitium or be present in sheets that completely replace normal elements. Like their benign counterparts, malignant plasma cells have a perinuclear clearing due to a prominent Golgi apparatus and an eccentrically placed nucleus (Fig. 13–17). Relatively normal-appearing plasma cells, **plasmablasts** with vesicular nuclear chromatin and a prominent single nucleolus, or **bizarre, multinucleated cells** may predominate. Other cytologic variants stem from the dysregulated synthesis and secretion of Ig, which often leads to intracellular accumulation of intact or partially degraded protein. Such variants include **flame cells** with fiery red cytoplasm, **Mott cells** with multiple grapelike cytoplasmic droplets, and cells containing a variety of other inclusions, including **fibrils, crystalline rods, and globules**. The globular inclusions are referred to as **Russell bodies** (if cytoplasmic) or **Dutcher bodies** (if nuclear). In advanced disease, plasma cell infiltrates may be present in the spleen, liver, kidneys, lungs, lymph nodes, and other soft tissues.

Commonly, the high level of M proteins causes red cells in peripheral blood smears to stick to one another in linear arrays, a finding referred to as **rouleaux formation**. Rouleaux formation is characteristic but not specific, in that it may be seen in other conditions in which Ig levels are elevated, such as lupus erythematosus and early HIV infection. Rarely, tumor cells flood the peripheral blood, giving rise to **plasma cell leukemia**.

Bence Jones proteins are excreted in the kidney and contribute to a form of renal disease called **myeloma kidney**. This important complication is discussed in detail in Chapter 20.

Clinical Features. The clinical features of multiple myeloma stem from (1) the effects of plasma cell growth in tissues, particularly the bones; (2) the production of excessive Igs, which often have abnormal physicochemical properties; and (3) the suppression of normal humoral immunity.

Bone resorption often leads to pathologic fractures and chronic pain. The attendant *hypercalcemia* can give rise to neurologic manifestations, such as confusion, weakness, lethargy, constipation, and polyuria, and contributes to renal dysfunction. Decreased production of normal Igs sets the stage for *recurrent bacterial infections.* Cellular immunity is relatively unaffected. *Of great significance is renal insufficiency, which trails only infections as a cause of death.* The pathogenesis of renal failure (discussed in Chapter 20), which occurs in up to 50% of patients, is multifactorial. However, the single most important factor seems to be *Bence Jones proteinuria*, since the excreted light chains are toxic to renal tubular epithelial cells. Certain light chains (particularly those of the $\lambda 6$ and $\lambda 3$ families) are prone to cause *amyloidosis* of the AL type (Chapter 6), which can exacerbate renal dysfunction and deposit in other tissue as well.

In 99% of patients, laboratory analyses reveal increased levels of Igs in the blood and/or light chains (Bence Jones proteins) in the urine. The monoclonal Igs are usually first detected as

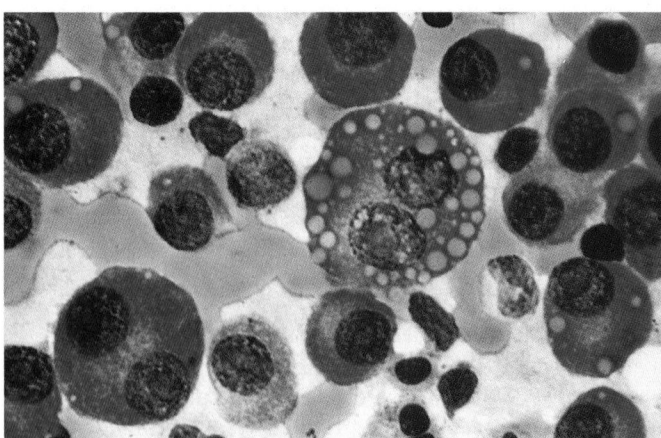

FIGURE 13–17 Multiple myeloma (bone marrow aspirate). Normal marrow cells are largely replaced by plasma cells, including forms with multiple nuclei, prominent nucleoli, and cytoplasmic droplets containing Ig.

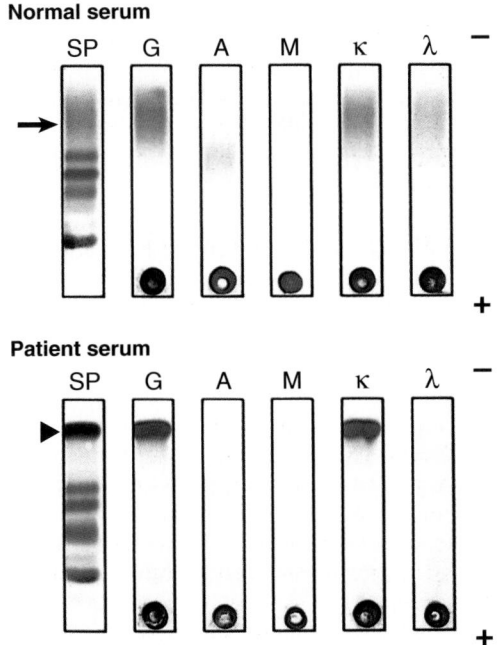

Normal serum

Patient serum

FIGURE 13–18 M protein detection in multiple myeloma. Serum protein electrophoresis (SP) is used to screen for a monoclonal immunoglobulin (M protein). Polyclonal IgG in normal serum (denoted by the *arrow*) appears as a broad band; in contrast, serum from a patient with multiple myeloma contains a single sharp protein band (denoted by the *arrowhead*) in this region of the electropherogram. The suspected monoclonal Ig is confirmed and characterized by immunofixation. In this procedure, proteins separated by electrophoresis within a gel are reacted with specific antisera. After extensive washing, proteins that are cross-linked by antisera are retained and detected with a protein stain. Note the sharp band in the patient serum is cross-linked by antisera specific for IgG heavy chain (G) and kappa light chain (κ), indicating the presence of an IgGκ M protein. Levels of polyclonal IgG, IgA (A), and lambda light chain (λ) are also decreased in the patient serum relative to normal, a finding typical of multiple myeloma. (Courtesy of Dr. David Sacks, Department of Pathology, Brigham and Women's Hospital, Boston, MA.)

abnormal protein "spikes" in serum or urine electrophoresis and then further characterized by immunofixation (Fig. 13–18). Most myelomas are associated with more than 3 gm/dL of serum Ig and/or more than 6 gm/dL of urine Bence Jones protein. The most common monoclonal Ig ("M protein") is IgG (~55% of patients), followed by IgA (~25% of cases). Myelomas expressing IgM, IgD, or IgE occur but are rare. Excessive production and aggregation of M proteins, usually of the IgA and or IgG$_3$ subtype, leads to symptoms related to hyperviscosity (described under lymphoplasmacytic lymphoma) in about 7% of patients. Both free light chains and a serum M protein are observed together in 60% to 70% of patients. However, in about 20% of patients only free light chains are present. Around 1% of myelomas are nonsecretory; hence, the absence of detectable M proteins does not completely exclude the diagnosis.

The clinicopathologic diagnosis of multiple myeloma rests on radiographic and laboratory findings. It can be strongly suspected when the distinctive radiographic changes are present, but definitive diagnosis requires a bone marrow examination. Marrow involvement often gives rise to a nor-

mocytic normochromic anemia, sometimes accompanied by moderate leukopenia and thrombocytopenia.

The prognosis is variable but generally poor. The median survival is 4 to 6 years, and cures have yet to be achieved. Patients with multiple bony lesions, if untreated, rarely survive for more than 6 to 12 months, whereas patients with "smoldering myeloma" may be asymptomatic for many years. Translocations involving cyclin D1 are associated with a good outcome, whereas deletions of 13q, deletions of 17p, and the t(4;14) all portend a more aggressive course.[41]

Cytotoxic agents induce remission in 50% to 70% of patients, and new therapeutic approaches are bringing hope. Myeloma cells are sensitive to inhibitors of the proteasome,[42] a cellular organelle that degrades unwanted and misfolded proteins. You will recall from Chapter 1 that misfolded proteins activate apoptotic pathways. Myeloma cells are prone to the accumulation of misfolded, unpaired Ig chains. Proteasome inhibitors may induce cell death by exacerbating this inherent tendency, and also seem to retard bone resorption through effects on stromal cells.[43] Thalidomide and related compounds also have activity against myeloma, apparently by altering interactions between myeloma cells and bone marrow stromal cells and by inhibiting angiogenesis.[35] Biphosphonates, drugs that inhibit bone resorption, reduce pathologic fractures and limit the hypercalcemia. Bone marrow transplantation prolongs life but has not yet proven to be curative.

Solitary Myeloma (Plasmacytoma). About 3% to 5% of plasma cell neoplasms present as a solitary lesion of bone or soft tissue. The bone lesions tend to occur in the same locations as in multiple myeloma. Extra-osseous lesions are often located in the lungs, oronasopharynx, or nasal sinuses. Modest elevations of M proteins in the blood or urine may be found in some patients. Solitary osseous plasmacytoma almost inevitably progresses to multiple myeloma, but this can take 10 to 20 years or longer. In contrast, extra-osseous plasmacytomas, particularly those involving the upper respiratory tract, are frequently cured by local resection.

Smoldering Myeloma. This entity defines a middle ground between multiple myeloma and monoclonal gammopathy of uncertain significance. Plasma cells make up 10% to 30% of the marrow cellularity, and the serum M protein level is greater than 3 gm/dL, but patients are asymptomatic. About 75% of patients progress to multiple myeloma over a 15-year period.[44]

Monoclonal Gammopathy of Uncertain Significance (MGUS). *MGUS is the most common plasma cell dyscrasia*,[45] occurring in about 3% of persons older than 50 years of age and in about 5% of individuals older than 70 years of age. By definition, patients are asymptomatic and the serum M protein level is less than 3 gm/dL. *Approximately 1% of patients with MGUS develop a symptomatic plasma cell neoplasm, usually multiple myeloma, per year*,[46] a rate of conversion that remains roughly constant over time. Of pathogenic interest, the clonal plasma cells in MGUS often contain the same chromosomal translocations and deletions that are found in full-blown multiple myeloma,[47] indicating that MGUS is an early stage of myeloma development. As in patients with smoldering myeloma, progression to multiple myeloma is unpredictable; hence, periodic assessment of serum M component levels and Bence Jones proteinuria is warranted.

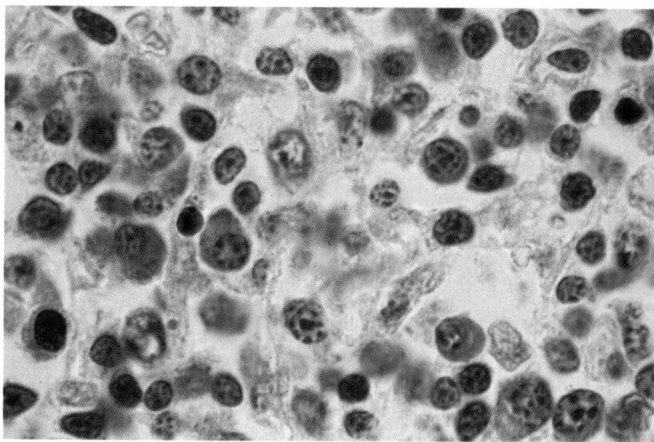

FIGURE 13–19 Lymphoplasmacytic lymphoma. Bone marrow biopsy shows a characteristic mixture of small lymphoid cells exhibiting various degrees of plasma cell differentiation. In addition, a mast cell with purplish red cytoplasmic granules is present at the left-hand side of the field.

Lymphoplasmacytic Lymphoma. Lymphoplasmacytic lymphoma is a B-cell neoplasm of older adults that usually presents in the sixth or seventh decade of life. Although bearing a superficial resemblance to CLL/SLL, it differs in that a substantial fraction of the tumor cells undergo terminal differentiation to plasma cells. *Most commonly, the plasma cell component secretes monoclonal IgM, often in amounts sufficient to cause a hyperviscosity syndrome known as Waldenström macroglobulinemia.* Unlike multiple myeloma, heavy- and light-chain synthesis is usually balanced and complications stemming from the secretion of free light chains (e.g., renal failure and amyloidosis) are rare. A further important distinction is that bone destruction is not observed in this disease.

> **Morphology.** Typically, the marrow contains a diffuse sparse-to-heavy infiltrate of lymphocytes, plasma cells, and plasmacytoid lymphocytes in varying proportions, often accompanied by mast cell hyperplasia (Fig. 13–19). Some tumors also contain a population of larger lymphoid cells with more vesicular nuclear chromatin and prominent nucleoli. Periodic acid–Schiff-positive inclusions containing Ig are frequently seen in the cytoplasm (**Russell bodies**) or the nucleus (**Dutcher bodies**) of some of the plasma cells. At diagnosis the tumor has usually disseminated to the lymph nodes, spleen, and liver. Infiltration of the nerve roots, meninges, and more rarely the brain can also occur with disease progression.

Immunophenotype and Molecular Pathogenesis. The lymphoid component expresses B-cell markers such as CD20 and surface Ig, whereas the plasma cell component secretes the same Ig that is expressed on the surface of the lymphoid cells. This is usually IgM but can also be IgG or IgA. These tumors usually lack chromosomal translocations; the most common cytogenetic abnormality is a deletion involving chromosome 6q.

Clinical Features. The dominant presenting complaints are nonspecific and include weakness, fatigue, and weight loss. Approximately half the patients have *lymphadenopathy, hepatomegaly, and splenomegaly.* Anemia caused by marrow infiltration is common. About 10% of patients have *autoimmune hemolysis* caused by *cold agglutinins*, IgM antibodies that bind to red cells at temperatures of less than 37°C (described in Chapter 14).

Patients with IgM-secreting tumors have additional complaints stemming from the physicochemical properties of IgM. Because of its large size, at high concentrations IgM greatly increases the viscosity of the blood, giving rise to a *hyperviscosity syndrome* characterized by the following:

- *Visual impairment* associated with venous congestion, which is reflected by striking tortuosity and distention of retinal veins; retinal hemorrhages and exudates can also contribute to the visual problems
- *Neurologic problems* such as headaches, dizziness, deafness, and stupor, all stemming from sluggish blood flow and sludging
- *Bleeding* related to the formation of complexes between macroglobulins and clotting factors as well as interference with platelet functions
- *Cryoglobulinemia* resulting from the precipitation of macroglobulins at low temperatures, which produces symptoms such as Raynaud phenomenon and cold urticaria

Lymphoplasmacytic lymphoma is an incurable progressive disease. Since most IgM is intravascular, symptoms caused by the high IgM levels (such as hyperviscosity and hemolysis) can be alleviated by plasmapheresis. Tumor growth can be controlled for a time with low doses of chemotherapeutic drugs and immunotherapy with anti-CD20 antibody. Transformation to large-cell lymphoma occurs but is uncommon. Median survival is about 4 years.

Mantle Cell Lymphoma

Mantle cell lymphoma is an uncommon lymphoid neoplasm that makes up about 2.5% of NHL in the United States and 7% to 9% of NHL in Europe. It usually presents in the fifth to sixth decades of life and shows a male predominance. As the name implies, *the tumor cells closely resemble the normal mantle zone B cells that surround germinal centers.*

> **Morphology.** Nodal tumor cells may surround reactive germinal centers to produce a nodular appearance at low power, or diffusely efface the node. **Typically, the proliferation consists of a homogeneous population of small lymphocytes with irregular to occasionally deeply clefted (cleaved) nuclear contours** (Fig. 13–20). Large cells resembling centroblasts and proliferation centers are absent, distinguishing mantle cell lymphoma from follicular lymphoma and CLL/SLL, respectively. In most cases the nuclear chromatin is condensed, nucleoli are inconspicuous, and the cytoplasm is scant. Occasionally, tumors composed of intermediate-sized cells

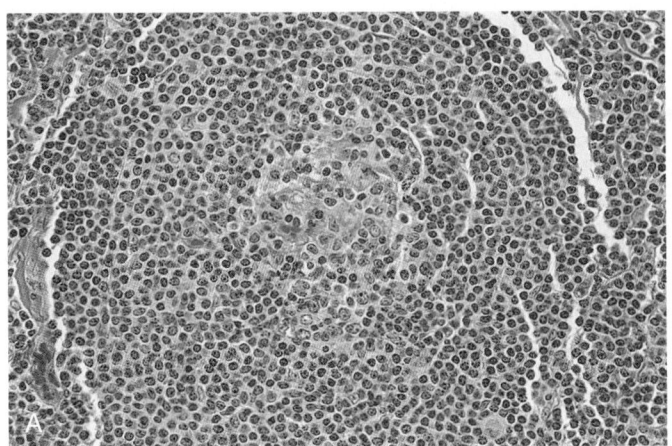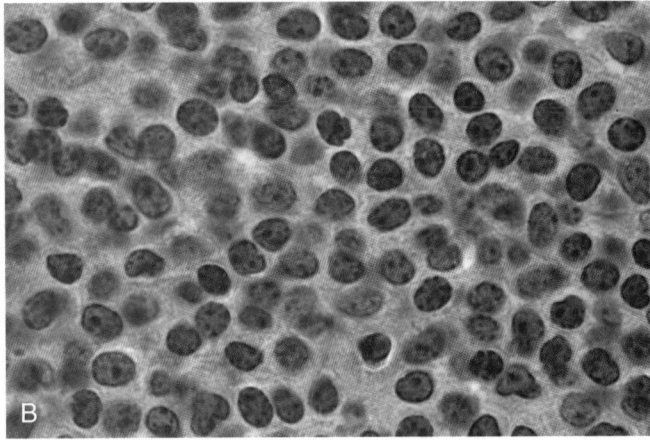

FIGURE 13–20   Mantle cell lymphoma. **A,** At low power, neoplastic lymphoid cells surround a small, atrophic germinal center, producing a mantle zone pattern of growth. **B,** High-power view shows a homogeneous population of small lymphoid cells with somewhat irregular nuclear outlines, condensed chromatin, and scant cytoplasm. Large cells resembling prolymphocytes (seen in chronic lymphocytic leukemia) and centroblasts (seen in follicular lymphoma) are absent.

with more open chromatin and a brisk mitotic rate are observed; immunophenotyping is necessary to distinguish these "blastoid" variants of mantle cell lymphoma from ALL.

At diagnosis the majority of patients have generalized lymphadenopathy, and 20% to 40% have peripheral blood involvement. Frequent sites of extranodal involvement include the bone marrow, spleen, liver, and gut. Occasionally, mucosal involvement of the small bowel or colon produces polyp-like lesions (lymphomatoid polyposis); of all forms of NHL, mantle cell lymphoma is most likely to spread in this fashion.

Immunophenotype. *Mantle cell lymphomas express high levels of cyclin D1.* Most tumors are also express CD19, CD20, and moderately high levels of surface Ig (usually IgM and IgD with κ or λ light chain). It is usually CD5+ and CD23−, which helps to distinguish it from CLL/SLL. The IgH genes lack somatic hypermutation, supporting an origin from a naive B cell.

Molecular Pathogenesis. *Cyclin D1 overexpression is caused by an (11;14) translocation involving the IgH locus on chromosome 14 and the cyclin D1 locus on chromosome 11.* This translocation is detected in about 70% of cases by standard karyotyping and in virtually all tumors by fluorescence in situ hybridization. The resulting up-regulation of cyclin D1 promotes G1- to S-phase progression during the cell cycle, as was described in Chapter 7.

Clinical Features. The most common presentation is painless lymphadenopathy. Symptoms related to involvement of the spleen (present in ~50% of cases) and the gut are also common. The prognosis is poor; the median survival is only 3 to 4 years. This lymphoma is not curable with conventional chemotherapy, and most patients eventually succumb to organ dysfunction caused by tumor infiltration. The blastoid variant and a "proliferative" expression profiling signature are associated with even shorter survivals.[26] Bone marrow transplantation and proteasome inhibitors are new therapeutic approaches showing some promise.

Marginal Zone Lymphomas

The category of marginal zone lymphoma encompasses a heterogeneous group of B-cell tumors that arise within lymph nodes, spleen, or extranodal tissues. The extranodal tumors were initially recognized at mucosal sites and are often referred to as mucosa-associated lymphoid tumors (or "maltomas"). In most cases, the tumor cells show evidence of somatic hypermutation and are considered to be of memory B-cell origin.

Although all marginal zone lymphomas share certain features, those occurring at extranodal sites deserve special attention because of their unusual pathogenesis and three exceptional characteristics.

- *They often arise within tissues involved by chronic inflammatory disorders of autoimmune or infectious etiology;* examples include the salivary gland in Sjögren disease, the thyroid gland in Hashimoto thyroiditis, and the stomach in *Helicobacter* gastritis.
- *They remain localized for prolonged periods, spreading systemically only late in their course.*
- *They may regress if the inciting agent (e.g., Helicobacter pylori) is eradicated.*

These characteristics suggest that extranodal marginal zone lymphomas arising in chronically inflamed tissues lie on a continuum between reactive lymphoid hyperplasia and full-blown lymphoma. The disease begins as a polyclonal immune reaction. With the acquisition of still-unknown initiating mutations, a B-cell clone emerges that still depends on antigen-stimulated T-helper cells for signals that drive growth and survival. At this stage, withdrawal of the responsible antigen causes tumor involution. A clinically relevant example is found in gastric "maltoma," in which antibiotic therapy directed against *H. pylori* often leads to tumor regression (Chapter 17). With time, however, tumors may acquire additional mutations that render their growth and survival antigen-independent, such as the (11;18), (14;18), or (1;14) chromosomal translocations, which are relatively specific for extranodal marginal zone lymphomas. All of these translocations up-regulate the expression and function of BCL10 or MALT1, protein components of a signaling complex that activates NF-κB and promotes the growth and survival of B cells.[5] With further clonal evolution, spread to distant sites and transformation to diffuse large B-cell lymphoma may occur. This theme of polyclonal to monoclonal transition during lymphomagenesis is also applicable to the pathogenesis of EBV-induced lymphoma and is discussed more fully in Chapter 7.

Hairy Cell Leukemia

This rare but distinctive B-cell neoplasm constitutes about 2% of all leukemias. It is predominantly a disease of middle-aged white males, with a median age of 55 and a male-to-female ratio of 5:1.

> **Morphology. Hairy cell leukemia derives its picturesque name from the appearance of the leukemic cells, which have fine hairlike projections that are best recognized under the phase-contrast microscope** (Fig. 13–21). On routine peripheral blood smears, hairy cells have round, oblong, or reniform nuclei and moderate amounts of pale blue cytoplasm with threadlike or bleblike extensions. The number of circulating cells is highly variable. The marrow is involved by a diffuse interstitial infiltrate of cells with oblong or reniform nuclei, condensed chromatin, and pale cytoplasm. Because these cells are enmeshed in an extracellular matrix composed of reticulin fibrils, they usually cannot be aspirated (a clinical difficulty referred to as a **"dry tap"**) and are only seen in marrow biopsies. The splenic red pulp is usually heavily infiltrated, leading to obliteration of white pulp and a beefy red gross appearance. Hepatic portal triads are also involved frequently.

Immunophenotype and Molecular Pathogenesis. Hairy cell leukemias typically express the pan-B-cell markers CD19 and CD20, surface Ig (usually IgG), and certain relatively distinctive markers, such as CD11c, CD25, and CD103. Analysis of Ig gene sequences has revealed a high incidence of somatic hypermutation, suggesting a post-germinal center memory B-cell origin.

Clinical Features. Clinical manifestations result largely from infiltration of the bone marrow, liver, and spleen. *Splenomegaly*, often massive, is the most common and sometimes the only abnormal physical finding. *Hepatomegaly* is less common and not as marked; lymphadenopathy is rare. *Pancytopenia* resulting from marrow involvement and splenic sequestration is seen in more than half the cases. About one third of those affected present with *infections.* There is an increased incidence of atypical mycobacterial infections, possibly related to frequent unexplained monocytopenia.

Hairy cell leukemia follows an indolent course. For unclear reasons, this tumor is exceptionally sensitive to "gentle" chemotherapeutic regimens, which produce long-lasting remissions. Tumors often relapse after 5 or more years, yet generally respond well when retreated with chemotherapy. The overall prognosis is excellent.

Peripheral T-Cell and NK-Cell Neoplasms

These categories include a heterogeneous group of neoplasms having phenotypes resembling mature T cells or NK cells. Peripheral T-cell tumors make up about 5% to 10% of NHLs in the United States and Europe, but are more common in Asia. NK-cell tumors are rare in the West, but also more common in the Far East. Only the most common diagnoses and those of particular pathogenetic interest will be discussed.

Peripheral T-Cell Lymphoma, Unspecified

Although the WHO classification includes a number of distinct peripheral T-cell neoplasms, many of these lymphomas are not easily categorized and are lumped into a "wastebasket" diagnosis, *peripheral T-cell lymphoma, unspecified.* As might be expected, no morphologic feature is pathognomonic, but certain findings are characteristic. These tumors efface lymph

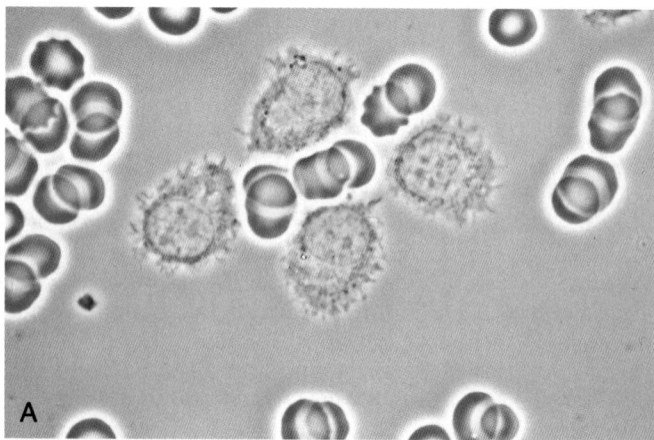
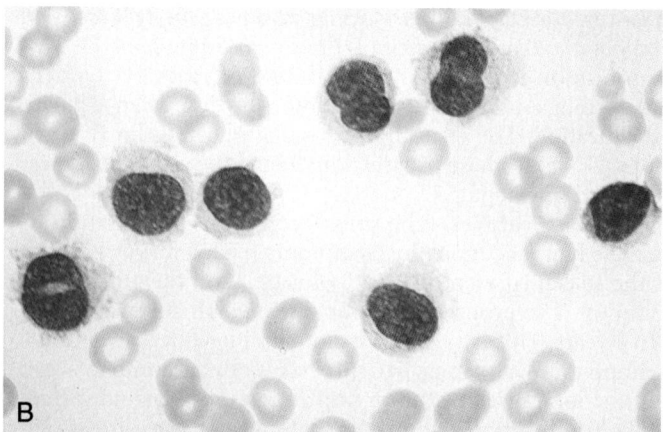

FIGURE 13–21 Hairy cell leukemia (peripheral blood smear). **A,** Phase-contrast microscopy shows tumor cells with fine hairlike cytoplasmic projections. **B,** In stained smears, these cells have round or folded nuclei and modest amounts of pale blue, agranular cytoplasm.

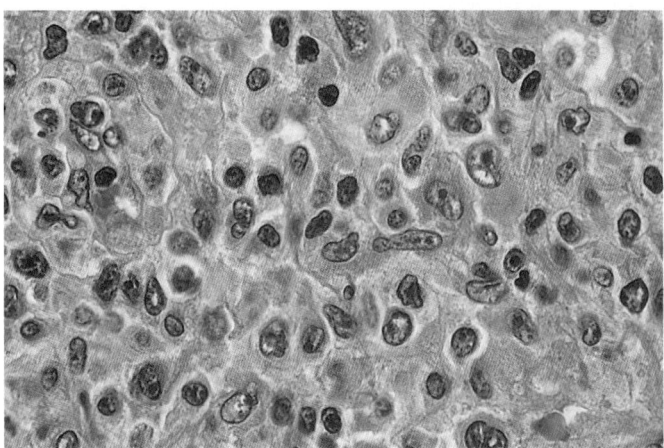

FIGURE 13–22 Peripheral T-cell lymphoma, unspecified (lymph node). A spectrum of small, intermediate, and large lymphoid cells, many with irregular nuclear contours, is visible.

nodes diffusely and are typically composed of a pleomorphic mixture of variably sized malignant T cells (Fig. 13–22). There is often a prominent infiltrate of reactive cells, such as eosinophils and macrophages, probably attracted by tumor-derived cytokines. Brisk neoangiogenesis may also be seen.

The diagnosis requires immunophenotyping. By definition, all peripheral T-cell lymphomas have a mature T-cell phenotype. They usually express CD2, CD3, CD5, and either αβ or γδ T-cell receptors. Some also express CD4 or CD8; such tumors are taken to be of helper or cytotoxic T-cell origin, respectively. However, many tumors have phenotypes that do not resemble any known normal T cell. In difficult cases where the differential diagnosis lies between lymphoma and a florid reactive process, DNA analysis can be used to confirm the presence of clonal T-cell receptor rearrangements.

Most patients present with generalized lymphadenopathy, sometimes accompanied by eosinophilia, pruritus, fever, and weight loss. Although cures of peripheral T-cell lymphoma have been reported, these tumors have a significantly worse prognosis than comparably aggressive mature B-cell neoplasms (e.g., diffuse large B-cell lymphoma).

Anaplastic Large-Cell Lymphoma (ALK Positive)

This uncommon entity is defined by the presence of rearrangements in the ALK gene on chromosome 2p23. These rearrangements break the *ALK* locus and lead to the formation of chimeric genes encoding ALK fusion proteins, constitutively active tyrosine kinases that trigger a number of signaling pathways, including the JAK/STAT pathway.[48]

As the name implies, this tumor is typically composed of large anaplastic cells, some containing horseshoe-shaped nuclei and voluminous cytoplasm (so-called hallmark cells) (Fig. 13–23A). The tumor cells often cluster about venules and infiltrate lymphoid sinuses, mimicking the appearance of metastatic carcinoma. ALK is not expressed in normal lymphocytes or other lymphomas; thus, the detection of ALK protein in tumor cells (Fig. 13–23B) is a reliable indicator of an *ALK* gene rearrangement.

T-cell lymphomas with ALK rearrangements tend to occur in children or young adults, frequently involve soft tissues, and carry a very good prognosis (unlike other aggressive peripheral T-cell neoplasms). The cure rate with chemotherapy is 75% to 80%. Inhibitors of ALK are under development and offer an excellent opportunity for the development of a selective, targeted therapy. Morphologically similar tumors lacking *ALK* rearrangements occur in older adults and have a poor prognosis, similar to that of peripheral T-cell lymphoma, unspecified.

Adult T-Cell Leukemia/Lymphoma

This neoplasm of CD4+ T cells is only observed in adults infected by human T-cell leukemia retrovirus type 1 (HTLV-1), which was discussed in Chapter 7. It occurs mainly in regions where HTLV-1 is endemic, namely southern Japan, West Africa, and the Caribbean basin. Common findings include skin lesions, generalized lymphadenopathy, hepatosplenomegaly,

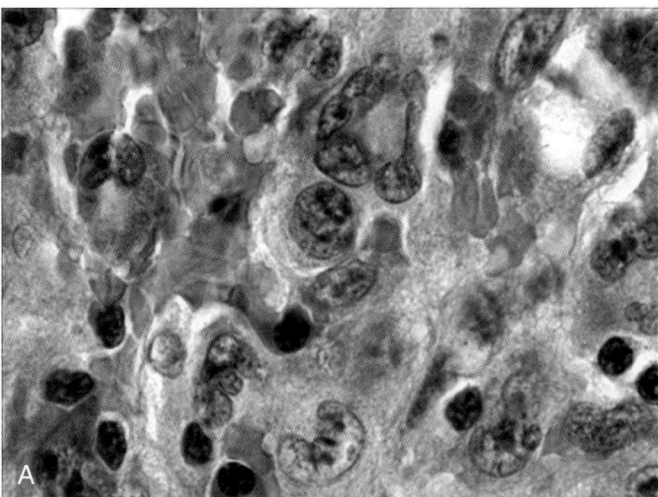
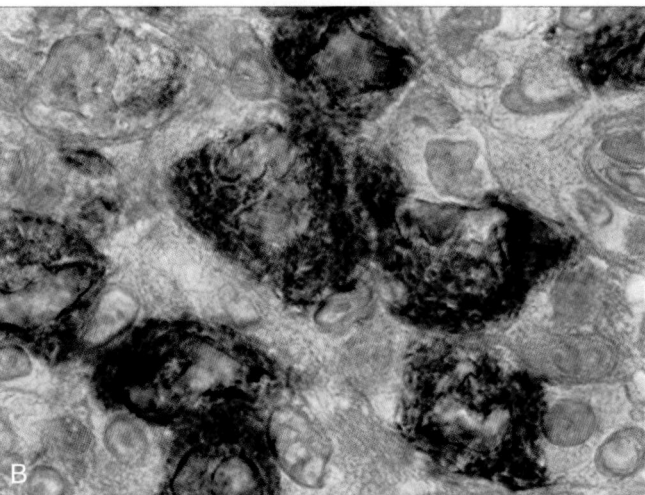

FIGURE 13–23 Anaplastic large-cell lymphoma. **A,** Several "hallmark" cells with horseshoe-like or "embryoid" nuclei and abundant cytoplasm lie near the center of the field. **B,** Immunohistochemical stain demonstrating the presence of ALK fusion protein. (Courtesy of Dr. Jeffrey Kutok, Department of Pathology, Brigham and Women's Hospital, Boston, MA.)

peripheral blood lymphocytosis, and hypercalcemia. The appearance of the tumor cells varies, but cells with multilobated nuclei ("cloverleaf" or "flower" cells) are frequently observed. *The tumor cells contain clonal HTLV-1 provirus, which is believed to play a critical pathogenic role.* Notably, HTLV-1 encodes a protein called Tax that is a potent activator of NF-κB,[49] which (as we have discussed) enhances lymphocyte growth and survival.

Most patients present with rapidly progressive disease that is fatal within months to 1 year despite aggressive chemotherapy. Less commonly, the tumor involves only the skin and follows a much more indolent course, like that of mycosis fungoides (described below). It should be noted that in addition to adult T-cell leukemia/lymphoma, HTLV-1 infection sometimes gives rise to a progressive demyelinating disease of the central nervous system and spinal cord (see Chapter 28).

Mycosis Fungoides/Sézary Syndrome

Mycosis fungoides and Sézary syndrome are different manifestations of a tumor of CD4+ helper T cells that home to the skin. Clinically, the cutaneous lesions of *mycosis fungoides* typically progress through three somewhat distinct stages, an inflammatory *premycotic phase*, a *plaque phase*, and a *tumor phase* (all discussed in more detail in Chapter 25). Histologically, the epidermis and upper dermis are infiltrated by neoplastic T cells, which often have a cerebriform appearance due to marked infolding of the nuclear membrane. Late disease progression is characterized by extracutaneous spread, most commonly to lymph nodes and bone marrow.

Sézary syndrome is a variant in which skin involvement is manifested as a *generalized exfoliative erythroderma*. In contrast to mycosis fungoides, the skin lesions rarely proceed to tumefaction, and *there is an associated leukemia of "Sézary" cells* with characteristic cerebriform nuclei.

The tumor cells characteristically express the adhesion molecule CLA and the chemokine receptors CCR4 and CCR10, all of which contribute to the homing of normal CD4+ T cells to the skin. Although cutaneous disease dominates the clinical picture, sensitive molecular analyses have shown that the tumor cells circulate through the blood, marrow, and lymph nodes even early in the course. Nevertheless, these are indolent tumors, with a median survival of 8 to 9 years. Transformation to aggressive T-cell lymphoma occurs occasionally as a terminal event.

Large Granular Lymphocytic Leukemia

T-cell and NK-cell variants of this rare neoplasm are recognized, both of which occur mainly in adults. Individuals with T-cell disease usually present with mild to moderate lymphocytosis and splenomegaly. Lymphadenopathy and hepatomegaly are usually absent. NK-cell disease often presents in an even more subtle fashion, with little or no lymphocytosis or splenomegaly.

The tumor cells are large lymphocytes with abundant blue cytoplasm and a few coarse azurophilic granules, best seen in peripheral blood smears. The marrow usually contains sparse interstitial lymphocytic infiltrates, which can be difficult to appreciate without immunohistochemical stains. Infiltrates are also usually present in the spleen and liver. As might be expected, T-cell variants are CD3+, whereas NK-cell large granular lymphocytic leukemias are CD3−, CD56+.

Despite the relative paucity of marrow infiltration, neutropenia and anemia dominate the clinical picture. Neutropenia is often accompanied by a striking decrease in late myeloid forms in the marrow. Rarely, pure red cell aplasia is seen. *There is also an increased incidence of rheumatologic disorders.* Some patients with Felty syndrome, a triad of rheumatoid arthritis, splenomegaly, and neutropenia, have this disorder as an underlying cause. The basis for these varied clinical abnormalities is unknown, but autoimmunity, provoked in some way by the tumor, seems likely.

The course is variable, being largely dependent on the severity of the cytopenias and their responsiveness to low-dose chemotherapy or steroids. In general, tumors of T-cell origin pursue an indolent course, whereas NK-cell tumors behave more aggressively.

Extranodal NK/T-Cell Lymphoma

This neoplasm is rare in the United States and Europe, but constitutes as many as 3% of NHLs in Asia. It presents most commonly as a destructive nasopharyngeal mass; less common sites of presentation include the testis and the skin. *The tumor cell infiltrate typically surrounds and invades small vessels, leading to extensive ischemic necrosis.* The tumor cell size is variable but usually includes a large-cell component. In touch preparations, *large azurophilic granules* are seen in the cytoplasm of the tumor cells that resemble those found in normal NK cells.

This form of lymphoma is highly associated with EBV. Within individual patients, all of the tumor cells contain identical EBV episomes, indicating that the tumor originates from a single EBV-infected cell. How EBV gains entry is uncertain, since the tumor cells fail to express CD21, a surface protein that serves as the B-cell EBV receptor. Most tumors are CD3− and lack T-cell receptor rearrangements and express NK-cell markers, including a restricted set of killer-cell Ig-like receptors, supporting an NK-cell origin. No consistent chromosome aberration has been described, and relatively little is known about the molecular pathogenesis beyond the involvement of EBV.

Most extranodal NK/T-cell lymphomas are highly aggressive neoplasms that respond well to radiation therapy but are resistant to chemotherapy. Thus, the prognosis is poor in patients with advanced disease.

This ends the discussion of the lymphocytic leukemias and the NHLs. We will now turn to the second major category of lymphoid neoplasms, Hodgkin lymphoma.

Hodgkin Lymphoma

Hodgkin lymphoma (HL) encompasses a group of lymphoid neoplasms that differ from NHL in several respects (Table 13–7). While NHLs frequently occur at extranodal sites and spread in an unpredictable fashion, *HL arises in a single node or chain of nodes and spreads first to anatomically contiguous lymphoid tissues.* For this reason, the staging of HL is much more important in guiding therapy than it is in NHL. HL also has distinctive morphologic features. It is characterized by the presence of neoplastic giant cells called *Reed-Sternberg cells*. These cells release factors that induce the accumulation of reactive lymphocytes, macrophages, and granulocytes, which typically make up greater than 90% of the tumor cellularity. In the

TABLE 13–7 Differences between Hodgkin and Non-Hodgkin Lymphomas	
Hodgkin Lymphoma	**Non-Hodgkin Lymphoma**
More often localized to a single axial group of nodes (cervical, mediastinal, para-aortic)	More frequent involvement of multiple peripheral nodes
Orderly spread by contiguity	Noncontiguous spread
Mesenteric nodes and Waldeyer ring rarely involved	Waldeyer ring and mesenteric nodes commonly involved
Extra-nodal presentation rare	Extra-nodal presentation common

vast majority of HLs, the neoplastic Reed-Sternberg cells are derived from germinal center or post-germinal center B cells.

Hodgkin lymphoma accounts for 0.7% of all new cancers in the United States; there are about 8000 new cases each year. The average age at diagnosis is 32 years. It is one of the most common cancers of young adults and adolescents, but also occurs in the aged. It was the first human cancer to be successfully treated with radiation therapy and chemotherapy, and is curable in most cases.

Classification. The WHO classification recognizes five subtypes of HL:

1. Nodular sclerosis
2. Mixed cellularity
3. Lymphocyte-rich
4. Lymphocyte depletion
5. Lymphocyte predominance

In the first four subtypes—nodular sclerosis, mixed cellularity, lymphocyte-rich, and lymphocyte depletion—the Reed-Sternberg cells have a similar immunophenotype. These subtypes are often lumped together as *classical* forms of HL. In the remaining subtype, lymphocyte predominance, the Reed-Sternberg cells have a distinctive B-cell immunophenotype that differs from that of the "classical" types.

Morphology. Identification of Reed-Sternberg cells and their variants is essential for the diagnosis. **Diagnostic Reed-Sternberg cells are large cells (≥45 μm in diameter) with multiple nuclei or a single nucleus with multiple nuclear lobes, each with a large inclusion-like nucleolus about the size of a small lymphocyte (5–7 μm in diameter)** (Fig. 13–24A). The cytoplasm

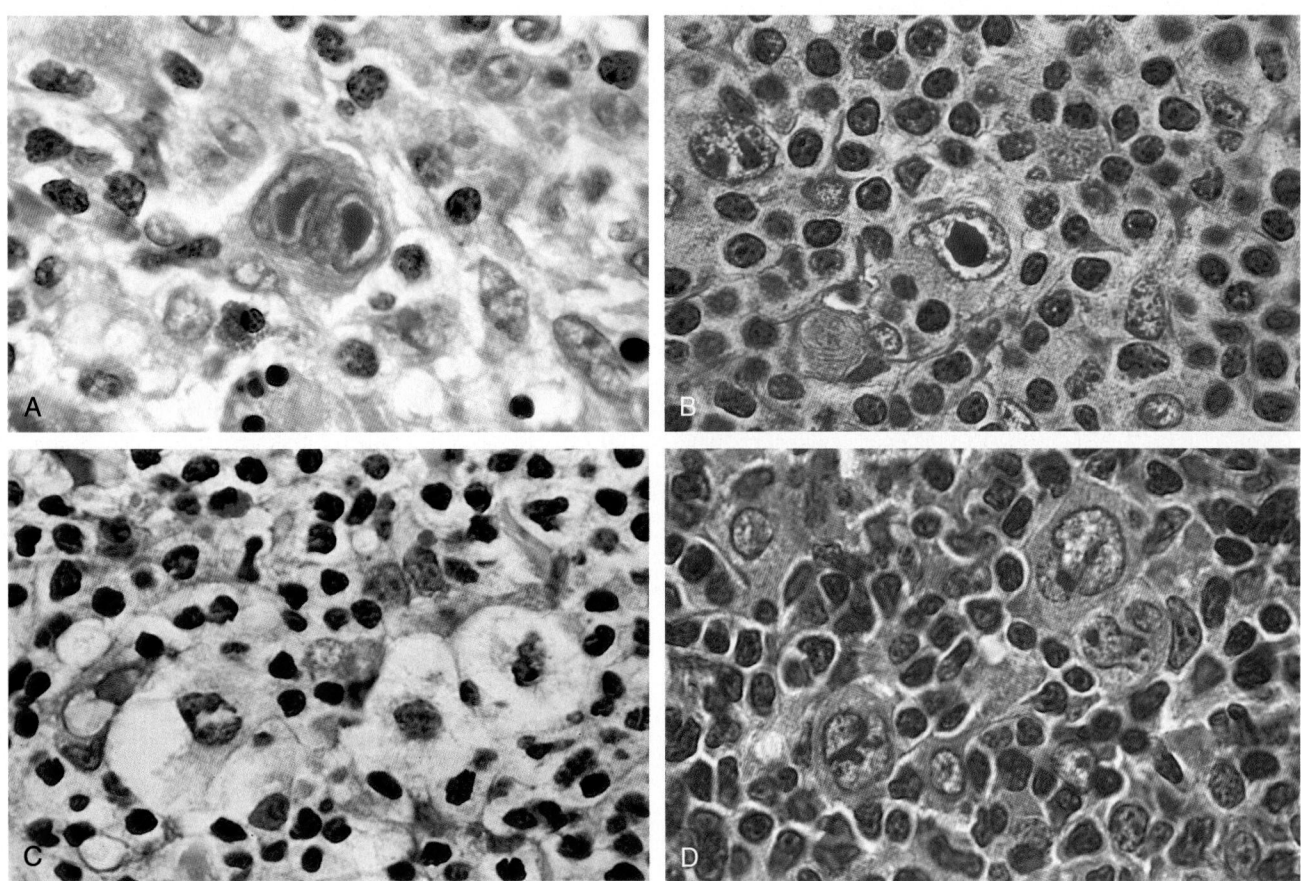

FIGURE 13–24 Reed-Sternberg cells and variants. **A,** Diagnostic Reed-Sternberg cell, with two nuclear lobes, large inclusion-like nucleoli, and abundant cytoplasm, surrounded by lymphocytes, macrophages, and an eosinophil. **B,** Reed-Sternberg cell, mononuclear variant. **C,** Reed-Sternberg cell, lacunar variant. This variant has a folded or multilobated nucleus and lies within a open space, which is an artifact created by disruption of the cytoplasm during tissue sectioning. **D,** Reed-Sternberg cell, lymphohistiocytic variant. Several such variants with multiply infolded nuclear membranes, small nucleoli, fine chromatin, and abundant pale cytoplasm are present. (**A,** Courtesy of Dr. Robert W. McKenna, Department of Pathology, University of Texas Southwestern Medical School, Dallas, TX.)

Table 13–8 Subtypes of Hodgkin Lymphoma		
Subtype	**Morphology and Immunophenotype**	**Typical Clinical Features**
Nodular sclerosis	Frequent lacunar cells and occasional diagnostic RS cells; background infiltrate composed of T lymphocytes, eosinophils, macrophages, and plasma cells; fibrous bands dividing cellular areas into nodules. RS cells CD15+, CD30+; usually EBV–	Most common subtype; usually stage I or II disease; frequent mediastinal involvement; equal occurrence in males and females (F = M), most patients young adults
Mixed cellularity	Frequent mononuclear and diagnostic RS cells; background infiltrate rich in T lymphocytes, eosinophils, macrophages, plasma cells; RS cells CD15+, CD30+; 70% EBV+	More than 50% present as stage III or IV disease; M greater than F; biphasic incidence, peaking in young adults and again in adults older than 55
Lymphocyte rich	Frequent mononuclear and diagnostic RS cells; background infiltrate rich in T lymphocytes; RS cells CD15+, CD30+; 40% EBV+	Uncommon; M greater than F; tends to be seen in older adults
Lymphocyte depletion	Reticular variant: Frequent diagnostic RS cells and variants and a paucity of background reactive cells; RS cells CD15+, CD30+; most EBV+	Uncommon; more common in older males, HIV-infected individuals, and in developing countries; often presents with advanced disease
Lymphocyte predominance	Frequent L&H (popcorn cell) variants in a background of follicular dendritic cells and reactive B cells; RS cells CD20+, CD15–, C30–; EBV–	Uncommon; young males with cervical or axillary lymphadenopathy; mediastinal

L&H, lymphohistiocytic; RS cell, Reed-Sternberg cell.

is abundant. Several Reed-Sternberg cell variants are also recognized. Mononuclear variants contain a single nucleus with a large inclusion-like nucleolus (Fig. 13–24B). Lacunar cells (seen in the nodular sclerosis subtype) have more delicate, folded, or multilobate nuclei and abundant pale cytoplasm that is often disrupted during the cutting of sections, leaving the nucleus sitting in an empty hole (a lacuna) (Fig. 13–24C). In classical forms of HL, Reed-Sternberg cells undergo a peculiar form of cell death in which the cells shrink and become pyknotic, a process described as "mummification." Lymphohistocytic variants (L&H cells) with polypoid nuclei, inconspicuous nucleoli, and moderately abundant cytoplasm are characteristic of the lymphocyte predominance subtype (Fig. 13–24D).

HL must be distinguished from other conditions in which cells resembling Reed-Sternberg cells can be seen, such as infectious mononucleosis, solid-tissue cancers, and large-cell NHLs. The diagnosis of HL depends on the identification of Reed-Sternberg cells in a typical prominent background of non-neoplastic inflammatory cells. The Reed-Sternberg cells of HL also have a characteristic immunohistochemical profile.

With this as background, we turn to the subclasses of HL, pointing out some of the salient morphologic and immunophenotypic features of each (summarized in Table 13–8). The clinical manifestations common to all will be presented later.

Nodular Sclerosis Type. This is the most common form of HL, constituting 65% to 70% of cases. It is characterized by the presence of **lacunar variant** Reed-Sternberg cells and the **deposition of collagen**

in bands that divide involved lymph nodes into circumscribed nodules (Fig. 13–25). The fibrosis may be scant or abundant. The Reed-Sternberg cells are found in a polymorphous background of T cells, eosinophils, plasma cells and macrophages. Diagnostic Reed-Sternberg cells are often uncommon. The Reed-Sternberg cells in this and other "classical" HL subtypes have a characteristic immunophenotype; they are positive for PAX5 (a B-cell transcription factor), CD15, and CD30, and negative for other B-cell markers, T-cell markers, and CD45 (leukocyte common antigen). As in other forms of HL, involvement of the spleen, liver, bone marrow, and other organs and

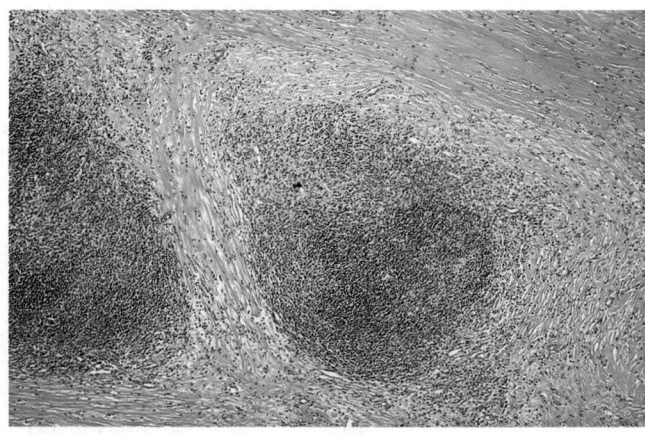

FIGURE 13–25 Hodgkin lymphoma, nodular sclerosis type. A low-power view shows well-defined bands of pink, acellular collagen that subdivide the tumor into nodules. (Courtesy of Dr. Robert W. McKenna, Department of Pathology, University of Texas Southwestern Medical School, Dallas, TX.)

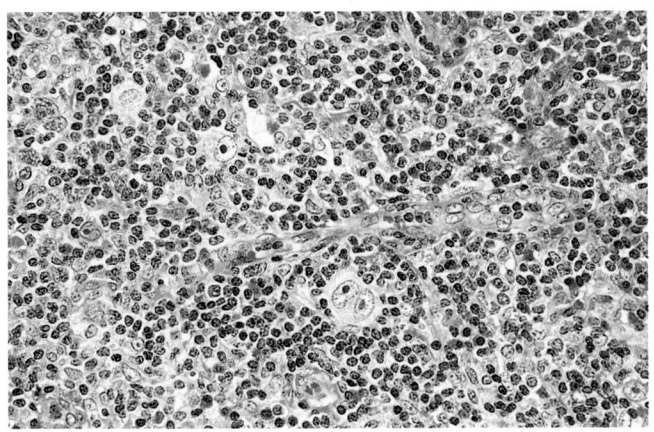

FIGURE 13–26 Hodgkin lymphoma, mixed-cellularity type. A diagnostic, binucleate Reed-Sternberg cell is surrounded by reactive cells, including eosinophils (bright red cytoplasm), lymphocytes, and histiocytes. (Courtesy of Dr. Robert W. McKenna, Department of Pathology, University of Texas Southwestern Medical School, Dallas, TX.)

tissues can appear in due course in the form of irregular tumor nodules resembling those seen in lymph nodes. This subtype is uncommonly associated with EBV.

The nodular sclerosis type occurs with equal frequency in males and females. It has a propensity to involve the lower cervical, supraclavicular, and mediastinal lymph nodes of adolescents or young adults. The prognosis is excellent.

Mixed-Cellularity Type. This form of HL constitutes about 20% to 25% of cases. Involved lymph nodes are diffusely effaced by a heterogeneous cellular infiltrate, which includes T cells, eosinophils, plasma cells, and benign macrophages admixed with Reed-Sternberg cells (Fig. 13–26). **Diagnostic Reed-Sternberg cells and mononuclear variants are usually plentiful. The Reed-Sternberg cells are infected with EBV in about 70% of cases.** The immunophenotype is identical to that observed in the nodular sclerosis type.

Mixed-cellularity HL is more common in males. Compared with the lymphocyte predominance and nodular sclerosis subtypes, it is more likely to be associated with older age, systemic symptoms such as night sweats and weight loss, and advanced tumor stage. Nonetheless, the overall prognosis is very good.

Lymphocyte-Rich Type. This is an uncommon form of classical HL in which reactive lymphocytes make up the vast majority of the cellular infiltrate. In most cases, involved lymph nodes are diffusely effaced, but vague nodularity due to the presence of residual B-cell follicles is sometimes seen. This entity is distinguished from the lymphocyte predominance type by the presence of frequent mononuclear variants and diagnostic Reed-Sternberg cells with a "classical" immunophenotypic profile. It is associated with

EBV in about 40% of cases and has a very good to excellent prognosis.

Lymphocyte Depletion Type. This is the least common form of HL, amounting to less than 5% of cases. It is characterized by a paucity of lymphocytes and a relative abundance of Reed-Sternberg cells or their pleomorphic variants. The immunophenotype of the Reed-Sternberg cells is identical to that seen in other classical types of HL. Immunophenotyping is essential, since most tumors suspected of being lymphocyte depletion HL actually prove to be large-cell NHLs. The Reed-Sternberg cells are infected with EBV in over 90% of cases.

Lymphocyte depletion HL occurs predominantly in the elderly, in HIV+ individuals of any age, and in nonindustrialized countries. Advanced stage and systemic symptoms are frequent, and the overall outcome is somewhat less favorable than in the other subtypes.

Lymphocyte Predominance Type. This uncommon "nonclassical" variant of HL accounts for about 5% of cases. Involved nodes are effaced by a nodular infiltrate of small lymphocytes admixed with variable numbers of macrophages (Fig. 13–27). "Classical" Reed-Sternberg cells are usually difficult to find. Instead, this tumor contains so-called L&H (lymphocytic and histiocytic) variants, which have a multilobed nucleus resembling a popcorn kernel ("popcorn cell"). Eosinophils and plasma cells are usually scant or absent.

In contrast to the Reed-Sternberg cells found in classical forms of HL, **L&H variants express B-cell markers typical of germinal-center B cells,** such as CD20 and BCL6, and are usually negative for CD15 and CD30. The typical nodular pattern of growth is due to the presence of expanded B-cell follicles, which are populated with L&H variants, numerous reactive

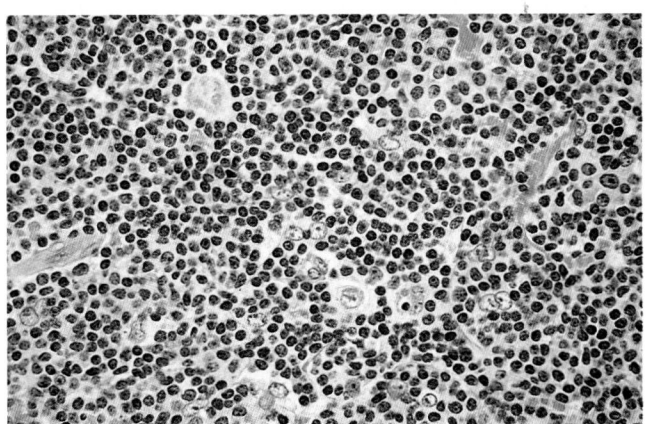

FIGURE 13–27 Hodgkin lymphoma, lymphocyte predominance type. Numerous mature-looking lymphocytes surround scattered, large, pale-staining lymphohistiocytic variants ("popcorn" cells). (Courtesy of Dr. Robert W. McKenna, Department of Pathology, University of Texas Southwestern Medical School, Dallas, TX.)

B cells, and follicular dendritic cells. The IgH genes of the L&H variants show evidence of ongoing somatic hypermutation, a modification that occurs only in germinal-center B cells. In 3% to 5% of cases, this type transforms into a tumor resembling diffuse large B-cell lymphoma. EBV is not associated with this subtype.

A majority of patients are males, usually younger than 35 years of age, who typically present with cervical or axillary lymphadenopathy. Mediastinal and bone marrow involvement is rare. In some series, this form of HL is more likely to recur than the classical subtypes, but the prognosis is excellent.

Molecular Pathogenesis. The origin of the neoplastic Reed-Sternberg cells of classical HL has been explained through elegant studies relying on molecular analysis of single isolated Reed-Sternberg cells and variants. In the vast majority of cases, *the Ig genes of Reed-Sternberg cells have undergone both V(D)J recombination and somatic hypermutation, establishing an origin from a germinal center or post-germinal-center B cell.*[50] Despite having the genetic signature of a B cell, the Reed-Sternberg cells of classical HL fail to express most B cell–specific genes, including the Ig genes. The cause of this wholesale reprogramming of gene expression has yet to be fully explained.[51]

Activation of the transcription factor NF-κB is a common event in classical HL. NF-κB is activated either by EBV infection or by some other mechanism and turns on genes that promote lymphocyte survival and proliferation. EBV+ tumor cells express latent membrane protein-1 (LMP-1), a protein encoded by the EBV genome that transmits signals that up-regulate NF-κB. Activation of NF-κB also occurs in EBV− tumors, in some instances as a result of acquired mutations in IκB,[52] a negative regulator of NF-κB. It is hypothesized that activation of NF-κB by EBV or other mechanisms rescues "crippled" germinal-center B cells that cannot express Igs from apoptosis, setting the stage for the acquisition of other unknown mutations that collaborate to produce Reed-Sternberg cells. Little is known about the basis for the morphology of Reed-Sternberg cells and variants, but it is intriguing that EBV-infected B cells resembling Reed-Sternberg cells are found in the lymph nodes of individuals with infectious mononucleosis, strongly suggesting that EBV-encoded proteins play a part in the remarkable metamorphosis of B cells into Reed-Sternberg cells.

The florid accumulation of reactive cells in tissues involved by classical HL occurs in response to a wide variety of *cytokines* (such as IL-5, IL-10, IL-13, and TGF-β) and *chemokines* (such as TARC, MDC, IP-10, and CCL28) that are secreted by Reed-Sternberg cells.[53] Once attracted, the reactive cells produce factors that support the growth and survival of the tumor cells and further modify the reactive cell response. For example, eosinophils and T cells express ligands that activate the CD30 and CD40 receptors found on Reed-Sternberg cells, producing signals that up-regulate NF-κB. Other examples of "cross-talk" between Reed-Sternberg cells and surrounding reactive cells are provided in Figure 13–28.

Reed-Sternberg cells are aneuploid and possess diverse clonal chromosomal aberrations. Copy number gains in the *c-REL* proto-oncogene on chromosome 2p are particularly common and may contribute to increases in NF-κB activity.[54]

Clinical Features. HL most commonly present as painless lymphadenopathy. Patients with the nodular sclerosis or lymphocyte predominance types tend to present with stage I–II disease and are usually free of systemic manifestations. Patients with disseminated disease (stages III–IV) or the mixed-cellularity or lymphocyte depletion subtypes are more likely to have constitutional symptoms, such as fever, night sweats, and weight loss. Cutaneous anergy resulting from depressed cell-mediated immunity is seen in most cases. The mix of factors released from Reed-Sternberg cells (see Fig. 13–28) suppress T_H1 immune responses and may contribute to immune dysregulation.

The spread of HL is remarkably stereotyped: nodal disease first, then splenic disease, hepatic disease, and finally involvement of the marrow and other tissues. Because of this behavior, radiation therapy can be curative for persons with early-stage disease. Thus, the staging of HL (Table 13–9) not only determines the prognosis, but also guides therapy. Staging involves physical examination, radiologic imaging of the abdomen, pelvis, and chest, and biopsy of the bone marrow. Systemic treatment is preferred whenever the staging is equivocal.

With current treatment protocols, tumor stage rather than histologic type is the most important prognostic variable. The cure rate of patients with stages I and IIA is close to 90%. Even with advanced disease (stages IVA and IVB), disease-free survival at 5 years is 60% to 70%.

Progress in the treatment of HL has created a new set of problems. Long-term survivors of chemotherapy and radiation therapy have an increased risk of developing second cancers. Myelodysplastic syndromes, AML, and lung cancer head the list, but also included are NHL, breast cancer, gastric cancer, sarcoma, and melanoma. Most of the risk of solid tumors is attributable to radiation therapy, which has also been linked to pulmonary fibrosis and accelerated atherosclerosis. The risk of breast cancer is particularly high in females treated with radiation to the chest during adolescence. Alkylating chemotherapeutic drugs seem to be responsible for the increased risk of AML and myelodysplasia. Fortunately, newer combinations of chemotherapeutic drugs and more judicious use of radiation therapy seem to largely avoid these complications and are equally curative.

MYELOID NEOPLASMS

The common feature of this heterogeneous group of neoplasms is an origin from hematopoietic progenitor cells. These diseases primarily involve the marrow and to a lesser degree the secondary hematopoietic organs (the spleen, liver, and lymph nodes), and usually present with symptoms related to altered hematopoiesis. Three broad categories of myeloid neoplasia exist:

- *Acute myeloid leukemias,* in which an accumulation of immature myeloid forms (blasts) in the bone marrow suppresses normal hematopoiesis
- *Myelodysplastic syndromes,* in which ineffective hematopoiesis leads to cytopenias

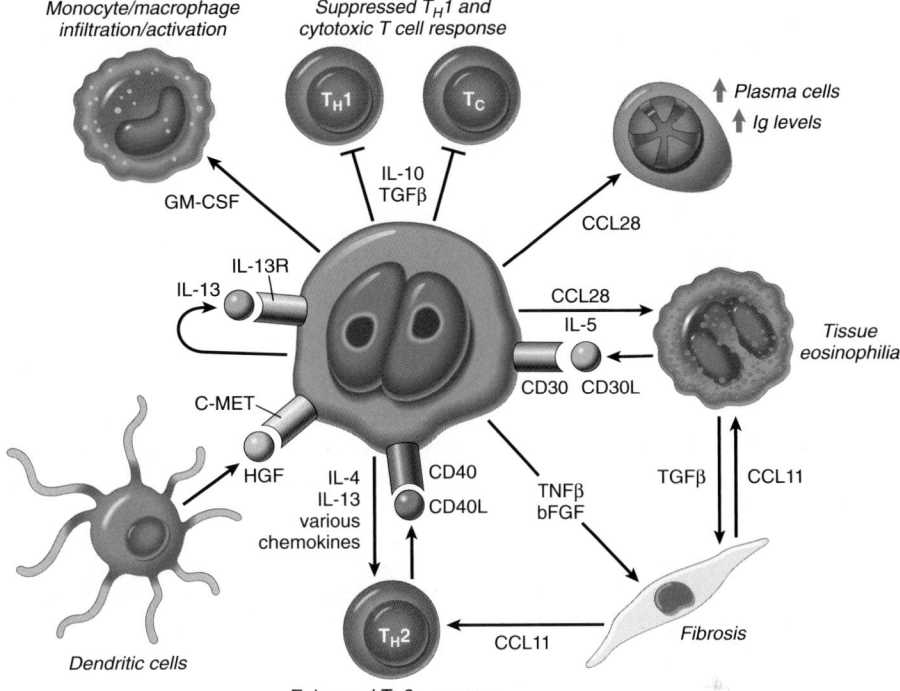

FIGURE 13–28 Proposed signals mediating "cross-talk" between Reed-Sternberg cells and surrounding normal cells in classical forms of Hodgkin lymphoma. CD30L, CD30 ligand; bFGF, basic fibroblast growth factor; GM-CSF, granulocyte-macrophage colony-stimulating factor; HGF, hepatocyte growth factor (binds to the c-MET receptor); TGFβ, transforming growth factor β; TNFβ, tumor necrosis factor β (lymphotoxin); T$_c$, CD8+ cytotoxic T cell; T$_H$1 and T$_H$2, CD4+ T helper cell subsets.

○ *Myeloproliferative disorders*, in which there is usually increased production of one or more types of blood cells

The pathogenesis of myeloid neoplasms is best understood in the context of normal hematopoiesis, which (you will remember from Fig. 13–1) involves a hierarchy of hematopoietic stem cells, committed progenitors, and more differentiated elements. Normal hematopoiesis is finely tuned by homeostatic feedback mechanisms involving cytokines and growth factors that modulate the production of red cells,

white cells, and platelets in the marrow. These mechanisms are deranged in marrows involved by myeloid neoplasms, which "escape" from normal homeostatic controls on growth and survival and suppress the function of residual normal stem cells. The specific manifestations of the different myeloid neoplasms are influenced by

○ *The position of the transformed cell within the hierarchy of progenitors* (i.e., a pluripotent hematopoietic stem cell versus a more committed progenitor)
○ *The effect of the transforming events on differentiation*, which may be inhibited, skewed, or deranged by particular oncogenic mutations

We will return to these themes as each type of myeloid neoplasm is discussed.

Given that all myeloid neoplasms originate from transformed hematopoietic progenitors, it is not surprising that divisions between these neoplasms are sometimes blurred. Myeloid neoplasms, like other malignancies, tend to evolve over time to more aggressive forms of disease. In particular, both myelodysplastic syndromes and myeloproliferative disorders often "transform" to AML. In one of the most important myeloproliferative disorders, chronic myeloid leukemia, transformation to acute lymphoblastic leukemia is also seen, indicating that it originates from a transformed pluripotent hematopoietic stem cell.

Acute Myeloid Leukemia

Acute myeloid leukemia (AML) is a tumor of hematopoietic progenitors caused by acquired oncogenic mutations that impede differentiation, leading to the accumulation of immature myeloid blasts in the marrow. The arrest in myeloid development leads

TBALE 13–9	Clinical Staging of Hodgkin and Non-Hodgkin Lymphomas (Ann Arbor Classification)
Stage	**Distribution of Disease**
I	Involvement of a single lymph node region (I) or a single extra-lymphatic organ or site (IE).
II	Involvement of two or more lymph node regions on the same side of the diaphragm alone (II) or localized involvement of an extra-lymphatic organ or site (IIE).
III	Involvement of lymph node regions on both sides of the diaphragm without (III) or with (IIIE) localized involvement of an extra-lymphatic organ or site.
IV	Diffuse involvement of one or more extra-lymphatic organs or sites with or without lymphatic involvement.
All stages are further divided on the basis of the absence (A) or presence (B) of the following symptoms: unexplained fever, drenching night sweats, and/or unexplained weight loss of greater than 10% of normal body weight.	

Data from Carbone PT et al.: Symposium (Ann Arbor): Staging in Hodgkin's disease. Cancer Res 31:1707, 1971.

to marrow failure and complications related to anemia, thrombocytopenia, and neutropenia. AML occurs at all ages, but the incidence rises throughout life, peaking after 60 years of age. There are about 13,000 new cases each year in the United States.

Classification. AML is quite heterogeneous, reflecting the complexities of myeloid cell differentiation. A new proposed classification from the WHO subdivides AML into four categories (Table 13–10).[11] The first includes forms of AML that are associated with particular genetic aberrations, which are important because they correlate with prognosis and guide therapy. Also included are categories of AML arising after a myelodysplastic disorder (MDS) or with MDS-like features, and therapy-related AML. AMLs in these two categories have distinct genetic features and respond poorly to therapy. A fourth "wastebasket" category includes AMLs lacking any of these features. These are classified according to the earlier French-American-British (FAB) classification, which divide AMLs into subtypes based on the degree of differentiation and the lineage of the leukemic blasts. Although it has limited utility, the FAB classification is still commonly referred to in practice. In recognition of this, Table 13–10 correlates (to the extent possible) the FAB and WHO classifications. Given the increasing role of cytogenetic and molecular features in directing therapy, a further shift toward genetic classification of AML is both inevitable and desirable.

> **Morphology. The diagnosis of AML is based on the presence of at least 20% myeloid blasts in the bone marrow.** Several types of myeloid blasts are recognized, and individual tumors may have more than one type of blast or blasts with hybrid features. **Myeloblasts** have delicate nuclear chromatin, two to

TABLE 13–10 Major Subtypes of AML in the WHO Classification

Class	Prognosis	FAB Subtype	Morphology/Comments
I. AML WITH GENETIC ABERRATIONS			
AML with t(8;21)(q22;q22); CBFα/ETO fusion gene	Favorable	M2	Full range of myelocytic maturation; Auer rods easily found; abnormal cytoplasmic granules
AML with inv(16)(p13;q22); CBFβ/MYH11 fusion gene	Favorable	M4eo	Myelocytic and monocytic differentiation; abnormal eosinophilic precursors with abnormal basophilic granules
AML with t(15;17)(q22;11-12); RARα/PML fusion gene	Intermediate	M3, M3v	Numerous Auer rods, often in bundles within individual progranulocytes; primary granules usually very prominent (M3 subtype), but inconspicuous in microgranular variant (M3v); high incidence of DIC
AML with t(11q23;v); diverse MLL fusion genes	Poor	M4, M5	Usually some degree of monocytic differentiation
AML with normal cytogenetics and mutated NPM	Favorable	Variable	Detected by immunohistochemical staining for NPM
II. AML WITH MDS-LIKE FEATURES			
With prior MDS	Poor	Variable	Diagnosis based on clinical history
AML with multilineage dysplasia	Poor	Variable	Maturing cells with dysplastic features typical of MDS
AML with MDS-like cytogenetic aberrations	Poor	Variable	Associated with 5q-, 7q-, 20q-aberrations
III. AML, THERAPY-RELATED	Very poor	Variable	If following alkylator therapy or radiation therapy, 2- to 8-year latency period, MDS-like cytogenetic aberrations (e.g., 5q-, 7q-); if following topoisomerase II inhibitor (e.g., etoposide) therapy, 1- to 3-year latency, translocations involving MLL (11q23)
IV. AML, NOT OTHERWISE SPECIFIED			
AML, minimally differentiated	Intermediate	M0	Negative for myeloperoxidase; myeloid antigens detected on blasts by flow cytometry
AML without maturation	Intermediate	M1	>3% of blasts positive for myeloperoxidase
AML with myelocytic maturation	Intermediate	M2	Full range of myelocytic maturation
AML with myelomonocytic maturation	Intermediate	M4	Myelocytic and monocytic differentiation
AML with monocytic maturation	Intermediate	M5a, M5b	In M5a subtype, nonspecific esterase-positive monoblasts and pro-monocytes predominate in marrow and blood; in M5b subtype, mature monocytes predominate in the blood
AML with erythroid maturation	Intermediate	M6a, M6b	Erythroid/myeloid subtype (M6a) defined by >50% dysplastic maturing erythroid precursors and >20% myeloblasts; pure erythroid subtype (M6b) defined by >80% erythroid precursors without myeloblasts
AML with megakaryocytic maturation	Intermediate	M7	Blasts of megakaryocytic lineage predominate; detected with antibodies against megakaryocyte-specific markers (GPIIb/IIIa or vWF); often associated with marrow fibrosis; most common AML in Down syndrome

AML, acute myeloid leukemia; DIC, disseminated intravascular coagulation; MDS, myelodysplasia; NPM, nucleophosmin; vWF, von Willebrand factor.

marrow examination is essential to exclude acute leukemia in pancytopenic patients.

Immunophenotype. Because it can be difficult to distinguish myeloblasts and lymphoblasts morphologically, the diagnosis of AML is confirmed by performing stains for myeloid-specific antigens (see Fig. 13–29B,C).

Cytogenetics. *Cytogenetic analysis has a central role in the classification of AML.* Karyotypic aberrations are detected in 50% to 70% of cases with standard techniques and in approximately 90% of cases using special high-resolution banding. Particular chromosomal abnormalities correlate with certain clinical features. AMLs arising de novo in younger adults are commonly associated with balanced chromosomal translocations, particularly t(8;21), inv(16), and t(15;17). In contrast, AMLs following MDS or exposure to DNA-damaging agents (such as chemotherapy or radiation therapy) often have

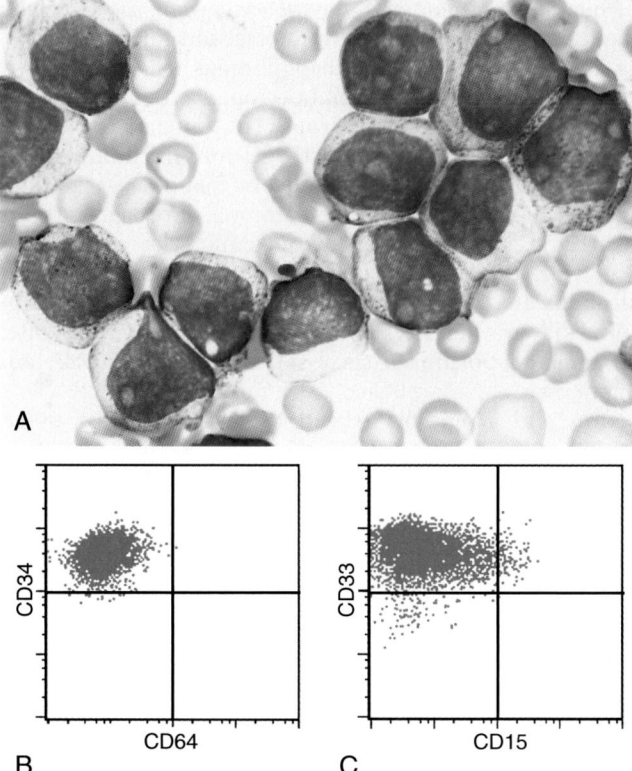

FIGURE 13–29 **A,** Acute myeloid leukemia without maturation (FAB M1 subtype). Myeloblasts have delicate nuclear chromatin, prominent nucleoli, and fine azurophilic granules in the cytoplasm. **B,** In the flow cytometric analysis shown, the myeloid blasts, represented by the red dots, express CD34, a marker of multipotent stem cells, but do not express CD64, a marker of mature myeloid cells. **C,** The same myeloid blasts express CD33, a marker of immature myeloid cells, and a subset express CD15, a marker of more mature myeloid cells. Thus, these blasts are myeloid cells showing limited maturation. (**A,** Courtesy of Dr. Robert W. McKenna Department of Pathology, University of Texas Southwestern Medical School, Dallas, TX; **B** and **C,** courtesy of Dr. Louis Picker, Oregon Health Science Center, Portland, OR.)

four nucleoli, and more voluminous cytoplasm than lymphoblasts (Fig. 13–29A). The cytoplasm often contains fine, peroxidase-positive azurophilic granules. **Auer rods**, distinctive needle-like azurophilic granules, are present in many cases; they are particularly numerous in AML with the t(15;17) (acute promyelocytic leukemia) (Fig. 13–30A). **Monoblasts** (Fig. 13–30B) have folded or lobulated nuclei, lack Auer rods, and are nonspecific esterase-positive. In some AMLs, blasts show megakaryocytic differentiation, which is often accompanied by marrow fibrosis caused by the release of fibrogenic cytokines. Rarely, the blasts of AML show erythroid differentiation.

The number of leukemic cells in the blood is highly variable. Blasts may be more than 100,000 per mm³, but are under 10,000 per mm³ in about 50% of patients. **Occasionally, blasts are entirely absent from the blood** (aleukemic leukemia). For this reason, a bone

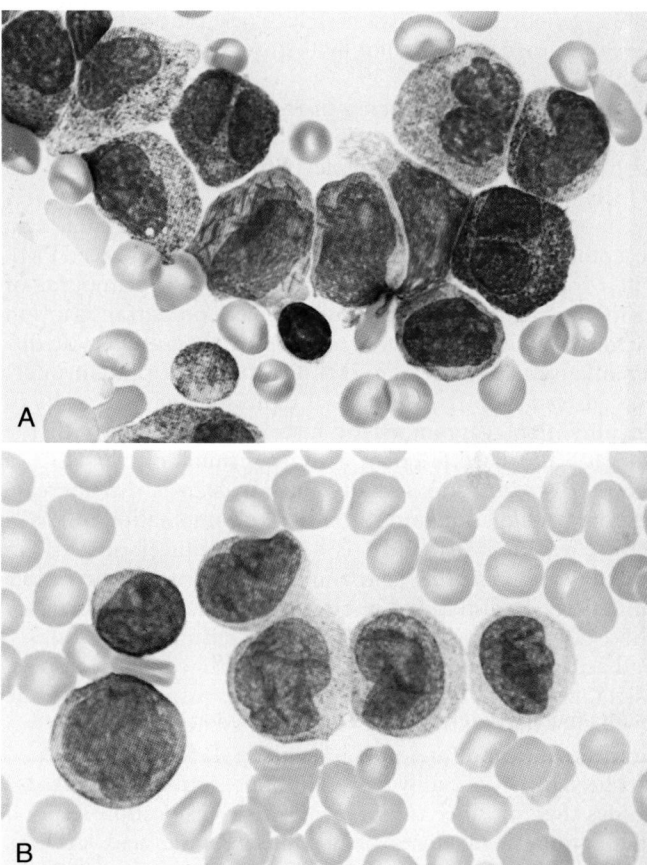

FIGURE 13–30 Acute myeloid leukemia subtypes. **A,** Acute promyelocytic leukemia with the t(15;17) (FAB M3 subtype). Bone marrow aspirate shows neoplastic promyelocytes with abnormally coarse and numerous azurophilic granules. Other characteristic findings include the presence of several cells with bilobed nuclei and a cell in the center of the field that contains multiple needle-like Auer rods. **B,** Acute myeloid leukemia with monocytic differentiation (FAB M5b subtype). Peripheral smear shows one monoblast and five promonocytes with folded nuclear membranes. (Courtesy of Dr. Robert W. McKenna, Department of Pathology, University of Texas Southwestern Medical School, Dallas, TX.)

deletions or monosomies involving chromosomes 5 and 7 and usually lack chromosomal translocations. The exception to this rule is AML occurring after treatment with topoisomerase II inhibitors, which is strongly associated with translocations involving the *MLL* gene on chromosome 11q23. AML in the elderly is also more likely to be associated with "bad" aberrations, such as deletions of chromosomes 5q and 7q.

Molecular Pathogenesis. *Many recurrent genetic aberrations seen in AML disrupt genes encoding transcription factors that are required for normal myeloid differentiation.* For example, the two most common chromosomal rearrangements, t(8;21) and inv(16), disrupt the *CBF1α* and *CBF1β* genes, respectively. These two genes encode polypeptides that bind one another to form a CBF1α/CBF1β transcription factor that is required for normal hematopoiesis.[55] The t(8;21) and the inv(16) create chimeric genes encoding fusion proteins that interfere with the function of CBF1α/CBF1β and block the maturation of myeloid cells. It should be noted, however, that "knockout" mice lacking either CBF1α or CBF1β and "knock-in" mice expressing the CBF1α or CBF1β fusion proteins succumb to hematopoietic failure, not leukemia. Thus, genetic lesions that merely block the maturation of myeloid progenitors are not by themselves sufficient to cause AML.

In line with this idea, *there is increasing evidence that mutated tyrosine kinases collaborate with transcription factor aberrations to produce AML.* One example is found in AML with the t(15;17), acute promyelocytic leukemia. The t(15;17) creates yet another fusion gene that encodes a part of the retinoic acid receptor-α (RARα) fused to a portion of a protein called PML (after the tumor). In the presence of physiologic amounts of retinoic acid, normal RARα interacts with other transcription factors to activate genes that are needed for granulocytic differentiation. However, the PML-RARα fusion protein interacts instead with transcriptional repressors, which results in an inhibition of granulocytic maturation.[56] AMLs with the t(15;17) also have frequent activating mutations in FLT3, a receptor tyrosine kinase that transmits signals that increase cellular proliferation and survival. The combination of PML-RARα and activated FLT3 is a potent inducer of AML in mice,[57] whereas neither gene alone is sufficient. Identical FLT3 mutations are also found in other forms of AML, particularly those associated with *NPM* (nucleophosmin) mutations,[58] and activating mutations in another tyrosine kinase receptor, c-KIT, are found in about 25% of AMLs associated with the inv(16) or the t(8;21).[59] Thus, aberrant tyrosine kinase activation is a common (and possibly universal) feature of AML.

The t(15;17) not only has pathogenic significance, but also guides therapy, since tumors with this translocation respond to pharmacologic doses of all-*trans* retinoic acid (ATRA). ATRA binds to the PML-RARα fusion protein and antagonizes its inhibitory effect on the transcription of target genes. Remarkably, the resulting activation of transcription overcomes the block in differentiation, and within 1 to 2 days the neoplastic promyelocytes begin to differentiate into neutrophils, which rapidly die. The response to ATRA proves that the major effect of PML-RARα is to block differentiation, and stands as one of the most successful uses of a targeted therapy in a human cancer.

Clinical Features. *Most patients present within weeks or a few months of the onset of symptoms with complaints related to* anemia, neutropenia, and thrombocytopenia, *most notably fatigue, fever, and spontaneous mucosal and cutaneous bleeding.* You will remember that these findings are very similar to those produced by ALL. Thrombocytopenia results in a bleeding diathesis, which is often prominent. Cutaneous petechiae and ecchymoses, serosal hemorrhages into the linings of the body cavities and viscera, and mucosal hemorrhages into the gingivae and urinary tract are common. Procoagulants and fibrinolytic factors released by leukemic cells, especially in AML with the t(15;17), exacerbate the bleeding tendency. Infections are frequent, particularly in the oral cavity, skin, lungs, kidneys, urinary bladder, and colon, and are often caused by opportunists such as fungi, *Pseudomonas*, and commensals.

Signs and symptoms related to involvement of tissues other than the marrow are usually less striking in AML than in ALL, but tumors with monocytic differentiation often infiltrate the skin (leukemia cutis) and the gingiva; this probably reflects the normal tendency of monocytes to extravasate into tissues. Central nervous system spread is less common than in ALL. AML occasionally presents as a localized soft-tissue mass known variously as a myeloblastoma, granulocytic sarcoma, or chloroma. Without systemic treatment, such tumors inevitably progress to full-blown AML over time.

Prognosis. AML is a difficult disease to treat. About 60% of patients achieve complete remission with chemotherapy, but only 15% to 30% remain free of disease for 5 years. AMLs with t(8;21) or inv(16) have a relatively good prognosis with conventional chemotherapy, particularly in the absence of c-KIT mutations.[59] In contrast, the prognosis is dismal for AMLs that follow MDS or genotoxic therapy, or that occur in the elderly, possibly because in these contexts the disease arises out of a background of hematopoietic stem cell damage or depletion. These "high-risk" forms of AML (as well as relapsed AML of all types) are treated with bone marrow transplantation when possible.

It is hoped that new approaches based on a better understanding of molecular pathogenesis will improve this situation. The best current example is AML with the t(15;17), which (as we have discussed) is treated with pharmacologic doses of ATRA combined with conventional chemotherapy, or, more recently, with arsenic salts, which appear to cause PML-RARα to be degraded. New therapies that target other molecular lesions in AML (e.g., the activated FLT3 and c-KIT tyrosine kinases) are being evaluated.

Myelodysplastic Syndromes

The term "myelodysplastic syndrome" (MDS) refers to a group of clonal stem cell disorders characterized by maturation defects that are associated with ineffective hematopoiesis and a high risk of transformation to AML. In MDS the bone marrow is partly or wholly replaced by the clonal progeny of a neoplastic multipotent stem cell that retains the capacity to differentiate but does so in an ineffective and disordered fashion. These abnormal cells stay within the bone marrow and hence the patients have peripheral blood cytopenias.

MDS may be either primary (idiopathic) or secondary to previous genotoxic drug or radiation therapy (t-MDS). t-MDS usually appears from 2 to 8 years after the genotoxic

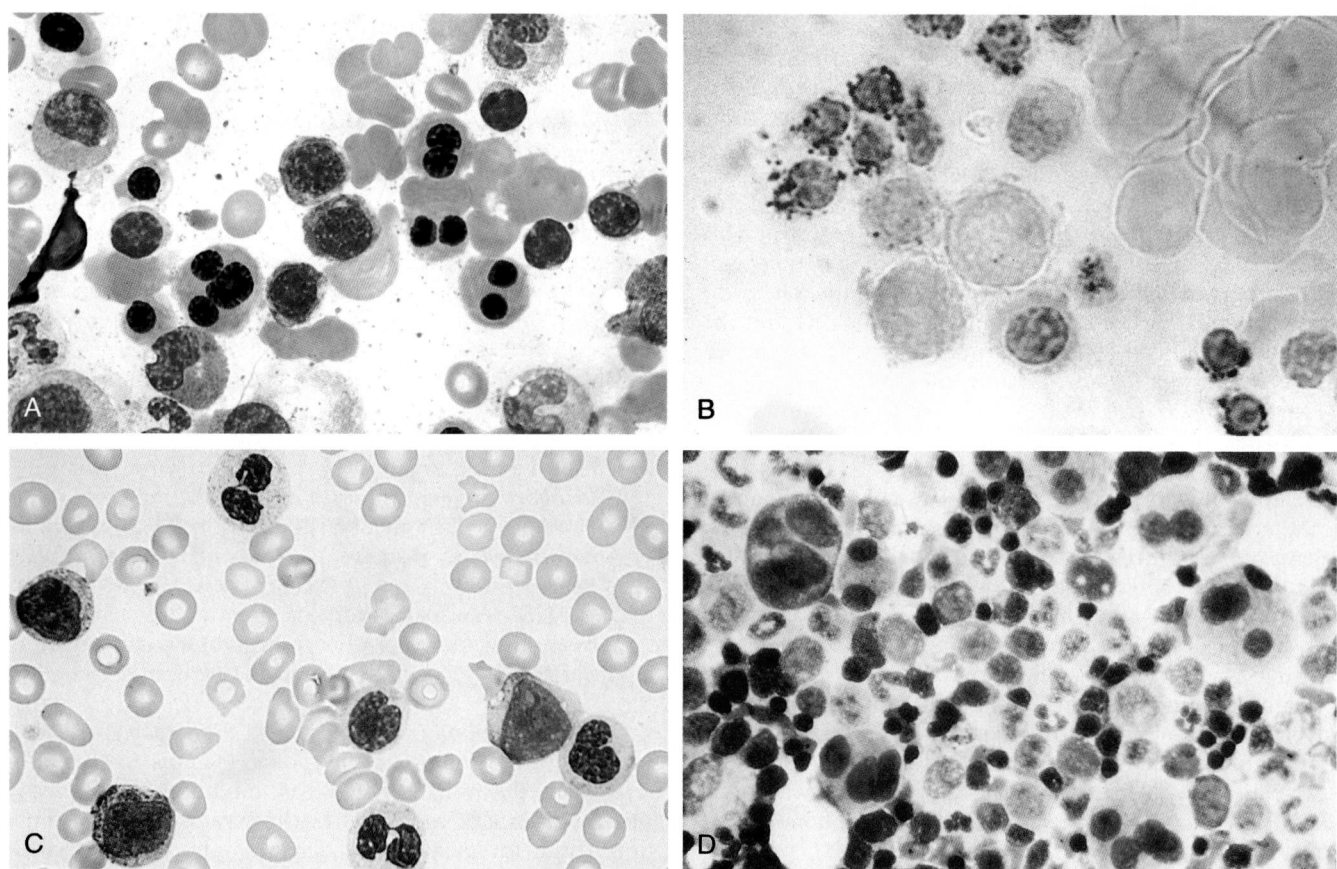

FIGURE 13–31 Myelodysplasia. Characteristic forms of dysplasia are shown. **A,** Nucleated red cell progenitors with multilobated or multiple nuclei. **B,** Ringed sideroblasts, erythroid progenitors with iron-laden mitochondria seen as blue perinuclear granules (Prussian blue stain). **C,** Pseudo-Pelger-Hüet cells, neutrophils with only two nuclear lobes instead of the normal three to four, are observed at the top and bottom of this field. **D,** Megakaryocytes with multiple nuclei instead of the normal single multilobated nucleus. (**A, B, D,** Marrow aspirates; **C,** peripheral blood smear.)

exposure. All forms of MDS can transform to AML, but transformation occurs with highest frequency and most rapidly in t-MDS. Although characteristic morphologic changes are typically seen in the marrow and the peripheral blood, the diagnosis frequently requires correlation with other laboratory tests. Cytogenetic analysis is particularly helpful, since certain chromosomal aberrations (discussed below) are often observed.

Molecular Pathogenesis. The pathogenesis is poorly understood.[60] In MDS, bone marrow progenitors undergo apoptotic cell death at an increased rate, the hallmark of ineffective hematopoiesis. Given this, it is difficult to understand how MDS progenitors gain a selective advantage over any remaining normal marrow progenitors, suggesting that the tumor may arise out of a background of stem cell damage or depletion. Both primary MDS and t-MDS are associated with similar clonal chromosomal abnormalities, including monosomies 5 and 7, deletions of 5q, 7q, and 20q, and trisomy 8.

Morphology. Although the marrow is usually hypercellular at diagnosis, it is sometimes normocellular or, less commonly, hypocellular. The most characteristic finding is disordered (dysplastic) differentiation affecting the erythroid, granulocytic, monocytic, and mega-

karyocytic lineages to varying degrees (Fig. 13–31). Within the erythroid series, common abnormalities include **ringed sideroblasts**, erythroblasts with iron-laden mitochondria visible as perinuclear granules in Prussian blue–stained aspirates or biopsies; **megaloblastoid maturation**, resembling that seen in vitamin B_{12} and folate deficiency (Chapter 14); and **nuclear budding abnormalities**, recognized as nuclei with misshapen, often polyploid, outlines. Neutrophils frequently contain decreased numbers of secondary granules, toxic granulations, and/or Döhle bodies. **Pseudo-Pelger-Hüet cells**, neutrophils with only two nuclear lobes, are commonly observed, and neutrophils are seen occasionally that completely lack nuclear segmentation. Megakaryocytes with single nuclear lobes or multiple separate nuclei **(pawn ball megakaryocytes)** are also characteristic. **Myeloid blasts** may be increased but make up less than 20% of the overall marrow cellularity. The blood often contains pseudo-Pelger-Hüet cells, giant platelets, macrocytes, and poikilocytes, accompanied by a relative or absolute monocytosis. Myeloid blasts usually make up less than 10% of the leukocytes in the blood.

Clinical Course. Primary MDS is predominantly a disease of the elderly; the mean age of onset is 70 years. In up to half of the cases, it is discovered incidentally on routine blood testing. When symptomatic, it presents with weakness, infections, and hemorrhages, all due to pancytopenia.

Primary MDS is divided into five morphologic categories in the WHO classification,[11] details of which are beyond our scope. Subtypes defined by having a higher proportion of blasts are associated with more severe cytopenias, an increased risk of progression to AML, and a worse prognosis. The presence of multiple clonal chromosomal abnormalities and the severity of peripheral blood cytopenias are independent risk factors also portending a worse outcome.

The median survival in primary MDS varies from 9 to 29 months, but some individuals in good prognostic groups may live for 5 years or more. Overall, progression to AML occurs in 10% to 40% of individuals and is usually accompanied by the appearance of additional cytogenetic abnormalities. Patients often succumb to the complications of thrombocytopenia (bleeding) and neutropenia (infection). The outlook is even grimmer in t-MDS, which has a median survival of only 4 to 8 months. In t-MDS, cytopenias tend to be more severe and progression to AML is often rapid.

Treatment options are fairly limited. In younger patients, allogeneic bone marrow transplantation offers hope for reconstitution of normal hematopoiesis and long-term survival. Older patients with MDS are treated supportively with antibiotics and blood product transfusions. Thalidomide-like drugs (which appear to alter the interaction of MDS progenitors with bone marrow stromal cells) and DNA methylase inhibitors improve the effectiveness of hematopoiesis and the peripheral blood counts in a subset of patients.[60]

Myeloproliferative Disorders

The common pathogenic feature of the myeloproliferative disorders is the presence of mutated, constitutively activated tyrosine kinases.[61,62] Hematopoietic growth factors act on normal progenitors by binding to surface receptors and activating tyrosine kinases, which turn on pathways that promote growth and survival. *The mutated tyrosine kinases found in the myeloproliferative disorders circumvent normal controls and lead to the growth factor–independent proliferation and survival of marrow progenitors.* Because the tyrosine kinase mutations underlying the various myeloproliferative disorders do not impair differentiation, the most common consequence is an increase in the production of one or more mature blood elements. Most myeloproliferative disorders originate in multipotent myeloid progenitors, whereas others arise in pluripotent stem cells that give rise to both lymphoid and myeloid cells.

There is a considerable degree of clinical and morphologic overlap among the myeloproliferative disorders. The common features include

- *Increased proliferative drive* in the bone marrow
- Homing of the neoplastic stem cells to secondary hematopoietic organs, producing *extramedullary hematopoiesis*
- Variable transformation to a spent phase characterized by marrow fibrosis and peripheral blood *cytopenias*
- Variable transformation to *acute leukemia*

Certain myeloproliferative disorders are strongly associated with activating mutations in specific tyrosine kinases. This insight and the availability of kinase inhibitors have increased the importance of molecular tests for tyrosine kinase mutations, both for purposes of diagnosis and the selection of therapy. We will confine our discussion to the more common myeloproliferative disorders, which are classified based on clinical, laboratory, and molecular criteria. Systemic mastocytosis, a distinctive myeloproliferative disorder that is associated with mutations in the c-KIT tyrosine kinase, is discussed under disorders of the skin (Chapter 25). The association of various myeloproliferative disorders with specific tyrosine kinase mutations (including several too rare to merit discussion) is summarized in Table 13–11.

TABLE 13–11	Tyrosine Kinase Mutations in Myeloproliferative Disorders		
Disorder	**Mutation**	**Frequency**[¶]	**Consequences***
Chronic myeloid leukemia	*BCR-ABL* fusion gene	100%	Constitutive ABL kinase activation[†]
Polycythemia vera	*JAK2* point mutations	>95%	Constitutive JAK2 kinase activation
Essential thrombocythemia	*JAK2* point muations *MPL* point mutations	50% to 60% 5% to 10%	Constitutive JAK2 kinase activation Constitutive MPL kinase activation
Primary myelofibrosis	*JAK2* point mutations *MPL* point mutations	50% to 60% 5% to 10%	Constitutive JAK2 kinase activation Constitutive MPL kinase activation
Systemic mastocytosis	*c-KIT* point mutations	>90%	Constitutive c-KIT kinase activation
Chronic eosinophilic leukemia[‖]	*FIP1L1-PDGFRα* fusion gene *PDE4DIP-PDGFRβ* fusion gene	Common Rare	Constitutive PDGFRα kinase activation Constitutive PDGFRβ kinase activation[†]
Stem cell leukemia[‡]	Various *FGFR1* fusion genes	100%	Constitutive FGFR1 kinase activation[§]

*All stimulate ligand-independent pro-growth and survival signals.
[†]Responds to imatinib therapy.
[‡]Rare disorder originating in pluripotent hematopoietic stem cells that presents with concomitant myeloproliferative disorder and lymphoblastic leukemia/lymphoma.
[§]Responds to PKC412 therapy.
[¶]Refers to frequency within a diagnostic category.
[‖]Associated with Loefflers endocarditis (Chapter 12).

Chronic Myeloid Leukemia

Chronic myeloid leukemia (CML) is distinguished from other myeloproliferative disorders by the presence of a chimeric BCR-ABL gene derived from portions of the BCR gene on chromosome 22 and the ABL gene on chromosome 9. BCR-ABL directs the synthesis of a constitutively active BCR-ABL tyrosine kinase (Fig. 13–32),[63] *which in CML is usually 210 kDa in size. In more than 90% of cases, BCR-ABL is created by a reciprocal (9;22)(q34;q11) translocation (the so-called Philadelphia chromosome [Ph]). In the remaining cases the BCR-ABL fusion gene is formed by cytogenetically complex or cryptic rearrangments and must be detected by other methods, such as fluorescence in situ hybridization or PCR-based tests. The cell of origin is a pluripotent hematopoietic stem cell.*

Molecular Pathogenesis. Tyrosine kinases are normally regulated by ligand-mediated dimerization and autophosphorylation, which creates an activated kinase capable of phosphorylating other protein substrates (discussed in Chapters 3 and 7). The BCR moiety of BCR-ABL contains a dimerization domain that self-associates, leading to the activation of the ABL tyrosine kinase moiety. The ABL kinase in turn phosphorylates proteins that induce signaling through the

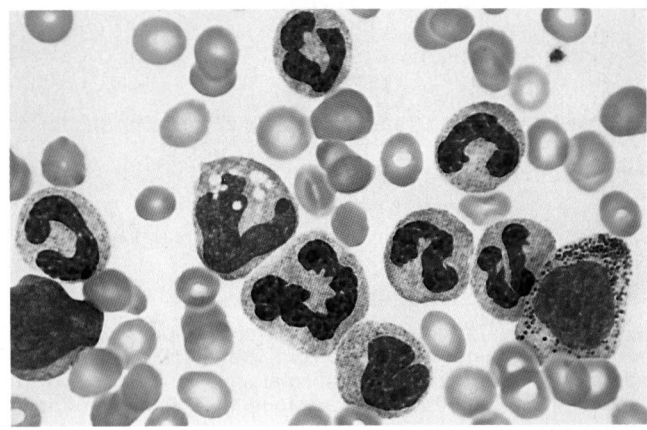

FIGURE 13–33 Chronic myeloid leukemia. Peripheral blood smear shows many mature neutrophils, some metamyelocytes, and a myelocyte. (Courtesy of Dr. Robert W. McKenna, Department of Pathology, University of Texas Southwestern Medical School, Dallas, TX.)

same pro-growth and pro-survival pathways that are turned on by hematopoietic growth factors, including the RAS, JAK/STAT, and AKT pathways. For unknown reasons, BCR-ABL preferentially drives the proliferation of granulocytic and megakaryocytic progenitors, and also causes the abnormal release of immature granulocytic forms from the marrow into the blood.

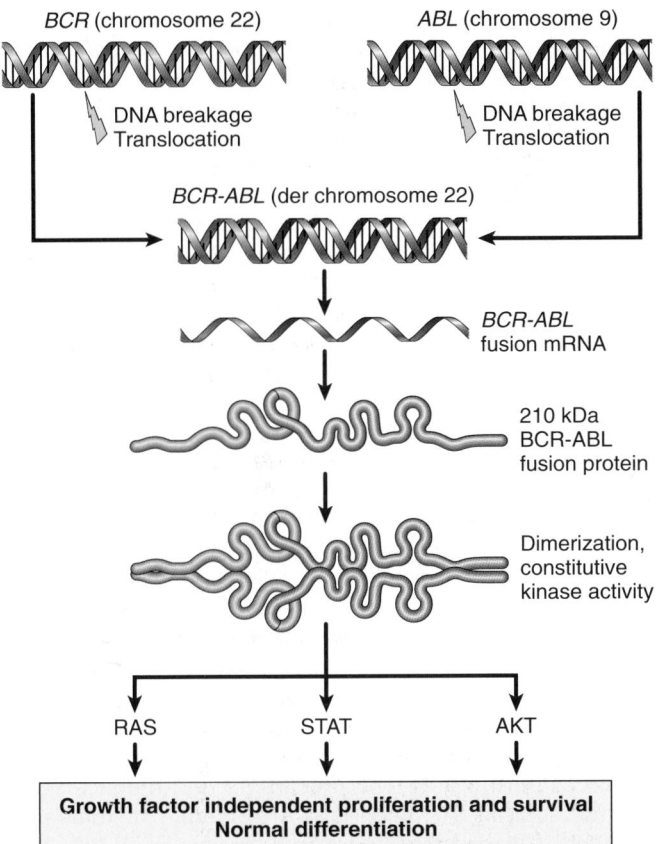

FIGURE 13–32 Molecular pathogenesis of chronic myeloid leukemia. Breakage and joining of *BCR* and *ABL* creates a chimeric *BCR-ABL* fusion gene that encodes a constitutively active BCR-ABL tyrosine kinase. BCR-ABL activates multiple downstream pathways, which drive growth factor–independent proliferation and survival of bone marrow progenitors. Because BCR-ABL does not interfere with differentiation, the net result is an increase in mature elements in the peripheral blood, particularly granulocytes and platelets.

Morphology. The marrow is markedly **hypercellular** because of massively increased numbers of maturing granulocytic precursors, which usually include an elevated proportion of eosinophils and basophils. Megakaryocytes are also increased and usually include small, dysplastic forms. Erythroid progenitors are present in normal or mildly decreased numbers. A characteristic finding is the presence of scattered macrophages with abundant wrinkled, green-blue cytoplasm so-called sea-blue histiocytes. Increased deposition of reticulin is typical, but overt marrow fibrosis is rare early in the course. The blood reveals a **leukocytosis, often exceeding 100,000 cells/mm³** (Fig. 13–33), which consists predominantly of neutrophils, band forms, metamyelocytes, myelocytes, eosinophils, and basophils. Blasts usually make up less than 10% of the circulating cells. Platelets are also usually increased, sometimes markedly. The spleen is often greatly enlarged as a result of extensive extramedullary hematopoiesis (Fig. 13–34) and often contains infarcts of varying age. Extramedullary hematopoiesis can also produce mild hepatomegaly and lymphadenopathy.

Clinical Features. CML is primarily a disease of adults but also occurs in children and adolescents. The peak incidence is in the fifth to sixth decades of life. There are about 4500 new cases per year in the United States.

The onset is insidious. Mild-to-moderate anemia and hypermetabolism due to increased cell turnover lead to fatigability, weakness, weight loss, and anorexia. Sometimes the first symptom is a dragging sensation in the abdomen caused by splenomegaly, or the acute onset of left upper quadrant

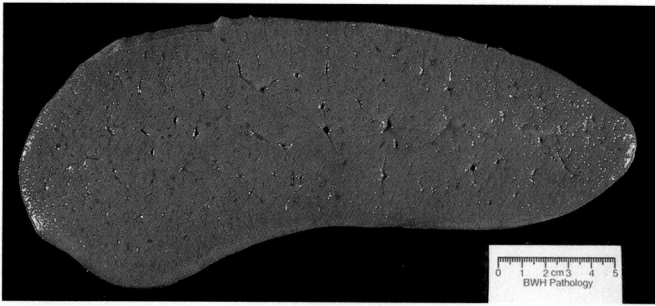

FIGURE 13–34 Chronic myeloid leukemia (spleen). Enlarged spleen (2630 gm; normal: 150–200 gm) with greatly expanded red pulp stemming from neoplastic hematopoiesis. (Courtesy of Dr. Daniel Jones, Department of Pathology, M.D. Anderson Cancer Center, Houston, TX.)

pain due to splenic infarction. CML is best differentiated from other myeloproliferative disorders by detection of the *BCR-ABL* fusion gene through either chromosomal analysis or PCR-based tests.

The natural history is one of slow progression; even without treatment, the median survival is about 3 years. After a variable period averaging 3 years, about 50% of patients enter an "accelerated phase" marked by increasing anemia and thrombocytopenia, sometimes accompanied by a rise in the number of basophils in the blood. Additional clonal cytogenetic abnormalities, such as trisomy 8, isochromosome 17q, or duplication of the Ph chromosome, often appear. Within 6 to 12 months, the accelerated phase terminates in a picture resembling acute leukemia (*blast crisis*). In the other 50% of patients, blast crises occur abruptly without an accelerated phase. In 70% of crises, the blasts are of myeloid origin (myeloid blast crisis), whereas in most of the remainder the blasts are of pre–B cell origin (lymphoid blast crisis). This is taken as evidence that CML orginates from a pluripotent stem cell with both myeloid and lymphoid potential. Recently, it has been observed that in greater than 85% of cases CML is associated with the appearance of mutations that interfere with the activity of Ikaros, a transcription factor that regulates the differentiation of hematopoietic progenitors.[64] The same types of Ikaros mutations are also seen in BCR-ABL-positive ALL, suggesting that these two varieties of aggressive leukemia have a similar pathogenic basis.

Understanding of the molecular pathogenesis of CML has led to the use of drugs that target BCR-ABL. Treatment with one BCR-ABL inhibitor, imatinib, results in sustained hematologic remissions in greater than 90% of patients, with few side effects.[65] Imatinib markedly decreases the number of BCR-ABL-positive cells in the marrow and elsewhere, but does not extinguish the CML "stem cell," a primitive cell that resembles a normal hematopoietic stem cell. As a result, it is not clear if imatinib is ever truly curative. However, imatinib therapy controls blood counts and substantially decreases the risk of transformation to the accelerated phase and blast crisis, which is the greatest threat to the patient. It is thought that by lowering the proliferative drive of the BCR-ABL-positive progenitors, imatinib decreases the rate at which these cells acquire mutations that lead to disease progression.[66] For relatively young patients, allogeneic bone marrow transplantation performed in the stable phase is curative in about 75% of cases

and remains the treatment of choice. The outlook is much more dire once the accelerated phase or blast crisis supervenes. Transplantation is not as effective, and (as in BCR-ABL-positive ALL) the disease rapidly becomes resistant to BCR-ABL inhibitors.

Polycythemia Vera

Polycythemia vera (PCV) is characterized by increased marrow production of red cells, granulocytes, and platelets (panmyelosis), but it is the increase in red cells (polycythemia) that is responsible for most of the clinical symptoms. PCV must be differentiated from relative polycythemia resulting from hemoconcentration and other causes of absolute polycythemia (discussed in Chapter 14). *PCV is strongly associated with activating point mutations in the tyrosine kinase JAK2.*[61,62] JAK2 participates in the JAK/STAT pathway, which lies downstream of multiple hematopoietic growth factor receptors, including the erythropoietin receptor.

Molecular Pathogenesis. In PCV the progenitor cells have markedly decreased requirements for erythropoietin and other hematopoietic growth factors due to constitutive JAK2 signaling. Accordingly, serum erythropoietin levels in PCV are very low, whereas secondary forms of absolute polycythemia have high erythropoietin levels. The elevated hematocrit leads to increased blood viscosity and sludging. These hemodynamic factors, together with thrombocytosis and abnormal platelet function, make patients with PCV prone to both thrombosis and bleeding.

More than 97% of cases are associated with a mutation in *JAK2* that results in a valine-to-phenylalanine substitution at residue 617; other *JAK2* mutations are found in most (and perhaps all) of the remaining cases. The mutated forms of JAK2 found in PCV render hematopoietic cell lines growth factor–independent, and when expressed in murine bone marrow progenitors cause a PCV-like syndrome that is associated with marrow fibrosis.[61,62] In 25% to 30% of cases the tumor cells contain two mutated copies of *JAK2*, a homozygous genotype that is associated with higher white cell counts, more significant splenomegaly, symptomatic pruritus, and a greater rate of progression to the spent phase.[67]

The proliferative drive in PCV (and other myeloproliferative disorders associated with JAK2 mutations) is less than in CML, which is associated with more pronounced marrow hypercellularity, leukocytosis, and splenomegaly. Presumably, JAK2 signals are quantitatively weaker or qualitatively different from those produced by BCR-ABL (see Fig. 13–32).

Morphology. The marrow is hypercellular, but some residual fat is usually present. The increase in red cell progenitors is subtle and usually accompanied by an increase in granulocytic precursors and megakaryocytes as well. At diagnosis, a moderate to marked increase in reticulin fibers is seen in about 10% of marrows. Mild organomegaly is common, being caused early in the course largely by congestion; at this stage extramedullary hematopoiesis is minimal. The peripheral blood often contains increased numbers of basophils and abnormally large platelets.

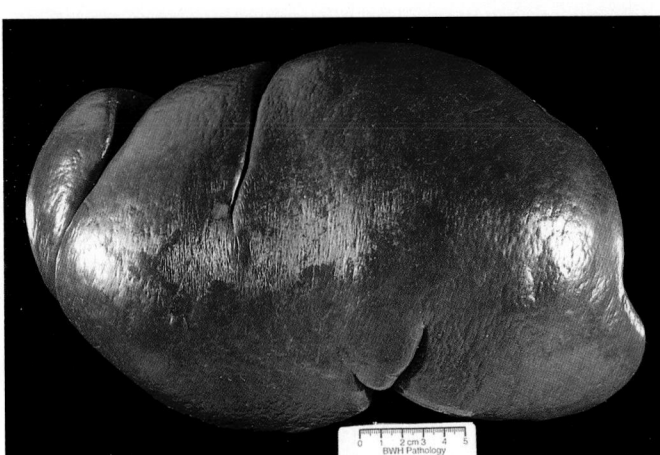

FIGURE 13–35 Polycythemia vera, spent phase. Massive spleno-megaly (3020 gm; normal: 150–200 gm) largely due to extramedullary hematopoiesis occurring in the setting of advanced marrow myelofibrosis. (Courtesy of Dr. Mark Fleming, Department of Pathology, Children's Hospital, Boston, MA.)

Late in the course, PCV often progresses to a spent phase characterized by extensive marrow fibrosis that displaces hematopoietic cells. This is accompanied by increased extramedullary hematopoiesis in the spleen and liver, often leading to prominent organomegaly (Fig. 13–35). Transformation to AML, with its typical features, occurs in about 1% of patients.

Clinical Features. PCV is uncommon, having an incidence of 1 to 3 per 100,000 per year. It appears insidiously, usually in adults of late middle age. *Most symptoms are related to the increased red cell mass and hematocrit.* Usually, there is also an increased total blood volume. Together, these factors cause abnormal blood flow, particularly on the low-pressure venous side of the circulation, which becomes greatly distended. Patients are plethoric and cyanotic due to stagnation and deoxygenation of blood in peripheral vessels. Headache, dizziness, hypertension, and gastrointestinal symptoms are common. Intense pruritus and peptic ulceration may occur, both possibly resulting from the release of histamine from basophils. High cell turnover gives rise to hyperuricemia; symptomatic gout is seen in 5% to 10% of cases.

More ominously, the abnormal blood flow and platelet function lead to an increased risk of both major bleeding and thrombotic episodes. About 25% of patients first come to attention due to deep venous thrombosis, myocardial infarction, or stroke. Thromboses sometimes also occur in the hepatic veins (producing Budd-Chiari syndrome) and the portal and mesenteric veins (leading to bowel infarction). It should be remembered that thrombotic complications sometimes precede the appearance of the typical hematologic findings.[68] Minor hemorrhages (epistaxis, bleeding gums) are common, and life-threatening hemorrhages occur in 5% to 10% of cases.

The hemoglobin concentration ranges from 14 to 28 gm/dL, and the hematocrit is usually 60% or more. Sometimes chronic bleeding leads to iron deficiency, which can suppress erythropoiesis sufficiently to lower the hematocrit into the

normal range, an example of two defects counteracting one another to "correct" a laboratory abnormality. The white cell count ranges from 12,000 to 50,000 cells/mm³, and the platelet count is often greater than 500,000 platelets/mm³. The platelets usually exhibit morphologic abnormalities such as giant forms and are often defective in functional aggregation studies.

Without treatment, death from bleeding or thrombosis occurs within months of diagnosis. However, simply maintaining the red cell mass at nearly normal levels by phlebotomy extends the median survival to about 10 years. JAK2 inhibitors are in preclinical development and represent a promising form of targeted therapy.

Extended survival with treatment has revealed that *PCV tends to evolve to a "spent phase," during which clinical and anatomic features of primary myelofibrosis develop.* The disease undergoes this transition in about 15% to 20% of patients after an average period of 10 years. It is marked by the appearance of obliterative fibrosis in the bone marrow (myelofibrosis) and extensive extramedullary hematopoiesis, principally in the spleen, which enlarges greatly. The mechanisms underlying the progression to the spent phase are not known.

In about 2% of patients, PCV transforms to AML. Surprisingly, the AML clone often lacks *JAK2* mutations,[69] suggesting that *JAK2* mutations are late secondary events, rather than early initiators of PCV. Unlike CML, transformation to ALL is rarely observed, consistent with the cell of origin being a progenitor committed to myeloid differentiation.

Essential Thrombocytosis

Essential thrombocytosis (ET) is often associated with activating point mutations in JAK2 (50% of cases) or MPL (5–10% of cases), a receptor tyrosine kinase that is normally activated by thrombopoietin.[61] It manifests clinically with elevated platelet counts and is separated from PCV and primary myelofibrosis based on the absence of polycythemia and marrow fibrosis, respectively. In those cases without tyrosine kinase mutations, causes of reactive thrombocytosis, such as inflammatory disorders and iron deficiency, must be excluded before the diagnosis can be established.

Constitutive JAK2 or MPL signaling renders the progenitors thrombopoietin-independent and leads to hyperproliferation. The *JAK2* mutation is the same as that found in almost all cases of PCV. Why some patients with *JAK2* mutations present with PCV and others with ET is not understood. Some cases of "ET" may in fact be PCV disguised by iron deficiency (which is more common in individuals diagnosed with ET), but this is probably true of only a small fraction of patients. Mutations in other tyrosine kinases are being sought in those cases in which *JAK2* and *MPL* are apparently normal.

Bone marrow cellularity is usually only mildly increased, but megakaryocytes are often markedly increased in number and include abnormally large forms. Delicate reticulin fibrils are often seen, but the overt fibrosis of primary myelofibrosis (see below) is absent. *Peripheral smears usually reveal abnormally large platelets* (Fig. 13–36), often accompanied by mild leukocytosis. Modest degrees of extramedullary hematopoiesis may occur, producing mild organomegaly in about 50% of patients. Uncommonly, a spent phase of marrow fibrosis or transformation to AML supervenes.

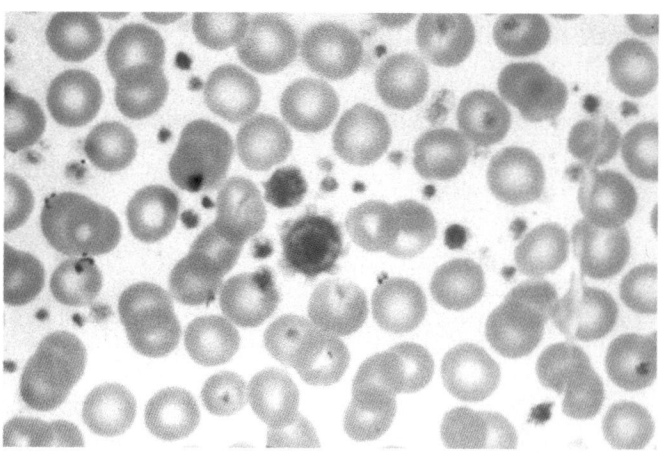

FIGURE 13–36 Essential thrombocytosis. Peripheral blood smear shows marked thrombocytosis, including giant platelets approximating the size of surrounding red cells.

The incidence of ET is 1 to 3 per 100,000 per year. It usually occurs past the age of 60 but may also be seen in young adults. *Dysfunctions of platelets derived from the neoplastic clone can lead to thrombosis and hemorrhage,* the major clinical manifestations. Platelets are not only increased in numbers but also frequently demonstrate qualitative abnormalities in functional tests. The types of thrombotic events resemble those observed in PCV; they include deep venous thrombosis, portal and hepatic vein thrombosis, and myocardial infarction. One characteristic symptom is *erythromelalgia,* a throbbing and burning of hands and feet caused by occlusion of small arterioles by platelet aggregates, which may also be seen in PCV.

ET is an indolent disorder with long asymptomatic periods punctuated by occasional thrombotic or hemorrhagic crises. Median survival times are 12 to 15 years. Thrombotic complications are most likely in patients with very high platelet counts and homozygous *JAK2* mutations.[67] Therapy consists of "gentle" chemotherapeutic agents that suppress thrombopoiesis.

Primary Myelofibrosis

The hallmark of primary myelofibrosis is the development of obliterative marrow fibrosis. The replacement of the marrow by fibrosis suppresses bone marrow hematopoiesis, leading to cytopenias and extensive neoplastic extramedullary hematopoiesis. Histologically, the appearance is identical to the spent phase that occurs occasionally late in the course of other myeloproliferative disorders. This similarity also extends to the underlying molecular pathogenesis.

Molecular Pathogenesis. *Activating JAK2 mutations are present in 50% to 60% of cases and activating MPL mutations in an additional 1% to 5% of cases.*[61] The chief pathologic feature is the extensive deposition of collagen in the marrow by non-neoplastic fibroblasts. The fibrosis inexorably displaces hematopoietic elements, including stem cells, from the marrow and eventually leads to marrow failure. It is probably caused by the inappropriate release of fibrogenic factors from neoplastic megakaryocytes. Two factors synthesized by megakaryocytes have been implicated: platelet-derived growth factor and TGF-β. As you recall, platelet-derived growth factor and TGF-β are fibroblast mitogens. In addition, TGF-β promotes collagen deposition and causes angiogenesis, both of which are observed in myelofibrosis. As marrow fibrosis progresses, circulating hematopoietic stem cells take up residence in niches in secondary hematopoietic organs, such as the spleen, the liver, and the lymph nodes, leading to the appearance of extramedullary hematopoiesis. For incompletely understood reasons, blood cell production at extramedullary sites is disordered. This factor and the concomitant suppression of marrow function result in moderate to severe cytopenias. It is not clear whether primary myelofibrosis (particularly when associated with *JAK2* or *MPL* mutations) is truly distinct from PCV and ET, or merely reflects unusually rapid progression of these MPDs to the spent phase.[61]

Morphology. Early in the course, the marrow is often hypercellular due to increases in maturing cells of all lineages, a feature reminiscent of PCV. Morphologically, the erythroid and granulocytic precursors appear normal, but megakaryocytes are large, dysplastic, and abnormally clustered. At this stage fibrosis is minimal, and the blood may show leukocytosis and thrombocytosis. With progression, the marrow becomes more hypocellular and diffusely fibrotic. Clusters of atypical megakaryocytes are seen, and hematopoietic elements are often found within dilated sinusoids, which is a manifestation of severe architectural distortion cause by the fibrosis. Very late in the course, the fibrotic marrow space may be converted into bone, a change called "osteosclerosis." These features are identical to those seen in the spent phase of other myeloproliferative disorders.

Fibrotic obliteration of the marrow space leads to extensive extramedullary hematopoiesis, principally in the spleen, which is usually markedly enlarged, sometimes up to 4000 gm. Grossly, such spleens are firm and diffusely red to gray. As in CML, subcapsular infarcts are common (see Fig. 13–40). Initially, extramedullary hematopoiesis is confined to the sinusoids, but later it expands into the cords. The **liver** may be enlarged moderately by sinusoidal foci of extramedullary hematopoiesis. Hematopoiesis can also appear within lymph nodes, but significant lymphadenopathy is uncommon.

The marrow fibrosis is reflected in several characteristic blood findings (Fig. 13–37). Marrow distortion leads to the premature release of nucleated erythroid and early granulocyte progenitors (**leukoerythroblastosis**), and immature cells also enter the circulation from sites of extramedullary hematopoiesis. **Teardrop-shaped red cells** (dacryocytes), cells that were probably damaged during the birthing process in the fibrotic marrow, are also often seen. Although characteristic of primary myelofibrosis, leukoerythroblastosis and teardrop red cells are seen in many infiltrative disorders of the marrow, including granulomatous diseases and metastatic tumors. Other common, albeit nonspecific, blood findings include abnormally large platelets and basophilia.

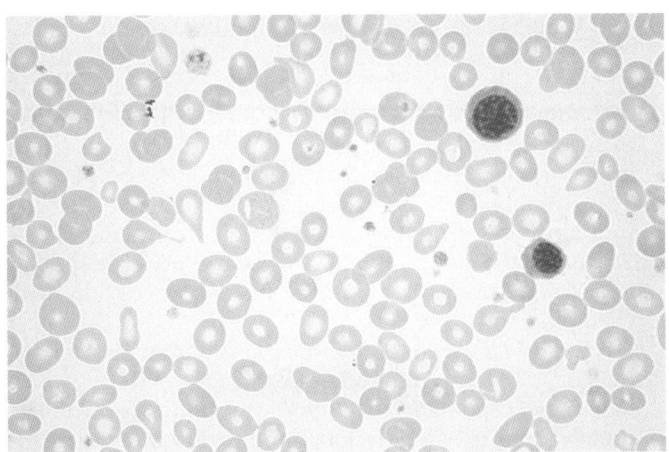

FIGURE 13–37 Primary myelofibrosis (peripheral blood smear). Two nucleated erythroid precursors and several teardrop-shaped red cells (dacryocytes) are evident. Immature myeloid cells were present in other fields. An identical picture can be seen in other diseases producing marrow distortion and fibrosis.

Clinical Features. Primary myelofibrosis is less common than PCV and ET and usually occurs in individuals older than 60 years of age. Except when preceded by another myeloproliferative disorder, it comes to attention because of progressive anemia and splenomegaly, which produces a sensation of fullness in the left upper quadrant. Nonspecific symptoms such as fatigue, weight loss, and night sweats result from an increase in metabolism associated with the expanding mass of hematopoietic cells. Hyperuricemia and secondary gout due to a high rate of cell turnover can complicate the picture.

Laboratory studies typically show a moderate to severe normochromic normocytic anemia accompanied by leukoerythroblastosis. The white cell count is usually normal or reduced, but can be markedly elevated (80,000–100,000 cells/mm³) early in the course. The platelet count is usually normal or elevated at the time of diagnosis, but thrombocytopenia supervenes as the disease progresses. These blood findings are not specific; bone marrow biopsy is essential for diagnosis.

Primary myelofibrosis is a much more difficult disease to treat than PCV or ET. The course is variable, but the median survival is in the range of 3 to 5 years. Threats to life include intercurrent infections, thrombotic episodes, bleeding related to platelet abnormalities, and transformation to AML, which occurs in 5% to 20% of cases. When myelofibrosis is extensive, AML sometimes arises at extramedullary sites, including lymph nodes and soft tissues. Bone marrow transplantation is being used in some younger patients, and kinase inhibitors represent a future hope for targeted therapy.

LANGERHANS CELL HISTIOCYTOSIS

The term *histiocytosis* is an "umbrella" designation for a variety of proliferative disorders of dendritic cells or macrophages. Some, such as rare "histiocytic" lymphomas, are clearly malignant, whereas others, such as reactive proliferations of macrophages in lymph nodes, are clearly benign. Lying between these two extremes are the Langerhans cell histiocytoses, a spectrum of proliferations of a special type of immature dendritic cell called the Langerhans cell (see Chapter 6). In most instances, these proliferations are monoclonal and therefore likely to be neoplastic in origin.

Regardless of the clinical picture, the proliferating Langerhans cells have abundant, often vacuolated cytoplasm and vesicular nuclei containing linear grooves or folds (Fig. 13–38A). *The presence of Birbeck granules in the cytoplasm is characteristic.* Birbeck granules are pentalaminar tubules, often with a dilated terminal end producing a tennis racket–like appearance (Fig. 13–38B), which contain the protein langerin. In addition, the tumor cells also typically express HLA-DR, S-100, and CD1a.

Langerhans cell histiocytosis presents as several clinicopathologic entities:

- *Multifocal multisystem Langerhans cell histiocytosis (Letterer-Siwe disease)* occurs most frequently before 2 years of age but occasionally affects adults. A dominant clinical

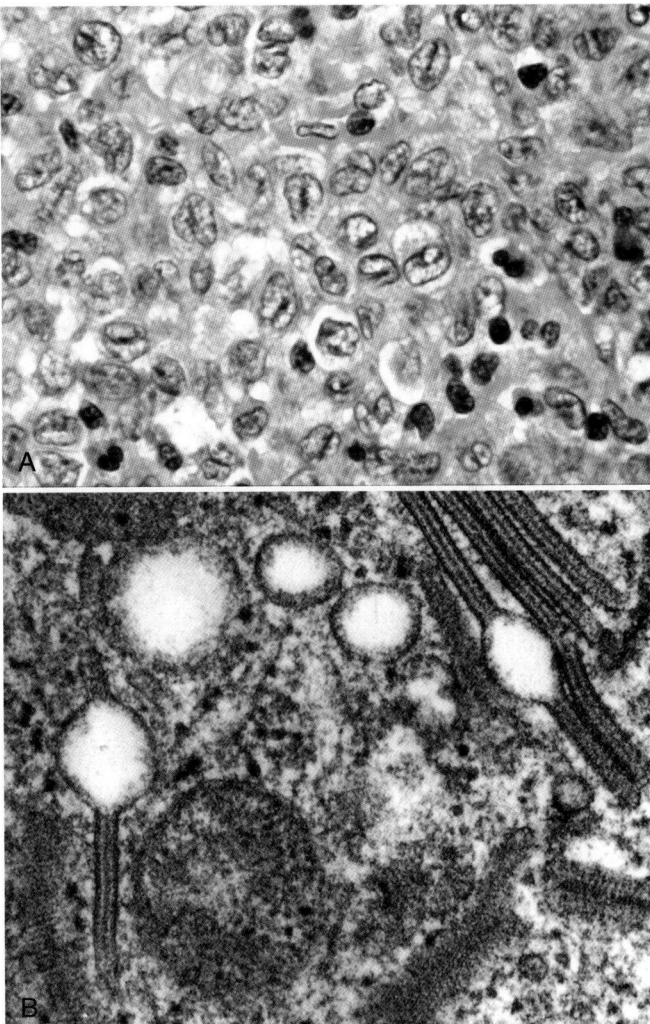

FIGURE 13–38 Langerhans cell histiocytosis. **A,** Langerhans cells with folded or grooved nuclei and moderately abundant pale cytoplasm are mixed with a few eosinophils. **B,** An electron micrograph shows rodlike Birbeck granules with characteristic periodicity and dilated terminal end. (**B,** Courtesy of Dr. George Murphy, Department of Pathology, Brigham and Women's Hospital, Boston, MA.)

feature is the development of cutaneous lesions resembling a seborrheic eruption, which is caused by infiltrates of Langerhans cells over the front and back of the trunk and on the scalp. Most of those affected have concurrent hepatosplenomegaly, lymphadenopathy, pulmonary lesions, and (eventually) destructive osteolytic bone lesions. Extensive infiltration of the marrow often leads to anemia, thrombocytopenia, and a predisposition to recurrent infections, such as otitis media and mastoiditis. In some instances the tumor cells are quite anaplastic; such tumors are sometimes referred to as Langerhans cell sarcoma. The course of untreated disease is rapidly fatal. With intensive chemotherapy, 50% of patients survive 5 years.

- *Unifocal and multifocal unisystem Langerhans cell histiocytosis (eosinophilic granuloma)* is characterized by proliferations of Langerhans cells admixed with variable numbers of eosinophils, lymphocytes, plasma cells, and neutrophils. Eosinophils are usually, but not always, a prominent component of the infiltrate. It typically arises within the medullary cavities of bones, most commonly the calvarium, ribs, and femur. Less commonly, unisystem lesions of identical histology arise in the skin, lungs, or stomach. *Unifocal lesions* most commonly affect the skeletal system in older children or adults. Bone lesions can be asymptomatic or cause pain, tenderness, and, in some instances, pathologic fractures. Unifocal disease is indolent and may heal spontaneously or be cured by local excision or irradiation. *Multifocal unisystem disease* usually affects young children, who present with multiple erosive bony masses that sometimes expand into adjacent soft tissue. Involvement of the posterior pituitary stalk of the hypothalamus leads to diabetes insipidus in about 50% of patients. The combination of calvarial bone defects, diabetes insipidus, and exophthalmos is referred to as the *Hand-Schuller-Christian* triad. Many patients experience spontaneous regression; others can be treated successfully with chemotherapy.

- *Pulmonary Langerhans cell histiocytosis* represents a special category of disease, most often seen in adult smokers, which may regress spontaneously upon cessation of smoking. It usually comprises a polyclonal population of Langerhans cells, suggesting that it is a reactive hyperplasia rather than a true neoplasm.

One factor that contributes to the homing of neoplastic Langerhans cells is the aberrant expression of chemokine receptors.[70,71] For example, while normal epidermal Langerhans cells express CCR6, their neoplastic counterparts express both CCR6 and CCR7. This allows the neoplastic cells to migrate into tissues that express the relevant chemokines—CCL20 (a ligand for CCR6) in skin and bone, and CCL19 and 21 (ligands for CCR7) in lymphoid organs.

SPLEEN

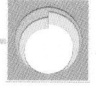

The spleen is an ingeniously designed filter for the blood and a site of immune responses to blood-borne antigens. Normally in the adult it weighs about 150 gm and is enclosed within a thin, glistening, slate-gray connective tissue capsule. Its cut surface reveals extensive red pulp dotted with gray specks, which are the white pulp follicles. These consist of an artery with an eccentric collar of T lymphocytes, the so-called periarteriolar lymphatic sheath. At intervals this sheath expands to form lymphoid nodules composed mainly of B lymphocytes, which are capable of developing into germinal centers identical to those seen in lymph nodes in response to antigenic stimulation (Fig. 13–39).

The red pulp of the spleen is traversed by numerous thin-walled vascular sinusoids, separated by the splenic cords or "cords of Billroth." The endothelial lining of the sinusoid is discontinuous, providing a passage for blood cells between the sinusoids and cords. The cords contain a labyrinth of macrophages loosely connected through long dendritic processes to create both a physical and a functional filter. As it traverses the red pulp, the blood takes two routes to reach the splenic veins. Some flows through capillaries into the cords, from which blood cells squeeze through gaps in the discontinuous basement of the endothelial lining to reach the sinusoids; this is the so-called open circulation or slow compartment. In the other "closed circuit," blood passes rapidly and directly from the capillaries to the splenic veins.

Although only a small fraction of the blood pursues the "open" route, during the course of a day the entire blood volume passes through the cords, where it is closely examined by macrophages.

The spleen has four functions that impact disease states:

1. *Phagocytosis of blood cells and particulate matter.* As will be discussed under the hemolytic anemias (Chapter 14), red cells undergo extreme deformation during passage from the cords into the sinusoids. In conditions in which red cell elasticity is decreased, red cells become trapped in the cords and are more readily phagocytosed by macrophages. Splenic macrophages are also responsible for "pitting" of red cells, the process by which inclusions such as Heinz bodies and Howell-Jolly bodies are excised, and for the removal of particles, such as bacteria, from the blood.

2. *Antibody production.* Dendritic cells in the periarterial lymphatic sheath trap antigens and present them to T lymphocytes. T- and B-cell interaction at the edges of white pulp follicles leads to the generation of antibody-secreting plasma cells, which are found mainly within the sinuses of the red pulp. The spleen seems to be an important source of antibodies directed against platelets and red cells in immune thrombocytopenia purpura and immunohemolytic anemias, both discussed in Chapter 14.

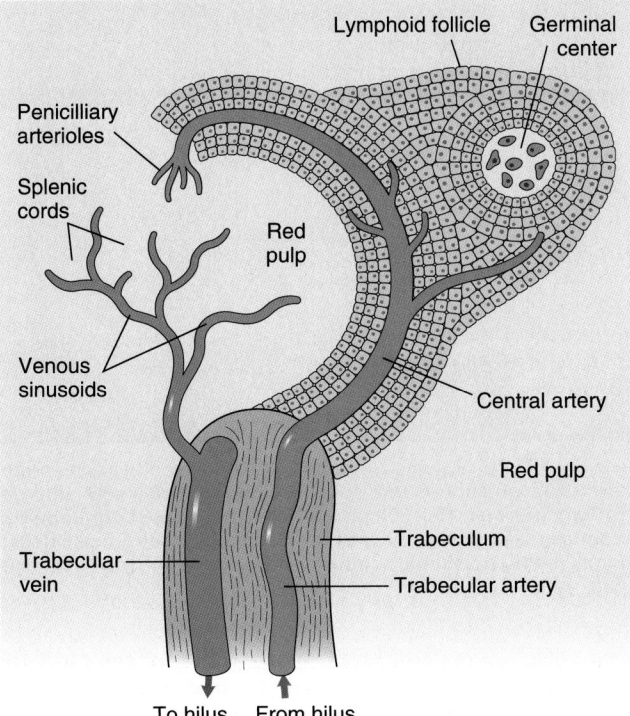

FIGURE 13–39 Normal splenic architecture. (Modified from Faller DV: Diseases of the spleen. In Wyngaarden JB, Smith LH (eds): Cecil Textbook of Medicine, 18th ed. Philadelphia, WB Saunders, 1988, p. 1036.)

3. *Hematopoiesis.* Splenic hematopoiesis normally ceases before birth, but can be reactivated in severe anemia. As we have seen, the spleen is also a prominent site of extramedullary hematopoiesis in myeloproliferative disorders, such as chronic myeloid leukemia.
4. *Sequestration of formed blood elements.* The normal spleen contains only about 30 to 40 mL of red cells, but this volume increases greatly with splenomegaly. The normal spleen also harbors approximately 30% to 40% of the total platelet mass in the body. *With splenomegaly up to 80% to 90% of the total platelet mass can be sequestered in the interstices of the red pulp, producing thrombocytopenia.* Similarly, the enlarged spleen can trap white cells and thereby induce leukopenia.

As the largest unit of the mononuclear phagocyte system, the spleen is involved in all systemic inflammations, generalized hematopoietic disorders, and many metabolic disturbances. In each, the spleen undergoes enlargement *(splenomegaly),* which is the major manifestation of disorders of this organ. It is rarely the primary site of disease. *Splenic insufficiency due to splenectomy or autoinfarction (as in sickle-cell disease) has one major clinical manifestation, an increased susceptibility to sepsis cause by encapsulated bacteria such as pneumococcus, meningococcus, and Haemophilus influenzae.* The loss of filtering and antibody production functions both contribute to the increased risk of sepsis, which may be fatal. All asplenic individuals should be vaccinated against these agents to reduce the risk of this tragic complication.

Splenomegaly

When sufficiently enlarged, the spleen causes a dragging sensation in the left upper quadrant and, through pressure on the stomach, discomfort after eating. In addition, enlargement can cause a syndrome known as *hypersplenism,* which is characterized by anemia, leukopenia, thrombocytopenia, alone or in combination. The probable cause of the cytopenias is increased sequestration of formed elements and the consequent enhanced phagocytosis by the splenic macrophages.

A list of the major disorders associated with splenomegaly is provided in Table 13–12. Splenomegaly in virtually all the conditions mentioned has been discussed elsewhere. There remain only a few disorders to consider.

NONSPECIFIC ACUTE SPLENITIS

Enlargement of the spleen occurs in any blood-borne infection. The nonspecific splenic reaction in these infections is

TABLE 13–12 Disorders Associated with Splenomegaly
I. INFECTIONS
Nonspecific splenitis of various blood-borne infections (particularly infectious endocarditis) Infectious mononucleosis Tuberculosis Typhoid fever Brucellosis Cytomegalovirus Syphilis Malaria Histoplasmosis Toxoplasmosis Kala-azar Trypanosomiasis Schistosomiasis Leishmaniasis Echinococcosis
II. CONGESTIVE STATES RELATED TO PORTAL HYPERTENSION
Cirrhosis of the liver Portal or splenic vein thrombosis Cardiac failure
III. LYMPHOHEMATOGENOUS DISORDERS
Hodgkin lymphoma Non-Hodgkin lymphomas and lymphocytic leukemias Multiple myeloma Myeloproliferative disorders Hemolytic anemias
IV. IMMUNOLOGICAL-INFLAMMATORY CONDITIONS
Rheumatoid arthritis Systemic lupus erythematosus
V. STORAGE DISEASES
Gaucher disease Niemann-Pick disease Mucopolysaccharidoses
VI. MISCELLANEOUS DISORDERS
Amyloidosis Primary neoplasms and cysts Secondary neoplasms

caused both by the microbiologic agents themselves and by cytokines that are released as part of the immune response.

> **Morphology.** The spleen is enlarged (200–400 gm) and soft. Microscopically, the major feature is acute congestion of the red pulp, which may encroach on and virtually efface the lymphoid follicles. Neutrophils, plasma cells, and occasionally eosinophils are usually present throughout the white and red pulp. At times the white pulp follicles may undergo necrosis, particularly when the causative agent is a hemolytic streptococcus. Rarely, abscess formation occurs.

CONGESTIVE SPLENOMEGALY

Chronic venous outflow obstruction causes a form of splenic enlargement referred to as *congestive splenomegaly.* Venous obstruction may be caused by intrahepatic disorders that retard portal venous drainage, or arise from extrahepatic disorders that directly impinge upon the portal or splenic veins. All of these disorders ultimately lead to portal or splenic vein hypertension. *Systemic, or central, venous congestion* is encountered in cardiac decompensation involving the right side of the heart, as can occur in tricuspid or pulmonic valvular disease, chronic cor pulmonale, or following left-sided heart failure. Systemic congestion is associated with only moderately enlarged spleens that rarely exceed 500 gm in weight.

Cirrhosis of the liver is the main cause of massive congestive splenomegaly. The "pipe-stem" hepatic fibrosis of schistosomiasis causes particularly severe congestive splenomegaly, while the diffuse fibrous scarring of alcoholic cirrhosis and pigment cirrhosis also evokes profound enlargements. Other forms of cirrhosis are less commonly implicated.

Congestive splenomegaly is also caused by obstruction of the extrahepatic portal vein or splenic vein. This can stem from *spontaneous portal vein thrombosis,* which is usually associated with some intrahepatic obstructive disease, or inflammation of the portal vein *(pylephlebitis),* such as follows intraperitoneal infections. Thrombosis of the splenic vein can be caused by infiltrating tumors arising in neighboring organs, such as carcinomas of the stomach or pancreas.

> **Morphology.** Long-standing splenic congestion produces marked enlargement (1000–5000 gm). The organ is firm, and the capsule is usually thickened and fibrous. Microscopically, the red pulp is congested early in the course but becomes increasingly fibrotic and cellular with time. The elevated portal venous pressure stimulates the deposition of collagen in the basement membrane of the sinusoids, which appear dilated because of the rigidity of their walls. The resultant slowing of blood flow from the cords to the sinusoids prolongs the exposure of the blood cells to macrophages, resulting in excessive destruction (hypersplenism).

SPLENIC INFARCTS

Splenic infarcts are common lesions caused by the occlusion of the major splenic artery or any of its branches. The spleen,

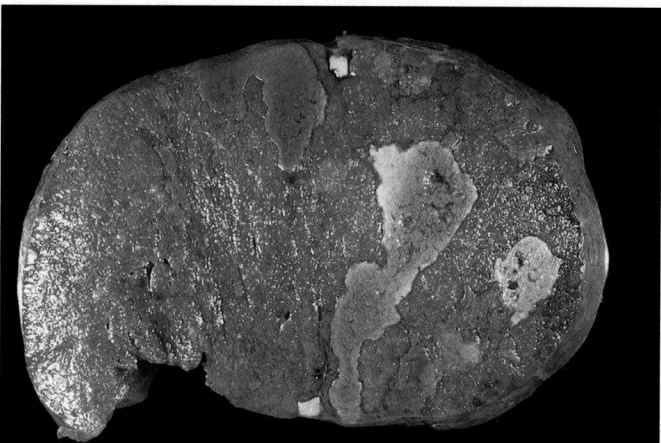

FIGURE 13–40 Splenic infarcts. Multiple well-circumscribed infarcts are present in this spleen, which is massively enlarged (2820 gm; normal: 150–200 gm) by extramedullary hematopoiesis secondary to a myeloproliferative disorder (myelofibrosis). Recent infarcts are hemorrhagic, whereas older, more fibrotic infarcts are a pale yellow-gray color.

along with kidneys and brain, ranks as one of the most frequent sites where emboli lodge. In normal-sized spleens, infarcts are most often caused by emboli that arise from the heart. The infarcts can be small or large, single or multiple, or even involve the entire organ. They are usually bland, except in individuals with infectious endocarditis of the mitral or aortic valves, in whom septic infarcts are common. Infarcts are also common in markedly enlarged spleens, regardless of cause, presumably because the blood supply is tenuous and easily compromised.

> **Morphology.** Bland infarcts are characteristically pale, wedge-shaped, and subcapsular in location. The overlying capsule is often covered with fibrin (Fig. 13–40). In septic infarcts this appearance is modified by the development of suppurative necrosis. In the course of healing, large depressed scars often develop.

Neoplasms

Neoplastic involvement of the spleen is rare except in myeloid and lymphoid tumors, which (as already discussed) often cause splenomegaly. Benign fibromas, osteomas, chondromas, lymphangiomas, and hemangiomas may arise in the spleen. Of these, lymphangiomas and hemangiomas are most common and often cavernous in type.

Congenital Anomalies

Complete absence of the spleen is rare and is usually associated with other congenital abnormalities, such as situs inversus and cardiac malformations. *Hypoplasia* is a more common finding.

Accessory spleens (spleniculi) are common, being present singly or multiply in 20% to 35% of postmortem examinations. They are small, spherical structures that are histologically and functionally identical to the normal spleen. They can be found at any place within the abdominal cavity. Accessory spleens are of great clinical importance in some hematologic disorders, such as hereditary spherocytosis and immune thrombocytopenia purpura, where splenectomy is used as a treatment. If an accessory spleen is overlooked, the therapeutic benefit of removal of the definitive spleen may be reduced or lost entirely.

Rupture

Splenic rupture is usually precipitated by blunt trauma. Much less often, it occurs in the apparent absence of a physical blow. Such "spontaneous ruptures" never involve truly normal spleens but rather stem from some minor physical insult to a spleen made fragile by an underlying condition. The most common predisposing conditions are infectious mononucleosis, malaria, typhoid fever, and lymphoid neoplasms. They cause the spleen to enlarge rapidly, producing a thin, tense capsule that is susceptible to rupture. This dramatic event often precipitates intraperitoneal hemorrhage, which must be treated by prompt splenectomy to prevent death from blood loss. Chronically enlarged spleens are unlikely to rupture because of the toughening effect of extensive reactive fibrosis.

THYMUS

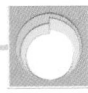

Once an organ buried in obscurity, the thymus has risen to a starring role in cell-mediated immunity (as detailed in Chapter 6). Here, our interest centers on the disorders of the gland itself.

The thymus is embryologically derived from the third and, inconstantly, the fourth pair of pharyngeal pouches. At birth it weighs 10 to 35 gm. It grows until puberty, when it achieves a maximum weight of 20 to 50 gm, and thereafter undergoes progressive involution to little more than 5 to 15 gm in the elderly. The thymus can also involute in children and young adults in response to severe illness and HIV infection.

The fully developed thymus is composed of two fused, well-encapsulated lobes. Fibrous extensions of the capsule divide each lobe into numerous lobules, each with an outer cortical layer enclosing the central medulla. Diverse types of cells populate the thymus, but thymic epithelial cells and immature T lymphocytes predominate. The cortical, peripheral, epithelial cells are polygonal in shape and have an abundant cytoplasm with dendritic extensions that contact adjacent cells. In contrast, the epithelial cells in the medulla are densely packed, often spindle-shaped, and have scant cytoplasm devoid of interconnecting processes. Whorls of medullary epithelial cells create *Hassall corpuscles*, with their characteristic keratinized cores.

As you know from the earlier consideration of the thymus in relation to immunity, progenitor cells of marrow origin migrate to the thymus and mature into T cells, which are exported to the periphery, but only after they have been educated in the "thymic university" to distinguish between self and non-self antigens. During adulthood the thymic production of T cells slowly declines as the organ atrophies.

Macrophages, dendritic cells, a minor population of B lymphocytes, rare neutrophils and eosinophils, and scattered myoid (muscle-like) cells are also found within the thymus. The myoid cells are of particular interest because of the suspicion that they play some role in the development of myasthenia gravis, a musculoskeletal disorder of immune origin.

Pathologic changes within the thymus are limited and will be described here. The changes associated with myasthenia gravis are considered in Chapter 27.

Developmental Disorders

Thymic hypoplasia or *aplasia* is seen in DiGeorge syndrome, which is marked by severe defects in cell-mediated immunity and variable abnormalities of parathyroid development associated with hypoparathyroidism. As discussed in Chapter 5, DiGeorge syndrome is often associated with other developmental defects as part of the 22q11 deletion syndrome.

Isolated *thymic cysts* are uncommon lesions that are usually discovered incidentally postmortem or during surgery. They rarely exceed 4 cm in diameter, can be spherical or arborizing, and are lined by stratified to columnar epithelium. The fluid contents can be serous or mucinous and are often modified by hemorrhage.

While isolated cysts are not clinically significant, neoplastic thymic masses (whatever their origin) compress and distort adjacent normal thymus and sometimes cause cysts to form. Therefore, the presence of a cystic thymic lesion in a symptomatic patient should provoke a thorough search for a neoplasm, particularly a lymphoma or a thymoma.

Thymic Hyperplasia

The term *thymic hyperplasia* is a bit misleading, since it usually applies to the appearance of B-cell germinal centers within the thymus, a finding that is referred to as *thymic follicular hyperplasia*. Such B-cell follicles are present in only small numbers in the normal thymus. Although follicular hyperplasia can occur in a number of chronic inflammatory and immunological states, it is most frequently encountered in myasthenia gravis, in which it is found in 65% to 75% of cases (see Chapter 27). Similar thymic changes are sometimes encountered in Graves' disease, systemic lupus erythematosus, scleroderma, rheumatoid arthritis, and other autoimmune disorders. In other instances, a morphologically normal thymus is simply large for the age of the patient. As mentioned, the size of the thymus varies widely, and whether this constitutes a true hyperplasia or is merely a variant of normal is unclear. The main significance of this form of thymic "hyperplasia" is that

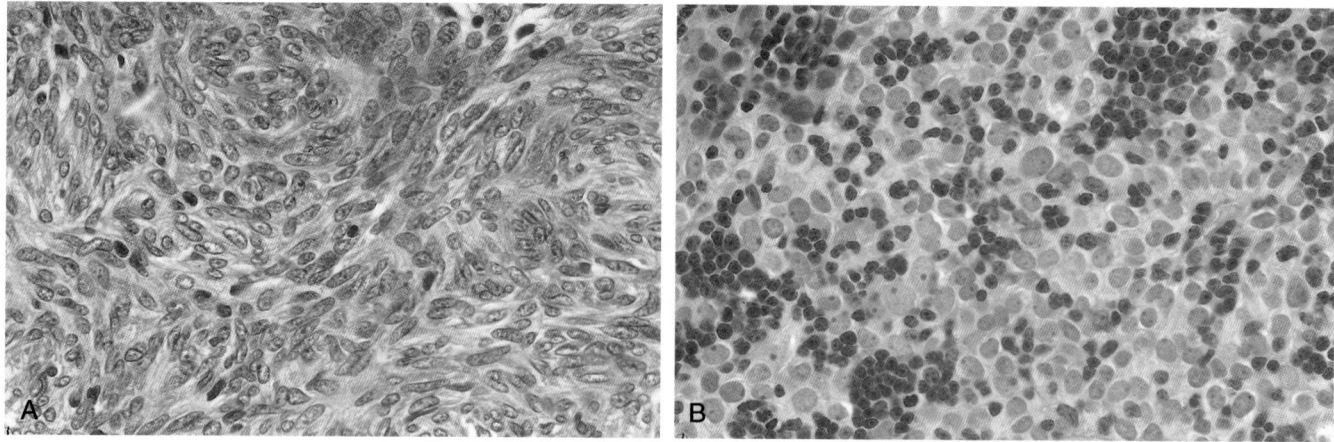

FIGURE 13–41   Thymoma. **A,** Benign thymoma (medullary type). The neoplastic epithelial cells are arranged in a swirling pattern and have bland, oval to elongated nuclei with inconspicuous nucleoli. Only a few small, reactive lymphoid cells are interspersed. **B,** Malignant thymoma, type I. The neoplastic epithelial cells are polygonal and have round to oval, bland nuclei with inconspicuous nucleoli. Numerous small, reactive lymphoid cells are interspersed. The morphologic appearance of this tumor is identical to that of benign thymomas of the cortical type. In this case, however, the tumor was locally aggressive, invading adjacent lung and pericardium.

it may be mistaken radiologically for a thymoma, leading to unnecessary surgical procedures.

Thymomas

A diversity of neoplasms may arise in the thymus—germ cell tumors, lymphomas, carcinoids, and others—but *the designation "thymoma" is restricted to tumors of thymic epithelial cells.* Such tumors typically also contain benign immature T cells (thymocytes).

The WHO has created a classification system based on histology for thymomas, but its clinical utility remains uncertain. We will instead use a classification that relies on the most important prognostic features, the surgical stage and the presence or absence of overt cytologic features of malignancy. In this simple system there are only three histologic subtypes:

- Tumors that are cytologically benign and noninvasive
- Tumors that are cytologically benign but invasive or metastatic
- Tumors that are cytologically malignant (thymic carcinoma)

In all categories, the tumors usually occur in adults older than 40 years of age; thymomas are rare in children. Males and females are affected equally. Most arise in the anterior superior mediastinum, but sometimes they occur in the neck, thyroid, pulmonary hilus, or elsewhere. They are uncommon in the posterior mediastinum. Thymomas account for 20% to 30% of tumors in the anterosuperior mediastinum, which is also a common location for certain lymphomas.

Morphology. Macroscopically, thymomas are lobulated, firm, gray-white masses of up to 15 to 20 cm in size. They sometimes have areas of cystic necrosis and calcification. Most are encapsulated, but 20% to 25% of the tumors penetrate the capsule and infiltrate perithymic tissues and structures.

Noninvasive thymomas are most often composed of medullary-type epithelial cells or a mixture of medullary- and cortical-type epithelial cells. The medullary-type epithelial cells are elongated or spindle-shaped (Fig. 13–41A). There is usually a sparse infiltrate of thymocytes, which often recapitulate the phenotype of medullary thymocytes. In mixed thymomas there is an admixture of polygonal cortical-type epithelial cells and a denser infiltrate of thymocytes. The medullary and mixed patterns together account for about 50% of all thymomas. Tumors that have a substantial proportion of medullary-type epithelial cells are usually noninvasive.

Invasive thymoma refers to a tumor that is cytologically benign but locally invasive. These tumors are much more likely to metastasize. The epithelial cells are most commonly of the cortical variety, with abundant cytoplasm and rounded vesicular nuclei (Fig. 13–41B), and are usually mixed with numerous thymocytes. In some cases, the neoplastic cells show cytologic atypia, a feature that correlates with a propensity for more aggressive behavior. These tumors account for about 20% to 25% of all thymomas. **By definition, invasive thymomas penetrate through the capsule into surrounding structures.** The extent of invasion has been subdivided into various stages, which are beyond our scope. With minimal invasion, complete excision yields a 5-year survival rate of greater than 90%, whereas extensive invasion is associated with a 5-year survival rate of less than 50%.

Thymic carcinoma represents about 5% of thymomas. Macroscopically, they are usually fleshy, obviously invasive masses, sometimes accompanied by metastases to sites such as the lungs. Microscopically, most are **squamous cell carcinomas.** The next most common variant is **lymphoepithelioma-like carcinoma,** a tumor composed of sheets of cells with indistinct borders that bears a close histologic resemblance to nasopharyngeal carcinoma. About 50% of lymphoepithelioma-like carcinomas contain monoclonal EBV genomes, consistent with a role for EBV in their pathogenesis. A variety of other less common histologic patterns of thymic carcinoma have been described; all exhibit cytologic atypia seen in other carcinomas.

Clinical Features. About 40% of thymomas present with symptoms stemming from impingement on mediastinal structures. Another 30% to 45% are detected in the course of evaluating patients with myasthenia gravis. The rest are discovered incidentally during imaging studies or cardiothoracic surgery. In addition to myasthenia gravis, other associated autoimmune disorders include hypogammaglobulinemia, pure red cell aplasia, Graves' disease, pernicious anemia, dermatomyositis-polymyositis, and Cushing syndrome. The basis for these associations is still obscure, but the thymocytes that arise within thymomas give rise to long-lived CD4+ and CD8+ T cells, and cortical thymomas rich in thymocytes are more likely to be associated with autoimmune disease. Hence, it seems likely that abnormalities in the selection or "education" of T cells maturing within the environment of the neoplasm contribute to the development of diverse autoimmune disorders.

REFERENCES

1. Dzierzak E, Speck NA: Of lineage and legacy: the development of mammalian hematopoietic stem cells. Nat Immunol 9:129, 2008.
2. Kiel MJ, Morrison SJ: Uncertainty in the niches that maintain haematopoietic stem cells. Nat Rev Immunol 8:290, 2008.
3. O'Malley DP: T-cell large granular leukemia and related proliferations. Am J Clin Pathol 127:850, 2007.
4. Mebius RE: Organogenesis of lymphoid tissues. Nat Rev Immunol 3:292, 2003.
5. Sagaert X et al.: The pathogenesis of MALT lymphomas: where do we stand? Leukemia 21:389, 2007.
6. Jost PJ, Ruland J: Aberrant NF-kappaB signaling in lymphoma: mechanisms, consequences, and therapeutic implications. Blood 109:2700, 2007.
7. Polo JM, Melnick A: B-cell lymphoma 6 and the molecular pathogenesis of diffuse large-B-cell lymphoma. Curr Opin Hematol 15:381, 2008.
8. Dorsett Y et al.: A role for AID in chromosome translocations between c-myc and the IgH variable region. J Exp Med 204:2225, 2007.
9. Ramiro AR et al.: Role of genomic instability and p53 in AID-induced c-myc-Igh translocations. Nature 440:105, 2006.
10. Pasqualucci L et al.: Hypermutation of multiple proto-oncogenes in B-cell diffuse large-cell lymphomas. Nature 412:341, 2001.
11. Harris NL et al.: World Health Organization classification of neoplastic diseases of the hematopoietic and lymphoid tissues: report of the Clinical Advisory Committee meeting–Airlie House, Virginia, November 1997. J Clin Oncol 17:3835, 1999.
12. Szczepanski T: Why and how to quantify minimal residual disease in acute lymphoblastic leukemia? Leukemia 21:622, 2007.
13. Nabhan C et al.: Minimal residual disease in chronic lymphocytic leukaemia: is it ready for primetime? Br J Haematol 136:379, 2007.
14. Aster JC et al.: Notch signaling in leukemia. Annu Rev Pathol 3:587, 2008.
15. Mullighan CG et al.: Genome-wide analysis of genetic alterations in acute lymphoblastic leukaemia. Nature 446:758, 2007.
16. Greaves MF et al.: Leukemia in twins: lessons in natural history. Blood 102:2321, 2003.
17. Schultz KR et al.: Risk- and response-based classification of childhood B-precursor acute lymphoblastic leukemia: a combined analysis of prognostic markers from the Pediatric Oncology Group (POG) and Children's Cancer Group (CCG). Blood 109:926, 2007.
18. Pfeifer H et al.: Kinase domain mutations of BCR-ABL frequently precede imatinib-based therapy and give rise to relapse in patients with de novo Philadelphia-positive acute lymphoblastic leukemia. Blood 110:727, 2007.
19. Calin GA, Croce CM: Genomics of chronic lymphocytic leukemia microRNAs as new players with clinical significance. Semin Oncol 33:167, 2006.
20. Bouley J et al.: New molecular markers in resistant B CLL. Leuk Lymphoma 47:791, 2006.
21. Endo T et al.: BAFF and APRIL support chronic lymphocytic leukemia B-cell survival through activation of the canonical NF-kappaB pathway. Blood 109:703, 2007.
22. Alinari L et al.: Alemtuzumab (Campath-1H) in the treatment of chronic lymphocytic leukemia. Oncogene 26:3644, 2007.
23. Tsimberidou AM, Keating MJ: Richter's transformation in chronic lymphocytic leukemia. Semin Oncol 33:250, 2006.
24. Dave SS et al.: Prediction of survival in follicular lymphoma based on molecular features of tumor-infiltrating immune cells. N Engl J Med 351:2159–2169, 2004.
25. Kuppers R: Prognosis in follicular lymphoma—it's in the microenvironment. N Engl J Med 351:2152, 2004.
26. Staudt LM, Dave S: The biology of human lymphoid malignancies revealed by gene expression profiling. Adv Immunol 87:163, 2005.
27. Abramson JS, Shipp MA: Advances in the biology and therapy of diffuse large B-cell lymphoma: moving toward a molecularly targeted approach. Blood 106:1164, 2005.
28. Parekh S et al.: BCL6 programs lymphoma cells for survival and differentiation through distinct biochemical mechanisms. Blood 10:2067, 2007.
29. Phan RT et al.: BCL6 interacts with the transcription factor Miz-1 to suppress the cyclin-dependent kinase inhibitor p21 and cell cycle arrest in germinal center B cells. Nat Immunol 6:1054, 2005.
30. Phan RT, Dalla-Favera R: The *BCL6* proto-oncogene suppresses p53 expression in germinal-centre B cells. Nature 432:635, 2004.
31. Hemann MT et al.: Evasion of the p53 tumour surveillance network by tumour-derived MYC mutants. Nature 436:807, 2005.
32. Dave SS et al.: Molecular diagnosis of Burkitt's lymphoma. N Engl J Med 354:2431, 2006.
33. Matsui W et al.: Characterization of clonogenic multiple myeloma cells. Blood 103:2332, 2004.
34. Peacock CD et al.: Hedgehog signaling maintains a tumor stem cell compartment in multiple myeloma. Proc Natl Acad Sci U S A 104:4048, 2007.
35. Anderson KC: Targeted therapy of multiple myeloma based upon tumor-microenvironmental interactions. Exp Hematol 35:155, 2007.
36. Terpos E et al.: Significance of macrophage inflammatory protein-1 alpha (MIP-1alpha) in multiple myeloma. Leuk Lymphoma 46:1699, 2005.
37. Hjertner O et al.: Bone disease in multiple myeloma. Med Oncol 23:431, 2006.
38. Bergsagel PL, Kuehl WM: Molecular pathogenesis and a consequent classification of multiple myeloma. J Clin Oncol 23:6333, 2005.
39. Terpos E et al.: Clinical implications of chromosomal abnormalities in multiple myeloma. Leuk Lymphoma 47:803, 2006.
40. Zhan F et al.: The molecular classification of multiple myeloma. Blood 108:2020, 2006.
41. Stewart AK, Fonseca R: Prognostic and therapeutic significance of myeloma genetics and gene expression profiling. J Clin Oncol 23:6339, 2005.
42. Rajkumar SV et al.: Proteasome inhibition as a novel therapeutic target in human cancer. J Clin Oncol 23:630, 2005.
43. Terpos E et al.: The effect of novel anti-myeloma agents on bone metabolism of patients with multiple myeloma. Leukemia 2007.
44. Kyle RA et al.: Clinical course and prognosis of smoldering (asymptomatic) multiple myeloma. N Engl J Med 356:2582, 2007.
45. Kyle RA et al.: Prevalence of monoclonal gammopathy of undetermined significance. N Engl J Med 354:1362, 2006.
46. Kyle RA et al.: A long-term study of prognosis in monoclonal gammopathy of undetermined significance. N Engl J Med 346:564, 2002.
47. Bergsagel PL, Kuehl WM: Chromosome translocations in multiple myeloma. Oncogene 20:5611 2001.
48. Chiarle R et al.: The anaplastic lymphoma kinase in the pathogenesis of cancer. Nat Rev Cancer 8:11, 2008.

49. Sun SC, Yamaoka S: Activation of NF-kappaB by HTLV-I and implications for cell transformation. Oncogene 24:5952, 2005.

50. Schmitz R et al.: Pathogenesis of classical and lymphocyte-predominant Hodgkin lymphoma. Annu Rev Pathol Mech Dis 4:151, 2009.

51. Kuppers R, Brauninger A: Reprogramming of the tumour B-cell phenotype in Hodgkin lymphoma. Trends Immunol 27:203, 2006.

52. Jungnickel B et al.: Clonal deleterious mutations in the IkappaBalpha gene in the malignant cells in Hodgkin's lymphoma. J Exp Med 191:395, 2000.

53. Re D et al.: Molecular pathogenesis of Hodgkin's lymphoma. J Clin Oncol 23:6379, 2005.

54. Joos S et al.: Classical Hodgkin lymphoma is characterized by recurrent copy number gains of the short arm of chromosome 2. Blood 99:1381, 2002.

55. de Bruijn MF, Speck NA: Core-binding factors in hematopoiesis and immune function. Oncogene 23:4238, 2004.

56. Scaglioni PP, Pandolfi PP: The theory of APL revisited. Curr Top Microbiol Immunol 313:85, 2007.

57. Kelly LM et al.: PML/RARalpha and FLT3-ITD induce an APL-like disease in a mouse model. Proc Natl Acad Sci U S A 99:8283, 2002.

58. Falini B et al.: Acute myeloid leukemia carrying cytoplasmic/mutated nucleophosmin (NPMc+ AML): biologic and clinical features. Blood 109:874, 2007.

59. Paschka P et al.: Adverse prognostic significance of KIT mutations in adult acute myeloid leukemia with inv(16) and t(8;21): a Cancer and Leukemia Group B Study. J Clin Oncol 24:3904, 2006.

60. Corey SJ et al.: Myelodysplastic syndromes: the complexity of stem-cell diseases. Nat Rev Cancer 7:118, 2007.

61. Campbell PJ, Green AR: The myeloproliferative disorders. N Engl J Med 355:2452, 2006.

62. Levine RL et al.: Role of JAK2 in the pathogenesis and therapy of myeloproliferative disorders. Nat Rev Cancer 7:673, 2007.

63. Goldman JM, Melo JV: Chronic myeloid leukemia—advances in biology and new approaches to treatment. N Engl J Med 349:1451, 2003.

64. Mullighan CG et al.: BCR-ABL1 lymphoblastic leukaemia is characterized by the deletion of Ikaros. Nature 453:110, 2008.

65. Druker BJ et al.: Five-year follow-up of patients receiving imatinib for chronic myeloid leukemia. N Engl J Med 355:2408, 2006.

66. Melo JV, Barnes DJ: Chronic myeloid leukaemia as a model of disease evolution in human cancer. Nat Rev Cancer 7:441, 2007.

67. Vannucchi AM et al.: Clinical profile of homozygous JAK2 617V > F mutation in patients with polycythemia vera or essential thrombocythemia. Blood 110:840, 2007.

68. Patel RK et al.: Prevalence of the activating JAK2 tyrosine kinase mutation V617F in the Budd-Chiari syndrome. Gastroenterology 130:2031, 2006.

69. Jelinek J et al.: JAK2 mutation 1849G > T is rare in acute leukemias but can be found in CMML, Philadelphia chromosome-negative CML, and megakaryocytic leukemia. Blood 106:3370, 2005.

70. Annels NE et al.: Aberrant chemokine receptor expression and chemokine production by Langerhans cells underlies the pathogenesis of Langerhans cell histiocytosis. J Exp Med 197:1385, 2003.

71. Fleming MD et al.: Coincident expression of the chemokine receptors CCR6 and CCR7 by pathologic Langerhans cells in Langerhans cell histiocytosis. Blood 101:2473, 2003.

14

Red Blood Cell and Bleeding Disorders

Anemias
  Anemias of Blood Loss
    Acute Blood Loss
    Chronic Blood Loss
  Hemolytic Anemias
    Hereditary Spherocytosis (HS)
    Hemolytic Disease Due to Red Cell
      Enzyme Defects: Glucose-6-Phosphate
      Dehydrogenase Deficiency
    Sickle Cell Disease
    Thalassemia Syndromes
    Paroxysmal Nocturnal
      Hemoglobinuria
    Immunohemolytic Anemia
    Hemolytic Anemia Resulting from
      Trauma to Red Cells
  Anemias of Diminished Erythropoiesis
    Megaloblastic Anemias
    Iron Deficiency Anemia
    Anemia of Chronic Disease
    Aplastic Anemia
    Pure Red Cell Aplasia
    Other Forms of Marrow Failure
Polycythemia
Bleeding Disorders: Hemorrhagic
  Diatheses

Bleeding Disorders Caused by Vessel Wall
  Abnormalities
Bleeding Related to Reduced Platelet
  Number: Thrombocytopenia
  Chronic Immune Thrombocytopenic
    Purpura
  Acute Immune Thrombocytopenic
    Purpura
  Drug-Induced Thrombocytopenia
  HIV-Associated Thrombocytopenia
  Thrombotic Microangiopathies:
    Thrombotic Thrombocytopenic
    Purpura (TTP) and Hemolytic-Uremic
    Syndrome (HUS)
Bleeding Disorders Related to Defective
  Platelet Functions
Hemorrhagic Diatheses Related to
  Abnormalities in Clotting
  Factors
  The Factor VIII-vWF Complex
  Von Willebrand Disease
  Hemophilia A (Factor VIII
    Deficiency)
  Hemophilia B (Christmas Disease,
    Factor IX Deficiency)
Disseminated Intravascular Coagulation
  (DIC)

In this chapter we will first consider diseases of red cells. Of these, by far the most important are the anemias, red cell deficiency states that most commonly have a non-neoplastic basis. We will then complete our review of blood diseases by discussing the major bleeding disorders.

Anemias

Anemia is defined as a reduction of the total circulating red cell mass below normal limits. Anemia reduces the oxygen-carrying capacity of the blood, leading to tissue hypoxia. In practice,

TABLE 14–1 Classification of Anemia According to Underlying Mechanism	
Mechanism	**Specific Examples**
BLOOD LOSS	
Acute blood loss	Trauma
Chronic blood loss	Gastrointestinal tract lesions, gynecologic disturbances*
INCREASED RED CELL DESTRUCTION (HEMOLYSIS)	
Inherited genetic defects	
Red cell membrane disorders	Hereditary spherocytosis, hereditary elliptocytosis
Enzyme deficiencies	
Hexose monophosphate shunt enzyme deficiencies	G6PD deficiency, glutathione synthetase deficiency
Glycolytic enzyme deficiencies	Pyruvate kinase deficiency, hexokinase deficiency
Hemoglobin abnormalities	
Deficient globin synthesis	Thalassemia syndromes
Structurally abnormal globins (hemoglobinopathies)	Sickle cell disease, unstable hemoglobins
Acquired genetic defects	
Deficiency of phosphatidylinositol-linked glycoproteins	Paroxysmal nocturnal hemoglobinuria
Antibody-mediated destruction	Hemolytic disease of the newborn (Rh disease), transfusion reactions, drug-induced, autoimmune disorders
Mechanical trauma	
Microangiopathic hemolytic anemias	Hemolytic uremic syndrome, disseminated intravascular coagulation, thrombotic thrombocytopenia purpura
Cardiac traumatic hemolysis	Defective cardiac valves
Repetitive physical trauma	Bongo drumming, marathon running, karate chopping
Infections of red cells	Malaria, babesiosis
Toxic or chemical injury	Clostridial sepsis, snake venom, lead poisoning
Membrane lipid abnormalities	Abetalipoproteinemia, severe hepatocellular liver disease
Sequestration	Hypersplenism
DECREASED RED CELL PRODUCTION	
Inherited genetic defects	
Defects leading to stem cell depletion	Fanconi anemia, telomerase defects
Defects affecting erythroblast maturation	Thalassemia syndromes
Nutritional deficiencies	
Deficiencies affecting DNA synthesis	B_{12} and folate deficiencies
Deficiencies affecting hemoglobin synthesis	Iron deficiency anemia
Erythropoietin deficiency	Renal failure, anemia of chronic disease
Immune-mediated injury of progenitors	Aplastic anemia, pure red cell aplasia
Inflammation-mediated iron sequestration	Anemia of chronic disease
Primary hematopoietic neoplasms	Acute leukemia, myelodysplasia, myeloproliferative disorders (Chapter 13)
Space-occupying marrow lesions	Metastatic neoplasms, granulomatous disease
Infections of red cell progenitors	Parvovirus B19 infection
Unknown mechanisms	Endocrine disorders, hepatocellular liver disase

G6PD, Glucose-6-phosphate dehydrogenase.
*Most often cause anemia due to iron deficiency, not bleeding per se.

the measurement of red cell mass is not easy, and anemia is usually diagnosed based on a reduction in the *hematocrit* (the ratio of packed red cells to total blood volume) and the *hemoglobin concentration* of the blood to levels that are below the normal range. These values correlate with the red cell mass except when there are changes in plasma volume caused by fluid retention or dehydration.

There are many classifications of anemia. We will follow one based on underlying mechanisms that is presented in Table 14–1. A second clinically useful approach classifies anemia according to alterations in red cell morphology, which often point to particular causes. Morphologic characteristics providing etiologic clues include red cell size (normocytic, microcytic, or macrocytic); degree of hemoglobinization, reflected in the color of red cells (normochromic or hypochromic); and shape. In general, microcytic hypochromic anemias are caused by disorders of hemoglobin synthesis (most often iron deficiency), while macrocytic anemias often stem from abnormalities that impair the maturation

of erythroid precursors in the bone marrow. Normochromic, normocytic anemias have diverse etiologies; in some of these anemias, specific abnormalities of red cell shape (best appreciated through visual inspection of peripheral smears) provide an important clue as to the cause. The other indices can also be assessed qualitatively in smears, but precise measurement is carried out in clinical laboratories with special instrumentation. The most useful red cell indices are as follows:

- *Mean cell volume*: the average volume of a red cell expressed in femtoliters (fL)
- *Mean cell hemoglobin*: the average content (mass) of hemoglobin per red cell, expressed in picograms
- *Mean cell hemoglobin concentration*: the average concentration of hemoglobin in a given volume of packed red cells, expressed in grams per deciliter
- *Red cell distribution width*: the coefficient of variation of red cell volume

TABLE 14–2 Adult Reference Ranges for Red Cells*

Measurement (units)	Men	Women
Hemoglobin (gm/dL)	13.6–17.2	12.0–15.0
Hematocrit (%)	39–49	33–43
Red cell count (×10^6/µL)	4.3–5.9	3.5–5.0
Reticulocyte count (%)		0.5–1.5
Mean cell volume (fL)		82–96
Mean cell hemoglobin (pg)		27–33
Mean cell hemoglobin concentration (gm/dL)		33–37
Red cell distribution width		11.5–14.5

*Reference ranges vary among laboratories. The reference ranges for the laboratory providing the result should always be used in interpreting the test result.

Adult reference ranges for red cell indices are shown in Table 14–2.

Whatever its cause, when sufficiently severe anemia leads to certain clinical features. Patients appear pale. Weakness, malaise, and easy fatigability are common complaints. The lowered oxygen content of the circulating blood leads to dyspnea on mild exertion. Hypoxia can cause fatty change in the liver, myocardium, and kidney. If fatty changes in the myocardium are sufficiently severe, cardiac failure can develop and compound the tissue hypoxia caused by the deficiency of O_2 in the blood. On occasion, the myocardial hypoxia manifests as angina pectoris, particularly when complicated by pre-existing coronary artery disease. With acute blood loss and shock, oliguria and anuria can develop as a result of renal hypoperfusion. Central nervous system hypoxia can cause headache, dimness of vision, and faintness.

ANEMIAS OF BLOOD LOSS

Acute Blood Loss

The effects of acute blood loss are mainly due to the loss of intravascular volume, which if massive can lead to cardiovascular collapse, shock, and death. The clinical features depend on the rate of hemorrhage and whether the bleeding is external or internal. If the patient survives, the blood volume is rapidly restored by the intravascular shift of water from the interstitial fluid compartment. This fluid shift results in hemodilution and a lowering of the hematocrit. The reduction in oxygenation triggers increased secretion of erythropoietin from the kidney, which stimulates the proliferation of committed erythroid progenitors (CFU-E) in the marrow (see Fig. 13–1). It takes about 5 days for the progeny of these CFU-Es to mature and appear as newly released red cells (reticulocytes) in the peripheral blood. The iron in hemoglobin is recaptured if red cells extravasate into tissues, whereas bleeding into the gut or out of the body leads to iron loss and possible iron deficiency, which can hamper the restoration of normal red cell counts.

Significant bleeding results in predictable changes in the blood involving not only red cells, but also white cells and platelets. If the bleeding is sufficiently massive to cause a decrease in blood pressure, the compensatory release of adrenergic hormones mobilizes granulocytes from the intravascular marginal pool and results in *leukocytosis* (see Fig. 13–2). Initially, red cells appear normal in size and color (normocytic, normochromic). However, as marrow production increases there is a striking *increase in the reticulocyte count* (reticulocytosis), which reaches 10% to 15% after 7 days. Reticulocytes are larger in size than normal red cells (macrocytes) and have a blue-red polychromatophilic cytoplasm. Early recovery from blood loss is also often accompanied by *thrombocytosis*, which results from an increase in platelet production.

Chronic Blood Loss

Chronic blood loss induces anemia only when the rate of loss exceeds the regenerative capacity of the marrow or when iron reserves are depleted and iron deficiency anemia appears; this will be discussed later.

HEMOLYTIC ANEMIAS

Hemolytic anemias share the following features:

- Premature destruction of red cells and a shortened red cell life span below the normal 120 days
- Elevated erythropoietin levels and a compensatory increase in erythropoiesis
- Accumulation of hemoglobin degradation products released by red cell breakdown derived from hemoglobin

The physiologic destruction of senescent red cells takes place within mononuclear phagocytes, which are abundant in the spleen, liver, and bone marrow. This process appears to be triggered by age-dependent changes in red cell surface proteins, which lead to their recognition and phagocytosis.[1] *In the great majority of hemolytic anemias the premature destruction of red cells also occurs within phagocytes*, an event that is referred to as *extravascular hemolysis*. If persistent, extravascular hemolysis leads to a hyperplasia of phagocytes manifested by varying degrees of *splenomegaly*.

Extravascular hemolysis is generally caused by alterations that render the red cell less deformable. Extreme changes in shape are required for red cells to navigate the splenic sinusoids successfully. Reduced deformability makes this passage difficult, leading to red cell sequestration and phagocytosis within the cords. *Regardless of the cause, the principal clinical features of extravascular hemolysis are (1) anemia, (2) splenomegaly, and (3) jaundice.* Some hemoglobin inevitably escapes from phagocytes, which leads to variable decreases in plasma haptoglobin, an α_2-globulin that binds free hemoglobin and prevents its excretion in the urine. Because much of the pathologic destruction of red cells occurs in the spleen, individuals with extravascular hemolysis often benefit from splenectomy.

Less commonly, *intravascular hemolysis* predominates. Intravascular hemolysis of red cells may be caused by mechanical injury, complement fixation, intracellular parasites (e.g., falciparum malaria, Chapter 8), or exogenous toxic factors. Causes of mechanical injury include trauma caused by cardiac valves, thrombotic narrowing of the microcirculation, or repetitive physical trauma (e.g., marathon running and bongo drum beating). Complement fixation occurs in a variety of situations in which antibodies recognize and bind red cell antigens. Toxic injury is exemplified by clostridial sepsis, which results in the release of enzymes that digest the red cell membrane.

Whatever the mechanism, *intravascular hemolysis is manifested by (1) anemia, (2) hemoglobinemia, (3) hemoglobinuria, (4) hemosiderinuria, and (5) jaundice.* The large amounts of free hemoglobin released from lysed red cells are promptly bound by haptoglobin, producing a complex that is rapidly cleared by mononuclear phagocytes. As serum haptoglobin is depleted, free hemoglobin oxidizes to methemoglobin, which is brown in color. The renal proximal tubular cells reabsorb and catabolize much of the filtered hemoglobin and methemoglobin, but some passes out in the urine, imparting a red-brown color. Iron released from hemoglobin can accumulate within tubular cells, giving rise to renal hemosiderosis. Concomitantly, heme groups derived from hemoglobin-haptoglobin complexes are catabolized to bilirubin within mononuclear phagocytes, leading to jaundice. Unlike in extravascular hemolysis, splenomegaly is not seen.

In all types of uncomplicated hemolytic anemias, the excess serum bilirubin is unconjugated. The level of hyperbilirubinemia depends on the functional capacity of the liver and the rate of hemolysis. When the liver is normal, jaundice is rarely severe. Excessive bilirubin excreted by the liver into the gastrointestinal tract leads to increased formation and fecal excretion of urobilin (Chapter 18), and often leads to the formation of gallstones derived from heme pigments.

> **Morphology.** Certain changes are seen in hemolytic anemias regardless of cause or type. Anemia and lowered tissue oxygen tension trigger the production of erythropoietin, which stimulates erythroid differentiation and leads to the appearance of **increased numbers of erythroid precursors (normoblasts) in the marrow** (Fig. 14–1). Compensatory increases in erythropoiesis result in a **prominent reticulocytosis in the peripheral blood**. The phagocytosis of red cells leads to hemosiderosis, which is most pronounced in the spleen, liver, and bone marrow. If the anemia is severe, extramedullary hematopoiesis can appear in the liver, spleen, and lymph nodes. With chronic hemolysis, elevated biliary excretion of bilirubin promotes the formation of pigment gallstones (cholelithiasis).

The hemolytic anemias can be classified in a variety of ways; here, we classify them according to underlying mechanisms (see Table 14–1). We begin by discussing the major inherited forms of hemolytic anemia, and then move on to the acquired forms that are most common or of particular pathophysiologic interest.

Hereditary Spherocytosis (HS)

This inherited disorder is caused by intrinsic defects in the red cell membrane skeleton that render red cells spheroid, less deformable, and vulnerable to splenic sequestration and destruction.[2] The prevalence of HS is highest in northern Europe, where rates of 1 in 5000 are reported. An autosomal dominant inher-

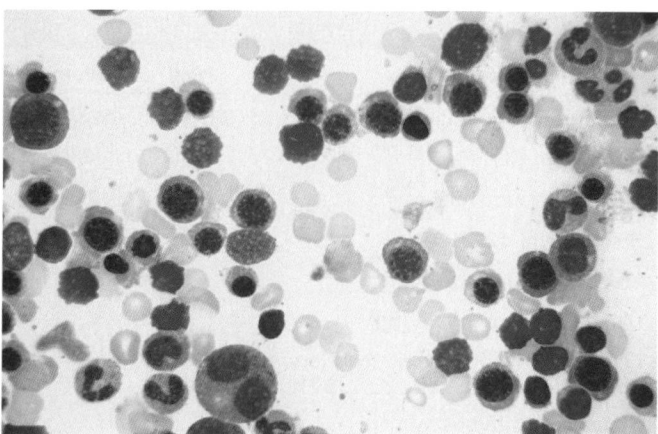

FIGURE 14–1   Marrow smear from a patient with hemolytic anemia. The marrow reveals greatly increased numbers of maturing erythroid progenitors (normoblasts). (Courtesy of Dr. Steven Kroft, Department of Pathology, University of Texas Southwestern Medical School, Dallas, TX.)

itance pattern is seen in about 75% of cases. The remaining patients have a more severe form of the disease that is usually caused by the inheritance of two different defects (a state known as compound heterozygosity).

Pathogenesis. The remarkable elasticity and durability of the normal red cell are attributable to the physicochemical properties of its specialized membrane skeleton (Fig. 14–2), which lies closely apposed to the internal surface of the plasma membrane. Its chief protein component, spectrin, consists of two polypeptide chains, α and β, which form intertwined (helical) flexible heterodimers. The "head" regions of spectrin dimers self-associate to form tetramers, while the "tails" associate with actin oligomers. Each actin oligomer can bind multiple spectrin tetramers, thus creating a two-dimensional spectrin-actin skeleton that is connected to the cell membrane by two distinct interactions. The first, involving the proteins ankyrin and band 4.2, binds spectrin to the transmembrane ion transporter, band 3. The second, involving protein 4.1, binds the "tail" of spectrin to another transmembrane protein, glycophorin A.

HS is caused by diverse mutations that lead to an insufficiency of membrane skeletal components. As a result of these alterations, the life span of the affected red cells is decreased on average to 10 to 20 days from the normal 120 days. The pathogenic mutations most commonly affect ankyrin, band 3, spectrin, or band 4.2, the proteins involved in the first of the two tethering interactions, presumably because this complex is particularly important in stabilizing the lipid bilayer. Most mutations cause shifts in reading frame or introduce premature stop codons, such that the mutated allele fails to produce any protein. The defective synthesis of the affected protein reduces the assembly of the skeleton as a whole and results in a decrease in the density of the membrane skeleton components. Compound heterozygosity for two defective alleles understandably results in a more severe membrane skeleton deficiency. Young HS red cells are normal in shape, but *the deficiency of membrane skeleton reduces the stability of the lipid bilayer, leading to the loss of membrane fragments as red cells age in the circulation.* The loss of membrane relative to cyto-

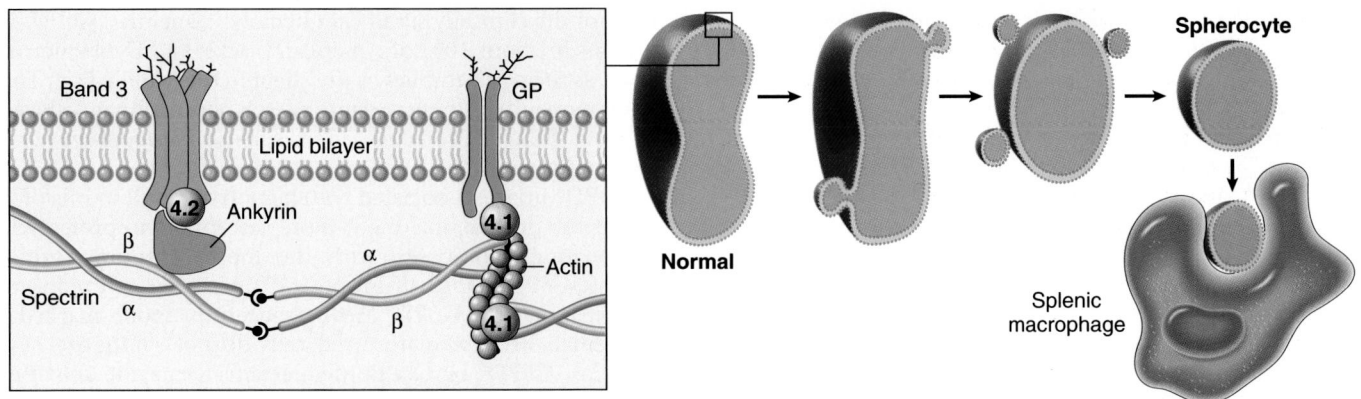

FIGURE 14–2 Role of the red cell membrane skeleton in hereditary spherocytosis. The left panel shows the normal organization of the major red cell membrane skeletal proteins. Various mutations involving α-spectrin, β-spectrin, ankyrin, band 4.2, or band 3 that weaken the interactions between these proteins cause red cells to lose membrane fragments. To accommodate the resultant change in the ratio of surface area to volume these cells adopt a spherical shape. Spherocytic cells are less deformable than normal ones and therefore become trapped in the splenic cords, where they are phagocytosed by macrophages. GP, glycophorin.

plasm "forces" the cells to assume the smallest possible diameter for a given volume, namely, a sphere.

The invariably beneficial effects of splenectomy prove that the spleen has a cardinal role in the premature demise of spherocytes. The travails of spherocytic red cells are fairly well defined. In the life of the portly inflexible spherocyte, the spleen is the villain. Normal red cells must undergo extreme deformation to leave the cords of Billroth and enter the sinusoids. Because of their spheroidal shape and reduced deformability, the hapless spherocytes are trapped in the splenic cords, where they provide a happy meal for phagocytes. The splenic environment also somehow exacerbates the tendency of HS red cells to lose membrane along with K^+ ions and H_2O; prolonged splenic exposure (erythrostasis), depletion of red cell glucose, and diminished red cell pH have all been suggested to contribute to these abnormalities (Fig. 14–3). After splenectomy the spherocytes persist, but the anemia is corrected.

Morphology. The most specific morphologic finding is spherocytosis, apparent on smears as abnormally small, dark-staining (hyperchromic) red cells lacking the central zone of pallor (Fig. 14–4). Spherocytosis is distinctive but not pathognomonic, since other forms of membrane loss, such as in autoimmune hemolytic anemias, also cause the formation of spherocytes. Other features are common to all hemolytic anemias. These include reticulocytosis, marrow erythroid hyperplasia, hemosiderosis, and mild jaundice. Cholelithiasis (pigment stones) occurs in 40% to 50% of affected adults. Moderate splenic enlargement is characteristic (500–1000 gm); in few other hemolytic anemias is the spleen enlarged as much or as consistently. Splenomegaly results from congestion of the cords of Billroth and increased numbers of phagocytes needed to clear the spherocytes.

Clinical Features. The diagnosis is based on family history, hematologic findings, and laboratory evidence. In two thirds of the patients the red cells are *abnormally sensitive to osmotic lysis* when incubated in hypotonic salt solutions, which causes

the influx of water into spherocytes with little margin for expansion. HS red cells also have an *increased mean cell hemoglobin concentration*, due to dehydration caused by the loss of K^+ and H_2O.

The characteristic clinical features are anemia, splenomegaly, and jaundice. The severity of HS varies greatly. In a small minority (mainly compound heterozygotes) HS presents at birth with marked jaundice and requires exchange transfusions. In 20% to 30% of patients the disease is so mild as to be virtually asymptomatic; here the decreased red cell survival is readily compensated for by increased erythropoiesis. In most, however, the compensatory changes are outpaced, producing a chronic hemolytic anemia of mild to moderate

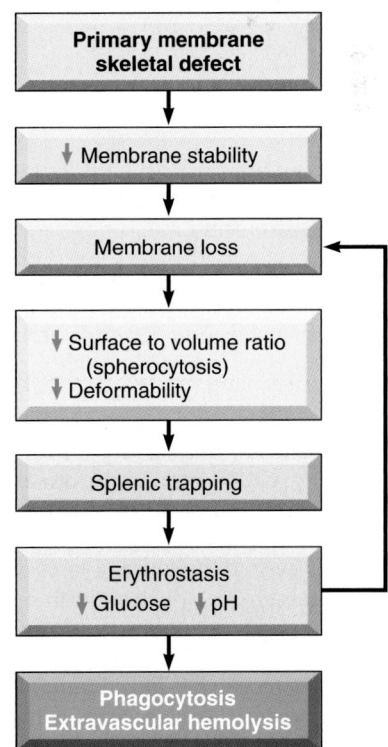

FIGURE 14–3 Pathophysiology of hereditary spherocytosis.

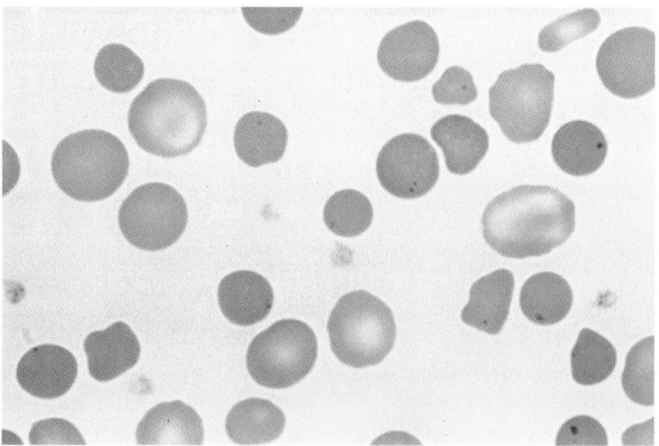

FIGURE 14–4 Hereditary spherocytosis (peripheral smear). Note the anisocytosis and several dark-appearing spherocytes with no central pallor. Howell-Jolly bodies (small dark nuclear remnants) are also present in red cells of this asplenic patient. (Courtesy of Dr. Robert W. McKenna, Department of Pathology, University of Texas Southwestern Medical School, Dallas, TX.)

severity. The generally stable clinical course is sometimes punctuated by *aplastic crises,* usually triggered by an acute parvovirus infection. Parvovirus infects and kills red cell progenitors, causing red cell production to cease until an effective immune response commences, generally in 1 to 2 weeks. Because of the reduced life span of HS red cells, cessation of erythropoiesis for even short time periods leads to sudden worsening of the anemia. Transfusions may be necessary to support the patient until the immune response clears the infection. *Hemolytic crises* are produced by intercurrent events leading to increased splenic destruction of red cells (e.g., infectious mononucleosis); these are clinically less significant than aplastic crises. Gallstones, found in many patients, can also produce symptoms. Splenectomy treats the anemia and its complications, but brings with it the risk of sepsis.

Hemolytic Disease Due to Red Cell Enzyme Defects: Glucose-6-Phosphate Dehydrogenase Deficiency

The red cell is vulnerable to injury by exogenous and endogenous oxidants. *Abnormalities in the hexose monophosphate shunt or glutathione metabolism resulting from deficient or impaired enzyme function reduce the ability of red cells to protect themselves against oxidative injuries and lead to hemolysis.* The most important of these enzyme derangements is the hereditary deficiency of glucose-6-phosphate dehydrogenase (G6PD) activity. G6PD reduces nicotinamide adenine dinucleotide phosphate (NADP) to NADPH while oxidizing glucose-6-phosphate (Fig. 14–5). NADPH then provides reducing equivalents needed for conversion of oxidized glutathione to reduced glutathione, which protects against oxidant injury by catalyzing the breakdown of compounds such as H_2O_2 (Chapter 1).

G6PD deficiency is a recessive X-linked trait, placing males at higher risk for symptomatic disease. Several hundred G6PD genetic variants are known, but most are harmless. Only two variants, designated G6PD⁻ and G6PD Mediterranean, cause

most of the clinically significant hemolytic anemias. G6PD⁻ is present in about 10% of American blacks; G6PD Mediterranean, as the name implies, is prevalent in the Middle East. The high frequency of these variants in each population is believed to stem from a protective effect against *Plasmodium falciparum* malaria.[3]

G6PD variants associated with hemolysis result in misfolding of the protein, making it more susceptible to proteolytic degradation. Compared with the most common normal variant, G6PD B, the half-life of G6PD⁻ is moderately reduced, whereas that of G6PD Mediterranean is more markedly abnormal. Because mature red cells do not synthesize new proteins, G6PD⁻ or G6PD Mediterranean enzyme activities fall quickly to levels inadequate to protect against oxidant stress as red cells age. Thus, older red cells are much more prone to hemolysis than younger ones.

The episodic hemolysis that is characteristic of G6PD deficiency is caused by exposures that generate oxidant stress. The most common triggers are *infections,* in which oxygen-derived free radicals are produced by activated leukocytes. Many infections can trigger hemolysis; viral hepatitis, pneumonia, and typhoid fever are among those most likely to do so. The other important initiators are *drugs* and certain *foods.* The oxidant drugs implicated are numerous, including antimalarials (e.g., primaquine and chloroquine), sulfonamides, nitrofurantoins, and others. Some drugs cause hemolysis only in individuals with the more severe Mediterranean variant. The most frequently cited food is the fava bean, which generates oxidants when metabolized. "Favism" is endemic in the Mediterranean, Middle East, and parts of Africa where consumption is prevalent. Uncommonly, G6PD deficiency presents as neonatal

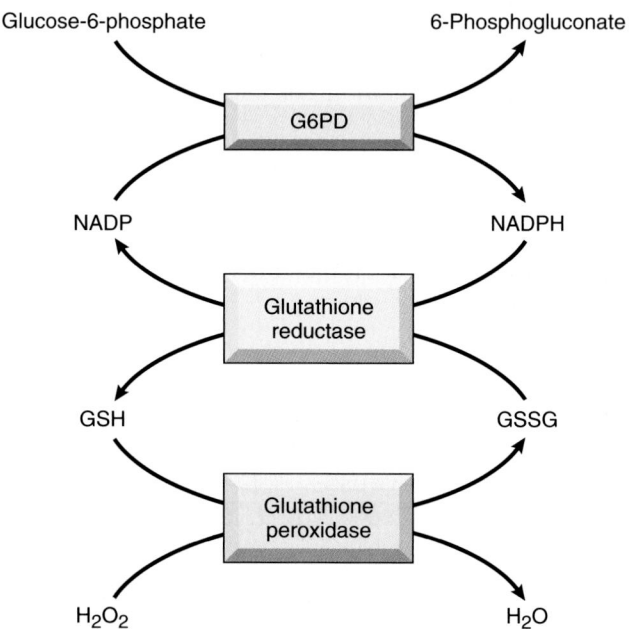

FIGURE 14–5 Role of glucose-6-phosphate dehydrogenase (G6PD) in defense against oxidant injury. The disposal of H_2O_2, a potential oxidant, is dependent on the adequacy of reduced glutathione (GSH), which is generated by the action of the reduced form of nicotinamide adenine dinucleotide (NADPH). The synthesis of NADPH is dependent on the activity of G6PD. GSSG, oxidized glutathione.

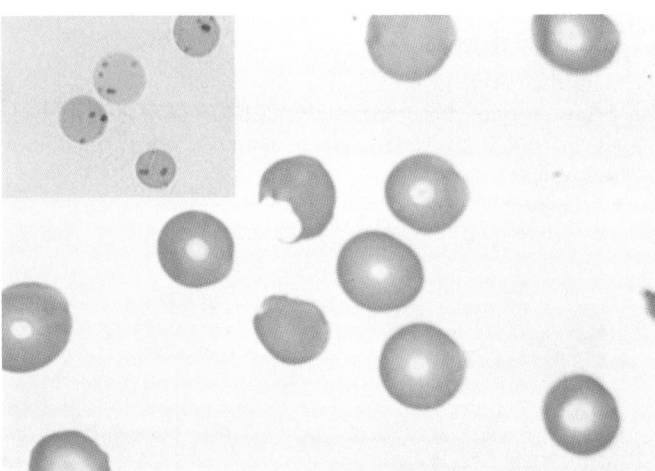

FIGURE 14–6   G6PD deficiency: effects of oxidant drug exposure (peripheral blood smear). *Inset,* Red cells with precipitates of denatured globin (Heinz bodies) revealed by supravital staining. As the splenic macrophages pluck out these inclusions, "bite cells" like the one in this smear are produced. (Courtesy of Dr. Robert W. McKenna, Department of Pathology, University of Texas Southwestern Medical School, Dallas, TX.)

jaundice or a chronic low-grade hemolytic anemia in the absence of infection or known environmental triggers.

Oxidants cause both intravascular and extravascular hemolysis in G6PD-deficient individuals. Exposure of G6PD-deficient red cells to high levels of oxidants causes the cross-linking of reactive sulfhydryl groups on globin chains, which become denatured and form membrane-bound precipitates known as *Heinz bodies.* These are seen as dark inclusions within red cells stained with crystal violet (Fig. 14–6). Heinz bodies can damage the membrane sufficiently to cause intravascular hemolysis. Less severe membrane damage results in decreased red cell deformability. As inclusion-bearing red cells pass through the splenic cords, macrophages pluck out the Heinz bodies. As a result of membrane damage, some of these partially devoured cells retain an abnormal shape, appearing to have a bite taken out of them (see Fig. 14–6). Other less severely damaged cells revert to a spherocytic shape due to loss of membrane surface area. Both bite cells and spherocytes are trapped in splenic cords and removed rapidly by phagocytes.

Acute intravascular hemolysis, marked by anemia, hemoglobinemia, and hemoglobinuria, usually begins 2 to 3 days following exposure of G6PD-deficient individuals to oxidants. The hemolysis tends to be greater in individuals with the highly unstable G6PD Mediterranean variant. Since only older red cells are at risk for lysis, the episode is *self-limited,* since hemolysis ceases when only younger G6PD-replete red cells remain (even if administration of an offending drug continues). The recovery phase is heralded by reticulocytosis. Since hemolytic episodes related to G6PD deficiency occur intermittently, features related to chronic hemolysis (e.g., splenomegaly, cholelithiasis) are absent.

Sickle Cell Disease

Sickle cell disease is a common hereditary hemoglobinopathy that occurs primarily in individuals of African descent. Several hundred different hemoglobinopathies caused by mutations

in globin genes are known, but only those associated with sickle cell disease are prevalent enough in the United States to merit discussion. Hemoglobin, as you recall, is a tetrameric protein composed of two pairs of globin chains, each with its own heme group. Normal adult red cells contain mainly HbA ($\alpha_2\beta_2$), along with small amounts of HbA$_2$ ($\alpha_2\delta_2$) and fetal hemoglobin (HbF; $\alpha_2\gamma_2$). Sickle cell disease is caused by a point mutation in the sixth codon of β-globin that leads to the replacement of a glutamate residue with a valine residue. The abnormal physiochemical properties of the resulting sickle hemoglobin (HbS) are responsible for the disease.

About 8% to 10% of African Americans, or roughly 2 million individuals, are heterozygous for HbS, a largely asymptomatic condition known as sickle cell trait. The offspring of two heterozygotes has a 1 in 4 chance of being homozygous for the sickle mutation, a state that produces symptomatic sickle cell disease. In such individuals, almost all the hemoglobin in the red cell is HbS ($\alpha_2\beta^s_2$). There are about 70,000 individuals with sickle cell disease in the United States. In certain populations in Africa the prevalence of heterozygosity is as high as 30%. This high frequency probably stems from protection afforded by HbS against falciparum malaria.[3]

Pathogenesis. *HbS molecules undergo polymerization when deoxygenated.* Initially the red cell cytosol converts from a freely flowing liquid to a viscous gel as HbS aggregates form. With continued deoxygenation aggregated HbS molecules assemble into long needle-like fibers within red cells, producing a distorted sickle or holly-leaf shape.

The presence of HbS underlies the major pathologic manifestations: (1) chronic hemolysis, (2) microvascular occlusions, and (3) tissue damage. Several variables affect the rate and degree of sickling:

- *Interaction of HbS with the other types of hemoglobin in the cell.* In heterozygotes with sickle cell trait, about 40% of the hemoglobin is HbS and the rest is HbA, which interferes with HbS polymerization. As a result, red cells in heterozygous individuals do not sickle except under conditions of profound hypoxia. HbF inhibits the polymerization of HbS even more than HbA; hence, infants do not become symptomatic until they reach 5 or 6 months of age, when the level of HbF normally falls. However, in some individuals HbF expression remains at relatively high levels, a condition known as hereditary persistence of HbF; in these individuals, sickle cell disease is much less severe. Another variant hemoglobin is HbC, in which lysine is substituted for glutamate in the sixth amino acid residue of β-globin. In HbSC cells the percentage of HbS is 50%, as compared with only 40% in HbAS cells. Moreover, HbSC cells tend to lose salt and water and become dehydrated, which increases the intracellular concentration of HbS. Both of these factors increase the tendency for HbS to polymerize. As a result, individuals with HbS and HbC have a symptomatic sickling disorder (termed *HbSC disease*), but it is milder than sickle cell disease. About 2% to 3% of American blacks are asymptomatic HbC heterozygotes, and about 1 in 1250 has HbSC disease.

- *Mean cell hemoglobin concentration* (MCHC). Higher HbS concentrations increase the probability that aggregation and polymerization will occur during any given period of deoxygenation. Thus, intracellular dehydration, which increases the MCHC, facilitates sickling. Conversely, conditions that decrease the MCHC reduce the disease severity. This occurs when the individual is homozygous for HbS but also has coexistent α-thalassemia, which reduces Hb synthesis and leads to milder disease.

○ *Intracellular pH.* A decrease in pH reduces the oxygen affinity of hemoglobin, thereby increasing the fraction of deoxygenated HbS at any given oxygen tension and augmenting the tendency for sickling.

○ *Transit time of red cells through microvascular beds.* As will be discussed, much of the pathology of sickle cell disease is related to vascular occlusion caused by sickling within microvascular beds. Transit times in most normal microvascular beds are too short for significant aggregation of deoxygenated HbS to occur, and as a result sickling is confined to microvascular beds with slow transit times. Transit times are slow in the normal spleen and bone marrow, which are prominently affected in sickle cell disease, and also in vascular beds that are inflamed. As you will recall from Chapter 2, the movement of blood through inflamed tissues is slowed because of the adhesion of leukocytes and red cells to activated endothelial cells and the transudation of fluid through leaky vessels. As a result, inflamed vascular beds are prone to sickling and occlusion. Sickle red cells may express elevated levels of several adhesion molecules that have been implicated in binding to endothelial cells.[4-6] There is also evidence suggesting that sickle red cells induce some degree of endothelial activation,[7] which may be related to the adhesion of red cells and granulocytes, vaso-occlusion–induced hypoxia, and other insults.

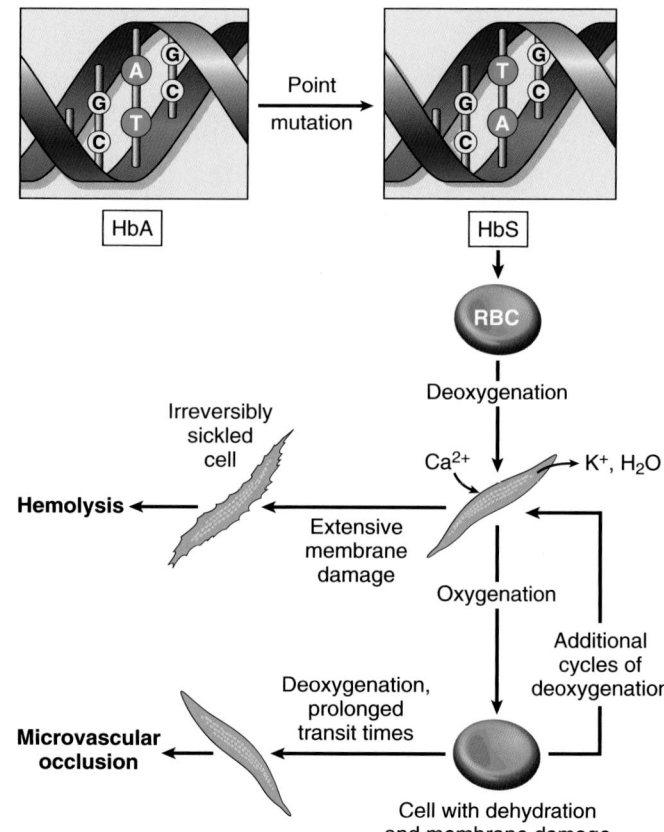

FIGURE 14–7   Pathophysiology of sickle cell disease.

Sickling causes cumulative damage to red cells through several mechanisms. As HbS polymers grow, they herniate through the membrane skeleton and project from the cell ensheathed by only the lipid bilayer. This severe derangement in membrane structure causes the influx of Ca^{2+} ions, which induce the cross-linking of membrane proteins and activate an ion channel that permits the efflux of K^+ and H_2O. *With repeated episodes of sickling, red cells become increasingly dehydrated, dense, and rigid* (Fig. 14–7). Eventually, the most severely damaged cells are converted to end-stage, nondeformable, irreversibly sickled cells, which retain a sickle shape even when fully oxygenated. *The severity of the hemolysis correlates with the percentage of irreversibly sickled cells,* which are rapidly sequestered and removed by mononuclear phagocytes (extravascular hemolysis). Sickled red cells are also mechanically fragile, leading to some intravascular hemolysis as well.

The pathogenesis of the *microvascular occlusions,* which are responsible for the most serious clinical features, is less certain. Microvascular occlusions are not related to the number of irreversibly sickled cells in the blood, but instead may be dependent upon more subtle red cell membrane damage and other factors, such as inflammation, that tend to slow or arrest the movement of red cells through microvascular beds (see Fig. 14–7). As mentioned above, sickle red cells express higher than normal levels of adhesion molecules and are sticky. Mediators released from granulocytes during inflammatory reactions up-regulate the expression of adhesion molecules on endothelial cells (Chapter 2) and further enhance the tendency for sickle red cells to get arrested during transit through

the microvasculature. A possible role for inflammatory cells is suggested by observations showing that the leukocyte count correlates with the frequency of pain crises and other measures of tissue damage. The stagnation of red cells within inflamed vascular beds results in extended exposure to low oxygen tension, sickling, and vascular obstruction. Once started, it is easy to envision how a vicious cycle of sickling, obstruction, hypoxia, and more sickling ensues. Depletion of nitric oxide (NO) may also play a part in the vascular occlusions. Free hemoglobin released from lysed sickle red cells can bind and inactivate NO, which is a potent vasodilator and inhibitor of platelet aggregation. Thus, reduced NO increases vascular tone (narrowing vessels) and enhances platelet aggregation, both of which may contribute to red cell stasis, sickling, and (in some instances) thrombosis.

Morphology. In full-blown sickle cell anemia, the peripheral blood demonstrates variable numbers of irreversibly sickled cells, reticulocytosis, and target cells, which result from red cell dehydration (Fig. 14–8). Howell-Jolly bodies (small nuclear remnants) are also present in some red cells due to the asplenia (see below). The bone marrow is hyperplastic as a result of a compensatory erythroid hyperplasia. Expansion of the marrow leads to bone resorption and secondary new bone formation, resulting in prominent cheekbones and changes in the skull that resemble a crew-cut in x-rays. Extramedullary hema-

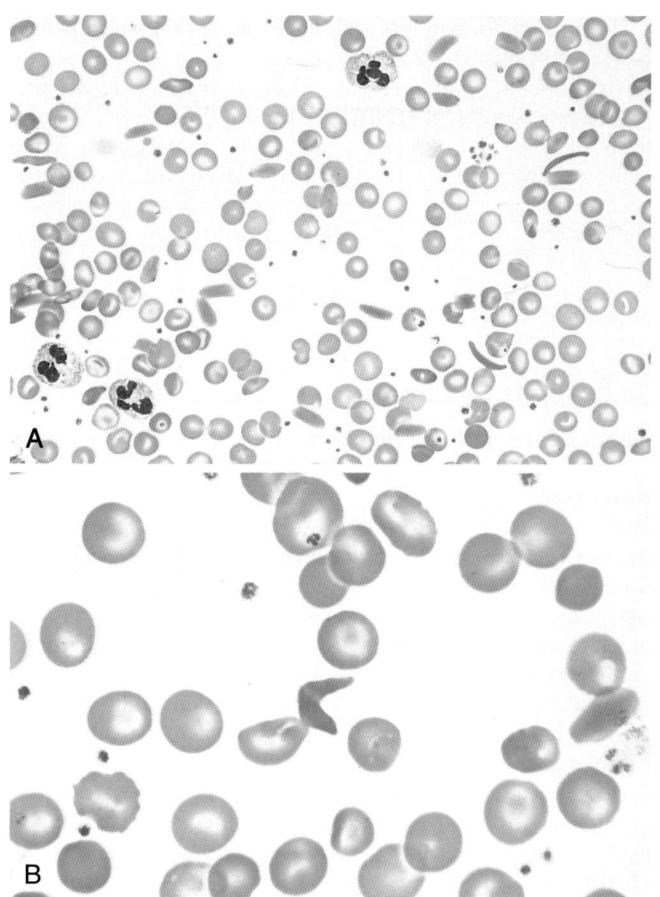

FIGURE 14–8 Sickle cell disease (peripheral blood smear). **A,** Low magnification shows sickle cells, anisocytosis, and poikilocytosis. **B,** Higher magnification shows an irreversibly sickled cell in the center. (Courtesy of Dr. Robert W. McKenna, Department of Pathology, University of Texas Southwestern Medical School, Dallas, TX.)

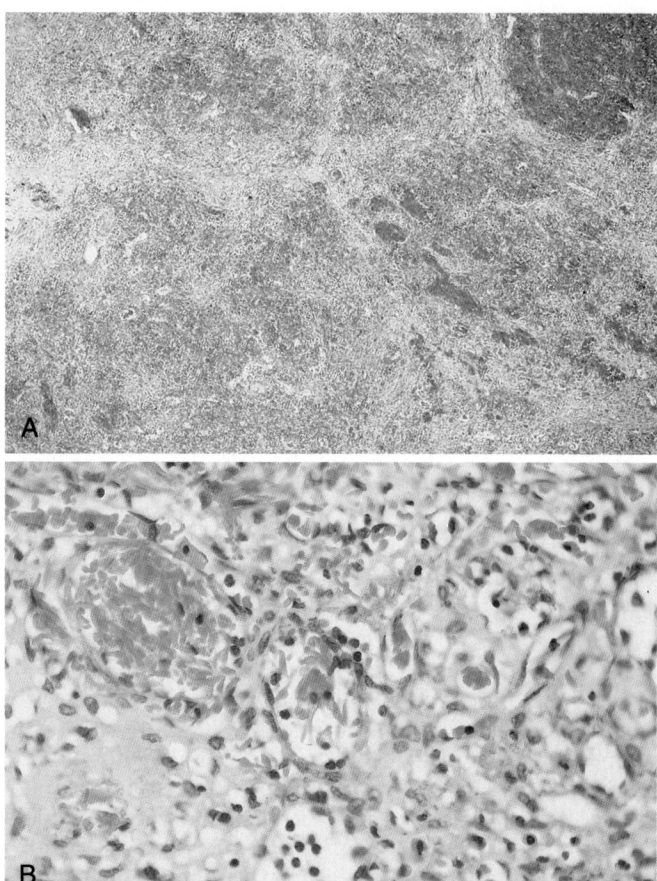

FIGURE 14–9 **A,** Spleen in sickle cell disease (low power). Red pulp cords and sinusoids are markedly congested; between the congested areas, pale areas of fibrosis resulting from ischemic damage are evident. **B,** Under high power, splenic sinusoids are dilated and filled with sickled red cells. (Courtesy of Dr. Darren Wirthwein, Department of Pathology, University of Texas Southwestern Medical School, Dallas, TX.)

topoiesis can also appear. The increased breakdown of hemoglobin can cause pigment gallstones and hyperbilirubinemia.

In early childhood, the spleen is enlarged up to 500 gm by red pulp congestion, which is caused by the trapping of sickled red cells in the cords and sinuses (Fig. 14–9). With time, however, the chronic erythrostasis leads to splenic infarction, fibrosis, and progressive shrinkage, so that by adolescence or early adulthood only a small nubbin of fibrous splenic tissue is left; this process is called **autosplenectomy** (Fig. 14–10). Infarctions caused by vascular occlusions can occur in many other tissues as well, including the bones, brain, kidney, liver, retina, and pulmonary vessels, the latter sometimes producing cor pulmonale. In adult patients, vascular stagnation in subcutaneous tissues often leads to leg ulcers; this complication is rare in children.

Clinical Features. Sickle cell disease causes a moderately severe hemolytic anemia (hematocrit 18% to 30%) that is associated with reticulocytosis, hyperbilirubinemia, and the presence of irreversibly sickled cells. Its course is punctuated

by a variety of "crises." *Vaso-occlusive crises,* also called *pain crises,* are episodes of hypoxic injury and infarction that cause severe pain in the affected region. Although infection, dehydration, and acidosis (all of which favor sickling) can act as triggers, in most instances no predisposing cause is identified.

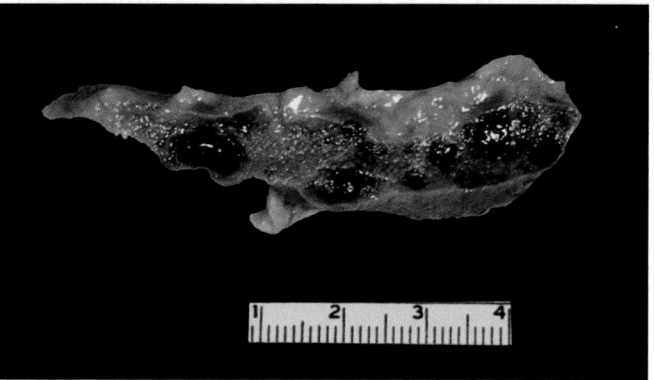

FIGURE 14–10 "Autoinfarcted" splenic remnant in sickle cell disease. (Courtesy of Dr. Dennis Burns and Dr. Darren Wirthwein, Department of Pathology, University of Texas Southwestern Medical School, Dallas, TX.)

The most commonly involved sites are the bones, lungs, liver, brain, spleen, and penis. *In children, painful bone crises are extremely common and often difficult to distinguish from acute osteomyelitis.* These frequently manifest as the hand-foot syndrome or dactylitis of the bones of the hands or feet, or both. *Acute chest syndrome* is a particularly dangerous type of vaso-occlusive crisis involving the lungs, which typically presents with fever, cough, chest pain, and pulmonary infiltrates. Pulmonary inflammation (such as may be induced by a simple infection) causes blood flow to become sluggish and "spleen-like," leading to sickling and vaso-occlusion. This compromises pulmonary function, creating a potentially fatal cycle of worsening pulmonary and systemic hypoxemia, sickling, and vaso-occlusion. Other forms of vascular obstruction, particularly stroke, can take a devastating toll. Factors proposed to contribute to stroke include the adhesion of sickle red cells to arterial vascular endothelium and vasoconstriction caused by the depletion of NO by free hemoglobin.[8]

Although occlusive crises are the most common cause of patient morbidity and mortality, several other acute events complicate the course. *Sequestration crises* occur in children with intact spleens. Massive entrapment of sickle red cells leads to rapid splenic enlargement, hypovolemia, and sometimes shock. These complications may be fatal in several cases. Survival from sequestration crises and the acute chest syndrome requires treatment with exchange transfusions. *Aplastic crises* stem from the infection of red cell progenitors by parvovirus B19, which causes a transient cessation of erythropoiesis and a sudden worsening of the anemia.

In addition to these dramatic crises, chronic tissue hypoxia takes a subtle but important toll. Chronic hypoxia is responsible for a generalized impairment of growth and development, as well as organ damage affecting spleen, heart, kidneys, and lungs. Sickling provoked by hypertonicity in the renal medulla causes damage that eventually leads to hyposthenuria (the inability to concentrate urine), which increases the propensity for dehydration and its attendant risks.

Increased susceptibility to infection with encapsulated organisms is another threat. This is due in large part to altered splenic function, which is severely impaired in children by congestion and poor blood flow, and completely absent in adults because of splenic infarction. Defects of uncertain etiology in the alternative complement pathway also impair the opsonization of bacteria. *Pneumococcus pneumoniae* and *Haemophilus influenzae* septicemia and meningitis, common causes of death, particularly in children, can be reduced by vaccination and prophylactic antibiotics.

It must be emphasized that there is great variation in the clinical manifestations of sickle cell disease. Some individuals are crippled by repeated vaso-occlusive crises, whereas others have only mild symptoms. The basis for this wide range in disease expression is not understood.

The diagnosis is suggested by the clinical findings and the presence of irreversibly sickled red cells and is confirmed by various tests for sickle hemoglobin. In general, these involve mixing a blood sample with an oxygen-consuming reagent, such as metabisulfite, which induces sickling of red cells if HbS is present. Hemoglobin electrophoresis is also used to demonstrate the presence of HbS and exclude other sickle syndromes, such as HbSC disease. Prenatal diagnosis is possible by analysis of fetal DNA obtained by amniocentesis or chorionic biopsy.

The outlook for patients with sickle cell disease has improved considerably over the last 10 to 20 years. About 90% of patients survive to age 20, and close to 50% survive beyond the fifth decade. A mainstay of treatment is an inhibitor of DNA synthesis, hydroxyurea, which has several beneficial effects. These include (1) an increase in red cell HbF levels, which occurs by unknown mechanisms; and (2) an anti-inflammatory effect, which stems from an inhibition of white cell production. These activities (and possibly others[9]) are believed to act in concert to decrease crises related to vascular occlusions in both children and adults.

Thalassemia Syndromes

The thalassemia syndromes are a heterogeneous group of disorders caused by inherited mutations that decrease the synthesis of adult hemoglobin, HbA ($\alpha_2\beta_2$). The two α chains in HbA are encoded by an identical pair of α-globin genes on chromosome 16, while the two β chains are encoded by a single β-globin gene on chromosome 11. β-Thalassemia is caused by deficient synthesis of β chains, whereas α-thalassemia is caused by deficient synthesis of α chains. The hematologic consequences of diminished synthesis of one globin chain stem not only from hemoglobin deficiency but also from a relative excess of the other globin chain, particularly in β-thalassemia. Thalassemia syndromes are endemic in the Mediterranean basin, the Middle East, tropical Africa, the Indian subcontinent, and Asia, and in aggregate are among the most common inherited disorders of humans. As with sickle cell disease and other common inherited red cell disorders, their prevalence seems to be explained by the protection they afford heterozygous carriers against malaria.[3] Although we will discuss the thalassemia syndromes with other inherited forms of anemia associated with hemolysis, *it is important to recognize that the defects in globin synthesis that underlie these disorders also impair red cell production and contribute to the pathogenesis of these disorders.*

β-Thalassemias

The β-thalassemias are caused by mutations that diminish the synthesis of β-globin chains. The clinical severity varies because of heterogeneity in the causative mutations. We will begin our discussion with the molecular lesions in β-thalassemia and then relate the clinical variants to specific underlying molecular defects.

Molecular Pathogenesis. The causative mutations fall into two categories: (1) β^0 *mutations,* associated with absent β-globin synthesis, and (2) β^+ *mutations,* characterized by reduced (but detectable) β-globin synthesis. Sequencing of β-thalassemia genes has revealed more than 100 different causative mutations, mostly consisting of point mutations. Details of these mutations and their effects are found in specialized texts. Figure 14–11 gives a few illustrative examples.

● *Splicing mutations. These are the most common cause of β^+-thalassemia.* Most of these mutations lie within introns, while a few are located within exons. Some of these mutations destroy the normal RNA splice junctions and completely prevent the production of normal β-globin mRNA, resulting in β^0-thalassemia. Others create an

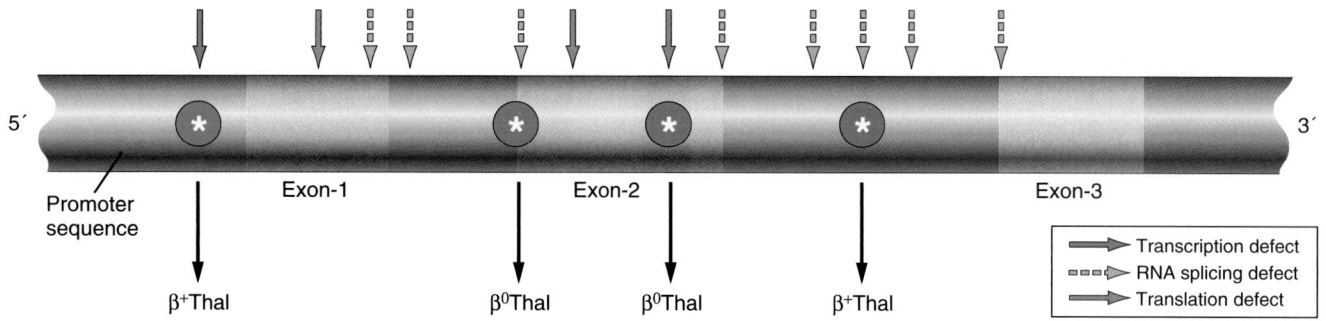

FIGURE 14–11 Distribution of β-globin gene mutations associated with β-thalassemia. Arrows denote sites where point mutations giving rise to β⁰ or β⁺ thalassemia have been identified.

"ectopic" splice site within an intron. Because the flanking normal splice sites remain, both normal and abnormal splicing occurs and some normal β-globin mRNA is made, resulting in β⁺-thalassemia.

○ *Promoter region mutations.* These mutations reduce transcription by 75% to 80%. Some normal β-globin is synthesized; thus, these mutations are associated with β⁺-thalassemia.

○ *Chain terminator mutations. These are the most common cause of β⁰-thalassemia.* Two subtypes of mutations fall into this category. The most common type creates a new stop codon within an exon; the second introduces small insertions or deletions that shift the mRNA reading frames (frameshift mutations; see Chapter 5). Both block translation and prevent the synthesis of any functional β-globin.

Impaired β-globin synthesis results in anemia by two mechanisms (Fig. 14–12). The deficit in HbA synthesis produces "underhemoglobinized" hypochromic, microcytic red cells with subnormal oxygen transport capacity. Even more important is the diminished survival of red cells and their precursors, which results from the imbalance in α- and β-globin synthesis. Unpaired α chains precipitate within red cell precursors, forming insoluble inclusions. These inclusions cause a variety of untoward effects, but *membrane damage is the proximal cause of most red cell pathology.* Many red cell precursors succumb to membrane damage and undergo apoptosis. In severe β-thalassemia, it is estimated that 70% to 85% of red cell precursors suffer this fate, which leads to *ineffective erythropoiesis.* Those red cells that are released from the marrow also bear inclusions and membrane damage and are prone to splenic sequestration and *extravascular hemolysis.*

In severe β-thalassemia, ineffective erythropoiesis creates several additional problems. Erythropoietic drive in the setting of severe uncompensated anemia leads to massive erythroid hyperplasia in the marrow and extensive extramedullary hematopoiesis. The expanding mass of red cell precursors erodes the bony cortex, impairs bone growth, and produces skeletal abnormalities (described later). Extramedullary hematopoiesis involves the liver, spleen, and lymph nodes, and in extreme cases produces extraosseous masses in the thorax, abdomen, and pelvis. The metabolically active erythroid progenitors steal nutrients from other tissues that are already oxygen-starved, causing severe cachexia in untreated patients.

Another serious complication of ineffective erythropoiesis is the excessive absorption of dietary iron. Ineffective erythropoi-esis suppresses the circulating levels of hepcidin, a critical negative regulator of iron absorption (described later under iron deficiency anemia). Low levels of hepcidin and the iron load of repeated blood transfusions inevitably lead to severe iron overload unless preventive steps are taken. Secondary injury to parenchymal organs, particularly the iron-laden liver, often follows and sometimes induces secondary hemochromatosis (Chapter 18).

Clinical Syndromes. The relationships of clinical phenotypes to underlying genotypes are summarized in Table 14–3. Clinical classification of β-thalassemia is based on the severity of the anemia, which in turn depends on the genetic defect (β⁺ or β⁰) and the gene dosage (homozygous or heterozygous). In general, individuals with two β-thalassemia alleles (β⁺/β⁺, β⁺/β⁰, or β⁰/β⁰) have a severe, transfusion-dependent anemia called β-*thalassemia major.* Heterozygotes with one β-thalassemia gene and one normal gene (β⁺/β or β⁰/β) usually have a mild asymptomatic microcytic anemia. This condition is referred to as β-*thalassemia minor* or β-*thalassemia trait.* A third genetically heterogeneous variant of moderate severity is called β-*thalassemia intermedia.* This category includes milder variants of β⁺/β⁺ or β⁺/β⁰-thalassemia and unusual forms of heterozygous β-thalassemia. Some patients with β-thalassemia intermedia have two defective β-globin genes and an α-thalassemia gene defect, which lessens the imbalance in α- and β-chain synthesis. In other rare but informative cases, individuals have a single β-globin defect and one or two extra copies of normal α-globin genes (stemming from a gene duplication event), which worsens the chain imbalance.[10] These unusual forms of the disease serve to emphasize the cardinal role of unpaired α-globin chains in the pathology. The clinical and morphologic features of β-thalassemia intermedia are not described separately but can be surmised from the following discussions of β-thalassemia major and β-thalassemia minor.

β-Thalassemia Major. β-thalassemia major is most common in Mediterranean countries, parts of Africa, and Southeast Asia. In the United States the incidence is highest in immigrants from these areas. The anemia manifests 6 to 9 months after birth as hemoglobin synthesis switches from HbF to HbA. In untransfused patients, hemoglobin levels are 3 to 6 gm/dL. The red cells may completely lack HbA (β⁰/β⁰ genotype) or contain small amounts (β⁺/β⁺ or β⁰/β⁺ genotypes). The major red cell hemoglobin is HbF, which is markedly elevated. HbA₂ levels are sometimes high but more often are normal or low.

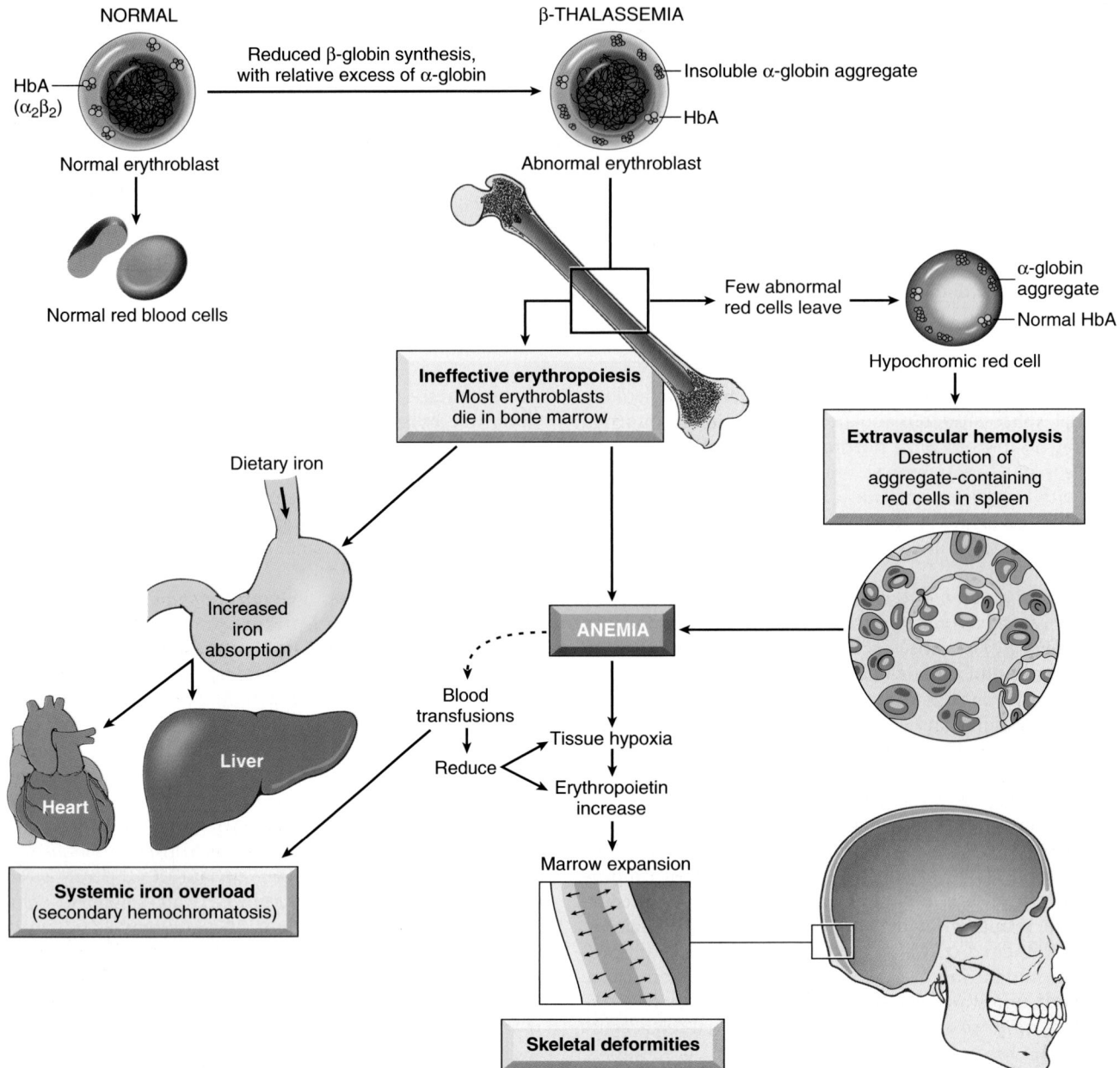

FIGURE 14–12 Pathogenesis of β-thalassemia major. Note that the aggregates of unpaired α-globin chains, a hallmark of the disease, are not visible in routinely stained blood smears. Blood transfusions are a double-edged sword, diminishing the anemia and its attendant complications, but also adding to the systemic iron overload.

Morphology. Blood smears show severe red cell abnormalities, including marked variation in size (anisocytosis) and shape (poikilocytosis), microcytosis, and hypochromia. Target cells (so called because hemoglobin collects in the center of the cell), basophilic stippling, and fragmented red cells are also common. Inclusions of aggregated α chains are efficiently removed by the spleen and not easily seen. The reticulocyte count is elevated, but it is lower than expected for the severity of anemia because of the ineffective erythropoiesis. Variable numbers of poorly hemoglobinized nucleated red cell precursors (nor-

moblasts) are seen in the peripheral blood as a result of "stress" erythropoiesis and abnormal release from sites of extramedullary hematopoiesis.

Other major alterations involve the bone marrow and spleen. In the untransfused patient there is a striking expansion of hematopoietically active marrow. In the bones of the face and skull the burgeoning marrow erodes existing cortical bone and induces new bone formation, giving rise to a "crew-cut" appearance on x-ray (Fig. 14–13). Both phagocyte hyperplasia and extramedullary hematopoiesis contribute to enlargement of the spleen, which can weigh as much as 1500 gm. The liver and the lymph nodes can also be enlarged by extramedullary hematopoiesis.

Hemosiderosis and secondary hemochromatosis, the two manifestations of iron overload (Chapter 18), occur in almost all patients. The deposited iron often damages organs, most notably the heart, liver, and pancreas.

The clinical course of β-thalassemia major is brief unless blood transfusions are given. Untreated children suffer from growth retardation and die at an early age from the effects of anemia. In those who survive long enough, the cheekbones and other bony prominences are enlarged and distorted. Hepatosplenomegaly due to extramedullary hematopoiesis is usually present. Although blood transfusions improve the anemia and suppress complications related to excessive erythropoiesis, they lead to complications of their own. Cardiac disease resulting from progressive iron overload and secondary hemochromatosis (Chapter 18) is an important cause of death, particularly in heavily transfused patients, who must be treated with iron chelators to prevent or reduce this complication. With transfusions and iron chelation, survival into the third decade is possible, but the overall outlook remains guarded. Bone marrow transplantation is the only therapy offering a cure and is being used increasingly.[11] Prenatal diagnosis is possible by molecular analysis of DNA.

β-Thalassemia Minor. β-Thalassemia minor is much more common than β-thalassemia major and understandably affects the same ethnic groups. Most patients are heterozygous carriers of a β^+ or β^0 allele. These patients are usually asymptomatic. Anemia, if present, is mild. The peripheral blood smear typically shows some red cell abnormalities, including hypochromia, microcytosis, basophilic stippling, and target cells. Mild erythroid hyperplasia is seen in the bone marrow. Hemoglobin electrophoresis usually reveals an increase in

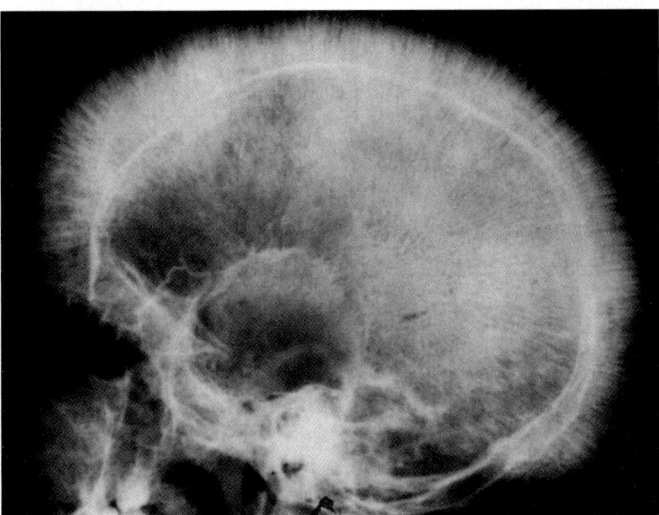

FIGURE 14–13 Thalassemia: x-ray film of the skull showing new bone formation on the outer table, producing perpendicular radiations resembling a crewcut. (Courtesy of Dr. Jack Reynolds, Department of Radiology, University of Texas Southwestern Medical School, Dallas, TX.)

HbA_2 ($\alpha_2\delta_2$) to 4% to 8% of the total hemoglobin (normal, 2.5% ± 0.3%), which is a reflection of an elevated ratio of δ-chain to β-chain synthesis. HbF levels are generally normal or occasionally slightly increased.

Recognition of β-thalassemia trait is important for two reasons: (1) differentiation from the hypochromic microcytic anemia of iron deficiency and (2) genetic counseling. Iron deficiency can usually be excluded through measurement of serum iron, total iron-binding capacity, and serum ferritin (as described later under iron deficiency anemia). The increase in HbA_2 is diagnostically useful, particularly in individuals (such as women of childbearing age) who are at risk for both β-thalassemia trait and iron deficiency.

α-Thalassemias

The α-thalassemias are caused by inherited deletions that result in reduced or absent synthesis of α-globin chains. Normally, there are four α-globin genes, and the severity of α-thalassemia depends on how many α-globin genes are affected. As in β-thalassemias, the anemia stems both from a lack of adequate hemoglobin and the effects of excess unpaired non-α chains (β, γ, and δ), which vary in type at different ages. In newborns with α-thalassemia, excess unpaired γ-globin chains form γ_4 tetramers known as hemoglobin Barts, whereas in older children and adults excess β-globin chains form β_4 tetramers known as HbH. Since free β and γ chains are more soluble than free α chains and form fairly stable homotetramers, hemolysis and ineffective erythropoiesis are less severe than in β-thalassemias. A variety of molecular lesions give rise to α-thalassemia, but gene deletion is the most common cause of reduced α-chain synthesis.

Clinical Syndromes. *The clinical syndromes are determined and classified by the number of α-globin genes that are deleted.* Each of the four α-globin genes normally contributes 25% of the total α-globin chains. α-Thalassemia syndromes stem from combinations of deletions that remove one to four α-globin genes. Not surprisingly, the severity of the clinical syndrome is proportional to the number of α-globin genes that are deleted. The different types of α-thalassemia and their salient clinical features are listed in Table 14–3.

Silent Carrier State. This is associated with the deletion of a single α-globin gene, which causes a barely detectable reduction in α-globin chain synthesis. These individuals are completely asymptomatic, but they have slight microcytosis.

α-Thalassemia Trait. This is caused by the deletion of two α-globin genes from a single chromosome (α/α –/–), or the deletion of one α-globin gene from each of the two chromosomes (α/– α/–) (see Table 14–3). The former genotype is more common in Asian populations, the latter in regions of Africa. Both genotypes produce similar quantitative deficiencies of α-globin and are clinically identical, but have different implications for the children of affected individuals, who are at risk of clinically significant α-thalassemia (HbH disease or hydrops fetalis) only when at least one parent has the –/– haplotype. As a result, symptomatic α-thalassemia is relatively common in Asian populations and rare in black African populations. The clinical picture in α-thalassemia trait is identical to that described for β-thalassemia minor, that is, small red cells (microcytosis), minimal or no anemia,

TABLE 14–3   Clinical and Genetic Classification of Thalassemias

Clinical Syndromes	Genotype	Clinical Features	Molecular Genetics
β-THALASSEMIAS			
β-Thalassemia major	Homozygous β-thalassemia (β^0/β^0, β^+/β^+, β^0/β^+)	Severe; requires blood transfusions	Mainly point mutations that lead to defects in the transcription, splicing, or translation of β-globin mRNA
β-Thalassemia intermedia	Variable (β^0/β^+, β^+/β^+, β^0/β, β^+/β)	Severe but does not require regular blood transfusions	
β-Thalassemia minor	Heterozygous β-thalassemia (β^0/β, β^+/β)	Asymptomatic with mild or absent anemia; red cell abnormalities seen	
α-THALASSEMIAS			
Silent carrier	$-/\alpha \ \alpha/\alpha$	Asymptomatic; no red cell abnormality	Mainly gene deletions
α-Thalassemia trait	$-/- \ \alpha/\alpha$ (Asian) $-/\alpha \ -/\alpha$ (black African, Asian)	Asymptomatic, like β-thalassemia minor	
HbH disease	$-/- \ -/\alpha$	Severe; resembles β-thalassemia intermedia	
Hydrops fetalis	$-/- \ -/-$	Lethal in utero without transfusions	

and no abnormal physical signs. HbA_2 levels are normal or low.

Hemoglobin H Disease. This is caused by deletion of three α-globin genes. As already discussed, HbH disease is most common in Asian populations. With only one normal α-globin gene, the synthesis of α chains is markedly reduced, and tetramers of β-globin, called HbH, form. HbH has an extremely high affinity for oxygen and therefore is not useful for oxygen delivery, leading to tissue hypoxia disproportionate to the level of hemoglobin. Additionally, HbH is prone to oxidation, which causes it to precipitate out and form intracellular inclusions that promote red cell sequestration and phagocytosis in the spleen. The result is a moderately severe anemia resembling β-thalassemia intermedia.

Hydrops Fetalis. This most severe form of α-thalassemia is caused by deletion of all four α-globin genes. In the fetus, excess γ-globin chains form tetramers (hemoglobin Barts) that have such a high affinity for oxygen that they deliver little to tissues. Survival in early development is due to the expression of ζ chains, an embryonic globin that pairs with γ chains to form a functional $\zeta_2\gamma_2$ Hb tetramer. Signs of fetal distress usually become evident by the third trimester of pregnancy. In the past, severe tissue anoxia led to death in utero or shortly after birth; with intrauterine transfusion many such infants are now saved. The fetus shows severe pallor, generalized edema, and massive hepatosplenomegaly similar to that seen in hemolytic disease of the newborn (Chapter 10). There is a lifelong dependence on blood transfusions for survival, with the associated risk of iron overload. Bone marrow transplantation can be curative.[11]

Paroxysmal Nocturnal Hemoglobinuria

Paroxysmal nocturnal hemoglobinuria (PNH) is a disease that results from acquired mutations in the phosphatidylinositol glycan complementation group A gene (PIGA), an enzyme that is essential for the synthesis of certain cell surface proteins. PNH has an incidence of 2 to 5 per million in the United States. Despite its rarity, it has fascinated hematologists because it is the only hemolytic anemia caused by an acquired genetic defect. Recall that proteins are anchored into the lipid bilayer in two ways. Most have a hydrophobic region that spans the cell membrane; these are called transmembrane proteins. The others are attached to the cell membrane through a covalent linkage to a specialized phospholipid called glycosylphosphatidylinositol (GPI). In PNH, these GPI-linked proteins are deficient because of somatic mutations that inactivate PIGA. PIGA is X-linked and subject to lyonization (random inactivation of one X chromosome in cells of females; Chapter 5). As a result, a single acquired mutation in the active *PIGA* gene of any given cell is sufficient to produce a deficiency state. Because the causative mutations occur in a hematopoietic stem cell, all of its clonal progeny (red cells, white cells, and platelets) are deficient in GPI-linked proteins. Typically the mutant clone coexists with the progeny of normal stem cells that are not PIGA deficient.

Remarkably, most normal individuals harbor small numbers of bone marrow cells with *PIGA* mutations identical to those that cause PNH. It is hypothesized that these cells increase in numbers (thus producing clinically evident PNH) only in rare instances where they have a selective advantage, such as in the setting of autoimmune reactions against GPI-linked antigens.[12] Such a scenario might explain the frequent association of PNH and aplastic anemia, a marrow failure syndrome (discussed later) that has an autoimmune basis in many individuals.

PNH blood cells are deficient in three GPI-linked proteins that regulate complement activity: (1) decay–accelerating factor, or CD55; (2) membrane inhibitor of reactive lysis, or CD59; and (3) C8 binding protein. Of these factors, the most important is CD59, a potent inhibitor of C3 convertase that prevents the spontaneous activation of the alternative complement pathway.

Red cells, platelets, and granulocytes deficient in these GPI-linked factors are abnormally susceptible to lysis or injury by complement. In red cells this manifests as *intravascular hemolysis*, which is caused by the C5b-C9 membrane attack complex. The hemolysis is paroxysmal and nocturnal in only 25% of cases; chronic hemolysis without dramatic hemoglobinuria is more typical. The tendency for red cells to lyse at night is explained by a slight decrease in blood pH during sleep, which increases the activity of complement. The anemia is variable but usually mild to moderate in severity. The loss of heme iron in the urine (hemosiderinuria) eventually leads to iron deficiency, which can exacerbate the anemia if untreated.

Thrombosis is the leading cause of disease-related death in individuals with PNH. About 40% of patients suffer from venous thrombosis, often involving the hepatic, portal, or cerebral veins. Dysfunction of platelets due to the absence of certain GPI-linked proteins contributes to the prothrombotic state, as does the absorption of NO by free hemoglobin (as discussed under sickle cell disease).[13] About 5% to 10% of patients eventually develop acute myeloid leukemia or a myelodysplastic syndrome, possibly because hematopoietic stem cells have suffered some type of genetic damage.

PNH is diagnosed by flow cytometry, which provides a sensitive means for detecting red cells that are deficient in GPI-linked proteins such as CD59 (Fig. 14–14). Several therapeutic approaches are available, none of which is entirely satisfactory. Infusion of a monoclonal antibody inhibitor of C5a greatly reduces the hemolysis but exposes patients to an increased risk of serious or fatal meningococcal infections (as is true of individuals with inherited complement defects). Immunosuppressive drugs are sometimes beneficial for those with evidence of marrow aplasia. The only cure is bone marrow transplantation.

Immunohemolytic Anemia

Hemolytic anemias in this category are caused by antibodies that bind to red cells, leading to their premature destruction. Although these disorders are commonly referred to as autoimmune hemolytic anemias, the designation immunohemolytic anemia is preferred because in some instances the immune reaction is initiated by an ingested drug. Immunohemolytic anemia can be classified based on the characteristics of the responsible antibody (Table 14–4).

The diagnosis of immunohemolytic anemia requires the detection of antibodies and/or complement on red cells from the patient. This is done using the *direct Coombs antiglobulin test*, in which the patient's red cells are mixed with sera con-

TABLE 14–4 Classification of Immunohemolytic Anemias
WARM ANTIBODY TYPE (IgG ANTIBODIES ACTIVE AT 37°C)
Primary (idiopathic)
Secondary
Autoimmune disorders (particularly systemic lupus erythematosus)
Drugs
Lymphoid neoplasms
COLD AGGLUTININ TYPE (IgM ANTIBODIES ACTIVE BELOW 37°C)
Acute (mycoplasmal infection, infectious mononucleosis)
Chronic
Idiopathic
Lymphoid neoplasms
COLD HEMOLYSIN TYPE (IgG ANTIBODIES ACTIVE BELOW 37°C)
Rare; occurs mainly in children following viral infections

taining antibodies that are specific for human immunoglobulin or complement. If either immunoglobulin or complement is present on the surface of the red cells, the multivalent antibodies cause agglutination, which is easily appreciated visually as clumping. In the *indirect Coombs antiglobulin test*, the patient's serum is tested for its ability to agglutinate commercially available red cells bearing particular defined antigens. This test is used to characterize the antigen target and temperature dependence of the responsible antibody. Quantitative immunological tests to measure such antibodies directly are also available.

Warm Antibody Type. *This is the most common form of immunohemolytic anemia.* About 50% of cases are idiopathic (primary); the others are related to a predisposing condition (see Table 14–4) or exposure to a drug. Most causative antibodies are of the IgG class; less commonly, IgA antibodies are culpable. The red cell hemolysis is mostly extravascular. IgG-coated red cells bind to Fc receptors on phagocytes, which remove red cell membrane during "partial" phagocytosis. As in hereditary spherocytosis, the loss of membrane converts the red cells to spherocytes, which are sequestered and removed in the spleen. Moderate splenomegaly due to hyperplasia of splenic phagocytes is usually seen.

As with other autoimmune disorders, the cause of primary immunohemolytic anemia is unknown. In many cases, the antibodies are directed against the Rh blood group antigens. The mechanisms of drug-induced immunohemolytic anemia are better understood. Two different mechanisms have been described.

○ *Antigenic drugs.* In this setting hemolysis usually follows large, intravenous doses of the offending drug and occurs 1 to 2 weeks after therapy is initiated. These drugs, exemplified by penicillin and cephalosporins, bind to the red cell membrane and are recognized by anti-drug antibodies. Sometimes the antibodies bind only to the drug, as in penicillin-induced hemolysis. In other cases, such as in quinidine-induced hemolysis, the antibodies recognize a complex of the drug and a membrane protein. The responsible antibodies sometimes fix complement and cause intravascular hemolysis, but more often they act as opsonins that promote extravascular hemolysis within phagocytes.

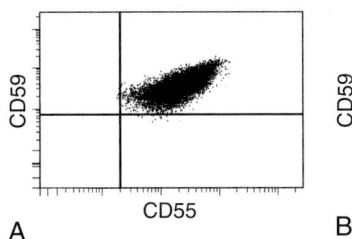
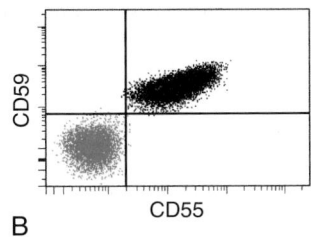

FIGURE 14–14 Paroxysmal nocturnal hemoglobinuria (PNH). **A,** Flow cytogram of blood from a normal individual shows that the red cells express two phosphatidylinositol glycan (PIG)–linked membrane proteins, CD55 and CD59, on their surfaces. **B,** Flow cytogram of blood from a patient with PNH shows a population of red cells that is deficient in both CD55 and CD59. As is typical of PNH, a second population of CD55+/CD59+ red cells that is derived from residual normal hematopoietic stem cells is also present. (Courtesy of Dr. Scott Rodig, Department of Pathology, Brigham and Women's Hospital, Boston, MA.)

● *Tolerance-breaking drugs.* These drugs, of which the antihypertensive agent α-methyldopa is the prototype, induce in some unknown manner the production of antibodies against red cell antigens, particularly the Rh blood group antigens. About 10% of patients taking α-methyldopa develop autoantibodies, as assessed by the direct Coombs test, and roughly 1% develop clinically significant hemolysis.

Cold Agglutinin Type. This form of immunohemolytic anemia is caused by IgM antibodies that bind red cells avidly at low temperatures (0°–4°C).[14] It is less common than warm antibody immunohemolytic anemia, accounting for 15% to 30% of cases. Cold agglutinin antibodies sometimes appear transiently following certain infections, such as with *Mycoplasma pneumoniae*, Epstein-Barr virus, cytomegalovirus, influenza virus, and human immunodeficiency virus (HIV). In these settings the disorder is self-limited and the antibodies rarely induce clinically important hemolysis. Chronic cold agglutinin immunohemolytic anemia occurs in association with certain B-cell neoplasms or as an idiopathic condition.

Clinical symptoms result from binding of IgM to red cells in vascular beds where the temperature may fall below 30°C, such as in exposed fingers, toes, and ears. IgM binding agglutinates red cells and fixes complement rapidly. As the blood recirculates and warms, IgM is released, usually before complement-mediated hemolysis can occur. However, the transient interaction with IgM is sufficient to deposit sublytic quantities of C3b, an excellent opsonin, which leads to the removal of affected red cells by phagocytes in the spleen, liver, and bone marrow. The hemolysis is of variable severity. Vascular obstruction caused by agglutinated red cells results in pallor, cyanosis, and Raynaud phenomenon (Chapter 11) in body parts exposed to cold temperature.

Cold Hemolysin Type. Cold hemolysins are autoantibodies responsible for an unusual entity known as *paroxysmal cold hemoglobinuria.* This rare disorder causes substantial, sometimes fatal, intravascular hemolysis and hemoglobinuria. The autoantibodies are IgGs that bind to the P blood group antigen on the red cell surface[14] in cool, peripheral regions of the body. Complement-mediated lysis occurs when the cells recirculate to warm central regions, since the complement cascade functions more efficiently at 37°C. Most cases are seen in children following viral infections; in this setting the disorder is transient, and most of those affected recover within 1 month.

Treatment of warm antibody immunohemolytic anemia centers on the removal of initiating factors (i.e., drugs); when this is not feasible, immunosuppressive drugs and splenectomy are the mainstays.[15] Chronic cold agglutinin immunohemolytic anemia caused by IgM antibodies is more difficult to treat.[14]

Hemolytic Anemia Resulting from Trauma to Red Cells

The most significant hemolysis caused by trauma to red cells is seen in individuals with cardiac valve prostheses and microangiopathic disorders. Artificial mechanical cardiac valves are more frequently implicated than are bioprosthetic porcine valves. The hemolysis stems from shear forces produced by turbulent blood flow and pressure gradients across damaged valves. Microangiopathic hemolytic anemia is most commonly seen with disseminated intravascular coagulation, but it also occurs in thrombotic thrombocytopenic purpura (TTP), hemolytic-uremic syndrome (HUS), malignant hypertension, systemic lupus erythematosus, and disseminated cancer. The common pathogenic feature in these disorders is a microvascular lesion that results in luminal narrowing, often due to the deposition of fibrin and platelets. These vascular changes produce shear stresses that mechanically injure passing red cells. Regardless of the cause, traumatic damage leads to the appearance of red cell fragments (schistocytes), "burr cells," "helmet cells," and "triangle cells" in blood smears (Fig. 14–15).

ANEMIAS OF DIMINISHED ERYTHROPOIESIS

Although the anemias that stem from the inadequate production of red cells are heterogeneous, they can be classified into several major categories based on pathophysiology (see Table 14–1). The most common and important anemias associated with red cell underproduction are those caused by nutritional deficiencies, followed by those that arise secondary to renal failure and chronic inflammation. Also included are less common disorders that lead to generalized bone marrow failure, such as aplastic anemia, primary hematopoietic neoplasms (discussed in Chapter 13), and infiltrative disorders that lead to marrow replacement (such as metastatic cancer and disseminated granulomatous disease). We will first discuss the extrinsic causes of diminished erythropoiesis, which are more common and clinically important, and then move to the non-neoplastic intrinsic causes.

Megaloblastic Anemias

The common theme among the various causes of megaloblastic anemia (Table 14–5) is an impairment of DNA synthesis that leads to distinctive morphologic changes, including abnormally large erythroid precursors and red cells. The following discussion first describes the common features and then turns to the two principal types: pernicious anemia (the major form

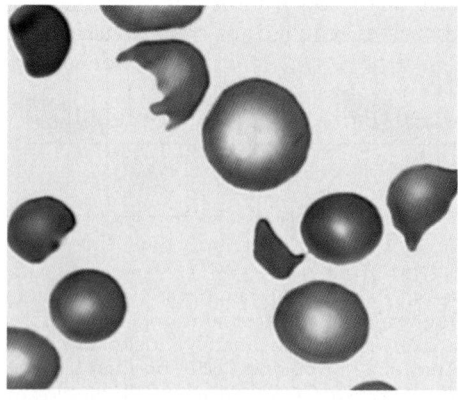

FIGURE 14–15 Microangiopathic hemolytic anemia. A peripheral blood smear from a person with hemolytic-uremic syndrome shows several fragmented red cells. (Courtesy of Dr. Robert W. McKenna, Department of Pathology, University of Texas Southwestern Medical School, Dallas, TX.)

TABLE 14–5 Causes of Megaloblastic Anemia

VITAMIN B₁₂ DEFICIENCY

Decreased Intake

Inadequate diet, vegetarianism

Impaired Absorption

Intrinsic factor deficiency
  Pernicious anemia
  Gastrectomy
Malabsorption states
Diffuse intestinal disease (e.g., lymphoma, systemic
  sclerosis)
Ileal resection, ileitis
  Competitive parasitic uptake
  Fish tapeworm infestation
Bacterial overgrowth in blind loops and diverticula of bowel

FOLIC ACID DEFICIENCY

Decreased Intake

Inadequate diet, alcoholism, infancy

Impaired Absorption

Malabsorption states
Intrinsic intestinal disease
Anticonvulsants, oral contraceptives

Increased Loss

Hemodialysis

Increased Requirement

Pregnancy, infancy, disseminated cancer, markedly
  increased hematopoiesis

Impaired Utilization

Folic acid antagonists

UNRESPONSIVE TO VITAMIN B₁₂ OR FOLIC ACID THERAPY

Metabolic inhibitors of DNA synthesis and/or folate
  metabolism (e.g., methotrexate)

Modified from Beck WS: Megaloblastic anemias. In Wyngaarden JB, Smith LH (eds): Cecil Textbook of Medicine, 18th ed. Philadelphia, WB Saunders, 1988, p. 900.

of vitamin B₁₂ deficiency anemia) and folate deficiency anemia.

Some of the metabolic roles of vitamin B₁₂ and folate are considered later. For now it suffices that vitamin B₁₂ and folic acid are coenzymes required for the synthesis of thymidine, one of the four bases found in DNA. A deficiency of these vitamins or impairment in their metabolism results in defective nuclear maturation due to deranged or inadequate DNA synthesis, with an attendant delay or block in cell division.

Morphology. Certain peripheral blood findings are shared by all megaloblastic anemias. **The presence of red cells that are macrocytic and oval (macro-ovalocytes) is highly characteristic.** Because they are larger than normal and contain ample hemoglobin, most macrocytes lack the central pallor of normal red cells and even appear "hyperchromic," but the MCHC is not elevated. There is marked variation in the size (anisocytosis) and shape (poikilocytosis) of red cells. The reticulocyte count is low. Nucleated red cell pro-

genitors occasionally appear in the circulating blood when anemia is severe. **Neutrophils are also larger than normal (macropolymorphonuclear) and hypersegmented, having five or more nuclear lobules instead of the normal three to four** (Fig. 14–16).

The marrow is usually markedly hypercellular as a result of increased hematopoietic precursors, which often completely replace the fatty marrow. **Megaloblastic changes are detected at all stages of erythroid development.** The most primitive cells (promegaloblasts) are large, with a deeply basophilic cytoplasm, prominent nucleoli, and a distinctive, fine nuclear chromatin pattern (Fig. 14–17, cell A). As these cells differentiate and begin to accumulate hemoglobin, the nucleus retains its finely distributed chromatin and fails to develop the clumped pyknotic chromatin typical of normoblasts. While nuclear maturation is delayed, cytoplasmic maturation and hemoglobin accumulation proceed at a normal pace, leading to nuclear-to-cytoplasmic asynchrony. Because DNA synthesis is impaired in all proliferating cells, granulocytic precursors also display dysmaturation in the form of **giant metamyelocytes and band forms.** Megakaryocytes, too, can be abnormally large and have bizarre, multilobate nuclei.

The marrow hyperplasia is a response to increased levels of growth factors, such as erythropoietin. However, the derangement in DNA synthesis causes most precursors to undergo apoptosis in the marrow (an example of ineffective hematopoiesis) and leads to pancytopenia. The anemia is further exacerbated by a mild degree of red cell hemolysis of uncertain etiology.

Anemias of Vitamin B₁₂ Deficiency: Pernicious Anemia

Pernicious anemia is a specific form of megaloblastic anemia caused by autoimmune gastritis and an attendant failure of

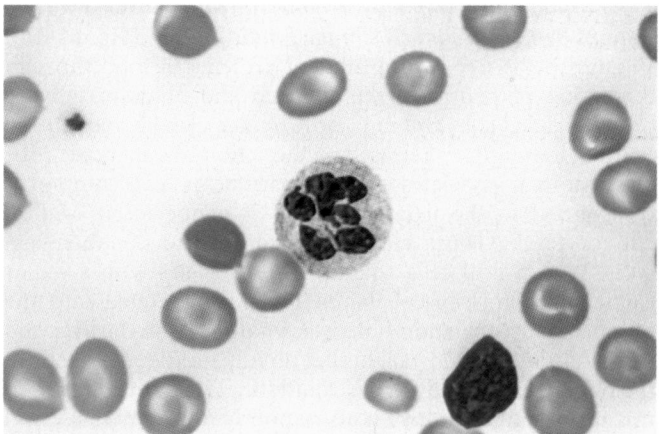

FIGURE 14–16 Megaloblastic anemia. A peripheral blood smear shows a hypersegmented neutrophil with a six-lobed nucleus. (Courtesy of Dr. Robert W. McKenna, Department of Pathology, University of Texas Southwestern Medical School, Dallas, TX.)

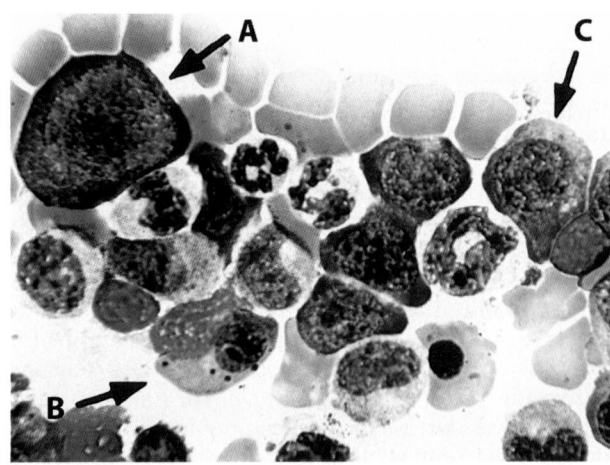

FIGURE 14–17 Megaloblastic anemia (bone marrow aspirate). **A** to **C,** Megaloblasts in various stages of differentiation. Note that the orthochromatic megaloblast (**B**) is hemoglobinized (as revealed by cytoplasmic color), but in contrast to normal orthochromatic normoblasts, the nucleus is not pyknotic. The early erythroid precursors (**A,C**) and the granulocytic precursors are also large and have abnormally immature chromatin. (Courtesy of Dr. Jose Hernandez, Department of Pathology, University of Texas Southwestern Medical School, Dallas, TX.)

intrinsic factor production, which leads to vitamin B_{12} deficiency. We first review vitamin B_{12} metabolism, since this helps to place pernicious anemia in perspective relative to the other causes of vitamin B_{12} deficiency anemia.

Normal Vitamin B_{12} Metabolism. Vitamin B_{12} is a complex organometallic compound known as cobalamin. Under normal circumstances humans are totally dependent on dietary vitamin B_{12}. Microorganisms are the ultimate origin of cobalamin in the food chain. Plants and vegetables contain little cobalamin, save that contributed by microbial contamination, and strictly vegetarian or macrobiotic diets do not provide adequate amounts of this essential nutrient. The daily requirement is 2 to 3 μg. A diet that includes animal products contains significantly larger amounts and normally results in the accumulation of intrahepatic stores of vitamin B_{12} that are sufficient to last for several years.

Absorption of vitamin B_{12} requires intrinsic factor, which is secreted by the parietal cells of the fundic mucosa (Fig. 14–18). Vitamin B_{12} is freed from binding proteins in food through the action of pepsin in the stomach and binds to salivary proteins called cobalophilins, or R-binders. In the duodenum, bound vitamin B_{12} is released by the action of pancreatic proteases. It then associates with intrinsic factor. This complex is transported to the ileum, where it is endocytosed by ileal enterocytes that express intrinsic factor receptors on their surfaces. Within ileal cells, vitamin B_{12} associates with a major carrier protein, transcobalamin II, and is secreted into the plasma. Transcobalamin II delivers vitamin B_{12} to the liver and other cells of the body, including rapidly proliferating cells in the bone marrow and the gastrointestinal tract. In addition to this major pathway, there is also a poorly understood alternative uptake mechanism that is not dependent on intrinsic factor or an intact terminal ileum. Up to 1% of a large oral dose can be absorbed by this pathway, making it feasible to treat pernicious anemia with high doses of oral vitamin B_{12}.

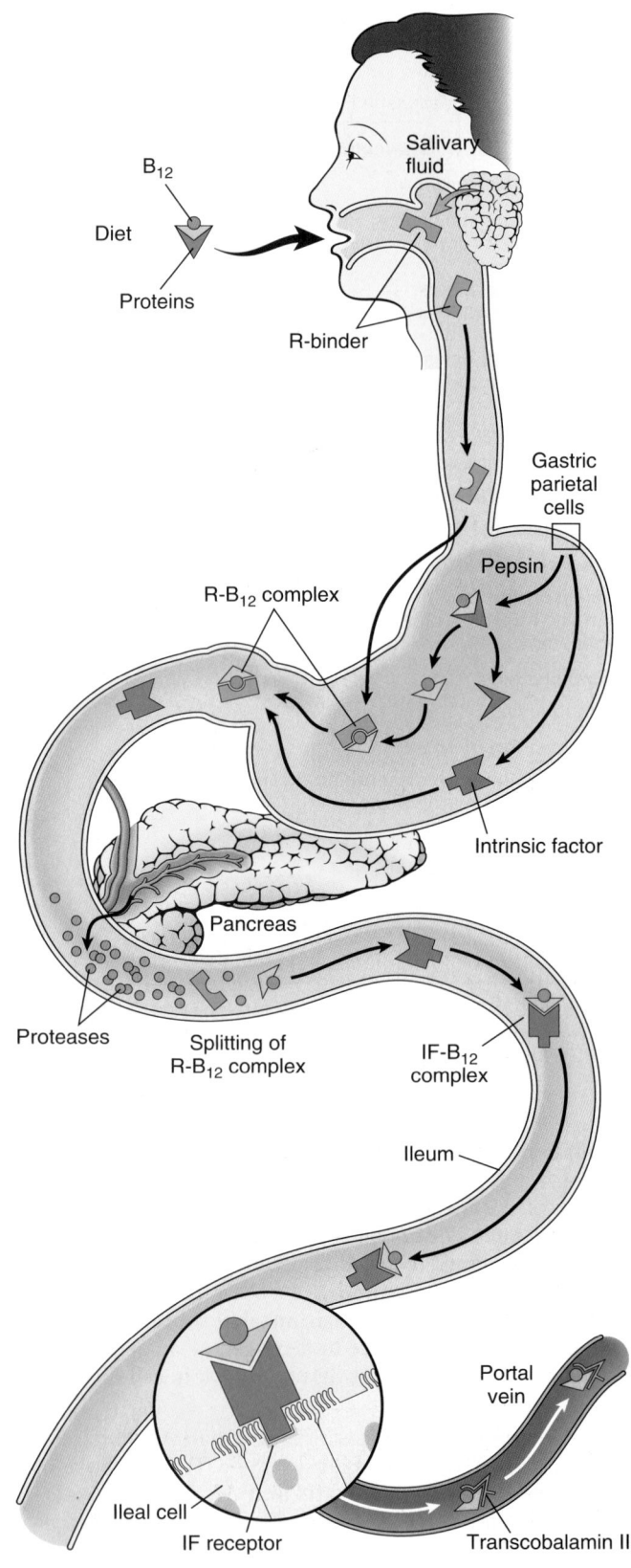

FIGURE 14–18 Schematic illustration of vitamin B_{12} absorption. IF, intrinsic factor; R-binders, cobalophilins (see text).

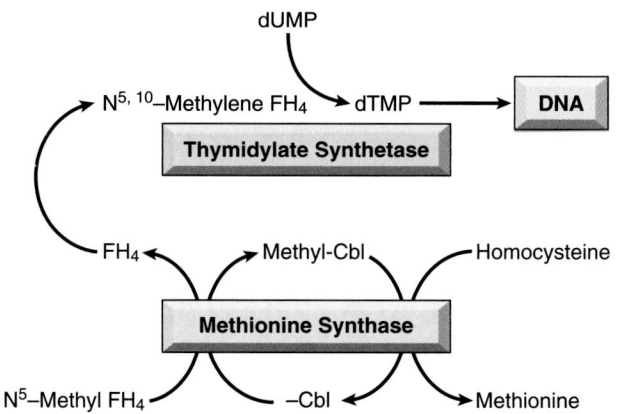

FIGURE 14–19 Relationship of N^5-methyl FH$_4$, methionine synthase, and thymidylate synthetase. In cobalamin (Cbl) deficiency, folate is sequestered as N^5-methyl FH$_4$. This ultimately deprives thymidylate synthetase of its folate coenzyme ($N^{5,10}$-methylene FH$_4$), thereby impairing DNA synthesis. FH$_4$, tetrahydrofolic acid.

Biochemical Functions of Vitamin B$_{12}$. Only two reactions in humans are known to require vitamin B$_{12}$. In one, methylcobalamin serves as an essential cofactor in the conversion of homocysteine to methionine by methionine synthase (Fig. 14–19). In the process, methylcobalamin yields a methyl group that is recovered from N^5-methyltetrahydrofolic acid (N^5-methyl FH$_4$), the principal form of folic acid in plasma. In the same reaction, N^5-methyl FH$_4$ is converted to tetrahydrofolic acid (FH$_4$). FH$_4$ is crucial, since it is required (through its derivative $N^{5,10}$-methylene FH$_4$) for the conversion of deoxyuridine monophosphate (dUMP) to deoxythymidine monophosphate (dTMP), an immediate precursor of DNA. *It is postulated that the fundamental cause of the impaired DNA synthesis in vitamin B$_{12}$ deficiency is the reduced availability of FH$_4$*, most of which is "trapped" as N^5-methyl FH$_4$. The FH$_4$ deficit may be further exacerbated by an "internal" folate deficiency caused by a failure to synthesize metabolically active polyglutamylated forms. This stems from the requirement for vitamin B$_{12}$ in the synthesis of methionine, which contributes a carbon group needed in the metabolic reactions that create folate polyglutamates (Fig. 14–20). Whatever the mechanism, *lack of folate is the proximate cause of anemia in vitamin B$_{12}$ deficiency*, since the anemia improves with administration of folic acid.

The neurologic complications associated with vitamin B$_{12}$ deficiency are more enigmatic, since they are not improved by folate administration. The other known reaction that depends on vitamin B$_{12}$ is the isomerization of methylmalonyl coenzyme A to succinyl coenzyme A, which requires adenosylcobalamin as a prosthetic group on the enzyme methylmalonyl–coenzyme A mutase. A deficiency of vitamin B$_{12}$ thus leads to increased plasma and urine levels of methylmalonic acid. Interruption of this reaction and the consequent buildup of methylmalonate and propionate (a precursor) could lead to the formation and incorporation of abnormal fatty acids into neuronal lipids. It has been suggested that this biochemical abnormality predisposes to myelin breakdown and thereby produces the neurologic complications of vitamin B$_{12}$ deficiency (Chapter 28). However, rare individuals with hereditary deficiencies of methylmalonyl–coenzyme A mutase, while having complications related to methylmalonyl acidemia, do not suffer from the neurologic abnormalities seen in vitamin

B$_{12}$ deficiency, casting doubt on this explanation.

Having completed our overview of vitamin B$_{12}$ metabolism, we can now turn to pernicious anemia.

Incidence. Although somewhat more prevalent in Scandinavian and other Caucasian populations, pernicious anemia occurs in all racial groups, including blacks and Hispanics. It is a disease of older adults; the median age at diagnosis is 60 years, and it is rare in people younger than 30. A genetic predisposition is strongly suspected, but no definable genetic pattern of transmission has been discerned. As described below, many affected individuals have a tendency to form antibodies against multiple self-antigens.

Pathogenesis. Pernicious anemia is believed to result from an autoimmune attack on the gastric mucosa. Histologically, there is a *chronic atrophic gastritis* marked by a loss of parietal cells, a prominent infiltrate of lymphocytes and plasma cells, and megaloblastic changes in mucosal cells similar to those found in erythroid precursors. *Three types of autoantibodies are present in many, but not all, patients.* About 75% of patients have a type I antibody that blocks the binding of vitamin B$_{12}$ to intrinsic factor. Type I antibodies are found in both plasma and gastric juice. Type II antibodies prevent binding of the intrinsic factor–vitamin B$_{12}$ complex to its ileal receptor. These antibodies are also found in a large proportion of patients with pernicious anemia. Type III antibodies, present in 85% to 90% of patients, recognize the α and β subunits of the gastric proton pump, which is normally localized to the microvilli of the canalicular system of the gastric parietal cell. These antibodies are not specific for pernicious anemia or other autoimmune diseases, since they are found in as many as 50% of elderly persons with idiopathic chronic gastritis not associated with pernicious anemia.

Autoantibodies are of diagnostic utility, but they are not thought to be the primary cause of the gastric pathology. Rather, it seems that an autoreactive T-cell response initiates gastric mucosal injury and triggers the formation of autoantibodies, which may exacerbate the epithelial injury. When the mass of intrinsic factor–secreting cells falls below a threshold (and reserves of stored vitamin B$_{12}$ are depleted), anemia develops. In an animal model of autoimmune gastritis mediated by CD4+ T cells, a pattern of autoantibodies resembling that seen

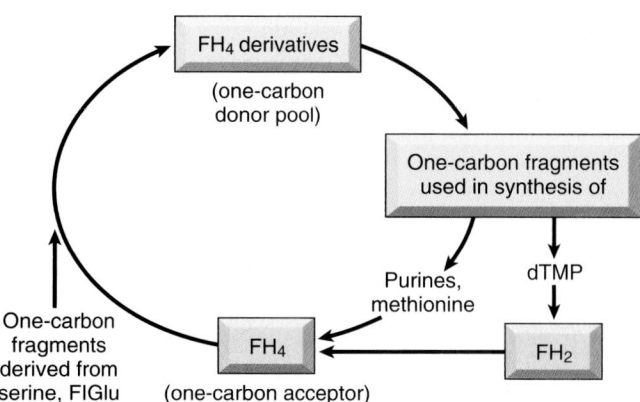

FIGURE 14–20 Role of folate derivatives in the transfer of one-carbon fragments for synthesis of biologic macromolecules. FH$_4$, tetrahydrofolic acid; FH$_2$, dihydrofolic acid; FIGlu, formiminoglutamate; dTMP, deoxythymidine monophosphate.

in pernicious anemia develops, thus supporting the primacy of T-cell autoimmunity. The common association of pernicious anemia with other autoimmune disorders, particularly autoimmune thyroiditis and adrenalitis, is also consistent with an underlying immune basis. The tendency to develop multiple autoimmune disorders, including pernicious anemia, is linked to specific sequence variants of NALP1,[16] an innate immune receptor that maps to chromosome 17p13.

Vitamin B_{12} deficiency is associated with disorders other than pernicious anemia. Most of these impair absorption of the vitamin at one of the steps outlined earlier (see Table 14–5). With achlorhydria and loss of pepsin secretion (which occurs in some elderly individuals), vitamin B_{12} is not readily released from proteins in food. With gastrectomy, intrinsic factor is not available for uptake in the ileum. With loss of exocrine pancreatic function, vitamin B_{12} cannot be released from R-binder–vitamin B_{12} complexes. Ileal resection or diffuse ileal disease can remove or damage the site of intrinsic factor–vitamin B_{12} complex absorption. Tapeworms compete with the host for B_{12} and can induce a deficiency state. In some settings, such as pregnancy, hyperthyroidism, disseminated cancer, and chronic infection, an increased demand for vitamin B_{12} can produce a relative deficiency, even with normal absorption.

Morphology. The findings in the **bone marrow and blood** in pernicious anemia are similar to those described earlier for all megaloblastic anemias. The stomach typically shows diffuse chronic gastritis (Chapter 17). **The most characteristic alteration is atrophy of the fundic glands,** affecting both chief cells and parietal cells, the latter being virtually absent. The glandular lining epithelium is replaced by mucus-secreting goblet cells that resemble those lining the large intestine, a form of metaplasia referred to as **intestinalization.** Some of the cells as well as their nuclei may increase to double the normal size, a form of "megaloblastic" change exactly analogous to that seen in the marrow. With time, the tongue may become shiny, glazed, and "beefy" (**atrophic glossitis**). The gastric atrophy and metaplastic changes are due to autoimmunity and not vitamin B_{12} deficiency; hence, parenteral administration of vitamin B_{12} corrects the megaloblastic changes in the marrow and the epithelial cells of the alimentary tract, but gastric atrophy and achlorhydria persist.

Central nervous system lesions are found in about three fourths of all cases of florid pernicious anemia but can also be seen in the absence of overt hematologic findings. **The principal alterations involve the spinal cord, where there is demyelination of the dorsal and lateral tracts,** sometimes followed by loss of axons. These changes give rise to spastic paraparesis, sensory ataxia, and severe paresthesias in the lower limbs. Less frequently, degenerative changes occur in the ganglia of the posterior roots and in peripheral nerves (Chapter 28).

Clinical Features. Pernicious anemia is insidious in onset, so the anemia is often quite severe by the time the affected

person seeks medical attention. The course is progressive unless halted by therapy.

The diagnosis is based on (1) a moderate to severe megaloblastic anemia, (2) leukopenia with hypersegmented granulocytes, (3) low serum vitamin B_{12}, and (4) elevated levels of homocysteine and methylmalonic acid in the serum. The diagnosis is confirmed by a striking increase in reticulocytes and an improvement in hematocrit levels beginning about 5 days after parenteral administration of vitamin B_{12}. Serum antibodies to intrinsic factor are highly specific for pernicious anemia. Their presence attests to the cause rather than the presence or absence of vitamin B_{12} deficiency.

Persons with atrophic and metaplastic changes in the gastric mucosa associated with pernicious anemia are at increased risk of developing gastric carcinoma (Chapter 17). As mentioned, serum homocysteine levels are raised in individuals with vitamin B_{12} deficiency. Elevated homocysteine levels are a risk factor for atherosclerosis and thrombosis, and it is suspected that vitamin B_{12} deficiency may increase the incidence of vascular disease. With parenteral or high-dose oral vitamin B_{12}, the anemia can be cured and the peripheral neurologic changes reversed or at least halted in their progression, but the changes in the gastric mucosa and the risk of carcinoma are unaffected.

Anemia of Folate Deficiency

A deficiency of folic acid (more properly, pteroylmonoglutamic acid) results in a megaloblastic anemia having the same characteristics as that caused by vitamin B_{12} deficiency. FH_4 derivatives act as intermediates in the transfer of one-carbon units such as formyl and methyl groups to various compounds (see Fig. 14–20). FH_4 serves as an acceptor of one-carbon fragments from compounds such as serine and formiminoglutamic acid. The FH_4 derivatives so generated in turn donate the acquired one-carbon fragments in reactions synthesizing various metabolites. FH_4, then, can be viewed as the biologic "middleman" in a series of swaps involving one-carbon moieties. The most important metabolic processes depending on such transfers are (1) purine synthesis; (2) the conversion of homocysteine to methionine, a reaction also requiring vitamin B_{12}; and (3) deoxythymidylate monophosphate synthesis. In the first two reactions, FH_4 is regenerated from its one-carbon carrier derivatives and is available to accept another one-carbon moiety and reenter the donor pool. In the synthesis of dTMP, a dihydrofolate is produced that must be reduced by dihydrofolate reductase for reentry into the FH_4 pool. The reductase step is significant, since this enzyme is susceptible to inhibition by various drugs. Among the molecules whose synthesis is dependent on folates, dTMP is perhaps the most important biologically, since it is required for DNA synthesis. It should be apparent from this discussion that suppressed synthesis of DNA, the common denominator of folic acid and vitamin B_{12} deficiency, is the immediate cause of megaloblastosis.

Etiology. *The three major causes of folic acid deficiency are (1) decreased intake, (2) increased requirements, and (3) impaired utilization* (see Table 14–5). Humans are entirely dependent on dietary sources for their folic acid requirement, which is 50 to 200 µg daily. Most normal diets contain ample amounts. The richest sources are green vegetables such as lettuce, spinach, asparagus, and broccoli. Certain fruits (e.g., lemons, bananas, melons) and animal sources (e.g., liver) contain lesser amounts. The folic acid in these foods is largely in the form of folylpolyglutamates. Despite their abundance in raw foods, polyglutamates are sensitive to heat; *boiling, steaming, or frying of foods for 5 to 10 minutes destroys up to 95% of the folate content.* Intestinal conjugases split the polyglutamates into monoglutamates that are readily absorbed in the proximal jejunum. During intestinal absorption they are modified to 5-methyltetrahydrofolate, the normal transport form of folate. The body's reserves of folate are relatively modest, and a deficiency can arise within weeks to months if intake is inadequate.

Decreased intake can result from either a nutritionally inadequate diet or impairment of intestinal absorption. A normal diet contains folate in excess of the minimal daily adult requirement. Inadequate dietary intakes are almost invariably associated with grossly deficient diets. *Such dietary inadequacies are most frequently encountered in chronic alcoholics, the indigent, and the very elderly.* In alcoholics with cirrhosis, other mechanisms of folate deficiency such as trapping of folate within the liver, excessive urinary loss, and disordered folate metabolism have also been implicated. Under these circumstances, the megaloblastic anemia is often accompanied by general malnutrition and manifestations of other avitaminoses, including cheilosis, glossitis, and dermatitis. Malabsorption syndromes, such as sprue, can lead to inadequate absorption of this nutrient, as can diffuse infiltrative diseases of the small intestine (e.g., lymphoma). In addition, certain drugs, particularly the anticonvulsant phenytoin and oral contraceptives, interfere with absorption.

Despite normal intake of folic acid, a *relative deficiency* can be encountered when requirements are increased. Conditions in which this is seen include pregnancy, infancy, hematologic derangements associated with hyperactive hematopoiesis (hemolytic anemias), and disseminated cancer. In all these circumstances the demands of increased DNA synthesis render normal intake inadequate.

Folic acid antagonists, such as methotrexate, inhibit dihydrofolate reductase and lead to a deficiency of FH_4. With inhibition of folate metabolism, all rapidly growing cells are affected, but particularly the cells of the bone marrow and the gastrointestinal tract. Many chemotherapeutic drugs used in the treatment of cancer damage DNA or inhibit DNA synthesis through other mechanisms; these can also cause megaloblastic changes in rapidly dividing cells.

As mentioned at the outset, the megaloblastic anemia that results from a deficiency of folic acid is identical to that encountered in vitamin B_{12} deficiency. Thus, the diagnosis of folate deficiency can be made only by demonstration of decreased folate levels in the serum or red cells. As in vitamin B_{12} deficiency, serum homocysteine levels are increased, but methylmalonate concentrations are normal. However, neurologic changes do not occur.

Although prompt hematologic response heralded by reticulocytosis follows the administration of folic acid, it should be remembered that the hematologic symptoms of vitamin B_{12} deficiency anemia also respond to folate therapy. However, *folate does not prevent (and may even exacerbate) the neurologic deficits typical of the vitamin B_{12} deficiency states.* It is thus essential to exclude vitamin B_{12} deficiency in megaloblastic anemia before initiating therapy with folate.

TABLE 14–6 Iron Distribution in Healthy Young Adults (mg)		
Pool	**Men**	**Women**
Total	3450	2450
Functional		
Hemoglobin	2100	1750
Myoglobin	300	250
Enzymes	50	50
Storage		
Ferritin, hemosiderin	1000	400

Iron Deficiency Anemia

Deficiency of iron is the most common nutritional disorder in the world. Although the prevalence of iron deficiency anemia is higher in developing countries, this form of anemia is also common in the United States, particularly in toddlers, adolescent girls, and women of childbearing age. The factors underlying the iron deficiency differ somewhat in various population groups and can be best considered in the context of normal iron metabolism.[17]

Iron Metabolism. The normal daily Western diet contains about 10 to 20 mg of iron, most in the form of heme contained in animal products, with the remainder being inorganic iron in vegetables. About 20% of heme iron (in contrast to 1% to 2% of nonheme iron) is absorbable, so the average Western diet contains sufficient iron to balance fixed daily losses. The total body iron content is normally about 2 gm in women and as high as 6 gm in men, and can be divided into functional and storage compartments (Table 14–6). About 80% of the functional iron is found in hemoglobin; myoglobin and iron-containing enzymes such as catalase and the cytochromes contain the rest. The storage pool represented by hemosiderin and ferritin contains about 15% to 20% of total body iron. Healthy young females have smaller stores of iron than do males, primarily because of blood loss during menstruation, and often develop iron deficiency due to excessive losses or increased demands associated with menstruation and pregnancy, respectively.

Iron in the body is recycled extensively between the functional and storage pools (Fig. 14–21). It is transported in plasma by an iron-binding glycoprotein called *transferrin,* which is synthesized in the liver. In normal individuals, transferrin is about one third saturated with iron, yielding serum iron levels that average 120 μg/dL in men and 100 μg/dL in women. The major function of plasma transferrin is to deliver iron to cells, including erythroid precursors, which require iron to synthesize hemoglobin. Erythroid precursors possess high-affinity receptors for transferrin, which mediate iron import through receptor-mediated endocytosis.

Free iron is highly toxic (as described in Chapter 18), and it is therefore important that storage iron be sequestered. This is achieved by binding iron in the storage pool tightly to either ferritin or hemosiderin. *Ferritin is a ubiquitous protein-iron complex* that is found at highest levels in the liver, spleen, bone marrow, and skeletal muscles. In the liver, most ferritin is stored within the parenchymal cells; in other tissues, such as the spleen and the bone marrow, it is found mainly in macrophages. Hepatocyte iron is derived from plasma transferrin,

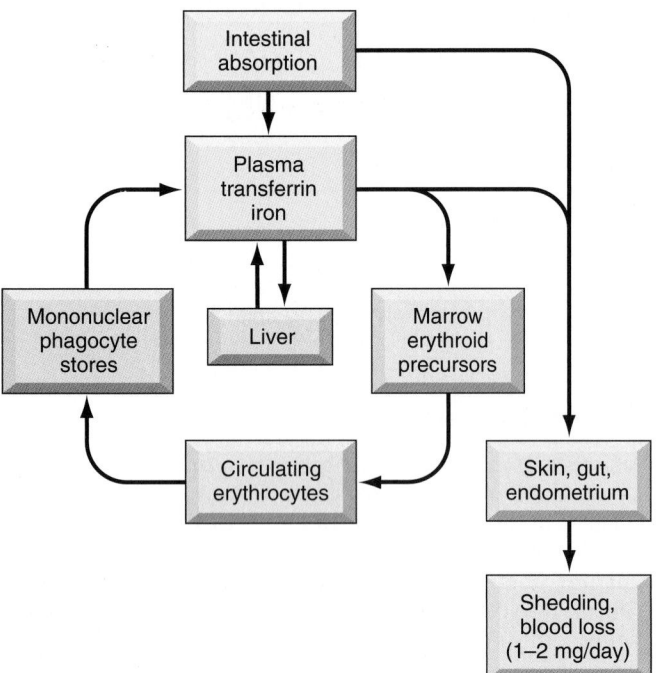

FIGURE 14–21 Iron metabolism. Iron absorbed from the gut is bound to plasma transferrin and transported to the marrow, where it is delivered to developing red cells and incorporated into hemoglobin. Mature red cells are released into the circulation and, after 120 days, are ingested by macrophages, primarily in the spleen, liver, and bone marrow. Here iron is extracted from hemoglobin and recycled to plasma transferrin. At equilibrium, iron absorbed from the gut is balanced by losses in shed keratinocytes, enterocytes, and (in women) endometrium.

whereas storage iron in macrophages is derived from the breakdown of red cells. Intracellular ferritin is located in the cytosol and in lysosomes, in which partially degraded protein shells of ferritin aggregate into *hemosiderin* granules. Iron in hemosiderin is chemically reactive and turns blue-black when exposed to potassium ferrocyanide, which is the basis for the Prussian blue stain. With normal iron stores, only trace amounts of hemosiderin are found in the body, principally in macrophages in the bone marrow, spleen, and liver. In iron-overloaded cells, most iron is stored in hemosiderin.

Since plasma ferritin is derived largely from the storage pool of body iron, its levels correlate well with body iron stores. In iron deficiency, serum ferritin is always below 12 μg/L, whereas in iron overload values approaching 5000 μg/L can be seen. Of physiologic importance, the storage iron pool can be readily mobilized if iron requirements increase, as may occur after loss of blood.

Iron balance is maintained largely by regulating the absorption of dietary iron in the proximal duodenum. Iron is both essential for cellular metabolism and highly toxic in excess, and total body iron stores must therefore be regulated meticulously. There is no regulated pathway for iron excretion, which is limited to the 1 to 2 mg lost each day through the shedding of mucosal and skin epithelial cells. In contrast, as body iron stores rise, absorption falls, and vice versa. The pathways responsible for the absorption of iron are now understood in reasonable detail (Fig. 14–22), and differ partially for nonheme and heme iron.[17] Luminal nonheme iron is mostly in the Fe^{3+} (ferric) state and must first be reduced to Fe^{2+} (ferrous) iron

by ferrireductases, such as b cytochromes and STEAP3. Fe^{2+} iron is then transported across the apical membrane by divalent metal transporter 1 (DMT1). The absorption of nonheme iron is variable and often inefficient, being inhibited by substances in the diet that bind and stabilize Fe^{3+} iron and enhanced by substances that stabilize Fe^{2+} iron (described below). Frequently, less than 5% of dietary nonheme iron is absorbed. In contrast, about 25% of the heme iron derived from hemoglobin, myoglobin, and other animal proteins is absorbed. Heme iron is moved across the apical membrane into the cytoplasm through transporters that are incompletely characterized. Here, it is metabolized to release Fe^{2+} iron, which enters a common pool with nonheme Fe^{2+} iron. Iron that enters the duodenal cells can follow one of two pathways: transport to the blood or storage as mucosal iron. This distribution is influenced by body iron stores, as we shall discuss below. Fe^{2+} iron destined for the circulation, is transported from the cytoplasm across the basolateral enterocyte membrane by ferriportin. This process is coupled to the oxidation of Fe^{2+} iron to Fe^{3+} iron, which is carried out by the iron oxidases hephaestin and ceruloplasmin. Newly absorbed Fe^{3+} iron binds rapidly to the plasma protein transferrin, which delivers iron to red cell progenitors in the marrow (see Fig. 14–21). Both DMT1 and ferriportin are widely distributed in the body and are involved in iron transport in other tissues as well. For example, DMT1 also mediates the uptake of "functional" iron (derived from endocytosed transferrin) across lysosomal membranes into the cytosol of red cell precursors in the bone marrow, and ferriportin plays an important role in the release of storage iron from macrophages.

Iron absorption is regulated by hepcidin, a small circulating peptide that is synthesized and released from the liver in response to increases in intrahepatic iron levels.[17] Hepcidin inhibits iron transfer from the enterocyte to plasma by binding to ferriportin and causing it to be endocytosed and degraded. As a result, as hepcidin levels rise, iron becomes trapped within duodenal cells in the form of mucosal ferritin and is lost as these cells are sloughed. Thus, when the body is replete with iron, high hepcidin levels inhibit its absorption into the blood. Conversely, with low body stores of iron, hepcidin synthesis falls and this in turn facilitates iron absorption. By inhibiting ferriportin, hepcidin not only reduces iron uptake from enterocytes but also suppresses iron release from macrophages, which are an important source of the iron that is used by erythroid precursors to make hemoglobin. This, as we shall see, is important in the pathogenesis of anemia of chronic diseases.

Alterations in hepcidin have a central role in diseases involving disturbances of iron metabolism. As will be described subsequently, the *anemia of chronic disease* is caused in part by inflammatory mediators that increase hepatic hepcidin production.[18] A rare form of microcytic anemia is caused by mutations that disable TMPRSS6, a hepatic transmembrane serine protease that normally suppresses hepcidin production when iron stores are low. Affected patients have high hepcidin levels, resulting in reduced iron absorption and failure to respond to iron therapy. Conversely, hepcidin activity is inappropriately low in both primary and secondary *hemochromatosis,* a syndrome caused by systemic iron overload. Secondary hemochromatosis can occur in diseases associated with *ineffective erythropoiesis,* such as β-thalassemia major and myelodysplastic syndromes (Chapter 13). Through incompletely understood mechanisms, ineffective erythropoiesis suppresses

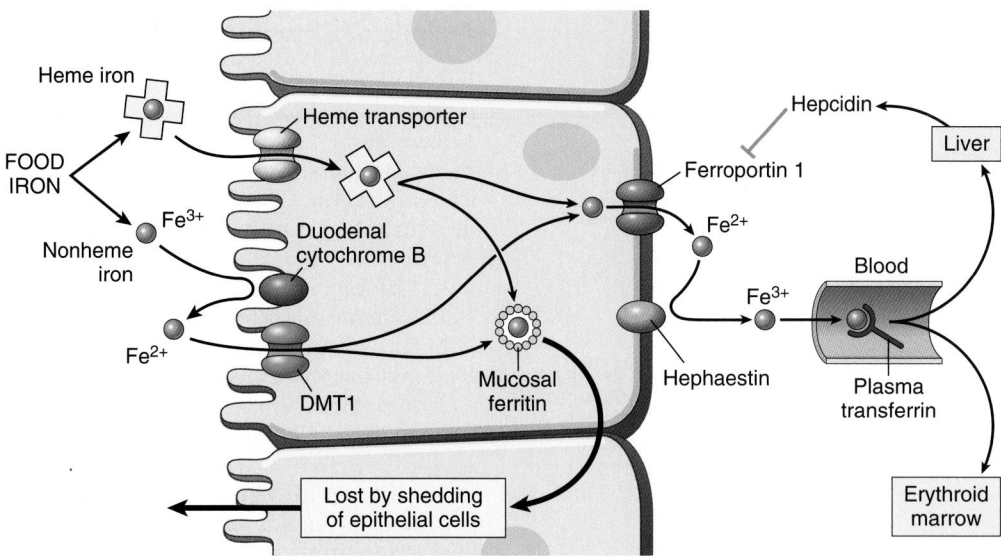

FIGURE 14–22 Regulation of iron absorption. Duodenal epithelial cell uptake of heme and nonheme iron is depicted. When the storage sites of the body are replete with iron and erythropoietic activity is normal, plasma hepcidin levels are high. This leads to down-regulation of ferriportin and trapping of most of the absorbed iron, which is lost when duodenal epithelial cells are shed into the gut. Conversely, when body iron stores decrease or when erythropoiesis is stimulated, hepcidin levels fall and ferriportin activity increases, allowing a greater fraction of the absorbed iron to be transferred to plasma transferrin. DMT1, divalent metal transporter 1.

hepatic hepcidin production, even when iron stores are high. As discussed in Chapter 18, the various inherited forms of primary hematochromatosis are associated with mutations in hepcidin or the genes that regulate hepcidin expression.

Etiology. *Iron deficiency can result from (1) dietary lack, (2) impaired absorption, (3) increased requirement, or (most importantly) (4) chronic blood loss.* To maintain a normal iron balance, about 1 mg of iron must be absorbed from the diet every day. Because only 10% to 15% of ingested iron is absorbed, the daily iron requirement is 7 to 10 mg for adult men and 7 to 20 mg for adult women. Since the average daily dietary intake of iron in the Western world is about 15 to 20 mg, most men ingest more than adequate iron, whereas many women consume marginally adequate amounts of iron. The bioavailability of dietary iron is as important as the overall content. Heme iron is much more absorbable than inorganic iron, the absorption of which is influenced by other dietary contents. Absorption of inorganic iron is enhanced by ascorbic acid, citric acid, amino acids, and sugars in the diet, and inhibited by tannates (found in tea), carbonates, oxalates, and phosphates.

Dietary lack is rare in developed countries, where on average about two thirds of the dietary iron is in the readily absorbed heme form provided by meat. The situation is different in developing countries, where food is less abundant and most iron in the diet is found in plants in the poorly absorbable inorganic form. Dietary iron inadequacy occurs in even privileged societies in the following groups:

- *Infants*, who are at high risk due to the very small amounts of iron in milk. Human breast milk provides only about 0.3 mg/L of iron. Cow's milk contains about twice as much iron, but its bioavailability is poor.
- *The impoverished*, who can have suboptimal diets for socioeconomic reasons at any age.
- *The elderly*, who often have restricted diets with little meat because of limited income or poor dentition.
- *Teenagers* who subsist on "junk" food.

Impaired absorption is found in sprue, other causes of fat malabsorption (steatorrhea), and chronic diarrhea. Gastrectomy impairs iron absorption by decreasing hydrochloric acid and transit time through the duodenum. Specific items in the diet, as is evident from the preceding discussion, can also affect absorption.

Increased requirement is an important cause of iron deficiency in growing infants, children, and adolescents, as well as premenopausal women, particularly during pregnancy. Economically deprived women having multiple, closely spaced pregnancies are at exceptionally high risk.

Chronic blood loss is the most common cause of iron deficiency in the Western world. External hemorrhage or bleeding into the gastrointestinal, urinary, or genital tracts depletes iron reserves. *Iron deficiency in adult men and postmenopausal women in the Western world must be attributed to gastrointestinal blood loss until proven otherwise.* To prematurely ascribe iron deficiency in such individuals to any other cause is to run the risk of missing an occult gastrointestinal cancer or other bleeding lesion. An alert clinician investigating unexplained iron deficiency anemia occasionally discovers an occult bleed or cancer and thereby saves a life.

Pathogenesis. *Whatever its basis, iron deficiency produces a hypochromic microcytic anemia.* At the outset of chronic blood loss or other states of negative iron balance, reserves in the form of ferritin and hemosiderin may be adequate to maintain normal hemoglobin and hematocrit levels as well as normal serum iron and transferrin saturation. Progressive depletion of these reserves first lowers serum iron and transferrin saturation levels without producing anemia. In this early stage there is increased erythroid activity in the bone marrow. Anemia appears only when iron stores are completely depleted and is accompanied by low serum iron, ferritin, and transferrin saturation levels.

Morphology. The bone marrow reveals a mild to moderate increase in erythroid progenitors. A diagnosti-

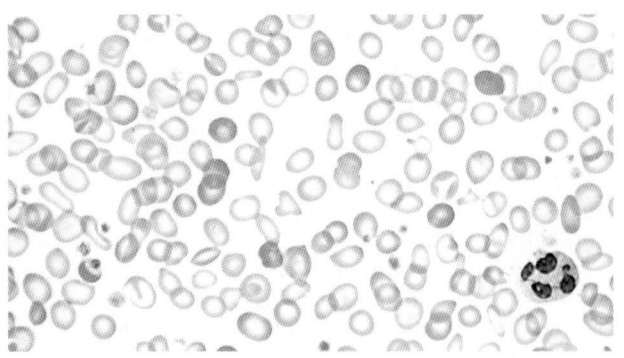

FIGURE 14–23 Hypochromic microcytic anemia of iron deficiency (peripheral blood smear). Note the small red cells containing a narrow rim of peripheral hemoglobin. Scattered fully hemoglobinized cells, present due to recent blood transfusion, stand in contrast. (Courtesy of Dr. Robert W. McKenna, Department of Pathology, University of Texas Southwestern Medical School, Dallas, TX.)

cally significant finding is the **disappearance of stainable iron from macrophages in the bone marrow**, which is best assessed by performing Prussian blue stains on smears of aspirated marrow. In peripheral blood smears, the red cells are small (**microcytic**) and pale (**hypochromic**). Normal red cells with sufficient hemoglobin have a zone of central pallor measuring about one third of the cell diameter. In established iron deficiency the zone of pallor is enlarged; hemoglobin may be seen only in a narrow peripheral rim (Fig. 14–23). Poikilocytosis in the form of small, elongated red cells (pencil cells) is also characteristically seen.

Clinical Features. The clinical manifestations of the anemia are nonspecific and were detailed earlier. The dominating signs and symptoms frequently relate to the underlying cause of the anemia, for example, gastrointestinal or gynecologic disease, malnutrition, pregnancy, and malabsorption. In severe and long-standing iron deficiency, depletion of iron-containing enzymes in cells throughout the body also causes other changes, including koilonychia, alopecia, atrophic changes in the tongue and gastric mucosa, and intestinal malabsorption. Depletion of iron from the central nervous system may lead to the appearance of pica, in which affected individuals consume non-foodstuffs such as clay or food ingredients such as flour, and periodically move their limbs during sleep. Esophageal webs appear together with microcytic hypochromic anemia and atrophic glossitis to complete the triad of major findings in the rare *Plummer-Vinson syndrome* (Chapter 17).

The diagnosis of iron deficiency anemia ultimately rests on laboratory studies. Both the hemoglobin and hematocrit are depressed, usually to a moderate degree, in association with hypochromia, microcytosis, and modest poikilocytosis. *The serum iron and ferritin are low, and the total plasma iron-binding capacity (reflecting elevated transferrin levels) is high. Low serum iron with increased iron-binding capacity results in a reduction of transferrin saturation to below 15%.* Reduced iron stores inhibit hepcidin synthesis, and its serum levels fall. In uncomplicated iron deficiency, oral iron supplementation produces an increase in reticulocytes in about 5 to 7 days that is followed by a steady increase in blood counts and the normalization of red cell indices.

Anemia of Chronic Disease

Impaired red cell production associated with chronic diseases is perhaps the most common cause of anemia among hospitalized patients in the United States. It is associated with a reduction in the proliferation of erythroid progenitors and impaired iron utilization. The chronic illnesses associated with this form of anemia can be grouped into three categories:

1. Chronic microbial infections, such as osteomyelitis, bacterial endocarditis, and lung abscess
2. Chronic immune disorders, such as rheumatoid arthritis and regional enteritis
3. Neoplasms, such as carcinomas of the lung and breast, and Hodgkin lymphoma

The anemia of chronic disease occurs in the setting of persistent systemic inflammation and is associated with low serum iron, reduced total iron-binding capacity, and abundant stored iron in tissue macrophages. Several effects of inflammation contribute to the observed abnormalities. *Most notably, certain inflammatory mediators, particularly interleukin-6 (IL-6), stimulate an increase in the hepatic production of hepcidin.*[17,18] As was discussed under the anemia of iron deficiency, hepcidin inhibits ferriportin function in macrophages and reduces the transfer of iron from the storage pool to developing erythroid precursors in the bone marrow. As a result, the erythroid precursors are starved for iron in the midst of plenty. In addition, these progenitors do not proliferate adequately because erythropoietin levels are inappropriately low for the degree of anemia. The precise mechanism underlying this alteration is uncertain, but transgenic mice expressing high levels of hepcidin develop a microcytic anemia associated with low erythropoietin levels,[19] suggesting that hepcidin directly or indirectly suppresses erythropoietin production.

What might be the reason for iron sequestration in the setting of inflammation? The best guess is that it serves to enhance the body's ability to fend off certain types of infection, particularly those caused by bacteria (such as *H. influenzae*) that require iron for pathogenicity. In this regard it is interesting to consider that hepcidin is structurally related to defensins, a family of peptides that have intrinsic antibacterial activity. This connection further highlights the uncertain but intriguing interrelationship between inflammation, innate immunity, and iron metabolism.

The anemia is usually mild, and the dominant symptoms are those of the underlying disease. The red cells can be normocytic and normochromic, or hypochromic and microcytic, as in anemia of iron deficiency. *The presence of increased storage iron in marrow macrophages, a high serum ferritin level, and a reduced total iron-binding capacity readily rule out iron deficiency as the cause of anemia.* Only successful treatment of the underlying condition reliably corrects the anemia. However, some patients, particularly those with cancer, benefit from administration of erythropoietin.

Aplastic Anemia

Aplastic anemia refers to a syndrome of chronic primary hematopoietic failure and attendant pancytopenia (anemia, neutro-

TABLE 14–7 Major Causes of Aplastic Anemia

ACQUIRED

Idiopathic

Acquired stem cell defects
Immune mediated

Chemical Agents

Dose related
  Alkylating agents
  Antimetabolites
Benzene
Chloramphenicol
Inorganic arsenicals

Idiosyncratic

Chloramphenicol
Phenylbutazone
Organic arsenicals
Methylphenylethylhydantoin
Carbamazepine
Penicillamine
Gold salts

Physical Agents

Whole-body irradiation

Viral Infections

Hepatitis (unknown virus)
Cytomegalovirus infections
Epstein-Barr virus infections
Herpes zoster (Varicella zoster)

INHERITED

Fanconi anemia
Telomerase defects

anomalies, such as hypoplasia of the kidney and spleen and bone anomalies, which most commonly involve the thumbs or radii. *Inherited defects in telomerase* are found in 5% to 10% of adult-onset aplastic anemia.[22] You will recall from Chapters 1 and 7 that telomerase is required for cellular immortality and limitless replication. It might be anticipated, therefore, that partial deficits in telomerase activity could result in premature hematopoietic stem cell exhaustion and marrow aplasia. Even more common than telomerase mutations are abnormally short telomeres, which are found in the marrow cells of as many as half of those affected with aplastic anemia. It is unknown whether this shortening is due to other unappreciated telomerase defects or is a consequence of excessive stem cell replication.

In most instances, however, no initiating factor can be identified; about 65% of cases fall into this *idiopathic* category.

Pathogenesis. The pathogenesis of aplastic anemia is not fully understood. Indeed, it is unlikely that a single mechanism underlies all cases. However, two major etiologies have been invoked: an extrinsic, immune-mediated suppression of marrow progenitors; and an intrinsic abnormality of stem cells (Fig. 14–24).

Experimental studies have increasingly focused on a model in which activated T cells suppress hematopoietic stem cells. Stem cells may first be antigenically altered by exposure to drugs, infectious agents, or other unidentified environmental insults. This provokes a cellular immune response, during which activated T_H1 cells produce cytokines such as interferon-γ (IFNγ) and TNF that suppress and kill hematopoietic progenitors. This scenario is supported by several

penia, and thrombocytopenia). In the majority of patients autoimmune mechanisms are suspected,[20] but inherited or acquired abnormalities of hematopoietic stem cells also seem to contribute in at least a subset of patients.

Etiology. The most common circumstances associated with aplastic anemia are listed in Table 14–7. *Most cases of "known" etiology follow exposure to chemicals and drugs.* Certain drugs and agents (including many cancer chemotherapy drugs and the organic solvent benzene) cause marrow suppression that is dose related and reversible. In other instances, aplastic anemia arises in an unpredictable, idiosyncratic fashion following exposure to drugs that normally cause little or no marrow suppression. The implicated drugs include chloramphenicol and gold salts.

Persistent marrow aplasia can also appear after a variety of viral infections, most commonly viral hepatitis of the non-A, non-B, non-C, non-G type, which is associated with 5% to 10% of cases. Why aplastic anemia develops in certain individuals is not understood.

Whole-body *irradiation* can destroy hematopoietic stem cells in a dose-dependent fashion. Persons who receive therapeutic irradiation or are exposed to radiation in nuclear accidents (e.g., Chernobyl) are at risk for marrow aplasia.

Inherited defects underlie some forms of aplastic aplasia. *Fanconi anemia* is a rare autosomal recessive disorder caused by defects in a multiprotein complex that is required for DNA repair (Chapter 7).[21] Marrow hypofunction becomes evident early in life and is often accompanied by multiple congenital

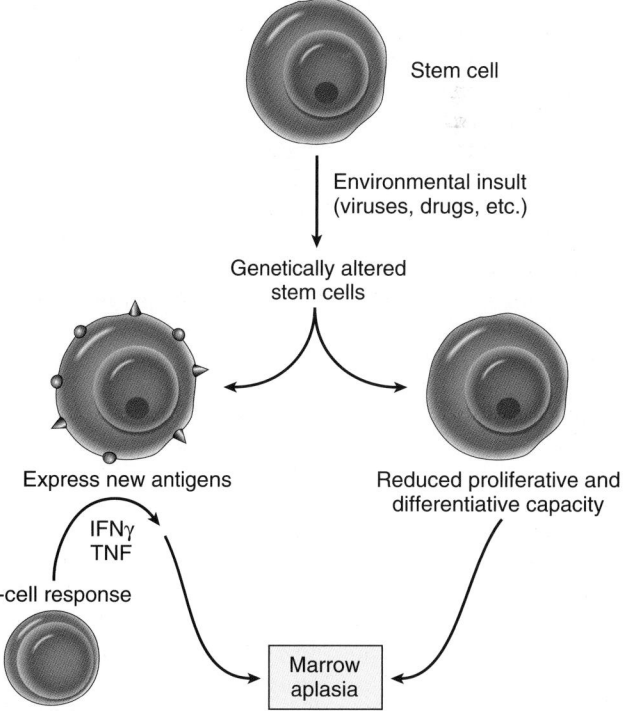

FIGURE 14–24 Pathophysiology of aplastic anemia. Damaged stem cells can produce progeny expressing neoantigens that evoke an autoimmune reaction, or give rise to a clonal population with reduced proliferative capacity. Either pathway could lead to marrow aplasia. See text for abbreviations.

observations. Expression analysis of the few remaining marrow stem cells from aplastic anemia marrows has revealed that genes involved in apoptosis and death pathways are up-regulated; of note, the same genes are up-regulated in normal stem cells exposed to interferon-γ. Even more compelling (and clinically relevant) evidence comes from experience with immunosuppressive therapy. Antithymocyte globulin and other immunosuppressive drugs such as cyclosporine produce responses in 60% to 70% of patients. It is proposed that these therapies work by suppressing or killing autoreactive T-cell clones. The antigens recognized by the autoreactive T cells are not well defined. In some instances GPI-linked proteins may be the targets, possibly explaining the previously noted association of aplastic anemia and PNH.

Alternatively, the notion that aplastic anemia results from a fundamental stem cell abnormality is supported by the presence of karyotypic aberrations in many cases; the occasional transformation of aplasias into myeloid neoplasms, typically myelodysplasia or acute myeloid leukemia; and the association with abnormally short telomeres. Some marrow insult (or a predisposition to DNA damage) presumably results in sufficient injury to limit the proliferative and differentiative capacity of stem cells. If the damage is extensive enough, aplastic anemia results. These two mechanisms are not mutually exclusive, since genetically altered stem cells might also express "neoantigens" that could serve as targets for a T-cell attack.

Morphology. The markedly hypocellular bone marrow is largely devoid of hematopoietic cells; often only fat cells, fibrous stroma, and scattered lymphocytes and plasma cells remain. Marrow aspirates often yield little material (a "dry tap"); hence, aplasia is best appreciated in marrow biopsies (Fig. 14–25). Other nonspecific pathologic changes are related to granulocytopenia and thrombocytopenia, such as mucocutaneous bacterial infections and abnormal bleeding, respectively. If the anemia necessitates multiple transfusions, systemic hemosiderosis can appear.

Clinical Features. Aplastic anemia can occur at any age and in either sex. The onset is usually insidious. Initial manifestations vary somewhat, depending on which cell line is predominantly affected, but pancytopenia ultimately appears, with the expected consequences. Anemia can cause progressive weakness, pallor, and dyspnea; thrombocytopenia is heralded by petechiae and ecchymoses; and neutropenia manifests as frequent and persistent minor infections or the sudden onset of chills, fever, and prostration. *Splenomegaly is characteristically absent; if it is present, the diagnosis of aplastic anemia should be seriously questioned.* The red cells are usually slightly macrocytic and normochromic. *Reticulocytopenia is the rule.*

The diagnosis rests on examination of a bone marrow biopsy. It is important to distinguish aplastic anemia from other causes of pancytopenia, such as "aleukemic" leukemia and myelodysplastic syndromes (Chapter 13), which can have identical clinical manifestations. In aplastic anemia, the marrow is hypocellular (and usually markedly so), whereas

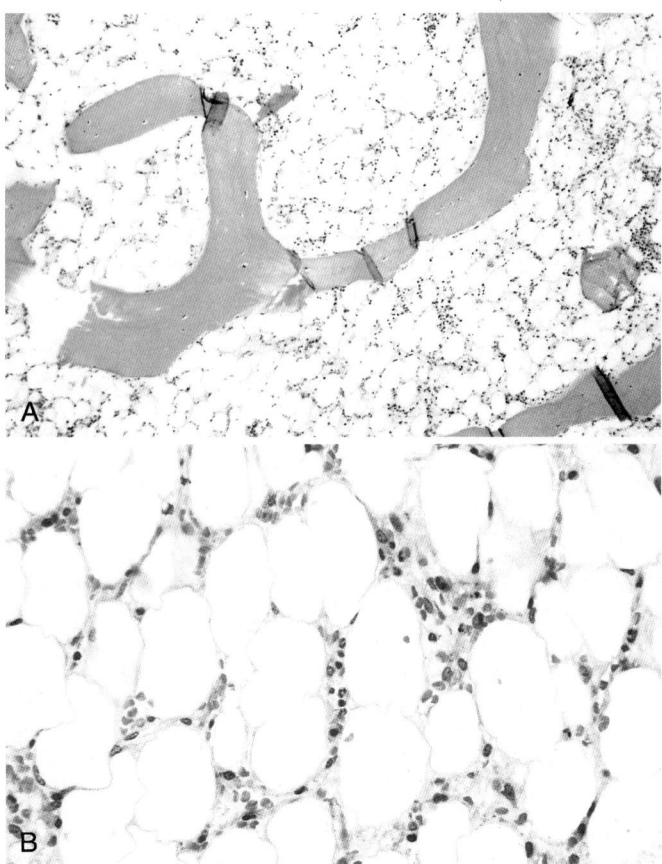

FIGURE 14–25 Aplastic anemia (bone marrow biopsy). Markedly hypocellular marrow contains mainly fat cells. **A,** Low power; **B,** high power. (Courtesy of Dr. Steven Kroft, Department of Pathology, University of Texas Southwestern Medical School, Dallas, TX.)

myeloid neoplasms are associated with hypercellular marrows filled with neoplastic progenitors.

The prognosis is variable.[20] Bone marrow transplantation is the treatment of choice in those with a suitable donor and provides a 5-year survival of over 75%. Older patients or those without suitable donors often respond well to immunosuppressive therapy.

Pure Red Cell Aplasia

As the name implies, pure red cell aplasia is a primary marrow disorder in which only erythroid progenitors are suppressed. In severe cases, red cell progenitors are completely absent from the marrow. It may occur in association with neoplasms, particularly thymoma and large granular lymphocytic leukemia (Chapter 13), drug exposures, autoimmune disorders, and parvovirus infection (a circumstance that is discussed below). With the exception of those with parvovirus infection, it is likely that most cases have an autoimmune basis. When a thymoma is present, resection leads to hematologic improvement in about half of the patients, possibly because the tumor is a source of marrow suppressive cells. In patients without thymoma, immunosuppressive therapy is often beneficial.

Plasmapheresis may also be helpful in unusual patients with pathogenic autoantibodies, such as neutralizing antibodies to erythropoietin that appear de novo or following the administration of recombinant erythropoietin.

A special form of red cell aplasia occurs in individuals infected with parvovirus B19, which preferentially infects and destroys red cell progenitors. Normal individuals clear parvovirus infections within 1 to 2 weeks; as a result, the aplasia is transient and clinically unimportant. However, in persons with moderate to severe hemolytic anemias, even a brief cessation of erythropoiesis results in rapid worsening of the anemia, producing an aplastic crisis. In those who are severely immunosuppressed (such as persons with advanced HIV infection), an ineffective immune response sometimes permits the infection to persist, leading to chronic red cell aplasia and a moderate to severe anemia.

Other Forms of Marrow Failure

Myelophthisic anemia describes a form of marrow failure in which space-occupying lesions replace normal marrow elements. The commonest cause is metastatic cancer, most often carcinomas arising in the breast, lung, and prostate. However, any infiltrative process (e.g., granulomatous disease) involving the marrow can produce identical findings. It should be remembered that myelophthisic anemia is also a feature of the spent phase of myeloproliferative disorders (Chapter 13). All of the responsible diseases cause marrow distortion and fibrosis, which act to displace normal marrow elements and disturb mechanisms that regulate the egress of red cells and granulocytes from the marrow. The latter effect causes the abnormal release of nucleated erythroid precursors and immature granulocytic forms *(leukoerythroblastosis)* into peripheral smears, and the appearance of *teardrop-shaped red cells*, which are believed to be deformed during their tortuous escape from the fibrotic marrow.

Chronic renal failure, whatever its cause, is almost invariably associated with an anemia that tends to be roughly proportional to the severity of the uremia. The basis of anemia in renal failure is multifactorial, but *the dominant cause is the diminished synthesis of erythropoietin by the damaged kidneys*, which leads to inadequate red cell production. Other contributors are an extracorpuscular defect that reduces red cell life span, and iron deficiency due to platelet dysfunction and increased bleeding, which is often encountered in uremia. Administration of recombinant erythropoietin results in a significant improvement of the anemia, although an optimal response may require concomitant iron replacement therapy. *Hepatocellular liver disease,* whether toxic, infectious, or cirrhotic, is associated with anemia attributed to decreased marrow function. Folate and iron deficiencies caused by poor nutrition and excessive bleeding often exacerbate anemia in this setting. Erythroid progenitors are preferentially affected; depression of the white cell count and platelets is less common but also occurs. The anemia is often slightly macrocytic due to lipid abnormalities associated with liver failure, which cause red cell membranes to acquire phospholipid and cholesterol as they circulate in the peripheral blood. *Endocrine disorders*, particularly hypothyroidism, may also be associated with a mild normochromic, normocytic anemia.

Polycythemia

Polycythemia denotes an abnormally high red cell count, usually with a corresponding increase in the hemoglobin level. The increase in red cell count is *relative* when there is hemoconcentration due to decreased plasma volume, or *absolute* when there is an increase in the total red cell mass. *Relative polycythemia* results from dehydration, such as occurs with deprivation of water, prolonged vomiting or diarrhea, or excessive use of diuretics. It is also associated with an obscure condition of unknown etiology called stress polycythemia, or Gaisböck syndrome. Affected individuals are usually hypertensive, obese, and anxious ("stressed"). *Absolute polycythemia* is *primary* when it results from an intrinsic abnormality of hematopoietic precursors and *secondary* when the red cell progenitors are responding to increased levels of erythropoietin. A pathophysiologic classification of polycythemia divided along these lines is given in Table 14–8.

The most common cause of primary polycythemia is *polycythemia vera*, a myeloproliferative disorder associated with mutations that lead to erythropoietin-independent growth of red cell progenitors (considered in Chapter 13). Another much less common form of primary polycythemia results from familial mutations in the erythropoietin receptor that induce erythropoietin-independent receptor activation. One such individual has won Olympic gold medals in cross-country skiing, having benefited from this natural form of blood doping! Secondary polycythemias are caused by compensatory or pathologic increases in erythropoietin secretion. Causes of the latter include erythropoietin-secreting tumors and rare, but illustrative, inherited defects that lead to the stabilization of HIF-1α, a hypoxia-induced factor that stimulates the transcription of the erythropoietin gene.[23]

TABLE 14–8 Pathophysiologic Classification of Polycythemia

RELATIVE

Reduced plasma volume (hemoconcentration)

ABSOLUTE

Primary (Low Erythropoietin)

Polycythemia vera
Inherited erythropoietin receptor mutations (rare)

Secondary (High Erythropoietin)

Compensatory
  Lung disease
  High-altitude living
  Cyanotic heart disease
Paraneoplastic
  Erythropoietin-secreting tumors (e.g., renal cell carcinoma, hepatocellular carcinoma, cerebellar hemangioblastoma)
Hemoglobin mutants with high O_2 affinity
Inherited defects that stabilize HIF-1α
  Chuvash polycythemia (homozygous *VHL* mutations)
  Prolyl hydroxylase mutations

HIF-1α, hypoxia-induced factor 1α.

Bleeding Disorders: Hemorrhagic Diatheses

Excessive bleeding can result from (1) increased fragility of vessels, (2) platelet deficiency or dysfunction, and (3) derangement of coagulation, alone or in combination. Before discussing specific bleeding disorders, it is helpful to review the common laboratory tests used in the evaluation of a bleeding diathesis. It should be recalled from the discussion in Chapter 4 that the normal hemostatic response involves the blood vessel wall, the platelets, and the clotting cascade. Tests used to evaluate different aspects of hemostasis are the following:

- *Prothrombin time (PT).* This test assesses the extrinsic and common coagulation pathways. The clotting of plasma after addition of an exogenous source of tissue thromboplastin (e.g., brain extract) and Ca^{2+} ions is measured in seconds. A prolonged PT can result from deficiency or dysfunction of factor V, factor VII, factor X, prothrombin, or fibrinogen.
- *Partial thromboplastin time (PTT).* This test assesses the intrinsic and common clotting pathways. The clotting of plasma after addition of kaolin, cephalin, and Ca^{2+} ions is measured in seconds. Kaolin activates the contact-dependent factor XII, and cephalin substitutes for platelet phospholipids. Prolongation of the PTT can be due to deficiency or dysfunction of factors V, VIII, IX, X, XI, or XII, prothrombin, or fibrinogen, or to interfering antibodies to phospholipid (described in Chapter 4).
- *Platelet counts.* These are obtained on anticoagulated blood using an electronic particle counter. The reference range is 150×10^3 to 300×10^3 platelets/μL. Counts well outside this range should be confirmed by a visual inspection of a peripheral blood smear, since clumping of platelets can cause spurious "thrombocytopenia" during automated counting, and high counts may be indicative of a myeloproliferative disorder, such as essential thrombocythemia (Chapter 13).
- *Tests of platelet function.* At present, no single test provides an adequate assessment of the complex functions of platelets. One older test, the bleeding time, which measures the time taken for a standardized skin puncture to stop bleeding, has some value but is time-consuming, difficult to perform well, and not a good predictor of bleeding during hemostatic stresses such as surgery. As a result of these limitations, the use of the bleeding time has declined considerably in recent years. Newer instrument-based assays designed to measure platelet function under conditions of high shear stress show promise but at present are also less than ideal screening tests. Other specialized tests that can be useful in particular clinical settings include tests of platelet aggregation, which measure the ability of platelets to aggregate in response to agonists like thrombin; and quantitative and qualitative tests of von Willebrand factor, which (as you will remember from Chapter 4) play an important role in platelet adhesion to the extracellular matrix.

More specialized tests are available to measure the levels of specific clotting factors, fibrinogen, fibrin split products, and the presence of circulating anticoagulants.

BLEEDING DISORDERS CAUSED BY VESSEL WALL ABNORMALITIES

Disorders within this category, sometimes called *nonthrombocytopenic purpuras,* are relatively common but do not usually cause serious bleeding problems. Most often, they induce small hemorrhages (petechiae and purpura) in the skin or mucous membranes, particularly the gingivae. On occasion, however, more significant hemorrhages can occur into joints, muscles, and subperiosteal locations, or take the form of menorrhagia, nosebleeds, gastrointestinal bleeding, or hematuria. *The platelet count, the bleeding time, and tests of coagulation (PT, PTT) usually yield normal results.*

The varied clinical conditions in which abnormalities in the vessel wall cause bleeding include the following:

- Many *infections* induce petechial and purpuric hemorrhages, particularly meningococcemia, other forms of septicemia, infective endocarditis, and several of the rickettsioses. The involved mechanisms include microbial damage to the microvasculature (vasculitis) and disseminated intravascular coagulation (DIC). Failure to recognize meningococcemia as a cause of petechiae and purpura can be catastrophic for the patient.
- *Drug reactions* sometimes induce cutaneous petechiae and purpura without causing thrombocytopenia. In many instances the vascular injury is mediated by the deposition of drug-induced immune complexes in vessel walls, which leads to hypersensitivity (leukocytoclastic) vasculitis (Chapter 11).
- *Scurvy and the Ehlers-Danlos syndrome* are associated with microvascular bleeding, which results from defects in collagen that weakens vessel walls. The same mechanism may account for the spontaneous purpura that are commonly seen in the elderly and the skin hemorrhages that are seen with *Cushing syndrome,* in which the protein-wasting effects of excessive corticosteroid production cause loss of perivascular supporting tissue.
- *Henoch-Schönlein purpura* is a systemic hypersensitivity disease of unknown cause that is characterized by a purpuric rash, colicky abdominal pain, polyarthralgia, and acute glomerulonephritis (Chapter 20). All these changes result from the deposition of circulating immune complexes within vessels throughout the body and within the glomerular mesangial regions.
- *Hereditary hemorrhagic telangiectasia* (also known as Weber-Osler-Rendu syndrome) is an autosomal dominant disorder characterized by dilated, tortuous blood vessels with thin walls that bleed readily. Bleeding can occur anywhere, but it is most common under the mucous membranes of the nose (epistaxis), tongue, mouth, and eyes, and throughout the gastrointestinal tract.
- *Perivascular amyloidosis* can weaken blood vessel walls and cause bleeding. This complication is most common with amyloid light-chain (AL) amyloidosis (Chapter 6) and often manifests as mucocutaneous petechiae.

Among these conditions, serious bleeding is most often associated with hereditary telangiectasia. The bleeding in each is nonspecific, and the diagnosis of these entities is based on the recognition of other more specific associated findings.

BLEEDING RELATED TO REDUCED PLATELET NUMBER: THROMBOCYTOPENIA

Reduction in platelet number constitutes an important cause of generalized bleeding. A count below 100,000 platelets/μL is generally considered to constitute thrombocytopenia. However, spontaneous bleeding does not become evident until platelet counts fall below 20,000 platelets/μL. Platelet counts in the range of 20,000 to 50,000 platelets/μL can aggravate post-traumatic bleeding. Bleeding resulting from thrombocytopenia is associated with a normal PT and PTT.

It hardly needs reiteration that platelets are critical for hemostasis, since they form temporary plugs that stop bleeding and promote key reactions in the coagulation cascade (as discussed in Chapter 4). Spontaneous bleeding associated with thrombocytopenia most often involves small vessels. Common sites for such hemorrhages are the skin and the mucous membranes of the gastrointestinal and genitourinary tracts. *Most feared, however, is intracranial bleeding, which is a threat to any patient with a markedly depressed platelet count.*

The many causes of thrombocytopenia can be classified into four major categories (Table 14–9).

- *Decreased platelet production.* This can result from conditions that depress marrow output generally (such as aplastic anemia and leukemia) or affect megakaryocytes

TABLE 14–9 Causes of Thrombocytopenia

DECREASED PRODUCTION OF PLATELETS

Selective impairment of platelet production
    Drug-induced: alcohol, thiazides, cytotoxic drugs
    Infections: measles, human immunodeficiency virus (HIV)
Nutritional deficiencies
    B_{12}, folate deficiency (megaloblastic leukemia)
Bone marrow failure
    Aplastic anemia (see Table 14–7)
Bone marrow replacement
    Leukemia, disseminated cancer, granulomatous disease
Ineffective hematopoiesis
    Myelodysplastic syndromes (Chapter 13)

DECREASED PLATELET SURVIVAL

Immunologic destruction
    Primary autoimmune
        Chromic immune thrombocytopenic purpura
        Acute immune thrombocytopenic purpura
    Secondary autoimmune
        Systemic lupus erythematosus, B-cell lymphoid neoplasms
    Alloimmune: post-transfusion and neonatal
    Drug-associated: quinidine, heparin, sulfa compounds
    Infections: HIV, infectious mononucleosis (transient, mild), dengue fever
Nonimmunologic destruction
    Disseminated intravascular coagulation
    Thrombotic microangiopathies
    Giant hemangiomas

SEQUESTRATION

Hypersplenism

DILUTION

Transfusions

somewhat selectively. Examples of the latter include certain drugs and alcohol, which may suppress platelet production through uncertain mechanisms when taken in large amounts; HIV, which may infect megakaryocytes and inhibit platelet production; and myelodysplastic syndromes (Chapter 13), which may occasionally present with isolated thrombocytopenia.

- *Decreased platelet survival.* This important mechanism of thrombocytopenia can have an immunological or nonimmunological basis. *In immune thrombocytopenia platelet destruction is caused by antibodies to platelets* or, less often, immune complexes that deposit on platelets. Antibodies to platelets can recognize self-antigens (autoantibodies) or non-self antigens (alloantibodies). Autoimmune thrombocytopenia is discussed in the following section. Alloantibodies can arise when platelets are transfused or cross the placenta from the fetus into the pregnant mother. In the latter case, IgG antibodies made in the mother can cause clinically significant thrombocytopenia in the fetus. This is reminiscent of hemolytic disease of the newborn, in which red cells are the target (Chapter 10). *The most important nonimmunological causes are disseminated intravascular coagulation (DIC) and the thrombotic microangiopathies,* in which unbridled, often systemic, platelet activation reduces platelet life span. Nonimmunological destruction of platelets may also be caused by *mechanical injury,* such as in individuals with prosthetic heart valves.
- *Sequestration.* The spleen normally sequesters 30% to 35% of the body's platelets, but this can rise to 80% to 90% when the spleen is enlarged, producing moderate degrees of thrombocytopenia.
- *Dilution.* Massive transfusions can produce a dilutional thrombocytopenia. With prolonged blood storage the number of viable platelets decreases; thus, plasma volume and red cell mass are reconstituted by transfusion, but the number of circulating platelets is relatively reduced.

Chronic Immune Thrombocytopenic Purpura (ITP)

Chronic ITP is caused by autoantibodies to platelets. It can occur in the setting of a variety of predisposing conditions and exposures (secondary) or in the absence of any known risk factors (primary or idiopathic). The contexts in which chronic ITP occurs secondarily are numerous and include individuals with systemic lupus erythematosus (Chapter 6), HIV infection, and B-cell neoplasms such as chronic lymphocytic leukemia (Chapter 13). The diagnosis of primary chronic ITP is made only after secondary causes are excluded.

Pathogenesis. The autoantibodies, most often directed against platelet membrane glycoproteins IIb-IIIa or Ib-IX, can be demonstrated in the plasma and bound to the platelet surface in about 80% of patients. In the overwhelming majority of cases, the antiplatelet antibodies are of the IgG class.

As in autoimmune hemolytic anemias, antiplatelet antibodies act as opsonins that are recognized by IgG Fc receptors expressed on phagocytes (Chapter 6), leading to increased platelet destruction. The thrombocytopenia is usually markedly improved by splenectomy, indicating that the spleen is the major site of removal of opsonized platelets. The splenic red pulp is also rich in plasma cells, and part of the benefit of splenectomy (a common treatment for chronic ITP) may stem from the removal of a source of autoantibodies. In some instances the autoantibodies may also bind to and damage megakaryocytes, leading to decreases in platelet production that further exacerbate the thrombocytopenia.

> **Morphology.** The principal changes of thrombocytopenic purpura are found in the spleen, bone marrow, and blood, but they are not specific. Secondary changes related to the bleeding diathesis may be found in any tissue or structure in the body.
>
> The **spleen** is of normal size. Typically, there is congestion of the sinusoids and enlargement of the splenic follicles, often associated with prominent reactive germinal centers. In many instances scattered megakaryocytes are found within the sinuses. This may represent a very mild form of extramedullary hematopoiesis that is driven by elevated levels of thrombopoietin. The **marrow** reveals a modestly increased number of megakaryocytes. Some are apparently immature, with large, nonlobulated, single nuclei. These findings are not specific for ITP but merely reflect accelerated thrombopoiesis, being found in most forms of thrombocytopenia resulting from increased platelet destruction. The importance of bone marrow examination is to rule out thrombocytopenias resulting from bone marrow failure or other primary bone marrow disorders. The secondary changes relate to the hemorrhages that are dispersed throughout the body. The **peripheral blood** often reveals abnormally large platelets (megathrombocytes), which are a sign of accelerated thrombopoiesis.

Clinical Features. Chronic ITP occurs most commonly in adult women typically under 40 years of age. The female-to-male ratio is 3 : 1. It is often insidious in onset and is characterized by bleeding into the skin and mucosal surfaces. Cutaneous bleeding is seen in the form of *pinpoint hemorrhages* (petechiae), which are especially prominent in the dependent areas where the capillary pressure is higher. Petechiae can become confluent, giving rise to *ecchymoses*. Often there is a history of easy bruising, nosebleeds, bleeding from the gums, and hemorrhages into soft tissues from relatively minor trauma. The disease may manifest first with melena, hematuria, or excessive menstrual flow. Subarachnoid hemorrhage and intracerebral hemorrhage are serious and sometimes fatal complications, but fortunately they are rare in treated patients. Splenomegaly and lymphadenopathy are uncommon in primary disease, and their presence should lead one to consider other diagnoses, such as ITP secondary to a B-cell neoplasm.

The clinical signs and symptoms are not specific but rather reflective of the thrombocytopenia. The findings of a low platelet count, normal or increased megakaryocytes in the bone marrow, and large platelets in the peripheral blood are taken as presumptive evidence of accelerated platelet destruction. The PT and PTT are normal. Tests for platelet autoantibodies are not widely available. *Therefore, the diagnosis is one of exclusion and can be made only after other causes of thrombocytopenia, such as those listed in Table 14–9, have been ruled out.*

Almost all patients respond to glucocorticoids (which inhibit phagocyte function), but many eventually relapse. In such individuals, splenectomy normalizes the platelet count in about two thirds of patients, but with the attendant increased risk of bacterial sepsis. Immunomodulatory agents such as intravenous immunoglobulin or anti-CD20 antibody (rituximab) are often effective in patients who relapse after splenectomy or for whom splenectomy is contraindicated.

Acute Immune Thrombocytopenic Purpura

Like chronic ITP, this condition is caused by autoantibodies to platelets, but its clinical features and course are distinct. Acute ITP is mainly a disease of childhood occurring with equal frequency in both sexes. Symptoms appear abruptly and usually follow a viral illness, which typically occurs about 2 weeks before the onset of the thrombocytopenia. Unlike chronic ITP, acute ITP is self-limited, usually resolving spontaneously within 6 months. Glucocorticoids are given only if the thrombocytopenia is severe. In about 20% of children, usually those without a viral prodrome, thrombocytopenia persists; these less fortunate children have a childhood form of chronic ITP that follows a course similar to the adult disease.

Drug-Induced Thrombocytopenia

Drugs can induce thrombocytopenia through direct effects on platelets and secondary to immunologically mediated platelet destruction. The drugs most commonly implicated are quinine, quinidine, and vancomycin, all of which bind platelet glycoproteins and in one way or another create antigenic determinants that are recognized by antibodies.[24] Much more rarely, drugs such as gold salts induce true autoantibodies through unknown mechanisms. Thrombocytopenia, which may be severe, is also a common consequence of platelet inhibitory drugs that bind glycoprotein IIb/IIIa; it is hypothesized that these drugs induce conformational changes in glycoprotein IIb/IIIa and create an immunogenic epitope.

Heparin-induced thrombocytopenia (HIT) has a distinctive pathogenesis and is of particular importance because of its potential for severe clinical consequences.[25] Thrombocytopenia occurs in about 5% of persons receiving heparin. Most develop so-called type I thrombocytopenia, which occurs rapidly after the onset of therapy and is of little clinical importance, sometimes resolving despite the continuation of therapy. It most likely results from a direct platelet-aggregating effect of heparin. Type II thrombocytopenia is less common but of much greater clinical significance. It occurs 5 to 14 days after therapy begins (or sooner if the person has been sensitized to heparin) and, paradoxically, often leads to life-threatening venous and arterial thrombosis. This severe form of HIT is caused by antibodies that recognize complexes of heparin and platelet factor 4, which is a normal component of platelet granules. *Binding of antibody to these complexes activates platelets and promotes thrombosis, even in the setting of thrombocytopenia.* Unless therapy is immediately discontinued and an alternative non-heparin anticoagulant instituted, clots within large arteries may lead to vascular insufficiency and limb loss, and emboli from deep venous thrombosis can cause fatal pulmonary thromboembolism. The risk of severe HIT is lowered, but not completely eliminated, by the use of low-molecular-weight heparin preparations. Unfortunately, once severe HIT develops even low-molecular-weight heparins exacerbate the thrombotic tendency and must be avoided.

HIV-Associated Thrombocytopenia

Thrombocytopenia is one of the most common hematologic manifestation of HIV infection. Both impaired platelet production and increased destruction contribute. CD4 and CXCR4, the receptor and coreceptor, respectively, for HIV, are found on megakaryocytes, allowing these cells to be infected. HIV-infected megakaryocytes are prone to apoptosis and their ability to produce platelets is impaired. HIV infection also causes B-cell hyperplasia and dysregulation, which predisposes to the development of autoantibodies. In some instances the antibodies are directed against platelet membrane glycoprotein IIb-III complexes. As in other immune cytopenias, the autoantibodies opsoninize platelets, promoting their destruction by mononuclear phagocytes in the spleen and elsewhere. The deposition of immune complexes on platelets may also contribute to the accelerated loss of platelets in some patients who are HIV infected.

Thrombotic Microangiopathies: Thrombotic Thrombocytopenic Purpura (TTP) and Hemolytic-Uremic Syndrome (HUS)

The term *thrombotic microangiopathy* encompasses a spectrum of clinical syndromes that includes TTP and HUS. According to its original description, TTP was defined as the pentad of fever, thrombocytopenia, microangiopathic hemolytic anemia, transient neurologic deficits, and renal failure. HUS is also associated with microangiopathic hemolytic anemia and thrombocytopenia but is distinguished by the absence of neurologic symptoms, the prominence of acute renal failure, and its frequent occurrence in children. With time, experience, and increased mechanistic insight, however, these distinctions have blurred. Many adult patients with "TTP" lack one or more of the five criteria, and some patients with "HUS" have fever and neurologic dysfunction. *It is now appreciated that HUS and TTP are both caused by insults that lead to the excessive activation of platelets, which deposit as thrombi in microcirculatory beds.* These intravascular thrombi cause a *microangiopathic hemolytic anemia* and widespread *organ dysfunction*, and the attendant consumption of platelets leads to *thrombocytopenia*. It is believed that the varied clinical manifestations of TTP and HUS are related to differing proclivities for thrombus formation in tissues.

Although certain features of the various thrombotic microangiopathies overlap, the triggers for the pathogenic platelet activation are distinctive and provide a more satisfying and clinically relevant way of thinking about these disorders; these are summarized in Table 14–10. *TTP is usually associated with a deficiency in a plasma enzyme called ADAMTS13,* also designated "vWF metalloprotease." ADAMTS13 normally degrades very high-molecular-weight multimers of von Willebrand factor (vWF). In its absence, these multimers accumulate in plasma and tend to promote platelet activation and aggregation. Superimposition of endothelial cell injury (caused by

TABLE 14–10	Thrombotic Microangiopathies: Causes and Associations

THROMBOTIC THROMBOCYTOPENIC PURPURA

Deficiency of ADAMTS13
  Inherited
  Acquired (autoantibodies)

HEMOLYTIC UREMIC SYNDROME

Epidemic: Escherichia coli strain O157:H7 infection
  Endothelial damage by Shiga-like toxin
Nonepidemic: alternative complement pathway inhibitor deficiencies (complement factor H, membrane cofactor protein (CD46), or factor I)
  Inherited
  Acquired (autoantibodies)
Miscellaneous associations
  Drugs (cyclosporine, chemotherapeutic agents)
  Radiation, bone marrow transplantation
  Other infections (HIV, pneumococcal sepsis)
  Conditions associated with autoimmunity (systemic lupus erythematosus, HIV infection, lymphoid neoplasms)

HIV, human immunodeficiency virus.

some other condition) may further promote the formation of platelet microaggregates, thus initiating or exacerbating clinically evident TTP.

The deficiency of ADAMTS13 can be inherited or acquired. In the acquired form, an autoantibody that inhibits the metalloprotease activity of ADAMTS13 is present.[26] Less commonly, patients inherit an inactivating mutation in *ADAMTS13*.[27] In those with hereditary ADAMTS13 deficiency, the onset is often delayed until adolescence and the symptoms are episodic. Thus, factors other than ADAMTS13 (e.g., some superimposed vascular injury or prothrombotic state) must be involved in triggering full-blown TTP.

TTP is an important diagnosis to consider in any patient presenting with thrombocytopenia and microangiopathic hemolytic anemia, since delays in diagnosis can be fatal. With plasma exchange, which removes autoantibodies and provides functional ADAMTS13, TTP (which once was uniformly fatal) can be treated successfully in more than 80% of patients.

In contrast, HUS is associated with normal levels of ADAMTS13 and is initiated by several other distinct defects.[28] *Epidemic, "typical" HUS is strongly associated with infectious gastroenteritis caused by Escherichia coli strain O157:H7, which elaborates a Shiga-like toxin.* This toxin is absorbed from the inflamed gastrointestinal mucosa into the circulation, where it alters endothelial cell function in some manner that results in platelet activation and aggregation. Children and the elderly are at highest risk. Those affected present with bloody diarrhea, and a few days later HUS makes its appearance. With appropriate supportive care complete recovery is possible, but irreversible renal damage and death can occur in more severe cases.

Nonepidemic, "atypical" HUS is often associated with defects in complement factor H, membrane cofactor protein (CD46), or factor I, three proteins that normally act to prevent excessive activation of the alternative complement pathway. Deficiencies of these proteins can be caused by inherited defects or acquired inhibitory autoantibodies and are associated with a remitting, relapsing course. Unlike TTP, the basis for the platelet activation in HUS is unclear; presumably, both Shiga-like toxin produced by pathogenic *E. coli* and defects in complement-regulatory proteins alter endothelial cell function in some way that promotes platelet activation.

Thrombotic microangiopathies resembling HUS can also be seen following exposures to other agents that damage endothelial cells (e.g., certain drugs and radiation therapy). The prognosis in these settings is guarded, because the HUS is often complicated by chronic, life-threatening conditions.

While DIC (discussed later) and thrombotic microangiopathies share features such as microvascular occlusion and microangiopathic hemolytic anemia, they are pathogenically distinct. In TTP and HUS (unlike in DIC), activation of the coagulation cascade is not of primary importance, and hence laboratory tests of coagulation, such as the PT and PTT, are usually normal.

BLEEDING DISORDERS RELATED TO DEFECTIVE PLATELET FUNCTIONS

Qualitative defects of platelet function can be inherited or acquired. Several inherited disorders characterized by abnormal platelet function and normal platelet count have been described. A brief discussion of these rare diseases is warranted because they provide excellent models for investigating the molecular mechanisms of platelet function.

Inherited disorders of platelet function can be classified into three pathogenically distinct groups: (1) *defects of adhesion,* (2) *defects of aggregation,* and (3) *disorders of platelet secretion (release reaction).*

- Bleeding resulting from defective adhesion of platelets to subendothelial matrix is best illustrated by the autosomal recessive disorder *Bernard-Soulier syndrome,* which is caused by an inherited deficiency of the platelet membrane glycoprotein complex Ib-IX. This glycoprotein is a receptor for vWF and is essential for normal platelet adhesion to the subendothelial extracellular matrix (Chapter 4).
- Bleeding due to *defective platelet aggregation* is exemplified by *Glanzmann thrombasthenia,* which is also transmitted as an autosomal recessive trait. Thrombasthenic platelets fail to aggregate in response to adenosine diphosphate (ADP), collagen, epinephrine, or thrombin because of deficiency or dysfunction of glycoprotein IIb-IIIa, an integrin that participates in "bridge formation" between platelets by binding fibrinogen.
- *Disorders of platelet secretion* are characterized by the defective release of certain mediators of platelet activation, such as thromboxanes and granule-bound ADP. The biochemical defects underlying these so-called *storage pool disorders* are varied, complex, and beyond the scope of our discussion.

Among the *acquired defects* of platelet function, two are clinically significant. The first is caused by *ingestion of aspirin and other nonsteroidal anti-inflammatory drugs.* Aspirin is a potent, irreversible inhibitor of the enzyme cyclooxygenase, which is required for the synthesis of thromboxane A_2 and prostaglandins (Chapter 2). These mediators play important roles in platelet aggregation and subsequent release reactions (Chapter 4). The antiplatelet effects of aspirin form the basis for its use in the prophylaxis of coronary thrombosis (Chapter

12). *Uremia* (Chapter 20) is the second condition exemplifying an acquired defect in platelet function. The pathogenesis of platelet dysfunction in uremia is complex and involves defects in adhesion, granule secretion, and aggregation.[29]

HEMORRHAGIC DIATHESES RELATED TO ABNORMALITIES IN CLOTTING FACTORS

Inherited or acquired deficiencies of virtually every coagulation factor have been reported as causes of bleeding diatheses. Unlike the petechial bleeding seen with thrombocytopenia, *bleeding due to isolated coagulation factor deficiencies most commonly manifests as large post-traumatic ecchymoses or hematomas, or prolonged bleeding after a laceration or any form of surgical procedure.* Bleeding into the gastrointestinal and urinary tracts, and particularly into weight-bearing joints (hemarthrosis), is common. Typical stories include the patient who oozes blood for days after a tooth extraction or who develops a hemarthrosis after minor stress on a knee joint.

Hereditary deficiencies typically affect a single clotting factor. The most common and important inherited deficiencies of coagulation factors affect factor VIII (hemophilia A), and factor IX (hemophilia B). Deficiencies of vWF (von Willebrand disease) are also discussed here, as this factor influences both coagulation and platelet function. Rare inherited deficiencies of each of the other coagulation factors have also been described. All cause bleeding except for factor XII deficiency; presumably, in vivo the extrinsic pathway and thrombin-mediated activation of factors XI and IX compensate for the absence of factor XII.

Acquired deficiencies usually involve multiple coagulation factors simultaneously and can be based on decreased protein synthesis or a shortened half-life. Vitamin K deficiency (Chapter 9) results in the impaired synthesis of factors II, VII, IX, and X and protein C. Many of these factors are made in the liver and are therefore deficient in severe parenchymal liver disease. Alternatively, in DIC, multiple coagulation factors are consumed and are therefore deficient. Acquired deficiencies of single factors occur, but they are rare. These are usually caused by inhibitory autoantibodies.

The Factor VIII-vWF Complex

The two most common inherited disorders of bleeding, hemophilia A and von Willebrand disease, are caused by qualitative or quantitative defects involving factor VIII and vWF, respectively. Before we discuss these disorders it will be helpful to review the structure and function of these two proteins, which exist together in the plasma as part of a single large complex.

Factor VIII and vWF are encoded by separate genes and are synthesized in different cells. Factor VIII is an essential cofactor of factor IX, which converts factor X to factor Xa (Fig. 14–26; also see Chapter 4). It is made in several tissues; sinusoidal endothelial cells and Kupffer cells in the liver, and tubular epithelial cells in the kidney, seem to be particularly important sources. Once factor VIII reaches the circulation, it binds to vWF, which is produced by endothelial cells and, to a lesser degree, by megakaryocytes, which are the source of the vWF that is found in platelet α-granules. vWF stabilizes factor VIII,

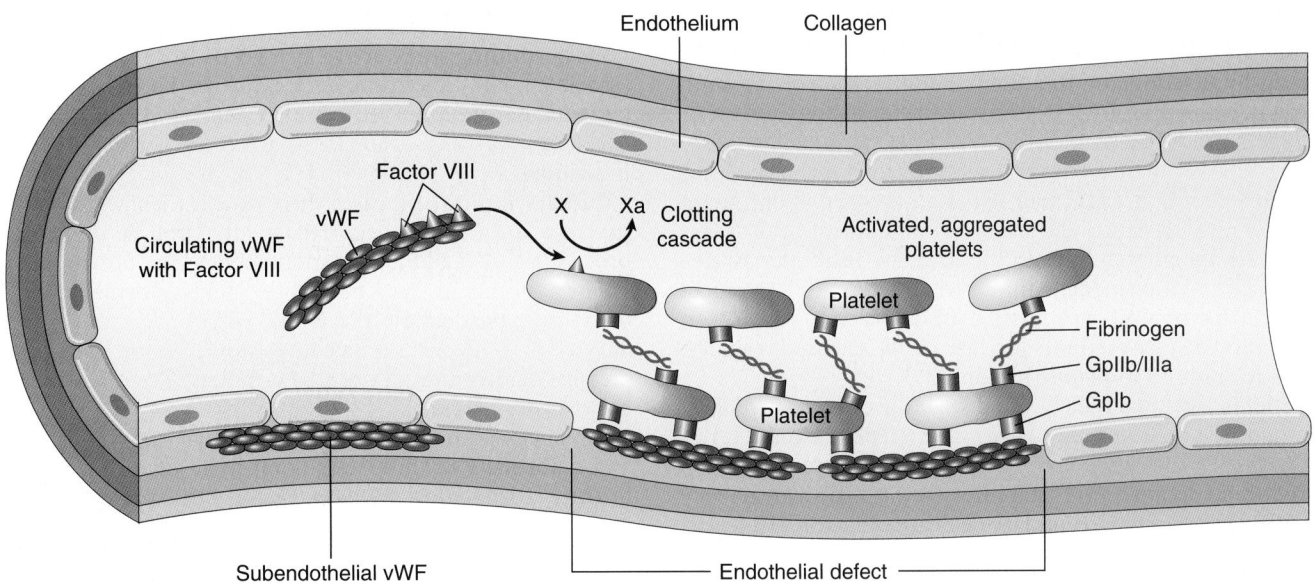

FIGURE 14–26 Structure and function of factor VIII–von Willebrand factor (vWF) complex. Factor VIII is synthesized in the liver and kidney, and vWF is made in endothelial cells and megakaryocytes. The two associate to form a complex in the circulation. vWF is also present in the subendothelial matrix of normal blood vessels and the α-granules of platelets. Following endothelial injury, exposure of subendothelial vWF causes adhesion of platelets, primarily via the glycoprotein Ib (GpIb) platelet receptor. Circulating vWF and vWF released from the α-granules of activated platelets can bind exposed subendothelial matrix, further contributing to platelet adhesion and activation. Activated platelets form hemostatic aggregates; fibrinogen (and possibly vWF) participates in aggregation through bridging interactions with the glycoprotein IIb/IIIa (GpIIb/IIIa) platelet receptor. Factor VIII takes part in the coagulation cascade as a cofactor in the activation of factor X on the surface of activated platelets.

which has a half-life of about 2.4 hours when free and 12 hours when bound to vWF in the circulation.

Circulating vWF exists as multimers containing as many as 100 subunits that can exceed 20×10^6 daltons in molecular mass. In addition to factor VIII, these multimers interact with several other proteins involved in hemostasis, including collagen, heparin, and possibly platelet membrane glycoproteins. The most important function of vWF is to promote the adhesion of platelets to the subendothelial matrix. This occurs through bridging interactions between platelet glycoprotein Ib-IX, vWF, and matrix components such as collagen. Some vWF is secreted from endothelial cells directly into the subendothelial matrix, where it lies ready to promote platelet adhesion if the endothelial lining is disrupted (see Fig. 14–26). Endothelial cells and platelets also release vWF into the circulation. Upon vascular injury, this second pool of vWF binds collagen in the subendothelial matrix to further augment platelet adhesion. vWF multimers may also promote platelet aggregation by binding to activated GpIIb/IIIa integrins; this activity may be of particular importance under conditions of high shear stress (such as occurs in small vessels).

Factor VIII and vWF protein levels are measured by immunological techniques. Factor VIII function is assessed by conducting coagulation assays with mixtures of patient plasma and factor VIII-deficient plasma. vWF function is assessed using the ristocetin agglutination test. This assay is performed by mixing the patient's plasma with formalin-fixed platelets and ristocetin, a small molecule that binds and "activates" vWF. Ristocetin induces multivalent vWF multimers to bind platelet glycoprotein Ib-IX and form interplatelet "bridges." The resulting clumping (agglutination) of platelets is mea-

sured in a device called an aggregometer. Thus, the degree to which patient plasma promotes ristocetin-dependent platelet agglutination is a measure of vWF activity.

Von Willebrand Disease

Von Willebrand disease is the most common inherited bleeding disorder of humans, affecting about 1% of adults in the United States. In most of those affected, the bleeding tendency is mild and often goes unnoticed until some hemostatic stress, such as surgery or a dental procedure, reveals its presence. The most common symptoms are spontaneous bleeding from mucous membranes (e.g., epistaxis); excessive bleeding from wounds; menorrhagia; and a prolonged bleeding time in the presence of a normal platelet count. It is usually transmitted as an autosomal dominant disorder, but rare autosomal recessive variants have been described.

Von Willebrand disease is molecularly heterogeneous.[30] More than 20 variants have been described, which can be grouped into two major categories:

Type 1 and type 3 von Willebrand disease are associated with a reduced quantity of circulating vWF. Type 1, an autosomal dominant disorder characterized by a mild to moderate quantitative vWF deficiency, accounts for about 70% of all cases. Incomplete penetrance and variable expressivity are commonly observed, but it generally is associated with mild disease. Type 3 (an autosomal recessive disorder) is associated with extremely low levels of functional vWF and correspondingly severe clinical manifestations. Because a severe deficiency of vWF has a marked effect on the stability of factor VIII, some of the bleeding characteristics resemble those seen in hemophilia. The nature of the mutations in the majority of individuals with type 1 disease is poorly defined. In some cases missense mutations have been found. Type 3 disease is usually caused by deletions or frameshift mutations involving both alleles.

Type 2 von Willebrand disease is characterized by qualitative defects in vWF; there are several subtypes, of which type 2A is the most common. It is inherited as an autosomal dominant disorder. vWF is expressed in normal amounts, but missense mutations are present that lead to defective multimer assembly. Large and intermediate multimers, representing the most active forms of vWF, are missing from plasma. Type 2 von Willebrand disease accounts for 25% of all cases and is associated with mild to moderate bleeding.

Patients with von Willebrand disease have *defects in platelet function* despite a *normal platelet count*. The plasma level of active vWF, measured as the ristocetin cofactor activity, is reduced. Because vWF stabilizes factor VIII, a deficiency of vWF gives rise to a secondary decrease in factor VIII levels. This may be reflected by a prolongation of the PTT in von Willebrand disease types 1 and 3. However, except in rare type 3 patients, adverse complications typical of severe factor VIII deficiency, such as bleeding into the joints, are not seen.

To summarize, in von Willebrand disease inherited defects in vWF lead to secondary abnormalities in platelet adhesion and clot formation. Even within families in which a single defective vWF allele is segregating, a wide variability in clinical expression is common. This is due in part to additional genetic factors that influence circulating levels of vWF, which vary greatly in normal populations. Persons facing hemostatic challenges (dental work, surgery) can be treated with desmopressin, which stimulates vWF release, or infusions of plasma concentrates containing factor VIII and vWF.

Hemophilia A (Factor VIII Deficiency)

Hemophilia A is the most common hereditary disease associated with life-threatening bleeding.[31] It is caused by mutations in factor VIII, which is an essential cofactor for factor IX in the coagulation cascade (Chapter 4). Hemophilia A is inherited as an X-linked recessive trait and thus affects mainly males and homozygous females. Rarely, excessive bleeding occurs in heterozygous females, presumably as a result of inactivation of the X chromosome bearing the normal factor VIII allele by chance in most cells (unfavorable lyonization). About 30% of patients have no family history; their disease is caused by new mutations.

Hemophilia A exhibits a wide range of clinical severity that correlates well with the level of factor VIII activity. Those with less than 1% of normal levels have severe disease; those with 2% to 5% of normal levels have moderately severe disease; and those with 6% to 50% of normal levels have mild disease. The varying degrees of factor VIII deficiency are largely explained by heterogeneity in the causative mutations. As with β-thalassemia, the genetic lesions include deletions, nonsense mutations that create stop codons, and mutations that cause errors in mRNA splicing. The most severe deficiencies result from an inversion involving the X chromosome that completely abolishes the synthesis of factor VIII. Less commonly, severe hemophilia A is associated with point mutations in factor VIII that impair the function of the protein. In such

cases factor VIII levels seem normal by immunoassay. Mutations permitting some active factor VIII to be synthesized are associated with mild to moderate disease. The disease in such patients may be modified by other genetic factors that influence factor VIII expression levels, which vary widely in normal individuals.

In all symptomatic cases there is a tendency toward easy bruising and massive hemorrhage after trauma or operative procedures. In addition, "spontaneous" hemorrhages frequently occur in regions of the body normally subject to trauma, particularly the joints, where they are known as *hemarthroses*. Recurrent bleeding into the joints leads to progressive deformities that can be crippling. *Petechiae are characteristically absent.*

Patients with hemophilia A typically have a prolonged PTT and a normal PT. These tests point to an abnormality of the intrinsic coagulation pathway. Factor VIII–specific assays are required for diagnosis.

Given that one arm of the coagulation cascade, the extrinsic pathway, is intact in hemophilia A, it is reasonable to ask: Why do patients bleed? Obviously, test tube assays of coagulation are imperfect surrogates for what occurs in vivo, and it must be that in the face of factor VIII deficiency, fibrin deposition is inadequate to achieve hemostasis. It is beyond our scope to discuss this issue in detail; it seems that the chief role of the extrinsic pathway in hemostasis is to initiate a limited burst of thrombin activation upon tissue injury. This initial procoagulant stimulus is reinforced and amplified by a critical feedback loop in which thrombin activates factors XI and IX of the intrinsic pathway (Chapter 4). In the absence of factor VIII, this feedback loop is inactive and insufficient thrombin (and fibrin) is generated to create a stable clot. In addition, high levels of thrombin are required to activate TAFI (thrombin-activated fibrinolysis inhibitor), a factor that inhibits fibrinolysis. Thus, both inadequate coagulation (fibrinogenesis) and inappropriate clot removal (fibrinolysis) contribute to the bleeding diathesis in hemophilia. The precise explanation for the tendency of hemophiliacs to bleed at particular sites (joints, muscles, and the central nervous system) remains uncertain.

Hemophilia A is treated with infusions of recombinant factor VIII. About 15% of patients with severe hemophilia A develop antibodies that bind and inhibit factor VIII, probably because the protein is perceived as foreign, having never been "seen" by the immune system. These antibody inhibitors can be a very difficult therapeutic challenge. Before the development of recombinant factor VIII therapy, thousands of hemophiliacs received plasma-derived factor VIII concentrates containing HIV, and many developed AIDS (Chapter 6). The risk of HIV transmission has been eliminated but tragically too late for an entire generation of hemophiliacs. Efforts to develop somatic gene therapy for hemophilia are continuing.

Hemophilia B (Christmas Disease, Factor IX Deficiency)

Severe factor IX deficiency produces a disorder clinically indistinguishable from factor VIII deficiency (hemophilia A). This should not be surprising, given that factors VIII and IX function together to activate factor X. A wide spectrum of mutations involving the gene that encodes factor IX is found in hemophilia B. Like hemophilia A it is inherited as an X-linked recessive trait and shows variable clinical severity. In about 15% of these patients, factor IX is present but nonfunctional. As with hemophilia A, the PTT is prolonged and the PT is normal. Diagnosis of Christmas disease (named after the first patient identified with this condition, and not the holiday) is possible only by assay of the factor levels. The disease is treated with infusions of recombinant factor IX.

DISSEMINATED INTRAVASCULAR COAGULATION (DIC)

DIC is an acute, subacute, or chronic thrombohemorrhagic disorder characterized by the excessive activation of coagulation, which leads to the formation of thrombi in the microvasculature of the body. It occurs as a secondary complication of many different disorders. Sometimes the coagulopathy is localized to a specific organ or tissue. As a consequence of the thrombotic diathesis there is consumption of platelets, fibrin, and coagulation factors and, secondarily, activation of fibrinolysis. DIC can present with signs and symptoms relating to the tissue hypoxia and infarction caused by the myriad microthrombi; with hemorrhage caused by the depletion of factors required for hemostasis and the activation of fibrinolytic mechanisms; or both.

Etiology and Pathogenesis. *At the outset, it must be emphasized that DIC is not a primary disease.* It is a coagulopathy that occurs in the course of a variety of clinical conditions. In discussing the general mechanisms underlying DIC, it is useful to briefly review the normal process of blood coagulation and clot removal (see Chapter 4 for more details).

Clotting can be initiated by either of two pathways: (1) the *extrinsic pathway*, which is triggered by the release of tissue factor ("tissue thromboplastin"); and (2) the *intrinsic pathway*, which involves the activation of factor XII by surface contact with collagen or other negatively charged substances. Both pathways, through a series of intermediate steps, result in the generation of thrombin, which in turn converts fibrinogen to fibrin. At the site of injury, thrombin further augments local fibrin deposition by directly activating the intrinsic pathway and factors that inhibit fibrinolysis.

Once clotting is initiated, it is critically important that it be limited to the site of injury. Remarkably, as thrombin is swept away in the bloodstream and encounters normal vessels, it is converted to an anticoagulant through binding to *thrombomodulin*, a protein found on the surface of endothelial cells. The thrombin-thrombomodulin complex activates protein C, which is an important inhibitor of two procoagulants, factor V and factor VIII. Other activated coagulation factors are removed from the circulation by the liver, and as you will recall, the blood also contains several potent fibrinolytic factors, such as plasmin. These and additional checks and balances normally ensure that just enough clotting occurs at the right place and time.

From this brief review it should be clear that DIC could result from pathologic activation of the extrinsic and/or intrinsic pathways of coagulation or the impairment of clot-inhibiting mechanisms. Since the latter rarely constitute primary mechanisms of DIC, we will focus on the abnormal initiation of clotting.

Two major mechanisms trigger DIC: (1) release of tissue factor or thromboplastic substances into the circulation, and (2) widespread injury to the endothelial cells. Thromboplastic substances can be derived from a variety of sources, such as the placenta in obstetric complications and the cytoplasmic granules of acute promyelocytic leukemia cells (Chapter 13). Mucus released from certain adenocarcinomas can directly activate factor X, independent of factor VII.

Endothelial injury can initiate DIC in several ways. Injuries that cause endothelial cell necrosis expose the subendothelial matrix, leading to the activation of platelets and both arms of the coagulation pathway. However, even subtle endothelial injuries can unleash procoagulant activity. One mediator of such effects is TNF, which is implicated in DIC occurring with sepsis. TNF induces endothelial cells to express tissue factor on their cell surfaces and to decrease the expression of thrombomodulin, shifting the checks and balances that govern hemostasis towards coagulation. In addition, TNF up-regulates the expression of adhesion molecules on endothelial cells, thereby promoting the adhesion of leukocytes, which can damage endothelial cells by releasing reactive oxygen species and preformed proteases. Widespread endothelial injury may also be produced by deposition of antigen-antibody complexes (e.g., systemic lupus erythematosus), temperature extremes (e.g., heat stroke, burns), or microorganisms (e.g., meningococci, rickettsiae). Even subtle endothelial injury can unleash procoagulant activity by enhancing membrane expression of tissue factor.

DIC is most likely to be associated with *obstetric complications, malignant neoplasms, sepsis, and major trauma.* The triggers in these conditions are often multiple and interrelated. For example, in bacterial infections *endotoxins* can injure endothelial cells and inhibit the expression of thrombomodulin directly or through production of TNF; stimulate the release of thromboplastins from inflammatory cells; and activate factor XII. Antigen-antibody complexes formed in response to the infection can activate the classical complement pathway, giving rise to complement fragments that secondarily activate both platelets and granulocytes. In *massive trauma, extensive surgery,* and *severe burns,* the major trigger is the release of tissue thromboplastins. In *obstetric conditions*, thromboplastins derived from the placenta, dead retained fetus, or amniotic fluid may enter the circulation. *Hypoxia, acidosis, and shock,* which often coexist in very ill patients, can also cause widespread endothelial injury, and supervening infections can complicate the problems further. *Among cancers, acute promyelocytic leukemia and adenocarcinomas* of the lung, pancreas, colon, and stomach are most frequently associated with DIC.

The possible consequences of DIC are twofold (Fig. 14–27). Firstly, there is *widespread deposition of fibrin* within the microcirculation. This leads to *ischemia* of the more severely affected or more vulnerable organs and a *microangiopathic hemolytic anemia,* which results from the fragmentation of red cells as they squeeze through the narrowed microvasculature. Secondly, the consumption of platelets and clotting factors and the activation of plasminogen leads to a *hemorrhagic diathesis.* Plasmin not only cleaves fibrin, but it also digests factors V and VIII, thereby reducing their concentration further. In addition, fibrin degradation products resulting from fibrinolysis inhibit platelet aggregation, fibrin polymerization, and

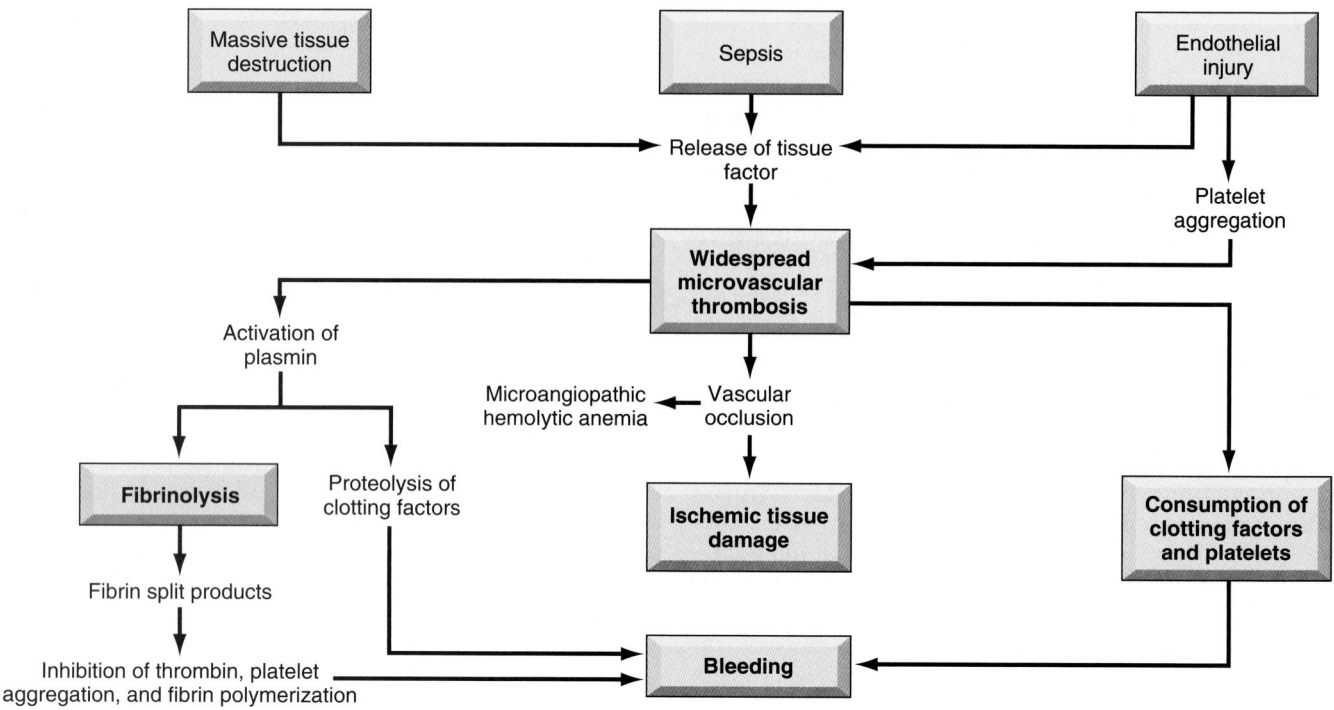

FIGURE 14–27 Pathophysiology of disseminated intravascular coagulation.

thrombin. All of these derangements contribute to the hemostatic failure seen in DIC.

Morphology. Thrombi are most often found in the brain, heart, lungs, kidneys, adrenals, spleen, and liver, in decreasing order of frequency, but any tissue can be affected. Affected kidneys may have small thrombi in the glomeruli that evoke only reactive swelling of endothelial cells or, in severe cases, microinfarcts or even bilateral renal cortical necrosis. Numerous fibrin thrombi may be found in alveolar capillaries, sometimes associated with pulmonary edema and fibrin exudation, creating "hyaline membranes" reminiscent of acute respiratory distress syndrome (Chapter 15). In the central nervous system, fibrin thrombi can cause microinfarcts, occasionally complicated by simultaneous hemorrhage, which can sometimes lead to variable neurologic signs and symptoms. The manifestations in the endocrine glands are of considerable interest. In meningococcemia, fibrin thrombi within the microcirculation of the adrenal cortex are the probable basis for the massive adrenal hemorrhages seen in **Waterhouse-Friderichsen syndrome** (Chapter 24). Similarly, **Sheehan postpartum pituitary necrosis** (Chapter 24) is a form of DIC complicating labor and delivery. In toxemia of pregnancy (Chapter 22) the placenta exhibits widespread microthrombi, providing a plausible explanation for the premature atrophy of the cytotrophoblast and syncytiotrophoblast that is encountered in this condition. An unusual form of DIC occurs in association with giant hemangiomas, in which thrombi form within the neoplasm because of stasis and recurrent trauma to fragile blood vessels.

Clinical Features. The onset can be fulminant, as in endotoxic shock or amniotic fluid embolism, or insidious and chronic, as in cases of carcinomatosis or retention of a dead fetus. Overall, about 50% of the affected are obstetric patients having complications of pregnancy. In this setting the disorder tends to be reversible with delivery of the fetus. About 33% of the affected patients have carcinomatosis. The remaining cases are associated with the various entities previously listed.

It is almost impossible to detail all the potential clinical presentations, but a few common patterns are worthy of description. These include microangiopathic hemolytic anemia; dyspnea, cyanosis, and respiratory failure; convulsions and coma; oliguria and acute renal failure; and sudden or progressive circulatory failure and shock. In general, *acute DIC, associated with obstetric complications or major trauma, for example, is dominated by a bleeding diathesis, whereas chronic DIC, such as occurs in cancer patients, tends to present with thrombotic complications.* The diagnosis is based on clinical observation and laboratory studies, including measurement of fibrinogen levels, platelets, the PT and PTT, and fibrin degradation products.

The prognosis is highly variable and largely depends on the underlying disorder. *The only definitive treatment is to remove or treat the inciting cause.* The management requires meticulous maneuvering between the Scylla of thrombosis and the Charybdis of bleeding diathesis. Administration of anticoagulants or procoagulants has been advocated in specific settings, but not without controversy.

REFERENCES

1. Kay M: Immunoregulation of cellular life span. Ann N Y Acad Sci 1057:85, 2005.

2. Eber S, Lux SE: Hereditary spherocytosis—defects in proteins that connect the membrane skeleton to the lipid bilayer. Semin Hematol 41:118, 2004.

3. Kwiatkowski DP: How malaria has affected the human genome and what human genetics can teach us about malaria. Am J Hum Genet 77:171, 2005.

4. Browne PV, Hebbel RP: CD36-positive stress reticulocytosis in sickle cell anemia. J Lab Clin Med 127:340, 1996.

5. Zennadi R et al: Epinephrine-induced activation of LW-mediated sickle cell adhesion and vaso-occlusion in vivo. Blood 110:2708, 2007.

6. El Nemer W et al: Endothelial Lu/BCAM glycoproteins are novel ligands for red blood cell alpha4beta1 integrin: role in adhesion of sickle red blood cells to endothelial cells. Blood 109:3544, 2007.

7. Belcher JD et al: Transgenic sickle mice have vascular inflammation. Blood 101:3953, 2003.

8. Kato GJ et al: Deconstructing sickle cell disease: reappraisal of the role of hemolysis in the development of clinical subphenotypes. Blood Rev 21:37, 2007.

9. Platt OS: Hydroxyurea for the treatment of sickle cell anemia. N Engl J Med 358:1362, 2008.

10. Premawardhena A et al: A novel molecular basis for beta thalassemia intermedia poses new questions about its pathophysiology. Blood 106:3251, 2005.

11. Schrier SL, Angelucci E: New strategies in the treatment of the thalassemias. Annu Rev Med 56:157, 2005.

12. Luzzatto L: Paroxysmal nocturnal hemoglobinuria: an acquired X-linked genetic disease with somatic-cell mosaicism. Curr Opin Genet Dev 16:317, 2006.

13. Hill A et al: Recent developments in the understanding and management of paroxysmal nocturnal haemoglobinuria. Br J Haematol 137:181, 2007.

14. Gertz MA: Management of cold haemolytic syndrome. Br J Haematol 138:422, 2007.

15. King KE, Ness PM: Treatment of autoimmune hemolytic anemia. Semin Hematol 42:131, 2005.

16. Jin Y et al: NALP1 in vitiligo-associated multiple autoimmune disease. N Engl J Med 356:1216, 2007.

17. Andrews NC, Schmidt PJ: Iron homeostasis. Annu Rev Physiol 69:69, 2007.

18. Roy CN, Andrews NC: Anemia of inflammation: the hepcidin link. Curr Opin Hematol 12:107, 2005.

19. Roy CN et al: Hepcidin antimicrobial peptide transgenic mice exhibit features of the anemia of inflammation. Blood 109:4038, 2007.

20. Young NS et al: Current concepts in the pathophysiology and treatment of aplastic anemia. Blood 108:2509, 2006.

21. Taniguchi T, D'Andrea AD: Molecular pathogenesis of Fanconi anemia: recent progress. Blood 107:4223, 2006.

22. Yamaguchi H et al: Mutations in TERT, the gene for telomerase reverse transcriptase, in aplastic anemia. N Engl J Med 352:1413, 2005.

23. Lee FS et al: Oxygen sensing: recent insights from idiopathic erythrocytosis. Cell Cycle 5:941, 2006.

24. Aster RH, Bougie DW: Drug-induced immune thrombocytopenia. N Engl J Med 357:580, 2007.

25. Levy JH, Husting JM: Heparin-induced thrombocytopenia, a prothrombotic disease. Hematol Oncol Clin North Am 21:65, 2007.

26. Zheng XL, Sadler JE: Pathogenesis of thrombotic microangiopathies. Annu Rev Pathol 3:249, 2008.

27. Kokame K, Miyata T: Genetic defects leading to hereditary thrombotic thrombocytopenic purpura. Semin Hematol 41:34, 2004.

28. Tsai HM: The molecular biology of thrombotic microangiopathy. Kidney Int 70:16, 2006.

29. Sohal AS et al: Uremic bleeding: pathophysiology and clinical risk factors. Thromb Res 118:417, 2006.

30. Sadler JE et al: Update on the pathophysiology and classification of von Willebrand disease: a report of the Subcommittee on von Willebrand Factor. J Thromb Haemost 4:2103, 2006.

31. Castaldo G et al: Haemophilia A: molecular insights. Clin Chem Lab Med 45:450, 2007.

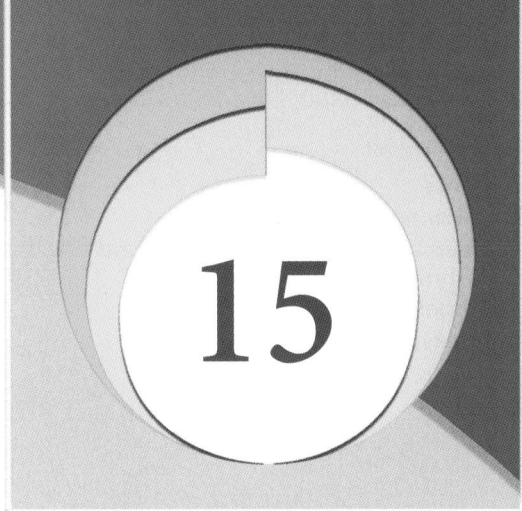

The Lung

ALIYA N. HUSAIN

Congenital Anomalies

Atelectasis (Collapse)

Pulmonary Edema
Hemodynamic Pulmonary Edema
Edema Caused by Microvascular Injury

Acute Lung Injury and Acute Respiratory Distress Syndrome (Diffuse Alveolar Damage)
Acute Interstitial Pneumonia

Obstructive versus Restrictive Pulmonary Diseases

Obstructive Pulmonary Diseases
Emphysema
Chronic Bronchitis
Asthma
Bronchiectasis

Chronic Diffuse Interstitial (Restrictive) Diseases
Fibrosing Diseases
Idiopathic Pulmonary Fibrosis
Nonspecific Interstitial Pneumonia
Cryptogenic Organizing Pneumonia
Pulmonary Involvement in Connective Tissue Diseases
Pneumoconioses
Complications of Therapies
Granulomatous Diseases
Sarcoidosis
Hypersensitivity Pneumonitis
Pulmonary Eosinophilia
Smoking-Related Interstitial Diseases
Desquamative Interstitial Pneumonia
Respiratory Bronchiolitis–Associated Interstitial Lung Disease
Pulmonary Alveolar Proteinosis

Diseases of Vascular Origin
Pulmonary Embolism, Hemorrhage, and Infarction
Pulmonary Hypertension
Diffuse Pulmonary Hemorrhage Syndromes
Goodpasture Syndrome
Idiopathic Pulmonary Hemosiderosis
Wegener Granulomatosis

Pulmonary Infections
Community-Acquired Acute Pneumonias
Streptococcus pneumoniae
Haemophilus influenzae
Moraxella catarrhalis
Staphylococcus aureus
Klebsiella pneumoniae
Pseudomonas aeruginosa
Legionella pneumophila
Community-Acquired Atypical (Viral and Mycoplasmal) Pneumonias
Influenza Infections
Human Metapneumovirus
Severe Acute Respiratory Syndrome
Hospital-Acquired Pneumonia
Aspiration Pneumonia
Lung Abscess
Chronic Pneumonia
Histoplasmosis
Blastomycosis
Coccidioidomycosis
Pneumonia in the Immunocompromised Host
Pulmonary Disease in Human Immunodeficiency Virus Infection

Lung Transplantation

Tumors
  Carcinomas
  Neuroendocrine Proliferations and
    Tumors
  Miscellaneous Tumors
  Metastatic Tumors
Pleura

Pleural Effusion
  Inflammatory Pleural Effusions
  Noninflammatory Pleural Effusions
Pneumothorax
Pleural Tumors
  Solitary Fibrous Tumor
  Malignant Mesothelioma

The lungs are ingeniously constructed to carry out their cardinal function: the exchange of gases between inspired air and blood. Developmentally, the respiratory system is an outgrowth from the ventral wall of the foregut. The midline trachea develops two lateral outpocketings, the lung buds. The right lung bud eventually divides into three branches—the lobar bronchi—and the left into two lobar bronchi, thus giving rise to three lobes on the right and two on the left. The right main stem bronchus is more vertical and more directly in line with the trachea. Consequently, aspirated foreign materials, such as vomitus, blood, and foreign bodies, tend to enter the right lung more than the left. The lobar right and left bronchi branch dichotomously, giving rise to progressively smaller airways. Accompanying the branching airways is the double arterial supply to the lungs, that is, the pulmonary and bronchial arteries.

Progressive branching of the bronchi forms *bronchioles*, which are distinguished from bronchi by the lack of cartilage and submucosal glands within their walls. Further branching of bronchioles leads to the *terminal bronchioles*, which are less than 2 mm in diameter. The part of the lung distal to the terminal bronchiole is called the *acinus*; it is roughly spherical, with a diameter of about 7 mm. An acinus is composed of *respiratory bronchioles* (which give off several alveoli from their sides), *alveolar ducts,* and *alveolar sacs,* the blind ends of the respiratory passages, whose walls are formed entirely of alveoli, which are the site of gas exchange. A cluster of three to five terminal bronchioles, each with its appended acinus, is referred to as the pulmonary *lobule.* This lobular architecture assumes importance in distinguishing the major forms of emphysema.

Except for the vocal cords, which are covered by stratified squamous epithelium, the entire respiratory tree, including the larynx, trachea, and bronchioles, is lined by pseudostratified, tall, columnar, ciliated epithelial cells. The bronchial mucosa also contains a population of neuroendocrine cells that have neurosecretory-type granules and can release a variety of factors, including serotonin, calcitonin, and gastrin-releasing peptide (bombesin). Numerous mucus-secreting goblet cells and submucosal glands are dispersed throughout the walls of the trachea and bronchi (but not the bronchioles).

The microscopic structure of the alveolar walls (or alveolar septa) consists, from blood to air, of the following (Fig. 15–1):

○ *Capillary endothelium* lining the intertwining network of anastomosing capillaries.

○ *Basement membrane and surrounding interstitial tissue* separating the endothelial cells from the alveolar lining epithelial cells. In thin portions of the alveolar septum, the basement membranes of epithelium and endothelium are fused, whereas in thicker portions they are separated by an interstitial space *(pulmonary interstitium)* containing fine elastic fibers, small bundles of collagen, a few fibroblast-like interstitial cells, smooth muscle cells, mast cells, and rarely lymphocytes and monocytes.

○ *Alveolar epithelium,* a continuous layer of two cell types: flattened, platelike *type I pneumocytes* covering 95% of the alveolar surface and rounded *type II pneumocytes.* Type II cells synthesize *surfactant,* contained in osmiophilic *lamellar bodies* seen with electron microscopy, and are involved in the repair of alveolar epithelium through their ability to give rise to type I cells.

○ *Alveolar macrophages,* loosely attached to the epithelial cells or lying free within the alveolar spaces, are derived from blood monocytes and belong to the mononuclear phagocyte system. Often, they are filled with carbon particles and other phagocytosed materials.

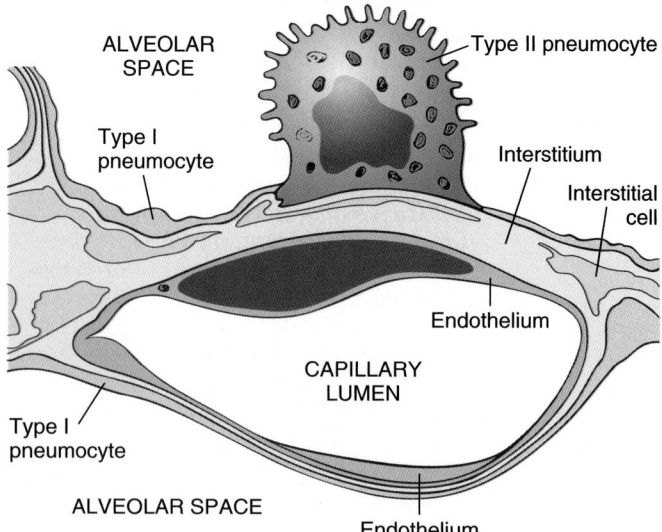

FIGURE 15–1 Microscopic structure of the alveolar wall. Note that the basement membrane *(yellow)* is thin on one side and widened where it is continuous with the interstitial space. Portions of interstitial cells are shown.

The alveolar walls are perforated by numerous *pores of Kohn*, which permit the passage of bacteria and exudate between adjacent alveoli (see Fig. 15–34B). Adjacent to the alveolar cell membrane is the pulmonary surfactant layer.

Primary respiratory infections, such as bronchitis and pneumonia, are commonplace in clinical and pathologic practice. With cigarette smoking, air pollution, and other environmental inhalants, chronic bronchitis and emphysema have become rampant. In men, malignancy of the lungs had been rising steadily but has now plateaued and is expected to decline in the future. Unfortunately, as more and more women are smoking, lung cancer has become the most common malignancy in women, surpassing even breast cancer and is now the most common lethal visceral malignancy in men and women. Although the lungs are secondarily involved in almost all forms of terminal disease, primary pulmonary diseases are emphasized in this chapter.

Congenital Anomalies

Developmental defects of the lung include the following[1]:

- Agenesis or hypoplasia of both lungs, one lung, or single lobes
- Tracheal and bronchial anomalies (atresia, stenosis, tracheoesophageal fistula)
- Vascular anomalies
- Congenital lobar overinflation (emphysema)
- Foregut cysts
- Congenital pulmonary airway malformation
- Pulmonary sequestrations

Only the more common anomalies are discussed here. *Pulmonary hypoplasia* is the defective development of both lungs (one may be more affected than the other) resulting in decreased weight, volume, and acini disproportional to the body weight and gestational age. It is caused by a variety of abnormalities that compress the lung(s) or impede normal lung expansion in utero such as congenital diaphragmatic hernia and oligohydramnions.

Foregut cysts arise from an abnormal detachment of primitive foregut and are most often located in the hilum or middle mediastinum. Depending on the wall structure, these cysts are classified as bronchogenic (most common), esophageal, or enteric. A bronchogenic cyst is rarely connected to the tracheobronchial tree. Microscopically, the cyst is lined by ciliated pseudostratified columnar epithelium with squamous metaplasia occurring in areas of inflammation. The wall contains bronchial glands, cartilage, and smooth muscle. Surgical resection is curative.

Pulmonary sequestration refers to the presence of a discrete mass of lung tissue *without normal connection to the airway system*. Blood supply to the sequestered area arises not from the pulmonary arteries but from the aorta or its branches. *Extralobar sequestrations* are external to the lung and may be located anywhere in the thorax or mediastinum. They most commonly come to attention in infants as abnormal mass lesions, and may be associated with other congenital anomalies. *Intralobar sequestrations* occur within the lung substance usually in older children and are often associated with recurrent localized infection or bronchiectasis.

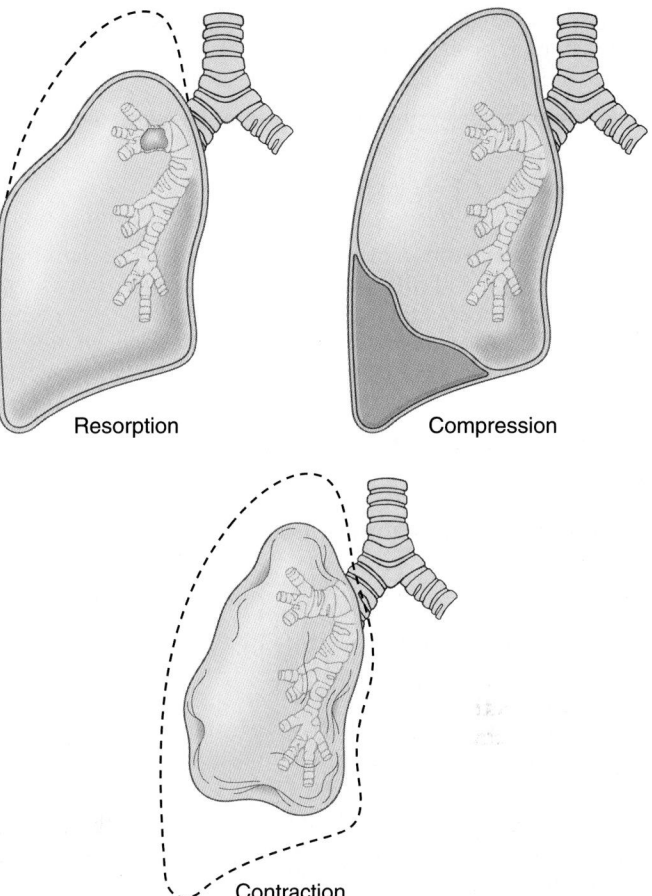

FIGURE 15–2 Various forms of acquired atelectasis. Dashed lines indicate normal lung volume.

Atelectasis (Collapse)

Atelectasis refers either to incomplete expansion of the lungs (neonatal atelectasis) or to the collapse of previously inflated lung, producing areas of relatively airless pulmonary parenchyma. Acquired atelectasis, encountered principally in adults, may be divided into *resorption* (or *obstruction*), *compression*, and *contraction atelectasis* (Fig. 15–2).

Resorption atelectasis is the consequence of complete obstruction of an airway, which in time leads to resorption of the oxygen trapped in the dependent alveoli, without impairment of blood flow through the affected alveolar walls. Since lung volume is diminished, the mediastinum shifts *toward* the atelectatic lung. Resorption atelectasis is caused principally by excessive secretions (e.g., mucus plugs) or exudates within smaller bronchi and is therefore most often found in bronchial asthma, chronic bronchitis, bronchiectasis, postoperative states, aspiration of foreign bodies and, rarely, bronchial neoplasms. *Compression atelectasis* results whenever the pleural cavity is partially or completely filled by fluid exudate, tumor, blood, or air (the last-mentioned constituting *pneumothorax*) or, with *tension pneumothorax*, when air pressure impinges on and threatens the function of the lung and mediastinum, especially the major vessels. With compressive atelectasis, the mediastinum shifts *away* from the affected lung. *Contraction atelectasis* occurs when local or generalized fibrotic changes in the lung or pleura prevent full expansion.

Significant atelectasis reduces oxygenation and predisposes to infection. Because the collapsed lung parenchyma can be re-expanded, *atelectasis is a reversible disorder* (except that caused by contraction).

Pulmonary Edema

A general consideration of edema is in Chapter 4, and pulmonary congestion and edema are described briefly in the context of congestive heart failure (Chapter 12). Pulmonary edema can result from *hemodynamic* disturbances *(hemodynamic or cardiogenic pulmonary edema)* or from direct *increases in capillary permeability,* as a result of microvascular injury (Table 15–1). Therapy and outcome depend on the underlying etiology.

Hemodynamic Pulmonary Edema

The most common *hemodynamic* cause of pulmonary edema is *increased hydrostatic pressure,* as occurs in left-sided congestive heart failure. Whatever the clinical setting, pulmonary congestion and edema are characterized by heavy, wet lungs. Fluid accumulates initially in the basal regions of the lower lobes because hydrostatic pressure is greater in these sites (dependent edema). Histologically, the alveolar capillaries are engorged, and an intra-alveolar granular pink precipitate is seen. Alveolar microhemorrhages and *hemosiderin-laden macrophages ("heart failure" cells)* may be present. In long-standing cases of pulmonary congestion, such as those seen in mitral stenosis, hemosiderin-laden macrophages are abundant, and fibrosis and thickening of the alveolar walls cause the soggy lungs to become firm and brown *(brown induration).* These changes not only impair normal respiratory function but also predispose to infection.

TABLE 15–1   Classification and Causes of Pulmonary Edema

HEMODYNAMIC EDEMA

Increased hydrostatic pressure (increased pulmonary venous pressure)
   Left-sided heart failure (common)
   Volume overload
   Pulmonary vein obstruction
Decreased oncotic pressure (less common)
   Hypoalbuminemia
   Nephrotic syndrome
   Liver disease
   Protein-losing enteropathies
Lymphatic obstruction (rare)

EDEMA DUE TO MICROVASCULAR INJURY (ALVEOLAR INJURY)

Infections: pneumonia, septicemia
Inhaled gases: oxygen, smoke
Liquid aspiration: gastric contents, near-drowning
Drugs and chemicals: chemotherapeutic agents (bleomycin), other medications (amphotericin B), heroin, kerosene, paraquat
Shock, trauma
Radiation
Transfusion related

EDEMA OF UNDETERMINED ORIGIN

High altitude
Neurogenic (central nervous system trauma)

Edema Caused by Microvascular Injury

The second mechanism leading to pulmonary edema is *injury to the capillaries of the alveolar septa.* Here the pulmonary capillary hydrostatic pressure is usually not elevated, and hemodynamic factors play a secondary role. The edema results from primary injury to the vascular endothelium or damage to alveolar epithelial cells (with secondary microvascular injury). This results in leakage of fluids and proteins first into the interstitial space and, in more severe cases, into the alveoli. In most forms of pneumonia the edema remains localized and is overshadowed by the manifestations of infection. When diffuse, however, alveolar edema is an important contributor to a serious and often fatal condition, *acute respiratory distress syndrome,* discussed in the following section.

Acute Lung Injury and Acute Respiratory Distress Syndrome (Diffuse Alveolar Damage)

Acute lung injury (ALI) (also called noncardiogenic pulmonary edema) is characterized by the abrupt onset of significant hypoxemia and diffuse pulmonary infiltrates in the absence of cardiac failure.[2] Acute respiratory distress syndrome (ARDS) refers to severe ALI. ARDS and ALI both have inflammation-associated increase in pulmonary vascular permeability, and epithelial and endothelial cell death. The histologic manifestation of these diseases is *diffuse alveolar damage* (DAD). Most cases of ALI are associated with an underlying etiology such as sepsis. In the absence of any etiologic association, such cases are called acute interstitial pneumonia (AIP).

ALI is a well-recognized complication of diverse conditions, including both direct injuries to the lungs and systemic disorders (Table 15–2). In many cases, a combination of predisposing conditions is responsible (e.g., shock, oxygen therapy, and sepsis). Nonpulmonary organ dysfunction may also be present in severe cases.

Morphology. In the acute stage, the lungs are heavy, firm, red, and boggy. They exhibit congestion, interstitial and intra-alveolar edema, inflammation, fibrin deposition, and **diffuse alveolar damage**. The alveolar walls become lined with waxy **hyaline membranes** (Fig. 15–3) that are morphologically similar to those seen in hyaline membrane disease of neonates (Chapter 10). Alveolar hyaline membranes consist of fibrin-rich edema fluid mixed with the cytoplasmic and lipid remnants of necrotic epithelial cells. In the organizing stage, type II pneumocytes undergo proliferation, and there is a granulation tissue response in the alveolar walls and in the alveolar spaces. In most cases the granulation tissue resolves, leaving minimal functional impairment. Sometimes, however, fibrotic thickening of the alveolar septa ensues, caused by proliferation of interstitial cells and deposition of collagen. Fatal cases often have superimposed bronchopneumonia.

TABLE 15–2 Conditions Associated with Development of Acute Respiratory Distress Syndrome
INFECTION
Sepsis*
Diffuse pulmonary infections*
Viral, *Mycoplasma*, and *Pneumocystis* pneumonia; miliary tuberculosis
Gastric aspiration*
PHYSICAL/INJURY
Mechanical trauma, including head injuries*
Pulmonary contusions
Near-drowning
Fractures with fat embolism
Burns
Ionizing radiation
INHALED IRRITANTS
Oxygen toxicity
Smoke
Irritant gases and chemicals
CHEMICAL INJURY
Heroin or methadone overdose
Acetylsalicylic acid
Barbiturate overdose
Paraquat
HEMATOLOGIC CONDITIONS
Multiple transfusions
Disseminated intravascular coagulation
PANCREATITIS
UREMIA
CARDIOPULMONARY BYPASS
HYPERSENSITIVITY REACTIONS
Organic solvents
Drugs

*More than 50% of cases of acute respiratory distress syndrome are associated with these four conditions.

Pathogenesis. The alveolar capillary membrane is formed by two separate barriers: the microvascular endothelium and the alveolar epithelium. *In ARDS the integrity of this barrier is compromised by either endothelial or epithelial injury or, more commonly, both.*[3] Markers of endothelial injury and activation such as endothelin and von Willebrand factor can be detected at high levels in the serum of patients with ARDS. Evidence of epithelial injury in the form of swelling, vacuolization, bleb formation, and frank necrosis is also noted early in the course of acute lung injury. The acute consequences of damage to the alveolar capillary membrane include increased vascular permeability and alveolar flooding, loss of diffusion capacity, and widespread surfactant abnormalities caused by damage to type II pneumocytes. Endothelial injury also triggers the formation of microthrombi that add the insult of ischemic injury (Fig. 15–4). Hyaline membranes so characteristic of ALI/ARDS result from inspissation of protein rich edema fluid that entraps debris of dead alveolar epithelial cells.

Although the cellular and molecular basis of acute lung injury and ARDS remains an area of active investigation, it appears that in ARDS, *lung injury is caused by an imbalance of pro-inflammatory and anti-inflammatory mediators.*[4] The most proximate signals leading to uncontrolled activation of the acute inflammatory response are not yet understood. However, *nuclear factor κB* (NF-κB), a transcription factor whose activation itself is tightly regulated under normal conditions, has emerged as a likely candidate shifting the balance in favor of a pro-inflammatory state. As early as 30 minutes after an acute insult, there is increased synthesis of interleukin-8 (IL-8), a potent neutrophil chemotactic and activating agent, by pulmonary macrophages. Release of this and similar compounds, such as IL-1 and tumor necrosis factor (TNF), leads to endothelial activation, and pulmonary microvascular sequestration and activation of neutrophils. *Neutrophils are thought to have an important role in the pathogenesis of ARDS.* Histologic examination of lungs early in the disease process shows increased numbers of neutrophils within the vascular space, the interstitium, and the alveoli. How neutrophils are sequestered in the lung is not entirely clear. There are two possible mechanisms. Firstly, neutrophils that are activated by cytokines like IL-8 and TNF upregulate the expression of adhesion molecules that allow them to bind to their ligands on activated endothelial cells. Secondly, activated neutrophils become "stiff" and less deformable and thus get trapped in the narrow capillary beds of the lung. Activated neutrophils release a variety of products (e.g., oxidants, proteases, platelet-activating factor, and leukotrienes) that cause damage to the alveolar epithelium and fuel the inflammatory cascade. Combined assault on the endothelium and epithelium perpetuate vascular leakiness and loss of surfactant that render the alveolar unit unable to expand. It should be noted that the destructive forces unleashed by neutrophils can be counteracted by an array of endogenous antiproteases, antioxidants, and anti-inflammatory cytokines (e.g., IL-10) that are upregulated by pro-inflammatory cytokines. Dysregulation of the coagulation system is also a feature of ARDS. Levels of tissue factor are increased and those of the anticoagulant, protein C, are decreased in the plasma and bronchoalveolar lavage fluid. The coagulation pathway itself is a powerful pro-inflammatory signal. Thrombin, for example, promotes adhesion of neutrophils to endothelium. In the end, it is the balance between the destructive and protective factors that determines the degree of tissue injury and clinical severity of ALI/ARDS.

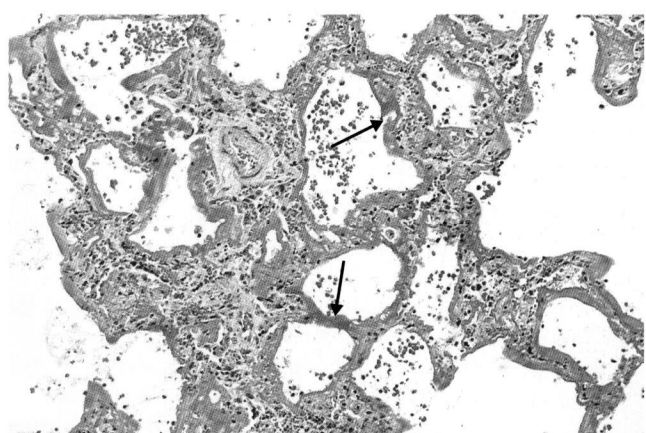

FIGURE 15–3 Diffuse alveolar damage (acute respiratory distress syndrome). Some of the alveoli are collapsed; others are distended, and many are lined by hyaline membranes *(arrows)*.

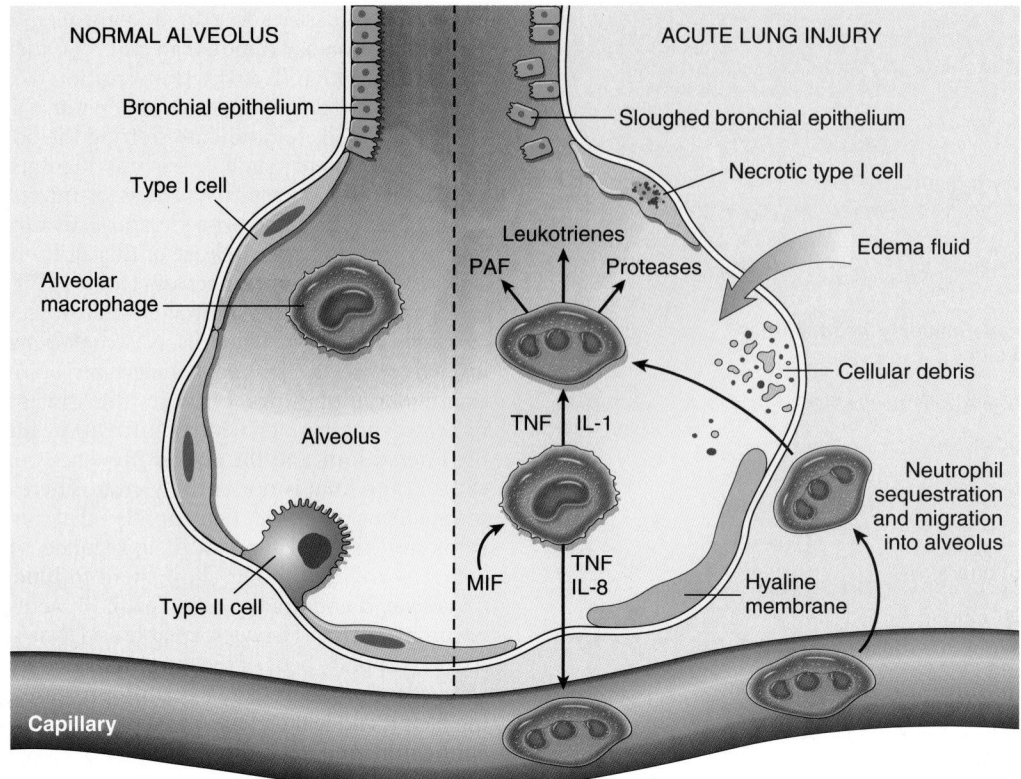

FIGURE 15–4 The normal alveolus *(left side)* compared with the injured alveolus in the early phase of acute lung injury and acute respiratory distress syndrome. Pro-inflammatory cytokines such as interleukin 8 (IL-8), interleukin 1 (IL-1), and tumor necrosis factor (TNF) (released by macrophages), cause neutrophils to adhere to pulmonary capillaries and extravasate into the alveolar space, where they undergo activation. Activated neutrophils release a variety of factors, such as leukotrienes, oxidants, proteases, and platelet-activating factor (PAF), which contribute to local tissue damage, accumulation of edema fluid in the airspaces, surfactant inactivation, and hyaline membrane formation. Macrophage migration inhibitory factor (MIF) released into the local milieu sustains the ongoing pro-inflammatory response. Subsequently, the release of macrophage-derived fibrogenic cytokines such as transforming growth factor β (TGF-β) and platelet-derived growth factor (PDGF) stimulate fibroblast growth and collagen deposition associated with the healing phase of injury. (Modified with permission from Ware LB, Matthay MA: The acute respiratory distress syndrome. N Engl J Med 342:1334, 2000.)

Resolution of ARDS requires resorption of the exudate, removal of dead cells, and their replacement by new endothelium and alveolar epithelial cells. Removal of exudates and tissue debris is accomplished by macrophages as in any other form of tissue injury. Epithelial cells are recovered by an initial proliferation of surviving type II pneumocytes that line the denuded basement membrane. The recently discovered bronchoalveolar stem cells may also participate. Type II cells then give rise to type I cells that constitute the majority of alveolar epithelium. Endothelial restoration occurs both by migration from uninjured capillaries and marrow-derived endothelial progenitor cells (Chapter 3); the latter can be detected in the circulation during recovery from ARDS.

Clinical Course. Individuals who develop ALI are usually hospitalized for one of the predisposing conditions listed earlier. Profound *dyspnea and tachypnea* herald ALI, followed by increasing *cyanosis and hypoxemia, respiratory failure*, and the appearance of *diffuse bilateral infiltrates* on radiographic examination. Hypoxemia can then become unresponsive to oxygen therapy, due to ventilation perfusion mismatching as described below, and respiratory acidosis can develop. Early in the course of the disease, lungs become stiff due to loss of functional surfactant. In a minority of patients, the exudate and diffuse tissue

destruction that occur with ALI-ARDS do not resolve and result in scarring. The interstitial fibrosis in such cases produces stiff lungs and chronic pulmonary disease.

The functional abnormalities in ALI are not evenly distributed throughout the lungs. The lungs can be divided into areas that are infiltrated, consolidated, or collapsed (and thus poorly aerated and poorly compliant) and regions that have nearly normal levels of compliance and ventilation. Poorly aerated regions continue to be perfused, producing *ventilation-perfusion mismatch* and hypoxemia. Due to improvements in therapy for sepsis, mechanical ventilation, and supportive care, the mortality rate among the 190,000 ALI cases seen yearly in the United States has decreased from 60% to about 40%.[5] The majority of deaths are attributable to sepsis or multi-organ failure and, in some cases, direct lung injury.[6]

ACUTE INTERSTITIAL PNEUMONIA

Acute interstitial pneumonia is a clinicopathologic term that is used to describe widespread ALI associated with a rapidly progressive clinical course that is of unknown etiology (sometimes referred to as idiopathic ALI-DAD). It is an uncommon disease occurring at a mean age of 50 years with no sex predilection.

TABLE 15–3	Disorders Associated with Airflow Obstruction: The Spectrum of Chronic Obstructive Pulmonary Disease			
Clinical Term	**Anatomic Site**	**Major Pathologic Changes**	**Etiology**	**Signs/Symptoms**
Chronic bronchitis	Bronchus	Mucous gland hyperplasia, hypersecretion	Tobacco smoke, air pollutants	Cough, sputum production
Bronchiectasis	Bronchus	Airway dilation and scarring	Persistent or severe infections	Cough, purulent sputum, fever
Asthma	Bronchus	Smooth muscle hyperplasia, excess mucus, inflammation	Immunological or undefined causes	Episodic wheezing, cough, dyspnea
Emphysema	Acinus	Airspace enlargement; wall destruction	Tobacco smoke	Dyspnea
Small-airway disease, bronchiolitis	Bronchiole	Inflammatory scarring/obliteration	Tobacco smoke, air pollutants, miscellaneous	Cough, dyspnea

Patients present with acute respiratory failure often following an illness of less than 3 weeks' duration that resembles an upper respiratory tract infection. The radiographic and pathologic features are identical to those of the organizing stage of ALI. The mortality rate varies from 33% to 74%, with most deaths occurring within 1 to 2 months.[7] In the surviving patients, recurrences and chronic interstitial disease may develop.[8–10]

Obstructive versus Restrictive Pulmonary Diseases

Based on pulmonary function tests, chronic noninfectious diffuse pulmonary diseases can be classified in one of two categories: (1) *obstructive diseases* (or *airway diseases*), characterized by an increase in resistance to airflow due to partial or complete obstruction at any level, from the trachea and larger bronchi to the terminal and respiratory bronchioles, and (2) *restrictive diseases*, characterized by reduced expansion of lung parenchyma and decreased total lung capacity. In individuals with diffuse obstructive disorders, pulmonary function tests show decreased maximal airflow rates during forced expiration, usually measured by forced expiratory volume at 1 second. Expiratory airflow obstruction may be caused by a variety of conditions listed in Table 15–3. They are distinguished by distinct anatomic lesions and hence different mechanisms for airflow obstruction. As discussed below, such neat distinctions are not always possible. In contrast, restrictive diseases are identified by a reduced total lung capacity, and an expiratory flow rate that is normal or reduced proportionately. Restrictive defects occur in two general conditions: (1) *chest wall disorders* (e.g., neuromuscular diseases such as poliomyelitis, severe obesity, pleural diseases, and kyphoscoliosis) and (2) *chronic interstitial and infiltrative diseases*, such as pneumoconioses and interstitial fibrosis of unknown etiology.

Obstructive Pulmonary Diseases

In their prototypical forms, these individual disorders—emphysema, chronic bronchitis, asthma, and bronchiectasis—have distinct anatomic and clinical characteristics (Table 15–3). Emphysema and chronic bronchitis are often clinically grouped together and referred to as *chronic obstructive pulmonary disease* (COPD), since many patients have overlapping features of damage at both the acinar level (emphysema) and bronchial level (bronchitis), almost certainly because one extrinsic trigger—cigarette smoking—is common to both. In addition, small-airway disease, a variant of chronic bronchiolitis, is now known to contribute to obstruction both in emphysema and chronic bronchitis.[11] While asthma is distinguished from chronic bronchitis and emphysema by the presence of reversible bronchospasm, some patients with otherwise typical asthma also develop an irreversible component (Fig. 15–5). Conversely, some patients with otherwise typical COPD have a reversible component. It is clinically common to label such patients as having COPD/asthma. In a recent study the overlap between these three disorders was found to be substantial.[12]

In most patients, COPD is the result of long-term heavy cigarette smoking; about 10% of patients are nonsmokers.[13,14] However, only a minority of smokers develop COPD, the reason for which is still unknown. Because of the increase in

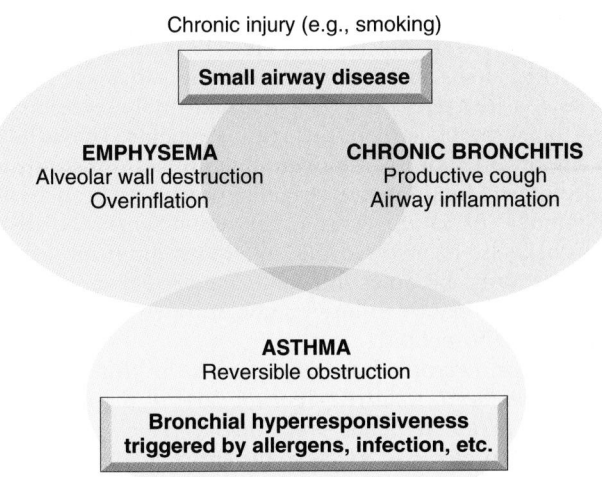

FIGURE 15–5 Schematic representation of overlap between chronic obstructive lung diseases.

smoking (smoking is decreasing in the United States but is increasing worldwide), environmental pollutants, and other noxious exposures, the incidence of COPD has increased markedly in the last few decades and now ranks fourth in the United States as a cause of morbidity and mortality.

Recognizing the overlap between various forms of COPD, each of the components and the features that characterize them in pure forms are discussed next, because it is essential to understand the pathophysiologic basis of different causes of airflow obstruction. While currently they are treated on the basis of symptoms, an understanding of pathogenesis may lead to therapies that target the mechanisms.

EMPHYSEMA

Emphysema is a condition of the lung characterized by *irreversible enlargement of the airspaces distal to the terminal bronchiole*, accompanied by destruction of their walls without obvious fibrosis.[15]

Incidence. COPD is a major public health problem. It is the fourth leading cause of morbidity and mortality in the United States[16] and is projected to rank fifth by 2020 as a worldwide burden of disease.[17] In one study there was a 50% combined incidence of panacinar and centriacinar emphysema at autopsy, and the pulmonary disease was considered to be responsible for death in 6.5% of these patients.[18] *There is a clear-cut association between heavy cigarette smoking and emphysema,* and women and African Americans are more susceptible than other groups.[19]

Types of Emphysema. Emphysema is classified according to its *anatomic distribution* within the lobule. Recall that the lobule is a cluster of acini, the terminal respiratory units. Although the term *emphysema* is sometimes loosely applied to diverse conditions, there are four major types: (1) *centriacinar*, (2) *panacinar*, (3) *paraseptal*, and (4) *irregular*. Of these, only the first two cause clinically significant airflow obstruction (Fig. 15–6). Centriacinar emphysema is far more common than the panacinar form, constituting more than 95% of cases.

Centriacinar (Centrilobular) Emphysema. In this type of emphysema *the central or proximal parts of the acini, formed by respiratory bronchioles, are affected, whereas distal alveoli are spared* (Figs. 15–6B and 15–7A). Thus, both emphysematous and normal airspaces exist within the same acinus and lobule. The lesions are more common and usually more severe in the upper lobes, particularly in the apical segments. The walls of the emphysematous spaces often contain large amounts of black pigment. Inflammation around bronchi and bronchioles is common. In severe centriacinar emphysema, the distal acinus may also be involved, and differentiation from panacinar emphysema becomes difficult. Centriacinar emphysema occurs predominantly in heavy smokers, often in association with chronic bronchitis.

Panacinar (Panlobular) Emphysema. In this type, the *acini are uniformly enlarged from the level of the respiratory bronchiole to the terminal blind alveoli* (Figs. 15–6C and 15–7B). The prefix "pan" refers to the entire acinus but not to the entire lung. In contrast to centriacinar emphysema, panacinar emphysema tends to occur more commonly in the lower zones and in the anterior margins of the lung, and it is usually most severe at the bases. This type of emphysema

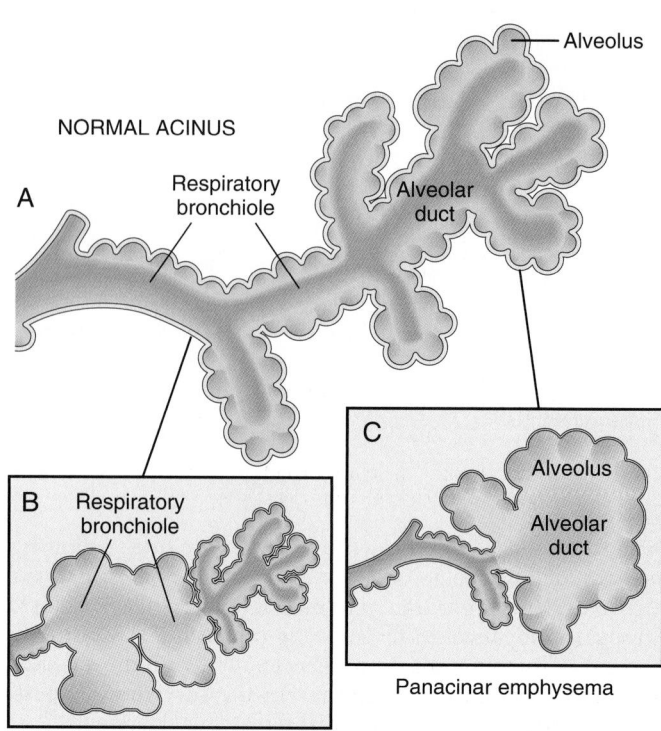

FIGURE 15–6 Major patterns of emphysema. **A,** Normal structure within the acinus. **B,** Centriacinar emphysema with dilation that initially affects the respiratory bronchioles. **C,** Panacinar emphysema with initial distention of the alveolus and alveolar duct.

is associated with α_1-antitrypsin (α_1-AT) deficiency (Chapter 18).

Distal Acinar (Paraseptal) Emphysema. In this type, the *proximal portion of the acinus is normal, and the distal part is predominantly involved.* The emphysema is more striking adjacent to the pleura, along the lobular connective tissue septa, and at the margins of the lobules. It occurs adjacent to areas of fibrosis, scarring, or atelectasis and is usually more severe in the upper half of the lungs. The characteristic findings are of multiple, continuous, enlarged airspaces from less than 0.5 cm to more than 2.0 cm in diameter, sometimes forming cystlike structures. This type of emphysema probably underlies many of the cases of spontaneous pneumothorax in young adults.

Airspace Enlargement with Fibrosis (Irregular Emphysema). *Irregular emphysema, so named because the acinus is irregularly involved, is almost invariably associated with scarring.* Thus, it may be the most common form of emphysema, because careful search of most lungs at autopsy shows one or more scars from a healed inflammatory process. In most instances, these foci of irregular emphysema are asymptomatic and clinically insignificant.

Pathogenesis. COPD is characterized by mild chronic inflammation throughout the airways, parenchyma, and pulmonary vasculature. Macrophages, CD8+ and CD4+ T lymphocytes, and neutrophils are increased in various parts of the lung. Activated inflammatory cells release a variety of mediators, including leukotriene B_4, IL-8, TNF, and others, that are capable of damaging lung structures or sustaining neutrophilic inflammation.[20] Although details of the genesis

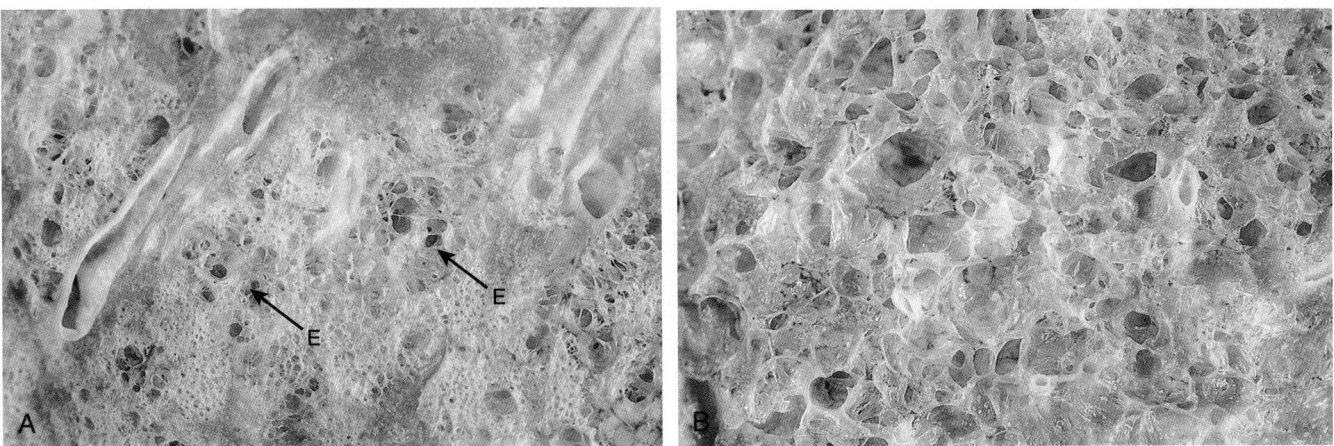

FIGURE 15–7 **A,** Centriacinar emphysema. Central areas show marked emphysematous damage (E), surrounded by relatively spared alveolar spaces. **B,** Panacinar emphysema involving the entire pulmonary lobule.

of the two common forms of emphysema—centriacinar and panacinar—remain unsettled, *the most plausible hypothesis to account for the destruction of alveolar walls is the protease-antiprotease mechanism, aided and abetted by imbalance of oxidants and antioxidants.*

The *protease-antiprotease imbalance* hypothesis is based on the observation that patients with a genetic deficiency of the antiprotease α1-antitrypsin have a markedly enhanced tendency to develop pulmonary emphysema, which is compounded by smoking (Fig. 15–8). About 1% of all patients with emphysema have this defect. α1-antitrypsin, normally present in serum, tissue fluids, and macrophages, is a major inhibitor of proteases (particularly elastase) secreted by neutrophils during inflammation. α1-antitrypsin is encoded by codominantly expressed genes on the proteinase inhibitor *(Pi)* locus on chromosome 14. The *Pi* locus is extremely polymorphic, with many different alleles. Most common is the normal *(M)* allele and the corresponding phenotype. Approximately 0.012% of the US population is homozygous for the *Z* allele, associated with markedly decreased serum levels of α1-

antitrypsin. More than 80% of these individuals develop symptomatic panacinar emphysema, which occurs at an earlier age and with greater severity if the individual smokes. The following sequence is postulated:

1. Neutrophils (the principal source of cellular proteases) are normally sequestered in peripheral capillaries, including those in the lung, and a few gain access to the alveolar spaces.
2. Any stimulus that increases either the number of leukocytes (neutrophils and macrophages) in the lung or the release of their protease-containing granules increases proteolytic activity.
3. With low levels of serum α1-antitrypsin, elastic tissue destruction is unchecked and emphysema results.

Thus, *emphysema is seen to result from the destructive effect of high protease activity in subjects with low antiprotease activity.* The protease-antiprotease imbalance hypothesis also helps explain the effect of cigarette smoking in the

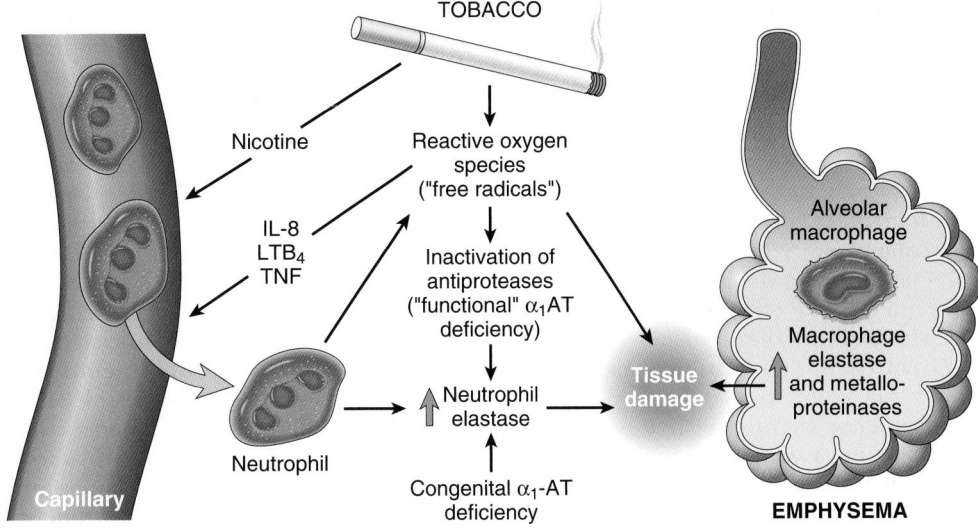

FIGURE 15–8 Pathogenesis of emphysema. Excessive protease activity and reactive oxygen species are additive in their effects and contribute to tissue damage. α1-antitrypsin (α1-AT) deficiency can be either congenital or "functional" as a result of oxidative inactivation. See text for details. IL-8, interleukin 8; LTB4, leukotriene B4; TNF, tumor necrosis factor.

development of emphysema, particularly the centriacinar form in subjects with normal amounts of α1-antitrypsin:

- *In smokers, neutrophils and macrophages accumulate in alveoli.* The mechanism of inflammation is not entirely clear, but possibly involves the direct chemoattractant effects of nicotine as well as the effects of reactive oxygen species contained in smoke. These activate the transcription factor NF-κB, which switches on genes that encode TNF and chemokines, including IL-8. These, in turn, attract and activate neutrophils.
- Accumulated neutrophils are activated and release their granules, rich in a variety of cellular proteases (neutrophil elastase, proteinase 3, and cathepsin G), resulting in tissue damage.
- Smoking also enhances elastase activity in macrophages; macrophage elastase is not inhibited by α1-antitrypsin) and, indeed, can proteolytically digest this antiprotease. There is increasing evidence that in addition to elastase, matrix metalloproteinases derived from macrophages and neutrophils have a role in tissue destruction.

In addition, smoking has a seminal role in perpetuating the *oxidant-antioxidant imbalance* in the pathogenesis of emphysema. Normally, the lung contains a healthy complement of antioxidants (superoxide dismutase, glutathione) that keep oxidative damage to a minimum. Tobacco smoke contains abundant reactive oxygen species (free radicals), which deplete these antioxidant mechanisms, thereby inciting tissue damage (Chapter 1). Activated neutrophils also add to the pool of reactive oxygen species in the alveoli. A secondary consequence of oxidative injury is inactivation of native antiproteases, resulting in "functional" α1-antitrypsin deficiency even in patients without enzyme deficiency.

Since small airways are normally tethered by the elastic recoil of the lung parenchyma, the loss of elastic tissue in the walls of alveoli that surround respiratory bronchioles reduces radial traction and thus causes the respiratory bronchioles to collapse during expiration. This leads to functional airflow obstruction despite the absence of mechanical obstruction.

Until recently loss of elastic recoil was considered to be the sole mechanism of airflow obstruction in emphysema. However, careful studies in young smokers who died in accidents have revealed that inflammation of small airways, defined as bronchioles less than 2 mm in diameter, occurs early in the evolution of COPD. Several changes are seen:

1. goblet cell metaplasia with mucus plugging of the lumen
2. inflammatory infiltration of the walls with neutrophils, macrophages, B cells (sometimes forming follicles), CD4 and CD8+ T cells
3. thickening of the bronchiolar wall due to smooth muscle hypertrophy and peribronchial fibrosis.

Together these changes narrow the bronchiolar lumen and contribute to airway obstruction.[21,25]

One of the perplexing features of COPD is that smoldering inflammation and slow progressive destruction of the lung parenchyma often continue for decades after cessation of smoking.[22] While there are no clear answers, there is emerging evidence that the initial insult in the form of tobacco smoke, or other irritants, triggers a maladaptive, self-perpetuating immune response in which both innate and adaptive components play a role. Fingers are pointing to pathogenic CD4+T$_H$17 cells similar to those that are involved in other immune-mediated inflammatory diseases such as Crohn disease, but much remains to be known.

Morphology. Advanced emphysema produces voluminous lungs, often overlapping the heart and hiding it when the anterior chest wall is removed. Generally, the upper two thirds of the lungs are more severely affected. Large apical blebs or bullae are more characteristic of irregular emphysema secondary to scarring and of distal acinar emphysema. Large alveoli can easily be seen on the cut surface of formalin-inflated fixed lung (see Fig. 15–7).

Microscopically, there are abnormally large alveoli separated by thin septa with only focal centriacinar fibrosis. There is loss of attachments of the alveoli to the outer wall of small airways. The pores of Kohn are so large that septa appear to be floating or protrude blindly into alveolar spaces with a club-shaped end. As alveolar walls are destroyed, there is decrease in the capillary bed. With advanced disease, there are even larger abnormal airspaces and possibly blebs or bullae, which often deform and compress the respiratory bronchioles and vasculature of the lung. Inflammatory changes in small airways were described earlier.

Clinical Course. The clinical manifestations of emphysema do not appear until at least one third of the functioning pulmonary parenchyma is damaged. *Dyspnea* is usually the first symptom; it begins insidiously but is steadily progressive. In some patients, cough or wheezing is the chief complaint, easily confused with asthma. Cough and expectoration are extremely variable and depend on the extent of the associated bronchitis. *Weight loss* is common and can be so severe as to suggest a hidden malignant tumor. Classically, the patient is barrel-chested and dyspneic, with obviously prolonged expiration, sits forward in a hunched-over position, and breathes through pursed lips. *Expiratory airflow limitation, best measured through spirometry, is the key to diagnosis.*

In individuals with severe emphysema, cough is often slight, overdistention is severe, diffusion capacity is low, and blood gas values are relatively normal at rest. Such patients may overventilate and remain well oxygenated, and therefore are somewhat ingloriously designated *pink puffers* (see Table 15–4). Development of cor pulmonale and eventually congestive heart failure, related to secondary pulmonary vascular hypertension, is associated with a poor prognosis. Death in most patients with emphysema is due to (1) respiratory acidosis and coma, (2) right-sided heart failure, and (3) massive collapse of the lungs secondary to pneumothorax. Treatment options include bronchodilators, steroids, bullectomy, and, in selected patients, lung volume reduction surgery and lung transplantation. Substitution therapy with α$_1$-AT is being evaluated.[23]

TABLE 15–4 Emphysema and Chronic Bronchitis		
	Predominant Bronchitis	Predominant Emphysema
Age (yr)	40–45	50–75
Dyspnea	Mild; late	Severe; early
Cough	Early; copious sputum	Late; scanty sputum
Infections	Common	Occasional
Respiratory insufficiency	Repeated	Terminal
Cor pulmonale	Common	Rare; terminal
Airway resistance	Increased	Normal or slightly increased
Elastic recoil	Normal	Low
Chest radiograph	Prominent vessels; large heart	Hyperinflation; small heart
Appearance	*Blue bloater*	*Pink puffer*

Other Forms of Emphysema. Now we come to some conditions in which the term *emphysema* is applied less stringently and to some closely related conditions.

Compensatory Hyperinflation (Emphysema). This term is sometimes used to designate dilation of alveoli but not destruction of septal walls in response to loss of lung substance elsewhere. It is best exemplified by the hyperexpansion of the residual lung parenchyma that follows surgical removal of a diseased lung or lobe.

Obstructive Overinflation. In this condition the lung expands because air is trapped within it. A common cause is subtotal obstruction by a tumor or foreign object. Another example is *congenital lobar overinflation* in infants, probably resulting from hypoplasia of bronchial cartilage and sometimes associated with other congenital cardiac and lung abnormalities. Overinflation in obstructive lesions occurs either (1) because of a ball-valve action of the obstructive agent, so that air enters on inspiration but cannot leave on expiration, or (2) because the bronchus may be totally obstructed but ventilation through *collaterals* may bring in air from behind the obstruction. These collaterals are the *pores of Kohn* and other direct accessory *bronchioloalveolar connections* (the canals of Lambert). Obstructive overinflation can be a life-threatening emergency, because the affected portion distends sufficiently to compress the remaining normal lung.

Bullous Emphysema. This is a descriptive term for large subpleural blebs or bullae (spaces more than 1 cm in diameter in the distended state) that can occur in any form of emphysema (Fig. 15–9). They represent localized accentuations of emphysema and occur near the apex, sometimes in relation to old tuberculous scarring. On occasion, rupture of the bullae may give rise to pneumothorax.

Interstitial Emphysema. The entrance of air into the connective tissue stroma of the lung, mediastinum, or subcutaneous tissue is called interstitial emphysema. In most instances, alveolar tears in pulmonary emphysema provide the avenue of entrance of air into the stroma of the lung, but rarely, a wound of the chest that allows air to be sucked in or a frac-

tured rib that punctures the lung substance may underlie this disorder. Alveolar tears usually occur when there is a combination of coughing plus some bronchiolar obstruction, producing sharply increased pressures within the alveolar sacs. Children with whooping cough and bronchitis, patients with obstruction to the airways (by blood clots, tissue, or foreign bodies) or who are being artificially ventilated, and individuals who suddenly inhale irritant gases are at risk.

CHRONIC BRONCHITIS

Chronic bronchitis is defined clinically as persistent cough with sputum production for at least 3 months in at least 2 consecutive years, in the absence of any other identifiable cause. Chronic bronchitis, so common among habitual smokers and inhabitants of smog-laden cities, is not nearly as trivial as was once thought. When persistent for years, it may (1) progress to COPD, (2) lead to cor pulmonale and heart failure, or (3) cause atypical metaplasia and dysplasia of the respiratory epithelium, providing a rich soil for cancerous transformation.

Pathogenesis. The primary or initiating factor in the genesis of chronic bronchitis seems to be long-standing irritation by inhaled substances such as *tobacco smoke* (90% of patients are smokers), and dust from grain, cotton, and silica. The earliest feature of chronic bronchitis is *hypersecretion of mucus* in the large airways, associated with hypertrophy of the submucosal glands in the trachea and bronchi.[24] Proteases released from neutrophils, such as neutrophil elastase and cathepsin, and matrix metalloproteinases, stimulate this mucus hypersecretion. As chronic bronchitis persists, there is also *a marked increase in goblet cells of small airways—small bronchi and bronchioles—*leading to excessive mucus production that contributes to airway obstruction. It is thought that both the submucosal gland hypertrophy and the increase in goblet cells are protective metaplastic reactions against tobacco smoke or other pollutants (e.g., sulfur dioxide and nitrogen dioxide).

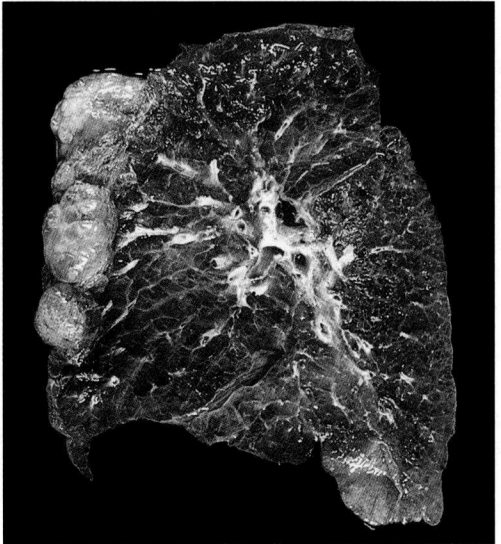

FIGURE 15–9 Bullous emphysema with large subpleural bullae *(upper left).*

Although mucus hypersecretion in large airways is the cause of sputum overproduction, it is now thought that accompanying *alterations in the small airways of the lung* (small bronchi and bronchioles, less than 2 to 3 mm in diameter) *can result in physiologically important and early manifestations of chronic airway obstruction.*[25,26] This feature is similar to that described earlier in emphysema and seems to be a common denominator in COPD.

The role of *infection* seems to be secondary. It is not responsible for the initiation of chronic bronchitis but is probably significant in maintaining it and may be critical in producing acute exacerbations. Cigarette smoke predisposes to infection in more than one way. It interferes with ciliary action of the respiratory epithelium, it may cause direct damage to airway epithelium, and it inhibits the ability of bronchial and alveolar leukocytes to clear bacteria. Viral infections can also cause exacerbations of chronic bronchitis.

Morphology. Grossly, there is hyperemia, swelling, and edema of the mucous membranes, frequently accompanied by excessive mucinous or mucopurulent secretions. Sometimes, heavy casts of secretions and pus fill the bronchi and bronchioles. The characteristic histologic features are chronic inflammation of the airways (predominantly lymphocytes) and enlargement of the mucus-secreting glands of the trachea and bronchi. Although the numbers of goblet cells increase slightly, the **major change is in the size of the mucous gland (hyperplasia)**. This increase can be assessed by the ratio of the thickness of the mucous gland layer to the thickness of the wall between the epithelium and the cartilage (**Reid index**). The Reid index (normally 0.4) is increased in chronic bronchitis, usually in proportion to the severity and duration of the disease. The bronchial epithelium may exhibit squamous metaplasia and dysplasia. There is marked narrowing of bronchioles caused by mucus plugging, inflammation, and fibrosis. In the most severe cases, there may be obliteration of lumen due to fibrosis (**bronchiolitis obliterans**).

Clinical Features. The cardinal symptom of chronic bronchitis is a persistent cough productive of sputum. For many years no other respiratory functional impairment is present, but eventually dyspnea on exertion develops. With the passage of time, and usually with continued smoking, other elements of COPD may appear, including hypercapnia, hypoxemia, and mild cyanosis (*"blue bloaters"*). Differentiation of pure chronic bronchitis from that associated with emphysema can be made in the classic case (see Table 15–4), but, as has been mentioned, many patients with COPD have both conditions. Longstanding severe chronic bronchitis commonly leads to cor pulmonale with cardiac failure. Death may also result from further impairment of respiratory function due to superimposed acute infections.

ASTHMA

Asthma is a chronic inflammatory disorder of the airways that causes recurrent episodes of wheezing, breathlessness, chest tightness, and cough, particularly at night and/or in the early morning. These symptoms are usually associated with widespread but variable bronchoconstriction and airflow limitation that is at least partly reversible, either spontaneously or with treatment. The hallmarks of the disease are: increased airway responsiveness to a variety of stimuli, resulting in episodic bronchoconstriction; inflammation of the bronchial walls; and increased mucus secretion. Some of the stimuli that trigger attacks in patients would have little or no effect in subjects with normal airways. Many cells play a role in the inflammatory response, in particular lymphocytes, eosinophils, mast cells, macrophages, neutrophils, and epithelial cells.[27]

Individuals with asthma experience attacks of varying severity of dyspnea, coughing, and wheezing due to sudden episodes of bronchospasm. Rarely, a state of unremitting attacks, called *status asthmaticus*, proves fatal; usually, such patients have had a long history of asthma. Between the attacks, patients may be virtually asymptomatic. *There has been a significant increase in the incidence of asthma in the Western world in the past four decades.*

Asthma may be categorized into *atopic* (evidence of allergen sensitization, often in a patient with a history of allergic rhinitis, eczema) and *non-atopic* (without evidence of allergen sensitization). In either type, episodes of bronchospasm can be triggered by diverse mechanisms, such as respiratory infections (especially viral infections), environmental exposure to irritants (e.g., smoke, fumes), cold air, stress, and exercise. Recent studies have suggested that the recognition of subphenotypes of asthma based on the pattern of airway inflammation may also be useful. There is emerging evidence for differing patterns of airway inflammation: eosinophilic, neutrophilic, mixed inflammatory, and pauci-granulocytic asthma. These subgroups may differ in their etiology, immunopathology, and response to treatment.[28] Asthma may also be classified according to the agents or events that trigger bronchoconstriction. These include seasonal, exercise-induced, drug-induced (e.g., aspirin), and occupational asthma, and asthmatic bronchitis in smokers.

Atopic Asthma. This most common type of asthma is a *classic example of type I IgE-mediated hypersensitivity reaction*, discussed in detail in Chapter 6. The disease usually begins in childhood and is triggered by environmental allergens, such as dusts, pollens, roach or animal dander, and foods. A positive family history of asthma is common, and a skin test with the offending antigen in these patients results in an immediate wheal-and-flare reaction. Atopic asthma may also be diagnosed based on evidence of allergen sensitization by serum radioallergosorbent tests (called RAST), which identify the presence of IgE specific for a panel of allergens.

Non-Atopic Asthma. The second group of individuals with asthma does not have evidence of allergen sensitization, and skin test results are usually negative. A positive family history of asthma is less common in these patients. Respiratory infections due to viruses (e.g., rhinovirus, parainfluenza virus) are common triggers in non-atopic asthma.[29] In these patients hyperirritability of the bronchial tree probably underlies their asthma. *It is thought that virus-induced inflammation of the respiratory mucosa lowers the threshold of the subepithelial vagal receptors to irritants.* Inhaled air pollutants, such as sulfur dioxide, ozone, and nitrogen dioxide, may also contribute to the chronic airway inflammation and hyperreactivity that are present in some cases.

Drug-Induced Asthma. Several pharmacologic agents provoke asthma. *Aspirin-sensitive asthma* is an uncommon yet fascinating type, occurring in individuals with recurrent rhinitis and nasal polyps. These individuals are exquisitely sensitive to small doses of aspirin as well as other nonsteroidal anti-inflammatory medications, and they experience not only asthmatic attacks but also urticaria. It is probable that aspirin triggers asthma in these patients by inhibiting the cyclooxygenase pathway of arachidonic acid metabolism without affecting the lipoxygenase route, thus tipping the balance toward elaboration of the bronchoconstrictor leukotrienes.

Occupational Asthma. This form of asthma is stimulated by fumes (epoxy resins, plastics), organic and chemical dusts (wood, cotton, platinum), gases (toluene), and other chemicals (formaldehyde, penicillin products). Minute quantities of chemicals are required to induce the attack, which usually occurs after repeated exposure. The underlying mechanisms vary according to stimulus and include type I reactions, direct liberation of bronchoconstrictor substances, and hypersensitivity responses of unknown origin.

Pathogenesis. The major etiologic factors in atopic asthma are a genetic predisposition to type I hypersensitivity ("atopy") and exposure to environmental triggers that remain poorly defined.[30] It is postulated that inheritance of susceptibility genes makes individuals prone to develop strong T_H2 reactions against environmental antigens (allergens) that are ignored or elicit harmless responses in most individuals. In the airways the scene for the reaction is set by initial sensitization to inhaled allergens, which stimulate induction of T_H2 cells (Fig. 15–10). T_H2 cells secrete cytokines that promote allergic inflammation and stimulate B cells to produce IgE and other antibodies. These cytokines include IL-4, which stimulates the production of IgE; IL-5, which activates locally recruited eosinophils; and IL-13, which stimulates mucus secretion from bronchial submucosal glands and also promotes IgE production by B cells. As in other allergic reactions (Chapter 6), IgE coats submucosal mast cells, and repeat exposure to the allergen triggers the mast cells to release granule contents and produce cytokines and other mediators, which collectively induce the *early-phase (immediate hypersensitivity) reaction and the late-phase reaction*. The early reaction is dominated by bronchoconstriction, increased mucus production, and variable degrees of vasodilation with increased vascular permeability. Bronchoconstriction is triggered by direct stimulation of subepithelial vagal (parasympathetic) receptors through both central and local reflexes (including those mediated by unmyelinated sensory C fibers).

The late-phase reaction consists largely of inflammation with recruitment of leukocytes, notably eosinophils, neutrophils, and more T cells. Leukocyte recruitment is stimulated by chemokines produced by mast cells, epithelial cells and T cells, and by other cytokines (Chapter 2). Epithelial cells are known to produce a large variety of cytokines in response to infectious agents, drugs, and gases as well as to inflammatory mediators.[31] This second wave of mediators stimulates the late reaction. For example, *eotaxin*, produced by airway epithelial cells, is a potent chemoattractant and activator of eosinophils.[32] *The major basic protein of eosinophils, in turn, causes epithelial damage*[31] and more *airway constriction*.[33] Many mediators have been implicated in the asthmatic response, but the relative importance of each putative mediator in actual human asthma has been difficult to establish. The long list of "suspects" in acute asthma can be subclassified by the clinical efficacy of pharmacologic intervention with inhibitors or antagonists of the mediators.

- The first (disappointingly small) group includes putative mediators whose role in bronchospasm is clearly supported by efficacy of pharmacologic intervention: (1) *leukotrienes* C_4, D_4, and E_4, extremely potent mediators that cause prolonged bronchoconstriction as well as increased vascular permeability and increased mucus secretion, and (2) *acetylcholine*, released from intrapulmonary motor nerves, which can cause airway smooth muscle constriction by directly stimulating muscarinic receptors.
- A second group includes agents present at the *scene of the crime* and with potent asthma-like effects but whose actual role in acute allergic asthma seems relatively minor on the basis of lack of efficacy of potent antagonists or synthesis inhibitors: (1) *histamine*, a potent bronchoconstrictor; (2) *prostaglandin* D_2, which elicits bronchoconstriction and vasodilatation; and (3) *platelet-activating factor*, which causes aggregation of platelets and release of histamine and serotonin from their granules. These mediators might yet prove important in other types of chronic or nonallergic asthma.
- Finally, a large third group comprises the *suspects* for whom specific antagonists or inhibitors are not available or have been insufficiently studied as yet. These include numerous cytokines, such as IL-1, TNF, and IL-6 (some of which exist in a preformed state within the mast cell granules),[34] chemokines (e.g., eotaxin), neuropeptides, nitric oxide, bradykinin, and endothelins.

It is thus clear that multiple mediators contribute to the acute asthmatic response. Moreover, the composition of this mediator soup might differ among different individuals or types of asthma. The appreciation of the importance of inflammatory cells and mediators in asthma has led to greater emphasis on anti-inflammatory drugs, such as corticosteroids, in the treatment of asthma.

Over time, repeated bouts of allergen exposure and immune reactions result in structural changes in the bronchial wall, referred to as "*airway remodeling*." These changes, described later in greater detail, include hypertrophy and hyperplasia of bronchial smooth muscle, epithelial injury, increased airway vascularity, increased subepithelial mucus gland hypertrophy/hyperplasia, and deposition of subepithelial collagen. The complex interactions between the immune system, airway epithelium, and mesenchymal tissues in the airways are poorly understood. Infections with common respiratory pathogens, such as respiratory syncytial virus and influenza, can exacerbate the chronic changes and cause serious worsening of the clinical manifestations of the disease.

Although infections are often triggers for asthma, paradoxically, some infections may be protective. Epidemiologic studies first suggested that the incidence of asthma was greater in populations not exposed to microbes than in those living in an environment with abundant microbes, and this relationship

A. NORMAL AIRWAY

B. AIRWAY IN ASTHMA

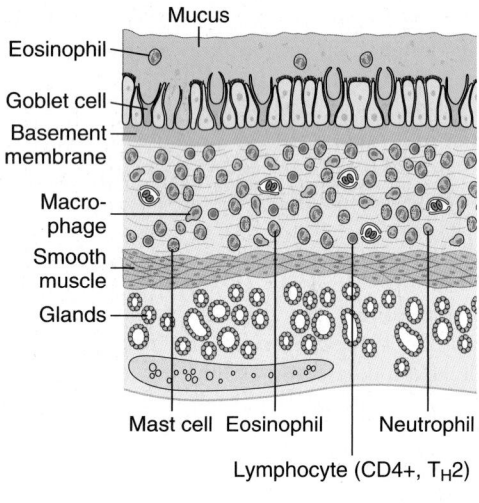

C. TRIGGERING OF ASTHMA

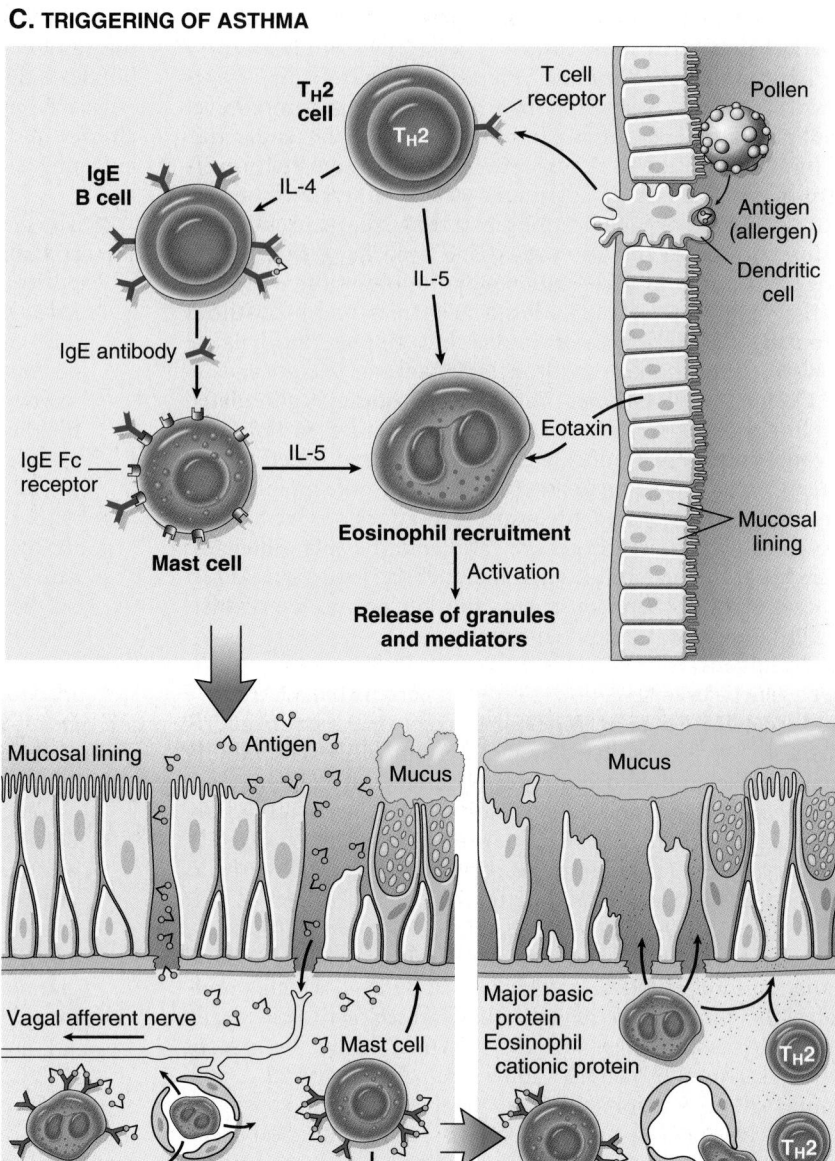

D. IMMEDIATE PHASE (MINUTES)

E. LATE PHASE (HOURS)

FIGURE 15–10 **A** and **B,** Comparison of a normal bronchus with that in a person with asthma. Note the accumulation of mucus in the bronchial lumen resulting from an increase in the number of mucus-secreting goblet cells in the mucosa and hypertrophy of submucosal glands. In addition, there is intense chronic inflammation due to recruitment of eosinophils, macrophages, and other inflammatory cells. Basement membrane underlying the mucosal epithelium is thickened, and there is hypertrophy and hyperplasia of smooth muscle cells. **C,** Inhaled allergens (antigen) elicit a T_H2-dominated response favoring IgE production and eosinophil recruitment (priming or sensitization). **D,** On re-exposure to antigen (Ag), the immediate reaction is triggered by Ag-induced cross-linking of IgE bound to IgE receptors on mast cells. These cells release preformed mediators. Collectively, either directly or via neuronal reflexes, the mediators induce bronchospasm, increased vascular permeability, and mucus production, and recruit additional mediator-releasing cells from the blood. **E,** The arrival of recruited leukocytes (neutrophils, eosinophils, and basophils; lymphocytes and monocytes) signals the initiation of the late phase of asthma and a fresh round of mediator release from leukocytes, endothelium, and epithelial cells. Factors, particularly from eosinophils (e.g., major basic protein, eosinophil cationic protein), also cause damage to the epithelium. GM-CSF, granulocyte-macrophage colony-stimulating factor.

may explain the increasing incidence of asthma in developed countries.[35] These findings have led to the "hygiene hypothesis," which states that eradication of infections may promote allergic and other harmful immune responses. Despite a fascination with this idea, there is no plausible explanation for the inverse relationship between infections and asthma.

Genetics of Asthma. Asthma is a complex genetic trait in which multiple susceptibility genes interact with environmental factors to initiate the pathologic reaction. As in other complex traits (Chapter 5), there is considerable variability in the expression of these genes and in the combinations of polymorphisms present in individual patients, and even in the significance and reproducibility of reported polymorphisms. Of the more than 100 genes that have been reported to be associated with the disease, relatively few have been replicated in multiple patient populations. Many of these affect the immune response or tissue remodeling. Some genes may influence the development of asthma, while others modify asthma severity or the patient's response to therapy.[36] A few of these are discussed below:

- One of the most replicated susceptibility loci for asthma is on chromosome 5q, near the gene cluster encoding the cytokines IL-3, IL-4, IL-5, IL-9, and IL-13 and the IL-4 receptor. The receptor for LPS (CD14), and another candidate gene, the β_2-adrenergic receptor, also map here. This region is of great interest because of the connection between several of the genes located here and the mechanisms of IgE regulation and mast cell and eosinophil growth and differentiation. Among the genes in this cluster, polymorphisms in the *IL13* gene have the strongest and most consistent associations with asthma or allergic disease.

  The association between asthma and other forms of atopy with a polymorphism in the gene encoding the monocyte receptor for endotoxin, *CD14*, is worthy of additional comments since it is paradigmatic for studies of gene-environment interactions. In some studies, the TT genotype of *CD14* has been associated with reduced levels of IgE and reduced risk for asthma and atopy. Other studies have revealed the opposite, i.e., an *increased* risk for atopy. Further analysis has revealed that the TT genotype is protective against asthma or allergic sensitization in individuals exposed to low (household) endotoxin levels, whereas the same genotype is associated with an increased risk for asthma or allergic sensitization in individuals exposed to high endotoxin levels (as may occur in those living on farms). These differences may relate to the influence of endotoxin levels on the regulation of T_H1 vs. T_H2 responses. In individuals with the TT genotype high endotoxin levels skew the response towards T_H2 type, thus favoring more brisk IgE production and a predisposition to allergy. These studies indicate that the relationship between genotype and phenotype is context dependent, and help explain some of the discrepant results of association studies in different populations.[37,38]

- The tendency to produce IgE antibodies against some but not all antigens, such as ragweed pollen, may be linked to particular class II HLA alleles.

- ADAM-33: ADAM-33 belongs to a subfamily of metalloproteinases related to the MMPs such as collagenases (Chapter 3). Although the precise function of ADAM-33 remains to be elucidated, it is known to be expressed by lung fibroblasts and bronchial smooth muscle cells. It is speculated that *ADAM-33 polymorphisms accelerate proliferation of bronchial smooth muscle cells and fibroblasts*, thus contributing to bronchial hyperreactivity and subepithelial fibrosis.[39] ADAM-33 is also associated with decline in lung functions.

- β_2-adrenergic receptor gene: This also maps to 5q and variations in this gene are associated with differential in vivo airway hyper-responsiveness and in vitro response to β-agonist stimulation. Thus, knowledge of the genotype can be of value in predicting response to treatment.[40]

- IL-4 receptor gene: Mutliple polymorphic variants in the gene encoding the alpha-chain of the IL-4 receptor are associated with atopy, elevated total serum IgE, and asthma.

- Mammalian chitinase family: *Chitinases* are enzymes that cleave chitin, a polysaccharide contained in many human parasites and the cell walls of fungi. In humans the chitinase family includes members with and without enzymic activity. One member with activity, acidic mammalian chitinase, is up-regulated in and contributes to T_H2 inflammation. Another chitinase family member with no enzymatic activity, YKL-40, is associated with asthma. Serum levels of YKL-40 correlate with the severity of asthma.[41]

Morphology. In patients dying of status asthmaticus the lungs are overdistended because of overinflation, with small areas of atelectasis. The most striking macroscopic finding is occlusion of bronchi and bronchioles by thick, tenacious mucus plugs. Histologically, the mucus plugs contain whorls of shed epithelium, which give rise to the well-known spiral shaped mucus plugs called **Curschmann spirals** (these result either from mucus plugging in subepithelial mucous gland ducts which later become extruded or from plugs in bronchioles). Numerous eosinophils and **Charcot-Leyden crystals** are present; the latter are collections of crystalloid made up of an eosinophil lysophospholipase binding protein called galectin-10.[42] The other characteristic histologic findings of asthma, collectively called *"airway remodeling"* (Fig. 15–10B), include:

- Overall thickening of airway wall
- Sub-basement membrane fibrosis (due to deposition of type I and III collagen beneath the classic basement membrane composed of type IV collagen and laminin) (Fig. 15–11)
- Increased vascularity
- An increase in size of the submucosal glands and mucous metaplasia of airway epithelial cells
- Hypertrophy and/or hyperplasia of the bronchial wall muscle (this has led to the novel therapy of bronchial thermoplasty in which radiofrequency

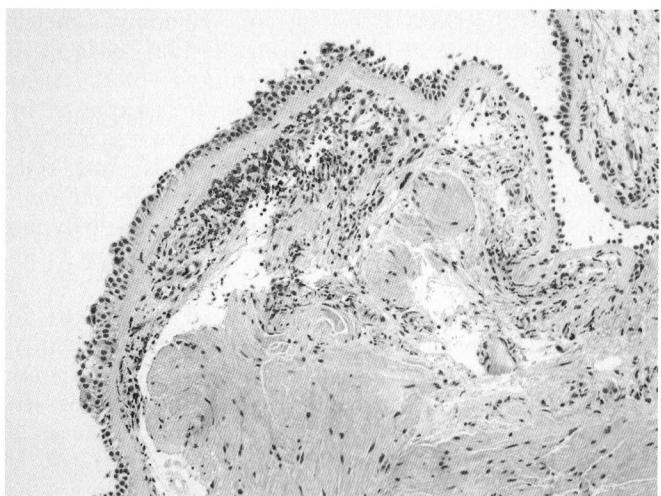

FIGURE 15–11 Bronchial biopsy specimen from an asthmatic patient showing sub-basement membrane fibrosis, eosinophilic inflammation, and muscle hyperplasia.

current is applied to the walls of the central airways through a bronchoscopically placed probe, which reduces airway hyper-responsiveness for up to at least a year).[43]

While acute airflow obstruction is primarily attributed to muscular bronchoconstriction, acute edema, and mucus plugging, airway remodeling may also contribute. Airway remodeling is commonly thought to contribute to chronic irreversible airway obstruction as well, although this is difficult to prove.

Clinical Course. The classic acute asthmatic attack lasts up to several hours. In some patients these symptoms of chest tightness, dyspnea, wheezing, and cough with or without sputum production, persist at a low level constantly. In its most severe form, *status asthmaticus*, the severe acute paroxysm persists for days and even weeks, and under these circumstances airflow obstruction might be so extreme as to cause severe cyanosis and even death. The clinical diagnosis is aided by the demonstration of an increase in airflow obstruction (from baseline levels), difficulty with exhalation (prolonged expiration, wheeze), and elevated eosinophil count in the peripheral blood and the finding of eosinophils, Curschmann spirals, and Charcot-Leyden crystals in the sputum (particularly in patients with atopic asthma). In the usual case, with intervals of freedom from respiratory difficulty, the disease is more discouraging and disabling than lethal, being more of a problem in adult women than men. With appropriate therapy to relieve the attacks, most individuals with asthma are able to maintain a productive life. Up to 50% of childhood asthma remits in adolescence only to return in adulthood in a significant number of patients. In other cases there is a variable decline in baseline lung function.

BRONCHIECTASIS

Bronchiectasis is a disease characterized by permanent dilation of bronchi and bronchioles caused by destruction of the muscle

and elastic tissue, resulting from or associated with chronic necrotizing infections. To be considered bronchiectasis the dilation must be permanent; reversible bronchial dilation often accompanies viral and bacterial pneumonia. Because of better control of lung infections, bronchiectasis is now an uncommon condition. Bronchiectasis develops in association with a variety of conditions, which include the following[44,45]:

- Congenital or hereditary conditions, including cystic fibrosis, intralobar sequestration of the lung, immunodeficiency states,[46] and primary ciliary dyskinesia and Kartagener syndromes
- *Postinfectious conditions*, including necrotizing pneumonia caused by bacteria (*Mycobacterium tuberculosis, Staphylococcus aureus, Haemophilus influenzae, Pseudomonas*), viruses (adenovirus, influenza virus, human immunodeficiency virus [HIV]), and fungi (*Aspergillus* species)
- *Bronchial obstruction*, due to tumor, foreign bodies, and occasionally mucus impaction, in which the bronchiectasis is localized to the obstructed lung segment
- Other conditions, including rheumatoid arthritis, systemic lupus erythematosus, inflammatory bowel disease, and post-transplantation (chronic lung rejection, and chronic graft-versus-host disease after bone marrow transplantation)

Etiology and Pathogenesis. *Obstruction* and *infection* are the major conditions associated with bronchiectasis, and it is likely that both are necessary for the development of full-fledged lesions, although either may come first. After bronchial obstruction, normal clearing mechanisms are impaired, there is pooling of secretions distal to the obstruction, and there is inflammation of the airway. Conversely, severe infections of the bronchi lead to inflammation, often with necrosis, fibrosis, and eventually dilation of airways.

These mechanisms, infection and obstruction, are most readily apparent in the severe form of bronchiectasis associated with cystic fibrosis (Chapter 10). In cystic fibrosis the primary defect in ion transport leads to defective mucociliary action, and accumulation of thick viscid secretions that obstruct the airways. This leads to a marked susceptibility to bacterial infections, which further damage the airways. With repeated infections there is widespread damage to airway walls, with destruction of supporting smooth muscle and elastic tissue, fibrosis, and further dilatation of bronchi. The smaller bronchioles become progressively obliterated as a result of fibrosis (bronchiolitis obliterans).[47]

In *primary ciliary dyskinesia*, an autosomal recessive syndrome with variable penetrance and a frequency of 1 in 15,000 to 40,000 births, poorly functioning cilia contribute to the retention of secretions and recurrent infections that in turn lead to bronchiectasis. There is an absence or shortening of the dynein arms that are responsible for the coordinated bending of the cilia. Approximately half of the patients with primary ciliary dyskinesia have *Kartagener syndrome* (bronchiectasis, sinusitis, and situs inversus or partial lateralizing abnormality).[48] The lack of ciliary activity interferes with bacterial clearance, predisposes the sinuses and bronchi to infection, and affects cell motility during embryogenesis, resulting in the situs inversus. Males with this condition tend to be infertile, as a result of sperm dysmotility.

Allergic bronchopulmonary aspergillosis is a condition that results from a hypersensitivity reaction to the fungus *Aspergillus fumigatus*. It is also an important complication of asthma and cystic fibrosis.[49] Characteristics are high serum IgE levels, serum antibodies to *Aspergillus*, intense airway inflammation with eosinophils, and the formation of mucus plugs, which play a primary role in its pathogenesis. There is evidence that neutrophil-mediated inflammation and a relative deficiency of anti-inflammatory cytokines such as IL-10 may also play a role.[50] Clinically, there are periods of exacerbation and remission that may lead to proximal bronchiectasis and fibrotic lung disease.

Morphology. Bronchiectasis usually affects the lower lobes bilaterally, particularly air passages that are vertical, and is most severe in the more distal bronchi and bronchioles. When tumors or aspiration of foreign bodies lead to bronchiectasis, the involvement may be sharply localized to a single segment of the lung. **The airways are dilated, sometimes up to four times normal size.** Characteristically, the bronchi and bronchioles are sufficiently dilated that they can be followed almost to the pleural surfaces. By contrast, in the normal lung, the bronchioles cannot be followed by ordinary gross dissection beyond a point 2 to 3 cm from the pleural surfaces. On the cut surface of the lung, the transected dilated bronchi appear as cysts filled with mucopurulent secretions (Fig. 15-12).

The histologic findings vary with the activity and chronicity of the disease. In the full-blown, active case there is an intense acute and chronic inflammatory exudation within the walls of the bronchi and bronchioles, associated with desquamation of the lining epithelium and extensive areas of necrotizing ulceration. There may be pseudostratification of the columnar cells or squamous metaplasia of the remaining epithelium. In some instances the necrosis completely destroys the bronchial or bronchiolar walls and forms a lung abscess. Fibrosis of the bronchial and bronchiolar walls and peribronchiolar fibrosis develop in the more chronic cases, leading to varying degrees of subtotal or total obliteration of bronchiolar lumens.

In the usual case of bronchiectasis, a mixed flora can be cultured from the involved bronchi, including staphylococci, streptococci, pneumococci, enteric organisms, anaerobic and microaerophilic bacteria, and (particularly in children) *Haemophilus influenzae* and *Pseudomonas aeruginosa*.[51] In allergic bronchopulmonary aspergillosis a few fungal hyphae can be seen on special stains within the muco-inflammatory contents of the cylindrically dilated segmental bronchi. In late stages the fungus may infiltrate the bronchial wall.

Clinical Course. Bronchiectasis causes severe, persistent cough; expectoration of foul-smelling, sometimes bloody sputum; dyspnea and orthopnea in severe cases; and occasional life-threatening hemoptysis. These symptoms are often

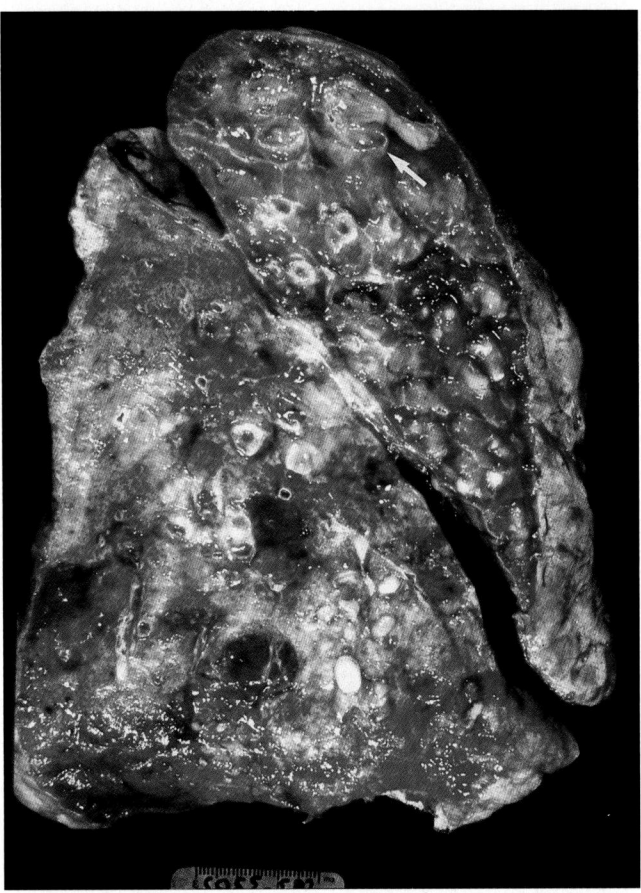

FIGURE 15-12 Bronchiectasis in a patient with cystic fibrosis, who underwent lung transplantation. Cut surface of lung shows markedly distended peripheral bronchi filled with mucopurulent secretions.

episodic and are precipitated by upper respiratory tract infections or the introduction of new pathogenic agents. Paroxysms of cough are particularly frequent when the patient rises in the morning, when changes in position lead to drainage of collections of pus and secretions into the bronchi. Obstructive respiratory insufficiency can lead to marked dyspnea and cyanosis. Cor pulmonale, brain abscesses, and amyloidosis are less frequent complications of bronchiectasis. However, due to current treatment with better antibiotics and physical therapy, outcome has improved considerably and life expectancy has almost doubled.

Chronic Diffuse Interstitial (Restrictive) Diseases

Chronic interstitial diseases are a heterogeneous group of disorders *characterized predominantly by inflammation and fibrosis of the pulmonary connective tissue, principally the most peripheral and delicate interstitium in the alveolar walls.* Many of the entities are of unknown cause and pathogenesis, some have an intra-alveolar as well as an interstitial component, and there is frequent overlap in histologic features among the different conditions. These disorders account for

TABLE 15–5   Major Categories of Chronic Interstitial Lung Disease

FIBROSING

Usual interstitial pneumonia (idiopathic pulmonary fibrosis)
Nonspecific interstitial pneumonia
Cryptogenic organizing pneumonia
Associated with connective tissue diseases
Pneumoconiosis
Drug reactions
Radiation pneumonitis

GRANULOMATOUS

Sarcoidosis
Hypersensitivity pneumonitis

EOSINOPHILIC

SMOKING RELATED

Desquamative interstitial pneumonia
Respiratory bronchiolitis-associated interstitial lung disease

OTHER

Pulmonary alveolar proteinosis

---

about 15% of noninfectious diseases seen by pulmonary physicians.

In general, the clinical and pulmonary functional changes are those of *restrictive lung disease* (see the earlier discussion of obstructive versus restrictive pulmonary diseases). Patients have dyspnea, tachypnea, end-inspiratory crackles, and eventual cyanosis, without wheezing or other evidence of airway obstruction. The classic physiologic features are reductions in carbon monoxide diffusing capacity, lung volume, and compliance. *Chest radiographs show bilateral infiltrative lesions in the form of small nodules, irregular lines, or ground-glass shadows*, hence the term *infiltrative*. Eventually, secondary pulmonary hypertension and right-sided heart failure with cor pulmonale may result. Although the entities can often be distinguished in the early stages, the advanced forms are hard to differentiate because they result in scarring and gross destruction of the lung, often referred to as *end-stage lung* or *honeycomb lung*. Diffuse restrictive diseases are categorized based on histology and clinical features (Table 15–5).

FIBROSING DISEASES

Idiopathic Pulmonary Fibrosis

The term *idiopathic pulmonary fibrosis* (IPF) refers to a clinicopathologic syndrome with characteristic radiologic, pathologic, and clinical features. In Europe the term *cryptogenic fibrosing alveolitis* is more popular. The histologic pattern of fibrosis is referred to as usual interstitial pneumonia (UIP), which is required for the diagnosis of IPF but can also be seen in other diseases, notably connective tissue diseases, chronic hypersensitivity pneumonia, and asbestosis. The International Multidisciplinary Consensus Classification is an excellent reference for definitions and understanding of idiopathic interstitial pneumonias.[52,53]

Pathogenesis. While the causative agent(s) of IPF remain unknown, our concepts of pathogenesis have evolved over the past several years.[54] The earlier view was that IPF is initiated

by an unidentified insult that gives rise to chronic inflammation resulting in fibrosis. The dismal failure of potent anti-inflammatory therapy in altering the course of the disease did not support this view. *The current concept is that IPF is caused by "repeated cycles" of epithelial activation/injury by some unidentified agent.* There is inflammation and induction of T_H2 type T cell response characterized by the presence of eosinophils, mast cells, IL-4 and IL-13 in the lesions. But the significance of this inflammatory response is unknown. Abnormal epithelial repair at these sites gives rise to exuberant fibroblastic/myofibroblastic proliferation, leading to the "fibroblastic foci" that are so characteristic of IPF (Fig. 15–13). The circuits that drive such aberrant epithelial repair are not fully understood, but all evidence points to *TGF-β1 as the driver of the process.* TGF-β1 is known to be fibrogenic and is released from injured type I alveolar epithelial cells (Fig. 15–13). It favors the transformation of fibroblasts into myofibroblasts and deposition of collagen and other extracellular matrix molecules.[55]

The concept that there is an intrinsic abnormality of tissue repair in IPF is supported by the finding that some patients with familial pulmonary fibrosis have mutations that shorten telomeres. Recall that telomeres control cell replications (see Chapters 1 and 7) and with shortening of telomeres alveolar epithelial cells undergo rapid senescence and apoptosis.[56,57] Interestingly, *TGF-β1 negatively regulates telomerase activity*, thus facilitating epithelial cell apoptosis and the cycle of death and repair.[58] Another molecule regulated by TGF-β1 is *caveolin-1*, the predominant structural protein of caveolae, flask-shaped invaginations of the plasma membrane present in many terminally differentiated cells. *Caveolin-1 acts as an endogenous inhibitor of pulmonary fibrosis* by limiting TGF-β1–induced production of extracellular matrix and restoring alveolar epithelial repair processes. Caveolin-1 is decreased in epithelial cells and fibroblasts of IPF patients, and overexpression of caveolin-1 in a mouse model limits fibrosis.[59] Such down-regulation may be mediated by the ability of TGF-β1 to attenuate the expression of caveolin-1 in fibroblasts. Thus, it

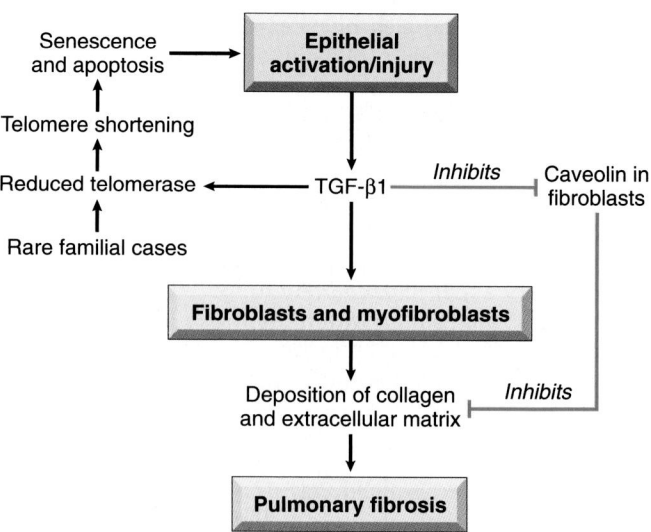

FIGURE 15–13 Schematic representation of current understanding of the pathogenesis of idiopathic pulmonary fibrosis.

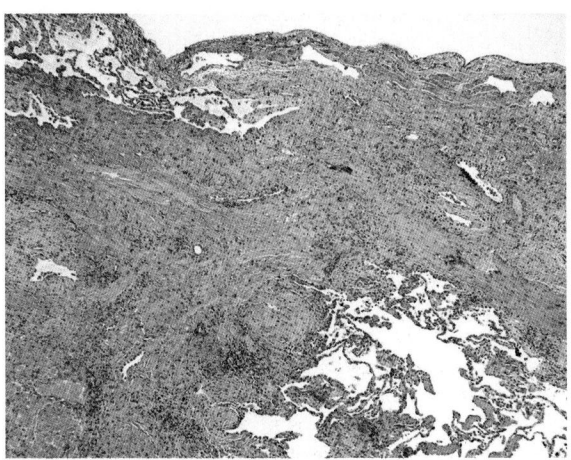

FIGURE 15–14 Usual interstitial pneumonia. The fibrosis is more pronounced in the subpleural region. (Courtesy of Dr. Nicole Cipriani, Department of Pathology, University of Chicago, Chicago, IL.)

seems that TGF-β1 has its fingerprints on multiple pathways that regulate pulmonary fibrosis. Therapeutics directed toward neutralizing TGF-β1, enhancing telomerase activity or delaying telomere shortening, or augmenting caveolin-1 may lead to novel treatments for IPF in the future.[60]

Morphology. Grossly, the pleural surfaces of the lung are cobblestoned as a result of the retraction of scars along the interlobular septa. The cut surface shows fibrosis (firm, rubbery white areas) of the lung parenchyma with lower-lobe predominance and a distinctive distribution in the **subpleural regions** and along the **interlobular septa**. Microscopically, the hallmark of UIP is **patchy interstitial fibrosis**, which varies in intensity (Fig. 15–14) and age. The earliest lesions contain exuberant fibroblastic proliferation **(fibroblastic foci)**. With time these areas become more collagenous and less cellular. Quite typical is the coexistence of both early and late lesions (Fig. 15–15).

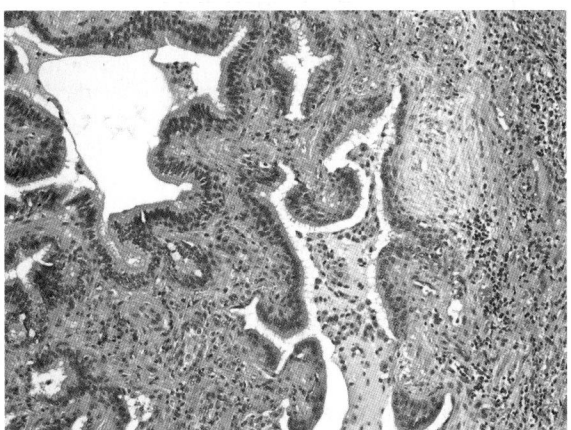

FIGURE 15–15 Usual interstitial pneumonia. Fibroblastic focus with fibers running parallel to surface and bluish myxoid extracellular matrix. Honeycombing is present on the *left*.

The dense fibrosis causes the destruction of alveolar architecture and formation of cystic spaces lined by hyperplastic type II pneumocytes or bronchiolar epithelium (**honeycomb fibrosis**). With adequate sampling, these diagnostic histologic changes (i.e., areas of dense collagenous fibrosis with relatively normal lung and fibroblastic foci) can be identified even in advanced IPF. There is mild to moderate inflammation within the fibrotic areas, consisting of mostly lymphocytes, and a few plasma cells, neutrophils, eosinophils, and mast cells. Foci of squamous metaplasia and smooth muscle hyperplasia may be present. Pulmonary arterial hypertensive changes (intimal fibrosis and medial thickening) are often present. In acute exacerbations diffuse alveolar damage is superimposed on the UIP pattern.[61]

Clinical Course. IPF begins insidiously, with gradually increasing *dyspnea on exertion* and dry cough. Most patients are 40 to 70 years old at the time of presentation. Hypoxemia, *cyanosis*, and clubbing occur late in the course. The progression in an individual patient is unpredictable. Most patients have a gradual deterioration of their pulmonary status, despite medical treatment (steroids, cyclophosphamide, or azathioprine). In some IPF patients, there are acute exacerbations of the underlying disease with a rapid downhill clinical course. The mean survival is 3 years or less. Lung transplantation is the only definitive therapy currently available.[62]

Nonspecific Interstitial Pneumonia

The concept of nonspecific interstitial pneumonia (NSIP) emerged when it was realized that there is a group of patients with diffuse interstitial lung disease of unknown etiology whose lung biopsies fail to show diagnostic features of any of the other well-characterized interstitial diseases. Despite its "nonspecific" name, NSIP has distinct radiologic and histologic features and is important to recognize, since these patients have a much better prognosis than do those with UIP.[63]

Morphology. On the basis of its histology, NSIP is divided into cellular and fibrosing patterns. The cellular pattern consists primarily of mild to moderate chronic interstitial inflammation, containing lymphocytes and a few plasma cells, in a uniform or patchy distribution. The fibrosing pattern consists of diffuse or patchy interstitial fibrosis without the temporal heterogeneity that is characteristic of UIP. Fibroblastic foci and honeycombing are absent. However, in some patients both NSIP and UIP patterns can be seen in different areas of the lung; the prognosis in these is the same as for UIP.[64]

Clinical Course. Patients present with dyspnea and cough of several months' duration. They are typically between 46 and 55 years of age. Those having the NSIP cellular pattern are somewhat younger than those with the fibrosing pattern or UIP. Patients with the cellular pattern have a better outcome than do those with fibrosing pattern and UIP.[65]

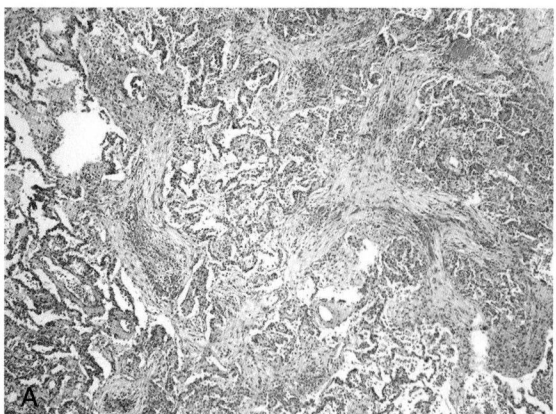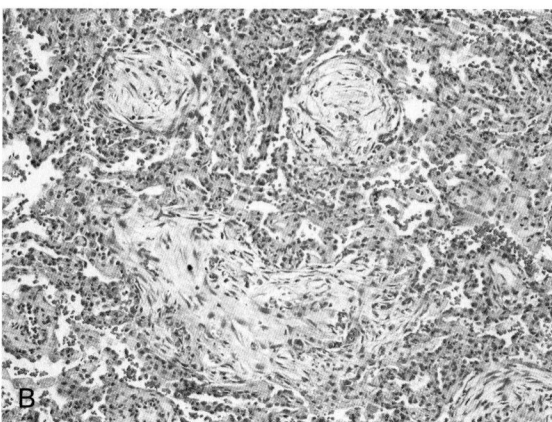

FIGURE 15–16   Cryptogenic organizing pneumonia. Some alveolar spaces are filled with balls of fibroblasts (Masson bodies), while the alveolar walls are relatively normal. **A,** Low power; **B,** high power.

Cryptogenic Organizing Pneumonia

Cryptogenic organizing pneumonia is synonymous with the popular term *bronchiolitis obliterans organizing pneumonia*; however, the former is now preferred, since it conveys the essential features of a clinicopathologic syndrome of unknown etiology and avoids confusion with airway diseases such as bronchiolitis obliterans. Patients present with cough and dyspnea and have subpleural or peribronchial patchy areas of airspace consolidation radiographically. Histologically, cryptogenic organizing pneumonia is characterized by the presence of polypoid plugs of loose organizing connective tissue (Masson bodies) within alveolar ducts, alveoli (Fig. 15–16), and often bronchioles. The connective tissue is all of the same age, and the underlying lung architecture is normal. There is no interstitial fibrosis or honeycomb lung. Some patients recover spontaneously, but most need treatment with oral steroids for 6 months or longer for complete recovery.

It is important to recognize that organizing pneumonia with intra-alveolar fibrosis is also often seen as a response to infections or inflammatory injury of the lungs.[66] These include viral and bacterial pneumonia, inhaled toxins, drugs, connective tissue disease, and graft-versus-host disease in bone marrow transplant recipients. The prognosis for these patients is the same as that for the underlying disorder.

Pulmonary Involvement in Connective Tissue Diseases

Many connective tissue diseases, notably systemic lupus erythematosus, rheumatoid arthritis, progressive systemic sclerosis (scleroderma), dermatomyositis-polymyositis, and mixed connective tissue disease, can involve the lung to a lesser or greater degree at some time in their course. Pulmonary involvement can occur in different patterns; NSIP, UIP (similar to that seen in IPF), vascular sclerosis, organizing pneumonia, and bronchiolitis are the most common.

- *Rheumatoid arthritis*: pulmonary involvement may occur in 30% to 40% of patients as (1) chronic pleuritis, with or without effusion; (2) diffuse interstitial pneumonitis and fibrosis; (3) intrapulmonary rheumatoid nodules; or (4) pulmonary hypertension

- *Systemic sclerosis* (scleroderma): diffuse interstitial fibrosis (NSIP pattern more common than UIP)
- *Lupus erythematosus*: patchy, transient parenchymal infiltrates, and occasionally severe lupus pneumonitis

Pulmonary involvement in these diseases is usually associated with a variable prognosis, partly dependent on the type of pulmonary disease, although it is still better than that of idiopathic UIP.[67]

Pneumoconioses

The term *pneumoconiosis* was originally coined to describe the non-neoplastic lung reaction to inhalation of mineral dusts encountered in the workplace. Now it also includes diseases induced by organic as well as inorganic particulates and chemical fumes and vapors. A simplified classification is presented in Table 15–6. Regulations limiting worker exposure have resulted in a marked decrease in dust-associated diseases.

Although the pneumoconioses result from well-defined occupational exposure to specific airborne agents, particulate air pollution also has deleterious effects on the general population, especially in urban areas. Studies have found increased morbidity (e.g., asthma incidence) and mortality rates in populations that are exposed to high ambient air particulate levels,[68,69] leading to calls for greater efforts to reduce the levels of particulates in urban air.

Pathogenesis. The development of a pneumoconiosis depends on (1) the amount of dust retained in the lung and airways; (2) the size, shape, and therefore buoyancy of the particles; (3) particle solubility and physiochemical reactivity; and (4) the possible additional effects of other irritants (e.g., concomitant tobacco smoking).

The amount of dust retained in the lungs is determined by the dust concentration in ambient air, the duration of exposure, and the effectiveness of clearance mechanisms. Any influence, such as cigarette smoking, that affects the integrity of the mucociliary apparatus significantly predisposes to the accumulation of dust. *The most dangerous particles range from 1 to 5 µm in diameter because they may reach the terminal small airways and air sacs and settle in their linings.* Under normal conditions there is a small pool of intra-alveolar macrophages, and this is expanded by recruitment of more macrophages when dust reaches the alveolar spaces. The protection pro-

TABLE 15–6	Lung Diseases Caused by Air Pollutants	
Agent	**Disease**	**Exposure**
MINERAL DUSTS		
Coal dust	Anthracosis	Coal mining (particularly hard coal)
	Macules	
	Progressive massive fibrosis	
	Caplan syndrome	
Silica	Silicosis	Foundry work, sandblasting, hard
	Caplan syndrome	rock mining, stone cutting, others
Asbestos	Asbestosis	Mining, milling, fabrication, and
	Pleural plaques	installation and removal of
	Caplan syndrome	insulation
	Mesothelioma	
	Carcinoma of the lung, larynx, stomach, colon	
Beryllium	Acute berylliosis	Mining, fabrication
	Beryllium granulomatosis	
	Lung carcinoma (?)	
Iron oxide	Siderosis	Welding
Barium sulfate	Baritosis	Mining
Tin oxide	Stannosis	Mining
ORGANIC DUSTS THAT INDUCE HYPERSENSITIVITY PNEUMONITIS		
Moldy hay	Farmer's lung	Farming
Bagasse	Bagassosis	Manufacturing wallboard, paper
Bird droppings	Bird-breeder's lung	Bird handling
ORGANIC DUSTS THAT INDUCE ASTHMA		
Cotton, flax, hemp	Byssinosis	Textile manufacturing
Red cedar dust	Asthma	Lumbering, carpentry
CHEMICAL FUMES AND VAPORS		
Nitrous oxide, sulfur dioxide, ammonia, benzene, insecticides	Bronchitis, asthma	Occupational and accidental exposure
	Pulmonary edema	
	ARDS	
	Mucosal injury	
	Fulminant poisoning	

ARDS, acute respiratory distress syndrome.

vided by phagocytosis of particles, however, can be overwhelmed by a large dust burden by specific chemical interactions of the particles with cells.

The *solubility and cytotoxicity of particles*, which are influenced to a considerable extent by their size, modify the nature of the pulmonary response. In general, the smaller the particle, the more likely it is to appear in the pulmonary fluids and reach toxic levels rapidly, depending, of course, on the solubility of the agent. Therefore, smaller particles tend to cause acute lung injury. Larger particles resist dissolution and so may persist within the lung parenchyma for years. These tend to evoke fibrosing collagenous pneumoconioses, such as is characteristic of silicosis. Some of the particles may be taken up by epithelial cells or may cross the epithelial cell lining and interact directly with fibroblasts and interstitial macrophages. Some may reach the lymphatics by direct drainage or within migrating macrophages and thereby initiate an immune response to components of the particulates or to self-proteins modified by the particles or both. This response amplifies the intensity and the duration of the local reaction. Although tobacco smoking worsens the effects of all inhaled mineral dusts, the effects of asbestos are particularly magnified by smoking. The effects of inhaled particles are not confined to the lung alone, since solutes from particles can enter the blood and lung inflammation invokes systemic responses.[70]

In general, only a small percentage of exposed people develop occupational respiratory diseases, implying a genetic predisposition to their development.[71] In one study, genetic variation of serum and erythrocytic proteins was shown to correlate with susceptibility to developing silicosis, chronic bronchitis, and occupational asthma.[72] Many of the diseases listed in Table 15–6 are quite uncommon. Hence only a selected few that cause fibrosis of the lung are presented next.

Coal Workers' Pneumoconiosis

Dust reduction measures in coal mines around the globe have drastically reduced the incidence of coal workers' pneumoconiosis (CWP). The spectrum of lung findings in coal workers is wide, varying from (1) asymptomatic anthracosis to (2) simple CWP with little to no pulmonary dysfunction to (3) complicated CWP, or progressive massive fibrosis (PMF), in which lung function is compromised.[73] The pathogenesis of complicated CWP, particularly what causes the lesions of simple CWP to progress to PMF, is incompletely understood. Contaminating silica in the coal dust can favor progressive disease. In most cases, carbon dust itself is the major culprit, and studies have shown that complicated lesions contain much more dust than simple lesions.

Morphology. Anthracosis is the most innocuous coal-induced pulmonary lesion in coal miners and is also seen to some degree in urban dwellers and tobacco smokers. Inhaled carbon pigment is engulfed by alveolar or interstitial macrophages, which then accumulate in the connective tissue along the lymphatics, including the pleural lymphatics, or in organized lymphoid tissue along the bronchi or in the lung hilus.

Simple CWP is characterized by **coal macules** (1 to 2 mm in diameter) and the somewhat larger **coal nodules**. The coal macule consists of carbon-laden macrophages; the nodule also contains small amounts of a delicate network of collagen fibers. Although these lesions are scattered throughout the lung, the upper lobes and upper zones of the lower lobes are more heavily involved. They are located primarily adjacent to respiratory bronchioles, the site of initial dust accumulation. In due course dilation of adjacent alveoli occurs, a condition sometimes referred to as **centrilobular emphysema**.

Complicated CWP (progressive massive fibrosis) occurs on a background of simple CWP and generally requires many years to develop. It is characterized by intensely blackened scars larger than 2 cm, sometimes up to 10 cm in greatest diameter. They are usually multiple (Fig. 15–17). Microscopically the lesions consist of dense collagen and pigment. The center of the lesion is often necrotic, most likely due to local ischemia.

Clinical Course. CWP is usually a benign disease that causes little decrement in lung function. Even mild forms of complicated CWP fail to demonstrate abnormalities of lung function. In a minority of cases (fewer than 10%), PMF develops, leading to increasing pulmonary dysfunction, pulmonary hypertension, and cor pulmonale. Once PMF develops, it may become progressive even if further exposure to dust is prevented. Unlike silicosis (discussed later), there is no convincing evidence that coal dust increases susceptibility to tuberculosis. There is some evidence that exposure to coal dust increases the incidence of chronic bronchitis and emphysema, independent of smoking. Thus far, however, there is no compelling evidence that CWP in the absence of smoking predisposes to cancer.

Silicosis

Silicosis is a lung disease caused by inhalation of crystalline silicon dioxide (silica).[74] *Currently the most prevalent chronic occupational disease in the world*, silicosis usually presents after decades of exposure as a slowly progressing, nodular, fibrosing pneumoconiosis. As shown in Table 15–6, workers in a large number of occupations are at risk, especially sandblasters and many mine workers. Less commonly, heavy exposure over months to a few years can result in acute silicosis, a disorder characterized by the accumulation of abundant lipoprotein-aceous material within alveoli (identical morphologically to alveolar proteinosis, which is discussed later).

Pathogenesis. Silica occurs in both crystalline and amorphous forms, but crystalline forms (including quartz, crysto-balite, and tridymite) are much more fibrogenic. Of these, quartz is most commonly implicated in silicosis. After inhala-

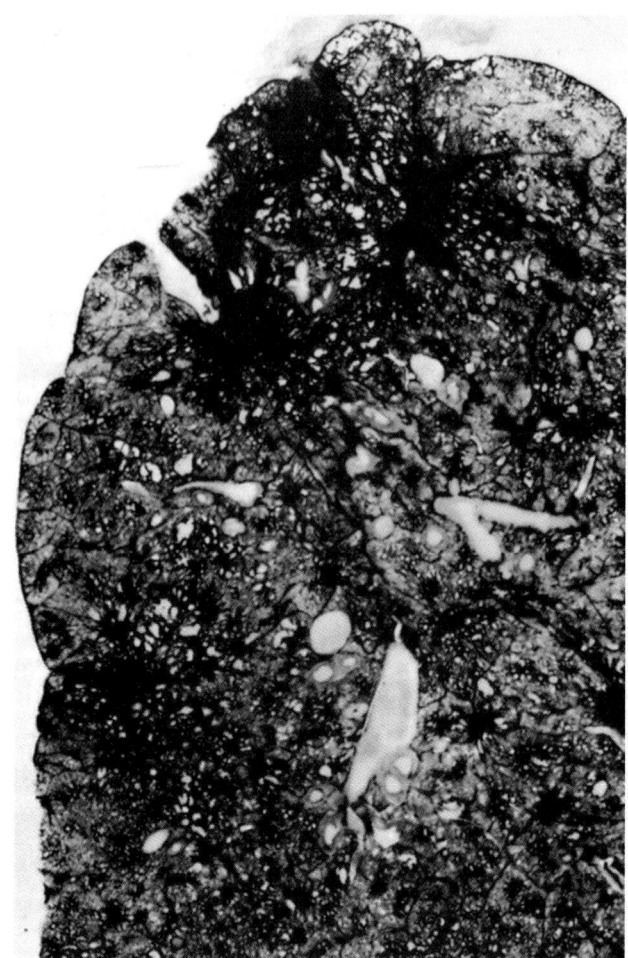

FIGURE 15–17 Progressive massive fibrosis superimposed on coal workers' pneumoconiosis. The large, blackened scars are located principally in the upper lobe. Note the extensions of scars into surrounding parenchyma and retraction of adjacent pleura. (Courtesy of Drs. Werner Laquer and Jerome Kleinerman, the National Institute of Occupational Safety and Health, Morgantown, WV.)

tion, the particles interact with epithelial cells and macrophages. Within the macrophages *silica causes activation and release of mediators*. Such mediators include IL-1, TNF, fibronectin, lipid mediators, oxygen-derived free radicals, and fibrogenic cytokines.[75,76] Especially compelling is evidence incriminating TNF, since anti-TNF monoclonal antibodies can block lung collagen accumulation in mice given silica intratracheally. It has been noted that when mixed with other minerals, quartz has a reduced fibrogenic effect. This phenomenon is of practical importance because quartz in the workplace is rarely pure. Thus, miners of the iron-containing ore hematite may have more quartz in their lungs than some quartz-exposed workers and yet have relatively mild lung disease because the hematite somehow provides a protective effect. Although amorphous silicates are biologically less active than crystalline silica, heavy lung burdens of these minerals may also produce lesions.

Morphology. Silicosis is characterized grossly in its early stages by tiny, barely palpable, discrete pale to

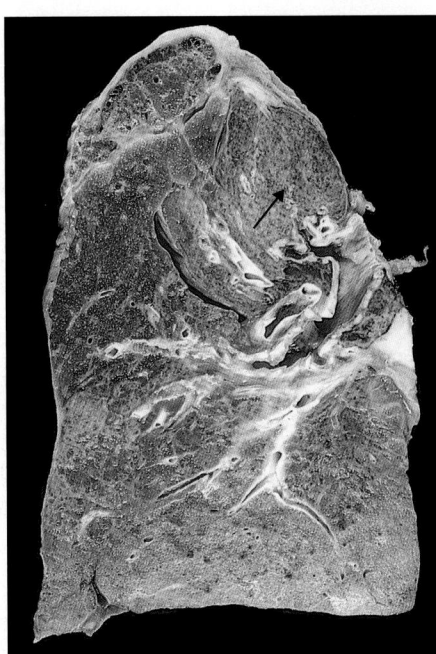

FIGURE 15–18 Advanced silicosis (transected lung). Scarring has contracted the upper lobe into a small dark mass *(arrow)*. Note the dense pleural thickening. (Courtesy of Dr. John Godleski, Brigham and Women's Hospital, Boston, MA.)

blackened (if coal dust is also present) nodules in the upper zones of the lungs. As the disease progresses, these nodules may coalesce into **hard, collagenous scars** (Fig. 15–18). Some nodules may undergo central softening and cavitation. This change may be due to superimposed tuberculosis or to ischemia. Fibrotic lesions may also occur in the hilar lymph nodes and pleura. Sometimes, thin sheets of calcification occur in the lymph nodes and are seen radiographically as **eggshell** calcification (i.e., calcium surrounding a zone lacking calcification). If the disease continues to progress, expansion and coalescence of lesions may produce progressive massive fibrosis. Histologic examination reveals that the nodular lesions consist of concentric layers of hyalinized collagen surrounded by a dense capsule of more condensed collagen (Fig. 15–19). Examination of the nodules by polarized microscopy reveals the birefringent silica particles.

Clinical Course. Chest radiographs typically show a fine nodularity in the upper zones of the lung, but pulmonary functions are either normal or only moderately affected. Most patients do not develop shortness of breath until late in the course, after progressive massive fibrosis is present. The disease may be progressive even if the patient is no longer exposed. The disease is slow to kill, but impaired pulmonary function may severely limit activity. Silicosis is associated with an increased susceptibility to *tuberculosis*. It is postulated that silicosis results in a depression of cell-mediated immunity, and crystalline silica may inhibit the ability of pulmonary macrophages to kill phagocytosed mycobacteria. Nodules of silicotuberculosis often display a central zone of caseation. The relationship between silica and *lung cancer* is contentious. In 1997, the International Agency for Research on Cancer (IARC) concluded that *crystalline silica from occupational sources is carcinogenic in humans.* However, this subject continues to be controversial.

Asbestos-Related Diseases

Asbestos is a family of crystalline hydrated silicates that form fibers. Use of asbestos is seriously restricted in many developed countries; however, there is little, if any, control in less developed parts of the world.[77] On the basis of epidemiologic studies, *occupational exposure* to asbestos is linked to[78]:

- Localized fibrous plaques or, rarely, diffuse pleural fibrosis
- Pleural effusions
- Parenchymal interstitial fibrosis *(asbestosis)*
- Lung carcinoma
- Mesotheliomas
- Laryngeal and perhaps other extrapulmonary neoplasms, including colon carcinomas

An increased incidence of asbestos-related cancer in family members of asbestos workers has alerted the general public to the potential hazards of asbestos in the environment. The proper public health policy toward low-level exposures that might be encountered in old buildings or schools is unsettled: some experts question the wisdom of expensive asbestos abatement programs for environments with airborne fiber counts that are as much as 100-fold lower than allowed by occupational standards.

Pathogenesis. Concentration, size, shape, and solubility of the different forms of asbestos dictate whether it causes disease.[79] There are two distinct geometric forms of asbestos: *serpentine* and *amphibole*. The serpentine chrysotile chemical form accounts for most of the asbestos used in industry. Amphiboles, even though less prevalent, are more pathogenic than chrysotiles particularly with respect to induction of malignant pleural tumors (mesotheliomas).

The greater pathogenicity of amphiboles is apparently related to their aerodynamic properties and solubility.

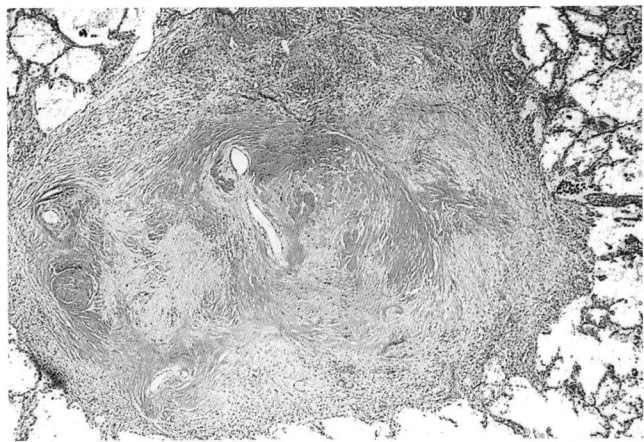

FIGURE 15–19 Several coalescent collagenous silicotic nodules. (Courtesy of Dr. John Godleski, Brigham and Women's Hospital, Boston, MA.)

Chrysotiles, with their more flexible, curled structure, are likely to become impacted in the upper respiratory passages and removed by the mucociliary elevator. Furthermore, once trapped in the lungs, chrysotiles are gradually leached from the tissues because they are more soluble than amphiboles. In contrast, the straight, stiff amphiboles may align themselves in the airstream and thus be delivered deeper into the lungs, where they can penetrate epithelial cells and reach the interstitium. *Both amphiboles and serpentines are fibrogenic,* and increasing doses are associated with a higher incidence of all asbestos-related diseases; however, serpentine chrysotile has lower carcinogenic potential than amphiboles.

In contrast to other inorganic dusts, asbestos can also act as a tumor initiator and promoter. Some of its *oncogenic effects* are mediated by reactive free radicals generated by asbestos fibers, which preferentially localize in the distal lung, close to the mesothelial layers. Potentially toxic chemicals adsorbed onto the asbestos fibers most likely contribute to the oncogenicity of the fibers. For example, the adsorption of carcinogens in tobacco smoke onto asbestos fibers may well contribute to the remarkable *synergy between tobacco smoking and the development of lung carcinoma* in asbestos workers. One study of asbestos workers found a fivefold increase of lung carcinoma with asbestos exposure alone, while asbestos exposure and smoking together led to a 55-fold increase in the risk of lung cancer.[80]

The occurrence of asbestosis, like the other pneumoconioses, depends on the interaction of inhaled fibers with lung macrophages and other parenchymal cells. The initial injury occurs at bifurcations of small airways and ducts, where the asbestos fibers land and penetrate. Macrophages, both alveolar and interstitial, attempt to ingest and clear the fibers and are activated to release chemotactic factors and fibrogenic mediators that amplify the response. Chronic deposition of fibers and persistent release of mediators eventually lead to generalized interstitial pulmonary inflammation and interstitial fibrosis.

Morphology. Asbestosis is marked by **diffuse pulmonary interstitial fibrosis**, which is indistinguishable from diffuse interstitial fibrosis resulting from other causes, except for the presence of multiple **asbestos bodies**. Asbestos bodies appear as **golden brown, fusiform or beaded rods with a translucent center and consist of asbestos fibers coated with an iron-containing proteinaceous material** (Fig. 15-20). They arise when macrophages attempt to phagocytose asbestos fibers; the iron is presumably derived from phagocyte ferritin. Other inorganic particulates may become coated with similar iron-protein complexes and are called **ferruginous bodies**. Rare single asbestos bodies can be found in the lungs of normal people.

Asbestosis begins as fibrosis around respiratory bronchioles and alveolar ducts and extends to involve adjacent alveolar sacs and alveoli. The fibrous tissue distorts the architecture, creating enlarged airspaces enclosed within thick fibrous walls; eventually the affected regions become honeycombed. The pattern of fibrosis is similar to that seen in UIP, with fibroblastic foci and varying degrees of fibrosis, the only

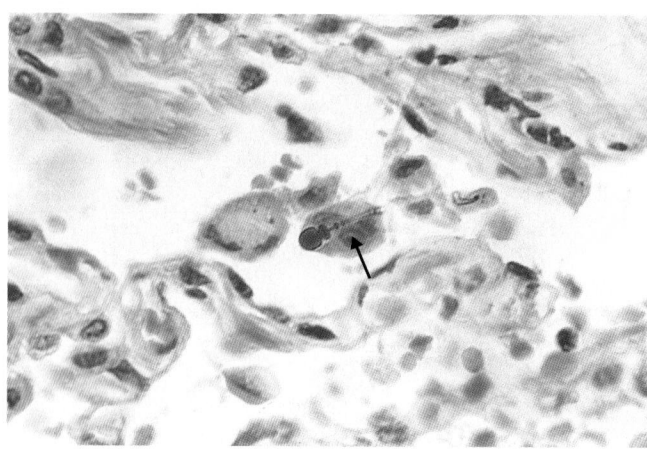

FIGURE 15–20   High-power detail of an asbestos body, revealing the typical beading and knobbed ends *(arrow).*

difference being the presence of numerous asbestos bodies. In contrast to CWP and silicosis, asbestosis begins in the lower lobes and subpleurally. The middle and upper lobes of the lungs become affected as fibrosis progresses. The scarring may trap and narrow pulmonary arteries and arterioles, causing pulmonary hypertension and cor pulmonale.

Pleural plaques, the most common manifestation of asbestos exposure, are well-circumscribed plaques of dense collagen (Fig. 15-21), often containing calcium. They develop most frequently on the anterior and posterolateral aspects of the **parietal pleura** and over the domes of the diaphragm. The size and number of pleural plaques do not correlate with the level of exposure to asbestos or the time since exposure.[81] They do not contain asbestos bodies; however, only rarely do they occur in individuals who have no history or evidence of asbestos exposure. Uncommonly, asbestos exposure induces pleural effusions, which are usually

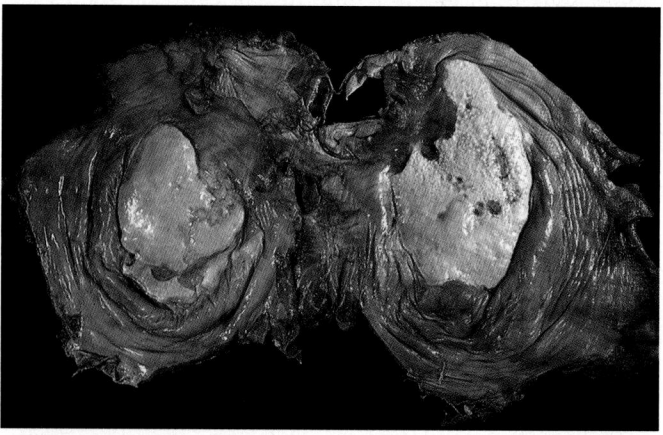

FIGURE 15–21   Asbestos-related pleural plaques. Large, discrete fibrocalcific plaques are seen on the pleural surface of the diaphragm. (Courtesy of Dr. John Godleski, Brigham and Women's Hospital, Boston, MA.)

serous but may be bloody. Rarely, diffuse visceral pleural fibrosis may occur and, in advanced cases, bind the lung to the thoracic cavity wall.

Both lung carcinomas and mesotheliomas (pleural and peritoneal) develop in workers exposed to asbestos. The risk of lung carcinoma is increased about fivefold for asbestos workers; the relative risk of mesotheliomas, normally a rare tumor (2 to 17 cases per 1 million persons), is more than 1000-fold greater. Concomitant cigarette smoking greatly increases the risk of lung carcinoma but not that of mesothelioma.

Clinical Course. The clinical findings in asbestosis are very similar to those caused by other diffuse interstitial lung diseases (discussed earlier). Dyspnea is usually the first manifestation; at first, it is provoked by exertion, but later it is present even at rest. The dyspnea is usually accompanied by a cough associated with production of sputum. These manifestations rarely appear fewer than 10 years after first exposure and are more common after 20 years or more. Chest x-rays reveal irregular linear densities, particularly in both lower lobes. With advancement of the pneumoconiosis, a honeycomb pattern develops. The disease may remain static or progress to respiratory failure, cor pulmonale, and death. Pleural plaques are usually asymptomatic and are detected on radiographs as circumscribed densities. Asbestosis complicated by lung or pleural cancer is associated with a particularly grim prognosis.

Complications of Therapies

Drug-Induced Lung Diseases. Drugs can cause a variety of both acute and chronic alterations in respiratory structure and function, interstitial fibrosis, bronchiolitis obliterans, and eosinophilic pneumonia (Table 15–7).[82] For example, cytotoxic drugs used in cancer therapy (e.g., bleomycin) cause pulmonary damage and fibrosis as a result of direct toxicity of the drug and by stimulating the influx of inflammatory cells into the alveoli. Amiodarone, a drug used to treat cardiac arrhythmias, is preferentially concentrated in the lung and causes significant pneumonitis in 5% to 15% of patients receiving it.

Radiation-Induced Lung Diseases. Radiation pneumonitis is a well-known complication of therapeutic radiation of

TABLE 15–7	Examples of Drug-Induced Pulmonary Disease
Drug	**Pulmonary Disease**
Bleomycin	Pneumonitis and fibrosis
Methotrexate	Hypersensitivity pneumonitis
Amiodarone	Pneumonitis and fibrosis
Nitrofurantoin	Hypersensitivity pneumonitis
Aspirin	Bronchospasm
β-Antagonists	Bronchospasm

thoracic tumors (lung, esophageal, breast, mediastinal).[83] It most often involves the lung within the radiation port but occasionally may extend to other areas of the same lung or even the contralateral lung. It occurs in acute and chronic forms. One to six months after fractionated irradiation, *acute radiation pneumonitis* (lymphocytic alveolitis or hypersensitivity pneumonitis) occurs in 10% to 20% of patients. It is manifest by fever, dyspnea out of proportion to the volume of lung irradiated, pleural effusion, and radiologic infiltrates that usually correspond to an area of previous irradiation. With steroid therapy, these symptoms may resolve completely in some patients without long-term effects,[84] while in others there is progression to *chronic radiation pneumonitis* (pulmonary fibrosis). The latter is a consequence of the repair of injured endothelial and epithelial cells within the radiation portal. Morphologic changes are those of diffuse alveolar damage, including severe atypia of hyperplastic type II cells and fibroblasts. Epithelial cell atypia and foam cells within vessel walls are also characteristic of radiation damage.

GRANULOMATOUS DISEASES

Sarcoidosis

Sarcoidosis is a systemic disease of unknown cause characterized by noncaseating granulomas in many tissues and organs. Sarcoidosis presents many clinical patterns, but bilateral hilar lymphadenopathy or lung involvement is visible on chest radiographs in 90% of cases. Eye and skin lesions occur next in frequency. Since other diseases, including mycobacterial and fungal infections and berylliosis, can also produce noncaseating *(hard)* granulomas, the histologic diagnosis of sarcoidosis is made by exclusion.[85]

The prevalence of sarcoidosis is higher in women than in men but varies widely in different countries and populations. In the United States the rates are highest in the Southeast; they are 10 times higher in American blacks than in whites. In contrast, the disease is rare among Chinese and Southeast Asians.

Etiology and Pathogenesis. Although the etiology of sarcoidosis remains unknown, several lines of evidence suggest that it is a disease of disordered immune regulation in genetically predisposed individuals exposed to certain environmental agents.[86] The role of each of these three contributory factors is summarized below.

Immunological Factors. There are several *immunological abnormalities* in the local milieu of sarcoid granulomas that suggest the development of a cell-mediated response to an unidentified antigen.[87] The process is driven by CD4+ helper T cells. These abnormalities include[88]:

- Intra-alveolar and interstitial accumulation of CD4+ T cells, resulting in CD4/CD8 T-cell ratios ranging from 5:1 to 15:1. There is oligoclonal expansion of T-cell subsets as determined by analysis of T-cell receptor rearrangement, suggesting an antigen-driven proliferation.
- Increased levels of T cell–derived T_H1 cytokines such as IL-2 and IFN-γ, resulting in T-cell expansion and macrophage activation, respectively.
- Increased levels of several cytokines in the local environment (IL-8, TNF, macrophage inflammatory protein 1α) that favor recruitment of additional T cells and monocytes

and contribute to the formation of granulomas. TNF in particular is released at high levels by activated alveolar macrophages, and the TNF concentration in the bronchoalveolar fluid is a marker of disease activity.

Additionally, there are *systemic immunological abnormalities* in individuals with sarcoidosis:

○ Anergy to common skin test antigens such as *Candida* or tuberculosis purified protein derivative (PPD)
○ Polyclonal hypergammaglobulinemia, another manifestation of helper T-cell dysregulation.

Genetic Factors. Evidence of genetic influences are the familial and racial clustering of cases and the association with certain HLA genotypes (e.g., HLA-A1 and HLA-B8).

Environmental Factors. These are possibly the most tenuous of all the associations in the pathogenesis of sarcoidosis. As with many other diseases of unknown etiology, suspicion falls on microbes. Indeed several putative microbes have been proposed as the inciting agent for sarcoidosis (e.g., mycobacteria, *Propionibacterium acnes,* and *Rickettsia* species).[89] Alas *there is no unequivocal evidence that sarcoidosis is caused by an infectious agent.*

Morphology. Histologically, all involved tissues show the classic well-formed **noncaseating granulomas** (Fig. 15–22), each composed of an aggregate of tightly clustered epithelioid cells, often with Langhans or foreign body–type giant cells. Central necrosis is unusual. With chronicity the granulomas may become enclosed within fibrous rims or may eventually be replaced by hyaline fibrous scars. Laminated concretions composed of calcium and proteins known as Schaumann bodies and stellate inclusions known as asteroid bodies enclosed within giant cells are found in approximately 60% of the granulomas. Though characteristic, these microscopic features are not

---

pathognomonic of sarcoidosis, because asteroid and Schaumann bodies may be encountered in other granulomatous diseases (e.g., tuberculosis). Pathologic involvement of virtually every organ in the body has been cited at one time or another.

The **lungs** are common sites of involvement.[90] Macroscopically there is usually no demonstrable alteration, although in advanced cases the coalescence of granulomas produces small nodules that are palpable or visible as 1 to 2 cm, noncaseating, noncavitated consolidations. Histologically, the lesions are distributed primarily along the lymphatics, around bronchi and blood vessels, although alveolar lesions are also seen. The relative frequency of granulomas in the bronchial submucosa accounts for the high diagnostic yield of bronchoscopic biopsies. There seems to be a strong tendency for lesions to heal in the lungs, so varying stages of fibrosis and hyalinization are often found. The pleural surfaces are sometimes involved.

Lymph nodes are involved in almost all cases, particularly the hilar and mediastinal nodes, but any other node in the body may be involved. Nodes are characteristically enlarged, discrete, and sometimes calcified. The tonsils are affected in about one quarter to one third of cases.

The **spleen** is affected microscopically in about three quarters of cases, but it is enlarged in only one fifth. On occasion, granulomas may coalesce to form small nodules that are barely visible macroscopically. The capsule is not involved. The **liver** is affected slightly less often than the spleen. It may also be moderately enlarged and contains scattered granulomas, more in portal triads than in the lobular parenchyma. Needle biopsy can be diagnostic.

The **bone marrow** is involved in about one fifth of cases of systemic sarcoidosis. The radiologically visible bone lesions have a particular tendency to involve phalangeal bones of the hands and feet, creating small circumscribed areas of bone resorption within the marrow cavity and a diffuse reticulated pattern throughout the cavity, with widening of the bony shafts or new bone formation on the outer surfaces.

Skin lesions are encountered in one third to one half of cases. Sarcoidosis of the skin assumes a variety of macroscopic appearances (e.g., discrete subcutaneous nodules; focal, slightly elevated, erythematous plaques; or flat lesions that are slightly reddened and scaling, and resemble those of lupus erythematosus). Lesions may also appear on the mucous membranes of the oral cavity, larynx, and upper respiratory tract. The **eye, its associated glands, and the salivary glands** are involved in about one fifth to one half of cases. The ocular involvement takes the form of iritis or iridocyclitis, either bilaterally or unilaterally. Consequently, corneal opacities, glaucoma, and total loss of vision may occur. These ocular lesions are frequently accompanied by inflammation

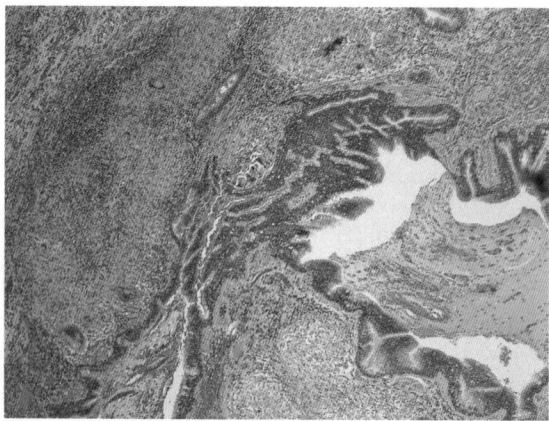

FIGURE 15–22 Characteristic sarcoid noncaseating granulomas, peribronchial, with many giant cells.

of the lacrimal glands, with suppression of lacrimation. Bilateral sarcoidosis of the parotid, submaxillary, and sublingual glands constitutes the combined uveoparotid involvement designated as Mikulicz syndrome (Chapter 16). **Muscle** involvement is often underdiagnosed, since it may be asymptomatic. Muscle weakness, aches, tenderness, and fatigue should prompt consideration of occult sarcoid myositis.[91] Muscle biopsy can be useful for diagnosis when clinical features point to sarcoidosis. Sarcoid granulomas occasionally occur in the heart, kidneys, central nervous system, and endocrine glands, particularly in the pituitary, as well as in other body tissues.

Clinical Course. Because of its varying severity and the inconstant distribution of the lesions, sarcoidosis is a protean clinical disease. It may be discovered unexpectedly on routine chest films as bilateral hilar adenopathy or may present with peripheral lymphadenopathy, cutaneous lesions, eye involvement, splenomegaly, or hepatomegaly. In the great majority of cases, however, individuals seek medical attention because of the insidious onset of respiratory abnormalities (shortness of breath, cough, chest pain, hemoptysis) or of constitutional signs and symptoms (fever, fatigue, weight loss, anorexia, night sweats).

Sarcoidosis follows an unpredictable course characterized by either progressive chronicity or periods of activity interspersed with remissions, sometimes permanent, that may be spontaneous or induced by steroid therapy. Overall, 65% to 70% of affected patients recover with minimal or no residual manifestations. Twenty percent have permanent loss of some lung function or some permanent visual impairment. Of the remaining 10% to 15%, some die of cardiac or central nervous system damage, but most succumb to progressive pulmonary fibrosis and cor pulmonale.

Hypersensitivity Pneumonitis

The term *hypersensitivity pneumonitis* describes a spectrum of immunologically mediated, predominantly interstitial, lung disorders caused by intense, often prolonged exposure to inhaled organic antigens.[92] Affected individuals have an abnormal sensitivity or heightened reactivity to the antigen, which, in contrast to that occurring in asthma, involves primarily the *alveoli* (thus the synonym "allergic alveolitis").[93] *It is important to recognize these diseases early in their course because progression to serious chronic fibrotic lung disease can be prevented by removal of the environmental agent.*

Most commonly, hypersensitivity results from the inhalation of organic dust containing antigens made up of spores of thermophilic bacteria, true fungi, animal proteins, or bacterial products. Numerous specifically named syndromes are described, depending on the occupation or exposure of the individual. *Farmer's lung* results from exposure to dusts generated from harvested humid, warm hay that permits the rapid proliferation of the spores of thermophilic actinomycetes. *Pigeon breeder's lung* (bird fancier's disease) is provoked by proteins from serum, excreta, or feathers of birds. *Humidifier* or *air-conditioner lung* is caused by thermophilic bacteria in heated water reservoirs.

Several lines of evidence suggest that hypersensitivity pneumonitis is an immunologically mediated disease:

- Bronchoalveolar lavage specimens obtained during the acute phase show increased levels of proinflammatory chemokines such as macrophage inflammatory protein 1α and IL-8.
- Bronchoalveolar lavage specimens also consistently demonstrate increased numbers of T lymphocytes of both CD4+ and CD8+ phenotypes.
- Most patients have specific antibodies in their serum, a feature that is suggestive of type III (immune complex) hypersensitivity.
- Complement and immunoglobulins have been demonstrated within vessel walls by immunofluorescence, also indicating a type III hypersensitivity.

Finally, the presence of noncaseating granulomas in two thirds of the patients suggests the development of a T cell–mediated (type IV) delayed-type hypersensitivity against the implicated antigen(s).

Morphology. Histologic changes in subacute and chronic forms are characteristically centered on bronchioles.[94] They include (1) interstitial pneumonitis consisting primarily of lymphocytes, plasma cells, and macrophages; (2) noncaseating granulomas in two thirds of patients (Fig. 15–23); and (3) interstitial fibrosis, honeycombing, and obliterative bronchiolitis (in late stages). In more than half the patients there is also evidence of an intra-alveolar infiltrate.

Clinical Features. The clinical manifestations are varied. Acute attacks, which follow inhalation of antigenic dust in sensitized patients, consist of recurring episodes of fever, dyspnea, cough, and leukocytosis. Diffuse and nodular infiltrates appear in the chest radiograph, and pulmonary function tests show an acute restrictive disorder. Symptoms usually appear 4 to 6 hours after exposure. If exposure is continuous

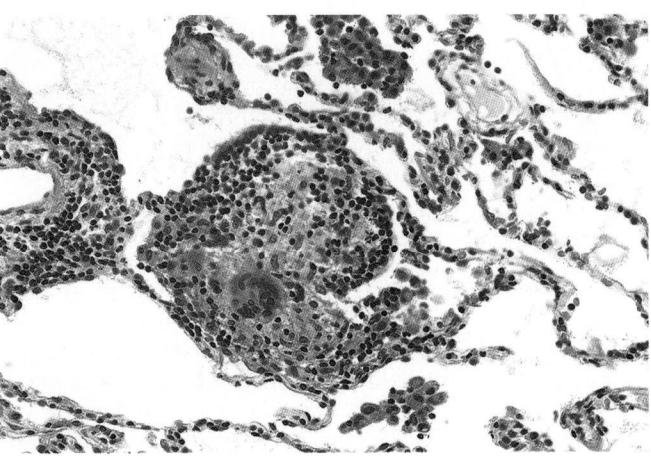

FIGURE 15–23 Hypersensitivity pneumonitis, histologic appearance. Loosely formed interstitial granulomas and chronic inflammation are characteristic.

and protracted, a chronic form of the disease supervenes with progressive respiratory failure, dyspnea, and cyanosis and a decrease in total lung capacity and compliance—a picture similar to other forms of chronic interstitial disease.

PULMONARY EOSINOPHILIA

Several clinical and pathologic pulmonary entities are characterized by an infiltration of eosinophils, recruited in part by elevated alveolar levels of eosinophil attractants such as IL-5.[95]

Pulmonary eosinophilia is divided into the following categories[96]:

- Acute eosinophilic pneumonia with respiratory failure
- Simple pulmonary eosinophilia or Löffler syndrome
- Tropical eosinophilia, caused by infection with microfilariae
- Secondary eosinophilia (which occurs in a number of parasitic, fungal, and bacterial infections; in hypersensitivity pneumonitis; in drug allergies; and in association with asthma, allergic bronchopulmonary aspergillosis, or vasculitis)
- So-called idiopathic chronic eosinophilic pneumonia

Acute eosinophilic pneumonia with respiratory failure is an acute illness of unknown cause. It has a rapid onset with fever, dyspnea, and hypoxemic respiratory failure. The chest radiograph shows diffuse infiltrates, and bronchoalveolar lavage fluid contains more than 25% eosinophils. There is a prompt response to corticosteroids.

Simple pulmonary eosinophilia is characterized by transient pulmonary lesions, eosinophilia in the blood, and a benign clinical course. CT scans are often quite striking, with shadows of varying size and shape in any of the lobes, suggesting irregular intrapulmonary densities. The alveolar septa are thickened by an infiltrate composed of eosinophils and occasional interspersed giant cells, but there is no vasculitis, fibrosis, or necrosis.

Chronic eosinophilic pneumonia is characterized by focal areas of cellular consolidation of the lung substance distributed chiefly in the periphery of the lung fields. Prominent in these lesions are heavy aggregates of lymphocytes and eosinophils within both the septal walls and the alveolar spaces. These patients have high fever, night sweats, and dyspnea, all of which respond to corticosteroid therapy. Chronic eosinophilic pneumonia is diagnosed when other causes of chronic pulmonary eosinophilia are excluded.

SMOKING-RELATED INTERSTITIAL DISEASES

Smoking-related diseases can be grouped into obstructive diseases (emphysema and chronic bronchitis, already discussed) and restrictive or interstitial diseases. A majority of individuals with idiopathic pulmonary fibrosis are smokers; however, the role of cigarette smoking in its pathogenesis has not been clarified yet. Desquamative interstitial pneumonia (DIP) and respiratory bronchiolitis-associated interstitial lung disease are thought to represent two ends of a spectrum of smoking-associated interstitial lung diseases.[97]

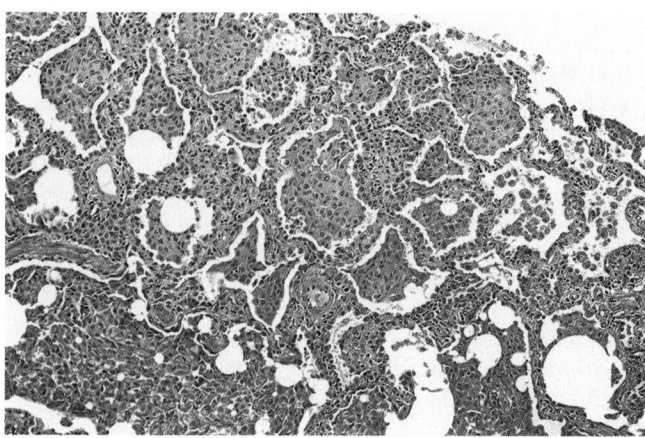

FIGURE 15–24 Desquamative interstitial pneumonia. Medium-power detail of lung demonstrates the accumulation of large numbers of macrophages within the alveolar spaces and only mild fibrous thickening of the alveolar walls.

Desquamative Interstitial Pneumonia

The large collections of airspace macrophages that characterize DIP were originally thought to be desquamated pneumocytes, thus the misnomer "desquamative interstitial pneumonia."

Morphology. The most striking histologic finding is the accumulation of a large number of macrophages with abundant cytoplasm containing dusty brown pigment **(smokers' macrophages)** in the airspaces. Finely granular iron may be seen in the macrophage cytoplasm. Some of the macrophages contain lamellar bodies (composed of surfactant) within phagocytic vacuoles, presumably derived from necrotic type II pneumocytes. The alveolar septa are thickened by a sparse inflammatory infiltrate of lymphocytes, plasma cells, and occasional eosinophils (Fig. 15–24). The septa are lined by plump, cuboidal pneumocytes. Interstitial fibrosis, when present, is mild. Emphysema is often present.

DIP usually presents in the fourth or fifth decade of life, and is more common in men than in women by a ratio of 2:1. Virtually all patients are cigarette smokers. Presenting symptoms include an insidious onset of dyspnea and dry cough over weeks or months, often associated with clubbing of digits. Pulmonary function tests usually show a mild restrictive abnormality with a moderate reduction of the diffusing capacity of carbon dioxide. Patients with DIP typically have a good prognosis with close to 100% response to steroid therapy and cessation of smoking.[65,98]

Respiratory Bronchiolitis-Associated Interstitial Lung Disease

Respiratory bronchiolitis is a common histologic lesion found in cigarette smokers. It is characterized by the presence of pigmented intraluminal macrophages within first- and second-order respiratory bronchioles. In its mildest form, it is seen most often as an incidental histologic finding in the lungs of smokers or ex-smokers.[99] The term *respiratory bronchiolitis-associated interstitial lung disease* is used for patients who develop significant pulmonary symptoms, abnormal pulmonary function, and imaging abnormalities.

> **Morphology.** The changes are patchy at low magnification and have a bronchiolocentric distribution. Respiratory bronchioles, alveolar ducts, and peribronchiolar spaces contain aggregates of dusty brown macrophages (**smokers' macrophages**) similar to those seen in DIP. There is a patchy submucosal and peribronchiolar infiltrate of lymphocytes and histiocytes. Mild peribronchiolar fibrosis is also seen, which expands contiguous alveolar septa. Centrilobular emphysema is common but not severe. Histologic overlap with DIP is often found in different parts of the same lung.

Symptoms are usually mild, consisting of gradual onset of dyspnea and cough in patients who are typically current smokers in the fourth or fifth decade of life with average exposures of over 30 pack-years of cigarette smoking. There is a 2:1 male predominance. Cessation of smoking usually results in improvement.

PULMONARY ALVEOLAR PROTEINOSIS

Pulmonary alveolar proteinosis (PAP) is a rare disease that is characterized radiologically by bilateral patchy asymmetric pulmonary opacifications and histologically by *accumulation of acellular surfactant in the intra-alveolar and bronchiolar spaces*. There are three distinct classes of this disease—acquired, congenital, and secondary PAP—each with a different pathogenesis but with a similar spectrum of histologic changes.

Acquired PAP represents 90% of all cases of PAP and lacks any familial predisposition. Unexpectedly, researchers working with knockout mice lacking the gene for the hematopoietic growth factor granulocyte-macrophage colony-stimulating factor (GM-CSF) found that these mice had impaired surfactant clearance by alveolar macrophages, leading to a condition that resembled human PAP. Subsequently, a GM-CSF–neutralizing autoantibody was found in the serum and bronchial fluid of individuals with acquired PAP that was not present in those with congenital or secondary PAP. Currently, it is thought that the *anti–GM-CSF antibody* is responsible for the development of the disease.[100] These antibodies inhibit the activity of endogenous GM-CSF, leading to a state of functional GM-CSF deficiency. The systemic production of the antibody also provides an explanation for the recurrence of PAP following bilateral-lung transplantation. Thus, acquired PAP is an autoimmune disorder.

Congenital PAP is a rare cause of immediate-onset neonatal respiratory distress. Thus far, mutations have been identified in multiple genes including those encoding ATP-binding cassette protein member A3 (ABCA3) (which may be the most frequent), surfactant protein B (SP-B), surfactant protein C (SP-C), GM-CSF, and GM receptor (GM-CSF/IL-3/IL-5) β chain. ABCA3 is localized to the lamellar body membrane and

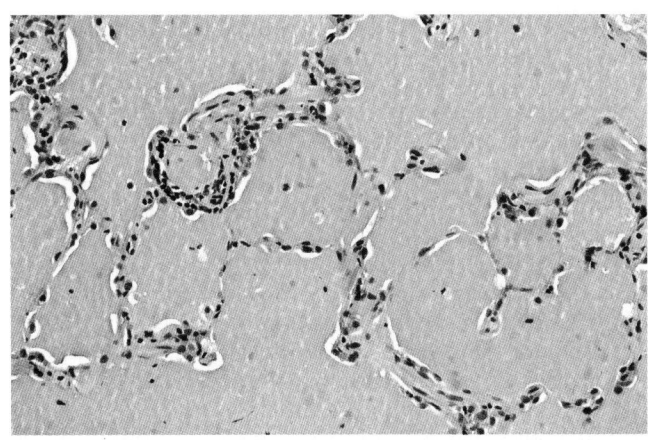

FIGURE 15–25 Pulmonary alveolar proteinosis, histologic appearance. The alveoli are filled with a dense, amorphous, protein-lipid granular precipitate, while the alveolar walls are normal.

is probably involved in transport of surfactant components.[101] SP-B deficiency is transmitted in an autosomal recessive manner and is most often caused by a frameshift mutation in the *SP-B* gene. This leads to an unstable SP-B messenger RNA, reduced or absent SP-B, secondary disturbances of SP-C, and intra-alveolar accumulation of SP-A and SP-C.

Secondary PAP is uncommon. The underlying causes include hematopoietic disorders, malignancies, immunodeficiency disorders, lysinuric protein intolerance, and acute silicosis and other inhalational syndromes.

> **Morphology.** The disease is characterized by a peculiar homogeneous, granular precipitate within the alveoli, causing focal-to-confluent consolidation of large areas of the lungs with minimal inflammatory reaction (Fig. 15–25). On section, turbid fluid exudes from these areas. As a consequence there is a marked increase in the size and weight of the lung. The alveolar precipitate is periodic acid–Schiff positive and also contains cholesterol clefts. Immunohistochemical stains show the presence of surfactant proteins A and C in congenital SP-B deficiency and all three proteins in the acquired form. Ultrastructurally, abnormalities in lamellar bodies in type II pneumocytes can be seen in mutations of *SP-B*, *SP-C*, and *ABCA3*.[102]

Adult patients, for the most part, present with nonspecific respiratory difficulty of insidious onset, cough, and abundant sputum that often contains chunks of gelatinous material. Some have symptoms lasting for years, often with febrile illnesses. These patients are at risk for developing secondary infections with a variety of organisms. Progressive dyspnea, cyanosis, and respiratory insufficiency may occur, but some patients tend to have a benign course, with eventual resolution of the lesions. Whole-lung lavage remains the current standard of care, while GM-CSF therapy is effective in 50% of patients.[103]

Congenital PAP is a fatal respiratory disorder that is usually immediately apparent in the newborn. Typically, the infant is full term and rapidly develops progressive respiratory distress shortly after birth. Without lung transplantation, death ensues between 3 and 6 months of age.

Diseases of Vascular Origin

PULMONARY EMBOLISM, HEMORRHAGE, AND INFARCTION

Blood clots that occlude the large pulmonary arteries are almost always embolic in origin. Large-vessel in situ thromboses are rare and develop only in the presence of pulmonary hypertension, pulmonary atherosclerosis, and heart failure. The usual source of pulmonary emboli—thrombi in the deep veins of the leg in more than 95% of cases—and the magnitude of the clinical problem were discussed in Chapter 4, in which the disturbing frequency of pulmonary embolism and infarction was emphasized. Pulmonary embolism causes more than 50,000 deaths in the United States each year. Its incidence at autopsy has varied from 1% in the general population of hospital patients to 30% in patients dying after severe burns, trauma, or fractures to 65% of hospitalized patients in one study in which special techniques were applied to discover emboli at autopsy. It is the sole or a major contributing cause of death in about 10% of adults who die acutely in hospitals.

Pulmonary embolism is a complication principally in patients who are already suffering from some underlying disorder, such as cardiac disease or cancer, or who are immobilized for several days or weeks, those with hip fracture being at high risk. Hypercoagulable states, either *primary* (e.g., factor V Leiden, prothrombin mutations, and antiphospholipid syndrome) or *secondary* (e.g., obesity, recent surgery, cancer, oral contraceptive use, pregnancy), are frequent risk factors. Indwelling central venous lines can be a nidus for right atrial thrombus, which can be a source of pulmonary embolism.

The pathophysiologic response and clinical significance of pulmonary embolism depend on the extent to which the pulmonary artery blood flow is obstructed, the size of the occluded vessel(s), the number of emboli, the overall status of the cardiovascular system, and the release of vasoactive factors such as thromboxane A_2 from platelets that accumulate at the site of the thrombus. Emboli result in two main pathophysiologic consequences: *respiratory compromise* due to the non-perfused, though ventilated, segment and *hemodynamic compromise* due to increased resistance to pulmonary blood flow engendered by the embolic obstruction.

> **Morphology.** Large emboli lodge in the main pulmonary artery or its major branches or at the bifurcation as a saddle embolus (Fig. 15–26). Sudden death often ensues, largely as a result of the blockage of blood flow through the lungs. Death may also be caused by acute failure of the right side of the heart (**acute cor pulmonale**). Smaller emboli travel out into the more peripheral vessels, where they may cause hemorrhage or infarction. In patients with adequate cardiovascular function, the bronchial arterial supply can sustain the lung parenchyma. Hemorrhages may occur, but there is no infarction. The underlying pul-

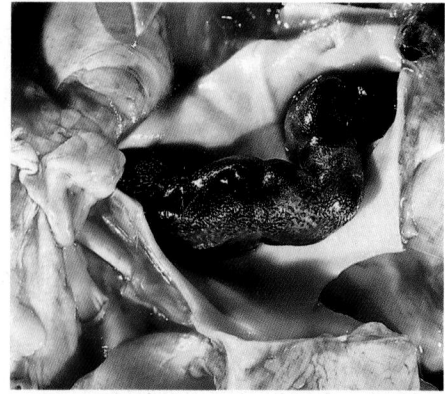

FIGURE 15–26 Large saddle embolus from the femoral vein lying astride the main left and right pulmonary arteries. (From the teaching collection of the Department of Pathology, University of Texas Southwestern Medical School, Dallas, TX.)

> monary architecture is preserved, and resorption of the blood permits reconstitution of the preexisting architecture.
>
> Only about 10% of emboli actually cause infarction, which occurs when the circulation is already inadequate, as in patients with heart or lung disease. Thus, pulmonary infarcts tend to be uncommon in the young. About three fourths of all infarcts affect the lower lobes, and in more than half, multiple lesions occur. They vary in size from lesions that are barely visible to the naked eye to massive involvement of large parts of an entire lobe. Typically, they extend to the periphery of the lung substance as a wedge with the apex pointing toward the hilus of the lung. In many cases, an occluded vessel can be identified near the apex of the infarct. Pulmonary embolus can be distinguished from a post-mortem clot by the presence of the lines of Zahn in the thrombus (Chapter 4).
>
> The pulmonary infarct is classically hemorrhagic and appears as a raised, red-blue area in the early stages (Fig. 15–27). Often, the apposed pleural surface is covered by a fibrinous exudate. The red cells begin to lyse within 48 hours, and the infarct becomes paler and eventually red-brown as hemosiderin is pro-

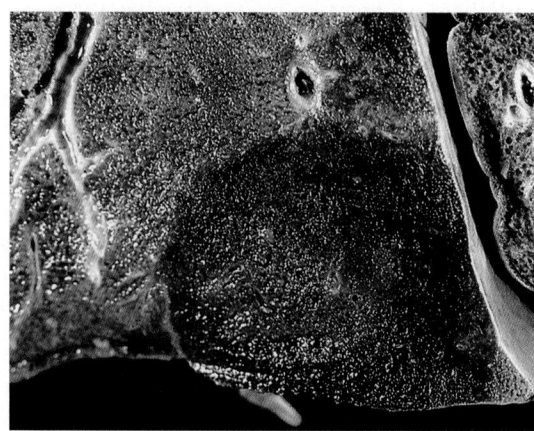

FIGURE 15–27 Recent, small, roughly wedge-shaped hemorrhagic pulmonary infarct.

duced. With the passage of time, fibrous replacement begins at the margins as a gray-white peripheral zone and eventually converts the infarct into a contracted scar. Histologically, the diagnostic feature of acute pulmonary infarction is the ischemic necrosis of the lung substance within the area of hemorrhage, affecting the alveolar walls, bronchioles, and vessels. If the infarct is caused by an infected embolus, it is modified by a more intense neutrophilic inflammatory reaction. Such lesions are referred to as **septic infarcts**, and some convert to abscesses.

Clinical Course. *A large pulmonary embolus is one of the few causes of virtually instantaneous death.* During cardiopulmonary resuscitation in such instances, the patient frequently is said to have *electromechanical dissociation,* in which the electrocardiogram has a rhythm but no pulses are palpated because no blood is entering the pulmonary arterial circulation. If the patient survives after a sizable pulmonary embolus, however, the clinical syndrome may mimic myocardial infarction, with severe chest pain, dyspnea, shock, fever, and increased levels of serum lactate dehydrogenase. Pulmonary hemorrhages due to *small emboli* induce only transient chest pain and cough. Infarcts manifest as dyspnea, tachypnea, fever, chest pain, cough, and hemoptysis. An overlying fibrinous pleuritis may produce a pleural friction rub.

Findings on *chest radiograph* are variable and can be normal or disclose a pulmonary infarct, usually 12 to 36 hours after it has occurred, as a *wedge-shaped infiltrate.* The diagnosis of pulmonary embolism is usually made with spiral computed tomographic angiography. Rarely, other diagnostic methods, such as ventilation perfusion scanning or pulmonary angiography are required. Alternatively, deep vein thrombosis can be diagnosed with duplex ultrasonography. After the initial acute insult, emboli often resolve via contraction and fibrinolysis, particularly in the relatively young. *Unresolved, multiple small emboli over the course of time may lead to pulmonary hypertension,* pulmonary vascular sclerosis, and chronic cor pulmonale. Perhaps most important is that a small embolus may presage a larger one. In the presence of an underlying predisposing condition, *patients with a pulmonary embolus have a 30% chance of developing a second embolus.* Repeated emboli can result in pulmonary arterial hypertension.

Prevention of pulmonary embolism constitutes a major clinical problem for which there is no easy solution. Prophylactic therapy includes early ambulation in postoperative and postpartum patients, elastic stockings and graduated compression stockings for bedridden patients, and anticoagulation in high-risk individuals. It is sometimes necessary to resort to insertion of a filter ("umbrella") into the inferior vena cava or to ligation of this vein, which are not minor procedures in an already seriously ill patient. Treatment of existing pulmonary embolism often includes anticoagulation, preceded by thrombolysis in some cases.

PULMONARY HYPERTENSION

The pulmonary circulation is normally one of low resistance, and pulmonary blood pressure is only about one eighth of systemic blood pressure. Pulmonary hypertension (PH) occurs when mean pulmonary pressure reaches one fourth of systemic levels. The clinical classification of PH groups entities that share similarities in pathophysiologic mechanisms, clinical presentation, and therapeutic options. The groups are (1) pulmonary arterial hypertension, (2) PH with left heart disease, (3) PH associated with lung diseases and/or hypoxemia, (4) PH due to chronic thrombotic and/or embolic disease, and (5) miscellaneous PH.[104]

PH is most frequently associated with structural cardiopulmonary conditions that increase pulmonary blood flow or pressure (or both), pulmonary vascular resistance, or left heart resistance to blood flow. These include the following:

- *Chronic obstructive or interstitial lung diseases:* Patients with these diseases have hypoxia as well as destruction of lung parenchyma and hence have fewer alveolar capillaries. This causes increased pulmonary arterial resistance and, secondarily, elevated pressure.
- *Antecedent congenital or acquired heart disease:* PH occurs in patients with mitral stenosis, for example, because of an increase in left atrial pressure that leads to an increase in pulmonary venous pressure and, consequently, to an increase in pulmonary artery pressure.
- *Recurrent thromboemboli:* Patients with recurrent pulmonary emboli may have PH primarily due to a reduction in the functional cross-sectional area of the pulmonary vascular bed brought about by the obstructing emboli, which, in turn, leads to an increase in pulmonary vascular resistance.
- *Connective tissue diseases:* Several of these diseases (most notably systemic sclerosis) involve the pulmonary vasculature, leading to inflammation, intimal fibrosis, medial hypertrophy, and PH.
- *Obstructive sleep apnea* is a common disorder that is associated with obesity and is now recognized to be a significant contributor to the development of pulmonary hypertension and cor pulmonate.

Uncommonly, PH is encountered sporadically in patients in whom all known causes of increased pulmonary pressure are excluded; this is referred to as *idiopathic pulmonary arterial hypertension.* Even less common is the familial form of pulmonary arterial hypertension with autosomal dominant mode of inheritance. Within these families, there is incomplete penetrance, and only 10% to 20% of the family members actually develop overt disease.

Pathogenesis. As is often the case, much has been learned about the pathogenesis of PH by investigating the molecular basis of the uncommon familial form of the disease. These studies have revealed that *familial PH is caused by mutations in the bone morphogenetic protein receptor type 2 (BMPR2) signaling pathway.*[105]

To understand how such a mutation causes PH, it is essential to review the vascular pathology of the disease and to understand the physiologic functions of BMPR2 signaling. PH is associated with obstruction to the vasculature caused by proliferation of endothelial, smooth muscle, and intimal cells accompanied by concentric laminar intimal fibrosis. How does BMPR2 cause these changes?

BMPR2 is a cell surface protein belonging to the TGF-β receptor superfamily, which binds a variety of cytokines, including TGF-β, bone morphogenetic protein (BMP), activin, and inhibin. Although originally described in the context of bone growth, BMP-BMPR2 signaling is now known to be important for embryogenesis, apoptosis, and cell proliferation and differentiation. The specific effects depend on the tissue and its microenvironment. *In vascular smooth muscle cells BMPR2 signaling causes inhibition of proliferation and favors apoptosis.* Thus, in the absence of such signaling, increased smooth muscle survival and proliferation may be expected. In keeping with this, *inactivating germline mutations in the BMPR2 gene are found in 50% of the familial cases of pulmonary arterial hypertension and 25% of sporadic cases.* In many families, even without mutations in the coding regions of the *BMPR2* gene, linkage to the *BMPR2* locus on chromosome 2q33 can be established, thus indicating that other possible lesions such as gene rearrangements, large deletions, or insertions could be involved.

Despite these discoveries, several questions remain unanswered. First, *how does loss of a single allele of the BMPR2 gene lead to complete loss of signaling?* Two possibilities exist: the mutation might act as a dominant negative (Chapter 5), or a secondary loss of the normal allele might occur in the vascular wall, thus leading to a homozygous loss of *BMPR2.* This is reminiscent of how germline mutations in tumor suppressor genes give rise to neoplasia. Interestingly, in some studies microsatellite instability has been reported in the proliferating endothelial cells within the vascular lesions. This could be a mechanism by which the normal allele is lost in the vasculature. Note that a similar mechanism can inactivate TGF-β receptors in hereditary nonpolyposis colon cancer (Chapters 7 and 17). The second unanswered question is why the phenotypic disease occurs only in 10% to 20% of individuals with *BMPR2* mutations. This strongly points toward the existence of *modifier genes and/or environmental triggers.* Among the modifier genes are those that control vascular tone, including endothelin, prostacyclin synthetase, and angiotensin-converting enzymes. The nature of the environmental factors remains unknown, but presumably they cause dysfunction of vasoregulatory mechanisms. Thus, as with tumor suppressor genes, a two-hit model has been proposed whereby a genetically susceptible individual with a *BMPR2* mutation requires additional genetic or environmental insults to develop the disease (Fig. 15–28).

In *secondary forms of PH*, endothelial cell dysfunction is produced by the process that initiates the disorder, such as the increased shear and mechanical injury associated with left-to-right shunts or the biochemical injury produced by fibrin in thromboembolism. Decreased elaboration of prostacyclin, decreased production of nitric oxide, and increased release of endothelin all promote pulmonary vasoconstriction. Also, decreased elaboration of prostacyclin and nitric oxide promotes platelet adhesion and activation. Moreover, endothelial activation, as detailed in Chapter 11, makes endothelial cells thrombogenic and promotes the persistence of fibrin. Finally, production and release of growth factors and cytokines induce the migration and replication of vascular smooth muscle cells and elaboration of extracellular matrix.

Some individuals with PH have a vasospastic component; in such patients, pulmonary vascular resistance can be rapidly decreased with vasodilators. Pulmonary arterial hypertension has also been reported after ingestion of certain plants or

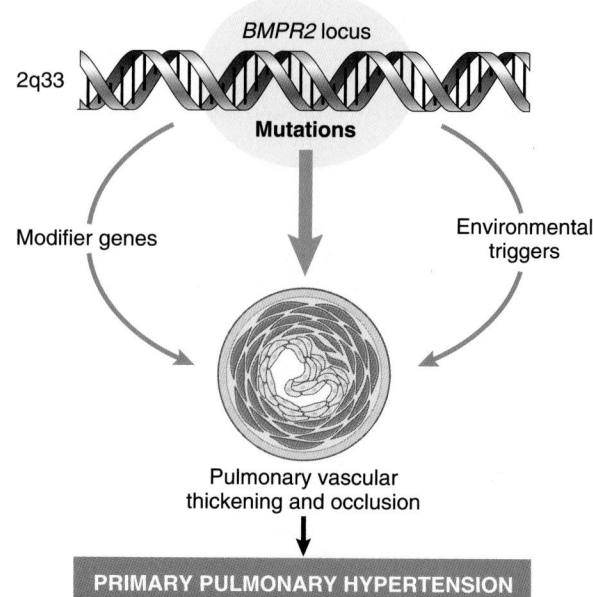

FIGURE 15–28 Pathogenesis of primary pulmonary hypertension. See text for details.

medicines, including the leguminous plant *Crotalaria spectabilis,* which is indigenous to the tropics and used medicinally in *bush tea*; the appetite depressant *aminorex*; adulterated olive oil; and the anti-obesity drugs fenfluramine and phentermine.[106] It has been suggested that such substances might act through effects on serotonin transporter expression or activity.

Morphology. All forms of PH have some common pathologic features regardless of their etiology, that is, **medial hypertrophy of muscular and elastic arteries, atheromas of pulmonary artery** and its major branches, and **right ventricular hypertrophy.**[107] The presence of many organizing or recanalized thrombi favors recurrent pulmonary emboli as the cause, and the coexistence of diffuse pulmonary fibrosis, or severe emphysema and chronic bronchitis, points to chronic hypoxia as the initiating event. The vessel changes can involve the entire arterial tree, from the main pulmonary arteries down to the arterioles (Fig. 15–29). In the most severe cases, atheromatous deposits form in the pulmonary artery and its major branches, resembling (but lesser in degree than) systemic atherosclerosis. The arterioles and small arteries (40 to 300 µm in diameter) are most prominently affected, with striking increases in the muscular thickness of the media (medial hypertrophy) and intimal fibrosis, sometimes narrowing the lumens to pinpoint channels. One extreme in the spectrum of pathologic changes, present most prominently in idiopathic and familial pulmonary arterial hypertension, unrepaired congenital heart disease with left-to-right shunts, and PH associated with drugs and HIV, is the **plexiform lesion,** so called because a tuft of capillary formations

young children. Clinical signs and symptoms of all forms of hypertension become evident only with advanced disease. In cases of idiopathic disease, the presenting features are usually dyspnea and fatigue, but some patients have chest pain of the anginal type. Over time, severe respiratory distress, cyanosis, and right ventricular hypertrophy occur, and death from decompensated cor pulmonale, often with superimposed thromboembolism and pneumonia, usually ensues within 2 to 5 years in 80% of patients.[109]

Conventional therapies (oxygen supplementation, calcium channel blockers, anticoagulation, digoxin, and diuretics) are helpful in the short course.[110] However, recently developed specific therapies such as prostacyclin analogues, endothelial receptor antagonists, inhaled nitric oxide, and phosphodiesterase-5 inhibitors[111–113] have improved the outcome in many patients. Lung transplantation provides definitive treatment for selected patients. Gene therapy has been successful in animals and may be possible for humans in the future.[114]

DIFFUSE PULMONARY HEMORRHAGE SYNDROMES

Hemorrhage from the lung is a dramatic complication of some interstitial lung disorders.[115,116] Among these so-called *pulmonary hemorrhage syndromes* (Fig. 15–30) are (1) Goodpasture syndrome, (2) idiopathic pulmonary hemosiderosis, and (3) vasculitis-associated hemorrhage, which is found in conditions such as hypersensitivity angiitis, Wegener granulomatosis, and lupus erythematosus (Chapter 11).

Goodpasture Syndrome

Goodpasture syndrome is an uncommon autoimmune disease in which kidney and lung injury are caused by circulating autoantibodies against the noncollagenous domain of the α3

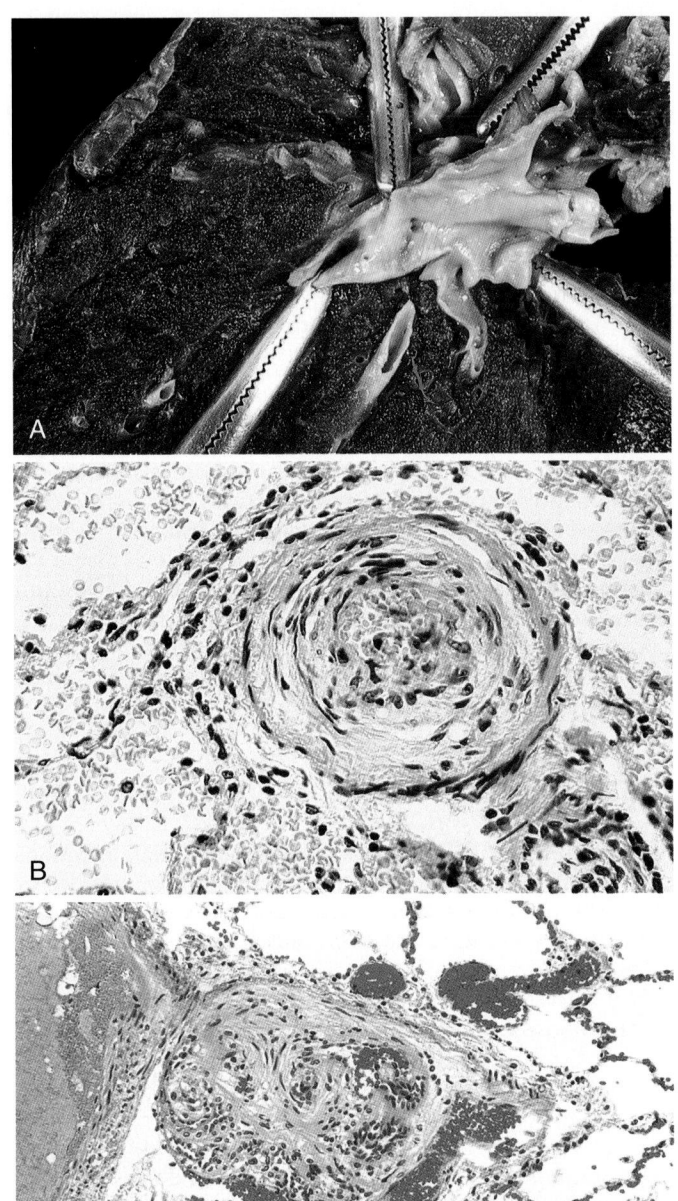

FIGURE 15–29 Vascular changes in pulmonary hypertension. **A,** Gross photograph of atheroma formation, a finding usually limited to large vessels. **B,** Marked medial hypertrophy. **C,** Plexiform lesion characteristic of advanced pulmonary hypertension seen in small arteries.

is present, producing a network, or web, that spans the lumens of dilated thin-walled, small arteries and may extend outside the vessel. Dilated vessels and arteritis may also be present. Rarely, extensive occlusion of the veins by fibrous tissue can be the cause of PH.[108]

Clinical Course. Idiopathic PH is most common in women who are 20 to 40 years of age and is also seen occasionally in

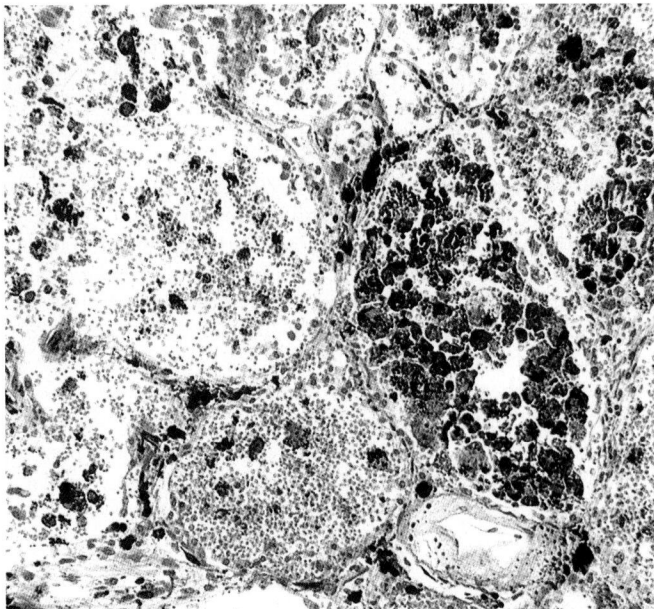

FIGURE 15–30 Diffuse pulmonary hemorrhage syndrome. Acute intra-alveolar hemorrhage and hemosiderin-laden macrophages, reflecting previous hemorrhage, are common features (Prussian blue stain for iron).

chain of collagen IV. The antibodies initiate inflammatory destruction of the basement membrane in renal glomeruli and pulmonary alveoli,[117] giving rise to *proliferative, usually rapidly progressive glomerulonephritis and a necrotizing hemorrhagic interstitial pneumonitis.* Most cases occur in the teens or 20s, and in contrast to many other autoimmune diseases, there is a male preponderance. In one study 89% of patients were active smokers.[118]

Pathogenesis. The immunopathogenesis of the syndrome and the nature of the Goodpasture antigens are described in Chapter 20. The trigger that initiates the anti–basement membrane antibodies is still unknown. Since the epitopes that evoke anti-collagen antibodies are normally hidden within the molecule, it is presumed that some environmental insult such as viral infection, exposure to hydrocarbon solvents (used in the dry cleaning industry), or smoking is required to unmask the cryptic epitopes. As in other autoimmune disorders, a genetic predisposition is indicated by association with certain HLA subtypes (e.g., HLA-DRB1*1501 and *1502).[115]

> **Morphology.** In the classic case, the lungs are heavy, with areas of red-brown consolidation. Histologically, there is focal necrosis of alveolar walls associated with intra-alveolar hemorrhages. Often the alveoli contain hemosiderin-laden macrophages (see Fig. 15–30). In later stages there may be fibrous thickening of the septae, hypertrophy of type II pneumocytes, and organization of blood in alveolar spaces. In many cases immunofluorescence studies reveal linear deposits of immunoglobulins along the basement membranes of the septal walls. The kidneys have the characteristic findings of focal proliferative glomerulonephritis in early cases or crescentic glomerulonephritis in patients with rapidly progressive glomerulonephritis. Diagnostic linear deposits of immunoglobulins and complement are seen by immunofluorescence studies along the glomerular basement membranes even in the few patients without renal disease.

Clinical Features. Most cases begin clinically with respiratory symptoms, principally hemoptysis, and radiographic evidence of focal pulmonary consolidations. Soon, manifestations of glomerulonephritis appear, leading to rapidly progressive renal failure. The most common cause of death is uremia. The once dismal prognosis for this disease has been markedly improved by intensive *plasmapheresis.* This procedure is thought to be beneficial by removing circulating anti–basement membrane antibodies as well as chemical mediators of immunological injury. Simultaneous immunosuppressive therapy inhibits further antibody production, ameliorating both lung hemorrhage and glomerulonephritis.

Idiopathic Pulmonary Hemosiderosis

Idiopathic pulmonary hemosiderosis is a rare disorder characterized by intermittent, diffuse alveolar hemorrhage. Most cases occur in young children, although the disease has been reported in adults as well.[119] It usually presents with an insidious onset of productive cough, hemoptysis, anemia, and weight loss associated with diffuse pulmonary infiltrations similar to Goodpasture syndrome.

The cause and pathogenesis are unknown, and no anti–basement membrane antibodies are detectable in serum or tissues. However, favorable response to long-term immunosuppression with prednisone and/or azathioprine indicates that an immunological mechanism could be involved in the pulmonary capillary damage underlying alveolar bleeding. In addition, long-term follow-up of patients shows that some of them develop other immune disorders.[120]

Wegener Granulomatosis

This autoimmune disease most often involves the upper respiratory tract and/or the lungs, with hemoptysis being the common presenting symptom. Its features are discussed in Chapter 11. Here, it is enough to emphasize that a transbronchial lung biopsy might provide the only tissue available for diagnosis. Since the amount of tissue is small, necrosis and granulomatous vasculitis might not be present. Rather, the diagnostically important features are *capillaritis and scattered, poorly formed granulomas* (unlike those of sarcoidosis, which are rounded and well-defined).

Pulmonary Infections

Respiratory tract infections are more frequent than infections of any other organ and account for the largest number of workdays lost in the general population. The vast majority are upper respiratory tract infections caused by viruses (common cold, pharyngitis), but bacterial, viral, mycoplasmal, and fungal infections of the lung (pneumonia) still account for an enormous amount of morbidity and are responsible for one sixth of all deaths in the United States.[121] Pneumonia can be very broadly defined as any infection of the lung parenchyma.

Pulmonary defense mechanisms are described in Chapter 8. Pneumonia can result whenever these local defense mechanisms are impaired or the systemic resistance of the host is lowered. Factors that affect resistance in general include chronic diseases, immunological deficiency, treatment with immunosuppressive agents, and leukopenia. The local defense mechanisms of the lung can be interfered with by many factors, such as the following:

- *Loss or suppression of the cough reflex,* as a result of coma, anesthesia, neuromuscular disorders, drugs, or chest pain (may lead to *aspiration* of gastric contents)
- *Injury to the mucociliary apparatus,* by either impairment of ciliary function or destruction of ciliated epithelium, due to cigarette smoke, inhalation of hot or corrosive gases, viral diseases, or genetic defects of ciliary function (e.g., the immotile cilia syndrome)
- *Accumulation of secretions* in conditions such as cystic fibrosis and bronchial obstruction
- *Interference with the phagocytic* or bactericidal action of alveolar macrophages by alcohol, tobacco smoke, anoxia, or oxygen intoxication
- Pulmonary *congestion and edema*

Defects in innate immunity (including neutrophil and complement defects) and humoral immunodeficiency typically lead to an increased incidence of infections with pyogenic bacteria. On the other hand, cell-mediated immune defects (congenital and acquired) lead to increased infections with intracellular microbes such as mycobacteria and herpesviruses as well as with microorganisms of very low virulence, such as *Pneumocystis jiroveci*.

Several other points should be emphasized. First, *one type of pneumonia sometimes predisposes to another, especially in debilitated patients.* For example, the most common cause of death in viral influenza epidemics is superimposed bacterial pneumonia. Second, although the portal of entry for most pneumonias is the respiratory tract, *hematogenous spread from one organ to other organs can occur,* and secondary seeding of the lungs may be difficult to distinguish from primary pneumonia. Finally, many *patients with chronic diseases acquire terminal pneumonias while hospitalized (nosocomial infection).* Bacteria common to the hospital environment may have acquired resistance to antibiotics; opportunities for spread are increased; invasive procedures, such as intubations and injections, are common; and bacteria may contaminate equipment used in respiratory care units.

Pneumonias are classified by the specific etiologic agent, which determines the treatment, or, if no pathogen can be isolated, by the clinical setting in which the infection occurs. The latter considerably narrows the list of suspected pathogens for administering empirical antimicrobial therapy. As Table 15–8 indicates, pneumonia can arise in seven distinct clinical settings ("pneumonia syndromes"), and the implicated pathogens are reasonably specific to each category.

COMMUNITY-ACQUIRED ACUTE PNEUMONIAS

Community-acquired pneumonias may be bacterial or viral. Often, the bacterial infection follows an upper respiratory tract viral infection. Bacterial invasion of the lung parenchyma causes the alveoli to be filled with an inflammatory exudate, thus causing consolidation ("solidification") of the pulmonary tissue. Many variables, such as the specific etiologic agent, the host reaction, and the extent of involvement, determine the precise form of pneumonia. Predisposing conditions include extremes of age, chronic diseases (congestive heart failure, COPD, and diabetes), congenital or acquired immune deficiencies, and decreased or absent splenic function (sickle cell disease or post-splenectomy, which puts the patient at risk for infection with encapsulated bacteria such as pneumococcus).

Streptococcus pneumoniae

Streptococcus pneumoniae, or *pneumococcus,* is the most common cause of community-acquired acute pneumonia. Examination of Gram-stained sputum is an important step in the diagnosis of acute pneumonia. The presence of numerous neutrophils containing the typical gram-positive, lancet-shaped diplococci supports the diagnosis of pneumococcal pneumonia, but it must be remembered that *S. pneumoniae* is a part of the endogenous flora in 20% of adults, and therefore false-positive results may be obtained. Isolation of pneumo-

TABLE 15–8 The Pneumonia Syndromes
COMMUNITY-ACQUIRED ACUTE PNEUMONIA
Streptococcus pneumoniae *Haemophilus influenzae* *Moraxella catarrhalis* *Staphylococcus aureus* *Legionella pneumophila* Enterobacteriaceae (*Klebsiella pneumoniae*) and *Pseudomonas* spp.
COMMUNITY-ACQUIRED ATYPICAL PNEUMONIA
Mycoplasma pneumoniae *Chlamydia* spp. (*C. pneumoniae, C. psittaci, C. trachomatis*) *Coxiella burnetii* (Q fever) Viruses: respiratory syncytial virus, parainfluenza virus (children); influenza A and B (adults); adenovirus (military recruits); SARS virus
HOSPITAL-ACQUIRED PNEUMONIA
Gram-negative rods, Enterobacteriaceae (*Klebsiella* spp., *Serratia marcescens, Escherichia coli*) and *Pseudomonas* spp. *Staphylococcus aureus* (usually penicillin resistant)
ASPIRATION PNEUMONIA
Anaerobic oral flora (*Bacteroides, Prevotella, Fusobacterium, Peptostreptococcus*), admixed with aerobic bacteria (*Streptococcus pneumoniae, Staphylococcus aureus, Haemophilus influenzae,* and *Pseudomonas aeruginosa*)
CHRONIC PNEUMONIA
Nocardia *Actinomyces* Granulomatous: *Mycobacterium tuberculosis* and atypical mycobacteria, *Histoplasma capsulatum, Coccidioides immitis, Blastomyces dermatitidis*
NECROTIZING PNEUMONIA AND LUNG ABSCESS
Anaerobic bacteria (extremely common), with or without mixed aerobic infection *Staphylococcus aureus, Klebsiella pneumoniae, Streptococcus pyogenes,* and type 3 pneumococcus (uncommon)
PNEUMONIA IN THE IMMUNOCOMPROMISED HOST
Cytomegalovirus *Pneumocystis jiroveci* *Mycobacterium avium-intracellulare* Invasive aspergillosis Invasive candidiasis "Usual" bacterial, viral, and fungal organisms (listed above)

SARS, severe acute respiratory syndrome.

cocci from blood cultures is more specific but less sensitive (in the early phase of illness, only 20% to 30% of patients have positive blood cultures). Pneumococcal vaccines containing capsular polysaccharides from the common serotypes are used in patients at high risk.

Haemophilus influenzae

Haemophilus influenzae is a pleomorphic, gram-negative organism that is a major cause of life-threatening acute lower respiratory tract infections and meningitis in young children. In adults it is a very common cause of community-acquired acute pneumonia.[122] This bacterium is a ubiquitous colonizer of the pharynx, where it exists in two forms: encapsulated (5%) and unencapsulated (95%). Typically, the encapsulated form dominates the unencapsulated forms by secreting an antibiotic called haemocin that kills the unencapsulated *H. influenzae*.[123] Although there are six serotypes of the encapsulated form (types a to f), type b, which has a polyribose-phosphate capsule, used to be the most frequent cause of severe invasive disease. With routine use of *H. influenzae* conjugate vaccines, the incidence of disease caused by the b serotype has declined significantly. By contrast, infections with nonencapsulated forms are increasing. Also called nontypeable forms, they spread along the surface of the upper respiratory tract and produce otitis media (infection of the middle ear), sinusitis, and bronchopneumonia.

Pili on the surface of *H. influenzae* mediate adherence of the organisms to the respiratory epithelium.[124] In addition, *H. influenzae* secretes a factor that disorganizes ciliary beating and a protease that degrades IgA, the major class of antibody secreted into the airways. Survival of *H. influenzae* in the bloodstream correlates with the presence of the capsule, which, like that of pneumococcus, prevents opsonization by complement and phagocytosis by host cells. Antibodies against the capsule protect the host from *H. influenzae* infection; hence the capsular polysaccharide b is incorporated in the vaccine against *H. influenzae* used for children.

H. influenzae pneumonia, which may follow a viral respiratory infection, is a pediatric emergency and has a high mortality rate. Descending laryngotracheobronchitis results in airway obstruction as the smaller bronchi are plugged by dense, fibrin-rich exudate of polymorphonuclear cells, similar to that seen in pneumococcal pneumonias. Pulmonary consolidation is usually lobular and patchy but may be confluent and involve the entire lung lobe. Before a vaccine became widely available, *H. influenzae* was a common cause of suppurative meningitis in children up to 5 years of age. *H. influenzae* also causes an acute, purulent conjunctivitis (pink eye) in children and, in predisposed older patients, may cause septicemia, endocarditis, pyelonephritis, cholecystitis, and suppurative arthritis. *H. influenzae* is the most common bacterial cause of acute exacerbation of COPD.

Moraxella catarrhalis

Moraxella catarrhalis is being increasingly recognized as a cause of bacterial pneumonia, especially in the elderly. It is the second most common bacterial cause of acute exacerbation of COPD. Along with *S. pneumoniae* and *H. influenzae*, *M. catarrhalis* constitutes one of the three most common causes of otitis media in children.

Staphylococcus aureus

Staphylococcus aureus is an important cause of secondary bacterial pneumonia in children and healthy adults following viral respiratory illnesses (e.g., measles in children and influenza in both children and adults). Staphylococcal pneumonia is associated with a high incidence of complications, such as lung abscess and empyema. *Intravenous drug abusers* are at high risk of developing staphylococcal pneumonia in association with endocarditis. It is also an important cause of hospital-acquired pneumonia, as will be discussed later.

Klebsiella pneumoniae

Klebsiella pneumoniae is the most frequent cause of gram-negative bacterial pneumonia. It commonly afflicts debilitated and malnourished people, particularly *chronic alcoholics*. Thick and gelatinous sputum is characteristic, because the organism produces an abundant viscid capsular polysaccharide, which the patient may have difficulty expectorating.

Pseudomonas aeruginosa

Although *Pseudomonas aeruginosa* most commonly causes hospital-acquired infections, it is mentioned here because of its occurrence in cystic fibrosis patients. It is common in patients who are neutropenic and it has a propensity to invade blood vessels with consequent extrapulmonary spread. *Pseudomonas* septicemia is a very fulminant disease.

Legionella pneumophila

Legionella pneumophila is the agent of Legionnaires' disease, an eponym for the epidemic and sporadic forms of pneumonia caused by this organism. It also causes Pontiac fever, a related self-limited upper respiratory tract infection. This organism flourishes in artificial aquatic environments, such as water-cooling towers and within the tubing system of domestic (potable) water supplies. The mode of transmission is either inhalation of aerosolized organisms or aspiration of contaminated drinking water. *Legionella* pneumonia is common in individuals with some predisposing condition such as cardiac, renal, immunological, or hematologic disease. *Organ transplant recipients are particularly susceptible.* It can be quite severe, frequently requiring hospitalization, and immunosuppressed patients may have fatality rates of up to 50%. Rapid diagnosis is facilitated by demonstration of *Legionella* antigens in the urine or by a positive fluorescent antibody test on sputum samples; culture remains the gold standard of diagnosis.

Morphology. Bacterial pneumonia has two patterns of anatomic distribution: lobular bronchopneumonia and lobar pneumonia (Fig. 15–31). Patchy consolidation of the lung is the dominant characteristic of **bronchopneumonia** (Fig. 15–32), while fibrinosuppurative consolidation of a large portion of a lobe or of an entire lobe defines **lobar pneumonia** (Fig. 15–33). These anatomic but still classic categorizations are often difficult to apply in individual cases because patterns overlap. The patchy involvement may become confluent, producing virtually total lobar consolidation; in contrast, effective antibiotic therapy for any form of pneumonia may limit involvement to a subtotal consolidation. Moreover, the same organisms may produce either pattern depending on patient susceptibility. **Most important from the clinical standpoint are identification of the causative agent and determination of the extent of disease.**

In **lobar pneumonia**, four stages of the inflammatory response have classically been described: congestion, red hepatization, gray hepatization, and

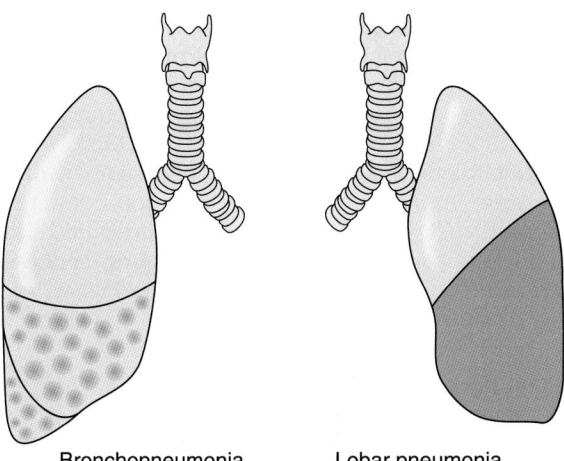

Bronchopneumonia   Lobar pneumonia

FIGURE 15–31 Comparison of bronchopneumonia and lobar pneumonia.

resolution. Current effective antibiotic therapy frequently slows or halts the progression. In the first stage of **congestion** the lung is heavy, boggy, and red. It is characterized by vascular engorgement, intra-alveolar fluid with few neutrophils, and often the presence of numerous bacteria. The stage of **red hepatization** that follows is characterized by massive confluent exudation with neutrophils, red cells, and fibrin filling the alveolar spaces (Fig. 15–34A). On gross examination, the lobe now appears distinctly red, firm, and airless, with a liver-like consistency, hence the term **hepatization**. The stage of **gray hepatization** follows with progressive disintegration of

red cells and the persistence of a fibrinosuppurative exudate (Fig. 15–34B), giving the gross appearance of a grayish brown, dry surface. In the final stage of **resolution** the consolidated exudate within the alveolar spaces undergoes progressive enzymatic digestion to produce granular, semifluid debris that is resorbed, ingested by macrophages, expectorated, or organized by fibroblasts growing into it (Fig. 15–34C). Pleural fibrinous reaction to the underlying inflammation, often present in the early stages if the consolidation extends to the surface (**pleuritis**), may similarly resolve. More often it undergoes organization, leaving fibrous thickening or permanent adhesions.

Foci of **bronchopneumonia** are consolidated areas of acute suppurative inflammation. The consolidation may be patchy through one lobe but is more often multilobar and frequently bilateral and basal because of the tendency of secretions to gravitate into the lower lobes. Well-developed lesions are slightly elevated, dry, granular, gray-red to yellow, and poorly delimited at their margins (see Fig. 15–32). Histologically, the reaction usually elicits a suppurative, neutrophil-rich exudate that fills the bronchi, bronchioles, and adjacent alveolar spaces (Fig. 15–34A).

Complications of pneumonia include (1) tissue destruction and necrosis, causing **abscess formation** (particularly common with type 3 pneumococci or *Klebsiella* infections); (2) spread of infection to the pleural cavity, causing the intrapleural fibrinosuppurative reaction known as **empyema**; and (3) **bacteremic dissemination** to the heart valves, pericardium, brain, kidneys, spleen, or joints, causing metastatic abscesses, endocarditis, meningitis, or suppurative arthritis.

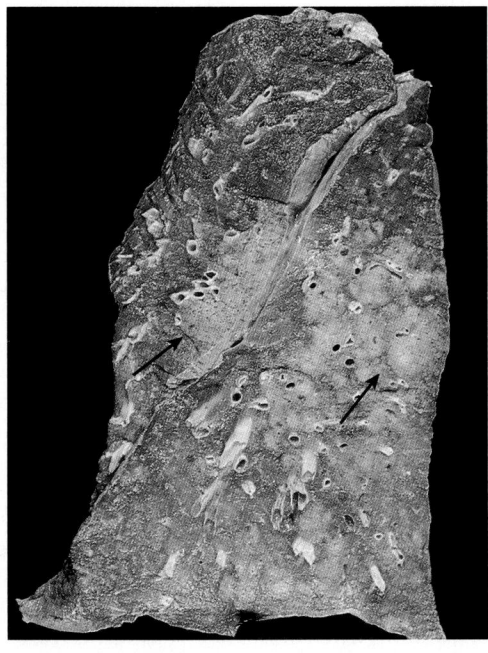

FIGURE 15–32 Bronchopneumonia. Gross section of lung showing patches of consolidation *(arrows)*.

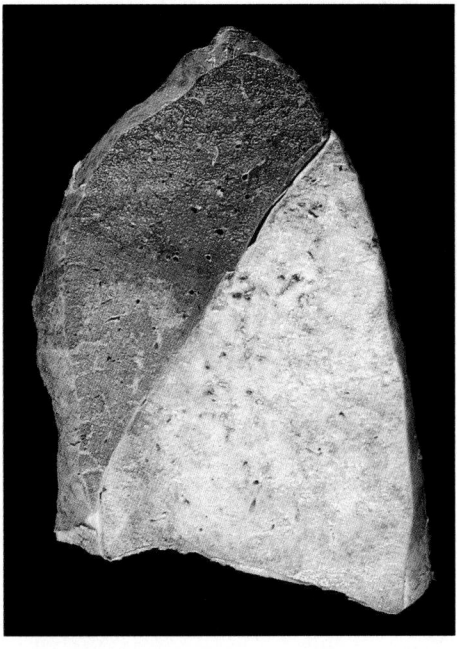

FIGURE 15–33 Lobar pneumonia—gray hepatization, gross photograph. The lower lobe is uniformly consolidated.

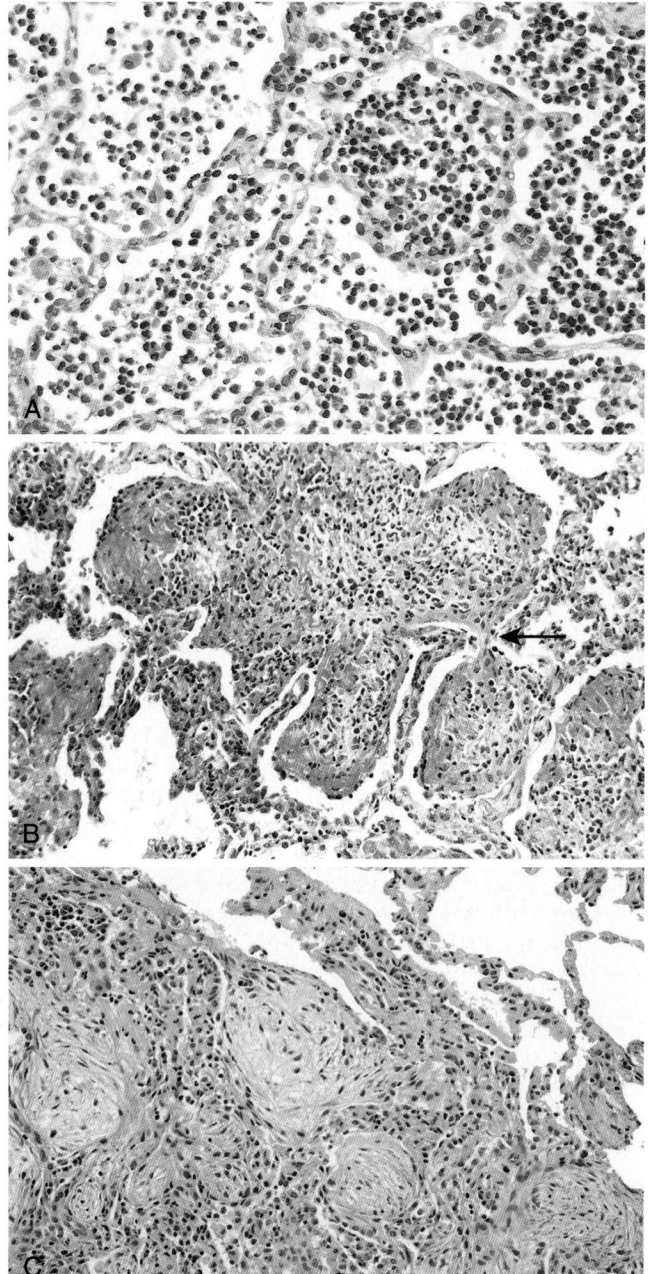

FIGURE 15–34 Stages of bacterial pneumonia. **A,** Acute pneumonia. The congested septal capillaries and extensive neutrophil exudation into alveoli corresponds to early red hepatization. Fibrin nets have not yet formed. **B,** Early organization of intra-alveolar exudate, seen in areas to be streaming through the pores of Kohn *(arrow).* **C,** Advanced organizing pneumonia featuring transformation of exudates to fibromyxoid masses richly infiltrated by macrophages and fibroblasts.

Clinical Course. The major symptoms of community-acquired acute pneumonia are abrupt onset of high fever, shaking chills, and cough productive of mucopurulent sputum; occasional patients may have hemoptysis. When fibrinosuppurative pleuritis is present it is accompanied by pleuritic pain and pleural friction rub. The whole lobe is radiopaque in lobar pneumonia, whereas there are focal opacities in bronchopneumonia.

The clinical picture is markedly modified by the administration of antibiotics. Treated patients may be relatively afebrile with few clinical signs 48 to 72 hours after the initiation of antibiotics. The identification of the organism and the determination of its antibiotic sensitivity are the keystones to appropriate therapy. Fewer than 10% of patients with pneumonia severe enough to merit hospitalization now succumb, and in most such instances death may be attributed either to a complication, such as empyema, meningitis, endocarditis, or pericarditis, or to some predisposing influence, such as debility or chronic alcoholism.

COMMUNITY-ACQUIRED ATYPICAL (VIRAL AND MYCOPLASMAL) PNEUMONIAS

The term *primary atypical pneumonia* was initially applied to an acute febrile respiratory disease characterized by patchy inflammatory changes in the lungs, largely confined to the alveolar septa and pulmonary interstitium. The term *atypical* denotes the moderate amount of sputum, no physical findings of consolidation, only moderate elevation of white cell count, and lack of alveolar exudate. The pneumonitis is caused by a variety of organisms, the most common being *Mycoplasma pneumoniae. Mycoplasma* infections are particularly common among children and young adults. They occur sporadically or as local epidemics in closed communities (schools, military camps, and prisons). Other etiologic agents are viruses, including influenza virus types A and B, the respiratory syncytial viruses, human metapneumovirus, adenovirus, rhinoviruses, rubeola, and varicella viruses; *Chlamydia pneumoniae*; and *Coxiella burnetii* (Q fever).[124,125] In some cases the cause cannot be determined. Any one of these agents can cause merely an upper respiratory tract infection, recognized as the common cold, or a more severe lower respiratory tract infection. Factors that favor such extension of the infection include extremes of age, malnutrition, alcoholism, and underlying debilitating illnesses.

The common pathogenetic mechanism is attachment of the organisms to the upper respiratory tract epithelium followed by necrosis of the cells and an inflammatory response. When the process extends to the alveoli there is usually interstitial inflammation, but there may also be some outpouring of fluid into alveolar spaces, so that on chest x-ray the changes may mimic bacterial pneumonia. Damage to and denudation of the respiratory epithelium inhibit mucociliary clearance and predispose to secondary bacterial infections.

Morphology. All causal agents produce essentially similar morphologic patterns. The lung involvement may be quite patchy or may involve whole lobes bilaterally or unilaterally. The affected areas are red-blue and congested. The pleura is smooth, and pleuritis or pleural effusions are infrequent.

The histologic pattern depends on the severity of the disease. **Predominant is the interstitial nature of the inflammatory reaction, virtually localized within the walls of the alveoli.** The alveolar septa are widened and edematous and usually have a mononuclear inflammatory infiltrate of lymphocytes, macrophages, and occasionally plasma cells. In acute cases neutrophils may also be present. The alveoli may be free from exudate, but in many patients there is intra-alveolar proteinaceous material and a cellular exudate. When complicated by ARDS, characteristically pink hyaline membranes lining the alveolar walls are present (see Fig. 15–3). Eradication of the infection is followed by reconstitution of the normal architecture of the lung.

Superimposed bacterial infection modifies the histologic picture by causing ulcerative bronchitis, bronchiolitis, and bacterial pneumonia. Some viruses, such as herpes simplex, varicella, and adenovirus, may be associated with necrosis of bronchial and alveolar epithelium and acute inflammation. Characteristic viral cytopathic changes are described in Chapter 8.

Clinical Course. The clinical course is extremely varied. Many cases masquerade as severe upper respiratory tract infections or as *chest colds*. Even individuals with well-developed atypical pneumonia have few localizing symptoms. Cough may be absent, and the major manifestations may consist only of fever, headache, muscle aches, and pains in the legs. The edema and exudation are both strategically located to cause mismatching of ventilation and blood flow and thus evoke symptoms out of proportion to the scanty physical findings.

The ordinary sporadic form of the disease is usually mild with a low mortality rate, below 1%. Interstitial pneumonia, however, may assume epidemic proportions with intensified severity and greater mortality, as documented in the devastating influenzal pandemics of 1915 and 1918 and the many smaller epidemics since then. Secondary bacterial infection by staphylococci or streptococci is common in such circumstances.

Influenza Infections

The genome of influenza virus is composed of eight helices of single-stranded RNA, each encoding a single gene and each bound by a nucleoprotein that determines the type of influenza virus (A, B, or C). The spherical surface of influenza virus is a lipid bilayer (envelope) containing the viral hemagglutinin and neuraminidase, which determine the subtype of the virus (H1 to H3; N1 or N2). Host antibodies to the hemagglutinin and neuraminidase prevent and ameliorate, respectively, future infection with the influenza virus. Two mechanisms account for the clearance of primary influenza virus infection: cytotoxic T cells kill virus-infected cells, and an intracellular anti-influenza protein (called Mx1) is induced in macrophages by the cytokines IFN-α and IFN-β.[126]

Influenza viruses of type A infect humans, pigs, horses, and birds and are the major cause of pandemic and epidemic influenza infections. A single subtype of influenza virus A predominates throughout the world at a given time.[127] Epidemics of influenza occur through mutations of the hemagglutinin and neuraminidase that allow the virus to escape most host antibodies *(antigenic drift)*. Pandemics, which are longer and more widespread than epidemics, may occur when both the hemagglutinin and the neuraminidase are replaced

through recombination of RNA segments with those of animal viruses, making all individuals susceptible to the new influenza virus *(antigenic shift)*. Polymerase chain reaction (PCR) analysis of influenza virus from the lungs of a soldier who died in the 1918 influenza pandemic that killed between 20 million and 40 million people worldwide identified a swine influenza virus belonging to the same family of influenza viruses causing illness today.[128] Current antiviral drugs are effective against recombinant influenza viruses bearing the 1918 hemagglutinin, neuraminidase, and matrix genes.[129] Influenza virus types B and C, which do not show antigenic drift or shift, infect mostly children, who develop antibodies that prevent reinfection. Rarely, influenza virus may cause interstitial myocarditis or, after aspirin therapy, Reye syndrome (Chapter 18).

Avian influenza refers to strains of influenza which primarily infect birds. One such strain with the *antigenic type H5N1 is of great concern* because infection is frequently lethal in humans (approximately 60%) and since 2003 the virus is spreading throughout the world in wild and domestic birds. As of the fall of 2008, a total of 387 H5N1 influenza virus infections in humans have been reported to the WHO. Nearly all cases of H5N1 influenza in humans have been acquired by close contact with domestic birds. The severity of the disease results from the ability of the virus to cause widespread infection in the human body, instead of infection being limited to the lung. *The tissue tropism of H5N1 influenza is increased due to the unusual structure of its hemagglutinin protein.* Cleavage of viral hemagglutinin by host proteases is required for the influenza virus to enter host cells. The hemagglutinin protein of H5N1 influenza virus, and other highly pathogenic influenza viruses, is unusual in that it can be cleaved by ubiquitous proteases in the human, while the hemagglutinin of less virulent influenza virus stains can only be cleaved by proteases found in limited organs, including the lung. Fortunately, the transmission of the current H5N1 virus is inefficient. Most patients with H5NI infection present with pneumonia. However, if antigenic recombination occurs between H5N1 influenza and a strain of influenza which is highly infectious for humans, sustained human-to-human transmission could give rise to a pandemic, similar to the Spanish pandemic of 1918. This concern has spurred efforts to develop a vaccine.[130]

> **Morphology.** Viral upper respiratory infections are marked by mucosal hyperemia and swelling with a predominantly lymphomonocytic and plasmacytic infiltration of the submucosa accompanied by overproduction of mucus secretions. The swollen mucosa and viscous exudate may plug the nasal channels, sinuses or the Eustachian tubes, and lead to suppurative secondary bacterial infection. Virus-induced tonsillitis with enlargement of the lymphoid tissue within the Waldeyer ring is frequent in children, although lymphoid hyperplasia is not usually associated with suppuration or abscess formation, such as is encountered with streptococci or staphylococci.
>
> In **laryngotracheobronchitis** and **bronchiolitis** there is vocal cord swelling and abundant mucus exudation. Impairment of bronchociliary function invites bacterial superinfection with more marked suppuration. Plugging of small airways may give rise to focal

lung atelectasis. In the more severe bronchiolar involvement widespread plugging of secondary and terminal airways by cell debris, fibrin, and inflammatory exudate may, when prolonged, cause organization and fibrosis, resulting in obliterative bronchiolitis and permanent lung damage.

Human Metapneumovirus (MPV)

Human MPV, a paramyxovirus discovered in 2001, is found worldwide and is associated with upper and lower respiratory tract infections, most commonly in young children, elderly subjects, and immunocompromised patients. Human MPV can cause severe infections such as bronchiolitis and pneumonia and is responsible for 5% to 10% of hospitalizations and 12% to 20% of outpatient visits of children suffering from acute respiratory tract infections. Such infections are clinically indistinguishable from those caused by human respiratory syncytial virus. The first human MPV infection occurs during early childhood, but reinfections are common throughout life, especially in older subjects. Molecular methods such as reverse transcriptase–PCR are the preferred diagnostic modality because of fastidious growth in cell culture. No commercial treatments are yet available for human MPV, although ribavirin has shown activity both in vitro and in animal models. Live attenuated vaccines produced by genetically altered virus have also shown good efficacy in animals.[131]

Severe Acute Respiratory Syndrome (SARS)

SARS first appeared in November 2002 in the Guangdong Province of China and subsequently spread to Hong Kong, Taiwan, Singapore, Vietnam, and Toronto, where large outbreaks also occurred.[132] The ease of travel between continents clearly contributed to this pandemic. Between Fall 2002 and Spring 2003, there were more than 8000 cases of SARS, including 774 deaths. The worldwide epidemic was halted, perhaps in part because of public health measures, and the last cases of SARS were laboratory-associated infections reported in April 2004.[125]

After an incubation period of 2 to 10 days, SARS begins with a dry cough, malaise, myalgias, fever, and chills. A third of patients improve and resolve the infection, but the rest progress to severe respiratory disease with shortness of breath, tachypnea, and pleurisy, and nearly 10% of patients die from the illness, for which there is no specific treatment.

The cause of SARS is a previously undiscovered coronavirus. Nearly a third of upper respiratory infections are caused by coronaviruses, but the SARS virus differs from previously known coronaviruses in that it infects the lower respiratory tract and spreads throughout the body. *The SARS virus seems to have been first transmitted to humans through contact with wild masked palm civets that are eaten in China.* Subsequent cases were spread person-to-person, mainly through infected respiratory secretions, although some cases may have been contracted from stool.

SARS can be diagnosed either by detection of the virus by PCR or by detection of antibodies to the virus. Levels of the virus are low initially and peak 10 days after onset of illness, so testing of different specimens (respiratory secretions, blood,

and stool) collected on several days may be needed to detect the virus. Detection of antibodies specific for the SARS virus is a very sensitive and specific test; however, patients may not have a measurable antibody response for up to 28 days after infection.

The pathophysiology of SARS is not understood, nor is it known why the virus moved from animals to humans. Most human SARS coronaviruses have a 29-nucleotide deletion in the RNA when compared to the virus found in wild animals, which may enhance its transmission or pathogenicity. In patients who have died of SARS the lungs show diffuse alveolar damage and multinucleated giant cells. Coronaviruses can be seen within pneumocytes by electron microscopy.

HOSPITAL-ACQUIRED PNEUMONIA

Hospital-acquired pneumonias are defined as pulmonary infections acquired in the course of a hospital stay. They are common in patients with severe underlying disease, immunosuppression, prolonged antibiotic therapy, or invasive access devices such as intravascular catheters. Patients on mechanical ventilation are at particularly high risk. Superimposed on an underlying disease (that caused hospitalization), hospital-acquired infections are serious and often life-threatening complications. Gram-negative rods (Enterobacteriaceae and *Pseudomonas* species) and *S. aureus* are the most common isolates; unlike community-acquired pneumonias, *S. pneumoniae* is not a major pathogen.

ASPIRATION PNEUMONIA

Aspiration pneumonia occurs in markedly debilitated patients or those who aspirate gastric contents either while unconscious (e.g., after a stroke) or during repeated vomiting. These patients have abnormal gag and swallowing reflexes that predispose to aspiration. The resultant pneumonia is partly chemical because of the extremely irritating effects of the gastric acid, and partly bacterial (from the oral flora). Typically, more than one organism is recovered on culture, aerobes being more common than anaerobes. This type of pneumonia is often necrotizing, pursues a fulminant clinical course, and is a frequent cause of death. In those who survive, lung abscess is a common complication.

LUNG ABSCESS

The term "pulmonary abscess" describes a local suppurative process within the lung, characterized by necrosis of lung tissue. Oropharyngeal surgical procedures, sinobronchial infections, dental sepsis, and bronchiectasis play important roles in their development.

Etiology and Pathogenesis. Although under appropriate circumstances any pathogen can produce an abscess, the commonly isolated organisms include aerobic and anaerobic streptococci, *S. aureus*, and a host of gram-negative organisms. Mixed infections often occur because of the important causal role played by inhalation of foreign material.[133] *Anaerobic organisms* normally found in the oral cavity, including members of the *Bacteroides*, *Fusobacterium*, and *Peptococcus* species, are the exclusive isolates in about 60% of cases. The causative organisms are introduced by the following mechanisms:

○ *Aspiration of infective material* (the most frequent cause): This is particularly common in acute alcoholism, coma, anesthesia, sinusitis, gingivodental sepsis, and debilitation in which the cough reflexes are depressed.

○ *Antecedent primary lung infection*: Post-pneumonic abscess formations are usually associated with *S. aureus*, *K. pneumoniae*, and the type 3 pneumococcus. Post-transplant or otherwise immunosuppressed individuals are at special risk.

○ *Septic embolism*: Infected emboli from thrombophlebitis in any portion of the systemic venous circulation or from the vegetations of infective bacterial endocarditis on the right side of the heart are trapped in the lung.

○ *Neoplasia*: Secondary infection is particularly common in the bronchopulmonary segment obstructed by a primary or secondary malignancy *(postobstructive pneumonia)*.

○ *Miscellaneous*: Direct traumatic penetrations of the lungs; spread of infections from a neighboring organ, such as suppuration in the esophagus, spine, subphrenic space, or pleural cavity; and hematogenous seeding of the lung by pyogenic organisms all may lead to lung abscess formation.

When all these causes are excluded, there are still cases in which no reasonable basis for the abscess formation can be identified. These are referred to as *primary cryptogenic lung abscesses*.

Morphology. Abscesses vary in diameter from lesions of a few millimeters to large cavities of 5 to 6 cm. They may affect any part of the lung and may be single or multiple. Pulmonary abscesses due to aspiration are more common on the right (because of the more vertical right main bronchus) and are most often single. Abscesses that develop in the course of pneumonia or bronchiectasis are usually multiple, basal, and diffusely scattered. Septic emboli and pyemic abscesses are multiple and may affect any region of the lungs.

The abscess cavity might be filled with suppurative debris. If there is communication with an air passage, the contained exudate may be partially drained to create an air-containing cavity. Superimposed saprophytic infections are prone to flourishing within the already necrotic debris of the abscess cavity. Continued infection leads to large, fetid, green-black, multilocular cavities with poor demarcation of their margins, designated **gangrene of the lung**. The **cardinal histologic change in all abscesses is suppurative destruction of the lung parenchyma within the central area of cavitation** (Fig. 15–35). In chronic cases considerable fibroblastic proliferation produces a fibrous wall.

Clinical Course. The manifestations of pulmonary abscesses are much like those of bronchiectasis and are characterized principally by cough, fever, and copious amounts of foul-smelling purulent or sanguineous sputum. Fever, chest pain, and weight loss are common. Clubbing of the fingers and toes may appear within a few weeks after the onset of an abscess. Diagnosis of this condition can be only suspected

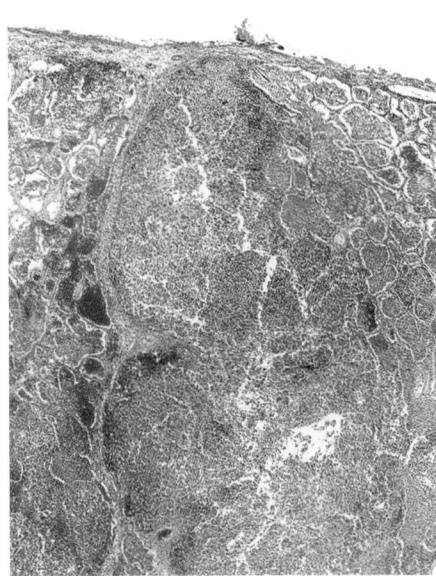

FIGURE 15–35 Pyemic lung abscess (center) with complete destruction of underlying parenchyma within the focus of involvement.

from the clinical findings and must be confirmed radiologically. Whenever an abscess is discovered in older individuals, it is important to rule out an underlying carcinoma, because this is present in 10% to 15% of cases.

The course of abscesses is variable. With antimicrobial therapy, most resolve leaving behind a scar. Complications include extension of the infection into the pleural cavity, hemorrhage, the development of *brain abscesses* or *meningitis* from septic emboli, and (rarely) secondary amyloidosis (type AA).

CHRONIC PNEUMONIA

Chronic pneumonia is most often a localized lesion in the immunocompetent patient, with or without regional lymph node involvement. Typically, the inflammatory reaction is granulomatous, and is caused by bacteria (e.g., *M. tuberculosis*) or fungi (e.g., *Histoplasma capsulatum*). Tuberculosis of the lung and other organs was described in Chapter 8. Here we will discuss chronic pneumonias caused by fungi.

Histoplasmosis, blastomycosis, and *coccidioidomycosis* are discussed together because (1) they are granulomatous diseases of the lungs that may resemble tuberculosis, (2) they are caused by fungi that are thermally dimorphic in that they grow as hyphae that produce spores at environmental temperatures but grow as yeasts (spherules or ellipses) at body temperature within the lungs, and (3) each fungus is geographic in that it causes disease primarily among immunocompetent individuals living along the Ohio and Mississippi rivers and in the Caribbean (*Histoplasma*), in the central and southeastern United States (*Blastomyces*), and in the Southwest and Far West of the United States and in Mexico (*Coccidioides*).

Histoplasmosis

Histoplasma capsulatum infection is acquired by inhalation of dust particles from soil contaminated with bird or bat droppings that contain small spores (microconidia), the infectious form of the fungus. Like *M. tuberculosis, H. capsulatum* is an intracellular parasite of macrophages. The *clinical presentations and morphologic lesions of histoplasmosis also strikingly resemble those of tuberculosis*, including (1) a self-limited and often latent primary pulmonary involvement, which may result in coin lesions on chest radiography; (2) chronic, progressive, secondary lung disease, which is localized to the lung apices and causes cough, fever, and night sweats; (3) localized lesions in extrapulmonary sites, including mediastinum, adrenals, liver, or meninges; and (4) a widely disseminated disease in immunocompromised patients.

The pathogenesis of histoplasmosis is incompletely understood. It is known that macrophages are the major target of infection. *H. capsulatum* may be internalized into macrophages after opsonization with antibody. *Histoplasma* yeasts can multiply within the phagosome, and lyse the host cells. *Histoplasma* infections are controlled by helper T cells that recognize fungal cell wall antigens and heat-shock proteins and subsequently secrete IFN-γ, which activates macrophages to kill intracellular yeasts. In addition, *Histoplasma* induces macrophages to secrete TNF, which recruits and stimulates other macrophages to kill *Histoplasma*. Lacking cellular immunity, patients with acquired immunodeficiency syndrome are susceptible to disseminated infection with *Histoplasma*, which is an opportunistic pathogen in this disease.

Morphology. In the lungs of otherwise healthy adults, *Histoplasma* infections produce epithelioid cell granulomas, which usually undergo caseation necrosis and coalesce to produce large areas of consolidation but may also liquefy to form cavities (seen in patients with COPD). With spontaneous or drug control of the infection, these lesions undergo fibrosis and concentric calcification (tree-bark appearance) (Fig. 15–36A). Histologic differentiation from tuberculosis, sarcoidosis, and coccidioidomycosis requires identification of the 3- to 5-μm thin-walled yeast forms that may persist in tissues for years.

In **fulminant disseminated histoplasmosis**, which occurs in immunosuppressed individuals, epithelioid cell granulomas are not formed; instead, there are focal accumulations of mononuclear phagocytes filled with fungal yeasts throughout the tissues and organs of the body (Fig. 15–36B).

The diagnosis of histoplasmosis is established by culture or identification of the fungus in tissue lesions. In addition, serologic tests for antibodies and antigen are also available. Antigen detection in body fluids is most useful in the early stages, because antibodies are formed 2 to 6 weeks after infection.[134]

Blastomycosis

Blastomyces dermatitidis is a soil-inhabiting, dimorphic fungus that is remarkably difficult to isolate. It is a cause of disease in people living in or visiting the central and southeastern United States; infection also occurs in Canada, Mexico, the Middle East, Africa, and India. *There are three clinical forms: pulmonary blastomycosis, disseminated blastomycosis, and a rare primary cutaneous* form that results from direct inoculation of organisms into the skin. Pulmonary blastomycosis most often presents as an abrupt illness with productive cough, headache, chest pain, weight loss, fever, abdominal pain, night sweats, chills, and anorexia. Chest radiographs reveal lobar consolidation, multilobar infiltrates, perihilar infiltrates, multiple nodules, or miliary infiltrates. The upper lobes are most frequently involved. The process may resolve spontaneously, persist, or progress to a chronic lesion.

Morphology. In the normal host the lung lesions of blastomycosis are suppurative granulomas. Macrophages have a limited ability to ingest and kill *B. dermatitidis*, and the persistence of the yeast cells leads to continued recruitment of neutrophils. In tissue, *B. dermatitidis* is a round, 5- to 15-μm yeast cell that divides by broad-based budding. It has a thick, double-

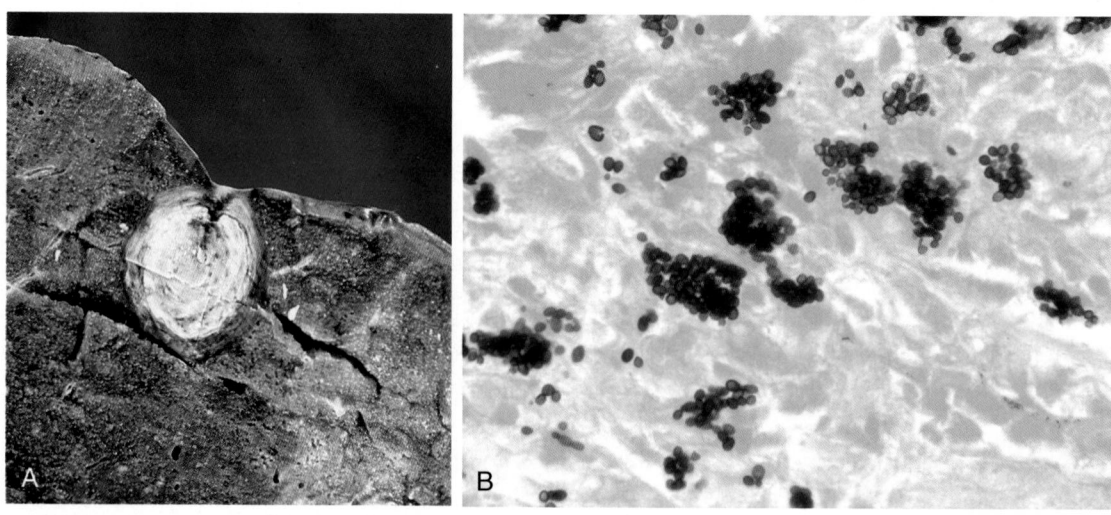

FIGURE 15–36 Histoplasmosis. **A,** Laminated *Histoplasma* granuloma of the lung. **B,** *Histoplasma capsulatum* yeast forms fill phagocytes in the lung of a patient with disseminated histoplasmosis (silver stain).

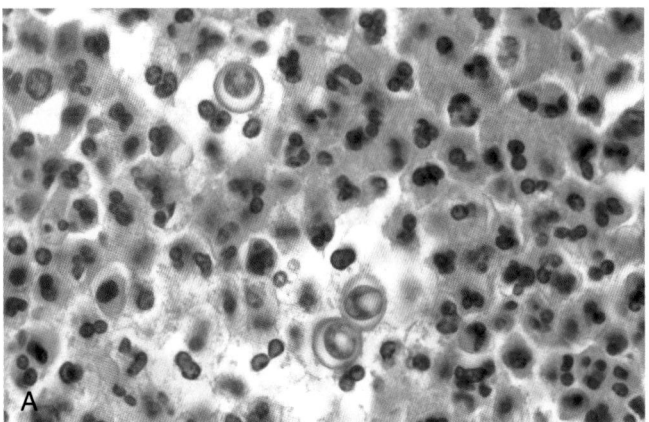
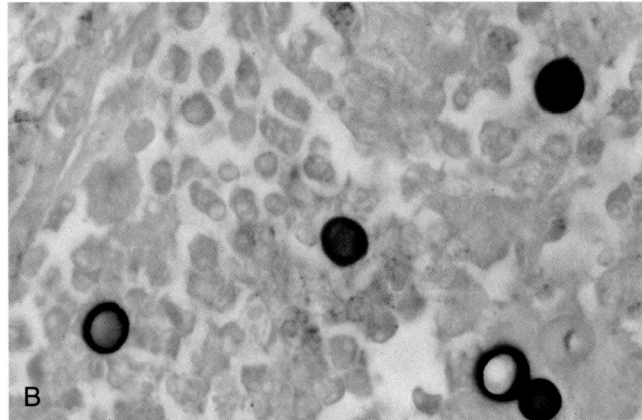

FIGURE 15–37 Blastomycosis. **A,** Rounded budding yeasts, larger than neutrophils, are present. Note the characteristic thick wall and nuclei (not seen in other fungi). **B,** Silver stain.

contoured cell wall and multiple nuclei (Fig. 15–37). Involvement of the skin and larynx is associated with marked epithelial hyperplasia, which may be mistaken for squamous cell carcinoma.

Coccidioidomycosis

Almost everyone who inhales the spores of *Coccidioides immitis* becomes infected and develops a delayed-type hypersensitivity to the fungus, so more than 80% of people in endemic areas of the southwestern and western United States have a positive skin test reaction. One reason for the high rate of infectivity by *C. immitis* is that infective arthroconidia, when ingested by alveolar macrophages, block fusion of the phagosome and lysosome and so resist intracellular killing. As is the case with *Histoplasma*, most primary infections with *C. immitis* are asymptomatic, but 10% of people have lung lesions, fever, cough, and pleuritic pains, accompanied by erythema nodosum or erythema multiforme (the San Joaquin Valley fever complex). Less than 1% of people develop disseminated *C. immitis* infection, which frequently involves the skin and meninges.

> **Morphology.** The primary and secondary lung lesions of *C. immitis* are similar to the granulomatous lesions of *Histoplasma*. Within macrophages or giant cells, *C. immitis* is present as thick-walled, nonbudding spherules 20 to 60 μm in diameter, often filled with small endospores. A pyogenic reaction is superimposed when the spherules rupture to release the endospores (Fig. 15–38). Rare progressive *C. immitis* disease involves the lungs, meninges, skin, bones, adrenals, lymph nodes, spleen, or liver. At all these sites, the inflammatory response may be purely granulomatous, pyogenic, or mixed. Purulent lesions dominate in patients with diminished resistance and with widespread dissemination.

PNEUMONIA IN THE IMMUNOCOMPROMISED HOST

The appearance of a pulmonary infiltrate, with or without signs of infection (e.g., fever), is one of the most common and serious complications in patients whose immune defenses are suppressed by disease, immunosuppressive therapy for organ transplants, chemotherapy for tumors, or irradiation.[135] A wide variety of so-called opportunistic infectious agents, many of which rarely cause infection in normal hosts, can cause these pneumonias, and often more than one agent is involved. Mortality from these opportunistic infections is high. Table 15–9 lists some of the opportunistic agents according to their prevalence and whether they cause local or diffuse pulmonary infiltrates. The differential diagnosis of such infiltrates includes drug reactions and involvement of the lung by tumor. The specific infections are discussed in Chapter 8. Of these, the ones that commonly involve the lung can be classified according to the etiologic agent: (1) bacteria (*P. aeruginosa*, *Mycobacterium* species, *L. pneumophila*, and *Listeria monocytogenes*), (2) viruses (cytomegalovirus [CMV] and herpesvirus), and (3) fungi (*P. jiroveci*, *Candida* species, *Aspergillus* species, the Phycomycetes, and *Cryptococcus neoformans*).

PULMONARY DISEASE IN HUMAN IMMUNODEFICIENCY VIRUS INFECTION

Pulmonary disease continues to be the leading cause of morbidity and mortality in HIV-infected individuals. Although the use of potent antiretroviral agents and effective chemoprophy-

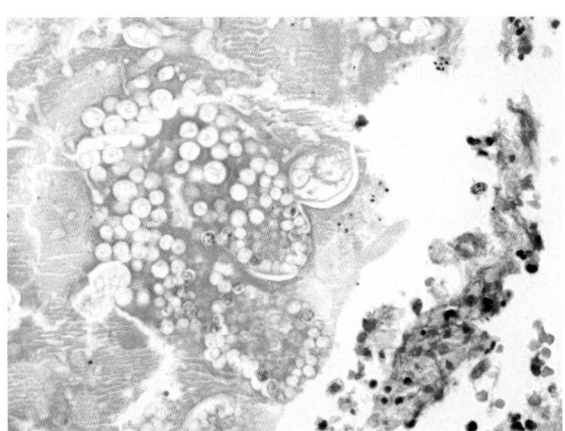

FIGURE 15–38 Coccidioidomycosis with intact and ruptured spherules.

TABLE 15–9   Causes of Pulmonary Infiltrates in Immunocompromised Hosts

Diffuse Infiltrate	Focal Infiltrate
COMMON	
Cytomegalovirus	Gram-negative rods
Pneumocystis jiroveci	*Staphylococcus aureus*
Drug reaction	*Aspergillus*
	Candida
	Malignancy
UNCOMMON	
Bacteria	*Cryptococcus*
Aspergillus	*Mucor*
Cryptococcus	*Pneumocystis jiroveci*
Malignancy	*Legionella pneumophila*

laxis has markedly altered the incidence and outcome of pulmonary disease in HIV-infected persons, the plethora of infectious agents and other pulmonary lesions make diagnosis and treatment a distinct challenge. Some of the individual microbial agents afflicting HIV-infected individuals have already been discussed; this section will focus only on the general principles of HIV-associated pulmonary disease.

○ Despite the emphasis on "opportunistic" infections, it must be remembered that bacterial lower respiratory tract infection caused by the "usual" pathogens is one of the most serious pulmonary disorders in HIV infection. The implicated organisms include *S. pneumoniae, S. aureus, H. influenzae,* and gram-negative rods. Bacterial pneumonias in HIV-infected persons are more common, more severe, and more often associated with bacteremia than in those without HIV infection.

○ Not all pulmonary infiltrates in HIV-infected individuals are infectious in etiology. A host of noninfectious diseases, including Kaposi sarcoma (Chapters 6 and 11), pulmonary non-Hodgkin lymphoma (Chapter 13), and primary lung cancer, occur with increased frequency and must be excluded.

○ *The CD4+ T-cell count can define the risk of infection with specific organisms.* As a rule of thumb, bacterial and tubercular infections are more likely at higher CD4+ counts (>200 cells/mm^3). *Pneumocystis* pneumonia usually strikes at CD4+ counts below 200 cells/mm^3, while cytomegalovirus and *Mycobacterium avium* complex infections are uncommon until the very late stages of immunosuppression (CD4+ counts <50 cells/mm^3).

Finally, it is useful to remember that pulmonary disease in HIV-infected persons may result from more than one cause, and even common pathogens may present with atypical manifestations. Therefore, the diagnostic work-up of these patients may be more extensive (and expensive) than would be necessary in an immunocompetent individual.

Lung Transplantation

Indications for transplantation may include almost all non-neoplastic terminal lung diseases, provided that the patient does not have any other serious disease, which would preclude lifelong immunosuppressive therapy. *The most common indications are end-stage emphysema, idiopathic pulmonary fibrosis, cystic fibrosis, and idiopathic/familial pulmonary arterial hypertension.* While bilateral lung and heart-lung transplants are possible, in many cases a single-lung transplant is performed, offering sufficient improvement in pulmonary function for each of two recipients from a single (and all too scarce) donor. When bilateral chronic infection is present (e.g., cystic fibrosis, bronchiectasis), both lungs of the recipient must be replaced to remove the reservoir of infection.

Morphology. With improving surgical and organ preservation techniques, postoperative complications (e.g., anastomotic dehiscence, vascular thrombosis, primary graft dysfunction) are fortunately becoming rare. The transplanted lung is subject to two major complications: infection and rejection.

Pulmonary infections in lung transplant patients are essentially those of any immunocompromised host, discussed earlier. In the early post-transplant period (the first few weeks), bacterial infections are most common. With ganciclovir prophylaxis and matching of donor-recipient CMV status, CMV pneumonia occurs less frequently and is less severe, although some resistant strains are emerging. Most infections occur in the third to twelfth month after transplantation. *Pneumocystis jiroveci* pneumonia is rare, since almost all patients receive adequate prophylaxis, usually with Bactrim (trimethoprim-sulfamethoxazole). Fungal infections are mostly due to *Candida* and *Aspergillus* species, and they involve the bronchial anastomotic site and/or the lung.

Acute rejection of the lung occurs to some degree in all patients despite routine immunosuppression. It often occurs during the early weeks to months after surgery but may occur years later whenever immunosuppression is decreased. Patients present with fever, dyspnea, cough, and radiologic infiltrates. Since these are similar to the picture of infections, diagnosis often relies on transbronchial biopsy. The morphologic features of acute rejection are primarily those of inflammatory infiltrates (lymphocytes, plasma cells, and few neutrophils and eosinophils), either around small vessels, in the submucosa of airways, or both.[136]

Chronic rejection is a significant problem in at least half of all lung transplant patients by 3 to 5 years. It is manifested by cough, dyspnea, and an irreversible decrease in lung function tests. The major morphologic correlate of chronic rejection is **bronchiolitis obliterans**, the partial or complete occlusion of small airways by fibrosis, with or without active inflammation (Fig. 15–39). Bronchiolitis obliterans is patchy and therefore difficult to diagnose via transbronchial biopsy. Bronchiectasis and pulmonary fibrosis may develop in long-standing cases.

Acute cellular airway rejection (the presumed forerunner of later, fibrous obliteration of these airways) is generally

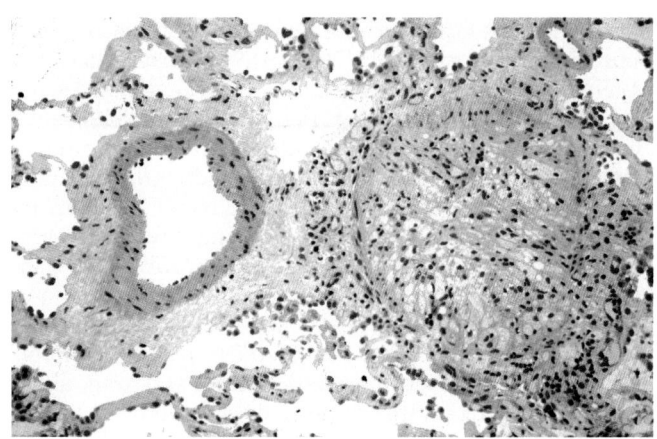

FIGURE 15–39 Chronic rejection of lung allograft, with total occlusion of bronchiole (bronchiolitis obliterans). Adjacent pulmonary artery branch is normal. (Courtesy of Dr. Thomas Krausz, Department of Pathology, The University of Chicago, Pritzker School of Medicine, Chicago, IL.)

responsive to therapy, but the treatment of established bronchiolitis obliterans has been disappointing. Its progress may be slowed or even halted for some time, but it cannot be reversed. Infrequent complications of lung transplantation include accelerated pulmonary arteriosclerosis in the graft and lymphoproliferative disease. With continuing improvement in surgical, immunosuppressive, and antimicrobial therapies, the short-term outcome of lung transplantation has improved considerably, although it is still not as good as that for renal or cardiac transplantation. One-, five-, and ten-year survival rates are 78%, 50%, and 26%, respectively.[137]

Tumors

A variety of benign and malignant tumors may arise in the lung, but 90% to 95% are carcinomas, about 5% are bronchial carcinoids, and 2% to 5% are mesenchymal and other miscellaneous neoplasms.[60]

CARCINOMAS

Lung cancer is currently the most frequently diagnosed major cancer in the world and the most common cause of cancer mortality worldwide. This is largely due to the carcinogenic effects of cigarette smoke. Over the coming decades, changes in smoking habits will greatly influence lung cancer incidence and mortality as well as the prevalence of various histologic types of lung cancer.[138]

The number of new cases of lung cancer occurring in 2008 in the United States is estimated to be 215,020 (note that in 1950 it was 18,000), accounting for about 15% of cancer diagnoses and 29% of cancer-related deaths. The annual number of deaths from lung cancer in the United States is estimated to be 161,840 in 2008.[139] Since the early 1990s lung cancer incidence and mortality rates have been decreasing in men, most likely from the decreased smoking rates over the past 30 years. However, decreases in smoking patterns among women lag behind those of men. Since 1987 more women have died

each year of lung cancer than of breast cancer, which for over 40 years had been the major cause of cancer death in women. Cancer of the lung occurs most often between ages 40 and 70 years, with a peak incidence in the 50s or 60s. Only 2% of all cases appear before the age of 40. The outlook for individuals diagnosed with lung cancer is dismal. The 1-year survival rate has increased from 34% in 1975 to 41% in 2007, largely because of improvements in surgical techniques. However, the 5-year rate for all stages combined is only 16%.

Etiology and Pathogenesis. Most carcinomas of the lung, similar to cancer at other sites, arise by a stepwise accumulation of genetic abnormalities that transform benign bronchial epithelium to neoplastic tissue. Unlike many other cancers, however, the major environmental insult that inflicts genetic damage is known. We begin our discussion with the well-known lung carcinogen—cigarette smoke.

Tobacco Smoking. The evidence provided by statistical and clinical observations establishing a positive relationship between tobacco smoking and lung cancer is overwhelming. Experimental data have also been pursued, but this approach is limited by species differences.

Statistical evidence is most compelling: 87% of lung carcinomas occur in active smokers or those who stopped recently. In numerous retrospective studies, there was an invariable statistical association between the frequency of lung cancer and (1) *the amount of daily smoking*, (2) *the tendency to inhale*, and (3) *the duration of the smoking habit*. Compared with nonsmokers, average smokers of cigarettes have a tenfold greater risk of developing lung cancer, and heavy smokers (more than 40 cigarettes per day for several years) have a 60-fold greater risk. Women have a higher susceptibility to tobacco carcinogens than men do. Cessation of smoking for 10 years reduces risk but never to control levels. It should be noted, however, that despite compelling evidence supporting the role of cigarette smoking, only 11% of heavy smokers develop lung cancer in their lifetime. Clearly, there are other (genetic) factors involved as will be discussed later. Epidemiologic studies also show an association between cigarette smoking and carcinoma of the mouth, pharynx, larynx, esophagus, pancreas, uterine cervix, kidney, and urinary bladder. *Secondhand smoke*, or environmental tobacco smoke, contains numerous human carcinogens for which there is no safe level of exposure. It is estimated that each year about 3000 nonsmoking adults die of lung cancer as a result of breathing secondhand smoke.[140] Cigar and pipe smoking also increase risk, although much more modestly than smoking cigarettes. The use of smokeless tobacco is not a safe substitute for smoking cigarettes or cigars, as these products cause oral cancers and can lead to nicotine addiction.

Clinical evidence is obtained largely through observations of histologic changes in the lining epithelium of the respiratory tract in habitual smokers. These sequential changes have been best documented for squamous cell carcinoma, but they may also be present in other histologic subtypes. In essence, there is a linear correlation between the intensity of exposure to cigarette smoke and the appearance of ever more worrisome epithelial changes that begin with squamous metaplasia and progress to squamous dysplasia, carcinoma in situ, and invasive carcinoma. Lung tumors of smokers frequently contain a typical, though not specific, molecular fingerprint in the form of $G:C > T:A$ mutations in the *p53* gene that are probably caused by benzo[*a*]pyrene, one of the many carcinogens in tobacco smoke.[138]

Experimental work has consisted mainly of attempts to induce cancer in experimental animals with extracts of tobacco smoke.[141] More than 1200 substances have been counted in cigarette smoke, many of which are potential carcinogens. They include both initiators (polycyclic aromatic hydrocarbons such as benzo[*a*]pyrene) and promoters, such as phenol derivatives. Radioactive elements may also be found (polonium-210, carbon-14, and potassium-40) as well as other contaminants, such as arsenic, nickel, molds, and additives. Protracted exposure of mice to these additives induces skin tumors. Efforts to produce lung cancer by exposing animals to tobacco smoke, however, have been unsuccessful. The few cancers that have developed have been bronchioloalveolar carcinomas, a type of tumor that is not strongly associated with smoking in humans.

Industrial Hazards. Certain industrial exposures increase the risk of developing lung cancer. High-dose ionizing *radiation* is carcinogenic. There was an increased incidence of lung cancer among survivors of the Hiroshima and Nagasaki atomic bomb blasts. *Uranium* is weakly radioactive, but lung cancer rates among nonsmoking uranium miners are four times higher than those in the general population, and among smoking miners they are about 10 times higher.

The risk of lung cancer is increased with *asbestos*. Lung cancer is the most frequent malignancy in individuals exposed to asbestos, particularly when coupled with smoking.[80] Asbestos workers who do not smoke have a five times greater risk of developing lung cancer than do nonsmoking control subjects, and those who smoke have a 50 to 90 times greater risk. The latent period before the development of lung cancer is 10 to 30 years.

Air Pollution. Atmospheric pollutants may play some role in the increased incidence of lung carcinoma today. Attention has been drawn to the potential problem of *indoor* air pollution, especially by radon.[142,143] Radon is a ubiquitous radioactive gas that has been linked epidemiologically to increased lung cancer in miners exposed to relatively high concentrations. The pathogenic mechanism is believed to be inhalation and bronchial deposition of radioactive decay products that become attached to environmental aerosols. These data have generated concern that low-level indoor exposure (e.g., in homes in areas of high radon in soil) could also lead to increased incidence of lung tumors; some attribute the bulk of lung cancers in nonsmokers to this insidious carcinogen (Chapter 9).[144]

Molecular Genetics. Ultimately, the exposures cited previously are thought to act by causing genetic alterations in lung cells, which accumulate and eventually lead to the neoplastic phenotype. It has been estimated that 10 to 20 genetic mutations have occurred by the time the tumor is clinically apparent.[145]

As will be discussed below, for all practical purposes lung cancers can be divided into two clinical subgroups: *small cell carcinoma* and *non-small cell carcinoma*. Some molecular lesions are common to both types, whereas others are relatively specific. The dominant oncogenes that are frequently involved in lung cancer include *c-MYC, KRAS, EGFR, c-MET,* and *c-KIT*. The commonly deleted or inactivated tumor suppressor genes include *p53, RB1, p16(INK4a),* and multiple loci on chromosome 3p. At this locale there are numerous candidate tumor suppressor genes, such as *FHIT, RASSF1A,* and others that remain to be identified. Of the various cancer associated genes, *C-KIT* (40–70%), *MYCN* and *MYCL* (20–30%), p53 (90%), 3p (100%), RB (90%), and *BCL2* (75–90%) are most commonly involved in small cell lung carcinoma. By comparison, *EGFR* (25%), *KRAS* (10–15%), *p53* (50%), *p16 INK4a* (70%) are the ones most commonly affected in non-small cell lung carcinoma. In addition recent studies show that *LKB1, PTEN,* and *TSC*, all relating to the m-TOR pathway are also mutated in up to 30% of lung cancers (mostly non-small cell lung carcinoma).[146] It should be noted that *C-KIT* is over expressed but only rarely mutated. Hence, drugs that target its tyrosine kinase domain (such as imatinib) are ineffective. Recall that in tumors with mutation of that kinase domain (e.g., gastrointestinal stromal tumor) this drug is useful for treatment. *Telomerase* activity is increased in over 80% of lung tumor tissues.

There are several signal transduction molecules that are activated in lung cancer, such as AKT, phosphatidylinositol-3-kinase, ERK1/2, STAT5, and focal adhesion proteins such as paxillin. Although certain genetic changes are known to be early (inactivation of chromosome 3p suppressor genes) or late (activation of *KRAS*), the temporal sequence is not yet well defined. More importantly, certain genetic changes such as loss of chromosome 3p material can be found in benign bronchial epithelium of individuals with lung cancer, as well as in the respiratory epithelium of smokers without lung cancers, suggesting that large areas of the respiratory mucosa are mutagenized after exposure to carcinogens ("field effect").[147] On this fertile soil, the cells that accumulate additional mutations ultimately develop into cancer.

Occasional *familial clustering* has suggested a genetic predisposition, as has the variable risk even among heavy smokers. Attempts at defining markers of genetic susceptibility are ongoing and have, for example, identified a role for polymorphisms in the cytochrome P-450 gene *CYP1A1* (Chapter 7).[148] People with certain alleles of *CYP1A1* have an increased capacity to metabolize procarcinogens derived from cigarette smoke and, conceivably, incur the greatest risk of developing lung cancer. Similarly, individuals whose peripheral blood lymphocytes undergo chromosomal breakages following exposure to tobacco-related carcinogens (mutagen sensitivity genotype) have a greater than tenfold risk of developing lung cancer compared with controls. In addition, large scale linkage studies point to an autosomal susceptibility locus on 6q23-25. More recently, genome-wide association studies have revealed an intriguing link to polymorphisms in the nicotine acetylcholine receptor gene located on chromosome 15q25 and lung cancer in both smokers and nonsmokers.[149]

It should also be pointed out that 25% of lung cancers worldwide arise in nonsmokers and these are pathogenetically distinct. They occur more commonly in women, and most are adenocarcinomas. They tend to have *EGFR* mutations, almost never have *KRAS* mutations and *p53* mutations, although common, occur less commonly. The nature of the *p53* mutations are also distinct.[150]

Precursor Lesions. Three types of precursor epithelial lesions are recognized: (1) squamous dysplasia and carcinoma in situ, (2) atypical adenomatous hyperplasia, and (3) diffuse idiopathic pulmonary neuroendocrine cell hyperplasia. It should be noted that the term *precursor* does not imply that progression to cancer will occur in all cases. Currently it is not possible to distinguish between precursor lesions that progress and those that remain localized or regress.

Classification. Tumor classification is important for consistency in patient treatment and because it provides a basis for epidemiologic and biologic studies. The most recent classification of the World Health Organization[138] has gained wide acceptance (Table 15–10). Several histologic variants of each type of lung cancer are described; however, their clinical significance is still undetermined, except as mentioned below. The relative proportions of the major categories are[151]:

- Adenocarcinoma (males 37%, females 47%)
- Squamous cell carcinoma (males 32%, females 25%)
- Small cell carcinoma (males 14%, females 18%)
- Large cell carcinoma (males 18%, females 10%)

The incidence of adenocarcinoma has increased significantly in the last two decades; it is now the most common form of lung cancer in women and, in many studies, men as well.[152] The basis for this change is unclear. A possible factor is the increase in women smokers, but this only highlights our lack of knowledge about why women tend to develop more adenocarcinomas. One interesting postulate is that changes in cigarette type (filter tips, lower tar and nicotine) have caused smokers to inhale more deeply and thereby expose more peripheral airways and cells (with a predilection to adenocarcinoma) to carcinogens.[153] There may be *mixtures of histologic patterns*, even in the same cancer. Thus, combined types of squamous cell carcinoma and adenocarcinoma or of small-cell and squamous cell carcinoma occur in about 10% of patients. For common clinical use, however, the various histologic types of lung cancer can be clustered into two groups on the basis of likelihood of metastases and response to available therapies: *small cell carcinomas* (almost always metastatic, high initial response to chemotherapy) versus *non-small cell carcinomas* (less often metastatic, less responsive). The strongest relationship to smoking is with squamous cell and small cell carcinoma.

Morphology. Lung carcinomas arise most often in and about the hilus of the lung. About three fourths of the lesions take their origin from first-order, second-order, and third-order bronchi. An increasing number of primary carcinomas of the lung arise in the periphery of the lung from the alveolar septal cells or terminal bronchioles. These are predominantly adenocarcinomas, including those of the bronchioloalveolar type, to be discussed separately.

The preneoplastic lesions that antedate, and usually accompany, invasive squamous cell carcinoma are well characterized. Squamous cell carcinomas are often preceded for years by **squamous metaplasia or dysplasia** in the bronchial epithelium, which then transforms to **carcinoma in situ,** a phase that may last for several years (Fig. 15–40). By this time, atypical cells may be identified in cytologic smears of sputum or in bronchial lavage fluids or brushings, although the lesion is asymptomatic and undetectable on radiographs. Eventually, the growing neoplasm reaches a symptomatic stage, when a well-defined tumor mass begins to obstruct the lumen of a major bronchus, often producing distal atelectasis and infection. The tumor may then follow a variety of paths. It may continue to fungate into the bronchial lumen to produce an intraluminal mass. It can also rapidly penetrate the wall of the bronchus to infiltrate along the peribronchial tissue (Fig. 15–41) into the adjacent region of the carina or mediastinum. In other instances, the tumor grows along a broad front to produce a cauliflower-like intraparenchymal mass that appears to push lung substance ahead of it. In almost all patterns the neoplastic tissue is gray-white and firm to hard. Especially when the tumors are bulky, focal areas of hemorrhage or necrosis may appear to produce red or yellow-white mottling and softening. Sometimes these necrotic foci cavitate. Often these tumors erode the bronchial epithelium and can be diagnosed by cytologic examination of sputum, bronchoalveolar lavage fluid, or fine-needle aspiration (Fig. 15–42).

Extension may occur to the pleural surface and then within the pleural cavity or into the pericardium. Spread to the tracheal, bronchial, and mediastinal nodes can be found in most cases. The frequency of nodal involvement varies slightly with the histologic pattern but averages greater than 50%.

Distant spread of lung carcinoma occurs through both lymphatic and hematogenous pathways. These tumors often spread early throughout the body except for squamous cell carcinoma, which metastasizes outside the thorax late. Metastasis may be the first manifestation of an underlying occult pulmonary lesion. No organ or tissue is spared in the spread of these lesions, but the adrenals, for obscure reasons, are involved in more than half the cases. The liver (30% to 50%), brain (20%), and bone (20%) are additional favored sites of metastases.

Adenocarcinoma. This is a malignant epithelial tumor with glandular differentiation or mucin production by the tumor cells. Adenocarcinomas grow in

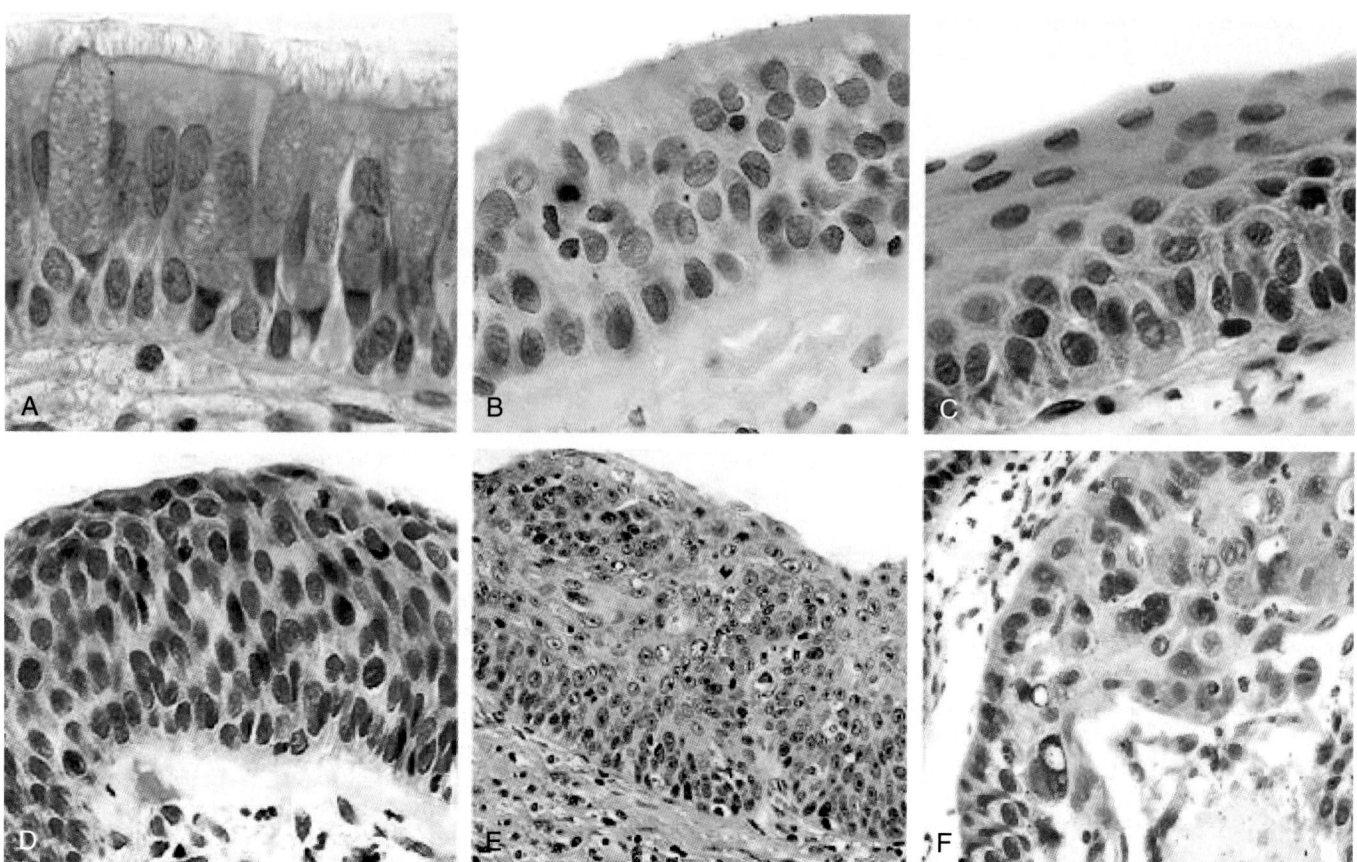

FIGURE 15–40 Precursor lesions of squamous cell carcinomas. Some of the earliest (and "mild") changes in smoking-damaged respiratory epithelium include goblet cell hyperplasia **(A)**, basal cell (or reserve cell) hyperplasia **(B)**, and squamous metaplasia **(C)**. More ominous changes include the appearance of squamous dysplasia **(D)**, characterized by the presence of disordered squamous epithelium, with loss of nuclear polarity, nuclear hyperchromasia, pleomorphism, and mitotic figures. Squamous dysplasia may, in turn, progress through the stages of mild, moderate, and severe dysplasia. Carcinoma-in-situ (CIS) **(E)** is the stage that immediately precedes invasive squamous carcinoma **(F)**, and apart from the lack of basement membrane disruption in CIS, the cytologic features are similar to those in frank carcinoma. Unless treated, CIS will eventually progress to invasive cancer. **(A–E,** Courtesy of Dr. Adi Gazdar, Department of Pathology, University of Texas, Southwestern Medical School, Dallas. **F,** reproduced with permission from Travis WD, et al [eds]: World Health Organization Histological Typing of Lung and Pleural Tumors. Heidelberg, Springer, 1999.)

various patterns, including acinar, papillary, bronchioloalveolar, and solid with mucin formation. Of these, only pure bronchioloalveolar carcinoma has distinct gross, microscopic, and clinical features and will be discussed separately.

Adenocarcinoma is the most common type of lung cancer in women and nonsmokers. As compared with squamous cell cancers, the lesions are usually more peripherally located, and tend to be smaller. They vary histologically from well-differentiated tumors with obvious glandular elements (Fig. 15–43A) to papillary lesions resembling other papillary carcinomas to solid masses with only occasional mucin-producing glands and cells. The majority are positive for thyroid transcription factor-1 (TTF-1) and about 80% contain mucin. At the periphery of the tumor there is often a bronchioloalveolar pattern of spread (see below). Adenocarcinomas grow more slowly than squamous cell carcinomas but tend to metastasize widely and earlier. Peripheral adenocarcinomas with a small central invasive component associated with

scarring and a predominantly peripheral bronchioloalveolar growth pattern may have a better outcome than invasive carcinomas of the same size. Adenocarcinomas, including bronchioloalveolar carcinomas, are less frequently associated with a history of smoking (still, greater than 75% are found in smokers) than are squamous or small cell carcinomas (>98% in smokers).

KRAS mutations occur primarily in adenocarcinoma, and are seen at a much lower frequency in nonsmokers (5%) than in smokers (30%). *p53*, *RB1*, and *p16* mutations and inactivation have the same frequency in adenocarcinoma as in squamous cell carcinoma. Mutations and amplifications in the epidermal growth factor receptor gene (*EGFR*) occur in patients with adenocarcinoma (mostly women, nonsmokers, and those of Asian origin).[154] A prospective trial has demonstrated that patients with *EGFR* mutations have improved survival with upfront EGFR inhibitor treatment. *KRAS* mutations highly correlate with worse outcome and resistance to EGFR inhibi-

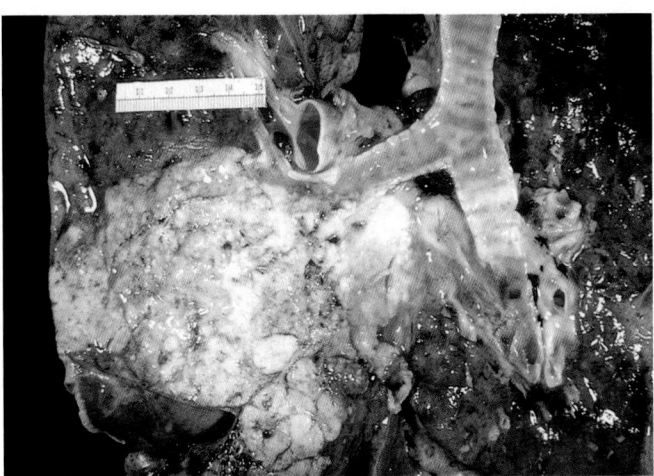

FIGURE 15–41 Lung carcinoma. The gray-white tumor tissue is seen infiltrating the lung substance. Histologically, this large tumor mass was identified as a squamous cell carcinoma.

tors.[154] Also, c-MET can be amplified or mutated in lung cancer, for which targeted therapies are being developed.

As the name implies, **bronchioloalveolar carcinoma** occurs in the pulmonary parenchyma in the terminal bronchioloalveolar regions. It represents, in various series, 1% to 9% of all lung cancers. Macroscopically, the tumor almost always occurs in the peripheral portions of the lung either as a single nodule or, more often, as multiple diffuse nodules that sometimes coalesce to produce a pneumonia-like consolidation. The parenchymal nodules have a mucinous, gray translucence when secretion is present but otherwise appear as solid, gray-white areas that can be confused with pneumonia on gross inspection.

Histologically, the tumor is characterized by a pure bronchioloalveolar growth pattern with no evidence of stromal, vascular, or pleural invasion. The key feature of bronchioloalveolar carcinomas is their growth along preexisting structures without destruction of alveolar architecture. This growth pattern has been termed *lepidic*, an allusion to the neoplastic cells resembling butterflies sitting on a fence. It has two subtypes: nonmucinous and mucinous. The former has columnar, peg-shaped, or cuboidal cells, while the latter has distinctive, tall, columnar cells with cytoplasmic and intra-alveolar mucin, growing along the alveolar septa (Fig. 15–44). Ultrastructurally, bronchioloalveolar carcinomas are a heterogeneous group, consisting of mucin-secreting bronchiolar cells, Clara cells, or, rarely, type II pneumocytes.[155]

Nonmucinous bronchioloalveolar carcinomas often consist of a peripheral lung nodule with only rare aerogenous spread and therefore are amenable to surgical resection with an excellent 5-year survival. Mucinous bronchioloalveolar carcinomas, on the other hand, tend to spread aerogenously, forming satellite tumors. These may present as a solitary nodule or as multiple nodules, or an entire lobe may be consolidated by tumor, resembling lobar pneumonia and thus are less likely to be cured by surgery.

Analogous to the adenoma-carcinoma sequence in the colon, it is proposed that adenocarcinoma of the lung arises from **atypical adenomatous hyperplasia progressing to bronchioloalveolar carcinoma**, which then transforms into invasive adenocarcinoma. This is supported by the observation that lesions of atypical adenomatous hyperplasia are monoclonal and they share many molecular aberrations such as *EGFR* mutations with nonmucinous bronchioloalveolar carcinomas and with invasive adenocarcinomas.[156] Microscopically, atypical adenomatous hyperplasia is recognized as a well-demarcated focus of epithelial proliferation composed of cuboidal to low columnar epithelium (Fig. 15–45). These cells demonstrate some cytologic atypia but not to the extent seen in frank adenocarcinoma. It should be pointed out, however, that not all adenocarcinomas arise in this manner, nor do all bronchioloalveolar carcinomas become invasive if left untreated.

Squamous Cell Carcinoma. Squamous cell carcinoma is most commonly found in men and is **closely correlated with a smoking history.** Histologically, this tumor is characterized by the presence of keratinization and/or intercellular bridges. Keratinization may take the form of squamous pearls or individual cells with markedly eosinophilic dense cytoplasm (see Fig. 15–43B). These features are prominent in the well-differentiated tumors, are easily seen but not extensive in moderately differentiated tumors, and are focally seen in poorly differentiated tumors. Mitotic activity is higher in poorly differentiated tumors. In the past, most squamous cell carcinomas were seen to arise centrally from the segmental or subsegmental bronchi. However, the incidence of squamous cell carcinoma of the peripheral lung is increasing. Squamous metaplasia, epithelial dysplasia, and foci of

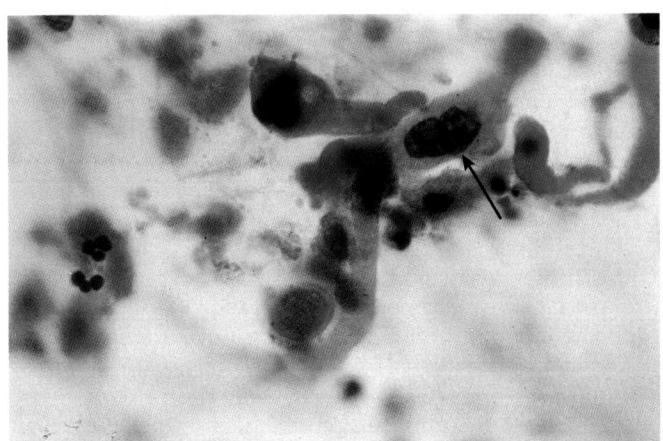

FIGURE 15–42 Cytologic diagnosis of lung cancer. A sputum specimen shows an orange-staining, keratinized squamous carcinoma cell with a prominent hyperchromatic nucleus *(arrow).* Note the size of the tumor cells compared with normal polymorphonuclear leukocytes in the *left lower corner.*

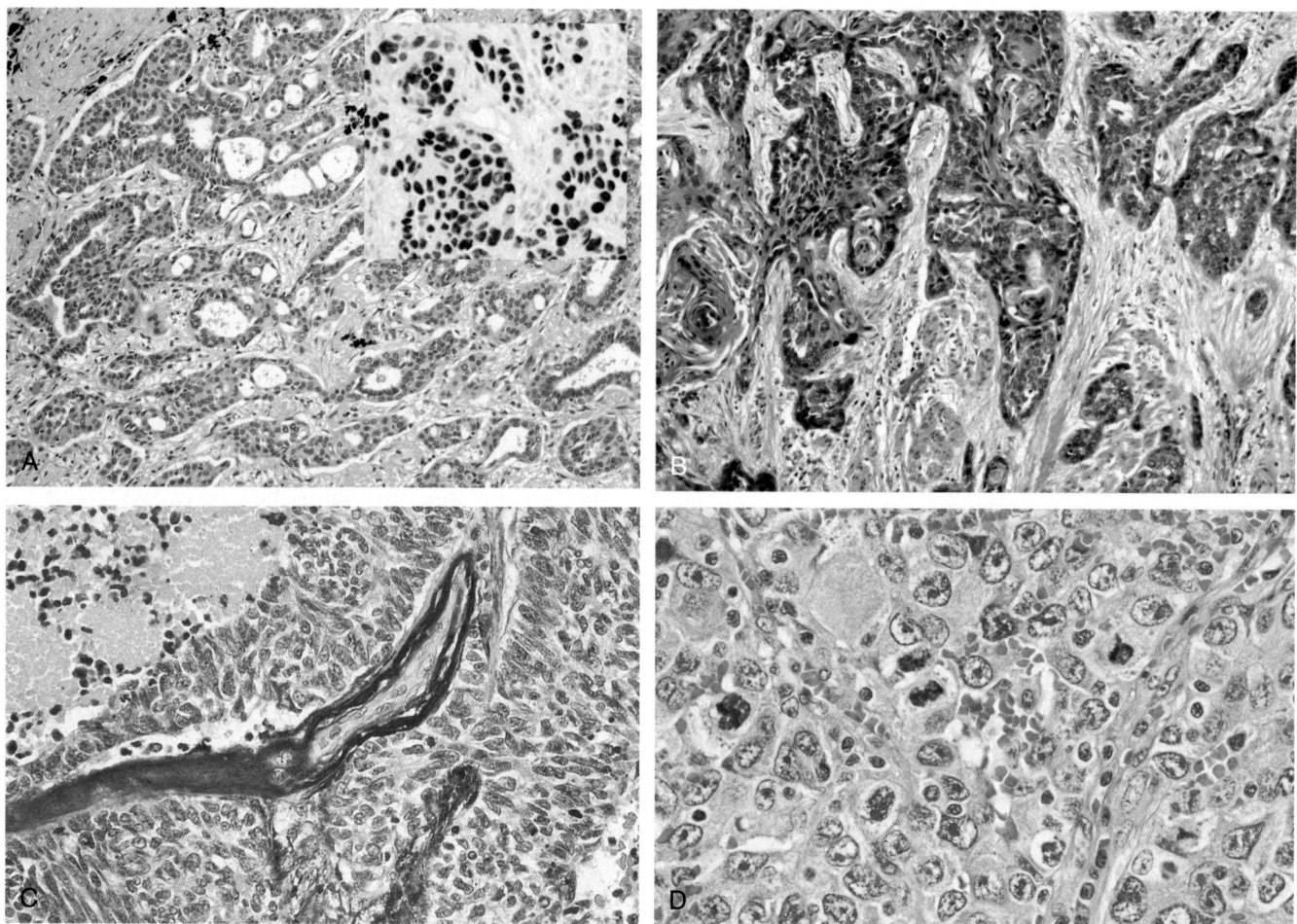

FIGURE 15–43   Histologic variants of lung carcinoma. **A,** Gland-forming adenocarcinoma, inset shows thyroid transcription factor 1 (TTF-1) positivity. **B,** Well-differentiated squamous cell carcinoma showing keratinization. **C,** Small cell carcinoma with islands of small deeply basophilic cells and areas of necrosis. **D,** Large cell carcinoma, featuring pleomorphic, anaplastic tumor cells with no squamous or glandular differentiation.

frank carcinoma in situ may be seen in bronchial epithelium adjacent to the tumor mass (see Fig. 15–40).

Squamous cell carcinomas show the highest frequency of *p53* mutations of all histologic types of lung carcinoma. p53 protein overexpression and, less commonly, mutations may precede invasion. Abnormal p53 accumulation is reported in 10% to 50% of dysplasias. There is increasing frequency and intensity of p53 immunostaining with higher grade dysplasia, and positivity can be seen in 60% to 90% of squamous cell carcinoma in situ. Loss of protein expression of the tumor suppressor gene *RB1* is detected by immunohistochemistry in 15% of squamous cell carcinomas. The cyclin-dependent kinase inhibitor *p16(INK4a)* is inactivated, and its protein product is lost in 65% of tumors. Multiple allelic losses are observed in squamous cell carcinomas at locations bearing tumor suppressor genes. These losses, especially those involving 3p, 9p, and 17p, may precede invasion and be detected in histologically normal cells in smokers. Overexpression of EGFR has

been detected in 80% of squamous cell carcinomas, but it is rarely mutated. HER-2/NEU is highly expressed in 30% of these cancers, but unlike in breast cancer, gene amplification is not the underlying mechanism.[157]

Small Cell Carcinoma. This highly malignant tumor has a distinctive cell type. The epithelial cells are relatively small, with scant cytoplasm, ill-defined cell borders, finely granular nuclear chromatin (salt and pepper pattern), and absent or inconspicuous nucleoli (see Fig. 15–43C). The cells are round, oval, or spindle-shaped, and nuclear molding is prominent. There is no absolute size for the tumor cells, but in general they are smaller than three small resting lymphocytes. The mitotic count is high. The cells grow in clusters that exhibit neither glandular nor squamous organization. Necrosis is common and often extensive. Basophilic staining of vascular walls due to encrustation by DNA from necrotic tumor cells (Azzopardi effect) is frequently present. All small cell carcinomas are high grade. A single variant of small cell carcinoma is recognized: combined small cell car-

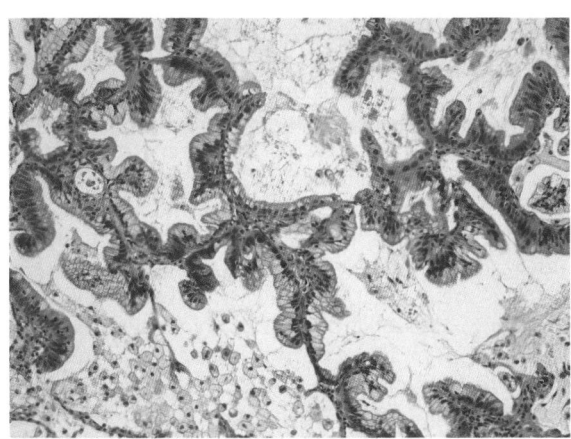

FIGURE 15–44 Bronchioloalveolar carcinoma, mucinous subtype, with characteristic growth along pre-existing alveolar septa, without invasion.

cinoma, in which there is a mixture of small cell carcinoma and any other non-small cell component, including large cell neuroendocrine carcinoma and sarcoma.

Electron microscopy shows dense-core neurosecretory granules, about 100 nm in diameter, in two thirds of cases. The granules are similar to those found in the neuroendocrine cells present along the bronchial epithelium, particularly in the fetus and neonate. Though distinctive, electron microscopy is not needed for diagnosis. The occurrence of neurosecretory granules, the ability of some of these tumors to secrete polypeptide hormones, and the presence of neuroendocrine markers such as chromogranin, synaptophysin, and CD57 (in 75% of cases) and parathormone-like and other hormonally active products suggest derivation of this tumor from neuroendocrine progenitor cells of the lining bronchial epithelium. This lung cancer type is most commonly associated with ectopic hormone production (discussed later).

Small cell carcinomas have a strong relationship to cigarette smoking; only about 1% occur in nonsmokers. They may arise in major bronchi or in the periphery of the lung. There is no known preinvasive phase or carcinoma in situ. They are the most aggressive of lung tumors, metastasize widely, and are virtually incurable by surgical means.

p53 and *RB1* tumor suppressor genes are frequently mutated (50% to 80% and 80% to 100% of small cell carcinomas, respectively). Immunohistochemistry demonstrates high levels of the anti-apoptotic protein BCL2 in 90% of tumors, in contrast with a low frequency of expression of the pro-apoptotic protein BAX.

Large Cell Carcinoma. This is an undifferentiated malignant epithelial tumor that lacks the cytologic features of small-cell carcinoma and glandular or squamous differentiation. The cells typically have large nuclei, prominent nucleoli, and a moderate amount of cytoplasm (see Fig. 15–43D). Large cell carcinomas

probably represent squamous cell carcinomas and adenocarcinomas that are so undifferentiated that they can no longer be recognized by light microscopy. Ultrastructurally, however, minimal glandular or squamous differentiation is common. One histologic variant is large cell neuroendocrine carcinoma. This is recognized by such features as organoid nesting, trabecular, rosette-like, and palisading patterns. These features suggest neuroendocrine differentiation, which can be confirmed by immunohistochemistry or electron microscopy. This tumor has the same molecular changes as small cell carcinoma.

Combined Carcinoma. Approximately 10% of all lung carcinomas have a combined histology, including two or more of the above types.

Secondary Pathology. Lung carcinomas cause related anatomic changes in the lung substance distal to the point of bronchial involvement. **Partial obstruction may cause marked focal emphysema; total obstruction may lead to atelectasis.** The impaired drainage of the airways is a common cause for **severe suppurative or ulcerative bronchitis or bronchiectasis. Pulmonary abscesses** sometimes call attention to a silent carcinoma that has initiated the chronic suppuration. Compression or invasion of the superior vena cava can cause venous congestion and edema of the head and arm, and, ultimately, circulatory compromise—the **superior vena cava syndrome.** Extension to the pericardial or pleural sacs may cause **pericarditis** (Chapter 12) or **pleuritis** with significant effusions.

Staging. A uniform TNM system for staging cancer according to its anatomic extent at the time of diagnosis is extremely useful, chiefly for comparing treatment results from different centers (Table 15–11).

Clinical Course. Lung cancer is one of the most insidious and aggressive neoplasms in the realm of oncology. In the usual case it is discovered in patients in their 50s whose symptoms are of several months' duration. *The major presenting*

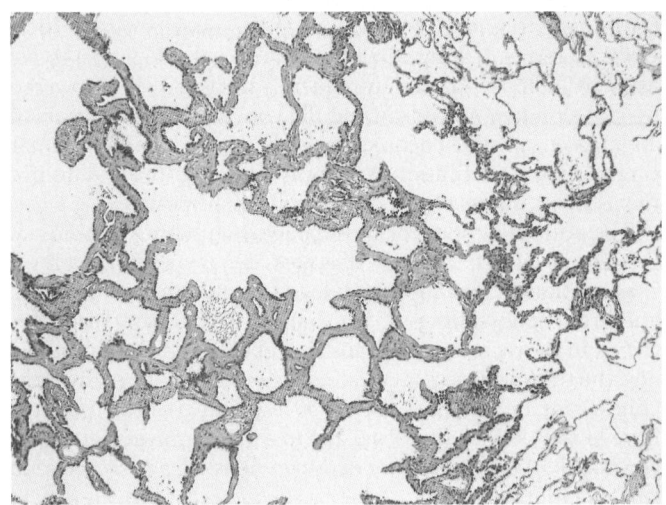

FIGURE 15–45 Atypical adenomatous hyperplasia with cuboidal epithelium and mild interstitial fibrosis.

TABLE 15–11   International Staging System for Lung Cancer

T1	Tumor <3 cm without pleural or main stem bronchus involvement (T1a, <2 cm; T1b, 2–3 cm)
T2	Tumor 3–7 cm or involvement of main stem bronchus 2 cm from carina, visceral pleural involvement, or lobar atelectasis (T2a, 3–5 cm; T2b, 5–7 cm)
T3	Tumor >7 cm or one with involvement of chest wall (including superior sulcus tumors), diaphragm, mediastinal pleura, pericardium, main stem bronchus 2 cm from carina, or entire lung atelectasis, or separate tumor nodule(s) in the same lobe
T4	Tumor with invasion of mediastinum, heart, great vessels, trachea, esophagus, vertebral body, or carina or separate tumor nodules in a different ipsilateral lobe
N0	No demonstrable metastasis to regional lymph nodes
N1	Ipsilateral hilar or peribronchial nodal involvement
N2	Metastasis to ipsilateral mediastinal or subcarinal lymph nodes
N3	Metastasis to contralateral mediastinal or hilar lymph nodes, ipsilateral or contralateral scalene, or supraclavicular lymph nodes
M0	No distant metastasis
M1	Distant metastasis (M1a, separate tumor nodule in contralateral lobe or pleural nodules or malignant pleural effusion; M1b, distant metastasis)

STAGE GROUPING

Stage Ia	T1	N0	M0
Stage Ib	T2	N0	M0
Stage IIa	T1	N1	M0
Stage IIb	T2	N1	M0
	T3	N0	M0
Stage IIIa	T1–3	N2	M0
	T3	N1	M0
Stage IIIb	Any T	N3	M0
	T3	N2	M0
	T4	Any N	M0
Stage IV	Any T	Any N	M1

Adapted from Goldstraw P, et al: The IASLC lung cancer staging project: proposals for the revision of the TNM stage groupings in the forthcoming (seventh) edition of the TNM classification of malignant tumors. J Thorac Oncol 2:706, 2007.

complaints are cough (75%), *weight loss* (40%), *chest pain* (40%), and *dyspnea* (20%). Some of the more common local manifestations of lung cancer and their pathologic bases are listed in Table 15–12. Not infrequently the tumor is discovered by its secondary spread during the course of investigation of an apparent primary neoplasm elsewhere. Bronchioloalveolar carcinomas, by definition, are noninvasive tumors and do not metastasize; unless resected, they kill by suffocation.

The outlook is poor for most patients with lung carcinoma. Despite all efforts at early diagnosis by frequent radiologic examination of the chest, cytologic examination of sputum, and bronchial washings or brushings and the many improvements in thoracic surgery, radiation therapy, and chemotherapy, the overall 5-year survival rate is only 15%. In many large clinics, not more than 20% to 30% of lung cancer patients have lesions sufficiently localized to even permit resection. *In general, the adenocarcinoma and squamous cell patterns tend to remain localized longer and have a slightly better prognosis than do the undifferentiated cancers, which are usually advanced by* the time they are discovered. The survival rate is 48% for cases detected when the disease is still localized. Only 15% of lung cancers are diagnosed at this early stage, some of which can be cured by lobectomy or pneumonectomy. Late-stage disease is usually treated with palliative chemotherapy and/or radiation therapy. Treatment of patients with adenocarcinoma and activating mutations in *EGFR* with inhibitors of EGFR prolongs survival. Many tumors that recur carry new mutations that generate resistance to these inhibitors, proving that these drugs are "hitting" their target. In contrast, activating *KRAS* mutations appear to be associated with a worse prognosis, regardless of treatment, in an already grim disease. Untreated, the survival time for patients with small-cell carcinoma is 6 to 17 weeks. This cancer is particularly sensitive to radiation therapy and chemotherapy, and potential cure rates of 15% to 25% for limited disease have been reported in some centers. Most patients have distant metastases at diagnosis. Thus, even with treatment, the mean survival after diagnosis is only about 1 year.

Paraneoplastic Syndromes. Lung carcinoma can be associated with several paraneoplastic syndromes[158] (Chapter 7), some of which may antedate the development of a detectable pulmonary lesion. The hormones or hormone-like factors elaborated include:

- *Antidiuretic hormone* (ADH), inducing hyponatremia due to inappropriate ADH secretion
- *Adrenocorticotropic hormone* (ACTH), producing Cushing syndrome
- *Parathormone, parathyroid hormone-related peptide, prostaglandin E, and some cytokines,* all implicated in the hypercalcemia often seen with lung cancer
- *Calcitonin,* causing hypocalcemia
- *Gonadotropins,* causing gynecomastia
- *Serotonin and bradykinin,* associated with the carcinoid syndrome

The incidence of clinically significant syndromes related to these factors ranges from 1% to 10% of all lung cancer patients,

TABLE 15–12   Local Effects of Lung Tumor Spread

Clinical Feature	Pathologic Basis
Pneumonia, abscess, lobar collapse	Tumor obstruction of airway
Lipoid pneumonia	Tumor obstruction; accumulation of cellular lipid in foamy macrophages
Pleural effusion	Tumor spread into pleura
Hoarseness	Recurrent laryngeal nerve invasion
Dysphagia	Esophageal invasion
Diaphragm paralysis	Phrenic nerve invasion
Rib destruction	Chest wall invasion
SVC syndrome	SVC compression by tumor
Horner syndrome	Sympathetic ganglia invasion
Pericarditis, tamponade	Pericardial involvement

SVC, superior vena cava.

although a much higher proportion of patients show elevated serum levels of these (and other) peptide hormones. Any one of the histologic types of tumors may occasionally produce any one of the hormones, but tumors that produce *ACTH and ADH are predominantly small cell carcinomas, whereas those that produce hypercalcemia are mostly squamous cell tumors.* The carcinoid syndrome is more common with carcinoid tumors, described later, and is only rarely associated with small cell carcinoma. However, small cell carcinoma occurs much more commonly; therefore, one is much more likely to encounter carcinoid syndrome in these patients.

Other systemic manifestations of lung carcinoma include the *Lambert-Eaton myasthenic syndrome* (Chapter 27), in which muscle weakness is caused by auto-antibodies (possibly elicited by tumor ionic channels) directed to the neuronal calcium channel[158]; *peripheral neuropathy*, usually purely sensory; dermatologic abnormalities, including *acanthosis nigricans* (Chapter 25); hematologic abnormalities, such as *leukemoid reactions*; and finally, a peculiar abnormality of connective tissue called *hypertrophic pulmonary osteoarthropathy*, associated with clubbing of the fingers.

Apical lung cancers in the superior pulmonary sulcus tend to invade the neural structures around the trachea, including the cervical sympathetic plexus, and produce a group of clinical findings that includes severe pain in the distribution of the ulnar nerve and *Horner syndrome* (enophthalmos, ptosis, miosis, and anhidrosis) on the same side as the lesion. Such tumors are also referred to as *Pancoast tumors.*

NEUROENDOCRINE PROLIFERATIONS AND TUMORS

The normal lung contains neuroendocrine cells within the epithelium as single cells or as clusters, the neuroepithelial bodies. While virtually all pulmonary neuroendocrine cell hyperplasias are secondary to airway fibrosis and/or inflammation, a rare disorder called diffuse idiopathic pulmonary neuroendocrine cell hyperplasia seems to be a precursor to the development of multiple tumorlets and typical or atypical carcinoids.

Neoplasms of neuroendocrine cells in the lung include benign *tumorlets*, small, inconsequential, hyperplastic nests of neuroendocrine cells seen in areas of scarring or chronic inflammation; *carcinoids*; and the (already discussed) highly aggressive small cell carcinoma and large cell neuroendocrine carcinoma of the lung. Neuroendocrine tumors are classified separately, since there are significant differences between them in incidence, clinical, epidemiologic, histologic, survival, and molecular characteristics. For example, in contrast to small cell and large cell neuroendocrine carcinomas, both typical and atypical carcinoids can occur in patients with multiple endocrine neoplasia type 1. Also note that neuroendocrine differentiation can be demonstrated by immunohistochemistry in 10% to 20% of lung carcinomas that do not show neuroendocrine morphology by light microscopy, the clinical significance of which is uncertain.

Carcinoid Tumors. Carcinoid tumors represent 1% to 5% of all lung tumors. Most patients with these tumors are younger than 40 years of age, and the incidence is equal for both sexes. Approximately 20% to 40% of patients are nonsmokers. Carcinoid tumors are low-grade malignant epithelial neoplasms that are subclassified into *typical* and *atypical carcinoids.* Typical carcinoids have no *p53* mutations or abnormalities of *BCL2* and *BAX* expression, while atypical carcinoids show these changes in 20% to 40% and 10% to 20% of tumors, respectively. Some carcinoids also show loss of heterozygosity at 3p, 13q14 (*RB1*), 9p, and 5q22, which are found in all neuroendocrine tumors with increasing frequency from typical to atypical carcinoid to large cell neuroendocrine and small cell carcinoma.

> **Morphology.** Carcinoids may arise centrally or may be peripheral. On gross examination, the central tumors grow as finger-like or spherical polypoid masses that commonly project into the lumen of the bronchus and are usually covered by an intact mucosa (Fig. 15–46A). They rarely exceed 3 to 4 cm in diameter. Most are confined to the main stem bronchi. Others, however, produce little intraluminal mass but instead penetrate the bronchial wall to fan out in the peribronchial tissue, producing the so-called **collar-**

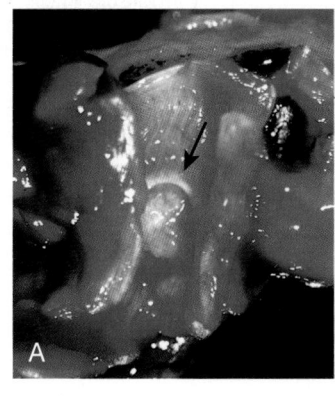
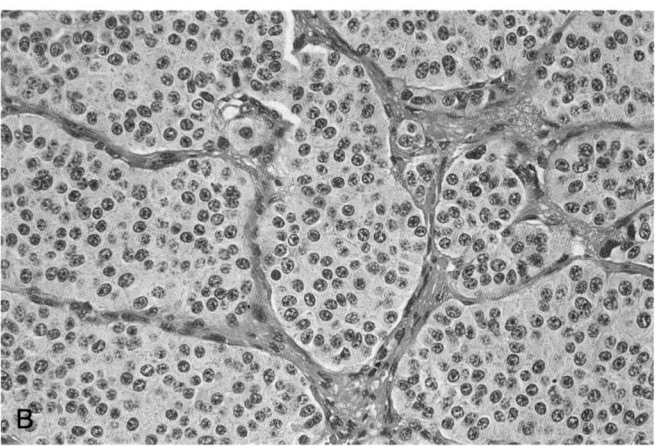

FIGURE 15–46 Bronchial carcinoid. **A,** Carcinoid growing as a spherical, pale mass *(arrow)* protruding into the lumen of the bronchus. **B,** Histologic appearance, demonstrating small, rounded, uniform nuclei and moderate cytoplasm. (Courtesy of Dr. Thomas Krausz, Department of Pathology, The University of Chicago, Pritzker School of Medicine, Chicago, IL.)

button lesion. Peripheral tumors are solid and nodular. Spread to local lymph nodes at the time of resection is more likely with atypical carcinoid.

Histologically, the tumor is composed of organoid, trabecular, palisading, ribbon, or rosette-like arrangements of cells separated by a delicate fibrovascular stroma. In common with the lesions of the gastrointestinal tract, the individual cells are quite regular and have uniform round nuclei and a moderate amount of eosinophilic cytoplasm (see Fig. 15–46B). Typical carcinoids have fewer than two mitoses per ten high-power fields and lack necrosis, while atypical carcinoids have between two and ten mitoses per ten high-power fields and/or foci of necrosis.[159] Atypical carcinoids also show increased pleomorphism, have more prominent nucleoli, and are more likely to grow in a disorganized fashion and invade lymphatics. On electron microscopy the cells exhibit the dense-core granules characteristic of other neuroendocrine tumors and, by immunohistochemistry, are found to contain serotonin, neuron-specific enolase, bombesin, calcitonin, or other peptides.

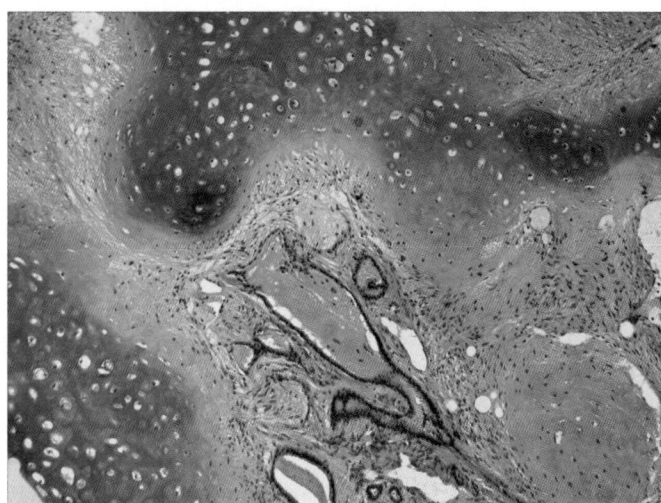

FIGURE 15–47 Pulmonary hamartoma. There are islands of cartilage and entrapped respiratory epithelium. (Courtesy of Dr. Justine A. Barletta, Department of Pathology, Brigham and Women's Hospital, Boston, MA.)

Clinical Features. The clinical manifestations of bronchial carcinoids emanate from their intraluminal growth, their capacity to metastasize, and the ability of some of the lesions to elaborate vasoactive amines. Persistent *cough, hemoptysis,* impairment of drainage of respiratory passages with *secondary infections, bronchiectasis, emphysema, and atelectasis* are all byproducts of the intraluminal growth of these lesions.

Most interesting, albeit rare, are functioning lesions capable of producing the classic carcinoid syndrome, that is, intermittent attacks of diarrhea, flushing, and cyanosis. Overall, most bronchial carcinoids do not have secretory activity and do not metastasize to distant sites but follow a relatively benign course for long periods and are therefore amenable to resection. The reported 5- to 10-year survival rates are 87% and 87% for typical carcinoids, 56% and 35% for atypical carcinoids, 27% and 9% for large cell neuroendocrine carcinoma, and 9% and 5% for small cell carcinoma, respectively.[159]

MISCELLANEOUS TUMORS

Lesions of the complex category of benign and malignant mesenchymal tumors, such as inflammatory myofibroblastic tumor, fibroma, fibrosarcoma, lymphangioleiomyomatosis, leiomyoma, leiomyosarcoma, lipoma, hemangioma, hemangiopericytoma, and chondroma, may occur but are rare. Benign and malignant hematopoietic tumors, similar to those described in other organs, may also affect the lung, either as isolated lesions or, more commonly, as part of a generalized disorder. These include Langerhans cell histiocytosis, non-Hodgkin and Hodgkin lymphomas, lymphomatoid granulomatosis, an unusual EBV-positive B cell lymphoma, and low-grade marginal zone B-cell lymphoma of the mucosa-associated lymphoid tissue (Chapter 13).

A lung *hamartoma* is a relatively common lesion that is usually discovered as an incidental, rounded focus of radio-opacity *(coin lesion)* on a routine chest film. The majority of these tumors are peripheral, solitary, less than 3 to 4 cm in diameter, and well circumscribed. Pulmonary hamartoma consists of nodules of connective tissue intersected by epithelial clefts. Cartilage is the most common connective tissue, but there may also be cellular fibrous tissue and fat. The epithelial clefts are lined by ciliated columnar epithelium or nonciliated epithelium and probably represent entrapment of respiratory epithelium (Fig. 15–47). The traditional term *hamartoma* is retained for this lesion, but several features suggest that it is a neoplasm rather than a malformation, such as its rarity in childhood, its increasing incidence with age, and the finding of chromosomal aberrations involving either 6p21 or 12q14–q15, indicating a clonal origin.[138]

Inflammatory myofibroblastic tumor, though rare, is more common in children, with an equal male-to-female ratio. Presenting symptoms include fever, cough, chest pain, and hemoptysis. It may also be asymptomatic. Imaging studies show a single (rarely multiple) round, well-defined, usually peripheral mass with calcium deposits in about a quarter of cases. Grossly, the lesion is firm, 3 to 10 cm in diameter, and grayish white. Microscopically, there is proliferation of spindle-shaped fibroblasts and myofibroblasts, lymphocytes, plasma cells, and peripheral fibrosis. The anaplastic lymphoma kinase (*ALK*) gene, located on 2p23, has been implicated in the pathogenesis of this tumor.

Tumors in the mediastinum either may arise in mediastinal structures or may be metastatic from the lung or other organs. They may also invade or compress the lungs. Table 15–13 lists the most common tumors in the various compartments of the mediastinum. Specific tumor types are discussed in appropriate sections of this book.

METASTATIC TUMORS

The lung is the most common site of metastatic neoplasms. Both carcinomas and sarcomas arising anywhere in the body may spread to the lungs via the blood or lymphatics or by direct continuity. Growth of contiguous tumors into the lungs occurs most often with esophageal carcinomas and mediastinal lymphomas.

TABLE 15–13   Mediastinal Tumors and Other Masses
SUPERIOR MEDIASTINUM
Lymphoma
Thymoma
Thyroid lesions
Metastatic carcinoma
Parathyroid tumors
ANTERIOR MEDIASTINUM
Thymoma
Teratoma
Lymphoma
Thyroid lesions
Parathyroid tumors
POSTERIOR MEDIASTINUM
Neurogenic tumors (schwannoma, neurofibroma)
Lymphoma
Gastroenteric hernia
MIDDLE MEDIASTINUM
Bronchogenic cyst
Pericardial cyst
Lymphoma

Morphology. The pattern of metastatic growth within the lungs is quite variable. In the usual case, multiple discrete nodules (cannonball lesions) are scattered throughout all lobes, more being at the periphery (Fig. 15–48). Other patterns include solitary nodule, endobronchial, pleural, pneumonic consolidation, and mixtures of the above. Foci of lepidic growth similar to bronchioloalveolar carcinoma are seen occasionally with metastatic carcinomas and may be associated with any of the patterns listed above.

Pleura

Pathologic involvement of the pleura is, most often, a secondary complication of some underlying disease. Secondary infections and pleural adhesions are particularly common

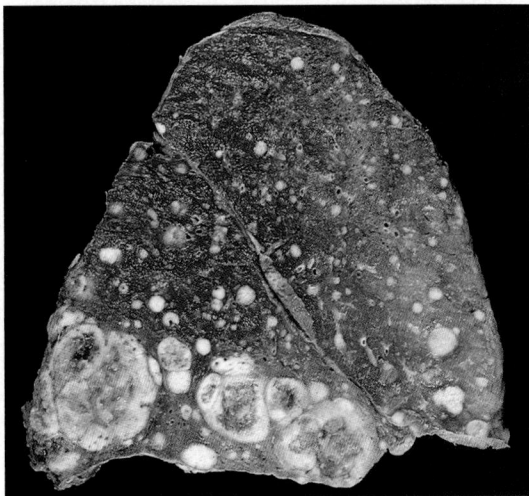

FIGURE 15–48 Numerous metastases to lung from a renal cell carcinoma. (Courtesy of Dr. Michelle Mantel, Brigham and Women's Hospital, Boston, MA.)

findings at autopsy. Important primary disorders include (1) primary intrapleural bacterial infections that imply seeding of this space as an isolated focus in the course of a transient bacteremia and (2) a primary neoplasm of the pleura: mesothelioma (discussed later).

PLEURAL EFFUSION

Pleural effusion is a common manifestation of both primary and secondary pleural diseases, which may be inflammatory or noninflammatory. Normally, no more than 15 mL of serous, relatively acellular, clear fluid lubricates the pleural surface. Accumulation of pleural fluid occurs in the following settings:

- Increased hydrostatic pressure, as in congestive heart failure
- Increased vascular permeability, as in pneumonia
- Decreased osmotic pressure, as in nephrotic syndrome
- Increased intrapleural negative pressure, as in atelectasis
- Decreased lymphatic drainage, as in mediastinal carcinomatosis

Inflammatory Pleural Effusions

Serous, *serofibrinous*, and fibrinous *pleuritis* all are caused by essentially the same processes. Fibrinous exudations generally reflect a later, more severe exudative reaction that, in an earlier developmental phase, might have presented as a serous or serofibrinous exudate.

The common causes of pleuritis are inflammatory diseases within the lungs, such as tuberculosis, pneumonia, lung infarcts, lung abscess, and bronchiectasis. Rheumatoid arthritis, disseminated lupus erythematosus, uremia, diffuse systemic infections, other systemic disorders, and metastatic involvement of the pleura can also cause serous or serofibrinous pleuritis. Radiation used in therapy for tumors in the lung or mediastinum often causes a serofibrinous pleuritis. In most instances the serofibrinous reaction is only minimal, and the fluid exudate is resorbed with either resolution or organization of the fibrinous component. Accumulation of large amounts of fluid can sufficiently encroach on lung space to cause respiratory distress.

A purulent pleural exudate *(empyema)* usually results from bacterial or mycotic seeding of the pleural space. Most commonly, this seeding occurs by contiguous spread of organisms from intrapulmonary infection, but occasionally, it occurs through lymphatic or hematogenous dissemination from a more distant source. Rarely, infections below the diaphragm, such as the subdiaphragmatic or liver abscess, may extend by continuity through the diaphragm into the pleural spaces, more often on the right side.

Empyema is characterized by loculated, yellow-green, creamy pus composed of masses of neutrophils admixed with other leukocytes. Although empyema may accumulate in large volumes (up to 500 to 1000 mL), usually the volume is small, and the pus becomes localized. Empyema may resolve, but this outcome is less common than organization of the exudate, with the formation of dense, tough fibrous adhesions that frequently obliterate the pleural space or envelop the lungs; either can seriously restrict pulmonary expansion.

True *hemorrhagic pleuritis* manifested by sanguineous inflammatory exudates is infrequent and is found in hemorrhagic diatheses, rickettsial diseases, and neoplastic involvement of the pleural cavity. The sanguineous exudate must be differentiated from hemothorax (discussed later). When hemorrhagic pleuritis is encountered, careful search should be made for the presence of exfoliated tumor cells.

Noninflammatory Pleural Effusions

Noninflammatory collections of serous fluid within the pleural cavities are called *hydrothorax*. The fluid is clear and straw colored. Hydrothorax may be unilateral or bilateral, depending on the underlying cause. The most common cause of hydrothorax is cardiac failure, and for this reason it is usually accompanied by pulmonary congestion and edema. Transudates may collect in any other systemic disease associated with generalized edema and are therefore found in renal failure and cirrhosis of the liver.

The escape of blood into the pleural cavity is known as *hemothorax*. It is almost invariably a fatal complication of a ruptured aortic aneurysm or vascular trauma or it may occur post-operatively. Pure hemothorax is readily identifiable by the large clots that accompany the fluid component of the blood.

Chylothorax is an accumulation of milky fluid, usually of lymphatic origin, in the pleural cavity. Chyle is milky white because it contains finely emulsified fats. Chylothorax is most often caused by thoracic duct trauma or obstruction that secondarily causes rupture of major lymphatic ducts. This disorder is encountered in malignant conditions arising within the thoracic cavity that cause obstruction of the major lymphatic ducts. More distant cancers may metastasize via the lymphatics and grow within the right lymphatic or thoracic duct to produce obstruction.

PNEUMOTHORAX

Pneumothorax refers to air or gas in the pleural cavities and may be spontaneous, traumatic, or therapeutic. Spontaneous pneumothorax may complicate any form of pulmonary disease that causes rupture of an alveolus. An abscess cavity that communicates either directly with the pleural space or with the lung interstitial tissue may also lead to the escape of air. In the latter circumstance the air may dissect through the lung substance or back through the mediastinum (interstitial emphysema), eventually entering the pleural cavity. *Pneumothorax is most commonly associated with emphysema, asthma, and tuberculosis.* Traumatic pneumothorax is usually caused by some perforating injury to the chest wall, but sometimes the trauma pierces the lung and thus provides two avenues for the accumulation of air within the pleural spaces. Resorption of the pleural space air occurs slowly in spontaneous and traumatic pneumothorax, provided that the original communication seals itself.

Of the various forms of pneumothorax, the one that attracts greatest clinical attention is so-called *spontaneous idiopathic pneumothorax.* This entity is encountered in relatively young people, seems to be due to rupture of small, peripheral, usually apical subpleural blebs, and usually subsides spontaneously as the air is resorbed. Recurrent attacks are common and can be quite disabling.

Pneumothorax may have as much clinical significance as a fluid collection in the lungs because it also causes compression, collapse, and atelectasis of the lung and may be responsible for marked respiratory distress. Occasionally the lung collapse is marked. When the defect acts as a flap valve and permits the entrance of air during inspiration but fails to permit its escape during expiration, it effectively acts as a pump that creates the progressively increasing pressures of *tension pneumothorax*, which may be sufficient to compress the vital mediastinal structures and the contralateral lung.

PLEURAL TUMORS

The pleura may be involved by primary or secondary tumors. Secondary metastatic involvement is far more common than are primary tumors. The most frequent metastatic malignancies arise from primary neoplasms of the lung and breast. In addition to these cancers, malignancy from any organ of the body may spread to the pleural spaces. Ovarian carcinomas, for example, tend to cause widespread implants in both the abdominal and thoracic cavities. In most metastatic involvements, a serous or serosanguineous effusion follows that often contains neoplastic cells. For this reason, careful cytologic examination of the sediment is of considerable diagnostic value.

Solitary Fibrous Tumor

Previously called "benign mesothelioma" or "benign fibrous mesothelioma" in the pleura and "fibroma" in the lung, solitary fibrous tumor is now recognized as a soft-tissue tumor with a propensity to occur in the pleura and, less commonly, in the lung, as well as other sites. The tumor is often attached to the pleural surface by a pedicle.[160] It may be small (1 to 2 cm in diameter) or may reach an enormous size, but it tends to remain confined to the surface of the lung (Fig. 15–49). Grossly, it consists of dense fibrous tissue with occasional cysts filled with viscid fluid; microscopically, the tumor shows whorls of reticulin and collagen fibers among which are interspersed spindle cells resembling fibroblasts. Rarely, this tumor

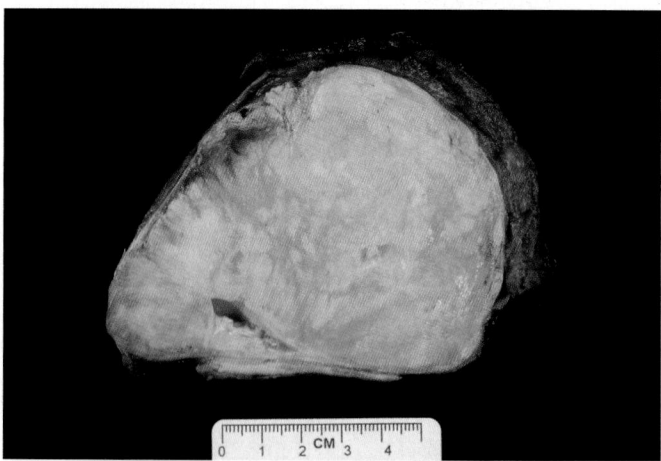

FIGURE 15–49   Solitary fibrous tumor. Cut surface is solid with a whorled appearance. (Courtesy of Dr. Justine A. Barletta, Department of Pathology, Brigham and Women's Hospital, Boston, MA.)

may be malignant, with pleomorphism, mitotic activity, necrosis, and large size (>10 cm). The tumor cells are CD34+ and keratin-negative by immunostaining. This feature can be diagnostically useful in distinguishing these lesions from malignant mesotheliomas (which show the opposite phenotype). The solitary fibrous tumor has no relationship to asbestos exposure.

Malignant Mesothelioma

Malignant mesotheliomas in the thorax arise from either the visceral or the parietal pleura.[161,162] Though uncommon, they have assumed great importance in the past few years because of their increased incidence among people with heavy exposure to asbestos (see "Pneumoconioses"). In coastal areas with shipping industries in the United States and Great Britain, and in Canadian, Australian, and South African mining areas, as many as 90% of reported mesotheliomas are asbestos-related. The lifetime risk of developing mesothelioma in heavily exposed individuals is as high as 7% to 10%. There is a long latent period of 25 to 45 years for the development of asbestos-related mesothelioma, and there seems to be no increased risk of mesothelioma in asbestos workers who smoke. *This is in contrast to the risk of asbestos-related lung carcinoma, already high, which is markedly magnified by smoking. Thus, for asbestos workers (particularly those who are also smokers), the risk of dying of lung carcinoma far exceeds that of developing mesothelioma.*

Asbestos bodies (see Fig. 15–20) are found in increased numbers in the lungs of patients with mesothelioma. Another marker of *asbestos exposure*, the *asbestos plaque*, has been previously discussed.

Cytogenetic studies have shown that approximately 60% to 80% of malignant mesotheliomas have deletions in chromosomes 1p, 3p, 6q, 9p, or 22q, and 31% have *p16* mutations. There is a low frequency of *p53* mutations, although p53 accumulation can be detected immunohistochemically

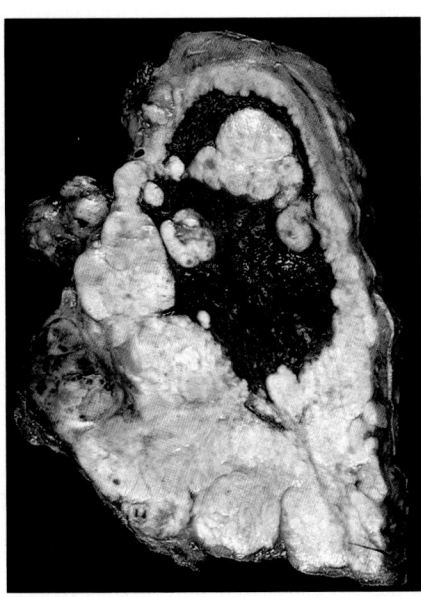

FIGURE 15–50 Malignant mesothelioma. Note the thick, firm, white pleural tumor tissue that ensheaths this bisected lung.

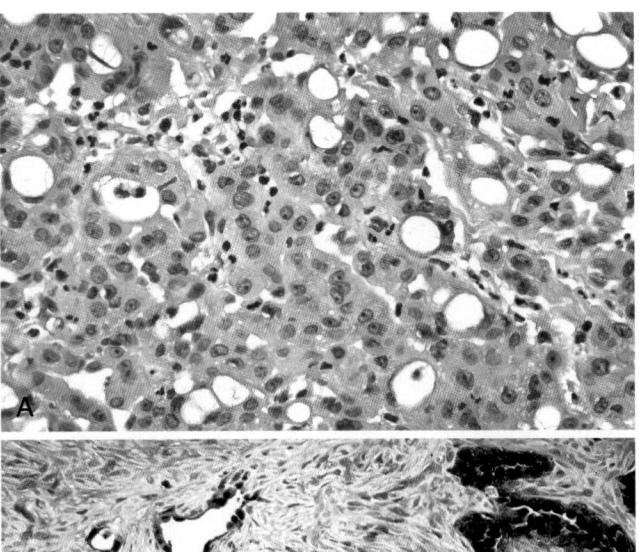
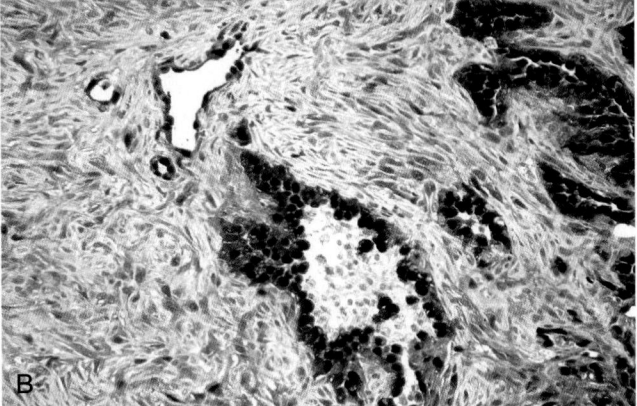

FIGURE 15–51 Histologic variants of malignant mesothelioma. **A,** Epithelioid type. **B,** Mixed type, stained for calretinin (immunoperoxidase method). The epithelial component is strongly positive (dark brown), while the sarcomatoid component is less so. (Courtesy of Dr. Thomas Krausz, Department of Pathology, The University of Chicago, Pritzker School of Medicine, Chicago, IL.)

in 70% of malignant mesotheliomas. Some but not all studies have demonstrated the presence of SV40 (simian virus 40) viral DNA sequences in 60% to 80% of pleural malignant mesotheliomas and in a smaller fraction of peritoneal mesotheliomas. The SV40 T-antigen is a potent carcinogen that binds to and inactivates several critical regulators of growth, such as p53 and RB. Whether SV40 is involved in the pathogenesis of mesothelioma remains controversial.[163]

Morphology. Malignant mesothelioma is a diffuse lesion that spreads widely in the pleural space and is usually associated with extensive pleural effusion and direct invasion of thoracic structures. The affected lung becomes ensheathed by a thick layer of soft, gelatinous, grayish pink tumor tissue (Fig. 15–50).

Microscopically, malignant mesotheliomas may be epithelioid (60%), sarcomatoid (20%), or mixed (20%). This is in keeping with the fact that mesothelial cells have the potential to develop as epithelium-like cells or mesenchymal stromal cells.

The **epithelioid type** of mesothelioma consists of cuboidal, columnar, or flattened cells forming tubular or papillary structures resembling adenocarcinoma (Fig. 15–51A). Epithelioid mesothelioma may at times

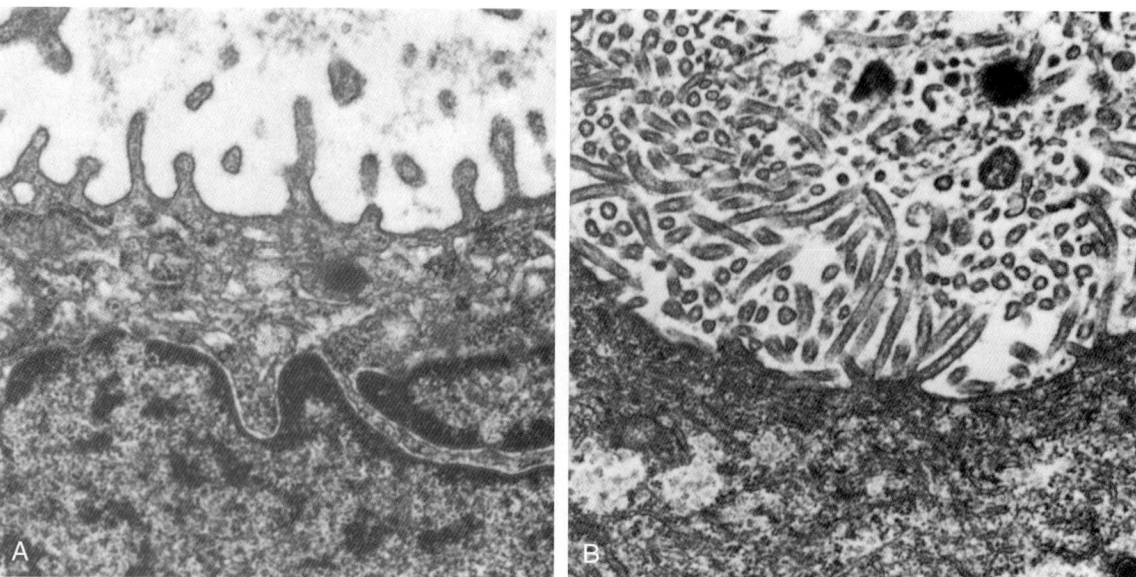

FIGURE 15–52 Ultrastructural features of pulmonary adenocarcinoma (**A**), characterized by short, plump microvilli, contrasted with those of mesothelioma (**B**), in which microvilli are numerous, long, and slender. (Courtesy of Dr. Noel Weidner, University of California, San Francisco, School of Medicine, San Francisco, CA.)

be difficult to differentiate grossly and histologically from pulmonary adenocarcinoma. Features that favor mesothelioma include (1) positive staining for acid mucopolysaccharide, which is inhibited by previous digestion by hyaluronidase; (2) lack of staining for carcinoembryonic antigen and other epithelial glycoprotein antigens, markers that are generally expressed by adenocarcinoma; (3) strong staining for keratin proteins, with accentuation of perinuclear rather than peripheral staining; (4) positive staining for calretinin (Fig. 15–51B), Wilms tumor 1 (WT-1), cytokeratin 5/6, and D2–40; and (5) on electron microscopy, the presence of long microvilli and abundant tonofilaments but absent microvillous rootlets and lamellar bodies (Fig. 15–52). The panel of special stains is diagnostic in a majority of cases when interpreted in the context of morphology and clinical presentation. The mesenchymal type of mesothelioma appears as a spindle cell sarcoma, resembling fibrosarcoma (**sarcomatoid type**). The **mixed type** of mesothelioma contains both epithelioid and sarcomatoid patterns (see Fig. 15–51B).

Clinical Course. The presenting complaints are chest pain, dyspnea, and, as noted, recurrent pleural effusions. Concurrent pulmonary asbestosis (fibrosis) is present in only 20% of individuals with pleural mesothelioma. The lung is invaded directly, and there is often metastatic spread to the hilar lymph nodes and, eventually, to the liver and other distant organs. Fifty percent of patients die within 12 months of diagnosis, and few survive longer than 2 years. Aggressive therapy (extrapleural pneumonectomy, chemotherapy, radiation therapy) seems to improve this poor prognosis in some patients with epithelioid mesothelioma.

Mesotheliomas also arise in the peritoneum, pericardium, tunica vaginalis, and genital tract (benign adenomatoid tumor;

see Chapter 21). *Peritoneal mesotheliomas* are particularly related to heavy asbestos exposure; 50% of such patients also have pulmonary fibrosis. Although in about 50% of cases the disease remains confined to the abdominal cavity, intestinal involvement frequently leads to death from intestinal obstruction or inanition.

REFERENCES

1. Askin FB: Potter's Pathology of the Fetus, Infant and Child, 2nd ed. St. Louis, Mosby/Elsevier, 2007.
2. Wheeler AP, Bernard GR: Acute lung injury and the acute respiratory distress syndrome: a clinical review. Lancet 369:1553, 2007.
3. Suratt BT, Parsons PE: Mechanisms of acute lung injury/acute respiratory distress syndrome. Clin Chest Med 27:579, 2006.
4. Ware LB: Pathophysiology of acute lung injury and the acute respiratory distress syndrome. Semin Respir Crit Care Med 27:337, 2006.
5. Rubenfeld GD et al.: Incidence and outcomes of acute lung injury. N Engl J Med 353:1685, 2005.
6. Ware LB, Matthay MA: The acute respiratory distress syndrome. N Engl J Med 342:1334, 2000.
7. Vouriekis JS et al.: Acute interstitial pneumonitis. Case series and review of the literature. Medicine 79:369, 2000.
8. Katzenstein AL et al.: Acute interstitial pneumonia. A clinicopathologic, ultrastructural, and cell kinetic study. Am J Surg Pathol 10:256, 1986.
9. Bouros D et al.: Acute interstitial pneumonia. Eur Respir J 15:412, 2000.
10. Katzenstein AL: Surgical Pathology of Non-Neoplastic Lung Disease, 4th ed. Philadelphia, Saunders/Elsevier, 2006.
11. Hogg JC et al.: The nature of small-airway obstruction in chronic obstructive pulmonary disease. N Eng J Med 350:2645, 2004.
12. Marsh SE et al.: Proportional classifications of COPD phenotypes. Thorax 63:761, 2008.
13. Shaw RJ et al.: The role of small airways in lung disease. Respir Med 96:67, 2002.
14. Barnes PJ: Novel approaches and targets for treatment of chronic obstructive pulmonary disease. Am J Respir Crit Care Med 160:S72, 1999.
15. Snider G: The definition of emphysema: report of the National Heart, Lung and Blood Institute, Division of Lung Diseases Workshop. Am Rev Respir Dis 132:182, 1985.
16. Morbidity and Mortality Chartbook on Cardiovascular Lung and Blood Disease. National Institutes of Health; 2007.

17. Rabe KF et al.: Global strategy for the diagnosis, management, and prevention of chronic obstructive pulmonary disease: GOLD executive summary. Am J Respir Crit Care Med 176:352, 2007.

18. Wright JL: Emphysema: concepts under change—a pathologist's perspective. Mod Pathol 8:873, 1995.

19. Cazzola M et al.: One hundred years of chronic obstructive pulmonary disease (COPD). Respir Med 101:1049, 2007.

20. Pauwels RA et al.: Global strategy for the diagnosis, management, and prevention of chronic obstructive pulmonary disease. NHLBI/WHO Global Initiative for Chronic Obstructive Lung Disease (GOLD) Workshop summary. Am J Respir Crit Care Med 163:1256, 2001.

21. Kim V et al.: New concepts in the pathobiology of chronic obstructive pulmonary disease. Proc Am Thorac Soc 5:478, 2008.

22. Taraseviciene-Stewart L, Voekel NF: Molecular pathogenesis of emphysema. J Clin Invest 118:394, 2008.

23. Kohnlein T, Welte T: Alpha-1 antitrypsin deficiency: pathogenesis, clinical presentation, diagnosis, and treatment. Am J Med 121:3, 2008.

24. deMello DE, Reid L: Pathology of Pulmonary Disease. Philadelphia, JB Lippincott, 1994.

25. Hogg JC, Timens W: The pathology of chronic obstructive pulmonary disease. Ann Rev Path Mech Dis 4:435, 2009.

26. Thurlbeck WM: Chronic Obstructive Pulmonary Disease. Philadelphia, WB Saunders, 1991.

27. Bloemen K et al.: The allergic cascade: review of the most important molecules in the asthmatic lung. Immunol Lett 113:6, 2007.

28. Green RH et al.: The reclassification of asthma based on subphenotypes. Curr Opin Allergy Clin Immunol 7:43, 2007.

29. Corne JM, Holgate ST: Mechanisms of virus induced exacerbations of asthma. Thorax 52:380, 1997.

30. Galli SJ et al.: The development of allergic inflammation. Nature 24:445, 2008.

31. Shelhamer JH et al.: NIH conference. Airway inflammation. Ann Intern Med 123:288, 1995.

32. Lilly CM et al.: Expression of eotaxin by human lung epithelial cells: induction by cytokines and inhibition by glucocorticoids. J Clin Invest 99:1767, 1997.

33. Costa JJ et al.: The cells of the allergic response: mast cells, basophils, and eosinophils. JAMA 278:1815, 1997.

34. Barnes PJ: Severe Asthma: Pathogenesis and Clinical Management. New York, Marcel Dekker, 1996.

35. Schaub B et al.: The many faces of hygiene hypothesis. J Allergy Clin Immunol 117:969, 2006.

36. Moffat MF: Genes in asthma: new genes and new ways. Curr Opin Allergy Clin Immunol 8:411, 2008.

37. Martinez FD: CD14, endotoxin, and asthma risk: Actions and interactions. Proc Am Thorac Soc 4:221, 2007.

38. Kabesch M: A glitch the switch? Of endotxin, CD14, and allergy. Am J Respir Crit Care Med 174:365, 2006.

39. Shapiro SD, Owen CA: ADAM-33 surfaces as an asthma gene. N Engl J Med 347:936, 2002.

40. Barnes KC: Genetics of asthma. Available at <http://www.uptodateonline.com/online/content/topic> (2008). Accessed March 2008.

41. Ober C et al.: Effect of variation in CHI3L1 on serum YKL-40 level, risk of asthma, and lung function. N Eng J Med 358:1682, 2008.

42. Ackerman SJ et al.: Charcot-Leyden crystal protein (galectin-10) is not a dual function galectin with lysophospholipase activity but binds a lysophospholipase inhibitor in a novel structural fashion. J Biol Chem 277:14859, 2002.

43. Solway J, Irvin CG: Airway smooth muscle as a target for asthma therapy. N Engl J Med 356:1367, 2007.

44. Luce L: Textbook of Respiratory Medicine. Philadelphia, WB Saunders, 1994.

45. Barker AF: Bronchiectasis. N Engl J Med 346:1383, 2002.

46. Notarangelo LD et al.: Genetic causes of bronchiectasis: primary immune deficiencies and the lung. Respiration 74:264, 2007.

47. Morrissey BM: Pathogenesis of bronchiectasis. Clin Chest Med 28:289, 2007.

48. Bush A et al.: Primary ciliary dyskinesia: current state of the art. Arch Dis Child 92:1136, 2007.

49. Al-Alawi A et al.: Aspergillus-related lung disease. Can Respir J 12:377, 2005.

50. Lazarus AA et al.: Allergic bronchopulmonary aspergillosis. Dis Mon 54:547, 2008.

51. Parameswaran GI, Murphy TF: Infections in chronic lung diseases. Infect Dis Clin North Am 21:673, 2007.

52. Collard HR, King TE, Jr.: Demystifying idiopathic interstitial pneumonia. Arch Intern Med 163:17, 2003.

53. American Thoracic Society/European Respiratory Society International Multidisciplinary Consensus Classification of the Idiopathic Interstitial Pneumonias. Am J Respir Crit Care Med 165:277, 2002.

54. Noble PW, Homer RJ: Idiopathic pulmonary fibrosis: new insights into pathogenesis. Clin Chest Med 25:749, 2004.

55. Scotton CJ, Chambers RC: Molecular targets in pulmonary fibrosis: the myofibroblast in focus. Chest 132:1311, 2007.

56. Tsakiri KD et al.: Adult-onset pulmonary fibrosis caused by mutations in telomerase. Proc Natl Acad Sci U S A 104:7552, 2007.

57. Armanios MY et al.:Telomerase mutations in families with idiopathic pulmonary fibrosis. N Engl J Med 356:1317, 2007.

58. Li H et al.: Transforming growth factor beta suppresses human telomerase reverse transcriptase (hTERT) by Smad3 interactions with c-Myc and the hTERT gene. J Biol Chem 281:25588, 2006.

59. Wang XM et al.: Caveolin-1: a critical regulator of lung fibrosis in idiopathic pulmonary fibrosis. J Exp Med 203:2895, 2006.

60. Verma S, Slutsky AS: Idiopathic pulmonary fibrosis—new insights. N Engl J Med 356:1370, 2007.

61. Visscher DW, Myers JL: Histologic spectrum of idiopathic interstitial pneumonias. Proc Am Thorac Soc 3:322, 2006.

62. Noth I, Martinez FJ: Recent advances in idiopathic pulmonary fibrosis. Chest 132:637, 2007.

63. Katzenstein AL, Fiorelli RF: Nonspecific interstitial pneumonia/fibrosis. Histologic features and clinical significance. Am J Surg Pathol 18:136, 1994.

64. du Bois R, King TE, Jr.: Challenges in pulmonary fibrosis × 5: the NSIP/UIP debate. Thorax 62:1008, 2007.

65. Travis WD et al.: Idiopathic nonspecific interstitial pneumonia: prognostic significance of cellular and fibrosing patterns: survival comparison with usual interstitial pneumonia and desquamative interstitial pneumonia. Am J Surg Pathol 24:19, 2000.

66. Cordier JF: Cryptogenic organising pneumonia. Eur Respir J 28:422, 2006.

67. Kim DS: Interstitial lung disease in rheumatoid arthritis: recent advances. Curr Opin Pulm Med 12:346, 2006.

68. Dockery DW et al.: An association between air pollution and mortality in six U.S. cities. N Engl J Med 329:1753, 1993.

69. Pope CA, 3rd et al.: Health effects of particulate air pollution: time for reassessment? Environ Health Perspect 103:472, 1995.

70. Borm PJ: Particle toxicology: from coal mining to nanotechnology. Inhal Toxicol 14:311, 2002.

71. Yucesoy B, Luster MI: Genetic susceptibility in pneumoconiosis. Toxicol Lett 168:249, 2007.

72. Izmerov NF et al.: Genetic-biochemical criteria for individual sensitivity in development of occupational bronchopulmonary diseases. Cent Eur J Public Health 10: 35, 2002.

73. Green F, Vallyathan V: Pathology of Occupational Lung Disease. Philadelphia, JB Lippincott, 1998.

74. Godleski JJ: Pathology of Pulmonary Disease. Philadelphia, JB Lippincott, 1994.

75. Vanhee D et al.: Cytokines and cytokine network in silicosis and coal workers' pneumoconiosis. Eur Respir J 8:834, 1995.

76. Ding M et al.: Diseases caused by silica: mechanisms of injury and disease development. Int Immunopharmacol 2:173, 2002.

77. Kazan-Allen L: Asbestos and mesothelioma: worldwide trends. Lung Cancer 49:S3, 2005.

78. Becklake MR et al.: Asbestos-related diseases of the lungs and pleura: uses, trends and management over the last century. Int J Tuberc Lung Dis 11:356, 2007.

79. Kamp DW, Weitzman SA: The molecular basis of asbestos induced lung injury. Thorax 54:638, 1999.

80. Hammond EC et al.: Asbestos exposure, cigarette smoking and death rates. Ann N Y Acad Sci 330:473, 1979.

81. Van Cleemput J, et al.: Surface of localized pleural plaques quantitated by computed tomography scanning: no relation with cumulative asbestos exposure and no effect on lung function. Am J Respir Crit Care Med 163:705, 2001.

82. Rossi SE et al.: Pulmonary drug toxicity: radiologic and pathologic manifestations. Radiographics 20:1245, 2000.

83. Movsas B et al.: Pulmonary radiation injury. Chest 111:1061, 1997.

84. Abratt RP, Morgan GW: Lung toxicity following chest irradiation in patients with lung cancer. Lung Cancer 35:103, 2002.

85. Rosen Y: Pathology of sarcoidosis. Semin Respir Crit Care Med 28:36, 2007.

86. Baughman RP et al.: Sarcoidosis. Lancet 361:1111, 2003.

87. Zissel G et al.: Sarcoidosis—immunopathogenetic concepts. Semin Respir Crit Care Med 28:3, 2007.

88. Ziegenhagen MW, Muller-Quernheim J: The cytokine network in sarcoidosis and its clinical relevance. J Intern Med 253:18, 2003.

89. du Bois RM et al.: Is there a role for microorganisms in the pathogenesis of sarcoidosis? J Intern Med 253:4, 2003.

90. Ma Y et al.: The pathology of pulmonary sarcoidosis: update. Semin Diagn Pathol 24:150, 2007.

91. Barnard J, Newman LS: Sarcoidosis: immunology, rheumatic involvement, and therapeutics. Curr Opin Rheumatol 13:84, 2001.

92. Sharma OP, Fujimura N: Hypersensitivity pneumonitis: a noninfectious granulomatosis. Semin Respir Infect 10:96, 1995.

93. Ismail T et al.: Extrinsic allergic alveolitis. Respirology 11:262, 2006.

94. Silva CI et al.: Hypersensitivity pneumonitis: spectrum of high-resolution CT and pathologic findings. AJR Am J Roentgenol 188:334, 2007.

95. Kita H et al.: Cytokine production at the site of disease in chronic eosinophilic pneumonitis. Am J Respir Crit Care Med 153:1437, 1996.

96. Jeong YJ et al.: Eosinophilic lung diseases: a clinical, radiologic, and pathologic overview. Radiographics 27:617, 2007.

97. Hidalgo A et al.: Smoking-related interstitial lung diseases: radiologic-pathologic correlation. Eur Radiol 16:2463, 2006.

98. Nicholson AG et al.: The prognostic significance of the histologic pattern of interstitial pneumonia in patients presenting with the clinical entity of cryptogenic fibrosing alveolitis. Am J Respir Crit Care Med 162:2213, 2000.

99. Fraig M et al.: Respiratory bronchiolitis: a clinicopathologic study in current smokers, ex-smokers, and never-smokers. Am J Surg Pathol 26:647, 2002.

100. Uchida K et al.: GM-CSF autoantibodies and neutrophil dysfunction in pulmonary alveolar proteinosis. N Engl J Med 356:567, 2007.

101. Garmany TH et al.: Surfactant composition and function in patients with *ABCA3* mutations. Pediatr Res 59:801, 2006.

102. Hamvas A et al.: Genetic disorders of surfactant proteins. Neonatology 91:311, 2007.

103. Ioachimescu OC, Kavuru MS: Pulmonary alveolar proteinosis. Chron Respir Dis 3:149, 2006.

104. Simonneau G et al.: Clinical classification of pulmonary hypertension. J Am Coll Cardiol 43:5S, 2004.

105. Runo JR, Loyd JE: Primary pulmonary hypertension. Lancet 361:1533, 2003.

106. Mark EJ et al.: Fatal pulmonary hypertension associated with short-term use of fenfluramine and phentermine. N Engl J Med 337:602, 1997.

107. Pietra GG et al.: Pathologic assessment of vasculopathies in pulmonary hypertension. J Am Coll Cardiol 43:25S, 2004.

108. Tuder RM et al.: Pathology of pulmonary hypertension. Clin Chest Med 28:23, 2007.

109. Fuster V et al.: Primary pulmonary hypertension: natural history and the importance of thrombosis. Circulation 70:580, 1984.

110. Alam S, Palevsky HI: Standard therapies for pulmonary arterial hypertension. Clin Chest Med 28:91, 2007.

111. Strauss WL, Edelman JD: Prostanoid therapy for pulmonary arterial hypertension. Clin Chest Med 28:127, 2007.

112. Langleben D: Endothelin receptor antagonists in the treatment of pulmonary arterial hypertension. Clin Chest Med 28:117, 2007.

113. Klinger JR: The nitric oxide/cGMP signaling pathway in pulmonary hypertension. Clin Chest Med 28:143, 2007.

114. O'Callaghan D, Gaine SP: Combination therapy and new types of agents for pulmonary arterial hypertension. Clin Chest Med 28:169, 2007.

115. Hudson BG et al.: Alport's syndrome, Goodpasture's syndrome, and type IV collagen. N Engl J Med 348:2543, 2003.

116. Travis WD, Fleming MV: Vasculitis of the lung. Pathology 4:23, 1996.

117. Gunnarsson A et al.: Molecular properties of the Goodpasture epitope. J Biol Chem 275:30844, 2000.

118. Lazor R et al.: Alveolar hemorrhage in anti-basement membrane antibody disease: a series of 28 cases. Medicine 86:181, 2007.

119. Collard HR, Schwarz MI: Diffuse alveolar hemorrhage. Clin Chest Med 25:583, 2004.

120. Nuesslein TG et al.: Pulmonary haemosiderosis in infants and children. Paediatr Respir Rev 7:45, 2006.

121. Pennington JE: Respiratory Infections: Diagnosis and Management, 3rd ed. New York, Raven Press, 1994.

122. Bartlett JG et al.: Community-acquired pneumonia in adults: guidelines for management. The Infectious Diseases Society of America. Clin Infect Dis 26:811, 1998.

123. Roche RJ, Moxon ER: Phenotypic variation of carbohydrate surface antigens and the pathogenesis of *Haemophilus influenzae* infections. Trends Microbiol 3:304, 1995.

124. Hasleton P: Spencer's Pathology of the Lung. New York, McGraw-Hill, 1996.

125. Kahn JS: Newly identified respiratory viruses. Pediatr Infect Dis J 26:745, 2007.

126. Arnheiter H et al.: Transgenic mice with intracellular immunity to influenza virus. Cell 62:51, 1990.

127. Gorman OT et al.: Evolutionary processes in influenza viruses: divergence, rapid evolution, and stasis. Curr Top Microbiol Immunol 176:75, 1992.

128. Taubenberger JK et al.: Initial genetic characterization of the 1918 "Spanish" influenza virus. Science 275:1793, 1997.

129. Tumpey TM et al.: Existing antivirals are effective against influenza viruses with genes from the 1918 pandemic virus. Proc Natl Acad Sci U S A 99:13849, 2002.

130. Gambotto A et al.: Human infection with highly pathogenic H5N1 influenza virus. Lancet 371:1464, 2008.

131. Deffrasnes C et al.: Human metapneumovirus. Semin Respir Crit Care Med 28:213, 2007.

132. Peiris JS et al.: The severe acute respiratory syndrome. N Engl J Med 349:2431, 2003.

133. Lomotan JR et al.: Aspiration pneumonia. Strategies for early recognition and prevention. Postgrad Med 102:225, 1997.

134. Joseph Wheat L: Current diagnosis of histoplasmosis. Trends Microbiol 11:488, 2003.

135. Rosenow EC, 3rd: Diffuse pulmonary infiltrates in the immunocompromised host. Clin Chest Med 11:55, 1990.

136. Yousem SA et al.: Revision of the 1990 working formulation for the classification of pulmonary allograft rejection: Lung Rejection Study Group. J Heart Lung Transplant 15:1, 1996.

137. Trulock EP et al.: Registry of the International Society for Heart and Lung Transplantation: twenty-fourth official adult lung and heart-lung transplantation report-2007. J Heart Lung Transplant 26:782, 2007.

138. Travis WD: World Health Organization Classification of Tumours. Lyon, IARC Press, 2004.

139. Jemal A et al.: Cancer statistics, 2008. CA Cancer J Clin 58:71, 2008.

140. US Environmental Protection Agency. Respiratory Health Effects of Passive Smoking: Lung Cancer and Other Disorders. Agency UEP. Washington, D.C., 1992.

141. Marchevsky A: Surgical Pathology of Lung Neoplasms. New York, Marcel Dekker, 1990.

142. Samet JM: Indoor radon and lung cancer. Estimating the risks. West J Med 156:25, 1992.

143. Pershagen G et al.: Residential radon exposure and lung cancer in Sweden. N Engl J Med 330:159, 1994.

144. Frumkin H, Samet JM: Radon. CA Cancer J Clin 51:337, 2001.

145. Mitsuo et al.: A translational view of molecular pathogenesis of lung cancer. J Thorac Oncol 2:327, 2007.

146. Makowski L, Hayes DN: Role of LKB1 in lung cancer development. Brit J Cancer 99:683, 2008.

147. Wistuba II, Gazdar AF: Lung cancer preneoplasia. Review in Advance 1:331, 2006.

148. Schwartz AG et al.: Molecular epidemiology of lung cancer. Carcinogenesis 28:507, 2007.

149. Hung RJ: A susceptibility locus for lung cancer maps to nicotinic acetylcholine receptor subunit genes on 15q25. Nature 452:633, 2008.

150. Sun S et al.: Lung cancer in never smokers—a different disease. Nat Rev Cancer 7:778, 2007.

151. Wahbah M et al.: Changing trends in the distribution of the histologic types of lung cancer: a review of 4,439 cases. Ann Diagn Pathol 11:89, 2007.

152. el-Torky M et al.: Significant changes in the distribution of histologic types of lung cancer. A review of 4928 cases. Cancer 65:2361, 1990.

153. Hoffmann D et al.: The biological significance of tobacco-specific N-nitrosamines: smoking and adenocarcinoma of the lung. Crit Rev Toxicol 26:199, 1996.

154. Herbst RS et al.: Molecular origins of cancer: Lung Cancer. N Eng J Med 359:1367, 2008.
155. Yousem SA, Beasley MB: Bronchioloalveolar carcinoma: a review of current concepts and evolving issues. Arch Pathol Lab Med 131:1027, 2007.
156. Sakuma Y et al.: Epidermal growth factor receptor gene mutations in atypical adenomatous hyperplasias of the lung. Mod Pathol 20:967, 2007.
157. Sekido Y et al.: Molecular genetics of lung cancer. Annu Rev Med 54:73, 2003.
158. Patel AM et al.: Paraneoplastic syndromes associated with lung cancer. Mayo Clin Proc 68:278, 1993.
159. Travis WD et al.: Survival analysis of 200 pulmonary neuroendocrine tumors with clarification of criteria for atypical carcinoid and its separation from typical carcinoid. Am J Surg Pathol 22:934, 1998.
160. Gold JS et al.: Clinicopathologic correlates of solitary fibrous tumors. Cancer 94:1057, 2002.
161. Corson JM: Pathology of diffuse malignant pleural mesothelioma. Semin Thorac Cardiovasc Surg 9:347, 1997.
162. Greillier L, Astoul P: Mesothelioma and asbestos-related pleural diseases. Respiration 76:1, 2008.
163. Rivera Z et al.: The relationship between simian virus 40 and mesothelioma. Curr Opin Pulmon Med 14:316, 2008.

Head and Neck

MARK W. LINGEN

■ **ORAL CAVITY**

Teeth and Supporting Structures
  Caries (Tooth Decay)
  Gingivitis
  Periodontitis

Inflammatory/Reactive Tumor-like Lesions
  Fibrous Proliferative Lesions
  Aphthous Ulcers (Canker Sores)
  Glossitis

Infections
  Herpes Simplex Virus Infections
  Other Viral Infections
  Oral Candidiasis (Thrush)
  Deep Fungal Infections

Oral Manifestations of Systemic Disease
  Hairy Leukoplakia

Tumors and Precancerous Lesions
  Leukoplakia and Erythroplakia
  Squamous Cell Carcinoma

Odontogenic Cysts and Tumors

■ **UPPER AIRWAYS**

Nose
  Inflammations
  Necrotizing Lesions of the Nose and Upper Airways

Nasopharynx
  Inflammations

Tumors of the Nose, Sinuses, and Nasopharynx

Larynx
  Inflammations
  Reactive Nodules (Vocal Cord Nodules and Polyps)
  Squamous Papilloma and Papillomatosis
  Carcinoma of the Larynx

■ **EARS**

Inflammatory Lesions

Otosclerosis

Tumors

■ **NECK**

Branchial Cyst (Cervical Lymphoepithelial Cyst)

Thyroglossal Duct Cyst

Paraganglioma (Carotid Body Tumor)

■ **SALIVARY GLANDS**

Xerostomia

Inflammation (Sialadenitis)

Neoplasms
  Pleomorphic Adenoma
  Warthin Tumor (Papillary Cystadenoma Lymphomatosum)
  Mucoepidermoid Carcinoma
  Other Salivary Gland Tumors

Diseases of the head and neck range from the common cold to uncommon neoplasms of the nose. Those selected for discussion are assigned, sometimes arbitrarily, to one of the following anatomic sites: (1) oral cavity; (2) upper airways, including the nose, pharynx, larynx, and nasal sinuses; (3) ears; (4) neck; and (5) salivary glands.

ORAL CAVITY

The oral cavity is a fearsome orifice guarded by ranks of upper and lower "horns" (lamentably, quite subject to erosion), demanding constant gratification, and teeming with microorganisms, some of which are potentially harmful. Among the many disorders that affect its various parts, only the more important or frequent conditions involving the teeth and supporting structures, oral mucous membranes, lips, and tongue are considered.

Teeth and Supporting Structures

Teeth contribute to several important functions, including mastication and proper speech. It is useful to briefly review normal dental anatomy before we delve into the common pathologic conditions affecting teeth. As is well known, teeth are firmly implanted in the jaw and are surrounded by the gingival mucosa (Fig. 16–1). The anatomic crown of the tooth projects into the mouth and is covered by *enamel*, a hard, inert, acellular tissue—the most highly mineralized tissue in the body. The enamel rests upon *dentin*, which is a specialized form of connective tissue that makes up most of the remaining hard-tissue portion of the tooth. Unlike enamel, dentin is cellular and contains numerous dentinal tubules, which contain the cytoplasmic extensions of odontoblasts. These cells line the interface between the dentin and the pulp and can, when properly stimulated, produce new (secondary) dentin within the interior of the tooth. The pulp chamber itself is surrounded by the dentin and consists of loose connective tissue stroma rich in nerve bundles, lymphatics, and capillaries.

To perform mastication, teeth must not only be composed of hard tissue but must also be firmly attached to the bones of the jaw. If this attachment were excessively firm, chewing would impose sufficient physical stress on the teeth to cause their loss or fracturing. Therefore, in mammals, teeth are attached to the alveolar ridge of the jaws by the *periodontal ligament*, which provides a strong yet flexible attachment that can withstand the forces of mastication. The periodontal ligament attaches to the alveolar bone of the jaw on one side and to *cementum*, present on the roots of the teeth, which acts as a "cement" to anchor the periodontal ligament to the tooth.

CARIES (TOOTH DECAY)

Dental caries, caused by focal degradation of the tooth structure, is one of the most common diseases throughout the world and is the most common cause of tooth loss before age 35. Carious lesions are the result of mineral dissolution of tooth structure by acid metabolic end products from bacteria that are present in the oral cavity and are capable of fermenting sugars. Traditionally, the rate of caries has been higher in industrialized countries, where there is ready access to processed foods containing large amounts of carbohydrates. However, global trends may change these demographics. First of all, the rate of caries has markedly dropped in countries such as the United States, where improved oral hygiene and fluoridation of the drinking water has become a standard practice. Fluoride incorporates into the crystalline structure of enamel, forming fluoroapatite, and contributes to resistance to degradation by bacterial acids. Second, with globalization of the world's economy, increased amounts of processed foods with high carbohydrate content are being imported into developing nations. With these trends, one can expect the rate of caries to increase dramatically in the less-developed world over the next several decades.

GINGIVITIS

Gingiva is the designation of the squamous mucosa in between the teeth and around them. Gingivitis is inflammation of the mucosa and the associated soft tissues. Typically, the development of gingivitis is the result of a lack of proper oral hygiene, leading to an accumulation of dental plaque and calculus. *Dental plaque* is a sticky, usually colorless, biofilm that builds in between and on the surface of the teeth. It is formed by a complex of the oral bacteria, proteins from the saliva, and desquamated epithelial cells. If plaque continues to build and

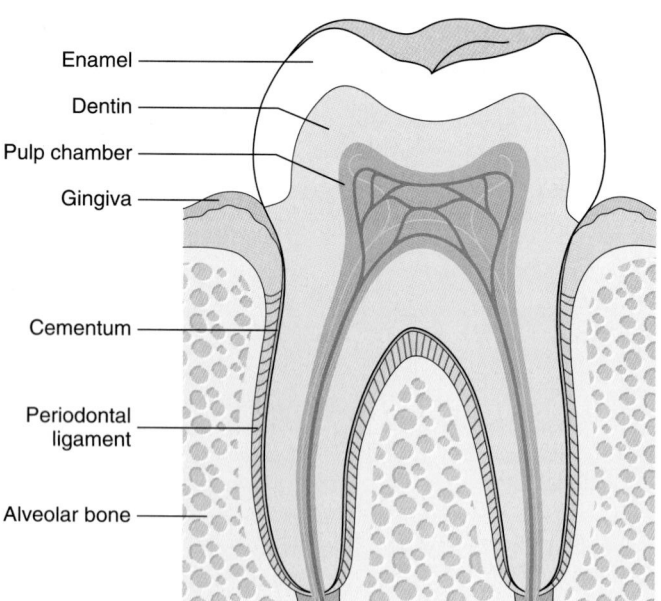

FIGURE 16–1 Schematic representation of the normal dental anatomy and surrounding supporting tissues.

Enamel
Dentin
Pulp chamber
Gingiva
Cementum
Periodontal ligament
Alveolar bone

is not removed, it becomes mineralized to form calculus (tartar). The bacteria in the plaque release acids from sugar-rich foods, which erode the enamel surface of the tooth. Repeated erosions lead to dental caries. Plaque build-up beneath the gumline can cause gingivitis. Chronic gingivitis is characterized by gingival erythema, edema, bleeding, changes in contour, and loss of soft-tissue adaptation to the teeth. Gingivitis occurs at any age but is most prevalent and severe in adolescence (ranging from 40% to 60%), after which the incidence tapers off. It is a reversible disease; therapy is primarily aimed at reducing the accumulation of plaque and calculus via brushing, flossing, and regular dental visits.[1]

PERIODONTITIS

Periodontitis refers to an inflammatory process that affects the supporting structures of the teeth: periodontal ligaments, alveolar bone, and cementum. With progression, periodontitis can lead to serious sequelae, including the loss of attachment caused by complete destruction of the periodontal ligament and alveolar bone. Loosening and eventual loss of teeth are possible. The pathogenesis of periodontal inflammation is not entirely clear. Until the 1960s it was believed that long-standing gingivitis uniformly progressed to periodontal disease. However, this is no longer thought to be the case. Rather, the development of periodontal disease is now considered to be an independent process, which, for reasons that are still unclear, is associated with a marked shift in the types and proportions of bacteria along the gingiva.[2] This shift, along with other environmental conditions such as poor oral hygiene, is believed to be important in the pathogenesis of periodontitis. This view is supported by significant differences in the content of dental plaque in areas of healthy and diseased periodontium. For the most part, facultative gram-positive organisms colonize healthy sites, while plaque within areas of active periodontitis contains anaerobic and microaerophilic gram-negative flora. Although 300 types of bacteria reside in the oral cavity, adult periodontitis is associated primarily with *Aggregatibacter (Actinobacillus) actinomycetemcomitans*, *Porphyromonas gingivalis*, and *Prevotella intermedia*.

While it typically presents without any associated disorders, periodontal disease can also be a component of several different systemic diseases, including acquired immunodeficiency syndrome (AIDS), leukemia, Crohn's disease, diabetes mellitus, Down syndrome, sarcoidosis, and syndromes associated with polymorphonuclear defects (Chédiak-Higashi syndrome, agranulocytosis, and cyclic neutropenia). In addition to being a component of certain systemic diseases, periodontal infections can also be etiologic factors in several important systemic diseases. These include, for example, infective endocarditis, pulmonary and brain abscesses, and adverse pregnancy outcomes.[3,4]

Inflammatory/Reactive Tumor-like Lesions

Several soft-tissue lesions of the oral cavity, which present as tumor masses or ulcerations, are reactive in nature and represent inflammations induced by irritation or by unknown mechanisms. All suspicious lesions, however, should be examined by biopsy. Reactive nodules of the oral cavity are fairly

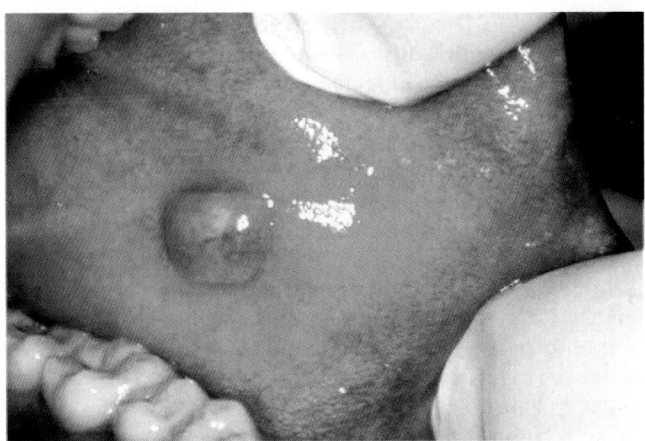

FIGURE 16–2 Fibroma. Smooth pink exophytic nodule on the buccal mucosa.

common and microscopically diverse. The most common fibrous proliferative lesions of the oral cavity include fibroma (61%), peripheral ossifying fibroma (22%), pyogenic granuloma (12%), and peripheral giant-cell granuloma (5%).[5] The most common inflammatory/reactive ulcerations of the oral cavity are traumatic and aphthous ulcers.

FIBROUS PROLIFERATIVE LESIONS

The so-called *irritation fibroma* (Fig. 16–2) primarily occurs in the buccal mucosa along the bite line or at the gingivodental margin. It consists of a nodular mass of fibrous tissue, with few inflammatory cells, covered by squamous mucosa. Treatment is complete surgical excision.

The *pyogenic granuloma* (Fig. 16–3) is a highly vascular pedunculated lesion, usually occurring in the gingiva of children, young adults, and, commonly, pregnant women (pregnancy tumor). The surface of the lesion is typically ulcerated and red to purple in color. In some cases growth is alarmingly rapid, raising the fear of a malignant neoplasm. Histologically these lesions demonstrate a highly vascular proliferation that is similar to granulation tissue. Because of this histologic picture, pyogenic granulomas are considered by some authorities to be a form of capillary hemangioma (Chapter 11). They

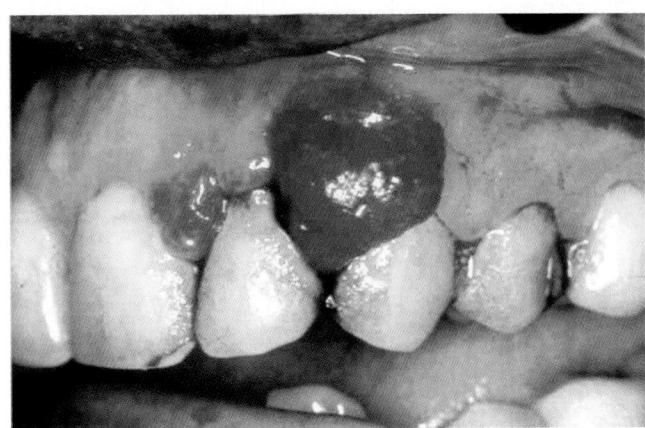

FIGURE 16–3 Pyogenic granuloma. Erythematous, hemorrhagic, and exophytic mass arising from the gingival mucosa.

either regress, particularly after pregnancy, or undergo fibrous maturation, and they may develop into a peripheral ossifying fibroma. Treatment is complete surgical excision.

The *peripheral ossifying fibroma* is a relatively common growth of the gingiva that is considered to be reactive in nature rather than neoplastic. However, the etiology of the lesion is unknown. Some may arise as a result of the maturation of a long-standing pyogenic granuloma. With a peak incidence in young and teenage females, peripheral ossifying fibromas appear as red, ulcerated, and nodular lesions of the gingiva. They are often mistaken clinically for pyogenic granulomas. Complete surgical excision down to the periosteum is the treatment of choice, since these lesions have a recurrence rate of 15% to 20%.

The *peripheral giant cell granuloma* is a relatively common lesion of the gingiva. It is generally covered by intact gingival mucosa, but it may be ulcerated. The clinical appearance of peripheral giant-cell granuloma can be similar to that of pyogenic granuloma, but which is generally more bluish purple in color while the pyogenic granuloma is more bright red. Histologically, however, these lesions are distinct. Peripheral giant-cell granuloma is made up of a striking aggregation of multinucleate, foreign body–like giant cells separated by a fibroangiomatous stroma. Although not encapsulated, these lesions are usually well delimited and easily excised. They should be differentiated from central giant-cell granulomas found within the maxilla or the mandible and from the histologically similar but frequently multiple "brown tumors" seen in hyperparathyroidism (Chapter 24).

APHTHOUS ULCERS (CANKER SORES)

These extremely common superficial ulcerations of the oral mucosa affect up to 40% of the population in the United States.[6] They are more common in the first two decades of life, are extremely painful and often recurrent, and tend to be prevalent within certain families.

The lesions appear as single or multiple, shallow, hyperemic ulcerations covered by a thin exudate and rimmed by a narrow zone of erythema (Fig. 16–4). The underlying inflammatory infiltrate is at first largely mononuclear, but secondary bacterial infection introduces numerous neutrophils. The lesions

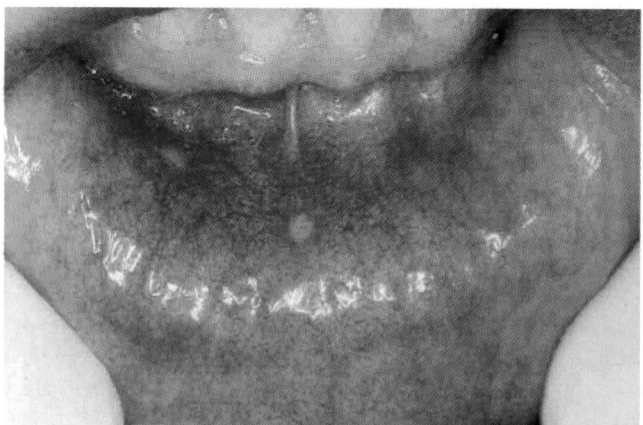

FIGURE 16–4 Aphthous ulcer. Single ulceration with an erythematous halo surrounding a yellowish fibrinopurulent membrane.

may spontaneously resolve in 7 to 10 days or be stubbornly persistent for weeks. The causation of these lesions is obscure. Most ulcers are more painful than serious and require only symptomatic treatment. Recurrent apthous ulcers may be associated with celiac disease and inflammatory bowel disease.

GLOSSITIS

Although the designation *glossitis* implies inflammation of the tongue, it is sometimes applied to the beefy-red tongue encountered in certain deficiency states; this change results from atrophy of the papillae of the tongue and thinning of the mucosa, exposing the underlying vasculature. In some instances the atrophic changes do indeed lead to inflammation and even shallow ulcerations. Such changes may be encountered in deficiencies of vitamin B_{12} (pernicious anemia), riboflavin, niacin, or pyridoxine. Similar alterations are sometimes encountered with sprue and iron-deficiency anemia, possibly complicated by deficiency in one of the B vitamins. *The combination of iron-deficiency anemia, glossitis, and esophageal dysphagia usually related to webs is known as the Plummer-Vinson or Paterson-Kelly syndrome.* Glossitis, characterized by ulcerative lesions (sometimes along the lateral borders of the tongue), may also be seen with jagged carious teeth, ill-fitting dentures, and, rarely, with syphilis, inhalation burns, or ingestion of corrosive chemicals.

Infections

The oral mucosa is highly resistant to its indigenous flora, having many defenses, including the competitive suppression of potential pathogens by organisms of low virulence, the elaboration of secretory IgA and other immunoglobulins by submucosal collections of lymphocytes and plasma cells, the antibacterial effects of saliva, and the irrigating effects of food and drink. Nonetheless, any lowering of these defenses, for example, with immunodeficiency or disruption of the microbiologic balance by antibacterial therapy, sets the stage for oral infections. Most of these infections are discussed in Chapter 8, and here we only briefly recapitulate the principal features of the oral lesions.

HERPES SIMPLEX VIRUS INFECTIONS

Most orofacial herpetic infections are caused by herpes simplex virus type 1 (HSV-1). However, because of changes in sexual habits, an increase in HSV-2 (genital herpes) has been observed in the oral cavity. Primary HSV infection typically occurs in children age 2 to 4 years, is often asymptomatic, and does not cause significant morbidity. Approximately 10% to 20% of the time, primary infection presents as *acute herpetic gingivostomatitis*, in which there is an abrupt onset of vesicles and ulcerations throughout the oral cavity, especially in the gingiva. These lesions are also accompanied by lymphadenopathy, fever, anorexia, and irritability.

Morphology. The vesicles range from lesions of a few millimeters to large bullae and are at first filled with a clear, serous fluid, but they often rupture to yield extremely painful, red-rimmed, shallow ulcerations. On microscopic examination there is intracellular and intercellular edema (acantholysis), yielding clefts that may become transformed into macroscopic vesicles. Individual epidermal cells in the margins of the vesicle or lying free within the fluid sometimes develop eosinophilic **intranuclear viral inclusions,** or several cells may fuse to produce giant cells **(multinucleate polykaryons),** changes that are demonstrated by the diagnostic **Tzanck test,** based on microscopic examination of the vesicle fluid. The vesicles and shallow ulcers usually spontaneously clear within 3 to 4 weeks, but the virus treks along the regional nerves and eventually becomes dormant in the local ganglia (e.g., the trigeminal).

The great preponderance of adults harbor latent HSV-1, but in some individuals, usually young adults, the virus becomes reactivated to produce the common but usually mild *cold sore.* The influences predisposing to activation are poorly understood but are thought to include trauma, allergies, exposure to ultraviolet light, upper respiratory tract infections, pregnancy, menstruation, immunosuppression, and exposure to extremes of temperature.

Recurrent herpetic stomatitis (in contrast to acute gingivostomatitis) occurs either at the site of primary inoculation or in adjacent mucosal areas that are associated with the same ganglion; it takes the form of groups of small (1–3 mm) vesicles. The lips (*Herpes labialis*), nasal orifices, buccal mucosa, gingiva, and hard palate are the most common locations for recurrent lesions. They resemble those already described in the primary infections but are much more limited in duration, are milder, usually dry up in 4 to 6 days, and heal within a week to 10 days.

OTHER VIRAL INFECTIONS

Additional viral infections that can be seen in the oral cavity as well as the head and neck region include herpes zoster, Epstein-Barr virus (EBV; mononucleosis), cytomegalovirus, enterovirus (herpangina, hand-foot-and-mouth disease, acute lymphonodular pharyngitis), and rubeola (measles).

ORAL CANDIDIASIS (THRUSH)

The many localizations of candidal infection are fully described in Chapter 8, and so this discussion is limited to presentation in the oral cavity. Candidiasis is by far the most common fungal infection in the oral cavity. *Candida albicans* is a normal component of the oral flora in approximately 50% of the population. Three factors seem to influence the likelihood of a clinical infection: (1) immune status of the individual; (2) the strain of *C. albicans* present; and (3) the composition of an individual's oral flora. There are three major clinical forms of oral candidiasis, including pseudo-membranous (thrush), erythematous, and hyperplastic, with several different variations within these groups. Only the pseudo-membranous form, the most common of these, is discussed here. Also known as "*thrush,*" pseudo-membranous candidiasis typically takes the form of a superficial, curdy, gray to white inflammatory membrane composed of matted organisms enmeshed in a fibrinosuppurative exudate that can be readily scraped off to reveal an underlying erythematous inflammatory base. This fungus causes mischief only in individuals who have some form of immunosuppression, as occurs in patients with diabetes mellitus, organ or bone marrow transplant recipients, those with neutropenia, chemotherapy-induced immunosuppression, or AIDS. In addition, broad-spectrum antibiotics that eliminate or alter the normal bacterial flora of the mouth can also result in the development of oral candidiasis.

DEEP FUNGAL INFECTIONS

In addition to their more common sites of infection, certain deep fungal infections have a significant predilection for the oral cavity and the head and neck region. Such fungi include histoplasmosis, blastomycosis, coccidioidomycosis, cryptococcosis, zygomycosis, and aspergillosis. With an increasing number of patients who are immunocompromised due to diseases such as AIDS or therapies for cancer and organ transplantation, the prevalence of fungal infections of the oral cavity has also increased in recent years.

Oral Manifestations of Systemic Disease

As oral clinicians are at pains to emphasize, the mouth is a part of the body and not merely a gateway for delicacies. Not surprisingly, then, many systemic diseases are associated with oral lesions. In fact, it is not uncommon for oral lesions to be the first sign of some underlying systemic condition. Some of the more common disease associations are cited in Table 16–1, with a few words about the associated oral changes. Only one—hairy leukoplakia—is characterized in more detail.

HAIRY LEUKOPLAKIA

Hairy leukoplakia is a distinctive oral lesion that is usually seen in immunocompromised patients. Approximately 80% of patients with hairy leukoplakia are infected with the human immunodeficiency virus (HIV); the presence of this lesion sometimes calls attention to the existence of HIV infection. However, 20% of lesions are seen in patients who are immunocompromised for other reasons, such as cancer therapy or transplant immunosuppression. Hairy leukoplakia takes the form of *white, confluent patches of fluffy ("hairy"), hyperkeratotic thickenings, almost always situated on the lateral border of the tongue.* Unlike thrush, the lesion cannot be scraped off. The distinctive microscopic appearance consists of *hyperparakeratosis* and *acanthosis with "balloon cells" in the upper spinous layer.* Sometimes there is koilocytosis of the superficial, nucleated epidermal cells, suggesting human papillomavirus (HPV) infection, and HPV transcripts have occasionally been found within the cells. However, EBV is present in most cells and is now accepted as the cause of the condition.[7] Sometimes there is superimposed candidal infection on the surface of the lesions, adding to the "hairiness." In HIV-positive individuals, with hairy leukoplarkia, symptoms of AIDS follow in 2 to 3 years.

TABLE 16–1 Oral Manifestantions of Some Systemic Diseases	
Systemic Disease	**Associated Oral Changes**
INFECTIOUS DISEASES	
Scarlet fever	Fiery red tongue with prominent papillae (raspberry tongue); white-coated tongue through which hyperemic papillae project (strawberry tongue)
Measles	Spotty enanthema in the oral cavity often precedes the skin rash; ulcerations on the buccal mucosa about Stensen duct produce Koplik spots
Infectious mononucleosis	Acute pharyngitis and tonsillitis that may cause coating with a gray-white exudative membrane; enlargement of lymph nodes in the neck, palatal petechiae
Diphtheria	Characteristic dirty white, fibrinosuppurative, tough, inflammatory membrane over the tonsils and retropharynx
Human immunodeficiency virus	Predisposition to opportunistic oral infections, particularly herpesvirus, *Candida*, and other fungi; oral lesions of Kaposi sarcoma and hairy leukoplakia (described in text)
DERMATOLOGIC CONDITIONS*	
Lichen planus	Reticulate, lacelike, white keratotic lesions that rarely become bullous and ulcerated; seen in more than 50% of patients with cutaneous lichen planus; rarely, is the sole manifestation
Pemphigus	Vesicles and bullae prone to rupture, leaving hyperemic erosions covered with exudates
Bullous pemphigoid	Oral lesions resemble macroscopically those of pemphigus but can be differentiated histologically
Erythema multiforme	Maculopapular, vesiculobullous eruption that sometimes follows an infection elsewhere, ingestion of drugs, development of cancer, or a collagen vascular disease; when it involves the lips and oral mucosa, it is referred to as *Stevens-Johnson syndrome*
HEMATOLOGIC DISORDERS	
Pancytopenia (agranulocytosis, aplastic anemia)	Severe oral infections in the form of gingivitis, pharyngitis, tonsillitis; may extend to produce cellulitis of the neck (*Ludwig angina*)
Leukemia	With depletion of functioning neutrophils, oral lesions may appear like those in pancytopenia
Monocytic leukemia	Leukemic infiltration and enlargement of the gingivae, often with accompanying periodontitis
MISCELLANEOUS	
Melanotic pigmentation	May appear in Addison disease, hemochromatosis, fibrous dysplasia of bone (Albright syndrome), and Peutz-Jegher syndrome (gastrointestinal polyposis)
Phenytoin (Dilantin) ingestion	Striking fibrous enlargement of the gingivae
Pregnancy	A friable, red, pyogenic granuloma protruding from the gingiva ("pregnancy tumor")
Rendu-Osler-Weber syndrome	Autosomal dominant disorder with multiple congenital aneurysmal telangiectasias beneath mucosal surfaces of the oral cavity and lips

*See Chapter 25 for details

Tumors and Precancerous Lesions

Many epithelial and connective tissue tumors of the head and neck region (e.g., papillomas, hemangiomas, lymphomas) also occur elsewhere in the body and are described adequately in other chapters. Therefore, this discussion will consider only oral squamous cell carcinoma and its associated precancerous lesions.

LEUKOPLAKIA AND ERYTHROPLAKIA

As is discussed in more detail below, oral cancers are common worldwide, with a fairly high mortality. Screening and early detection in populations at risk have been proposed to decrease the morbidity and mortality associated with oral cancer.[8,9] However, the visual detection of definitive premalignant oral lesions is problematic. This is in stark contrast to skin lesions, where visual screening for melanomas of the skin has been shown to have sensitivity and specificity rates of 93% and 98%.[10,11] One explanation for this discrepancy is that the early lesions frequently do not demonstrate any of the clinical characteristics observed in advanced oral cancer such as ulceration, induration, pain, or cervical lymphadenopathy.[12] In addition, the clinical presentation of potentially premalignant lesions in the oral cavity is highly heterogeneous. We begin our discussion with two premalignant lesions: leukoplakia and erythroplakia.

The term *leukoplakia* is defined by the World Health Organization as "a white patch or plaque that cannot be scraped off and cannot be characterized clinically or pathologically as any other disease." Simply put, if a white lesion in the oral cavity can be given a specific diagnosis it is not a leukoplakia. This clinical term is reserved for lesions that are present in the oral cavity for no apparent reason. As such, white patches

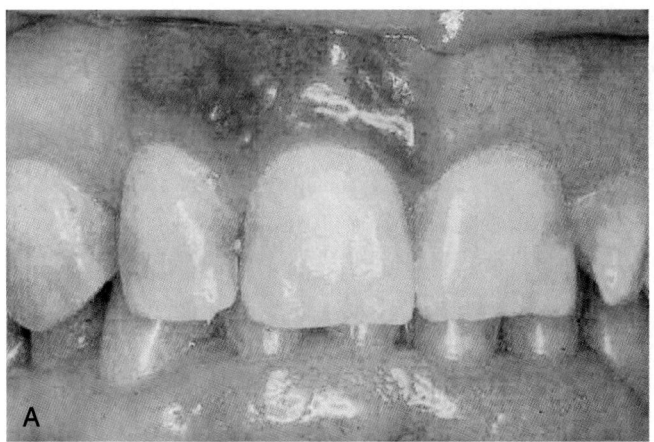
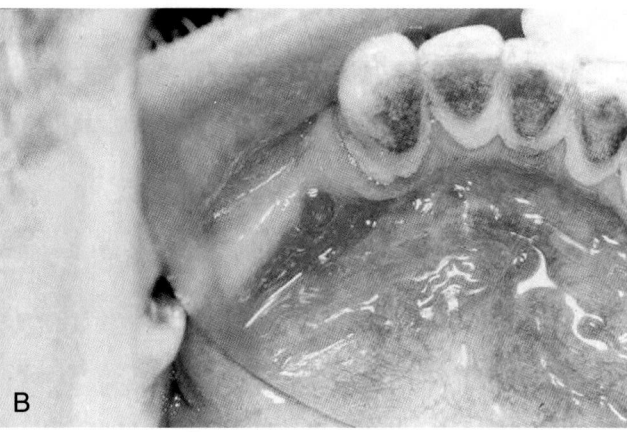

FIGURE 16–5   Erythroplakia. **A,** Lesion of the maxillary gingiva. **B,** Red lesion of the mandibular alveolar ridge. Biopsy of both lesions revealed carcinoma in situ.

caused by entities such as lichen planus and candidiasis are not leukoplakias. Approximately 3% of the world's population have leukoplakic lesions, and somewhere between 5% and 25% of these lesions are premalignant.[13] *Thus, until it is proved otherwise via histologic evaluation, all leukoplakias must be considered precancerous.*

Related to leukoplakia, but much less common and much more ominous, is *erythroplakia*. It represents a red, velvety, possibly eroded area within the oral cavity that usually remains level with or may be slightly depressed in relation to the surrounding mucosa (Fig. 16–5). The epithelium in such lesions tends to be markedly atypical, incurring a much higher risk of malignant transformation than that seen with leukoplakia. Intermediate forms are occasionally encountered that have the characteristics of both leukoplakia and erythroplakia, termed *speckled leukoerythroplakia.*

Both leukoplakia and erythroplakia may be seen in adults at any age, but they are usually found between ages 40 and 70, with a 2:1 male preponderance. *Although these lesions have multifactorial origins, the use of tobacco (cigarettes, pipes, cigars, and chewing tobacco) is the most common antecedent.*

> **Morphology. Leukoplakias** may occur anywhere in the oral cavity (favored locations are buccal mucosa, floor of the mouth, ventral surface of the tongue, palate, and gingiva). They appear as solitary or multiple white patches or plaques, often with sharply demarcated borders. They may be slightly thickened and smooth or wrinkled and fissured, or they may appear as raised, sometimes corrugated, verrucous plaques (Fig. 16–6). On histologic examination they present a spectrum of epithelial changes ranging from hyperkeratosis overlying a thickened, acanthotic but orderly mucosal epithelium to lesions with markedly dysplastic changes sometimes merging into carcinoma in situ (Fig. 16–7). The more dysplastic or anaplastic the lesion, the more likely that a subjacent inflammatory infiltrate of lymphocytes and macrophages will be present.
>
> The histologic changes in **erythroplakia** only rarely consist of orderly epidermal maturation; virtually all

> (approximately 90%) disclose superficial erosions with dysplasia, carcinoma in situ, or already developed carcinoma in the surrounding margins. Often, an intense subepithelial inflammatory reaction with vascular dilation is seen that likely contributes to the reddish clinical appearance.

SQUAMOUS CELL CARCINOMA

At least 95% of cancers of the head and neck are squamous cell carcinomas (HNSCCs), arising most commonly in the oral cavity. The remainder includes adenocarcinomas (of salivary gland origin), melanomas, various carcinomas, and other rarities. Biologically, squamous cell carcinomas in the oral cavity are fairly similar to those elsewhere in the head and neck, hence they are described together here. Features that apply to squamous cell cancer at specific sites in the head and neck are mentioned in the following discussion. Laryngeal squamous cell cancers are described later.

HNSCC is an aggressive epithelial malignancy that is the sixth most common neoplasm in the world today. At current rates, approximately 45,000 cases in the United States and more than 650,000 cases worldwide will be diagnosed each year.[14,15–17] Despite numerous advances in treatment taking advantage of the most recent protocols for surgery, radiation therapy, and chemotherapy, the overall long-term survival has remained at less than 50% for the past 50 years.[16] The 5-year survival rate of early-stage oral cancer is approximately 80%, while survival drops to 19% for late-stage disease. This dismal outlook is due to several factors, including the fact that oral cancer is often diagnosed when the disease has already reached an advanced stage. In addition, the frequent development of multiple primary tumors markedly decreases survival. The rate of second primary tumors in these patients has been reported to be 3% to 7% per year, which is higher than for any other malignancy.[18,19] This observation has led to the concept of "field cancerization." It is postulated that multiple individual primary tumors develop independently in the upper aerodigestive tract as a result of years of chronic exposure of the mucosa to carcinogens.[20,21] Because of such field cancerization, an individual who is fortunate to live 5 years

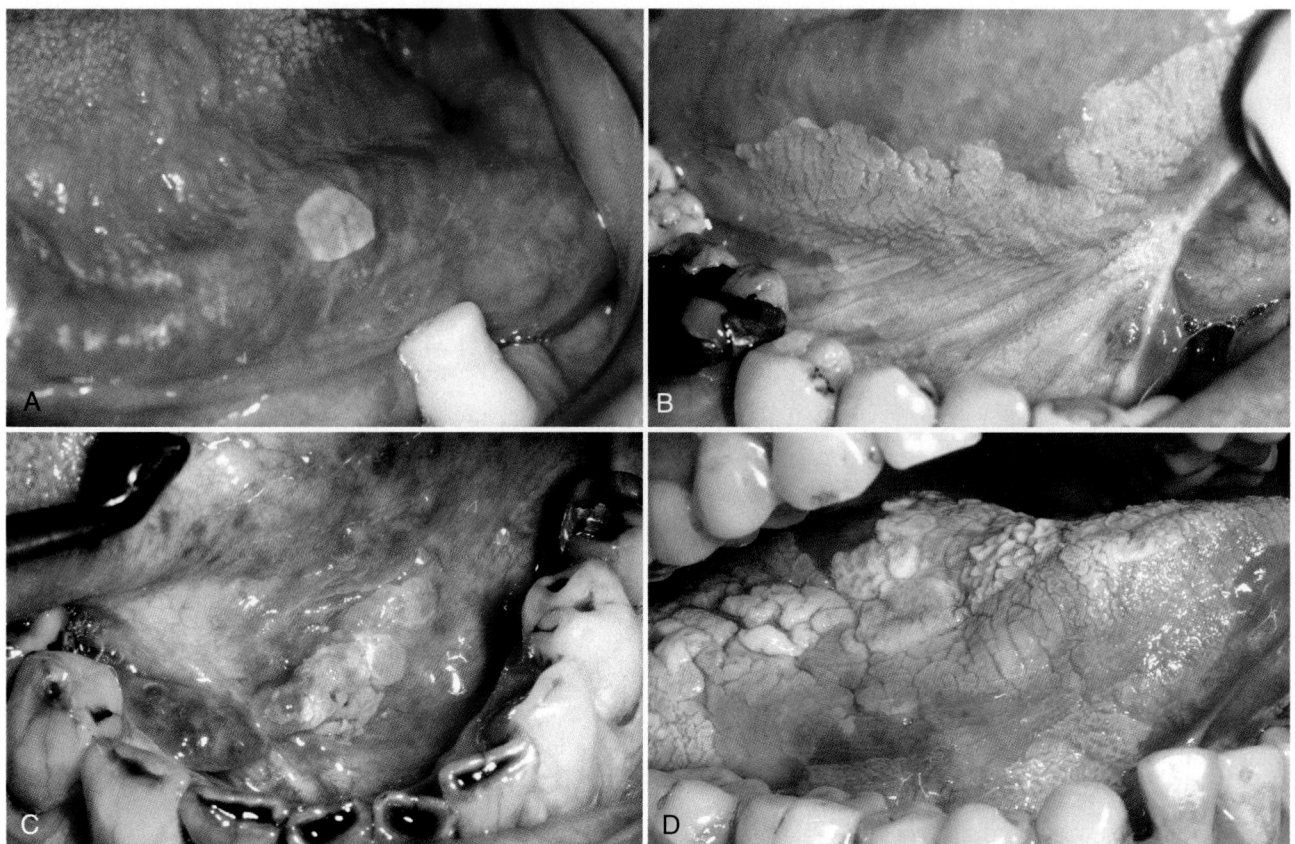

FIGURE 16–6 Leukoplakia. Clinical appearance of leukoplakias is highly variable and can range from (**A**) smooth and thin with well-demarcated borders, (**B**) diffuse and thick, (**C**) irregular with a granular surface, to (**D**) diffuse and corrugated. (Courtesy of Drs. Neville, Damm, Allen, Bouquot [eds], Oral and Maxillofacial Pathology. Philadelphia, WB Saunders, 2008.)

after the initial primary tumor has up to a 35% chance of developing at least one new primary tumor within that period of time. The occurrence of new primary tumors can be particularly devastating for individuals whose initial lesions were small. The 5-year survival rate for the first primary tumor is considerably better than 50%, but in such individuals, second primary tumors are the most common cause of death.[22] Therefore, the early detection of all premalignant lesions is critical for the long-term survival of these patients.

Pathogenesis. The pathogenesis of squamous cell carcinoma is multifactorial. Within North America and Europe it has classically been considered to be a disease of middle-aged men who have been chronic abusers of *smoked tobacco* and *alcohol*. The risk is magnified in those who smoke as well as consume alochol. Not unexpectedly, therefore, and concurrent with increased cigarette usage, the incidence of oral cancer in women is on the rise.

It is now known that at least 50% of oropharyngeal cancers, particularly those involving the tonsils, the base of the tongue, and the oropharynx harbor oncogenic variants of HPV.[23] It is predicted that the incidence of HPV-associated HNSCC will surpass that of cervical cancer in the next decade, in part because the anatomic sites of origin (tonsillar crypts, base of tongue, and oropharynx) are not readily accessible or amenable to cytologic screening (unlike the cervix). It should be noted, however, that *patients with HPV-positive HNSCC do better than those with HPV-negative tumors.* The HPV vaccine, which is protective against cervical cancer, offers hope to stem the tide of HPV-associated HNSCC, although it is not yet approved for this use.

There is increasing epidemiologic evidence that a family history of head and neck cancer is a risk factor for the disease, thought to be due to inherited genomic instability.[24] Finally, *actinic radiation* (sunlight) and, particularly, pipe smoking are known predisposing influences for cancer of the lower lip. Outside of North America and Europe, a major regional predisposing influence is the chewing of betel quid and paan in India and parts of Asia. The betel quid is a "witches' brew" that contains several ingredients such as areca nut, slaked lime, and tobacco, which are wrapped in a betel leaf. While protracted irritation from ill-fitting dentures, jagged teeth, or chronic infections is no longer thought to be a direct antecedent to oral cancer, chronic irritation of the mucosa could act as a "promoter" of cancer in much the same way as alcohol does.

The incidence of oral cancer in individuals under age 40 who have no known risk factors has been on the rise for the past several years.[25–27] The pathogenesis of this group of patients who are nonsmokers and not infected with HPV is unknown.

Molecular Biology of Squamous Cell Carcinoma. Like all epithelial neoplasms, the development of squamous cell carcinoma is thought to be a multi-step process involving the sequential activation of oncogenes and inactivation of tumor

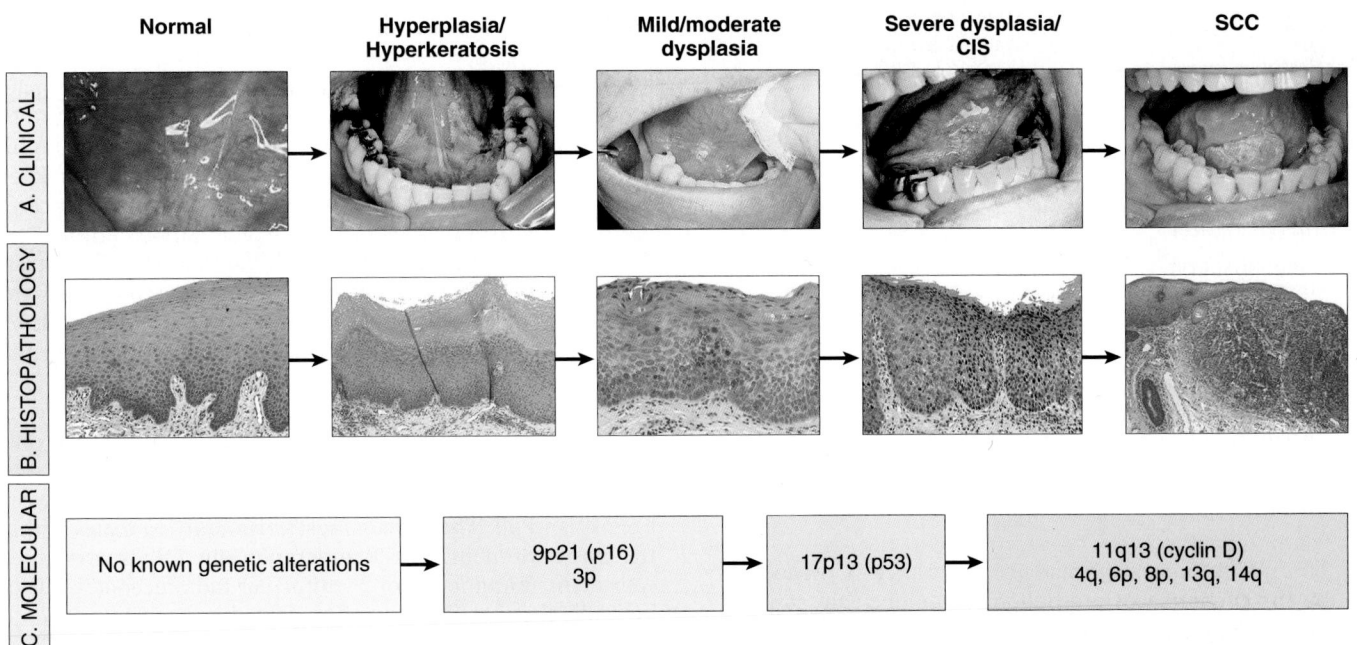

	Normal	Hyperplasia/ Hyperkeratosis	Mild/moderate dysplasia	Severe dysplasia/ CIS	SCC

FIGURE 16–7 Clinical, histologic, and molecular progression of oral cancer. **A,** The typical clinical progression of oral cancer. **B,** The histologic progression of squamous epithelium from normal, to hyperkeratosis, to mild/moderate dysplasia, to severe dysplasia, to cancer. **C,** The sites of the most common genetic alterations identified as important for cancer development. CIS, carcinoma in situ; SCC, squamous cell carcinoma. (Clinical photographs courtesy of Sol Silverman, MD, from Silverman S: Oral Cancer. Hamilton, Ontario, Canada, BD Dekker, 2003.)

suppressor genes in a clonal population of cells. Several genetic alterations, some definitively identified and some inferred from tumor-specific chromosomal alterations, have been found in HNSCC. While not all of the specific mutations required for progression have been delineated, a working molecular model has been established (see Fig. 16–7). The first change is the loss of chromosomal regions of 3p and 9p21.[28] Loss of heterozygosity (LOH) in conjunction with promoter hypermethylation at this locus results in the inactivation of the *p16* gene, an inhibitor of cyclin-dependent kinase (Chapter 7). This alteration is associated with the transition from normal to hyperplasia/hyperkeratosis and occurs before the development of histologic atypia, thus underscoring the histologic limitations for early diagnosis. Subsequent LOH at 17p with mutation of the *p53* tumor suppressor gene is associated with progression to dysplasia.[29] Recently it has been demonstrated that gross genomic alterations as well as deletions on 4q, 6p, 8p, 11q, 13q, and 14q may act as predictors of progression to frank malignancy.[30] Ultimately, amplification and overexpression of the cyclin D1 gene (located on chromosome 11q13), which constitutively activates cell cycle progression, is a common late event. Data suggest that alterations of this gene confer the ability to invade in certain clones.[31,32]

However, while this model is a good working draft of the molecular changes involved in development of HNSCC, it is incomplete. First, while some of the gross genomic alterations correlate with genes known to be important in HNSCC (such as *p16*, *p53*, and *CyclinD1*), many of the specific genes are still unknown. Second, this model does not take into account alterations in genes such as the epidermal growth factor receptor (EFGR), which is overexpressed in a high percentage of HNSCC and has been successfully targeted in the treatment

of this disease. Finally, as indicated above, it is increasingly clear that HNSCC is a heterogeneous disease in terms of etiology and its molecular mechanisms of development.

Morphology. Squamous cell carcinoma may arise anywhere in the oral cavity, but the favored locations are the ventral surface of the tongue, floor of the mouth, lower lip, soft palate, and gingiva (Fig. 16–8).

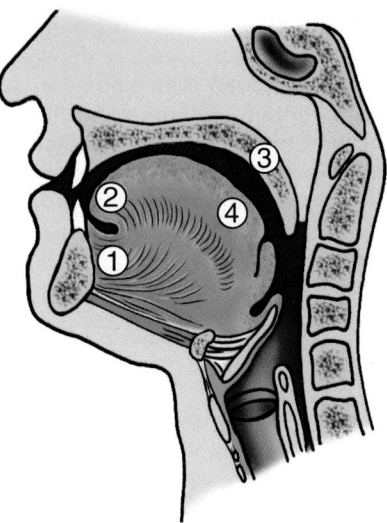

FIGURE 16–8 Schematic representation of the sites of origin of squamous cell carcinoma of the oral cavity, in numerical order of frequency.

TABLE 16–2 Histologic Classification of Odontogenic Cysts
1. INFLAMMATORY
Periapical cyst
Residual cyst
Paradental cyst
2. DEVELOPMENTAL
Dentigerous cyst
Odontogenic keratocyst
Gingival cyst of newborn
Gingival cyst of adult
Eruption cyst
Lateral periodontal cyst
Glandular odontogenic cyst
Calcifying epithelial odontogenic cyst (Gorlin cyst)

The malignancies themselves are typically preceded by the presence of premalignant lesions that can be very heterogeneous in presentation (see above).

In the early stages, cancers of the oral cavity appear either as raised, firm, pearly plaques or as irregular, roughened, or verrucous areas of mucosal thickening, possibly mistaken for leukoplakia. Either pattern may be superimposed on a background of apparent leukoplakia or erythroplakia. As these lesions enlarge, they typically create ulcerated and protruding masses that have irregular and indurated (rolled) borders.

On histologic examination, these cancers begin as dysplastic lesions, which may or may not progress to full-thickness dysplasia (carcinoma in situ) before invading the underlying connective tissue stroma (Fig. 16–7). This difference in progression should be contrasted with cervical cancer (Chapter 22), in which, typically, full-thickness dysplasia, representing carcinoma in situ, develops before invasion. Squamous cell carcinomas range from well-differentiated keratinizing neoplasms to anaplastic, sometimes sarcomatoid, tumors, and from slowly to rapidly growing lesions. However, the degree of histologic differentiation, as determined by the relative degree of keratinization, is not correlated with behavior. As a group these tumors tend to infiltrate locally before they metastasize to other sites. The routes of extension depend on the primary site. The favored sites of local metastasis are the cervical lymph nodes, while the most common sites of distant metastasis are mediastinal lymph nodes, lungs, liver, and bones. Unfortunately, such distant metastases are often occult at the time of discovery of the primary lesion.

Odontogenic Cysts and Tumors

In contrast to the rest of the skeleton, epithelial-lined cysts are quite common in the jaws. The overwhelming majority of these cysts are derived from remnants of odontogenic epithelium present within the jaws. In general, these cysts are subclassified as either inflammatory or developmental (Table 16–2). Only the most common of these lesions are described below.

The *dentigerous cyst* is defined as a cyst that originates around the crown of an unerupted tooth and is thought to be the result of a degeneration of the dental follicle. Radiographically, they are unilocular lesions and are most often associated with impacted third molar (wisdom) teeth. Histologically they are lined by a thin layer of stratified squamous epithelium. Often, there is a very dense chronic inflammatory cell infiltrate in the connective tissue stroma. Complete removal of the lesion is curative. This is important, since incomplete excision may result in recurrence or, very rarely, neoplastic transformation into an ameloblastoma or a squamous cell carcinoma.

The *odontogenic keratocyst (OKC)* is an important entity to differentiate from other odontogenic cysts because it is locally aggressive and has a high rate of recurrence. OKCs can be seen at any age but are most often diagnosed in patients between ages 10 and 40. They occur most commonly in males within the posterior mandible. Radiographically, OKCs present as well-defined unilocular or multilocular radiolucencies. Histologically, the cyst lining consists of a thin layer of parakeratinized or orthokeratinized stratified squamous epithelium with a prominent basal cell layer and a corrugated appearance of the epithelial surface. Treatment requires aggressive and complete removal of the lesion, because recurrence rates for inadequately removed lesions can reach 60%. Multiple OKCs may occur; these patients should be evaluated for nevoid basal cell carcinoma syndrome (Gorlin syndrome), which, as we shall see, is related to mutations in the tumor suppressor gene *PTCH* located on chromosome 9q22 (Chapter 25).

TABLE 16–3 Histologic Classification of Odontogenic Tumors
1. TUMORS OF ODONTOGENIC EPITHELIUM
Benign
Ameloblastoma
Calcifying epithelial odontogenic tumor (Pindborg tumor)
Squamous odontogenic tumor
Malignant
Ameloblastic carcinoma
Malignant ameloblastoma
Clear-cell odontogenic carcinoma
2. TUMORS OF ODONTOGENIC ECTOMESENCHYME
Odontogenic fibroma
Odontogenic myxoma
Cementoblastoma
3. TUMORS OF ODONTOGENIC EPITHELIUM AND ECTOMESENCHYME
Benign
Ameloblastic fibroma
Ameloblastic fibro-odontoma
Ameloblastic fibrosarcoma
Adenomatoid odontogenic tumor
Odontoameloblastoma
Complex odontoma
Compound odontoma
Malignant
Ameloblastic fibrosarcoma

The *periapical cyst,* in contrast to the developmental cysts described above, is inflammatory in origin. These are extremely common lesions found at the apex of teeth. They develop as a result of long-standing pulpitis, which may be caused by advanced carious lesions or by trauma to the tooth in question. The inflammatory process may result in necrosis of the pulpal tissue, which can traverse the length of the root and exit the apex of the tooth into the surrounding alveolar bone, giving rise to a periapical abscess. Over time, like any chronic inflammatory process, a lesion with granulation tissue (with or without an epithelial lining) may develop. While the term *periapical granuloma* is not the most appropriate terminology (as the lesion does not show true granulomatous inflammation), old terminology, like bad habits, is difficult to shed. Periapical inflammatory lesions persist as a result of the continued presence of bacteria or other offensive agents in the area. Successful treatment, therefore, necessitates the complete removal of offending material and appropriate restoration of the tooth or extraction.

Odontogenic tumors are a complex group of lesions with diverse histologic appearances and clinical behavior.[33] Some are true neoplasms (both benign and malignant), while others are more likely hamartomas. Odontogenic tumors are derived from odontogenic epithelium, ectomesenchyme, or both (Table 16–3). The two most common and clinically significant tumors are:

- *Ameloblastoma,* which arises from odontogenic epithelium and shows *no* ectomesenchymal differentiation. It is commonly cystic, slow growing, and locally invasive but has an indolent course in most cases.
- *Odontoma,* the most common type of odontogenic tumor, arises from epithelium but shows extensive depositions of enamel and dentin. Odontomas are probably hamartomas rather than true neoplasms and are cured by local excision.

UPPER AIRWAYS

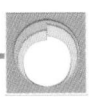

The term *upper airways* is used here to include the nose, pharynx, and larynx and their related parts. Disorders of these structures are among the most common afflictions of humans, but fortunately the overwhelming majority are more nuisances than threats.

Nose

Inflammatory diseases, mostly in the form of the common cold, as everyone knows, are the most common disorders of the nose and accessory air sinuses. Most of these inflammatory conditions are viral in origin, but they are often complicated by superimposed bacterial infections having considerably greater significance. Much less common are a few destructive inflammatory nasal diseases and tumors primary in the nasal cavity or paranasal sinuses.

INFLAMMATIONS

Infectious Rhinitis. Infectious rhinitis, the more elegant way of saying "common cold," is in most instances caused by one or more viruses. Major offenders are adenoviruses, echoviruses, and rhinoviruses. They evoke a profuse catarrhal discharge that is familiar to all and the bane of the kindergarten teacher. During the initial acute stages, the nasal mucosa is thickened, edematous, and red; the nasal cavities are narrowed; and the turbinates are enlarged. These changes may extend, producing a concomitant pharyngotonsillitis. Secondary bacterial infection enhances the inflammatory reaction and produces an essentially mucopurulent or sometimes frankly suppurative exudate. But as all have learned from experience, these infections soon clear up—as the saying goes, in a week if treated but in 7 days if ignored.

Allergic Rhinitis. Allergic rhinitis (hay fever) is initiated by hypersensitivity reactions to one of a large group of allergens, most commonly the plant pollens, fungi, animal allergens, and dust mites.[34] It affects 20% of the US population. As is the case with asthma, allergic rhinitis is an IgE–mediated immune reaction with an early- and late-phase response (see "Immediate (Type I) Hypersensitivity" in Chapter 6). The allergic reaction is characterized by marked mucosal edema, redness, and mucus secretion, accompanied by a leukocytic infiltration in which eosinophils are prominent.

Nasal Polyps. Recurrent attacks of rhinitis may eventually lead to focal protrusions of the mucosa, producing so-called *nasal polyps,* which may reach 3 to 4 cm in length. On histologic examination these polyps consist of edematous mucosa having a loose stroma, often harboring hyperplastic or cystic mucous glands, infiltrated with a variety of inflammatory cells, including neutrophils, eosinophils, and plasma cells with occasional clusters of lymphocytes (Fig. 16–9). In the absence of bacterial infection, the mucosal covering of these polyps is intact, but with chronicity it may become ulcerated or infected. When multiple or large, the polyps may encroach on the airway and impair sinus drainage. Although the features of nasal polyps point to an allergic etiology, most people with nasal polyps are not atopic, and only 0.5% of atopic patients develop polyps.[35]

Chronic Rhinitis. Chronic rhinitis is a sequel to repeated attacks of acute rhinitis, either microbial or allergic in origin, with the eventual development of superimposed bacterial infection. A deviated nasal septum or nasal polyps with impaired drainage of secretions contribute to the likelihood of microbial invasion. Frequently, there is superficial desquamation or ulceration of the mucosal epithelium and a variable inflammatory infiltrate of neutrophils, lymphocytes, and

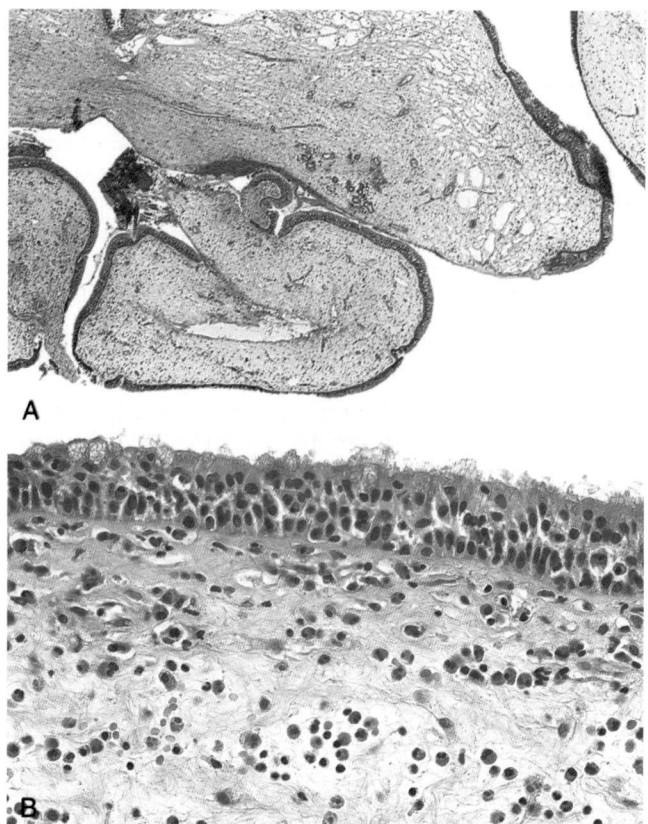

FIGURE 16–9 **A,** Nasal polyps. Low-power magnification showing edematous masses lined by epithelium. **B,** High-power view showing edema and eosinophil-rich inflammatory infiltrate.

plasma cells subjacent to the epithelium. These suppurative infections sometimes extend into the air sinuses.

Sinusitis. Acute sinusitis is most commonly preceded by acute or chronic rhinitis, but maxillary sinusitis occasionally arises by extension of a periapical infection through the bony floor of the sinus. The offending agents are usually inhabitants of the oral cavity, and the inflammatory reaction is entirely nonspecific. Impairment of drainage of the sinus by inflammatory edema of the mucosa is an important contributor to the process and, when complete, may impound the suppurative exudate, producing *empyema* of the sinus. Obstruction of the outflow, most often from the frontal and less commonly from the anterior ethmoid sinuses, occasionally leads to an accumulation of mucous secretions in the absence of direct bacterial invasion, producing a so-called *mucocele*. Acute sinusitis may, in time, give rise to *chronic sinusitis*, particularly when there is interference with drainage. There is usually a mixed microbial flora, largely of normal inhabitants of the oral cavity. Particularly severe forms of chronic sinusitis are caused by fungi (e.g., mucormycosis), especially in diabetics. Uncommonly, sinusitis is a component of *Kartagener syndrome*, which also includes bronchiectasis and situs inversus (Chapter 15). All these features are secondary to defective ciliary action. Although most instances of chronic sinusitis are more uncomfortable than disabling or serious, the infections have the potential of spreading into the orbit or of penetrating into the surrounding bone to give rise to osteomyelitis or

spreading into the cranial vault, causing septic thrombophlebitis of a dural venous sinus.

NECROTIZING LESIONS OF THE NOSE AND UPPER AIRWAYS

Necrotizing ulcerating lesions of the nose and upper respiratory tract may be produced by

- Acute fungal infections (including mucormycosis; Chapter 8), particularly in diabetic and immunosuppressed patients
- Wegener granulomatosis (discussed in Chapter 11)
- A condition once called *lethal midline granuloma* or *polymorphic reticulosis* and now known to be a lymphoma of natural killer cells infected with EBV[36] (Chapter 14). Ulceration and superimposed bacterial infection frequently complicate the process. At one time these lesions were almost always rapidly fatal as a result of uncontrolled growth of the lymphoma, possibly with penetration into the cranial vault, or because of tumor necrosis with secondary bacterial infection and blood-borne dissemination of the infection. Currently, localized cases can often be controlled with radiotherapy, but once the tumors spread, they are difficult to treat. Most of those affected die of the disease.

Nasopharynx

Although the nasopharyngeal mucosa, related lymphoid structures, and glands may be involved in a wide variety of specific infections (e.g., diphtheria, infectious mononucleosis) and by neoplasms, the only disorders mentioned here are nonspecific inflammations; tumors are discussed separately.

INFLAMMATIONS

Pharyngitis and *tonsillitis* are frequent in the usual viral upper respiratory infections. Most commonly implicated are the multitudinous rhinoviruses, echoviruses, and adenoviruses, and, less frequently, respiratory syncytial viruses and the various strains of influenza virus. In the usual case, there is reddening and slight edema of the nasopharyngeal mucosa, with reactive enlargement of the related lymphoid structures. Bacterial infections may be superimposed on these viral involvements, or may be primary invaders. The most common offenders are the β-hemolytic streptococci, but sometimes *Staphylococcus aureus* or other pathogens may be implicated. The inflamed nasopharyngeal mucosa may be covered by an exudative membrane (pseudomembrane), and the nasopalatine and palatine tonsils may be enlarged and covered by exudate. A typical appearance is of enlarged, reddened tonsils (due to reactive lymphoid hyperplasia) dotted by pinpoints of exudate emanating from the tonsillar crypts, so-called *follicular tonsillitis*.

The major importance of streptococcal "sore throats" lies in the possible development of late sequelae, such as, rheumatic fever (Chapter 12) and glomerulonephritis (Chapter 20). Whether recurrent episodes of acute tonsillitis favor the development of chronic tonsillitis (true chronic tonsillitis is extremely rare) is open to debate, but the result is residual

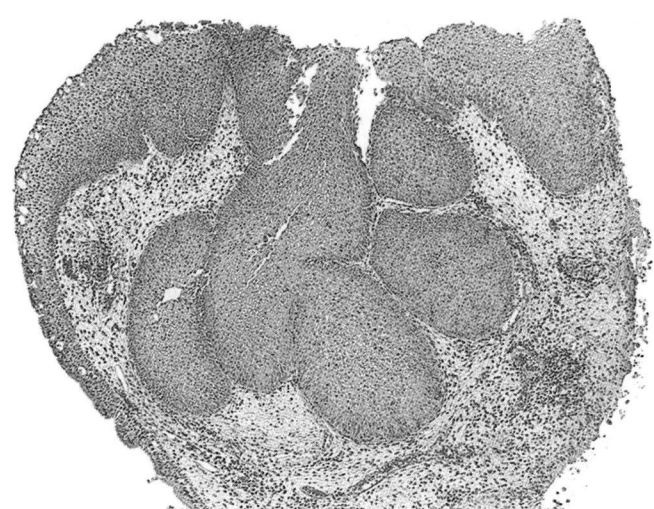

FIGURE 16–10   Inverted papilloma. The masses of squamous epithelium are growing inward; hence, the term *inverted*. (Courtesy of Dr. James Gulizia, Brigham and Women's Hospital, Boston, MA.)

enlargement of the lymphoid tissue, inviting the tender mercies of the otolaryngologist.

Tumors of the Nose, Sinuses, and Nasopharynx

Tumors in these locations are infrequent but include the entire category of mesenchymal and epithelial neoplasms.[36,37] Brief mention is made of some distinctive types.

Nasopharyngeal Angiofibroma. This is a highly vascular tumor that occurs almost exclusively in adolescent males. Despite its benign nature, it may cause serious clinical problems because of its tendency to bleed profusely during surgery.

Sinonasal (Schneiderian) Papilloma. These are benign neoplasms arising from the sinonasal mucosa and are composed of squamous or columnar epithelium. Although their etiology is still unproven, HPV types 6 and 11 have been identified in the lesions. These lesions occur in three forms: *exophytic* (most common), *inverted* (most important biologically), and *cylindrical*. Because of its uniquely aggressive biologic behavior, only inverted papilloma is discussed here. Inverted papillomas are benign but locally aggressive neoplasms occurring in both the nose and the paranasal sinuses. As the name implies, the papillomatous proliferation of squamous epithelium, instead of producing an exophytic growth (like the septal and cylindrical papillomas), extends into the mucosa, that is, it is inverted (Fig. 16–10). If not adequately excised, it has a high rate of recurrence, with the potentially serious complication of invasion of the orbit or cranial vault; rarely, frank carcinoma may also develop.

Olfactory Neuroblastoma (Esthesioneuroblastoma). These are uncommon, malignant tumors composed of small round cells, resembling neuroblasts, which form lobular nests encircled by vascularized connective tissue. They arise most often superiorly and laterally in the nose from the neuroendocrine cells dispersed in the olfactory mucosa. The differential diagnosis of these neoplasms includes all other small-cell tumors (Chapter 10), such as lymphoma, Ewing sarcoma, and embryonal rhabdomyosarcoma.[38] The cells are of neuroendocrine origin and thus exhibit membrane-bound secretory granules on electron microscopy and express neuron-specific enolase, synaptophysin, CD56, and chromogranin by immunohistochemistry. While the name implies that they are primitive neuroectodermal tumors, many do not share the 11;22 translocation or fusion-gene products typical of Ewing sarcoma of bone (Chapter 26) and other primitive neuroectodermal tumors. Some of these tumors reveal trisomy 8. Depending on the stage and grade of a particular neoplasm, combinations of surgery, radiation therapy, and chemotherapy yield 5-year survival rates of 40% to 90%.[39]

Nasopharyngeal Carcinoma. This tumor is characterized by a distinctive geographic distribution, a close anatomic relationship to lymphoid tissue, and an association with EBV infection.[40] The nomenclature for nasopharyngeal carcinomas is in constant flux. However, at present the disease is thought to take one of three patterns: (1) keratinizing squamous cell carcinomas, (2) nonkeratinizing squamous cell carcinomas, and (3) undifferentiated carcinomas that have an abundant non-neoplastic, lymphocytic infiltrate. The last pattern has often been called *lymphoepithelioma*. However, while widely used in clinical practice, this highly descriptive term should be avoided.

Three factors affect the origins of these neoplasms: (1) heredity, (2) age, and (3) infection with EBV. Nasopharyngeal carcinomas are particularly common in some parts of Africa, where they are the most frequent childhood cancer. In contrast, in southern China, they are very common in adults but rarely occur in children. In the United States they are rare in both adults and children. In addition to EBV infection, diets high in nitrosamines, such as fermented foods and salted fish, as well as other environmental factors such as smoking and chemical fumes, have been linked to the disease. Components of the EBV genome such as EBNA-1 can be identified in the tumor epithelial cells (not the lymphocytes) of most undifferentiated and nonkeratinizing squamous cell nasopharyngeal carcinomas, particularly when in situ hybridization is performed.[41]

Morphology. On histologic examination, the keratinizing and nonkeratinizing squamous cell lesions resemble usual well-differentiated and poorly differentiated squamous cell carcinomas arising in other locations. The undifferentiated variant is composed of large epithelial cells with oval or round vesicular nuclei, prominent nucleoli, and indistinct cell borders disposed in a syncytium-like array (Fig. 16–11). Admixed with the epithelial cells are abundant, mature, normal-appearing lymphocytes, which are predominantly T cells.

Primary nasopharyngeal carcinomas are often clinically occult for long periods, and present as metastases in the cervical lymph nodes in as many as 70% of the patients. Radiotherapy is the standard modality of treatment, yielding 50% to 70% 3-year survival rate. The undifferentiated carcinoma is the most radiosensitive and the keratinizing squamous cell carcinoma is the least radiosensitive.

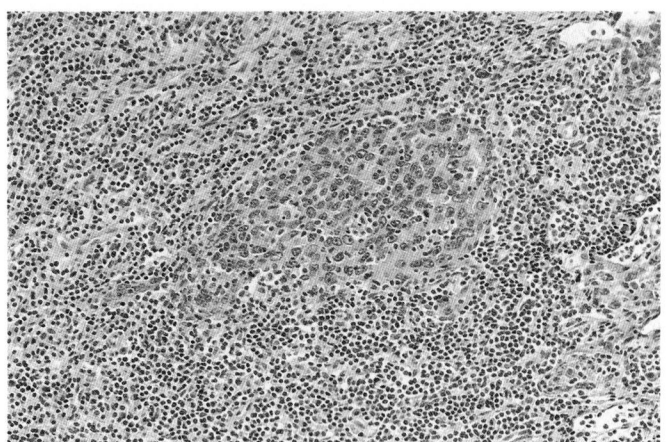

FIGURE 16–11 Nasopharyngeal carcinoma, undifferentiated type. The syncytium-like nests of epithelium are surrounded by lymphocytes. (Courtesy of Dr. James Gulizia, Brigham and Women's Hospital, Boston, MA.)

Larynx

The most common disorder that affects the larynx is inflammation. Tumors are uncommon but are amenable to resection, though often at the price of loss of natural voice.

INFLAMMATIONS

Laryngitis may occur as the sole manifestation of allergic, viral, bacterial, or chemical insult, but it is more commonly part of a generalized upper respiratory tract infection or the result of heavy exposure to environmental toxins such as tobacco smoke. It may also occur in association with gastroesophageal reflux due to the irritating effect of gastric contents. The larynx may also be affected in systemic infections, such as tuberculosis and diphtheria. Although most infections are self-limited, they may at times be serious, especially in infancy or childhood, when mucosal congestion, exudation, or edema may cause laryngeal obstruction. In particular, laryngoepiglottitis, caused by respiratory syncytial virus, *Haemophilus influenzae*, or β-hemolytic streptococci in infants and young children with their small airways, may induce such sudden swelling of the epiglottis and vocal cords that a potentially lethal medical emergency is created. This form of disease is uncommon in adults because of the larger size of the larynx and the stronger accessory muscles of respiration. *Croup* is the name given to laryngotracheobronchitis in children, in which the inflammatory narrowing of the airway produces the inspiratory stridor so frightening to parents. The most common form of laryngitis, encountered in heavy smokers, predisposes to squamous epithelial metaplasia and sometimes overt carcinoma.

REACTIVE NODULES (VOCAL CORD NODULES AND POLYPS)

Reactive nodules, also called polyps, sometimes develop on the vocal cords, most often in heavy smokers or in individuals who impose great strain on their vocal cords (*singers' nodules*) (Fig. 16–12). By convention, singers' nodules are bilateral lesions and polyps are unilateral. Adults, predominantly men, are most often affected. These nodules are smooth, rounded, sessile or pedunculated excrescences, generally only a few millimeters in the greatest dimension, located usually on the true vocal cords. They are typically covered by squamous epithelium that may become keratotic, hyperplastic, or even slightly dysplastic. The core of the nodule is a loose myxoid connective tissue that may be variably fibrotic or punctuated by numerous vascular channels. When nodules on opposing vocal cords impinge on each other, the mucosa may undergo ulceration. Because of their strategic location and accompanying inflammation, they characteristically change the character of the voice and often cause progressive hoarseness. They virtually never give rise to cancers.

SQUAMOUS PAPILLOMA AND PAPILLOMATOSIS

Laryngeal squamous papillomas are benign neoplasms, usually located on the true vocal cords, that form soft, raspberry-like excrescences rarely more than 1 cm in diameter (Fig. 16–12). On histologic examination, the papillomas are made up of multiple slender, finger-like projections supported by central fibrovascular cores and covered by an orderly stratified squamous epithelium. When the papillomas are on the free edge of the vocal cord, trauma may lead to ulceration that can be accompanied by hemoptysis.

Papillomas are usually single in adults but are often multiple in children, in whom they are referred to as *juvenile laryngeal papillomatosis*.[42] However, multiple recurring papillomas also occur in adults. *The lesions are caused by HPV types 6 and 11.* They do not become malignant, but frequently recur. They often spontaneously regress at puberty, but some affected patients endure numerous surgeries before this occurs. Cancerous transformation is rare.

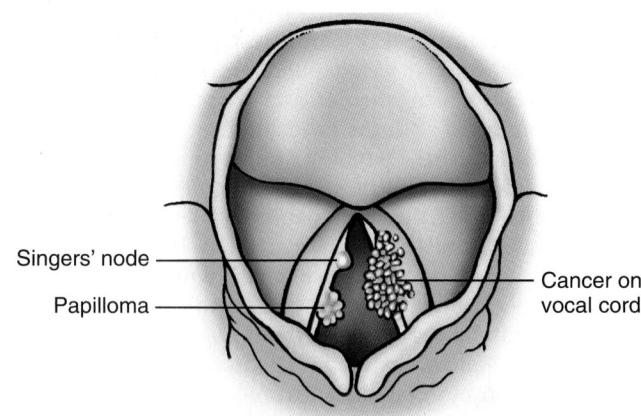

Singers' node
Papilloma
Cancer on vocal cord

FIGURE 16–12 Diagrammatic comparison of a benign papilloma and an exophytic carcinoma of the larynx to highlight their quite different appearances.

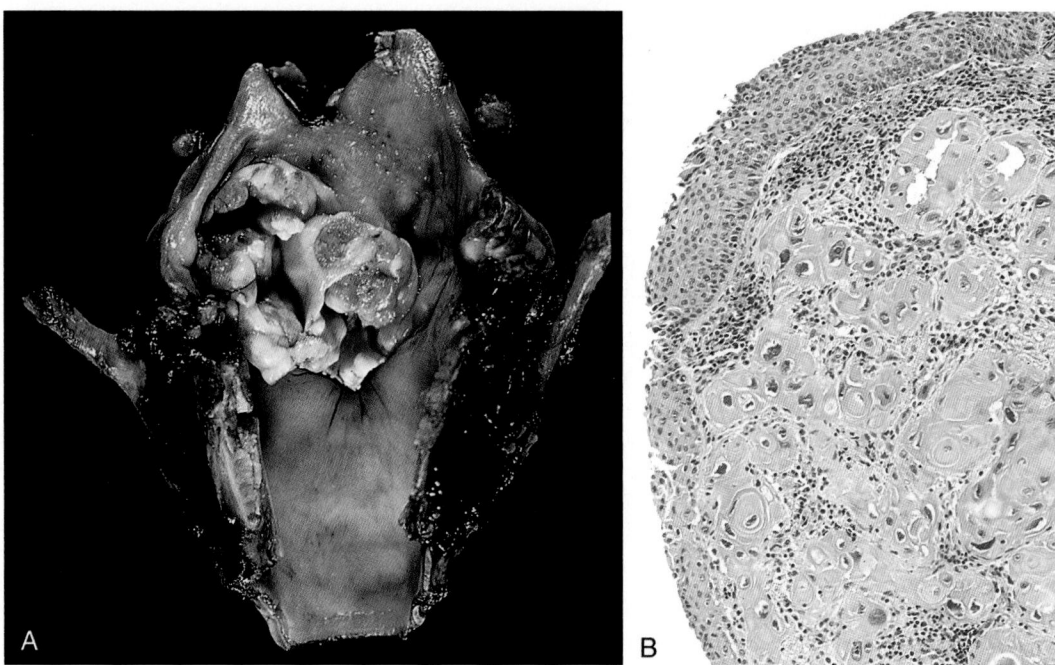

FIGURE 16–13 **A,** Laryngeal carcinoma. Note the large, ulcerated, fungating lesion involving the vocal cord and pyriform sinus. **B,** Histologic appearance of laryngeal squamous cell carcinoma. Note the atypical lining epithelium and invasive keratinizing cancer cells in the submucosa.

CARCINOMA OF THE LARYNX

Sequence of Hyperplasia-Dysplasia-Carcinoma. A spectrum of epithelial alterations is seen in the larynx. They range from *hyperplasia, atypical hyperplasia, dysplasia, carcinoma in situ, to invasive carcinoma.*[43] Macroscopically, the epithelial changes vary from smooth, white or reddened focal thickenings, sometimes roughened by keratosis, to irregular verrucous or ulcerated white-pink lesions that are similar in appearance to carcinoma.

There are all gradations of epithelial hyperplasia of the true vocal cords, and the likelihood of the development of an overt carcinoma is directly proportional to the level of atypia when the lesion is first seen. Orderly hyperplasias have almost no potential for malignant transformation, but the risk rises to 1% to 2% during the span of 5 to 10 years with mild dysplasia and 5% to 10% with severe dysplasia. Only histologic evaluation can determine the gravity of the changes.

The various changes described are most often related to tobacco smoke, the risk being proportional to the level of exposure. Indeed, up to the point of frank cancer, the changes often regress after cessation of smoking. Alcohol is also clearly a risk factor. Together smoking and alochol increase the risk substantially. Other factors that may contribute to increased risk include nutritional factors, exposure to asbestos, irradiation, and infection with HPV.[44,45]

Morphology. About 95% of laryngeal carcinomas are typical squamous cell tumors. The tumor usually develops directly on the vocal cords, but it may arise above or below the cords, on the epiglottis or aryepiglottic folds, or in the pyriform sinuses. Those confined within the larynx proper are termed **intrinsic**, whereas those that arise or extend outside the larynx are called **extrinsic**. Squamous cell carcinomas of the larynx follow the growth pattern of other squamous cell carcinomas. They begin as in situ lesions that later appear as pearly gray, wrinkled plaques on the mucosal surface, ultimately ulcerating and fungating (Fig. 16–13). The degree of anaplasia of the laryngeal tumors is highly variable. Sometimes massive tumor giant cells and multiple bizarre mitotic figures are seen. As expected with lesions arising from recurrent exposure to environmental carcinogens, adjacent mucosa may demonstrate squamous cell hyperplasia with foci of dysplasia or even carcinoma in situ.

Carcinoma of the larynx manifests itself clinically by persistent hoarseness. At presentation, about 60% of these cancers are confined to the larynx. The prognosis for these is better than for those tumors that have spread into adjacent structures. Later, laryngeal tumors may produce pain, dysphagia, and hemoptysis. Patients are also extremely vulnerable to secondary infection of the ulcerating lesion. With surgery, irradiation, or combination therapy, many patients can be cured, but about one third die of the disease. The usual causes of death are infection of the distal respiratory passages or widespread metastases and cachexia.

EARS

Although disorders of the ear rarely shorten life, many impair its quality. The most common aural disorders, in descending order of frequency, are (1) acute and chronic otitis (most often involving the middle ear and mastoid), sometimes leading to a cholesteatoma; (2) symptomatic otosclerosis; (3) aural polyps; (4) labyrinthitis; (5) carcinomas, largely of the external ear; and (6) paragangliomas, found mostly in the middle ear. Only those conditions that have distinctive morphologic features (save for labyrinthitis) are described. Paragangliomas are discussed later.

Inflammatory Lesions

Inflammations of the ear—*otitis media, acute or chronic*—occur mostly in infants and children. These lesions are typically viral in nature and produce a serous exudate but may become suppurative with superimposed bacterial infection. The most common offenders are *Streptococcus pneumoniae,* non-typeable *H. influenzae,* and *Moraxella catarrhalis.*[46]

Repeated bouts of acute otitis media with failure of resolution lead to chronic disease. The causative agents of chronic disease are usually *Pseudomonas aeruginosa, Staphylococcus aureus,* or a fungus; sometimes a mixed flora is the cause. Chronic infection has the potential to perforate the eardrum, encroach on the ossicles or labyrinth, spread into the mastoid spaces, and even penetrate into the cranial vault to produce a temporal cerebritis or abscess. Otitis media in the diabetic person, when caused by *P. aeruginosa,* is especially aggressive and spreads widely causing destructive necrotizing otitis media.

Cholesteatomas, associated with chronic otitis media, are not neoplasms, nor do they always contain cholesterol. Rather, they are cystic lesions 1 to 4 cm in diameter, lined by keratinizing squamous epithelium or metaplastic mucus-secreting epithelium, and filled with amorphous debris (derived largely from desquamated epithelium). Sometimes they contain spicules of cholesterol. The precise events involved in their development are not clear, but it is proposed that chronic inflammation and perforation of the eardrum with ingrowth of the squamous epithelium or metaplasia of the secretory epithelial lining of the middle ear are responsible for the formation of a squamous cell nest that becomes cystic. A chronic inflammatory reaction surrounds the keratinous cyst. Sometimes, the cyst ruptures, increasing the inflammatory reaction and inducing the formation of giant cells that enclose partially necrotic squames and other particulate debris. These lesions, by progressive enlarge-

ment, can erode into the ossicles, the labyrinth, the adjacent bone, or the surrounding soft tissue and sometimes produce visible neck masses.

Otosclerosis

As the name implies, otosclerosis refers to abnormal bone deposition in the middle ear about the rim of the oval window into which the footplate of the stapes fits. Both ears are usually affected. At first there is fibrous ankylosis of the footplate, followed in time by bony overgrowth anchoring it into the oval window. The degree of immobilization governs the severity of the hearing loss. This condition usually begins in the early decades of life; minimal degrees of this derangement are exceedingly common in the United States in young to middle-aged adults, but fortunately more severe symptomatic otosclerosis is relatively uncommon. In most instances it is familial, following autosomal dominant transmission with variable penetrance. The basis for the osseous overgrowth is completely obscure, but it appears to represent uncoupling of normal bone resorption and bone formation. Thus, it begins with bone resorption, followed by fibrosis and vascularization of the temporal bone in the immediate vicinity of the oval window, in time replaced by dense new bone anchoring the footplate of the stapes. In most instances the process is slowly progressive over the span of decades, leading eventually to marked hearing loss.

Tumors

A large variety of epithelial and mesenchymal tumors that arise in the ear—external, middle, internal—all are rare save for basal cell or squamous cell carcinomas of the pinna (external ear). These carcinomas tend to occur in elderly men and are thought to be associated with actinic radiation. By contrast, those within the canal tend to be squamous cell carcinomas, which occur in middle-aged to elderly women and are not associated with sun exposure. Wherever they arise they morphologically resemble their counterparts in other skin locations, beginning as papules that extend and eventually erode and invade locally. Basal cell and squamous cell lesions of the pinna are locally invasive but they rarely spread. Squamous cell carcinomas arising in the external canal may invade the cranial cavity or metastasize to regional nodes accounting for a 5-year mortality of about 50%.

NECK

Most of the conditions that involve the neck are described elsewhere (e.g., squamous cell and basal cell carcinomas of the skin, melanomas, lymphomas), or they are a component of a systemic disorder (e.g., generalized rashes, the lymphadenopathy of infectious mononucleosis or tonsillitis). What remains for consideration here are a few uncommon lesions unique to the neck.

Branchial Cyst (Cervical Lymphoepithelial Cyst)

These benign cysts usually appear on the upper lateral aspect of the neck along the sternocleidomastoid muscle. The vast majority of these cysts are thought to arise from remnants of the second branchial arch and are most commonly observed in young adults between the ages of 20 and 40. Clinically, the cysts are well circumscribed, 2 to 5 cm in diameter, with fibrous walls usually lined by stratified squamous or pseudostratified columnar epithelium. The cyst wall typically contains lymphoid tissue with prominent germinal centers. The cystic contents may be clear, watery to mucinous fluid or may contain desquamated, granular cellular debris. The cysts enlarge slowly, are rarely the site of malignant transformation, and generally are readily excised. Similar lesions sometimes appear in the parotid gland or in the oral cavity beneath the tongue.

Thyroglossal Duct Cyst

Embryologically, the thyroid anlage begins in the region of the foramen cecum at the base of the tongue; as the gland develops it descends to its definitive location in the anterior neck. Remnants of this developmental tract may persist, producing cysts, 1 to 4 cm in diameter, which may be lined by stratified squamous epithelium, when located near the base of the tongue, or by pseudostratified columnar epithelium in lower locations. Transitional patterns are also encountered. The connective tissue wall of the cyst may harbor lymphoid aggregates or remnants of recognizable thyroid tissue. The treatment is excision. Malignant transformation within the lining epithelium has been reported but is rare.

Paraganglioma (Carotid Body Tumor)

Paraganglia are clusters of neuroendocrine cells associated with the sympathetic and parasympathetic nervous systems. As a result, these neoplasms can be seen throughout various regions of the body. While the most common location of these tumors is within the adrenal medulla, where they give rise to pheochromocytomas (Chapter 24), approximately 70% of extra-adrenal paragangliomas occur in the head and neck region.[47] The pathogenesis of paragangliomas is not fully understood. However, alterations in genes encoding subunits of succinate oxidoreductase, an enzyme involved in mitochondrial respiration, have been reported in both hereditary and spontaneous paragangliomas. Paragangliomas typically develop in two locations:

- Paravertebral paraganglia (e.g., organs of Zuckerkandl and, rarely, bladder). Such tumors have sympathetic connections and are chromaffin-positive, a stain that detects catecholamines.
- Paraganglia related to the great vessels of the head and neck, the so-called aorticopulmonary chain, including the *carotid*

bodies (most common); aortic bodies; jugulotympanic ganglia; ganglion nodosum of the vagus nerve; and clusters located about the oral cavity, nose, nasopharynx, larynx, and orbit. These are innervated by the parasympathetic nervous system and infrequently release catecholamines.

Morphology. The **carotid body tumor** is a prototype of a parasympathetic paraganglioma. It rarely exceeds 6 cm in diameter and arises close to or envelops the bifurcation of the common carotid artery. The tumor tissue is red-pink to brown. The microscopic features of all paragangliomas, wherever they arise, are remarkably uniform. They are chiefly composed of nests (**Zellballen**) of round to oval chief cells (neuroectodermal in origin) that are surrounded by delicate vascular septae. The tumor cells contain abundant, clear or granular, eosinophilic cytoplasm and uniform, round to ovoid, sometimes vesicular, nuclei (Fig. 16–14).[48] In most tumors there is little cellular pleomorphism, and mitoses are scant. The chief cells stain strongly for neuroendocrine markers such as chromogranin, synaptophysin, neuron-specific enolase, CD56, and CD57. In addition, there is a supporting network of spindle-shaped stromal cells, collectively

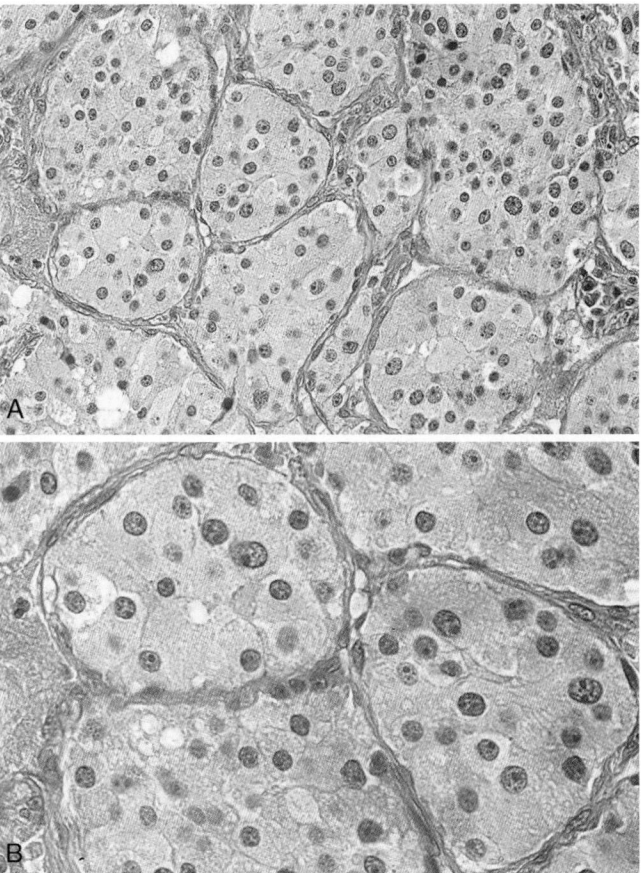

FIGURE 16–14   Carotid body tumor. **A,** Low-power view showing tumor clusters separated by septa (Zellballen). **B,** High-power view of large, eosinophilic, slightly vacuolated tumor cells with elongated sustentacular cells in the septa.

called sustentacular cells, that are positive for S-100 protein. Electron microscopy often discloses well-demarcated neuroendocrine granules in paravertebral tumors, but their number can be highly variable and they tend to be scant in nonfunctioning tumors.

Carotid body tumors (and paragangliomas in general) are rare. They are slow-growing and painless masses that usually arise in the fifth and sixth decades of life. They commonly occur singly and sporadically but may be familial, with autosomal dominant transmission in the multiple endocrine neoplasia 2 syndrome (Chapter 24); in this setting they are often multiple and sometimes bilaterally symmetric. Carotid body tumors frequently recur after incomplete resection and, despite their benign appearance, may metastasize to regional lymph nodes and distant sites. About 50% ultimately prove fatal, largely because of infiltrative growth. Unfortunately, it is almost impossible histologically to judge the clinical course of a carotid body tumor—mitoses, pleomorphism, and even vascular invasion are not reliable indicators.[47]

SALIVARY GLANDS

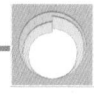

There are three major salivary glands—parotid, submandibular, and sublingual—as well as innumerable minor salivary glands distributed throughout the mucosa of the oral cavity. All these glands are subject to inflammation or to the development of neoplasms.

Xerostomia

Xerostomia is defined as a *dry mouth* resulting from a decrease in the production of saliva. Its incidence among various populations has been reported to be as high as 29%.[48] It is a major feature of the autoimmune disorder Sjögren syndrome, in which it is usually accompanied by dry eyes (Chapter 6). A lack of salivary secretions is also a major complication of radiation therapy. However, xerostomia is most frequently observed as a result of many commonly prescribed classes of medications including: anticholinergic, antidepressant/antipsychotic, diuretic, antihypertensive, sedative, muscle relaxant, analgesic, and antihistamine agents.[48–50] The oral cavity may merely reveal dry mucosa and/or atrophy of the papillae of the tongue, with fissuring and ulcerations, or in Sjögren syndrome, concomitant inflammatory enlargement of the salivary glands. Complications of xerostomia include increased rates of dental caries, candidiasis, as well as difficulty in swallowing and speaking.

Inflammation (Sialadenitis)

Sialadenitis may be of traumatic, viral, bacterial, or autoimmune origin. Mucoceles are the most common type of inflammatory salivary gland lesion. The most common form of viral sialadenitis is *mumps*, in which the major salivary glands, particularly the parotids, are affected (Chapter 8). Other glands (e.g., the pancreas and testes) may also be involved. Autoimmune disease underlies the inflammatory salivary gland changes of Sjögren syndrome, discussed in Chapter 6. In this condition the widespread involvement of the salivary glands and the mucus-secreting glands of the mucosa induces xerostomia. Associated involvement of the lacrimal glands produces dry eyes—*keratoconjunctivitis sicca*.

Mucocele. This is the most common lesion of the salivary glands. It results from either blockage or rupture of a salivary gland duct, with consequent leakage of saliva into the surrounding connective tissue stroma. Mucoceles are most often found on the lower lip and are the result of trauma (Fig. 16–15A). As such, they are typically seen in toddlers and young adults as well as the geriatric population (as a result of falling). Clinically, they present as fluctuant swellings of the lower lip and have a blue translucent hue to them. Patients may report a history of changes in the size of the lesion, particularly in association with meals. Histologically, mucoceles demonstrate a cystlike space that is lined by inflammatory granulation tissue or by fibrous connective tissue. The cystic spaces are filled with mucin as well as inflammatory cells, particularly macrophages (Fig. 16–15B). Complete excision of the cyst with the minor salivary gland lobule of origin is required. Incomplete excision can result in recurrence.

A *ranula* is histologically identical to a mucocele. However, this term is reserved for mucoceles that arise when the duct of the sublingual gland has been damaged. A *ranula* can become extremely large and develop into a "plunging ranula" when it dissects its way through the connective tissue stroma connecting the two bellies of the mylohyoid muscle.

Sialolithiasis and Nonspecific Sialadenitis. Nonspecific bacterial sialadenitis, most often involving the major salivary glands, particularly the submandibular glands, is a common condition, usually secondary to ductal obstruction produced by stones *(sialolithiasis)*. The common offenders are *S. aureus* and *Streptococcus viridans*. The stone formation is sometimes related to obstruction of the orifices of the salivary glands by impacted food debris or by edema about the orifice after some injury. Frequently, the stones are of obscure origin. Dehydration and decreased secretory function may also predispose to secondary bacterial invasion, as sometimes occurs in patients receiving long-term phenothiazines that suppress salivary secretion. Dehydration with decreased secretion may lead to the development of bacterial suppurative parotitis in elderly patients with a recent history of major thoracic or abdominal surgery.

Whatever the origin, the obstructive process and bacterial invasion lead to a nonspecific inflammation of the affected glands that may be largely interstitial or, when induced by

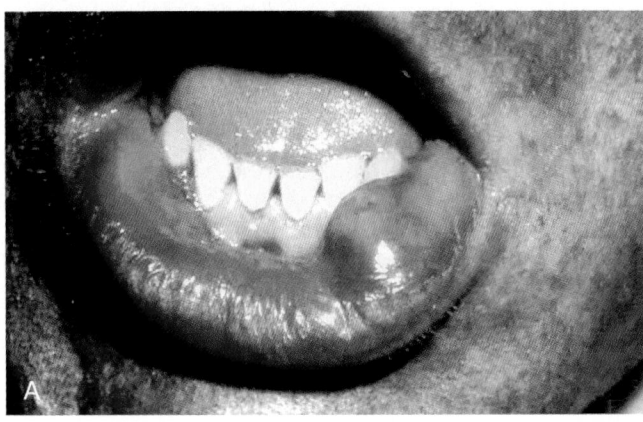

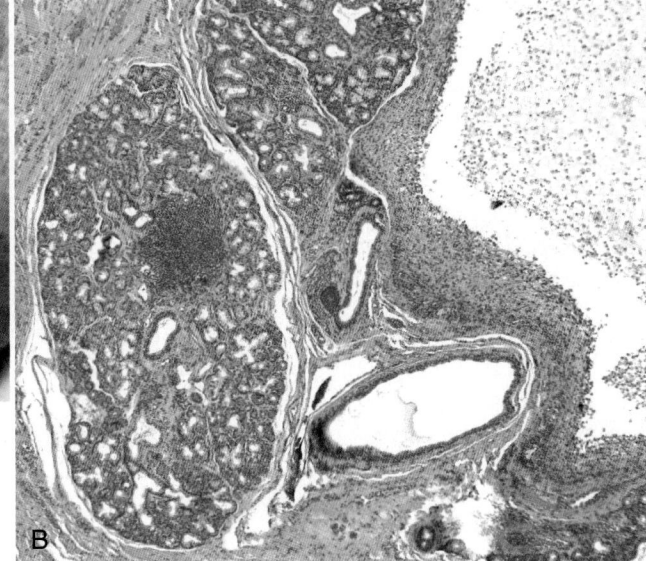

FIGURE 16–15 Mucocele. **A,** Fluctuant fluid-filled lesion on the lower lip subsequent to trauma. **B,** Cystlike cavity filled with mucinous material and lined by organizing granulation tissue.

staphylococcal or other pyogens, may be associated with overt suppurative necrosis and abscess formation. Unilateral involvement of a single gland is the rule. The inflammatory involvement causes painful enlargement and sometimes a purulent ductal discharge.

Neoplasms

Despite their relatively simple morphology, the salivary glands give rise to no fewer than 30 histologically distinct tumors.[51–53] A classification and the relative incidence of benign and malignant tumors is shown in Table 16–4; not included are the rare benign and malignant mesenchymal neoplasms.

As indicated in Table 16–4, a small number of neoplasms makes up more than 90% of salivary gland tumors, and so our discussion is restricted to these. Overall, these neoplasms are relatively uncommon and represent less than 2% of all tumors in humans. *About 65% to 80% arise within the parotid, 10% in the submandibular gland,* and the remainder in the minor salivary glands, including the sublingual glands. Approximately 15% to 30% of tumors in the parotid glands are malignant. In contrast, approximately 40% of submandibular, 50% of minor salivary gland, and 70% to 90% of sublingual tumors are cancerous. *The likelihood, then, of a salivary gland tumor being malignant is more or less inversely proportional to the size of the gland.*

These tumors usually occur in adults, with a slight female predominance, but about 5% occur in children younger than age 16 years. For unknown reasons, Warthin tumors occur much more often in males than in females. The benign tumors most often appear in the fifth to seventh decades of life. The malignant ones tend, on average, to appear somewhat later. Whatever the histologic pattern, neoplasms in the parotid glands produce distinctive swellings in front of and below the ear. In general, when they are first diagnosed, both benign and malignant lesions range from 4 to 6 cm in diameter and are mobile on palpation except in the case of neglected malignant tumors. Although benign tumors are known to have been present usually for many months to several years before coming to clinical attention, cancers seem to demand attention more promptly, probably because of their more rapid growth. Ultimately, however, there are no reliable criteria to differentiate, on clinical grounds, the benign from the malignant lesions, and morphologic evaluation is necessary.

TABLE 16–4 Histologic Classification and Incidence of Benign and Malignant Tumors of the Salivary Glands

Benign	Malignant
Pleomorphic adenoma (50%) (mixed tumor)	Mucoepidermoid carcinoma (15%)
Warthin tumor (5% to 10%)	Adenocarcinoma (NOS) (10%)
Oncocytoma (1%)	Acinic cell carcinoma (5%)
Other adenomas (5% to 10%) Basal cell adenoma Canalicular adenoma	Adenoid cystic carcinoma (5%) Malignant mixed tumor (3% to 5%) Squamous cell carcinoma (1%)
Ductal papillomas	Other carcinomas (2%)

NOS, not otherwise specified.
Data from Ellis GL, Auclair PL: Tumors of the Salivary Glands. Atlas of Tumor Pathology, Third Series. Washington, DC, Armed Forces Institute of Pathology, 1996.

PLEOMORPHIC ADENOMA

Because of their remarkable histologic diversity, these neoplasms have also been called *mixed tumors.* They represent about *60% of tumors in the parotid,* are less common in the submandibular glands, and are relatively rare in the minor salivary glands. They are benign tumors that consist of a mixture of ductal (epithelial) and myoepithelial cells, and

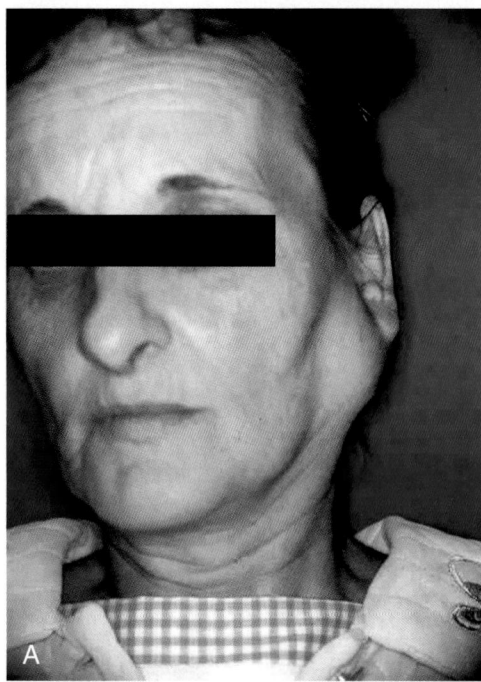

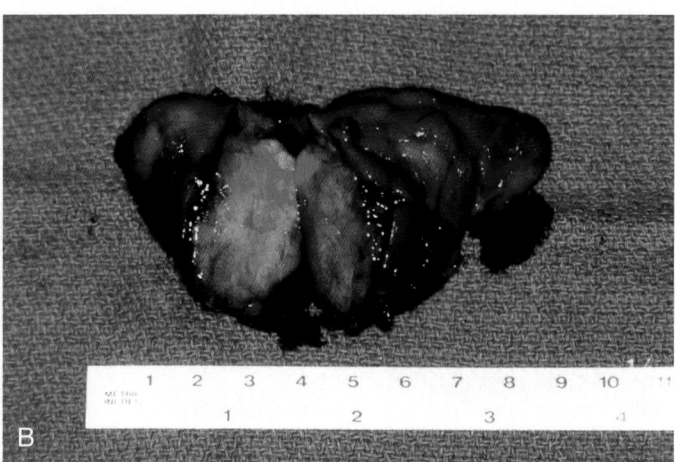

FIGURE 16–16 Pleomorphic adenoma. **A,** Slowly enlarging neoplasm in the parotid gland of many years duration. **B,** The bisected, sharply circumscribed, yellow-white tumor can be seen surrounded by normal salivary gland tissue.

therefore they show both epithelial and mesenchymal differentiation. They reveal epithelial elements dispersed throughout the matrix along with varying degrees of myxoid, hyaline, chondroid (cartilaginous), and even osseous tissue. In some tumors the epithelial elements predominate; in others they are present only in widely dispersed foci.

Little is known about the origins of these neoplasms, except that radiation exposure increases the risk. Equally uncertain is the histogenesis of the various components. A currently popular view is that all neoplastic elements, including those that appear mesenchymal, are of either myoepithelial or ductal reserve cell origin (hence the designation *pleomorphic adenoma*).

Morphology. Most pleomorphic adenomas present as rounded, well-demarcated masses rarely exceeding 6 cm in the greatest dimension (Fig. 16–16). Although they are encapsulated, in some locations (particularly the palate) the capsule is not fully developed, and expansile growth produces protrusions into the surrounding gland, rendering enucleation of the tumor hazardous. The cut surface is gray-white with myxoid and blue translucent areas of chondroid (cartilage-like).

The dominant histologic feature is the great heterogeneity mentioned. The epithelial elements resembling ductal cells or myoepithelial cells are arranged in duct formations, acini, irregular tubules, strands, or sheets of cells. These elements are typically dispersed within a mesenchyme-like background of loose myxoid tissue containing islands of chondroid and, rarely, foci of bone (Fig. 16–17). Sometimes the epithelial cells form well-developed ducts lined by cuboidal to columnar cells with an underlying layer

of deeply chromatic, small myoepithelial cells. In other instances there may be strands or sheets of myoepithelial cells. Islands of well-differentiated squamous epithelium may also be present. In most cases there is no epithelial dysplasia or evident mitotic activity. There is no difference in biologic behavior between the tumors composed largely of epithelial elements and those composed largely of seemingly mesenchymal elements.

Clinical Features. These tumors present as painless, slow-growing, mobile discrete masses within the parotid (Fig. 16–16) or submandibular areas or in the buccal cavity. The recurrence rate (perhaps months to years later) with parotidectomy is about 4% but, with simple enucleation, approaches 25%. This high recurrence is because of failure to recognize minute protrusions from the main mass, into the surrounding tissue, at the time of surgery.

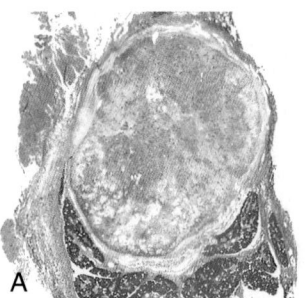
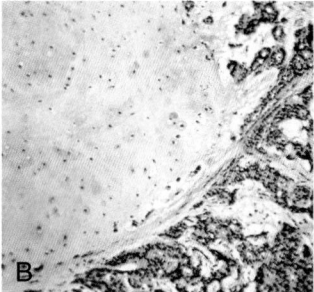

FIGURE 16–17 Pleomorphic adenoma. **A,** Low-power view showing a well-demarcated tumor with adjacent normal salivary gland parenchyma. **B,** High-power view showing epithelial cells as well as myoepithelial cells found within a chondroid matrix material.

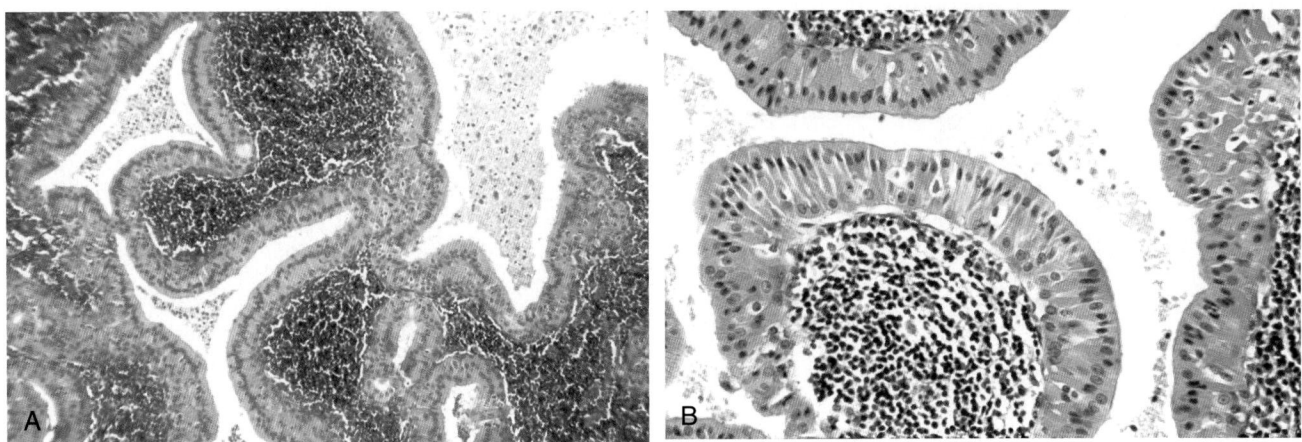

FIGURE 16–18 Warthin tumor. **A,** Low-power view showing epithelial and lymphoid elements. Note the follicular germinal center beneath the epithelium. **B,** Cystic spaces separate lobules of neoplastic epithelium consisting of a double layer of eosinophilic epithelial cells based on a reactive lymphoid stroma.

A carcinoma arising in a pleomorphic adenoma is referred to variously as a *carcinoma ex pleomorphic adenoma* or a *malignant mixed tumor.* The incidence of malignant transformation increases with the duration of the tumor, being about 2% for tumors present less than 5 years and almost 10% for those of more than 15 years' duration. The cancer usually takes the form of an adenocarcinoma or undifferentiated carcinoma, and often it virtually completely overgrows the last vestiges of the preexisting pleomorphic adenoma; but to substantiate the diagnosis of carcinoma ex pleomorphic adenoma, recognizable traces of the latter must be found. Regrettably, these cancers, when they appear, are among the most aggressive of all salivary gland malignant neoplasms, producing mortality rates of 30% to 50% at 5 years.

WARTHIN TUMOR (PAPILLARY CYSTADENOMA LYMPHOMATOSUM)

This curious benign neoplasm with its intimidating histologic name is the second most common salivary gland neoplasm. It arises almost *exclusively in the parotid gland* (the only tumor virtually restricted to the parotid) and occurs more commonly in males than in females, usually in the fifth to seventh decades of life. About 10% are multifocal and 10% bilateral. Smokers have eight times the risk of nonsmokers for developing these tumors.

Morphology. Most Warthin tumors are round to oval, encapsulated masses, 2 to 5 cm in diameter, usually arising in the superficial parotid gland, where they are readily palpable. Transection reveals a pale gray surface punctuated by narrow cystic or cleftlike spaces filled with a mucinous or serous secretion. On microscopic examination these spaces are lined by a double layer of neoplastic epithelial cells resting on a dense lymphoid stroma sometimes bearing germinal centers (Fig. 16–18). The spaces are frequently narrowed by polypoid projections of the lymphoepithelial elements. The double layer of lining cells is distinctive; it consists of a surface palisade of columnar cells

having an abundant, finely granular, eosinophilic cytoplasm, that imparts an oncocytic appearance, which rests on a layer of cuboidal to polygonal cells. Oncocytes are epithelial cells stuffed with mitochondria, which impart the granular appearance to the cytoplasm. Secretory cells are dispersed in the columnar cell layer, accounting for the secretions within the cystically dilated lumens. On occasion, there are foci of squamous metaplasia.

The histogenesis of these tumors has long been disputed. The occasional finding of small salivary gland rests in lymph nodes in the neck suggests that these tumors arise from the aberrant incorporation of similar inclusion-bearing lymphoid tissue in the parotids. Indeed, rarely, Warthin tumors have arisen within cervical lymph nodes, a finding that should not be mistaken for metastases. These neoplasms are benign, with recurrence rates of only 2% after resection.

MUCOEPIDERMOID CARCINOMA

These neoplasms are composed of variable mixtures of squamous cells, mucus-secreting cells, and intermediate cells. They represent about 15% of all salivary gland tumors, and while they occur mainly (60% to 70%) in the parotids, they account for a large fraction of salivary gland neoplasms in the other glands, particularly the minor salivary glands. In more than half the cases, this tumor is associated with a balanced (11;19) (q21;p13) chromosomal translocation that creates a fusion gene composed of portions of the *MECT1* and *MAML2* genes. The *MECT1-MAML2* gene is believed to play a key role in the genesis of this tumor, possibly by perturbing the notch and cAMP-dependent signaling pathways.[54,55] Overall, they are the most common form of primary *malignant* tumor of the salivary glands.

Morphology. Mucoepidermoid carcinomas can grow as large as 8 cm in diameter and although they are apparently circumscribed, they lack well-defined capsules and are often infiltrative at the margins. Pale

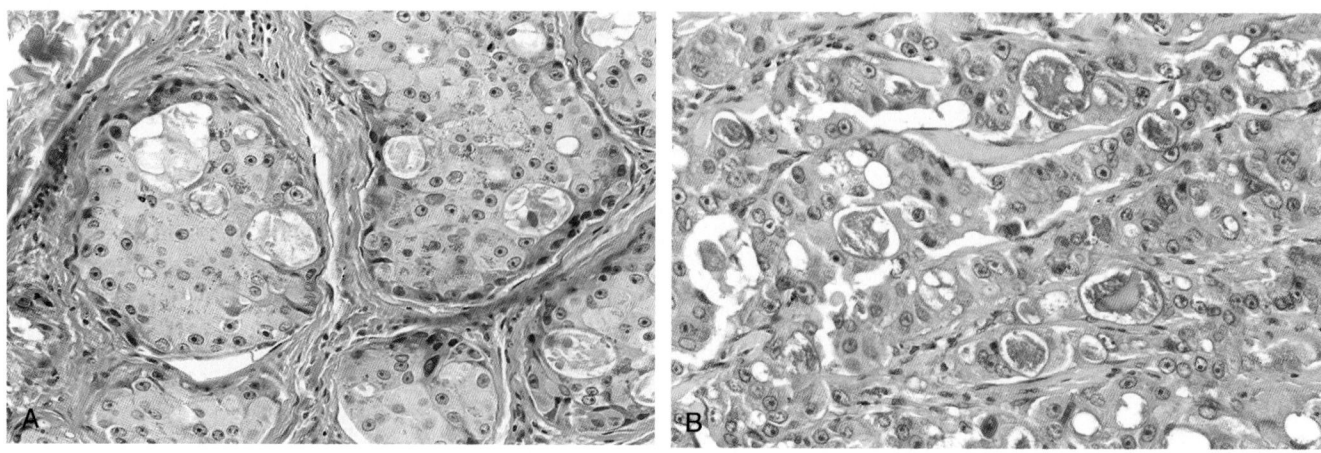

FIGURE 16–19   **A,** Mucoepidermoid carcinoma growing in nests composed of squamous cells as well as clear vacuolated cells containing mucin. **B,** Mucicarmine stains the mucin reddish pink. (Courtesy of Dr. James Gulizia, Brigham and Women's Hospital, Boston, MA.)

and gray-white on transection, they frequently contain small, mucin-containing cysts. The basic histologic pattern is that of cords, sheets, or cystic configurations of squamous, mucous, or intermediate cells. The hybrid cell types often have squamous features, with small to large mucus-filled vacuoles, best seen when highlighted with mucin stains (Fig. 16–19). The tumor cells may be regular and benign appearing or, alternatively, highly anaplastic and unmistakably malignant. Accordingly, mucoepidermoid carcinomas are subclassified into low, intermediate, or high grade.

The clinical course and prognosis depend on the grade of the neoplasm. Low-grade tumors may invade locally and recur in about 15% of cases, but only rarely do they metastasize and so yield a 5-year survival rate of more than 90%. By contrast, high-grade neoplasms and, to a lesser extent, intermediate-grade tumors are invasive and difficult to excise and so recur in about 25% to 30% of cases and, in 30% of cases, metastasize to distant sites. The 5-year survival rate in patients with these tumors is only 50%.

OTHER SALIVARY GLAND TUMORS

Two less common neoplasms merit brief description: adenoid cystic carcinoma and acinic cell tumor.

Adenoid cystic carcinoma is a relatively uncommon tumor, which in approximately 50% of cases is found in the minor salivary glands (in particular the palate). Among the major salivary glands, the parotid and submandibular glands are the most common locations. Similar neoplasms have been reported in the nose, sinuses, and upper airways and elsewhere.

Morphology. In gross appearance, they are generally small, poorly encapsulated, infiltrative, gray-pink lesions. On histologic evaluation, they are composed of small cells having dark, compact nuclei and scant cytoplasm. These cells tend to be disposed in tubular, solid, or cribriform patterns reminiscent of cylindromas arising in the adnexa of the skin. The spaces between the tumor cells are often filled with a hyaline material thought to represent excess basement membrane (Fig. 16–20A). Other less common histologic patterns have been designated as tubular and solid variants.

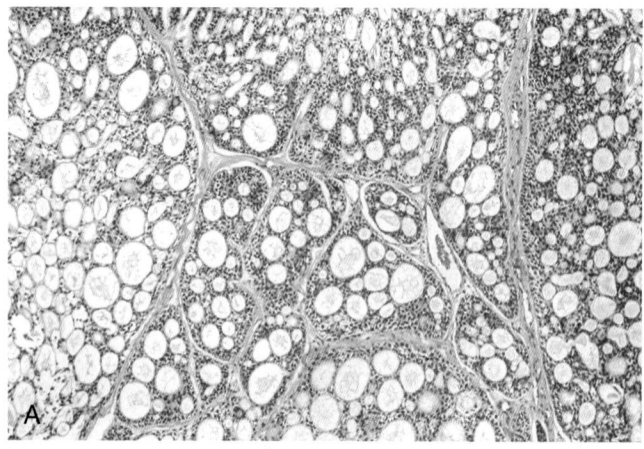
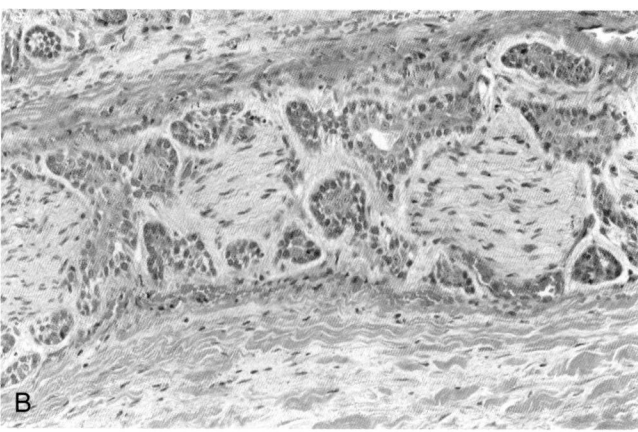

FIGURE 16–20   Adenoid cystic carcinoma in a salivary gland. **A,** Low-power view. The tumor cells have created a cribriform pattern enclosing secretions. **B,** Perineural invasion by tumor cells.

Although slow growing, adenoid cystic carcinomas are relentless and unpredictable tumors with a tendency to invade perineural spaces (Fig. 16–20B), and they are stubbornly recurrent. Eventually, 50% or more disseminate widely to distant sites such as bone, liver, and brain, sometimes decades after attempted removal. Thus, although the 5-year survival rate is about 60% to 70%, it drops to about 30% at 10 years and 15% at 15 years. Neoplasms arising in the minor salivary glands have, on average, a poorer prognosis than those primary in the parotids.

The *acinic cell tumor* is composed of cells resembling the normal serous acinar cells of salivary glands. They are relatively uncommon, representing only 2% to 3% of salivary gland tumors. Most arise in the parotids; the remainder arise in the submandibular glands. They rarely involve the minor glands, which normally have only a scant number of serous cells. Like Warthin tumor, they are sometimes bilateral or multicentric. They are generally small, discrete lesions that may appear encapsulated. On histologic examination, they reveal a variable architecture and cell morphology. Most characteristically, the cells have clear cytoplasm but the cells are sometimes solid and at other times vacuolated. The cells are disposed in sheets or microcystic, glandular, follicular, or papillary patterns. There is usually little anaplasia and few mitoses, but some tumors are occasionally slightly more pleomorphic.

The clinical course of these neoplasms is somewhat dependent on the level of pleomorphism. Overall, recurrence after resection is uncommon, but about 10% to 15% of these neoplasms metastasize to lymph nodes. The survival rate is in the range of 90% at 5 years and 60% at 20 years.

REFERENCES

1. Research, Science and Therapy Committee of the American Academy of Periodontology: Treatment of plaque-induced gingivitis, chronic periodontitis, and other clinical conditions. J Periodontol 72:1790, 2001.
2. Research, Science and Therapy Committee of the American Academy of Periodontology: Epidemiology of periodontal disease. J Periodontol 76:1406, 2005.
3. Kinane D: Periodontal disease and health: Consensus report of the sixth European workshop on Periodontology. J Clin Periodontol 35:333, 2008.
4. Persson GR, Persson RE: Cardiovascular disease and periodontitis: an update on the associations and risk. J Clin Periodontol 35:362, 2008.
5. Cawson RA et al. (eds): Lucas's Pathology of Tumors of the Oral Tissues. London, Churchill Livingstone, 1998.
6. Scully C: The diagnosis and management of recurrent aphthous stomatitis: a consensus approach. J Am Dent Assoc 134:200, 2003.
7. Hille JJ et al: Mechanisms of expression of HHV8, EBV and HPV in selected HIV-associated oral lesions. Oral Dis 8:161, 2002.
8. Silverman S: Early diagnosis of oral cancer. Cancer 62:1796, 1988.
9. Shugars DC, Patton LL: Detecting, diagnosing, and preventing oral cancer. Nurse Pract 22:109, 1997.
10. Whited JD, Grichnick JM: Does this patient have a mole or a melanoma? JAMA 279:696, 1998.
11. Rampen FH et al.: False-negative findings in skin cancer and melanoma screening. J Am Acad Dermatol 33:59, 1995.
12. Mashberg A, Feldman LJ: Clinical criteria for identifying early oral and oropharyngeal carcinoma: erythroplasia revisted. Am J Surg 156:273, 1988.
13. Neville BW et al. (eds): Oral and Maxillofacial Pathology. Philadelphia, WB Saunders, 2008.
14. Jemal A et al: Cancer statistics, 2008. CA Cancer J Clin 58:71, 2008.
15. Parkin DM et al: Global cancer statistics, 2002. CA Cancer J Clin 55:74, 2005.
16. Haddad RI, Shin DM: Recent advances in head and neck cancer. N Engl J Med 359:1143, 2008.
17. Pai SI, Westia WH: Molecular pathology of head and neck cancer: implication for diagnosis and treatment. Ann Rev Pathol Mech Dis 4:49, 2009.
18. Anderson WF et al.: Secondary chemoprevention of upper aerodigestive tract tumors. Semin Oncol 28:106, 2001.
19. Day GL, Blot WJ: Second primary tumors in patients with oral cancer. Cancer 70:14, 1992.
20. Slaughter DP et al.: "Field cancerization" in oral stratified squamous epithelium. Cancer 6:962, 1953.
21. Braakhuis BJM et al.: A genetic explanation of Slaughter's concept of field cancerization: evidence and clinical implications. Cancer Res 63:1727, 2003.
22. Lippman SM, Hong WK: Second malignant tumors in head and neck squamous cell carcinoma: the overshadowing threat for patients with early-stage disease. Int J Radiat Oncol Biol Phys 17:691, 1989.
23. Chaturvedi AK et al: Incidence trends for human papillomavirus-related and -unrelated oral squamous cell carcinomas in the United States. JCO 26:612, 2008.
24. Jefferies S, Foulkes WD: Genetic mechanisms in squamous cell carcinoma of the head and neck. Oral Oncol 37:115, 2001.
25. Koch WM et al.: Head and neck cancer in nonsmokers: a distinct clinical and molecular entity. Laryngoscope 109:1544, 1999.
26. Lingen MW et al.: Overexpression of *p53* in squamous cell carcinoma of the tongue in young patients with no known risk factors is not associated with mutations in exons 5–9. Head Neck 22:328, 2000.
27. Schantz SP, Yu GP: Head and neck cancer incidence trends in young Americans, 1973–1997, with a special analysis for tongue cancer. Arch Otolaryngol Head Neck Surg 128:268, 2002.
28. Mao L et al.: Frequent microsatellite alterations at chromosomes 9p21 and 3p14 in oral premalignant lesions and their value in cancer risk assessment. Nat Med 2:682, 1996.
29. Boyle JO et al.: The incidence of *p53* mutations increases with progression of head and neck cancer. Cancer Res 53:4477, 1993.
30. Rosin MP et al.: Use of allelic loss to predict malignant risk for low-grade oral epithelial dysplasia. Clin Cancer Res 6:357, 2000.
31. Michalides R et al.: Overexpression of cyclin D1 correlates with recurrence in a group of forty-seven operable squamous cell carcinomas of the head and neck. Cancer Res 55:975, 1995.
32. Izzo JG et al.: Dysregulated cyclin D1 expression early in head and neck tumorigenesis: in vivo evidence for an association with subsequent gene amplification. Oncogene 17:2313, 1998.
33. El-Mofty S (ed): Odontogenic tumors. Semin Diagn Pathol 16:269, 1999.
34. Pinto JM, Naclerio RM: Environmental and allergic factors in chronic rhinosinusitis. Clin Allergy Immunol 20:25, 2007.
35. Slavin RG: Nasal polyps and sinusitis. JAMA 278:1845, 1997.
36. Thompson LDR: Malignant neoplasms of the nasal cavity, paranasal sinuses, and nasopharynx. In Thompson LDR (Ed): Head and Neck Pathology. London, Churchill Livingtone, 2006, pp 155–213.
37. Perez-Ordonez B, Huvos AG: Nonsquamous lesions of the nasal cavity, paranasal sinuses and nasopharynx. In Gnepp DR (ed): Diagnostic Surgical Pathology of the Head and Neck. Philadelphia, W.B. Saunders, 2001, pp 79–139.
38. Meyers LL, Oxford LE: Differential diagnosis and treatment options in paranasal sinus cancers Surg Oncol Clin N Am 13:167, 2004.
39. Klepin HD et al: Esthesioneuroblastoma. Curr Treat Options Oncol 6:509, 2005.
40. Rabb-Traub N: Epstein-Barr virus in the pathogenesis of NPC. Semin Cancer Biol 12:431, 2002.
41. Thompson LDR: Malignant neoplasms of the nasal cavity, paranasal sinuses, and nasopharynx. In Thompson LDR (ed): Head and Neck Pathology. Philadelphia, Churchill Livingstone, 2006, pp 155–215.
42. Juvenile recurrent respiratory papillomatosis: still a mystery disease with difficult management. Head Neck 29:155, 2007.
43. Kristt D et al.: The spectrum of laryngeal neoplasia: the pathologist's view. Pathol Res Pract 198:709, 2002.
44. Loyo M, Pai SI: The molecular genetics of laryngeal cancer. Otolaryngol Clin North Am 41:657, 2008.
45. Hobbs CG et al: Human papillomavirus and head and neck cancer: a systematic review and meta-analysis. Clin Otolaryngol. 31:259, 2006.
46. Rovers MM et al.: Otitis media. Lancet 363:465, 2004.

47. Capella C et al.: Histopathology, cytology, and cytochemistry of pheochromocytomas and paragangliomas including chemodectomas. Pathol Res Pract 186:176, 1988.

48. Guggenheimer J, Moore PA: Xerostomia: etiology, recognition and treatment. J Am Dent Assoc 134:61, 2003.

49. Ciancio SG: Medications' impact on oral health. J Am Dent Assoc 135:1440, 2004.

50. Scully C: Drug effects on salivary glands: dry mouth. Oral Dis 9:165, 2003.

51. Ellis GL et al.: Surgical Pathology of Salivary Glands. Philadelphia, WB Saunders, 1991.

52. Ellis GL, Auclair PL: Tumors of the salivary glands. In Atlas of Tumor Pathology, Third Series, Fascicle 17. Washington, DC, Armed Forces Institute of Pathology, 1996.

53. Dardick I: Color Atlas/Text of Salivary Gland Pathology. New York, Igaku-Shoin, 1996.

54. Tonon G et al: t(11;19)(q21;p13) translocation in mucoepidermoid carcinoma creates a novel fusion product that disrupts a Notch signaling pathway. Nat Genet 33:208, 2003.

55. Coxon A et al: Mect1-Maml2 fusion oncogene linked to the aberrant activation of cyclic AMP/CREB regulated genes. Cancer Res 65:7137, 2005.

17

The Gastrointestinal Tract

JERROLD R. TURNER

■ **CONGENITAL ABNORMALITIES**

Atresia, Fistulae, and Duplications

Diaphragmatic Hernia, Omphalocele, and Gastroschisis

Ectopia

Meckel Diverticulum

Pyloric Stenosis

Hirschsprung Disease

■ **ESOPHAGUS**

Esophageal Obstruction
  Achalasia

Esophagitis
  Lacerations
  Chemical and Infectious Esophagitis
  Reflux Esophagitis
  Eosinophilic Esophagitis

Barrett Esophagus
  Esophageal Varices

Esophageal Tumors
  Adenocarcinoma
  Squamous Cell Carcinoma
  Uncommon Esophageal Tumors

■ **STOMACH**

Acute Gastritis
  Acute Gastric Ulceration

Chronic Gastritis
  Helicobacter Pylori Gastritis
  Autoimmune Gastritis
  Uncommon Forms of Gastritis

Complications of Chronic Gastritis
  Peptic Ulcer Disease
  Mucosal Atrophy and Intestinal Metaplasia
  Dysplasia
  Gastritis Cystica

Hypertrophic Gastropathies
  Ménétrier Disease
  Zollinger-Ellison Syndrome

Gastric Polyps and Tumors
  Inflammatory and Hyperplastic Polyps
  Fundic Gland Polyps
  Gastric Adenoma
  Gastric Adenocarcinoma
  Lymphoma
  Carcinoid Tumor
  Gastrointestinal Stromal Tumor

■ **SMALL INTESTINE AND COLON**

Intestinal Obstruction
  Hernias
  Adhesions
  Volvulus
  Intussusception

Ischemic Bowel Disease

Angiodysplasia

Malabsorption and Diarrhea
  Cystic Fibrosis
  Celiac Disease
  Tropical Sprue
  Autoimmune Enteropathy

Lactase (Disaccharidase) Deficiency
Abetalipoproteinemia

Infectious Enterocolitis
  Cholera
  Campylobacter Enterocolitis
  Shigellosis
  Salmonellosis
  Typhoid Fever
  Yersinia
  Escherichia Coli
  Pseudomembranous Colitis
  Whipple Disease
  Viral Gastroenteritis
  Parasitic Enterocolitis

Irritable Bowel Syndrome

Inflammatory Bowel Disease
  Crohn Disease
  Ulcerative Colitis
    Indeterminate Colitis
    Colitis-Associated Neoplasia

Other Causes of Colitis
  Diversion Colitis
  Microscopic Colitis
  Graft-versus-Host Disease

Sigmoid Diverticulitis

Polyps
  Inflammatory Polyps
  Hamartomatous Polyps
    Juvenile Polyps
    Peutz-Jeghers Syndrome
    Cowden Syndrome and Bannayan-Ruvalcaba-Riley Syndrome
    Cronkhite-Canada Syndrome
  Hyperplastic Polyps
  Neoplastic Polyps

Familial Syndromes
  Familial Adenomatous Polyposis
  Hereditary Non-Polyposis Colorectal Cancer

Adenocarcinoma

Tumors of the Anal Canal

Hemorrhoids

Acute Appendicitis

Tumors of the Appendix

■ **PERITONEAL CAVITY**

Inflammatory Disease
  Peritoneal Infection
  Sclerosing Retroperitonitis
  Cysts

Tumors

The gastrointestinal (GI) tract is a hollow tube extending from the oral cavity to the anus that consists of anatomically distinct segments, including the esophagus, stomach, small intestine, colon, rectum, and anus. Each of these segments has unique, complementary, and highly integrated functions, which together serve to regulate the intake, processing, and absorption of ingested nutrients and the disposal of waste products.

The regional variations in structure and function are reflected in diseases of the GI tract, which often affect one or another segment preferentially. Accordingly, following consideration of several important congenital abnormalities, the discussion will be organized anatomically. Disorders affecting more than one segment of the GI tract, such as Crohn disease, will be discussed with the region that is involved most frequently.

CONGENITAL ABNORMALITIES

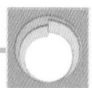

Depending on both the nature and timing of the insult, a variety of developmental anomalies can affect the GI tract. Importantly, because many organs develop simultaneously during embryogenesis, the presence of congenital GI disorders should prompt evaluation of other organs. Some defects are commonly associated with GI lesions.

Atresia, Fistulae, and Duplications

Atresia, fistulae, and duplications may occur in any part of the GI tract. When present within the esophagus they are discovered shortly after birth, usually because they cause regurgitation during feeding. These must be corrected promptly, since

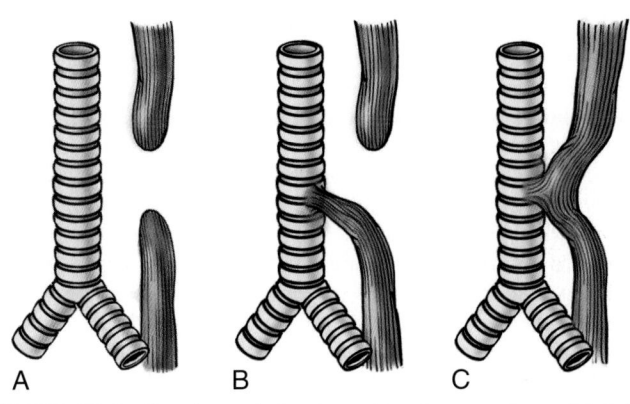

FIGURE 17–1 Esophageal atresia and tracheoesophageal fistula. **A,** Blind upper and lower esophageal segments. **B,** Blind upper segment with fistula between lower segment and trachea. **C,** Fistula between patent esophagus and trachea. Type **B** is the most common. (Adapted from Morson BC, Dawson IMP, eds: Gastrointestinal Pathology. Oxford, Blackwell Scientific Publications, 1972, p 8.)

they are incompatible with life. Absence, or *agenesis*, of the esophagus is extremely rare, but *atresia*, in which development is incomplete, is more common. In esophageal atresia a thin, noncanalized cord replaces a segment of esophagus, causing a mechanical obstruction (Fig. 17–1A). Proximal and distal blind pouches connect to the pharynx and stomach, respectively. Atresia occurs most commonly at or near the tracheal bifurcation and is usually associated with a *fistula* connecting the upper or lower esophageal pouches to a bronchus or the trachea (17–1B). Fistulae can lead to aspiration, suffocation, pneumonia, and severe fluid and electrolyte imbalances (Fig. 17–1B,C). Esophageal atresia is associated with congenital heart defects, genitourinary malformations, and neurologic disease. Intestinal atresia is less common than esophageal atresia but frequently involves the duodenum and is characterized by a segment of bowel lacking a lumen.

Stenosis is an incomplete form of atresia in which the lumen is markedly reduced in caliber as a result of fibrous thickening of the wall, resulting in partial or complete obstruction. Stenosis may involve any part of the GI tract, although the esophagus and small intestine are affected most often. *Imperforate anus*, the most common form of congenital intestinal atresia, is due to a failure of the cloacal diaphragm to involute. Stenosis can also be caused by inflammatory scarring, as may occur with chronic gastroesophageal reflux, irradiation, scleroderma, or caustic injury.

Congenital duplication cysts are saccular or elongated cystic masses that contain redundant smooth muscle layers. These may be present in the esophagus, small intestine, or colon.

Diaphragmatic Hernia, Omphalocele, and Gastroschisis

Diaphragmatic hernia occurs when incomplete formation of the diaphragm allows the abdominal viscera to herniate into the thoracic cavity. When severe, the space-filling effect of the displaced viscera can cause pulmonary hypoplasia that is incompatible with life after birth. *Omphalocele* occurs when closure of the abdominal musculature is incomplete and the abdominal viscera herniate into a ventral membranous sac. This may be repaired surgically, but as many as 40% of infants with an omphalocele have other birth defects, including diaphragmatic hernia and cardiac anomalies. *Gastroschisis* is another ventral wall defect similar to omphalocele except that it involves all of the layers of the abdominal wall, from the peritoneum to the skin.

Ectopia

Ectopic tissues *(developmental rests)* are common in the GI tract. The most frequent site of *ectopic gastric mucosa* is the upper third of the esophagus, where it is referred to as an *inlet patch*. While generally asymptomatic, acid released by gastric mucosa within the esophagus can result in dysphagia, esophagitis, Barrett esophagus, or, rarely, adenocarcinoma. *Ectopic pancreatic tissue* occurs less frequently and can be found in the esophagus or stomach. Like inlet patches, these nodules are most often asymptomatic but can produce damage and local inflammation. When ectopic pancreatic tissue is present in the pylorus, inflammation and scarring may lead to obstruction. Because the rests may be present within any layer of the gastric wall, they can mimic invasive cancer. *Gastric heterotopia,* small patches of ectopic gastric mucosa in the small bowel or colon, may present with occult blood loss due to peptic ulceration of adjacent mucosa.[1]

Meckel Diverticulum

A true diverticulum is a blind outpouching of the alimentary tract that is lined by mucosa, communicates with the lumen, and includes all three layers of the bowel wall. The most common type is the *Meckel diverticulum*, which occurs in the ileum.

The Meckel diverticulum occurs as a result of failed involution of the vitelline duct, which connects the lumen of the developing gut to the yolk sac. This solitary diverticulum is a small pouch extending from the antimesenteric side of the bowel (Fig. 17–2). It is a true diverticulum with a wall that

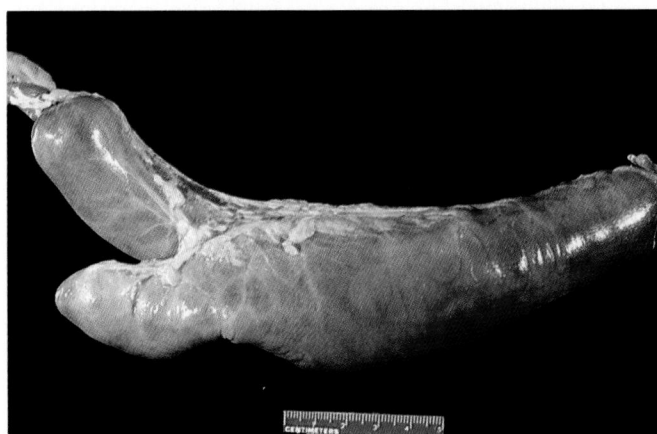

FIGURE 17–2 Meckel diverticulum. The blind pouch is located on the antimesenteric side of the small bowel.

includes mucosa, submucosa, and muscularis propria. Meckel diverticulae occur in approximately 2% of the population, are generally present within 2 feet (85 cm) of the ileocecal valve, are approximately 2 inches (5 cm) long, are twice as common in males as in females, and are most often symptomatic by age 2 (although only ~4% of Meckel diverticulae are symptomatic). These facts comprise the "rule of 2s" that is often used to help remember characteristics of Meckel diverticulae. The mucosal lining of Meckel diverticulae may resemble that of normal small intestine, but ectopic pancreatic or gastric tissue may also be present. The latter may result in *peptic ulceration* of adjacent small intestinal mucosa and present with occult bleeding or abdominal pain resembling acute appendicitis or intestinal obstruction.

Less commonly, congenital diverticulae occur in other parts of the small intestine and ascending colon. Virtually all other diverticulae are acquired and either lack muscularis entirely or have an attenuated muscularis propria. Although acquired diverticulae may occur in the esophagus, stomach, and duodenum, the most common site is the sigmoid colon (discussed later).

Pyloric Stenosis

Congenital hypertrophic pyloric stenosis is three to four times more common in males and occurs once in 300 to 900 live births. Monozygotic twins have a high rate of corcordance, suggesting a genetic basis. Family studies suggest a complex polygenic inheritance. Turner syndrome and trisomy 18 are also associated with the disease. *Congenital hypertrophic pyloric stenosis generally presents in the second or third week of life as new-onset regurgitation and persistent, projectile, nonbilious vomiting.* Physical examination reveals hyperperistalsis and a firm, ovoid abdominal mass. These findings stem from hyperplasia of the pyloric muscularis propria, which obstructs the gastric outflow tract. Edema and inflammatory changes in the mucosa and submucosa may aggravate the narrowing. Surgical splitting of the muscularis (myotomy) is curative. Acquired pyloric stenosis occurs in adults as a consequence of antral gastritis or peptic ulcers close to the pylorus. Carcinomas of the distal stomach and pancreas may also narrow the pyloric channel due to fibrosis or malignant infiltration.

Hirschsprung Disease

Hirschsprung disease occurs in approximately 1 of 5000 live births. It may be isolated or occur in combination with other developmental abnormalities; 10% of all cases occur in children with Down syndrome and serious neurologic abnormalities are present in another 5%.

Pathogenesis. You may recall that the enteric neuronal plexus develops from neural crest cells that migrate into the bowel wall during embryogenesis. Hirschsprung disease, also known as *congenital aganglionic megacolon*, results when the normal migration of neural crest cells from cecum to rectum is arrested prematurely or when the ganglion cells undergo premature death. This produces a distal intestinal segment that lacks both the Meissner submucosal and the Auerbach myenteric plexus ("aganglionosis"). Coordinated peristaltic

contractions are absent and functional obstruction occurs, resulting in dilation proximal to the affected segment.

The mechanisms underlying defective neural crest cell migration in Hirschsprung disease are unknown, but a genetic component is present in nearly all cases and 4% of patients' siblings are affected.[2] However, simple Mendelian inheritance is not involved in most cases. *Heterozygous loss-of-function mutations in the receptor tyrosine kinase RET account for the majority of familial cases* and approximately 15% of sporadic cases.[3] Mutations also occur in at least seven other genes encoding proteins involved in enteric neurodevelopment, including the RET ligand glial-derived neurotrophic factor, endothelin, and the endothelin receptor, but, in aggregate, these account for fewer than 30% of patients, suggesting that other defects are yet to be discovered. Because penetrance is incomplete, modifying genes or environmental factors must also be important. In addition, it is clear that sex-linked factors exist, since males are affected preferentially while disease tends to be more extensive in females.

Morphology. Diagnosis of Hirschsprung disease requires documenting the absence of ganglion cells within the affected segment. Because migration of neural crest cells in the Meissner and Auerbach plexi are linked, it is possible to establish the diagnosis preoperatively by examining suction biopsy specimens. In addition to their characteristic morphology in hematoxylin and eosin (H&E)-stained sections, ganglion cells can be identified using immunohistochemical stains for acetylcholinesterase.

The rectum is always affected, but the length of the additional involved segments varies widely. Most cases are limited to the rectum and sigmoid colon, but severe cases can involve the entire colon. The aganglionic region may have a grossly normal or contracted appearance, while the normally innervated proximal colon may undergo progressive dilation (Fig. 17–3). With time the proximal colon may

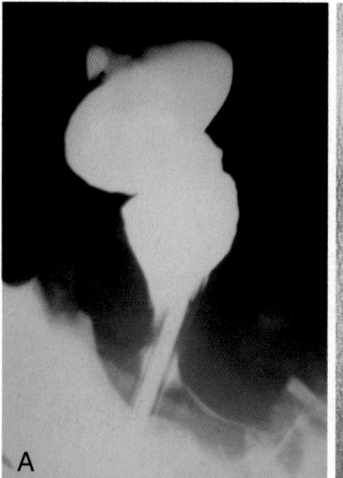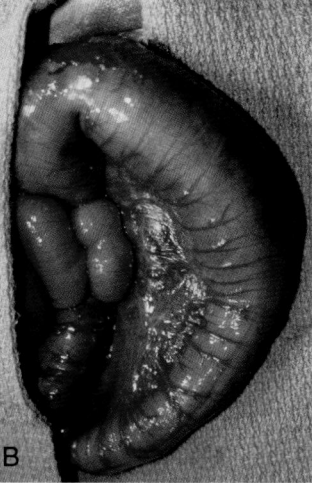

FIGURE 17–3 Hirschsprung disease. **A,** Preoperative barium enema study showing constricted rectum *(bottom of the image)* and dilated sigmoid colon. **B,** Corresponding intraoperative photograph showing constricted rectum and dilation of the sigmoid colon. (Courtesy of Dr. Aliya Husain, The University of Chicago, Chicago, IL.)

become massively distended **(megacolon)**, reaching diameters of as much as 20 cm. Dilation may stretch and thin the colonic wall to the point of rupture, which occurs most frequently near the cecum. Mucosal inflammation or shallow ulcers may also be present. These changes proximal to the diseased segment can make gross identification of the extent of aganglionosis difficult. Hence, intraoperative frozen-section analysis of transmural sections is commonly used to confirm the presence of ganglion cells at the anastamotic margin.

Clinical Features. Patients typically present neonatally, often with a failure to pass meconium in the immediate post-

natal period. Obstructive constipation follows, although in cases where only a few centimeters of the rectum are involved there may be occasional passage of stool. The major threats to life are enterocolitis, fluid and electrolyte disturbances, perforation, and peritonitis. The primary mode of treatment is surgical resection of the aganglionic segment and anastamosis of the normal colon to the rectum. Even after successful surgery, it may take years for patients to attain normal bowel function and continence.

In contrast to the congenital megacolon of Hirschsprung disease, *acquired megacolon* may occur at any age as a result of Chagas disease, obstruction by a neoplasm or inflammatory stricture, *toxic megacolon* complicating ulcerative colitis, visceral myopathy, or in association with functional psychosomatic disorders. Of these, only Chagas disease (discussed later) is associated with loss of ganglia.

ESOPHAGUS

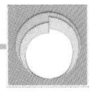

The esophagus develops from the cranial portion of the foregut and is recognizable by the third week of gestation. It is a hollow, highly distensible muscular tube that extends from the epiglottis in the pharynx to the gastroesophageal junction. Acquired diseases of the esophagus run the gamut from highly lethal cancers to the persistent "heartburn" that may be chronic and incapacitating or merely an occasional annoyance.

Esophageal Obstruction

For food and fluids to be delivered efficiently from the esophagus to the stomach, swallowing must be accompanied by a coordinated wave of peristaltic contractions. Esophageal dysmotility interferes with this process and can take several forms. High-amplitude esophageal contractions in which the outer longitudinal layer of smooth muscle contracts before the inner circular layer occur in some patients. Such lack of coordination results in a syndrome termed *nutcracker esophagus* that can cause periodic short-lived esophageal obstruction.[4] Other motor disorders of the esophagus include *diffuse esophageal spasm*, which can also result in functional obstruction. Because it increases esophageal wall stress, diffuse esophageal spasm can cause small *diverticulae* to form. These small mucosal outpouchings, which are more accurately described as pseudodiverticulae because they lack a true muscularis, are uncommon, probably because of the dense and continuous esophageal musculature. The *Zenker diverticulum (pharyngoesophageal diverticulum)* is located immediately above the upper esophageal sphincter; the *traction diverticulum* occurs near the midpoint of the esophagus; and the *epiphrenic diverticulum* is immediately above the lower esophageal sphincter. Zenker diverticulae may reach several centimeters in size and accumulate significant amounts of food, producing a mass and symptoms that include regurgitation.

Passage of food can also be impeded by esophageal *stenosis*, or narrowing of the lumen. This is generally caused by fibrous thickening of the submucosa and is associated with atrophy of the muscularis propria as well as secondary epithelial damage. Although occasionally congenital, *stenosis is most often due to inflammation and scarring that may be caused by chronic gastroesophageal reflux, irradiation, or caustic injury.* The dysphagia associated with stenosis is usually progressive, first affecting the ability to eat solids and only later interfering with ingestion of liquids. Because obstruction develops slowly, patients may subconsciously modify their diet to favor soft foods and liquids and be unaware of their condition until the obstruction is nearly complete.

Esophageal mucosal webs are uncommon ledge-like protrusions of mucosa that may cause obstruction. The pathogenesis is unknown, but webs are encountered most frequently in women over age 40. Webs are often associated with gastroesophageal reflux, chronic graft-versus-host disease, or blistering skin diseases. Upper esophageal webs accompanied by iron-deficiency anemia, glossitis, and cheilosis are part of the *Paterson-Brown-Kelly* or *Plummer-Vinson syndrome.* Esophageal webs are most common in the upper esophagus, where they are generally semicircumferential, eccentric lesions that protrude less than 5 mm and have a thickness of 2 to 4 mm. Microscopically, webs are composed of a fibrovascular connective tissue and overlying epithelium. The main symptom of webs is dysphagia associated with incompletely chewed food.

Esophageal rings, or *Schatzki rings,* are similar to webs, but are circumferential and thicker. Rings include mucosa, submucosa, and, in some cases, hypertrophic muscularis propria. When present in the distal esophagus, above the gastroesophageal junction, they are termed *A rings* and are covered by squamous mucosa; in contrast those located at the squamocolumnar junction of the lower esophagus are designated *B rings* and may have gastric cardia-type mucosa on their undersurface.

ACHALASIA

Increased tone of the *lower esophageal sphincter* (LES), as a result of impaired smooth muscle relaxation, is an important cause of esophageal obstruction. Release of nitric oxide and vasoactive intestinal polypeptide from inhibitory neurons, along with interruption of normal cholinergic signaling, allows the LES to relax during swallowing. *Achalasia is characterized by the triad of incomplete LES relaxation, increased LES tone, and aperistalsis of the esophagus.* Primary achalasia is caused by failure of distal esophageal inhibitory neurons and is, by definition, idiopathic.[5] Degenerative changes in neural innervation, either intrinsic to the esophagus or within the extraesophageal vagus nerve or the dorsal motor nucleus of the vagus, may also occur. Secondary achalasia may arise in Chagas disease, in which *Trypanosoma cruzi* infection causes destruction of the myenteric plexus, failure of peristalsis, and esophageal dilatation. Duodenal, colonic, and ureteric myenteric plexi can also be affected in Chagas disease. Achalasia-like disease may be caused by diabetic autonomic neuropathy; infiltrative disorders such as malignancy, amyloidosis, or sarcoidosis; and lesions of dorsal motor nuclei, particularly polio or surgical ablation. Treatment options for primary and secondary achalasia include laparoscopic myotomy and pneumatic balloon dilatation. Botulinum neurotoxin (Botox) injection, to inhibit LES cholinergic neurons, can also be effective.

Esophagitis

LACERATIONS

Longitudinal tears in the esophagus near the gastroesophageal junction are termed *Mallory-Weiss tears,* and are most often associated with severe retching or vomiting secondary to acute alcohol intoxication. Normally, a reflex relaxation of the gastroesophageal musculature precedes the antiperistaltic contractile wave associated with vomiting. It is speculated that this relaxation fails during prolonged vomiting, with the result that refluxing gastric contents overwhelm the gastric inlet and cause the esophageal wall to stretch and tear. The roughly *linear lacerations of Mallory-Weiss syndrome are longitudinally oriented and range in length from millimeters to several centimeters.* These tears usually cross the gastroesophageal junction but may also be located in the proximal gastric mucosa. Up to 10% of upper GI bleeding, which often presents as hematemesis (Table 17–1), is due to superficial esophageal lacerations such as those associated with Mallory-Weiss syndrome. These do not generally require surgical intervention, and healing tends to be rapid and complete. In contrast, *Boerhaave syndrome,* characterized by distal esophageal rupture and mediastinitis, occurs rarely and is a catastrophic event.

CHEMICAL AND INFECTIOUS ESOPHAGITIS

The stratified squamous mucosa of the esophagus may be damaged by a variety of irritants including alcohol, corrosive

TABLE 17–1   **Esophageal Causes of Hematemesis**
Lacerations (Mallory-Weiss syndrome)
Esophageal perforation (cancer or Boerhaave syndrome)
Varices (cirrhosis)
Esophageal-aortic fistula (usually with cancer)
Chemical and pill esophagitis
Infectious esophagitis (*Candida*, Herpes)
Benign strictures
Vasculitis (autoimmune, cytomegalovirus)
Reflux esophagitis (erosive)
Eosinophilic esophagitis
Esophageal ulcers (many etiologies)
Barrett esophagus
Adenocarcinoma
Squamous cell carcinoma
Hiatal hernia

acids or alkalis, excessively hot fluids, and heavy smoking. The esophageal mucosa may also be injured when medicinal pills lodge and dissolve in the esophagus rather than passing into the stomach intact, a condition termed *pill-induced esophagitis.* Esophagitis due to chemical injury generally only causes self-limited pain, particularly *dysphagia* (pain with swallowing). Hemorrhage, stricture, or perforation may occur in severe cases. Iatrogenic esophageal injury may be caused by cytotoxic *chemotherapy, radiation therapy,* or *graft-versus-host disease.*

Infections may occur in otherwise healthy individuals but are most frequent in those who are debilitated or immunosuppressed as a result of disease or therapy. In these patients, esophageal infection by *Herpes simplex viruses, cytomegalovirus (CMV), or fungal organisms* is common. Among fungi, *candidiasis* is most common, although *mucormycosis* and *aspergillosis* may occur. The esophagus may also be involved by the desquamative skin diseases *bullous pemphigoid* and *epidermolysis bullosa* and, rarely, *Crohn disease.*

> **Morphology.** The morphology of **chemical and infectious esophagitis** varies with etiology. Dense infiltrates of neutrophils are present in most cases but may be absent following injury induced by chemicals (lye, acids, or detergent), which may result in outright necrosis of the esophageal wall. Pill-induced esophagitis frequently occurs at the site of strictures that impede passage of luminal contents. When present, ulceration is accompanied by superficial necrosis with granulation tissue and eventual fibrosis.
>
> Esophageal irradiation causes damage similar to that seen in other tissues and includes intimal proliferation and luminal narrowing of submucosal and mural blood vessels. The mucosal damage is, in part, often secondary to radiation-induced vascular injury as discussed in Chapter 9.
>
> Infection by fungi or bacteria can either cause damage or complicate a preexisting ulcer. Nonpathogenic oral bacteria are frequently found in ulcer beds, while pathogenic organisms, which account for about 10% of infectious esophagitis, may invade the lamina

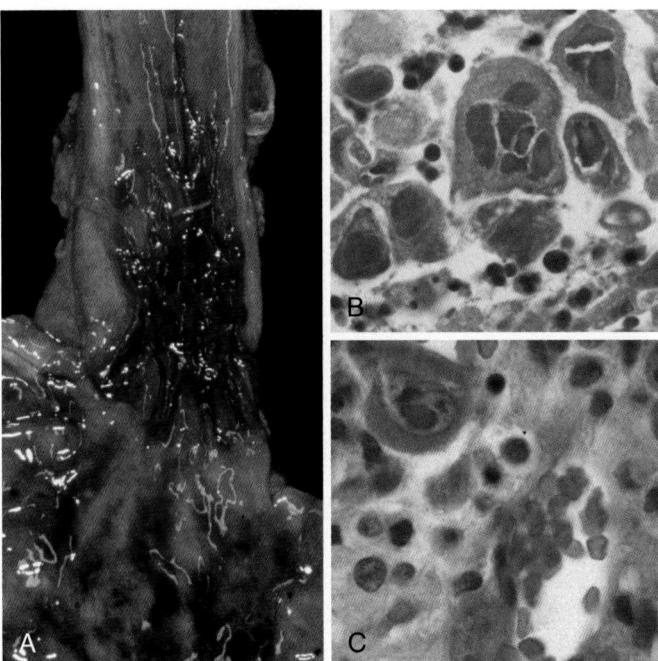

FIGURE 17–4 Viral esophagitis. **A,** Postmortem specimen with multiple herpetic ulcers in the distal esophagus. **B,** Multinucleate squamous cells containing Herpesvirus nuclear inclusions. **C,** Cytomegalovirus-infected endothelial cells with nuclear and cytoplasmic inclusions.

propria and cause necrosis of overlying mucosa. Candidiasis, in its most advanced form, is characterized by adherent, gray-white **pseudomembranes** composed of densely matted fungal hyphae and inflammatory cells covering the esophageal mucosa.

The endoscopic appearance often provides a clue as to the infectious agent in viral esophagitis. Herpesviruses typically cause punched-out ulcers (Fig. 17–4A). Biopsy specimens demonstrate nuclear viral inclusions within a rim of degenerating epithelial cells at the margin of the ulcer (Fig. 17–4B). In contrast, CMV causes shallower ulcerations and characteristic nuclear and cytoplasmic inclusions within capillary endothelium and stromal cells (Fig. 17–4C). Although the histologic appearance is characteristic, immunohistochemical stains for virus-specific antigens are a sensitive and specific ancillary diagnostic tool.

Histologic features of esophageal **graft-versus-host disease** are similar to those in the skin and include basal epithelial cell apoptosis, mucosal atrophy, and submucosal fibrosis without significant acute inflammatory infiltrates. The microscopic appearances of esophageal involvement in bullous pemphigoid, epidermolysis bullosa, and Crohn disease are also similar to those in the skin (Chapter 25).

REFLUX ESOPHAGITIS

The stratified squamous epithelium of the esophagus is resistant to abrasion from foods but is sensitive to acid. Submuco-

sal glands, which are most abundant in the proximal and distal esophagus, contribute to mucosal protection by secreting mucin and bicarbonate. More importantly, constant lower esophageal sphincter tone prevents reflux of acidic gastric contents, which are under positive pressure and would otherwise enter the esophagus. Reflux of gastric contents into the lower esophagus is the most frequent cause of esophagitis and the most common outpatient GI diagnosis in the United States.[6] The associated clinical condition is termed *gastroesophageal reflux disease (GERD)*.

Pathogenesis. Reflux of gastric juices is central to the development of mucosal injury in GERD. In severe cases, reflux of bile from the duodenum may exacerbate the damage. Conditions that decrease lower esophageal sphincter tone or increase abdominal pressure contribute to GERD and include alcohol and tobacco use, obesity, central nervous system depressants, pregnancy, hiatal hernia (discussed below), delayed gastric emptying, and increased gastric volume. In many cases, no definitive cause is identified.

> **Morphology.** Simple **hyperemia**, evident to the endoscopist as redness, may be the only alteration. In mild GERD the mucosal histology is often unremarkable. With more significant disease, **eosinophils** are recruited into the squamous mucosa followed by neutrophils, which are usually associated with more severe injury (Fig. 17–5A). **Basal zone hyperplasia** exceeding 20% of the total epithelial thickness and elongation of lamina propria papillae, such that they extend into the upper third of the epithelium, may also be present.

Clinical Features. GERD is most common in adults over age 40 but also occurs in infants and children. The most common clinical symptoms are dysphagia, heartburn, and, less frequently, noticeable regurgitation of sour-tasting gastric contents. Rarely, chronic GERD is punctuated by attacks of

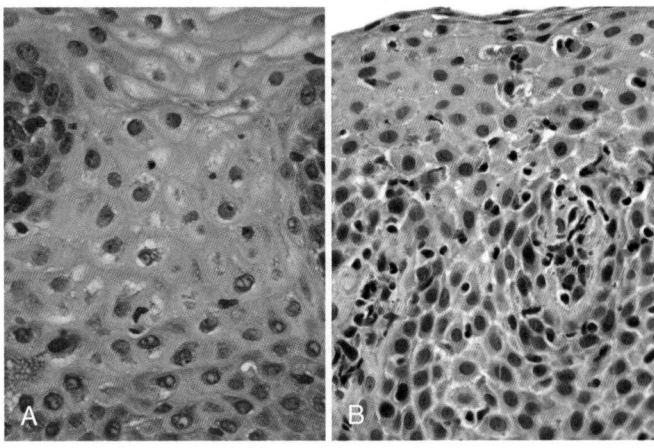

FIGURE 17–5 Esophagitis. **A,** Reflux esophagitis with scattered intraepithelial eosinophils. Although mild basal zone expansion can be appreciated, squamous cell maturation is relatively normal. **B,** Eosinophilic esophagitis is characterized by numerous intraepithelial eosinophils. Abnormal squamous maturation is also apparent.

severe chest pain that may be mistaken for heart disease. Treatment with proton pump inhibitors or H$_2$ histamine receptor antagonists, which reduce gastric acidity, typically provides symptomatic relief. While the severity of symptoms is not closely related to the degree of histologic damage, the latter tends to increase with disease duration. Complications of reflux esophagitis include esophageal ulceration, hematemesis, melena, stricture development, and Barrett esophagus.

Hiatal hernia is characterized by separation of the diaphragmatic crura and protrusion of the stomach into the thorax through the resulting gap. Congenital hiatal hernias are recognized in infants and children, but many are acquired in later life. Hiatal hernia is symptomatic in fewer than 10% of adults, and these cases are generally associated with other causes of LES incompetence. Symptoms, including heartburn and regurgitation of gastric juices, are similar to GERD.

EOSINOPHILIC ESOPHAGITIS

The incidence of eosinophilic esophagitis is increasing markedly.[7] Symptoms include food impaction and dysphagia in adults and feeding intolerance or GERD-like symptoms in children. The cardinal histologic feature is large numbers of intraepithelial eosinophils, particularly superficially (Fig. 17–5B). Their abundance can help to differentiate eosinophilic esophagitis from GERD, Crohn disease, and other causes of esophagitis. Clinical characteristics, particularly failure of high-dose proton pump inhibitor treatment and the absence of acid reflux, are also necessary for diagnosis. The majority of individuals with eosinophilic esophagitis are atopic and many have atopic dermatitis, allergic rhinitis, asthma, or modest peripheral eosinophilia. Treatments include dietary restrictions to prevent exposure to food allergens, such as cow's milk and soy products, and topical or systemic corticosteroids.

Barrett Esophagus

Barrett esophagus is a complication of chronic GERD that is characterized by *intestinal metaplasia within the esophageal squamous mucosa.* The incidence of Barrett esophagus is rising, and it is estimated to occur in as many as 10% of individuals with symptomatic GERD. Barrett esophagus is most common in white males and it typically presents between 40 and 60 years of age. The greatest concern in Barrett esophagus is that *it confers an increased risk of esophageal adenocarcinoma.* Molecular studies suggest that Barrett epithelium may be more similar to adenocarcinoma than to normal esophageal epithelium, consistent with the view that Barrett esophagus is a pre-malignant condition. In keeping with this, epithelial *dysplasia,* considered to be a pre-invasive lesion, is detected in 0.2% to 2.0% of persons with Barrett esophagus each year and is associated with prolonged symptoms and increased patient age. Although the vast majority of esophageal adenocarcinomas are associated with Barrett esophagus, it is important to remember that most individuals with Barrett esophagus do not develop esophageal tumors.

Morphology. Barrett esophagus can be recognized as one or several tongues or patches of red, velvety

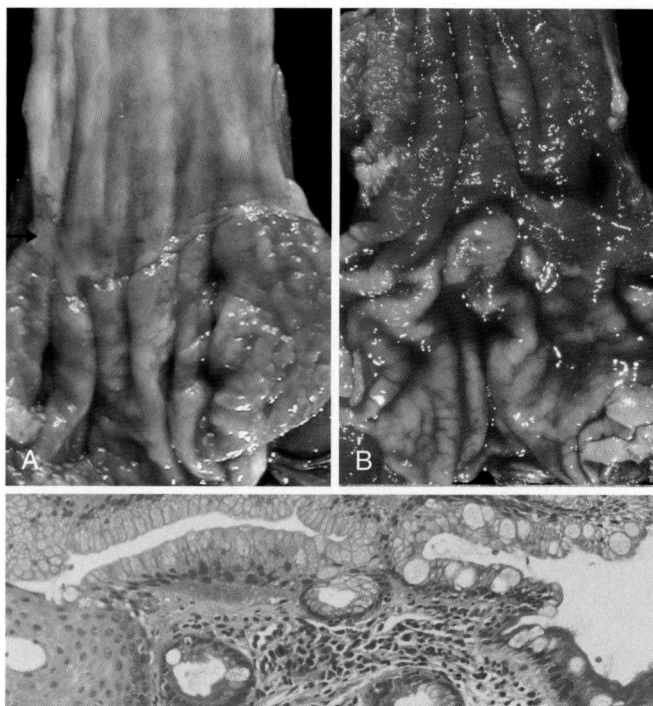

FIGURE 17–6   Barrett esophagus. **A,** Normal gastroesophageal junction. **B,** Barrett esophagus. Note the small islands of paler squamous mucosa within the Barrett mucosa. **C,** Histologic appearance of the gastroesophageal junction in Barrett esophagus. Note the transition between esophageal squamous mucosa *(left)* and Barrett metaplasia, with abundant metaplastic goblet cells *(right).*

mucosa extending upward from the gastroesophageal junction. This metaplastic mucosa alternates with residual smooth, pale squamous (esophageal) mucosa and interfaces with light-brown columnar (gastric) mucosa distally (Fig. 17–6A, B). High-resolution endoscopes have increased the sensitivity of Barrett esophagus detection. This has led to subclassification of Barrett esophagus as long segment, in which 3 cm or more of esophagus is involved, or short segment, in which less than 3 cm is involved. It is not yet clear if the risk of dysplasia in short segment disease is less than in long segment Barrett esophagus.

Diagnosis of Barrett esophagus requires both endoscopic evidence of abnormal mucosa above the gastroesophageal junction and histologically documented intestinal metaplasia. **Goblet cells**, which have distinct mucous vacuoles that stain pale blue by H&E and impart the shape of a wine goblet to the remaining cytoplasm, define **intestinal metaplasia** and are necessary for diagnosis of Barrett esophagus (Fig. 17–6C). The requirement for intestinal metaplasia reflects the fact that this feature correlates with neoplastic risk. Foveolar mucus cells, which do not have distinct mucous vacuoles are insufficient for diagnosis. The requirement for an endoscopic abnormality helps to prevent misdiagnosis if metaplastic

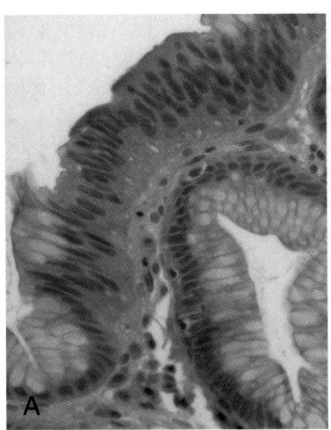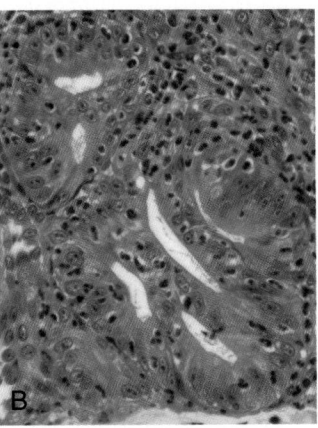

FIGURE 17–7 Dysplasia in Barrett esophagus. **A,** Abrupt transition from Barrett metaplasia to low-grade dysplasia. Note the nuclear stratification and hyperchromasia. **B,** Architectural irregularities, including gland-within-gland, or cribriform, profiles in high-grade dysplasia.

goblet cells within the cardia are included in the biopsy.

When **dysplasia** is present, it is classified as low grade or high grade. Increased epithelial proliferation, often with atypical mitoses, nuclear hyperchromasia and stratification, irregularly clumped chromatin, increased nuclear-to-cytoplasmic ratio, and a failure of epithelial cells to mature as they migrate to the esophageal surface are present in both grades of dysplasia (Fig. 17–7A). Gland architecture is frequently abnormal and is characterized by budding, irregular shapes, and cellular crowding (Fig. 17–7B). High-grade dysplasia exhibits more severe cytologic and architectural changes. Intramucosal carcinoma is characterized by invasion of neoplastic epithelial cells into the lamina propria.

Clinical Features. Barrett esophagus can only be identified thorough endoscopy and biopsy, which are usually prompted by GERD symptoms. Once diagnosed, the best course of management in Barrett esophagus is a matter of debate. However, most agree that periodic endoscopy with biopsy, for detection of dysplasia, has an important role. Nevertheless, uncertainties about the potential of dysplasia to regress, either spontaneously or in response to therapy, complicate clinical decisions when dysplasia is identified. In contrast, intramucosal carcinoma requires therapeutic intervention. Treatment options include surgical resection, or *esophagectomy*, as well as newer modalities such as photodynamic therapy, laser ablation, and endoscopic mucosectomy. Multifocal high-grade dysplasia, which carries a significant risk of progression to intramucosal or invasive carcinoma, is treated similarly to intramucosal carcinoma. Many physicians follow low-grade dysplasia or a single focus of high-grade dysplasia with endoscopy and biopsy at frequent intervals. However, management of esophageal dysplasia is evolving, and it is hoped that improved molecular understanding of neoplastic progression may allow development of chemopreventive approaches that reduce incidence of esophageal adenocarcinoma.[8]

ESOPHAGEAL VARICES

Instead of returning directly to the heart, venous blood from the GI tract is delivered to the liver via the portal vein before reaching the inferior vena cava. This circulatory pattern is responsible for the *first-pass effect* in which drugs and other materials absorbed in the intestines are processed by the liver before entering the systemic circulation. Diseases that impede this flow cause portal hypertension and can lead to the development of esophageal varices, an important cause of esophageal bleeding.

Pathogenesis. Portal hypertension results in the development of collateral channels at sites where the portal and caval systems communicate. Although these collateral veins allow some drainage to occur, they lead to development of a congested subepithelial and submucosal venous plexus within the distal esophagus. These vessels, termed *varices*, develop in 90% of cirrhotic patients, most commonly in association with alcoholic liver disease. Worldwide, hepatic schistosomiasis is the second most common cause of varices. A more detailed consideration of portal hypertension is given in Chapter 18.

Morphology. Varices can be detected by venogram (Fig. 17–8A) and appear as tortuous dilated veins lying primarily within the submucosa of the distal esophagus and proximal stomach. Venous channels directly beneath the esophageal epithelium may also become massively dilated. Varices may not be grossly obvious in surgical or postmortem specimens, because they collapse in the absence of blood flow (Fig. 17–8B) and, when they are not ruptured, the overlying mucosa is intact (Fig. 17–8C). Variceal rupture results in hemorrhage into the lumen or esophageal wall, in which case the overlying mucosa appears ulcerated and necrotic. If rupture has occurred in the past, venous thrombosis, inflammation, and evidence of prior therapy may also be present.

Clinical Features. While varices are often asymptomatic, they may rupture, causing massive hematemesis. The factors that lead to rupture are not well defined, but inflammatory erosion of thinned overlying mucosa, increased tension in progressively dilated veins, and increased vascular hydrostatic pressure associated with vomiting are likely to contribute. In any case, hemorrhage due to variceal rupture is a medical emergency that is treated by any of several methods: sclerotherapy by endoscopic injection of thrombotic agents; endoscopic balloon tamponade; or endoscopic rubber band ligation. Despite these interventions, as many as half of patients die from the first bleeding episode either as a direct consequence of hemorrhage or following hepatic coma triggered by hypovolemic shock. Among those who survive, additional instances of hemorrhage occur in over 50% within 1 year. Each episode has a similar rate of mortality. Thus, over half of deaths among individuals with advanced cirrhosis result from variceal rupture. It must be remembered, however, that even when varices are present, they are only one of several causes of hematemesis.

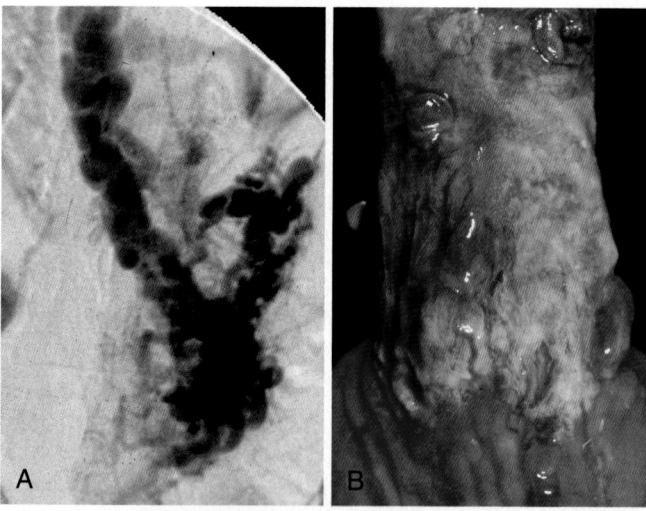

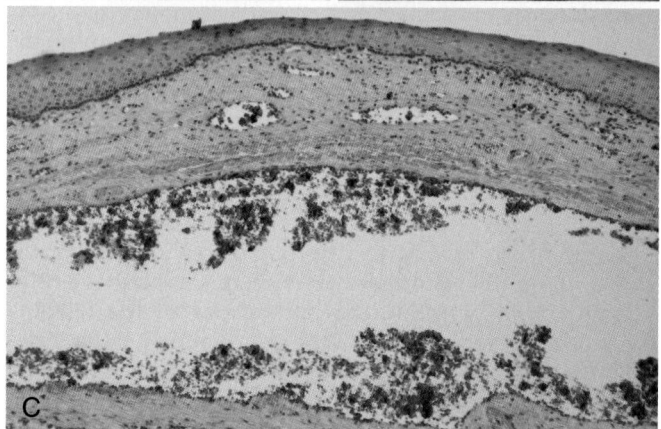

FIGURE 17–8 Esophageal varices. **A,** This angiogram shows several tortuous esophageal varices. **B,** Collapsed varices are present in this postmortem specimen corresponding to the angiogram in **A**. The polypoid areas represent previous sites of variceal hemorrhage that have been ligated with bands. **C,** Dilated varice beneath intact squamous mucosa.

Esophageal Tumors

Two morphologic variants comprise the majority of esophageal cancers: adenocarcinoma and squamous cell carcinoma. Worldwide, squamous cell carcinoma is more common, but in the United States and other Western countries adenocarcinoma is on the rise. The potential reasons for these increases are discussed below.

ADENOCARCINOMA

Adenocarcinoma of the esophagus typically arises in a background of Barrett esophagus and long-standing GERD. Risk of adenocarcinoma is greater in those with documented dysplasia and is further increased by tobacco use, obesity, and prior radiation therapy.[9] Conversely, risk of adenocarcinoma is reduced by diets rich in fresh fruits and vegetables. Some *Helicobacter pylori* serotypes are associated with a decreased risk of adenocarcinoma, perhaps by causing gastric atrophy and reducing acid reflux.

Esophageal adenocarcinoma occurs most frequently in Caucasians and shows a strong gender bias, being sevenfold more common in men. However, the incidence varies 60-fold worldwide, with rates being highest in certain developed Western countries, including the United States, the United Kingdom, Canada, Australia, the Netherlands, and Brazil and lowest in Korea, Thailand, Japan, and Ecuador. In countries where esophageal adenocarcinoma is more common, the incidence has increased markedly since 1970, more rapidly than almost any other cancer. As a result, esophageal adenocarcinoma, which represented less than 5% of esophageal cancers before 1970, now accounts for half of all esophageal cancers in the United States.

Pathogenesis. Molecular studies suggest that the progression of Barrett esophagus to adenocarcinoma occurs over an extended period through the stepwise acquisition of genetic and epigenetic changes. This model is supported by the observation that epithelial clones identified in nondysplastic Barrett metaplasia persist and accumulate mutations during progression to dysplasia and invasive carcinoma. Chromosomal abnormalities and mutation or overexpression of p53 are present at early stages of esophageal adenocarcinoma. Additional genetic changes include amplification of *c-ERB-B2*, *cyclin D1*, and *cyclin E* genes; mutation of the retinoblastoma tumor suppressor gene; and allelic loss of the cyclin-dependent kinase inhibitor *p16/INK4a*. In other instances *p16/INK4a* is epigenetically silenced by hypermethylation. Increased epithelial expression of tumor necrosis factor (TNF)- and nuclear factor (NF)-κB–dependent genes suggests that inflammation may also contribute to neoplastic progression.

Morphology. Esophageal adenocarcinoma usually occurs in the distal third of the esophagus and may invade the adjacent gastric cardia (Fig. 17–9A). Initially appearing as flat or raised patches in otherwise intact mucosa, large masses of 5 cm or more in diameter may develop. Alternatively, tumors may infiltrate diffusely or ulcerate and invade deeply. Microscopically, Barrett esophagus is frequently present adjacent to the tumor. Tumors most commonly produce mucin and form glands (Fig. 17–10A), often with intestinal-type morphology; less frequently tumors are composed of diffusely infiltrative signet-ring cells (similar to those seen in diffuse gastric cancers) or, in rare cases, small poorly differentiated cells (similar to small-cell carcinoma of the lung).

Clinical Features. Although esophageal adenocarcinomas are occasionally discovered in evaluation of GERD or surveillance of Barrett esophagus, they more commonly present with pain or difficulty in swallowing, progressive weight loss, hematemesis, chest pain, or vomiting. By the time symptoms appear, the tumor has usually spread to submucosal lymphatic vessels. As a result of the advanced stage at diagnosis, overall 5-year survival is less than 25%. In contrast, 5-year survival approximates 80% in the few patients with adenocarcinoma limited to the mucosa or submucosa.

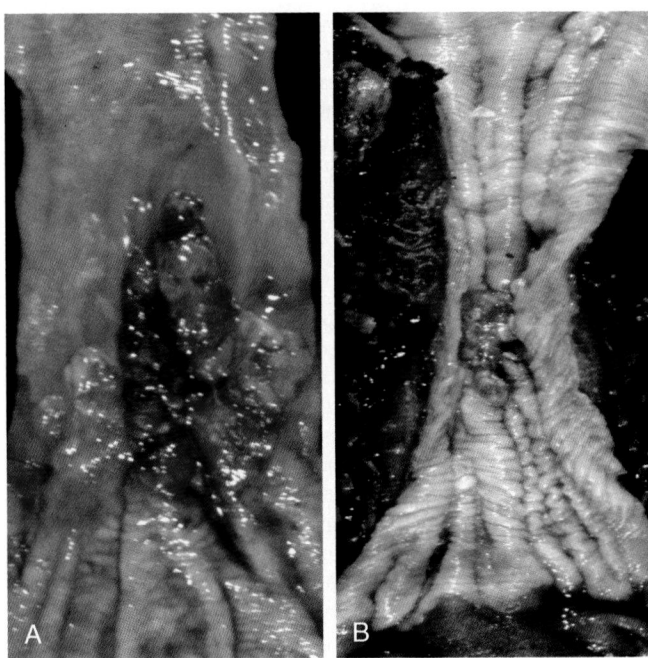

FIGURE 17–9 Esophageal cancer. **A,** Adenocarcinoma usually occurs distally and, as in this case, often involves the gastric cardia. **B,** Squamous cell carcinoma is most frequently found in the mid-esophagus, where it commonly causes strictures.

SQUAMOUS CELL CARCINOMA

In the United States, esophageal squamous cell carcinoma occurs in adults over age 45 and affects males four times more frequently than females.[10] Risk factors include alcohol and tobacco use, poverty, caustic esophageal injury, achalasia, tylosis, Plummer-Vinson syndrome, and frequent consumption of very hot beverages.[9] It is nearly sixfold more common in African-Americans than Caucasians, a striking risk disparity that reflects differences in rates of alcohol and tobacco use as well as other poorly understood factors.[11] Previous radiation therapy to the mediastinum also predisposes individuals to esophageal carcinoma, typically 10 or more years after exposure.[9]

Esophageal squamous cell carcinoma incidence varies up to 180-fold between and within countries, being more common in rural and underdeveloped areas. The regions with highest incidences are Iran, central China, Hong Kong, Brazil, and South Africa.

Pathogenesis. The majority of esophageal squamous cell carcinomas in Europe and the United States are at least partially attributable to the use of alcohol and tobacco, which synergize to increase risk. However, esophageal squamous cell carcinoma is also common in some regions where alcohol and tobacco use is uncommon. Thus, nutritional deficiencies, as well as polycyclic hydrocarbons, nitrosamines, and other mutagenic compounds, such as those found in fungus-contaminated foods, must be considered. Human papillomavirus (HPV) infection has also been implicated in esophageal squamous cell carcinoma in high-risk areas but not in low-risk regions.[12] The molecular pathogenesis of esophageal squamous cell carcinoma remains incompletely defined, but loss

of several tumor suppressor genes, including *p53* and *p16/INK4a*, is involved.

Morphology. In contrast to adenocarcinoma, half of squamous cell carcinomas occur in the middle third of the esophagus (see Fig. 17–9B). Squamous cell carcinoma begins as an in situ lesion termed **squamous dysplasia** (this lesion is referred to as intraepithelial neoplasia or carcinoma in situ at other sites). Early lesions appear as small, gray-white, plaque-like thickenings. Over months to years they grow into tumor masses that may be polypoid or exophytic and protrude into and obstruct the lumen. Other tumors are either ulcerated or diffusely infiltrative lesions that spread within the esophageal wall and cause thickening, rigidity, and luminal narrowing. These may invade surrounding structures including the respiratory tree, causing pneumonia; the aorta, causing catastrophic exsanguination; or the mediastinum and pericardium.

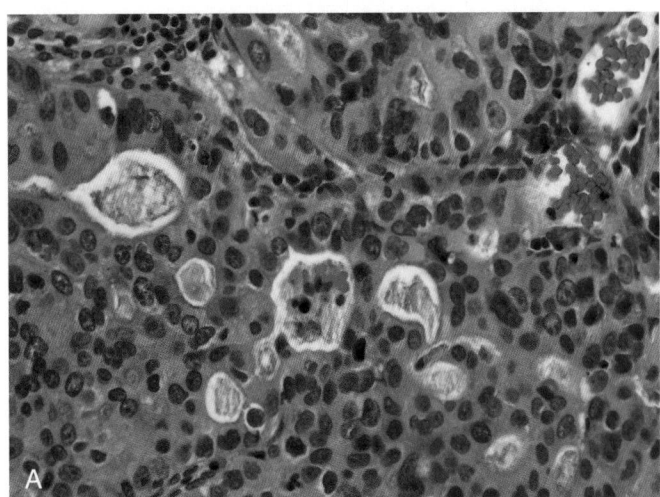

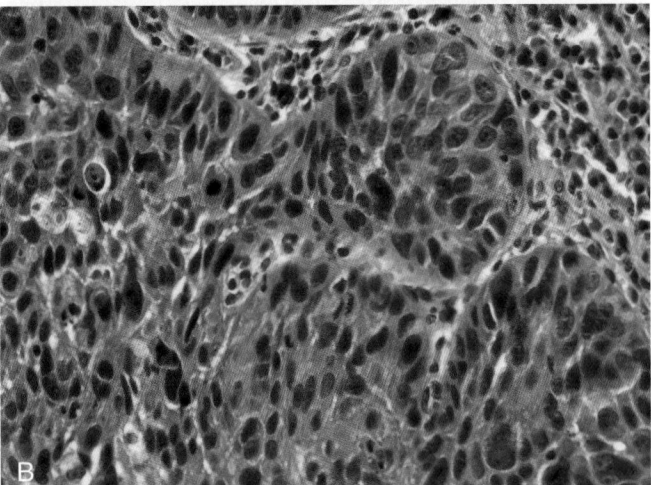

FIGURE 17–10 Esophageal cancer. **A,** Esophageal adenocarcinoma organized into back-to-back glands. **B,** Squamous cell carcinoma composed of nests of malignant cells that partially recapitulate the organization of squamous epithelium.

Most squamous cell carcinomas are moderately to well-differentiated (see Fig. 17–10B). Less common histologic variants include verrucous squamous cell carcinoma, spindle cell carcinoma, and basaloid squamous cell carcinoma. Regardless of histology, symptomatic tumors are generally very large at diagnosis and have already invaded the esophageal wall. The rich submucosal lymphatic network promotes circumferential and longitudinal spread, and intramural tumor nodules may be present several centimeters away from the principal mass. The sites of lymph node metastases vary with tumor location: cancers in the upper third of the esophagus favor cervical lymph nodes; those in the middle third favor mediastinal, paratracheal, and tracheobronchial nodes; and those in the lower third spread to gastric and celiac nodes.

Clinical Features. The onset of esophageal squamous cell carcinoma is insidious and ultimately produces dysphagia, odynophagia (pain on swallowing), and obstruction. Patients subconsciously adjust to the progressively increasing obstruction by altering their diet from solid to liquid foods. Extreme weight loss and debilitation result from both impaired nutrition and effects of the tumor itself. Hemorrhage and sepsis may accompany tumor ulceration. Occasionally, the first symptoms are caused by aspiration of food via a tracheoesophageal fistula.

Increased prevalence of endoscopic screening has led to earlier detection of esophageal squamous cell carcinoma. This is critical, because 5-year survival rates are 75% in individuals with superficial esophageal carcinoma but much lower in patients with more advanced tumors. Lymph node metastases, which are common, are associated with poor prognosis. The overall 5-year survival remains a dismal 9%.

UNCOMMON ESOPHAGEAL TUMORS

Other malignancies of the esophagus include unusual forms of adenocarcinoma, undifferentiated carcinoma, carcinoid tumor, melanoma, lymphoma, and sarcoma.

Benign tumors of the esophagus are generally mesenchymal in origin and arise within the esophageal wall. Tumors of smooth muscle origin, *leiomyomas*, are most common; fibromas, lipomas, hemangiomas, neurofibromas, and lymphangiomas also occur. Some benign tumors take the form of mucosal polyps. These are usually composed of fibrous and vascular tissue, or adipose tissue, and are known as *fibrovascular polyps* or *pedunculated lipomas*, respectively. *Squamous papillomas* are sessile lesions with a central core of connective tissue and a hyperplastic papilliform squamous mucosa. Uncommonly, papillomas are associated with HPV infection, in which case the term *condyloma* applies. In rare instances a mass of inflamed granulation tissue, growing either as an *inflammatory polyp* or an infiltrative mass in the wall of the esophagus, may resemble a malignant lesion. These benign lesions are called *inflammatory pseudotumors*.

STOMACH

Disorders of the stomach are a frequent cause of clinical disease, with inflammatory and neoplastic lesions being particularly common. In the United States, diseases related to gastric acid account for nearly one third of all health care spending on GI disease. In addition, despite a decreasing incidence in certain locales such as the United States, gastric cancer remains a leading cause of death worldwide.

The stomach is divided into four major anatomic regions: the cardia, fundus, body, and antrum. The cardia and antrum are lined mainly by mucin-secreting foveolar cells that form small glands. The antral glands are similar but also contain endocrine cells, such as G cells, that release gastrin to stimulate luminal acid secretion by parietal cells within the gastric fundus and body. The well-developed glands of the body and fundus also contain chief cells that produce and secrete digestive enzymes such as pepsin.

Acute Gastritis

Acute gastritis is a transient mucosal inflammatory process that may be asymptomatic or cause variable degrees of epigastric pain, nausea, and vomiting. In more severe cases there

may be mucosal erosion, ulceration, hemorrhage, hematemesis, melena, or, rarely, massive blood loss.

Pathogenesis. The gastric lumen is strongly acidic with pH close to 1, more than a million times more acidic than the blood. This harsh environment contributes to digestion but also has the potential to damage the gastric mucosa. Multiple mechanisms have evolved to protect the gastric mucosa (Fig. 17–11). Mucin secreted by surface *foveolar cells* forms a thin layer of mucus that prevents large food particles from directly touching the epithelium. The mucus layer also promotes formation of an "unstirred" layer of fluid over the epithelium that protects the mucosa and has a neutral pH as a result of bicarbonate ion secretion by surface epithelial cells. Finally, the rich vascular supply to the gastric mucosa delivers oxygen, bicarbonate, and nutrients while washing away acid that has back-diffused into the lamina propria. Acute or chronic gastritis can occur following disruption of any of these protective mechanisms. For example, reduced mucin synthesis in the elderly has been suggested as one factor that may explain their increased susceptibility to gastritis. Nonsteroidal anti-inflammatory drugs (NSAIDs) may interfere with cytoprotection normally provided by prostaglandins or reduce bicarbonate secretion, either of which increases the susceptibility of the

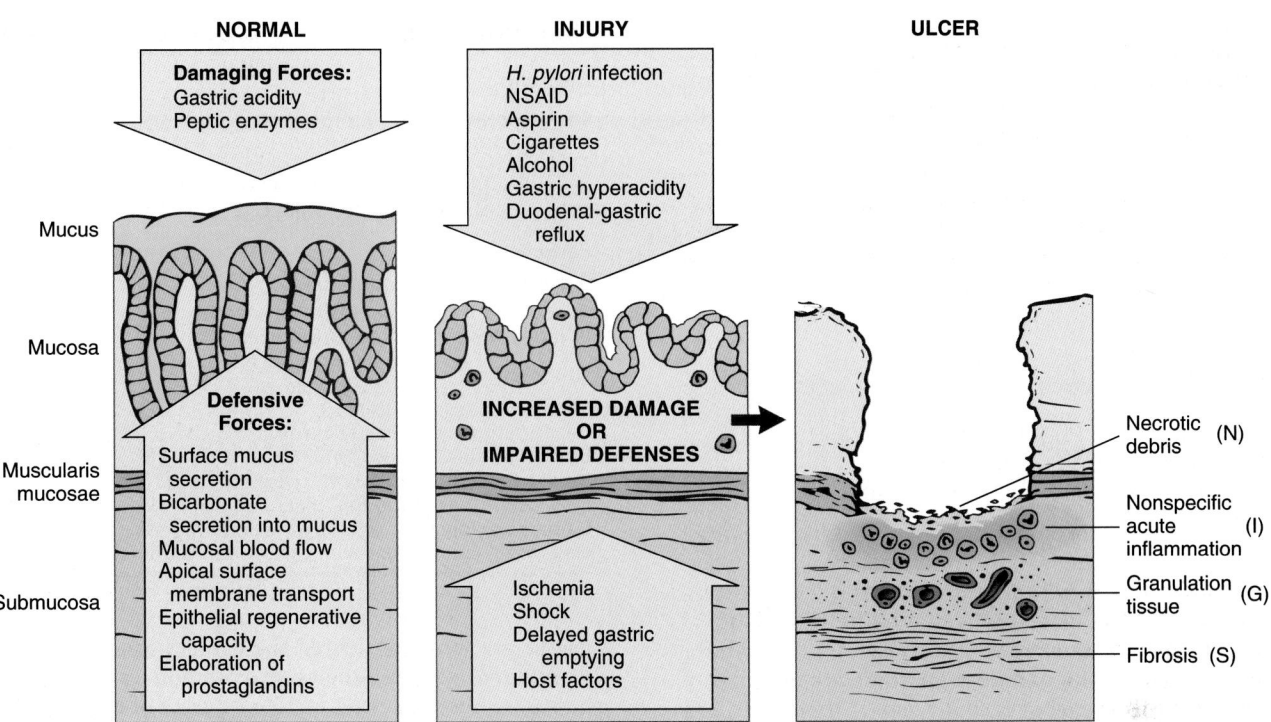

NORMAL

Damaging Forces:
Gastric acidity
Peptic enzymes

INJURY

H. pylori infection
NSAID
Aspirin
Cigarettes
Alcohol
Gastric hyperacidity
Duodenal-gastric
reflux

ULCER

Mucus

Mucosa

**Defensive
Forces:**

**INCREASED DAMAGE
OR
IMPAIRED DEFENSES**

Muscularis
mucosae

Surface mucus
secretion
Bicarbonate
secretion into mucus
Mucosal blood flow
Apical surface
membrane transport
Epithelial regenerative
capacity
Elaboration of
prostaglandins

Submucosa

Ischemia
Shock
Delayed gastric
emptying
Host factors

Necrotic (N)
debris

Nonspecific
acute (I)
inflammation

Granulation (G)
tissue

Fibrosis (S)

FIGURE 17–11   Mechanisms of gastric injury and protection. This diagram illustrates the progression from more mild forms of injury to ulceration that may occur with acute or chronic gastritis. Ulcers include layers of necrosis (N), inflammation (I), and granulation tissue (G), but a fibrotic scar (S), which takes time to develop, is only present in chronic lesions.

gastric mucosa to injury. Similarly, the gastric injury that occurs in uremic patients and those infected with urease-secreting *H. pylori* may be due to inhibition of gastric bicarbonate transporters by ammonium ions. Ingestion of harsh chemicals, particularly acids or bases, either accidentally or as a suicide attempt, also results in severe gastric injury, predominantly as a result of direct injury to mucosal epithelial and stromal cells. Direct cellular injury is also implicated in gastritis due to excessive alcohol consumption, NSAIDs, radiation therapy, and chemotherapy. Since the entire gastric mucosal surface is replaced every 2 to 6 days, mitotic inhibitors, including those used in cancer chemotherapy, cause generalized mucosal damage due to insufficient epithelial regeneration. Finally, decreased oxygen delivery may explain increased incidence of acute gastritis at high altitudes.

Morphology. Histologically, mild acute gastritis may be difficult to recognize, since the lamina propria shows only moderate edema and slight vascular congestion. The **surface epithelium is intact**, although scattered neutrophils may be present among the epithelial cells or within mucosal glands. In contrast, an abundance of lymphocytes or plasma cells suggests chronic disease. The presence of neutrophils above the basement membrane in direct contact with epithelial cells is abnormal in all parts of the GI tract and signifies **active inflammation**. This term is preferred over acute inflammation, since active inflammation may be present in both acute and chronic disease states. With more severe mucosal damage, erosions and hemorrhage develop. An **erosion**

denotes loss of the superficial epithelium, generating a defect in the mucosa that is limited to the lamina propria. It is accompanied by a pronounced neutrophilic infiltrate within the mucosa and a fibrin-containing purulent exudate in the lumen. Hemorrhage may occur and cause dark punctae in an otherwise hyperemic mucosa. Concurrent erosion and hemorrhage is termed **acute erosive hemorrhagic gastritis**. Large areas of the gastric surface may be denuded, although the involvement is typically superficial. When erosions extend deeply, they may progress to ulcers, as described below.

ACUTE GASTRIC ULCERATION

Focal, acutely developing gastric mucosal defects are a well-known complication of therapy with NSAIDs. They may also appear after severe physiologic stress. Some of these are given specific names, based on location and clinical associations. For example:

- *Stress ulcers* are most common in individuals with shock, sepsis, or severe trauma.
- Ulcers occurring in the proximal duodenum and associated with severe burns or trauma are called *Curling ulcers.*
- Gastric, duodenal, and esophageal ulcers arising in persons with intracranial disease are termed *Cushing ulcers* and carry a high incidence of perforation.

Pathogenesis. The pathogenesis of acute ulceration is complex and incompletely understood. NSAID-induced ulcers are related to cyclooxygenase inhibition. This prevents synthesis of prostaglandins, which enhance bicarbonate secretion, inhibit acid secretion, promote mucin synthesis, and increase vascular perfusion. Lesions associated with intracranial injury are thought to be caused by direct stimulation of vagal nuclei, which causes hypersecretion of gastric acid. Systemic acidosis, a frequent finding in these settings, may also contribute to mucosal injury by lowering the intracellular pH of mucosal cells. Hypoxia and reduced blood flow caused by stress-induced splanchnic vasoconstriction also contribute to the pathogenesis of acute ulcers.

> **Morphology.** Lesions described as acute gastric ulcers range in depth from shallow erosions caused by superficial epithelial damage to deeper lesions that penetrate the depth of the mucosa. Acute ulcers are rounded and less than 1 cm in diameter. The ulcer base is frequently stained brown to black by acid digestion of extravasated blood and may be associated with transmural inflammation and local serositis. Unlike peptic ulcers, which arise in the setting of chronic injury, acute stress ulcers are found anywhere in the stomach. The gastric rugal folds are essentially normal, and the margins and base of the ulcers are not indurated. While they may occur singly, more often there are multiple ulcers throughout the stomach and duodenum. Microscopically, acute stress ulcers are sharply demarcated, with essentially normal adjacent mucosa. Depending on the duration of the ulceration, there may be a suffusion of blood into the mucosa and submucosa and some inflammatory reaction. Conspicuously absent are the scarring and thickening of blood vessels that characterize chronic peptic ulcers. Healing with complete re-epithelialization occurs after the injurious factors are removed. The time required for healing varies from days to several weeks.

Clinical Features. Most critically ill patients admitted to hospital intensive care units have histologic evidence of gastric mucosal damage. Bleeding from superficial gastric erosions or ulcers that may require transfusion develops in 1% to 4% of these patients. Other complications, including perforation, can also occur (Table 17–2). Prophylactic H_2 histamine receptor antagonists or proton pump inhibitors may blunt the impact of stress ulceration, but the most important determinant of clinical outcome is the ability to correct the underlying conditions. The gastric mucosa can recover completely if the patient does not succumb to their primary disease.

Chronic Gastritis

In contrast to acute gastritis, the symptoms associated with chronic gastritis are typically less severe but more persistent. Nausea and upper abdominal discomfort may occur, sometimes with vomiting, but hematemesis is uncommon. *The most common cause of chronic gastritis is infection with the bacillus Helicobacter pylori.* Before the acceptance of the central role of *H. pylori* infection in chronic gastritis, other chronic irritants, including psychologic stress, caffeine, alcohol, and

TABLE 17–2	Complications of Gastric Ulcers

Bleeding

Occurs in 15% to 20% of patients
Most frequent complication
May be life-threatening
Accounts for 25% of ulcer deaths
May be the first indication of an ulcer

Perforation

Occurs in up to 5% of patients
Accounts for two thirds of ulcer deaths
Is rarely first indication of an ulcer

Obstruction

Mostly in chronic ulcers
Secondary to edema or scarring
Occurs in about 2% of patients
Most often associated with pyloric channel ulcers
May occur with duodenal ulcers
Causes incapacitating, crampy abdominal pain
Can rarely cause total obstruction and intractable vomiting

tobacco use were considered the primary causes of gastritis. *Autoimmune gastritis*, the most common cause of *atrophic gastritis*, represents less than 10% of cases of chronic gastritis and is the most common form of chronic gastritis in patients without *H. pylori* infection. Less common etiologies include radiation injury, chronic bile reflux, mechanical injury, and involvement by systemic disease such as Crohn disease, amyloidosis, or graft-versus-host disease.

HELICOBACTER PYLORI GASTRITIS

The discovery of *H. pylori* has revolutionized our understanding of chronic gastritis.[13] *These spiral-shaped or curved bacilli are present in gastric biopsy specimens of almost all patients with duodenal ulcers and the majority of individuals with gastric ulcers or chronic gastritis.*[13] In a now-famous experiment, the Nobel laureate Barry Marshall ingested *H. pylori* cultures and developed mild gastritis. While not a recommended approach to infectious disease investigation, this experiment did demonstrate the pathogenicity of *H. pylori*. Acute *H. pylori* infection does not produce sufficient symptoms to require medical attention in most cases; it is the chronic gastritis that ultimately causes the individual to seek treatment. *H. pylori* organisms are present in 90% of individuals with chronic gastritis affecting the antrum. In addition, *H. pylori* has important roles in other gastric and duodenal diseases. For example, the increased acid secretion that occurs in *H. pylori* gastritis may result in peptic ulcer disease, and *H. pylori* infection also confers increased risk of gastric cancer.

Epidemiology. In the United States, *H. pylori* infection is associated with poverty, household crowding, limited education, African-American or Mexican-American ethnicity, residence in rural areas, and birth outside of the United States. Colonization rates exceed 70% in some groups and vary from less than 10% to more than 80% worldwide. In high-prevalence areas infection is often acquired in childhood and then persists for decades, explaining the direct correlation between colonization rate and patient age.

The mode of *H. pylori* transmission is not well defined, but humans are the only known host, making oral-oral, fecal-oral, and environmental spread the most likely routes of infection.

The related organism *Helicobacter heilmannii* causes similar disease and has reservoirs in cats, dogs, pigs, and nonhuman primates. While the morphologic differences between *H. pylori* and *H. heilmannii* organisms are subtle, recognition of *H. heilmannii* infection can be important since it may prompt treatment of household pets to prevent re-infection of the human companion.

Pathogenesis. *H. pylori* infection is the most common cause of chronic gastritis. The disease most often presents as a *predominantly antral gastritis with high acid production, despite hypogastrinemia.* The risk of duodenal ulcer is increased in these patients and, in most, gastritis is limited to the antrum with occasional involvement of the cardia. In a subset of patients the gastritis progresses to involve the gastric body and fundus. This pangastritis is associated with multifocal mucosal atrophy, reduced acid secretion, intestinal metaplasia, and increased risk of gastric adenocarcinoma.

H. pylori organisms have adapted to the ecologic niche provided by gastric mucus. Although *H. pylori* may invade the gastric mucosa, this is not evident histologically and the contribution of invasion to disease is not known. Four features are linked to *H. pylori* virulence:

- *Flagella*, which allow the bacteria to be motile in viscous mucus
- *Urease*, which generates ammonia from endogenous urea and thereby elevates local gastric pH
- *Adhesins* that enhance their bacterial adherence to surface foveolar cells
- *Toxins*, such as cytotoxin-associated gene A *(CagA)*, that may be involved in ulcer or cancer development by poorly defined mechanisms

Although the mechanisms by which *H. pylori* cause gastritis are incompletely defined, it is clear that infection results in increased acid production and disruption of normal gastric and duodenal protective mechanisms, as described earlier (see Fig. 17–11). *H. pylori* gastritis is, therefore, the result of an imbalance between gastroduodenal mucosal defenses and damaging forces that overcome those defenses.

Over time chronic antral *H. pylori* gastritis may progress to pangastritis, resulting in *multifocal atrophic gastritis.* The underlying mechanisms contributing to this progression are not clear, but interactions between the host and bacterium seem to be critical. For example, particular polymorphisms in the gene encoding the pro-inflammatory cytokine interleukin-1β (IL-1β) correlate with the development of pangastritis after *H. pylori* infection. Polymorphisms in TNF and a variety of other genes associated with the inflammatory response also influence the clinical outcome in *H. pylori* infection.[14] Severity of disease may also be influenced by genetic variation among *H. pylori* strains. For example, the *CagA* gene, a marker for a pathogenicity island of approximately 20 genes, is present in 50% of *H. pylori* isolates overall but in 90% of *H. pylori* isolates found in populations with elevated gastric cancer risk.

> **Morphology.** Gastric biopsy specimens generally demonstrate *H. pylori* in infected individuals. The organism is concentrated within the superficial mucus overlying epithelial cells in the surface and neck regions. The distribution can be irregular, with areas

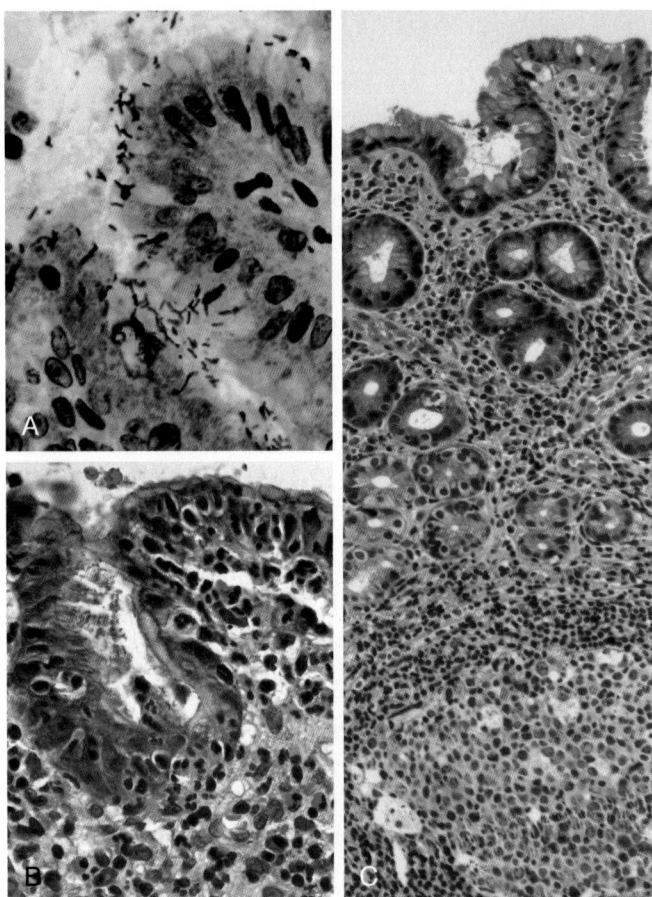

FIGURE 17–12 *Helicobacter pylori* gastritis. **A,** Spiral-shaped *H. pylori* are highlighted in this Warthin-Starry silver stain. Organisms are abundant within surface mucus. **B,** Intraepithelial and lamina propria neutrophils are prominent. **C,** Lymphoid aggregates with germinal centers and abundant subepithelial plasma cells within the superficial lamina propria are characteristic of *H. pylori* gastritis.

> of heavy colonization adjacent to those with few organisms. In extreme cases, the organisms carpet the luminal surfaces of foveolar and mucous neck cells, and can even extend into the gastric pits. Organisms are most easily demonstrated with a variety of special stains (Fig. 17–12A). *H. pylori* shows tropism for gastric epithelia and is generally not found in association with gastric intestinal metaplasia or duodenal epithelium. However, *H. pylori* may be present in foci of pyloric metaplasia within chronically injured duodenum or gastric-type mucosa within Barrett esophagus.
>
> Within the stomach, *H. pylori* are typically found in the antrum (Table 17–3). Although there is a good concordance between colonization of the antrum and cardia, infection of the cardia occurs at somewhat lower rates. *H. pylori* are uncommon in **oxyntic** (acid-producing) mucosa of the fundus and body except in heavy colonization. Thus, an antral biopsy is preferred for evaluation of *H. pylori* gastritis. When viewed endoscopically, *H. pylori*–infected antral mucosa is usually **erythematous** and has a coarse or

TABLE 17–3 Characteristics of *Helicobacter pylori*–Associated and Autoimmune Gastritis

	H. pylori–Associated	Autoimmune
Location	Antrum	Body
Inflammatory infiltrate	Neutrophils, subepithelial plasma cells	Lymphocytes, macrophages
Acid production	Increased to slightly decreased	Decreased
Gastrin	Normal to decreased	Increased
Other lesions	Hyperplastic/inflammatory polyps	Neuroendocrine hyperplasia
Serology	Antibodies to *H. pylori*	Antibodies to parietal cells (H^+,K^+-ATPase, intrinsic factor)
Sequelae	Peptic ulcer, adenocarcinoma	Atrophy, pernicious anemia, adenocarcinoma, carcinoid tumor
Associations	Low socioeconomic status, poverty, residence in rural areas	Autoimmune disease; thyroiditis, diabetes mellitus, Graves disease

even nodular appearance. The inflammatory infiltrate generally includes variable numbers of neutrophils within the lamina propria, including some that cross the basement membrane to assume an **intraepithelial** location (Fig. 17–12B) and accumulate in the lumen of gastric pits to create **pit abscesses**. In addition, the superficial lamina propria includes large numbers of plasma cells, often in clusters or sheets, and increased numbers of lymphocytes and macrophages. **Intraepithelial neutrophils** and **subepithelial plasma cells** are characteristic of *H. pylori* gastritis. When intense, inflammatory infiltrates may create thickened rugal folds, mimicking early infiltrative lesions. Long-standing *H. pylori* gastritis may extend to involve the body and fundus, and the mucosa can become **atrophic**. Lymphoid aggregates, some with germinal centers, are frequently present (Fig. 17–12C) and represent an induced form of **mucosa-associated lymphoid tissue**, or MALT, that has the potential to transform into lymphoma.

Clinical Features. In addition to histologic identification of the organism, several diagnostic tests have been developed including a noninvasive serologic test for antibodies to *H. pylori*, fecal bacterial detection, and the urea breath test based on the generation of ammonia by the bacterial urease. Gastric biopsy specimens can also be analyzed by the rapid urease test, bacterial culture, or bacterial DNA detection by PCR.

Effective treatments for *H. pylori* infection include combinations of antibiotics and proton pump inhibitors. Individuals with *H. pylori* gastritis usually improve after treatment, although relapses can occur after incomplete eradication or re-infection. Prophylactic and therapeutic vaccine development is still at an early stage of development. Peptic ulcer disease, a complication of chronic *H. pylori* gastritis, is described later.

AUTOIMMUNE GASTRITIS

Autoimmune gastritis accounts for less than 10% of cases of chronic gastritis. In contrast to that caused by *H. pylori*, auto-immune gastritis typically spares the antrum and includes *hypergastrinemia* (see Table 17–3). Autoimmune gastritis is characterized by:

- Antibodies to parietal cells and intrinsic factor that can be detected in serum and gastric secretions
- Reduced serum pepsinogen I concentration
- Antral endocrine cell hyperplasia
- Vitamin B_{12} deficiency
- Defective gastric acid secretion *(achlorhydria)*

Pathogenesis. Autoimmune gastritis is associated with loss of parietal cells, which are responsible for secretion of gastric acid and intrinsic factor. The absence of acid production stimulates gastrin release, resulting in hypergastrinemia and hyperplasia of antral gastrin-producing G cells. Lack of intrinsic factor disables ileal vitamin B_{12} absorption, leading to B_{12} deficiency and a slow-onset megaloblastic anemia *(pernicious anemia)*. The reduced serum pepsinogen I concentration results from chief cell destruction. In contrast, although *H. pylori* can cause hypochlorhydria, it is not associated with achlorhydria or pernicious anemia because the parietal and chief cell damage is not as severe as in autoimmune gastritis.

It was initially thought that the autoantibodies to parietal cell components, most prominently the H^+,K^+-ATPase, or proton pump, and intrinsic factor were involved in the pathogenesis of autoimmune gastritis. However, this is unlikely because neither secreted intrinsic factor nor the luminally oriented proton pump are accessible to circulating antibodies, and passive transfer of these antibodies does not produce gastritis in experimental animals. It is more likely that CD4+ T cells directed against parietal cell components, including the H^+,K^+-ATPase, are the principal agents of injury. This is supported by the observation that transfer of H^+,K^+-ATPase-reactive CD4+ T cells into naive mice results in gastritis and production of H^+,K^+-ATPase autoantibodies. There is no evidence of an autoimmune reaction to chief cells, suggesting that these are lost through gastric gland destruction during autoimmune attack on parietal cells. If autoimmune destruction is controlled by immunosuppression, the glands can repopulate, demonstrating that gastric stem cells survive and are able to differentiate into parietal and chief cells.

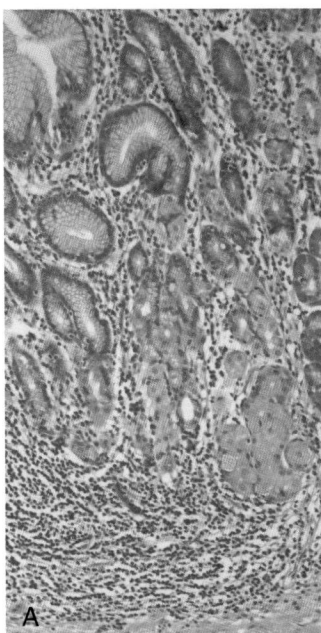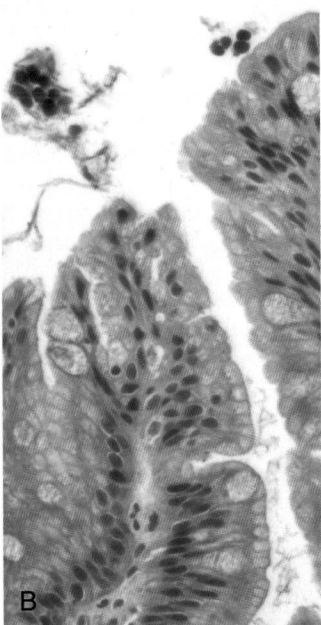

FIGURE 17–13 Autoimmune gastritis. **A,** Low-magnification image of gastric body demonstrating deep inflammatory infiltrates, primarily composed of lymphocytes, and glandular atrophy. **B,** Intestinal metaplasia, recognizable as the presence of goblet cells admixed with gastric foveolar epithelium.

Morphology. Autoimmune gastritis is characterized by diffuse mucosal **damage of the oxyntic (acid-producing) mucosa** within the body and fundus. Damage to the antrum and cardia is typically absent or mild. With **diffuse atrophy**, the oxyntic mucosa of the body and fundus appears markedly thinned, and rugal folds are lost. If vitamin B$_{12}$ deficiency is severe, nuclear enlargement (megaloblastic change) occurs within epithelial cells. Neutrophils may be present, but the inflammatory infiltrate is more often composed of lymphocytes, macrophages, and plasma cells. Lymphoid aggregates may be present. The superficial lamina propria plasma cells of *H. pylori* gastritis are typically absent, and the inflammatory reaction is most often deep and centered on the gastric glands (Fig. 17–13A). Loss of parietal and chief cells can be extensive. When atrophy is incomplete residual islands of oxyntic mucosa may give the appearance of multiple small polyps or nodules. Small surface elevations may be apparent, and these correlate with areas of **intestinal metaplasia**, characterized by the presence of goblet cells and columnar absorptive cells (Fig. 17–13B). The **antral endocrine cell hyperplasia** that develops in most patients can be difficult to appreciate on H&E-stained sections, since the endocrine cells, which are also referred to as enterochromaffin-like (ECL) cells, are not easily recognized. This hyperplasia parallels the degree of mucosal atrophy and is a physiologic response to decreased acid production. Over time, hypergastrinemia can stimulate endocrine cell hyperplasia in the fundus and body. Rarely, this may progress to form small, multicentric, low-grade neuroendocrine, or carcinoid, tumors.

Clinical Features. Antibodies to parietal cells and to intrinsic factor are present early in the disease course. Progression to gastric atrophy probably occurs over 2 to 3 decades, and anemia is seen in only a few patients. Because of the slow onset and variable progression, patients are generally diagnosed only after being affected for many years; the median age at diagnosis is 60 years. Slightly more women than men are affected. Pernicious anemia and autoimmune gastritis are often associated with other autoimmune diseases including Hashimoto thyroiditis, insulin-dependent (type I) diabetes mellitus, Addison disease, primary ovarian failure, primary hypoparathyroidism, Graves disease, vitiligo, myasthenia gravis, and Lambert-Eaton syndrome. These associations, along with concordance in some monozygotic twins and clustering of disease in families, support a genetic predisposition. In general, about 20% of relatives of individuals with pernicious anemia also have autoimmune gastritis, although they may be asymptomatic. Despite this strong genetic influence, autoimmune gastritis stands apart from other autoimmune diseases in that there is little evidence of linkage to specific HLA alleles.

Clinical presentation may be linked to symptoms of anemia.[15] In addition, vitamin B$_{12}$ deficiency may cause *atrophic glossitis*, in which the tongue becomes smooth and beefy red, epithelial megaloblastosis, and malabsorptive diarrhea. Vitamin B$_{12}$ deficiency may also cause peripheral neuropathy, spinal cord lesions, and cerebral dysfunction. Neuropathic changes include demyelination, axonal degeneration, and neuronal death. The most frequent manifestations of peripheral neuropathy are paresthesias and numbness. The spinal lesions may be associated with a mixture of loss of vibration and position sense, sensory ataxia with positive Romberg sign, limb weakness, spasticity, and extensor plantar responses. Cerebral manifestations range from mild personality changes and memory loss to psychosis. In contrast to anemia, neurologic changes are not reversed by vitamin B$_{12}$ replacement therapy.

UNCOMMON FORMS OF GASTRITIS

Reactive Gastropathy. This group of disorders is marked by foveolar hyperplasia, glandular regenerative changes, and mucosal edema. Neutrophils are not abundant. Causes of reactive gastropathy include chemical injury, NSAID use, bile reflux, and mucosal trauma secondary to prolapse. Notably, reactive gastropathy and bile reflux are common after gastric surgeries that bypass the pylorus. Gastric antral trauma induces a grossly characteristic lesion referred to as *gastric antral vascular ectasia* (GAVE). Endoscopy shows longitudinal stripes of edematous erythematous mucosa alternating with less severely injured mucosa that is sometimes referred to as *watermelon stomach*. Histologically, the antral mucosa shows reactive gastropathy with dilated capillaries containing fibrin thrombi.[16]

Eosinophilic Gastritis. As indicated by the name, this form of gastritis is characterized by tissue damage associated with dense infiltrates of eosinophils in the mucosa and muscularis, usually in the antral or pyloric region. The lesion is often present in other areas of the GI tract as well and is associated with peripheral eosinophilia and increased serum IgE levels. Allergic reactions are one cause of eosinophilic gastritis. In children, the allergens include cow's milk and soy protein, while drugs are common allergens in children and adults. Eosinophilic gastritis can also occur in association with systemic collagen-vascular disease, such as systemic sclerosis and polymyositis. Parasitic infections and *H. pylori* infection are other causes of eosinophilic gastritis.

Lymphocytic Gastritis. This disease preferentially affects women and produces nonspecific symptoms such as abdominal pain, anorexia, nausea, and vomiting. It is idiopathic, but approximately 40% of cases are associated with celiac disease, suggesting an immune-mediated pathogenesis. Lymphocytic gastritis is also referred to as *varioliform gastritis* based on the distinctive endoscopic appearance (thickened folds covered by small nodules with central aphthous ulceration).[17] The entire stomach is affected in most cases, but disease is occasionally limited to the body. Histologically there is a marked increase in the number of intraepithelial T lymphocytes, mostly CD8+ cells, within surface and pit regions.

Granulomatous Gastritis. This descriptive term is applied to any gastritis that contains granulomas, or aggregates of epithelioid histiocytes (tissue macrophages). It encompasses a diverse group of diseases with widely varying clinical and pathologic features. Correlation with clinical, endoscopic, radiologic, and serologic data is generally necessary for diagnosis. In Western populations, gastric involvement by Crohn disease is the most common specific cause of granulomatous gastritis.[18] Sarcoidosis is the second most common cause, followed by a variety of infections including mycobacteria, fungi, CMV, and *H. pylori*. In addition to the presence of histologically evident granulomas, narrowing and rigidity of the gastric antrum may occur secondary to transmural granulomatous inflammation.

Complications of Chronic Gastritis

PEPTIC ULCER DISEASE

Peptic ulcer disease (PUD) is most often associated with *H. pylori*–induced hyperchlorhydric chronic gastritis, which is present in 85% to 100% of individuals with duodenal ulcers and in 65% with gastric ulcers. The presence of chronic gastritis can help to distinguish peptic ulcers from acute erosive gastritis or stress ulcers, since the mucosa adjacent to the ulcer is generally normal in the latter two conditions. PUD may occur in any portion of the GI tract exposed to acidic gastric juices, but is most common in the gastric antrum and first portion of the duodenum. PUD may also occur in the esophagus as a result of GERD or acid secretion by ectopic gastric mucosa. Gastric mucosa within a Meckel diverticulum can result in peptic ulceration of adjacent mucosa.

Epidemiology. PUD is common and ranks fourth in both annual physician visits and costs among all GI diseases.[19] In the United States, the lifetime risk of developing an ulcer is approximately 10% for males and 4% for females; the latter are typically affected during or after menopause. PUD affects more than 300 million people and is responsible for treatment and ongoing care of over 3 million people, 190,000 hospitalizations, and 5000 deaths in the United States each year.[19]

Pathogenesis. *The imbalances of mucosal defenses and damaging forces that cause chronic gastritis are also responsible for PUD.* Thus, PUD generally develops on a background of chronic gastritis. The reasons why some people develop only chronic gastritis while others develop PUD are poorly understood.

H. pylori infection and NSAID use are the primary underlying causes of PUD, and both compromise mucosal defense while causing mucosal damage. Although more than 70% of individuals with PUD are infected by *H. pylori*, fewer than 20% of *H. pylori*–infected individuals develop peptic ulcer. It is probable that host factors as well as variation among *H. pylori* strains determine the clinical outcomes.

The gastric hyperacidity that drives PUD may be caused by *H. pylori* infection, parietal cell hyperplasia, excessive secretory responses, or impaired inhibition of stimulatory mechanisms such as gastrin release. For example, *Zollinger-Ellison syndrome*, in which there are multiple peptic ulcerations in the stomach, duodenum, and even jejunum, is caused by uncontrolled release of gastrin by a tumor and the resulting massive acid production. More common cofactors in peptic ulcerogenesis include chronic NSAID use, which causes direct chemical irritation while suppressing prostaglandin synthesis necessary for mucosal protection; cigarette smoking, which impairs mucosal blood flow and healing; and high-dose corticosteroids that suppress prostaglandin synthesis and impair healing. Duodenal ulcers are more frequent in individuals with alcoholic cirrhosis, chronic obstructive pulmonary disease, chronic renal failure, and hyperparathyroidism. In the latter two conditions, hypercalcemia stimulates gastrin production and therefore increases acid secretion. Finally, self-imposed or exogenous psychologic stress may increase gastric acid production.

Morphology. Peptic ulcers are four times more common in the proximal duodenum than in the stomach. Duodenal ulcers usually occur within a few centimeters of the pyloric valve and involve the anterior duodenal wall. Gastric peptic ulcers are predominantly located along the lesser curvature near the interface of the body and antrum.

Peptic ulcers are solitary in more than 80% of patients. Lesions less than 0.3 cm in diameter tend to be shallow while those over 0.6 cm are likely to be deeper ulcers. The classic peptic ulcer is a round to oval, **sharply punched-out defect** (Fig. 17–14A). The mucosal margin may overhang the base slightly, particularly on the upstream side, but is usually level with the surrounding mucosa. In contrast, **heaped-up margins are more characteristic of cancers**. The depth of ulcers may be limited by the thick gastric muscularis propria or by adherent pancreas, omental fat, or the liver. Hemorrhage and fibrin deposition are often present on the gastric serosa. **Perforation** into the peritoneal cavity is a surgical emergency that may be

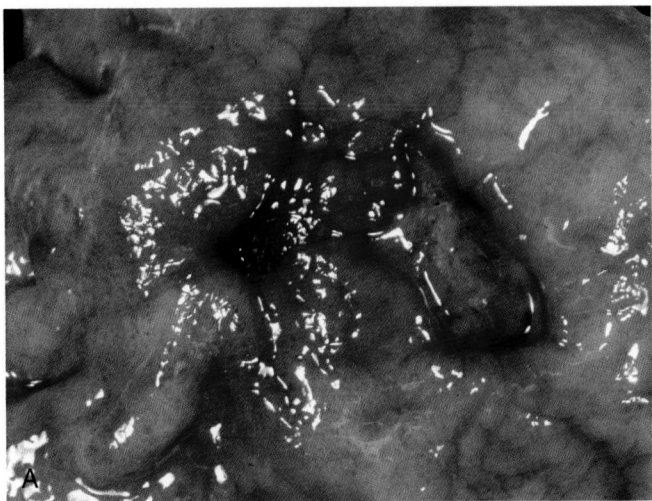

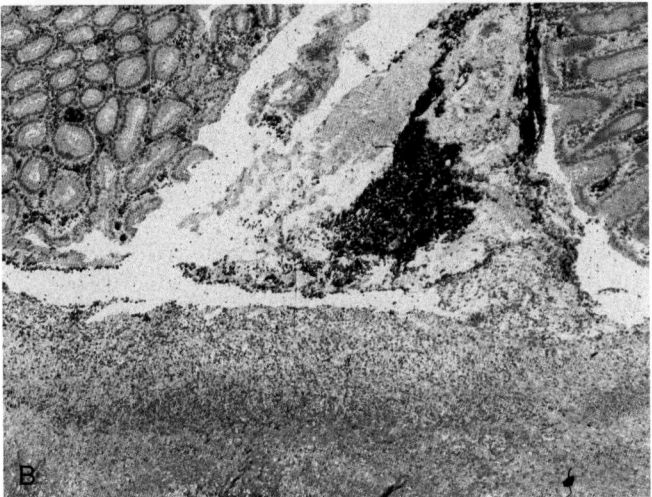

FIGURE 17–14   Acute gastric perforation in a patient presenting with free air under the diaphragm. **A,** Mucosal defect with clean edges. **B,** The necrotic ulcer base is composed of granulation tissue.

identified by the presence of free air under the diaphragm on upright radiographs of the abdomen.

The base of peptic ulcers is smooth and clean as a result of peptic digestion of exudate, and blood vessels may be evident. In active ulcers the base may have a thin layer of fibrinoid debris underlaid by a predominantly neutrophilic inflammatory infiltrate. Beneath this, active granulation tissue infiltrated with mononuclear leukocytes and a fibrous or collagenous scar forms the ulcer base (Fig. 17–14B). Vessel walls within the scarred area are typically thickened and are occasionally thrombosed. Ongoing bleeding within the ulcer base may cause life-threatening hemorrhage. Scarring may involve the entire thickness of the wall and pucker the surrounding mucosa into folds that radiate outward.

Size and location do not differentiate benign and malignant ulcers. However, the gross appearance of chronic peptic ulcers is virtually diagnostic. **Malig-**nant transformation of peptic ulcers is very rare, and reports of transformation probably represent cases wherein a lesion thought to be benign was actually an ulcerated carcinoma from the start.

Clinical Features. Peptic ulcers are notoriously chronic, recurring lesions with much greater morbidity than mortality. They may present in young adults but are most often diagnosed in middle-aged to older adults without obvious precipitating conditions. After a period of weeks to months of active disease, healing may occur with or without therapy, but the tendency to develop peptic ulcers remains. The majority of peptic ulcers come to clinical attention because of *epigastric burning or aching pain*, although a significant fraction present with complications such as *iron deficiency anemia*, *frank hemorrhage*, or *perforation*. The pain tends to occur 1 to 3 hours after meals during the day, is worse at night, and is relieved by alkali or food. Nausea, vomiting, bloating, belching, and significant weight loss are additional manifestations. With penetrating ulcers the pain is occasionally referred to the back, the left upper quadrant, or the chest, where it may be misinterpreted as cardiac in origin.

Current therapies for PUD are aimed at *H. pylori* eradication and neutralization of gastric acid, primarily with proton pump inhibitors or H_2 histamine receptor antagonists.[20] A variety of surgical approaches were formerly used, including antrectomy to remove gastrin-producing cells and vagotomy to remove the acid-stimulatory effects mediated by the vagus nerve. Proton pump inhibitors and *H. pylori* eradication have markedly reduced the need for surgical intervention, which is primarily reserved for treatment of bleeding or perforated peptic ulcers.

MUCOSAL ATROPHY AND INTESTINAL METAPLASIA

Long-standing chronic gastritis that involves the body and fundus may ultimately lead to significant loss of parietal cell mass. This oxyntic atrophy may be associated with intestinal metaplasia, recognized by the presence of goblet cells, and is *strongly associated with increased risk of gastric adenocarcinoma*. The risk of adenocarcinoma is greatest in autoimmune gastritis. This may be because achlorhydria of gastric mucosal atrophy permits overgrowth of bacteria that produce carcinogenic nitrosamines. Intestinal metaplasia also occurs in chronic *H. pylori* gastritis and may regress after clearance of the organism.

DYSPLASIA

Chronic gastritis exposes the epithelium to inflammation-related free radical damage and proliferative stimuli. Over time this combination of stressors can lead to the accumulation of genetic alterations that result in carcinoma. Pre-invasive in situ lesions can be recognized histologically as *dysplasia*. The morphologic hallmarks of dysplasia are variations in epithelial size, shape, and orientation along with coarse chromatin texture, hyperchromasia, and nuclear enlargement. The distinction between dysplasia and *regenerative epithelial changes* induced by active inflammation can be a challenge for the pathologist, since increased epithelial proliferation and mitotic figures may be prominent in both. However, reactive epithelial cells mature as they reach the mucosal surface, while dysplastic lesions remain cytologically immature.

GASTRITIS CYSTICA

Gastritis cystica refers to an exuberant reactive epithelial proliferation associated with entrapment of epithelial-lined cysts. These may be found within the submucosa (gastritis cystica polyposa) or deeper layers of the gastric wall (gastritis cystica profunda). Because of the association with chronic gastritis and partial gastrectomy, it is presumed that gastritis cystica is trauma-induced, but the reasons for the development of epithelial cysts within deeper portions of the gastric wall are not clear. Regenerative epithelial changes can be prominent in the entrapped epithelium, and gastritis cystica can therefore mimic invasive adenocarcinoma.

Hypertrophic Gastropathies

Hypertrophic gastropathies are uncommon diseases characterized by giant cerebriform enlargement of the rugal folds due to epithelial hyperplasia without inflammation. As might be expected, the hypertrophic gastropathies are linked to excessive growth factor release. The two most well-understood examples are Ménétrier disease and Zollinger-Ellison syndrome, the morphologic features of which are compared with other gastric proliferations in Table 17–4.

MÉNÉTRIER DISEASE

Ménétrier disease is a rare disorder caused by *excessive secretion of transforming growth factor α* (TGF-α)[21] The disease is characterized by diffuse hyperplasia of the foveolar epithelium of the body and fundus and hypoproteinemia due to protein-losing enteropathy. Secondary symptoms, such as weight loss, diarrhea, and peripheral edema, are commonly present. Symptoms and pathologic features of Ménétrier disease in children are similar to those in adults, but pediatric disease is usually self-limited and often follows respiratory infection. Risk of gastric adenocarcinoma is increased in adults with Ménétrier disease.

> **Morphology.** Ménétrier disease is characterized by irregular enlargement of the gastric rugae. Some areas may appear polypoid. Enlarged rugae are present in the body and fundus (Fig. 17–15A), but the antrum is generally spared. Histologically, the most characteristic feature is **hyperplasia of foveolar mucous cells.** The glands are elongated with a corkscrew-like appearance and cystic dilation is common (Fig. 17–15B). Inflammation is usually only modest, although some cases show marked intraepithelial lymphocytosis. Diffuse or patchy glandular atrophy, evident as hypoplasia of parietal and chief cells, is typical.

Treatment of Ménétrier disease is supportive, with intravenous albumin and parenteral nutritional supplementation. In severe cases gastrectomy may be performed. More recently, agents that block TGF-α–mediated activation of the epidermal growth factor receptor have shown promise.[22]

ZOLLINGER-ELLISON SYNDROME

Zollinger-Ellison syndrome is caused by gastrin-secreting tumors, gastrinomas, that are most commonly found in the small intestine or pancreas. Patients often present with duo-

TABLE 17–4	Hypertrophic Gastropathies and Gastric Polyps					
Parameter	**Ménétrier Disease (adult)**	**Zollinger-Ellison Syndrome**	**Inflammatory and Hyperplastic Polyps**	**Gastritis Cystica**	**Fundic Gland Polyps**	**Gastric Adenomas**
Mean patient age (yr)	30–60	50	50–60	Variable	50	50–60
Location	Body and fundus	Fundus	Antrum > body	Body	Body and fundus	Antrum > body
Predominant cell type	Mucous	Parietal > mucous, endocrine	Mucous	Mucous, cyst-lining	Parietal and chief	Dysplastic, intestinal
Inflammatory infiltrate	Limited, lymphocytes	Neutrophils	Neutrophils and lymphocytes	Neutrophils and lymphocytes	None	Variable
Symptoms	Hypoproteinemia, weight loss, diarrhea	Peptic ulcers	Chronic gastritis	Chronic gastritis	None, nausea	Chronic gastritis
Risk factors	None	Multiple endocrine neoplasia	Chronic gastritis, *H. pylori*	Trauma, prior surgery	PPIs, FAP	Chronic gastritis, atrophy, intestinal metaplasia
Association with adenocarcinoma	Yes	No	Occasional	No	No	Frequent

FAP, familial aderomatous polyposis; PPIs, proton pump inhibitors.

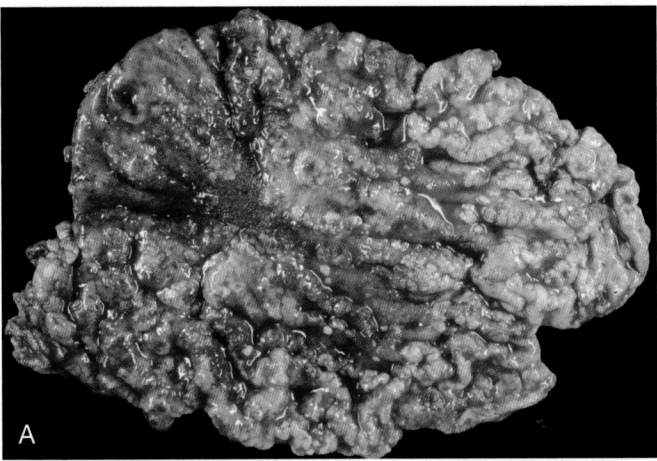

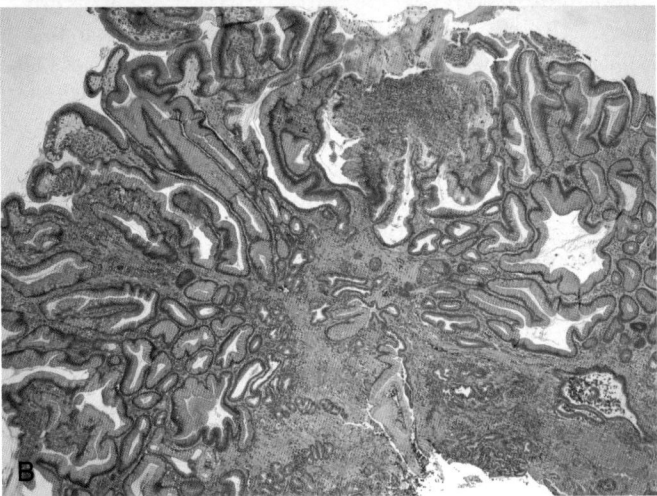

FIGURE 17–15 Ménétrier disease. **A,** Marked enlargement of rugal folds. **B,** Foveolar hyperplasia with elongated and focally dilated glands. (Courtesy of Dr. M. Kay Washington, Vanderbilt University, Nashville, TN.)

denal ulcers or chronic diarrhea. Within the stomach, the most remarkable feature is a doubling of oxyntic mucosal thickness due to a fivefold *increase in the number of parietal cells.* Gastrin also induces hyperplasia of mucous neck cells, mucin hyperproduction, and proliferation of endocrine cells within oxyntic mucosa. In some cases these endocrine cells can form small dysplastic nodules or, rarely, true carcinoid tumors.

Treatment of individuals with Zollinger-Ellison syndrome includes blockade of acid hypersecretion, which is accomplished in almost all patients with proton pump inhibitors or high-dose H_2 histamine receptor antagonists. Acid suppression allows peptic ulcers to heal and prevents gastric perforation, allowing treatment to focus on the gastrinoma, which becomes the main determinant of long-term survival.

Although they grow slowly, 60% to 90% of gastrinomas are malignant. Tumors are sporadic in 75% of patients. These tend to be solitary tumors and can be surgically resected. The remaining 25% of patients with gastrinomas have multiple endocrine neoplasia type I. These individuals often have multiple tumors or metastatic disease and may benefit from treatment with somatostatin analogues.[23] Clinical identification of tumors may be enhanced by somatostatin receptor scintigraphy and endoscopic ultrasonography.

Gastric Polyps and Tumors

Polyps, nodules or masses that project above the level of the surrounding mucosa, are identified in up to 5% of upper GI endoscopies. Polyps may develop as a result of epithelial or stromal cell hyperplasia, inflammation, ectopia, or neoplasia. Only the most common types of polyps will be discussed here (Peutz-Jeghers and juvenile polyps are discussed with intestinal polyps). This is followed by a presentation of gastric tumors, including *adenocarcinomas, lymphomas, carcinoid tumors, and stromal tumors.*

INFLAMMATORY AND HYPERPLASTIC POLYPS

Approximately 75% of all gastric polyps are *inflammatory* or *hyperplastic polyps.* They are most common in individuals between 50 and 60 years of age. These polyps usually develop in association with chronic gastritis, which initiates the injury and reactive hyperplasia that leads to polyp growth. Inflammatory or hyperplastic polyps are most common in individuals between 50 and 60 years of age. Among individuals with *H. pylori* gastritis, polyps may regress after bacterial eradication. Because the risk of dysplasia correlates with size, polyps larger than 1.5 cm should be resected and examined histologically.

> **Morphology.** The majority of inflammatory or hyperplastic polyps are smaller than 1 cm in diameter and are frequently multiple, particularly in individuals with atrophic gastritis. These polyps are ovoid in shape and have a smooth surface, though superficial erosions are common. Microscopically, polyps have irregular, cystically dilated, and elongated foveolar glands (Fig. 17–16A). The lamina propria is typically edematous with variable degrees of acute and chronic inflammation, and surface ulceration may be present (Fig. 17–16B).

FUNDIC GLAND POLYPS

Fundic gland polyps occur sporadically and in individuals with familial adenomatous polyposis (FAP). The prevalence of fundic gland polyps has increased markedly in recent years as a result of proton pump inhibitor therapy. This likely reflects increased gastrin secretion, in response to reduced gastric acidity, and the resulting glandular hyperplasia. These polyps are five times more common in women and are discovered at an average age of 50 years. Fundic gland polyps may be asymptomatic or associated with nausea, vomiting, or epigastric pain.

> **Morphology.** Fundic gland polyps occur in the gastric body and fundus and are well-circumscribed lesions with a smooth surface. They may be single or multiple and are composed of cystically dilated, irregular glands lined by flattened parietal and chief cells. Inflammation is typically absent or minimal (Fig. 17–16C).

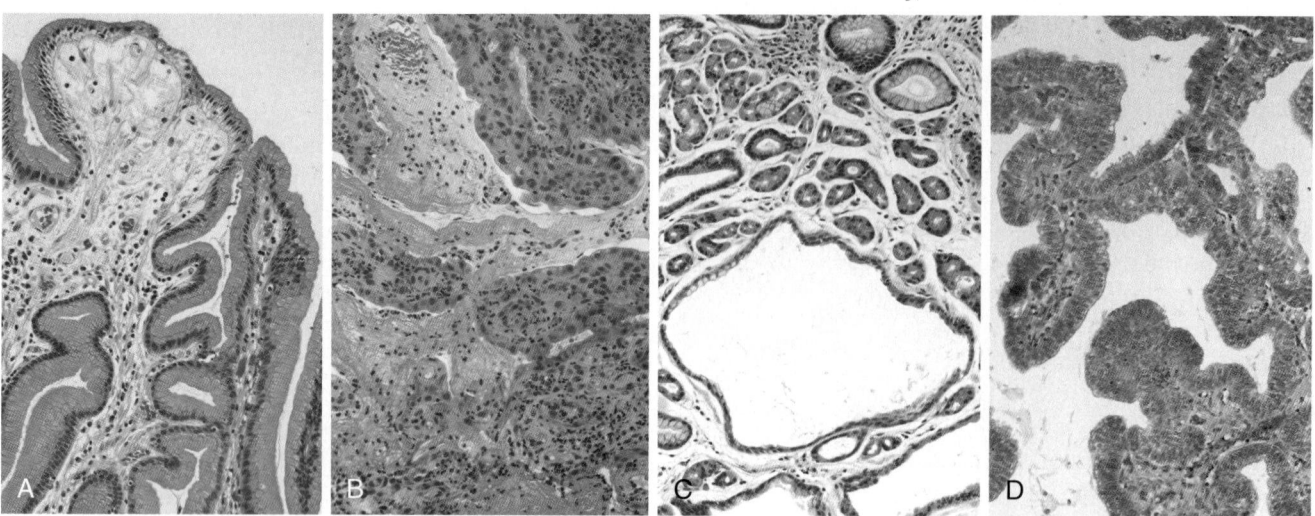

FIGURE 17–16   Gastric polyps. **A,** Hyperplastic polyp containing corkscrew-shaped foveolar glands. **B,** Hyperplastic polyp with ulceration. **C,** Fundic gland polyp composed of cystically dilated glands lined by parietal, chief, and foveolar cells. **D,** Gastric adenoma recognized by the presence of epithelial dysplasia.

GASTRIC ADENOMA

Gastric adenomas represent as many as 10% of all gastric polyps (Table 17–4). Their incidence increases progressively with age,[24] and there is a marked variation in rate among different populations that parallels the incidence of gastric adenocarcinoma. Patients are usually between 50 and 60 years of age, and males are affected three times more often than females. Like fundic gland polyps, the incidence of adenomas is increased in individuals with FAP. *Similar to other forms of gastric dysplasia, adenomas almost always occur on a background of chronic gastritis with atrophy and intestinal metaplasia.* The risk of adenocarcinoma in gastric adenomas is related to the size of the lesion and is particularly elevated in lesions greater than 2 cm in diameter. Overall, carcinoma may be present in up to 30% of gastric adenomas.[24]

> **Morphology.** Gastric adenomas are usually solitary lesions less than 2 cm in diameter, most commonly located in the antrum. The majority of adenomas are composed of intestinal-type columnar epithelium. By definition, all GI adenomas have epithelial dysplasia (Fig. 17–16D) that can be classified as low or high grade. Both grades may include enlargement, elongation, and hyperchromasia of epithelial cell nuclei, epithelial crowding, and pseudostratification. High-grade dysplasia is characterized by more severe cytologic atypia and irregular architecture, including glandular budding and gland-within-gland, or cribriform, structures.[25]

GASTRIC ADENOCARCINOMA

Adenocarcinoma is the most common malignancy of the stomach, comprising over 90% of all gastric cancers. Early symptoms resemble those of chronic gastritis, including dyspepsia, dysphagia, and nausea. As a result, these tumors are often discovered at advanced stages, when symptoms such as weight loss, anorexia, altered bowel habits, anemia, and hemorrhage trigger further diagnostic evaluation.

Epidemiology. Gastric cancer incidence varies markedly with geography. In Japan, Chile, Costa Rica, and Eastern Europe the incidence is up to 20-fold higher than in North America, northern Europe, Africa, and Southeast Asia. Mass endoscopic screening programs can be successful in regions where the incidence is high, such as Japan, where 35% of newly detected cases are *early gastric cancer,* tumors limited to the mucosa and submucosa. Unfortunately, mass screening programs are not cost-effective in regions where the incidence is low, and fewer than 20% of cases are detected at an early stage in North America and northern Europe.

In the United States, *gastric cancer rates dropped by over 85% during the twentieth century.*[26] Adenocarcinoma of the stomach was the most common cause of cancer death in the United States in 1930 and remains a leading cause of cancer death worldwide, but now accounts for fewer than 2.5% of cancer deaths in the United States. Similar declines have been reported in many other Western countries, suggesting that environmental and dietary factors are responsible.[26] Consistent with this conclusion, studies of migrants from high-risk to low-risk regions have shown that gastric cancer rates in second-generation immigrants are similar to those in their new country of residence.

The cause of the overall reduction in gastric cancer is unknown. One possible explanation is the decreased consumption of dietary carcinogens, such as N-nitroso compounds and benzo[a]pyrene, because of reduced use of salt and smoking for food preservation and the widespread availability of food refrigeration. Conversely, intake of green, leafy vegetables and citrus fruits, which contain antioxidants such as vitamin C, vitamin E, and beta-carotene, and is correlated with reduced risk of gastric cancers, may have increased as a result of improved food transportation networks.

Gastric cancer is more common in lower socioeconomic groups and in individuals with *multifocal mucosal atrophy and intestinal metaplasia.* PUD does not impart an increased risk of gastric cancer, but patients who have had *partial gastrecto-*

mies for PUD have a slightly higher risk of developing cancer in the residual gastric stump as a result of hypochlorhydria, bile reflux, and chronic gastritis.

Although overall incidence of gastric adenocarcinoma is falling, *cancer of the gastric cardia is on the rise*. This is probably related to Barrett esophagus and may reflect the increasing incidence of chronic GERD and obesity.[10] Consistent with this presumed common pathogenesis, distal esophageal adenocarcinomas and gastric cardia adenocarcinomas are similar in morphology, clinical behavior, and therapeutic response.[27–29]

Pathogenesis. While the majority of gastric cancers are not hereditary, the mutations identified in familial gastric cancer have provided important insights into mechanisms of carcinogenesis in sporadic cases. Germline mutations in *CDH1*, which encodes E-cadherin, a protein that contributes to epithelial intercellular adhesion, are associated with familial gastric cancers, which are usually of the diffuse type. Mutations in *CDH1* are present in about 50% of sporadic cases of diffuse gastric tumors, while E-cadherin expression is drastically decreased in the rest, often by methylation of the *CDH1* promoter. *Thus, the loss of E-cadherin function seems to be a key step in the development of diffuse gastric cancer.* Notably, *CDH1* mutations are also common in sporadic and familial lobular carcinoma of the breast, which also tends to infiltrate as single cells, and individuals with *BRCA2* mutations are at increased risk of developing diffuse gastric cancer.

In contrast to diffuse gastric tumors, there is an increased risk of intestinal-type gastric cancer in individuals with FAP, particularly in Japan. This implies an interaction between host genetic background and environmental factors, since gastric cancer risk is less markedly elevated in individuals with FAP residing in areas of low gastric cancer incidence. Mutations in β-catenin, a protein that binds to both E-cadherin and adenomatous polyposis coli (APC), as well as microsatellite instability and hypermethylation of several genes including *TGFβRII*, *BAX*, *IGFRII*, and *p16/INK4a* have also been described in sporadic intestinal-type gastric cancer.

Genetic variants of pro-inflammatory and immune response genes, including those that encode IL-1β, TNF, IL-10, IL-8, and Toll-like receptor 4 (TLR4), are associated with elevated risk of gastric cancer when accompanied by *H. pylori* infection, and *p53* mutations are present in the majority of sporadic gastric cancers of both histologic types. Thus, although specific sequences of events have not been defined, it is clear that chronic inflammation promotes neoplastic progression. Other associations between chronic inflammation and cancer were discussed in Chapter 7.

Morphology. Gastric adenocarcinomas are classified according to their location in the stomach, and most importantly, according to gross and histologic morphology. Most gastric adenocarcinomas involve the gastric antrum; the lesser curvature is involved more often than the greater curvature.[28] Gastric tumors with an **intestinal** morphology tend to form bulky tumors (Fig. 17–17A) composed of glandular structures (Fig. 17–18A), while cancers with a **diffuse** infiltrative growth pattern (see Fig. 17–17B) are more often composed of

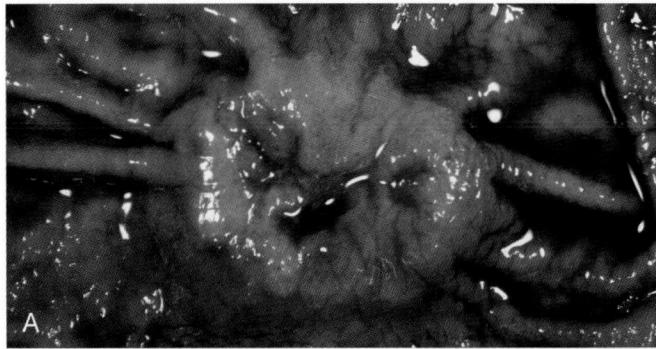
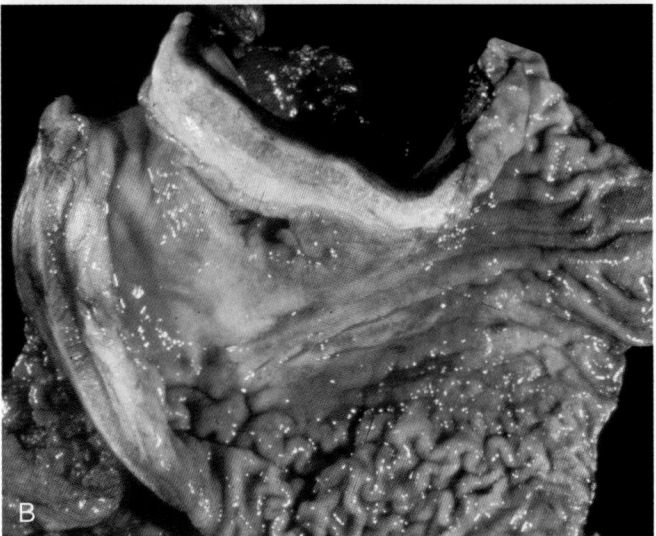

FIGURE 17–17   Gastric adenocarcinoma. **A,** Intestinal-type adenocarcinoma consisting of an elevated mass with heaped-up borders and central ulceration. Compare to the peptic ulcer in Figure 17–14A. **B,** Linitis plastica. The gastric wall is markedly thickened, and rugal folds are partially lost.

signet-ring cells (see Fig. 17–18B). Although intestinal-type adenocarcinomas may penetrate the gastric wall, they typically grow along broad cohesive fronts to form either an exophytic mass or an ulcerated tumor. The neoplastic cells often contain apical mucin vacuoles, and abundant mucin may be present in gland lumens. In contrast, diffuse gastric cancer is generally composed of discohesive cells that do not form glands but instead have large mucin vacuoles that expand the cytoplasm and push the nucleus to the periphery, creating a **signet-ring cell** morphology. These cells permeate the mucosa and stomach wall individually or in small clusters, which makes tumor cells easy to confuse with inflammatory cells, such as macrophages, at low magnification. Extracellular mucin release in either type of gastric cancer can result in formation of large **mucin lakes** that dissect tissue planes.

A mass may be difficult to appreciate in diffuse gastric cancer, but these infiltrative tumors often evoke a **desmoplastic** reaction that stiffens the gastric wall and may provide a valuable diagnostic clue. When there are large areas of infiltration,

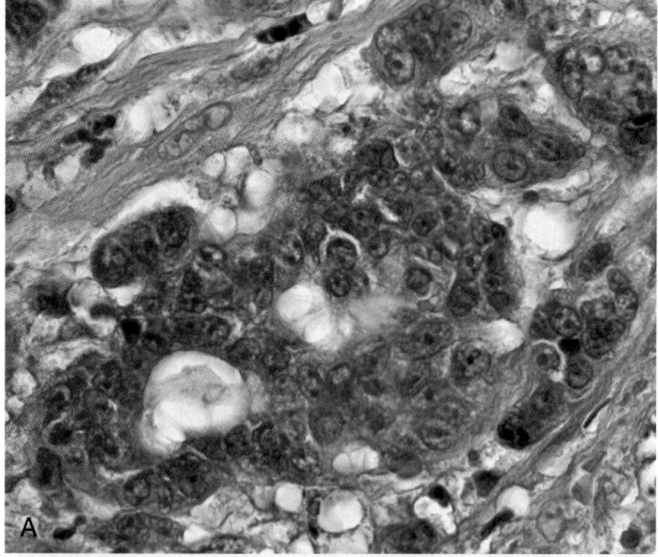

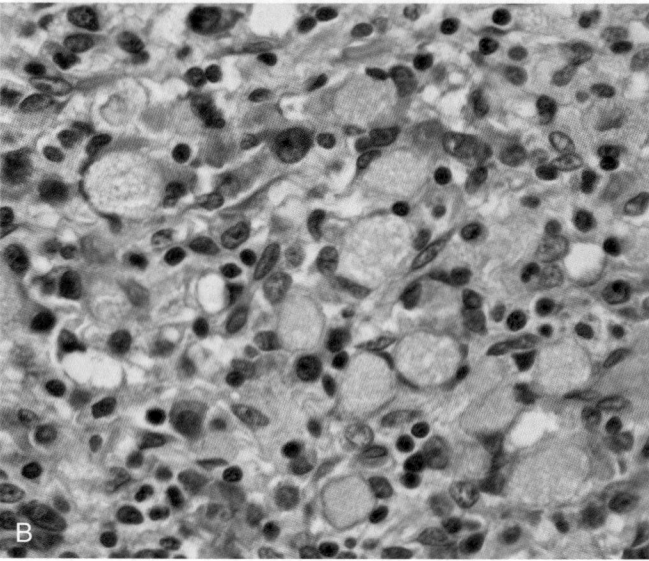

FIGURE 17–18　Gastric adenocarcinoma. **A,** Intestinal-type adenocarcinoma composed of columnar, gland-forming cells infiltrating through desmoplastic stroma. **B,** Signet-ring cells can be recognized by their large cytoplasmic mucin vacuoles and peripherally displaced, crescent-shaped nuclei.

diffuse rugal flattening and a rigid, thickened wall may impart a **leather bottle** appearance termed **linitis plastica** (see Fig. 17–17B). Breast and lung cancers that metastasize to the stomach may also create a linitis plastica–like appearance.

Clinical Features. Intestinal-type gastric cancer predominates in high-risk areas and develops from precursor lesions including flat dysplasia and adenomas. The mean age of presentation is 55 years, and the male-to-female ratio is 2:1. In contrast, the incidence of diffuse gastric cancer is relatively uniform across countries, there are no identified precursor lesions, and the disease occurs at similar frequencies in males and females. Notably, *the remarkable decrease in gastric cancer incidence applies only to the intestinal type*, which is most closely associated with atrophic gastritis and intestinal meta-

plasia. As a result, the incidences of intestinal and diffuse types of gastric cancers are now similar.

The depth of invasion and the extent of nodal and distant metastasis at the time of diagnosis remain the most powerful prognostic indicators for gastric cancer.[30] In advanced cases gastric carcinoma may first be detected as metastases to the supraclavicular sentinel lymph node, also called *Virchow's node*. Gastric tumors can also metastasize to the periumbilical region to form a subcutaneous nodule, termed a *Sister Mary Joseph nodule*, after the nurse who first noted this lesion as a marker of metastatic carcinoma. Local invasion into the duodenum, pancreas, and retroperitoneum is also characteristic. In such cases efforts are usually focused on chemotherapy or radiation therapy and palliative care. However, when possible, surgical resection remains the preferred treatment for gastric adenocarcinoma. After surgical resection, the 5-year survival rate of early gastric cancer can exceed 90%, even if lymph node metastases are present. In contrast, the 5-year survival rate for advanced gastric cancer remains below 20%.[28] Because of the advanced stage at which most gastric cancers are discovered in the United States, the overall 5-year survival is less than 30%.[28,31]

LYMPHOMA

Although extra-nodal lymphomas can arise in virtually any tissue, they do so most commonly in the GI tract, particularly the stomach. In allogeneic bone marrow transplant and organ transplant recipients, the bowel is also the most frequent site for Epstein-Barr virus–positive B-cell lymphoproliferations,[32] because the deficits in T-cell function caused by oral immunosuppressive agents (e.g., cyclosporine) are greatest at intestinal sites of drug absorption. Nearly 5% of all gastric malignancies are primary lymphomas, the most common of which are indolent extra-nodal marginal zone B-cell lymphomas. In the gut these tumors are often referred to as lymphomas of *mucosa-associated lymphoid tissue (MALT)*, or *MALTomas*.[33] This entity and the second most common primary lymphoma of the gut, diffuse large B-cell lymphoma, are also discussed in Chapter 13.

Pathogenesis. Extra-nodal marginal zone B-cell lymphomas usually arise at sites of chronic inflammation. They can originate in the GI tract at sites of preexisting MALT, such as the Peyer's patches of the small intestine, but more commonly arise within tissues that are normally devoid of organized lymphoid tissue. The most common cause of "pro-lymphomatous" inflammation in the stomach is chronic *H. pylori* infection, which is found in association with most cases of gastric MALToma.[34] As with other low-grade lymphomas, MALTomas can transform into more aggressive tumors that are histologically identical to diffuse large B-cell lymphomas.

The most striking evidence linking *H. pylori* gastritis to MALToma is that eradication of the infection with antibiotics induces durable remissions with low rates of recurrence in most patients.[35] Histologic features that predict antibiotic treatment failures include transformation to large-cell lymphoma, tumor invasion to the muscularis propria or beyond, and lymph node involvement.

Three translocations are associated with gastric MALToma, the t(11;18)(q21;q21) and the less common t(1;14)(p22;q32) and t(14;18)(q32;q21). They are also highly predictive of response failure.[36,37] The t(11;18)(q21;q21) translocation brings together the apoptosis inhibitor 2 *(API2)* gene on chromosome 11 with the "mutated in MALT lymphoma," or *MLT*, gene on chromosome 18. This creates a chimeric *API2-MLT* fusion gene that encodes an API2-MLT fusion protein. The t(14;18)(q32;q21) and t(1;14)(p22;q32) translocations cause increased expression of intact MLT and BCL-10 proteins, respectively.

Although some details remain uncertain, each of the three translocations has the same net effect, the constitutive activation of NF-κB, a transcription factor that promotes B-cell growth and survival. Remarkably, antigen-dependent activation of NF-κB in normal B and T cells requires both BCL-10 and MLT, which work together in a pathway down-stream of the B- and T-cell antigen receptors. In MALTomas that lack these translocations, *H. pylori*–induced inflammation may trigger NF-κB activation through the MLT/BCL-10 pathway. In these tumors elimination of the immune stimulus *(H. pylori)* down-regulates NF-κB, resulting in tumor regression. In contrast, NF-κB is constitutively active in tumors bearing translocations involving *MLT* or *BCL10*, and as a result the elimination of *H. pylori* has no effect. Additional genetic changes, such as inactivation of the tumor suppressor genes that encode p53 and p16, may lead to transformation of gastric MALToma into aggressive diffuse large B-cell lymphoma.[38]

> **Morphology.** Histologically, gastric MALToma takes the form of a dense lymphocytic infiltrate in the lamina propria (Fig. 17–19A). Characteristically, the neoplastic lymphocytes infiltrate the gastric glands focally to create diagnostic **lymphoepithelial lesions** (Fig. 17–19A, inset). Reactive-appearing B-cell follicles may be present, and, in about 40% of tumors, plasmacytic differentiation is observed. Occasionally the tumor cells accumulate large amounts of pale cytoplasm, a feature referred to as **"monocytoid"** change.
>
> Like other tumors of mature B cells, MALTomas express the B-cell markers CD19 and CD20. They do not express CD5 and CD10, and are positive for CD43 in about 25% of cases, an unusual feature that can be diagnostically helpful. In cases lacking lymphoepithelial lesions, monoclonality may be demonstrated by restricted expression of either κ or λ immunoglobulin light chain or by molecular detection of clonal IgH rearrangements. Molecular cytogenetic analysis (e.g., fluorescent in situ hybridization) is being used increasingly to identify tumors with translocations that predict resistance to therapy.

Clinical Features. The most common presenting symptoms are dyspepsia and epigastric pain. Hematemesis, melena, and constitutional symptoms such as weight loss can also be present. Because gastric MALTomas and *H. pylori* gastritis often coexist and have overlapping clinical symptoms and endoscopic appearances, diagnostic difficulties sometimes arise, particularly in small biopsy specimens. GI lymphomas may also disseminate as discrete small nodules (Fig. 17–19B) or infiltrate the wall diffusely (Fig. 17–19C).

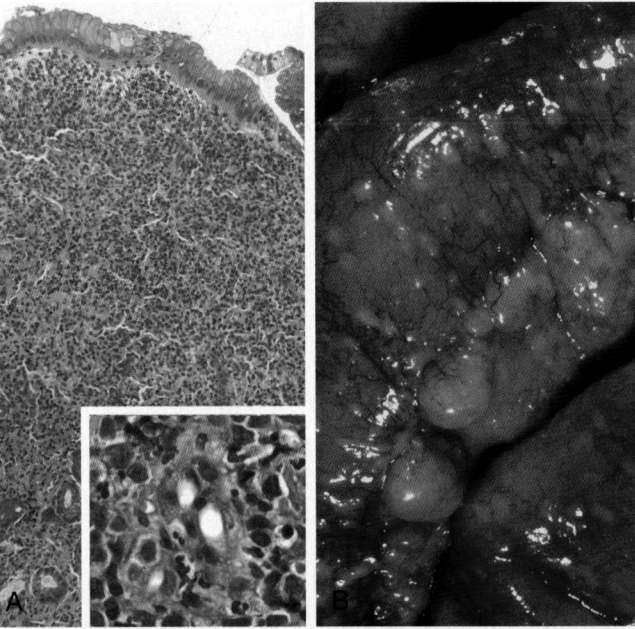
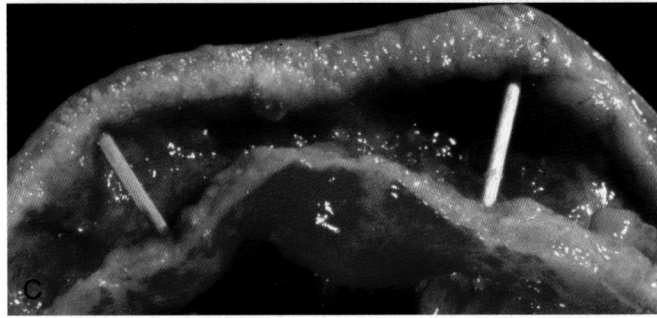

FIGURE 17–19 GI lymphoma. **A,** Gastric MALT lymphoma replacing much of the gastric epithelium. Inset shows lymphoepithelial lesions with neoplastic lymphocytes surrounding and infiltrating gastric glands. **B,** Disseminated lymphoma within the small intestine with numerous small serosal nodules. **C,** Large B-cell lymphoma infiltrating the small intestinal wall and producing diffuse thickening.

CARCINOID TUMOR

Carcinoid tumors arise from the diffuse components of the endocrine system. The majority are found in the GI tract, and more than 40% occur in the small intestine (Table 17–5).[39] The tracheobronchial tree and lungs are the next most commonly sites involved. Gastric carcinoids may be associated with endocrine cell hyperplasia, chronic atrophic gastritis, and Zollinger-Ellison syndrome. The term *carcinoid*, or "carcinoma-like," was applied because these tumors tend to have a more indolent clinical course than GI carcinomas. Carcinoid tumors are best considered to be *well-differentiated neuroendocrine carcinomas*. Carcinoids within the GI tract arise from the endocrine cells that release peptide and nonpeptide hormones to coordinate gut function.

> **Morphology.** Grossly, carcinoids are intramural or submucosal masses that create small polypoid lesions (Fig. 17–20A). The overlying mucosa may be intact or ulcerated, and the tumors may invade deeply to

TABLE 17–5   Features of Gastrointestinal Carcinoid Tumors

Feature	Esophagus	Stomach	Proximal Duodenum	Jejunum and Ileum	Appendix	Colorectum
Fraction of GI carcinoids	<1%	<10%	<10%	>40%	<25%	>25%
Mean patient age (yr)	Rare	55	50	65	All ages	60
Location	Distal	Body and fundus	Proximal third, peri-ampullary	Throughout	Tip	Rectum > cecum
Size	Limited data	1–2 cm, multiple; >2 cm, solitary	0.5–2 cm	<3.5 cm	0.2–1 cm	>5 cm (cecum); <1 cm (rectum)
Secretory product(s)	Limited data	Histamine, somatostatin, serotonin	Gastrin, somatostatin, cholecystokinin	Serotonin, substance P, polypeptide YY	Serotonin, polypeptide YY	Serotonin, polypeptide YY
Symptoms	Dysphagia, weight loss, reflux	Gastritis, ulcer, incidental	Peptic ulcer, biliary obstruction, abdominal pain	Asymptomatic, obstruction, metastatic disease	Asymptomatic, incidental	Abdominal pain, weight loss, incidental
Behavior	Limited data	Variable	Variable	Aggressive	Benign	Variable
Disease associations	None	Atrophic gastritis, MEN-I	Zollinger-Ellison syndrome, NF-1, sporadic	None	None	None

MEN-I, multiple endocrine neoplasia type I; NF-1, neurofibromatosis type I.

involve the mesentery. Carcinoids tend to be yellow or tan in color and are very firm as a consequence of an intense desmoplastic reaction, which may cause kinking of the bowel and obstruction. Histologically, carcinoid tumors are composed of islands, trabeculae, strands, glands, or sheets of uniform cells with scant, pink granular cytoplasm and a round to oval stippled nucleus (Fig. 17–20). In most tumors there is minimal pleomorphism, but anaplasia, mitotic activity, and necrosis may be present in rare cases. Immunohistochemical stains are typically positive for endocrine granule markers, such as synaptophysin and chromogranin A.

Clinical Features. The peak incidence of carcinoid tumors is in the sixth decade, but they may appear at any age. Symp-

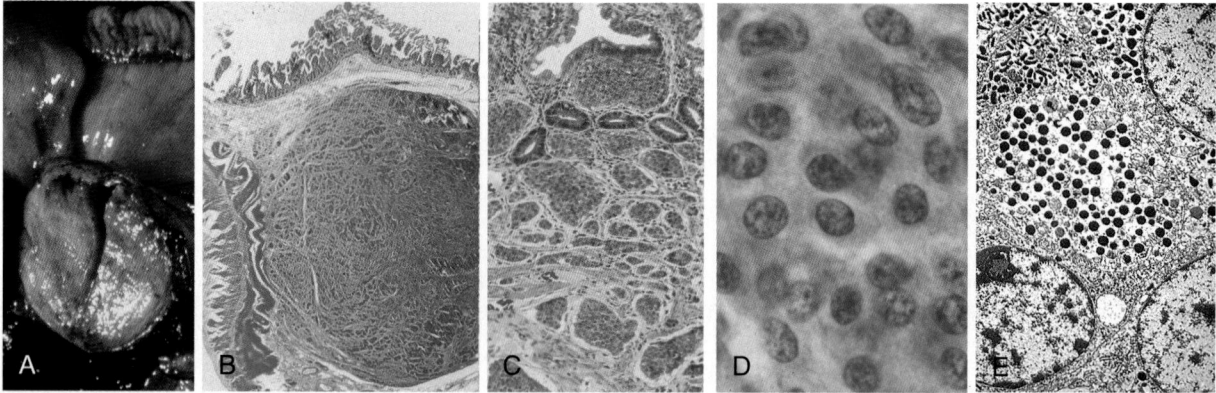

FIGURE 17–20 GI carcinoid tumor (neuroendocrine carcinoma). **A,** Gross cross-section of a submucosal tumor nodule. **B,** Microscopically the nodule is composed of tumor cells embedded in dense fibrous tissue. **C,** In other areas, the tumor has spread extensively within mucosal lymphatic channels. **D,** High magnification shows the bland cytology of carcinoid tumors. The chromatin texture, with fine and coarse clumps, is frequently described as a "salt and pepper" pattern. Despite their innocuous appearance, carcinoids can be extremely aggressive clinically. **E,** Electron microscopy reveals cytoplasmic dense core neurosecretory granules.

toms are determined by the hormones produced. For example, tumors that produce gastrin may cause Zollinger-Ellison syndrome, while ileal tumors may cause carcinoid syndrome, which is characterized by cutaneous flushing, sweating, bronchospasm, colicky abdominal pain, diarrhea, and right-sided cardiac valvular fibrosis. *Carcinoid syndrome occurs in fewer than 10% of patients and is caused by vasoactive substances secreted by the tumor into the systemic circulation.* When tumors are confined to the intestine, the vasoactive substances released are metabolized to inactive forms by the liver, a "first-pass" effect similar to that exerted on oral drugs. Carcinoid syndrome generally requires tumors to secrete hormones into a non-portal venous circulation and therefore is *strongly associated with metastatic disease.*

The most important prognostic factor for GI carcinoid tumors is location.

- *Foregut carcinoid tumors*, those found within the stomach, duodenum proximal to the ligament of Treitz, and esophagus, rarely metastasize and are generally cured by resection. This is particularly true for gastric carcinoid tumors that arise in association with atrophic gastritis, while gastric carcinoid tumors without predisposing factors are more aggressive.
- *Midgut carcinoid tumors* that arise in the jejunum and ileum are often multiple and tend to be aggressive. In these tumors, greater depth of local invasion, increased size, and presence of necrosis and mitosis are associated with poor outcome.
- *Hindgut carcinoids* arising in the appendix and colorectum are typically discovered incidentally. Those in the appendix occur at any age and are generally located at the tip. These tumors are rarely more than 2 cm in diameter and are almost uniformly benign. Rectal carcinoid tumors tend to produce polypeptide hormones and, when symptomatic, present with abdominal pain and weight loss. Metastasis of rectal carcinoid tumors is uncommon. In contrast, tumors of the proximal colon are uncommon but may grow to large size and metastasize.

GASTROINTESTINAL STROMAL TUMOR

A wide variety of mesenchymal neoplasms may arise in the stomach. Many are named according to the cell type they most resemble; for example, smooth muscle tumors are called *leiomyomas* or *leiomyosarcomas*, nerve sheath tumors are termed *schwannomas*, and those resembling glomus bodies in the nailbeds and at other sites are termed *glomus tumors*. These are all rare and are discussed in greater detail in Chapter 26. *GI stromal tumor (GIST)* is the most common mesenchymal tumor of the abdomen, and more than half of these tumors occur in the stomach. As will be discussed below, the term *stromal* reflects historical confusion about the origin of this tumor.

Epidemiology. Overall, GISTs are slightly more common in males. The peak age of GIST diagnosis in the stomach is approximately 60 years, with fewer than 10% occurring in individuals under 40 years of age. Of the uncommon GISTs in children, some are related to the *Carney triad*, a nonhereditary syndrome seen primarily in young females that includes

gastric GIST, paraganglioma, and pulmonary chondroma. There is also an increased incidence of GIST in individuals with neurofibromatosis type 1.[40]

Pathogenesis. Approximately *75% to 80% of all GISTs have oncogenic, gain-of-function mutations of the gene encoding the tyrosine kinase c-KIT,* which is the receptor for stem cell

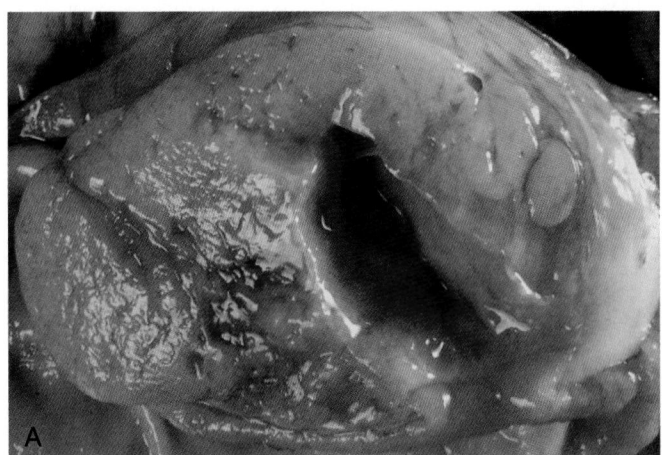
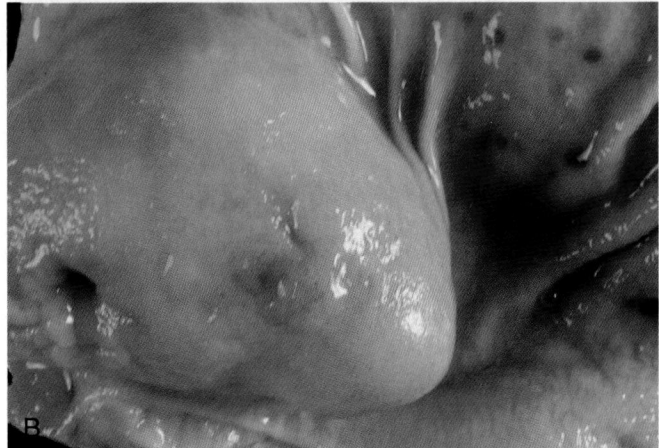
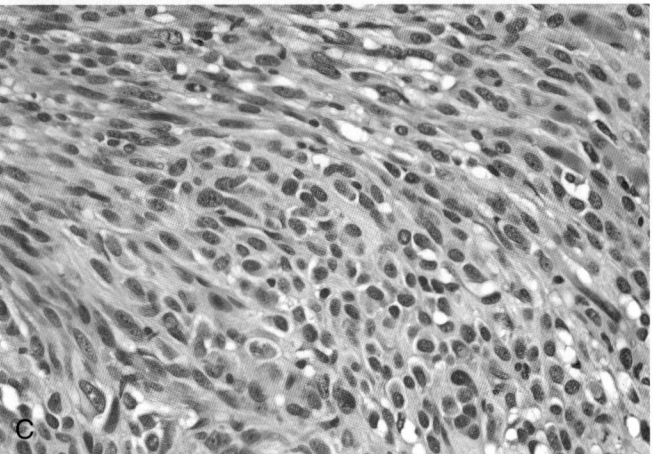

FIGURE 17–21 GI stromal tumor. **A,** On cross-section a whorled texture is evident within the white, fleshy tumor. **B,** The mass is covered by intact mucosa. **C,** Histologically the tumor is primarily composed of bundles, or fascicles, of spindle-shaped tumor cells. (Courtesy of Dr. Christopher Weber, The University of Chicago, Chicago, IL.)

factor. Approximately 8% of GISTs have mutations that activate a related tyrosine kinase, platelet-derived growth factor receptor α (PDGFRA).[41] In sporadic GISTs, *c-KIT* and *PDGFRA* gene mutations are mutually exclusive.[21] GISTs appear to arise from, or share a common stem cell with, the interstitial cells of Cajal, which are located in the muscularis propria and serve as pacemaker cells for gut peristalsis. Like GISTs, Cajal cells express c-KIT (also known as CD117) and CD34. Interestingly, familial GIST, which is rare, is associated with germline *c-KIT* or *PDGFRA* mutations; these patients, who develop multiple GISTs, may also have diffuse hyperplasia of Cajal cells.[42] Mutation of *c-KIT* or *PDGFRA* is an early event in sporadic GISTs and is detectable in lesions as small as 3 mm. The constitutively active c-KIT and PDGFRA receptor tyrosine kinases produce intracellular signals that activate the RAS and PI3K/AKT pathways and thereby promote tumor cell proliferation and survival.[21]

Morphology. Primary gastric GISTs can be quite large, as much as 30 cm in diameter. They usually form a solitary, well-circumscribed, fleshy mass (Fig. 17–21A) covered by ulcerated or intact mucosa (Fig. 17–21B), but can also project outward toward the serosa. Metastases may take the form of multiple serosal nodules throughout the peritoneal cavity or as one or more nodules in the liver; spread outside of the abdomen is uncommon. GISTs composed of thin elongated cells are classified as **spindle cell type** (Fig. 17–21C), whereas tumors dominated by epithelial-appearing cells are termed **epithelioid type**; mixtures of the two patterns also occur. The most useful diagnostic marker is c-KIT, which is immunohistochemically detectable in 95% of gastric GISTs.

Clinical Features. Symptoms of GISTs at presentation may be related to mass effects. Mucosal ulceration can cause blood loss, and approximately half of individuals with GIST present with anemia or related symptoms. GISTs may also be discovered as an incidental finding during radiologic imaging, endoscopy, or abdominal surgery performed for other reasons. Complete surgical resection is the primary treatment for localized gastric GIST. The prognosis correlates with tumor size, mitotic index, and location, *with gastric GISTs being somewhat less aggressive than those arising in the small intestine.* Recurrence or metastasis is rare for gastric GISTs under 5 cm but common for mitotically active tumors larger than 10 cm.

Patients with unresectable, recurrent, or metastatic disease often respond to *imatinib*, a tyrosine kinase inhibitor that inhibits c-KIT and PDGFRA, and is also effective in suppressing BCR-ABL kinase activity in chronic myeloid leukemia (Chapter 13).[43] Development of resistance to imatinib is most often related to secondary *c-KIT* mutations that limit drug efficacy.

SMALL INTESTINE AND COLON

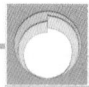

The small intestine and colon account for the majority of GI tract length and are the sites of a broad array of diseases. Some of these relate to nutrient and water transport. Perturbation of these processes can cause malabsorption and diarrhea. The intestines are also the principal site where the immune system interfaces with a diverse array of antigens present in food and gut microbes. Indeed, intestinal bacteria outnumber eukaryotic cells in our bodies by tenfold. Thus, it is not surprising that the small intestine and colon are frequently involved by infectious and inflammatory processes. Finally, the colon is the most common site of GI neoplasia in Western populations.

Intestinal Obstruction

Obstruction of the GI tract may occur at any level, but the small intestine is most often involved because of its relatively narrow lumen. Collectively, *hernias, intestinal adhesions, intussusception, and volvulus* account for 80% of mechanical obstructions (Fig. 17–22), while tumors and infarction account for only about 10% to 15% of small bowel obstructions. The clinical manifestations of intestinal obstruction include abdominal pain and distention, vomiting, and constipation.

Surgical intervention is usually required in cases of mechanical obstruction or severe infarction.

HERNIAS

Any weakness or defect in the wall of the peritoneal cavity may permit protrusion of a serosa-lined pouch of peritoneum called a *hernia sac*. Acquired hernias most commonly occur anteriorly, via the inguinal and femoral canals or umbilicus, or at sites of surgical scars. These are of concern because of visceral protrusion *(external herniation)*. This is particularly true of inguinal hernias, which tend to have narrow orifices and large sacs. Small bowel loops are involved most often, but portions of omentum or large bowel also protrude, and any of these may become entrapped. Pressure at the neck of the pouch may impair venous drainage of the entrapped viscus. The resultant stasis and edema increase the bulk of the herniated loop, leading to permanent entrapment, or *incarceration*, and, over time, arterial and venous compromise *(strangulation)* develops that can result in infarction (Fig. 17–23A).

ADHESIONS

Surgical procedures, infection, or other causes of peritoneal inflammation, such as endometriosis, may result in develop-

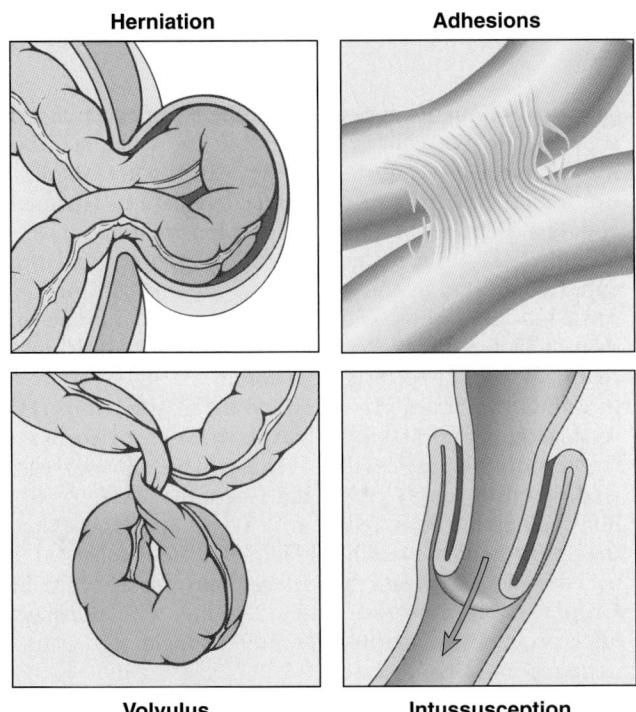

Herniation   **Adhesions**

Volvulus   **Intussusception**

FIGURE 17–22 Intestinal obstruction. The four major causes of intestinal obstruction are (1) herniation of a segment in the umbilical or inguinal regions, (2) adhesion between loops of intestine, (3) volvulus, and (4) intussusception.

ment of *adhesions* between bowel segments, the abdominal wall, and operative sites. These fibrous bridges can create closed loops through which other viscera may slide and become entrapped, resulting in *internal herniation*. Sequelae, including obstruction and strangulation, are much the same as with external hernias. Though rare, fibrous adhesions may be congenital, therefore, internal herniation must be considered even in the absence of a history of peritonitis or surgery.

VOLVULUS

Complete twisting of a loop of bowel about its mesenteric base of attachment is called *volvulus* and produces both luminal and vascular compromise. Thus, presentation includes features of obstruction and infarction. Volvulus occurs most often in large redundant loops of sigmoid colon, followed in frequency by the cecum, small bowel, stomach, or, rarely, transverse colon. Because it is rare, volvulus is often missed clinically.

INTUSSUSCEPTION

Intussusception occurs when a segment of the intestine, constricted by a wave of peristalsis, telescopes into the immediately distal segment. Once trapped, the invaginated segment is propelled by peristalsis and pulls the mesentery along. Untreated intussusception may progress to intestinal obstruction, compression of mesenteric vessels, and infarction.

When encountered in infants and children, there is usually no underlying anatomic defect and the patient is otherwise

healthy, although some cases are associated with rotavirus infection. In older children and adults an intraluminal mass or tumor generally serves as the point of traction that causes intussusception (Fig. 17–23B). Barium enema may effectively reduce the intussusception in infants and young children, but surgical intervention is usually necessary in older patients.

Ischemic Bowel Disease

The majority of the GI tract is supplied by the celiac, superior mesenteric, and inferior mesenteric arteries. As they approach the intestinal wall the superior and inferior mesenteric arteries ramify into the mesenteric arcades. Interconnections between arcades, as well as collateral supplies from the proximal celiac

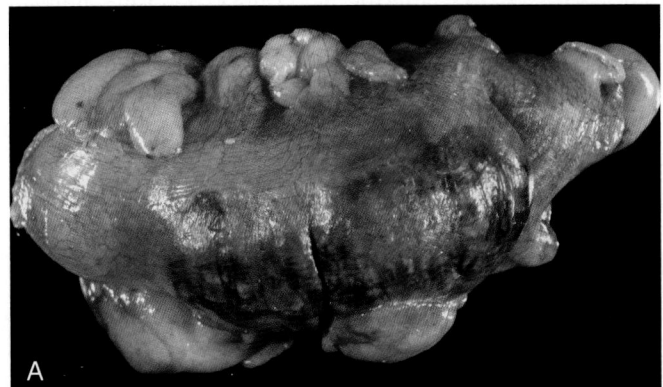

A

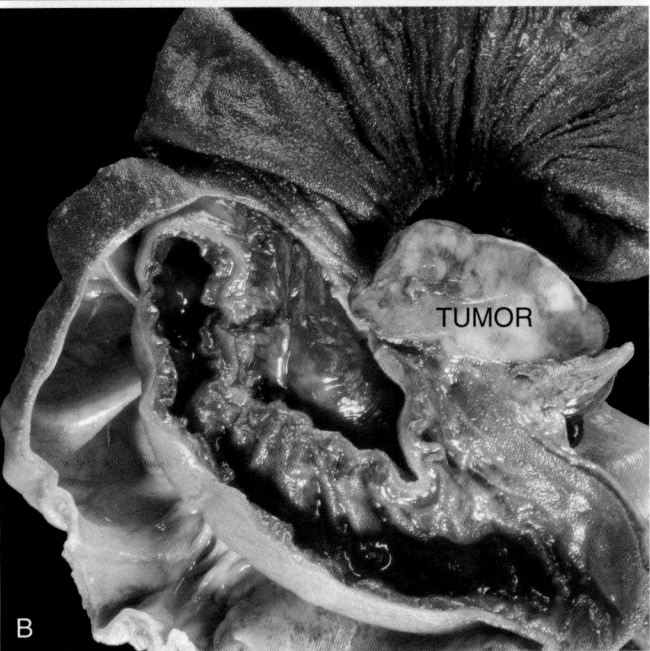

TUMOR

B

FIGURE 17–23 Intestinal obstruction. **A,** Portion of bowel incarcerated within an inguinal hernia. Note dusky serosa and hemorrhage that indicate ischemic damage. **B,** Intussusception caused by a tumor. The outermost layer of intestine with external serosa has been removed, leaving the mucosa of the second layer exposed. The serosa of the second layer is apposed to the serosa of the intussuscepted intestine. A tumor mass *(right, labelled* **tumor***)* is present at the leading edge of the intussusception. Compare to Figure 17–22. (**B,** Courtesy of Dr. Christopher Weber, The University of Chicago, Chicago, IL.)

and distal pudendal and iliac circulations, make it possible for the small intestine and colon to tolerate slowly progressive loss of the blood supply from one artery. In contrast, acute compromise of any major vessel can lead to infarction of several meters of intestine. Damage can range from *mucosal infarction,* extending no deeper than the muscularis mucosa; to *mural infarction* of mucosa and submucosa; to *transmural infarction* involving all three wall layers. While mucosal or mural infarctions are often secondary to acute or chronic *hypoperfusion,* transmural infarction is generally caused by acute vascular obstruction. Important causes of acute arterial obstruction include severe *atherosclerosis* (which is often prominent at the origin of mesenteric vessels), *aortic aneurysm, hypercoagulable states, oral contraceptive use,* and *embolization of cardiac vegetations or aortic atheromas.* Intestinal hypoperfusion can also be associated with *cardiac failure, shock, dehydration,* or *vasoconstrictive drugs.* Systemic *vasculitides,* such as polyarteritis nodosum, Henoch-Schönlein purpura, or Wegener granulomatosis, may also damage intestinal arteries. Mesenteric venous thrombosis, which can also lead to ischemic disease, is uncommon but can result from inherited or acquired hypercoagulable states, invasive neoplasms, cirrhosis, trauma, or abdominal masses that compress the portal drainage.

Pathogenesis. Intestinal responses to ischemia occur in two phases. The initial *hypoxic injury* occurs at the onset of vascular compromise. While some damage occurs during this phase, the epithelial cells lining the intestine are relatively resistant to transient hypoxia. The second phase, *reperfusion injury,* is initiated by restoration of the blood supply and it is at this time that the greatest damage occurs. In severe cases this may trigger multiorgan failure. While the underlying mechanisms of reperfusion injury are incompletely understood, they involve free radical production, neutrophil infiltration, and release of inflammatory mediators, such as complement proteins and TNF (Chapter 1). Activation of intracellular signaling molecules and transcription factors, including hypoxia-inducible factor 1 (HIF-1) and NF-κB, also contribute to intestinal ischemia-reperfusion injury.[44,45]

The severity of vascular compromise, the time frame during which it develops, and the vessels affected are the major variables in ischemic bowel disease. Two aspects of intestinal vascular anatomy also contribute to the distribution of ischemic damage.

○ Intestinal segments at the end of their respective arterial supplies are particularly susceptible to ischemia. These *watershed zones* include the splenic flexure, where the superior and inferior mesenteric arterial circulations terminate, and, to a lesser extent, the sigmoid colon and rectum where inferior mesenteric, pudendal, and iliac arterial circulations end. Generalized hypotension or hypoxemia can therefore cause localized injury, and ischemic disease should be considered in the differential diagnosis of focal colitis of the splenic flexure or rectosigmoid colon.

○ Intestinal capillaries run alongside the glands, from crypt to surface, before making a hairpin turn at the surface to empty into the post-capillary venules. This allows oxygenated blood to supply crypts but leaves the surface epithelium vulnerable to ischemic injury. This anatomy protects the crypts, which contain the epithelial stem cells that are necessary to repopulate the surface. Thus, surface epithelial atrophy, or even necrosis and sloughing, with normal or hyperproliferative crypts is a morphologic signature of ischemic intestinal disease.

Morphology. Despite the increased susceptibility of watershed zones, **mucosal and mural infarction** may involve any level of the gut from stomach to anus. The lesions may be continuous but are more often segmental and patchy (Fig. 17–24A). The mucosa is hemorrhagic and may be ulcerated and dark red or purple as a result of luminal hemorrhage (Fig. 17–24B). The bowel wall is also thickened by edema that may involve the mucosa or extend into the submucosa and muscularis propria. When severe, there is extensive mucosal and submucosal hemorrhage and necrosis, but serosal hemorrhage and serositis are generally absent.

Substantial portions of the bowel are generally involved in **transmural infarction** due to acute arterial obstruction. For reasons described above, the

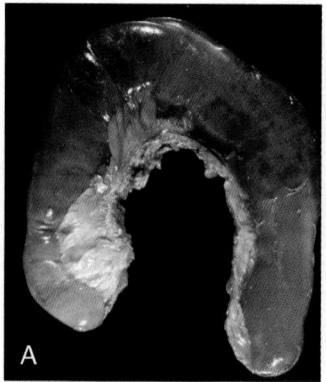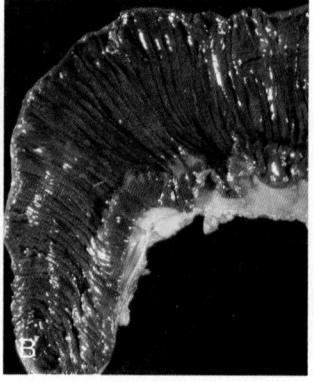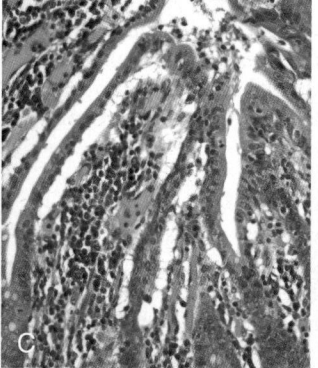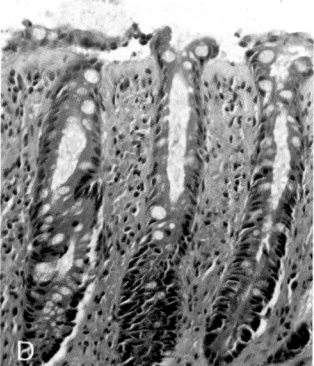

FIGURE 17–24   Ischemia. **A,** Jejunal resection with dusky serosa. **B,** Mucosa is stained with blood after hemorrhage. **C,** Characteristic attenuated villous epithelium in this case of acute jejunal ischemia. **D,** Chronic colonic ischemia with atrophic surface epithelium and fibrotic lamina propria.

splenic flexure is the site at greatest risk. The demarcation between normal and ischemic bowel is sharply defined and the infarcted bowel is initially intensely congested and dusky to purple-red. Later, blood-tinged mucus or frank blood accumulates in the lumen and the wall becomes edematous, thickened, and rubbery. There is coagulative necrosis of the muscularis propria within 1 to 4 days, and perforation may occur. Serositis, with purulent exudates and fibrin deposition, may be prominent.

In mesenteric venous thrombosis arterial blood continues to flow for a time, resulting in a less abrupt transition from affected to normal bowel. However, propagation of the thrombus may lead to secondary involvement of the splanchnic bed. The ultimate result is similar to that produced by acute arterial obstruction because impaired venous drainage eventually prevents oxygenated arterial blood from entering the capillaries.

Microscopic examination of ischemic intestine demonstrates **atrophy or sloughing of surface epithelium** (Fig. 17–24C). In contrast, crypts may be hyperproliferative. Inflammatory infiltrates are initially absent in acute ischemia, but neutrophils are recruited within hours of reperfusion. Chronic ischemia is accompanied by fibrous scarring of the lamina propria (Fig. 17–24D) and, uncommonly, stricture formation. In acute phases of ischemic damage bacterial superinfection and enterotoxin release may induce pseudomembrane formation that can resemble *Clostridium difficile*–associated pseudomembranous colitis (discussed later).

Clinical Features. Ischemic bowel disease tends to occur in older individuals with coexisting cardiac or vascular disease. Acute transmural infarction typically presents with sudden, severe abdominal pain and tenderness, sometimes accompanied by nausea, vomiting, bloody diarrhea, or grossly melanotic stool. Patients may progress to shock and vascular collapse within hours as a result of blood loss. Peristaltic sounds diminish or disappear, and muscular spasm creates board-like rigidity of the abdominal wall. Because these physical signs overlap with those of other abdominal emergencies, including acute appendicitis, perforated ulcer, and acute cholecystitis, the diagnosis of intestinal necrosis may be delayed or missed, with disastrous consequences. As the mucosal barrier breaks down, bacteria enter the circulation and sepsis can develop; mortality may exceed 50%. The overall progression of ischemic enteritis depends on the underlying cause and severity of injury.

○ *Mucosal and mural infarctions* by themselves may not be fatal. However, these may progress to more extensive infarction if the vascular supply is not restored by correction of the insult or, in chronic disease, by development of adequate collateral supplies. The diagnosis of nonocclusive ischemic enteritis and colitis can be particularly difficult because there may be a confusing array of nonspecific abdominal symptoms, including intermittent bloody diarrhea and intestinal pseudo-obstruction.

○ *Chronic ischemia* may masquerade as inflammatory bowel disease, with episodes of bloody diarrhea interspersed with periods of healing.

○ *CMV infection* causes ischemic GI disease due to the viral tropism for and infection of endothelial cells. CMV infection, which can be a complication of immunosuppressive therapy, is discussed further in Chapter 8.

○ *Radiation enterocolitis* occurs when the GI tract is irradiated. In addition to epithelial damage, radiation-induced vascular injury may be significant and produce changes that are similar to ischemic disease. In addition to clinical history, the presence of bizarre "radiation fibroblasts" within the stroma may provide an important clue to the etiology. Acute radiation enteritis manifests as anorexia, abdominal cramps, and a malabsorptive diarrhea, while chronic radiation enteritis or colitis is often more indolent and may present as an inflammatory colitis.

○ *Necrotizing enterocolitis* (NEC) is an acute disorder of the small and large intestines that can result in transmural necrosis. It is the most common acquired GI emergency of neonates, particularly those who are premature or of low birth weight, and occurs most often at the time of oral feeding. NEC is discussed in more detail in Chapter 10, but is noted here because ischemic injury is generally considered to contribute to the pathogenesis.

Angiodysplasia

Angiodysplasia is characterized by malformed submucosal and mucosal blood vessels. It occurs *most often in the cecum or right colon*, usually after the sixth decade of life. Although the prevalence of angiodysplasia is less than 1% in the adult population, *it accounts for 20% of major episodes of lower intestinal bleeding; intestinal hemorrhage may be chronic and intermittent or acute and massive.*

The pathogenesis of angiodysplasia remains undefined but has been attributed to mechanical and congenital factors. Normal distention and contraction may intermittently occlude the submucosal veins that penetrate through the muscularis propria and can lead to focal dilation and tortuosity of overlying submucosal and mucosal vessels. Because the cecum has the largest diameter of any colonic segment, it develops the greatest wall tension. This may explain the preferential distribution of angiodysplastic lesions in the cecum and right colon. Degenerative vascular changes related to aging may also have some role. Finally, some data link angiodysplasia with aortic stenosis and Meckel diverticulum, suggesting the possibility of a developmental component.

Lesions of angiodysplasia are ectatic nests of tortuous veins, venules, and capillaries. The vascular channels may be separated from the intestinal lumen by only the vascular wall and a layer of attenuated epithelial cells; limited injury may therefore result in significant hemorrhage.

Malabsorption and Diarrhea

Malabsorption, which presents most commonly as *chronic diarrhea*, is characterized by defective absorption of fats, fat- and water-soluble vitamins, proteins, carbohydrates, electro-

TABLE 17–6	Defects in Malabosorptive and Diarrheal Disease			
Disease	**Intraluminal Digestion**	**Terminal Digestion**	**Transepithelial Transport**	**Lymphatic Transport**
Celiac disease		+	+	
Tropical sprue		+	+	
Chronic pancreatitis	+			
Cystic fibrosis	+			
Primary bile acid malabsorption	+		+	
Carcinoid syndrome			+	
Autoimmune enteropathy		+	+	
Disaccharidase deficiency		+		
Whipple disease				+
Abetalipoproteinemia			+	
Viral gastroenteritis		+	+	
Bacterial gastroenteritis		+	+	
Parasitic gastroenteritis		+	+	
Inflammatory bowel disease	+	+	+	

+ indicates that the process is abnormal in the disease indicated. Other processes are not affected.

lytes and minerals, and water. Chronic malabsorption can be accompanied by weight loss, anorexia, abdominal distention, borborygmi, and muscle wasting. A hallmark of malabsorption is *steatorrhea*, characterized by excessive fecal fat and bulky, frothy, greasy, yellow or clay-colored stools. *The chronic malabsorptive disorders most commonly encountered in the United States are pancreatic insufficiency, celiac disease, and Crohn disease* (Table 17–6). Intestinal graft-versus-host disease is an important cause of malabsorption and diarrhea after allogeneic bone marrow transplantation.

Malabsorption results from disturbance in at least one of the four phases of nutrient absorption: (1) *intraluminal digestion*, in which proteins, carbohydrates, and fats are broken down into forms suitable for absorption; (2) *terminal digestion*, which involves the hydrolysis of carbohydrates and peptides by disaccharidases and peptidases, respectively, in the brush border of the small intestinal mucosa; (3) *transepithelial transport*, in which nutrients, fluid, and electrolytes are transported across and processed within the small intestinal epithelium; and (4) *lymphatic transport* of absorbed lipids.

In many malabsorptive disorders a defect in one of these processes predominates, but more than one usually contributes. As a result, malabsorption syndromes resemble each other more than they differ. General symptoms include *diarrhea* (from nutrient malabsorption and excessive intestinal secretion), *flatus*, *abdominal pain*, and *weight loss*. Inadequate absorption of vitamins and minerals can result in anemia and mucositis due to pyridoxine, folate, or vitamin B_{12} deficiency; bleeding, due to vitamin K deficiency; osteopenia and tetany due to calcium, magnesium, or vitamin D deficiencies; or peripheral neuropathy due to vitamin A or B_{12} deficiencies. A variety of endocrine and skin disturbances may also occur.

Diarrhea is defined as an increase in stool mass, frequency, or fluidity, typically greater than 200 g per day. In severe cases

stool volume can exceed 14 L per day and, without fluid resuscitation, result in death. Painful, bloody, small-volume diarrhea is known as *dysentery*. Diarrhea can be classified according to four major categories:

- *Secretory diarrhea* is characterized by isotonic stool and persists during fasting.
- *Osmotic diarrhea*, such as that which occurs with lactase deficiency, is due to the excessive osmotic forces exerted by unabsorbed luminal solutes. The diarrhea fluid is over 50 mOsm more concentrated than plasma and abates with fasting.
- *Malabsorptive diarrhea* follows generalized failures of nutrient absorption and is associated with steatorrhea and is relieved by fasting.
- *Exudative diarrhea* is due to inflammatory disease and characterized by purulent, bloody stools that continue during fasting.

CYSTIC FIBROSIS

Cystic fibrosis is discussed in greater detail elsewhere (Chapter 10). Only the malabsorption associated with cystic fibrosis is considered here. Due to the absence of the epithelial cystic fibrosis transmembrane conductance regulator (CFTR), individuals with cystic fibrosis have defects in intestinal chloride ion secretion. This interferes with bicarbonate, sodium, and water secretion, ultimately resulting in defective luminal hydration. Formation of intraductal concretions can begin in utero, leading to duct obstruction, low-grade chronic autodigestion of the pancreas, and eventual *exocrine pancreatic insufficiency in more than 80% of patients*. The result is failure of the intraluminal phase of nutrient absorption, which can be effectively treated in most patients with oral enzyme supplementation.

CELIAC DISEASE

Celiac disease is also known as *celiac sprue* or *gluten-sensitive enteropathy*. It is an immune-mediated enteropathy triggered by the ingestion of gluten-containing cereals, such as wheat, rye, or barley, in genetically predisposed individuals. In countries where most people are Caucasians of European ancestry, celiac disease is a common disorder, with an estimated prevalence of 0.5% to 1%.

Pathogenesis. Celiac disease is a unique intestinal immune disorder because the environmental precipitant, *gluten*, is known. Gluten is the major storage protein of wheat and similar grains, and the alcohol-soluble fraction of gluten, *gliadin*, contains most of the disease-producing components. Gluten is digested by luminal and brush-border enzymes into amino acids and peptides, including a 33–amino acid α-gliadin peptide that is resistant to degradation by gastric, pancreatic, and small intestinal proteases (Fig. 17–25). The network of immune reactions to gliadin that are thought to result in celiac disease is illustrated below. Some gliadin peptides induce epithelial cells to express IL-15, which in turn triggers activation and proliferation of CD8+ intraepithelial lymphocytes that are induced to express NKG2D, a natural killer cell marker. These lymphocytes become cytotoxic and kill enterocytes with surface MIC-A, an HLA class I–like protein expressed in response to stress. NKG2D is the receptor for MIC-A. Thus, unlike the CD4+ T cells, these NKG2D+ CD8+ T cells do not recognize gliadin. The resulting epithelial damage may contribute to the process by which other gliadin peptides cross the epithelium to be deamidated by tissue transglutaminase. Deamidated gliadin peptides are then able to interact with HLA-DQ2 or HLA-DQ8 on antigen-presenting cells and be presented to CD4+ T cells. These T cells produce cytokines that contribute to tissue damage and the characteristic mucosal pathology.

While nearly all people eat grain and are exposed to gluten and gliadin, most do not develop celiac disease. Thus, host factors determine whether disease develops. Among these, HLA proteins seem to be critical, since almost all people with celiac disease carry the class II HLA-DQ2 or HLA-DQ8 allele. However, the HLA locus accounts for less than half of the genetic component of celiac disease. Remaining genetic factors may include polymorphisms of immune-regulatory genes, such as those encoding IL-2, IL-21, CCR3, and SH2B3,[46] and genes that determine epithelial polarity.[47,48] There is also an association of celiac disease with other immune diseases including type 1 diabetes, thyroiditis, and Sjögren syndrome, as well as ataxia, autism, depression, some forms of epilepsy, IgA nephropathy, Down syndrome, and Turner syndrome.

Morphology. Biopsy specimens from the second portion of the duodenum or proximal jejunum, which are exposed to the highest concentrations of dietary gluten, are generally diagnostic in celiac disease. The histopathology is characterized by increased numbers of intraepithelial CD8+ T lymphocytes (**intraepithelial lymphocytosis**), **crypt hyperplasia**, and **villous atrophy** (Fig. 17–26). This loss of mucosal and brush-border surface area probably accounts for the malabsorption. In addition, increased rates of epithelial turnover, reflected in increased crypt mitotic activity, may limit the ability of absorptive enterocytes to fully differentiate and contribute to defects in terminal digestion and transepithelial transport. Other features of fully developed celiac disease include increased numbers of plasma cells, mast cells, and eosinophils, especially within the upper part of the lamina propria. With increased frequency of serologic screening and early detection of disease-associated antibodies, it is now appreciated that an increase in the number of intraepithelial lymphocytes, particularly within the

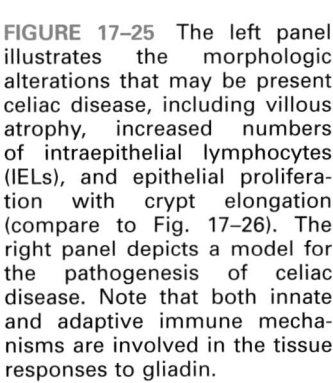

FIGURE 17–25 The left panel illustrates the morphologic alterations that may be present celiac disease, including villous atrophy, increased numbers of intraepithelial lymphocytes (IELs), and epithelial proliferation with crypt elongation (compare to Fig. 17–26). The right panel depicts a model for the pathogenesis of celiac disease. Note that both innate and adaptive immune mechanisms are involved in the tissue responses to gliadin.

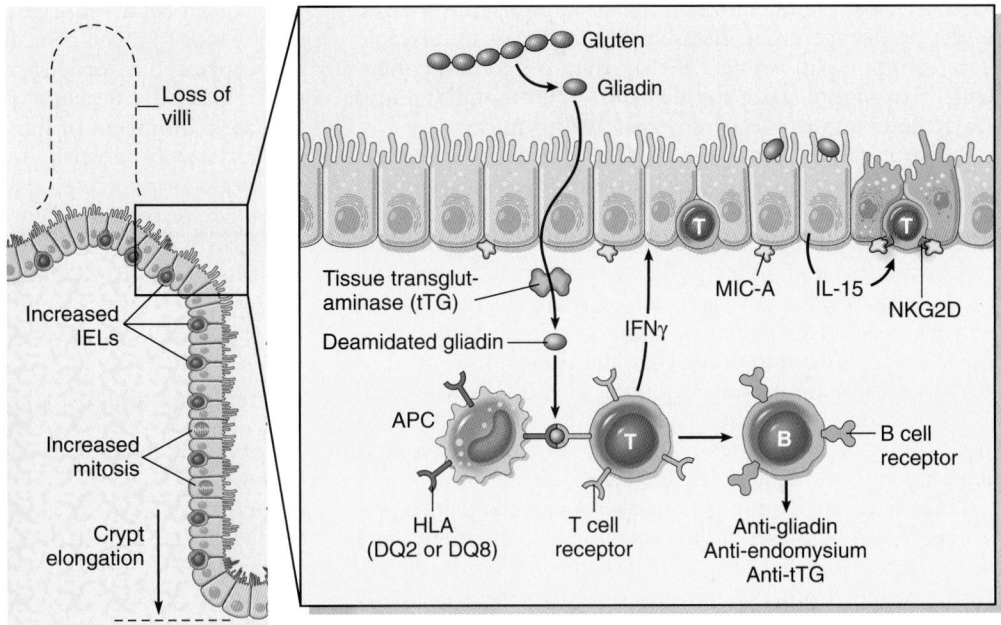

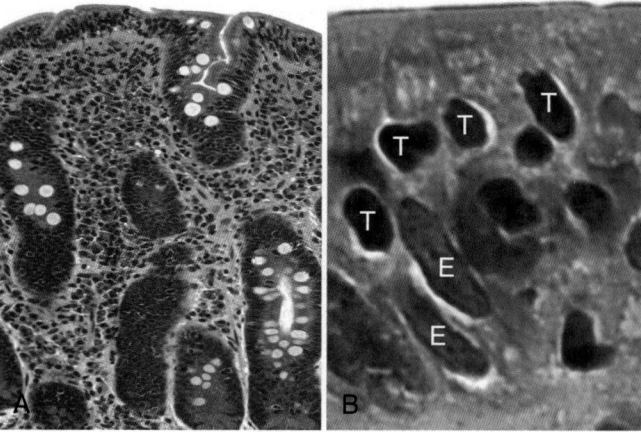

FIGURE 17–26 Celiac disease. **A,** Advanced cases of celiac disease show complete loss of villi, or total villous atrophy. Note the dense plasma cell infiltrates in the lamina propria. **B,** Infiltration of the surface epithelium by T lymphocytes, which can be recognized by their densely stained nuclei (labelled **T**). Compare to elongated, pale-staining epithelial nuclei (labelled **E**).

villus, is a marker of less advanced celiac disease.[49] However, intraepithelial lymphocytosis and villous atrophy are not specific for celiac disease and can be present in other diseases, including viral enteritis. The combination of histology and serology is most specific for diagnosis of celiac disease.

Clinical Features. In adults, celiac disease presents most commonly between the ages of 30 and 60. However, many cases escape clinical attention for extended periods because of atypical presentations. Some patients may have *silent* celiac disease, defined as positive serology and villous atrophy without symptoms, or *latent* celiac disease, in which positive serology is not accompanied by villous atrophy. Symptomatic adult celiac disease is often associated with anemia, chronic diarrhea, bloating, or chronic fatigue. Although there is no gender preference, celiac disease is detected two- to threefold more commonly in women, perhaps because monthly menstrual bleeding increases the demand for iron and vitamins and accentuates the effects of impaired absorption.

Pediatric celiac disease, which affects males and females equally, may present with malabsorption or atypical symptoms affecting almost any organ.[50] In those with *classic symptoms*, disease typically begins between ages of 6 and 24 months, after introduction of gluten to the diet, and includes irritability, abdominal distention, anorexia, chronic diarrhea, failure to thrive, weight loss, or muscle wasting.[50] Children with *nonclassic symptoms* tend to present at older ages with complaints of abdominal pain, nausea, vomiting, bloating, or constipation. Common extra-intestinal complaints include arthritis or joint pain, seizure disorders, aphthous stomatitis, iron deficiency anemia, pubertal delay, and short stature.

A characteristic itchy, blistering skin lesion, *dermatitis herpetiformis*, can be present in as many as 10% of patients, and the incidence of *lymphocytic gastritis* and *lymphocytic colitis* is also increased. Unfortunately, the only treatment currently available for celiac disease is a *gluten-free diet*, but, despite the

challenges of adhering to this diet, it does result in symptomatic improvement for most patients. A gluten-free diet may also reduce the risk of long-term complications including anemia, female infertility, osteoporosis, and cancer.

Noninvasive serologic tests are generally performed prior to biopsy.[51] The most sensitive tests are the presence of IgA antibodies to tissue transglutaminase or IgA or IgG antibodies to deamidated gliadin. Anti-endomysial antibodies are highly specific but less sensitive than other antibodies. In cases with negative IgA tests, IgA deficiency, which is more common in celiac patients, should be ruled out. If IgA deficiency is present, titers of IgG antibodies to tissue transglutaminase and deamidated gliadin should be measured. The absence of HLA-DQ2 or HLA-DQ8 is useful for its high negative predictive value, but the presence of these alleles is not helpful in confirming the diagnosis.

Individuals with celiac disease have a higher than normal rate of malignancy. The most common celiac disease–associated cancer is *enteropathy-associated T-cell lymphoma*, an aggressive lymphoma of intraepithelial T lymphocytes. *Small intestinal adenocarcinoma* is also more frequent in individuals with celiac disease. Thus, when symptoms such as abdominal pain, diarrhea, and weight loss develop despite a strict gluten-free diet, cancer or *refractory sprue*, in which the response to a gluten-free diet is lost, must be considered. It is, however, important to remember that failure to adhere to a gluten-free diet is the most common cause of recurrent symptoms, and that most people with celiac disease do well with dietary restrictions and die of unrelated causes.

TROPICAL SPRUE

Tropical sprue is a malabsorption syndrome that occurs almost exclusively in people living in or visiting the tropics, including Puerto Rico, the Caribbean, northern South America, West Africa, India, and Southeast Asia. Inexplicably, it is uncommon in Jamaica. The disease is generally endemic, although epidemics have occurred.

Histologic changes of tropical sprue are similar to celiac disease, but total villous atrophy is uncommon, and tropical sprue tends to involve the distal small bowel. The latter probably explains the frequency of folate or vitamin B_{12} deficiencies with enlarged (megaloblastic) nuclei within epithelial cells that are reminiscent of those seen in pernicious anemia.

Malabsorption usually becomes apparent within days or a few weeks of an acute diarrheal enteric infection in visitors. Although no definite causal organism has been identified, overgrowth of aerobic enteric bacteria has been documented, and broad-spectrum antibiotics usually effect rapid recovery. Various infections, including *Cyclospora* or enterotoxigenic bacteria, have been suggested as etiologic factors.

AUTOIMMUNE ENTEROPATHY

Autoimmune enteropathy is an X-linked disorder characterized by severe persistent diarrhea and autoimmune disease that occurs most often in young children. A particularly severe familial form, termed *IPEX*, an acronym denoting immune dysregulation, polyendocrinopathy, enteropathy, and X-linkage, is due to a germline mutation in the *FOXP3* gene, which is located on the X chromosome.[52] FOXP3 is a transcription factor expressed in CD4+ regulatory T cells,[53] and individuals with IPEX and *FOXP3* mutations have defective T-regulatory function. Other defects in regulatory T cell function have also been linked to less severe forms of autoimmune enteropathy. Autoantibodies to enterocytes and goblet cells are common, and some patients may have antibodies to parietal or islet cells. Within the small intestine intraepithelial lymphocytes may be increased, but not to the extent seen in celiac disease, and neutrophils are often present. Therapy includes immunosuppressive drugs such as cyclosporine and, in rare cases, bone marrow transplantation.[54]

LACTASE (DISACCHARIDASE) DEFICIENCY

The disaccharidases, including lactase, are located in the apical brush-border membrane of the villus absorptive epithelial cells. Because the defect is biochemical, biopsy histology is generally unremarkable. Lactase deficiency is of two types:

○ *Congenital lactase deficiency*, caused by a mutation in the gene encoding lactase,[55] is an autosomal recessive disorder. The disease is rare and presents as explosive diarrhea with watery, frothy stools and abdominal distention upon milk ingestion. Symptoms abate when exposure to milk and milk products is terminated, thus removing the osmotically active but unabsorbable lactose from the lumen.
○ *Acquired lactase deficiency* is caused by down-regulation of lactase gene expression and is particularly common among Native Americans, African-Americans, and Chinese populations. Disease presents after childhood, perhaps reflecting the fact that, before farming of dairy animals, lactase was unnecessary after children stopped drinking mothers' milk. Onset of acquired lactose deficiency is sometimes associated with enteric viral or bacterial infections. Symptoms, including abdominal fullness, diarrhea, and flatulence, due to fermentation of the unabsorbed sugars by colonic bacteria, are triggered by ingestion of lactose-containing dairy products.

ABETALIPOPROTEINEMIA

Abetalipoproteinemia is a rare autosomal recessive disease characterized by an inability to secrete triglyceride-rich lipoproteins. It is caused by a mutation in the *microsomal triglyceride transfer protein* (MTP) that catalyzes transport of triglycerides, cholesterol esters, and phospholipids. MTP-deficient enterocytes are unable to export lipoproteins and free fatty acids. As a result, monoglycerides cannot be assembled into chylomicrons and triglycerides accumulate within the epithelial cells. The malabsorption of abetalipoproteinemia is therefore a failure of transepithelial transport. Lipid vacuolization of small intestinal epithelial cells is evident under the light microscope and can be highlighted by special stains, such as oil red-O, particularly after a fatty meal.

Abetalipoproteinemia presents in infancy and the clinical picture is dominated by failure to thrive, diarrhea, and steatorrhea. Patients also have a complete absence of all plasma lipoproteins containing apolipoprotein B, although the gene that encodes apolipoprotein B itself is not affected. Failure to absorb essential fatty acids leads to deficiencies of fat-soluble vitamins as well as lipid membrane defects that can be recognized by the presence of acanthocytic red cells (burr cells) in peripheral blood smears.

Infectious Enterocolitis

Enterocolitis can present with a broad range of symptoms including diarrhea, abdominal pain, urgency, perianal discomfort, incontinence, and hemorrhage (Table 17–7). This global problem is responsible for more than 12,000 deaths per day among children in developing countries and half of all deaths before age 5 worldwide. Bacterial infections, such as enterotoxigenic *Escherichia coli*, are frequently responsible, but the most common pathogens vary with age, nutrition, and host immune status as well as environmental influences (Table 17–7). For example, epidemics of cholera are common in areas with poor sanitation, as a result of inadequate public health measures, or as a consequence of natural disasters or war. Pediatric infectious diarrhea, which may result in severe dehydration and metabolic acidosis, is commonly caused by enteric viruses.

CHOLERA

Vibrio cholerae are comma-shaped, Gram-negative bacteria that cause cholera, a disease that has been endemic in the Ganges Valley of India and Bangladesh for all of recorded history. Since 1817, seven great pandemics have spread along trade routes to large parts of Europe, Australia, and the Americas,[56] but, for unknown reasons these pandemics resolved and cholera retreated back to the Ganges Valley. Cholera also persists within the Gulf of Mexico.

V. cholerae is primarily transmitted by contaminated drinking water. However, it can also be present in food and causes sporadic cases of seafood-associated disease in North America. There is a marked seasonal variation in most climates due to rapid growth of *Vibrio* bacteria at warm temperatures; the only animal reservoirs are shellfish and plankton. Relatively few *V. cholerae* serotypes are pathogenic, but other species of *Vibrio* can also cause disease. For example, *V. parahaemolyticus* is the most common cause of seafood-associated gastroenteritis in North America.[57]

Pathogenesis. Despite the severe diarrhea, *Vibrio* organisms are non-invasive and remain within the intestinal lumen. A *preformed enterotoxin*, cholera toxin, encoded by a virulence phage and released by the *Vibrio* organism, causes disease, but flagellar proteins, which are involved in motility and attachment, are necessary for efficient bacterial colonization. Hemagglutinin, a metalloproteinase, is important for bacterial detachment and shedding in the stool. The mechanism by which cholera toxin induces diarrhea is well understood (Fig. 17–27). Cholera toxin is composed of five B subunits and a single A subunit. The B subunit binds GM1 ganglioside on the surface of intestinal epithelial cells, and is carried by endocytosis to the endoplasmic reticulum, a process called *retrograde transport*.[58] Here, the A subunit is reduced by protein disulfide isomerase, and a fragment of the A subunit is unfolded and released. This peptide fragment is then transported into the cytosol using host cell machinery that moves misfolded proteins from the endoplasmic reticulum to the cytosol. Such unfolded proteins are normally disposed of via the proteasome, but the A subunit refolds to avoid degradation. The refolded A

TABLE 17-7 Features of Bacterial Enterocolitides

Infection Type	Geography	Reservoir	Transmission	Epidemiology	Affected GI Sites	Symptoms	Complications
Cholera	India, Africa	Shellfish	Fecal-oral, water	Sporadic, endemic, epidemic	Small intestine	Severe watery diarrhea	Dehydration, electrolyte imbalances
***Campylobacter* spp.**	Developed countries	Chickens, sheep, pigs, cattle	Poultry, milk, other foods	Sporadic; children, travelers	Colon	Watery or bloody diarrhea	Arthritis, Guillain-Barré syndrome
Shigellosis	Developing countries	Humans	Fecal-oral, food, water	Children	Left colon, ileum	Bloody diarrhea	Reiter syndrome, hemolytic-uremic syndrome
Salmonellosis	Worldwide	Poultry, farm animals, reptiles	Meat, poultry, eggs, milk	Children, elderly	Colon and small intestine	Watery or bloody diarrhea	Sepsis, abscess
Enteric (typhoid) fever	India, Mexico, Phillipines	Humans	Fecal-oral, water	Children, adolescents, travelers	Small intestine	Bloody diarrhea, fever	Chronic infection, carrier state, encephalopathy, myocarditis
***Yersinia* spp.**	Northern and central Europe	Pigs	Pork, milk, water	Clustered cases	Ileum, appendix, right colon	Abdominal pain, fever, diarrhea	Autoimmune, e.g., Reiter syndrome
Escherichia coli							
Enterotoxigenic (ETEC)	Developing countries	Unknown	Food or fecal-oral	Infants, adolescents, travelers	Small intestine	Severe watery diarrhea	Dehydration, electrolyte imbalances
Enterohemorrhagic (EHEC)	Worldwide	Widespread, includes cattle	Beef, milk, produce	Sporadic and epidemic	Colon	Bloody diarrhea	Hemolytic-uremic syndrome
Enteroinvasive (EIEC)	Developing countries	Unknown	Cheese, other foods, water	Young children	Colon	Bloody diarrhea	Unknown
Enteroaggregative (EAEC)	Worldwide	Unknown	Unknown	Children, adults, travelers	Colon	Nonbloody diarrhea, afebrile	Poorly defined
Pseudomembranous colitis (*C. difficile*)	Developing countries	Humans, hospitals	Antibiotics allow emergence	Immunosuppressed, antibiotic-treated	Colon	Watery diarrhea, fever	Relapse
Whipple disease	Rural > urban	Unknown	Unknown	Rare	Small intestine	Malabsorption	Arthritis, CNS disease
Mycobacterial infection	Worldwide	Unknown	Unknown	Immunosuppressed	Small intestine	Malabsorption	Pneumonia, infection at other sites

CNS, central nervous system; GI, gastrointestinal.

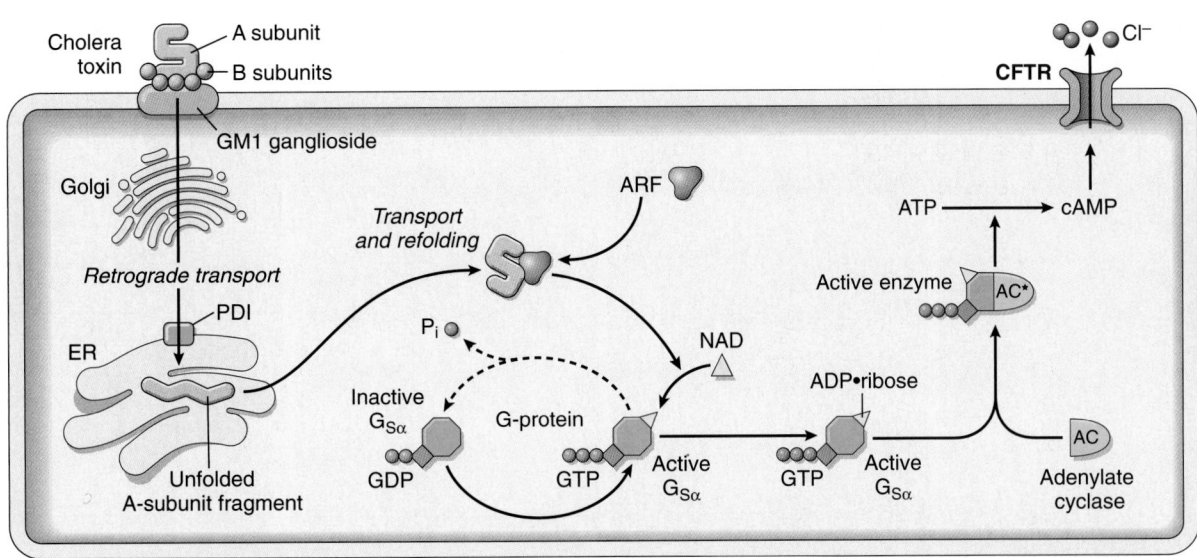

FIGURE 17–27 Mechanisms of cholera toxin transport and signaling. After retrograde toxin transport to the endoplasmic reticulum (ER), the A subunit is released by the action of protein disulfide isomerase (PDI) and is then able to access the epithelial cell cytoplasm. In concert with an ADP-ribosylation factor (ARF), the A subunit then ADP-ribosylates $G_{s\alpha}$, which locks it in the active, GTP-bound state. This leads to adenylate cyclase (AC) activation, and the cAMP produced opens CFTR to drive chloride secretion and diarrhea.

subunit peptide then interacts with cytosolic ADP ribosylation factors (ARFs) to ribosylate and activate the stimulatory G protein $G_{s\alpha}$. This stimulates adenylate cyclase and the resulting increases in intracellular cAMP open the cystic fibrosis transmembrane conductance regulator, CFTR, which releases chloride ions into the lumen. This causes secretion of bicarbonate, sodium, and water, leading to massive diarrhea. Chloride and sodium absorption are also inhibited by cAMP. Remarkably, mucosal biopsies show only minimal alterations.

Clinical Features. Most exposed individuals are asymptomatic or develop only mild diarrhea. In those with severe disease there is an abrupt onset of watery diarrhea and vomiting following an incubation period of 1 to 5 days. The voluminous stools resemble rice water and are sometimes described as having a fishy odor. The rate of diarrhea may reach 1 liter per hour, leading to dehydration, hypotension, muscular cramping, anuria, shock, loss of consciousness, and death. Most deaths occur within the first 24 hours after presentation. Although the mortality for severe cholera is about 50% without treatment, timely fluid replacement can save more than 99% of patients. Oral rehydration is often sufficient.[59] Because of an improved understanding of the host and *Vibrio* proteins involved, new therapies are being developed including CFTR inhibitors that block chloride secretion and prevent diarrhea.[60] Prophylactic vaccination is a long-term goal.[61]

CAMPYLOBACTER ENTEROCOLITIS

Campylobacter jejuni is the most common bacterial enteric pathogen in developed countries[57] and is an important cause of traveler's diarrhea. Most infections are associated with ingestion of improperly cooked chicken, but outbreaks can also be caused by unpasteurized milk or contaminated water.

Pathogenesis. The pathogenesis of *Campylobacter* infection remains poorly defined, but four major virulence properties contribute: motility, adherence, toxin production, and

invasion. Flagella allow *Campylobacter* to be motile. This facilitates adherance and colonization, which are necessary for mucosal invasion. Cytotoxins that cause epithelial damage and a cholera toxin–like enterotoxin are also released by some *C. jejuni* isolates. *Dysentery* is generally associated with invasion and only occurs with a small minority of *Campylobacter* strains. *Enteric fever* occurs when bacteria proliferate within the lamina propria and mesenteric lymph nodes.

Campylobacter infection can result in reactive arthritis, primarily in patients with HLA-B27. Other extra-intestinal complications, including erythema nodosum and Guillain-Barré syndrome, a flaccid paralysis caused by autoimmune-induced inflammation of peripheral nerves, are not HLA-linked.[62] Molecular mimicry has been implicated in the pathogenesis of Guillain-Barré syndrome, as serum antibodies to *C. jejuni* lipopolysaccharide cross-react with peripheral and central nervous system gangliosides. Moreover, 15% to 50% of individuals with Guillain-Barré syndrome have positive stool cultures or circulating antibodies to *Campylobacter*.[63] Fortunately, Guillain-Barré syndrome develops in 0.1% or less of those infected with *Campylobacter*.

Morphology. *Campylobacter* are comma-shaped, flagellated, Gram-negative organisms. Diagnosis is primarily by stool culture, since biopsy findings are nonspecific, and reveal **acute self-limited colitis** with features common to many forms of infectious colitis.[64] Mucosal and intraepithelial neutrophil infiltrates are prominent, particularly within the superficial mucosa (Fig. 17–28A); **cryptitis** (neutrophil infiltration of the crypts) and **crypt abscesses** (crypts with accumulations of luminal neutrophils) may also be present. Importantly, crypt architecture is preserved (Fig. 17–28D), although this can be difficult to assess in cases with severe mucosal damage.

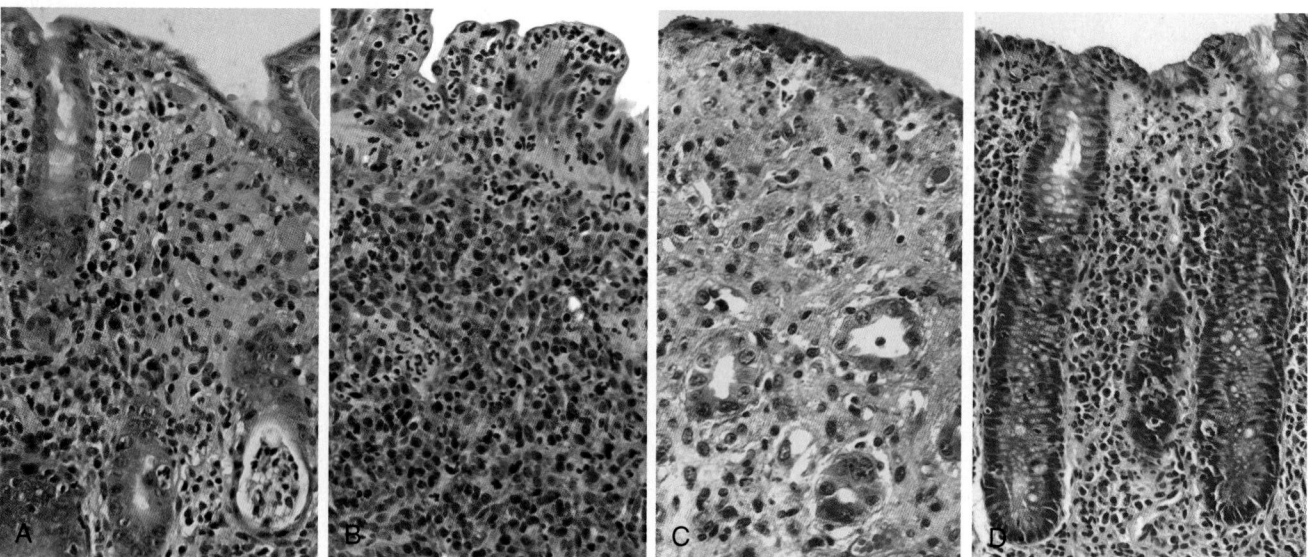

FIGURE 17–28 Bacterial enterocolitis. **A,** *Campylobacter jejuni* infection produces acute, self-limited colitis. Neutrophils can be seen within surface and crypt epithelium and a crypt abscess is present at the *lower right*. **B,** In *Yersinia* infection the surface epithelium can be eroded by neutrophils and the lamina propria is densely infiltrated by sheets of plasma cells admixed with lymphocytes and neutrophils. **C,** Enterohemorrhagic *E. coli* O157:H7 results in an ischemia-like morphology with surface atrophy and erosion. **D,** Enteroinvasive *E. coli* infection is a similar to other acute, self-limited colitides. Note the maintenance of normal crypt architecture and spacing, despite abundant intraepithelial neutrophils.

Clinical Features. Ingestion of as few as 500 *C. jejuni* organisms can cause disease after an incubation period of up to 8 days. Watery diarrhea, either acute or following an influenza-like prodrome, is the primary symptom, and dysentery develops in 15% of patients. Patients may shed bacteria for 1 month or more after clinical resolution. Antibiotic therapy is generally not required.

SHIGELLOSIS

Shigella are Gram-negative bacilli that were initially isolated during the Japanese red diarrhea epidemic of 1897. Four major strains are now recognized. *Shigella* are unencapsulated, nonmotile, facultative anaerobes that belong to the Enterobacteriaceae and are closely related to *enteroinvasive E. coli*. Although humans are the only known reservoir, *Shigella* spp. remain one of the most common causes of bloody diarrhea. It is estimated that 165 million cases occur worldwide each year.[65] Given the *infective dose of fewer than several hundred organisms* and the presence of as many as 10^9 organisms in each gram of stool during acute disease, *Shigella* are highly transmissible by the fecal-oral route or via contaminated water and food.

In the United States and Europe, children in daycare centers, migrant workers, travelers to developing countries, and those in nursing homes are most commonly affected.[66,67] Most *Shigella* infections and deaths occur in children under 5 years of age, and in countries where *Shigella* is endemic it is responsible for approximately 10% of all pediatric diarrheal disease and as many as 75% of diarrheal deaths.[65,68]

Pathogenesis. *Shigella* are resistant to the harsh acidic environment of the stomach, which translates into an extremely low infective dose. Once in the intestine, organisms are taken up by M, or microfold, epithelial cells, which are specialized for sampling and presentation of luminal antigens. *Shigella* prolif-

erate intracellularly, escape into the lamina propria, and are phagocytosed by macrophages, in which they induce apoptosis. The ensuing inflammatory process damages surface epithelia and allows *Shigella* within the intestinal lumen to gain access to the colonocyte basolateral membrane, which is the only surface through which infection can occur in epithelial cells (other than M cells). All *Shigella* spp. carry virulence plasmids, some of which encode a type III secretion system capable of directly injecting bacterial proteins into the host cytoplasm. *S. dysenteriae* serotype 1 also release the Shiga toxin Stx, which inhibits eukaryotic protein synthesis resulting in host cell damage and death.[69]

Morphology. *Shigella* infections are most prominent in the left colon, but the ileum may also be involved, perhaps reflecting the abundance of M cells in the dome epithelium over the Peyer's patches. The mucosa is hemorrhagic and ulcerated, and pseudomembranes may be present. The histology of early cases is similar to other acute self-limited colitides, such as *Campylobacter* colitis, but because of the tropism for M cells, aphthous-appearing ulcers similar to those seen in Crohn disease may occur. The potential for confusion with chronic inflammatory bowel disease is significant, particularly if there is distortion of crypt architecture.

Clinical Features. After an incubation period of as long as 4 days, *Shigella* causes self-limited disease characterized by about 6 days of diarrhea, fever, and abdominal pain. The initially watery diarrhea progresses to a dysenteric phase in approximately 50% of patients, and constitutional symptoms can persist for as long as 1 month. The subacute presentation that develops in a minority of adults is characterized by several weeks of waxing and waning diarrhea that can mimic new-onset ulcerative colitis.[68] While duration is typically shorter in children, severity is often much greater. Confirmation of *Shigella* infection requires stool culture.

Complications of *Shigella* infection are uncommon and include *Reiter syndrome*, a triad of sterile arthritis, urethritis, and conjunctivitis that preferentially affects HLA-B27-positive men between 20 and 40 years of age. Hemolytic-uremic syndrome, which is typically associated with *enterohemorrhagic E. coli* (EHEC), may also occur after infection with *S. dysenteriae* serotype 1 that secrete Shiga toxin[69–71]; only *Shigella* organisms that secrete the toxin are associated with hemolytic-uremic syndrome (Chapter 20). Antibiotic treatment shortens the clinical course and reduces the duration over which organisms are shed in the stool, but antidiarrheal medications are contraindicated because they can prolong symptoms and delay *Shigella* clearance.

SALMONELLOSIS

Salmonella, which are classified within the Enterobacteriaceae family of Gram-negative bacilli, are divided into *Salmonella typhi*, the causative agent of typhoid fever (discussed in the next section) and nontyphoid *Salmonella*. Nontyphoid *Salmonella* infection is usually due to *S. enteritidis*; more than 1 million cases occur each year in the United States, and the prevalence is even greater in other countries. Infection is most common in young children and the elderly, with peak incidence in summer and fall. Transmission is usually through contaminated food, particularly raw or undercooked meat, poultry, eggs, and milk.

Pathogenesis. Very few viable *Salmonella* are necessary to cause infection, and the absence of gastric acid, as in individuals with atrophic gastritis or those on acid-suppressive therapy, further reduces the required inoculum. *Salmonella* possess *virulence genes that encode a type III secretion system* capable of transferring bacterial proteins into M cells and enterocytes. The transferred proteins activate host cell Rho GTPases, thereby triggering actin rearrangement and bacterial uptake that allow bacterial growth within phagosomes. In addition, *flagellin*, the core protein of bacterial flagellae, activates TLR5 on host cells and increases the local inflammatory response.[72] Similarly, bacterial *lipopolysaccharide* activates TLR4, although some *Salmonella* strains express a virulence factor that prevents TLR4 activation from occurring. *Salmonella* also secrete a molecule that induces epithelial release of the eicosanoid hepoxilin A3, thereby drawing neutrophils into the intestinal lumen and potentiating mucosal damage.[73] Mucosal T_H17 immune responses limit infection to the colon.

> **Morphology.** The gross and microscopic features of *Salmonella* enteritis are non-specific and are similar to the acute self-limited colitis of *Campylobacter* and *Shigella*. Stool cultures are essential for diagnosis.

Clinical Features. *Salmonella* infections are clinically indistinguishable from those caused by other enteric pathogens, and symptoms range from loose stools to cholera-like profuse diarrhea to dysentery. Fever often resolves within

2 days, but diarrhea can persist for a week and organisms can be shed in the stool for several weeks after resolution. Antibiotic therapy is not recommended in most cases, because it can prolong the carrier state or even cause relapse and does not typically shorten the duration of diarrhea.[74] Most *Salmonella* infections are self-limited, but deaths do occur. The risk of severe illness and complications is increased in patients with malignancies, immunosuppression, alcoholism, cardiovascular dysfunction, sickle cell disease, and hemolytic anemia.

TYPHOID FEVER

Typhoid fever, also referred to as *enteric fever*, is caused by *Salmonella typhi* and *Salmonella paratyphi*. It affects up to 30 million individuals worldwide each year. The majority of cases in endemic countries are due to *S. typhi*, while infection by *S. paratyphi* is more common among travelers,[75] perhaps because travelers tend to be vaccinated against *S. typhi* (there are no effective *S. paratyphi* vaccines). In endemic areas children and adolescents are affected most often, but there is no age preference in developed countries. Infection is strongly associated with travel to India, Mexico, the Philippines, Pakistan, El Salvador, and Haiti.[76] Like *Shigella*, humans are the sole reservoir for *S. typhi* and *S. paratyphi* and transmission occurs from person to person or via food or contaminated water. Gallbladder colonization with *S. typhi* or *S. paratyphi* may be associated with gallstones and the chronic carrier state.

Pathogenesis. *S. typhi* are able to survive in gastric acid and, once in the small intestine, are taken up by and invade M cells. Organisms are then engulfed by mononuclear cells in the underlying lymphoid tissue. Unlike *S. enteritidis*, *S. typhi* can then disseminate via lymphatic and blood vessels. This causes reactive hyperplasia of phagocytes and lymphoid tissues throughout the body.

> **Morphology.** Infection causes Peyer's patches in the terminal ileum to enlarge into sharply delineated, plateau-like elevations up to 8 cm in diameter. Draining mesenteric lymph nodes are also enlarged. Neutrophils accumulate within the superficial lamina propria, and macrophages containing bacteria, red blood cells, and nuclear debris mix with lymphocytes and plasma cells in the lamina propria. Mucosal shedding creates **oval ulcers, oriented along the axis of the ileum,** that may perforate. The draining lymph nodes also harbor organisms and are enlarged due to phagocyte accumulation.
>
> The spleen is enlarged and soft, with uniformly pale red pulp, obliterated follicular markings, and prominent phagocyte hyperplasia. The liver shows small, randomly scattered foci of parenchymal necrosis in which hepatocytes are replaced by macrophage aggregates, called **typhoid nodules**, that may also develop in the bone marrow and lymph nodes.

Clinical Features. Patients experience anorexia, abdominal pain, bloating, nausea, vomiting, and bloody diarrhea followed by a short asymptomatic phase that gives way to bacteremia and fever with flu-like symptoms.[77] *Blood cultures are positive in more than 90% of affected individuals during the febrile phase*, which may prompt antibiotic treatment and prevent further disease progression.[76] In patients who do not receive treatment the febrile phase is followed by up to 2 weeks of sustained high fevers and abdominal tenderness that may mimic appendicitis. *Rose spots*, small erythematous maculopapular lesions, are seen on the chest and abdomen.[77] Symptoms abate after several weeks in those who survive, although relapse can occur.[77] Systemic dissemination may cause *extra-intestinal complications* including encephalopathy, meningitis, seizures, endocarditis, myocarditis, pneumonia, and cholecystitis. Patients with sickle cell disease are particularly susceptible to *Salmonella* osteomyelitis.

YERSINIA

Three *Yersinia* species are human pathogens. *Y. enterocolitica* and *Y. pseudotuberculosis* cause GI disease and are discussed here; *Y. pestis*, the agent of pulmonic and bubonic plague, is discussed in Chapter 8. GI *Yersinia* infections are more common in Europe than North America and are most frequently linked to ingestion of pork, raw milk, and contaminated water. *Y. enterocolitica* is far more common than *Y. pseudotuberculosis*, and infections tend to cluster in the winter, possibly related to inadequately cooked foods served at holiday gatherings.

Pathogenesis. *Yersinia* invade M cells and use bacterial adhesion proteins, *adhesins*, to bind to host cell β1 integrins. A pathogenicity island encodes an iron uptake system that mediates iron capture and transport; similar iron transport systems are also present in *E. coli*, *Klebsiella*, *Salmonella*, and enterobacteria. In *Yersinia*, iron enhances virulence and stimulates systemic dissemination, explaining why individuals with hemolytic anemia or hemochromatosis are more likely to develop sepsis and are at greater risk of death.[78]

> **Morphology.** *Yersinia* infections preferentially involve the ileum, appendix, and right colon (Fig. 17–28B). The organisms multiply extracellularly in lymphoid tissue, resulting in regional **lymph node and Peyer's patch hyperplasia** and bowel wall thickening.[79] The mucosa overlying lymphoid tissue may become hemorrhagic, and aphthous-appearing ulcers may develop, along with neutrophil infiltrates (see Fig. 17–28B) and granulomas, increasing the potential for diagnostic confusion with Crohn disease.

Clinical Features. People infected with *Yersinia* generally present with abdominal pain, but fever and diarrhea may also occur. Nausea, vomiting, and abdominal tenderness are common, and Peyer's patch invasion with subsequent involvement of regional lymphatics can mimic acute appendicitis in teenagers and young adults. Enteritis and colitis predominate in younger children. *Extra-intestinal symptoms of pharyngitis, arthralgia, and erythema nodosum* occur frequently. *Yersinia* can be detected in stool cultures on *Yersinia*-selective agar or, in cases with extra-intestinal disease, cultures of lymph nodes or blood.[80] Postinfectious complications, including sterile arthritis, Reiter syndrome, myocarditis, glomerulonephritis, and thyroiditis, have been reported.

ESCHERICHIA COLI

Escherichia coli are Gram-negative bacilli that colonize the healthy GI tract; most are nonpathogeneic, but a subset cause human disease. The latter are classified according to morphology, mechanism of pathogenesis, and in vitro behavior. Subgroups with major clinical relevance include enterotoxigenic *E. coli* (ETEC), enterohemorrhagic *E. coli* (EHEC), enteroinvasive *E. coli* (EIEC), and enteroaggregative *E. coli* (EAEC).

Enterotoxigenic E. Coli. *ETEC organisms are the principal cause of traveler's diarrhea* and spread via contaminated food or water. Infection is common in underdeveloped regions, and children younger than 2 years of age are particularly susceptible. ETEC produce heat-labile toxin (LT) and heat-stable toxin (ST), and both induce chloride and water secretion while inhibiting intestinal fluid absorption. The LT toxin is similar to cholera toxin and activates adenylate cyclase, resulting in increased intracellular cAMP. This stimulates chloride secretion and, simultaneously, inhibits absorption. ST toxins, which have homology to the mammalian regulatory protein guanylin, bind to guanylate cyclase and increase intracellular cGMP with resulting effects on transport that are similar to those produced by LT. Like cholera, the histopathology induced by ETEC infection is limited. Clinical symptoms include secretory, noninflammatory diarrhea, dehydration, and, in severe cases, shock.

Enterohemorrhagic E. Coli. EHEC are categorized as *E. coli* O157:H7 and non-O157:H7 serotypes. Large outbreaks of *E. coli* O157:H7 in developed countries have been associated with the consumption of inadequately cooked ground beef, sometimes from fast-food establishments. Contaminated milk and vegetables are also vehicles for infection. Both O157:H7 and non-O157:H7 serotypes produce Shiga-like toxins, and the morphology (see Fig. 17–28C) and clinical symptoms are thus similar to *S. dysenteriae*. O157:H7 strains of EHEC are more likely than non-O157:H7 serotypes to cause large outbreaks, bloody diarrhea, and hemolytic-uremic syndrome.

Enteroinvasive E. Coli. EIEC organisms are bacteriologically similar to *Shigella* and are transmitted via food, water, or by person-to-person contact. While EIEC do not produce toxins, they invade epithelial cells and cause nonspecific features of acute self-limited colitis (see Fig. 17–28D). EIEC infections are most common among young children in developing countries and are occasionally associated with outbreaks in developed countries.

Enteroaggregative E. Coli. EAEC organisms were identified on the basis of their unique pattern of adherence to epithelial cells. These organisms are now recognized as a cause of diarrhea in children and adults in developed as well as developing countries. These can also be a cause of traveler's diarrhea.[81] EAEC attach to enterocytes via *adherence fimbriae* and are aided by *dispersin*, a bacterial surface protein that neutralizes the negative surface charge of lipopolysaccharide. While the bacteria do produce enterotoxins related to *Shigella* enterotoxin and ETEC ST toxin, histologic damage is minimal and the characteristic adherence lesions are only visible by electron microscopy.[82] EAEC organisms cause nonbloody diarrhea that may be prolonged in individuals with the acquired immunodeficiency syndrome (AIDS).

PSEUDOMEMBRANOUS COLITIS

Pseudomembranous colitis, generally caused by *Clostridium difficile*, is also known as antibiotic-associated colitis or antibiotic-associated diarrhea. The latter terms apply to diarrhea developing during or after a course of antibiotic therapy and may be due to *C. difficile* as well as *Salmonella, C. perfringens* type A, or *Staphylococcus aureus*. The latter two organisms produce enterotoxins and are common agents of food poisoning.

Pathogenesis. It is likely that disruption of the normal colonic flora by antibiotics allows *C. difficile* overgrowth. Although almost any antibiotic may be responsible, third-generation cephalosporins are implicated most frequently. Immunosuppression is also a predisposing factor for *C. difficile* colitis. Toxins released by *C. difficile* cause the ribosylation of small GTPases, such as Rho, and lead to disruption of the epithelial cytoskeleton, tight junction barrier loss, cytokine release, and apoptosis.[83] The mechanisms by which these processes lead to the characteristic morphology of pseudomembranous colitis are incompletely understood.

> **Morphology.** Fully developed *C. difficile*–associated colitis is accompanied by formation of **pseudomembranes** (Fig. 17–29A, B), made up of an adherent layer of inflammatory cells and debris at sites of colonic mucosal injury. While pseudomembranes are not specific and may occur in ischemia and necrotizing infections, the histopathology of *C. difficile*–associated colitis is striking. The surface epithelium is denuded, and the superficial lamina propria contains a dense infiltrate of neutrophils and occasional fibrin thrombi within capillaries. Superficially damaged crypts are distended by a mucopurulent exudate that forms an **eruption reminiscent of a volcano** (Fig. 17–29C). These exudates coalesce to form the pseudomembranes.

Clinical Features. Risk factors for *C. difficile*–associated colitis include advanced age, hospitalization, and antibiotic treatment. The organism is particularly prevalent in hospitals; as many as 30% of hospitalized adults are colonized with *C. difficile* (a rate tenfold greater than the general population), but most colonized patients are free of disease. Individuals with *C. difficile*–associated colitis present with fever, leukocytosis, abdominal pain, cramps, hypoalbuminemia, watery diarrhea, and dehydration. Fecal leukocytes and occult blood may be present, but grossly bloody diarrhea is rare. Diagnosis of *C. difficile*–associated colitis is usually accomplished by detection of *C. difficile* toxin, rather than culture, and is supported by the characteristic histopathology. Metronidazole or vancomycin are generally effective therapies, but antibiotic-resistant and hypervirulent *C. difficile* strains as well as recurrent disease are increasingly common.[84]

WHIPPLE DISEASE

Whipple disease is a rare, multivisceral chronic disease first described as intestinal lipodystrophy in 1907 by George Hoyt Whipple. A mere 27 years later the pathologist went on to win

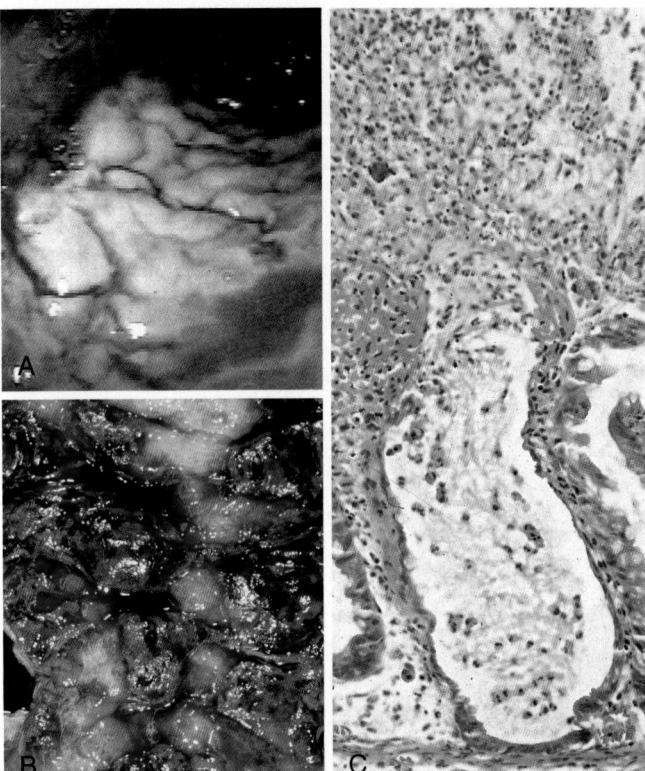

FIGURE 17–29   *Clostridium difficile* colitis. **A,** The colon is coated by tan pseudomembranes composed of neutrophils, dead epithelial cells, and inflammatory debris (endoscopic view). **B,** Pseudomembranes are easily appreciated on gross examination. **C,** Typical pattern of neutrophils emanating from a crypt is reminiscent of a volcanic eruption.

the Nobel Prize for his work on pernicious anemia. He was a contemporary, but not a relative, of Allen Oldfather Whipple, the surgeon who pioneered the pancreatoduodenectomy.

Pathogenesis. Whipple's original case report described an individual with malabsorption, lymphadenopathy, and arthritis of undefined origin. Postmortem examination demonstrated the presence of foamy macrophages and large numbers of argyrophilic rods in the lymph nodes, providing evidence that the disease was infectious.[85] The Gram-positive actinomycete, named *Tropheryma whippelii*, that is responsible for Whipple disease was identified by PCR in 1992 and finally cultured in 2000.[86] Clinical symptoms occur because organism-laden macrophages accumulate within the small intestinal lamina propria and mesenteric lymph nodes, causing lymphatic obstruction. Thus, the *malabsorptive diarrhea* of Whipple disease is due to *impaired lymphatic transport*.

> **Morphology.** The morphologic hallmark of Whipple disease is a dense accumulation of **distended, foamy macrophages** in the small intestinal lamina propria (Fig. 17–30A). The macrophages contain periodic acid–Schiff (PAS)-positive, diastase-resistant granules that represent lysosomes stuffed with partially digested bacteria (Fig. 17–30B). Intact rod-shaped bacilli can also be identified by electron microscopy

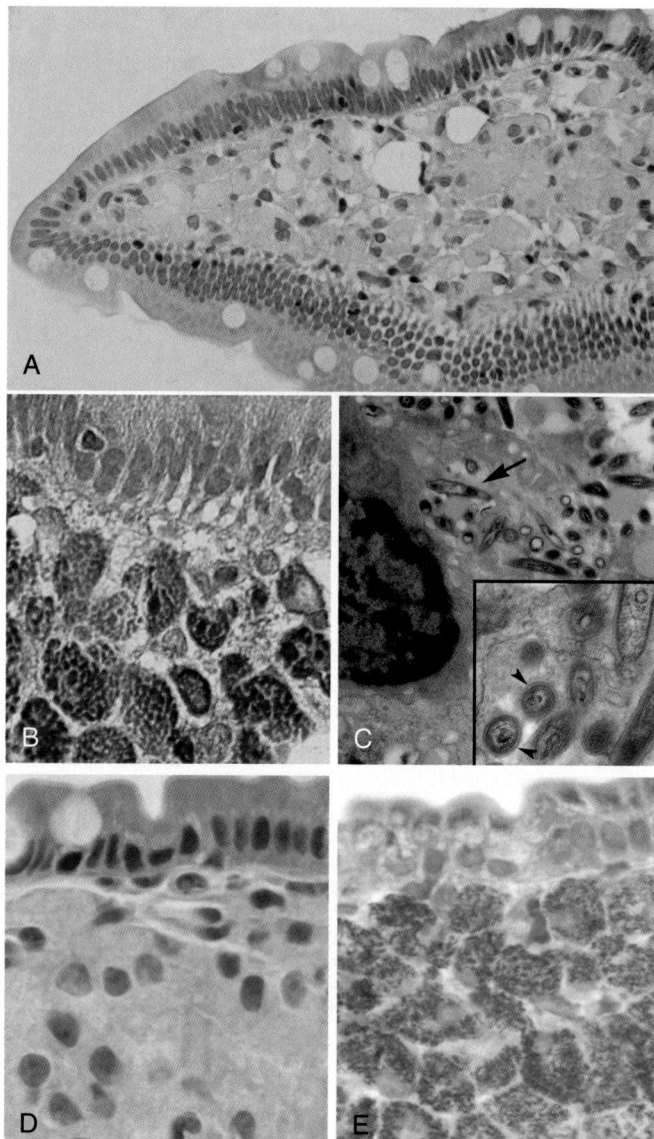

FIGURE 17–30 Whipple disease and mycobacterial infection. **A,** H&E staining shows effacement of normal lamina propria by a sheet of swollen macrophages. **B,** PAS stain highlights macrophage lysosomes full of bacilli. Note the positive staining of mucous vacuoles in the overlying goblet cells. **C,** An electron micrograph of one lamina propria macrophage shows these bacilli within the cell *(top)* and at higher magnification *(inset)*. **D,** The morphology of mycobacterial infection can be similar to Whipple disease, particularly in the immunocompromised host. Compare with **A**. **E,** Mycobacteria are positive with stains for acid-fast bacteria. (**C,** Courtesy of George Kasnic and Dr. William Clapp, University of Florida, Gainesville, FL.)

(Fig. 17–30C). A similar infiltrate of foamy macrophages is present in intestinal tuberculosis (Fig. 17–30D), and in both diseases the organisms are PAS-positive. However, the acid-fast stain can be used to distinguish between these, since mycobacteria stain positively (Fig. 17–30E) while *T. whippelii* do not.

The **villous expansion** caused by the dense macrophage infiltrate imparts a shaggy gross appearance to the mucosal surface. Lymphatic dilatation and mucosal lipid deposition account for the common endoscopic detection of white to yellow mucosal plaques. In Whipple disease, bacteria-laden macrophages can accumulate within **mesenteric lymph nodes, synovial membranes of affected joints, cardiac valves, the brain,** and other sites.

The clinical presentation of Whipple disease is usually a triad of *diarrhea, weight loss, and malabsorption*. Extraintestinal symptoms, which can exist for months or years before malabsorption, include arthritis, arthralgia, fever, lymphadenopathy, and neurologic, cardiac, or pulmonary disease.

Mycobacterial infections are considered in detail in Chapter 8.

VIRAL GASTROENTERITIS

Symptomatic human infection is caused by several distinct groups of viruses. The most common are discussed here.

Norovirus. This was previously known as *norwalk-like virus* and is a common cause of nonbacterial infectious gastroenteritis.[87] These are small icosahedral viruses with a single-stranded RNA genome that forms a genus within the Caliciviridae family. *Norovirus causes approximately half of all gastroenteritis outbreaks worldwide and is a common cause of sporadic gastroenteritis in developed countries.* Local outbreaks are usually related to contaminated food or water, but person-to-person transmission underlies most sporadic cases. Infections spread easily within schools, hospitals, nursing homes, and, most recently, cruise ships. Following a short incubation period, affected individuals develop nausea, vomiting, watery diarrhea, and abdominal pain. Biopsy morphology is nonspecific. When detected, abnormalities are most evident in the small intestine and include mild villous shortening, epithelial vacuolization, loss of the microvillus brush border, crypt hypertrophy, and lamina propria infiltration by lymphocytes (Fig. 17–31A). The disease is self-limited.

Rotavirus. This encapsulated virus with a segmented double-stranded RNA genome infects 140 million people and causes 1 million deaths each year, making rotavirus *the most common cause of severe childhood diarrhea and diarrheal mortality worldwide*. Children between 6 and 24 months of age are most vulnerable. Protection in the first 6 months of life is probably due to the presence of antibodies to rotavirus in breast milk, while protection beyond 2 years is due to immunity that develops following the first infection.[88] Outbreaks in hospitals and daycare centers are common, and infection spreads easily; the estimated minimal infective inoculum is only 10 viral particles. *Rotavirus selectively infects and destroys mature enterocytes in the small intestine, and the villus surface is repopulated by immature secretory cells.* This results in loss of absorptive function and net secretion of water and electrolytes that is compounded by an osmotic diarrhea from incompletely absorbed nutrients. Like norovirus, rotavirus has a short incubation period followed by several days of vomiting and watery diarrhea. Vaccines are now available, and their use will probably change the epidemiology of rotavirus infection.

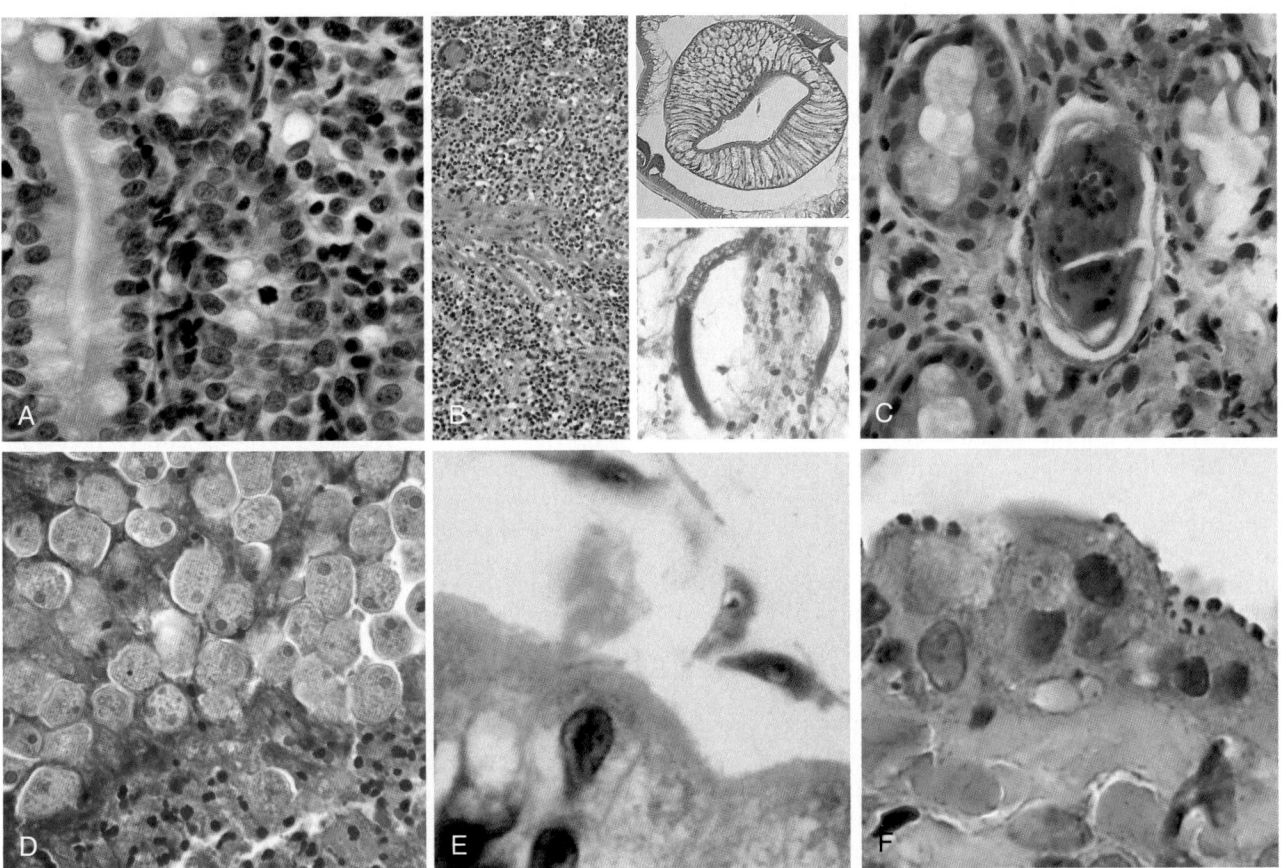

FIGURE 17–31 Infectious enteritis. **A,** Histologic features of viral enteritis include increased numbers of intraepithelial and lamina propria lymphocytes and crypt hypertrophy. **B,** Diffuse eosinophilic infiltrates in parasitic infection. This case was caused by *Ascaris (upper inset),* but a similar tissue reaction could be caused by *Strongyloides (lower inset).* **C,** Schistosomiasis can induce an inflammatory reaction to eggs trapped within the lamina propria. **D,** *Entamoeba histolytica* in a colon biopsy specimen. Note some organisms ingesting red blood cells. **E,** *Giardia lamblia,* which are present in the luminal space over nearly normal-appearing villi, are easily overlooked. **F,** *Cryptosporidia* organisms are seen as small blue spheres that appear to lay on top of the brush border but are actually enveloped by a thin layer of host cell cytoplasm.

Adenovirus. The second most common cause of pediatric diarrhea (after rotavirus), adenovirus also affects immunocompromised patients.[89] Small intestinal biopsy specimens can show epithelial degeneration but more often exhibit nonspecific villous atrophy and compensatory crypt hyperplasia. Viral nuclear inclusions are uncommon. Disease typically presents after an incubation period of 1 week with nonspecific symptoms that include diarrhea, vomiting, and abdominal pain. Fever and weight loss may also be present. Symptoms generally resolve within 10 days.

PARASITIC ENTEROCOLITIS

Although viruses and bacteria are the predominant enteric pathogens in the United States, parasitic disease and protozoal infections affect over one half of the world's population on a chronic or recurrent basis. The small intestine can harbor as many as 20 species of parasites, including nematodes, such as the roundworms *Ascaris* and *Strongyloides*; hookworms and pinworms; cestodes, including flatworms and tapeworms; trematodes, or flukes; and protozoa. Parasitic infections are covered in Chapter 8, and we will briefly discuss only those that are common in the intestinal tract.

Ascaris lumbricoides. This nematode infects over a billion individuals worldwide as a result of human fecal-oral contamination. Ingested eggs hatch in the intestine and larvae penetrate the intestinal mucosa, but disease is caused when larvae migrate from the splanchnic circulation to the systemic circulation and create hepatic abscess or *Ascaris* pneumonitis. In the latter case, larvae migrate up the trachea, are swallowed, and arrive again in the intestine to mature into adult worms. Adult worm masses induce an eosinophil-rich inflammatory reaction (Fig. 17–31B) that can physically obstruct the intestine or biliary tree. Diagnosis is usually made by detection of eggs in stool samples.

Strongyloides. The larvae of *Strongyloides* live in fecally contaminated ground soil and can penetrate unbroken skin. They migrate through the lungs, where they induce inflammatory infiltrates, and then reside in the intestine while maturing into adult worms. Unlike other intestinal worms, which require an ova or larval stage outside the human, the eggs of *Strongyloides* can hatch within the intestine and release larvae that penetrate the mucosa, causing autoinfection (see Fig. 17–31B). Hence, *Strongyloides* infection can persist for life, and immunosuppressed individuals can develop overwhelming autoinfection. *Strongyloides* incite a strong tissue reaction and induce peripheral eosinophilia.

Necator duodenale and Ancylostoma duodenale. These hookworms infect 1 billion people worldwide and cause significant morbidity. Infection is initiated by larval penetration through the skin and, after further development in the lungs the larvae migrate up the trachea and are swallowed. Once in the duodenum the worms attach to the mucosa, suck blood, and reproduce. This causes multiple superficial erosions, focal hemorrhage, and inflammatory infiltrates and, in chronic infection, iron deficiency anemia. Diagnosis can be made by detection of the eggs in fecal smears.

Enterobius vermicularis. Also known as pinworms, these parasites infect people in industrialized and developing countries; in the United States more than 60 million people have pinworms. Because they do not invade host tissue and live their entire life within the intestinal lumen, they rarely cause serious illness. Infection by *E. vermicularis*, or enterobiasis, is primarily by the fecal-oral route. Adult worms living in the intestine migrate to the anal orifice at night, where the female deposits eggs on the perirectal mucosa. The eggs cause intense irritation. Rectal and perineal pruritus ensues and leads to contamination of the fingers, which promotes human-to-human transmission. Both eggs and adult pinworms remain viable outside the body, and repeat infection is common. Diagnosis can be made by applying cellophane tape to the perianal skin and examining the tape for eggs under a microscope.

Trichuris trichiura. Whipworms primarily infect young children. Similar to *E. vermicularis*, *Trichuris trichiura* does not penetrate the intestinal mucosa and rarely cause serious disease. Heavy infections, however, may cause bloody diarrhea and rectal prolapse.

Schistosomiasis. This disease involving the intestines most commonly takes the form of adult worms residing within the mesenteric veins. Symptoms of intestinal schistosomiasis are caused by trapping of eggs within the mucosa and submucosa (Fig. 17–31C). The resulting immune reaction is often granulomatous and can cause bleeding and even obstruction. More details are presented in Chapter 8.

Intestinal cestodes. The three primary species of cestodes that affect humans are *Diphyllobothrium latum*, fish tapeworms; *Taenia solium*, pork tapeworms; and *Hymenolepsis nana*, dwarf tapeworms. They reside exclusively within the intestinal lumen and are transmitted by ingestion of raw or undercooked fish, meat, or pork that contain encysted larvae. Release of the larvae allows attachment to the intestinal mucosa through its head, or scolex. The worm derives its nutrients from the food stream and enlarges by formation of egg-filled segments termed *proglottids*. Humans are usually infected by a single worm, and, since the worm does not penetrate the intestinal mucosa, peripheral eosinophilia does not generally occur. Nevertheless, the parasite burden can be staggering, since adult worms can grow to many meters in length. Large numbers of proglottids or individual eggs are shed in the feces. Clinical symptoms include abdominal pain, diarrhea, and nausea. Diagnosis is established by stool examination.

Entamoeba histolytica. This protozoan that causes amebiasis is spread by fecal-oral transmission. *E. histolytica* infects approximately 500 million people in developing countries such as India, Mexico, and Colombia, and causes 40 million cases of dysentery and liver abscess annually. *E. histolytica*

cysts, which have a chitin wall and four nuclei, are resistant to gastric acid, a characteristic that allows them to pass through the stomach without harm. Cysts then colonize the epithelial surface of the colon and release *trophozoites*, ameboid forms that reproduce under anaerobic conditions.

Amebiasis is seen most frequently in the cecum and ascending colon, although the sigmoid colon, rectum, and appendix can also be involved. Dysentery develops when the amebae attach to the colonic epithelium, induce apoptosis, invade crypts, and burrow laterally into the lamina propria. This recruits neutrophils, causes tissue damage, and creates a *flask-shaped ulcer* with a narrow neck and broad base. Histologic diagnosis can be difficult, since amebae are similar to macrophages in size and general appearance (see Fig. 17–31D). Parasites may penetrate splanchnic vessels and embolize to the liver to produce abscesses in about 40% of patients with amebic dysentery. *Amebic liver abscesses*, which can exceed 10 cm in diameter, have a scant inflammatory reaction at their margins and a shaggy fibrin lining. The abscesses persist after the acute intestinal illness has passed and may, rarely, reach the lung and the heart by direct extension from the liver. Amebae may also spread via the bloodstream into the kidneys and brain.

Individuals with amebiasis may present with abdominal pain, bloody diarrhea, or weight loss. Occasionally, acute necrotizing colitis and megacolon occur, and both are associated with significant mortality. The parasites lack mitochondria or Krebs cycle enzymes and are thus obligate fermenters of glucose. Therefore, metronidazole, which inhibits the enzyme pyruvate oxidoreductase that is required for fermentation, is the most effective treatment.

Giardia lamblia. These organisms, also referred to as *G. duodenalis* or *G. intestinalis*, were initially described by van Leeuwenhoek, the inventor of the microscope, who discovered the pathogen in his own stool. They are the *most common pathogenic parasitic infection in humans* and are spread by fecally contaminated water or food. Infection may occur after ingestion of as few as 10 cysts. Because cysts are resistant to chlorine, *Giardia* are endemic in unfiltered public water supplies. They are commonly present in rural streams, explaining infection in campers who use these as a water source. Infection may also occur by the fecal-oral route and, because the cysts are stable, they may be accidentally swallowed while swimming in contaminated water.

Giardia are flagellated protozoans that cause decreased expression of brush-border enzymes, including lactase; microvillous damage; and apoptosis of small intestinal epithelial cells. Secretory IgA and mucosal IL-6 responses are important for clearance of *Giardia* infections, and immunosuppressed, agammaglobulinemic, or malnourished individuals are often severely affected.[90] *Giardia* can evade immune clearance through continuous modification of the major surface antigen, variant surface protein, and can persist for months or years while causing intermittent symptoms.

Giardia trophozoites can be identified in duodenal biopsies by their characteristic pear shape with two nuclei of equal size, each of which contains a complete copy of the genome. Despite large numbers of trophozoites, which are sickle-shaped in profile and tightly bound to the brush border of villous enterocytes, there is no invasion and small intestinal morphology may be normal by light microscopy (see Fig.

17–31E). Villous blunting with increased numbers of intraepithelial lymphocytes and mixed lamina propria inflammatory infiltrates may be present in patients with heavy infections.

Giardiasis may be subclinical or accompanied by acute or chronic diarrhea, malabsorption, and weight loss.[90] Infection is usually documented by *immunofluorescent detection of cysts in stool samples*. Although oral antimicrobial therapy is effective, recurrence is common.

Cryptosporidium. Like *Giardia, Cryptosporidia* are an important cause of diarrhea worldwide. Cryptosporidiosis was first discovered in the 1980s as an agent of *chronic diarrhea in AIDS patients* and is now recognized as a cause of acute, self-limited disease in immunologically normal hosts. Cryptosporidiosis causes traveler's diarrhea as well as persistent diarrhea in residents of developing countries. The organisms are present worldwide, with the exception of Antarctica, perhaps because the oocysts are killed by freezing. The oocysts are resistant to chlorine and may, therefore, persist in treated, but unfiltered, water. *Contaminated drinking water continues to be the most common means of transmission*. The largest documented outbreak, a result of inadequate water purification, occurred in 1993 in Milwaukee, Wisconsin, and affected more than 400,000 people. Like giardiasis, cryptosporidiosis can be spread to water sport participants via contaminated water. Food-borne infection occurs less frequently.

Humans are infected by several different *Cryptosporidium* species, including *C. hominis* and *C. parvum*. All are able to go through an entire life cycle, with asexual and sexual reproductive phases, in a single host. The ingested encysted oocyte, of which 10 are sufficient to cause symptomatic infection, is activated by acid in the stomach to produce proteases that allow release of sporozoites from the oocysts. The sporozoites are motile and have a specialized organelle for attachment to the enterocyte brush border, where they induce actin polymerization. This drives extension of the epithelial cell membrane to engulf the parasite and form a vacuole within the microvilli. Sodium malabsorption, chloride secretion, and increased tight junction permeability are responsible for the nonbloody, watery diarrhea that ensues.

Mucosal histology is often only minimally altered, but persistent cryptosporidiosis in children is associated with villous atrophy. Heavy infection in immunosuppressed patients may be associated with villous atrophy, crypt hyperplasia, and variable inflammatory infiltrates. Although the sporozoite is intracellular, it appears, by light microscopy, to sit on top of the epithelial apical membrane (Fig. 17–31F). Organisms are typically most concentrated in the terminal ileum and proximal colon, but can be present throughout the gut, biliary tract, and even the respiratory tract of immunodeficient hosts. Diagnosis is based on finding oocysts in the stool.

Irritable Bowel Syndrome

Irritable bowel syndrome (IBS) is characterized by chronic, relapsing abdominal pain, bloating, and changes in bowel habits.[91] Despite very real symptoms, the gross and microscopic evaluation is normal in most IBS patients. Thus, the diagnosis depends on clinical symptoms.

Pathogenesis. The pathogenesis of IBS remains poorly defined, although there is clearly an interplay between psychologic stressors, diet, and abnormal GI motility. Data showing disturbances of intestinal motility and enteric sensory function suggest that impairment of signaling in the brain-gut axis contributes to IBS. A small subgroup of IBS patients also relate onset to a bout of infectious gastroenteritis, suggesting an immune or neuroimmune contribution.

Clinical Features. The peak prevalence of IBS is between 20 and 40 years of age, and there is a significant female predominance. Variability in diagnostic criteria makes it difficult to establish the incidence, but most authors report a *prevalence in developed countries of between 5% and 10%*. IBS is presently diagnosed using clinical criteria that require the occurrence of abdominal pain or discomfort at least 3 days per month over 3 months, improvement with defecation, and a change in stool frequency or form. Many patients also report fibromyalgia or other chronic pain disorders, visceral hypersensitivity, backache, headache, urinary symptoms, dyspareunia, lethargy, and depression. In those with diarrhea, microscopic colitis, celiac disease, giardiasis, lactose intolerance, small bowel bacterial overgrowth, bile salt malabsorption, *colon cancer*, and *inflammatory bowel disease must be excluded* (although IBS is common in inflammatory bowel disease patients). IBS is not associated with serious long-term sequelae, but affected patients may undergo unnecessary abdominal surgery due to chronic pain and their ability to function socially may be compromised. The prognosis of IBS is most closely related to symptom duration, with longer duration correlating with reduced likelihood of improvement. Ongoing life stressors also reduce the chance of symptom resolution. Consistent with the uncertain mechanisms of disease, diverse treatments are used including psychotherapy, dietary fiber supplementation, tricyclic antidepressants, selective serotonin reuptake inhibitors, probiotics, and antibiotics. In addition, a chloride channel agonist may provide benefit in a subset of patients whose primary manifestation is constipation.

Inflammatory Bowel Disease

Inflammatory bowel disease (IBD) is a chronic condition resulting from inappropriate mucosal immune activation. The two disorders that comprise IBD are *Crohn disease* and *ulcerative colitis*. Descriptions of ulcerative colitis and Crohn disease date back to antiquity and at least the sixteenth century, respectively, but it took modern bacteriologic techniques to exclude conventional infectious etiologies for these diseases.[92] As will be discussed below, however, commensal bacteria normally present in the intestinal lumen are probably involved in IBD pathogenesis.

The distinction between ulcerative colitis and Crohn disease is based, in large part, on the distribution of affected sites (Fig. 17–32) and the morphologic expression of disease (Table 17–8) at those sites. *Ulcerative colitis is a severe ulcerating inflammatory disease that is limited to the colon and rectum and extends only into the mucosa and submucosa. In contrast, Crohn disease, which has also been referred to as regional enteritis (because of frequent ileal involvement) may involve any area of the GI tract and is typically transmural.*

Epidemiology. Both Crohn disease and ulcerative colitis are more common in females and frequently present in the

CROHN DISEASE   ULCERATIVE COLITIS

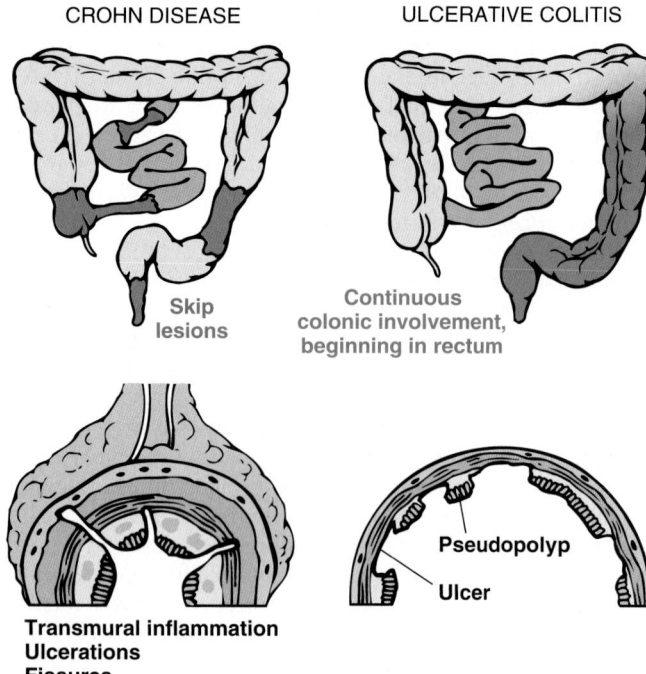

Skip lesions

Continuous colonic involvement, beginning in rectum

Pseudopolyp

Ulcer

**Transmural inflammation
Ulcerations
Fissures**

FIGURE 17–32 Distribution of lesions in inflammatory bowel disease. The distinction between Crohn disease and ulcerative colitis is primarily based on morphology.

teens and early 20s. In Western industrialized nations IBD is most common among Caucasians and, in the United States, occurs 3 to 5 times more often among eastern European (Ashkenazi) Jews. This is at least partly due to genetic factors, as discussed below. The geographic distribution of IBD is highly variable, but it is most common in North America, northern Europe, and Australia. However, IBD incidence worldwide is on the rise, and it is becoming more common in regions such as Africa, South America, and Asia, where the prevalence was historically low. The *hygiene hypothesis* suggests that this increasing incidence may be related to improved food storage conditions and decreased food contamination. This hypothesis suggests that reduced frequency of enteric infections has resulted in inadequate development of regulatory processes to limit mucosal immune responses, allowing pathogens that should cause self-limited disease to trigger overwhelming immune responses and chronic inflammatory disease in susceptible hosts. Although many details to support this hypothesis are lacking, the observation that helminth infection, which is endemic in regions where IBD incidence is low, can prevent IBD development in animal models and reduce disease in some patients lends support to this idea. The observation that an episode of acute infectious gastroenteritis may precede onset of IBD in some individuals is also consistent with the hygiene hypothesis.

Pathogenesis. IBD is an *idiopathic disorder* and the responsible processes are only beginning to be understood. Although there is limited epidemiologic association of IBD with autoimmunity, neither Crohn disease nor ulcerative colitis is thought to be an autoimmune disease. Rather, *most investigators believe that the two diseases result from a combination of defects in host interactions with intestinal microbiota, intestinal epithelial dysfunction, and aberrant mucosal immune responses.* This view is supported by epidemiologic, genetic, and clinical

studies as well as data from laboratory models of IBD (Fig. 17–33).

○ **Genetics.** Genetic factors contribute to IBD.[93] Risk of disease is increased when there is an affected family member and, in Crohn disease, the concordance rate for monozygotic twins is approximately 50%. The same factors may also contribute to disease phenotype, because twins affected by Crohn disease tend to present within 2 years of each other and develop disease in similar regions of the GI tract. The concordance of monozygotic twins for ulcerative colitis is only 16%, suggesting that genetic factors are less dominant than in Crohn disease. Concordance for dizygotic twins is less than 10% for both Crohn disease and ulcerative colitis.

Molecular linkage analyses of affected families have identified *NOD2* (nucleotide oligomerization binding domain 2) as a susceptibility gene in Crohn disease. Specific *NOD2* polymorphisms confer at least a four-fold increase in Crohn disease risk among Caucasians of European ancestry. *NOD2* encodes a protein that binds to intracellular bacterial peptidoglycans and subsequently activates NF-κB. It has been postulated that disease-associated *NOD2* variants are less effective at recognizing and combating luminal microbes, which are then able to enter the lamina propria and trigger inflammatory reactions. Other data suggest that *NOD2* may regulate immune responses to prevent excessive activation by luminal microbes. Whatever the mechanism by which *NOD2* polymorphisms contribute to Crohn disease pathogenesis, it should be remembered that fewer than 10% of individuals carrying *NOD2* mutations develop disease. Furthermore, *NOD2* mutations are uncommon in African and Asian Crohn disease patients. Thus, defective

TABLE 17–8 Features That Differ between Crohn Disease and Ulcerative Colitis		
Feature	**Crohn Disease**	**Ulcerative Colitis**
MACROSCOPIC		
Bowel region	Ileum ± colon	Colon only
Distribution	Skip lesions	Diffuse
Stricture	Yes	Rare
Wall appearance	Thick	Thin
MICROSCOPIC		
Inflammation	Transmural	Limited to mucosa
Pseudopolyps	Moderate	Marked
Ulcers	Deep, knife-like	Superficial, broad-based
Lymphoid reaction	Marked	Moderate
Fibrosis	Marked	Mild to none
Serositis	Marked	Mild to none
Granulomas	Yes (~35%)	No
Fistulae/sinuses	Yes	No
CLINICAL		
Perianal fistula	Yes (in colonic disease)	No
Fat/vitamin malabsorption	Yes	No
Malignant potential	With colonic involvement	Yes
Recurrence after surgery	Common	No
Toxic megacolon	No	Yes

Note: All features may not be present in a single case.

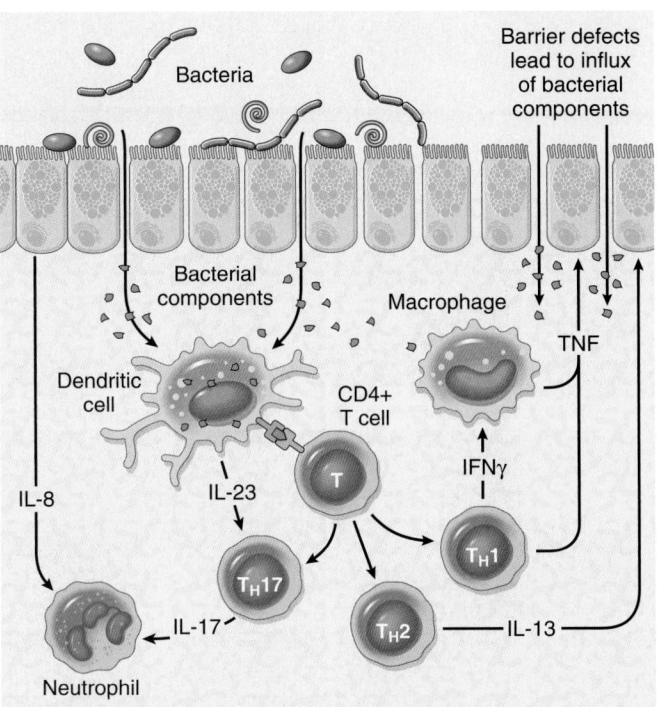

FIGURE 17–33 One model of IBD pathogenesis. Aspects of both Crohn disease and ulcerative colitis are shown.

NOD2 signaling is only one of many genetic factors that contribute to Crohn disease pathogenesis.

More recently, the search for IBD-associated genes has used genome-wide association studies (GWAS) that assess single-nucleotide polymorphisms, as described in Chapter 5.[94] The number of genes identified by GWAS is increasing rapidly (already numbering more than 30), but along with *NOD2*, two Crohn disease–related genes of particular interest are *ATG16L1* (autophagy-related 16-like), a part of the autophagosome pathway that is critical to host cell responses to intracellular bacteria and, perhaps, epithelial homeostasis, and *IRGM* (immunity-related GTPase M), which is also involved in autophagy and clearance of intracellular bacteria. *NOD2*, *ATG16L1*, and *IRGM* are expressed in multiple cell types, and their precise roles in Crohn disease pathogenesis have yet to be defined. However, like *NOD2*, *ATG16L1* and *IRGM* are related to recognition and response to intracellular pathogens, supporting the hypothesis that inappropriate immune reactions to luminal bacteria are an important component of IBD pathogenesis. None of these genes are associated with ulcerative colitis. However, some polymorphisms of the IL-23 receptor are protective in both Crohn disease and ulcerative colitis (discussed later).[95]

● ***Mucosal immune responses.*** Although the mechanisms by which mucosal immunity contributes to ulcerative colitis and Crohn disease pathogenesis are still being deciphered, immunosuppression remains the mainstay of IBD therapy. Polarization of helper T cells to the T_H1 type (see Chapter 6) is well-recognized in Crohn disease, and emerging data suggest that T_H17 T cells also contribute to disease pathogenesis. Consistent with this, certain polymorphisms of the IL-23 receptor confer protection from Crohn disease and ulcerative colitis.[95] IL-23 is involved in the development and maintenance of T_H17 cells, suggesting that the protective

IL-23 receptor polymorphisms may attenuate pro-inflammatory T_H17 responses in Crohn disease and ulcerative colitis.

Some data suggest that ulcerative colitis is a T_H2-mediated disease, and this is consistent with observations of increased mucosal IL-13 in ulcerative colitis patients. However, the protection afforded by IL-23 receptor polymorphisms and effectiveness of anti-TNF therapy in some ulcerative colitis patients seems to support roles for T_H1 and T_H17 cells. A recent report linking polymorphisms near the *IL-10* gene to ulcerative colitis, but not Crohn disease, further emphasizes the importance of immunoregulatory signals in IBD pathogenesis.[96] Overall it is likely that some combination of derangements that activate mucosal immunity and suppress immunoregulation contribute to the development of ulcerative colitis and Crohn disease. The relative roles of innate and adaptive arms of the immune system are presently the subject of intense scrutiny.

● ***Epithelial defects.*** A variety of epithelial defects have been described in both Crohn disease and ulcerative colitis. For example, defects in intestinal epithelial tight junction barrier function are present in Crohn disease patients and a subset of their healthy first-degree relatives.[97] In patients with Crohn disease and their relatives, this barrier dysfunction is associated with *NOD2* polymorphisms,[98] and experimental models demonstrate that barrier dysfunction can activate innate and adaptive mucosal immunity and sensitize subjects to disease.[99] Moreover, mutation of the organic cation transporter *SLC22A4* in Crohn disease suggests that defective transepithelial transport may also be related to IBD pathogenesis. Defects in the extracellular barrier formed by secreted mucin may also contribute.[100] Interestingly, polymorphisms in *ECM1* (extracellular matrix protein 1), which inhibits matrix metalloproteinase 9, are associated with ulcerative colitis but not Crohn disease.[101] While the pathogenic relevance of *ECM1* mutations is not understood, it is notable that inhibition of matrix metalloproteinase 9 reduces the severity of colitis in experimental models. Finally, the Paneth cell granules, which contain antibacterial peptides termed defensins, are abnormal in Crohn disease patients carrying *ATG16L1* mutations,[102] suggesting that defective epithelial anti-microbial function contributes to IBD. Thus, while the details are incompletely defined and probably differ between Crohn disease and ulcerative colitis, deranged epithelial function is a critical component of IBD pathogenesis.

● ***Microbiota.*** The abundance of microbiota in the GI lumen is overwhelming, amounting to as much as 10^{12} organisms per milliliter in the colon and 50% of fecal mass. In total, these organisms greatly outnumber human cells in our bodies, meaning that, at a cellular level, we are only about 10% human. Although the composition of this dense microbial population tends to be stable within individuals over at least several years, it can be modified by diet and there is significant variation between individuals. In addition to the luminal microbiota, the more limited microbial population that inhabits the intestinal mucous layer may have the greatest impact on health. Despite growing evidence that intestinal microbiota contribute to IBD pathogenesis,[103] their precise role remains to be defined and is probably different in ulcerative colitis and Crohn disease. For example, antibodies against the bacterial protein flagellin are associated with *NOD2* polymorphisms as well as stricture formation, perforation, and small-bowel involvement in patients with Crohn disease, but are uncommon in ulcerative colitis patients. In addition, some antibiotics, e.g. metronidazole, can be helpful in management of Crohn disease, and broad-spectrum antibiotics can prevent disease in some experimental models of IBD.[104] Ongoing studies suggest that ill-defined mixtures containing probiotic, or beneficial, bacteria may combat disease in experimental models as well as some IBD patients, although the mechanisms responsible are not well understood.[105]

One model that unifies the roles of intestinal microbiota, epithelial function, and mucosal immunity suggests a cycle by which transepithelial flux of luminal bacterial components activates innate and adaptive immune responses.[106] In a genetically susceptible host, the subsequent release of TNF and other immune-mediated signals direct epithelia to increase tight junction permeability, which causes further increases in the flux of luminal material. These events may establish a self-amplifying cycle in which a stimulus at any site may be sufficient to initiate IBD.[107] Although this model is helpful in advancing our understanding of IBD pathogenesis, it is important to recognize that a variety of factors are associated with disease for unknown reasons. For example, an episode of appendicitis is associated with reduced risk of developing ulcerative colitis. Tobacco also modifies IBD epidemiology, but, paradoxically, the risk of Crohn disease is increased by smoking while that of ulcerative colitis is reduced.

CROHN DISEASE

Crohn disease, an eponym based on the 1932 description by Crohn, Ginzburg, and Oppenheimer, has existed for centuries. Louis XIII of France (1601–1643) suffered relapsing bloody diarrhea, fever, rectal abscess, small intestinal and colonic ulcers, and fistulae beginning at age 20 years, most likely due to Crohn disease.

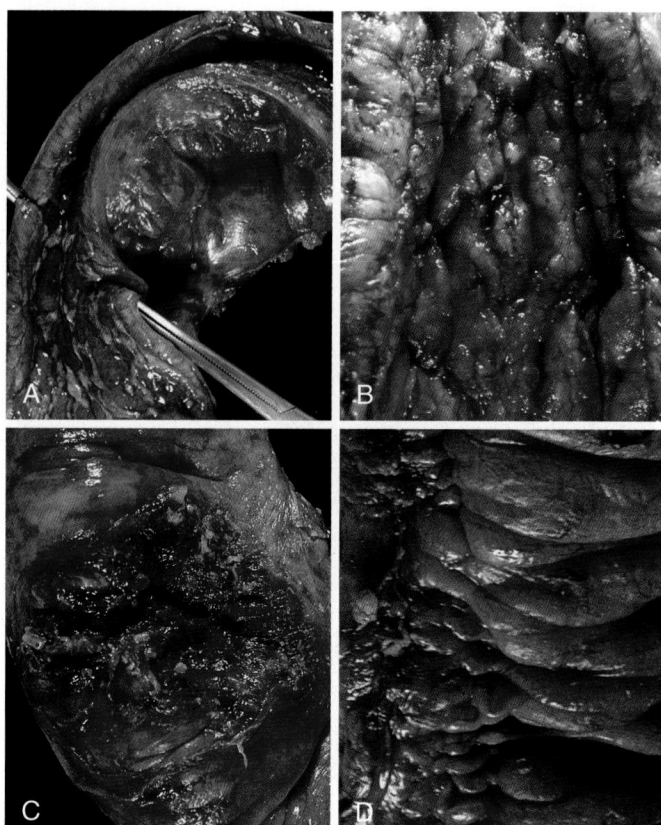

FIGURE 17–34 Gross pathology of Crohn disease. **A,** Small-intestinal stricture. **B,** Linear mucosal ulcers and thickened intestinal wall. **C,** Perforation and associated serositis. **D,** Creeping fat.

> **Morphology.** Crohn disease may occur in any area of the GI tract, but the most common sites involved at presentation are the **terminal ileum, ileocecal valve, and cecum.** Disease is limited to the small intestine alone in about 40% of cases; the small intestine and colon are both involved in 30% of patients; and the remainder have only colonic involvement. The presence of multiple, separate, sharply delineated areas of disease, resulting in **skip lesions,** is characteristic of Crohn disease and may help in the differentiation from ulcerative colitis. Strictures are common (Fig. 17–34A).
>
> The earliest Crohn disease lesion, the **aphthous ulcer,** may progress, and multiple lesions often coalesce into elongated, serpentine ulcers oriented along the axis of the bowel. Edema and loss of the normal mucosal texture are common. Sparing of interspersed mucosa, a result of the patchy distribution of Crohn disease, results in a coarsely textured, **cobblestone** appearance in which diseased tissue is depressed below the level of normal mucosa (Fig. 17–34B). **Fissures** frequently develop between
>
> mucosal folds and may extend deeply to become fistula tracts or sites of perforation (Fig. 17–34C). The intestinal wall is thickened and rubbery as a consequence of transmural edema, inflammation, submucosal fibrosis, and hypertrophy of the muscularis propria, all of which contribute to stricture formation. In cases with extensive transmural disease, mesenteric fat frequently extends around the serosal surface **(creeping fat)** (Fig. 17–34D).
>
> The microscopic features of active Crohn disease include abundant neutrophils that infiltrate and damage crypt epithelium. Clusters of neutrophils within a crypt are referred to as **crypt abscesses** and are often associated with crypt destruction. Ulceration is common in Crohn disease, and there may be an abrupt transition between ulcerated and adjacent normal mucosa. Even in areas where gross examination suggests diffuse disease, microscopic pathology can appear patchy. Repeated cycles of crypt destruction and regeneration lead to **distortion of mucosal architecture;** the normally straight and parallel crypts take on bizarre branching shapes and unusual orientations to one another (Fig. 17–35A). Epithelial metaplasia, another consequence of chronic relapsing injury, often takes the form of gastric antral-appearing glands, and is called pseudopyloric metaplasia. **Paneth cell metaplasia** may also occur in

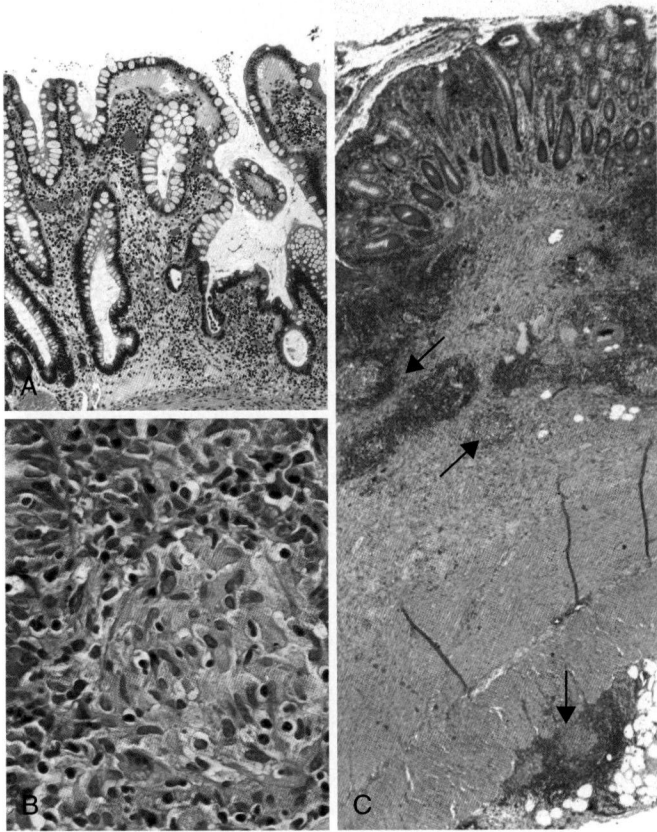

FIGURE 17–35 Microscopic pathology of Crohn disease. **A,** Haphazard crypt organization results from repeated injury and regeneration. **B,** Noncaseating granuloma. **C,** Transmural Crohn disease with submucosal and serosal granulomas (*arrows*).

the left colon, where Paneth cells are normally absent. These architectural and metaplastic changes may persist even when active inflammation has resolved. Mucosal atrophy, with loss of crypts, may occur after years of disease. **Noncaseating granulomas** (Fig. 17–35B), a hallmark of Crohn disease, are found in approximately 35% of cases and may occur in areas of active disease or uninvolved regions in any layer of the intestinal wall (Fig. 17–35C). Granulomas may also be present in mesenteric lymph nodes. Cutaneous granulomas form nodules that are referred to as **metastatic Crohn disease.** The absence of granulomas does not preclude a diagnosis of Crohn disease.

Clinical Features. The clinical manifestations of Crohn disease are extremely variable. In most patients *disease begins with intermittent attacks of relatively mild diarrhea, fever, and abdominal pain.* Approximately 20% of patients present acutely with right lower quadrant pain, fever, and bloody diarrhea that may mimic acute appendicitis or bowel perforation. Periods of active disease are typically interrupted by asymptomatic periods that last for weeks to many months. Disease re-activation can be associated with a variety of external triggers, including physical or emotional stress, specific dietary items, and cigarette smoking. The latter is a strong exogenous risk factor for development of Crohn disease and, in some

cases, disease onset is associated with initiation of smoking. Unfortunately, smoking cessation does not result in disease remission.

Iron-deficiency anemia may develop in individuals with colonic disease, while extensive small bowel disease may result in serum protein loss and hypoalbuminemia, generalized nutrient malabsorption, or malabsorption of vitamin B_{12} and bile salts. Fibrosing strictures, particularly of the terminal ileum, are common and require surgical resection. Disease often recurs at the site of anastamosis, and as many as 40% of patients require additional resections within 10 years. Fistulae develop between loops of bowel and may also involve the urinary bladder, vagina, and abdominal or perianal skin. Perforations and peritoneal abscesses are common.

Extra-intestinal manifestations of Crohn disease include uveitis, migratory polyarthritis, sacroiliitis, ankylosing spondylitis, erythema nodosum, and clubbing of the fingertips, any of which may develop before intestinal disease is recognized. Pericholangitis and primary sclerosing cholangitis occur in Crohn disease but are more common in ulcerative colitis (see Chapter 18). As discussed below, risk of colonic adenocarcinoma is increased in patients with long-standing colonic disease.

ULCERATIVE COLITIS

Ulcerative colitis is closely related to Crohn disease. However, intestinal disease in ulcerative colitis is limited to the colon and rectum. Common extra-intestinal manifestations of ulcerative colitis overlap with those of Crohn disease and include migratory polyarthritis, sacroiliitis, ankylosing spondylitis, uveitis, skin lesions, pericholangitis, and primary sclerosing cholangitis (Chapter 18). Approximately 2.5% to 7.5% of individuals with ulcerative colitis also have primary sclerosis cholangitis. The long-term outlook for ulcerative colitis patients depends on the severity of active disease and disease duration.

Morphology. Grossly, ulcerative colitis always involves the rectum and extends proximally in a continuous fashion to involve part or all of the colon. Skip lesions are not seen (although focal appendiceal or cecal inflammation may occasionally be present in ulcerative colitis). Disease of the entire colon is termed **pancolitis** (Fig. 17–36A), while **left-sided disease** extends no farther than the transverse colon. Limited distal disease may be referred to descriptively as **ulcerative proctitis** or **ulcerative proctosigmoiditis.** The small intestine is normal, although mild mucosal inflammation of the distal ileum, **backwash ileitis,** may be present in severe cases of pancolitis.

Grossly, involved colonic mucosa may be slightly red and granular or have extensive, **broad-based ulcers,** and there can be an abrupt transition between diseased and uninvolved colon (Fig. 17–36B). Ulcers are aligned along the long axis of the colon but do not typically replicate the serpentine ulcers of Crohn disease. Isolated islands of regenerating mucosa often bulge into the lumen to create **pseudopolyps** (Fig. 17–36C), and the tips of these polyps may fuse to create **mucosal bridges** (Fig. 17–36D). Chronic

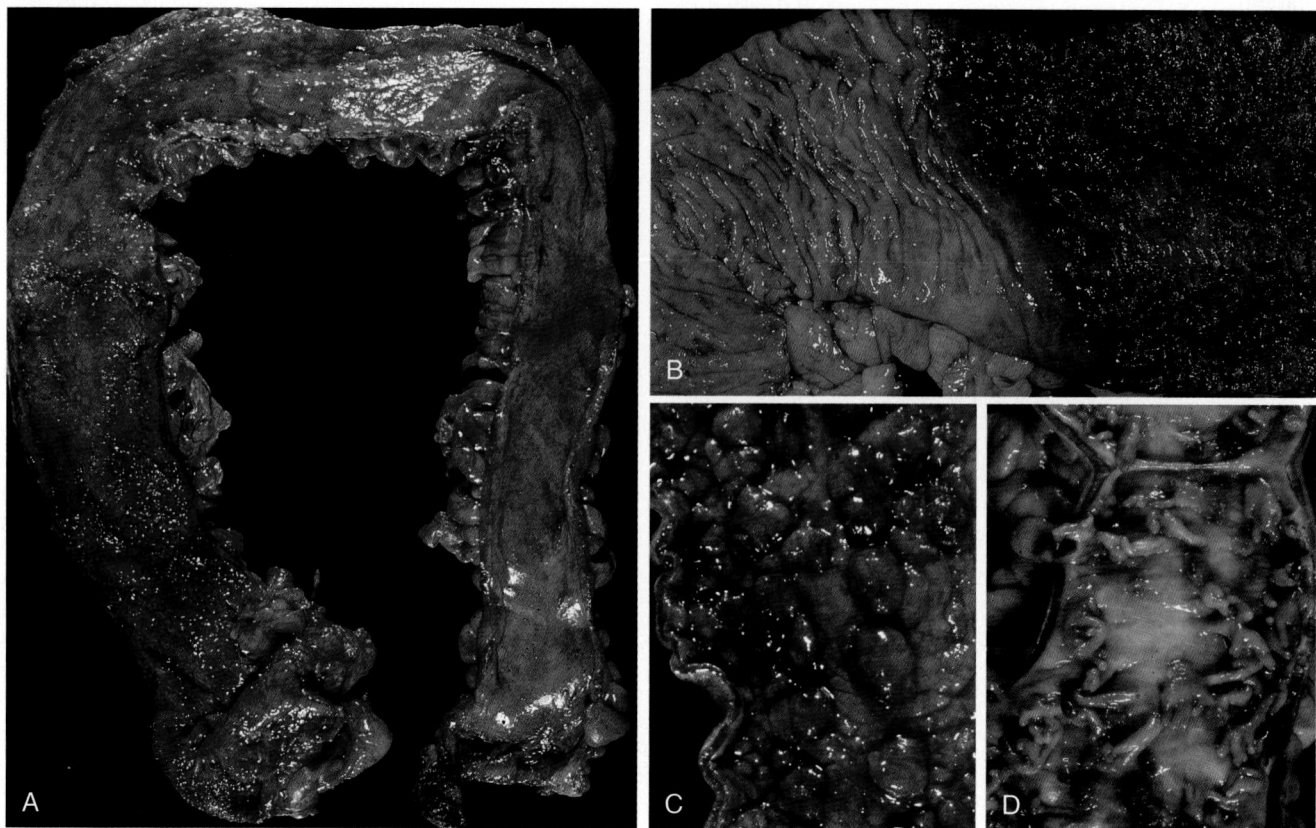

FIGURE 17–36 Gross pathology of ulcerative colitis. **A,** Total colectomy with pancolitis showing active disease, with red, granular mucosa in the cecum *(left)* and smooth, atrophic mucosa distally *(right)*. **B,** Sharp demarcation between active ulcerative colitis *(right)* and normal *(left)*. **C,** Inflammatory polyps. **D,** Mucosal bridges.

disease may lead to **mucosal atrophy** with a flat and smooth mucosal surface that lacks normal folds. Unlike Crohn disease, **mural thickening is not present, the serosal surface is normal, and strictures do not occur**. However, inflammation and inflammatory mediators can damage the muscularis propria and disturb neuromuscular function leading to colonic dilation and **toxic megacolon**, which carries a significant risk of perforation.

Histologic features of mucosal disease in ulcerative colitis are similar to colonic Crohn disease and include inflammatory infiltrates, crypt abscesses (Fig. 17–37A), architectural crypt distortion, and epithelial metaplasia (Fig. 17–37B). However, **the inflammatory process is diffuse and generally limited to the mucosa** and superficial submucosa (Fig. 17–37C). In severe cases, extensive mucosal destruction may be accompanied by ulcers that extend more deeply into the submucosa, but the muscularis propria is rarely involved. Submucosal fibrosis, mucosal atrophy, and distorted mucosal architecture remain as residua of healed disease but histology may also revert to near normal after prolonged remission. **Granulomas are not present** in ulcerative colitis.

Clinical Features. Ulcerative colitis is a relapsing disorder characterized by attacks of bloody diarrhea with stringy, mucoid material, lower abdominal pain, and cramps that are temporarily relieved by defecation. These symptoms may persist for days, weeks, or months before they subside, and, occasionally, the initial attack may be severe enough to constitute a medical or surgical emergency. More than half of patients have clinically mild disease, although almost all experience at least one relapse during a 10-year period, and up to 30% require colectomy within the first 3 years after presentation because of uncontrollable symptoms. Colectomy effectively cures intestinal disease in ulcerative colitis, but extra-intestinal manifestations may persist.

The factors that trigger ulcerative colitis are not known, but, as noted above, infectious enteritis precedes disease onset in some cases. In other cases the first attack is preceded by psychologic stress, which may also be linked to relapse during remission. The initial onset of symptoms has also been reported to occur shortly after smoking cessation in some patients, and smoking may partially relieve symptoms. Unfortunately, studies of nicotine as a therapeutic agent have been disappointing.

Indeterminate Colitis

There is extensive pathologic and clinical overlap between ulcerative colitis and Crohn disease (Table 17–8); definitive diagnosis is not possible in approximately 10% of IBD patients. These cases, termed *indeterminate colitis*, do not involve the small bowel and have colonic disease in a continuous pattern

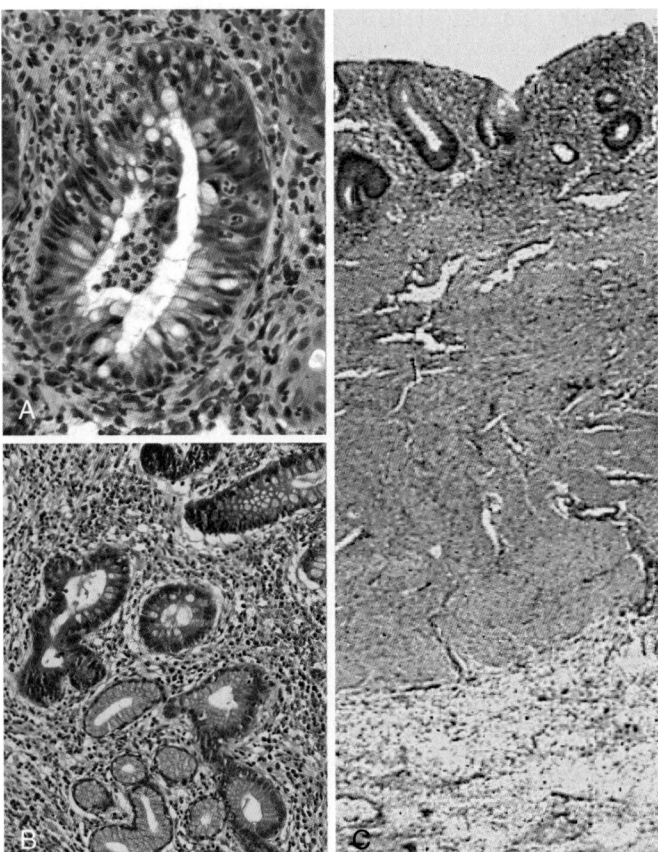

FIGURE 17–37 Microscopic pathology of ulcerative colitis. **A,** Crypt abscess. **B,** Pseudopyloric metaplasia *(bottom)*. **C,** Disease is limited to the mucosa. Compare to Figure 17–35C.

that would typically indicate ulcerative colitis. However, patchy histologic disease, fissures, a family history of Crohn disease, perianal lesions, onset after initiating use of cigarettes, or other features that are not typical of ulcerative colitis may prompt more detailed endoscopic, radiographic, and histologic examination. Serologic studies can be useful in these cases, because perinuclear anti-neutrophil cytoplasmic antibodies are positive in 75% of individuals with ulcerative colitis but only 11% with Crohn disease. In contrast, ulcerative colitis patients tend to lack antibodies to *Saccharomyces cerevisiae*, which are often present in those with Crohn disease. Even after extensive evaluation, IBD in approximately 10% of patients defies classification. In some of these cases features that develop over time (e.g., strictures or fistulae) ultimately establish the diagnosis; classification remains impossible in other patients. Because of extensive overlap in medical management of ulcerative colitis and Crohn disease, patients carrying a diagnosis of indeterminate colitis can be treated effectively. However, it is preferable to definitively categorize patients, when possible, as evolving medical therapies and surgical management differ in ulcerative colitis and Crohn disease.

Colitis-Associated Neoplasia

One of the most feared long-term complications of ulcerative colitis and colonic Crohn disease is the development of neoplasia. This begins as dysplasia, which, just as in Barrett esophagus

and chronic gastritis, represents in situ transformation. The risk of dysplasia is related to several factors:

- Risk increases sharply 8 to 10 years after disease initiation.
- Patients with pancolitis are at greater risk than those with only left-sided disease.
- Greater frequency and severity of active inflammation (characterized by the presence of neutrophils) may increase risk.

The role of inflammation in promoting dysplasia is emphasized by the observation that anti-TNF antibody treatment can suppress the development of colitis-associated cancers in experimental animals.

To facilitate early detection of neoplasia, patients are typically enrolled in surveillance programs approximately 8 years after diagnosis of IBD. The major exception to this is patients with primary sclerosing cholangitis, who have an even greater risk of dysplasia and are generally enrolled for surveillance at the time of diagnosis. Surveillance requires regular and extensive mucosal biopsy, making it a costly practice. Research efforts have therefore included a search for molecular markers of dysplasia in nondysplastic mucosa. Genomic instability in rectal mucosa has the potential to be such a marker, but biopsy surveillance remains the best tool currently available.

In many cases dysplasia occurs in flat areas of mucosa that are not grossly recognized as abnormal. Thus, advanced endoscopic imaging techniques including chromoendoscopy and confocal endoscopy are beginning to be used experimentally to increase sensitivity of detection. IBD-associated dysplasia is classified histologically as low grade or high grade (Fig. 17–38A, B) and may be multifocal. High-grade dysplasia may be associated with invasive carcinoma at the same site (Fig. 17–38C) or elsewhere in the colon and, therefore typically prompts colectomy. Low-grade dysplasia may be treated with colectomy or followed closely, depending on a variety of factors including patient age and the number of dysplastic foci present. Colonic adenomas (discussed below) also occur in IBD patients, and in some cases these may be difficult to differentiate from a polypoid focus of IBD-associated dysplasia.[108]

Other Causes of Chronic Colitis

DIVERSION COLITIS

Surgical treatment of ulcerative colitis, Hirschsprung disease, and other intestinal disorders sometimes requires creation of a temporary or permanent ostomy and a blind distal segment of colon, such as a Hartmann's pouch, from which the normal fecal flow is diverted. Colitis can develop within the diverted segment, particularly in ulcerative colitis patients. Besides mucosal erythema and friability, the most striking feature of *diversion colitis* is the development of numerous mucosal lymphoid follicles (Fig. 17–39A). Increased numbers of lamina propria lymphocytes, monocytes, macrophages, and plasma cells may also be present. In severe cases the histopathology may resemble IBD and include crypt abscesses, mucosal architectural distortion, or, rarely, granulomas. The pathogenic mechanisms responsible for diversion colitis are not well understood, but changes in the luminal microbiota and diversion of the fecal stream that provides nutrients to colonic

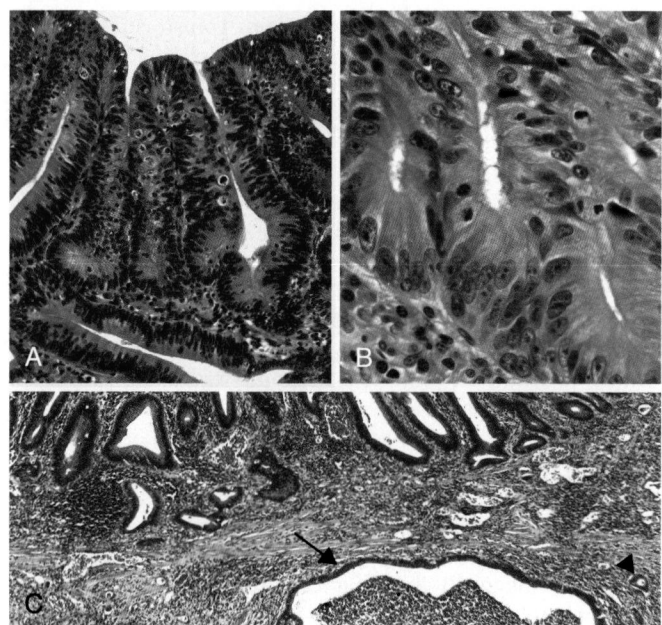

FIGURE 17–38 Colitis-associated dysplasia. **A,** Dysplasia with extensive nuclear stratification and marked nuclear hyperchromasia. **B,** Cribriform glandular arrangement in high-grade dysplasia. **C,** Colectomy specimen with high-grade dysplasia on the surface and underlying invasive adenocarcinoma. A large cystic, neutrophil-filled space lined by invasive adenocarcinoma is apparent at the bottom right (*arrow*) beneath the muscularis mucosa, and is surrounded by small invasive glands (*arrowhead*).

epithelial cells have been proposed. Consistent with this, enemas containing short-chain fatty acids, a product of bacterial digestion in the colon and an important energy source for colonic epithelial cells, can promote mucosal recovery in some cases. The ultimate cure is reanastomosis of the diverted segment.

MICROSCOPIC COLITIS

Microscopic colitis encompasses two entities, *collagenous colitis* and *lymphocytic colitis*. These idiopathic diseases both present with chronic, nonbloody, watery diarrhea without weight loss. Radiologic and endoscopic studies are typically normal. Collagenous colitis, which occurs primarily in middle-aged and older women, is characterized by the presence of a dense subepithelial collagen layer, increased numbers of intraepithelial lymphocytes, and a mixed inflammatory infiltrate within the lamina propria (Fig. 17–39B). Lymphocytic colitis is histologically similar, but the subepithelial collagen layer is of normal thickness and the increase in intraepithelial lymphocytes may be greater, frequently exceeding one T lymphocyte per five colonocytes (Fig. 17–39C). Lymphocytic colitis shows a strong association with celiac disease and autoimmune diseases, including thyroiditis, arthritis, and autoimmune or lymphocytic gastritis.

GRAFT-VERSUS-HOST DISEASE

Graft-versus-host disease occurs following allogeneic bone marrow transplantation. The small bowel and colon are involved in most cases. Although graft-versus-host disease is

secondary to donor T cells targeting antigens on the recipient's GI epithelial cells, the lamina propria lymphocytic infiltrate is typically sparse. Epithelial apoptosis, particularly of crypt cells, is the most common histologic finding. Rarely, total gland destruction occurs, although endocrine cells may persist. Intestinal graft-versus-host disease often presents as a watery diarrhea.

Sigmoid Diverticulitis

In general, diverticular disease refers to acquired pseudodiverticular outpouchings of the colonic mucosa and submucosa. Such *colonic diverticula* are rare in persons under age 30, but the prevalence approaches 50% in Western adult populations over age 60. Diverticulae are generally multiple and the condition is referred to as *diverticulosis*. This disease is much less common in Japan and nonindustrialized tropical countries, probably because of dietary differences.

Pathogenesis. Colonic diverticula result from the unique structure of the colonic muscularis propria and elevated intraluminal pressure in the sigmoid colon. Where nerves, arterial vasa recta, and their connective tissue sheaths penetrate the inner circular muscle coat, focal discontinuities in the muscle wall are created. In other parts of the intestine these gaps are reinforced by the external longitudinal layer of the muscularis propria, but, in the colon, this muscle layer is gathered into

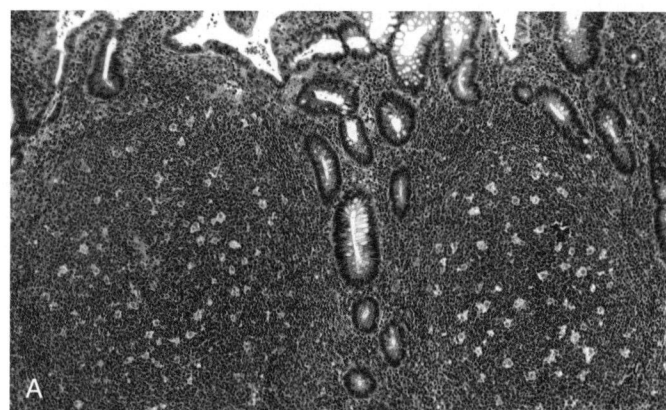

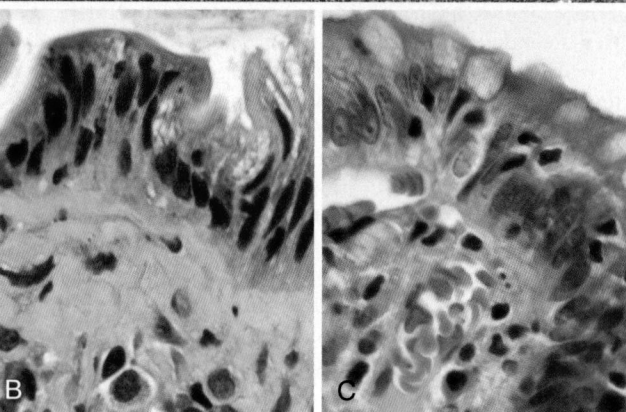

FIGURE 17–39 Uncommon causes of colitis. **A,** Diversion colitis in a Hartmann's pouch. Note the large lymphoid aggregates with germinal centers. **B,** Collagenous colitis with intraepithelial lymphocytes and a dense subepithelial collagen band. **C,** Lymphocytic colitis.

the three bands termed *taeniae coli*. Increased intraluminal pressure is probably due to exaggerated peristaltic contractions, with spasmodic sequestration of bowel segments, and may be enhanced by diets low in fiber, which reduce stool bulk, particularly in the sigmoid colon.

Morphology. Anatomically, colonic diverticula are small, flask-like outpouchings, usually 0.5 to 1 cm in diameter, that occur in a regular distribution alongside the taeniae coli (Fig. 17–40A). These are most common in the sigmoid colon, but more extensive areas may be affected in severe cases. Because diverticulae are compressible, easily emptied of fecal contents, and often surrounded by the fat-containing **epiploic appendices** on the surface of the colon, they may be missed on casual inspection. Colonic diverticula have a thin wall composed of a flattened or atrophic mucosa, compressed submucosa, and attenuated or, most often, totally absent muscularis propria (Fig. 17–40B, C). Hypertrophy of the circular layer of the muscularis propria in the affected bowel segment is common. Obstruction of diverticulae leads to inflammatory changes, producing **diverticulitis** and peri-diverticulitis. Because the wall of the diverticulum is supported only by the muscularis mucosa and a thin layer of subserosal adipose tissue, inflammation and increased pressure within an obstructed diverticulum can lead to **perforation**. With or without perforation, diverticulitis may cause segmental diver-ticular disease–associated colitis, fibrotic thickening in and around the colonic wall, or stricture formation. Perforation can result in pericolonic abscesses, sinus tracts, and, occasionally, peritonitis.

Clinical Features. Most individuals with diverticular disease remain asymptomatic throughout their lives, and the lesions are most often discovered incidentally. About 20% of those affected develop manifestations of disease including intermittent cramping, continuous lower abdominal discomfort, constipation, distention, and a sensation of never being able to completely empty the rectum. Patients sometimes experience alternating constipation and diarrhea. Occasionally there may be minimal chronic or intermittent blood loss, or, in extremely rare cases, massive hemorrhage. Longitudinal studies have shown that diverticulae can regress early in their development or, more commonly, become more numerous and prominent over time. Whether a high-fiber diet prevents such progression or protects against diverticulitis is unclear, but diets supplemented with fiber may provide symptomatic improvement. Even when diverticulitis occurs, it most often resolves spontaneously and relatively few patients require surgical intervention.

Polyps

Polyps are most common in the colon but may occur in the esophagus, stomach, or small intestine. Most, if not all, polyps begin as small elevations of the mucosa. These are referred to as *sessile*, a term borrowed from botanists who use it to describe flowers and leaves that grow directly from the stem without a stalk. As sessile polyps enlarge, several processes, including proliferation of cells adjacent to the mass and the effects of traction on the luminal protrusion, may combine to create a stalk. Polyps with stalks are termed *pedunculated*. In general, intestinal polyps can be classified as non-neoplastic or neoplastic in nature. The most common neoplastic polyp is the adenoma, which has the potential to progress to cancer. The non-neoplastic polyps can be further classified as inflammatory, hamartomatous, or hyperplastic.

INFLAMMATORY POLYPS

The polyp that forms as part of the *solitary rectal ulcer syndrome* is an example of a purely inflammatory lesion. Patients present with a clinical triad of rectal bleeding, mucus discharge, and an inflammatory lesion of the anterior rectal wall. The underlying cause is impaired relaxation of the anorectal sphincter that creates a sharp angle at the anterior rectal shelf and leads to recurrent abrasion and ulceration of the overlying rectal mucosa. An inflammatory polyp may ultimately form as a result of chronic cycles of injury and healing. Entrapment of this polyp in the fecal stream leads to mucosal prolapse. Thus, the distinctive histologic features are those of a typical inflammatory polyp with superimposed mucosal prolapse and include lamina propria fibromuscular hyperplasia, mixed

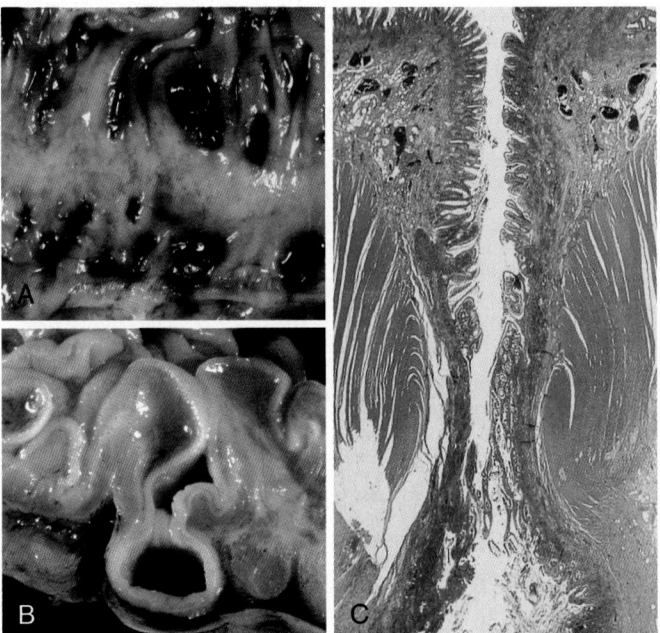

FIGURE 17–40 Sigmoid diverticular disease. **A,** Stool-filled diverticula are regularly arranged. **B,** Cross-section showing the outpouching of mucosa beneath the muscularis propria. **C,** Low-power photomicrograph of a sigmoid diverticulum showing protrusion of the mucosa and submucosa through the muscularis propria.

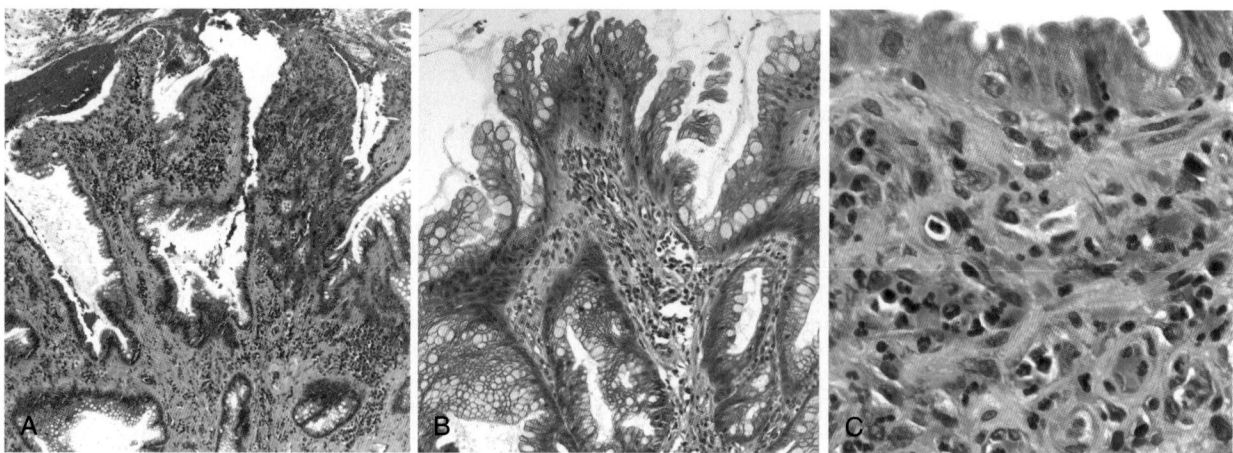

FIGURE 17–41 Solitary rectal ulcer syndrome. **A,** The dilated glands, proliferative epithelium, superficial erosions, and inflammatory infiltrate are typical of an inflamatory polyp. However, the smooth muscle hyperplasia within the lamina propria suggests that mucosal prolapse has also occurred. **B,** Epithelial hyperplasia. **C,** Granulation tissue-like capillary proliferation within the lamina propria caused by repeated erosion and re-epithelialization.

inflammatory infiltrates, erosion, and epithelial hyperplasia (Fig. 17–41).

HAMARTOMATOUS POLYPS

Hamartomatous polyps occur sporadically and in the context of various genetically determined or acquired syndromes (Table 17–9). Recall that hamartomas are tumor-like growths composed of mature tissues that are normally present at the site in which they develop. Although hamartomatous polyposis syndromes are rare, they are important to recognize because of associated intestinal and extra-intestinal manifestations and the possibility that other family members are affected.

Juvenile Polyps

Juvenile polyps are focal malformations of the mucosal epithelium and lamina propria. These may be *sporadic or syndromic*, but the morphology of the two forms may be indistinguish-

Syndrome	Mean Age at Presentation (yr)	Mutated Gene	Gastrointestinal Lesions	Selected Extra-Gastrointestinal Manifestations
Peutz-Jeghers syndrome	10–15	LKB1/STK11	Arborizing polyps; Small intestine > colon > stomach; colonic adenocarcinoma	Skin macules; increased risk of thyroid, breast, lung, pancreas, gonadal, and bladder cancers
Juvenile polyposis	<5	SMAD4, BMPR1A	Juvenile polyps; risk of gastric, small intestinal, colonic, and pancreatic adenocarcinoma	Pulmonary arteriovenous malformations, digital clubbing
Cowden syndrome, Bannayan-Ruvalcaba-Riley syndrome	<15	PTEN	Hamartomatous polyps, lipomas, ganglioneuromas, inflammatory polyps, risk of colon cancer	Benign skin tumors, benign and malignant thyroid and breast lesions
Cronkhite-Canada syndrome	>50	Nonhereditary	Hamartomatous colon polyps, crypt dilatation and edema in nonpolypoid mucosa	Nail atrophy, hair loss, abnormal skin pigmentation, cachexia, and anemia
Tuberous sclerosis		TSC1, TSC2	Hamartomatous polyps (rectal)	Facial angiofibroma, cortical tubers, renal angiomyolipoma
Familial adenomatous polyposis (FAP)				
Classic FAP	10–15	APC, MUTYH	Multiple adenomas	Congenital RPE hypertrophy
Attenuated FAP	40–50	APC, MUTYH	Multiple adenomas	
Gardner syndrome	10–15	APC, MUTYH	Multiple adenomas	Osteomas, desmoids, skin cysts
Turcot syndrome	10–15	APC, MUTYH	Multiple adenomas	CNS tumors, medulloblastoma

TABLE 17–9　Gastrointestinal Polyposis Syndromes

CNS, central nervous system; RPE, retinal pigmented epithelium.

able. The vast majority of juvenile polyps occur in children less than 5 years of age. When present in adults, polyps with identical morphology are sometimes confusingly referred to as *inflammatory polyps. The majority of juvenile polyps are located in the rectum* and most present with rectal bleeding. In some cases prolapse occurs and the polyp protrudes through the anal sphincter. Sporadic juvenile polyps are usually solitary lesions and may be referred to as *retention polyps.* In contrast, individuals with the autosomal dominant syndrome of juvenile polyposis have from 3 to as many as 100 hamartomatous polyps and may require colectomy to limit the chronic and sometimes severe hemorrhage associated with polyp ulceration. A minority of patients also have polyps in the stomach and small bowel. Pulmonary arteriovenous malformations are a recognized extra-intestinal manifestation of the syndrome.

> **Morphology.** Most juvenile polyps are less than 3 cm in diameter. They are typically pedunculated, smooth-surfaced, reddish lesions with characteristic cystic spaces apparent after sectioning. Microscopic examination shows these cysts to be dilated glands filled with mucin and inflammatory debris (Fig. 17–42). The remainder of the polyp is composed of lamina propria expanded by mixed inflammatory infiltrates. The muscularis mucosa may be normal or attenuated.

Although the morphogenesis of juvenile polyps is incompletely understood, some have suggested that mucosal hyperplasia is the initiating event. This hypothesis is consistent with the discovery that mutations in pathways that regulate cellular growth cause autosomal dominant juvenile polyposis. The most common mutation identified is of *SMAD4*, which encodes a cytoplasmic intermediate in the TGF-β signaling pathway. *BMPR1A*, a kinase that is a member of the TGF-β superfamily, may be mutated in other cases (see Table 17–9). However, these mutations account for fewer than half of patients, suggesting that changes in other genes can also cause juvenile polyposis. Dysplasia occurs in a small proportion of juvenile polyps, and the juvenile polyposis syndrome is associated with an increased risk of colonic adenocarcinoma.

Peutz-Jeghers Syndrome

This rare autosomal dominant syndrome presents at a median age of 11 years with *multiple GI hamartomatous polyps and mucocutaneous hyperpigmentation.* The latter takes the form of dark blue to brown macules around the mouth, eyes, nostrils, buccal mucosa, palmar surfaces of the hands, genitalia, and perianal region. These lesions are similar to freckles but are distinguished by their presence in the buccal mucosa. Peutz-Jeghers polyps can initiate intussusception, which is occasionally fatal. Of greater importance, *Peutz-Jeghers syndrome is associated with an increased risk of several malignancies,* including cancers of the colon, pancreas, breast, lung, ovaries, uterus, and testicles, as well as other unusual neoplasms, such as sex cord tumors.

Pathogenesis. Germline heterozygous loss-of-function mutations in the gene *LKB1/STK11* are present in approximately half of individuals with familial Peutz-Jeghers syn-

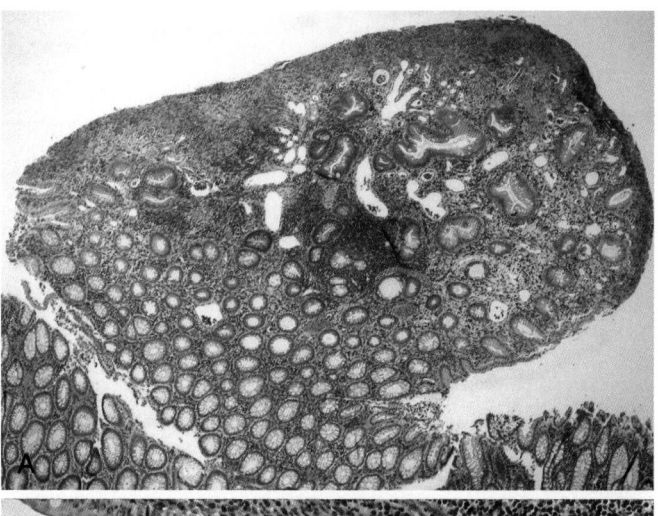
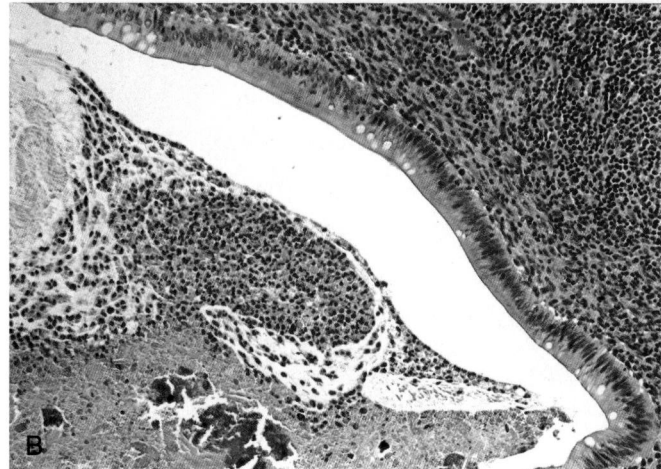

FIGURE 17–42 Juvenile polyposis. **A,** Juvenile polyp. Note the surface erosion and cystically dilated crypts. **B,** Inspissated mucous, neutrophils, and inflammatory debris can accumulate within dilated crypts.

drome as well as a subset of patients with sporadic Peutz-Jeghers syndrome. LKB1/STK11 is a kinase that regulates cell polarization, growth, and metabolism. The function of the second "normal" copy of *LKB1/STK11* is often lost through somatic mutation in cancers occurring in Peutz-Jeghers syndrome, consistent with the view that *LKB1/STK11* is a tumor suppressor gene and providing an explanation for the high risk of neoplasia in affected patients. The GI adenocarcinomas arise independently of the hamartomatous polyps, indicating that the hamartomas are not preneoplastic precursor lesions.

> **Morphology.** The polyps of Peutz-Jeghers syndrome are most common in the small intestine, although they may occur in the stomach and colon, and, with much lower frequency, in the bladder and lungs. Grossly, the polyps are large and pedunculated with a lobulated contour. Histologic examination demonstrates a characteristic arborizing network of connective tissue, smooth muscle, lamina propria, and glands lined by normal-appearing intestinal

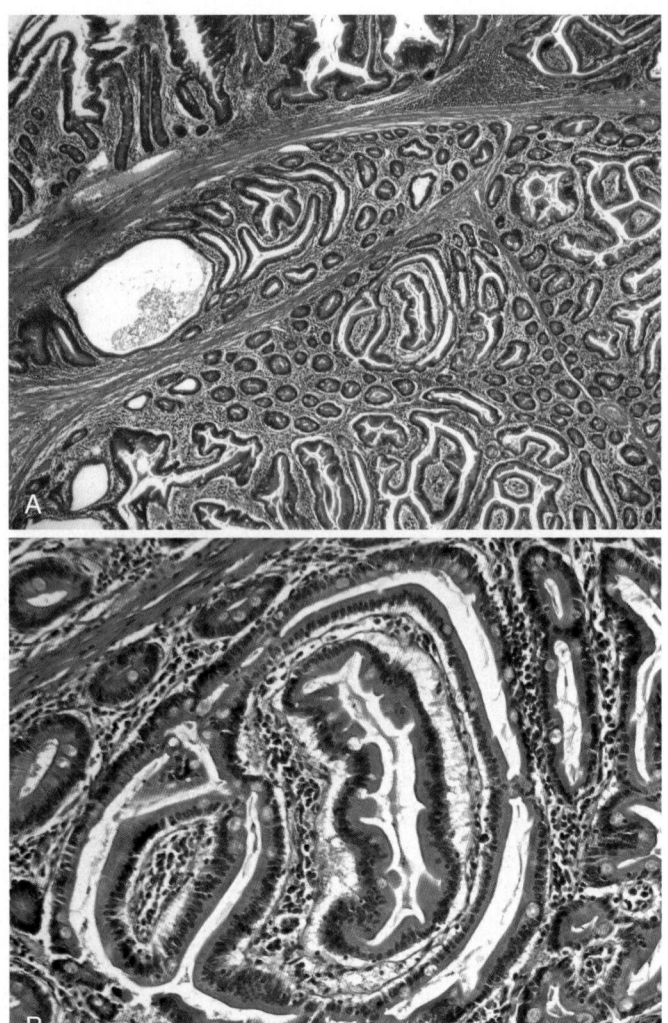

FIGURE 17–43 Peutz-Jeghers polyp. **A,** Polyp surface *(top)* overlies stroma composed of smooth muscle bundles cutting through the lamina propria. **B,** Complex glandular architecture and the presence of smooth muscle are features that distinguish Peutz-Jeghers polyps from juvenile polyps. Compare to Figure 17–42.

epithelium (Fig. 17–43). The arborization and presence of smooth muscle intermixed with lamina propria are helpful in distinguishing polyps of Peutz-Jeghers syndrome from juvenile polyps.

Clinical Features. Because the morphology of Peutz-Jeghers polyps can overlap with that of sporadic hamartomatous polyps, the presence of multiple polyps in the small intestine, mucocutaneous hyperpigmentation, and a positive family history are key to the diagnosis. Detection of *LKB1/STK11* mutations can be helpful diagnostically in patients with polyps who lack mucocutaneous hyperpigmentation. However, the absence of *LKB1/STK11* mutations does not exclude the diagnosis, since mutations in other presently unknown genes can also cause the syndrome. Because of the increased risk of cancer, routine surveillance of the GI tract, pelvis, and gonads is typically recommended.

Cowden Syndrome and Bannayan-Ruvalcaba-Riley Syndrome

Cowden syndrome and *Bannayan-Ruvalcaba-Riley syndrome* are autosomal dominant hamartomatous polyp syndromes associated with loss-of-function mutations in *PTEN*, a gene encoding a lipid phosphatase that inhibits signaling through the PI3K/AKT pathway. *PTEN*, a well-characterized tumor suppressor, is also mutated in a small number of patients presenting with juvenile polyposis. The multiple syndromes associated with *PTEN* mutations are sometimes grouped together under the heading "PTEN hamartoma syndrome." The basis for the differing presentations of these syndromes is not understood; interaction of PTEN loss-of-function mutations with other unknown modifying genes is suspected.

Cowden syndrome is characterized by macrocephaly, intestinal hamartomatous polyps, and benign skin tumors, typically trichilemmomas, papillomatous papules, and acral keratoses. A variety of other lesions derived from all three embryologic layers, including subcutaneous lipomas, leiomyomas, and hemangiomas, also occur. While individuals with Cowden syndrome do not have increased risk of GI malignancy, they are predisposed to breast carcinoma, follicular carcinoma of the thyroid, and endometrial carcinoma. Bannayan-Ruvalcaba-Riley syndrome can be distinguished from Cowden syndrome on clinical grounds; for example, mental deficiencies and developmental delays are only seen with the Bannayan-Ruvalcaba-Riley syndrome, which also seems to be associated with a lower incidence of neoplasia than Cowden syndrome. Features shared by these two syndromes include GI hamartomatous polyps, lipomas, macrocephaly, hemangiomas, and, in males, pigmented macules on the glans penis.

Cronkhite-Canada Syndrome

Cronkhite-Canada syndrome contrasts sharply with other hamartomatous polyposis syndromes in that it is nonhereditary and most often develops in individuals over 50 years of age. The clinical symptoms are nonspecific and include diarrhea, weight loss, abdominal pain, and weakness. The most characteristic feature is the presence of hamartomatous polyps of the stomach, small intestine, and colorectum that are histologically indistinguishable from juvenile polyps. However, the nonpolypoid intervening mucosa also shows cystic crypt dilatation and lamina propria edema and inflammation. Associated abnormalities include nail atrophy and splitting, hair loss, and areas of cutaneous hyperpigmentation and hypopigmentation. The cause of Cronkhite-Canada syndrome is unknown, and no specific therapies are available. Supportive nutritional therapy, which alleviates cachexia and anemia, can occasionally induce remission. Nonetheless, as many as 50% of cases are fatal.

HYPERPLASTIC POLYPS

Colonic hyperplastic polyps are common epithelial proliferations that are typically discovered in the sixth and seventh decades of life. The pathogenesis of hyperplastic polyps is incompletely understood, but they are thought to result from decreased epithelial cell turnover and delayed shedding of surface epithelial cells, leading to a "piling up" of goblet cells and absorptive cells. It is now appreciated that these lesions are without malignant potential. Their chief significance is that *they must be distinguished from sessile serrated adenomas, histologically similar lesions that have malignant potential*, as described later. It is also important to remember that epithelial hyperplasia can occur as a nonspecific reaction adjacent to or overlying any mass or inflammatory lesion and, therefore, can be a clue to the presence of an adjacent, clinically important lesion.

> **Morphology.** Hyperplastic polyps are most commonly found in the left colon and are typically less than 5 mm in diameter. They are smooth, nodular protrusions of the mucosa, often on the crests of mucosal folds. They may occur singly but are more frequently multiple, particularly in the sigmoid colon and rectum. Histologically, hyperplastic polyps are composed of mature goblet and absorptive cells. The delayed shedding of these cells leads to crowding that creates the serrated surface architecture that is the morphologic hallmark of these lesions (Fig. 17–44).

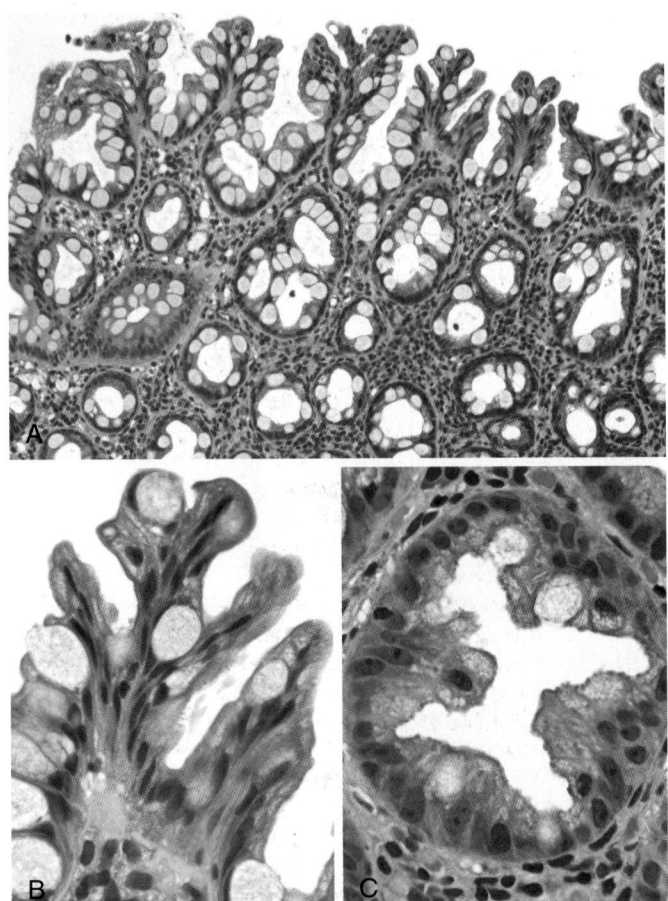

FIGURE 17–44 Hyperplastic polyp. **A,** Polyp surface with irregular tufting of epithelial cells. **B,** Tufting results from epithelial overcrowding. **C,** Epithelial crowding produces a serrated architecture when glands are cut in cross-section.

NEOPLASTIC POLYPS

Any neoplastic mass lesion in the GI tract may produce a mucosal protrusion, or polyp. This includes carcinoid tumors, stromal tumors, lymphomas, and even metastatic cancers from distant sites. However, the most common and clinically important neoplastic polyps are *colonic adenomas, benign polyps that are precursors to the majority of colorectal adenocarcinomas.*

Adenomas are intraepithelial neoplasms that range from small, often pedunculated polyps to large sessile lesions. There is no gender preference, and they are present in nearly 50% of adults living in the Western world by age 50. These polyps are precursors to colorectal cancer and it is recommended that all adults in the United States undergo surveillance colonoscopy by age 50. Because those with a family history are at risk for developing colon cancer earlier in life, these patients are typically screened at least 10 years before the youngest age at which a relative was diagnosed.[109] While adenomas are less common in Asia, their frequency has risen (in parallel with an increasing incidence of colorectal adenocarcinoma) in these populations as Western diets and lifestyles become more common.

Colorectal adenomas are characterized by the presence of epithelial dysplasia. Consistent with their role as precursor lesions, the prevalence of colorectal adenomas correlates with that of colorectal carcinoma and the distributions of adenomas and adenocarcinoma within the colon are similar. Large studies have demonstrated that regular surveillance colonoscopy and polyp removal reduces the incidence of colorectal adenocarcinoma. Despite this strong relationship, it must be emphasized that the majority of adenomas do not progress to become adenocarcinoma. However, there are no tools presently available to distinguish between those that will or will not undergo malignant transformation. Most adenomas are clinically silent, with the exception of large polyps that produce occult bleeding and anemia and rare villous adenomas that cause hypoproteinemic hypokalemia by secreting large amounts of protein and potassium.

> **Morphology.** Typical adenomas range from 0.3 to 10 cm in diameter and can be **pedunculated** (Fig. 17–45A) or **sessile**, with the surface of both types having a texture resembling velvet (Fig. 17–45B) or a raspberry, due to the abnormal epithelial growth pattern. Histologically, the cytologic hallmark of epithelial **dysplasia** is nuclear hyperchromasia, elongation, and stratification. These changes are most easily appreciated at the surface of the adenoma and are often accompanied by the presence of large nucleoli, eosinophilic cytoplasm, and a reduction in the number of goblet cells. Notably, the epithelium fails to mature as cells migrate from crypt to surface. Pedunculated adenomas have slender fibromuscular stalks (Fig. 17–45C) containing prominent blood vessels derived from the submucosa. The stalk is usually covered by non-neoplastic epithelium, but dysplastic epithelium is sometimes present.
>
> Adenomas can be classified as **tubular, tubulovillous,** or **villous** based on their architecture. These

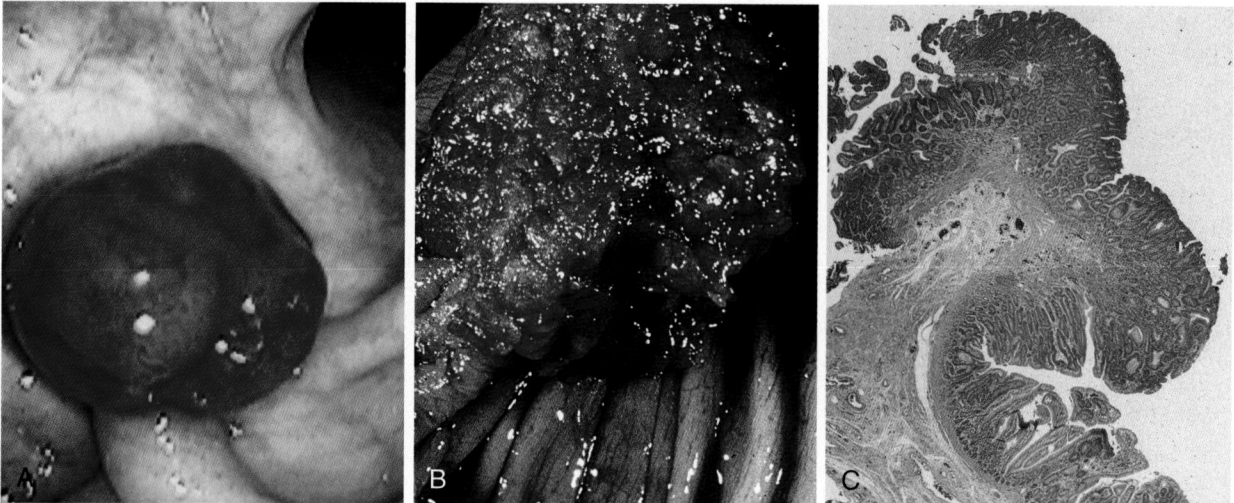

FIGURE 17–45 Colonic adenomas. **A,** Pedunculated adenoma (endoscopic view). **B,** Adenoma with a velvety surface. **C,** Low-magnification photomicrograph of a pedunculated tubular adenoma.

categories, however, have little clinical significance in isolation. Tubular adenomas tend to be small, pedunculated polyps composed of small rounded, or tubular, glands (Fig. 17–46A). In contrast, villous adenomas, which are often larger and sessile, are covered by slender villi (Fig. 17–46B). Tubulovillous adenomas have a mixture of tubular and villous elements. Although villous adenomas contain foci of invasion more frequently than tubular adenomas, villous architecture alone does not increase cancer risk when polyp size is considered.

Sessile serrated adenomas overlap histologically with hyperplastic polyps, but are more commonly found in the right colon.[110] Despite their malignant potential, sessile serrated adenomas lack typical cytologic features of dysplasia that are present in other adenomas (Fig. 17–46C). Histologic criteria include serrated architecture throughout the full length of the glands, including the crypt base, associated with lateral growth and crypt dilation (Fig. 17–46D). In contrast, serrated architecture is typically confined to the surface of hyperplastic polyps.

Intramucosal carcinoma occurs when dysplastic epithelial cells breach the basement membrane to invade the lamina propria or muscularis mucosa. Because lymphatic channels are absent in the colonic mucosa, intramucosal carcinoma has little or no metastatic potential and complete polypectomy is effective therapy (Fig. 17–47A). Invasion beyond the muscularis mucosa, including into the submucosal stalk of a pedunculated polyp (Fig. 17–47B), constitutes invasive adenocarcinoma and carries a risk of spread to other sites. In such cases several factors, including the histologic grade of the invasive component, the presence of vascular or lymphatic invasion, and the distance of the invasive component from the margin of resection, must be considered in planning further therapy. Invasive adenocarcinoma in a polyp requires resection.

Although most colorectal adenomas are benign lesions, a small proportion may harbor invasive cancer at the time of detection. *Size is the most important characteristic that correlates with risk of malignancy.* For example, while cancer is extremely rare in adenomas less than 1 cm in diameter, some studies suggest that nearly 40% of lesions larger than 4 cm in diameter contain foci of cancer. In addition to size, high-grade dysplasia is a risk factor for cancer in an individual polyp (but not other polyps in the same patient).

Familial Syndromes

Several syndromes characterized by the presence of colonic polyps and increased rates of colon cancer have been described. The genetic basis of these disorders has been established and has greatly enhanced our understanding of sporadic colon cancer (Table 17–10).

FAMILIAL ADENOMATOUS POLYPOSIS

Familial adenomatous polyposis (FAP) is an autosomal dominant disorder in which patients develop numerous colorectal adenomas as teenagers. It is caused by mutations of the *adenomatous polyposis coli*, or *APC*, gene.

At least *100 polyps are necessary for a diagnosis* of classic FAP, and as many as several thousand may be present (Fig. 17–48). Except for their remarkable numbers, these growths are *morphologically indistinguishable from sporadic adenomas.* In addition, however, flat or depressed adenomas are also prevalent in FAP, and microscopic adenomas, consisting of only one or two dysplastic glands, are frequently observed in otherwise normal-appearing mucosa.

Colorectal adenocarcinoma develops in 100% of untreated FAP patients, often before age 30. As a result, prophylactic colectomy is the standard therapy for individuals carrying *APC* mutations.[111] Colectomy prevents colorectal cancer, but patients remain at risk for neoplasia at other sites. For example,

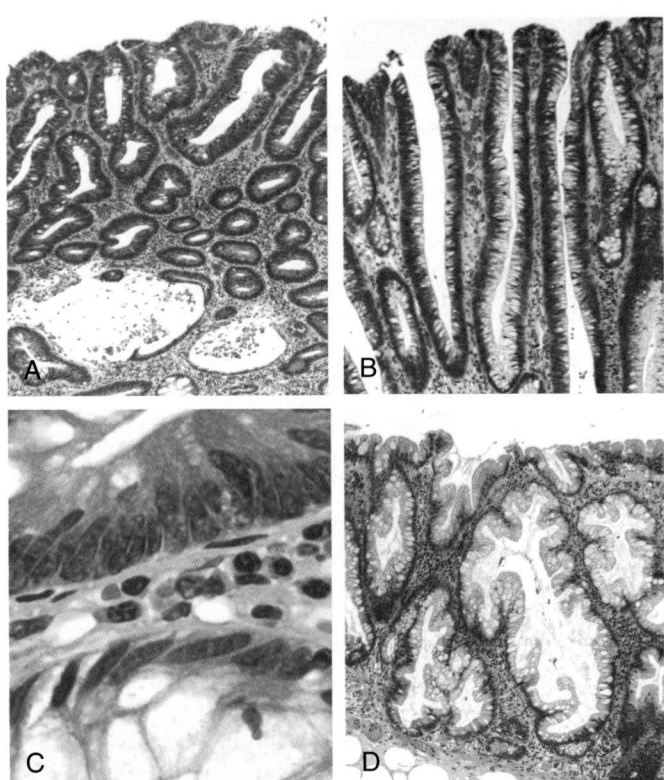

FIGURE 17–46 Histologic appearance of colonic adenomas. **A,** Tubular adenoma with a smooth surface and rounded glands. Active inflammation is occasionally present in adenomas, in this case, crypt dilation and rupture can be seen at the bottom of the field. **B,** Villous adenoma with long, slender projections that are reminiscent of small intestinal villi. **C,** Dysplastic epithelial cells *(top)* with an increased nuclear-to-cytoplasmic ratio, hyperchromatic and elongated nuclei, and nuclear pseudostratification. Compare to the nondysplastic epithelium below. **D,** Sessile serrated adenoma lined by goblet cells without typical cytologic features of dysplasia. This lesion is distinguished from a hyperplastic polyp by extension of the neoplastic process to the crypts, resulting in lateral growth. Compare to the hyperplastic polyp in Figure 17–44A.

adenomas may develop elsewhere in the GI tract, particularly adjacent to the ampulla of Vater and in the stomach.

FAP is associated with a variety of *extra-intestinal manifestations* including congenital hypertrophy of the retinal pigment epithelium, which can generally be detected at birth and can be an adjunct to early screening. Specific *APC* mutations have been associated with the development of other manifestations of FAP and explain variants such as Gardner syndrome and Turcot syndrome. In addition to intestinal polyps, *Gardner syndrome* families have osteomas of mandible, skull, and long bones, epidermal cysts, desmoid tumors, thyroid tumors, and dental abnormalities, including unerupted and supernumerary teeth. *Turcot syndrome* is rarer and characterized by intestinal adenomas and tumors of the central nervous system. Two thirds of patients with Turcot syndrome have *APC* gene mutations and develop medulloblastomas. The remaining one third have mutations in one of several genes involved in DNA repair and develop glioblastomas.

Some FAP patients without *APC* loss have mutations of the base-excision repair gene *MUTYH*.[112] The role of these genes

in tumor development is discussed below. In addition, certain *APC* and *MUTYH* mutations are associated with attenuated forms of FAP, which are characterized by delayed polyp development, the presence of fewer than 100 adenomas, and the delayed appearance of colon cancer, often to ages of 50 or above.[113]

HEREDITARY NON-POLYPOSIS COLORECTAL CANCER

Hereditary non-polyposis colorectal cancer (HNPCC), also known as Lynch syndrome, was originally described based on familial clustering of cancers at several sites including the colorectum, endometrium, stomach, ovary, ureters, brain, small bowel, hepatobiliary tract, and skin. Colon cancers in HNPCC patients tend to occur at *younger ages* than sporadic colon cancers and are often located in the *right colon* (see Table 17–10). Just as identification of *APC* mutations in FAP has provided molecular insights into the pathogenesis of the majority of sporadic colon cancers, dissection of the defects

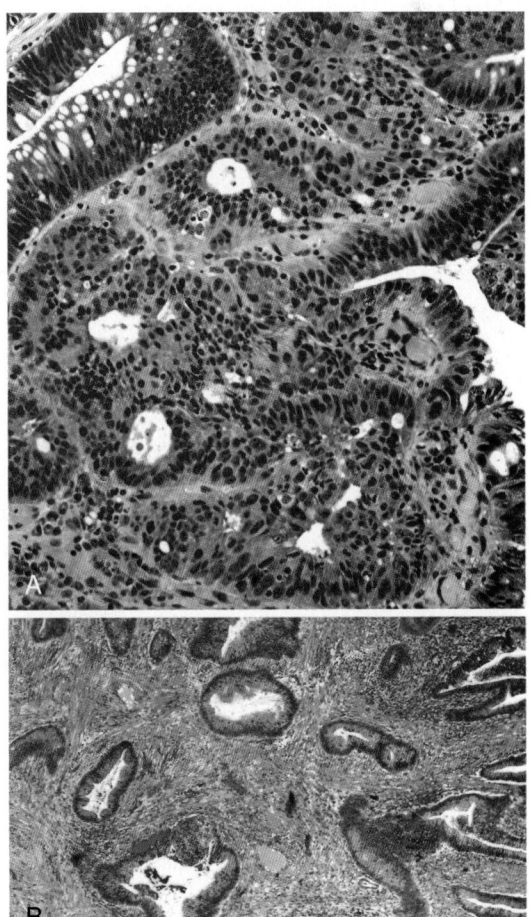

FIGURE 17–47 Adenoma with intramucosal carcinoma. **A,** Cribriform glands interface directly with the lamina propria without an intervening basement membrane. **B,** Invasive adenocarcinoma (left) beneath a villous adenoma (right). Note the desmoplastic response to the invasive components.

TABLE 17–10   Common Patterns of Sporadic and Familial Colorectal Neoplasia

Etiology	Molecular Defect	Target Gene(s)	Transmission	Predominant Site(s)	Histology
Familial adenomatous polyposis (70% of FAP)	APC/WNT pathway	*APC*	Autosomal dominant	None	Tubular, villous; typical adenocarcinoma
Familial adenomatous polyposis (<10% of FAP)	DNA mismatch repair	*MUTYH*	None, recessive	None	Sessile serrated adenoma; mucinous adenocarcinoma
Hereditary nonpolyposis colorectal cancer	DNA mismatch repair	*MSH2, MLH1*	Autosomal dominant	Right side	Sessile serrated adenoma; mucinous adenocarcinoma
Sporadic colon cancer (80%)	APC/WNT pathway	*APC*	None	Left side	Tubular, villous; typical adenocarcinoma
Sporadic colon cancer (10% to 15%)	DNA mismatch repair	*MSH2, MLH1*	None	Right side	Sessile serrated adenoma; mucinous adenocarcinoma

in HNPCC has shed light on the mechanisms responsible for most of the remaining sporadic cases. HNPCC is caused by inherited mutations in genes that encode proteins responsible for the detection, excision, and repair of errors that occur during DNA replication (Chapter 7). There are at least five such mismatch repair genes, but the majority of HNPCC cases involve *MSH2* and *MLH1*. Patients with HNPCC inherit one mutated DNA repair gene and one normal allele. When the second copy is lost through mutation or epigenetic silencing,

defects in mismatch repair lead to the accumulation of mutations at rates up to 1000 times higher than normal, mostly in regions containing short repeating DNA sequences referred to as microsatellite DNA. The human genome contains approximately 50,000 to 100,000 microsatellites, which are prone to undergo expansion during DNA replication and represent the most frequent sites of mutations in HNPCC. The consequences of mismatch repair deficiency and the resulting *microsatellite instability* are discussed in the context of colonic adenocarcinoma.

Adenocarcinoma

Adenocarcinoma of the colon is the most common malignancy of the GI tract and is a major cause of morbidity and mortality worldwide. In contrast, the small intestine, which accounts for 75% of the overall length of the GI tract, is an uncommon site for benign and malignant tumors. Among malignant small intestinal tumors, adenocarcinomas and carcinoid tumors have roughly equal incidence, followed by lymphomas and sarcomas. Hence, our discussion is focused on colorectal adenocarcinomas.

Epidemiology. Each year in the United States there are more than 130,000 new cases and 55,000 deaths from colorectal adenocarcinoma. This represents nearly 15% of all cancer-related deaths, and is second only to lung cancer. Colorectal cancer incidence peaks at 60 to 70 years of age, and fewer than 20% of cases occur before age 50. Males are affected slightly more often than females. Colorectal carcinoma is most prevalent in the United States, Canada, Australia, New Zealand, Denmark, Sweden, and other developed countries. The incidence of this cancer is as much as 30-fold lower in India, South America, and Africa. In Japan, where incidence was previously very low, rates have now risen to intermediate levels (similar to those in the United Kingdom), presumably as a result of changes in lifestyle and diet.

The dietary factors most closely associated with increased colorectal cancer rates are low intake of unabsorbable vegetable fiber and high intake of refined carbohydrates and fat. Although these associations are clear, the mechanistic relationship between diet and risk remains poorly understood. However, it is theorized that reduced fiber content leads to

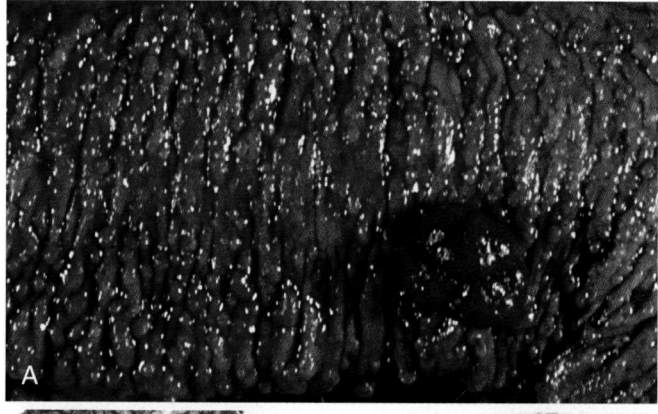
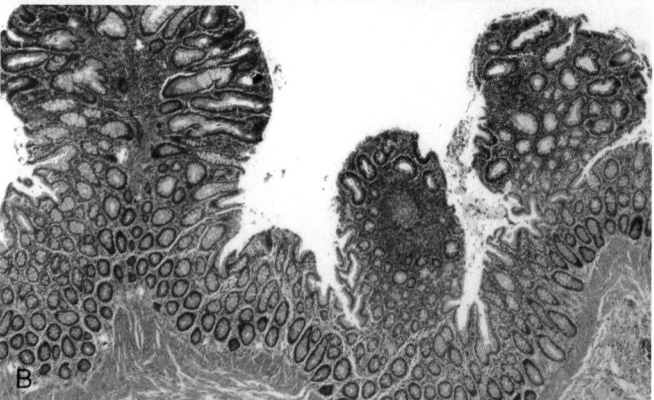

FIGURE 17–48   Familial adenomatous polyposis. **A,** Hundreds of small polyps are present throughout this colon with a dominant polyp *(right)*. **B,** Three tubular adenomas are present in this single microscopic field.

decreased stool bulk and altered composition of the intestinal microbiota. This change may increase synthesis of potentially toxic oxidative by-products of bacterial metabolism, which would be expected to remain in contact with the colonic mucosa for longer periods of time as a result of reduced stool bulk. Deficiencies of vitamins A, C, and E, which act as free-radical scavengers, may compound damage caused by oxidants. High fat intake enhances the hepatic synthesis of cholesterol and bile acids, which can be converted into carcinogens by intestinal bacteria.

In addition to dietary modification, pharmacologic chemoprevention has become an area of great interest. Several epidemiologic studies suggest that aspirin or other NSAIDs have a protective effect. This is consistent with studies showing that some NSAIDs cause polyp regression in FAP patients in whom the rectum was left in place after colectomy. It is suspected that this effect is mediated by inhibition of the enzyme cyclooxygenase-2 (COX-2), which is highly expressed in 90% of colorectal carcinomas and 40% to 90% of adenomas. COX-2 is necessary for production of prostaglandin E_2, which promotes epithelial proliferation, particularly after injury.[114] Of further interest, COX-2 expression is regulated by TLR4, which recognizes lipopolysaccharide and is also overexpressed in adenomas and carcinomas.[115]

Pathogenesis. Studies of colorectal carcinogenesis have provided fundamental insights into the general mechanisms of cancer evolution. These were discussed in Chapter 7; concepts that pertain specifically to colorectal carcinogenesis will be reviewed here.

The combination of molecular events that lead to colonic adenocarcinoma is heterogeneous and includes genetic and epigenetic abnormalities. At least two distinct genetic pathways have been described. In simplest terms, these are the *APC/β-catenin pathway*, which is associated with *WNT* and the classic adenoma-carcinoma sequence; and the *microsatellite instability pathway*, which is associated with defects in DNA mismatch repair (see Table 17–10). Both pathways involve the stepwise accumulation of multiple mutations, but the genes involved and the mechanisms by which the mutations accumulate differ. Epigenetic events, the most common of which is methylation-induced gene silencing, may enhance progression along both pathways.

The classic *adenoma-carcinoma sequence*, which accounts for as much as 80% of sporadic colon tumors, typically includes mutation of *APC* early in the neoplastic process (Fig. 17–49). Both copies of the *APC* gene must be functionally inactivated, either by mutation or epigenetic events, for adenomas to develop. *APC is a key negative regulator of β-catenin, a component of the WNT signaling pathway* (see Chapter 7). The APC protein normally binds to and promotes degradation of β-catenin. With loss of APC function, β-catenin accumulates and translocates to the nucleus, where it activates the transcription of genes, such as those encoding MYC and cyclin D1, which promote proliferation. This is followed by additional mutations, including activating mutations in *KRAS*, which also promote growth and prevent apoptosis. The conclusion that mutation of *KRAS* is a late event is supported by the observation that mutations are present in fewer than 10% of adenomas less than 1 cm in diameter but are found in 50% of adenomas greater than 1 cm in diameter and 50% of invasive adenocarcinomas. Neoplastic progression is also associated with mutations in other tumor suppressor genes such as those encoding SMAD2 and SMAD4, which are effectors of TGF-β signaling. Because TGF-β signaling normally inhibits the cell cycle, loss of these genes may allow unrestrained cell growth. The tumor suppressor *p53* is mutated in 70% to

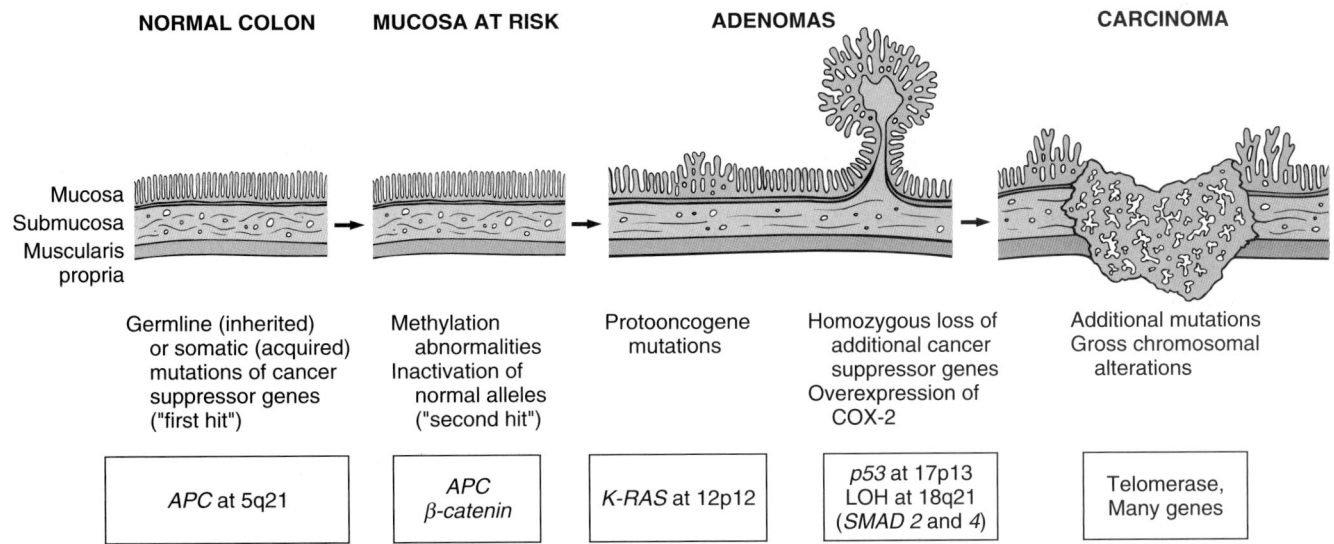

FIGURE 17–49 Morphologic and molecular changes in the adenoma-carcinoma sequence. It is postulated that loss of one normal copy of the tumor suppressor gene *APC* occurs early. Individuals may be born with one mutant allele, making them extremely prone to develop colon cancer, or inactivation of *APC* may occur later in life. This is the "first hit" according to Knudson's hypothesis (Chapter 7). The loss of the intact copy of *APC* follows ("second hit"). Other mutations include those on *KRAS*, losses at 18q21 involving *SMAD2* and *SMAD4*, and inactivation of the tumor suppressor gene *p53*, lead to the emergence of carcinoma, in which additional mutations occur. Although there seems to be a temporal sequence of changes, the accumulation of mutations, rather than their occurrence in a specific order, is most critical.

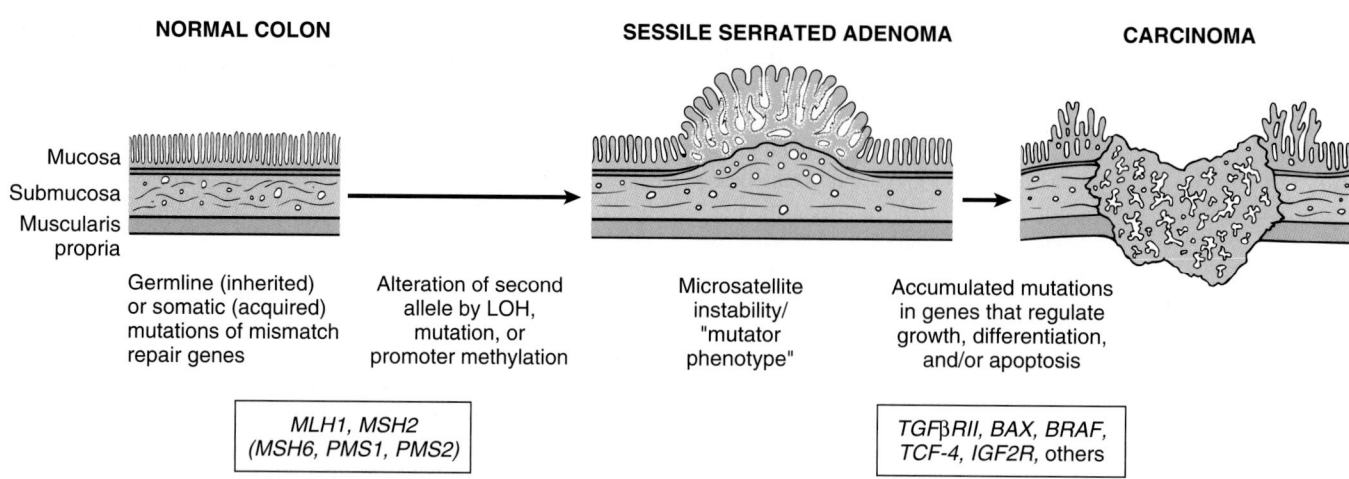

FIGURE 17–50 Morphologic and molecular changes in the mismatch repair pathway of colon carcinogenesis. Defects in mismatch repair genes result in microsatellite instability and permit accumulation of mutations in numerous genes. If these mutations affect genes involved in cell survival and proliferation, cancer may develop.

80% of colon cancers, but is uncommonly affected in adenomas, suggesting that *p53* mutations also occur at late stages of tumor progression. "Loss of function" of *p53* and other tumor suppressor genes is often caused by chromosomal deletions, pointing out that chromosomal instability is a hallmark of the APC/β-catenin pathway. Alternatively, tumor suppressor genes may be silenced by methylation of a CpG-rich zone, or CpG island, a 5′ region of some genes that frequently includes the promoter and transcriptional start site. Expression of telomerase also increases as lesions become more advanced.

○ In patients with DNA mismatch repair deficiency (due to loss of mismatch repair genes, as discussed earlier) mutations accumulate in microsatellite repeats, a condition referred to as *microsatellite instability*. While these mutations are generally silent because microsatellites are typically in noncoding regions, some microsatellite sequences are located in the coding or promoter region of genes involved in regulation of cell growth, such as those encoding the type II TGF-β receptor and the pro-apoptotic protein BAX (Fig. 17–50). Because TGF-β inhibits colonic epithelial cell proliferation, type II TGF-β receptor mutants can contribute to uncontrolled cell growth, while loss of *BAX* may enhance the survival of genetically abnormal clones. Mutations in the oncogene *BRAF* and silencing of distinct groups of genes due to CpG island hypermethylation are also common in cancers that develop through DNA mismatch repair defects. In contrast, *KRAS* and *p53* are not typically mutated. Thus, the combination of microsatellite instability, *BRAF* mutation, and methylation of specific targets, such as *MLH1*, is the signature of this pathway of carcinogenesis.[116]

○ A third group of colon cancers with increased CpG island methylation in the absence of microsatellite instability also exists. Many of these tumors harbor *KRAS* mutations, but *p53* and *BRAF* mutations are uncommon. In contrast, *p53* mutations are common in colon cancers that do not display a CpG island methylator phenotype.[116,117]

While morphology cannot reliably predict the underlying molecular events that led to carcinogenesis, certain correlations have been associated with mismatch repair deficiency and microsatellite instability. These molecular alterations are common in sessile serrated adenomas. In addition, invasive carcinomas with microsatellite instability often have prominent mucinous differentiation and peritumoral lymphocytic infiltrates. These tumors, as well as those with a CpG island methylator phenotype, are frequently located in the right colon. Tumors with microsatellite instability can be recognized by the absence of immunohistochemical staining for mismatch repair proteins or by molecular genetic analysis of microsatellite sequences. It is important to identify those with HNPCC because of the implications for genetic counseling, the elevated risk of a second malignancy of the colon and other organs, and, in some settings, differences in prognosis and therapy.

Morphology. Overall, adenocarcinomas are distributed approximately equally over the entire length of the colon. Tumors in the proximal colon often grow as polypoid, exophytic masses that extend along one wall of the large-caliber cecum and ascending colon; these tumors rarely cause obstruction. In contrast, carcinomas in the distal colon tend to be annular lesions that produce "napkin-ring" constrictions and luminal narrowing (Fig. 17–51), sometimes to the point that obstruction occurs. Both forms grow into the bowel wall over time and may be palpable as firm masses. The general microscopic characteristics of right- and left-sided colonic adenocarcinomas are similar. Most tumors are composed of tall columnar cells that resemble dysplastic epithelium found in adenomas (Fig. 17–52A). The invasive component of these tumors elicits a strong stromal desmoplastic response, which is responsible for their characteristic firm consistency. Some poorly differentiated tumors form few glands (Fig. 17–52B). Others may produce abundant mucin that accumulates within the intesti-

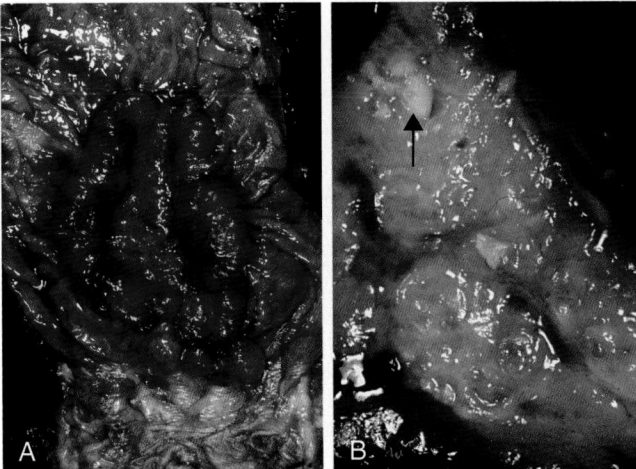

FIGURE 17–51 Colorectal carcinoma. **A,** Circumferential, ulcerated rectal cancer. Note the anal mucosa at the bottom of the image. **B,** Cancer of the sigmoid colon that has invaded through the muscularis propria and is present within subserosal adipose tissue *(left)*. Areas of chalky necrosis are present within the colon wall *(arrow)*.

nal wall, and these are associated with poor prognosis. Tumors may also be composed of signet-ring cells that are similar to those in gastric cancer (Fig. 17–52C). Others may display features of neuroendocrine differentiation.

Clinical Features. The availability of endoscopic screening combined with the knowledge that most carcinomas arise within adenomas presents a unique opportunity for cancer prevention. Unfortunately, colorectal cancers develop insidiously and may therefore go undetected for long periods. Cecal and other *right-sided colon cancers* are most often called to clinical attention by the appearance of *fatigue and weakness due to iron deficiency anemia.* Thus, it is a clinical maxim that the underlying cause of iron deficiency anemia in an older man or postmenopausal woman is GI cancer until proven

otherwise. *Left-sided colorectal adenocarcinomas* may produce *occult bleeding, changes in bowel habits, or cramping* left lower quadrant discomfort.

Although poorly differentiated and mucinous histologies are associated with poor prognosis, *the two most important prognostic factors are depth of invasion and the presence or absence of lymph node metastases.* Invasion into the muscularis propria confers significantly reduced survival that is decreased further by the presence of lymph node metastases (Fig. 17–53A).[118] These factors were originally recognized by Dukes and Kirklin and form the core of the TNM (tumor-nodes-metastasis) classification (Table 17–11) and staging system (Table 17–12) from the American Joint Committee on Cancer. Regardless of stage, it must be remembered that some patients with small numbers of metastases do well for years following resection of distant tumor nodules. This, once again, emphasizes the clinical and molecular heterogeneity of colorectal carcinomas. Metastases may involve regional lymph nodes, lungs (Fig. 17–53B) and bones, but as a result of portal drainage of the colon, the liver is the most common site of metastatic lesions (Fig. 17–53C). The rectum does not drain via the portal circulation, and carcinomas of the anal region that metastasize often circumvent the liver.

Tumors of the Anal Canal

The anal canal can be divided into thirds. The upper zone is lined by columnar rectal epithelium; the middle third by transitional epithelium; and the lower third by stratified squamous epithelium. Carcinomas of the anal canal may have typical glandular or squamous (Fig. 17–54A) patterns of differentiation, recapitulating the normal epithelium of the upper and lower thirds, respectively. An additional differentiation pattern, termed *basaloid*, is present in tumors populated by immature cells derived from the basal layer of transitional epithelium (Fig. 17–54B). When the entire tumor displays a basaloid pattern, the archaic term *cloacogenic carcinoma* is still often applied. Alternatively, basaloid differentiation may be mixed with squamous or mucinous differentiation. All are considered variants of anal canal carcinoma. Pure squamous cell

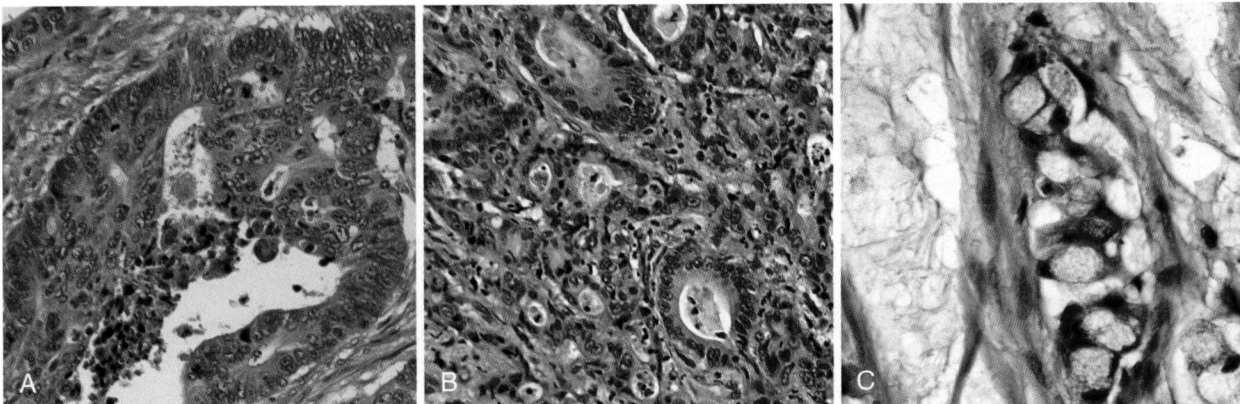

FIGURE 17–52 Histologic appearance of colorectal carcinoma. **A,** Well-differentiated adenocarcinoma. Note the elongated, hyperchromatic nuclei. Necrotic debris, present in the gland lumen, is typical. **B,** Poorly differentiated adenocarcinoma forms a few glands but is largely composed of infiltrating nests of tumor cells. **C,** Mucinous adenocarcinoma with signet-ring cells and extracellular mucin pools.

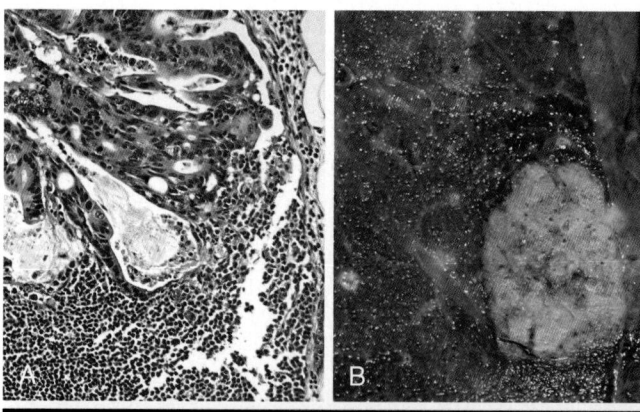

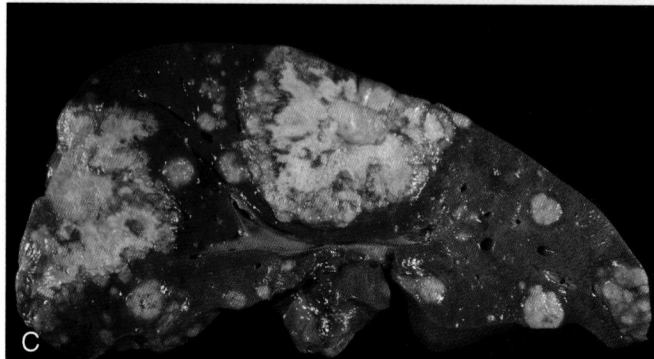

FIGURE 17–53 Metastatic colorectal carcinoma. **A,** Lymph node metastasis. Note the glandular structures within the subcapsular sinus. **B,** Solitary subpleural nodule of colorectal carcinoma metastatic to the lung. **C,** Liver containing two large and many smaller metastases. Note the central necrosis within metastases.

carcinoma of the anal canal is frequently associated with HPV infection, which also causes precursor lesions such as *condyloma accuminatum* (Fig. 17–54C).

Hemorrhoids

Hemorrhoids affect about 5% of the general population and develop secondary to persistently elevated venous pressure within the hemorrhoidal plexus. The most frequent predisposing influences are straining at stool because of constipation and the venous stasis of pregnancy.

Pathogenesis. The pathogenesis of hemorrhoids (anal varices) is similar to that of esophageal varices, although anal varices are both more common and less serious. Variceal dilations of the anal and perianal venous plexuses form collaterals that connect the portal and caval venous systems, thereby relieving the venous hypertension.

Morphology. Collateral vessels within the inferior hemorrhoidal plexus are located below the anorectal line and are termed **external hemorrhoids**, while those that result from dilation of the superior hemorrhoidal plexus within the distal rectum are referred to as **internal hemorrhoids**. Histologically, hemorrhoids consist of thin-walled, dilated, submucosal vessels that protrude beneath the anal or rectal mucosa. In

their exposed position, they are subject to trauma and tend to become inflamed, thrombosed, and, in the course of time, recanalized. Superficial ulceration may occur.

Clinical Features. Hemorrhoids often present with pain and rectal bleeding, particularly bright red blood seen on toilet tissue. Except for pregnant women, hemorrhoids are rarely encountered in persons under age 30. Hemorrhoids may also develop as a result of portal hypertension, where the implications are more ominous. Hemorrhoidal bleeding is not generally a medical emergency and can be treated by sclerotherapy, rubber band ligation, or infrared coagulation. Extensive or severe internal or external hemorrhoids may be removed surgically by *hemorrhoidectomy*.

Acute Appendicitis

The appendix is a normal true diverticulum of the cecum that is prone to acute and chronic inflammation. Acute appendicitis is most common in adolescents and young adults, but may occur in any age group. The lifetime risk for appendicitis is 7%; males are affected slightly more often than females. Despite the prevalence of acute appendicitis, the diagnosis can be difficult to confirm preoperatively and may be confused with mesenteric lymphadenitis (often secondary to unrecognized *Yersinia* infection or viral enterocolitis), acute salpingitis, ectopic pregnancy, mittelschmerz (pain caused by minor pelvic bleeding at the time of ovulation), and Meckel diverticulitis.

TABLE 17–11	American Joint Committee on Cancer (AJCC) TNM Classification of Colorectal Carcinoma
TNM	
TUMOR	
Tis	In situ dysplasia or intramucosal carcinoma
T1	Tumor invades submucosa
T2	Tumor invades into, but not through, muscularis propria
T3	Tumor invades through muscularis propria
T3a	Invasion <0.1 cm beyond muscularis propria
T3b	Invasion 0.1 to 0.5 cm beyond muscularis propria
T3c	Invasion >0.5 to 1.5 cm beyond muscularis propria
T3d	Invasion >1.5 cm beyond muscularis propria
T4	Tumor invades adjacent organs or visceral peritoneum
T4a	Invasion into other organs or structures
T4b	Invasion into visceral peritoneum
REGIONAL LYMPH NODES	
NX	Lymph nodes cannot be assessed
N0	No regional lymph node metastasis
N1	Metastasis in one to three regional lymph nodes
N2	Metastasis in four or more regional lymph nodes
DISTANT METASTASIS	
MX	Distant metastasis cannot be assessed
M0	No distant metastasis
M1	Distant metastasis or seeding of abdominal organs

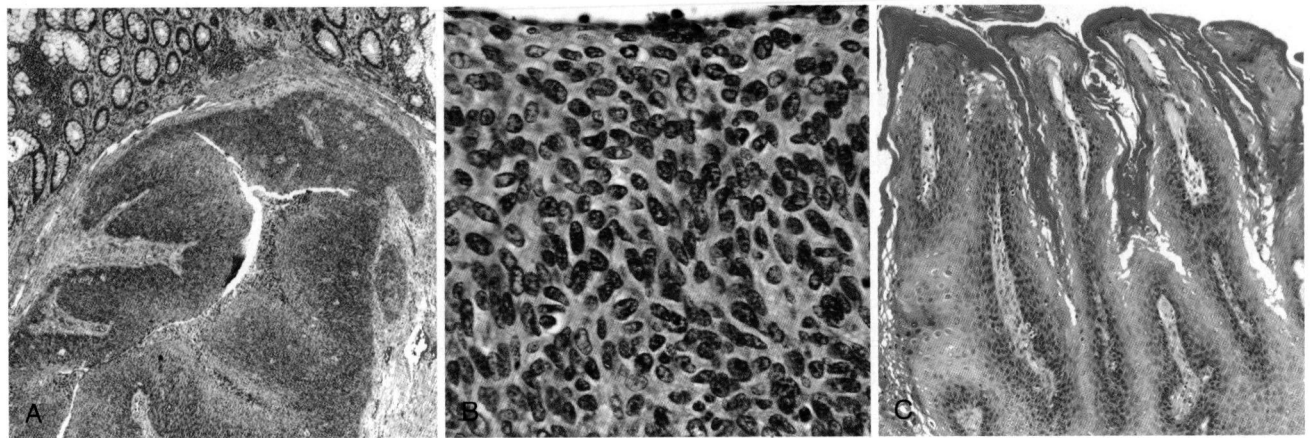

FIGURE 17–54 Anal tumors. **A,** This squamous anal transition zone tumor forms nests with central necrosis. The adjacent rectal mucosa is intact. **B,** This basaloid anal transition zone tumor is composed of hyperchromatic cells that resemble the basal layer of normal squamous mucosa. **C,** Condyloma accuminatum with verrucous architecture.

Pathogenesis. Acute appendicitis is thought to be initiated by progressive increases in intraluminal pressure that compromise venous outflow. In 50% to 80% of cases, acute appendicitis is associated with overt luminal obstruction, usually caused by a small stone-like mass of stool, or *fecalith*, or, less commonly, a gallstone, tumor, or mass of worms *(oxyuriasis vermicularis)*. Ischemic injury and stasis of luminal contents, which favor bacterial proliferation, trigger inflammatory responses including tissue edema and neutrophilic infiltration of the lumen, muscular wall, and periappendiceal soft tissues.

> **Morphology.** In early acute appendicitis subserosal vessels are congested and there is a modest perivascular neutrophilic infiltrate within all layers of the wall. The inflammatory reaction transforms the normal glistening serosa into a dull, granular, erythematous surface. Diagnosis of acute appendicitis requires neutrophilic infiltration of the muscularis propria. Although mucosal neutrophils and focal superficial ulceration are often present, these are not specific markers of acute appendicitis. In more severe cases a prominent neutrophilic exudate generates a serosal fibrinopurulent reaction. As the process continues, focal abscesses may form within the wall **(acute suppurative appendicitis).** Further appendiceal compromise leads to large areas of hemorrhagic ulceration and gangrenous necrosis that extends to the serosa creating **acute gangrenous appendicitis**, which is often followed by rupture and suppurative peritonitis.

Clinical Features. Typically, early acute appendicitis produces periumbilical pain that ultimately localizes to the right lower quadrant, followed by nausea, vomiting, low-grade fever, and a mildly elevated peripheral white cell count. A classic physical finding is *McBurney's sign*, deep tenderness located two thirds of the distance from the umbilicus to the right anterior superior iliac spine (McBurney's point). Regrettably, these signs and symptoms are often absent, creating difficulty in clinical diagnosis. In some cases, a retrocecal appendix may generate right flank or pelvic pain, while a malrotated colon may give rise to appendicitis in the left upper quadrant. In other cases the peripheral leukocytosis may be minimal or, alternatively, so great that other causes are considered. The diagnosis of acute appendicitis in young children and the very elderly is particularly problematic, since other causes of abdominal emergencies are prevalent in these populations, and the very young and old are also more likely to have atypical clinical presentations. Given these diagnostic challenges, it should be no surprise that even highly skilled surgeons remove normal appendices. This is preferred to delayed resection of a diseased appendix, given the significant morbidity and mortality associated with appendiceal perforation. Other complications of appendicitis include pyelophlebitis, portal venous thrombosis, liver abscess, and bacteremia.

TABLE 17–12 American Joint Committee on Cancer (AJCC) Colorectal Cancer Staging and Survival

	T	N	M	5-YEAR SURVIVAL (%)
STAGE*				
I	T1, T2	N0	M0	93
II				
IIA	T3	N0	M0	85
IIB	T4	N0	M0	72
III				
IIIA	T1, T2	N1	M0	83
IIIB	T3, T4	N1	M0	64
IIIC	Any T	N2	M0	44
IV	Any T	Any N	M1	8

*Colorectal cancer staging is based on the TNM classification (Table 17–11). For example, a T3 tumor without nodal or distant metastases is classified as stage IIA and is associated with a 5-year survival rate of 85%.

Tumors of the Appendix

The most common tumor of the appendix is the *carcinoid*. It is usually discovered incidentally at the time of surgery or examination of a resected appendix. This neoplasm most frequently involves the distal tip of the appendix, where it produces a solid bulbous swelling up to 2 to 3 cm in diameter. Although intramural and transmural extension may be evident, nodal metastases are very infrequent, and distant spread is exceptionally rare. Conventional adenomas or non-mucin-producing adenocarcinomas also occur in the appendix and may cause obstruction and enlargement that mimics acute appendicitis. *Mucocele*, a dilated appendix filled with mucin, may simply represent an obstructed appendix containing inspissated mucin or be a consequence of *mucinous cystadenoma* or *mucinous cystadenocarcinoma*. In the latter instance, invasion through the appendiceal wall can lead to intraperitoneal seeding and spread. In women the resulting peritoneal implants may be mistaken for mucinous ovarian tumors. In the most advanced cases the abdomen fills with tenacious, semisolid mucin, a condition called *pseudomyxoma peritoneii* (Chapter 22). This disseminated intraperitoneal disease may be held in check for years by repeated debulking but, in most instances, follows an inexorably fatal course.

PERITONEAL CAVITY

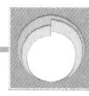

The peritoneal cavity houses the abdominal viscera and is lined by a single layer of mesothelial cells; these cover the visceral and parietal surfaces and are supported by a thin layer of connective tissue to form the peritoneum. Here we discuss inflammatory, infectious, and neoplastic disorders of the peritoneal cavity and retroperitoneal space. Although they are less common than inflammatory and infectious processes, tumors can carry a grave prognosis and, thus, deserve discussion.

Inflammatory Disease

Peritonitis may result from bacterial invasion or chemical irritation and is most often due to:

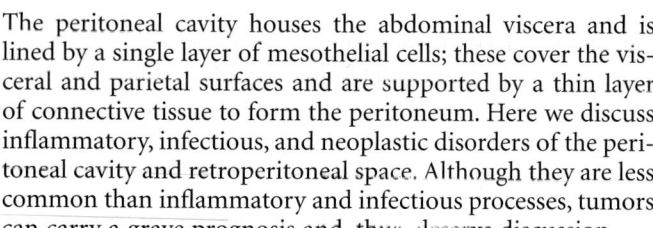

- Leakage of bile or pancreatic enzymes, which produces *sterile peritonitis*
- *Perforation or rupture of the biliary system* that evokes a highly irritating peritonitis, usually complicated by bacterial superinfection
- *Acute hemorrhagic pancreatitis* (see Chapter 19), which is associated with leakage of pancreatic enzymes and fat necrosis. Globules of fat may be found in the peritoneal fluid. Damage to the bowel wall may allow bacteria to spread to the peritoneal cavity, leading to a frank suppurative exudate after 24 to 48 hours.
- *Foreign material*, including that introduced surgically (e.g., talc and sutures), that induces foreign body–type granulomas and fibrous scarring
- *Endometriosis*, which causes hemorrhage into the peritoneal cavity, where it acts as an irritant
- *Ruptured dermoid cysts* release keratins that invoke an intense granulomatous reaction
- *Perforation* of abdominal viscera, as described below

PERITONEAL INFECTION

Bacterial peritonitis occurs when bacteria from the gastrointestinal lumen are released into the abdominal cavity, typically following perforation. This occurs most commonly as a complication of *acute appendicitis, peptic ulcer, cholecystitis, diverticulitis,* and *intestinal ischemia. Acute salpingitis, abdominal trauma,* and *peritoneal dialysis* are other potential sources of contaminating bacteria. Although *E. coli,* streptococci, *S. aureus,* enterococci, and *C. perfringens* are implicated most often, virtually any bacteria can be associated with bacterial peritonitis.

Spontaneous bacterial peritonitis develops in the absence of an obvious source of contamination. It is an uncommon disorder that is seen most often in patients with cirrhosis and ascites; 10% of such individuals develop spontaneous bacterial peritonitis. Children, particularly those with nephrotic syndrome, may also develop spontaneous bacterial peritonitis. The manner by which bacteria gain access to the peritoneal cavity is unknown, but the organisms identified most often are *E. coli* and pneumococci, suggesting sources in the GI tract or the lungs, respectively.

Morphology. Normally glistening serosal and peritoneal surfaces become dull and lusterless, and serous or slightly turbid fluid begins to accumulate within 2 to 4 hours of infection. As the infection progresses, creamy suppurative material that may be extremely viscous accumulates. The volume of fluid varies enormously; it may be localized by the omentum and viscera to a small area or may fill the abdominal cavity. Exudate may collect around the liver to form subhepatic and subdiaphragmatic abscesses.

The cellular inflammatory response is composed primarily of dense collections of neutrophils and fibrinopurulent debris that coat the viscera and abdominal wall. The reaction usually remains superficial and does not penetrate deeply. One exception is tuberculous peritonitis, which typically studs the serosal and peritoneal surfaces with small, pale granulomas.

While bacterial peritonitis can be fatal, the inflammatory process can also heal, either spontaneously or as a result of therapy. It may resolve completely; undergo organization into fibrous adhesions; or become walled off in abscesses that may persist (potentially serving as new sources of infection) or heal.

SCLEROSING RETROPERITONITIS

Sclerosing retroperitonitis, also known as *idiopathic retroperitoneal fibrosis* or *Ormond disease,* is characterized by dense fibrosis that may extend to involve the mesentery. Although the cause of sclerosing retroperitonitis is unknown, it is thought to be an inflammatory process. Because the process frequently compresses the ureters, this entity is described in more detail in Chapter 21.

CYSTS

Cysts may develop within the abdominal cavity and are frequently attached to the peritoneum. They can be quite large, sometimes presenting as palpable abdominal masses. The origins of such cysts are diverse; they can develop from "blind" lymphatic channels; foregut or hindgut diverticulae that pinch off during development; the urogenital ridge or its derivatives (i.e., the urinary tract and male and female genital tracts); walled-off infections; or as a sequela of pancreatitis *(pseudocysts).*

Tumors

Most tumors of the peritoneum are malignant and can be divided into primary and secondary forms.

Primary tumors arising from peritoneal lining are *mesotheliomas* that are similar to tumors of the pleura and pericardium. Peritoneal mesotheliomas are almost always associated with significant asbestos exposure. It has been hypothesized that swallowed asbestos fibers somehow penetrate through the intestinal wall to reach the peritoneum. As with pleural mesothelioma, the histopathologic diagnosis can be difficult. The differential diagnosis includes metastatic adenocarcinoma, which can be distinguished from mesothelioma using a variety of immunohistochemical markers (Chapter 15).

Rarely, primary benign and malignant soft-tissue tumors develop within the peritoneum and retroperitoneum. The most common of these is *desmoplastic small round cell tumor.* This aggressive tumor occurs in children and young adults. The neoplasm is characterized by a reciprocal chromosomal translocation, t(11;22)(p13;q12) that results in fusion of genes associated with Ewing sarcoma *(EWS)* and Wilms tumor *(WT1).* Morphologically, the tumor bears a resemblance to Ewing sarcoma and related tumors.

Secondary tumors of the peritoneum are, in contrast, quite common. In any form of advanced cancer, direct spread to the serosal surface or metastatic seeding (peritoneal carcinomatosis) may occur. The most common tumors producing diffuse serosal implants are ovarian and pancreatic adenocarcinoma. Appendiceal mucinous carcinomas may produce *pseudomyxoma peritoneii.* However, any intra-abdominal malignancy, as well as a wide variety of tumors of extra-abdominal origin, may spread to the peritoneum.

REFERENCES

1. Bueno RC et al.: Intraoperative localization of ectopic gastric mucosa in the nonduplicated intestinal lumen with technetium 99m pertechnetate scanning. J Pediatr Surg 36:1720, 2001.
2. Emison ES et al.: A common sex-dependent mutation in a RET enhancer underlies Hirschsprung disease risk. Nature 434:857, 2005.
3. Gabriel SB et al.: Segregation at three loci explains familial and population risk in Hirschsprung disease. Nat Genet 31:89, 2002.
4. Dogan I, Mittal RK: Esophageal motor disorders: recent advances. Curr Opin Gastroenterol 22:417, 2006.
5. Dantas RO, Aprile LR: Esophageal contractions in Chagas' disease and in idiopathic achalasia. J Clin Gastroenterol 39:863, 2005.
6. Shaheen NJ et al.: The burden of gastrointestinal and liver diseases, 2006. Am J Gastroenterol 101:2128, 2006.
7. Furuta GT et al.: Eosinophilic esophagitis in children and adults: a systematic review and consensus recommendations for diagnosis and treatment. Gastroenterology 133:1342, 2007.
8. Izzo JG et al.: Molecular mechanisms in Barrett's metaplasia and its progression. Semin Oncol 34:S2, 2007.
9. Enzinger PC, Mayer RJ: Esophageal cancer. N Engl J Med 349:2241, 2003.
10. Devesa SS et al.: Changing patterns in the incidence of esophageal and gastric carcinoma in the United States. Cancer 83:2049, 1998.
11. Polednak AP: Secular trend in U.S. black-white disparities in selected alcohol-related cancer incidence rates. Alcohol Alcohol 42:125, 2007.
12. Turner JR et al.: Low prevalence of human papillomavirus infection in esophageal squamous cell carcinomas from North America: analysis by a highly sensitive and specific polymerase chain reaction–based approach. Hum Pathol 28:174, 1997.
13. Marshall BJ, Warren JR: Unidentified curved bacilli in the stomach of patients with gastritis and peptic ulceration. Lancet 1:1311, 1984.
14. Wilson KT, Crabtree JE: Immunology of *Helicobacter pylori*: insights into the failure of the immune response and perspectives on vaccine studies. Gastroenterology 133:288, 2007.
15. Toh BH et al.: Pernicious anemia. N Engl J Med 337:1441, 1997.
16. Suit PF et al.: Gastric antral vascular ectasia. A histologic and morphometric study of "the watermelon stomach". Am J Surg Pathol 11:750, 1987.
17. Haot J et al.: Lymphocytic gastritis: a newly described entity: a retrospective endoscopic and histological study. Gut 29:1258, 1988.
18. Shapiro JL et al.: A clinicopathologic study of 42 patients with granulomatous gastritis. Is there really an "idiopathic" granulomatous gastritis? Am J Surg Pathol 20:462, 1996.
19. Sandler RS et al.: The burden of selected digestive diseases in the United States. Gastroenterology 122:1500, 2002.
20. Louw JA: Peptic ulcer disease. Curr Opin Gastroenterol 22:607, 2006.
21. Coffey RJ et al.: Menetrier disease and gastrointestinal stromal tumors: hyperproliferative disorders of the stomach. J Clin Invest 117:70, 2007.
22. Burdick JS et al.: Treatment of Menetrier's disease with a monoclonal antibody against the epidermal growth factor receptor. N Engl J Med 343:1697, 2000.
23. Tomassetti P et al.: Treatment of type II gastric carcinoid tumors with somatostatin analogues. N Engl J Med 343:551, 2000.
24. Ming SC, Goldman H: Gastric polyps: a histogenetic classification and its relation to carcinoma. Cancer 18:721, 1965.
25. Goldstein NS, Lewin KJ: Gastric epithelial dysplasia and adenoma: historical review and histological criteria for grading. Hum Pathol 28:127, 1997.
26. Wingo PA et al.: Long-term trends in cancer mortality in the United States, 1930–1998. Cancer 97:3133, 2003.
27. El-Serag HB et al.: Epidemiological differences between adenocarcinoma of the oesophagus and adenocarcinoma of the gastric cardia in the USA. Gut 50:368, 2002.
28. Hundahl SA et al.: The National Cancer Data Base report on poor survival of U.S. gastric carcinoma patients treated with gastrectomy. Cancer 88:921, 2000.
29. Hansen S et al.: Two distinct aetiologies of cardia cancer; evidence from premorbid serological markers of gastric atrophy and *Helicobacter pylori* status. Gut 56:918, 2007.
30. Rohatgi PR et al.: Surgical pathology stage by American Joint Commission on Cancer criteria predicts patient survival after preoperative chemoradiation for localized gastric carcinoma. Cancer 107:1475, 2006.
31. Lau M et al.: Noncardia gastric adenocarcinoma remains an important and deadly cancer in the United States: secular trends in incidence and survival. Am J Gastroenterol 101:2485, 2006.

32. Gurbuxani S, Anastasi J: What to do when you suspect gastrointestinal lymphoma: a pathologist's perspective. Clin Gastroenterol Hepatol 5:417, 2007.

33. Sagaert X et al.: The pathogenesis of MALT lymphomas: where do we stand? Leukemia 21:389, 2007.

34. Suarez F et al.: Infection-associated lymphomas derived from marginal zone B cells: a model of antigen-driven lymphoproliferation. Blood 107:3034, 2006.

35. Hsi ED et al.: Classification of primary gastric lymphomas according to histologic features. Am J Surg Pathol 22:17, 1998.

36. Ye H et al.: High incidence of t(11;18)(q21;q21) in *Helicobacter pylori*–negative gastric MALT lymphoma. Blood 101:2547, 2003.

37. Ye H et al.: Strong BCL10 nuclear expression identifies gastric MALT lymphomas that do not respond to *H. pylori* eradication. Gut 55:137, 2006.

38. Ruefli-Brasse AA et al.: Regulation of NF-κB–dependent lymphocyte activation and development by paracaspase. Science 302:1581, 2003.

39. Levy AD, Sobin LH: From the archives of the AFIP: gastrointestinal carcinoids: imaging features with clinicopathologic comparison. Radiographics 27:237, 2007.

40. Lasota J, Miettinen M: *KIT* and *PDGFRA* mutations in gastrointestinal stromal tumors (GISTs). Semin Diagn Pathol 23:91, 2006.

41. Hirota S et al.: Gain-of-function mutations of platelet-derived growth factor receptor alpha gene in gastrointestinal stromal tumors. Gastroenterology 125:660, 2003.

42. Hirota S et al.: Gain-of-function mutations of c-KIT in human gastrointestinal stromal tumors. Science 279:577, 1998.

43. Demetri GD et al.: Efficacy and safety of imatinib mesylate in advanced gastrointestinal stromal tumors. N Engl J Med 347:472, 2002.

44. Taylor CT, Colgan SP: Hypoxia and gastrointestinal disease. J Mol Med 85:1295, 2007.

45. Chen LW et al.: The two faces of IKK and NF-κB inhibition: prevention of systemic inflammation but increased local injury following intestinal ischemia-reperfusion. Nat Med 9:575, 2003.

46. Hunt KA et al.: Newly identified genetic risk variants for celiac disease related to the immune response. Nat Genet 40:395, 2008.

47. Wapenaar MC et al.: Associations with tight junction genes *PARD3* and *MAGI2* in Dutch patients point to a common barrier defect for coeliac disease and ulcerative colitis. Gut 57:463, 2008.

48. Wolters VM et al.: The *MYO9B* gene is a strong risk factor for developing refractory celiac disease. Clin Gastroenterol Hepatol 5:1399, 2007.

49. Goldstein NS, Underhill J: Morphologic features suggestive of gluten sensitivity in architecturally normal duodenal biopsy specimens. Am J Clin Pathol 116:63, 2001.

50. Fasano A: Clinical presentation of celiac disease in the pediatric population. Gastroenterology 128:S68, 2005.

51. Rostom A et al.: American Gastroenterological Association (AGA) Institute technical review on the diagnosis and management of celiac disease. Gastroenterology 131:1981, 2006.

52. Bennett CL et al.: The immune dysregulation, polyendocrinopathy, enteropathy, X-linked syndrome (IPEX) is caused by mutations of *FOXP3*. Nat Genet 27:20, 2001.

53. Hori S et al.: Control of regulatory T cell development by the transcription factor Foxp3. Science 299:1057, 2003.

54. Baud O et al.: Treatment of the immune dysregulation, polyendocrinopathy, enteropathy, X-linked syndrome (IPEX) by allogeneic bone marrow transplantation. N Engl J Med 344:1758, 2001.

55. Kuokkanen M et al.: Mutations in the translated region of the lactase gene (*LCT*) underlie congenital lactase deficiency. Am J Hum Genet 78:339, 2006.

56. Sack DA et al.: Cholera. Lancet 363:223, 2004.

57. Mead PS et al.: Food-related illness and death in the United States. Emerg Infect Dis 5:607, 1999.

58. Lencer WI, Tsai B: The intracellular voyage of cholera toxin: going retro. Trends Biochem Sci 28:639, 2003.

59. Ramakrishna BS et al.: Amylase-resistant starch plus oral rehydration solution for cholera. N Engl J Med 342:308, 2000.

60. Li C et al.: Lysophosphatidic acid inhibits cholera toxin-induced secretory diarrhea through CFTR-dependent protein interactions. J Exp Med 202:975, 2005.

61. Zuckerman JN et al.: The true burden and risk of cholera: implications for prevention and control. Lancet Infect Dis 7:521, 2007.

62. Pope JE et al.: *Campylobacter* reactive arthritis: a systematic review. Semin Arthritis Rheum 37:48, 2007.

63. Ang CW et al.: Structure of *Campylobacter jejuni* lipopolysaccharides determines antiganglioside specificity and clinical features of Guillain-Barré and Miller Fisher patients. Infect Immun 70:1202, 2002.

64. Schneider EN et al.: Molecular diagnosis of *Campylobacter jejuni* infection in cases of focal active colitis. Am J Surg Pathol 30:782, 2006.

65. Kotloff KL et al.: Global burden of *Shigella* infections: implications for vaccine development and implementation of control strategies. Bull World Health Organ 77:651, 1999.

66. Svenungsson B et al.: Enteropathogens in adult patients with diarrhea and healthy control subjects: a 1-year prospective study in a Swedish clinic for infectious diseases. Clin Infect Dis 30:770, 2000.

67. Crockett CS et al.: Prevalence of shigellosis in the U.S.: consistency with dose-response information. Int J Food Microbiol 30:87, 1996.

68. Niyogi SK: Shigellosis. J Microbiol 43:133, 2005.

69. Fontaine A et al.: Role of Shiga toxin in the pathogenesis of bacillary dysentery, studied by using a Tox- mutant of *Shigella dysenteriae* 1. Infect Immun 56:3099, 1988.

70. O'Brien AO et al.: *Escherichia coli* O157:H7 strains associated with haemorrhagic colitis in the United States produce a *Shigella dysenteriae* 1 (SHIGA) like cytotoxin. Lancet 1:702, 1983.

71. Riley LW et al.: Hemorrhagic colitis associated with a rare *Escherichia coli* serotype. N Engl J Med 308:681, 1983.

72. Gewirtz AT et al.: *Salmonella typhimurium* translocates flagellin across intestinal epithelia, inducing a proinflammatory response. J Clin Invest 107:99, 2001.

73. Mrsny RJ et al.: Identification of hepoxilin A3 in inflammatory events: a required role in neutrophil migration across intestinal epithelia. Proc Natl Acad Sci U S A 101:7421, 2004.

74. Thielman NM, Guerrant RL: Clinical practice. Acute infectious diarrhea. N Engl J Med 350:38, 2004.

75. Connor BA, Schwartz E: Typhoid and paratyphoid fever in travellers. Lancet Infect Dis 5:623, 2005.

76. O'Brien D et al.: Fever in returned travelers: review of hospital admissions for a 3-year period. Clin Infect Dis 33:603, 2001.

77. Parry CM et al.: Typhoid fever. N Engl J Med 347:1770, 2002.

78. Rabson AR et al.: Generalized *Yersinia enterocolitica* infection. J Infect Dis 131:447, 1975.

79. Lamps LW et al.: Molecular biogrouping of pathogenic *Yersinia enterocolitica*: development of a diagnostic PCR assay with histologic correlation. Am J Clin Pathol 125:658, 2006.

80. Bottone EJ: *Yersinia enterocolitica*: overview and epidemiologic correlates. Microbes Infect 1:323, 1999.

81. Cohen MB et al.: Prevalence of diarrheagenic *Escherichia coli* in acute childhood enteritis: a prospective controlled study. J Pediatr 146:54, 2005.

82. Harrington SM et al.: Pathogenesis of enteroaggregative *Escherichia coli* infection. FEMS Microbiol Lett 254:12, 2006.

83. Farrell RJ, LaMont JT: Pathogenesis and clinical manifestations of *Clostridium difficile* diarrhea and colitis. Curr Top Microbiol Immunol 250:109, 2000.

84. Kuijper EJ et al.: *Clostridium difficile*: changing epidemiology and new treatment options. Curr Opin Infect Dis 20:376, 2007.

85. Whipple GH: A hitherto undescribed disease characterized anatomically by deposits of fat and fatty acids in the intestinal mesenteric lymphatic tissue. Johns Hopkins Hosp Bull 18:382, 1907.

86. Raoult D et al.: Cultivation of the bacillus of Whipple's disease. N Engl J Med 342:620, 2000.

87. Lopman BA et al.: Viral gastroenteritis outbreaks in Europe, 1995–2000. Emerg Infect Dis 9:90, 2003.

88. Anderson EJ, Weber SG: Rotavirus infection in adults. Lancet Infect Dis 4:91, 2004.

89. Forrest G: Gastrointestinal infections in immunocompromised hosts. Curr Opin Gastroenterol 20:16, 2004.

90. Huang DB, White AC: An updated review on *Cryptosporidium* and *Giardia*. Gastroenterol Clin North Am 35:291, 2006.

91. Spiller R et al.: Guidelines on the irritable bowel syndrome: mechanisms and practical management. Gut 56:1770, 2007.

92. Sands BE: Inflammatory bowel disease: past, present, and future. J Gastroenterol 42:16, 2007.

93. Cho JH, Weaver CT: The genetics of inflammatory bowel disease. Gastroenterology 133:1327, 2007.

94. Genome-wide association study of 14,000 cases of seven common diseases and 3,000 shared controls. Nature 447:661, 2007.

95. Duerr RH et al.: A genome-wide association study identifies *IL23R* as an inflammatory bowel disease gene. Science 314:1461, 2006.

96. Franke A et al.: Sequence variants in *IL10, ARPC2* and multiple other loci contribute to ulcerative colitis susceptibility. Nat Genet 40:1319, 2008.

97. Turner JR: Molecular basis of epithelial barrier regulation: from basic mechanisms to clinical application. Am J Pathol 169:1901, 2006.

98. Buhner S et al.: Genetic basis for increased intestinal permeability in families with Crohn's disease: role of *CARD15* 3020insC mutation? Gut 55:342, 2006.

99. Su L, Turner JR: Got guts? Need nerve! Gastroenterology 132:1615, 2007.

100. An G et al.: Increased susceptibility to colitis and colorectal tumors in mice lacking core 3-derived O-glycans. J Exp Med 204:1417, 2007.

101. Fisher SA et al.: Genetic determinants of ulcerative colitis include the *ECM1* locus and five loci implicated in Crohn's disease. Nat Genet 40:710, 2008.

102. Cadwell K et al.: A key role for autophagy and the autophagy gene *Atg16l1* in mouse and human intestinal Paneth cells. Nature 13:259, 2008.

103. Sartor RB: Microbial influences in inflammatory bowel diseases. Gastroenterology 134:577, 2008.

104. Kang SS et al.: An antibiotic-responsive mouse model of fulminant ulcerative colitis. PLoS Med 5:e41, 2008.

105. Bibiloni R et al.: VSL#3 probiotic-mixture induces remission in patients with active ulcerative colitis. Am J Gastroenterol 100:1539, 2005.

106. Su L et al.: Targeted epithelial tight junction dysfunction causes immune activation and contributes to development of experimental colitis. Gastroenterol 136:551, 2009.

107. Clayburgh DR et al.: A porous defense: the leaky epithelial barrier in intestinal disease. Lab Invest 84:282, 2004.

108. Rubin DT, Turner JR: Surveillance of dysplasia in inflammatory bowel disease: the gastroenterologist-pathologist partnership. Clin Gastroenterol Hepatol 4:1309, 2006.

109. Winawer SJ et al.: Guidelines for colonoscopy surveillance after polypectomy: a consensus update by the US Multi-Society Task Force on Colorectal Cancer and the American Cancer Society. Gastroenterology 130:1872, 2006.

110. Farris AB et al.: Sessile serrated adenoma: challenging discrimination from other serrated colonic polyps. Am J Surg Pathol 32:30, 2008.

111. Hes FJ et al.: Somatic APC mosaicism: an underestimated cause of polyposis coli. Gut 57:71, 2008.

112. Sieber OM et al.: Multiple colorectal adenomas, classic adenomatous polyposis, and germ-line mutations in *MYH*. N Engl J Med 348:791, 2003.

113. Galiatsatos P, Foulkes WD: Familial adenomatous polyposis. Am J Gastroenterol 101:385, 2006.

114. Brown SL et al.: Myd88-dependent positioning of Ptgs2-expressing stromal cells maintains colonic epithelial proliferation during injury. J Clin Invest 117:258, 2007.

115. Fukata M et al.: Toll-like receptor-4 promotes the development of colitis-associated colorectal tumors. Gastroenterology 133:1869, 2007.

116. Shen L et al.: Integrated genetic and epigenetic analysis identifies three different subclasses of colon cancer. Proc Natl Acad Sci U S A 104:18654, 2007.

117. Lassmann S et al.: Array CGH identifies distinct DNA copy number profiles of oncogenes and tumor suppressor genes in chromosomal- and microsatellite-unstable sporadic colorectal carcinomas. J Mol Med 85:293, 2007.

118. O'Connell JB et al.: Colon cancer survival rates with the new American Joint Committee on Cancer Sixth Edition Staging. J Natl Cancer Inst 96:1420, 2004.

18

Liver and Biliary Tract

JAMES M. CRAWFORD · CHEN LIU

■ THE LIVER

General Features of Hepatic Disease
  Patterns of Hepatic Injury
  Hepatic Failure
  Cirrhosis
  Portal Hypertension
  Jaundice and Cholestasis
    Bilirubin and Bile Formation
    Pathophysiology of Jaundice
    Cholestasis

Infectious Disorders
  Viral Hepatitis
    Hepatitis A Virus
    Hepatitis B Virus
    Hepatitis C Virus
    Hepatitis D Virus
    Hepatitis E Virus
    Hepatitis G Virus
    Clinicopathologic Syndromes of Viral Hepatitis
  Bacterial, Parasitic, and Helminthic Infections

Autoimmune Hepatitis

Drug- and Toxin-Induced Liver Disease
  Alcoholic Liver Disease

Metabolic Liver Disease
  Nonalcoholic Fatty Liver Disease
  Hemochromatosis
  Wilson Disease
  α_1-Antitrypsin Deficiency
  Neonatal Cholestasis

Intrahepatic Biliary Tract Disease
  Secondary Biliary Cirrhosis
  Primary Biliary Cirrhosis (PBC)

Primary Sclerosing Cholangitis (PSC)
Anomalies of the Biliary Trees (Including Liver Cysts)

Circulatory Disorders
  Impaired Blood Flow into the Liver
    Hepatic Artery Compromise
    Portal Vein Obstruction and Thrombosis
  Impaired Blood Flow through the Liver
    Passive Congestion and Centrilobular Necrosis
    Peliosis Hepatis
  Hepatic Venous Outflow Obstruction
    Hepatic Vein Thrombosis and Inferior Vena Cava Thrombosis
    Sinusoidal Obstruction Syndrome (Veno-Occlusive Disease)

Hepatic Complications of Organ or Bone Marrow Transplantation
  Graft-Versus-Host Disease and Liver Rejection

Hepatic Disease Associated with Pregnancy
  Preeclampsia and Eclampsia
  Acute Fatty Liver of Pregnancy
  Intrahepatic Cholestasis of Pregnancy

Nodules and Tumors
  Nodular Hyperplasias
  Benign Neoplasms
    Hepatic Adenoma
  Malignant Tumors
    Hepatoblastoma
    Hepatocellular Carcinoma (HCC)
    Cholangiocarcinoma (CCA)
  Metastatic Tumors

■ **THE BILIARY TRACT**

Congenital Anomalies

Disorders of the Gallbladder
　Cholelithiasis (Gallstones)
　Cholecystitis
　　Acute Cholecystitis
　　Chronic Cholecystitis

Disorders of the Extrahepatic Bile Ducts
　Choledocholithiasis and Ascending Cholangitis
　Biliary Atresia
　Choledochal Cysts

Tumors
　Carcinoma of the Gallbladder

THE LIVER

The normal adult liver weighs 1400 to 1600 gm, constituting approximately 2.5% of body weight. The liver has a dual blood supply: the portal vein provides 60% to 70% of hepatic blood flow, and the hepatic artery supplies 30% to 40%. The portal vein and the hepatic artery enter the liver through the hilum, also called *porta hepatis*, which is a transverse fissure in the inferior surface of the liver. Within the liver, the branches of the portal veins, hepatic arteries, and bile ducts travel in parallel in *portal tracts*, ramifying variably through 17 to 20 orders of branches.

Terminology of the hepatic microarchitecture is based on two different concepts: the hepatic lobule and the hepatic acinus. According to the lobular model, the liver is divided into 1- to 2-mm diameter hexagonal *lobules* oriented around the terminal tributaries of the hepatic vein *(terminal hepatic veins)*, with portal tracts at the periphery of the lobule. The hepatocytes in the vicinity of the terminal hepatic vein are called "centrilobular"; those near the portal tract are "periportal" (Fig. 18–1). In the acinar model the hepatocytes near the terminal hepatic veins are the distal apices of roughly triangular *acini*, whose bases are formed by the penetrating septal venules from the portal vein extending out from the portal tracts.[1] In the acinus the parenchyma is divided into three zones, zone 1 being closest to the vascular supply, zone 3 abutting the terminal hepatic venule and most remote from the afferent blood supply, and zone 2 being intermediate. Regardless of the model used, zonation of the parenchyma is an important concept because of the gradient of activity displayed by many hepatic enzymes, and the zonal distribution of certain types of hepatic injury. While the acinar model best describes the physiologic relationships between hepatocytes and their vascular supply, *the histopathology of the liver is usually discussed on the basis of a lobular architecture.*

Hepatocytes are organized into cribriform, anastomosing sheets or "plates" extending from portal tracts to the terminal hepatic veins. Between the plates of hepatocytes are vascular sinusoids. Blood traverses the sinusoids and exits into the terminal hepatic veins through numerous orifices in the vein wall. Hepatocytes are thus bathed on two sides by well-mixed portal venous and hepatic arterial blood, making hepatocytes among the most richly perfused cells in the body. The sinusoids are lined by fenestrated and discontinuous endothelial cells. Deep to the endothelial cells lies the *space of Disse*, into which protrude abundant microvilli of hepatocytes. Scattered *Kupffer cells* of the mononuclear phagocyte system are attached to the luminal face of endothelial cells, and fat-containing

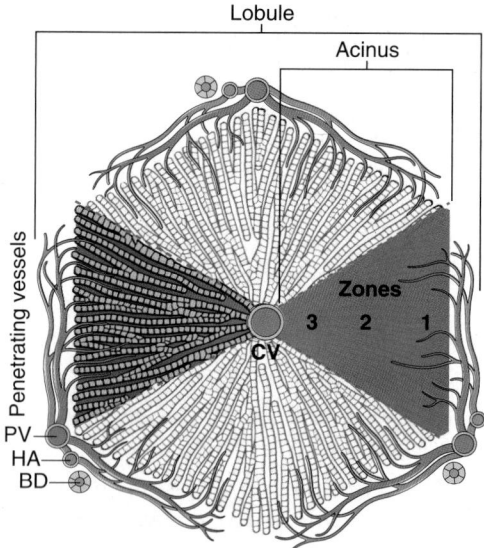

FIGURE 18–1 Microscopic anatomy of the liver; the two models, hepatic lobular model and acinar model, are illustrated. In the lobular model the terminal hepatic vein (CV) is at the center of a "lobule," while the portal tracts (PV) are at the periphery. Pathologists refer to the regions of the parenchyma as "periportal and centrilobular." In the acinar model, on the basis of blood flow, three zones can be defined, zone 1 being the closest to the blood supply and zone 3 being the farthest. BD, bile duct; HA, hepatic artery.

hepatic stellate cells (HSCs) are found in the space of Disse. Between abutting hepatocytes are *bile canaliculi*, which are channels 1 to 2 μm in diameter, formed by grooves in the plasma membranes of facing hepatocytes and separated from the vascular space by tight junctions. These channels drain into the *canals of Hering*, ductular structures that connect the bile canaliculi to *bile ductules* in the periportal region. The ductules empty into the *terminal bile ducts* within the portal tracts.[2] The liver also contains lymphocytes, including relatively large numbers of natural killer cells, and NK-T cells (Chapter 6).

General Features of Hepatic Disease

The liver is vulnerable to a wide variety of metabolic, toxic, microbial, circulatory, and neoplastic insults. The major primary diseases of the liver are viral hepatitis, alcoholic liver disease, nonalcoholic fatty liver disease (NAFLD), and hepatocellular carcinoma (HCC). Hepatic damage also occurs secondary to some of the most common diseases in humans, such as cardiac decompensation, disseminated cancer, and extrahepatic infections. The enormous functional reserve of the liver masks the clinical impact of mild liver damage, but with progression of diffuse disease or disruption of bile flow, the consequences of deranged liver function may become life-threatening.

With the rare exception of fulminant hepatic failure, liver disease is an insidious process in which clinical detection and symptoms of hepatic decompensation may occur weeks, months, or many years after the onset of injury. The ebb and flow of hepatic injury may be imperceptible to the patient and detectable only by abnormal laboratory tests (Table 18–1), and liver injury and healing may also occur without clinical detection. Hence, individuals with hepatic abnormalities who are referred to hepatologists most frequently have chronic liver disease. Surveillance studies in the United States document an annual incidence of newly diagnosed chronic liver disease of 72 per 100,000 population.[3] Liver disease accounts for over 27,000 deaths per year in the United States (1.1% of all deaths).

PATTERNS OF HEPATIC INJURY

The liver has a relatively limited repertoire of cellular and tissue responses to injury, regardless of cause. The most common are:

- Hepatocyte degeneration and intracellular accumulations
- Hepatocyte necrosis and apoptosis
- Inflammation
- Regeneration
- Fibrosis

Clinically, a few common syndromes occur that are a consequence of many different diseases. Before considering specific diseases, we will discuss some of these syndromes, which include hepatic failure, cirrhosis, portal hypertension, and disturbances of bilirubin metabolism causing jaundice and cholestasis.

TABLE 18–1	Laboratory Evaluation of Liver Disease
Test Category	**Serum Measurement***
Hepatocyte integrity	Cytosolic hepatocellular enzymes[†] *Serum aspartate aminotransferase* (AST) *Serum alanine aminotransferase* (ALT) Serum lactate dehydrogenase (LDH)
Biliary excretory function	Substances normally secreted in bile[†] *Serum bilirubin* *Total:* unconjugated plus conjugated *Direct:* conjugated only *Delta:* covalently linked to albumin Urine bilirubin Serum bile acids Plasma membrane enzymes (from damage to bile canaliculus)[†] *Serum alkaline phosphatase* Serum γ-glutamyl transpeptidase Serum 5′-nucleotidase
Hepatocyte function	Proteins secreted into the blood *Serum albumin*[†] *Prothrombin time*[†] (factors V, VII, X, prothrombin, fibrinogen) Hepatocyte metabolism Serum ammonia[†] Aminopyrine breath test (hepatic demethylation)[‡] Galactose elimination (intravenous injection)[‡]

* The most common tests are in italics.
[†] An elevation implicates liver disease.
[‡] A decrease implicates liver disease.

HEPATIC FAILURE

The most severe clinical consequence of liver disease is *hepatic failure*. It may be the result of sudden and massive hepatic destruction (fulminant hepatic failure), which accounts for about 2000 cases per year in the United States, or, more often, represents the end stage of progressive chronic damage to the liver. End-stage liver disease may occur by insidious destruction of hepatocytes or by repetitive discrete waves of parenchymal damage. In cases of severe hepatic dysfunction, hepatic failure is often triggered by intercurrent diseases. Whatever the sequence, 80% to 90% of hepatic functional capacity must be lost before hepatic failure ensues. When the liver can no longer maintain homeostasis, transplantation offers the best hope for survival; the mortality of hepatic failure without liver transplantation is about 80%.

The alterations that cause liver failure fall into three categories:[4]

1. *Acute liver failure.* This is defined as an acute liver illness that is associated with encephalopathy within 6 months after the initial diagnosis. The condition is known as *fulminant liver failure* when the encephalopathy develops rapidly, within 2 weeks of the onset of jaundice, and as sub-fulminant liver failure when the encephalopathy develops within 3 months of the onset of jaundice. Acute liver failure is caused by massive hepatic necrosis, most often induced by drugs or toxins (discussed later). Accidental or deliberate ingestion of acetaminophen (Chapter 9)

accounts for almost 50% of cases in the United States. Exposure to halothane, antimycobacterial drugs (rifampin, isoniazid), antidepressant monoamine oxidase inhibitors, industrial chemicals such as carbon tetrachloride, and mushroom poisoning (*Amanita phalloides*) collectively accounts for an additional 14% of cases. Hepatitis A virus (HAV) infection accounts for an additional 4% of cases and hepatitis B (HBV) infection for 8%. Autoimmune hepatitis and unknown causes (15% of cases) account for the remaining cases. Hepatitis C (HCV) infection only rarely causes massive hepatic necrosis. The mechanism of hepatocellular necrosis may be direct toxic damage (e.g., acetaminophen, mushroom toxins) but more often is a variable combination of toxicity and immune-mediated hepatocyte destruction (e.g., hepatitis virus infection).[5]

2. *Chronic liver disease.* This is the most common route to hepatic failure and is the end point of relentless chronic hepatitis ending in *cirrhosis*, described later.

3. *Hepatic dysfunction without overt necrosis.* Hepatocytes may be viable but unable to perform normal metabolic function, as with tetracycline toxicity and acute fatty liver of pregnancy.

Clinical Features. The clinical signs of hepatic failure are much the same regardless of cause, and are the result of hepatocytes failing to perform their homeostatic functions. *Jaundice* is an almost invariable finding. *Hypoalbuminemia*, which predisposes to peripheral edema, and *hyperammonemia*, which plays a major role in cerebral dysfunction, are worrisome developments. *Fetor hepaticus* is a characteristic body odor that is variously described as "musty" or "sweet and sour." It is related to the formation of mercaptans by the action of gastrointestinal bacteria on the sulfur-containing amino acid methionine, and shunting of splanchnic blood from the portal into the systemic circulation (portosystemic shunting). Impaired estrogen metabolism and consequent hyperestrogenemia are the putative causes of *palmar erythema* (a reflection of local vasodilatation) and *spider angiomas* of the skin. Each angioma is a central, pulsating, dilated arteriole from which small vessels radiate. In the male, hyperestrogenemia also leads to *hypogonadism* and *gynecomastia*.

Hepatic failure is life-threatening, because *with severely impaired liver function, patients are highly susceptible to encephalopathy and failure of multiple organ systems.* Respiratory failure with pneumonia, and sepsis combined with renal failure, claim the lives of many individuals with hepatic failure. A *coagulopathy* develops, attributable to impaired hepatic synthesis of several blood clotting factors. These defects can lead to massive gastrointestinal bleeding. Intestinal absorption of blood places a further metabolic load on the liver, which worsens the extent of hepatic failure. A rapid downhill course is usual, death occurring within weeks to a few months. A fortunate few survive acute episodes of hepatic failure, and hepatic function can be restored by hepatocellular regeneration if the liver does not have advanced fibrosis. As noted, liver transplantation may be life-saving.

Three particular complications associated with hepatic failure merit separate consideration, since they have grave implications.

● *Hepatic encephalopathy* is manifested by a spectrum of disturbances in consciousness, ranging from subtle behavioral abnormalities, to marked confusion and stupor, to deep coma and death. These changes may progress over hours or days in acute hepatic failure, or more insidiously in a person with marginal hepatic function due to chronic liver disease. Associated fluctuating neurologic signs include rigidity, hyper-reflexia, and asterixis: nonrhythmic, rapid extension-flexion movements of the head and extremities, best seen when the arms are held in extension with dorsiflexed wrists. *Hepatic encephalopathy is regarded as a disorder of neurotransmission in the central nervous system and neuromuscular system,* and seems to be associated with elevated ammonia levels in blood and the central nervous system, which impair neuronal function and promote generalized brain edema.[6] *In the great majority of instances there are only minor morphologic changes in the brain, such as astrocyte swelling.* The encephalopathy is reversible if the underlying hepatic condition can be corrected.

● *Hepatorenal syndrome* refers to the appearance of renal failure in individuals with severe chronic liver disease in whom there are no intrinsic morphologic or functional causes for the renal failure. Sodium retention, impaired free-water excretion, and decreased renal perfusion and glomerular filtration rate are the main renal functional abnormalities.[7] The incidence of this syndrome is about 8% per year among patients who have cirrhosis and ascites. Several factors are involved in its development, including decreased renal perfusion pressure due to systemic vasodilation, activation of the renal sympathetic nervous system with vasoconstriction of the afferent renal arterioles, and increased synthesis of renal vasoactive mediators, which further decrease glomerular filtration. The onset of this syndrome is typically heralded by a drop in urine output, associated with rising blood urea nitrogen and creatinine. Rapid development of renal failure is usually associated with a precipitating stress factor such as infection, gastrointestinal hemorrhage, or a major surgical procedure. The prognosis is poor, with a median survival of only 2 weeks in the rapid-onset form and 6 months with the insidious-onset form. The treatment of choice is liver transplantation.

● *Hepatopulmonary syndrome* (HPS) is characterized by the clinical triad of chronic liver disease, hypoxemia, and intrapulmonary vascular dilations (IVPD).[8] The possible causes of hypoxemia are: ventilation perfusion mismatch (the predominant cause), because of lack of uniform blood flow in the presence of stable alveolar ventilation; limitation of oxygen diffusion ("diffusion-perfusion" defect), which occurs because there is inadequate time for oxygen exchange at the alveolo-capillary junction due to rapid flow of blood in the dilated vessels; and shunting of blood from pulmonary arteries to pulmonary veins. Many vasoactive substances have been implicated in the pathogenesis of this syndrome, although enhanced production of nitric oxide (NO) by the lung appears to be the key mediator. Clinically, patients may have decreased arterial oxygen saturation and increased dyspnea on moving from supine to upright position (known, respectively, as orthodeoxia and platypnea); cutaneous spider nevi may be present in patients with IVPD. Most patients respond to oxygen therapy, although liver transplantation is the only curative treatment.

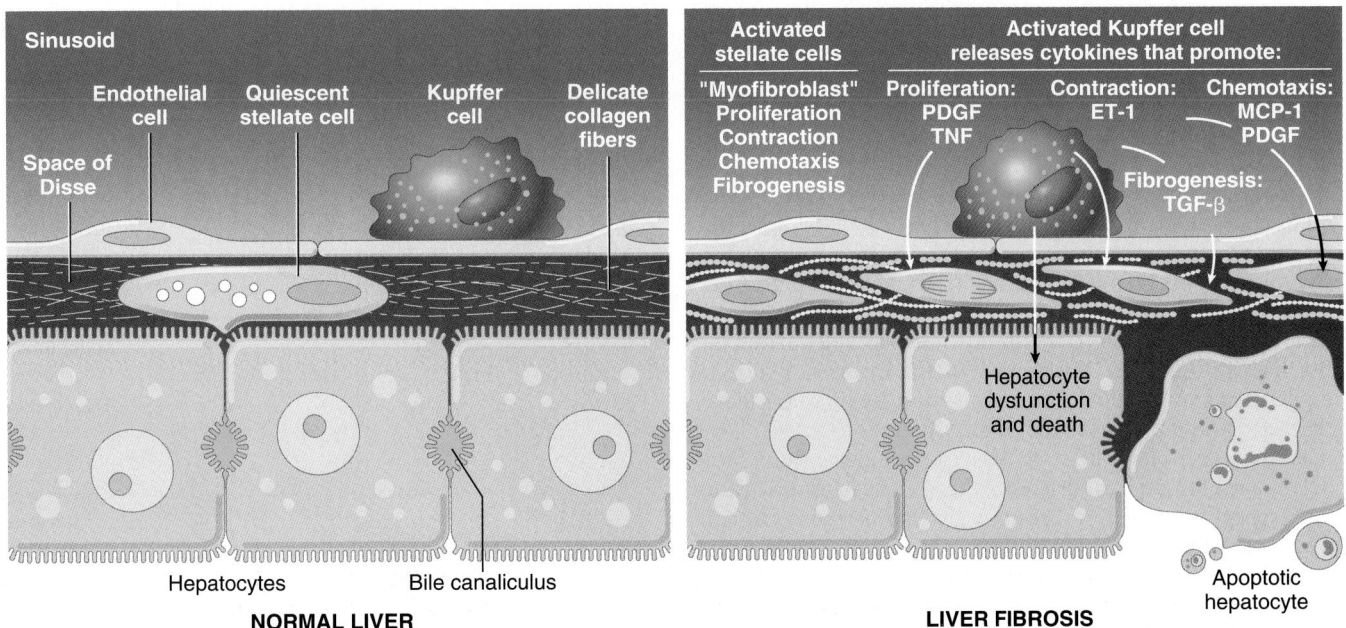

FIGURE 18–2   Stellate cell activation and liver fibrosis. Kupffer cell activation leads to secretion of multiple cytokines. Platelet-derived growth factor (PDGF) and tumor necrosis factor (TNF) activate stellate cells, and contraction of the activated stellate cells is stimulated by endothelin-1 (ET-1). Fibrogenesis is stimulated by transforming growth factor β (TGF-β). Chemotaxis of activated stellate cells to areas of injury is promoted by PDGF and monocyte chemotactic protein-1 (MCP-1). See text for details.

CIRRHOSIS

Cirrhosis is the twelfth most common cause of death in the United States, accounting for most liver-related deaths. The chief worldwide causes of cirrhosis are alcohol abuse, viral hepatitis, and non-alcoholic steatohepatitis (NASH). Other etiologies include biliary disease and iron overload. Cirrhosis, as the end stage of chronic liver disease, is defined by three main morphologic characteristics:

- *Bridging fibrous septa* in the form of delicate bands or broad scars linking portal tracts with one another and portal tracts with terminal hepatic veins. *Fibrosis is the key feature of progressive damage to the liver.* As discussed in Chapter 3, fibrosis is a dynamic process of collagen deposition and remodeling.[9]
- *Parenchymal nodules* containing hepatocytes encircled by fibrosis, with diameters varying from very small (<0.3 cm, micronodules) to large (several centimeters, macronodules). *Nodularity* results from cycles of hepatocyte regeneration and scarring.
- *Disruption of the architecture of the entire liver. The parenchymal injury and consequent fibrosis are diffuse,* extending throughout the liver. Focal injury with scarring does not constitute cirrhosis, nor does diffuse nodular transformation without fibrosis.

Pathogenesis. *The central pathogenic processes in cirrhosis are death of hepatocytes, extracellular matrix (ECM) deposition, and vascular reorganization.*[10] In the normal liver, interstitial collagens (types I and III) are concentrated in portal tracts and around central veins, and thin strands of type IV collagen are present in the space of Disse. In cirrhosis, types I and III col-

lagen are deposited in the space of Disse, creating fibrotic septal tracts. The vascular architecture of the liver is disrupted by the parenchymal damage and scarring, with the formation of new vascular channels in the fibrotic septa that connect the vessels in the portal region (hepatic arteries and portal veins) to terminal hepatic veins, shunting blood from the parenchyma. The deposition of collagen in the space of Disse is accompanied by the loss of fenestrations of sinusoidal endothelial cells *(capillarization of sinusoids)*, impairing the function of sinusoids as channels that permit the exchange of solutes between hepatocytes and plasma (Fig. 18–2).

The predominant mechanism of fibrosis is the *proliferation of hepatic stellate cells and their activation into highly fibrogenic cells*, but other cell types, such as portal fibroblasts, fibrocytes, and cells derived from epithelium-mesenchymal transitions may also produce collagen. Proliferation of hepatic stellate cells and their activation into myofibroblasts is initiated by a series of changes that include an increase in the expression of platelet-derived growth factor receptor β (PDGFR-β) in the stellate cells. At the same time, Kupffer cells and lymphocytes release cytokines and chemokines that modulate the expression of genes in stellate cells that are involved in fibrogenesis. These include transforming growth factor β (TGF-β) and its receptors, metalloproteinase 2 (MMP-2), and tissue inhibitors of metalloproteinases 1 and 2 (TIMP-1 and -2). As they are converted into myofibroblasts, the cells release chemotactic and vasoactive factors, cytokines, and growth factors. Myofibroblasts are contractile cells, capable of constricting sinusoidal vascular channels and increasing vascular resistance within the liver parenchyma; their contraction is stimulated by endothelin-1 (ET-1). The stimuli for stellate cell activation may originate from several sources (Fig 18–2): (a) chronic inflammation, with production of inflammatory cytokines such as tumor necrosis factor (TNF), lymphotoxin, and interleukin 1β (IL-1β), and lipid peroxidation products; (b) cytokine and chemokine production by Kupffer cells, endothelial cells, hepatocytes, and bile duct epithelial cells; in response to (c) disruption of the ECM; and (d) direct stimulation of stellate cells by toxins.

Throughout the process of liver damage and fibrosis in the development of cirrhosis, the surviving hepatocytes are stimulated to regenerate and proliferate as spherical nodules within the confines of the fibrous septa. The net outcome is a fibrotic, nodular liver in which delivery of blood to hepatocytes is severely compromised, as is the ability of hepatocytes to secrete substances into plasma. Disruption of the interface between the parenchyma and portal tracts may also obliterate biliary channels, leading to the development of jaundice.

Clinical Features. About 40% of individuals with cirrhosis are asymptomatic until late in the course of the disease. When symptomatic, they present with nonspecific clinical manifestations: anorexia, weight loss, weakness, and, in advanced disease, symptoms and signs of hepatic failure discussed earlier. Incipient or overt hepatic failure may develop, usually precipitated by a superimposed metabolic load on the liver, usually from systemic infection or gastrointestinal hemorrhage. Imbalances of pulmonary blood flow may lead to severely impaired oxygenation (hepatopulmonary syndrome, already discussed under liver failure), further stressing the patient. *The ultimate mechanism of deaths in most cirrhotic patients is (1) progressive liver failure, (2) a complication related to portal hypertension, or (3) the development of hepatocellular carcinoma.* In a small number of cases, cessation of liver injury may give the necessary time for resorption of the fibrous tissue and "reversal" of the cirrhosis.[11] Even in such instances, the portal hypertension and risk of hepatocellular carcinoma remain.

PORTAL HYPERTENSION

Increased resistance to portal blood flow may develop in a variety of circumstances, which can be divided into *prehepatic, intrahepatic, and posthepatic causes.* The major *prehepatic conditions* are obstructive thrombosis, narrowing of the portal vein before it ramifies within the liver, or massive splenomegaly with increased splenic vein blood flow. The main *posthepatic causes* are severe right-sided heart failure, constrictive pericarditis, and hepatic vein outflow obstruction. *The dominant intrahepatic cause is cirrhosis, accounting for most cases of portal hypertension.* Far less frequent intrahepatic causes are schistosomiasis, massive fatty change, diffuse fibrosing granulomatous disease such as sarcoidosis, and diseases affecting the portal microcirculation such as nodular regenerative hyperplasia (discussed later).

The pathophysiology of portal hypertension is complex and involves the resistance to portal flow at the level of sinusoids and the increase in portal flow caused by hyperdynamic circulation.

- *The increased resistance to portal flow* at the level of the sinusoids is caused by contraction of vascular smooth muscle cells and myofibroblasts, and disruption of blood flow by scarring and the formation of parenchymal nodules. Sinusoidal endothelial cells contribute to intrahepatic vasoconstriction associated with portal hypertension

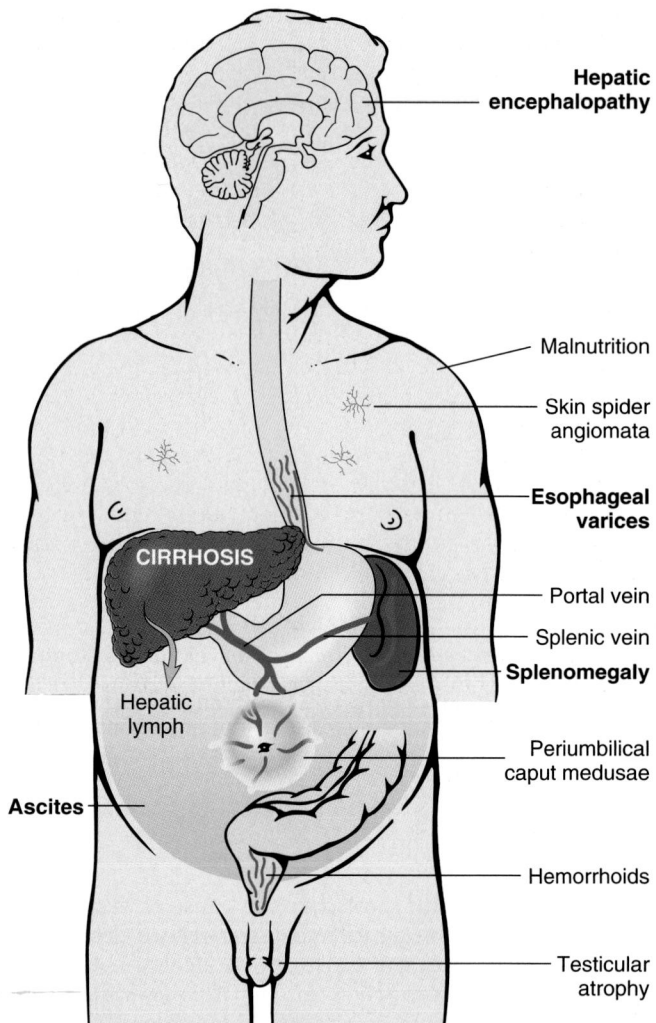

FIGURE 18–3 The major clinical consequences of portal hypertension in the setting of cirrhosis, shown for the male. In women, oligomenorrhea, amenorrhea, and sterility are frequent, as a result of hypogonadism.

through a decrease in nitric oxide production, the release of endothelin-1 (ET-1), angiotensinogen, and eicosanoids.[10] Sinusoidal remodeling and anastomosis between the arterial and portal system in the fibrous septa contribute to portal hypertension by imposing arterial pressures on the low pressure portal venous system. Sinusoidal remodeling and intrahepatic shunts also interfere with the metabolic exchange between sinusoidal blood and hepatocytes.

- Another major factor in the development of portal hypertension is an *increase in portal venous blood flow resulting from a hyperdynamic circulation.*[13,14] This is caused by arterial vasodilation, primarily in the splanchnic circulation. The increased splanchnic arterial blood flow in turn leads to increased venous efflux into the portal venous system. While various mediators such as prostacyclin and TNF have been implicated in the causation of the splanchnic arterial vasodilation, NO has emerged as the most significant one. It is thought that NO production is stimulated by reduced clearance of bacterial DNA absorbed from the gut, due to decreased function of the mononuclear phagocyte system and shunting of blood from the portal to systemic circulation, thereby bypassing the vast pool of Kupffer cells in the liver. In keeping with this hypothesis, treatment with antibiotics appears to be beneficial in experimental models of portal hypertension.

The four major clinical consequences of portal hypertension are (1) ascites, (2) the formation of portosystemic venous shunts, (3) congestive splenomegaly, and (4) hepatic encephalopathy (discussed earlier). These are illustrated in Figure 18–3.

Ascites. *Ascites is the accumulation of excess fluid in the peritoneal cavity.* In 85% of cases, ascites is caused by cirrhosis. Ascites usually becomes clinically detectable when at least 500 mL have accumulated. The fluid is generally serous, having less than 3 gm/dL of protein (largely albumin), and a serum to ascites albumin gradient of ≥1.1 gm/dL. The concentration of solutes such as glucose, sodium, and potassium are similar to that in the blood. The fluid may contain a scant number of mesothelial cells and mononuclear leukocytes. Influx of neutrophils suggests secondary infection, whereas the presence of blood cells points to possible disseminated intra-abdominal cancer. With long-standing ascites, seepage of peritoneal fluid through transdiaphragmatic lymphatics may produce hydrothorax, more often on the right side.

The *pathogenesis of ascites* is complex, involving the following mechanisms:[11,12]

- *Sinusoidal hypertension*, altering Starling's forces and driving fluid into the space of Disse, which is then removed by hepatic lymphatics; this movement of fluid is also promoted by *hypoalbuminemia*.
- *Percolation of hepatic lymph into the peritoneal cavity*: Normal thoracic duct lymph flow approximates 800 to 1000 mL/day. With cirrhosis, hepatic lymphatic flow may approach 20 L/day, exceeding thoracic duct capacity. Hepatic lymph is rich in proteins and low in triglycerides, which explains the presence of protein in the ascitic fluid.
- *Splanchnic vasodilation and hyperdynamic circulation.* These conditions were described earlier, in relationship to the pathogenesis of portal hypertension. Arterial vasodilation in the splanchnic circulation tends to reduce arterial blood pressure. With worsening of the vasodilation, the heart rate and cardiac output are unable to maintain the blood pressure. This triggers the activation of vasoconstrictors, including the renin-angiotensin system, and also increases the secretion of antidiuretic hormone. The combination of portal hypertension, vasodilation, and sodium and water retention increases the perfusion pressure of interstitial capillaries, causing extravasation of fluid into the abdominal cavity.

Portosystemic Shunts. With the rise in portal system pressure, the flow is reversed from portal to systemic circulation by dilation of collateral vessels and development of new vessels. Venous bypasses develop wherever the systemic and portal circulation share common capillary beds (see Fig. 18–3). Principal sites are veins around and within the rectum (manifest as hemorrhoids), the esophagogastric junction (producing varices), the retroperitoneum, and the falciform ligament of the liver (involving periumbilical and abdominal wall collaterals). Although hemorrhoidal bleeding may occur, it is rarely massive or life-threatening. *Much more important are the esophagogastric varices that appear in about 40% of*

individuals with advanced cirrhosis of the liver and cause massive hematemesis and death in about half of them. Each episode of bleeding is associated with a 30% mortality. Abdominal wall collaterals appear as dilated subcutaneous veins extending from the umbilicus toward the rib margins (*caput medusae*) and constitute an important clinical hallmark of portal hypertension.

Splenomegaly. Long-standing congestion may cause congestive splenomegaly. The degree of splenic enlargement varies widely and may reach as much as 1000 gm, but it is not necessarily correlated with other features of portal hypertension. The massive splenomegaly may secondarily induce hematologic abnormalities attributable to hypersplenism, such as thrombocytopenia or even pancytopenia.

JAUNDICE AND CHOLESTASIS

The common causes of jaundice are bilirubin overproduction, hepatitis, and obstruction of the flow of bile. Hepatic bile serves two major functions: (1) the emulsification of dietary fat in the lumen of the gut through the detergent action of bile salts, and (2) the elimination of bilirubin, excess cholesterol, xenobiotics, and other waste products that are insufficiently water-soluble to be excreted into urine. Alterations of bile formation become clinically evident as yellow discoloration of the skin and sclera (*jaundice* and *icterus*, respectively) due to retention of bilirubin, and as *cholestasis*, characterized by systemic retention of not only bilirubin but also other solutes eliminated in bile. To understand the pathophysiology of jaundice it is important first to become familiar with the major aspects of bile formation and metabolism. The metabolism of bilirubin by the liver consists of four separate but interrelated events: uptake from the circulation; intracellular storage; conjugation with glucoronic acid; and biliary excretion. These are described next.

Bilirubin and Bile Formation

Bilirubin is the end product of heme degradation (Fig. 18–4). The majority of daily production (0.2 to 0.3 gm, 85%) is derived from breakdown of senescent red cells by the mononuclear phagocytic system, especially in the spleen, liver, and bone marrow. Most of the remainder (15%) of bilirubin is derived from the turnover of hepatic heme or hemoproteins (e.g., the P-450 cytochromes) and from premature destruction of red cell precursors in the bone marrow (Chapter 13). Whatever the source, intracellular heme oxygenase oxidizes heme to biliverdin (step 1 in Fig. 18–4), which is immediately reduced to bilirubin by biliverdin reductase. Bilirubin thus formed outside the liver is released and bound to serum albumin (step 2). Albumin binding is necessary to transport bilirubin because bilirubin is virtually insoluble in aqueous solutions at physiologic pH. Hepatic processing of bilirubin involves carrier-mediated uptake at the sinusoidal membrane (step 3), conjugation with one or two molecules of glucuronic acid by bilirubin uridine diphosphate (UDP)–glucuronyltransferase (UGT1A1, step 4) in the endoplasmic reticulum, and excretion of the water-soluble, nontoxic bilirubin glucuronides into bile. Most bilirubin glucuronides are deconjugated in the gut lumen by bacterial β-glucuronidases and degraded to colorless urobilinogens (step 5). The urobilinogens and the residue of intact pigment are largely excreted in

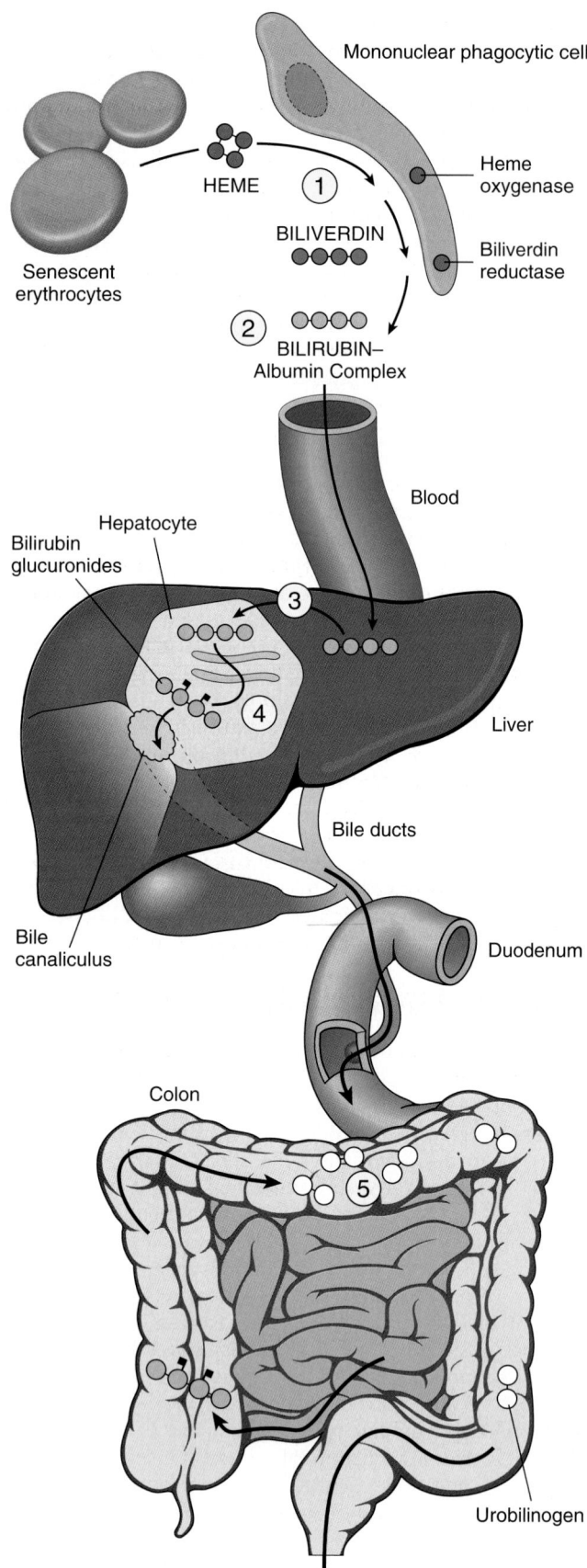

FIGURE 18–4 Bilirubin metabolism and elimination. (1) Normal bilirubin production from heme (0.2–0.3 gm/day) is derived primarily from the breakdown of senescent circulating erythrocytes. (2) Extrahepatic bilirubin is bound to serum albumin and delivered to the liver. (3) Hepatocellular uptake and (4) glucuronidation in the endoplasmic reticulum generate bilirubin monoglucuronides and diglucuronides, which are water soluble and readily excreted into bile. (5) Gut bacteria deconjugate the bilirubin and degrade it to colorless urobilinogens. The urobilinogens and the residue of intact pigments are excreted in the feces, with some reabsorption and excretion into urine.

feces. Approximately 20% of the urobilinogens formed are reabsorbed in the ileum and colon, returned to the liver, and re-excreted into bile. A small amount of reabsorbed urobilinogen is excreted in the urine.

The hepatic conjugating enzyme UGT1A1 is a product of the *UGT1* gene located on chromosome 2q37. It is a member of a family of enzymes that catalyze the glucuronidation of an array of substrates such as steroid hormones, carcinogens, and drugs. In humans, UGT1A1, generated from the exon 1A of the *UGT1* gene, is the only isoform responsible for bilirubin glucuronidation. Mutations of *UGT1A1* cause hereditary unconjugated hyperbilirubinemias: Crigler-Najjar syndrome types I and II, and Gilbert syndrome.

Two thirds of the organic materials in bile are bile salts, which are formed by the conjugation of bile acids with taurine or glycine. Bile acids, the major catabolic products of cholesterol, are a family of water-soluble sterols with carboxylated side chains. The primary human bile acids are cholic acid and chenodeoxycholic acid. Bile acids in bile salts act as highly effective detergents. Their primary physiologic role is to solubilize water-insoluble lipids secreted by hepatocytes into bile, and also to solubilize dietary lipids in the gut lumen. Ninety-five percent of secreted bile acids, conjugated or unconjugated, are reabsorbed from the gut lumen and recirculate the liver *(enterohepatic circulation)*, thus helping to maintain a large endogenous pool of bile acids for digestive and excretory purposes.

Pathophysiology of Jaundice

Both unconjugated bilirubin and conjugated bilirubin (bilirubin glucuronides) may accumulate systemically. There are two important pathophysiologic differences between the two forms of bilirubin. *Unconjugated bilirubin is virtually insoluble in water at physiologic pH and exists in tight complexes with serum albumin. This form cannot be excreted in the urine even when blood levels are high.* Normally, a very small amount of unconjugated bilirubin is present as an albumin-free anion in plasma. This fraction of unbound bilirubin may diffuse into tissues, particularly the brain in infants, and produce toxic injury. The unbound plasma fraction may increase in severe hemolytic disease or when protein-binding drugs displace bilirubin from albumin. Hence, *hemolytic disease of the newborn (erythroblastosis fetalis) may lead to accumulation of unconjugated bilirubin in the brain, which can cause severe neurologic damage, referred to as kernicterus* (Chapter 10). In contrast, *conjugated bilirubin is water-soluble, nontoxic, and only loosely bound to albumin. Because of its solubility and weak association with albumin, excess conjugated bilirubin in plasma*

TABLE 18–2   Causes of Jaundice

PREDOMINANTLY UNCONJUGATED HYPERBILIRUBINEMIA

Excess production of bilirubin
  Hemolytic anemias
  Resorption of blood from internal hemorrhage (e.g.,
    alimentary tract bleeding, hematomas)
  Ineffective erythropoiesis (e.g., pernicious anemia,
    thalassemia)
Reduced hepatic uptake
  Drug interference with membrane carrier systems
  Some cases of Gilbert syndrome
Impaired bilirubin conjugation
  Physiologic jaundice of the newborn (decreased UGT1A1
    activity, decreased excretion)
  Breast milk jaundice (β-glucuronidases in milk)
  Genetic deficiency of UGT1A1 activity (Crigler-Najjar
    syndrome types I and II)
  Gilbert syndrome
  Diffuse hepatocellular disease (e.g., viral or drug-induced
    hepatitis, cirrhosis)

PREDOMINANTLY CONJUGATED HYPERBILIRUBINEMIA

Deficiency of canalicular membrane transporters (Dubin-
  Johnson syndrome, Rotor syndrome)
Impaired bile flow

UGT, uridine diphosphate–glucuronyltransferase.

can be excreted in urine. With prolonged conjugated hyperbilirubinemia, a portion of circulating pigment may become covalently bound to albumin; this is termed the *bilirubin delta fraction.*

Serum bilirubin levels in the normal adult vary between 0.3 and 1.2 mg/dL, and the rate of systemic bilirubin production is equal to the rates of hepatic uptake, conjugation, and biliary excretion. Jaundice becomes evident when the serum bilirubin levels rise above 2.0 to 2.5 mg/dL; levels as high as 30 to 40 mg/dL can occur with severe disease. *Jaundice occurs when the equilibrium between bilirubin production and clearance is disturbed* by one or more of the following mechanisms (Table 18–2): *(1) excessive extrahepatic production of bilirubin; (2) reduced hepatocyte uptake; (3) impaired conjugation; (4)*

decreased hepatocellular excretion; and (5) impaired bile flow. The first three mechanisms produce unconjugated hyperbilirubinemia, and the latter two produce predominantly conjugated hyperbilirubinemia. Although more than one mechanism may be operative, generally one mechanism predominates, so knowledge of the major form of plasma bilirubin is of value in evaluating possible causes of hyperbilirubinemia.

Two conditions result from specific defects in hepatocellular bilirubin metabolism.

Neonatal Jaundice. Because the hepatic machinery for conjugating and excreting bilirubin does not fully mature until about 2 weeks of age, almost every newborn develops transient and mild unconjugated hyperbilirubinemia, termed neonatal jaundice or *physiologic jaundice of the newborn.* This may be exacerbated by breastfeeding, as a result of the presence of bilirubin-deconjugating enzymes in breast milk. Nevertheless, sustained jaundice in the newborn is abnormal, discussed later under *neonatal hepatitis.*

Hereditary Hyperbilirubinemias. Multiple genetic mutations can cause hereditary hyperbilirubinemia[15] (Table 18–3). In *Crigler-Najjar syndrome type I* hepatic UGT1A1 (described earlier) is completely absent, and the colorless bile contains only trace amounts of unconjugated bilirubin. *The liver is morphologically normal by light and electron microscopy.* However, serum unconjugated bilirubin reaches very high levels, producing severe jaundice and icterus. Without liver transplantation, this condition is invariably fatal, causing death secondary to kernicterus within 18 months of birth.

Crigler-Najjar syndrome type II is a less severe, nonfatal disorder in which UGT1A1 enzyme activity is greatly reduced, and the enzyme is capable of forming only monoglucuronidated bilirubin. Unlike Crigler-Najjar syndrome type I, the only major consequence is extraordinarily yellow skin. Phenobarbital treatment can improve bilirubin glucuronidation by inducing hypertrophy of the hepatocellular endoplasmic reticulum.

Gilbert syndrome is a relatively common, benign, inherited condition presenting with mild, fluctuating hyperbilirubinemia, in the absence of hemolysis or liver disease. It affects 3%

TABLE 18–3   Hereditary Hyperbilirubinemias

Disorder	Inheritance	Defects in Bilirubin Metabolism	Liver Pathology	Clinical Course
UNCONJUGATED HYPERBILIRUBINEMIA				
Crigler-Najjar syndrome type I	Autosomal recessive	Absent UGT1A1 activity	None	Fatal in neonatal period
Crigler-Najjar syndrome type II	Autosomal dominant with variable penetrance	Decreased UGT1A1 activity	None	Generally mild, occasional kernicterus
Gilbert syndrome	Autosomal recessive	Decreased UGT1A1 activity	None	Innocuous
CONJUGATED HYPERBILIRUBINEMIA				
Dubin-Johnson syndrome	Autosomal recessive	Impaired biliary excretion of bilirubin glucuronides due to mutation in canalicular multidrug resistance protein 2 (MRP2)	Pigmented cytopasmic globules; ?epinephrine metabolites	Innocuous
Rotor syndrome	Autosomal recessive	Decreased hepatic uptake and storage? Decreased biliary excretion?	None	Innocuous

UGT, uridine diphosphate–glucuronyltransferase.

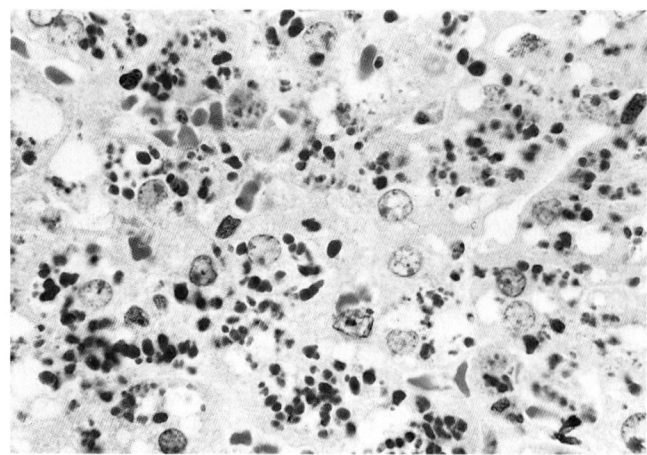

FIGURE 18–5 Dubin-Johnson syndrome, showing abundant pigment inclusions in otherwise normal hepatocytes.

to 10% of the U.S. population. In Gilbert syndrome, hepatic bilirubin-glucuronidating activity is about 30% of normal, a less severe reduction than in Crigler-Najjar syndromes. It is caused in most patients by the homozygous insertion of two extra bases in the 5′ promoter region of the *UGT1* gene, leading to reduced transcription. The mild hyperbilirubinemia may go undiscovered for years and is not associated with functional derangements. When detected in adolescence or adult life it is typically in association with stress, such as an intercurrent illness, strenuous exercise, or fasting. Gilbert syndrome itself has no clinical consequence except for the anxiety that a jaundiced sufferer might justifiably experience with this otherwise innocuous condition. However, individuals who have Gilbert syndrome may be more susceptible to adverse effects of drugs that are metabolized by UGT1A1.

Dubin-Johnson syndrome is an autosomal recessive disorder characterized by chronic conjugated hyperbilirubinemia. It is caused by a defect in hepatocellular excretion of bilirubin glucuronides across the canalicular membrane. The molecular basis for this syndrome is absence of the canalicular protein, *multidrug resistance protein 2*, which is responsible for transport of bilirubin glucuronides and related organic anions into bile.[16] The liver is darkly pigmented because of coarse pigmented granules within the cytoplasm of hepatocytes (Fig. 18–5). Electron microscopy reveals that the pigment is located in lysosomes: it appears to be composed of polymers of epinephrine metabolites. The liver is otherwise normal. Apart from chronic or recurrent jaundice of fluctuating intensity, most patients are asymptomatic and have a normal life expectancy.

Rotor syndrome is a rare form of asymptomatic conjugated hyperbilirubinemia associated with multiple defects in hepatocellular uptake and excretion of bilirubin pigments. The precise molecular basis for this syndrome is unknown. The liver is morphologically normal. As with Dubin-Johnson syndrome, patients with Rotor syndrome have jaundice but otherwise have normal lives.

Cholestasis

Cholestasis denotes a pathologic condition of impaired bile formation and bile flow, leading to accumulation of bile pigment in the hepatic parenchyma.[17] *It can be caused by extra-*

hepatic or intrahepatic obstruction of bile channels, or by defects in hepatocyte bile secretion. Patients may have jaundice, pruritus, skin xanthomas (focal accumulation of cholesterol), or symptoms related to intestinal malabsorption, including nutritional deficiencies of the fat-soluble vitamins A, D, or K. *A characteristic laboratory finding is elevated serum alkaline phosphatase and γ-glutamyl transpeptidase (GGT),* enzymes present on the apical membranes of hepatocytes and bile duct epithelial cells.

Morphology. The morphologic features of cholestasis depend on its severity, duration, and underlying cause. **Common to both obstructive and nonobstructive cholestasis is the accumulation of bile pigment within the hepatic parenchyma** (Figs. 18–6 and 18–7). Elongated green-brown plugs of bile are visible in dilated bile canaliculi (Fig. 18–7B). Rupture of canaliculi leads to extravasation of bile, which is quickly phagocytosed by Kupffer cells. Droplets of bile pigment also accumulate within hepatocytes, which can take on a fine, foamy appearance (**feathery degeneration**).

Obstruction of the biliary tree, either intrahepatic or extrahepatic, causes distention of upstream bile ducts

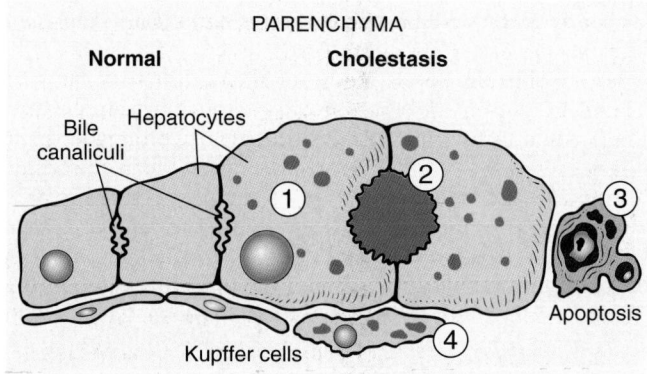

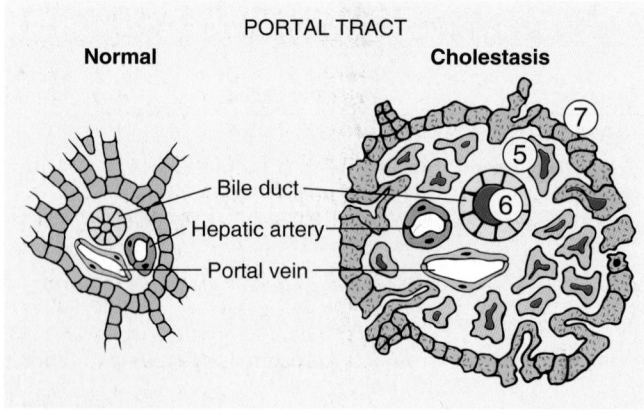

FIGURE 18–6 Morphologic features of cholestasis *(right)* and comparison with normal liver *(left)*. In the parenchyma *(upper panel)* cholestatic hepatocytes (1) are enlarged with dilated canalicular spaces (2). Apoptotic cells (3) may be seen, and Kupffer cells (4) frequently contain regurgitated bile pigments. In the portal tracts of obstructed liver *(lower panel)* there is also bile ductular proliferation (5), edema, bile pigment retention (6), and eventually neutrophilic inflammation (not shown). Surrounding hepatocytes (7) are swollen and undergoing degeneration.

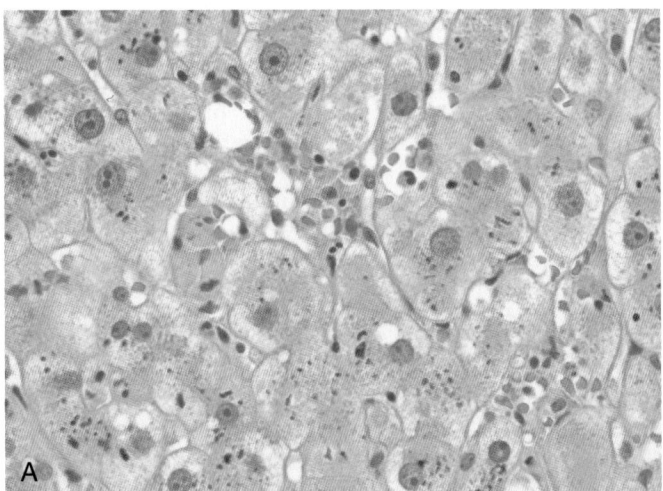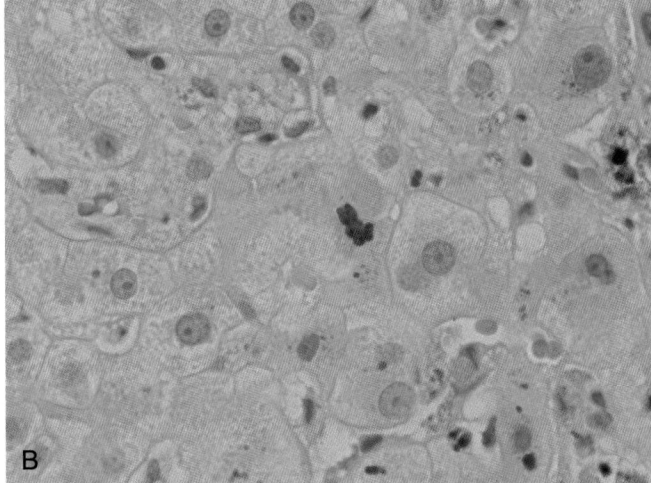

FIGURE 18–7 Histology of cholestasis. **A,** Intracellular cholestasis showing the bile pigments in the cytoplasm; **B,** bile plug showing the expansion of bile canaliculus by bile.

and ductules by bile. The bile stasis and back-pressure induce proliferation of the duct epithelial cells, and looping and reduplication of ducts and ductules in the portal tracts. The labyrinthine ductules reabsorb secreted bile salts, serving to protect the downstream obstructed bile ducts from the toxic detergent action of bile salts. Associated histologic findings include portal tract edema and periductular infiltrates of neutrophils. Prolonged obstructive cholestasis leads not only to feathery change of hepatocytes but also to focal dissolution of hepatocytes by detergents, giving rise to bile lakes filled with cellular debris and pigment. Unrelieved obstruction leads to portal tract fibrosis, and ultimately, to biliary cirrhosis.

Since extrahepatic biliary obstruction is frequently amenable to surgical alleviation, correct and prompt diagnosis is imperative. In contrast, cholestasis due to diseases of the intrahepatic biliary tree or hepatocellular secretory failure (collectively termed *intrahepatic cholestasis*) is not benefited by surgery (short of transplantation), and the patient's condition may be worsened by an operative procedure. *There is thus some urgency in making a correct diagnosis of the cause of jaundice and cholestasis.*

Progressive Familial Intrahepatic Cholestasis (PFIC). Here we discuss a striking but heterogeneous group of autosomal-recessively inherited cholestatic conditions known as PFICs.[17] PFIC-1 (also known as Byler disease as it was first identified in the descendents of Jacob Byler, an Amish patient), PFIC-2, and PFIC-3 are caused by mutations of three different genes. PFIC-1 and PFIC-2 share a similar phenotype, which includes normal or near normal GGT activity, and lack of bile ductular proliferation in portal tracts.

Progressive familial intrahepatic cholestasis 1 (PFIC-1) is characterized by cholestasis beginning in infancy, with severe pruritus due to high serum bile acid levels, and relentlessly progresses to liver failure before adulthood. The genetic defect is usually a mutation in the *ATP8B1* gene on chromosome 18q21 that causes impaired bile secretion, through mecha-

nisms that are not yet fully elucidated.[18] In the mild form of PFIC-1 called *benign recurrent intrahepatic cholestasis,* there are intermittent attacks of cholestasis over life without progression to chronic liver disease.

Progressive familial intrahepatic cholestasis 2 (PFIC-2) is caused by mutations in the hepatocyte canalicular bile salt export pump (BSEP), encoded by the *ABCB11* gene. BSEP is a member of the adenosine triphosphate–binding cassette (ABC) family of transporters.[19] Mutations of the *ABCB11* gene cause severely impaired bile salt secretion into bile. Patients suffer extreme pruritus, growth failure, and progression to cirrhosis in the first decade of life. These patients also have higher risk for cholangiocarcinoma.

Progressive familial intrahepatic cholestasis 3 (PFIC-3) is caused by mutations in the *ABCB4* gene, and is characterized by cholestasis with a *high* serum GGT.[20] The *ABCB4*-encoded protein, MDR3, is a liver-specific canalicular transport protein. In individuals with PFIC-3, there is absence of secreted phosphatidylcholine in bile, which leaves the apical surfaces of the biliary tree epithelia subject to the full detergent action of secreted bile salts, with resultant toxic destruction of these epithelia and release of GGT into the circulation.

Infectious Disorders

Inflammatory disorders of the liver dominate the clinical practice of hepatology. This is partly because virtually any insult to the liver can kill hepatocytes and recruit inflammatory cells, but also because inflammatory diseases are frequently long-term chronic conditions. Among inflammatory disorders, viral infection is by far the most frequent.

VIRAL HEPATITIS

Systemic viral infections can involve the liver as in (1) infectious mononucleosis (Epstein-Barr virus), which may cause a mild hepatitis during the acute phase; (2) cytomegalovirus infection, particularly in the newborn or immunosuppressed patient; and (3) yellow fever (yellow fever virus), which has been a major and serious cause of hepatitis in tropical countries. Infrequently, in children and immunosuppressed patients, the liver is affected in the course of rubella, adenovirus, herpesvirus, or enterovirus infections. However, unless otherwise specified, *the term viral hepatitis is applied for hepatic infections caused by a group of viruses known as hepatotropic virus (hepatitis viruses A, B, C, D, and E) that have a particular affinity for the liver* (Table 18–4). We first present the main features of each hepatotropic virus, followed by a discussion of the clinicopathologic characteristics of acute and chronic viral hepatitis.

Hepatitis A Virus

Hepatitis A virus (HAV), the scourge of military campaigns since antiquity, is a benign, self-limited disease with an incubation period of 3 to 6 weeks. *HAV does not cause chronic hepatitis or a carrier state and only rarely causes fulminant hepatitis, so the fatality rate associated with HAV is about 0.1%.* HAV occurs throughout the world and is endemic in countries with substandard hygiene and sanitation, where populations may have detectable antibodies to HAV by the age of 10 years. Clinical disease tends to be mild or asymptomatic, and is rare after childhood. In developed countries, the prevalence of seropositivity (indicative of previous exposure) increases gradually with age, reaching 50% by age 50 years in the United States. In this population acute HAV tends to be a sporadic febrile illness. Affected individuals have nonspecific symptoms such as fatigue and loss of appetite, and often develop jaundice. Overall, HAV accounts for about 25% of clinically evident acute hepatitis worldwide and an estimated 30,000 to 50,000 new cases per year in the United States.

HAV, discovered in 1973, is a small, nonenveloped, positive-strand RNA picornavirus that occupies its own genus, *Hepatovirus*. Ultrastructurally, HAV is an icosahedral capsid 27 nm in diameter and can be cultured in vitro. The receptor for HAV is HAVcr-1, a 451–amino acid class I integral-membrane mucin-like glycoprotein of unknown normal function.[21] HAV is spread by ingestion of contaminated water and foods and is shed in the stool for 2 to 3 weeks before and 1 week after the onset of jaundice. Thus, close personal contact with an infected individual or fecal-oral contamination during this period accounts for most cases and explains the outbreaks in institutional settings such as schools and nurseries, and the water-borne epidemics in places where people live in overcrowded, unsanitary conditions. HAV can also be detected in serum and saliva. *Because HAV viremia is transient, blood-borne transmission of HAV occurs only rarely; therefore, donated blood is not specifically screened for this virus.* In developed countries, sporadic infections may be contracted by the consumption of raw or steamed shellfish (oysters, mussels, clams), which concentrate the virus from seawater contaminated with human sewage. Infected workers in the food industry may also be the source of outbreaks. HAV itself does not seem to be cytopathic. Cellular immunity, particularly CD8+ T cells, plays a key role in hepatocellular injury during HAV infection.[22]

Specific IgM antibody against HAV appears in blood at the onset of symptoms, constituting a reliable marker of acute infection (Fig. 18–8). Fecal shedding of the virus ends as the IgM titer rises. The IgM response usually begins to decline in a few months and is followed by the appearance of IgG anti-HAV. The latter persists for years, perhaps conferring lifelong immunity against reinfection by all strains of HAV. However, there are no routinely available tests for IgG anti-HAV. The presence of this antibody is inferred from the difference between total and IgM anti-HAV. HAV vaccine, available since 1992, is effective in preventing infection.[23]

TABLE 18-4	The Hepatitis Viruses				
Virus	**Hepatitis A**	**Hepatitis B**	**Hepatitis C**	**Hepatitis D**	**Hepatitis E**
Type of virus	ssRNA	partially dsDNA	ssRNA	Circular defective ssRNA	ssRNA
Viral family	Hepatovirus; related to picornavirus	Hepadnavirus	Flaviridae	Subviral particle in Deltaviridae family	Calicivirus
Route of transmission	Fecal-oral (contaminated food or water)	Parenteral, sexual contract, perinatal	Parenteral; intranasal cocaine use is a risk factor	Parenteral	Fecal-oral
Mean incubation period	2–4 weeks	1–4 months	7–8 weeks	Same as HBV	4–5 weeks
Frequency of chronic liver disease	Never	10%	~80%	5% (coinfection); ≤70% for superinfection	Never
Diagnosis	Detection of serum IgM antibodies	Detection of HBsAg or antibody to HBcAg	PCR for HCV RNA; 3rd-generation ELISA for antibody detection	Detection of IgM and IgG antibodies; HDV RNA serum; HDAg in liver	PCR for HEV RNA; detection of serum IgM and IgG antibodies

dsDNA, double-stranded DNA; ELISA, enzyme-linked immunosorbent assay; HBcAg, hepatitis B core antigen; HBsAg, hepatitis B surface antigen; HBV, hepatitis B virus; HCV, hepatitis C virus; HDAg, hepatitis D antigen; HDV, hepatitis D virus; HEV, hepatitis E virus; IV, intravenous; PCR, polymerase chain reaction; ssRNA, single stranded RNA.

From Washington K: Inflammatory and infectious diseases of the liver. In Iacobuzio-Donahue CA, Montgomery EA (eds): Gastrointestinal and Liver Pathology. Philadelphia, Churchill Livingstone; 2005.

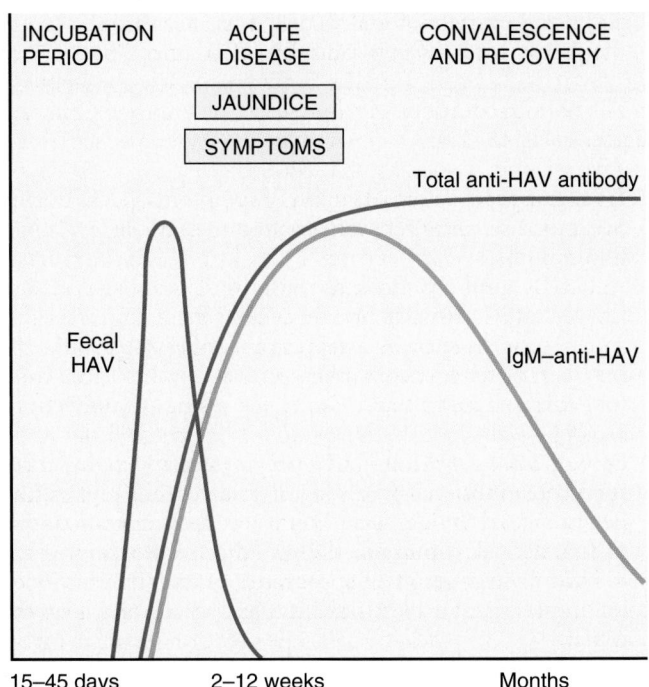

FIGURE 18–8 The sequence of serologic markers in acute hepatitis A infection. HAV, hepatitis A virus.

Hepatitis B Virus (HBV)

HBV can produce (1) acute hepatitis with recovery and clearance of the virus, (2) nonprogressive chronic hepatitis, (3) progressive chronic disease ending in cirrhosis, (4) fulminant hepatitis with massive liver necrosis, and (5) an asymptomatic carrier state. HBV-induced chronic liver disease is an important precursor for the development of hepatocellular carcinoma.[24] The approximate frequencies of clinical outcomes of HBV infection are depicted in Figure 18–9.

Liver disease due to HBV is an enormous global health problem. One third of the world population (2 billion people)

have been infected with HBV, and 400 million people have chronic infection. Seventy-five percent of all chronic carriers live in Asia and the Western Pacific rim. The global prevalence of chronic hepatitis B infection varies widely, from high (>8%) in Africa, Asia, and the Western Pacific to intermediate (2% to 7%) in southern and eastern Europe to low (<2%) in western Europe, North America, and Australia. As will be discussed later, the carrier rate is largely dictated by the age at infection, being the highest when infection occurs in children perinatally and the lowest when adults are infected. In the United States, incidence of HBV infection has dramatically decreased; there are now an estimated 46,000 new infections per year with about 5,000 acute symptomatic cases.

The mode of transmission of HBV varies with geographical areas. In high prevalence regions of the world, perinatal transmission during childbirth accounts for 90% of cases. In areas with intermediate prevalence, horizontal transmission, especially in early childhood, is the dominant mode of transmission. Such spread occurs through minor cuts and breaks in the skin or mucous membranes among children with close bodily contact. In low prevalence areas such as the United States, unprotected heterosexual or homosexual intercourse and intravenous drug abuse (sharing of needles and syringes) are the chief modes of spread. The incidence of transfusion-related spread has dwindled greatly in recent years due to screening of donated blood and HBsAg and exclusion of paid blood donors.

HBV has a prolonged incubation period (4–26 weeks). Unlike HAV, HBV remains in the blood until and during active episodes of acute and chronic hepatitis. In the United States acute HBV infection mostly affects adults. Approximately 70% have mild or no symptoms and do not develop jaundice. The remaining 30% have nonspecific constitutional symptoms such as anorexia, fever, jaundice, and upper right quadrant pain. In almost all cases the infection is self-limited and resolves without treatment. Chronic disease rarely occurs in adults in non-endemic areas. Fulminant hepatitis is also rare, occurring in approximately 0.1 to 0.5% of cases.

HBV was first linked to hepatitis in the 1960s when Australia antigen (later known as HBV surface antigen) was

FIGURE 18–9 Potential outcomes of hepatitis B infection in adults, with their approximate frequencies in the United States. *Recovery from acute hepatitis refers to complete recovery as well as latent infections with maintenance of T cell response. **Recovery from chronic hepatitis is indicated by negative test for HBsAg. ***Healthy carrier state is indicated by positive HBsAg >6 months; HBeAg negative; serum HBV DNA <10⁵ copies/mL; persistently normal AST and ALT levels; absence of significant inflammation and necrosis on liver biopsy.

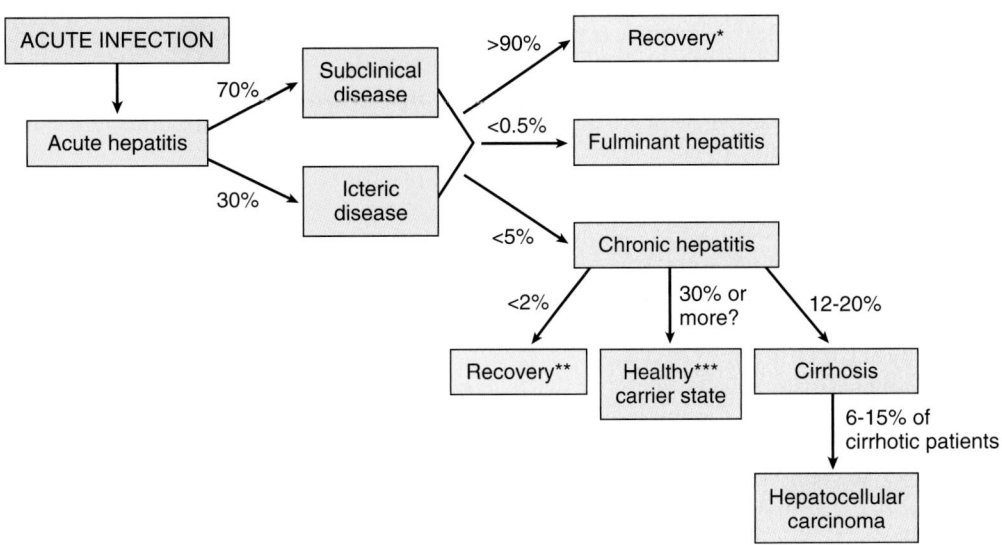

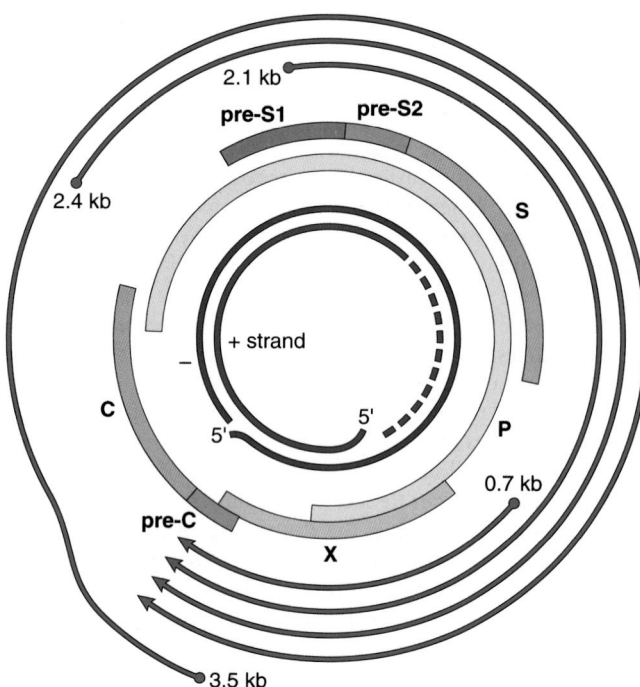

FIGURE 18–10 Diagrammatic representation of genomic structure and transcribed components of the hepatitis B virion. The innermost circles represent the DNA (+) strand and the DNA (–) strand of the virion. The thick bars labeled P, X, pro-C, C, pre-SI, pre-S2, and S denote the peptides derived from the virion. The outermost lines denote the mRNA transcripts of the virion.

identified.[25] The virus is a member of the *Hepadnaviridae*, a family of DNA viruses that cause hepatitis in multiple animal species. There are eight HBV genotypes with geographic distribution around the globe. The mature HBV virion is a 42-nm, spherical double-layered "Dane particle" that has an outer surface envelope of protein, lipid, and carbohydrate enclosing an electron-dense, 28-nm, slightly hexagonal core. The genome of HBV is a partially double-stranded circular DNA molecule having 3200 nucleotides (Fig. 18–10). The HBV genome contains four open reading frames coding for:[26]

- A nucleocapsid "core" protein (HBcAg, hepatitis B core antigen) and a longer polypeptide transcript with a precore and core region, designated HBeAg (hepatitis B "e" antigen). The precore region directs the HBeAg polypeptide toward secretion into blood, whereas HBcAg remains in hepatocytes for the assembly of complete virions.
- Envelope glycoproteins (HBsAg, hepatitis B surface antigen), which consist of three related proteins: large HBsAg (containing Pre-S1, Pre-S2, and S), middle HBsAg (containing Pre-S2 and S), and small HBsAg (containing S only). Infected hepatocytes are capable of synthesizing and secreting massive quantities of noninfective surface protein (mainly small HBsAg).
- A polymerase (Pol) that exhibits both DNA polymerase activity and reverse transcriptase activity. Genomic replication occurs via an intermediate RNA template, through a unique replication cycle: DNA → RNA → DNA.
- HBx protein, which is necessary for virus replication and may act as a transcriptional transactivator of the viral genes

and a wide variety of host genes. It has been implicated in the pathogenesis of liver cancer in HBV infection.

The natural course of the disease can be followed by serum markers (Fig 18–11).

- HBsAg appears before the onset of symptoms, peaks during overt disease, and then declines to undetectable levels in 3 to 6 months.
- Anti-HBs antibody does not rise until the acute disease is over and is usually not detectable for a few weeks to several months after the disappearance of HBsAg. Anti-HBs may persist for life, conferring protection; this is the basis for current vaccination strategies using noninfectious HBsAg.
- HBeAg, HBV-DNA, and DNA polymerase appear in serum soon after HBsAg, and all signify active viral replication. Persistence of HBeAg is an important indicator of continued viral replication, infectivity, and probable progression to chronic hepatitis. The appearance of anti-HBe antibodies implies that an acute infection has peaked and is on the wane.
- IgM anti-HBc becomes detectable in serum shortly before the onset of symptoms, concurrent with the onset of elevated serum aminotransferase levels (indicative of hepatocyte destruction). Over a period of months the IgM anti-HBc antibody is replaced by IgG anti-HBc. As in the case of anti-HAV, there is no direct assay for IgG anti-HBc, but its presence is inferred from decline of IgM anti-HBc in the face of rising levels of total anti-HBc.

Occasionally, mutated strains of HBV emerge that do not produce HBeAg but are replication competent and express HBcAg. In such patients, the HBeAg may be low or undetectable despite the presence of HBV viral load. A second ominous development is the appearance of vaccine-induced escape mutants, which replicate in the presence of vaccine-induced immunity. For instance, in one such viral mutant, replacement of arginine at amino acid 145 of HBsAg with glycine significantly alters recognition of HBsAg by anti-HBsAg antibodies.

Despite the self-limited nature of acute HBV infection, recent studies show that very low levels of HBV DNA can be detected by PCR analysis in the blood of some individuals who may have anti-HBe antibodies. It is unclear at this time whether the viral material detected is composed of virus fragments, infectious virus, or non-infectious virus, but the material persists for many years.

The host immune response to the virus is the main determinant of the outcome of the infection.[27] The mechanisms of innate immunity protect the host during the initial phases of the infection, and a strong response by virus-specific CD4+ and CD8+ interferon γ-producing cells is associated with the resolution of acute infection. There are several reasons to believe that HBV does not cause direct hepatocyte injury. Most importantly, many chronic carriers have virions in their hepatocytes with no evidence of cell injury. Hepatocyte damage is believed to result from damage to the virus-infected cells by CD8+ cytotoxic T cells.

Hepatitis B can prevented by vaccination and by the screening of donor blood, organs, and tissues. The vaccine is pre-

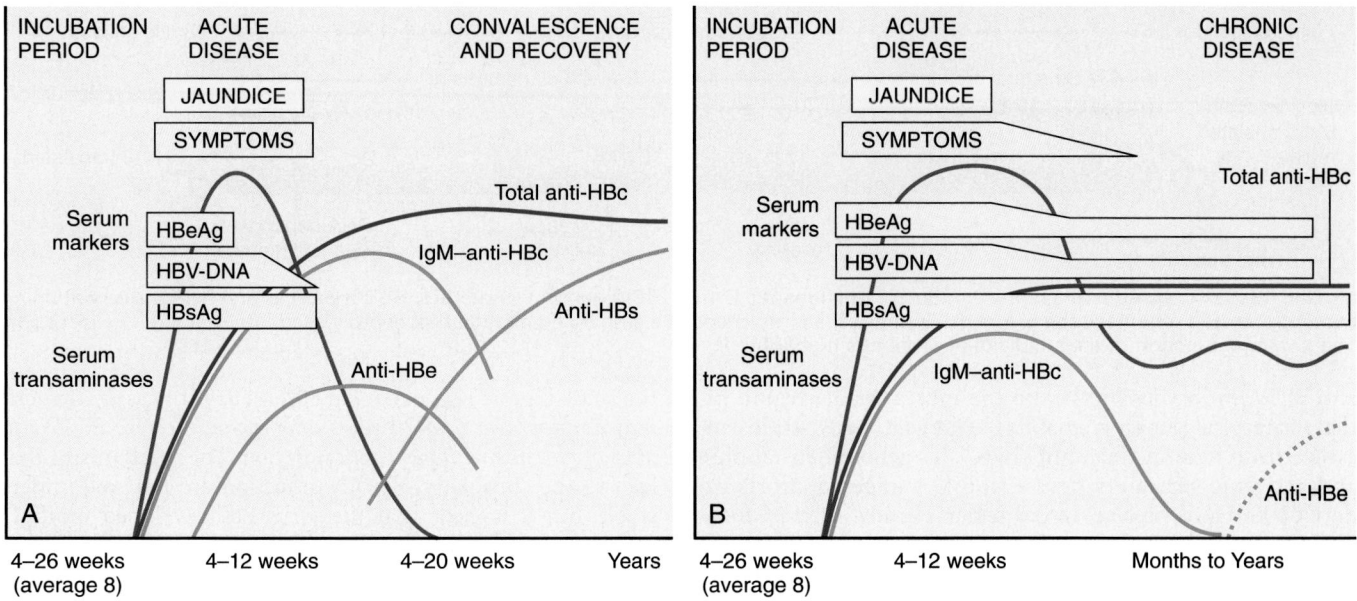

FIGURE 18–11 Sequence of serologic markers for hepatitis B viral hepatitis demonstrating (**A**) acute infection with resolution and (**B**) progression to chronic infection.

pared from purified HbsAg produced in yeast. Vaccination induces a protective anti-HBs antibody response in 95% of infants, children, and adolescents. Universal vaccination has had notable success in Taiwan and Gambia, but unfortunately, it has not been adopted worldwide.

Hepatitis C Virus

Hepatitis C virus (HCV) is a major cause of liver disease worldwide, with approximately 170 million people affected. Approximately 4.1 million Americans, or 1.6% of the population, have chronic HCV infection. This makes HCV the most common chronic blood-borne infection and accounts for almost half of all US individuals with chronic liver disease. Notably, there has been a decrease in the annual incidence of infection from its mid-1980s peak of over 230,000 new infections per year to a current 19,000 new infections per year. This welcome decline resulted primarily from a marked reduction in transfusion-associated causes as a result of screening procedures. Nevertheless, the number of patients with chronic infection will continue to increase, as a result of potential lifelong persistence of HCV infection. *In contrast to HBV, progression to chronic disease occurs in the majority of HCV-infected individuals, and cirrhosis eventually occurs in 20% to 30% of individuals with chronic HCV infection.* Thus, HCV is the most common cause of chronic liver disease in the United States and the most common indication for liver transplantation.

According to the 2008 data from the USA Centers for Disease Control, the most common risk factors for HCV infection are:

- Intravenous drug abuse (54%)
- Multiple sex partners (36%)
- Having had surgery within the last 6 month (16%)
- Needle stick injury (10%)
- Multiple contacts with an HCV-infected person (10%)

- Employment in medical or dental fields (1.5%)
- Unknown (32%)

Currently, transmission of HCV by blood transfusion is close to zero in the United States; the risk of acquiring HCV by needle sticks is about six times higher than that for HIV (1.8 vs 0.3%). For children, the major route of infection is perinatal, but is much lower than for HBV (6% vs. 20%). Note that patients may have multiple risk factors (the total of the listed risks above is >100%).

HCV, discovered in 1989, is a member of the Flaviviridae family. It is a small, enveloped, single-stranded RNA virus with a 9.6-kilobase (kb) genome that codes for a single polyprotein with one open reading frame, which is subsequently processed into functional proteins (Fig. 18–12). We review, briefly, the genomic structure of HCV because this has a bearing on the pathogenesis of hepatitis C. The 5′ end of the genome encodes a highly conserved nucleocapsid core protein, followed by envelope proteins E1 and E2. Two hypervariable regions (HVR 1 and 2) are present in the E2 sequence. A protein, p7, is believed to function as an ion channel. Toward the 3′ end are six less conserved nonstructural proteins: NS2, NS3, NS4A, NS4B, NS5A, and NS5B. NS5B is the viral RNA-dependent RNA polymerase. The 3′ sequences of both the positive- and negative-strand RNAs contribute *cis*-acting functions that are essential for viral replication. The secondary structure and protein-binding properties of these highly conserved nontranslated regions are thought to promote HCV RNA synthesis and genome stability through the binding of various host and viral proteins.

Because of the poor fidelity of the HCV RNA polymerase (NS5B), the virus is inherently unstable, giving rise to multiple genotypes and subtypes. Indeed, within any given patient HCV circulates as a population of divergent but closely related variants known as *quasispecies*.[28] Over time, dozens of quasispecies can be detected within one individual and mapped as derivative strains of the original HCV strain that infected the patient. The E2 protein of the envelope is the target of many

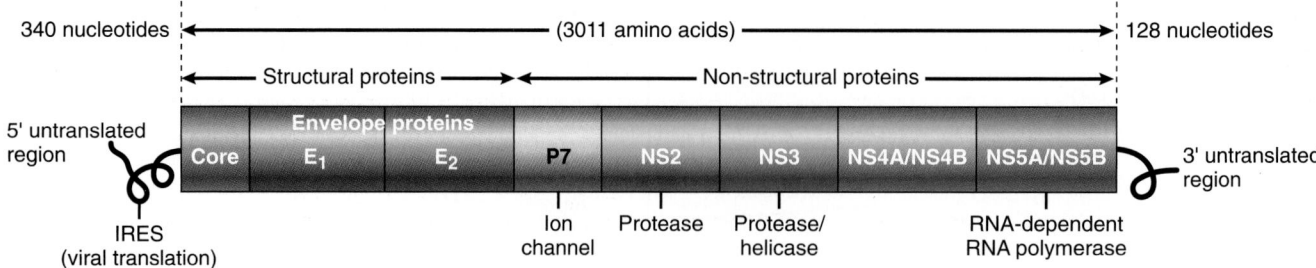

FIGURE 18–12 Diagrammatic representation of the hepatitis C viral (HCV) genomic structure. HCV is a (+) strand RNA virus containing two untranslated regions at the 5′ and the 3′ ends. The virus encodes a single polypeptide that is processed into multiple viral proteins. The potential function of each individual protein is highlighted.

anti-HCV antibodies but is also the most variable region of the entire viral genome, enabling emergent virus strains to escape from neutralizing antibodies. This genomic instability and antigenic variability have seriously hampered efforts to develop an HCV vaccine. In particular, *elevated titers of anti-HCV IgG occurring after an active infection do not consistently confer effective immunity.* A characteristic feature of HCV infection, therefore, is repeated bouts of hepatic damage, the result of reactivation of a preexisting infection or emergence of an endogenous, newly mutated strain.

The incubation period for HCV hepatitis ranges from 2 to 26 weeks, with a mean between 6 and 12 weeks. In about 85% of individuals, the clinical course of the acute infection is asymptomatic and easily missed. HCV RNA is detectable in blood for 1 to 3 weeks, coincident with elevations in serum transaminases. In symptomatic acute HCV infection, anti-HCV antibodies are detected in only 50% to 70% of patients; in the remaining patients, the anti-HCV antibodies emerge after 3 to 6 weeks. The clinical course of acute HCV hepatitis is milder than that of HBV; rare cases may be severe and indistinguishable from HAV or HBV hepatitis. Strong immune responses involving CD4+ and CD8+ T cells are associated with self-limited HCV infections, but it is not known why only a small minority of individuals are capable of clearing HCV infection.

Persistent infection and chronic hepatitis are the hallmarks of HCV infection, despite the generally asymptomatic nature of the acute illness. This occurs in 80% to 85% of cases. *Cirrhosis may develop over 5 to 20 years after acute infection in 20% to 30% of patients with persistent infection.* The mechanisms that lead to the chronicity of HCV infection are not well understood, but it is clear that the virus has developed multiple strategies to evade host antiviral immunity.[29] HCV is able to actively inhibit the interferon (IFN)-mediated cellular antiviral response at multiple steps, including Toll-like receptor signaling in response to viral RNA recognition and signaling downstream of IFN receptors that confers on cells an antiviral state.

In chronic HCV infection, circulating HCV RNA persists in many patients despite the presence of neutralizing antibodies, including more than 90% of patients with chronic disease (Fig. 18–13). Hence, in persons with chronic hepatitis, HCV RNA testing must be performed to assess viral replication and to confirm the diagnosis of HCV infection. *A clinical feature that is quite characteristic of chronic HCV infection is episodic elevations in serum aminotransferases, with intervening normal or near-normal periods. Fulminant hepatic failure rarely occurs.*

Hepatitis D Virus

Also called "hepatitis D virus," hepatitis D virus (HDV) is a unique RNA virus that is dependent for its life cycle on HBV. Infection with HDV arises in the following settings.[30]

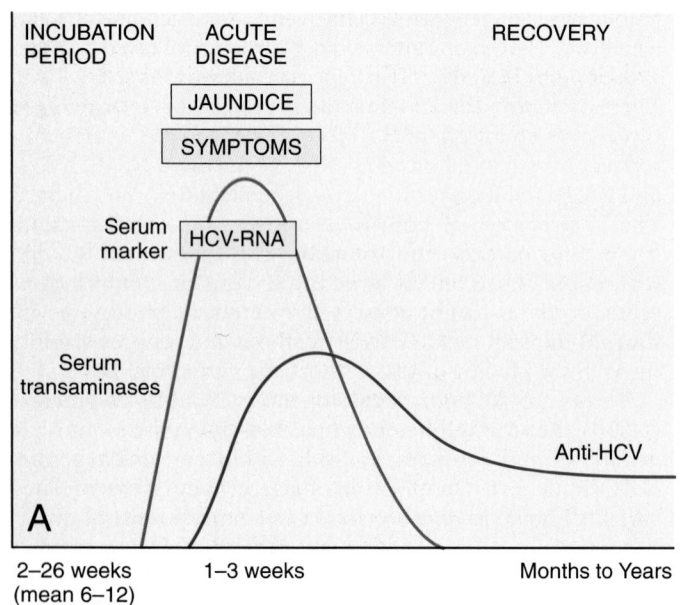

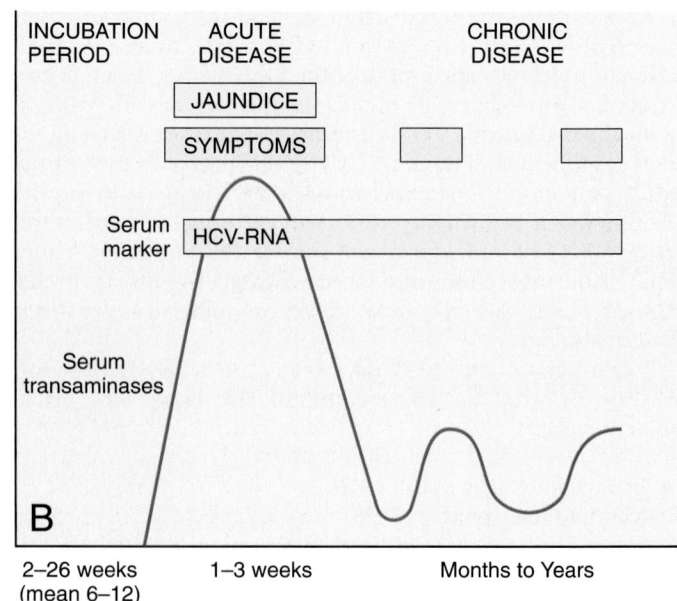

FIGURE 18–13 Sequence of serologic markers for HCV hepatitis. **A,** Acute infection with resolution; **B,** progression to chronic infection.

- *Acute coinfection* occurs following exposure to serum containing both HDV and HBV. The HBV must become established first to provide the HBsAg necessary for development of complete HDV virions.
- *Superinfection* occurs when a chronic carrier of HBV is exposed to a new inoculum of HDV. This results in disease 30–50 days later.
- *Helper-independent latent infection* observed in the liver transplant setting.

Coinfection of HBV and HDV results in acute hepatitis B + D which is clinically indistinguishable from classical acute hepatitis B and is usually transient and self-limited. Elimination of hepatitis B leads to elimination of HDV. The rate of progression to chronic infection is not different from that observed after classical acute hepatitis B. However, a high incidence of liver failure has been reported among drug addicts.

Superinfection with HDV in a chronic HBsAg carrier may present as severe acute hepatitis in a previously unrecognized HBV carrier, or as an exacerbation of preexisting chronic hepatitis B. Chronic HDV infection occurs in 80% to 90% of such patients. The superinfection may have two phases; an acute phase with active HDV replication and suppression of HBV with high ALT levels; and a chronic phase in which HDV replication decreases, HBV replication increases, ALT levels fluctuate, and the disease progresses to cirrhosis and hepatocellular cancer (HCC).

Helper-independent latent infection may be seen in liver transplants. HDV can be detected in nuclei of the grafted liver within a few hours after transplantation without evidence of productive HDV infection or HBV reinfection. This likely occurs due to infection of the allograft by HDV alone, while concomitant infection by HBV is prevented by hepatitis B immunoglobulin administered to prevent HBV reinfection. During this latent phase, there is no evidence of liver disease. HD viremia and hepatitis ensues only when HBV escapes neutralization and coinfection of the graft with high levels of HBV replication occurs, leading to activation of the HDV by the helper virus.

Infection by HDV is worldwide with an estimate of 15 million affected individuals (about 5% of 300 million of HBV infected persons). The prevalence varies widely in different countries. It is high in the Amazonian basin, and in Africa, the Middle East and southern Italy. Twenty to forty percent of HbsAg carriers may have anti-HDV antibody, although there has been a definite decline in recent years. In the United States HDV has virtually disappeared from hemophiliacs and other individuals who receive blood transfusion, because of the HBV screening procedures. Surprisingly HDV infection is uncommon in the large population of HBsAg carriers in Southeast Asia and China.

HDV, discovered in 1977, is a 35-nm, double-shelled particle that by electron microscopy resembles the "Dane particle" of HBV. The external coat antigen of HBsAg surrounds an internal polypeptide assembly, designated delta antigen (HDAg), the only protein produced by the virus. Associated with HDAg is a small circular molecule of single-stranded RNA, whose length is smaller than the genome of any known animal virus. Replication of the virus is through RNA-directed RNA synthesis by host RNA polymerase, mainly Pol II.

Diagnosis. HDV RNA is detectable in the blood and liver just before and in the early days of acute symptomatic disease. IgM anti-HDV is the most reliable indicator of recent HDV exposure, although its appearance is late and frequently short-lived. Nevertheless, acute co-infection by HDV and HBV is best indicated by detection of IgM against both HDAg and HBcAg (denoting new infection with hepatitis B). With chronic delta hepatitis arising from HDV superinfection, HBsAg is present in serum, and anti-HDV antibodies (IgG and IgM) persist for months or longer. Treatment of HDV infection is limited to IFN-α.[30] Other antiviral agents for HBV have not shown effectiveness. Vaccination for HBV can also prevent HDV infection.

Hepatitis E Virus

Hepatitis E virus (HEV) hepatitis is an enterically transmitted, water-borne infection that occurs primarily in young to middle-aged adults; sporadic infection and overt illness in children are rare. HEV is a zoonotic disease with animal reservoirs, such as monkeys, cats, pigs, and dogs.[31] Epidemics have been reported in Asia and the Indian subcontinent, sub-Saharan Africa, and Mexico. Sporadic infection may occur in travelers to these regions, but, most importantly, HEV infection accounts for more than 30% to 60% of cases of sporadic acute hepatitis in India, exceeding the frequency of HAV. *A characteristic feature of HEV infection is the high mortality rate among pregnant women, approaching 20%.* In most cases the disease is self-limiting; HEV is not associated with chronic liver disease or persistent viremia. The average incubation period following exposure is 6 weeks.

Discovered in 1983, HEV is an unenveloped, positive-stranded RNA virus in the *Hepevirus* genus.[31] Viral particles are 32 to 34 nm in diameter, and the RNA genome is approximately 7.3 kb in size. A specific antigen (HEV Ag) can be identified in the cytoplasm of hepatocytes during active infection, and virions are shed in stool during the acute illness.

Diagnosis. Before the onset of clinical illness, HEV RNA and HEV virions can be detected by PCR in stool and serum. The onset of rising serum aminotransferases, clinical illness, and elevated IgM anti-HEV titers are virtually simultaneous. Symptoms resolve in 2 to 4 weeks, during which time the IgM is replaced with a persistent IgG anti-HEV titer.

Hepatitis G Virus

A flavivirus bearing similarities to HCV was cloned in 1995 and designated hepatitis G virus (HGV, also referred to as GBV-C). HGV is transmitted by contaminated blood or blood products, and via sexual contact. However, HGV is inappropriately named: *it is not hepatotropic and does not cause elevations in serum aminotransferases.* Instead, the virus appears to replicate in the bone marrow and spleen. The prevalence of HGV RNA in American blood donors ranges from 1% to 4%; but since the virus does not cause known human disease, blood donors do not need screening. HGV commonly co-infects individuals infected with the human immunodeficiency virus (HIV; prevalence 35%); curiously this dual infection is somewhat protective against HIV disease.[32]

Clinicopathologic Syndromes of Viral Hepatitis

Several clinical syndromes may develop following exposure to hepatitis viruses: (1) acute asymptomatic infection with recovery (serologic evidence only); (2) acute symptomatic hepatitis with recovery, anicteric or icteric; (3) chronic hepatitis, without or with progression to cirrhosis; and (4) fulminant hepatitis with massive to submassive hepatic necrosis.

Each of the hepatotropic viruses can cause acute asymptomatic or symptomatic infection. A small number of HBV-infected adult patients develop chronic hepatitis. In contrast, HCV is notorious for chronic infection. HAV and HEV do not cause chronic hepatitis. Fulminant hepatitis is unusual and is seen primarily with HBV. Although HBV and HCV are responsible for most cases of chronic hepatitis, there are many other causes of chronic hepatitis (described later), including chronic alcoholism, drugs (e.g., isoniazid, α-methyldopa, methotrexate), toxins, Wilson disease, $α_1$-antitrypsin deficiency, and autoimmunity. Therefore, serologic and molecular studies are essential for the diagnosis of viral hepatitis, and for distinguishing between the various types.

Acute Asymptomatic Infection with Recovery. Patients in this group are identified only incidentally on the basis of minimally elevated serum transaminases or, after the fact, by the presence of antiviral antibodies. Worldwide, HAV and HBV infection are frequently subclinical events in childhood, verified only in adulthood by the presence of anti-HAV or anti-HBV antibodies.

Acute Symptomatic Infection with Recovery. Any one of the hepatotropic viruses can cause symptomatic acute viral hepatitis. Whatever the agent, the disease is more or less the same and can be divided into four phases: (1) an incubation period, (2) a symptomatic preicteric phase, (3) a symptomatic icteric phase, and (4) convalescence. The incubation period for the different viruses is given in Table 18–4. Peak infectivity occurs during the last asymptomatic days of the incubation period and the early days of acute symptoms.

Chronic Hepatitis. Chronic hepatitis is defined as symptomatic, biochemical, or serologic evidence of continuing or relapsing hepatic disease for more than 6 months. As mentioned earlier, HCV infection causes chronic hepatitis at a high frequency while only a small number of patients with HBV infection develop chronic disease. The clinical features of chronic hepatitis are extremely variable and are not predictive of outcome. In some patients the only signs of chronic disease are persistent elevations of serum transaminases. The most common symptom is fatigue; less common symptoms are malaise, loss of appetite, and occasional bouts of mild jaundice. Physical findings are few, the most common being spider angiomas, palmar erythema, mild hepatomegaly, hepatic tenderness, and mild splenomegaly. Laboratory studies may reveal prolongation of the prothrombin time and, in some instances, hyperglobulinemia, hyperbilirubinemia, and mild elevations in alkaline phosphatase levels. Occasionally, in cases of HBV and HCV, immune complex disease may develop secondary to the presence of circulating antibody-antigen complexes, in the form of vasculitis (subcutaneous or visceral, Chapter 11) and glomerulonephritis (Chapter 20). Cryoglobulinemia is found in about 35% of individuals with chronic hepatitis C.

The development of chronic infection after exposure to HBV is an important clinical problem. *Age at the time of infec-*

tion is the best determinant of chronicity. The younger the age at the time of infection, the higher the probability of chronicity. In many endemic areas, maternal-to-infant transmission is a major risk factor for chronic HBV infection. Though uncommon, patients can recover completely from chronic HBV infection.[33] Despite progress in the treatment of chronic HBV infection, complete cure is extremely difficult to achieve. Thus, the goal of the treatment of chronic hepatitis B is to slow disease progression, reduce liver damage, and prevent liver cirrhosis or liver cancer. The major problems associated with the current treatment regimens are viral resistance and side effects.

HCV is by far the most common cause of chronic viral hepatitis. The clinical diagnosis may not be apparent because patients with chronic HCV infection often have mild or no symptoms. However, even patients with normal transaminases are at high risk of developing permanent liver damage. Therefore, *any individual with detectable HCV RNA in the serum needs medical attention.*

HCV infection is potentially curable. Treatment is currently based on combination of pegylated IFN-α and ribavirin. The response to therapy depends on the viral genotype; patients with genotype 2 or 3 infection generally have the best responses. Several new drugs targeting viral protease and polymerase are under investigation.

The Carrier State. A "carrier" is an individual who harbors and can transmit an organism, but has no manifest symptoms. In the case of hepatotropic virus this definition is somewhat confusing, as it can be interpreted to mean: (1) individuals who carry one of the viruses but have no liver disease; (2) those who harbor one of the viruses and have non-progressive liver damage, but are essentially free of symptoms or disability. In both cases, particularly the latter, these individuals constitute reservoirs for infection. In the case of HBV infection a "healthy carrier" is often defined as an individual without HBeAg, but with presence of anti-HBe, normal aminotransferases, low or undetectable serum HBV DNA, and a liver biopsy showing a lack of significant inflammation and necrosis (Fig. 18–9). In non-endemic areas such as the United States, less than 1% of HBV infections acquired by adults produces a carrier state. This frequency is larger in those who have chronic hepatitis B (Fig. 18–9). In contrast, HBV infection acquired early in life in endemic areas (such as Southeast Asia, China, and Sub-Saharan Africa) gives rise to a carrier state of the two categories described above, in more than 90% of cases. It has been estimated that HCV infection in the United States may yield a carrier state in 10% to 40% of cases, but in most of the studies, absence of liver disease was assessed by persistent normal levels of aminotransferases, rather than liver biopsy. This is a limitation of such studies.

HIV and Chronic Viral Hepatitis. Because of the similar transmission mode and the similar high-risk patient population, co-infection of HIV and hepatitis viruses is becoming a common clinical problem. Among HIV patients, 10% are infected with HBV and 30% with HCV. Chronic HBV and HCV infection is now a leading cause of morbidity and mortality for HIV-infected patients, and liver disease is the second most common cause of death in individuals with acquired immunodeficiency syndrome (AIDS).[34] It is clear that HIV infection significantly exacerbates the severity of liver disease caused by HBV or HCV. Less clear is the impact of HBV or

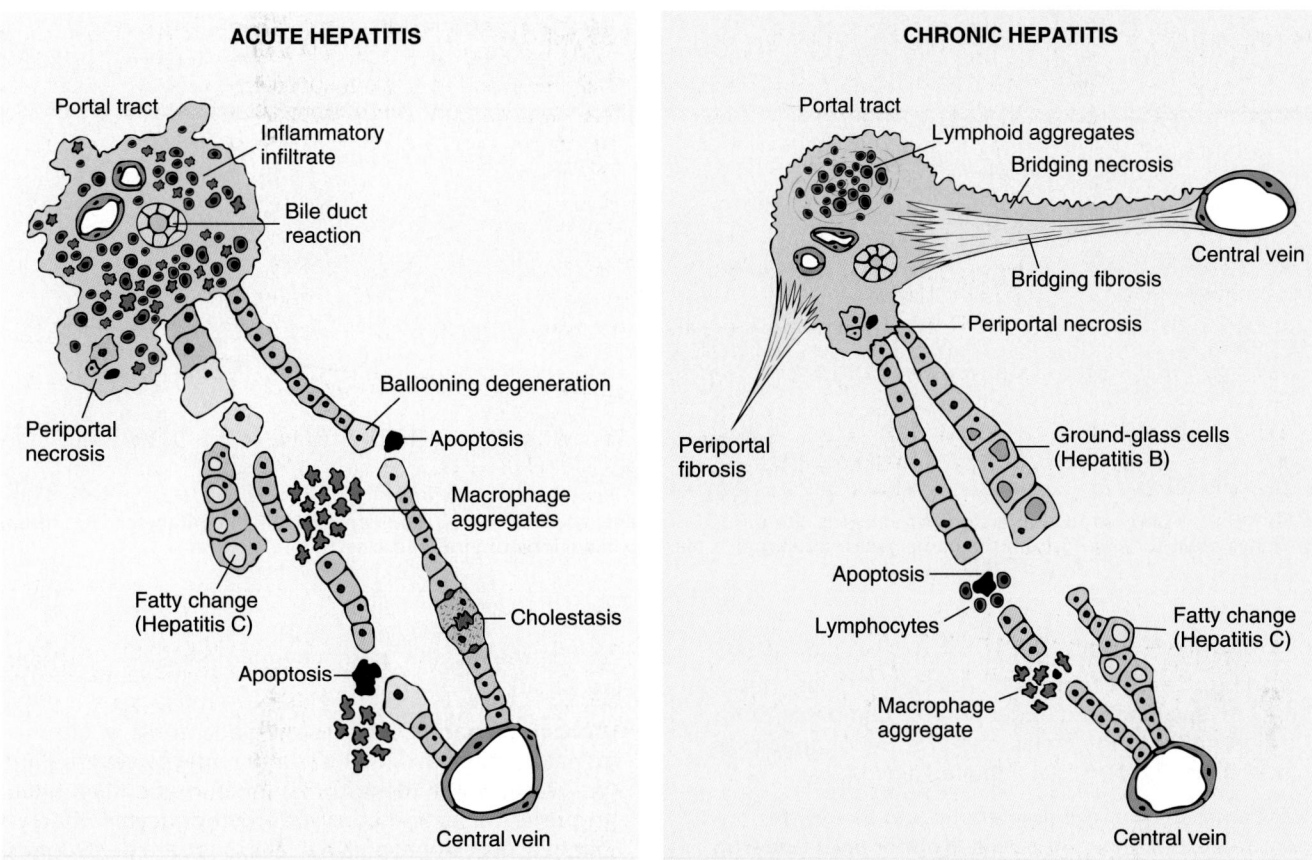

FIGURE 18–14 Diagrammatic representation of the morphologic features of acute and chronic hepatitis. Bridging necrosis (and fibrosis) is shown only for chronic hepatitis but may also occur in acute hepatitis (not shown).

HCV on the course of HIV infection. In addition, anti-HIV agents may cause hepatotoxicity in some patients with HBV or HCV co-infection.

Morphology of Acute and Chronic Hepatitis. The general morphologic features of viral hepatitis are depicted schematically in Figure 18–14. The morphologic changes in acute and chronic viral hepatitis are shared among the hepatotropic viruses and can be mimicked by drug reactions or autoimmune liver disease. Tissue alterations caused by acute infection with HAV, HBV, HCV, and HEV are generally similar, as is the chronic hepatitis caused by HBV, HCV, and HBV + HDV. A few histologic changes may be indicative of a particular type of virus. HBV-infected hepatocytes may show a cytoplasm packed with spheres and tubules of HBsAg, producing a finely granular cytoplasm ("ground-glass hepatocytes," Fig. 18–15). HCV-infected livers frequently show lymphoid aggregates within portal tracts and focal lobular regions of hepatocyte macrovesicular steatosis, which are to be distinguished from the extensive panlobular microvesicular and macrovesicular steatosis seen in many forms of toxic hepatitis (e.g., alcohol-induced).

Acute Hepatitis. With acute hepatitis (Fig. 18–16) hepatocyte injury takes the form of diffuse swelling (**"ballooning degeneration"**), so the cytoplasm looks empty and contains only scattered eosinophilic remnants of cytoplasmic organelles. An inconstant finding is **cholestasis**, with bile plugs in canaliculi and brown pigmentation of hepatocytes. The canalicular bile plugs result from cessation of the contractile activity of the hepatocyte pericanalicular actin microfilament web. Several patterns of hepatocyte cell death are seen.

- Rupture of the cell membrane leads to cell death and focal loss of hepatocytes. The sinusoidal collagen reticulin framework collapses where the cells have disappeared, and scavenger **macrophage aggregates** mark sites of hepatocyte loss.
- **Apoptosis**, caused by anti-viral cytotoxic (effector) T cells. Apoptotic hepatocytes shrink, become intensely eosinophilic, and have fragmented nuclei; effector T cells may still be present in the immediate vicinity. Apoptotic cells are rapidly phagocytosed by macrophages and hence might be difficult to find, despite a brisk rate of hepatocyte injury.
- In severe cases of acute hepatitis, confluent necrosis of hepatocytes may lead to **bridging necrosis**

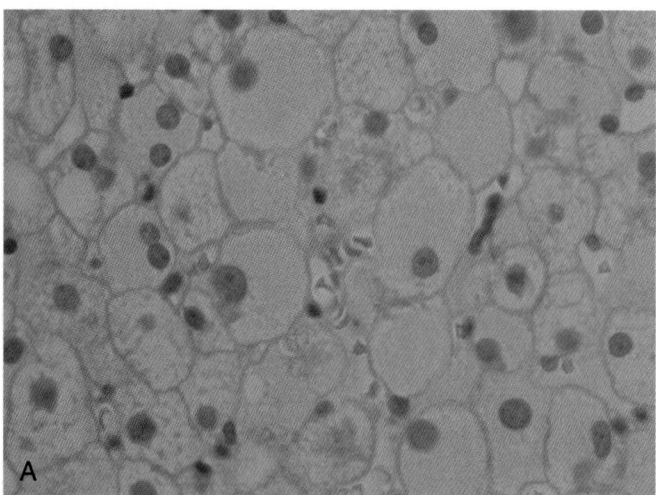
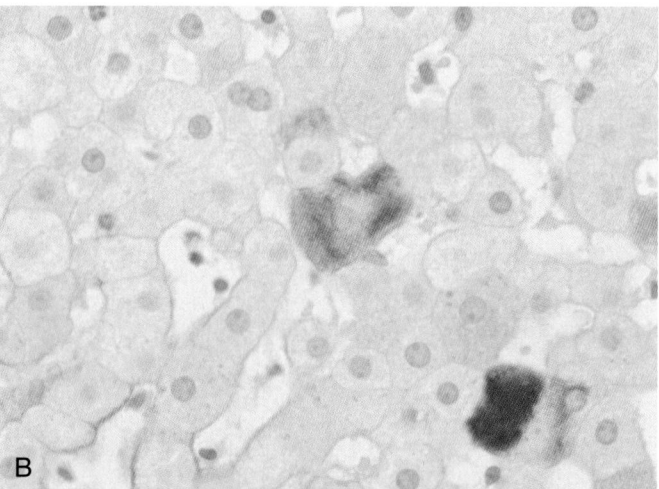

FIGURE 18–15 Chronic HBV infection. **A,** Showing the diffuse granular cytoplasm, so-called ground-glass hepatocytes. **B,** Immunoperoxidase stain for HBsAg from the same case, showing cytoplasmic inclusions of viral particles.

connecting portal-to-portal, central-to-central, or portal-to-central regions of adjacent lobules. Hepatocyte swelling and regeneration compress sinusoids, and the more or less radial array of hepatocyte plates around terminal hepatic veins is lost.

Inflammation is a characteristic and usually prominent feature of acute hepatitis. **Kupffer cells undergo hypertrophy and hyperplasia** and are often laden with lipofuscin pigment as a result of phagocytosis of hepatocellular debris. **The portal tracts are usually infiltrated with a mixture of inflammatory cells.** The inflammatory infiltrate may spill over into the adjacent parenchyma, causing apoptosis of periportal hepatocytes. This is known as **interface hepatitis,** which can occur in acute and chronic hepatitis. Cells in the canals of Hering proliferate, forming ductular

structures at the parenchymal interface (ductular reaction).

Chronic Hepatitis. The histologic features of chronic hepatitis range from exceedingly mild to severe (Fig. 18–17). In the mildest forms, inflammation is limited to portal tracts and consists of lymphocytes, macrophages, occasional plasma cells, and rare neutrophils or eosinophils. Liver architecture is usually well preserved, but smoldering hepatocyte apoptosis throughout the lobule may occur in all forms of chronic hepatitis. In chronic HCV infection, common findings (occurring in 55% of HCV infections) are **lymphoid aggregates** and **bile duct reactive changes** in the portal tracts, and focal mild to moderate macrovesicular **steatosis.** The steatosis is more prevalent and

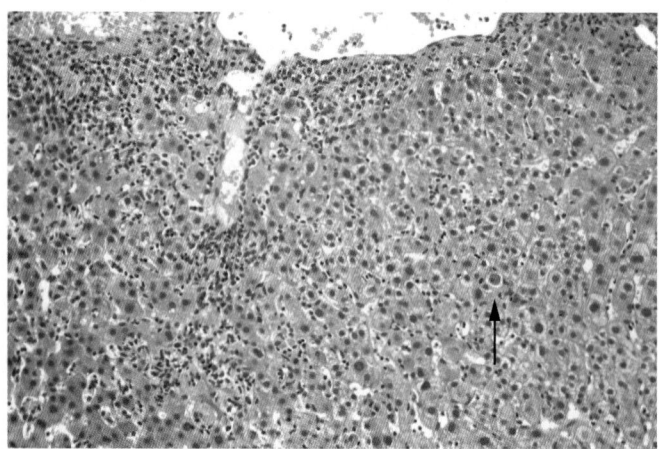

FIGURE 18–16 Acute viral hepatitis showing disruption of lobular architecture, inflammatory cells in the sinusoids, and hepatocyte apoptosis *(arrow).*

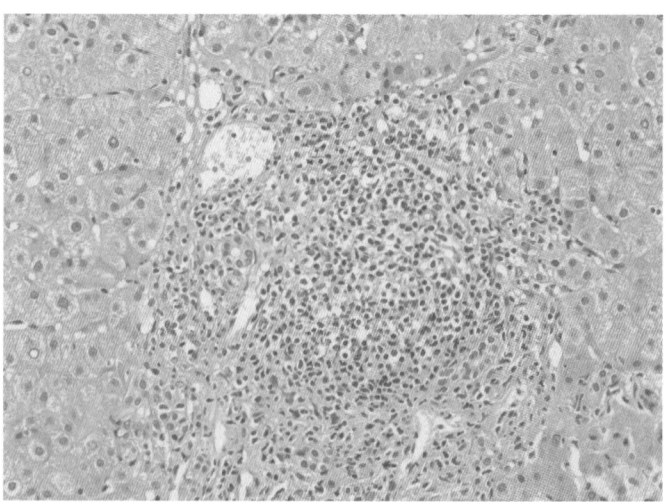

FIGURE 18–17 Chronic viral hepatitis due to HCV, showing portal tract expansion with inflammatory cells and fibrous tissue and interface hepatitis with spillover of inflammation into the adjacent parenchyma. A lymphoid aggregate is present.

prominent in HCV genotype 3 infections. In all forms of chronic hepatitis, continued **interface hepatitis** and **bridging necrosis** between portal tracts and portal tracts-to-terminal hepatic veins, are harbingers of progressive liver damage.

The hallmark of chronic liver damage is the deposition of fibrous tissue. At first, only portal tracts show increased fibrosis, but with time periportal septal fibrosis occurs, followed by linking of fibrous septa (bridging fibrosis), especially between portal tracts. In clinical practice, several systems have been used to score the severity and progression of liver damage due to HBV and HCV infection.[35] In each system the key elements are inflammation and hepatocyte destruction (grade), and the severity of fibrosis (stage)

Continued loss of hepatocytes and fibrosis results in cirrhosis. It is characterized by irregularly sized nodules separated by variable but mostly broad scars, and is often referred to as post-necrotic cirrhosis (Fig. 18–18). However, this term is not specific to viral etiology, and is applied to all forms of cirrhosis in which the liver shows large, irregular-sized nodules with broad scars. In addition to viral hepatitis, autoimmune hepatitis, hepatotoxins (carbon tetrachloride, mushroom poisoning), pharmaceutical drugs (acetaminophen, α-methyldopa), and even alcohol (discussed later) can give rise to cirrhotic livers with irregular-sized large nodules. In about 20% of cases the inciting cause of the cirrhosis cannot be determined, and these are labeled as **cryptogenic cirrhosis.** Thus, the morphology of the end-stage cirrhotic liver is often not helpful in determining the basis of the liver injury.

The clinical course of viral hepatitis is unpredictable. Patients may experience spontaneous remission or may have

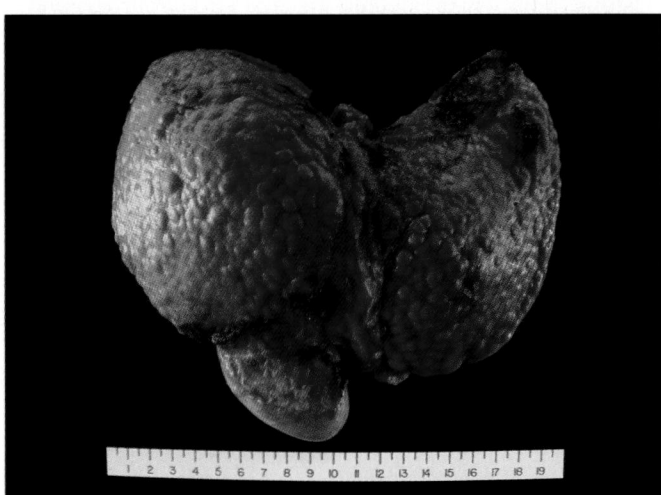

FIGURE 18–18 Cirrhosis resulting from chronic viral hepatitis. Note the broad scar and coarse nodular surface.

indolent disease without progression for many years. Conversely, some patients have rapidly progressive disease and develop cirrhosis within a few years. The major causes of death from cirrhosis are: liver failure and hepatic encephalopathy, massive hematemesis from esophageal varices, and HCC in those with long-standing HBV (particularly neonatal) or HCV infection.

Fulminant Hepatic Failure. Hepatic insufficiency that progresses from onset of symptoms to hepatic encephalopathy within 2 to 3 weeks in individuals who do not have chronic liver disease is termed *fulminant hepatic failure.* Viral hepatitis is responsible for about 12% of cases of fulminant hepatic failure; of these 8% are caused by HBV infection and the rest by HAV. Occasionally, HCV, herpesvirus infection, and Dengue virus cause fulminant hepatitis. Noninfectious causes, such as acetaminophen toxicity, were mentioned earlier. In about 15% of cases, the cause of fulminant hepatic failure is unknown.

The pathogenesis of fulminant hepatic failure varies depending on etiology. In the case of HBV-induced fulminant hepatitis, there is massive apoptosis.[36]

Morphology of Fulminant Hepatitis. Viral hepatitis and all other causative agents produce essentially identical morphologic changes that vary with the severity of the necrotizing process. The distribution of liver destruction is extremely capricious, since **the entire liver or only random areas may be involved.** With massive loss of mass, the liver may shrink to as little as 500 to 700 gm, and becomes a limp, red organ covered by a wrinkled, too-large capsule. On transection (Fig. 18–19A), necrotic areas have a muddy red, mushy appearance with hemorrhage. Microscopically, complete destruction of hepatocytes in contiguous lobules leaves only a collapsed reticulin framework and preserved portal tracts. There may be surprisingly little inflammatory reaction. Alternatively, with survival for several days, there is a massive influx of inflammatory cells to begin the phagocytic cleanup process (Fig. 18–19B).

Survival for more than a week may permit the replication of residual hepatocytes. The proliferation and differentiation of a quiescent stem/progenitor cell population in the canals of Hering, known as oval cells (Chapter 3), creates a *ductular reaction.* Maturation of these proliferating cells can generate both hepatocytes and bile duct cells. If the parenchymal framework is preserved, regeneration resulting mostly from hepatocyte replication can completely restore the liver architecture. With more massive destruction of confluent lobules, regeneration is disorderly, yielding nodular masses of liver cells that produce a more irregular liver on healing. Fibrous scarring may occur in patients with a protracted course of submassive or patchy necrosis, leading to cirrhosis.

The treatment for fulminant hepatic failure is to correct the underlying liver abnormality and provide supportive care. Liver transplantation is the only option for patients whose disease does not resolve before secondary infection and other organ failure develop. The mortality of fulminant hepatic failure is approximately 80% without liver transplantation, and about 35% with transplantation.

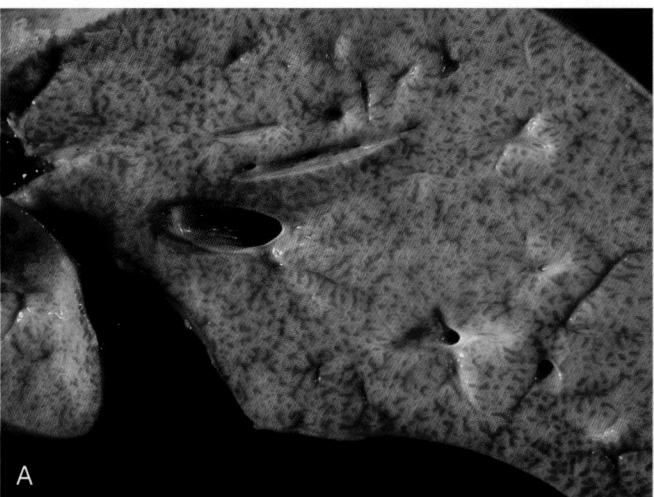
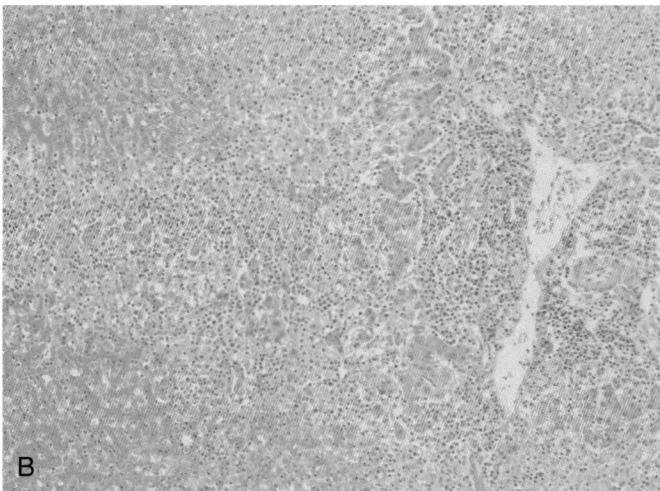

FIGURE 18-19 Massive necrosis. **A,** Cut section of liver. The liver is small (700 gm), bile-stained, and soft. The capsule is wrinkled. **B,** Microscopic section. Portal tracts and terminal hepatic veins are closer together than normal, as a result of necrosis and collapse of the intervening parenchyma. The rudimentary ductal structures are the result of early ductular regeneration. An infiltrate of mononuclear inflammatory cells is present.

BACTERIAL, PARASITIC, AND HELMINTHIC INFECTIONS

Extrahepatic bacterial infections, particularly sepsis, can induce mild hepatic inflammation and varying degrees of hepatocellular cholestasis. The latter effect is attributable to the effects of pro-inflammatory cytokines released by Kupffer cells and endothelial cells, in response to circulating endotoxin. Several bacteria can infect the liver directly, including *Staphylococcus aureus* in the setting of toxic shock syndrome, *Salmonella typhi* in the setting of typhoid fever, and *T. pallidum* in secondary or tertiary syphilis. Alternatively, bacteria may proliferate in a biliary tree especially when outflow is compromised by partial or complete obstruction. The intrabiliary bacterial composition reflects the gut flora, and the severe acute inflammatory response within the intrahepatic biliary tree is called *ascending cholangitis*.

Parasitic and helminthic infections are major causes of morbidity worldwide, and the liver is frequently involved (Chapter 8). These diseases include malaria, schistosomiasis, strongyloidiasis, cryptosporidiosis, leishmaniasis, echinococcosis, and infections by the liver flukes *Fasciola hepatica* and *Clonorchis sinensis*.

Liver abscesses, a form of liver infection that is common in developing countries, deserve special mention. They are usually caused by echinococcal and amebic infections (Chapter 8), and less commonly, by other protozoal and helminthic organisms. In developed countries liver abscesses are uncommon; the incidence of amebic infections is low and is usually present in immigrants from endemic regions. Most such abscesses are pyogenic, representing a complication of a bacterial infection elsewhere. The organisms reach the liver by (1) the portal vein, (2) arterial supply, (3) ascending infection in the biliary tract (ascending cholangitis), (4) direct invasion of the liver from a nearby source, or (5) a penetrating injury. The majority of hepatic abscesses used to result from portal spread of intra-abdominal infections (e.g., appendicitis, diverticulitis, colitis). With improved management of these conditions, spread now occurs primarily through the biliary tree or

the arterial supply in patients suffering from some form of immune deficiency (e.g., old age with debilitating disease, immunosuppression, or cancer chemotherapy with marrow failure). In these settings, abscesses may develop without a primary focus elsewhere.

Morphology. Liver abscesses may occur as solitary or multiple lesions, ranging in size from millimeters to massive lesions many centimeters in diameter. Bacteremic spread through the arterial or portal system tends to produce multiple small abscesses, whereas direct extension and trauma usually cause solitary large abscesses. Biliary abscesses, which are usually multiple, may contain purulent material from adjacent bile ducts. Gross and microscopic features are similar to those seen in any abscess. The causative organism can occasionally be identified in the case of fungal or parasitic abscesses. On rare occasions, abscesses located in the subdiaphragmatic region, particularly amebic, may burrow into the thoracic cavity to produce empyema or a lung abscess. Rupture of subcapsular liver abscesses can lead to peritonitis or localized peritoneal abscesses. Echinococcal infection has a characteristic cystic structure; the wall is laminated, and hooklets and intact organisms can be identified (Fig. 18-20). Calcification in the cystic wall is common.

Liver abscesses are associated with fever and, in many instances, right upper quadrant pain and tender hepatomegaly. Jaundice may result from extrahepatic biliary obstruction. Although antibiotic therapy may control smaller lesions, surgical drainage is often necessary for the larger lesions. Because diagnosis is frequently delayed since the patients are elderly and have serious coexistent disease, the mortality rate of patients with large liver abscesses ranges from 30% to 90%. With early recognition and management as many as 80% of patients can survive. In the case of echinococcal cysts, rupture

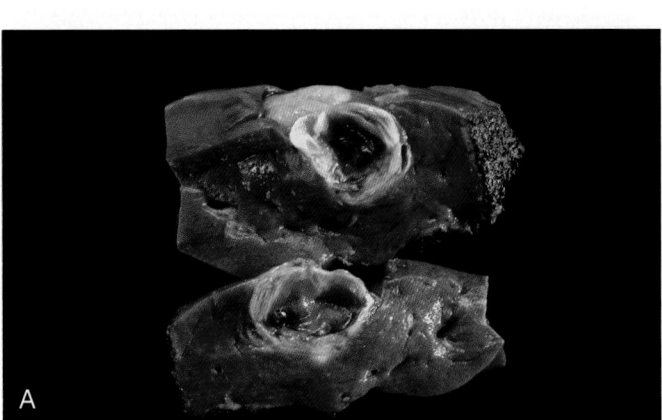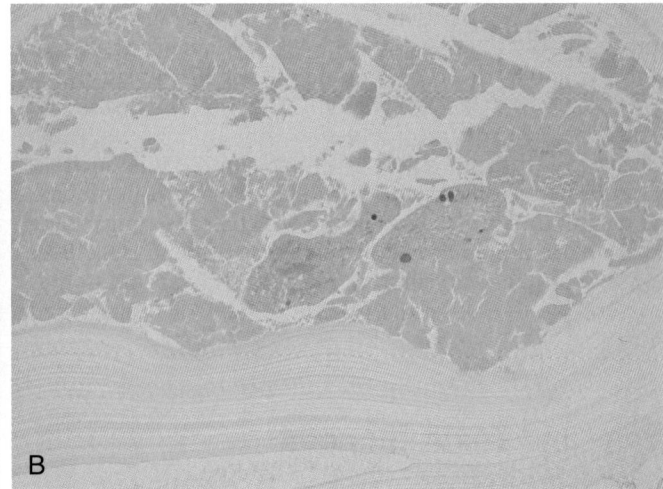

FIGURE 18–20 Echinococcal infection (**A**) demonstrating the cyst and (**B**) showing the laminated cystic wall with hooklet.

of this cyst has severe clinical consequences, including systemic spread of the organism and resultant shock from massive immune response.

Autoimmune Hepatitis

Autoimmune hepatitis is a chronic and progressive hepatitis of unknown etiology.[37] The pathogenesis is attributed to T cell–mediated autoimmunity, in which hepatocyte injury is caused by IFN-γ produced by CD4+ and CD8+ T cells and by CD8+ T-cell–mediated cytotoxicity. A defect in regulatory T-cells may underlie the uncontrolled activation of pathogenic, self-reactive lymphocytes. Genetic factors likely play a role in the autoimmunity (Chapter 6). The injurious immune reaction may be triggered by viral infections, certain drugs such as minocycline, atorvastatin, simvastatin, methyldopa, interferons, nitrofurantoin, and pemoline, and herbal products (such as black cohosh). Autoimmune hepatitis commonly occurs concurrently with other autoimmune disorders, such as celiac disease, systemic lupus erythematosus, rheumatoid arthritis, thyroiditis, Sjögren syndrome, and ulcerative colitis.

Clinicopathologic Features. The disease may run an indolent or severe course (including fulminant hepatitis). There is a *female predominance* (78%), particularly in young and perimenopausal women. The annual incidence is highest among white northern Europeans at 1.9 per 100,000, but all ethnic groups are susceptible. The salient features[38] include the absence of serologic markers of viral infection, elevated serum IgG and γ-globulin levels (1.2 to 3.0 times normal), and high serum titers of autoantibodies. *Autoimmune hepatitis is classified into types 1 and 2, based on the patterns of circulating antibodies.* Type 1 is characterized by the presence of antinuclear (ANA), anti–smooth muscle (SMA), anti–actin (AAA), and anti–soluble liver antigen/liver-pancreas antigen (anti-SLA/LP) antibodies. The main antibodies detected in Type 2 autoimmune hepatitis are anti–liver kidney microsome-1 (ALKM-1) antibodies, which are mostly directed against CYP2D6, and anti–liver cytosol-1 (ACL-1). Type 1 is much more common than Type 2 in the United States and is associated with the HLA-DR3 serotype. There is a female predomi-

nance, but the disease occurs in children and adults of both sexes.

The entire histologic spectrum of chronic hepatitis may be seen in autoimmune hepatitis, but it is marked by prominent inflammatory infiltrates of lymphocytes and plasma cells. *Clusters of plasma cells in the interface of portal tracts and hepatic lobules are fairly characteristic for autoimmune hepatitis* (Fig. 18–21). Symptomatic patients with autoimmune hepatitis tend to show substantial liver destruction and scarring at the time of diagnosis. Alternatively, autoimmune hepatitis may present in an atypical fashion with symptoms primarily from involvement of other organ systems, or may be asymptomatic and progress to cirrhosis without clinical diagnosis. An acute appearance of clinical illness is common (40%), and a fulminant presentation with onset of hepatic encephalopathy within 8 weeks of disease onset is possible. In a small subset of patients, autoimmune hepatitis diagnosed clinically may show histologic destruction of bile ducts ("autoimmune cholangitis"), making distinction from primary biliary cirrhosis (PBC) or primary sclerosing cholangitis (PSC) quite difficult. In some cases there is overlap of the clinical and histologic features of autoimmune hepatitis with those of PBC or PSC.

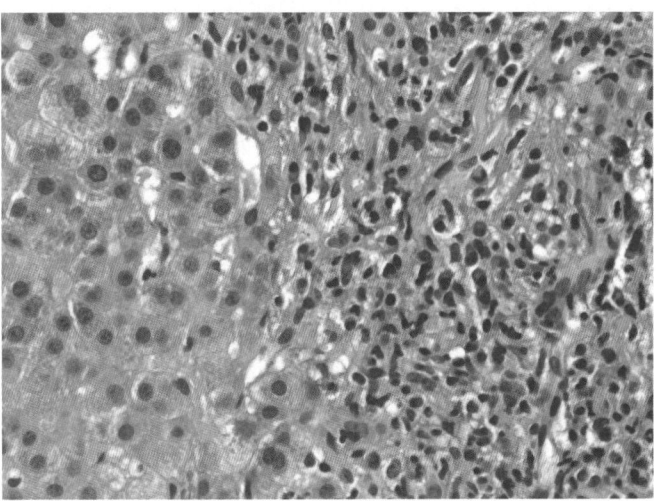

FIGURE 18–21 Autoimmune hepatitis. The photograph shows the interface hepatitis with prominent plasma cells.

The mortality of patients with severe untreated autoimmune hepatitis is approximately 40% within 6 months of diagnosis, and cirrhosis develops in at least 40% of survivors. Hence, diagnosis and intervention are clinical imperatives. Prednisone alone or in combination with azathioprine is the mainstay of therapy. Other immunosuppressants such as cyclosporine, tacrolimus, azathioprine, mycophenolate mofetil, and rapamycin are also used in various clinical settings. Liver transplantation is indicated for patients with end-stage liver disease. The ten-year survival rate after transplantation is 75%, but the disease recurs in 22% to 42% of transplanted patients.

Drug- and Toxin-Induced Liver Disease

The liver is subject to potential damage from an enormous array of pharmaceutical and environmental chemicals.[39] Drug-induced liver injury accounts for about 10% of adverse drug reactions, and is the *most common cause of fulminant hepatitis in the United States.* The incidence of liver injury induced by prescribed drugs is estimated to be between 14 and 40 per 100,000 patients. Genetic variability is a critical factor that influences the susceptibility to drug-induced injury. Injury may result (1) from direct toxicity to hepatocytes or biliary epithelial cells, causing necrosis, apoptosis, or disruption of cellular function; (2) through hepatic conversion of a xenobiotic to an active toxin; or (3) through immune mechanisms, usually by a drug or a metabolite acting as a hapten to convert a cellular protein into an immunogen.[40]

The main principles of drug and toxic injury are discussed in Chapter 9. Here it suffices to recall that drug reactions may be *predictable (intrinsic)* or *unpredictable (idiosyncratic).* Predictable drug reactions can occur in anyone who receives a sufficient dose of an agent. Unpredictable reactions depend on idiosyncrasies of the host, particularly the rate at which the host metabolizes the agent, and the intensity of the immune response. Idiosyncratic drug reaction should be considered in any patient receiving a therapeutic drug who develops evidence of liver damage. Generally, adults are more susceptible than children, and women are affected more than men. Important examples include chlorpromazine, an agent that causes cholestasis in patients who are slow to metabolize it to an innocuous byproduct, and halothane, which can cause a fatal immune-mediated hepatitis in some patients who are exposed to this anesthetic on multiple occasions. Table 18–5 lists more common offending agents, grouped according to the type of morphologic injury. It should be noted that the injury may be immediate or may take weeks to months to develop, presenting only after severe liver damage has developed. It may take the form of *hepatocyte necrosis, cholestasis,* or *insidious onset of liver dysfunction. Drug-induced chronic hepatitis is clinically and histologically indistinguishable from chronic viral hepatitis; hence, serologic markers of viral infection are critical for making the distinction.*

Among the agents listed in Table 18–5, hepatic injury is considered predictable with overdoses of acetaminophen, exposure to *Amanita phalloides* toxin, carbon tetrachloride, and, to a certain extent, alcohol. However, individual genetic

TABLE 18–5 Patterns of Injury in Drug- and Toxin-Induced Hepatic Injury

Pattern of Injury	Morphologic Findings	Examples of Associated Agents
Cholestatic	Bland hepatocellular cholestasis, without inflammation	Contraceptive and anabolic steroids; estrogen replacement therapy
Cholestatic hepatitis	Cholestasis with lobular necroinflammatory activity; may show bile duct destruction	Numerous antibiotics; phenothiazines
Hepatocellular necrosis	Spotty hepatocyte necrosis Submassive necrosis, zone 3 Massive necrosis	Methyldopa, phenytoin Acetaminophen, halothane Isoniazid, phenytoin
Steatosis	Macrovesicular	Ethanol, methotrexate, corticosteroids, total parenteral nutrition
Steatohepatitis	Microvesicular, Mallory bodies	Amiodarone, ethanol
Fibrosis and cirrhosis	Periportal and pericellular fibrosis	Methotrexate, isoniazid, enalapril
Granulomas	Noncaseating epithelioid granulomas	Sulfonamides, numerous other agents
Vascular lesions	Sinusoidal obstruction syndrome (veno-occlusive disease): obliteration of central veins Budd-Chiari syndrome Sinusoidal dilatation Peliosis hepatis: blood-filled cavities, not lined by endothelial cells	High-dose chemotherapy, bush teas Oral contraceptives Oral contraceptives, numerous other agents Anabolic steroids, tamoxifen
Neoplasms	Hepatic adenoma Hepatocellular carcinoma Cholangiocarcinoma Angiosarcoma	Oral contraceptives, anabolic steroids Thorotrast Thorotrast Thorotrast, vinyl chloride

From Washington K: Metabolic and toxic conditions of the liver. In Iacobuzio-Donahue CA, Montgomery EA (eds): Gastrointestinal and Liver Pathology. Philadelphia, Churchill Livingstone; 2005.

differences in the hepatic metabolism of xenobiotics through activating and detoxification pathways play a major role in individual susceptibility to even "predictable" hepatotoxins. Many other xenobiotics, such as sulfonamides, α-methyldopa, and allopurinol, cause idiosyncratic reactions. As already mentioned (in this chapter and in Chapter 9), *acetaminophen is the leading cause of drug-induced acute liver failure.* The most common prescription drugs causing idiosyncratic injury (that is, drug toxicity unrelated to drug dosage) include antibiotics and, in particular, isonazid, nonsteroidal analgesics, and antiseizure medications. Idiosyncratic reactions evolve with a subacute course and are usually characterized by high bilirubin levels. Herbal preparations can be responsible for both predictable and idiosyncratic liver damage. *Reye syndrome,* a rare and potentially fatal syndrome of mitochondrial dysfunction in liver, brain, and elsewhere, occurs predominantly in children and is characterized morphologically by extensive accumulation of fat droplets within hepatocytes (microvesicular steatosis). Its development has been associated with the administration of acetylsalicylic acid (aspirin) for the relief of fever, but a causal relationship between aspirin and Reye syndrome has not been established. Nevertheless, aspirin should be avoided in children with febrile illness. Long-term methotrexate administration, an effective treatment for moderate to severe psoriasis, can cause liver injury, including hepatic steatosis and fibrosis.[41]

Drug-induced liver disease is usually followed by recovery upon removal of the drug. *Exposure to a toxin or therapeutic agent should always be included in the differential diagnosis of liver disease.*

ALCOHOLIC LIVER DISEASE

Excessive alcohol (ethanol) consumption is the leading cause of liver disease in most Western countries. In the United States, 50% of the population 18 years of age or older drink alcohol. A subset of these individuals suffer serious health consequences associated with alcoholism (Chapter 9). Of greatest impact is alcoholic liver disease, which affects more than 2 million Americans and causes 27,000 deaths a year. There are three distinctive, albeit overlapping, forms of alcoholic liver disease: (1) *hepatic steatosis (fatty liver disease),* (2) *alcoholic hepatitis,* and (3) *cirrhosis* (Fig. 18–22). The morphology of the three forms of alcoholic liver disease is presented first, followed by a discussion of their pathogenesis.

> **Morphology.**
>
> ***Hepatic Steatosis (Fatty Liver).*** After even moderate intake of alcohol, **microvesicular** lipid droplets accumulate in hepatocytes. With chronic intake of alcohol, lipid accumulates creating large, clear **macrovesicular** globules that compress and displace the hepatocyte nucleus to the periphery of the cell. Macroscopically, the fatty liver of chronic alcoholism is a

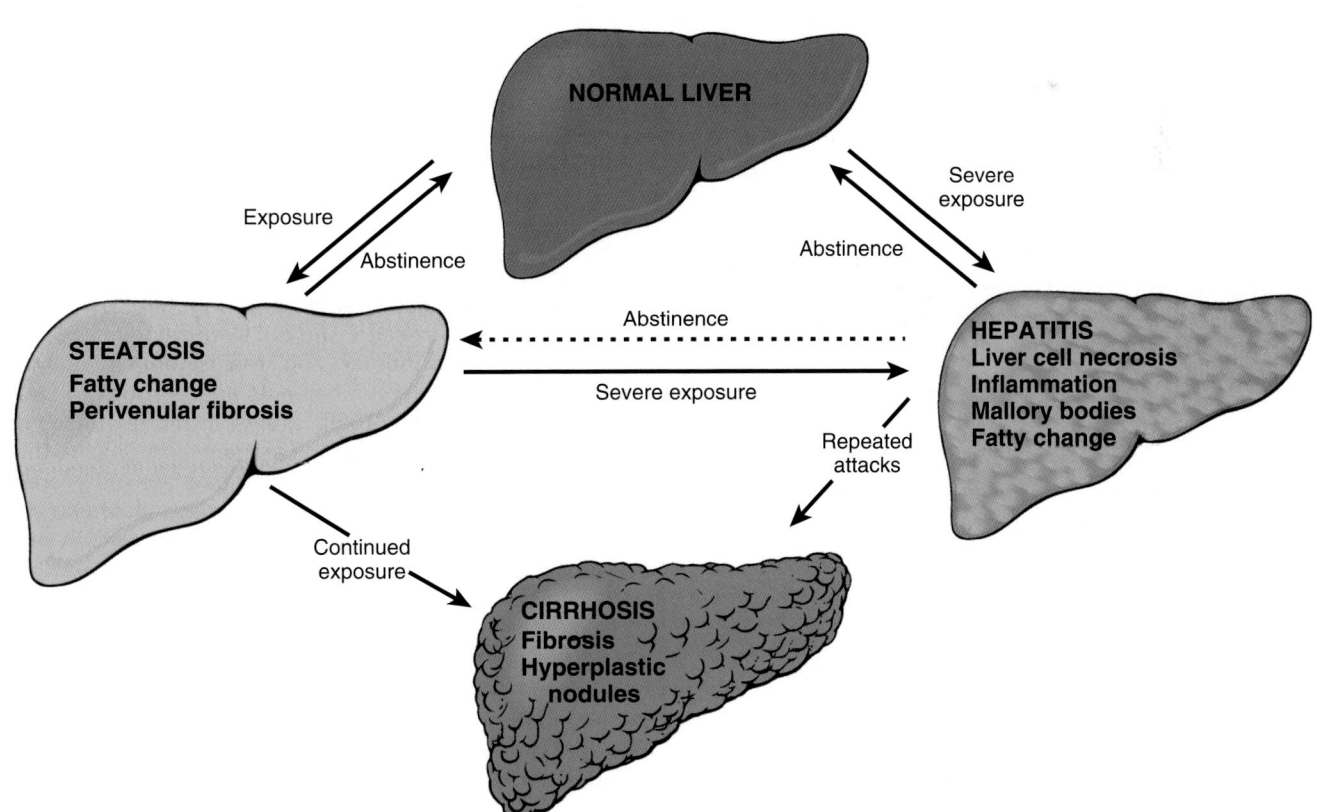

FIGURE 18–22 Alcoholic liver disease. The interrelationships among hepatic steatosis, hepatitis, and cirrhosis are shown, depicting key morphologic features.

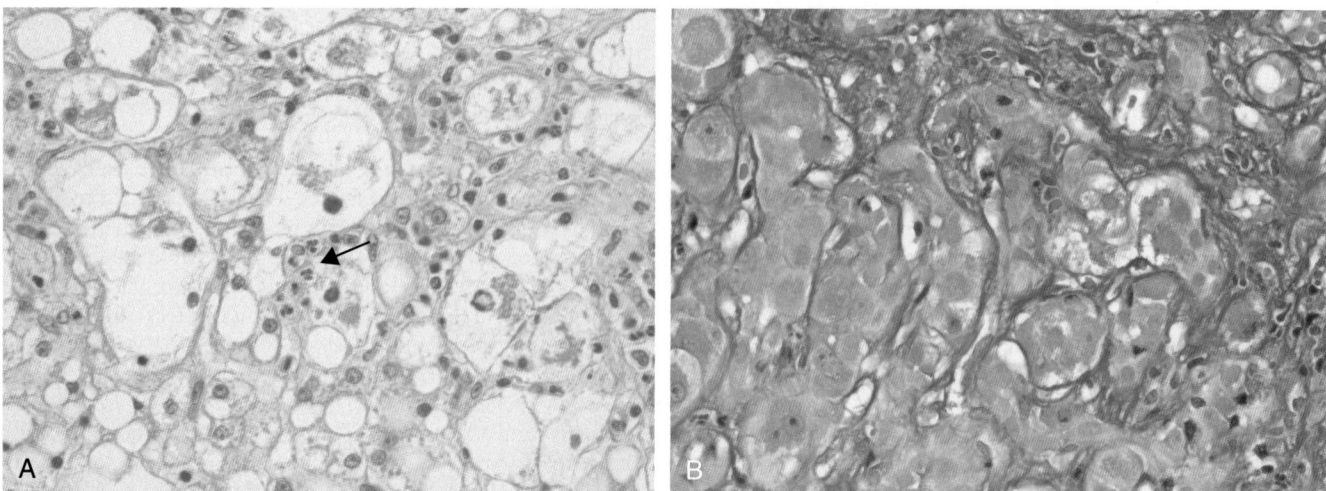

FIGURE 18–23   Alcoholic hepatitis. **A,** The cluster of inflammatory cells marks the site of a necrotic hepatocyte *(arrow).* **B,** Eosinophilic Mallory bodies are seen in hepatocytes, which are surrounded by fibrous (Masson stain) tissue.

large (as heavy as 4 to 6 kg), soft organ that is yellow and greasy. Although there is little or no fibrosis at the outset, with continued alcohol intake fibrous tissue develops around the terminal hepatic veins and extends into the adjacent sinusoids. **The fatty change is completely reversible if there is abstention from further intake of alcohol.**

Alcoholic Hepatitis (Alcoholic Steatohepatitis). Alcoholic hepatitis is characterized by:

1. **Hepatocyte swelling and necrosis:** Single or scattered foci of cells undergo swelling (ballooning) and necrosis. The swelling results from the accumulation of fat and water, as well as proteins that normally are exported. In some cases there is cholestasis in surviving hepatocytes and mild deposition of hemosiderin (iron) in hepatocytes and Kupffer cells.
2. **Mallory bodies:** Scattered hepatocytes accumulate tangled skeins of cytokeratin intermediate filaments such as cytokeratin 8 and 18, in complex with other proteins such as ubiquitin. Mallory bodies are visible as eosinophilic cytoplasmic clumps in hepatocytes (Fig. 18–23). These inclusions are a characteristic but not specific feature of alcoholic liver disease, since they also present in NAFLD, PBC, Wilson disease, chronic cholestatic syndromes, and hepatocellular tumors.
3. **Neutrophilic reaction:** Neutrophils permeate the hepatic lobule and accumulate around degenerating hepatocytes, particularly those having Mallory bodies. Lymphocytes and macrophages also enter portal tracts and spill into the parenchyma.
4. **Fibrosis:** Alcoholic hepatitis is almost always accompanied by prominent activation of sinusoidal stellate cells and portal tract fibroblasts, giving rise to fibrosis. Most frequently fibrosis is sinusoidal and perivenular, separating parenchymal cells; occasionally, periportal fibrosis may predominate, par-

ticularly with repeated bouts of heavy alcohol intake.

Cirrhosis. The final and irreversible form of alcoholic liver disease usually evolves slowly and insidiously but may develop in 1 or 2 years in some cases. At first the cirrhotic liver is yellow-tan, fatty, and enlarged, usually weighing over 2 kg. Over the span of years, it is transformed into a brown, shrunken, nonfatty organ, sometimes less than 1 kg in weight. Initially the developing fibrous septa are delicate and extend through sinusoids from central to portal regions as well as from portal tract to portal tract. Regenerative activity of entrapped parenchymal hepatocytes generates uniform micronodules. With time the nodularity becomes more prominent; scattered larger nodules create a "hobnail" appearance on the surface of the liver (Fig. 18–24A). As fibrous septa dissect and surround nodules, the liver becomes more fibrotic, loses fat, and shrinks progressively in size. Parenchymal islands are engulfed by wider bands of fibrous tissue, and the liver is converted into a mixed micronodular and macronodular pattern (Fig. 18–24B). Ischemic necrosis and fibrous obliteration of nodules eventually create broad expanses of tough, pale scar tissue ("Laennec cirrhosis"). Bile stasis often develops; Mallory bodies are only rarely evident at this stage. Thus, **end-stage alcoholic cirrhosis comes to resemble, both macroscopically and microscopically, the cirrhosis developing from viral hepatitis and other causes.**

Pathogenesis. Short-term ingestion of as much as 80 gm of alcohol (six beers or 8 ounces of 80-proof liquor) over one to several days generally produces mild, reversible hepatic steatosis. Daily intake of 80 gm or more of ethanol generates significant risk for severe hepatic injury, and daily ingestion of 160 gm or more for 10 to 20 years is associated more consistently with severe injury. *Only 10% to 15% of alcoholics, however, develop cirrhosis.* Thus, other factors must also influ-

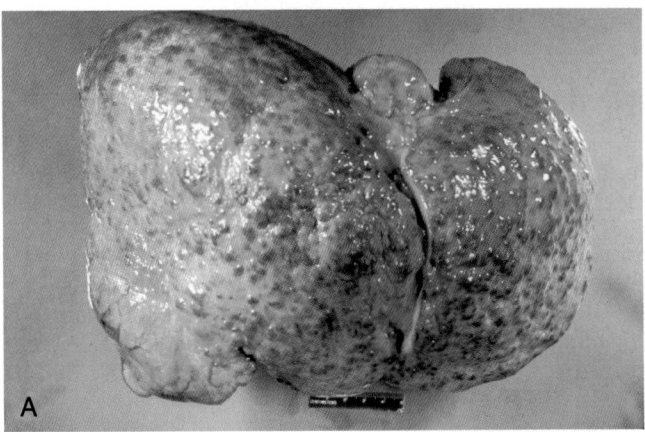

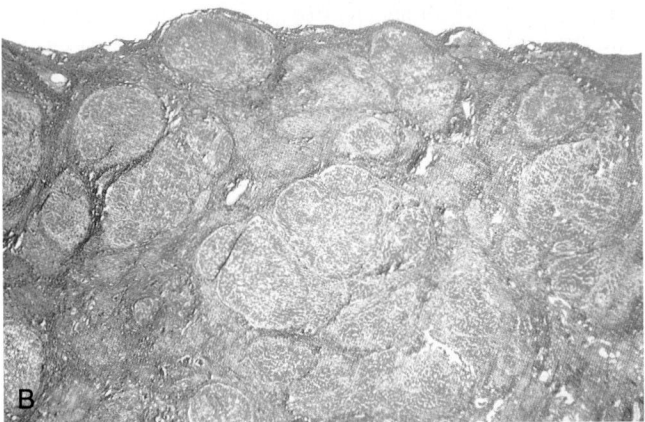

FIGURE 18–24 Alcoholic cirrhosis. **A,** The characteristic diffuse nodularity of the surface reflects the processes of nodular regeneration and scarring. The greenish tint of some nodules is due to bile stasis. A hepatocellular carcinoma is present as a budding mass at the lower edge of the right lobe *(lower left).* **B,** The microscopic view shows nodules of varying sizes entrapped in bluestaining fibrous tissue. The liver capsule is at the top (Masson trichrome).

ence the development and severity of alcoholic liver disease. These factors include:

- *Gender.* Women seem to be more susceptible to hepatic injury than men are, although the majority of patients are men. This difference may be related to alcohol pharmacokinetics and metabolism, and the estrogen-dependent response to gut-derived endotoxin (LPS) in the liver.[42] Estrogen increases gut permeability to endotoxins, which, in turn, increase the expression of the LPS receptor CD14 in Kupffer cells. This predisposes to increased production of pro-inflammatory cytokines and chemokines.
- *Ethnic differences.* In the United States, cirrhosis rates are higher for African Americans than for white Americans. The difference cannot be explained by the amount of alcohol consumption, since there is no significant difference in consumption among the ethnic groups.
- *Genetic factors.* Studies with twins suggest that there is a genetic component in alcohol-induced liver disease. There is also a strong family association, but in these cases it is difficult to separate genetic from environmental influences. Current attention is being given to genetic polymorphisms in detoxifying enzymes and some cytokine promoters. ALDH*2,

a genetic variant of aldehyde-dehydrogenase (ALDH), found in 50% of Asians, has a very low activity (Chapter 9). Individuals who are homozygous for ALDH*2 are unable to oxidize acetaldehyde and do not tolerate alcohol.
- *Co-morbid conditions.* Iron overload and infections with HCV and HBV increase the severity of alcoholic liver disease.

The pharmacokinetics and metabolism of alcohol were described in Chapter 9. Pertinent to our discussion here are the detrimental effects of alcohol and its byproducts on hepatocellular function. *Exposure to alcohol causes steatosis, dysfunction of mitochondrial and cellular membranes, hypoxia, and oxidative stress.* At millimolar concentrations, alcohol directly affects microtubular and mitochondrial function and membrane fluidity.

Hepatocellular steatosis results from (1) shunting of normal substrates away from catabolism and toward lipid biosynthesis, as a result of generation of excess reduced nicotinamide adenine dinucleotide ($NADH + H^+$) by the two major enzymes of alcohol metabolism, alcohol dehydrogenase and acetaldehyde dehydrogenase; (2) impaired assembly and secretion of lipoproteins; and (3) increased peripheral catabolism of fat.

The causes of *alcoholic hepatitis* are uncertain but some of the factors in its pathogenesis are discussed next. *Acetaldehyde* (the major intermediate metabolite of alcohol) induces lipid peroxidation and acetaldehyde-protein adduct formation, further disrupting cytoskeletal and membrane function. Cytochrome P-450 metabolism produces *reactive oxygen species (ROS)* that react with cellular proteins, damage membranes, and alter hepatocellular function. In addition, alcohol-induced impaired hepatic metabolism of methionine leads to decreased intrahepatic glutathione levels, thereby sensitizing the liver to oxidative injury. The induction of CYP2E1 and other cytochrome P-450 enzymes in the liver by alcohol increases alcohol catabolism in the endoplasmic reticulum and enhances the conversion of other drugs (e.g., acetaminophen) to toxic metabolites.

Alcohol can become a major source of calories in the diet of an alcoholic, displacing other nutrients and leading to *malnutrition and deficiencies of vitamins* (such as thiamine). This is compounded by impaired digestive function, primarily related to chronic gastric and intestinal mucosal damage, and pancreatitis.

Alcohol causes the *release of bacterial endotoxin from the gut* into the portal circulation, inducing inflammatory responses in the liver, such as the activation of NF-κB, and release of TNF, IL-6, and TGF-α. In addition, alcohol stimulates the *release of endothelins* from sinusoidal endothelial cells, causing vasoconstriction and the contraction of activated stellate cells ("myofibroblasts"), leading to a decrease in hepatic sinusoidal perfusion (already discussed under "Portal Hypertension").

In summary, alcoholic liver disease is a chronic disorder featuring steatosis, hepatitis, progressive fibrosis, cirrhosis, and marked derangement of vascular perfusion. It can be regarded as a maladaptive state in which cells in the liver respond in an increasingly pathologic manner to a stimulus (alcohol) that originally was only marginally harmful. For some unknown reason, cirrhosis develops in only a small fraction of chronic alcoholics.

Clinical Features. *Hepatic steatosis* (fatty liver) may become evident as hepatomegaly, with mild elevation of serum bilirubin and alkaline phosphatase levels. Severe hepatic dysfunction is unusual. Alcohol withdrawal and the provision of an adequate diet are sufficient treatment. In contrast, *alcoholic hepatitis* tends to appear acutely, usually following a bout of heavy drinking. Symptoms and laboratory manifestations may range from minimal to fulminant hepatic failure. Between these two extremes are the nonspecific symptoms of malaise, anorexia, weight loss, upper abdominal discomfort, tender hepatomegaly, and the laboratory findings of hyperbilirubinemia, elevated alkaline phosphatase, and often a neutrophilic leukocytosis. An acute cholestatic syndrome may appear, resembling large bile duct obstruction. The outlook is unpredictable; each bout of hepatitis incurs about a 10% to 20% risk of death. With repeated bouts, cirrhosis appears in about one third of patients within a few years. Alcoholic hepatitis also may be superimposed on established cirrhosis. With proper nutrition and total cessation of alcohol consumption, the alcoholic hepatitis may clear slowly. However, in some patients, the hepatitis persists, despite abstinence, and progresses to cirrhosis.

The manifestations of *alcoholic cirrhosis* are similar to those of other forms of cirrhosis. Laboratory findings reflect the hepatic dysfunction, with elevated serum aminotransferase, hyperbilirubinemia, variable elevation of serum alkaline phosphatase, hypoproteinemia (globulins, albumin, and clotting factors), and anemia. In some instances, liver biopsy may be indicated, since in about 10% to 20% of cases of presumed alcoholic cirrhosis, another disease process is found. Finally, cirrhosis may be clinically silent, discovered only at autopsy or when stress such as infection or trauma tips the balance toward hepatic insufficiency.

The long-term outlook for alcoholics with liver disease is variable. Five-year survival approaches 90% in abstainers who are free of jaundice, ascites, or hematemesis; it drops to 50% to 60% in those who continue to imbibe. In the end-stage alcoholic the proximate causes of death are (1) hepatic coma, (2) massive gastrointestinal hemorrhage, (3) intercurrent infection (to which these patients are predisposed), (4) hepatorenal syndrome following a bout of alcoholic hepatitis, and (5) hepatocellular carcinoma (the risk of developing this tumor in alcoholic cirrhosis is 1% to 6% of cases annually).

Metabolic Liver Disease

A distinct group of liver diseases is attributable to disorders of metabolism, either acquired or inherited. The most common acquired metabolic disorder is non-alcoholic fatty liver disease. Among inherited metabolic diseases, hemochromatosis, Wilson disease, and α_1-antitrypsin deficiency are most prominent. Also included among liver metabolic diseases is neonatal hepatitis, a broad disease category encompassing rare inherited diseases and neonatal infections.

NONALCOHOLIC FATTY LIVER DISEASE (NAFLD)

NAFLD is a group of conditions that have in common the presence of hepatic steatosis (fatty liver), in individuals who do not consume alcohol, or do so in very small quantities (less than 20 g of ethanol/week). It has become *the most common cause of chronic liver disease in the United States*, and in its various forms, probably affects more than 30% of the population. However, these estimates are approximate, because fatty liver without other complications may not be detected clinically. NAFLD includes simple *hepatic steatosis, steatosis accompanied by minor, non-specific inflammation, and non-alcoholic steatohepatitis (NASH).*[43] Steatosis with or without non-specific inflammation is generally a stable condition without significant clinical problems. In contrast, NASH is a condition in which there is hepatocyte injury that may progress to cirrhosis in 10% to 20% of cases. The main components of NASH are hepatocyte ballooning, lobular inflammation, and steatosis.[44] With progressive disease fibrosis occurs. NASH affects men and women equally and the condition is strongly associated with obesity and the other components of the metabolic syndrome, such as dyslipidemia, hyperinsulinemia and insulin resistance. It is estimated that more than 70% of obese individuals have some form of NAFLD. It is the most common cause of so-called cryptogenic cirrhosis, namely cirrhosis of "unknown" origin. NAFLD contributes to the progression of other liver diseases such as HCV infection and HCC. The epidemic of obesity in the United States heightens concern that NAFLD will increase in prevalence.

Pathogenesis. The precise mechanisms of steatosis and hepatocellular damage in NAFLD are not entirely known, but genetics and environment play a role in the pathogenesis.[44] A "two-hit" model of pathogenesis has been proposed, encompassing two sequential events: (1) hepatic fat accumulation and, (2) hepatic oxidative stress.[45] The oxidative stress acts upon the accumulated hepatic lipids, resulting in lipid peroxidation and the release of lipid peroxides, which can produce reactive oxygen species.

Clinical Features. Individuals with simple steatosis are generally asymptomatic. Clinical presentation is often related to other metabolic derangements, such as obesity, insulin resistance, and diabetes.[46] Imaging studies may reveal fat accumulation in the liver. However, liver biopsy is the most reliable diagnostic tool for NASH and helps determine the extent of steatosis, presence of steatohepatitis, and degree of fibrosis. Serum AST and ALT are elevated in about 90% of patients with NASH. The AST/ALT ratio is usually less than 1, in contrast to alcoholic steatohepatitis in which the ratio is generally above 2.0 to 2.5. Despite the enzyme elevations, patients may be asymptomatic. Others have general symptoms such as fatigue and right-sided abdominal discomfort caused by hepatomegaly. Because of the association between NASH and the metabolic syndrome, cardiovascular disease is a frequent cause of death in patients with NASH. The goal of treating individuals with NASH is to reverse the steatosis and prevent cirrhosis. The current management strategy seeks to correct the underlying risk factors, such as obesity and hyperlipidemia, and to treat insulin resistance.

Morphology. Steatosis usually involves more than 5% of the hepatocytes and sometimes more than 90%. Large (macrovesicular) and small (microvesicular) droplets of fat, predominantly triglycerides, accumulate within hepatocytes (Fig. 18–25A). At the most

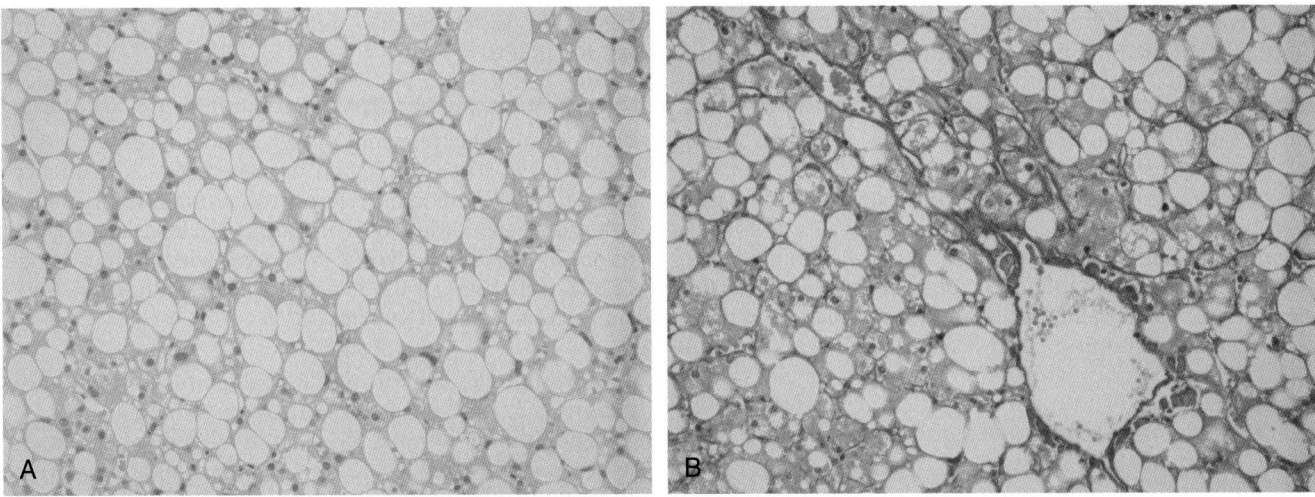

FIGURE 18–25 Histologic appearance of nonalcoholic fatty liver disease. **A,** Liver tissue with macrovesicular steatosis (H&E stain). **B,** NASH, showing perivenular fibrosis and perisinusoidal fibrosis *(blue fibers)* in this trichrome stain.

clinically benign end of the spectrum, there is no appreciable hepatic inflammation, hepatocyte death, or scarring, despite persistent elevation of serum liver enzymes. **Steatohepatitis** (NASH) is characterized by steatosis and multifocal parenchymal inflammation, mainly neutrophils, Mallory bodies, hepatocyte death (both ballooning degeneration and apoptosis), and sinusoidal fibrosis. Fibrosis also occurs within portal tracts and around terminal hepatic venules (Fig. 18–25B). These histological changes are similar to those of alcoholic steatohepatitis. **Cirrhosis** may develop, presumably the result of years of subclinical progression of the necroinflammatory and fibrotic processes. When cirrhosis is established, the steatosis or steatohepatitis tends to be reduced and sometimes is not identifiable.

HEMOCHROMATOSIS

Hemochromatosis was first described by von Recklinghausen in 1889. It is characterized by the excessive accumulation of body iron, most of which is deposited in parenchymal organs such as the liver and pancreas. Iron can also accumulate in the heart, joints, or endocrine organs. Hemochromatosis (also known as primary or hereditary hemochromatosis) is a homozygous-recessive inherited disorder[47] that is caused by excessive iron absorption. Accumulation of iron in tissues, which may occur as a consequence of parenteral administration of iron, usually in the form of transfusions, or other causes (Table 18–6), is variably known as secondary hemochromatosis, acquired hemochromatosis, or *hemosiderosis*. We will use the terms *hemochromatosis* for the hereditary disease and *hemosiderosis* for the acquired deposition of iron in some tissues.

As was discussed in Chapter 14, the total body iron pool ranges from 2 to 6 gm in normal adults; about 0.5 gm is stored in the liver, 98% of which is in hepatocytes. In hemochromatosis, total iron accumulation may exceed 50 gm, over one third of which accumulates in the liver. The following features characterize this disease:

- Fully developed cases exhibit (1) *micronodular cirrhosis* in all patients; (2) *diabetes mellitus* in 75% to 80% of patients; and (3) *skin pigmentation* in 75% to 80% of patients.
- Iron accumulation is lifelong but the injury caused by excessive iron is slow and progressive; hence symptoms usually first appear in the fifth to sixth decades of life.
- Males predominate (5 to 7:1) with slightly earlier clinical presentation, partly because physiologic iron loss (menstruation, pregnancy) delays iron accumulation in women.

TABLE 18–6 Classification of Iron Overload
I. HEREDITARY HEMOCHROMATOSIS
Mutations of genes encoding HFE, transferrin receptor 2 (TfR2), or hepcidin
Mutations of genes encoding HJV (hemojuvelin: juvenile hemochromatosis)
(Neonatal hemochromatosis)*
II. HEMOSIDEROSIS (SECONDARY HEMOCHROMATOSIS)

A. Parenteral iron overload
     Transfusions
     Long-term hemodialysis
     Aplastic anemia
     Sickle cell disease
     Myelodysplastic syndromes
     Leukemias
     Iron-dextran injections

B. Ineffective erythropoiesis with increased erythroid activity
     β-Thalassemia
     Sideroblastic anemia
     Pyruvate kinase deficiency

C. Increased oral intake of iron   African iron overload (Bantu siderosis)
D. Congenital atransferrinemia

E. Chronic liver disease
     Chronic alcoholic liver disease
     Porphyria cutanea tarda

F. Neonatal hemochromatosis

*Neonatal hemochromatosis develops in utero and does not appear to be a hereditary condition.

Pathogenesis. Because there is no regulated iron excretion from the body, the total body content of iron is tightly regulated by intestinal absorption as described below. *In hemochromatosis, regulation of intestinal absorption of dietary iron is abnormal, leading to net iron accumulation of 0.5 to 1.0 gm/ year, mainly in the liver.* The disease manifests itself typically after 20 gm of stored iron have accumulated. *Excessive iron appears to be directly toxic to host tissues,* by the following mechanisms: (1) lipid peroxidation via iron-catalyzed free radical reactions, (2) stimulation of collagen formation by activation of hepatic stellate cells, and (3) interaction of reactive oxygen species and of iron itself with DNA, leading to lethal cell injury or predisposition to hepatocellular carcinoma. The actions of iron are reversible in cells that are not fatally injured, and removal of excess iron with therapy promotes recovery of tissue function.

The main regulator of iron absorption is the protein hepcidin (also known as liver expressed antimicrobial peptide or LEAP1), encoded by the *HAMP* gene. Hepcidin, which also has antibacterial activity, is produced in hepatocytes as an 84 amino acid propeptide that is cleaved into a mature form of 25 amino acids and smaller circulating forms of 20 and 23 amino acids. *Transcription of hepcidin is increased by inflammatory cytokines and iron, and decreased by iron deficiency, hypoxia and ineffective erythropoiesis.* Hepcidin binds to the cellular iron efflux channel ferroportin (FPN), causing internalization and proteolysis of the channel. This prevents the release of iron from intestinal cells and macrophages; *thus hepcidin lowers plasma iron levels. Conversely, a deficiency in hepcidin causes iron overload.*

Other proteins involved in iron metabolism, do so by regulating hepcidin levels. These include: (1) hemojuvelin (HJV), which is expressed in the liver, heart, and skeletal muscle; (2) transferrin receptor 2 (TfR2), which is highly expressed in hepatocytes, where it mediates the uptake of transferrin-bound iron, and (3) HFE, the product of the hemochromatosis gene. *Lack of hepcidin expression caused by mutations in hepcidin, HJV, TfR2, and HFE cause hemochromatosis.* Of these mutations, those in HFE are the most common, as discussed below. Mutations of *HAMP* and *HJV* cause a severe form of hereditary hemochromatosis, known as juvenile hemochromatosis. Mutations of *HFE* and *TfR2* cause the classic form of hereditary adult hemochromatosis, a milder disease than the juvenile form. Mutations of ferroportin cause a distinctive iron storage disease that is different from hereditary hemochromatosis. The precise mechanisms by which HFE, HJV, and TfR2 regulate hepcidin and ferroportin remain to be determined. A serine protease (TMPRSS6) was recently identified as an iron sensor that suppresses *HAMP expression.*[48]

The adult form of hemochromatosis is almost always caused by mutations of HFE, a gene located on the short arm of chromosome 6 at 6p21.3, close to the *HLA* gene locus. It encodes an HLA class I-like molecule that regulates intestinal absorption of dietary iron. The most common *HFE* mutation is a cysteine-to-tyrosine substitution at amino acid 282 (called C282Y), due to a single G to A transition at nucleotide 845 (G845A). This mutation, which causes inactivation of the protein, is present in 70% to 100% of the patients diagnosed with hereditary hemochromatosis. The other common mutation is H63D (histidine at position 63 to aspartate). The H63D homozygous state and C282Y/H63D compound heterozygous mutations often cause only mild iron accumulation.

The C282Y mutation is largely confined to white populations of European origin, while the H63D has a worldwide distribution. The frequency of C282Y homozygosity is 0.45% (1 of every 220 persons), and the heterozygous frequency is 11%, making hereditary hemochromatosis one of the most common genetic disorders in humans. However, the penetrance of this disorder is low in patients with the homozygous C282Y mutation, so the genetic condition does not lead to clinical disease in all individuals.

Morphology. The morphologic changes in hereditary hemochromatosis are characterized principally by: (1) **deposition of hemosiderin** in the following organs (in decreasing order of severity): liver, pancreas, myocardium, pituitary gland, adrenal gland, thyroid and parathyroid glands, joints, and skin (detected by the Prussian blue histologic reaction or by atomic absorption analysis of tissue); (2) **cirrhosis**; and (3) **pancreatic fibrosis**. In the liver, iron becomes evident first as golden-yellow hemosiderin granules in the cytoplasm of periportal hepatocytes, which stain blue with the Prussian blue stain (Fig. 18–26). With increasing iron load, there is progressive involvement of the rest of the lobule, along with bile duct epithelium and Kupffer cell pigmentation. Iron is a direct hepatotoxin, and inflammation is characteristically absent. At this stage, the liver is typically slightly larger than normal, dense, and chocolate brown. Fibrous septa develop slowly, leading ultimately to a micronodular pattern of cirrhosis in an intensely pigmented liver.

Biochemical determination of hepatic tissue iron concentration is the standard for quantitating hepatic iron content. In normal individuals, the iron content of liver tissue is less than 1000 μg per gram dry weight of liver. Adult patients with hereditary hemochromatosis exhibit over 10,000 μg iron per gram dry weight; hepatic iron concentrations in excess of 22,000 μg per gram dry weight are associated with the development of fibrosis and cirrhosis.

The **pancreas** becomes intensely pigmented, has diffuse interstitial fibrosis, and may exhibit some parenchymal atrophy. Hemosiderin is found in both the acinar and the islet cells, and sometimes in the interstitial fibrous stroma. The **heart** is often enlarged and has hemosiderin granules within the myocardial fibers, producing a striking brown coloration to the myocardium. A delicate interstitial fibrosis may appear. Although **skin** pigmentation is partially attributable to hemosiderin deposition in dermal macrophages and fibroblasts, most of the pigmentation results from increased epidermal melanin production. The combination of these pigments imparts a characteristic slate-gray color to the skin. With hemosiderin deposition in the **joint synovial linings**, an acute synovitis may develop. Excessive deposition of calcium pyrophosphate damages the articular cartilage, producing a disabling polyarthritis referred to as **pseudo-gout**. The **testes** may be small and atrophic but are not usually significantly pigmented. It is

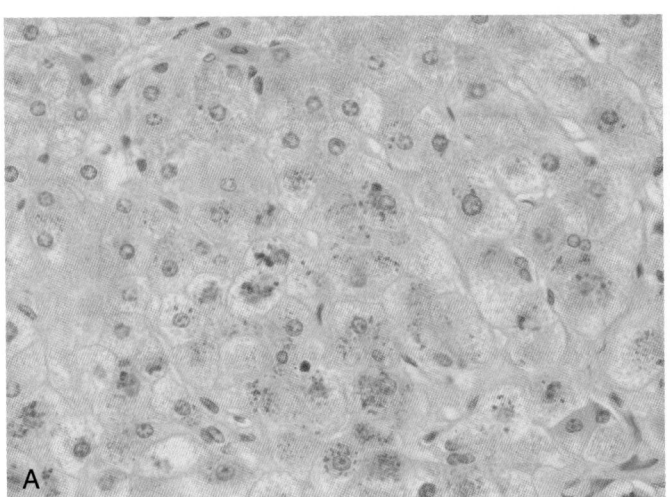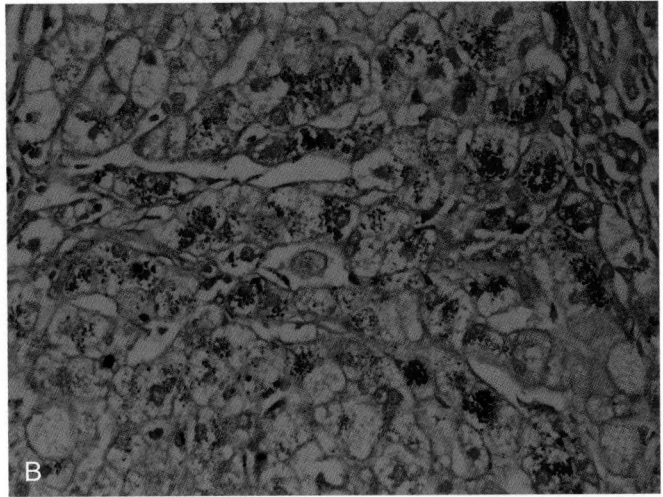

FIGURE 18-26   Histologic appearance of hereditary hemochromatosis. Hepatocellular iron deposition is dark-brown in H&E stain (**A**) and blue in Prussian blue–stained section (**B**). This is a section from an early stage of the disease, in which parenchymal architecture is normal.

thought that the atrophy is secondary to a derangement in the hypothalamic-pituitary axis resulting in reduced gonadotropin and testosterone levels.

Clinical Features. Classical hemochromatosis is more often a disease of males and rarely becomes evident before age 40. The principal manifestations include hepatomegaly, abdominal pain, skin pigmentation (particularly in sun-exposed areas), deranged glucose homeostasis or frank diabetes mellitus due to destruction of pancreatic islets, cardiac dysfunction (arrhythmias, cardiomyopathy), and atypical arthritis. In some patients, the presenting complaint is hypogonadism (e.g., amenorrhea in the female, impotence and loss of libido in the male). *The classic triad of pigment cirrhosis with hepatomegaly, skin pigmentation, and diabetes mellitus might not develop until late in the course of the disease.* Death may result from cirrhosis or cardiac disease. A significant cause of death is hepatocellular carcinoma; the risk is 200-fold greater than in the general population, and treatment for iron overload does not remove the risk for this tumor.

Fortunately, hemochromatosis can be diagnosed long before irreversible tissue damage has occurred. Screening involves demonstration of very high levels of serum iron and ferritin, exclusion of secondary causes of iron overload, and liver biopsy if indicated. *Screening of family members of probands is important.* Heterozygotes also accumulate excessive iron, but not to a level that causes significant tissue damage. Currently most patients with hemochromatosis are diagnosed in the subclinical, precirrhotic stage due to routine serum iron measurements (as part of other diagnostic workup). They are treated by regular phlebotomy and have a normal life expectancy.

Neonatal hemochromatosis (also called congenital hemochromatosis) is a disease of unknown origin manifested by severe liver disease and extrahepatic hemosiderin deposition.[49] Neonatal hemochromatosis is not an inherited disease; liver injury, leading to hemosiderin accumulation, occurs in utero, and might be related to maternal alloimmune injury to the fetal liver. Extrahepatic hemosiderin deposition, detected by

buccal biopsy, needs to be documented for the correct diagnosis. There is no specific treatment, except for supportive care, and liver transplantation in severe cases.

The most common causes of *hemosiderosis* (secondary or acquired hemochromatosis) are disorders associated with ineffective erythropoiesis, such as severe forms of thalassemia (Chapter 14) and myelodysplastic syndromes (Chapter 13). In these disorders, the excess iron results not only from transfusions, but also from increased absorption. Transfusions alone, when given repeatedly over a period of years (such as in patients with chronic hemolytic anemias), can also lead to systemic hemosiderosis and parenchymal organ injury. *Alcoholic cirrhosis* is often associated with a modest increase in stainable iron within liver cells. However, this represents alcohol-induced redistribution of iron, since total body iron is not significantly increased. A rather unusual form of iron overload resembling hereditary hemochromatosis occurs in sub-Saharan Africa, the result of ingesting large quantities of alcoholic beverages fermented in iron utensils (Bantu siderosis). Home brewing in steel drums continues to this day, and genetic susceptibility to this disease, such as mutations of ferroportin has been proposed in these populations.[50] Lastly, chronic HBV and HCV infection may increase iron storage within hepatocytes.

WILSON DISEASE

Wilson disease is an autosomal recessive disorder caused by mutation of the *ATP7B* gene, resulting in impaired copper excretion into bile and a failure to incorporate copper into *ceruloplasmin*.[51] This disorder is marked by *the accumulation of toxic levels of copper in many tissues and organs, principally the liver, brain, and eye.* Normally, 40% to 60% of ingested copper (2 to 5 mg/day) is absorbed in the duodenum and proximal small intestine, and is transported to the portal circulation complexed with albumin and histidine. Free copper dissociates and is taken up by hepatocytes. Copper is incorporated into enzymes and also binds to a α_2-globulin (apoceruloplasmin) to form ceruloplasmin, which is secreted into the blood. Excess copper is transported into the bile.

Ceruloplasmin accounts for 90% to 95% of plasma copper. Circulating ceruloplasmin is eventually desialylated, endocytosed by the liver, and degraded within lysosomes, after which the released copper is excreted into bile. This degradation/excretion pathway is the primary route for copper elimination. The estimated total body copper is only 50 to 150 mg.

The *ATP7B* gene, located on chromosome 13, encodes a transmembrane copper-transporting ATPase, expressed on the hepatocyte canalicular membrane. More than 300 mutations in the *ATP7B* gene have been identified, but not all genes cause the disease. *The overwhelming majority of patients are compound heterozygotes containing different mutations on each ATP7B allele.* The overall frequency of mutated alleles is 1 : 100, and the prevalence of the disease of approximately 1 : 30,000 to 1 : 50,000 (approximately 9000 patients in the United States). *Deficiency in the ATP7B protein causes a decrease in copper transport into bile, impairs its incorporation into ceruloplasmin, and inhibits ceruloplasmin secretion into the blood.* These changes cause copper accumulation in the liver and a decrease in circulating ceruloplasmin. The copper causes toxic liver injury, through the production of ROS by the Fenton reaction (Chapter 1). Although there is a latent period of variable duration for the disease, once the hepatic capacity for incorporating copper into ceruloplasmin is exceeded, there may be sudden onset of critical systemic illness. Specifically, non-ceruloplasmin–bound copper spills over from the liver into the circulation, causing hemolysis and pathologic changes at other sites such as the brain, corneas, kidneys, bones, joints, and parathyroids. Concomitantly, urinary excretion of copper markedly increases from its normal minuscule levels.

Morphology. The liver often bears the brunt of injury, but the disease may also present as a neurologic disorder. The hepatic changes are variable, ranging from relatively minor to massive damage. **Fatty change (steatosis)** may be mild to moderate, with vacuolated nuclei (glycogen or water) and occasionally, focal hepatocyte necrosis. An **acute hepatitis** can show features mimicking acute viral hepatitis, except possibly for the accompanying fatty change. The **chronic hepatitis** of Wilson disease exhibits moderate to severe inflammation and hepatocyte necrosis, with the particular features of macrovesicular steatosis, vacuolated hepatocellular nuclei, and Mallory bodies. With progression of chronic hepatitis, **cirrhosis** will develop. **Massive liver necrosis** is a rare manifestation that is indistinguishable from that caused by viruses or drugs. Excess copper deposition can often be demonstrated by special stains (rhodamine stain for copper, orcein stain for copper-associated protein). Because copper also accumulates in chronic obstructive cholestasis and because histology cannot reliably distinguish Wilson disease from viral- and drug-induced hepatitis, demonstration of hepatic copper content in excess of 250 μg per gram dry weight is most helpful for making a diagnosis.

In the **brain**, toxic injury primarily affects the basal ganglia, particularly the putamen, which shows atrophy and even cavitation. Nearly all patients with neurologic involvement develop **eye lesions** called

Kayser-Fleischer rings, green to brown deposits of copper in Descemet's membrane in the limbus of the cornea.

Clinical Features. The age at onset and the clinical presentation of Wilson disease are extremely variable (average age is 11.4 years), but the disorder usually manifests in affected individuals between 6 and 40 years of age. The most common presentation is *acute or chronic liver disease.* Neuropsychiatric manifestations, including mild behavioral changes, frank psychosis, or a *Parkinson disease–like syndrome* (such as tremor), are the initial features in most of the remaining cases. The biochemical diagnosis of Wilson disease is based on *a decrease in serum ceruloplasmin, an increase in hepatic copper content (the most sensitive and accurate test), and increased urinary excretion of copper (the most specific screening test).* Serum copper levels are of no diagnostic value, since they may be low, normal, or elevated, depending on the stage of evolution of the disease. Demonstration of Kayser-Fleischer rings further favors the diagnosis. Early recognition and long-term copper chelation therapy (as with D-penicillamine, or Trientine) or zinc-based therapy has dramatically altered the usual progressive downhill course. Individuals with hepatitis or unmanageable cirrhosis require liver transplantation for survival, which can also lead to eventual cure.

α₁-ANTITRYPSIN DEFICIENCY

α_1-Antitrypsin deficiency is an autosomal recessive disorder marked by very low levels of α_1-antitrypsin. The major function of this protein is the inhibition of proteases, particularly neutrophil elastase, cathepsin G, and proteinase 3, which are normally released from neutrophils at sites of inflammation. α_1-Antitrypsin deficiency leads to the development of pulmonary emphysema, because the activity of destructive proteases is not inhibited (discussed in Chapter 15). It also causes liver disease, as a consequence of the accumulation of this protein in hepatocytes.[52] In addition, cutaneous panniculitis, arterial aneurysm, bronchiectasis, and Wegener's granulomatosis can occur in α_1-antitrypsin deficiency.

α_1-Antitrypsin is a small 394–amino acid plasma glycoprotein synthesized predominantly by hepatocytes. It is a member of the serine protease inhibitor (serpin) family. The gene, located on chromosome 14, is very polymorphic, and at least 75 α_1-antitrypsin forms have been identified, denoted alphabetically by their relative migration on an isoelectric gel. The general notation is "Pi" for "protease inhibitor" and an alphabetic letter for the position on the gel; two letters denote the genotype of the two alleles. The most common genotype is PiMM, occurring in 90% of individuals (in the traditional sense, this would be the wild-type genotype). Most allelic variants show substitutions in the polypeptide chain but produce normal levels of functional α_1-antitrypsin. Some *deficiency variants*, including the PiS variant, result in a moderate reduction in serum concentrations of α_1-antitrypsin without clinical manifestations. Rare variants termed *Pi-null* have no detectable serum α_1-antitrypsin. The most common clinically significant mutation is PiZ; homozygotes for the PiZZ protein have circulating α_1-antitrypsin levels that are only 10% of

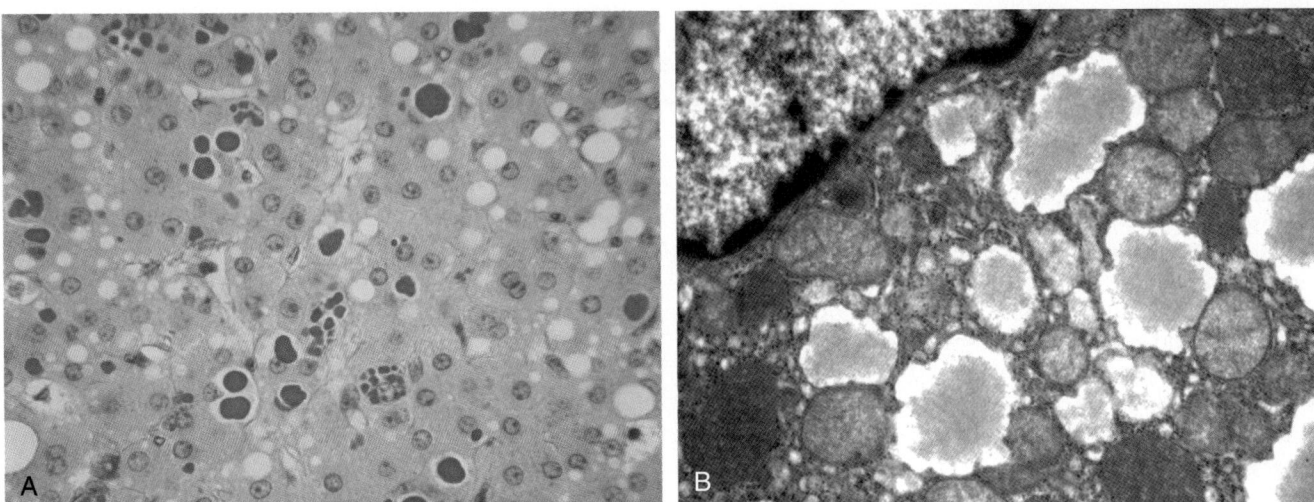

FIGURE 18–27 α_1-Antitrypsin deficiency. **A,** Periodic acid–Schiff (PAS) stain of the liver, highlighting the characteristic red cytoplasmic granules. **B,** Electron micrograph showing the dilatation of the endoplasmic reticulum.

normal. These individuals are at high risk for developing clinical disease. Expression of alleles is autosomal codominant, and consequently, PiMZ heterozygotes have intermediate plasma levels of α_1-antitrypsin. Among people of northern European descent the PiS frequency is 6% and the PiZ frequency is 4%; the PiZZ state affects 1 in 1800 live births. Because of its occasionally early presentation for liver disease, α_1-antitrypsin deficiency is the most commonly diagnosed genetic hepatic disorder in infants and children.

Pathogenesis. With most allelic variants, the mRNA is transcribed, and the protein is synthesized and secreted normally. Deficiency variants show a selective defect in migration of this secretory protein from the endoplasmic reticulum to Golgi apparatus; this is most marked for the PiZ polypeptide, attributable to a single amino acid substitution of Glu342 to Lys342. *The mutant polypeptide (α_1AT-Z) is abnormally folded and polymerizes,* creating endoplasmic reticulum stress and leading to apoptosis (Chapter 1; see Fig. 1–27). The precise mechanisms of liver disease with α_1AT-Z are not well defined. The accumulated α_1AT-Z in the endoplasmic reticulum triggers a series of events, including an autophagocytic response, mitochondrial dysfunction, and possible activation of proinflammatory NF-κB, causing hepatocyte damage.[53] All individuals with the PiZZ genotype accumulate α_1AT-Z in the endoplasmic reticulum of hepatocytes, but only 10% to 15% of PiZZ individuals develop overt clinical liver disease. Other genetic factors or environmental factors are thus posited to play a role in the development of liver disease.

Morphology. α_1-Antitrypsin deficiency is characterized by the presence of round-to-oval cytoplasmic globular inclusions in hepatocytes, which in routine H&E stains are acidophilic and indistinctly demarcated from the surrounding cytoplasm. They are strongly periodic acid–Schiff (PAS)-positive and diastase-resistant (Fig. 18–27). The globules are also present but in diminished size and number in the PiMZ and PiSZ genotypes. For unknown reasons

most of the globules are in hepatocytes surrounding the portal tracts. Moreover, the number of globule-containing hepatocytes in a patient's liver is not correlated with the severity of pathologic findings. The hepatic pathology associated with PiZZ homozygosity is extremely varied, ranging from neonatal hepatitis (Fig. 18–28) without or with cholestasis and fibrosis (discussed below), to childhood cirrhosis, to a smoldering chronic inflammatory hepatitis or cirrhosis that becomes apparent only late in life. For the most part the only distinctive feature of the hepatic disease is the PAS-positive globules; infrequently, fatty change and Mallory bodies are present. The diagnostic α_1-antitrypsin globules may be absent in the young infant; steatosis may be present as a tip-off to the possibility of α_1-antitrypsin deficiency.

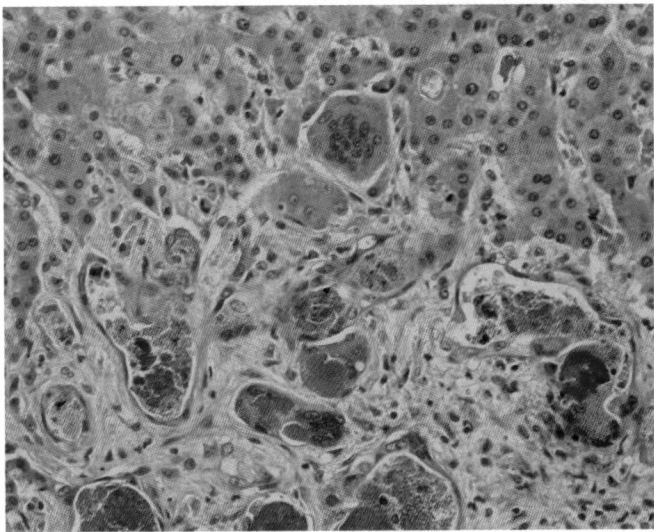

FIGURE 18–28 Neonatal hepatitis caused by α_1-antitrypsin deficiency. Note the severe cholestasis.

Clinical Features. Neonatal hepatitis with cholestatic jaundice appears in 10% to 20% of newborns with the deficiency. In adolescence, presenting symptoms may be related to hepatitis or cirrhosis. Attacks of hepatitis may subside with apparent complete recovery, or they may become chronic and lead progressively to cirrhosis. Finally, the disease may remain silent until cirrhosis appears in middle to later life. HCC develops in 2% to 3% of PiZZ adults, usually but not always in the setting of cirrhosis. The treatment, and the cure, for severe hepatic disease is orthotopic liver transplantation. In patients with pulmonary disease the single most important treatment is avoidance of cigarette smoking, because smoking markedly accelerates emphysema and the destructive lung disease associated with α_1-antitrypsin deficiency.

NEONATAL CHOLESTASIS

Prolonged conjugated hyperbilirubinemia in the neonate, termed *neonatal cholestasis*, affects approximately 1 in 2500 live births. The major conditions causing it are (1) cholangiopathies, primarily *biliary atresia* (discussed later), and (2) a variety of disorders causing conjugated hyperbilirubinemia in the neonate, collectively referred to as *neonatal hepatitis*. *Neonatal cholestasis and hepatitis are not specific entities, nor are the disorders necessarily inflammatory.* Instead, the finding of "neonatal cholestasis" should evoke a diligent search for recognizable toxic, metabolic, and infectious liver diseases, the more common of which are listed in Table 18–7. Once identifiable causes have been excluded, one is left with the syndrome of "idiopathic" neonatal hepatitis, which shows considerable clinical overlap with biliary atresia. Despite the long list of disorders associated with neonatal cholestasis, most are quite rare. "Idiopathic" neonatal hepatitis represents as many as 50% of cases, biliary atresia represents another 20%, and α_1-antitrypsin deficiency represents 15%. Differentiation of biliary atresia from nonobstructive neonatal cho-

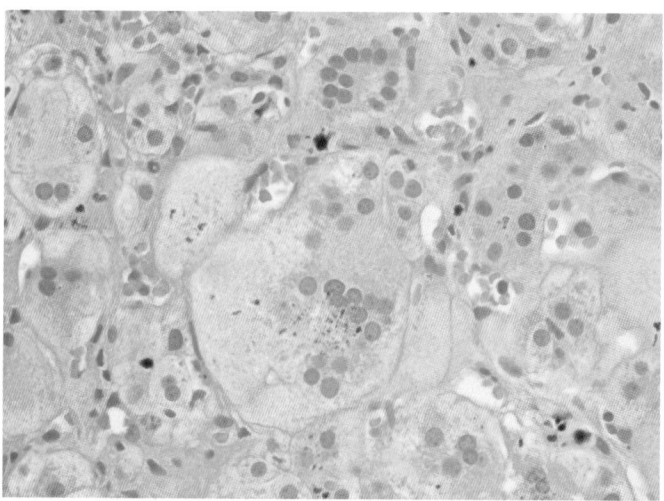

FIGURE 18–29   Neonatal hepatitis. Note the multinucleated giant hepatocytes.

lestasis assumes great importance, since definitive treatment of biliary atresia requires surgical intervention (Kasai procedure), whereas surgery may adversely affect the clinical course of a child with other disorders. Fortunately, discrimination can be made with clinical data in about 90% of cases, with or without liver biopsy. Affected infants have jaundice, dark urine, light or acholic stools, and hepatomegaly. Variable degrees of hepatic synthetic dysfunction may be identified, such as hypoprothrombinemia. Thus, liver biopsy is critical in distinguishing neonatal hepatitis from an identifiable cholangiopathy.

> **Morphology.** The morphologic features of neonatal hepatitis include lobular disarray with focal liver cell apoptosis and necrosis, panlobular giant-cell transformation of hepatocytes (Fig. 18–29), prominent hepatocellular and canalicular cholestasis, mild mononuclear infiltration of the portal areas, reactive changes in Kupffer cells, and extramedullary hematopoiesis. This predominantly parenchymal pattern of injury may blend imperceptibly into a ductal pattern of injury, with bile ductular proliferation and fibrosis of portal tracts. In these cases distinction from an obstructive biliary atresia may therefore be difficult.

Intrahepatic Biliary Tract Disease

In this section we discuss three disorders of intrahepatic bile ducts: *secondary biliary cirrhosis, primary biliary cirrhosis,* and *primary sclerosing cholangitis* (summarized in Table 18–8). Secondary biliary cirrhosis is a condition resulting most often from uncorrected obstruction of the extrahepatic biliary tree. Primary biliary cirrhosis is a destructive disorder of the intrahepatic biliary tree. Primary sclerosing cholangitis involves both the extrahepatic and intrahepatic biliary tree. It should also be noted that intrahepatic bile ducts are frequently damaged as part of more general liver diseases as in drug toxicity, viral hepatitis, liver transplantation, and graft-versus-host disease after bone marrow transplantation.

TABLE 18–7 Major Causes of Neonatal Cholestasis
Bile duct obstruction   Extrahepatic biliary atresia

Neonatal infection
   Cytomegalovirus
   Bacterial sepsis
   Urinary tract infection
   Syphilis

Toxic
   Drugs
   Parenteral nutrition

Metabolic disease
   Tyrosinemia
   Niemann-Pick disease
   Galactosemia
   Defective bile acid synthetic pathways
   α_1-Antitrypsin deficiency
   Cystic fibrosis

Miscellaneous
   Shock/hypoperfusion
   Indian childhood cirrhosis
   Alagille syndrome (paucity of bile ducts)

Idiopathic neonatal hepatitis

TABLE 18–8 Distinguishing Features of the Major Intrahepatic Bile Duct Disorders

	Secondary Biliary Cirrhosis	Primary Biliary Cirrhosis	Primary Sclerosing Cholangitis
Etiology	Extrahepatic bile duct obstruction: biliary atresia, gallstones, stricture, carcinoma of pancreatic head	Possibly autoimmune	Unknown, possibly autoimmune; 50% to 70% associated with inflammatory bowel disease
Sex predilection	None	Female to male, 6:1	Female to male, 1:2
Symptoms and signs	Pruritus, jaundice, malaise, dark urine, light stools, hepatosplenomegaly	Same as secondary biliary cirrhosis; insidious onset	Same as secondary biliary cirrhosis; insidious onset
Laboratory findings	Conjugated hyperbilirubinemia, increased serum alkaline phosphatase, bile acids, cholesterol	Same as secondary biliary cirrhosis, plus elevated serum IgM autoantibodies (especially M2 form of anti-mitochondrial antibody)	Same as secondary biliary cirrhosis, plus elevated serum IgM, hypergammaglobulinemia
Important pathologic findings before cirrhosis develops	Prominent bile stasis in bile ducts, bile ductular proliferation with surrounding neutrophils, portal tract edema	Dense lymphocytic infiltrate in portal tracts with granulomatous destruction of bile ducts	Periductal portal tracts fibrosis, segmental stenosis of extrahepatic and intrahepatic bile ducts

SECONDARY BILIARY CIRRHOSIS

Prolonged obstruction of the extrahepatic biliary tree results in profound hepatic alterations. The most common cause of obstruction in adults is *extrahepatic cholelithiasis* (gallstones, described later), followed by *malignancies* of the biliary tree or head of the pancreas, and strictures resulting from previous *surgical procedures*. Obstructive conditions in children include biliary atresia, cystic fibrosis, choledochal cysts (a cystic anomaly of the extrahepatic biliary tree, discussed later), and syndromes in which there are insufficient intrahepatic bile ducts (paucity of bile duct syndromes). The initial morphologic features of *cholestasis* were described earlier and are entirely reversible with correction of the obstruction. However, secondary inflammation resulting from biliary obstruction initiates periportal fibrosis, which eventually leads to hepatic scarring and nodule formation, generating secondary biliary cirrhosis. Subtotal obstruction may promote secondary bacterial infection of the biliary tree *(ascending cholangitis)*, which aggravates the inflammatory injury. Enteric organisms such as coliforms and enterococci are common culprits.

Morphology. The end-stage obstructed liver shows yellow-green pigmentation that is accompanied by marked icteric discoloration of body tissues and fluids. On cut surface the liver is hard, with a finely granular appearance (Fig. 18–30). The histology is characterized by coarse fibrous septa that subdivide the liver in a jigsaw-like pattern. Embedded in the septa are distended small and large bile ducts, which frequently contain inspissated pigmented material. There is extensive **proliferation of smaller bile ductules**, particularly at the interface between septa in former portal tracts and the parenchyma. Cholestatic features in the parenchyma may be severe, with extensive **feathery degeneration** and formation of **bile lakes**. However, once regenerative nodules have formed, bile stasis may become less conspicuous. Ascending bacterial infection incites a robust neutrophilic infiltration of bile ducts; severe pylephlebitis and cholangitic abscesses may develop.

PRIMARY BILIARY CIRRHOSIS (PBC)

PBC is an inflammatory autoimmune disease mainly affecting the intrahepatic bile ducts. *The primary feature of this disease is a nonsuppurative, inflammatory destruction of medium-sized intrahepatic bile ducts.* It is accompanied by portal inflammation, scarring, and eventual development of cirrhosis and liver failure.[54] Because cirrhosis develops only after many years, the

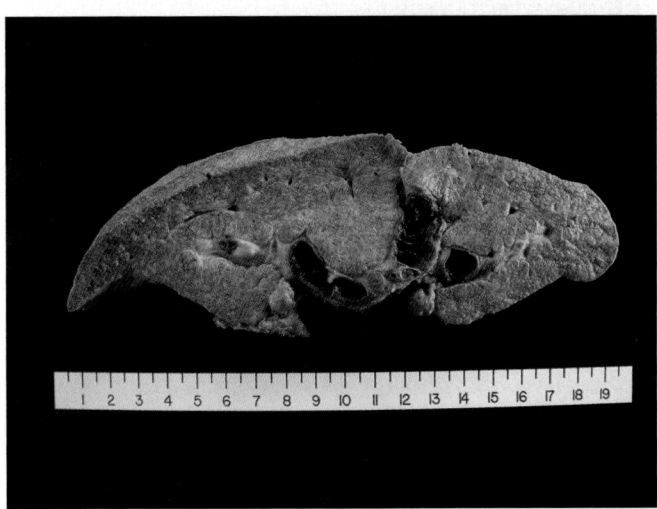

FIGURE 18–30 Biliary cirrhosis. Sagittal section through the liver demonstrates the fine nodularity and bile staining of end-stage biliary cirrhosis.

disease name is somewhat misleading for patients diagnosed early at a pre-cirrhotic stage.

This is primarily a disease of middle-aged women, with a female predominance over males in excess of 6:1. It may occur between the ages of 20 and 80 years, with peak incidence between 40 and 50 years of age. The incidence of this disease in the United States is approximately 27 per million people (7 and 45 per million in males and females, respectively). Both the incidence and prevalence of PBC are increasing and geographic clustering has been reported, suggesting that genetic and environmental factors are important in the pathogenesis of the disease. Family members of PBC patients have an increased risk of developing the disease. The onset is insidious, usually presenting with fatigue and pruritus. Hepatomegaly is a typical finding, and eyelid xanthelasmas arise as a result of infiltration of the nasal area of the eyelid by cholesterol-rich macrophages. Hyperpigmentation due to melanin deposition and an inflammatory arthropathy are seen in 25% to 40% of cases. Signs and symptoms of chronic liver disease, such as spider nevi, are late features. Over a period of two or more decades, patients develop cirrhosis and complications that include portal hypertension with variceal bleeding, and hepatic encephalopathy.

Serum *alkaline phosphatase and cholesterol are almost always elevated*, even at onset; hyperbilirubinemia is a late development and usually signifies incipient hepatic decompensation. *Antimitochondrial* antibodies are present in 90% to 95% of patients. They are highly characteristic of PBC and an essential element for diagnosis, together with the elevation of alkaline phosphatase and γ-glutamyltransferase, which are markers of cholestasis.

Pathogenesis. PBC is thought to be an autoimmune disorder, but its pathogenesis is still unknown. Many potential mechanisms have been proposed, including aberrant expression of MHC class II molecules on bile duct epithelial cells, accumulation of autoreactive T cells around bile ducts, reaction of antimitochondrial antibodies to hepatocytes, or of other antibodies against cellular components (nuclear pore proteins, and centromeric proteins, among others).[55] The antimitochondrial antibodies, the characteristic autoantibodies in PBC, target the E2 component of the pyrurate dehydrogenase complex (PDC-E2). PDC-E2–specific T cells are also present in these patients, supporting the notion of immune-mediated pathogenesis.[56]

Morphology. PBC is the prototype of conditions leading to **small-duct biliary fibrosis and cirrhosis**. PBC is a focal and variable disease, showing different degrees of severity in different portions of the liver. During the pre-cirrhotic stage portal tracts are **infiltrated by a dense accumulation of lymphocytes, macrophages, plasma cells, and occasional eosinophils**. Interlobular bile ducts are infiltrated by lymphocytes and may show noncaseating granulomatous inflammation (Fig. 18–31) and undergo progressive destruction. With time the obstruction to intrahepatic bile flow leads to progressive secondary hepatic damage. Portal tracts upstream from damaged bile ducts show bile ductular proliferation, inflammation,

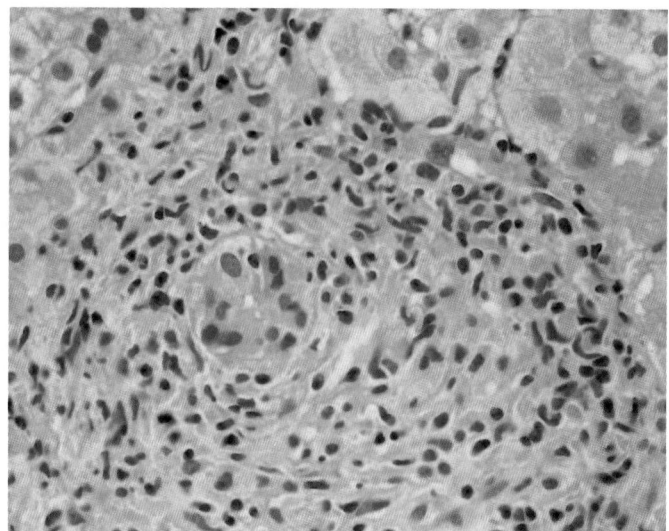

FIGURE 18–31   Primary biliary cirrhosis. A portal tract is markedly expanded by an infiltrate of lymphocytes and plasma cells. There is a granulomatous reaction to a bile duct undergoing destruction (florid duct lesion).

and necrosis of the adjacent periportal hepatic parenchyma. The parenchyma develops generalized cholestasis. Over years to decades, relentless portal tract scarring and bridging fibrosis lead to cirrhosis.

Macroscopically, the liver does not at first appear abnormal, but as the disease progresses bile stasis stains the liver green. The capsule remains smooth and glistening until a fine granularity appears, representing deposition of fibrous septa. This process culminates in a well-developed, uniform micronodular cirrhosis. Liver weight is at first normal to increased (because of inflammation) but is ultimately decreased. **In most cases the end-stage picture is indistinguishable from secondary biliary cirrhosis or the cirrhosis that follows chronic hepatitis from other causes.**

Clinical Features. The onset is extremely insidious, and patients may be symptom-free for many years. Eventually, *pruritus, fatigue,* and abdominal discomfort develop, followed in time by secondary features: skin pigmentation, xanthelasmas, steatorrhea, and vitamin D malabsorption–related osteomalacia and/or osteoporosis. More general features of jaundice and hepatic decompensation, including portal hypertension and variceal bleeding, mark entry into the end stages of the disease. PBC patients have an *increased risk to develop hepatocellular carcinomas.* The major cause of death is liver failure, followed in order by massive variceal hemorrhage and intercurrent infection. Individuals with PBC may also have extrahepatic manifestations of autoimmunity, including the sicca complex of dry eyes and mouth (Sjögren syndrome; from the Latin *sicca,* meaning dryness), systemic sclerosis, thyroiditis, rheumatoid arthritis, Raynaud phenomenon, membranous glomerulonephritis, and celiac disease. There is no specific therapy for PBC but treatment with ursodeoxycholic acid, if started early, can provide complete remission and prolong survival is 25% to 30% of cases. Its mechanism of action is not well understood. Liver transplantation is the best form of treatment for persons with end-stage liver disease.

PRIMARY SCLEROSING CHOLANGITIS (PSC)

PSC is characterized by inflammation and obliterative fibrosis of intrahepatic and extrahepatic bile ducts, with dilation of preserved segments. Characteristic "beading" of a contrast medium in radiographs of the intrahepatic and extrahepatic biliary tree is attributable to the irregular strictures and dilations of affected bile ducts. *PSC is commonly seen in association with inflammatory bowel disease* (see Chapter 17), particularly chronic ulcerative colitis, which coexists in approximately 70% of individuals with primary sclerosing cholangitis. Conversely, the prevalence of PSC in persons with ulcerative colitis is about 4%. PSC tends to occur in the third through fifth decades of life, and males predominate 2:1. (See Table 18–8 for comparisons with primary and secondary biliary cirrhosis.)

Pathogenesis. Primary sclerosing cholangitis is a chronic cholestatic disorder characterized by non-specific inflammation, fibrosis and strictures of intra- and extrahepatic bile ducts.[57] Several features of the disease suggest that it results from immunologically mediated injury to bile ducts. These include the detection of T cells in the periductal stroma, the presence of a plethora of circulating autoantibodies, and the association with ulcerative colitis. It has been proposed that T cells activated in the gut mucosa travel to the liver where they recognize a bile duct antigen that cross-reacts with gut antigens. Another proposed etiology is that the bile duct lesions are a consequence of cross-reaction of bile duct antigens with enteric bacteria or bacterial products. Antibodies commonly found in patients with primary sclerosing cholangitis include anti-smooth muscle antibodies, anti-nuclear antibodies (ANAs), rheumatoid factor, and an atypical p-ANCA which shows a perinuclear staining pattern but is directed against a nuclear envelope protein, instead of myeloperoxidase as is typical of p-ANCA antibodies. The atypical p-ANCA is found in up to 80% of patients, but its relationship with the pathogenesis of the disease is unknown. First degree relatives of patients with primary sclerosing cholangitis have an increased risk of developing the disease. As with many other immunologically mediated diseases, primary sclerosing cholangitis is associated with an increased prevalence of certain MHC class I and class II haplotypes.[58]

Morphology. PSC is a fibrosing cholangitis of bile ducts, with a lymphocytic infiltrate, progressive atrophy of the bile duct epithelium, and obliteration of the lumen (Fig. 18–32). The concentric periductal fibrosis around affected ducts ("onion-skin fibrosis") is followed by their disappearance, leaving behind a solid, cordlike fibrous scar. In between areas of progressive stricture, bile ducts become ectatic and inflamed, presumably the result of downstream obstruction. As the disease progresses the liver becomes markedly cholestatic, culminating in biliary cirrhosis much like that seen with primary and secondary biliary cirrhosis.

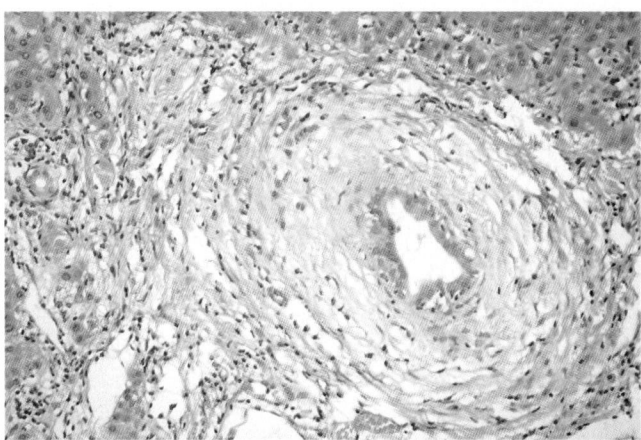

FIGURE 18–32 Primary sclerosing cholangitis. A bile duct undergoing degeneration is entrapped in a dense, "onion-skin" concentric scar.

Clinical Features. Asymptomatic patients may come to attention only because of persistent elevation of serum alkaline phosphatase. Alternatively, progressive fatigue, pruritus, and jaundice may develop. The disease follows a protracted course of 5 to 17 years, and the severely afflicted patients have the usual symptoms of chronic liver disease, including weight loss, ascites, variceal bleeding, and encephalopathy. Approximately 7% of individuals with PSC develop *cholangiocarcinoma*, a very high frequency relative to that of the general population. The incidence of *chronic pancreatitis* and *hepatocellular carcinoma* also seems to be increased in PSC patients. A distinctive type of sclerosing cholangitis, with elevated IgG4 and associated with autoimmune pancreatitis, has been recognized recently.[59] There is no specific medical therapy for PSC. Cholestyramine has been used for pruritus, and endoscopic dilation with sphincterotomy or stenting is used for relieving symptoms. *Liver transplantation* is the definitive treatment for persons with end-stage liver disease.

ANOMALIES OF THE BILIARY TREES (INCLUDING LIVER CYSTS)

A heterogeneous group of lesions exist in which the primary abnormality is altered architecture or paucity of the intrahepatic biliary tree. Lesions may be found incidentally during radiographic studies, surgery, or at autopsy. Such conditions may become manifest as hepatosplenomegaly and portal hypertension in the absence of hepatic dysfunction, starting in late childhood or adolescence. There are five distinct conditions: von Meyenburg complexes, polycystic liver disease, congenital hepatic fibrosis, Caroli disease, and Alagille syndrome.

Von Meyenburg Complexes. These are small clusters of modestly dilated bile ducts embedded in a fibrous, sometimes hyalinized, stroma located close to or within portal tracts. These lesions are often referred to as "bile duct hamartomas" (Fig. 18–33). Von Meyenburg complexes are common and without clinical significance except in the differential diagnosis of metastases to the liver.

Polycystic Liver Disease. In this disease there are multiple diffuse cystic lesions in the liver, varying in number from a

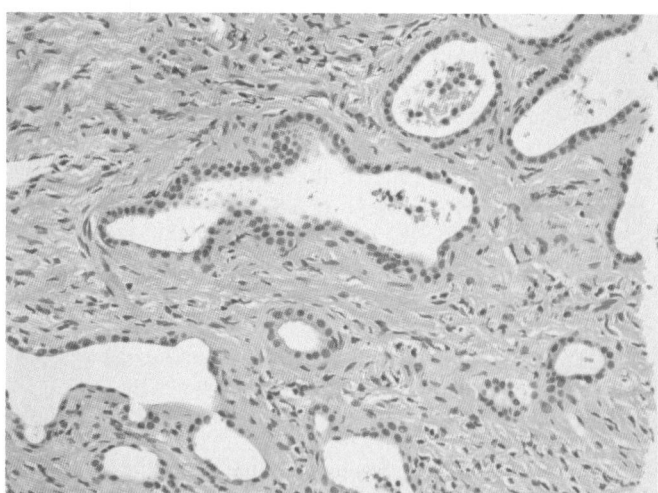

FIGURE 18–33 Bile duct hamartoma (von Meyenburg complexes). Note the dilated and irregularly shaped bile ducts.

scattered few to hundreds (Fig. 18–34). The cysts, lined by cuboidal or flattened biliary epithelium, contain straw-colored fluid.

Congenital Hepatic Fibrosis. In this condition portal tracts are enlarged by irregular, broad bands of collagenous tissue, forming septa that divide the liver into irregular islands. Variable numbers of abnormally shaped bile ducts are embedded in the fibrous tissue, and are in continuity with the biliary tree. This anomaly arises because of persistence of the embryonic form of the biliary tree, with ensuing portal tract fibrosis over the individual's lifetime. Although individuals with congenital hepatic fibrosis rarely develop cirrhosis, they may still face complications of portal hypertension, particularly bleeding varices.

Caroli Disease. In this disease the larger ducts of the intrahepatic biliary tree are segmentally dilated and may contain

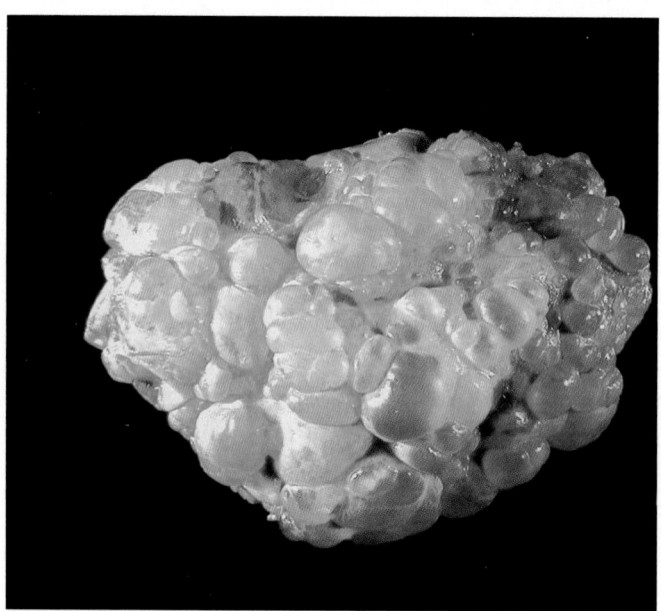

FIGURE 18–34 Polycystic liver disease.

inspissated bile. Pure forms are rare; this disease is usually associated with portal tract fibrosis of the congenital hepatic fibrosis type. The disease is frequently complicated by intrahepatic cholelithiasis (described later), cholangitis, hepatic abscesses, and portal hypertension. Persons with Caroli disease and congenital hepatic fibrosis have an increased risk of developing cholangiocarcinomas.

Each of the four conditions discussed above can be associated with polycystic kidney disease. Single or multiple liver cysts are the most frequent extrarenal manifestation of autosomal-dominant polycystic kidney disease caused by a mutation in *PKD1* (Chapter 20), and occur in 75% to 90% of patients with this type of kidney disease.[60] A form of polycystic liver disease caused by mutations of the *PRKCSH* gene (which encodes a protein kinase C substrate 80K-H) does not coexist with polycystic kidney disease.[61] Congenital hepatic fibrosis is strongly associated with the autosomal recessive form of polycystic kidney disease, which is caused by mutations of the *PKHD1* (polycystic kidney and hepatic disease) gene.[62] The exact pathogenesis of these biliary lesions and the basis of their association with polycystic kidney disorders remain unclear.

Alagille Syndrome (Syndromatic Paucity of Bile Ducts; Arteriohepatic Dysplasia). This is a rare autosomal dominant multi-organ disorder, in which *the liver pathology is characterized by absence of bile ducts in portal tracts.* The syndrome is caused by mutations or deletion of the gene encoding *Jagged1*, which is located on chromosome 20p. Jagged1 is a cell surface protein that functions as a ligand for Notch receptors (Chapter 3). Mutations in Jagged can be detected in as many as 94% of individuals with a clinical diagnosis of Alagille syndrome, and some of the remaining patients have mutations in the Notch 2 receptor.[63] The Jagged1-Notch signaling pathway regulates cell fate and is involved in the development of the organ systems affected in Alagille syndrome. Affected patients have five major clinical features: chronic cholestasis, peripheral stenosis of the pulmonary artery, butterfly-like vertebral arch defects, an eye defect known as posterior embryotoxon, and a peculiar hypertelic facies. Patients can survive into adulthood but are at risk for hepatic failure and hepatocellular carcinoma.

Circulatory Disorders

Given the enormous flow of blood through the liver, it is not surprising that circulatory disturbances have considerable impact on the liver. In most instances, however, clinically significant abnormalities of liver function do not develop, but hepatic morphology may be strikingly affected. These disorders can be grouped according to whether blood flow into, through, or from the liver is impaired (Fig. 18–35).

IMPAIRED BLOOD FLOW INTO THE LIVER

Hepatic Artery Compromise

Liver infarcts are rare, thanks to the double blood supply to the liver. Nonetheless, thrombosis or compression of an intrahepatic branch of the hepatic artery by embolism (Fig. 18–36), neoplasia, polyarteritis nodosa (Chapter 11), or sepsis may result in a localized infarct that is usually anemic and pale tan,

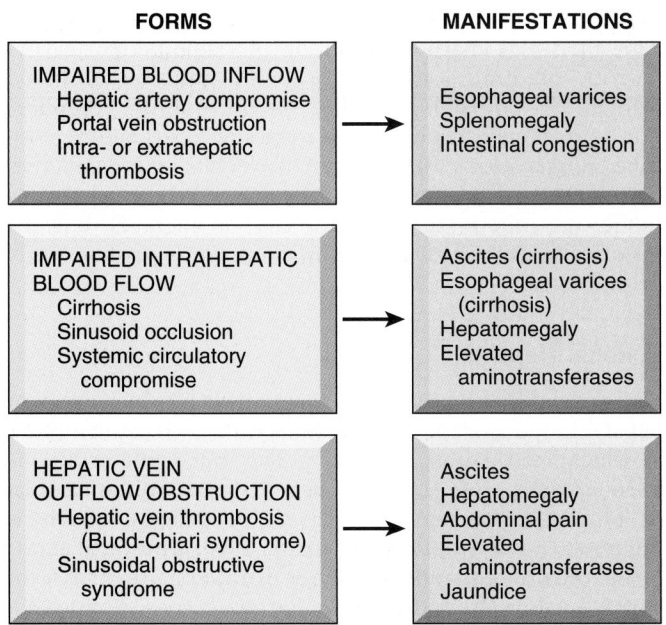

FORMS	MANIFESTATIONS
IMPAIRED BLOOD INFLOW Hepatic artery compromise Portal vein obstruction Intra- or extrahepatic thrombosis	Esophageal varices Splenomegaly Intestinal congestion
IMPAIRED INTRAHEPATIC BLOOD FLOW Cirrhosis Sinusoid occlusion Systemic circulatory compromise	Ascites (cirrhosis) Esophageal varices (cirrhosis) Hepatomegaly Elevated aminotransferases
HEPATIC VEIN OUTFLOW OBSTRUCTION Hepatic vein thrombosis (Budd-Chiari syndrome) Sinusoidal obstructive syndrome	Ascites Hepatomegaly Abdominal pain Elevated aminotransferases Jaundice

FIGURE 18–35 Hepatic circulatory disorders. Forms and clinical manifestations of compromised hepatic blood flow.

or sometimes hemorrhagic, as a result of suffusion of portal blood. Interruption of the main hepatic artery does not always produce ischemic necrosis of the organ, particularly if the liver is otherwise normal. Retrograde arterial flow through accessory vessels, when coupled with the portal venous supply, is usually sufficient to sustain the liver parenchyma. The one exception is hepatic artery thrombosis in a transplanted liver, which generally leads to infarction of the major ducts of the biliary tree and loss of the organ.

Portal Vein Obstruction and Thrombosis

Blockage of the extrahepatic portal vein may be insidious and well tolerated, or may be a catastrophic and potentially lethal event; most cases fall somewhere in between. Occlusive disease of the portal vein or its major radicles typically produces abdominal pain and, in most instances, other manifestations of portal hypertension, principally esophageal varices that are prone to rupture. Ascites is not common (because the block is presinusoidal), but when present, is often massive and intractable. As discussed earlier, ascites is common in cirrhosis due to sinusoidal block and hyperdynamic circulation. Acute impairment of visceral blood flow leads to profound congestion and bowel infarction.

Extrahepatic portal vein obstruction may arise from the following conditions, but in about one third of cases no cause can be implicated:

- Subclinical occlusion of the portal vein, from neonatal umbilical sepsis or umbilical vein catheterization, presents as variceal bleeding and ascites years later
- Intra-abdominal sepsis, caused by acute diverticulitis or appendicitis leading to *pylephlebitis* in the splanchnic circulation
- Inherited or acquired hypercoagulable disorders, including postsurgical thromboses and myeloproliferative syndromes

- Trauma
- Pancreatitis and pancreatic cancer that initiate splenic vein thrombosis, which propagates into the portal vein
- Invasion of the portal vein by hepatocellular carcinoma
- Cirrhosis, which is associated with portal vein thrombosis in about 25% of patients with thrombosis

Intrahepatic portal vein radicles may be obstructed by acute thrombosis. The thrombosis does not cause ischemic infarction but instead results in a sharply demarcated area of red-blue discoloration called *infarct of Zahn*. There is no necrosis, only severe hepatocellular atrophy and marked hemostasis in distended sinusoids. Invasion of the portal vein system by primary or secondary cancer in the liver can progressively occlude portal inflow to the liver; tongues of HCC can even occlude the extrahepatic portal vein.

Noncirrhotic Portal Fibrosis and Idiopathic Portal Hypertension. These conditions are similar and characterized by portal hypertension and a moderate degree of portal fibrosis without cirrhosis.[64] Noncirrhotic portal fibrosis is common in India and generally presents with upper gastrointestinal bleeding. Idiopathic portal hypertension, described in Japan, has a female predominance, and usually presents with splenomegaly. The pathogenesis of these conditions is unknown. It has been proposed that they may result from bacterial infection of the gut causing septic embolization of the portal vein. Another proposed mechanism is the fibrosis of portal vein branches associated with the increased expression of vascular cell adhesion molecule-1 (VCAM-1). Histologically there is a variable involvement of portal tracts, only some of which have increased connective tissue deposition and fibrosis. In addition, there is obliteration of small branches of the portal veins. This histological picture is sometimes referred to as *hepatic sclerosis* or obliterative portal venopathy.

IMPAIRED BLOOD FLOW THROUGH THE LIVER

The most common *intrahepatic cause* of blood flow obstruction is *cirrhosis*, as described earlier. In addition, physical

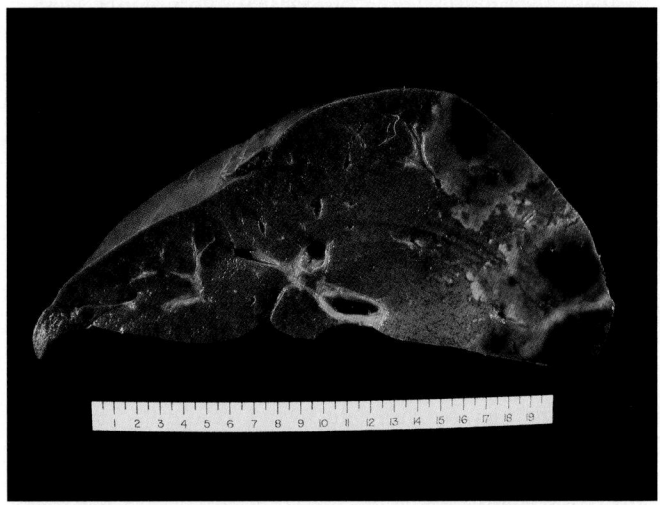

FIGURE 18–36 Liver infarct. A thrombus is lodged in a peripheral branch of the hepatic artery and compresses the adjacent portal vein; the distal hepatic tissue is pale, with a hemorrhagic margin.

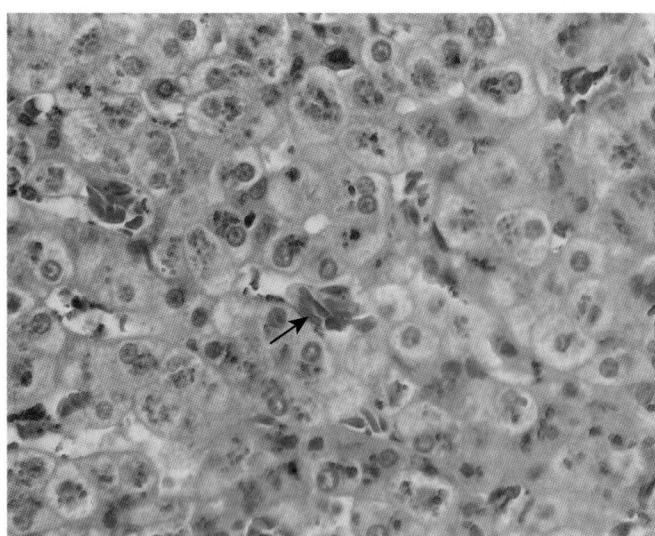

FIGURE 18-37 Sickle cell crisis in liver. The photomicrograph shows several aggregates of red blood cells, with some of them showing "sickle cell" appearance *(arrow)*.

occlusion of the *sinusoids* occurs in a small but striking group of diseases. In *sickle cell disease* the hepatic sinusoids may become packed with sickled erythrocytes, free in the sinusoids or phagocytosed by Kupffer cells (Fig. 18-37), leading to panlobular parenchymal necrosis. *Disseminated intravascular coagulation* may occlude sinusoids. This is usually inconsequential except for the periportal sinusoidal occlusion and parenchymal necrosis that may arise in pregnancy as part of *eclampsia* (discussed later). Finally, metastatic tumor cells (e.g., breast carcinoma, lymphoma, malignant melanoma) may fill the hepatic sinusoids in the absence of a mass lesion. The attendant obstruction to blood flow and massive necrosis of hepatocytes can lead to fulminant hepatic failure.

Passive Congestion and Centrilobular Necrosis

These hepatic manifestations of systemic circulatory compromise are considered together because they represent a morphologic continuum. Both changes are commonly seen at autopsy because there is an element of preterminal circulatory failure with virtually every nontraumatic death.

Right-sided cardiac decompensation leads to passive congestion of the liver. The liver is slightly enlarged, tense, and cyanotic, with rounded edges. Microscopically there is congestion of centrilobular sinusoids. With time, centrilobular hepatocytes become atrophic, resulting in markedly attenuated liver cell plates. *Left-sided cardiac failure* or *shock* may lead to hepatic hypoperfusion and hypoxia, causing ischemic coagulative necrosis of hepatocytes in the central region of the lobule *(centrilobular necrosis).* In most instances the only clinical evidence of centrilobular necrosis or its variants is transient elevation of serum aminotransferases, but the parenchymal damage may be sufficient to induce mild to moderate jaundice.

The combination of hypoperfusion and retrograde congestion acts synergistically to cause *centrilobular hemorrhagic necrosis.* The liver takes on a variegated mottled appearance, reflecting hemorrhage and necrosis in the centrilobular

regions, known as the *nutmeg liver* (Fig. 18-38). By microscopy there is a sharp demarcation of viable periportal and necrotic pericentral hepatocytes, with suffusion of blood through the centrilobular region. An uncommon complication of sustained chronic severe congestive heart failure is so-called *cardiac sclerosis.* The pattern of liver fibrosis is distinctive, inasmuch as it is mostly centrilobular. The damage rarely fulfills the criteria for the diagnosis of cirrhosis, but the historically sanctified term *cardiac cirrhosis* cannot easily be dislodged.

Peliosis Hepatis

Sinusoidal dilation occurs in any condition in which efflux of hepatic blood is impeded. *Peliosis hepatis* is a rare condition in which the dilation is primary. The liver contains blood-filled cystic spaces, either unlined or lined with sinusoidal endothelial cells. The pathogenesis of peliosis hepatis is unknown. Focal apoptosis of hepatocytes or sinusoidal endothelial cells, and disruption of liver extracellular matrix seem to play a role in the pathogenesis. *Bartonella* species have been seen in the sinusoidal endothelial cells in AIDS-associated peliosis.[65] Clinically, peliosis hepatis is associated with many diseases, including cancer, tuberculosis, AIDS, or post-transplantation immunodeficiency. It is also associated with exposure to anabolic steroids and, rarely, oral contraceptives and danazol. Clinical signs are generally absent even in advanced peliosis, but potentially fatal intra-abdominal hemorrhage or hepatic failure may occur. Peliotic lesions usually disappear after correction of the underlying causes.

HEPATIC VENOUS OUTFLOW OBSTRUCTION

Hepatic Vein Thrombosis and Inferior Vena Cava Thrombosis

Obstruction of a single main hepatic vein by thrombosis is clinically silent. The obstruction of two or more major hepatic veins produces liver enlargement, pain, and ascites, a condition known as *Budd-Chiari syndrome.* Hepatic damage is the

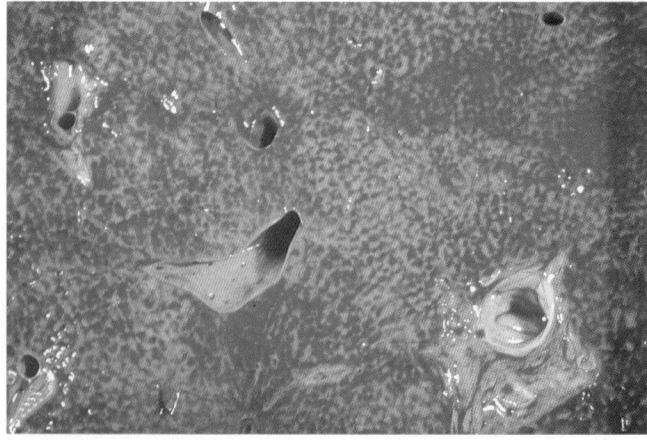

FIGURE 18-38 Centrilobular hemorrhagic necrosis. The cut liver section, in which major blood vessels are visible, is notable for a variegated, mottled, red appearance (nutmeg liver).

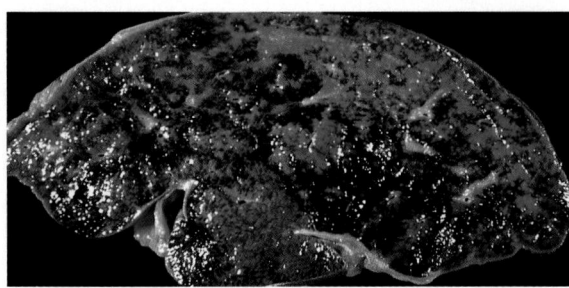

FIGURE 18-39 Budd-Chiari syndrome. Thrombosis of the major hepatic veins has caused extreme blood retention in the liver.

consequence of increased intrahepatic blood pressure, and an inability of the massive hepatic blood flow to shunt around the blocked outflow tract. *Hepatic vein thrombosis* is associated with primary myeloproliferative disorders (including polycythemia vera), inherited disorders of coagulation (e.g., deficiencies in antithrombin, protein S, or protein C, or mutations of factor V; see Chapter 4), antiphospholipid syndrome, paroxysmal nocturnal hemoglobinuria, and intra-abdominal cancers, particularly HCC. The occurrence of hepatic vein thrombosis in the setting of pregnancy or oral contraceptive use is usually through interaction with an underlying thrombogenic disorder. About 10% of cases are idiopathic in origin, presumably unrecognized thrombogenic disorders.

A separate distinction is made for *inferior vena cava obstruction at its hepatic portion (obliterative hepatocavopathy)*. This disorder is caused by inferior vena cava thrombosis or membranous obstruction of the inferior vena cava. It is endemic in Nepal, with a suspected association with infections.

Morphology. In the Budd-Chiari syndrome, acutely developing thrombosis of the major hepatic veins or the hepatic portion of the inferior vena cava, the liver is swollen and red-purple and has a tense capsule (Fig. 18-39). Microscopically the affected hepatic parenchyma reveals severe centrilobular congestion and necrosis. Centrilobular fibrosis develops in instances in which the thrombosis is more slowly developing. The major veins may contain totally occlusive fresh thrombi, subtotal occlusion, or, in chronic cases, organized adherent thrombi.

The mortality of untreated acute hepatic vein thrombosis is high. Prompt surgical creation of a portosystemic venous shunt permits reverse flow through the portal vein and considerably improves the prognosis. In the case of vena caval thrombosis, direct dilation of caval obstruction may be possible during angiography. The chronic forms of these thrombotic syndromes are far less lethal, and more than two thirds of patients are alive after 5 years.

Sinusoidal Obstruction Syndrome (Veno-Occlusive Disease)

Originally described in Jamaican drinkers of pyrrolizidine alkaloid–containing bush tea and named veno-occlusive

disease, the disease is now called sinusoidal obstruction syndrome, and occurs primarily following allogeneic bone marrow transplantation, usually within the first 3 weeks. The incidence approaches 25% in recipients of allogeneic marrow transplants. Sinusoidal obstruction syndrome can occur in cancer patients receiving chemotherapy, especially with agents such as gemtuzumad and ozagamicin, used in the treatment of acute myeloid leukemia, actinomycin D in the treatment of Wilms' tumors, dacarbazine (a drug activated by sinusoidal endothelial cells), and in patients who receive cytotoxic agents such as cyclophosphamide before bone marrow transplantation (discussed below). The mortality rates can be higher than 30%. Although histology is the gold standard for the diagnosis, a diagnosis of sinusoidal obstruction syndrome is frequently made on clinical grounds only (tender hepatomegaly, ascites, weight gain, and jaundice), because of the high risk of liver biopsy in these patients.

Morphology. Sinusoidal obstruction syndrome is characterized by obliteration of hepatic vein radicles by varying amounts of subendothelial swelling and finely reticulated collagen. In acute disease there is striking centrilobular congestion with hepatocellular necrosis and accumulation of hemosiderin-laden macrophages. As the disease progresses, obliteration of the lumen of the venule is easily identified with special stains for connective tissue (Fig. 18-40). In chronic or healed sinusoidal obstruction syndrome, dense perivenular fibrosis radiating out into the parenchyma may be present, frequently with total obliteration of the venule; hemosiderin deposition is evident in the scar tissue, and congestion is minimal.

Sinusoidal obstruction syndrome arises from toxic injury to the sinusoidal endothelium.[66] Endothelial lining cells round up and slough off the sinusoidal wall, embolizing downstream

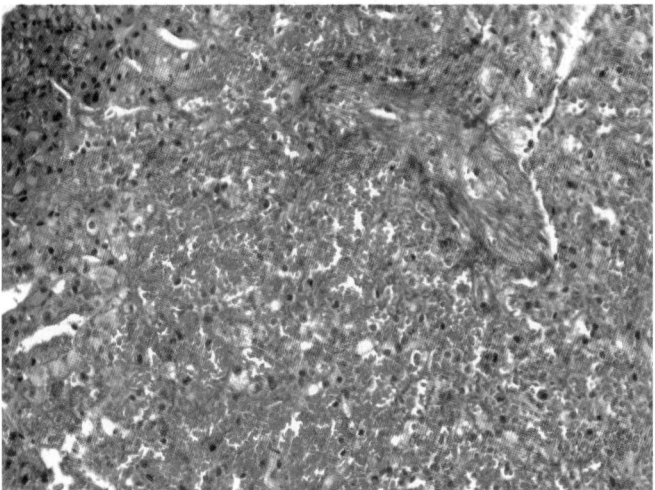

FIGURE 18-40 Sinusoidal obstruction syndrome (previously known as veno-occlusive disease). Reticulin stain reveals the parenchyma framework of the lobule and the marked deposition of collagen within the lumen of the central vein.

and obstructing sinusoidal blood flow. This is accompanied by entry of erythrocytes into the space of Disse, necrosis of perivenular hepatocytes, and downstream accumulation of cellular debris in the terminal hepatic vein. Proliferation of perisinusoidal stellate cells and subendothelial fibroblasts in the terminal hepatic vein follows, with fibrosis and deposition of extracellular matrix in the sinusoids.

Hepatic Complications of Organ or Bone Marrow Transplantation

The use of transplantation for bone marrow, renal, hepatic and other organ disorders has generated a challenging group of hepatic complications. The liver may be damaged by toxic drugs or graft-versus-host disease in patients undergoing bone marrow transplantation, whereas patients receiving a liver transplant may have graft failure or rejection, and may develop sinusoidal obstruction syndrome, as already discussed. Although the clinical settings are obviously different for each patient population, the common themes of toxic or immunologically mediated liver damage, infection of immunosuppressed hosts, recurrent disease, and post-transplant lymphoproliferative disorder are readily apparent. The following focuses on post-transplant graft-versus-host disease and liver rejection.

GRAFT-VERSUS-HOST DISEASE AND LIVER REJECTION

The liver has the unenviable position of being attacked by graft-versus-host and host-versus-graft mechanisms, in the setting of bone marrow transplantation and liver transplantation, respectively. These processes are discussed in detail in Chapter 6. More than other solid organs, liver transplants are reasonably well tolerated by recipients. That being said, the hepatic morphologic features that are peculiar to immunological attack after transplantation deserve comment.

> **Morphology.** Liver damage after bone marrow transplantation is the consequence of acute or chronic **graft-versus-host disease. In acute graft-versus-host disease,** which occurs 10 to 50 days after bone marrow transplantation, donor lymphocytes attack the epithelial cells of the liver. This results in hepatitis with necrosis of hepatocytes and bile duct epithelial cells, and inflammation of the parenchyma and portal tracts. In **chronic hepatic graft-versus-host disease** (usually more than 100 days after transplantation), there is portal tract inflammation, selective bile duct destruction, and eventual fibrosis. Portal vein and hepatic vein radicles may show endothelitis, a process in which a subendothelial lymphocytic infiltrate lifts the endothelium from its basement membrane. Cholestasis may be observed in both acute and chronic graft-versus-host disease.
>
> In **transplanted livers, acute rejection** is characterized by infiltration of a mixed population of inflammatory cells that include eosinophils into portal tracts,

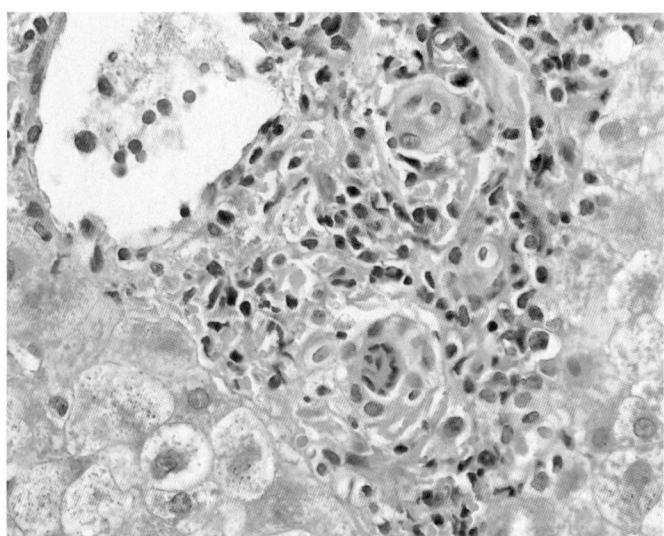

FIGURE 18–41 Transplanted liver with acute cellular rejection. Note the mixed inflammatory cell infiltration including eosinophils in portal tracts, bile duct damage, and endotheliitis.

> bile duct and hepatocyte injury, and endothelitis (Fig. 18–41). The severity of the rejection is graded according to the BANFF scheme, which is important for clinical management.[67] With **chronic rejection** a severe obliterative arteritis of small and larger arterial vessels (arteriopathy) results in ischemic changes in the liver parenchyma. Alternatively, bile ducts are progressively destroyed, because of either direct immunological attack or obliteration of their arterial supply, resulting in loss of the graft.

Hepatic Disease Associated with Pregnancy

Hepatic diseases may occur in women with chronic liver disease who become pregnant, or they may develop during pregnancy in women who were not affected by liver disease. Abnormal liver tests occur in 3% to 5% of pregnancies.[68] Viral hepatitis (HAV, HBV, HCV, and even HBV + HDV) is the most common cause of jaundice in pregnancy. While these women require careful clinical management, pregnancy does not specifically alter the course of the liver disease. The one exception is HEV infection, which, for unknown reasons, runs a more severe course in pregnant patients, with fatality rates of 10% to 20%.

A very small subgroup of pregnant women (0.1%) develops hepatic complications directly attributable to pregnancy: preeclampsia and eclampsia, acute fatty liver of pregnancy, and intrahepatic cholestasis of pregnancy. In extreme cases of the first two conditions, the outcome is fatal.

PREECLAMPSIA AND ECLAMPSIA

Preeclampsia affects 3% to 5% of pregnancies and is characterized by maternal hypertension, proteinuria, peripheral

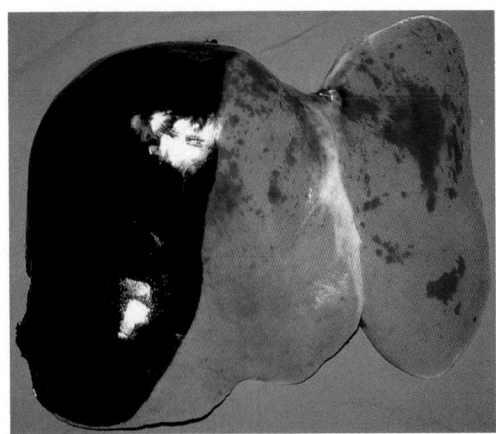

FIGURE 18–42 Eclampsia. Subcapsular hematoma dissecting under Glisson's capsule in a fatal case of eclampsia. (Courtesy of Dr. Brian Blackbourne, Office of the Medical Examiner, San Diego, CA.)

edema, coagulation abnormalities, and varying degrees of disseminated intravascular coagulation (Chapter 22). When hyper-reflexia and convulsions occur the condition is called *eclampsia* and may be life-threatening. Alternatively, subclinical hepatic disease may be the primary manifestation of preeclampsia, as part of a syndrome of hemolysis, elevated liver enzymes, and low platelets, dubbed the *HELLP syndrome*.[69]

> **Morphology.** The affected liver in preeclampsia is normal in size, firm, and pale, with small red patches due to hemorrhage. Occasionally, yellow or white patches of ischemic infarction can be seen. Microscopically, **the periportal sinusoids contain fibrin deposits with hemorrhage into the space of Disse**, leading to periportal hepatocellular coagulative necrosis. Blood under pressure may coalesce and expand to form a **hepatic hematoma; dissection of blood under Glisson's capsule may lead to catastrophic hepatic rupture** (Fig. 18–42). Patients with hepatic involvement in preeclampsia may show modest to severe elevation of serum aminotransferases and mild elevation of serum bilirubin. Hepatic dysfunction sufficient to cause a coagulopathy signifies far-advanced and potentially lethal disease. **Definitive treatment in severe cases requires termination of the pregnancy.** In mild cases patients may be managed conservatively. Women who survive mild or severe preeclampsia recover without sequelae.

ACUTE FATTY LIVER OF PREGNANCY (AFLP)

AFLP presents with a spectrum ranging from modest or even subclinical hepatic dysfunction (evidenced by elevated serum aminotransferase levels) to hepatic failure, coma, and death. It is a rare disease affecting 1 in 13,000 deliveries. Affected women present in the latter half of pregnancy, usually in the third trimester. Symptoms are directly attributable to incipient hepatic failure, including bleeding, nausea and vomiting,

jaundice, and coma. In 20% to 40% of cases the presenting symptoms may be those of coexistent preeclampsia.

> **Morphology.** The diagnosis of acute fatty liver rests on biopsy identification of the characteristic microvesicular fatty transformation of hepatocytes. In severe cases there may be lobular disarray with hepatocyte dropout, reticulin collapse, and portal tract inflammation, making distinction from viral hepatitis difficult. Diagnosis depends on (1) a high index of suspicion and (2) confirmation of microvesicular steatosis using special stains for fat (oil-red-O or Sudan black) on frozen tissue sections; electron microscopy may also be used to demonstrate the steatosis.

While this condition most commonly runs a mild course, women with AFLP can progress within days to hepatic failure and death. *The primary treatment for AFLP is termination of the pregnancy.* The pathogenesis of this disease is unknown, but mitochondrial dysfunction has been implicated. In a subset of patients, both mother and father carry a heterozygous deficiency in mitochondrial long-chain 3-hydroxyacyl coenzyme A (CoA) dehydrogenase. The homozygous-deficient fetuses fare well during pregnancy but cause hepatic dysfunction in the mother, because long-chain 3-hydroxylacyl metabolites produced by the fetus or placenta are washed away into the maternal circulation and cause hepatic toxicity. This is a rare instance of the fetus causing metabolic disease in the mother.[70]

INTRAHEPATIC CHOLESTASIS OF PREGNANCY

The onset of pruritus in the third trimester, followed by darkening of the urine and occasionally light stools and jaundice, heralds the development of this enigmatic syndrome. Serum bilirubin (mostly conjugated) rarely exceeds 5 mg/dL; alkaline phosphatase may be slightly elevated. Liver biopsy reveals mild cholestasis without necrosis. The altered hormonal state of pregnancy seems to combine with biliary defects in the secretion of bile salts or sulfated progesterone metabolites to engender cholestasis. Although this is generally a benign condition, the mother is at risk for gallstones and malabsorption, and the incidence of fetal distress, stillbirths, and prematurity is modestly increased. Perhaps most importantly, the pruritus can be extremely distressing for the pregnant mother.

Nodules and Tumors

Hepatic masses may come to attention for a variety of reasons. They may generate epigastric fullness and discomfort or be detected by routine physical examination or radiographic studies for other indications. Nodular hyperplasias are not neoplasms; the remaining lesions discussed in this section are true neoplasms.

NODULAR HYPERPLASIAS

Solitary or multiple hyperplastic hepatocellular nodules may develop in the noncirrhotic liver. Two such conditions, having

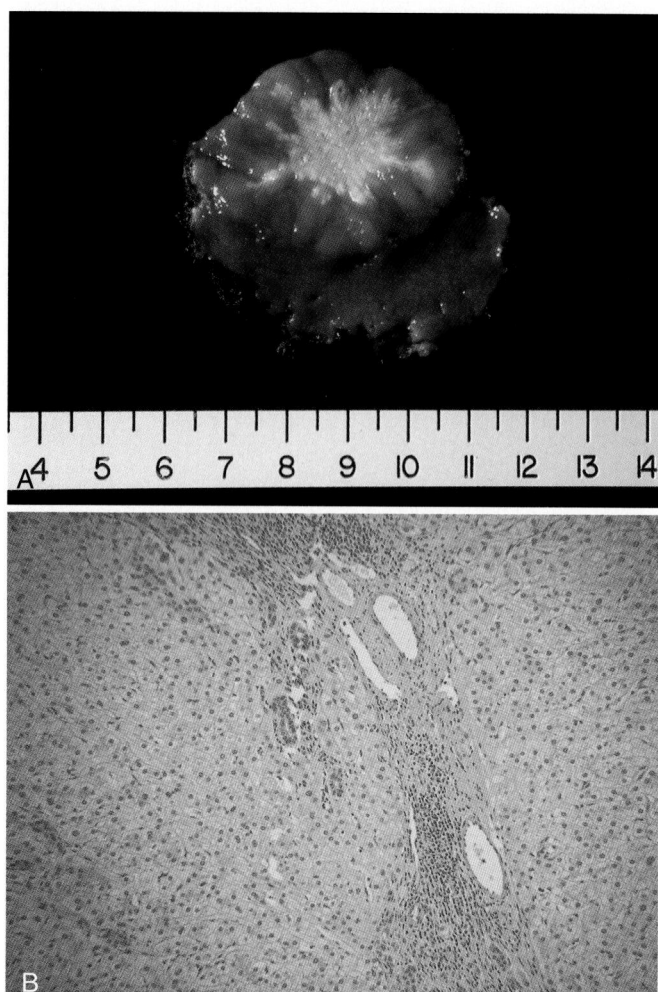

FIGURE 18–43 Focal nodular hyperplasia. **A,** Resected specimen showing lobulated contours and a central stellate scar. **B,** Low-power photomicrograph showing a broad fibrous scar with hepatic arterial and bile duct elements and chronic inflammation, present within hepatic parenchyma that lacks the normal sinusoidal plate architecture.

fibromuscular hyperplasia with eccentric or concentric narrowing of the lumen. The radiating septa show foci of intense lymphocytic infiltrates and exuberant bile duct proliferation along septal margins. The parenchyma between the septa shows essentially normal hepatocytes but with a thickened plate architecture characteristic of regeneration. Long-term use of anabolic hormones or of contraceptives have been implicated in the development of focal nodular hyperplasia.

Nodular regenerative hyperplasia denotes a liver entirely transformed into roughly spherical nodules, in the absence of fibrosis. Microscopically, plump hepatocytes are surrounded by rims of atrophic hepatocytes. The variation in parenchymal architecture may be missed on an H&E stain, and reticulin staining is required to appreciate the changes in hepatocellular architecture. Nodular regenerative hyperplasia can lead to the development of portal hypertension and occurs in association with conditions affecting intrahepatic blood flow, including solid-organ (particularly renal) transplantation, bone marrow transplantation, and vasculitis. It also occurs in HIV-infected persons.[71]

BENIGN NEOPLASMS

Cavernous hemangiomas, blood vessel tumors identical to those occurring elsewhere (see Chapter 11), are the most common benign liver tumors. They appear as discrete red-blue, soft nodules, usually less than 2 cm in diameter, generally located directly beneath the capsule. Histologically, the tumor consists of vascular channels in a bed of fibrous connective tissue (Fig. 18–44). Their chief clinical significance is that they should not be mistaken for metastatic tumors, and that blind percutaneous biopsies not be performed on them.

confusingly overlapping names, are *focal nodular hyperplasia* and *nodular regenerative hyperplasia*. The common factor in both types of nodules seems to be either focal or diffuse alterations in hepatic blood supply, arising from obliteration of portal vein radicles and compensatory augmentation of arterial blood supply.

Morphology. Focal nodular hyperplasia appears as a well-demarcated but poorly encapsulated nodule, ranging up to many centimeters in diameter (Fig. 18–43A). It presents as a spontaneous mass lesion in an otherwise normal liver, most frequently in young to middle-aged adults. The lesion is generally lighter than the surrounding liver and is sometimes yellow. Typically, there is a central gray-white, depressed stellate scar from which fibrous septa radiate to the periphery (Fig. 18–43B). The central scar contains large vessels, usually arterial, that typically show

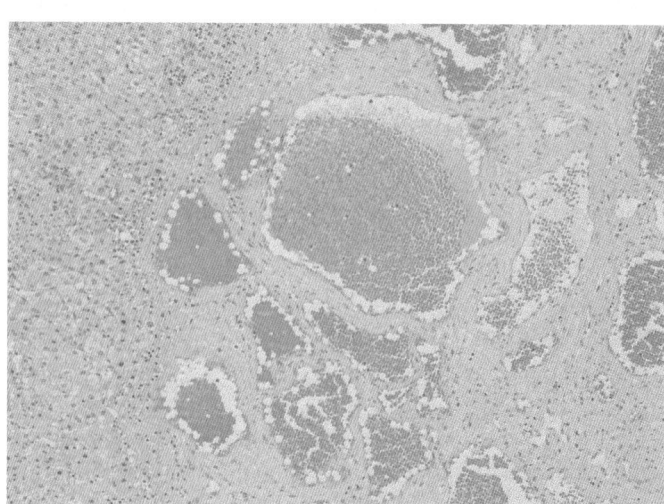

FIGURE 18–44 Hemangioma. The photomicrograph shows the vesicular channels embedded in fibrous stroma.

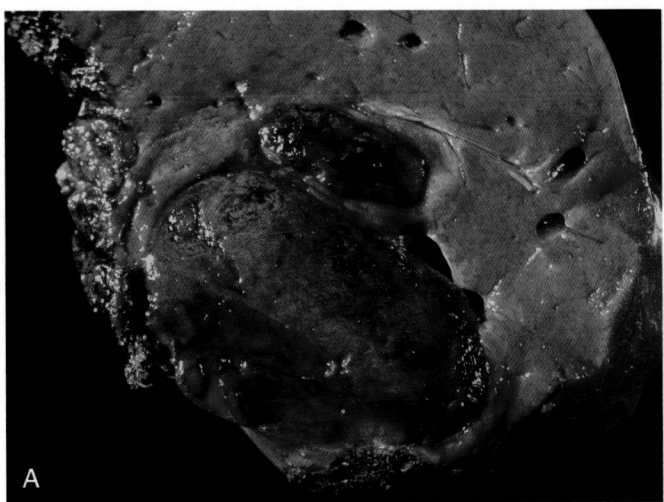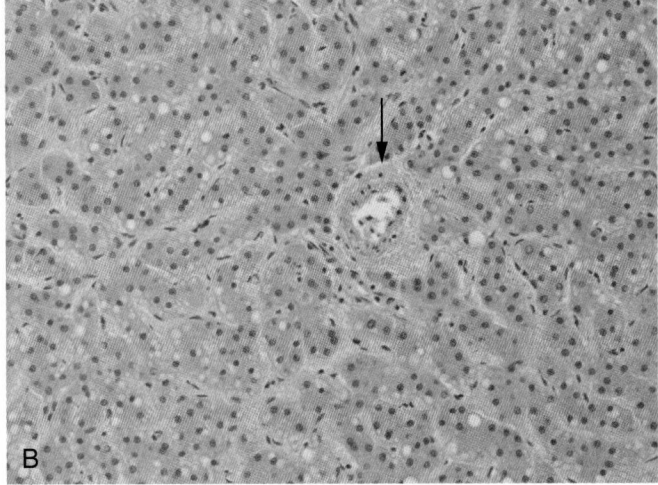

FIGURE 18–45 Liver cell adenoma. **A,** Resected specimen presenting as a pendulous mass arising from the liver. **B,** Microscopic view showing cords of hepatocytes, with an arterial vascular supply *(arrow)* and no portal tracts.

Hepatic Adenoma

Benign neoplasms developing from hepatocytes are called *hepatic adenomas* or *liver cell adenomas.* Although they may occur in men, hepatic adenomas most frequently occur in young women who have used oral contraceptives; tumors generally regress if contraceptive use is terminated. The incidence of adenoma is approximately 1 in 100,000. Hepatic adenomas have clinical significance for three reasons: (1) when they present as an intrahepatic mass they may be mistaken for the more ominous hepatocellular carcinomas; (2) subcapsular adenomas have a tendency to rupture, particularly during pregnancy (under estrogen stimulation), causing life-threatening intraperitoneal hemorrhage; (3) rarely, they may transform into carcinomas, particularly, when the adenoma arises in an individual with glycogen storage disease, and adenomas in which mutations of the β-catenin gene are present.

Pathogenesis. Although hormonal stimulation is clearly associated with the development of solitary hepatic adenoma, the causal events are unknown. Mutations in the genes encoding the transcription factor HNF1α and β-catenin have been identified in 50% and 15% of the hepatic adenomas, respectively.[72] Multiple hepatic adenoma (adenomatosis) syndromes can occur in individuals with maturity-onset diabetes of young (MODY3), with *HNF1* mutations.[73]

> **Morphology. Liver cell adenomas** are pale, yellow-tan, and frequently bile-stained nodules, found anywhere in the hepatic substance but often beneath the capsule (Fig. 18–45A). They may reach 30 cm in diameter. Although they are usually well demarcated, encapsulation might not be present. The tumor commonly presents as a solitary lesion, but multiple lesions (adenomatosis) can occur. Histologically, liver cell adenomas are composed of sheets and cords of cells that may resemble normal hepatocytes or have some variation in cell and nuclear size (Fig. 18–45B). Abundant glycogen may generate large hepatocytes with a clear cytoplasm. Steatosis is commonly present. Portal tracts are absent; instead, prominent solitary arterial vessels and draining veins are distributed through the substance of the tumor.

MALIGNANT TUMORS

Malignant tumors occurring in the liver can be primary or metastatic. Most of the discussion in this section deals with primary hepatic tumors. Primary carcinomas of the liver are relatively uncommon in North America and western Europe (0.5% to 2% of all cancers) but represent 20% to 40% of cancers in many other countries. Most primary liver cancers arise from hepatocytes and are termed *hepatocellular carcinoma* (HCC). Much less common are carcinomas of bile duct origin, *cholangiocarcinomas.* The incidence of these two cancers is increasing in the United States.

Before embarking on a discussion of the major forms of malignancy affecting the liver, two rare forms of primary liver cancer deserve brief mention: hepatoblastomas and angiosarcomas. *Angiosarcoma* of the liver resembles those occurring elsewhere. The primary liver form is of interest because of its association with exposure to vinyl chloride, arsenic, or Thorotrast (Chapters 9 and 11). The latency period after exposure to the putative carcinogen may be several decades. These highly aggressive neoplasms metastasize widely and generally kill within a year. The major features of hepatoblastoma are discussed next.

Hepatoblastoma

Hepatoblastoma is the most common liver tumor of young childhood. Its incidence, which is increasing, is approximately 1 to 2 in 1 million births.[74] The tumor is usually fatal within a few years if not treated. This tumor has two anatomic variants:

- The *epithelial type,* composed of small polygonal fetal cells or smaller embryonal cells forming acini, tubules,

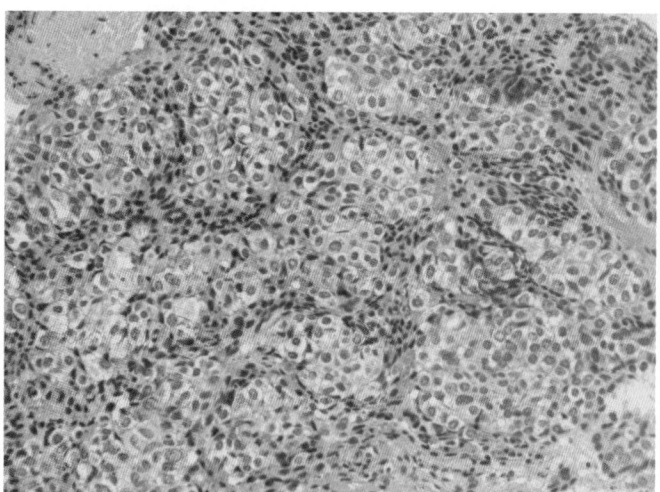

FIGURE 18–46 Hepatoblastoma. The photograph shows proliferating hepatoblasts.

or papillary structures vaguely recapitulating liver development (Fig. 18–46)

⊙ The *mixed epithelial and mesenchymal type*, which contains foci of mesenchymal differentiation that may consist of primitive mesenchyme, osteoid, cartilage, or striated muscle

A characteristic feature of hepatoblastomas is the frequent activation of the WNT/β-catenin signaling pathway.[75] Chromosomal abnormalities are common in hepatoblastomas, and FOXG1, a regulator of the TGF-β pathway, is highly expressed in some subsets of the tumor.[76] Hepatoblastoma may be associated with familial adenomatous polyposis syndrome and Beckwith-Wiedmann syndrome. The treatment is chemotherapy and complete surgical resection. The therapy has raised the 5-year survival to 80%.

Hepatocellular Carcinoma (HCC)

On a global basis, there are more than 626,000 new cases per year of primary liver cancer, almost all being HCC, and approximately 598,000 patients die from this cancer every year,[77] the third most frequent cause of cancer deaths. About 82% of HCC cases occur in developing countries with high rates of chronic HBV infection, such as in southeast Asian and African countries; 52% of all HCC cases occur in China. In the United States the incidence of liver cancer increased by 25% between 1993 and 1998, mainly due to HCV and HBV chronic infection. There is a clear predominance of males with a ratio of 2.4:1.

Pathogenesis. Several general factors relevant to the pathogenesis of HCC were discussed in Chapter 7. Some issues specifically related to HCC deserve emphasis here.

Four major etiologic factors associated with HCC have been established: chronic viral infection (HBV, HCV), chronic alcoholism, non-alcoholic steatohepatitis (NASH), and food contaminants (primarily aflatoxins). Other conditions include tyrosinemia, glycogen storage disease, hereditary hemochromatosis, non-alcoholic fatty liver disease, and α_1-antitrypsin deficiency. Many factors, including genetic factors, age, gender, chemicals, hormones, and nutrition, interact in the develop-

ment of HCC. The disease that is most likely to give rise to HCC is the extremely rare hereditary tyrosinemia, in which almost 40% of patients develop the tumor despite adequate dietary control.

The pathogenesis of HCC may be different in high-incidence, HBV-prevalent populations versus low-incidence Western populations, in which other chronic liver diseases such as alcoholism, non-alcoholic steatohepatitis, chronic HCV infection, and hemochromatosis are more common. In high-prevalence regions the HBV infection begins in infancy by the vertical transmission of virus from infected mothers, which confers a 200-fold increased risk for HCC development by adulthood. Cirrhosis may be absent in as many as half of these patients, and the cancer often occurs between 20 and 40 years of age. In the Western world where HBV is not prevalent, cirrhosis is present in 75% to 90% of cases of HCC, usually in the setting of other chronic liver diseases. Thus, cirrhosis seems to be a prerequisite contributor to the emergence of HCC in Western countries but may have a different role in HCC that develops in endemic areas. In China and southern Africa, where HBV is endemic, there may also be exposure to aflatoxin, a toxin produced by the fungus *Aspergillus flavus*, which contaminates peanuts and grains. Aflatoxin can bind covalently with cellular DNA and cause a specific mutation in codon 249 of *p53* (Chapter 9).

Although the precise mechanisms of carcinogenesis are unknown, several events have been implicated. Repeated cycles of cell death and regeneration, as occurs in chronic hepatitis from any cause, are important in the pathogenesis of HCCs (Chapter 7). It is thought that the accumulation of mutations during continuous cycles of cell division may damage DNA repair mechanisms and eventually transform hepatocytes. Preneoplastic changes can be recognized morphologically by the occurrence of hepatocyte dysplasia. Progression to HCC might result from point mutations in selected cellular genes such as *KRAS* and *p53*, and constitutive expression of c-MYC, c-MET (the receptor for hepatocyte growth factor), TGF-α, and insulin-like growth factor 2. Recent global gene expression studies revealed that approximately 50% of HCC cases are associated with activation of WNT or AKT pathways. A subgroup of tumors expresses a high proportion of genes present in fetal liver and liver progenitor cells, suggesting that at least some HCCs may be generated from liver stem cells (Chapter 3).

Molecular analysis of tumor cells in HBV-infected individuals showed that most nodules are clonal with respect to the HBV DNA integration pattern, suggesting that viral integration precedes or accompanies a transforming event. In HBV-induced carcinogenesis not only the disruption of cell genome caused by virus integration but also the site of integration can be important. Depending on the integration site, HBV integration may activate proto-oncogenes that contribute to tumorigenicity. Alternatively, it has been proposed that the HBV X-protein, a transcriptional activator of multiple genes, might be the main cause of cell transformation. The situation is even more uncertain regarding the mechanisms of HCV carcinogenesis. HCV is a RNA virus that does not disrupt DNA, and it does not produce oncogenic proteins. However, there are indications that the HCV core and NS5A proteins may participate in the development of HCC.[78]

Universal vaccination of children against HBV in endemic areas can dramatically decrease the incidence of HBV infec-

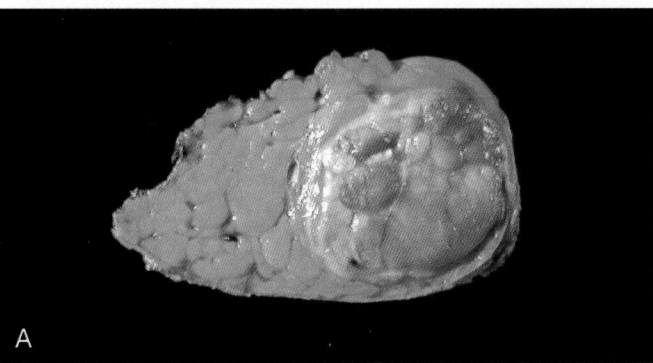

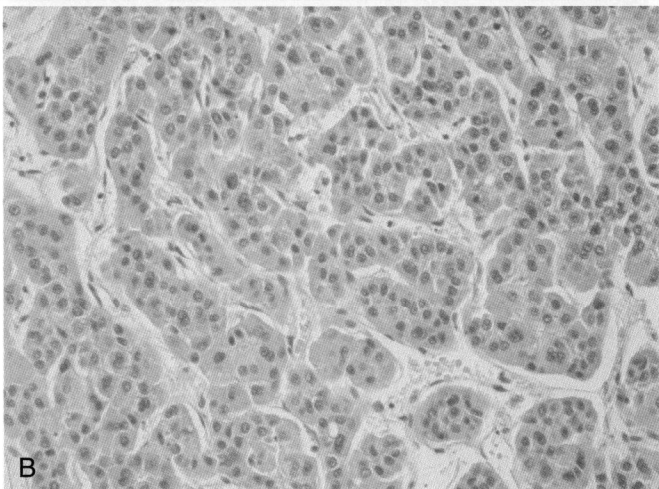

FIGURE 18-47 Hepatocellular carcinoma. **A,** Liver removed at autopsy showing a unifocal, massive neoplasm replacing most of the right hepatic lobe in a noncirrhotic liver; a satellite tumor nodule is directly adjacent. **B,** Microscopic view of a well-differentiated lesion; tumor cells are arranged in nests, sometimes with a central lumen.

tion, and most likely, the incidence of HCC. Such a program, started in Taiwan in 1984, has reduced HBV infection rates from 10% to less than 1% in 20 years.[79]

Morphology. HCC may appear grossly as (1) a **unifocal** (usually large) mass (Fig. 18-47A); (2) **multifocal**, widely distributed nodules of variable size; or (3) a **diffusely infiltrative** cancer, permeating widely and sometimes involving the entire liver. All three patterns may cause liver enlargement, particularly the large unifocal and multinodular patterns. The diffusely infiltrative tumor may blend imperceptibly into a cirrhotic liver background.

HCCs are usually paler than the surrounding liver, and sometimes take on a green hue when composed of well-differentiated hepatocytes capable of secreting bile. **All patterns of HCCs have a strong propensity for invasion of vascular structures**. Extensive intrahepatic metastases ensue, and occasionally, long, snakelike masses of tumor invade the portal vein (with occlusion of the portal circulation) or inferior vena cava, extending even into the right side of the heart. HCC spreads extensively within the liver by

obvious contiguous growth and by the development of satellite nodules, which can be shown by molecular methods to be derived from the parent tumor. Metastasis outside the liver is primarily via vascular invasion, especially into the hepatic vein system, but hematogenous metastases, especially to the lung, tend to occur late in the disease. Lymph node metastases to the perihilar, peripancreatic, and para-aortic nodes above and below the diaphragm are found in fewer than half of HCCs that spread beyond the liver. If HCC with venous invasion is identified in explanted livers at the time of liver transplantation, tumor recurrence is likely to occur in the transplanted donor liver.

HCCs range from well-differentiated to highly anaplastic undifferentiated lesions. In well-differentiated and moderately differentiated tumors, cells that are recognizable as hepatocytic in origin are disposed either in a trabecular pattern (recapitulating liver cell plates) (Fig. 18-47B) or in an acinar, pseudoglandular pattern. In poorly differentiated forms, tumor cells can take on a pleomorphic appearance with numerous anaplastic giant cells, can be small and completely undifferentiated, or may even resemble a spindle cell sarcoma.

A distinctive variant of HCC is the **fibrolamellar carcinoma**, which was first described in 1956. This variant constitutes 5% of HCCs. It occurs in young male and female adults (20 to 40 years of age) with equal incidence. Patients usually do not have underlying chronic liver diseases, and so the prognosis is better than the conventional HCC.[80] The etiology of fibrolamellar carcinoma is unknown. It usually presents as single large, hard "scirrhous" tumor with fibrous bands coursing through it. On microscopic examination it is composed of well-differentiated polygonal cells growing in nests or cords, and separated by parallel lamellae of dense collagen bundles. The tumor cells have abundant eosinophilic cytoplasm and prominent nucleoli (Fig. 18-48).

Clinical Features. The clinical manifestations of HCC are seldom characteristic and, in the Western population, often are masked by those related to the underlying cirrhosis or chronic hepatitis. In areas of high incidence such as tropical Africa, patients usually have no clinical history of liver disease, although cirrhosis may be detected at autopsy. In both populations most patients have ill-defined upper abdominal pain, malaise, fatigue, weight loss, and sometimes awareness of an abdominal mass or abdominal fullness. In many cases the enlarged liver can be felt on palpation, with sufficient irregularity or nodularity to permit differentiation from cirrhosis. Jaundice, fever, and gastrointestinal or esophageal variceal bleeding are inconstant findings.

Laboratory studies may be helpful but are rarely conclusive. Elevated levels of *serum α-fetoprotein* are found in 50% of persons with HCC. However, false-positive results are encountered with yolk-sac tumors and many non-neoplastic conditions, including cirrhosis, massive liver necrosis (with compensatory liver cell regeneration), chronic hepatitis

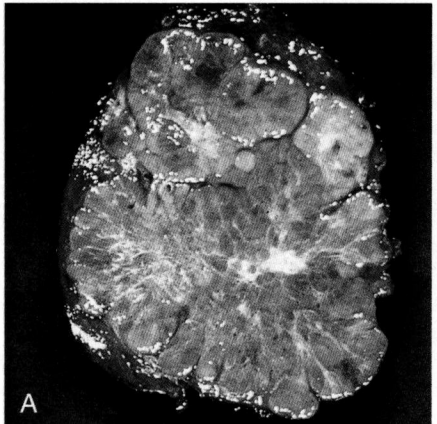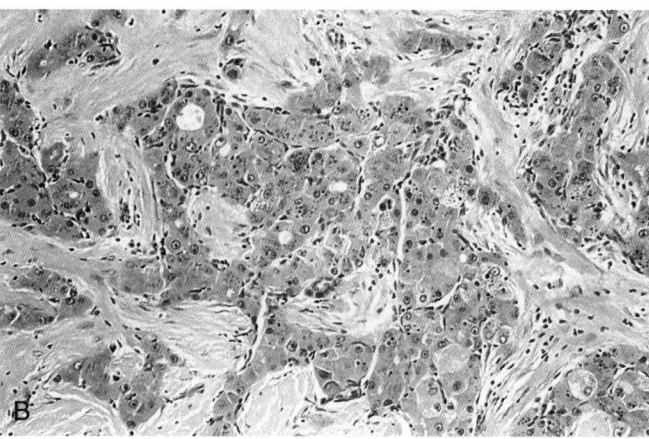

FIGURE 18–48   Fibrolamellar carcinoma. **A,** Resected specimen showing a demarcated nodule in an otherwise normal liver. **B,** Microscopic view showing nests and cords of malignant-appearing hepatocytes separated by dense bundles of collagen.

(especially HCV infection), normal pregnancy, fetal distress or death, and fetal neural tube defects such as anencephaly and spina bifida. Laboratory testing for α-fetoprotein and other proteins (such as serum carcinoembryonic antigen levels) often fails to detect small HCC lesions. Recently, staining for Glypican-3 has been used to distinguish early HCC from dysplastic nodules. Most valuable for detection of small tumors are imaging studies: ultrasonography, hepatic angiography, computed tomography, and magnetic resonance imaging. Molecular analysis of HCC is actively being pursued and will most likely lead to new HCC classifications that can help determine treatment options. As already mentioned, some molecular signatures of HCC have already been identified.[81]

The natural course of HCC involves the progressive enlargement of the primary mass until it seriously disturbs hepatic function, or metastasizes, generally first to the lungs and then to other sites. Overall, death usually occurs from (1) cachexia, (2) gastrointestinal or esophageal variceal bleeding, (3) liver failure with hepatic coma, or, rarely, (4) rupture of the tumor with fatal hemorrhage. The 5-year survival of large tumors is dismal, with the majority of patients dying within the first 2 years. With implementation of screening procedures and advances in imaging, the detection of HCCs less than 2 cm in diameter has increased in countries where such facilities are available. These small tumors can be removed surgically with good prognostic outcomes. Radiofrequency ablation is used for local control of large tumors, and chemoembolization can also be used, according to a clinical algorithm that has been widely adopted.[82] Recent findings show that the kinase inhibitor sorafenib can prolong the life of individuals with advanced-stage HCC.[83]

Cholangiocarcinoma (CCA)

Cholangiocarcinoma, the second most common hepatic malignant tumor after HCC, is a malignancy of the biliary tree, arising from bile ducts within and outside of the liver.[84] It accounts for 7.6% of cancer deaths worldwide and 3% of cancer deaths in the United States. The prevalence of the disease in the United States is variable, the highest being in Hispanics (1.22 per 100,000 population), and the lowest in

African-Americans (0.17–0.5 per 100,000). The risk factors for development of CCA include primary sclerosing cholangitis (PSC), congenital fibropolycystic diseases of the biliary system (particularly Caroli disease and choledochal cysts that will be discussed later), HCV infection, and previous exposure to Thorotrast (formerly used in radiography of the biliary tract). Most cholangiocarcinomas in the Western world, however, arise without evidence of such antecedent conditions. In southeast Asia, where the incidence rates are higher, a major risk factor is chronic infection of the biliary tract by the liver fluke *Opisthorchis sinensis* and its close relatives. *According to their localization, CCAs are classified into intrahepatic and extrahepatic forms.* Eighty to 90% of the tumors are extrahepatic. However, the incidence of intrahepatic tumors has increased during the last two decades in the United States, western Europe, and Japan, while the incidence of extrahepatic CCA has remained constant. The extrahepatic forms include perihilar tumors known as *Klatskin tumors,* which are located at the junction of the right and left hepatic ducts forming the common hepatic duct, and distal bile duct tumors. A subgroup of distal tumors arise in the immediate vicinity of the ampulla of Vater. Tumors of this region also include adenocarcinoma of the duodenal mucosa and pancreatic carcinoma (discussed in Chapters 17 and 19, respectively) and are collectively referred to as *periampullary carcinomas.*

Fifty to 60% of all CCAs are perihilar (Klatskin) tumors, 20% to 30% are distal tumors, and about 10% are intrahepatic. In any case the prognosis is dismal, with survival rates of about 15% at 2 years after diagnosis. The median time from diagnosis to death for intrahepatic CCAs is 6 months, even after surgery. Intrahepatic CCAs are not usually detected until late in their course, and come to the attention because of obstruction of bile flow, or as a symptomatic liver mass. In contrast, hilar and distal tumors present with symptoms of biliary obstruction, cholangitis, and right upper quadrant pain.

Morphology. Extrahepatic CCAs are generally small lesions at the time of diagnosis. Most tumors appear as firm, gray nodules within the bile duct wall; some may be diffusely infiltrative lesions; others are papil-

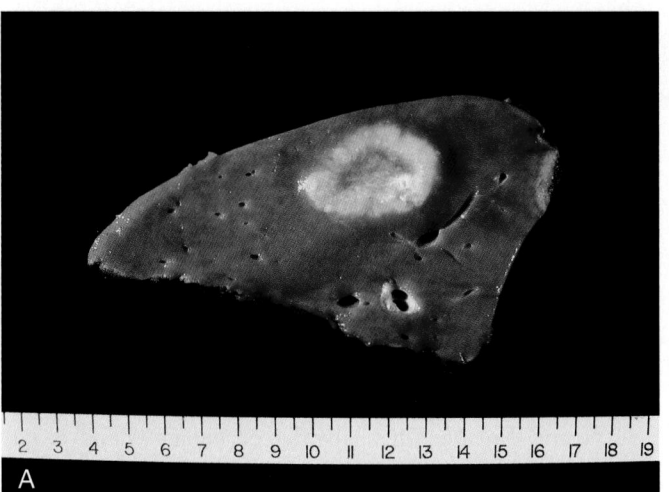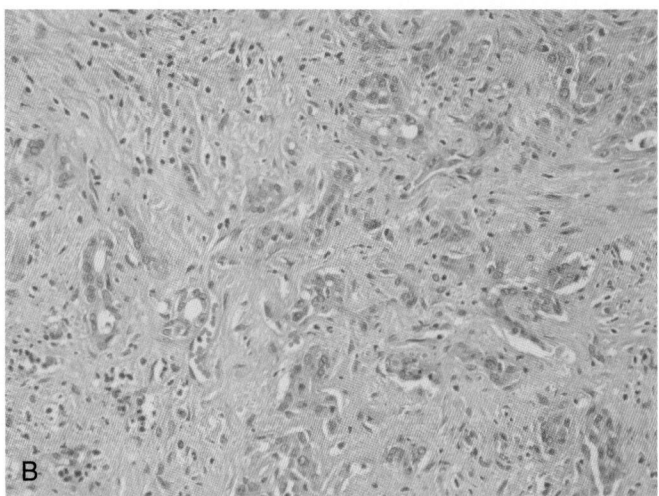

FIGURE 18–49 Cholangiocarcinoma. **A,** Liver removed at autopsy showing a massive neoplasm in the right hepatic lobe and innumerable metastases permeating the entire liver. **B,** Microscopic view showing tubular glandular structures embedded in a dense sclerotic stroma.

lary, polypoid lesions. Most are adenocarcinomas that may or may not secrete mucin. Uncommonly, squamous features are present. For the most part, an abundant fibrous stroma accompanies the epithelial proliferation. Klatskin tumors generally have slower growth than other CCAs, show prominent fibrosis, and infrequently involve distal metastases.

Intrahepatic CCAs occur in the noncirrhotic liver and may track along the intrahepatic portal tract system to create a treelike tumorous mass within a portion of the liver. Alternatively, a massive tumor nodule may develop. In either instance, vascular invasion and propagation along portal lymphatics may be prominent features, giving rise to extensive intrahepatic metastasis (Fig. 18–49A). By microscopy, CCAs resemble adenocarcinomas arising in other parts of the body, and they may show the full range of morphologic variation. Most are well- to moderately differentiated sclerosing adenocarcinomas with clearly defined glandular and tubular structures lined by cuboidal to low columnar epithelial cells (Fig. 18–49B). These neoplasms are usually markedly desmoplastic, with dense collagenous stroma separating the glandular elements. As a result, the tumor substance is extremely firm and gritty. Lymph node metastasis and hematogenous metastases to the lungs, bones (mainly vertebrae), adrenals, brain, or elsewhere are present at autopsy in about 50% of cases. Mixed variants occur, in which elements of both HCC and CCA are present. Three forms are recognized: (1) separate tumor masses of HCC and CCA within the same liver; (2) "collision tumors," in which tumorous masses of HCC and CCA commingle at an identifiable interface; and (3) tumors in which elements of HCC and CCA are intimately mixed at the microscopic level. These "mixed tumors" are infrequent, but careful microscopic examination of CCAs

can often reveal small foci of hepatocellular differentiation. The HCC-CCA may be generated from a common bipotential precursor cell (oval cells, Chapter 3), capable of producing both hepatocytes and bile duct epithelial cells (cholangiocytes).

Pathogenesis. Several signaling pathways, some listed here, are involved in the pathogenesis of CCA. Among these is IL-6 overexpression that leads to activation of AKT and the anti-apoptotic protein MCL-1. Also increased in CCAs is the expression of COX-2, ERB-2, and c-MET. *KRAS* expression is increased in 20% to 100% of cases in different studies, and *p53* expression is decreased in about 40% of cases. Other alterations involve amplification of epidermal growth factor receptors, and decreases in the expression of the cell cycle regulator and tumor suppressor p16/ink4A. In addition to cytologic diagnosis, fluorescence in situ hybridization using specific probes for epidermal growth factor receptors and digital image analysis to determine ploidy are now being used to improve diagnostic accuracy. Surgery, when possible, is the only treatment that is potentially curative.

METASTATIC TUMORS

Involvement of the liver by metastatic malignancy is far more common than primary hepatic neoplasia. The liver and lungs share the dubious distinction of being the visceral organs that are most often involved in the metastatic spread of cancers. Although the most common primary sources producing hepatic metastases are those of the colon, breast, lung, and pancreas, any cancer in any site of the body may spread to the liver, including leukemias, melanomas, and lymphomas. Typically, multiple nodular metastases are found that often cause striking hepatomegaly and may replace over 80% of existent hepatic parenchyma. The liver weight can exceed several kilograms. Metastasis may also appear as a single nodule, in which case it may be resected surgically. There is a tendency for metastatic nodules to outgrow their blood supply, producing central necrosis and umbilication when viewed from the surface of the liver. Always surprising is the amount of metastatic involvement that may be present in the absence of clinical or laboratory evidence of hepatic functional insufficiency.

Often the only telltale clinical sign is hepatomegaly, sometimes with nodularity of the free edge. However, with massive destruction of liver substance or direct obstruction of major bile ducts, jaundice and abnormal elevations of liver enzymes may appear.

THE BILIARY TRACT

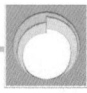

Disorders of the biliary tract affect a significant portion of the world's population. Over 95% of biliary tract disease is attributable to cholelithiasis (gallstones). In the United States, gallstones affect 20 million people, and more than 700,000 cholecystectomies are performed annually at a cost of approximately $6 billion.

As much as 1 L of bile is secreted by the liver per day. Between meals bile is stored in the gallbladder, where it is concentrated. The adult gallbladder has a capacity of about 50 mL. The organ is not essential for biliary function, since humans do not suffer from indigestion or malabsorption of fat after cholecystectomy.

Congenital Anomalies

The gallbladder may be *congenitally absent*, or there may be gallbladder *duplication* with conjoined or independent cystic ducts. A longitudinal or transverse septum may create a *bilobed gallbladder*. *Aberrant locations* of the gallbladder occur in 5% to 10% of the population, most commonly partial or complete embedding in the liver substance. A *folded fundus* is the most common anomaly, creating a *phrygian cap* (Fig. 18–50). *Agenesis* of all or any portion of the hepatic or common bile ducts and *hypoplastic* narrowing of biliary channels (true "biliary atresia") may also occur.

Disorders of the Gallbladder

CHOLELITHIASIS (GALLSTONES)

Gallstones afflict 10% to 20% of adult populations in developed countries. It is estimated that more than 20 million persons in the United States have gallstones, totaling some 25 to 50 tons in weight! The vast majority of gallstones (>80%) are "silent," and most individuals remain free of biliary pain or other complications for decades. There are two main types of gallstones. In the West, about 90% are *cholesterol stones*, containing more than 50% of crystalline cholesterol monohydrate. The rest are *pigment stones* composed predominantly of bilirubin calcium salts.[85]

Prevalence and Risk Factors. Certain populations are far more prone than others to develop gallstones. The major risk factors are listed in Table 18–9 and discussed below.

Cholesterol gallstones are more prevalent in the United States and western Europe and uncommon in developing countries. The prevalence rates of cholesterol gallstones approach 75% in Native Americans of the Pima, Hopi, and Navajo groups; pigment stones are rare in these populations. Pigment gallstones, the predominant type of gallstone in non-Western populations, arise primarily in the setting of bacterial infections of the biliary tree and parasitic infestations.

The risk factors most commonly associated with the *development of cholesterol stones* are:

- **Age and Sex.** The prevalence of cholesterol gallstones increases throughout life. In the United States, fewer than 5% to 6% of people under age 40 have stones, in contrast to 25% to 30% of those older than age 80. The prevalence in Caucasian women is about twice as high as in men. With both aging and gender, hypersecretion of biliary cholesterol seems to play the major role. In aging populations there is an increase in patients with gallstone disease associated with the metabolic syndrome and obesity.
- **Environmental Factors.** Estrogenic influence, including oral contraceptives and pregnancy, increases the expression of hepatic lipoprotein receptors and stimulates hepatic HMG-CoA reductase activity, enhancing both cholesterol uptake and biosynthesis, respectively. Clofibrate, used to

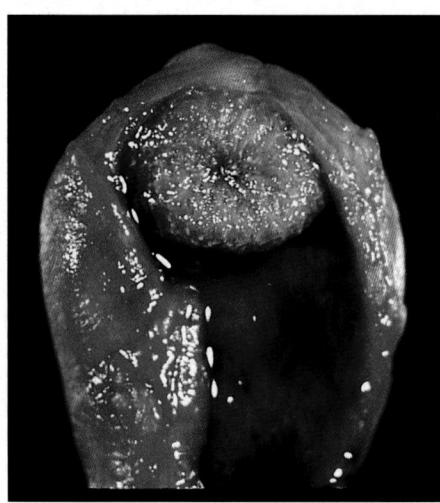

FIGURE 18–50 Phrygian cap of the gallbladder; the fundus is folded inward.

TABLE 18–9 Risk Factors for Gallstones

CHOLESTEROL STONES

Demography: northern Europeans, North and South Americans, Native Americans, Mexican-Americans
Advancing age
Female sex hormones
  Female gender
  Oral contraceptives
  Pregnancy
Obesity and metabolic syndrome
Rapid weight reduction
Gallbladder stasis
Inborn disorders of bile acid metabolism
Hyperlipidemia syndromes

PIGMENT STONES

Demography: Asians more than Westerners, rural more than urban
Chronic hemolytic syndromes
Biliary infection
Gastrointestinal disorders: ileal disease (e.g., Crohn disease), ileal resection or bypass, cystic fibrosis with pancreatic insufficiency

lower blood cholesterol, increases hepatic HMG-CoA reductase and decreases conversion of cholesterol to bile acids by reducing cholesterol 7-α-hydroxylase activity. The net result of these influences is excess biliary secretion of cholesterol. Obesity and rapid weight loss also are strongly associated with increased biliary cholesterol secretion.

● *Acquired Disorders.* Gallbladder stasis, either neurogenic or hormonal, fosters a local environment that is favorable for both cholesterol and pigment gallstone formation.

● *Hereditary Factors.* Much progress has been made recently in identifying susceptibility factors for cholesterol gallstones. These investigations have focused on genes encoding hepatocyte proteins that transport biliary lipids, known as ATP-binding cassette (ABC) transporters. In particular, a common variant of the protein heterodimer encoded by the *ABCG5* and *ABG2* genes that participates in biliary cholesterol secretion, confers a genetic risk for the development of cholesterol gallstones. The variant is known as D19H, and it is estimated that it may contribute 8% to 11% of the risk for the formation of cholesterol gallstones. (The odds ratios are 2–3 for heterozygous carriers of D19H, and 7 for homozygous carriers). Individuals with the D19H variant absorb less, but synthesize more, cholesterol, suggesting that HMG-CoA inhibitors (statins) may decrease the risk of gallstone formation in these individuals.

Pathogenesis of Cholesterol Stones. Cholesterol is rendered soluble in bile by aggregation with water-soluble bile salts and water-insoluble lecithins, both of which act as detergents. *When cholesterol concentrations exceed the solubilizing capacity of bile (supersaturation), cholesterol can no longer remain dispersed and nucleates into solid cholesterol monohydrate crystals.* Cholesterol gallstone formation involves four simultaneous conditions (Fig. 18–51): (1) The bile must be supersaturated with cholesterol; (2) hypomotility of the gallbladder promotes nucleation; (3) cholesterol nucleation in the bile is accelerated; (4) hypersecretion of mucus in the gallblad-

der traps the nucleated crystals, leading to their aggregation into stones.

Pathogenesis of Pigment Stones. Pigment gallstones are complex mixtures of abnormal insoluble calcium salts of unconjugated bilirubin along with inorganic calcium salts. Disorders that are associated with elevated levels of unconjugated bilirubin in bile such as hemolytic syndromes, severe ileal dysfunction (or bypass), and bacterial contamination of the biliary tree, increase the risk of developing pigment stones. Unconjugated bilirubin is normally a minor component of bile, but it increases when infection of the biliary tract leads to release of microbial β-glucuronidases, which hydrolyze bilirubin glucuronides. Thus, infection of the biliary tract with *Escherichia coli, Ascaris lumbricoides,* or the liver fluke *O.*

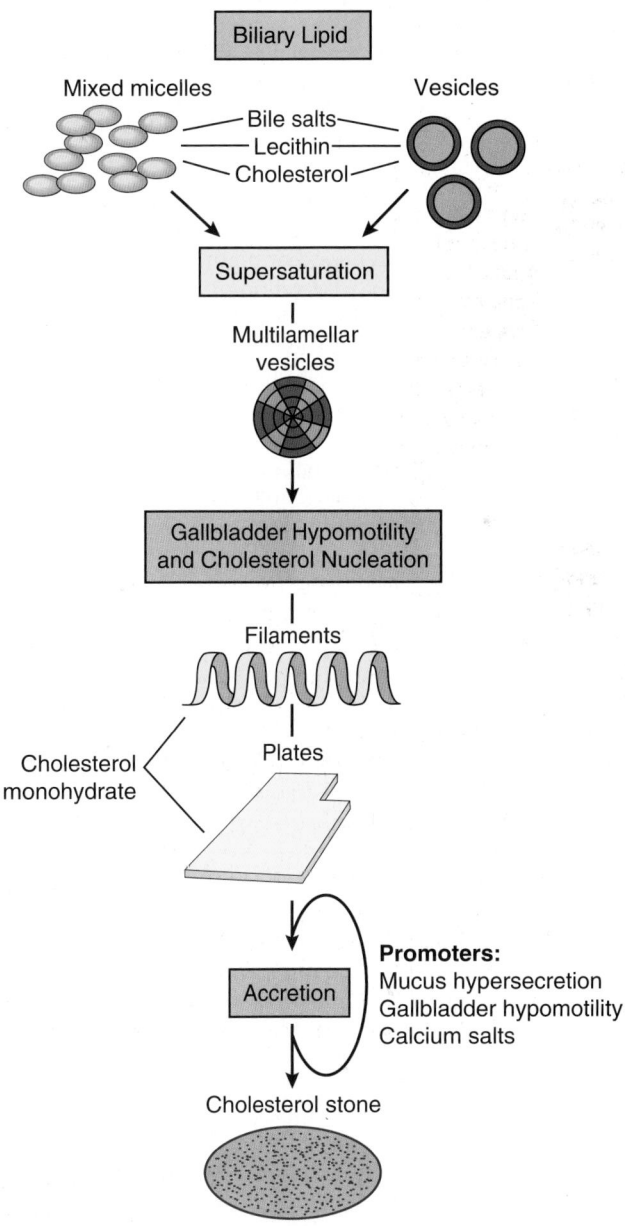

FIGURE 18–51 The four contributing factors for cholelithiasis: supersaturation, gallbladder hypomotility, crystal nucleation, and accretion within the gallbladder mucous layer.

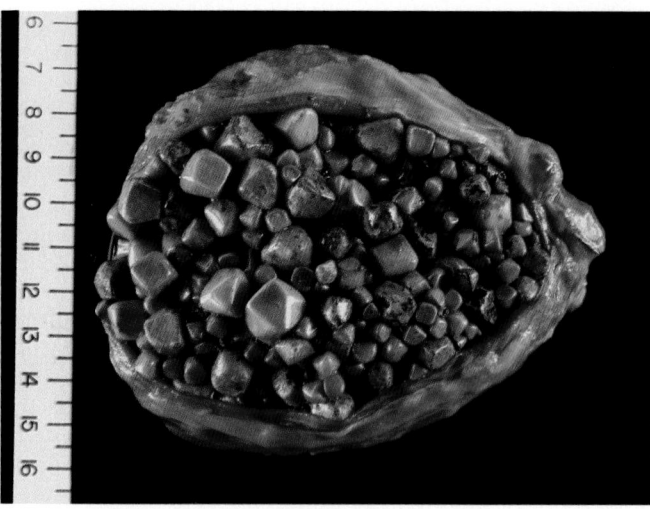

FIGURE 18–52 Cholesterol gallstones. Mechanical manipulation during laparoscopic cholecystectomy has caused fragmentation of several cholesterol gallstones, revealing interiors that are pigmented because of entrapped bile pigments. The gallbladder mucosa is reddened and irregular as a result of coexistent chronic cholecystitis.

sinensis, increases the likelihood of pigment stone formation. In hemolytic syndromes the secretion of conjugated bilirubin into the bile increases. However, because about 1% of bilirubin glucuronides are deconjugated in the biliary tree, the large amounts of unconjugated bilirubin produced may exceed its solubility.

> **Morphology. Cholesterol stones** arise exclusively in the gallbladder and are composed of cholesterol, ranging from 100% pure (which is rare) down to around 50%. **Pure cholesterol stones** are pale yellow, round to ovoid, and have a finely granular, hard external surface (Fig. 18–52), which on transection reveals a glistening radiating crystalline palisade. With increasing proportions of calcium carbonate, phosphates, and bilirubin, the stones show discoloration and may be lamellated and gray-white to black. Most often, multiple stones are present that range up to several centimeters in diameter. Rarely, there is a single much larger stone that may virtually fill the fundus. Surfaces of multiple stones may be rounded or faceted, because of tight apposition. **Stones composed largely of cholesterol are radiolucent; sufficient calcium carbonate is found in 10% to 20% of cholesterol stones to render them radiopaque.**
>
> **Pigment gallstones** are trivially classified as "black" and "brown." In general, black pigment stones are found in sterile gallbladder bile, and brown stones are found in infected intrahepatic or extrahepatic ducts. "Black" pigment stones contain oxidized polymers of the calcium salts of unconjugated bilirubin, small amounts of calcium carbonate, calcium phosphate, and mucin glycoprotein, and some cholesterol monohydrate crystals. "Brown" pigment stones contain pure calcium salts of unconjugated bilirubin,

mucin glycoprotein, a substantial cholesterol fraction, and calcium salts of palmitate and stearate. The black stones are rarely greater than 1.5 cm in diameter, are almost invariably present in great number (with an inverse relationship between size and number; Fig. 18–53), and may crumble to the touch. Their contours are usually spiculated and molded. Brown stones tend to be laminated and soft and may have a soaplike or greasy consistency. Because of calcium carbonates and phosphates, **approximately 50% to 75% of black stones are radiopaque.** Brown stones, which contain calcium soaps, are radiolucent. Mucin glycoproteins constitute the scaffolding and interparticle cement of all stones, whether pigment or cholesterol.

Clinical Features. Gallstones may be present for decades before symptoms develop, and 70% to 80% of patients remain asymptomatic throughout their lives. It has been estimated that asymptomatic patients convert to symptomatic ones at the rate of 1% to 4% per year, and the risk diminishes with time. Prominent among symptoms is *biliary pain*, which tends to be excruciating and constant or "colicky" (spasmodic), as a result of the obstructive nature of gallstones in the biliary tree and perhaps in the gallbladder itself. Inflammation of the gallbladder (cholecystitis, discussed below), in association with stones, also generates pain. More severe complications include empyema, perforation, fistulas, inflammation of the biliary tree (cholangitis), and obstructive cholestasis or pancreatitis with ensuing problems. The larger the calculi, the less likely they are to enter the cystic or common ducts to produce obstruction; it is the very small stones, or "gravel," that are the more dangerous. Occasionally a large stone may erode directly into an adjacent loop of small bowel, generating intestinal obstruction ("gallstone ileus" or Bouveret's syndrome). Most notable is the *increased risk for carcinoma* of the gallbladder, discussed later.

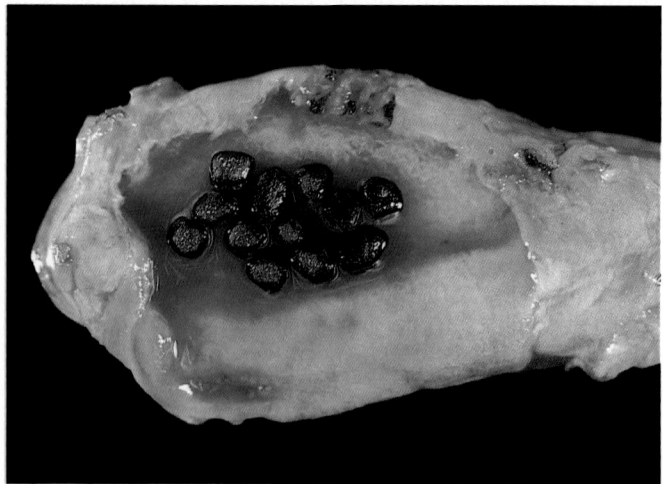

FIGURE 18–53 Pigment gallstones. Several faceted black gallstones are present in this otherwise unremarkable gallbladder from a patient with a mechanical mitral valve prosthesis, leading to chronic intravascular hemolysis.

CHOLECYSTITIS

Inflammation of the gallbladder may be acute, chronic, or acute superimposed on chronic. It almost always occurs in association with gallstones. In the United States cholecystitis is one of the most common indications for abdominal surgery. Its epidemiologic distribution closely parallels that of gallstones.

Acute Cholecystitis

Acute calculous cholecystitis is an acute inflammation of the gallbladder, precipitated 90% of the time by obstruction of the neck or cystic duct.[86] It is the primary complication of gallstones and the most common reason for emergency cholecystectomy. Cholecystitis without gallstones called acalculous cholecystitis may occur in severely ill patients and accounts for about 10% of patients with cholecystitis.[87]

Pathogenesis. Acute *calculous cholecystitis* results from chemical irritation and inflammation of the obstructed gallbladder. The action of mucosal phospholipases hydrolyzes luminal lecithins to toxic lysolecithins. The normally protective glycoprotein mucus layer is disrupted, exposing the mucosal epithelium to the direct detergent action of bile salts. Prostaglandins released within the wall of the distended gallbladder contribute to mucosal and mural inflammation. Gallbladder dysmotility develops; distention and increased intraluminal pressure compromise blood flow to the mucosa. *These events occur in the absence of bacterial infection*; only later in the course may bacterial contamination develop. Acute calculous cholecystitis frequently develops in diabetic patients who have symptomatic gallstones.

Acute *acalculous cholecystitis* is thought to result from ischemia. The cystic artery is an end artery with essentially no collateral circulation. Contributing factors may include inflammation and edema of the wall compromising blood flow, gallbladder stasis, and accumulation of microcrystals of cholesterol (biliary sludge), viscous bile, and gallbladder mucus, causing cystic duct obstruction in the absence of frank stone formation. It occurs in patients who are hospitalized for unrelated conditions. Risk factors for acute acalculous cholecystitis include: (1) sepsis with hypotension and multisystem organ failure; (2) immunosuppression; (3) major trauma and burns; (4) diabetes mellitus; and (5) infections.

> **Morphology.** In **acute cholecystitis** the gallbladder is usually enlarged and tense, and it may assume a bright red or blotchy, violaceous to green-black discoloration, imparted by subserosal hemorrhages. The serosal covering is frequently layered by fibrin and, in severe cases, by a definite suppurative, coagulated exudate. There are no specific morphologic differences between acute acalculous and calculous cholecystitis, except for the absence of macroscopic stones in the acalculous form. In calculous cholecystitis, an obstructing stone is usually present in the neck of the gallbladder or the cystic duct. The gallbladder lumen may contain one or more stones and is filled with a cloudy or turbid bile that may contain large amounts of fibrin, pus, and hemorrhage. When the contained exudate is virtually pure pus, the condition is referred to as **empyema of the gallbladder**. In mild cases the gallbladder wall is thickened, edematous, and hyperemic. In more severe cases it is transformed into a green-black necrotic organ, termed **gangrenous cholecystitis**, with small-to-large perforations. The invasion of gas-forming organisms, notably clostridia and coliforms, may cause an acute "emphysematous" cholecystitis. The inflammatory reactions are not histologically distinctive and consist of the usual patterns of acute inflammation.

Clinical Features. An attack of acute cholecystitis begins with progressive right upper quadrant or epigastric pain, frequently associated with mild fever, anorexia, tachycardia, sweating, nausea, and vomiting. Most patients are free of jaundice; the presence of hyperbilirubinemia suggests obstruction of the common bile duct. Mild to moderate leukocytosis may be accompanied by mild elevations in serum alkaline phosphatase values.

Individuals with acute calculous cholecystitis usually, but not always, have experienced previous episodes of pain. *Acute calculous cholecystitis may appear with remarkable suddenness and constitute an acute surgical emergency or may present with mild symptoms that resolve without medical intervention.* In the absence of medical attention, the attack usually subsides in 7 to 10 days and frequently within 24 hours. However, as many as 25% of patients progressively develop more severe symptoms, requiring immediate surgical intervention. Recurrence is common in patients who recover.

Clinical symptoms of acute acalculous cholecystitis tend to be more insidious, since symptoms are obscured by the underlying conditions precipitating the attacks. A higher proportion of patients have no symptoms referable to the gallbladder; diagnosis therefore rests on a high index of suspicion. In the severely ill patient, early recognition of the condition is crucial, since failure to do so almost ensures a fatal outcome. As a result of either delay in diagnosis or the disease itself, the incidence of gangrene and perforation is much higher in acalculous than in calculous cholecystitis. In rare instances, primary bacterial infection can give rise to acute acalculous cholecystitis, including agents such as *Salmonella typhi* and staphylococci. A more indolent form of acute acalculous cholecystitis may occur in the outpatient population in the setting of systemic vasculitis, severe atherosclerotic ischemic disease in the elderly, in patients with AIDS, and with biliary tract infection.

Chronic Cholecystitis

Chronic cholecystitis may be a sequel to repeated bouts of mild to severe acute cholecystitis, but in many instances it develops in the apparent absence of antecedent attacks. Since it is associated with *cholelithiasis in more than 90% of cases*, the patient populations are the same as those for gallstones. The evolution of chronic cholecystitis is obscure, in that it is not clear that gallstones play a direct role in the initiation of inflammation or the development of pain, particularly since chronic acalculous cholecystitis shows symptoms and histology similar to those of the calculous form. Rather, supersaturation of bile predisposes to both chronic inflammation and, in most instances, stone formation. Microorganisms, usually *E. coli* and enterococci, can be cultured from the bile in about one third of cases. Unlike acute calculous cholecystitis, obstruction of gallbladder outflow is not a requisite. Nevertheless, the symptoms of calculous chronic cholecystitis are similar to those of the acute form and range from *biliary colic* to indolent *right upper quadrant pain* and *epigastric distress*. Since most gallbladders that are removed at elective surgery for gallstones show features of chronic cholecystitis, one must conclude that biliary symptoms often emerge following long-term coexistence of gallstones and low-grade inflammation.

Morphology. The morphologic changes in chronic cholecystitis are extremely variable and sometimes minimal. The serosa is usually smooth and glistening but may be dulled by subserosal fibrosis. Dense fibrous adhesions may remain as sequelae of preexistent acute inflammation. On sectioning, the wall is variably thickened, and has an opaque gray-white appearance. In the uncomplicated case the lumen contains fairly clear, green-yellow, mucoid bile and usually stones (Fig. 18–54). The mucosa itself is generally preserved.

On histologic examination the degree of inflammation is variable. In the mildest cases, only scattered lymphocytes, plasma cells, and macrophages are found in the mucosa and in the subserosal fibrous tissue. In more advanced cases there is marked subepithelial and subserosal fibrosis, accompanied by mononuclear cell infiltration. Reactive proliferation of the mucosa and fusion of the mucosal folds may give rise to buried crypts of epithelium within the gallbladder wall. Outpouchings of the mucosal epithelium through the wall (**Rokitansky-Aschoff sinuses**) may be quite prominent. Superimposition of acute inflammatory changes implies acute exacerbation of an already chronically injured gallbladder.

In rare instances extensive dystrophic calcification within the gallbladder wall may yield a **porcelain gallbladder**, notable for a markedly increased incidence of associated cancer. **Xanthogranulomatous cholecystitis** is also a rare condition in which the gallbladder has a massively thickened wall, is shrunken, nodular, and chronically inflamed with foci of necrosis and hemorrhage. Finally, an atrophic, chronically obstructed gallbladder may contain only clear secretions, a condition known as **hydrops of the gallbladder**.

Clinical Features. Chronic cholecystitis does not have the striking manifestations of the acute forms and is usually characterized by recurrent attacks of either steady or colicky epigastric or right upper quadrant pain. Nausea, vomiting, and intolerance for fatty foods are frequent accompaniments.

Diagnosis of both acute and chronic cholecystitis is important because of the following complications:

- Bacterial superinfection with cholangitis or sepsis
- Gallbladder perforation and local abscess formation
- Gallbladder rupture with diffuse peritonitis
- Biliary enteric (cholecystenteric) fistula, with drainage of bile into adjacent organs, entry of air and bacteria into the biliary tree, and potentially, gallstone-induced intestinal obstruction (ileus)
- Aggravation of preexisting medical illness, with cardiac, pulmonary, renal, or liver decompensation

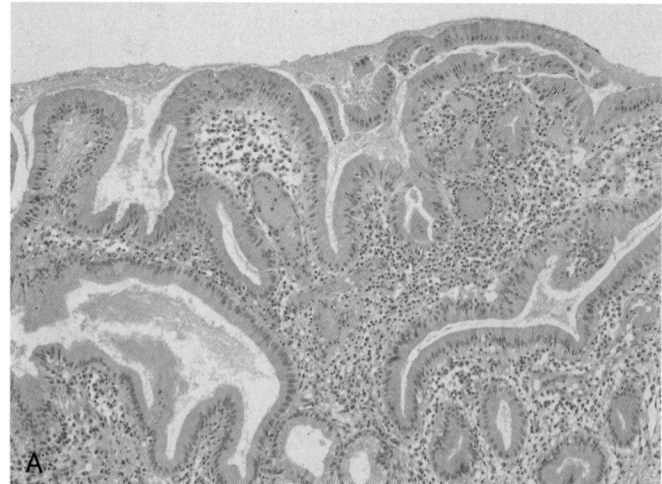
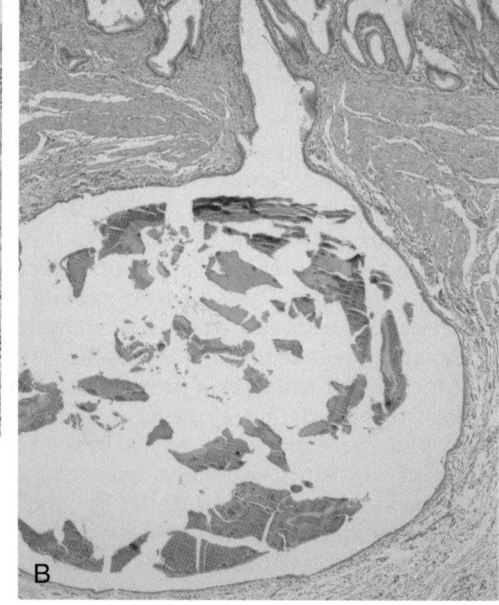

FIGURE 18–54 Chronic cholecystitis with Rokitansky-Aschoff sinus. **A,** The gallbladder mucosa is infiltrated by inflammatory cells. **B,** Outpouching of the mucosa through the wall forms Rokitansky-Aschoff sinus (contains bile).

• Porcelain gallbladder, with increased risk of cancer, although surveys of this risk have yielded widely discrepant frequencies.

Disorders of the Extrahepatic Bile Ducts

CHOLEDOCHOLITHIASIS AND ASCENDING CHOLANGITIS

These conditions are considered together, since they frequently go hand in hand. *Choledocholithiasis is defined as the presence of stones within the bile ducts of the biliary tree*, as opposed to cholelithiasis (stones in the gallbladder). In Asia, there is a much higher incidence of primary stone formation within the biliary tree than in Western countries. The stones are usually pigmented and associated with biliary tract infections, as noted earlier in the discussion of gallstones. Choledocholithiasis may be asymptomatic or may cause symptoms from (1) obstruction, (2) pancreatitis, (3) cholangitis, (4) hepatic abscess, (5) secondary biliary cirrhosis, and (6) acute calculous cholecystitis.

Cholangitis is the term used for bacterial infection of the bile ducts. Cholangitis can result from any lesion that creates obstruction to bile flow, most commonly choledocholithiasis and biliary strictures. Less common causes include indwelling stents or catheters, tumors, acute pancreatitis, and rarely, fungi, viruses, or parasites. Bacteria most likely enter the biliary tract through the sphincter of Oddi; infection of intrahepatic biliary radicles is termed *ascending cholangitis*. The bacteria are usually enteric gram-negative aerobes such as *E. coli, Klebsiella, Interococcus*, or *Enterobacter. Clostridium* and *Bacteroides* are usually present as a mixed infection. Cholangitis usually presents with fever, chills, abdominal pain, and jaundice, accompanied by acute inflammation of the wall of the bile ducts with entry of neutrophils into the luminal space. The most severe form of cholangitis is suppurative cholangitis, in which purulent bile fills and distends bile ducts. Since sepsis rather than cholestasis tends to dominate the picture, prompt diagnostic evaluation and intervention are imperative in these seriously ill patients.

BILIARY ATRESIA

The infant presenting with neonatal cholestasis has been discussed already in the context of intrahepatic disorders. A major contributor to neonatal cholestasis is *biliary atresia*, representing one third of infants with neonatal cholestasis and occurring in approximately 1:12,000 live births. *Biliary atresia is defined as a complete or partial obstruction of the lumen of the extrahepatic biliary tree within the first 3 months of life.* It is characterized by progressive inflammation and fibrosis of intrahepatic or extrahepatic bile ducts.[88] Biliary atresia is the single most frequent cause of death from liver disease in early childhood and accounts for 50% to 60% of children referred for liver transplantation, as a result of the rapidly progressing secondary biliary cirrhosis.

Pathogenesis. Two major forms of biliary atresia are recognized; they are based on the presumed timing of luminal obliteration. The *fetal form* accounts for as many as 20% of cases and is commonly associated with other anomalies resulting from ineffective establishment of laterality of thoracic and abdominal organ development. These include malrotation of abdominal viscera, interrupted inferior vena cava, polysplenia, and congenital heart disease. The presumed cause is aberrant intrauterine development of the extrahepatic biliary tree. Much more common is the *perinatal form* of biliary atresia, in which a presumed normally developed biliary tree is destroyed following birth. Although the etiology of perinatal biliary atresia remains unknown, viral infection and autoimmunity presumably play a critical role in the pathogenesis. Reovirus, rotavirus, and cytomegalovirus have been implicated in different cases.[89]

Morphology. The salient features of biliary atresia include inflammation and fibrosing stricture of the hepatic or common bile ducts, periductular inflammation of intrahepatic bile ducts, and progressive destruction of the intrahepatic biliary tree. On liver biopsy, florid features of extrahepatic biliary obstruction are evident in about two thirds of cases, that is, marked bile ductular proliferation, portal tract edema and fibrosis, and parenchymal cholestasis. In the remainder, inflammatory destruction of intrahepatic ducts leads to paucity of bile ducts and absence of edema or bile ductular proliferation on liver biopsy. When biliary atresia is unrecognized or uncorrected, cirrhosis develops within 3 to 6 months of birth.

There is considerable variability in the anatomy of biliary atresia. When the disease is limited to the common duct (type I) or hepatic bile ducts (type II) with patent proximal branches, the disease is surgically correctable (Kasai procedure). Unfortunately, 90% of patients have type III biliary atresia, in which there also is obstruction of bile ducts at or above the porta hepatis. These cases are noncorrectable, since there are no patent bile ducts amenable to surgical anastomosis. Moreover, in most patients, bile ducts within the liver are initially patent but are progressively destroyed.

Clinical Features. Infants with biliary atresia present with neonatal cholestasis, discussed earlier. These infants exhibit normal birth weight and postnatal weight gain, a slight female preponderance, and the progression of initially normal stools to acholic stools as the disease evolves. At the time of presentation, serum bilirubin values are usually in the range of 6 to 12 mg/dL, with only moderately elevated aminotransferase and alkaline phosphatase levels. The success of surgical resection and bypass of the biliary tree is limited by subsequent bacterial contamination of the intrahepatic biliary tree and intrahepatic progression of the disease. Liver transplantation with accompanying donor bile ducts remains the primary hope for salvage of these young patients. Without surgical intervention, death usually occurs within 2 years of birth.

CHOLEDOCHAL CYSTS

Choledochal cysts are congenital dilations of the common bile duct, presenting most often in children before age 10 with the nonspecific symptoms of jaundice and/or recurrent abdominal pain that are typical of biliary colic.[90] Approximately 20% of cases become symptomatic only in adulthood; these sometimes occur in conjunction with cystic dilation of the intrahepatic biliary tree (Caroli disease, discussed earlier). The female-to-male ratio is 3:1 to 4:1. These uncommon cysts may take the form of segmental or cylindric dilation of the common bile duct, diverticuli of the extrahepatic ducts, or choledochoceles, which are cystic lesions that protrude into the duodenal lumen. Choledochal cysts predispose to stone formation, stenosis and stricture, pancreatitis, and obstructive biliary complications within the liver. In the older patient the risk of bile duct carcinoma is elevated.

Tumors

Although heterotopic tissues and carcinoids, fibromas, myomas, neuromas, hemangiomas, and their malignant counterparts have been described in the biliary tract, the neoplasms of primary clinical importance are those derived from the epithelium lining the biliary tree. Adenomas are benign epithelial tumors, representing localized neoplastic growth of the lining epithelium. Adenomas are classified as tubular, papillary, and tubulopapillary and are similar to adenomas found elsewhere in the alimentary tract. *Inflammatory polyps* are sessile mucosal projections with a surface stroma infiltrated with chronic inflammatory cells and lipid-laden macrophages. These lesions may be difficult to differentiate from neoplasms on imaging studies. *Adenomyosis* of the gallbladder is characterized by hyperplasia of the muscle layer, containing intramural hyperplastic glands.

Malignant tumors of the extrahepatic bile ducts have already been discussed under "Cholangiocarcinomas."

CARCINOMA OF THE GALLBLADDER

Carcinoma of the gallbladder is the most common malignancy of the extrahepatic biliary tract. It is slightly more common in women and occurs most frequently in the seventh decade of life. The incidence in the United States is 1 in 50,000. Only rarely is it discovered at a resectable stage, and the mean 5-year survival rate has remained for many years at about 5% to 12% despite surgical intervention. The most important risk factor associated with gallbladder carcinoma is gallstones (cholelithiasis), which are present in 95% of cases.[91] However, it should be noted that only 0.5% of patients with gallstones develop gallbladder cancer after twenty or more years. In Asia, where pyogenic and parasitic diseases of the biliary tree are common, the coexistence of gallstones in gallbladder cancer is much lower. Presumably, gallbladders containing stones or infectious agents develop cancer as a result of irritative trauma and chronic inflammation. Carcinogenic derivatives of bile acids are believed to play a role.

> **Morphology.** Carcinomas of the gallbladder show two patterns of growth: **infiltrating** and **exophytic**. The infiltrating pattern is more common and usually appears as a poorly defined area of diffuse thickening and induration of the gallbladder wall that may cover

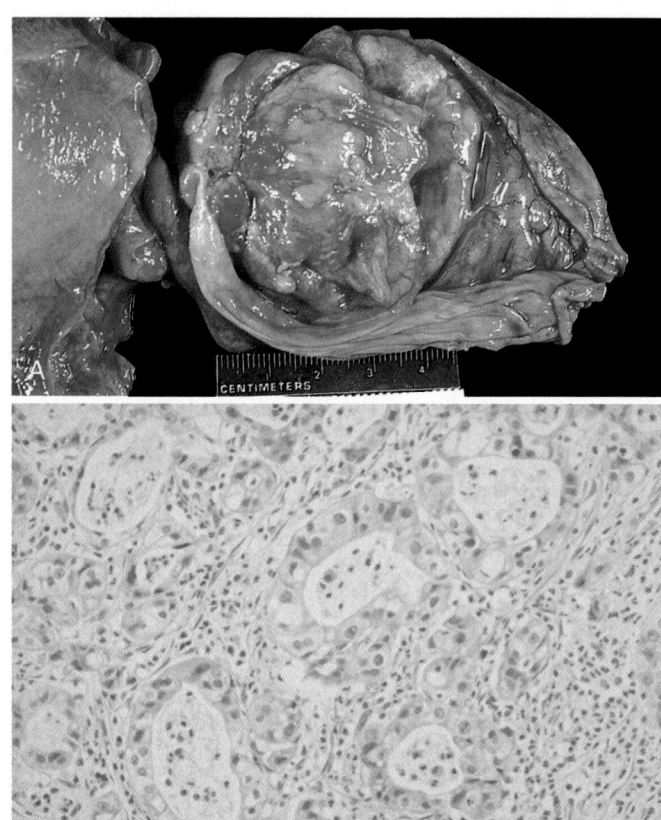

FIGURE 18–55 Gallbladder adenocarcinoma. **A,** The opened gallbladder contains a large, exophytic tumor that virtually fills the lumen. **B,** Malignant glandular structures are present within a densely fibrotic gallbladder wall.

several square centimeters or may involve the entire gallbladder. Deep ulceration can cause direct penetration of the gallbladder wall or fistula formation to adjacent viscera into which the neoplasm has grown. These tumors are scirrhous and have a very firm consistency. The exophytic pattern grows into the lumen as an irregular, cauliflower mass but at the same time invades the underlying wall. The luminal portion may be necrotic, hemorrhagic, and ulcerated (Fig. 18–55A). The most common sites of involvement are the fundus and the neck; about 20% involve the lateral walls.

Most carcinomas of the gallbladder are adenocarcinomas. They may be derived from adenomas, which are present in 1% of cholecystectomy specimens. Some of the carcinomas are papillary in architecture and are well to moderately differentiated; others are infiltrative and poorly differentiated to undifferentiated (Fig. 18–55B). About 5% are squamous cell carcinomas or have adenosquamous differentiation. A minority may show carcinoid or a variety of mesenchymal features (carcinosarcoma). Papillary tumors generally have a better prognosis than other tumors. By the time these neoplasms are discovered, **most**

have invaded the liver centrifugally, and many have extended to the cystic duct and adjacent bile ducts and portal-hepatic lymph nodes. The peritoneum, gastrointestinal tract, and lungs are common sites of seeding.

Clinical Features. Preoperative diagnosis of carcinoma of the gallbladder is the exception rather than the rule, occurring in fewer than 20% of patients. Presenting symptoms are insidious and typically indistinguishable from those associated with cholelithiasis: abdominal pain, jaundice, anorexia, and nausea and vomiting. Early detection of the tumor may be possible in patients who develop a palpable gallbladder and acute cholecystitis before extension of the tumor into adjacent structures, or when the carcinoma is an incidental finding during a cholecystectomy for symptomatic gallstones. Surgical resection, often including adjacent liver, is the only effective treatment, when possible, but chemotherapy regimens are also used.

REFERENCES

1. MacSween R et al.: Developmental anatomy and normal structure. In MacSween R (ed): Pathology of the Liver, 4th ed. 2002.
2. Crawford JM: Development of the intrahepatic biliary tree. Semin Liver Dis 22:213, 2002.
3. Lim YS, Kim WR: The global impact of hepatic fibrosis and end-stage liver disease. Clin Liver Dis 12:733, 2008.
4. Lee WM: Etiologies of acute liver failure. Semin Liver Dis 28:142, 2008.
5. Fontana RJ: Acute liver failure due to drugs. Semin Liver Dis 28:175, 2008.
6. Haussinger D, Schliess F: Pathogenetic mechanisms of hepatic encephalopathy. Gut 57:1156, 2008.
7. Munoz SJ: The hepatorenal syndrome. Med Clin N Am 92:813, 2008.
8. Rodriguez-Rosin R, Krowka MJ: Hepatopulmonary syndrome—a liver induced lung vascular disease. N Engl J Med 358:2378, 2008.
9. Friedman SE: Mechanisms of hepatic fibrogenesis. Gastroenterology 134:1655, 2008.
10. Sanyal AJ et al.: Portal hypertension and its complications. Gastroenterology 134:1715, 2008.
11. Schuppan D, Afdhal NH: Liver cirrhosis. Lancet 371:838, 2008.
12. Desmet VJ, Roskams T: Cirrhosis reversal: a duel between dogma and myth. J Hepatol 40:860, 2004.
13. Iwakiri Y, Groszmann RJ: Vascular endothelial dysfunction in cirrhosis. J Hepatol 46:927, 2007.
14. Bosch J: Vascular deterioration in cirrhosis: The big picture. J Clin Gastroenterol 41:S247, 2007.
15. Servedio V et al.: Spectrum of *UGT1A1* mutations in Crigler-Najjar (CN) syndrome patients: identification of twelve novel alleles and genotype-phenotype correlation. Hum Mutat 25:325, 2005.
16. Kartenbeck J et al.: Absence of the canalicular isoform of the *MRP* gene-encoded conjugate export pump from the hepatocytes in Dubin-Johnson syndrome. Hepatology 23:1061, 1996.
17. O'Leary JG, Pratt DS: Cholestasis and cholestatic syndromes. Curr Opin Gastroenterol 23:232, 2007.
18. Paulusma CC et al.: ATP8B1 requires an accessory protein for endoplasmic reticulum exit and plasma membrane lipid flippase activity. Hepatology 47:268, 2008.
19. Suchy FJ, Ananthanarayanan M: Bile salt excretory pump: biology and pathobiology. J Pediatr Gastroenterol Nutr 43 (Suppl 1):S10, 2006.
20. Sundaram SS, Sokol RJ: The multiple facets of ABCB4 (MDR3) deficiency. Current Treat Options Gastroenterol 101:495, 2007.
21. Feigelstock D et al.: The human homolog of HAVcr-1 codes for a hepatitis A virus cellular receptor. J Virol 72:6621, 1998.
22. Martin A, Lemon SM: Hepatitis A virus: from discovery to vaccines. Hepatology 43:S164, 2006.
23. Andre FE: Universal mass vaccination against hepatitis A. Curr Top Microbiol Immunol 304:95, 2006.
24. Pungpapong S et al.: Natural history of hepatitis B infection: an update for clinicians. May Clin Proc 82:967, 2007.
25. Blumberg BS et al.: A "new" antigen in leukemia sera. JAMA 191:541, 1965.
26. Block TM et al.: Molecular virology of hepatitis B virus for clinicians. Clin Liver Dis 11:685, 2007.
27. Bertoletti A, Gehring AJ: The immune response during hepatitis B virus infection. J Gen Virol 87:1439, 2006.
28. Pawlotsky JM: Hepatitis C virus population dynamics during infection. Curr Top Microbiol Immunol 299:261, 2006.
29. Missiha SB et al.: Disease progression in chronic hepatitis C: modifiable and nonmodifiable factors. Gastroenterology 134:1699, 2008.
30. Koytak ES, Yurdaydin C, Glenn JS: Hepatitis D. Current Treat Options Gastroenterol 10:456, 2007.
31. Purcell RH, Emerson SU: Hepatitis E: an emerging awareness of an old disease. J Hepatol 48:494, 2008.
32. Williams CF et al.: Persistent GB virus C infection and survival in HIV-infected men. N Engl J Med 350:981, 2004.
33. Yim HJ, Lok AS: Natural history of chronic hepatitis B virus infection: what we knew in 1981 and what we know in 2005. Hepatology 43:S173, 2006.
34. Weber R, et al.: Liver-related deaths in persons infected with the human immunodeficiency virus: the D:A:D study. Arch Intern Med 166:1632, 2006.
35. Goodman ZD: Grading and staging systems for inflammation and fibrosis in chronic liver diseases. J Hepatol 47:598, 2007.
36. Leifeld L et al.: Intrahepatic activation of caspases in human fulminant hepatic failure. Liver Int 26:872, 2006.
37. Krawitt EL: Autoimmune hepatitis. N Engl J Med 354:54, 2006.
38. Czaja AJ: Autoimmune liver disease. Curr Opin Gastroenterol 23:255, 2007.
39. Arundel C, Lewis JH: Drug-induced liver disease in 2006. Curr Opin Gastroenterol 23:244, 2007.
40. Bleibel W et al.: Drug-induced liver injury: review article. Dig Dis Sci 52:2463, 2007.
41. Aithal GP: Dangerous liaisons: drug, host and the environment. J Hepatol 46:995, 2007.
42. Gramenzi A et al.: Review article: alcoholic liver disease—pathophysiological aspects and risk factors. Aliment Pharmacol Ther 24:1151, 2006.
43. Ongi JP, Younossi ZM: Epidemiology and natural history of NAFLD and NASH. Clin Liv Dis 11:1, 2007.
44. Yeh MM, Brunt EM: Pathology of non-alcoholic fatty liver disease. Am J Clin Pathol 128:837, 2007.
45. Farrell GC, Larter CZ: Nonalcoholic fatty liver disease: from steatosis to cirrhosis. Hepatology 43:S99, 2006.
46. Greenfield V, Cheung O, Sanyal AJ: Recent advances in non-alcoholic fatty liver. Curr Opin Gastroenterol 24:320, 2008.
47. Pietrangelo A: Hereditary hemochromatosis. Annu Rev Nutr 26:251, 2006.
48. Du X et al.: The serine protease TMPRSS6 is required to sense iron deficiency. Science 320:1088, 2008.
49. Whitington PF: Neonatal hemochromatosis: a congenital alloimmune hepatitis. Semin Liver Dis 27:243, 2007.
50. Gordeuk VR et al.: Iron overload in Africans and African-Americans and a common mutation in the *SCL40A1* (ferroportin 1) gene. Blood Cells Mol Dis 31:299, 2003.
51. Pfeiffer RF: Wilson's disease. Semin Neurol 27:123, 2007.
52. Ioachimescu OC, Stoller JK: A review of alpha-1 antitrypsin deficiency. COPD 2:263, 2005.
53. Perlmutter DH: Pathogenesis of chronic liver injury and hepatocellular carcinoma in alpha-1-antitrypsin deficiency. Pediatr Res 60:233, 2006.
54. Kaplan MM, Gershwin ME: Primary biliary cirrhosis. N Engl J Med 353:1261, 2005.
55. Jones DE: Pathogenesis of primary biliary cirrhosis. Gut 56:1615, 2007.
56. Abe M, Onji M: Natural history of primary biliary cirrhosis. Hepatology Res 38:639, 2008.
57. Weismüller TJ et al.: The challenges in primary sclerosing cholangitis—Aetiopathogenesis, autoimmunity, management and malignancy. J Hepatol 48:S38, 2008.
58. Maggs JL, Champamn RW: An update on primary sclerosing cholangitis. Curr Opin Gastroenter 24:377, 2008.

59. Nakanuma Y, Zen Y: Pathology and immunopathology of immunoglobulin G4-related sclerosing cholangitis: the latest addition to the sclerosing cholangitis family. Hepatol Res 37 (Suppl 3):S478, 2007.

60. Everson GT, et al.: Advances in the management of polycycstic liver disease. Expert Rev Gastroenterol Hepatol 2:563, 2008.

61. Masyuk T, LaRusso N: Polycystic liver disease: New insights into disease pathogenesis. Hepatology 43:906, 2006.

62. Gunay-Aygun M et al.: Autosomal recessive polycystic kidney disease and congenital hepatic fibrosis: summary statement of a first National Institutes of Health/Office of Rare Diseases conference. J Pediatr 149:159, 2006.

63. Warthen DM et al.: Jagged1 (*JAG1*) mutations in Alagille syndrome: increasing the mutation detection rate. Hum Mutat 27:436, 2006.

64. Chawla Y, Dhiman RK: Intrahepatic portal venopathy and related disorders of the liver. Semin Liv Dis 208:270, 2008.

65. Pulliainen AT, Dehio C: *Bartonella henselae:* Subversion of vascular endothelial cell functions by translocated bacterial effector proteins. Int J Biochem Cell Biol 2008, epub.

66. DeLeve LD: Hepatic microvasculature in liver injury. Semin Liver Dis 27:390, 2007.

67. Demetris A et al.: Update of the International Banff Schema for Liver Allograft Rejection: working recommendations for the histopathologic staging and reporting of chronic rejection. An International Panel. Hepatology 31:792, 2000.

68. Hay JE: Liver disease in pregnancy. Hepatology 47:1067, 2008.

69. Baxter JK, Weinstein L: HELLP syndrome: the state of the art. Obstet Gynecol Surv 59:838, 2004.

70. Browning MF et al.: Fetal fatty acid oxidation defects and maternal liver disease in pregnancy. Obstet Gynecol 107:115, 2006.

71. Mallet V et al.: Nodular regenerative hyperplasia is a new cause of chronic liver disease in HIV-infected patients. AIDS 21:187, 2007.

72. Zucman-Rossi J et al.: Genotype-phenotype correlation in hepatocellular adenoma: new classification and relationship with HCC. Hepatology 43:515, 2006.

73. Reznik Y et al.: Hepatocyte nuclear factor-1 alpha gene inactivation: cosegregation between liver adenomatosis and diabetes phenotypes in two maturity-onset diabetes of the young (MODY)3 families. J Clin Endocrinol Metab 89:1476, 2004.

74. Linabery AM, Ross JA: Trends in childhood cancer incidence in the U.S. (1992–2004). Cancer 112:416, 2008.

75. Cairo S et al.: Hepatic stem-like phenotype and interplay of Wnt/beta catenin and Myc signaling in aggressive childhood liver cancer. Cancer Cell 9:14, 2008.

76. Adesina AM et al.: FOXG1 is overexpressed in hepatoblastoma. Hum Pathol 38:400, 2007.

77. Parkin DM et al.: Global cancer statistics, 2002. CA Cancer J Clin 55:74, 2005.

78. Levrero M: Viral hepatitis and liver cancer: the case of hepatitis C. Oncogene 25:3834, 2006.

79. Ni YH et al.: Two decades of universal hepatitis B vaccination in Taiwan: impact and implication for future strategies. Gastroenterology 132:1287, 2007.

80. Torbenson M: Review of the clinicopathologic features of fibrolamellar carcinoma. Adv Anat Pathol 14:217, 2007.

81. Lee JS et al.: A novel prognostic subtype of human hepatocellular carcinoma derived from hepatic progenitor cells. Nat Med 12:410, 2006.

82. Llovet JM et al.: Design and endpoints of clinical trials in hepatocellular carcinoma. J Nat Cancer Inst 100:698, 2008.

83. Llovet JM et al.: Sorafenib in advanced hepatocellular carcinoma. N Eng J Med 359:378, 2008.

84. Gores GJ, Blechacz B: Cholangiocarcinoma: Advances in pathogenesis, diagnosis and treatment. Hepatology 48:308, 2008.

85. Lammert F, Miguel JF: Gallstone disease: from genes to evidence based therapy. J Hepatol 48:S124, 2008.

86. Strasberg SM: Acute calculous cholecystitis. New Engl J Med 358:2804, 2008.

87. Elwood DR: Cholecystitis. Surg Clin N Am 88:1241, 2008.

88. Petersen C: Pathogenesis and treatment opportunities for biliary atresia. Clin Liver Dis 10:73, vi, 2006.

89. Mack CL: The pathogenesis of biliary atresia: evidence for a virus-induced autoimmune disease. Semin Liver Dis 27:233, 2007.

90. Kerkar N et al.: The hepatic fibrocystic diseases. Clin Liver Dis 10:55, v–vi, 2006.

91. Randi G et al.: Gallbladder cancer worldwide: geographical distribution and risk factors. Int J Cancer 118:1591, 2006.

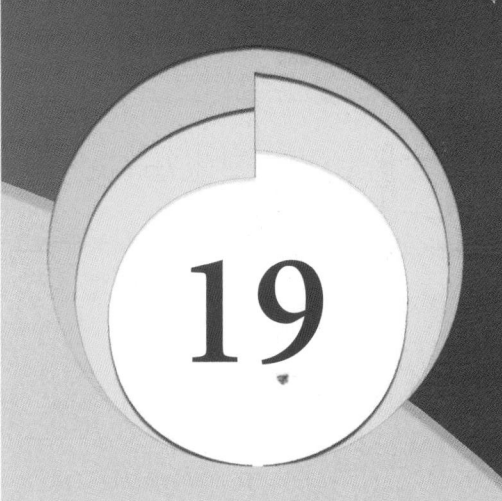

19

The Pancreas

RALPH H. HRUBAN · CHRISTINE IACOBUZIO-DONAHUE

Congenital Anomalies
  Agenesis
  Pancreas Divisum
  Annular Pancreas
  Ectopic Pancreas
Pancreatitis
  Acute Pancreatitis
  Chronic Pancreatitis
Non-Neoplastic Cysts
	Congenital Cysts
	Pseudocysts
	Neoplasms
	  Cystic Neoplasms
	  Pancreatic Carcinoma
	    Precursors to Pancreatic Cancer
	    Molecular Carcinogenesis
	  Acinar Cell Carcinoma
	  Pancreatoblastoma

The adult pancreas is a transversely oriented retroperitoneal organ extending from the "C" loop of the duodenum to the hilum of the spleen (Fig. 19–1). On average, the pancreas measures 20 cm in length and weighs 90 gm in men and 85 gm in women.[1] The vasculature adjacent to the pancreas can be used to separate the pancreas into four parts: the head, neck, body, and tail.

The pancreatic duct system is highly variable. The main pancreatic duct, also known as the duct of Wirsung, most commonly drains into the duodenum at the papilla of Vater, whereas the accessory pancreatic duct, also known as the duct of Santorini, most often drains into the duodenum through a separate minor papilla approximately 2 cm cephalad (proximal) to the major papilla of Vater (Fig. 19–1A). In most adults the main pancreatic duct joins the common bile duct proximal to the papilla of Vater, thus creating the ampulla of Vater, a common channel for biliary and pancreatic drainage. This ductal architecture can differ significantly from person to person.

The pancreas arises from the fusion of dorsal and ventral outpouchings of the foregut, which fuse to form a single organ.[2,3] The majority of the gland, including the body, the tail, the superior/anterior aspect of the head, and the accessory duct of Santorini, is derived from the dorsal primordium. The ventral primordium gives rise to the posterior/inferior part of the head of the pancreas, and drains into the papilla of Vater.

Although the organ gets its name from the Greek *pankreas*, meaning "all flesh," the pancreas is, in fact, a complex lobulated organ with distinct exocrine and endocrine components. The exocrine portion, which produces digestive enzymes, constitutes 80% to 85% of the pancreas. The endocrine portion is composed of about 1 million clusters of cells, the islets of Langerhans. The islet cells secrete insulin, glucagon, and somatostatin and constitute only 1% to 2% of the organ. Diseases of the endocrine pancreas are described in detail in Chapter 24.

The exocrine pancreas is composed of acinar cells, which produce the enzymes needed for digestion, and a series of ductules and ducts that convey secretions to the duodenum.[1] Acinar cells are pyramidally shaped epithelial cells that are radially oriented around a central lumen (Fig. 19–2). Acinar

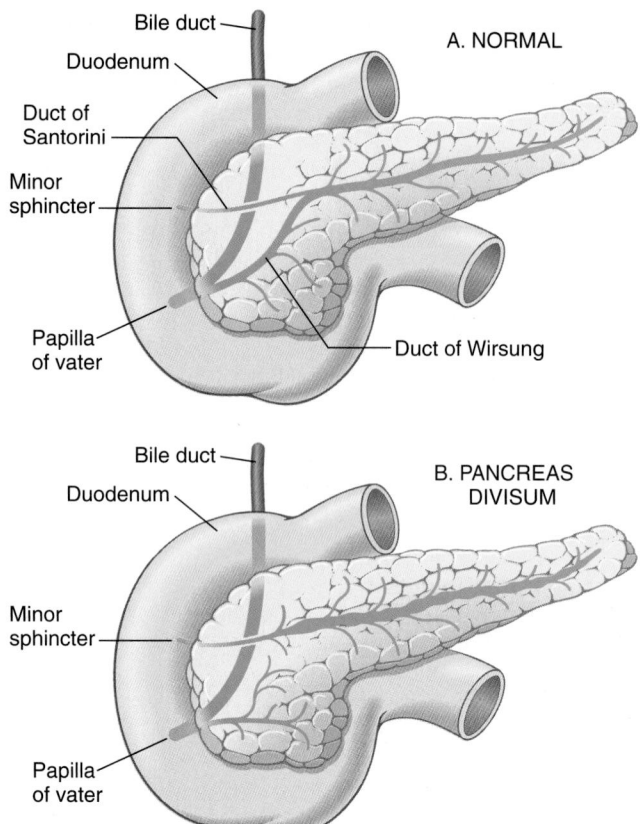

FIGURE 19–1 Pancreatic ductal anatomy. **A,** The normal ductal anatomy. **B,** The ductal anatomy in pancreatic divisum. (Adapted from Gregg JA et al.: Pancreas divisum: results of surgical intervention. Am J Surg 145:488–492, 1983.)

cells contain membrane-bound zymogen granules rich in digestive enzymes.

The pancreas secretes its exocrine products as enzymatically inert proenzymes. They include trypsinogen, chymotrypsinogen, procarboxypeptidase, proelastase, kallikreinogen, and prophospholipase A and B.[1] Self-digestion of pancreatic tissue is prevented by several mechanisms:

- The majority of the enzymes are synthesized as inactive proenzymes (with the exception of amylase and lipase).
- The enzymes are sequestered in membrane-bound zymogen granules in the acinar cells.
- Activation of proenzymes requires conversion of inactive trypsinogen to active trypsin by duodenal enteropeptidase (enterokinase). Trypsin cleaves proenzymes to yield products such as chymotrypsin, elastases, and phospholipases.
- Trypsin inhibitors including serine protease inhibitor Kazal type l (SPINK1, also known as pancreatic secretory trypsin inhibitor, PSTI) are present within acinar and ductal secretions.
- Acinar cells are remarkably resistant to the action of trypsin, chymotrypsin, and phospholipase A_2.

The most significant disorders of the *exocrine* pancreas include cystic fibrosis, congenital anomalies, acute and chronic pancreatitis, pseudocysts, and neoplasms. Cystic fibrosis is discussed in detail in Chapter 10.

Congenital Anomalies

The complex process by which the dorsal and ventral pancreatic primordia fuse during pancreatic development frequently gives rise to congenital variations in pancreatic anatomy.[3] Most of these do not directly cause disease; however, such variations, especially in ductal anatomy, may present particular problems to endoscopists and surgeons. For example, failure to recognize aberrant ductal anatomy may lead to the inadvertent ligation of a pancreatic duct during surgery, causing serious sequelae such as pancreatitis.

AGENESIS

Very rarely the pancreas may be totally absent (agenesis), a condition associated with other severe malformations that are usually incompatible with life. *PDX1* (pancreatic and duodenal homeobox-1 gene) encodes a transcription factor critical for the development of the pancreas.[3] Homozygous *PDX1* mutations on chromosome 13q12.1 have been reported in a person with pancreatic agenesis.[3,4]

PANCREAS DIVISUM

Pancreas divisum is the most common congenital anomaly of the pancreas, with an incidence of 3% to 10%.[4] This anomaly is caused by a failure of fusion of the fetal duct systems of the dorsal and ventral pancreatic primordia.[4] As a result, the bulk of the pancreas (formed by the dorsal pancreatic primordium) drains through the dorsal pancreatic duct and the *small-caliber minor papilla* (see Fig. 19–1B).[4] The duct of Wirsung in persons with divisum, normally the main pancreatic duct, is very short (1 to 2 cm) and drains only a small portion of the head of the gland through the larger caliber major papilla of Vater. Although controversy exists about the clinical significance of pancreatic divisum, it has been suggested that the relative stenosis caused by the bulk of the pancreatic secretions passing through the minor papilla predisposes individuals to the development of chronic pancreatitis.[4,5]

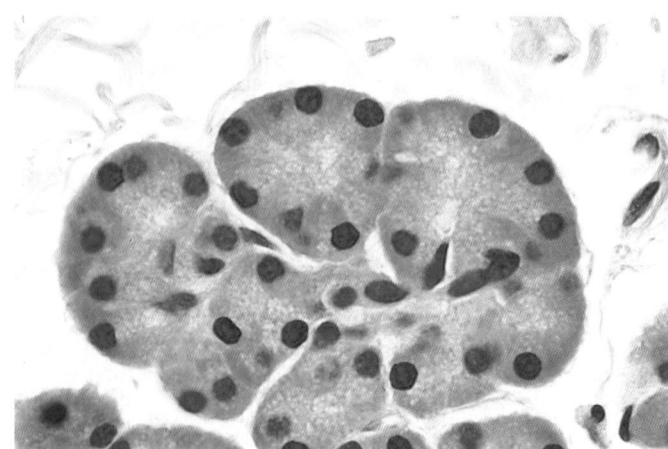

FIGURE 19–2 Pancreatic acini, showing the radial orientation of the pyramidal exocrine acinar cells. The cytoplasm is devoted to the synthesis and packaging of digestive enzymes for secretion into a central lumen.

ANNULAR PANCREAS

Annular pancreas is a band-like ring of normal pancreatic tissue that completely encircles the second portion of the duodenum. Annular pancreas is often associated with other congenital anomalies and may present early in life or in adults with signs and symptoms of duodenal obstruction such as gastric distention and vomiting.[4,6]

ECTOPIC PANCREAS

Aberrantly situated, or *ectopic*, pancreatic tissue is found in about 2% of careful routine postmortem examinations. The favored sites for ectopia are the stomach and duodenum, followed by the jejunum, Meckel diverticula, and ileum.[4] These embryologic rests are a few millimeters to centimeters in size and are located in the submucosa. Histologic examination reveals that they are composed of normal-appearing pancreatic acini, glands, and sometimes islets of Langerhans. Though usually incidental, ectopic pancreas may cause pain from localized inflammation, or, rarely, may incite mucosal bleeding. Approximately 2% of islet cell neoplasms (Chapter 24) arise in ectopic pancreatic tissue. The pathogenesis of ectopic pancreas has not been established.

Pancreatitis

Pancreatitis is inflammation in the pancreas associated with injury to the exocrine parenchyma. The clinical manifestations range in severity from a mild, self-limited disease to a life-threatening acute inflammatory process, and the duration of the disease can range from a transient attack to a permanent loss of function.[7,8] In *acute pancreatitis* the gland can return to normal if the underlying cause of the pancreatitis is removed.[9,10] By contrast, *chronic pancreatitis* is defined by the irreversible loss of exocrine pancreatic parenchyma.[7,11]

ACUTE PANCREATITIS

Acute pancreatitis is reversible pancreatic parenchymal injury associated with inflammation. Acute pancreatitis is relatively common, with an annual incidence rate in Western countries of 10 to 20 cases per 100,000 people. Biliary tract disease and alcoholism account for approximately 80% of cases in Western countries (Table 19–1).[8–10,12] Gallstones are present in 35% to 60% of cases of acute pancreatitis, and about 5% of patients with gallstones develop pancreatitis. The proportion of cases of acute pancreatitis caused by excessive alcohol intake varies from 65% in the United States to 20% in Sweden to 5% or less in southern France and the United Kingdom.[13] The male-to-female ratio is 1:3 in the group with biliary tract disease and 6:1 in those with alcoholism.

Less common causes of acute pancreatitis include the following:

- Obstruction of the pancreatic duct system. Reasons for obstruction other than gallstones include periampullary neoplasms (such as pancreatic cancer), pancreas divisum (although its role is controversial), choledochoceles (congenital cystic dilatation of the common bile duct), biliary

"sludge," and parasites (particularly the *Ascaris lumbricoides* and *Clonorchis sinensis* organisms).[10,14]

- Medications. More than 85 drugs have been implicated. These include furosemide, azathioprine, 2′,3′-dideoxyinosine, estrogens, and many others.[10,15]
- Infections, including mumps, can lead to acute pancreatitis.
- Metabolic disorders, such as hypertriglyceridemia, hyperparathyroidism, and other hypercalcemic states.
- Ischemic injury from shock, vascular thrombosis, embolism, and vasculitis.
- Trauma. Both blunt abdominal trauma and iatrogenic injury during surgery or endoscopic retrograde cholangiopancreatography.
- Inherited alterations in genes encoding pancreatic enzymes and their inhibitors, including germline mutations in the cationic trypsinogen (*PRSS1*) and trypsin inhibitor (*SPINK1*) genes.[16–19] These are discussed below.

Hereditary Pancreatitis. Notably, 10% to 20% of individuals with acute pancreatitis have no known associated processes. Although this condition is currently termed *idiopathic*, a growing body of evidence suggests that some of these cases actually have a genetic basis. The genetic alterations associated with the development of pancreatitis therefore deserve special note.[17] Hereditary pancreatitis is characterized by recurrent attacks of severe pancreatitis usually beginning in childhood.[16,17] Most cases are caused by germline (inherited) mutations in the *cationic trypsinogen* gene (also known as *PRSS1*).[16] These mutations abrogate a critical fail-safe mechanism by altering a site on the cationic trypsinogen molecule that is essential for the cleavage (inactivation) of trypsin by trypsin itself.[17] When this site is mutated, trypsin becomes resistant to cleavage by another trypsin molecule, and if a small amount of this tryspin is inappropriately activated in the pancreas, it can activate other digestive

TABLE 19–1 Etiologic Factors in Acute Pancreatitis
METABOLIC
Alcoholism
Hyperlipoproteinemia
Hypercalcemia
Drugs (e.g., azathioprine)
GENETIC
Mutations in the cationic trypsinogen (*PRSS1*) and trypsin inhibitor (*SPINK1*) genes
MECHANICAL
Gallstones
Trauma
Iatrogenic injury
Operative injury
Endoscopic procedures with dye injection
VASCULAR
Shock
Atheroembolism
Vasculitis
INFECTIOUS
Mumps

proenzymes, resulting in the development of pancreatitis. Only one mutated allele is required for cleavage-resistant trypsin to be produced; thus, this form of hereditary pancreatitis has an autosomal dominant mode of inheritance.

The *serine protease inhibitor Kazal type 1 (SPINK1)* gene codes for a pancreatic secretory trypsin inhibitor that, as the name suggests, inhibits trypsin activity, helping to prevent the autodigestion of the pancreas by activated trypsin.[17] As one might suspect, inherited inactivating mutations in the *SPINK1* gene can also lead to the development of pancreatitis. This form of hereditary pancreatitis has an autosomal recessive mode of inheritance, as both alleles must be inactivated.

Morphology. The morphology of acute pancreatitis ranges from trivial inflammation and edema to severe extensive necrosis and hemorrhage. The basic alterations are **(1) microvascular leakage causing edema, (2) necrosis of fat by lipolytic enzymes, (3) acute inflammation, (4) proteolytic destruction of pancreatic parenchyma, and (5) destruction of blood vessels and subsequent interstitial hemorrhage**. The extent of each of these alterations depends on the duration and severity of the process.

In the milder form, acute interstitial pancreatitis, histologic alterations are limited to mild inflammation, interstitial edema, and focal areas of fat necrosis in the substance of the pancreas and in peripancreatic fat (Fig. 19–3). Fat necrosis, as we have seen, results from enzymatic activity of lipase. The released fatty acids combine with calcium to form insoluble salts that impart a granular blue microscopic appearance to the fat cells (Chapter 1).

In the more severe form, **acute necrotizing pancreatitis**, the acinar and ductal tissues as well as the islets of Langerhans are necrotic. Vascular injury can lead to hemorrhage into the parenchyma of the pancreas. Macroscopically, the pancreatic substance shows areas of red-black hemorrhage interspersed with foci of yellow-white, chalky fat necrosis (Fig. 19–4). Foci of fat necrosis may also be found in extra-

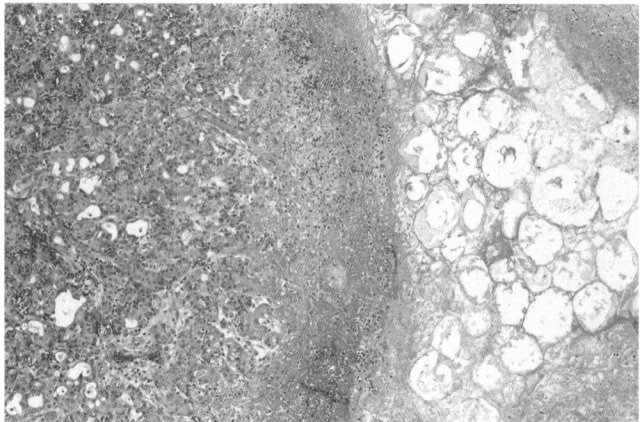

FIGURE 19–3 Acute pancreatitis. The microscopic field shows a region of fat necrosis on the right and focal pancreatic parenchymal necrosis *(center)*.

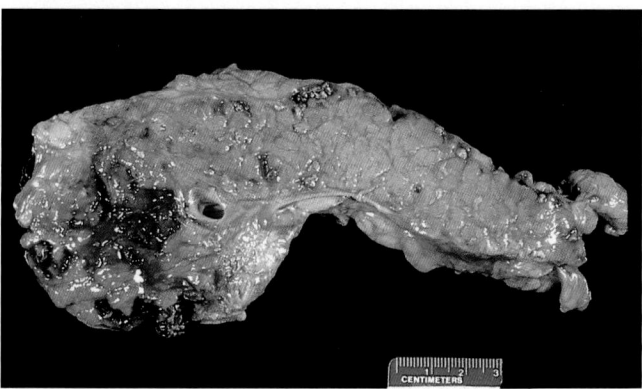

FIGURE 19–4 Acute pancreatitis. The pancreas has been sectioned longitudinally to reveal dark areas of hemorrhage in the head of the pancreas and a focal area of pale fat necrosis in the peripancreatic fat *(upper left)*.

pancreatic collections of fat, such as the omentum and the mesentery of the bowel, and even outside the abdominal cavity, such as in the subcutaneous fat. In the majority of cases the peritoneal cavity contains a serous, slightly turbid, brown-tinged fluid in which globules of fat (derived from the action of enzymes on adipose tissue) can be identified. In its most severe form, **hemorrhagic pancreatitis**, extensive parenchymal necrosis is accompanied by dramatic hemorrhage within the substance of the gland.[20,21]

Pathogenesis. The anatomic changes of acute pancreatitis strongly suggest *autodigestion of the pancreatic substance by inappropriately activated pancreatic enzymes*. This hypothesis is supported by the hereditary forms of pancreatitis described above. Here we focus on the more common, acquired forms of acute pancreatitis.

As has been discussed, pancreatic enzymes, including trypsin, are synthesized in an inactive proenzyme form. If trypsin is inappropriately activated it can in turn activate other proenzymes such as prophospholipase and proelastase, which then degrade fat cells and damage the elastic fibers of blood vessels, respectively.[8–10,12] Trypsin also converts prekallikrein to its activated form, thus bringing into play the kinin system and, by activation of Hageman factor (factor XII), the clotting and complement systems as well (Chapters 2 and 4). In this way inflammation and small-vessel thromboses (which may lead to congestion and rupture of already weakened vessels) are amplified. Thus, the *inappropriate activation of trypsinogen is an important triggering event in acute pancreatitis*.

The mechanisms by which the activation of pancreatic enzymes is initiated are not entirely clear, but there is evidence for three possible events (Fig. 19–5):

1. *Pancreatic duct obstruction.* Gallstones or biliary sludge impacted in the region of the ampulla of Vater can raise intrapancreatic ductal pressure and lead to the accumulation of enzyme-rich fluid in the interstitium. Since lipase is one of the few enzymes secreted in an active form, this can cause local fat necrosis. Injured tissues, periacinar myofibroblasts, and leukocytes then release proinflamma-

CAUSES: **DUCT OBSTRUCTION**   **ACINAR CELL INJURY**   **DEFECTIVE INTRACELLULAR TRANSPORT**

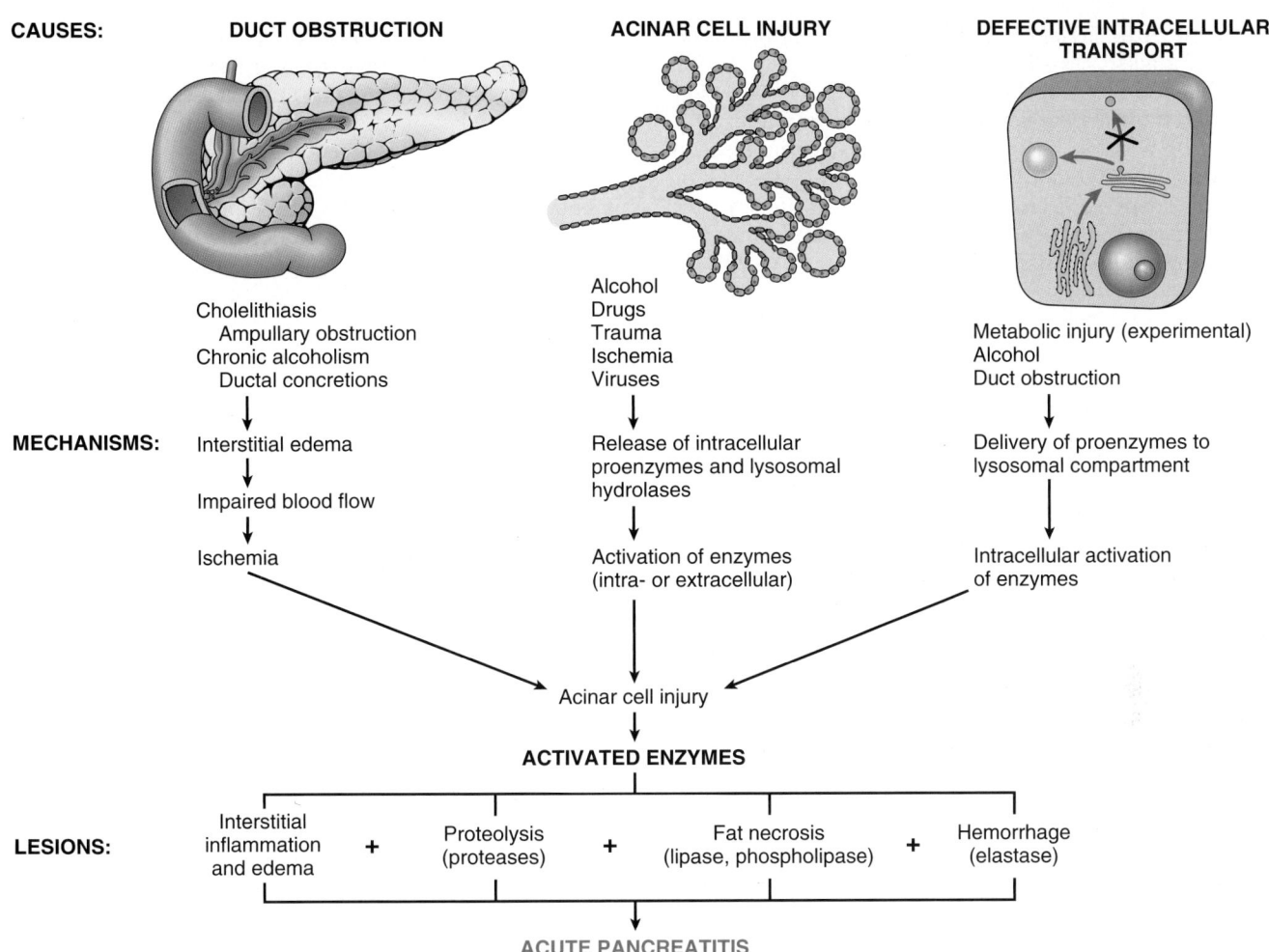

Cholelithiasis
   Ampullary obstruction
Chronic alcoholism
   Ductal concretions

Alcohol
Drugs
Trauma
Ischemia
Viruses

Metabolic injury (experimental)
Alcohol
Duct obstruction

MECHANISMS: Interstitial edema

Impaired blood flow

Ischemia

Release of intracellular
proenzymes and lysosomal
hydrolases

Activation of enzymes
(intra- or extracellular)

Delivery of proenzymes to
lysosomal compartment

Intracellular activation
of enzymes

Acinar cell injury

ACTIVATED ENZYMES

LESIONS: Interstitial
inflammation   +   Proteolysis   +   Fat necrosis   +   Hemorrhage
and edema   (proteases)   (lipase, phospholipase)   (elastase)

ACUTE PANCREATITIS

FIGURE 19–5 Three proposed pathways in the pathogenesis of acute pancreatitis.

tory cytokines including IL-1β, IL-6, tumor necrosis factor, platelet-activating factor, and substance P, initiating local inflammation and promoting the development of interstitial edema through a leaky microvasculature (see Fig. 19–5).[22–25] Edema may further compromise local blood flow, causing vascular insufficiency and ischemic injury to acinar cells.[26]

2. *Primary acinar cell injury.* This mechanism is most clearly involved in the pathogenesis of acute pancreatitis caused by certain viruses (e.g., mumps), drugs, and direct trauma to the pancreas, as well as pancreatitis following ischemia or shock.

3. *Defective intracellular transport of proenzymes within acinar cells.*[27] In normal acinar cells, digestive enzymes and lysosomal hydrolases are transported in separate pathways. In animal models of acinar injury, the pancreatic proenzymes are inappropriately delivered to the intracellular compartment containing lysosomal hydrolases. Proenzymes are then activated, the lysosomes disrupted, and activated enzymes released. The role of this mechanism in human acute pancreatitis is not clear.[28]

Alcohol consumption may cause pancreatitis by several mechanisms. Chronic alcohol ingestion results in the secre-

tion of protein-rich pancreatic fluid, which leads to the deposition of inspissated protein plugs and obstruction of small pancreatic ducts. Alcohol also transiently increases pancreatic exocrine secretion and contraction of the sphincter of Oddi (the muscle at the ampulla of Vater), and it has direct toxic effects on acinar cells.[29]

Clinical Features. *Abdominal pain* is the cardinal manifestation of acute pancreatitis.[8–10,12] Characteristically, the pain is constant and intense and is often referred to the upper back and occasionally can be associated with referred pain to the left shoulder. Its severity varies from mild and uncomfortable to severe and incapacitating. Anorexia, nausea, and vomiting frequently accompany the pain. Suspected acute pancreatitis is primarily diagnosed by the presence of elevated plasma levels of amylase and lipase and the exclusion of other causes of abdominal pain.

Full-blown acute pancreatitis is a medical emergency. These patients usually have the sudden calamitous onset of an "acute abdomen." Many of the systemic features of severe acute pancreatitis can be attributed to release of toxic enzymes, cytokines, and other mediators into the circulation and explosive activation of the systemic inflammatory response, resulting in *leukocytosis, hemolysis, disseminated intravascular coagulation, fluid sequestration, acute respiratory distress syndrome, and diffuse fat necrosis. Peripheral vascular collapse and shock with acute renal tubular necrosis may occur.*[8–10,12]

Laboratory findings include marked elevation of serum amylase levels during the first 24 hours, followed within 72 to 96 hours by a rising serum lipase level. Glycosuria occurs in 10% of cases. Hypocalcemia may result from precipitation of calcium soaps in necrotic fat; if persistent, it is a poor prognostic sign. Direct visualization of the enlarged inflamed pancreas by radiography is useful in the diagnosis of pancreatitis.

The key to the management of acute pancreatitis is "resting" the pancreas by total restriction of oral intake and by supportive therapy with intravenous fluids and analgesia. Although most individuals with acute pancreatitis recover fully, about 5% with severe acute pancreatitis die from shock during the first week of illness. Acute respiratory distress syndrome and acute renal failure are ominous complications.[8–10,12] Sequelae can include a sterile *pancreatic abscess* and a *pancreatic pseudocyst* (discussed later). In 40% to 60% of patients with acute necrotizing pancreatitis the necrotic debris becomes infected, usually by gram-negative organisms from the alimentary tract, further complicating the clinical course.

CHRONIC PANCREATITIS

Chronic pancreatitis is defined as inflammation of the pancreas with irreversible destruction of exocrine parenchyma, fibrosis, and, in the late stages, the destruction of endocrine parenchyma.[11,30] Although chronic pancreatitis may present as repeated bouts of acute pancreatitis, the chief distinction between acute and chronic pancreatitis is the irreversible impairment in pancreatic function that is characteristic of chronic pancreatitis. The prevalence of chronic pancreatitis ranges between 0.04% and 5%.[7] There is significant overlap in the causes of acute and chronic pancreatitis. By far *the most common cause of chronic pancreatitis is long-term alcohol abuse,* and these patients are usually middle-aged males.

Less common causes of chronic pancreatitis include the following:

● Long-standing *obstruction* of the pancreatic duct by pseudocysts, calculi, trauma, neoplasms, or pancreas divisum. There is often dilation of the pancreatic duct.
● *Tropical pancreatitis,* which is a poorly characterized heterogeneous disease seen in Africa and Asia.[31] Some cases have a genetic basis.
● *Hereditary pancreatitis,* which is caused by germline mutations in *PRSS1* (cationic trypsinogen gene) or *SPINK1* (serine protease inhibitor Kazal type 1 gene), and is associated with the development of both acute and chronic pancreatitis.[16,17]
● *CFTR gene mutations.* As was discussed in detail in Chapter 10, cystic fibrosis is caused by bi-allelic inherited mutations in the cystic fibrosis transmembrane conductance regulator (*CFTR*) gene. Mutations in *CFTR* decrease bicarbonate secretion by pancreatic ductal cells, thereby promoting protein plugging and the development of chronic pancreatitis.[19] Mutations in the *CFTR* gene occur in 25% to 30% of patients with idiopathic pancreatitis, a rate that is approximately 5 times higher than that of the general population.

As many as 40% of individuals with chronic pancreatitis have no recognizable predisposing factor, but as is true for acute pancreatitis, a growing number of these "idiopathic" cases can now be shown to be caused by inherited mutations in pancreatitis-associated genes.[19]

Pathogenesis. The pathogenesis of chronic pancreatitis is not well understood. Almost all individuals with repeated episodes of acute pancreatitis later develop chronic pancreatitis. It has been proposed that acute pancreatitis initiates a sequence of perilobular fibrosis, duct distortion, and altered pancreatic secretions. Over time and with multiple episodes, this can lead to loss of pancreatic parenchyma and fibrosis.[32] The events that have been proposed to account for the development of chronic pancreatitis include:[32,33]

1. *Ductal obstruction by concretions.* Some of the agents responsible for the development of chronic pancreatitis are believed to increase protein concentrations in the pancreatic juice. These proteins form ductal plugs. Such plugs are particularly prominent in alcoholic chronic pancreatitis.[34] The ductal plugs may calcify, forming calculi composed of calcium carbonate precipitates that can further obstruct the pancreatic ducts and contribute to the development of chronic pancreatitis.
2. *Toxic effects.* Toxins, including alcohol and its metabolites, can exert a direct toxic effect on acinar cells.
3. *Oxidative stress.* Alcohol-induced oxidative stress may generate free radicals in acinar cells, leading to membrane lipid oxidation and the activation of transcription factors, including AP1 and NF-κB, which in turn induce the expression of chemokines that attract mononuclear cells.[32,33] Oxidative stress may promote the fusion of lysosomes and zymogen granules, acinar cell necrosis, inflammation, and fibrosis.

A variety of chemokines have been identified in chronic pancreatitis, including IL-8 and monocyte chemoattractant protein.[35] In addition, transforming growth factor β (TGF-β) and platelet-derived growth factor induce the activation and proliferation of periacinar myofibroblasts (pancreatic stellate cells), resulting in the deposition of collagen and ultimately fibrosis (Fig. 19–6).[36–38] While the chemokines produced during chronic pancreatitis are similar to those produced in acute pancreatitis, the profibrogenic chemokines tend to predominate in chronic pancreatitis.[39]

Morphology. Chronic pancreatitis is characterized by parenchymal fibrosis, reduced number and size of acini with relative sparing of the islets of Langerhans, and variable dilation of the pancreatic ducts (Fig. 19–7A). These changes are usually accompanied by a chronic inflammatory infiltrate around lobules and ducts. The interlobular and intralobular ducts are frequently dilated and contain protein plugs in their lumens. The ductal epithelium may be atrophied or hyperplastic or may show squamous metaplasia, and ductal concretions may be evident (Fig. 19–7B). Acinar loss is a constant feature. The remaining islets of Langerhans become embedded in the sclerotic tissue and may fuse and appear enlarged. Eventually, they

FIGURE 19–6 Comparison of the mediators in acute and chronic pancreatitis. In acute pancreatitis acinar injury results in release of proteolytic enzymes, leading to a cascade of events including activation of the clotting cascade, acute and chronic inflammation, vascular injury, and edema. In most patients, complete resolution of the acute injury occurs with restoration of acinar cell mass. In chronic pancreatitis, repeated episodes of acinar cell injury lead to the production of profibrogenic cytokines such as transforming growth factor β (TGF-β) and platelet-derived growth factor (PDGF), resulting in the proliferation of myofibroblasts, the secretion of collagen, and remodeling of the extracellular matrix (ECM). Repeated injury produces irreversible loss of acinar cell mass, fibrosis, and pancreatic insufficiency.

too disappear. Grossly, the gland is hard, sometimes with extremely dilated ducts and visible calcified concretions. **Lymphoplasmacytic sclerosing pancreatitis** (autoimmune pancreatitis) is a distinct form of chronic pancreatitis characterized by a duct-centric mixed inflammatory cell infiltrate, venulitis, and increased numbers of IgG4-producing plasma cells.[40] It is important to recognize lymphoplasmacytic sclerosing pancreatitis, since it can clinically mimic pancreatic cancer and also because it responds to steroid therapy.

Clinical Features. Chronic pancreatitis may present in many different forms. It may be associated with repeated attacks of moderately severe abdominal pain, recurrent attacks of mild pain, or persistent abdominal and back pain. The disease may be entirely silent until pancreatic insufficiency and diabetes mellitus develop, the latter from associated destruction of islets of Langerhans. In still other instances, recurrent attacks of jaundice or vague attacks of indigestion may hint at pancreatic disease. Attacks may be precipitated by alcohol abuse, overeating (which increases demand on the pancreas), or the use of opiates and other drugs that increase the tone of the sphincter of Oddi.

The diagnosis of chronic pancreatitis requires a high degree of suspicion. During an attack of abdominal pain there may be mild fever and mild-to-moderate elevations of serum amylase. When the disease has been present for a long time, however,

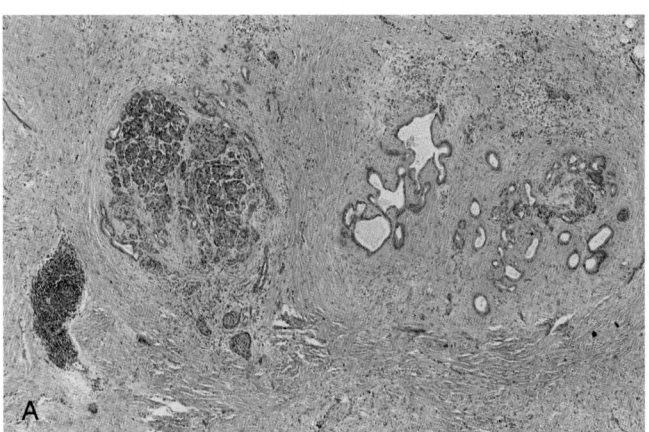
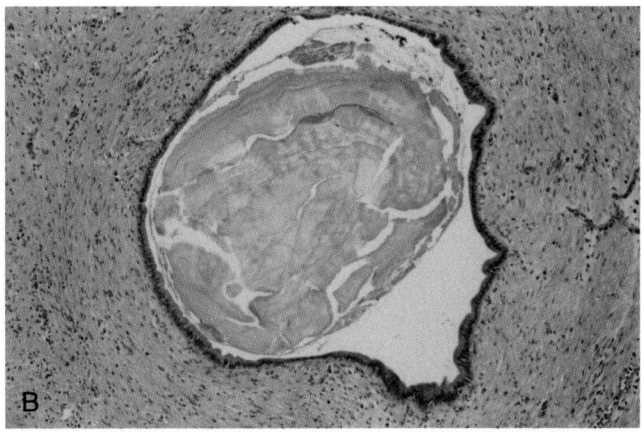

FIGURE 19–7 Chronic pancreatitis. **A,** Extensive fibrosis and atrophy has left only residual islets *(left)* and ducts *(right)*, with a sprinkling of chronic inflammatory cells and acinar tissue. **B,** A higher power view demonstrating dilated ducts with inspissated eosinophilic ductal concretions in a person with alcoholic chronic pancreatitis.

the destruction of acinar cells may preclude such diagnostic clues. Gallstone-induced obstruction may be evident as jaundice or elevations in serum levels of alkaline phosphatase. A very helpful finding is visualization of calcifications within the pancreas by computed tomography and ultrasonography. Weight loss and hypoalbuminemic edema from malabsorption caused by pancreatic exocrine insufficiency may point toward the disease.

Although chronic pancreatitis is usually not an immediately life-threatening condition, the long-term outlook for individuals with chronic pancreatitis is poor, with a 20- to 25-year mortality rate of 50%. Severe *pancreatic exocrine insufficiency* and chronic malabsorption may develop, as can *diabetes mellitus*. In other patients *severe chronic pain* may become the dominant problem. *Pancreatic pseudocysts* (described below) develop in about 10% of patients. While patients with hereditary pancreatitis have a 40% lifetime risk of developing pancreatic cancer, the degree to which other forms of chronic pancreatitis predispose to the development of pancreatic cancer is unclear.[41,42]

Non-Neoplastic Cysts

A variety of cysts can arise in the pancreas. Most are non-neoplastic pseudocysts (discussed later), but congenital cysts and neoplastic cysts also occur.

CONGENITAL CYSTS

Congenital cysts are believed to result from anomalous development of the pancreatic ducts. Cysts in the kidney, liver, and pancreas frequently coexist in *polycystic disease* (discussed in Chapter 20). Congenital cysts are usually unilocular, thin-walled, and range from microscopic lesions to 5 cm in diameter. They are lined by a glistening, uniform cuboidal epithelium or, if the intracystic pressure is high, by a flattened and attenuated cell layer; they are enclosed in a thin, fibrous capsule and are filled with a clear serous fluid. Congenital cysts may be sporadic, or part of *autosomal-dominant polycystic*

kidney disease and *von Hippel-Lindau disease.*[4] In von Hippel-Lindau disease (Chapter 20) vascular neoplasms are found in the retina and cerebellum or brain stem in association with congenital cysts (and also neoplasms) in the pancreas, liver, and kidney.

PSEUDOCYSTS

Pseudocysts are localized collections of necrotic-hemorrhagic material rich in pancreatic enzymes.[43] Such cysts lack an epithelial lining (hence the prefix "pseudo"), and account for approximately 75% of cysts in the pancreas.[43] Pseudocysts usually arise after an episode of acute pancreatitis, often in the setting of chronic alcoholic pancreatitis. Traumatic injury to the pancreas can also give rise to pseudocysts.

> **Morphology.** Pseudocysts are usually solitary and may be situated within the substance of the pancreas, or, more commonly, involve the lesser omental sac or lie in the retroperitoneum between the stomach and transverse colon or between the stomach and liver. They can even be subdiaphragmatic[43] (Fig. 19–8A). Pseudocysts are formed by the walling off of areas of peripancreatic hemorrhagic fat necrosis with fibrous tissue. As such, they usually are composed of central necrotic-hemorrhagic material rich in pancreatic enzymes surrounded by non-epithelial-lined fibrous walls of granulation tissue (Fig. 19–8B).[43] They can range in size from 2 to 30 cm in diameter.

While many pseudocysts spontaneously resolve, they may become secondarily infected, and larger pseudocysts may compress or even perforate into adjacent structures.

Neoplasms

A broad spectrum of exocrine neoplasms can arise in the pancreas. They may be cystic or solid; some are benign, while others are among the most lethal of all malignancies.

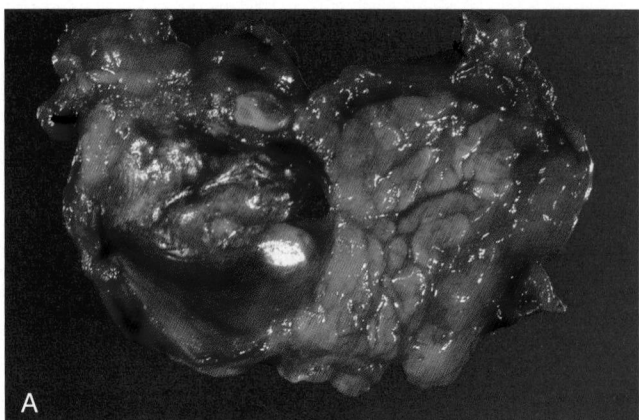
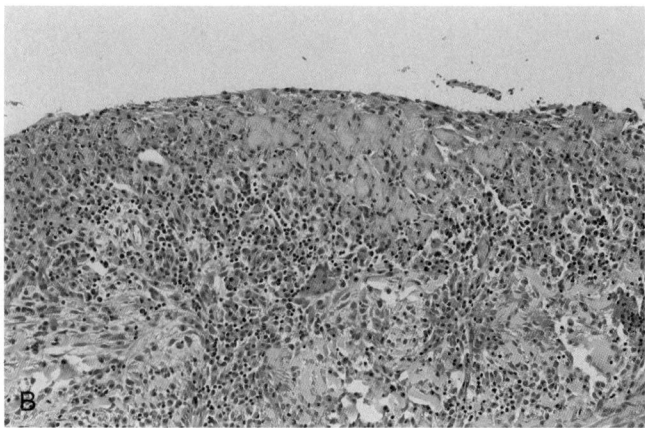

FIGURE 19–8 Pancreatic pseudocyst. **A,** Cross-section through this previously bisected lesion revealing a poorly defined cyst with a necrotic brown-black wall. **B,** Histologically, the cyst lacks a true epithelial lining and instead is lined by fibrin and granulation tissue.

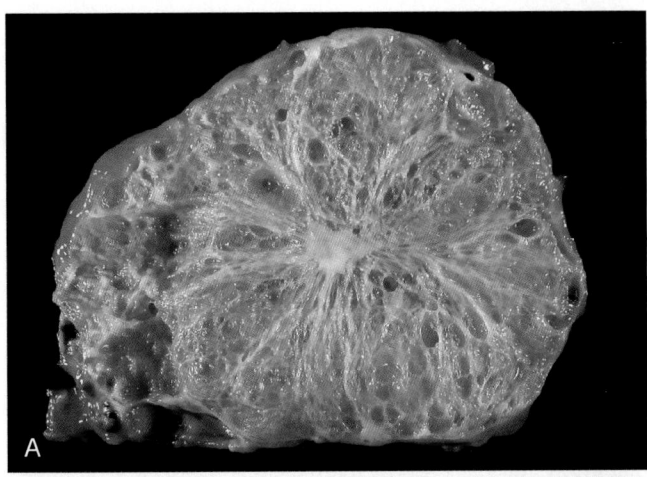

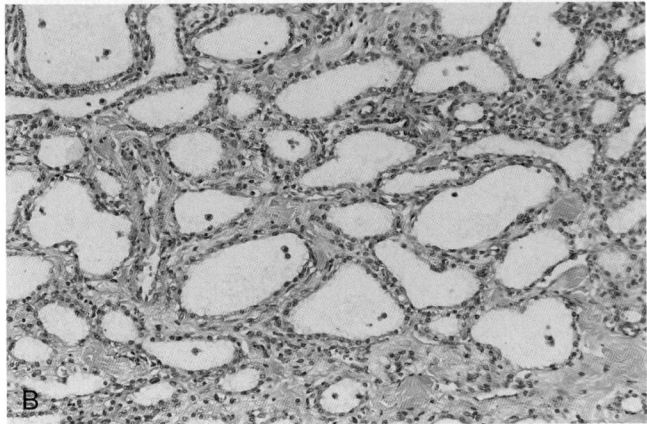

FIGURE 19–9 Serous cystadenoma. **A,** Cross-section through a serous cystadenoma. Only a thin rim of normal pancreatic parenchyma remains. The cysts are relatively small and contain clear, straw-colored fluid. **B,** The cysts are lined by cuboidal epithelium without atypia.

CYSTIC NEOPLASMS

Only 5% to 15% of all pancreatic cysts are neoplastic (most cysts are pseudocysts; see the previous section), and cystic neoplasms make up fewer than 5% of all pancreatic neoplasms. While some, such as the serous cystadenoma, are entirely benign, others, such as mucinous cystic neoplasms, can be benign or malignant.

Serous cystadenomas are benign cystic neoplasms composed of glycogen-rich cuboidal cells surrounding small (1- to 3-mm) cysts containing clear, thin, straw-colored fluid (Fig. 19–9).[1] They account for about 25% of all cystic neoplasms of the pancreas. These neoplasms arise twice as often in women as in men and typically present in the seventh decade of life with nonspecific symptoms such as abdominal pain. They may also present as palpable abdominal masses. Serous cystadenomas are almost always benign, and surgical resection is curative in the vast majority of patients.[44]

Close to 95% of *mucinous cystic neoplasms* arise in women, and, in contrast to serous cystadenomas, they can be associated with an invasive carcinoma.[1,45,46] Mucinous cystic neoplasms usually arise in the body or tail of the pancreas and present as painless, slow-growing masses. The cysts are larger than those formed in serous cystadenomas; they are filled with thick, tena-

cious mucin and lined by a columnar mucin-producing epithelium with an associated dense stroma similar to ovarian stroma (Fig. 19–10).[1] One third of surgically resected mucinous cystic neoplasms harbor an associated invasive adenocarcinoma. The best way to distinguish the entirely benign form (mucinous cystadenoma) from its malignant counterpart (invasive adenocarcinoma arising in association with a mucinous cystic neoplasm) is pathologic assessment after complete surgical removal, usually by distal pancreatectomy.[45]

Intraductal papillary mucinous neoplasms (IPMNs) are mucin-producing intraductal neoplasms.[1,47,48] In contrast to mucinous cystic neoplasms, IPMNs arise more frequently in men than in women, and they involve the head of the pancreas more often than the tail. Ten to twenty percent are multifocal. Two features are useful in distinguishing IPMNs from mucinous cystic neoplasms: IPMNs lack the dense "ovarian" stroma seen in mucinous cystic neoplasms, and involve a larger pancreatic duct (Fig. 19–11), while mucinous cystic neoplasms do not connect to the pancreatic duct system. Just as with mucinous cystic neoplasms, benign IPMNs are distinguished from malignant IPMNs by the lack of tissue invasion.

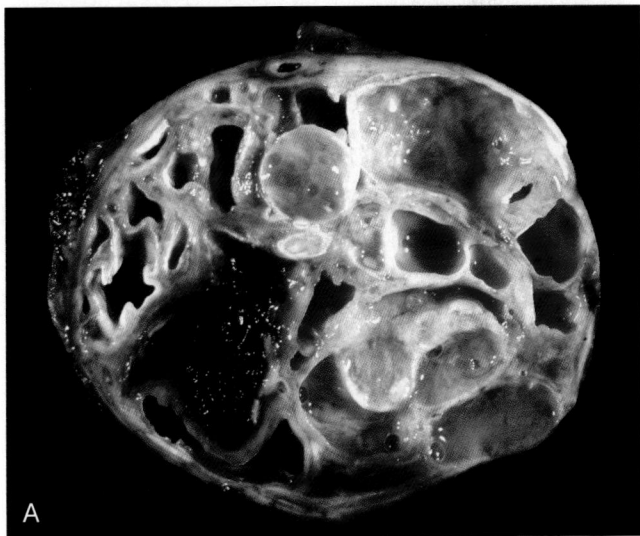

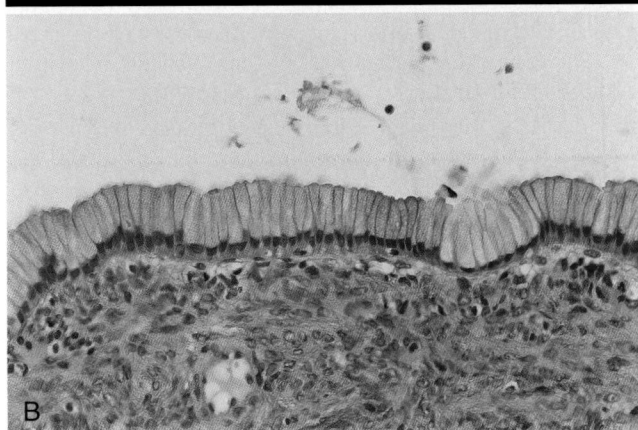

FIGURE 19–10 Pancreatic mucinous cystadenoma. **A,** Cross-section through a mucinous multiloculated cyst in the tail of the pancreas. The cysts are large and filled with tenacious mucin. **B,** The cysts are lined by columnar mucinous epithelium, and a dense "ovarian" stroma is noted.

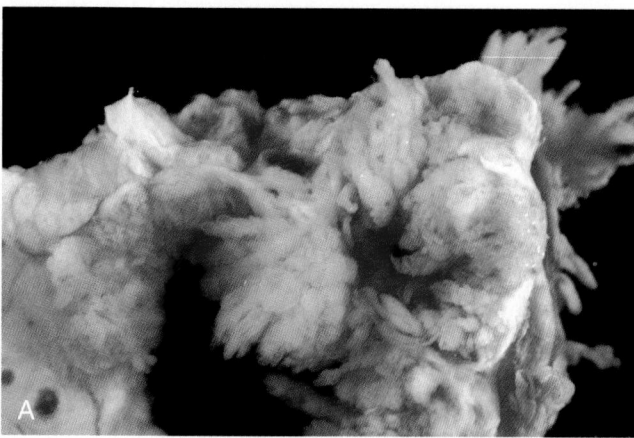
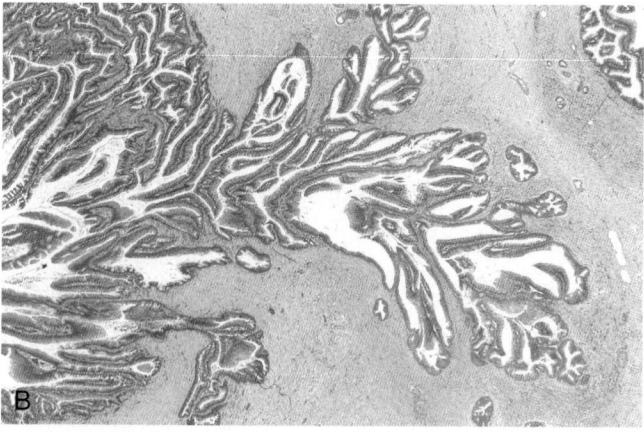

FIGURE 19–11 Intraductal papillary mucinous neoplasm. **A,** Cross-section through the head of the pancreas showing a prominent papillary neoplasm distending the main pancreatic duct. **B,** The papillary mucinous neoplasm involved the main pancreatic duct *(left)* and extending down into the smaller ducts and ductules *(right)*.

The unusual *solid-pseudopapillary neoplasm* is seen mainly in young women.[1,49] These large, well-circumscribed masses have solid and cystic components. The cystic areas are filled with hemorrhagic debris, and on histologic examination the neoplastic cells can be seen to grow in solid sheets or, as the name suggests, as papillary projections. These neoplasms often cause abdominal discomfort because of their large size. Of note, the β-catenin/adenomatous polyposis coli genetic pathway (Chapter 7) seems to be almost universally altered in these neoplasms often due to the presence of activating mutations of β-catenin.[49] Surgical resection is the treatment of choice. Although some solid-pseudopapillary neoplasms are locally aggressive, most patients are cured following complete surgical resection of the neoplasm.

PANCREATIC CARCINOMA

Infiltrating ductal adenocarcinoma of the pancreas, more commonly known as "pancreatic cancer," is the fourth leading cause of cancer deaths in the United States, preceded only by lung, colon, and breast cancers.[50] Pancreatic cancer has one of the highest mortality rates of any cancer. It is estimated that in 2008 approximately 37,000 Americans were diagnosed with pancreatic cancer, and that virtually all of them will die from their disease. The 5-year survival rate is dismal, less than 5%.

Precursors to Pancreatic Cancer

Just as there is a progression in the colorectum from non-neoplastic epithelium to adenoma to invasive carcinoma (Chapters 7 and 17), there is a progression in the pancreas from non-neoplastic epithelium to histologically well-defined noninvasive lesions in small ducts and ductules to invasive carcinoma.[51] These precursor lesions are called "pancreatic intraepithelial neoplasias" (PanINs). The PanIN-invasive carcinoma sequence is supported by the following observations:

- The distribution of PanINs within the pancreas parallels that of invasive cancer.
- PanINs are often found in pancreatic parenchyma adjacent to infiltrating carcinomas.

- Isolated case reports have documented individuals with PanINs who later developed an invasive pancreatic cancer.

The genetic and epigenetic alterations identified in PanINs are similar to those present in invasive cancers. The epithelial cells in PanINs show dramatic telomere shortening. A critical shortening of telomere length in PanINs may predispose these lesions to accumulate progressive chromosomal abnormalities and to develop invasive carcinoma.[52]

Based on these observations, a model for progression of PanINs has been proposed (Fig. 19–12).[51]

Molecular Carcinogenesis

Multiple genes are often altered in a single pancreatic cancer, and the patterns of genetic alterations differ from those seen in other malignancies.[53] Molecular alterations in pancreatic carcinogenesis are summarized in Table 19–2 and include the following:

KRAS. The *KRAS* gene (chromosome 12p) is the most frequently altered oncogene in pancreatic cancer. This oncogene is activated by point mutation in 80% to 90% of cases. These point mutations impair the intrinsic guanosine triphosphatase activity of the K-ras protein, resulting in a protein that is constitutively active. Ras in turn activates several intracellular signal transduction pathways that, among other effects, culminate in the activation of the transcription factors Fos and Jun.

CDKN2A (p16). The *p16/CDKN2A* gene (chromosome 9p) is inactivated in 95% of the cases, making *p16/CDKN2A* the most frequently inactivated tumor suppressor gene in pancreatic cancer.[54] The p16 protein plays a critical role in the control of the cell cycle, and inactivation of *p16* abrogates an important cell cycle checkpoint.

SMAD4. The *SMAD4* tumor suppressor gene (chromosome 18q) is inactivated in 55% of pancreatic cancers.[55] *SMAD4* encodes a protein that plays an important role in signal transduction from the TGF-β family of cell surface receptors. *SMAD4* is only rarely inactivated in other cancer types.

p53. Inactivation of the *p53* tumor suppressor gene (chromosome 17p) is seen in 50% to 70% of pancreatic cancers.[56]

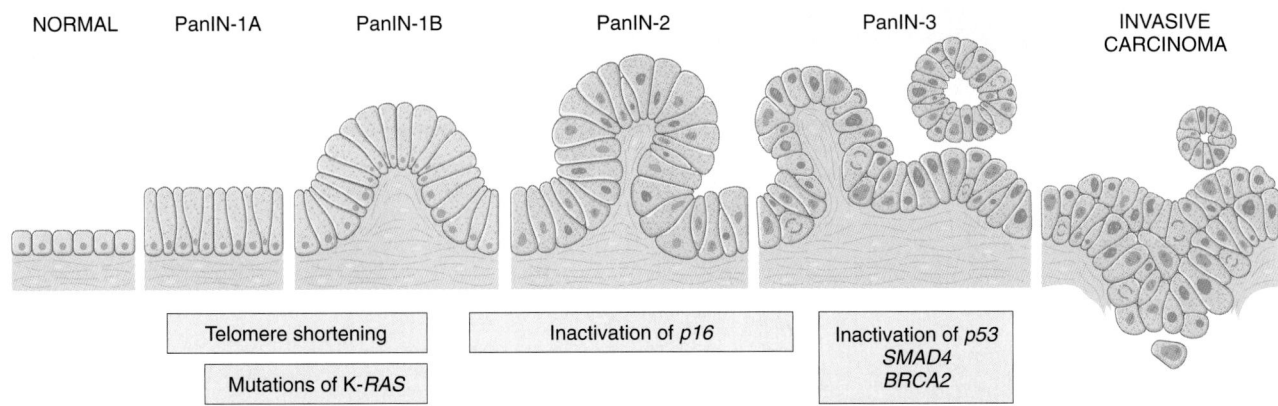

NORMAL   PanIN-1A   PanIN-1B   PanIN-2   PanIN-3   INVASIVE CARCINOMA

Telomere shortening   Inactivation of *p16*   Inactivation of *p53* SMAD4 BRCA2

Mutations of K-*RAS*

FIGURE 19–12   Progression model for the development of pancreatic cancer. It is postulated that telomere shortening and mutations of the oncogene *KRAS* occur at early stages, that inactivation of the *p16* tumor suppressor gene occurs at intermediate stages, and the inactivation of the *TP53*, *SMAD4* (*DPC4*), and *BRCA2* tumor suppressor genes occur at late stages. It is important to note that while there is a general temporal sequence of changes, the accumulation of multiple mutations is more important than their occurrence in a specific order. (Adapted from Wilentz RE et al.: Loss of expression of DPC4 in pancreatic intraepithelial neoplasia: evidence that *DPC4* inactivation occurs late in neoplastic progression. Cancer Res 60:2002, 2000.)

As you recall, the p53 protein is a nuclear DNA-binding protein that acts both as a cell cycle checkpoint, as an inducer of cell death (apoptosis), and cellular senescence (Chapter 7).

Other Genes. A growing number of less common, but nonetheless important, genetic loci have been reported to be damaged in pancreatic cancer (see Table 19–2). For example, the *AKT2* gene (chromosome 19q) is amplified in 10% to 20%, the *MYB* gene (6q) in 10%, the *GATA-6* gene (chromosome 18q) in 10%, and the *NCOA3/AIB1* gene (chromosome 20q) in 10%.[58] The *BRCA2* (chromosome 13q), *LKB1/STK11* (chromosome 19p), *MAP2K4/MKK4* (chromosome 17p), *TGFβ-R1* (chromosome 9q), *TGFβ-R2* (chromosome 3p), and *RB1* (chromosome 13q) tumor suppressor genes are inactivated in fewer than 10% of pancreatic cancers.

Methylation Abnormalities. Several methylation abnormalities also occur in pancreatic cancer. Hypermethylation of the promoter of several tumor suppressor genes is associated with transcriptional silencing of the genes.

Gene Expression. In addition to DNA alterations, global analyses of gene expression have identified several genes that are highly expressed in pancreatic cancers.[54,59] These genes are potential targets for novel therapeutics and may form the basis of future screening tests. For example, the hedgehog signaling pathway has been shown to be activated in pancreatic cancer, and inhibition of this pathway with the drug cyclopamine blocks growth of pancreatic cancers in experimental systems.[60]

Epidemiology, Etiology, and Pathogenesis. Pancreatic cancer is primarily a disease in the elderly, 80% of cases occurring between the ages of 60 and 80 years.[61] It is more common in blacks than in whites, and it is slightly more common in individuals of Ashkenazi Jewish descent.

The strongest environmental influence is *cigarette smoking*, which is believed to double the risk of pancreatic cancer.[59] Even though the magnitude of this increased risk is not great, the impact of smoking on pancreatic cancer is significant because of the large number of people who smoke. Consumption of a diet rich in fats has also been implicated, but less consistently. Chronic pancreatitis and diabetes mellitus have both been associated with an increased risk of pancreatic cancer. Pancreatic cancer arises with greater frequency in patients with chronic pancreatitis,[42] but a causal role for pancreatitis, with the exception of hereditary pancreatitis, is not well established. Smoking and alcohol use in individuals with chronic pancreatitis may underlie some of the association.[42] In an individual patient it can be difficult to sort out whether chronic pancreatitis is the cause of pancreatic cancer or an effect of the disease, since small pancreatic cancers may block the pancreatic duct and produce chronic pancreatitis. A similar argument applies to the association of diabetes mellitus with pancreatic cancer, since diabetes may develop as a consequence of pancreatic cancer. New-onset diabetes mellitus in an elderly patient may be the first sign that the patient has pancreatic cancer.[62]

TABLE 19–2   Molecular Alterations in Invasive Pancreatic Adenocarcinoma

Gene	Chromosomal Region	Percentage of Carcinoma with Genetic Alteration
KRAS	12p	90
p16/CDKN2A	9p	95
TP53	17p	50–70
SMAD4	18q	55
AKT2	19q	10–20
MYB	6q	10
NCOA3/AIB1	20q	10
BRCA2	13q	7–10
GATA-6	18q	10
STK11	19p	5
MAP2K4/MKK4	17p	5
TGFβ-R1	9q	2
TGFβ-R2	3p	2
RB1	13q	5

TABLE 19-3 Inherited Predisposition to Pancreatic Cancer

Disorder	Gene (Chromosome Location)	Increased Risk of Pancreatic Cancer fold	Risk of Pancreatic Cancer by Age 70 (%)
Hereditary breast and ovarian cancer	BRCA2 (13q12–q13)	4–10	5
Familial atypical multiple-mole melanoma syndrome	p16/CDKN2A (9p21)	20–35	10–17
Strong family history (3 or more relatives with pancreatic cancer)	Unknown	14–32	8–16
Hereditary pancreatitis	PRSS1 (7q35) and SPINK1	50–80	25–40
Peutz-Jeghers syndrome	LKB1 (19p13)	130	30–60

Familial clustering of pancreatic cancer has been reported, and a growing number of inherited genetic defects are recognized to increase pancreatic cancer risk (Table 19–3).[63] BRCA2 mutations account for approximately 10% of pancreatic cancer cases in Ashkenazi Jews. Patients with these mutations may not have a family history of breast or ovarian cancers. Mutations in CDKN2A (p16) in pancreatic cancer almost always occur in individuals from melanoma-prone families.

A mutation in the PALLD gene, which encodes the extracellular matrix protein palladin, was reported in one family with high incidence of pancreatic cancer. The mutation was not found in other families, but palladin is highly expressed in the surrounding stroma of pancreatic cancers.

Morphology. Approximately 60% of cancers of the pancreas arise in the head of the gland, 15% in the body, and 5% in the tail; in 20% the neoplasm diffusely involves the entire gland. Carcinomas of the pancreas are usually hard, stellate, gray-white, poorly defined masses (Fig. 19–13A).

The vast majority of carcinomas are ductal adenocarcinomas that recapitulate to some degree normal ductal epithelium by forming glands and secreting mucin. Two features are characteristic of pancreatic cancer: It is highly invasive (even "early" invasive pancreatic cancers extensively invade peripancreatic tissues), and elicits an intense non-neoplastic host reaction composed of fibroblasts, lymphocytes, and extracellular matrix (called a "desmoplastic response").

Most carcinomas of the head of the pancreas obstruct the distal common bile duct as it courses through the head of the pancreas. As a consequence there is marked distention of the biliary tree in about 50% of patients with carcinoma of the head of the pancreas, and most develop jaundice. In marked contrast, **carcinomas of the body and tail of the pancreas do not impinge on the biliary tract and hence remain silent for some time. They may be quite large and most are widely disseminated by the time they are discovered.** Pancreatic cancers often grow along nerves and invade into the retroperitoneum. They can directly invade the spleen, adrenals, vertebral column, transverse colon, and stomach. Peripancre-

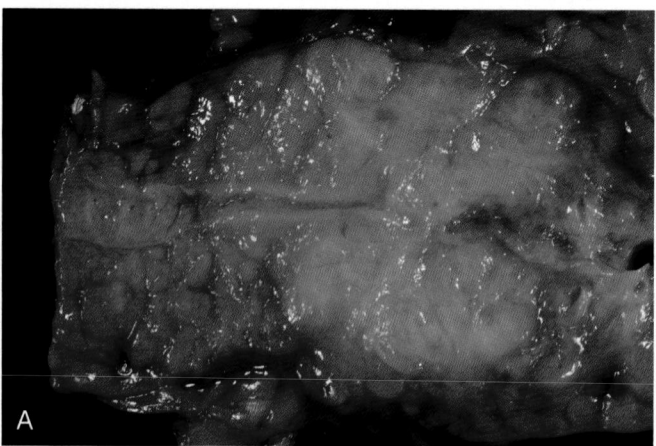
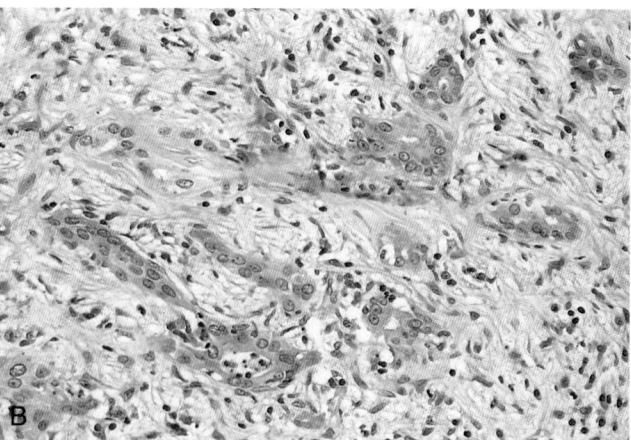

FIGURE 19–13 Carcinoma of the pancreas. **A,** A cross-section through the tail of the pancreas showing normal pancreatic parenchyma and a normal pancreatic duct *(left)*, an ill-defined mass in the pancreatic substance *(center)* with narrowing of the pancreatic duct, and dilatation of the pancreatic duct upstream *(right)* from the mass. **B,** Poorly formed glands are present in densely fibrotic stroma within the pancreatic substance; there are some inflammatory cells.

atic, gastric, mesenteric, omental, and portahepatic lymph nodes are frequently involved. Distant metastases occur, principally to the liver, lungs, and bones.

Microscopically, there is no difference between carcinomas of the head of the pancreas and those of the body and tail of the pancreas. The appearance is usually that of a **moderately to poorly differentiated adenocarcinoma forming abortive tubular structures or cell clusters and showing an aggressive, deeply infiltrative growth pattern** (Fig. 19–13B). Dense stromal fibrosis accompanies the invasive cancer, and there is a proclivity for perineural invasion within and beyond the organ. Lymphatic and large vessel invasion are also commonly seen. The malignant glands are poorly formed and are usually lined by pleomorphic cuboidal-to-columnar epithelial cells. Well-differentiated carcinomas are the exception.

Less common variants of pancreatic cancer include **adenosquamous carcinomas, colloid carcinoma, hepatoid carcinoma, medullary carcinoma, signet-ring cell carcinoma, undifferentiated carcinoma, and undifferentiated carcinomas with osteoclast-like giant cells.**[1] Adenosquamous carcinomas have focal squamous differentiation in addition to glandular differentiation, and undifferentiated carcinomas may contain large multinucleated osteoclast-like giant cells.

Clinical Features. From the preceding discussion it should be evident that *carcinomas of the pancreas remain silent until they invade into adjacent structures.* Pain is usually the first symptom, but by the time pain appears these cancers are usually beyond cure. *Obstructive jaundice* is associated with most cases of carcinoma of the head of the pancreas, but it rarely draws attention to the invasive cancer soon enough. Weight loss, anorexia, and generalized malaise and weakness tend to be signs of advanced disease. *Migratory thrombophlebitis,* known as the *Trousseau sign,* occurs in about 10% of patients and is attributable to the elaboration of platelet-aggregating factors and procoagulants from the carcinoma or its necrotic products (Chapter 4). On a sad note, Armand Trousseau (1801–1867, physician at Hotel Dieu, Paris) suspected that he had cancer when he developed spontaneously appearing and disappearing (migratory) thrombosis, and his autopsy revealed that he had pancreatic cancer.

The course of pancreatic carcinoma is typically brief and progressive. Despite the tendency of lesions of the head of the pancreas to obstruct the biliary system, fewer than 20% of pancreatic cancers overall are resectable at the time of diagnosis. There has long been a search for tests that could be useful in the early detection of pancreatic cancer. Serum levels of many enzymes and antigens (e.g., carcinoembryonic antigen and CA19–9 antigen) are often elevated in individuals with pancreatic cancer. These markers, while useful in following a patient's response to treatment, are too nonspecific and lack the sensitivity needed to be used as screening tests. Several imaging techniques, such as endoscopic ultrasonography and computed tomography, have proved of great value in establishing the diagnosis once it is suspected, but are not useful as screening tests.

ACINAR CELL CARCINOMA

Acinar cell carcinomas, by definition, show prominent acinar cell differentiation, including the formation of zymogen granules and the production of exocrine enzymes including trypsin and lipase.[64] Fifteen percent of individuals with acinar cell carcinoma develop the syndrome of metastatic fat necrosis caused by the release of lipase into the circulation.

PANCREATOBLASTOMA

Pancreatoblastomas are rare neoplasms that occur primarily in children aged 1 to 15 years.[65] They have a distinct microscopic appearance with squamous islands admixed with acinar cells. These are fully malignant neoplasms, although survival may be better than that for pancreatic ductal adenocarcinomas.

REFERENCES

1. Hruban RH et al.: Tumors of the pancreas. Atlas of tumor pathology. Fourth Series, Fascicle 6 ed. Washington, DC, American Registry of Pathology and Armed Forces Institute of Pathology, 2007.
2. Oertel JE: The pancreas. Nonneoplastic alterations. Am J Surg Pathol 13:50, 1989.
3. Zaret KS, Grompe M: Generation and regeneration of cells of the liver and pancreas. Science 322:1490, 2008.
4. Cano DA et al.: Pancreatic development and disease. Gastroenterology 132:745, 2007.
5. Spicak J et al.: Pancreas divisum does not modify the natural course of chronic pancreatitis. J Gastroenterol 42:135, 2007.
6. Jimenez JC et al.: Annular pancreas in children: a recent decade's experience. J Pediatr Surg 39:1654, 2004.
7. Mitchell RM et al.: Pancreatitis. Lancet 361:1447, 2003.
8. Frossard JL et al.: Acure pancreatitis. Lancet 371:143, 2008.
9. Cappell MS: Acute pancreatitis: etiology, clinical presentation, diagnosis and therapies. Med Clin North Am 92:889, 2008.
10. Carroll JK et al.: Acute pancreatitis: diagnosis, prognosis, and treatment. Am Fam Physician 75:1513, 2007.
11. Witt H et al.: Chronic pancreatitis: challenges and advances in pathogenesis, genetics, diagnosis, and therapy. Gastroenterology 132:1557, 2007.
12. Granger J, Remick D: Acute pancreatitis: models, markers, and mediators. Shock 24 (Suppl 1):45, 2005.
13. Sand J et al.: Alcohol consumption in patients with acute or chronic pancreatitis. Pancreatology 7:147, 2007.
14. Pazzi P et al.: Biliary sludge: the sluggish gallbladder. Dig Liver Dis 35: S39, 2003.
15. Scarpelli DG: Toxicology of the pancreas. Toxicol Appl Pharmacol 101:543, 1989.
16. Whitcomb DC et al.: Hereditary pancreatitis is caused by a mutation in the cationic trypsinogen gene. Nat Genet 14:141, 1996.
17. Grendell JH: Genetic factors in pancreatitis. Curr Gastroenterol Rep 5:105, 2003.
18. Witt H et al.: Mutations in the gene encoding the serine protease inhibitor, Kazal type 1 are associated with chronic pancreatitis. Nat Genet 25:213, 2000.
19. Noone PG et al.: Cystic fibrosis gene mutations and pancreatitis risk: relation to epithelial ion transport and trypsin inhibitor gene mutations. Gastroenterology 121:1310, 2001.
20. Phat VN et al.: Early histological changes in acute necrotizing hemorrhagic pancreatitis. Pathol Res Pract 178:273, 1984.
21. Pandol SJ, Raraty M: Pathobiology of alcoholic pancreatitis. Pancreatology 7:105, 2007.
22. Norman J: The role of cytokines in the pathogenesis of acute pancreatitis. Am J Surg 175:76, 1998.
23. Saluja AK, Steer MLP: Pathophysiology of pancreatitis. Role of cytokines and other mediators of inflammation. Digestion 60 (Suppl 1):27, 1999.

24. Rau B et al.: Differential effects of caspase-1/interleukin-1beta-converting enzyme on acinar cell necrosis and apoptosis in severe acute experimental pancreatitis. Lab Invest 81:1001, 2001.
25. Shimada M et al.: IL-6 secretion by human pancreatic periacinar myofibroblasts in response to inflammatory mediators. J Immunol 168:861, 2002.
26. Blackstone MO: Hypothesis: vascular compromise is the central pathogenic mechanism for acute hemorrhagic pancreatitis. Perspect Biol Med 39:56, 1995.
27. Steer ML: Pathogenesis of acute pancreatitis. Digestion 58 (Suppl 1):46, 1997.
28. Whitcomb DC: Early trypsinogen activation in acute pancreatitis. Gastroenterology 116:770, 1999.
29. Pitchumoni CS, Bordalo O: Evaluation of hypotheses on pathogenesis of alcoholic pancreatitis. Am J Gastroenterol 91:637, 1996.
30. Vonlaufen A et al.: Molecular mechanisms of pancreatitis: current opinion. J Gastroenterol Hepatol 23:1339, 2008.
31. Witt H, Bhatia E: Genetic aspects of tropical calcific pancreatitis. Rev Endocr Metab Disord 9:213, 2008.
32. Klopel G: Chronic pancreatitis, pseudotumors and tumor-like lesions. Mod Pathol 20:S113, 2007.
33. Pitchumoni CS: Pathogenesis of alcohol-induced chronic pancreatitis: facts, perceptions, and misperceptions. Surg Clin North Am 81:379, 2001.
34. Tattersal SJN et al.: A fire inside: current concepts in chronic pancreatitis. Int Med J 38:592, 2008.
35. Saurer L et al.: Differential expression of chemokines in normal pancreas and in chronic pancreatitis. Gastroenterology 118:356, 2000.
36. Whitcomb DC: Hereditary pancreatitis: new insights into acute and chronic pancreatitis. Gut 45:317, 1999.
37. Luttenberger T et al.: Platelet-derived growth factors stimulate proliferation and extracellular matrix synthesis of pancreatic stellate cells: implications in pathogenesis of pancreas fibrosis. Lab Invest 80:47, 2000.
38. Van Laethem JL et al.: Localization of transforming growth factor beta 1 and its latent binding protein in human chronic pancreatitis. Gastroenterology 108:1873, 1995.
39. Detlefsen S et al.: Fibrogenesis in alcoholic chronic pancreatitis: the role of tissue necrosis, macrophages, myofibroblasts and cytokines. Mod Pathol 19:1019, 2006.
40. Hamano H et al.: High serum IgG4 concentrations in patients with sclerosing pancreatitis. N Engl J Med 344:732, 2001.
41. Treiber M et al.: Genetics of pancreatitis: a guide for clinicians. Curr Gastroenterol Rep 10:122, 2008.
42. Rebours V et al.: Risk of pancreatic adenocarcinoma in patients with hereditary pancreatitis: a national exhaustive series. Am J Gastroenterol 103:111, 2008.
43. Klöppel G: Pseudocysts and other non-neoplastic cysts of the pancreas. Semin Diagn Pathol 17:7, 2000.
44. Galanis C et al.: Resected serous cystic neoplasms of the pancreas: a review of 158 patients with recommendations for treatment. J Gastrointest Surg 11:820, 2007.
45. Wilentz RE et al.: Pathologic examination accurately predicts prognosis in mucinous cystic neoplasms of the pancreas. Am J Surg Pathol 23:1320, 1999.
46. Zamboni G et al.: Mucinous cystic tumors of the pancreas: clinicopathological features, prognosis, and relationship to other mucinous cystic tumors. Am J Surg Pathol 23:410, 1999.
47. Hruban RH et al.: An illustrated consensus on the classification of pancreatic intraepithelial neoplasia and intraductal papillary mucinous neoplasms. Am J Surg Pathol 28:977, 2004.
48. Chari ST et al.: Study of recurrence after surgical resection of intraductal papillary mucinous neoplasm of the pancreas. Gastroenterology 123:1500, 2002.
49. Abraham SC et al.: Solid-pseudopapillary tumors of the pancreas are genetically distinct from pancreatic ductal adenocarcinomas and almost always harbor beta-catenin mutations. Am J Pathol 160:1361, 2002.
50. American Cancer Society: Cancer Facts & Figures. Cancer 1–68. 2008. New York, American Cancer Society.
51. Hruban RH et al.: Pancreatic intraepithelial neoplasia: a new nomenclature and classification system for pancreatic duct lesions. Am J Surg Pathol 25:579, 2001.
52. van Heek NT et al.: Telomere shortening is nearly universal in pancreatic intraepithelial neoplasia. Am J Pathol 161:1541, 2002.
53. Bardeesy N, DePinho RA: Pancreatic cancer biology and genetics. Nat Rev Cancer 2:897, 2002.
54. Jones S et al.: Core signaling pathways in human pancreatic cancers revealed by global analyses. Science 321:1801, 2008.
55. Caldas C et al.: Frequent somatic mutations and homozygous deletions of the p16 (*MTS1*) gene in pancreatic adenocarcinoma. Nat Genet 8:27, 1994.
56. Hahn SA et al.: *DPC4*, a candidate tumor suppressor gene at human chromosome 18q21.1. Science 271:350, 1996.
57. Redston MS et al.: *p53* mutations in pancreatic carcinoma and evidence of common involvement of homocopolymer tracts in DNA microdeletions. Cancer Res 54:3025, 1994.
58. Fu B et al.: Frequent genomic copy number gain and overexpression of GATA-6 in parcreatic caroinoma. Cancer Biol Ther 7, 2008 [epub ahead of print].
59. Iacobuzio-Donahue CA et al.: Highly expressed genes in pancreatic ductal adenocarcinomas: a comprehensive characterization and comparison of the transcription profiles obtained from three major technologies. Cancer Res 63:8614, 2003.
60. Berman DM et al.: Widespread requirement for Hedgehog ligand stimulation in growth of digestive tract tumours. Nature 425:846, 2003.
61. Gold EB: Epidemiology of and risk factors for pancreatic cancer. Surg Clin North Am 75:819, 1995.
62. Chari ST et al.: Probability of pancreatic cancer following diabetes: a population-based study. Gastroenterology 129:504, 2005.
63. Foulkes WD: Inherited susceptibility to common cancers. N Engl J Med 359:2143, 2008.
64. Klimstra DS et al.: Acinar cell carcinoma of the pancreas. A clinicopathologic study of 28 cases. Am J Surg Pathol 16:815, 1992.
65. Klimstra DS et al.: Pancreatoblastoma. A clinicopathologic study and review of the literature. Am J Surg Pathol 19:1371, 1995.

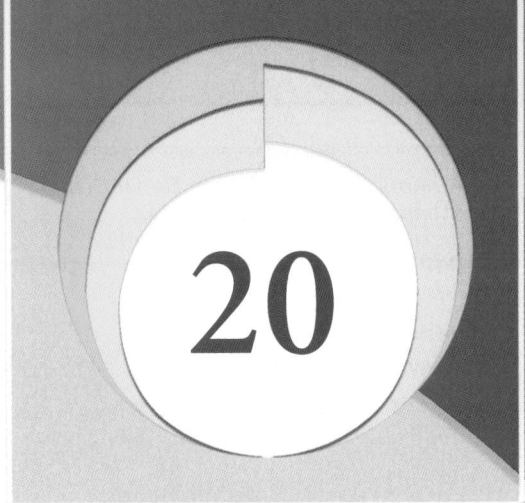

The Kidney

CHARLES E. ALPERS

Clinical Manifestations of Renal Diseases

Glomerular Diseases
  Clinical Manifestations
  Histologic Alterations
  Pathogenesis of Glomerular Injury
    Immune Complex Deposition Involving Intrinsic and in Situ Renal Antigens
    Circulating Immune Complex Glomerulonephritis
    Antibodies to Glomerular Cells
    Cell-Mediated Immunity in Glomerulonephritis
    Other Mechanisms of Glomerular Injury
    Activation of Alternative Complement Pathway
    Epithelial Cell Injury
    Mediators of Glomerular Injury
  Mechanisms of Progression in Glomerular Diseases
  Nephritic Syndrome
    Acute Proliferative (Poststreptococcal, Postinfectious) Glomerulonephritis
  Rapidly Progressive (Crescentic) Glomerulonephritis
  Nephrotic Syndrome
    Membranous Nephropathy
    Minimal-Change Disease
    Focal Segmental Glomerulosclerosis
    Membranoproliferative Glomerulonephritis
  Isolated Urinary Abnormalities
    IgA Nephropathy (Berger Disease)
    Alport Syndrome
    Thin Basement Membrane Disease (Benign Familial Hematuria)

Chronic Glomerulonephritis

Glomerular Lesions Associated with Systemic Diseases
  Lupus Nephritis
  Henoch-Schönlein Purpura
  Bacterial Endocarditis–Associated Glomerulonephritis
  Diabetic Nephropathy
  Amyloidosis
  Fibrillary Glomerulonephritis and Immunotactoid Glomerulopathy
  Other Systemic Disorders

Tubular and Interstitial Diseases
  Acute Kidney Injury (Acute Tubular Necrosis)
  Tubulointerstitial Nephritis
    Pyelonephritis and Urinary Tract Infection
    Acute Pyelonephritis
    Chronic Pyelonephritis and Reflux Nephropathy
    Tubulointerstitial Nephritis Induced by Drugs and Toxins
    Other Tubulointerstitial Diseases

Vascular Diseases
  Benign Nephrosclerosis
  Malignant Hypertension and Accelerated Nephrosclerosis
  Renal Artery Stenosis
  Thrombotic Microangiopathies
    Epidemic Hemolytic-Uremic Syndrome
    Non-Epidemic Hemolytic-Uremic Syndrome
    Thrombotic Thrombocytopenic Purpura
  Other Vascular Disorders

Atherosclerotic Ischemic Renal Disease
Atheroembolic Renal Disease
Sickle-Cell Disease Nephropathy
Diffuse Cortical Necrosis
Renal Infarcts

Congenital Anomalies
  Multicystic Renal Dysplasia

Cystic Diseases of the Kidney
  Autosomal-Dominant (Adult) Polycystic Kidney Disease
  Autosomal-Recessive (Childhood) Polycystic Kidney Disease
  Cystic Diseases of Renal Medulla
    Medullary Sponge Kidney
    Nephronophthisis and Adult-Onset Medullary Cystic Disease

Acquired (Dialysis-Associated) Cystic Disease
Simple Cysts
Urinary Tract Obstruction (Obstructive Uropathy)
Urolithiasis (Renal Calculi, Stones)
Tumors of the Kidney
  Benign Tumors
    Renal Papillary Adenoma
    Angiomyolipoma
    Oncocytoma
  Malignant Tumors
    Renal Cell Carcinoma (Adenocarcinoma of the Kidney)
    Urothelial Carcinomas of the Renal Pelvis

What is a human but an ingenious machine designed to turn, with "infinite artfulness, the red wine of Shiraz into urine"? So said the storyteller in Isak Dinesen's *Seven Gothic Tales*.[1] More accurately but less poetically, human kidneys serve to convert more than 1700 liters of blood per day into about 1 liter of a highly specialized concentrated fluid called urine. In so doing the kidney excretes the waste products of metabolism, precisely regulates the body's concentration of water and salt, maintains the appropriate acid balance of plasma, and serves as an endocrine organ, secreting such hormones as erythropoietin, renin, and prostaglandins. The physiologic mechanisms that the kidney has developed to carry out these functions require a high degree of structural complexity.

Renal diseases are responsible for a great deal of morbidity but, fortunately, are not equally major causes of mortality. To place the problem in some perspective, approximately 45,000 deaths are attributed yearly to renal disease in the United States, in contrast to about 650,000 to heart disease, 560,000 to cancer, and 145,000 to stroke.[2] Morbidity, however, is by no means insignificant. Millions of people are affected annually by nonfatal kidney diseases, most notably infections of the kidney or lower urinary tract, kidney stones, and urinary obstruction. Twenty percent of all women suffer from infection of the urinary tract or kidney at some time in their lives, and as many as 5% of the U.S. population develops renal stones. Similarly, modern treatments, notably dialysis and transplantation, keep many patients alive who earlier would have died of renal failure, adding to the pool of renal morbidity. Further, people with even mild chronic kidney disease have greatly enhanced risk for cardiovascular disease.

The study of kidney diseases is facilitated by dividing them into those that affect the four basic morphologic components: glomeruli, tubules, interstitium, and blood vessels. This traditional approach is useful, since the early manifestations of disease affecting each of these components tend to be distinct. Further, some components seem to be more vulnerable to specific forms of renal injury; for example, *most glomerular diseases are immunologically mediated, whereas tubular and interstitial disorders are frequently caused by toxic or infectious agents.* Nevertheless, some agents affect more than one structure. In addition, the anatomic and functional interdependence of the components of the kidney implies that damage to one almost always secondarily affects the others. Disease primarily in the blood vessels, for example, inevitably affects all the structures that depend on this blood supply. Severe glomerular damage impairs the flow through the peritubular vascular system and also delivers potentially toxic products to tubules; conversely, tubular destruction, by increasing intraglomerular pressure, may induce glomerular injury. Thus, whatever the origin, there is a tendency for all forms of chronic kidney disease ultimately to destroy all four components of the kidney, culminating in chronic renal failure and what has been called end-stage kidneys. The functional reserve of the kidney is large, and much damage may occur before there is evident functional impairment. For these reasons the early signs and symptoms are particularly important clinically.

Clinical Manifestations of Renal Diseases

The clinical manifestations of renal disease can be grouped into reasonably well-defined syndromes. Some are peculiar to glomerular diseases, and others are present in diseases that affect any one of the components. Before we list the syndromes, a few terms must be clarified.

Azotemia is a biochemical abnormality that refers to an elevation of the blood urea nitrogen (BUN) and creatinine levels, and is related largely to a decreased glomerular filtration rate (GFR). Azotemia is a consequence of many renal disorders, but it also arises from extrarenal disorders. *Prerenal azotemia* is encountered when there is hypoperfusion of the kidneys (e.g., in hemorrhage, shock, volume depletion, and congestive heart failure) that impairs renal function in the absence of parenchymal damage. *Postrenal azotemia* is seen whenever urine flow is obstructed beyond the level of the kidney. Relief of the obstruction is followed by correction of the azotemia.

When azotemia becomes associated with a constellation of clinical signs and symptoms and biochemical abnormalities, it is termed *uremia*. Uremia is characterized not only by failure of renal excretory function but also by a host of metabolic and endocrine alterations resulting from renal damage. Uremic patients frequently manifest secondary involvement of the gastrointestinal system (e.g., uremic gastroenteritis), peripheral nerves (e.g., peripheral neuropathy), and heart (e.g., uremic fibrinous pericarditis).

We can now turn to a brief description of the clinical presentations of renal disease:

- *Nephritic syndrome* is due to glomerular disease and is dominated by the acute onset of usually grossly visible hematuria (red blood cells in urine), mild to moderate proteinuria, and hypertension; it is the classic presentation of acute poststreptococcal glomerulonephritis.
- *Rapidly progressive glomerulonephritis* is characterized as a nephritic syndrome with rapid decline (hours to days) in GFR.
- The *nephrotic syndrome*, also due to glomerular disease, is characterized by heavy proteinuria (more than 3.5 gm/day), hypoalbuminemia, severe edema, hyperlipidemia, and lipiduria (lipid in the urine).
- *Asymptomatic hematuria or proteinuria*, or a combination of these two, is usually a manifestation of subtle or mild glomerular abnormalities.
- *Acute renal failure* is dominated by oliguria or anuria (reduced or no urine flow), and recent onset of azotemia. It can result from glomerular, interstitial, or vascular injury or acute tubular injury.
- *Chronic renal failure*, characterized by prolonged symptoms and signs of uremia, is the end result of all chronic renal parenchymal diseases.
- Renal tubular defects are dominated by polyuria (excessive urine formation), nocturia, and electrolyte disorders (e.g., metabolic acidosis). They are the result of diseases that either directly affect tubular structure (e.g., medullary cystic disease) or cause defects in specific tubular functions. The latter can be inherited (e.g., familial nephrogenic diabetes, cystinuria, renal tubular acidosis) or acquired (e.g., lead nephropathy).
- Urinary tract infection is characterized by bacteriuria and pyuria (bacteria and leukocytes in the urine). The infection may be symptomatic or asymptomatic, and it may affect the kidney (pyelonephritis) or the bladder (cystitis).
- Nephrolithiasis (renal stones) is manifested by severe spasms of pain (renal colic) and hematuria, often with recurrent stone formation.
- Urinary tract obstruction and renal tumors have varied clinical manifestations based on the specific anatomic location and nature of the lesion.

Renal Failure. *Acute renal failure* implies a rapid and frequently reversible deterioration of renal function. It is discussed in the section on "Acute Kidney Injury (Acute Tubular Necrosis)," because it commonly occurs in this disorder. Here, the discussion is limited to chronic renal failure, which is the end result of a variety of renal diseases and the major cause of death from renal disease.

Although exceptions abound, the evolution from normal renal function to symptomatic *chronic renal failure* broadly progresses through a series of four stages that merge into one another.

1. In *diminished renal reserve* the GFR is about 50% of normal. Serum BUN and creatinine values are normal, and the patients are asymptomatic. However, they are more susceptible to developing azotemia with an additional renal insult.
2. In *renal insufficiency* the GFR is 20% to 50% of normal. Azotemia appears, usually associated with anemia and hypertension. Polyuria and nocturia can occur as a result of decreased concentrating ability. Sudden stress (e.g., with nephrotoxins) may precipitate uremia.
3. In *chronic renal failure* the GFR is less than 20% to 25% of normal. The kidneys cannot regulate volume and solute composition, and patients develop edema, metabolic acidosis, and hyperkalemia. Overt uremia may ensue, with neurologic, gastrointestinal, and cardiovascular complications.
4. In *end-stage renal disease* the GFR is less than 5% of normal; this is the terminal stage of uremia. Recent clinical classifications of chronic kidney disease, adopted in part to better stratify patients in clinical trials, adhere to this schema of progressive injury but divide patients into five classes based on levels of GFR.

The details of the pathophysiology of chronic renal failure are beyond the scope of this book and are well covered in various nephrology texts. Table 20–1 lists the major systemic abnormalities in chronic kidney failure.

Glomerular Diseases

Glomerular diseases constitute some of the major problems in nephrology; indeed, chronic glomerulonephritis is one of the most common causes of chronic kidney disease in humans. Glomeruli may be injured by a variety of factors and in the course of several systemic diseases. Systemic immunological diseases such as systemic lupus erythematosus (SLE), vascular disorders such as hypertension, metabolic diseases such as diabetes mellitus, and some hereditary conditions such as Fabry disease often affect the glomerulus. These are termed *secondary glomerular diseases* to differentiate them from disorders in which the kidney is the only or predominant organ involved. The latter constitute the various types of *primary glomerulonephritis* or, because some do not have a cellular inflammatory component, *glomerulopathy. However, both the clinical manifestations and glomerular histologic changes in primary and secondary forms can be similar.*

Here we discuss the various types of primary glomerulopathies and briefly review the secondary forms covered in other parts of this book. Table 20–2 lists the most common forms of glomerulonephritis that have reasonably well defined morphologic and clinical characteristics.

TABLE 20-1 Principal Systemic Manifestations of Chronic Kidney Disease and Uremia

FLUID AND ELECTROLYTES

Dehydration
Edema
Hyperkalemia
Metabolic acidosis

CALCIUM PHOSPHATE AND BONE

Hyperphosphatemia
Hypocalcemia
Secondary hyperparathyroidism
Renal osteodystrophy

HEMATOLOGIC

Anemia
Bleeding diathesis

CARDIOPULMONARY

Hypertension
Congestive heart failure
Cardiomyopathy
Pulmonary edema
Uremic pericarditis

GASTROINTESTINAL

Nausea and vomiting
Bleeding
Esophagitis, gastritis, colitis

NEUROMUSCULAR

Myopathy
Peripheral neuropathy
Encephalopathy

DERMATOLOGIC

Sallow color
Pruritus
Dermatitis

TABLE 20-2 Glomerular Diseases

PRIMARY GLOMERULOPATHIES

Acute proliferative glomerulonephritis
  Post-infectious
  Other
Rapidly progressive (crescentic) glomerulonephritis
Membranous glomerulopathy
Minimal-change disease
Focal segmental glomerulosclerosis
Membranoproliferative glomerulonephritis
IgA nephropathy
Chronic glomerulonephritis

SYSTEMIC DISEASES WITH GLOMERULAR INVOLVEMENT

Systemic lupus erythematosus
Diabetes mellitus
Amyloidosis
Goodpasture syndrome
Microscopic polyarteritis/polyangiitis
Wegener granulomatosis
Henoch-Schönlein purpura
Bacterial endocarditis

HEREDITARY DISORDERS

Alport syndrome
Thin basement membrane disease
Fabry disease

CLINICAL MANIFESTATIONS

The clinical manifestations of glomerular disease are clustered into the five major glomerular syndromes summarized in Table 20-3. Both the primary glomerulopathies and the systemic diseases affecting the glomerulus can result in these syndromes. Because glomerular diseases are often associated with systemic disorders, mainly *diabetes mellitus, SLE, vasculitis,* and *amyloidosis,* in any patient with manifestations of glomerular disease it is essential to consider these systemic conditions.

Many clinical manifestations of glomerular disease result from perturbations of specific components of the glomerular tuft, so we present key anatomic structures that are subject to alteration in disease. The glomerulus consists of an anastomosing network of capillaries lined by fenestrated endothelium invested by two layers of epithelium (Fig. 20-1). The visceral epithelium is incorporated into and becomes an intrinsic part of the capillary wall, separated from endothelial cells by a basement membrane. The parietal epithelium, situated on the Bowman capsule, lines the urinary space, the cavity in which plasma filtrate first collects.

The glomerular capillary wall is the filtering membrane and consists of the following structures[3,4] (Fig. 20-2):

- There is a thin layer of fenestrated *endothelial cells*, each fenestrum being about 70 to 100 nm in diameter.
- A *glomerular basement membrane* (GBM) with a thick electron-dense central layer, the *lamina densa*, and thinner electron-lucent peripheral layers, the *lamina rara interna* and *lamina rara externa*. The GBM consists of collagen (mostly type IV), laminin, polyanionic proteoglycans (mostly heparan sulfate), fibronectin, entactin, and several other glycoproteins. Type IV collagen forms a network suprastructure to which other glycoproteins attach. The

TABLE 20-3 The Glomerular Syndromes	
Syndrome	**Manifestations**
Nephritic syndrome	Hematuria, azotemia, variable proteinuria, oliguria, edema, and hypertension
Rapidly progressive glomerulonephritis	Acute nephritis, proteinuria, and acute renal failure
Nephrotic syndrome	>3.5 gm/day proteinuria, hypoalbuminemia, hyperlipidemia, lipiduria
Chronic renal failure	Azotemia → uremia progressing for months to years
Isolated urinary abnormalities	Glomerular hematuria and/or subnephrotic proteinuria

CL
MES
EP
END
CL
MES
A

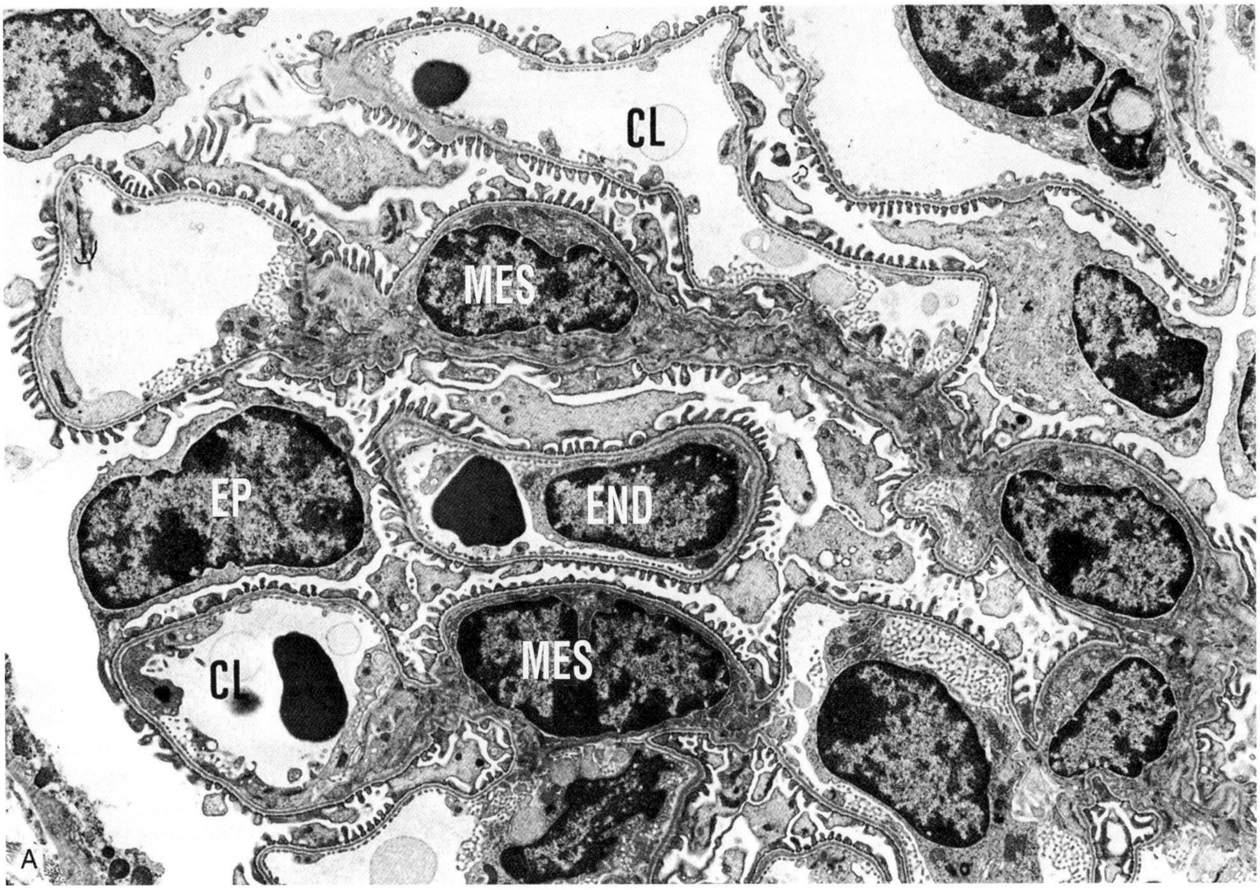

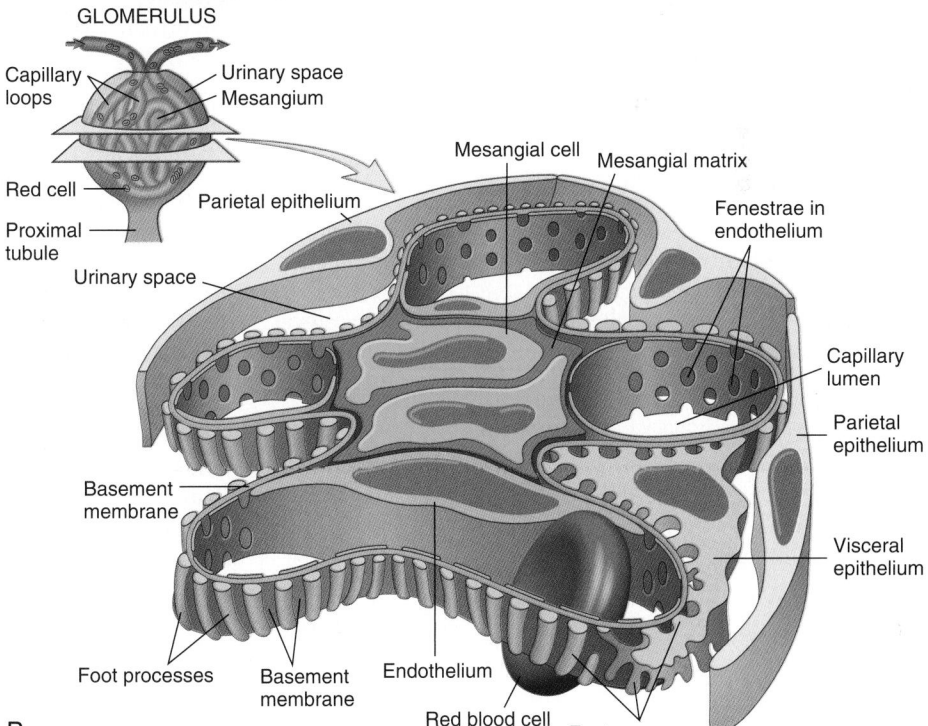

GLOMERULUS
Capillary loops
Urinary space
Mesangium
Red cell
Proximal tubule
Parietal epithelium
Urinary space
Mesangial cell
Mesangial matrix
Fenestrae in endothelium
Capillary lumen
Parietal epithelium
Basement membrane
Visceral epithelium
Foot processes
Basement membrane
Endothelium
Red blood cell
Foot processes
B

FIGURE 20–1 **A,** Low-power electron micrograph of renal glomerulus. CL, capillary lumen; EP, visceral epithelial cells with foot processes; END, endothelium; MES, mesangium. **B,** Schematic representation of a glomerular lobe. (**A,** Courtesy of Dr. Vicki Kelley, Brigham and Women's Hospital, Boston, MA.)

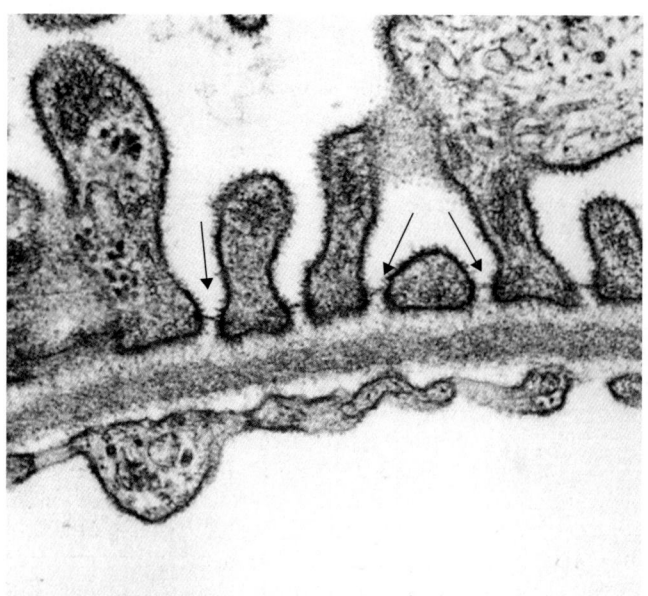

FIGURE 20–2 Glomerular filter consisting, from bottom to top, of fenestrated endothelium, basement membrane, and foot processes of epithelial cells. Note the filtration slits *(arrows)* and diaphragm situated between the foot processes. Note also that the basement membrane consists of a central lamina densa, sandwiched between two looser layers, the lamina rara interna and lamina rara externa. (Courtesy of Dr. Helmut Rennke, Brigham and Women's Hospital, Boston, MA.)

building block (monomer) of this network is a triple-helical molecule made up of three α chains, composed of one or more of six types of α chains (α₁ to α₆ or COL4A1 to COL4A6), the most common consisting of α₁, α₂, α₁.[3,5] Each molecule consists of a 7S domain at the N terminus, a triple-helical domain in the middle, and a globular noncollagenous domain (NC1) at the C terminus. The NC1 domain is important for helix formation and for assembly of collagen monomers into the basement membrane suprastructure. Glycoproteins (laminin, entactin) and proteoglycans (heparan sulfate, perlecan) attach to the collagenous suprastructure. These biochemical determinants are critical

to understanding glomerular diseases. For example, as we shall see, the antigens in the NC1 domain are the targets of antibodies in anti-GBM nephritis; genetic defects in the α-chains underlie some forms of hereditary nephritis; and the proteoglycan content of the GBM may contribute to its permeability characteristics.

- The *visceral epithelial cells* (podocytes) are structurally complex cells that possess interdigitating processes embedded in and adherent to the lamina rara externa of the basement membrane. Adjacent *foot processes* (pedicels) are separated by 20- to 30-nm-wide *filtration slits*, which are bridged by a thin diaphragm (see Fig. 20–2).
- The entire glomerular tuft is supported by *mesangial cells* lying between the capillaries. Basement membrane–like *mesangial matrix* forms a meshwork through which the mesangial cells are centered (see Fig. 20–1). These cells, of mesenchymal origin, are contractile, phagocytic, and capable of proliferation, of laying down both matrix and collagen, and of secreting several biologically active mediators. Biologically, they are most akin to vascular smooth muscle cells and pericytes. They are, as we shall see, important players in many forms of human glomerulonephritis.

The major characteristics of normal glomerular filtration are an extraordinarily high permeability to water and small solutes, because of the highly fenestrated nature of the endothelium, and impermeability to proteins, such as molecules of the size of albumin (~3.6-nm radius; 70 kilodaltons [kD] molecular weight) or larger. The latter property of the *glomerular filtration barrier* allows discrimination among various protein molecules, depending on their size (the larger, the less permeable) and charge (the more cationic, the more permeable). This size- and charge-dependent barrier function is accounted for by the complex structure of the capillary wall, the collagenous porous and charged structure of the GBM, and the many anionic moieties present within the wall, including the acidic proteoglycans of the GBM and the sialoglycoproteins of epithelial and endothelial cell coats (also called glycocalyx). The charge-dependent restriction is important in the virtually complete exclusion of albumin from the filtrate, because albumin is an anionic molecule of a pI 4.5. The visceral epithelial cell, also known as a podocyte, is important for the maintenance of glomerular barrier function; its slit diaphragm presents a size-selective distal diffusion barrier to the filtration of proteins, and it is the cell type that is largely responsible for synthesis of GBM components. Proteins located in the slit diaphragm control glomerular permeability. Three of the most important slit diaphragm proteins are depicted in Figure 20–3. Nephrin is a transmembrane protein with a large extracellular portion made up of immunoglobulin (Ig)-like domains. Nephrin molecules extend toward each other from neighboring foot processes and dimerize across the slit diaphragm. Within the cytoplasm of the foot processes, nephrin forms molecular connections with podocin, CD2-associated protein, and ultimately the actin cytoskeleton. The number of identified slit diaphragm proteins continues to grow rapidly, and more comprehensive descriptions of their complex localization and interactions have been published.[6,7] The importance of these proteins in maintaining glomerular permeability is demonstrated by the observation that mutations in the genes encoding them give rise to nephrotic

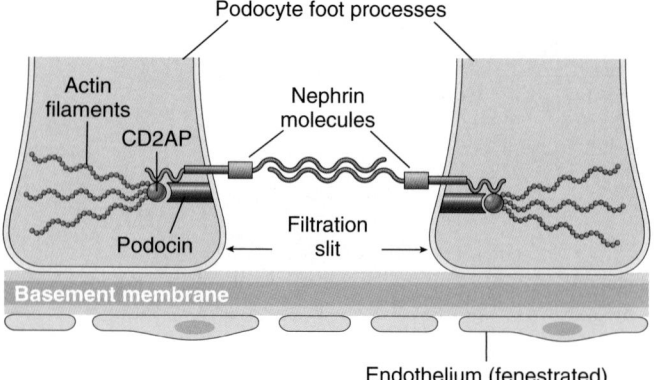

FIGURE 20–3 A simplified schematic diagram of some of the best-studied proteins of the glomerular slit diaphragm. CD2AP, CD2-associated protein.

syndrome (discussed later). This has resulted in renewed appreciation of the importance of the slit diaphragm in glomerular barrier function and its contribution to protein leakage in disease states.[8]

HISTOLOGIC ALTERATIONS

Various types of glomerulopathies are characterized by one or more of four basic tissue reactions.

Hypercellularity. Some *inflammatory diseases* of the glomerulus are characterized by an increase in the number of cells in the glomerular tufts. This hypercellularity is characterized by one or more combinations of the following:

○ *Cellular proliferation* of mesangial or endothelial cells.
○ *Leukocytic infiltration* consisting of neutrophils, monocytes, and, in some diseases, lymphocytes.
○ *Formation of crescents.* These are accumulations of cells composed of proliferating parietal epithelial cells and infiltrating leukocytes. The epithelial cell proliferation that characterizes crescent formation occurs following an immune/inflammatory injury (see later). Fibrin, which leaks into the urinary space, often through ruptured basement membranes, has been long thought to be the molecule that elicits the crescentic response. In support of this, fibrin can be demonstrated immunohistochemically in the glomerular tufts and urinary spaces of glomeruli that contain crescents. Mice that are deficient in fibrinogen are protected to a degree from crescent formation, and mice that are deficient in molecules important in fibrinolysis (e.g., plasminogen activators) exhibit enhanced crescent formation in models of anti-GBM antibody–mediated crescentic glomerulonephritis.[9] Other molecules that have been implicated in crescent formation and recruitment of leukocytes into crescents include procoagulants such as tissue factor and cytokines such as interleukin-1 (IL-1), tumor necrosis factor (TNF), and interferon-γ.

Basement Membrane Thickening. By light microscopy, this change appears as thickening of the capillary walls, best seen in sections stained with periodic acid–Schiff (PAS). By electron microscopy such thickening takes one of two forms:

○ Deposition of amorphous electron-dense material, most often immune complexes, on the endothelial or epithelial side of the basement membrane or within the GBM itself. Fibrin, amyloid, cryoglobulins, and abnormal fibrillary proteins may also deposit in the GBM.
○ Thickening of the basement membrane due to increased synthesis of its protein components, as occurs in diabetic glomerulosclerosis.

Hyalinosis and Sclerosis. *Hyalinosis,* as applied to the glomerulus, denotes the accumulation of material that is homogeneous and eosinophilic by light microscopy. By electron microscopy the hyalin is extracellular and amorphous. It is made up of plasma proteins that have insudated from the circulation into glomerular structures. When extensive, this change contributes to obliteration of the capillary lumens of the glomerular tuft. Hyalinosis is usually a consequence of endothelial or capillary wall injury and typically the end result of various forms of glomerular damage. It is a common feature of focal segmental glomerulosclerosis.

Sclerosis is characterized by accumulations of extracellular collagenous matrix, either confined to mesangial areas as is often the case in diabetic glomerulosclerosis, or involving the capillary loops, or both. The sclerosing process may also result in obliteration of some or all of the capillary lumens in affected glomeruli, which in turn can result in formation of fibrous adhesions between the sclerotic portions of glomeruli and the nearby parietal epithelium and Bowman capsules.

Because many of the primary glomerulopathies are of unknown cause, they are often classified by their histology, as can be seen in Table 20–2. The histologic changes can be further subdivided by their distribution into *diffuse,* involving all glomeruli; *global,* involving the entire glomerulus; *focal,* involving only a proportion of the glomeruli; *segmental,* affecting a part of each glomerulus; and by either *capillary loop* or *mesangial,* affecting predominantly capillary or mesangial regions. These terms are sometimes appended to the histologic classifications.

PATHOGENESIS OF GLOMERULAR INJURY

Although much is not known about etiologic agents and triggering events, it is clear that immune mechanisms underlie most forms of primary glomerulopathy and many of the secondary glomerular disorders[10,11] (Table 20–4). Glomerulonephritis can be readily induced experimentally by antigen-antibody reactions. Furthermore, glomerular deposits of immunoglobulins, often with components of complement, are found in the majority of individuals with glomerulonephritis. Cell-mediated immune reactions also may play a role, usually in concert with antibody-mediated events. We begin this discussion with a review of antibody-instigated injury.

TABLE 20–4 Immune Mechanisms of Glomerular Injury

ANTIBODY-MEDIATED INJURY

IN SITU IMMUNE COMPLEX DEPOSITION

Fixed intrinsic tissue antigens
  NC1 domain of collagen type IV antigen (anti-GBM nephritis)
  Heymann antigen (membranous glomerulopathy)
  Mesangial antigens
  Others
Planted antigens
  Exogenous (infectious agents, drugs)
  Endogenous (DNA, nuclear proteins, immunoglobulins, immune complexes, IgA)

CIRCULATING IMMUNE COMPLEX DEPOSITION

Endogenous antigens (e.g., DNA, tumor antigens)
Exogenous antigens (e.g., infectious products)

CYTOTOXIC ANTIBODIES

CELL-MEDIATED IMMUNE INJURY

ACTIVATION OF ALTERNATIVE COMPLEMENT PATHWAY

GBM, glomerular basement membrane.

Two forms of antibody-associated injury have been established: (1) injury by *antibodies reacting in situ within the glomerulus, either binding to insoluble fixed (intrinsic) glomerular antigens or to molecules planted within the glomerulus,* and (2) injury resulting from *deposition of circulating antigen-antibody complexes* in the glomerulus. In addition, there is experimental evidence that *cytotoxic antibodies* directed against glomerular cell components may cause glomerular injury. These pathways are not mutually exclusive, and in humans, all may contribute to injury.

Immune Complex Deposition Involving Intrinsic and in Situ Renal Antigens

In these forms of injury, antibodies react directly with intrinsic tissue antigen, or antigens "planted" in the glomerulus from the circulation. The best established experimental models for anti–glomerular antibody–mediated glomerular injury, for which there are counterparts in human disease, are anti–glomerular basement membrane (anti-GBM) antibody–induced glomerulonephritis and Heymann nephritis.

Heymann Nephritis

The Heymann model of rat glomerulonephritis is induced by immunizing animals with an antigen contained within preparations of proximal tubular brush border (Fig. 20–4C). The rats develop antibodies to this antigen, and a membranous nephropathy, resembling human membranous nephropathy, develops (discussed later; see also Fig. 20–13). On electron microscopy the glomerulopathy is characterized by the presence of numerous discrete electron-dense deposits (made up largely of immune reactants) along the *subepithelial aspect* of the basement membrane. The pattern of immune deposition by immunofluorescence microscopy is *granular* rather than linear. It is now clear that this type of disease results largely from the reaction of antibody with an antigen complex located on the basal surface of visceral epithelial cells and cross-reacting with the brush-border antigen used in the original experiments. This so-called Heymann antigen in rats is a large 330-kD protein called *megalin*, which has homology to the low-density lipoprotein receptor (Chapter 5); the corresponding antigen in human membranous nephropathy has not yet been identified.[12] Antibody binding to glomerular epithelial cell membrane is followed by complement activation and then shedding of the immune aggregates from the cell surface to form the characteristic subepithelial deposits (see Fig. 20–4C).

In humans, anti-GBM antibody–induced disease and membranous nephropathy are autoimmune diseases, caused by antibodies to endogenous tissue components. What triggers these autoantibodies is unclear, but any one of the several mechanisms responsible for autoimmunity, discussed in Chapter 6, may be involved. Several forms of autoimmune glomerulonephritis can be experimentally induced by drugs (e.g., mercuric chloride), infectious products (endotoxin), and the graft-versus-host reaction (Chapter 6). In such models there is an alteration of immune regulation associated with B-cell activation and the induction of an array of autoantibodies that react with renal antigens.

Antibodies against Planted Antigens

Antibodies can react in situ with antigens that are not normally present in the glomerulus but are "planted" there. There is increasing experimental support for such a mechanism of glomerulonephritis. Such antigens may localize in the kidney by interacting with various intrinsic components of the glomerulus. Planted antigens include cationic molecules that bind to anionic components of the glomerulus; DNA, nucleosomes, and other nuclear proteins, which have an affinity for GBM components; bacterial products; large aggregated proteins (e. g., aggregated immunoglobulins, which deposit in the mesangium because of their size; and immune complexes themselves, since they continue to have reactive sites for further interactions with free antibody, free antigen, or complement. There is no dearth of other possible planted antigens, including viral, bacterial, and parasitic products and drugs. Antibodies that bind to most of these planted antigens induce a discrete pattern of Ig deposition detected as granular staining by immunofluorescence microscopy, similar to the pattern found in circulating immune complex nephritis.

Anti-GBM Antibody–Induced Glomerulonephritis

In this type of injury *antibodies are directed against intrinsic fixed antigens that are normal components of the GBM proper.* It has its experimental counterpart in so-called Masugi or nephrotoxic nephritis, produced in rats by injections of anti-rat kidney antibodies prepared in rabbits by immunization with rat kidney tissue. The injected antibodies bind along the entire length of the GBM, *resulting in a diffuse linear pattern of staining for the antibodies by immunofluorescent techniques* (see Fig. 20–4B and E*).* This is contrasted with the granular lumpy pattern of immunofluorescent staining seen in other in situ models, such as the Heymann model of membranous glomerulopathy, or after deposition of circulating immune complexes.

In the Masugi model the injected anti-GBM antibody is rabbit Ig, which is foreign to the host and thus acts as an antigen eliciting anti-Ig antibody in the rat. The rat antibodies then react with the rabbit Ig deposited in the basement membrane, leading to further glomerular injury. Often the anti-GBM antibodies cross-react with other basement membranes, especially those in the lung alveoli, resulting in simultaneous lung and kidney lesions (*Goodpasture syndrome*). *The GBM antigen that is responsible for classic anti-GBM antibody–induced glomerulonephritis and Goodpasture syndrome is a component of the noncollagenous domain (NC1) of the α_3 chain of collagen type IV that is critical for maintenance of GBM suprastructure.*[5] Anti-GBM antibody–induced glomerulonephritis accounts for fewer than 5% of cases of human glomerulonephritis. It is solidly established as the cause of injury in Goodpasture syndrome, discussed later. Most instances of anti-GBM antibody–induced glomerulonephritis are characterized by severe crescentic glomerular damage and the clinical syndrome of rapidly progressive glomerulonephritis.

Circulating Immune Complex Glomerulonephritis

In this type of nephritis glomerular injury is caused by the trapping of circulating antigen-antibody complexes within

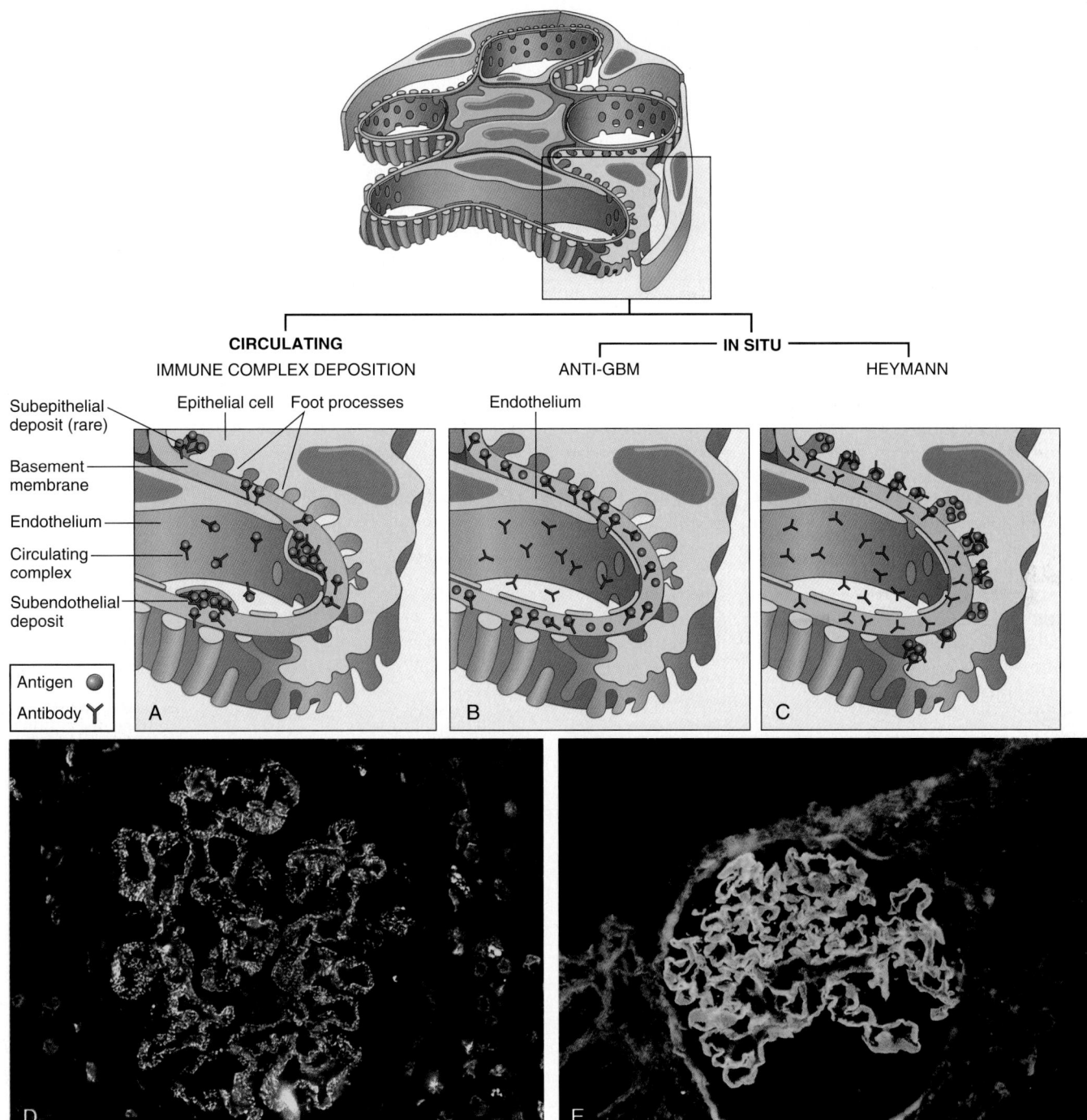

FIGURE 20–4 Antibody-mediated glomerular injury can result either from the deposition of circulating immune complexes (**A**) or, more commonly, from in situ formation of complexes exemplified by anti-GBM disease (**B**) or Heymann nephritis (**C**). **D** and **E**, Two patterns of deposition of immune complexes as seen by immunofluorescence microscopy: granular, characteristic of circulating and in situ immune complex nephritis (**D**), and linear, characteristic of classic anti-GBM disease (**E**).

glomeruli. The antibodies have no immunological specificity for glomerular constituents, and the complexes localize within the glomeruli because of their physicochemical properties and the hemodynamic factors peculiar to the glomerulus (see Fig. 20–4A).

The pathogenesis of immune complex diseases was discussed in Chapter 6. Here we briefly review the salient features that relate to glomerular injury.

The antigens that trigger the formation of circulating immune complexes may be of endogenous origin, as in the glomerulonephritis associated with SLE, or they may be exogenous, as is likely in the glomerulonephritis that follows certain infections. Microbial antigens that are implicated include bacterial products (streptococci), the surface antigen of hepatitis B virus, hepatitis C virus antigens, and antigens of *Treponema pallidum, Plasmodium falciparum,* and several viruses. Some tumor antigens are also thought to cause immune complex–mediated nephritis. In many cases the inciting antigen is unknown.

Whatever the antigen may be, antigen-antibody complexes are formed in the circulation and then trapped in the glomeruli, where they produce injury. It has long been thought that this injury is mediated and amplified by the binding of complement, but recent studies in knockout mice also point to the importance of engagement of Fc receptors on leukocytes and perhaps intrinsic renal cells as mediators of the injury process.[13] The glomerular lesions usually exhibit leukocytic infiltration and proliferation of mesangial and endothelial cells. Electron microscopy reveals the immune complexes as electron-dense deposits that lie in the mesangium, between the endothelial cells and the GBM (subendothelial deposits), or between the outer surface of the GBM and the podocytes (subepithelial deposits). Deposits may be located at more than one site in a given case. By immunofluorescence microscopy the immune complexes are seen as granular deposits along the basement membrane, in the mesangium, or in both locations (see Fig. 20–4D). Once deposited in the kidney, immune complexes may eventually be degraded, mostly by infiltrating neutrophils and monocytes/macrophages, mesangial cells, and endogenous proteases, and the inflammatory reaction may then subside. Such a course occurs when the exposure to the inciting antigen is short-lived and limited, as in most cases of poststreptococcal glomerulonephritis. However, if a continuous shower of antigens develops, as may be seen in SLE or viral hepatitis, repeated cycles of immune complex formation, deposition, and injury may occur, leading to a more chronic membranous or membranoproliferative type of glomerulonephritis.

Several factors affect glomerular localization of antigen, antibody, or complexes of both. The molecular charge and size of these reactants are clearly important. Highly cationic immunogens tend to cross the GBM, and the resultant complexes eventually reside in a subepithelial location. Highly anionic macromolecules are excluded from the GBM and either are trapped subendothelially or are not nephritogenic at all. Molecules of neutral charge and immune complexes containing these molecules tend to accumulate in the mesangium. Large circulating complexes are not usually nephritogenic, because they are cleared by the mononuclear phagocyte system and do not enter the GBM in sufficient quantities. The pattern of localization is also affected by changes in glomerular hemodynamics, mesangial function, and integrity of the charge-selective barrier in the glomerulus. These influences may underlie the variable pattern of immune reactant deposition in various forms of glomerulonephritis, as shown in Figure 20–5. In turn, the distinct patterns of localization of immune complexes is a key determinant of the injury response and the histologic features that subsequently develop.

Antibodies to Glomerular Cells

In addition to causing immune deposits, antibodies against glomerular cell antigens may react with cellular components and cause injury by cytotoxic or other mechanisms. Antibodies to mesangial cell antigens, for example, can cause mesangiolysis followed by mesangial cell proliferation; anti-

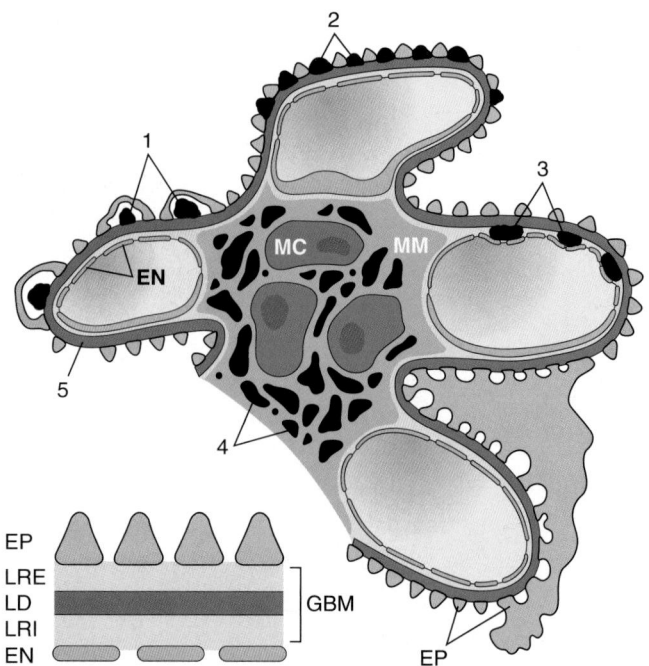

FIGURE 20–5 Localization of immune complexes in the glomerulus: (1) subepithelial humps, as in acute glomerulonephritis; (2) epimembranous deposits, as in membranous nephropathy and Heymann glomerulonephritis; (3) subendothelial deposits, as in lupus nephritis and membranoproliferative glomerulonephritis; (4) mesangial deposits, as in IgA nephropathy; (5) basement membrane. EN, endothelium; EP, epithelium; LD, lamina densa; LRE, lamina rara externa; LRI, lamina rara interna; MC, mesangial cell; MM, mesangial matrix. (Modified from Couser WG: Mediation of immune glomerular injury. J Am Soc Nephrol 1:13, 1990.)

bodies to endothelial cell antigens cause endothelial injury and intravascular thrombosis; and antibodies to certain visceral epithelial cell components cause proteinuria in experimental animals. This mechanism may play a role in certain human immune disorders that are without demonstrable immune deposits.

In summary, *most cases of human glomerulonephritis are a consequence of deposits of discrete immune complexes, which are visualized by granular immunofluorescence staining along the basement membranes or in the mesangium.* However, it may be difficult to determine whether the deposition has occurred in situ, by circulating complexes, or by both mechanisms because, as was discussed earlier, trapping of circulating immune complexes can initiate further in situ complex formation. Single etiologic agents, such as hepatitis B and C viruses, can cause either a membranous pattern of glomerulonephritis, suggesting in situ deposition, or a membranoproliferative pattern, more indicative of circulating complexes. It is best then to consider that *antigen-antibody deposition in the glomerulus is a major pathway of glomerular injury and that in situ immune reactions, trapping of circulating complexes, interactions between these two events, and local hemodynamic and structural determinants in the glomerulus all contribute to the diverse morphologic and functional alterations in glomerulonephritis.*

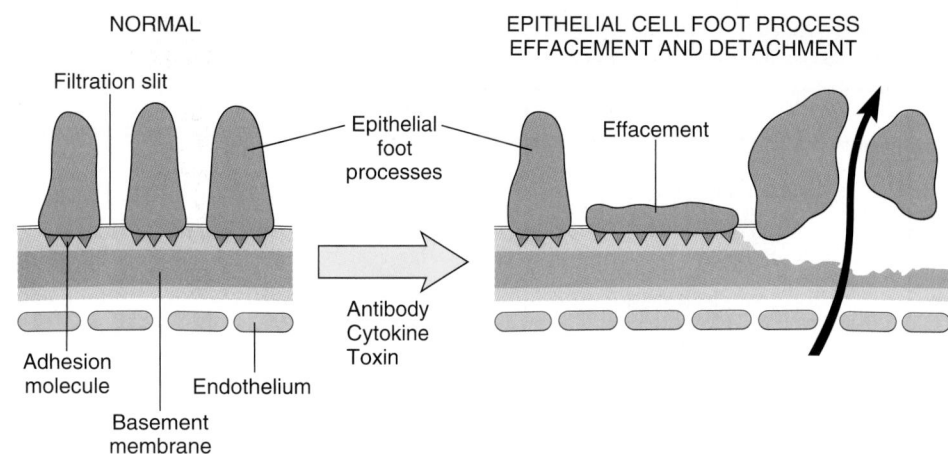

NORMAL

Filtration slit

EPITHELIAL CELL FOOT PROCESS
EFFACEMENT AND DETACHMENT

Epithelial
foot
processes

Effacement

Antibody
Cytokine
Toxin

Adhesion
molecule

Endothelium

Basement
membrane

FIGURE 20–6 Epithelial cell injury. The postulated sequence is a consequence of antibodies specific to epithelial cell antigens, toxins, cytokines, or other factors causing injury; this results in foot process effacement and sometimes detachment of epithelial cells and protein leakage through defective GBM and filtration slits.

Cell-Mediated Immunity in Glomerulonephritis

Although antibody-mediated mechanisms may initiate many forms of glomerulonephritis, there is now considerable evidence that sensitized T cells cause some forms of glomerular injury and are involved in the progression of many glomerulonephritides.[14] Clues to the role of cellular immunity include the presence of activated macrophages and T cells and their products in the glomerulus in some forms of human and experimental glomerulonephritis;[15] in vitro and in vivo evidence of lymphocyte activation on exposure to antigen in human and experimental glomerulonephritis; abrogation of glomerular injury by lymphocyte depletion; and successful attempts to induce glomerular injury by transfer of T cells from nephritic animals to normal recipients. The evidence is most compelling for certain types of experimental crescentic glomerulonephritis in which antibodies to GBM may initiate glomerular injury but activated T lymphocytes may propogate the inflammation.[15]

Activation of Alternative Complement Pathway

Alternative complement pathway activation occurs in the clinicopathologic entity called dense-deposit disease, also referred to as *membranoproliferative glomerulonephritis (MPGN type II)*. It may also occur in some forms of proliferative glomerulonephritis. This mechanism is discussed later.

Epithelial Cell Injury

This can be induced by antibodies to visceral epithelial cell antigens; by toxins, as in an experimental model of proteinuria induced by puromycin aminonucleoside; conceivably by certain cytokines; or by still poorly characterized factors, as in the case of human minimal-change disease and focal segmental glomerulosclerosis, discussed later. Such injury is reflected morphologically by changes in the visceral epithelial cells, which include effacement of foot processes, vacuolization, retraction, and detachment of cells from the GBM, and functionally by proteinuria. It is hypothesized that the detachment of visceral epithelial cells is caused by loss of adhesive interactions with the basement membrane and that this detachment contributes to protein leakage (Fig. 20–6).

Mediators of Glomerular Injury

Once immune reactants or sensitized T cells have localized in the glomerulus, how does the glomerular damage ensue? The mediators—both cells and molecules—are the usual suspects involved in acute and chronic inflammation, described in Chapter 2, and only a few are highlighted here (Fig. 20–7).

Cells

- *Neutrophils* and *monocytes* infiltrate the glomerulus in certain types of glomerulonephritis, largely as a result of activation of complement, resulting in generation of chemotactic agents (mainly C5a), but also by Fc-mediated adherence and activation. Neutrophils release proteases, which cause GBM degradation; oxygen-derived free radicals, which cause cell damage; and arachidonic acid metabolites, which contribute to the reductions in GFR.
- *Macrophages, T lymphocytes,* and *natural killer cells,* which infiltrate the glomerulus in antibody- and cell-mediated reactions, when activated release a vast number of biologically active molecules.
- *Platelets* aggregate in the glomerulus during immune-mediated injury. Their release of eicosanoids and growth factors may contribute to the manifestations of glomerulonephritis. Antiplatelet agents have beneficial effects in both human and experimental glomerulonephritis.
- *Resident glomerular cells,* particularly mesangial cells, can be stimulated to produce several inflammatory mediators, including reactive oxygen species (ROS), cytokines, chemokines, growth factors, eicosanoids, nitric oxide, and endothelin. In the absence of leukocytic infiltration, they may initiate inflammatory responses in the glomerulus.

Soluble Mediators

Virtually all the known inflammatory chemical mediators have been implicated in glomerular injury.

- The *chemotactic complement components* induce leukocyte influx (complement-neutrophil–dependent injury) and lead to formation of C5b-C9, the membrane attack complex. C5b-C9 causes cell lysis but, in addition, stimulates mesan-

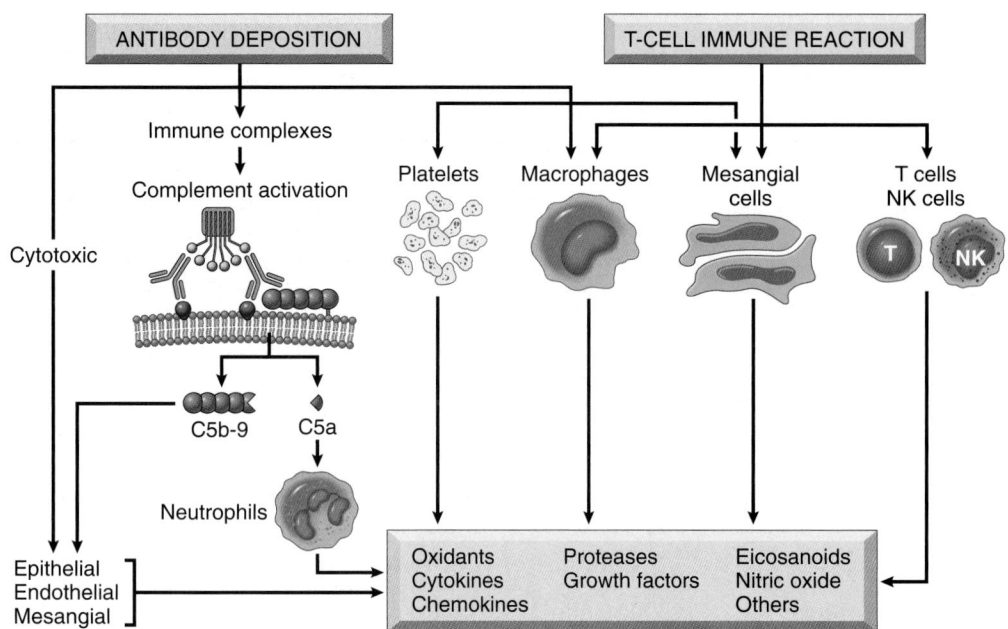

FIGURE 20–7 Mediators of immune glomerular injury including cells and soluble mediators (see text).

gial cells to produce oxidants, proteases, and other mediators. Thus, even in the absence of neutrophils, C5b-C9 can cause proteinuria, as has been postulated in membranous glomerulopathy.

- *Eicosanoids, nitric oxide, angiotensin,* and *endothelin* are involved in the hemodynamic changes.
- *Cytokines,* particularly IL-1 and TNF, which may be produced by infiltrating leukocytes and resident glomerular cells, induce leukocyte adhesion and a variety of other effects.
- *Chemokines* such as monocyte chemoattractant protein 1 and CCL5 promote monocyte and lymphocyte influx. *Growth factors* such as platelet-derived growth factor (PDGF) are involved in mesangial cell proliferation.[16] TGF-β, connective tissue growth factor, and fibroblast growth factor seem to be critical in the ECM deposition and hyalinization leading to glomerulosclerosis in chronic injury.[17] Vascular endothelial growth factor (VEGF) seems to maintain endothelial integrity and may help regulate capillary permeability.
- The *coagulation system* is also a mediator of glomerular damage. Fibrin is frequently present in the glomeruli in glomerulonephritis, and fibrin may leak into Bowman space, serving as a stimulus for parietal epithelial cell proliferation (crescent formation). Fibrin deposition is mediated largely by stimulation of macrophage procoagulant activity. Plasminogen activator inhibitor-1 is linked to increased thrombosis and fibrosis by inhibiting degradation of fibrin and matrix proteins.

MECHANISMS OF PROGRESSION IN GLOMERULAR DISEASES

Thus far we have discussed the immunological mechanisms and mediators that *initiate* glomerular injury. The outcome of such injury depends on several factors, including the initial severity of renal damage, the nature and persistence of the antigens, and the immune status, age, and genetic predisposition of the host.

It has long been known that once any renal disease, glomerular or otherwise, destroys functioning nephrons and reduces the GFR to about 30% to 50% of normal, progression to end-stage renal failure proceeds at a relatively constant rate, independent of the original stimulus or activity of the underlying disease. The secondary factors that lead to progression are of great clinical interest, since they can be targets of therapy that delays or even prevents the inexorable journey to dialysis or transplantation.

The two major histologic characteristics of such progressive renal damage are *focal segmental glomerulosclerosis* and *tubulointerstitial fibrosis*; we discuss these separately.[18–20]

Focal Segmental Glomerulosclerosis (FSGS). Patients with this secondary change develop proteinuria, even if the primary disease was nonglomerular. The glomerulosclerosis seems to be initiated by the *adaptive change* that occurs in the relatively unaffected glomeruli of diseased kidneys.[19,21] Such a mechanism is suggested by experiments in rats subjected to ablation of renal mass by subtotal nephrectomy. *Compensatory hypertrophy* of the remaining glomeruli serves to maintain renal function in these animals, but proteinuria and segmental glomerulosclerosis soon develop, leading eventually to total glomerular sclerosis and uremia. The glomerular hypertrophy is associated with *hemodynamic changes*, including increases in glomerular blood flow, filtration, and transcapillary pressure (glomerular hypertension), and often with systemic hypertension. The sequence of events (Fig. 20–8) that is thought to lead to sclerosis in this setting entails endothelial and epithelial cell injury, increased glomerular permeability to proteins, and accumulation of proteins in the mesangial matrix. This is followed by proliferation of mesangial cells, infiltration by macrophages, increased accumulation of extracellular matrix (ECM), and segmental and eventually global

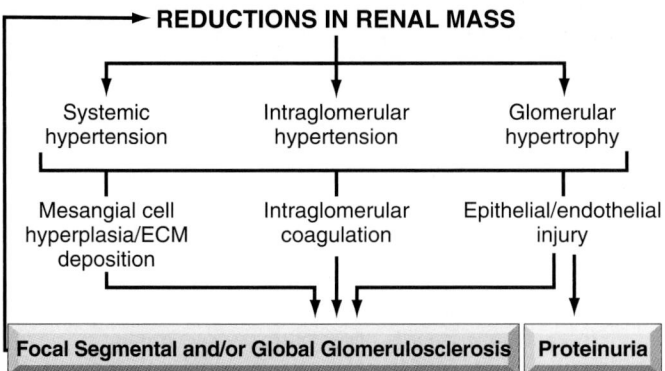

REDUCTIONS IN RENAL MASS

Systemic hypertension	Intraglomerular hypertension	Glomerular hypertrophy
Mesangial cell hyperplasia/ECM deposition	Intraglomerular coagulation	Epithelial/endothelial injury

Focal Segmental and/or Global Glomerulosclerosis **Proteinuria**

FIGURE 20–8 Focal segmental glomerulosclerosis associated with loss of renal mass. The adaptive changes in glomeruli (hypertrophy and glomerular capillary hypertension), as well as systemic hypertension, cause epithelial and endothelial injury and resultant proteinuria. The mesangial response, involving mesangial cell proliferation and ECM production together with intraglomerular coagulation, causes the glomerulosclerosis. This results in further loss of functioning nephrons and a vicious circle of progressive glomerulosclerosis.

sclerosis of glomeruli. This results in further reductions in nephron mass, ongoing activation of these compensatory changes, and a vicious circle of continuing glomerulosclerosis. Most of the mediators of chronic inflammation and fibrosis, particularly TGF-β, play a role in the induction of sclerosis. Currently, the most successful interventions to interrupt these mechanisms of progressive glomerulosclerosis involve treatment with inhibitors of the renin-angiotensin system, which not only reduce intraglomerular hypertension, but also have direct effects on each of the mechanisms identified above.[21] Importantly, these agents have been shown to ameliorate progression of sclerosis in both animal and human studies.[20]

Contributing to the progressive injury of focal and segmental glomerulosclerosis is the inability of mature visceral epithelial cells (podocytes) to proliferate after injury. This can lead to a decrease in glomerular podocyte number after a severe injury resulting in loss of some of these cells, leading in turn to a process whereby remaining podocytes are either abnormally stretched to maintain an appropriate filtration barrier or unable to cover portions of the GBM, which become denuded of the overlying podocyte foot processes. These alterations lead to abnormal protein filtration as well as loss of structural support for the glomerular capillary walls. This latter alteration in turn may lead to segmental loop dilation because of now incompletely opposed intracapillary pressures, with subsequent formation of a fibrous attachment to Bowman capsule by the bulging capillary segment, and eventual sclerosis of this segment.[22]

Tubulointerstitial Fibrosis. Tubulointerstitial injury, manifested by tubular damage and interstitial inflammation, is a component of many acute and chronic glomerulonephritides. Tubulointerstitial fibrosis contributes to progression in both immune and nonimmune glomerular diseases, for example, diabetic nephropathy. *Indeed, there is often a much better correlation of decline in renal function with the extent of tubulointerstitial damage than with the severity of glomerular injury.*[18] Many factors may lead to such tubulointerstitial injury, including ischemia of tubule segments downstream

from sclerotic glomeruli, acute and chronic inflammation in the adjacent interstitium, and damage or loss of the peritubular capillary blood supply. Current work also points to the effects of *proteinuria* on tubular cell structure and function[23]. On the basis of in vitro and animal studies, proteinuria is thought to cause *direct injury to and activation of tubular cells.* Activated tubular cells in turn express adhesion molecules and elaborate pro-inflammatory cytokines, chemokines, and growth factors that contribute to interstitial fibrosis. Filtered proteins that may produce these tubular effects include cytokines, complement products, the iron in transferrin, immunoglobulins, lipid moieties, and oxidatively modified plasma proteins.

Having discussed factors in the initiation and progression of glomerular injury, we now turn to a discussion of individual glomerular diseases. Table 20–5 summarizes the main clinical and pathologic features of the major forms of primary glomerulopathies.

NEPHRITIC SYNDROME

Glomerular diseases presenting with a nephritic syndrome are often *characterized by inflammation in the glomeruli.* The nephritic patient usually presents with hematuria, red cell casts in the urine, azotemia, oliguria, and mild to moderate hypertension. Proteinuria and edema are common, but these are not as severe as those encountered in the nephrotic syndrome, discussed later. The acute nephritic syndrome may occur in such multisystem diseases as SLE and microscopic polyangiitis. Typically, however, it is characteristic of acute proliferative glomerulonephritis and is an important component of crescentic glomerulonephritis, which is described later.

Acute Proliferative (Poststreptococcal, Postinfectious) Glomerulonephritis

As the name implies, this cluster of diseases is characterized histologically by diffuse proliferation of glomerular cells, associated with influx of leukocytes. These lesions are typically caused by immune complexes. The inciting antigen may be exogenous or endogenous. The prototypic exogenous antigen-induced disease pattern is postinfectious glomerulonephritis, whereas an example of an endogenous antigeninduced disease is the nephritis of SLE, described in Chapter 6. The most common underlying infections are streptococcal, but the disorder also has been associated with other infections.

Poststreptococcal Glomerulonephritis

This glomerular disease is decreasing in frequency in the United States but continues to be a fairly common disorder worldwide.[24] It usually appears 1 to 4 weeks after a streptococcal infection of the pharynx or skin (impetigo). Skin infections are commonly associated with overcrowding and poor hygiene. Poststreptococcal glomerulonephritis occurs most frequently in children 6 to 10 years of age, but adults of any age can also be affected.

Etiology and Pathogenesis. Only certain strains of group A β-hemolytic streptococci are nephritogenic, more than 90%

TABLE 20–5 Summary of Major Primary Glomerulonephritides

Disease	Most Frequent Clinical Presentation	Pathogenesis	Glomerular Pathology		
			Light Microscopy	Fluorescence Microscopy	Electron Microscopy
Postinfectious glomerulonephritis	Nephritic syndrome	Immune complex mediated; circulating or planted antigen	Diffuse endocapillary proliferation; leukocytic infiltration	Granular IgG and C3 in GBM and mesangium	Subepithelial humps
Goodpasture syndrome	Rapidly progressive glomerulonephritis	Anti-GBM COL4-A3 antigen	Extracapillary proliferation with crescents; necrosis	Linear IgG and C3; fibrin in crescents	No deposits; GBM disruptions; fibrin
Chronic glomerulonephritis	Chronic renal failure	Variable	Hyalinized glomeruli	Granular or negative	
Membranous glomerulopathy	Nephrotic syndrome	In situ immune complex formation; antigens mostly unknown	Diffuse capillary wall thickening	Granular IgG and C3; diffuse	Subepithelial deposits
Minimal-change disease	Nephrotic syndrome	Unknown; loss of glomerular polyanion; podocyte injury	Normal; lipid in tubules	Negative	Loss of foot processes; no deposits
Focal segmental glomerulosclerosis	Nephrotic syndrome; non-nephrotic proteinuria	Unknown Ablation nephropathy Plasma factor (?); podocyte injury	Focal and segmental sclerosis and hyalinosis	Focal; IgM + C3	Loss of foot processes; epithelial denudation
Membranoproliferative glomerulonephritis (MPGN) type I	Nephrotic/nephrotic syndrome	Immune complex		IgG + C3; C1q + C4	Subendothelial deposits
Dense-deposit disease (MPGN type II)	Hematuria Chronic renal failure	Autoantibody; alternative complement pathway	Mesangial and endocapillary proliferation; GBM thickening; splitting	C3 ± IgG; no C1q or C4	Dense deposits
IgA nephropathy	Recurrent hematuria or proteinuria	Unknown	Focal mesangial proliferative glomerulonephritis; mesangial widening	IgA ± IgG, IgM, and C3 in mesangium	Mesangial and paramesangial dense deposits

GBM, glomerular basement membrane.

of cases being traced to types 12, 4, and 1, which can be identified by typing of M protein of the cell wall.

Poststreptococcal glomerulonephritis is an immunologically mediated disease. The latent period between infection and onset of nephritis is compatible with the time required for the production of antibodies and the formation of immune complexes. Elevated titers of antibodies against one or more streptococcal antigens are present in a great majority of patients. Serum complement levels are low, compatible with activation of the complement system and consumption of complement components. There are granular immune deposits in the glomeruli, supporting an immune complex–mediated mechanism. The streptococcal antigenic component responsible for the immune reaction has eluded identification for years. Several *cationic antigens*, including a nephritis-associated streptococcal plasmin receptor (NAPlr), unique to nephritogenic strains of streptococci, can be found in affected glomeruli. Other evidence suggests that

streptococcal pyogenic exotoxin B (SpeB) and its zymogen precursor (zSpeB), another protein that functions as a plasmin receptor, are the principal antigenic determinants in most cases of poststreptococcal glomerulonephritis.[25] It is not known if these represent antigens planted in the GBM, or parts of circulating immune complexes, or both. GBM proteins altered by streptococcal enzymes have also been implicated as antigens.

Morphology. The classic diagnostic picture is one of **enlarged, hypercellular glomeruli** (Fig. 20–9). The hypercellularity is caused by (1) infiltration by leukocytes, both neutrophils and monocytes; (2) proliferation of endothelial and mesangial cells; and (3) in severe cases by crescent formation. The proliferation and leukocyte infiltration are diffuse, that is, involving all lobules of all glomeruli. There is also swelling of

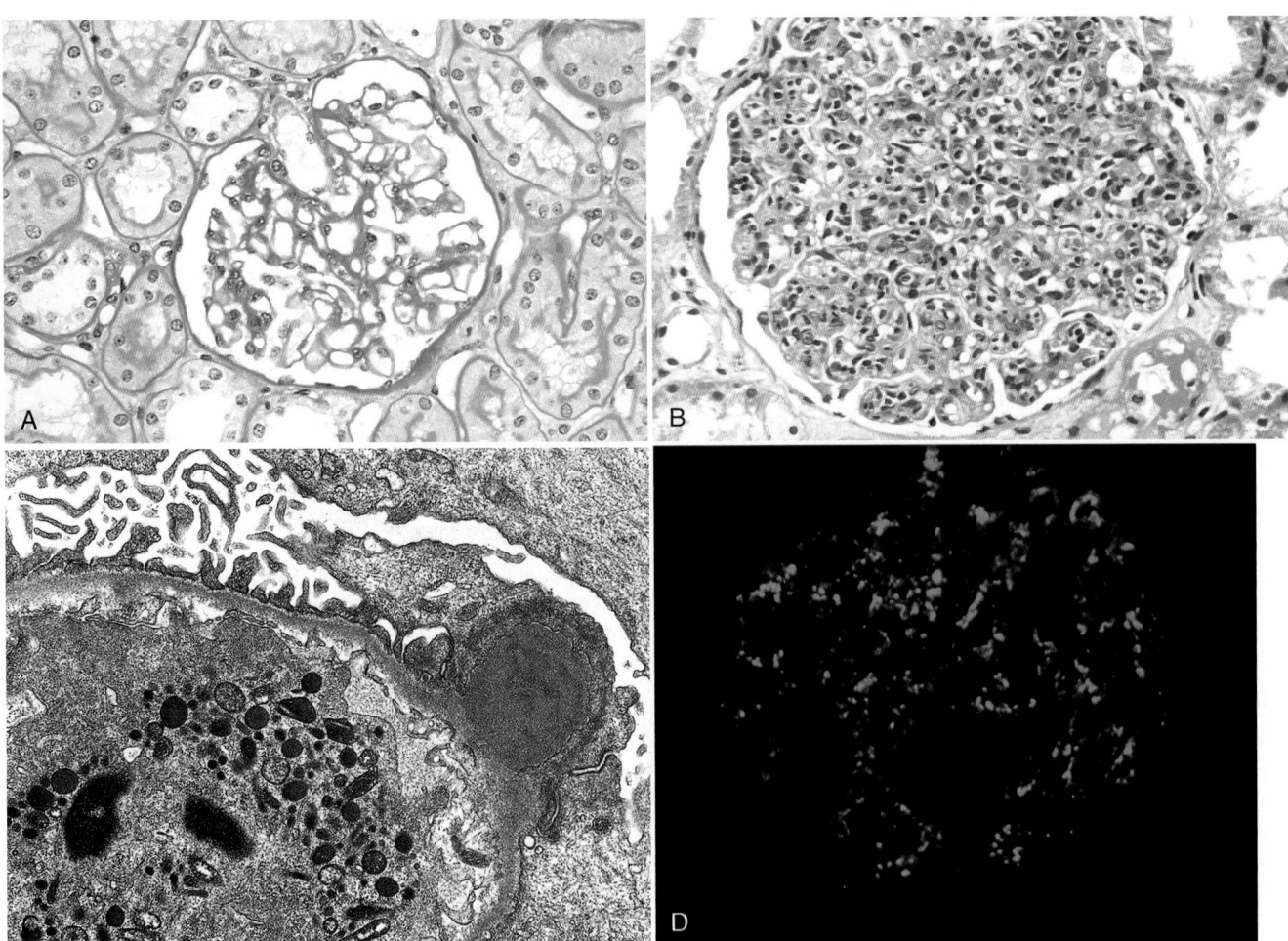

FIGURE 20–9   Acute proliferative glomerulonephritis. **A,** Normal glomerulus. **B,** Glomerular hypercellularity is due to intracapillary leukocytes and proliferation of intrinsic glomerular cells. **C,** Typical electron-dense subepithelial "hump" and a neutrophil in the lumen. **D,** Immunofluorescent stain demonstrates discrete, coarsely granular deposits of complement protein C3, corresponding to "humps" illustrated in part C. (**A–C,** courtesy of Dr. H. Rennke, Brigham and Women's Hospital, Boston, MA. **D,** courtesy of D. J. Kowaleska, University of Washington, Seattle, WA.)

endothelial cells, and the combination of proliferation, swelling, and leukocyte infiltration obliterates the capillary lumens. There may be interstitial edema and inflammation, and the tubules often contain red cell casts.

By **immunofluorescence microscopy,** there are granular deposits of IgG, IgM, and C3 in the mesangium and along the GBM (Fig. 20–9D). Although immune complex deposits are almost universally present, they are often focal and sparse. The characteristic **electron microscopic findings** are discrete, amorphous, electron-dense deposits on the epithelial side of the membrane, often having the appearance of "humps" (Fig. 20–9C), presumably representing the antigen-antibody complexes at the epithelial cell surface. Subendothelial and intramembranous deposits are also commonly seen, and mesangial deposits may be present.

Clinical Course.   In the classic case, a young child abruptly develops malaise, fever, nausea, oliguria, and hematuria (smoky or cola-colored urine) 1 to 2 weeks after recovery from a sore throat. The patients have red cell casts in the urine, mild proteinuria (usually less than 1 gm/day), periorbital edema, and mild to moderate hypertension. In adults the onset is more likely to be atypical, such as the sudden appearance of hypertension or edema, frequently with elevation of BUN. During epidemics caused by nephritogenic streptococcal infections, glomerulonephritis may be asymptomatic, discovered only on screening for microscopic hematuria. Important laboratory findings include elevations of antistreptococcal antibody titers and a decline in the serum concentration of C3 and other components of the complement cascade.

More than 95% of affected children eventually recover totally with conservative therapy aimed at maintaining sodium and water balance. A small minority of children (perhaps fewer than 1%) do not improve, become severely oliguric, and develop a rapidly progressive form of glomerulonephritis (described later). Some of the remaining patients may undergo slow progression to chronic glomerulonephritis with or without recurrence of an active nephritic picture. Prolonged and persistent heavy proteinuria and abnormal GFR mark patients with an unfavorable prognosis.

In adults the disease is less benign. Although the overall prognosis in epidemics is good, in only about 60% of *sporadic cases* do the patients recover promptly. In the remainder the glomerular lesions fail to resolve quickly, as manifested by persistent proteinuria, hematuria, and hypertension. In some of these patients, the lesions eventually clear totally, but others develop chronic glomerulonephritis. Some patients will develop a syndrome of rapidly progressive glomerulonephritis.

Nonstreptococcal Acute Glomerulonephritis (Postinfectious Glomerulonephritis)

A similar form of glomerulonephritis occurs sporadically in association with other infections, including bacterial (e.g., staphylococcal endocarditis, pneumococcal pneumonia, and meningococcemia), viral (e.g., hepatitis B, hepatitis C, mumps, human immunodeficiency virus [HIV] infection, varicella, and infectious mononucleosis), and parasitic (malaria, toxoplasmosis). In these settings, granular immunofluorescent deposits and subepithelial humps characteristic of immune complex nephritis are present.

RAPIDLY PROGRESSIVE (CRESCENTIC) GLOMERULONEPHRITIS

Rapidly progressive glomerulonephritis (RPGN) is a syndrome associated with severe glomerular injury and does not denote a specific etiologic form of glomerulonephritis. It is characterized clinically by rapid and progressive loss of renal function associated with severe oliguria and signs of nephritic syndrome; if untreated, death from renal failure occurs within weeks to months. *The most common histologic picture is the presence of crescents in most of the glomeruli* (crescentic glomerulonephritis). As discussed earlier, these are produced by the proliferation of the parietal epithelial cells lining Bowman capsule and by the infiltration of monocytes and macrophages.

Classification and Pathogenesis. RPGN may be caused by a number of different diseases, some restricted to the kidney and others systemic. Although no single mechanism can explain all cases, there is little doubt that in most cases the glomerular injury is immunologically mediated. A practical classification divides RPGN into three groups on the basis of immunological findings (Table 20–6). In each group the disease may be associated with a known disorder, or it may be idiopathic.

The first type of RPGN is *anti-GBM antibody–induced disease*, characterized by linear deposits of IgG and, in many cases, C3 in the GBM that are visualized by immunofluorescence.[26] In some of these patients, the anti-GBM antibodies cross-react with pulmonary alveolar basement membranes to produce the clinical picture of pulmonary hemorrhage associated with renal failure (*Goodpasture syndrome*). Plasmapheresis to remove the pathogenic circulating antibodies is usually part of the treatment, which also includes therapy to suppress the underlying immune response.

The Goodpasture antigen is a peptide within the noncollagenous portion of the α_3 chain of collagen type IV.[5] What triggers the formation of these antibodies is unclear in most patients. Exposure to viruses or hydrocarbon solvents (found in paints and dyes) has been implicated in some patients, as

TABLE 20–6 Rapidly Progressive Glomerulonephritides
TYPE I (ANTI-GBM ANTIBODY)
Renal limited
Goodpasture syndrome
TYPE II (IMMUNE COMPLEX)
Idiopathic
Post-infectious glomerulonephritis
Lupus nephritis
Henoch-Schönlein purpura (IgA nephropathy)
Others
TYPE III (PAUCI-IMMUNE)
ANCA-associated
Idiopathic
Wegener granulomatosis
Microscopic polyangiitis

ANCA, antineutrophil cytoplasmic antibodies; GBM, glomerular basement membrane.

have various drugs and cancers. There is a high prevalence of certain HLA subtypes and haplotypes (e.g., HLA-DRB1) in affected patients, a finding consistent with the genetic predisposition to autoimmunity.[27]

The second type of RPGN is the result of *immune complex deposition*. It can be a complication of any of the immune complex nephritides, including postinfectious glomerulonephritis, lupus nephritis, IgA nephropathy, and Henoch-Schönlein purpura. In all these cases, immunofluorescence studies reveal the granular pattern of staining characteristic of immune complex deposition. This type of RPGN frequently demonstrates cellular proliferation within the glomerular tuft, in addition to crescent formation. These patients cannot usually be helped by plasmapheresis, and they require treatment for the underlying disease.

The third type of RPGN, also called *pauci-immune type*, is defined by the lack of anti-GBM antibodies or immune complexes by immunofluorescence and electron microscopy. Most patients with this type of RPGN have circulating *antineutrophil cytoplasmic antibodies* (ANCAs) that produce cytoplasmic (c) or perinuclear (p) staining patterns and, as we have seen (Chapter 11), play a role in some vasculitides. Hence, in some cases this type of RPGN is a component of a systemic vasculitis such as Wegener granulomatosis or microscopic polyangiitis. In many cases, however, pauci-immune crescentic glomerulonephritis is isolated and hence *idiopathic*. More than 90% of such idiopathic cases have c-ANCAs or p-ANCAs in the sera.[26] The presence of circulating ANCAs in both idiopathic crescentic glomerulonephritis and cases of crescentic glomerulonephritis that occur as a component of systemic vasculitis, and the similar pathologic features in either setting, have led to the idea that these disorders are pathogenetically related. According to this concept, all cases of crescentic glomerulonephritis of the pauci-immune type are manifestations of small-vessel vasculitis or polyangiitis, which is limited to glomerular and perhaps peritubular capillaries in cases of idiopathic crescentic glomerulonephritis. The clinical distinction between systemic vasculitis with pauci-immune renal involvement and idiopathic crescentic glomerulonephritis accordingly has become de-emphasized, since these entities are viewed as part of a spectrum of vasculitic disease. ANCAs have proved to be invaluable as a highly sensitive diagnostic marker for pauci-immune crescentic glomerulonephritis, but proof of their role as a direct cause of this glomerulonephritis has been elusive. Recent strong evidence of their pathogenic potential has been obtained by studies in mice showing that transferring antibodies against myeloperoxidase (the target antigen of most p-ANCAs) induces a form of RPGN.[28]

To summarize, all three types of RPGN may be associated with a well-defined renal or extrarenal disease, but in many cases (~50%), the disorder is idiopathic. Of the patients with this syndrome, about one fifth have anti–GBM antibody–mediated glomerulonephritis without lung involvement; another one fourth have immune complex–mediated crescentic glomerulonephritis; and the remainder are of the pauci-immune type. *The common denominator in all types of RPGN is severe glomerular injury.*

Morphology. The kidneys are enlarged and pale, often with petechial hemorrhages on the cortical surfaces. Depending on the underlying cause, the glomeruli may show focal necrosis, diffuse or focal endothelial proliferation, and mesangial proliferation. The histologic picture, however, is dominated by distinctive **crescents** (Fig. 20–10). Crescents are formed by proliferation of parietal cells and by migration of monocytes and macrophages into the urinary space. Neutrophils and lymphocytes may be present. The crescents eventually obliterate Bowman space and compress the glomerular tuft. **Fibrin strands are frequently prominent between the cellular layers in the crescents;** indeed, as discussed earlier, the escape of fibrinogen into Bowman space and its conversion to fibrin are an important contributor to crescent formation. By immunofluorescence microscopy, immune complex–mediated cases show granular immune deposits; Goodpasture syndrome cases show linear GBM fluorescence for Ig and complement, and pauci-immune cases have little or no deposition of immune reactants. Electron microscopy discloses deposits in

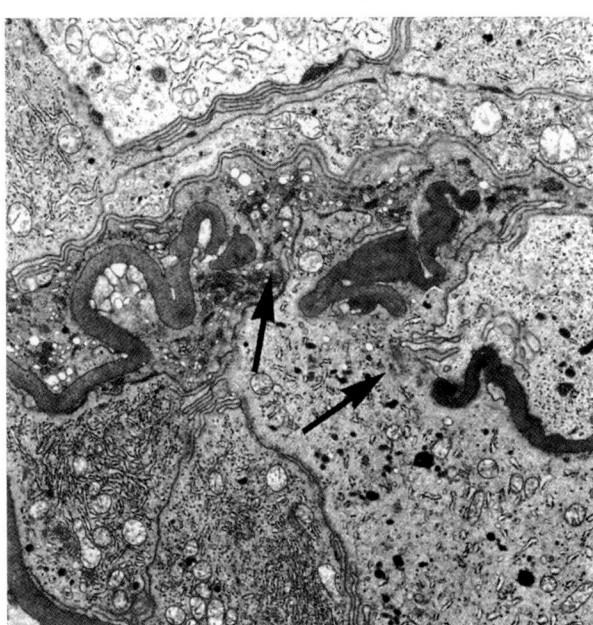

FIGURE 20–11   Crescentic glomerulonephritis. Electron micrograph showing characteristic wrinkling of GBM with focal disruptions *(arrows)*.

those cases due to immune complex deposition (type II). Regardless of type, electron microscopy may show distinct **ruptures in the GBM**, the severe injury that allows leukocytes, proteins, and inflammatory mediators to reach the urinary space, where they trigger the crescent formation (Fig. 20–11). In time, most crescents undergo sclerosis, but restoration of normal glomerular architecture may be achieved with early aggressive therapy.

Clinical Course.   The renal manifestations of all forms of crescentic glomerulonephritis include hematuria with red blood cell casts in the urine, moderate proteinuria occasionally reaching the nephrotic range, and variable hypertension and edema. In Goodpasture syndrome the course may be dominated by recurrent hemoptysis or even life-threatening pulmonary hemorrhage. Serum analyses for anti-GBM antibodies, antinuclear antibodies, and ANCAs are helpful in the diagnosis of specific subtypes. Although milder forms of glomerular injury may subside, the renal involvement is usually progressive over a matter of weeks and culminates in severe oliguria. Recovery of renal function may follow early intensive plasmapheresis (plasma exchange) combined with steroids and cytotoxic agents in Goodpasture syndrome. This therapy can reverse both pulmonary hemorrhage and renal failure. Other forms of RPGN also respond well to steroids and cytotoxic agents. However, despite therapy, some patients may eventually require chronic dialysis or transplantation, particularly if the disease is discovered at a late stage.

NEPHROTIC SYNDROME

Certain glomerular diseases virtually always produce the nephrotic syndrome. In addition, many other forms of primary and secondary glomerulopathies discussed in this chapter may

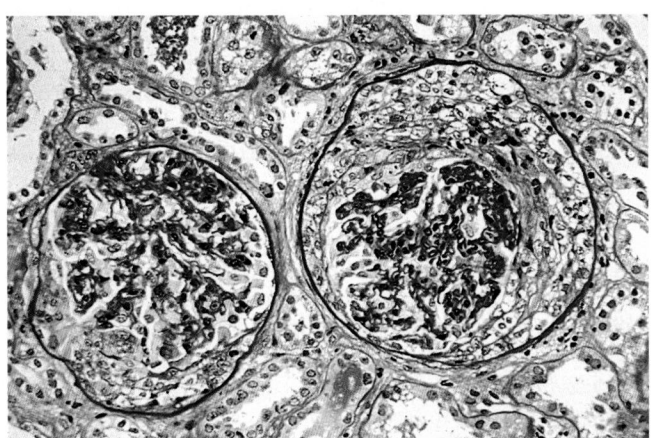

FIGURE 20–10   Crescentic glomerulonephritis (PAS stain). Note the collapsed glomerular tufts and the crescent-shaped mass of proliferating parietal epithelial cells and leukocytes internal to Bowman capsule. (Courtesy of Dr. M.A. Venkatachalam, University of Texas Health Sciences Center, San Antonio, TX.)

underlie the syndrome. Before the major diseases associated with nephrotic syndrome are presented, the causes and pathophysiology of this clinical complex are briefly discussed.

Pathophysiology. The manifestations of the nephrotic syndrome include:

1. *Massive proteinuria*, with the daily loss of 3.5 gm or more of protein (less in children)
2. *Hypoalbuminemia*, with plasma albumin levels less than 3 gm/dL
3. *Generalized edema*
4. *Hyperlipidemia and lipiduria*

The various components of nephrotic syndrome bear a logical relationship to one another. The initial event is a derangement in glomerular capillary walls resulting in *increased permeability to plasma proteins.* The glomerular capillary wall, with its endothelium, GBM, and visceral epithelial cells, acts as a size and charge barrier through which the plasma filtrate passes. Increased permeability resulting from either structural or physicochemical alterations allows protein to escape from the plasma into the urinary space. *Massive proteinuria results.*

The heavy proteinuria depletes serum albumin levels at a rate beyond the compensatory synthetic capacity of the liver, resulting in hypoalbuminemia and a reversed albumin-to-globulin ratio. Increased renal catabolism of filtered albumin also contributes to the hypoalbuminemia. The generalized edema is, in turn, the consequence of decreased colloid osmotic pressure of the blood with subsequent accumulation of fluid in the interstitial tissues. There is also *sodium and water retention*, which aggravates the edema (Chapter 4). This seems to be due to several factors, including compensatory secretion of aldosterone, mediated by the hypovolemia-enhanced renin secretion; stimulation of the sympathetic system; and a reduction in the secretion of natriuretic factors such as atrial peptides. Edema is characteristically soft and pitting, most marked in the periorbital regions and dependent portions of the body. It may be massive, with pleural effusions and ascites.

The largest proportion of protein lost in the urine is albumin, but globulins are also excreted in some diseases. The ratio of low- to high-molecular-weight proteins in the urine in various cases of nephrotic syndrome is a manifestation of the *selectivity* of proteinuria. A *highly selective proteinuria* consists mostly of low-molecular-weight proteins (albumin, 70 kD; transferrin, 76 kD molecular weight), whereas a *poorly selective proteinuria* consists of higher molecular-weight globulins in addition to albumin.

The genesis of the *hyperlipidemia* is complex. Most patients with nephritic syndrome have increased blood levels of cholesterol, triglyceride, very-low-density lipoprotein, low-density lipoprotein, Lp(a) lipoprotein, and apoprotein, and there is a decrease in high-density lipoprotein concentration in some patients. These defects seem to be due in part to *increased synthesis of lipoproteins in the liver, abnormal transport of circulating lipid particles, and decreased catabolism.* Lipiduria follows the hyperlipidemia, because lipoproteins also leak across the glomerular capillary wall. The lipid appears in the urine either as free fat or as *oval fat bodies*, representing lipoprotein resorbed by tubular epithelial cells and then shed along with the degenerated cells.

Nephrotic patients are particularly vulnerable to *infection*, especially staphylococcal and pneumococcal, probably related to loss of immunoglobulins in the urine. *Thrombotic and thromboembolic complications* are also common in nephrotic syndrome, due in part to loss of endogenous anticoagulants (e.g., antithrombin III) and antiplasmins in the urine. *Renal vein thrombosis*, once thought to be a cause of nephrotic syndrome, is most often a *consequence* of this hypercoagulable state, particularly in patients with membranous nephropathy (see below).

Causes. The relative frequencies of the several causes of the nephrotic syndrome vary according to age and geography. In children younger than 17 years in North America, for example, the nephrotic syndrome is almost always caused by a lesion primary to the kidney; among adults, in contrast, it may often be associated with a systemic disease. Table 20–7 represents a composite derived from several studies of the causes of the nephrotic syndrome and is therefore only approximate. The most frequent *systemic causes* of the nephrotic syndrome are diabetes, amyloidosis, and SLE. The most important of the *primary glomerular lesions* are *minimal-change disease, membranous glomerulopathy*, and *focal segmental glomerulosclerosis.* The first is most common in children in North America, the second is most common in older adults, and focal segmental glomerulosclerosis occurs at all ages.[29] These three lesions are discussed individually in the following sections. Other primary causes, the various proliferative glomerulonephritides including MPGN, frequently present as a mixed syndrome with nephrotic and nephritic features.

Membranous Nephropathy

Membranous nephropathy is a common cause of the nephrotic syndrome in adults. It is characterized by diffuse thickening of the glomerular capillary wall due to the accumulation of electron-dense, Ig-containing deposits along the subepithelial side of the basement membrane.[30]

Membranous glomerulopathy occurring in association with other systemic diseases and a variety of identifiable etiologic agents is referred to as secondary membranous glomerulopathy. The most notable such associations are as follows:

- *Drugs* (penicillamine, captopril, gold, nonsteroidal anti-inflammatory drugs [NSAIDs]): 1% to 7% of patients with rheumatoid arthritis treated with penicillamine or gold (drugs now used infrequently for this purpose) develop membranous glomerulopathy. NSAIDs, as we shall see, also cause minimal-change disease.
- *Underlying malignant tumors*, particularly carcinomas of the lung and colon, and melanoma. According to some investigators, these are present in as many as 5% to 10% of adults with membranous glomerulopathy.[31]
- *SLE*. About 10% to 15% of glomerulonephritis in SLE is of the membranous type.
- *Infections* (chronic hepatitis B, hepatitis C, syphilis, schistosomiasis, malaria).
- *Other autoimmune disorders* such as thyroiditis can underlie secondary membranous glomerulopathy.

In about 85% of patients no associated condition can be uncovered, and the disease is considered idiopathic.

Causes	Prevalence (%)* Children	Adults
PRIMARY GLOMERULAR DISEASE		
Membranous glomerulopathy	5	30
Minimal-change disease	65	10
Focal segmental glomerulosclerosis	10	35
Membranoproliferative glomerulonephritis[†]	10	10
Other proliferative glomerulonephritides (focal, "pure mesangial," IgA nephropathy)[†]	10	15
SYSTEMIC DISEASES		
Diabetes mellitus		
Amyloidosis		
Systemic lupus erythematosus		
Drugs (nonsteroidal anti-inflammatory, penicillamine, "street heroin")		
Infections (malaria, syphilis, hepatitis B and C, HIV)		
Malignant disease (carcinoma, lymphoma)		
Miscellaneous (bee-sting allergy, hereditary nephritis)		

*Approximate prevalence of primary disease = 95% of nephrotic syndrome in children, 60% in adults. Approximate prevalence of systemic disease = 5% in children, 40% in adults.
[†]Membranoproliferative and other proliferative glomerulonephritides may have mixed nephrotic/nephritic syndromes.

Pathogenesis. Membranous glomerulopathy is a form of chronic immune complex–mediated disease. In secondary membranous glomerulopathy, the inciting antigens can sometimes be identified in the immune complexes. For example, membranous glomerulopathy in SLE is associated with deposition of autoantigen-antibody complexes. Antigens that have been identified in the deposits in some patients include exogenous antigens (e.g., hepatitis B, *Treponema*), endogenous nonrenal antigens (e.g., thyroglobulin), and endogenous renal antigens (e.g., the membrane protein neutral endopeptidase recognized by placental transfer of maternal antibodies in cases of neonatal membranous nephropathy and possibly the phospholipase A_2 receptor in adult cases).[12]

The lesions bear a striking resemblance to those of experimental Heymann nephritis, which, as you might recall, is induced by antibodies to a *megalin* antigenic complex. It is still not known if a similar antigen is present in most cases of idiopathic membranous glomerulopathy in humans. Susceptibility to Heymann nephritis in rats and membranous glomerulopathy in humans is linked to the major histocompatibility complex locus, which can influence the ability to produce antibodies to the nephritogenic antigen. Thus, idiopathic membranous glomerulopathy, like Heymann nephritis, is considered *an autoimmune disease linked to susceptibility genes and caused most likely by antibodies to a renal autoantigen.*

How does the glomerular capillary wall become leaky in membranous glomerulopathy? There is a paucity of neutrophils, monocytes, or platelets in glomeruli. The virtually uniform presence of complement and corroborating experimental work suggest a direct action of C5b-C9, the pathway leading to the formation of the membrane attack complex. It

is postulated that C5b-C9 activates glomerular epithelial and mesangial cells, inducing them to liberate proteases and oxidants, which cause capillary wall injury and increased protein leakage.[32]

Morphology. By light microscopy the glomeruli either appear normal in the early stages of the disease or exhibit **uniform, diffuse thickening of the glomerular capillary wall** (Fig. 20–12A). By electron microscopy the thickening is seen to be caused by irregular dense deposits of immune complexes between the basement membrane and the overlying epithelial cells, the latter having effaced foot processes (Fig. 20–12B and D). Basement membrane material is laid down between these deposits, appearing as irregular spikes protruding from the GBM. These spikes are best seen by silver stains, which color the basement membrane, but not the deposits, black. In time, these spikes thicken to produce domelike protrusions and eventually close over the immune deposits, burying them within a markedly thickened, irregular membrane. Immunofluorescence microscopy demonstrates that the granular deposits contain both immunoglobulins and complement (see Fig. 20–12C). As the disease advances sclerosis may occur; in the course of time glomeruli may become totally sclerosed. The epithelial cells of the proximal tubules contain protein reabsorption droplets, and there may be considerable interstitial mononuclear cell inflammation.

Clinical Features. In a previously healthy individual, this disorder usually begins with the insidious onset of the nephrotic syndrome or, in 15% of patients, with non-nephrotic proteinuria. Hematuria and mild hypertension are present in 15% to 35% of cases. It is necessary in any patient to first rule out the secondary causes described earlier, since treatment of the underlying condition (malignant neoplasm, infection, or SLE) or discontinuance of the offending drug can reverse the injury.

The course of the disease is variable but generally indolent. In contrast to minimal-change disease, described later, the proteinuria is nonselective and usually does not respond well to corticosteroid therapy. Progression is associated with increasing sclerosis of glomeruli, rising serum creatinine reflecting renal insufficiency, and development of hypertension. Although proteinuria persists in more than 60% of patients, only about 10% die or progress to renal failure within 10 years, and no more than 40% eventually develop renal insufficiency. Concurrent sclerosis of glomeruli in the renal biopsy at the time of diagnosis is a predictor of poor prognosis. Spontaneous remissions and a relatively benign outcome occur more commonly in women and in those with proteinuria in the non-nephrotic range. Because of the variable course of the disease, it has been difficult to evaluate the overall effectiveness of corticosteroids or other immunosuppressive therapy in controlling the proteinuria or progression.

Minimal-Change Disease

This relatively benign disorder is the *most frequent cause of nephrotic syndrome in children*, but it is less common in adults

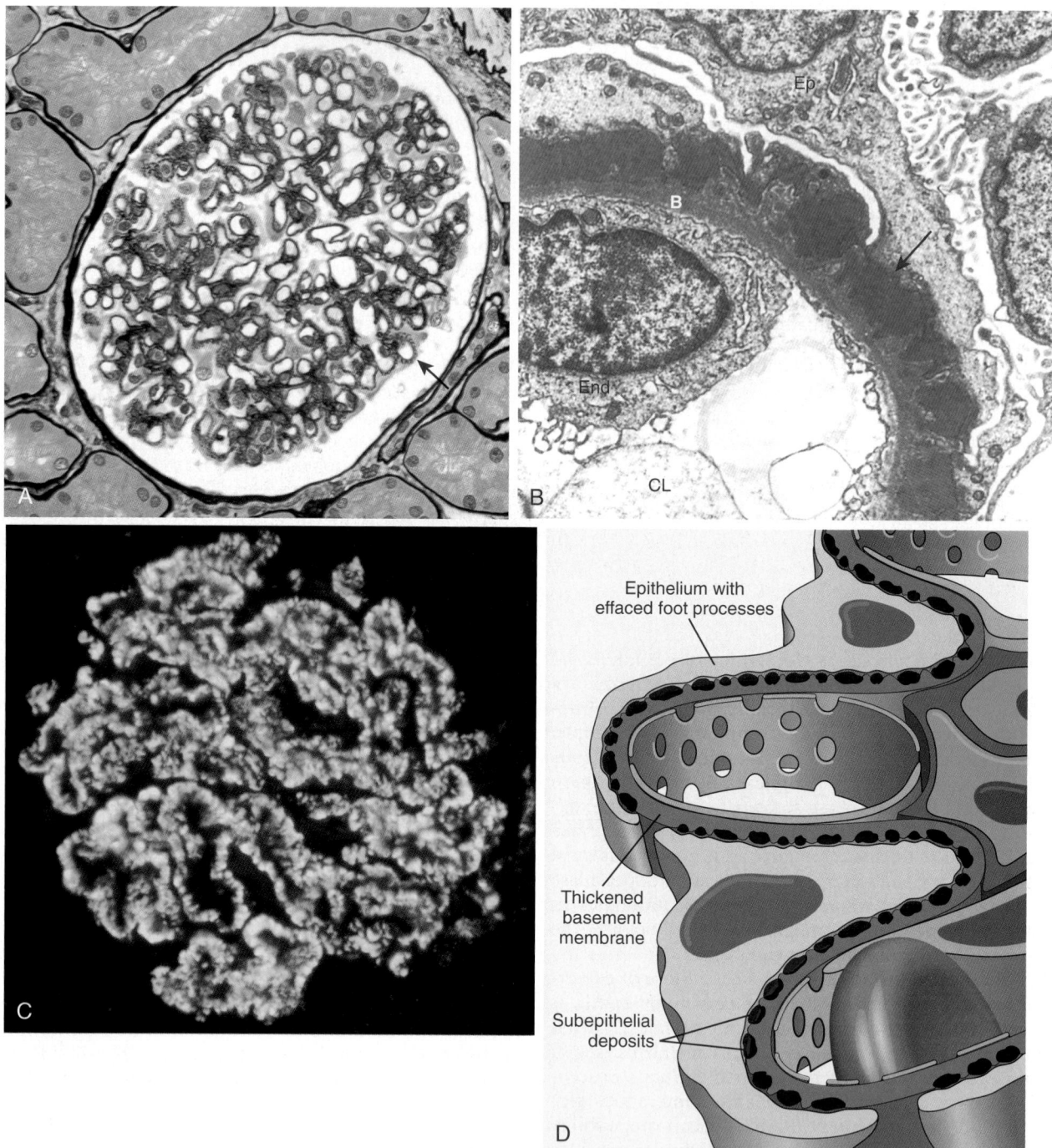

FIGURE 20–12 Membranous nephropathy. **A,** Silver methenamine stain. Note the marked diffuse thickening of the capillary walls without an increase in the number of cells. There are prominent "spikes" of silver-staining matrix *(arrow)* projecting from the basement membrane lamina densa toward the urinary space, which separate and surround deposited immune complexes that lack affinity for the silver stain. **B,** Electron micrograph showing electron-dense deposits *(arrow)* along the epithelial side of the basement membrane (B). Note the effacement of foot processes overlying deposits. CL, capillary lumen; End, endothelium; Ep, epithelium. **C,** Characteristic granular immunofluorescent deposits of IgG along GBM. **D,** Diagrammatic representation of membranous nephropathy. (**A,** Courtesy of Dr. Charles Lassman, UCLA School of Medicine, Los Angeles, CA.)

(see Table 20–7). *It is characterized by diffuse effacement of foot processes of visceral epithelial cells (podocytes) in glomeruli that appear virtually normal by light microscopy.* The peak incidence is between 2 and 6 years of age. The disease sometimes follows a respiratory infection or routine prophylactic immunization. *Its most characteristic feature is its usually dramatic response to corticosteroid therapy.*[33]

Etiology and Pathogenesis. Although the absence of immune deposits in the glomerulus excludes classic immune complex mechanisms, several features of the disease point to an immunological basis,[34] including (1) the clinical association with respiratory infections and prophylactic immunization; (2) the response to corticosteroids and/or other immunosuppressive therapy; (3) the association with other atopic disorders (e.g., eczema, rhinitis); (4) the increased prevalence of certain HLA haplotypes in patients with minimal-change disease associated with atopy (suggesting a genetic predisposition); (5) the increased incidence of minimal-change disease in patients with Hodgkin lymphoma, in whom defects in T cell–mediated immunity are well recognized; and (6) reports of proteinuria-inducing factors in the plasma or lymphocyte supernatants of patients with minimal-change disease.

The current leading hypothesis is that minimal-change disease involves some immune dysfunction, eventually resulting in the elaboration of a cytokine that damages visceral epithelial cells and causes proteinuria. The ultrastructural changes point to a primary *visceral epithelial cell injury*, and studies in animal models suggest the loss of glomerular polyanions. Thus, defects in the charge barrier may contribute to the proteinuria. The actual route by which protein traverses the epithelial cell portion of the capillary wall remains an enigma. Possibilities include transcellular passage through the epithelial cells, passage through residual spaces between remaining but damaged foot processes or through abnormal spaces developing underneath the portion of the foot process that directly abuts the basement membrane, or leakage through foci in which the epithelial cells have become detached from the basement membrane.

Additional insight into mechanisms by which epithelial cell injury results in proteinuria in minimal-change disease, focal segmental glomerulosclerosis, and related entities comes from the discovery of mutations in several podocyte proteins, including *nephrin and podocin*, discussed in the section on focal glomerulosclerosis below. These structural proteins are localized to the slit diaphragm, and nephrotic syndrome resulting from mutations in these proteins illustrates that structural defects of the podocyte are sufficient to cause marked proteinuria in the absence of an immune injury. A mutation in the nephrin gene causes a hereditary form of congenital nephrotic syndrome (Finnish type) with minimal-change glomerular morphology.[8]

Morphology. The glomeruli are normal by light microscopy (Fig. 20–13). By electron microscopy the GBM appears normal, and no electron-dense material is deposited. **The principal lesion is in the visceral epithelial cells, which show a uniform and diffuse effacement of foot processes,** these being replaced by a rim of cytoplasm often showing vacuolization,

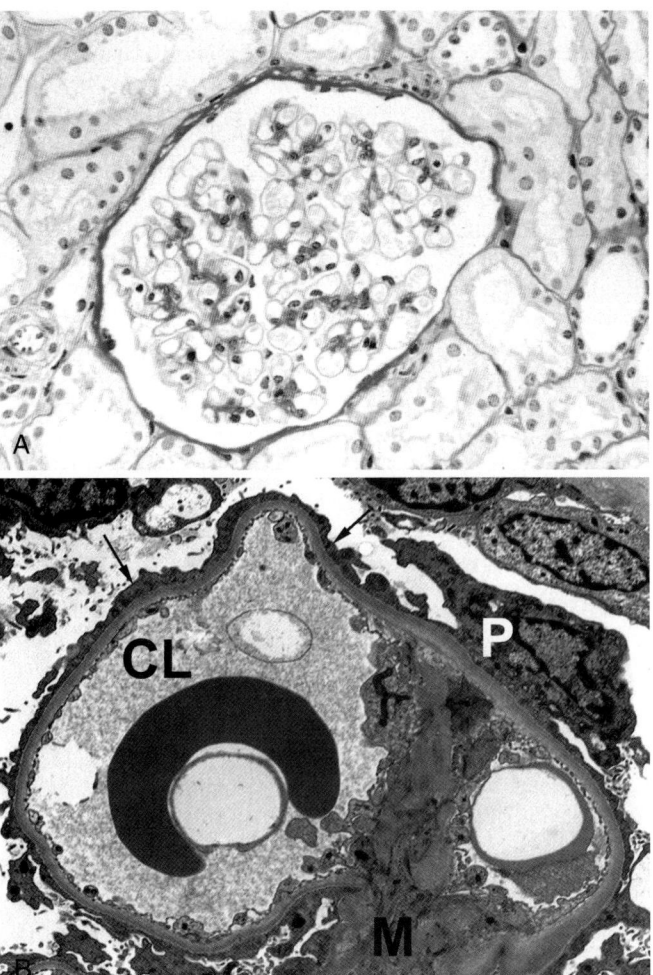

FIGURE 20–13 Minimal-change disease. **A,** Glomerulus stained with PAS. Note normal basement membranes and absence of proliferation. **B,** Ultrastructural characteristics of minimal-change disease include effacement of foot processes *(arrows)* and absence of deposits. CL, capillary lumen; M, mesangium; P, podocyte cell body.

swelling, and hyperplasia of villi (see Fig. 20–13). This change, often incorrectly termed "fusion" of foot processes, actually represents simplification of the epithelial cell architecture with flattening, retraction, and swelling of foot processes. Foot process effacement is also present in other proteinuric states (e.g., membranous glomerulopathy, diabetic nephropathy); it is only when effacement is associated with normal glomeruli by light microscopy that the diagnosis of minimal-change disease can be made. The visceral epithelial changes are completely reversible after corticosteroid therapy, concomitant with remission of the proteinuria. The cells of the proximal tubules are often laden with lipid and protein, reflecting tubular reabsorption of lipoproteins passing through diseased glomeruli (thus, the historical name **lipoid nephrosis** for this disease). Immunofluorescence studies show no Ig or complement deposits.

Clinical Features. Despite massive proteinuria, renal function remains good, and there is commonly no hypertension or hematuria. The proteinuria usually is highly selective, most of the protein being albumin. Most children (>90%) with minimal-change disease respond rapidly to corticosteroid therapy. However, proteinuria may recur, and some patients may become steroid-dependent or resistant. Nevertheless, the long-term prognosis for patients is excellent, and even steroid-dependent disease resolves when children reach puberty. Although adults are slower to respond, their long-term prognosis is also excellent.

As has been noted, minimal-change disease in adults can be associated with Hodgkin lymphoma and, less frequently, other lymphomas and leukemias. In addition, secondary minimal-change disease may follow NSAID therapy, usually in association with acute interstitial nephritis, to be described later in this chapter.

Focal Segmental Glomerulosclerosis

As the name implies, *this lesion is characterized by sclerosis of some, but not all, glomeruli (thus, it is focal); and in the affected glomeruli, only a portion of the capillary tuft is involved (thus, it is segmental)*. Focal segmental glomerulosclerosis is frequently manifest clinically by the nephrotic syndrome or heavy proteinuria.

Classification and Types. Focal segmental glomerulosclerosis (FSGS) occurs in the following settings[35]:

- As a primary disease (idiopathic focal segmental glomerulosclerosis)
- In association with other known conditions, such as HIV infection (HIV-associated nephropathy), heroin addiction (heroin nephropathy), sickle-cell disease, and massive obesity
- As a secondary event, reflecting scarring of previously active necrotizing lesions, in cases of focal glomerulonephritis (e.g., IgA nephropathy)
- As a component of the adaptive response to loss of renal tissue (renal ablation, described earlier) in advanced stages of other renal disorders, such as reflux nephropathy, hypertensive nephropathy, or with unilateral renal agenesis
- In uncommon inherited forms of nephrotic syndrome where the disease, in some pedigrees, is caused by mutations in genes that encode proteins localized to the slit diaphragm, e.g., podocin, α-actinin 4, and TRPC6 (transient receptor potential calcium channel-6)

Idiopathic focal segmental glomerulosclerosis accounts for as many as 10% and 35% of cases of nephrotic syndrome in children and adults in many series, respectively. FSGS (both primary and secondary forms) has increased in incidence and is now the most common cause of nephrotic syndrome in adults in the United States,[29] particularly in Hispanic and African-American patients. The clinical signs differ from those of minimal-change disease in the following respects: (1) there is a higher incidence of hematuria, reduced GFR, and hypertension; (2) proteinuria is more often nonselective; (3) there is poor response to corticosteroid therapy; and (4) there is progression to chronic kidney disease, with at least 50% developing end-stage renal disease within 10 years.

Pathogenesis. Whether idiopathic FSGS represents a distinct disease or is simply a phase in the evolution of a subset of patients with minimal-change disease remains unresolved. The characteristic degeneration and focal disruption of visceral epithelial cells are thought to represent an accentuation of the diffuse epithelial cell change typical of minimal-change disease. *It is this epithelial damage that is the hallmark of FSGS.* Multiple different mechanisms can cause this epithelial damage, including circulating cytokines and genetically determined defects affecting components of the slit diaphragm complex. The hyalinosis and sclerosis stem from entrapment of plasma proteins in extremely hyperpermeable foci and increased ECM deposition. The recurrence of proteinuria, sometimes within 24 hours after transplantation, with subsequent progression to overt lesions of FSGS, suggests that a circulating factor, perhaps a cytokine, may be the cause of the epithelial damage in some patients. An approximately 50-kD non-Ig factor causing proteinuria has been isolated from sera of such patients, but more precise characterization of this factor has not been achieved.[36]

Morphology. By light microscopy the focal and segmental lesions may involve only a minority of the glomeruli and may be missed if the biopsy specimen contains an insufficient number of glomeruli (Fig. 20–14A). The lesions initially tend to involve the juxtamedullary glomeruli, although they subsequently become more generalized. In the sclerotic segments there is collapse of capillary loops, increase in matrix, and segmental deposition of plasma proteins along the capillary wall (hyalinosis), which may become so pronounced as to occlude capillary lumens. Lipid droplets and foam cells are often present (Fig. 20–14B). Glomeruli that do not show segmental lesions usually appear normal on light microscopy but may show increased mesangial matrix. On electron microscopy both sclerotic and nonsclerotic areas show diffuse effacement of foot processes, and there may also be focal detachment of the epithelial cells and denudation of the underlying GBM. By immunofluorescence microscopy IgM and C3 may be present in the sclerotic areas and/or in the mesangium. In addition to the focal sclerosis, there may be pronounced hyalinosis and thickening of afferent arterioles. With the progression of the disease, increased numbers of glomeruli become involved and sclerosis spreads within each glomerulus. In time, this leads to total (i.e., global) sclerosis of glomeruli, with pronounced tubular atrophy and interstitial fibrosis.

A morphologic variant of FSGS, called **collapsing glomerulopathy**, is characterized by retraction and/or collapse of the entire glomerular tuft, with or without additional FSGS lesions of the type described above (Fig. 20–15). A characteristic feature is proliferation and hypertrophy of glomerular visceral epithelial cells. This lesion may be idiopathic, but it is the most characteristic lesion of HIV-associated nephropathy. In both cases there is associated prominent tubular injury with formation of microcysts. It has a particularly poor prognosis.[37,38]

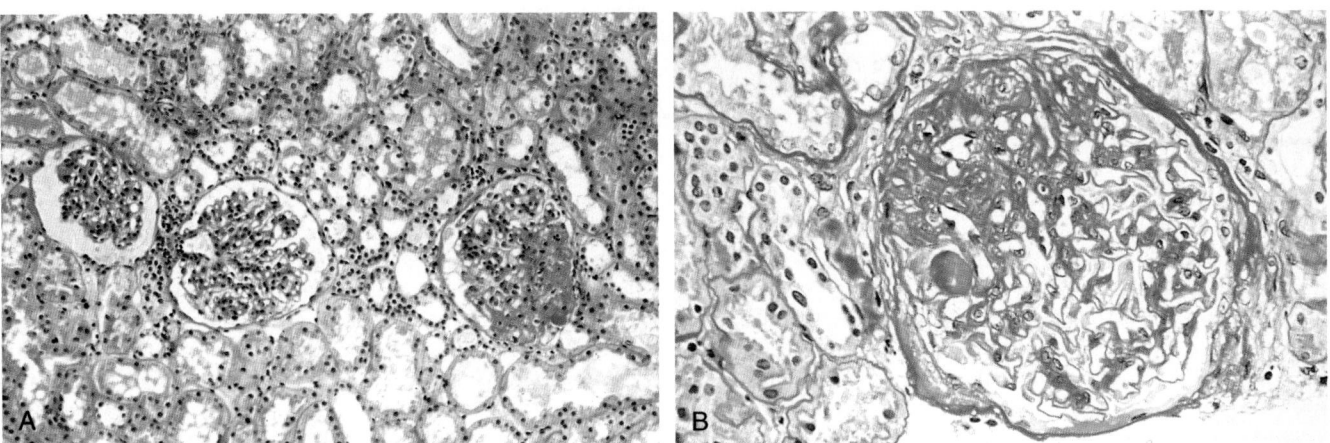

FIGURE 20–14 Focal segmental glomerulosclerosis, PAS stain. **A,** Low-power view showing segmental sclerosis in one of three glomeruli (at 3 o'clock). **B,** High-power view showing hyaline insudation and lipid (small vacuoles) in sclerotic area.

The discovery of a genetic basis for some cases of FSGS and other causes of the nephrotic syndrome has improved the understanding of the pathogenesis of proteinuria in the nephrotic syndrome and has provided new methods for diagnosis and prognosis of affected patients. The first relevant gene to be identified, *NPHS1*, maps to chromosome 19q13 and encodes the protein *nephrin*.[8] Nephrin is a key component of the slit diaphragm (see Fig. 20–3), the zipper-like structure between podocyte foot processes that might control glomerular permeability. Several mutations of the *NPHS1* gene have been identified that give rise to *congenital nephrotic syndrome* of the Finnish type, producing a minimal-change disease–like glomerulopathy with extensive foot process effacement. Prenatal diagnosis of congenital nephrotic syndrome is possible by analysis of the *NPHS1* gene.

A distinctive pattern of autosomal recessive FSGS results from mutations in the *NPHS2* gene, which maps to chromosome 1q25–q31 and encodes the protein product *podocin*. Podocin has also been localized to the slit diaphragm. Mutations in *NPHS2* result in a syndrome of steroid-resistant nephrotic syndrome of childhood onset. Affected children usually show pathologic features of FSGS. Podocin mutations may account for as many as 30% of cases of steroid-resistant nephrotic syndrome in children.[8,39] A third set of mutations in the gene encoding the podocyte actin-binding protein α-actinin 4 underlies some cases of autosomal dominant FSGS, which can be insidious in onset but has a high rate of progression to renal insufficiency.[39]

A fourth type of mutation was found in some kindreds with adult-onset FSGS, in the gene encoding TRPC6. This protein is widely expressed, including in podocytes, and the pathogenic mutations may perturb podocyte function by increasing calcium flux in these cells.

What these proteins have in common is their localization to the slit diaphragm and to adjacent podocyte cytoskeletal structures. Their specific functions and interactions are incompletely understood, but it is clear that the integrity of each is necessary to maintain the normal glomerular filtration barrier. Additional components of the podocyte/slit diaphragm apparatus, such as CD2-associated protein (CD2AP), have been identified that may also contribute to proteinuria,

as has been suggested in studies of knockout mice (but only rarely demonstrated in humans).[6] While identification of these genetic defects has clarified the pathogenesis of some cases of the so-called idiopathic nephrotic syndrome, many other factors contribute to permeability defects. These include cell-cell and cell-matrix interactions, particularly those mediated by $\alpha_3\beta_1$ integrins, dystroglycans, and laminins. Defects in these interactions may also cause a loss of podocyte adhesion to the GBM.

Renal ablation FSGS, a secondary form of FSGS, occurs as a complication of glomerular and nonglomerular diseases

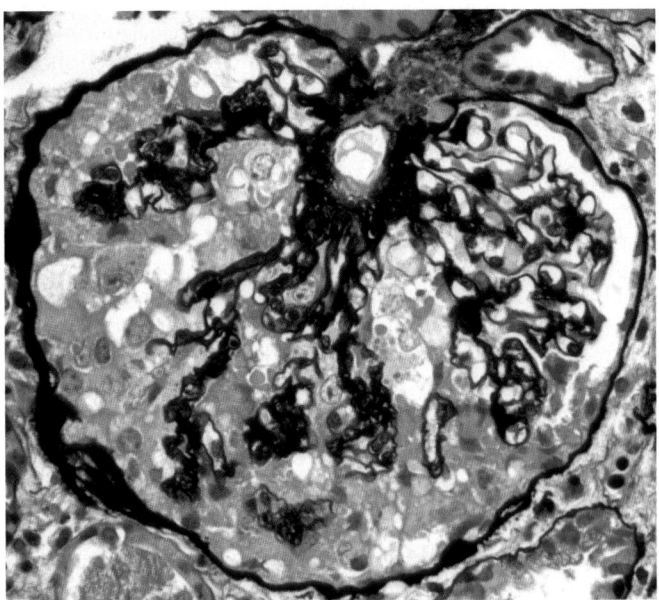

FIGURE 20–15 Collapsing glomerulopathy. Visible are retraction of the glomerular tuft, narrowing of capillary lumens, proliferation and swelling of visceral epithelial cells, and prominent accumulation of intracellular protein absorption droplets in the visceral epithelial cells. The appearance is identical in cases wherein the etiology is idiopathic to cases associated with HIV infection. Silver methenamine stain. (Courtesy of Dr. Jolanta Kowalewska, University of Washington, Seattle, WA.)

causing reduction in functioning renal tissue, particularly reflux nephropathy and unilateral agenesis. These may lead to progressive glomerulosclerosis and renal failure. The pathogenesis of FSGS in this setting has been described earlier in this chapter.

Clinical Course. There is little tendency for spontaneous remission in idiopathic FSGS, and responses to corticosteroid therapy are variable. In general, children have a better prognosis than adults do. Progression of renal failure occurs at variable rates. About 20% of patients follow an unusually rapid course, with intractable massive proteinuria ending in renal failure within 2 years. Recurrences are seen in 25% to 50% of patients receiving allografts.

HIV-Associated Nephropathy

HIV infection can result directly or indirectly in several renal complications, including acute renal failure and/or acute interstitial nephritis induced by drugs or infection, thrombotic microangiopathies, postinfectious glomerulonephritis, and, *most commonly, a severe form of the collapsing variant of FSGS.*[40] The latter occurs in 5% to 10% of HIV-infected individuals in some series, more frequently in blacks than in whites. In rare cases the nephrotic syndrome may precede the development of acquired immunodeficiency syndrome. The morphologic features are characterized by

- A high frequency of the collapsing variant of FSGS (see Fig. 20–16)
- A striking focal cystic dilation of tubule segments, which are filled with proteinaceous material, and inflammation and fibrosis
- The presence of large numbers of tubuloreticular inclusions within endothelial cells, detected by electron microscopy. Such inclusions, also present in SLE, have been shown to be modifications of endoplasmic reticulum induced by circulating interferon-α. They are not present in idiopathic FSGS and therefore may have diagnostic value in a biopsy specimen.

The pathogenesis of HIV-related FSGS and tubular injury is probably due to infection of glomerular and tubular cells by HIV, which has been detected in a few cases by very sensitive polymerase chain reaction methods. Studies from animal models indicate that the glomerular lesion is most specifically the result of podocyte expression of the HIV gene products *vpr* and *nef*. Altered systemic or local release of cytokines may also modify and promote this particular renal injury.

Membranoproliferative Glomerulonephritis

MPGN is characterized histologically by *alterations in the glomerular basement membrane, proliferation of glomerular cells, and leukocyte infiltration.* Because the proliferation is predominantly in the mesangium but also may involve the capillary loops, a frequently used synonym is *mesangiocapillary glomerulonephritis.* MPGN accounts for 10% to 20% of cases of nephrotic syndrome in children and young adults. Some patients present only with hematuria or proteinuria in the non-nephrotic range, but many others have a combined nephrotic-nephritic picture. Like many other glomerulone-

phritides, MPGN either can be associated with other systemic disorders and known etiologic agents (secondary MPGN) or may be idiopathic (primary MPGN).[41]

Primary MPGN is divided into two major types on the basis of distinct ultrastructural, immunofluorescent, and pathologic findings: type I and type II MPGN (*dense-deposit disease*).

Pathogenesis. *In most cases of type I MPGN there is evidence of immune complexes in the glomerulus and activation of both classical and alternative complement pathways.*[42] The antigens involved in idiopathic MPGN are unknown. In many cases they are believed to be proteins derived from infectious agents such as hepatitis C and B viruses, which presumably behave either as "planted" antigens after first binding to or becoming trapped within glomerular structures or are contained in preformed immune complexes deposited from the circulation.

Most patients with dense-deposit disease (type II MPGN) have abnormalities that suggest activation of the alternative complement pathway.[43] These patients have a consistently decreased serum C3 but normal C1 and C4, the immune complex–activated early components of complement. They also have diminished serum levels of factor B and properdin, components of the alternative complement pathway. In the glomeruli, C3 and properdin are deposited, but IgG is not. Recall that in the alternative complement pathway, C3 is directly cleaved to C3b (Fig. 20–16; see also Chapter 2, Fig. 2–14). The reaction depends on the initial interaction of C3 with such substances as bacterial polysaccharides, endotoxin, and aggregates of IgA in the presence of factors B and D. This leads to the generation of C3bBb, the alternative pathway C3 convertase. This C3 convertase is labile, being degraded by factors I and H, but it can be stabilized by properdin. More than 70% of patients with dense-deposit disease have a circulating antibody termed *C3 nephritic factor (C3NeF)*, which is an autoantibody that binds to the alternative pathway C3 convertase (see Fig. 20–16). Binding of the antibody stabilizes the convertase, protecting it from enzymatic degradation and thus favoring persistent C3 activation and hypocomplementemia. There is also decreased C3 synthesis by the liver, further con-

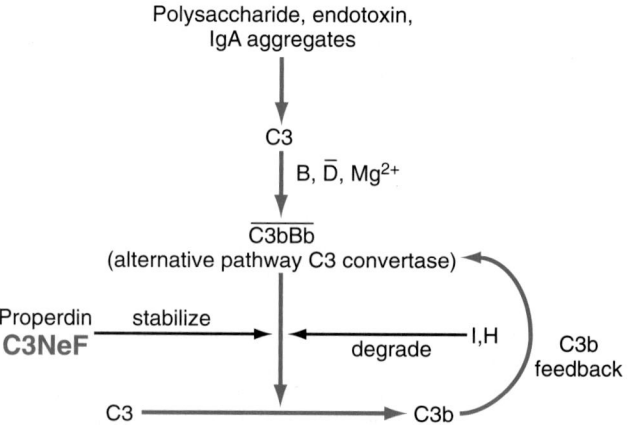

FIGURE 20–16 The alternative complement pathway in MPGN. Note that C3NeF, an antibody present in the serum of individuals with membranoproliferative glomerulonephritis, acts at the same step as properdin, serving to stabilize the alternative pathway C3 convertase, thus enhancing C3 activation and consumption, causing hypocomplementemia.

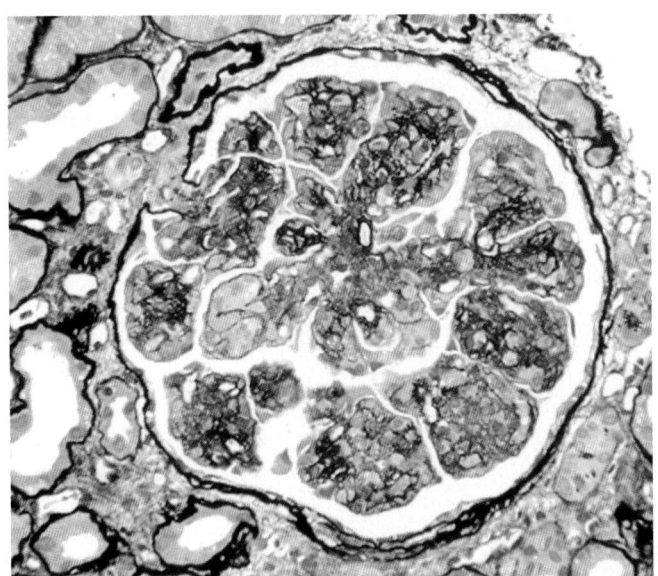

FIGURE 20–17 Membranoproliferative glomerulonephritis, showing mesangial cell proliferation, increased mesangial matrix (staining black with silver stain), basement membrane thickening with segmental splitting, accentuation of lobular architecture, swelling of cells lining peripheral capillaries, and influx of leukocytes (endocapillary proliferation).

tributing to the profound hypocomplementemia. Precisely how C3NeF is related to glomerular injury and the nature of the dense deposits is unknown. C3NeF activity also occurs in some patients with a genetically determined disease, *partial lipodystrophy*, some of whom develop dense-deposit disease (type II MPGN).

Morphology. By light microscopy both types of MPGN are similar. The glomeruli are large and hypercellular. The hypercellularity is produced both by proliferation of cells in the mesangium and so-called endocapillary proliferation involving capillary endothelium and infiltrating leukocytes. Crescents are present in many cases. The glomeruli have an accentuated "lobular" appearance due to the proliferating mesangial cells and increased mesangial matrix (Fig. 20–17). The GBM is thickened, often segmentally; this is most evident in the peripheral capillary loops. The glomerular capillary wall often shows a "double-contour" or "tram-track" appearance, especially evident in silver or PAS stains. This is caused by "duplication" of the basement membrane (also commonly referred to as splitting), usually as the result of new basement membrane synthesis in response to the subendothelial deposits of immune complexes. Within the duplicated basement membranes there is inclusion or interposition of cellular elements, which can be of mesangial, endothelial, or leukocytic origin. Such interposition also gives rise to the appearance of "split" basement membranes (Fig. 20–18A).

Types I and II MPGN differ in their ultrastructural and immunofluorescent features (Fig. 20–18).

Type I MPGN (the great majority of cases) is characterized by the presence of discrete **subendothelial electron-dense deposits**. Mesangial and occasional subepithelial deposits may also be present (see Fig. 20–18A). By immunofluorescence, C3 is deposited in a granular pattern, and IgG and early complement components (C1q and C4) are often also present, suggesting an immune complex pathogenesis.

In **dense-deposit disease (type II MPGN)** (Fig. 20–18B), a relatively rare entity, the lamina densa of the GBM is transformed into an irregular, ribbon-like, extremely electron-dense structure due to the **deposition of dense material** of unknown composition in the GBM proper. C3 is present in irregular granular or linear foci in the basement membranes on either side but not within the dense deposits. C3 is also present in the mesangium in characteristic circular aggregates (mesangial rings). IgG is usually absent, as are the early-acting complement components (C1q and C4).

Clinical Features. Most patients present in adolescence or as young adults with nephrotic syndrome and a nephritic component manifested by hematuria or, more insidiously, as mild proteinuria. Few remissions occur spontaneously in either type, and the disease follows a slowly progressive but unremitting course. Some patients develop numerous crescents and a clinical picture of RPGN. About 50% develop chronic renal failure within 10 years. Treatments with steroids, immunosuppressive agents, and antiplatelet drugs have not been proved to be materially effective. There is a high incidence of recurrence in transplant recipients, particularly in dense-deposit disease; dense deposits may recur in 90% of such patients, although renal failure in the allograft is much less common.

Secondary MPGN

Secondary MPGN (invariably type I) is more common in adults and arises in the following settings[41]:

○ Chronic immune complex disorders, such as SLE; hepatitis B infection; hepatitis C infection, usually with cryoglobulinemia; endocarditis; infected ventriculoatrial shunts; chronic visceral abscesses; HIV infection; and schistosomiasis
○ α_1-Antitrypsin deficiency
○ Malignant diseases (chronic lymphocytic leukemia and lymphoma)
○ Hereditary deficiencies of complement regulatory proteins

The mechanisms underlying the process of immune complex deposition in the last three categories above remain unknown.

ISOLATED URINARY ABNORMALITIES

IgA Nephropathy (Berger Disease)

This form of glomerulonephritis is characterized by the presence of prominent IgA deposits in the mesangial regions, detected by immunofluorescence microscopy. The disease can be suspected

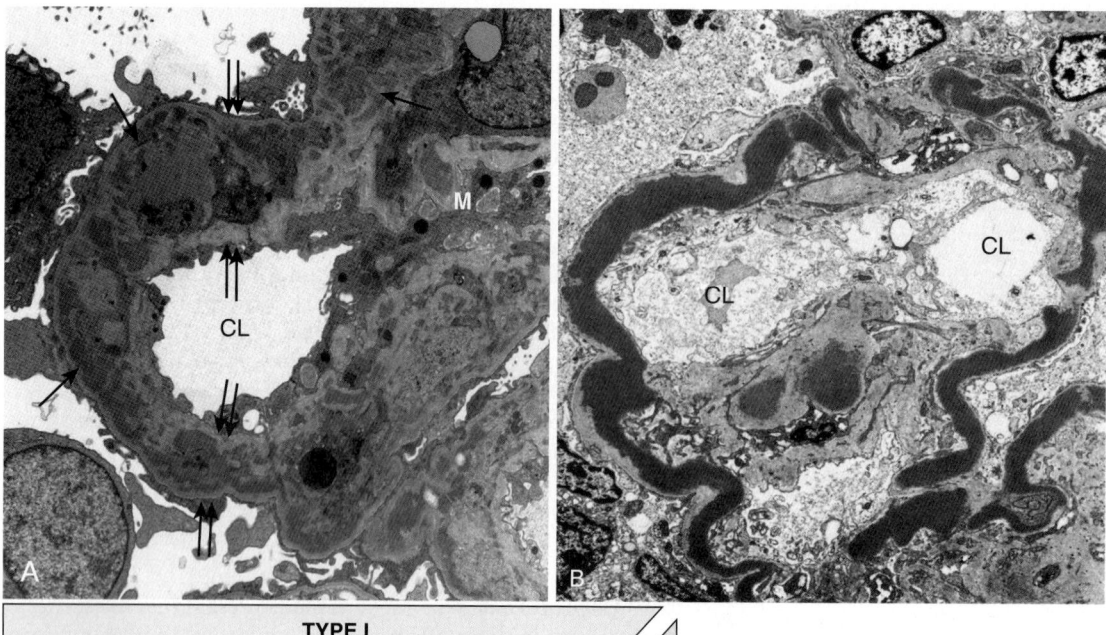

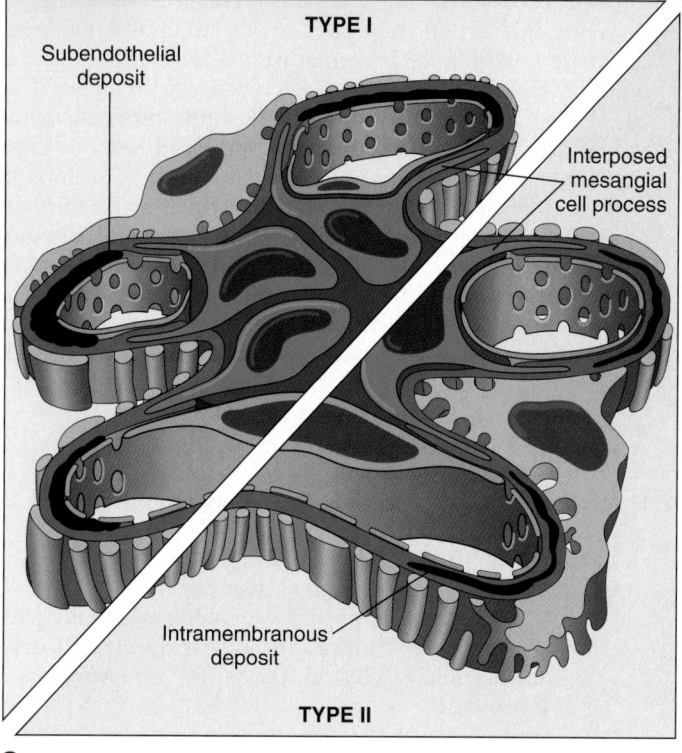

FIGURE 20–18   A, Membranoproliferative glomerulonephritis, type I. Note discrete electron-dense deposits *(arrows)* incorporated into the glomerular capillary wall between duplicated (split) basement membranes *(double arrows)*, and in mesangial regions (M); CL, capillary lumen. **B,** Dense-deposit disease (type II membranoproliferative glomerulonephritis). There are markedly dense homogeneous deposits within the basement membrane proper. CL, capillary lumen. In both, mesangial interposition gives the appearance of split basement membranes when viewed in the light microscope. **C,** Schematic representation of patterns in the two types of membranoproliferative GN. In type I there are subendothelial deposits; type II is characterized by intramembranous dense deposits (dense-deposit disease). In both, mesangial interposition gives the appearance of split basement membranes when viewed in the light microscope. (**A,** Courtesy of Dr. Jolanta Kowalewska, University of Washington, Seattle, WA.)

by light microscopic examination, but the diagnosis is made only by immunocytochemical techniques (Fig. 20–19). *IgA nephropathy is a frequent cause of recurrent gross or microscopic hematuria and is probably the most common type of glomerulonephritis worldwide.*[44] Mild proteinuria is usually present, and the nephrotic syndrome may occasionally develop. Rarely, patients may present with cresentic RPGN.

Whereas IgA nephropathy is typically an isolated renal disease, similar IgA deposits are present in a systemic disorder of children, *Henoch-Schönlein purpura,* to be discussed later, which has many overlapping features with IgA nephropathy.

In addition, *secondary IgA nephropathy* occurs in patients with liver and intestinal diseases, as discussed below.

Pathogenesis. IgA, the main Ig in mucosal secretions, is present in plasma at low concentrations, mostly in monomeric form, the polymeric forms being catabolized in the liver. In patients with IgA nephropathy, plasma polymeric IgA is increased, and circulating IgA-containing immune complexes are present in some patients. However, it is clear that increased production of IgA cannot itself cause this disease. Although there are two subclasses of IgA molecules in humans (IgA1 and IgA2), only IgA1 forms the nephritogenic deposits of IgA

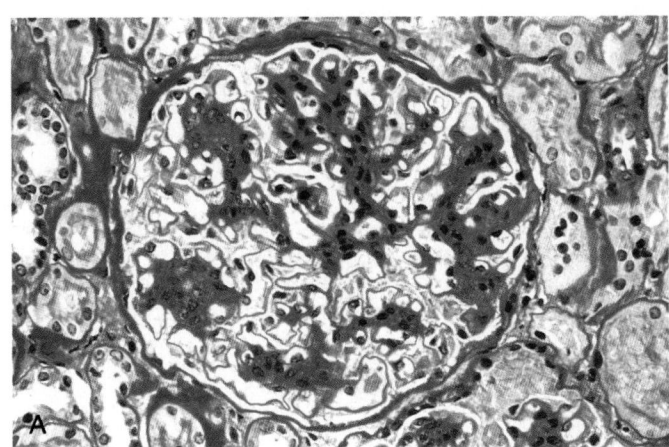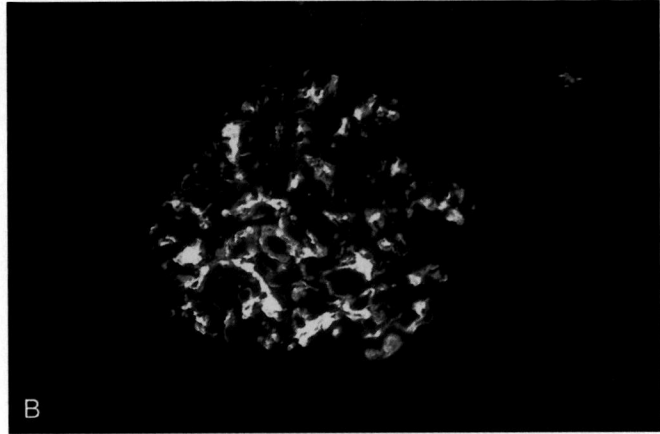

FIGURE 20–19 IgA nephropathy. **A,** Light microscopy showing mesangial proliferation and matrix increase. **B,** Characteristic deposition of IgA, principally in mesangial regions, detected by immunofluorescence.

nephropathy. The prominent mesangial deposition of IgA suggests entrapment of IgA immune complexes in the mesangium, and the presence of C3 combined with the absence of C1q and C4 in glomeruli points to activation of the alternative complement pathway. A genetic influence is suggested by the occurrence of this condition in families and in HLA-identical brothers and the increased frequency of certain HLA and complement genotypes in some populations.

Taken together, these clues suggest a genetic or acquired abnormality of immune regulation leading to increased IgA synthesis in response to respiratory or gastrointestinal exposure to environmental agents (e.g., viruses, bacteria, food proteins). IgA1 and IgA1-containing immune complexes are then trapped in the mesangium, where they activate the alternative complement pathway and initiate glomerular injury. In support of this scenario, IgA nephropathy occurs with increased frequency in individuals with *gluten enteropathy* (celiac disease), in whom intestinal mucosal defects are well defined, and in *liver disease*, in which there is defective hepatobiliary clearance of IgA complexes (*secondary IgA nephropathy*).

The nature of the initiating antigens is unknown, and several infectious agents and food products have been implicated. The deposited IgA appears to be polyclonal, and it may be that a variety of antigens are involved in the course of the disease. Alternatively, there is evidence for qualitative alterations in the IgA1 molecule itself, specifically a defect in normal galactosylation that makes it immunogenic, giving rise to autoantibodies against the IgA1 that form immune complexes that deposit in the mesangium.[45]

> **Morphology.** On histologic examination the lesions vary considerably. The glomeruli may be normal or may show mesangial widening and endocapillary proliferation (mesangioproliferative glomerulonephritis), segmental proliferation confined to some glomeruli (focal proliferative glomerulonephritis), or rarely, overt crescentic glomerulonephritis. The presence of leukocytes within glomerular capillaries is a variable feature. The mesangial widening may be the result of cell proliferation, accumulation of matrix,

> immune deposits, or some combination of these abnormalities. Healing of the focal proliferative lesion may lead to secondary focal segmental sclerosis. The characteristic immunofluorescent picture is of **mesangial deposition of IgA** (Fig. 20–19B), often with C3 and properdin and lesser amounts of IgG or IgM. Early complement components are usually absent. Electron microscopy confirms the presence of electron-dense deposits in the mesangium.

Clinical Features. The disease affects people of any age, but older children and young adults are most commonly affected. Many patients present with gross hematuria after an infection of the respiratory or, less commonly, gastrointestinal or urinary tract; 30% to 40% have only microscopic hematuria, with or without proteinuria; and 5% to 10% develop a typical acute nephritic syndrome. The hematuria typically lasts for several days and then subsides, only to return every few months. The subsequent course is highly variable. Many patients maintain normal renal function for decades. Slow progression to chronic renal failure occurs in 15% to 40% of cases over a period of 20 years. Onset in old age, heavy proteinuria, hypertension, and the extent of glomerulosclerosis on biopsy are clues to an increased risk of progression. Recurrence of IgA deposits in transplanted kidneys is frequent. In approximately 15% of those with recurrent IgA deposits, there is resulting clinical disease, which most frequently runs the same slowly progressive course as that of the primary IgA nephropathy.

Alport Syndrome

Hereditary nephritis refers to a group of heterogeneous familial renal diseases associated primarily with glomerular injury. Two deserve discussion: *Alport syndrome*, because the lesions and genetic defects have been well studied,[46] and *thin basement membrane lesion*, the most common cause of *benign familial hematuria*.[47]

Alport syndrome, when fully developed, is manifest by hematuria with progression to chronic renal failure, accompanied by nerve deafness and various eye disorders, including lens disloca-

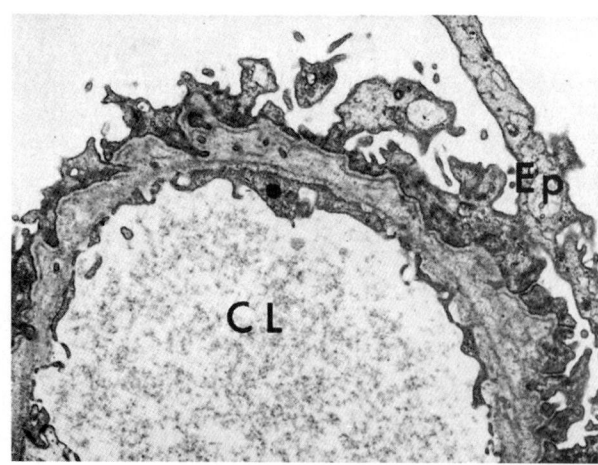

FIGURE 20–20 Hereditary nephritis (Alport syndrome). Electron micrograph of glomerulus with irregular thickening of the basement membrane, lamination of the lamina densa, and foci of rarefaction. Such changes may be present in other diseases but are most pronounced and widespread in hereditary nephritis. CL, capillary lumen; Ep, epithelium.

tion, posterior cataracts, and corneal dystrophy.[48] The disease is inherited as an X-linked trait in approximately 85% of cases. In this X-linked form, males express the full syndrome, and females are carriers in whom manifestations of disease are typically limited to hematuria. Autosomal recessive and autosomal dominant pedigrees also exist, in which males and females are equally susceptible to the full syndrome.

Pathogenesis. The disease manifestations are due to abnormal α_3 (COL4A3), α_4 (COL4A4), or α_5 (COL4A5) chain of type IV collagen. This is due to mutation of COL4A5 in the classic X-linked form and COL4A3 or COL4A4 in the autosomal forms. In all cases, the result is defective assembly of type IV collagen, which is crucial for function of the GBM, the lens of the eye, and the cochlea. Because the GBM consists of networks of trimeric collagen molecules composed of α_3, α_4, and α_5 chains, mutations in COL4A5 also result in defective assembly of the collagen network.[46] The α_3 chain includes the Goodpasture antigen, and glomeruli from patients with Alport syndrome who lack the α_3 chain fail to react with anti-GBM antibodies from patients with Goodpasture syndrome.

Morphology. On histologic examination the glomeruli are always involved. The early lesion is detectable only by electron microscopy and consists of diffuse GBM thinning. Interstitial foam cells stuffed with neutral fats and mucopolysaccharides are a nonspecific finding consequent to proteinuria that for unknown reasons can be unusually prominent in this disorder. As the disease progresses there is development of focal segmental and global glomerulosclerosis and other changes of progressive renal injury, including vascular sclerosis, tubular atrophy, and interstitial fibrosis.

The characteristic electron microscopic findings of fully developed disease are found in most individuals with hereditary nephritis. The GBM shows irregular foci of thickening alternating with attenuation (thin-ning), and pronounced splitting and lamination of the lamina densa, often producing a distinctive basketweave appearance (Fig. 20–20). Similar alterations can be found in the tubular basement membranes.

Immunohistochemistry can be helpful in cases with absent or borderline basement membrane lesions, because antibodies to α_3, α_4, and α_5 collagen fail to stain both glomerular and tubular basement membranes in the classic X-linked form. There is also absence of α_5 staining in skin biopsy specimens from these patients.

Clinical Features. The most common presenting sign is gross or microscopic hematuria, frequently accompanied by red cell casts. Proteinuria may develop later, and rarely, the nephrotic syndrome develops. Symptoms appear at ages 5 to 20 years, and the onset of overt renal failure is between ages 20 and 50 years in men. The auditory defects may be subtle, requiring sensitive testing.

Thin Basement Membrane Lesion (Benign Familial Hematuria)

This is a fairly common hereditary entity manifested *clinically by familial asymptomatic hematuria*—usually uncovered on routine urinalysis—*and morphologically by diffuse thinning of the GBM* to between 150 and 250 nm (compared with 300–400 nm in normal adult individuals). Although mild or moderate proteinuria may also be present, renal function is normal and prognosis is excellent.

The disorder should be distinguished from IgA nephropathy, another common cause of hematuria, and X-linked Alport syndrome. In contrast to Alport syndrome, hearing loss, ocular abnormalities, and a family history of renal failure are absent.

The anomaly in thin basement membrane lesion has also been traced to mutations in genes encoding α_3 or α_4 chains of type IV collagen.[46,47] Most patients are heterozygous for the defective gene and thus may be carriers. The disorder in homozygotes resembles autosomal recessive Alport syndrome. Homozygotes or compound heterozygotes may progress to renal failure. Thus, these diseases illustrate a continuum of changes resulting from mutations in collagen type IV genes.

CHRONIC GLOMERULONEPHRITIS

Chronic glomerulonephritis is best considered a pool of end-stage glomerular disease fed by several streams of specific types of glomerulonephritis (Fig. 20–21). Most of these diseases were described earlier in this chapter. Poststreptococcal glomerulonephritis is a rare antecedent of chronic glomerulonephritis, except in adults. Patients with crescentic glomerulonephritis, if they survive the acute episode, usually progress to chronic glomerulonephritis. Membranous nephropathy, MPGN, IgA nephropathy, and FSGS all may progress to chronic renal failure. *Nevertheless, in any series of individuals with chronic glomerulonephritis, a variable percentage of cases arise mysteriously with no antecedent history of any of the well-recognized forms of acute glomerulonephritis.* These cases must represent the end result of relatively asymptomatic forms of glomeru-

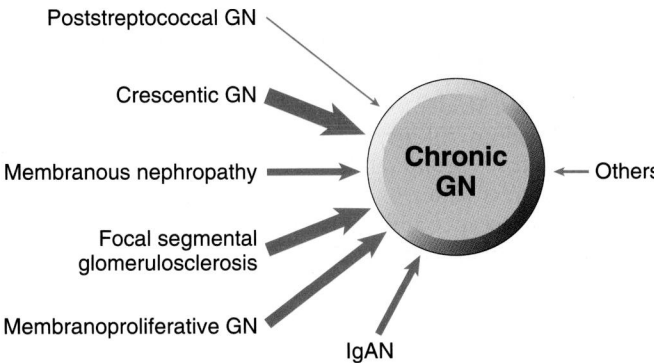

Poststreptococcal GN

Crescentic GN

Membranous nephropathy

Focal segmental
glomerulosclerosis

Membranoproliferative GN

Chronic
GN

Others

IgAN

FIGURE 20–21 Primary glomerular diseases leading to chronic glomerulonephritis (GN). The thickness of the arrows reflects the approximate proportion of patients in each group who progress to chronic GN: poststreptococcal (1% to 2%); rapidly progressive (crescentic) (90%), membranous (30% to 50%), focal segmental glomerulosclerosis (50% to 80%), membranoproliferative GN (50%), IgA nephropathy (IgAN, 30% to 50%).

lonephritis, either known or still unrecognized, that progress to uremia. Clearly, the proportion of such unexplained cases depends on the availability of renal biopsy material from patients early in their disease.

Morphology. The kidneys are symmetrically contracted and have diffusely granular cortical surfaces. On section, **the cortex is thinned**, and there is an increase in peripelvic fat. The glomerular histology depends on the stage of the disease. In early cases, the glomeruli may still show evidence of the primary disease (e.g., membranous nephropathy or MPGN). However, there eventually ensues **obliteration of glomeruli**, transforming them into acellular eosinophilic masses, representing a combination of trapped plasma proteins, increased mesangial matrix, basement membrane–like material, and collagen (Fig. 20–22). Because hypertension is an accompaniment of chronic glomerulonephritis, **arterial and arteriolar sclerosis may be conspicuous. Marked atrophy of associated tubules**, irregular interstitial fibrosis, and mononuclear leukocytic infiltration of the interstitium also occur.

Dialysis Changes. Kidneys from patients with end-stage disease on long-term dialysis show a variety of changes that are unrelated to the primary disease. These include **arterial intimal thickening** caused by accumulation of smooth muscle–like cells and a loose, proteoglycan-rich stroma; focal calcification, usually within residual tubular segments; **extensive deposition of calcium oxalate crystals** in tubules and interstitium; **acquired cystic disease,** discussed later; and increased numbers of renal adenomas and adenocarcinomas.

Uremic Complications. Individuals dying with chronic glomerulonephritis also exhibit pathologic changes outside the kidney that are related to the uremic state

and are also present in other forms of chronic renal failure. Often clinically important, these include uremic **pericarditis**, uremic gastroenteritis, **secondary hyperparathyroidism** with nephrocalcinosis and renal osteodystrophy, **left ventricular hypertrophy** due to hypertension, and pulmonary changes of diffuse alveolar damage often ascribed to uremia (uremic pneumonitis).

Clinical Course. In most individuals, chronic glomerulonephritis develops insidiously and slowly progresses to renal insufficiency or death from uremia during a span of years or possibly decades (see the discussion of chronic renal failure). Not infrequently, patients present with such nonspecific complaints as loss of appetite, anemia, vomiting, or weakness. In some, the renal disease is suspected with the discovery of proteinuria, hypertension, or azotemia on routine medical examination. In others, the underlying renal disorder is discovered in the course of investigation of edema. *Most patients are hypertensive, and sometimes the dominant clinical manifestations are cerebral or cardiovascular.* In all, the disease is relentlessly progressive, though at widely varying rates. In nephrotic patients, as glomeruli become obliterated and therefore the GFR decreases, the protein loss in the urine diminishes. If patients with chronic glomerulonephritis do not recieve dialysis or if they do not receive a renal transplant, they invariably succumb to their disease.

GLOMERULAR LESIONS ASSOCIATED WITH SYSTEMIC DISEASES

Many immunologically mediated, metabolic, or hereditary systemic disorders are associated with glomerular injury; in some (e.g., SLE and diabetes mellitus), the glomerular involvement is a major clinical manifestation. Most of these diseases are discussed elsewhere in this book. Here we briefly recall some of the lesions and discuss only those not considered in other sections.

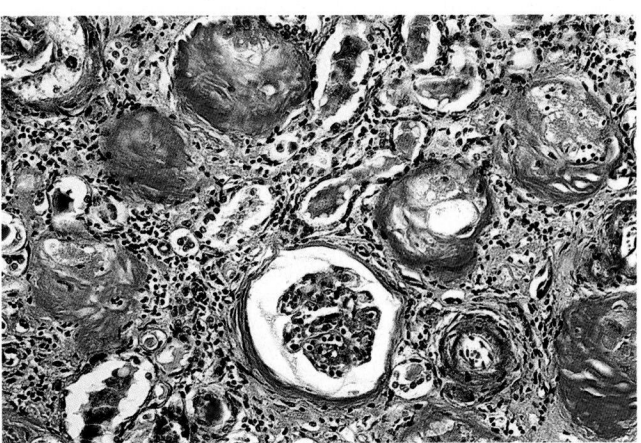

FIGURE 20–22 Chronic glomerulonephritis. A Masson trichrome preparation shows complete replacement of virtually all glomeruli by blue-staining collagen. (Courtesy of Dr. M.A. Venkatachalam, Department of Pathology, University of Texas Health Sciences Center, San Antonio, TX.)

Lupus Nephritis

The various types of lupus nephritis were described and illustrated in Chapter 6. As discussed, SLE gives rise to a heterogeneous group of lesions and clinical presentations. The clinical manifestations can include recurrent microscopic or gross hematuria, the nephritic syndrome, the nephrotic syndrome, chronic renal failure, and hypertension.

Henoch-Schönlein Purpura

This syndrome consists of *purpuric skin lesions characteristically involving the extensor surfaces of arms and legs as well as buttocks; abdominal manifestations including pain, vomiting, and intestinal bleeding; nonmigratory arthralgia; and renal abnormalities.* The renal manifestations occur in one third of patients and include gross or microscopic hematuria, nephritic syndrome, and nephrotic syndrome, or some combination of these. A small number of patients, mostly adults, develop a rapidly progressive form of glomerulonephritis with many crescents. Not all components of the syndrome need to be present, and individual patients may have purpura, abdominal pain, or urinary abnormalities as the dominant feature. The disease is most common in children 3 to 8 years old, but it also occurs in adults, in whom the renal manifestations are usually more severe. There is a strong background of atopy in about one third of patients, and onset often follows an upper respiratory infection. IgA is deposited in the glomerular mesangium in a distribution similar to that of IgA nephropathy. This has led to the concept that *IgA nephropathy and Henoch-Schönlein purpura are manifestations of the same disease.*[49]

Morphology. On histologic examination, the renal lesions vary from mild focal mesangial proliferation to diffuse mesangial proliferation and/or endocapillary to crescentic glomerulonephritis. Whatever the histologic lesions, the prominent feature by fluorescence microscopy is the **deposition of IgA, sometimes with IgG and C3, in the mesangial region**. The skin lesions consist of subepidermal hemorrhages and a necrotizing vasculitis involving the small vessels of the dermis. IgA deposits are also present in such vessels. Vasculitis also occurs in other organs, such as the gastrointestinal tract, but is rare in the kidney.

The course of the disease is variable, but recurrences of hematuria may persist for many years after onset. Most children have an excellent prognosis. Patients with the more diffuse lesions, crescents, or the nephrotic syndrome have a somewhat poorer prognosis.

Bacterial Endocarditis–Associated Glomerulonephritis

Glomerular lesions occurring in the course of bacterial endocarditis represent a type of immune complex nephritis initiated by complexes of bacterial antigen and antibody. Hematuria and proteinuria of various degrees characterize this entity

clinically, but an acute nephritic presentation is not uncommon, and even RPGN may occur in rare instances. The histologic lesions, when present, generally reflect these clinical manifestations. Milder forms have a more focal and segmental necrotizing glomerulonephritis, whereas more severe ones show a diffuse proliferative glomerulonephritis, and the rapidly progressive forms show large numbers of crescents. Immunofluorescence and electron microscopy show the presence of glomerular immune deposits.

Diabetic Nephropathy

Diabetes mellitus is a major cause of renal morbidity and mortality, and diabetic nephropathy is one of the leading causes of chronic kidney failure in the United States (see Chapter 24). Advanced or end-stage kidney disease occurs in as many as 40% of both insulin-dependent type 1 diabetics and type 2 diabetics. By far the most common lesions involve the glomeruli and are associated clinically with three glomerular syndromes: non-nephrotic proteinuria, nephrotic syndrome, and chronic renal failure.[50] However, diabetes also affects the arterioles (causing *hyalinizing arteriolar sclerosis*), increases susceptibility to the development of pyelonephritis and particularly *papillary necrosis*, and causes a variety of tubular lesions. The term *diabetic nephropathy* is applied to the conglomerate of lesions that often occur concurrently in the diabetic kidney.

The morphologic changes in the glomeruli include (1) capillary basement membrane thickening, (2) diffuse mesangial sclerosis, and (3) nodular glomerulosclerosis. The morphologic manifestations of diabetic nephropathy are identical in type 1 and type 2 diabetes and are described below as a single entity.[51,52]

Pathogenesis. The pathogenesis of diabetic glomerulosclerosis is intimately linked with that of generalized diabetic microangiopathy, discussed in Chapter 24. The principal points are as follows[53]:

- The bulk of the evidence suggests that diabetic glomerulosclerosis *is caused by the metabolic defect*, that is, the insulin deficiency, the resultant hyperglycemia, or some other aspects of glucose intolerance. These metabolic defects are responsible for biochemical alterations in the GBM, including increased amounts of collagen type IV and fibronectin and decreased heparan sulfate proteoglycan, and for increased production of reactive oxygen species, which may further damage the glomerular filter.
- *Nonenzymatic glycosylation* of proteins, which is known to occur in diabetics and gives rise to advanced glycosylation end products, may contribute to the glomerulopathy.[54] The mechanisms by which advanced glycosylation end products cause their effects are discussed in Chapter 24.
- One hypothesis implicates *hemodynamic changes* in the initiation and progression of diabetic glomerulosclerosis. It is well known that the early stages of diabetic nephropathy are characterized by an increased GFR, increased glomerular capillary pressure, *glomerular hypertrophy*, and an increased glomerular filtration area.[51,55] Hemodynamic alterations and glomerular hypertrophy also occur in experimental streptozotocin-induced diabetes in rats, in which they are associated with proteinuria and can be

reversed or inhibited by diabetic control and angiotensin inhibition. It has been speculated that the subsequent morphologic alterations discussed above are somehow influenced by the glomerular hypertrophy and hemodynamic changes, akin to the adaptive responses to ablation of renal mass, discussed earlier.

To sum up, two processes seem to play a role in the fully developed diabetic glomerular lesions: a metabolic defect, probably linked to advanced glycosylation end products, that accounts for the thickened GBM and increased mesangial matrix that occur in patients; and hemodynamic effects, associated with glomerular hypertrophy, which also contribute to the development of glomerulosclerosis. Both of these processes contribute also to the loss of podocytes, which may undergo apoptosis in response to the metabolic abnormalities and exposure to reactive oxygen species, or become detached from the basement membranes as a consequence of these metabolic changes and/or stretching induced by hemodynamic perturbations.[56] The morphologic alterations and clinical features of diabetic nephropathy are described in Chapter 24.

Amyloidosis

The various forms of amyloidosis and their pathogenesis are discussed in Chapter 6. Most types of disseminated amyloidosis may be associated with deposits of amyloid within the glomeruli; most commonly renal amyloid is of light-chain (AL) or AA type. The typical Congo red–positive fibrillary amyloid deposits are present within the mesangium and capillary walls and rarely are localized to the subepithelial space. Eventually, they obliterate the glomerulus completely. Deposits of amyloid also appear in blood vessel walls and in the kidney interstitium. Patients with glomerular amyloid may present with the nephrotic syndrome and later, as a result of destruction of the glomeruli, die of uremia. Characteristically, kidney size tends to be either normal or increased.

Fibrillary Glomerulonephritis and Immunotactoid Glomerulopathy

Fibrillary glomerulonephritis is a morphologic variant of glomerulonephritis associated with characteristic fibrillar deposits in the mesangium and glomerular capillary walls that resemble amyloid fibrils superficially but differ ultrastructurally and do not stain with Congo red.[60] The fibrils most often are 18 to 24 nm in diameter and hence are larger than the 10 to 12 nm fibrils characteristic of amyloid. The glomerular lesions usually show membranoproliferative or mesangioproliferative patterns by light microscopy, and by immunofluorescence microscopy, there is selective deposition of polyclonal IgG, often of the IgG4 subclass, complement C3, and Igκ and Igλ light chains. Clinically, patients develop nephrotic syndrome, hematuria, and progressive renal insufficiency. The disease recurs in kidney transplants.

In *immunotactoid glomerulopathy*, a much rarer condition, the deposits are microtubular in structure and 30 to 50 nm in width. Patients often have circulating paraproteins and/or monoclonal Ig deposition in glomeruli.[57]

The pathogenesis of both of these entities is unknown.

Other Systemic Disorders

Goodpasture syndrome (Chapter 15), *microscopic polyangiitis*, and *Wegener granulomatosis* (Chapter 11) are commonly associated with glomerular lesions, as described in the discussion of these diseases. Suffice it to say here that the glomerular lesions in these three conditions can be histologically similar and are principally characterized by foci of glomerular necrosis and crescent formation. In the early or mild forms of involvement, there is focal and segmental, sometimes necrotizing, glomerulonephritis, and most of these patients will have hematuria with mild decline in GFR. In the more severe cases associated with RPGN, there is more extensive necrosis, fibrin deposition, and extensive formation of epithelial (cellular) crescents, which can become organized to form fibrocellular and fibrous crescents if the glomerular injury evolves into segmental or global scarring (sclerosis).

Essential mixed cryoglobulinemia is another systemic condition in which deposits of cryoglobulins composed principally of IgG-IgM complexes induce cutaneous vasculitis, synovitis, and a proliferative glomerulonephritis, typically MPGN. Most cases of essential mixed cryoglobulinemia have been associated with infection with hepatitis C virus, and this condition in particular is associated with glomerulonephritis, usually MPGN type I.

Plasma cell dyscrasias may also induce glomerular lesions. *Multiple myeloma* and other dyscrasias producing circulating monoclonal immunoglobulins are associated with (1) amyloidosis, in which the fibrils are usually composed of monoclonal λ light chains, (2) deposition of monoclonal immunoglobulins or light chains in the GBM, and (3) distinctive nodular glomerular lesions resulting from the deposition of *nonfibrillar* light chains. This so-called *light-chain* or *monoclonal Ig deposition disease* sometimes occurs in the absence of overt myeloma and is usually characterized by deposition of monoclonal Igκ or Igλ light chains in glomeruli. The glomeruli show PAS-positive mesangial nodules, lobular accentuation, and mild mesangial hypercellularity. These lesions must be differentiated from diabetic nodular glomerulosclerosis and other glomerulopathies that can cause nodular mesangial expansion, such as MPGN. These patients usually present with proteinuria or the nephrotic syndrome, hypertension, and progressive azotemia. Other renal manifestations of multiple myeloma are discussed later.

Tubular and Interstitial Diseases

Most forms of tubular injury involve the interstitium as well; therefore, diseases affecting these two components are discussed together. Under this heading we consider two major groups of processes: (1) ischemic or toxic tubular injury, leading to *acute kidney injury (AKI)* and acute renal failure, and (2) inflammatory reactions of the tubules and interstitium *(tubulointerstitial nephritis)*.

ACUTE KIDNEY INJURY (AKI) (ACUTE TUBULAR NECROSIS, ATN)

AKI, a term increasingly favored over the often synonymously used terms acute tubular necrosis (ATN) and acute tubular injury, is a clinicopathologic entity characterized clinically by acute diminution of renal function and often, but not invariably, morphologic evidence of tubular injury. It is the most common cause of acute renal failure,[58,59] which signifies rapid reduction of renal function and urine flow, falling within 24 hours to less than 400 mL per day. It can be caused by a variety of conditions, including

- *Ischemia, due to decreased or interrupted blood flow,* examples of which include diffuse involvement of the intrarenal blood vessels such as in microscopic polyangiitis, malignant hypertension, microangiopathies and systemic conditions associated with thrombosis (e.g., hemolytic uremic syndrome [HUS], thrombotic thrombocytopenic pupura [TTP], and disseminated intravascular coagulation [DIC]), or decreased effective circulating blood volume
- *Direct toxic injury to the tubules* (e.g., by drugs, radiocontrast dyes, myoglobin, hemoglobin, radiation)
- *Acute tubulointerstitial nephritis,* most commonly occurring as a hypersensitivity reaction to drugs
- *Urinary obstruction* by tumors, prostatic hypertrophy, or blood clots (so-called postrenal acute renal failure)

AKI accounts for some 50% of cases of acute renal failure in hospitalized patients. Other causes of acute renal failure are discussed elsewhere in this chapter.

AKI is a reversible renal lesion that arises in a variety of clinical settings. Most of these, ranging from severe trauma to acute pancreatitis, have in common a period of inadequate blood flow to the peripheral organs, usually accompanied by marked hypotension and shock. This pattern of AKI is called *ischemic AKI.* The second pattern, called *nephrotoxic AKI,* is caused by a multitude of drugs, such as gentamicin and other antibiotics; radiographic contrast agents; poisons, including heavy metals (e.g., mercury); and organic solvents (e.g., carbon tetrachloride). Combinations of ischemic and nephrotoxic AKI also can occur, exemplified by mismatched blood transfusions and other hemolytic crises causing *hemoglobinuria* and skeletal muscle injuries causing *myoglobinuria.* Such injuries result in characteristic intratubular hemoglobin or myoglobin casts, respectively; the toxic iron content of these globin molecules contributes to the AKI. In addition to its frequency, the potential reversibility of AKI adds to its clinical importance. Proper management means the difference between full recovery and death.

Pathogenesis. The critical events in both ischemic and nephrotoxic AKI are believed to be (1) tubular injury and (2) persistent and severe disturbances in blood flow[60] (Fig. 20–23).

- *Tubule cell injury:* Tubular epithelial cells are particularly sensitive to ischemia and are also vulnerable to toxins. Several factors predispose the tubules to toxic injury, including a vast charged surface for tubular reabsorption, active transport systems for ions and organic acids, a high metabolic rate and oxygen consumption requirement so as to perform these transport and reabsorption functions, and the capability for effective concentration.

Ischemia causes numerous structural and functional alterations in epithelial cells, as discussed in Chapter 1. The structural changes include those of reversible injury (such

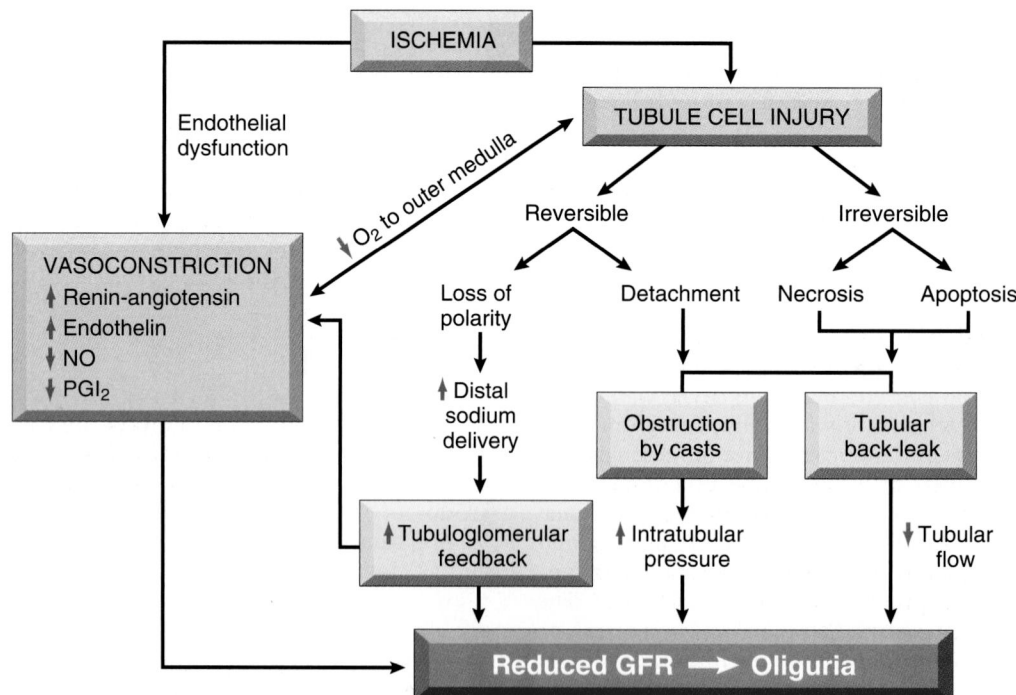

FIGURE 20–23 Postulated sequence in acute kidney injury. GFR, glomerular filtration rate; NO, nitric oxide; PGI₂, prostaglandin I2 (prostacyclin). (Modified from Brady HR et al.: Acute renal failure. In Brenner BM [ed]: Brenner and Rector's The Kidney, 5th ed, Vol II. Philadelphia, WB Saunders, 1996, p 1210).

as cellular swelling, loss of brush border and polarity, blebbing, and cell detachment) and those associated with lethal injury (necrosis and apoptosis). Biochemically there is depletion of ATP; accumulation of intracellular calcium; activation of proteases (e.g., calpain), which cause cytoskeletal disruption; activation of phospholipases, which damage membranes; generation of reactive oxygen species; and activation of caspases, which induce apoptotic cell death. One early reversible result of ischemia is *loss of cell polarity* due to redistribution of membrane proteins (e.g., the enzyme Na$^+$,K$^+$-ATPase) from the basolateral to the luminal surface of the tubular cells, resulting in abnormal ion transport across the cells, and *increased sodium delivery to distal tubules*. The latter incites vasoconstriction via *tubuloglomerular feedback*, which will be discussed below. In addition, ischemic tubular cells express cytokines (such as monocyte chemoattractant protein 1) and adhesion molecules (such as intercellular adhesion molecule 1), thus recruiting leukocytes that appear to participate in the subsequent injury. In time, injured cells detach from the basement membranes and cause *luminal obstruction*, increased intratubular pressure, and decreased GFR. In addition, fluid from the damaged tubules leaks into the interstitium, resulting in interstitial edema, increased interstitial pressure, and further damage to the tubule. All these effects, as shown in Figure 20–23, contribute to the decreased GFR.

- *Disturbances in blood flow:* Ischemic renal injury is also characterized by *hemodynamic alterations* that cause reduced GFR. The major one is *intrarenal vasoconstriction*, which results in both reduced glomerular blood flow and reduced oxygen delivery to the functionally important tubules in the outer medulla (thick ascending limb and straight segment of the proximal tubule). Several vasoconstrictor pathways have been implicated, including the renin-angiotensin system, stimulated by increased distal sodium delivery (via *tubuloglomerular feedback*), and *sublethal endothelial injury*, leading to increased release of the vasoconstrictor *endothelin* and decreased production of the vasodilators *nitric oxide* and *prostacyclin (prostaglandin I$_2$)*. There is also some evidence of a direct effect of ischemia or toxins on the glomerulus, causing a reduced glomerular ultrafiltration coefficient, possibly due to mesangial contraction.

The patchiness of tubular necrosis and maintenance of the integrity of the basement membrane along many segments allow ready repair of the necrotic foci and recovery of function if the precipitating cause is removed. This repair is dependent on the capacity of reversibly injured epithelial cells to proliferate and differentiate. Re-epithelialization is mediated by a variety of growth factors and cytokines produced locally by the tubular cells themselves (autocrine stimulation) or by inflammatory cells in the vicinity of necrotic foci (paracrine stimulation).[61] Of these, epidermal growth factor, TGF-α, insulin-like growth factor type 1, and hepatocyte growth factor have been shown to be particularly important in renal tubular repair. Growth factors, indeed, are being explored as possible therapeutic agents to enhance re-epithelialization in AKI, although clinical trials to date have been disappointing.[61]

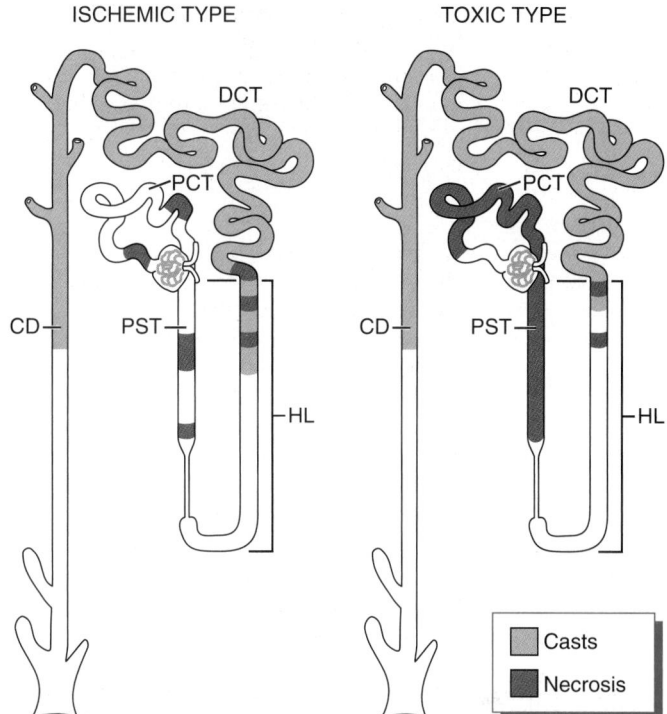

FIGURE 20–24   Patterns of tubular damage in ischemic and toxic acute kidney injury. In the ischemic type, tubular necrosis is patchy, relatively short lengths of tubules are affected, and straight segments of proximal tubules (PST) and ascending limbs of Henle's loop (HL) are most vulnerable. In toxic acute kidney injury, extensive necrosis is present along the proximal convoluted tubule segments (PCT) with many toxins (e.g., mercury), but necrosis of the distal tubule, particularly ascending HL, also occurs. In both types, lumens of the distal convoluted tubules (DCT) and collecting ducts (CD) contain casts.

Morphology. Ischemic AKI is characterized by focal tubular epithelial necrosis at multiple points along the nephron, with large skip areas in between, often accompanied by rupture of basement membranes (tubulorrhexis) and occlusion of tubular lumens by casts[62] (Figs. 20–24 and 20–25). The straight portion of the proximal tubule and the ascending thick limb in the renal medulla are especially vulnerable, but focal lesions may also occur in the distal tubule, often in conjunction with casts. Paradoxically, the clinical syndrome of AKI is often associated with lesser degrees of tubular injury. This includes attenuation or loss of proximal tubule brush borders, simplification of cell structure, cell swelling and vacuolization, and sloughing of non-necrotic tubular cells into the tubular lumina (see Fig. 20–25). The severity of the morphologic findings often does not correlate well with the severity of the clinical manifestations.

Eosinophilic hyaline casts, as well as pigmented granular casts, are common, particularly in distal tubules and collecting ducts. These casts consist principally of Tamm-Horsfall protein (a urinary glycoprotein normally secreted by the cells of ascending thick limb and distal tubules) in conjunction with other

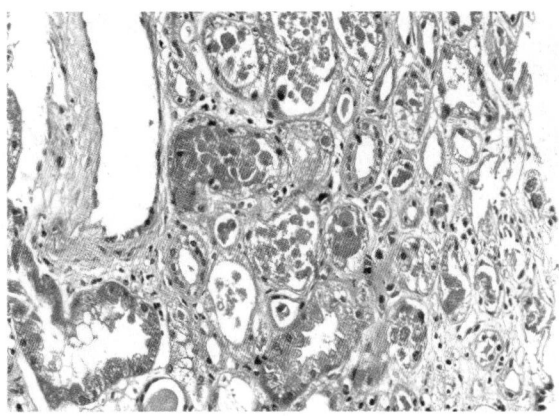

FIGURE 20–25 Acute kidney injury. Some of the tubular epithelial cells in the tubules are necrotic, and many have become detached (from their basement membranes) and been sloughed into the tubular lumens, whereas others are swollen, vacuolated, and regenerating. (Courtesy of Dr. Agnes Fogo, Vanderbilt University, Nashville, TN.)

plasma proteins. Other findings in ischemic AKI are interstitial edema and accumulations of leukocytes within dilated vasa recta. There is also evidence of epithelial regeneration: flattened epithelial cells with hyperchromatic nuclei and mitotic figures are often present. In the course of time this regeneration repopulates the tubules so that, no residual evidence of damage is seen.

Toxic AKI is manifested by acute tubular injury, most obvious in the proximal convoluted tubules. On histologic examination the tubular necrosis may be entirely nonspecific, but it is somewhat distinctive in poisoning with certain agents. With mercuric chloride, for example, severely injured cells may contain large acidophilic inclusions. Later, these cells become totally necrotic, are desquamated into the lumen, and may undergo calcification. Carbon tetrachloride poisoning, in contrast, is characterized by the accumulation of neutral lipids in injured cells; again, such fatty change is followed by necrosis. Ethylene glycol produces marked ballooning and hydropic or vacuolar degeneration of proximal convoluted tubules. Calcium oxalate crystals are often found in the tubular lumens in such poisoning.

Clinical Course. The clinical course of AKI is highly variable, but the classic case may be divided into *initiation*, *maintenance*, and *recovery* stages. The *initiation phase*, lasting for about 36 hours, is dominated by the inciting medical, surgical, or obstetric event in the ischemic form of AKI. The only indication of renal involvement is a slight decline in urine output with a rise in BUN. At this point, oliguria could be explained on the basis of a transient decrease in blood flow and declining GFR.

The *maintenance phase* is characterized by sustained decreases in urine output to between 40 and 400 mL/day (oliguria), salt and water overload, rising BUN concentrations, hyperkalemia, metabolic acidosis, and other manifestations of uremia. With appropriate attention to the balance of water and blood electrolytes, including dialysis, the patient can be supported through this oliguric crisis.

The *recovery phase* is ushered in by a steady increase in urine volume that may reach up to 3 L/day. The tubules are still damaged, so large amounts of water, sodium, and potassium are lost in the flood of urine. *Hypokalemia, rather than hyperkalemia, becomes a clinical problem.* There is a peculiar increased vulnerability to infection at this stage. Eventually, renal tubular function is restored and concentrating ability improves. At the same time, BUN and creatinine levels begin to return to normal. Subtle tubular functional impairment may persist for months, but most patients who reach this phase eventually recover completely.

The prognosis of AKI depends on the clinical setting. Recovery is expected with nephrotoxic AKI when the toxin has not caused serious damage to other organs, such as the liver or heart. With current supportive care, 95% of those who do not succumb to the precipitating cause recover. Conversely, in shock related to sepsis, extensive burns, or other causes of multi-organ failure, the mortality rate can rise to more than 50%.

Up to 50% of patients with AKI do not have oliguria and instead often have increased urine volumes. This so-called *nonoliguric AKI* occurs particularly often with nephrotoxins, and it generally tends to follow a more benign clinical course.

TUBULOINTERSTITIAL NEPHRITIS

This group of renal diseases is characterized by histologic and functional alterations that involve predominantly the tubules and interstitium. We have previously seen that chronic tubulointerstitial injury may occur in diseases that primarily affect the glomerulus (see Fig. 20–22) and that such injury may be an important cause of progression in these diseases.[18] *Secondary tubulointerstitial nephritis* is also present in a variety of vascular, cystic (polycystic kidney disease), and metabolic (diabetes) renal disorders, in which it may also contribute to progressive damage. Here we discuss disorders in which tubulointerstitial injury seems to be a primary event. *These disorders have diverse causes and different pathogenetic mechanisms* (Table 20–8). Glomerular and vascular abnormalities may also be present but either are mild or occur only in advanced stages of these diseases.

Tubulointerstitial nephritis can be acute or chronic. Acute tubulointerstitial nephritis has a rapid clinical onset and is characterized histologically by interstitial edema, often accompanied by leukocytic infiltration of the interstitium and tubules, and focal tubular necrosis. In *chronic interstitial nephritis* there is infiltration with predominantly mononuclear leukocytes, prominent interstitial fibrosis, and widespread tubular atrophy. Morphologic features that are helpful in separating acute from chronic tubulointerstitial nephritis include edema and, when present, eosinophils and neutrophils in the acute form, while fibrosis and tubular atrophy characterize the chronic form.

These conditions are distinguished clinically from the glomerular diseases by the absence, in early stages, of such hallmarks of glomerular injury as nephritic or nephrotic syndrome and by the presence of defects in tubular function. The latter may be subtle and include impaired ability

TABLE 20–8 Causes of Tubulointerstitial Nephritis

INFECTIONS

Acute bacterial pyelonephritis
Chronic pyelonephritis (including reflux nephropathy)
Other infections (e.g., viruses, parasites)

TOXINS

Drugs
Acute-hypersensitivity interstitial nephritis
Analgesics
Heavy metals
Lead, cadmium

METABOLIC DISEASES

Urate nephropathy
Nephrocalcinosis (hypercalcemic nephropathy)
Acute phosphate nephropathy
Hypokalemic nephropathy
Oxalate nephropathy

PHYSICAL FACTORS

Chronic urinary tract obstruction

NEOPLASMS

Multiple myeloma (light-chain cast nephropathy)

IMMUNOLOGIC REACTIONS

Transplant rejection
Sjögren syndrome
Sarcoidosis

VASCULAR DISEASES

MISCELLANEOUS

Balkan nephropathy
Nephronophthisis–medullary cystic disease complex
"Idiopathic" interstitial nephritis

to concentrate urine, evidenced clinically by polyuria or nocturia; salt wasting; diminished ability to excrete acids (metabolic acidosis); and isolated defects in tubular reabsorption or secretion. The advanced forms, however, may be difficult to distinguish clinically from other causes of renal insufficiency.

Some of the specific conditions listed in Table 20–8 are discussed elsewhere in this book. In this section we deal principally with pyelonephritis and interstitial diseases induced by drugs.

Pyelonephritis and Urinary Tract Infection

Pyelonephritis is a renal disorder affecting the tubules, interstitium, and renal pelvis and is one of the most common diseases of the kidney. It occurs in two forms. *Acute pyelonephritis* is caused by bacterial infection and is the renal lesion associated with urinary tract infection. *Chronic pyelonephritis* is a more complex disorder; bacterial infection plays a dominant role, but other factors (vesicoureteral reflux, obstruction) are involved in its pathogenesis. Pyelonephritis is a serious complication of *urinary tract infections* that affect the bladder (cystitis), the kidneys and their collecting systems (pyelonephritis), or both. Bacterial infection of the lower urinary tract may be completely asymptomatic (asymptomatic bacteriuria) and most often remains localized to the bladder without the devel-

opment of renal infection. However, lower urinary tract infection always carries the potential of spread to the kidney.

Etiology and Pathogenesis. The dominant etiologic agents, accounting for more than 85% of cases of urinary tract infection, are the gram-negative bacilli that are normal inhabitants of the intestinal tract.[63] By far the most common is *Escherichia coli*, followed by *Proteus*, *Klebsiella*, and *Enterobacter*. *Streptococcus faecalis*, also of enteric origin, staphylococci, and virtually every other bacterial and fungal agent can also cause lower urinary tract and renal infection. In immunocompromised persons, particularly those with transplanted organs, viruses such as *Polyomavirus*, cytomegalovirus, and adenovirus can also be a cause of renal infection.

In most patients with urinary tract infection, the infecting organisms are derived from the patient's own fecal flora. This is thus a form of endogenous infection. There are two routes by which bacteria can reach the kidneys: (1) through the bloodstream (hematogenous infection) and (2) from the lower urinary tract (ascending infection) (Fig. 20–26). The hematogenous route is the less common of the two and results from seeding of the kidneys by bacteria from distant foci in the course of septicemia or infective endocarditis. Hematogenous infection is more likely to occur in the presence of ureteral obstruction, in debilitated patients, in patients receiving immunosuppressive therapy, and with nonenteric organisms, such as staphylococci and certain fungi and viruses.

Ascending infection is the most common cause of clinical pyelonephritis. Normal human bladder and bladder urine are sterile; therefore, a number of steps must occur for renal infection to occur:

- The first step in ascending infection seems to be the *colonization of the distal urethra and introitus* (in the female) by coliform bacteria. This colonization is influenced by the ability of bacteria to adhere to urethral mucosal epithelial cells. Such bacterial adherence, as discussed in Chapter 8, involves adhesive molecules (adhesins) on the P-fimbriae (pili) of bacteria that interact with receptors on the surface of uroepithelial cells. Specific adhesins (e.g., that encoded by the pyelonephritis-associated pili [*pap*] gene[64]) are associated with infection. In addition, certain types of fimbriae promote renal tropism, persistence of infection, or an enhanced inflammatory response.[64]

- *From the urethra to the bladder*, organisms gain entrance during urethral catheterization or other instrumentation. Long-term catheterization, in particular, carries a risk of infection. In the absence of instrumentation, *urinary infections are much more common in females*, and this has been ascribed to the shorter urethra in females, as well as the absence of antibacterial properties such as are found in prostatic fluid, hormonal changes affecting adherence of bacteria to the mucosa, and urethral trauma during sexual intercourse, or a combination of these factors.

- *Urinary tract obstruction and stasis of urine.* Ordinarily, organisms introduced into the bladder are cleared by the continual flushing of voiding and by antibacterial mechanisms. However, outflow obstruction or bladder dysfunction results in incomplete emptying and increased residual volume of urine. In the presence of stasis, bacteria introduced into the bladder can multiply unhindered without being flushed out or destroyed. Accordingly, urinary tract

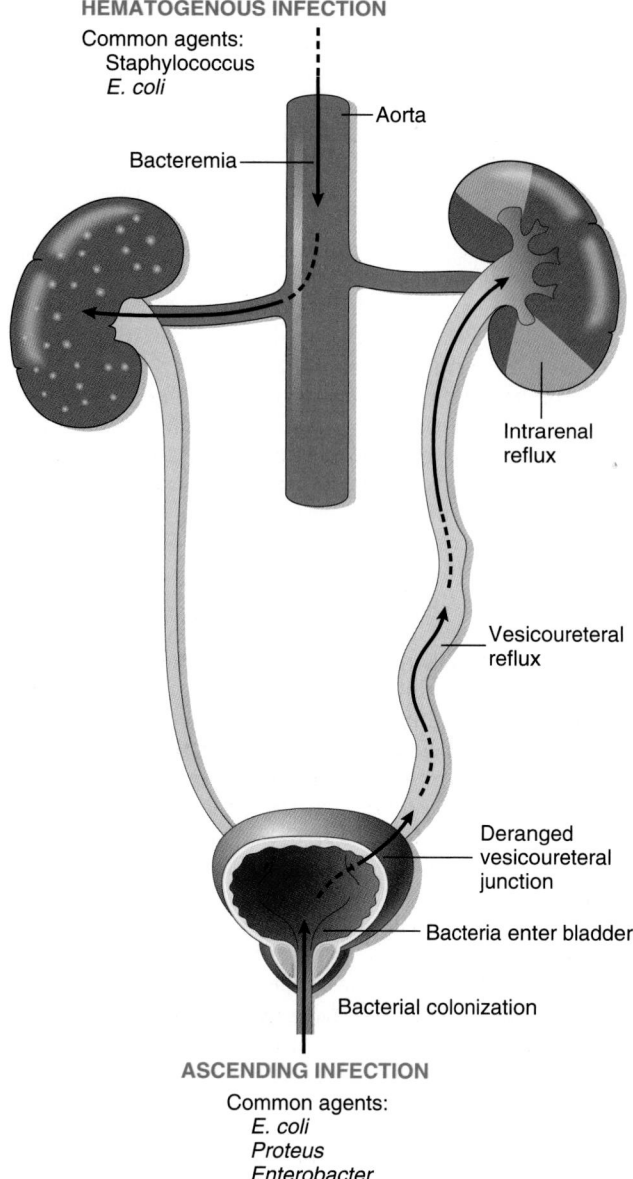

HEMATOGENOUS INFECTION
Common agents:
Staphylococcus
E. coli

Aorta

Bacteremia

Intrarenal
reflux

Vesicoureteral
reflux

Deranged
vesicoureteral
junction

Bacteria enter bladder

Bacterial colonization

ASCENDING INFECTION
Common agents:
E. coli
Proteus
Enterobacter

FIGURE 20–26 Schematic representation of pathways of renal infection. Hematogenous infection results from bacteremic spread. More common is ascending infection, which results from a combination of urinary bladder infection, vesicoureteral reflux, and intrarenal reflux.

infection is particularly frequent among patients with lower urinary tract obstruction, such as may occur with benign prostatic hypertrophy, tumors, or calculi, or with neurogenic bladder dysfunction caused by diabetes or spinal cord injury.

○ *Vesicoureteral reflux.* Although obstruction is an important predisposing factor in ascending infection, it is *incompetence of the vesicoureteral valve* that allows bacteria to ascend the ureter into the renal pelvis. The normal ureteral insertion into the bladder is a competent one-way valve that prevents retrograde flow of urine, especially during micturition, when the intravesical pressure rises. An incompetent vesicoureteral orifice allows the reflux of bladder urine into the ureters (*vesicoureteral reflux*) (Fig. 20–27). Reflux is

most often due to a congenital absence or shortening of the intravesical portion of the ureter, such that the ureter is not compressed during micturition. In addition, bladder infection itself, probably as a result of the action of bacterial or inflammatory products on ureteral contractility, can cause or accentuate vesicoureteral reflux, particularly in children. Vesicoureteral reflux is not uncommon; it is estimated to affect 1% to 2% of otherwise normal children.[65] *Acquired vesicoureteral reflux* in adults can result from persistent bladder atony caused by spinal cord injury. The effect of vesicoureteral reflux is similar to that of an obstruction in that there is residual urine in the urinary tract after voiding, which favors bacterial growth.

○ *Intrarenal reflux.* Vesicoureteral reflux also affords a ready mechanism by which the infected bladder urine can be propelled up to the renal pelvis and deep into the renal parenchyma through open ducts at the tips of the papillae (intrarenal reflux). Intrarenal reflux is most common in the upper and lower poles of the kidney, where papillae tend to have flattened or concave tips rather than the convex pointed type present in the midzones of the kidney (and depicted in most textbooks). Reflux can be demonstrated radiographically by a voiding cystourethrogram: The bladder is filled with a radiopaque dye, and films are taken during micturition. Vesicoureteral reflux can be demonstrated in about 30% of infants and children with urinary tract infection (see Fig. 20–27).

In the absence of vesicoureteral reflux, infection usually remains localized in the bladder. Thus, the majority of indi-

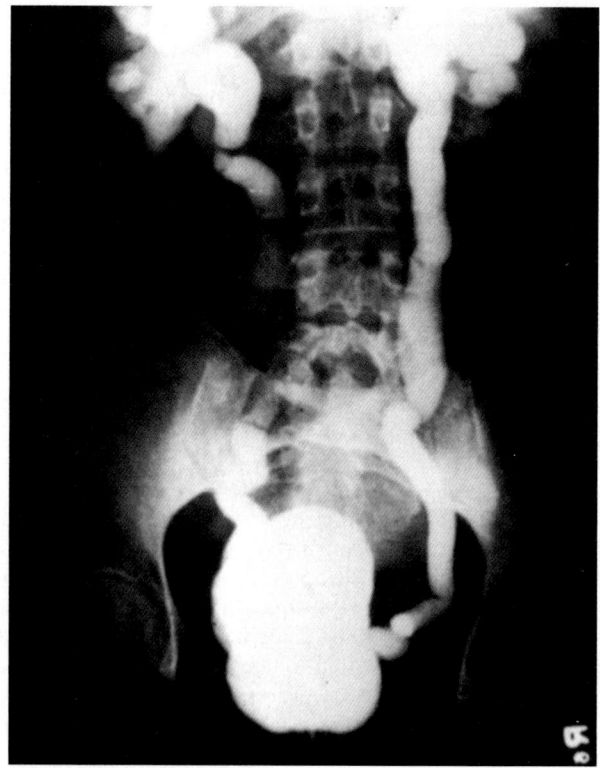

FIGURE 20–27 Vesicoureteral reflux demonstrated by a voiding cystourethrogram. Dye injected into the bladder refluxes into both dilated ureters, filling the pelvis and calyces.

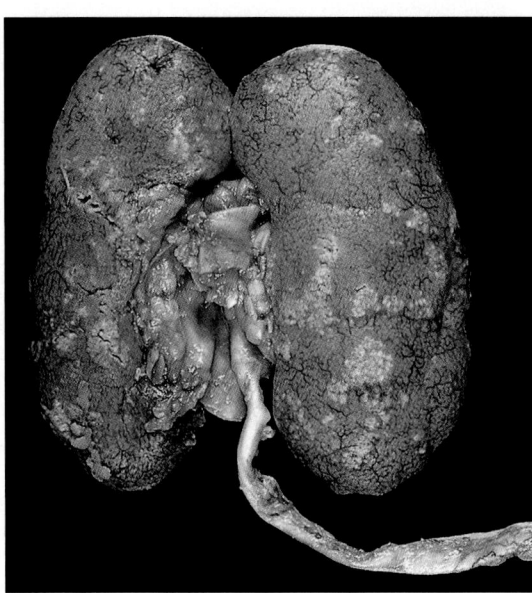

FIGURE 20–28 Acute pyelonephritis. Cortical surface shows grayish white areas of inflammation and abscess formation.

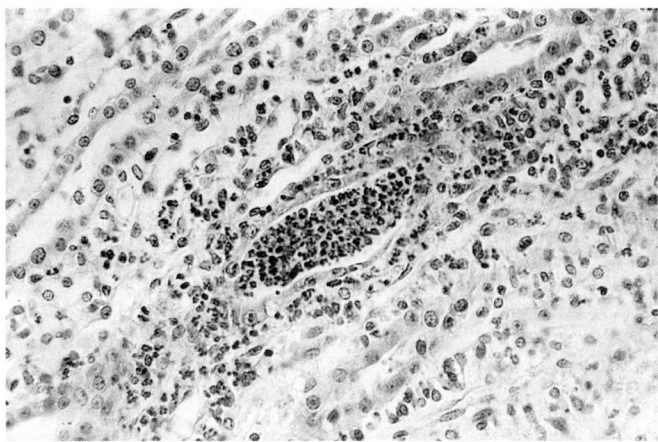

FIGURE 20–29 Acute pyelonephritis marked by an acute neutrophilic exudate within tubules and interstitial inflammation.

viduals with repeated or persistent bacterial colonization of the urinary tract suffer from cystitis and urethritis *(lower urinary tract infection)* rather than pyelonephritis.

Acute Pyelonephritis

Acute pyelonephritis is an acute suppurative inflammation of the kidney caused by bacterial and sometimes viral (e.g., polyomavirus) infection, whether hematogenous and induced by septicemic spread or ascending and associated with vesicoureteral reflux.[66]

Morphology. The hallmarks of acute pyelonephritis are **patchy interstitial suppurative inflammation, intratubular aggregates of neutrophils, and tubular necrosis.** The suppuration may occur as discrete focal abscesses involving one or both kidneys, which can extend to large wedge-shaped areas of suppuration (Fig. 20–28). The distribution of these lesions is unpredictable and haphazard, but in pyelonephritis associated with reflux, damage occurs most commonly in the lower and upper poles.

In the early stages, the neutrophilic infiltration is limited to the interstitial tissue. Soon, however, the reaction involves tubules and produces a characteristic abscess with the destruction of the engulfed tubules (Fig. 20–29). Since the tubular lumens present a ready pathway for the extension of the infection, large masses of intraluminal neutrophils frequently extend along the involved nephron into the collecting tubules. Characteristically, glomeruli seem to be relatively resistant to the infection. Large areas of severe necrosis, however, eventually destroy the glomeruli, and fungal pyelonephritis (e.g., *Candida*) often affects glomeruli.

Three complications of acute pyelonephritis are encountered in special circumstances.

- **Papillary necrosis** is seen mainly in diabetics and in those with urinary tract obstruction. Papillary necrosis is usually bilateral but may be unilateral. One or all of the pyramids of the affected kidney may be involved. On cut section, the tips or distal two thirds of the pyramids have areas of gray-white to yellow necrosis (Fig. 20–30). On microscopic examination the necrotic tissue shows characteristic coagulative necrosis, with preservation of outlines of tubules. The leukocytic response is limited to the junctions between preserved and destroyed tissue.
- **Pyonephrosis** is seen when there is total or almost complete obstruction, particularly when it is high in the urinary tract. The suppurative exudate is unable to drain and thus fills the renal pelvis, calyces, and ureter with pus.
- **Perinephric abscess** is an extension of suppurative inflammation through the renal capsule into the perinephric tissue.

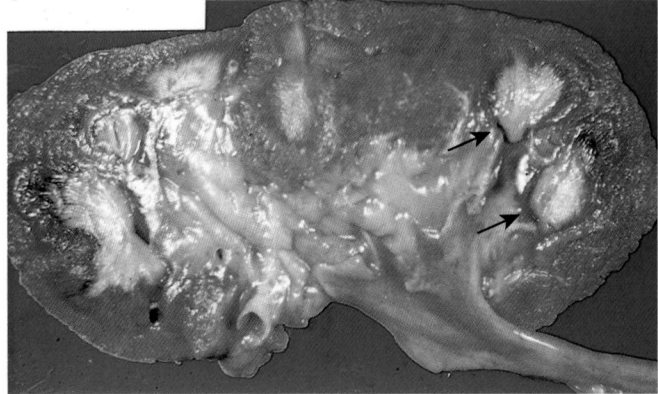

FIGURE 20–30 Papillary necrosis. Areas of pale-gray necrosis involve the papillae *(arrows)*.

After the acute phase of pyelonephritis, healing occurs. The neutrophilic infiltrate is replaced by one that is predominantly composed of macrophages, plasma cells, and (later) lymphocytes. The inflammatory foci are eventually replaced by irregular scars that can be seen on the cortical surface as fibrous depressions. Such scars are characterized microscopically by tubular atrophy, interstitial fibrosis, and a lymphocytic infiltrate in a characteristic patchy, jigsaw pattern with intervening preserved parenchyma. **The pyelonephritic scar is almost always associated with inflammation, fibrosis, and deformation of the underlying calyx and pelvis**, reflecting the role of ascending infection and vesicoureteral reflux in the pathogenesis of the disease.

Clinical Features. Acute pyelonephritis is often associated with predisposing conditions, some of which were mentioned before. These include the following:

- *Urinary tract obstruction,* either congenital or acquired
- *Instrumentation* of the urinary tract, most commonly catheterization
- *Vesicoureteral reflux*
- *Pregnancy.* Between 4% and 6% of pregnant women develop bacteriuria sometime during pregnancy, and 20% to 40% of these eventually develop symptomatic urinary infection if not treated.
- *Gender and age.* After the first year of life (when congenital anomalies in males commonly become evident) and up to around age 40 years, infections are much more frequent in females. With increasing age the incidence in males rises as a result of prostatic hypertrophy and instrumentation.
- *Preexisting renal lesions,* causing intrarenal scarring and obstruction
- *Diabetes mellitus,* in which increased susceptibility to infection, neurogenic bladder dysfunction, and more frequent instrumentation are predisposing factors
- *Immunosuppression and immunodeficiency*

When acute pyelonephritis is clinically apparent, the onset is usually sudden, with pain at the costovertebral angle and systemic evidence of infection, such as fever and malaise. There are usually indications of bladder and urethral irritation, such as dysuria, frequency, and urgency. The urine contains many leukocytes (pyuria) derived from the inflammatory infiltrate, but pyuria does not differentiate upper from lower urinary tract infection. The finding of leukocyte *casts,* typically rich in neutrophils (pus casts), indicates renal involvement, because casts are formed only in tubules. The diagnosis of infection is established by quantitative urine culture.

Uncomplicated acute pyelonephritis usually follows a benign course, and the symptoms disappear within a few days after the institution of appropriate antibiotic therapy. Bacteria, however, may persist in the urine, or there may be recurrence of infection with new serologic types of *E. coli* or other organisms. Such bacteriuria then either disappears or may persist, sometimes for years. In the presence of unrelieved urinary obstruction, diabetes mellitus, or immunodeficiency, acute pyelonephritis may be more serious, leading to repeated septicemic episodes. The superimposition of *papillary necrosis* may lead to acute renal failure.

An emerging viral pathogen causing pyelonephritis in kidney allografts is *polyomavirus.* Latent infection with polyomavirus is widespread in the general population, but immunosuppression of the allograft recipient can lead to reactivation of latent infection and the development of a nephropathy resulting in allograft failure in as many as 1% to 5% of kidney transplant recipients.[67] This form of pyelonephritis, now referred to as *polyomavirus nephropathy,* is characterized by viral infection of tubular epithelial cell nuclei, leading to nuclear enlargement and intranuclear inclusions visible by light microscopy (viral cytopathic effect). The inclusions are composed of virions arrayed in distinctive crystalline-like lattices when visualized by electron microscopy (Fig. 20–31). An interstitial inflammatory response is invariably present. Treatment consists of a reduction in immunosuppression.

Chronic Pyelonephritis and Reflux Nephropathy

Chronic pyelonephritis is a disorder in which *chronic tubulointerstitial inflammation and renal scarring are associated with pathologic involvement of the calyces and pelvis* (Fig. 20–32). Pelvocalyceal damage is important in that virtually all the disease etiologies listed in Table 20–8 produce chronic tubulointerstitial alterations, but with the exception of chronic pyelonephritis and analgesic nephropathy, none affect the calyces. Chronic pyelonephritis is an important cause of end-stage kidney disease; at one time it accounted for as many as 10% to 20% of patients in renal transplant or dialysis units, until predisposing conditions such as reflux became better recognized. This condition remains an important cause of kidney destruction in children with severe lower urinary tract abnormalities.

Chronic pyelonephritis can be divided into two forms: chronic reflux-associated and chronic obstructive.

Reflux Nephropathy. This is by far the more common form of chronic pyelonephritic scarring. Renal involvement in reflux nephropathy occurs early in childhood as a result of superimposition of a urinary infection on congenital vesicoureteral reflux and intrarenal reflux. Reflux may be unilateral or bilateral; thus, the resultant renal damage may cause scarring and atrophy of one kidney or involve both, leading to chronic renal insufficiency. Vesicoureteral reflux occasionally causes renal damage in the absence of infection (sterile reflux), but only when obstruction is severe.

Chronic Obstructive Pyelonephritis. We have seen that obstruction predisposes the kidney to infection. Recurrent infections superimposed on diffuse or localized obstructive lesions lead to recurrent bouts of renal inflammation and scarring, resulting in a picture of chronic pyelonephritis. In this condition, the effects of obstruction contribute to the parenchymal atrophy; indeed, it is sometimes difficult to differentiate the effects of bacterial infection from those of obstruction alone. The disease can be bilateral, as with posterior urethral valves, resulting in renal insufficiency unless the anomaly is corrected, or unilateral, such as occurs with calculi and unilateral obstructive anomalies of the ureter.

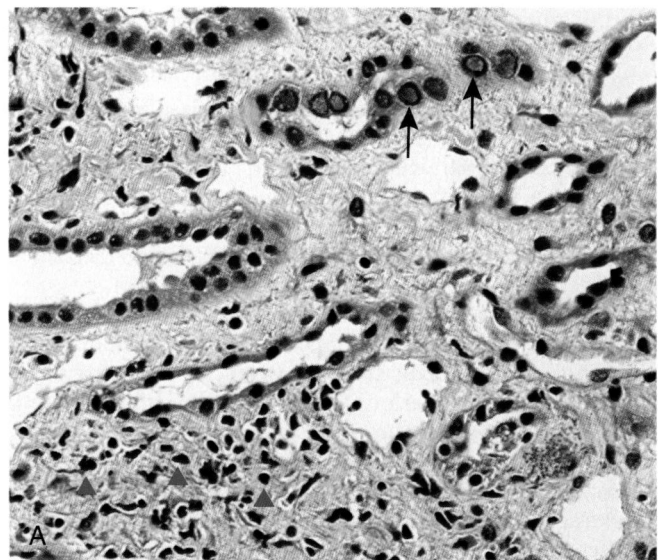 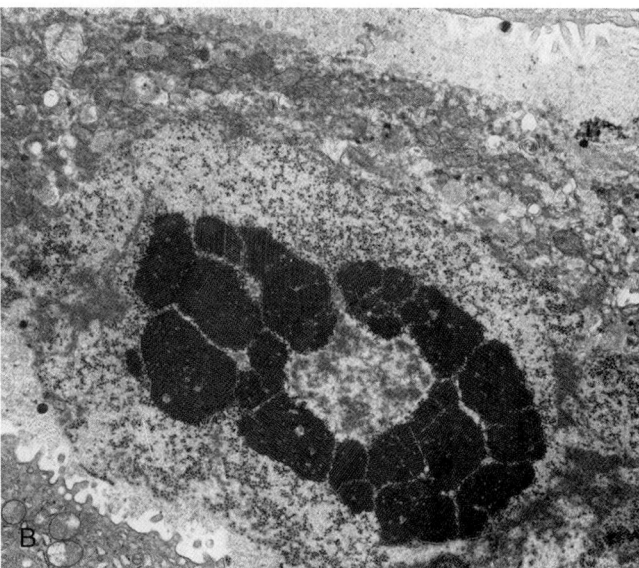

FIGURE 20–31 Polyomavirus nephropathy. **A,** The kidney shows enlarged tubular epithelial cells with nuclear inclusions *(arrows)* and interstitial inflammation *(arrowheads)*. **B,** Intranuclear viral inclusions visualized by electron microscopy. (Courtesy of Dr. Jean Olson, Department of Pathology, University of California San Francisco, San Francisco, CA.)

Morphology. The characteristic changes of chronic pyelonephritis are seen on gross examination (Figs. 20–32 and 20–33). The kidneys usually are irregularly scarred; if bilateral, the involvement is asymmetric. This contrasts with chronic glomerulonephritis, in which both kidneys are diffusely and symmetrically scarred. The hallmarks of chronic pyelonephritis are coarse, discrete, corticomedullary scars overlying dilated, blunted, or deformed calyces, and flattening of the papillae (see Fig. 20–33). The scars can vary from one to several in number and may affect one or both kidneys. Most are in the upper and lower poles, consistent with the frequency of reflux in these sites.

The microscopic changes involve predominantly tubules and interstitium. The tubules show atrophy in some areas and hypertrophy or dilation in others. Dilated tubules with flattened epithelium may be filled with colloid casts (thyroidization). There are varying degrees of chronic interstitial inflammation and fibrosis in the cortex and medulla. In the presence of active infection there may be neutrophils in the interstitium and pus casts in the tubules. Arcuate and interlobular vessels demonstrate obliterative intimal sclerosis in the scarred areas; and in the presence of hypertension, hyaline arteriosclerosis is seen in the entire kidney. There is often fibrosis around the calyceal epithelium as well as a marked chronic inflammatory infiltrate. Glomeruli may appear normal except for periglomerular fibrosis, or exhibit a variety of changes, including ischemic fibrous obliteration and secondary changes related to hypertension. Individuals with chronic pyelonephritis and reflux nephropathy who develop proteinuria in advanced stages show secondary focal segmental glomerulosclerosis, as described later.

Xanthogranulomatous pyelonephritis is an unusual and relatively rare form of chronic pyelonephritis characterized by accumulation of foamy macrophages intermingled with plasma cells, lymphocytes, polymorphonuclear leukocytes, and occasional giant cells. Often associated with *Proteus* infections and obstruction, the lesions sometimes produce large, yellowish orange nodules that may be grossly confused with renal cell carcinoma.

Clinical Features. Chronic obstructive pyelonephritis may be insidious in onset or present with clinical manifestations of acute recurrent pyelonephritis, such as back pain, fever, frequent pyuria, and bacteriuria. Chronic pyelonephritis associated with reflux may have a silent onset. These patients come to medical attention relatively late in the course of their disease because of the gradual onset of renal insufficiency and hypertension or because of the discovery of pyuria or bacteriuria on routine examination. Reflux nephropathy is often discovered when hypertension in children is investigated. Loss of tubular function—in particular of concentrating ability—gives rise to polyuria and nocturia. Radiographic studies show asymmetrically contracted kidneys with characteristic coarse scars and blunting and deformity of the calyceal system. Significant bacteriuria may be present, but it is often absent in the late stages.

Although proteinuria is usually mild, some individuals with pyelonephritic scars develop secondary *focal segmental glomerulosclerosis* with significant proteinuria, even in the nephrotic range, usually several years after the scarring has occurred and often in the absence of continued infection or persistent vesicoureteral reflux. The appearance of proteinuria and focal segmental glomerulosclerosis is a poor prognostic sign, and patients with these findings may proceed to chronic or end-stage renal failure. The glomerulosclerosis, as we have

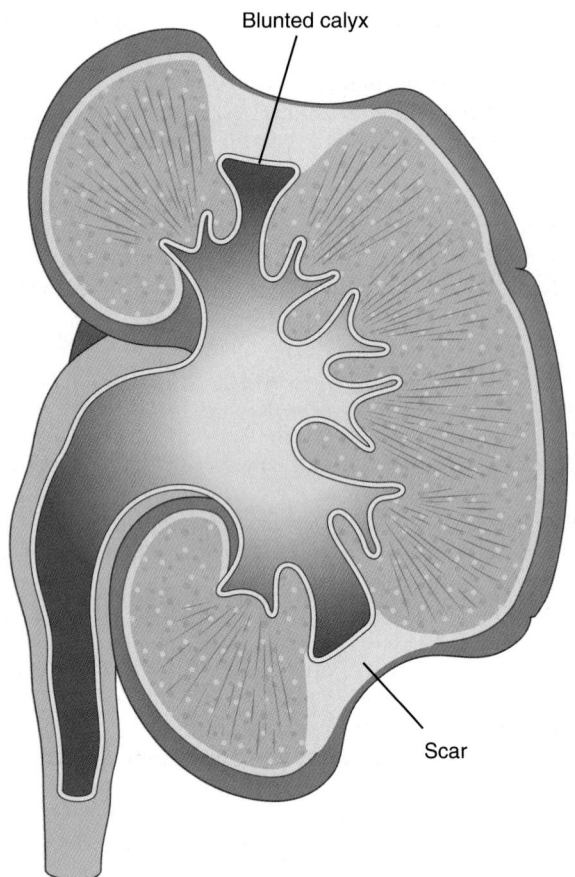

FIGURE 20–32 Typical coarse scars of chronic pyelonephritis associated with vesicoureteral reflux. The scars are usually polar and are associated with underlying blunted calyces.

discussed, may be attributable to the adaptive glomerular alterations secondary to loss of renal mass caused by pyelonephritic scarring (renal ablation nephropathy).

Tubulointerstitial Nephritis Induced by Drugs and Toxins

Toxins and drugs can produce renal injury in at least three ways: (1) They may trigger an interstitial immunological reaction, exemplified by the acute hypersensitivity nephritis induced by such drugs as methicillin; (2) they may cause acute renal failure, as described earlier; and (3) they may cause subtle but cumulative injury to tubules that takes years to become manifest, resulting in chronic renal insufficiency.[68] The last type of damage is especially treacherous, because it may be clinically unrecognized until significant renal damage has occurred. Such is the case with analgesic abuse nephropathy, which is usually detected only after the onset of chronic renal insufficiency.

Acute Drug-Induced Interstitial Nephritis

This is a well-recognized adverse reaction to a constantly increasing number of drugs. First reported after the use of sulfonamides, acute tubulointerstitial nephritis most frequently occurs with synthetic penicillins (methicillin, ampicil-

lin), other synthetic antibiotics (rifampin), diuretics (thiazides), NSAIDs, and miscellaneous drugs (allopurinol, cimetidine). The disease begins about 15 days (range: 2–40) after exposure to the drug and is characterized by *fever, eosinophilia* (which may be transient), *a rash* in about 25% of patients, and *renal abnormalities.* The latter take the form of hematuria, mild proteinuria, and leukocyturia (often including eosinophils). A *rising serum creatinine level or acute renal failure with oliguria develops in about 50% of cases,* particularly in older patients.

Pathogenesis. Many features of the disease suggest an immune mechanism. The immune response is idiosyncratic and not dose-related. Clinical evidence of hypersensitivity includes the latent period, the eosinophilia and rash, the fact that the onset of nephropathy is not dose-related, and the recurrence of hypersensitivity after re-exposure to the same or a cross-reactive drug. In some patients, serum IgE levels are increased, and IgE-containing plasma cells and basophils are present in the lesions, suggesting that the *late-phase reaction of an IgE-mediated (type I) hypersensitivity* may be involved in the pathogenesis (Chapter 6). In other cases, mononuclear or granulomatous infiltrate, together with positive results of skin

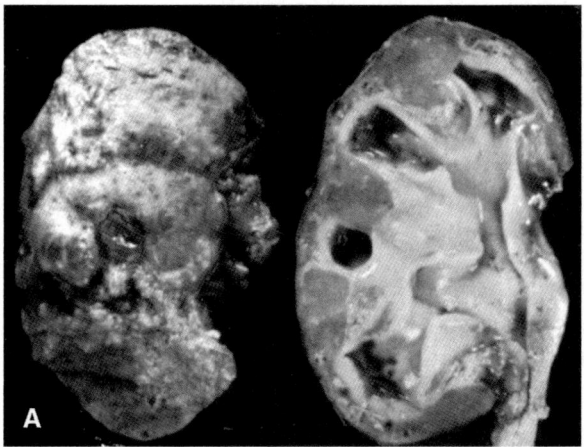

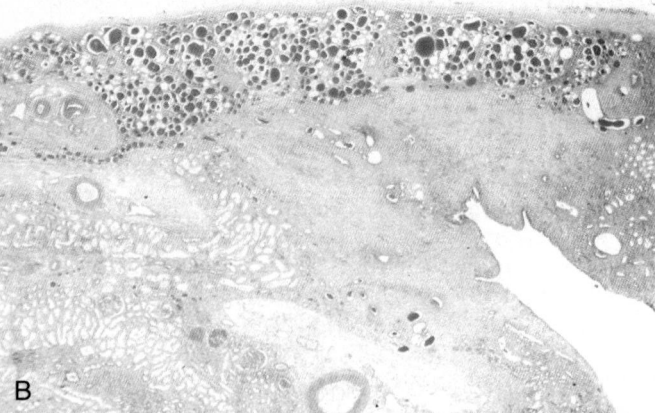

FIGURE 20–33 **A,** Chronic pyelonephritis. The surface *(left)* is irregularly scarred. The cut section *(right)* reveals characteristic dilation and blunting of calyces. The ureter is dilated and thickened, a finding that is consistent with chronic vesicoureteral reflux. **B,** Low-power view showing a corticomedullary renal scar with an underlying dilated deformed calyx. Note the thyroidization of tubules in the cortex.

tests to drug haptens, suggest a T cell–mediated delayed-hypersensitivity reaction (type IV).

The most likely sequence of events is that the drugs act as haptens, which covalently bind to some cytoplasmic or extracellular component of tubular cells and become immunogenic. The resultant injury is then due to IgE and/or cell-mediated immune reactions to tubular cells or their basement membranes.

> **Morphology.** On histologic examination the abnormalities are in the interstitium, which shows variable but frequently pronounced edema and infiltration by mononuclear cells, principally lymphocytes and macrophages. Eosinophils and neutrophils may be present (Fig. 20–34), often in clusters and large numbers, and plasma cells and basophils are sometimes found in small numbers. With some drugs (e.g., methicillin, thiazides), interstitial non-necrotizing granulomas containing giant cells may be seen. "Tubulitis," the infiltration of tubules by lymphocytes, is common. Variable degrees of tubular necrosis and regeneration are present. The glomeruli are normal except in some cases caused by NSAIDs, when minimal-change disease and the nephrotic syndrome develop concurrently (see the discussion of NSAIDs later in the chapter).

Clinical Features. It is important to recognize drug-induced renal failure because withdrawal of the offending drug is followed by recovery, although it may take several months, and irreversible damage occurs occasionally in older subjects. It is also important to remember that while drugs are the leading identifiable cause of acute interstitial nephritis, in many affected patients (approximately 30% to 40%) an offending drug or mechanism cannot be identified.

Analgesic Nephropathy

This is a form of chronic renal disease caused by excessive intake of analgesic mixtures and characterized morphologically by chronic tubulointerstitial nephritis and renal papillary necrosis.[69]

The incidence of analgesic nephropathy reflects the consumption of analgesics in various populations throughout the world. In some parts of Australia, it ranked as one of the most common causes of chronic renal insufficiency until public health measures reduced its incidence. Its incidence in the United States is relatively low but varies among states, being highest in the southeast. Overall, it accounted for 9%, 3%, and 1% of patients undergoing dialysis in Australia, Europe, and the United States, respectively, before the recent surge in end-stage renal disease attributable to diabetes reduced these relative percentages. The renal damage was first ascribed to phenacetin, but the analgesic mixtures that are consumed often contain, in addition, aspirin, caffeine, acetaminophen (a metabolite of phenacetin), and codeine. Patients who develop this disease usually ingest large quantities of mixtures of at least two antipyretic analgesics. Most patients consume phenacetin-containing mixtures, and cases ascribed to ingestion of aspirin, phenacetin, or acetaminophen alone are uncommon. In most countries, restriction of over-the-counter sale of phenacetin or analgesic mixtures has reduced the incidence of the disorder but has not eradicated it, presumably because non-phenacetin-containing mixtures are available.

Pathogenesis. Papillary necrosis is readily induced experimentally by a mixture of aspirin and phenacetin, usually combined with water depletion. It is now clear that in the sequence of events leading to renal damage, *papillary necrosis occurs first, and cortical tubulointerstitial nephritis follows as a consequence of impeded urine outflow.* The phenacetin metabolite acetaminophen, which can deplete cells of glutathione, then injures these cells by subsequent generation of *oxidative metabolites.* Aspirin induces its potentiating effect by inhibiting the vasodilatory effects of prostaglandins, predisposing the papillae to ischemia. Thus, the papillary damage may be due to a combination of direct toxic effects of phenacetin metabolites and ischemic injury to both tubular cells and vessels.

> **Morphology.** In gross appearance the kidneys are either normal or slightly reduced in size, and the cortex shows depressed areas representing cortical atrophy overlying necrotic papillae. The papillae show various stages of necrosis, calcification, fragmentation, and sloughing. This gross appearance contrasts with the papillary necrosis seen in diabetic patients, in which all papillae are at the same stage of injury. On microscopic examination the papillary changes may take one of several forms. In early cases there is patchy necrosis, but in the advanced form the entire papilla is necrotic, often remaining in place as a structureless mass containing "ghosts" of tubules and foci of dystrophic calcification (Fig. 20–35). Segments of entire portions of the papilla may then be sloughed and excreted in the urine.
>
> The cortical changes consist of loss and atrophy of tubules and interstitial fibrosis and inflammation. These changes are mainly due to obstructive atrophy caused by the tubular damage in the papillae. The cortical columns of Bertin are characteristically spared from this atrophy.

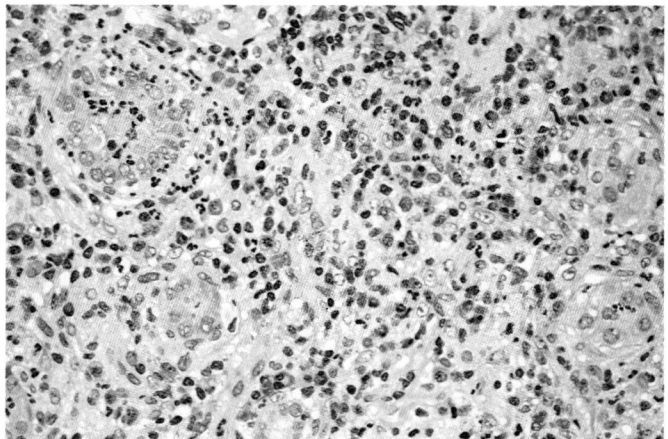

FIGURE 20–34 Drug-induced interstitial nephritis, with prominent eosinophilic and mononuclear cell infiltrate. (Courtesy of Dr. H. Rennke, Brigham and Women's Hospital, Boston, MA.)

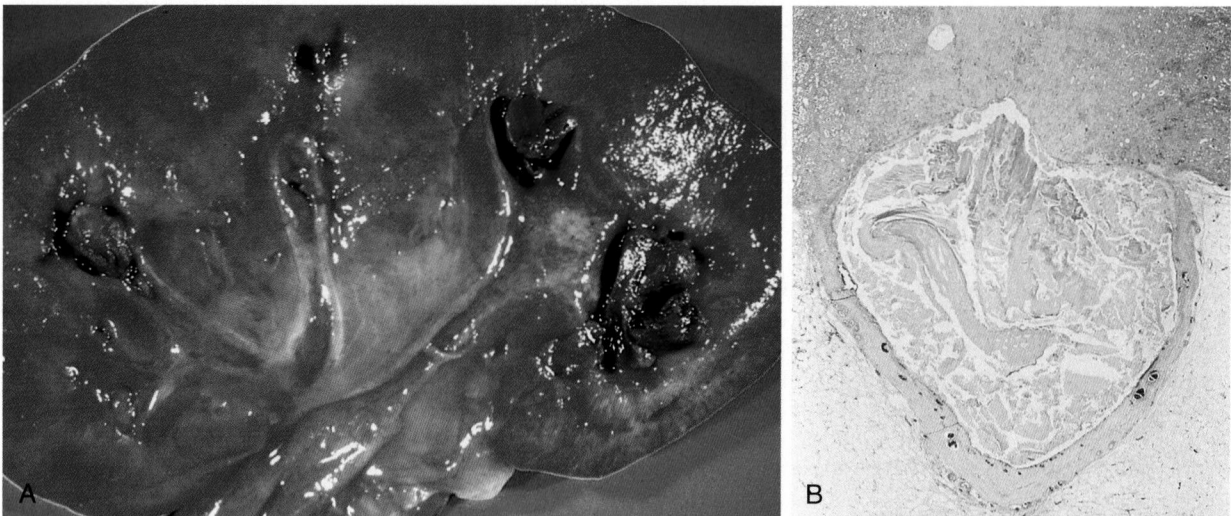

FIGURE 20–35   Analgesic nephropathy. A, The brownish necrotic papilla, transformed to a necrotic, structureless mass, fills the pelvis. B, Microscopic view. Note the fibrosis in the medulla. (Courtesy of Dr. F.J. Gloor, Institut für Pathologie, Kantonsspital, St. Gallen, Switzerland.)

Clinical Features.   Analgesic nephropathy is more common in women than in men and is particularly prevalent in individuals with recurrent headaches and muscle pain, in psychoneurotic patients, and in factory workers. Early renal findings include inability to concentrate the urine (hyposthenuria), as would be expected for papillary lesions. Acquired distal renal tubular acidosis contributes to the development of renal stones. Headache, anemia, gastrointestinal symptoms, and hypertension are common accompaniments of analgesic nephropathy. Urinary tract infection complicates about 50% of cases. On occasion, entire tips of necrotic papillae are excreted, and these may cause gross hematuria or renal colic due to obstruction of the ureter by necrotic fragments. Magnetic resonance and computed tomographic imaging are helpful in detecting papillary necrosis and calcifications. Progressive impairment of renal function may lead to chronic renal failure, but *with drug withdrawal, renal function may either stabilize or actually improve.*

Unfortunately, a small percentage of patients with analgesic nephropathy develop *transitional papillary carcinoma of the renal pelvis.* Whether the carcinogenic effect is due to a metabolite of phenacetin or to some other component of the analgesic compounds is unsettled.

Papillary necrosis is not specific for analgesic nephropathy. It is also seen in diabetes mellitus, as was mentioned earlier, as well as in urinary tract obstruction, sickle cell disease or trait (described later), and focally in renal tuberculosis. Table 20–9 lists certain features of papillary necrosis in these conditions.

Nephropathy Associated with NSAIDs

NSAIDs, one of the most common classes of drugs currently in use, produce several forms of renal injury. Although these complications are uncommon, they should be kept in mind since NSAIDs are frequently administered to patients with other potential causes of renal disease. Many NSAIDs are non-

selective cyclooxygenase inhibitors, and their adverse renal effects are related to their ability to inhibit cyclooxygenase-dependent prostaglandin synthesis. The selective COX-2 inhibitors, while sparing the gastrointestinal tract, do affect the kidneys because COX-2 is expressed in human kidneys.[70] NSAID-associated renal syndromes include

- Hemodynamically induced *acute renal failure,* due to the decreased synthesis of vasodilatory prostaglandins. This is particularly likely to occur in the setting of other renal diseases or conditions causing volume depletion.
- *Acute hypersensitivity interstitial nephritis,* resulting in acute renal failure, as described earlier.
- *Acute interstitial nephritis and minimal-change disease.* This curious association of two diverse renal conditions, one leading to renal failure and the other to nephrotic syndrome, suggests a hypersensitivity reaction affecting the interstitium and possibly the glomeruli, but also is consistent with injury to podocytes mediated by cytokines released as part of the inflammatory process.
- *Membranous nephropathy,* with the nephrotic syndrome, is a recently appreciated association, also of unclear pathogenesis.

Aristolochic Nephropathy

A syndrome of chronic tubulointerstitial nephritis caused by aristolochic acid, a supplement found in some herbal remedies, has been recognized recently. The drug forms covalent adducts with DNA and causes a distinctive picture of renal failure and interstitial fibrosis associated with a relative paucity of infiltrating leukocytes. As with analgesic nephropathy, there is an increased incidence of carcinoma in the kidney and urinary tract. Ingestion of aristolochic acid has also been identified as the cause of Balkan nephropathy, a chronic tubulointerstitial nephritis common in that part of the world.[71]

TABLE 20–9 Causes of Papillary Necrosis				
	Diabetes Mellitus	**Analgesic Nephropathy**	**Sickle-Cell Disease**	**Obstruction**
Male-to-female ratio	1:3	1:5	1:1	9:1
Time course	10 years	7 years of abuse	Variable	Variable
Infection	80%	25%	±	90%
Calcification	Rare	Frequent	Rare	Frequent
Number of papillae affected	Several; all of same stage	Almost all; different stages of necrosis	Few	Variable

Data from Seshan S et al. (eds): Classification and Atlas of Tubulointerstitial and Vascular Diseases. Baltimore, Williams & Wilkins, 1999.

Other Tubulointerstitial Diseases

Urate Nephropathy

Three types of nephropathy can occur in persons with hyperuricemic disorders:

- *Acute uric acid nephropathy* is caused by the precipitation of uric acid crystals in the renal tubules, principally in collecting ducts, leading to obstruction of nephrons and the development of acute renal failure. This type is particularly likely to occur in individuals with leukemias and lymphomas who are undergoing chemotherapy; the drugs increase the death of tumor cells, and uric acid is produced as released nucleic acids are broken down. Precipitation of uric acid is favored by the acidic pH in collecting tubules.
- *Chronic urate nephropathy*, or gouty nephropathy, occurs in patients with more protracted forms of hyperuricemia. The lesions are ascribed to the deposition of monosodium urate crystals in the acidic milieu of the distal tubules and collecting ducts as well as in the interstitium. *These deposits have a distinct histologic appearance and may form variably birefringent needle-like crystals either in the tubular lumens or in the interstitium* (Fig. 20–36). The urates induce a *tophus* consisting of foreign-body giant cells, other mononuclear cells, and a fibrotic reaction (Chapter 26). Tubular obstruction by the urates causes cortical atrophy and scarring. Renal arterial and arteriolar thickening is common as a result of the relatively high frequency of hypertension in patients with gout. Clinically, urate nephropathy is a subtle disease associated with tubular defects that may progress slowly. Individuals with gout who actually develop a chronic nephropathy commonly have evidence of increased exposure to lead, sometimes by way of drinking "moonshine" whiskey contaminated with lead.
- The third renal syndrome in hyperuricemia is *nephrolithiasis*; uric acid stones are present in 22% of individuals with gout and 42% of those with secondary hyperuricemia (see later discussion of renal stones).

Hypercalcemia and Nephrocalcinosis

Disorders associated with hypercalcemia, such as hyperparathyroidism, multiple myeloma, vitamin D intoxication, metastatic cancer, or excess calcium intake (milk-alkali syndrome), may induce the formation of calcium stones and deposition of calcium in the kidney (nephrocalcinosis). Extensive degrees of calcinosis, under certain conditions, may lead to chronic tubulointerstitial disease and renal insufficiency. The earliest damage induced by the hypercalcemia is to the tubular epithelial cells in the form of mitochondrial distortion and other signs of cell injury. Subsequently, calcium deposits appear within the mitochondria, cytoplasm, and basement membrane. Calcified cellular debris may obstruct tubular lumens and cause obstructive atrophy of nephrons and secondary interstitial fibrosis and inflammation. Atrophy of entire cortical areas drained by calcified tubules may occur, accounting for the alternating areas of normal and scarred parenchyma seen in such kidneys.

The earliest functional defect is an inability to concentrate the urine. Other tubular defects, such as tubular acidosis and salt-losing nephritis, may also occur. With further damage, a slowly progressive renal insufficiency develops. This is usually due to nephrocalcinosis, but many of these patients also have calcium stones and secondary pyelonephritis.

Acute Phosphate Nephropathy

Extensive accumulations of calcium phosphate crystals in tubules can occur in patients consuming high doses of oral

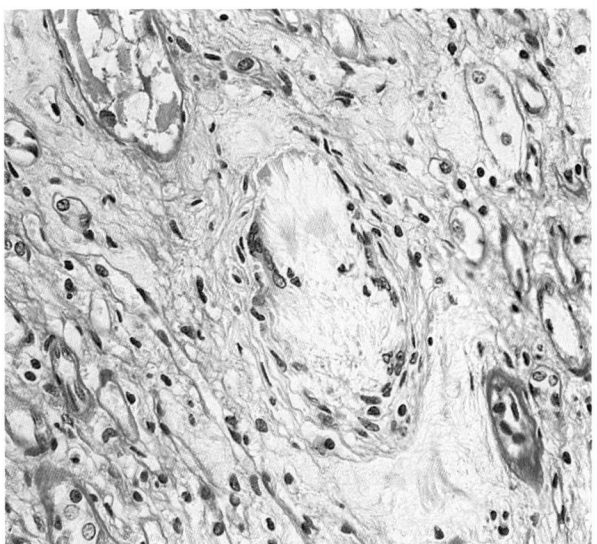

FIGURE 20–36 Urate crystals in the renal medulla. Note the giant cells and fibrosis around the crystals.

TABLE 20–10   Renal Disease Related to Nonrenal Neoplasms
Direct tumor invasion of renal parenchyma Ureters (obstruction) Artery (renovascular hypertension)
Hypercalcemia
Hyperuricemia
Amyloidosis (AL, light-chain type)
Excretion of abnormal proteins (multiple myeloma)
Glomerulopathies Membranous nephropathy, secondary (carcinomas) Minimal-change disease (Hodgkin's disease) Membranoproliferative glomerulonephritis (leukemias and lymphomas) Monoclonal immunoglobin/light-chain deposition disease (multiple myeloma)
Effects of radiation therapy, chemotherapy, secondary infection

phosphate solutions in preparation for colonoscopy.[72] These patients are not hypercalcemic, but excess phosphate load, perhaps complicated by dehydration, causes marked precipitation of calcium phosphate, typically presenting as renal insufficiency several weeks after the exposure. Patients typically only partially recover renal function.

Light-Chain Cast Nephropathy ("Myeloma Kidney")

Nonrenal malignant tumors, particularly those of hematopoietic origin, affect the kidneys in several ways (Table 20–10). The most common involvements are tubulointerstitial, caused by complications of the tumor (hypercalcemia, hyperuricemia, obstruction of ureters) or therapy (irradiation, hyperuricemia, chemotherapy, infections in immunosuppressed patients). As the survival rate of persons with malignant neoplasms increases, so do these renal complications. We limit the discussion here to the tubulointerstitial lesions in *multiple myeloma* that sometimes dominate the clinical picture in people with this disease.

Overt renal insufficiency occurs in half of those with multiple myeloma and related lymphoplasmacytic disorders. Several factors contribute to renal damage:

- *Bence Jones proteinuria and cast nephropathy.* The main cause of renal dysfunction is related to Bence Jones (light-chain) proteinuria. Renal failure correlates well with the presence and amount of such proteinuria and is uncommon in its absence. Two mechanisms seem to account for the renal toxicity of Bence Jones proteins. First, some light chains are directly toxic to epithelial cells, apparently because of their intrinsic physicochemical properties. Second, Bence Jones proteins combine with the urinary glycoprotein (Tamm-Horsfall protein) under acidic conditions to form large, histologically distinct tubular casts that obstruct the tubular lumens and induce a characteristic inflammatory reaction around the casts (light-chain cast nephropathy).

- *Amyloidosis,* of AL type formed from free light chains (usually of λ type), which occurs in 6% to 24% of individuals with myeloma.

- *Light-chain deposition disease.* In some patients, light chains (usually of κ type) deposit in GBMs and mesangium in nonfibrillar forms, causing a glomerulopathy (described earlier), or in tubular basement membranes, which may cause tubulointerstitial nephritis.

- *Hypercalcemia and hyperuricemia* are often present in these patients.

Morphology. The tubulointerstitial changes in light-chain cast nephropathy are fairly characteristic. The Bence Jones tubular casts appear as pink to blue amorphous masses, sometimes concentrically laminated and often fractured, which fill and distend the tubular lumens. Some of the casts are surrounded by multinucleate giant cells that are derived from mononuclear phagocytes (Fig. 20–37). The adjacent interstitial tissue usually shows a nonspecific inflammatory response and fibrosis. On occasion, the casts erode their way from the tubules into the interstitium and here evoke a granulomatous inflammatory reaction. Amyloidosis, light-chain deposition disease, nephrocalcinosis, and infection may also be present.

Clinical Features. Clinically, the renal manifestations are of several types. In the most common form, *chronic renal failure* develops insidiously and usually progresses slowly during a period of several months to years. Another form occurs suddenly and is manifested by *acute renal failure* with oliguria. Precipitating factors in these patients include dehydration, hypercalcemia, acute infection, and treatment with nephrotoxic antibiotics. *Bence Jones proteinuria* occurs in 70% of individuals with multiple myeloma; the presence of significant non–light-chain proteinuria (e.g., albuminuria) suggests AL amyloidosis or light-chain deposition disease.

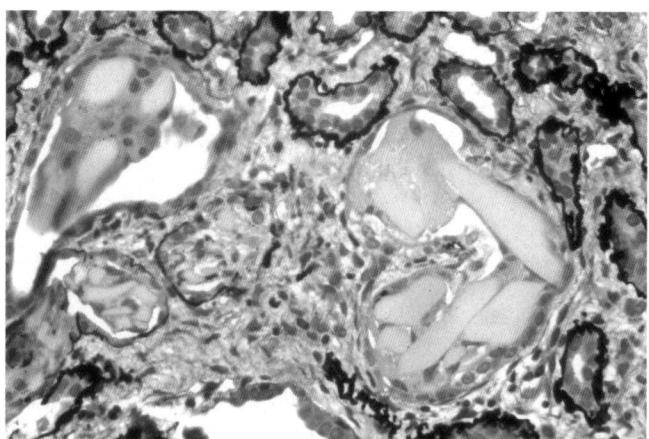

FIGURE 20–37   Light-chain cast nephropathy. Note the angulated and tubular casts, surrounded by macrophages, including multinucleate cells.

Vascular Diseases

Nearly all diseases of the kidney involve the renal blood vessels secondarily. Systemic vascular diseases, such as various forms of vasculitis, also affect renal vessels, and their effects on the kidney are often clinically important. Hypertension, as we discussed in Chapter 11, is intimately linked with the kidney, because kidney disease can be both the cause and consequence of increased blood pressure.[73] In this chapter we discuss benign and malignant nephrosclerosis and renal artery stenosis, lesions associated with hypertension, and sundry lesions involving mostly smaller vessels of the kidney.

BENIGN NEPHROSCLEROSIS

Benign nephrosclerosis is the term used for the renal pathology associated with sclerosis of renal arterioles and small arteries. The resultant effect is focal ischemia of parenchyma supplied by vessels with thickened walls and consequent narrowed lumens. The parenchymal effects include glomerulosclerosis and chronic tubulointersititial injury, producing a reduction in functional renal mass. Nephrosclerosis at autopsy is associated with increasing age, more frequent in blacks than whites, and may be seen in the absence of hypertension.[74,75] Hypertension and diabetes mellitus, however, increase the incidence and severity of the lesions.

Pathogenesis. Two processes participate in the arterial lesions:

- Medial and intimal thickening, as a response to hemodynamic changes, aging, genetic defects, or some combination of these
- Hyaline deposition in arterioles, caused partly by extravasation of plasma proteins through injured endothelium and partly by increased deposition of basement membrane matrix

Morphology. The kidneys are either normal or moderately reduced in size, with average weights between 110 and 130 gm. The cortical surfaces have a fine, even granularity that resembles grain leather (Fig. 20–38). The loss of mass is due mainly to cortical scarring and shrinking.

On histologic examination there is narrowing of the lumens of arterioles and small arteries, caused by thickening and hyalinization of the walls **(hyaline arteriolosclerosis)** (Fig. 20–39). Corresponding to the fine surface granulations are microscopic subcapsular scars with sclerotic glomeruli and tubular dropout, alternating with better preserved parenchyma. In addition, the interlobular and arcuate arteries show a characteristic lesion that consists of medial hypertrophy, reduplication of the elastic lamina, and increased myofibroblastic tissue in the intima, which combine to narrow the lumen. This change, called fibroelastic hyperplasia, often accompanies hyaline arteriolosclerosis and increases in severity with age and in the presence of hypertension.

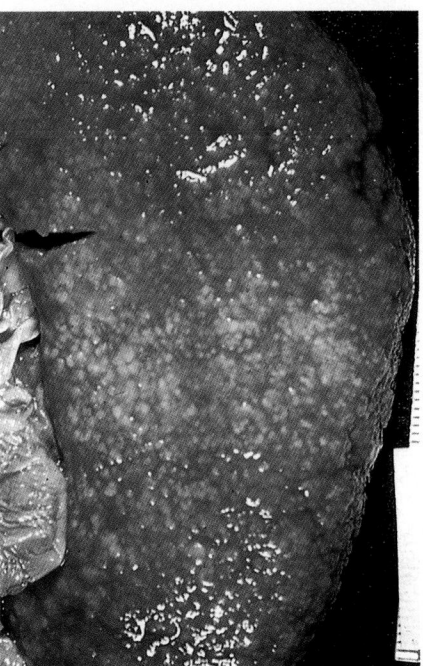

FIGURE 20–38 Close-up of the gross appearance of the cortical surface in benign nephrosclerosis illustrating the fine, leathery granularity of the surface.

Consequent to the vascular narrowing, there is patchy ischemic atrophy, which consists of (1) foci of tubular atrophy and interstitial fibrosis and (2) a variety of glomerular alterations. The latter include collapse of the GBM, deposition of collagen within the Bowman space, periglomerular fibrosis, and total sclerosis of glomeruli. When the ischemic changes are pronounced and affect large areas of parenchyma, they can produce regional scars and histologic alterations that may resemble those seen in renal ablation injury, mentioned earlier.

Clinical Features. It is unusual for uncomplicated benign nephrosclerosis to cause renal insufficiency or uremia. There are usually moderate reductions in renal blood flow, but the GFR is normal or only slightly reduced. On occasion, there is mild proteinuria. However, three groups of hypertensive patients with benign nephrosclerosis are at increased risk of developing renal failure: people of African descent, people with more severe blood pressure elevations, and persons with a second underlying disease, especially diabetes. In these groups renal insufficiency may supervene after prolonged benign hypertension, but more rapid renal failure results from the development of the malignant or accelerated phase of hypertension, discussed next.

MALIGNANT HYPERTENSION AND ACCELERATED NEPHROSCLEROSIS

Malignant nephrosclerosis is the form of renal disease associated with the malignant or accelerated phase of hypertension.[76] This dramatic pattern of hypertension may occasionally develop in previously normotensive individuals but often is superimposed

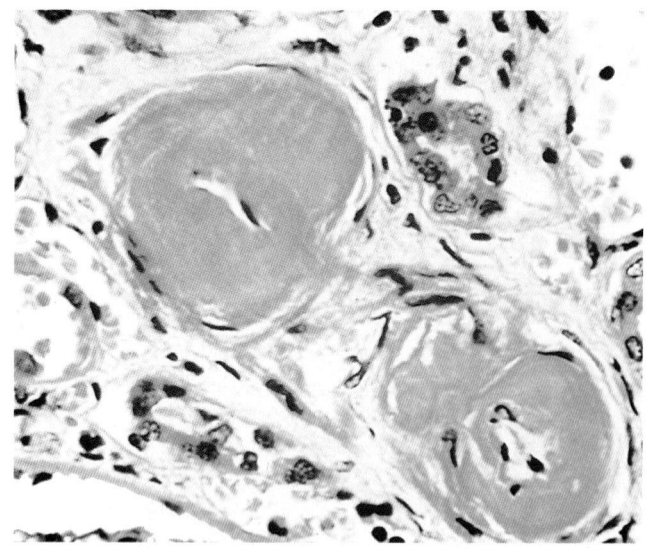

FIGURE 20–39 Hyaline arteriolosclerosis. High-power view of two arterioles with hyaline deposition, marked thickening of the walls, and a narrowed lumen. (Courtesy of Dr. M.A. Venkatachalam, Department of Pathology, University of Texas Health Sciences Center, San Antonio, TX.)

increased permeability of the small vessels to fibrinogen and other plasma proteins, endothelial injury, focal death of cells of the vascular wall, and platelet deposition. This leads to the appearance of *fibrinoid necrosis* of arterioles and small arteries, swelling of the vascular intima, and intravascular thrombosis. Mitogenic factors from platelets (e.g., PDGF), plasma, and other cells cause hyperplasia of intimal smooth muscle of vessels, resulting in the hyperplastic arteriolosclerosis that is typical of malignant hypertension and further narrowing of the lumens. The kidneys become markedly ischemic. With severe involvement of the renal afferent arterioles, the renin-angiotensin system receives a powerful stimulus; indeed, *patients with malignant hypertension have markedly elevated levels of plasma renin*. This sets up a self-perpetuating cycle in which angiotensin II causes intrarenal vasoconstriction, and the attendant renal ischemia perpetuates renin secretion. Other vasoconstrictors (e.g., endothelin) and loss of vasodilators (nitric oxide) may also contribute to vasoconstriction. Aldosterone levels are also elevated, and salt retention undoubtedly contributes to the elevation of blood pressure. The consequences of the markedly elevated blood pressure on the blood vessels throughout the body are known as *malignant arteriosclerosis*, and the renal disorder is malignant nephrosclerosis.

on preexisting essential benign hypertension, secondary forms of hypertension, or an underlying chronic renal disease, particularly glomerulonephritis or reflux nephropathy (Chapter 11). It is also a frequent cause of death from uremia in individuals with scleroderma. Malignant hypertension is relatively uncommon, occurring in 1% to 5% of all people with elevated blood pressure. In its pure form it usually affects younger individuals, and occurs more often in men and in blacks.

Pathogenesis. The basis for this turn for the worse in hypertensive subjects is unclear, but the following sequence of events is suggested. The initial insult seems to be some form of vascular damage to the kidneys. This might result from long-standing benign hypertension, with eventual injury to the arteriolar walls, or the initiating injury may spring de novo from arteritis, a coagulopathy, or some injury causing acute exacerbation of the hypertension. In any case, the result is

Morphology. On gross inspection the kidney size depends on the duration and severity of the hypertensive disease. Small, pinpoint petechial hemorrhages may appear on the cortical surface from rupture of arterioles or glomerular capillaries, giving the kidney a peculiar "flea-bitten" appearance.

Two histologic alterations characterize blood vessels in malignant hypertension (Fig. 20–40):

- **Fibrinoid necrosis of arterioles.** This appears as an eosinophilic granular change in the blood vessel wall, which stains positively for fibrin by histochemical or immunofluorescence techniques. This change represents an acute event; it may be accompanied by limited inflammatory infiltrate within the

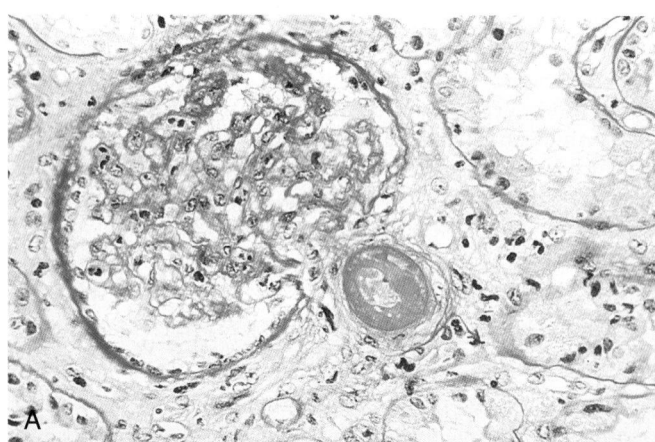
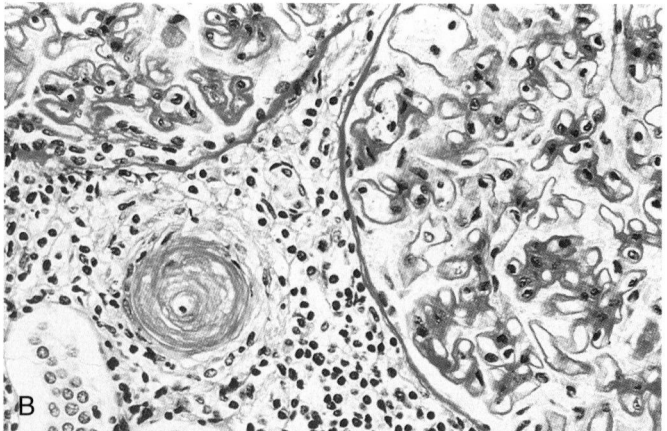

FIGURE 20–40 Malignant hypertension. **A,** Fibrinoid necrosis of afferent arteriole (PAS stain). **B,** Hyperplastic arteriolitis (onion-skin lesion). (Courtesy of Dr. H. Rennke, Brigham and Women's Hospital, Boston, MA.)

wall, but prominent inflammation is not seen. Sometimes the glomeruli become necrotic and infiltrated with neutrophils, and the glomerular capillaries may thrombose.

- In the interlobular arteries and arterioles, there is intimal thickening caused by a proliferation of elongated, concentrically arranged smooth muscle cells, together with fine concentric layering of collagen and accumulation of pale-staining material that probably represents accumulations of proteoglycans and plasma proteins. This alteration has been referred to as **onion-skinning** because of its concentric appearance. The lesion, also called hyperplastic arteriolitis, correlates well with renal failure in malignant hypertension. There may be superimposed intraluminal thrombosis. The arteriolar and arterial lesions result in considerable narrowing of all vascular lumens, ischemic atrophy and, at times, infarction distal to the abnormal vessels.

Clinical Features. The full-blown syndrome of malignant hypertension is characterized by systolic pressures greater than 200 mm Hg and diastolic pressures greater than 120 mm Hg, papilledema, retinal hemorrhages, encephalopathy, cardiovascular abnormalities, and renal failure. Most often, the early symptoms are related to increased intracranial pressure and include headaches, nausea, vomiting, and visual impairments, particularly scotomas or spots before the eyes. "Hypertensive crises" are sometimes encountered, characterized by episodes of loss of consciousness or even convulsions. At the onset of rapidly mounting blood pressure, there is marked proteinuria and microscopic or sometimes macroscopic hematuria but no significant alteration in renal function. Soon, however, renal failure makes its appearance. The syndrome is a true medical emergency requiring the institution of aggressive and prompt antihypertensive therapy to prevent the development of irreversible renal lesions. Before the introduction of current antihypertensive drugs, malignant hypertension was associated with a 50% mortality rate within 3 months of onset, progressing to 90% within a year. At present, however, about 75% of patients survive 5 years, and 50% survive with restoration of pre-crisis renal function.

RENAL ARTERY STENOSIS

Unilateral renal artery stenosis is a relatively uncommon cause of hypertension, responsible for 2% to 5% of cases, but is important because it represents a potentially curable form of hypertension with surgical treatment. Furthermore, important insights into renal mechanisms of hypertension came from studies of experimental and human renal artery stenosis.

Pathogenesis. The classic experiments of Goldblatt and colleagues[78] showed that constriction of one renal artery in dogs results in hypertension and that the magnitude of the effect is roughly proportional to the amount of constriction. Later experiments in rats confirmed these results, and in time it was shown that the hypertensive effect, at least initially, is due to stimulation of renin secretion by cells of the juxtaglomerular apparatus and the subsequent production of the

vasoconstrictor angiotensin II. *A large proportion of individuals with renovascular hypertension have elevated plasma or renal vein renin levels*, and almost all show a reduction of blood pressure when given drugs that block the activity of angiotensin II. Furthermore, unilateral renal renin hypersecretion can be normalized after renal revascularization, usually resulting in a decrease in blood pressure. Other factors, however, may contribute to the maintenance of renovascular hypertension after the renin-angiotensin system has initiated it, including *sodium retention* and possibly endothelin and loss of nitric oxide.

Morphology. The most common cause of renal artery stenosis (70% of cases) is occlusion by an atheromatous plaque at the origin of the renal artery. This lesion occurs more frequently in men, and the incidence increases with advancing age and diabetes mellitus. The plaque is usually concentrically placed, and superimposed thrombosis often occurs.

The second type of lesion leading to stenosis is so-called **fibromuscular dysplasia** of the renal artery. This is a heterogeneous group of lesions characterized by fibrous or fibromuscular thickening and may involve the intima, the media, or the adventitia of the artery. These lesions are thus subclassified into intimal, medial, and adventitial hyperplasia, the medial type being by far the most common (Fig. 20–41). The stenoses, as a whole, are more common in women and tend to occur in younger age groups (i.e., in the third and fourth decades). The lesions may consist of a single well-defined constriction or a series of narrowings, usually in the middle or distal portion of the renal artery. They may also involve the segmental branches and may be bilateral.

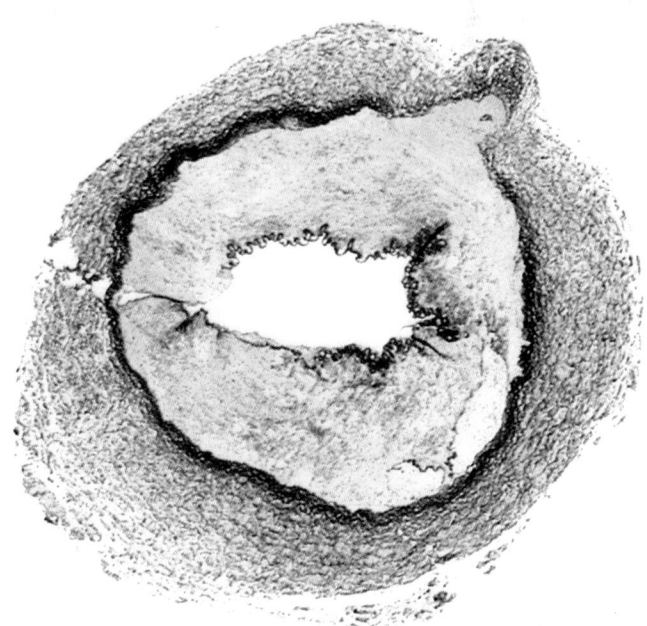

FIGURE 20–41 Fibromuscular dysplasia of the renal artery, medial type (elastic tissue stain). The media shows marked fibrous thickening, and the lumen is stenotic. (Courtesy of Dr. Seymour Rosen, Beth Israel Hospital, Boston, MA.)

The ischemic kidney is usually reduced in size and shows signs of diffuse ischemic atrophy, with crowded glomeruli, atrophic tubules, interstitial fibrosis, and focal inflammatory infiltrates. The arterioles in the ischemic kidney are usually protected from the effects of high pressure, thus showing only mild arteriolosclerosis. In contrast, the contralateral nonischemic kidney may show more severe arteriolosclerosis, depending on the severity of the hypertension.

Clinical Course. Few distinctive features suggest the presence of renal artery stenosis, and in general, these patients resemble those with essential hypertension. On occasion, a bruit can be heard on auscultation of the affected kidneys. Elevated plasma or renal vein renin, response to angiotensin-converting enzyme inhibitor, renal scans, and intravenous pyelography may aid with diagnosis, but arteriography is required to localize the stenotic lesion. The cure rate after surgery is 70% to 80% in well-selected cases.

THROMBOTIC MICROANGIOPATHIES

As was described in Chapter 14, *this group of disorders is characterized clinically by microangiopathic hemolytic anemia, thrombocytopenia, and (in many cases) renal failure, and morphologically by thrombotic lesions in capillaries and arterioles in various tissue beds, including those of the kidney* (Fig. 20–42).[79,80] Schistocytes (fragmented red cells) in peripheral blood smears provide an important clue to the diagnosis. Unlike DIC, these disorders are generally associated with normal coagulation times and normal or only slightly elevated fibrin split products.

The classification of these disorders has been muddied by the fact that the two main forms, hemolytic-uremic syndrome (HUS) and thrombotic thrombocytopenic purpura (TTP), show considerable overlap in their clinical features.[80,81] However, it is now evident that the category of HUS/TTP includes several entities with distinct causes, natural histories, and therapeutic approaches. We will thus classify these disorders according to our current understanding of their causes or associations, as follows:

1. *Typical HUS (synonyms: epidemic, classic, diarrhea-positive)*, most frequently associated with consumption of food contaminated by bacteria producing Shiga-like toxins
2. *Atypical HUS (synonyms: non-epidemic, diarrhea-negative)*, associated with:
   a. Inherited mutations of complement-regulatory proteins
   b. Diverse acquired causes of endothelial injury, including: antiphospholipid antibodies; complications of pregnancy and oral contraceptives; vascular renal diseases such as scleroderma and hypertension; chemotherapeutic and immunosuppressive drugs; and radiation
3. *TTP*, which is often associated with inherited or acquired deficiencies of ADAMTS13, a plasma metalloprotease that regulates the function of von Willebrand factor (vWF)

Pathogenesis. Within the thrombotic microangiopathies, two pathogenetic triggers dominate: (1) *endothelial injury*,

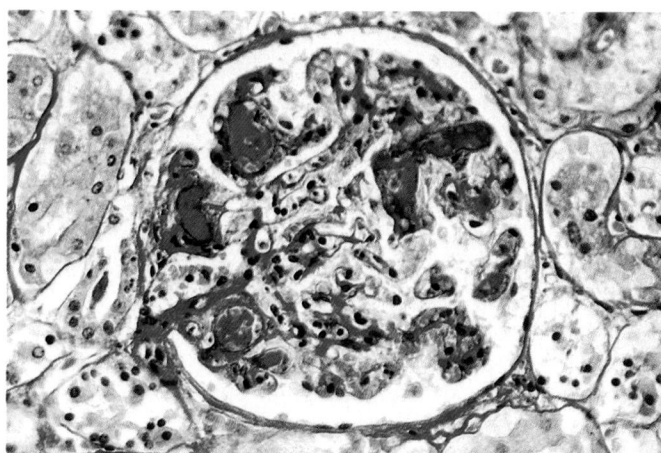

FIGURE 20–42   Fibrin stain showing platelet-fibrin thrombi (*red*) in the glomerular capillaries, characteristic of thrombotic microangiopathic disorders.

and (2) *platelet activation and aggregation*. As will be discussed, endothelial injury appears to be the primary cause of HUS, whereas platelet activation may be the inciting event in TTP.

Endothelial Injury. In typical (epidemic, classic, diarrhea-positive) HUS, the trigger for endothelial injury and activation is usually a Shiga-like toxin, while in inherited forms of atypical HUS the cause of the endothelial injury appears to be excessive, inappropriate activation of complement. Many other exposures and conditions can occasionally precipitate a HUS-like picture, presumably also by injuring the endothelium. The endothelial injury in HUS appears to cause platelet activation and thrombosis within microvascular beds. There is evidence that reduced endothelial production of prostaglandin I$_2$ and NO (both inhibitors of platelet aggregation) contributes to thrombosis. The reduction in these two factors and increased production of endothelium-derived endothelin may also promote vasoconstriction, exacerbating the hypoperfusion of tissues. Finally, adhesion molecules expressed on injured endothelium result in the recruitment of leukocytes, which may also contribute to thrombosis, as described in Chapter 4.

Platelet Aggregation. In contrast to HUS, in TTP the initiating event appears to be platelet aggregation induced by very large multimers of vWF, which accumulate due to a deficiency of ADAMTS13, a plasma protease that cleaves vWF multimers into smaller sizes. The deficiency of ADAMTS13 is most often caused by autoantibodies that inhibit ADAMTS13 function. Less commonly, a chronic relapsing and remitting form of TTP is associated with inherited deficiencies of ADAMTS13. Very large vWF multimers can bind platelet surface glycoproteins and activate platelets spontaneously, providing a pathophysiologic explanation for the microthrombi that are observed in vascular beds.[80,82]

Regardless of the trigger, tissue dysfunction in all forms of HUS/TTP appears to result from the formation of microthrombi, *vascular obstruction*, and tissue ischemia.[80] We will first describe the various subtypes of HUS/TTP, and then return to the morphologic features that are common to all.

Typical (epidemic, classic, diarrhea-positive) Hemolytic-Uremic Syndrome. This is the best-characterized form of

HUS. Most cases occur following intestinal infection with strains of *E. coli* (the most common being O157:H7) that produce Shiga-like toxins,[83] so-called because they resemble those made by *Shigella dysenteriae* (Chapter 17). Epidemics have been traced to various sources, most commonly the ingestion of contaminated ground meat (as in hamburgers), but also drinking water, raw milk, and person-to-person transmission. However, most cases of typical HUS caused by *E. coli* are sporadic. Less commonly, infections by other agents, including *Shigella dysenteriae*, can give rise to a similar clinical picture.

Typical HUS can occur in adults, particularly the elderly, but it affects children preferentially, in whom it is one of the main causes of acute renal failure. Following a prodrome of influenza-like or diarrheal symptoms, there is a *sudden onset of bleeding manifestations (especially hematemesis and melena), severe oliguria, and hematuria, associated with microangiopathic hemolytic anemia, thrombocytopenia, and (in some patients) prominent neurologic changes.* Hypertension is present in about half the patients.

Shiga-like toxin injures endothelial cells, inducing increased expression of leukocyte adhesion molecules; increased endothelin and decreased nitric oxide production; and in the presence of cytokines such as TNF, endothelial apoptosis. These alterations lead to platelet activation and induce vasoconstriction, resulting in the characteristic microangiopathy. There is also some evidence that Shiga-like toxins bind and directly activate platelets.

In typical HUS, if the renal failure is managed properly with dialysis, most patients recover normal renal function in a matter of weeks. However, due to underlying renal damage the long-term (15 to 25 year) outlook is more guarded. In one study, only 10 of 25 patients with prior epidemic HUS had normal renal function, and 7 had chronic kidney disease.

Atypical (non-epidemic, diarrhea-negative) Hemolytic-Uremic Syndrome. Atypical HUS occurs mainly in adults in a number of different settings. More than half of those affected have an inherited deficiency of complement-regulatory proteins, most commonly factor H, which normally breaks down the alternative pathway C3 convertase and protects cells from damage by uncontrolled complement activation (Chapter 2).[82] A small number of patients have mutations in two other proteins that regulate complement, complement factor I and CD46 (membrane cofactor protein). Patients with genetic mutations in complement-regulatory proteins may develop HUS at any age. Roughly half of affected individuals have a course marked by multiple relapses and progression to end-stage renal disease. As the deficiencies in complement-regulatory factors are life-long, it is a mystery why the onset of HUS is delayed; additional unknown co-factors that trigger the development of HUS are suspected.

A variety of miscellaneous conditions or exposures are occasionally associated with atypical forms of HUS. These include:

1. The *antiphospholipid syndrome*, either primary or secondary to SLE (lupus anticoagulant). The syndrome is described in detail in Chapter 4. In this setting the microangiopathy tends to follow a chronic course.
2. Complications of pregnancy or the postpartum period. So-called *postpartum renal failure* is a form of HUS that usually

occurs after an uneventful pregnancy, 1 day to several months after delivery. The condition has a grave prognosis, although recovery can occur in milder cases.
3. *Vascular diseases affecting the kidney*, such as systemic sclerosis and malignant hypertension.
4. Chemotherapeutic and immunosuppressive drugs, such as mitomycin, cyclosporine, cisplatin, and gemcitabine.
5. Irradiation of the kidney.

Patients with atypical HUS do not fare as well as those with typical HUS, in large part because the underlying conditions may be chronic and difficult to treat.[80] As in typical HUS, some patients have neurologic symptoms; the disease in these patients can be distinguished from TTP by the presence of normal ADAMTS13 levels in the plasma (see below).

Thrombotic Thrombocytopenic Purpura. TTP is classically manifested by the pentad of fever, neurologic symptoms, microangiopathic hemolytic anemia, thrombocytopenia, and renal failure.[80] As discussed above, it is usually caused by antibodies (either autoimmune or drug-induced) or genetic defects that lead to functional deficits in ADAMTS13.[82] The most common cause of deficient ADAMTS13 activity is inhibitory autoantibodies, and the majority of those with such antibodies are women. Regardless of cause, most patients present as adults at ages younger than 40.

In TTP, central nervous system involvement is the dominant feature, whereas renal involvement occurs in only about 50% of patients. The clinical findings are dictated by the distribution of the microthrombi, which are found in arterioles throughout the body. Untreated, the disease was once highly fatal, but in those with autoantibodies exchange transfusions and immunosuppressive therapy have reduced the mortality to less than 50%. As in HUS associated with inherited deficiencies of complement regulatory proteins, it is not understood why those with life-long genetic deficiency of ADAMTS13 present in adulthood. Such patients tend to follow a relapsing and remitting course.

Morphology. The morphological findings in the various forms of HUS/TTP show considerable overlap, and vary mainly according to chronicity rather than cause. In acute, active disease the kidney may show patchy or diffuse cortical necrosis (described later) and subcapsular petechiae. On microscopic examination, the glomerular capillaries are occluded by thrombi composed of aggregated platelets and to a lesser extent fibrin. The capillary walls are thickened due to endothelial cell swelling and subendothelial deposits of cell debris and fibrin. Disruption of the mesangial matrix and damage to the mesangial cells often results in mesangiolysis. Interlobular arteries and arterioles often show fibrinoid necrosis of the wall and occlusive thrombi. Chronic disease is confined to patients with atypical HUS or TTP, and has features that stem from continued injury and attempts at healing. The renal cortex reveals various degrees of scarring. By light microscopy the glomeruli are mildly hypercellular and have marked thickening of the capillary walls associated with splitting or reduplication of the basement membrane (so called double contours or tram tracks). The walls of arteries and arterioles often exhibit increased layers of cells and connective tissue ("onion-skinning") that narrow the vessel lumens. These changes lead to persistent hypoperfusion and ischemic atrophy of the parenchyma, which manifests clinically as renal failure and hypertension.

OTHER VASCULAR DISORDERS

Atherosclerotic Ischemic Renal Disease

We have seen that atherosclerotic unilateral renal artery stenosis can lead to hypertension. *Bilateral renal artery disease,* usually diagnosed definitively by arteriography, now seems to be a fairly common cause of chronic ischemia with renal insufficiency in older individuals, sometimes in the absence of hypertension.[84,85] The importance of recognizing this condition is that surgical revascularization is beneficial in reversing further decline in renal function.

Atheroembolic Renal Disease

Embolization of fragments of atheromatous plaques from the aorta or renal artery into intraparenchymal renal vessels occurs in elderly patients with severe atherosclerosis, especially after surgery on the abdominal aorta, aortography, or intra-aortic cannulization. These emboli can be recognized in the lumens and walls of arcuate and interlobular arteries by their content of cholesterol crystals, which appear as rhomboid clefts (Fig. 20–43). The clinical consequences of atheroemboli vary according to the number of emboli and the preexisting state of renal function. Frequently they have no functional significance. However, acute renal failure may develop in elderly patients in whom renal function is already compromised, principally after abdominal surgery on atherosclerotic aneurysms.

Sickle-Cell Disease Nephropathy

Sickle-cell disease (homozygous) or trait (heterozygous) may lead to a variety of alterations in renal morphology and func-

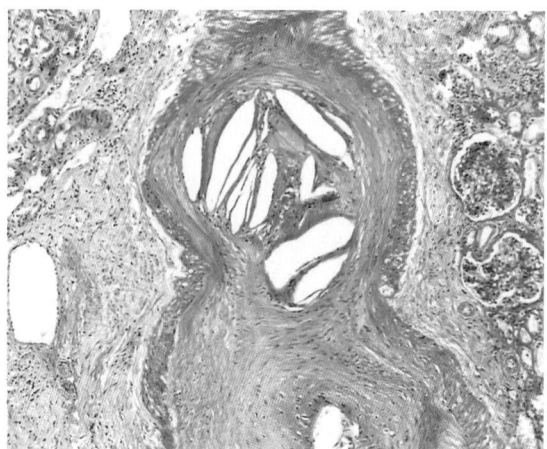

FIGURE 20–43 Atheroemboli with typical cholesterol clefts in an interlobar artery.

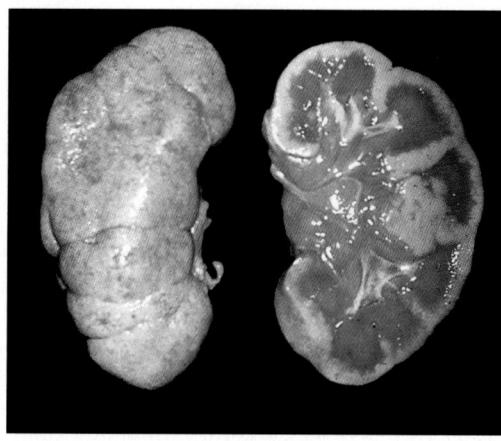

FIGURE 20–44 Diffuse cortical necrosis. The pale ischemic necrotic areas are confined to the cortex and columns of Bertin.

tion, some of which produce clinically significant abnormalities. The various manifestations are termed *sickle-cell nephropathy*.

The most common clinical and functional abnormalities are *hematuria* and a *diminished concentrating ability* (hyposthenuria). These are thought to be due largely to accelerated sickling in the hypertonic hypoxic milieu of the renal medulla; the hyperosmolarity dehydrates red cells and increases intracellular HbS concentrations, which likely explains why even those with sickle trait are affected. Patchy *papillary necrosis* may occur in both homozygotes and heterozygotes; this is sometimes associated with cortical scarring. *Proteinuria* is also common in sickle-cell disease, occurring in about 30% of patients. It is usually mild to moderate, but on occasion the overt nephrotic syndrome arises, associated with sclerosing glomerular lesions.

Diffuse Cortical Necrosis

This is an uncommon condition that occurs most frequently after an obstetric emergency, such as abruptio placentae (premature separation of the placenta), septic shock, or extensive surgery. When bilateral and symmetric, it is fatal in the absence of supportive therapy. The cortical destruction has the features of ischemic necrosis. Glomerular and arteriolar microthrombi are found in most cases, and clearly contribute to the necrosis and renal damage. The morphologic features have considerable overlap with thrombotic microangiopathy and disseminated intravascular coagulation, but the pathogenetic sequence of events in this injury remains obscure.

Morphology. The gross alterations of massive ischemic necrosis are sharply limited to the cortex (Fig. 20–44). The histologic appearance is that of acute ischemic infarction. The lesions may be patchy, with areas of coagulative necrosis and apparently better preserved cortex. Intravascular and intraglomerular thromboses may be prominent but are usually focal, and acute necroses of small arterioles and capillaries may occasionally be present. Hemorrhages occur into the glomeruli, together with the formation of fibrin plugs in the glomerular capillaries.

Massive acute cortical necrosis is of grave significance, since it gives rise to sudden anuria, terminating rapidly in uremic death. Instances of unilateral or patchy involvement are compatible with survival.

Renal Infarcts

The kidneys are favored sites for the development of infarcts. Contributing to this predisposition is the extensive blood flow to the kidneys (one fourth of the cardiac output), but probably more important is the "end-organ" nature of the arterial blood supply and the extremely limited collateral circulation from extrarenal sites (essentially small blood vessels penetrating from the renal capsule). Although thrombosis in advanced atherosclerosis and the acute vasculitis of polyarteritis nodosa may occlude arteries, most infarcts are due to embolism. A major source of such emboli is mural thrombosis in the left atrium and ventricle as a result of myocardial infarction. Vegetative endocarditis, aortic aneurysms, and aortic atherosclerosis are less frequent sources of emboli.

> **Morphology.** Because of the end-organ type of arterial supply, most renal infarcts are of the "white" anemic variety. They may be solitary lesions or may be multiple and bilateral. Within 24 hours infarcts become sharply demarcated, pale, yellow-white areas that may contain small irregular foci of hemorrhagic discoloration. They are usually ringed by a zone of intense hyperemia.
>
> On section the infarcts are wedge-shaped, with the base against the cortical surface and the apex pointing toward the medulla. There may be a narrow rim of preserved subcortical tissue that has been spared by the collateral capsular circulation. In time these acute areas of ischemic necrosis undergo progressive fibrous scarring, giving rise to depressed, pale, gray-white scars that assume a V-shape on section. The histologic changes in renal infarction are those of ischemic coagulative necrosis, described in Chapter 1.

Many renal infarcts are clinically silent. Sometimes, pain with tenderness localized to the costovertebral angle occurs, associated with showers of red cells in the urine. Large infarcts of one kidney are probably associated with narrowing of the renal artery or one of its major branches, which in turn may be a cause of hypertension.

Congenital Anomalies

About 10% of all people are born with potentially significant malformations of the urinary system. Renal dysplasias and hypoplasias account for 20% of chronic renal failure in children.

Congenital renal disease can be hereditary but is most often the result of an acquired developmental defect that arises during gestation. As was discussed in Chapter 10, defects in genes involved in development, including the Wilms tumor–associated genes, cause urogenital anomalies. As a rule, developmental abnormalities involve structural components of the kidney and urinary tract, causing syndromes termed CAKUT (congenital abnormalities of the kidney and urinary tract). However, genetic abnormalities also cause enzymatic or metabolic defects in tubular transport, such as cystinuria and renal tubular acidosis. Here, we restrict the discussion to structural anomalies involving primarily the kidney. All except horseshoe kidney are uncommon. Anomalies of the lower urinary tract are discussed in Chapter 21.

Agenesis of the Kidney. Bilateral agenesis, which is incompatible with life, is usually encountered in stillborn infants. It is often associated with many other congenital disorders (e.g., limb defects, hypoplastic lungs) and leads to early death. Unilateral agenesis is an uncommon anomaly that is compatible with normal life if no other abnormalities exist. The opposite kidney is usually enlarged as a result of compensatory hypertrophy. Some patients eventually develop progressive glomerular sclerosis in the remaining kidney as a result of the adaptive changes in hypertrophied nephrons, discussed earlier in the chapter, and in time, chronic kidney disease ensues.

Hypoplasia. Renal hypoplasia refers to failure of the kidneys to develop to a normal size. This anomaly may occur bilaterally, resulting in renal failure in early childhood, but it is more commonly encountered as a unilateral defect. True renal hypoplasia is extremely rare; most cases reported probably represent acquired scarring due to vascular, infectious, or other parenchymal diseases rather than an underlying developmental failure. Differentiation between congenital and acquired atrophic kidneys may be impossible, but *a truly hypoplastic kidney shows no scars and has a reduced number of renal lobes and pyramids*, usually six or fewer. In one form of hypoplastic kidney, *oligomeganephronia*, the kidney is small with fewer nephrons that are markedly hypertrophied.

Ectopic Kidneys. The development of the definitive metanephros may occur in ectopic foci, usually at abnormally low levels. These kidneys lie either just above the pelvic brim or sometimes within the pelvis. They are usually normal or slightly small in size but otherwise are not remarkable. Because of their abnormal position, kinking or tortuosity of the ureters may cause some obstruction to urinary flow, which predisposes to bacterial infections.

Horseshoe Kidneys. Fusion of the upper or lower poles of the kidneys produces a horseshoe-shaped structure that is continuous across the midline anterior to the great vessels. This anatomic anomaly is common and is found in about 1 in 500 to 1000 autopsies. Ninety percent of such kidneys are fused at the lower pole, and 10% are fused at the upper pole.

MULTICYSTIC RENAL DYSPLASIA

This sporadic disorder is due to an abnormality in metanephric differentiation *characterized histologically by the persistence in the kidney of abnormal structures—cartilage, undifferentiated mesenchyme, and immature collecting ductules—and by abnormal lobar organization.* Most cases are associated with ureteropelvic obstruction, ureteral agenesis or atresia, and other anomalies of the lower urinary tract.

Dysplasia can be unilateral or bilateral and is almost always cystic. The kidney is usually enlarged, extremely irregular, and multicystic (Fig. 20–45A). The cysts vary in size from microscopic structures to some that are several centimeters in diameter. On histologic examination, they are lined by flattened epithelium. Although normal nephrons are present, many have immature collecting ducts. The characteristic histologic

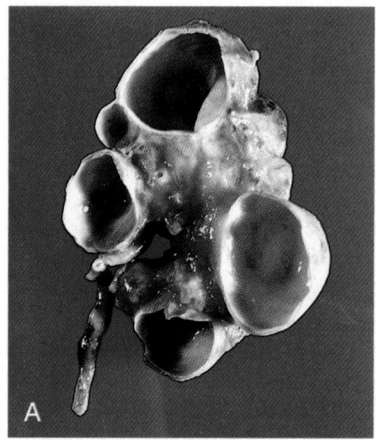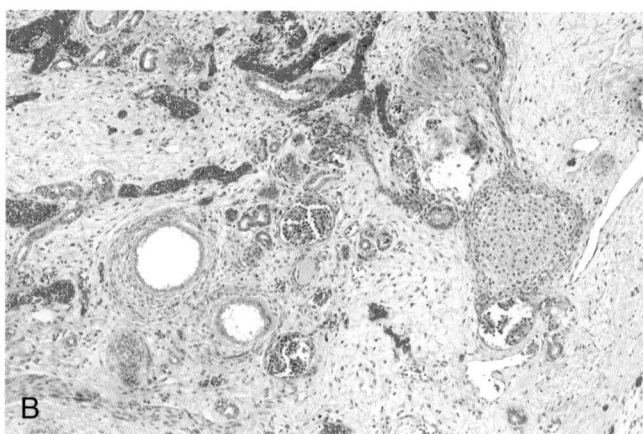

FIGURE 20–45 Multicystic renal dysplasia. **A,** Gross appearance. **B,** Histologic section showing disorganized architecture, dilated tubules with cuffs of primitive stroma, and an island of cartilage (H & E stain). (**A,** Courtesy of Dr. D. Schofield, Children's Hospital, Los Angeles, CA; **B,** courtesy of Dr. Laura Finn, Children's Hospital, Seattle, WA.)

feature is the *presence of islands of undifferentiated mesenchyme, often with cartilage, and immature collecting ducts* (Fig. 20–45B).

When unilateral, the dysplasia is discovered by the appearance of a flank mass that leads to surgical exploration and nephrectomy. The function of the opposite kidney is normal, and such patients have an excellent prognosis after surgical removal of the affected kidney. In bilateral multicystic renal dysplasia, renal failure may ultimately result.

Cystic Diseases of the Kidney

Cystic diseases of the kidney are heterogeneous, comprising hereditary, developmental, and acquired disorders. As a group, they are important for several reasons: (1) They are reasonably common and often represent diagnostic problems for clinicians, radiologists, and pathologists; (2) some forms, such as adult polycystic kidney disease, are major causes of chronic kidney disease; and (3) they can occasionally be confused with malignant tumors. A useful classification of renal cysts is as follows:[86]

1. Multicystic renal dysplasia
2. Polycystic kidney disease
   a. Autosomal-dominant (adult) polycystic disease
   b. Autosomal-recessive (childhood) polycystic disease
3. Medullary cystic disease
   a. Medullary sponge kidney
   b. Nephronophthisis
4. Acquired (dialysis-associated) cystic disease
5. Localized (simple) renal cysts
6. Renal cysts in hereditary malformation syndromes (e.g., tuberous sclerosis)
7. Glomerulocystic disease
8. Extraparenchymal renal cysts (pyelocalyceal cysts, hilar lymphangitic cysts)

Only the more important of the cystic diseases are discussed below. Table 20–11 summarizes the characteristic features of the principal renal cystic diseases.

AUTOSOMAL-DOMINANT (ADULT) POLYCYSTIC KIDNEY DISEASE

Autosomal-dominant (adult) polycystic kidney disease (ADPKD) is a hereditary disorder characterized by multiple expanding cysts of both kidneys that ultimately destroy the renal parenchyma and cause renal failure.[87] It is a common condition affecting roughly 1 of every 400 to 1000 live births and accounting for about 5% to 10% of cases of chronic renal failure requiring transplantation or dialysis. The pattern of inheritance is autosomal dominant, with high penetrance. Despite the autosomal dominant inheritance, as will be described later, the manifestation of the disease requires mutation of both alleles of either PKD gene. The disease is universally bilateral; reported unilateral cases probably represent multicystic dysplasia. The cysts initially involve only portions of the nephrons, so renal function is retained until about the fourth or fifth decade of life. ADPKD is genetically heterogeneous. Family studies show that the disease is caused by mutations in genes located on chromosome 16p13.3 (*PKD1*) and 4q21 (*PKD2*), and rare unlinked families point toward the presence of at least one additional disease-associated gene. Mutations of *PKD1* account for about 85% of cases (most of the remainder involving *PKD2*) and are associated with a more severe disease, end-stage renal disease or death occurring at an average age of 53 years as compared with 69 years for *PKD2*.[88] For *PKD1* mutations, the likelihood of developing renal failure is less than 5% by 40 years of age, rising to more than 35% by 50 years, more than 70% at 60 years of age, and more than 95% by 70 years of age.[89] Corresponding figures for *PKD2* are less than 5% at 50 years of age, about 15% at 60 years of age, and about 45% at 70 years of age.[87,90] Although the major pathologic process is in the kidneys, adult polycystic kidney disease is a systemic disorder in which cysts and other anomalies also arise in other organs (discussed later).

Genetics and Pathogenesis. A wide range of different mutations in *PKD1* and *PKD2* has been described, and this allelic heterogeneity has complicated genetic diagnosis of this disorder.

- The *PKD1* gene encodes a large (460-kD) integral membrane protein named *polycystin-1*, which has a large extra-

TABLE 20–11 Summary of Renal Cystic Diseases

	Inheritance	Pathologic Features	Clinical Features or Complications	Typical Outcome	Diagrammatic Representation
Adult polycystic kidney disease	Autosomal dominant	Large multicystic kidneys, liver cysts, berry aneurysms	Hematuria, flank pain, urinary tract infection, renal stones, hypertension	Chronic renal failure beginning at age 40–60 years	
Childhood polycystic kidney disease	Autosomal recessive	Enlarged, cystic kidneys at birth	Hepatic fibrosis	Variable, death in infancy or childhood	
Medullary sponge kidney	None	Medullary cysts on excretory urography	Hematuria, urinary tract infection, recurrent renal stones	Benign	
Familial juvenile nephronophthisis	Autosomal recessive	Corticomedullary cysts, shrunken kidneys	Salt wasting, polyuria, growth retardation, anemia	Progressive renal failure beginning in childhood	
Adult-onset medullary cystic disease	Autosomal dominant	Corticomedullary cysts, shrunken kidneys	Salt wasting, polyuria	Chronic renal failure beginning in adulthood	
Simple cysts	None	Single or multiple cysts in normal-sized kidneys	Microscopic hematuria	Benign	
Acquired renal cystic disease	None	Cystic degeneration in end-stage kidney disease	Hemorrhage, erythrocytosis, neoplasia	Dependence on dialysis	

cellular region, multiple transmembrane domains, and a short cytoplasmic tail.[90] It has been localized to tubular epithelial cells, particularly those of the distal nephron. At present its precise function is not known, but it contains domains that are usually involved in cell-cell and cell-matrix interactions.

- The *PKD2* gene product *polycystin-2* is an integral membrane protein.[90] It has been localized to all segments of the renal tubules and is also expressed in many extrarenal tissues. Polycystin-2 functions as a Ca2+-permeable cation channel, and a basic defect in ADPKD is a disruption in the regulation of intracellular Ca2+ levels.

The pathogenesis of polycystic disease is not established, but the hypothesis that is currently favored places the cilia-centrosome complex of tubular epithelial cells at the center of the disorder (Fig. 20–46).[91–93] The epithelial cells of the kidney each contain a single nonmotile primary cilium, a 2–3 μm long hairlike organelle that projects into the tubular lumen from the apical surface of tubular cells. The cilium is made up of microtubules, and arises from and is attached to a basal body derived from the centriole. The cilia are part of a system of organelles and cellular structures that sense mechanical signals. It is believed that the apical cilia function in the kidney tubule as a mechanosensor to monitor changes in fluid flow and shear stress, while intercellular junctional complexes monitor forces between cells, and focal adhesions sense attachment to extracellular matrices. In response to external signals, these sensors regulate ion flux (cilia can

induce Ca2+ flux in cultured kidney epithelial cells) and cellular behavior, including cell polarity and proliferation. The hypothesis that defects in mechanosensing, Ca2+ flux, and signal transduction underlie cyst formation is supported several observations.

- Both polycystin-1 and polycystin-2 are localized to the primary cilium.[91,93] Other genes that are mutated in cystic diseases (such as the *NPHP* genes described below) encode proteins that are also localized to cilia and/or basal bodies.
- Knockout of the PKD1 gene in one model organism (the worm *C. elegans*) results in ciliary abnormalities and cyst formation.[92]
- Tubular cells obtained from mice with a deletion of the *PKD1* gene (which causes embryonic lethality in this species) have normal cilia architecture but not the flow-induced Ca2+ flux that occurs in normal tubular cells.[92]

Polycystin-1 and polycystin-2 may form a protein complex that acts to regulate intracellular Ca2+ in response to fluid flow, perhaps because fluid moving through the kidney tubules causes ciliary bending that opens Ca2+ channels.[91,93] Mutation of either of the *PKD* genes would lead to loss of the polycystin complex or the formation of an aberrant complex. The consequent disruption of normal polycystin activity then leads to changes in intracellular Ca2+ level and, given the second-messenger effects of Ca2+, to changes in *cellular proliferation, basal levels of apoptosis, interactions with the ECM, and*

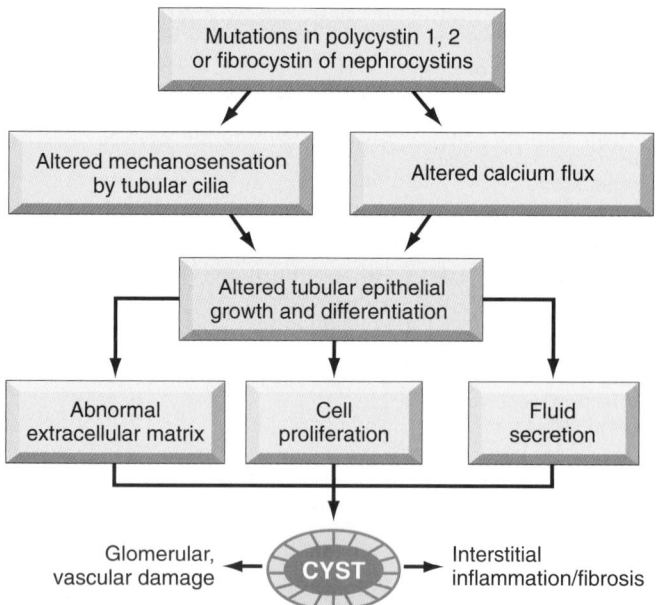

FIGURE 20-46 Possible mechanisms of cyst formation in polycystic kidney disease (see text).

secretory function of the epithelia that together result in the characteristic feature of ADPKD. The interaction of *PKD1* and *PKD2* gene products probably accounts for the similar phenotype in the disease induced by mutations in either of the two genes.[91] The increase in the number of cells caused by abnormal proliferation, and the expanding volume of intraluminal fluid caused by abnormal secretion from epithelial cells lining the cysts, result in progressive cyst enlargement. In addition, cyst fluids have been shown to harbor mediators, derived from epithelial cells, that enhance fluid secretion and induce inflammation. These abnormalities contribute to further enlargement of cysts and the interstitial fibrosis characteristic of progressive polycystic kidney disease.

Morphology. In gross appearance, the kidneys are usually bilaterally enlarged and may achieve enormous sizes; weights as high as 4 kg for each kidney have been reported. The external surface appears to be composed solely of a mass of cysts, up to 3 to 4 cm in diameter, with no intervening parenchyma (Fig. 20–47A and B). However, microscopic examination reveals functioning nephrons dispersed between the cysts. The cysts may be filled with a clear, serous fluid or, more usually, with turbid, red to brown, sometimes hemorrhagic fluid. As these cysts enlarge, they may encroach on the calyces and pelvis to produce pressure defects. The cysts arise from the tubules throughout the nephron and therefore have variable lining epithelia. On occasion, papillary epithelial formations and polyps project into the lumen. Bowman capsules are occasionally involved in cyst formation, and glomerular tufts may be seen within the cystic space.

Clinical Features. Many of these patients remain asymptomatic until renal insufficiency announces the presence of the disease. In others, hemorrhage or progressive dilation of cysts may produce pain. Excretion of blood clots causes renal colic. The enlarged kidneys, usually apparent on abdominal palpation, may induce a dragging sensation. The disease occasionally begins with the insidious onset of hematuria, followed by other features of progressive chronic kidney disease, such as proteinuria (rarely more than 2 gm/day), polyuria, and hypertension. Patients with *PKD2* mutations tend to have an older age at onset and later development of renal failure. Both genetic and environmental factors influence disease severity.

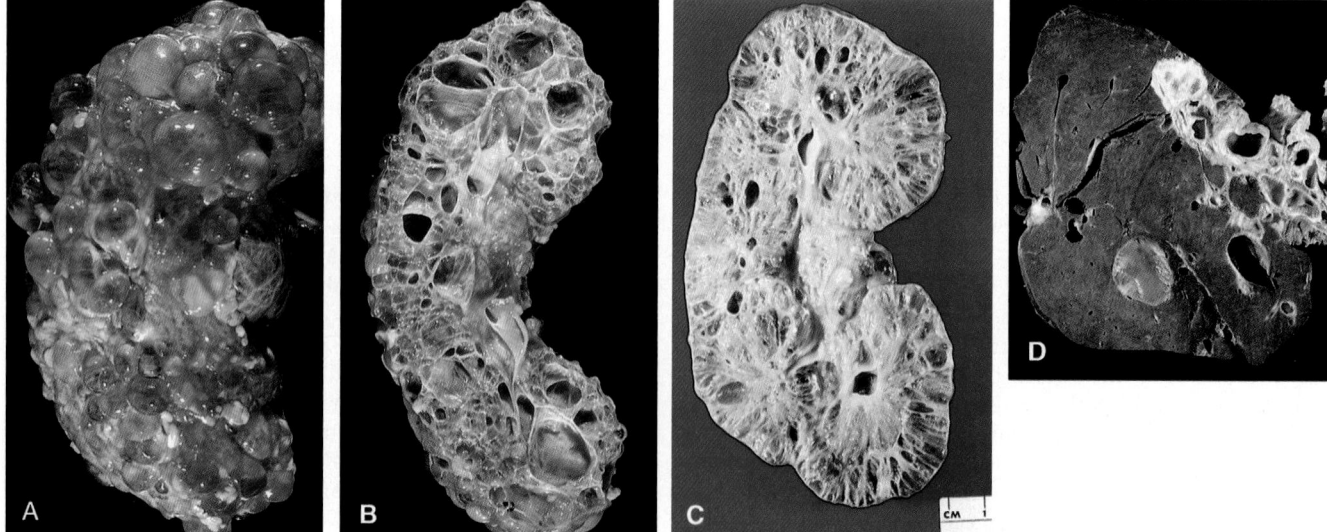

FIGURE 20-47 **A** and **B,** Autosomal-dominant adult polycystic kidney disease (ADPKD) viewed from the external surface and bisected. The kidney is markedly enlarged and contains numerous dilated cysts. **C,** Autosomal-recessive childhood PKD, showing smaller cysts and dilated channels at right angles to the cortical surface. **D,** Liver cysts in adult PKD.

Progression is accelerated in blacks (largely correlated with sickle-cell trait), in males, and in the presence of hypertension.

Individuals with polycystic kidney disease also tend to have extrarenal congenital anomalies.[87] *About 40% have one to several cysts in the liver (polycystic liver disease) that are usually asymptomatic.* The cysts are derived from biliary epithelium. Cysts occur much less frequently in the spleen, pancreas, and lungs. Intracranial berry aneurysms, presumably from altered expression of polycystin in vascular smooth muscle, arise in the circle of Willis, and subarachnoid hemorrhages from these account for death in about 4% to 10% of individuals. *Mitral valve prolapse* and other cardiac valvular anomalies occur in 20% to 25% of patients, but most are asymptomatic. The clinical diagnosis is made by radiologic imaging techniques.

This form of chronic renal failure is remarkable in that patients may survive for many years with azotemia slowly progressing to uremia. Ultimately, about 40% of adult patients die of coronary or hypertensive heart disease, 25% of infection, 15% of a ruptured berry aneurysm or hypertensive intracerebral hemorrhage, and the rest of other causes.

AUTOSOMAL-RECESSIVE (CHILDHOOD) POLYCYSTIC KIDNEY DISEASE

Autosomal-recessive (childhood) polycystic kidney disease (ARPKD) is genetically distinct from adult polycystic kidney disease. *Perinatal, neonatal, infantile,* and *juvenile* subcategories have been defined, depending on the time of presentation and presence of associated hepatic lesions. The first two are the most common; serious manifestations are usually present at birth, and the young infant might succumb rapidly to renal failure.

In most cases, the disease is caused by mutations of the *PKHD1* gene, which maps to chromosome region 6p21–p23. The *PKHD1* gene encodes a large novel protein, *fibrocystin.*[94] The gene is highly expressed in adult and fetal kidney and also in liver and pancreas. Fibrocystin is a 447-kD integral membrane protein with a large extracellular region, a single transmembrane component, and a short cytoplasmic tail. The extracellular region contains multiple copies of a domain forming an Ig-like fold. Like polycystins 1 and 2, fibrocystin also has been localized to the primary cilium of tubular cells.[93] The function of fibrocystin is unknown, but its putative conformational structure indicates it may be a cell surface receptor with a role in collecting-duct and biliary differentiation.

Analysis of ARPKD patients has revealed a wide range of different mutations. The vast majority of cases are compound heterozygotes (i.e. inherit a different mutant allele from each of the two parents). This complicates molecular diagnosis of ARPKD.

Morphology. The kidneys are enlarged and have a smooth external appearance. On cut section, numerous small cysts in the cortex and medulla give the kidney a spongelike appearance. Dilated elongated channels are present at right angles to the cortical surface, completely replacing the medulla and cortex (Fig. 20–47C). On microscopic examination, there is cylindrical or, less commonly, saccular dilation of all collecting tubules. The cysts have a uniform lining of cuboidal cells, reflecting their origin from the collecting ducts. In almost all cases the liver has cysts associated with portal fibrosis (Fig. 20–47D) and proliferation of portal bile ducts.

Patients who survive infancy (infantile and juvenile forms) may develop a peculiar type of hepatic fibrosis characterized by bland periportal fibrosis and the proliferation of well-differentiated biliary ductules, a condition now termed *congenital hepatic fibrosis.* In older children the hepatic disease is the predominant clinical concern. Such patients may develop portal hypertension with splenomegaly. Curiously, congenital hepatic fibrosis sometimes occurs in the absence of polycystic kidneys and has been reported occasionally in the presence of adult polycystic kidney disease.

CYSTIC DISEASES OF RENAL MEDULLA

The three major types of medullary cystic disease are *medullary sponge kidney,* a relatively common and usually innocuous structural change, and *nephronophthisis and adult-onset medullary cystic disease,* which are almost always associated with renal dysfunction.

Medullary Sponge Kidney

The term medullary sponge kidney should be restricted to lesions consisting of multiple cystic dilations of the collecting ducts in the medulla. The condition occurs in adults and is usually discovered radiographically, either as an incidental finding or sometimes in relation to secondary complications. The latter include calcifications within the dilated ducts, hematuria, infection, and urinary calculi. Renal function is usually normal. On gross inspection the papillary ducts in the medulla are dilated, and small cysts may be present. The cysts are lined by cuboidal epithelium or occasionally by transitional epithelium. Unless there is superimposed pyelonephritis, cortical scarring is absent. The pathogenesis is unknown.

Nephronophthisis and Adult-Onset Medullary Cystic Disease

This is a group of progressive renal disorders. The common characteristic is the presence of a variable number of *cysts in the medulla, usually concentrated at the corticomedullary junction.* Initial injury probably involves the distal tubules with tubular basement membrane disruption, followed by chronic and progressive tubular atrophy involving both medulla and cortex and interstitial fibrosis. Although the presence of medullary cysts is important, the *cortical tubulointerstitial damage is the cause of the eventual renal insufficiency.*

Three variants of the nephronophthisis disease complex are recognized: (1) sporadic, nonfamilial; (2) familial juvenile nephronophthisis (most common); and (3) renal-retinal dysplasia (15%) in which the kidney disease is accompanied by ocular lesions. The familial forms are inherited as autosomal recessive traits and usually become manifest in childhood or adolescence. As a group, the nephronophthisis complex is now thought to be the most common genetic cause of end-stage

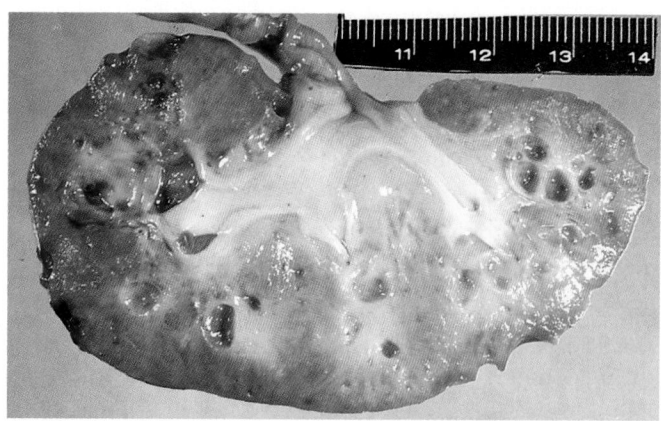

FIGURE 20–48 Medullary cystic disease. Cut section of kidney showing cysts at the corticomedullary junction and in the medulla.

renal disease in children and young adults. Adult-onset medullary cystic disease, at one time considered to be part of the nephronophthisis spectrum, has an autosomal dominant pattern of transmission and is now considered a distinct entity.

Affected children present first with polyuria and polydipsia, which reflect a marked defect in the concentrating ability of renal tubules. Sodium wasting and tubular acidosis are also prominent. Some variants of juvenile nephronophthisis can have extrarenal associations, including ocular motor abnormalities, retinal dystrophy, liver fibrosis, and cerebellar abnormalities. The expected course is progression to terminal renal failure during a period of 5 to 10 years.

Pathogenesis. At least seven responsible gene loci have been identified. Three genes, *NPH1*, *NPH2*, and *NPH3*, are mutated in the juvenile forms of nephronophthisis.[95] The protein products of NPH1 and NPH3–NPH6 have been identified (collectively called *nephrocystins*), but their functions are not yet known. As discussed earlier, these proteins are present in the primary cilia, basal bodies attached to these cilia, or the centrosome organelle from which the basal bodies originate. The NPHP2 gene product has been identified as *inversin*, which mediates left-right patterning during embryogenesis.[91] Two genes (*MCKD1* and *MCKD2*), with autosomal dominant transmission, have been identified as causing medullary cystic disease that is characterized by progression to end-stage kidney disease in adult life.[87]

Morphology. The kidneys are small, have contracted granular surfaces, and show cysts in the medulla, most prominently at the corticomedullary junction (Fig. 20–48). Small cysts are also seen in the cortex. The cysts are lined by flattened or cuboidal epithelium and are usually surrounded by either inflammatory cells or fibrous tissue. In the cortex there is widespread atrophy and thickening of the basement membranes of the proximal and distal tubules, together with interstitial fibrosis. Some glomeruli may be hyalinized, but in general, glomerular structure is preserved.

There are few specific clues to diagnosis, because the medullary cysts might be too small to be visualized radiographically.

The disease should be strongly considered in children or adolescents with otherwise unexplained chronic renal failure, a positive family history, and chronic tubulointerstitial nephritis on biopsy.

ACQUIRED (DIALYSIS-ASSOCIATED) CYSTIC DISEASE

The kidneys from patients with end-stage renal disease who have undergone prolonged dialysis sometimes show numerous cortical and medullary cysts. The cysts measure 0.5 to 2 cm in diameter, contain clear fluid, are lined by either hyperplastic or flattened tubular epithelium, and often contain calcium oxalate crystals. They probably form as a result of obstruction of tubules by interstitial fibrosis or by oxalate crystals.

Most are asymptomatic, but sometimes the cysts bleed, causing hematuria. The most ominous complication is the development of renal cell carcinoma in the walls of these cysts, occurring in 7% of dialyzed patients observed for 10 years.

SIMPLE CYSTS

These occur as multiple or single, usually cortical, cystic spaces that vary widely in diameter. They are commonly 1 to 5 cm but may reach 10 cm or more in size. They are translucent, lined by a gray, glistening, smooth membrane, and filled with clear fluid. On microscopic examination these membranes are composed of a single layer of cuboidal or flattened cuboidal epithelium, which in many instances may be completely atrophic.

Simple cysts are common postmortem findings without clinical significance. On occasion, hemorrhage into them may cause sudden distention and pain, and calcification of the hemorrhage may give rise to bizarre radiographic shadows. The main importance of cysts lies in their differentiation from kidney tumors when they are discovered either incidentally or because of hemorrhage and pain. Radiologic studies show that in contrast to renal tumors, renal cysts have smooth contours, are almost always avascular, and give fluid rather than solid signals on ultrasonography.

Urinary Tract Obstruction (Obstructive Uropathy)

Recognition of urinary obstruction is important because *obstruction increases susceptibility to infection and to stone formation, and unrelieved obstruction almost always leads to permanent renal atrophy,* termed *hydronephrosis* or *obstructive uropathy.* Fortunately, many causes of obstruction are surgically correctable or medically treatable.

Obstruction may be sudden or insidious, partial or complete, unilateral or bilateral; it may occur at any level of the urinary tract from the urethra to the renal pelvis. It can be caused by lesions that are *intrinsic* to the urinary tract or *extrinsic* lesions that compress the ureter.[96] The common causes are as follows (Fig. 20–49):

1. *Congenital anomalies:* posterior urethral valves and urethral strictures, meatal stenosis, bladder neck obstruction;

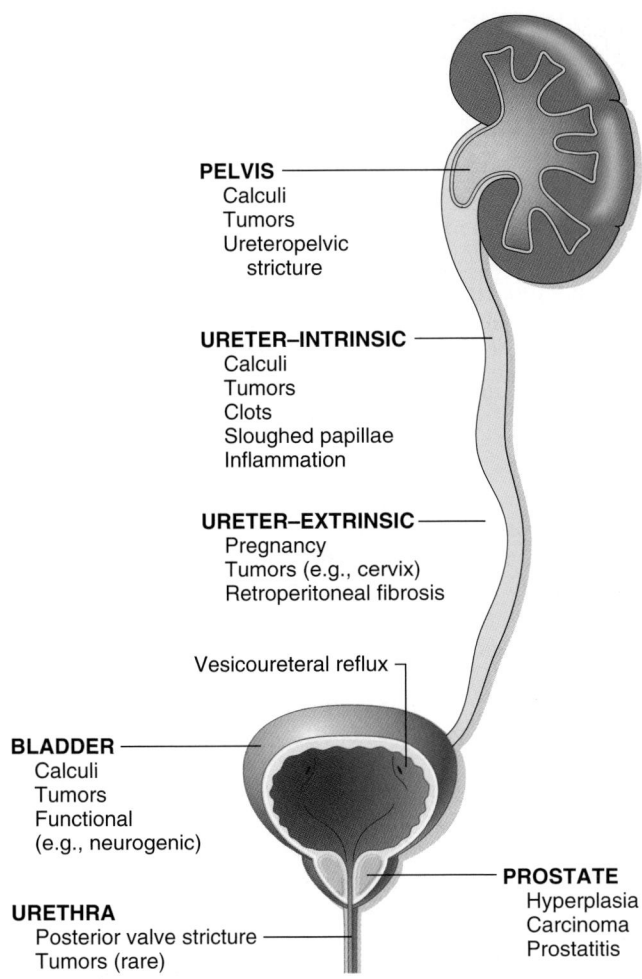

PELVIS
Calculi
Tumors
Ureteropelvic
    stricture

URETER–INTRINSIC
Calculi
Tumors
Clots
Sloughed papillae
Inflammation

URETER–EXTRINSIC
Pregnancy
Tumors (e.g., cervix)
Retroperitoneal fibrosis

Vesicoureteral reflux

BLADDER
Calculi
Tumors
Functional
(e.g., neurogenic)

URETHRA
Posterior valve stricture
Tumors (rare)

PROSTATE
Hyperplasia
Carcinoma
Prostatitis

FIGURE 20–49 Obstructive lesions of the urinary tract.

dilated, often markedly so. The high pressure in the pelvis is transmitted back through the collecting ducts into the cortex, causing renal atrophy, but it also compresses the renal vasculature of the medulla, causing a diminution in inner medullary blood flow. The medullary vascular defects are initially reversible, but lead to medullary functional disturbances. Accordingly, the initial functional alterations caused by obstruction are largely tubular, manifested primarily by impaired concentrating ability. Only later does the GFR begin to fall. *Obstruction also triggers an interstitial inflammatory reaction, leading eventually to interstitial fibrosis*, by mechanisms similar to those discussed earlier (see Fig. 20–9).

Morphology. When the obstruction is sudden and complete, glomerular filtration is reduced. It leads to mild dilation of the pelvis and calyces and sometimes to atrophy of the renal parenchyma. When the obstruction is subtotal or intermittent, glomerular filtration is not suppressed, and progressive dilation ensues. Depending on the level of urinary block, the dilation may affect the bladder first, or the ureter and then the kidney.

The kidney may be slightly to massively enlarged, depending on the degree and the duration of the obstruction. The earlier features are those of simple dilation of the pelvis and calyces, but in addition there is often significant interstitial inflammation, even in the absence of infection. In chronic cases the picture is one of cortical tubular atrophy with marked diffuse interstitial fibrosis. Progressive blunting of the apices of the pyramids occurs, and these eventually become cupped. In far-advanced cases the kidney may become transformed into a thin-walled cystic structure having a diameter of up to 15 to 20 cm (Fig. 20–50) with striking parenchymal atrophy, total obliteration of the pyramids, and thinning of the cortex.

ureteropelvic junction narrowing or obstruction; severe vesicoureteral reflux
2. *Urinary calculi*
3. *Benign prostatic hypertrophy*
4. *Tumors:* carcinoma of the prostate, bladder tumors, contiguous malignant disease (retroperitoneal lymphoma), carcinoma of the cervix or uterus
5. *Inflammation:* prostatitis, ureteritis, urethritis, retroperitoneal fibrosis
6. *Sloughed papillae or blood clots*
7. *Pregnancy*
8. *Uterine prolapse and cystocele*
9. *Functional disorders:* neurogenic (spinal cord damage or diabetic nephropathy) and other functional abnormalities of the ureter or bladder (often termed *dysfunctional obstruction*)

Hydronephrosis is the term used to describe dilation of the renal pelvis and calyces associated with progressive atrophy of the kidney due to obstruction to the outflow of urine. Even with complete obstruction, glomerular filtration persists for some time because the filtrate subsequently diffuses back into the renal interstitium and perirenal spaces, where it ultimately returns to the lymphatic and venous systems. Because of this continued filtration, the affected calyces and pelvis become

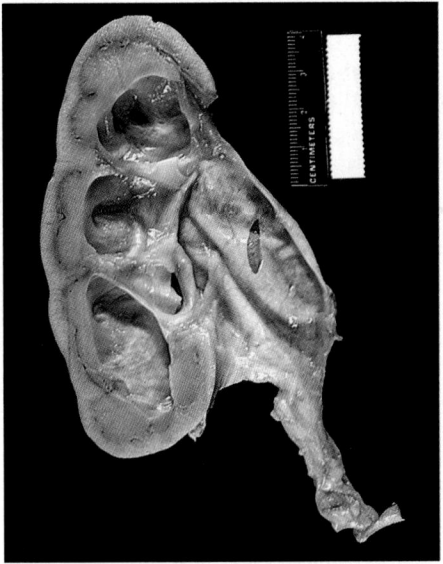

FIGURE 20–50 Hydronephrosis of the kidney, with marked dilation of the pelvis and calyces and thinning of the renal parenchyma.

Clinical Features. *Acute obstruction* may provoke pain attributed to distention of the collecting system or renal capsule. Most of the early symptoms are produced by the underlying cause of the hydronephrosis. Thus, calculi lodged in the ureters may give rise to renal colic, and prostatic enlargements may give rise to bladder symptoms.

Unilateral complete or partial hydronephrosis may remain silent for long periods, since the unaffected kidney can maintain adequate renal function. Sometimes its existence first becomes apparent in the course of intravenous pyelography. It is regrettable that this disease tends to remain asymptomatic, because in its early stages, perhaps the first few weeks, relief of obstruction leads to reversion to normal function. *Ultrasonography* is a useful noninvasive technique in the diagnosis of obstructive uropathy.

In *bilateral partial obstruction* the earliest manifestation is inability to concentrate the urine, reflected by polyuria and nocturia. Some patients have acquired distal tubular acidosis, renal salt wasting, secondary renal calculi, *and a typical picture of chronic tubulointerstitial nephritis* with scarring and atrophy of the papilla and medulla. Hypertension is common in such patients.

Complete bilateral obstruction results in oliguria or anuria and is incompatible with survival unless the obstruction is relieved. Curiously, after relief of complete urinary tract obstruction, postobstructive *diuresis* occurs. This can often be massive, with the kidney excreting large amounts of urine that is rich in sodium chloride.

Urolithiasis (Renal Calculi, Stones)

Stones may form at any level in the urinary tract, but most arise in the kidney. Urolithiasis is a frequent clinical problem, affecting 5% to 10% of Americans in their lifetime.[97] Men are affected more often than women, and the peak age at onset is between 20 and 30 years. Familial and hereditary predisposition to stone formation has long been known. Many inborn errors of metabolism, such as gout, cystinuria, and primary hyperoxaluria, provide examples of hereditary disease characterized by excessive production and excretion of stone-forming substances.

Cause and Pathogenesis. There are four main types of calculi[98] (Table 20–12): (1) *calcium stones (about 70%),* composed largely of calcium oxalate or calcium oxalate mixed with calcium phosphate; (2) another 15% are so-called *triple stones* or *struvite stones,* composed of magnesium ammonium phosphate; (3) 5% to 10% are *uric acid stones;* and (4) 1% to 2% are *made up of cystine.* An organic mucoprotein matrix, making up 1% to 5% of the stone by weight, is present in all calculi. Although there are many causes for the initiation and propagation of stones, *the most important determinant is an increased urinary concentration of the stones' constituents, such that it exceeds their solubility (supersaturation). A low urine volume* in some metabolically normal patients may also favor supersaturation.

Calcium oxalate stones (Table 20–12) are associated in about 5% of patients with *hypercalcemia* and *hypercalciuria,* such as occurs with hyperparathyroidism, diffuse bone disease, sarcoidosis, and other hypercalcemic states. About 55% have *hypercalciuria without hypercalcemia.* This is caused by several

TABLE 20–12	Prevalence of Various Types of Renal Stones	
Stone Type	**Percentage of All Stones**
CALCIUM OXALATE AND PHOSPHATE	70
Idiopathic hypercalciuria (50%) Hypercalciuria and hypercalcemia (10%) Heperoxaluria (5%) Enteric (4.5%) Primary (0.5%) Hyperuricosuria (20%) Hypocitraturia No known metabolic abnormality (15% to 20%)	
MAGNESIUM AMMONIUM PHOSPHATE (STRUVITE)	15–20
URIC ACID	5–10
Associated with hyperuricemia Associated with hyperuricosuria Idiopathic (50% of uric stones)	
CYSTINE	1–2
OTHERS OR UNKNOWN	±5

factors, including hyperabsorption of calcium from the intestine (absorptive hypercalciuria), an intrinsic impairment in renal tubular reabsorption of calcium (renal hypercalciuria), or idiopathic fasting hypercalciuria with normal parathyroid function. As many as 20% of calcium oxalate stones are associated with increased uric acid secretion *(hyperuricosuric calcium nephrolithiasis),* with or without hypercalciuria. The mechanism of stone formation in this setting involves "nucleation" of calcium oxalate by uric acid crystals in the collecting ducts. Five percent are associated with *hyperoxaluria,* either hereditary (primary oxaluria) or, more commonly, acquired by intestinal overabsorption in patients with enteric diseases. The latter, so-called enteric hyperoxaluria, also occurs in vegetarians, because much of their diet is rich in oxalates. *Hypocitraturia,* associated with acidosis and chronic diarrhea of unknown cause, may produce calcium stones. *In a variable proportion of individuals with calcium stones,* no cause can be found (idiopathic calcium stone disease).

Magnesium ammonium phosphate stones are formed largely after infections by bacteria (e.g., *Proteus* and some staphylococci) that convert urea to ammonia. The resultant alkaline urine causes the precipitation of magnesium ammonium phosphate salts. These form some of the largest stones, as the amounts of urea excreted normally are huge. Indeed, so-called *staghorn calculi* occupying large portions of the renal pelvis are almost always a consequence of infection.

Uric acid stones are common in individuals with hyperuricemia, such as gout, and diseases involving rapid cell turnover, such as the leukemias. However, *more than half of all patients with uric acid calculi have neither hyperuricemia nor increased urinary excretion of uric acid.* In this group, it is thought that an unexplained tendency to excrete urine of pH below 5.5 may predispose to uric acid stones, because uric acid is insoluble in acidic urine. In contrast to the radiopaque calcium stones, uric acid stones are radiolucent.

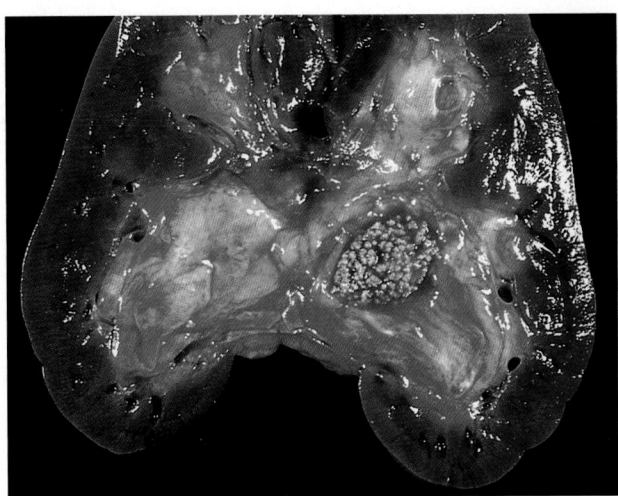

FIGURE 20–51 Nephrolithiasis. A large stone impacted in the renal pelvis. (Courtesy of Dr. E. Mosher, Brigham and Women's Hospital, Boston, MA.)

Cystine stones are caused by genetic defects in the renal reabsorption of amino acids, including cystine, leading to cystinuria. Stones form at low urinary pH.

It can therefore be appreciated that increased concentration of stone constituents, changes in urinary pH, decreased urine volume, and the presence of bacteria influence the formation of calculi. *However, many calculi occur in the absence of these factors; conversely, individuals with hypercalciuria, hyperoxaluria, and hyperuricosuria often do not form stones.* It has therefore been postulated that stone formation is enhanced by a *deficiency in inhibitors of crystal formation in urine.* The list of such inhibitors is long, including pyrophosphate, diphosphonate, citrate, glycosaminoglycans, osteopontin, and a glycoprotein called *nephrocalcin.*

Morphology. Stones are unilateral in about 80% of patients. The favored sites for their formation are within the renal calyces and pelves (Fig. 20–51) and in the bladder. If formed in the renal pelvis they tend to remain small, having an average diameter of 2 to 3 mm. These may have smooth contours or may take the form of an irregular, jagged mass of spicules. Often many stones are found within one kidney. On occasion, progressive accretion of salts leads to the development of branching structures known as staghorn calculi, which create a cast of the pelvic and calyceal system.

Clinical Features. Stones are of importance when they obstruct urinary flow or produce ulceration and bleeding. They may be present without producing any symptoms or they may cause significant renal damage. In general, smaller stones are most hazardous, because they may pass into the ureters, producing colic, one of the most intense forms of pain, and ureteral obstruction. Larger stones cannot enter the ureters and are more likely to remain silent within the renal pelvis. Commonly, these larger stones first manifest themselves by hematuria. Stones also predispose to superimposed

infection, both by their obstructive nature and by the trauma they produce.

Tumors of the Kidney

Both benign and malignant tumors occur in the kidney. With the exception of oncocytoma, the benign tumors rarely cause clinical problems. Malignant tumors on the other hand, are of great importance clinically and deserve considerable emphasis. By far the most common of these malignant tumors is renal cell carcinoma, followed by Wilms tumor, which is found in children and is described in Chapter 10, and finally urothelial tumors of the calyces and pelves.

BENIGN TUMORS

Renal Papillary Adenoma

Small, discrete adenomas arising from the renal tubular epithelium are found commonly (7% to 22%) at autopsy. They are most frequently papillary and are therefore called *papillary adenomas* in the most recent classifications.[99]

Morphology. These are small tumors, usually less than 0.5 cm in diameter. They are present invariably within the cortex and appear grossly as pale yellow-gray, discrete, well-circumscribed nodules. On microscopic examination, they are composed of complex, branching, papillomatous structures with numerous complex fronds. Cells may also grow as tubules, glands, cords, and sheets of cells. The cells are cuboidal to polygonal in shape and have regular, small central nuclei, scanty cytoplasm, and no atypia.

By histologic criteria, these tumors do not differ from low-grade papillary renal cell adenocarcinoma and indeed share some immunohistochemical and cytogenetic features (trisomies 7 and 17) with papillary cancers, to be discussed later. The size of the tumor is used as a prognostic feature, with a cutoff of 3 cm separating those that metastasize from those that rarely do.[99] However, because of occasional reports of small tumors that have metastasized, the current view is to regard all adenomas, regardless of size, as potentially malignant until an unequivocal marker of benignity is discovered.

Angiomyolipoma

This is a benign tumor consisting of vessels, smooth muscle, and fat. *Angiomyolipomas are present in 25% to 50% of patients with tuberous sclerosis,* a disease caused by loss-of-function mutations in the TSC1 or TSC2 tumor suppressor genes. It is characterized by lesions of the cerebral cortex that produce epilepsy and mental retardation, a variety of skin abnormalities, and unusual benign tumors at other sites, such as the heart (Chapters 12 and 28). The clinical importance of angiomyolipoma is due largely to their susceptibility to spontaneous hemorrhage.

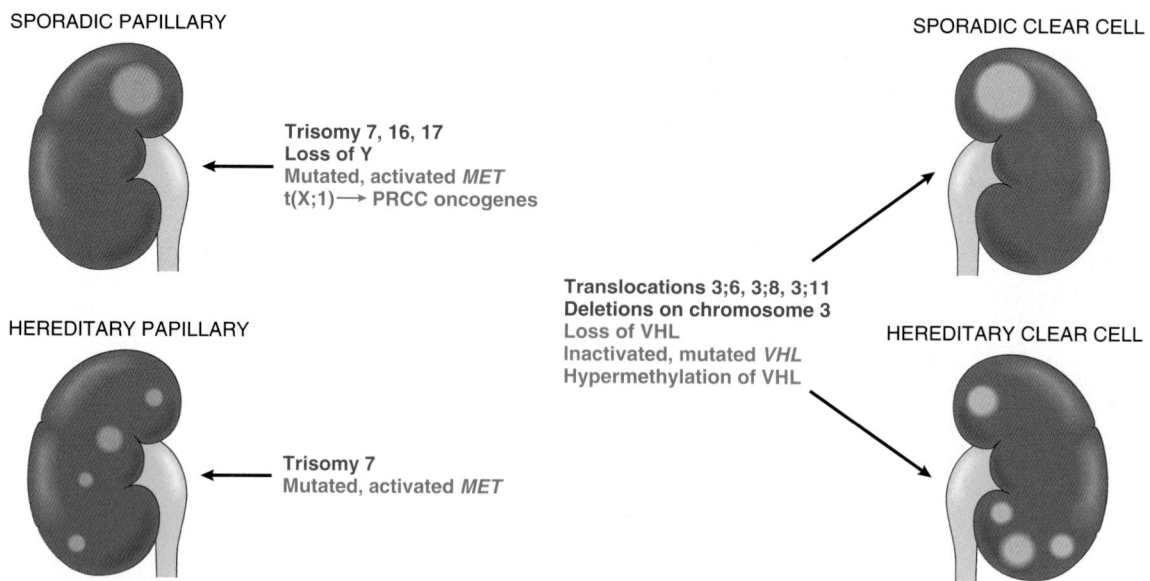

FIGURE 20–52 Cytogenetics (blue) and genetics (red) of clear cell versus papillary renal cell carcinoma. (Courtesy of Dr. Keith Ligon, Brigham and Women's Hospital, Boston, MA.)

Oncocytoma

This is an epithelial tumor composed of large eosinophilic cells having small, round, benign-appearing nuclei that have large nucleoli. It is thought to arise from the intercalated cells of collecting ducts. It is not an uncommon tumor, accounting for approximately 5% to 15% of surgically resected renal neoplasms. *Ultrastructurally the eosinophilic cells have numerous mitochondria.* In gross appearance the tumors are tan or mahogany brown, relatively homogeneous, and usually well encapsulated. However, they may achieve a large size (up to 12 cm in diameter). There are some familial cases in which these tumors are multicentric rather than solitary.

MALIGNANT TUMORS

Renal Cell Carcinoma (Adenocarcinoma of the Kidney)

Renal cell carcinomas represent about 3% of all newly diagnosed visceral cancers in the United States and account for 85% of renal cancers in adults. There are approximately 30,000 new cases per year and 12,000 deaths from the disease.[100] The tumors occur most often in older individuals, usually in the sixth and seventh decades of life, and show a 2:1 male preponderance. Because of their gross yellow color and the resemblance of the tumor cells to clear cells of the adrenal cortex, they were at one time called *hypernephroma.* It is now clear that all these tumors arise from tubular epithelium and are therefore renal adenocarcinomas.

Epidemiology. Tobacco is the most significant risk factor. Cigarette smokers have double the incidence of renal cell carcinoma, and pipe and cigar smokers are also more susceptible. An international study has identified additional risk factors, including obesity (particularly in women); hypertension; unopposed estrogen therapy; and exposure to asbestos, petro-

leum products, and heavy metals.[101,102] There is also an increased incidence in patients with chronic renal failure and acquired cystic disease (see earlier) and in tuberous sclerosis.

Most renal cancer is sporadic, but unusual forms of autosomal dominant familial cancers occur, usually in younger individuals. Although they account for only 4% of renal cancers, familial variants have been enormously instructive in studying renal carcinogenesis.

- *Von Hippel-Lindau (VHL) syndrome:* Half to two thirds of individuals with VHL (nearly all, if they live long enough) (Chapter 28) develop renal cysts and bilateral, often multiple, renal cell carcinomas. As we shall see, *current studies implicate the VHL gene in the development of both familial and sporadic clear cell tumors.*
- *Hereditary (familial) clear cell carcinoma,* without the other manifestations of VHL but with abnormalities involving the same or a related gene, is another familial variant.
- *Hereditary papillary carcinoma.* This autosomal dominant form is manifested by multiple bilateral tumors with papillary histology. These tumors show a series of cytogenetic abnormalities and, as will be described, mutations in the *MET* proto-oncogene.

Classification of renal cell carcinoma: histology, cytogenetics, and genetics. The classification of renal cell carcinoma is based on correlative cytogenetic, genetic, and histologic studies of both familial and sporadic tumors.[103,104] The major types of tumor are as follows (Fig. 20–52):

1. *Clear cell carcinoma.* This is the most common type, accounting for 70% to 80% of renal cell cancers. The tumors are made up of cells with clear or granular cytoplasm and are *nonpapillary.* They can be familial, but in most cases (95%) are sporadic. In 98% of these tumors,

whether familial, sporadic, or associated with VHL, there is loss of sequences on the short arm of chromosome 3. This occurs by deletion (3p–) or by unbalanced chromosomal translocation (3;6, 3;8, 3;11) resulting in loss of chromosome 3 spanning 3p12 to 3p26. This region harbors the *VHL* gene (3p25.3).[105] A second nondeleted allele of the *VHL* gene shows somatic mutations or hypermethylation-induced inactivation in up to 80% of clear cell cancers, indicating that the *VHL* gene acts as a tumor suppressor gene in both sporadic and familial cancers (Chapter 7).[106] The *VHL* gene encodes a protein that is part of a ubiquitin ligase complex involved in targeting other proteins for degradation.[106] Important among the targets of the VHL protein is hypoxia-inducible factor-1 (HIF-1). When *VHL* is mutated, HIF-1 levels remain high, and this constitutively active protein increases the transcription and production of hypoxia-inducible, pro-angiogenic proteins such as VEGF, PDGF, TGF-α, and TGF-β. In addition, insulin-like growth factor 1, another VHL target, is upregulated. Thus, both cell growth and angiogenesis are stimulated. At least two other tumor suppressor genes have also been mapped to 3p.[107]

2. *Papillary carcinoma* accounts for 10% to 15% of renal cancers. It is characterized by a papillary growth pattern and also occurs in both familial and sporadic forms. These tumors are not associated with 3p deletions. The most common cytogenetic abnormalities are trisomies 7, 16, and 17 and loss of Y in male patients in the sporadic form, and trisomy 7 in the familial form. The gene for the familial form has been mapped to a locus on chromosome 7, encompassing the locus for *MET*, a proto-oncogene that serves as the tyrosine kinase receptor for *hepatocyte growth factor*.[108] This gene has also been shown to be mutated in a proportion of the sporadic cases of papillary carcinoma. Described in Chapter 3, hepatocyte growth factor (also called scatter factor) mediates growth, cell mobility, invasion, and morphogenetic differentiation. Unlike clear cell carcinomas, papillary carcinomas are frequently multifocal in origin.

3. *Chromophobe renal carcinoma* represents 5% of renal cell cancers and is composed of cells with prominent cell membranes and pale eosinophilic cytoplasm, usually with a halo around the nucleus. On cytogenetic examination these tumors show multiple chromosome losses and extreme hypodiploidy. They are, like the benign oncocytoma, thought to grow from intercalated cells of collecting ducts and have an excellent prognosis compared with that of the clear cell and papillary cancers. Histologic distinction from oncocytoma can be difficult.

4. *Collecting duct (Bellini duct) carcinoma* represents approximately 1% or less of renal epithelial neoplasms. They arise from collecting duct cells in the medulla. Several chromosomal losses and deletions have been described for this tumor, but a distinct pattern has not been identified. Histologically these tumors are characterized by nests of malignant cells enmeshed within a prominent fibrotic stroma, typically in a medullary location.

New variants of renal cell carcinoma that are distinctive (histologically, genetically, and clinically) are being recognized as a result of molecular profiling, illustrating how application

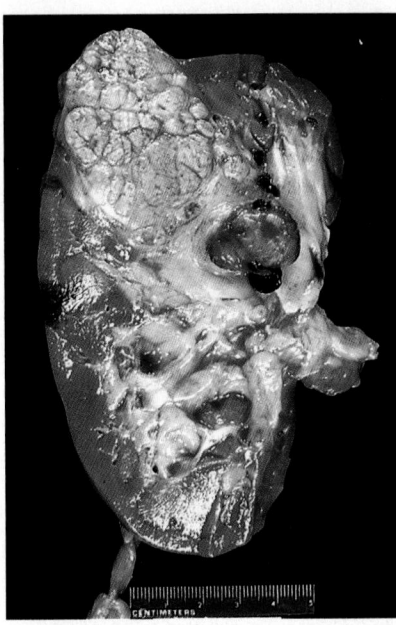

FIGURE 20–53 Renal cell carcinoma. Typical cross-section of yellowish, spherical neoplasm in one pole of the kidney. Note the tumor in the dilated thrombosed renal vein.

of these techniques may improve our clinical understanding and management of these neoplasms.[109]

Morphology. Renal cell carcinomas may arise in any portion of the kidney, but more commonly affects the poles. Clear cell carcinomas arise most likely from proximal tubular epithelium, and usually occur as solitary unilateral lesions. They are spherical masses, which can vary in size, composed of bright yellow-gray-white tissue that distorts the renal outline. The yellow color is a consequence of the prominent lipid accumulations in tumor cells. There are commonly large areas of ischemic, opaque, gray-white necrosis, and foci of hemorrhagic discoloration. The margins are usually sharply defined and confined within the renal capsule (Fig. 20–53). **Papillary tumors**, thought to arise from distal convoluted tubules, can be multi-focal and bilateral. They are typically hemorrhagic and cystic, especially when large. Papillary carcinomas are the most common type of renal cancer in patients who develop dialysis-associated cystic disease.

As tumors enlarge they may bulge into the calyces and pelvis and eventually may fungate through the walls of the collecting system to extend into the ureter. One of the striking characteristics of renal cell carcinoma is its tendency to invade the renal vein (see Fig. 20–53) and grow as a solid column of cells within this vessel. Further growth may produce a continuous cord of tumor in the inferior vena cava that may extend into the right side of the heart.

In **clear cell carcinoma** the growth pattern varies from solid to trabecular (cordlike) or tubular (resembling tubules). The tumor cells have a rounded or

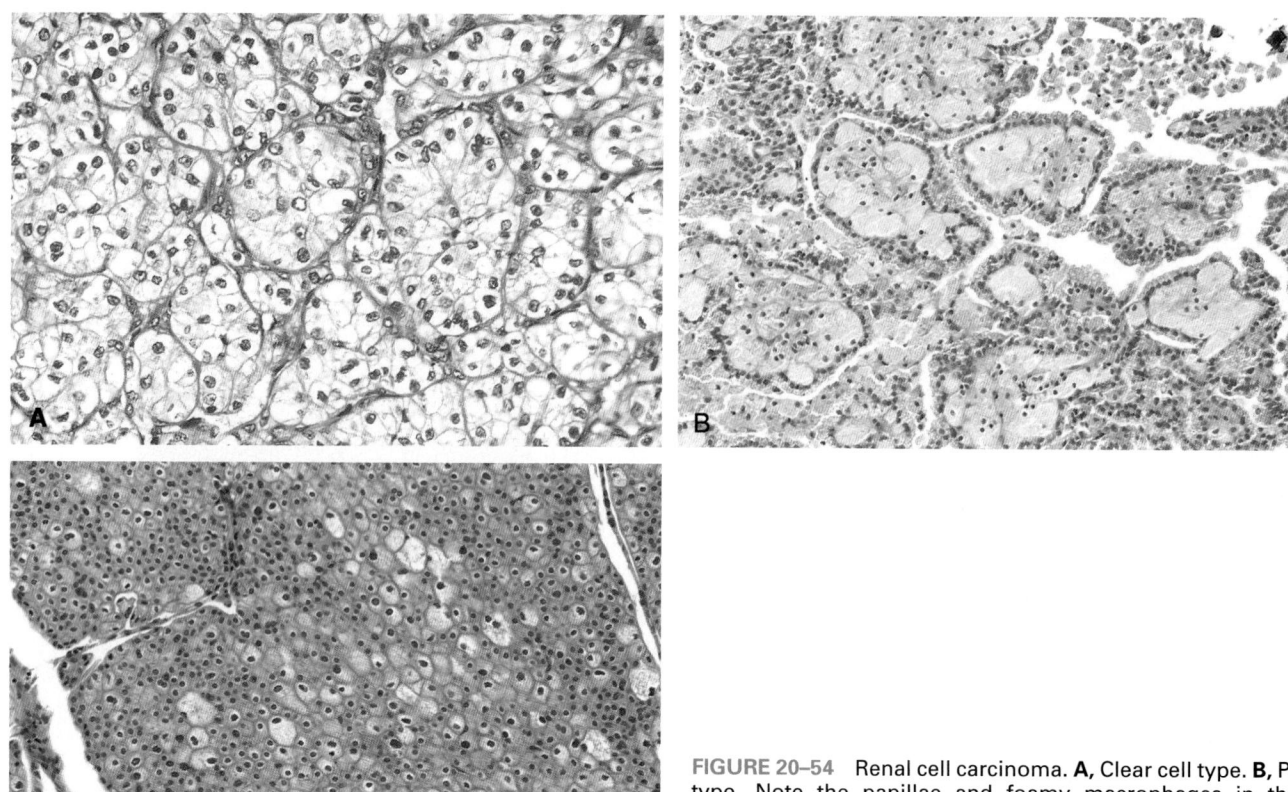

FIGURE 20–54 Renal cell carcinoma. **A,** Clear cell type. **B,** Papillary type. Note the papillae and foamy macrophages in the stalk. **C,** Chromophobe type. (Courtesy of Dr. A. Renshaw, Baptist Hospital, Miami, FL.)

polygonal shape and abundant clear or granular cytoplasm, which contains glycogen and lipids (Fig. 20–54A). The tumors have delicate branching vasculature and may show cystic as well as solid areas. Most tumors are well differentiated, but some show marked nuclear atypia with formation of bizarre nuclei and giant cells. **Papillary carcinoma** is composed of cuboidal or low columnar cells arranged in papillary formations. Interstitial foam cells are common in the papillary cores (Fig. 20–54B). Psammoma bodies may be present. The stroma is usually scanty but highly vascularized. **Chromophobe renal carcinoma** is made up of pale eosinophilic cells, often with a perinuclear halo, arranged in solid sheets with a concentration of the largest cells around blood vessels (Fig. 20–54C). **Collecting duct carcinoma** is a rare variant showing irregular channels lined by highly atypical epithelium with a hobnail pattern. Sarcomatoid changes arise infrequently in all types of renal cell carcinoma and are a decidedly ominous feature.

Clinical Features. The three classic diagnostic features of renal cell carcinoma are *costovertebral pain, palpable mass,* and *hematuria,* but these are seen in only 10% of cases. The most reliable of the three is hematuria, but it is usually intermittent and may be microscopic; thus, the tumor may remain silent until it attains a large size. At this time it is often associated with generalized constitutional symptoms, such as fever,

malaise, weakness, and weight loss. This pattern of asymptomatic growth occurs in many patients, so the tumor may have reached a diameter of more than 10 cm when it is discovered. Currently, an increasing number of tumors are being discovered in the asymptomatic state by incidental radiologic studies (e.g., computed tomographic scan or magnetic resonance imaging) usually performed for nonrenal indications.

Renal cell carcinoma is classified as one of the great mimics in medicine, because it tends to produce a diversity of systemic symptoms not related to the kidney. In addition to fever and constitutional symptoms mentioned earlier, renal cell carcinomas produce a number of paraneoplastic syndromes (Chapter 7), ascribed to abnormal hormone production, including *polycythemia, hypercalcemia, hypertension, hepatic dysfunction, feminization or masculinization, Cushing syndrome, eosinophilia, leukemoid reactions,* and *amyloidosis.*

One of the common characteristics of this tumor is its *tendency to metastasize widely before giving rise to any local symptoms or signs.* In 25% of new patients with renal cell carcinoma, there is radiologic evidence of metastases at the time of presentation. The most common locations of metastasis are the lungs (more than 50%) and bones (33%), followed in frequency by the regional lymph nodes, liver, adrenal, and brain.

The average 5-year survival rate of persons with renal cell carcinoma is about 45% and as high as 70% in the absence of distant metastases. With renal vein invasion or extension into the perinephric fat, the figure is reduced to approximately 15% to 20%. Nephrectomy has been the treatment of choice,

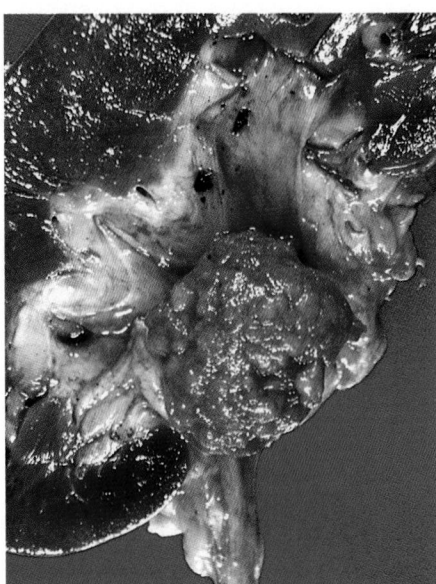

FIGURE 20–55 Urothelial carcinoma of the renal pelvis. The pelvis has been opened to expose the nodular irregular neoplasm, just proximal to the ureter.

but partial nephrectomy to preserve renal function is being done with increasing frequency and similar outcome.

Urothelial Carcinomas of the Renal Pelvis

Approximately 5% to 10% of primary renal tumors originate from the urothelium of the renal pelvis (Fig. 20–55). These tumors span the range from apparently benign papillomas to invasive urothelial (transitional cell) carcinomas.

Renal pelvic tumors usually become clinically apparent within a relatively short time, because they lie within the pelvis and, by fragmentation, produce noticeable hematuria. They are almost invariably small when discovered. These tumors may block the urinary outflow and lead to palpable hydronephrosis and flank pain. On histologic examination, pelvic tumors are the exact counterpart of those found in the urinary bladder; further details are in Chapter 21.

Urothelial tumors may occasionally be multiple, involving the pelvis, ureters, and bladder. In 50% of renal pelvic tumors there is a preexisting or concomitant bladder urothelial tumor. On histologic examination, there are also foci of atypia or carcinoma in situ in grossly normal urothelium remote from the pelvic tumor. As already mentioned, there is an increased incidence of urothelial carcinomas of the renal pelvis and bladder in individuals with analgesic nephropathy and Balkan nephropathy.

Infiltration of the wall of the pelvis and calyces is common. For this reason, despite their apparently small, deceptively benign appearance, the prognosis for these tumors is not good. Reported 5-year survival rates vary from 50% to 100% for low-grade noninvasive lesions to 10% with high-grade infiltrating tumors.

REFERENCES

1. Dinesen I: Seven Gothic Tales. New York, Modern Library, 1939.
2. National Center for Health Statistics: National Vital Statistics Report, 2002.
3. Miner JH: Renal basement membrane components. Kidney Int 56:2016, 1999.
4. Tryggvason K, Wartiovaara J. Molecular basis of glomerular permselectivity. Curr Opin Nephrol Hypertens 10:543, 2001.
5. Hudson BG et al.: Alport's syndrome, Goodpasture's syndrome, and type IV collagen. N Engl J Med 348:2543, 2003.
6. Kwoh C et al.: Pathogenesis of nonimmune glomerulopathies. Annu Rev Pathol 1:349, 2006.
7. Pavenstadt H et al.: Cell biology of the glomerular podocyte. Physiol Rev 83:253, 2003.
8. Tryggvason K et al.: Hereditary proteinuria syndromes and mechanisms of proteinuria. N Engl J Med 354:1387, 2006.
9. Drew AF et al.: Crescentic glomerulonephritis is diminished in fibrinogen-deficient mice. Am J Physiol Renal Physiol 281:F1157, 2001.
10. Couser WG: Glomerulonephritis. Lancet 353:1509, 1999.
11. Neilson EG, Couser WG (eds): Immunologic Renal Diseases, 2nd ed. Philadelphia, Lippincott-Raven, 2001.
12. Ronco P, Debiec H: Target antigens and nephritogenic antibodies in membranous nephropathy: of rats and men. Semin Immunopathol 29:445, 2007.
13. Nimmerjahn F, Ravetch JV: Fc-receptors as regulators of immunity. Adv Immunol 96:179, 2007.
14. Kurts C, Heymann F et al.: Role of T cells and dendritic cells in glomerular immunopathology. Semin Immunopathol 29:317, 2007.
15. Tipping PG, Holdsworth SR: T cells in glomerulonephritis. Springer Semin Immunopathol 24:377, 2003.
16. Floege J et al.: A new look at platelet-derived growth factor in renal disease. J Am Soc Nephrol 19:12, 2008.
17. Bottinger EP: TGF-beta in renal injury and disease. Semin Nephrol 27:309, 2007.
18. Eddy AA: Progression in chronic kidney disease. Adv Chronic Kidney Dis 12:353, 2005.
19. Fogo AB: Progression and potential regression of glomerulosclerosis. Kidney Int 59:804, 2001.
20. Remuzzi G et al.: Mechanisms of progression and regression of renal lesions of chronic nephropathies and diabetes. J Clin Invest 116:288, 2006.
21. Brenner BM: Remission of renal disease: recounting the challenge, acquiring the goal. J Clin Invest 110:1753, 2002.
22. Shankland SJ: The podocyte's response to injury: role in proteinuria and glomerulosclerosis. Kidney Int 69:2131, 2006.
23. Abbate M et al.: How does proteinuria cause progressive renal damage? J Am Soc Nephrol 17:2974, 2006.
24. Couser WG Jr, Alpers CE: Postinfectious glomerulonephritis. In Neilson EG, Couser WG (eds): Immunologic Renal Diseases, 2nd ed. Philadelphia, Lippincott, Williams and Wilkins, 2001, p 899.
25. Rodriguez-Iturbe B, Batsford S: Pathogenesis of poststreptococcal glomerulonephritis a century after Clemens von Pirquet. Kidney Int 71:1094, 2007.
26. Jennette JC: Rapidly progressive crescentic glomerulonephritis. Kidney Int 63:1164, 2003.
27. Phelps RG, Rees AJ: The HLA complex in Goodpasture's disease: a model for analyzing susceptibility to autoimmunity. Kidney Int 56:1638, 1999.
28. Jennette JC et al.: Pathogenesis of vascular inflammation by anti-neutrophil cytoplasmic antibodies. J Am Soc Nephrol 17:1235, 2006.
29. Kitiyakara C et al.: Trends in the epidemiology of focal segmental glomerulosclerosis. Semin Nephrol 23:172, 2003.
30. Cattran DC: Idiopathic membranous glomerulonephritis. Kidney Int 59:1983, 2001.
31. Ponticelli C: Membranous nephropathy. J Nephrol 20:268, 2007.
32. Couser WG, Nangaku M: Cellular and molecular biology of membranous nephropathy. J Nephrol 19:699, 2006.
33. Saha TC, Singh H: Minimal change disease: a review. South Med J 99:1264, 2006.
34. Grimbert P et al.: Recent approaches to the pathogenesis of minimal-change nephrotic syndrome. Nephrol Dial Transplant 18:245, 2003.
35. D'Agati V: The many masks of focal segmental glomerulosclerosis. Kidney Int 46:1223, 1994.
36. Sharma M et al.: "The FSGS factor:" enrichment and in vivo effect of activity from focal segmental glomerulosclerosis plasma. J Am Soc Nephrol 10:552, 1999.
37. Albaqumi M et al.: Collapsing glomerulopathy. J Am Soc Nephrol 17:2854, 2006.

38. Laurinavicius A, Rennke HG: Collapsing glomerulopathy—a new pattern of renal injury. Semin Diagn Pathol 19:106, 2002.

39. Pollak MR: Focal segmental glomerulosclerosis: recent advances. Curr Opin Nephrol Hypertens 17:138, 2008.

40. Wyatt CM, Klotman PE: HIV-1 and HIV-associated nephropathy 25 years later. Clin J Am Soc Nephrol 2 (Suppl 1):S20, 2007.

41. Rennke HG: Secondary membranoproliferative glomerulonephritis. Kidney Int 47:643, 1995.

42. Smith KD, Alpers CE: Pathogenic mechanisms in membranoproliferative glomerulonephritis. Curr Opin Nephrol Hypertens 14:396, 2005.

43. Appel GB et al.: Membranoproliferative glomerulonephritis type II (dense deposit disease): an update. J Am Soc Nephrol 16:1392, 2005.

44. Barratt J, Feehally J: IgA nephropathy. J Am Soc Nephrol 16:2088, 2005.

45. Barratt J et al.: Immunopathogenesis of IgAN. Semin Immunopathol 29:427, 2007.

46. Gubler MC: Inherited diseases of the glomerular basement membrane. Nat Clin Pract Nephrol 4:24, 2008.

47. Thorner PS: Alport syndrome and thin basement membrane nephropathy. Nephron Clin Pract 106:c82, 2007.

48. Kashtan CE: Alport syndromes: phenotypic heterogeneity of progressive hereditary nephritis. Pediatr Nephrol 14:502, 2000.

49. Donadio JV, Grande JP: IgA nephropathy. N Engl J Med 347:738, 2002.

50. Ibrahim HN, Hostetter TH: Diabetic nephropathy. J Am Soc Nephrol 8:487, 1997.

51. Sheetz MJ, King GL: Molecular understanding of hyperglycemia's adverse effects for diabetic complications. JAMA 288:2579, 2002.

52. Bohlender JM et al.: Advanced glycation end products and the kidney. Am J Physiol Renal Physiol 289:F645, 2005.

53. Wolf G, Ziyadeh FN: Molecular mechanisms of diabetic renal hypertrophy. Kidney Int 56:393, 1999.

54. Dalla Vestra M et al.: Structural involvement in type 1 and type 2 diabetic nephropathy. Diabetes Metab 26 (Suppl 4):8, 2000.

55. Wolf G et al.: From the periphery of the glomerular capillary wall toward the center of disease: podocyte injury comes of age in diabetic nephropathy. Diabetes 54:1626, 2005.

56. Fioretto P, Mauer M: Histopathology of diabetic nephropathy. Semin Nephrol 27:195, 2007.

57. Alpers CE, Kowalewska J: Fibrillary glomerulonephritis and immunotactoid glomerulopathy. J Am Soc Nephrol 19:34, 2008.

58. American Society of Nephrology: Renal Research Report. J Am Soc Nephrol 16:1886, 2005.

59. Schrier RW et al.: Acute renal failure: definitions, diagnosis, pathogenesis, and therapy. J Clin Invest 114:5, 2004.

60. Abuelo JG: Normotensive ischemic acute renal failure. N Engl J Med 357:797, 2007.

61. Jo SK et al.: Pharmacologic treatment of acute kidney injury: why drugs haven't worked and what is on the horizon. Clin J Am Soc Nephrol 2:356, 2007.

62. Oliver J et al.: The pathogenesis of acute renal failure associated with traumatic and toxic injury; renal ischemia, nephrotoxic damage and the ischemic episode. J Clin Invest 30:1307, 1951.

63. Ronald A: The etiology of urinary tract infection: traditional and emerging pathogens. Am J Med 113 (Suppl 1A):14S, 2002.

64. Lane MC, Mobley HL: Role of P-fimbrial-mediated adherence in pyelonephritis and persistence of uropathogenic Escherichia coli (UPEC) in the mammalian kidney. Kidney Int 72:19, 2007.

65. Gargollo PC, Diamond DA: Therapy insight: what nephrologists need to know about primary vesicoureteral reflux. Nat Clin Pract Nephrol 3:551, 2007.

66. Piccoli G et al.: Acute pyelonephritis: a new approach to an old clinical entity. J Nephrol 18:474, 2005.

67. Nickeleit V, Mihatsch MJ: Polyomavirus nephropathy in native kidneys and renal allografts: an update on an escalating threat. Transpl Int 19:960, 2006.

68. Choudhury D, Ahmed Z: Drug-associated renal dysfunction and injury. Nat Clin Pract Nephrol 2:80, 2006.

69. Fored CM et al.: Acetaminophen, aspirin, and chronic renal failure. N Engl J Med 345:1801, 2001.

70. Gambaro G, Perazella MA: Adverse renal effects of anti-inflammatory agents: evaluation of selective and nonselective cyclooxygenase inhibitors. J Intern Med 253:643, 2003.

71. Grollman AP et al.: Aristolochic acid and the etiology of endemic (Balkan) nephropathy. Proc Natl Acad Sci U S A 104:12129, 2007.

72. Markowitz GS et al.: Acute phosphate nephropathy following oral sodium phosphate bowel purgative: an underrecognized cause of chronic renal failure. J Am Soc Nephrol 16:3389, 2005.

73. Kurokawa K et al.: Hypertension: causes and consequences of renal injury. Kidney Int 49:S1, 1997.

74. Meyrier A et al.: Ischemic renal diseases: new insights into old entities. Kidney Int 54:2, 1998.

75. Marcantoni C, Fogo AB: A perspective on arterionephrosclerosis: from pathology to potential pathogenesis. J Nephrol 20:518, 2007.

76. Kitiyakara C, Guzman NJ: Malignant hypertension and hypertensive emergencies. J Am Soc Nephrol 9:133, 1998.

77. Safian RD, Textor SC: Renal-artery stenosis. N Engl J Med 344:431, 2001.

78. Goldblatt H et al.: Studies on experimental hypertension: I. Production of persistent elevation of systolic blood pressure by means of renal ischemia. J Exp Med 59:347, 1934.

79. Besbas N et al.: A classification of hemolytic uremic syndrome and thrombotic thrombocytopenic purpura and related disorders. Kidney Int 70:423, 2006.

80. Moake JL: Thrombotic microangiopathies. N Engl J Med 347:589, 2002.

81. Desch K, Motto D: Is there a shared pathophysiology for thrombotic thrombocytopenic purpura and hemolytic-uremic syndrome? J Am Soc Nephrol 18:2457, 2007.

82. Tsai HM: The molecular biology of thrombotic microangiopathy. Kidney Int 70:16, 2006.

83. Grabowski EF: The hemolytic-uremic syndrome—toxin, thrombin, and thrombosis. N Engl J Med 346:58, 2002.

84. Textor SC, Wilcox CS: Ischemic nephropathy/azotemic renovascular disease. Semin Nephrol 20:489, 2000.

85. Foley RN, Collins AJ: End-stage renal disease in the United States: an update from the United States Renal Data System. J Am Soc Nephrol 18:2644, 2007.

86. Gardner KD Jr. BJ: The Cystic Kidney. Dordrecht, Kluwer Academic Publishers, 1990.

87. Torres VE et al.: Autosomal dominant polycystic kidney disease. Lancet 369:1287, 2007.

88. Rossetti S, Harris PC: Genotype-phenotype correlations in autosomal dominant and autosomal recessive polycystic kidney disease. J Am Soc Nephrol 18:1374, 2007.

89. Rossetti S et al.: The position of the polycystic kidney disease 1 (PKD1) gene mutation correlates with the severity of renal disease. J Am Soc Nephrol 13:1230, 2002.

90. Wilson PD, Goilav B: Cystic disease of the kidney. Annu Rev Pathol 2:341, 2007.

91. Guay-Woodford LM: Renal cystic diseases: diverse phenotypes converge on the cilium/centrosome complex. Pediatr Nephrol 21:1369, 2006.

92. Wilson PD: Polycystic kidney disease. N Engl J Med 350:151, 2004.

93. Yoder BK: Role of primary cilia in the pathogenesis of polycystic kidney disease. J Am Soc Nephrol 18:1381, 2007.

94. Ward CJ et al.: The gene mutated in autosomal recessive polycystic kidney disease encodes a large, receptor-like protein. Nat Genet 30:259, 2002.

95. Hildebrandt F, Zhou W: Nephronophthisis-associated ciliopathies. J Am Soc Nephrol 18:1855, 2007.

96. Chevalier RL: Obstructive nephropathy: towards biomarker discovery and gene therapy. Nat Clin Pract Nephrol 2:157, 2006.

97. Coe FL et al.: Kidney stone disease. J Clin Invest 115:2598, 2005.

98. Pak CY: Kidney stones. Lancet 351:1797, 1998.

99. Eble JN, Moch H: Papillary adenoma of the kidney. In Eble JN, Sauter G, et al. WHO Classification of Tumours: Pathology and Genetics of Tumours of the Urinary System and Male Genital Organs. Lyon, France, IARC Press, 2004, p41.

100. Jemal A et al.: Cancer statistics, 2008. CA Cancer J Clin 58:71, 2008.

101. McLaughlin JK, Lipworth L: Epidemiologic aspects of renal cell cancer. Semin Oncol 27:115, 2000.

102. Moore LE et al.: Lifestyle factors, exposures, genetic susceptibility, and renal cell cancer risk: a review. Cancer Invest 23:240, 2005.

103. Eble JN, Sauter G, et al.: WHO Classification of Tumours: Pathology and Genetics of Tumours of the Urinary System and Male Genital Organs. Lyon, France, IARC Press, 2004.

104. Cohen HT, McGovern FJ: Renal-cell carcinoma. N Engl J Med 353:2477, 2005.
105. Bodmer D et al.: Understanding familial and non-familial renal cell cancer. Hum Mol Genet 11:2489, 2002.
106. Kaelin WG, Jr: The von Hippel-Lindau tumor suppressor protein and clear cell renal carcinoma. Clin Cancer Res 13:680s, 2007.
107. Pavlovich CP et al.: The genetic basis of renal cell carcinoma. Urol Clin North Am 30:437, 2003.
108. Linehan WM et al.: Identification of the genes for kidney cancer: opportunity for disease-specific targeted therapeutics. Clin Cancer Res 13:671s, 2007.
109. Young AN et al.: Renal epithelial neoplasms: diagnostic applications of gene expression profiling. Adv Anat Pathol 15:28, 2008.

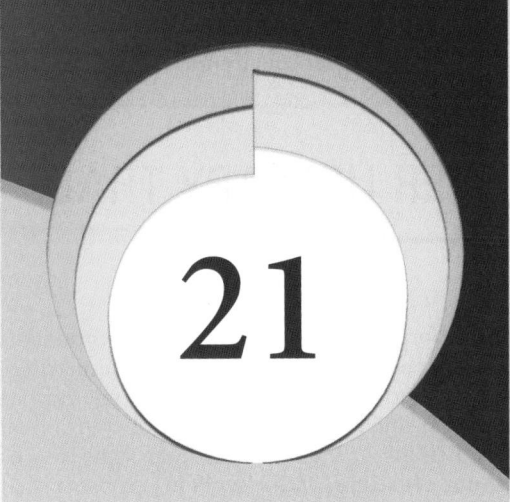

The Lower Urinary Tract and Male Genital System

JONATHAN I. EPSTEIN

■ THE LOWER URINARY TRACT

Ureters
  Congenital Anomalies
  Inflammation
  Tumors and Tumor-like Lesions
  Obstructive Lesions

Urinary Bladder
  Congenital Anomalies
  Inflammation
    Acute and Chronic Cystitis
    Special Forms of Cystitis
  Metaplastic Lesions
  Neoplasms
    Urothelial Tumors
    Mesenchymal Tumors
    Secondary Tumors
  Obstruction

Urethra
  Inflammation
  Tumors and Tumor-like Lesions

■ THE MALE GENITAL TRACT

Penis
  Congenital Anomalies
    Hypospadias and Epispadias
    Phimosis
  Inflammation
  Tumors
    Benign Tumors
    Malignant Tumors

Testis and Epididymis
  Congenital Anomalies
    Cryptorchidism
  Regressive Changes
    Atrophy and Decreased Fertility
  Inflammation
    Nonspecific Epididymitis and Orchitis
    Granulomatous (Autoimmune) Orchitis
    Specific Inflammations
  Vascular Disorders
    Torsion
  Spermatic Cord and Paratesticular Tumors
  Testicular Tumors
    Germ Cell Tumors
    Tumors of Sex Cord–Gonadal Stroma
    Gonadoblastoma
    Testicular Lymphoma
  Miscellaneous Lesions of Tunica Vaginalis

Prostate
  Inflammation
  Benign Enlargement
    Benign Prostatic Hyperplasia (BPH) or Nodular Hyperplasia
  Tumors
    Adenocarcinoma
    Miscellaneous Tumors and Tumor-like Conditions

THE LOWER URINARY TRACT

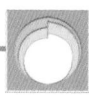

Despite differing embryonic origins, the various components of the lower urinary tract have many morphologic similarities. The renal pelves, ureters, bladder, and urethra (save for its terminal portion) are lined by a special form of transitional epithelium (urothelium). The surface layer consists of large, flattened "umbrella cells" with abundant cytoplasm that horizontally cover several underlying cells. The umbrella cells have a trilaminar asymmetric unit membrane and possess apical plaques composed of specific proteins called *uroplakins*. The underlying urothelium is composed of several layers of cells with oval smaller nuclei often with linear nuclear grooves and less cytoplasm. This epithelium rests on a well-developed basement membrane, beneath which is a lamina propria. The lamina propria in the urinary bladder contains wisps of smooth muscle that form a discontinuous muscularis mucosae. It is important to differentiate the muscularis mucosae from the deeper well-defined larger muscle bundles of the detrusor muscle (muscularis propria), since bladder cancers are staged on the basis of invasion of the latter. The bladder musculature is capable, with obstruction to the flow of urine, of great thickening.

The ureters lie throughout their course in a retroperitoneal position. Retroperitoneal tumors or fibrosis may trap the ureters in neoplastic or dense, fibrous tissue, sometimes obstructing them. As ureters enter the pelvis, they pass anterior to either the common iliac or the external iliac artery. In the female pelvis they lie close to the uterine arteries and are therefore vulnerable to injury in operations on the female genital tract. There are three points of slight narrowing—at the ureteropelvic junction, where they enter the bladder, and where they cross the iliac vessels— all providing loci where renal calculi may become impacted when they pass from the kidney to the bladder. As the ureters enter the bladder they pursue an oblique course, terminating in a slitlike orifice. The obliquity of this intramural segment of the ureteral orifice permits the enclosing bladder musculature to act like a sphincteric valve, blocking the upward reflux of urine even in the presence of marked distention of the urinary bladder. As discussed in Chapter 20, a defect in the intravesical portion of the ureter leads to vesicoureteral reflux.

The close relationship of the female genital tract to the bladder makes possible the spread of disease from one tract to the other. In middle-aged and elderly women, relaxation of pelvic support leads to prolapse (descent) of the uterus, pulling with it the floor of the bladder. In this fashion the bladder is protruded into the vagina, creating a pouch (cystocele) that fails to empty readily with micturition. In males the seminal vesicles and prostate have similar close relationships, being situated just posterior and inferior to the neck of the bladder. Thus, enlargement of the prostate, so common in middle to later life, constitutes an important cause of urinary tract obstruction. In the subsequent sections we discuss the major pathologic lesions in the ureters, urinary bladder, and urethra separately.

Ureters

CONGENITAL ANOMALIES

Congenital anomalies of the ureters are found in about 2% or 3% of all autopsies. Although most have little clinical significance, certain anomalies may contribute to obstruction to the flow of urine and thus cause clinical disease. Anomalies of the ureterovesical junction that potentiate reflux are discussed with pyelonephritis in Chapter 20.

Double and bifid ureters. Double ureters are almost invariably associated either with totally distinct double renal pelves or with the anomalous development of a large kidney having a partially bifid pelvis terminating in separate ureters. Double ureters may pursue separate courses to the bladder but commonly are joined within the bladder wall and drain through a single ureteral orifice. The majority of double ureters are unilateral and of no clinical significance.

Ureteropelvic junction (UPJ) obstruction, a congenital disorder, results in hydronephrosis. It usually presents in infants or children, much more commonly in boys. However, it is bilateral in 20% of cases and may be associated with other congenital anomalies. It is the most common cause of hydronephrosis in infants and children. In adults, UPJ obstruction is more common in women and is most often unilateral. The condition has been ascribed to abnormal organization of smooth muscle bundles at the UPJ, to excess stromal deposition of collagen between smooth muscle bundles, or rarely to congenitally extrinsic compression by polar renal vessels. There is agenesis of the kidney on the opposite side in a significant number of cases, probably resulting from obstructive lesions in utero.

Diverticula, saccular outpouchings of the ureteral wall, are uncommon lesions that are usually asymptomatic and are found on imaging studies. They appear as congenital or acquired defects and are of importance as pockets of stasis and secondary infections. Dilation *(hydroureter)*, elongation, and tortuosity of the ureters may occur as congenital anomalies or as acquired defects.

INFLAMMATION

Ureteritis, though associated with inflammation, is typically not associated with infection and is of little clinical consequence.

Morphology. The accumulation or aggregation of lymphocytes forming germinal centers in the subepithelial region may cause slight elevations of the mucosa and produce a fine granular mucosal surface **(ureteritis follicularis)**. At other times the mucosa may become sprinkled with fine cysts varying in diameter from 1 to 5 mm lined by flattened urothelium **(ureteritis cystica)** (Fig. 21–1).

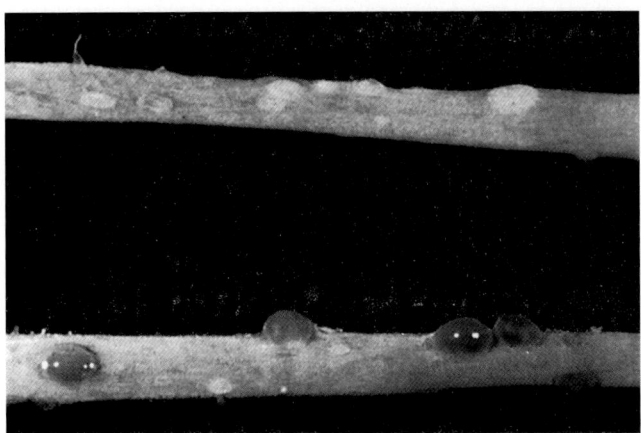

FIGURE 21–1 Opened ureters showing ureteritis cystica. Note smooth cysts projecting from the mucosa.

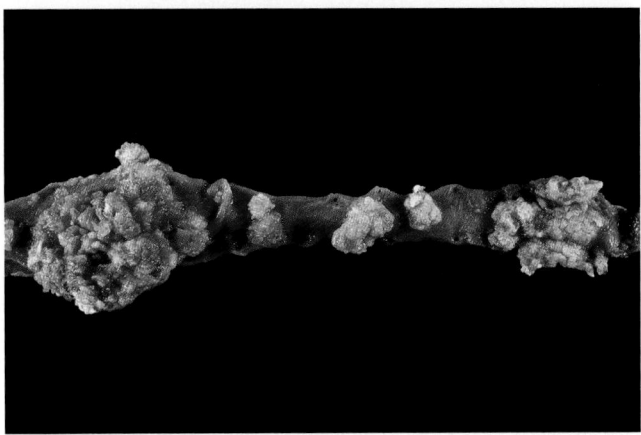

FIGURE 21–2 Papillary transitional cell carcinoma extensively involving the ureter. (Courtesy of Dr. Cristina Magi-Galluzzi, The Johns Hopkins Hospital, Baltimore, MD.)

TUMORS AND TUMOR-LIKE LESIONS

Primary tumors of the ureter are rare. Small *benign tumors* of the ureter are generally of mesenchymal origin. *Fibroepithelial polyp* is a tumor-like lesion that grossly presents as a small mass projecting into the lumen, often in children. The lesion occurs more commonly in the ureters but may also appear in the bladder, renal pelves, and urethra. The polyp is composed of a loose, vascularized connective tissue mass lying beneath the mucosa.

Primary *malignant tumors* of the ureter resemble those arising in the renal pelvis, calyces, and bladder. The majority are urothelial carcinomas (Fig. 21–2). They are found most frequently during the sixth and seventh decades of life and cause obstruction of the ureteral lumen. They are sometimes multiple and commonly occur concurrently with similar neoplasms in the bladder or renal pelvis.

OBSTRUCTIVE LESIONS

A great variety of pathologic lesions may obstruct the ureters and give rise to *hydroureter, hydronephrosis,* and sometimes *pyelonephritis* (Chapter 20). It is not the ureteral dilation that is of significance in these cases, but the consequent involvement of the kidneys. The more important causes, divided into those of intrinsic or extrinsic origin, are listed in Table 21–1. Unilateral obstruction typically results from proximal causes, whereas bilateral obstruction arises from distal causes, such as nodular hyperplasia of the prostate. Only sclerosing retroperitoneal fibrosis is discussed further.

Sclerosing Retroperitoneal Fibrosis. This refers to an uncommon cause of ureteral narrowing or obstruction characterized by a *fibrous proliferative inflammatory process encasing the retroperitoneal structures and causing hydronephrosis.*[1] The disorder occurs in middle to late age. In some cases specific causes can be identified, such as drugs (ergot derivatives, β-adrenergic blockers), adjacent inflammatory conditions (vasculitis, diverticulitis, Crohn disease), or malignant disease (lymphomas, urinary tract carcinomas). However, 70% of cases have no obvious cause and are considered primary or idiopathic (Ormond disease). Several cases have been reported with similar fibrotic changes in other sites (such as mediastinal fibrosis, sclerosing cholangitis, and Riedel

TABLE 21–1 Major Causes of Ureteral Obstruction	
Type of Obstruction	**Cause**
INTRINSIC	
Calculi	Of renal origin, rarely more than 5 mm in diameter
	Larger renal stones cannot enter ureters
	Impact at loci of ureteral narrowing—ureteropelvic junction, where ureters cross iliac vessels, and where they enter bladder—and cause excruciating "renal colic"
Strictures	Congenital or acquired (inflammations)
Tumors	Transitional cell carcinomas arising in ureters
	Rarely, benign tumors or fibroepithelial polyps
Blood clots	Massive hematuria from renal calculi, tumors, or papillary necrosis
Neurogenic	Interruption of the neural pathways to the bladder
EXTRINSIC	
Pregnancy	Physiologic relaxation of smooth muscle or pressure on ureters at pelvic brim from enlarging fundus
Periureteral inflammation	Salpingitis, diverticulitis, peritonitis, sclerosing retroperitoneal fibrosis
Endometriosis	With pelvic lesions, followed by scarring
Tumors	Cancers of the rectum, bladder, prostate, ovaries, uterus, cervix; lymphomas, sarcomas

fibrosing thyroiditis), suggesting that the disorder is systemic in distribution but preferentially involves the retroperitoneum. Thus, an autoimmune reaction, sometimes triggered by drugs, has been proposed as the immediate cause of the systemic disease.

On microscopic examination the inflammatory fibrosis is marked by a prominent infiltrate of lymphocytes, often with germinal centers, plasma cells, and eosinophils. Treatment involves surgical extrication of the ureters from the surrounding fibrous tissue (ureterolysis).

Urinary Bladder

Diseases of the bladder, particularly inflammation (cystitis), constitute an important source of clinical signs and symptoms. Usually, however, these disorders are more disabling than lethal. Cystitis is particularly common in young women of reproductive age. Tumors of the bladder are an important source of both morbidity and mortality.

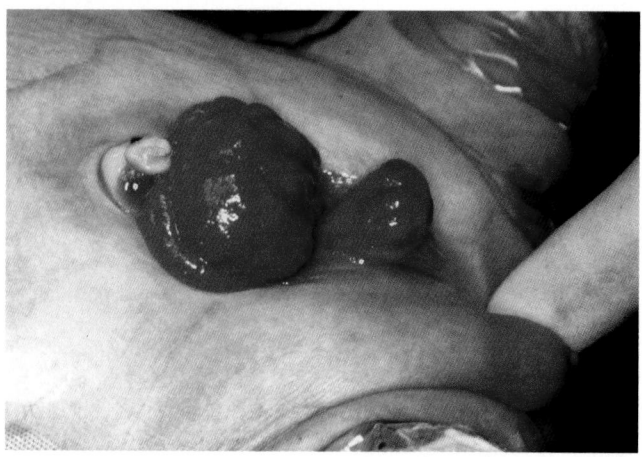

FIGURE 21–3 Exstrophy of the bladder in a newborn boy. The tied umbilical cord is seen above the hyperemic mucosa of the everted bladder. Below is an incompletely formed penis with marked epispadias. (Courtesy of Dr. John Gearhart, The Johns Hopkins Hospital, Baltimore, MD.)

CONGENITAL ANOMALIES

Diverticula. A bladder or vesical diverticulum consists of a pouchlike evagination of the bladder wall. Diverticula may arise as congenital defects but more commonly are acquired lesions caused by persistent urethral obstruction.

The *congenital form* may be due to a focal failure of development of the normal musculature or to some urinary tract obstruction during fetal development. *Acquired diverticula* are most often seen with prostatic enlargement (hyperplasia or neoplasia), producing obstruction to urine outflow and marked muscle thickening of the bladder wall. The increased intravesical pressure causes outpouching of the bladder wall and the formation of diverticula. They are frequently multiple and have narrow necks located between the interweaving hypertrophied muscle bundles. In both the congenital and the acquired forms, the diverticulum usually consists of a round to ovoid, saclike pouch that varies from less than 1 cm to 5 to 10 cm in diameter.

Although most diverticula are small and asymptomatic, they may be clinically significant, since they constitute sites of urinary stasis and predispose to infection and the formation of bladder calculi. They may also predispose to vesicoureteral reflux as a result of impingement on the ureter. Rarely, carcinomas may arise in bladder diverticuli. When invasive cancers arise in diverticula, they tend to be more advanced in stage as a result of the thin or absent muscle wall of a diverticulum.

Exstrophy. Exstrophy of the bladder is a developmental failure in the anterior wall of the abdomen and the bladder, so that the bladder either communicates directly through a large defect with the surface of the body or lies as an opened sac (Fig. 21–3). The exposed bladder mucosa may undergo colonic glandular metaplasia and is subject to infections that often spread to upper levels of the urinary system. Patients have an increased risk of adenocarcinoma arising in the bladder remnant.[2] These lesions are amenable to surgical correction, and long-term survival is possible.

Miscellaneous Anomalies. *Vesicoureteral reflux* is the most common and serious anomaly. As a major contributor to renal infection and scarring, it was discussed earlier, in Chapter 20,

in the consideration of pyelonephritis. Abnormal connections between the bladder and the vagina, rectum, or uterus may create *congenital vesicouterine fistulas*.

Rarely, the *urachus* (the canal that connects the fetal bladder with the allantois) may remain patent in part or in whole. When totally patent, a fistulous urinary tract is created that connects the bladder with the umbilicus. At times, only the central region of the urachus persists, giving rise to *urachal cysts,* lined by either urothelium or metaplastic glandular epithelium. *Carcinomas*, mostly glandular tumors, may arise from such cysts (see "Neoplasms"). These account for only a minority of all bladder cancers (0.1% to 0.3%) but 20% to 40% of bladder adenocarcinomas.

INFLAMMATION

Acute and Chronic Cystitis

The pathogenesis of cystitis and the common bacterial etiologic agents are discussed in Chapter 20 in the consideration of urinary tract infections. As emphasized earlier, bacterial pyelonephritis is frequently preceded by infection of the urinary bladder, with retrograde spread of microorganisms into the kidneys and their collecting systems. The common etiologic agents of cystitis are the coliforms: *Escherichia coli,* followed by *Proteus, Klebsiella,* and *Enterobacter.* Women are more likely to develop cystitis as a result of their shorter urethras. *Tuberculous cystitis* is almost always a sequel to renal tuberculosis. *Candida albicans* and, much less often, cryptococcal agents cause cystitis, particularly in immunosuppressed patients or those receiving long-term antibiotics. Schistosomiasis *(Schistosoma haematobium)* is rare in the United States but is common in certain Middle Eastern countries, notably Egypt. Viruses (e.g., adenovirus), *Chlamydia,* and *Mycoplasma* may also cause cystitis. Predisposing factors include bladder calculi, urinary obstruction, diabetes mellitus, instrumentation, and immune deficiency. Finally, irradiation of the bladder region gives rise to *radiation cystitis.*

Morphology. Most cases of cystitis take the form of nonspecific acute or chronic inflammation of the bladder. In gross appearance there is hyperemia of the mucosa, sometimes associated with exudate. Patients receiving **cytotoxic antitumor drugs**, such as cyclophosphamide, may develop **hemorrhagic cystitis.**[3] Adenovirus infection also causes a hemorrhagic cystitis.

Persistence of the infection leads to **chronic cystitis**, which differs from the acute form only in the character of the inflammatory infiltrate. **Follicular cystitis**, characterized by the aggregation of lymphocytes into lymphoid follicles within the bladder mucosa and underlying wall, is not necessarily associated with infection. **Eosinophilic cystitis**, manifested by infiltration with submucosal eosinophils, typically also represents nonspecific subacute inflammation, although rarely it is a manifestation of a systemic allergic disorder. The ubiquitous presence of mild chronic inflammation in the bladder unaccompanied by clinical symptoms should not be given the diagnosis of chronic cystitis.

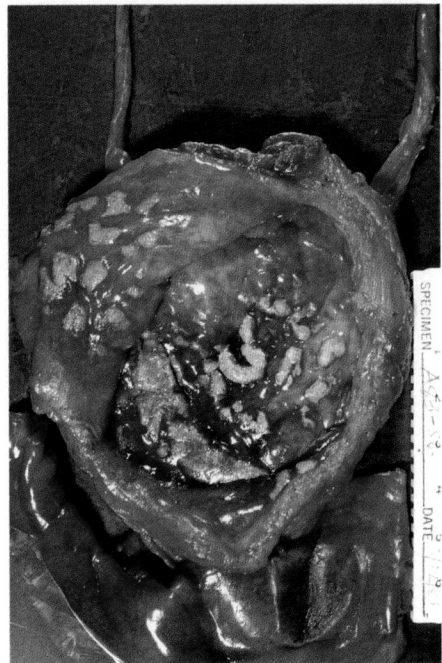

FIGURE 21-4 Cystitis with malacoplakia of bladder showing inflammatory exudate and broad, flat plaques.

All forms of cystitis are characterized by a triad of symptoms: (1) frequency, which in acute cases may necessitate urination every 15 to 20 minutes; (2) lower abdominal pain localized over the bladder region or in the suprapubic region; and (3) dysuria—pain or burning on urination.

The local symptoms of cystitis may be disturbing, but these infections are also important as antecedents to pyelonephritis. Cystitis is sometimes a secondary complication of some underlying disorder such as prostatic enlargement, cystocele of the bladder, calculi, or tumors. These primary diseases must be corrected before the cystitis can be relieved.

Special Forms of Cystitis

Several variants of cystitis are distinctive by their morphologic appearance or causation.

Interstitial Cystitis (Chronic Pelvic Pain Syndrome). This is a *persistent, painful form of chronic cystitis occurring most frequently in women.*[4] It is characterized clinically by intermittent, often severe suprapubic pain, urinary frequency, urgency, hematuria and dysuria without evidence of bacterial infection, and cystoscopic findings of fissures and punctate hemorrhages (glomerulations) in the bladder mucosa after luminal distention. Some but not all patients show morphologic features of chronic mucosal ulcers *(Hunner ulcers)*; this is termed the *late (classic, ulcerative) phase.* Although mast cells are characteristic of this disease, there is no uniformity in the literature about their specificity and diagnostic utility. Late in the disease, transmural fibrosis may ensue, leading to a contracted bladder. The major role of biopsy is not to specifically diagnose the disease as much as it is to rule out carcinoma in situ, which may mimic interstitial cystitis clinically. Its etiology is unknown, its evaluation and diagnosis remain controversial, and its treatment is largely empiric.[5]

Malacoplakia. This designation refers to a *peculiar pattern of vesical inflammatory reaction characterized macroscopically by soft, yellow, slightly raised mucosal plaques 3 to 4 cm in* diameter (Fig. 21-4), and *histologically by infiltration with large, foamy macrophages mixed with occasional multinucleate giant cells and interspersed lymphocytes.*[6] The macrophages have an abundant granular cytoplasm due to phagosomes stuffed with particulate and membranous debris of bacterial origin. In addition, laminated mineralized concretions resulting from deposition of calcium in enlarged lysosomes, known as Michaelis-Gutmann bodies, are typically present within the macrophages (Fig. 21-5). Similar lesions have been described in the colon, lungs, bones, kidneys, prostate, and epididymis.

Malacoplakia is clearly related to chronic bacterial infection, mostly by *E. coli* or occasionally *Proteus* species. It occurs with increased frequency in immunosuppressed transplant recipients. The unusual-appearing macrophages and giant phagosomes point to defects in phagocytic or degradative function of macrophages, such that phagosomes become overloaded with undigested bacterial products.

Polypoid Cystitis. Polypoid cystitis is an inflammatory condition resulting from irritation to the bladder mucosa.[7,8] Although indwelling catheters are the most commonly cited culprits, any injurious agent may give rise to this lesion. The urothelium is thrown into broad bulbous polypoid projections as a result of marked submucosal edema. Polypoid cystitis may be confused with papillary urothelial carcinoma both clinically and histologically.

METAPLASIC LESIONS

Cystitis Glandularis and Cystitis Cystica. These terms refer to common lesions of the urinary bladder in which nests of urothelium (Brunn nests) grow downward into the lamina propria and undergo transformation of their central epithelial cells into cuboidal or columnar epithelium lining *(cystitis*

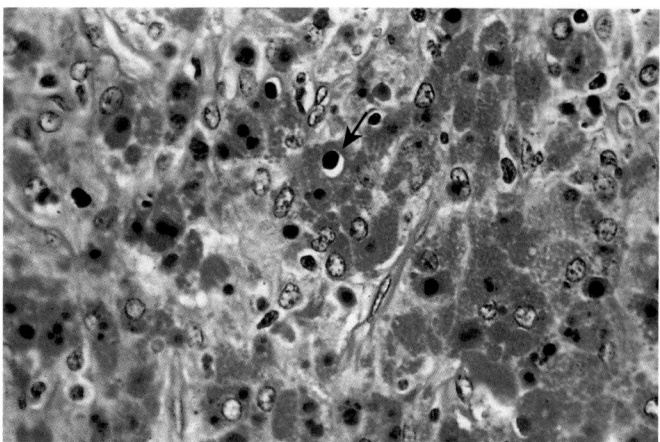

FIGURE 21–5 Malacoplakia, periodic acid–Schiff (PAS) stain. Note the large macrophages with granular PAS-positive cytoplasm and several dense, round Michaelis-Gutmann bodies surrounded by artifactual cleared holes in the upper middle field *(arrow)*.

glandularis) or cystic spaces filled with clear fluid lined by flattened urothelium *(cystitis cystica)*. Because the two processes often coexist, the condition is typically referred to as *cystitis cystica et glandularis*. In a variant of cystitis glandularis goblet cells are present, and the epithelium resembles intestinal mucosa *(intestinal or colonic metaplasia)*. Both variants are common microscopic incidental findings in relatively normal bladders, although they can also arise from inflammation and metaplasia. In contrast to earlier reports, lesions showing extensive intestinal metaplasia are not associated with an increased risk for the development of adenocarcinoma (except when associated with exstrophy).[9]

Squamous Metaplasia. As a response to injury, the urothelium is often replaced by squamous epithelium, which is a more durable lining. This should be distinguished from glycogenated squamous epithelium that is normally found in women at the trigone.

Nephrogenic Adenoma. Nephrogenic adenoma is an unusual lesion that in the past was believed to represent metaplasia of the urothelium in response to injury.[10,11] It has now been demonstrated to result from shed renal tubular cells that implant in sites of injured urothelium.[12] The term *nephrogenic adenoma* was originally given because the lesion resembles renal tubules histologically, but the term also reflects the pathogenesis of the lesion. The overlying urothelium may be focally replaced by cuboidal epithelium, which can assume a papillary growth pattern. In addition, a tubular proliferation in the underlying lamina propria and superficial detrusor muscle can mimic a malignant process.[13] Although typically less than a centimeter, lesions may be sizable, and may resemble cancer clinically.

NEOPLASMS

Bladder cancer accounts for approximately 7% of cancers and 3% of cancer mortality in the United States.[14] About 95% of bladder tumors are of epithelial origin, the remainder being mesenchymal tumors (Table 21–2). Most epithelial tumors are composed of urothelial (transitional cell) type and are thus

interchangeably called *urothelial or transitional tumors*, but squamous and glandular carcinomas also occur. Here we focus on urothelial tumors and touch briefly on the others.

Urothelial Tumors

Urothelial tumors represent about 90% of all bladder tumors and run the gamut from small benign lesions that may never recur to aggressive cancers associated with a high risk of death. Many of these tumors are multifocal at presentation. Though most commonly seen in the bladder, any of the urothelial lesions described below may be seen at any site where there is urothelium, from the renal pelvis to the distal urethra.

There are two distinct precursor lesions to invasive urothelial carcinoma: non-invasive papillary tumors, and flat non-invasive urothelial carcinoma. The most common precursor lesions are the non-invasive papillary tumors, which originate from papillary urothelial hyperplasia.[15] These tumors have a range of atypical changes, and are graded according to their biological behavior. The other precursor lesion to invasive carcinoma, flat non-invasive urothelial carcinoma is referred to as carcinoma in situ or CIS. As discussed in Chapter 7, CIS is a histologic term used to describe epithelial lesions that have cytologic changes of malignancy, but are confined to the epithelium, without basement membrane invasion.[16] Such lesions are considered to be high grade. In about one half of individuals with invasive bladder cancer, the tumor has already invaded the bladder wall, at the time of presentation, and no precursor lesions may be detected. It is presumed that the precursor lesion has been destroyed by the high-grade invasive component, which typically appears as a large frequently ulcerated mass. Although invasion into the lamina propria worsens the prognosis, the major decrease in survival is associated with invasion of the muscularis propria (detrusor muscle). Once muscularis propria invasion occurs, there is a 30% 5-year mortality rate.

In Table 21–3, we have listed two of the most common grading systems of these tumors. The World Health Organization (WHO) 1973 classification grades tumors into a rare totally benign papilloma and three grades of transitional cell carcinoma (grades I, II, and III). A more recent classification, based on a consensus reached at a conference by the International Society of Urological Pathology (ISUP) in 1998 and adopted by the WHO in 2004, recognizes a rare benign papil-

TABLE 21–2   Tumors of the Urinary Bladder
Urothelial (transitional) tumors

Exophytic papilloma
   Inverted papilloma
   Papillary urothelial neoplasms of low malignant potential
   Low grade and high grade papillary urothelial cancers
   Carcinoma in situ (CIS, or flat non-invasive urothelial carcinoma)

Mixed carcinoma
Adenocarcinoma
Small-cell carcinoma
Sarcomas

TABLE 21–3 Grading of Urothelial (Transitional Cell) Tumors
WHO/ISUP Grades
Urothelial papiloma
Urothelial neoplasm of low malignant potential
Papillary urothelial carcinoma, low grade
Papillary urothelial carcinoma, high grade
WHO Grades
Urothelial papilloma
Urothelial neoplasm of low malignant potential
Papillary urothelial carcinoma, grade 1
Papillary urothelial carcinoma, grade 2
Papillary urothelial carcinoma, grade 3

WHO, World Health Organization; ISUP, International Society of Urological Pathology.

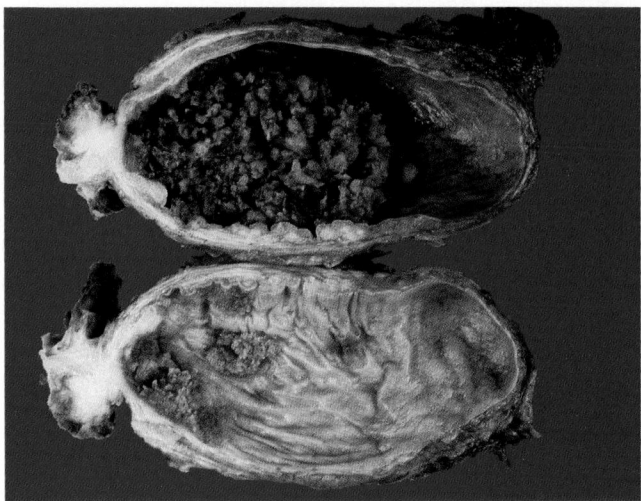

FIGURE 21–7 Cross-section of bladder with upper section showing a large papillary tumor. The lower section demonstrates multifocal smaller papillary neoplasms. (Courtesy of Dr. Fred Gilkey, Sinai Hospital, Baltimore, MD.)

loma, a group of papillary urothelial neoplasms of low malignant potential, and two grades of carcinoma (low and high grade).[16,17]

Morphology. The gross patterns of urothelial tumors vary from purely papillary to nodular or flat (Fig. 21–6). Papillary lesions appear as red, elevated excrescences varying in size from less than 1 cm in diameter to large masses up to 5 cm in diameter (Fig. 21–7). Multicentric origins may produce separate tumors. As noted, the histologic changes encompass a spectrum from benign papilloma to highly aggressive anaplastic cancers. Overall, the majority of papillary tumors are low grade. Most arise from the lateral or posterior walls at the bladder base.

- **Papillomas** represent 1% or less of bladder tumors, and are usually seen in younger patients.[18] The tumors typically arise singly as small (0.5 to 2.0 cm), delicate, structures, superficially attached to the mucosa by a stalk and are referred to as **exophytic**

papillomas. The individual finger-like papillae have a central core of loose fibrovascular tissue covered by epithelium that is **histologically identical to normal urothelium** (Fig. 21–8). Recurrences and progression rarely occur, yet patients still need long-term follow-up. In contrast to exophytic papillomas, **inverted papillomas** are benign lesions, cured by excision and consist of inter-anastomosing cords of cytologically bland urothelium that extend down into the lamina propria.[19,20]

- **Papillary urothelial neoplasms of low malignant potential (PUNLMPs)** share many histologic features with papilloma, the only differences being either thicker urothelium or diffuse nuclear enlargement in PUNLMPs. Mitotic figures are rare. At cystoscopy, PUNLMPs tend to be larger than papillomas and may be indistinguishable from low- and high-grade papillary cancers. PUNLMPs may recur

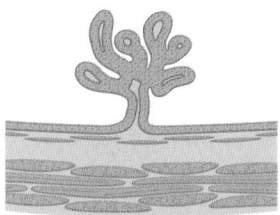

Papilloma– papillary carcinoma

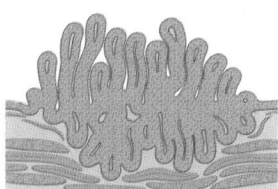

Invasive papillary carcinoma

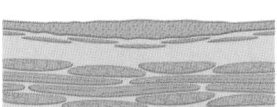

Flat noninvasive carcinoma (CIS)

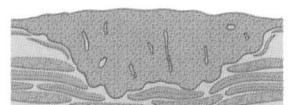

Flat invasive carcinoma

FIGURE 21–6 Four morphologic patterns of bladder tumors. CIS, carcinoma in situ.

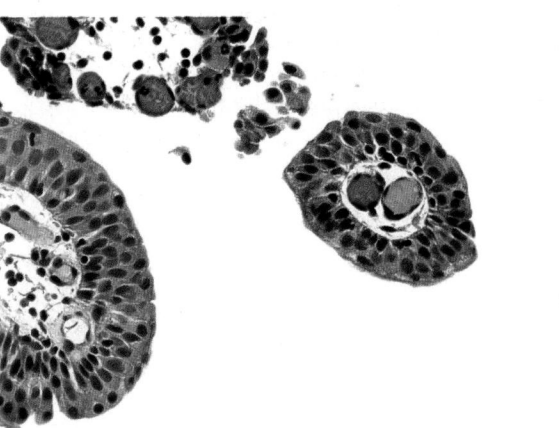

FIGURE 21–8 Papilloma consisting of small papillary fronds lined by normal-appearing urothelium.

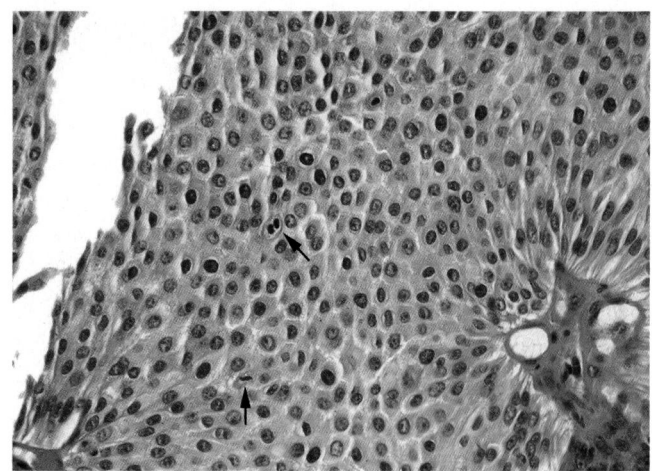

FIGURE 21–9 Low-grade papillary urothelial carcinoma with an overall orderly appearance, with a thicker lining than papilloma and scattered hyperchromatic nuclei and mitotic figures *(arrows)*.

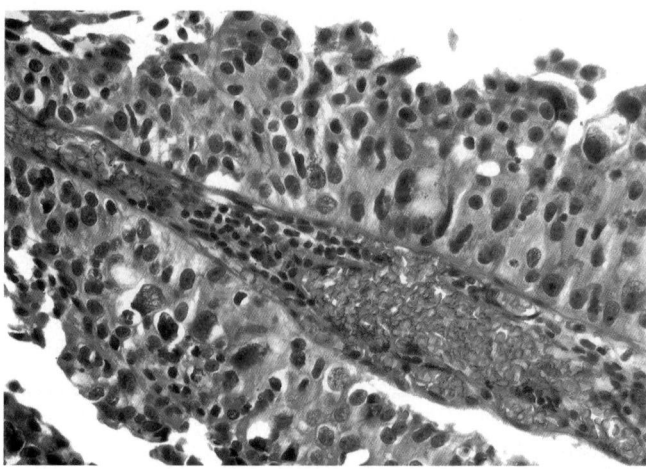

FIGURE 21–10 High-grade papillary urothelial carcinoma with marked cytologic atypia.

with the same morphology, are not associated with invasion, and only rarely recur as higher grade tumors associated with invasion and progression.

- **Low-grade papillary urothelial carcinomas** are characterized by an orderly appearance both architecturally and cytologically. The cells are evenly spaced (i.e., maintain polarity) and cohesive. There is minimal but definite evidence of nuclear atypia consisting of scattered hyperchromatic nuclei, infrequent mitotic figures predominantly toward the base, and mild variation in nuclear size and shape (Fig. 21–9). Low-grade cancers can recur and, though infrequent, can invade. Only rarely do these tumors pose a threat to the patient's life.

- **High-grade papillary urothelial cancers** contain cells that may be dyscohesive with large hyperchromatic nuclei. Some of the tumor cells show frank anaplasia (Fig. 21–10). Mitotic figures, including atypical ones, are frequent. Architecturally, there is disarray and loss of polarity. These tumors have a much higher incidence of invasion into the muscular layer, a higher risk of progression than low-grade lesions, and, when associated with invasion, a significant metastatic potential.

In most analyses, less than 10% of low-grade cancers invade, but as many as 80% of high-grade urothelial carcinomas are invasive.[21,22] Aggressive tumors may extend not only into the bladder wall, but, in more advanced stages, invade the adjacent prostate, seminal vesicles, ureters, and retroperitoneum. Some tumors produce fistulous communications to the vagina or rectum. About 40% of these deeply invasive tumors metastasize to regional lymph nodes. Hematogenous dissemination, principally to the liver, lungs, and bone marrow, may result.

Carcinoma in situ (CIS or flat urothelial carcinoma) is defined by the presence of cytologically malignant

cells within a flat urothelium.[16,23–26] CIS may range from full-thickness cytologic atypia to scattered malignant cells in an otherwise normal urothelium, the latter termed **pagetoid spread** (Fig. 21–11). A common feature similar to high-grade papillary urothelial carcinoma is the lack of cohesiveness, which leads to the shedding of malignant cells into the urine. When shedding is widespread, it may result in a denuded urothelium with only a few CIS cells clinging to the basement membrane. CIS usually appears grossly as an area of mucosal reddening, granularity, or thicken-

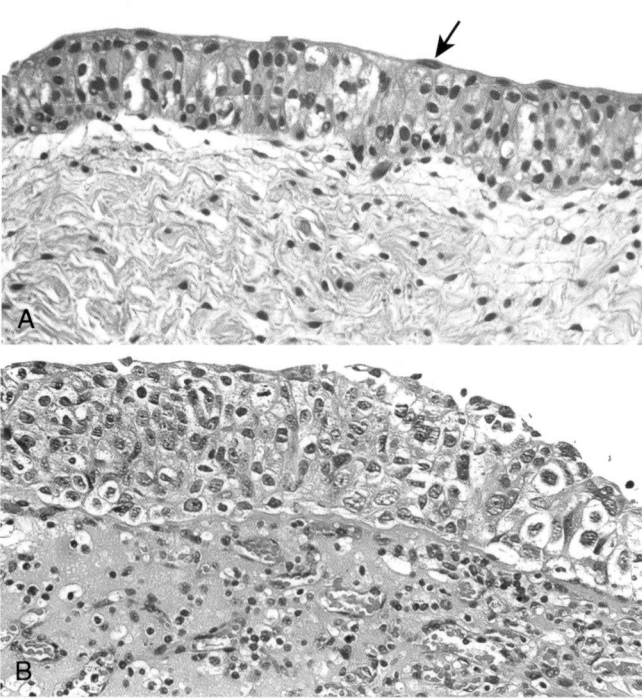

FIGURE 21–11 **A**, Normal urothelium with uniform nuclei and well-developed umbrella cell layer *(arrow)*. **B**, Flat carcinoma in situ with numerous cells having enlarged and pleomorphic nuclei.

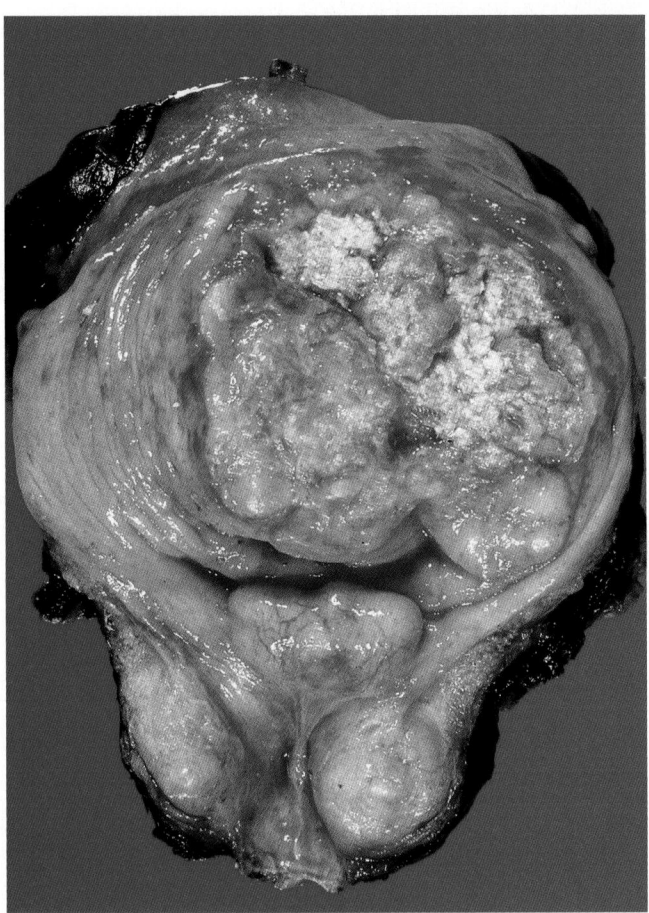

FIGURE 21–12 Opened bladder showing a high-grade invasive transitional cell carcinoma at an advanced stage. The aggressive multinodular neoplasm has fungated into the bladder lumen and spread over a wide area. The yellow areas represent areas of ulceration and necrosis.

ing without producing an evident intraluminal mass. It is commonly multifocal and may involve most of the bladder surface and extend into the ureters and urethra. If untreated, 50% to 75% of CIS cases progress to muscle-invasive cancer.

Invasive urothelial cancer (Fig. 21–12) may be associated with papillary urothelial cancer, usually high grade, or CIS. The extent of the invasion into the muscularis mucosae is of prognostic significance, and understaging on biopsy is a significant problem. The extent of spread **(staging)** at the time of initial diagnosis is the most important factor in determining the outlook for a patient (Table 21–4). Almost all infiltrating urothelial carcinomas are high grade, such that grading of the infiltrating component is not critical, as opposed to the importance of grading noninvasive papillary urothelial carcinoma.

Variants of Urothelial Carcinoma. Unusual variants of urothelial cancer include the nested variant with deceptively bland cytology, lymphoepithelioma-like carcinoma, and micropapillary carcinoma.[27–32]

Other Epithelial Tumors. **Squamous cell carcinomas** represent about 3% to 7% of bladder cancers in the United States, but in countries where urinary schistosomiasis is endemic, they occur much more frequently.[33,34] Pure squamous cell carcinomas are nearly always associated with chronic bladder irritation and infection. **Mixed urothelial carcinomas with areas of squamous carcinoma** are more frequent than pure squamous cell carcinomas. Most are invasive, fungating tumors or are infiltrative and ulcerative. The level of cytologic differentiation varies widely, from highly differentiated lesions producing abundant keratin to more anaplastic tumors with only focal evidence of squamous differentiation.

Adenocarcinomas of the bladder are rare and histologically identical to adenocarcinomas seen in the gastrointestinal tract.[35,36] Some arise from urachal remnants or in association with extensive intestinal metaplasia (discussed earlier).

Small-cell carcinomas, indistinguishable from small-cell carcinomas of the lung, arise in the bladder often in association with urothelial, squamous, or adenocarcinoma.[37]

Epidemiology and Pathogenesis. The incidence of carcinoma of the bladder is higher in men than in women, in developed than in developing nations, and in urban than in rural dwellers. The male-to-female ratio for urothelial tumors is approximately 3:1. About 80% of patients are between the ages of 50 and 80 years. Bladder cancer, with rare exceptions, is not familial.

Several factors have been implicated in the causation of urothelial carcinoma. Some of the more important contributors include the following:

○ *Cigarette smoking* is clearly the most important influence, increasing the risk threefold to sevenfold, depending on the pack-years and smoking habits. Between 50% and 80% of all bladder cancers among men are associated with the use of cigarettes. Cigars, pipes, and smokeless tobacco are associated with a smaller risk.

○ *Industrial exposure to arylamines,* particularly 2-naphthylamine as well as related compounds, as pointed out in the discussion of chemical carcinogenesis (Chapter 7). The cancers appear 15 to 40 years after the first exposure.

○ *Schistosoma haematobium* infections in endemic areas (Egypt, Sudan) are an established risk. The ova are

TABLE 21–4	Pathologic T (Primary Tumor) Staging of Bladder Carcinoma
Depth of Invasion	**AJCC/UICC**
Ta	Noninvasive, papillary
Tis	Carcinoma in situ (noninvasive, flat)
T1	Lamina propria invasion
T2	Muscularis propria invasion
T3a	Microscopic extra-vesicle invasion
T3b	Grossly apparent extra-vesicle invasion
T4	Invades adjacent structures

AJCC/UICC, American Joint Commission on Cancer/Union Internationale Contre le Cancer.

deposited in the bladder wall and incite a brisk chronic inflammatory response that induces progressive mucosal squamous metaplasia and dysplasia and, in some instances, neoplasia. Seventy percent of the cancers are squamous, the remainder being urothelial or, least commonly, glandular.

- Long-term use of analgesics is implicated, as it is in analgesic nephropathy (Chapter 20).
- Heavy long-term exposure to cyclophosphamide, an immunosuppressive agent, induces, as noted, hemorrhagic cystitis, and increases the risk of bladder cancer.
- Prior exposure of the bladder to irradiation, often administered for other pelvic malignancies, increases the risk of urothelial carcinoma. In this setting, bladder cancer occurs many years after the irradiation.

Several genetic alterations have been observed in urothelial carcinoma.[38-42] Particularly common (occurring in 30% to 60% of tumors) are chromosome 9 monosomy or deletions of 9p and 9q as well as deletions of 17p, 13q, 11p, and 14q. The *chromosome 9 deletions are the only genetic changes present frequently in superficial papillary tumors and occasionally in noninvasive flat tumors.* The 9p deletions (9p21) involve the tumor suppressor gene *p16 (INK4a)*, which encodes an inhibitor of a cyclin-dependent kinase (Chapter 7), and also the related tumor suppressor gene *p15*. The identity of the putative second tumor suppressor locus on chromosome 9q is not yet known. On the other hand, many invasive urothelial carcinomas show *deletions of 17p*, including the region of the *p53* gene, as well as mutations in *p53*, suggesting that alterations in p53 contribute to the progression of urothelial carcinoma. Mutations in *p53* are also found in CIS.

On the basis of these findings, a model for bladder carcinogenesis has been proposed. In this two-pathway model the first pathway is *initiated by deletions of tumor suppressor genes* on 9p and 9q, leading to superficial papillary tumors, a few of which may then acquire p53 mutations and progress to invasion; a second pathway, possibly *initiated by p53 mutations*, leads to CIS and, with loss of chromosome 9, progression to invasion (Chapter 7).

Clinical Course of Bladder Cancer. Bladder tumors classically produce *painless hematuria*. This is their dominant and sometimes only clinical manifestation. Frequency, urgency, and dysuria occasionally accompany the hematuria. When the ureteral orifice is involved, pyelonephritis or hydronephrosis may follow. About 60% of neoplasms, when first discovered, are single, and 70% are localized to the bladder.

Individuals with urothelial tumors, whatever their grade, have a tendency to develop new tumors after excision, and *recurrences* may show a higher grade. The risk of recurrence and progression is related to several variables, including tumor size, stage, grade, multifocality, prior recurrence rate, and associated dysplasia and/or CIS in the surrounding mucosa.[43-48] Although the term recurrence is used, most of the subsequent tumors arise at different sites from the original lesion. Recurrent tumors reflect in some cases new tumors, and in other instances they share the same clonal abnormalities as the initial tumor and represent a true recurrence of the initial lesion caused by shedding and implantation of the original tumor cells.

The prognosis depends on the histologic grade of the papillary tumor and the stage at diagnosis. Papillomas, papillary urothelial neoplasms of low malignant potential, and low-grade papillary urothelial cancer yield a 98% 10-year survival rate regardless of the number of recurrences; only a few patients (<10%) have progression of their disease to higher grade lesions. High-grade papillary urothelial carcinomas invade and lead to death in about 25% of cases. Patients with primary (de novo) CIS, as opposed to CIS associated with infiltrating urothelial carcinoma, are less likely to progress to muscle-invasive cancer (28% versus 59%) or die of disease (7% versus 45%).[49] Invasive urothelial carcinoma is associated with a 30% mortality rate once tumor invades into the lamina propria. Overall, squamous cell carcinoma and adenocarcinoma are associated with a worse prognosis than urothelial carcinoma, yet stage for stage they are all similar.

The clinical challenge with these neoplasms is early detection and adequate follow-up. A significant issue is that 50% of invasive bladder cancers present with muscle-invasive disease and a relatively poor prognosis despite therapy. For tumors detected at an earlier stage, cystoscopy and biopsy are the mainstays of diagnosis. Of value in these circumstances are *cytologic examinations* and newer urine tests that detect the presence of various markers such as human complement factor H–related protein, telomerase, fibrin-fibrinogen degradation products, mucins, carcinoembryonic antigen, hyaluronic acid, hyaluronidase, nuclear matrix proteins, and chromosomal abnormalities detected by fluorescent in situ hybridization in cells in the urine.[50,51] The major limitation of cytologic examination is the under-recognition of low-grade papillary neoplasms, whereas tests measuring urine markers have relatively low specificity, due to positive results caused by other conditions associated with injured urothelium.

The treatment for bladder cancer depends on the grade, stage, and whether the lesion is flat or papillary.[52] For small, localized papillary tumors that are not high grade, the initial diagnostic transurethral resection is the only surgical procedure done. Patients are closely followed with periodic cystoscopies and urine cytologies for the rest of their lives to detect recurrence. Research is ongoing to determine whether less invasive urine marker studies can be used as follow-up tests to increase the interval between cystoscopic procedures. After the biopsy site has healed, patients at high risk of recurrence and/or progression (CIS; papillary tumors that are high grade, multifocal, have a history of rapid recurrence, or are associated with lamina propria invasion) receive topical immunotherapy consisting of intravesicle instillation of an attenuated strain of tuberculous bacillus called bacillus Calmette-Guérin (BCG). The bacteria elicit a local inflammatory reaction that destroys the tumor. Radical cystectomy is typically performed for (1) tumor invading the muscularis propria, (2) CIS or high-grade papillary cancer refractory to BCG, and (3) CIS extending into the prostatic urethra and extending down the prostatic ducts, where BCG will not come into contact with the neoplastic cells. Advanced bladder cancer is treated by chemotherapy.

Mesenchymal Tumors

Benign Tumors. A great variety of benign mesenchymal tumors may arise in the bladder, having the histologic features of their counterparts elsewhere. Collectively, they are rare. The most common is *leiomyoma*.[53] They all tend to grow as isolated, intramural, encapsulated, oval-to-spherical masses, varying in diameter up to several centimeters.

Sarcomas. True sarcomas are distinctly uncommon in the bladder. Inflammatory myofibroblastic tumors and various carcinomas may assume sarcomatoid growth patterns and be mistaken histologically for sarcomas.[54,55] As a group, sarcomas tend to produce large masses (varying up to 10 to 15 cm in diameter) that protrude into the vesicle lumen. Their soft, fleshy, gray-white gross appearance suggests their sarcomatous nature. The most common sarcoma in infancy or childhood is *embryonal rhabdomyosarcoma*.[56] In some of these cases they manifest as a polypoid grapelike mass *(sarcoma botryoides)*. The most common sarcoma in the bladder in adults is leiomyosarcoma[53] (Chapter 26).

Secondary Tumors

Secondary malignant involvement of the bladder is most often by direct extension from primary lesions in nearby organs, cervix, uterus, prostate, and rectum. Lymphomas may involve the bladder as a component of systemic disease, but also, rarely, as primary bladder lymphoma.[57]

OBSTRUCTION

Obstruction to the bladder neck is of major clinical importance, mainly because of its eventual effect on the kidney. In males the most important lesion is enlargement of the prostate gland due to nodular hyperplasia (Fig. 21–13). Bladder obstruction is somewhat less common in females and is most often caused by cystocele of the bladder. Infrequent causes are (1) congenital urethral strictures, (2) inflammatory urethral strictures, (3) inflammatory fibrosis and contraction of the bladder, (4) bladder tumors, either benign or malignant, (5) invasion of the bladder neck by tumors arising in contiguous organs, (6) mechanical obstructions caused by foreign bodies and calculi, and (7) injury to the innervation of the bladder causing neurogenic bladder.

Morphology. In the early stages there is only some thickening of the bladder wall due to smooth muscle hypertrophy. With progressive hypertrophy the individual muscle bundles greatly enlarge and produce trabeculation of the bladder wall. In the course of time, crypts form and may then become converted into diverticula.

In some cases of acute obstruction or in terminal disease when the patient's normal reflex mechanisms are depressed, the bladder may become extremely dilated. The enlarged bladder may reach the brim of the pelvis or even the level of the umbilicus. In these cases the bladder wall is markedly thinned and without trabeculations.

Urethra

INFLAMMATION

Urethritis is classically divided into gonococcal and nongonococcal. *Gonococcal urethritis* is one of the earliest manifestations of this venereal infection. *Nongonococcal urethritis* is common and can be caused by a variety of bacteria, among which *E. coli* and other enteric organisms predominate. Urethritis is often accompanied by cystitis in women and by prostatitis in men. In many instances bacteria cannot be isolated. Various strains of *Chlamydia* (e.g., *C. trachomatis*) are the cause of 25% to 60% of nongonococcal urethritis in men and about 20% in women. *Mycoplasma (Ureaplasma urealyticum)* also accounts for the symptoms of urethritis in many cases. Urethritis is also one component of *Reiter syndrome*, which comprises the clinical triad of arthritis, conjunctivitis, and urethritis (Chapter 26).

The morphologic changes are entirely typical of inflammation in other sites within the urinary tract. The urethral involvement is not itself a serious clinical problem but may cause considerable local pain, itching, and frequency, and may represent a forerunner of more serious disease at higher levels of the urogenital tract.

TUMORS AND TUMOR-LIKE LESIONS

Urethral caruncle is an inflammatory lesion presenting as a small, red, painful mass about the external urethral meatus, typically in older females. It may be covered by an intact mucosa but is extremely friable, and the slightest trauma may cause ulceration of the surface and bleeding. On histologic examination, it is composed of an inflamed granulation tissue polyp. Surgical excision affords prompt relief and cure.

Benign epithelial tumors of the urethra include squamous and urothelial papillomas, inverted urothelial papillomas, and condylomas.

Peyronie disease results in fibrous bands involving the corpus cavernosum of the penis. Although some classify it as a variant of fibromatosis, its etiology remains an enigma. Clinically, the lesion results in penile curvature and pain during intercourse.

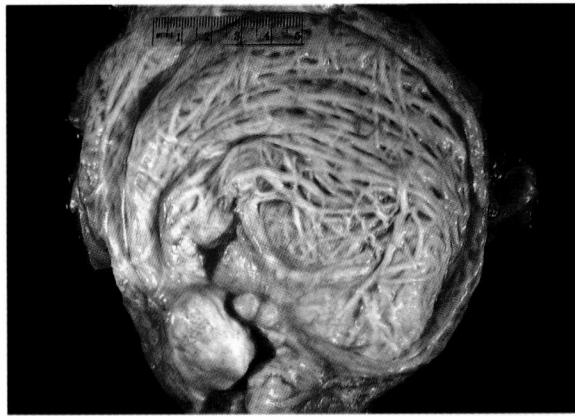

FIGURE 21–13 Hypertrophy and trabeculation of bladder wall secondary to polypoid hyperplasia of the prostate.

Primary *carcinoma of the urethra* is an uncommon lesion (Fig. 21–14). Tumors arising within the proximal urethra tend to show urothelial differentiation and are analogous to those occurring within the bladder. Those lesions found within the distal urethra are more typically squamous carcinomas. Glandular carcinomas occur less frequently in the urethra generally in women. A rare variant is clear cell adenocarcinoma. Some neoplastic lesions of the urethra are similar to those described in the bladder, arising through metaplasia or, less commonly, from periurethral glands. Cancers arising within the prostatic urethra are dealt with in the section on the prostate.

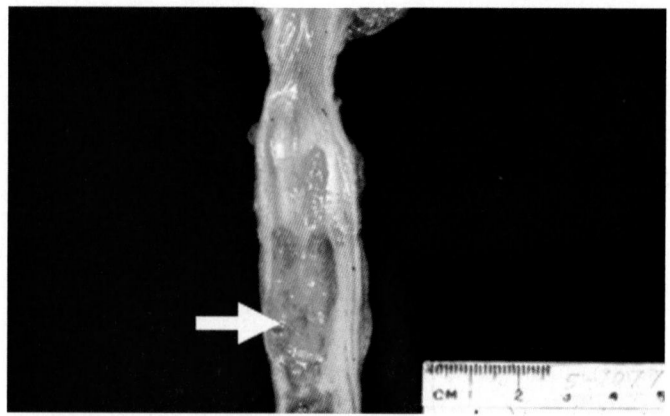

FIGURE 21–14 Carcinoma of urethra with typical fungating growth.

THE MALE GENITAL TRACT

Penis

The penis can be affected by congenital anomalies, inflammations, and tumors, inflammations and tumors being the most important. The venereal infections (e.g., syphilis and gonorrhea) usually begin with penile lesions. Carcinoma of the penis is an uncommon neoplasm in North America.

CONGENITAL ANOMALIES

The penis is the site of many forms of congenital anomalies, only some of which have clinical significance.

Hypospadias and Epispadias

Malformation of the urethral groove and urethral canal may create abnormal openings either on the *ventral surface of the penis (hypospadias)* or on the *dorsal surface (epispadias)*.[58] Though more frequent with epispadias, either of these two anomalies may be associated with failure of normal descent of the testes and with malformations of the urinary tract. Hypospadias, the more common of the two, occurs in approximately 1 in 300 live male births.[59] Even when isolated, these urethral defects may have clinical significance, because the abnormal opening is often constricted, resulting in urinary tract obstruction and an increased risk of ascending urinary tract infections. When the orifices are situated near the base of the penis, normal ejaculation and insemination are hampered or totally blocked. These lesions therefore are possible causes of sterility in men.

Phimosis

When the orifice of the prepuce is too small to permit its normal retraction, the condition is designated *phimosis*. Such an abnormally small orifice may result from anomalous development but is more frequently the result of repeated attacks of infection that cause scarring of the preputial ring.[60] Phimosis is important because it interferes with cleanliness and permits the accumulation of secretions and detritus under the prepuce, favoring the development of secondary infections and possibly carcinoma.

INFLAMMATION

Inflammations of the penis almost invariably involve the glans and prepuce and include a wide variety of specific and nonspecific infections. The specific infections—syphilis, gonorrhea, chancroid, granuloma inguinale, lymphopathia venerea, genital herpes—are sexually transmitted and are discussed in Chapter 8. Only the nonspecific infections causing so-called balanoposthitis require description here.

Balanoposthitis refers to infection of the glans and prepuce caused by a wide variety of organisms. Among the more common agents are *Candida albicans*, anaerobic bacteria, *Gardnerella*, and pyogenic bacteria.[61] Most cases occur as a consequence of poor local hygiene in uncircumcised males, with accumulation of desquamated epithelial cells, sweat, and debris, termed *smegma*, acting as local irritant. Persistence of such infections leads to inflammatory scarring and, as mentioned earlier, is a common cause of phimosis.

TUMORS

Tumors of the penis are, on the whole, uncommon. The most frequent neoplasms are carcinomas and a benign epithelial tumor, condyloma acuminatum.

Benign Tumors

Condyloma Acuminatum

Condyloma acuminatum is a benign sexually transmitted tumor caused by human papillomavirus (HPV). It is related

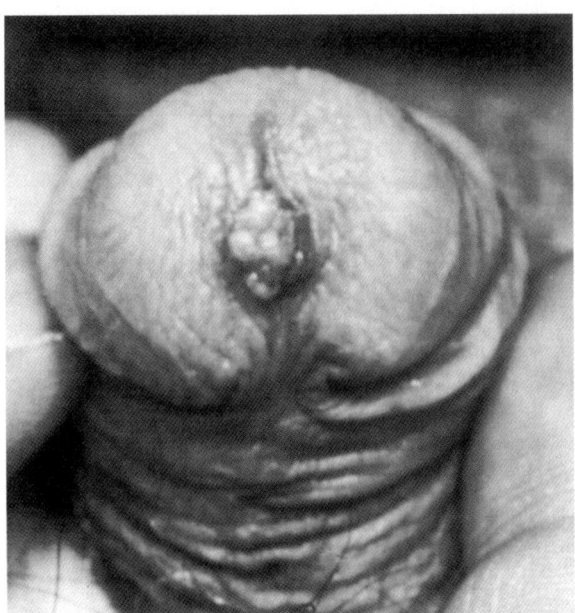

FIGURE 21–15 Condyloma acuminatum of the penis.

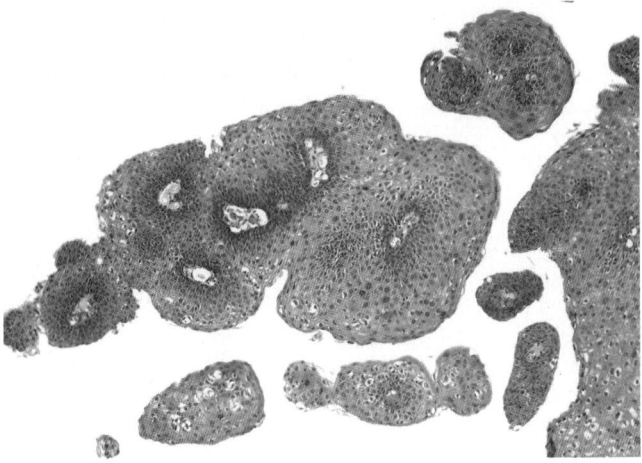

FIGURE 21–16 Condyloma acuminatum of the penis. Low magnification reveals the papillary (villous) architecture, and thickening of the epidermis.

to the common wart and may occur on any moist mucocutaneous surface of the external genitals in either sex. HPV type 6, and less frequently type 11, are the most frequent agents that cause condylomata acuminata.

> **Morphology.** Condylomata acuminata may occur on the external genitalia or perineal areas. On the penis these lesions occur most often about the coronal sulcus and inner surface of the prepuce. They consist of single or multiple sessile or pedunculated, red papillary excrescences that vary from 1 mm to several millimeters in diameter (Fig. 21–15). Histologically a branching, villous, papillary connective tissue stroma is covered by epithelium that may have considerable superficial hyperkeratosis and thickening of the underlying epidermis (acanthosis) (Fig. 21–16). The normal orderly maturation of the epithelial cells is preserved. Cytoplasmic vacuolization of the squamous cells (koilocytosis), characteristic of HPV infection, is noted in these lesions (Fig. 21–17). Cells may have degenerative (viral) atypia but true dysplasia is rare. Condylomata acuminata tend to recur but only rarely progress into in situ or invasive cancers.

Malignant Tumors

Carcinoma in Situ (CIS)

In the external male genitalia, two distinct lesions display histologic features of CIS: *Bowen disease* and *bowenoid papulosis*. These lesions have a strong association with infection by HPV, most commonly type 16.[62]

Bowen disease occurs in the genital region of both men and women, usually in those over the age of 35 years. In men it tends to involve the skin of the shaft of the penis and the scrotum. Grossly it appears as a solitary, thickened, gray-white, opaque plaque. It can also manifest on the glans and prepuce as single or multiple shiny red, sometimes velvety plaques.

Histologically the epidermis shows proliferation with numerous mitoses, some atypical. The cells are markedly dysplastic with large hyperchromatic nuclei and lack of orderly maturation (Fig. 21–18). Nevertheless, *the dermal-epidermal border is sharply delineated by an intact basement membrane.* Over the span of years, Bowen disease may transform into infiltrating squamous cell carcinoma in approximately 10% of patients. Bowen disease may also be associated with visceral cancer, such as that of the colon or breast, but not as frequently as initially reported.

Bowenoid papulosis occurs in sexually active adults. Clinically, it differs from Bowen disease by the younger age of patients and the presence of multiple (rather than solitary) reddish brown papular lesions. Histologically, bowenoid papulosis is indistinguishable from Bowen disease and is also related to HPV type 16. However, in contrast to Bowen disease, bowenoid papulosis virtually never develops into an invasive carcinoma and in many cases spontaneously regresses.

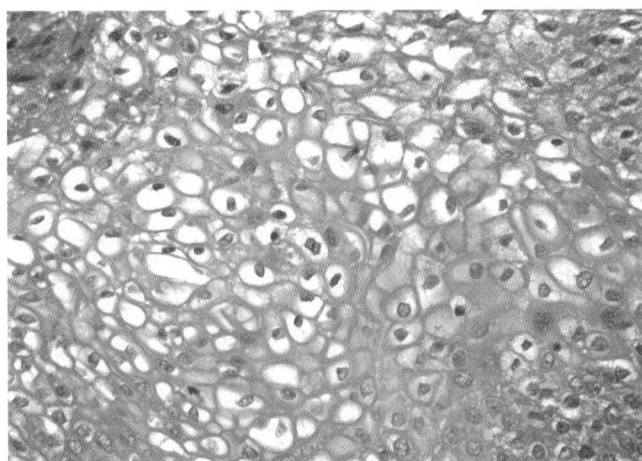

FIGURE 21–17 Condyloma acuminatum of the penis. The epithelium shows vacuolization (koilocytosis) characteristic of human papillomavirus infection.

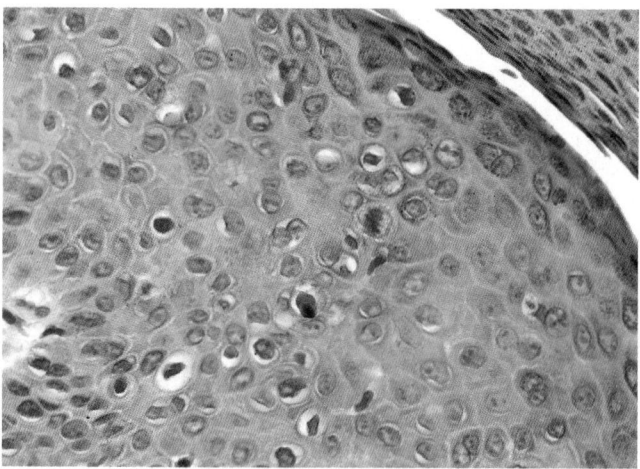

FIGURE 21–18 Bowen disease (carcinoma in situ) of the penis. Note the hyperchromatic, dysplastic dyskeratotic epithelial cells with scattered mitoses above the basal layer. The intact basement membrane is not readily seen in this picture.

Invasive Carcinoma

Squamous cell carcinoma of the penis is an uncommon malignancy in the United States, accounting for fewer than 1% of cancers in males. By contrast, in some parts of Asia, Africa, and South America the incidence of squamous cell carcinoma of the penis ranges from 10% to 20% of male malignancies. Circumcision confers protection, and hence this cancer is extremely rare among Jews and Moslems and is correspondingly more common in populations in which circumcision is not routinely practiced. It is postulated that circumcision is associated with better genital hygiene, which, in turn, reduces exposure to carcinogens that may be concentrated in smegma and decreases the likelihood of infection with potentially oncogenic types of HPV. HPV DNA can be detected in penile squamous cancer in approximately 50% of patients.[62] HPV type 16 is the most frequent culprit, but HPV 18 is also implicated. Cigarette smoking elevates the risk of developing cancer of the penis.[63] Carcinomas are usually found in patients between the ages of 40 and 70.

Morphology. Squamous cell carcinoma of the penis usually begins on the glans or inner surface of the prepuce near the coronal sulcus. Two macroscopic patterns are seen—papillary and flat. The papillary lesions simulate condylomata acuminata and may produce a cauliflower-like fungating mass. Flat lesions appear as areas of epithelial thickening accompanied by graying and fissuring of the mucosal surface. With progression, an ulcerated papule develops (Fig. 21–19). Histologically, both the papillary and the flat lesions are squamous cell carcinomas with varying degrees of differentiation. **Verrucous carcinoma** is an exophytic well-differentiated variant of squamous cell carcinoma that has low malignant potential. These tumors are locally invasive, but they rarely metastasize. Other, less common, subtypes of penile squamous carcinoma include basaloid, warty, and papillary variants.[64,65]

Clinical Features. Invasive squamous cell carcinoma of the penis is a slowly growing, locally invasive lesion that often has been present for a year or more before it is brought to medical attention.[66] The lesions are nonpainful until they undergo secondary ulceration and infection. Metastases to inguinal lymph nodes characterize the early stage, but widespread dissemination is extremely uncommon until the lesion is far advanced. Clinical assessment of regional lymph node involvement is notoriously inaccurate; 50% of men with penile squamous cell carcinoma and clinically enlarged inguinal nodes have only reactive lymphoid hyperplasia when examined histologically. The prognosis is related to the stage of the tumor. In persons with limited lesions without invasion of the inguinal lymph nodes, there is a 66% 5-year survival rate, whereas metastasis to the lymph nodes carries a grim 27% 5-year survival.

Testis and Epididymis

Distinct pathological conditions affect the testis and epididymis. In the epididymis, the most important and frequent conditions are inflammatory diseases, whereas in the testis the major lesions are tumors.

CONGENITAL ANOMALIES

With the exception of undescended testes (cryptorchidism), congenital anomalies are extremely rare and include absence of one or both testes and fusion of the testes (so-called *synorchism*).

Cryptorchidism

Cryptorchidism is found in approximately 1% of 1-year-old boys.[67] This anomaly represents a complete or incomplete failure of the intra-abdominal testes to descend into the scrotal sac. It usually occurs as an isolated anomaly but may be accompanied by other malformations of the genitourinary tract, such as hypospadias.

Testicular descent occurs in two morphologically and hormonally distinct phases.[68] During the first, the transabdomi-

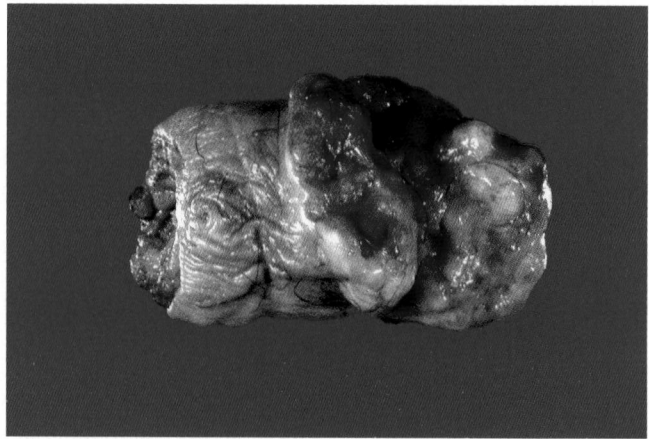

FIGURE 21–19 Carcinoma of the penis. The glans penis is deformed by a firm, ulcerated, infiltrative mass.

nal, phase, the testis comes to lie within the lower abdomen or brim of the pelvis. This phase is believed to be controlled by a hormone called *müllerian-inhibiting substance.* In the second, or the inguinoscrotal, phase, the testes descend through the inguinal canal into the scrotal sac. This phase is androgen dependent and is possibly mediated by androgen-induced release of calcitonin gene–related peptide, from the genito-femoral nerve. Although testes may be arrested anywhere along their pathway of descent, defects in transabdominal descent are uncommon, accounting for approximately 5% to 10% of cases. In most patients the undescended testis is palpable in the inguinal canal. *Even though testicular descent is controlled by hormonal factors, cryptorchidism is only rarely associated with a well-defined hormonal disorder.* The condition is completely asymptomatic, and it is found by the patient or the examining physician only when the scrotal sac is discovered not to contain the testis.

> **Morphology.** Cryptorchidism is unilateral in most cases, but it may be bilateral in 25% of patients. Histologic changes in the malpositioned testis begin as early as 2 years of age. They are characterized by an arrest in the development of germ cells associated with marked hyalinization and thickening of the basement membrane of the spermatic tubules (Fig. 21–20). Eventually the tubules appear as dense cords of hyaline connective tissue outlined by prominent basement membranes. There is concomitant increase in interstitial stroma. Because Leydig cells are spared, they appear to be prominent. As might be expected with progressive tubular atrophy, the cryptorchid testis is small in size and is firm in consistency as a result of fibrotic changes. Histologic deterioration, associated with a paucity of germ cells, has also been noted in the contralateral (descended) testis in males with unilateral cryptorchidism, supporting an intrinsic defect in testicular development.

In addition to sterility, cryptorchidism can be associated with other morbidity. When the testis lies in the inguinal canal, it is particularly exposed to trauma and crushing against the ligaments and bones. A concomitant inguinal hernia accompanies the undescended testis in about 10% to 20% of cases. In addition, the undescended testis is at a greater risk of developing testicular cancer than is the descended testis.[69] During the first year of life the majority of inguinal cryptorchid testes descend spontaneously into the scrotum. Those that remain undescended require surgical correction, preferably before histologic deterioration sets in at around 2 years of age.[70] Orchiopexy (placement in the scrotal sac) does not guarantee fertility; deficient spermatogenesis has been reported in 10% to 60% of patients in whom surgical repositioning was performed.[67,70] To what extent the risk of cancer is reduced after orchiopexy is also unclear. According to some studies, orchiopexy of unilateral cryptorchidism before 10 years of age protects against cancer development.[71] This is not universally accepted, however.[72] Malignant change may occur in the contralateral, normally descended testis. These observations suggest that cryptorchidism is associated with a defect in testicular development and cellular differentiation that is unrelated to anatomic position.

REGRESSIVE CHANGES

Atrophy and Decreased Fertility

Atrophy is a regressive change that affects the scrotal testis and can have any of several causes, including (1) progressive atherosclerotic narrowing of the blood supply in old age, (2) the end stage of an inflammatory orchitis, (3) cryptorchidism, (4) hypopituitarism, (5) generalized malnutrition or cachexia, (6) irradiation, (7) prolonged administration of antiandrogens (treatment for advanced carcinoma of the prostate), and (8) exhaustion atrophy, which may follow the persistent stimulation produced by high levels of follicle-stimulating pituitary hormone. The gross and microscopic alterations follow the pattern already described for cryptorchidism. *Atrophy*

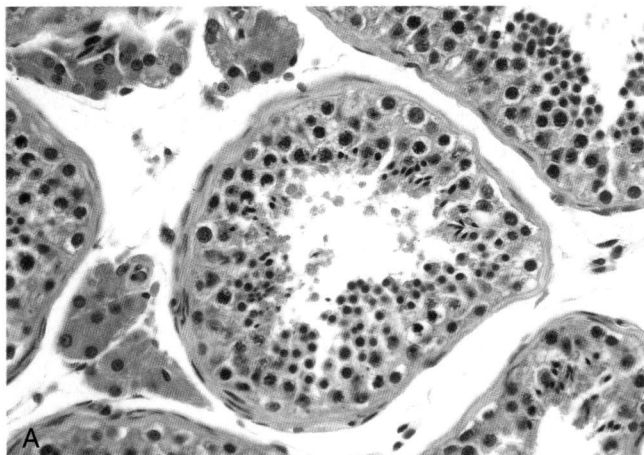
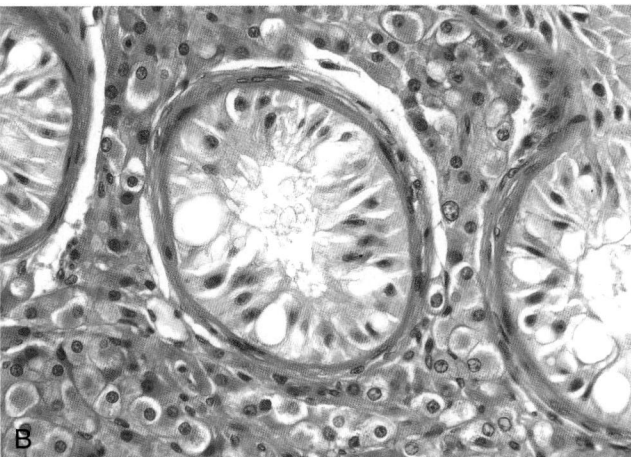

FIGURE 21–20 **A,** Normal testis shows tubules with active spermatogenesis. **B,** Testicular atrophy in cryptorchidism. The tubules show Sertoli cells but no spermatogenesis. There is thickening of basement membranes and an apparent increase in interstitial Leydig cells.

occasionally occurs as a primary failure of genetic origin, such as in Klinefelter syndrome (discussed in Chapter 5).

Atrophy is an end-stage pattern of testicular injury. Before this terminal histologic appearance is reached, several other patterns are associated with decreased fertility.[73] These include hypospermatogenesis, maturation arrest, and findings associated with vas deferens obstruction. In some instances a specific cause for the testicular injury can be found, and if it can be removed before the development of atrophy, testicular function can be restored.

INFLAMMATION

Inflammations are distinctly more common in the epididymis than in the testis. Of the three major specific inflammatory states that affect the testis and epididymis, *gonorrhea and tuberculosis almost invariably arise in the epididymis, whereas syphilis affects first the testis.*

Nonspecific Epididymitis and Orchitis

Epididymitis and possible subsequent orchitis are commonly related to infections in the urinary tract (cystitis, urethritis, prostatitis), which reach the epididymis and the testis through either the vas deferens or the lymphatics of the spermatic cord.

The cause of epididymitis varies with the age of the patient. Though uncommon in children, epididymitis in childhood is usually associated with a congenital genitourinary abnormality and infection with gram-negative rods. In sexually active men younger than age 35 years, the sexually transmitted pathogens *C. trachomatis* and *Neisseria gonorrhoeae* are the most frequent culprits. In men older than age 35 the common urinary tract pathogens, such as *E. coli* and *Pseudomonas*, are responsible for most infections.

> **Morphology.** The bacterial invasion induces nonspecific acute inflammation characterized by congestion, edema, and infiltration by neutrophils, macrophages, and lymphocytes. Although the infection, in the early stage, is more or less limited to the interstitial connective tissue, it rapidly extends to involve the tubules and may progress to frank abscess formation or complete suppurative necrosis of the entire epididymis (Fig. 21–21). Usually, having involved the epididymis, the infection extends into the testis to evoke a similar inflammatory reaction. Such inflammatory involvement of the epididymis and testis is often followed by fibrous scarring, which in many cases leads to sterility. Usually the interstitial cells of Leydig are not totally destroyed, so sexual activity is not disturbed.

Granulomatous (Autoimmune) Orchitis

Idiopathic granulomatous orchitis presents in middle age as a moderately tender testicular mass of sudden onset sometimes associated with fever. It may appear insidiously, however, as a painless testicular mass mimicking a testicular tumor, hence its importance. Histologically the orchitis is distinguished by granulomas restricted to spermatic tubules. The lesions closely

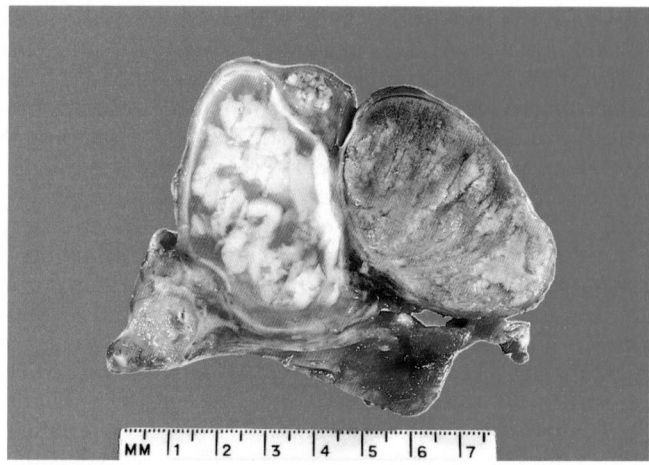

FIGURE 21–21 Acute epididymitis caused by gonococcal infection. The epididymis is replaced by an abscess. Normal testis is seen on the *right.*

resemble tubercles but differ in that the granulomatous reaction is present diffusely throughout the testis and is confined to the seminiferous tubules. Although an autoimmune basis is suspected, the cause of these lesions remains unknown.

Specific Inflammations

Gonorrhea

Extension of infection from the posterior urethra to the prostate, seminal vesicles, and then to the epididymis is the usual course of a neglected gonococcal infection. Inflammatory changes similar to those described for nonspecific infections occur, with the development of frank abscesses in the epididymis, which may lead to extensive destruction of this organ. In neglected cases, the infection may spread to the testis and produce suppurative orchitis.

Mumps

Mumps is a systemic viral disease that most commonly affects school-aged children. Testicular involvement is extremely uncommon in this age group. In postpubertal males, however, orchitis may develop and has been reported in 20% to 30% of male patients. Most often, acute interstitial orchitis develops about 1 week after the onset of swelling of the parotid glands.

Tuberculosis

Tuberculosis almost invariably begins in the epididymis and may spread to the testis. The infection invokes the classic morphologic reactions of caseating granulomatous inflammation characteristic of tuberculosis elsewhere.

Syphilis

The testis and epididymis are affected in both acquired and congenital syphilis, but *almost invariably the testis is involved first by the infection.* In many cases, the orchitis is not accompanied by epididymitis. The morphologic pattern of the reaction takes two forms: the production of gummas or a diffuse interstitial inflammation characterized by edema and lymphocytic and plasma cell infiltration with the characteristic hallmark of all syphilitic infections (i.e., obliterative endarteritis with perivascular cuffing of lymphocytes and plasma cells).

VASCULAR DISORDERS

Torsion

Twisting of the spermatic cord typically cuts off the venous drainage of the testis. The thick-walled arteries remain patent, so that the intense vascular engorgement may be followed by hemorrhagic infarction. There are two types of testicular torsion. Neonatal torsion occurs either in utero or shortly after birth. It lacks any associated anatomic defect to account for its occurrence. Adult torsion is typically seen in adolescence presenting as sudden onset of testicular pain. It often occurs without any inciting injury; sudden pain heralding the torsion may even occur during sleep. *Torsion is one of the few urologic emergencies.* If the testis is explored surgically and manually untwisted within approximately 6 hours after the onset of torsion, there is a good chance that the testis will remain viable. In contrast to neonatal torsion, adult torsion results from a bilateral anatomic defect where the testis has increased mobility, giving rise to what is termed the *bell-clapper abnormality.* To prevent the catastrophic occurrence of subsequent torsion in the contralateral testis, the testis unaffected by torsion is surgically fixed to the scrotum (orchiopexy).

> **Morphology.** Depending on the duration of the process, the morphologic changes range from intense congestion to widespread extravasation of blood into the interstitial tissue to hemorrhagic testicular infarction (Fig. 21–22). In these late stages the testis is markedly enlarged and is converted virtually into a sac of soft, necrotic, hemorrhagic tissue.

SPERMATIC CORD AND PARATESTICULAR TUMORS

Lipomas are common lesions involving the proximal spermatic cord, identified at the time of inguinal hernia repair.

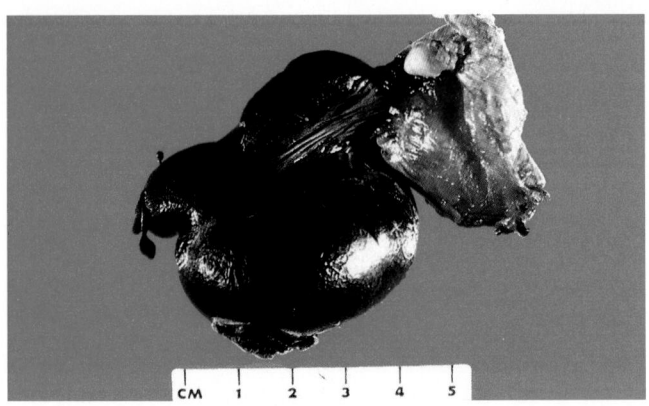

FIGURE 21–22   Torsion of testis.

TABLE 21–5   **Pathologic Classification of Common Testicular Tumors**
Germ Cell Tumors
Seminomatous tumors
Seminoma
Spermatocytic seminoma
Non-seminomatous tumors
Embryonal carcinoma,
Yolk sac (endodermal sinus) tumor
Choriocarcinoma
Teratoma
Sex Cord-Stromal Tumors
Leydig cell tumor
Sertoli cell tumor

Although diagnosed as "lipomas," many of these lesions probably represent retroperitoneal adipose tissue that has been pulled into the inguinal canal along with the hernia sac, rather than a true neoplasm.

The most common benign paratesticular tumor is *adenomatoid tumor.* Although these lesions are mesothelial in nature, they are not referred to as mesotheliomas to distinguish them from other mesothelial lesions that may occur at this site. Adenomatoid tumors are usually small nodules, typically occurring near the upper pole of the epididymis. Although grossly well circumscribed, microscopically they may be minimally invasive into the adjacent testis. The importance of this lesion is that it is one of the few benign tumors that occur near the testis. If the pathologist can identify the nature of this lesion in intraoperative frozen sections, local excision of the adenomatoid tumor can spare the patient orchiectomy.

The most common malignant paratesticular tumors located at the distal end of the spermatic cord are rhabdomyosarcomas in children and liposarcomas in adults.

TESTICULAR TUMORS

Testicular neoplasms span an amazing gamut of anatomic types.[17,74] They are divided into two major categories: germ cell tumors and sex cord–stromal tumors (Table 21–5). Approximately 95% of testicular tumors arise from germ cells. Germ cell tumors are subdivided into seminomas and nonseminomas. Most germ cell tumors are aggressive cancers capable of rapid, wide dissemination, although with current therapy most can be cured.[75] Sex cord–stromal tumors, in contrast, are generally benign.

Germ Cell Tumors

The incidence of testicular tumors in the United States is approximately 6 per 100,000, resulting in approximately 300 deaths per year. For unexplained reasons there is a worldwide increase in the incidence of these tumors. In the 15- to 34-year age group, they constitute the most common tumor of men and cause approximately 10% of all cancer deaths. In the United States these tumors are much more common in whites than in blacks (ratio 5 : 1).

Environmental Factors and Genetic Predisposition. Environmental factors play a role in the incidence of testicular germ cell tumors, as demonstrated by population migration studies. The incidence of testicular germ cell tumors in Finland is about two times lower than in Sweden; second generation Finnish immigrants to Sweden, have a tumor incidence that approaches that of the Swedish population. Testicular germ cell tumors are associated with a spectrum of disorders known as *testicular dysgenesis syndrome (TDS)*. This syndrome includes cryptorchidism, hypospadias, and poor sperm quality, and it has been proposed that some of these conditions might be influenced by in utero exposures to pesticides and nonsteroidal estrogens. Cryptorchidism, which is associated with approximately 10% of testicular germ cell tumors, is the most important risk factor. Klinefelter syndrome (a TDS condition) is associated with an increased risk (50 times greater than normal) for the development of mediastinal germ cell tumors, but these patients do not develop testicular tumors.

There is a strong family predisposition associated with the development of testicular germ cell tumors. The relative risk of development of these tumors in fathers and sons of patients with testicular germ cell tumors is four times higher than normal, and is 8 to 10 times higher between brothers. It is possible that genetic polymorphisms at the Xq27 locus may be responsible for this susceptibility, but further studies are needed to validate this hypothesis.

Classification and Pathogenesis. A simple classification of the most common types of testicular tumors is presented in Table 21–5. Two broad groups are recognized. *Seminomatous tumors* are composed of cells that ressemble primordial germ cells or early gonocytes. The *non-seminomatous tumors* may be composed of undifferentiated cells that resemble embryonic stem cells, as in the case of embryonal carcinoma, but the malignant cells can differentiate into various lineages generating yolk sac tumors, choriocarcinomas and teratomas. Germ cell tumors may have a single tissue component, but in approximately 60% of cases, the tumors contain *mixtures of seminomatous and non-seminomatous components* and multiple tissues. In teratomas, tissues of the three germ layers are represented as a result of the differentiation of embryonal carcinoma cells. Seminomas constitute approximately 50% of all testicular germ cell neoplasms and are the most common testicular tumor.

Most testicular germ cell tumors originate from lesions called *intratubular germ cell neoplasia (ITGCN)*, which is also referred to as *intratubular germ cell neoplasia unclassified (ITGCNU)*.[76,77] However, ITGCN has not been implicated as a precursor lesion of pediatric yolk sac tumors and teratomas, or of adult spermatocytic seminoma. ITGCN is believed to occur in utero and stay dormant until puberty, when it may progress into seminomas or non-seminomatous tumors. The lesion consists of atypical primordial germ cells with large nuclei and clear cytoplasm, which are about twice the size of normal germ cells. These cells retain the expression of the transcription factors *OCT3/4* and *NANOG*, which are associated with pluripontentiality (Chapter 3), and are expressed in normal embryonic stem cells. ITGCN share some of the genetic alterations found in germ cell tumors such as the gain of additional copies of the short arm of chromosome 12 (12p) in the form of an isochromosome of its short arm, i(12p). This change is invariably found in invasive tumors regardless of histological type. Activating mutations of c-KIT, which may be present in seminomas, are also present in ITGCN. About

50% of individuals with ITGCN develop invasive germ cell tumors within five years after diagnosis, and it has been proposed that practically all patients with ITGCN eventually develop invasive tumors. ITGCN is essentially a type of carcinoma in situ (CIS), although the term *CIS* is not frequently used to refer to this lesion.

Seminoma

Seminomas are the most common type of germ cell tumor, making up about 50% of these tumors. The peak incidence is the third decade and they almost never occur in infants. An identical tumor arises in the ovary, where it is called *dysgerminoma* (Chapter 22). Seminomas contain an isochromosome 12p, and express *OCT3/4* and *NANOG*. Approximately 25% of these tumors have c-KIT activating mutations. c-KIT amplification has also been repeated, but increased *c-KIT* expression may occur without genetic defects.

> **Morphology.** If not otherwise specified, "seminoma" refers to "classical" or "typical" seminoma that consists of a uniform population of cells. Spermatocytic seminoma, despite its nosologic similarity, is a distinct tumor discussed later. Seminomas produce bulky masses, sometimes ten times the size of the normal testis. The typical seminoma has a homogeneous, gray-white, lobulated cut surface, usually devoid of hemorrhage or necrosis (Fig. 21–23). Generally the tunica albuginea is not penetrated, but occasionally extension to the epididymis, spermatic cord, or scrotal sac occurs.
>
> Microscopically the typical seminoma is composed of sheets of uniform cells divided into poorly demarcated lobules by delicate septa of fibrous tissue containing a moderate amount of lymphocytes (Fig. 21–24A). **The classic seminoma cell is large and round to polyhedral and has a distinct cell membrane; a clear or watery-appearing cytoplasm; and a large, central nucleus with one or two prominent nucleoli** (Fig. 21–24B). Mitoses vary in frequency. The cytoplasm contains varying amounts of glycogen. Seminoma cells are diffusely positive for *c-KIT*, (regardless of c-KIT mutational status) *OCT4*, and placental

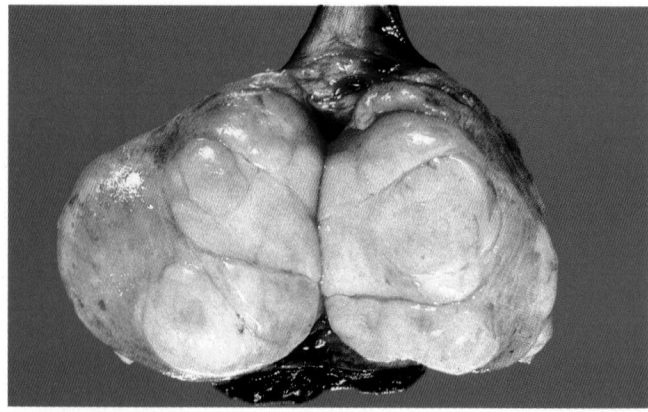

FIGURE 21–23 Seminoma of the testis appears as a fairly well-circumscribed, pale, fleshy, homogeneous mass.

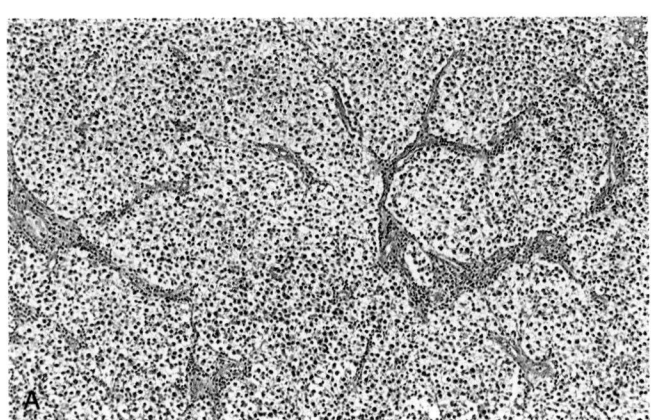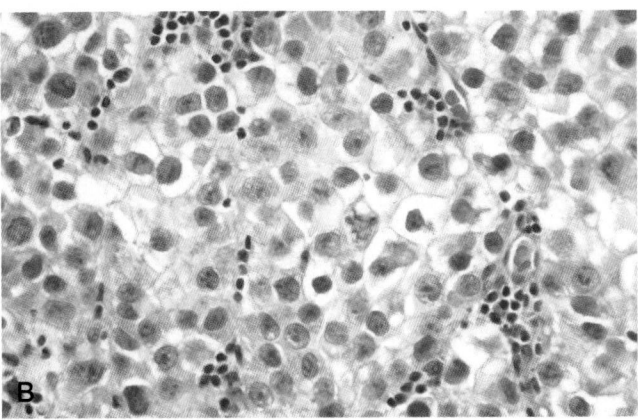

FIGURE 21–24   Seminoma. **A,** Low magnification shows clear seminoma cells divided into poorly demarcated lobules by delicate septa. **B,** Microscopic examination reveals large cells with distinct cell borders, pale nuclei, prominent nucleoli, and a sparse lymphocytic infiltrate.

alkaline phosphatase (PLAP), with sometimes scattered keratin-positive cells.

Approximately 15% of seminomas contain syncytiotrophoblasts. In this subset of patients, serum human chorionic gonadotropin (HCG) levels are elevated, though not to the extent seen in patients with choriocarcinoma. Seminomas may also be accompanied by an ill-defined granulomatous reaction, in contrast to the well-formed discrete granulomas seen with tuberculosis.

The term **anaplastic seminoma** is used by some to indicate greater cellular and nuclear irregularity with more frequent tumor giant cells and many mitoses. However, since "anaplastic seminoma" is not associated with a worse prognosis when matched stage for stage with classic seminoma and is not treated differently, most authorities do not recognize anaplastic seminoma as a distinct entity.

Spermatocytic Seminoma

Though related by name to seminoma, spermatocytic seminoma is a distinctive tumor both clinically and histologically.[78] Spermatocytic seminoma is an uncommon tumor, representing 1% to 2% of all testicular germ cell neoplasms. The age of involvement is much later than for most testicular tumors: Affected individuals are generally over the age of 65 years. In contrast to classic seminoma, it is a slow-growing tumor that does not produce metastases, and hence the prognosis is excellent. In contrast to typical seminomas, spermatocytic seminomas lack lymphocytes, granulomas, syncytiotrophoblasts, extra-testicular sites of origin, admixture with other germ cell tumors, and association with ITGCN (see "Clinical Features of Testicular Tumors" discussed later).

Morphology. Grossly, spermatocytic seminoma tends to have a soft, pale gray, cut surface that sometimes reveal mucoid cysts. Spermatocytic seminomas contain three cell populations, all intermixed: (1) medium-sized cells, the most numerous, containing a round nucleus and eosinophilic cytoplasm; (2) smaller cells with a narrow rim of eosinophilic cytoplasm resembling secondary spermatocytes; and (3) scattered giant cells, either uninucleate or multinucleate. The chromatin in some intermediate-sized cells is similar to that seen in the meiotic phase of non-neoplastic spermatocytes (spireme chromatin).

Embryonal Carcinoma

Embryonal carcinomas occur mostly in the 20- to 30-year age group. These tumors are more aggressive than seminomas.

Morphology. Grossly, the tumor is smaller than seminoma and usually does not replace the entire testis. On cut surfaces the mass is often variegated, poorly demarcated at the margins, and punctuated by foci of hemorrhage or necrosis (Fig. 21–25). Extension through the tunica albuginea into the epididymis or cord frequently occurs. **Histologically the cells grow in alveolar or tubular patterns, sometimes with papillary convolutions** (Fig. 21–26). Embryonal carcinomas lack the well-formed glands with basally situated nuclei and apical cytoplasm seen in teratomas. **More undifferentiated lesions may display sheets of cells.** The neoplastic cells have an epithelial appearance, are large and anaplastic, and have hyperchromatic nuclei with prominent nucleoli. In contrast to seminoma, the cell borders are usually indistinct, and there is considerable variation in cell and nuclear size and shape. Mitotic figures and tumor giant cells are frequently seen. Embryonal carcinomas share some markers with seminomas such as OCT 3/4 and PLAP, but differ by being positive for cytokeratin and CD30, and negative for c-KIT.[79]

Yolk Sac Tumor

Also known as *endodermal sinus tumor*, yolk sac tumor is of interest because it is the most common testicular tumor in

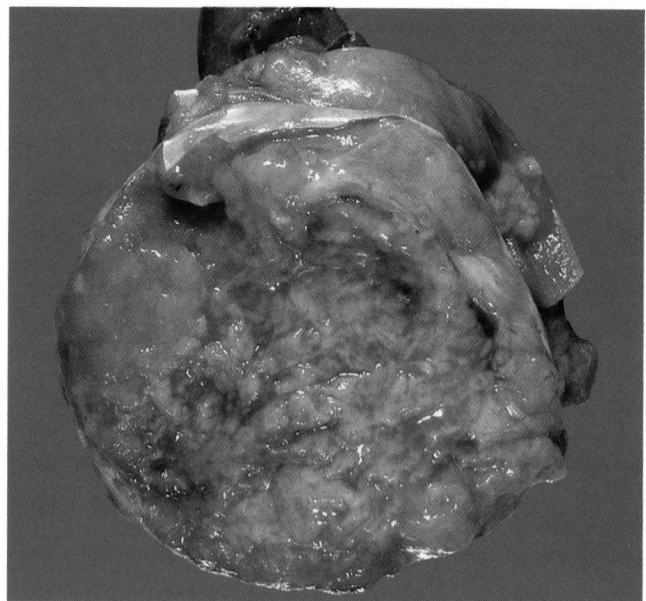

FIGURE 21–25 Embryonal carcinoma. In contrast to the seminoma illustrated in Figure 21–23, the embryonal carcinoma is a hemorrhagic mass.

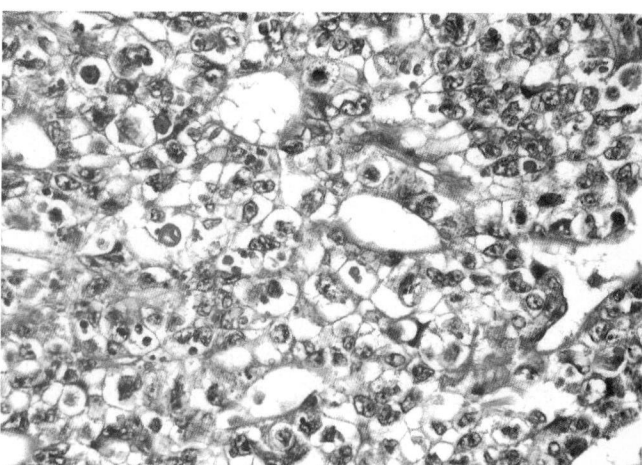

FIGURE 21–26 Embryonal carcinoma shows sheets of undifferentiated cells as well as primitive glandular differentiation. The nuclei are large and hyperchromatic.

infants and children up to 3 years of age. In this age group it has a very good prognosis. In adults the pure form of this tumor is rare; instead, yolk sac elements frequently occur in combination with embryonal carcinoma.

Morphology. Grossly, the tumor is nonencapsulated, and on cross-section it presents a homogeneous, yellow-white, mucinous appearance. Characteristic on microscopic examination is a lacelike (reticular) network of medium-sized cuboidal or flattened cells. In addition, papillary structures, solid cords of cells, and a multitude of other less common patterns may be found. In approximately 50% of tumors, structures resembling endodermal sinuses (Schiller-Duval bodies) may be seen; these consist of a mesodermal core with a central capillary and a visceral and parietal layer of cells resembling primitive glomeruli. Present within and outside the cytoplasm are eosinophilic, hyaline-like globules in which α-fetoprotein (AFP) and α₁-antitrypsin can be demonstrated by immunocytochemical staining. The presence of AFP in the tumor cells is highly characteristic, and it underscores their differentiation into yolk sac cells.

Choriocarcinoma

Choriocarcinoma is a highly malignant form of testicular tumor. In its "pure" form choriocarcinoma is rare, constituting less than 1% of all germ cell tumors.

Morphology. Often they cause no testicular enlargement and are detected only as a small palpable nodule. Typically, these tumors are small, rarely larger than 5 cm in diameter. Hemorrhage and necro-

sis are extremely common. Histologically the tumors contain two cell types (Fig. 21–27). The syncytiotrophoblastic cells are large and have many irregular or lobular hyperchromatic nuclei and an abundant eosinophilic vacuolated cytoplasm. HCG can be readily demonstrated in the cytoplasm. The cytotrophoblastic cells are more regular and tend to be polygonal, with distinct borders and clear cytoplasm; they grow in cords or masses and have a single, fairly uniform nucleus. More anatomic details are available in the discussion of these neoplasms in the female genital tract (Chapter 22).

Teratoma

The designation *teratoma* refers to a group of complex testicular tumors having various cellular or organoid components reminiscent of normal derivatives from more than one germ

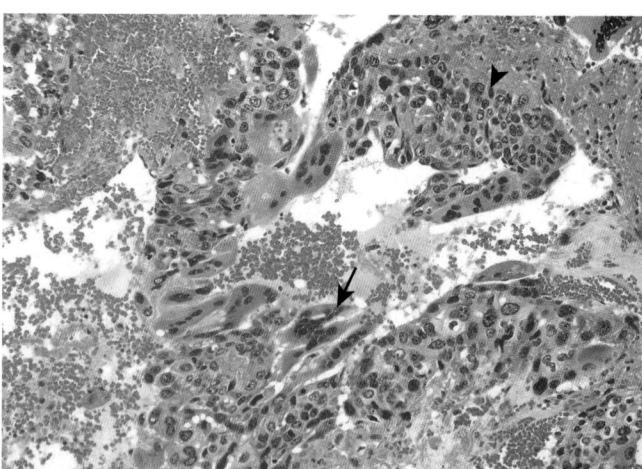

FIGURE 21–27 Choriocarcinoma shows clear cytotrophoblastic cells (arrowhead) with central nuclei and syncytiotrophoblastic cells (arrow) with multiple dark nuclei embedded in eosinophilic cytoplasm. Hemorrhage and necrosis are seen in the *upper right field*.

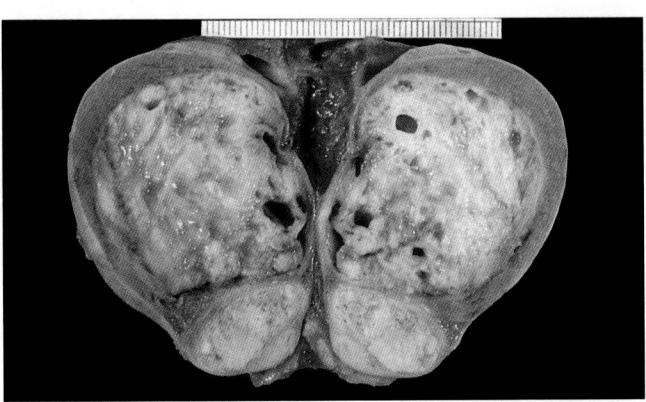

FIGURE 21–28 Teratoma of testis. The variegated cut surface with cysts reflects the multiplicity of tissue found histologically.

layer. They may occur at any age from infancy to adult life. Pure forms of teratoma are fairly common in infants and children, second in frequency only to yolk sac tumors. In adults, pure teratomas are rare, constituting 2% to 3% of germ cell tumors. However, the frequency of teratomas mixed with other germ cell tumors is approximately 45%.

Morphology. Grossly, teratomas are usually large, ranging from 5 to 10 cm in diameter. Because they are composed of various tissues, the gross appearance is heterogeneous with solid, sometimes cartilaginous, and cystic areas (Fig. 21–28). Hemorrhage and necrosis usually indicate admixture with embryonal carcinoma, choriocarcinoma, or both.

Teratomas are composed of a heterogeneous, helter-skelter collection of differentiated cells or organoid structures, such as neural tissue, muscle bundles, islands of cartilage, clusters of squamous epithelium, structures reminiscent of thyroid gland, bronchial or bronchiolar epithelium, and bits of intestinal wall or brain substance, all embedded in a fibrous or myxoid stroma (Fig. 21–29). Elements may be mature (resembling various adult tissues) or immature (sharing histologic features with fetal or embryonal tissue). Dermoid cysts and epidermoid cysts, are a form of teratoma that are common in the ovary (Chapter 22), but rare in the testis. Unlike testicular teratomas, they have a uniformly benign behavior.

Rarely, a malignant non–germ cell tumors may arise in teratoma.[80] This phenomenon is referred to as "teratoma with malignant transformation," where there is malignancy in derivatives of one or more germ cell layers. Thus, there may be a focus of squamous cell carcinoma, mucin-secreting adenocarcinoma, or sarcoma. The importance of recognizing a non–germ cell malignancy arising in a teratoma is that the non–germ cell component does not respond to chemotherapy when it spreads outside of the testis. In this case, the only hope for cure resides in the resectability of the tumor. These non–germ cell malignancies have an isochromosome 12p, similar to the germ cell tumors from which they arose.

In the child, differentiated mature teratomas usually follow a benign course. *In the postpubertal male all teratomas are regarded as malignant*, capable of metastatic behavior whether the elements are mature or immature. Consequently, it is not critical to detect immaturity in a testicular teratoma of a postpubertal male.

Mixed Tumors

About 60% of testicular tumors are composed of more than one of the "pure" patterns. Common mixtures include: teratoma, embryonal carcinoma, and yolk sac tumor; seminoma with embryonal carcinoma; and embryonal carcinoma with teratoma *(teratocarcinoma)*. In most instances the prognosis is worsened by the inclusion of the more aggressive element.

Clinical Features of Germ Cell Testicular Tumors. Although *painless enlargement of the testis* is a characteristic feature of germ cell neoplasms, *any solid testicular mass should be considered neoplastic unless proved otherwise.* Biopsy of a testicular neoplasm is associated with a risk of tumor spillage, which would necessitate excision of the scrotal skin in addition to orchiectomy. Consequently, the standard management of a solid testicular mass is radical orchiectomy based on the presumption of malignancy.

Testicular tumors have a characteristic mode of spread. *Lymphatic spread* is common to all forms of testicular tumors. In general retroperitoneal para-aortic nodes are the first to be involved. Subsequent spread may occur to mediastinal and supraclavicular nodes. *Hematogenous spread* is primarily to the lungs, but liver, brain, and bones may also be involved. The histology of metastases may sometimes be different from that of the testicular lesion. For example, an embryonal carcinoma may present a teratomatous picture in the secondary deposits. As discussed earlier, because all these tumors are derived from pluripotent germ cells, the apparent "forward" and "backward" differentiation seen in different locations is not entirely surprising. Another explanation for the differing morphologic patterns in the primary and metastatic site is that minor components in the primary tumor that were unresponsive to

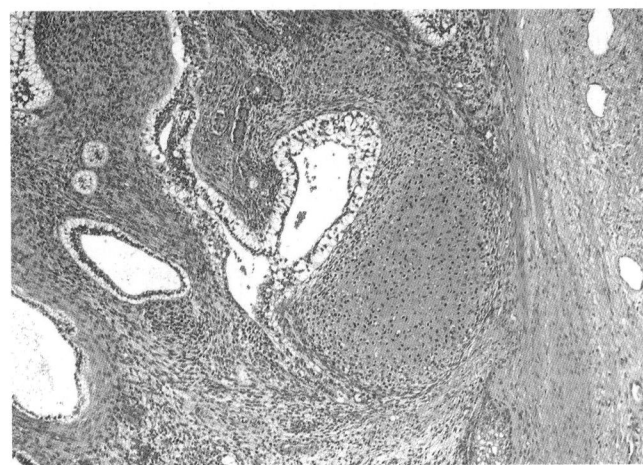

FIGURE 21–29 Teratoma of the testis consisting of a disorganized collection of glands, cartilage, smooth muscle, and immature stroma.

chemotherapy survive, resulting in the dominant metastatic pattern.

From a clinical standpoint, tumors of the testis are segregated into two broad categories: *seminoma* and *nonseminomatous germ cell tumors* (NSGCTs). Seminomas tend to remain localized to the testis for a long time, and hence approximately 70% present in clinical stage I (see later). In contrast, approximately 60% of males with NSGCTs present with advanced clinical disease (stages II and III). Metastases from seminomas typically involve lymph nodes. Hematogenous spread occurs later in the course of dissemination. NSGCTs not only metastasize earlier but also use the hematogenous route more frequently. The rare pure choriocarcinoma is the most aggressive NSGCT. It may not cause any testicular enlargement but instead spreads predominantly and rapidly by the bloodstream. Therefore, lungs and liver are involved early in virtually every case. From a therapeutic viewpoint, seminomas are extremely radiosensitive, whereas NSGCTs are relatively radioresistant. *To summarize, as compared with seminomas, NSGCTs are biologically more aggressive and in general have a poorer prognosis.*

In the United States, three clinical stages of testicular tumors are defined:

- Stage I: tumor confined to the testis, epididymis, or spermatic cord
- Stage II: distant spread confined to retroperitoneal nodes below the diaphragm
- Stage III: metastases outside the retroperitoneal nodes or above the diaphragm

Germ cell tumors of the testis often secrete polypeptide hormones and certain enzymes that can be detected in blood by sensitive assays.[81] Such biologic markers include HCG, AFP, and lactate dehydrogenase, which are valuable in the diagnosis and management of testicular cancer. The elevation of lactate dehydrogenase correlates with the mass of tumor cells, and provides a tool to assess tumor burden. Marked elevation of serum AFP or HCG levels are produced by yolk sac tumor and choriocarcinoma elements, respectively. Both of these markers are elevated in more than 80% of individuals with NSGCT at the time of diagnosis. As stated earlier, approximately 15% of seminomas have syncytiotrophoblastic giant cells and minimal elevation of HCG levels, which does not affect prognosis. In the context of testicular tumors, the value of serum markers is fourfold:

- In the evaluation of testicular masses
- In the staging of testicular germ cell tumors. For example, after orchiectomy, persistent elevation of HCG or AFP concentrations indicates stage II disease even if the lymph nodes appear of normal size by imaging studies.
- In assessing tumor burden
- In monitoring the response to therapy. After eradication of tumors there is a rapid fall in serum AFP and HCG. With serial measurements it is often possible to predict recurrence before the patients become symptomatic or develop any other clinical signs of relapse.

The therapy and prognosis of testicular tumors depend largely on clinical stage and on the histologic type. Seminoma, which is extremely radiosensitive and tends to remain localized for long periods, has the best prognosis. More than 95% of patients with stage I and II disease can be cured. Among NSGCTs, the histologic subtype does not influence the prognosis significantly, and hence these are treated as a group. Approximately 90% of patients with NSGCTs can achieve complete remission with aggressive chemotherapy, and most can be cured. Pure choriocarcinoma has a poor prognosis. However, when it is a minor component of a mixed germ cell tumor, the prognosis is less adversely affected. With all testicular tumors, distant metastases, if present, usually occur within the first 2 years after treatment.

Tumors of Sex Cord–Gonadal Stroma

As indicated in Table 21–5, sex cord–gonadal stroma tumors are subclassified based on their presumed histogenesis and differentiation. The two most important members of this group—Leydig cell tumors and Sertoli cell tumors—are described here. Details of other tumors in this group can be found in a review.[82]

Leydig Cell Tumors

Tumors of Leydig cells are particularly interesting, because they may elaborate androgens and in some cases both androgens and estrogens, and even corticosteroids.[83,84] They may arise at any age, although most cases occur between 20 and 60 years of age. As with other testicular tumors, the most common presenting feature is testicular swelling, but in some patients gynecomastia may be the first symptom. In children, hormonal effects, manifested primarily as sexual precocity, are the dominating features.

Morphology. These neoplasms form circumscribed nodules, usually less than 5 cm in diameter. They have a distinctive golden brown, homogeneous cut surface. Histologically, neoplastic Leydig cells usually are remarkably similar to their normal counterparts in that they are large and round or polygonal, and they have an abundant granular eosinophilic cytoplasm with a round central nucleus. The cytoplasm frequently contains lipid granules, vacuoles, or lipofuscin pigment, and, most characteristically, rod-shaped crystalloids of Reinke occur in about 25% of the tumors. Approximately 10% of the tumors in adults are invasive and produce metastases; most are benign.

Sertoli Cell Tumors

Most Sertoli cell tumors are hormonally silent and present as a testicular mass.[85]

Morphology. These neoplasms appear as firm, small nodules with a homogeneous gray-white to yellow cut surface. Histologically the tumor cells are arranged in distinctive trabeculae that tend to form cordlike structures and tubules. Most Sertoli cell tumors are benign, but occasional tumors (~10%) pursue a malignant course.

Gonadoblastoma

Gonadoblastomas are rare neoplasms containing a mixture of germ cells and gonadal stromal elements, that almost always arise in gonads with some form of testrcular dysgenesis (discussed earlier). In some cases the germ cell component becomes malignant, giving rise to seminoma.

Testicular Lymphoma

Although an uncommon tumor of the testis, testicular lymphoma is included here because affected patients present with only a testicular mass, mimicking other, more common, testicular tumors. Aggressive non-Hodgkin lymphomas account for 5% of testicular neoplasms, *and are the most common form of testicular neoplasms in men over the age of 60.* In most cases, the disease is already disseminated at the time of detection. The most common testicular lyphomas, in decreasing order of frequency, are diffuse large B cell lymphoma, Burkitt Lymphoma, and EBV-positive extranodal NK/T cell lymphoma (Chapter 13). Patients with testicular lymphomas have a higher incidence of central nervous system involvement than those similar tumors located elsewhere.

MISCELLANEOUS LESIONS OF TUNICA VAGINALIS

Brief mention should be made of the tunica vaginalis, which is a mesothelial-lined surface exterior to the testis that may accumulate serous fluid *(hydrocele)* causing considerable enlargement of the scrotal sac. By transillumination it is usually possible to define the clear, translucent character of the contained fluid. Hydrocele sacs are frequently lined by mesothelial cells. Rarely, malignant mesotheliomas also can be seen arising from the tunica vaginalis.

Hematocele indicates the presence of blood in the tunica vaginalis. It is an uncommon condition usually encountered only when there has been either direct trauma to the testis or torsion of the testis with hemorrhagic suffusion into the surrounding tunica vaginalis or in hemorrhagic diseases associated with widespread bleeding diatheses. *Chylocele* refers to the accumulation of lymph in the tunica and is almost always found in patients with elephantiasis who have widespread, severe lymphatic obstruction caused, for example, by filariasis (Chapter 8). *Spermatocele* refers to a small cystic accumulation of semen in dilated efferent ducts or ducts of the rete testis. *Varicocele* is a dilated vein in the spermatic cord. Varicoceles may be asymptomatic but have also been implicated in some men as a contributing factor to infertility. They can be corrected by surgical repair.

Prostate

In the normal adult the prostate weighs approximately 20 gm. The prostate is a retroperitoneal organ encircling the neck of the bladder and urethra, and is devoid of a distinct capsule. In the adult, prostatic parenchyma can be divided into four biologically and anatomically distinct zones or regions: the peripheral, central, and transitional zones, and the region of the anterior fibromuscular stroma (Fig. 21–30).[87] The types of

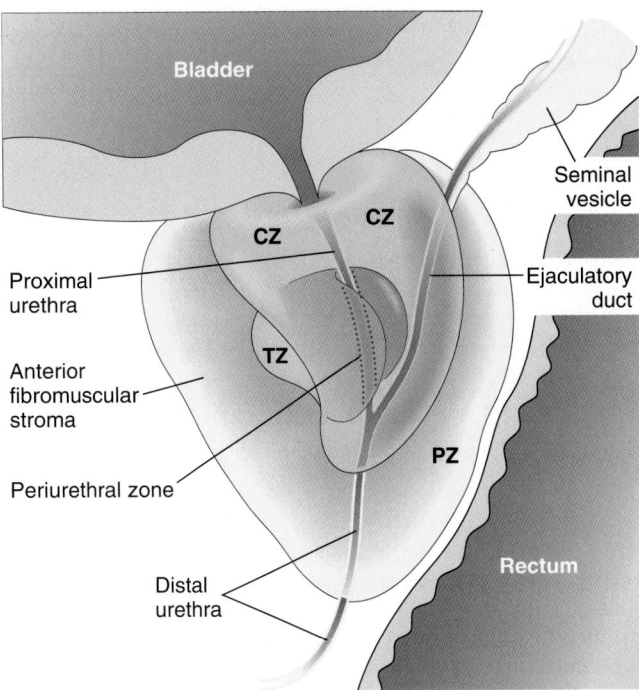

FIGURE 21–30 Adult prostate. The normal prostate contains several distinct regions, including a central zone (CZ), a peripheral zone (PZ), a transitional zone (TZ), and a periurethral zone. Most carcinomas arise from the peripheral glands of the organ and may be palpable during digital examination of the rectum. Nodular hyperplasia, in contrast, arises from more centrally situated glands and is more likely to produce urinary obstruction early than is carcinoma.

proliferative lesions are different in each region. For example, most hyperplasias arise in the transitional zone, whereas most carcinomas originate in the peripheral zone.

Histologically the prostate is composed of glands lined by two layers of cells: a basal layer of low cuboidal epithelium covered by a layer of columnar secretory cells (Fig. 21–31). In many areas there are small papillary infoldings of the epithelium. These glands are separated by abundant fibromuscular stroma. Testicular androgens control the growth and survival of prostatic cells. Castration leads to atrophy of the prostate caused by widespread apoptosis.

Only three pathologic processes affect the prostate gland with sufficient frequency to merit discussion: inflammation, benign nodular enlargement, and tumors. Of these three, the benign nodular enlargements are by far the most common and occur so often in advanced age that they can almost be construed as a "normal" aging process. Prostatic carcinoma is also an extremely common lesion in men and therefore merits careful consideration. We begin our discussion with consideration of the inflammatory processes.

INFLAMMATION

Prostatitis may be divided into several categories: acute and chronic bacterial prostatitis, chronic abacterial prostatitis, and granulomatous prostatitis.

Acute bacterial prostatitis typically results from bacteria similar to those that cause urinary tract infections. Thus, most cases are caused by various strains of *E. coli*, other gram-negative rods, enterococci, and staphylococci. The organisms

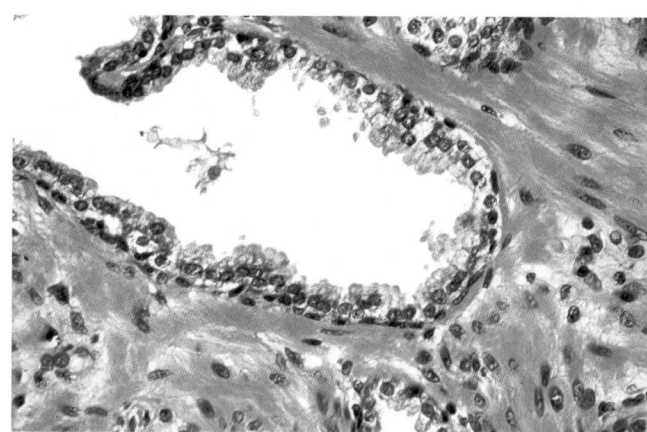

FIGURE 21–31 Benign prostate gland with basal cell and secretory cell layer.

become implanted in the prostate usually by intraprostatic reflux of urine from the posterior urethra or from the urinary bladder, but occasionally they seed the prostate by lymphohematogenous routes from distant foci of infection. Prostatitis sometimes follows surgical manipulation of the urethra or prostate gland itself, such as catheterization, cystoscopy, urethral dilation, or resection procedures on the prostate. Clinically, acute bacterial prostatitis is associated with fever, chills, and dysuria. On rectal examination the prostate is exquisitely tender and boggy. The diagnosis can be established by urine culture and clinical features.

Chronic bacterial prostatitis is difficult to diagnose and treat. It may present with low back pain, dysuria, and perineal and suprapubic discomfort. Alternatively, it may be virtually asymptomatic. *Patients often have a history of recurrent urinary tract infections (cystitis, urethritis) caused by the same organism.* Because most antibiotics penetrate the prostate poorly, bacteria find safe haven in the parenchyma and constantly seed the urinary tract. Diagnosis of chronic bacterial prostatitis depends on the demonstration of leukocytosis in the expressed prostatic secretions, along with positive bacterial cultures. In most cases, there is no antecedent acute attack, and the disease appears insidiously and without obvious provocation. The implicated organisms are the same as those cited as causes of acute prostatitis.

Chronic abacterial prostatitis is the most common form of prostatitis seen today. *Clinically, it is indistinguishable from chronic bacterial prostatitis. There is no history, however, of recurrent urinary tract infection.* Expressed prostatic secretions contain more than 10 leukocytes per high-power field, but bacterial cultures are uniformly negative.

Granulomatous prostatitis may be specific, where an etiologic infectious agent may be identified or non-specific.[88] In the United States the most common cause is related to instillation of BCG within the bladder for treatment of superficial bladder cancer, discussed earlier in this chapter.[89,90] BCG is an attenuated mycobacterial strain that gives rise to a histologic picture indistinguishable from that seen with systemic tuberculosis. However, in this setting the finding of granulomas in the prostate is of no clinical significance, and requires no treatment. Fungal granulomatous prostatitis is typically seen only in immunocompromised hosts. Nonspecific granulomatous prostatitis is relatively common and represents a reaction to

secretions from ruptured prostatic ducts and acini.[91] Although some of these men have a recent history of urinary tract infection, bacteria are not seen within the tissue in nonspecific granulomatous prostatitis.

> **Morphology. Acute prostatitis** may appear as minute, disseminated abscesses; as large, coalescent focal areas of necrosis; or as diffuse edema, congestion, and boggy suppuration of the entire gland.
>
> In men with symptoms of acute or chronic prostatitis, biopsy or surgical specimens are uncommonly examined microscopically, because the disease is diagnosed on clinical and laboratory findings. In fact biopsy of a man with acute prostatitis is contraindicated, as it may lead to sepsis. It is common in prostate specimens removed surgically to find histologic evidence of acute or chronic inflammation in men with no clinical symptoms of acute or chronic prostatitis. In these instances etiologic infectious agents have yet to be identified.[92] So as not to be confused with the clinical syndromes of acute and chronic prostatitis, these prostate specimens are instead diagnosed in descriptive terms as showing "acute inflammation" or "chronic inflammation" and not as "prostatitis."

BENIGN ENLARGEMENT

Benign Prostatic Hyperplasia (BPH) or Nodular Hyperplasia

BPH is an extremely common disorder in men over age 50.[94] It is characterized by hyperplasia of prostatic stromal and epithelial cells, resulting in the formation of large, fairly discrete nodules in the periurethral region of the prostate. When sufficiently large, the nodules compress and narrow the urethral canal to cause partial, or sometimes virtually complete, obstruction of the urethra.

Incidence. Histologic evidence of BPH can be seen in approximately 20% of men 40 years of age, a figure that increases to 70% by age 60 and to 90% by age 80. There is no direct correlation, however, between histologic changes and clinical symptoms. Only 50% of those who have microscopic evidence of BPH have clinically detectable enlargement of the prostate, and of these individuals, only 50% develop clinical symptoms. BPH is a problem of enormous magnitude, with approximately 30% of white American males over 50 years of age having moderate to severe symptoms.

Etiology and Pathogenesis. Despite the fact that there is an increased number of epithelial cells and stromal components in the periurethral area of the prostate, there is no clear evidence of increased epithelial cell proliferation in human BPH. Instead, it is believed that the main component of the "hyperplastic" process is impaired cell death. It has been proposed that there is an overall reduction of the rate of cell death, resulting in the accumulation of senescent cells in the prostate.[94] In keeping with this androgens (discussed below), which are required for the development of BPH, can not only increase cellular proliferation, but also inhibit cell death.

The main androgen in the prostate, constituting 90% of total prostatic androgens, is dihydrotestosterone (DHT). It is formed in the prostate from the conversion of testosterone by the enzyme type 2 5α-reductase.[93–96] This enzyme is located almost entirely in stromal cells; epithelial cells of the prostate do not contain type 2 5α reductase, with the exception of a few basal cells. *Thus stromal cells are responsible for androgen-dependent prostatic growth.* Type 1 5α-reductase is not detected in the prostate, or is present at very low levels. However this enzyme may produce DHT from testosterone in liver and skin, and circulating DHT may act in the prostate by an endocrine mechanism.

DHT binds to the nuclear androgen receptor (AR) present in both stromal and epithelial prostate cells. DHT is more potent than testosterone because it has a higher affinity for AR and forms a more stable complex with the receptor. Binding of DHT to AR activates the transcription of androgen-dependent genes. DHT is not a direct mitogen for prostate cells, instead DHT-mediated transcription of genes results in the increased production of several growth factors and their receptors. Most important among these are members of the fibroblast growth factor (FGF) family, and particularly FGF-7 (keratinocyte growth factor; Chapter 3). FGF-7, produced by stromal cells, is probably the most important factor mediating the paracrine regulation of androgen-stimulated prostatic growth. Other growth factors produced in BPH are FGFs 1 and 2, and TGFβ, which promote fibroblast proliferation. Although the ultimate cause of BPH is unknown, it is believed that DHT-induced growth factors act by increasing the proliferation of stromal cells and decreasing the death of epithelial cells.

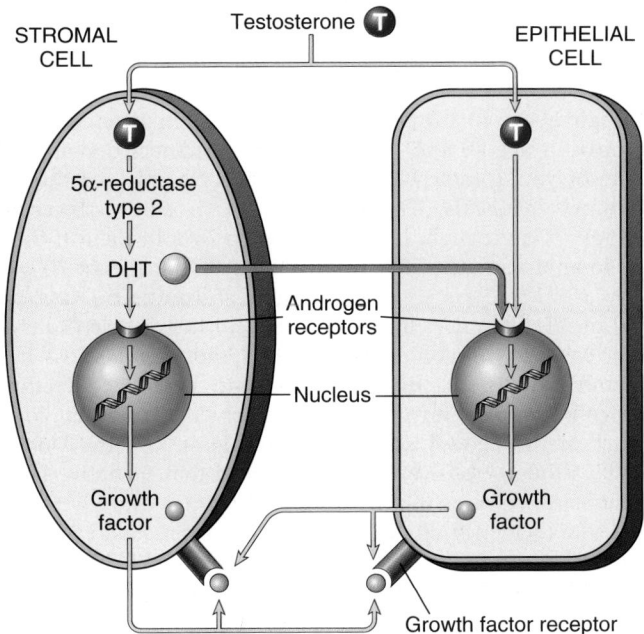

FIGURE 21–32 Simplified scheme of the pathogenesis of prostatic hyperplasia. The central role of the stromal cells in generating dihydrotestosterone (DHT) should be noted. DHT may also be produced in skin and liver by both type 1 and 2 5α-reductase.

Morphology. In the usual case of prostatic enlargement, the prostate weighs between 60 and 100 gm. Nodular hyperplasia of the prostate originates almost exclusively in the inner aspect of the prostate gland (transition zone). The early nodules are composed almost entirely of stromal cells, and later predominantly epithelial nodules arise. From their origin in this strategic location the nodular enlargements may encroach on the lateral walls of the urethra to compress it to a slitlike orifice (Fig. 21–33). In some cases, nodular enlargement may project up into the floor of the urethra as a hemispheric mass directly beneath the mucosa of the urethra, which is termed **median lobe hypertrophy** by clinicians.

On cross-section, the nodules vary in color and consistency. In nodules that contain mostly glands, the tissue is yellow-pink with a soft consistency, and a milky-white prostatic fluid oozes out of these areas. In nodules composed primarily of fibromuscular stroma, each nodule is pale gray, is tough, does not exude fluid, and is less clearly demarcated from the surrounding uninvolved prostatic tissue. Although the nodules do not have true capsules, the compressed surrounding prostatic tissue creates a plane of cleavage about them.

Microscopically, the hallmark of BPH is nodularity (Fig. 21–33B). The composition of the nodules ranges from purely stromal fibromuscular nodules to fibro-epithelial nodules with a glandular predominance. Glandular proliferation takes the form of aggregations of small to large to cystically dilated glands, lined by two layers, an inner columnar and an outer cuboidal or flattened epithelium (Fig. 21–33C). The diagnosis of BPH cannot usually be made on needle biopsy, since the histology of glandular or mixed glandular-stromal nodules of BPH cannot be appreciated in limited samples. Also, needle biopsies do not typically sample the transition zone where BPH occurs. Occasionally foci of reactive squamous metaplasia histologically mimicking urothelial carcinoma can be seen adjacent to prostatic infarcts in prostates with prominent BPH.

Clinical Features. The pathophysiology of BPH is complex, as it involves several factors. The increased size of the gland, and the smooth muscle-mediated contraction of the prostate cause urethral obstruction. The increased resistance to urinary outflow leads to bladder hypertrophy and distension, accompanied by urine retention. The inability to empty the bladder completely creates a reservoir of residual urine that is a common source of infection. Patients experience increased urinary frequency, nocturia, difficulty in starting and stopping the stream of urine, overflow dribbling, dysuria (painful micturition), and have an increased risk of developing bacterial infections of the bladder and kidney. In many cases, sudden, acute urinary retention appears for unknown reasons that requires emergency catheterization.

Mild cases of BPH may be treated without medical or surgical therapy, such as by decreasing fluid intake, especially before

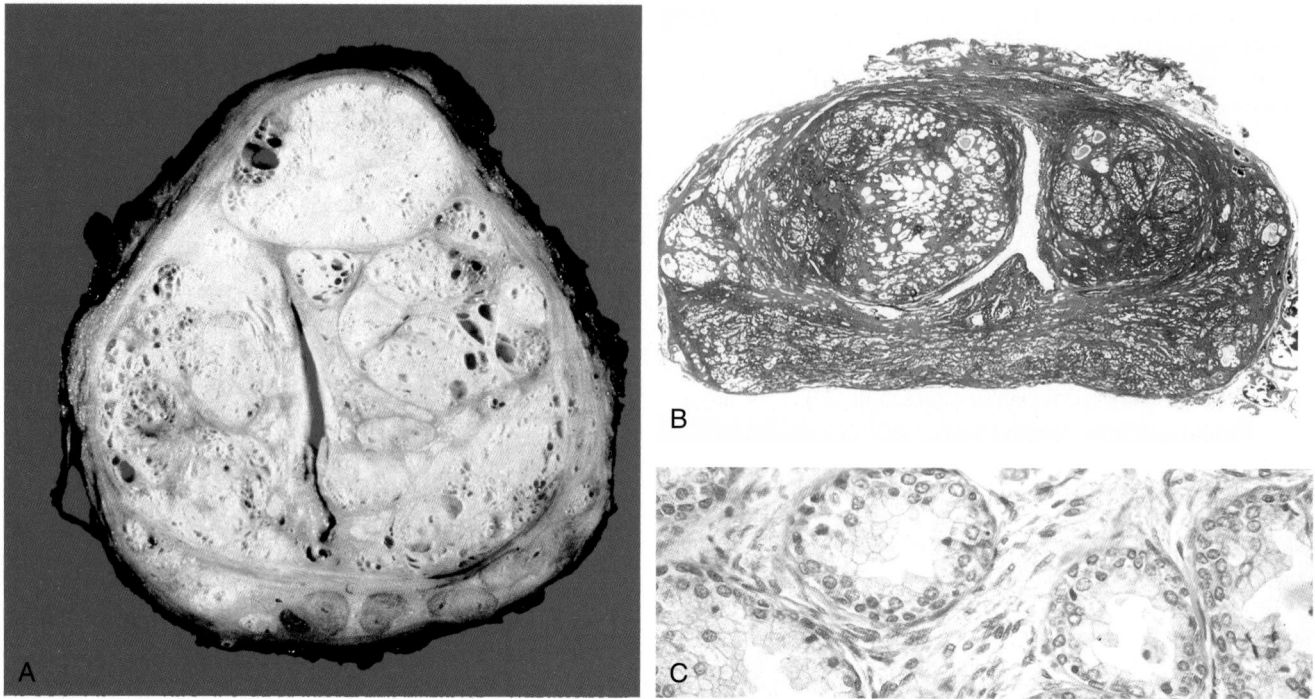

FIGURE 21–33 Nodular prostatic hyperplasia. **A,** Well-defined nodules of BPH compress the urethra into a slitlike lumen. **B,** A microscopic view of a whole mount of the prostate shows nodules of hyperplastic glands on both sides of the urethra. **C,** Under high power the characteristic dual cell population: the inner columnar and outer flattened basal cell can be seen.

bedtime; moderating the intake of alcohol and caffeine-containing products; and following timed voiding schedules. The most commonly used and effective medical therapy for symptoms relating to BPH are α-blockers, which decrease prostate smooth muscle tone via inhibition of α_1-adrenergic receptors.[97,98] Another common pharmacologic therapy aims to decrease symptoms by physically shrinking the prostate with an agent that inhibits the synthesis of DHT. Inhibitors of 5-α-reductase fall into this category. For moderate to severe cases recalcitrant to medical therapy, a wide range of more invasive procedures exist. Transurethral resection of the prostate (TURP) has been the gold standard in terms of reducing symptoms, improving flow rates, and decreasing post-voiding residual urine. It is indicated as a first line of therapy in certain circumstances, such as recurrent urinary retention. As a result of its morbidity and cost, alternative procedures have been developed. These include high-intensity focused ultrasound, laser therapy, hyperthermia, transurethral electrovaporization, and transurethral needle ablation using radiofrequency. Nodular hyperplasia is not considered to be a premalignant lesion.

TUMORS

Adenocarcinoma

Adenocarcinoma of the prostate is the most common form of cancer in men, accounting for 29% of cancer in the United States in 2007.[99] However, prostate cancer is tied with colorectal cancer in terms of cancer mortality, causing 9% of cancer deaths in the United States in 2007. There is a one in six life-time probability of being diagnosed with prostate cancer. Over the last 20 years there has been a significant drop in prostate cancer mortality. It is one of the most remarkable tumors, exhibiting a wide range of clinical behaviors from very aggressive lethal cancers to incidentally discovered clinically insignificant cancers.

Incidence. Cancer of the prostate is typically a disease of men over age 50. However, in men who are at increased risk (see "Etiology"), screening for prostate cancer is recommended to begin at age 40. Consideration has also been given to screen all men at age 40 and again at age 45 to detect uncommon cases of young men with prostate cancer before the disease becomes incurable. The incidence of prostatic cancer at autopsy is quite high. It increases from 20% in men in their 50s to approximately 70% in men between the ages of 70 and 80 years. There are some remarkable and puzzling national and racial differences in the incidence of the disease.[100] Prostatic cancer is uncommon in Asians and occurs most frequently among blacks. In addition to hereditary factors, environment plays a role, as evidenced by the rise in the incidence of the disease in Japanese immigrants to the United States, though not nearly to the level of that of native-born Americans. Also, as the diet in Asia becomes more westernized, the incidence of clinically significant prostate cancer in this region of the world seems to be increasing. Whether this is due to dietary factors or other lifestyle changes is not clear.

Etiology and Pathogenesis. Our knowledge of the causes of prostate cancer is far from complete. Several factors, including age, race, family history, hormone levels, and environmental influences are suspected to play a role.

The increased incidence of this disease upon migration from a low-incidence region to one with a high incidence is consistent with a role for environmental influences. There are many candidate environmental factors, but none has been proven to be causative. For example, increased consumption of fats has been implicated. Other dietary products suspected of preventing or delaying prostate cancer development include lycopenes (found in tomatoes), selenium, soy products, and vitamin D.[101]

Androgens play an important role in prostate cancer. Like their normal counterparts, the growth and survival of prostate cancer cells depends on androgens, which bind to the androgen receptor (AR) and induce the expression of pro-growth and pro-survival genes. Of interest with respect to differences in prostate cancer risk among races, the X-linked AR gene contains a polymorphic sequence composed of repeats of the codon CAG (which codes for glutamine). Very large expansions of this stretch of CAGs cause a rare neurodegenerative disorder, Kennedy disease, characterized by muscle cramping and weakness. However, even in normal individuals, there is sufficient variation in the length of the CAG repeats to affect AR function. ARs with the shortest stretches of polyglutamine have the highest sensitivity to androgens. The shortest polyglutamine repeats on average are found in African Americans, while Caucasians have an intermediate length and Asians have the longest, paralleling the incidence and mortality of prostate cancer in these groups. More directly, the length of the repeats is inversely related to rate at which prostate cancer develops in mouse models.[102]

The importance of androgens in maintaining the growth and survival of prostate cancer cells can be seen in the therapeutic effect of castration or treatment with anti-androgens, which usually induce disease regression. Unfortunately, *most tumors eventually become resistant to androgen blockade.* Tumors escape through a variety of mechanisms, including acquisition of hypersensitivity to low levels of androgen (e.g., through AR gene amplification); mutations in AR that allow it to be activated by non-androgen ligands; and other mutations or epigenetic changes that activate alternative signaling pathways, which may bypass the need for AR altogether.[103] Among the latter are changes that lead to increased activation of the P1-3 kinase/AKT signaling pathway, which is observed most often in tumors that have become resistant to anti-androgen therapy.

There is much interest in the role of other *inherited polymorphisms* in the development of prostate cancer.[104–108] Compared with men with no family history, men with one first-degree relative with prostate cancer have twice the risk and those with two first-degree relatives have five times the risk of developing prostate cancer. Men with a strong family history of prostate cancer also tend to develop the disease at an earlier age. Men with germline mutations of the tumor suppressor *BRCA2* have a 20-fold increased risk of prostate cancer, but the vast majority of familial prostate cancers are due to variation in other loci that confer a small increase in cancer risk. Family and genome-wide association studies have identified a number of risk-associated loci, including one at 8q24 that appears to selectively increase the risk among African American men.[108] Of possible interest, a number of the candidate genes in these regions are involved in innate immunity, leading to speculation that inflammation may set the stage for the development of prostate carcinoma, as has been shown with respect to other human cancers (Chapter 7).

Other work is focused on the role of tumor-specific acquired somatic mutations and epigenetic changes. One very common type of somatic mutation in prostate cancer gives rise to *chromosomal rearrangements that juxtapose the coding sequence of an ETS family transcription factor gene (most commonly ERG or ETV1) next to the androgen-regulated TMPRSS2 promoter.*[110] These rearrangements place the involved ETS gene under the control of the *TMPRSS2* promoter and lead to their over-expression in an androgen-dependent fashion. Over-expression of ETS transcription factors makes normal prostate epithelial cells more invasive, possibly through the upregulation of matrix metalloproteases. In addition, tumors with rearranged ETS genes have certain distinctive morphologic features[111] and a different gene expression signature than those lacking ETS gene rearrangements,[112] suggesting that ETS gene rearrangements define a specific molecular sub-class of prostate cancer. ETS rearrangements may also have implications for prostate cancer screening and early diagnosis, as it is possible to detect ETS fusion genes in the urine using sensitive PCR assays.

The most common epigenetic alteration in prostate cancer is hypermethylation of glutathione *S*-transferase (*GSTP1*) gene which down-regualtes GSTP1 expression. The *GSTP1* gene is located on chromosome 11q13 and is an important part of the pathway that prevents damage from a wide range of carcinogens.[113] Other genes silenced by epigenetic modifications in a subset of prostate cancers include a number of tumor suppressor genes, including *PTEN*, *RB*, *p16/INK4a*, *MLH1*, *MSH2*, and *APC*.

In addition to prostate specific antigen (PSA, discussed below), other genes and proteins that may serve as biomarkers in prostate cancer have emerged, and some of these appear to play a direct role in the biology of the disease. Three worthy of brief mention are EZH-2 (enhancer of zeste-2), alpha-methylacyl-CoA racemase (AMACR), and *PCA3*. Prostate cancers show a relatively frequent loss of E-cadherin,[114] an adhesion protein that is also down-regulated in invasive signet ring carcinoma of the stomach and lobular carcinoma of the breast. Loss of E-cadherin from prostate cancer cells is associated with expression of high levels of EZH-2, a transcriptional repressor that may contribute to prostate cancer progression.[115] AMACR, an enzyme involved in the beta-oxidation of branched chain amino acids, is selectively upregulated in prostate cancer and its possible precursor lesions as compared to normal prostate (described below)[116,117], as is *PCA3*, a gene on chromosome 9q that appears to encode a regulatory RNA.[118,119]

As can be surmised from the multiplicity of abnormalities, prostate carcinoma (like other cancers) is the product of some critical combination of acquired somatic mutations and epigenetic changes. A putative precursor lesion, prostatic intraepithelial neoplasia (PIN), has been described. Prostates containing cancer have a higher frequency and a greater extent of PIN, which is also often seen in proximity to cancer. Studies have revealed that many of the molecular changes seen in invasive cancers are present in PIN (for example, rearrangements involving *ETS* genes are found in a subset[120,121]), strongly supporting the argument that PIN is a precursor of invasive cancer. What remains unclear is whether PIN inevitably

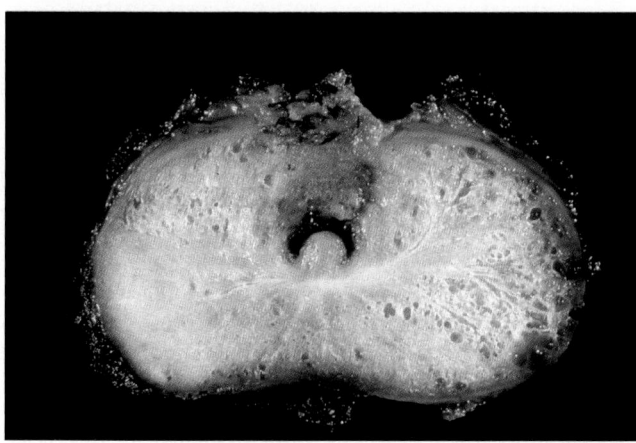

FIGURE 21–34 Adenocarcinoma of the prostate. Carcinomatous tissue is seen on the posterior aspect *(lower left)*. Note solid whiter tissue of cancer in contrast to spongy appearance of benign peripheral zone in the contralateral side.

progresses to cancer, or instead sometimes remains latent or even regresses.[122]

Morphology. When the terms **"prostate cancer"** or **"prostate adenocarcinoma"** are used without qualifications it refers to the common or acinar variant of prostate cancer. In approximately 70% of cases, carcinoma of the prostate arises in the peripheral zone of the gland, classically in a posterior location, where it may be palpable on rectal examination (Fig. 21–34). Characteristically, on cross-section of the prostate **the neoplastic tissue is gritty and firm, but when embedded within the prostatic substance it may be extremely difficult to visualize and be more readily apparent on palpation**. Local extension most commonly involves periprostatic tissue, seminal vesicles, and the base of the urinary bladder, which in advanced disease may result in ureteral obstruction. Metastases first spread via lymphatics initially to the obturator nodes and eventually to the para-aortic nodes. Hematogenous spread occurs chiefly to the bones, particularly the axial skeleton, but some lesions spread widely to viscera. Massive visceral dissemination is an exception rather than the rule. The bony metastases are typically osteoblastic and in men point strongly to prostatic cancer (Fig. 21–35). The bones commonly involved, in descending order of frequency, are lumbar spine, proximal femur, pelvis, thoracic spine, and ribs.

Histologically, most lesions are adenocarcinomas that produce well-defined, readily demonstrable gland patterns.[123,124] The glands are typically smaller than benign glands and are lined by a single uniform layer of cuboidal or low columnar epithelium. In contrast to benign glands, prostate cancer glands are more crowded, and characteristically lack branching and papillary infolding. **The outer basal cell layer typical of benign glands is absent.** The cytoplasm of the tumor cells ranges from pale-clear as seen in

benign glands to a distinctive amphophilic appearance. Nuclei are large and often contain one or more large nucleoli. There is some variation in nuclear size and shape, but in general pleomorphism is not marked. Mitotic figures are uncommon.

The histologic diagnosis of prostate cancer on biopsy specimens is one of the more difficult challenges for pathologists.[125] In part, difficulty stems not only from the scant amount of tissue available for histologic examination removed by the needle biopsy, but also that biopsy often only samples a few malignant glands among many benign glands (Fig. 21–36). Morphologically, prostate cancer is difficult to diagnose in that the clues to malignancy may be subtle, increasing the likelihood of underdiagnosis. There are also many benign mimickers of cancer that can lead the unwary pathologist to a misdiagnosis of cancer. Although there are a few histologic findings on biopsy that are specific for prostate cancer, such as perineural invasion, in general the diagnosis is made based on a constellation of architectural, cytologic, and ancillary findings (Fig. 21–37). As discussed earlier, one distinguishing feature between benign and malignant prostate glands is that benign glands contain basal cells whereas they are absent in cancer (compare benign and malignant glands in Fig. 21–36A, and benign glands in Fig.

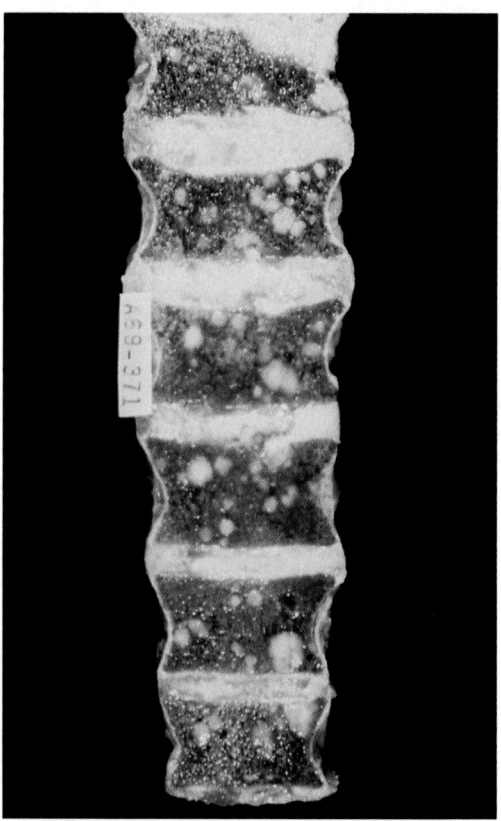

FIGURE 21–35 Metastatic osteoblastic prostatic carcinoma within vertebral bodies.

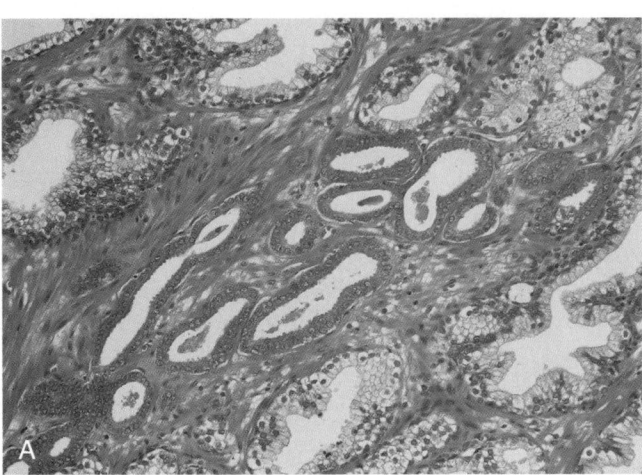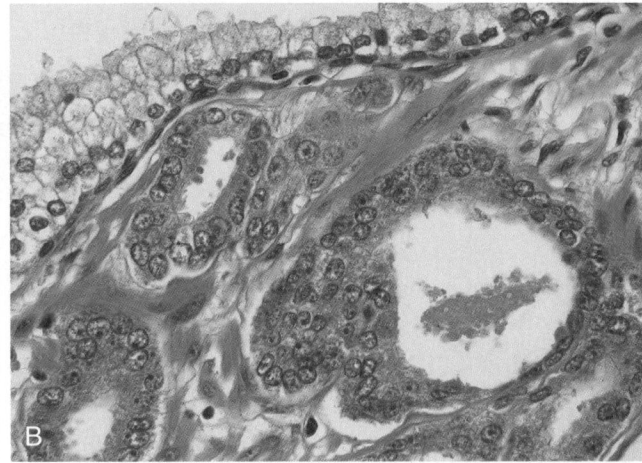

FIGURE 21-36   **A,** Photomicrograph of small focus of adenocarcinoma of the prostate demonstrating small glands crowded in between larger benign glands. **B,** Higher magnification shows several small malignant glands with enlarged nuclei, prominent nucleoli, and dark cytoplasm, as compared with larger benign gland *(top)*.

21-33C with cancerous glands in Fig. 21-36B).[126] Pathologists have exploited this finding, by using various immunohistologic markers to label basal cells. α-methylacyl-coenzyme A-racemase (AMACR) is up-regulated in prostate cancer and can be detected by immunohistochemistry. The majority of prostate cancers are positive for AMACR, the sensitivity varying among studies from 82% to 100%. The use of all of these markers, while improving the accuracy of the diagnosis of prostate cancer, have their limitations with false positive and false negatives and must be used in conjunction with the routine H&E-stained sections.

In approximately 80% of cases, prostatic tissue removed for carcinoma also harbors presumptive precursor lesions, referred to as **high-grade prostatic intraepithelial neoplasia (PIN)**.[127-128] PIN consists of architecturally benign prostatic acini lined by cytologically atypical cells with prominent nucleoli. Cyto-logically PIN and carcinoma may be identical, yet architecturally PIN involves larger branching glands with papillary infolding, in contrast to invasive cancer that is typically characterized by small crowded glands with straight luminal borders. PIN glands are surrounded by a patchy layer of basal cells and an intact basement membrane. There are several lines of evidence relating PIN to invasive cancer. First, both PIN and cancer typically predominate in the peripheral zone and are relatively uncommon in other zones. If one compares prostates without cancer to those with cancer, prostates containing cancer have a higher frequency and a greater extent of PIN. PIN is also often seen in proximity to cancer, in some cases the cancer appearing to bud off of the PIN. Many of the molecular changes seen in invasive cancers are also present in PIN, supporting the view that PIN is an intermediate lesion between normal and invasive cancer. Despite all this evidence, we do not know the natural history of PIN, and in particular how often it progresses to cancer. Thus, unlike in cancer of the cervix, the term **"Carcinoma in situ"** is not used for PIN. There are many other secrets about prostate cancer that have yet to be revealed.

Grading and Staging. The grading schema used for prostate cancer is the Gleason system.[129,130] According to this system, prostate cancers are stratified into five grades on the basis of glandular patterns of differentiation. Grade 1 represents the most well-differentiated tumors, in which the neoplastic glands are uniform and round in appearance and are packed into well-circumscribed nodules (Fig. 21-38A). By contrast, grade 5 tumors show no glandular differentiation, and the tumor cells infiltrate the stroma in the form of cords, sheets, and nests (Fig. 21-38C). The other grades fall in between. Most tumors contain more than one pattern, where one assigns a primary grade to the dominant pattern and a secondary grade to the second most frequent pattern. The two numeric grades are then added to obtain a combined Gleason grade or score. Thus, for example, a tumor with a dominant grade 3 and a

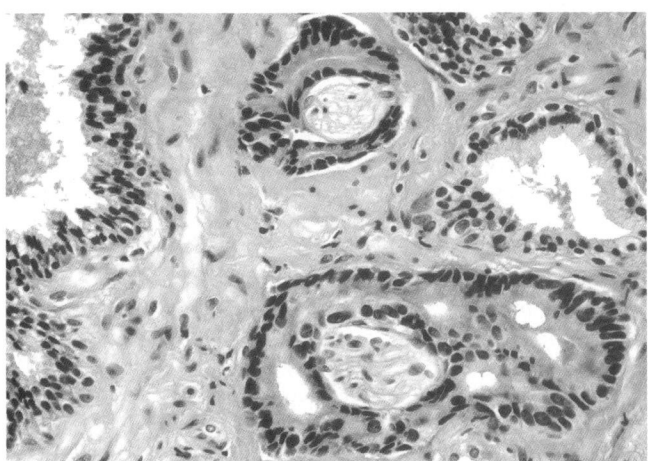

FIGURE 21-37   Carcinoma of prostate showing perineural invasion by malignant glands. Compare to benign gland *(left)*.

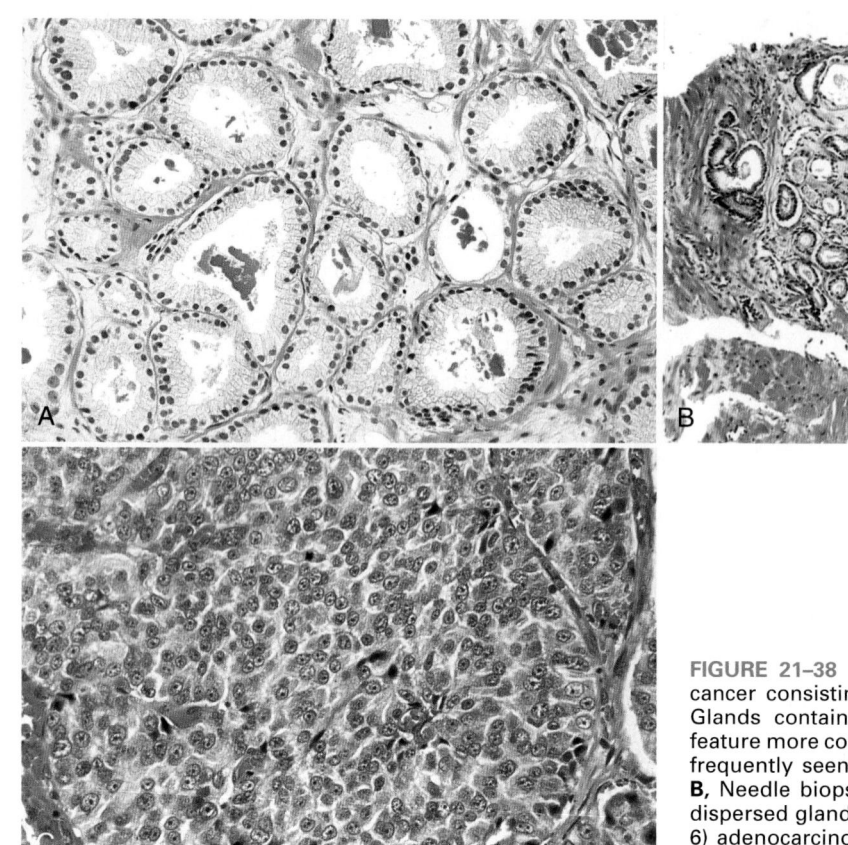

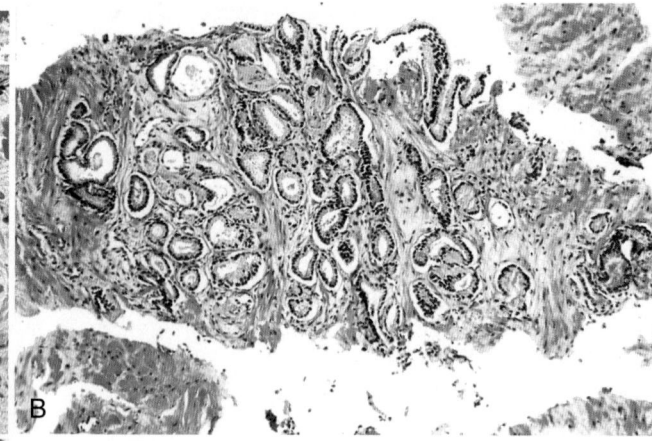

FIGURE 21–38 **A,** Low-grade (Gleason score 1 + 1 = 2) prostate cancer consisting of back-to-back uniform-sized malignant glands. Glands contain eosinophilic intraluminal prostatic crystalloids, a feature more commonly seen in cancer than benign glands and more frequently seen in lower grade than higher grade prostate cancer. **B,** Needle biopsy of the prostate with variably sized, more widely dispersed glands of moderately differentiated Gleason score 3 + 3 = 6) adenocarcinoma. **C,** Poorly differentiated (Gleason score 5 + 5 = 10) adenocarcinoma composed of sheets of malignant cells.

secondary grade 4 would achieve a Gleason score of 7. Tumors with only one pattern are treated as if their primary and secondary grades are the same, and hence, the number is doubled. An exception to the rule is if three patterns are present on biopsy, the most common and highest grades are added together to arrive at the Gleason score. Thus, under this schema the most well-differentiated tumors have a Gleason score of 2 (1 + 1), and the least-differentiated tumors merit a score of 10 (5 + 5). Gleason scores are often combined into groups with similar biologic behavior, with grades 2 through 4 representing well-differentiated cancer, 5 and 6 intermediate-grade tumor, 7 moderate to poorly differentiated cancer, and 8 through 10 high-grade tumor. Gleason scores of 2 through 4 are typically found in small tumors within the transition zone. In surgical specimens, such low-grade cancer is typically an incidental finding on TURP performed for symptoms of BPH. The majority of potentially treatable cancers detected on needle biopsy as a result of screening have Gleason scores of 5 through 7. Tumors with Gleason scores 8 through 10 tend to be advanced cancers that are unlikely to be cured. Although there is some evidence that prostate cancers can become more aggressive with time, most commonly, the Gleason score remains stable over a period of several years. *Grading is of particular importance in prostatic cancer, because grade and stage are the best prognostic predictors.*

Staging of prostatic cancer is also important in the selection of the appropriate form of therapy (Table 21–6). Stage T1 refers to incidentally found cancer, either on TURP done for BPH symptoms (T1a and T1b depending on the extent and grade) or on needle biopsy typically performed for elevated serum prostate-specific antigen (PSA) levels (stage T1c).[131–133] Stage T2 is organ-confined cancer. Stage T3a and T3b tumors show extra-prostatic extension, with and without seminal vesicle invasion, respectively. Stage T4 reflects direct invasion of contiguous organs. Any spread of tumor to the lymph nodes regardless of extent is eventually associated with a fatal outcome, such that the staging system merely records the presence or absence of this finding (N0/N1).

Clinical Course. It is generally accepted that most men with incidentally discovered focal (stage T1a) cancer found on TURP do not show evidence of progression when followed for 10 or more years. Older patients with stage T1a disease are typically followed, but younger men with a longer life expectancy may undergo needle biopsy to look for additional cancer in the peripheral zone of the prostate. Stage T1b lesions are more ominous and are treated the same as tumors that are found on needle biopsy, since they have a mortality of 20% if left untreated.

Localized prostate cancer is asymptomatic, and is usually discovered by the detection of a suspicious nodule on rectal examination or elevated serum PSA level (discussed later). Most prostatic cancers arise peripherally away from the urethra, and therefore urinary symptoms occur late. Patients with clinically advanced prostatic cancer may present with urinary symptoms, such as difficulty in starting or stopping the stream, dysuria, frequency, or hematuria. Today it is uncommon for patients to come to attention because of

Table 21–6	Staging of Prostatic Adenocarcinoma Using the TNM System
TNM Designation	**Anatomic Findings**
Extent of Primary Tumor (T)	
T1	**CLINICALLY INAPPARENT LESION (BY PALPATION/IMAGING STUDIES)**
T1a	Involvement of ≤5% of resected tissue
T1b	Involvement of >5% of resected tissue
T1c	Carcinoma present on needle biopsy (following elevated PSA)
T2	**PALPABLE OR VISIBLE CANCER CONFINED TO PROSTATE**
T2a	Involvement of ≤5% of one lobe
T2b	Involvement of >5% of one lobe, but unilateral
T2c	Involvement of both lobes
T3	**LOCAL EXTRAPROSTATIC EXTENSION**
T3a	Extracapsular extension
T3b	Seminal vesical invasion
T4	**INVASION OF CONTIGUOUS ORGANS AND/OR SUPPORTING STRUCTURES INCLUDING BLADDER NECK, RECTUM, EXTERNAL SPHINCTER, LEVATOR MUSCLES, OR PELVIC FLOOR**
Status of Regional Lymph Nodes (N)	
N0	**NO REGIONAL NODAL METASTASES**
N1	**METASTASIS IN REGIONAL LYMPH NODES**
Distant Metastases (M)	
M0	**NO DISTANT METASTASES**
M1	**DISTANT METASTASES PRESENT**
M1a	Metastases to distant lymph nodes
M1b	Bone metastases
M1c	Other distant sites

PSA, prostate-specific antigen.

back pain caused by vertebral metastases. *The finding of osteoblastic metastases by skeletal surveys or the much more sensitive radionuclide bone scanning is virtually diagnostic of this form of cancer in men.* These patients have a universally fatal outcome.

Digital rectal examination may detect some early prostatic carcinomas because of their posterior location, although the test suffers from both low sensitivity and specificity. Although there are characteristic findings of prostate cancer on transrectal ultrasonography and other imaging modalities, the poor sensitivity and specificity of these tests also limit their diagnostic utility. Typically a transrectal needle *biopsy is required to confirm the diagnosis.*

PSA is the most important test used in the diagnosis and management of prostate cancer.[134] PSA is a product of prostatic epithelium and is normally secreted in the semen. It is a serine protease whose function is to cleave and liquefy the seminal coagulum formed after ejaculation. In normal men, only minute amounts of PSA circulate in the serum. Elevated blood levels of PSA occur in association with localized as well as advanced cancer. In most laboratories a serum level of 4 ng/mL is used as a cutoff point between normal and abnormal. However, as discussed below, this simplified approach to serum PSA tests is not appropriate, and has led to the delay in diagnosis of many prostate cancers.

PSA is organ-specific, yet not cancer-specific. Although serum levels of PSA are elevated to a lesser extent in BPH, there is considerable overlap. Other factors such as prostatitis, infarct, instrumentation of the prostate, and ejaculation also increase serum PSA levels. Furthermore, 20% to 40% of patients with organ-confined prostate cancer have a PSA value of 4.0 ng/mL or less.

Whereas most readers of this text will not directly practice pathology, almost all will be confronted with evaluation of a serum PSA test, either as a treating primary care physician, in addressing the results of a family member's or friend's test, or for the male readers reviewing one's own test results. The widespread use of this test, along with its complexity and the corresponding increased risk of it being interpreted incorrectly, warrant a detailed discussion of this topic. This test differs from most other laboratory tests that a physician may order in that it is a cancer detection test. Consequently, physicians should ensure that tests come back from the laboratory, abnormal values are recorded, and patients are contacted for follow-up of elevated levels. Numerous medical malpractice cases result from the mishandling of serum PSA test results and the subsequent delay in diagnosis.

Several refinements in the estimation and interpretation of PSA values have been proposed. These include the ratio between the serum PSA value and volume of prostate gland (PSA density), the rate of change in PSA value with time (PSA velocity), the use of age-specific reference ranges, and the ratio of free and bound PSA in the serum. Men with enlarged hyperplastic prostate glands have higher total serum PSA levels than men with small glands. The measurement of serum *PSA density* factors out the contribution of benign prostatic tissue to serum PSA levels. It is calculated by dividing the total serum PSA level by the estimated gland volume (usually determined by transrectal ultrasound measurements) to estimate the PSA produced per gram of prostate tissue. As men age, their prostates tend to enlarge with BPH. One would then anticipate that overall older men would have higher serum PSA levels than younger men. The upper *age-specific PSA* reference ranges are 2.5 ng/mL for men 40 to 49 years of age, 3.5 ng/mL for men 50 to 59 years, 4.5 ng/mL for men 60 to 69 years, and 6.5 ng/mL for men 70 to 79 years. Consequently, a serum PSA value of 3.5, while it will appear as a normal value on a laboratory test, is a worrisome finding in a man in his 40s, warranting additional evaluation. Another means of interpreting serum PSA tests is by assessing *PSA velocity* or the rate of change of PSA. Men with prostate cancer demonstrate an increased rate of rise in PSA as compared with men who do not have prostate cancer. The rate of change in PSA that best distinguishes between men with and without prostate cancer is 0.75 ng/mL per year. If this test is to be valid, there must be at least three PSA measurements available over a period of 1.5 to 2 years, as there is substantial short-term variability (up to 20%) between repeat PSA measurements. A man who has a significant rise in serum PSA levels even though the latest serum PSA test may be below the normal cutoff (<4 ng/mL), should undergo additional work-up. Studies have revealed that immunoreactive PSA (the form detected by the widely used antibody test) exists in two forms: a major fraction bound to α_1-antichymotrypsin and a minor free fraction. The *percentage of free PSA* (free PSA/total PSA × 100) is lower in men with prostate cancer than in men with benign prostatic diseases. Free PSA higher than 25% indicates a lower risk of cancer, as compared with free PSA values of less than 10%, which are of concern for cancer.

Because many small cancers localized to the prostate may never progress to clinically significant invasive cancers, there is considerable uncertainty regarding the management of small lesions that are detected because of an elevated PSA level. This has created some controversy about the role of widespread screening for prostate cancer. Much effort is therefore focused in devising criteria by which those localized lesions most likely to advance can be distinguished from those that may remain innocuous.

Serial measurements of PSA are of great value in assessing the response to therapy. For example, a rising PSA level after radical prostatectomy or radiotherapy for localized disease is indicative of recurrent or disseminated disease. Immunohistochemical localization of PSA on tissue sections can also help the pathologist to determine whether a metastatic tumor originated in the prostate.[135]

Cancer of the prostate is treated by surgery, radiation therapy, and hormonal manipulations. More than 90% of patients who receive such therapy can expect to live for 15 years. Currently, the most common treatment for clinically localized prostate cancer is radical prostatectomy. The prognosis following radical prostatectomy is based on the pathologic stage, margin status, and Gleason grade. Alternative treatments for localized prostate cancer are either external-beam radiation therapy or interstitial radiation therapy, the latter consisting of placing radioactive seeds throughout the prostate (brachytherapy). External-beam radiation therapy is also used to treat prostate cancer that is too locally advanced to be cured by surgery. Since some prostate cancers have a relatively indolent course, wherein it may take 10 years to see benefit from surgery or radiation therapy, active surveillance is appropriate for many older men or those with significant co-morbidity or even some younger men with low serum PSA values and limited lower grade cancer on biopsy. Advanced, metastatic carcinoma is treated by androgen deprivation either by orchiectomy or by administration of synthetic agonists of luteinizing hormone–releasing hormone (LHRH). Long-term administration of LHRH agonists suppresses normal LHRH, achieving in effect a pharmacologic orchiectomy. Although anti-androgen therapy induces remissions, eventually tumors develop testosterone-resistance, followed by a rapid progression of disease and death.

Miscellaneous Tumors and Tumor-like Conditions

Prostate adenocarcinomas may also arise from prostatic ducts. Ductal adenocarcinomas arising in peripheral ducts may present in a similar fashion to ordinary prostate cancer, whereas those arising in the larger periurethral ducts may show signs and symptoms similar to urothelial cancer, causing hematuria and urinary obstructive symptoms.[136,137] Ductal adenocarcinomas are associated with a relatively poor prognosis. Prostate cancer may show squamous differentiation, either following hormone therapy or de novo, resulting in either adenosquamous or pure squamous cancer. Prostate cancer that reveal abundant mucinous secretions are termed *colloid carcinoma of the prostate*.[138] The most aggressive variant of prostate cancer is small-cell cancer.[139] Almost all cases are rapidly fatal, only a few surviving with aggressive combination chemotherapy.

The most common tumor to secondarily involve the prostate is urothelial cancer.[139] Two distinct patterns of involvement exist. Large invasive urothelial cancers can directly invade from the bladder into the prostate. Alternatively, CIS of the bladder can extend into the prostatic urethra and down into the prostatic ducts and acini.

The same mesenchymal tumors described earlier that involve the bladder may also manifest in the prostate.[140–142] In addition, there exist unique mesenchymal tumors of the prostate derived from the prostatic stroma.[143] Although lymphomas may appear to first arise in the prostate, most patients shortly thereafter demonstrate systemic disease.[144]

REFERENCES

1. Kottra JJ, Dunnick NR: Retroperitoneal fibrosis. Radiol Clin North Am 34:1259, 1996.
2. Smeulders N, Woodhouse CR: Neoplasia in adult exstrophy patients. BJU Int 87:623, 2001.
3. deVries CR, Freiha FS: Hemorrhagic cystitis: a review. J Urol 143:1, 1990.
4. Nickel JC: Interstitial cystitis. Etiology, diagnosis, and treatment. Can Fam Physician 46:2430, 2000.
5. Wyndaele JJ: Evaluation of patients with painful bladder syndrome/interstitial cystitis. Sci World J 5:942, 2005.
6. Long JP, Jr, Althausen AF: Malacoplakia: a 25-year experience with a review of the literature. J Urol 141:1328, 1989.
7. Young RH: Papillary and polypoid cystitis. A report of eight cases. Am J Surg Pathol 12:542, 1988.
8. Lane Z, Epstein JI: Polypoid/papillary cystitis: a series of 41 cases misdiagnosed as papillary urothelial neoplasia. Am J Surg Pathol. 32:758, 2008.
9. Corica FA et al.: Intestinal metaplasia is not a strong risk factor for bladder cancer: study of 53 cases with long-term follow-up. Urology 50:427, 1997.
10. Young RH, Scully RE: Nephrogenic adenoma. A report of 15 cases, review of the literature, and comparison with clear cell adenocarcinoma of the urinary tract. Am J Surg Pathol 10:268, 1986.
11. Allan CH, Epstein JI: Nephrogenic adenoma of the prostatic urethra: a mimicker of prostate adenocarcinoma. Am J Surg Pathol 25:802, 2001.
12. Mazal PR et al.: Derivation of nephrogenic adenomas from renal tubular cells in kidney-transplant recipients. N Engl J Med 347:653, 2002.
13. Allan CH, Epstein JI: Nephrogenic adenoma of the prostatic urethra: a mimicker of prostate adenocarcinoma. Am J Surg Pathol 25:802, 2001.
14. Jemal A et al.: Cancer statistics, 2007. CA Cancer J Clin 57:43, 2007.
15. Taylor DC et al.: Papillary urothelial hyperplasia. A precursor to papillary neoplasms. Am J Surg Pathol 20:1481, 1996.
16. Epstein JI et al.: The World Health Organization/International Society of Urological Pathology consensus classification of urothelial (transitional cell) neoplasms of the urinary bladder. Bladder Consensus Conference Committee. Am J Surg Pathol 22:1435, 1998.
17. Eble JN et al.: The World Health Organization Classification of Tumours of the Urinary System and Male Genital System. Lyon, IARC Press, 2004.
18. Magi-Galluzzi C, Epstein JI: Urothelial papilloma of the bladder: a review of 34 de novo cases. Am J Surg Pathol 28:1615, 2004.
19. Cheville JC et al.: Inverted urothelial papilloma: is ploidy, MIB-1 proliferative activity, or p53 protein accumulation predictive of urothelial carcinoma? Cancer 88:632, 2000.
20. Witjes JA et al.: The prognostic value of a primary inverted papilloma of the urinary tract. J Urol 158:1500, 1997.
21. Gilbert HA et al.: The natural history of papillary transitional cell carcinoma of the bladder and its treatment in an unselected population on the basis of histologic grading. J Urol 119:488, 1978.
22. Heney NM et al.: Superficial bladder cancer: progression and recurrence. J Urol 130:1083, 1983.

23. Melamed MR et al.: Natural history and clinical behavior of in situ carcinoma of the human urinary bladder. 1964. CA Cancer J Clin 43:348, 1993.
24. Elliott GB et al.: "Denuding cystitis" and in situ urothelial carcinoma. Arch Pathol 96:91, 1973.
25. Farrow GM et al.: Clinical observations on sixty-nine cases of in situ carcinoma of the urinary bladder. Cancer Res 37:2794, 1977.
26. Melicow MM, Hollowell JW: Intra-urothelial cancer: carcinoma in situ, Bowen's disease of the urinary system: discussion of thirty cases. J Urol 68:763, 1952.
27. Drew PA et al.: The nested variant of transitional cell carcinoma: an aggressive neoplasm with innocuous histology. Mod Pathol 9:989, 1996.
28. Volmar KE et al.: Florid von Brunn nests mimicking urothelial carcinoma: a morphologic and immunohistochemical comparison to the nested variant of urothelial carcinoma. Am J Surg Pathol 27:1243, 2003.
29. Amin MB et al.: Lymphoepithelioma-like carcinoma of the urinary bladder. Am J Surg Pathol 18:466, 1994.
30. Talbert ML, Young RH: Carcinomas of the urinary bladder with deceptively benign-appearing foci. A report of three cases. Am J Surg Pathol 13:374, 1989.
31. Tamas EF et al.: Lymphoepithelioma-like carcinoma of the urinary tract: a clinicopathological study of 30 pure and mixed cases. Mod Pathol 20:828, 2007.
32. Kamat AM et al.: Micropapillary bladder cancer: a review of the University of Texas M. D. Anderson Cancer Center experience with 100 consecutive patients. Cancer 110:62, 2007.
33. Sakamoto N et al.: Urinary bladder carcinoma with a neoplastic squamous component: a mapping study of 31 cases. Histopathology 21:135, 1992.
34. El-Bolkainy MN et al.: The impact of schistosomiasis on the pathology of bladder carcinoma. Cancer 48:2643, 1981.
35. Grignon DJ et al.: Primary adenocarcinoma of the urinary bladder. A clinicopathologic analysis of 72 cases. Cancer 67:2165, 1991.
36. Xiaoxu L et al.: Bladder adenocarcinoma: 31 reported cases. Can J Urol 8:1380, 2001.
37. Trias I et al.: Small cell carcinoma of the urinary bladder. Presentation of 23 cases and review of 134 published cases. Eur Urol 39:85, 2000.
38. Brandau S, Bohle A: Bladder cancer. I. Molecular and genetic basis of carcinogenesis. Eur Urol 39:491, 2000.
39. Jung I, Messing E: Molecular mechanisms and pathways in bladder cancer development and progression. Cancer Control 7:325, 2000.
40. Gibas Z, Gibas L: Cytogenetics of bladder cancer. Cancer Genet Cytogenet 95:108, 1997.
41. Spruck CH et al.: Two molecular pathways to transitional cell carcinoma of the bladder. Cancer Res 54:784, 1994.
42. Luis NM et al.: Molecular biology of bladder cancer. Clin Transl Oncol 9:5, 2007.
43. Holmang S et al.: Stage progression in Ta papillary urothelial tumors: relationship to grade, immunohistochemical expression of tumor markers, mitotic frequency and DNA ploidy. J Urol 165:1124, 2001.
44. Malmstrom PU et al.: Recurrence, progression and survival in bladder cancer. A retrospective analysis of 232 patients with greater than or equal to 5-year follow-up. Scand J Urol Nephrol 21:185, 1987.
45. Koss LG: Mapping of the urinary bladder: its impact on the concepts of bladder cancer. Hum Pathol 10:533, 1979.
46. Melicow MM: Histological study of vesical urothelium intervening between gross neoplasms in total cystectomy. J Urol 68:261, 1952.
47. Smith G et al.: Prognostic significance of biopsy results of normal-looking mucosa in cases of superficial bladder cancer. Br J Urol 55:665, 1983.
48. Murphy WM, Soloway MS: Developing carcinoma (dysplasia) of the urinary bladder. Pathol Annu 17 (Pt 1):197, 1982.
49. Orozco RE et al.: Carcinoma in situ of the urinary bladder. Clues to host involvement in human carcinogenesis. Cancer 74:115, 1994.
50. Murphy WM et al.: Urinary cytology and bladder cancer. The cellular features of transitional cell neoplasms. Cancer 53:1555, 1984.
51. Nielsen ME et al.: Urinary markers in the detection of bladder cancer: what's new? Curr Opin Urol 16:350, 2006.
52. Herr HW et al.: Bacillus Calmette-Guérin therapy for superficial bladder cancer: a 10-year followup. J Urol 147:1020, 1992.
53. Martin SA et al.: Smooth muscle neoplasms of the urinary bladder: a clinicopathologic comparison of leiomyoma and leiomyosarcoma. Am J Surg Pathol 26:292, 2002.
54. Montgomery EA et al.: Inflammatory myofibroblastic tumors of the urinary tract: a clinicopathologic study of 46 cases, including a malignant example inflammatory fibrosarcoma and a subset associated with high-grade urothelial carcinoma. Am J Surg Pathol 30:1502, 2006.
55. Lopez-Beltran A et al.: Carcinosarcoma and sarcomatoid carcinoma of the bladder: clinicopathological study of 41 cases. J Urol 159:1497, 1998.
56. Scholtmeijer RJ et al.: Embryonal rhabdomyosarcoma of the urogenital tract in childhood. Eur Urol 9:69, 1983.
57. Kempton CL et al.: Malignant lymphoma of the bladder: evidence from 36 cases that low-grade lymphoma of the MALT-type is the most common primary bladder lymphoma. Am J Surg Pathol 21:1324, 1997.
58. Diamond DA, Ransley PG: Male epispadias. J Urol 154:2150, 1995.
59. Belman AB: Hypospadias update. Urology 49:166, 1997.
60. Davenport M: ABC of general surgery in children. Problems with the penis and prepuce. BMJ 312:299, 1996.
61. Edwards S: Balanitis and balanoposthitis: a review. Genitourin Med 72:155, 1996.
62. Cupp MR et al.: The detection of human papillomavirus deoxyribonucleic acid in intraepithelial, in situ, verrucous and invasive carcinoma of the penis. J Urol 154:1024, 1995.
63. Dillner J et al.: Etiology of squamous cell carcinoma of the penis. Scand J Urol Nephrol Suppl 205:189, 2000.
64. Cubilla AL et al.: Morphological features of epithelial abnormalities and precancerous lesions of the penis. Scand J Urol Nephrol Suppl 205:215, 2000.
65. Cubilla AL et al.: Histologic classification of penile carcinoma and its relation to outcome in 61 patients with primary resection. Int J Surg Pathol 9:111, 2001.
66. Burgers JK et al.: Penile cancer. Clinical presentation, diagnosis, and staging. Urol Clin North Am 19:247, 1992.
67. Rozanski TA, Bloom DA: The undescended testis. Theory and management. Urol Clin North Am 22:107, 1995.
68. Hutson JM et al.: Normal testicular descent and the aetiology of cryptorchidism. Adv Anat Embryol Cell Biol 132:1, 1996.
69. Swerdlow AJ et al.: Risk of testicular cancer in cohort of boys with cryptorchidism. BMJ 314:1507, 1997.
70. Davenport M: ABC of general paediatric surgery. Inguinal hernia, hydrocele, and the undescended testis. BMJ 312:564, 1996.
71. United Kingdom Testicular Cancer Study Group: Aetiology of testicular cancer: association with congenital abnormalities, age at puberty, infertility, and exercise. BMJ 308:1393, 1994.
72. Buetow SA: Epidemiology of testicular cancer. Epidemiol Rev 17:433, 1995.
73. Nistal M, Paniagua R: Testicular biopsy. Contemporary interpretation. Urol Clin North Am 26:555, 1999.
74. Ulbright TM: Germ cell neoplasms of the testis. Am J Surg Pathol 17:1075, 1993.
75. Bosl GJ, Motzer RJ: Testicular germ-cell cancer. N Engl J Med 337:242, 1997.
76. McIntyre A et al.: Genes, chromosomes and the development of testicular germ cell tumors of adolescents and adults. Genes, Chromosomes, Cancer 47:547, 2008.
77. Looijenga LHS et al.: Chromosomes and expression in human testicular germ-cell tumors. Insight into their origin and pathogenesis. Ann NY Acad Sci 1120:187, 2007.
78. Eble JN: Spermatocytic seminoma. Hum Pathol 25:1035, 1994.
79. Emerson RE, Ulbright TM: The use of immunohistochemistry in the differential diagnosis of tumors of the testis and paratestis. Semin Diagn Pathol 22:33, 2005.
80. Motzer RJ et al.: Teratoma with malignant transformation: diverse malignant histologies arising in men with germ cell tumors. J Urol 159:133, 1998.
81. Doherty AP et al.: The role of tumour markers in the diagnosis and treatment of testicular germ cell cancers. Br J Urol 79:247, 1997.
82. Dilworth JP et al.: Non–germ cell tumors of testis. Urology 37:399, 1991.
83. Kim I et al.: Leydig cell tumors of the testis. A clinicopathological analysis of 40 cases and review of the literature. Am J Surg Pathol 9:177, 1985.
84. Cheville JC et al.: Leydig cell tumor of the testis: a clinicopathologic, DNA content, and MIB-1 comparison of nonmetastasizing and metastasizing tumors. Am J Surg Pathol 22:1361, 1998.
85. Young RH et al.: Sertoli cell tumors of the testis, not otherwise specified: a clinicopathologic analysis of 60 cases. Am J Surg Pathol 22:709, 1998.

86. Ferry JA et al.: Malignant lymphoma of the testis, epididymis, and spermatic cord. A clinicopathologic study of 69 cases with immunophenotypic analysis. Am J Surg Pathol 18:376, 1994.

87. McNeal JE: Normal and pathologic anatomy of prostate. Urology 17:11, 1981.

88. Wise GJ, Silver DA: Fungal infections of the genitourinary system. J Urol 149:1377, 1993.

89. Oates RD et al.: Granulomatous prostatitis following bacillus Calmette-Guerin immunotherapy of bladder cancer. J Urol 140:751, 1988.

90. Mukamel E et al.: Clinical and pathological findings in prostates following intravesical bacillus Calmette-Guérin instillations. J Urol 144:1399, 1990.

91. Epstein JI, Hutchins GM: Granulomatous prostatitis: distinction among allergic, nonspecific, and post-transurethral resection lesions. Hum Pathol 15:818, 1984.

92. Kohnen PW, Drach GW: Patterns of inflammation in prostatic hyperplasia: a histologic and bacteriologic study. J Urol 121:755, 1979.

93. Roehrborn CG, McConnell: Benign prostatic hyperplasia: etiology, pathophysiology, epidemiology and natural history. In: Wein AJ eds., Campbell-Walsh Urology, Philadelphia, WB Saunders, 2007, vol XVI: 2727.

94. Umtergasser G et al.: Benign prostatic hyperplasia: age related tissue-remodeling. Exp Gerontol 40:121, 2005.

95. Marks LS et al.: Prostate tissue androgens: history and current clinical relevance. Urology 72:247, 2008.

96. Heracek J et al.: Tissue and serum levels of principal androgens in benign prostatic hyperplasia and prostate cancer. Steroids 72:375, 2007.

97. Roehrborn GC: Current medical therapies for men with lower urinary tract symptoms and benign prostatic hyperplasia: achievements and limitations. Rev Urol 10:14, 2008.

98. Barkin J: management of benign prostatic hyperplasia by primary care physicians in the 21st century: the new paradigm. Can J Urol Suppl 1:21, 2008.

99. Jemal A et al.: Cancer statistics, 2007. CA Cancer J Clin 57:43, 2007.

100. Ekman P: Genetic and environmental factors in prostate cancer genesis: identifying high-risk cohorts. Eur Urol 35:362, 1999.

101. Holick MF: Vitamin D deficiency. N Engl J Med 357:266, 2007.

102. Albertelli MA et al.: Replacing the mouse androgen receptor with human alleles demonstrates glutamine tract length-dependent effects on physiology and tumorigenesis in mice. Mol Endocrin 20:1248, 2006.

103. Nieto M et al.: Prostate cancer: Refocusing on androgen receptor signaling. Int J Biochem Cell Biol 39:1562, 2007.

104. DeMarzo AM et al.: Pathological and molecular aspects of prostate cancer. Lancet 361:955, 2003.

105. Nelson WG et al.: Prostate cancer. N Engl J Med 349:366, 2003.

106. Prowatke I et al.: Expression analysis of imbalanced genes in prostate carcinoma using tissue microarrays. Br J Cancer 96:82, 2007.

107. Tomlins SA, Rubin MA, Chinnaiyan AM: Integrative biology of prostate cancer progression. Annu Rev Pathol 1:243, 2006.

108. Wiklund F, Gillanders EM, Albertus JA, Bergh A, Damber JE, Emanuelsson M, et al.: Genome-wide scan of Swedish families with hereditary prostate cancer: suggestive evidence of linkage at 5q11.2 and 19p13.3. Prostate 57:290, 2003.

109. Freedman ML et al.: Admixture mapping identifies 8q24 as a prostate cancer risk locus in African-American men. Proc Natl Acad Sci USA 103:14068, 2006.

110. Kumar-Sinha C, Tomlins SA, Chinnaiyan AM: Recurrent gene fusions in prostate cancer. Nature Rev Cancer 8:497, 2008.

111. Mosquera JM et al.: Morphologic features of *TMPRSS2-ERG* gene fusion prostate cancer. J Pathol 212:91, 2007.

112. Iljin K et al.: TMRPSS2 fusions with oncogenic ETS factors in prostate cancer involve unbalanced genomic rearrangements and are associated with HDAC1 and epigenetic reprogramming. Cancer Res 66:10658, 2006.

113. Carmen J et al.: Quantitation of GSTP1 methylation in non-neoplastic prostatic tissue and organ-confined prostate adenocarcinoma. J Natl Cancer Inst 93:1671, 2001.

114. Schalken JA et al.: Molecular prostate cancer pathology: current issues and achievements. Scand J Urol Nephrol Suppl 216:82, 2005.

115. Varambally S et al.: The polycomb group protein EZH2 is involved in progression of prostate cancer. Nature 419:624, 2002.

116. Jiang Z et al.: Discovery and clinical application of a novel prostate cancer marker: alpha-methylacyl CoA racemase (P504S). Am J Clin Pathol 122:275, 2004.

117. Luo J et al.: Alpha-methylacyl-CoA racemase: a new molecular marker for prostate cancer. Cancer Res 62:2220, 2002.

118. Groskopf J et al.: APTIMA PCA3 molecular urine test: development of a method to aid in the diagnosis of prostate cancer. Clin Chem 52:1089, 2006.

119. Marks LS et al.: PCA3 molecular urine assay for prostate cancer in men.

120. Cerveira N et al.: *TMPRSS2-ERG* gene fusion causing ERG overexpression precedes chromosome copy number changes in prostate carcinomas and paired HGPIN lesions. Neoplasia 8:826, 2006.

121. Perner S et al.: *TMPRSS2: ERG* fusion prostate cancer: an early molecular event associated with invasion. Am J Surg Pathol 31:882, 2007.

122. Epstein JI, Herawi M: Prostate needle biopsies containing prostatic intraepithelial neoplasia or atypical foci suspicious for carcinoma: implications for patient care. J Urol 175:820, 2006.

123. Epstein JI, Netto GJ: Biopsy Interpretation of the Prostate. Philadelphia, JB Lippincott Williams & Wilkins, 2008.

124. Eble JN et al.: Pathology and Genetics: Tumors of the urinary system and male genital organs. WHO classification of tumors. World Health Organization, Geneva, 2004.

125. Epstein JI: Diagnostic criteria of limited adenocarcinoma of the prostate on needle biopsy. Hum Pathol 26:223, 1995.

126. Wojno KJ, Epstein JI: The utility of basal cell-specific anti-cytokeratin antibody (34 beta E12) in the diagnosis of prostate cancer. A review of 228 cases. Am J Surg Pathol 19:251, 1995.

127. McNeal JE: Significance of duct-acinar dysplasia in prostatic carcinogenesis. Urology 34:9, 1989.

128. McNeal JE, Bostwick DG: Intraductal dysplasia: a premalignant lesion of the prostate. Hum Pathol 17:64, 1986.

129. Epstein JI et al.: Update on the Gleason grading system for prostate cancer: results of an international consensus conference of urologic pathologists. Adv Anat Pathol 13:57, 2006.

130. Gleason DF, Mellinger GT: Prediction of prognosis for prostatic adenocarcinoma by combined histological grading and clinical staging. J Urol 111:58, 1974.

131. Epstein JI et al.: Pathologic and clinical findings to predict tumor extent of nonpalpable (stage T1c) prostate cancer. JAMA 271:368, 1994.

132. Matzkin H et al.: Stage T1A carcinoma of prostate. Urology 43:11, 1994.

133. Eble JN, Epstein JI: Stage A carcinoma of the prostate. In Roth LM (ed): Pathology of the Prostate, Seminal Vesicles, and Male Urethra. New York, Churchill Livingstone, 1990, pp 61–82.

134. Gretzer MB, Partin AW: PSA markers in prostate cancer detection. Urol Clin North Am 30:677, 2003.

135. Epstein JI: PSAP and PSA as immunohistochemical markers. Urol Clin North Am 20:757, 1993.

136. Brinker DA et al.: Ductal adenocarcinoma of the prostate diagnosed on needle biopsy: correlation with clinical and radical prostatectomy findings and progression. Am J Surg Pathol 23:1471, 1999.

137. Ro JY et al.: Mucinous adenocarcinoma of the prostate: histochemical and immunohistochemical studies. Hum Pathol 21:593, 1990.

138. Wang W, Epstein JI: Small cell carcinoma of the prostate: a morphological and immunohistochemical study of 95 cases. Am J Surg Pathol, 32:65, 2008.

139. Oliai BR et al.: A clinicopathologic analysis of urothelial carcinomas diagnosed on prostate needle biopsy. Am J Surg Pathol 25:794, 2001.

140. Sexton WJ et al.: Adult prostate sarcoma: the M.D. Anderson Cancer Center Experience. J Urol 166:521, 2001.

141. Raney RB et al.: Rhabdomyosarcoma and undifferentiated sarcoma in the first two decades of life: a selective review of intergroup rhabdomyosarcoma study group experience and rationale for Intergroup Rhabdomyosarcoma Study V. J Pediatr Hematol Oncol 23:215, 2001.

142. Hansel DE, Epstein JI: Sarcomatoid carcinoma of the prostate: a study of 42 cases. Am J Surg Pathol 30:1316, 2006.

143. Herawi M, Epstein JI: Specialized stromal tumors of the prostate: a clinicopathologic study of 50 cases. Am J Surg Pathol 30:694, 2006.

144. Bostwick DG, Mann RB: Malignant lymphomas involving the prostate. A study of 13 cases. Cancer 56:2932, 1985.

The Female Genital Tract*

LORA HEDRICK ELLENSON · EDYTA C. PIROG

Development

Anatomy

Infections of the Female Genital Tract
  Infections of the Lower Genital Tract
  Infections Involving the Lower and
    Upper Genital Tract

■ VULVA

Bartholin Cyst

Non-Neoplastic Epithelial Disorders
  Lichen Sclerosus
  Squamous Cell Hyperplasia

Benign Exophytic Lesions
  Condyloma Acuminatum

Squamous Neoplastic Lesions
  Vulvar Intraepithelial Neoplasia and
    Vulvar Carcinoma

Glandular Neoplastic Lesions
  Papillary Hidradenoma
  Extramammary Paget Disease

Malignant Melanoma

■ VAGINA

Development Anomalies

Premalignant and Malignant
  Neoplasms
  Vaginal Intraepithelial Neoplasia and
    Squamous Cell Carcinoma
  Embryonal Rhabdomyosarcoma

■ CERVIX

Inflammations
  Acute and Chronic Cervicitis

Endocervical Polyps

Premalignant and Malignant
  Neoplasms
  Cervical Intraepithelial Neoplasia
  Cervical Carcinoma
    Cervical Cancer Screening And
      Prevention

■ BODY OF UTERUS AND
  ENDOMETRIUM

Endometrial Histology in the
  Menstrual Cycle

Functional Endometrial Disorders
  (Dysfunctional Uterine Bleeding)
  Anovulatory Cycle
  Inadequate Luteal Phase
  Endometrial Changes Induced by Oral
    Contraceptives
  Menopausal and Postmenopausal
    Changes

Inflammation
  Acute Endometritis
  Chronic Endometritis

Endometriosis and Adenomyosis

Endometrial Polyps

Endometrial Hyperplasia

*The contributions of Dr. Christopher Crum to this chapter over the past
many editions are gratefully acknowledged.

Malignant Tumors of the Endometrium
Carcinoma of the Endometrium
Malignant Mixed Müllerian Tumors

Tumors of the Endometrium with Stromal Differentiation
Adenosarcomas
Stromal Tumors

Tumors of the Myometrium
Leiomyomas
Leiomyosarcomas

■ **FALLOPIAN TUBES**

Inflammations

Tumors and Cysts

■ **OVARIES**

Non-Neoplastic and Functional Cysts
Follicle and Luteal Cysts
Polycystic Ovaries and Stromal Hyperthecosis

Ovarian Tumors
Tumors of Surface (Müllerian) Epithelium
Serous Tumors
Mucinous Tumors
Endometrioid Tumors
Clear Cell Adenocarcinoma
Cystadenofibroma
Brenner Tumor
Clinical Course, Detection, and Prevention of Surface Epithelial Tumors

Germ Cell Tumors
Teratomas
Dysgerminoma
Endodermal Sinus (Yolk Sac) Tumor
Choriocarcinoma
Other Germ Cell Tumors
Sex Cord–Stromal Tumors
Granulosa–Theca Cell Tumors
Fibromas, Thecomas, and Fibrothecomas
Sertoli–Leydig Cell Tumors (Androblastomas)
Other Sex Cord–Stromal Tumors
Metastatic Tumors

■ **GESTATIONAL AND PLACENTAL DISORDERS**

Disorders of Early Pregnancy
Spontaneous Abortion
Ectopic Pregnancy

Disorders of Late Pregnancy
Twin Placentas
Abnormalities of Placental Implantation
Placental Infections
Preeclampsia and Eclampsia

Gestational Trophoblastic Disease
Hydatidiform Mole
Complete Mole
Partial Mole
Invasive Mole
Choriocarcinoma
Placental Site Trophoblastic Tumor (PSTT)

Development

The development of the female genital tract is relevant to both anomalies in this region and the histogenesis of various tumors. The primordial germ cells arise in the wall of the yolk sac by the fourth week of gestation; by the fifth or sixth week they migrate into the urogenital ridge. The mesodermal epithelium of the urogenital ridge then proliferates, to eventually produce the epithelium and stroma of the gonad. The dividing germ cells, which are of endodermal origin, are incorporated into the proliferating mesodermal epithelium to form the ovary.[1]

A second component of female genital development is the *müllerian duct.* At about the sixth week, invagination and subsequent fusion of the coelomic lining epithelium forms the lateral müllerian (or paramesonephric) ducts. Müllerian ducts progressively grow caudally to enter the pelvis, where they swing medially to fuse with the urogenital sinus at the müllerian tubercle (Fig. 22–1A). Further caudal growth brings these fused ducts into contact with the urogenital sinus, formed when the cloaca is subdivided by the urorectal septum. The

urogenital sinus eventually becomes the vestibule of the external genitalia (Fig. 22–1B). Normally the unfused portions mature into the fallopian tubes, the fused caudal portion develop into the uterus and upper vagina, and the urogenital sinus forms the lower vagina and vestibule. Consequently, the entire lining of the uterus and tubes as well as the ovarian surface is ultimately derived from coelomic epithelium (mesothelium). This close embryologic relationship between the mesothelium and müllerian system may be reflected in adult life in the form of benign (endometriosis) and malignant (endometrioid and serous neoplasia) lesions, which may arise in both the surface of the ovaries and the peritoneal surfaces. In addition, it explains the morphologic overlap of tumors arising in the various parts of the female genital tract (e.g., serous, endometrioid, clear cell).

The epithelium of the vagina, cervix, and urinary tract is formed by induction of basal cells from the underlying stroma, which undergo squamous and urothelial differentiation.[2] A portion of these cells remains uncommitted, forming the reserve cells of the cervix. The latter are capable of both squamous and columnar cell differentiation.[3]

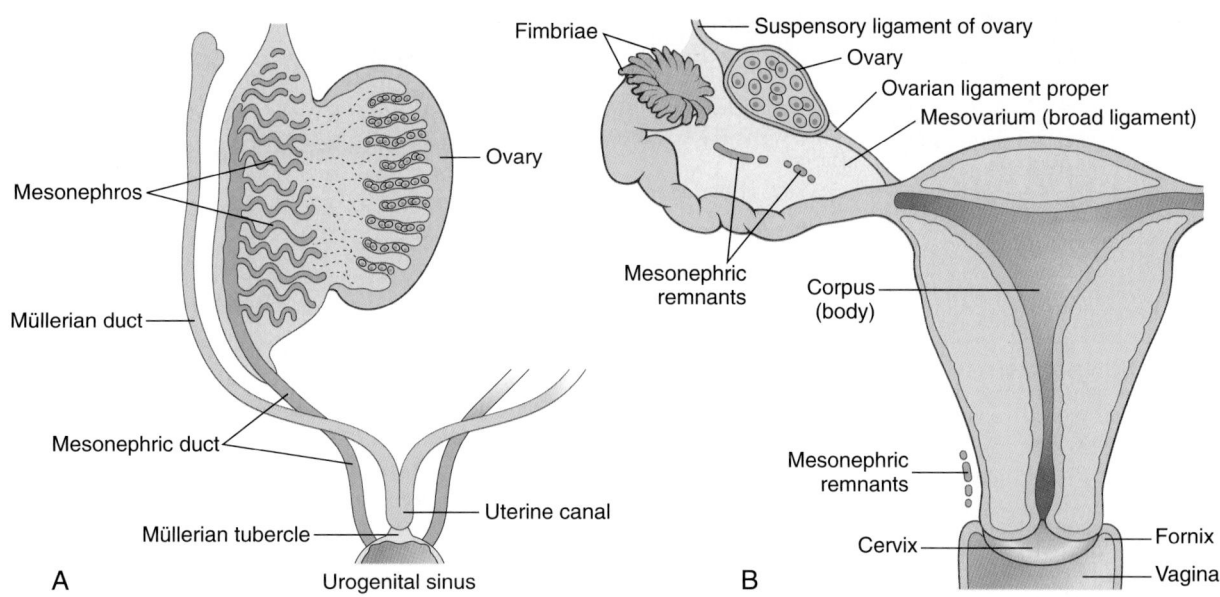

FIGURE 22–1 Embryology and anatomy of the female genital tract. **A,** Early in development the mesonephric *(blue)* and müllerian *(red)* ducts merge at the urogenital sinus to form the müllerian tubercle. **B,** By birth the müllerian ducts have fused to form the fallopian tubes, uterus, and endocervix *(red),* merging with the vaginal squamous mucosa. The mesonephric ducts regress but may be found as a remnant in the ovary, adnexa, and cervix (Gartner duct). (Adapted from Langman J: Medical Embryology. Baltimore, Williams and Wilkins, 1981.)

In males, müllerian inhibitory substance[4] from the developing testis causes regression of the müllerian ducts, and the paired wolffian (or mesonephric) ducts form the epididymis and the vas deferens. Normally the mesonephric duct regresses in the female, but remnants may persist into adult life as epithelial inclusions adjacent to the ovaries, tubes, and uterus. In the cervix and vagina these rests may be cystic and are termed *Gartner duct cysts.* Many of the events in the formation of the internal and external genitalia and their epithelial coverings result from reciprocal epithelial-stromal signaling, leading to mesenchymal remodeling and changes in epithelial cell fate.[2,5]

Anatomy

During active reproductive life, the ovaries measure about 4 × 2.5 × 1.5 cm in dimension. The ovary is divided into a cortex and a medulla. The cortex consists of a layer of closely packed stromal cells and a thin covering of relatively acellular collagenous connective tissue. Follicles in varying stages of maturation are found within the outer cortex. With each menstrual cycle, one follicle develops into a graafian follicle, which is transformed into a corpus luteum following ovulation. Corpora lutea ranging from recent to senescent (corpora albicans) may be found in the cortex of the adult ovary.

The medulla of the ovary consists of loosely arranged mesenchymal tissue and contains remnants of the mesonephric duct (rete ovarii) and small clusters of round to polygonal, epithelioid cells (hilus cells) around vessels and nerves. These hilus cells are vestigial remains of the gonad from its primitive "ambisexual" phase, are steroid producing, and resemble the interstitial cells of the testis. Rarely, these cells give rise to masculinizing tumors (hilar cell tumors).

The fallopian tube mucosa is composed of numerous delicate papillary folds (plica) consisting of three cell types: ciliated columnar cells; nonciliated, columnar secretory cells; and so-called intercalated cells, which may simply represent inactive secretory cells.

The uterus varies in size depending on the age and parity of the individual. It weighs about 50 gm and measures about 8.0 × 6.0 × 3.0 cm in nulliparous reproductive age women. Following pregnancies, uteri are slightly larger (up to 70 gm in weight), then diminish to half their weight and dimension following menopause.

The uterus has three distinctive anatomic and functional regions: the cervix, the lower uterine segment, and the corpus. The cervix is further divided into the vaginal portio (ectocervix) and the endocervix. The portio is visible to the naked eye on vaginal examination and is covered by a stratified nonkeratinizing squamous epithelium continuous with the vaginal vault. The squamous epithelium converges centrally at a small opening termed the *external os.* In the nulliparous woman, this os is virtually closed. Just cephalad from the os is the endocervix, which is lined by columnar, mucus-secreting epithelium that dips down into the underlying stroma to produce endocervical glands. The point at which the squamous and endocervical mucinous columnar epithelium meet is termed the *squamocolumnar junction* (Fig. 22–2). The position of the junction is variable because of both the cervical anatomy and age-related hormonal influences. The differentiation of basal/reserve cells at the squamocolumnar junction into either squamous or glandular cell type governs the microanatomy of this region and results in a progressive upward migration of the squamocolumnar junction with age. The area of the cervix where the columnar epithelium is ultimately replaced by squamous epithelium is termed the *transformation zone* (see Fig. 22–2). Metaplasia of glandular epithelium to squamous

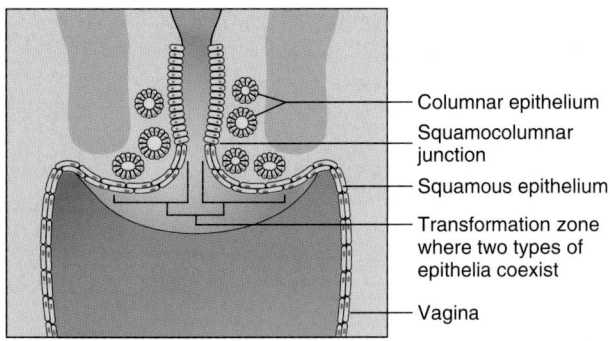

Columnar epithelium
Squamocolumnar junction
Squamous epithelium
Transformation zone where two types of epithelia coexist
Vagina

FIGURE 22–2 Schematic of the cervical transformation zone where squamous and endocervical columnar epithelia coexist undergoing metaplasia ("transformation") from glandular to squamous differentiation.

epithelium at the squamocolumnar junction produces multi-layered, initially immature, squamous epithelium known as "squamous metaplasia." These immature squamous cells are susceptible to human papillomavirus (HPV) infection and, as discussed below, it is at the squamocolumnar junction where precancerous lesions and cervical carcinomas develop.[6]

The corpus consists of the endometrium surrounded by the myometrium. Changes in the endometrium that occur during the menstrual cycle (discussed below) are keyed to the rise and fall in the levels of ovarian hormones, and the reader should be familiar with the complex but fascinating interactions among hypothalamic, pituitary, and ovarian factors underlying maturation of ovarian follicles, ovulation, and the menstrual cycle.

Diseases of the female genital tract are extremely common and include complications of pregnancy, infections, tumors, and hormonally induced effects. The following discussion presents the pathology of the major diseases that result in clinical problems. Details can be found in current textbooks of gynecologic pathology and clinical obstetrics and gynecology.[7,8] The pathologic conditions peculiar to each segment of the female genital tract are discussed separately, but first we briefly review infections and pelvic inflammatory disease because they can affect many of the various anatomic structures concomitantly.

Infections of the Female Genital Tract

A large variety of organisms can infect the female genital tract. Infections with some microorganisms, such as *Candida*, *Trichomonas*, and *Gardnerella*, are extremely common and may cause significant discomfort with no serious sequelae. Others, such as *Neisseria gonorrhoeae* and *Chlamydia* infections, are major causes of female infertility, and others still, such as *Ureaplasma urealyticum* and *Mycoplasma hominis* infections, are implicated in preterm deliveries. Viruses, especially herpes simplex viruses (HSVs) and human papillomaviruses (HPVs), also account for considerable morbidity; HSVs cause painful genital ulcerations, whereas HPVs are involved in the pathogenesis of cervical, vaginal, and vulvar cancers.

Many of these infections are sexually transmitted, including trichomoniasis, gonorrhea, chancroid, granuloma inguinale,

lymphogranuloma venereum, syphilis, mycoplasma, chlamydia, HSV, and HPV.[9] Most of these conditions have been considered in Chapter 8. Here we touch only on selected aspects relevant to the female genital tract, including pathogens confined to the lower genital tract (vulva, vagina, and cervix) and those that involve the entire genital tract and are implicated in pelvic inflamatory disease. Papillomaviruses are also discussed in Chapter 7.

Infections of the Lower Genital Tract

Genital *herpes simplex virus* infection is common and involves, in the order of frequency, the cervix, vagina, and vulva. HSVs are DNA viruses that include two serotypes, HSV-1 and HSV-2. *HSV-1 typically results in oropharyngeal infection, whereas HSV-2 usually involves genital mucosa and skin;* however, depending on the sexual practices HSV-1 may be detected in the genital region and HSV-2 may cause oral infections as well (see also Chapter 8). The frequency of genital herpes has increased dramatically in the past decades, particularly in teenagers and young women. *By the age of 40, 20% of women are seropositive for antibodies against HSV-2.*[10]

Clinical symptoms are seen in about one third of infected individuals. The initial lesions typically develop 3 to 7 days after sexual transmission and consist of red papules that progress to vesicles and then to painful coalescent ulcers. Such lesions are clinically apparent on vulvar skin and mucosa, while cervical or vaginal lesions present with severe purulent discharge and pelvic pain. Lesions around the urethra may cause painful urination and urine retention. The initial infection typically produces systemic symptoms such as fever, malaise, and tender inguinal lymph nodes. The vesicles and ulcers contain numerous viral particles, accounting for the high transmission rate during active infection. The mucosal and skin lesions heal spontaneously in 1 to 3 weeks, but as with herpetic infections elsewhere, the virus migrates to the regional lumbosacral nerve ganglia establishing a latent infection. Because of viral latency, HSV infections persist indefinitely and any decrease in immune system surveillance, as well as stress, trauma, ultraviolet radiation, and hormonal changes, can trigger reactivation of the virus and recurrence of the skin and mucosal lesions.[9] As expected, recurrences are much more common in immunosuppressed individuals. In addition, *HSV-2 infections are more likely to recur than HSV-1 infections.*

Transmission of HSV may occur during both the active and latent phases (subclinical virus shedding), although it is much less likely in asymptomatic carriers. Condoms offer limited protection against HSV infection, since a large genital area may be affected by the virus. As with other sexually transmitted diseases, women are more susceptible to transmission than men. Previous infection with HSV-1 seems to reduce susceptibility to HSV-2 infection. The gravest consequence of HSV infection is transmission to the neonate during birth. This risk is highest if the infection is active during delivery and particularly if it is a primary (initial) infection in the mother. Cesarian section is warranted in such cases.

The diagnosis is based on typical clinical findings and HSV detection. For diagnosis the purulent exudate is aspirated from the lesions and inoculated into a tissue culture. After 48 to 72 hours the *viral cytopathic effect* can be seen, and the virus may then be isolated and serotyped. In addition, some laboratories offer more sensitive *polymerase chain reaction,* enzyme-linked immunosorbent assays, and direct immunofluorescent antibody tests for detection of HSV in the lesional secretions. Individuals with primary, acute-phase HSV infection do not have serum anti-HSV antibodies. Detection of *anti-HSV antibodies in the serum is indicative of recurrent/ latent infection.*

There is no effective treatment for latent HSV; however, antiviral agents like acyclovir or famciclovir may shorten the length of the initial and recurrent symptomatic phase. Several prophylactic and therapeutic vaccine strategies have been developed using animal models, and several clinical trials are currently underway.[11]

Molluscum contagiosum is a poxvirus infection of the skin and the mucous membranes. There are four types of *molluscum contagiosum viruses* (MCVs), MCV-1 to -4, with MCV-1 being the most prevalent and MCV-2 being most often sexually transmitted. The infections are common in young children between 2 and 12 years of age and are transmitted through direct contact or shared articles (e.g., towels). Molluscum may affect any area of the skin but is most common on the trunk, arms, and legs. In adults, molluscum infections are typically sexually transmitted and affect the genitals, lower abdomen, buttocks, and inner thighs. The average incubation period is 6 weeks. Diagnosis is based on the characteristic clinical appearance of pearly, dome-shaped papules with a dimpled center. The papules measure 1 to 5 mm in diameter, and their central waxy core contains cells with *intracytoplasmic viral inclusions* (Fig. 22–3).

Fungal infections, especially those caused by yeasts (*Candida*), are extremely common; in fact, yeasts are part of many women's normal vaginal microflora and the development of symptomatic candidiasis is typically a result of a disturbance in the patient's vaginal microbial ecosystem. *Diabetes mellitus, antibiotics, pregnancy, and conditions resulting in compromised cell-mediated immunity are permissive to symptomatic infection,* which manifests itself by marked vulvovaginal pruritus, erythema, swelling, and curdlike vaginal discharge. Severe infection may result in mucosal ulcerations. The diagnosis is made by finding the pseudospores or filamentous fungal hyphae in wet KOH mounts of the discharge or on Pap smear. Even though sexual transmission of yeast infection has been documented, candidiasis is not considered a sexually transmitted disease.

Trichomonas vaginalis is a large, flagellated ovoid protozoan that can be readily identified in wet mounts of vaginal discharge or Pap smear of infected patients. The infection is usually transmitted by sexual contact and develops within 4 days to 4 weeks. The patients may be asymptomatic or may complain of yellow, frothy vaginal discharge, vulvovaginal discomfort, dysuria (painful urination), and dyspareunia (painful intercourse). The vaginal and cervical mucosa typically has a fiery-red appearance, with marked dilatation of cervical mucosal vessels resulting in characteristic colposcopic appearance of "strawberry cervix."

Gardnerella vaginalis is a gram-negative bacillus that is implicated as the main cause of bacterial vaginosis (vaginitis). Patients typically present with thin, green-gray, malodorous (fishy) vaginal discharge. Pap smears reveal superficial and intermediate squamous cells covered by a shaggy coat of multiple coccobacilli. Bacterial cultures in such cases reveal *G. vaginalis* and other bacteria including anaerobic peptostreptococci and aerobic α-hemolytic streptococci. In pregnant patients, bacterial vaginosis has been implicated in premature labor.

Ureaplasma urealyticum and *Mycoplasma hominis* species account for some cases of vaginitis and cervicitis, and have been implicated in chorioamnionitis and premature delivery in pregnant patients.[12]

Most *Chlamydia trachomatis* infections take the form of cervicitis. However, in some patients it ascends to the uterus and fallopian tubes, resulting in endometritis and salpingitis, and thus is one of the causes of pelvic inflammatory disease, as discussed below.

For description of genital lesions caused by *Treponema pallidium*, see Chapter 8. Description of HPV infections is presented in this chapter under "Cervix", and gonorrhea infections are described below.

Infections Involving The Lower and Upper Genital Tract

Pelvic Inflammatory Disease (PID)

PID is an ascending infection that begins in the vulva or vagina and spreads upward to involve most of the structures in the female genital system, resulting in pelvic pain, adnexal tenderness, fever, and vaginal discharge. Gonococcus continues to be a common cause of PID, the most serious complication of gonorrhea in women. *Chlamydia* infection is another well-recognized cause of PID. Besides these two organisms, infections after spontaneous or induced abortions and normal or abnormal deliveries (called puerperal infections) are important causes of PID. In these situations the infections are typically polymicrobial and may be caused by staphylococci, streptococci, coliform bacteria, and *Clostridium perfringens.*

With gonococcus, inflammatory changes start to appear approximately 2 to 7 days after inoculation. Endocervical mucosa is the most common site of initial involvement.

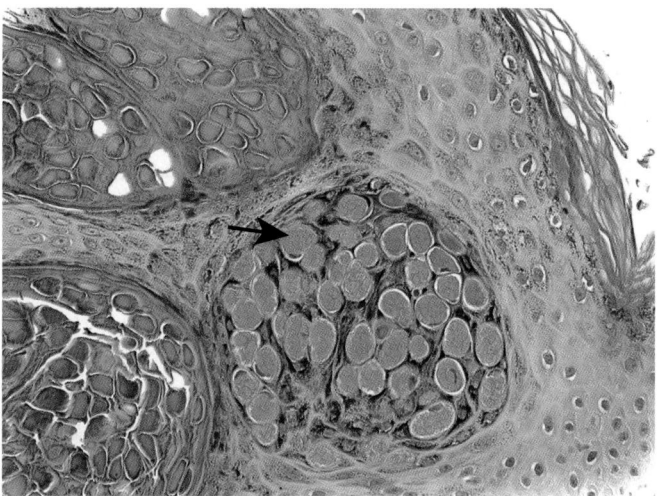

FIGURE 22–3 Lesion caused by molluscum contagiosum infection. *Arrow* points to intracytoplasmic viral inclusions.

Gonococcal inflammation may also begin in the Bartholin gland and other vestibular, or periurethral, glands. From any of these sites, the organisms may spread upward to involve the fallopian tubes and tubo-ovarian region. The non-gonococcal bacterial infections that follow induced abortion, dilation and curettage of the uterus, and other surgical procedures of the female genital tract are thought to spread from the uterus upward through the lymphatics or venous channels rather than on the mucosal surfaces. Therefore, these infections tend to produce less mucosal involvement but more reaction within the deeper layers of the organs.

Morphology. Wherever it occurs, gonococcal disease is characterized by marked acute inflammation largely confined to the superficial mucosa. Smears of the inflammatory exudate disclose the intracellular gram-negative diplococcus; however, definitive diagnosis requires culture, or detection of gonoccocal RNA or DNA. If spread occurs, the endometrium is usually spared for unclear reasons. Once the infection reaches the tubes, an **acute suppurative salpingitis** ensues. The tubal mucosa becomes congested and diffusely infiltrated by neutrophils, plasma cells, and lymphocytes. Gonococcal lipopolysaccharide and inflammatory mediators such as TNF cause epithelial injury and sloughing of the plicae. The tubal lumen fills with purulent exudate that may leak out of the fimbriated end. The infection may further spill over to the ovary to create a **salpingo-oophoritis**. Collections of pus within the ovary and tube (**tubo-ovarian abscesses**) or tubal lumen (**pyosalpinx**) may occur (Fig. 22–4). In the course of time the infecting organisms may disappear, leaving the sequelae of **chronic follicular salpingitis** and **hydrosalpinx** (dilated, fluid-filled fallopian tube). The tubal plicae, denuded of epithelium, adhere to one another and slowly fuse in a reparative, scar-ring process that forms glandlike spaces and blind pouches, referred to as chronic follicular salpingitis. The lumen of such tubes may be impenetrable for the oocyte, resulting in infertility or ectopic pregnancy. Hydrosalpinx develops as a consequence of the fusion of the fimbriae and the subsequent accumulation of the tubal secretions and tubal distention. Hydrosalpinx is another cause of post-PID infertility, since lack of flexible tubal fimbriae prevents uptake of the oocyte after ovulation.

PID caused by staphylococci, streptococci, and the other puerperal invaders tends to have less exudation within the lumen of the tube and less involvement of the mucosa, but a greater inflammatory response within the deeper tissue layers. These infections often spread throughout the wall to involve the serosa and the broad ligaments, pelvic structures, and peritoneum. Bacteremia is a more frequent complication of streptococcal or staphylococcal PID than of gonococcal infections.

The acute complications of PID include peritonitis and bacteremia, which in turn may result in endocarditis, meningitis, and suppurative arthritis. The remote sequelae of PID include infertility and tubal obstruction, increased risk of ectopic pregnancy, pelvic pain, as well as intestinal obstruction due to adhesions between the bowel and pelvic organs.

In the early stages, gonococcal infections are readily controlled with antibiotics, although penicillin-resistant strains have regrettably emerged. When the infection becomes walled off in tubo-ovarian abscesses, it is difficult to achieve sufficient levels of antibiotics within such infectious foci and it sometimes becomes necessary to remove the organs surgically. Postabortion and postpartum PIDs are also amenable to treatment with antibiotics but are far more difficult to control than the gonococcal infections because of the broad spectrum of pathogens that may be involved.

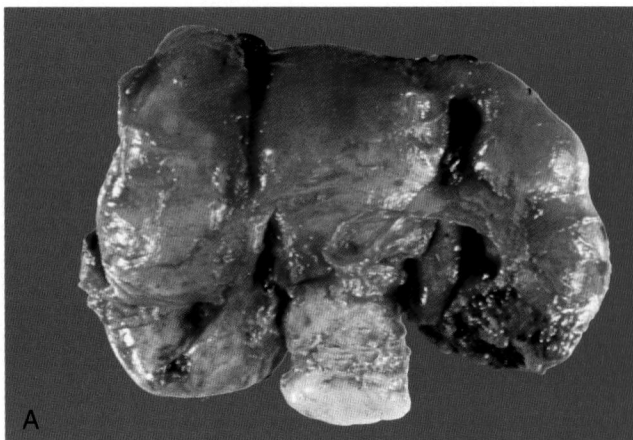
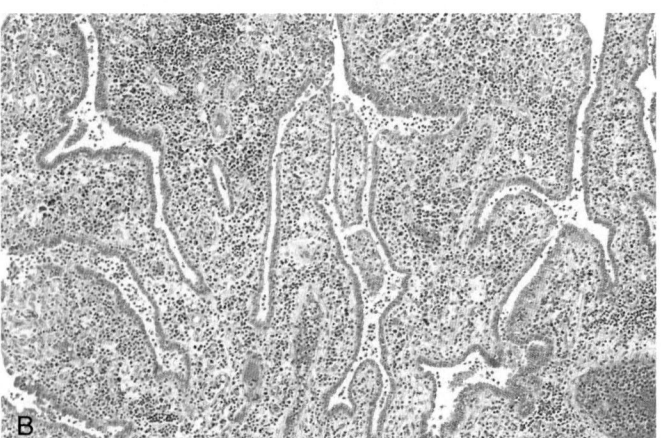

FIGURE 22–4   **A,** Acute salpingo-oophoritis, with tubo-ovarian abscess. The fallopian tubes and ovaries have coalesced into an inflammatory mass adherent to the uterus. **B,** Salpingitis with edematous tubal plicae expanded by inflammatory cell infiltrates.

VULVA

Diseases of the vulva in the aggregate constitute only a small fraction of gynecologic practice. Many inflammatory dermatologic diseases that affect skin elsewhere on the body may also occur on the vulva, such as psoriasis, eczema, and allergic dermatitis. The vulva is more prone to skin infections, because it is constantly exposed to secretions and moisture. Nonspecific vulvitis is particularly likely to occur in the setting of immunosuppression. Most skin cysts (epidermal inclusion cysts) and skin tumors can also occur in the vulva. Here we discuss disorders particular to the vulva, including Bartholin cyst, non-neoplastic epithelial disorders, benign exophytic lesions, and tumors of the vulva.

Bartholin Cyst

Infection of the Bartholin gland produces an acute inflammation within the gland (adenitis) and may result in an abscess. Bartholin duct cysts are relatively common, occur at all ages, and result from obstruction of the duct by an inflammatory process. The resulting cysts are lined by the ductal squamous metaplastic and/or epithelium. They may become large, up to 3 to 5 cm in diameter, and produce pain and local discomfort. Bartholin duct cysts are either excised or opened permanently (marsupialization).

Non-Neoplastic Epithelial Disorders

A heterogeneous group of lesions of the vulva presents as opaque, white, plaquelike mucosal thickening that may produce itching (pruritus) and scaling. Because of their appearance, these disorders have traditionally been termed *leukoplakia* by clinicians. This is a non-specific descriptive term, as *white plaques may represent a variety of benign, premalignant, or malignant lesions* including (1) inflammatory dermatoses (e.g., psoriasis, chronic dermatitis); (2) vulvar intraepithelial neoplasia, Paget disease, or even invasive carcinoma; and (3) epithelial disorders of unknown etiology. Excluding neoplasms and specific disease entities, non-neoplastic epithelial disorders of unknown etiology are classified into two categories: (1) *lichen sclerosus* and (2) *squamous cell hyperplasia (also known as lichen simplex chronicus)*. The two disorders may coexist and the lesions are often multiple, making their clinical management particularly difficult.

LICHEN SCLEROSUS

This lesion is characterized by thinning of the epidermis and disappearance of rete pegs, hydropic degeneration of the basal cells, superficial hyperkeratosis, and dermal fibrosis with a scant perivascular, mononuclear inflammatory cell infiltrate (Fig. 22–5). The lesions appear clinically as smooth, white plaques or papules that in time may extend and coalesce. The surface is smoothed out and sometimes resembles parchment.

When the entire vulva is affected, the labia become somewhat atrophic and stiffened, and the vaginal orifice is constricted. It occurs in all age groups but is most common in postmenopausal women. It may also be encountered elsewhere on the skin. The pathogenesis is uncertain, but the presence of activated T cells in the subepithelial inflammatory infiltrate and the increased frequency of autoimmune disorders in these women suggests an autoimmune reaction may be involved. Although the lesion in lichen sclerosus is not pre-malignant by itself, women with symptomatic lichen sclerosus have a somewhat increased chance of developing squamous cell carcinoma in their lifetime.[13]

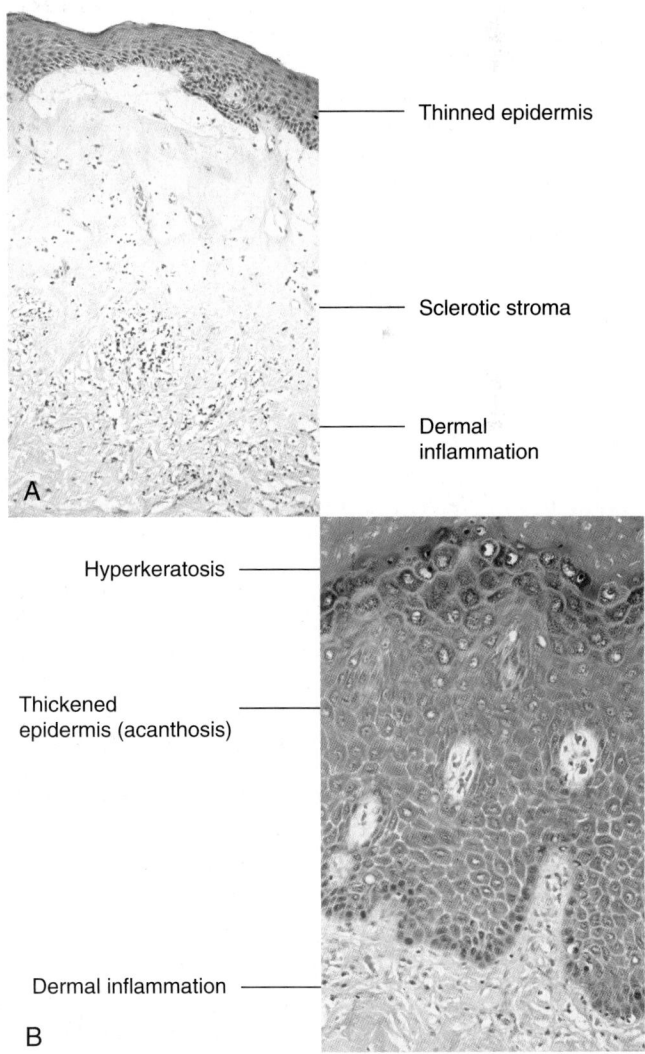

Thinned epidermis

Sclerotic stroma

Dermal inflammation

A

Hyperkeratosis

Thickened epidermis (acanthosis)

Dermal inflammation

B

FIGURE 22–5 Non-neoplastic epithelial vulvar disorders. **A,** Lichen sclerosus. **B,** Squamous cell hyperplasia. The main features of the lesions are indicated in the figures.

SQUAMOUS CELL HYPERPLASIA

Previously called hyperplastic dystrophy, or *lichen simplex chronicus*, squamous cell hyperplasia is a nonspecific condition resulting from rubbing or scratching of the skin to relieve pruritus. It is marked by epithelial thickening, expansion of the stratum granulosum, and significant surface hyperkeratosis. It appears clinically as an area of leukoplakia. The epithelium may show increased mitotic activity in both the stratum basalis and spinosum. Leukocytic infiltration of the dermis is sometimes pronounced. The hyperplastic epithelial changes show no atypia (see Fig. 22–5B). There is generally no increased predisposition to cancer, but suspiciously, lichen simplex chronicus is often present at the margins of established cancer of the vulva.

Benign Exophytic Lesions

Benign raised (exophytic) or wartlike conditions of the vulva may be caused by an infection or are of unknown etiology. *Condyloma acuminatum*, a papillomavirus-induced lesion, also called a genital wart, and syphilitic *condyloma latum* (described in Chapter 8) are consequences of sexually transmitted infections. Vulvar *fibroepithelial polyps*, or skin tags, are similar to skin tags occurring elsewhere on the skin. Vulvar *squamous papillomas* are benign exophytic proliferations covered by nonkeratinized squamous epithelium, which develop on vulvar mucosal surfaces and may be single or numerous (vulvar papillomatosis). The etiology of *fibroepithelial polyps* and *squamous papillomas* is unknown; however, these lesions are not related to any known infectious agent.

CONDYLOMA ACUMINATUM

Condylomata acuminata are sexually transmitted, benign lesions that have a distinct *verrucous gross appearance* (Fig. 22–6A). Although they may be solitary, they are more frequently multifocal: they may involve vulvar, perineal, and perianal regions as well as the vagina and, less commonly, the cervix. The lesions are identical to those found on the penis and around the anus in males (Chapter 21). On histologic examination, they consist of branching, treelike cores of stroma covered by squamous epithelium with characteristic viral cytopathic changes referred to as *koilocytic atypia* (Fig. 22–6B). Condylomata acuminata are caused by low oncogenic risk HPVs, principally types 6 and 11, and represent productive viral infection in which HPV replicates in the squamous cells. The virus life cycle is completed in the mature superficial cells, resulting in distinct cytologic changes—*koilocytotic atypia*—characterized by nuclear enlargement and atypia as well as a cytoplasmic perinuclear halo (see also "Cervix"). Condylomata acuminata are not considered precancerous lesions.

Squamous Neoplastic Lesions

VULVAR INTRAEPITHELIAL NEOPLASIA AND VULVAR CARCINOMA

Carcinoma of the vulva is an uncommon malignant neoplasm (approximately one eighth as frequent as cervical cancer) rep-

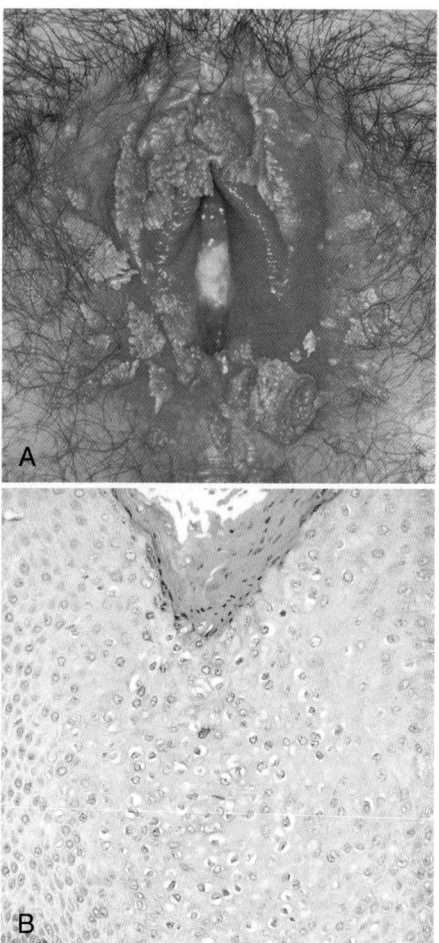

FIGURE 22–6 **A,** Numerous condylomas of the vulva encircling the introitus. **B,** Histopathology of condyloma acuminatum showing acanthosis, hyperkeratosis, and koilocytic atypia with enlarged, atypical nuclei and cytoplasmic vacuolation *(center of microphotograph).* (**A,** Courtesy of Dr. Alex Ferenczy, McGill University, Montreal, PQ, Canada.)

resenting about 3% of all genital cancers in the female; approximately two thirds occur in women older than 60 years. Squamous cell carcinoma is the most common histologic type of vulvar cancer. In terms of etiology, pathogenesis, and histologic features, vulvar squamous cell carcinomas are divided into two groups: *basaloid and warty carcinomas* related to infection with high oncogenic risk HPVs (30% of cases) and *keratinizing squamous cell carcinomas*, not related to HPV infection (70% of cases).[14]

Invasive *basaloid and warty carcinomas* develop from a precancerous in situ lesion called *classic vulvar intraepithelial neoplasia* (classic VIN). This form of VIN includes lesions designated formerly as carcinoma in situ or Bowen disease. Classic VIN is characterized by nuclear atypia of the squamous cells, increased mitoses, and lack of cellular maturation (Fig. 22–7A). It is analogous to cervical squamous intraepithelial lesions (SILs, see under "Cervix"). It most commonly occurs in reproductive-age women, and the risk factors are the same as those associated with cervical squamous intraepithelial lesions (e.g., young age at first intercourse, multiple sexual partners, male partner with multiple sexual partners), since

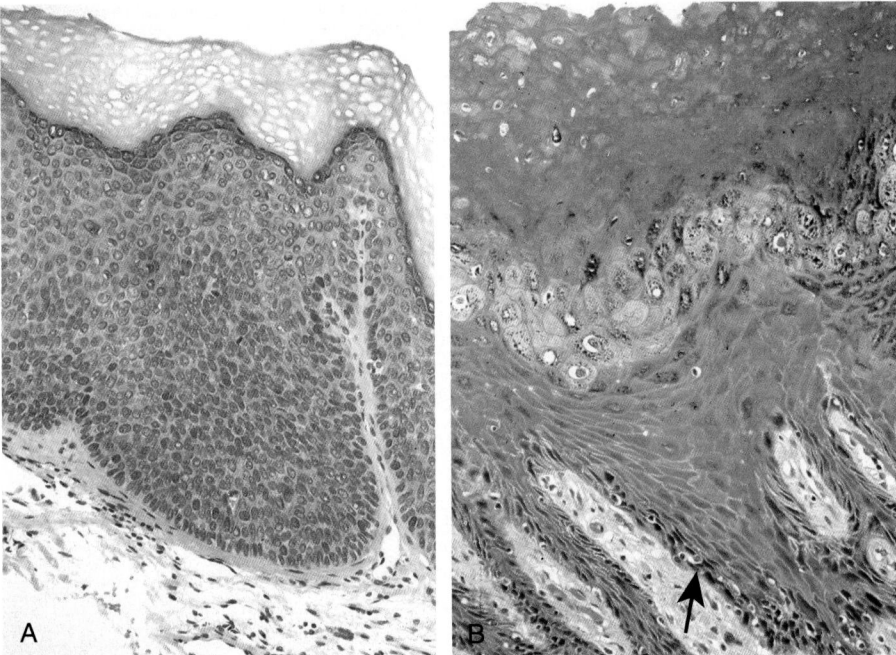

FIGURE 22–7   **A,** Histopathology of classic vulvar intraepithelial neoplasia (HPV positive) with diffuse cellular atypia, immaturity, nuclear crowding, and increased mitotic activity. **B,** Differentiated VIN (HPV negative), showing maturation of the superficial layers, hyperkeratosis, and basal cell atypia *(arrow)*.

both cervical squamous intraepithelial lesions and classic VIN are related to HPV infection. VIN is frequently multicentric in the vulva, and 10% to 30% of patients with VIN also have vaginal or cervical HPV-related lesions. The majority of cases of classic VIN are positive for HPV 16, and less frequently for other high-risk HPV types, like HPV 18 or 31. Spontaneous regression of VIN lesions has been reported, usually in younger women; the risk of progression to invasive carcinoma is higher in women older than 45 years of age or in women with immunosuppression.

Morphology. HPV-associated vulvar squamous cell carcinomas begin as classic VIN lesions, which present as discrete white (hyperkeratotic), flesh-colored or pigmented, slightly raised lesions. Coexisting carcinomas may be exophytic or indurated, frequently with ulceration. On histologic examination, basaloid carcinoma (Fig. 22–8A) shows an infiltrating tumor characterized by nests and cords of small, tightly packed malignant squamous cells

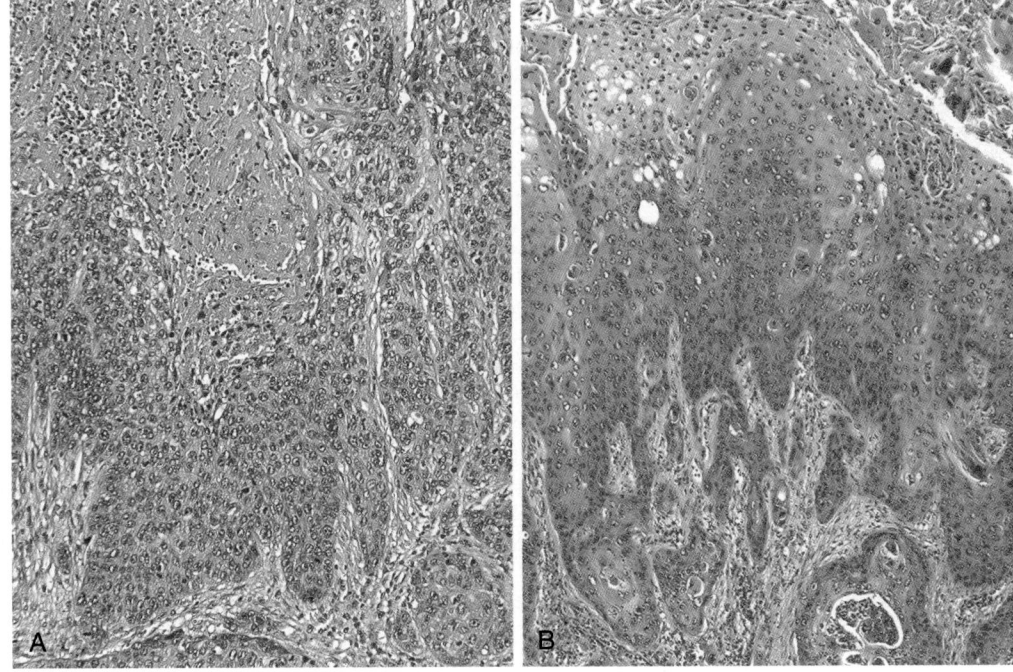

FIGURE 22–8 **A,** Basaloid vulvar carcinoma (HPV positive). **B,** Warty vulvar carcinoma (HPV positive).

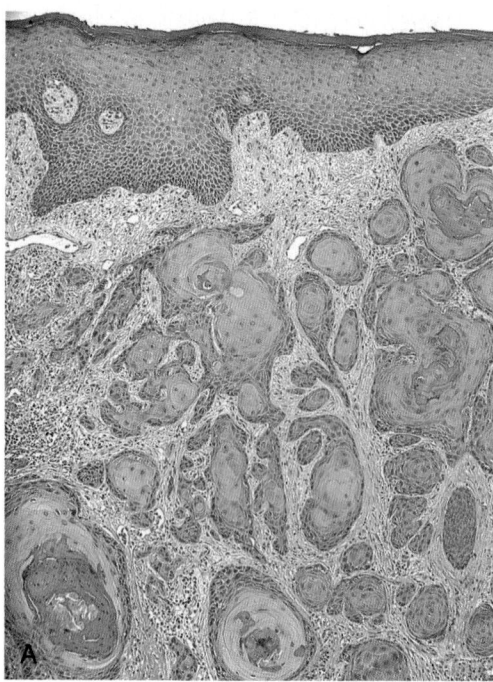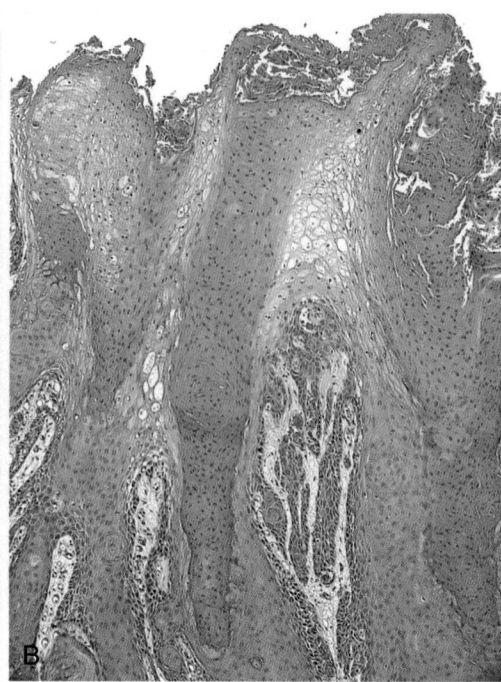

FIGURE 22–9   A, Well-differentiated, keratinizing squamous cell carcinoma of the vulva (HPV negative). **B,** Verrucous carcinoma of the vulva (HPV negative).

lacking maturation that resemble immature cells from the basal layer of the normal epithelium. The tumor may have foci of central necrosis.

Warty carcinoma is characterized by exophytic, papillary architecture and prominent koilocytic atypia (Fig. 22–8B).

Non-HPV-related *keratinizing squamous cell carcinomas* frequently arise in individuals with long-standing lichen sclerosus or squamous cell hyperplasia. The mean age of the patients is 76 years. The immediate premalignant lesion is referred to as *differentiated vulvar intraepithelial neoplasia* (differentiated VIN) or VIN *simplex* (see Fig. 22–7B).[14] Differentiated VIN is characterized by marked atypia of the basal layer of the squamous epithelium with apparently normal epithelial maturation and differentiation in the superfical layers, thus the designation "differentiated VIN." The etiology of differentiated VIN is unknown, but it is postulated that chronic epithelial irritation in lichen sclerosus or squamous cell hyperplasia may contribute to a gradual evolution of the malignant phenotype. The putative molecular events leading to malignant transformation in lichen sclerosus, squamous cell hyperplasia, and differentiated VIN are under investigation. A report of allelic imbalance in lichen sclerosus and squamous cell hyperplasia supports the hypothesis that both conditions pose a risk for neoplasia despite the lack of morphologic evidence of atypia. Rare cases of lichen sclerosus, differentiated VIN, and adjacent carcinoma with identical *p53* gene mutations have been reported. Overall, however, *p53* gene mutation is an infrequent and rather late event in vulvar carcinogenesis.[15]

Morphology. Carcinomas associated with lichen sclerosus, squamous cell hyperplasia, and differentiated VIN may develop as nodules in a background of vulvar inflammation. The often-subtle emergence of cancer may be misinterpreted as dermatitis, eczema, or leukoplakia for long periods. The clinical manifestations are nonspecific, including local discomfort, itching, and exudation because of superficial secondary infection, and underscore the importance of repeated examination in women with vulvar inflammatory disorders. Histologic examination reveals infiltrating tumor characterized by nests and tongues of malignant squamous epithelium with prominent central keratin pearls (Fig. 22–9A).

Risk of cancer development in VIN is principally a function of age, extent, and immune status.[16] Once invasive cancer develops, metastatic spread is linked to the size of tumor, depth of invasion, and involvement of lymphatic vessels. The initial spread is to inguinal, pelvic, iliac, and periaortic lymph nodes. Ultimately, lymphohematogenous dissemination to the lungs, liver, and other internal organs may occur. Patients with lesions less than 2 cm in diameter have a 60% to 80% 5-year survival after treatment with vulvectomy and lymphadenectomy; however, larger lesions with lymph node involvement have a 5-year survival rate of less than 10%.

Rare variants of squamous cell carcinoma include *verrucous carcinomas* (Fig. 22–9B), which are fungating tumors resembling condyloma acuminatum, and *basal cell carcinomas*, which are identical to their counterparts in the skin. Neither tumor is associated with papillomaviruses. Both tumors rarely metastasize and are successfully cured by wide excision.

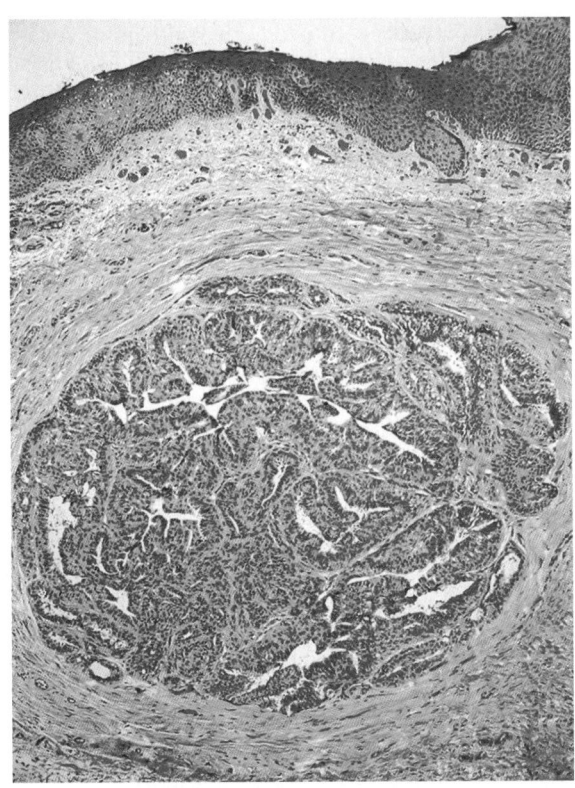

FIGURE 22–10 Papillary hidradenoma of the vulva, a well-circumscribed tumor nodule composed of benign papillary projections covered with columnar secretory epithelium and underlying myoepithelial cells.

Glandular Neoplastic Lesions

PAPILLARY HIDRADENOMA

Like the breast, the vulva contains modified apocrine sweat glands. In fact, the vulva may contain tissue closely resembling breast ("ectopic breast") and develop two tumors with counterparts in the breast, namely papillary hidradenoma and extramammary Paget disease. Papillary hidradenoma presents as a sharply circumscribed nodule, most commonly on the labia majora or interlabial folds, and may be confused clinically with carcinoma because of its tendency to ulcerate.

> **Morphology.** On histologic examination hidradenoma is identical in appearance to intraductal papillomas of the breast and consists of papillary projections covered with two layers of cells: the top columnar, secretory cells and an underlying layer of flattened "myoepithelial cells." These myoepithelial elements are characteristic of sweat glands and sweat gland tumors (Fig. 22–10).

EXTRAMAMMARY PAGET DISEASE

This curious and rare lesion of the vulva, and sometimes the perianal region, is similar in its manifestations to Paget disease of the breast (Chapter 23). As a vulvar neoplasm, it presents as a pruritic, red, crusted, sharply demarcated, maplike area, occurring usually on the labia majora. It may be accompanied by a palpable submucosal thickening or nodule.

> **Morphology.** Paget disease is a distinctive intraepithelial proliferation of malignant cells. The diagnostic microscopic feature is the presence of large tumor cells lying singly or in small clusters within the epidermis and its appendages. These cells are distinguished by a clear separation ("halo") from the surrounding epithelial cells (Fig. 22–11) and a finely granular cytoplasm containing mucopolysaccharide that stains with periodic acid–Schiff (PAS), Alcian blue, or mucicarmine stains. Ultrastructurally, Paget cells display apocrine, eccrine, and keratinocyte differentiation and presumably arise from primitive germinal cells of the mammary-like gland ducts of the vulvar skin.[17,18]

In contrast to Paget disease of the nipple, in which 100% of patients show an underlying ductal breast carcinoma, vulvar lesions are most frequently confined to the epidermis of the skin and adjacent hair follicles and sweat glands. Paget disease is treated with wide local excision and shows a high recurrence rate. Typically, Paget cells spread beyond the confines of the grossly visible lesion, and therefore are frequently present beyond the margins of surgical excision. Intraepidermal Paget disease may persist for many years, even decades, without invasion or metastases. Invasion develops rarely, and in such patients the prognosis is poor.

Malignant Melanoma

Melanomas of the vulva are rare, representing less than 5% of all vulvar cancers and 2% of all melanomas in women. Their peak incidence is in the sixth or seventh decade; they tend to have the same biologic and histologic characteristics as melanomas occurring elsewhere in the skin and are capable of

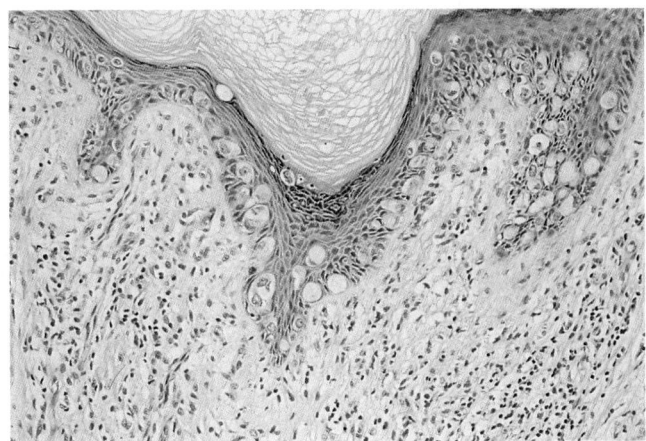

FIGURE 22–11 Paget disease of the vulva with clusters and single pale tumor cells spreading along the basal portion of the squamous epithelium. There is inflammation in the underlying dermis.

widespread metastatic dissemination. The 5-year survival rate is less than 32%, presumably because of delays in detection and because the majority of these tumors rapidly enter a vertical growth phase following inception (Chapter 25). Prognosis is linked principally to depth of invasion, with greater than 60% mortality for lesions invading deeper than 1 mm.

Because it is initially confined to the epithelium, melanoma may resemble Paget disease, both grossly and histologically. It can usually be differentiated by its uniform reactivity with antibodies to S100 protein, absence of reactivity with antibodies to cytokeratin, and lack of mucopolysaccharides, both of which are present in Paget disease.

VAGINA

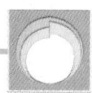

The vagina is a portion of the female genital tract that is remarkably free from primary disease. In the adult, inflammations often affect the vulva and perivulvar structures and spread to the cervix without significant involvement of the vagina. Primary lesions of the vagina are rare; the most serious of which is primary vaginal carcinoma. Thus, they are discussed only briefly.

Developmental Anomalies

Septate, or double, vagina is an uncommon anomaly that arises from failure of total fusion of the müllerian ducts and accompanies a double uterus (uterus didelphys). These and other anomalies of the external genitalia may be the manifestations of genetic syndromes, in utero exposure to diethylstilbestrol (DES) used to prevent threatened abortions in the 1940s through 1960s, or other disturbances associated with abnormalities in reciprocal epithelial-stromal signaling during fetal development.[19]

Vaginal adenosis is a remnant of columnar, endocervical-type epithelium that during embryonal development extends from the endocervix and covers the ectocervix as well as the upper vagina and is subsequently replaced by the squamous epithelium advancing upwardly from the urogenital sinus. Small patches of unreplaced glandular epithelium may persist focally into adult life. Adenosis presents clinically as red, granular areas contrasting with the normal pale-pink vaginal mucosa. On microscopic examination, adenosis consists of columnar mucinous epithelium indistinguishable from endocervical epithelium. Adenosis, while normally present in a small percentage of adult women, has been reported in 35% to 90% of women exposed to DES in utero. Rare cases of clear cell carcinoma (Fig. 22–12) arising in DES-related adenosis were recorded in teens and young women in the 1970s and 1980s, resulting in discontinuation of DES treatment.

Gartner duct cysts are relatively common lesions found along the lateral walls of the vagina and derived from wolffian (mesonephric) duct rests. They are 1- to 2-cm fluid-filled cysts that occur in the submucosal location. Other cysts, including mucus cysts, which occur in the proximal vagina, are derived from müllerian epithelium. Another müllerian-derived lesion, endometriosis (described later), may occur in the vagina and simulate a neoplasm.

Premalignant and Malignant Neoplasms

Most of the benign tumors of the vagina occur in reproductive-age women and include stromal tumors (stromal polyps), leiomyomas, and hemangiomas. The most common malignant tumor of the vagina is carcinoma metastatic from the cervix, followed by a primary squamous cell carcinoma of the vagina. Infants may develop a unique, rare malignancy—embryonal rhabdomyosarcoma (sarcoma botryoides).

VAGINAL INTRAEPITHELIAL NEOPLASIA AND SQUAMOUS CELL CARCINOMA

Primary carcinoma of the vagina is an extremely uncommon cancer (about 0.6 per 100,000 women yearly) accounting for about 1% of malignant neoplasms in the female genital tract. Almost all of these tumors are squamous cell carcinomas associated with *high oncogenic risk HPVs*. The greatest risk factor is a previous carcinoma of the cervix or vulva; 1% to 2% of women with an invasive cervical carcinoma eventually develop a vaginal squamous cell carcinoma. Squamous cell carcinoma of the vagina arises from a premalignant lesion, *vaginal*

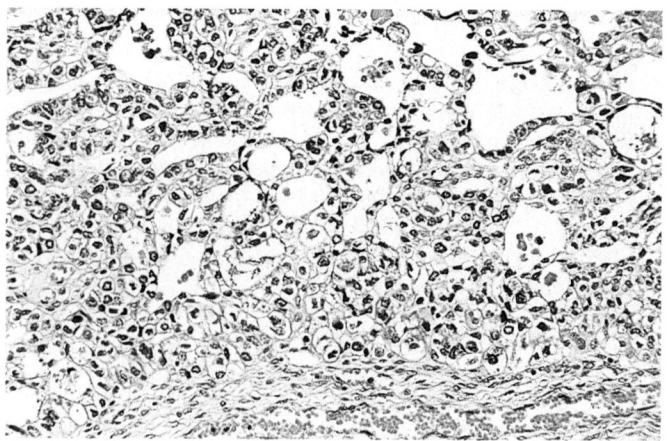

FIGURE 22–12 Clear cell adenocarcinoma of the vagina showing vacuolated tumor cells in clusters and glandlike structures.

intraepithelial neoplasia, analogous to cervical squamous intraepithelial lesions (SILs, see under "Cervix"). Most often the invasive tumor affects the upper posterior vagina, particularly along the posterior wall at the junction with the ectocervix. The lesions in the lower two thirds of the vagina metastasize to the inguinal nodes, whereas upper lesions tend to involve the regional iliac nodes.

EMBRYONAL RHABDOMYOSARCOMA

Also called *sarcoma botryoides,* this uncommon vaginal tumor is most frequently found in infants and in children younger than 5 years of age and consists predominantly of malignant embryonal rhabdomyoblasts.[20] These tumors tend to grow as *polypoid, rounded, bulky masses that sometimes fill and project out of the vagina;* they have the appearance and consistency of grapelike clusters (hence the designation botryoides = grapelike) (Fig. 22–13). On histologic examination, the tumor cells are small and have oval nuclei, with small protrusions of cytoplasm from one end, resembling a tennis racket. Rarely, striations can be seen within the cytoplasm. Beneath the vaginal epithelium, the tumor cells are crowded in a so-called cambium layer, but in the deep regions they lie within a loose fibromyxomatous stroma that is edematous and may contain many inflammatory cells. For this reason the lesions can be mistaken for benign inflammatory polyps, leading to unfortunate delays in diagnosis and treatment. These tumors tend to invade locally and cause death by pen-

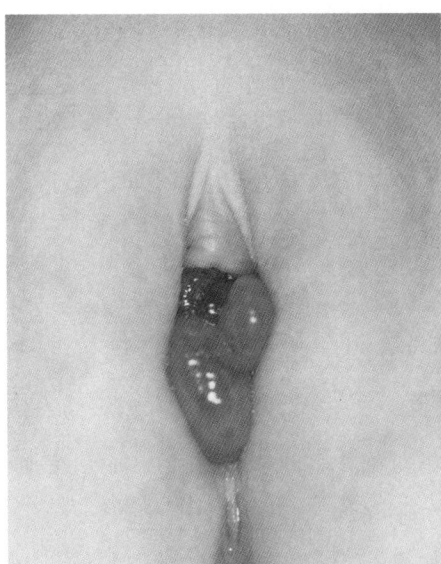

FIGURE 22–13 Sarcoma botryoides (embryonal rhabdomyosarcoma) of the vagina appearing as a polypoid mass protruding from the vagina. (Courtesy of Dr. Michael Donovan, Children's Hospital, Boston, MA.)

etration into the peritoneal cavity or by obstruction of the urinary tract. Conservative surgery, coupled with chemotherapy, seems to offer the best results in cases diagnosed sufficiently early.

CERVIX

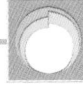

The cervix is both a sentinel for potentially serious upper genital tract infections and a target for viruses and other carcinogens, which may lead to invasive carcinoma. Worldwide, cervical carcinoma is the second most common cancer in women, with an estimated 493,000 new cases each year, over half of which are fatal. In the United States, 11,150 women were diagnosed with cervical cancer and 3670 women died from this disease in 2007. The potential threat of cancer is central to Papanicolaou (Pap) smear screening programs and histologic interpretation of biopsy specimens by the pathologist.

Inflammations

ACUTE AND CHRONIC CERVICITIS

At the onset of menarche, the production of estrogens by the ovary stimulates maturation of the cervical and vaginal squamous mucosa and formation of intracellular glycogen vacuoles in the squamous cells. As these cells are shed, the glycogen provides a substrate for endogenous vaginal aerobes and anaerobes, including streptococci, enterococci, *Escherichia coli,* and staphylococci; however, the normal vaginal and cervical flora is largely dominated by lactobacilli. Lactobacilli produce lactic acid that maintains the vaginal pH below 4.5, suppressing the growth of other saprophytic and pathogenic organisms. In addition, at low pH, lactobacilli produce bacteriotoxic hydrogen peroxide (H_2O_2).[21] At higher, more alkaline pH caused by bleeding, sexual intercourse, vaginal douching as well as during antibiotic treatment, lactobacilli decrease H_2O_2 production, permitting the overgrowth of other microorganisms, which may result in clinically apparent cervicitis or vaginitis. Some degree of cervical inflammation may be found in virtually all women, and it is usually of little clinical consequence. However, infections by *gonococci, chlamydiae, mycoplasmas,* and *herpes simplex virus* may produce significant acute or chronic cervicitis and are important to identify due to their association with upper genital tract disease, complications during pregnancy, and sexual transmission. Marked cervical inflammation produces reparative and reactive changes of the epithelium and shedding of atypical-appearing squamous cells, and therefore may cause a nonspecific, abnormal Pap test result.

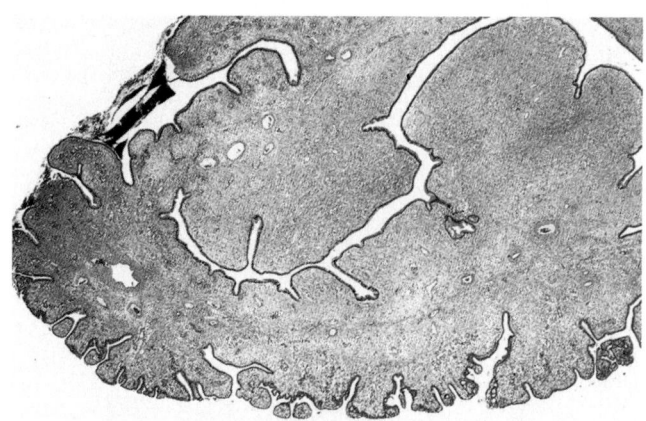

FIGURE 22–14 Endocervical polyp composed of a dense fibrous stroma covered with endocervical columnar epithelium.

Endocervical Polyps

Endocervical polyps are benign exophytic growths that occur in 2% to 5% of adult women. Perhaps the major significance of polyps lies in their production of irregular vaginal "spotting" or bleeding that arouses suspicion of some more ominous lesion. Most polyps arise within the endocervical canal and vary from small and sessile to large, 5-cm masses that may protrude through the cervical os. All are soft, almost mucoid, lesions composed of a loose fibromyxomatous stroma harboring dilated, mucus-secreting endocervical glands, often accompanied by inflammation (Fig. 22–14). Simple curettage or surgical excision effects a cure.

Premalignant and Malignant Neoplasms

No form of cancer better documents the remarkable effects of screening, early diagnosis, and curative therapy on the mortality rate than does cancer of the cervix. Fifty years ago, carcinoma of the cervix was the leading cause of cancer deaths in women in the United States, but the death rate has declined by two thirds to its present rank as the eighth leading cause of cancer mortality. In sharp contrast to this reduced mortality, the detection frequency of early cancers and precancerous lesions is high. Much credit for these dramatic gains belongs to the effectiveness of the Pap test in detecting cervical precancers and to the accessibility of the cervix to colposcopy (visual examination of the cervix with a magnifying glass) and biopsy. While there are an estimated 11,000 new cases of invasive cervical cancer in the United States annually, there are nearly 1 million precancerous lesions of varying grade that are discovered yearly by cytologic examinations. Thus, it is evident that Pap smear screening not only has increased the detection of potentially curable, low-stage cancers but has also allowed the detection and eradication of preinvasive lesions, some of which would have progressed to cancer if not discovered and treated.

Pathogenesis. The pathogenesis of cervical carcinoma has been delineated by a series of epidemiologic, clinicopatho-

logic, and molecular genetic studies. Epidemiologic data have long implicated a sexually transmitted agent, which is now established to be HPV. For his discovery of HPV as a cause of cervical cancer, Harald zur Hausen was awarded the Nobel Prize in 2008. HPVs are DNA viruses that are typed based on their DNA sequence and subgrouped into high and low oncogenic risk. *High oncogenic risk HPVs are currently considered to be the single most important factor in cervical oncogenesis.* High oncogenic risk HPVs have also been detected in vaginal squamous cell carcinomas and in a subset of vulvar, penile, anal, tonsillar, and other oropharyngeal carcinomas, as detailed in Chapter 7. As noted earlier, low oncogenic risk HPVs are the cause of the sexually transmitted vulvar, perineal, and perianal condyloma acuminatum. There are 15 high oncogenic risk HPVs that are currently identified. From the point of view of cervical pathology, HPV 16 and HPV 18 are the most important. HPV 16 alone accounts for almost 60% of cervical cancer cases, and HPV 18 accounts for another 10% of cases; other HPV types contribute to less than 5% of cases, individually.[22] The risk factors for cervical cancer are related to both host and viral characteristics such as HPV exposure, viral oncogenicity, inefficiency of immune response, and presence of co-carcinogens.[23] These include:

1. Multiple sexual partners
2. A male partner with multiple previous or current sexual partners
3. Young age at first intercourse
4. High parity
5. Persistent infection with a high oncogenic risk HPV, e.g., HPV 16 or HPV18
6. Immunosuppression
7. Certain HLA subtypes
8. Use of oral contraceptives
9. Use of nicotine

Genital HPV infections are extremely common; most of them are asymptomatic, do not cause any tissue changes, and therefore are not detected on Pap test. Figure 22–15 shows age-dependent prevalence of HPVs in cervical smears in women with normal Pap test results. The high peak of HPV

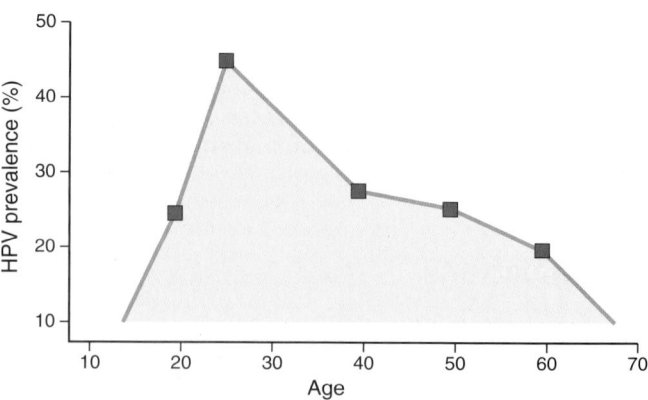

FIGURE 22–15 Age-dependent prevalence of HPVs in cervical smears in women with normal Pap test results in the US population. (Adapted from Dunne EF et al.: Prevalence of HPV infection among females in the United States. JAMA 297:813, 2007.)

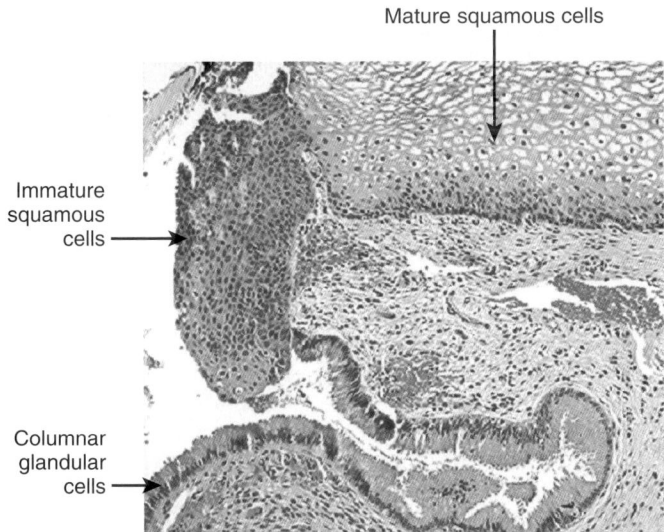

FIGURE 22–16 Cervical squamocolumnar junction showing mature, glycogenized *(pale)* squamous epithelium, immature *(dark pink)* squamous metaplastic cells, and columnar endocervical glandular epithelium.

Mature squamous cells

Immature squamous cells

Columnar glandular cells

prevalence in 20-year-olds is related to sexual début, while the subsequent decrease in prevalence reflects acquisition of immunity and monogamous relationships. Most HPV infections are transient and are eliminated by the immune response in the course of months. On average, 50% of HPV infections are cleared within 8 months, and 90% of infections are cleared within 2 years. The duration of the infection is related to HPV type; on average, infections with high oncogenic risk HPVs last longer than infections with low oncogenic risk HPVs, 13 months versus 8 months, respectively.[24] Persistent infection increases the risk of the development of cervical precancer and subsequent carcinoma.

HPVs infect immature basal cells of the squamous epithelium in areas of epithelial breaks, or immature metaplastic squamous cells present at the squamocolumnar junction (Fig. 22–16). HPVs cannot infect the mature superficial squamous cells that cover the ectocervix, vagina, or vulva. Establishing HPV infection in these sites requires damage to the surface epithelium, which gives the virus access to the immature cells in the basal layer of the epithelium. The cervix, with its relatively large areas of immature squamous metaplastic epithelium, is particularly vulnerable to HPV infection as compared, for example, with vulvar skin and mucosa that are covered by mature squamous cells. This difference in epithelial susceptibility to HPV infection accounts for the marked difference in incidence of HPV-related cancers arising in different sites, and explains the high frequency of cervical cancer in women or anal cancer in homosexual men and a relatively low frequency of vulvar and penile cancer.

Although the virus can *infect* only the immature squamous cells, *replication* of HPV occurs in the maturing squamous cells and results in a cytopathic effect, "*koilocytic atypia*," consisting of nuclear atypia and a cytoplasmic perinuclear halo. To replicate, HPV has to induce DNA synthesis in the host cells. Since HPV replicates in maturing, nonproliferating squamous cells, it must reactivate the mitotic cycle in

such cells. Experimental studies have shown that HPV activates the cell cycle by interfering with the function of *Rb* and *p53*, two important tumor suppressor genes (Chapter 7).

Viral E6 and E7 proteins are critical for the oncogenic effects of HPV. They can promote cell cycle by binding to RB and up-regulation of cyclin E (E7); interrupt cell death pathways by binding to p53 (E6); induce centrosome duplication and genomic instability (E6, E7); and prevent replicative senescence by up-regulation of telomerase (E6) (Chapter 7). HPV E6 induces rapid degradation of p53 via ubiquitin-dependent proteolysis, reducing p53 levels by two- to three-fold. E7 complexes with the hypophosphorylated (active) form of RB, promoting its proteolysis via the proteosome pathway. Because hypophosphorylated RB normally inhibits S-phase entry via binding to the E2F transcription factor, the two viral oncogenes cooperate to promote DNA synthesis while interrupting p53-mediated growth arrest and apoptosis of genetically altered cells. Thus, the viral oncogenes are critical in extending the life span of epithelial cells—a necessary component of tumor development.

The physical state of the virus differs in different lesions, being integrated into the host DNA in cancers, and present as free (episomal) viral DNA in condylomata and most precancerous lesions. Certain chromosome abnormalities, including deletions at 3p and amplifications of 3q, have been associated with cancers containing specific (HPV-16) papillomaviruses.

Even though HPV has been firmly established as a causative factor for cancer of the cervix, the evidence does not implicate HPV as the only factor. A high percentage of young women are infected with one or more HPV types during their reproductive years, and only a few develop cancer. Other co-carcinogens, the immune status of the individual, and hormonal and other factors influence whether the HPV infection will regress or persist and eventually progress to cancer.[23]

In addition to infecting squamous cells, HPVs may also infect glandular cells or neuroendocrine cells present in the cervical mucosa and cause malignant transformation, resulting in adenocarcinomas, and adenosquamous and neuroendocrine carcinomas; these tumor subtypes, however, are less common since glandular and neuroendocrine cells do not support effective HPV replication.

CERVICAL INTRAEPITHELIAL NEOPLASIA

The classification of cervical precancerous lesions has evolved over time and the terms from the different classification systems are currently used interchangeably. Hence a brief review of the terminology is warranted. The oldest classification system classified lesions as having mild dysplasia on one end and severe dysplasia/carcinoma in situ on the other. This was followed by *cervical intraepithelial neoplasia* (CIN) classification, with mild dysplasia termed *CIN I*, moderate dysplasia *CIN II*, and severe dysplasia termed *CIN III*. Because the decision with regard to patient management is two-tiered (observation versus surgical treatment), the three-tier classification system has been recently simplified to a two-tiered system, with CIN I renamed low-grade squamous intraepithelial lesion (LSIL) and CIN II and CIN III combined into one category referred to as high-grade squamous intraepithelial lesion (HSIL) (Table 22–1).

TABLE 22–1	**Classification Systems for Premalignant Squamous Cervical Lesions**	
Dysplasia/Carcinoma in Situ	**Cervical Intraepithelial Neoplasia (CIN)**	**Squamous Intraepithelial Lesion (SIL), Current Classification**
Mild dysplasia	CIN I	Low-grade SIL (LSIL)
Moderate dysplasia	CIN II	High-grade SIL (HSIL)
Severe dysplasia	CIN III	High-grade SIL (HSIL)
Carcinoma in situ	CIN III	High-grade SIL (HSIL)

LSILs are associated with productive HPV infection, but show no significant disruption or alteration of the host cell cycle. Most LSILs regress spontaneously, with only a small percentage progressing to HSIL. LSIL does not progress directly to invasive carcinoma. For these reasons LSIL is not treated like a premalignant lesion. In HSIL, there is a progressive deregulation of the cell cycle by HPV, which results in increased cellular proliferation, decreased or arrested epithelial maturation, and a lower rate of viral replication, as compared with LSIL. HSILs are one tenth as common as LSILs.

Morphology. Figure 22–17 illustrates a spectrum of morphologic alterations that range from normal to high grade dysplasia. The diagnosis of SIL is based on identification of nuclear atypia characterized by nuclear enlargement, hyperchromasia (dark staining), presence of coarse chromatin granules, and variation of nuclear sizes and shapes. The nuclear changes may be accompanied by cytoplasmic halos indicating disruption of the cytoskeleton before release of the virus into the environment. Nuclear alterations and perinuclear halo are termed *koilocytic atypia*. The grading of SIL into low or high grade is based on expansion of the immature cell layer from its normal, basal location. If the atypical, immature squamous cells are confined to the lower one third of the epithelium, the lesion is graded as LSIL; if they expand to two thirds of the epithelial thickness, it is graded as HSIL.

Figure 22–18A illustrates the histologic features of LSIL. The adjacent panel, Figure 22–18B, shows detection of HPV DNA using an in situ hybridization test. The staining is most intense in the superficial layers of the epithelium, which contain the highest viral load. Figures 22–18C and D show immunostaining for Ki-67 and p16. Ki-67 is a marker of cellular proliferation, and in normal squamous mucosa is confined to the basal layer of the epithelium. In contrast, in SILs, Ki-67 positivity is seen throughout the entire thickness of epithelium, indicating abnormal expansion of the epithelial proliferative zone (see Fig. 22–18C). p16, a cyclin kinase inhibitor, is a cell cycle–regulatory protein, which inhibits the cell cycle by preventing the phosphorylation of RB. It has been shown that in cells infected with oncogenic HPVs, there is overexpression of p16 (see Fig. 22–18D). Despite high levels of p16, however, the HPV-infected cells continue to proliferate because RB, the target of p16 inhibitory activity, is inactivated by the E7 HPV oncoprotein. Both Ki-67 and p16 staining are highly correlated with HPV infection and are useful for confirmation of the diagnosis in equivocal cases of SIL.

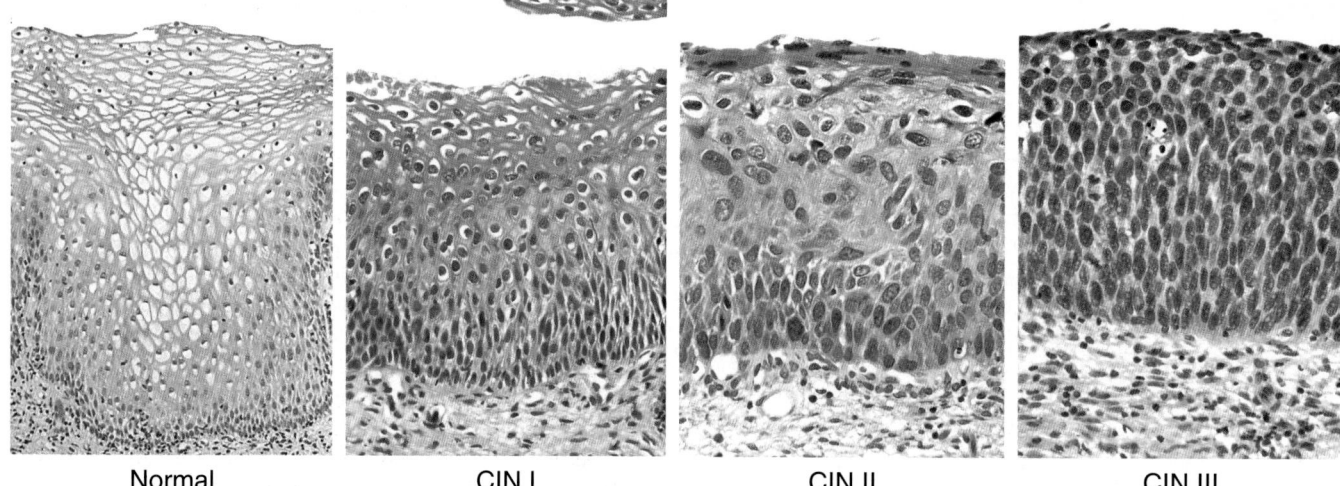

Normal   CIN I   CIN II   CIN III

FIGURE 22–17 Spectrum of cervical intraepithelial neoplasia: normal squamous epithelium for comparison; LSIL (CIN I) with koilocytic atypia; HSIL (CIN II) with progressive atypia and expansion of the immature basal cells above the lower third of the epithelial thickness; HSIL (CIN III) with diffuse atypia, loss of maturation, and expansion of the immature basal cells to the epithelial surface.

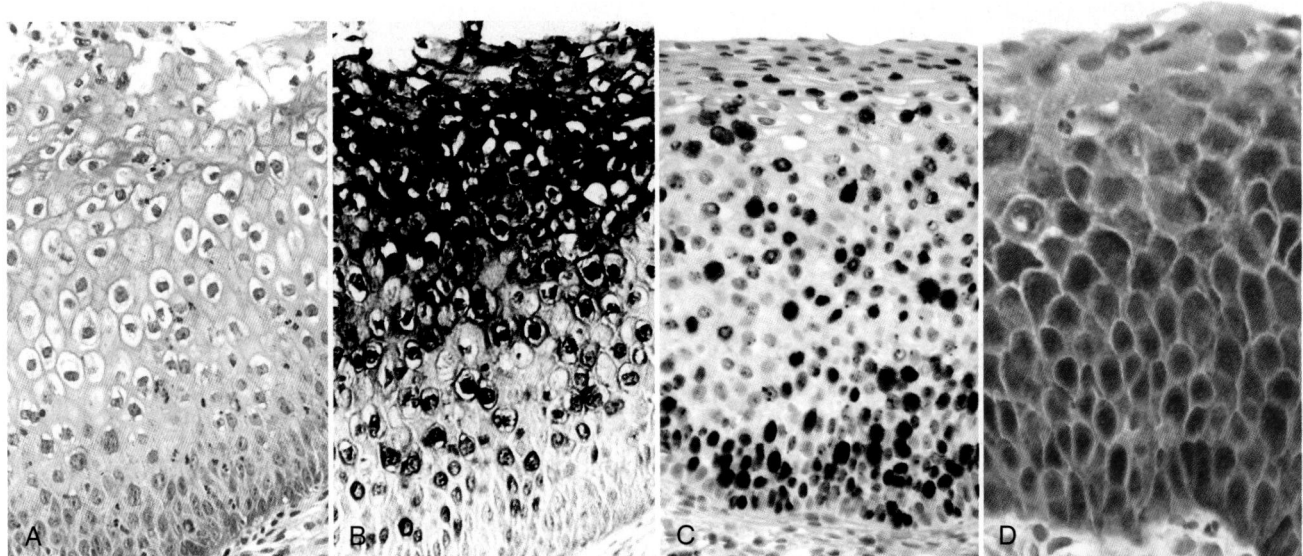

FIGURE 22-18   **A,** LSIL—routine H&E staining. **B,** In situ hybridization test for HPV DNA. The dark granular staining denotes HPV DNA, which is typically most abundant in the koilocytes. **C,** Diffuse immunostaining for the proliferation marker Ki-67, illustrating abnormal expansion of the proliferating cells from the normal basal location to the superficial layers of the epithelium. **D,** Up-regulation of p16INK4 (seen as intense brown immunostaining) characterizes high oncogenic risk HPV infections.

More than 80% of LSILs and 100% of HSILs are associated with high oncogenic risk HPVs. HPV 16 is the single most common HPV type detected in both categories of lesions. Table 22-2 shows rates of regression and progression of SILs within 2-year follow-up.[25] Although the majority of HSILs develop from LSILs, approximately 20% of cases of HSIL develop de novo, without the preexisting LSIL.[26] The rates of progression are by no means uniform, and although HPV type—especially HPV 16—is associated with increased risk, it is difficult to predict the outcome in an individual patient. These findings underscore that the *risk of developing precancer and cancer is conferred only in part by HPV type*, and depends also on immune status and environmental factors. Progression to invasive carcinoma, when it occurs, may take place in a few months to more than a decade.

CERVICAL CARCINOMA

Squamous cell carcinoma is the most common histologic subtype of cervical cancer, accounting for approximately 80% of cases. As outlined above, HSIL is an immediate precursor of cervical squamous cell carcinoma. The second most common tumor type is cervical adenocarcinoma, which constitutes about 15% of cervical cancer cases and develops from

a precursor lesion called adenocarcinoma in situ. Adenosquamous and neuroendocrine carcinomas are rare cervical tumors that account for the remaining 5% of cases. All of the above tumor types are caused by high oncogenic risk HPVs. The clinical characteristics and risk factors are the same for each tumor type, with the exception that adenocarcinomas and adenosquamous and neuroendocrine carcinomas typically present with advanced-stage disease. This unfortunate outcome occurs because Pap screening is less effective in detecting these cancers. Patients with adenosquamous and neuroendocrine carcinomas, therefore, have a less favorable prognosis than patients with squamous cell carcinomas or adenocarcinomas. The peak incidence of invasive cervical carcinoma is 45 years. With the advent of widespread screening, many cervical carcinomas are detected at a subclinical stage, during evaluation of an abnormal Pap smear.

TABLE 22-2 Natural History of Squamous Intraepithelial Lesions (SILs) with Approximate 2-Year Follow-up			
Lesion	Regress	Persist	Progress
LSIL	60%	30%	10% to HSIL
HSIL	30%	60%	10% to carcinoma*

HSIL, high-grade SIL; LSIL, low-grade SIL.
*Progression within 2–10 years.

Morphology. Invasive cervical carcinoma may manifest as either fungating (exophytic) or infiltrative cancers.

On histologic examination, squamous cell carcinomas are composed of nests and tongues of malignant squamous epithelium, either keratinizing or nonkeratinizing, invading the underlying cervical stroma (Fig. 22–19). Adenocarcinomas are characterized by proliferation of glandular epithelium composed of malignant endocervical cells with large, hyperchromatic nuclei and relatively mucin-depleted cytoplasm, resulting in dark appearance of the glands, as compared with the normal endocervical epithelium (Fig. 22–20A). Adenosquamous carcinomas are tumors composed of intermixed malignant glandular and malignant squamous epithelium. Neuroendocrine cervical carcinomas typically have an appearance

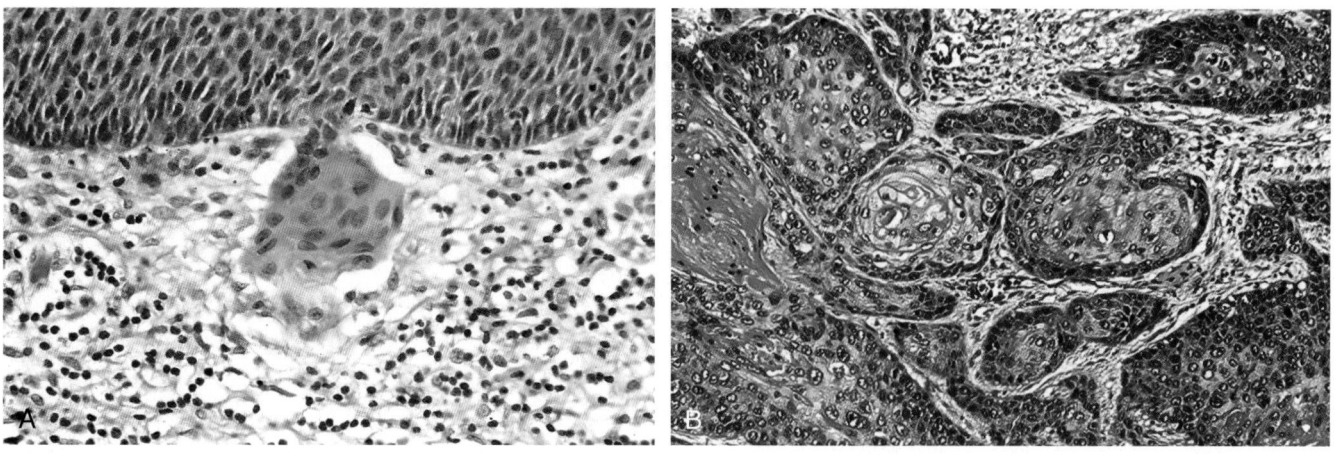

FIGURE 22–19 Squamous cell carcinoma of the cervix. **A,** Microinvasive squamous cell carcinoma with invasive nest breaking through the basement membrane of HSIL. **B,** Invasive squamous cell carcinoma.

similar to small-cell carcinoma of the lung (see Chapter 15); however, in contrast to the lung tumor, which is not related to HPV infection, cervical small-cell carcinomas are positive for high oncogenic risk HPVs.

Advanced cervical carcinoma extends by direct spread to involve contiguous tissues, including the paracervical tissues, urinary bladder, ureters, rectum, and vagina. Local and distant lymph nodes are also involved. Distant metastases may be found in the liver, lungs, bone marrow, and other structures.

Cervical cancer is staged as follows:

Stage 0. Carcinoma in situ (CIN III, HSIL)
Stage I. Carcinoma confined to the cervix
    Ia. Preclinical carcinoma, that is, diagnosed only by microscopy
    Ia1. Stromal invasion no deeper than 3 mm and no wider than 7 mm (so-called **microinvasive carcinoma**) (see Fig. 22–19A)
    Ia2. Maximum depth of invasion of stroma deeper than 3 mm and no deeper than 5 mm taken from base of epithelium; horizontal invasion not more than 7 mm
    Ib. Histologically invasive carcinoma confined to the cervix and greater than stage Ia2
Stage II. Carcinoma extends beyond the cervix but not to the pelvic wall. Carcinoma involves the vagina but not the lower third.
Stage III. Carcinoma has extended to the pelvic wall. On rectal examination there is no cancer-free space between the tumor and the pelvic wall. The tumor involves the lower third of the vagina.
Stage IV. Carcinoma has extended beyond the true pelvis or has involved the mucosa of the bladder or rectum. This stage also includes cancers with metastatic dissemination.

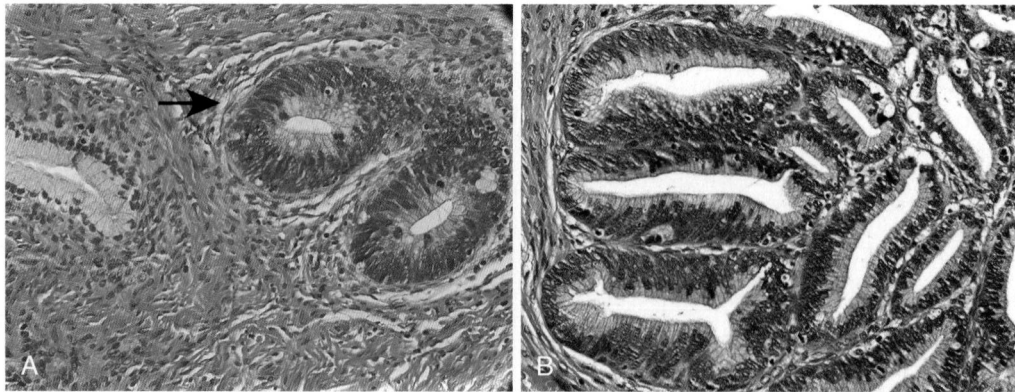

FIGURE 22–20 Adenocarcinoma of the cervix. **A,** Adenocarcinoma in situ *(arrow)* showing dark glands adjacent to normal, pale endocervcial glands. **B,** Invasive adenocarcinoma.

Clinical Features. More than half of invasive cervical cancers are detected in women who did not participate in regular screening. While early invasive cancers of the cervix (microinvasive carcinomas) may be treated by cone biopsy alone, most invasive cancers are managed by hysterectomy with lymph node dissection and, for advanced lesions, irradiation. The prognosis and survival for invasive carcinomas depend largely on the stage at which cancer is first discovered and to some degree on the cell type, with small-cell neuroendocrine tumors having a very poor prognosis. With current methods of treatment there is a 5-year survival rate of at least 95% for stage Ia (including microinvasive) carcinomas, about 80% to 90% with stage Ib, 75% with stage II, and less than 50% for stage III and higher. Most patients with stage IV cancer die as a consequence of local extension of the tumor (e.g., into and about the urinary bladder and ureters, leading to ureteral obstruction, pyelonephritis, and uremia) rather than distant metastases. However, as mentioned above, early detection has reduced the number of patients with stage IV cancer by more than two thirds in the past 50 years.

Cervical Cancer Screening and Prevention

Cervical cancer prevention and control can be divided into several components. One includes cytologic screening and management of Pap smear abnormalities. Another is the histologic diagnosis and removal of precancerous lesions. Still another component is surgical removal of invasive cancers, with adjunctive radiation therapy and chemotherapy. A new aspect is an HPV vaccination program, approved by the US Food and Drug Administration (FDA) for preventing HPV infection. HPV vaccines are also being evaluated for effectiveness as a therapeutic tool in cervical precancers.

The reason that cytologic screening is so effective in preventing cervical cancer is that the majority of cancers are preceded by a long-standing precancerous lesion. This lesion may exist in the noninvasive stage for years and shed abnormal cells that can be detected on cytologic examination. Pap tests are cytologic preparations of exfoliated cells from the cervical transformation zone that are stained with the Papanicolaou method. Using a spatula or brush, the transformation zone of the cervix is circumferentially scraped and the cells are smeared or spun down onto a slide. Following fixation and staining, the cytotechnologist, a person specifically trained to identify cytologic abnormalities, screens the smears. The cellular changes on Pap test illustrating the spectrum from normal, through LSIL to HSIL, are shown in Figure 22–21.

The false-negative error rate of the Pap test is around 10% to 20%. Most of these false-negative tests stem from sampling

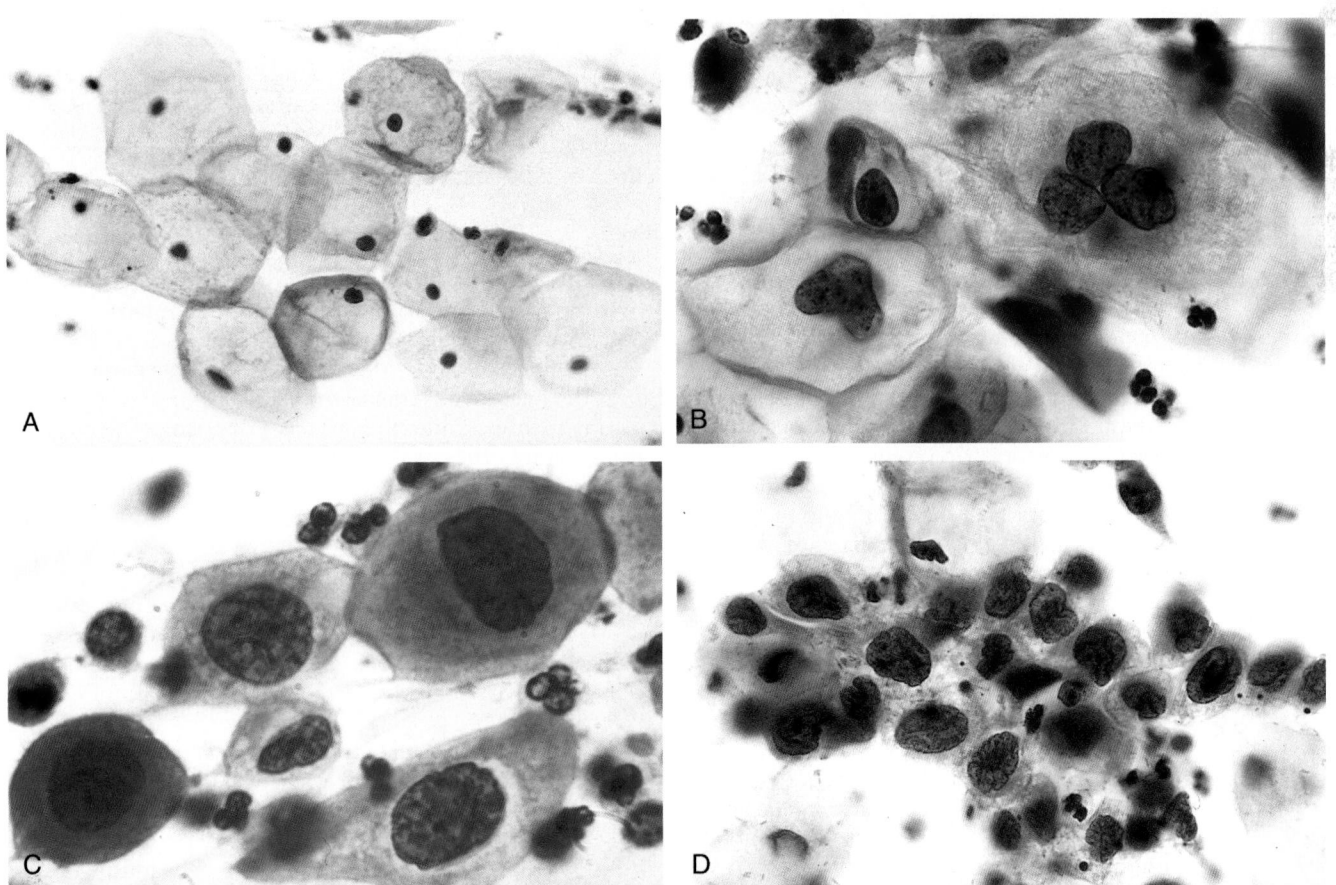

FIGURE 22–21   The cytology of cervical intraepithelial neoplasia as seen on the Papanicolaou smear. Normal cytoplasmic staining in superficial cells (**A** and **B**) may be either red or blue. **A,** Normal exfoliated superficial squamous cells. **B,** LSIL—koilocytes. **C,** HSIL (CIN II). **D,** HSIL (CIN III). Note the reduction in cytoplasm and the increase in the nucleus-to-cytoplasm ratio, which occurs as the grade of the lesion increases. This reflects the progressive loss of cellular differentiation on the surface of the lesions from which these cells are exfoliated. (Courtesy of Dr. Edmund S. Cibas, Brigham and Women's Hospital, Boston, MA.)

errors. Recommendations for the frequency of Pap screening vary, but in general the first smear should be at age 21 years or within 3 years of onset of sexual activity, and thereafter on an annual basis. After age 30, women who have had three consecutive normal cytology results may be screened every 2 to 3 years.[27]

As an adjunct to cytology, HPV DNA testing may be added to cervical cytology for screening in women aged 30 years or older. Women with normal cytology result and negative HPV DNA testing may be rescreened every 3 years. Women with a normal cytology result, but who are high-risk HPV DNA–positive, should have cervical cytology repeated at 6 to 12 months.[28] HPV testing of women younger than 30 is not recommended because of the high prevalence of HPV infection in this age group and the low specificity of the positive result (see Fig. 22–15).

When the Pap test is abnormal, a colposcopic examination of the cervix and vagina is performed to delineate the extent of the lesion and to target the areas to be biopsied. Application of acetic acid to the cervix highlights abnormal areas. After confirmation by tissue biopsy, women with LSIL can be followed in a conservative fashion with repeat smears and close follow-up. Some gynecologists use local ablative measures based upon their experience with the disease and reliability of patient follow-up. HSILs are treated with cervical conization (excision).[29] Follow-up smears and clinical examinations should continue for life, since vaginal, vulvar, or cervical precancers and cancers may later develop.

In 2006 the FDA licensed a quadrivalent, prophylactic HPV vaccine for HPV types 6, 11, 16, and 18. This vaccine is designed to reduce the incidence of cervical cancer caused by HPV 16 and HPV 18 (together accounting for approximately 70% of cervical cancer cases[22]) and vulvar condylomas (HPV 6 and 11). In phase III trials the vaccine prevented 100% of HPV 16/18–associated HSILs. The vaccine is prepared from noninfectious, DNA-free virus-like particles produced by recombinant technology. It induces high levels of serum antibodies in all vaccinated individuals. In women who have no evidence of past or current infection with the HPV genotypes included in the vaccine, there is protection from HPV infection for up to 5 years after vaccination; longer follow-up studies are still pending. Since the HPV vaccine does not eliminate the risk of cervical cancer due to other oncogenic HPV types, cervical cancer screening should still continue according to past guidelines to minimize cancer incidence.[30]

BODY OF UTERUS AND ENDOMETRIUM

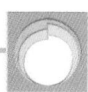

The uterus has two major components: the myometrium and the endometrium. The myometrium is composed of tightly interwoven bundles of smooth muscle that form the wall of the uterus. The internal cavity of the uterus is lined by the endometrium composed of glands embedded in a cellular stroma. The uterus is subject to a variety of disorders, the most common of which result from endocrine imbalances, complications of pregnancy, and neoplastic proliferation. Together with the lesions that affect the cervix (causing abnormal Pap smears), the lesions of the corpus of the uterus and the endometrium (causing abnormal vaginal bleeding) account for most patient visits to gynecologic practices.

Endometrial Histology in the Menstrual Cycle

The endometrium is a dynamic tissue that undergoes physiologic and characteristic morphologic changes during the menstrual cycle as a result of the effect of sex steroid hormones coordinately produced in the ovary. The ovary, in turn, is influenced by hormones produced by the pituitary. Together the hypothalamic, pituitary, and ovarian factors and their interactions regulate maturation of ovarian follicles, ovulation, and menstruation.

"Dating" the endometrium by its histologic appearance is often used clinically to assess hormonal status, document ovulation, and determine causes of endometrial bleeding and infertility (Fig. 22–22). The cycle begins with the shedding of the upper half to two thirds of the endometrium, referred to as the functionalis (the hormonally responsive upper zone), during menses. Under the influence of estrogen, produced by the granulosa cells of the developing follicle in the ovary, the remaining third (basalis) of the endometrium undergoes extremely rapid growth of both glands and stroma (*proliferative phase*). During the proliferative phase the glands are straight, tubular structures lined by regular, tall, pseudostratified columnar cells. Mitotic figures are numerous, and there is no evidence of mucus secretion or vacuolation. The endometrial stroma is composed of thickly compacted spindle cells that have scant cytoplasm but abundant mitotic activity (Fig. 22–22A).

At the time of ovulation the endometrium slows in its growth, and it ceases mitotic activity within days after ovulation, at which time the corpus luteum is producing progesterone in addition to estrogen. The postovulatory endometrium is initially marked by secretory vacuoles beneath the nuclei in the glandular epithelium (Fig. 22–22B). This *secretory activity* is most prominent during the third week of the menstrual cycle, when the basal vacuoles progressively push past the nuclei. By the fourth week, the secretions are discharged into

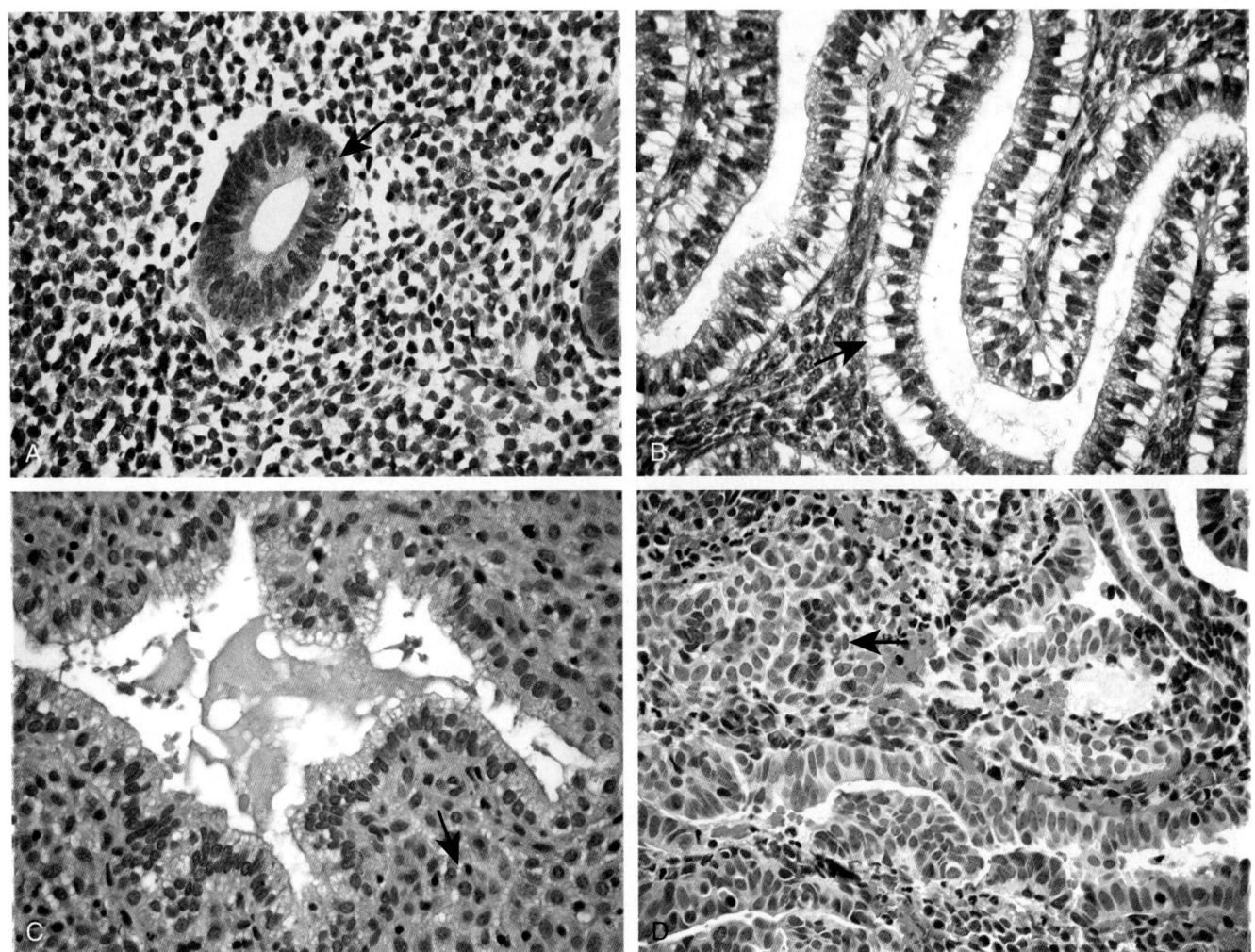

FIGURE 22–22 Histology of the menstrual cycle. **A,** Proliferative phase with mitoses *(arrow)*. **B,** Early secretory phase with subnuclear vacuoles *(arrow)*. **C,** Late secretory exhaustion and predecidual changes *(arrow)*. **D,** Menstrual endometrium with stromal breakdown *(arrow)* (see text).

the gland lumens. When secretion is maximal, between 18 and 24 days, the glands are dilated. By the fourth week the glands are tortuous, producing a serrated appearance when they are cut in their long axis. This serrated or "saw-toothed" appearance is accentuated by secretory exhaustion and shrinking of the glands.

The stromal changes in late secretory phase, due predominantly to progesterone, are important for dating the endometrium and consist of the development of prominent spiral arterioles by days 21 to 22. A considerable increase in ground substance and edema between the stromal cells occurs and is followed in days 23 to 24 by stromal cell hypertrophy with accumulation of cytoplasmic eosinophilia (predecidual change) and resurgence of stromal mitoses (Fig. 22–22C). Predecidual changes spread throughout the functionalis during days 24 to 28 and are accompanied by scattered neutrophils and occasional lymphocytes, which in this context do not imply inflammation. With the dissolution of the corpus luteum and the subsequent lack of progesterone, the disintegration of the functionalis begins with the escape of blood into the stroma, marking the beginning of menstrual shedding (Fig. 22–22D).

Although the molecular mechanism(s) by which estrogen and progesterone cause these profound changes in the endometrium are not well understood, it is known that these hormones induce local production of molecules that act in an autocrine and paracrine fashion.[31] Much of the hormonal action occurs through their cognate nuclear receptors (estrogen receptor α, progesterone receptor A, and progesterone receptor B). However, they may also act through alternate receptors or perhaps even by receptor-independent pathways.[32] In addition, there is considerable cross-talk between the glands and stroma. For example, much of the effect of estrogen on glandular proliferation occurs via stromal cells, which in response to estrogen produce growth factors (e.g., insulin-like growth factor 1 and epidermal growth factor) that bind receptors expressed on the epithelial cells. In the secretory phase, progesterone initially inhibits proliferation in both the glands and the stroma. It also promotes differentiation of the glands and causes profound alterations of the stroma. Interestingly, progesterone secretion leads to a decrease in estrogen receptor expression in both the glands and stroma, making the endometrium relatively unresponsive to estrogen still being produced by the ovary. To further elucidate the

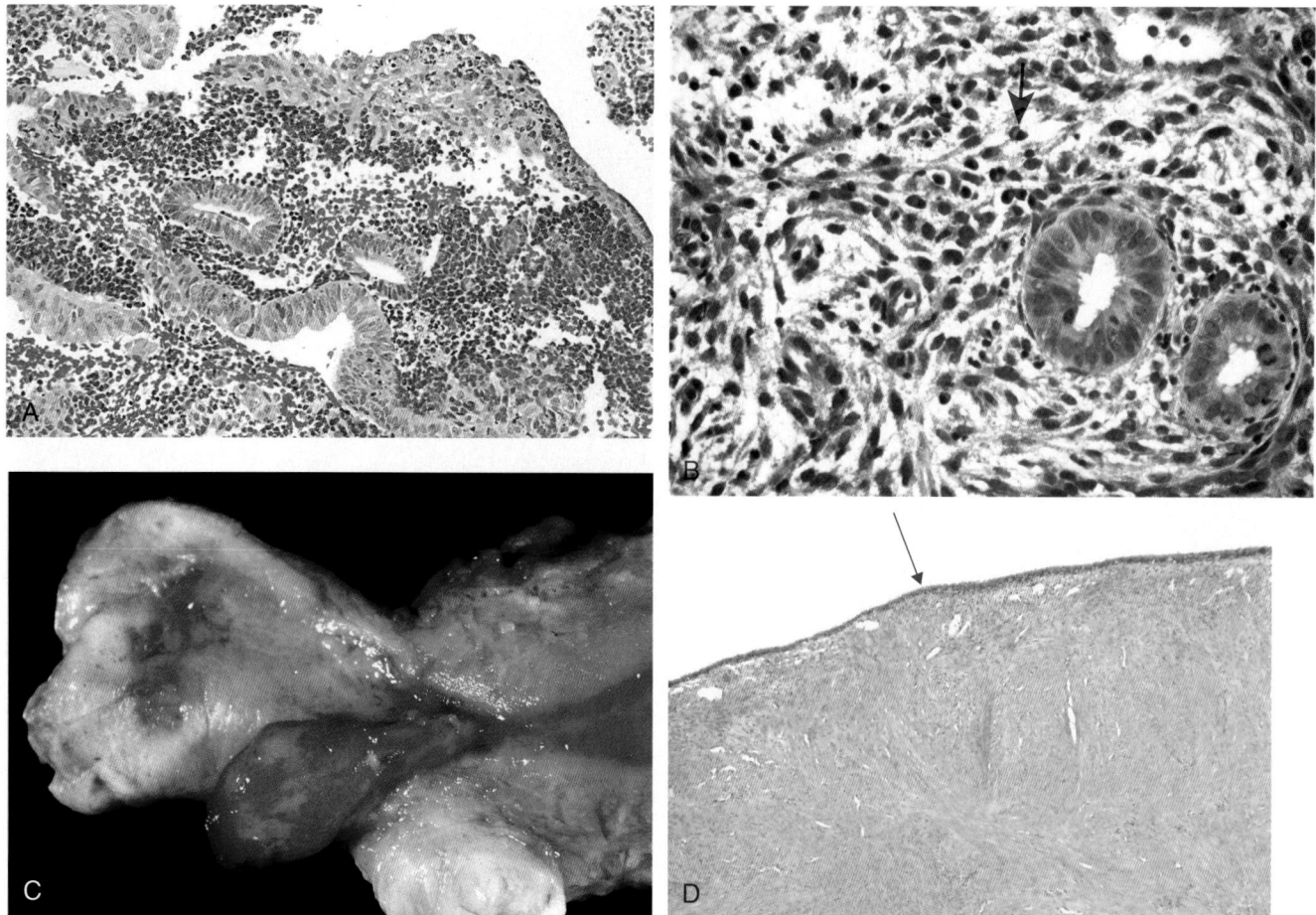

FIGURE 22–23 Common causes of abnormal uterine bleeding. **A,** The most common is dysfunctional uterine bleeding, seen here as anovulatory endometrium with stromal breakdown. Note breakdown associated with proliferative glands. **B,** Chronic endometritis with numerous plasma cells *(arrow).* **C,** Endometrial polyp. **D,** Submucosal leiomyoma with attenuation of the endometrial lining *(arrow).*

mechanisms responsible for the hormonal effects, global gene expression studies are being used.[33] It is thought that such information will aid in the treatment of women with disorders of the endometrium that range from infertility to cancer, as discussed below.

Functional Endometrial Disorders (Dysfunctional Uterine Bleeding)

During active reproductive life, the endometrium is in a dynamic state of proliferation, differentiation, and shedding, in preparation for implantation of an embryo. As discussed above, this cycle is exquisitely controlled by the rise and fall of pituitary and ovarian hormones, which is executed by proper timing of hormone release in both absolute and relative amounts. Abnormalities in this system result in abnormal uterine bleeding.

Although abnormal uterine bleeding can be caused by well-defined organic pathologic conditions, such as chronic endometritis, endometrial polyp (see Fig. 22–23C), submucosal leiomyomas (see Fig. 22–23D), or endometrial neoplasms, the largest single group encompasses functional disturbances, referred to as dysfunctional uterine bleeding (DUB; Table 22–3). DUB is a clinical term for uterine bleeding not caused by any underlying organic (structural) abnormality. The most common causes of DUB are discussed.

ANOVULATORY CYCLE

In most instances, dysfunctional bleeding is due to the occurrence of an anovulatory cycle. Anovulation results in excessive and prolonged estrogenic stimulation without the counteractive effect of the progestational phase that regularly follows ovulation. In most women anovulatory cycles have no obvious cause, occurring most likely due to subtle hormonal imbalances. Anovulatory cycles are most common at menarche and in the perimenopausal period. Less commonly, lack of ovulation is the result of (1) an endocrine disorder, such as thyroid disease, adrenal disease, or pituitary tumors; (2) a primary lesion of the ovary, such as a functioning ovarian tumor (granulosa-theca cell tumors) or polycystic ovaries (see "Ovaries"); or (3) a generalized metabolic disturbance, such as marked obesity, severe malnutrition, or any chronic systemic disease.

TABLE 22–3	Causes of Abnormal Uterine Bleeding by Age Group
Age Group	**Causes**
Prepuberty	Precocious puberty (hypothalamic, pituitary, or ovarian origin)
Adolescence	Anovulatory cycle, coagulation disorders

Reproductive age	Complications of pregnancy (abortion, trophoblastic disease, ectopic pregnancy)
	Organic lesions (leiomyoma, adenomyosis, polyps, endometrial hyperplasia, carcinoma)
	Dysfunctional uterine bleeding
	    Anovulatory cycle
	    Ovulatory dysfunctional bleeding (e.g., inadequate luteal phase)

Perimenopausal	Dysfunctional uterine bleeding
	    Anovulatory cycle
	    Irregular shedding
	Organic lesions (carcinoma, hyperplasia, polyps)

Postmenopausal	Endometrial atrophy Organic lesions (carcinoma, hyperplasia, polyps)

Failure of ovulation results in prolonged, excessive endometrial stimulation by estrogens. Under these circumstances the endometrial glands undergo mild architectural changes, including cystic dilation, that are usually self-limited by the occurrence of the next ovulatory cycle. Unscheduled breakdown of the stroma may also occur ("anovulatory menstruation"), with no evidence of endometrial secretory activity (see Fig. 22–23A). More severe consequences of repeated anovulation are discussed under "Endometrial Hyperplasia."

INADEQUATE LUTEAL PHASE

This term refers to a condition that is thought to stem from inadequate corpus luteum function resulting in low progesterone output, with subsequent early menses. The condition often manifests clinically as infertility, with either increased bleeding or amenorrhea. Endometrial biopsy performed at an estimated postovulatory date shows secretory endometrium, which, however, lags in its secretory characteristics expected at that date.

ENDOMETRIAL CHANGES INDUCED BY ORAL CONTRACEPTIVES

As might be suspected, oral contraceptives containing synthetic or derivative ovarian steroids induce a wide variety of endometrial changes, depending on the steroids used, the method of administration (combined or sequential regimen), and the dose. A common response pattern is a discordant appearance between glands and stroma, usually with inactive glands amid a stroma showing large cells with abundant cytoplasm reminiscent of the decidua of pregnancy. When such therapy is discontinued, the endometrium reverts to normal. All these changes have been minimized with newer low-dose contraceptives.

MENOPAUSAL AND POSTMENOPAUSAL CHANGES

Because the menopause is characterized by anovulatory cycles, architectural alterations in the endometrial glands may be present transiently, followed by ovarian failure and atrophy of the endometrium. As discussed later in this chapter, anovulatory cycles and uninterrupted estrogen production can induce mild hyperplasias with cystic dilation of glands. If this is followed by complete ovarian atrophy and loss of stimulus, the cystic dilation may remain, while the ovarian stroma and gland epithelium undergo atrophy. In this case, so-called cystic atrophy results. Such cystic changes should not be confused with simple hyperplasia, which shows evidence of glandular and stromal proliferation.

Inflammation

The endometrium and myometrium are relatively resistant to infections, primarily because the endocervix normally forms a barrier to ascending infection. Thus, although chronic inflammation in the cervix is an expected and frequently insignificant finding, it is of concern in the endometrium, excluding the menstrual phase.

ACUTE ENDOMETRITIS

Acute endometritis is uncommon and limited to bacterial infections that arise after delivery or miscarriage. Retained products of conception are the usual predisposing influence; the causative agents include group A hemolytic streptococci, staphylococci, and other bacteria. The inflammatory response is chiefly limited to the interstitium and is entirely nonspecific. Removal of the retained gestational fragments by curettage, accompanied by antibiotic therapy, is promptly followed by remission of the infection.

CHRONIC ENDOMETRITIS

Chronic inflammation of the endometrium occurs in the following settings: (1) in patients suffering from chronic PID; (2) in postpartum or post-abortion patients with retained gestational tissue; (3) in women with intrauterine contraceptive devices; and (4) in women with tuberculosis, either from miliary spread or, more commonly, from drainage of tuberculous salpingitis. The last is distinctly rare in Western countries.

The chronic endometritis in all these cases is secondary to another underlying cause.

In about 15% of cases no cause is obvious, yet plasma cells (which are not present in normal endometrium) are seen together with macrophages and lymphocytes (see Fig. 22–23B). Some women with this so-called nonspecific chronic endometritis have gynecologic complaints such as abnormal bleeding, pain, discharge, and infertility. *Chlamydia* may be involved and is commonly associated with both acute (e.g., polymorphonuclear leukocytes) and chronic (e.g., lymphocytes, plasma cells) inflammatory cell infiltrates. The organisms may or may not be successfully cultured.[34] Importantly, antibiotic therapy is indicated because it may prevent other sequelae (e.g., salpingitis).

Endometriosis and Adenomyosis

Endometriosis is the presence of endometrial tissue outside of the uterus. It most commonly consists of both endometrial glands and stroma, but rarely consists only of endometrial stroma. It occurs in the following sites, in descending order of frequency: (1) ovaries; (2) uterine ligaments; (3) rectovaginal septum; (4) cul de sac; (5) pelvic peritoneum; (6) large and small bowel and appendix; (7) mucosa of the cervix, vagina, and fallopian tubes; and (8) laparotomy scars.

Endometriosis is an important clinical condition; it often causes *infertility, dysmenorrhea (painful menstruation), pelvic pain*, and other problems. The disorder is principally a disease of women in active reproductive life, most often in the third and fourth decades, affecting approximately 10% of women. Uncommonly, endometriosis can show features (metastasis and invasion) similar to malignant tumors. When these features are present they often contribute to significant complications. For example, invasion of the muscular wall of the bowel can result in intestinal symptoms (Fig. 22–24).

Two major theories for the development of endometriosis have been proposed.[7]

1. *The metastatic theory.* According to this, endometrial tissue is implanted at abnormal locations. Retrograde menstrua-tion through the fallopian tubes occurs regularly even in normal women and could mediate spread of endometrial tissue to the peritoneal cavity. Endometriosis is also found in cervical mucosa, particularly following surgical procedures, supporting implantation from above. In addition, this theory can explain the "spread" of endometriosis to distant sites via hematogenous and lymphatic "metastases." In the context of endometriosis, the term *metastatic* simply refers to the appearance of endometrial tissue in extrauterine locations but does not imply an underlying mechanism.

2. *The metaplastic theory.* Endometrium could arise directly from coelomic epithelium (mesothelium of pelvis or abdomen), from which the müllerian ducts and ultimately the endometrium itself originate during embryonic development.

The metaplastic theory is most widely accepted and provides a plausible explanation for the majority of cases of endometriosis. However, it fails to explain some situations in which endometriosis arises. For example, the presence of endometriosis in women who are amenorrheic because of a variety of underlying etiologies (e.g., gonadal dysgenesis) cannot be due to displaced menstrual endometrium. In addition, the relatively low incidence of endometriosis despite the common occurrence of retrograde menstruation (76% to 90% of women) suggests that specific individual factors must predispose women. Other factors that have been postulated include genetic, hormonal, and immune factors.[35] Molecular analysis, including gene expression profiling, have provided novel insights into pathogenesis of endometriosis. Some of the specific abnormalities that distinguish normal endometrium from endometriotic tissue are highlighted below[35]:

○ There is a profound activation of the *inflammatory cascade* in endometriosis, characterized by high levels of prostaglandin E2, IL-1β, TNF and IL-6. The key role played by prostaglandins in endometriosis is supported by the beneficial effects of COX-2 inhibitors on pelvic pain, an important clinical feature of this disorder.

○ *Estrogen production* by endometriotic stromal cells is markedly upregulated, due in large part to high levels of the key

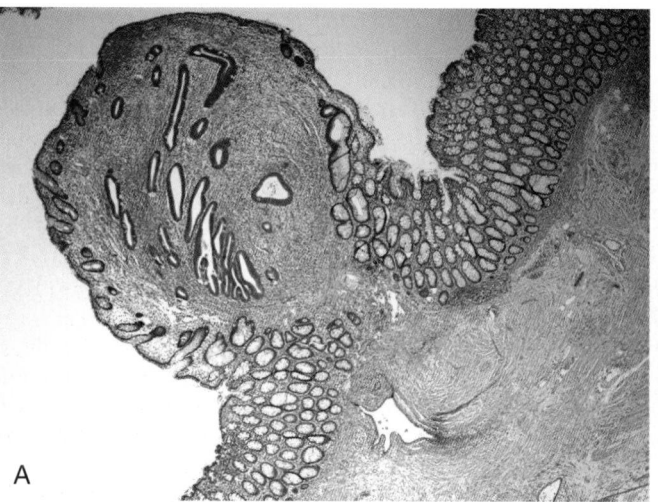
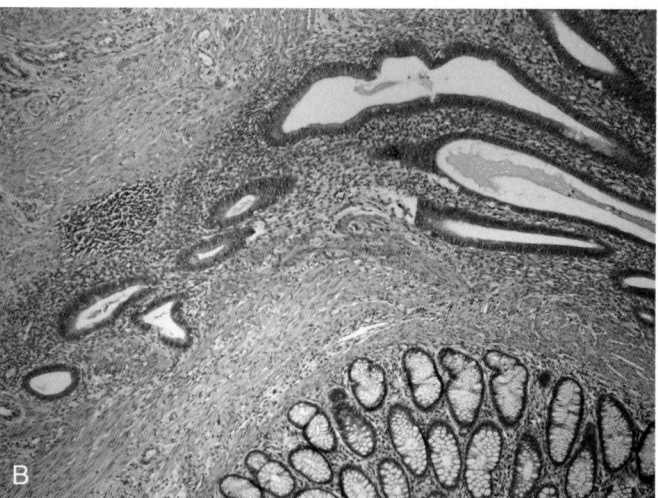

FIGURE 22–24 Endometriosis. **A,** Endometriosis is present in the mucosa of the colon. **B,** Higher magnification reveals the presence of both endometrial glands and stroma.

steroidogenic enzyme aromatase.[36] This enzyme is absent in normal endometrial stroma. Estrogen enhances the survival and persistence of endometriotic tissue; in keeping with this, inhibitors of aromatase are beneficial in the treatment of endometriosis. A linkage between activation of inflammation and estrogen production is suggested by the ability of prostaglandin E_2 to stimulate local synthesis of estrogen. Interestingly, endometriotic tissue is resistant to the anti-estrogenic effect of progesterone,[37] suggesting that progesterone resistance also plays a role in endometriosis.

These abnormalities seem related to epigenetic changes in key genes that encode two nuclear receptors: steroidogenic factor-1, and estrogen receptor-β. Substantially decreased methylation of the promoters of these genes cause their pathologic overexpression leading to activation of a downstream molecular cascade favoring overproduction of estrogen and prostaglandin and resistance to progesterone action. These defects are present not only in ectopic endometriotic tissue, but, to a lesser degree, also in the endometrium lining the uterus in patients with endometriosis suggesting that they are not secondary to abnormal location.

Some studies have suggested that endometriosis is clonal, yet other studies have demonstrated polyclonality.[38,39] Moreover, recent studies have detected mutations in endometriotic cysts that are similar to those found in ovarian endometrioid adenocarcinoma,[40] and clinicopathologic studies have long reported an association between the two. Collectively, these findings suggest that endometriosis can give rise to carcinoma.

> **Morphology.** The foci of endometriosis respond to both extrinsic cyclic (ovarian) and intrinsic hormonal stimulation with periodic bleeding. This produces nodules with a red-blue to yellow-brown appearance on or just beneath the mucosal and/or serosal surfaces in the site of involvement. When the disease is extensive, organizing hemorrhage causes extensive fibrous adhesions between tubes, ovaries, and other structures and obliterates the pouch of Douglas. The ovaries may become markedly distorted by large cystic masses (3 to 5 cm in diameter) filled with brown fluid resulting from previous hemorrhage; these are often referred to clinically as chocolate cysts or endometriomas. Aggressive forms of endometriosis can infiltrate tissues and cause fibrosis and subsequent adhesions.
>
> The histologic diagnosis of endometriosis is usually straightforward but may be difficult in long-standing cases in which the endometrial tissue is obscured by the secondary fibrosis. A histologic diagnosis of endometriosis is readily made when both endometrial glands and stroma are present (Fig. 22–24B), with or without the presence of hemosiderin. In rare cases only stroma is identified; however, if only glands are present it must be distinguished from other entities, such as endosalpingiosis, that have different clinical ramifications.

Clinical Features. Clinical signs and symptoms usually consist of severe dysmenorrhea, dyspareunia (pain with intercourse), and pelvic pain due to the intrapelvic bleeding and

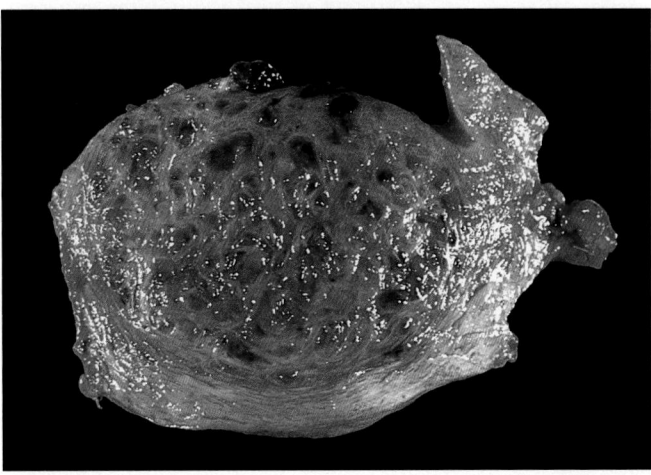

FIGURE 22–25   Adenomyosis. This disorder is characterized by functional endometrial nests within the myometrium, producing foci of hemorrhagic cysts within the uterine wall.

periuterine adhesions. Pain on defecation indicates rectal wall involvement, and dysuria results from involvement of the serosa of the bladder. Intestinal disturbances may appear when the small intestine is affected. Menstrual irregularities are common, and infertility is the presenting complaint in 30% to 40% of women. In addition, though uncommon, malignancies can develop in this setting, suggesting that endometriosis contains "at-risk" epithelium.

A closely related disorder, *adenomyosis*, is defined as the *presence of endometrial tissue within the uterine wall* (myometrium). Adenomyosis remains in continuity with the endometrium, presumably signifying downgrowth of endometrial tissue into and between the smooth muscle fascicles of the myometrium. Adenomyosis occurs in up to 20% of uteri (Fig. 22–25). On microscopic examination, irregular nests of endometrial stroma, with or without glands, are arranged within the myometrium, separated from the basalis by at least 2 to 3 mm. Like endometriosis, the clinical symptoms of adenomyosis include menometrorrhagia (irregular and heavy menses), colicky dysmenorrhea, dyspareunia, and pelvic pain, particularly during the premenstrual period.

Endometrial Polyps

Endometrial polyps are exophytic masses of variable size that project into the endometrial cavity. They may be single or multiple and are usually sessile, measuring from 0.5 to 3 cm in diameter, but are occasionally large and pedunculated. Polyps may be asymptomatic or may cause abnormal bleeding (intramenstrual, menometrorrhagia, or postmenopausal) if they ulcerate or undergo necrosis. Most commonly the glands within polyps are hyperplastic or atrophic, but they can occasionally demonstrate secretory changes (functional polyps). Hyperplastic polyps may develop in association with generalized endometrial hyperplasia and are responsive to the growth effect of estrogen but show little or no progesterone response (see Fig. 22–23C). Atrophic polyps, which largely occur in postmenopausal women, most likely represent atrophy of a hyperplastic polyp. Rarely, adenocarcinomas arise within endometrial polyps. Endometrial polyps have been observed in association with the administration of tamoxifen. This drug is often used in the therapy of breast cancer due to its anti-estrogenic activity on the breast.[41] However, tamoxifen has weak estrogenic effects in the endometrium. Cytogenetic studies indicate that the stromal cells in endometrial polyps contain chromosome (6p21) rearrangements involving the *HMGIY* gene, which is also rearranged in a variety of other benign mesenchymal tumors.[42]

Endometrial Hyperplasia

Endometrial hyperplasia, an important cause of abnormal bleeding, is defined as an increased proliferation of the endometrial glands relative to the stroma, resulting in an increased gland-to-stroma ratio when compared with normal proliferative endometrium. Endometrial hyperplasia deserves special attention because of its *relationship with endometrial carcinoma.* Clinicopathologic and epidemiologic studies have supported the malignant potential of endometrial hyperplasia and the concept of a continuum of proliferative glandular lesions culminating, in some cases, in carcinoma.[43] Molecular studies have confirmed this relationship, since endometrial hyperplasia and carcinoma share specific molecular genetic alterations.

Endometrial hyperplasia is associated with *prolonged estrogen stimulation of the endometrium*, which can be due to anovulation, increased estrogen production from endogenous sources, or exogenous estrogen. Thus, conditions associated with hyperplasia include obesity, menopause, polycystic ovarian disease (including Stein-Leventhal syndrome), functioning granulosa cell tumors of the ovary, excessive cortical function (cortical stromal hyperplasia), and prolonged administration of estrogenic substances (estrogen replacement therapy). These are the same influences postulated to be of pathogenetic significance in some endometrial carcinomas, discussed later.

A common genetic alteration found in a significant number of hyperplasias and related endometrial carcinomas is *inactivation of the PTEN tumor suppressor gene.*[44] *PTEN* is located on chromosome 10q23.3 and encodes a dual-specificity phosphatase capable of dephosphorylating both lipid and protein molecules. Its main function in tumorigenesis, as presently understood, is dephosphorylation of the lipid molecule phosphatidylinositol (3,4,5)-trisphosphate (PIP_3), which blocks the phosphorylation of AKT, a central factor in the phosphatidylinositol 3-kinase (PI3K) growth-regulatory pathway. When PTEN is inactive, AKT phosphorylation is enhanced, and it stimulates protein synthesis and cell proliferation and inhibits apoptosis. Mutations in *PTEN* have been found in more than 20% of hyperplasias, both with and without atypia, and in 30% to 80% of endometrial carcinomas, suggesting that alterations in *PTEN* occur at a relatively early stage in endometrial tumorigenesis.[45,46] You will also recall that patients with Cowden syndrome, which is caused by germline mutations in PTEN, have a high incidence of endometrial carcinoma. Although it is clear that PTEN plays a central role in the development of hyperplasia and carcinoma, the mechanism by which its loss contributes to endometrial tumorigenesis is not yet well understood. It has been shown that loss of PTEN, resulting in the activation of AKT, can lead to phosphorylation of the estrogen receptor in a ligand (estrogen)-independent manner.[47] Thus,

loss of PTEN function may activate pathways normally activated by estrogen.

Morphology. Based on architectural and cytologic features, endometrial hyperplasia is divided into four major categories:

Simple hyperplasia without atypia, also known as cystic or mild hyperplasia, is characterized by glands of various sizes and irregular shapes with cystic dilatation. There is a mild increase in the gland-to-stroma ratio. The epithelial growth pattern and cytology are similar to those of proliferative endometrium, although mitoses are not as prominent (Fig. 22–26A). These lesions uncommonly progress to adenocarcinoma (approximately 1%) and largely reflect a response to persistent estrogen stimulation. Simple hyperplasia may evolve into cystic atrophy when the estrogen stimulation is withdrawn.

Simple hyperplasia with atypia is uncommon. Architecturally it has the appearance of simple hyperplasia, but there is cytologic atypia within the glandular epithelial cells, as defined by loss of polarity, vesicular nuclei, and prominent nucleoli. Morphologically the cells become rounded and lose the normal perpendicular orientation to the basement membrane. In addition, the nuclei have an open chromatin pattern and conspicuous nucleoli. Approximately 8% of such lesions progress to carcinoma.

Complex hyperplasia without atypia shows an increase in the number and size of endometrial glands, marked gland crowding, and branching of glands. As a result, the glands may be crowded back-to-back with little intervening stroma and abundant mitotic figures (Fig. 22–26B). However, the glands remain distinct and nonconfluent, and the epithelial cells remain cytologically normal. This class of lesions has about a 3% progression to carcinoma, lower than that of simple hyperplasia with atypia.

Complex hyperplasia with atypia has considerable morphologic overlap with well-differentiated endometrioid adenocarcinoma (as discussed below), and an accurate distinction between complex hyperplasia with atypia and cancer may not be possible without hysterectomy (Fig. 22–26C and D).[48] It has been found that approximately 23% to 48% of women with a diagnosis of complex hyperplasia with atypia have carcinoma when a hysterectomy is performed shortly after the endometrial biopsy or curettage.[49] In one study, in which women with complex hyperplasia with atypia were treated with progestin therapy alone, 50% had persistent disease, 25% recurred, and 25% progressed to carcinoma.[50] Currently, complex hyperplasia with atypia is managed by hysterectomy or, in young women, a trial of progestin therapy and close follow-up. The low rate of regression usually requires the removal of the uterus.

A proportion of endometrial hyperplasias are less easily classified, including complex lesions without cellular atypia (uncommon) and those with altered cellular differentiation

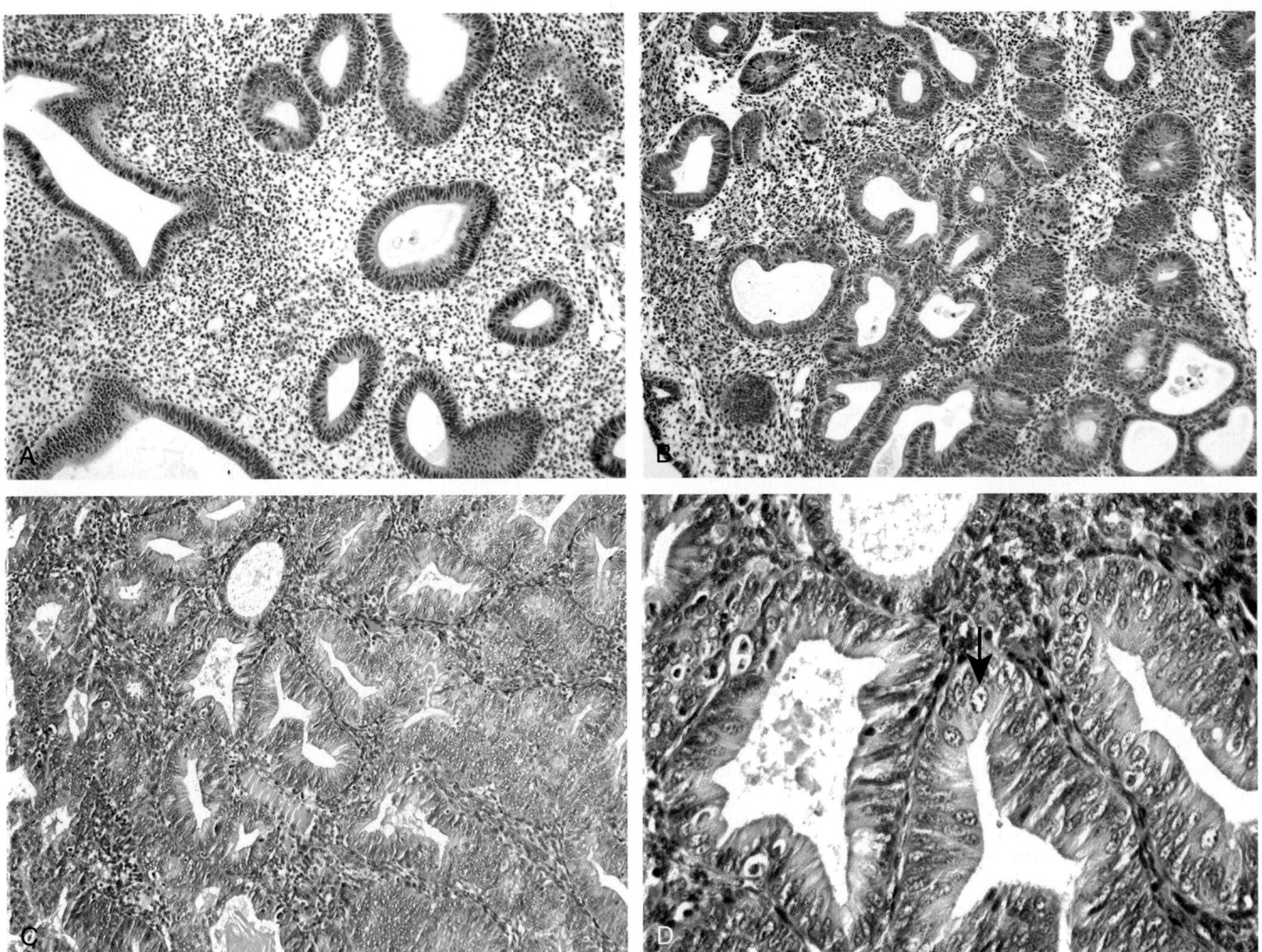

FIGURE 22–26 **A,** Simple hyperplasia without atypia with architectural abnormalities including mild glandular crowding and cystic glandular dilatation. **B,** Complex hyperplasia without atypia demonstrates increased glandular crowding with areas of back-to-back glands with cytologic features similar to proliferative endometrium. **C,** Complex hyperplasia with atypia has architectural features similar to complex hyperplasia without atypia, but the cytologic features have changed. **D,** High magnification of complex hyperplasia with atypia showing rounded, vesicular nuclei with prominent nucleoli *(arrow).*

(metaplasia), such as squamous, ciliated cell, and mucinous metaplasia. The latter may result from alterations in epithelial-stromal interactions inducing the basal endometrial cells to follow different differentiation pathways.[51] Because of these nuances of cell growth and differentiation, interpretation of endometrial hyperplasia may be highly subjective, and thus precise classification of every change is not possible. Any assessment of a suspected hyperplasia should include the degree of atypia in a manner clearly understandable by the clinician because the impact on therapy is great. For the patient it may mean the difference between cyclic progestin therapy on one hand and continuous high-dose progestin therapy or hysterectomy (or both) on the other.

Malignant Tumors of the Endometrium

CARCINOMA OF THE ENDOMETRIUM

Endometrial carcinoma is the most common invasive cancer of the female genital tract and accounts for 7% of all invasive

cancer in women, excluding skin cancer. At one time, it was far less common than cancer of the cervix, but earlier detection and eradication of squamous intraepithelial lesions and an increase in endometrial carcinomas in younger age groups have reversed this ratio. There are now 39,000 new endometrial cancers per year, compared with 11,000 new invasive cervical cancers. Although they occur at a high frequency, endometrial cancers arise mainly in postmenopausal women. Because they cause abnormal (postmenopausal) bleeding, early detection and cures are possible.

Molecular Pathogenesis. Carcinoma of the endometrium is uncommon in women younger than 40 years of age. The peak incidence is in 55- to 65-year-old women. Clinico-pathologic studies and molecular analyses support the classification of endometrial carcinoma into two broad categories, referred to as type I and type II, as summarized in Table 22–4.[52] Because of their distinct pathogenesis they will be discussed separately.

Type I carcinomas. These are the most common type, accounting for greater than 80% of all cases. The majority are well differentiated and mimic proliferative endometrial glands

TABLE 22–4 Characteristics of Type I and Type II Endometrial Carcinoma

Characteristics	Type I	Type II
Age	55–65 yr	65–75 yr
Clinical setting	Unopposed estrogen Obesity Hypertension Diabetes	Atrophy Thin physique
Morphology	Endometrioid	Serous Clear cell Mixed müllerian tumor
Precursor	Hyperplasia	Endometrial intraepithelial carcinoma
Molecular genetics	*PTEN* *PIK3CA* *KRAS* MSI* *β-catenin* *p53*	*p53* Aneuploidy *PIK3CA*
Behavior	Indolent Spreads via lymphatics	Aggressive Intraperitoneal and lymphatic spread

*MSI, microsatellite instability.

and, as such, are referred to as *endometrioid carcinoma*. As discussed above, they typically arise in the setting of endometrial hyperplasia and like endometrial hyperplasia they are associated with (1) obesity, (2) diabetes (abnormal glucose tolerance is found in more than 60%), (3) hypertension, (4) infertility (women who develop cancer of the endometrium tend to be nulliparous and have a history of functional menstrual irregularities consistent with anovulatory cycles), and (5) unopposed estrogen stimulation. Recent molecular studies have provided further evidence that endometrial hyperplasia is a precursor to endometrioid carcinoma (Fig. 22–27).[53]

As mentioned earlier, *mutations in the PTEN tumor suppressor gene have been identified in 30% to 80% of endometrioid carcinomas and in approximately 20% of endometrial hyperplasias*, both with and without atypia. In hysterectomy specimens containing complex hyperplasia with atypia and carcinoma, identical *PTEN* mutations have been identified in each component.[54] These findings support complex hyperplasia with atypia as a precursor to carcinoma and demonstrate that *PTEN* mutations occur before the development of invasion. Of interest, *PIK3CA* mutations have recently been reported in approximately 39% of endometrioid carcinomas, and they have been found in tumors with and without *PTEN* mutations.[55] PIK3CA is the catalytic subunit of PI3K, a lipid kinase that phosphorylates PIP_2 to PIP_3, directly antagonizing the action of *PTEN*. However, in contrast to *PTEN* mutations, *PIK3CA* mutations rarely occur in complex hyperplasia with atypia, suggesting that mutations in *PIK3CA* play a role in invasion.[56] Additional molecular changes that are common in type I carcinomas include microsatellite instability and mutations in the *KRAS* and β-catenin oncogenes. Microsatellite instability occurs in about 20% of sporadic tumors but is also found in tumors in women from families with hereditary nonpolyposis colorectal carcinoma (HNPCC), as discussed in Chapter 17. While microsatellite instability in HNPCC-related carcinomas is caused by germline mutations, in sporadic endometrioid carcinomas it is most commonly due to epigenetic silencing (via promoter hypermethylation) of one of the DNA mismatch repair genes. Mutations in *KRAS* are found in approximately 25% of cases and have also, but less commonly, been found in complex atypical hyperplasia. These molecular genetic alterations in endometrioid carcinoma, are rarely, if ever, found in type II carcinomas. One of the genes altered in both tumor types is *p53*. In the more poorly differentiated endometrioid carcinomas, mutations in *p53* can be found in up to 50% of cases. They are not identified in well-differentiated tumors or in complex atypical hyperplasias. Thus, it is thought that *p53* mutations are a late-occurring event in endometrioid carcinoma, in contrast to what is seen in serous endometrial carcinoma, as discussed below.

Morphology. On gross inspection, endometrial carcinoma can be either a localized polypoid tumor or a diffuse tumor involving the endometrial surface (Fig. 22–28A). Spread generally occurs by direct myometrial invasion with eventual extension to the periuterine structures by direct continuity. Spread into the broad ligaments may create a palpable mass. Dissemination to the regional lymph nodes eventually

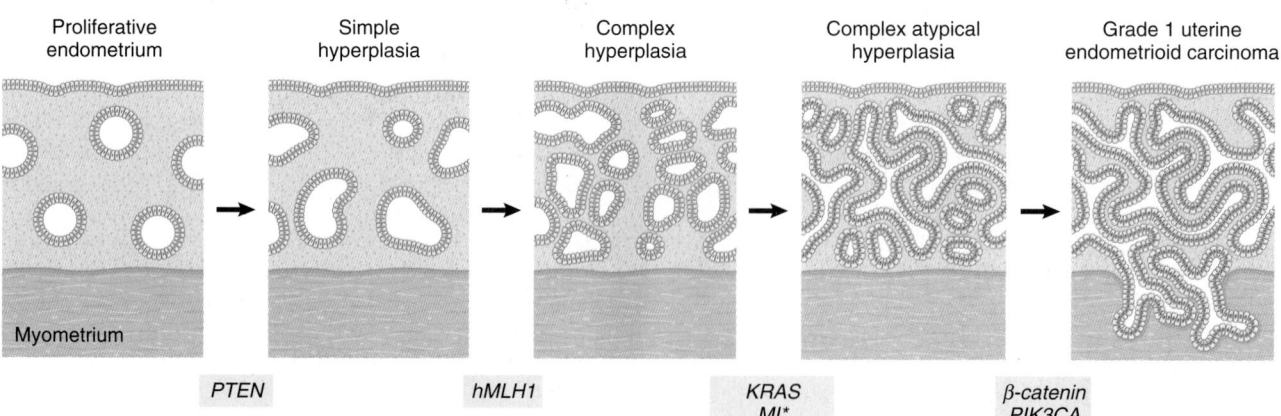

FIGURE 22–27 Schematic diagram depicting the development of type I endometrial carcinoma arising in the setting of hyperplasia. The most common molecular genetic alterations are shown at the time they are most likely to occur during the progression of the disease. *MI, microsatellite instability.

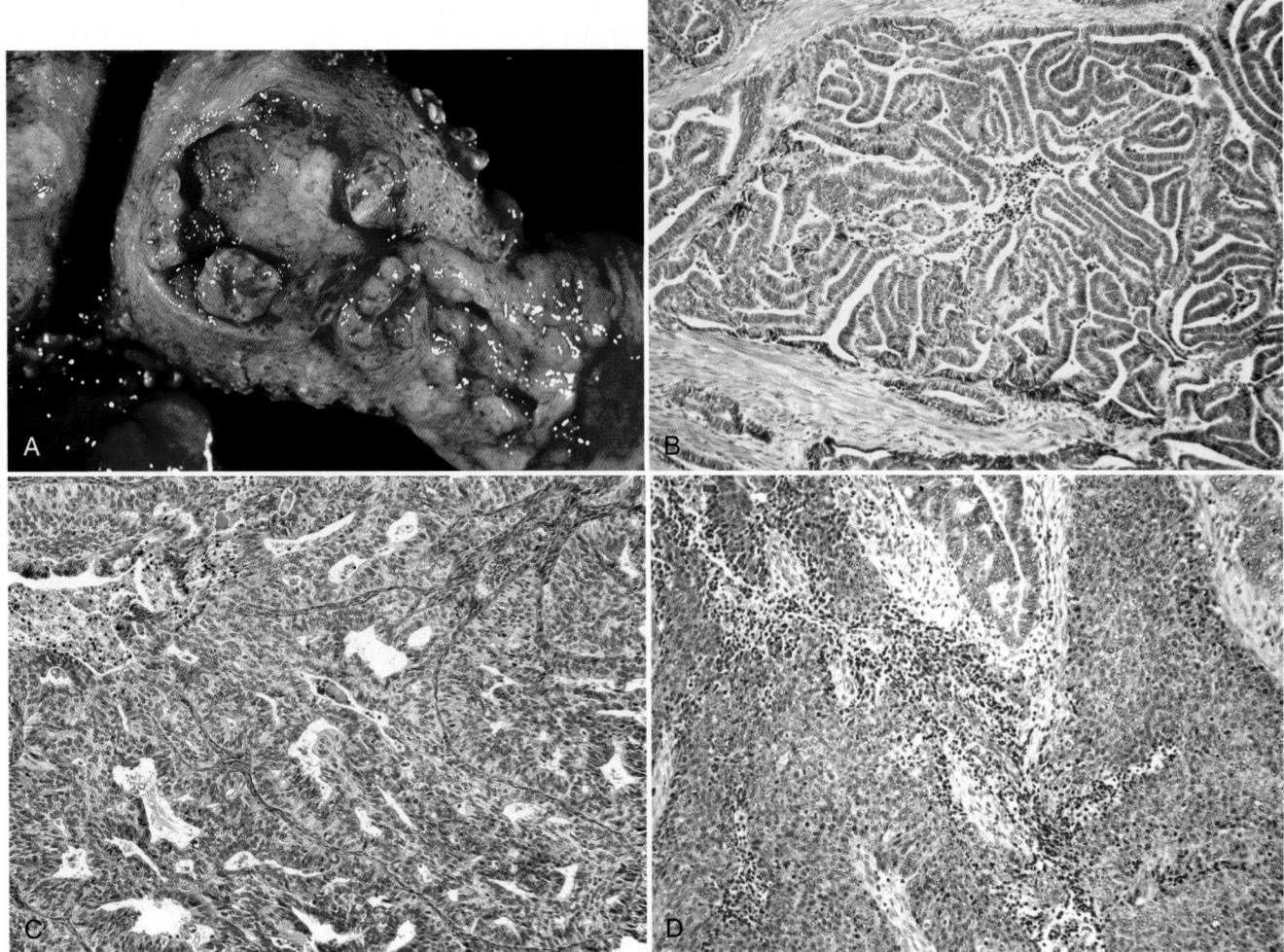

FIGURE 22–28 Type I carcinoma. **A,** Endometrial adenocarcinoma presenting as a fungating mass in the fundus of the uterus. **B,** Well-differentiated (grade 1) endometrioid adenocarcinoma with preserved glandular architecture but lack of intervening stroma, distinguishing it from hyperplasia. **C,** Moderately differentiated (grade 2) endometrioid adenocarcinoma with glandular architecture admixed with solid areas. **D,** Poorly differentiated (grade 3) endometrioid adenocarcinoma with predominantly solid growth.

occurs, and in the late stages, the tumor may metastasize to the lungs, liver, bones, and other organs.

On histologic examination, most endometrial carcinomas (about 85%) are **endometrioid adenocarcinomas** characterized by gland patterns resembling normal endometrial epithelium. A three-step grading system is applied to endometrioid tumors and includes well differentiated (grade 1) (Fig. 22–28B), with easily recognizable glandular patterns; moderately differentiated (grade 2) (Fig. 22–28C), showing well-formed glands mixed with solid sheets of malignant cells; or poorly differentiated (grade 3) (Fig. 22–28D), characterized by solid sheets of cells with barely recognizable glands and a greater degree of nuclear atypia and mitotic activity (see below).

G1. Well-differentiated adenocarcinoma, less than 5% solid growth

G2. Moderately differentiated adenocarcinoma with partly (less than 50%) solid growth

G3. Poorly differentiated adenocarcinoma with predominantly solid growth (greater than 50%)

Up to 20% of endometrioid carcinomas contain foci of squamous differentiation. Squamous elements may be histologically benign-appearing when they are associated with well-differentiated adenocarcinomas. Less commonly, moderately or poorly differentiated endometrioid carcinomas contain squamous elements that appear frankly malignant. Current classification systems grade the carcinomas based on glandular differentiation alone and do not include areas of solid squamous differentiation when considering grading.

Type II carcinomas. These generally occur in women a decade later than type I carcinoma, and in contrast to type I carcinoma they *usually arise in the setting of endometrial atrophy* (Fig. 22–29). Type II tumors are by definition poorly differentiated (grade 3) tumors and account for approximately 15% of cases of endometrial carcinoma. The most common subtype is serous carcinoma, referred to as such because of morphologic and biologic overlap with ovarian serous carcinoma. There are less common histologic subtypes (clear cell

Atrophic endometrium   Endometrial intraepithelial   Serous carcinoma
                                                  carcinoma

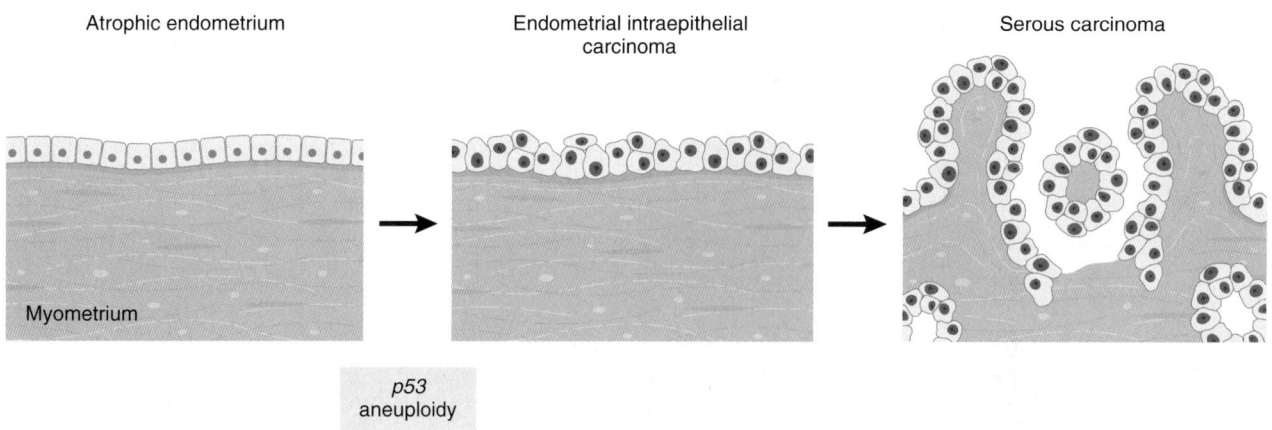

p53
aneuploidy

FIGURE 22–29   Schematic diagram of the development of type II endometrial carcinoma.

carcinoma and malignant mixed müllerian tumor) within this category, but very little is known about their pathogenesis. The most frequent alteration described thus far in serous endometrial carcinoma is mutation of the *p53* tumor suppressor gene. Alterations in other genes have been described, but at much lower frequency. Mutations in *p53* are present in at least 90% of serous endometrial carcinoma.[57] The majority of mutations are missense mutations that result in an accumulation of the altered protein that can be detected with immunohistochemistry as strong, diffuse staining of the tumor cell nuclei (Fig. 22–30B and D).

The precursor of serous carcinoma, endometrial intraepithelial carcinoma (EIC), consists of cells identical to those of serous carcinoma but lacks identifiable stromal invasion. Mutations in *p53* are found in approximately 75% of these lesions, suggesting that *mutation of p53 is an early event in serous endometrial carcinoma*. Thus, serous carcinoma presumably begins as a surface epithelial neoplasm that extends into adjacent gland structures and later invades endometrial stroma. Their generally poorer prognosis is thought to be a consequence of a propensity to exfoliate, undergo transtubal spread, and implant on peritoneal surfaces like their ovarian counterparts. They have often spread outside of the uterus at the time of diagnosis.

Morphology. Generally, serous carcinomas arise in small atrophic uteri and are often large bulky tumors or deeply invasive into the myometrium. The precursor lesion, endometrial intraepithelial carcinoma, consists of malignant cells identical to those of serous carcinoma but they remain contained to the gland surface without identifiable stromal invasion (see Fig. 22–30A and B). The invasive lesions may have a papillary growth pattern composed of cells with marked cytologic atypia including high nuclear-to-cytoplasmic ratio, atypical mitotic figures, heterochromasia, and prominent nucleoli (see Fig. 22–30C and D). However, they can also have a predominantly glandular growth pattern that can be distinguished from endometroid carcinoma by the marked cytologic atypia. All of the non-endometrioid carcinomas are classified as grade 3 irrespective of histologic pattern.

Serous carcinoma, despite relatively superficial endometrial involvement, may be associated with extensive peritoneal disease, suggesting spread by routes (i.e., tubal or lymphatic transmission) other than direct invasion.

Clinical Course. There is no currently available screening test for carcinoma of the endometrium. Although it may be asymptomatic for a period of time, it usually produces irregular or postmenopausal vaginal bleeding with excessive leukorrhea. Uterine enlargement may be absent in the early stages. The diagnosis of endometrial cancer must ultimately be established by biopsy or curettage and histologic examination of the tissue.

As would be anticipated, the prognosis depends heavily on the clinical stage of the disease when it is discovered, and its histologic grade and type. In the United States, most women (about 80%) present in stage I and have well-differentiated or moderately differentiated endometrioid carcinomas. Surgery, alone or in combination with irradiation, gives about 90% 5-year survival in stage I (grade 1 or 2) disease. This rate drops to approximately 75% for grade 3/stage I and to 50% or less for stage II and III endometrial carcinomas.

As mentioned, serous carcinoma has a propensity for extrauterine (lymphatic or transtubal) spread, even when apparently confined to the endometrium or its surface epithelium. Overall, fewer than 50% of patients with these tumors are alive 3 years after diagnosis and 35% after 5 years. If peritoneal cytology and adnexal histologic exam are negative, the 5-year survival of those with stage I disease is approximately 80% to 85%.[58] The additional advantage of prophylactic radiation or chemotherapy in early-stage disease is unclear.[59,60]

MALIGNANT MIXED MÜLLERIAN TUMORS

MMMTs (previously referred to as carcinosarcomas) consist of endometrial adenocarcinomas with malignant changes in the stroma.[61] The stroma tends to differentiate into a variety of malignant mesodermal components, including muscle, cartilage, and even osteoid. The epithelial and stromal components are presumably derived from the same cell, a concept

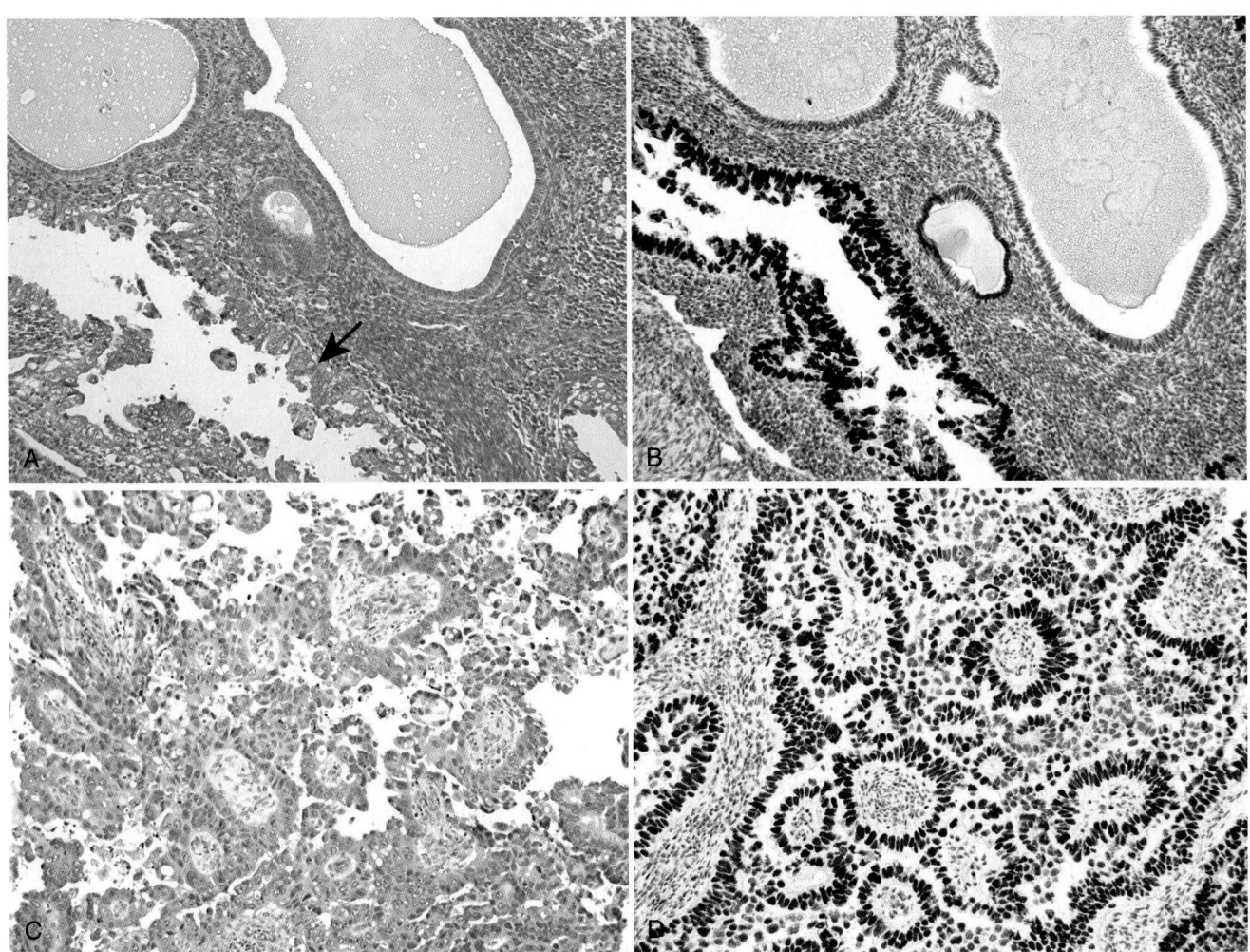

FIGURE 22–30   Type II carcinoma. **A,** Endometrial intraepithelial carcinoma, the precursor to serous carcinoma showing malignant cells *(arrow)* with morphologic features identical to serous carcinoma lining the surfaces of the endometrial glands without obvious stromal invasion. **B,** Strong, diffuse expression of p53 as detected by immunohistochemistry in endometrial intraepithelial carcinoma. **C,** Serous carcinoma of the endometrium with papillary growth pattern consisting of malignant cells with marked cytologic atypia including high nuclear-to-cytoplasmic ratio, atypical mitotic figures, and hyperchromasia. **D,** As with the previous lesion, there is an accumulation of p53 protein in the nucleus.

supported by immunohistochemical and molecular studies.[62] Both clinicopathologic and molecular studies suggest that the vast majority of these tumors are carcinomas with sarcomatous differentiation. The mechanisms underlying the sarcomatous transformation are unknown. MMMTs occur in postmenopausal women and present with postmenopausal bleeding.

Morphology. In gross appearance, MMMTs are fleshier than adenocarcinomas, may be bulky and polypoid, and sometimes protrude through the cervical os. On histology, the tumors consist of adenocarcinoma (endometrioid, serous, or clear cell) mixed with the malignant mesenchymal (sarcoma) elements (Fig. 22–31A); alternatively, the tumor may contain two distinct and separate epithelial and mesenchymal components. Sarcomatous components may also mimic extrauterine tissues (e.g., striated muscle, cartilage, adipose tissue, and bone). Metastases

usually contain only epithelial components (Fig. 22–31B).

Outcome of MMMTs is determined primarily by depth of invasion and stage. As with endometrial carcinomas, the prognosis is influenced by the grade and type of the adenocarcinoma, being poorest with serous differentiation. These tumors are highly malignant, with 5-year survival rate of 25% to 30%.[61]

Staging of types I and II of endometrial adenocarcinoma and MMMTs is as follows:

Stage I.   Carcinoma is confined to the corpus uteri itself.

Stage II.   Carcinoma involves the corpus and the cervix.

Stage III.   Carcinoma extends outside the uterus but not outside the true pelvis.

Stage IV.   Carcinoma extends outside the true pelvis or involves the mucosa of the bladder or the rectum.

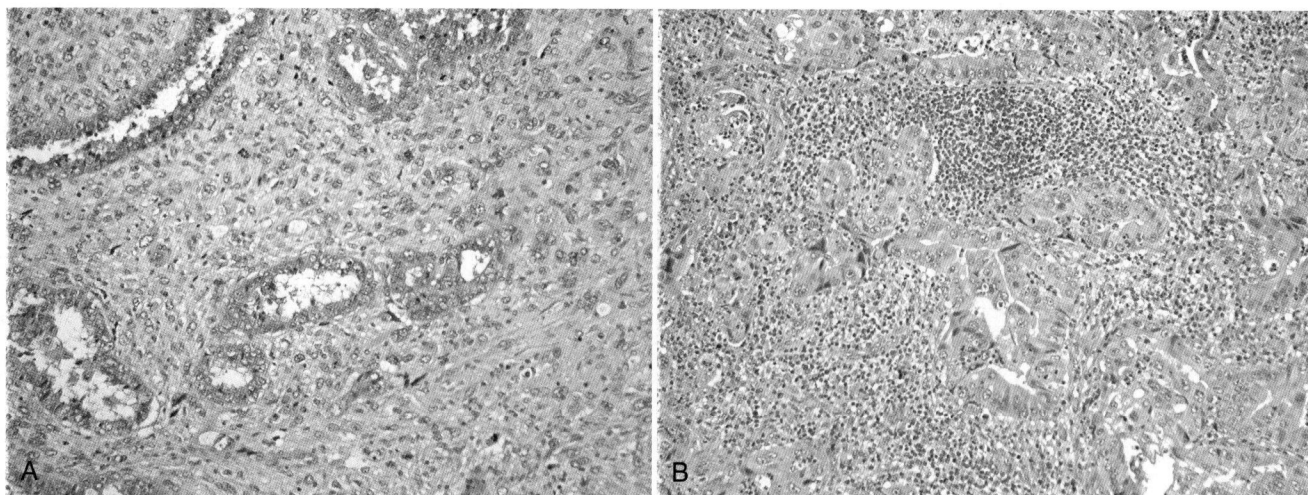

FIGURE 22–31   A, Malignant mixed müllerian tumor (MMMT), showing both malignant epithelial and stromal components. **B,** Lymph node metastasis from a MMMT showing only the epithelial component as is typically seen.

Tumors of the Endometrium with Stromal Differentiation

These are relatively uncommon tumors and comprise less than 5% of endometrial cancers. One group is composed of stromal neoplasias in association with benign glands (adenosarcomas). The other group consists of pure stromal neoplasms, ranging from benign (stromal nodule) to malignant (stromal sarcoma).

ADENOSARCOMAS

Adenosarcomas present most commonly as large broad-based endometrial polypoid growths that may prolapse through the cervical os. The diagnosis is based on malignant-appearing stroma, which coexists with benign but abnormally shaped endometrial glands. These tumors predominate in women between the fourth and fifth decades and are generally considered to be a low-grade malignancy; recurrences develop in one fourth and are nearly always confined to the pelvis.[63] The principal diagnostic dilemma is distinguishing these tumors from large benign polyps. The distinction is important, because oophorectomy is typically performed in cases of adenosarcoma, since they are estrogen-sensitive.

STROMAL TUMORS

The endometrial stroma occasionally gives rise to neoplasms that may resemble normal stromal cells. Similar to most neoplasms, they may be well or poorly differentiated. Stromal neoplasms are divided into two categories: (1) benign stromal nodules and (2) endometrial stromal sarcomas.

> **Morphology. Stromal nodule** is a well-circumscribed aggregate of endometrial stromal cells in the myometrium that does not penetrate the myometrium and is of little consequence. **Stromal sarcoma** consists of neoplastic endometrial stroma lying between muscle bundles of the myometrium and is distinguished from stromal nodules by either diffuse infiltration of myometrial tissue or the invasion of lymphatic channels (previously termed **endolymphatic stromal myosis**).

About half of stromal sarcomas recur, with relapse rates of 36% to over 80% for stage I and stage III/IV tumor, respectively; relapse cannot be predicted by either mitotic index or degree of cytologic atypia.[64] Distant metastases may occur decades after initial diagnosis, and death from metastatic tumor occurs in about 15% of cases. Five-year survival rates average 50%. A recurrent chromosomal translocation, t(7;17)(p15;q21), occurs in endometrial stromal sarcoma. This translocation leads to the fusion of two polycomb group genes, *JAZF1* and *JJAZ1*, with production of a fusion transcript with anti-apoptotic properties.[65] Interestingly, even normal endometrial stromal cells express the fusion gene, derived not by translocation, but by the "stitching" together of m-RNAs. Thus, it appears that a pro-survival gene in the normal endometrium is somehow subverted to become pro-neoplastic.

Tumors of the Myometrium

LEIOMYOMAS

Uterine leiomyomas (commonly called *fibroids*) are perhaps the most common tumor in women. They are benign smooth muscle neoplasms that may occur singly, but most often are multiple. Most leiomyomas have normal karyotypes, but approximately 40% have a simple chromosomal abnormality. Several cytogenetic subgroups have been recognized: a balanced translocation between chromosomes 12 and 14 (i.e., t(12;14)(q14–q15;q23–q24)), partial deletions of the long arm of chromosome 7 (i.e., del(7)(q22–q32)), trisomy 12, and rearrangements of 6p, 3q, and 10q. The rearrangements of 12q14 and 6p involving the *HMGIC* and *HMGIY* genes, respectively, which are also implicated in a variety of other benign neoplasms. Both genes encode closely related DNA-binding factors that regulate chromatin structure.[66,67]

> **Morphology.** Leiomyomas are sharply circumscribed, discrete, round, firm, gray-white tumors varying in size from small, barely visible nodules to massive tumors that fill the pelvis. Except in rare instances, they are found within the myometrium of the corpus. Only infrequently do they involve the uterine ligaments, lower uterine segment, or cervix. They can occur within the myometrium (intramural), just beneath the endometrium (submucosal) (Fig. 22–32A; see also Fig. 22–23D), or beneath the serosa (subserosal).
>
> Whatever their size, the characteristic whorled pattern of smooth muscle bundles on cut section usually makes these lesions readily identifiable on gross inspection. Large tumors may develop areas of yellow-brown to red softening (red degeneration).
>
> On histologic examination, the leiomyoma is composed of whorled bundles of smooth muscle cells that resemble the uninvolved myometrium (Fig. 22–32B). Usually, the individual muscle cells are uniform in size and shape and have the characteristic oval nucleus and long, slender bipolar cytoplasmic processes. Mitotic figures are scarce. Benign variants of leiomyoma include atypical or bizarre (symplastic) tumors with nuclear atypia and giant cells, and cellular leiomyomas. Importantly, both have a low mitotic index. An extremely rare variant, **benign metastasizing leiomyoma**, consists of a uterine tumor that extends into vessels and migrates to other sites, most commonly the lung. Another variant, **disseminated peritoneal leiomyomatosis**, presents as multiple small nodules on the peritoneum. Both are considered benign despite their unusual behavior.

Leiomyomas of the uterus, even when they are extensive, may be asymptomatic. The most important symptoms are abnormal bleeding, compression of the bladder (urinary frequency), sudden pain if disruption of blood supply occurs, and impaired fertility. Myomas in pregnant women increase the frequency of spontaneous abortion, fetal malpresentation, uterine inertia, and postpartum hemorrhage. Malignant transformation (leiomyosarcoma) within a leiomyoma is extremely rare.

LEIOMYOSARCOMAS

These uncommon malignant neoplasms arise de novo from the myometrium or endometrial stromal precursor cells. In contrast to leiomyomas, leiomyosarcomas have complex, highly variable karyotypes that frequently include deletions.[68]

> **Morphology.** Leiomyosarcomas grow within the uterus in two somewhat distinctive patterns: bulky, fleshy masses that invade the uterine wall, or polypoid masses that project into the uterine lumen (Fig. 22–33A). On histologic examination, they contain a wide range of atypia, from those that are extremely well differentiated to highly anaplastic, pleomorphic lesions (Fig. 22–33B). The distinction from leiomyomas is based on nuclear atypia, mitotic index, and

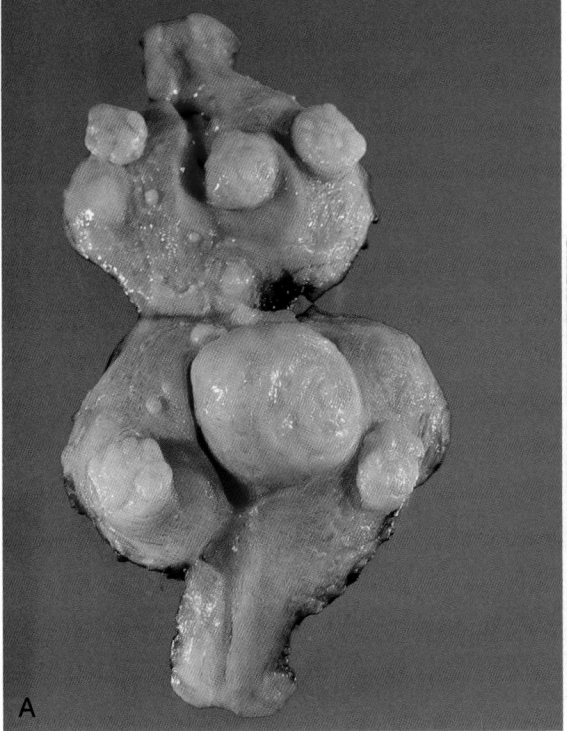

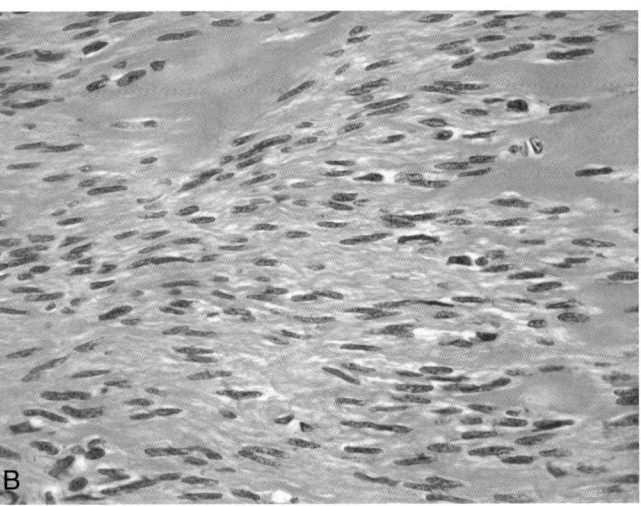

FIGURE 22–32   **A,** Leiomyomas of the myometrium. The uterus is opened to reveal multiple tumors in submucosal (bulging into the endometrial cavity), intramural, and subserosal locations that display a firm white appearance on sectioning. **B,** Leiomyoma showing well-differentiated, regular, spindle-shaped smooth muscle cells associated with hyalinization.

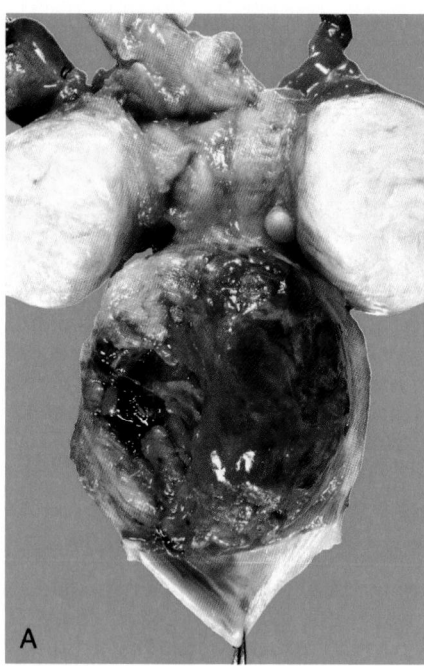
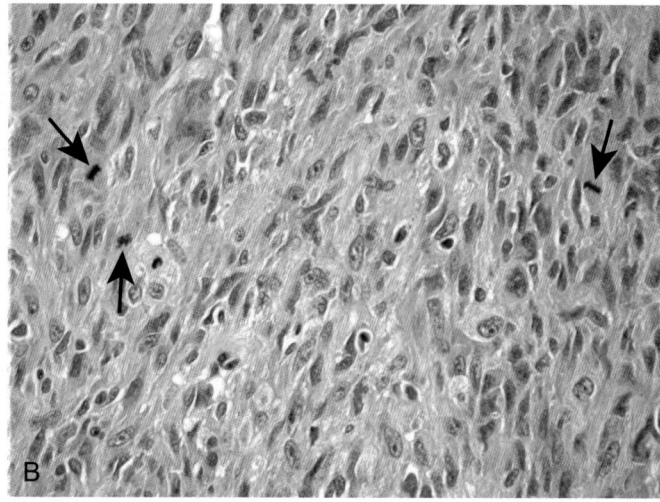

FIGURE 22–33 Leiomyosarcoma. **A,** A large hemorrhagic tumor mass distends the lower corpus and is flanked by two leiomyomas. (A courtesy of Dr. Anna Walker, Mercer University, Macon, Georgia.) **B,** The tumor cells are irregular in size and have hyperchromatic nuclei with numerous mitotic figures *(arrows).*

zonal necrosis. With few exceptions, the presence of 10 or more mitoses per 10 high-power (400×) fields indicates malignancy, particularly if accompanied by cytologic atypia and/or necrosis. If the tumor contains nuclear atypia or large (epithelioid) cells, 5 mitoses per 10 high-power (400×) fields are sufficient to justify a diagnosis of malignancy.[69] Rare exceptions include mitotically active leiomyomas in young or pregnant women, and caution should be exercised in interpreting such neoplasms as malignant. A proportion of smooth muscle neoplasms may be impossible to classify and are called smooth muscle tumors of "uncertain malignant potential."[69]

Leiomyosarcomas are equally common before and after menopause, and have a peak incidence at 40 to 60 years of age. These tumors have a striking tendency to recur after removal, and more than half eventually metastasize through the bloodstream to distant organs, such as lungs, bone, and brain. Dissemination throughout the abdominal cavity is also encountered. The 5-year survival rate averages about 40%. The well-differentiated lesions have a better prognosis than the anaplastic lesions, which have a 5-year survival rate of only 10% to 15%.[69]

FALLOPIAN TUBES

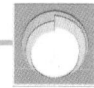

The most common disorders in these structures are infections leading to inflammatory conditions, followed in frequency by ectopic (tubal) pregnancy (see discussion later in this chapter) and endometriosis.

Inflammations

Suppurative salpingitis may be caused by any of the pyogenic organisms; often more than one is involved. The gonococcus still accounts for more than 60% of cases of suppurative salpingitis, with chlamydiae less often a factor. These tubal infections are a part of pelvic inflammatory disease, described earlier in this chapter.

Tuberculous salpingitis is extremely uncommon in the United States and accounts for probably not more than 1% to 2% of all forms of salpingitis. It is more common, however, in parts of the world where tuberculosis is prevalent and is an important cause of infertility in these areas.

Tumors and Cysts

The most common primary lesions of the fallopian tube (excluding endometriosis) are minute, 0.1- to 2-cm translucent cysts filled with clear serous fluid, called *paratubal cysts.* Larger varieties are found near the fimbriated end of the tube or in the broad ligaments and are referred to as *hydatids of Morgagni.* These cysts are presumed to arise in remnants of the müllerian duct and are of little significance.

Tumors of the fallopian tube are uncommon. Benign tumors include *adenomatoid tumors* (mesotheliomas), which occur subserosally on the tube or sometimes in the mesosalpinx. These small nodules are the exact counterparts of those already described in relation to the testes or epididymus (Chapter 21) and are benign. Primary *adenocarcinoma* of the fallopian tubes is rare and is defined as an adenocarcinoma with a dominant tubal mass and luminal and mucosal involvement. These tumors are detected by pelvic examination, abnormal discharge, or bleeding, and occasionally, cervical cytology. Approximately one half are stage I at diagnosis, but nearly 40% of these patients do not survive 5 years. Higher stage tumors have a poorer prognosis.[70] Patients are typically managed with ovarian cancer chemotherapy protocols. Recently, occult carcinoma of the fallopian tube has been associated with germline *BRCA* mutations, as discussed below.[71]

OVARIES

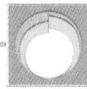

The most common types of lesions encountered in the ovary include functional or benign cysts and tumors. Intrinsic inflammations of the ovary (oophoritis) are uncommon, and usually accompany tubal inflammation. Rarely, a primary inflammatory disorder involving ovarian follicles (autoimmune oophoritis) occurs and is associated with infertility. The ovary has three main histologic compartments: (1) the surface müllerian epithelium, (2) the germ cells, and (3) the sex cord–stromal cells. Each compartment gives rise to distinct non-neoplastic and neoplastic entities, as discussed below.

Non-Neoplastic and Functional Cysts

FOLLICLE AND LUTEAL CYSTS

Cystic follicles in the ovary are so common that they are considered virtually normal. They originate in unruptured graafian follicles or in follicles that have ruptured and immediately sealed.

> **Morphology.** These cysts are usually multiple. They range in size up to 2 cm in diameter, are filled with a clear serous fluid, and are lined by a gray, glistening membrane. On occasion, larger cysts exceeding 2 cm (follicle cysts) may be diagnosed by palpation or ultrasonography; these may cause pelvic pain. Granulosa lining cells can be identified histologically if the intraluminal pressure has not been too great. The outer theca cells may be conspicuous due to increased amounts of pale cytoplasm (luteinized). As discussed subsequently, when this alteration is pronounced (hyperthecosis), it may be associated with increased estrogen production and endometrial abnormalities.
>
> Granulosa **luteal cysts** (corpora lutea) are normally present in the ovary. These cysts are lined by a rim of bright yellow tissue containing luteinized granulosa cells. They occasionally rupture and cause a peritoneal reaction. Sometimes the combination of old hemorrhage and fibrosis may make their distinction from endometriotic cysts difficult.

POLYCYSTIC OVARIES AND STROMAL HYPERTHECOSIS

Polycystic ovarian disease (PCOD; formerly termed *Stein-Leventhal syndrome*) affects 3% to 6% of reproductive-age women. The central pathologic abnormality is numerous cystic follicles or follicle cysts, often associated with oligomenorrhea. Women with PCOD have persistent anovulation, obesity (40%), hirsutism (50%), and, rarely, virilism.[72,73]

> **Morphology.** The ovaries are usually twice normal size and have a smooth, gray-white outer cortex studded with subcortical cysts 0.5 to 1.5 cm in diameter. On histologic examination, there is a thickened, fibrotic superficial cortex beneath which are innumerable follicle cysts associated with hyperplasia of the theca interna (follicular hyperthecosis) (Fig. 22–34). Corpora lutea are frequently but not invariably absent.

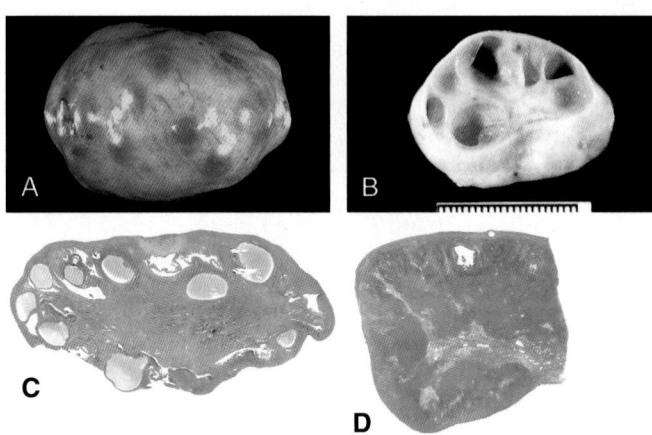

FIGURE 22–34 Polycystic ovarian disease and cortical stromal hyperplasia. **A,** The ovarian cortex reveals numerous clear cysts. **B,** Sectioning of the cortex reveals several subcortical cystic follicles. **C,** Cystic follicles seen in a low-power microphotograph. **D,** Cortical stromal hyperplasia manifests as diffuse stromal proliferation with symmetric enlargement of the ovary.

The initiating event in PCOD is not clear. Increased secretion of luteinizing hormone may stimulate the theca-lutein cells of the follicles, to produce excessive androgen (androstenedione), which is converted to estrone. For years, these endocrine abnormalities were attributed to primary ovarian dysfunction because large wedge resections of the ovaries sometimes restored fertility. It is now believed that *a variety of enzymes involved in androgen biosynthesis are poorly regulated in PCOD*. Recent studies link PCOD, like type 2 diabetes, to insulin resistance. Treatment of the insulin resistance sometimes results in resumption of ovulation.[74]

Stromal hyperthecosis, also called cortical stromal hyperplasia, is a disorder of ovarian stroma most commonly seen in postmenopausal women, but it may blend with PCOD in younger women. The disorder is characterized by uniform enlargement of the ovary (up to 7 cm), which has a white to tan appearance on sectioning. The involvement is usually bilateral and microscopically shows hypercellular stroma and luteinization of the stromal cells, which are visible as discrete nests of cells with vacuolated cytoplasm. The clinical presentation and effects on the endometrium are similar to those of PCOD, although virilization may be striking.[72]

A physiologic condition mimicking the above syndromes is *theca lutein hyperplasia of pregnancy*. In response to pregnancy hormones (gonadotropins), proliferation of theca cells and expansion of the perifollicular zone occurs. As the follicles regress, the concentric theca-lutein hyperplasia may appear nodular. This change is not to be confused with true luteomas of pregnancy (see below).

Ovarian Tumors

There are numerous types of ovarian tumors, and overall they fall into benign, borderline, and malignant categories. About 80% are benign, and these occur mostly in young women between the ages of 20 and 45 years. Borderline tumors occur at slightly older ages. Malignant tumors are more common in older women, between the ages of 45 and 65 years. Ovarian cancer accounts for 3% of all cancers in females and is the fifth most common cause of death due to cancer in women in the United States. Among cancers of the female genital tract, the incidence of ovarian cancer ranks below only carcinoma of the cervix and the endometrium. In addition, because *most ovarian cancers are detected when they have spread beyond the ovary, they account for a disproportionate number of deaths from cancer of the female genital tract*.

Classification. The classification of ovarian tumors given in Table 22–5 and Figure 22–35 is a simplified version of the World Health Organization Histological Classification, which separates ovarian neoplasms according to the most probable tissue of origin. It is now believed that tumors of the ovary arise ultimately from one of three ovarian components: (1) surface epithelium derived from the coelomic epithelium; (2) the germ cells, which migrate to the ovary from the yolk sac and are pluripotent; and (3) the stroma of the ovary, including the sex cords, which are forerunners of the endocrine apparatus of the postnatal ovary. There is also a group of tumors that defy classification, and finally there are secondary or metastatic tumors to the ovary.

TABLE 22–5 WHO Classification of Ovarian Neoplasms

SURFACE EPITHELIAL-STROMAL TUMORS

Serous tumors
  Benign (cystadenoma)
  Borderline tumors (serous borderline tumor)
  Malignant (serous adenocarcinoma)
Mucinous tumors, endocervical-like and intestinal type
  Benign (cystadenoma)
  Borderline tumors (mucinous borderline tumor)
  Malignant (mucinous adenocarcinoma)
Endometrioid tumors
  Benign (cystadenoma)
  Borderline tumors (endometrioid borderline tumor)
  Malignant (endometrioid adenocarcinoma)
Clear cell tumors
  Benign
  Borderline tumors
  Malignant (clear cell adenocarcinoma)
Transitional cell tumors
  Brenner tumor
  Brenner tumor of borderline malignancy
  Malignant Brenner tumor
  Transitional cell carcinoma (non-Brenner type)
Epithelial-stromal
  Adenosarcoma
  Malignant mixed müllerian tumor

SEX CORD–STROMAL TUMORS

Granulosa tumors
Fibromas
Fibrothecomas
Thecomas
Sertoli cell tumors
Leydig cell tumors
Sex cord tumor with annular tubules
Gynandroblastoma
Steroid (lipid) cell tumors

GERM CELL TUMORS

Teratoma
  Immature
  Mature
    Solid
    Cystic (dermoid cyst)
  Monodermal (e.g., struma ovarii, carcinoid)
Dysgerminoma
Yolk sac tumor (endodermal sinus tumor)
Mixed germ cell tumors

MALIGNANT, NOT OTHERWISE SPECIFIED

METASTATIC CANCER FROM NONOVARIAN PRIMARY

Colonic, appendiceal
Gastric
Breast

Although some of the specific tumors have distinctive features and are hormonally active, most are nonfunctional and tend to produce relatively mild symptoms until they reach a large size. Malignant tumors have usually spread outside the ovary by the time a definitive diagnosis is made. Some of these tumors, principally epithelial tumors, tend to be bilateral. Table 22–6 lists the tumors and their subtypes. Abdominal pain and distention, urinary and gastrointestinal tract symptoms due to compression by the tumor or cancer invasion, and vaginal bleeding are the most common symptoms. The benign forms may be entirely asymptomatic and occasionally are

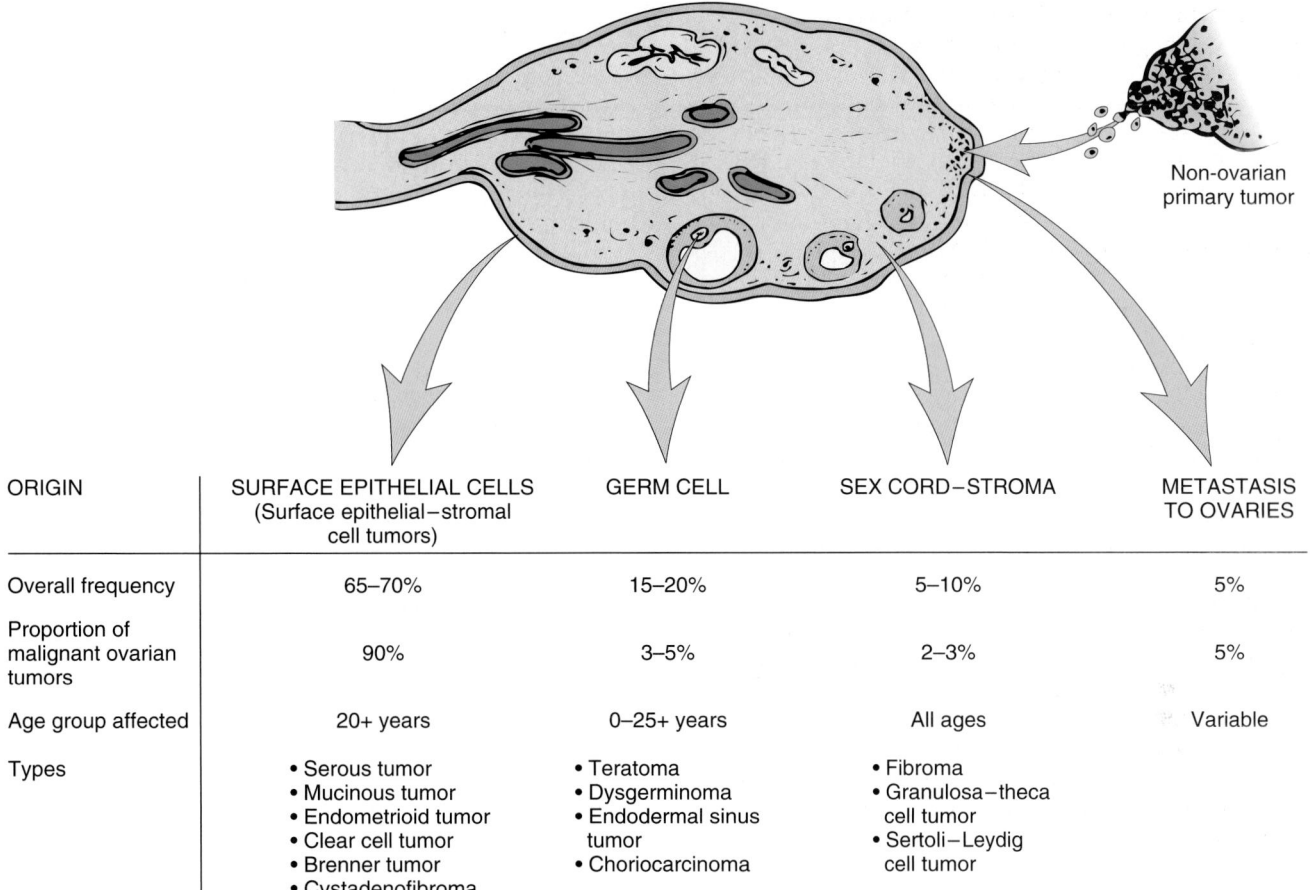

ORIGIN	SURFACE EPITHELIAL CELLS (Surface epithelial–stromal cell tumors)	GERM CELL	SEX CORD–STROMA	METASTASIS TO OVARIES
Overall frequency	65–70%	15–20%	5–10%	5%
Proportion of malignant ovarian tumors	90%	3–5%	2–3%	5%
Age group affected	20+ years	0–25+ years	All ages	Variable
Types	• Serous tumor • Mucinous tumor • Endometrioid tumor • Clear cell tumor • Brenner tumor • Cystadenofibroma	• Teratoma • Dysgerminoma • Endodermal sinus tumor • Choriocarcinoma	• Fibroma • Granulosa–theca cell tumor • Sertoli–Leydig cell tumor	

FIGURE 22–35 Derivation of various ovarian neoplasms and some data on their frequency and age distribution.

TABLE 22–6 Frequency of Major Ovarian Tumors

Type	Percentage of Malignant Ovarian Tumors	Percentage That Are Bilateral
Serous		
Benign (60%)		25
Borderline (15%)		30
Malignant (25%)	45	65
Mucinous		
Benign (80%)		5
Borderline (10%)		10
Malignant (10%)	5	<5
Endometrioid carcinoma	20	40
Undifferentiated carcinoma	10	—
Clear cell carcinoma	6	40
Granulosa cell tumor	5	5
Teratoma		15
Benign (96%)		
Malignant (4%)	1	Rare
Metastatic	5	>50
Others	3	—

found unexpectedly on abdominal or pelvic examination or during surgery.

TUMORS OF SURFACE (MÜLLERIAN) EPITHELIUM

Most primary neoplasms in the ovary fall within this category. The classification of epithelial tumors of the ovary is based on both differentiation and extent of proliferation of the epithelium. There are *three major histologic types based on the differentiation of the neoplastic epithelium: serous, mucinous, and endometrioid tumors.*[75] The extent of epithelial proliferation is associated with the biologic behavior of the tumor and is classified as benign (minimal epithelial proliferation), borderline (moderate epithelial proliferation), and malignant (marked epithelial proliferation with stromal invasion). The benign tumors are often further classified based on the components of the tumors, which may include cystic areas (cystadenomas), cystic and fibrous areas (cystadenofibromas), and predominantly fibrous areas (adenofibromas). The borderline tumors and the malignant tumors can also have a cystic component, and when malignant they are sometimes referred to as cystadenocarcinomas. The tumors can be relatively small, or they can grow to fill the entire pelvis before they are detected.

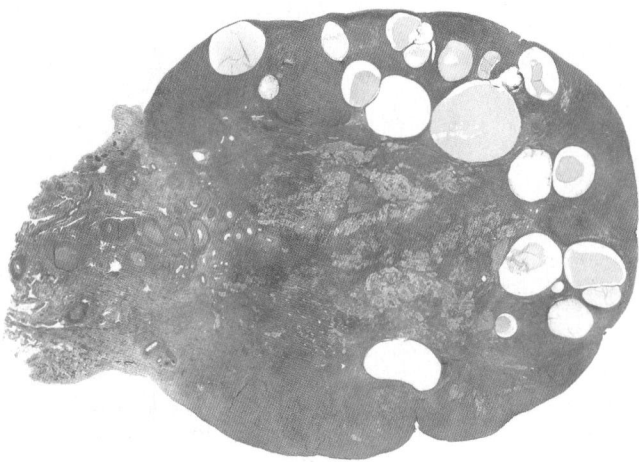

FIGURE 22–36 Cortical inclusion cysts of the ovary. These cysts appear to arise from the overlying mesothelium and are presumed to be the site of origin for many ovarian epithelial neoplasms.

The origin of ovarian epithelial tumors is, at present, unresolved. This is in large part because most tumors are detected relatively late, interfering with the identification of a precursor lesion. The most widely accepted theory for the derivation of müllerian epithelial tumors is the transformation of coelomic epithelium. This view is based on the embryologic pathway by which the müllerian *ducts are formed from the coelomic epithelium and evolve into serous (tubal), endometrioid (endometrial), and mucinous (cervical) epithelia present* in the normal female genital tract. Such tumors are thought to occur predominantly in the ovary, because coelomic epithelium is incorporated into the ovarian cortex to form epithelial inclusion cysts (also known as mesothelial, cortical, or germinal inclusion cysts) (Fig. 22–36). The exact mechanism by which the cysts develop is not known, but they are thought to result from invaginations of the surface epithelium that subsequently loses its connection to the surface.[76] The cysts are most often lined by either mesothelial or tubal-type epithelium. The close association of ovarian carcinomas with either the ovarian surface epithelium or inclusion cysts may explain the development of extra-ovarian carcinomas of similar histology from coelomic epithelial rests (so-called endosalpingiosis) in the mesentery.[75] However, this is clearly an oversimplification of the pathogenesis of ovarian cancer.

Regardless of their specific origin(s), ovarian epithelial tumors composed of serous, mucinous, and endometrioid cell types are emblematic of the plasticity of müllerian epithelium and range from clearly benign to malignant tumors.[75] Several recent studies have suggested that ovarian carcinomas may be broadly categorized into two different types based on pathogenesis: (1) those that arise in association with borderline tumors, and (2) those that arise as "de novo" carcinomas. Clinicopathologic studies have shown that well-differentiated serous, endometrioid, and mucinous carcinomas often contain areas of borderline tumors of the same epithelial cell type, whereas this association is rarely seen for moderately to poorly differentiated serous carcinoma or MMMTs. Recent molecular studies have provided support for this classification scheme, as will be discussed below in the relevant sections.

Serous Tumors

These common *cystic neoplasms are lined by tall, columnar, ciliated and nonciliated epithelial cells* and are filled with clear serous fluid. Although the term *serous* appropriately describes the cyst fluid, it has become synonymous with the tubal-like epithelium in these tumors. Together the benign, borderline, and malignant types account for about 30% of all ovarian tumors and just over 50% of ovarian epithelial tumors. About 70% are benign or borderline, and 30% are malignant. *Serous carcinomas account for approximately 40% of all cancers of the ovary and are the most common malignant ovarian tumors.* Benign and borderline tumors are most common between the ages of 20 and 45 years. Serous carcinomas occur later in life on average, though somewhat earlier in familial cases.

Molecular Pathogenesis. Little is known about the risk factors for the development of the benign and borderline tumors. Risk factors for malignant serous tumors (serous carcinomas) are also much less clear than for other genital tumors, but nulliparity, family history, and heritable mutations play a role in tumor development.[71,77] There is a higher frequency of carcinoma in women with low parity. Gonadal dysgenesis in children is associated with a higher risk of ovarian cancer. Women 40 to 59 years of age who have taken oral contraceptives or undergone tubal ligation have a reduced risk of developing ovarian cancer.[78,79] The most intriguing risk factors are genetic. As discussed in Chapters 7 and 23, mutations in both *BRCA1* and *BRCA2* increase susceptibility to ovarian cancer.[71,77] *BRCA1* mutations occur in about 5% of patients younger than 70 years of age with ovarian cancer. The estimated risk of ovarian cancer in women bearing *BRCA1* or *BRCA2* mutations is 20% to 60% by the age of 70 years.[77]

Based on both clinicopathologic and molecular studies it has recently been proposed that serous ovarian carcinoma be divided into two major groups: (1) low-grade (well-differentiated) carcinoma and (2) high-grade (moderately to poorly differentiated) carcinoma. This distinction can be made on the basis of nuclear atypia and correlates with patient survival.[80] Some low-grade carcinomas arise in association with serous borderline tumors, while most high-grade carcinomas appear to arise "de novo" without a recognizable precursor lesion.[81]

Molecular studies of low- and high-grade serous carcinoma have revealed distinct molecular genetic changes in the two types of carcinoma.[82] The low-grade tumors arising in serous borderline tumors have mutations in the *KRAS* or *BRAF* oncogenes, with only rare mutations in *p53*. In contrast, the high-grade tumors have a high frequency of mutations in the *p53* gene but lack mutations in either *KRAS* or *BRAF*. Almost all reported cases of ovarian carcinomas arising in women with *BRCA1* or *BRCA2* mutations are high-grade serous carcinoma and commonly have *p53* mutations. Close examination of these tumors has suggested that *a significant percentage of BRCA1- and BRCA2-related tumors arise from the epithelium lining the fimbriated end of the fallopian tube.* This finding has led investigators to speculate that at least some sporadic high-grade ovarian and so-called *primary peritoneal* serous carcinomas may also originate from the distal fallopian tube, an area of current investigation.

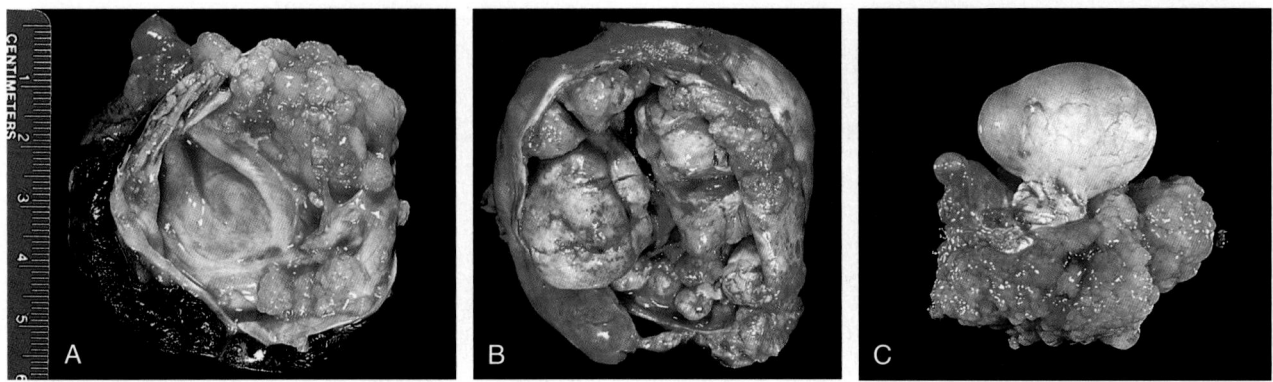

FIGURE 22–37   **A,** Serous borderline tumor opened to display a cyst cavity lined by delicate papillary tumor growths. **B,** Cystadeno-carcinoma. The cyst is opened to reveal a large, bulky tumor mass. **C,** Another borderline tumor growing on the ovarian surface *(lower)*.

Morphology. The characteristic serous tumor may present on gross examination as either a cystic lesion in which the papillary epithelium is contained within a few fibrous walled cysts (intracystic) (Fig. 22–37A), or projecting from the ovarian surface. Benign tumors typically present with a smooth glistening cyst wall with no epithelial thickening or with small papillary projections. Borderline tumors contain an increased number of papillary projections (Fig. 22–37A and C). Bilaterality is common, occurring in 20% of benign serous cystadenomas, 30% of serous borderline tumors, and approximately 66% of serous carcinomas. A significant proportion of both serous border-line tumors and malignant serous tumors involve (or originate from) the surface of the ovary (Fig. 22–37C). On histologic examination, the cysts are lined by columnar epithelium, which has abundant cilia in benign tumors (Fig. 22–38A). Microscopic papillae may be found. Serous borderline tumors exhibit increased complexity of the stromal papillae,

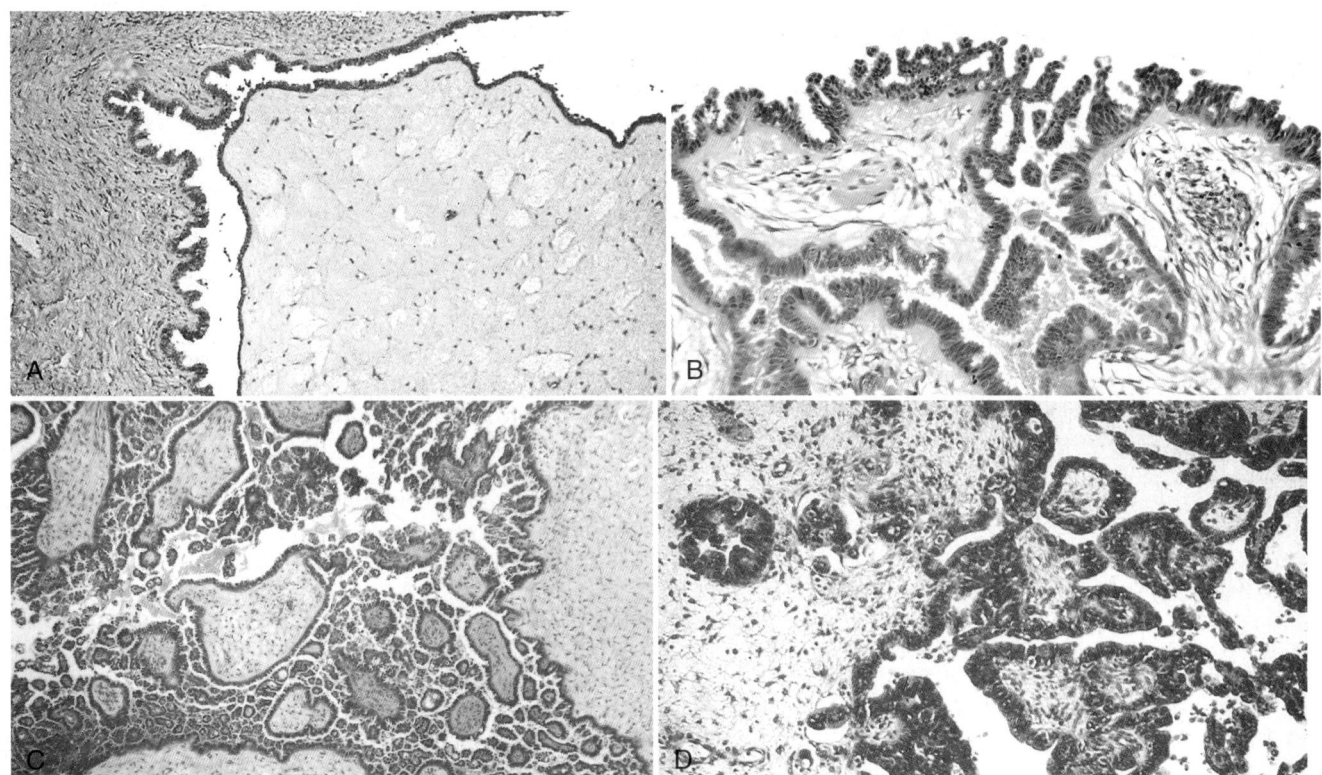

FIGURE 22–38   Serous cystadenomas. **A,** Papillary serous cystadenoma revealing stromal papillae with a columnar epithelium. **B,** Borderline serous tumor showing increased architectural complexity and epithelial cell stratification. **C,** Complex micropapillary growth defines a low-grade "micropapillary" serous carcinoma. **D,** Papillary serous cystadenocarcinoma of the ovary with invasion of underlying stroma.

stratification of the epithelium and mild nuclear atypia, but destructive infiltrative growth into the stroma is not seen (Fig. 22–38B).[75] This epithelial proliferation often grows in a delicate, papillary pattern referred to as "micropapillary carcinoma" and is thought to be the precursor to low-grade serous carcinoma (Fig. 22–38C). Larger amounts of solid or papillary tumor mass, irregularity in the tumor mass, and fixation or nodularity of the capsule are important indicators of probable malignancy (see Fig. 22–37B). These features are characteristic of high-grade serous carcinoma, which microscopically exhibits even more complex growth patterns and infiltration or frank effacement of the underlying stroma (Fig. 22–38D). The individual tumor cells in the high-grade carcinomas display marked nuclear atypia, including pleomorphism, atypical mitotic figures, and multinucleation. The cells may even become so undifferentiated that serous features are no longer recognizable. Concentric calcifications (psammoma bodies) characterize serous tumors, but are not specific for neoplasia. Ovarian serous tumors, both low- and high-grade, have a propensity to spread to the peritoneal surfaces and omentum and are commonly associated with the presence of ascites. As with other tumors, the extent of the spread outside the ovary determines the stage of the disease.

The biologic behavior of serous tumors depends on degree of differentiation, distribution, and characteristics of the disease in the peritoneum, if present. Importantly, serous tumors may occur on the surface of the ovaries and, rarely, as primary tumors of the peritoneal surface, which are referred to as primary peritoneal serous carcinoma. Predictably, unencapsulated serous tumors of the ovarian surface are more likely to extend to the peritoneal surfaces, and prognosis is closely related to the histologic appearance of the tumor and its growth pattern on the peritoneum. Borderline serous tumors may arise from or extend to the peritoneal surfaces as noninvasive implants, remaining localized and causing no symptoms, or slowly spread, producing intestinal obstruction or other complications after many years. As discussed above, low-grade serous carcinomas can arise in borderline serous tumors and may be associated with what are often referred to as "invasive implants" because they demonstrate destructive, infiltrative growth, similar to metastatic carcinoma. However, the low-grade carcinomas even when spread outside the ovary often progress slowly, and patients may survive for relatively long periods before dying of disease. In contrast, high-grade tumors are often widely metastatic throughout the abdomen at the time of presentation. These findings are associated with rapid clinical deterioration.[75] Consequently, careful pathologic classification of the tumor, even if it has extended to the peritoneum, is relevant to both prognosis and selection of therapy.[75,83] The 5-year survival rate for borderline and malignant tumors confined within the ovarian mass is, respectively, 100% and 70%, whereas the 5-year survival rate for the same tumors involving the peritoneum is about 90% and 25%, respectively. Because of their protracted course, borderline

tumors may recur after many years, and 5-year survival is not synonymous with cure.[75]

Mucinous Tumors

Mucinous tumors are less common than serous tumors, *accounting for about 30% of all ovarian neoplasms*. They occur principally in middle adult life and are rare before puberty and after menopause. *Eighty percent are benign or borderline, and about 15% are malignant.* Primary ovarian mucinous carcinomas are relatively uncommon and account for fewer than 5% of all ovarian cancers.

Molecular Pathogenesis. Like serous tumors, little is known about the pathogenesis of mucinous ovarian tumors. Most of the studies analyzing risk factors have not segregated the different histologic types of ovarian cancer, so it is not clear how they relate to the individual types. However, recent studies have suggested that mucinous tumors may have different risk factors, including smoking, which is not a risk factor for serous ovarian tumors. Although several molecular studies have been done over the years, very few molecular genetic alterations have been identified in mucinous tumors. The one consistent alteration that has been identified is mutation of the *KRAS* proto-oncogene. Mutations in *KRAS* are common in benign mucinous cystadenomas (58%), mucinous borderline tumors (75% to 86%), and in primary ovarian mucinous carcinomas (85%).[84,85] Interestingly, one study showed that several tumors with distinct areas of epithelium showing benign, borderline, and carcinoma had identical *KRAS* mutations from each area.[85] Thus, *KRAS* mutations may occur early in the development of these neoplasms.

Morphology. In gross appearance, the mucinous tumors differ from the serous variety in several ways. They are characterized by rarity of surface involvement and are less frequently bilateral. Only 5% of primary mucinous cystadenomas and mucinous cystadenocarcinomas are bilateral. Mucinous tumors tend to produce larger cystic masses; some have been recorded with weights of more than 25 kg. They appear grossly as multiloculated tumors filled with sticky, gelatinous fluid rich in glycoproteins (Fig. 22–39A). On histologic examination, benign mucinous tumors are characterized by a lining of tall, columnar epithelial cells with apical mucin and the absence of cilia, akin to benign cervical or intestinal epithelia (Fig. 22–39B). One group of typically benign or borderline mucinous tumors arises in endometriosis and is termed *müllerian mucinous cystadenoma*, resembling endometrial or cervical epithelium.[75] The second, more common group includes tumors showing abundant glandlike or papillary growth with nuclear atypia and stratification, an appearance strikingly similar to tubular adenomas or villous adenomas of the intestine. These tumors are presumed precursors to most cystadenocarcinomas. Cystadenocarcinomas contain areas of solid growth and conspicuous epithelial cell atypia and stratification, loss of gland architecture, and necrosis; these tumors are similar to colonic cancer in appearance. Because both

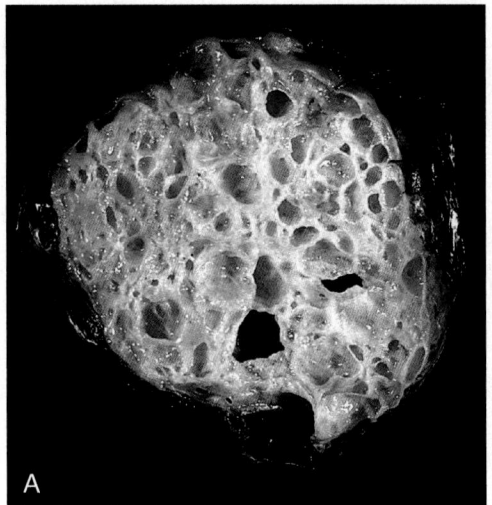
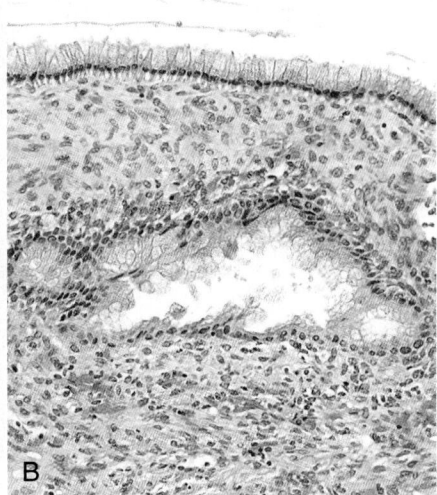

FIGURE 22–39 **A,** A mucinous cystadenoma with its multicystic appearance and delicate septa. Note the presence of glistening mucin within the cysts. **B,** Columnar cell lining of mucinous cystadenoma.

borderline and malignant mucinous cystadenomas form complex glands in the stroma, the documentation of clear-cut stromal invasion, which is easily ascertained in serous tumors, is more difficult. Some authors describe a category of "noninvasive" mucinous carcinomas (intraepithelial carcinomas) for those tumors with marked epithelial atypia without obvious stromal alterations.[86] Approximate 10-year survival rates for stage I, noninvasive "intraepithelial carcinomas," and frankly invasive malignant tumors are greater than 95% and 90%, respectively.[87] Mucinous carcinomas that have spread beyond the ovary are usually fatal, but as previously stated, these tumors are uncommon.

A clinical condition referred to as *pseudomyxoma peritonei* is defined by extensive mucinous ascites, cystic epithelial implants on the peritoneal surfaces, adhesions, and frequently mucinous tumor involving the ovaries (Fig. 22–40). Pseudo-

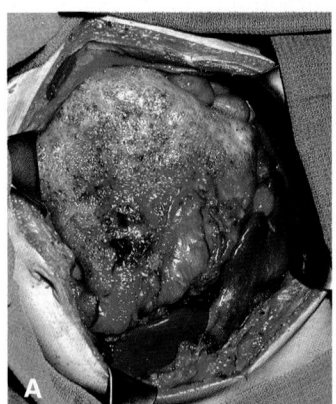
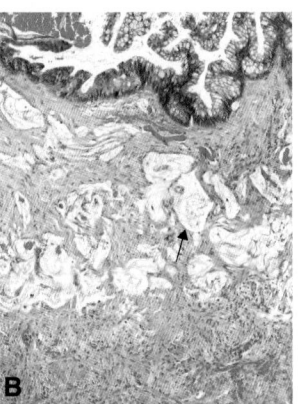

FIGURE 22–40 **A,** Pseudomyxoma peritonei viewed at laparotomy revealing massive overgrowth of a gelatinous metastatic tumor originating from the appendix. **B,** Histology of peritoneal implants from an appendiceal tumor, showing mucin-producing epithelium and free mucin *(arrow).* (**A,** Courtesy of Dr. Paul H. Sugarbaker, Washington Hospital Cancer Center, Washington, DC.)

myxoma peritonei, if extensive, may result in intestinal obstruction and death. Historically, it was thought that many cases of pseudomyxoma peritonei in women were due to primary ovarian mucinous neoplasms. However, recent evidence points to the presence, in most cases, of extraovarian (usually appendiceal) primary mucinous tumor with secondary ovarian and peritoneal spread (Chapter 17).[88] Because the majority of primary mucinous ovarian tumors are unilateral, bilateral presentation of mucinous tumors always requires exclusion of a non-ovarian origin.

Endometrioid Tumors

Benign endometrioid tumors, called *endometrioid adenofibromas*, and borderline endometrioid tumors are uncommon. However, *endometrioid carcinomas account for approximately 20% of all ovarian cancers*. Endometrioid tumors are distinguished from serous and mucinous tumors by the presence of tubular glands bearing a close resemblance to benign or malignant endometrium. Endometrioid carcinomas may arise in the setting of endometriosis and are occasionally associated with areas of borderline tumor. Although these tumors are less common than either serous or mucinous tumors, more is known about the molecular genetic alterations associated with their development. This is due to the recent development of mouse models that closely mimic the human disease and molecular genetic overlap with endometrioid carcinomas of the endometrium. In fact, 15% to 30% of ovarian endometrioid carcinomas are accompanied by carcinoma of the endometrium, and the relatively good prognosis in such cases suggests that the two may arise independently rather than by metastatic spread from one another.[89]

Pathogenesis. *About 15% to 20% of cases with endometrioid carcinoma coexist with endometriosis*, although an origin directly from ovarian surface epithelium is also possible. The women with associated endometriosis are usually about a decade younger than women with endometrioid carcinoma that is not associated with endometriosis. Molecular studies have found relatively frequent mutations in the *PTEN tumor suppressor gene and in the KRAS and β-catenin oncogenes, as well as microsatellite instability.*[90] Similar to endometrioid carcinomas of the endometrium, *p53* mutations are common in the poorly differentiated tumors. Interestingly, in endometrioid carcinomas associated with endometriosis, identical *PTEN* mutations have been detected in both the carcinoma and the endometriosis, suggesting that *PTEN* mutations may precede the development of malignancy.[91]

> **Morphology.** In gross appearance, endometrioid carcinomas present as a combination of solid and cystic areas, similar to other cystadenocarcinomas. Forty percent involve both ovaries, and such bilaterality usually, though not always, implies extension of the neoplasm beyond the genital tract. These are low-grade tumors that reveal glandular patterns bearing a strong resemblance to those of endometrial origin. The 5-year survival rate for patients with stage I tumors is approximately 75%.

Clear Cell Adenocarcinoma

Benign and borderline clear cell tumors are exceedingly rare, and clear cell carcinomas are uncommon. They are characterized by large epithelial cells with abundant clear cytoplasm similar to hypersecretory gestational endometrium. Because these tumors sometimes occur in association with endometriosis or endometrioid carcinoma of the ovary and resemble clear cell carcinoma of the endometrium, they are now thought to be of müllerian origin and variants of endometrioid adenocarcinoma.[75] Little is currently known about the molecular alterations that underlie the pathogenesis of these tumors. The clear cell tumors of the ovary can be predominantly solid or cystic. In the solid neoplasm, the clear cells are arranged in sheets or tubules. In the cystic variety, the neoplastic cells line the spaces. The 5-year survival rate is approximately 65% when the tumors are confined to the ovaries; however, these tumors tend to be aggressive, and with spread beyond the ovary, a survival of 5 years is exceptional.

Cystadenofibroma

Cystadenofibromas are variants in which there is more pronounced proliferation of the fibrous stroma that underlies the columnar lining epithelium. These benign tumors are usually small and multilocular and have simple papillary processes that do not become as complicated and branching as those found in the ordinary cystadenoma. They may be composed of mucinous, serous, endometrioid, and transitional (Brenner tumors) epithelium. Borderline lesions with cellular atypia and, rarely, tumors with focal carcinoma occur, but metastatic spread of either is extremely uncommon.

Brenner Tumor

Brenner tumors are classified as *adenofibromas in which the epithelial component consists of nests of transitional-type epithelial cells resembling those lining the urinary bladder.* Less frequently, the nests contain microcysts or glandular spaces lined by columnar, mucin-secreting cells.

> **Morphology.** These neoplasms may be solid or cystic, are usually unilateral (approximately 90%), and vary in size from small lesions less than 1 cm in diameter to massive tumors up to 20 and 30 cm (Fig. 22–41A). The fibrous stroma, resembling that of the normal ovary, is marked by sharply demarcated nests of epithelial cells resembling the epithelium of the urinary tract, often with mucinous glands in their center (Fig. 22–41B). Infrequently, the stroma is composed of somewhat plump fibroblasts resembling theca cells; such neoplasms may have hormonal activity. Most Brenner tumors are benign, but borderline (proliferative Brenner tumor) and malignant counterparts have been reported.

Several reports have emphasized the occurrence of ovarian tumors that are composed in part or entirely of neoplastic epithelium similar to transitional carcinoma of the bladder but without a coexisting Brenner component. Though often referred to as *transitional cell carcinoma*, these tumors are frequently seen in association with conventional serous or endometrioid carcinomas and probably represent altered differentiation patterns of the tumor cells.

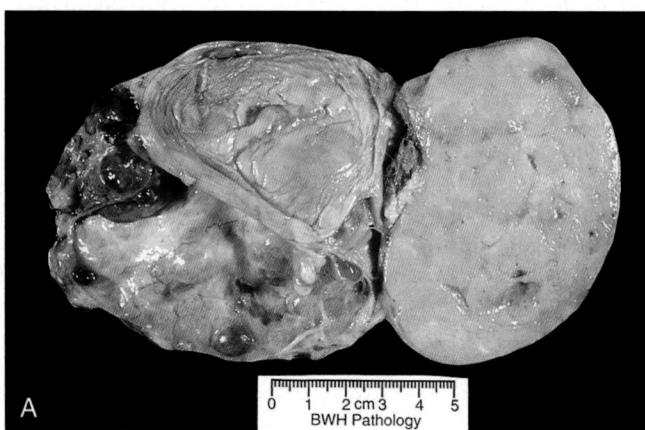
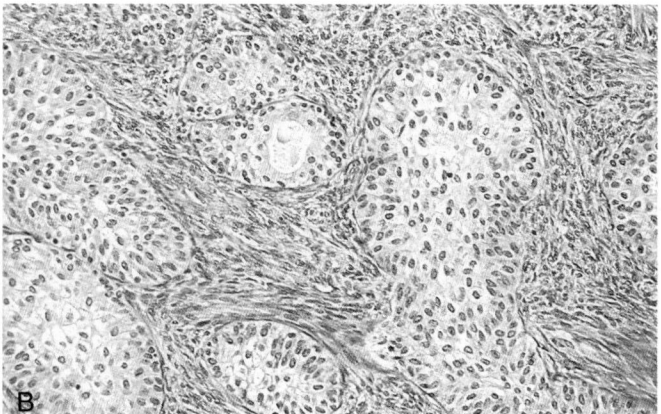

FIGURE 22–41   A, Brenner tumor *(right)* associated with a benign cystic teratoma *(left).* **B,** Histologic detail of characteristic epithelial nests within the ovarian stroma. (Courtesy of Dr. M. Nucci, Brigham and Women's Hospital, Boston, MA.)

Clinical Course, Detection, and Prevention of Surface Epithelial Tumors

All ovarian epithelial carcinomas produce similar clinical manifestations, most commonly lower abdominal pain and abdominal enlargement. Gastrointestinal complaints, urinary frequency, dysuria, pelvic pressure, and many other symptoms may appear. Benign lesions are easily resected and cured. The malignant forms tend to cause progressive weakness, weight loss, and cachexia characteristic of all malignant neoplasms. If the carcinomas extend through the capsule of the tumor to seed the peritoneal cavity, massive ascites is common. Characteristically, the ascitic fluid is filled with diagnostic exfoliated tumor cells. The peritoneal pattern of spread is distinctive: all serosal surfaces are diffusely seeded with 0.1- to 0.5-cm nodules of tumor. These surface implants rarely invade deeply into the underlying parenchyma. The regional nodes are often involved, and metastases may be found in the liver, lungs, gastrointestinal tract, and elsewhere. Metastasis across the midline to the opposite ovary is discovered in about half the cases by the time of laparotomy and heralds a progressive downhill course to death within a few months or years.

Because ovarian carcinomas often remain undiagnosed until they are large, or originate on the ovarian surface from where they readily spread to the pelvis, many patients are first seen with lesions that are no longer confined to the ovary. This is perhaps the primary reason for the relatively *poor 5- and 10-year survival rates* for these patients, compared with rates in cervical and endometrial carcinoma. For these reasons, both early diagnosis and prevention are top priorities. Specific biochemical markers for tumor antigens or tumor products in the plasma of these patients are being sought vigorously. One such marker, known as CA-125, is a high-molecular-weight glycoprotein present in the serum of more than 80% of patients with serous and endometrioid carcinomas. Although this marker is often used to monitor disease progression after diagnosis, it has not proven to be a reliable marker because elevations in CA-125 can occur with nonspecific irritation of the peritoneum (e.g., endometriosis, inflammation).[92] Newly identified biomarkers such as osteopontin, which is expressed at significantly higher levels in ovarian cancer patients, may improve early detection.[93] Other attempts to distinguish cancer patients from nonaffected individuals are based on patterns of circulating proteins generated by mass spectroscopic analysis of patient sera.[94] These and other approaches may in the future create a more cost-effective, noninvasive approach to ovarian cancer screening.

Prevention of ovarian cancer remains an elusive goal, but both fallopian tubal ligation and oral contraceptive therapy are associated with significant reductions in relative risk. Long-term contraceptive use has reduced risk by half in women with a family history of ovarian cancer.[78] Tubal ligation reduces risk by more than half and may be effective in subsets of women with *BRCA* mutations and family history of ovarian cancer.[77,79,95] Screening strategies based on identifying women at risk (positive for *BRCA* mutations) and using prophylactic salpingo-oophorectomy are currently standard, but the long-term impact of these approaches on ovarian cancer death rates remains to be determined.

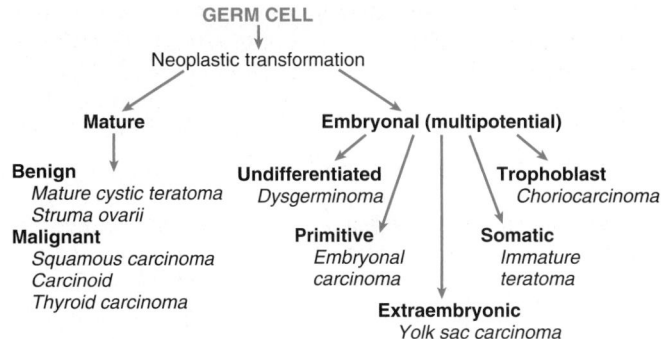

FIGURE 22–42 Histogenesis and interrelationships of tumors of germ cell origin.

GERM CELL TUMORS

Germ cell tumors constitute 15% to 20% of all ovarian tumors.[75] *Most are benign cystic teratomas*, but the remainder, which are found principally in children and young adults, have a higher incidence of malignant behavior and pose problems in histologic diagnosis and in therapy. They bear a remarkable similarity to germ cell tumors in the male testis (Chapter 21) and arise in a similar manner (Fig. 22–42).

Teratomas

Teratomas are divided into three categories: (1) mature (benign), (2) immature (malignant), and (3) monodermal or highly specialized.

Mature (Benign) Teratomas. Most benign teratomas are cystic and are better known in clinical parlance as *dermoid cysts*. Cystic teratomas are usually found in young women during the active reproductive years.[75] They may be discovered incidentally, but are occasionally associated with clinically important paraneoplastic syndromes, such as inflammatory limbic encephalititis, which may remit upon removal of the tumor.

> **Morphology.** Benign teratomas are bilateral in 10% to 15% of cases. Characteristically they are unilocular cysts containing hair and cheesy sebaceous material (Fig. 22–43). On section, they reveal a thin wall lined by an opaque, gray-white, wrinkled epidermis. From this epidermis, hair shafts frequently protrude. Within the wall, it is common to find tooth structures and areas of calcification.
>
> On histologic examination the cyst wall is composed of stratified squamous epithelium with underlying sebaceous glands, hair shafts, and other skin adnexal structures (Fig. 22–44). In most cases structures from other germ layers can be identified, such as cartilage, bone, thyroid tissue, and neural tissues. Dermoid cysts are sometimes incorporated within the wall of a mucinous cystadenoma. **About 1% of the dermoids undergo malignant transformation (e.g., thyroid carcinoma, melanoma, but most commonly, squamous cell carcinoma).**
>
> In rare instances a benign teratoma is solid and composed entirely of benign-looking heterogeneous col-

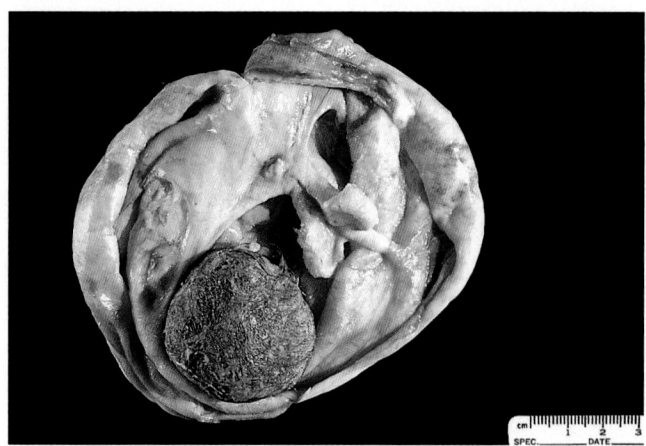

FIGURE 22–43 Opened mature cystic teratoma (dermoid cyst) of the ovary. Hair *(bottom)* and a mixture of tissues are evident.

lections of tissues and organized structures derived from all three germ layers. These tumors presumably have the same histogenetic origin as dermoid cysts but lack preponderant differentiation into ectodermal derivatives. These neoplasms may be difficult to differentiate, on gross inspection, from the malignant, immature teratomas.

The origin of teratomas has been a matter of fascination for centuries. Some common beliefs blamed witches, nightmares, or adultery with the devil. The karyotype of almost all benign ovarian teratomas is 46,XX. From the results of chromosome banding techniques and the distribution of electrophoretic variants of enzymes in normal and teratoma cells, it has been suggested that the tumors arise from an ovum after the first meiotic division.[96] Other derivations have also been proposed.[97]

Monodermal or Specialized Teratomas. The specialized teratomas are a remarkable, rare group of tumors, *the most common of which are struma ovarii and carcinoid.* They are always unilateral, although a contralateral teratoma may be present. Struma ovarii is composed entirely of mature thyroid tissue. Interestingly, these thyroidal neoplasms may hyperfunction, causing hyperthyroidism. The ovarian carcinoid, which presumably arises from intestinal epithelium in a teratoma, may also be functional, particularly large (>7 cm) tumors, producing 5-hydroxytryptamine and the carcinoid syndrome. Primary ovarian carcinoid can be distinguished from metastatic intestinal carcinoid, which is virtually always bilateral. Even rarer is the strumal carcinoid, a combination of struma ovarii and carcinoid in the same ovary. Only about 2% of carcinoids metastasize.

Immature Malignant Teratomas. These are rare tumors that differ from benign teratomas in that the component tissues resemble embryonal and immature fetal tissue. The tumor is found chiefly in prepubertal adolescents and young women, the mean age being 18 years.[98]

Morphology. The tumors are bulky and have a smooth external surface. On section they have a solid (or predominantly solid) structure. There are areas of necrosis and hemorrhage. Hair, sebaceous material, cartilage, bone, and calcification may be present. On microscopic examination there are varying amounts of immature neuroepithelium, cartilage, bone, muscle, and others. An important risk for subsequent extraovarian spread is the histologic grade of tumor (I through III), which is based on the proportion of tissue containing immature neuroepithelium (Fig. 22–45).

Immature teratomas grow rapidly, frequently penetrate the capsule, and spread either locally or distantly. Stage I tumors, however, particularly those with low-grade (grade 1) histology, have an excellent prognosis. Higher grade tumors confined to the ovary are generally treated with prophylactic chemotherapy. Most recurrences develop in the first 2 years, and absence of disease beyond this period carries an excellent chance of cure.

Dysgerminoma

The dysgerminoma is best considered as the *ovarian counterpart of the seminoma of the testis.* Similar to the seminoma, it

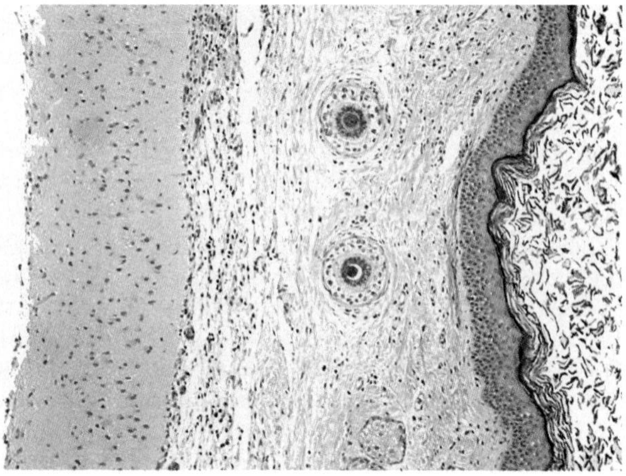

FIGURE 22–44 Benign cystic teratoma. Low-power view of skin *(right edge),* beneath which there is brain tissue *(left edge).*

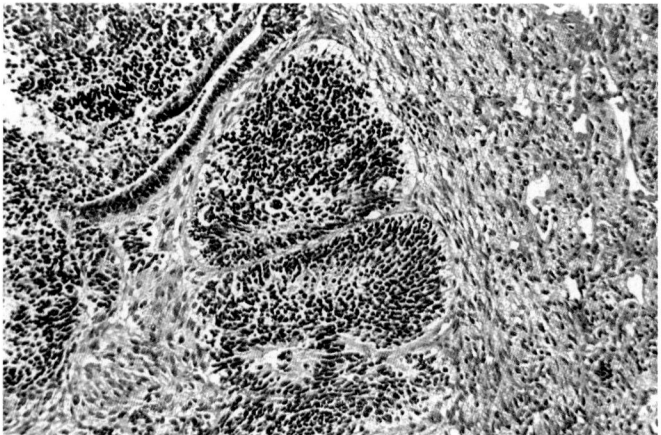

FIGURE 22–45 Immature teratoma of the ovary illustrating primitive neuroepithelium.

is composed of large vesicular cells having a clear cytoplasm, well-defined cell boundaries, and centrally placed regular nuclei. Dysgerminomas account for about 2% of all ovarian cancers yet form about half of malignant germ cell tumors. They may occur in childhood, but 75% occur in the second and third decades. Some occur in patients with gonadal dysgenesis, including pseudohermaphroditism. Most of these tumors have no endocrine function. A few produce elevated levels of chorionic gonadotropin and may have syncytiotrophoblastic giant cells on histologic examination. Like seminomas, dysgerminomas express Oct3, Oct4, and Nanog.[99] These transcription factors are implicated in maintenance of pluripotency. They also express the receptor tyrosine kinase *c-KIT*. These proteins are useful diagnostic markers and, in the case of c-KIT, may also serve as a therapeutic target.[100]

Morphology. Usually unilateral (80% to 90%), most are solid tumors ranging in size from barely visible nodules to masses that virtually fill the entire abdomen. On cut surface they have a yellow-white to gray-pink appearance and are often soft and fleshy. On histologic examination the dysgerminoma cells are dispersed in sheets or cords separated by scant fibrous stroma (Fig. 22–46). As in the seminoma, the fibrous stroma is infiltrated with mature lymphocytes and occasional granulomas. On occasion, small nodules of dysgerminoma are encountered in the wall of an otherwise benign cystic teratoma; conversely, a predominantly dysgerminomatous tumor may contain a small cystic teratoma.

All dysgerminomas are malignant, but the degree of histologic atypia is variable, and only about one third are aggressive. Thus, a unilateral tumor that has not broken through the capsule and has not spread has an excellent prognosis (up to 96% cure rate) after simple salpingo-oophorectomy. *These neoplasms are responsive to chemotherapy*, and even those that have extended beyond the ovary can often be cured.[101] Overall survival exceeds 80%.

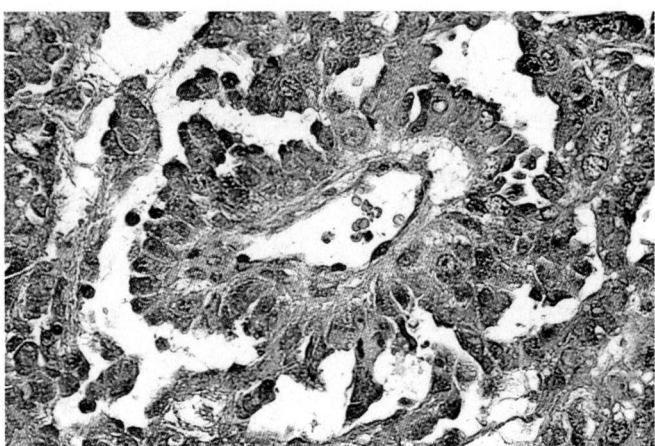

FIGURE 22–47　A Schiller-Duval body in yolk sac carcinoma.

Endodermal Sinus (Yolk Sac) Tumor

This tumor is rare but is the second most common malignant tumor of germ cell origin. It is thought to be derived from differentiation of malignant germ cells along the extra-embryonic yolk sac lineage (see Fig. 22–42). Similar to the normal yolk sac, the tumor is *rich in α-fetoprotein and α₁-antitrypsin*. Its characteristic histologic feature is a glomerulus-like structure composed of a central blood vessel enveloped by germ cells within a space lined by germ cells (Schiller-Duval body) (Fig. 22–47). Conspicuous intracellular and extracellular hyaline droplets are present in all tumors, and some of these stain for α-fetoprotein by immunoperoxidase techniques.

Most patients are children or young women presenting with abdominal pain and a rapidly developing pelvic mass. The tumors usually appear to involve a single ovary but grow rapidly and aggressively. These tumors were once almost uniformly fatal within 2 years of diagnosis, but combination chemotherapy has measurably improved the outcome.

Choriocarcinoma

More commonly of placental origin, the choriocarcinoma, like the endodermal sinus tumor, is an example of extra-embryonic differentiation of malignant germ cells. It is generally held that a germ cell origin can be confirmed only in the prepubertal girl, because after this age an origin from an ovarian ectopic pregnancy cannot be excluded.

Most ovarian choriocarcinomas exist in combination with other germ cell tumors, and pure choriocarcinomas are extremely rare. They are histologically identical to the more common placental lesions, described later. The ovarian primaries are *aggressive tumors* that generally have metastasized widely through the bloodstream to the lungs, liver, bone, and other viscera by the time of diagnosis. Like all choriocarcinomas they elaborate *high levels of chorionic gonadotropins*, which is sometimes helpful in establishing the diagnosis or detecting recurrences. In contrast to choriocarcinomas arising in placental tissue, those arising in the ovary are generally unresponsive to chemotherapy and are often fatal.

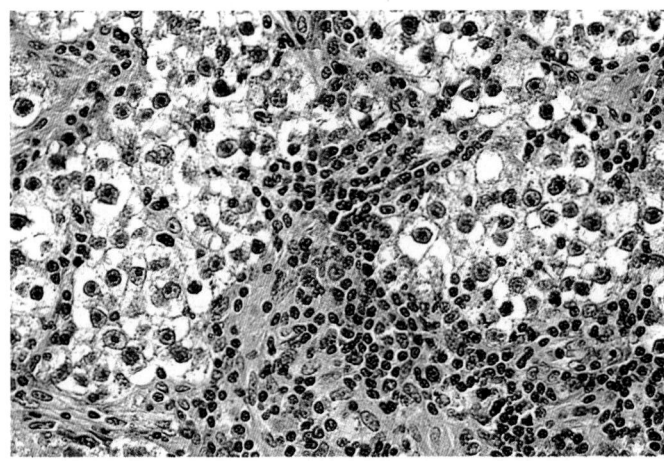

FIGURE 22–46　Dysgerminoma showing polyhedral tumor cells with round nuclei and adjacent inflammation.

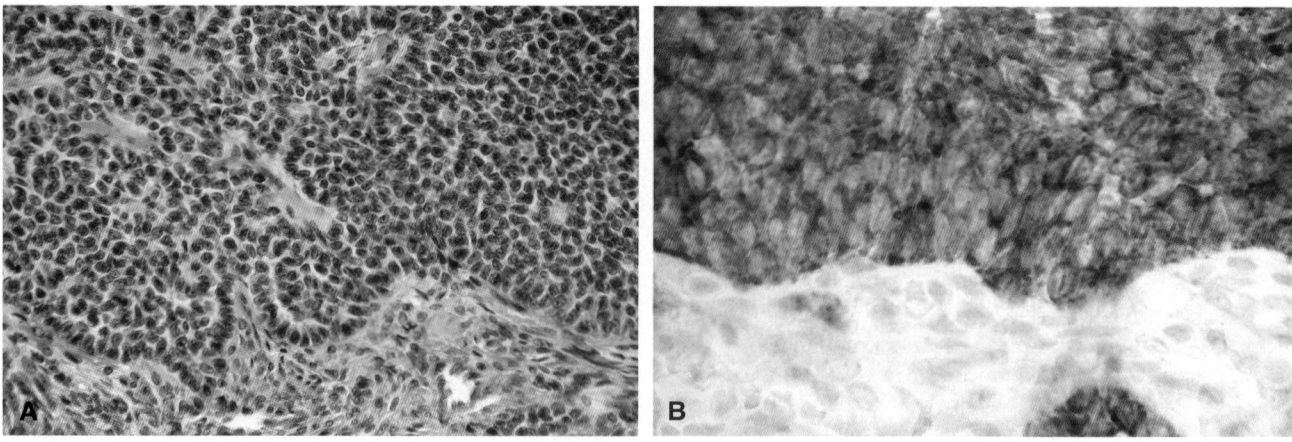

FIGURE 22–48 Granulosa cell tumor. **A,** The tumor cells are arranged in sheets punctuated by small follicle-like structures (Call-Exner bodies). **B,** Strong immunohistochemical positivity with an antibody to inhibin characterizes these tumors.

Other Germ Cell Tumors

These include (1) embryonal carcinoma, another highly malignant tumor of primitive embryonal elements, histologically similar to tumors arising in the testes (Chapter 21)[75]; (2) polyembryoma, a malignant tumor containing so-called embryoid bodies; and (3) mixed germ cell tumors containing various combinations of dysgerminoma, teratoma, endodermal sinus tumor, and choriocarcinoma.

SEX CORD–STROMAL TUMORS

These ovarian neoplasms are derived from the ovarian stroma, which in turn is derived from the sex cords of the embryonic gonad. Because the undifferentiated gonadal mesenchyme eventually produces structures of specific cell type in both male (Sertoli and Leydig) and female (granulosa and theca) gonads, tumors resembling all of these cell types can be identified in the ovary.[102] Moreover, because some of these cells normally secrete estrogens (granulosa and theca cells) or androgens (Leydig cells), their corresponding tumors may be either feminizing (granulosa–theca cell tumors) or masculinizing (Leydig cell tumors).

Granulosa–Theca Cell Tumors

This designation embraces ovarian neoplasms composed of varying proportions of granulosa and theca cell differentiation. They may be composed almost entirely of granulosa cells or a mixture of granulosa and theca cells. Collectively, these neoplasms account for about 5% of all ovarian tumors. Although they may be discovered at any age, approximately two thirds occur in postmenopausal women.

Morphology. Granulosa cell tumors are usually unilateral and vary from microscopic foci to large, solid, and cystic encapsulated masses. Tumors that are hormonally active have a yellow coloration to their cut surfaces, due to intracellular lipids. The pure thecomas are solid, firm tumors.

The granulosa cell component of these tumors takes one of many histologic patterns. The small, cuboidal to polygonal cells may grow in anastomosing cords, sheets, or strands (Fig. 22–48A). In occasional cases small, distinctive, gland-like structures filled with an acidophilic material recall immature follicles (Call-Exner bodies). When these structures are evident the diagnosis is straightforward. The thecoma component consists of clusters or sheets of cuboidal to polygonal cells. In some tumors, the granulosa or theca cells may appear plumper and have ample cytoplasm characteristic of luteinization (i.e., luteinized granulosa–theca cell tumors).

Granulosa cell tumors have clinical importance for two reasons: (1) *their potential to elaborate large amounts of estrogen* and (2) *the small but distinct hazard of malignancy* in the granulosa cell forms. Functionally active tumors in young girls (juvenile granulosa cell tumors) may produce precocious sexual development in prepubertal girls. In adult women they may be associated with endometrial hyperplasia, cystic disease of the breast, and endometrial carcinoma. About 10% to 15% of women with steroid-producing tumors eventually develop an endometrial carcinoma. Occasionally, granulosa cell tumors produce androgens, masculinizing the patient.

All granulosa cell tumors are potentially malignant. It is difficult to predict their biologic behavior from histology.[102] The estimates of malignancy (recurrence, extension) range from 5% to 25%. In general, malignant tumors pursue an indolent course in which local recurrences may be amenable to surgical therapy. Recurrences within the pelvis and abdomen may appear 10 to 20 years after removal of the original tumor. The 10-year survival rate is approximately 85%. Tumors composed predominantly of theca cells are almost never malignant.

Elevated tissue and serum levels of *inhibin*, a product of granulosa cells, are associated with granulosa cell tumors. This biomarker may be useful for identifying granulosa and other sex cord–stromal tumors, and for monitoring patients being treated for these neoplasms (Fig. 22–48B).[103]

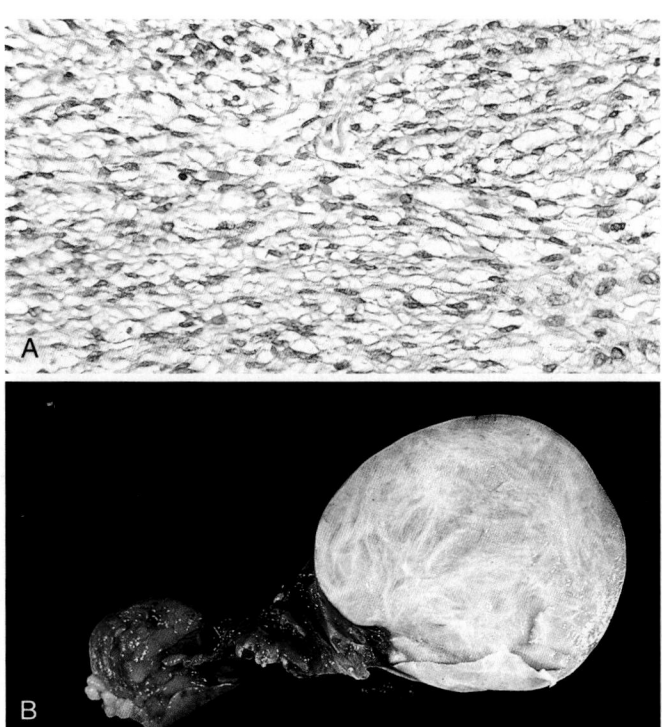

FIGURE 22–49 **A,** Thecoma-fibroma composed of plump, differentiated stromal cells with thecal appearance. **B,** Large bisected fibroma of the ovary apparent as a white, firm mass *(right)*. The fallopian tube is attached.

Fibromas, Thecomas, and Fibrothecomas

Tumors arising in the ovarian stroma that are composed of either fibroblasts (fibromas) or plump spindle cells with lipid droplets (thecomas) are relatively common and account for about 4% of all ovarian tumors (Fig. 22–49A). Many tumors contain a mixture of these cells and are termed *fibromathecomas*. Pure thecomas are rare, but tumors in which these cells predominate may be hormonally active.

Fibromas of the ovary are unilateral in about 90% of cases and are usually solid, spherical or slightly lobulated, encapsulated, hard, gray-white masses covered by glistening, intact ovarian serosa (Fig. 22–49B). On histologic examination, they are composed of well-differentiated fibroblasts and a scant interspersed collagenous connective tissue. Focal areas of thecal differentiation may be identified.

Most of these tumors are pure fibromas and are hormonally inactive. These tumors usually come to attention as a pelvic mass, sometimes accompanied by pain and through two other curious associations. The first is ascites, which is found in about 40% of cases in which the tumors measure more than 6 cm in diameter. Uncommonly there is also a hydrothorax, usually only of the right side. *This combination of findings (i.e., ovarian tumor, hydrothorax, and ascites) is designated Meigs syndrome.* Its genesis is unknown. The second association is with the basal cell nevus syndrome, described in Chapter 25. The vast majority of fibromas, fibrothecomas, and thecomas are benign. Rarely, cellular fibromas with mitotic activity and increased nuclear-to-cytoplasmic ratio are identified; because they may pursue a malignant course, they are termed *fibrosarcomas*.[104]

Sertoli–Leydig Cell Tumors (Androblastomas)

These tumors recapitulate, to a certain extent, the cells of the testis at various stages of development.[105] They commonly produce *masculinization or at least defeminization, but a few have estrogenic effects.* They occur in women of all ages, although the peak incidence is in the second and third decades. The embryogenesis of such male-directed stromal cells remains a puzzle. These tumors are *unilateral* and may resemble granulosa–theca cell neoplasms.

Morphology. The cut surface is usually solid and varies from gray to golden brown in appearance (Fig. 22–50A). On histologic examination the well-differentiated tumors show tubules composed of Sertoli cells or Leydig cells interspersed with stroma (Fig. 22–50B). The intermediate forms show only outlines of immature tubules and large eosinophilic Leydig cells. The poorly differentiated tumors have a sarcomatous pattern with a disorderly disposition of epithelial cell

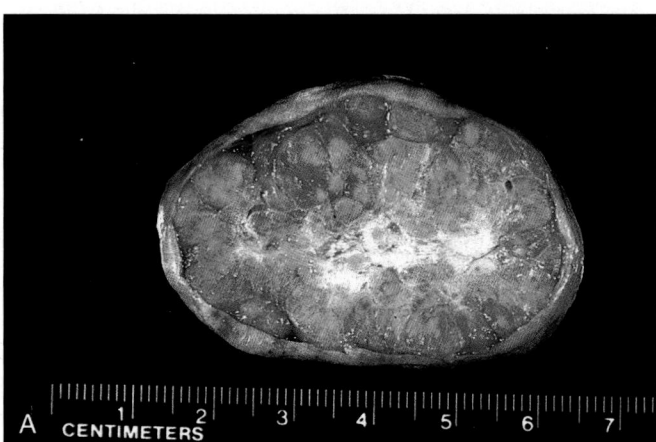
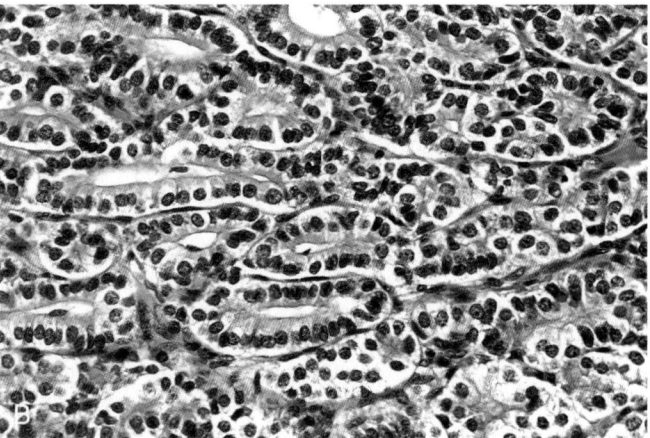

FIGURE 22–50 Sertoli cell tumor. **A,** Gross photograph illustrating characteristic golden-yellow appearance of the tumor. **B,** Photomicrograph showing well-differentiated Sertoli cell tubules. (Courtesy of Dr. William Welch, Brigham and Women's Hospital, Boston, MA.)

cords. Leydig cells may be absent. Heterologous elements, such as mucinous glands, bone, and cartilage, may be present in some tumors.

The incidence of recurrence or metastasis by Sertoli–Leydig cell tumors is less than 5%. These neoplasms may block normal female sexual development in children and may cause defeminization of women, manifested by atrophy of the breasts, amenorrhea, sterility, and loss of hair. The syndrome may progress to striking virilization (hirsutism) associated with male distribution of hair, hypertrophy of the clitoris, and voice changes.

Other Sex Cord–Stromal Tumors

The ovarian hilum normally contains clusters of polygonal cells arranged around vessels (hilar cells). *Hilus cell tumors (pure Leydig cell tumors)* are derived from these cells and are rare, unilateral, and characterized histologically by large lipid-laden cells with distinct borders. A typical cytoplasmic structure characteristic of Leydig cells (Reinke crystalloids) is usually present. Women with hilus cell tumors usually present with evidence of masculinization, hirsutism, voice changes, and clitoral enlargement. The tumors are unilateral. The most consistent laboratory finding is an elevated 17-ketosteroid excretion level unresponsive to cortisone suppression. Treatment is surgical excision. True hilus cell tumors are almost always benign. On occasion, histologically identical tumors occur in the cortical stroma *(nonhilar Leydig cell tumors)*.

In addition to Leydig cell tumors, the stroma may rarely give rise to tumors composed of pure luteinized cells, producing small benign tumors generally less than 3 cm in diameter.

The tumor may produce the clinical effects of androgen, estrogen, or progesterone stimulation.

As mentioned before, the ovary in pregnancy may show microscopic nodular proliferation of theca cells in response to gonadotropins. Rarely, a frank tumor may develop (termed *pregnancy luteoma*) that closely resembles a corpus luteum of pregnancy. These tumors have been associated with virilization in pregnant patients and in their respective female infants.

Gonadoblastoma is an uncommon tumor thought to be composed of germ cells and sex cord–stroma derivatives. It occurs in individuals with abnormal sexual development and in gonads of indeterminate nature. Eighty percent of patients are phenotypic females, and 20% are phenotypic males with undescended testicles and female internal secondary organs. On microscopic examination the tumor consists of a mixture of germ cells and sex cord derivatives resembling immature Sertoli and granulosa cells arranged in nests. A coexistent dysgerminoma occurs in 50% of the cases. The prognosis is excellent if the tumor is completely excised.[106]

Metastatic Tumors

The most common metastatic tumors of the ovary are derived from tumors of müllerian origin: the uterus, fallopian tube, contralateral ovary, or pelvic peritoneum. The most common extra-müllerian tumors metastatic to the ovary are carcinomas of the breast and gastrointestinal tract, including colon, stomach, biliary tract, and pancreas. Also included in this group are the rare cases of pseudomyxoma peritonei, derived from appendiceal tumors. A classic example of metastatic gastrointestinal neoplasia to the ovaries is termed *Krukenberg tumor*, characterized by bilateral metastases composed of mucin-producing, signet-ring cancer cells, most often of gastric origin.[7]

GESTATIONAL AND PLACENTAL DISORDERS

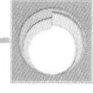

Diseases of pregnancy and pathologic conditions of the placenta are important causes of intrauterine or perinatal death, congenital malformations, intrauterine growth retardation, maternal death, and a great deal of morbidity for both mother and child.[8] Here we discuss only a limited number of the disorders in which knowledge of the morphologic lesions contributes to an understanding of the clinical problem. This discussion is divided into selected disorders of early pregnancy, late pregnancy, and trophoblastic neoplasia. But first we will review the unique structure of the placenta to facilitate an understanding of placental changes that underlie various conditions.

The placenta is composed of chorionic villi (Fig. 22–51) that sprout from the chorion to provide a large contact area

between the fetal and maternal circulations. In the mature placenta, the maternal blood enters the intervillous space through endometrial arteries (spiral arteries) and circulates around the villi allowing for gaseous and nutrient exchange (Fig. 22–52). The deoxygenated blood flows back from the intervillous space to the decidua and enters the endometrial veins. Deoxygenated fetal blood enters the placenta through two umbilical arteries that branch radially to form chorionic arteries. Chorionic arteries additionally branch as they enter the villi. In the chorionic villi they form an extensive capillary system, bringing fetal blood in close proximity to maternal blood. The gas and nutrient diffusion occurs through the villous capillary endothelial cells and thinned-out syncytiotrophoblast and cytotrophoblast. Under normal circumstances

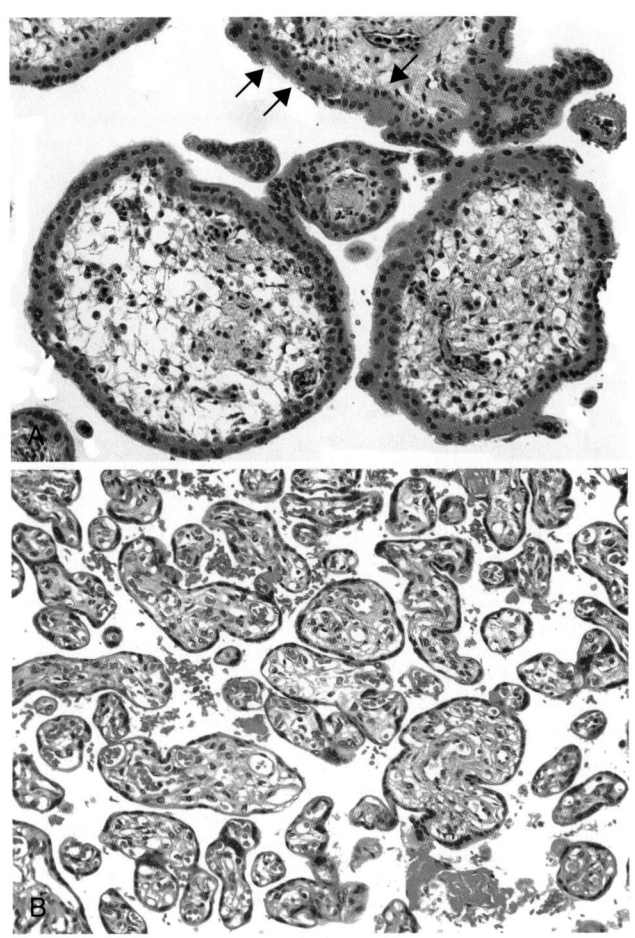

FIGURE 22–51　**A,** First-trimester chorionic villi composed of delicate mesh of central stroma surrounded by two discrete layers of epithelium—the outer layer consisting of syncytiotrophoblast *(two arrows)* and the inner layer consisting of cytotrophoblast *(arrow).* **B,** Third-trimester chorionic villi composed of stroma with dense network of dilated capillaries surrounded by markedly thinned-out syncytiotrophoblast and cytotrophoblast (same magnification as **A.**)

there is no mixing between the fetal and maternal blood. Blood oxygenated in the placenta returns to the fetus through the single umbilical vein.

Disorders of Early Pregnancy

SPONTANEOUS ABORTION

Spontaneous abortion, or "miscarriage," is defined as pregnancy loss before 20 weeks of gestation. Most of these occur before 12 weeks. Ten to fifteen percent of clinically recognized pregnancies terminate in spontaneous abortion. However, using sensitive chorionic gonadotropin assays, it has been identified that an additional 22% of early pregnancies in otherwise healthy women terminate spontaneously.[107] The causes of spontaneous abortion are both fetal and maternal. Chromosomal anomalies such as aneuploidy, polyploidy, and translocations are present in approximately 50% of early abor-

tuses. More subtle genetic defects, for which routine genetic testing is not readily available, account for an additional fraction of abortions. Maternal factors include luteal-phase defect, poorly controlled diabetes, and other uncorrected endocrine disorders. Physical defects of the uterus, such as submucosal leiomyomas, uterine polyps, or uterine malformations may prevent implantation adequate to support fetal development. Systemic disorders affecting maternal vasculature, such as antiphospholipid antibody syndrome, coagulopathies, and hypertension, may predispose to miscarriage. Finally, infections with bacteria such as *Toxoplasma*, *Mycoplasma*, and *Listeria*, as well as viral infections, have also been implicated as causes of abortion. Ascending infection is particularly common in second-trimester losses.[8] In many cases, however, the mechanisms leading to early loss of pregnancy are still unknown.

ECTOPIC PREGNANCY

Ectopic pregnancy is the term applied to implantation of the fetus in any site other than a normal intrauterine location. *The most common site is within the fallopian tubes (~90%).* Other sites include the ovary, the abdominal cavity, and the intrauterine portion of the fallopian tube (cornual pregnancy). Ectopic pregnancies occur about once in every 150 pregnancies. The most important predisposing condition, present in 35% to 50% of patients, is prior pelvic inflammatory disease resulting in fallopian tube scarring (chronic follicular salpingitis). Other factors leading to peritubal scarring and adhesions are appendicitis, endometriosis, and previous surgery. In some cases, however, the fallopian tubes are apparently normal. Intrauterine contraceptive devices also increase the risk of ectopic pregnancy by about 2.5 fold.[108]

Ovarian pregnancy is presumed to result from the rare fertilization and trapping of the ovum within the follicle just at the time of its rupture. Abdominal pregnancies may develop when the fertilized ovum fails to enter or drops out of the fimbriated end of the tube. In all these abnormal locations, the fertilized ovum undergoes its usual development with the formation of placental tissue, amniotic sac, and fetus, and the host implantation site may develop decidual changes.

Morphology. Tubal pregnancy is the most common cause of **hematosalpinx** (blood-filled fallopian tube) and should always be suspected when a tubal hematoma is present. Initially the embryonal sac, surrounded by placental tissue composed of immature chorionic villi, implants in the lumen of the fallopian tube. With time trophoblastic cells and chorionic villi start to invade the fallopian tube wall as they do in the uterus during normal pregnancy. However, proper decidualization is lacking in the fallopian tube, and growth of the gestational sac distends the fallopian tube causing thinning and rupture. Fallopian tube rupture frequently results in massive intraperitoneal hemorrhage. Less commonly the tubal pregnancy may undergo spontaneous regression and resorption of the entire conceptus. Still less commonly, the tubal pregnancy is extruded through the fimbriated end into the abdominal cavity (tubal abortion).

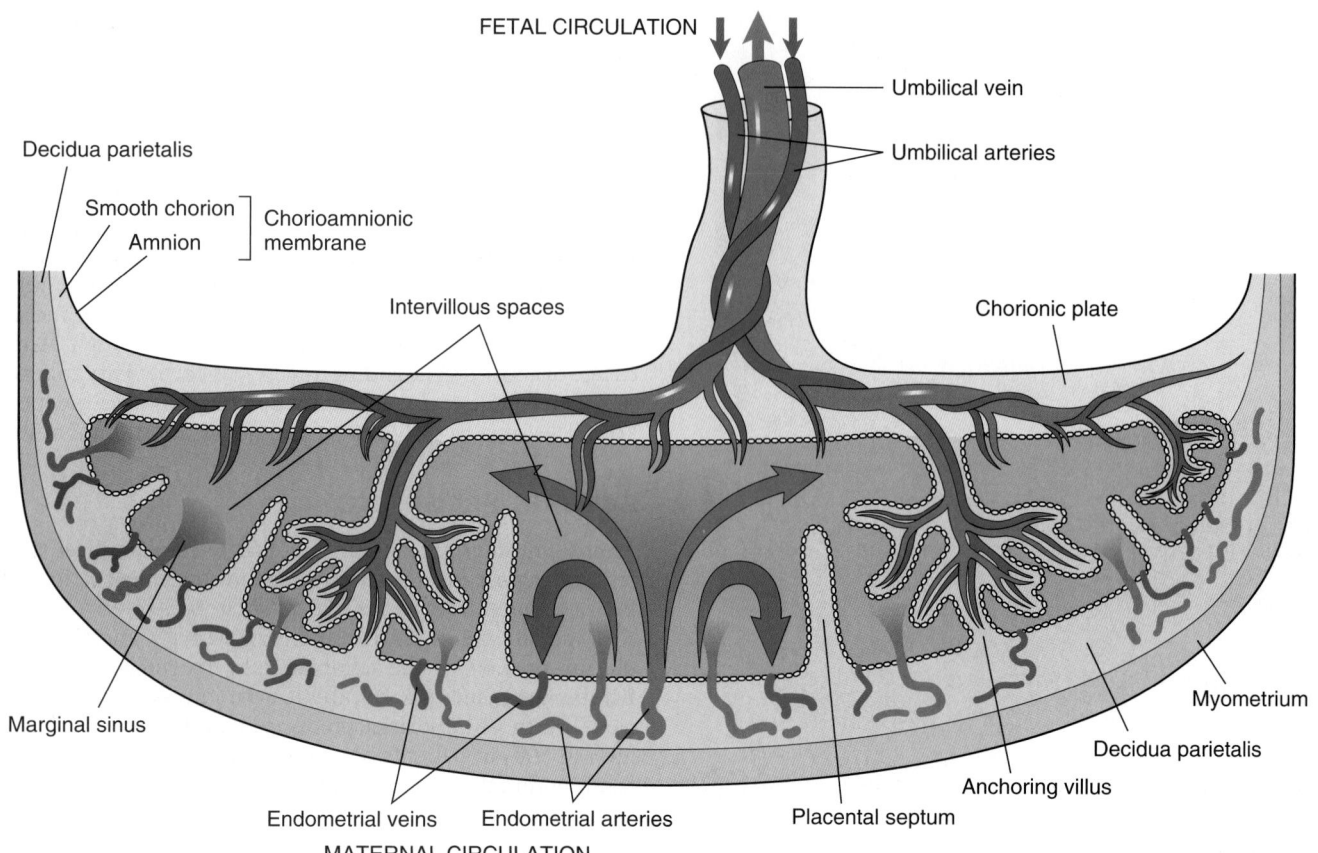

FETAL CIRCULATION

Umbilical vein

Umbilical arteries

Decidua parietalis

Smooth chorion ⎤ Chorioamnionic
Amnion ⎦ membrane

Intervillous spaces

Chorionic plate

Myometrium

Decidua parietalis

Marginal sinus

Endometrial veins   Endometrial arteries   Placental septum   Anchoring villus

MATERNAL CIRCULATION

FIGURE 22–52   Diagram of placental anatomy. Within the outer boundary of myometrium is a layer of decidua, from which the maternal vessels originate and deliver blood to and from the intervillous spaces. Umbilical vessels branch and terminate in placental villi, where nutrient exchange takes place.

Clinical Features. The clinical course of ectopic pregnancy is punctuated by the onset of *severe abdominal pain*, most commonly about 6 weeks after a previous normal menstrual period, when rupture of the tube leads to pelvic hemorrhage. *Rupture* of a tubal pregnancy constitutes a medical emergency. In such cases the patient may rapidly develop *hemorrhagic shock* with signs of an acute abdomen, and early diagnosis is critical. Chorionic gonadotropin assays, ultrasound studies, and laparoscopy may be helpful. Endometrial biopsy specimens may or may not disclose decidual changes, but—excluding the extremely rare dual pregnancy—do not exhibit chorionic villi or evidence of an implantation site.

Disorders of Late Pregnancy

The multitude of disorders that can occur in the third trimester are related to the complex anatomy of the maturing placenta. Complete interruption of blood flow through the umbilical cord from any cause (such as constricting knots or compression) can be lethal to the fetus. Ascending infections involving the chorioamnionic membranes may lead to premature rupture and delivery. Retroplacental hemorrhage at the interface of placenta and myometrium (abruptio placentae) threatens both mother and fetus. Disruption of the fetal vessels in terminal villi may produce a significant loss of fetal blood

with resultant fetal injury or death. Uteroplacental malperfusion can be precipitated by abnormal placental implantation or development, or maternal vascular disease; the effects may range from mild intrauterine growth retardation to severe uteroplacental ischemia, and maternal preeclampsia.

TWIN PLACENTAS

Twin pregnancies arise from fertilization of two ova (dizygotic) or from division of one fertilized ovum (monozygotic). There are three basic types of twin placentas (Fig. 22–53): diamnionic dichorionic (which may be fused), diamnionic monochorionic, and monoamnionic monochorionic. Monochorionic placentas imply monozygotic (identical) twins, and the time at which splitting occurs determines whether one or two amnions are present. Dichorionic placentation may occur with either monozygotic or dizygotic twins and is not specific.

One complication of monochorionic twin pregnancy is twin-twin transfusion syndrome. In all monochorionic twin placentas there are vascular anastomoses, which connect the circulations of the twins. In some cases there is an abnormal sharing of fetal circulations through an arteriovenous shunt. If an imbalance in blood flow occurs, a marked disparity in fetal blood volumes may result in twin-twin transfusion syndrome and the death of one or both fetuses.

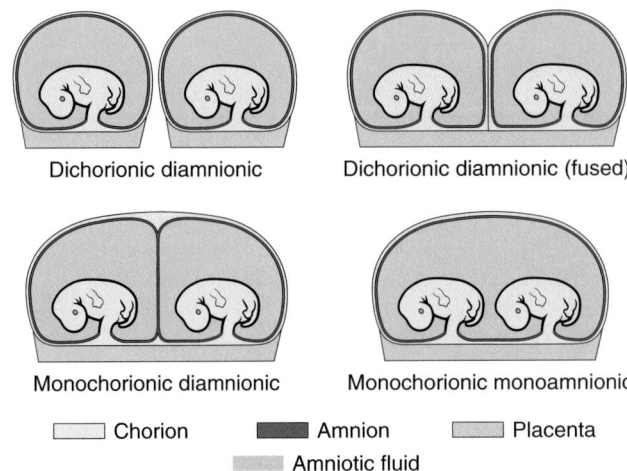

Dichorionic diamnionic

Dichorionic diamnionic (fused)

Monochorionic diamnionic

Monochorionic monoamnionic

☐ Chorion   ■ Amnion   ▨ Placenta

▨ Amniotic fluid

FIGURE 22–53 Diagrammatic representation of the various types of twin placentation and their membrane relationships. (Adapted from Gersell D et al.: Diseases of the placenta. In Kurman R (ed): Blaustein's Pathology of the Female Genital Tract. New York, Springer-Verlag, 1994.)

ABNORMALITIES OF PLACENTAL IMPLANTATION

Abnormal placental implantations may have significant consequences for the pregnancy outcome. *Placenta previa* is a condition in which the placenta implants in the lower uterine segment or cervix, often with serious third-trimester bleeding. A complete placenta previa covers the internal cervical os and thus requires delivery via cesarean section to avert placental rupture and fatal maternal hemorrhage during vaginal delivery. *Placenta accreta* is caused by partial or complete absence of the decidua with adherence of the placental villous tissue directly to the myometrium and failure of placental separation. It is an important cause of postpartum bleeding, which

often may be life-threatening to the mother. Common predisposing factors are placenta previa (in up to 60% of cases) and history of previous cesarean section.

PLACENTAL INFECTIONS

Infections in the placenta develop by two pathways: (1) ascending infection through the birth canal and (2) hematogenous (transplacental) infection. Ascending infections are by far the most common and are virtually always bacterial; in many such instances, localized infection of the membranes by an organism produces premature rupture of membranes and preterm delivery. The amniotic fluid may be cloudy with purulent exudate, and histologically the chorion-amnion contains a polymorphonuclear leukocytic infiltrate accompanied by edema and congestion of the vessels (Fig. 22–54A and B). The infection frequently elicits a fetal response with "vasculitis" of umbilical and fetal chorionic plate vessels. Uncommonly, bacterial infections may arise by the hematogenous spread of bacteria directly to the placenta. The villi will then show acute inflammatory cells (acute villitis) (Fig. 22–54C).

Several hematogenous infections, classically TORCH (toxoplasmosis and others [syphilis, tuberculosis, listeriosis], rubella, cytomegalovirus, herpes simplex), can affect the placenta. They give rise to inflammatory infiltrates in the chorionic villi, usually of chronic inflammatory cells (chronic villitis). Often, the cause of chronic villitis is obscure and may involve immunological phenomena[8] (see also Chapter 10).

PREECLAMPSIA AND ECLAMPSIA

Preeclampsia refers to a *systemic syndrome characterized by widespread maternal endothelial dysfunction presenting clinically with hypertension, edema, and proteinuria during pregnancy*. It occurs in about 3% to 5% of pregnant women, usually in the last trimester and more commonly in primiparas

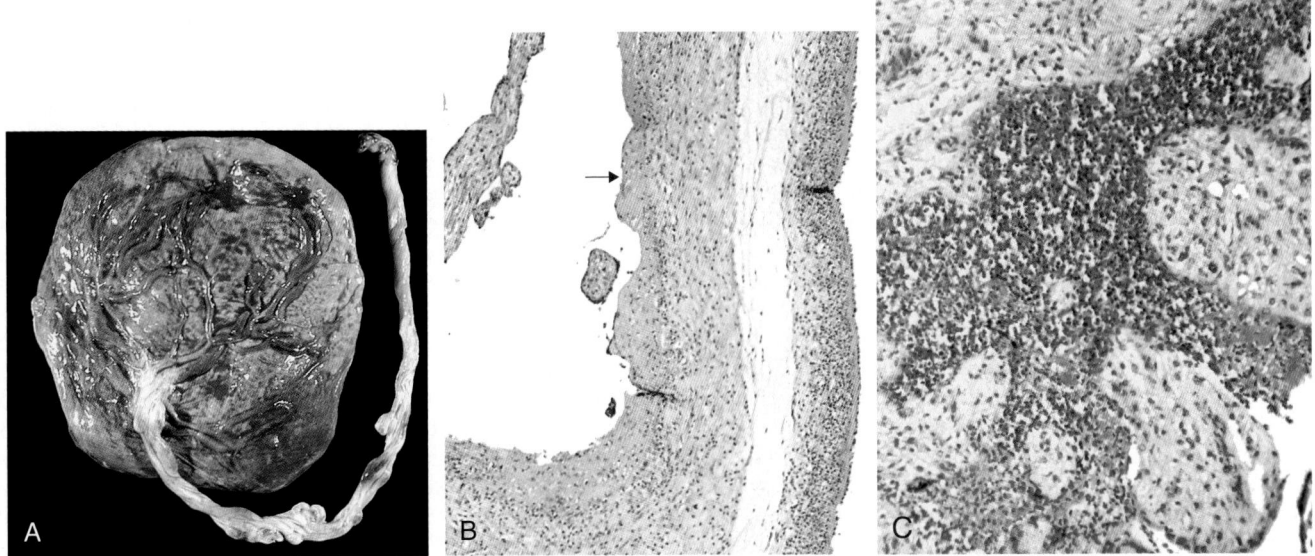

FIGURE 22–54 Placental infections derived from ascending and blood-borne routes. Acute chorioamnionitis. **A,** On gross examination the placenta contains greenish opaque membranes. **B,** A photomicrograph illustrates a dense bandlike inflammatory exudate on the amniotic surface *(arrow)*. **C,** Acute necrotizing intervillositis, from a fetal-maternal infection by *Listeria*.

(women pregnant for the first time). Some of these women become more seriously ill, developing convulsions; this more severe form is termed *eclampsia*. Other complications stemming from systemic endothelial dysfunction include hypercoaguability, acute renal failure and pulmonary edema. Approximately 10% of women with severe preeclampsia develop hemolysis, elevated liver enzymes, and low platelets, referred to as the HELLP syndrome (Chapter 18). Preeclampsia should be distinguished from gestational hypertension that can develop in pregnancy without proteinuria.

Pathogenesis. The exact mechanisms leading to development of preeclampsia are still being investigated; however, *it is clear that the placenta plays a central role in the pathogenesis of the syndrome*, since the symptoms disappear rapidly after delivery of the placenta. *The critical abnormalities in preeclampsia are diffuse endothelial dysfunction, vasoconstriction (leading to hypertension), and increased vascular permeability (resulting in proteinuria and edema).* Recent work has demonstrated that these effects are most likely mediated by placenta derived factor(s) released into the maternal circulation. Although the release of these factors and the clinical syndrome develop late in gestation, the pathogenesis of the disease appears to be closely tied to the earliest events of pregnancy and placentation. The principal pathophysiologic aberrations appear to be the following.

○ *Abnormal placental vasculature.* The initial event in the pathogenesis of preeclampsia is abnormal trophoblastic implantation and lack of development of physiologic alterations in the maternal vessels required for adequate perfusion of the placental bed.[109] In normal pregnancy, fetal extravillous trophoblastic cells (trophoblastic cells not associated with chorionic villi) at the implantation site invade the maternal decidua and decidual vessels, destroy the vascular smooth muscle and replace the maternal endothelial cells with fetal trophoblastic cells (forming hybrid feto-maternal blood vessels). *This process converts the decidual spiral arteries from small-caliber resistance vessels to large capacity uteroplacental vessels lacking a smooth muscle coat* (Fig. 22–55). In preeclampsia this remodeling fails to occur, leaving the placenta ill equipped to meet the increased circulatory demands of late gestation and setting the stage for the development of placental ischemia.

○ *Endothelial dysfunction and imbalance of angiogenic and anti-angiogenic factors.* Although not formally proven, it is postulated that in response to hypoxia, the ischemic placenta releases factors into the maternal circulation that cause an imbalance in circulating angiogenic and anti-angiogenic factors; this in turn leads to systemic maternal endothelial dysfunction and the clinical symptoms of the disease.[110,111] In support of this, the blood levels of two placenta-derived *anti-angiogenic factors*, soluble fms-like tyrosine kinase (sFltl) and endoglin, are several orders of magnitude higher in women with preeclampsia than in healthy controls. Placental hypoxia causes overproduction of sFlt1 from the villous trophoblast; sFltl is a truncated soluble form of VEGF receptor that acts as a decoy receptor, binding VEGF and placental growth factor in circulation and thereby neutralizing their pro-angiogenic activity. Similarly circulating endoglin, a soluble form of a TGF-β receptor, can bind TGF-β and inhibit signaling via cellular

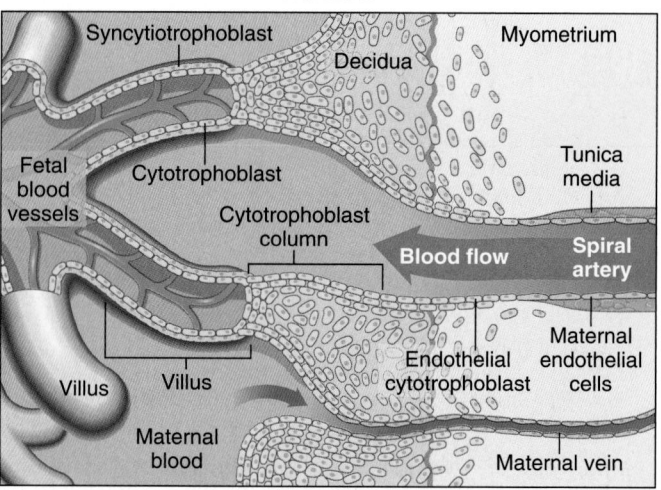

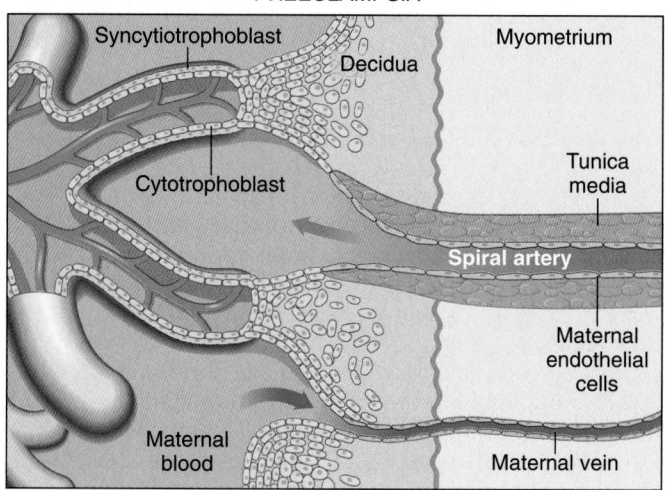

FIGURE 22–55 The physiologic alterations in the uterine spiral arteries and the failure of their remodeling in preeclampsia (Modified from Maynard S, Epstein FH, Karumanchi, SA: Preeclampsia and angiogenic imbalance. Ann Rev Med. *59*: 61, 2008.)

TGF-β receptors. Normally, in late gestation, levels of sFltl and soluble endoglin in the blood increase while placental growth factor and vascular endothelial growth factor decrease, leading to a reduction in angiogenic activity. *In preeclampsia, high levels of sFlt1 and soluble endoglin bring about a decrease in angiogenesis much earlier than in normal pregnancy. The result is defective vascular development in the placenta.*

Studies in animal models also implicate sFltl and soluble endoglin in the pathogenesis of endothelial dysfunction. When sFlt and endoglin are overexpressed together, rats develop nephrotic-range proteinuria, severe hypertension, and fetal growth restriction, the hallmarks of severe preeclampsia, as well as features of the HELLP syndrome, including elevated liver enzymes, decreased platelet counts, and hemolysis. Thus, it seems that *sFlt1 and soluble endoglin are key mediators that link the placenta to the characteristic maternal endothelial dysfunction of preeclampsia.*[112] These effects of sFltl and endoglin appear to be related to their inhibition of VEGF and TGF-β-mediated production of endothelial-dependent nitric oxide (NO) and prostacyclin (PGI₂). The capillary endothelium of the kidney is extremely sensitive to locally produced VEGF, which may explain why proteinuria and renal dysfunction are early markers of preeclampsia.

- *Coagulation abnormalities.* Preeclampsia is associated with a hypercoaguable state; thrombosis of arterioles and capillaries may occur throughout the body, particularly in the liver, kidneys, brain, and pituitary. This hypercoaguability is likely related to the reduced endothelial production of PGI₂, a potent antithrombotic factor, and increased release of procoagulant factors. Production of PGI₂ is stimulated by both VEGF and TGF-β, and women with preeclampsia have been shown to have decreased endothelial production of PGI₂.

Morphology. The **placenta** reveals various microscopic changes, most of which reflect malperfusion, ischemia, and vascular injury. These include: (1) Placental infarcts—small, peripheral ones that may occur in normal full-term placentas—are larger and more numerous in preeclampsia. There is also an exaggeration of ischemic changes in the chorionic villi and trophoblast. This includes increased syncytial knots and the appearance of accelerated villous maturity. (2) There is increased frequency of retroplacental hematomas due to bleeding and instability of uteroplacental vessels. (3) The most characteristic finding is in the decidual vessels, reflecting abnormal implantation. This can be in the form of thrombosis, lack of normal physiologic conversion (described earlier), fibrinoid necrosis, or intraintimal lipid deposition (acute atherosis) (Fig. 22–56).

The **liver** lesions, when present, take the form of irregular, focal, subcapsular, and intraparenchymal hemorrhages. On histologic examination there are fibrin thrombi in the portal capillaries and foci of hemorrhagic necrosis.

The **kidney** lesions are variable. Glomerular lesions are diffuse, when assessed by electron microscopy. They consist of marked swelling of endothelial cells, the deposition of fibrinogen-derived amorphous dense deposits on the endothelial side of the basement membrane, and mesangial cell hyperplasia. Immunofluorescent studies show an abundance of fibrin in glomeruli. In the better defined cases, fibrin thrombi are present in the glomeruli and capillaries of the cortex. When the lesion is far advanced, it may produce complete destruction of the cortex in the pattern referred to as bilateral renal cortical necrosis (Chapter 20). The **brain** may have gross or microscopic foci of hemorrhage along with small-vessel thromboses. Similar changes are often found in the **heart** and the **anterior pituitary**.

Clinical Feature. *Preeclampsia* most commonly starts after 34 weeks of gestation but begins earlier in women with hydatidiform mole (discussed below) or preexisting kidney disease, hypertension, or coagulopathies. The onset is typically insidious, characterized by hypertension and edema, with protein-

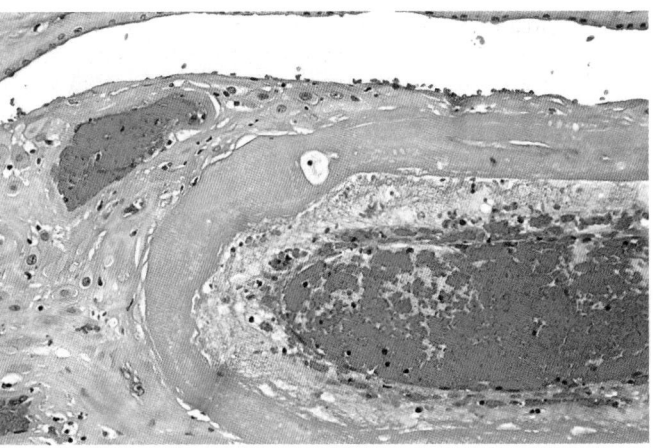

FIGURE 22–56 Acute atherosis of uterine vessels in eclampsia. Note fibrinoid necrosis of the vessel walls, subendothelial macrophages, and perivascular lymphocytic infiltrate. (Courtesy of Dr. Drucilla J. Roberts, Massachusetts General Hospital, Boston, MA.)

uria following within several days. Headaches and visual disturbances are serious events and are indicative of severe preeclampsia, often requiring delivery. *Eclampsia* is heralded by central nervous system involvement, including convulsions and eventual coma. Management of preeclampsia differs depending upon the gestational age and severity of disease. For term pregnancies, delivery is the treatment of choice regardless of disease severity. In preterm pregnancies, where delivery may not be in the best interest of the fetus, patients with mild disease can be managed expectantly with close monitoring of the mother and fetus. However, eclampsia, severe preeclampsia with maternal end-organ dysfunction, fetal compromise, or the HELLP syndrome are indications for delivery regardless of gestational age. Antihypertensive therapy does not affect the disease course or improve outcomes. Proteinuria and hypertension usually disappear within 1 to 2 weeks after delivery except when they predate the pregnancy. Although it is typically believed that preeclampsia has no lasting sequelae, recent studies indicate that about 20% of women develop hypertension and microalbuminuria within 7 years of a pregnancy complicated by preeclampsia. There is also a two-fold increase in the long-term risk of vascular diseases of the heart and the brain.

Gestational Trophoblastic Disease

Gestational trophoblastic disease constitutes a spectrum of tumors and tumor-like conditions characterized by proliferation of placental tissue, either villous or trophoblastic. The lesions include hydatidiform mole (complete and partial), invasive mole, and the frankly malignant choriocarcinoma and placental-site trophoblastic tumor.

HYDATIDIFORM MOLE

Hydatidiform mole is characterized histologically by cystic swelling of the chorionic villi, accompanied by variable trophoblastic proliferation. The most important reason for the

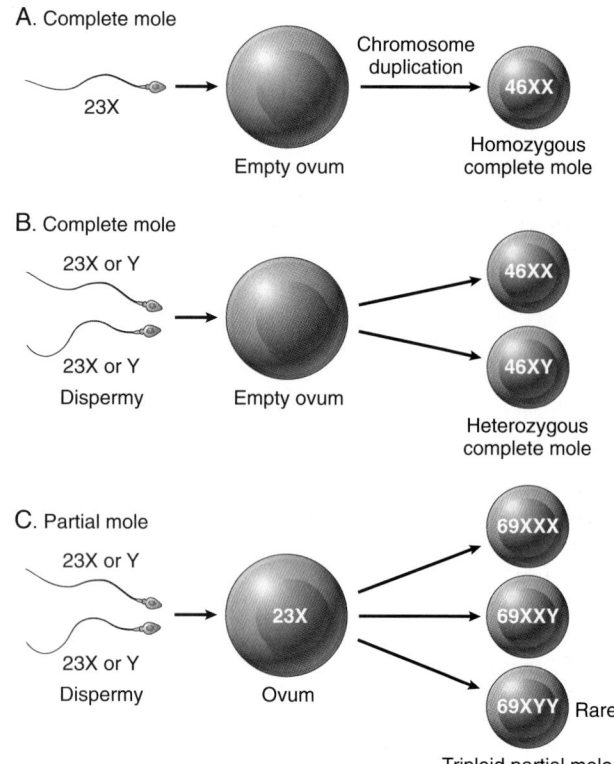

FIGURE 22–57 Origin of complete and partial hydatidiform moles. **A,** Complete moles most commonly arise from fertilization of an empty ovum by a single sperm that undergoes duplication of its chromosomes. **B,** Less commonly, complete moles arise from dispermy in which two sperm fertilize an empty ovum. **C,** Partial moles arise from two sperm fertilizing a single ovum.

correct recognition of moles is that they are associated with an increased risk of persistent trophoblastic disease (invasive mole) or choriocarcinoma. In the past, most patients presented in the fourth or fifth month of pregnancy with vaginal bleeding. Currently, hydatidiform moles are being diagnosed at earlier gestational ages (8.5 versus 17.0 weeks) due to routine ultrasound and close monitoring of early pregnancy. Molar pregnancy can develop at any age, but the risk is higher at the far ends of reproductive life: in teens and between the ages of 40 and 50 years. For poorly explained reasons, the incidence varies considerably in different regions of the world. Hydatidiform mole is a rather infrequent complication of gestation in the United States, occurring about once in every 1000 to 2000 pregnancies, but is quite common in the Far East; the incidence is 1 in 100 in Indonesia.[114] Two types of benign, noninvasive moles—complete and partial—can be identified by cytogenetic (Fig. 22–57) and histologic studies.

Complete Mole

Complete mole results from fertilization of an egg that has lost its chromosomes, and the genetic material is completely paternally derived (Fig. 22–57A and B). Ninety percent have a 46,XX diploid pattern, all derived from duplication of the genetic material of one sperm (a phenomenon called androgenesis). The remaining 10% are from the fertilization of an empty egg by two sperm (46,XX and 46,XY). Histologically, in complete mole all or most of the villi are enlarged and

edematous, and there is diffuse trophoblast hyperplasia. Although fetal vessels and fetal parts are extremely rare in complete moles since the embryo dies very early in development, they do occur. Patients have 2.5% risk of subsequent choriocarcinoma.

Partial Mole

Partial moles result from fertilization of an egg with two sperm (Fig. 22–57C). In these moles the karyotype is triploid (e.g., 69,XXY) or even occasionally tetraploid (92,XXXY). Fetal parts are more commonly present than in complete moles. In partial moles some of the villi are edematous, and other villi show only minor changes; the trophoblastic proliferation is focal and less marked. Although partial moles have an increased risk of persistent molar disease, they are not considered to have an increased risk for choriocarcinoma.

Morphology. The classic gross appearance is of a delicate, friable mass of thin-walled, translucent, cystic, grapelike structures consisting of swollen edematous (hydropic) villi (Figs. 22–58 and 22–59). Fetal parts are frequently seen in partial moles. On histologic examination **complete moles** show abnormalities that involve all or most of the villous tissue. The chorionic villi are enlarged, scalloped in shape with central cavitation (cisterns), and lack adequately developed vessels. The most impressive abnormality is, however, an extensive trophoblast proliferation that involves the entire circumference of the villi, in addition to "extravillous" islands of trophoblast proliferation. The implantation site often displays atypia and an exuberant proliferation of implantation trophoblast. In contrast, **partial moles** demonstrate villous enlargement and architectural disturbances in only a proportion of villi. The trophoblastic proliferation is moderate but still may be circumferential.

Histologic distinction of complete mole from partial molar gestations is important. In equivocal cases

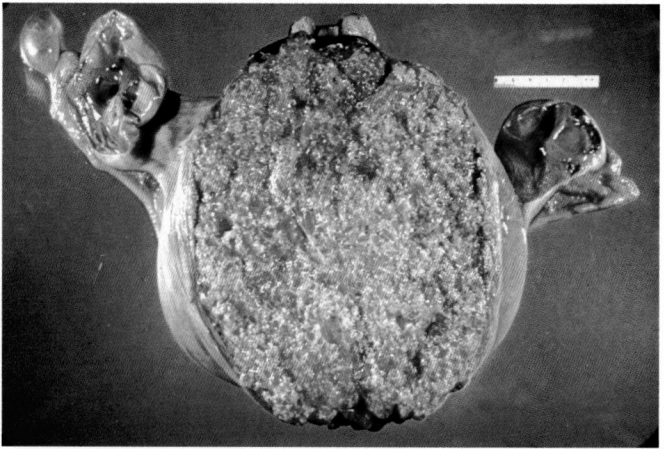

FIGURE 22–58 Complete hydatidiform mole. Note marked distention of the uterus by vesicular chorionic villi. Adnexa (ovaries and fallopian tubes) are visible on the *left* and *right side* of the uterus.

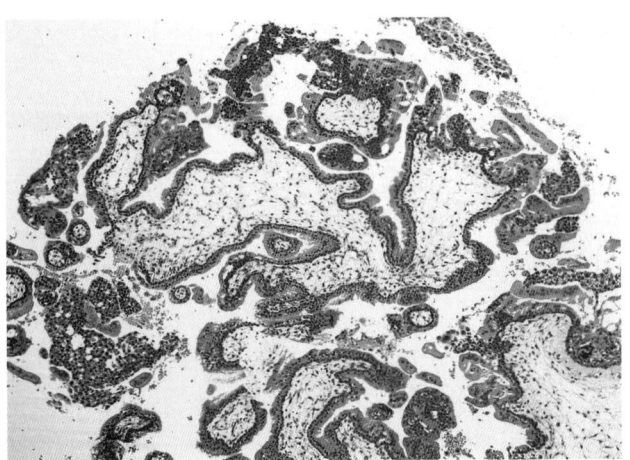

FIGURE 22–59 Complete hydatidiform mole demonstrating marked villous enlargement, edema, and circumferential trophoblast proliferation.

immunostaining for p57, a cell cycle inhibitor, may aid the diagnosis. The *p57KIP2* gene is maternally transcribed but **paternally imprinted**, and shows expression in maternal decidual tissue as well as cytotrophoblast and stromal cells of the villi, when maternal genetic material is present in the conceptus (Fig. 22–60A). In contrast, since both the X chromosomes in complete moles are derived from the father, there is no expression of p57 protein in the cytotrophoblast or stromal cells of the villi in complete moles (Fig. 22–60B).

Clinical Features. Most women with partial and early complete moles present with spontaneous pregnancy loss or undergo curettage because of abnormalities in ultrasound showing diffuse villous enlargement. In complete moles quantitative analysis of human chorionic gonadotropin (HCG) shows levels of hormone greatly exceeding those produced during a normal pregnancy of similar gestational age. Serial

hormone determination indicates a rapidly mounting level that climbs faster than for the usual normal single or even multiple pregnancy. The vast majority of moles are removed by thorough curettage. Monitoring serum concentrations of HCG is necessary to determine the early development of persistent trophoblastic disease, since up to 10% of moles develop into persistent or invasive moles.[115] In addition, 2.5% of complete moles evolve into gestational choriocarcinoma. Therefore, serum HCG levels are usually followed until they fall to and remain at zero for 6 months to a year.

INVASIVE MOLE

This is defined as a mole that penetrates or even perforates the uterine wall (Fig. 22–61). There is invasion of the myometrium by hydropic chorionic villi, accompanied by proliferation of both cytotrophoblast and syncytiotrophoblast. The tumor is locally destructive and may invade parametrial tissue and blood vessels. Hydropic villi may embolize to distant sites, such as lungs and brain, but do not grow in these organs as true metastases, and even without chemotherapy they eventually regress. The tumor is manifested clinically by vaginal bleeding and irregular uterine enlargement. It is always associated with a persistently elevated serum HCG and varying degrees of luteinization of the ovaries. The tumor responds well to chemotherapy but may result in uterine rupture and necessitate hysterectomy.

CHORIOCARCINOMA

Gestational choriocarcinoma is a malignant neoplasm of trophoblastic cells derived from a previously normal or abnormal pregnancy, which can even include extrauterine ectopic pregnancy. Choriocarcinoma is rapidly invasive and metastasizes widely, but once identified responds well to chemotherapy.

Incidence. This is an uncommon condition that arises in 1 in 20,000 to 30,000 pregnancies in the United States. It is much more common in some African countries; for example, it occurs in 1 in 2500 pregnancies in Ibadan, Nigeria. It is

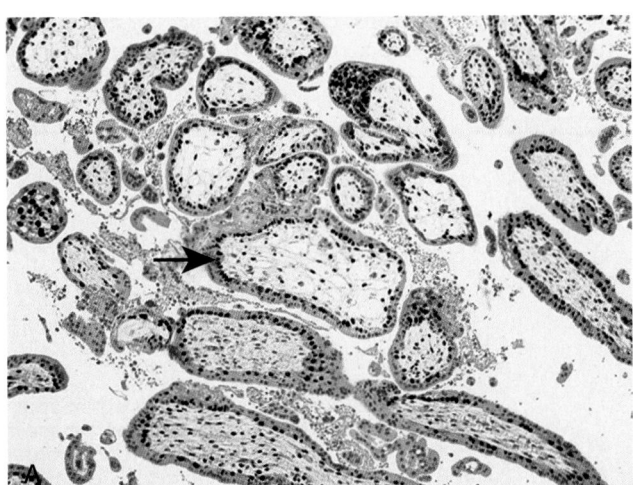
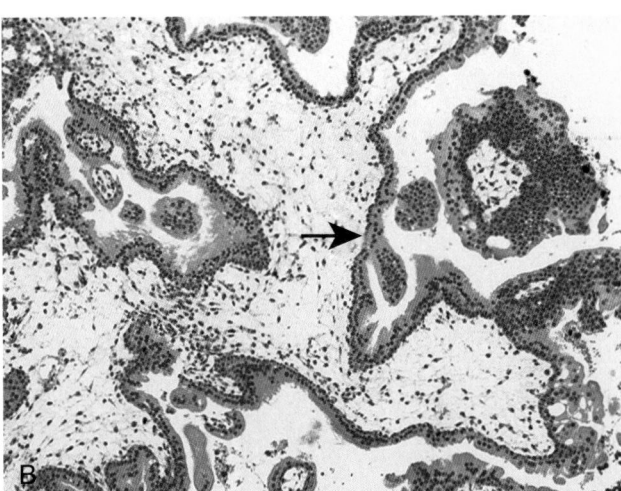

FIGURE 22–60 **A,** Normal chorionic villi immunostained for p57 exhibit staining in both stromal and cytotrophoblast *(arrow)* nuclei. **B,** Complete moles lack expression of p57 in the cytotrophoblast *(arrow)* and villous stroma.

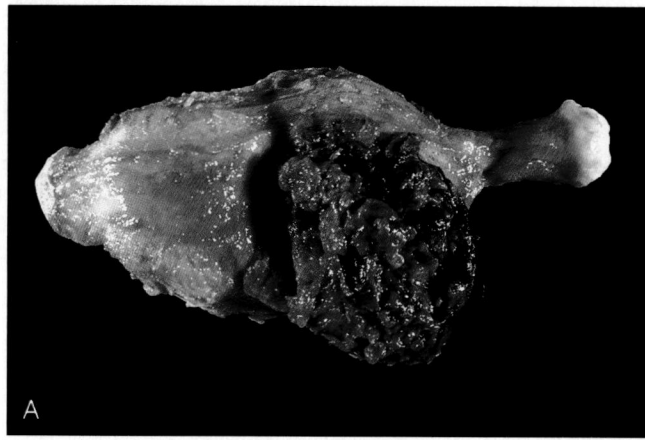
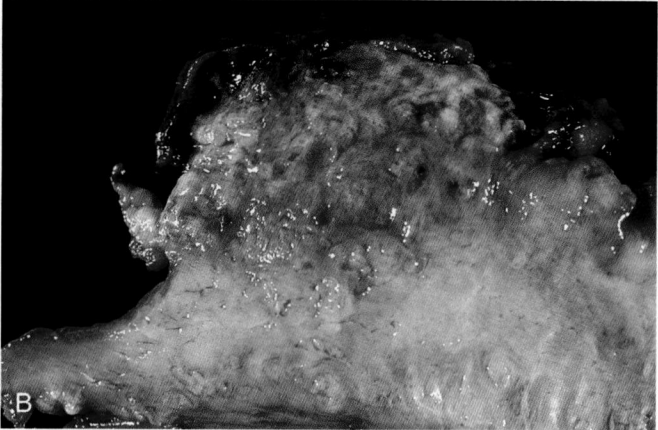

FIGURE 22–61   A, Invasive mole presenting as a hemorrhagic mass adherent to the uterine wall. **B,** On cross-section, the tumor invades into the myometrium. (Courtesy of Dr. David R. Genest, Brigham and Women's Hospital, Boston, MA.)

preceded by several conditions; 50% arise in hydatidiform moles, 25% in previous abortions, approximately 22% in normal pregnancies (intraplacental choriocarcinoma), with the remainder occuring in ectopic pregnancies. Very rarely, a nongestational choriocarcinoma may develop from germ cells in the ovaries or the mediastinum. About 1 in 40 complete hydatidiform moles may be expected to give rise to a choriocarcinoma, in contrast to 1 in approximately 150,000 normal pregnancies.

Morphology. Choriocarcinoma is classically a soft, fleshy, yellow-white tumor with a marked tendency to form large pale areas of ischemic necrosis, foci of cystic softening, and extensive hemorrhage (Fig. 22–62A). Histologically, it does not produce chorionic villi and consists entirely of a mixed proliferation of syncytiotrophoblasts and cytotrophoblasts (Fig. 22–62B). Mitoses are abundant and sometimes abnormal. The tumor invades the underlying myometrium, frequently penetrates blood vessels and lymphatics, and in some cases extends out onto the uterine serosa and into adjacent structures. Due to rapid growth it is subject to hemorrhage, ischemic necrosis, and secondary inflammation. In fatal cases metastases are found in the lungs, brain, bone marrow, liver, and other organs. On occasion, metastatic choriocarcinoma is discovered without a detectable primary in the uterus (or ovary), presumably because the primary has undergone complete necrosis.

Clinical Features. Uterine choriocarcinoma usually does not produce a large, bulky mass, but it manifests as irregular vaginal spotting of a bloody, brown fluid. This discharge may appear in the course of an apparently normal pregnancy, after a miscarriage, or after curettage. Sometimes the tumor does not appear until months after these events. Usually, by the time the tumor is discovered, radiographs of the chest and bones already disclose the presence of metastatic lesions. The titers of HCG are elevated to levels above those encountered in hydatidiform moles. Occasionally, tumors produce little hormone, and some tumors become so necrotic as to become functionally inactive. Widespread metastases are characteristic. Frequent sites of involvement are the lungs (50%) and vagina (30% to 40%), followed in descending order of frequency by the brain, liver, and kidney.

The treatment of gestational choriocarcinoma (and other trophoblastic neoplasms) depends on the type and stage of the tumor and includes evacuation of the contents of the uterus,

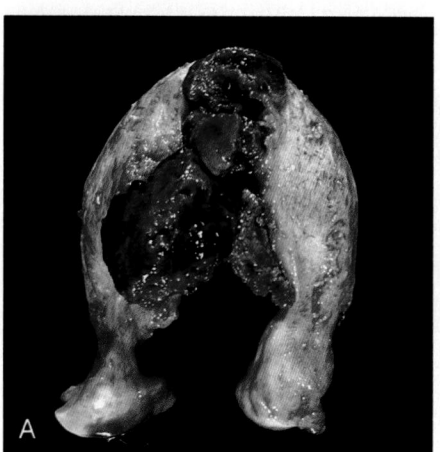
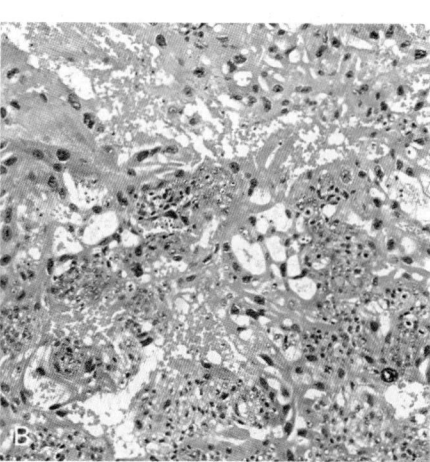

FIGURE 22–62 A, Choriocarcinoma presenting as a bulky hemorrhagic mass invading the uterine wall. **B,** Photomicrograph of choriocarcinoma illustrating both neoplastic cytotrophoblast and syncytiotrophoblast. (Courtesy of Dr. David R. Genest, Brigham and Women's Hospital, Boston, MA.)

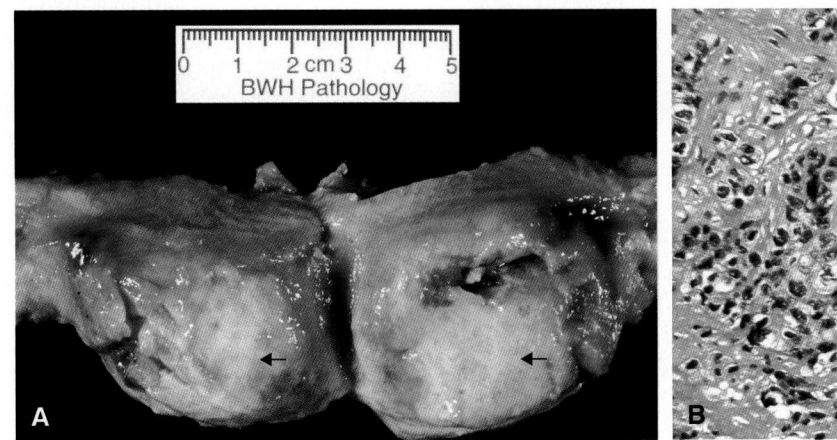
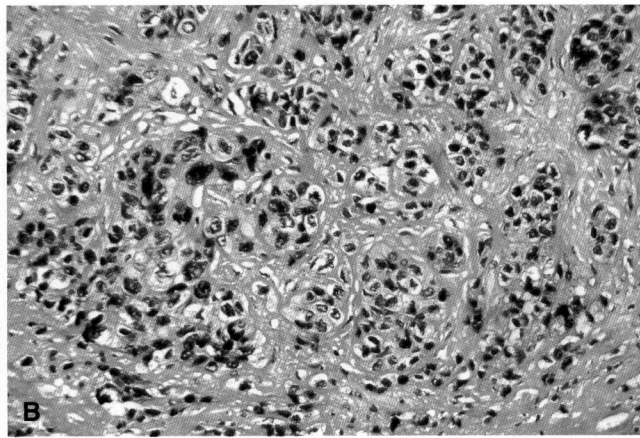

FIGURE 22–63   **A,** Placental-site trophoblastic tumor (PSTT), presenting as a discrete mass in the myometrium. **B,** Histology of PSTT. (Courtesy of Dr. Bradley J. Quade, Brigham and Women's Hospital, Boston, MA.)

surgery, and chemotherapy. The results of chemotherapy for gestational choriocarcinoma are spectacular and result in nearly 100% remission and a high rate of cures. Many of the cured patients have had normal subsequent pregnancies and deliveries. By contrast, nongestational choriocarcinomas are much more resistant to therapy. The difference is believed to be due to the expression of paternal antigens in gestational choriocarcinomas that can evoke an immune response from the mother.

PLACENTAL-SITE TROPHOBLASTIC TUMOR (PSTT)

PSTTs compose less than 2% of gestational trophoblastic neoplasms and represent neoplastic proliferation of extravillous trophoblast, also called intermediate trophoblast. In normal pregnancy, extravillous (intermediate) trophoblast is found in nonvillous sites such as the implantation site, in islands of cells within the placental parenchyma, in the chorionic plate, and in the placental membranes. In contrast, syncytiotrophoblast and cytotrophoblast are present on the chorionic villi. Normal extravillous trophoblasts are polygonal mononuclear cells that have abundant cytoplasm and produce human placental lactogen. Malignant transformation of extravillous trophoblast gives rise to PSTT, which presents as a uterine mass (Fig. 22–63A), accompanied by either abnormal uterine bleeding or amenorrhea and moderate elevation of β-HCG. Histologically, PSTT is composed of malignant trophoblastic cells diffusely infiltrating the endomyometrium (Fig. 22–63B). PSTTs may be preceded by a normal pregnancy (one half), spontaneous abortion (one sixth), or hydatidiform mole (one fifth).[116,117] Patients with localized disease or a less than 2-year interval from the prior pregnancy to diagnosis have an excellent prognosis. Tumors diagnosed at advanced stage, or diagnosed 2 or more years following pregnancy, have a poor prognosis; overall, about 10% to 15% of women with PSTT die of disseminated disease.[118]

REFERENCES

1. Robboy S et al. (eds): Embryology of the Female Genital Tract, 5th ed. New York, Springer-Verlag, 2002.
2. Kurita T et al.: Epithelial-stromal tissue interaction in paramesonephric (müllerian) epithelial differentiation. Dev Biol 240:194, 2001.
3. Quade BJ et al.: Expression of the p53 homologue p63 in early cervical neoplasia. Gynecol Oncol 80:24, 2001.
4. Malasanos TH: Sexual development of the fetus and pubertal child. Clin Obstet Gynecol 40:153, 1997.
5. Ince TA et al.: p63 coordinates anogenital modeling and epithelial cell differentiation in the developing female urogenital tract. Am J Pathol 161:1111, 2002.
6. Richart RM: Cervical intraepithelial neoplasia. Pathol Annu 8:301, 1973.
7. Kurman R (ed): Blaustein's Pathology of the Female Genital Tract, 5th ed. New York, Springer-Verlag, 2002.
8. Benirschke KP, Baergen RN: Pathology of the Human Placenta, 5th ed. New York, Springer, 2006.
9. McMillan A et al. (eds): Clinical Practice in Sexually Transmissible Infections. London, WB Saunders, 2002.
10. Xu F et al.: Seroprevalence and coinfection with herpes simplex virus type 1 and type 2 in the United States, 1988–1994. J Infect Dis 185:1019, 2002.
11. Stanberry LR et al.: Prospects for control of herpes simplex virus disease through immunization. Clin Infect Dis 30:549, 2000.
12. Pararas MV et al.: Preterm birth due to maternal infection: causative pathogens and modes of prevention. Eur J Clin Microbiol Infect Dis 25:562, 2006.
13. Pinto AP et al.: Allelic imbalance in lichen sclerosus, hyperplasia, and intraepithelial neoplasia of the vulva. Gynecol Oncol 77:171, 2000.
14. de Koning MN et al.: Prevalence of mucosal and cutaneous human papillomaviruses in different histologic subtypes of vulvar carcinoma. Mod Pathol 21:334, 2008.
15. Vanin K et al.: Overexpression of wild-type p53 in lichen sclerosus adjacent to human papillomavirus-negative vulvar cancer. J Invest Dermatol 119:1027, 2002.
16. Jones RW et al.: Vulvar intraepithelial neoplasia: aspects of the natural history and outcome in 405 women. Obstet Gynecol 106:1319, 2005.
17. Belousova IE et al.: Vulvar Toker cells: the long-awaited missing link: a proposal for an origin-based histogenetic classification of extramammary Paget disease. Am J Dermatopathol 28:84, 2006.
18. Willman JH et al.: Vulvar clear cells of Toker: precursors of extramammary Paget's disease. Am J Dermatopathol 27:185, 2005.
19. Schrager S, Potter BE: Diethylstilbestrol exposure. Am Fam Physician 69:2395, 2004.
20. Hilgers RD et al.: Embryonal rhabdomyosarcoma (botryoid type) of the vagina. A clinicopathologic review. Am J Obstet Gynecol 107:484, 1970.
21. Kaewsrichan J et al.: Selection and identification of anaerobic *Lactobacilli* producing inhibitory compounds against vaginal pathogens. FEMS Immunol Med Microbiol 48:75, 2006.
22. Munoz N et al.: Epidemiologic classification of human papillomavirus types associated with cervical cancer. N Engl J Med 348:518, 2003.

23. Schiffman M et al.: Human papillomavirus and cervical cancer. Lancet 370:890, 2007.

24. Franco EL et al.: Epidemiology of acquisition and clearance of cervical human papillomavirus infection in women from a high-risk area for cervical cancer. J Infect Dis 180:1415, 1999.

25. Ostor AG: Natural history of cervical intraepithelial neoplasia: a critical review. Int J Gynecol Pathol 12:186, 1993.

26. Moscicki AB et al.: Risk of high-grade squamous intraepithelial lesion in HIV-infected adolescents. J Infect Dis 190:1413, 2004.

27. Saslow D et al.: American Cancer Society guideline for the early detection of cervical neoplasia and cancer. J Low Genit Tract Dis 7:67, 2003.

28. Wright TC, Jr. et al.: Interim guidance for the use of human papillomavirus DNA testing as an adjunct to cervical cytology for screening. Obstet Gynecol 103:304, 2004.

29. Wright TC, Jr. et al.: 2006 consensus guidelines for the management of women with abnormal cervical cancer screening tests. Am J Obstet Gynecol 197:346, 2007.

30. Cutts FT et al.: Human papillomavirus and HPV vaccines: a review. Bull World Health Organ 85:719, 2007.

31. Jabbour HN et al.: Endocrine regulation of menstruation. Endocr Rev 27:17, 2006.

32. Hou X et al.: Canonical Wnt signaling is critical to estrogen-mediated uterine growth. Mol Endocrinol 18:3035, 2004.

33. Groothuis PG et al.: Estrogen and the endometrium: lessons learned from gene expression profiling in rodents and human. Hum Reprod Update 13:405, 2007.

34. Kiviat NB et al.: Endometrial histopathology in patients with culture-proved upper genital tract infection and laparoscopically diagnosed acute salpingitis. Am J Surg Pathol 14:167, 1990.

35. Bulun SE: Mechanisms of disease: Endometriosis. New Engl J Med 360:268, 2009.

36. Noble LS et al.: Prostaglandin E2 stimulates aromatase expression in endometriosis-derived stromal cells. J Clin Endocrinol Metab 82:600, 1997.

37. Burney RO et al.: Gene expression analysis of endometrium reveals progesterone resistance and candidate susceptibility genes in women with endometriosis. Endocrinology 148:3814, 2007.

38. Nabeshima H et al.: Analysis of the clonality of ectopic glands in peritoneal endometriosis using laser microdissection. Fertil Steril 80:1144, 2003.

39. Wu Y et al.: Resolution of clonal origins for endometriotic lesions using laser capture microdissection and the human androgen receptor (HUMARA) assay. Fertil Steril 79 (Suppl 1):710, 2003.

40. Wells M: Recent advances in endometriosis with emphasis on pathogenesis, molecular pathology, and neoplastic transformation. Int J Gynecol Pathol 23:316, 2004.

41. Corley D et al.: Postmenopausal bleeding from unusual endometrial polyps in women on chronic tamoxifen therapy. Obstet Gynecol 79:111, 1992.

42. Kazmerczak B et al.: HMGIY is the target of 6p21.3 rearrangements in various benign mesenchymal tumors. Genes Chromosome Cancer 23:279, 1998.

43. Kurman RJ et al.: The behavior of endometrial hyperplasia. A long-term study of "untreated" hyperplasia in 170 patients. Cancer 56:403, 1985.

44. Di Cristofano A, Ellenson LH: Endometrial carcinoma. Annu Rev Pathol 2:57, 2007.

45. Tashiro H et al.: Mutations in PTEN are frequent in endometrial carcinoma but rare in other common gynecological malignancies. Cancer Res 57:3935, 1997.

46. Maxwell GL et al.: Mutation of the PTEN tumor suppressor gene in endometrial hyperplasias. Cancer Res 58:2500, 1998.

47. Vilgelm A et al.: Akt-mediated phosphorylation and activation of estrogen receptor alpha is required for endometrial neoplastic transformation in Pten$^{+/-}$ mice. Cancer Res 66:3375, 2006.

48. Silverberg SG: Problems in the differential diagnosis of endometrial hyperplasia and carcinoma. Mod Pathol 13:309, 2000.

49. Trimble CL et al.: Concurrent endometrial carcinoma in women with a biopsy diagnosis of atypical endometrial hyperplasia: a Gynecologic Oncology Group study. Cancer 106:812, 2006.

50. Ferenczy A, Gelfand M: The biologic significance of cytologic atypia in progestogen-treated endometrial hyperplasia. Am J Obstet Gynecol 160:126, 1989.

51. O'Connell JT et al.: Identification of a basal/reserve cell immunophenotype in benign and neoplastic endometrium: a study with the p53 homologue p63. Gynecol Oncol 80:30, 2001.

52. Sherman ME: Theories of endometrial carcinogenesis: a multidisciplinary approach. Mod Pathol 13:295, 2000.

53. Mutter GL et al.: Allelotype mapping of unstable microsatellites establishes direct lineage continuity between endometrial precancers and cancer. Cancer Res 56:4483, 1996.

54. Levine RL et al.: PTEN mutations and microsatellite instability in complex atypical hyperplasia, a precursor lesion to uterine endometrioid carcinoma. Cancer Res 58:3254, 1998.

55. Oda K et al.: High frequency of coexistent mutations of PIK3CA and PTEN genes in endometrial carcinoma. Cancer Res 65:10669, 2005.

56. Hayes MP et al.: PIK3CA and PTEN mutations in uterine endometrioid carcinoma and complex atypical hyperplasia. Clin Cancer Res 12:5932, 2006.

57. Tashiro H et al.: p53 gene mutations are common in uterine serous carcinoma and occur early in their pathogenesis. Am J Pathol 150:177, 1997.

58. Grice J et al.: Uterine papillary serous carcinoma: evaluation of long-term survival in surgically staged patients. Gynecol Oncol 69:69, 1998.

59. Tay EH, Ward BG: The treatment of uterine papillary serous carcinoma (UPSC): are we doing the right thing? Int J Gynecol Cancer 9:463, 1999.

60. Lim P et al.: Early stage uterine papillary serous carcinoma of the endometrium: effect of adjuvant whole abdominal radiotherapy and pathologic parameters on outcome. Cancer 91:752, 2001.

61. Silverberg SG et al.: Carcinosarcoma (malignant mixed mesodermal tumor) of the uterus. A Gynecologic Oncology Group pathologic study of 203 cases. Int J Gynecol Pathol 9:1, 1990.

62. Abeln EC et al.: Molecular genetic evidence for the conversion hypothesis of the origin of malignant mixed müllerian tumours. J Pathol 183:424, 1997.

63. Clement PB, Scully RE: Müllerian adenosarcoma of the uterus: a clinicopathologic analysis of 100 cases with a review of the literature. Hum Pathol 21:363, 1990.

64. Chang KL et al.: Primary uterine endometrial stromal neoplasms. A clinicopathologic study of 117 cases. Am J Surg Pathol 14:415, 1990.

65. Li H et al.: Gene fusion and RNA trans-splicing in normal and neoplastic cells. Cell Cycle 8:218, 2009.

66. Ligon AH, Morton CC: Leiomyomata: treatability and cytogenetic studies. Human Reproduction update 7:8, 2008.

67. Ligon AH, Morton CC: Genetics of uterine leiomyomata. Genes Chromosomes Cancer 28:235, 2000.

68. Quade BJ et al.: Frequent loss of heterozygosity for chromosome 10 in uterine leiomyosarcoma in contrast to leiomyoma. Am J Pathol 154:945, 1999.

69. Bell SW et al.: Problematic uterine smooth muscle neoplasms. A clinicopathologic study of 213 cases. Am J Surg Pathol 18:535, 1994.

70. Obermair A et al.: Primary fallopian tube carcinoma: the Queensland experience. Int J Gynecol Cancer 11:69, 2001.

71. Aziz S et al.: A genetic epidemiological study of carcinoma of the fallopian tube. Gynecol Oncol 80:341, 2001.

72. Young RHS, Scully RE, (ed): Ovarian pathology in infertility. In Krausz FT (ed): Pathology of Reproductive Failure. Baltimore, Williams and Wilkins, p. 104–139, 1991.

73. Homburg R: Polycystic ovary syndrome—from gynaecological curiosity to multisystem endocrinopathy. Hum Reprod 11:29, 1996.

74. Ovalle F, Azziz R: Insulin resistance, polycystic ovary syndrome, and type 2 diabetes mellitus. Fertil Steril 77:1095, 2002.

75. Young RH et al. (eds): The Ovary. In Steinberg S et al. (eds.): Diagnostic Surgical Pathology. New York, Raven Press, 1994.

76. Scully RE: Pathology of ovarian cancer precursors. J Cell Biochem Suppl 23:208, 1995.

77. Narod SA, Boyd J: Current understanding of the epidemiology and clinical implications of BRCA1 and BRCA2 mutations for ovarian cancer. Curr Opin Obstet Gynecol 14:19, 2002.

78. Narod SA et al.: Tubal ligation and risk of ovarian cancer in carriers of BRCA1 or BRCA2 mutations: a case-control study. Lancet 357:1467, 2001.

79. Ness RB et al.: Oral contraceptives, other methods of contraception, and risk reduction for ovarian cancer. Epidemiology 12:307, 2001.

80. Malpica A et al.: Interobserver and intraobserver variability of a two-tier system for grading ovarian serous carcinoma. Am J Surg Pathol 31:1168, 2007.
81. Bell DA: Origins and molecular pathology of ovarian cancer. Mod Pathol 18:S19, 2005.
82. Shih IeM, Kurman RJ. Ovarian tumorigenesis: a proposed model based on morphological and molecular genetic analysis. Am J Pathol 164:1511, 2004.
83. Werness BA et al.: Histopathology of familial ovarian tumors in women from families with and without germline *BRCA1* mutations. Hum Pathol 31:1420, 2000.
84. Szych C et al.: Molecular genetic evidence supporting the clonality and appendiceal origin of pseudomyxoma peritonei in women. Am J Pathol 154:1849, 1999.
85. Cuatrecasas M et al.: *K-RAS* mutations in mucinous ovarian tumors: a clinicopathologic and molecular study of 95 cases. Cancer 79:1581, 1997.
86. Lee KR, Scully RE: Mucinous tumors of the ovary: a clinicopathologic study of 196 borderline tumors (of intestinal type) and carcinomas, including an evaluation of 11 cases with "pseudomyxoma peritonei." Am J Surg Pathol 24:1447, 2000.
87. Watkin W et al.: Mucinous carcinoma of the ovary. Pathologic prognostic factors. Cancer 69:208, 1992.
88. Ronnett BM et al.: Immunohistochemical evidence supporting the appendiceal origin of pseudomyxoma peritonei in women. Int J Gynecol Pathol 16:1, 1997.
89. Eifel P et al.: Simultaneous presentation of carcinoma involving the ovary and the uterine corpus. Cancer 50:163, 1982.
90. Catasus L et al.: Molecular genetic alterations in endometrioid carcinomas of the ovary: similar frequency of β-catenin abnormalities but lower rate of microsatellite instability and *PTEN* alterations than in uterine endometrioid carcinomas. Hum Pathol 35:1360, 2004.
91. Sato N et al.: Loss of heterozygosity on 10q23.3 and mutation of the tumor suppressor gene *PTEN* in benign endometrial cyst of the ovary: possible sequence progression from benign endometrial cyst to endometrioid carcinoma and clear cell carcinoma of the ovary. Cancer Res 60:7052, 2000.
92. Berek JS, Bast RC, Jr.: Ovarian cancer screening. The use of serial complementary tumor markers to improve sensitivity and specificity for early detection. Cancer 76 (10 Suppl):2092, 1995.
93. Kim JH et al.: Osteopontin as a potential diagnostic biomarker for ovarian cancer. JAMA 287:1671, 2002.
94. Petricoin EF et al.: Use of proteomic patterns in serum to identify ovarian cancer. Lancet 359:572, 2002.
95. Hankinson SE et al.: Tubal ligation, hysterectomy, and risk of ovarian cancer. A prospective study. JAMA 270:2813, 1993.
96. Linder D et al.: Pathenogenic origin of benign ovarian teratomas. N Engl J Med 292:63, 1975.
97. Mutter GL: Teratoma genetics and stem cells: a review. Obstet Gynecol Surv 42:661, 1987.
98. O'Connor DM, Norris HJ: The influence of grade on the outcome of stage I ovarian immature (malignant) teratomas and the reproducibility of grading. Int J Gynecol Pathol 13:283, 1994.
99. Hole-Hansen CE et al.: Ovarian dysgerminomas are characterized by frequent KIT mutations and abundant expression of pluripotency markers. Mol Cancer 6:12, 2007.
100. Sever M et al.: Expression of CD117 (*C-KIT*) receptor in dysgerminoma of the ovary: diagnostic and therapeutic implications. Mod Pathol 18:1411, 2005.
101. Williams S et al.: Adjuvant therapy of ovarian germ cell tumors with cisplatin, etoposide, and bleomycin: a trial of the Gynecologic Oncology Group. J Clin Oncol 12:701, 1994.
102. Young RH, Scully RE: Ovarian sex cord–stromal tumors: recent progress. Int J Gynecol Pathol 1:101, 1982.
103. Robertson DM et al.: Inhibins/activins as diagnostic markers for ovarian cancer. Mol Cell Endocrinol 191:97, 2002.
104. Prat J, Scully RE: Cellular fibromas and fibrosarcomas of the ovary: a comparative clinicopathologic analysis of seventeen cases. Cancer 47:2663, 1981.
105. Roth LM et al.: Sertoli–Leydig cell tumors: a clinicopathologic study of 34 cases. Cancer 48:187, 1981.
106. Hart WR, Burkons DM: Germ cell neoplasms arising in gonadoblastomas. Cancer 43:669, 1979.
107. Wilcox AJ et al.: Incidence of early loss of pregnancy. N Engl J Med 319:189, 1988.
108. Rossing MA et al.: Past use of an intrauterine device and risk of tubal pregnancy. Epidemiology 4:245, 1993.
109. Schmidt M et al.: Altered angiogenesis in preeclampsia: evaluation of a new test system for measuring placental growth factor. Clin Chem Lab Med 45:1504, 2007.
110. Baumwell S, Karumanchi SA: Pre-eclampsia: clinical manifestations and molecular mechanisms. Nephron Clin Pract 106:c72, 2007.
111. Venkatesha S et al.: Soluble endoglin contributes to the pathogenesis of preeclampsia. Nat Med 12:642, 2006.
112. Maynard S, Epstein FH, Karumanchi SA: Preeclampsia and angiogenic imbalance. Ann Rev Med 59:61, 2008.
113. Clark BA et al.: Urinary cyclic GMP, endothelin, and prostaglandin E2 in normal pregnancy and preeclampsia. Am J Perinatol 14:559, 1997.
114. Bracken MB et al.: Epidemiology of hydatidiform mole and choriocarcinoma. Epidemiol Rev 6:52, 1984.
115. Lurain JR et al.: Natural history of hydatidiform mole after primary evacuation. Am J Obstet Gynecol 145:591, 1983.
116. Papadopoulos AJ et al.: Twenty-five years' clinical experience with placental site trophoblastic tumors. J Reprod Med 47:460, 2002.
117. Chang YL et al.: Prognostic factors and treatment for placental site trophoblastic tumor—report of 3 cases and analysis of 88 cases. Gynecol Oncol 73:216, 1999.
118. Baergen RN et al.: Placental site trophoblastic tumor: a study of 55 cases and review of the literature emphasizing factors of prognostic significance. Gynecol Oncol 100:511, 2006.

The Breast

SUSAN C. LESTER

■ THE FEMALE BREAST

Disorders of Development

Clinical Presentations of Breast Disease

Inflammatory Disorders
- **Acute Mastitis**
- **Periductal Mastitis**
- **Mammary Duct Ectasia**
- **Fat Necrosis**
- **Lymphocytic Mastopathy (Sclerosing Lymphocytic Lobulitis)**
- **Granulomatous Mastitis**

Benign Epithelial Lesions
- **Nonproliferative Breast Changes (Fibrocystic Changes)**
- **Proliferative Breast Disease without Atypia**
- **Proliferative Breast Disease with Atypia**
- **Clinical Significance of Benign Epithelial Changes**

Carcinoma of the Breast
- **Incidence and Epidemiology**
- **Etiology and Pathogenesis**

Hereditary Breast Cancer
Sporadic Breast Cancer
Overview of Carcinogenesis and Tumor Progression

Classification of Breast Carcinoma
Carcinoma in Situ
Invasive (Infiltrating) Carcinoma
Invasive Carcinoma, No Special Type (NST; Invasive Ductal Carcinoma)
Invasive Lobular Carcinoma
Medullary Carcinoma
Mucinous (Colloid) Carcinoma
Tubular Carcinoma
Invasive Papillary Carcinoma
Metaplastic Carcinoma

Prognostic and Predictive Factors

Stromal Tumors
Fibroadenoma
Phyllodes Tumor
Benign Stromal Lesions
Malignant Stromal Tumors

Other Malignant Tumors of the Breast

■ THE MALE BREAST

Gynecomastia

Carcinoma

THE FEMALE BREAST

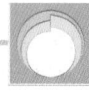

The class Mammalia is distinguished from other animals by highly evolved modified skin appendages, known as mammary glands or breasts, that provide a complete source of nourishment and an important degree of immunological protection for offspring. In humans, paired mammary glands rest on the pectoralis muscle on the upper chest wall. The breasts are composed of specialized epithelium and stroma that may give rise to both benign and malignant lesions (Fig. 23–1).

Diseases of the breast are best understood in the context of its normal anatomy. The human breast contains six to ten major ductal systems. The keratinizing squamous epithelium of the overlying skin dips into the orifices at the nipple and then abruptly changes to a double-layered cuboidal epithelium lining the ducts. Successive branching of the large ducts eventually leads to the terminal duct lobular unit. In adult women the terminal duct branches into a grapelike cluster of small acini to form a lobule (Figs. 23–1 and 23–2B). Each ductal system typically occupies more than one quadrant of the breast, and the systems extensively overlap one another. In some women, ducts extend into the subcutaneous tissue of the chest wall and into the axilla.

Two cell types line the ducts and lobules. Contractile myoepithelial cells containing myofilaments lie in a meshlike pattern on the basement membrane. These cells assist in milk ejection during lactation and provide structural support to the lobules. Luminal epithelial cells overlay the myoepithelial cells. Only the lobular luminal cells are capable of producing milk. A committed stem cell in the terminal duct is postulated to give rise to both luminal and myoepithelial cells.[1]

There are also two types of breast stroma. The interlobular stroma consists of dense fibrous connective tissue admixed with adipose tissue. The intralobular stroma envelopes the acini of the lobules and consists of breast-specific hormonally responsive fibroblast-like cells admixed with scattered lymphocytes. There is important cross-talk between breast epithelium and stroma that promotes the normal structure and function of the breast.[2]

In the prepubertal breast in males and females, the large duct system ends in terminal ducts with minimal lobule formation. Changes in the breast are most dynamic and profound during the reproductive years (Fig. 23–2). Just as the endometrium grows and ebbs with each menstrual cycle, so does the breast.[3] In the first half of the menstrual cycle the lobules are relatively quiescent. After ovulation, under the influence of estrogen and rising progesterone levels, cell proliferation increases, as does the number of acini per lobule. The intralobular stroma also becomes markedly edematous. Upon menstruation, the fall in estrogen and progesterone levels induces the regression of the lobules and the disappearance of the stromal edema.

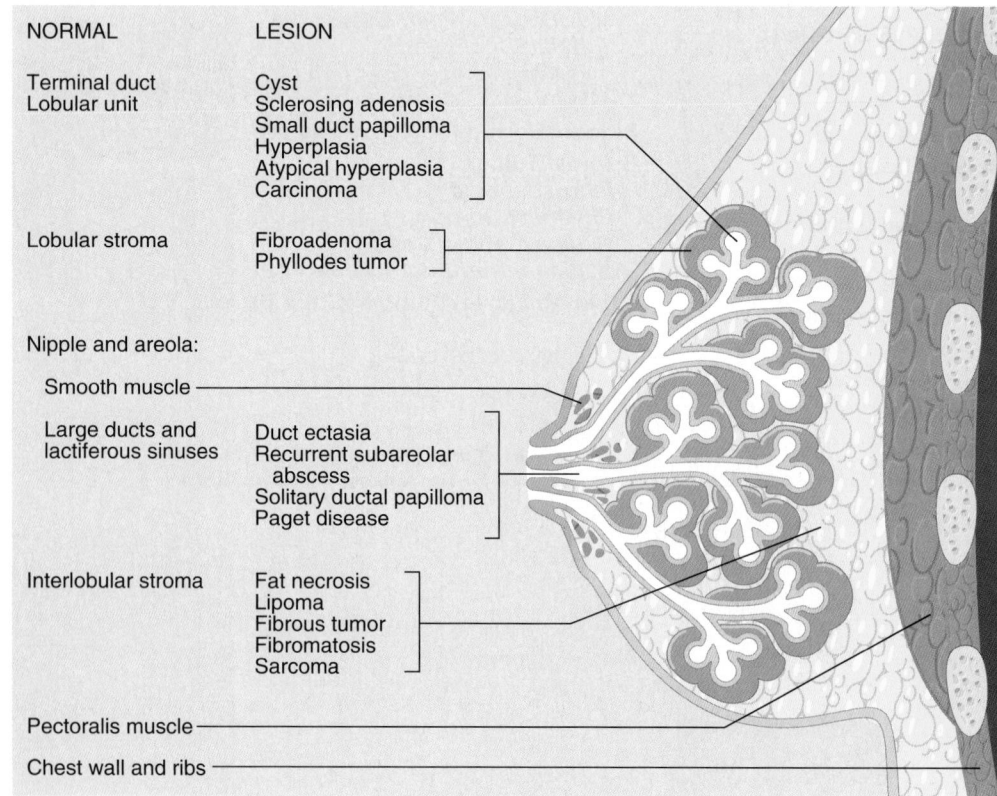

FIGURE 23–1 Anatomic origins of common breast lesions.

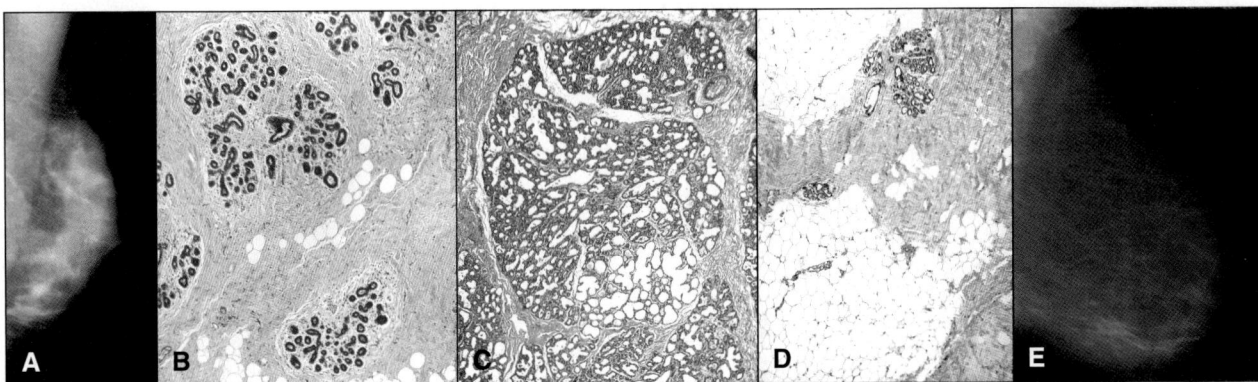

FIGURE 23–2 Life cycle changes. **A,** Mammograms in young women are typically radiodense or white in appearance, making mass-forming lesions or calcifications (which are also radiodense) difficult to detect. **B,** The density of a young woman's breast stems from the predominance of fibrous interlobular stroma and the paucity of adipose tissue. Before pregnancy the lobules are small and are invested by loose cellular intralobular stroma. Larger ducts connect lobules. **C,** During pregnancy, branching of terminal ducts produces more numerous, larger lobules. Luminal cells within lobules undergo lactational change, a precursor to milk formation. **D,** With increasing age the lobules decrease in size and number, and the interlobular stroma is replaced by adipose tissue. **E,** Mammograms become more radiolucent with age as a result of the increase in adipose tissue, which facilitates the detection of radiodense mass-forming lesions and calcifications. (**A, E,** Courtesy of Dr. Darrell Smith, Brigham and Women's Hospital, Boston, MA.)

Only with the onset of pregnancy does the breast become completely mature and functional. Lobules increase progressively in number and size. As a consequence, by the end of the pregnancy the breast is composed almost entirely of lobules separated by relatively scant stroma (Fig. 23–2C).

Immediately after delivery of the baby the luminal cells of the lobules produce colostrum (high in protein), which changes to milk (higher in fat and calories) over the next 10 days as progesterone levels drop. Not surprisingly, given these profound morphologic changes, the terminally differentiated breast has a specific pattern of gene expression.[4]

Breast milk not only provides complete nourishment from birth until several years of age, but it also provides protection against infection, allergies, and some autoimmune diseases. Maternal antibodies (chiefly secretory IgA), vitamins, enzymes, and numerous other mediators (e.g., cytokines, antioxidants, fibronectin, and lysozyme) augment the infant's own developing immune defenses. However, certain drugs, radioactive compounds given during diagnostic procedures, and viruses can also be passed to the infant through breast milk.

Upon the cessation of lactation, the breast epithelium and stroma undergo extensive remodeling.[5] Epithelial cells undergo apoptosis, lobules regress and atrophy, and the total breast size is diminished. However, full regression does not occur, and as a result pregnancy causes a permanent increase in the size and number of lobules.

After the third decade, long before menopause, lobules and their specialized stroma start to involute. Lobular atrophy may be almost complete in elderly females (Fig. 23–2D). The interlobular stroma also changes, since the radiodense fibrous stroma of the young female (see Fig. 23–2A) is progressively replaced by radiolucent adipose tissue (Fig. 23–2E).

Disorders of Development

Milkline Remnants. Supernumerary nipples or breasts result from the persistence of epidermal thickenings along the milk line, which extends from the axilla to the perineum. The disorders that affect the normally situated breast rarely arise in these heterotopic, hormone-responsive foci, which most commonly come to attention as a result of painful premenstrual enlargements.

Accessory Axillary Breast Tissue. In some women the normal ductal system extends into the subcutaneous tissue of the chest wall or the axillary fossa (the "axillary tail of Spence"). This epithelium can undergo lactational changes (resulting in a palpable mass) or give rise to carcinomas outside the breast proper. Therefore, prophylactic mastectomies markedly reduce, but do not completely eliminate, the risk of breast cancer.

Congenital Nipple Inversion. The failure of the nipple to evert during development is common and may be unilateral. Congenitally inverted nipples usually correct spontaneously during pregnancy, or can sometimes be everted by simple traction. Acquired nipple retraction is of more concern, since it may indicate the presence of an invasive cancer or an inflammatory disorder (e.g., recurrent subareolar abscess or duct ectasia).

Clinical Presentations of Breast Disease

The most common symptoms reported by women are pain, a palpable mass, "lumpiness" (without a discrete mass), or nipple discharge (Fig. 23–3). Asymptomatic women with abnormal findings on mammographic screening also require further evaluation.

Pain (mastalgia or mastodynia) is a common symptom that may be cyclic with menses or noncyclic. Diffuse cyclic pain has no pathologic correlate, and most effective treatments target hormone levels. Noncyclic pain is usually localized to one area of the breast. Causes include ruptured cysts, physical injury, and infections, but most often no specific lesion is identified. Although roughly 95% of painful masses are benign, it must be remembered that about 10% of breast cancers are painful.

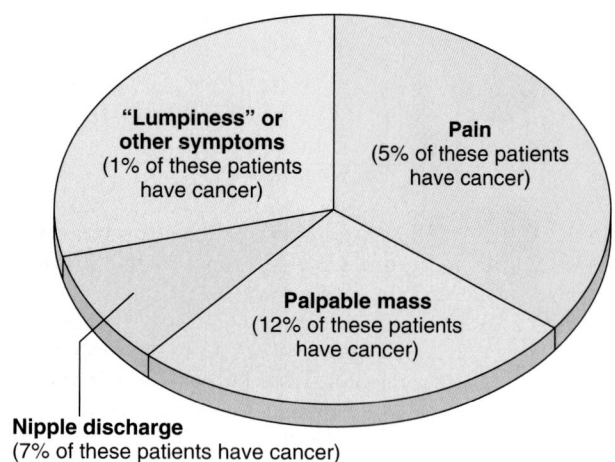

FIGURE 23–3   Common clinical symptoms of breast disease.

Discrete *palpable masses* are also common and must be distinguished from the normal nodularity (or "lumpiness") of the breast. The most common palpable lesions are invasive carcinomas, fibroadenomas, and cysts. A breast mass generally becomes palpable when it is at least 2 cm in size. Palpable masses are most common in premenopausal women (Fig. 23–4), but the likelihood of a palpable mass being malignant increases with age. For example, only 10% of breast masses in women under age 40 are malignant as compared with 60% of masses in women over age 50. Approximately 50% of carcinomas arise in the upper outer quadrant, 10% in each of the remaining quadrants, and about 20% in the central or subareolar region.

Nipple discharge is a less common finding that is most worrisome when it is spontaneous and unilateral, since it might be from an underlying carcinoma. A small discharge is often produced by the manipulation of normal breasts. Milky discharges (galactorrhea) are associated with elevated prolactin levels (e.g., by a pituitary adenoma), hypothyroidism, or endocrine anovulatory syndromes, and can also occur in patients taking oral contraceptives, tricyclic antidepressants, methyldopa, or phenothiazines. Repeated nipple stimulation can also induce lactation (a method sometimes used by women who wish to breastfeed adopted infants). Galactorrhea is not associated with malignancy.

Bloody or serous discharges are also most commonly associated with benign conditions, but in a significant minority of cases can be a sign of malignancy. The most common etiologies are solitary large duct papillomas and cysts. Benign bloody discharges may also occur during pregnancy, possibly as a result of the rapid growth and remodeling of the breast. The risk of malignancy with discharge increases with age, since it is associated with carcinoma in 7% of women younger than 60 years and in 30% of women older than 60 years (see Fig. 23–4). There is considerable interest in using induced nipple discharges as a source of cells and DNA for noninvasive cytologic and molecular breast cancer screening tests.[6]

Mammographic screening was introduced in the 1980s as a means to detect small, nonpalpable, asymptomatic breast carcinomas (discussed later). The sensitivity and specificity of mammography increase with age, as a result of replacement

of the fibrous, radiodense tissue of youth with the fatty, radiolucent tissue of the elderly (see Fig. 23–2). At age 40, the probability that a mammographic lesion is cancer is only 10%, but this rises to greater than 25% in women over 50 (see Fig. 23–4). *The principal mammographic signs of breast carcinoma are densities and calcifications:*

○ *Densities.* Mammographic densities are produced most commonly by invasive carcinomas, fibroadenomas, or cysts (see Fig. 23–4). Most neoplasms are radiologically denser than the intermingled normal breast tissue. The value of mammography lies in its ability to identify small, nonpalpable cancers. For example, the average size of an invasive carcinoma detected by mammography (1.1 cm) is less than half that of carcinomas detected by palpation (2.4 cm).

○ *Calcifications.* Calcifications form on secretions, necrotic debris, or hyalinized stroma. Benign calcifications are often associated with clusters of apocrine cysts, hyalinized fibroadenomas, and sclerosing adenosis. Calcifications associated with malignancy are usually small, irregular, numerous, and clustered. Ductal carcinoma in situ (DCIS) is most commonly detected as mammographic calcifications, which are often deposited in a linear, branching pattern as the carcinoma fills the ductal system. Mammographic screening has increased the number of breast cancers diagnosed as DCIS (see Fig. 23–13). Invasive carcinomas presenting as calcifications without an accompanying radiodensity are uncommon, generally small in size, and rarely associated with lymph node metastases.

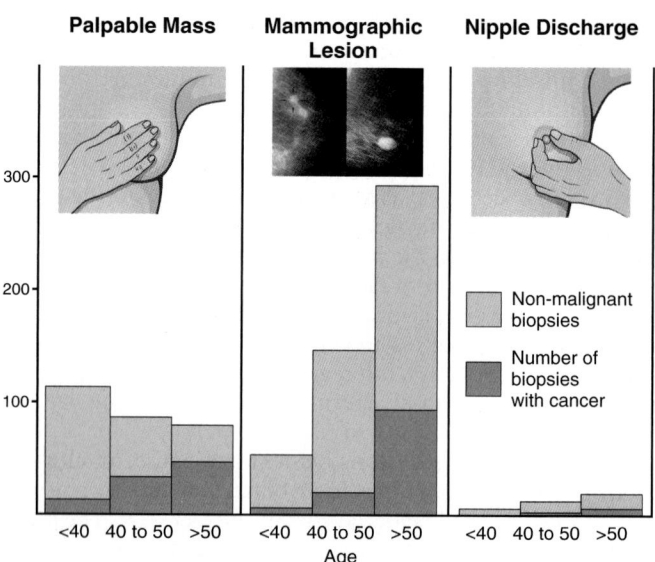

Most frequently diagnosed lesions according to clinical presentation:

Carcinoma (33%)	Carcinoma (23%)	Papilloma (50%)
Fibroadenoma (23%)	Fibroadenoma (20%)	Carcinoma (10%)
Cysts (10%)	Cysts (22%)	Cysts (20%)

FIGURE 23–4   Frequency of pathologically diagnosed benign and malignant breast lesions by clinical presentation and age. Based on 914 women undergoing diagnostic breast surgery at Brigham and Women's Hospital (Boston, MA) from January to June 2001.

In about 10% of cases, carcinomas are missed by mammography. The principal causes of these failures are the presence of surrounding radiodense tissue (especially in younger women) that obscures the tumor, the absence of calcifications, small size, a diffuse infiltrative pattern with little or no desmoplastic response, or a location close to the chest wall or in the periphery of the breast. The inability to image a palpable mass does not indicate that it is benign, and all palpable masses require further investigation.

Other imaging modalities are useful adjuncts. Ultrasonography distinguishes between solid and cystic lesions and can define more precisely the borders of solid lesions. Most palpable masses that are not imaged by mammography are detectable by ultrasound. Magnetic resonance imaging (MRI) detects cancers by the rapid uptake of contrast agents due to increased tumor vascularity and blood flow. It is useful in screening for cancer in women with dense breasts or at very high risk for cancer, in determining the extent of chest wall invasion by locally advanced cancers, and in the evaluation of breast implant rupture. A high rate of false-positive results limits its usefulness in screening women outside of these groups.

Inflammatory Disorders

Inflammatory diseases of the breast are uncommon, accounting for less than 1% of women with breast symptoms. Women usually present with an erythematous swollen painful breast. "Inflammatory breast cancer" mimics inflammation by obstructing dermal vasculature with tumor emboli, resulting in an enlarged erythematous breast, and should always be suspected in a nonlactating woman with the clinical appearance of mastitis.

ACUTE MASTITIS

Almost all cases of acute mastitis occur during the first month of breastfeeding. During this time the breast is vulnerable to bacterial infection because of the development of cracks and fissures in the nipples. From this portal of entry, *Staphylococcus aureus* or, less commonly, streptococci invade the breast tissue. The breast is erythematous and painful, and fever is often present. At the outset only one duct system or sector of the breast is involved. If not treated the infection may spread to the entire breast.

Morphology. Staphylococcal infections usually produce a localized area of acute inflammation that may progress to the formation of single or multiple abscesses. Streptococcal infections tend to cause (as elsewhere) a diffuse spreading infection that eventually involves the entire breast. The involved breast tissue is infiltrated by neutrophils and may be necrotic.

Most cases of lactational mastitis are easily treated with appropriate antibiotics and continued expression of milk from the breast. Rarely, surgical drainage is required.

PERIDUCTAL MASTITIS

This condition is known by a variety of names, including recurrent subareolar abscess, squamous metaplasia of lactiferous ducts, and Zuska disease. Women, and sometimes men, present with a painful erythematous subareolar mass that clinically appears to be an infectious process. More than 90% of the afflicted are smokers. This condition is not associated with lactation, a specific reproductive history, or age. In recurrent cases, a fistula tract often tunnels under the smooth muscle of the nipple and opens onto the skin at the edge of the areola. Many women with this condition have an inverted nipple, most likely as a secondary effect of the underlying inflammation. The strong association with cigarette smoking is intriguing. It has been suggested that the vitamin A deficiency associated with smoking or toxic substances in tobacco smoke alter the differentiation of the ductal epithelium.[7]

Morphology. The key histologic feature is keratinizing squamous metaplasia of the nipple ducts (Fig. 23–5). Keratin shed from these cells plugs the ductal system, causing dilation and eventually rupture of the duct. An intense chronic and granulomatous inflammatory response develops once keratin spills into the surrounding periductal tissue. Sometimes a secondary bacterial infection supervenes and causes acute inflammation.

In most cases en bloc surgical removal of the involved duct and contiguous fistula tract is curative.[7] Simple incision drains the abscess cavity, but the offending keratinizing epithelium remains and recurrences are common. When bacterial infection is present, antibiotics also have a therapeutic role.

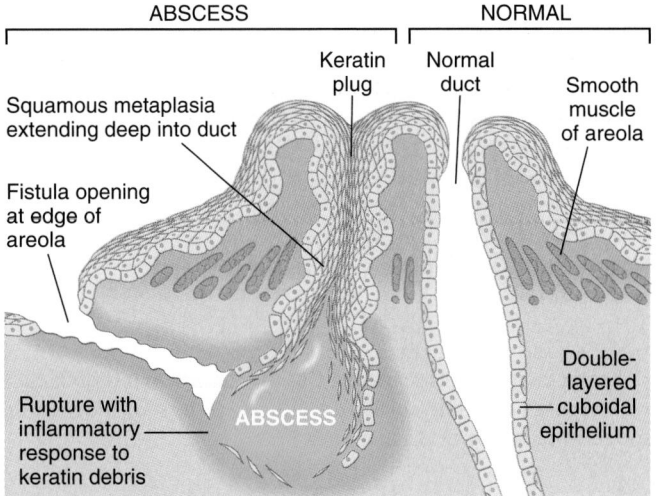

FIGURE 23–5 Recurrent subareolar abscess. When squamous metaplasia extends deep into a nipple duct, keratin becomes trapped and accumulates. If the duct ruptures, the ensuing intense inflammatory response to keratin results in an erythematous painful mass. A fistula tract may burrow beneath the smooth muscle of the nipple to open at the edge of the areola.

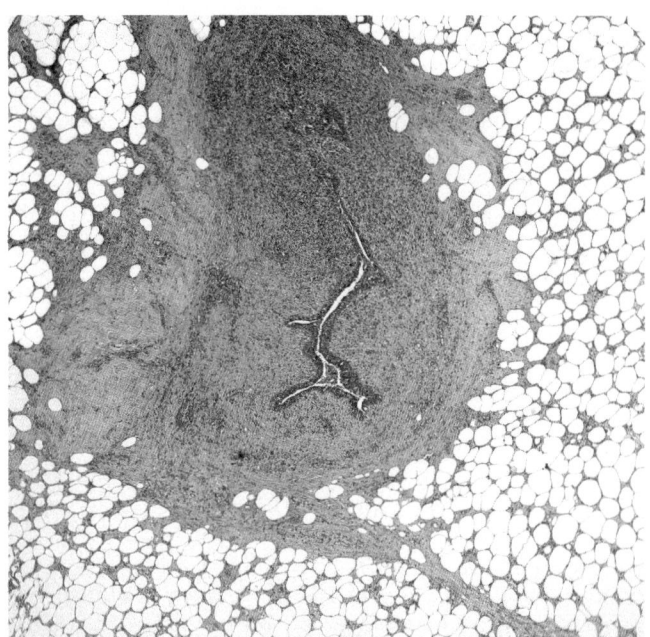

FIGURE 23–6 Mammary duct ectasia. Chronic inflammation and fibrosis surround an ectatic duct filled with inspissated debris. The fibrotic response can produce a firm irregular mass that mimics invasive carcinoma on palpation or mammogram.

MAMMARY DUCT ECTASIA

This disorder tends to occur in the fifth or sixth decade of life, usually in multiparous women. Unlike periductal mastitis, it is not associated with cigarette smoking. Patients present with a poorly defined palpable periareolar mass that is often associated with thick, white nipple secretions and sometimes with skin retraction. Pain and erythema are uncommon.

> **Morphology.** This lesion is characterized chiefly by dilation of ducts, inspissation of breast secretions, and a marked periductal and interstitial chronic granulomatous inflammatory reaction (Fig. 23–6). The dilated ducts are filled by granular debris that contains numerous lipid-laden macrophages. The periductal and interductal tissue contains dense infiltrates of lymphocytes and macrophages, and variable numbers of plasma cells. On occasion, granulomatous inflammation forms around cholesterol deposits. Fibrosis may eventually produce skin and nipple retraction. Squamous metaplasia of nipple ducts is absent.

The principal significance of this disorder is that it produces an irregular palpable mass that mimics the mammographic appearance of carcinoma.

FAT NECROSIS

Fat necrosis can present as a painless palpable mass, skin thickening or retraction, a mammographic density, or mammographic calcifications. The majority of affected women have a history of breast trauma or prior surgery.

> **Morphology.** Acute lesions may be hemorrhagic and contain central areas of liquefactive fat necrosis. In subacute lesions the areas of fat necrosis take on the appearance of ill-defined, firm, gray-white nodules containing small chalky-white foci or dark hemorrhagic debris. The central region of necrotic fat cells is initially associated with an intense neutrophilic infiltrate mixed with macrophages. Over the next few days proliferating fibroblasts associated with new vessels and chronic inflammatory cells surround the injured area. Subsequently, giant cells, calcifications, and hemosiderin make their appearance, and eventually the focus is replaced by scar tissue or is encircled and walled off by fibrous tissue.

As with other inflammatory breast disorders, the major clinical significance of the condition is its possible confusion with breast cancer.

LYMPHOCYTIC MASTOPATHY (SCLEROSING LYMPHOCYTIC LOBULITIS)

This condition presents with single or multiple hard palpable masses. The masses may be bilateral and may be detected as mammographic densities. The lesions are so hard that it can be difficult to obtain tissue with a needle biopsy. Microscopically, they show collagenized stroma surrounding atrophic ducts and lobules. The epithelial basement membrane is often thickened. A prominent lymphocytic infiltrate surrounds the epithelium and small blood vessels. This condition is most common in women with type 1 (insulin-dependent) diabetes or autoimmune thyroid disease. Based on this association, it is hypothesized to have an autoimmune basis. Its only clinical significance is that it must be distinguished from breast cancer.

GRANULOMATOUS MASTITIS

Granulomatous inflammation is present in less than 1% of all breast biopsy specimens. The causes include systemic granulomatous diseases (e.g., Wegener granulomatosis or sarcoidosis) that occasionally involve the breast, and granulomatous infections caused by mycobacteria or fungi. Infections of this type are most common in immunocompromised patients or adjacent to foreign objects such as breast prostheses or nipple piercings. *Granulomatous lobular mastitis* is an uncommon breast-limited disease that only occurs in parous women. The granulomatous inflammation is confined to the lobules, suggesting that it is caused by a hypersensitivity reaction to antigens expressed by lobular epithelium during lactation.

Benign Epithelial Lesions

A wide variety of benign alterations in ducts and lobules are observed in the breast. Most come to clinical attention when detected by mammography or as incidental findings in surgical specimens. These lesions have been divided into three groups, according to the subsequent risk of developing breast cancer: (1) nonproliferative breast changes, (2) proliferative breast disease, and (3) atypical hyperplasia.

NONPROLIFERATIVE BREAST CHANGES (FIBROCYSTIC CHANGES)

This group includes a number of very common morphologic alterations that are often grouped under the term *fibrocystic changes*. To the clinician the term might mean "lumpy bumpy" breasts on palpation; to the radiologist, a dense breast with cysts; and to the pathologist, benign histologic findings. These lesions are termed *nonproliferative* to distinguish them from "proliferative" changes, which are associated with an increased risk of breast cancer.

Morphology. There are three principal morphologic changes: (1) cystic change, often with apocrine metaplasia; (2) fibrosis; and (3) adenosis.

- *Cysts.* Small cysts form by the dilation and unfolding of lobules, and in turn may coalesce to form larger cysts. Unopened cysts contain turbid, semi-translucent fluid that produces a brown or blue color (blue-dome cysts) (Fig. 23–7B). Cysts are lined either by a flattened atrophic epithelium or by metaplastic apocrine cells. The latter cells, which have an abundant granular, eosinophilic cytoplasm and round nuclei, closely resemble the normal apocrine epithelium of sweat glands (Fig. 23–7C). Calcifications are common and may be detected by mammography (see Fig. 23–7A). "Milk of calcium" is a term mammographers use to describe calcifications that line the bottom of a rounded cyst. Cysts are alarming when they are solitary and firm to palpation. The diagnosis is confirmed by the disappearance of the cyst after fine-needle aspiration of its contents.

- *Fibrosis.* Cysts frequently rupture, releasing secretory material into the adjacent stroma. The resulting chronic inflammation and fibrosis contribute to the palpable firmness of the breast.

- *Adenosis.* Adenosis is defined as an increase in the number of acini per lobule. A normal physiologic adenosis occurs during pregnancy. In nonpregnant women, adenosis can occur as a focal change. The acini are often enlarged (blunt-duct adenosis), but are not distorted as is seen in sclerosing adenosis, described later. Calcifications are occasionally present within the lumens. The acini are lined by columnar cells, which may appear benign or show atypical features ("flat epithelial atypia"). These lesions may be the earliest recognizable precursor of epithelial neoplasia.[8–10]

Lactational adenomas present as palpable masses in pregnant or lactating women. They are formed by normal-appearing breast tissue with physiologic adenosis and lactational changes. These lesions are probably not true neoplasms but an exaggerated focal response to hormonal influences.

PROLIFERATIVE BREAST DISEASE WITHOUT ATYPIA

These changes are commonly detected as mammographic densities, calcifications, or as incidental findings in specimens from biopsies performed for other reasons. Although each can be found in isolation, typically more than one lesion is present, frequently in association with nonproliferative breast changes.

These lesions are characterized by proliferation of ductal epithelium and/or stroma without cytologic or architectural features suggestive of carcinoma in situ.

Morphology

Epithelial Hyperplasia. Normal breast ducts and lobules are lined by a double layer of myoepithelial cells and luminal cells (Fig. 23–8A). Epithelial hyperplasia is defined by the presence of more than two cell layers. The additional cells consist of both luminal and myoepithelial cell types that fill and distend ducts and lobules. Irregular lumens can often be discerned at the periphery of the cellular masses (Fig. 23–8B). Epithelial hyperplasia is usually an incidental finding.

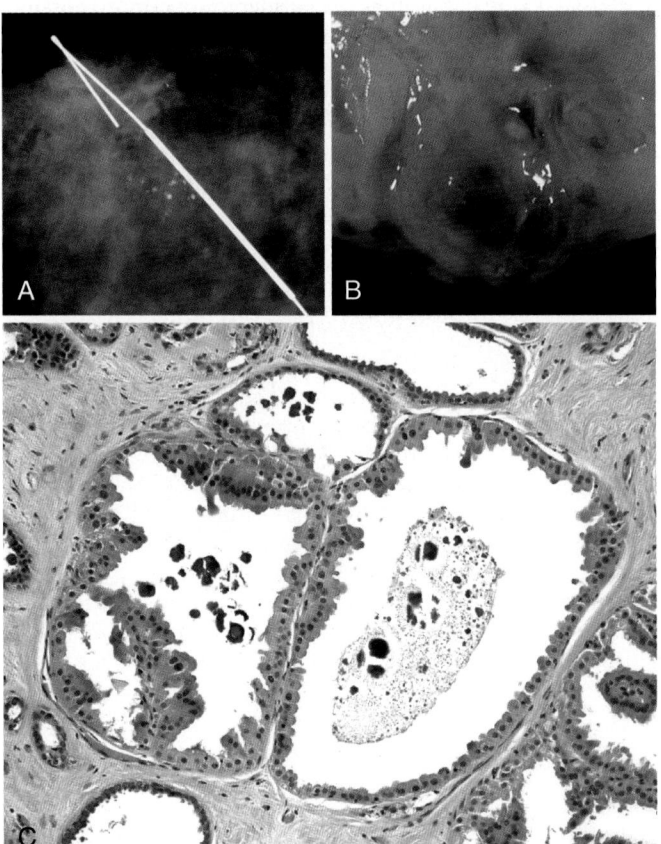

FIGURE 23–7 Apocrine cysts. **A,** Clustered, rounded calcifications are seen in a radiograph. **B,** Gross appearance of typical cysts filled with dark, turbid fluid contents. **C,** Cysts are lined by apocrine cells with round nuclei and abundant granular cytoplasm. Note the luminal calcifications, which form on secretory debris.

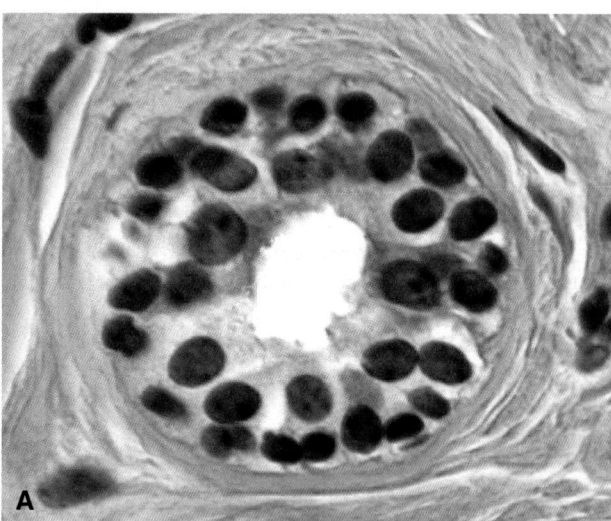 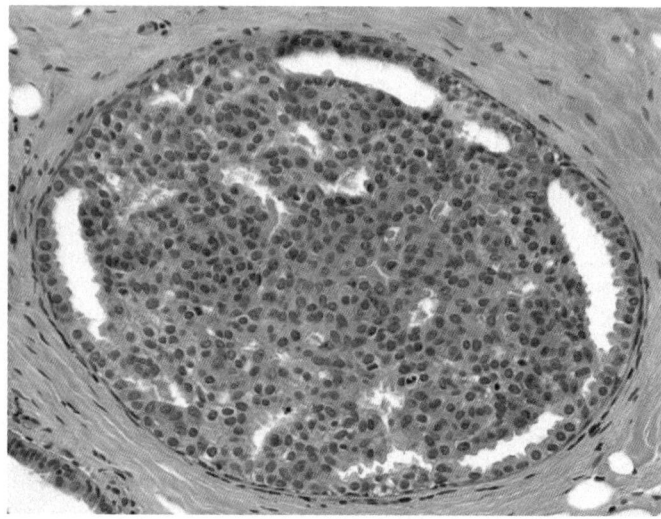

FIGURE 23–8 **A,** A normal duct or acinus with a single basally located myoepithelial cell layer (cells with dark, compact nuclei and scant cytoplasm) and a single luminal cell layer (cells with larger open nuclei, small nucleoli, and more abundant cytoplasm). **B,** Epithelial hyperplasia. The lumen is filled by a heterogeneous, mixed population of luminal and myoepithelial cell types. Irregular slitlike fenestrations are prominent at the periphery.

Sclerosing Adenosis. The number of acini per terminal duct is increased to at least double the number found in uninvolved lobules. The normal lobular arrangement is maintained. The acini are compressed and distorted in the central portions of the lesion but characteristically dilated at the periphery. Myoepithelial cells are usually prominent. On occasion, stromal fibrosis may completely compress the lumens to create the appearance of solid cords or double strands of cells lying within dense stroma, a histologic pattern that at times closely mimics the appearance of invasive carcinoma (Fig. 23–9). Sclerosing adenosis can come to attention as a palpable mass, a radiologic density, or calcifications.

Complex Sclerosing Lesion. Complex sclerosing lesions have components of sclerosing adenosis, papillomas, and epithelial hyperplasia. One member of this group, the radial sclerosing lesion ("radial scar"), is the only commonly occurring benign lesion that forms irregular masses and can closely mimic invasive carcinoma mammographically, grossly, and histologically (Fig. 23–10). There is a central nidus of entrapped glands in a hyalinized stroma with long radiating projections into stroma. The term *radial scar* is a misnomer, as these lesions are not associated with prior trauma or surgery.

Papillomas. Papillomas are composed of multiple branching fibrovascular cores, each having a connective tissue axis lined by luminal and myoepithelial cells (Fig. 23–11). Growth occurs within a dilated duct. Epithelial hyperplasia and apocrine metaplasia are frequently present. Large duct papillomas are usually solitary and situated in the lactiferous sinuses of the nipple. Small duct papillomas are commonly multiple and located deeper within the ductal system.

More than 80% of large duct papillomas produce a nipple discharge. Large papillomas may undergo infarction, possibly because of torsion on the stalk, resulting in a bloody discharge. Nonbloody discharge probably results from intermittent blockage and release of normal breast secretions or irritation of the duct by the papilloma. The remaining large duct papillomas and most small duct papillomas come to clinical attention as small palpable masses, or as densities or calcifications seen on mammograms.

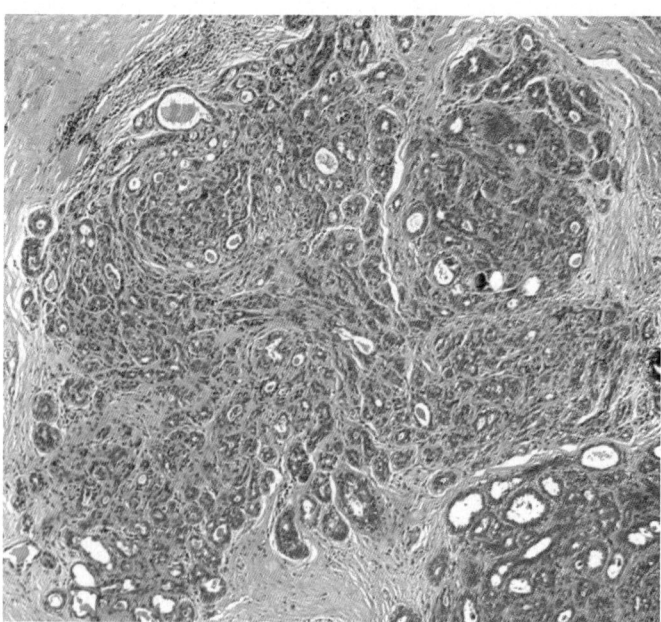

FIGURE 23–9 Sclerosing adenosis. The involved terminal duct lobular unit is enlarged, and the acini are compressed and distorted by dense stroma. Calcifications are present within some of the lumens. Unlike carcinomas, the acini are arranged in a swirling pattern, and the outer border is well circumscribed.

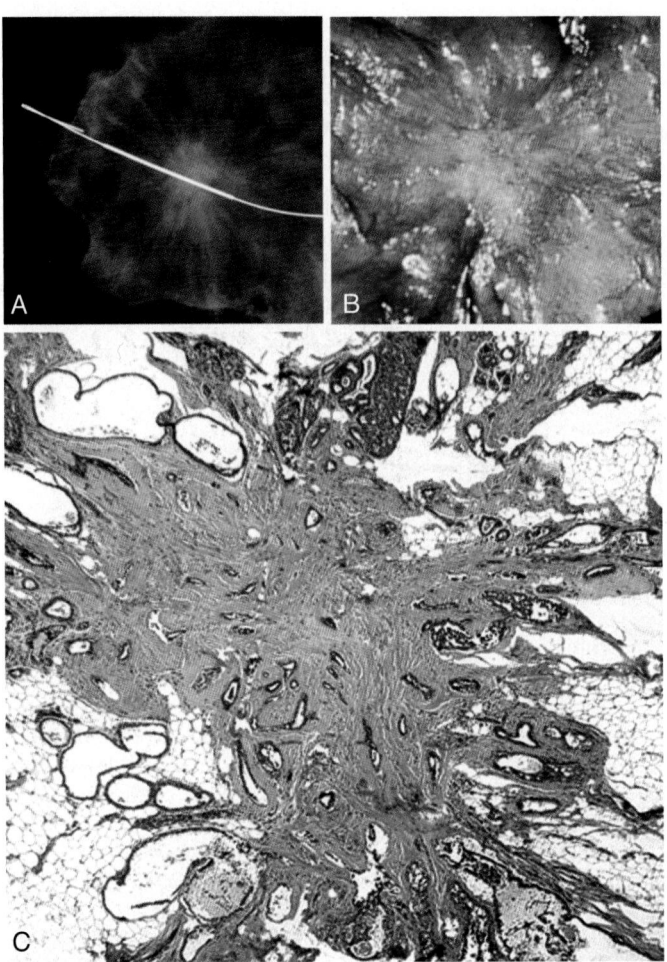

FIGURE 23–10   Radial sclerosing lesion. **A,** The radiograph shows an irregular central mass with long radiodense projections. **B,** Grossly the mass appears solid and has irregular borders, but it is not as firm as an invasive carcinoma. **C,** The mass consists of a central nidus of small tubules entrapped in a densely fibrotic stroma and numerous projections containing epithelium with varying degrees of cyst formation and hyperplasia.

PROLIFERATIVE BREAST DISEASE WITH ATYPIA

Proliferative disease with atypia includes atypical ductal hyperplasia and atypical lobular hyperplasia. Atypical ductal hyperplasia is present in 5% to 17% of specimens from biopsies performed for calcifications and is found less frequently in specimens from biopsies for mammographic densities or palpable masses. Occasionally, atypical ductal hyperplasia is associated with radiologic calcifications; more commonly it is adjacent to another calcifying lesion. Atypical lobular hyperplasia is an incidental finding and is found in fewer than 5% of specimens from biopsies performed for any reason.

> **Morphology.** Atypical hyperplasia is a cellular proliferation resembling carcinoma in situ but lacking sufficient qualitative or quantitative features for diagnosis as carcinoma. Unlike other benign changes, atypical hyperplasias harbor some of the same acquired genetic losses and gains that are present in carcinoma in situ.

> **Atypical ductal hyperplasia** is recognized by its histologic resemblance to ductal carcinoma in situ (DCIS). It consists of a relatively monomorphic proliferation of regularly spaced cells, sometimes with cribriform spaces. It is distinguished from DCIS by being limited in extent and only partially filling ducts (Fig. 23–12A).
>
> **Atypical lobular hyperplasia** is defined as a proliferation of cells identical to those of lobular carcinoma in situ (LCIS, described later), but the cells do not fill or distend more than 50% of the acini within a lobule (Fig. 23–12B). Atypical lobular hyperplasia can also involve contiguous ducts through pagetoid spread, in which atypical lobular cells lie between the ductal basement membrane and overlying normal ductal epithelial cells.

CLINICAL SIGNIFICANCE OF BENIGN EPITHELIAL CHANGES

Multiple epidemiologic studies have classified benign histologic changes in the breast and determined their association with the later development of invasive cancer[11–13] (Table 23–1). Nonproliferative changes do not increase the risk of cancer. Proliferative disease is associated with a mild increase in risk, while proliferative disease with atypia confers a moderate increase in risk. Both breasts are at increased risk, although a few more subsequent carcinomas occur in the same breast.[14] Risk reduction can be achieved by bilateral prophylactic mastectomy or treatment with estrogen antagonists, such as tamoxifen.[15] However, more than 80% of women with atypical hyperplasia will not develop breast cancer, and many choose careful clinical and radiologic surveillance over intervention.

Carcinoma of the Breast

Carcinoma of the breast is the most common non-skin malignancy in women. A woman who lives to age 90 has a one in

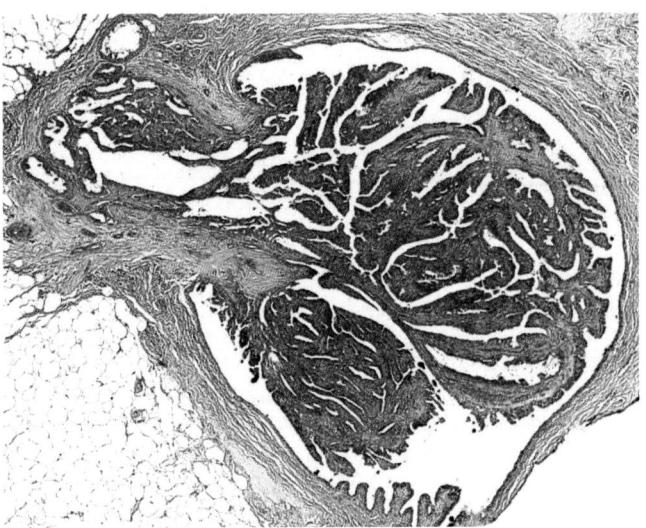

FIGURE 23–11   Intraductal papilloma. A central fibrovascular core extends from the wall of a duct. The papillae arborize within the lumen and are lined by myoepithelial and luminal cells.

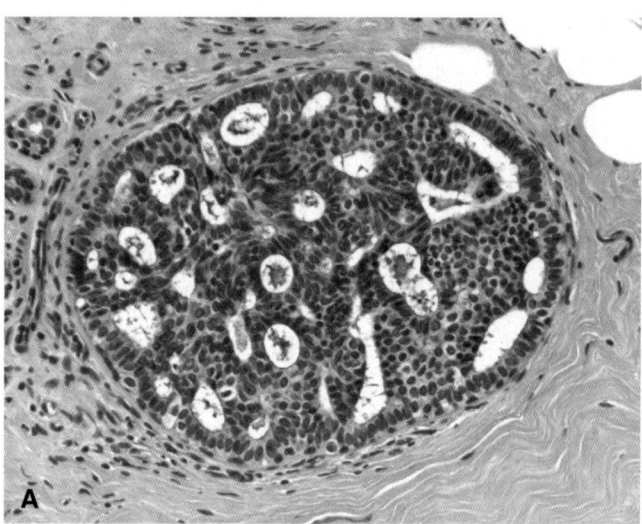
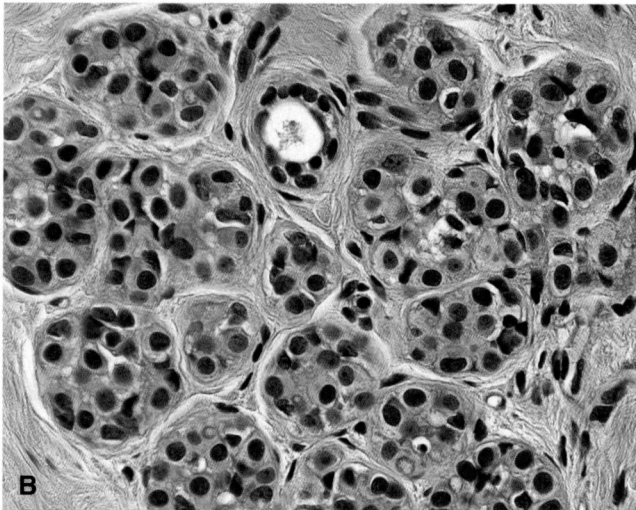

FIGURE 23–12 **A,** Atypical ductal hyperplasia. A duct is filled with a mixed population of cells consisting of oriented columnar cells at the periphery and more rounded cells within the central portion. Although some of the spaces are round and regular, the peripheral spaces are irregular and slitlike. These features are highly atypical, but fall short of a diagnosis of DCIS. **B,** Atypical lobular hyperplasia. A population of monomorphic small, round, loosely cohesive cells partially fill a lobule. Some intracellular lumens can be seen. Although the cells are morphologically identical to the cells of LCIS, the extent of involvement is not sufficient for this diagnosis.

eight chance of developing breast cancer. In 2007 an estimated 178,480 women were diagnosed with invasive breast cancer, 62,030 with carcinoma in situ, and over 40,000 women died of the disease (Surveillance Epidemiology and End Results

TABLE 23–1	Epithelial Breast Lesions and the Risk of Developing Invasive Carcinoma
Pathologic Lesion	**Relative Risk (Absolute Lifetime Risk)***
NONPROLIFERATIVE BREAST CHANGES (Fibrocystic changes)	1.0 (3%)
Duct ectasia Cysts Apocrine change Mild hyperplasia Adenosis Fibroadenoma w/o complex features	
PROLIFERATIVE DISEASE WITHOUT ATYPIA	1.5 to 2.0 (5% to 7%)
Moderate or florid hyperplasia Sclerosing adenosis Papilloma Complex sclerosing lesion (radial scar) Fibroadenoma with complex features	
PROLIFERATIVE DISEASE WITH ATYPIA	4.0 to 5.0 (13% to 17%)
Atypical ductal hyperplasia (ADH) Atypical lobular hyperplasia (ALH)	
CARCINOMA IN SITU Lobular carcinoma in situ (LCIS) Ductal carcinoma in situ (DCIS)	8.0 to 10.0 (25% to 30%)

*Relative risk is the risk compared to women without any risk factors. Absolute lifetime risk is the percentage of patients expected to develop invasive carcinoma if untreated.

[SEER] data at http://seer.cancer.gov/). As the demographic bulge of the "baby boomers" continues to grow older, the number of women with breast cancer is expected to increase by about a third over the next 20 years. It is both ironic and tragic that a neoplasm arising in an exposed organ, readily accessible to self-examination and clinical diagnosis, continues to exact such a heavy toll. Only lung cancer causes more cancer deaths in women living in the United States.

It has long been appreciated that breast cancer is a heterogeneous disease with a wide array of histologic appearances. Recent gene profiling studies have confirmed that there are many types of cancers but also show that most carcinomas cluster into several major groups with important biologic and clinical differences. The majority of carcinomas are estrogen receptor (ER) positive and are characterized by a gene signature dominated by the dozens of genes under the control of estrogen. Among the ER-negative tumors, many fall into a distinctive "basal-like" group that is discussed later.

ER-positive and ER-negative carcinomas show striking differences with regard to patient characteristics, pathologic features, treatment response, and outcome. In the past, most studies grouped all breast cancers together, but it is now widely recognized that the diagnosis of breast cancer encompasses multiple molecular subclasses of disease, as discussed later.

INCIDENCE AND EPIDEMIOLOGY

After remaining constant for many years (except for a transient rise in 1974 attributed to increased awareness surrounding the recurrence of breast cancer in Betty Ford and Happy Rockefeller), the incidence of breast cancer began to increase in older women (Fig. 23–13). What seemed to be an alarming trend was, in part, due to the introduction of mammographic screening in the early 1980s. Rates of screening gradually increased but have recently reached a plateau of 60% to 80% of eligible women. The main benefit of screening is the detection of small, predominantly ER-positive invasive carcinomas and in situ carcinomas. DCIS is almost exclusively detected by

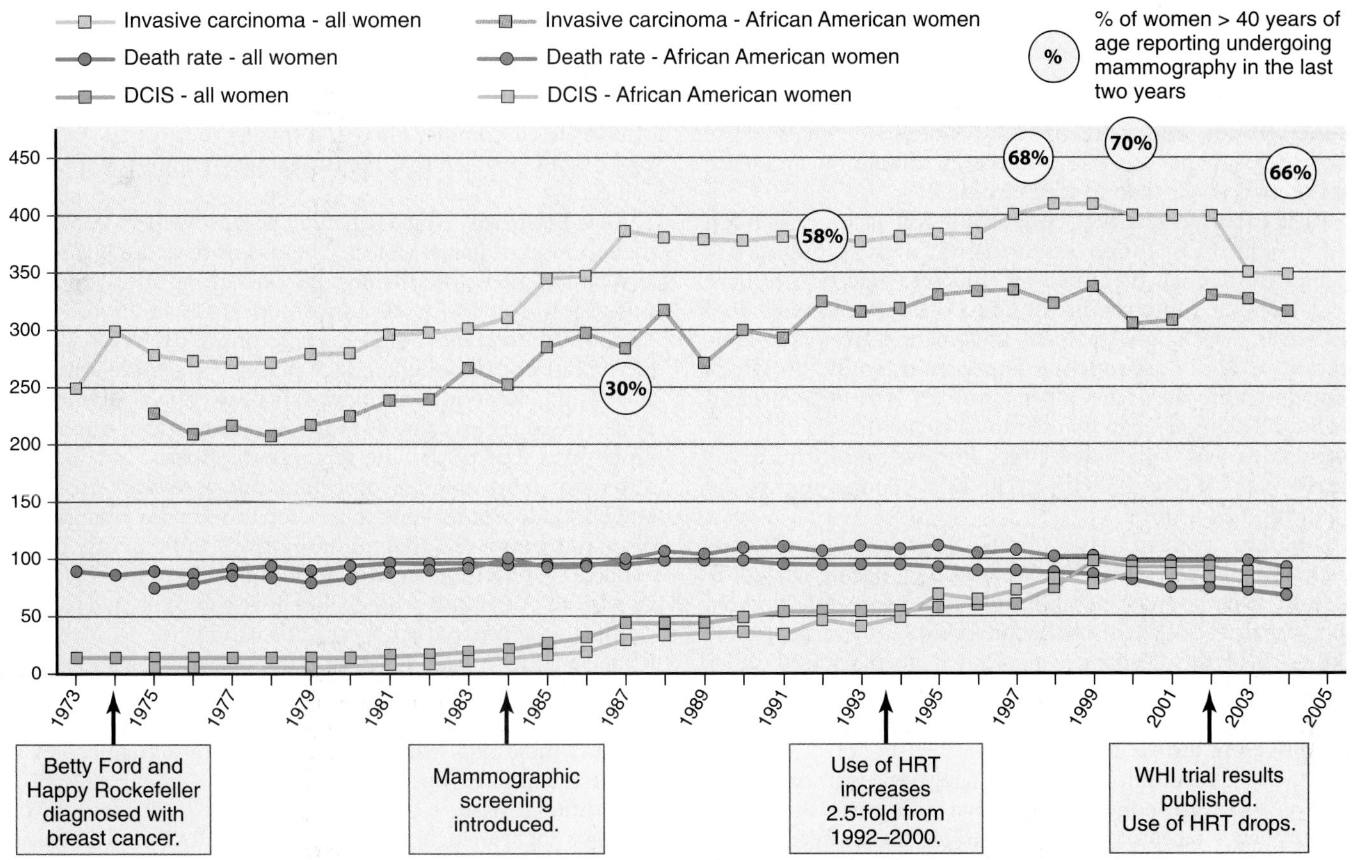

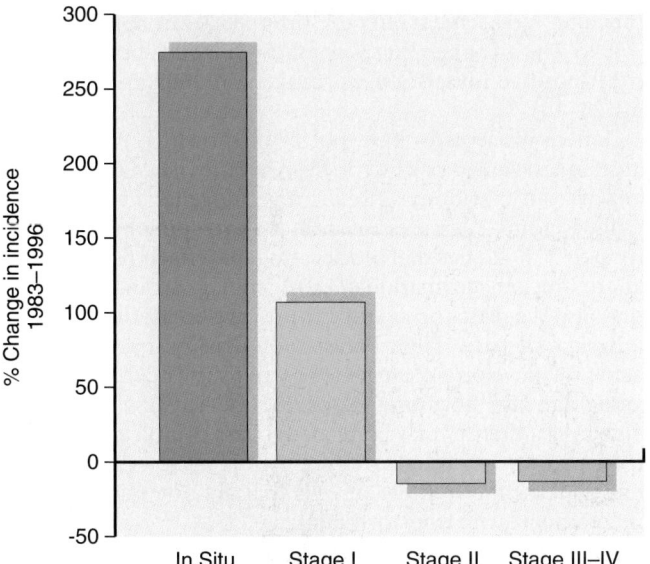

FIGURE 23–13 Breast cancer incidence and mortality rates for women over 50 years of age. Rates are per 100,000 women and are age-adjusted to the 2000 US standard million population. (SEER Cancer Statistics Review; http://seer.cancer.gov/)

mammography, providing an explanation for the sharp increase in the diagnosis of DCIS since 1980 (see Fig. 23–13). Small node-negative carcinomas (stage I), which are best detected by mammography, increased in frequency as the

number of large, advanced-stage breast carcinomas (stages II to IV) diminished modestly (Fig. 23–14). Over the same time period the incidence of breast carcinoma in younger women, for whom screening is not recommended, did not change.

From 2001 to 2004, the incidence of ER-positive invasive cancer decreased. The reasons for this trend are probably multifactorial. The plateau in the number of women screened should be associated with a decrease in incidence back to prescreening levels. In addition, in 2002 many women stopped using postmenopausal hormone replacement therapy after the results of the Women's Health Initiative trial showed that this treatment had limited benefits.[16] It is possible that this treatment stimulated the growth or development of ER-positive cancers. During the same time period the incidence of breast cancer for African American women remained stable and the number of ER-negative cancers increased, suggesting that these cancers are not affected by hormonal treatment. Finally, there may have been changes in modifiable risk factors (e.g., the frequency and length of breastfeeding) or the use of chemopreventive agents that can lower risk. Whatever the reason or reasons, the decrease in breast cancers is a promising trend that hopefully will continue.

During the 1980s the number of women dying of breast cancer remained constant, while the incidence of breast cancer was increasing. Since 1994 the breast cancer mortality rate for all women has slowly declined from 30% to 20% (Fig. 23–13). The decrease is attributed to the detection of clinically significant cancers at a curable stage due to screening, as well as

FIGURE 23–14 Change in stage of breast cancer at presentation from 1983 to 1996. (SEER Cancer Statistics Review, http://seer.cancer.gov/)

better and more effective treatment modalities. The number of women dying from their breast cancer has decreased from 30% to 20%. However, the decline in the death rate has been less impressive for African American women, women in other ethnic groups, and women with ER-negative cancers. The mortality is higher in these groups even though the incidence of cancer is lower than in white women.

Risk Factors. The most important risk factor is gender; only 1% of breast cancer cases occur in men. Common risk factors for women identified by epidemiologic studies have been combined into the Breast Cancer Risk Assessment Tool (BCRAT), which now includes information from the Contraceptive and Reproductive Experiences study,[17,18] which provides more accurate information for African American women. The model can be used to calculate the absolute risk of an individual woman developing invasive cancer within the next 5 years or over a lifetime. The BCRAT incorporates the following risk factors.

Age. The incidence rises throughout a woman's lifetime, peaking at the age of 75–80 years and then declining slightly thereafter. The average age at diagnosis is 61 for white women, 56 for Hispanic women, and 46 for African American women. Only 20% of non-Hispanic white women are diagnosed under the age of 50, compared with 35% of African American women and 31% of Hispanic women. Breast cancer is very rare in all groups before the age of 25.

Although carcinoma is uncommon in young women, almost half of these are either ER negative or human epidermal growth factor receptor 2 (HER2/neu) positive, whereas these cancers make up less than a third of cancers in women over the age of 40.

Age at Menarche. Women who reach menarche when younger than 11 years of age have a 20% increased risk compared with women who are more than 14 years of age at menarche. Late menopause also increases risk.

Age at First Live Birth. Women who experience a first full-term pregnancy at ages younger than 20 years have half the risk of nulliparous women or women over the age of 35 at their first birth. It is hypothesized that pregnancy results in terminal differentiation of milk-producing luminal cells, removing them from the potential pool of cancer precursors.[4] This protective effect might be overshadowed in older women by stimulation of proliferation early in pregnancy of cells that have already undergone preneoplastic changes. It is also possible that the changes in stroma that allow the growth and expansion of lobules during pregnancy facilitate the transition from in situ to invasive carcinoma. These pregnancy-related changes may help explain the transient increase in cancer risk that follows a pregnancy, an effect that is most pronounced in older women.[5] Age at first live birth is not a strong risk factor for African American women.

First-Degree Relatives with Breast Cancer. The risk of breast cancer increases with the number of affected first-degree relatives (mother, sister, or daughter), especially if the cancer occurred at a young age. However, most women do not have a family history. Only 13% of women with breast cancer have one affected first-degree relative, and only 1% have two or more. In turn, over 87% of women with a family history will not develop breast cancer. Most family risk is probably due to the interaction of low-risk susceptibility genes and nongenetic factors. The BCRAT is not designed to calculate the risk for women with a mutation in a high-risk breast cancer gene, such as *BRCA1* or *BRCA2* (see the section "Hereditary Breast Cancer" below).

Atypical Hyperplasia. A history of prior breast biopsies, especially if revealing atypical hyperplasia, increases the risk of invasive carcinoma. There is a smaller increase in risk associated with proliferative breast changes without atypia (see Table 23–1).

Race/Ethnicity. Non-Hispanic white women have the highest rates of breast cancer. The risk of developing an invasive carcinoma within the next 20 years at age 50 is 1 in 15 for this group, 1 in 20 for African Americans, 1 in 26 for Asian/Pacific Islanders, and 1 in 27 for Hispanics.[19] However, women of African or Hispanic ancestry present at a more advanced stage and have an increased mortality rate. Social factors such as decreased access to health care and lower use of mammography may well contribute to these disparities, but biologic differences also play an important role.[20] African American and Hispanic women tend to develop cancers at a younger age, prior to menopause, that are more likely to be poorly differentiated and ER negative. Mutations in *p53* are more common in African American women but less common in Hispanic women, as compared with non-Hispanic white women. It is suspected that variation in breast cancer risk genes across ethnic groups is responsible, at least in part, for these differences. One known example is the incidence of *BRCA1* and *BRCA2* mutations, which occur at different frequencies in different ethnic groups.[21]

Additional risk factors (listed below) are recognized, but have not been incorporated into the BCRAT model because of their rarity or uncertainties about quantifying the magnitude of risk.

Estrogen Exposure. Postmenopausal hormone replacement therapy increases the risk of breast cancer 1.2- to 1.7-fold, and adding progesterone increases the risk further. Most excess cancers are ER-positive carcinomas, including invasive lobular carcinomas, that tend to be of small size when detected. As a result, any effect on the death rate is expected to be small. After publication of the Women's Health Initiative trial in 2002, the number of postmenopausal women receiving hormone replacement therapy dropped from approximately 17% to 7%, a change that was followed by a substantial drop in ER-positive invasive breast cancers in 2003 and 2004 (see Fig. 23–13).[16]

Oral contraceptives have not been shown convincingly to affect breast cancer risk but do decrease the risk of endometrial and ovarian carcinomas. Reducing endogenous estrogens by oophorectomy decreases the risk of developing breast cancer by up to 75%. Drugs that block estrogenic effects (e.g., tamoxifen) or block the formation of estrogen (e.g., aromatase inhibitors) also decrease the risk of ER-positive breast cancer.

Breast Density. High breast radiodensity is a strong risk factor for developing cancer. High density is correlated with young age and hormone exposure, and clusters in families. High breast density may be related to less complete involution of lobules at the end of each menstrual cycle, which in turn may increase the number of cells that are potentially susceptible to neoplastic transformation.

Dense breasts also make detection of cancer more difficult by mammography. Other modalities, such as MRI, may be helpful in such women.

Radiation Exposure. Radiation to the chest, whether due to cancer therapy, atomic bomb exposure, or nuclear accidents, results in a higher rate of breast cancer. The risk is greatest with exposure at young ages and with high radiation doses. For example, women in their teens and early 20s who received radiation to the chest for Hodgkin lymphoma have a 20% to 30% risk of developing breast cancer over 10 to 30 years. Recognition of this iatrogenic complication has led to a much more judicious use of radiation therapy in adolescents and young women undergoing cancer treatment. The risks of radiation exposure are substantially lower in women over the age of 25. Current mammographic screening uses low doses of radiation and is unlikely to have an effect on the risk of breast cancer.

Carcinoma of the Contralateral Breast or Endometrium. Approximately 1% of women with breast cancer develop a second contralateral breast carcinoma per year. The risk is higher for women with germline mutations in high-risk breast cancer genes such as *BRCA1* and *BRCA2*, who frequently develop multiple cancers. Breast and endometrial carcinomas have several risk factors in common, the most important of which is exposure to prolonged estrogenic stimulation.

Geographic Influence. Breast cancer incidence rates in the United States and Europe are four to seven times higher than those in other countries. Unfortunately, the rates are rising worldwide, and by 2020 it is estimated that 70% of cases will be in developing countries.

The risk of breast cancer increases in immigrants to the United States with each generation. The factors responsible for this increase are of considerable interest because they are likely to include modifiable risk factors. Reproductive history (number and timing of pregnancies), breastfeeding, diet, obesity, physical activity, and environmental factors all probably play a role.

Diet. Large studies have failed to find strong correlations between breast cancer risk and dietary intake of any specific type of food. Coffee addicts will be pleased to know that caffeine consumption may decrease the risk of breast cancer. On the other hand, moderate or heavy alcohol consumption increases risk. Higher estrogen levels and lower folate levels may underlie this association.

Obesity. There is decreased risk in obese women younger than 40 years as a result of the association with anovulatory cycles and lower progesterone levels late in the cycle. In contrast, the risk is increased for postmenopausal obese women, which is attributed to the synthesis of estrogens in fat depots.

Exercise. There is a probable small protective effect for women who are physically active. The decrease in risk is greatest for premenopausal women, women who are not obese, and women who have had full-term pregnancies.

Breastfeeding. The longer women breastfeed, the greater the reduction in risk. Lactation suppresses ovulation and may trigger terminal differentiation of luminal cells.[4] The lower incidence of breast cancer in developing countries largely can be explained by the more frequent and longer nursing of infants.[22]

Environmental Toxins. There is concern that environmental contaminants, such as organochlorine pesticides, have estrogenic effects on humans. Possible links to breast cancer risk are being investigated intensively, but definitive associations have yet to be made.

Tobacco. Cigarette smoking has not been clearly associated with breast cancer but is associated with the development of periductal mastitis (subareolar abscess; discussed earlier). Breast cancer was the leading cause of cancer deaths in women until the early 1990s, when lung cancer deaths surged ahead. Currently, twice as many women die from lung cancer—surely a good reason to avoid tobacco use.

ETIOLOGY AND PATHOGENESIS

The major risk factors for the development of breast cancer are hormonal and genetic. Breast carcinomas can therefore be divided into sporadic cases, probably related to hormonal exposure, and hereditary cases, associated with germline mutations. Hereditary carcinoma has received intense scrutiny in the hopes that the specific genetic mutations can be identified and that these alterations will illuminate the causes of nonfamilial breast cancers as well. Recent studies have borne out these hopes. We begin our discussion with hereditary breast cancer and follow with sporadic breast cancer.

Hereditary Breast Cancer

The inheritance of a susceptibility gene or genes is the primary cause of approximately 12% of breast cancers.[23,24] The probability of a hereditary etiology increases with multiple affected first-degree relatives, when individuals are affected before menopause and/or have multiple cancers, or there are family members with other specific cancers (discussed below).

In some families the increased risk is the result of a single mutation in a highly penetrant breast cancer gene (Table 23–2). Mutations in *BRCA1* and *BRCA2* account for the majority of cancers attributable to single mutations and about 3% of all breast cancers. Penetrance (the percentage of carriers who develop breast cancer) varies from 30% to 90% depending on the specific mutation present. Mutations in *BRCA1* also markedly increase the risk of developing ovarian carcinoma, which occurs in as many as 20% to 40% of carriers. *BRCA2* confers a smaller risk for ovarian carcinoma (10% to 20%) but is associated more frequently with male breast cancer. *BRCA1* and *BRCA2* carriers are also at higher risk for other epithelial cancers, such as prostatic and pancreatic carcinomas.

BRCA1 and *BRCA2* are both large genes over 80 kilobases in size. Hundreds of different mutations distributed throughout the coding regions have been reported for each. The frequency of mutations that increase breast cancer risk is only 0.1% to 0.2% in the general population, and inconsequential polymorphisms are common. As a result, genetic testing is difficult and generally restricted to individuals with a strong family history or those belonging to certain ethnic groups. For example, 2% to 3% of people of Ashkenazi Jewish descent carry one of three specific mutations, two in *BRCA1* and one in *BRCA2*. Identification of carriers is important, since increased surveillance, prophylactic mastectomy, and oophorectomy can reduce cancer-related morbidity and mortality.

BRCA1-associated breast cancers are commonly poorly differentiated, have "medullary features" (a syncytial growth pattern with pushing margins and a lymphocytic response), and do not express hormone receptors or overexpress HER2/ neu (the so-called "triple negative" phenotype). Their gene profiling signature is very similar to basal-like breast cancers, a distinct molecular subtype that is discussed later. *BRCA1*

TABLE 23–2 Most Common "Single Gene" Mutations Associated with Hereditary Susceptibility to Breast Cancer

GENE (location) Syndrome (Incidence)*	% of "Single Gene" Hereditary Cancers†	Breast Cancer Risk by Age 70‡	Changes in Sporadic Breast Cancer	Other Associated Cancers	Functions	Comments
BRCA1 (17q21) Familial breast and ovarian cancer (1 in 860)	52% (~2% of all breast cancers)	40% to 90%	Mutations rare; inactivated in 50% of some subtypes (e.g. medullary and metaplastic) by methylation	Ovarian, male breast cancer (but lower than BRCA2), prostate, pancreas, fallopian tube	Tumor suppressor, transcriptional regulation, repair of double-stranded DNA breaks	Breast carcinomas are commonly poorly differentiated and triple negative (basal-like), and have *P53* mutations.
BRCA2 (13q12-13) Familial breast and ovarian cancer (1 in 740)	32% (~1% of all breast cancers)	30% to 90%	Mutations and loss of expression rare	Ovarian, male breast cancer, prostate, pancreas, stomach, melanoma, gallbladder, bile duct, pharynx	Tumor suppressor, transcriptional regulation, repair of double-stranded DNA breaks	Biallelic germline mutations cause a rare form of Fanconi anemia (Chapter 7)
p53 (17p13.1) Li-Fraumeni (1 in 5,000)	3% (<1% of all breast cancers)	>90%	Mutations in 20%, LOH in 30% to 42%; most frequent in triple negative cancers	Sarcoma, leukemia, brain tumors, adrenocortical carcinoma, others	Tumor suppressor with critical roles in cell cycle control, DNA replication, DNA repair, and apoptosis	*p53* is the most commonly mutated gene in sporadic breast cancers
CHEK2 (22q12.1) Li-Fraumeni variant (1 in 100)	5% (~1% of all breast cancers)	10% to 20%	Mutations rare (<5%); loss of protein expression in at least one third by unknown mechanism(s)	Prostate, thyroid, kidney, colon	Cell cycle checkpoint kinase, recognition and repair of DNA damage, activates BRCA1 and p53 by phosphorylation	May increase risk for breast cancer after radiation exposure

*Frequency of heterozygotes in the U.S. population; the incidence of gene mutations is higher in some ethnic populations (e.g., *BRCA1* and *BRCA2* mutations occur at high frequencies in Askenazi Jews).

†Defined as familial breast cancers showing a pattern of inheritance consistent with a major effect of a single gene.

‡Risk varies with specific mutations and is likely modified by other genes.

cancers are also frequently associated with loss of the inactive X chromosome and reduplication of the active X, resulting in the absence of the Barr body.[25] *BRCA2*-associated breast carcinomas also tend to be relatively poorly differentiated, but are more often ER positive than *BRCA1* cancers.

Other known susceptibility genes are much less commonly implicated; together, this group accounts for fewer than 10% of hereditary breast carcinomas (see Table 23–2). Li-Fraumeni syndrome (due to germline mutations in *p53*) and Li-Fraumeni variant syndrome (due to germline mutations in *CHEK2*) together account for about 8% of breast cancers caused by single genes. Three other tumor suppressor genes, *PTEN* (Cowden syndrome), *LKBI/STK11* (Peutz-Jeghers syndrome), and *ATM* (ataxia telangiectasia), are mutated in less than 1% of all breast cancers and are described elsewhere.

The known high-risk breast cancer genes account for only about one quarter of familial breast cancers. The search for a high-risk "BRCA3" gene has been unsuccessful, and other highly penetrant genes may not exist. As a result, it is likely that the remaining familial cancers are caused by multiple genes with weak effects. As with other multigenic diseases, genome-wide association studies (GWAS) have commenced and have identified a number of candidate genes associated with risk, including the fibroblast growth factor receptor-2 (FGFR2).[24] Such studies will need to take into account genetic variation across different ethnic groups, which (as we have seen) correlates with both overall breast cancer risk and susceptibility to particular molecular subtypes.

The major susceptibility genes for breast cancer are tumor suppressors that have normal roles in DNA repair, cell cycle control, and the regulation of apoptosis in many tissues (Chapter 7). Except for *p53*, mutations in genes implicated in hereditary breast cancer are uncommon in sporadic breast cancers. However, decreased expression of *BRCA1* and *CHEK2* is common in sporadic cancers, particularly those that are "triple-negative" or poorly differentiated, and basal-like cancers, which comprise a large subset of the triple-negative group, have a gene expression profile that bears a striking resemblance to hereditary cancers arising in *BRCA1* carriers. Based on these observations, it is suspected that the pathways that these genes participate in are frequently disrupted in sporadic cancers through currently unknown mechanisms.

Sporadic Breast Cancer

The major risk factors for sporadic breast cancer are related to hormone exposure: gender, age at menarche and menopause, reproductive history, breastfeeding, and exogenous estrogens. The majority of sporadic cancers occur in postmenopausal women and are ER positive.

Hormonal exposure increases the number of potential target cells by stimulating breast growth during puberty, menstrual cycles, and pregnancy. Exposure also drives cycles of proliferation that place cells at risk for DNA damage. Once premalignant or malignant cells are present, hormones can stimulate their growth, as well as the growth of normal epithelial and stromal cells that may aid and abet tumor development.

Estrogen may also play a more direct role in carcinogenesis. Metabolites of estrogen can cause mutations or generate DNA-damaging free radicals in cell and animal model systems.[26] It also has been proposed that variants of genes involved in estrogen synthesis and metabolism could increase the risk of breast cancer. Such variants would be analogous to cytochrome P-450 alleles that alter the metabolism of tamoxifen in some women.[27]

Overview of Carcinogenesis and Tumor Progression

The diverse histologic appearances of carcinomas and putative precursor lesions are the outward manifestations of the complex genetic and epigenetic changes that drive carcinogenesis. One model of carcinogenesis postulates that a normal cell must acquire several new capabilities to become malignant (see Chapter 7).[28,29] Each may be achieved by a change in the activity of one of many different genes that regulate common cellular activities.

Populations of cells that harbor some, but not all, of the genetic and epigenetic changes that are required for carcinogenesis give rise to morphologically recognizable breast lesions (discussed earlier) that are associated with an increased risk of progression to cancer. The earliest such alterations are proliferative changes, which may stem from the loss of growth-inhibiting signals, aberrant increases in pro-growth signals, or decreased apoptosis. For example, most early lesions (such as atypical ductal hyperplasia and atypical lobular hyperplasia) show increased expression of hormone receptors and abnormal regulation of proliferation.[10,30] LOH is rarely detected in typical proliferative change but becomes more frequent in atypical hyperplasias and is almost universally present in carcinoma in situ. Profound DNA instability in the form of aneuploidy, which manifests morphologically by nuclear enlargement, irregularity, and hyperchromasia, is observed only in high-grade DCIS and some invasive carcinomas. At some point during tumor progression the malignant clone also becomes immortalized and acquires the ability to drive neo-angiogenesis. The morphologic and biologic features of carcinomas are usually established at the in situ stage, since in the majority of cases the in situ lesion closely resembles the accompanying invasive carcinoma.

The cell of origin of breast cancers is of interest, since this has important implications for etiology and treatment. The "cancer stem cell hypothesis" proposes that malignant changes occur in a stem cell population that has unique properties distinguishing them from more differentiated cells.[31,32] Although the majority of tumor cells would consist of non–stem cell progeny, only the malignant stem cells would contribute to tumor progression or recurrence. Effective treatment would need to target only this population, which to date has been difficult to define.

The most likely cell type of origin for the majority of carcinomas is the ER-expressing luminal cell, since the majority of cancers are ER-positive and precursor lesions, such as atypical hyperplasias, are most similar to this type of cell (Fig. 23–15). ER-negative carcinomas may arise from ER-negative myoepithelial cells.[33,34] This would explain why many proteins found in myoepithelial cells are shared by the "triple-negative" or basal-like cancers. An alternative possibility is an origin from an ER-positive precursor that loses ER expression.[10,35] The precursor lesion for ER-negative tumors is unknown (see Fig. 23–15).

The final step of carcinogenesis, the transition of carcinoma in situ to invasive carcinoma, is the most important and unfortunately the least understood. Genetic markers specific for invasive carcinomas have been difficult to identify. It is important to remember that the structure and function of the normal breast depend on a complex interplay between luminal cells, myoepithelial cells, and stromal cells. The same molecular events that allow for the normal formation of new ductal branch points and lobules during puberty and pregnancy— abrogation of the basement membrane, increased proliferation, escape from growth inhibition, angiogenesis, and invasion of stroma—may be recapitulated during carcinogenesis.[2] Remodeling of the breast, which involves inflammatory and "wound healing–like" tissue reactions, could explain the transient increase in breast cancers during and shortly after pregnancy, since such changes could facilitate the transition of carcinoma in situ to invasive cancer.[5,36,37]

As can be surmised from this discussion, there are many paths that can lead to the development of breast cancer. Breast cancer is not one disease, but many, each with its own clinical characteristics and optimal prevention and treatment strategies. This recognition has led to the introduction of molecular classification systems, which are discussed below.

CLASSIFICATION OF BREAST CARCINOMA

Greater than 95% of breast malignancies are adenocarcinomas, which are divided into in situ carcinomas and invasive carcinomas. Carcinoma in situ refers to a neoplastic proliferation that is limited to ducts and lobules by the basement membrane. Invasive carcinoma (synonymous with "infiltrating" carcinoma) has penetrated through the basement membrane into stroma. Here, the cells have the potential to invade into the vasculature and thereby reach regional lymph nodes and distant sites.

Despite evidence that all breast carcinomas arise from cells in the terminal duct lobular unit[38], the use of the terms *lobular* and *ductal* to describe both in situ and invasive carcinomas persists. Carcinoma in situ was originally classified as ductal or lobular based on the resemblance of the involved spaces to normal ducts or lobules. However, it is now recognized that varied patterns of growth in situ are not related to the site or cell of origin, but rather reflect differences in tumor cell biology, such as whether the tumor cells express the cell

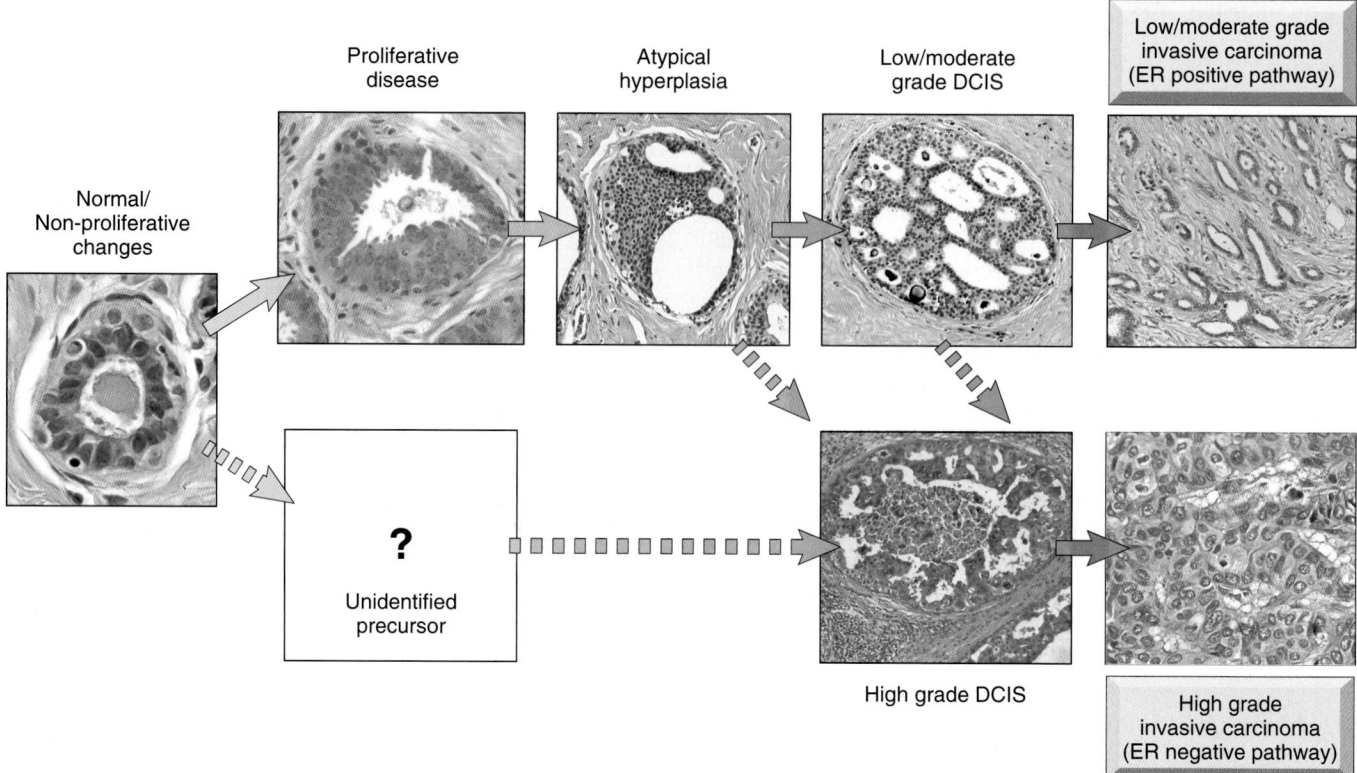

FIGURE 23–15 Proposed precursor-carcinoma sequences in breast cancer. Morphologic changes are displayed from left to right according to the risk for subsequent invasive carcinoma.

adhesion protein E-cadherin or not. By current convention, "lobular" refers to carcinomas of a specific type, and "ductal" is used more generally for adenocarcinomas that have no other designation.

Carcinoma in Situ

Ductal Carcinoma in Situ (DCIS; Intraductal Carcinoma)

With the advent of mammographic screening, the diagnosis of DCIS rapidly increased from fewer than 5% of all carcinomas to 15% to 30% of carcinomas in well-screened populations (see Fig. 23–13).[39] Among cancers detected mammographically, almost half are DCIS. Most are detected as a result of calcifications; less commonly, periductal fibrosis surrounding DCIS forms a mammographic density or a vaguely palpable mass. Rarely, DCIS (often of micropapillary type) produces a nipple discharge or is detected as an incidental finding upon biopsy for another lesion.

DCIS consists of a malignant clonal population of cells limited to ducts and lobules by the basement membrane. The myoepithelial cells are preserved, although they may be diminished in number. DCIS can spread throughout ducts and lobules and produce extensive lesions involving an entire sector of a breast. When DCIS involves lobules, the acini are usually distorted and unfolded and take on the appearance of small ducts.

Morphology. Historically, DCIS has been divided into five architectural subtypes: comedocarcinoma, solid,

cribriform, papillary, and micropapillary. Some cases of DCIS have a single growth pattern, but the majority show a mixture of patterns.

Comedocarcinoma is characterized by the presence of solid sheets of pleomorphic cells with "high-grade" hyperchromatic nuclei and areas of central necrosis (see Fig. 23–16C). The necrotic cell membranes commonly calcify and are detected on mammography as clusters or linear and branching microcalcifications (Fig. 23–16A). Periductal concentric fibrosis and chronic inflammation are common, and extensive lesions are sometimes palpable as an area of vague nodularity (Fig. 23–16B).

Noncomedo DCIS consists of a monomorphic population of cells with nuclear grades ranging from low to high. Several morphologic variants can be seen. In cribriform DCIS, intraepithelial spaces are evenly distributed and regular in shape (cookie cutter–like) (Fig. 23–17A). Solid DCIS completely fills the involved spaces (Fig. 23–17B). Papillary DCIS grows into spaces along fibrovascular cores that typically lack the normal myoepithelial cell layer (Fig. 23–18A). Micropapillary DCIS is recognized by bulbous protrusions without a fibrovascular core, often arranged in complex intraductal patterns (Fig. 23–18B). Calcifications may be associated with central necrosis but more commonly form on intraluminal secretions.

Paget disease of the nipple is a rare manifestation of breast cancer (1% to 4% of cases) and presents as

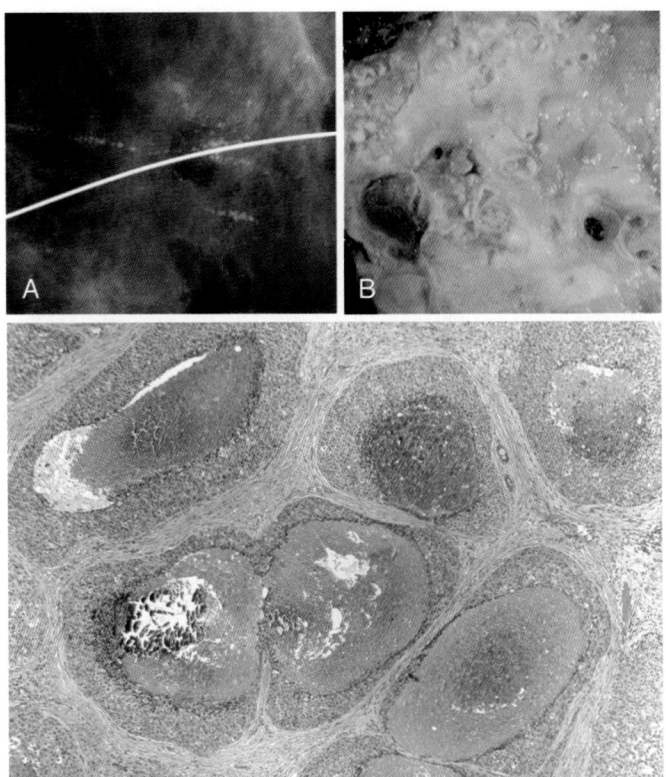

FIGURE 23–16 Ductal carcinoma in situ (DCIS) comedo type. **A,** The specimen radiogram reveals linear and branching calcifications within the ductal system. **B,** Ducts filled with punctate areas of necrosis ("comedone" like) and surrounded by periductal fibrosis are seen. **C,** DCIS with large central zones of necrosis and calcifications fills several adjacent ducts.

a unilateral erythematous eruption with a scale crust. Pruritus is common, and the lesion may be mistaken for eczema. Malignant cells (Paget cells) extend from DCIS within the ductal system, via the lactiferous sinuses, into nipple skin without crossing the base-

ment membrane (Fig. 23–19). The tumor cells disrupt the normal epithelial barrier, allowing extracellular fluid to seep out onto the nipple surface. The Paget cells are readily detected by nipple biopsy or cytologic preparations of the exudate.

A palpable mass is present in 50% to 60% of women with Paget disease, and almost all of these women have an invasive carcinoma deeper in the breast, in addition to DCIS. In contrast, the majority of women without a palpable mass have only DCIS in the underlying breast. The carcinomas are usually poorly differentiated, ER negative, and over express HER2/neu.

Prognosis of Paget disease depends on the features of the underlying carcinoma and is not affected by the presence or absence of DCIS involving the skin when matched for other prognostic factors.

DCIS with microinvasion is diagnosed when there is an area of invasion through the basement membrane into stroma measuring no more than 0.1 cm. Microinvasion is most commonly seen in association with comedocarcinoma. If only one or a few foci of microinvasion are present, the prognosis is very similar to DCIS.

The natural history of DCIS has been difficult to determine because, until recently, all women were treated with mastectomy, and the current practice of surgical excision, usually followed by radiation, is largely curative. If untreated, women with small, low-grade DCIS develop invasive cancer at a rate of about 1% per year.[40] The majority of these cancers are in the same quadrant and have a similar grade and expression pattern of ER and HER2/neu as the DCIS. It is assumed that women with high-grade or extensive DCIS progress to invasive carcinoma at higher rates. Specific biologic features that predict recurrence or progression to invasion are being sought so as to target treatment to these patients.[35]

Mastectomy for DCIS is curative for over 95% of patients. Rare recurrences and/or death are usually due to residual DCIS in ducts in subcutaneous adipose tissue that was not removed during surgery, or occult foci of invasion that were not detected at the time of diagnosis.

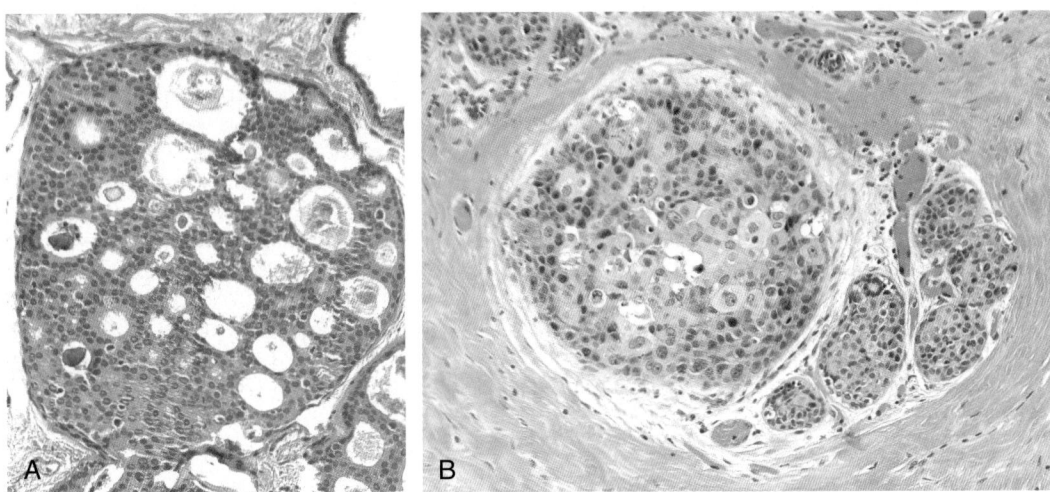

FIGURE 23–17 Noncomedo DCIS. **A,** Cribriform DCIS composed of cells forming round, regular ("cookie cutter") spaces. The lumens are filled with calcifying secretory material. **B,** This solid DCIS has almost completely filled and distorted this lobule with only a few remaining normal luminal cells visible. This type of DCIS is not usually associated with calcifications and may be clinically occult.

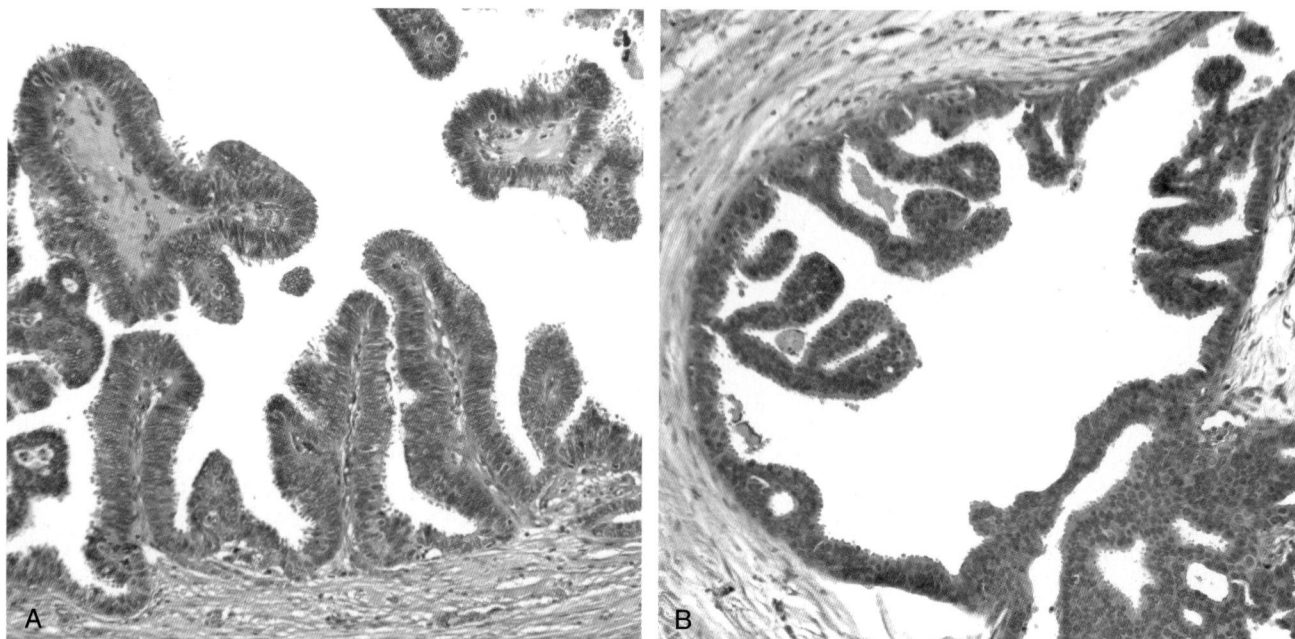

FIGURE 23–18 Noncomedo DCIS. **A,** Papillary DCIS. Delicate fibrovascular cores extend into a duct and are lined by a monomorphic population of tall columnar cells. Myoepithelial cells are absent. **B,** Micropapillary DCIS. The papillae are connected to the duct wall by a narrow base and often have bulbous or complex outgrowths. The papillae are solid and lack fibrovascular cores.

Breast conservation is appropriate for most women with DCIS but results in a slightly higher risk of recurrence. The major risk factors for recurrence are (1) grade, (2) size, and (3) margins. However, if wide margins (i.e., at least 1 cm) can be achieved, the rate of recurrence is quite low. Complete excision of DCIS presents a challenge, since its extent can only be reli-ably predicted by pathologic evaluation. Postoperative radia-tion therapy and tamoxifen also reduce the risk of recurrence. The benefit of tamoxifen may be restricted to women with ER-positive DCIS.[41] If DCIS is treated adequately, the risk of recur-rence in the same breast is only slightly higher than the risk in the contralateral breast for subsequent carcinoma.[42] Whatever the treatment, deaths from breast cancer are very uncommon, occurring in fewer than 2% of women with DCIS.

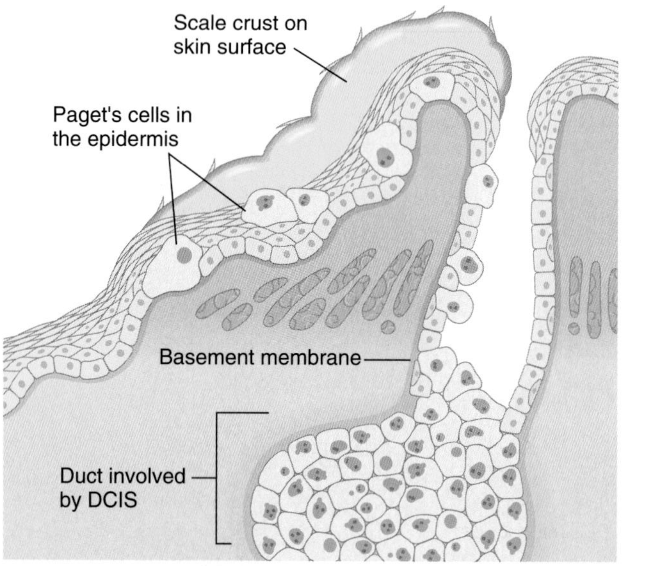

Lobular Carcinoma in Situ (LCIS)

LCIS is always an incidental biopsy finding, since it is not associated with calcifications or stromal reactions that produce mammographic densities. As a result, its incidence (1% to 6% of all carcinomas) has not been affected by the introduction of mammographic screening. When both breasts are biopsied, LCIS is bilateral in 20% to 40% of cases, com-pared with 10% to 20% of cases of DCIS. LCIS is more common in young women, with 80% to 90% of cases occur-ring before menopause.

The cells of LCIS and invasive lobular carcinoma are identi-cal in appearance and share genetic abnormalities, such as those that lead to loss of expression of E-cadherin, a trans-membrane cell adhesion protein that contributes to the cohe-sion of normal breast epithelial cells.

FIGURE 23–19 Paget disease of the nipple. DCIS arising within the ductal system of the breast can extend up the lactiferous ducts and into the skin of the nipple without crossing the basement membrane. The malignant cells disrupt the normally tight squa-mous epithelial cell barrier, allowing extracellular fluid to seep out and form an oozing scaly crust.

Scale crust on skin surface

Paget's cells in the epidermis

Basement membrane

Duct involved by DCIS

Morphology. Atypical lobular hyperplasia, LCIS, and invasive lobular carcinoma all consist of dyscohesive cells with oval or round nuclei and small nucleoli (Fig. 23–20A). The cells lack the cell adhesion protein E-cadherin, resulting in the cells appearing rounded without attachment to adjacent cells (Fig. 23–20B). Mucin-positive signet-ring cells are commonly

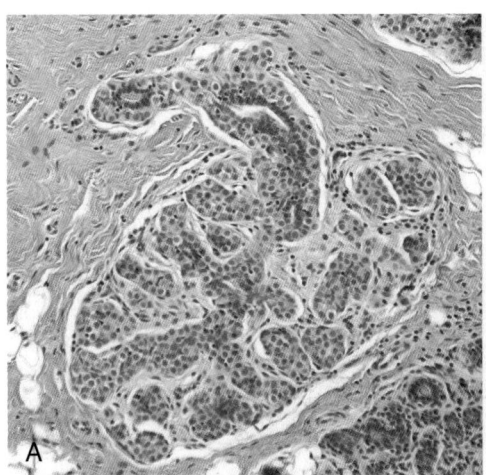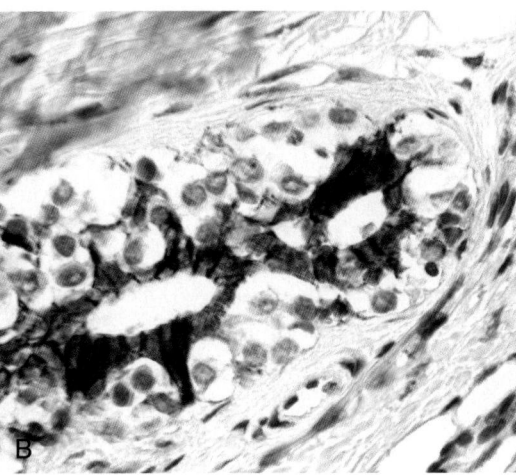

FIGURE 23–20 Lobular carcinoma in situ. **A,** A monomorphic population of small, rounded, loosely cohesive cells fills and expands the acini of a lobule. The underlying lobular architecture can still be recognized. The cells extend into the adjacent lobule by pagetoid spread. **B,** An immunoperoxidase study shows E-cadherin-positive normal luminal cells that have been undermined by E-cadherin-negative LCIS cells spreading along the basement membrane.

present. LCIS rarely distorts the underlying architecture, and the involved acini remain recognizable as lobules. LCIS almost always expresses ER and PR. Overexpression of HER2/neu is not observed.

Women with LCIS develop invasive carcinomas at a frequency similar to that of women with untreated DCIS. In patients observed for more than 20 years, invasive carcinoma develops in 25% to 35%, or at about 1% per year. Although both breasts are at increased risk, the risk is slightly higher in the ipsilateral breast.[42–44] Invasive carcinomas developing in women after a diagnosis of LCIS are threefold more likely to be of the lobular type, but the majority do not show specific lobular morphology. Treatment choices include bilateral prophylactic mastectomy, tamoxifen, or, more typically, close clinical follow-up and mammographic screening.

Rare cases of carcinoma in situ that lack E-cadherin have high-grade nuclei and/or central necrosis. The cells may be ER negative, and some overexpress HER2/neu. The natural history of this type of CIS is not known and may well be different from typical LCIS.[44]

Invasive (Infiltrating) Carcinoma

In the absence of mammographic screening, invasive carcinoma almost always presents as a palpable mass. *Palpable tumors are associated with axillary lymph node metastases in over 50% of patients.* Larger carcinomas may be fixed to the chest wall or cause dimpling of the skin. When the tumor involves the central portion of the breast, retraction of the nipple may develop. Lymphatics may become so involved as to block the local area of skin drainage and cause lymphedema and thickening of the skin. In such cases, tethering of the skin to the breast by Cooper ligaments mimics the appearance of an orange peel, an appearance referred to as *peau d'orange.*

In older women undergoing mammography, invasive carcinomas most commonly present as a radiodense mass (Fig. 23–21A). Mammographically detected cancers are, on average,

half the size of palpable cancers. Fewer than 20% will have nodal metastases. Invasive carcinomas presenting as mammographic calcifications without an associated density are very small in size, and metastases are unusual.

The term *inflammatory carcinoma* is reserved for tumors that present with a swollen, erythematous breast. This gross appearance is caused by extensive invasion and obstruction of dermal lymphatics by tumor cells. The underlying carcinoma is usually diffusely infiltrative and typically does not form a discrete palpable mass. This can result in confusion with true inflammatory conditions and a delay in diagnosis. Many patients have metastases at diagnosis or recur rapidly, and the overall prognosis is poor.[45]

Rarely, breast cancer presents as an axillary nodal metastasis or distant metastasis before cancer is detected in the breast. In most cases, the primary carcinoma is either small or obscured by dense breast tissue. The number of primary carcinomas that remain occult in such cases has been minimized with imaging using mammography, ultrasound, and MRI.

The most common histologic types of breast adenocarcinoma are listed in Table 23–3. These special types are important to recognize because of their specific clinical associations.

Invasive Carcinoma, No Special Type (NST; Invasive Ductal Carcinoma)

Invasive carcinomas of no special type include the majority of carcinomas (70% to 80%).

Morphology. On gross examination, most tumors are firm to hard and have an irregular border (Fig. 23–21B). When cut or scraped, they typically produce a characteristic grating sound (similar to cutting a water chestnut) due to small, central pinpoint foci or streaks of chalky-white elastotic stroma and occasional small foci of calcification. Less frequently, carcinomas have a well-circumscribed border and a softer consistency.

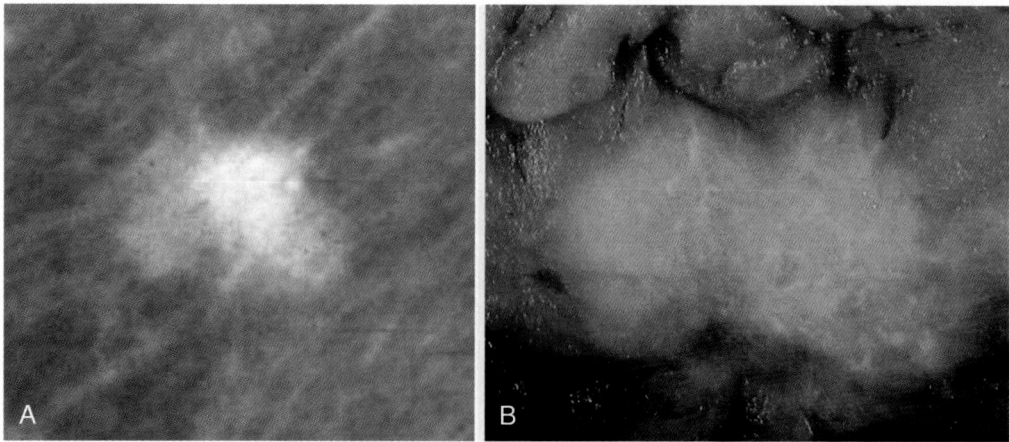

FIGURE 23–21 Invasive ductal carcinoma. **A,** The radiograph shows an invasive cancer with a characteristic irregular border. **B,** Grossly, the irregular firm white mass contains chalky areas of elastotic stroma that extend out into the surrounding yellow adipose tissue. (**B,** Courtesy of Dr. Anna Laury, Brigham and Women's Hospital, Boston, MA.)

There is a wide range of histologic appearances. Well-differentiated carcinomas show prominent tubule formation, small round nuclei, and rare mitotic figures (Fig. 23–22A). Moderately differentiated carcinomas may have tubules, but solid clusters or single infiltrating cells are also present. These tumors have a greater degree of nuclear pleomorphism and contain mitotic figures (Fig. 23–22B). Poorly differentiated carcinomas often invade as ragged nests or solid sheets of cells with enlarged irregular nuclei. A high proliferation rate and areas of tumor necrosis are common (Fig. 23–22C).

Recently developed techniques that examine the DNA, RNA, and proteins of carcinomas globally have provided a framework for new molecular classifications of this group of

TABLE 23–3 Distribution of Histologic Types of Breast Cancer

Total Cancers	Percentage
CARCINOMA IN SITU*	**15–30**
Ductal carcinoma in situ	80
Lobular carcinoma in situ	20
INVASIVE CARCINOMA	**70–85**
No-special-type carcinoma ("ductal")	79
Lobular carcinoma	10
Tubular/cribriform carcinoma	6
Mucinous (colloid) carcinoma	2
Medullary carcinoma	2
Papillary carcinoma	1
Metaplastic carcinoma	<1

*The proportion of in situ carcinomas detected depends on the percentage of women undergoing mammographic screening and ranges from less than 5% in unscreened populations to almost 50% in populations that are well screened. Current observed numbers are between these two extremes.

The data on invasive carcinomas are modified from Dixon JM et al.: Long-term survivors after breast cancer. Br J Surg 72:445, 1985.

breast cancers (Fig. 23–23). Gene expression profiling, which can measure the relative quantities of mRNA for essentially every gene, has identified five major patterns of gene expression in the NST group: luminal A, luminal B, normal, basal-like, and HER2 positive.[46] These molecular classes correlate with prognosis and response to therapy, and thus have taken on clinical importance.

○ *"Luminal A"* (40% to 55% of NST cancers): This is the largest group and consists of cancers that are ER positive and HER2/neu negative. The gene signature is dominated by the dozens of genes under the control of ER (see Fig. 23–23). ER-positive carcinomas also show increased transcription of genes thought to be characteristic of normal luminal cells. The majority are well- or moderately differentiated, and most occur in postmenopausal women.

These cancers are generally slow growing and respond well to hormonal treatments. Conversely, only a small number will respond to standard chemotherapy. Commercial tests, some already available for use with formalin-fixed tissues, have been developed to identify this and other molecular classes.[47] In addition, clinical trials are attempting to identify different types or combinations of chemotherapeutic agents that may be efficacious for ER-positive cancers.

○ *"Luminal B"* (15% to 20% of NST cancers): This group of cancers also expresses ER but is generally of higher grade, has a higher proliferative rate, and often overexpresses HER2/neu. They are sometimes referred to as *triple-positive* cancers. They compose a major group of ER-positive cancers that are more likely to have lymph node metastases and that may respond to chemotherapy.

○ *"Normal breast–like"* (6% to 10% of NST cancers): This is a small group of usually well-differentiated ER-positive, HER2/neu-negative cancers characterized by the similarity of their gene expression pattern to normal tissue. It is not yet clear whether or not this is a specific tumor expression pattern.

○ *"Basal-like"* (13% to 25% of NST cancers): These cancers are notable for the absence of ER, PR, and HER2/neu and

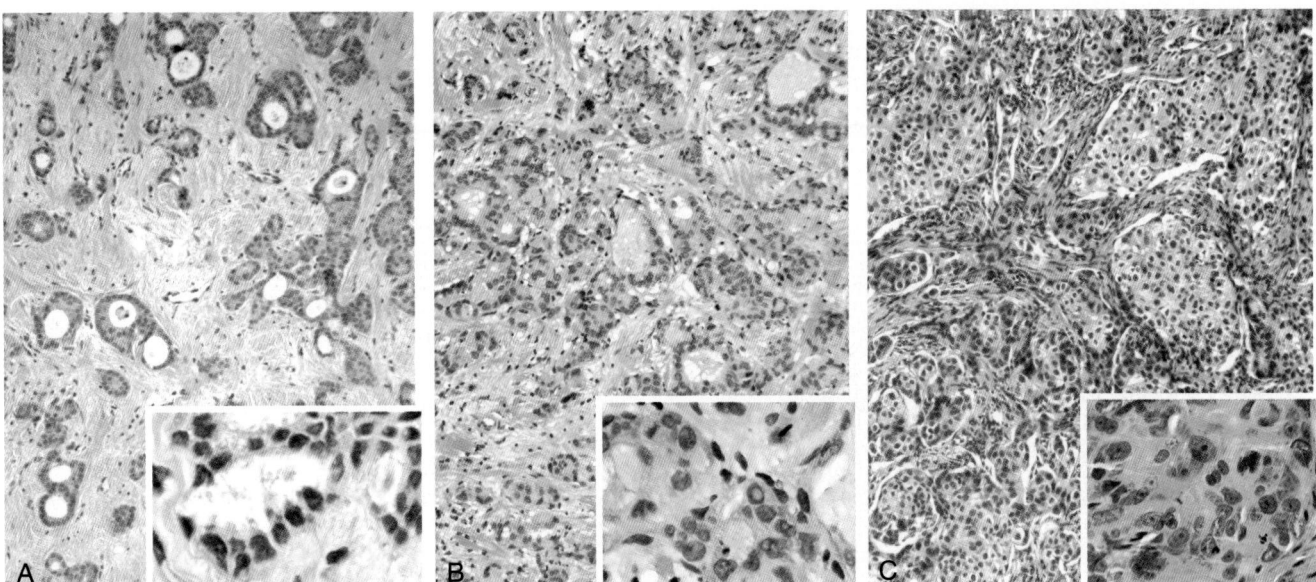

FIGURE 23–22 **A,** A well-differentiated invasive carcinoma of no special type consists of tubules or a cribriform pattern of cells with small monomorphic nuclei. **B,** A moderately differentiated carcinoma shows less tubule formation and more solid nests of cells and pleomorphic nuclei. **C,** This poorly differentiated invasive carcinoma of no special type infiltrates as ragged sheets of pleomorphic cells with numerous mitotic figures and central areas of tumor necrosis.

the expression of markers typical of myoepithelial cells (e.g., basal keratins, P-cadherin, p63, or laminin), progenitor cells, or putative stem cells (e.g., cytokeratins 5 and 6) (see Fig. 23–23). "Basal" was chosen as a general term that covers all of these cell types.

By strict definition this group is defined by their gene expression profile. Basal-like cancers are a subgroup of ER-PR-HER2/neu "triple-negative" carcinomas.[48,49] Members of this group include medullary carcinomas, metaplastic carcinomas (e.g., spindle cell carcinomas or matrix-producing carcinomas), and carcinomas with a central fibrotic focus.

Basal-like cancers are of particular interest because of their distinct genetic and epidemiologic features. Many carcinomas arising in women with *BRCA1* mutations are of this type. There is also an increased incidence in certain ethnic populations and in young women.

These cancers are generally high grade and have a high proliferation rate. They are associated with an aggressive course, frequent metastasis to viscera and the brain, and a poor prognosis. However, approximately 15% to 20% will have a pathologic complete response to chemotherapy; cure may be possible in this chemosensitive subgroup.

○ "*HER2 positive*" (7% to 12% of NST cancers): This group comprises ER-negative carcinomas that overexpress HER2/neu protein. In over 90% of HER2/neu positive cancers, overexpression is due to amplification of the segment of DNA on 17q21 that includes the *HER2/neu* gene and varying numbers of adjacent genes. This amplicon dominates the gene signature of this group (see Fig. 23–23). HER2/neu assays, which include measurement of gene copy number by fluorescence in situ hybridization, mRNA level by gene arrays, and protein by immunohistochemistry, are all abnormal in the majority of these cancers. In rare cases,

HER2/neu protein overexpression may occur as a result of mechanisms other than gene amplification.[50] These cancers are usually poorly differentiated, have a high proliferation rate, and are associated with a high frequency of brain metastasis.

Trastuzumab (Herceptin) is a humanized monoclonal antibody specific to HER2/neu. The combination of trastuzumab and chemotherapy is highly effective in treating carcinomas that overexpress HER2/neu. Demonstrating the first gene-targeted therapeutic agent for a solid tumor, these results have created great excitement within the community of physicians and scientists involved with treating cancer patients. Unfortunately, trastuzumab does not cross the blood-brain barrier, leaving patients susceptible to metastatic disease to this site. Newer agents, such as the dual tyrosine kinase inhibitor lapatinib, that targets both EGFR and HER2/neu, will hopefully overcome these limitations.[51] Other genes on the same segment of amplified DNA may influence the sensitivity of HER2 tumors to these agents.

Invasive Lobular Carcinoma

Invasive lobular carcinomas usually present as a palpable mass or a mammographic density with irregular borders. However, in about one fourth of cases the tumor infiltrates the tissue diffusely and causes little desmoplasia. Such tumors are difficult to detect by palpation and may cause only very subtle mammographic changes. Metastases can also be difficult to detect clinically and radiologically because of this type of invasion.

Lobular carcinomas have been reported to have a greater incidence of bilaterality. However, many studies have been biased by the greater likelihood of performing contralateral

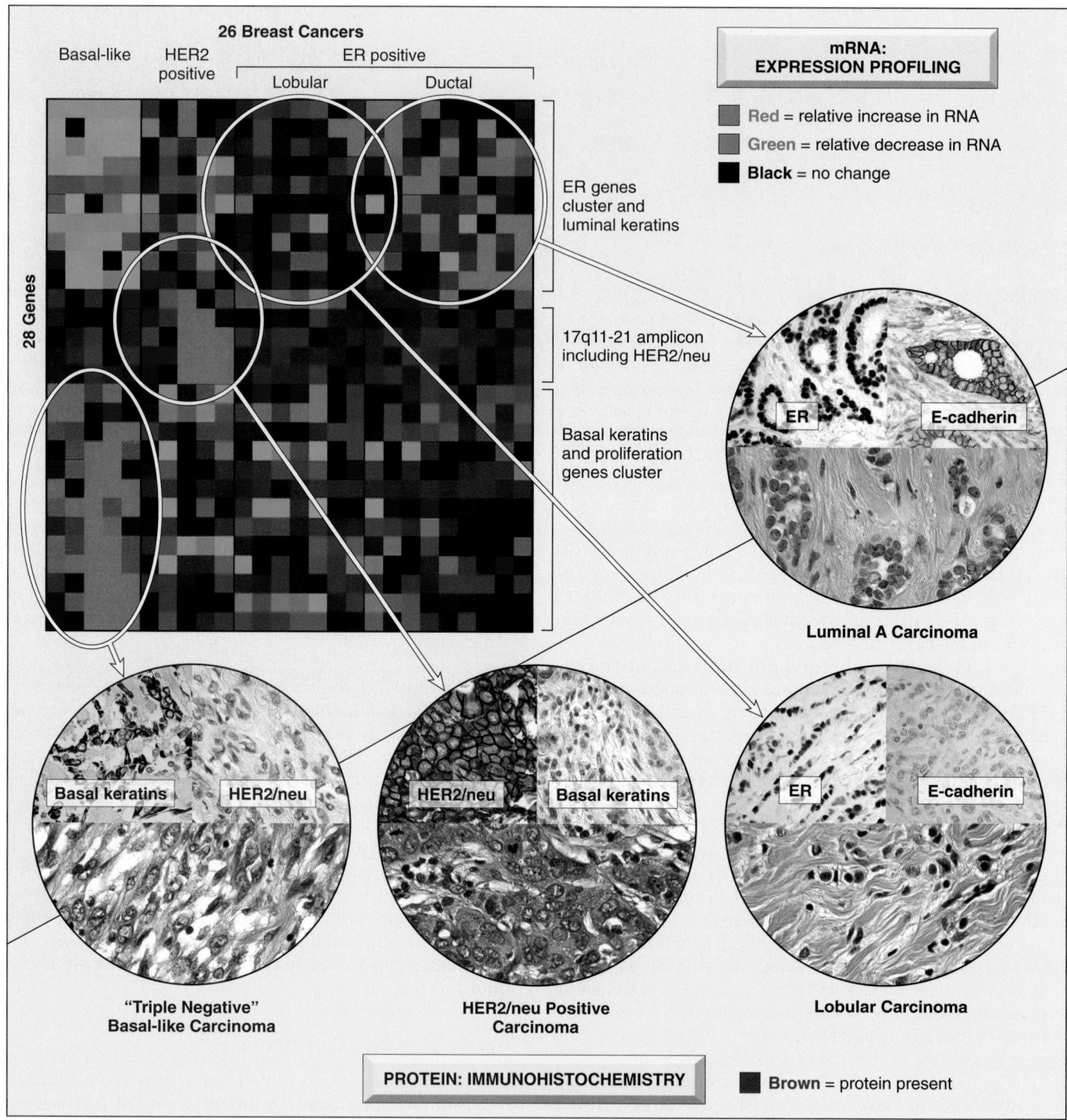

FIGURE 23–23 Gene expression portraits of breast carcinomas. Alterations in DNA, messenger RNA (mRNA), and protein expression identify breast cancer subtypes previously recognized by morphology (e.g., lobular carcinomas) and define new subtypes ("luminal A," "HER2/neu positive," and "basal-like").

(Array data courtesy of Dr. Andrea Richardson, Brigham and Women's Hospital, Boston, MA, as modified from Signoretti S et al.: Oncogenic role of the ubiquitin ligase subunit skp2 in human breast cancer. J Clin Invest 110:633, 2002.)

surgery in women with lobular carcinoma. The actual fraction of women who develop invasive carcinomas in the contralateral breast is only 5% to 10%, which is similar to the incidence for NST carcinomas.

> **Morphology.** The histologic hallmark is the presence of dyscohesive infiltrating tumor cells, often arranged in single file or in loose clusters or sheets (see Fig. 23–23). Tubule formation is absent. The cytologic appearance is identical to the cells of atypical lobular hyperplasia and LCIS. Signet-ring cells containing an intracytoplasmic mucin droplet are common. Desmoplasia may be minimal or absent.

Invasive lobular carcinoma is graded using the same criteria as those applied to other breast carcinomas.[52] Well-differentiated and moderately differentiated invasive lobular carcinomas are usually diploid, ER positive, and associated with LCIS. HER2/neu overexpression is very rare. These cancers have a gene expression profile similar to luminal A cancers (see Fig. 23–23).[53] In contrast, poorly differentiated lobular carcinomas are generally aneuploid, often lack hormone receptors, and may overexpress HER2/neu. If matched by grade and stage, lobular carcinomas have the same prognosis as NST carcinomas.

Lobular carcinomas have a different pattern of metastasis than other breast cancers. Metastasis tends to occur to the peritoneum and retroperitoneum, the leptomeninges (carcinoma meningitis), the gastrointestinal tract, and the ovaries and uterus.[53] In some cases, metastatic lobular carcinoma may be mistaken for signet ring carcinoma of the GI tract, which it closely resembles. The morphologic resemblance of these two tumors is not coincidental, but rather reflects a common underlying molecular etiology. Both lobular carcinoma and signet ring carcinoma of the gastrointestinal tract are characterized by the loss of E-cadherin, a cell adhesion molecule that functions as a tumor suppressor. In lobular carcinoma, biallelic loss of expression of *CDH1*, the gene that encodes E-cadherin, stems from a combination of deletions, mutations, and promoter silencing via methylation. Loss of E-cadherin is also seen in atypical lobular hyperplasia and LCIS, indicating that this alteration is a relatively early event in the development of lobular carcinoma. Rare patients with heterozygous germline mutations in *CDH1* are at very high risk of developing lobular carcinoma (if female) and gastric signet ring carcinoma (males and females), emphasizing the close molecular relationship between these two tumors and the importance of E-cadherin loss in their pathogenesis.[54,55]

Medullary Carcinoma

Medullary carcinoma is most common in women in the sixth decade and presents as a well-circumscribed mass. It may closely mimic a benign lesion clinically and radiologically, or present as a rapidly growing mass.

> **Morphology.** These tumors produce little desmoplasia and are distinctly more yielding on palpation and cutting than typical breast carcinomas. The tumor is soft, fleshy (*medulla* is Latin for "marrow"), and well circumscribed. Histologically, the carcinoma is characterized by (1) solid, syncytium-like sheets of large cells with vesicular, pleomorphic nuclei, and prominent nucleoli, which compose more than 75% of the tumor mass; (2) frequent mitotic figures; (3) a moderate to marked lymphoplasmacytic infiltrate surrounding and within the tumor; and (4) a pushing (noninfiltrative) border (Fig. 23–24C). All medullary carcinomas are poorly differentiated. DCIS is minimal or absent.

Medullary carcinomas have a slightly better prognosis than do NST carcinomas, despite the almost universal presence of poor prognostic factors, including high nuclear grade, aneuploidy, absence of hormone receptors, and high proliferative rates. HER2/neu overexpression is not observed. Lymph node metastases are infrequent and rarely involve multiple nodes. The syncytial growth pattern and pushing borders may stem from the overexpression of adhesion molecules, such as intercellular cell adhesion molecule and E-cadherin, which could potentially limit metastatic potential.[53]

Medullary carcinomas have a basal-like gene expression profile.[56] Among cancers arising in *BRCA1* carriers, 13% are of medullary type, and up to 60% have a subset of medullary features (see Table 23–3). Although, the majority of medullary carcinomas are not associated with germline *BRCA1* mutations, hypermethylation of the *BRCA1* promoter is observed in 67% of medullary carcinomas, suggesting an association of this morphology with underlying gene expression.

Mucinous (Colloid) Carcinoma

These carcinomas occur in older women (median age 71) and tend to grow slowly over the course of many years.

> **Morphology.** The tumor is soft or rubbery and has the consistency and appearance of pale gray-blue gelatin. The borders are pushing or circumscribed. The tumor cells are arranged in clusters and small islands of cells within large lakes of mucin (Fig. 23–24D).

Mucinous carcinomas are usually diploid, well to moderately differentiated, and ER positive. Lymph node metastases are uncommon. The overall prognosis is slightly better than that of NST carcinomas.

Tubular Carcinoma

Tubular carcinomas are typically detected as small irregular mammographic densities in women in their late 40s. They are uncommon, but constitute up to 10% of tumors that are smaller than 1 cm in size. In a significant minority of cases, tumors are multifocal within one breast or detected bilaterally.

> **Morphology.** These tumors consist exclusively of well-formed tubules and are sometimes mistaken for

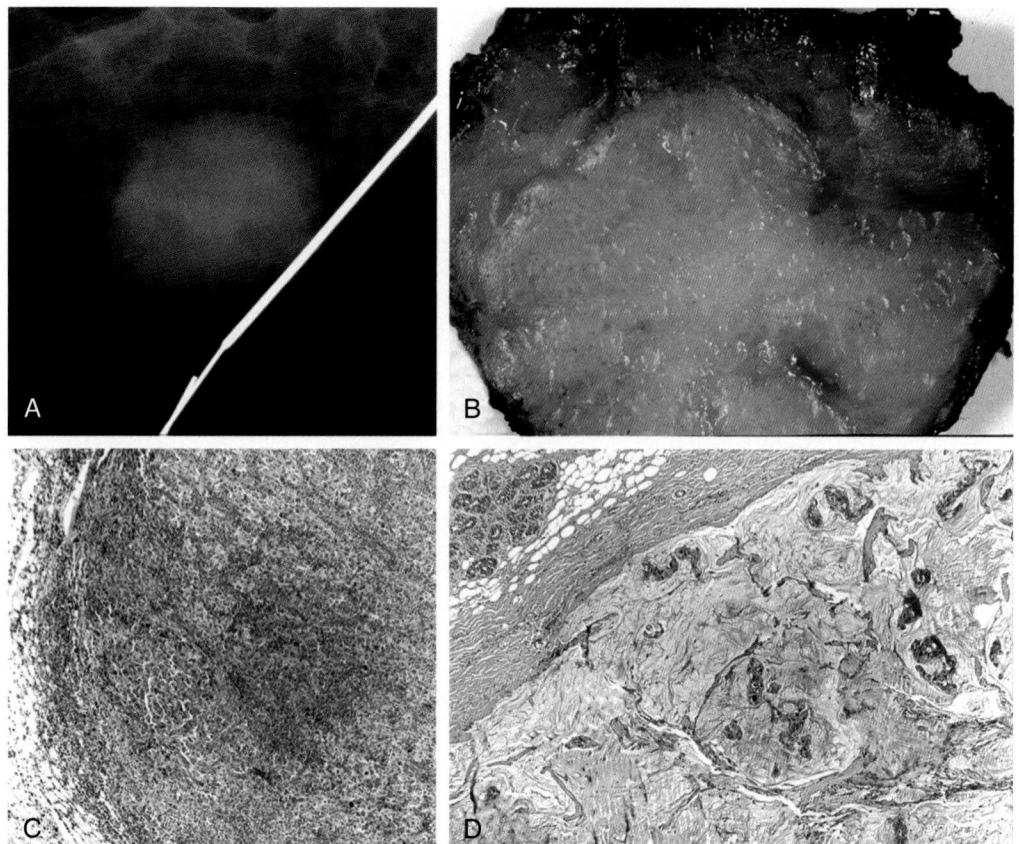

FIGURE 23–24 Invasive carcinoma variants. **A,** The specimen radiogram shows a well-circumscribed mass. The majority of such masses are benign, but approximately 6% are carcinomas. **B,** Grossly, this carcinoma has a pushing border and a fleshy appearance. **C,** Medullary carcinoma. Note the pushing border, the sheetlike growth of the pleomorphic tumor cells, and the prominent lympho-plasmacytic infiltrate. **D,** Mucinous (colloid) carcinoma. The malignant cells lie within pools of extracellular mucin. The tumor also has a pushing border and is very deceptively soft in texture.

benign sclerosing lesions (Fig. 23–25). However, the myoepithelial cell layer is absent, placing the tumor cells in direct contact with the stroma. A cribriform pattern is sometimes seen. Apocrine snouts are typical, and calcifications may be present within the lumens. Tubular carcinomas are frequently associated with atypical lobular hyperplasia, LCIS, or low-grade DCIS.[8]

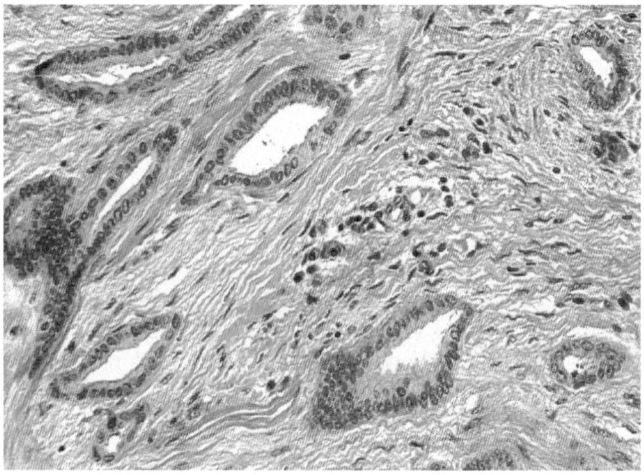

More than 95% of all tubular carcinomas are diploid, ER positive, and HER2/neu negative. By definition, all are well differentiated. Axillary metastases occur in fewer than 10% of cases unless multiple foci of invasion are present. This subtype is important to recognize because of its excellent prognosis.

Invasive Papillary Carcinoma

Invasive papillary carcinomas and invasive micropapillary carcinomas are rare, representing 1% or fewer of all invasive cancers. Papillary or micropapillary architecture is more commonly seen in DCIS. Invasive papillary carcinomas are usually ER positive and have a favorable prognosis. In contrast, invasive micropapillary carcinomas are more likely to be ER negative and HER2 positive. Lymph node metastases are very common, and the prognosis is poor.

Metaplastic Carcinoma

"Metaplastic carcinoma" includes a variety of rare types of breast cancer (<1% of all cases), such as matrix-producing

FIGURE 23–25 Tubular carcinoma. This carcinoma is composed of well-formed angulated tubules lined by a single layer of cells with small uniform nuclei.

carcinomas, squamous cell carcinomas, and carcinomas with a prominent spindle cell component. They are ER-PR-HER2/neu "triple negative," often express myoepithelial proteins, and appear to be related to the basal-like carcinomas. Lymph node metastases are infrequent, but the prognosis is generally poor.

PROGNOSTIC AND PREDICTIVE FACTORS

The outcome for women with breast cancer varies widely. Many women have a normal life expectancy, whereas others have only a 10% chance of being alive in 5 years. Except in women who present with distant metastasis (<10%) or with inflammatory carcinoma (<5%) (in whom the prognosis is poor regardless of other findings), *prognosis is determined by the pathologic examination of the primary carcinoma and the axillary lymph nodes.* Prognostic information is important in counseling patients about the likely outcome of their disease, choosing appropriate treatment, and the design of clinical trials.

Major prognostic factors that are the strongest predictors of death from breast cancer are incorporated into the American Joint Committee on Cancer (AJCC) staging system,[57] which is used to divide patients into five stages (0 to IV) that are correlated with survival (Table 23–4). The major prognostic factors are as follows:

1. **Invasive carcinoma versus in situ disease.** By definition, in situ carcinoma is confined to the ductal system and cannot metastasize. Breast cancer deaths associated with DCIS are due to the subsequent development of invasive carcinoma or areas of invasion that were not detected at the time of diagnosis. The great majority of women with adequately treated DICS are cured. In contrast, at least half of invasive carcinomas have metastasized locally or distantly at the time of diagnosis.
2. **Distant metastases.** Once distant metastases are present, cure is unlikely, although long-term remissions and palliation can be achieved, especially in women with hormonally responsive tumors. As mentioned earlier, the tumor type influences the timing and location of metastases.[58,59]
3. **Lymph node metastases.** *Axillary lymph node status is the most important prognostic factor for invasive carcinoma in the absence of distant metastases.* The clinical assessment of lymph node status is unreliable due to both false positives (e.g., palpable reactive nodes) and false negatives (e.g., lymph nodes with small metastatic deposits). Therefore, biopsy is necessary for accurate assessment. With no nodal involvement, the 10-year disease-free survival rate is close to 70% to 80%; the rate falls to 35% to 40% with one to three positive nodes, and to 10% to 15% when more than 10 nodes are positive.

   Lymphatic vessels in most breast carcinomas drain first to one or two *sentinel nodes,* which can be identified with radiotracer or colored dyes. If a biopsy restricted to the sentinel nodes is negative for metastasis, it is unlikely that other more distant nodes will be involved and the patient can be spared the morbidity of a complete axillary dissection. For these reasons, sentinel node biopsy has been adopted in many centers as part of the assessment of lymph node status. In some tumors of the medial breast, the sentinel node is an intrathoracic internal mammary node.

These nodes are generally not biopsied owing to the morbidity associated with the procedure.

Macrometastases (greater than 0.2 cm) are of proven prognostic importance. Through more sensitive approaches, including serial sectioning of lymph nodes, immunohistochemistry for keratins, and RT-PCR–based detection of tumor-specific mRNA, increased numbers of women with micrometastases (0.2 cm or less) are being identified. The clinical significance of these small metastases is unclear and is being addressed by current clinical trials.

Approximately 10% to 20% of women without axillary lymph node metastases have a recurrence outside of the breast and about the same number die from breast cancer. In these patients, metastasis may occur via the internal mammary lymph nodes or hematogenously.

4. **Tumor size.** The size of an invasive carcinoma is the second most important prognostic factor. The risk of axillary lymph node metastases increases with the size of the primary tumor, but both are independent prognostic factors. Women with node-negative carcinomas <1 cm in size have a 10-year survival rate of over 90%, whereas survival drops to 77% for cancers >2 cm.

   Unfortunately, breast self-examination does not lower breast cancer mortality,[60] suggesting that by the time breast cancers become palpable (typically when at least 2 to 3 cm), tumors capable of metastasizing have already done so. Mammographically detected cancers are smaller and less likely to have metastasized.
5. **Locally advanced disease.** Carcinomas invading into skin or skeletal muscle are usually large and may be difficult to treat surgically. With increased awareness of breast cancer detection, such cases have fortunately decreased in frequency and are now rare at initial presentation.
6. **Inflammatory carcinoma.** Breast cancers presenting with breast swelling and skin thickening due to dermal lymphatic involvement have a particularly poor prognosis. The 3-year survival rate is only 3% to 10%. Less than 3% of cancers are in this group, but the incidence is higher in African American women and younger women.[61]

Minor Prognostic and Predictive Factors

In addition to the six factors used by the AJCC, a number of other factors are predictive of outcome; some of these also direct therapies against particular molecular targets.

- **Histologic subtype.** The 30-year survival rate of women with special types of invasive carcinomas (tubular, mucinous, medullary, lobular, and papillary) is greater than 60%, compared with less than 20% for women with NST cancers. With the exception of medullary carcinoma, most of these carcinomas will be well to moderately differentiated, ER positive, and HER2/neu negative. This favorable prognosis probably does not apply to unusual special-type carcinomas without these characteristics.
- **Histologic grade.** The most commonly used grading system, the Nottingham Histologic Score (also referred to as Scarff-Bloom-Richardson), combines nuclear grade, tubule formation, and mitotic rate to classify invasive carcinomas into three groups that are highly correlated with survival.[52] Survival for patients with well-differentiated grade 1 carcinomas (approximately 20% of the total) grad-

TABLE 23–4   AJCC Staging*

Stage	T: Primary Cancer	Lymph Nodes (LNs)	M: Distant Metastasis	5-Year Survival (%)
0	DCIS or LCIS	No metastases	Absent	92
I	Invasive carcinoma ≤2 cm	No metastases	Absent	87
II	Invasive carcinoma >2 cm Invasive carcinoma <5 cm	No metastases 1 to 3 positive LNs	Absent Absent	75
III	Invasive carcinoma >5 cm Any size invasive carcinoma Invasive carcinoma with skin or chest wall involvement or inflammatory carcinoma	1 to 3 positive LNs ≥4 positive LNs 0 to >10 positive LNs	Absent Absent Absent	46
IV	Any size invasive carcinoma	Negative or positive lymph nodes	Present	13

DCIS, ductal carcinoma in situ; LCIS, lobular carcinoma in situ.
*The groups listed in the table are based on the characteristics of the primary carcinoma and the axillary lymph nodes. For rare women with involved internal mammary lymph nodes or supraclavicular lymph nodes, there are additional staging criteria.[57]

ually declines to 70% at 24 years. In contrast, most deaths for poorly differentiated grade 3 carcinomas (approximately 46% of the total) occur in the first 10 years, and 45% of patients survive long-term. Women with moderately differentiated grade 2 carcinomas (approximately 35% of the total) have better survival initially, but their long-term survival is only slightly better than grade 3 carcinomas.

○ **Estrogen and progesterone receptors.** Current assays use immunohistochemistry to detect nuclear hormone receptors, a finding that is correlated with a better outcome and is an important predictor of response to hormonal therapy (see Fig. 23–23). Eighty percent of carcinomas that are ER and PR positive respond to hormonal manipulation, whereas only about 40% of those with either ER or PR alone respond. ER-positive cancers are less likely to respond to chemotherapy. Conversely, cancers that fail to express either ER or PR have a less than 10% likelihood of responding to hormonal therapy but are more likely to respond to chemotherapy.

○ **HER2/neu.** HER2/neu overexpression is associated with poorer survival, but its main importance is as a predictor of response to agents that target this transmembrane protein (e.g., trastuzumab or lapatinib). Several different assays are used to determine *HER/neu* gene amplification and protein overexpression (see Fig. 23–23).

○ **Lymphovascular invasion.** Tumor cells are present within vascular spaces (either lymphatics or small capillaries) in about half of all invasive carcinomas. This finding is strongly associated with the presence of lymph node metastases. It is a poor prognostic factor for overall survival in women without lymph node metastases and a risk factor for local recurrence. As already mentioned, extensive plugging of the lymphovascular spaces of the dermis with carcinoma cells (inflammatory carcinoma) bodes a very poor prognosis.

○ **Proliferative rate.** Proliferation can be measured by mitotic counts (e.g., as part of histologic grading), by immunohistochemical detection of cellular proteins produced during the cell cycle (e.g., cyclins, Ki-67), by flow cytometry (as the S-phase fraction), or by thymidine labeling index. Carcino-

mas with high proliferation rates have a poorer prognosis but may respond better to chemotherapy.

○ **DNA content.** The amount of DNA per tumor cell can be determined by flow-cytometric analysis or by image analysis of tissue sections. Tumors with a DNA index of 1 have the same total amount of DNA as normal diploid cells, although marked karyotypic changes may be present. Aneuploid tumors are those with abnormal DNA indices and have a slightly worse prognosis.

○ **Response to neoadjuvant therapy.** Most patients complete their surgery and subsequently receive systemic treatment (referred to as adjuvant therapy). Neoadjuvant therapy is an alternative approach in which the patient is treated before surgery. Although this approach does not improve survival, the degree that the tumor responds to chemotherapy is a strong prognostic factor. Clinical and radiologic examinations are useful to monitor changes during treatment, but often underestimate or overestimate the amount of residual carcinoma. Cancers most likely to respond well are poorly differentiated, ER negative, and have areas of necrosis. The subgroup of patients who achieve a pathologic complete response (i.e., no residual cancer in the breast or lymph nodes) have a greater than 95% long-term survival, in contrast to the poor prognosis of this group as a whole.[62] Pathologic response can be used as a short-term end point for clinical trials (which thus can yield useful information with fewer patients in shorter periods of time) and is being linked to research studies investigating the molecular basis of tumor sensitivity or resistance to therapy.

○ **Gene expression profiling.** Expression profiling has been shown to predict survival and recurrence-free interval, and also identifies patients who are most likely to benefit from particular types of chemotherapy. Methods that require rapidly frozen tissue will be difficult to apply in clinical practice, but alternative approaches that use formalin-fixed paraffin-embedded tissues are beginning to enter clinical practice.[47]

Although gene expression profiles provide a vast amount of information about carcinomas, they are not well correlated with tumor size or lymph node status—two of the strongest prognostic factors.[63] This suggests that while patterns of gene expression likely determine metastatic potential, time and chance also influence whether and when metastasis occurs. It is likely that future means of estimating prognosis will involve some combination of these "old" and "new" factors.

Current therapeutic approaches directed at local and regional control consist of combinations of surgery (mastectomy or breast conservation) and postoperative radiation, whereas attempts at systemic control rely on hormonal treatment, chemotherapy, or both. Axillary node dissection or sentinel node sampling is performed for prognostic purposes, but the axilla can also be treated with radiation alone. Newer therapeutic strategies include inhibitors of membrane-bound growth factor receptors (e.g., HER2/neu), stromal proteases, and angiogenesis.

Such therapies are based on models of breast cancer dissemination that have evolved as our understanding of its biology has changed. Earlier models proposed that breast cancer spreads in a contiguous fashion by direct extension from breast to nodes and could therefore be cured by en bloc surgical resection. However, radical surgery, including mastectomies with removal of pectoralis muscles, internal mammary nodes, and even supraclavicular nodes, failed to decrease mortality. A subsequent model, based on studies demonstrating that breast-conserving surgery and radiation were equivalent to radical mastectomy, postulated that all cancers had spread systemically by the time of diagnosis and that local or regional treatment was unimportant for overall survival. In the current era of increased detection of early-stage carcinomas by mammography, a third model that combines the first two is thought to be a more appropriate guide to therapy.[64]

STROMAL TUMORS

The two types of stroma in the breast, intralobular and interlobular (see the introductory section on the normal female breast), give rise to distinct types of neoplasms. The breast-specific biphasic tumors fibroadenoma and phyllodes tumor arise from intralobular stroma. This specialized stroma may elaborate growth factors for epithelial cells, resulting in the proliferation of the non-neoplastic epithelial component of these tumors. Interlobular stroma is the source of the same types of tumors found in connective tissue in other sites of the body (e.g., lipomas and angiosarcomas) as well as tumors arising more commonly in the breast (e.g., pseudoangiomatous stromal hyperplasia, myofibroblastomas, and fibrous tumors).

Fibroadenoma

This is the most common benign tumor of the female breast. Most occur in women in their 20s and 30s, and they are frequently multiple and bilateral. Young women usually present with a palpable mass and older women with a mammographic density (Fig. 23–26A) or mammographic calcifications. The epithelium of the fibroadenoma is hormonally responsive, and an increase in size due to lactational changes during pregnancy, which may be complicated by infarction and inflammation, can mimic carcinoma. The

stroma often becomes densely hyalinized after menopause and may calcify. Large lobulated ("popcorn") calcifications have a characteristic mammographic appearance, but small calcifications may appear clustered and require biopsy to exclude carcinoma.

Morphology. Fibroadenomas grow as spherical nodules that are usually sharply circumscribed and freely movable. They vary in size from less than 1 cm to large tumors that can replace most of the breast. The tumors are well-circumscribed, rubbery, grayish white nodules that bulge above the surrounding tissue and often contain slitlike spaces (Fig. 23–26B).

The delicate, cellular, and often myxoid stroma resembles normal intralobular stroma. The epithelium may be surrounded by stroma or compressed and distorted by it (Fig. 23–26C). In older women, the stroma typically becomes densely hyalinized and the epithelium atrophic.

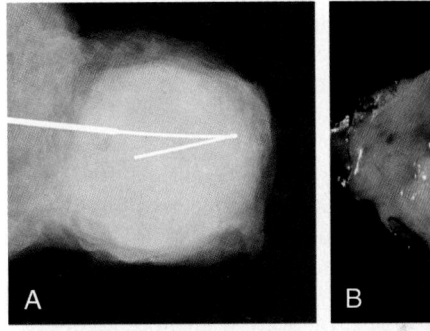
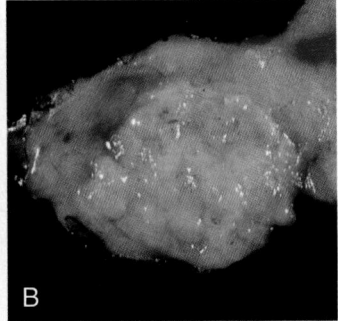
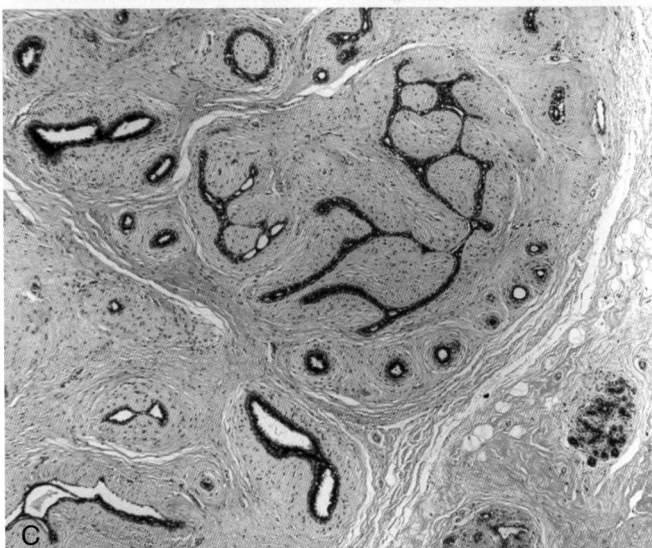

FIGURE 23–26   Fibroadenoma. **A,** The radiogram shows a characteristically well-circumscribed mass. **B,** Grossly, a rubbery, white, well-circumscribed mass is clearly demarcated from the surrounding yellow adipose tissue. The absence of adipose tissue accounts for the radiodensity of the lesion. **C,** The proliferation of intralobular stroma surrounds, pushes, and distorts the associated epithelium. The border is sharply delimited from the surrounding tissue.

Some fibroadenomas are polyclonal hyperplasias of lobular stroma due to some type of stimulus. For example, almost half of women receiving cyclosporin A after renal transplantation develop fibroadenomas. In this setting the tumors are frequently multiple and bilateral. Regression may occur after cessation of cyclosporin treatment. Other fibroadenomas are benign neoplasms associated with clonal cytogenetic aberrations that are confined to the stromal component. No consistent cytogenetic changes have been found.

Fibroadenomas were originally grouped with other "proliferative changes without atypia" in conferring a mild increase in the risk of subsequent cancer. However, in one study the increased risk was limited to fibroadenomas associated with cysts larger than 0.3 cm, sclerosing adenosis, epithelial calcifications, or papillary apocrine change ("complex fibroadenomas") (see Table 23–1).[65]

Phyllodes Tumor

Phyllodes tumors, like fibroadenomas, arise from intralobular stroma. Although they can occur at any age, most present in the sixth decade, 10 to 20 years later than the peak age for fibroadenomas.[66] The majority are detected as palpable masses, but a few are found by mammography. The term *cystosarcoma phyllodes* is sometimes used for these lesions. However, the term *phyllodes tumor* is preferred, since the majority of these tumors behave in a relatively benign fashion, and most are not cystic.

Morphology. The tumors vary in size from a few centimeters to massive lesions involving the entire breast. The larger lesions often have bulbous protrusions (*phyllodes* is Greek for "leaflike") due to the presence of nodules of proliferating stroma covered by epithelium (Fig. 23–27). In some tumors these protrusions extend into a cystic space. This growth pattern can also occasionally be seen in larger fibroadenomas and is not an indication of malignancy. Phyllodes tumors are distinguished from the more common fibroadenomas on the basis of cellularity, mitotic rate, nuclear pleomorphism, stromal overgrowth, and infiltrative borders. Low-grade lesions resemble fibroadenomas but are more cellular and contain mitotic figures. High-grade lesions may be difficult to distinguish from other soft-tissue sarcomas and may have foci of mesenchymal differentiation (e.g., rhabdomyosarcoma or liposarcoma). The frequency of chromosomal changes increases with grade and the majority of high-grade lesions are reported to have amplification of EGFR.[67] Recurrent phyllodes tumors are often of a higher grade than the presenting lesion.

Phyllodes tumors must be excised with wide margins or by mastectomy to avoid local recurrences. Axillary lymph node dissection is not indicated, because the incidence of nodal metastases (as for other stromal malignancies) is exceedingly small. The majority are low-grade tumors that may recur locally but only rarely metastasize. Rare high-grade lesions behave aggressively, with frequent local recurrences and distant hematogenous metastases in about one third of cases. Only the stromal component metastasizes.

Benign Stromal Lesions

Tumors of the interlobular stroma of the breast are composed of stromal cells without an accompanying epithelial component. Pseudoangiomatous stromal hyperplasia and fibrous tumors present as circumscribed palpable masses or mammographic densities in premenopausal women or older women on hormone replacement therapy and are benign proliferations of interlobular fibroblasts and myofibroblasts. Myofibroblastoma consists of myofibroblasts and is unusual in that it is the only breast tumor that is more common in males. Lipomas and hamartomas are often palpable but can also be detected mammographically as fat-containing lesions. The only importance of these lesions is to distinguish them from malignancies.

Fibromatosis is a clonal proliferation of fibroblasts and myofibroblasts. It presents as an irregular, infiltrating mass that can involve both skin and muscle. Though locally aggressive, this lesion does not metastasize. Most cases are sporadic, but some occur as part of familial adenomatous polyposis, hereditary desmoid syndrome, and Gardner syndrome. You will recall that familial adenomatous polyposis is caused by mutations in the adenomatosis polyposis coli (*APC*) gene, which negatively regulates the nuclear translocation of β-catenin. The abnormal presence of β-catenin in the nucleus is a useful diagnostic feature.[68]

Malignant Stromal Tumors

Malignant stromal tumors include angiosarcoma, rhabdomyosarcoma, liposarcoma, leiomyosarcoma, chondrosarcoma, and osteosarcoma. Sarcomas usually present as bulky palpable

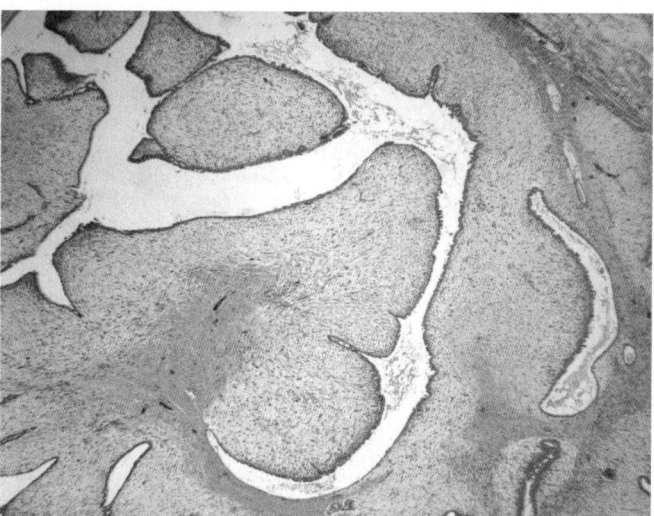

FIGURE 23–27 Phyllodes tumor. Compared to a fibroadenoma, there is increased stromal cellularity, cytologic atypia, and stromal overgrowth, giving rise to the typical leaflike architecture.

masses. Lymph node metastases are rare; hematogenous spread to the lung is commonly seen.

Angiosarcomas of the breast can be sporadic or arise as a complication of radiation therapy.[69] Most sporadic angiosarcomas occur in young women (mean age 35), are of high grade, and have a poor prognosis. There is an approximate 0.3% risk of sarcoma after radiation therapy for breast cancer, with most cases arising 5 to 10 years after treatment. Two thirds are angiosarcomas, most of which arise in the overlying skin. Angiosarcomas can also arise in the skin of an arm rendered chronically lymphedematous by prior mastectomy and lymph node dissection (Stewart-Treves syndrome). Fortunately, this complication has become much less common with better surgical techniques.

OTHER MALIGNANT TUMORS OF THE BREAST

Malignant tumors may arise from the skin of the breast, sweat glands, sebaceous glands, and hair shafts; these tumors are identical to their counterparts found in skin elsewhere. Lymphomas may arise primarily in the breast, or the breasts may be secondarily involved by systemic lymphomas. Most are of diffuse large B-cell type. Young women with Burkitt lymphoma may present with massive bilateral breast involvement and are often pregnant or lactating. Metastases to the breast are rare, and most commonly arise from a contralateral breast carcinoma. The most frequent nonmammary metastases are from melanomas and lung cancers.

THE MALE BREAST

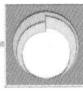

The normal male breast consists of the nipple and a rudimentary duct system ending in terminal buds without lobule formation. Only two processes occur with sufficient frequency to merit consideration.

Gynecomastia

Gynecomastia (enlargement of the male breast) may be unilateral or bilateral and presents as a button-like subareolar enlargement. In advanced cases, the swelling can simulate the adolescent female breast. The lesion must be differentiated only from rare carcinomas of the male breast.

> **Morphology.** There is an increase in dense collagenous connective tissue and marked micropapillary epithelial hyperplasia of the duct lining (Fig. 23–28). The individual epithelial cells are fairly regular, columnar to cuboidal cells with regular nuclei. Lobule formation is rare.

Like the female breast, the male breast is subject to hormonal influences, and gynecomastia may occur as a result of an imbalance between estrogens, which stimulate breast tissue, and androgens, which counteract these effects. It is encountered under a variety of normal and abnormal circumstances, including puberty, in the very aged, or at any time during adult life when there is cause for hyperestrinism. The most important of these is cirrhosis of the liver, since this organ is responsible for metabolizing estrogen. In older males, gynecomastia may be due to a relative increase in adrenal estrogens as the androgenic function of the testis fails. Drugs such as alcohol, marijuana, heroin, antiretroviral therapy, anabolic steroids used by some athletes and body builders, and some psychoactive agents have also been associated with gynecomastia. Rarely, gynecomastia may occur as part of Klinefelter syndrome (XXY karyotype) or in association with functioning testicular neoplasms, such as Leydig cell and, rarely, Sertoli cell tumors.

Carcinoma

Carcinoma arising in the male breast is a rare occurrence.[70] The overall incidence in men is only 1% of that in women, which translates to a lifetime risk of 0.11% (as compared with about 13% in women). There are about 1500 cases and 400 deaths each year. Risk factors are similar to those in women and include first-degree relatives with breast cancer, decreased testicular function (e.g., Klinefelter syndrome),

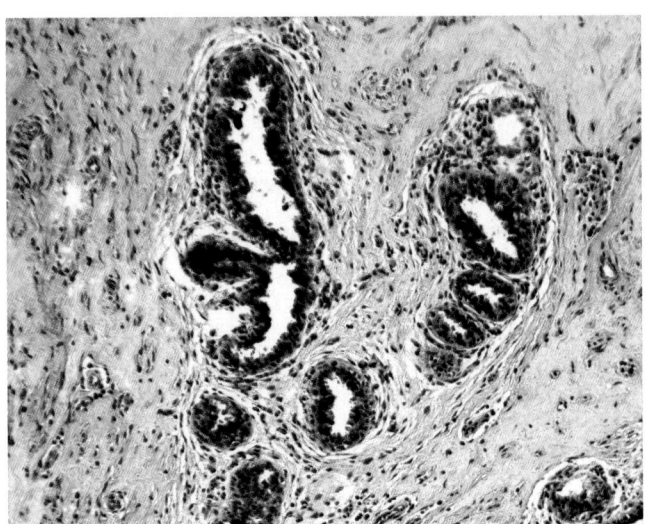

FIGURE 23–28 Gynecomastia. Terminal ducts (without lobule formation) are lined by a multilayered epithelium with small papillary tufts. There is typically surrounding periductal hyalinization and fibrosis.

exposure to exogenous estrogens, increasing age, infertility, obesity, prior benign breast disease, exposure to ionizing radiation, and residency in Western countries. Gynecomastia does not seem to be a risk factor. From 4% to 14% of cases in males are attributed to germline *BRCA2* mutations. There is a 60% to 76% chance of a *BRCA2* mutation in families with at least one affected male. Male breast cancer is also observed in *BRCA1* families, though not as frequently (see Table 23–2). From 3% to 8% of cases are associated with Klinefelter syndrome.

The pathology of male breast cancer is remarkably similar to that of cancers seen in women. The same histologic subtypes of invasive cancer are present, although papillary carcinomas (both invasive and in situ) are more common and lobular carcinomas are less common. The expression of molecular markers is similar, with the exception that ER positivity is more common in male breast cancer (81% of tumors). Unlike in women, the incidence of ER-positive tumors does not increase with age. Prognostic factors are similar in men and women.

Because breast epithelium in men is limited to large ducts near the nipple, carcinomas usually present as a palpable subareolar mass, 2 to 3 cm in size. Nipple discharge is a common symptom. The carcinoma is situated close to the overlying skin and underlying thoracic wall, and even small carcinomas can invade these structures and ulcerate through the skin. Dissemination follows the same pattern as in women, and axillary lymph node involvement is present in about half of cases at the time of diagnosis. Distant metastases to the lungs, brain, bone, and liver are common. Although men present at higher stages, prognosis is similar in men and women when they are matched by stage. Most cancers are treated locally with mastectomy and axillary node dissection. The same systemic treatment guidelines are used for men and women, and response rates are similar.

REFERENCES

1. Bocker W et al.: Common adult stem cells in the human breast give rise to glandular and myoepithelial cell lineages: a new cell biological concept. Lab Invest 82:737, 2002.
2. Wiseman BS, Werb Z: Stromal effects on mammary gland development and breast cancer. Science 296:1046, 2002.
3. Longacre TA, Bartow SA: A correlative morphologic study of human breast and endometrium in the menstrual cycle. Am J Surg Pathol 10:382, 1986.
4. Russo J et al.: Full-term pregnancy induces a specific genomic signature in the human breast. Cancer Epidemiol Biomarkers Prev 17:51, 2008.
5. Schedin P: Pregnancy-associated breast cancer and metastasis. Nat Rev Cancer 4:281, 2006.
6. Lang JE, Kuerer HM: Breast ductal secretions: clinical features, potential uses, and possible applications. Cancer Control 14:350, 2007.
7. Meguid M et al.: Pathogenesis-based treatment of recurring subareolar breast abscesses. Surgery 118:775, 1995.
8. Abdel-Fatah TMA et al.: High frequency of coexistence of columnar cell lesions, lobular neoplasia, and low grade ductal carcinoma in situ with invasive tubular carcinoma and invasive lobular carcinoma. Am J Surg Pathol 31:417, 2007.
9. Abdel-Fatah TM et al.: Morphologic and molecular evolutionary pathways of low nuclear grade invasive breast cancers and their putative precursor lesions: further evidence to support the concept of low nuclear grade breast neoplasia family. Am J Surg Pathol 2008;32:513, 2008.
10. Allred DC et al.: Ductal carcinoma in situ and the emergence of diversity during breast cancer evolution. Clin Cancer Res 14:370, 2008.
11. Fitzgibbons PL et al.: Benign breast changes and the risk for subsequent breast cancer: an update of the 1985 consensus statement. Arch Pathol Lab Med 122:1053, 1998.
12. Schnitt SJ: Benign breast disease and breast cancer risk: morphology and beyond. Am J Surg Pathol 27:836, 2003.
13. Hartmann LC et al.: Benign breast disease and the risk of breast cancer. N Engl J Med 353:229, 2005.
14. Collins LC et al.: Magnitude and laterality of breast cancer risk according to histologic type of atypical hyperplasia. Results from the Nurses' Health Study. Cancer 109:180, 2007.
15. Reeder JG, Vogel VG: Breast cancer risk management. Clin Breast Cancer 7:833, 2007.
16. Rossouw JE et al.: Risks and benefits of estrogen plus progestin in healthy postmenopausal women: principal results from the Women's Health Initiative randomized controlled trial. JAMA 288:321, 2002.
17. Gail MH et al.: Projecting individualized probabilities of developing breast cancer for white females who are being examined annually. J Natl Cancer Inst 81:1879, 1989.
18. Gail MH et al.: Projecting individualized absolute invasive breast cancer risk in African American women. J Natl Cancer Inst 99:1782, 2007.
19. Morris CR et al.: The risk of developing breast cancer within the next 5, 10, or 20 years of a woman's life. Am J Prev Med 20:213, 2001.
20. Hayanga AJ, Newman LA: Investigating the phenotypes and genotypes of breast cancer in women with African ancestry: the need for more genetic epidemiology. Surg Clin North Am 87:551, 2007.
21. John EM et al.: Prevalence of pathogenic *BRCA1* mutation carriers in 5 US racial/ethnic groups. JAMA 298:2910, 2007.
22. Collaborative Group on Hormonal Factors in Breast Cancer, Beral V: Breast cancer and breastfeeding: collaborative reanalysis of individual data from 47 epidemiological studies in 30 countries, including 50,302 women with breast cancer and 96,973 women without the disease. Lancet 360:187, 2002.
23. Bradbury AR, Olopade OI: Genetic susceptibility to breast cancer. Rev Endocr Metab Disord 8:225, 2007.
24. Garcia-Closas M et al.: Heterogeneity of breast cancer associations with five susceptibility loci by clinical and pathological characteristics. PLOS Genetics 4:e10000054, 2008.
25. Pageau GJ et al.: The disappearing Barr body in breast and ovarian cancers. Nat Rev Cancer 7:628, 2007.
26. Yager JD, Davidson NE: Estrogen carcinogenesis in breast cancer. N Engl J Med 354:270, 2006.
27. Desta Z, Flockhart DA: Germline pharmacogenetics of tamoxifen response: have we learned enough? J Clin Oncol 25:5147, 2007.
28. Hanahan D, Weinberg RA: The hallmarks of cancer. Cell 100:57, 2000.
29. Hahn WC, Weinberg RA: Rules for making human tumor cells. N Engl J Med 347:1593, 2002.
30. Iqbal M et al.: Subgroups of non-atypical hyperplasia of breast defined by proliferation of oestrogen receptor-positive cells. J Pathol 193:333, 2001.
31. Campbell LL, Polyak K: Breast tumor heterogeneity. Cancer stem cells or clonal evolution? Cell Cycle 6:2332, 2007.
32. Stingl J, Caldas C: Molecular heterogeneity of breast carcinomas and the cancer stem cell hypothesis. Nat Rev Cancer 10:791, 2007.
33. Murad TM: A proposed histochemical and electron microscopic classification of human breast cancer according to cell of origin. Cancer 27:288, 1971.
34. Shipitsin M et al.: Molecular definition of breast tumor heterogeneity. Cancer Cell 11:259, 2007.
35. Gauthier ML et al.: Abrogated response to cellular stress identifies DCIS associated with subsequent tumor events and defines basal-like breast tumors. Cancer Cell 12:479, 2007.
36. Tlsty T, Coussens LM: Tumor stroma and regulation of cancer development. Ann Rev Pathol Mech Dis 1:119, 2006.
37. Patocs A et al.: Breast-cancer stromal cells with *TP53* mutations and nodal metastases. N Engl J Med 357:2543, 2007.
38. Wellings SR: A hypothesis of the origin of human breast cancer from the terminal ductal lobular unit. Pathol Res Pract 166:515, 1980.
39. Burstein HJ et al.: Ductal carcinoma in situ of the breast. N Engl J Med 350:1430, 2004.
40. Page DL et al.: Continued local recurrence of carcinoma 15–25 years after a diagnosis of low grade ductal carcinoma in situ of the breast treated only by biopsy. Cancer 76:1197, 1995.
41. O'Sullivan MJ, Morrow M: Ductal carcinoma in situ—current management. Surg Clin North Am 87:333, 2007.

42. Li CI et al.: Risk of invasive breast carcinoma among women diagnosed with ductal carcinoma in situ and lobular carcinoma in situ, 1988–2001. Cancer 106:2104, 2006.

43. Lakhani SR et al.: The management of lobular carcinoma in situ (LCIS). Is LCIS the same as ductal carcinoma in situ (DCIS)? Eur J Cancer 42:2205, 2006.

44. Hanby AM, Hughes TA: In situ and invasive lobular neoplasia of the breast. Histopathology 52:58, 2008.

45. Cristofanilli M et al.: Inflammatory breast cancer (IBC) and patterns of recurrence. Understanding the biology of a unique disease. Cancer 110:1436, 2007.

46. Peppercorn J et al.: Molecular subtypes in breast cancer evaluation and management: divide and conquer. Cancer Invest 26:1, 2008.

47. Harris L et al.: American Society of Clinical Oncology 2007 update of recommendations for the use of tumor markers in breast cancer. J Clin Oncol 25:5287, 2007.

48. Kang SP et al.: Triple negative breast cancer: current understanding of biology and treatment options. Curr Opin Obstet Gynecol 20:40, 2008.

49. Reis-Filho JS, Tutt ANJ: Triple negative tumours: a critical review. Histopathology 52:108, 2008.

50. Bempt IV et al.: The complexity of genotypic alterations underlying HER2-positive breast cancer: an explanation for its clinical heterogeneity. Curr Opin Oncol 19:552, 2007.

51. Pal SK, Pegram M: HER2 targeted therapy in breast cancer . . . beyond Herceptin. Rev Endocr Metab Disord 8:269, 2007.

52. Ellis IO, Elston CW: Histologic grade. In O'Malley FP, Pinder SE (eds): Breast Pathology. Elsevier, 2006, pp 225–233.

53. Yoder BJ et al.: Molecular and morphologic distinctions between infiltrating ductal and lobular carcinoma of the breast. Breast J 13:172, 2007.

54. Schrader KA et al.: Hereditary diffuse gastric cancer: association with lobular breast cancer. Fam Cancer 7:73, 2008.

55. Masciari S et al.: Germline E-cadherin mutations in familial lobular breast cancer. J Med Genet 44:726, 2007.

56. Bertucci F et al.: Gene expression profiling shows medullary breast cancer is a subgroup of basal breast cancers. Cancer Res 66:4636, 2006.

57. American Joint Committee on Cancer: AJCC Cancer Staging Manual, 6th ed. New York, Springer, 2002.

58. Kang Y: New tricks against an old foe: molecular dissection of metastasis tissue tropism in breast cancer. Breast Dis 26:129, 2006.

59. Luck AA et al.: The influence of basal phenotype on the metastatic pattern of breast cancer. Clin Oncol 20:40, 2008.

60. Hackshaw AK, Paul EA: Breast self-examination and death from breast cancer: a meta-analysis. Br J Cancer 88:1047, 2003.

61. Levine PH, Veneroso C: The epidemiology of inflammatory breast cancer. Semin Oncol 35:11, 2008.

62. Gralow JR et al.: Preoperative therapy in invasive breast cancer: pathologic assessment and systemic therapy issues in operable disease. J Clin Oncol 26:814, 2008.

63. Lu X et al.: Predicting features of breast cancer with gene expression patterns. Breast Cancer Res Treat 108:191, 2008.

64. Hellman S: Natural history of small breast cancers. J Clin Oncol 12:2229, 1994.

65. Dupont WD et al.: Long-term risk of breast cancer in women with fibroadenoma. N Engl J Med 331:10, 1994.

66. Telli ML et al.: Phyllodes tumors of the breast: natural history, diagnosis, and treatment. J Natl Compr Canc Netw 5:324, 2007.

67. Agelopoulos K et al.: EGFR amplification specific gene expression in phyllodes tumours of the breast. Cell Oncol 29:443, 2007.

68. Lee AH: Recent developments in the histological diagnosis of spindle cell carcinoma, fibromatosis and phyllodes tumour of the breast. Histopathology 52:45, 2008.

69. Brodie C, Provenzano E: Vascular proliferations of the breast. Histopathology 52:30, 2008.

70. Agrawal A et al.: Male breast cancer: a review of clinical management. Breast Cancer Res Treat 103:11, 2007.

24

The Endocrine System

ANIRBAN MAITRA

■ PITUITARY GLAND

Clinical Manifestations of Pituitary
  Disease

Pituitary Adenomas and
  Hyperpituitarism
  Prolactinomas
  Growth Hormone Cell (Somatotroph)
    Adenomas
  ACTH Cell (Corticotroph) Adenomas
  Other Anterior Pituitary Adenomas

Hypopituitarism

Posterior Pituitary Syndromes

Hypothalamic Suprasellar Tumors

■ THYROID GLAND

Hyperthyroidism

Hypothyroidism
  Cretinism
  Myxedema

Thyroiditis
  Hashimoto Thyroiditis
  Subacute (Granulomatous) Thyroiditis
  Subacute Lymphocytic (Painless)
    Thyroiditis

Graves Disease

Diffuse and Multinodular Goiters
  Diffuse Nontoxic (Simple) Goiter
  Multinodular Goiter

Neoplasms of the Thyroid
  Adenomas
  Carcinomas

Pathogenesis
Papillary Carcinoma
Follicular Carcinoma
Anaplastic (Undifferentiated) Carcinoma
Medullary Carcinoma

Congenital Anomalies

■ PARATHYROID GLANDS

Hyperparathyroidism
  Primary Hyperparathyroidism
  Secondary Hyperparathyroidism

Hypoparathyroidism

Pseudohypoparathyroidism

■ THE ENDOCRINE PANCREAS

Diabetes Mellitus
  Diagnosis
  Classification
  Glucose Homeostasis
    Regulation of Insulin Release
    Insulin Action and Insulin Signaling
      Pathways
  Pathogenesis of Type 1 Diabetes Mellitus
    Genetic Susceptibility
    Environmental Factors
    Mechanisms of β-Cell Destruction
  Pathogenesis of Type 2 Diabetes Mellitus
    Insulin Resistance
    β-Cell Dysfunction
  Monogenic Forms of Diabetes
  Pathogenesis of the Complications of
    Diabetes
  Morphology of Diabetes and Its Late
    Complications
  Clinical Features of Diabetes

Pancreatic Endocrine Neoplasms
  Hyperinsulinism (Insulinoma)
  Zollinger-Ellison Syndrome (Gastrinomas)
  Other Rare Pancreatic Endocrine
    Neoplasms

■ **ADRENAL GLANDS**

Adrenal Cortex
  Adrenocortical Hyperfunction
    (Hyperadrenalism)
    Hypercortisolism (Cushing Syndrome)
    Primary Hyperaldosteronism
    Adrenogenital Syndromes
  Adrenocortical Insufficiency
    Primary Acute Adrenocortical
      Insufficiency
    Waterhouse-Friderichsen Syndrome

  Primary Chronic Adrenocortical
    Insufficiency (Addison Disease)
  Secondary Adrenocortical Insufficiency
  Adrenocortical Neoplasms
  Other Lesions of the Adrenal

Adrenal Medulla
  Pheochromocytoma

■ **MULTIPLE ENDOCRINE NEOPLASIA**
  SYNDROMES
  Multiple Endocrine Neoplasia, Type 1
  Multiple Endocrine Neoplasia, Type 2

■ **PINEAL GLAND**
Pinealomas

The endocrine system consists of a highly integrated and widely distributed group of organs that orchestrate a state of metabolic equilibrium, or homeostasis, among the various organs of the body. Signaling by extracellular secreted molecules can be classified into three types—autocrine, paracrine, or endocrine—on the basis of the distance over which the signal acts. In endocrine signaling, the secreted molecules, which are frequently called *hormones*, act on target cells that are distant from their site of synthesis. An endocrine hormone is frequently carried by the blood from its site of release to its target. In response, the target tissue often secretes factors that down-regulate the activity of the gland that produces the stimulating hormone, a process known as *feedback inhibition*.

Several processes can disturb the normal activity of the endocrine system, including impaired synthesis or release of hormones, abnormal interactions between hormones and their target tissues, and abnormal responses of target organs. Endocrine diseases can be generally classified as (1) diseases of *underproduction or overproduction* of hormones and their resulting biochemical and clinical consequences and (2) diseases associated with the development of *mass lesions*. Such lesions might be nonfunctional, or they might be associated with overproduction or underproduction of hormones. The study of endocrine diseases requires integration of morphologic findings with biochemical measurements of the levels of hormones, their regulators, and other metabolites.

PITUITARY GLAND

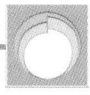

The pituitary gland is composed of two morphologically and functionally distinct components: the anterior lobe (adenohypophysis) and the posterior lobe (neurohypophysis). The *anterior pituitary* constitutes about 80% of the gland. The production of most pituitary hormones is controlled predominantly by positive-acting releasing factors from the hypothalamus (Fig. 24–1), which are carried to the anterior pituitary by a portal vascular system. Prolactin is the major exception; its primary hypothalamic control is inhibitory, through the action of dopamine. Pituitary growth hormone also differs in that it receives both stimulatory and inhibitory influences via the hypothalamus. In routine histologic sections of the anterior pituitary, a colorful array of cells is present that contain eosinophilic cytoplasm (acidophil), basophilic cytoplasm (basophil), or poorly staining cytoplasm (chromophobe) cells

(Fig. 24–2). Specific antibodies against the pituitary hormones identify five cell types:

1. *Somatotrophs*, producing growth hormone (GH): These acidophilic cells constitute half of all the hormone-producing cells in the anterior pituitary.
2. *Lactotrophs* (mammotrophs), producing prolactin: These acidophilic cells secrete prolactin, which is essential for lactation.
3. *Corticotrophs:* These basophilic cells produce adrenocorticotropic hormone (ACTH), pro-opiomelanocortin (POMC), melanocyte-stimulating hormone (MSH), endorphins, and lipotropin.
4. *Thyrotrophs:* These pale basophilic cells produce thyroid-stimulating hormone (TSH).

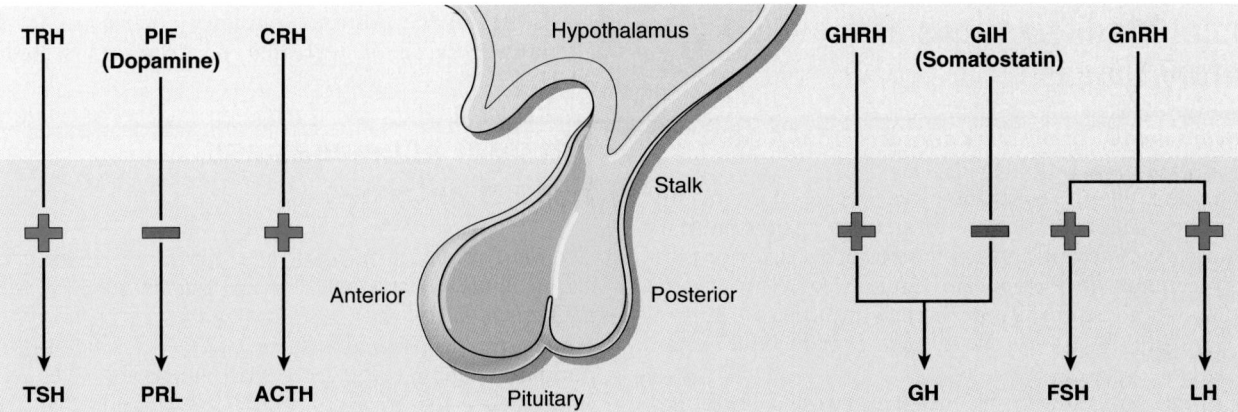

FIGURE 24–1 Hormones released by the anterior pituitary. The adenohypophysis (anterior pituitary) releases five hormones that are in turn under the control of various stimulatory and inhibitory hypothalamic releasing factors. TSH, thyroid-stimulating hormone (thyrotropin); PRL, prolactin; ACTH, adrenocorticotropic hormone (corticotropin); GH, growth hormone (somatotropin); FSH, follicle-stimulating hormone; LH, luteinizing hormone. The stimulatory releasing factors are TRH (thyrotropin-releasing hormone), CRH (corticotropin-releasing hormone), GHRH (growth hormone–releasing hormone), GnRH (gonadotropin-releasing hormone). The inhibitory hypothalamic influences comprise PIF (prolactin inhibitory factor or dopamine) and growth hormone inhibitory factor (GIH or somatostatin).

5. *Gonadotrophs:* These basophilic cells produce both follicle-stimulating hormone (FSH) and luteinizing hormone (LH). FSH stimulates the formation of graafian follicles in the ovary, and LH induces ovulation and the formation of corpora lutea in the ovary. The same two hormones also regulate spermatogenesis and testosterone production in males.

The *posterior pituitary* consists of modified glial cells (termed *pituicytes*) and axonal processes extending from the hypothalamus through the pituitary stalk to the posterior lobe (*axon terminals*). The two peptide hormones secreted from the posterior pituitary—oxytocin and *antidiuretic hormone* (ADH, also called *vasopressin*)—are actually synthesized in the hypothalamus and are stored within the axon terminals residing in the posterior pituitary. In response to appropriate stimuli, the pre-formed hormones are released directly into the systemic circulation through the venous channels of the pituitary. For example, dilatation of the cervix in pregnancy results in massive oxytocin release, leading to contraction of the uterine smooth muscle, facilitating parturition (uterine labor). Similarly, oxytocin released upon nipple stimulation in the postnatal period acts on the smooth muscles surrounding the lactiferous ducts of the mammary glands and facilitates lactation. Synthetic oxytocin can be administered during pregnancy for artificial induction of labor. The most important function of ADH is to conserve water by restricting diuresis during periods of dehydration and hypovolemia. Decreased blood pressure, sensed by *baroreceptors* (pressure-sensing receptors) in the cardiac atria and carotids, stimulates ADH release. An increase in plasma osmotic pressure detected by *osmoreceptors* also tiggers ADH secretion. In contrast, states of hypervolemia and increased atrial distention result in inhibition of ADH secretion.

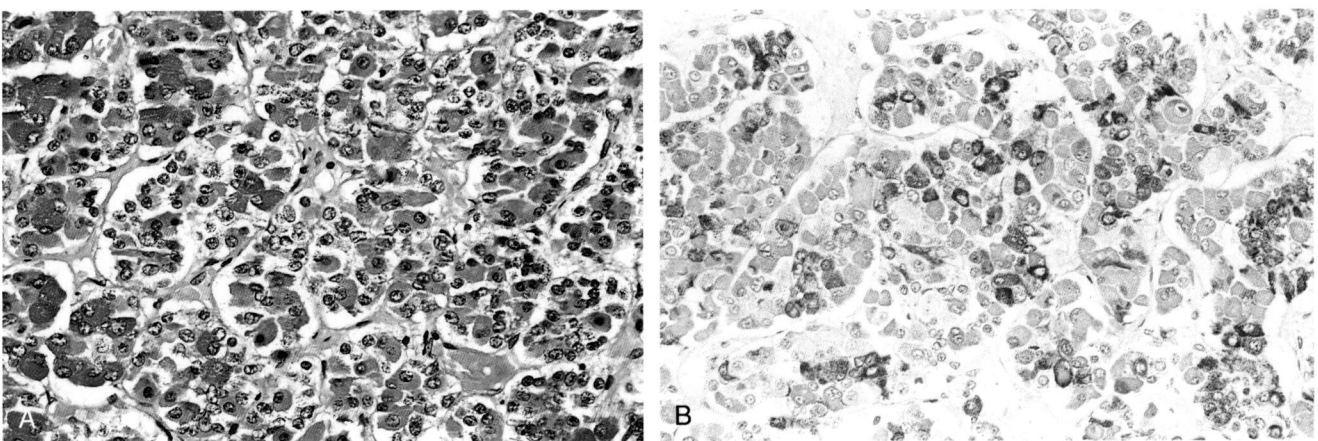

FIGURE 24–2 **A,** Photomicrograph of normal pituitary. The gland is populated by several distinct cell populations containing a variety of stimulating (tropic) hormones. Each of the hormones has different staining characteristics, resulting in a mixture of cell types in routine histologic preparations. **B,** Immunostain for human growth hormone.

Clinical Manifestations of Pituitary Disease

The manifestations of pituitary disorders are as follows:

Hyperpituitarism: Arising from excess secretion of trophic hormones. The causes of hyperpituitarism include pituitary adenoma, hyperplasia and carcinomas of the anterior pituitary, secretion of hormones by nonpituitary tumors, and certain hypothalamic disorders. The symptoms of hyperpituitarism are discussed in the context of individual tumors below.

Hypopituitarism: Arising from deficiency of trophic hormones. This may be caused by destructive processes, including *ischemic injury, surgery or radiation, inflammatory reactions,* and *nonfunctional pituitary adenomas.*

Local mass effects: Among the earliest changes referable to mass effect are *radiographic abnormalities of the sella turcica,* including sellar expansion, bony erosion, and disruption of the diaphragma sella. Because of the close proximity of the optic nerves and chiasm to the sella, expanding pituitary lesions often compress decussating fibers in the optic chiasm. This gives rise to *visual field abnormalities,* classically in the form of defects in the lateral (temporal) visual fields, so-called *bitemporal hemianopsia.* In addition, a variety of other visual field abnormalities may be caused by asymmetric growth of many tumors. Like any expanding intracranial mass, pituitary adenomas can produce signs and symptoms of *elevated intracranial pressure,* including headache, nausea, and vomiting. On occasion, acute hemorrhage into an adenoma is associated with clinical evidence of rapid enlargement of the lesion, a situation appropriately termed *pituitary apoplexy.* Acute pituitary apoplexy is a neurosurgical emergency, since it can cause sudden death (see below).

Diseases of the posterior pituitary often come to clinical attention because of increased or decreased secretion of ADH.

Pituitary Adenomas and Hyperpituitarism

The most common cause of hyperpituitarism is an adenoma arising in the anterior lobe. Pituitary adenomas are classified on the basis of hormone(s) produced by the neoplastic cells, which are detected by immunohistochemical stains (Table 24–1). Some pituitary adenomas can secrete two hormones (GH and prolactin being the most common combination), and rarely, pituitary adenomas are plurihormonal. Pituitary adenomas can be *functional* (i.e., associated with hormone excess and clinical manifestations thereof) or *nonfunctioning* (i.e., immunohistochemical and/or ultrastructural demonstration of hormone production at the tissue level, without clinical symptoms of hormone excess). Less common causes of hyperpituitarism include pituitary carcinomas and some hypothalamic disorders. Large pituitary adenomas, and particularly nonfunctioning ones, may cause hypopituitarism as they encroach on and destroy adjacent anterior pituitary parenchyma.

Pituitary adenomas are usually found in adults, with a peak incidence from 35 to 60 years of age. They are designated, somewhat arbitrarily, *microadenomas* if they are less than 1 cm in diameter and *macroadenomas* if they exceed 1 cm in diameter. Silent and hormone-negative adenomas are likely to come to clinical attention at a later stage than those associated with endocrine abnormalities and are therefore more likely to be macroadenomas. A meta-analysis of autopsy studies estimates the population prevalence of pituitary adenomas to be about 14%, although the vast majority of these lesions are incidentally diagnosed microadenomas ("pituitary incidentaloma").[1]

TABLE 24–1	Classification of Pituitary Adenomas		
Pituitary Cell Type	**Hormone**	**Tumor Type**	**Associated Syndrome***
Corticotroph	ACTH and other POMC-derived peptides	ACTH cell (corticotroph) adenoma	Cushing syndrome Nelson syndrome
Somatotroph	GH	GH cell (somatotroph) adenoma	Gigantism (children) Acromegaly (adults)
Lactotroph	Prolactin	Prolactin cell (lactotroph) adenoma	Galactorrhea and amenorrhea (in females) Sexual dysfunction, infertility
Mammosomatotroph	Prolactin, GH	Mammosomatotroph	Combined features of GH and prolactin excess
Thyrotroph	TSH	TSH cell (thyrotroph) adenoma	Hyperthyroidism
Gonadotroph	FSH, LH	Gonadotroph, "null cell," oncocytic adenomas	Hypogonadism, mass effects, and hypopituitarism

ACTH, adrenocorticotrophic hormone; FSH, follicle-stimulating hormone; GH, growth hormone; LH, luteinizing hormone; POMC, pro-opiomelanocortin; TSH, thyroid-stimulating hormone.
*Note that nonfunctional adenomas in each category typically present with *mass effects* accompanied by *hypopituitarism* due to destruction of normal pituitary parenchyma. These features are particularly common with gonadotroph adenomas.
Adapted from Ezzat S, Asa SL: Mechanisms of disease: the pathogenesis of pituitary tumors. Nat Clin Prac Endocrinol Metab 2:200–230, 2006.

TABLE 24–2 Genetic Alterations in Pituitary Tumors

Gene	Mechanism of Alteration	Pituitary Tumor Subtype
GAIN OF FUNCTION		
$G_s\alpha$	Activating mutation	GH adenomas
Protein kinase A (PKA)*	Germline inactivating mutations of *PRKARIA* (Carney complex), a negative regulator of PKA	GH and prolactin adenomas
Cyclin D1	Overexpression	Aggressive adenomas
HRAS	Activating mutation	Pituitary carcinomas
LOSS OF FUNCTION		
Menin*	Germline inactivating mutations of *MEN1* (multiple endocrine neoplasia, type 1)	GH, prolactin, and ACTH adenomas
CDKN1B (p27/KIP1)*	Germline inactivating mutations of CDKN1B ("MEN-1-like" syndrome)	ACTH adenomas
Aryl hydrocarbon receptor interacting protein (AIP)*	Germline mutations of *AIP* (pituitary adenoma predisposition [PAP] syndrome)	GH adenomas
Retinoblastoma (RB) protein	Methylation of *RB* gene promoter	Aggressive adenomas

ACTH, adrenocorticotrophic hormone; GH, growth hormone.
*Genetic alterations associated with *familial* predisposition to pituitary adenomas.
Adapted from Boikos SA, Stratakis CA: Molecular genetics of the cAMP-dependent protein kinase pathway and of sporadic pituitary tumorigenesis. Hum Mol Genet 16:R80–R87, 2007.

With recent advances in molecular techniques, substantial insight has been gained into *the genetic abnormalities associated with pituitary adenomas*[2] (Table 24–2):

- G-protein mutations are possibly the best-characterized molecular abnormalities in pituitary adenomas. G proteins are described in Chapter 3; here we will review their function in the context of endocrine neoplasms. G proteins play a critical role in signal transduction, transmitting signals from particular *cell surface receptors* (e.g., GHRH receptor) to *intracellular effectors* (e.g., adenyl cyclase), which then generate *second messengers* (e.g., cyclic adenosine monophosphate, cAMP). These are heterotrimeric proteins, composed of a specific α-subunit that binds guanine nucleotide and interacts with both cell surface receptors and intracellular effectors (Fig. 24–3); the β- and γ-subunits are noncovalently bound to the specific α-subunit. G_s is a stimulatory G protein that has a pivotal role in signal transduction in several endocrine organs, including the pituitary. The α-subunit of G_s ($G_s\alpha$) is encoded by the *GNAS* gene, located on chromosome 20q13. In the basal state, G_s exists in an inactive state, with guanosine diphosphate (GDP) bound to the guanine nucleotide-binding site of $G_s\alpha$. On interaction with the ligand-bound cell surface receptor, GDP dissociates, and guanosine triphosphate (GTP) binds to $G_s\alpha$, activating the G protein. The activation of $G_s\alpha$ results in the generation of cAMP, which acts as a potent mitogenic stimulus for a variety of endocrine cell types (such as pituitary somatotrophs and corticotrophs, thyroid follicular cells, parathyroid cells), promoting cellular proliferation and hormone synthesis and secretion. The activation of $G_s\alpha$, and resultant generation of cAMP, are *transient* because of an intrinsic GTPase activity in the α-subunit, which hydrolyzes GTP into GDP. *A mutation in the α-subunit that interferes with its intrinsic GTPase activity will therefore result in constitutive activation of $G_s\alpha$, persistent generation of cAMP, and unchecked cellular proliferation* (see Fig. 24–3). Approximately 40% of somatotroph cell adenomas bear *GNAS* mutations that abrogate the GTPase activ-

ity of $G_s\alpha$. In addition, *GNAS* mutations have also been described in a minority of corticotroph adenomas; in contrast, *GNAS* mutations are absent in thyrotroph, lactotroph, and gonadotroph adenomas, since their respective hypothalamic release hormones do not mediate their action via cAMP-dependent pathways.

- The overwhelming majority of pituitary adenomas are sporadic in nature, and only approximately 5% of cases arise as a result of an inherited predisposition. *Four genes have been identified thus far as a cause of familial pituitary adenomas: MEN1, CDKN1B, PRKAR1A, and AIP.*[3] Germline inactivating mutations of the *MEN1* gene on chromosome 11q13 are responsible for multiple endocrine neoplasia syndrome, type 1 (MEN-1, discussed in detail below). The gene product of *MEN1* is the tumor suppressor protein menin, and individuals with MEN-1 syndrome develop tumors in multiple endocrine organs, including the pituitary. Approximately a third of patients with MEN-1 develop pituitary adenomas, most commonly GH-, prolactin-, or ACTH-secreting tumors. In contrast, somatic mutations of *MEN1* are rare in sporadic pituitary tumors. The gene product of *CDKN1B* on chromosome 12p13 is the cell cycle checkpoint regulator p27 or KIP1; germline mutations of *CDKN1B* are responsible for a subset of patients with a "MEN-1 like" syndrome who lack *MEN1* abnormalities.[4] The *protein kinase A regulatory subunit 1α (PRKAR1A)* gene on chromosome 17q24 is mutated in patients with Carney complex, an autosomal-dominant disorder characterized by pituitary and other endocrine tumors. This gene encodes a tumor suppressor that regulates the activity of protein kinase A, a downstream mediator of cAMP-dependent signaling. Thus, loss of PRKAR1A protein function leads to inappropriate activation of cAMP cellular targets, further underscoring the importance of this second-messenger pathway in pituitary neoplasia. The *aryl hydrocarbon receptor interacting protein (AIP)* on chromosome 11q is a recently described pituitary adenoma predisposition gene. Patients with germline *AIP* mutations often present with acromegaly due to an underlying GH-

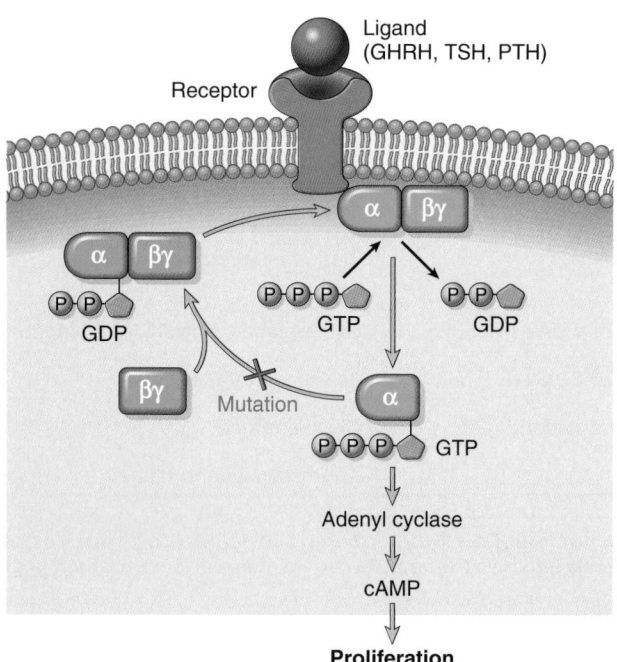

FIGURE 24–3 G-protein signaling in endocrine neoplasia. Mutations that lead to G-protein hyperactivity are seen in a variety of endocrine neoplasms, including pituitary, thyroid, and parathyroid adenomas. G proteins play a critical role in signal transduction, transmitting signals from cell surface receptors (GHRH, TSH, or PTH receptor) to intracellular effectors (e.g., adenyl cyclase), which then generate second messengers (cAMP, cyclic adenosine monophosphate). GDP, guanosine diphosphate; GTP, guanosine triphosphate; P_i, inorganic phosphate. See Figure 24–1 for other abbreviations.

secreting adenoma, and are typically younger (<35 years of age) at the time of diagnosis than sporadic GH adenoma patients.[5] The precise mechanism by which the AIP protein acts as a tumor suppressor in the pituitary is not known. Not all persons with germline *AIP* mutations have a positive family history of pituitary tumors, as a result of incomplete penetrance. Immunohistochemistry for AIP is recommended in GH adenomas arising in younger patients, as mutations associated with adenoma typically cause absence of protein expression. Somatic mutations of these four genes are rarely encountered in sporadic pituitary adenomas.

○ Molecular abnormalities associated with aggressive behavior include aberrations in cell cycle checkpoint genes, such as overexpression of cyclin D1, mutations of *p53*, and epigenetic silencing of the retinoblastoma gene (*RB1*). In addition, activating mutations of the *HRAS* oncogene are observed in rare *pituitary carcinomas* (see below).

Morphology. The **typical pituitary adenoma** is a soft, well-circumscribed lesion that may be confined to the sella turcica. Larger lesions typically extend superiorly through the diaphragm sella into the suprasellar region, where they often compress the optic chiasm

and adjacent structures, such as some of the cranial nerves (Fig. 24–4). As these adenomas expand, they frequently erode the sella turcica and anterior clinoid processes. In as many as 30% of cases, the adenomas are not grossly encapsulated and infiltrate neighboring tissues such as the cavernous and sphenoid sinuses, dura, and on occasion, the brain itself. Such lesions are termed **invasive adenomas**. Not unexpectedly, macroadenomas tend to be invasive more frequently than smaller tumors. Foci of hemorrhage and necrosis are also more common in these larger adenomas.

Histologically, typical pituitary adenomas are composed of relatively uniform, polygonal cells arrayed in sheets or cords. Supporting connective tissue, or reticulin, is sparse, accounting for the soft, gelatinous consistency of many of these lesions. Mitotic activity is usually sparse. The cytoplasm of the constituent cells may be acidophilic, basophilic, or chromophobic, depending on the type and amount of secretory product within the cells, but it is generally uniform throughout the tumor. **This cellular monomorphism and the absence of a significant reticulin network distinguish pituitary adenomas from nonneoplastic anterior pituitary parenchyma** (Fig. 24–5). The biologic behavior of the adenoma cannot always be reliably predicted from its histologic appearance. A subset of pituitary adenomas demonstrates brisk mitotic activity and staining of greater than 3% of the nuclei with the proliferation marker Ki-67; these tumors typically also demonstrate extensive nuclear p53 immunoreactivity in the neoplastic cells, a feature that correlates with the presence of *p53* mutations. It is recommended that adenomas with this profile be classified as **atypical adenomas**, since these tumors have a higher propensity for aggressive behavior, including invasion and recurrence.

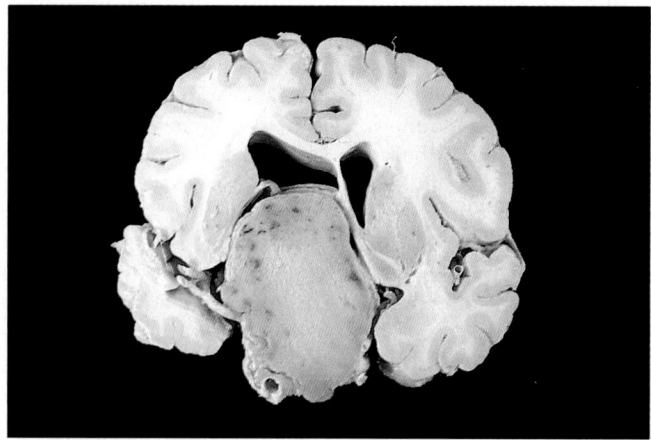

FIGURE 24–4 Pituitary adenoma. This massive, nonfunctional adenoma has grown far beyond the confines of the sella turcica and has distorted the overlying brain. Nonfunctional adenomas tend to be larger at the time of diagnosis than those that secrete a hormone.

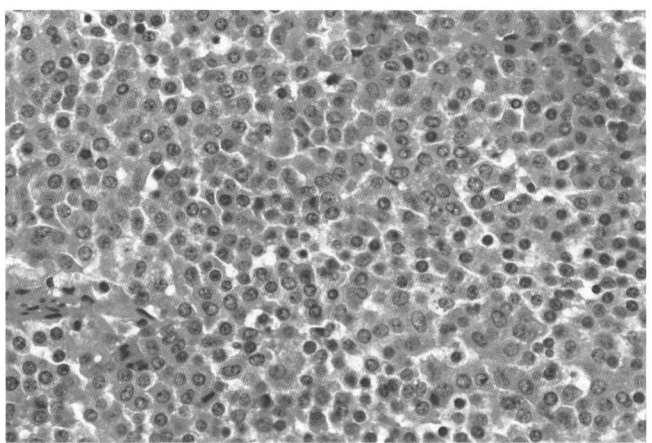

FIGURE 24–5 Pituitary adenoma. The monomorphism of these cells contrasts markedly with the mixture of cells seen in the normal anterior pituitary. Note also the absence of reticulin network.

Clinical Course. The signs and symptoms of pituitary adenomas include endocrine abnormalities and mass effects. The effects of excessive secretion of anterior pituitary hormones are mentioned below, when the specific types of pituitary adenoma are described. Local mass effects may be encountered in any type of pituitary tumor and have been discussed previously under clinical manifestations of pituitary disease. Briefly, these include *radiographic abnormalities of the sella turcica*, *visual field abnormalities*, signs and symptoms of elevated *intracranial pressure*, and occasionally *hypopituitarism*. Acute hemorrhage into an adenoma is sometimes associated with *pituitary apoplexy*, as was noted above.

With this general introduction to pituitary adenomas, we proceed to a discussion of the individual types of tumors.

PROLACTINOMAS

Prolactinomas (lactotroph adenomas) are the most frequent type of hyperfunctioning pituitary adenoma, accounting for about 30% of all clinically recognized cases. These lesions range from small microadenomas to large, expansile tumors associated with substantial mass effect. Microscopically, the overwhelming majority of prolactinomas are composed of weakly acidophilic or chromophobic cells *(sparsely granulated prolactinoma)*; rare prolactinomas are strongly acidophilic *(densely granulated prolactinoma)* (Fig. 24–6). Prolactin can be demonstrated within the secretory granules in the cytoplasm of the cells using immunohistochemical stains. Prolactinomas have a propensity to undergo dystrophic calcification, ranging from isolated psammoma bodies to extensive calcification of virtually the entire tumor mass ("pituitary stone"). Prolactin secretion by functioning adenomas is usually efficient (even microadenomas secrete sufficient prolactin to cause hyperprolactinemia) and *proportional*, in that serum prolactin concentrations tend to correlate with the size of the adenoma.

Increased serum levels of prolactin, or *prolactinemia*, cause amenorrhea, galactorrhea, loss of libido, and infertility. The diagnosis of an adenoma is made more readily in women than in men, especially between the ages of 20 and 40 years, presumably because of the sensitivity of menses to disruption by hyperprolactinemia. Prolactinoma underlies almost a quarter of cases of amenorrhea. In contrast, in men and older women, the hormonal manifestations may be subtle, allowing the tumors to reach considerable size (macroadenomas) before being detected clinically.

Hyperprolactinemia may result from causes other than prolactin-secreting pituitary adenomas. Physiologic hyperprolactinemia occurs in pregnancy; serum prolactin levels increase throughout pregnancy, reaching a peak at delivery. Prolactin levels are also elevated by nipple stimulation, as occurs during suckling in lactating women, and as a response

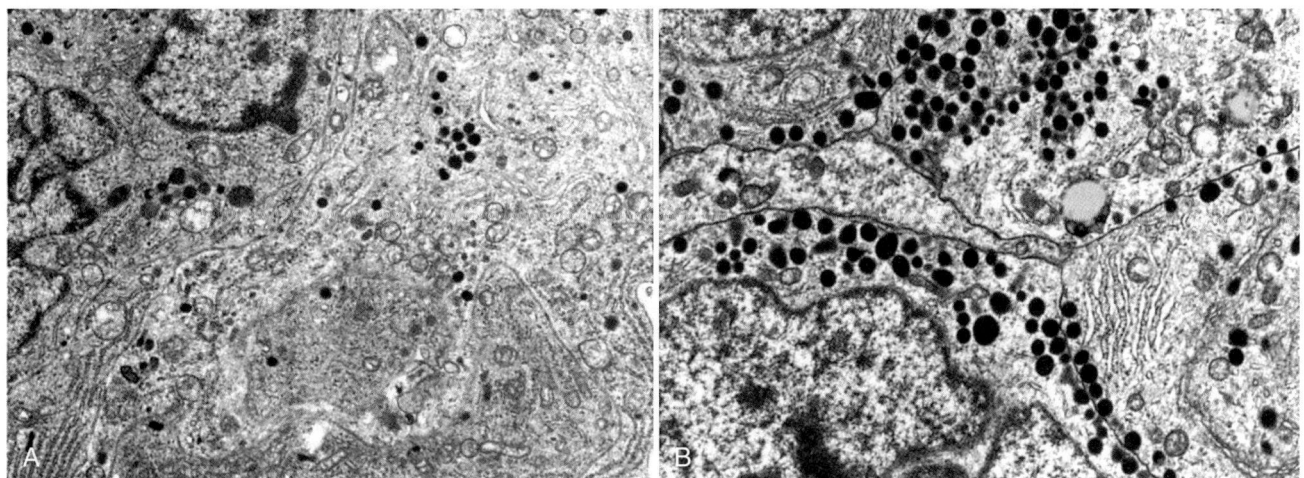

FIGURE 24–6 Ultrastructural features of prolactinomas. **A,** Electron micrograph of a sparsely granulated prolactinoma. The tumor cells contain abundant granular endoplasmic reticulum (indicative of active protein synthesis) and small numbers of electron-dense secretory granules. **B,** Electron micrograph of densely granulated growth hormone–secreting adenoma. The tumor cells are filled with numerous large, electron-dense secretory granules. (Courtesy of Dr. Eva Horvath, St. Michael's Hospital, Toronto, ON, Canada.)

to many types of stress. Pathologic hyperprolactinemia can also result from *lactotroph hyperplasia*, such as when there is interference with normal dopamine inhibition of prolactin secretion. This may occur as a result of damage to the dopaminergic neurons of the hypothalamus, damage to the pituitary stalk (e.g., due to head trauma), or drugs that block dopamine receptors on lactotroph cells. Any mass in the suprasellar compartment may disturb the normal inhibitory influence of the hypothalamus on prolactin secretion, resulting in hyperprolactinemia. *Therefore, a mild elevation in serum prolactin in a person with a pituitary adenoma does not necessarily indicate a prolactin-secreting tumor.* Other causes of hyperprolactinemia include several classes of drugs (such as dopamine antagonists), estrogens, renal failure, and hypothyroidism. Prolactinomas are treated by surgery or, more commonly, with bromocriptine, a dopamine receptor agonist that causes the lesions to diminish in size.

GROWTH HORMONE CELL (SOMATOTROPH) ADENOMAS

GH-secreting tumors are the second most common type of functioning pituitary adenoma. Somatotroph cell adenomas may be quite large by the time they come to clinical attention because the manifestations of excessive GH may be subtle. Histologically, pure GH cell–containing adenomas are also classified into two subtypes: *densely granulated* and *sparsely granulated*. The densely granulated adenomas are composed of cells that are monomorphic and acidophilic in routine sections, retain strong cytoplasmic GH reactivity on immunohistochemistry, and demonstrate cytokeratin staining in a perinuclear distribution. In contrast, the sparsely granulated variants are composed of chromophobe cells with considerable nuclear and cytologic pleomorphism and focal, weak staining for GH. Bihormonal *mammosomatotroph* adenomas that express both GH and prolactin are being increasingly recognized with the availability of better immunohistochemical reagents; morphologically, most bihormonal adenomas resemble the densely granulated pure somatotroph adenomas.

Persistently elevated levels of GH stimulate the hepatic secretion of insulin-like growth factor 1 (IGF-1 or somatomedin C), which causes many of the clinical manifestations. If a somatotrophic adenoma appears in children before the epiphyses have closed, the elevated levels of GH (and IGF-1) result in *gigantism*. This is characterized by a generalized increase in body size with disproportionately long arms and legs. If the increased levels of GH are present after closure of the epiphyses, patients develop *acromegaly*. In this condition, growth is most conspicuous in skin and soft tissues; viscera (thyroid, heart, liver, and adrenals); and bones of the face, hands, and feet. Bone density may be increased (hyperostosis) in both the spine and the hips. Enlargement of the jaw results in protrusion (prognathism), with broadening of the lower face. The hands and feet are enlarged with broad, sausage-like fingers. In most instances gigantism is also accompanied by evidence of acromegaly. These changes develop for decades before being recognized, hence the opportunity for the adenomas to reach substantial size. GH excess is also correlated with a variety of other disturbances, including gonadal dysfunction, diabetes mellitus, generalized muscle weakness, hypertension, arthritis,

congestive heart failure, and an increased risk of gastrointestinal cancers.

The diagnosis of pituitary GH excess relies on documentation of elevated serum GH and IGF-1 levels. *In addition, failure to suppress GH production in response to an oral load of glucose is one of the most sensitive tests for acromegaly.* The underlying pituitary adenoma can be either removed surgically or treated via pharmacologic means. The latter includes somatostatin analogs (recall that somatostatin has an inhibitory effect on pituitary GH secretion) or the use of GH receptor antagonists, which prevent hormone binding to target organs such as the liver. When effective control of high GH levels is achieved, the characteristic tissue overgrowth and related symptoms gradually recede, and the metabolic abnormalities improve.

ACTH CELL (CORTICOTROPH) ADENOMAS

Corticotroph adenomas are usually small microadenomas at the time of diagnosis. These tumors are most often basophilic *(densely granulated)* and occasionally chromophobic *(sparsely granulated)*. Both variants stain positively with periodic acid–Schiff (PAS) because of the presence of carbohydrate in POMC, the ACTH precursor molecule; in addition, they demonstrate variable immunoreactivity for POMC and its derivatives, including ACTH and β-endorphin.

Excess production of ACTH by the corticotroph adenoma leads to adrenal hypersecretion of cortisol and the development of *hypercortisolism* (also known as *Cushing syndrome*). This syndrome is discussed in more detail later with the diseases of the adrenal gland. It can be caused by a wide variety of conditions in addition to ACTH-producing pituitary tumors. When the hypercortisolism is due to excessive production of ACTH by the pituitary, the process is designated *Cushing disease*. Large destructive adenomas can develop in patients after surgical removal of the adrenal glands for treatment of Cushing syndrome. This condition, known as *Nelson syndrome*, occurs most often because of a loss of the inhibitory effect of adrenal corticosteroids on a preexisting corticotroph microadenoma. Because the adrenals are absent in persons with this disorder, hypercortisolism does not develop. In contrast, patients present with mass effects of the pituitary tumor. In addition, there can be hyperpigmentation because of the stimulatory effect of other products of the ACTH precursor molecule on melanocytes.

OTHER ANTERIOR PITUITARY ADENOMAS

Pituitary adenomas may elaborate more than one hormone. For example, prolactin may be demonstrable by immunolabeling of somatotroph adenomas. In other cases, unusual plurihormonal adenomas are capable of secreting multiple hormones; these tumors are usually aggressive. A few comments are made about several of the less frequent functioning tumors.

Gonadotroph (LH-producing and FSH-producing) adenomas can be difficult to recognize because they secrete hormones inefficiently and variably, and the secretory products usually do not cause a recognizable clinical syndrome (*nonfunctioning adenomas*, see below). Gonadotroph adenomas are most frequently found in middle-aged men and women when they become large enough to cause neurologic symptoms, such as impaired vision, headaches, diplopia, or pituitary apoplexy. Pituitary hormone deficiencies can also be found, most commonly impaired secretion of LH. This causes decreased energy and libido in men (due to reduced testosterone) and amenorrhea in premenopausal women. Thus, gonadotroph adenomas are paradoxically associated with secondary gonadal hypofunction. The neoplastic cells usually demonstrate immunoreactivity for the common gonadotropin α-subunit and the specific β-FSH and β-LH subunits; FSH is usually the predominant secreted hormone.

Thyrotroph (TSH-producing) adenomas are rare, accounting for approximately 1% of all pituitary adenomas. Thyrotroph adenomas are a rare cause of hyperthyroidism.

Nonfunctioning pituitary adenomas are a heterogeneous group that constitutes approximately 25% to 30% of all pituitary tumors. Their lineage can be established by immunohistochemical staining for hormones or by biochemical demonstration of cell type-specific transcription factors. In the past, many such tumors have been called *silent variants* or *null-cell adenomas.* Not surprisingly, the typical presentation of nonfunctioning adenomas is mass effects. These lesions may also compromise the residual anterior pituitary sufficiently to cause hypopituitarism. This may occur as a result of gradual enlargement of the adenoma or after abrupt enlargement of the tumor because of acute hemorrhage (pituitary apoplexy).

Pituitary carcinomas are quite rare, accounting for less than 1% of pituitary tumors. The demonstration of craniospinal or systemic metastases is a sine qua non of a pituitary carcinoma. The majority of pituitary carcinomas are functional neoplasms, with prolactin and ACTH being the most common secreted products. Metastases usually appear late in the course, following multiple local recurrences.

Hypopituitarism

Hypopituitarism refers to decreased secretion of pituitary hormones, which can result from diseases of the hypothalamus or of the pituitary. Hypofunction of the anterior pituitary occurs when approximately 75% of the parenchyma is lost or absent. This may be congenital or the result of a variety of acquired abnormalities that are intrinsic to the pituitary. *Hypopituitarism accompanied by evidence of posterior pituitary dysfunction in the form of diabetes insipidus (see below) is almost always of hypothalamic origin.* Most cases of hypofunction arise from destructive processes directly involving the anterior pituitary, although other mechanisms have been identified.

- *Tumors and other mass lesions:* Pituitary adenomas, other benign tumors arising within the sella, primary and metastatic malignancies, and cysts can cause hypopituitarism. Any mass lesion in the sella can cause damage by exerting pressure on adjacent pituitary cells.
- *Traumatic brain injury and subarachnoid hemorrhage* are among the most common causes of pituitary hypofunction.
- *Pituitary surgery or radiation:* Surgical excision of a pituitary adenoma may inadvertently extend to the nonadeno-

matous pituitary. Radiation of the pituitary, used to prevent regrowth of residual tumor after surgery, can damage the nonadenomatous pituitary.

- *Pituitary apoplexy:* As has been mentioned, this is a sudden hemorrhage into the pituitary gland, often occurring into a pituitary adenoma. In its most dramatic presentation, apoplexy causes the sudden onset of excruciating headache, diplopia due to pressure on the oculomotor nerves, and hypopituitarism. In severe cases, it can cause cardiovascular collapse, loss of consciousness, and even sudden death. Thus, pituitary apoplexy is a neurosurgical emergency.
- *Ischemic necrosis of the pituitary and Sheehan syndrome: Sheehan syndrome,* or postpartum necrosis of the anterior pituitary, is the most common form of clinically significant ischemic necrosis of the anterior pituitary. During pregnancy the anterior pituitary enlarges to almost twice its normal size. This physiologic expansion of the gland is not accompanied by an increase in blood supply from the low-pressure venous system; hence, there is relative anoxia. Further reduction in blood supply caused by obstetric hemorrhage or shock may precipitate infarction of the anterior lobe. The posterior pituitary, because it receives its blood directly from arterial branches, is much less susceptible to ischemic injury and is therefore usually not affected. Pituitary necrosis may also be encountered in other conditions, such as disseminated intravascular coagulation and (more rarely) sickle cell anemia, elevated intracranial pressure, traumatic injury, and shock of any origin. Whatever the pathogenesis, the ischemic area is resorbed and replaced by a nubbin of fibrous tissue attached to the wall of an empty sella.
- *Rathke cleft cyst:* These cysts, lined by ciliated cuboidal epithelium with occasional goblet cells and anterior pituitary cells, can accumulate proteinaceous fluid and expand, compromising the normal gland.
- *Empty sella syndrome:* Any condition that destroys part or all of the pituitary gland, such as ablation of the pituitary by surgery or radiation, can result in an *empty sella.* The *empty sella syndrome* refers to the presence of an enlarged, empty sella turcica. There are two types: (1) In a *primary* empty sella, there is a defect in the diaphragma sella that allows the arachnoid mater and cerebrospinal fluid to herniate into the sella, resulting in expansion of the sella and compression of the pituitary. Classically, affected patients are obese women with a history of multiple pregnancies. The empty sella syndrome may be associated with visual field defects and occasionally with endocrine anomalies, such as *hyperprolactinemia,* as a result of interruption of inhibitory hypothalamic effects. Loss of functioning parenchyma can be severe enough to result in hypopituitarism. (2) In a *secondary* empty sella, a mass, such as a pituitary adenoma, enlarges the sella, but then it is either surgically removed or undergoes spontaneous necrosis, leading to loss of pituitary function. Hypopituitarism can result from the treatment or spontaneous infarction.
- *Genetic defects:* Congenital deficiency of transcription factors required for normal pituitary function is a rare cause of hypopituitarism. For example, mutation of the pituitary-specific homeobox gene *POU1F1* (previously known as *PIT-1*) results in combined pituitary hormone

deficiency, characterized by deficiencies of GH, prolactin, and TSH.

○ *Hypothalamic lesions*: As mentioned above, hypothalamic lesions can also affect the pituitary by interfering with the delivery of pituitary hormone–releasing factors. In contrast to diseases that involve the pituitary directly, hypothalamic abnormalities can also diminish the secretion of ADH, resulting in diabetes insipidus (discussed later). Hypothalamic lesions that cause hypopituitarism include *tumors*, including benign lesions that arise in the region of the hypothalamus, such as craniopharyngiomas, and malignant tumors that metastasize to this site, such as breast and lung carcinomas. Hypothalamic hormone deficiency can ensue when brain or nasopharyngeal tumors are treated with radiation.

○ *Inflammatory disorders and infections*, such as sarcoidosis or tuberculous meningitis, can cause deficiencies of anterior pituitary hormones and diabetes insipidus.

The clinical manifestations of anterior pituitary hypofunction can be protean, and depend on the specific hormone(s) that are lacking. Children can develop growth failure (*pituitary dwarfism*) due to growth hormone deficiency. Gonadotropin (LH and FSH) deficiency leads to amenorrhea and infertility in women and decreased libido, impotence, and loss of pubic and axillary hair in men. TSH and ACTH deficiencies result in symptoms of hypothyroidism and hypoadrenalism, respectively, and are discussed later in the chapter. Prolactin deficiency results in failure of postpartum lactation. The anterior pituitary is also a rich source of MSH, synthesized from the same precursor molecule that produces ACTH; therefore, one of the manifestations of hypopituitarism includes pallor due to a loss of stimulatory effects of MSH on melanocytes.

Posterior Pituitary Syndromes

The clinically relevant posterior pituitary syndromes involve ADH and include *diabetes insipidus* and *secretion of inappropriately high levels of ADH*.

○ *Diabetes insipidus*. ADH deficiency causes diabetes insipidus, a condition characterized by excessive urination (polyuria) due to an inability of the kidney to resorb water properly from the urine. It can result from a variety of processes, including head trauma, tumors, and inflammatory disorders of the hypothalamus and pituitary as well as surgical procedures involving these organs. The condition can also arise spontaneously, in the absence of an underlying disorder. Diabetes insipidus from ADH deficiency is designated as *central* to differentiate it from *nephrogenic* diabetes insipidus, which is a result of renal tubular unresponsiveness to circulating ADH. The clinical manifestations of the two diseases are similar and include the excretion of large volumes of dilute urine with an inappropriately low specific gravity. Serum sodium and osmolality are increased as a result of excessive renal loss of free water, resulting in thirst and polydipsia. Patients who can drink water can generally compensate for urinary losses; patients who are obtunded, bedridden, or otherwise limited in their

ability to obtain water may develop life-threatening dehydration.

○ *Syndrome of inappropriate ADH (SIADH) secretion*. ADH excess causes resorption of excessive amounts of free water, resulting in *hyponatremia*. The most frequent causes of SIADH include the secretion of ectopic ADH by malignant neoplasms (particularly small-cell carcinomas of the lung), drugs that increase ADH secretion, and a variety of central nervous system disorders, including infections and trauma.[6] The clinical manifestations of SIADH are dominated by hyponatremia, cerebral edema, and resultant neurologic dysfunction. Although total body water is increased, blood volume remains normal, and peripheral edema does not develop.

Hypothalamic Suprasellar Tumors

Neoplasms in this location may induce hypofunction or hyperfunction of the anterior pituitary, diabetes insipidus, or combinations of these manifestations. The most commonly implicated lesions are *gliomas* (sometimes arising in the chiasm; see Chapter 28) and *craniopharyngiomas*. The craniopharyngioma is thought to be derived from vestigial remnants of Rathke pouch. These slow-growing tumors account for 1% to 5% of intracranial tumors; a small minority of these lesions arise within the sella, but most are suprasellar, with or without intrasellar extension. A bimodal age distribution is observed, with one peak in childhood (5 to 15 years) and a second peak in adults 65 years or older. Patients usually come to attention because of headaches and visual disturbances, while children might present with growth retardation due to pituitary hypofunction and GH deficiency. Abnormalities of the *WNT signaling pathway*, including activating β-catenin mutations, have been reported in craniopharyngiomas.

Morphology. Craniopharyngiomas average 3 to 4 cm in diameter; they may be encapsulated and solid, but more commonly they are cystic and sometimes multiloculated. In their strategic location, they often encroach on the optic chiasm or cranial nerves, and not infrequently they bulge into the floor of the third ventricle and base of the brain. Two distinct histologic variants are recognized: **adamantinomatous craniopharyngioma** (most often observed in children) and **papillary craniopharyngioma** (most often observed in adults). The adamantinomatous type frequently contains radiologically demonstrable calcifications; the papillary variant calcifies only rarely.

Adamantinomatous craniopharyngioma consists of nests or cords of stratified squamous epithelium embedded in a spongy "reticulum" that becomes more prominent in the internal layers. "Palisading" of the squamous epithelium is frequently observed at the periphery. Compact, lamellar keratin formation ("wet keratin") is a diagnostic feature of this tumor (Fig. 24–7). As was mentioned above, **dystrophic calcification** is a frequent finding. Additional features include cyst formation, fibrosis, and chronic inflammatory reaction. The cysts of adamantinomatous cra-

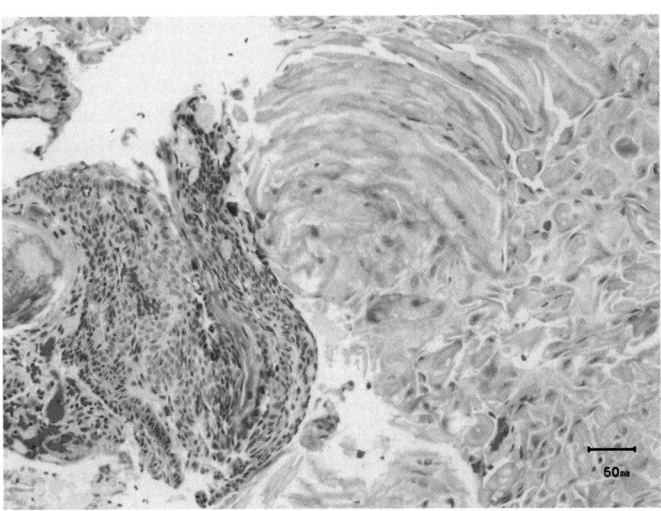

FIGURE 24–7 Adamantinomatous craniopharyngioma, demonstrating characteristic compact, lamellar "wet" keratin (right half of photomicrograph) and cords of squamous epithelium with peripheral palisading on the left. (Courtesy of Dr. Charles Eberhart, Department of Pathology, Johns Hopkins University, Baltimore, MD.)

niopharyngiomas often contain a cholesterol-rich, thick brownish-yellow fluid that has been compared to "machine oil." These tumors extend fingerlets of epithelium into adjacent brain, where they elicit a brisk glial reaction.

Papillary craniopharyngiomas contain both solid sheets and papillae lined by well-differentiated squamous epithelium. These tumors usually lack keratin, calcification, and cysts. The squamous cells of the solid sections of the tumor lack the peripheral palisading and do not typically generate a spongy reticulum in the internal layers.

Patients with craniopharyngiomas, especially those <5 cm in diameter, have an excellent recurrence-free and overall survival. Larger lesions are more invasive but this does not impact on the prognosis. Malignant transformation of craniopharyngiomas into squamous carcinomas is exceptionally rare and usually occurs after irradiation.

THYROID GLAND

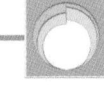

The thyroid gland consists of two bulky lateral lobes connected by a relatively thin isthmus, usually located below and anterior to the larynx. The thyroid is divided by thin fibrous septae into lobules composed of about 20 to 40 evenly dispersed follicles, lined by a cuboidal to low columnar epithelium, and filled with PAS-positive thyroglobulin. In response to hypothalamic factors, TSH *(thyrotropin)* is released by thyrotrophs in the anterior pituitary into the circulation. The binding of TSH to its receptor on the thyroid follicular epithelium results in conformational change and activation of the receptor, allowing it to associate with a G_s protein (Fig. 24–8). Activation of the G protein eventually results in an increase in intracellular cAMP levels, which stimulates thyroid growth, and hormone synthesis and release via cAMP-dependent protein kinases. The dissociation of thyroid hormone synthesis and release from the controlled influence of TSH-signaling pathways results in so-called *thyroid autonomy* and hyperfunction (see below).

Thyroid follicular epithelial cells convert thyroglobulin into *thyroxine (T_4)* and lesser amounts of *triiodothyronine (T_3)*. T_4 and T_3 are released into the systemic circulation, where most of these peptides are reversibly bound to circulating plasma proteins, such as thyroxine-binding globulin and transthyretin, for transport to peripheral tissues. The binding proteins serve to maintain the serum unbound ("free") T_3 and T_4 concentrations within narrow limits yet ensure that the hormones are readily available to the tissues. In the periphery, the majority of free T_4 is deiodinated to T_3; the latter binds to thyroid hormone nuclear receptors in target cells with tenfold greater

affinity than does T_4 and has proportionately greater activity. *The interaction of thyroid hormone with its nuclear thyroid hormone receptor (TR) results in the formation of a multiprotein hormone-receptor complex that binds to thyroid hormone response elements (TREs) in target genes, regulating their transcription (see Fig. 24–8).* Thyroid hormone has diverse cellular effects, including up-regulation of carbohydrate and lipid catabolism and stimulation of protein synthesis in a wide range of cells. The net result of these processes is an increase in the basal metabolic rate. One of the most important functions of thyroid hormone is its critical role in brain development in the fetus and neonate (see below).

The function of the thyroid gland can be inhibited by a variety of chemical agents, collectively referred to as *goitrogens*. Because they suppress T_3 and T_4 synthesis, the level of TSH increases, and subsequent hyperplastic enlargement of the gland *(goiter)* follows. The antithyroid agent *propylthiouracil* inhibits the oxidation of iodide and thus blocks production of the thyroid hormones; parenthetically, propylthiouracil also inhibits the peripheral deiodination of circulating T_4 into T_3, thus ameliorating symptoms of thyroid hormone excess (see below). Iodide, when given to individuals with thyroid hyperfunction, also blocks the release of thyroid hormones but through different mechanisms. Iodides in large doses inhibit proteolysis of thyroglobulin. Thus, thyroid hormone is synthesized and incorporated within increasing amounts of colloid, but it is not released into the blood.

The thyroid gland follicles also contain a population of *parafollicular cells*, or C cells, which synthesize and secrete the

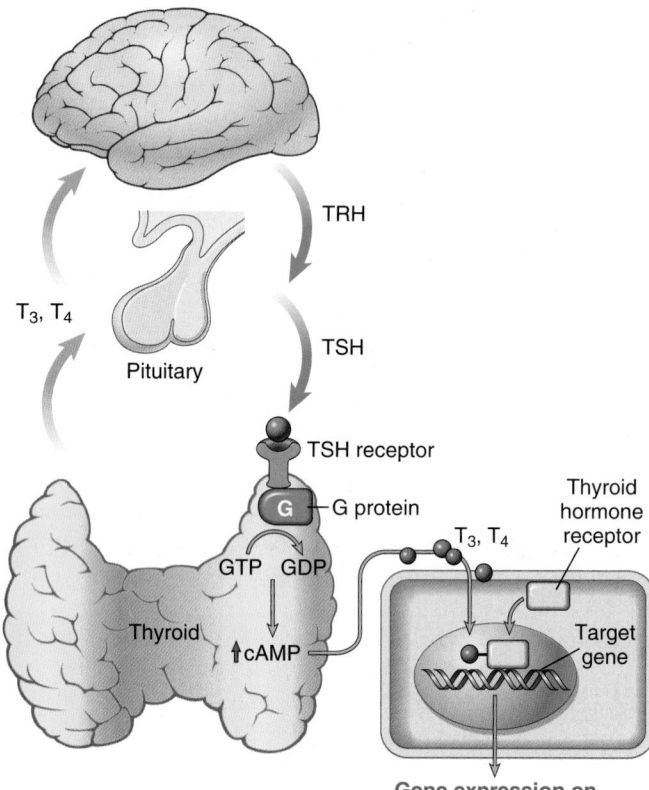

FIGURE 24–8 Homeostasis in the hypothalamus-pituitary-thyroid axis and mechanism of action of thyroid hormones. Secretion of thyroid hormones (T_3 and T_4) is controlled by trophic factors secreted by both the hypothalamus and the anterior pituitary. Decreased levels of T_3 and T_4 stimulate the release of thyrotropin-releasing hormone (TRH) from the hypothalamus and thyroid-stimulating hormone (TSH) from the anterior pituitary, causing T_3 and T_4 levels to rise. Elevated T_3 and T_4 levels, in turn, feed back to suppress the secretion of both TRH and TSH. TSH binds to the TSH receptor on the thyroid follicular epithelium, which causes activation of G proteins, and cAMP-mediated synthesis and release of thyroid hormones (T_3 and T_4). In the periphery, T_3 and T_4 interact with the thyroid hormone receptor (TR) to form a hormone-receptor complex that translocates to the nucleus and binds to so-called thyroid response elements (TREs) on target genes to initiate transcription.

hormone *calcitonin.* This hormone promotes the absorption of calcium by the skeletal system and inhibits the resorption of bone by osteoclasts.

Diseases of the thyroid include conditions associated with excessive release of thyroid hormones (hyperthyroidism), those associated with thyroid hormone deficiency (hypothyroidism), and mass lesions of the thyroid. We first consider the clinical consequences of disturbed thyroid function, then focus on the disorders that generate these problems.

Hyperthyroidism

Thyrotoxicosis is a hypermetabolic state caused by elevated circulating levels of free T_3 and T_4. Because it is caused most commonly by hyperfunction of the thyroid gland, it is often referred to as *hyperthyroidism.* However, in certain conditions

the oversupply is related to either excessive release of preformed thyroid hormone (e.g., in thyroiditis) or to an extrathyroidal source, rather than hyperfunction of the gland (Table 24–3). *Thus, strictly speaking, hyperthyroidism is only one (albeit the most common) cause of thyrotoxicosis.* The terms *primary* and *secondary hyperthyroidism* are sometimes used to designate hyperthyroidism arising from an intrinsic thyroid abnormality and that arising from processes outside of the thyroid, such as a TSH-secreting pituitary tumor. With this caveat, we will follow the common practice of using the terms *thyrotoxicosis* and *hyperthyroidism* interchangeably. The three most common causes of thyrotoxicosis are also associated with hyperfunction of the gland and include the following:

- *Diffuse hyperplasia* of the thyroid associated with Graves disease (accounts for 85% of cases)
- Hyperfunctional *multinodular goiter*
- Hyperfunctional *adenoma* of the thyroid

Clinical Course. The clinical manifestations of hyperthyroidism are protean and include changes referable to the *hypermetabolic state* induced by excess thyroid hormone and to overactivity of the *sympathetic nervous system* (i.e., an increase in the β-adrenergic "tone").

Excessive levels of thyroid hormone result in *an increase in the basal metabolic rate.* The *skin* of thyrotoxic patients tends to be soft, warm, and flushed because of increased blood flow and peripheral vasodilation to increase heat loss. *Heat intolerance* is common. Sweating is increased because of higher levels of calorigenesis. Increased basal metabolic rate also results in characteristic *weight loss despite increased appetite.*

Cardiac manifestations are among the earliest and most consistent features of hyperthyroidism. Individuals with hyperthyroidism can have an increase in cardiac output, due to both increased cardiac contractility and increased peripheral oxygen requirements. Tachycardia, palpitations, and cardiomegaly are common. Arrhythmias, particularly atrial fibrillation, occur frequently and are more common in older patients. Conges-

TABLE 24–3 Disorders Associated with Thyrotoxicosis
ASSOCIATED WITH HYPERTHYROIDISM
Primary
Diffuse toxic hyperplasia (Graves disease)
Hyperfunctioning ("toxic") multinodular goiter
Hyperfunctioning ("toxic") adenoma
Iodine-induced hyperthyroidism
Neonatal thyrotoxicosis associated with maternal Graves disease
Secondary
TSH-secreting pituitary adenoma (rare)*
NOT ASSOCIATED WITH HYPERTHYROIDISM
Granulomatous (de Quervain) thyroiditis (*painful*)
Subacute lymphocytic thyroiditis (*painless*)
Struma ovarii (ovarian teratoma with ectopic thyroid)
Factitious thyrotoxicosis (exogenous thyroxine intake)

*Associated with increased thyroid-stimulating hormone (TSH); all other causes of thyrotoxicosis associated with decreased TSH.

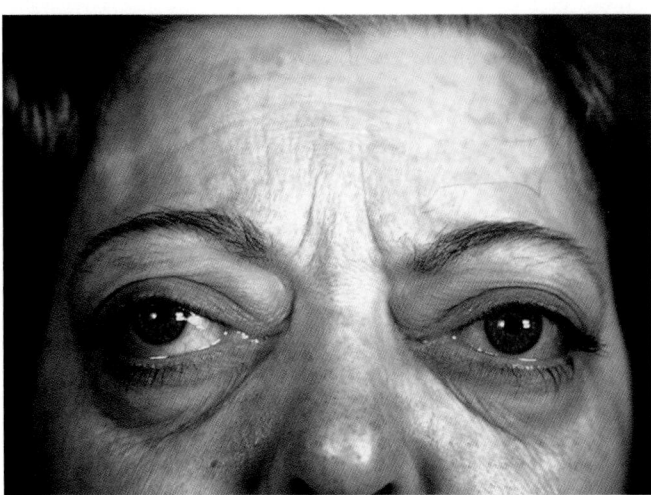

FIGURE 24–9 A person with hyperthyroidism. A wide-eyed, staring gaze, caused by overactivity of the sympathetic nervous system, is one of the features of this disorder. In Graves disease, one of the most important causes of hyperthyroidism, accumulation of loose connective tissue behind the eyeballs, also adds to the protuberant appearance of the eyes.

tive heart failure may develop, particularly in elderly patients with preexisting cardiac disease. Myocardial changes, such as foci of lymphocytic and eosinophilic infiltration, mild fibrosis in the interstitium, fatty changes in myofibers, and an increase in size and number of mitochondria, have been described. Some individuals with thyrotoxicosis develop reversible *left ventricular dysfunction* and "low-output" heart failure, so-called *thyrotoxic or hyperthyroid cardiomyopathy.*

In the *neuromuscular system,* overactivity of the sympathetic nervous system produces tremor, hyperactivity, emotional lability, anxiety, inability to concentrate, and insomnia. Proximal muscle weakness and decreased muscle mass are common *(thyroid myopathy).*

Ocular changes often call attention to hyperthyroidism. A wide, staring gaze and lid lag are present because of sympathetic overstimulation of the levator palpebrae superioris (Fig. 24–9). However, true *thyroid ophthalmopathy* associated with proptosis is seen only in Graves disease (see below).

In the *gastrointestinal system,* sympathetic hyperstimulation of the gut results in hypermotility, malabsorption, and diarrhea.

The *skeletal system* is also affected. Thyroid hormone stimulates bone resorption, increasing porosity of cortical bone and reducing the volume of trabecular bone. The net effect is osteoporosis and an increased risk of fractures in patients with chronic hyperthyroidism.

Other findings include atrophy of skeletal muscle, with fatty infiltration and focal interstitial lymphocytic infiltrates; minimal liver enlargement due to fatty changes in the hepatocytes; and generalized lymphoid hyperplasia and lymphadenopathy in patients with Graves disease.

Thyroid storm is used to designate the abrupt onset of severe hyperthyroidism. This condition occurs most commonly in patients with underlying Graves disease and probably results from an acute elevation in catecholamine levels, as might be encountered during infection, surgery, cessation of antithyroid medication, or any form of stress. Patients are often febrile and present with tachycardia out of proportion to the fever. Thyroid storm is a medical emergency: A significant number of untreated patients die of cardiac arrhythmias.

Apathetic hyperthyroidism refers to thyrotoxicosis occurring in the elderly, in whom advanced age and various co-morbidities may blunt the typical features of thyroid hormone excess seen in younger patients. The diagnosis of thyrotoxicosis in these individuals is often made during laboratory work-up for unexplained weight loss or worsening cardiovascular disease.

A diagnosis of hyperthyroidism is made using both clinical and laboratory findings. The measurement of serum TSH concentration using sensitive TSH assays provides the most useful single screening test for hyperthyroidism, since its levels are decreased even at the earliest stages, when the disease may still be subclinical. A low TSH value is usually confirmed with measurement of free T_4, which is expectedly increased. In an occasional patient, hyperthyroidism results predominantly from increased circulating levels of T_3 ("T_3 toxicosis"). In these cases, free T_4 levels may be decreased, and direct measurement of serum T_3 may be useful. In rare cases of pituitary-associated (secondary) hyperthyroidism, TSH levels are either normal or raised. Determining TSH levels after the injection of thyrotropin-releasing hormone (TRH stimulation test) is used in the evaluation of cases of suspected hyperthyroidism with equivocal changes in the baseline serum TSH level. A normal rise in TSH after administration of TRH excludes secondary hyperthyroidism. Once the diagnosis of thyrotoxicosis has been confirmed by a combination of TSH assays and free thyroid hormone levels, measurement of radioactive iodine uptake by the thyroid gland may be valuable in determining the etiology. For example, there may be diffusely increased uptake in the whole gland (Graves' disease), increased uptake in a solitary nodule (toxic adenoma), or decreased uptake (thyroiditis).

The therapeutic options for hyperthyroidism include multiple medications, each of which has a different mechanism of action. Typically, these include a β-blocker to control symptoms induced by increased adrenergic tone, a thionamide to block new hormone synthesis, an iodine solution to block the release of thyroid hormone, and agents that inhibit peripheral conversion of T_4 to T_3. Radioiodine, which is incorporated into thyroid tissues, resulting in ablation of thyroid function over a period of 6 to 18 weeks, may also be used.

Hypothyroidism

Hypothyroidism is caused by any structural or functional derangement that interferes with the production of adequate levels of thyroid hormone. Hypothyroidism is a fairly common disorder, and by some estimates the population prevalence of overt hypothyroidism is 0.3%, while subclinical hypothyroidism can be found in greater than 4%.[7] The prevalence of hypothyroidism increases with age, and it is nearly tenfold more common in women than in men. It can result from a defect anywhere in the hypothalamic-pituitary-thyroid axis. As in the case of hyperthyroidism, this disorder is divided into *primary* and *secondary* categories, depending on whether the hypothyroidism arises from an intrinsic abnormality in the

TABLE 24–4   Causes of Hypothyroidism
PRIMARY
Developmental (thyroid dysgenesis: *PAX8, FOXE1*, TSH receptor mutations)
Thyroid hormone resistance syndrome (*THRB* mutations)
Postablative
Surgery, radioiodine therapy, or external irradiation
Autoimmune hypothyroidism
Hashimoto thyroiditis*
Iodine deficiency*
Drugs (lithium, iodides, *p*-aminosalicylic acid)*
Congenital biosynthetic defect (dyshormonogenetic goiter)*
SECONDARY (CENTRAL)
Pituitary failure
Hypothalamic failure (rare)

*Associated with enlargement of thyroid ("goitrous hypothyroidism"). Hashimoto thyroiditis and postablative hypothyroidism account for the majority of cases of hypothyroidism in developed countries. *FOXE1*, forkhead box E1; *PAX8*, paired box 8; *THRB*, thyroid hormone receptor β.

thyroid itself, or occurs as a result of pituitary and hypothalamic disease (Table 24–4). Primary hypothyroidism accounts for the vast majority of cases of hypothyroidism, and can be accompanied by an enlargement in the size of the thyroid gland (goiter). Primary hypothyroidism can be congenital, acquired, or autoimmune.

Worldwide, *congenital hypothyroidism* is most often the result of *endemic iodine deficiency* in the diet (see below). Other less common forms of congenital hypothyroidism include *inborn errors of thyroid metabolism (dyshormonogenetic goiter)*, wherein any one of the multiple steps leading to thyroid hormone synthesis may be deficient, such as (1) iodide transport into thyrocytes, (2) iodide "organification" (binding of iodide to tyrosine residues of the storage protein, thyroglobulin), and (3) iodotyrosine coupling to form hormonally active T_3 and T_4. Mutations in the *thyroid peroxidase (TPO)* gene are the most common cause of dyshormonogenetic goiter. *Pendred syndrome*, characterized by hypothyroidism and sensorineural deafness, is caused by mutations in the *SLC26A4* gene, whose product, pendrin, is an anion transporter expressed on the apical surface of thyrocytes and in the inner ear.[8] In rare instances there may be complete absence of thyroid parenchyma *(thyroid agenesis)*, or the gland may be greatly reduced in size *(thyroid hypoplasia)*. Germline mutations in transcription factors that are expressed in the developing thyroid and regulate follicular differentiation, such as *thyroid transcription factor-2 (TTF-2)*, also known as *FOXE1*, and *paired box-8 (PAX-8)*, have been reported in individuals with thyroid agenesis. These patients typically present with a constellation of extra-thyroidal malformations. Inactivating germline mutations of the *TSH receptor (TSHR)* is a rare genetic cause of isolated hypothyroidism (note that *activating* somatic mutations of *TSHR* are found in autonomous thyroid nodules, see below). *Thyroid hormone resistance syndrome* is a rare autosomal-dominant disorder caused by inherited mutations in the thyroid hormone receptor, which abolish the ability of the receptor to bind thyroid hormones. Patients demonstrate a generalized resistance to thyroid hormone, despite high circulating levels of T_3 and T_4. Since the pituitary

is also resistant to feedback from thyroid hormones, TSH levels tend to be high as well.

Acquired hypothyroidism can be caused by *surgical or radiation-induced ablation* of thyroid parenchyma. A large resection of the gland (total thyroidectomy) for the treatment of hyperthyroidism of a primary neoplasm can lead to hypothyroidism. The gland may also be ablated by radiation, whether in the form of radioiodine administered for the treatment of hyperthyroidism, or exogenous irradiation, such as external radiation therapy to the neck. *Drugs* given intentionally to decrease thyroid secretion (e.g., methimazole and propylthiouracil) can cause acquired hypothyroidism, as can agents used to treat nonthyroid conditions (e.g., lithium, *p*-aminosalicylic acid).

Autoimmune hypothyroidism is the most common cause of hypothyroidism in iodine-sufficient areas of the world. The vast majority of cases of autoimmune hypothyroidism are due to Hashimoto thyroiditis. Circulating autoantibodies, including *anti-microsomal, anti-thyroid peroxidase,* and *anti-thyroglobulin* antibodies, are found in this disorder, and the thyroid is typically enlarged (goitrous). Autoimmune hypothyroidism can occur in isolation or in conjunction with autoimmune polyendocrine syndrome (APS), types 1 and 2 (see discussion in "Adrenal Glands").

Secondary (or central) hypothyroidism is caused by deficiency of TSH, and far more uncommonly, that of TRH. Any of the causes of hypopituitarism (for example, pituitary tumor, postpartum pituitary necrosis, trauma, and nonpituitary tumors), or of hypothalamic damage from tumors, trauma, radiation therapy, or infiltrative diseases can cause central hypothyroidism.

Classic clinical manifestations of hypothyroidism include cretinism and myxedema.

CRETINISM

Cretinism refers to hypothyroidism that develops in infancy or early childhood. The term *cretin* was derived from the French *chrétien*, meaning "Christian" or "Christlike," and was applied to these unfortunates because they were considered to be so mentally retarded as to be incapable of sinning. In the past this disorder occurred fairly commonly in areas of the world where dietary iodine deficiency is endemic, such as the Himalayas, inland China, Africa, and other mountainous areas. It has become much less frequent in recent years, as a result of the widespread supplementation of foods with iodine. On rare occasions, cretinism may also result from inborn errors in metabolism that interfere with the biosynthesis of normal levels of thyroid hormone (dyshormonogenetic goiter, see above).

Clinical features of cretinism include impaired development of the skeletal system and central nervous system, manifested by severe mental retardation, short stature, coarse facial features, a protruding tongue, and umbilical hernia. The severity of the mental impairment in cretinism seems to be related to the time at which thyroid deficiency occurs in utero. Normally, maternal hormones, including T_3 and T_4, cross the placenta and are critical to fetal brain development. If there is maternal thyroid deficiency before the development of the fetal thyroid gland, mental retardation is severe. In contrast, reduction in maternal thyroid hormones later in pregnancy, after the fetal thyroid has developed, allows normal brain development.

MYXEDEMA

The term *myxedema* is applied to hypothyroidism developing in the older child or adult. Myxedema, or Gull disease, was first linked with thyroid dysfunction in 1873 by Sir William Gull in an article addressing the development of a "cretinoid state" in adults.[9] The clinical manifestations vary with the age of onset of the deficiency. The older child shows signs and symptoms intermediate between those of the cretin and those of the adult with hypothyroidism. In the adult the condition appears insidiously and may take years to reach the level of clinical suspicion.

Clinical features of myxedema are characterized by a slowing of physical and mental activity. The initial symptoms include generalized fatigue, apathy, and mental sluggishness, which may mimic depression in the early stages of the disease. Speech and intellectual functions become slowed. Patients with myxedema are listless, cold intolerant, and frequently overweight. Decreased sympathetic activity results in constipation and decreased sweating. The skin of these patients is cool and pale because of decreased blood flow. Reduced cardiac output probably contributes to shortness of breath and decreased exercise capacity, two frequent complaints in individuals with hypothyroidism. Thyroid hormones regulate the transcription of several sarcolemmal genes, such as *calcium ATPases*, whose encoded products are critical in maintaining efficient cardiac output. In addition, hypothyroidism promotes an atherogenic profile—an increase in total cholesterol and low-density lipoprotein (LDL) levels—probably contributing toward the adverse cardiovascular mortality rates in this disease. Histologically, there is an accumulation of matrix substances, such as glycosaminoglycans and hyaluronic acid, in skin, subcutaneous tissue, and a number of visceral sites. This results in non-pitting edema, a broadening and coarsening of facial features, enlargement of the tongue, and deepening of the voice.

Laboratory evaluation plays a vital role in the diagnosis of suspected hypothyroidism because of the nonspecific nature of symptoms. Patients with unexplained increase in body weight or hypercholesterolemia should be assessed for potential hypothyroidism. *Measurement of the serum TSH level is the most sensitive screening test for this disorder.* The TSH level is increased in primary hypothyroidism as a result of a loss of feedback inhibition of TRH and TSH production by the hypothalamus and pituitary, respectively. The TSH level is not increased in persons with hypothyroidism due to primary hypothalamic or pituitary disease. T_4 *levels are decreased* in individuals with hypothyroidism of any origin.

Thyroiditis

Thyroiditis, or inflammation of the thyroid gland, encompasses a diverse group of disorders characterized by some form of thyroid inflammation. These diseases include conditions that result in acute illness with severe thyroid pain (e.g., infectious thyroiditis, subacute granulomatous thyroiditis) and disorders in which there is relatively little inflammation and the illness is manifested primarily by thyroid dysfunction—subacute lymphocytic thyroiditis and fibrous (Reidel) thyroiditis.

Infectious thyroiditis may be either acute or chronic. Acute infections can reach the thyroid by hematogenous spread or through direct seeding of the gland, such as through a fistula from the piriform sinus adjacent to the larynx. Other infections of the thyroid, including mycobacterial, fungal, and *Pneumocystis* infections, are more chronic and frequently occur in immunocompromised patients. Whatever the cause, the inflammatory involvement may cause sudden onset of neck pain and tenderness in the area of the gland and is accompanied by fever, chills, and other signs of infection. Infectious thyroiditis can be self-limited or can be controlled with appropriate therapy. Thyroid function is usually not significantly affected, and there are few residual effects except for possible small foci of scarring. This section focuses on the more common and clinically significant types of thyroiditis: (1) Hashimoto thyroiditis, (2) granulomatous (de Quervain) thyroiditis, and (3) subacute lymphocytic thyroiditis.

HASHIMOTO THYROIDITIS

Hashimoto thyroiditis is the most common cause of hypothyroidism in areas of the world where iodine levels are sufficient. The name *Hashimoto thyroiditis* is derived from the 1912 report by Hashimoto describing patients with goiter and intense lymphocytic infiltration of the thyroid *(struma lymphomatosa)*.[10] Hashimoto thyroiditis and Graves disease (see below) are the two most common immunologically mediated disorders of the thyroid. Hashimoto thyroiditis is characterized by gradual thyroid failure because of autoimmune destruction of the thyroid gland. This disorder is most prevalent between 45 and 65 years of age and is more common in women than in men, with a female predominance of 10:1 to 20:1. Although it is primarily a disease of older women, it can occur in children and is a major cause of nonendemic goiter in the pediatric population.

Akin to other autoimmune diseases, Hashimoto thyroiditis has a strong genetic component. This is supported by the concordance of disease in as many as 40% of monozygotic twins, as well as the presence of circulating antithyroid antibodies in approximately 50% of asymptomatic siblings of Hashimoto patients. Increased susceptibility to Hashimoto thyroiditis is associated with polymorphisms in multiple immune regulation–associated genes, the most significant of which is the linkage to *cytotoxic T lymphocyte–associated antigen-4 (CTLA4)* polymorphisms.[11] CTLA4 is a negative regulator of T-cell responses, and not surprisingly, polymorphisms of the *CTLA4* gene that result in reduced protein level or function are associated with a predisposition to autoimmune disease. Another recently described genetic determinant of susceptibility to Hashimoto thyroiditis is a functional polymorphism in *protein tyrosine phosphatase-22 (PTPN22)* gene that encodes a lymphoid tyrosine phosphatase, which is also thought to inhibit T-cell function.[12] Susceptibility to other autoimmune diseases, such as type 1 diabetes (see below), has been associated with polymorphisms in both *CTLA4* and *PTPN22*.

Pathogenesis. Hashimoto thyroiditis is caused by a breakdown in self-tolerance to thyroid auto-antigens. This is exemplified by the presence of circulating autoantibodies

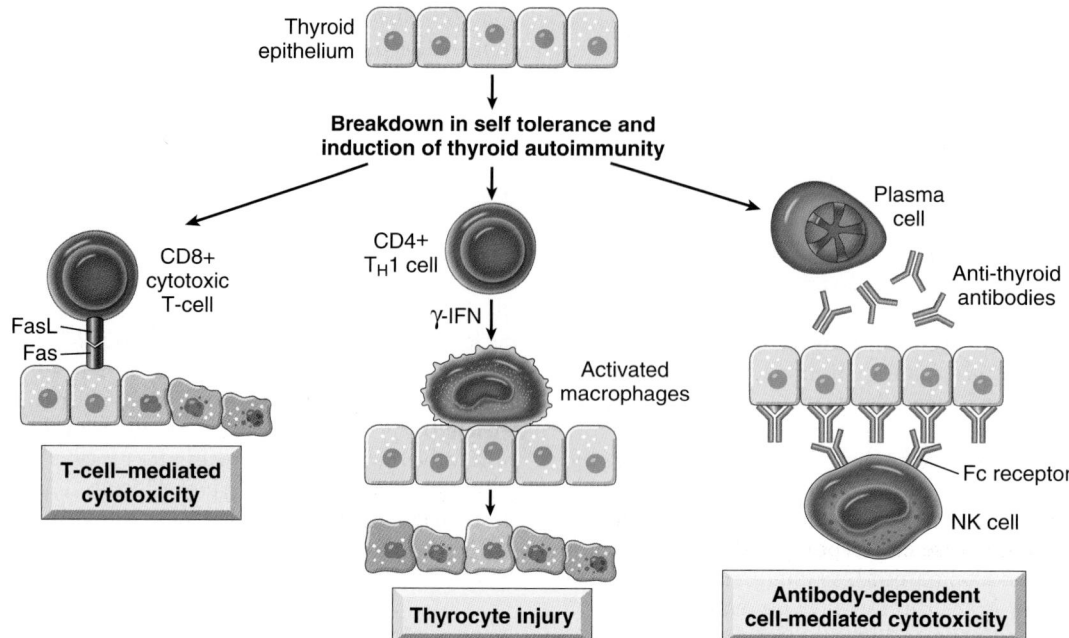

FIGURE 24–10 Pathogenesis of Hashimoto thyroiditis. Breakdown of peripheral tolerance to thyroid auto-antigens, results in progressive autoimmune destruction of thyrocytes by infiltrating cytotoxic T cells, locally released cytokines, or by antibody-dependent cytotoxicity.

against thyroglobulin and thyroid peroxidase in the vast majority of Hashimoto patients. The inciting events leading to breakdown in self-tolerance in Hashimoto patients have not been fully elucidated, but possibilities include abnormalities of regulatory T cells (Tregs)[13], or exposure of normally sequestered thyroid antigens (Chapter 6). Induction of thyroid autoimmunity is accompanied by a progressive depletion of thyrocytes by apoptosis and replacement of the thyroid parenchyma by mononuclear cell infiltration and fibrosis. Multiple immunologic mechanisms may contribute to thyroid cell death, including (Fig. 24–10):

- *CD8+ cytotoxic T cell–mediated cell death:* CD8+ cytotoxic T cells may cause thyrocyte destruction.
- *Cytokine-mediated cell death:* Excessive T-cell activation leads to the production of T_H1 inflammatory cytokines such as interferon-γ in the thyroid gland, with resultant recruitment and activation of macrophages and damage to follicles.
- Binding of anti-thyroid antibodies (anti-thyroglobulin, and anti-thyroid peroxidase antibodies) followed by antibody-dependent cell-mediated cytotoxicity (Chapter 6).

Morphology. The thyroid is often diffusely enlarged, although more localized enlargement may be seen in some cases. The capsule is intact, and the gland is well demarcated from adjacent structures. The cut surface is pale, yellow-tan, firm, and somewhat nodular. Microscopic examination reveals extensive infiltration of the parenchyma by a **mononuclear inflammatory infiltrate** containing small lymphocytes, plasma cells, and well-developed **germinal centers** (Fig. 24–11). The thyroid follicles are atrophic and are

lined in many areas by epithelial cells distinguished by the presence of abundant eosinophilic, granular cytoplasm, termed **Hürthle cells**. This is a metaplastic response of the normally low cuboidal follicular epithelium to ongoing injury. In fine-needle aspiration biopsy samples, the presence of Hürthle cells in conjunction with a heterogeneous population of lymphocytes is characteristic of Hashimoto thyroiditis. In "classic" Hashimoto thyroiditis, interstitial connective tissue is increased and may be abundant. A **fibrous variant** is characterized by severe thyroid follicular atrophy and dense "keloid-like" fibrosis, broad bands

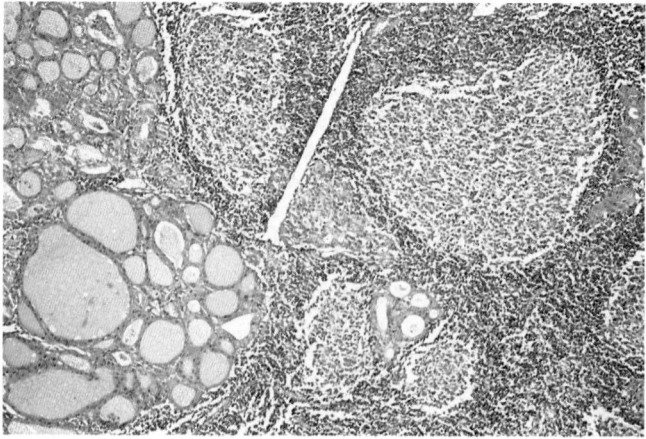

FIGURE 24–11 Hashimoto thyroiditis. The thyroid parenchyma contains a dense lymphocytic infiltrate with germinal centers. Residual thyroid follicles lined by deeply eosinophilic Hürthle cells are also seen.

of acellular collagen encompassing residual thyroid tissue. Unlike Reidel thyroiditis (see below), the fibrosis does not extend beyond the capsule of the gland. The remnant thyroid parenchyma demonstrates features of chronic lymphocytic thyroiditis.

Clinical Course. Hashimoto thyroiditis most often comes to clinical attention as painless enlargement of the thyroid, usually associated with some degree of hypothyroidism, in a middle-aged woman. The enlargement of the gland is usually symmetric and diffuse, but in some cases it may be sufficiently localized to raise a suspicion of neoplasm. In the usual clinical course, hypothyroidism develops gradually. In some cases, however, it may be preceded by transient thyrotoxicosis caused by disruption of thyroid follicles, with secondary release of thyroid hormones ("hashitoxicosis"). During this phase, free T_4 and T_3 levels are elevated, TSH is diminished, and radioactive iodine uptake is decreased. As hypothyroidism supervenes, T_4 and T_3 levels fall, accompanied by a compensatory increase in TSH. Individuals with Hashimoto thyroiditis are at increased risk for developing other autoimmune diseases, both endocrine (type 1 diabetes, autoimmune adrenalitis) and nonendocrine (systemic lupus erythematosus, myasthenia gravis, and Sjögren syndrome; see Chapter 6). They are also at increased risk for the development of B-cell non-Hodgkin lymphomas, especially marginal zone lymphomas of mucosa-associated lymphoid tissues (MALT lymphomas; see Chapter 13). The relationship between Hashimoto disease and thyroid epithelial cancers remains controversial, with some morphologic and molecular studies suggesting a predisposition to papillary carcinomas.

SUBACUTE (GRANULOMATOUS) THYROIDITIS

Subacute thyroiditis, which is also referred to as *granulomatous thyroiditis* or *De Quervain thyroiditis*, occurs much less frequently than does Hashimoto disease. The disorder is most common between the ages of 40 and 50 and, like other forms of thyroiditis, affects women considerably more often than men (4:1).

Pathogenesis. Subacute thyroiditis is believed to be triggered by a *viral infection*. The majority of patients have a history of an upper respiratory infection just before the onset of thyroiditis. The disease has a seasonal incidence, with occurrences peaking in the summer, and clusters of cases have been reported in association with coxsackievirus, mumps, measles, adenovirus, and other viral illnesses. Although the pathogenesis of the disease is unclear, one model suggests that it results from a viral infection that leads to exposure to a viral or thyroid antigen, which is released secondary to virus-induced host tissue damage. This antigen stimulates cytotoxic T lymphocytes, which then damage thyroid follicular cells. In contrast to autoimmune thyroid disease, the immune response is virus-initiated and not self-perpetuating, so the process is limited.

Morphology. The gland may be unilaterally or bilaterally enlarged and firm, with an intact capsule. It

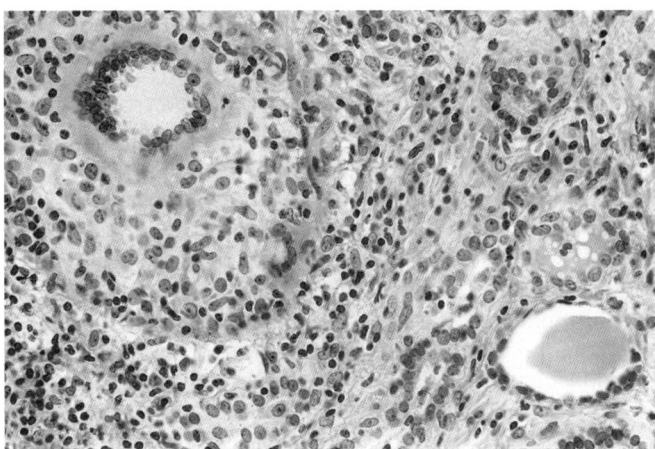

FIGURE 24–12 Granulomatous thyroiditis. The thyroid parenchyma contains a chronic inflammatory infiltrate with a multinucleate giant cell *(above left)* and a colloid follicle *(bottom right)*.

may be slightly adherent to surrounding structures. On cut section, the involved areas are firm and yellow-white and stand out from the more rubbery, normal brown thyroid substance. Histologically, the changes are patchy and depend on the stage of the disease. Early in the active inflammatory phase, scattered follicles may be entirely disrupted and replaced by neutrophils forming microabscesses. Later, the more characteristic features appear in the form of aggregates of lymphocytes, activated macrophages, and plasma cells about collapsed and damaged thyroid follicles. **Multinucleate giant cells** enclose naked pools or fragments of colloid (Fig. 24–12), hence the designation **granulomatous thyroiditis**. In later stages of the disease a chronic inflammatory infiltrate and fibrosis may replace the foci of injury. Different histologic stages are sometimes found in the same gland, suggesting waves of destruction over a period of time.

Clinical Course. Granulomatous (de Quervain) thyroiditis is the most common cause of *thyroid pain*. There is a variable enlargement of the thyroid. The thyroid inflammation and hyperthyroidism are transient, usually diminishing in 2 to 6 weeks, even if the patient is not treated. Nearly all patients have high serum T_4 and T_3 levels and low serum TSH levels during this phase. However, unlike in hyperthyroid states such as Graves disease, radioactive iodine uptake is diminished. After recovery, generally in 6 to 8 weeks, normal thyroid function returns.

SUBACUTE LYMPHOCYTIC (PAINLESS) THYROIDITIS

Subacute lymphocytic thyroiditis, which is also referred to as *painless thyroiditis*, usually comes to clinical attention because of mild hyperthyroidism, goitrous enlargement of the gland, or both. Although it can occur at any age, it is most often seen in middle-aged adults and is more common in women. A disease process resembling painless thyroiditis can occur during the postpartum period in up to 5% of women *(postpartum thyroiditis)*. Painless and postpartum thyroiditides are variants of Hashimoto thyroiditis, since the majority of patients have circulating anti-thyroid peroxidase antibodies or a family history of other autoimmune disorders. As many as a third of cases can evolve into overt hypothyroidism over time, and the thyroid histology is also reminiscent of Hashimoto thyroiditis (see below).

> **Morphology.** Except for possible mild symmetric enlargement, the thyroid appears normal on gross inspection. The most specific histologic features consist of lymphocytic infiltration with hyperplastic germinal centers within the thyroid parenchyma and patchy disruption and collapse of thyroid follicles. Unlike in frank Hashimoto thyroiditis, however, fibrosis and Hürthle cell metaplasia are not prominent features.

Clinical Course. Individuals with painless thyroiditis can present with a painless goiter, transient overt hyperthyroidism, or both. Some patients transition from a hyperthyroid state to hypothyroidism before recovery. The vast majority (~80%) of individuals with postpartum thyroiditis are euthyroid by 1 year. Postpartum thyroiditis can resemble Graves disease, the incidence of which is also increased in the setting of pregnancy. Infiltrative ophthalmopathy and other manifestations of Graves disease (see below) are, however, not present in the former. As stated, as many as a third of affected individuals eventually progress to overt hypothyroidism over a 10-year period.

Other, less common forms of thyroiditis include *Riedel thyroiditis*, a rare disorder of unknown etiology characterized by extensive fibrosis involving the thyroid and contiguous neck structures. The presence of a hard and fixed thyroid mass clinically simulates a thyroid carcinoma. It may be associated with idiopathic fibrosis in other sites in the body, such as the retroperitoneum. The presence of circulating anti-thyroid antibodies in most patients suggests an autoimmune etiology.

Graves Disease

Graves reported in 1835 his observations of a disease characterized by "violent and long continued palpitations in females" associated with enlargement of the thyroid gland.[14] *Graves disease is the most common cause of endogenous hyperthyroidism.* It is characterized by a *triad* of clinical findings:

1. *Hyperthyroidism* due to diffuse, hyperfunctional enlargement of the thyroid
2. Infiltrative *ophthalmopathy* with resultant exophthalmos
3. Localized, infiltrative *dermopathy*, sometimes called *pretibial myxedema*, which is present in a minority of patients

Graves disease has a peak incidence between 20 and 40 years of age. *Women are affected as much as 10 times more frequently than men.* This disorder is said to be present in 1.5% to 2.0%

of women in the United States. As previously mentioned, Graves disease (hyperthyroidism) and Hashimoto thyroiditis (hypothyroidism) span two extremes of autoimmune thyroid disorders, and not surprisingly share many underlying tenets. For example, akin to Hashimoto thyroiditis, genetic factors are also important in the etiology of Graves disease, with a concordance rate in monozygotic twins of 30% to 40%, as compared with less than 5% among dizygotic individuals. Like Hashimoto thyroiditis, genetic susceptibility for Graves disease has been linked to polymorphisms in immune-function genes like *CTLA4* and *PTPN22* and the HLA-DR3 allele.[15]

Pathogenesis. *Graves disease is characterized by a breakdown in self-tolerance to thyroid auto-antigens, most importantly the TSH receptor.* The result is the production of multiple autoantibodies, including:

- *Thyroid-stimulating immunoglobulin:* This IgG antibody binds to the TSH receptor and mimics the action of TSH, stimulating adenyl cyclase and increasing the release of thyroid hormones. Almost all individuals with Graves disease have detectable levels of this autoantibody. Thyroid-stimulating immunoglobulin is relatively specific for Graves disease, in contrast to thyroglobulin and thyroid peroxidase antibodies.
- *Thyroid growth-stimulating immunoglobulins:* Also directed against the TSH receptor, thyroid growth-stimulating immunoglobulins have been implicated in the proliferation of thyroid follicular epithelium.
- *TSH-binding inhibitor immunoglobulins:* These anti–TSH receptor antibodies prevent TSH from binding normally to its receptor on thyroid epithelial cells. In so doing, some forms of TSH-binding inhibitor immunoglobulins mimic the action of TSH, resulting in the stimulation of thyroid epithelial cell activity, whereas other forms may actually *inhibit* thyroid cell function. It is not unusual to find the coexistence of stimulating *and* inhibiting immunoglobulins in the serum of the same patient, a finding that could explain why some patients with Graves disease have episodes of hypothyroidism.

The key role of anti–TSH receptor antibodies in the pathogenesis of hyperthyroidism is supported by animal models of Graves disease. Immunization of mice with the TSH receptor results in generation of antibodies that cause thyroid stimulation, thyroid enlargement with lymphocytic infiltration, elevated thyroxine levels, and, in a subset of mice, ocular signs reminiscent of Graves ophthalmopathy (see below).

Autoimmunity also plays a role in the development of the *infiltrative ophthalmopathy* that is characteristic of Graves disease. In Graves ophthalmopathy, the volume of the retro-orbital connective tissues and extraocular muscles is increased for several reasons, including (1) marked infiltration of the retro-orbital space by mononuclear cells, predominantly T cells; (2) inflammatory edema and swelling of extraocular muscles; (3) accumulation of extracellular matrix components, specifically hydrophilic glycosaminoglycans such as hyaluronic acid and chondroitin sulfate; and (4) increased numbers of adipocytes (fatty infiltration). These changes displace the eyeball forward and can interfere with the function of the extraocular muscles. Recent evidence suggests that *orbital preadipocyte fibroblasts* express the TSH receptor and

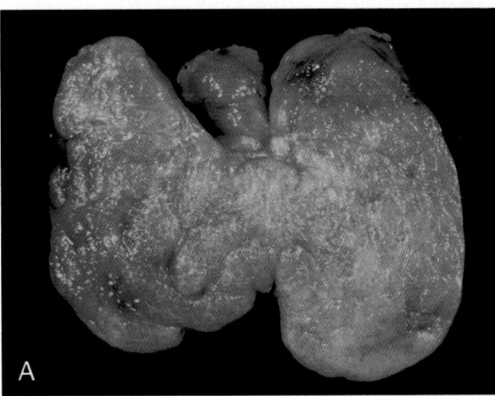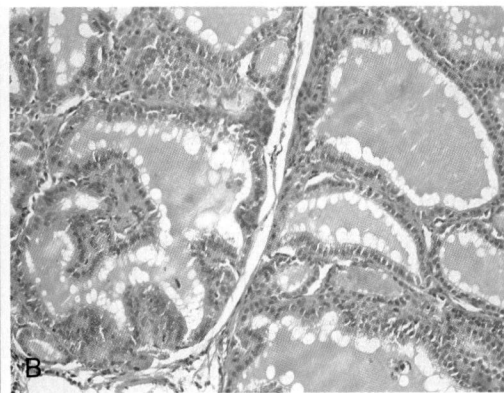

FIGURE 24–13   Graves disease. **A,** There is diffuse symmetric enlargement of the gland and a beefy deep red parenchyma. Compare with gross photograph of multinodular goiter in Figure 24–15. **B,** Diffusely hyperplastic thyroid in a case of Graves' disease. The follicles are lined by tall, columnar epithelium. The crowded, enlarged epithelial cells project into the lumens of the follicles. These cells actively resorb the colloid in the centers of the follicles, resulting in the scalloped appearance of the edges of the colloid. (**A,** Reproduced with permission from Lloyd RV et al. (eds): Atlas of Nontumor Pathology: Endocrine Diseases. Washington, DC, American Registry of Pathology, 2002.)

thus become targets of an autoimmune attack. T cells reactive against these fibroblasts secrete cytokines, which stimulate fibroblast proliferation and synthesis of extracellular matrix proteins (glycosaminoglycans) and increase surface TSH receptor expression, perpetuating the autoimmune response. The result is progressive infiltration of the retro-orbital space and ophthalmopathy.

Morphology. The thyroid gland is usually symmetrically enlarged because of **diffuse hypertrophy and hyperplasia** of thyroid follicular epithelial cells (Fig. 24–13A). Increases in weight to over 80 gm are not uncommon. On cut section, the parenchyma has a soft, meaty appearance resembling normal muscle. Histologically, the follicular epithelial cells in untreated cases are tall and more crowded than usual. This crowding often results in the formation of small papillae, which project into the follicular lumen and encroach on the colloid, sometimes filling the follicles (Fig. 24–13B). Such papillae lack fibrovascular cores, in contrast to those of papillary carcinoma (see below). The colloid within the follicular lumen is pale, with scalloped margins. Lymphoid infiltrates, consisting predominantly of T cells, with fewer B cells and mature plasma cells, are present throughout the interstitium; germinal centers are common.

Preoperative therapy alters the morphology of the thyroid in Graves disease. Preoperative administration of iodine causes involution of the epithelium and the accumulation of colloid by blocking thyroglobulin secretion. Treatment with the antithyroid drug propylthiouracil exaggerates the epithelial hypertrophy and hyperplasia by stimulating TSH secretion. Thus, in pretreated patients it is impossible from histologic examination of surgical specimens to evaluate the functional activity of the gland.

Changes in extra-thyroidal tissue include generalized lymphoid hyperplasia. The heart may be hypertrophied, and ischemic changes may be present,

particularly in patients with preexisting coronary artery disease. In patients with ophthalmopathy, the tissues of the orbit are edematous because of the presence of hydrophilic mucopolysaccharides. In addition, there is infiltration by lymphocytes and fibrosis. Orbital muscles are edematous initially but may undergo fibrosis late in the course of the disease. The dermopathy, if present, is characterized by thickening of the dermis due to deposition of glycosaminoglycans and lymphocyte infiltration.

Clinical Course. The clinical findings in Graves disease include changes referable to *thyrotoxicosis* as well as those associated uniquely with Graves disease, *diffuse hyperplasia of the thyroid*, *ophthalmopathy*, and *dermopathy*. The degree of thyrotoxicosis varies from case to case and is sometimes less conspicuous than other manifestations of the disease. Diffuse enlargement of the thyroid is present in all cases. The *thyroid enlargement* may be accompanied by increased flow of blood through the hyperactive gland, often producing an audible "bruit." *Sympathetic overactivity* produces a characteristic wide, staring gaze and lid lag. The ophthalmopathy of Graves disease results in abnormal protrusion of the eyeball (*exophthalmos*). The extraocular muscles are often weak. The exophthalmos may persist or progress despite successful treatment of the thyrotoxicosis, sometimes resulting in corneal injury. The infiltrative dermopathy, or *pretibial myxedema*, is most common in the skin overlying the shins, where it presents as scaly thickening and induration. However, it is present only in a minority of patients. Sometimes individuals spontaneously develop thyroid hypofunction. Patients are at increased risk for other autoimmune diseases, such as systemic lupus erythematosus, pernicious anemia, type 1 diabetes, and Addison disease.

Laboratory findings in Graves disease include *elevated free T_4 and T_3 levels* and *depressed TSH* levels. Because of ongoing stimulation of the thyroid follicles by thyroid-stimulating immunoglobulins, *radioactive iodine uptake is increased, and radioiodine scans show a diffuse uptake of iodine.*

Graves disease is treated with β-blockers, which address symptoms related to the increased β-adrenergic tone (e.g., tachycardia, palpitations, tremulousness, and anxiety), and by measures aimed at decreasing thyroid hormone synthesis, such as the administration of thionamides (e.g., propylthiouracil), radioiodine ablation, and surgical intervention.

Diffuse and Multinodular Goiters

Enlargement of the thyroid, or *goiter*, is the most common manifestation of thyroid disease. *Diffuse and multinodular goiters reflect impaired synthesis of thyroid hormone,* which is most often caused by dietary iodine deficiency. Impairment of thyroid hormone synthesis leads to a compensatory rise in the serum TSH level, which, in turn, causes hypertrophy and hyperplasia of thyroid follicular cells and, ultimately, gross enlargement of the thyroid gland. The compensatory increase in functional mass of the gland is able to overcome the hormone deficiency, ensuring a *euthyroid* metabolic state in most individuals. If the underlying disorder is sufficiently severe (e.g., a congenital biosynthetic defect or endemic iodine deficiency, see below), the compensatory responses may be inadequate to overcome the impairment in hormone synthesis, resulting in *goitrous hypothyroidism.* The degree of thyroid enlargement is proportional to the level and duration of thyroid hormone deficiency.

DIFFUSE NONTOXIC (SIMPLE) GOITER

Diffuse nontoxic (simple) goiter causes enlargement of the entire gland without producing nodularity. Because the enlarged follicles are filled with colloid, the term *colloid goiter* has been applied to this condition. This disorder occurs in both an endemic and a sporadic distribution.

Endemic goiter occurs in geographic areas where the soil, water, and food supply contain low levels of iodine. The term *endemic* is used when goiters are present in more than 10% of the population in a given region. Such conditions are particularly common in mountainous areas of the world, including the Andes and Himalayas, where iodine deficiency is widespread. The lack of iodine leads to decreased synthesis of thyroid hormone and a compensatory increase in TSH, leading to follicular cell hypertrophy and hyperplasia and goitrous enlargement. With increasing dietary iodine supplementation, the frequency and severity of endemic goiter have declined significantly, although as many as 200 million people worldwide continue to be at risk for severe iodine deficiency.

Variations in the prevalence of endemic goiter in regions with similar levels of iodine deficiency point to the existence of other causative influences, particularly dietary substances, referred to as *goitrogens.* The ingestion of substances that interfere with thyroid hormone synthesis at some level, such as vegetables belonging to the Brassicaceae (Cruciferae) family (e.g., cabbage, cauliflower, Brussels sprouts, turnips, and cassava), has been documented to be goitrogenic. Native populations subsisting on cassava root are particularly at risk. Cassava contains a thiocyanate that inhibits iodide transport within the thyroid, worsening any possible concurrent iodine deficiency.

Sporadic goiter occurs less frequently than does endemic goiter. There is a striking female preponderance and a peak incidence at puberty or in young adult life. Sporadic goiter can be caused by several conditions, including the ingestion of substances that interfere with thyroid hormone synthesis. In other instances, goiter may result from hereditary enzymatic defects that interfere with thyroid hormone synthesis, all transmitted as autosomal-recessive conditions (dyshormonogenetic goiter; see above). In most cases, however, the cause of sporadic goiter is not apparent.

Morphology. Two phases can be identified in the evolution of diffuse nontoxic goiter: the **hyperplastic phase** and the phase of **colloid involution**. In the hyperplastic phase, the thyroid gland is diffusely and symmetrically enlarged, although the increase is usually modest, and the gland rarely exceeds 100 to 150 gm. The follicles are lined by crowded columnar cells, which may pile up and form projections similar to those seen in Graves disease. The accumulation is not uniform throughout the gland, and some follicles are hugely distended, whereas others remain small. If dietary iodine subsequently increases or if the demand for thyroid hormone decreases, the stimulated follicular epithelium involutes to form an enlarged, colloid-rich gland (**colloid goiter**). In these cases the cut surface of the thyroid is usually brown, somewhat glassy, and translucent. Histologically the follicular epithelium is flattened and cuboidal, and colloid is abundant during periods of involution.

Clinical Course. As stated above, the vast majority of persons with simple goiters are clinically euthyroid. Therefore, the clinical manifestations are primarily related to *mass effects* from the enlarged thyroid gland (Fig. 24–14). Although serum T_3 and T_4 levels are normal, the serum TSH is usually elevated or at the upper range of normal, as is expected in marginally euthyroid individuals. In children, dyshormonogenetic goiter, caused by a congenital biosynthetic defect, may induce cretinism.

MULTINODULAR GOITER

With time, recurrent episodes of hyperplasia and involution combine to produce a more irregular enlargement of the thyroid, termed *multinodular goiter.* Virtually all long-standing simple goiters convert into multinodular goiters. *Multinodular goiters produce the most extreme thyroid enlargements and are more frequently mistaken for neoplastic involvement than any other form of thyroid disease.* Because they derive from simple goiter, they occur in both sporadic and endemic forms, having the same female-to-male distribution and presumably the same origins but affecting older individuals because they are late complications.

It is believed that multinodular goiters arise because of variations among follicular cells in their response to external stimuli, such as trophic hormones. If some cells in a follicle have a growth advantage, perhaps because of intrinsic genetic abnormalities similar to those that give rise to adenomas, those cells can give rise to clones of proliferating cells. This

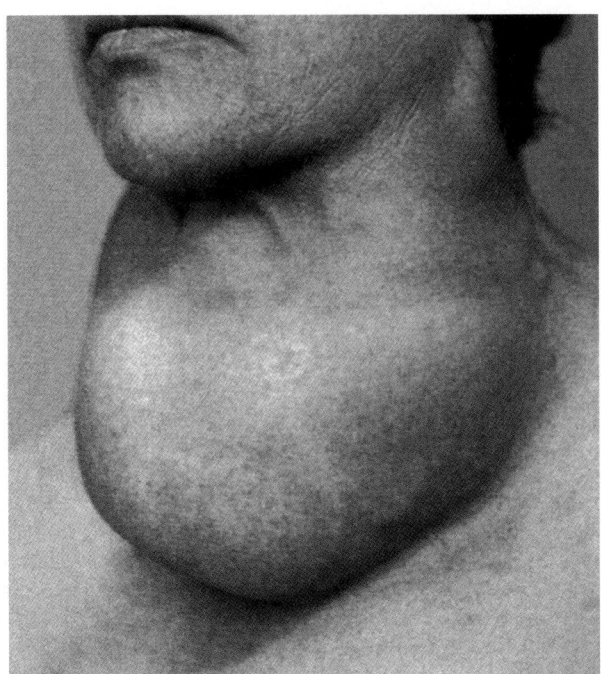

FIGURE 24–14 A 52-year-old woman with a huge colloid goiter who developed compressive symptoms. (Reproduced with permission from Lloyd RV et al. (eds): Atlas of Nontumor Pathology: Endocrine Diseases. Washington, DC, American Registry of Pathology, 2002.)

stress that leads to rupture of follicles and vessels followed by hemorrhages, scarring, and sometimes calcifications. With scarring, nodularity appears, which may be accentuated by the preexisting stromal framework of the gland.

> **Morphology.** Multinodular goiters are multilobulated, asymmetrically enlarged glands that can reach weights of more than 2000 gm. The pattern of enlargement is quite unpredictable and may involve one lobe far more than the other, producing lateral pressure on midline structures, such as the trachea and esophagus. In other instances the goiter grows behind the sternum and clavicles to produce the so-called **intrathoracic** or **plunging goiter**. Occasionally, most of it is hidden behind the trachea and esophagus; in other instances one nodule may so stand out as to impart the clinical appearance of a solitary nodule. On cut section, irregular nodules containing variable amounts of brown, gelatinous colloid are present (Fig. 24–15A). Older lesions have areas of hemorrhage, fibrosis, calcification, and cystic change. The microscopic appearance includes colloid-rich follicles lined by flattened, inactive epithelium and areas of **follicular hyperplasia**, accompanied by the degenerative changes noted previously. In contrast to follicular neoplasms, a prominent capsule between the hyperplastic nodules and residual compressed thyroid parenchyma is not present (Fig. 24–15B).

may result in the formation of a nodule whose continued growth is autonomous, without the external stimulus. Consistent with this model, both polyclonal and monoclonal nodules coexist within the same multinodular goiter, the latter presumably having arisen because of the acquisition of a genetic abnormality favoring growth. Not surprisingly, *mutations affecting proteins of the TSH-signaling pathway that lead to constitutive activation of this pathway have been identified in a subset of autonomous thyroid nodules* (TSH-signaling pathway mutations and their implications are discussed under "Adenomas"). The uneven follicular hyperplasia, generation of new follicles, and uneven accumulation of colloid produce physical

Clinical Course. The dominant clinical features of multinodular goiter are those caused by the *mass effects* of the enlarged gland. In addition to the obvious cosmetic effects of a large neck mass, goiters may cause airway obstruction, dysphagia, and compression of large vessels in the neck and upper thorax *(superior vena cava syndrome)*. Most patients are euthyroid or have subclinical hyperthyroidism (identified only by reduced TSH levels), but in a substantial minority of patients an autonomous nodule may develop within a long-standing goiter and produce hyperthyroidism *(toxic multinodular goiter)*. This condition, known as *Plummer syndrome*, is not accompanied by the infiltrative ophthalmopathy and

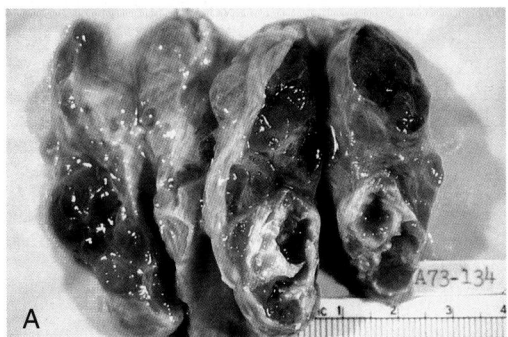
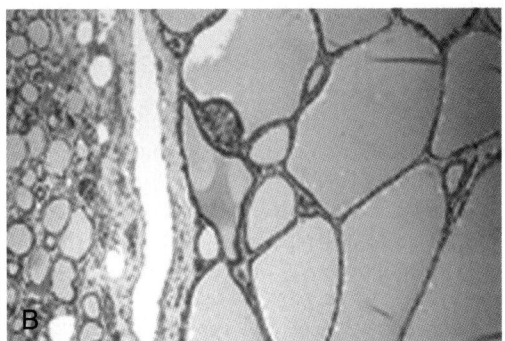

FIGURE 24–15 Multinodular goiter. **A,** Gross morphology demonstrating a coarsely nodular gland, containing areas of fibrosis and cystic change. **B,** Photomicrograph of a hyperplastic nodule, with compressed residual thyroid parenchyma on the periphery. Note absence of a prominent capsule, a distinguishing feature from follicular neoplasms. (**B,** Courtesy of Dr. William Westra, Department of Pathology, Johns Hopkins University, Baltimore, MD.)

dermopathy of Graves disease. It is estimated that clinically apparent autonomous nodules can develop in approximately 10% of multinodular goiters over a 10-year follow-up. The incidence of malignancy in long-standing multinodular goiters is low (<5%) but not zero, and concern for malignancy arises in goiters that demonstrate sudden changes in size or symptoms (e.g., hoarseness). Dominant nodules in a multinodular goiter can present as a "solitary thyroid nodule" (see below), mimicking a thyroid neoplasm. A radioiodine scan demonstrates uneven iodine uptake (including the occasional "hot" autonomous nodule) consistent with the diffuse parenchymal involvement, and an admixture of hyperplastic and involuting nodules in multinodular goiter. A fine-needle aspiration biopsy is helpful and can often, albeit not always, facilitate the distinction of follicular hyperplasia from a follicular neoplasm (see below).[16]

Neoplasms of the Thyroid

The solitary thyroid nodule is a palpably discrete swelling within an otherwise apparently normal thyroid gland. The estimated incidence of solitary palpable nodules in the adult population of the United States varies between 1% and 10%, although it is significantly higher in endemic goitrous regions. Single nodules are about four times more common in women than in men. The incidence of thyroid nodules increases throughout life.

From a clinical standpoint, the possibility of neoplastic disease is of major concern in persons who present with thyroid nodules. Fortunately, the overwhelming majority of solitary nodules of the thyroid prove to be localized, non-neoplastic conditions (e.g., a dominant nodule in multinodular goiter, simple cysts, or foci of thyroiditis) or benign neoplasms such as follicular adenomas. In fact, *benign neoplasms outnumber thyroid carcinomas by a ratio of nearly 10:1.* While under 1% of solitary thyroid nodules are malignant, this still represents about 15,000 new cases of thyroid carcinoma per year in the United States. Fortunately, most of these cancers are indolent, permitting a 90% survival at 20 years. Several clinical criteria provide clues to the nature of a given thyroid nodule:

- *Solitary nodules,* in general, are more likely to be neoplastic than are multiple nodules.
- *Nodules in younger patients* are more likely to be neoplastic than are those in older patients.
- *Nodules in males* are more likely to be neoplastic than are those in females.
- A history of *radiation* treatment to the head and neck region is associated with an increased incidence of thyroid malignancy.
- Functional nodules that take up radioactive iodine in imaging studies *(hot nodules)* are significantly more likely to be benign than malignant.

Such general trends and statistics, however, are of little significance in the evaluation of a given patient, in whom the timely recognition of a malignancy can be lifesaving. Ultimately, it is the morphologic evaluation of a given thyroid nodule, by fine-needle aspiration and histologic study of sur-

gically resected thyroid parenchyma, that provides the most definitive information about its nature. In the following sections we consider the major thyroid neoplasms, including adenoma and carcinoma in its various forms.

ADENOMAS

Adenomas of the thyroid are typically discrete, solitary masses, derived from follicular epithelium, and hence they are also known as *follicular adenomas.* Clinically, follicular adenomas can be difficult to distinguish from dominant nodules of follicular hyperplasia or from the less common follicular carcinomas. In general, follicular adenomas are *not* forerunners to carcinomas; nevertheless, shared genetic alterations support the possibility that at least of subset of follicular carcinomas arise in preexisting adenomas (see below). Although the vast majority of adenomas are nonfunctional, a small proportion produces thyroid hormones and causes clinically apparent thyrotoxicosis. Hormone production in functional adenomas ("toxic adenomas") is independent of TSH stimulation and represents another example of *thyroid autonomy*, analogous to toxic multinodular goiters. Not surprisingly, both of these benign processes share altered genetic pathways.

Pathogenesis. A minority (<20%) of *nonfunctioning* follicular adenomas have mutations of *RAS or phosphotidylinositol-3-kinase subunit (PIK3CA),*[17] or bear a *PAX8-PPARG* fusion gene,[18] all of which are genetic alterations shared with follicular carcinomas. These are discussed in further detail under "Carcinomas" (see below).

Somatic mutations of the *TSH receptor signaling pathway* have been found in toxic adenomas, as well as in toxic multinodular goiter. Gain-of-function mutations in one of two components of this signaling system—most often *TSHR* itself or the α-subunit of G_s (*GNAS*)—allow follicular cells to secrete thyroid hormone independent of TSH stimulation ("thyroid autonomy"). This causes symptoms of hyperthyroidism and produces a "hot" thyroid nodule on imaging. Overall, mutations in the TSH receptor signaling pathway seem to be present in slightly over half of toxic thyroid nodules. Notably, *TSHR* and *GNAS* mutations are rare in follicular carcinomas; thus toxic adenomas and toxic multinodular goiter do not seem to be forerunners of malignancy.

Morphology. The typical thyroid adenoma is a solitary, spherical, encapsulated lesion that is well demarcated from the surrounding thyroid parenchyma (Fig. 24–16A). Follicular adenomas average about 3 cm in diameter, but some are much larger (≥10 cm in diameter). In freshly resected specimens the adenoma bulges from the cut surface and compresses the adjacent thyroid. The color ranges from gray-white to red-brown, depending on the cellularity of the adenoma and its colloid content. The neoplastic cells are demarcated from the adjacent parenchyma by a well-defined, intact capsule. **These features are important in making the distinction from multinodular goiters,** which contain multiple nodules on their cut surface even though the patient may present clinically with a solitary dominant nodule. Areas of hemorrhage, fibrosis, calcification, and cystic change,

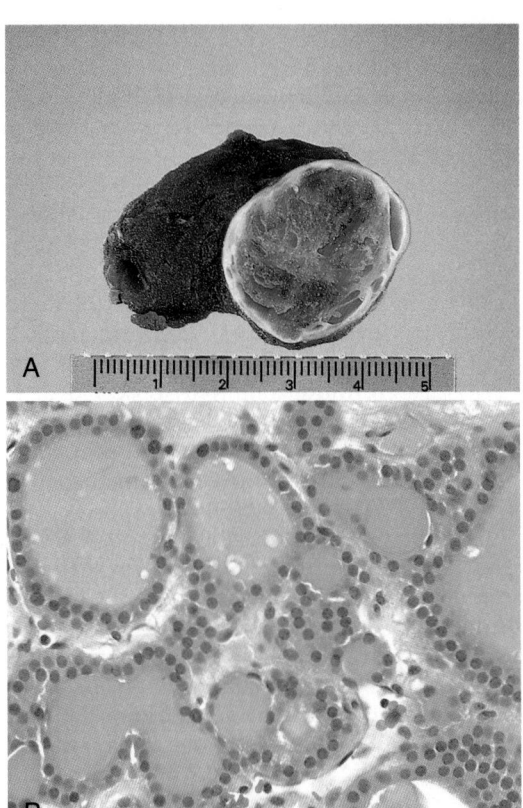

FIGURE 24–16 Follicular adenoma of the thyroid. **A,** A solitary, well-circumscribed nodule is seen. **B,** The photomicrograph shows well-differentiated follicles resembling normal thyroid parenchyma.

similar to those encountered in multinodular goiters, are common in follicular adenomas, particularly within larger lesions.

Microscopically, the constituent cells often form uniform-appearing follicles that contain colloid (Fig. 24–16B). The follicular growth pattern within the adenoma is usually quite distinct from the adjacent non-neoplastic thyroid. The epithelial cells composing the follicular adenoma reveal little variation in cell and nuclear morphology, and mitotic figures are rare. Extensive mitotic activity, necrosis, or high cellularity warrants careful examination of the capsule to exclude a follicular carcinoma, as well as of the nuclear features to exclude a follicular variant of papillary carcinoma (see below). Occasionally the neoplastic cells acquire brightly eosinophilic granular cytoplasm (oxyphil or Hürthle cell change) (Fig. 24–17); the clinical presentation and behavior of a follicular adenoma with oxyphilia (**Hürthle cell adenoma**) is no different from that of a conventional adenoma. The hallmark of all follicular adenomas is the presence of an intact, well-formed capsule encircling the tumor. **Careful evaluation of the integrity of the capsule is therefore critical in distinguishing follicular adenomas from follicular carcinomas,** which demonstrate capsular and/or vascular invasion (see below).

Clinical Features. Many follicular adenomas present as a unilateral painless mass, often discovered during a routine physical examination. Larger masses may produce local symptoms, such as difficulty in swallowing. Nonfunctioning adenomas take up less radioactive iodine than does normal thyroid parenchyma. On radionuclide scanning, therefore, nonfunctioning adenomas usually appear as *cold* nodules relative to the adjacent thyroid tissue. As many as 10% of cold nodules eventually prove to be malignant on histologic analysis. By contrast, malignancy is rare in *hot* nodules (toxic adenomas). Other techniques used in the preoperative evaluation of suspected adenomas are ultrasonography and fine-needle aspiration biopsy. *Because of the need for evaluating capsular integrity, the definitive diagnosis of adenomas can be made only after careful histologic examination of the resected specimen.* Suspected adenomas of the thyroid are therefore removed surgically to exclude malignancy. Follicular adenomas have an excellent prognosis and do not recur or metastasize.

CARCINOMAS

Carcinomas of the thyroid are relatively uncommon in the United States, accounting for about 1.5% of all cancers. A female predominance has been noted among patients who develop thyroid carcinoma in the early and middle adult years. In contrast, cases presenting in childhood and late adult life are distributed equally among males and females. Most thyroid carcinomas (except medullary carcinomas) are derived from the thyroid follicular epithelium, and of these, the vast majority are well-differentiated lesions. The major subtypes of thyroid carcinoma and their relative frequencies include the following:

- Papillary carcinoma (>85% of cases)
- Follicular carcinoma (5% to 15% of cases)
- Anaplastic (undifferentiated) carcinoma (<5% of cases)
- Medullary carcinoma (5% of cases)

Because of the unique clinical and biologic features associated with each variant of thyroid carcinoma, these subtypes

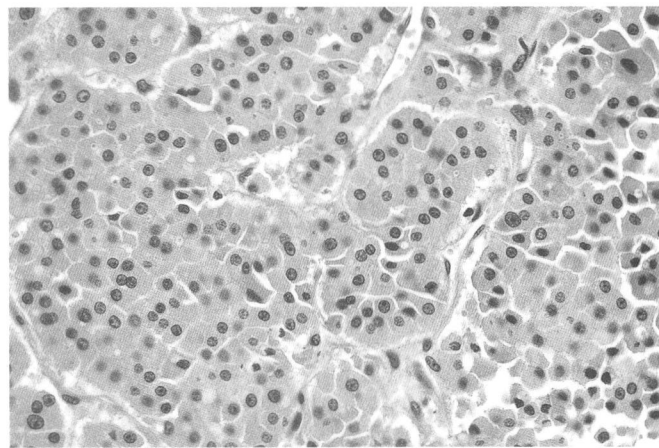

FIGURE 24–17 Hürthle cell (oxyphil) adenoma. A high-power view showing that the tumor is composed of cells with abundant eosinophilic cytoplasm and small regular nuclei. (Courtesy of Dr. Mary Sunday, Duke University, Durham, NC.)

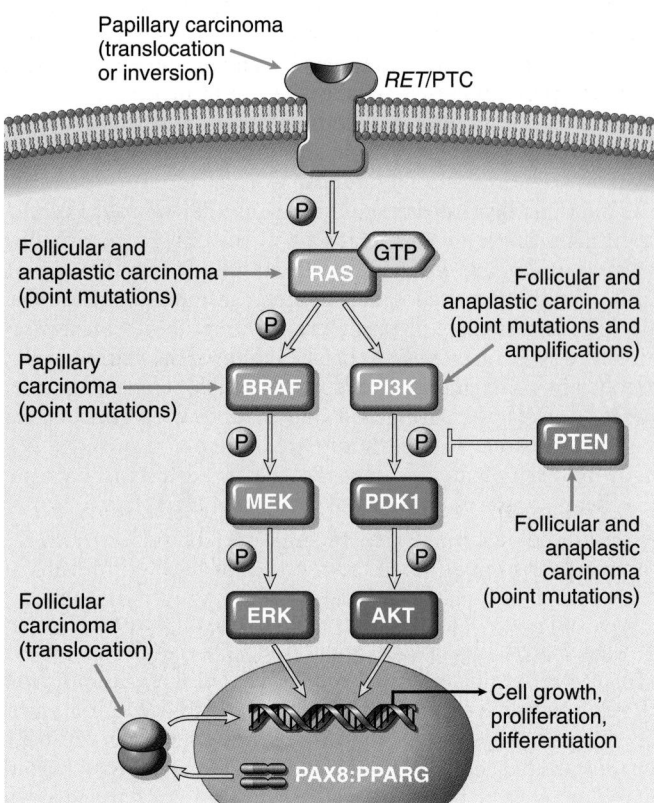

FIGURE 24–18 Genetic alterations in follicular cell–derived malignancies of the thyroid gland.

are described separately. We begin with a discussion of the molecular pathogenesis of all thyroid cancers.

Pathogenesis

Genetic Factors. Distinct genetic events are involved in the pathogenesis of the four major histologic variants of thyroid cancer. As stated, medullary carcinomas do not arise from the follicular epithelium. Genetic alterations in the three follicular cell–derived malignancies are clustered along two oncogenic pathways—the mitogen-activated protein (MAP) kinase pathway and the phosphatidylinositol-3-kinase (PI-3K)/AKT pathway (Fig. 24–18). In normal cells, these pathways are transiently activated by binding of soluble growth factor ligands to the extracellular domain of receptor tyrosine kinases, which results in autophosphorylation of the cytoplasmic domain of the receptor, permitting intracellular signal transduction. In thyroid carcinomas, as with many solid cancers (see Chapter 7), gain-of-function mutations along components of these pathways lead to constitutive activation even in the absence of ligand and thus promote carcinogenesis.[17]

Papillary Carcinomas. Activation of the MAP kinase pathway is a feature of most papillary carcinomas and can occur by one of two major mechanisms. The first mechanism involves rearrangements of *RET* or *NTRK1* (neurotrophic tyrosine kinase receptor 1), both of which encode transmembrane receptor tyrosine kinases, and the second mechanism involves activating point mutations in *BRAF*, whose product is an intermediate signaling component in the MAP kinase

pathway (see Fig. 24–18). The *RET* gene is located on chromosome 10q11, and the receptor tyrosine kinase it encodes is normally not expressed in thyroid follicular cells. In papillary cancers, either a paracentric inversion of chromosome 10 or a reciprocal translocation between chromosomes 10 and 17 places the tyrosine kinase domain of *RET* under the transcriptional control of genes that are constitutively expressed in the thyroid epithelium. The novel fusion proteins that are so formed are known as *RET/PTC* (*RET*/papillary thyroid carcinoma) and are present in approximately 20% to 40% of papillary thyroid cancers. There are more than 15 fusion partners of *RET*, and two—designated as *RET/PTC1* and *RET/PTC2*—are most commonly observed in sporadic papillary cancers. The frequency of *RET/PTC* rearrangements is significantly higher in papillary cancers arising in the backdrop of radiation exposure. Irrespective of frequency, the presence of a RET/PTC fusion protein leads to constitutive expression of the tyrosine kinase in thyroid follicular cells, with resultant activation of the MAP kinase pathway. Similarly, paracentric inversions or translocations of *NTRK1* on chromosome 1q21 are present in 5% to 10% of papillary thyroid cancers, and the resultant fusion proteins are constitutively expressed in thyroid cells, leading to activation of MAP kinase and other oncogenic signaling pathways. One third to one half of papillary thyroid carcinomas harbor a gain-of-function mutation in the *BRAF* gene, which is most commonly a valine-to-glutamate change on codon 600 ($BRAF^{V600E}$).[19] The presence of *BRAF* mutations in papillary carcinomas correlates with adverse prognostic factors like metastatic disease and extra-thyroidal extension. The histologic variants of papillary carcinoma demonstrate some unique characteristics vis-à-vis the frequency or nature of *BRAF* mutation (see below). Since chromosomal rearrangements of the *RET* or *NTRK1* genes and mutations of *BRAF* have redundant effects on the thyroid epithelium (both mechanisms result in activation of the MAP kinase signaling pathway), papillary thyroid carcinomas demonstrate either one or the other molecular abnormality, but not both. *RET/PTC* rearrangements and *BRAF* point mutations are not observed in follicular adenomas or carcinomas.

Follicular Carcinomas. Approximately one third to one half of follicular thyroid carcinomas harbor mutations in the PI-3K/AKT signaling pathway, resulting in constitutive activation of this oncogenic pathway. This subset of cases includes tumors with gain-of-function point mutations of *RAS* and *PIK3CA*, tumors with amplification of *PIK3CA*, and those with loss-of-function mutations of *PTEN*, a tumor suppressor gene and negative regulator of this pathway (see Fig. 24–18). The genetic alterations activating the PI-3K/AKT pathway are almost always mutually exclusive in follicular carcinomas, in line with their functional equivalence. The progressive increase in the prevalence of *RAS* and *PIK3CA* mutations from benign follicular adenomas to follicular carcinomas to anaplastic carcinomas (see below) suggests a shared histogenesis and molecular evolution among these follicular cell–derived tumors. A unique (2;3)(q13;p25) translocation has been described in one third to one half of follicular carcinomas. This translocation creates a fusion gene composed of portions of *PAX8*, a paired homeobox gene that is important in thyroid development, and the peroxisome proliferator-activated receptor gene (*PPARG*), whose gene product is a nuclear hormone receptor implicated in terminal differentiation of cells. Fewer than 10% of follicular adenomas harbor *PAX8-PPARG* fusion genes, and these have not been documented thus far in other thyroid neoplasms.

Anaplastic (Undifferentiated) Carcinomas. These highly aggressive and lethal tumors can arise de novo, or more commonly, by "dedifferentiation" of a well-differentiated papillary or follicular carcinoma. Molecular alterations present in anaplastic carcinomas include those also seen in well-differentiated carcinomas (e.g., *RAS* or *PIK3CA* mutations), albeit at a significantly higher rate, suggesting that the presence of these mutations might predispose existing thyroid neoplasms to transform.[20] Other genetic "hits," such as inactivation of *p53* or activating mutations of β-catenin, are essentially restricted to anaplastic carcinomas, and might also relate to their aggressive behavior.

Medullary Thyroid Carcinomas. Familial medullary thyroid carcinomas occur in multiple endocrine neoplasia type 2 (MEN-2, see below) and are associated with germline *RET* proto-oncogene mutations that lead to constitutive activation of the receptor. *RET* mutations are also seen in approximately one half of nonfamilial (sporadic) medullary thyroid cancers. Chromosomal rearrangements involving *RET*, such as the *RET/PTC* translocations reported in papillary cancers, are not seen in medullary carcinomas.

Environmental Factors. The major risk factor predisposing to thyroid cancer is exposure to *ionizing radiation*, particularly during the first 2 decades of life. In keeping with this, there was a marked increase in the incidence of papillary car-

cinomas among children exposed to ionizing radiation after the Chernobyl nuclear disaster in 1986.[21] *Deficiency of dietary iodine* (and by extension, an association with goiter) is linked with a higher frequency of follicular carcinomas.

Papillary Carcinoma

Papillary carcinomas are the most common form of thyroid cancer, accounting for nearly 85% of primary thyroid malignancies in the United States. They occur throughout life but most often between the ages of 25 and 50, and account for the majority of thyroid carcinomas associated with previous exposure to ionizing radiation. The incidence of papillary carcinoma has increased markedly in the last 30 years, partly because of the recognition of follicular variants (see below) that were misdiagnosed in the past.

> **Morphology.** Papillary carcinomas are solitary or multifocal lesions. Some tumors may be well circumscribed and even encapsulated; others may infiltrate the adjacent parenchyma with ill-defined margins. The lesions may contain areas of fibrosis and calcification and are often cystic. The cut surface sometimes reveals papillary foci that may point to the diagnosis. The microscopic hallmarks of papillary neoplasms include the following (Fig. 24–19):

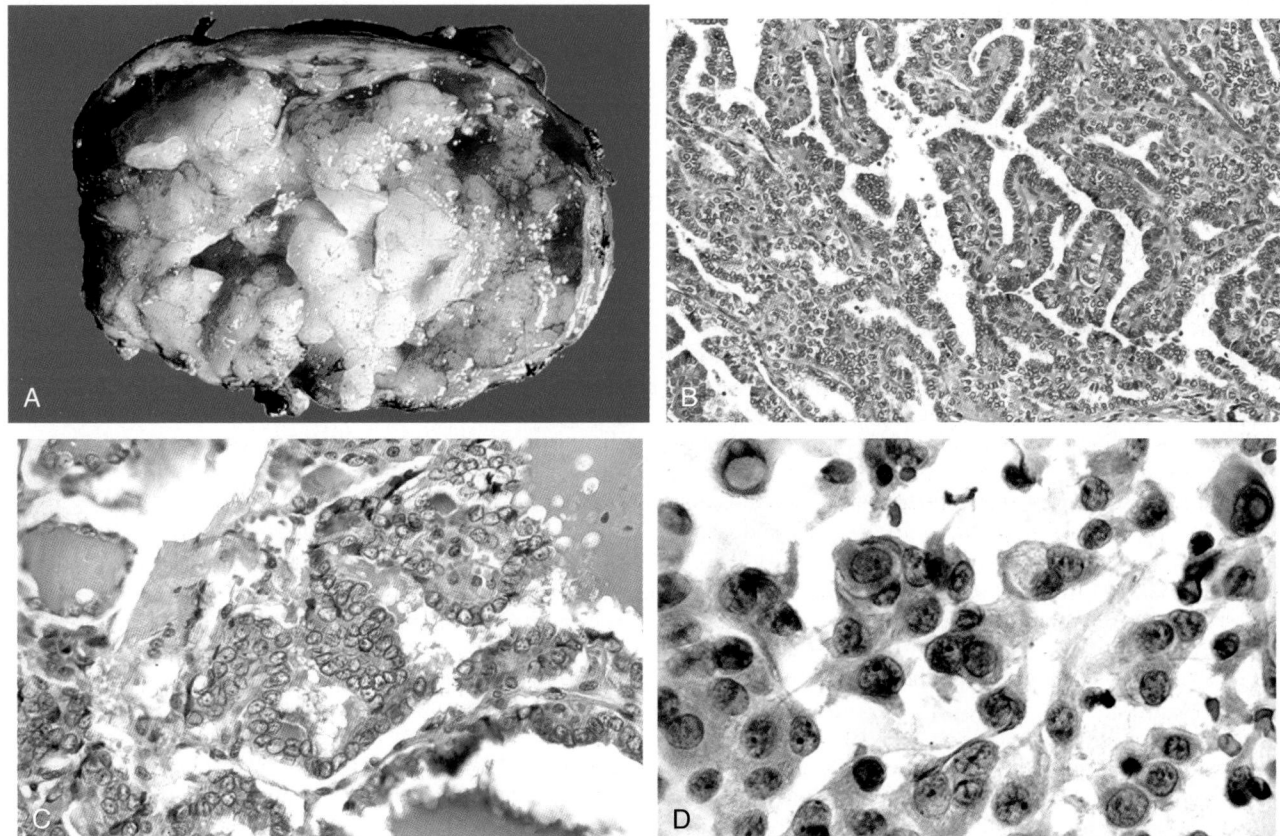

FIGURE 24–19 Papillary carcinoma of the thyroid. **A,** The macroscopic appearance of a papillary carcinoma with grossly discernible papillary structures. This particular example contains well-formed papillae (**B**), lined by cells with characteristic empty-appearing nuclei, sometimes called "Orphan Annie eye" nuclei (**C**). **D,** Cells obtained by fine-needle aspiration of a papillary carcinoma. Characteristic intranuclear inclusions are visible in some of the aspirated cells.

- Papillary carcinomas can contain branching **papillae** having a fibrovascular stalk covered by a single to multiple layers of cuboidal epithelial cells. In most neoplasms, the epithelium covering the papillae consists of well-differentiated, uniform, orderly cuboidal cells, but at the other extreme are those with fairly anaplastic epithelium showing considerable variation in cell and nuclear morphology. When present, the papillae of papillary carcinoma differ from those seen in areas of hyperplasia in being more complex and having dense fibrovascular cores.
- The nuclei of papillary carcinoma cells contain finely dispersed chromatin, which imparts an **optically clear** or **empty** appearance, giving rise to the designation **ground-glass** or **Orphan Annie eye nuclei**. In addition, invaginations of the cytoplasm may in cross-sections give the appearance of intranuclear inclusions ("pseudo-inclusions") or intranuclear grooves. **The diagnosis of papillary carcinoma is made based on these nuclear features,** even in the absence of papillary architecture.
- Concentrically calcified structures termed **psammoma bodies** are often present within the lesion, usually within the cores of papillae. These structures are almost never found in follicular and medullary carcinomas, and so, when present in fine-needle aspiration material, they are a strong indication that the lesion is a papillary carcinoma.
- Foci of lymphatic invasion by tumor are often present, but involvement of blood vessels is relatively uncommon, particularly in smaller lesions. Metastases to adjacent cervical lymph nodes are estimated to occur in up to half the cases.

There are over a dozen histologic variants of papillary carcinoma that can mimic other lesions of the thyroid or harbor distinct prognostic implications[22]; their discussion is beyond the scope of this book. The most common variant, and the one most liable to misdiagnosis, is the **follicular variant,** which has the characteristic nuclei of papillary carcinoma but has an almost totally follicular architecture. The incidence of this variant has sharply increased in recent years with greater recognition of its existence among pathologists. The genetic alterations in the follicular variant demonstrate several distinctions from conventional papillary carcinomas, including a lower frequency of *RET/PTC* rearrangements and a significantly higher frequency of *RAS* mutations.[23] Further, the follicular variant often harbors a distinct mutation in *BRAF,* which results in a lower degree of BRAF kinase activation than the mutation present in conventional papillary carcinomas.[24] The follicular variant is more frequently encapsulated and has a lower incidence of lymph node metastases and extra-thyroidal extension than conventional papillary carcinomas. Recent studies suggest that encapsulated follicular variant carcinomas have a favorable prognosis and can be managed with conservative surgical excision, while the more infiltrative tumors associated with metastases should be treated more aggressively.

A **tall-cell variant** is marked by tall columnar cells with intensely eosinophilic cytoplasm lining the papillary structures. These tumors tend to occur in older individuals and have higher frequencies of vascular invasion, extra-thyroidal extension, and cervical and distant metastases than conventional papillary thyroid carcinoma. Tall-cell variant papillary carcinomas harbor *BRAF* mutations in most (55% to 100%) cases, and often have a *RET/PTC* translocation. The occurrence of these together may be responsible for the aggressive behavior of this variant.

An unusual **diffuse sclerosing variant** of papillary carcinoma occurs in younger individuals, including children. The tumor demonstrates a prominent papillary growth pattern, intermixed with solid areas containing nests of squamous metaplasia. As the name suggests, there is extensive, diffuse fibrosis throughout the thyroid gland, often associated with a prominent lymphocytic infiltrate, simulating Hashimoto thyroiditis. Lymph node metastases are present in almost all cases. The diffuse sclerosing variant carcinomas lack *BRAF* mutations, but *RET/PTC* translocations are found in approximately half the cases.

In passing, we should mention the **papillary microcarcinoma**, which is defined as an otherwise conventional papillary carcinoma less than 1 cm in size, and usually confined to the thyroid gland. These lesions are most often observed as an incidental finding upon surgery. These might well be precursors of the usual papillary cancers.

Clinical Course. Most conventional papillary carcinomas present as asymptomatic thyroid nodules, but the first manifestation may be a mass in a cervical lymph node. Interestingly, the presence of isolated cervical nodal metastases does not seem to have a significant influence on the generally good prognosis of these lesions. The carcinoma, which is usually a single nodule, moves freely during swallowing and is not distinguishable from a benign nodule. Hoarseness, dysphagia, cough, or dyspnea suggests advanced disease. In a minority of patients, hematogenous metastases are present at the time of diagnosis, most commonly in the lung.

A variety of diagnostic tests have been used to help separate benign from malignant thyroid nodules, including radionuclide scanning and fine-needle aspiration. Papillary carcinomas are *cold* masses on scintiscans. Improvements in cytologic analysis have made fine-needle aspiration cytology a reliable test for distinguishing between benign and malignant nodules. The nuclear features are often nicely demonstrable in aspirated specimens.

Papillary thyroid cancers have an excellent prognosis, with a 10-year survival rate in excess of 95%. Between 5% and 20% of patients have local or regional recurrences, and 10% to 15% have distant metastases. The prognosis of someone with papillary thyroid cancers is dependent on several factors including age (in general, the prognosis is less favorable among patients older than 40 years), the presence of extra-thyroidal extension, and presence of distant metastases (stage).

Follicular Carcinoma

Follicular carcinomas account for 5% to 15% of primary thyroid cancers. They are more common in women (3:1) and present at an older age than do papillary carcinomas, with a peak incidence between 40 and 60 years of age. Follicular carcinoma is more frequent in areas with dietary iodine deficiency (25% to 40% of thyroid cancers), while its incidence has either decreased or remained stable in iodine-sufficient areas of the world.

> **Morphology.** Follicular carcinomas are single nodules that may be well circumscribed or widely infiltrative (Fig. 24–20A). Sharply demarcated lesions may be exceedingly difficult to distinguish from follicular adenomas by gross examination. Larger lesions may penetrate the capsule and infiltrate well beyond the thyroid capsule into the adjacent neck. They are gray to tan to pink on cut section and, on occasion, are somewhat translucent due to the presence of large, colloid-filled follicles. Degenerative changes, such as central fibrosis and foci of calcification, are sometimes present.
>
> Microscopically, most follicular carcinomas are composed of fairly uniform cells forming small follicles containing colloid, quite reminiscent of normal thyroid (Fig. 24–20B). In other cases follicular differentiation may be less apparent, and there may be nests or sheets of cells without colloid. Occasional tumors are dominated by cells with abundant granular, eosinophilic cytoplasm (**Hürthle cell or oncocytic variant of follicular carcinoma**). Whatever the pattern, the nuclei lack the features typical of papillary carcinoma, and psammoma bodies are not present. It is important to note the absence of these details, because some papillary carcinomas appear almost entirely follicular. Follicular lesions in which the nuclear features are typical of papillary carcinomas should be treated as papillary cancers. While nuclear features are helpful in distinguishing papillary from follicular neoplasms, they are of little value in distinguishing follicular adenomas from **minimally invasive follicular carcinomas**. This distinction requires extensive histologic sampling of the tumor-capsule-thyroid interface to exclude capsular and/or vascular invasion (Fig. 24–21). The criterion for vascular invasion is applicable only to capsular vessels and vascular spaces beyond the capsule; the presence of tumor plugs within intra-tumoral blood vessels has little prognostic significance. Unlike in papillary cancers, lymphatic spread is uncommon in follicular cancers.
>
> In contrast to minimally invasive follicular cancers, the diagnosis of carcinoma is obvious in **widely invasive follicular carcinomas,** which infiltrate the thyroid parenchyma and extra-thyroidal soft tissues. Histologically, these cancers tend to have a greater proportion of solid or trabecular growth pattern, less evidence of follicular differentiation, and increased mitotic activity.

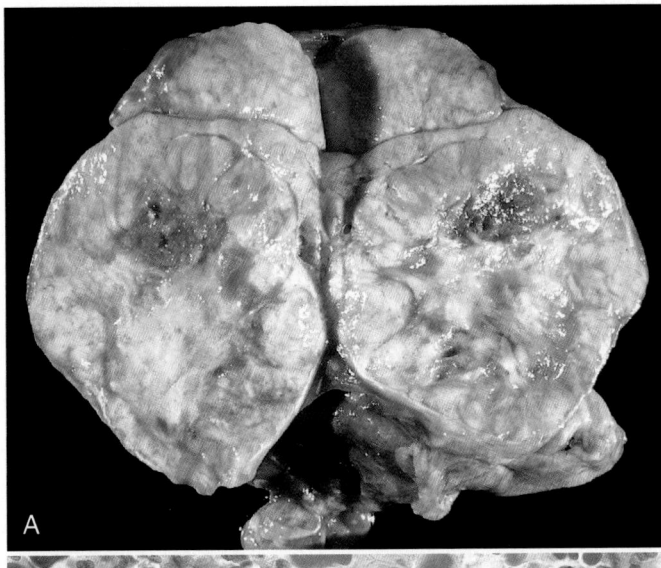

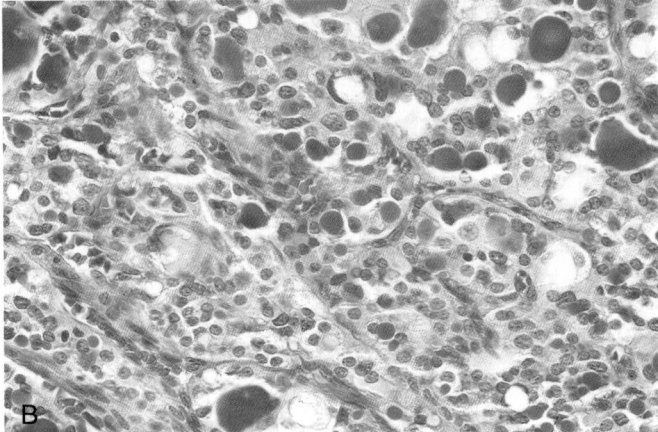

FIGURE 24–20 Follicular carcinoma. **A,** Cut surface of a follicular carcinoma with substantial replacement of the lobe of the thyroid. The tumor has a light-tan appearance and contains small foci of hemorrhage. **B,** A few of the glandular lumens contain recognizable colloid.

Clinical Course. Follicular carcinomas present as slowly enlarging painless nodules. Most frequently they are *cold nodules* on scintigrams, although rare, better differentiated lesions may be hyperfunctional, take up radioactive iodine and appear *warm* on scintiscan. Follicular carcinomas have little propensity for invading lymphatics; therefore, regional lymph nodes are rarely involved, but vascular (hematogenous) dissemination is common, with metastases to bone, lungs, liver, and elsewhere. The prognosis is largely dependent on the extent of invasion and stage at presentation. Widely invasive follicular carcinomas not infrequently present with systemic metastases, and as many as half the patients succumb to their disease within 10 years. This is in stark contrast to minimally invasive follicular carcinoma, with which the 10-year survival rate is greater than 90%. Most follicular carcinomas are treated with total thyroidectomy followed by the administration of radioactive iodine, the rationale being that metastases are likely to take up the radioactive element, which can be used

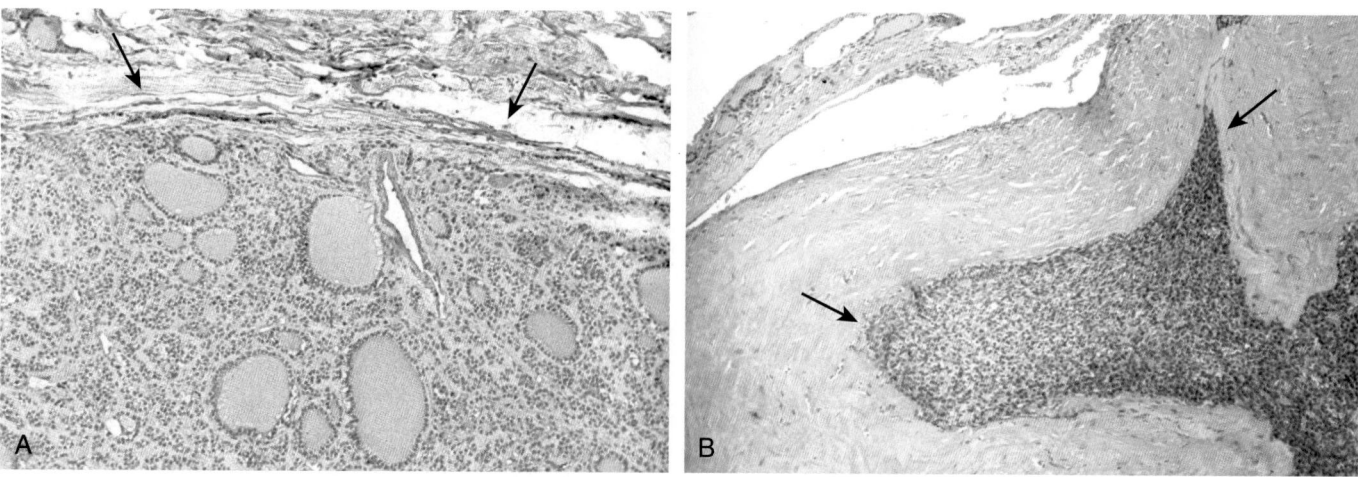

FIGURE 24–21 Capsular integrity in follicular neoplasms. In adenomas (**A**), a fibrous capsule, usually thin but occasionally more prominent, circumferentially surrounds the neoplastic follicles and no capsular invasion is seen *(arrows)*; compressed normal thyroid parenchyma is usually present external to the capsule *(top of the panel)*. In contrast, follicular carcinomas demonstrate capsular invasion (**B**, *arrows*) that may be minimal, as in this case, or widespread. The presence of vascular invasion is another feature of follicular carcinomas.

to identify and ablate such lesions. In addition, because any residual follicular carcinoma may respond to TSH stimulation, patients are usually treated with thyroid hormone after surgery to suppress endogenous TSH. Serum thyroglobulin levels are used for monitoring tumor recurrence, since this product should be barely detectable in a patient who is free of disease.

Anaplastic (Undifferentiated) Carcinoma

Anaplastic carcinomas are undifferentiated tumors of the thyroid follicular epithelium, accounting for less than 5% of thyroid tumors. They are aggressive, with a mortality rate approaching 100%. Patients with anaplastic carcinoma are older than those with other types of thyroid cancer, with a mean age of 65 years. Approximately a quarter of patients with anaplastic thyroid carcinomas have a past history of a well-differentiated thyroid carcinoma, and another quarter harbor a concurrent well-differentiated tumor in the resected specimen.

Morphology. Microscopically, these neoplasms are composed of highly anaplastic cells, with variable morphology, including: (1) large, pleomorphic **giant** cells, including occasional osteoclast-like multinucleate giant cells; (2) **spindle** cells with a sarcomatous appearance; and (3) **mixed** spindle and giant cells. Foci of papillary or follicular differentiation may be present in some tumors, suggesting an origin from a better differentiated carcinoma. The neoplastic cells express epithelial markers like cytokeratin, but are usually negative for markers of thyroid differentiation, like thyroglobulin.

Clinical Course. Anaplastic carcinomas usually present as a rapidly enlarging bulky neck mass. In most cases, the disease

has already spread beyond the thyroid capsule into adjacent neck structures or has metastasized to the lungs at the time of presentation. Symptoms related to compression and invasion, such as dyspnea, dysphagia, hoarseness, and cough, are common. There are no effective therapies, and the disease is almost uniformly fatal. Although metastases to distant sites are common, in most cases death occurs in less than 1 year as a result of aggressive growth and compromise of vital structures in the neck.

Medullary Carcinoma

Medullary carcinomas of the thyroid are *neuroendocrine* neoplasms derived from the parafollicular cells, or C cells, of the thyroid, and account for approximately 5% of thyroid neoplasms. Medullary carcinomas, similar to normal C cells, secrete *calcitonin*, the measurement of which plays an important role in the diagnosis and postoperative follow-up of patients. In some instances the tumor cells elaborate other polypeptide hormones, such as serotonin, ACTH, and vasoactive intestinal peptide (VIP). About 70% of tumors arise sporadically. The remainder occurs in the setting of MEN syndrome 2A or 2B or as familial tumors without an associated MEN syndrome (familial medullary thyroid carcinoma, or FMTC; see "Multiple Endocrine Neoplasia Syndromes"). Recall that *activating point mutations in the RET proto-oncogene* play an important role in the development of both familial and sporadic medullary carcinomas. Cases associated with MEN types 2A or 2B occur in younger patients, and may even arise during the first decade of life. In contrast, sporadic as well as familial medullary carcinomas are lesions of adulthood, with a peak incidence in the 40s and 50s.

Morphology. Sporadic medullary thyroid carcinomas present as a solitary nodule (Fig. 24–22A). In contrast, **bilaterality and multicentricity are common in famil-**

ial cases. Larger lesions often contain areas of necrosis and hemorrhage and may extend through the capsule of the thyroid. The tumor tissue is firm, pale gray to tan, and infiltrative. There may be foci of hemorrhage and necrosis in the larger lesions.

Microscopically, medullary carcinomas are composed of polygonal to spindle-shaped cells, which may form nests, trabeculae, and even follicles. Small, more anaplastic cells are present in some tumors and may be the predominant cell type. Acellular **amyloid deposits,** derived from altered calcitonin polypeptides, are present in the adjacent stroma in many cases (Fig. 24–22B). Calcitonin is readily demonstrable within the cytoplasm of the tumor cells as well as in the stromal amyloid by immunohistochemical methods. As with all neuroendocrine tumors, electron microscopy reveals variable numbers of mem-

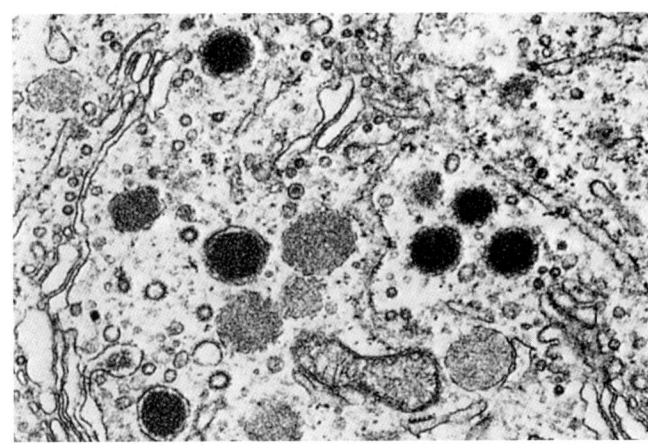

FIGURE 24–23 Electron micrograph of medullary thyroid carcinoma. These cells contain membrane-bound secretory granules that are the sites of storage of calcitonin and other peptides.

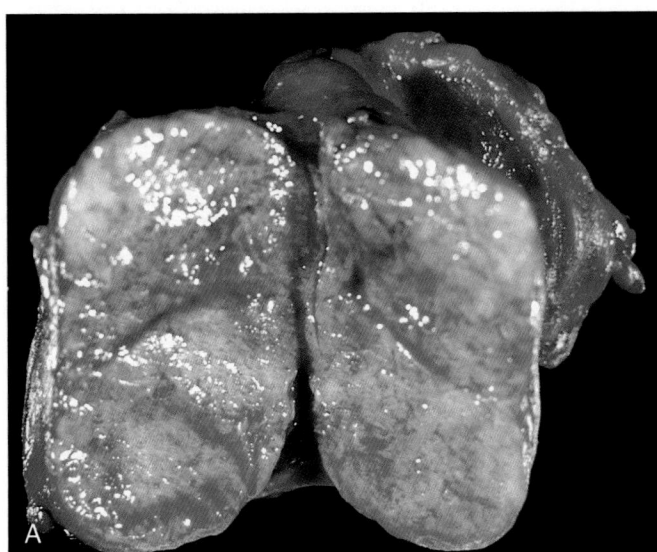

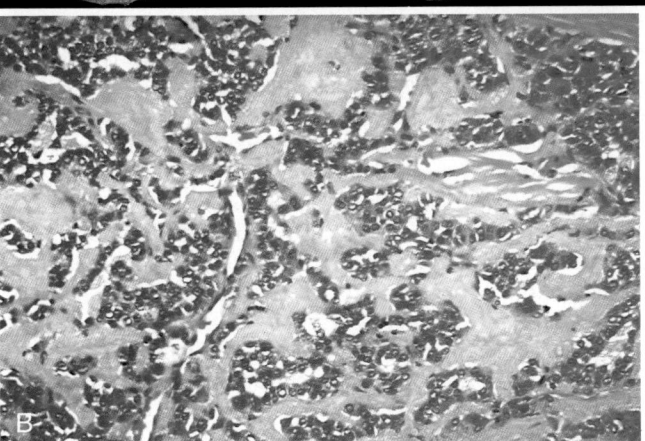

FIGURE 24–22 Medullary carcinoma of thyroid. **A,** These tumors typically show a solid pattern of growth and do not have connective tissue capsules. **B,** Histology demonstrates abundant deposition of amyloid, visible here as homogeneous extracellular material, derived from calcitonin molecules secreted by the neoplastic cells. (**A,** Courtesy of Dr. Joseph Corson, Brigham and Women's Hospital, Boston, MA.)

brane-bound electron-dense granules within the cytoplasm of the neoplastic cells (Fig. 24–23). One of the peculiar features of familial medullary cancers is the presence of multicentric **C-cell hyperplasia** in the surrounding thyroid parenchyma, a feature that is usually absent in sporadic lesions. While the precise criteria for defining C-cell hyperplasia are not established, the presence of multiple prominent clusters of C cells scattered throughout the parenchyma should raise the specter of a familial tumor, even if that history is not explicitly present. Foci of C-cell hyperplasia are believed to represent the precursor lesions from which medullary carcinomas arise.

Clinical Course. *Sporadic* cases of medullary carcinoma come to medical attention most often as a mass in the neck, sometimes associated with local effects such as dysphagia or hoarseness. In some instances, the initial manifestations are those of a paraneoplastic syndrome, caused by the secretion of a peptide hormone (e.g., diarrhea due to the secretion of VIP, or Cushing syndrome due to ACTH). Notably, hypocalcemia is not a prominent feature, despite the presence of raised calcitonin levels. In addition to circulating calcitonin, secretion of carcinoembryonic antigen by the neoplastic cells is a useful biomarker, especially for presurgical assessment of tumor load and in calcitonin-negative tumors. Patients with *familial syndromes* may come to attention because of symptoms localized to the thyroid or as a result of endocrine neoplasms in other organs (e.g., adrenal or parathyroid glands). Medullary carcinomas arising in the context of MEN-2B are generally more aggressive and metastasize more frequently than those occurring in patients with sporadic tumors, MEN-2A, or FMTC. As will be discussed later, all asymptomatic MEN-2 kindred carrying germline *RET* mutations are offered prophylactic thyroidectomy as early as possible to protect against the inevitable development of medullary carcinomas, the major risk factor for poor outcome in these families. Sometimes the only histologic finding in the resected thyroid of asymptomatic carriers is the presence of C-cell hyperplasia or small (<1 cm) "micromedullary" carcinomas. Several promising small-molecule inhibitors of RET tyrosine kinase have recently been developed, and are being tested in individuals with medullary carcinomas.[25]

Congenital Anomalies

Thyroglossal duct or cyst is the most common clinically significant congenital anomaly of the thyroid. A persistent sinus tract may remain as a vestigial remnant of the tubular development of the thyroid gland. Parts of this tube may be obliterated, leaving small segments to form cysts. These occur at any age and might not become evident until adult life.

Mucinous, clear secretions may collect within these cysts to form either spherical masses or fusiform swellings, rarely over 2 to 3 cm in diameter. These are present in the midline of the neck anterior to the trachea. Segments of the duct and cysts that occur high in the neck are lined by stratified squamous epithelium, which is essentially identical with that covering the posterior portion of the tongue in the region of the foramen cecum. The anomalies that occur in the lower neck more proximal to the thyroid gland are lined by epithelium resembling the thyroidal acinar epithelium. Characteristically, subjacent to the lining epithelium, there is an intense lymphocytic infiltrate. Superimposed infection may convert these lesions into abscess cavities, and rarely, they give rise to cancers.

PARATHYROID GLANDS

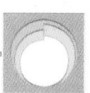

The four parathyroid glands are composed mainly of *chief cells*. The chief cells vary from light to dark pink with hematoxylin and eosin stains, depending on their glycogen content. They are polygonal, 12 to 20 μm in diameter, and have central, round, uniform nuclei. In addition, they have secretory granules containing *parathyroid hormone (PTH)*. Sometimes these cells have a *water-clear* appearance due to lakes of glycogen. *Oxyphil cells* and transitional oxyphils are found throughout the normal parathyroid, either singly or in small clusters. They are slightly larger than the chief cells, have acidophilic cytoplasm, and are tightly packed with mitochondria. Glycogen granules are also present in these cells, but secretory granules are sparse or absent. In early infancy and childhood, the parathyroid glands are composed almost entirely of solid sheets of chief cells. The amount of stromal fat increases up to age 25, reaching a maximum of approximately 30% of the gland, and then plateaus.

The activity of the parathyroid glands is controlled by the level of free (ionized) calcium in the bloodstream rather than by trophic hormones secreted by the hypothalamus and pituitary. Normally, decreased levels of free calcium stimulate the synthesis and secretion of PTH. The metabolic functions of PTH in regulating serum calcium levels can be summarized as follows:

- It increases the renal tubular reabsorption of calcium, thereby conserving free calcium.
- It increases the conversion of vitamin D to its active dihydroxy form in the kidneys.
- It increases urinary phosphate excretion, thereby lowering serum phosphate levels.
- It augments gastrointestinal calcium absorption.

The net result of these activities is an increase in the level of free calcium, which, in turn, inhibits further PTH secretion in a classic feedback loop.

Hypercalcemia is one of a number of changes induced by elevated levels of PTH. As was discussed in Chapter 7, hypercalcemia is also a relatively common complication of malignancy, occurring both with solid tumors, such as lung, breast, head and

neck, and renal cancers, and with hematologic malignancies, notably multiple myeloma. In fact, *malignancy is the most common cause of clinically apparent hypercalcemia*, while primary hyperparathyroidism (see below) is a more common cause of asymptomatic elevated blood calcium *(incidental hypercalcemia)*. The prognosis of individuals with malignancy-associated hypercalcemia is generally poor, because it more frequently occurs with advanced cancers. Hypercalcemia of malignancy is due to increased bone resorption and subsequent release of calcium. Bone resorption can occur in tumors that have not metastasized to the bone, as well as in tumors with *osteolytic metastases*. This is because many solid cancers secrete PTH-related protein (PTHrP) (Chapter 7), which promotes the expression of receptor activator of nuclear factor κB ligand (RANKL) on osteoblasts. RANKL is an osteoclast differentiation factor, which binds to its receptor, RANK, on the surface of osteoclast progenitor cells, and promotes their differentiation into mature osteoclasts, capable of bone resorption. Calcium homeostasis in bones is maintained by the secretion of *osteoprotegerin*, a *decoy receptor* of RANKL, capable of "siphoning" off excess ligand, and thereby preventing unbalanced bone resorption (Chapter 26). PTHrP inhibits osteoprotegerin secretion by osteoblastic cells, thereby altering the RANKL/osteoprotegerin ratio in a direction favoring osteoclastogenesis.[26] Thus, administration of soluble osteoprotegerin and monoclonal antibodies against RANKL have both emerged as promising therapeutic strategies in cancer patients with hypercalcemia of malignancy.

Similar to the other endocrine organs, abnormalities of the parathyroid glands include both hyperfunction and hypofunction. Tumors of the parathyroid glands, in contrast to thyroid tumors, usually come to attention because of excessive secretion of PTH rather than mass effects.

Hyperparathyroidism

Hyperparathyroidism occurs in two major forms—*primary* and *secondary*—and, less commonly, *tertiary*. The first condition represents an autonomous, spontaneous over-

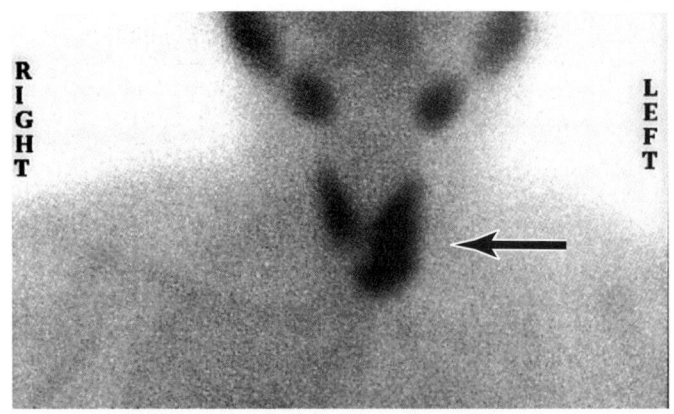

FIGURE 24–24 Parathyroid adenomas are almost always solitary lesions. Technetium-99m-sestamibi radionuclide scan demonstrates an area of increased uptake corresponding to the left inferior parathyroid gland *(arrow)*. This person had a parathyroid adenoma. Preoperative scintigraphy is useful in localizing and distinguishing adenomas from parathyroid hyperplasia, where more than one gland would demonstrate increased uptake.

production of PTH; the latter two conditions typically occur as secondary phenomena in individuals with chronic renal insufficiency.

PRIMARY HYPERPARATHYROIDISM

Primary hyperparathyroidism is one of the most common endocrine disorders, and it is an important cause of *hypercalcemia*. The frequency of the various parathyroid lesions underlying the hyperfunction is as follows:

- Adenoma: 85% to 95%
- Primary hyperplasia (diffuse or nodular): 5% to 10%
- Parathyroid carcinoma: ~1%

Primary hyperparathyroidism is usually a disease of adults and is more common in women than in men by a ratio of nearly 4:1. The annual incidence is now estimated to be about 25 cases per 100,000 in the United States and Europe; as many as 80% of patients with this condition are identified in the outpatient setting, when hypercalcemia is discovered incidentally on a serum electrolyte panel. Most cases occur in the 50s or later in life.

The most common cause of primary hyperparathyroidism is a solitary parathyroid adenoma arising in the sporadic (nonfamilial) setting (Fig. 24–24). Although familial syndromes are a distant second, they have provided a unique insight into the pathogenesis of primary hyperparathyroidism. The genetic syndromes associated with *familial primary hyperparathyroidism* include the following:

- *Multiple endocrine neoplasia-1 (MEN-1):* The *MEN1* gene on chromosome 11q13 is a tumor suppressor gene inactivated in a variety of MEN-1–related parathyroid lesions, including parathyroid adenomas and hyperplasia. In addition to familial cases, *MEN1* mutations have also been described in sporadic parathyroid tumors. The MEN-1 syndrome is discussed in further detail below.
- *Multiple endocrine neoplasia-2 (MEN-2):* The MEN-2 syndrome is caused by activating mutations in the tyrosine

kinase receptor, *RET*, on chromosome 10q. Primary hyperparathyroidism occurs as a component of MEN-2A, which is discussed in further detail below. *RET* mutations have not been described in sporadic parathyroid lesions outside the context of MEN-2.
- *Familial hypocalciuric hypercalcemia* is an autosomal-dominant disorder characterized by enhanced parathyroid function due to decreased sensitivity to extracellular calcium. Inactivating mutations in the parathyroid *calcium-sensing receptor gene (CASR)* on chromosome 3q are a primary cause for this disorder.[27] *CASR* mutations have not been described in sporadic parathyroid tumors.

Most, if not all, *sporadic parathyroid adenomas* are monoclonal, suggesting that they are true neoplasms. Sporadic parathyroid hyperplasia is also monoclonal in many instances, particularly when associated with a persistent stimulus for parathyroid growth (refractory secondary or tertiary parathyroidism; see below). Among the sporadic adenomas there are two molecular defects that have an established role in pathogenesis:

- *Cyclin D1 gene inversions.* Cyclin D1 is a major regulator of the cell cycle. A pericentromeric inversion on chromosome 11 results in relocation of the *cyclin D1* gene (normally on 11q), so that it is positioned adjacent to the 5′-flanking region of the *PTH* gene (on 11p). As a consequence of these changes, a regulatory element from the *PTH* gene 5′-flanking sequence directs overexpression of cyclin D1 protein, forcing the cells to proliferate. Between 10% and 20% of adenomas have this clonal genetic defect. In addition, cyclin D1 is overexpressed in approximately 40% of parathyroid adenomas, suggesting that mechanisms other than *cyclin D1* gene inversion can lead to its activation.
- *MEN1 mutations:* Approximately 20% to 30% of parathyroid tumors not associated with the MEN-1 syndrome have mutations in both copies of the *MEN1* gene. The spectrum of *MEN1* mutations in the sporadic tumors is virtually identical to that in familial parathyroid adenomas.

Morphology. The morphologic changes seen in primary hyperparathyroidism include those in the parathyroid glands as well as those in other organs affected by elevated levels of PTH and calcium. Parathyroid **adenomas** are almost always solitary and, similar to the normal parathyroid glands, may lie in close proximity to the thyroid gland or in an ectopic site (e.g., the mediastinum). The typical parathyroid adenoma averages 0.5 to 5.0 gm; is a well-circumscribed, soft, tan to reddish-brown nodule; and is invested by a delicate capsule. In contrast to primary hyperplasia, the glands outside the adenoma are usually normal in size or somewhat shrunken because of feedback inhibition by elevated levels of serum calcium. Microscopically, parathyroid adenomas are mostly composed of fairly uniform, polygonal chief cells with small, centrally placed nuclei (Fig. 24–25). At least a few nests of larger oxyphil cells are present as well; uncommonly, entire adenomas may be composed of this cell type (**oxyphil adenomas**). These may resemble Hürthle cell tumors in the thyroid. A

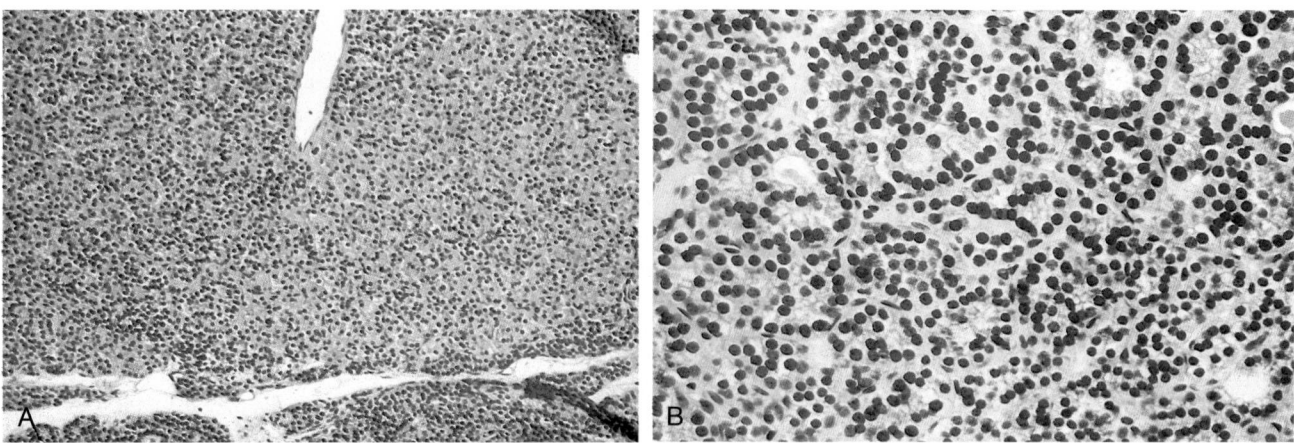

FIGURE 24–25 Parathyroid adenoma. **A,** Solitary chief cell parathyroid adenoma (low-power photomicrograph) revealing clear delineation from the residual gland below. **B,** High-power detail of a chief cell parathyroid adenoma. There is some slight variation in nuclear size but no anaplasia and some slight tendency to follicular formation.

rim of compressed, non-neoplastic parathyroid tissue, generally separated by a fibrous capsule, is often visible at the edge of the adenoma. Mitotic figures are rare, but it is not uncommon to find bizarre and pleomorphic nuclei even within adenomas (so-called **endocrine atypia**); this is not a criterion for malignancy. In contrast to the normal parathyroid parenchyma, adipose tissue is inconspicuous.

Primary hyperplasia may occur sporadically or as a component of MEN syndrome. Although classically all four glands are involved, there is frequently asymmetry with apparent sparing of one or two glands, making the distinction between hyperplasia and adenoma difficult. The combined weight of all glands rarely exceeds 1.0 gm and is often less. Microscopically, the most common pattern seen is that of chief cell hyperplasia, which may involve the glands in a diffuse or multinodular pattern. Less commonly, the constituent cells contain abundant water-clear cells ("water-clear cell hyperplasia"). In many instances there are islands of oxyphils, and poorly developed, delicate fibrous strands may envelop the nodules. As in the case of adenomas, stromal fat is inconspicuous within the foci of hyperplasia.

Parathyroid carcinomas may be circumscribed lesions that are difficult to distinguish from adenomas, or they may be clearly invasive neoplasms. These tumors enlarge one parathyroid gland and consist of gray-white, irregular masses that sometimes exceed 10 gm in weight. The cells are usually uniform and resemble normal parathyroid cells. They are arrayed in nodular or trabecular patterns with a dense, fibrous capsule enclosing the mass. There is general agreement that a **diagnosis of carcinoma based on cytologic detail is unreliable, and invasion of surrounding tissues and metastasis are the only reliable criteria.** Local recurrence occurs in one third of cases, and more distant dissemination occurs in another third.

Morphologic changes in other organs deserving special mention include skeletal and renal lesions.

Skeletal changes include increased numbers of osteoclasts, which erode bone matrix and mobilize calcium salts, particularly in the metaphyses of long tubular bones. Bone resorption is accompanied by increased osteoblastic activity and the formation of new bony trabeculae. In many cases the resultant bone contains widely spaced, delicate trabeculae reminiscent of those seen in osteoporosis. In more severe cases the cortex is grossly thinned, and the marrow contains increased amounts of fibrous tissue accompanied by foci of hemorrhage and cyst formation (**osteitis fibrosa cystica**) (Chapter 26). Aggregates of osteoclasts, reactive giant cells, and hemorrhagic debris occasionally form masses that may be mistaken for neoplasms (**brown tumors** of hyperparathyroidism). PTH-induced hypercalcemia favors formation of **urinary tract stones** (nephrolithiasis) as well as calcification of the renal interstitium and tubules (nephrocalcinosis). Metastatic calcification secondary to hypercalcemia may also be seen in other sites, including the stomach, lungs, myocardium, and blood vessels.

Clinical Course. Primary hyperparathyroidism may be: (1) asymptomatic and identified after a routine chemistry profile, or (2) associated with the classic clinical manifestations of primary hyperparathyroidism.

Asymptomatic Hyperparathyroidism. Because serum calcium levels are routinely assessed in the work-up of most patients who need blood tests, clinically silent hyperparathyroidism is often detected early. Hence, many of the classic manifestations, particularly those referable to bone and renal disease, are now seen infrequently in clinical practice. Primary hyperparathyroidism is the most common cause of *asymptomatic* hypercalcemia and indeed the most common manifestation of primary hyperparathyroidism is hypercalcemia. Among many other less common causes of hypercalcemia (Table 24–5), malignancy stands out as the most frequent cause of *clinically apparent* hypercalcemia in adults and must be excluded by appropriate clinical and laboratory investigations in patients with suspected hyperparathyroidism. *In individuals*

TABLE 24–5	Causes of Hypercalcemia
Raised [PTH]	**Decreased [PTH]**
Hyperparathyroidism	Hypercalcemia of malignancy*
Primary (adenoma >	Vitamin D toxicity
hyperplasia)*	
Secondary†	Immobilization
Tertiary†	Thiazide diuretics
Familial hypocalciuric	Granulomatous disease
hypercalcemia	(sarcoidosis)

[PTH], parathyroid hormone concentration.
*Primary hyperparathyroidism is the most common cause of hyper-calcemia overall. Malignancy is the most common cause of *symptomatic* hypercalcemia. Primary hyperparathyroidism and malignancy account for nearly 90% of cases of hypercalcemia.
†Secondary and teriary hyperparathyroidism are most commonly associated with progressive renal failure.

with primary hyperparathyroidism, *serum PTH levels are inappropriately elevated for the level of serum calcium, whereas PTH levels are low to undetectable in hypercalcemia caused by of nonparathyroid diseases* (see Table 24–5). In persons with hypercalcemia caused by secretion of PTHrP by certain non-parathyroid tumors, radioimmunoassays specific for PTH and PTHrP can distinguish between the two molecules. Other laboratory alterations referable to PTH excess include hypophosphatemia and increased urinary excretion of both calcium and phosphate. Secondary renal disease may lead to phosphate retention with normalization of serum phosphates.

Symptomatic Primary Hyperparathyroidism. The signs and symptoms of hyperparathyroidism reflect the combined effects of increased PTH secretion and hypercalcemia. Primary hyperparathyroidism is associated with "painful bones, renal stones, abdominal groans, and psychic moans." The constellation of symptoms includes:

- *Bone disease* and bone pain secondary to fractures of bones weakened by osteoporosis or osteitis fibrosa cystica.
- *Nephrolithiasis* (renal stones) in 20% of newly diagnosed patients, with attendant pain and obstructive uropathy. Chronic renal insufficiency and abnormalities in renal function lead to polyuria and secondary polydipsia.
- Gastrointestinal disturbances, including constipation, nausea, peptic ulcers, pancreatitis, and gallstones.
- Central nervous system alterations, including depression, lethargy, and eventually seizures.
- Neuromuscular abnormalities, including weakness and fatigue.
- Cardiac manifestations, including aortic or mitral valve calcifications (or both).

The abnormalities most directly related to hyperparathyroidism are nephrolithiasis and bone disease, whereas those attributable to hypercalcemia include fatigue, weakness, and constipation. The pathogenesis of many of the other manifestations of the disorder remains poorly understood.

SECONDARY HYPERPARATHYROIDISM

Secondary hyperparathyroidism is caused by any condition that gives rise to chronic hypocalcemia, which in turn leads to compensatory overactivity of the parathyroid glands. *Renal*

failure is by far the most common cause of secondary hyperparathyroidism, although several other diseases, including inadequate dietary intake of calcium, steatorrhea, and vitamin D deficiency, may also cause this disorder. The mechanisms by which chronic renal failure induces secondary hyperparathyroidism are complex and not fully understood. Chronic renal insufficiency is associated with decreased phosphate excretion, which in turn results in hyperphosphatemia. The elevated serum phosphate levels directly depress serum calcium levels and thereby stimulate parathyroid gland activity. In addition, loss of renal substance reduces the availability of α-1-hydroxylase necessary for the synthesis of the active form of vitamin D, which in turn reduces intestinal absorption of calcium (Chapter 9). Because vitamin D has suppressive effects on parathyroid growth and PTH secretion, its relative deficiency compounds the hyperparathyroidism in renal failure.

Morphology. The **parathyroid glands in secondary hyperparathyroidism are hyperplastic.** As in primary hyperparathyroidism, the degree of glandular enlargement is not necessarily symmetric. Microscopically, the hyperplastic glands contain an increased number of chief cells, or cells with more abundant, clear cytoplasm (so-called water-clear cells) in a diffuse or multinodular distribution. Fat cells are decreased in number. **Bone changes** similar to those seen in primary hyperparathyroidism may also be present. **Metastatic calcification** may be seen in many tissues, including lungs, heart, stomach, and blood vessels.

Clinical Course. The clinical features of secondary hyperparathyroidism are usually dominated by symptoms of chronic renal failure. Bone abnormalities (*renal osteodystrophy*) and other changes associated with PTH excess are, in general, less severe than are those seen in primary hyperparathyroidism. The vascular calcification associated with secondary hyperparathyroidism may occasionally result in significant ischemic damage to skin and other organs, a process sometimes referred to as *calciphylaxis*. Patients with secondary hyperparathyroidism often respond to dietary vitamin D supplementation, as well as phosphate binders to decrease the prevailing hyperphosphatemia.

In a minority of patients, parathyroid activity may become autonomous and excessive, with resultant hypercalcemia, a process that is sometimes termed *tertiary hyperparathyroidism.* Parathyroidectomy may be necessary to control the hyperparathyroidism in such patients.

Hypoparathyroidism

Hypoparathyroidism is far less common than is hyperparathyroidism. Acquired hypoparathyroidism is almost always an inadvertent consequence of surgery; in addition, there are several genetic causes of hypoparathyroidism.

- *Surgically induced hypoparathyroidism* occurs with inadvertent removal of all the parathyroid glands during thyroidectomy, excision of the parathyroid glands in the mistaken belief that they are lymph nodes during radical neck dissection for some form of malignant disease, or removal of too large a proportion of parathyroid tissue in the treatment of primary hyperparathyroidism.

- *Autoimmune hypoparathyroidism* is often associated with chronic mucocutaneous candidiasis and primary adrenal insufficiency; this syndrome is known as autoimmune polyendocrine syndrome type 1 (APS1) and is caused by mutations in the *autoimmune regulator (AIRE)* gene. The syndrome typically presents in childhood with the onset of candidiasis, followed several years later by hypoparathyroidism and then adrenal insufficiency during adolescence. APS1 is discussed further under "Adrenal Glands."
- *Autosomal-dominant hypoparathyroidism* is caused by gain-of-function mutations in the *calcium-sensing receptor (CASR)* gene. Inappropriate CASR activity due to abnormal calcium sensing suppresses PTH, resulting in *hypocalcemia* and *hypercalciuria*.
- *Familial isolated hypoparathyroidism* (FIH) is a rare condition with either autosomal dominant or autosomal recessive patterns of inheritance. Autosomal-dominant FIH is caused by a mutation in the gene encoding PTH precursor peptide, which impairs its processing to the mature hormone. Autosomal-recessive FIH is caused by loss-of-function mutations in the transcription factor gene *glial cells missing-2 (GCM2)*, which is essential for development of the parathyroid.
- *Congenital absence* of parathyroid glands can occur in conjunction with other malformations, such as thymic aplasia and cardiovascular defects, or as a component of the 22q11 deletion syndrome.[28] As discussed in Chapter 5, when thymic defects are present, the condition is called DiGeorge syndrome.

The major clinical manifestations of hypoparathyroidism are related to the severity and chronicity of the hypocalcemia.

- The hallmark of hypocalcemia is *tetany,* which is characterized by *neuromuscular irritability,* resulting from decreased serum ionized calcium concentration. These symptoms range from circumoral numbness or paresthesias (tingling) of the distal extremities and carpopedal spasm, to life-threatening laryngospasm and generalized seizures. The classic findings on physical examination are *Chvostek sign* and *Trousseau sign.* Chvostek sign is elicited in subclinical disease by tapping along the course of the facial nerve, which induces contractions of the muscles of the eye, mouth, or nose. Trousseau sign refers to carpal spasms produced by occlusion of the circulation to the forearm and hand with a blood pressure cuff for several minutes.
- *Mental status changes* include emotional instability, anxiety and depression, confusional states, hallucinations, and frank psychosis.
- *Intracranial manifestations* include calcifications of the basal ganglia, parkinsonian-like movement disorders, and increased intracranial pressure with resultant papilledema. The paradoxical association of hypocalcemia with calcifications may be because of an increase in phosphate levels, resulting in tissue deposits with locally produced calcium.
- *Ocular disease* takes the form of calcification of the lens and cataract formation.
- *Cardiovascular manifestations* include a conduction defect that produces a characteristic prolongation of the QT interval in the electrocardiogram.
- *Dental abnormalities* occur when hypocalcemia is present during early development. These findings are highly characteristic of hypoparathyroidism and include dental hypoplasia, failure of eruption, defective enamel and root formation, and abraded carious teeth.

Pseudohypoparathyroidism

In this condition, hypoparathyroidism occurs because of end-organ resistance to the actions of PTH. Indeed, serum PTH levels are normal or elevated. In one form of pseudohypoparathyroidism, there is multi-hormone end-organ resistance to TSH and FSH/LH, besides PTH. All these hormones signal via G-protein–triggered second messengers, and the disorder results from genetic defects in this pathway. The PTH resistance is the most obvious clinical manifestation, presenting as hypocalcemia, hyperphosphatemia, and elevated circulating PTH. TSH resistance is generally mild, while LH/FSH resistance manifests as hypergonadotropic hypogonadism in females.

THE ENDOCRINE PANCREAS

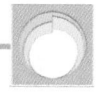

The endocrine pancreas consists of about 1 million clusters of cells, the *islets of Langerhans,* which contain four major and two minor cell types. The four main types are β, α, δ, and PP (pancreatic polypeptide) cells. They can be differentiated by the ultrastructural characteristics of their granules, and by their hormone content (Fig. 24–26). *The β cell produces insulin,* as will be detailed in the discussion of diabetes. The insulin-containing intracellular granules contain a rectangular crystalline matrix, surrounded by a halo. *The α cell secretes glucagon,* inducing hyperglycemia by its glycogenolytic activity in the liver. α-cell granules are round, with closely applied membranes and a dense center. δ cells contain somatostatin, which suppresses both insulin and glucagon release; they have large, pale granules with closely applied membranes. *PP cells contain a unique pancreatic polypeptide that exerts several gastrointestinal effects,* such as stimulation of secretion of gastric and intestinal enzymes and inhibition of intestinal motility. These cells have small, dark granules and not only are present in islets but also are scattered in the exocrine pancreas. The two rare cell types are *D1 cells* and *enterochromaffin cells.* D1 cells elaborate vasoactive intestinal polypeptide (*VIP*), a hormone that induces glycogenolysis and hyperglycemia; it also stimulates gastrointestinal fluid secretion and causes secretory diarrhea. *Enterochromaffin cells synthesize serotonin*

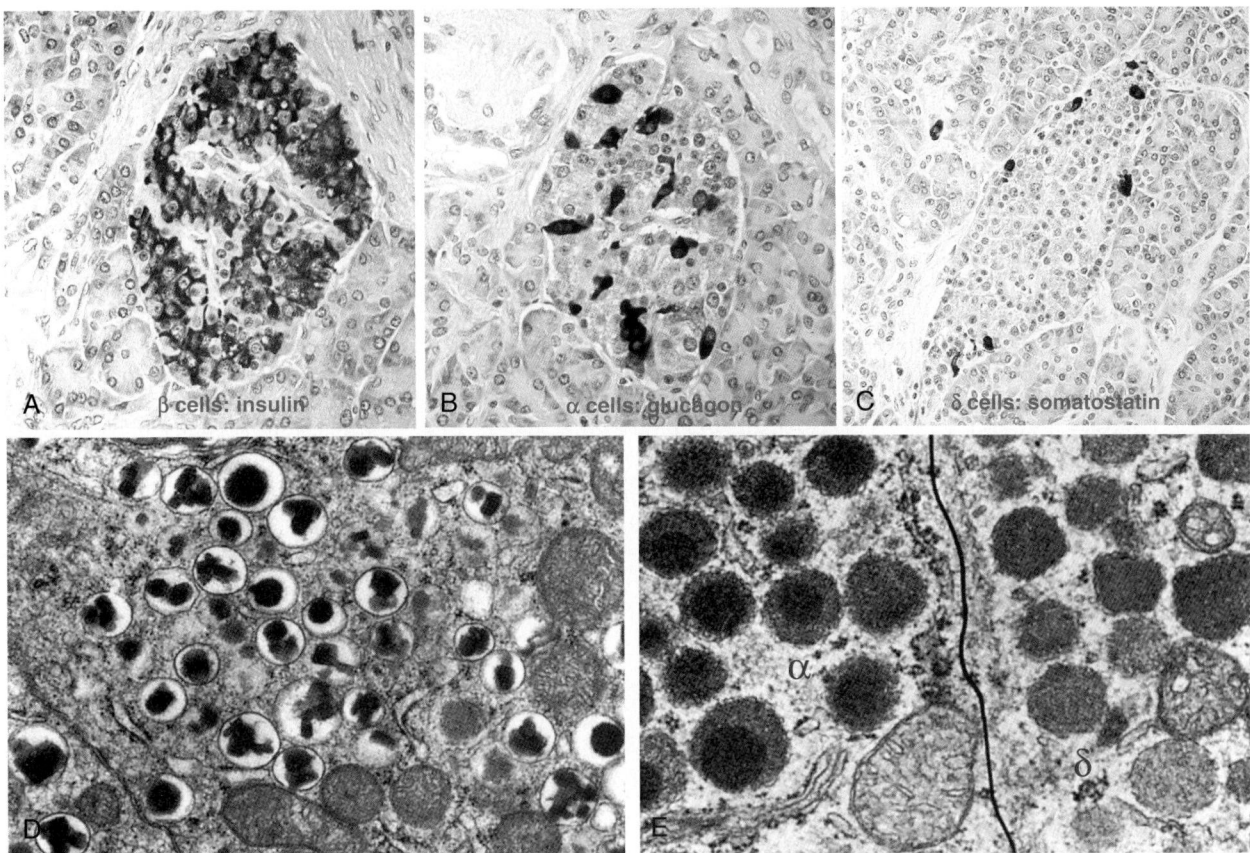

FIGURE 24–26 Hormone production in pancreatic islet cells. Immunoperoxidase staining shows a dark reaction product for insulin in β cells (**A**), glucagon in α cells (**B**), and somatostatin in δ cells (**C**). **D,** Electron micrograph of a β cell shows the characteristic membrane-bound granules, each containing a dense, often rectangular core and distinct halo. **E,** Portions of an α cell *(left)* and a δ cell *(right)* also show granules, but with closely apportioned membranes. The α-cell granule shows a dense, round center. (Electron micrographs courtesy of Dr. Arthur Like, University of Massachusetts Medical School, Worcester, MA.)

and are the source of pancreatic tumors that cause the carcinoid syndrome (Chapter 19).

We now turn to the two main disorders of islet cells: diabetes mellitus and pancreatic endocrine tumors.

Diabetes Mellitus

Diabetes mellitus is not a single disease entity but rather a *group of metabolic disorders sharing the common underlying feature of hyperglycemia.* Hyperglycemia in diabetes results from defects in insulin secretion, insulin action, or, most commonly, both. The chronic hyperglycemia and attendant metabolic dysregulation may be associated with secondary damage in multiple organ systems, especially the kidneys, eyes, nerves, and blood vessels. According to the American Diabetes Association, diabetes affects over 20 million children and adults, or 7% of the population, in the United States, nearly a third of whom are currently unaware that they have hyperglycemia. Approximately 1.5 million new cases of diabetes are diagnosed each year in the United States, and diabetes is the leading cause of end-stage renal disease, adult-onset blindness, and non-traumatic lower extremity amputations. A staggering 54 million adults in this country have "pre-diabetes," which is defined as elevated blood sugar that does not reach the criterion accepted for an outright diagnosis of diabetes (see below);

individuals with pre-diabetes have an elevated risk for developing frank diabetes. Compared to non-Hispanic whites, Native Americans, African Americans, and Hispanics are 1.5 to 2 times more likely to develop diabetes over their lifetime. The total number of people with diabetes worldwide was estimated to be between 151 million and 171 million at the turn of the century, and is expected to rise to 366 million by 2030. The prevalence of diabetes is increasingly sharply in the developing world as people adopt more sedentary life styles, with India and China being the largest contributors to the world's diabetic load.

DIAGNOSIS

Blood glucose values are normally maintained in a very narrow range, usually 70 to 120 mg/dL. *The diagnosis of diabetes is established by noting elevation of blood glucose by any one of three criteria:*

1. A random glucose concentration greater than 200 mg/dL, with classical signs and symptoms (discussed below)
2. A fasting glucose concentration greater than 126 mg/dL on more than one occasion
3. An abnormal oral glucose tolerance test (OGTT), in which the glucose concentration is greater than 200 mg/dL 2 hours after a standard carbohydrate load

Levels of blood glucose proceed along a continuum. Individuals with fasting glucose concentrations less than 100 mg/dL, or less than 140 mg/dL following an OGTT, are considered to be euglycemic. However, those with fasting glucose concentrations greater than 100 mg/dL but less than 126 mg/dL, or OGTT values greater than 140 mg/dL but less than 200 mg/dL, are considered to have impaired glucose tolerance, also known as "pre-diabetes." Pre-diabetic individuals have a significant risk of progressing to overt diabetes over time, with as many as 5% to 10% advancing to diabetes mellitus per year. In addition, pre-diabetics are at risk for cardiovascular disease, as a result of the abnormal carbohydrate metabolism as well as the coexistence of other risk factors such as low levels of high-density lipoprotein, hypertriglyceridemia, and increased plasminogen activator inhibitor-1 (PAI-1) (see Chapter 11).

CLASSIFICATION

Although all forms of diabetes mellitus share hyperglycemia as a common feature, the underlying abnormalities involved in the development of hyperglycemia vary widely. The previous classification schemes of diabetes mellitus were based on the age at onset of the disease or on the mode of therapy; in contrast, the etiologic classification reflects our greater understanding of the pathogenesis of each variant (Table 24–6). *The vast majority of cases of diabetes fall into one of two broad classes:*

Type 1 diabetes is an autoimmune disease characterized by pancreatic β-cell destruction and an absolute deficiency of insulin. It accounts for approximately 5% to 10% of all cases, and is the most common subtype diagnosed in patients younger than 20 years of age.

Type 2 diabetes is caused by a combination of peripheral resistance to insulin action and an inadequate secretory response by the pancreatic β cells ("relative insulin deficiency"). Approximately 90% to 95% of diabetic patients have type 2 diabetes, and the vast majority of such individuals are overweight. Although classically considered "adult-onset," the prevalence of type 2 diabetes in children and adolescents is increasing at an alarming pace.[29]

A variety of monogenic and secondary causes are responsible for the remaining cases, and these will be discussed later. It should be stressed that while the major types of diabetes have different pathogenic mechanisms, *the long-term complications affecting the kidneys, eyes, nerves, and blood vessels are the same, as are the principal causes of morbidity and death.* The pathogenesis of the two major types is discussed separately, but first we briefly review normal insulin secretion and the mechanism of insulin signaling, since these aspects are critical to understanding the pathogenesis of diabetes.

GLUCOSE HOMEOSTASIS

Normal glucose homeostasis is tightly regulated by three interrelated processes: glucose production in the liver; glucose uptake and utilization by peripheral tissues, chiefly skeletal muscle; and actions of insulin and counter-regulatory hormones, including glucagon, on glucose uptake and metabolism.

Insulin and glucagon have opposing regulatory effects on glucose homeostasis. During fasting states, low insulin and

---

TABLE 24–6   Classification of Diabetes Mellitus

1. **Type 1 diabetes** (β-cell destruction, usually leading to absolute insulin deficiency)

   Immune-mediated
   Idiopathic

2. **Type 2 diabetes** (combination of insulin resistance and β-cell dysfunction)

3. **Genetic defects of β-cell function**

   Maturity-onset diabetes of the young (MODY), caused by mutations in:
   Hepatocyte nuclear factor 4α (*HNF4A*), MODY1
   Glucokinase (*GCK*), MODY2
   Hepatocyte nuclear factor 1α (*HNF1A*), MODY3
   Pancreatic and duodenal homeobox 1 (*PDX1*), MODY4
   Hepatocyte nuclear factor 1β (*HNF1B*), MODY5
   Neurogenic differentiation factor 1 (*NEUROD1*), MODY6
   Neonatal diabetes (activating mutations in *KCNJ11* and *ABCC8*, encoding Kir6.2 and SUR1, respectively)
   Maternally inherited diabetes and deafness (MIDD) due to mitochondrial DNA mutations (m.3243A→G)
   Defects in proinsulin conversion
   Insulin gene mutations

4. **Genetic defects in insulin action**

   Type A insulin resistance
   Lipoatrophic diabetes, including mutations in *PPARG*

5. **Exocrine pancreatic defects**

   Chronic pancreatitis
   Pancreatectomy/trauma
   Neoplasia
   Cystic fibrosis
   Hemachromatosis
   Fibrocalculous pancreatopathy

6. **Endocrinopathies**

   Acromegaly
   Cushing syndrome
   Hyperthyroidism
   Pheochromocytoma
   Glucagonoma

7. **Infections**

   Cytomegalovirus
   Coxsackie B virus
   Congenital rubella

8. **Drugs**

   Glucocorticoids
   Thyroid hormone
   Interferon-α
   Protease inhibitors
   β-adrenergic agonists
   Thiazides
   Nicotinic acid
   Phenytoin (Dilantin)
   Vacor

9. **Genetic syndromes associated with diabetes**

   Down syndrome
   Kleinfelter syndrome
   Turner syndrome
   Prader-Willi syndrome

10. **Gestational diabetes mellitus**

American Diabetes Association: Position statement from the American Diabetes Association on the diagnosis and classification of diabetes mellitus. Diabetes Care 31 (Suppl. 1):S55–S60, 2008.

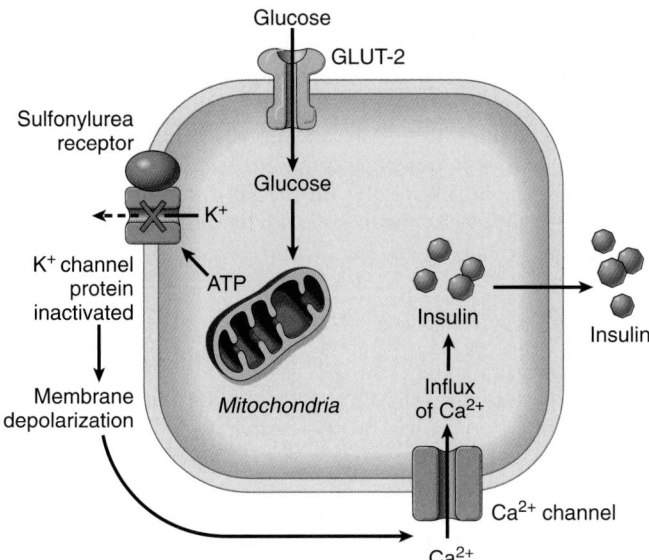

FIGURE 24–27 Insulin synthesis and secretion. Intracellular transport of glucose is mediated by GLUT-2, an insulin-independent glucose transporter in β cells. Glucose undergoes oxidative metabolism in the β cell to yield ATP. ATP inhibits an inward rectifying K⁺ channel receptor on the β-cell surface; the receptor itself is a dimeric complex of the sulfonylurea receptor (SUR1) and a K⁺-channel protein (Kir6.2). Inhibition of this receptor leads to membrane depolarization, influx of Ca²⁺ ions, and release of stored insulin from β cells. The sulfonylurea class of oral hypoglycemic agents bind to the SUR1 receptor protein.

high glucagon levels facilitate hepatic gluconeogenesis and glycogenolysis (glycogen breakdown) while decreasing glycogen synthesis, thereby preventing hypoglycemia. Thus, fasting plasma glucose levels are determined primarily by hepatic glucose output. Following a meal, insulin levels rise and glucagon levels fall in response to the large glucose load. Insulin promotes glucose uptake and utilization in tissues (discussed later). The skeletal muscle is the major insulin-responsive site for postprandial glucose utilization, and is critical for preventing hyperglycemia and maintaining glucose homeostasis.

Regulation of Insulin Release

The insulin gene is expressed in the β cells of the pancreatic islets (see Fig. 24–26). Preproinsulin is synthesized in the rough endoplasmic reticulum from insulin mRNA and delivered to the Golgi apparatus. There, a series of proteolytic cleavage steps generate mature insulin and a cleavage peptide, *C-peptide*. Both insulin and C-peptide are then stored in secretory granules and secreted in equimolar quantities after physiologic stimulation; thus, C-peptide levels serve as a surrogate for β-cell function, decreasing with loss of β-cell mass in type 1 diabetes, or increasing with insulin resistance–associated hyperinsulinemia.

The most important stimulus for insulin synthesis and release is glucose itself.[30] A rise in blood glucose levels results in glucose uptake into pancreatic β cells, facilitated by an insulin-independent glucose-transporter, GLUT-2 (Fig. 24–27). β cells express an ATP-sensitive K⁺ channel on the membrane, which comprises two subunits: an inward rectifying K⁺ channel (Kir6.2) and the sulfonylurea receptor (SUR1), the latter being

the binding site for oral hypoglycemic agents (sulfonylureas) used in the treatment of diabetes (see below). Metabolism of glucose by glycolysis generates ATP, resulting in an increase in β-cell cytoplasmic ATP/ADP ratios. This inhibits the activity of the ATP-sensitive K⁺ channel, leading to membrane depolarization and the influx of extracellular Ca²⁺ through voltage-dependent Ca²⁺ channels. The resultant increase in intracellular Ca²⁺ stimulates secretion of insulin, presumably from stored hormone within the β-cell granules. This is the phase of *immediate release of insulin*. If the secretory stimulus persists, a delayed and protracted response follows that involves *active synthesis of insulin*. Other factors, including intestinal hormones and certain amino acids (leucine and arginine), also stimulate insulin release, but not its synthesis.

Insulin Action and Insulin Signaling Pathways

Insulin is the most potent anabolic hormone known, with multiple synthetic and growth-promoting effects (Fig. 24–28).[31] *Its principal metabolic function is to increase the rate of glucose transport into certain cells in the body, thus providing an increased source of energy*. These cells are the *striated muscle cells* (including myocardial cells) and to a lesser extent, *adipocytes*, which together represent about two thirds of the entire body weight. Glucose uptake in other peripheral tissues, most notably the brain, is insulin independent. In muscle cells, glucose is then either stored as glycogen or oxidized to generate ATP. In adipose tissue, glucose is primarily stored as lipid. Besides promoting lipid synthesis, insulin also inhibits lipid degradation in adipocytes. Similarly, insulin promotes amino acid uptake and protein synthesis, while inhibiting protein degradation. *Thus, the anabolic effects of insulin are attribut-*

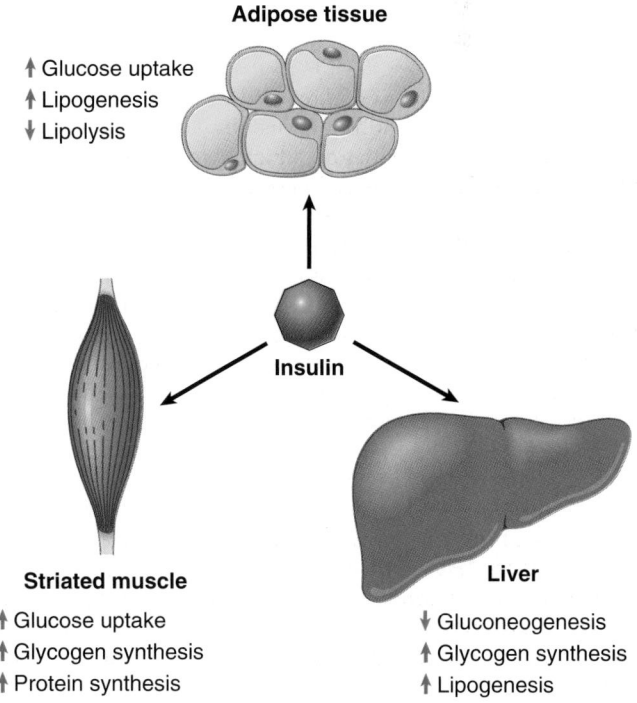

FIGURE 24–28 Metabolic actions of insulin in striated muscle, adipose tissue, and liver.

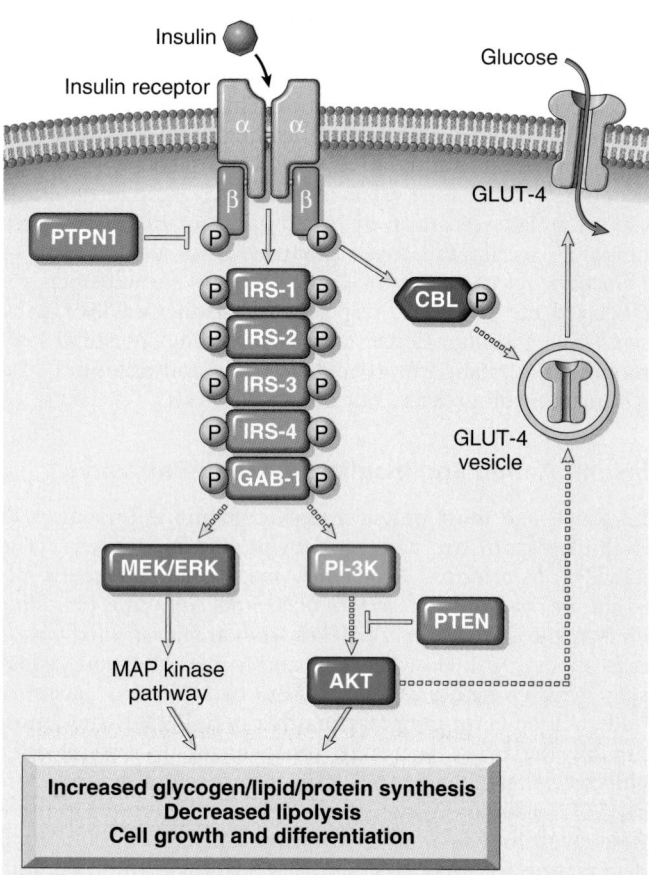

FIGURE 24–29 Insulin action on a target cell. The metabolic actions of insulin include promoting glycogen synthesis by activating glycogen synthase, and enhancing protein synthesis and lipogenesis while inhibiting lipolysis (see text). Dashed arrows represent intermediate proteins and binding partners that are not shown in this overview diagram.

able to increased synthesis and reduced degradation of glycogen, lipids, and proteins. In addition, insulin has several *mitogenic* functions, including initiation of DNA synthesis in certain cells and stimulation of their growth and differentiation.

Elucidation of the insulin signaling pathway has been central to our understanding of the pathogenesis of diabetes. The complete description of this intricate network is beyond the scope of this book, and we will only summarize some of the more pertinent mediators (Fig. 24–29). The *insulin receptor* is a tetrameric protein composed of two α- and two β-subunits. The β-subunit cytosolic domain possesses tyrosine kinase activity. Insulin binding to the α-subunit extracellular domain activates the β-subunit tyrosine kinase, resulting in autophosphorylation of the receptor and the phosphorylation (activation) of several intracellular substrate proteins, such as the family of insulin receptor substrate (IRS) proteins, which includes IRS1–IRS4 and GAB1. The substrate proteins, in turn, activate multiple downstream signaling cascades, including the PI-3K and the MAP kinase pathways, which mediate the metabolic and mitogenic activities of insulin on the cell. Insulin signaling facilitates the trafficking and docking of vesicles containing the glucose transporter protein GLUT-4 to the plasma membrane, which promotes glucose uptake. This process is mediated by AKT, the principal effector of the PI-3K pathway, but also independently by the cytoplasmic protein CBL, which is a direct phosphorylation target of the insulin receptor. Insulin signaling is attenuated in vivo by several endogenous inhibitors that act along components of the pathway. For example, protein tyrosine phosphatase 1B (PTPN1B) dephosphorylates the insulin receptor and inhibits insulin signaling. The phosphatase PTEN can attenuate insulin signaling by blocking AKT activation by the PI-3K pathway.

PATHOGENESIS OF TYPE 1 DIABETES MELLITUS

Type 1 diabetes is an autoimmune disease in which islet destruction is caused primarily by immune effector cells reacting against endogenous β-cell antigens. Type 1 diabetes most commonly develops in childhood, becomes manifest at puberty, and progresses with age. Since the disease can develop at any age, including late adulthood, the appellation "juvenile diabetes" is now considered obsolete. Similarly, the older moniker "insulin-dependent diabetes mellitus" has been excluded from the recent classification of diabetes because insulin dependence is not a consistent distinguishing feature. Nevertheless, most patients with type 1 diabetes depend on insulin for survival; without insulin they develop serious metabolic complications such as ketoacidosis and coma. A rare form of "idiopathic" type 1 diabetes has been described in which the evidence for autoimmunity is not definitive.[32] Here we will focus on the typical immune-mediated type 1 diabetes.

As with most autoimmune diseases, the pathogenesis of type 1 diabetes represents interplay of genetic susceptibility and environmental factors.

Genetic Susceptibility. Epidemiologic studies, such as those demonstrating higher concordance rates for disease in monozygotic vs dizygotic twins, have convincingly established a genetic basis for type 1 diabetes. More recently, genome-wide association studies have identified multiple genetic susceptibility loci for type 1 diabetes, as well as for type 2 diabetes (see below). Over a dozen susceptibility loci for type 1 diabetes are now known.[33,34] Of these, by far the most important is the *HLA locus* on chromosome 6p21; according to some estimates, the HLA locus contributes as much as 50% of the genetic susceptibility to type 1 diabetes. Ninety to 95% of Caucasians with this disease have either a HLA-DR3 or HLA-DR4 haplotype, in contrast to about 40% of normal subjects; moreover, 40% to 50% of type 1 diabetics are combined DR3/DR4 heterozygotes, in contrast to 5% of normal subjects. Individuals who have either DR3 or DR4 concurrently with a DQ8 haplotype (which corresponds to *DQA1*0301-DQB1*0302* alleles) demonstrate one of the highest inherited risks for type 1 diabetes in sibling studies.[35] Predictably, the polymorphisms in the HLA molecules are located in or adjacent to the peptide-binding pockets, consistent with the notion that disease-associated alleles code for molecules that have particular features of antigen display. However, as we discussed in Chapter 6, it is still not known if these HLA-disease associations reflect the ability of specific HLA molecules to present self antigens or if they are related to T-cell selection and tolerance.

Several *non-HLA genes* also confer susceptibility to type 1 diabetes. The first disease-associated non-MHC gene to be identified was *insulin*, with variable number of tandem repeats (VNTRs) in the promoter region being associated with disease susceptibility.[36] The mechanism underlying this association is unknown. It is possible that these polymorphisms influence the level of expression of insulin in the thymus, thus altering the negative selection of insulin-reactive T cells (Chapter 6). We have previously mentioned the association between polymorphisms in *CTLA4* and *PTPN22* and autoimmune thyroiditis (see above); both genes are also linked with susceptibility to type 1 diabetes. Both CTLA-4 and PTPN-22 are thought to inhibit T-cell responses, so polymorphisms that interfere with their functional activity are expected to set the stage for excessive T-cell activation. Whether this is the only mechanism of action of these proteins in the development of autoimmune diseases remains an open question. Another recently identified polymorphism is in *CD25*, which encodes the α chain of the IL-2 receptor. It is postulated that the polymorphism reduces the activity of this receptor, which is critical for the maintenance of functional regulatory T cells.[37] Many of the other susceptibility loci identified in type 1 diabetes have been linked to various chromosomal regions but the involved genes are not defined.

Environmental Factors. There is evidence that environmental factors, especially viral infections, may be involved in triggering islet cell destruction in type 1 diabetes. Epidemiologic associations have been reported between type 1 diabetes and infection with mumps, rubella, coxsackie B, or cytomegalovirus, among others. At least three different mechanisms have been proposed to explain the role of viruses in the induction of autoimmunity. The first is "bystander" damage, wherein viral infections induce islet injury and inflammation, leading to the release of sequestered β-cell antigens and the activation of autoreactive T cells. The second possibility is that the viruses produce proteins that mimic β-cell antigens, and the immune response to the viral protein cross-reacts with the self-tissue ("molecular mimicry"). The third hypothesis suggests that viral infections incurred early in life ("predisposing virus") might persist in the tissue of interest, and subsequent re-infection with a related virus ("precipitating virus") that shares antigenic epitopes leads to an immune response against the infected islet cells. This last mechanism, also known as "viral déjà vu," might explain the latency between infections and the onset of diabetes. It is unclear whether any of these mechanisms contribute to β-cell damage, and no causative viral infection is established. In fact, some epidemiologic data and studies of experimental models suggest that infections may be protective; the underlying mechanisms of such a protective effect are unknown. An epidemiologic study has also established no causal association between childhood vaccinations and the risk of developing type 1 diabetes.[38]

Mechanisms of β-Cell Destruction

Although the clinical onset of type 1 diabetes is often abrupt, the autoimmune process usually starts many years before the disease becomes evident, with progressive loss of insulin reserves over time[39] (Fig. 24–30). The classic manifestations of the disease (hyperglycemia and ketosis) occur late in its course, after more than 90% of the β cells have been destroyed. Many of the advances in type 1 diabetes pathogenesis have emerged from studies of the nonobese diabetic (NOD) mouse model,

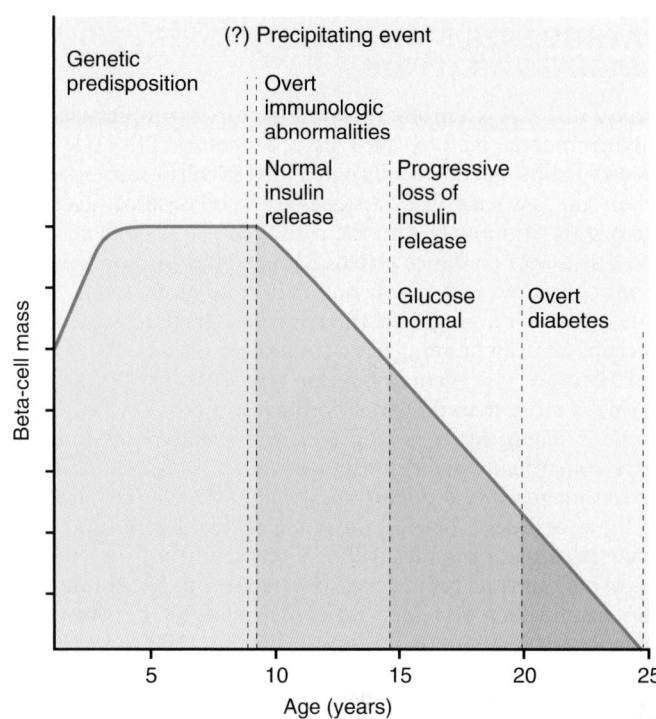

FIGURE 24–30 Stages in the development of type 1 diabetes mellitus. The stages are listed from left to right, and hypothetical β-cell mass is plotted against age. (From Eisenbarth GE: Type 1 diabetes: a chronic autoimmune disease. N Engl J Med 314:1360, 1986. Copyright © 1986, Massachusetts Medical Society. All rights reserved.)

which shares features of autoimmune islet destruction observed in the human disease. *The fundamental immune abnormality in type 1 diabetes is a failure of self-tolerance in T-cells.*[40] This failure of tolerance may be a result of some combination of defective clonal deletion of self-reactive T cells in the thymus, as well as defects in the functions of regulatory T cells or resistance of effector T cells to suppression by regulatory cells. Thus, autoreactive T-cells not only survive but are poised to respond to self-antigens. The initial activation of these cells is thought to occur in the peripancreatic lymph nodes, perhaps in response to antigens that are released from damaged islets. The activated T cells then traffic to the pancreas, where they cause β cell injury. Multiple T-cell populations have been implicated in this damage, including T$_H$1 cells (which may injure β cells by secreted cytokines, including IFN-γ and TNF), and CD8+ CTLs (which directly kill β cells). The islet auto-antigens that are the targets of immune attack may include insulin itself, as well as the β-cell enzyme glutamic acid decarboxylase (GAD), and islet cell autoantigen 512 (ICA512).[41]

A role for antibodies in type 1 diabetes is suspected because of the observation that autoantibodies against islet antigens are found in the vast majority of patients with type 1 diabetes, as well as in asymptomatic family members at risk for progression to overt disease; in fact, the presence of islet cell antibodies is used as a predictive marker for the disease.[42] However, it is not clear if the autoantibodies are involved in causing injury or are produced as a consequence of islet injury.

PATHOGENESIS OF TYPE 2 DIABETES MELLITUS

Type 2 diabetes is a prototypic multifactorial complex disease. Environmental factors, such as a sedentary life style and dietary habits, unequivocally play a role, as will become evident when the association with obesity is considered. Genetic factors are also involved in the pathogenesis, as evidenced by the disease concordance rate of 35% to 60% in monozygotic twins compared with nearly half that in dizygotic twins. Such concordance is even greater than in type 1 diabetes, suggesting perhaps an even larger genetic component in type 2 diabetes. Furthermore, the lifetime risk for type 2 diabetes in an off-spring is more than double if both parents are affected. *Additional evidence for a genetic basis has emerged from recent large-scale genome-wide association studies, which have identified over a dozen susceptibility loci.*[43,44] The detailed description of these analyses is beyond the scope of this chapter, and only a few pertinent examples will be discussed here. Not surprisingly, polymorphisms in genes associated with β-cell function and insulin secretion seem to confer some of the strongest genetic risk for developing type 2 diabetes. The most reproducible association occurs with *transcription factor 7–like-2 (TCF7L2)* on chromosome 10q, which encodes a transcription factor in the *WNT* signaling pathway. Unlike type 1 diabetes, however, the disease is not linked to genes involved in immune tolerance and regulation (*HLA, CTLA4*, etc.), and there is no evidence of an autoimmune basis.

The two metabolic defects that characterize type 2 diabetes are (1) a decreased response of peripheral tissues to insulin (insulin resistance) and (2) β-cell dysfunction that is manifested as inadequate insulin secretion in the face of insulin resistance and hyperglycemia. Insulin resistance predates the development of hyperglycemia and is usually accompanied by compensatory β-cell hyperfunction and hyperinsulinemia in the early stages of the evolution of diabetes (Fig. 24–31).

Insulin Resistance

Insulin resistance is defined as the failure of target tissues to respond normally to insulin. It leads to decreased uptake of glucose in muscle, reduced glycolysis and fatty acid oxidation in the liver, and an inability to suppress hepatic gluconeogenesis. Studies in tissue-specific insulin receptor knockout mice suggest that *loss of insulin sensitivity in the hepatocytes is likely to be the largest contributor to the pathogenesis of insulin resistance in vivo.*[45] A variety of functional defects have been reported in the insulin signaling pathway in states of insulin resistance (for example, reduced tyrosine phosphorylation and increased serine phosphorylation of the insulin receptor and IRS proteins), which attenuate signal transduction.[46] *Few factors play as important a role in the development of insulin resistance as obesity.*

Obesity and Insulin Resistance. The epidemiologic association of obesity with type 2 diabetes has been recognized for decades, with visceral obesity observed in greater than 80% of patients. Obesity has profound effects on sensitivity of tissues to insulin, and as consequence, on systemic glucose homeostasis. Insulin resistance is present even in simple obesity unaccompanied by hyperglycemia, indicating a fundamental abnormality of insulin signaling in states of fatty excess (see

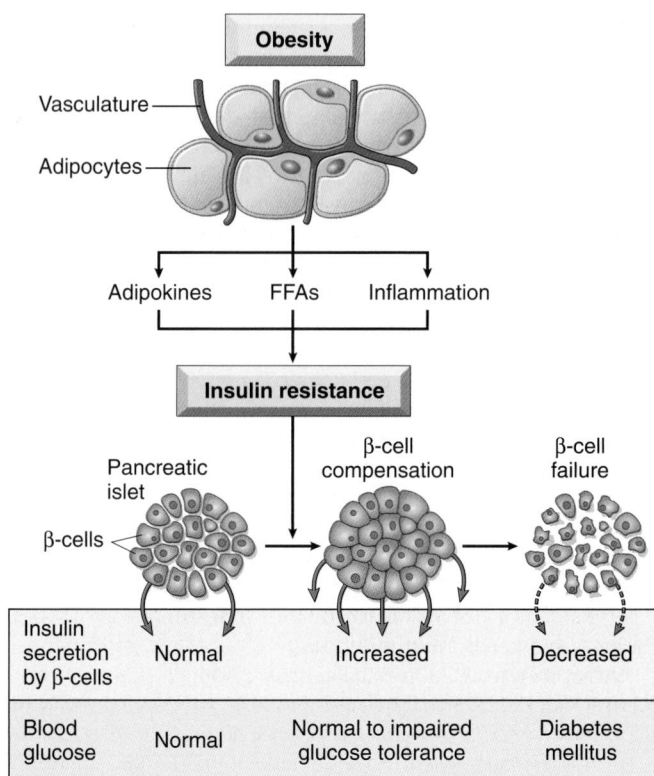

FIGURE 24–31 Development of type 2 diabetes. Insulin resistance associated with obesity is induced by adipokines, free fatty acids, and chronic inflammation in adipose tissue. Pancreatic β cells compensate for insulin resistance by hypersecretion of insulin. However, at some point, β-cell compensation is followed by β-cell failure, and diabetes ensues. (Reproduced with permission from Kasuga M: Insulin resistance and pancreatic β-cell failure. J Clin Invest 116:1756, 2006.)

metabolic syndrome, below). The risk for diabetes increases as the body mass index (a measure of body fat content) increases. It is not only the absolute amount but also the distribution of body fat that has an effect on insulin sensitivity: central obesity (abdominal fat) is more likely to be linked with insulin resistance than are peripheral (gluteal/subcutaneous) fat depots. *Obesity can adversely impact insulin sensitivity in numerous ways* (see Fig. 24–31).[47]

- *Nonesterified fatty acids (NEFAs)*: Cross-sectional studies have demonstrated an inverse correlation between fasting plasma NEFAs and insulin sensitivity. The level of intracellular triglycerides is often markedly increased in muscle and liver tissues of obese individuals, presumably because excess circulating NEFAs are deposited in these organs. Central adipose tissue is more "lipolytic" than peripheral sites, which might explain the particularly deleterious consequences of this pattern of fat distribution. Excess intracellular NEFAs overwhelm the fatty acid oxidation pathways, leading to accumulation of cytoplasmic intermediates like diacylglycerol (DAG) and ceramide. These "toxic" intermediates can activate serine/threonine kinases, which cause aberrant serine phosphorylation of the insulin receptor and IRS proteins. Recall that, unlike tyrosine modification, phosphorylation at serine residues *attenuates* insulin signaling. Insulin normally inhibits hepatic gluconeogenesis by blocking the activity of phosphoenolpyruvate carboxykinase, the first enzymatic step in this process. Attenuated insulin signaling allows phosphoenolpyruvate carboxykinase to "ramp up" gluconeogenesis. Excess NEFAs also compete with glucose for substrate oxidation, leading to feedback inhibition of glycolytic enzymes, and thereby further exacerbating the existing glucose imbalance.

○ *Adipokines:* It is recognized that adipose tissue is not merely a passive storage depot for fat but is a functional endocrine organ that releases hormones in response to changes in the metabolic status. A variety of proteins secreted into the systemic circulation by adipose tissue have been identified, and these are collectively termed *adipokines* (or adipose cytokines). Both pro-hyperglycemic adipokines (e.g., resistin, retinol binding protein 4 [RBP4]) and anti-hyperglycemic adipokines (leptin, adiponectin) have been identified. Leptin and adiponectin improve insulin sensitivity by directly enhancing the activity of the AMP-activated protein kinase (AMPK), an enzyme that promotes fatty acid oxidation, in liver and skeletal muscle. Adiponectin levels are reduced in obesity, thus contributing to insulin resistance. Notably, AMPK is also the target for metformin, a commonly used oral antidiabetic medication.[48]

○ *Inflammation:* Adipose tissue also secretes a variety of pro-inflammatory cytokines like tumor necrosis factor, interleukin-6, and macrophage chemoattractant protein-1, the last attracting macrophages to fat deposits. Studies in experimental models have demonstrated that reducing the levels of pro-inflammatory cytokines enhances insulin sensitivity. These cytokines induce insulin resistance by increasing cellular "stress," which in turn, activates multiple signaling cascades that antagonize insulin action on peripheral tissues.

○ *Peroxisome proliferator-activated receptor γ (PPARγ):* PPARγ is a nuclear receptor and transcription factor expressed in adipose tissue, and plays a seminal role in adipocyte differentiation. A class of antidiabetic medications known as thiazolidinediones acts as agonist ligands for PPARγ and improves insulin sensitivity. Activation of PPARγ promotes secretion of anti-hyperglycemic adipokines like adiponectin, and shifts the deposition of NEFAs toward adipose tissue and away from liver and skeletal muscle. As discussed below, rare mutations of *PPARG* that cause profound loss of protein function can result in monogenic diabetes.

β-Cell Dysfunction

In type 2 diabetes, β cells seemingly exhaust their capacity to adapt to the long-term demands of peripheral insulin resistance. In states of insulin resistance like obesity, insulin secretion is initially higher for each level of glucose than in controls. This hyperinsulinemic state is a compensation for peripheral resistance and can often maintain normal plasma glucose for years. Eventually, however, β-cell compensation becomes inadequate, and there is progression to hyperglycemia. *The observation that not all obese individuals with insulin resistance develop overt diabetes suggests that an intrinsic predisposition to β-cell failure must also exist.* For example, recent studies have shown that allelic variants associated with the highest risk for type 2 diabetes in the diabetogenic gene *TCF7L2* (see above) are associated with reduced insulin secretion from islets, indi-

cating a preexisting propensity toward β-cell failure.[49] The molecular mechanisms underlying β-cell dysfunction in type 2 diabetes are multifactorial and in many instances overlap with those implicated in insulin resistance. Thus, the excess NEFAs and attenuated insulin signaling ("lipotoxicity") predispose to both insulin resistance and β-cell failure. Agents like metformin that enhance fatty acid oxidation through AMPK activation (see above) also improve β-cell function, further highlighting the shared pathogenetic mechanisms between insulin resistance and β-cell failure. Amyloid replacement of islets is a characteristic finding in individuals with long-standing type 2 diabetes and is present in more than 90% of diabetic islets examined. Some believe that the islet amyloid protein is directly cytotoxic to islets, analogous to the role played by amyloid plaques implicated in the pathogenesis of Alzheimer disease (Chapter 28).

MONOGENIC FORMS OF DIABETES

Although genetically defined causes of diabetes are uncommon, they have been intensively studied in the hope of gaining insights into the disease. As Table 24–6 illustrates, monogenic forms of diabetes are classified separately from types 1 and 2. These forms of diabetes result from either a primary defect in β-cell function or a defect in insulin–insulin receptor signaling, as described below.

Genetic Defects in β-Cell Function. Approximately 1% to 2% of diabetics harbor a *primary defect in β-cell function that occurs without β-cell loss, affecting either β-cell mass and/or insulin production.* This form of monogenic diabetes is caused by a heterogeneous group of genetic defects, and is characterized by (1) autosomal-dominant inheritance, with high penetrance; (2) early onset, usually before age 25 and even in the neonatal period, as opposed to after age 40 for most patients with type 2 diabetes; (3) absence of obesity; and (4) absence of β-cell autoantibodies. Because of genetic heterogeneity, the clinical features vary widely from mild persistent hyperglycemia to severe diabetes requiring insulin for survival.

The largest subgroup of patients in this category was traditionally designated as having "maturity-onset diabetes of the young" (MODY) because of its superficial resemblance to type 2 diabetes and its occurrence in younger patients. MODY can result from hemizygous loss-of-function mutations in one of six genes (see Table 24–6). Glucokinase, implicated in MODY2, is an enzyme that catalyzes the transfer of phosphate from ATP to glucose, which is the first and rate-limiting step in glucose metabolism. β-cell glucokinase controls the entry of glucose into the glycolytic cycle, which, in turn, is coupled to insulin secretion. Mutations of the *glucokinase (GCK)* gene increase the glucose threshold that triggers insulin release, causing mild increases in fasting blood glucose (*familial mild fasting hyperglycemia*). As many as 50% of carriers of glucokinase mutations develop gestational diabetes mellitus, defined as any degree of glucose intolerance during pregnancy; conversely, approximately 2% to 5% of women with gestational diabetes mellitus and a first-degree relative with diabetes carry a mutation in the glucokinase gene. The other five genes mutated in MODY encode transcription factors that control insulin expression in β cells and β-cell mass; one such factor, *IPF1* (also known as *PDX1*), plays a central role in the development of the pancreas.

Permanent neonatal diabetes (to be distinguished from transient neonatal hyperglycemic states) occurs as a result of mutations of *KCNJ11* and *ABCC8* genes, which encode the Kir6.2 and SUR1 subunits, respectively, of the ATP-sensitive K^+ channel (see Fig. 24–27).[50,51] You will recall that inactivation of this channel is required for membrane depolarization and physiologic insulin secretion from β cells. Gain-of-function *KCNJ11* or *ABCC8* mutations cause constitutive activation of the K^+ channel, membrane hyperpolarization, and hypoinsulinemic diabetes. Permanent neonatal diabetes presents with severe hyperglycemia and ketoacidosis, and a fifth of such patients also demonstrate concurrent neurologic symptoms like epilepsy. *Maternally inherited diabetes and deafness* results from mitochondrial DNA mutations.[52] Impairment of mitochondrial ATP synthesis in metabolically active islet cells results in decreased insulin secretion. Mitochondrial diabetes is associated with bilateral sensorineural deafness. Finally, mutations within the *insulin gene* itself have recently been described as a form of monogenic diabetes, most commonly presenting in the neonatal period, but also in childhood and adolescence.[53]

Genetic Defects in Insulin Action. Rare instances of *insulin receptor* mutations that affect receptor synthesis, insulin binding, or receptor tyrosine kinase activity can cause severe insulin resistance, accompanied by hyperinsulinemia and diabetes (type A insulin resistance). Such patients often show a velvety hyperpigmentation of the skin, known as *acanthosis nigricans*. Females with type A insulin resistance frequently have polycystic ovaries and elevated androgen levels. *Lipoatrophic diabetes*, as the name suggests, is hyperglycemia accompanied by loss of adipose tissue, the latter occurring selectively in the subcutaneous fat. This rare group of genetic disorders has in common insulin resistance, diabetes, hypertriglyceridemia, acanthosis nigricans, and abnormal fat deposition in the liver (hepatic steatosis). Multiple subtypes of lipoatrophic diabetes, each ascribed to a different causal mutation, have been reported. Dominant-negative mutations in the DNA-binding domain of PPARG are found in a subset of patients, which interfere with the function of wild-type PPARγ in the nucleus, leading to severe insulin resistance.[54] As discussed above, common *PPARG* polymorphisms are associated with susceptibility to type 2 diabetes, while PPARγ has emerged as a target for therapies that aim to improve insulin sensitivity in this disease.

PATHOGENESIS OF THE COMPLICATIONS OF DIABETES

The morbidity associated with long-standing diabetes of either type results from several serious complications, caused mainly by lesions involving both large- and medium-sized muscular arteries *(macrovascular disease)* and capillary dysfunction in target organs *(microvascular disease)*. Macrovascular disease causes *accelerated atherosclerosis* among diabetics, resulting in increased risk of myocardial infarction, stroke, and lower extremity gangrene. The effects of microvascular disease are most profound in the retina, kidneys, and peripheral nerves, resulting in *diabetic retinopathy, nephropathy,* and *neuropathy,* respectively.

The pathogenesis of the long-term complications of diabetes is multifactorial, although persistent hyperglycemia ("glucotoxic-ity") seems to be a key mediator. Much of the evidence supporting a role for glycemic control in ameliorating the long-term complications of diabetes has come from large randomized trials. The assessment of glycemic control in these trials has been based on the percentage of *glycosylated hemoglobin,* also known as Hb_{A1C}, which is formed by nonenzymatic covalent addition of glucose moieties to hemoglobin in red cells. Unlike blood glucose levels, Hb_{A1C} provides a measure of glycemic control over the lifespan of a red cell (120 days) and is little affected by day-to-day variations. The American Dietetic Association recommends that Hb_{A1C} be maintained below 7% in diabetic patients. It is important to stress that hyperglycemia is not the only factor responsible for the long-term complications of diabetes, and that other underlying abnormalities, such as insulin resistance, and co-morbidities like obesity, also play an important role.

At least three distinct metabolic pathways have been implicated in the deleterious effects of persistent hyperglycemia on peripheral tissues, although the primacy of any one over the others is unclear. The pathways are discussed below.

Formation of Advanced Glycation End Products. *Advanced glycation end products* (AGEs) are formed as a result of nonenzymatic reactions between intracellular glucose-derived dicarbonyl precursors (glyoxal, methylglyoxal, and 3-deoxyglucosone) with the amino groups of both intracellular and extracellular proteins. The natural rate of AGE formation is greatly accelerated in the presence of hyperglycemia. AGEs bind to a specific receptor (RAGE), which is expressed on inflammatory cells (macrophages and T cells), endothelium, and vascular smooth muscle. The detrimental effects of the AGE-RAGE signaling axis within the vascular compartment include (1) release of pro-inflammatory *cytokines and growth factors* from intimal macrophages; (2) generation of *reactive oxygen species* in endothelial cells; (3) increased *procoagulant activity* on endothelial cells and macrophages; and (4) enhanced *proliferation of vascular smooth muscle cells and synthesis of extracellular matrix.* Not surprisingly, endothelial-specific overexpression of RAGE in diabetic mice accelerates large vessel injury and microangiopathy, while RAGE-null mice show attenuation of these features.[55,56] Antagonists of RAGE have emerged as a therapeutic strategy in diabetes and are being tested in clinical trials.

In addition to receptor-mediated effects, *AGEs can directly cross-link extracellular matrix proteins.* Cross-linking of collagen type I molecules in large vessels decreases their elasticity, which may predispose these vessels to shear stress and endothelial injury (Chapter 11). Similarly, AGE-induced cross-linking of type IV collagen in basement membrane decreases endothelial cell adhesion and increases extravasation of fluid. Proteins cross-linked by AGEs are resistant to proteolytic digestion. Thus, cross-linking decreases protein removal while enhancing protein deposition. AGE-modified matrix components also trap nonglycated plasma or interstitial proteins. In large vessels, trapping of LDL, for example, retards its efflux from the vessel wall and enhances the deposition of cholesterol in the intima, thus accelerating atherogenesis (Chapter 11). In capillaries, including those of renal glomeruli, plasma proteins such as albumin bind to the glycated basement membrane, accounting in part for the basement membrane thickening that is characteristic of diabetic microangiopathy.

Activation of Protein Kinase C. Activation of intracellular protein kinase C (PKC) by Ca^{2+} ions and the second messenger diacyl glycerol (DAG) is an important signal transduction pathway in many cellular systems. Intracellular hyperglycemia stimulates the de novo synthesis of DAG from glycolytic intermediates, and hence causes activation of PKC. The downstream effects of PKC activation are numerous and include the following.

- Production of proangiogenic vascular endothelial growth factor (VEGF), implicated in the neovascularization characterizing diabetic retinopathy (Chapter 29)
- Elevated levels of the vasoconstrictor endothelin-1 and decreased levels of the vasodilator NO, due to decreased expression of endothelial nitric oxide synthase
- Production of profibrogenic factors like TGF-β, leading to increased deposition of extracellular matrix and basement membrane material
- Production of PAI-1, leading to reduced fibrinolysis and possible vascular occlusive episodes
- Production of pro-inflammatory cytokines by the vascular endothelium

It should be evident that some effects of AGEs and activated PKC are overlapping, and both contribute to the long-term complications of diabetic microangiopathy. Clinical trials using a PKC inhibitor (ruboxistaurin) have yielded promising results in diabetic retinopathy,[57] and this pathway is also under investigation as a therapeutic target in diabetic nephropathy.

Intracellular Hyperglycemia and Disturbances in Polyol Pathways. In some tissues that do not require insulin for glucose transport (e.g., nerves, lenses, kidneys, blood vessels), persistent hyperglycemia in the extracellular milieu leads to an increase in intracellular glucose. This excess glucose is metabolized by the enzyme aldose reductase to sorbitol, a polyol, and eventually to fructose, in a reaction that uses NADPH (the reduced form of nicotinamide dinucleotide phosphate) as a cofactor. NADPH is also required by the enzyme glutathione reductase in a reaction that regenerates reduced glutathione (GSH). You will recall that GSH is one of the important antioxidant mechanisms in the cell (Chapter 1), and any reduction in GSH increases cellular susceptibility to oxidative stress. In the face of sustained hyperglycemia, progressive depletion of intracellular NADPH by aldol reductase compromises GSH regeneration, increasing cellular susceptibility to oxidative stress. In neurons, persistent hyperglycemia appears to be the major underlying cause of diabetic neuropathy (*"glucose neurotoxicity"*).[58] Although clinical trials with aldose reductase inhibitors have been disappointing to date, targeting this pathway as a means for amelioration of diabetic complications remains on the horizon.

MORPHOLOGY OF DIABETES AND ITS LATE COMPLICATIONS

Pathologic findings in the pancreas are variable and not necessarily dramatic. The important morphologic changes are related to the many late systemic complications of diabetes. There is great variability among patients in the time of onset of these complications, their severity, and the particular organ or organs involved. In individuals with tight control of diabetes, the onset might be delayed. In most patients, however, morphologic changes are likely to be found in arteries (*macrovascular disease*), basement membranes of small vessels (*microangiopathy*), kidneys (*diabetic nephropathy*), retina (*retinopathy*), nerves (*neuropathy*), and other tissues (Fig. 24–32). These changes are seen in both type 1 and type 2 diabetes.

Morphology

Pancreas. Lesions in the pancreas are inconstant and rarely of diagnostic value. Distinctive changes are more commonly associated with type 1 than with type 2 diabetes. One or more of the following alterations may be present:

- **Reduction in the number and size of islets.** This is most often seen in type 1 diabetes, particularly with rapidly advancing disease. Most of the islets are small and inconspicuous.
- **Leukocytic infiltrates in the islets** (insulitis) are principally composed of T lymphocytes, as is also seen in animal models of autoimmune diabetes (Fig. 24–33A). Lymphocytic infiltrates may be present in type 1 diabetics at the time of clinical presentation. The distribution of insulitis may be strikingly uneven. Eosinophilic infiltrates may also be found, particularly in diabetic infants who fail to survive the immediate postnatal period.
- **In type 2 diabetes there may be a subtle reduction in islet cell mass,** demonstrated only by special morphometric studies.
- **Amyloid deposition within islets in type 2 diabetes** begins in and around capillaries and between cells. At advanced stages, the islets may be virtually obliterated (Fig. 24–33B); fibrosis may also be observed. Similar lesions may be found in elderly nondiabetics, apparently as part of normal aging.
- **An increase in the number and size of islets** is especially characteristic of nondiabetic newborns of diabetic mothers. Presumably, fetal islets undergo hyperplasia in response to the maternal hyperglycemia.

Diabetic Macrovascular Disease. Diabetes exacts a heavy toll on the vascular system. **Endothelial dysfunction** (see Chapter 11), which predisposes to atherosclerosis and other cardiovascular morbidities, is widespread in diabetes, as a consequence of the deleterious effects of persistent hyperglycemia and insulin resistance on the vascular compartment. The hallmark of diabetic macrovascular disease is **accelerated atherosclerosis** involving the aorta and large- and medium-sized arteries. Except for its greater severity and earlier age at onset, atherosclerosis in diabetics is indistinguishable from that in nondiabetics (Chapter 11). **Myocardial infarction, caused by atherosclerosis of the coronary arteries, is the most common cause of death in diabetics**, and an elevated

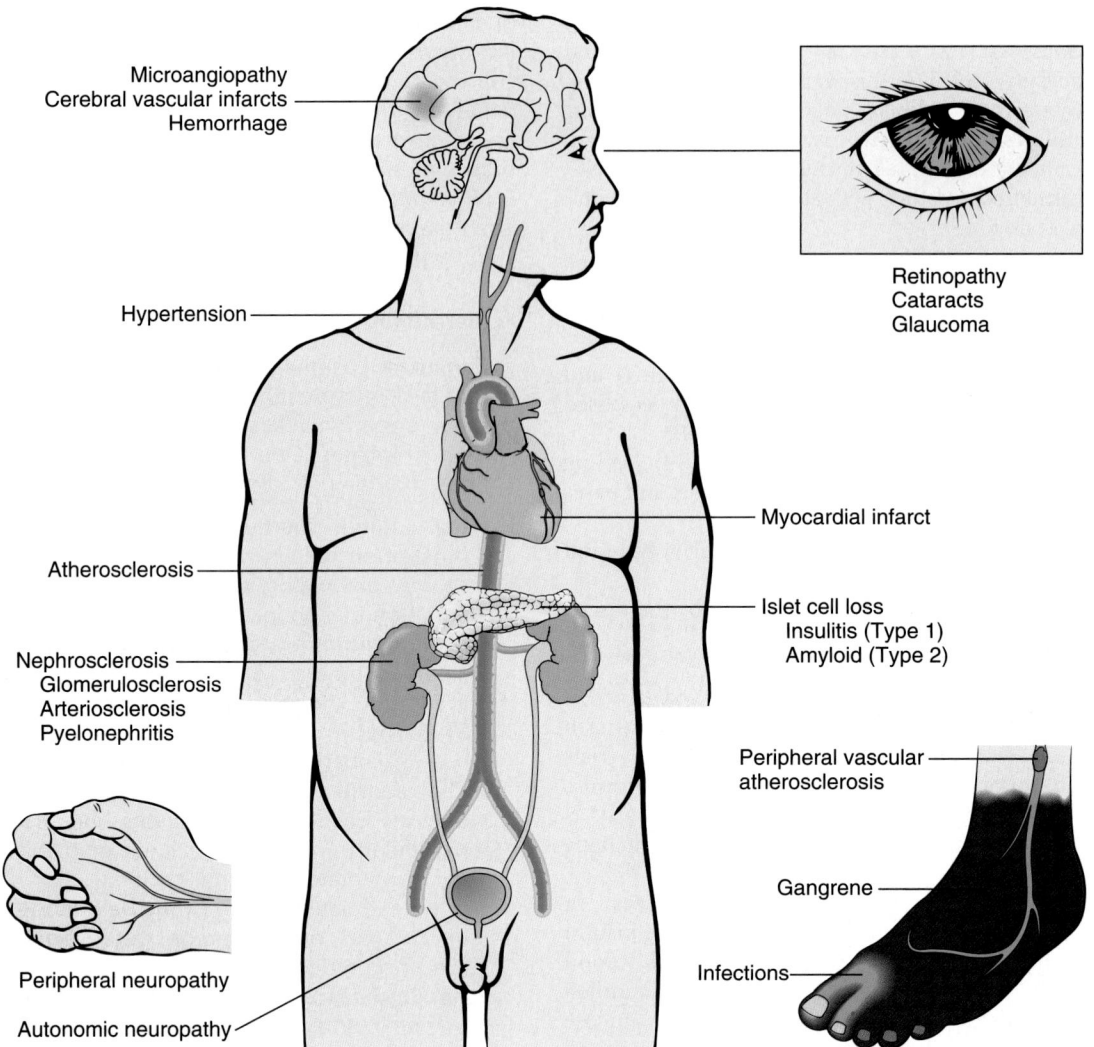

Microangiopathy
Cerebral vascular infarcts
Hemorrhage

Hypertension

Atherosclerosis

Nephrosclerosis
Glomerulosclerosis
Arteriosclerosis
Pyelonephritis

Peripheral neuropathy

Autonomic neuropathy

Retinopathy
Cataracts
Glaucoma

Myocardial infarct

Islet cell loss
Insulitis (Type 1)
Amyloid (Type 2)

Peripheral vascular
atherosclerosis

Gangrene

Infections

FIGURE 24–32   Long-term complications of diabetes.

risk for cardiovascular disease is even observed in pre-diabetics. Significantly, myocardial infarction is almost as common in diabetic women as in diabetic men. In contrast, myocardial infarction is uncommon in nondiabetic women of reproductive age. **Gangrene of the lower extremities,** as a result of advanced vascular disease, is about 100 times more common in diabetics than in the general population. The larger renal arteries are also subject to severe atherosclerosis, but the most damaging effect of diabetes on the kidneys is exerted at the level of the glomeruli and the microcirculation. This is discussed later.

Hyaline arteriolosclerosis, the vascular lesion associated with hypertension (Chapters 11 and 20), is both more prevalent and more severe in diabetics than in nondiabetics, but it is not specific for diabetes and may be seen in elderly nondiabetics without hypertension. It takes the form of an amorphous, hyaline thickening of the wall of the arterioles, which causes narrowing of the lumen (Fig. 24–34). Not sur-

prisingly, in diabetics it is related not only to the duration of the disease but also to the level of blood pressure.

Diabetic Microangiopathy. One of the most consistent morphologic features of diabetes is **diffuse thickening of basement membranes**. The thickening is most evident in the capillaries of the skin, skeletal muscle, retina, renal glomeruli, and renal medulla. However, it may also be seen in such nonvascular structures as renal tubules, the Bowman capsule, peripheral nerves, and placenta. It should be noted that despite the increase in the thickness of basement membranes, **diabetic capillaries are more leaky than normal to plasma proteins. The microangiopathy underlies the development of diabetic nephropathy, retinopathy, and some forms of neuropathy.** An indistinguishable microangiopathy can be found in aged nondiabetic patients but rarely to the extent seen in patients with long-standing diabetes.

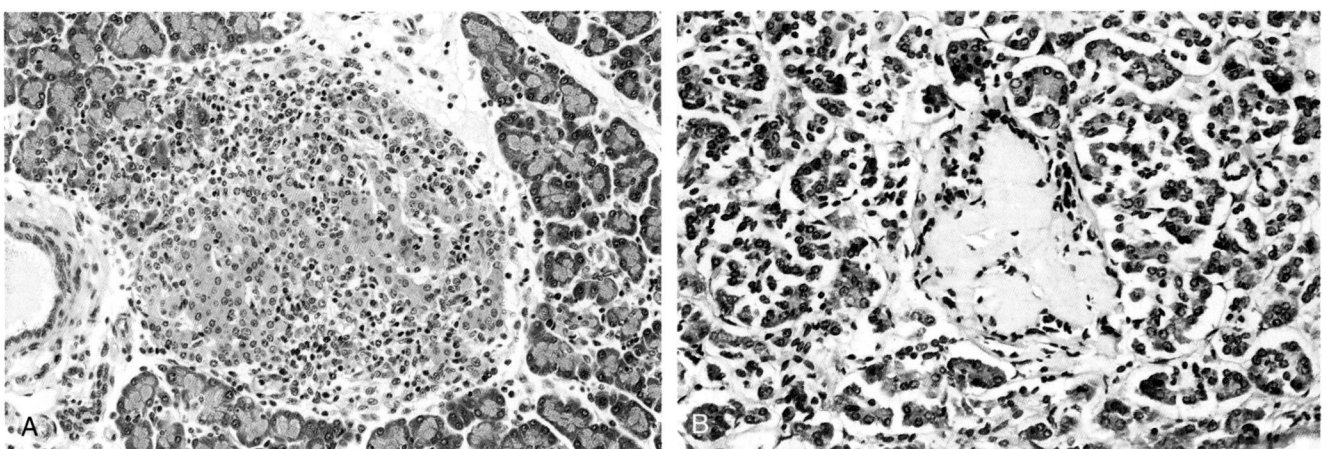

FIGURE 24–33   **A,** Insulitis, shown here from a rat (BB) model of autoimmune diabetes, also seen in type 1 human diabetes. **B,** Amyloidosis of a pancreatic islet in type 2 diabetes. (**A,** Courtesy of Dr. Arthur Like, University of Massachusetts, Worchester, MA.)

Diabetic Nephropathy. The kidneys are prime targets of diabetes. Renal failure is second only to myocardial infarction as a cause of death from this disease. **Three lesions are encountered: (1) glomerular lesions; (2) renal vascular lesions, principally arteriolosclerosis; and (3) pyelonephritis, including necrotizing papillitis.**

The most important glomerular lesions are capillary basement membrane thickening, diffuse mesangial sclerosis, and nodular glomerulosclerosis.

Capillary Basement Membrane Thickening. **Widespread thickening of the glomerular capillary basement membrane (GBM)** occurs in virtually all cases of diabetic nephropathy and is part and parcel of the diabetic microangiopathy. Pure capillary basement membrane thickening can be detected only by electron microscopy (Fig. 24–35). Careful morphometric

studies demonstrate that this thickening begins as early as 2 years after the onset of type 1 diabetes and by 5 years amounts to about a 30% increase. The thickening continues progressively and usually concurrently with mesangial widening. Simultaneously, there is thickening of the tubular basement membranes (Fig 24–36).

Diffuse Mesangial Sclerosis. This lesion consists of **diffuse increase in mesangial matrix.** There can be mild proliferation of mesangial cells early in the disease process, but cell proliferation is not a prominent part of this injury. The mesangial increase is

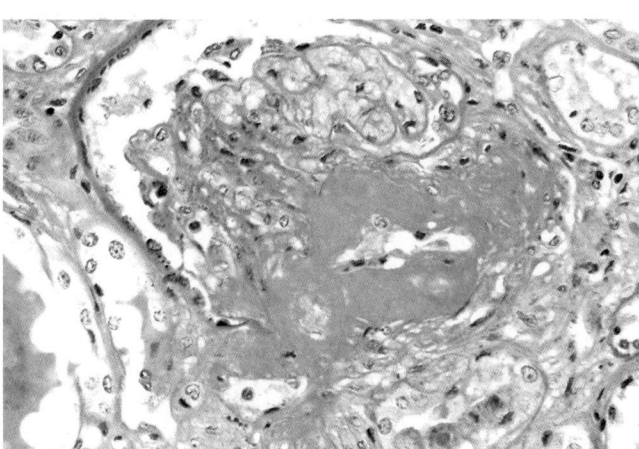

FIGURE 24–34   Severe renal hyaline arteriolosclerosis. Note a markedly thickened, tortuous afferent arteriole. The amorphous nature of the thickened vascular wall is evident. (PAS stain). (Courtesy of M.A. Venkatachalam, MD, Department of Pathology, University of Texas Health Science Center at San Antonio, TX.)

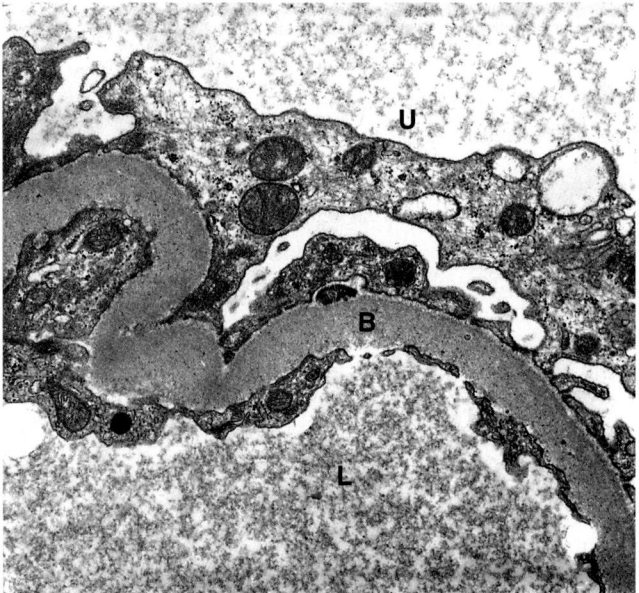

FIGURE 24–35   Electron micrograph of a renal glomerulus showing markedly thickened glomerular basement membrane (B) in a diabetic. L, glomerular capillary lumen; U, urinary space. (Courtesy of Dr. Michael Kashgarian, Department of Pathology, Yale University School of Medicine, New Haven, CT.)

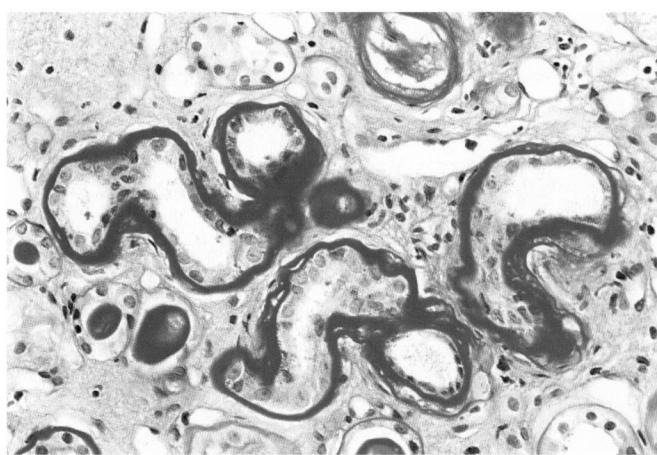

FIGURE 24–36 Renal cortex showing thickening of tubular basement membranes in a diabetic patient (PAS stain).

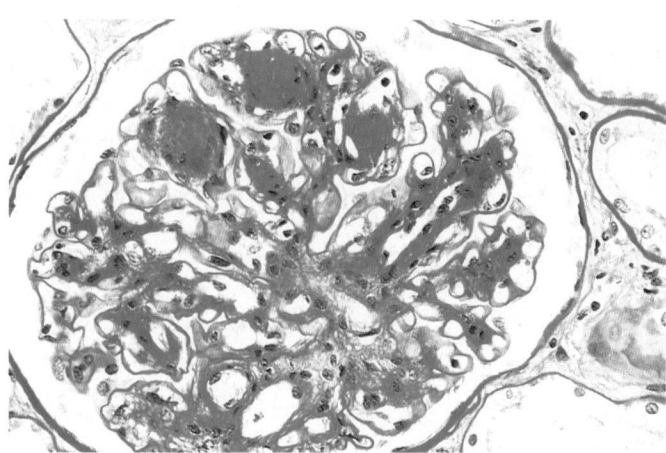

FIGURE 24–37 Diffuse and nodular diabetic glomerulosclerosis (PAS stain). Note the diffuse increase in mesangial matrix and characteristic acellular PAS-positive nodules.

typically associated with the overall thickening of the GBM. The matrix depositions are PAS-positive (Fig. 24–37). As the disease progresses, the expansion of mesangial areas can extend to nodular configurations. The progressive expansion of the mesangium has been shown to correlate well with measures of deteriorating renal function such as increasing proteinuria.

Nodular Glomerulosclerosis. This is also known as **intercapillary glomerulosclerosis or Kimmelstiel-Wilson disease**. The glomerular lesions take the form of ovoid or spherical, often laminated, nodules of matrix situated in the periphery of the glomerulus. The nodules are PAS-positive. They lie within the mesangial core of the glomerular lobules and can be surrounded by patent peripheral capillary loops (Fig 24–37) or loops that are markedly dilated. The nodules often show features of mesangiolysis with fraying of the mesangial/capillary lumen interface, disruption of sites at which the capillaries are anchored into the mesangial stalks, and resultant capillary microaneurysm formation as the untethered capillaries distend outward as a result of intracapillary pressures and flows. Usually, not all the lobules in the individual glomerulus are involved by nodular lesions, but even uninvolved lobules and glomeruli show striking diffuse mesangial sclerosis. As the disease advances, the individual nodules enlarge and may eventually compress and engulf capillaries, obliterating the glomerular tuft. These nodular lesions are frequently accompanied by prominent accumulations of hyaline material in capillary loops ("fibrin caps") or adherent to Bowman's capsules ("capsular drops"). Both afferent and efferent glomerular hilar arterioles show hyalinosis. As a consequence of the glomerular and arteriolar lesions, the kidney suffers from ischemia, develops tubular atrophy and interstitial fibrosis, and usually undergoes overall contraction in size (Fig. 24–38). Approximately 15% to 30% of individuals with

long-term diabetes develop nodular glomerulosclerosis, and in most instances it is associated with renal failure.

Renal atherosclerosis and arteriolosclerosis constitute part of the macrovascular disease in diabetics. The kidney is one of the most frequently and severely affected organs; however, the changes in the arteries and arterioles are similar to those found throughout the body. Hyaline arteriolosclerosis affects not only the afferent but also the efferent arteriole. Such efferent arteriolosclerosis is rarely, if ever, encountered in individuals who do not have diabetes.

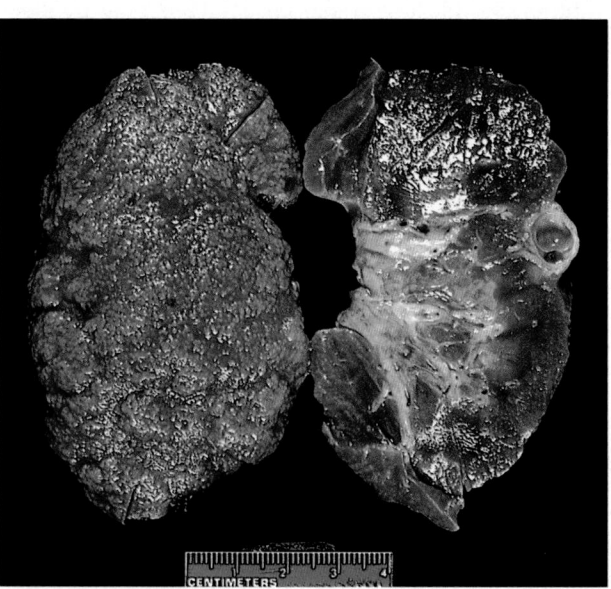

FIGURE 24–38 Nephrosclerosis in a patient with long-standing diabetes. The kidney has been bisected to demonstrate both diffuse granular transformation of the surface *(left)* and marked thinning of the cortical tissue *(right)*. Additional features include some irregular depressions, the result of pyelonephritis, and an incidental cortical cyst *(far right)*.

Pyelonephritis is an acute or chronic inflammation of the kidneys that usually begins in the interstitial tissue and then spreads to affect the tubules. Both the acute and chronic forms of this disease occur in nondiabetics as well as in diabetics but are more common in diabetics than in the general population, and, once affected, diabetics tend to have more severe involvement. One special pattern of acute pyelonephritis, **necrotizing papillitis** (or papillary necrosis), is much more prevalent in diabetics than in nondiabetics.

Diabetic Ocular Complications. The ocular involvement may take the form of retinopathy, cataract formation, or glaucoma. The morphologic features are discussed further in Chapter 29.

Diabetic Neuropathy. The central and peripheral nervous systems are not spared by diabetes. The morphology of diabetes in the nervous system is described further in Chapter 27.

CLINICAL FEATURES OF DIABETES

It is difficult to sketch with brevity the diverse clinical presentations of diabetes mellitus. Only a few characteristic patterns will be presented.

Type 1 diabetes was formerly thought to occur primarily in those under age 18 but is now known to occur at any age. In the initial 1 or 2 years following the onset of overt type 1 diabetes, the exogenous insulin requirements may be minimal because of ongoing endogenous insulin secretion (referred to as the *honeymoon period*). Thereafter, any residual β-cell reserve is exhausted and insulin requirements increase dramatically. Although β-cell destruction is a prolonged process, the transition from impaired glucose tolerance to overt diabetes may be abrupt, and is often brought on by an event, such as infection, that is also associated with increased insulin requirements.

The onset is marked by polyuria, polydipsia, polyphagia, and, when severe, ketoacidosis, all resulting from metabolic derangements. Since insulin is a major anabolic hormone in the body, *deficiency of insulin results in a catabolic state that affects not only glucose metabolism but also fat and protein metabolism.* Unopposed secretion of counter-regulatory hormones (glucagon, growth hormone, epinephrine) also plays a role in these metabolic derangements. The assimilation of glucose into muscle and adipose tissue is sharply diminished or abolished. Not only does storage of glycogen in liver and muscle cease, but also reserves are depleted by glycogenolysis. The resultant hyperglycemia exceeds the renal threshold for reabsorption, and glycosuria ensues. The glycosuria induces an osmotic diuresis and thus *polyuria*, causing a profound loss of water and electrolytes (Fig. 24–39). The obligatory renal water loss combined with the hyperosmolarity resulting from the increased levels of glucose in the blood tends to deplete intracellular water, triggering the osmoreceptors of the thirst centers of the brain. In this manner, intense thirst *(polydipsia)* appears. With a deficiency of insulin the scales swing from insulin-promoted anabolism to catabolism of proteins and fats. Proteolysis follows, and the gluconeogenic amino acids

are removed by the liver and used as building blocks for glucose. The catabolism of proteins and fats tends to induce a negative energy balance, which in turn leads to increasing appetite *(polyphagia)*, thus completing the classic triad of diabetes: *polyuria*, *polydipsia*, and *polyphagia*. Despite the increased appetite, catabolic effects prevail, resulting in weight loss and muscle weakness. *The combination of polyphagia and weight loss is paradoxical and should always raise the suspicion of diabetes.*

Diabetic ketoacidosis is a serious complication of type 1 diabetes but may also occur in type 2 diabetes, though not as commonly and not to as marked an extent. These patients have marked insulin deficiency, and the release of the catecholamine hormone *epinephrine* blocks any residual insulin action and stimulates the secretion of glucagon. The insulin deficiency coupled with glucagon excess decreases peripheral utilization of glucose while increasing gluconeogenesis, severely exacerbating hyperglycemia (the plasma glucose levels are usually in the range of 500 to 700 mg/dL). The hyperglycemia causes an osmotic diuresis and dehydration characteristic of the ketoacidotic state. The second major effect of an alteration in the insulin-to-glucagon ratio is activation of the ketogenic machinery. Insulin deficiency stimulates lipoprotein lipase, with resultant breakdown of adipose stores, and an increase in levels of free fatty acids. When these free fatty acids reach the liver, they are esterified to fatty acyl coenzyme A. Oxidation of fatty acyl coenzyme A molecules within the hepatic mitochondria produces *ketone bodies* (acetoacetic acid and β-hydroxybutyric acid). The rate at which ketone bodies are formed may exceed the rate at which acetoacetic acid and β-hydroxybutyric acid can be utilized by peripheral tissues, leading to *ketonemia* and *ketonuria*. If the urinary excretion of ketones is compromised by dehydration, systemic *metabolic ketoacidosis* results. Release of ketogenic amino acids by protein catabolism aggravates the ketotic state.

Type 2 diabetes mellitus may also present with polyuria and polydipsia, but unlike in type 1 diabetes, patients are often older (over 40 years) and frequently obese. However, with the increase in obesity and sedentary life style in our society, type 2 diabetes is now seen in children and adolescents with increasing frequency. In some cases medical attention is sought because of unexplained weakness or weight loss. *Most frequently, however, the diagnosis is made after routine blood or urine testing in asymptomatic persons.* The infrequency of ketoacidosis and milder presentation in type 2 diabetes is presumably because of higher portal vein insulin levels in these patients than in type 1 diabetics, which prevents unrestricted hepatic fatty acid oxidation and keeps the formation of ketone bodies in check. In the decompensated state, these patients may develop *hyperosmolar nonketotic coma* due to severe dehydration resulting from sustained osmotic diuresis (particularly in patients who do not drink enough water to compensate for urinary losses from chronic hyperglycemia). Typically, the patient is an elderly diabetic who is disabled by a stroke or an infection and is unable to maintain adequate water intake. Furthermore, the absence of ketoacidosis and its symptoms (nausea, vomiting, respiratory difficulties) delays the seeking of medical attention until severe dehydration and coma occur. Table 24–7 summarizes some of the pertinent clinical, genetic, and histopathologic features that distinguish type 1 and type 2 diabetes.

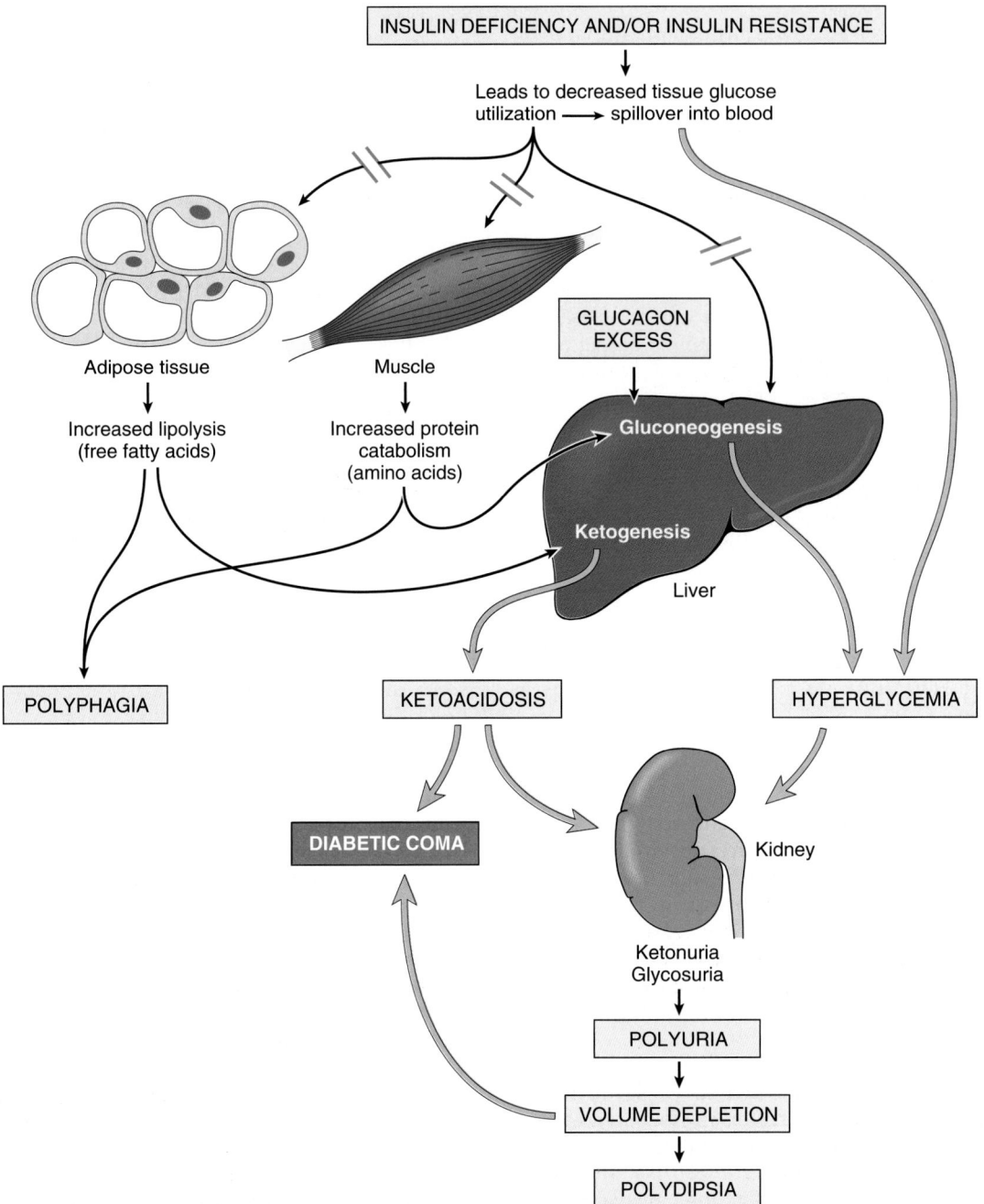

FIGURE 24–39 Sequence of metabolic derangements underlying the clinical manifestations of diabetes. An absolute insulin deficiency leads to a catabolic state, culminating in ketoacidosis and severe volume depletion. These cause sufficient central nervous system compromise to lead to coma and eventual death if left untreated.

In both types it is the long-term effects of diabetes, more than the acute metabolic complications, that are responsible for the overwhelming majority of the morbidity and mortality.[59,60] In most instances these complications appear approximately 15 to 20 years after the onset of hyperglycemia.

- *Macrovascular complications such as myocardial infarction, renal vascular insufficiency, and cerebrovascular accidents are the most common causes of mortality in long-standing diabetes.*[61] Diabetics have a two to four times greater incidence

of coronary artery disease, and a fourfold higher risk of dying from cardiovascular complications than nondiabetics. Diabetes is often accompanied by underlying conditions that favor the development of adverse cardiovascular events. For example, *hypertension* is found in approximately 75% of individuals with type 2 diabetes and potentiates the effects of hyperglycemia and insulin resistance on endothelial dysfunction and atherosclerosis. Another cardiovascular risk frequently seen in diabetics is *dyslipidemia*, which includes both increased triglycerides and LDL levels and

TABLE 24–7   Type 1 Versus Type 2 Diabetes Mellitus

	Type 1 Diabetes Mellitus	Type 2 Diabetes Mellitus
CLINICAL		
	Onset: usually childhood and adolescence	Onset: usually adult; increasing incidence in childhood and adolescence
	Normal weight or weight loss preceding diagnosis	Vast majority are obese (80%)
	Progressive decrease in insulin levels	Increased blood insulin (early); normal or moderate decrease in insulin (late)
	Circulating islet autoantibodies (anti-insulin, anti-GAD, anti-ICA512)	No islet auto-antibodies
	Diabetic ketoacidosis in absence of insulin therapy	Nonketotic hyperosmolar coma more common
GENETICS		
	Major linkage to MHC class I and II genes; also linked to polymorphisms in *CTLA4* and *PTPN22*, and insulin gene VNTRs	No HLA linkage; linkage to candidate diabetogenic and obesity-related genes (*TCF7L2, PPARG, FTO,* etc.)
PATHOGENESIS		
	Dysfunction in regulatory T cells (Tregs) leading to breakdown in self-tolerance to islet auto-antigens	Insulin resistance in peripheral tissues, failure of compensation by β-cells Multiple obesity-associated factors (circulating nonesterified fatty acids, inflammatory mediators, adipocytokines) linked to pathogenesis of insulin resistance
PATHOLOGY		
	Insulitis (inflammatory infiltrate of T cells and macrophages)	No insulitis; amyloid deposition in islets
	β-cell depletion, islet atrophy	Mild β-cell depletion

HLA, human leukocyte antigen; MHC, major histocompatibility complex; VNTRs, variable number of tandem repeats.

decreased levels of the "protective" lipoprotein, high-density lipoprotein (Chapter 11). Insulin resistance is believed to contribute to "diabetic dyslipidemia" by favoring the hepatic production of atherogenic lipoproteins and by suppressing the uptake of circulating lipids in peripheral tissues. Finally, diabetics have elevated levels of PAI-1, which is an inhibitor of fibrinolysis and therefore acts as a procoagulant in the formation of atherosclerotic plaques.

○ *Diabetic nephropathy* is a leading cause of end-stage renal disease in the United States. Approximately 30% to 40% of all diabetics develop clinical evidence of nephropathy, but a considerably smaller fraction of patients with type 2 diabetes progress to end-stage renal disease. However, because of the much greater prevalence of type 2 diabetes, these patients constitute slightly over half the diabetic patients starting dialysis each year. The frequency of diabetic nephropathy is greatly influenced by the genetic makeup of the population in question; for example, Native Americans, Hispanics, and African Americans have a greater risk of developing end-stage renal disease than do non-Hispanic whites with type 2 diabetes. The earliest manifestation of diabetic nephropathy is the appearance of low amounts of albumin in the urine (>30 mg/day, but <300 mg/day), that is, *microalbuminuria*. Notably, microalbuminuria is also a marker for greatly increased cardiovascular morbidity and mortality for persons with either type 1 or type 2 diabetes. Therefore, all patients with microalbuminuria should be screened for macrovascular disease, and aggressive intervention should be undertaken to reduce cardiovascular risk factors. Without specific interventions, approximately 80% of type 1 diabetics and 20% to 40% of type 2 diabetics will develop *overt nephropathy with macroalbuminuria* (>300 mg of urinary albumin per day) over 10 to 15 years, usually accompanied by the appearance of hypertension. The progression from overt nephropathy to end-stage renal disease can be highly variable. By 20 years, more than 75% of type 1 diabetics and approximately 20% of type 2 diabetics with overt nephropathy will develop end-stage renal disease, requiring dialysis or renal transplantation. Diabetic nephropathy is also discussed in Chapter 20.

○ *Visual impairment,* sometimes even total blindness, is one of the more feared consequences of long-standing diabetes. Approximately 60% to 80% of patients develop some form of *diabetic retinopathy* approximately 15 to 20 years after diagnosis. The fundamental lesion of retinopathy—neovascularization—is attributable to hypoxia-induced overexpression of VEGF in the retina. Indeed, current treatment for this condition includes intravitreous injection of anti-angiogenic agents. Diabetic retinopathy, described in Chapter 29, consists of a constellation of changes that together are considered by many ophthalmologists to be virtually diagnostic of the disease. In addition to retinopathy, diabetics also have an increased propensity for *glaucoma* and *cataract formation,* both of which contribute to visual impairment in diabetes.

○ *Diabetic neuropathy* can elicit a variety of clinical syndromes, afflicting the central nervous system, peripheral sensorimotor nerves, and the autonomic nervous system (Chapter 27). The most frequent pattern of involvement is a *distal symmetric polyneuropathy* of the lower extremities that affects both motor and sensory function, but particularly the latter. Over time the upper extremities may be involved as well, thus approximating a "glove and stocking" pattern of polyneuropathy. Other forms include *autonomic neuropathy*, which produces disturbances in bowel and bladder function and sometimes sexual impotence, and *diabetic mononeuropathy*, which may manifest as sudden footdrop, wristdrop, or isolated cranial nerve palsies.

○ *Diabetics are plagued by enhanced susceptibility to infections of the skin and to tuberculosis, pneumonia, and pyelonephritis.* Such infections cause the deaths of about 5% of diabetics. In an individual with diabetic neuropathy, a trivial infection in a toe may be the first event in a long succession of complications (gangrene, bacteremia, pneumonia) that may ultimately lead to death. The basis of enhanced susceptibility is multifactorial, and includes decreased neutrophil functions (chemotaxis, adherence to the endothelium, phagocytosis, and microbicidal activity), and impaired cytokine production by macrophages. The vascular compromise also reduces delivery of circulating cells and molecules that are required for host defense.

In recent years increasingly sedentary life styles and poor eating habits have contributed to the simultaneous escalation of diabetes and obesity worldwide, which some have termed as the *diabesity* epidemic.[62] Sadly, obesity and diabetes have now percolated even to children exposed to "junk" food and lacking adequate exercise. The term *metabolic syndrome* (previously called "syndrome X") has been applied to an increasingly common condition wherein abdominal obesity and insulin resistance are accompanied by a constellation of risk factors for cardiovascular disease like abnormal lipid profiles.[63] Persons with metabolic syndrome benefit greatly from changes in their life style, including dietary modification and weight reduction; a similar benefit is observed in individuals with frank type 2 diabetes.[64] As the incidence of communicable diseases has declined and expected life span has increased, diabetes has become a major public health problem, and it continues to be one of the top 10 "killers" in the United States. The American Diabetes Association estimates that the total costs from diabetes to the United States economy is an astounding $132 billion dollars, including $92 billion from direct medical costs and the additional $40 billion from indirect costs such as disability, work loss, and premature mortality. There is hope, however, since the role of primary prevention of type 2 diabetes by lifestyle and dietary alterations, and secondary prevention of diabetic complications by strict glycemic control, has become increasingly recognized. It is also hoped that islet cell transplantation, stem cell therapies, and immune modulators may result in a cure for those afflicted with type 1 diabetes.

Pancreatic Endocrine Neoplasms

The preferred term for tumors of the pancreatic islet cells ("islet cell tumors") is *pancreatic endocrine neoplasms*. They are rare in comparison with tumors of the exocrine pancreas, accounting for only 2% of all pancreatic neoplasms. They are most common in adults and can occur anywhere along the length of the pancreas, embedded in the substance of the pancreas or arising in the immediate peripancreatic tissues. They resemble in appearance their counterparts, carcinoid tumors, found elsewhere in the alimentary tract (Chapter 17). These tumors may be single or multiple and benign or malig-

nant. Pancreatic endocrine neoplasms often elaborate pancreatic hormones, but some may be totally nonfunctional.

Like any other endocrine neoplasms in the body (see below), it is difficult to predict the biologic behavior of a pancreatic endocrine neoplasm based on light microscopic criteria alone. *Unequivocal criteria for malignancy* include metastases, vascular invasion, and local infiltration. The functional status of the tumor has some impact on prognosis, since approximately 90% of insulinomas are benign, while 60% to 90% of other functioning and nonfunctioning pancreatic endocrine neoplasms are malignant. Fortunately, insulinomas are the most common subtype of pancreatic endocrine neoplasms.

The three most common and distinctive clinical syndromes associated with functional pancreatic endocrine neoplasms are (1) *hyperinsulinism*, (2) *hypergastrinemia and the Zollinger-Ellison syndrome*, and (3) *MEN* (described in detail later).

HYPERINSULINISM (INSULINOMA)

β-cell tumors (insulinomas) are the most common of pancreatic endocrine neoplasms. They may be responsible for the elaboration of sufficient insulin to induce clinically significant hypoglycemia. The characteristic clinical picture is dominated by hypoglycemic episodes, which (1) occur with blood glucose levels below 50 mg/dL of serum; (2) consist principally of central nervous system manifestations such as confusion, stupor, and loss of consciousness; and (3) are precipitated by fasting or exercise and are promptly relieved by feeding or parenteral administration of glucose.

> **Morphology.** Insulinomas are most often found within the pancreas and are generally benign. Most are solitary, although multiple tumors may be encountered. Bona fide carcinomas, making up only about 10% of cases, are diagnosed on the basis of local invasion and distant metastases. On rare occasions an insulinoma may arise in ectopic pancreatic tissue. In such cases, electron microscopy reveals the distinctive granules of β-cells (see Fig. 24–26).
>
> **Solitary tumors** are usually small (often <2 cm in diameter) and are encapsulated, pale to red-brown nodules located anywhere in the pancreas. Histologically, these benign tumors look remarkably like giant islets, with preservation of the regular cords of monotonous cells and their orientation to the vasculature. Not even the malignant lesions present much evidence of anaplasia, and they may be deceptively encapsulated. **Deposition of amyloid** in the extracellular tissue is a characteristic feature of many insulinomas (Fig. 24–40).
>
> Hyperinsulinism may also be caused by **focal or diffuse hyperplasia of the islets**. This change is found occasionally in adults but is far more commonly encountered as congenital hyperinsulinism with hypoglycemia in neonates and infants. Several clinical scenarios may result in islet hyperplasia (previously known as *nesidioblastosis*), including maternal diabetes, Beckwith-Wiedemann syndrome (Chapter 10), and rare mutations in the β-cell K⁺-channel protein or sulfonylurea receptor.[65] In maternal diabetes, the fetal islets respond to the hyperglycemia by increas-

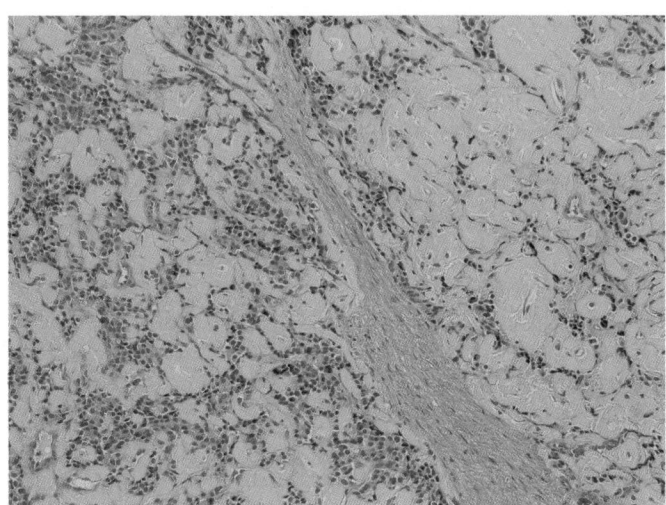

FIGURE 24–40 Pancreatic endocrine neoplasm ("islet cell tumor"). The neoplastic cells are monotonous and demonstrate minimal pleomorphism or mitotic activity. There is abundant amyloid deposition, characteristic of an insulinoma. Clinically, the patient had episodic hypoglycemia.

ing their size and number. In the postnatal period, these hyperactive islets may be responsible for serious episodes of hypoglycemia. This phenomenon is usually transient.

Clinical Features. While up to 80% of islet cell tumors may demonstrate excessive insulin secretion, the hypoglycemia is mild in all but about 20%, and many cases never become clinically symptomatic. The critical laboratory findings in insulinomas are high circulating levels of insulin and a high insulin-to-glucose ratio. Surgical removal of the tumor is usually followed by prompt reversal of the hypoglycemia.

It is important to note that *there are many other causes of hypoglycemia besides insulinomas.* The differential diagnosis of this metabolic abnormality includes such conditions as abnormal insulin sensitivity, diffuse liver disease, inherited glycogenoses, and ectopic production of insulin by certain retroperitoneal fibromas and fibrosarcomas. Depending on the clinical circumstances, hypoglycemia induced by self-injection of insulin should also be considered.

ZOLLINGER-ELLISON SYNDROME (GASTRINOMAS)

Marked hypersecretion of gastrin usually has its origin in gastrin-producing tumors *(gastrinomas)*, which are just as likely to arise in the duodenum and peripancreatic soft tissues as in the pancreas (so-called gastrinoma triangle). There has been lack of agreement regarding the cell of origin for these tumors, although it seems likely that endocrine cells of either the gut or the pancreas could be the source. Zollinger and Ellison first called attention to the *association of pancreatic islet cell lesions, hypersecretion of gastric acid and severe peptic ulceration,* which are present in 90% to 95% of patients.

Morphology. Gastrinomas may arise in the pancreas, the peripancreatic region, or the wall of the duode-

num. **Over half of gastrin-producing tumors are locally invasive or have already metastasized at the time of diagnosis.** In approximately 25% of patients, gastrinomas arise in conjunction with other endocrine tumors, as part of the MEN-1 syndrome (see below); MEN-1–associated gastrinomas are frequently multifocal, while sporadic gastrinomas are usually single. As with insulin-secreting tumors of the pancreas, gastrin-producing tumors are histologically bland and rarely show marked anaplasia.

In the Zollinger-Ellison syndrome, hypergastrinemia gives rise to extreme gastric acid secretion, which in turn causes **peptic ulceration** (Chapter 17). The duodenal and gastric ulcers are often multiple; although they are identical to those found in the general population, they are often unresponsive to therapy. In addition, ulcers may occur in unusual locations such as the jejunum; when intractable jejunal ulcers are found, Zollinger-Ellison syndrome should be considered.

Clinical Features. More than 50% of the patients have diarrhea; in 30%, it is the presenting symptom. Treatment of Zollinger-Ellison syndrome involves control of gastric acid secretion by use of H^+,K^+-ATPase inhibitors (Chapter 17) and excision of the neoplasm. Total resection of the neoplasm, when possible, eliminates the syndrome. Patients with hepatic metastases have a significantly shortened life expectancy, with progressive tumor growth leading to liver failure usually within 10 years.

OTHER RARE PANCREATIC ENDOCRINE NEOPLASMS

α-cell tumors (glucagonomas) are associated with increased serum levels of glucagon and a syndrome consisting of mild diabetes mellitus, a characteristic skin rash (necrolytic migratory erythema), and anemia. They occur most frequently in perimenopausal and postmenopausal women and are characterized by extremely high plasma glucagon levels.

δ-cell tumors (somatostatinomas) are associated with diabetes mellitus, cholelithiasis, steatorrhea, and hypochlorhydria. They are exceedingly difficult to localize preoperatively. High plasma somatostatin levels are required for diagnosis.

VIPoma (watery diarrhea, hypokalemia, achlorhydria, or WDHA syndrome) is an endocrine tumor that induces a characteristic syndrome, caused by release of vasoactive intestinal peptide (VIP) from the tumor. Some of these tumors are locally invasive and metastatic. A VIP assay should be performed on all patients with severe secretory diarrhea. Neural crest tumors, such as neuroblastomas, ganglioneuroblastomas, and ganglioneuromas (Chapter 10) and pheochromocytomas (see below) can also be associated with the VIPoma syndrome.

Pancreatic carcinoid tumors producing serotonin and an atypical carcinoid syndrome are exceedingly rare. *Pancreatic polypeptide-secreting endocrine tumors* are endocrinologically asymptomatic, despite the presence of high levels of the hormone in plasma.

Some pancreatic and extra-pancreatic endocrine tumors produce two or more hormones. In addition to insulin, glucagon, and gastrin, pancreatic endocrine tumors may produce

ACTH, MSH, ADH, serotonin, and norepinephrine. These *multihormonal tumors* are to be distinguished from the MEN syndromes (discusssed later), in which a multiplicity of hormones is produced by tumors in several different glands.

ADRENAL GLANDS

Adrenal Cortex

The *adrenal glands* are paired endocrine organs consisting of both cortex and medulla, which differ in their development, structure, and function. Beneath the capsule of the adrenal is the narrow layer of zona glomerulosa. An equally narrow zona reticularis abuts the medulla. Intervening is the broad zona fasciculata, which makes up about 75% of the total cortex. The *adrenal cortex* synthesizes three different types of steroids: (1) *glucocorticoids* (principally cortisol), which are synthesized primarily in the zona fasciculata and to a lesser degree in the zona reticularis; (2) *mineralocorticoids*, the most important being aldosterone, which is generated in the zona glomerulosa; and (3) *sex steroids* (estrogens and androgens), which are produced largely in the zona reticularis. The *adrenal medulla* is composed of chromaffin cells, which synthesize and secrete *catecholamines*, mainly epinephrine. Catecholamines have many effects that allow rapid adaptations to changes in the environment.

Diseases of the adrenal cortex can be conveniently divided into those associated with hyperfunction and those associated with hypofunction.

ADRENOCORTICAL HYPERFUNCTION (HYPERADRENALISM)

Just as there are three basic types of corticosteroids elaborated by the adrenal cortex, so there are three distinctive hyperadrenal syndromes: (1) *Cushing syndrome*, characterized by an excess of cortisol; (2) *hyperaldosteronism*; and (3) *adrenogeni-tal* or virilizing syndromes caused by an excess of androgens. The clinical features of these syndromes overlap somewhat because of the overlapping functions of some of the adrenal steroids.

Hypercortisolism (Cushing Syndrome)

Pathogenesis. This disorder is caused by any condition that produces elevated glucocorticoid levels. Cushing syndrome can be broadly divided into *exogenous* and *endogenous* causes. *The vast majority of cases of Cushing syndrome are the result of the administration of exogenous glucocorticoids* ("iatrogenic" Cushing syndrome).[66] The endogenous causes can, in turn, be divided into those that are *ACTH dependent* and those that are *ACTH independent* (Table 24–8).

ACTH-secreting pituitary adenomas account for approximately 70% of cases of endogenous hypercortisolism. In recognition of Harvey Cushing, the neurosurgeon who first published the full description of this syndrome, the pituitary form is referred to as *Cushing disease*.[67] The disorder affects women about four times more frequently than men and occurs most frequently in young adults. In the vast majority of cases it is caused by an *ACTH-producing pituitary microadenoma*; some corticotroph tumors qualify as macroadenomas (>10 mm). Rarely, the anterior pituitary contains areas of *corticotroph cell hyperplasia* without a discrete adenoma. Corticotroph cell hyperplasia may be primary or arise secondarily from excessive stimulation of ACTH release by a hypothalamic corticotrophin-releasing hormone (CRH)–producing tumor. The adrenal glands in individuals with Cushing disease are

TABLE 24–8 Endogenous Causes of Cushing Syndrome		
Cause	**Relative Frequency (%)**	**Ratio of Females to Males**
ACTH-DEPENDENT		
Cushing disease (pituitary adenoma; rarely CRH-dependent pituitary hyperplasia)	70	3.5 : 1.0
Ectopic corticotropin syndrome (ACTH-secreting pulmonary small-cell carcinoma, bronchial carcinoid)	10	1 : 1
ACTH-INDEPENDENT		
Adrenal adenoma	10	4 : 1
Adrenal carcinoma	5	1 : 1
Macronodular hyperplasia (ectopic expression of hormone receptors, including GIPR, LHR, vasopressin and serotonin receptors)	<2	1 : 1
Primary pigmented nodular adrenal disease (*PRKARIA* and *PDE11* mutations)	<2	1 : 1
McCune-Albright syndrome (*GNAS* mutations)	<2	1 : 1

ACTH, adrenocorticotropic hormone; GIPR, gastric inhibitory polypeptide receptor; LHR, luteinizing hormone receptor; *PRKAR1A*, protein kinase A regulatory subunit 1α; *PDE11*, phosphodiesterase 11A.
Note: These etiologies are responsible for endogenous Cushing syndrome. The most common overall cause of Cushing syndrome is exogenous glucocorticoid administration (iatrogenic Cushing syndrome).
Adapted with permission from Newell-Price J et al.: Cushing syndrome. Lancet 367:1605–1616, 2006.

characterized by variable degrees of nodular cortical hyperplasia (discussed later), caused by the elevated levels of ACTH. The cortical hyperplasia, in turn, is responsible for hypercortisolism.

Secretion of ectopic ACTH by nonpituitary tumors accounts for about 10% of ACTH-dependent Cushing syndrome. In many instances the responsible tumor is a *small-cell carcinoma of the lung*, although other neoplasms, including carcinoids, medullary carcinomas of the thyroid, and islet cell tumors, have been associated with the syndrome. In addition to tumors that elaborate ectopic ACTH, an occasional neuroendocrine neoplasm produces ectopic CRH, which, in turn, causes ACTH secretion and hypercortisolism. As in the pituitary variant, the adrenal glands undergo bilateral cortical hyperplasia, but the rapid downhill course of patients with these cancers often cuts short the adrenal enlargement. This variant of Cushing syndrome is more common in men and usually occurs in the 40s and 50s.

Primary adrenal neoplasms, such as adrenal adenoma (~10%) and carcinoma (~5%) are the most common underlying causes for *ACTH-independent* Cushing syndrome. The biochemical sine qua non of ACTH-independent Cushing syndrome is elevated serum levels of cortisol with low levels of ACTH. Cortical carcinomas tend to produce more marked hypercortisolism than adenomas or hyperplasias. In instances of a unilateral neoplasm, the uninvolved adrenal cortex and the cortex in the opposite gland undergo atrophy because of suppression of ACTH secretion.

The overwhelming majority of hyperplastic adrenals are ACTH dependent, and *primary cortical hyperplasia (i.e., ACTH-independent hyperplasia) is uncommon*. In *macronodular hyperplasia* the nodules are usually greater than 3 mm in diameter. Macronodular hyperplasia is typically a sporadic (nonsyndromic) condition observed in adults. It is now known that, although the condition is ACTH independent, it is not entirely "autonomous." Specifically, cortisol production is regulated by non-ACTH circulating hormones, as a result of ectopic overexpression of their corresponding receptors in the adrenocortical cells. For example, overexpression of the receptors for gastric inhibitory peptide, LH, ADH, and serotonin are often found within the hyperplastic tissues.[68] The mechanism by which these receptors for non-ACTH hormones are overexpressed in adrenocortical tissues is, however, not known. A subset of macronodular hyperplasia arises in the setting of McCune-Albright syndrome, characterized by germline activating mutations in *GNAS*, which encodes a stimulatory $G_s\alpha$ (Chapter 26). In addition, primary cortical hyperplasias may result from mutations in other genes that control intracellular levels of cAMP. These include the *PRKR1A* gene (see below) and the *phosphodiesterase 11A (PDE11A)* gene.[69]

> **Morphology.** The main lesions of Cushing syndrome are found in the pituitary and adrenal glands. The **pituitary** shows changes regardless of the cause. The most common alteration, resulting from high levels of endogenous or exogenous glucocorticoids, is termed **Crooke hyaline change.** In this condition the normal granular, basophilic cytoplasm of the ACTH-producing cells in the anterior pituitary becomes homogeneous and paler. This alteration is the result

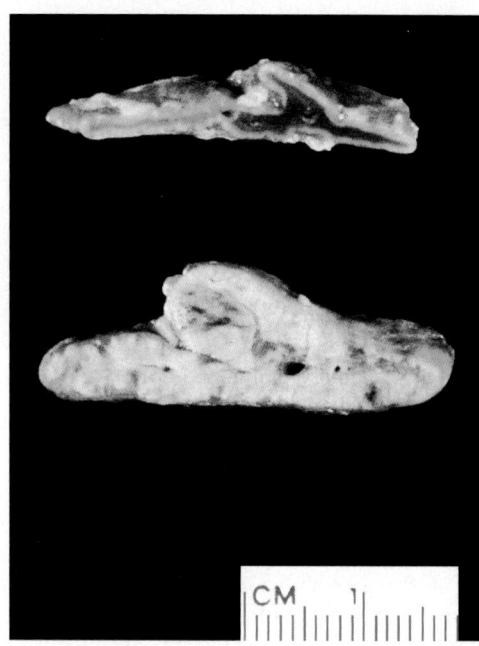

FIGURE 24–41 Diffuse hyperplasia of the adrenal contrasted with normal adrenal gland. In cross-section the adrenal cortex is yellow and thickened, and a subtle nodularity is seen (contrast with Figure 24–46). Both adrenal glands were diffusely hyperplastic in this patient with ACTH-dependent Cushing syndrome.

> of the accumulation of intermediate keratin filaments in the cytoplasm.
>
> Depending on the cause of the hypercortisolism the **adrenals** have one of the following abnormalities: (1) cortical atrophy, (2) diffuse hyperplasia, (3) macronodular or micronodular hyperplasia, and (4) an adenoma or carcinoma. In patients in whom the syndrome results from exogenous glucocorticoids, suppression of endogenous ACTH results in bilateral **cortical atrophy,** due to a lack of stimulation of the zonae fasciculata and reticularis by ACTH. The zona glomerulosa is of normal thickness in such cases, because this portion of the cortex functions independently of ACTH. In contrast, in cases of endogenous hypercortisolism, the adrenals either are hyperplastic or contain a cortical neoplasm. **Diffuse hyperplasia** is found in individuals with ACTH-dependent Cushing syndrome (Fig. 24–41). Both glands are enlarged, either subtly or markedly, weighing up to 30 gm. The adrenal cortex is diffusely thickened and variably nodular, although the latter is not as pronounced as seen in cases of ACTH-independent nodular hyperplasia. Microscopically, the hyperplastic cortex demonstrates an expanded "lipid-poor" zona reticularis, comprising compact, eosinophilic cells, surrounded by an outer zone of vacuolated "lipid-rich" cells, resembling those seen in the zona fasciculata. Any nodules present are usually composed of vacuolated "lipid-rich" cells, which accounts for the yellow color of diffusely hyperplastic glands. In contrast, in **macronodular hyperplasia** the adrenals are almost entirely replaced by prominent nodules of varying sizes

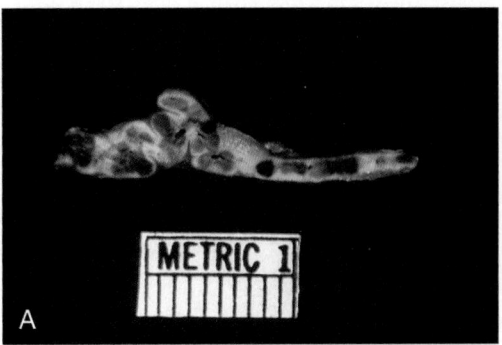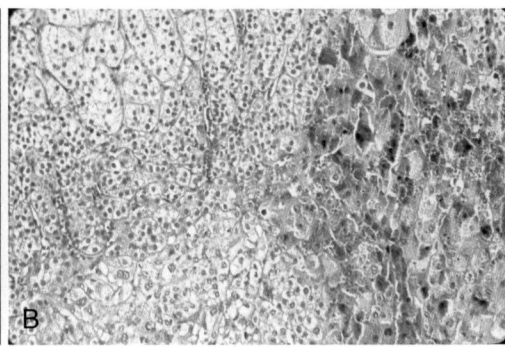

FIGURE 24–42 **A,** Primary pigmented nodular adrenocortical disease showing prominent pigmented nodules in the adrenal gland. **B,** On histologic examination the nodules are composed of cells containing lipofuscin pigment, seen in the right part of the field. (Photographs courtesy of Dr. Aidan Carney, Department of Medicine, Mayo Clinic, Rochester, MN.)

(≤3 cm), which contain an admixture of lipid-poor and lipid-rich cells. Unlike diffuse hyperplasia, the areas between the macroscopic nodules also demonstrate evidence of microscopic nodularity. **Micronodular hyperplasia** is composed of 1- to 3-mm darkly pigmented (brown to black) micronodules, with atrophic intervening areas (Fig. 24–42). The pigment is believed to be lipofuscin, a wear-and-tear pigment (Chapter 1).

Primary adrenocortical neoplasms causing Cushing syndrome may be malignant or benign. Functional adenomas or carcinomas of the adrenal cortex as the source of cortisol are not morphologically distinct from nonfunctioning adrenal neoplasms (described later). Both the benign and the malignant lesions are more common in women in their 30s to 50s. Adrenocortical **adenomas** are yellow tumors surrounded by thin or well-developed capsules, and most weigh less than 30 gm. Microscopically, they are composed of cells that are similar to those encountered in the normal zona fasciculata. The **carcinomas** associated with Cushing syndrome, by contrast, tend to be larger than the adenomas. These tumors are unencapsulated masses frequently exceeding 200 to 300 gm in weight, having all of the anaplastic characteristics of cancer, as will be detailed later. With functioning tumors, both benign and malignant, the adjacent adrenal cortex and that of the contralateral adrenal gland are atrophic, as a result of suppression of endogenous ACTH by high cortisol levels.

Clinical Course. Developing slowly over time, Cushing syndrome can be quite subtle in its early manifestations. Early stages of the disorder may present with hypertension and weight gain (Table 24–9). With time the more characteristic central pattern of adipose tissue deposition becomes apparent in the form of truncal obesity, moon facies, and accumulation of fat in the posterior neck and back *(buffalo hump)*. Hypercortisolism causes selective atrophy of fast-twitch (type 2) myofibers, resulting in decreased muscle mass and proximal limb weakness. Glucocorticoids induce gluconeogenesis and inhibit the uptake of glucose by cells, with resultant *hyperglycemia, glucosuria* and *polydipsia (secondary diabetes)*. The catabolic effects cause loss of collagen and resorption of bones.

Consequently the *skin is thin, fragile, and easily bruised*; wound healing is poor; and cutaneous striae are particularly common in the abdominal area (Fig. 24–43). Bone resorption results in the development of *osteoporosis*, with consequent backache and increased susceptibility to fractures. Persons with Cushing syndrome are at increased risk for a variety of infections, because glucocorticoids suppress the immune response. Additional manifestations include several *mental disturbances*, including mood swings, depression, and frank psychosis, as well as *hirsutism* and *menstrual abnormalities*.

Cushing syndrome is diagnosed in the laboratory with the following: (1) the 24-hour urine free-cortisol concentration, which is increased, and (2) loss of normal diurnal pattern of cortisol secretion. Determining the cause of Cushing syndrome depends on the serum ACTH and measurement of urinary steroid excretion after administration of dexamethasone (dexamethasone suppression test). The results of these tests fall into three general patterns:

TABLE 24–9 Clinical Features of Cushing Syndrome	
Obesity or weight gain	95%*
Facial plethora	90%
Rounded face	90%
Decreased libido	90%
Thin skin	85%
Decrease in linear growth in children	70–80%
Menstrual irregularity	80%
Hypertension	75%
Hirsutism	75%
Depression/emotional liability	70%
Easy bruising	65%
Glucose intolerance	60%
Weakness	60%
Osteopenia or fracture	50%
Nephrolithiasis	50%

*100% in children.
Adapted from Newell-Price J et al.: Cushing syndrome. Lancet 367:1605–1616, 2006.

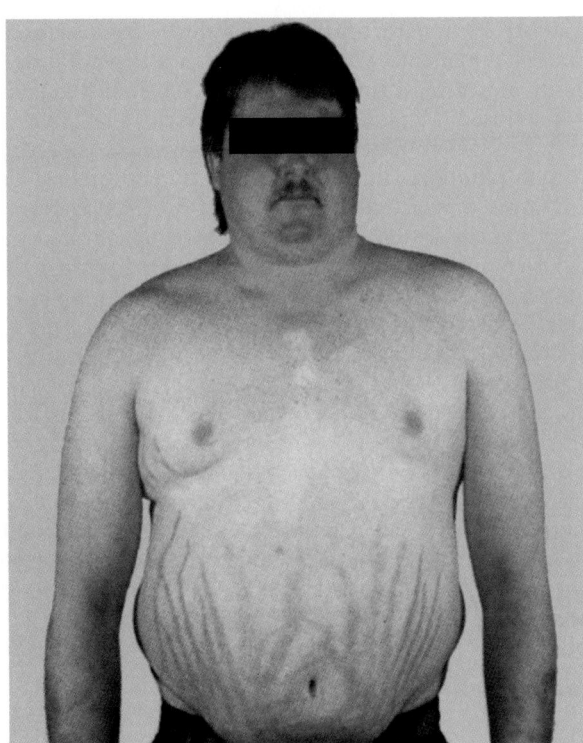

FIGURE 24–43 A patient with Cushing syndrome demonstrating central obesity, "moon facies," and abdominal striae. (Reproduced with permission from Lloyd RV et al.: Atlas of Nontumor Pathology: Endocrine Diseases. Washington, DC, American Registry of Pathology, 2002.)

1. In pituitary Cushing syndrome, the most common form, ACTH levels are elevated and cannot be suppressed by the administration of a low dose of dexamethasone. Hence, there is no reduction in urinary excretion of 17-hydroxycorticosteroids. After higher doses of injected dexamethasone, however, the pituitary responds by reducing ACTH secretion, which is reflected by suppression of urinary steroid secretion.
2. Ectopic ACTH secretion results in an elevated level of ACTH, but its secretion is completely insensitive to low or high doses of exogenous dexamethasone.
3. When Cushing syndrome is caused by an adrenal tumor, the ACTH level is quite low because of feedback inhibition of the pituitary. As with ectopic ACTH secretion, both low-dose and high-dose dexamethasone fail to suppress cortisol excretion.

Primary Hyperaldosteronism

Hyperaldosteronism is the generic term for a group of closely related conditions characterized by chronic excess aldosterone secretion. Hyperaldosteronism may be primary, or it may be secondary to an extra-adrenal cause. *Primary hyperaldosteronism* stems from an autonomous overproduction of aldosterone, with resultant suppression of the renin-angiotensin system and *decreased plasma renin activity*. Blood pressure elevation is the most common manifestation of primary hyperaldosteronism, which is caused by one of three mechanisms (Fig. 24–44):

- *Bilateral idiopathic hyperaldosteronism* (IHA), characterized by bilateral nodular hyperplasia of the adrenal glands, is the most common underlying cause of primary hyperaldosteronism, accounting for about 60% of cases. Individuals with IHA tend to be older and to have less severe hypertension than those presenting with adrenal neoplasms. The pathogenesis of IHA remains unclear.
- *Adrenocortical neoplasm*, either an aldosterone-producing adenoma (the most common cause) or, rarely, an adrenocortical carcinoma. In approximately 35% of cases, primary hyperaldosteronism is caused by a solitary aldosterone-secreting adenoma, a condition referred to as *Conn syndrome*.[70] This syndrome occurs most frequently in adult middle life and is more common in women than in men (2:1). Multiple adenomas may be present in an occasional patient.
- *Glucocorticoid-remediable hyperaldosteronism* is an uncommon cause of primary familial hyperaldosteronism. In some families, it is caused by a chimeric gene resulting from fusion between *CYP11B1* (the *11β-hydroxylase* gene) and *CYP11B2* (the *aldosterone synthase* gene). This leads to a sustained production of hybrid steroids in addition to both cortisol and aldosterone. The activation of aldosterone secretion is under the influence of ACTH and hence is suppressible by exogenous administration of dexamethasone.

In *secondary hyperaldosteronism*, in contrast, aldosterone release occurs in response to activation of the renin-angiotensin system (Chapter 11). It is characterized by *increased levels of plasma renin* and is encountered in conditions such as the following:

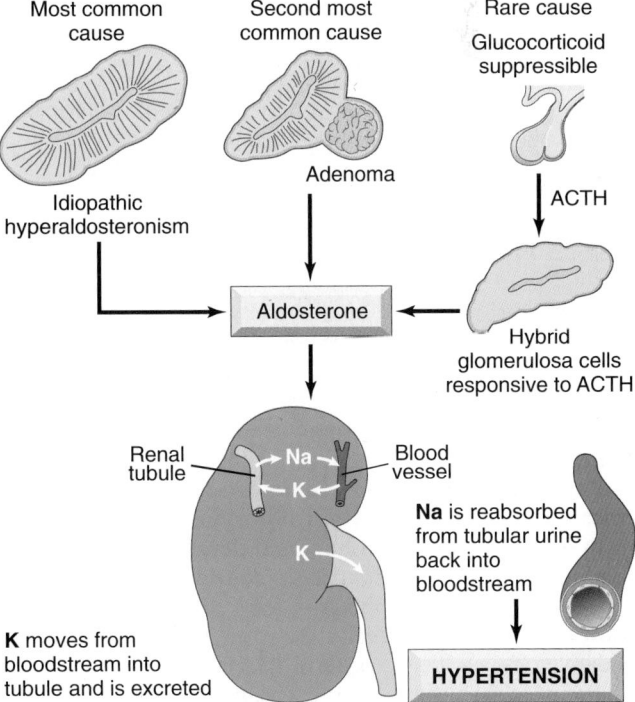

FIGURE 24–44 The major causes of primary hyperaldosteronism and its principal effects on the kidney.

- Decreased renal perfusion (arteriolar nephrosclerosis, renal artery stenosis)
- Arterial hypovolemia and edema (congestive heart failure, cirrhosis, nephrotic syndrome)
- Pregnancy (due to estrogen-induced increases in plasma renin substrate)

Morphology. Aldosterone-producing adenomas are almost always solitary, small (<2 cm in diameter), well-circumscribed lesions, more often found on the left than on the right. They tend to occur in the 30s and 40s, and in women more often than in men. These lesions are often buried within the gland and do not produce visible enlargement, a point to be remembered in interpreting sonographic or scanning images. They are bright yellow on cut section and, surprisingly, are composed of lipid-laden cortical cells that more closely resemble fasciculata cells than glomerulosa cells (the normal source of aldosterone). In general, the cells tend to be uniform in size and shape and resemble mature cortical cells; occasionally, there is modest nuclear and cellular pleomorphism (see Fig. 24–50). A characteristic feature of aldosterone-producing adenomas is the presence of eosinophilic, laminated cytoplasmic inclusions, known as **spironolactone bodies**, found after treatment with the antihypertensive drug spironolactone. In contrast to cortical adenomas associated with Cushing syndrome, those associated with hyperaldosteronism do not usually suppress ACTH secretion. Therefore, the adjacent adrenal cortex and that of the contralateral gland are not atrophic.

Bilateral idiopathic hyperplasia is marked by diffuse and focal hyperplasia of cells resembling those of the normal zona glomerulosa. The hyperplasia is often wedge-shaped, extending from the periphery toward the center of the gland. Bilateral enlargement can be subtle in idiopathic hyperplasia, and as a rule, an adrenocortical adenoma should be carefully excluded as the cause for hyperaldosteronism.

Clinical Course. *The clinical sine qua non of hyperaldosteronism is hypertension.* With an estimated prevalence rate of 5% to 10% among nonselected hypertensive patients, primary hyperaldosteronism may be the most common cause of secondary hypertension (i.e., hypertension secondary to an identifiable cause). The prevalence of hyperaldosteronism increases with the severity of hypertension, reaching nearly 20% in patients who are classified as having treatment-resistant hypertension. Through its effects on the renal mineralocorticoid receptor, aldosterone promotes sodium reabsorption, which secondarily increases the reabsorption of water, expanding the extracellular fluid volume and elevating cardiac output. In addition, *aldosterone contributes to endothelial dysfunction* by decreasing glucose-6-phospate dehydrogenase levels, which, in turn, reduces endothelial nitric oxide synthesis and causes oxidative stress.[71] The long-term effects of hyperaldosteronism-induced hypertension are cardiovascular compromise (e.g., left ventricular hypertrophy and reduced diastolic volumes) and an increase in the prevalence of adverse events

such as stroke and myocardial infarction. *Hypokalemia* was considered a mandatory feature of primary hyperaldosteronism, but increasing numbers of normokalemic patients are now diagnosed. Hypokalemia results from renal potassium wasting and, when present, can cause a variety of neuromuscular manifestations, including weakness, paresthesias, visual disturbances, and occasionally frank tetany. The diagnosis of primary hyperaldosteronism is confirmed by elevated ratios of plasma aldosterone concentration to plasma renin activity; if this screening test is positive, a confirmatory *aldosterone suppression test* must be performed, since many unrelated causes can alter the plasma aldosterone and renin ratios.

In primary hyperaldosteronism, the therapy varies according to cause. Adenomas are amenable to surgical excision. In contrast, surgical intervention is not very beneficial in patients with primary hyperaldosteronism due to bilateral hyperplasia, which often occurs in children and young adults. These patients are best managed medically with an aldosterone antagonist such as spironolactone. The treatment of secondary hyperaldosteronism rests on correcting the underlying cause stimulating the renin-angiotensin system.

Adrenogenital Syndromes

Disorders of sexual differentiation, such as virilization or feminization, can be caused by primary gonadal disorders (Chapter 22) and several primary adrenal disorders. The adrenal cortex secretes two compounds—dehydroepiandrosterone and androstenedione—that can be converted to testosterone in peripheral tissues. Unlike gonadal androgens, ACTH regulates adrenal androgen formation (Fig. 24–45); thus, excess secretion can occur either as a "pure" syndrome or as a component of Cushing disease. The adrenal causes of androgen excess include *adrenocortical neoplasms* and a group of disorders that have been designated *congenital adrenal hyperplasia (CAH)*.

Adrenocortical neoplasms associated with virilization are more likely to be *androgen-secreting adrenal carcinomas* than adenomas. Such tumors are often also associated with hypercortisolism ("mixed syndrome"). They are morphologically identical to other cortical neoplasms and will be discussed later.

CAH represents a group of autosomal-recessive, inherited metabolic errors, each characterized by a deficiency or total lack of a particular enzyme involved in the biosynthesis of cortical steroids, particularly cortisol. Steroidogenesis is then channeled into other pathways, leading to increased production of androgens, which accounts for virilization. Simultaneously, the deficiency of cortisol results in increased secretion of ACTH, resulting in adrenal hyperplasia. Certain enzyme defects may also impair aldosterone secretion, adding *salt wasting* to the virilizing syndrome. Other enzyme deficiencies may be incompatible with life or, in rare instances, may involve only the aldosterone pathway without involving cortisol synthesis. Thus, there is a spectrum of these syndromes; the following remarks focus on the most common.

21-Hydroxylase Deficiency. The defective conversion of progesterone to 11-deoxycorticosterone by 21-hydroxylase (the product of *CYP21A2*) accounts for over 90% of cases of CAH. Figure 24–45 illustrates normal adrenal steroidogenesis and the consequences of 21-hydroxylase deficiency, which

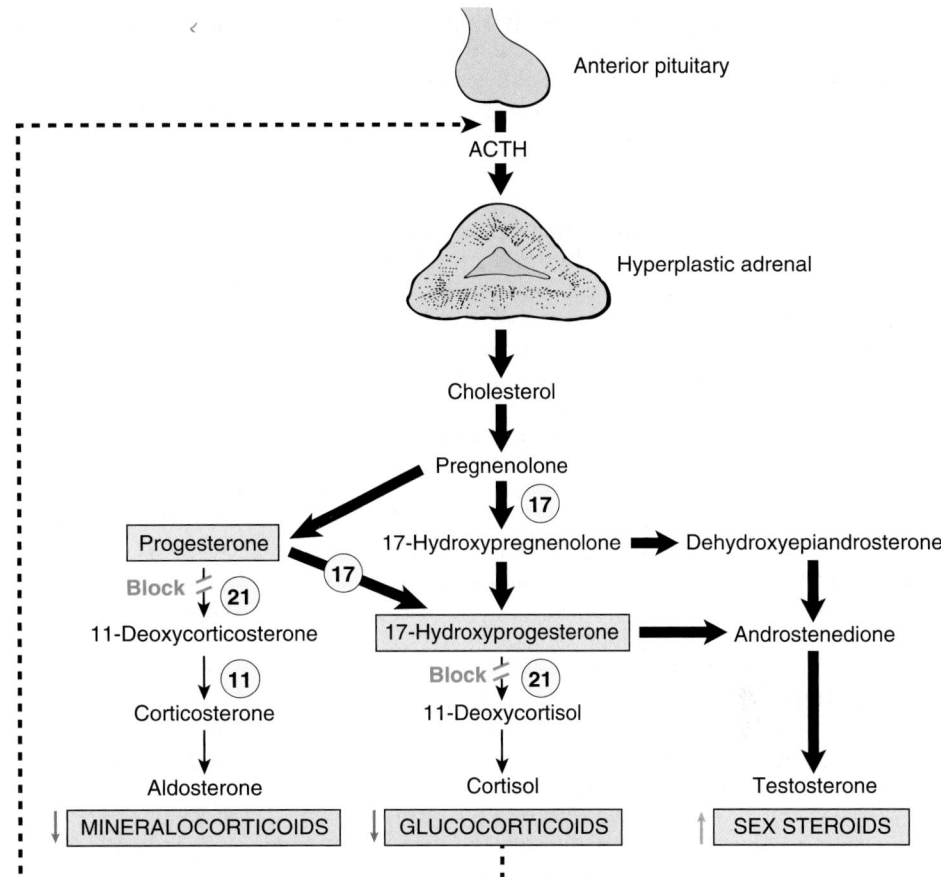

Anterior pituitary

ACTH

Hyperplastic adrenal

Cholesterol

Pregnenolone

17

Progesterone

Block 21

11-Deoxycorticosterone

11

Corticosterone

Aldosterone

↓ MINERALOCORTICOIDS

17

17-Hydroxypregnenolone → Dehydroxyepiandrosterone

17-Hydroxyprogesterone → Androstenedione

Block 21

11-Deoxycortisol

Cortisol

↓ GLUCOCORTICOIDS

Testosterone

↑ SEX STEROIDS

FIGURE 24–45 Consequences of C-21 hydroxylase deficiency. 21-Hydroxylase deficiency impairs the synthesis of both cortisol and aldosterone. The resultant decrease in feedback inhibition *(dashed line)* causes increased secretion of ACTH, resulting ultimately in adrenal hyperplasia and increased synthesis of testosterone. The sites of action of 11-, 17-, and 21-hydroxylase are shown by the numbers in circles.

may range from a total lack to a mild loss, depending on the nature of the *CYP21A2* mutation. Three distinctive syndromes have been described: (1) salt-wasting (classic) adrenogenitalism, (2) simple virilizing adrenogenitalism, and (3) nonclassic adrenogenitalism, a mild disease that may be entirely asymptomatic or associated only with symptoms of androgen excess during childhood or puberty.

The carrier frequency of the classic form is approximately 1 in 120, while the carrier frequency of the nonclassic or mild form may be higher, depending on the ethnic group; Hispanics and Ashkenazi Jewish populations have the highest carrier frequencies. The incidence of classic 21-hydroxylase deficiency varies somewhat between populations, with a worldwide mean of around 1 in 13,000 newborns. The mechanism of *CYP21A2* gene inactivation in 21-hydroxylase deficiency involves recombination with a neighboring pseudogene on chromosome 6p21 called *CYP21A1* (a *pseudogene* is an inactive homologous gene created by ancestral duplication in a localized region of the genome).[72] In the majority of cases of CAH, portions of the *CYP21A1* pseudogene replace all or part of the active *CYP21A2* gene. The introduction of nonfunctional sequences from *CYP21A1* into the *CYP21A2* sequence has the same effect as inactivating mutations in *CYP21A2*.

The *salt-wasting syndrome* results from an inability to convert progesterone into deoxycorticosterone because of a total lack of the hydroxylase. Thus, there is virtually no synthesis of mineralocorticoids, and concomitantly, there is a block in the conversion of hydroxyprogesterone into deoxycortisol resulting in deficient cortisol synthesis. This pattern usually comes to light soon after birth, because in utero the electrolytes and fluids can be maintained by the maternal kidneys. There is *salt wasting, hyponatremia,* and *hyperkalemia,* which induce acidosis, *hypotension,* cardiovascular collapse, and possibly death. The concomitant block in cortisol synthesis and excess production of androgens, however, lead to virilization, which is easily recognized in the female at birth or in utero but is difficult to recognize in the male. Males with this disorder are generally unrecognized at birth but come to clinical attention 5 to 15 days later because of some salt-losing crisis.

Simple virilizing adrenogenital syndrome without salt wasting (presenting as genital ambiguity) occurs in approximately a third of patients with 21-hydroxylase deficiency. These patients generate sufficient mineralocorticoid for salt reabsorption and prevent a salt-wasting "crisis." However, the lowered glucocorticoid level fails to cause feedback inhibition of ACTH secretion. Thus, the level of testosterone is increased, with resultant progressive virilization.

Nonclassic or late-onset adrenal virilism is significantly more common than the classic patterns already described. There is only a partial deficiency in 21-hydroxylase function, which accounts for the later onset. Individuals with this syndrome may be virtually asymptomatic or have mild manifestations, such as hirsutism, acne, and menstrual irregularities.

Nonclassic CAH cannot be diagnosed on routine newborn screening, and the diagnosis is usually rendered by demonstration of biosynthetic defects in steroidogenesis.

> **Morphology.** In all cases of CAH the adrenals are bilaterally hyperplastic, sometimes increasing to 10 to 15 times their normal weights because of the sustained elevation in ACTH. The adrenal cortex is thickened and nodular, and on cut section the widened cortex appears brown, because of total depletion of all lipid. The proliferating cells are mostly compact, eosinophilic, lipid-depleted cells, intermixed with lipid-laden clear cells. Hyperplasia of corticotroph (ACTH-producing) cells is present in the anterior pituitary in most persons with CAH.

Clinical Course. The clinical features of these disorders are determined by the specific enzyme deficiency and include abnormalities related to *androgen excess*, with or without *aldosterone* and *glucocorticoid deficiency*. CAH affects not only adrenal cortical enzymes but also products synthesized in the medulla. High levels of intra-adrenal glucocorticoids are required to facilitate medullary catecholamine (epinephrine and norepinephrine) synthesis. In patients with severe salt-wasting 21-hydroxylase deficiency, a combination of low cortisol levels and developmental defects of the medulla *(adrenomedullary dysplasia)* profoundly affects catecholamine secretion, further predisposing these individuals to hypotension and circulatory collapse.[73]

Depending on the nature and severity of the enzymatic defect, the onset of clinical symptoms may occur in the perinatal period, later childhood, or, less commonly, adulthood. For example, in 21-hydroxylase deficiency excessive androgenic activity causes signs of masculinization in females, ranging from clitoral hypertrophy and pseudohermaphroditism in infants, to oligomenorrhea, hirsutism, and acne in postpubertal females. In males, androgen excess is associated with enlargement of the external genitalia and other evidence of precocious puberty in prepubertal patients and oligospermia in older males.

CAH should be suspected in any neonate with ambiguous genitalia; severe enzyme deficiency in infancy can be a life-threatening condition with vomiting, dehydration, and salt wasting. Individuals with CAH are treated with exogenous glucocorticoids, which, in addition to providing adequate levels of glucocorticoids, also suppress ACTH levels and thus decrease the excessive synthesis of the steroid hormones responsible for many of the clinical abnormalities. Mineralocorticoid supplementation is required in the salt-wasting variants of CAH. With the availability of routine neonatal metabolic screens for CAH and the feasibility of molecular testing for antenatal detection of 21-hydroxylase mutations, the outcome for even the most severe variants has improved significantly.

ADRENOCORTICAL INSUFFICIENCY

Adrenocortical insufficiency, or hypofunction, may be caused by either primary adrenal disease (primary hypoadrenalism)

TABLE 24–10 Adrenocortical Insufficiency
PRIMARY INSUFFICIENCY
Loss of Cortex
Congenital adrenal *hypo*plasia
X-linked adrenal hypoplasia (*DAX1* gene on Xp21)
"Miniature"-type adrenal hypoplasia (unknown cause)
Adrenoleukodystrophy (*ALD* gene on Xq28)
Autoimmune adrenal insufficiency
Autoimmune polyendocrinopathy syndrome type 1 (*AIRE1* gene on 21q22)
Autoimmune polyendocrinopathy syndrome type 2 (polygenic)
Isolated autoimmune adrenalitis (polygenic)
Infection
Acquired immune deficiency syndrome
Tuberculosis
Fungi
Acute hemorrhagic necrosis (*Waterhouse-Friderichsen syndrome*)
Amyloidosis, sarcoidosis, hemochromatosis
Metastatic carcinoma
Metabolic Failure in Hormone Production
Congenital adrenal *hyper*plasia (cortisol and aldosterone deficiency with virilization)
Drug- and steroid-induced inhibition of ACTH or cortical cell function
SECONDARY INSUFFICIENCY
Hypothalamic Pituitary Disease
Neoplasm, inflammation (sarcoidosis, tuberculosis, pyogens, fungi)
Hypothalamic Pituitary Suppression
Long-term steroid administration
Steroid-producing neoplasms

ACTH, adrenocorticotropic hormone.

---

or decreased stimulation of the adrenals due to a deficiency of ACTH (secondary hypoadrenalism) (Table 24–10). The patterns of adrenocortical insufficiency can be considered under the following headings: (1) primary *acute* adrenocortical insufficiency (adrenal crisis), (2) primary *chronic* adrenocortical insufficiency *(Addison disease)*, and (3) secondary adrenocortical insufficiency.

Primary Acute Adrenocortical Insufficiency

Acute adrenal cortical insufficiency occurs in a variety of clinical settings.

- As a *crisis* in individuals with chronic adrenocortical insufficiency precipitated by any form of stress that requires an immediate increase in steroid output from glands incapable of responding
- In patients maintained on exogenous corticosteroids, in whom *rapid withdrawal of steroids* or failure to increase steroid doses in response to an acute stress may precipitate an adrenal crisis, as a result of the inability of the atrophic adrenals to produce glucocorticoid hormones
- As a result of *massive adrenal hemorrhage*, which damages the adrenal cortex sufficiently to cause acute adrenocortical insufficiency—as occurs in newborns following prolonged and difficult delivery with considerable trauma and hypoxia.

Newborns are particularly vulnerable because they are often deficient in prothrombin for at least several days after birth. It also occurs in some patients maintained on anticoagulant therapy, in postsurgical patients who develop disseminated intravascular coagulation and consequent hemorrhagic infarction of the adrenals, and as a complication of bacteremic infection; in this last setting, it is called *Waterhouse-Friderichsen syndrome.*[74,75]

Waterhouse-Friderichsen Syndrome

This uncommon but catastrophic syndrome is characterized by the following:

- Overwhelming bacterial infection, classically *Neisseria meningitidis* septicemia but occasionally caused by other highly virulent organisms, such as *Pseudomonas* species, pneumococci, *Haemophilus influenzae*, or even staphylococci
- Rapidly progressive hypotension leading to shock
- Disseminated intravascular coagulation associated with widespread purpura, particularly of the skin
- Rapidly developing adrenocortical insufficiency associated with massive bilateral adrenal hemorrhage

Waterhouse-Friderichsen syndrome can occur at any age but is somewhat more common in children. The basis for the adrenal hemorrhage is uncertain but could be attributable to direct bacterial seeding of small vessels in the adrenal, the development of disseminated intravascular coagulation, endotoxin-induced vasculitis, or some form of hypersensitivity vasculitis. *Whatever the basis, the adrenals are converted to sacs of clotted blood, which virtually obscures all underlying detail* (Fig. 24–46). Histologic examination reveals that the hemorrhage starts within the medulla near thin-walled venous sinusoids, then suffuses peripherally into the cortex, often leaving islands of recognizable cortical cells (Fig. 24–47). When it is recognized promptly and treated effectively with antibiotics, recovery is possible, but the clinical course is usually abrupt and devastating. Prompt recognition and appropriate therapy must be instituted immediately, or death follows within hours to a few days.

Primary Chronic Adrenocortical Insufficiency (Addison Disease)

In an article published in 1855, Thomas Addison described a group of patients suffering from a constellation of symptoms, including "general languor and debility, remarkable feebleness of the heart's action, and a peculiar change in the color of the skin" associated with disease of the "suprarenal capsules" or, in more current terminology, the adrenal glands.[76] Addison disease, or chronic adrenocortical insufficiency, is an uncommon disorder resulting from progressive destruction of the adrenal cortex. In general, clinical manifestations of adrenocortical insufficiency do not appear until at least 90% of the adrenal cortex has been compromised. The causes of chronic adrenocortical insufficiency are listed in Table 24–10. Although all races and both sexes may be affected, certain causes of Addison disease (such as autoimmune adrenalitis) are much more common in whites and in women.

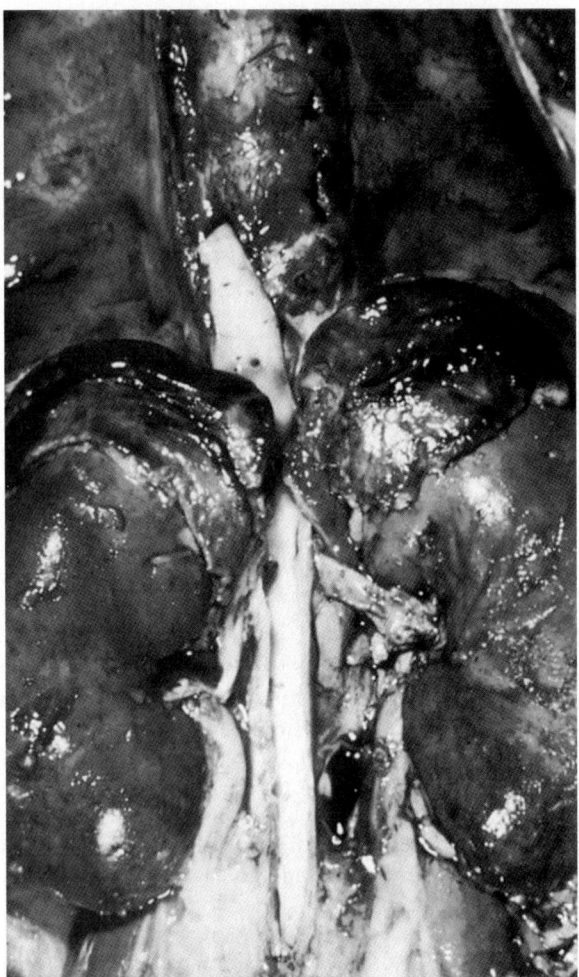

FIGURE 24–46 Waterhouse-Friderichsen syndrome in a child. The dark, hemorrhagic adrenal glands are distended with blood.

Pathogenesis. A large number of diseases may affect the adrenal cortex, including lymphomas, amyloidosis, sarcoidosis, hemochromatosis, fungal infections, and adrenal hemorrhage, but more than 90% of all cases are attributable to one of four disorders: *autoimmune adrenalitis, tuberculosis, AIDS, or metastatic cancers.*

Autoimmune adrenalitis accounts for 60% to 70% of cases; it is by far the most common cause of primary adrenal insufficiency in developed countries. As the name implies, there is autoimmune destruction of steroidogenic cells. Autoantibodies to several key steroidogenic enzymes (21-hydroxylase, 17-hydroxylase) have been detected in these patients. Autoimmune adrenalitis can occur in one of two clinical settings:

- *Autoimmune polyendocrine syndrome type 1* (APS1) is also known as autoimmune polyendocrinopathy, candidiasis, and ectodermal dystrophy. APS1 is characterized by chronic mucocutaneous candidiasis and abnormalities of skin, dental enamel, and nails (ectodermal dystrophy) occurring in association with a combination of organ-specific autoimmune disorders (autoimmune adrenalitis, autoimmune hypoparathyroidism, idiopathic hypogonadism, pernicious

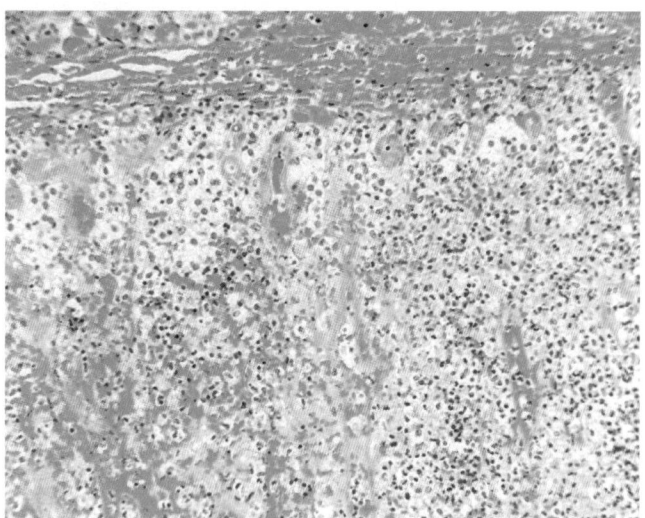

FIGURE 24–47 Waterhouse-Friderichsen syndrome. At autopsy, the adrenals were grossly hemorrhagic and shrunken; microscopically, little residual cortical architecture is discernible.

anemia) that result in immune destruction of target organs. APS1 is caused by mutations in the autoimmune regulator *(AIRE)* gene on chromosome 21q22. AIRE is expressed primarily in the thymus, where it functions as a transcription factor that promotes the expression of many peripheral tissue antigens. Self-reactive T cells that recognize these antigens undergo clonal deletion (Chapter 6).[77] In the absence of AIRE function, central tolerance to peripheral tissue antigens is compromised, promoting autoimmunity.

● *Autoimmune polyendocrine syndrome type 2* (APS2) usually starts in early adulthood and presents as a combination of adrenal insufficiency and autoimmune thyroiditis or type 1 diabetes. Unlike in APS1, mucocutaneous candidiasis, ectodermal dysplasia, and autoimmune hypoparathyroidism do not occur.

Infections, particularly tuberculosis and those produced by fungi, may also cause primary chronic adrenocortical insufficiency. Tuberculous adrenalitis, which once accounted for as much as 90% of Addison disease, has become less common with the development of antituberculous agents. With the resurgence of tuberculosis in most urban centers and the persistence of the disease in developing countries, however, this cause of adrenal insufficiency must be kept in mind. When present, tuberculous adrenalitis is usually associated with active infection in other sites, particularly in the lungs and genitourinary tract. Among the fungi, disseminated infections caused by *Histoplasma capsulatum* and *Coccidioides immitis* may result in chronic adrenocortical insufficiency. AIDS sufferers are at risk for developing adrenal insufficiency from several infectious (cytomegalovirus, *Mycobacterium avium-intercellulare*) and noninfectious (Kaposi sarcoma) complications.

Metastatic neoplasms involving the adrenals are another cause of adrenal insufficiency. The adrenals are a fairly common site for metastases in patients with disseminated carcinomas. Although adrenal function is preserved in most

such patients, the metastatic tumors occasionally destroy enough adrenal cortex to produce a degree of adrenal insufficiency. Carcinomas of the lung and breast are the source of a majority of metastases, although many other neoplasms, including gastrointestinal carcinomas, malignant melanoma, and hematopoietic neoplasms, may also metastasize to the adrenals.

Genetic causes of adrenal insufficiency include congenital adrenal hypoplasia *(adrenal hypoplasia congenita)* and *adrenoleukodystrophy*. Adrenoleukodystrophy is described in Chapter 28. Congenital adrenal hypoplasia is a rare X-linked disease caused by mutations in a gene that encodes a transcription factor implicated in adrenal development.

Morphology. The anatomic changes in the adrenal glands depend on the underlying disease. **Primary autoimmune adrenalitis** is characterized by irregularly shrunken glands, which may be difficult to identify within the suprarenal adipose tissue. Histologically the cortex contains only scattered residual cortical cells in a collapsed network of connective tissue. A variable lymphoid infiltrate is present in the cortex and may extend into the adjacent medulla, although the medulla is otherwise preserved (Fig. 24–48). In cases of **tuberculous and fungal disease** the adrenal architecture is effaced by a granulomatous inflammatory reaction identical to that encountered in other sites of infection. When hypoadrenalism is caused by **metastatic carcinoma**, the adrenals are enlarged, and their normal architecture is obscured by the infiltrating neoplasm.

Clinical Course. Addison disease begins insidiously and does not come to attention until the levels of circulating glucocorticoids and mineralocorticoids are significantly decreased. The initial manifestations include *progressive weakness and easy fatigability*, which may be dismissed as nonspecific complaints. *Gastrointestinal* disturbances are common and include anorexia, nausea, vomiting, weight loss, and diarrhea. In individuals with primary adrenal disease, *hyperpigmentation* of

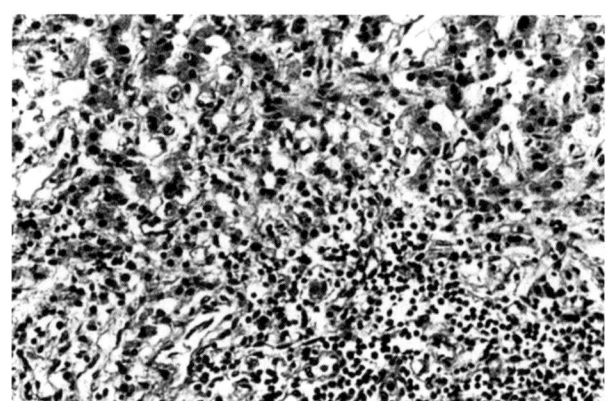

FIGURE 24–48 Autoimmune adrenalitis. In addition to loss of all but a subcapsular rim of cortical cells, there is an extensive mononuclear cell infiltrate.

the skin, particularly of sun-exposed areas and at pressure points, such as the neck, elbows, knees, and knuckles, is quite characteristic. This is caused by elevated levels of pro-opi-omelanocortin (POMC), which is derived from the anterior pituitary and is a precursor of both ACTH and melanocyte stimulating hormone (MSH). By contrast, hyperpigmentation is not seen in persons with adrenocortical insufficiency caused by primary pituitary or hypothalamic disease. Decreased mineralocorticoid activity in persons with primary adrenal insufficiency results in potassium retention and sodium loss, with consequent *hyperkalemia, hyponatremia, volume depletion, and hypotension.* Hypoglycemia may occasionally occur as a result of glucocorticoid deficiency and impaired gluconeogenesis. Stresses such as infections, trauma, or surgical procedures in such patients can precipitate an acute adrenal crisis, manifested by intractable vomiting, abdominal pain, hypotension, coma, and vascular collapse. Death occurs rapidly unless corticosteroid therapy begins immediately.

Secondary Adrenocortical Insufficiency

Any disorder of the hypothalamus and pituitary, such as metastatic cancer, infection, infarction, or irradiation, that reduces the output of ACTH leads to a syndrome of hypoadrenalism that has many similarities to Addison disease. Analogously, prolonged administration of exogenous glucocorticoids suppresses the output of ACTH and adrenal function. *With secondary disease the hyperpigmentation of primary Addison disease is lacking, because levels of melanocyte-stimulating hormone are not elevated.* The manifestations also differ in that secondary hypoadrenalism is characterized by deficient cortisol and androgen output but normal or near-normal aldosterone synthesis. Thus, in adrenal insufficiency secondary to pituitary malfunction, marked hyponatremia and hyperkalemia are not seen.

ACTH deficiency can occur alone, but in some instances, it is only one component of panhypopituitarism, associated with multiple primary trophic hormone deficiencies. Secondary disease can be differentiated from Addison disease by demonstration of low levels of plasma ACTH. In patients with primary disease the destruction of the adrenal cortex precludes a response to exogenously administered ACTH, whereas in those with secondary hypofunction there is a prompt rise in plasma cortisol levels.

> **Morphology.** In cases of hypoadrenalism secondary to hypothalamic or pituitary disease (**secondary hypoadrenalism**), depending on the severity of ACTH deficiency, the adrenals may be moderately to markedly decreased in size. The small, flattened glands usually retain their yellow color as a result of a small amount of residual lipid. The cortex may be reduced to a thin ribbon composed largely of zona glomerulosa. The medulla is unaffected.

ADRENOCORTICAL NEOPLASMS

It should be evident from the preceding sections that functional adrenal neoplasms may be responsible for any of the various forms of hyperadrenalism. Adenomas and carcinomas are about equally common in adults; in children, carcinomas predominate. While most cortical neoplasms are sporadic, two familial cancer syndromes are associated with a predisposition for developing adrenocortical carcinomas: Li-Fraumeni syndrome, wherein patients harbor germline *p53* mutations (Chapter 7), and Beckwith-Wiedemann syndrome, an imprinting disorder (Chapter 10). *Functional adenomas are most commonly associated with hyperaldosteronism and Cushing syndrome, whereas a virilizing neoplasm is more likely to be a carcinoma.* However, not all adrenocortical neoplasms elaborate steroid hormones. *Functional and nonfunctional adrenocortical neoplasms cannot be distinguished on the basis of morphologic features.* Determination of functionality is based on clinical evaluation, and measurement of hormones or hormone metabolites in the blood.

> **Morphology.** Most **adrenocortical adenomas** are clinically silent and are usually incidental findings at autopsy or during abdominal imaging for an unrelated cause (see the discussion of adrenal "incidentalomas" below). Some experts believe that all adrenal adenomas should, by definition, demonstrate clinical or biochemical evidence of hyperfunction and that incidentally discovered "tumors" are best classified as hyperplasia. In either case the typical cortical adenoma is a well-circumscribed, nodular lesion up to 2.5 cm in diameter that expands the adrenal (Fig. 24–49). In contrast to functional adenomas, which are associated with atrophy of the adjacent cortex, the cortex adjacent to nonfunctional adenomas is normal. On cut surface, adenomas are usually yellow to yellow-brown because of the presence of lipid. Microscopically, adenomas are composed of cells similar to those populating the normal adrenal cortex. The nuclei tend to be small, although some degree of pleomorphism may be encountered even in benign

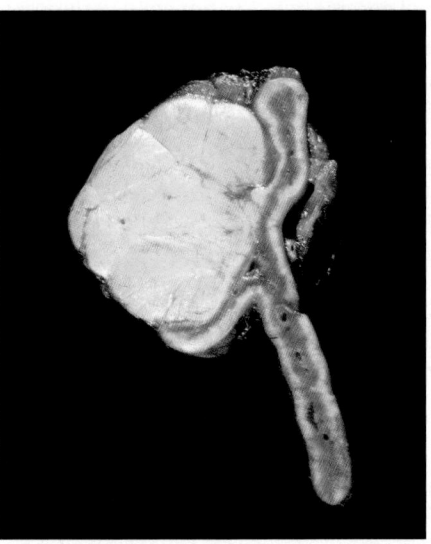

FIGURE 24–49 Adrenal cortical adenoma. The adenoma is distinguished from nodular hyperplasia by its solitary, circumscribed nature. The functional status of an adrenal cortical adenoma cannot be predicted from its gross or microscopic appearance.

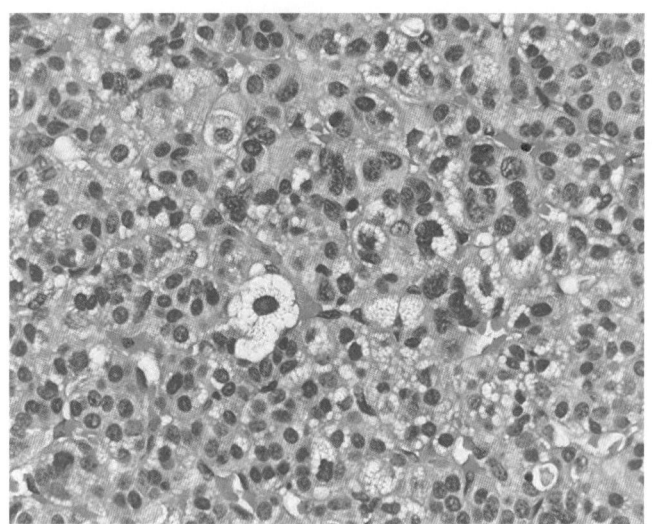

FIGURE 24–50 Histologic features of an adrenal cortical adenoma. The neoplastic cells are vacuolated because of the presence of intracytoplasmic lipid. There is mild nuclear pleomorphism. Mitotic activity and necrosis are not seen.

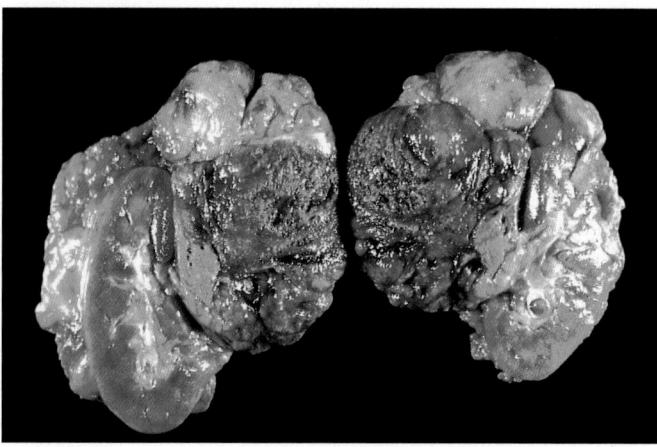

FIGURE 24–51 Adrenal carcinoma. The hemorrhagic and necrotic tumor dwarfs the kidney and compresses the upper pole.

lesions ("endocrine atypia"). The cytoplasm of the neoplastic cells ranges from eosinophilic to vacuolated, depending on their lipid content (Fig. 24–50). Mitotic activity is generally inconspicuous.

Adrenocortical carcinomas are rare neoplasms that can occur at any age, including childhood. They are more likely to be functional than adenomas and are often associated with virilism or other clinical manifestations of hyperadrenalism. In most cases adrenocortical carcinomas are large, invasive lesions, many exceeding 20 cm in diameter, which efface the native adrenal gland (Fig. 24–51). The less common, smaller, and better circumscribed lesions may be difficult to distinguish from an adenoma. On cut surface, adrenocortical carcinomas are typically variegated, poorly demarcated lesions containing areas of necrosis,

hemorrhage, and cystic change. Adrenal cancers have a strong tendency to invade the adrenal vein, vena cava, and lymphatics. Metastases to regional and periaortic nodes are common, as is distant hematogenous spread to the lungs and other viscera. Bone metastases are unusual. The median patient survival is about 2 years. Microscopically, adrenocortical carcinomas may be composed of well-differentiated cells, resembling those seen in cortical adenomas, or bizarre, monstrous giant cells (Fig. 24–52), which may be difficult to distinguish from those of an undifferentiated carcinoma metastatic to the adrenal. Between these extremes are found cancers with moderate degrees of anaplasia, some composed predominantly of spindle cells. Carcinomas, particularly those of bronchogenic origin, may metastasize to the adrenals, and may be difficult to differentiate from primary cortical carcinomas. Of note, carcinomas metastatic to the adrenal cortex are significantly more frequent than a primary adrenocortical carcinoma.

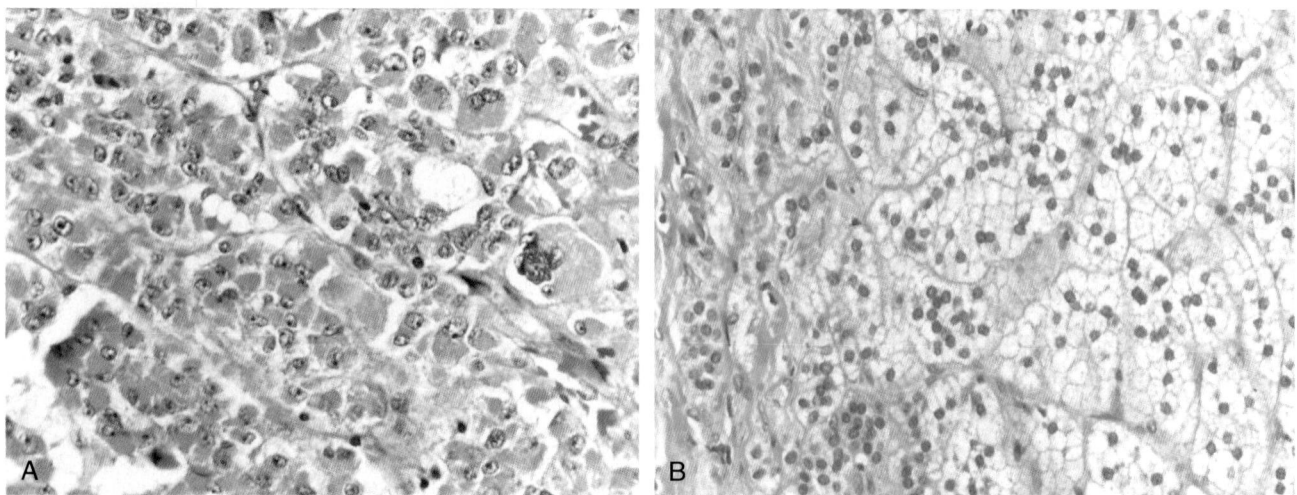

FIGURE 24–52 Adrenal carcinoma (**A**) revealing marked anaplasia, contrasted with normal adrenal cortical cells (**B**).

OTHER LESIONS OF THE ADRENAL

Adrenal cysts are relatively uncommon; however, with the use of sophisticated abdominal imaging techniques, the frequency of detection of these lesions seems to be increasing. Larger cysts may produce an abdominal mass and flank pain. Both cortical and medullary neoplasms may undergo necrosis and cystic degeneration and may present as "nonfunctional cysts."

Adrenal myelolipomas are unusual benign lesions composed of mature fat and hematopoietic cells. Although most of these lesions represent incidental findings, occasional myelolipomas may reach massive proportions. Histologically, mature adipocytes are admixed with aggregates of hematopoietic cells belonging to all three lineages. Foci of myelolipomatous change may be seen in cortical tumors and in adrenals with cortical hyperplasia.

The term *adrenal incidentaloma* is a half-facetious moniker that has crept into the medical lexicon as advancements in medical imaging have led to the incidental discovery of adrenal masses in asymptomatic individuals or in individuals in whom the presenting complaint is not directly related to the adrenal gland.[78] The estimated population prevalence of "incidentalomas" discovered by imaging is approximately 4%, with an age-dependent increase in prevalence. Fortunately, *the vast majority of adrenal incidentalomas are small nonsecreting cortical adenomas of no clinical importance.*

Adrenal Medulla

The adrenal medulla is developmentally, functionally, and structurally distinct from the adrenal cortex. It is composed of specialized neural crest (neuroendocrine) cells, termed *chromaffin* cells, and their supporting (sustentacular) cells. The adrenal medulla is the major source of catecholamines (epinephrine, norepinephrine) in the body. Neuroendocrine cells similar to chromaffin cells are widely dispersed in an extra-adrenal system of clusters and nodules that, together with the adrenal medulla, make up the *paraganglion system*. These extra-adrenal paraganglia are closely associated with the autonomic nervous system and can be divided into three groups based on their anatomic distribution: (1) branchiomeric, (2) intravagal, and (3) aorticosympathetic. The branchiomeric and intravagal paraganglia associated with the parasympathetic system are located close to the major arteries and cranial nerves of the head and neck and include the carotid bodies (Chapter 16). The intravagal paraganglia, as the term implies, are distributed along the vagus nerve. The aorticosympathetic chain is found in association with segmental ganglia of the sympathetic system and therefore is distributed mainly alongside of the abdominal aorta. The organs of Zuckerkandl, close to the aortic bifurcation, belong to this group.

The most important diseases of the adrenal medulla are neoplasms, which include neoplasms of chromaffin cells *(pheochromocytomas)* and neuronal neoplasms *(neuroblastic tumors)*. Neuroblastomas and other neuroblastic tumors are further discussed in Chapter 10.

PHEOCHROMOCYTOMA

Pheochromocytomas are neoplasms composed of chromaffin cells, which synthesize and release catecholamines and in some instances peptide hormones. It is important to recognize these tumors because they are a rare cause of surgically correctable hypertension. Traditionally, pheochromocytomas have been associated with a *"rule of 10s".*

- *10% of pheochromocytomas are extra-adrenal,* occurring in sites such as the organs of Zuckerkandl and the carotid body. Pheochromocytomas that develop in extra-adrenal paraganglia are designated *paragangliomas* and are discussed in Chapter 16.
- *10% of sporadic adrenal pheochromocytomas are bilateral;* this figure may rise to as high as 50% in cases that are associated with familial syndromes (see below).
- *10% of adrenal pheochromocytomas are biologically malignant,* defined by the presence of metastatic disease. Notably, malignancy is more common (20% to 40%) in extra-adrenal paragangliomas, and in tumors arising in the setting of certain germline mutations (see below).
- *10% of adrenal pheochromocytomas are not associated with hypertension.* Of the 90% that present with hypertension, approximately two thirds have "paroxysmal" episodes associated with sudden rise in blood pressure and palpitations, which can, on occasion, be fatal.
- One "traditional" 10% rule that has now been modified pertains to familial cases. It is now recognized that *as many as 25% of individuals with pheochromocytomas and paragangliomas harbor a germline mutation* in one of at least six known genes (Table 24–11).[79] Patients with germline mutations are typically younger at presentation than those with sporadic tumors and more often harbor bilateral disease. The incidence of malignancy is higher (~30%) in tumors that arise on the backdrop of germline *SDHB* mutations. The three succinate dehydrogenase complex subunit genes (*SDHB, SDHC,* and *SDHD*) encode proteins involved in mitochondrial electron transport and oxygen sensing. It is postulated that loss of function in one or more of these subunits leads to stabilization of the oncogenic transcription factor hypoxia-inducible factor 1α (HIF-1α), promoting tumorigenesis.[80] Notably, stabilization of HIF-1α is also the most likely mechanism underlying cancer predisposition in patients with von Hippel-Lindau (VHL) syndrome, since the VHL protein normally targets HIF-1α for destruction.

Morphology. Pheochromocytomas range from small, circumscribed lesions confined to the adrenal (Fig. 24–53) to large hemorrhagic masses weighing kilograms. The average weight of a pheochromocytoma is 100 gm, but weights from just over 1 gm to almost 4000 gm have been reported. The larger tumors are well demarcated by either connective tissue or compressed cortical or medullary tissue. Richly vascularized fibrous trabeculae within the tumor produce a lobular pattern. In many tumors, remnants of the adrenal gland can be seen, stretched over the surface or attached at one pole. On section, the cut surfaces of smaller pheochromocytomas are yellow-tan. Larger lesions tend to be hemorrhagic, necrotic, and cystic and typically efface the adrenal gland. Incubation of fresh tissue with a potassium dichromate solution turns the tumor a dark brown color due to

TABLE 24–11   Familial Syndromes Associated with Pheochromocytoma and Extra-Adrenal Paragangliomas

Syndrome	Gene	Associated Lesion	Other Features
Multiple endocrine neoplasia, type 2A (MEN-2A)	*RET*	Pheochromocytoma	Medullary thyroid carcinoma Parathyroid hyperplasia
Multiple endocrine neoplasia, type 2B (MEN-2B)	*RET*	Pheochromocytoma	Medullary thyroid carcinoma Marfanoid habitus Mucocutaneous GNs
Neurofibromatosis, type 1 (NF1)	*NF1*	Pheochromocytoma	Neurofibromatosis Café-au-lait spots Optic nerve glioma
Von Hippel-Lindau (VHL)	*VHL*	Pheochromocytoma, paraganglioma *(uncommon)*	Renal cell carcinoma Hemangioblastoma Pancreatic endocrine neoplasm
Familial paraganglioma 1	*SDHD*	Pheochromocytoma, paraganglioma	
Familial paraganglioma 3	*SDHC*	Paraganglioma	
Familial paraganglioma 4	*SDHB*	Pheochromocytoma, paraganglioma	

GN, ganglioneuroma; *NF1*, neurofibromin; *SDHB*, succinate dehydrogenase complex, subunit B; *SDHC*, succinate dehydrogenase complex, subunit C; *SDHD*, succinate dehydrogenase complex, subunit D.
Adapted with permission from Elder EE et al.: Pheochromocytoma and functional paraganglioma syndrome: no longer the 10% tumor. J Surg Oncol 89:193–201, 2005.

oxidation of stored catecholamines, thus the term **chromaffin**.

The histologic pattern in pheochromocytoma is quite variable. The tumors are composed of polygonal to spindle-shaped chromaffin cells or chief cells, clustered with the sustentacular cells into small nests or alveoli (**zellballen**) by a rich vascular network (Fig. 24–54). Uncommonly, the dominant cell type is a spindle or small cell; various patterns can be found in any one tumor. The cytoplasm has a finely granular appearance, best demonstrated with silver stains, due to the presence of granules containing catecholamines. The nuclei are usually round to ovoid, with a stippled "salt and pepper" chromatin that is char-

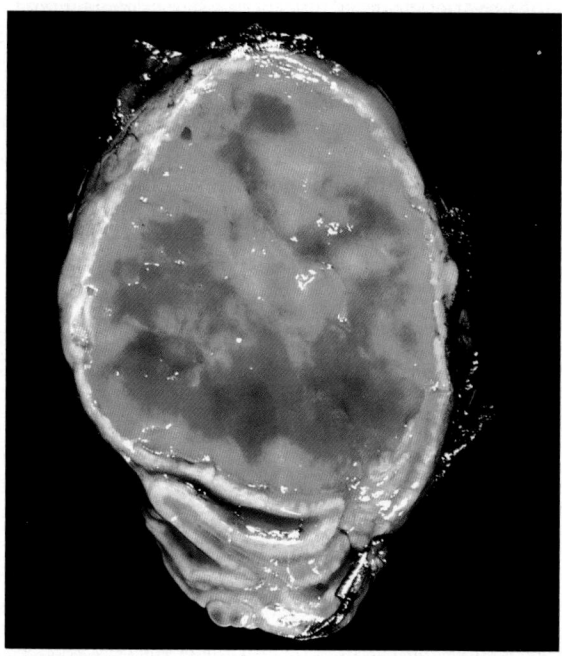

FIGURE 24–53 Pheochromocytoma. The tumor is enclosed within an attenuated cortex and demonstrates areas of hemorrhage. The comma-shaped residual adrenal is seen below. (Courtesy of Dr. Jerrold R. Turner, Department of Pathology, University of Chicago Hospitals, Chicago, IL.)

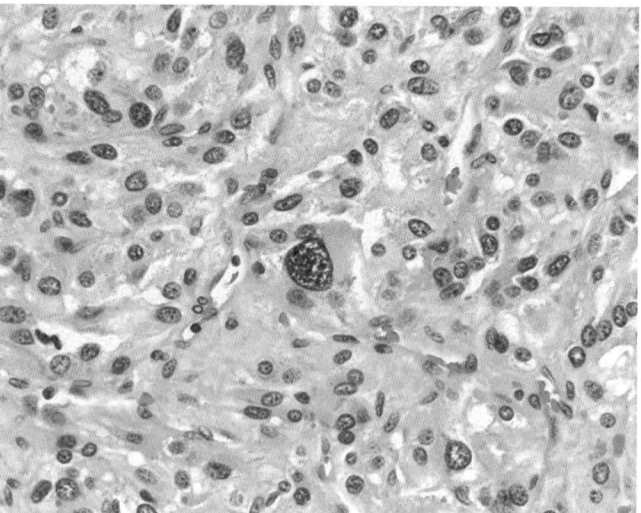

FIGURE 24–54 Pheochromocytoma demonstrating characteristic nests of cells ("zellballen") with abundant cytoplasm. Granules containing catecholamine are not visible in this preparation. It is not uncommon to find bizarre cells even in pheochromocytomas that are biologically benign. (Courtesy of Dr. Jerrold R. Turner, Department of Pathology, University of Chicago Hospitals, Chicago, IL.)

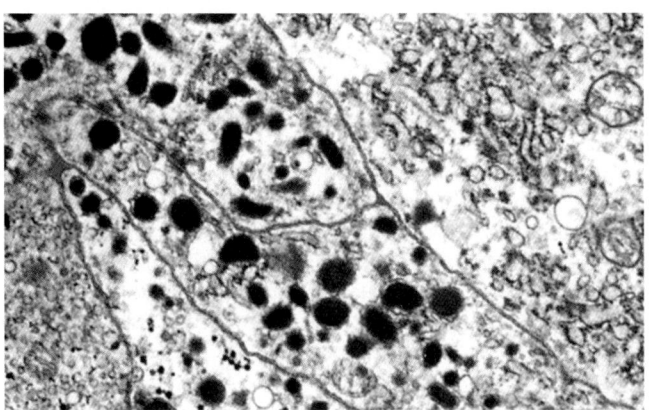

FIGURE 24–55 Electron micrograph of pheochromocytoma. This tumor contains membrane-bound secretory granules in which catecholamines are stored (30,000×).

acteristic of neuroendocrine tumors. Electron microscopy reveals variable numbers of membrane-bound, electron-dense secretory granules (Fig. 24–55). Immunoreactivity for neuroendocrine markers (chromogranin and synaptophysin) is seen in the chief cells, while the peripheral sustentacular cells stain with antibodies against S-100, a calcium-binding protein expressed by a variety of mesenchymal cell types.

Determining malignancy in pheochromocytomas can be vexing. **There is no histologic feature that reliably predicts clinical behavior.** Several histologic features, such as numbers of mitoses, confluent tumor necrosis, and spindle cell morphology, have been associated with an aggressive behavior and increased risk of metastasis, but these are not entirely reliable. Tumors with "benign" histologic features may metastasize, while bizarrely pleomorphic tumors may remain confined to the adrenal gland. In fact, cellular and nuclear pleomorphism, including the presence of giant cells, and mitotic figures are often seen in benign pheochromocytomas, while cellular monotony is paradoxically associated with an aggressive behavior. Even capsular and vascular invasion may be encountered in benign lesions. **Therefore, the definitive diagnosis of malignancy in pheochromocytomas is based**

exclusively on the presence of metastases. These may involve regional lymph nodes as well as more distant sites, including liver, lung, and bone.

Clinical Course. The dominant clinical manifestation of pheochromocytoma is *hypertension*, observed in 90% of patients. Approximately two thirds of patients with hypertension demonstrate *paroxysmal episodes*, which are described as an abrupt, precipitous elevation in blood pressure, associated with tachycardia, palpitations, headache, sweating, tremor, and a sense of apprehension. These episodes may also be associated with pain in the abdomen or chest, nausea, and vomiting. *Isolated* paroxysmal episodes of hypertension occur in fewer than half of patients; more commonly, patients demonstrate chronic, sustained elevation in blood pressure punctuated by the aforementioned paroxysms. The paroxysms may be precipitated by emotional stress, exercise, changes in posture, and palpation in the region of the tumor; patients with urinary bladder paragangliomas occasionally precipitate a paroxysm during micturition. The elevations of blood pressure are induced by the sudden release of catecholamines that may acutely precipitate congestive heart failure, pulmonary edema, myocardial infarction, ventricular fibrillation, and cerebrovascular accidents. The cardiac complications have been attributed to what has been called *catecholamine cardiomyopathy*, or catecholamine-induced myocardial instability and ventricular arrhythmias. Nonspecific myocardial changes, such as focal necrosis, mononuclear infiltrates, and interstitial fibrosis, have been attributed either to ischemic damage secondary to the catecholamine-induced vasomotor constriction of the myocardial circulation or to direct catecholamine toxicity. In some cases pheochromocytomas secrete other hormones, such as ACTH and somatostatin, and may therefore be associated with clinical features related to the secretion of these or other peptide hormones. The laboratory diagnosis of pheochromocytoma is based on the demonstration of increased urinary excretion of free catecholamines and their metabolites, such as vanillylmandelic acid and metanephrines.

Isolated benign tumors are treated with surgical excision, after preoperative and intraoperative medication of patients with adrenergic-blocking agents to prevent a hypertensive crisis. Multifocal lesions require long-term medical treatment for hypertension.

MULTIPLE ENDOCRINE NEOPLASIA SYNDROMES

The MEN syndromes are a group of genetically inherited diseases resulting in proliferative lesions (hyperplasia, adenomas, and carcinomas) of multiple endocrine organs. Like other inherited cancer disorders (Chapter 7), endocrine tumors arising in the context of MEN syndromes have certain distinct features that contrast with their sporadic counterparts.

- Tumors occur at a *younger age* than sporadic tumors.
- They arise in *multiple endocrine organs*, either *synchronously* (at the same time) or *metachronously* (at different times).
- Even in one organ, the tumors are often *multifocal*.
- The tumors are usually preceded by an *asymptomatic stage of endocrine hyperplasia* involving the cell of origin. For

example, individuals with MEN-2 almost universally demonstrate C-cell hyperplasia in the thyroid parenchyma adjacent to medullary thyroid carcinomas.

- These tumors are usually *more aggressive* and *recur* in a higher proportion of cases than do similar sporadic endocrine tumors.

MULTIPLE ENDOCRINE NEOPLASIA, TYPE 1

MEN-1, or *Wermer syndrome*, is a rare heritable disorder with a prevalence of about 2 per 100,000. MEN-1 is characterized by abnormalities involving the *parathyroid*, *pancreas*, and *pituitary glands*; thus the mnemonic device, the *3Ps*:

- *Parathyroid:* Primary *hyperparathyroidism* is the most common manifestation of MEN-1 (80% to 95% of patients) and is the initial manifestation of the disorder in most patients, appearing in almost all patients by age 40 to 50. Parathyroid abnormalities include both hyperplasia and adenomas. Hyperplasias arising in the context of MEN-1 are monoclonal.
- *Pancreas:* Endocrine tumors of the pancreas are a leading cause of morbidity and mortality in persons with MEN-1. These tumors are usually aggressive and often present with metastatic disease. It is not uncommon to find multiple "microadenomas" scattered throughout the pancreas in conjunction with one or two dominant lesions. Pancreatic endocrine tumors are often functional; however, since pancreatic polypeptide is the most commonly secreted product, these tumors might not be accompanied by an endocrine hypersecretion syndrome. Among symptomatic pancreatic tumors, gastrinomas associated with Zollinger-Ellison syndrome and insulinomas associated with hypoglycemia and neurologic manifestations are the most common subtypes.
- *Pituitary:* The most frequent anterior pituitary tumor encountered in MEN-1 is a *prolactinoma*; some patients develop acromegaly from somatotrophin-secreting tumors.

It is now recognized that the spectrum of this disease extends beyond the *3Ps*. The *duodenum is the most common site of gastrinomas in individuals with MEN-1* (far in excess of the frequency of pancreatic gastrinomas), and synchronous duodenal and pancreatic tumors may be present in the same individual. In addition, carcinoid tumors, thyroid and adrenocortical adenomas, and lipomas are more frequent than in the general population.

MEN-1 syndrome is caused by germline mutations in the *MEN1* tumor suppressor gene, which encodes a 610–amino acid product known as *menin*. How menin acts is poorly understood, but it is clear that it plays a part in regulating normal gene transcription.[81] Menin is a component of several different transcription factor complexes, which (depending on the other constituent proteins) may either activate or inhibit gene expression. For example, some complexes containing menin activate the expression of cell cycle inhibitors, such as p16 and p27, whereas menin interferes with the ability of the transcription factor JunD to activate transcription.[82] As with many other ubiquitously expressed tumor sup-

pressors and oncogenes that are preferentially associated with specific kinds of tumors, why defects in menin selectively increase the frequency of neuroendocrine tumors is unknown.

The dominant clinical manifestations of MEN-1 usually result from the peptide hormones that are overproduced and include such abnormalities as recurrent hypoglycemia due to insulinomas, intractable peptic ulcers in persons with Zollinger-Ellison syndrome, nephrolithiasis caused by PTH-induced hypercalcemia, or symptoms of prolactin excess from a pituitary tumor. As expected, malignant behavior by one or more of the endocrine tumors arising in these patients is often the proximate cause of death.

MULTIPLE ENDOCRINE NEOPLASIA, TYPE 2

MEN-2 is subclassified into three distinct syndromes: MEN-2A, MEN-2B, and familial medullary thyroid cancer.

- *MEN-2A,* or *Sipple syndrome,* is characterized by *pheochromocytoma, medullary carcinoma,* and *parathyroid hyperplasia* (see Table 24–11). Medullary carcinomas of the thyroid occur in almost 100% of patients. They are usually multifocal and are virtually always associated with foci of C-cell hyperplasia in the adjacent thyroid. The medullary carcinomas may elaborate calcitonin and other active products and are usually clinically aggressive. Among individuals with MEN-2A, 40% to 50% have pheochromocytomas, which are often bilateral and may arise in extra-adrenal sites. Parathyroid hyperplasia and evidence of hypercalcemia or renal stones occur in 10% to 20% of patients. MEN-2A is clinically and genetically distinct from MEN-1 and has been linked to germline mutations in the *RET* proto-oncogene on chromosome 10q11.2. As was noted earlier, the *RET* proto-oncogene encodes a receptor tyrosine kinase that binds *glial-derived neurotrophic factor* (GDNF) and other ligands in the GDNF family and transmits growth and differentiation signals (Chapter 7). *Loss-of-function* mutations in *RET* result in intestinal aganglionosis and Hirschsprung disease (Chapter 17). In contrast, in MEN-2A (as well as in MEN-2B), germline mutations constitutively activate the *RET* receptor, resulting in *gain of function.*
- *MEN-2B* has significant clinical overlap with MEN-2A. Patients develop medullary thyroid carcinomas, which are usually multifocal and more aggressive than in MEN-2A, and pheochromocytomas. However, unlike in MEN-2A, primary hyperparathyroidism is not present. In addition, MEN-2B is accompanied by *neuromas* or ganglioneuromas involving the skin, oral mucosa, eyes, respiratory tract, and gastrointestinal tract, and a *marfanoid habitus,* with long axial skeletal features and hyperextensible joints (see Table 24–11). A single amino acid change in *RET,* distinct from the mutations that are seen in MEN-2A, seems to be responsible for virtually all cases of MEN-2B and affects a critical region of the tyrosine kinase catalytic domain of the protein.[83] The resulting conformational change leads to autophosphorylation and constitutive activation of RET in the absence of ligand. Of note, approximately a third of sporadic medullary thyroid carcinomas harbor an identical

somatic mutation, and these cases are associated with aggressive disease and an adverse prognosis.

○ *Familial medullary thyroid cancer* is a variant of MEN-2A, in which there is a strong predisposition to medullary thyroid cancer but not the other clinical manifestations of MEN-2A or MEN-2B. A substantial majority of cases of medullary thyroid cancer are sporadic, but as many as 20% may be familial. Familial medullary thyroid cancers develop at an older age than those occurring in the full-blown MEN-2 syndrome and follow a more indolent course.

In contrast to MEN-1, in which the long-term benefit of early diagnosis by genetic screening is not well established, diagnosis via screening of at-risk family members in MEN-2A kindred is important because medullary thyroid carcinoma is a life-threatening disease that can be prevented by early thyroidectomy. Now, routine genetic testing identifies *RET* mutation carriers earlier and more reliably in MEN-2 kindred; *all individuals carrying germline RET mutations are advised to undergo prophylactic thyroidectomy to prevent the inevitable development of medullary carcinomas.*

PINEAL GLAND

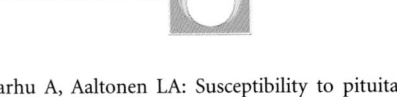

The rarity of clinically significant lesions (virtually only tumors) justifies brevity in the consideration of the pineal gland. It is a minute, pinecone-shaped organ (hence its name), weighing 100 to 180 mg and lying between the superior colliculi at the base of the brain. It is composed of a loose, neuroglial stroma enclosing nests of epithelial-appearing *pineocytes*, cells with photosensory and neuroendocrine functions (hence the designation of the pineal gland as the "third eye"). Silver impregnation stains reveal that these cells have long, slender processes reminiscent of primitive neuronal precursors intermixed with the processes of astrocytic cells. The principal secretory product of the pineal gland is melatonin, which is involved in the control of circadian rhythms, including the sleep–wake cycle; hence the popular use of melatonin for the treatment of jet lag.

All tumors involving the pineal are rare; most (50% to 70%) arise from sequestered embryonic germ cells (Chapter 28). They most commonly take the form of so-called *germinomas*, resembling testicular seminoma (Chapter 21) or ovarian dysgerminoma (Chapter 22). Other lines of germ cell differentiation include embryonal carcinomas; choriocarcinomas; mixtures of germinoma, embryonal carcinoma, and choriocarcinoma; and, uncommonly, typical teratomas (usually benign). Whether to characterize these germ cell neoplasms as pinealomas is still a subject of debate, but most "pinealophiles" favor restricting the term *pinealoma* to neoplasms arising from the pineocytes.

Pinealomas

These neoplasms are divided into two categories, pineoblastomas and pineocytomas, based on their level of differentiation, which, in turn, correlates with their aggressiveness. These tumors are rare, and are described in specialized texts.

REFERENCES

1. Ezzat S, Asa SL, Couldwell WT, et al.: The prevalence of pituitary adenomas: a systematic review. Cancer 101:613, 2004.
2. Asa SL, Ezzat S: The pathogenesis of pituitary tumors. Annu Rev Pathol Mech Dis 4:97, 2009.
3. Karhu A, Aaltonen LA: Susceptibility to pituitary neoplasia related to MEN-1, CDKN1B and AIP mutations: an update. Hum Mol Genet 16 (Spec No 1):R73, 2007.
4. Pellegata NS, et al.: Germ-line mutations in p27Kip1 cause a multiple endocrine neoplasia syndrome in rats and humans. Proceedings of the National Academy of Sciences of the United States of America 103:15558, 2006.
5. Vierimaa O, et al.: Pituitary adenoma predisposition caused by germline mutations in the AIP gene. Science 312:1228, 2006.
6. Ellison DH, Berl T: Clinical practice. The syndrome of inappropriate antidiuresis. N Engl J Med 356:2064, 2007.
7. Devdhar M et al.: Hypothyroidism. Endocrinol Metab Clin North Am 36:595, 2007.
8. Kere J: Overview of the SLC26 family and associated diseases. Novartis Found Symp 273:2, 2006.
9. Gull WW: On a cretinoid state supervening in adult life in women. Transactions of the Clinical Society of London 7:180, 1873.
10. Hashimoto H: Zur Kenntnis der lymphomatösen Veränderung der Schilddrüse (Struma lymphatosa). Arch Klin 97, 1912.
11. Kavvoura FK, Akamizu T, Awata T, et al.: Cytotoxic T-lymphocyte associated antigen 4 gene polymorphisms and autoimmune thyroid disease: a meta-analysis. The Journal of Clinical Endocrinology and Metabolism 92:3162, 2007.
12. Jacobson EM, Tomer Y: The CD40, CTLA-4, thyroglobulin, TSH receptor, and PTPN22 gene quintet and its contribution to thyroid autoimmunity: back to the future. J Autoimmun 28:85, 2007.
13. McLachlan SM, Nagayama Y, Pichurin PN, et al.: The link between Graves' disease and Hashimoto's thyroiditis: a role for regulatory T cells. Endocrinology 148:5724, 2007.
14. Graves RJ: A newly observed affection of the thyroid gland in females. London Med Surg J 7:516, 1835.
15. Jacobson EM, Huber A, Tomer Y: The HLA gene complex in thyroid autoimmunity: from epidemiology to etiology. J Autoimmun 30:58, 2008.
16. Baloch ZW, LaVolsi VA: Our approach to follicular-patterned lesions of the thyroid. J Clin Pathol 60:244, 2007.
17. Kondo T, Ezzat S, Asa SL: Pathogenetic mechanisms in thyroid follicular-cell neoplasia. Nat Rev Cancer 6:292, 2006.
18. Marques AR, Espadinha C, Catarino AL, et al.: Expression of PAX8-PPAR gamma 1 rearrangements in both follicular thyroid carcinomas and adenomas. J Clin Endocrinol Metab 87:3947, 2002.
19. Xing M: BRAF mutation in papillary thyroid cancer: pathogenic role, molecular bases, and clinical implications. Endocr Rev 28:742, 2007.
20. Santarpia L, El-Naggar AK, Cote GJ, Myers JN, Sherman SI: Phosphatidylinositol 3-kinase/akt and ras/raf-mitogen-activated protein kinase pathway mutations in anaplastic thyroid cancer. J Clin Endocrinol Metab 93:278, 2008.
21. Williams ED: Chernobyl and thyroid cancer. J Surg Oncol 94:670, 2006.
22. Albores-Saavedra J, Wu J: The many faces and mimics of papillary thyroid carcinoma. Endocr Pathol 17:1, 2006.

23. Adeniran AJ, Zhu Z, Gandhi M, et al.: Correlation between genetic alterations and microscopic features, clinical manifestations, and prognostic characteristics of thyroid papillary carcinomas. Am J Surg Pathol 30:216, 2006.

24. Wan PT, Garnett MJ, Roe SM, et al.: Mechanism of activation of the RAF-ERK signaling pathway by oncogenic mutations of B-RAF. Cell 116:855, 2004.

25. Santoro M, Carlomagno F: Drug insight: Small-molecule inhibitors of protein kinases in the treatment of thyroid cancer. Nat Clin Pract Endocrinol Metab 2:42, 2006.

26. Roodman GD, Dougall WC: RANK ligand as a therapeutic target for bone metastases and multiple myeloma. Cancer Treat Rev 34:92, 2008.

27. Brown EM: Clinical lessons from the calcium-sensing receptor. Nat Clin Pract Endocrinol Metab 3:122, 2007.

28. Kobrynski LJ, Sullivan KE: Velocardiofacial syndrome, DiGeorge syndrome: the chromosome 22q11.2 deletion syndromes. Lancet 370:1443, 2007.

29. Pinhas-Hamiel O, Zeitler P: Acute and chronic complications of type 2 diabetes mellitus in children and adolescents. Lancet 369:1823, 2007.

30. Herman MA, Kahn BB: Glucose transport and sensing in the maintenance of glucose homeostasis and metabolic harmony. J Clin Invest 116:1767, 2006.

31. Youngren JF: Regulation of insulin receptor signaling. Cell Mol Life Sci 64:873, 2007.

32. Imagawa A, Hanafusa T, Miyagawa J, Matsuzawa Y: A novel subtype of type 1 diabetes mellitus characterized by a rapid onset and an absence of diabetes-related antibodies. Osaka IDDM Study Group. N Engl J Med 342:301, 2000.

33. Wellcome Trust Case Control Consortium. Genome-wide association study of 14,000 cases of seven common diseases and 3,000 shared controls. Nature 447:661, 2007.

34. Todd JA, Walker NM, Cooper JD, et al.: Robust associations of four new chromosome regions from genome-wide analyses of type 1 diabetes. Nat Genet 39:857, 2007.

35. Jones EY, Fugger L, Strominger JL, Siebold C: MHC class II proteins and disease: a structural perspective. Nat Rev Immunol 6:271, 2006.

36. Park Y: Functional evaluation of the type 1 diabetes (T1D) susceptibility genes. Diabetes Res Clin Pract 77 Suppl 1:S110, 2007.

37. Chistiakov et al.: The crucial role of IL-2/IL-2RA-mediated immune regulation in the pathogenesis of type 1 diabetes, an evidence coming from genetic and animal model studies. Immunol Lett 118:1, 2008.

38. Hviid A, Stellfeld M, Wohlfahrt J, Melbye M: Childhood vaccination and type 1 diabetes. N Engl J Med 350:1398, 2004.

39. Eisenbarth GS: Type I diabetes mellitus. A chronic autoimmune disease. N Engl J Med 314:1360, 1986.

40. Knip M, Siljander H: Autoimmune mechanisms in type 1 diabetes. Autoimm Rev 7:550, 2008.

41. Zhang L et al.: Insulin as an autoantigen in NOD/human diabetes. Curr Opin Immunol 20:111, 2008.

42. Taplin CE, Barker JM: Autoantibodies in type 1 diabetes. Autoimmunity 41:11, 2008.

43. Frayling TM: Genome-wide association studies provide new insights into type 2 diabetes aetiology. Nat Rev Genet 8:657, 2007.

44. Zeggini E, et al.: Meta-analysis of genome-wide association data and large-scale replication identifies additional susceptibility loci for type 2 diabetes. Nat Genet 2008.

45. Michael MD, et al.: Loss of insulin signaling in hepatocytes leads to severe insulin resistance and progressive hepatic dysfunction. Molecular Cell 6:87, 2000.

46. Muoio DM, Newgard CB: Mechanisms of disease: molecular and metabolic mechanisms of insulin resistance and beta-cell failure in type 2 diabetes. Nat Rev Mol Cell Biol 9:193, 2008.

47. Kahn SE, Hull RL, Utzschneider KM: Mechanisms linking obesity to insulin resistance and type 2 diabetes. Nature 444:840, 2006.

48. Long YC, Zierath JR: AMP-activated protein kinase signaling in metabolic regulation. J Clin Invest 116:1776, 2006.

49. Lyssenko V, Lupi R, Marchetti P, et al.: Mechanisms by which common variants in the TCF7L2 gene increase risk of type 2 diabetes. J Clin Invest 117:2155, 2007.

50. Babenko AP, et al.: Activating mutations in the ABCC8 gene in neonatal diabetes mellitus. N Engl J Med 355:456, 2006.

51. Gloyn AL, et al.: Activating mutations in the gene encoding the ATP-sensitive potassium-channel subunit Kir6.2 and permanent neonatal diabetes. N Engl J Med 350:1838, 2004.

52. Murphy R, et al.: Clinical features, diagnosis and management of maternally inherited diabetes and deafness (MIDD) associated with the 3243A>G mitochondrial point mutation. Diabet Med 2008.

53. Stoy J, et al.: Insulin gene mutations as a cause of permanent neonatal diabetes. Proc Nat Acad Sci USA 104:15040, 2007.

54. Agostini M, et al.: Non-DNA binding, dominant-negative, human PPAR-gamma mutations cause lipodystrophic insulin resistance. Cell Metab 4:303, 2006.

55. Harja E, et al.: Vascular and inflammatory stresses mediate atherosclerosis via RAGE and its ligands in apoE-/- mice. J Clin Invest 118:183, 2008.

56. Yamamoto Y, et al.: Development and prevention of advanced diabetic nephropathy in RAGE-overexpressing mice. J Clin Invest 108:261, 2001.

57. Clarke M, Dodson PM: PKC inhibition and diabetic microvascular complications. Best Pract Res Clin Endocrinol Metab 21:573, 2007.

58. Tomlinson DR, Gardiner NJ: Glucose neurotoxicity. Nat Rev Neurosci 9:36, 2008.

59. Daneman D: Type 1 diabetes. Lancet 367:847, 2006.

60. Stumvoll M, et al.: Type 2 diabetes: principles of pathogenesis and therapy. Lancet 365:1333, 2005.

61. Boyle PJ: Diabetes mellitus and macrovascular disease: mechanisms and mediators. Am J Med 120:S12, 2007.

62. Zimmet P, et al.: Global and societal implications of the diabetes epidemic. Nature 414:782, 2001.

63. Despres JP, Lemieux I: Abdominal obesity and metabolic syndrome. Nature 444:881, 2006.

64. Pi-Sunyer X, et al.: Reduction in weight and cardiovascular disease risk factors in individuals with type 2 diabetes: one-year results of the look AHEAD trial. Diabetes Care 30:1374, 2007.

65. Delonlay P, et al.: Neonatal hyperinsulinism: clinicopathologic correlation. Hum Pathol 38:387, 2007.

66. Newell-Price J, et al.: Cushing's syndrome. Lancet 367:1605, 2006.

67. Cushing HW: The basophil adenomas of the pituitary body and their clinical manifestations (pituitary basophilism). Bull Johns Hopkins Hosp 50:137, 1932.

68. Mazzuco TL, et al.: Aberrant GPCR expression is a sufficient genetic event to trigger adrenocortical tumorigenesis. Mol Cell Endocrinol 265–266:23, 2007.

69. Horvath A, et al.: A genome-wide scan identifies mutations in the gene encoding phosphodiesterase 11A4 (PDE11A) in individuals with adrenocortical hyperplasia. Nat Genet 38:794, 2006.

70. Conn JW, Louis LH: Primary aldosteronism: a new clinical entity. Trans Assoc Am Physicians 68:215, 1955.

71. Leopold JA, et al.: Aldosterone impairs vascular reactivity by decreasing glucose-6-phosphate dehydrogenase activity. Nature Medicine 13:189, 2007.

72. Goncalves J, et al.: Congenital adrenal hyperplasia: focus on the molecular basis of 21-hydroxylase deficiency. Expert Rev Mol Med 9:1, 2007.

73. Merke DP, et al.: Adrenomedullary dysplasia and hypofunction in patients with classic 21-hydroxylase deficiency. N Engl J Med 343:1362, 2000.

74. Waterhouse R: A case of suprarenal apoplexy. Lancet 1:577, 1911.

75. Friderichsen C: Nebennierenapoplexie bei kleinen Kindern. Jahrbuch für Kinderhilkunde 87:109, 1918.

76. Addison T: On the constitutional and local effects of disease of the suprarenal capsules. London: Samuel Highley; 1855.

77. Mathis D, Benoist C: A decade of AIRE. Nat Rev Immunol 7:645, 2007.

78. Young WF, Jr: Clinical practice. The incidentally discovered adrenal mass. N Engl J Med 356:601, 2007.

79. Elder EE, et al.: Pheochromocytoma and functional paraganglioma syndrome: no longer the 10% tumor. J Surg Oncol 89:193, 2005.

80. Kaelin WG: Von hippel-lindau disease. Annu Rev Pathol 2:145, 2007.

81. Scacheri PC, et al.: Genome-wide analysis of menin binding provides insights into MEN1 tumorigenesis. PLoS Genet 2:e51, 2006.

82. Agarwal SK, et al.: Transcription factor JunD, deprived of menin, switches from growth suppressor to growth promoter. Proc Nat Acad Sci USA 100:10770, 2003.

83. Gujral TS, et al.: Molecular mechanisms of RET receptor-mediated oncogenesis in multiple endocrine neoplasia 2B. Cancer Res 66:10741, 2006.

The Skin

ALEXANDER J.F. LAZAR · GEORGE F. MURPHY

The Skin: More Than a Mechanical Barrier
Definitions of Macroscopic Terms
Definitions of Microscopic Terms
Disorders of Pigmentation and Melanocytes
Freckle (Ephelis)
Lentigo
Melanocytic Nevus (Pigmented Nevus, Mole)
Dysplastic Nevi
Melanoma
Benign Epithelial Tumors
Seborrheic Keratoses
Acanthosis Nigricans
Fibroepithelial Polyp
Epithelial Cyst (Wen)
Adnexal (Appendage) Tumors
Premalignant and Malignant Epidermal Tumors
Actinic Keratosis
Squamous Cell Carcinoma
Basal Cell Carcinoma
Tumors of the Dermis
Benign Fibrous Histiocytoma (Dermatofibroma)
Dermatofibrosarcoma Protuberans
Tumors of Cellular Migrants to the Skin
Mycosis Fungoides (Cutaneous T-Cell Lymphoma)
Mastocytosis

Disorders of Epidermal Maturation
Ichthyosis
Acute Inflammatory Dermatoses
Urticaria
Acute Eczematous Dermatitis
Erythema Multiforme
Chronic Inflammatory Dermatoses
Psoriasis
Seborrheic Dermatitis
Lichen Planus
Blistering (Bullous) Diseases
Inflammatory Blistering Disorders
Pemphigus
Bullous Pemphigoid
Dermatitis Herpetiformis
Noninflammatory Blistering Disorders
Epidermolysis Bullosa and Porphyria
Disorders of Epidermal Appendages
Acne Vulgaris
Rosacea
Panniculitis
Erythema Nodosum and Erythema Induratum
Infection
Verrucae (Warts)
Molluscum Contagiosum
Impetigo
Superficial Fungal Infections

The Skin: More Than a Mechanical Barrier

Little more than a century ago, the noted pathologist Rudolph Virchow considered the skin as a mere protective covering for more delicate and functionally sophisticated internal viscera.[1] Then, and for the century that followed, the skin was considered primarily a passive protective barrier to both fluid loss and mechanical injury. Over the last few decades, however, studies have demonstrated the skin to be a complex organ— the largest in the body—in which precisely regulated cellular and molecular interactions govern many crucial responses to our environment.

Like other complex organs, the skin is composed of several interdependent cell types and structures that are functionally cooperative (Fig. 25–1).

- *Squamous epithelial cells (keratinocytes)*, in addition to producing protective keratin protein, are major sites for the biosynthesis of soluble molecules (cytokines) that regulate adjacent epidermal cells as well as cells in the dermis.
- *Melanocytes* within the epidermis are cells responsible for the production of melanin, a brown pigment that protects against potentially injurious ultraviolet (UV) radiation in sunlight.

- *Dendritic cells*. Skin is constantly battered with microbial and nonmicrobial antigens that are processed by intraepidermal dendritic *Langerhans cells*, which interact with the systemic immune system by migrating to regional lymph nodes. Specialized *dendrocytes* within the dermis perform similar functions there.
- *Lymphocytes*. Both the innate and adaptive immune systems respond to these signals (Fig. 25–2), including a subset of lymphocytes programmed to home to the skin through expression of cutaneous lymphocyte-associated antigen (CLA). As elsewhere in the body, cutaneous T cells are divided into helper (CD4+) and cytotoxic (CD8+) populations (Chapter 6). The local tissue response to cytokines produced by these T cells mediates the microscopic patterns and clinical expressions of cutaneous inflammatory and infectious diseases.[2]
- *Neural end organs* and *axonal processes* warn of potentially damaging physical factors in the environment and have recently been found to assist in regulation of immunocompetent cells, indicating important neuroimmune modulation.[3] Among the neural network are neuroendocrine *Merkel cells* residing within the epithelial basal cell layer. These may serve as mechanoreceptors or possibly provide neuroendocrine function in skin.[4]
- *Adnexal components. Sweat glands* guard against deleterious variations in body temperature, and *hair follicles*, in addi-

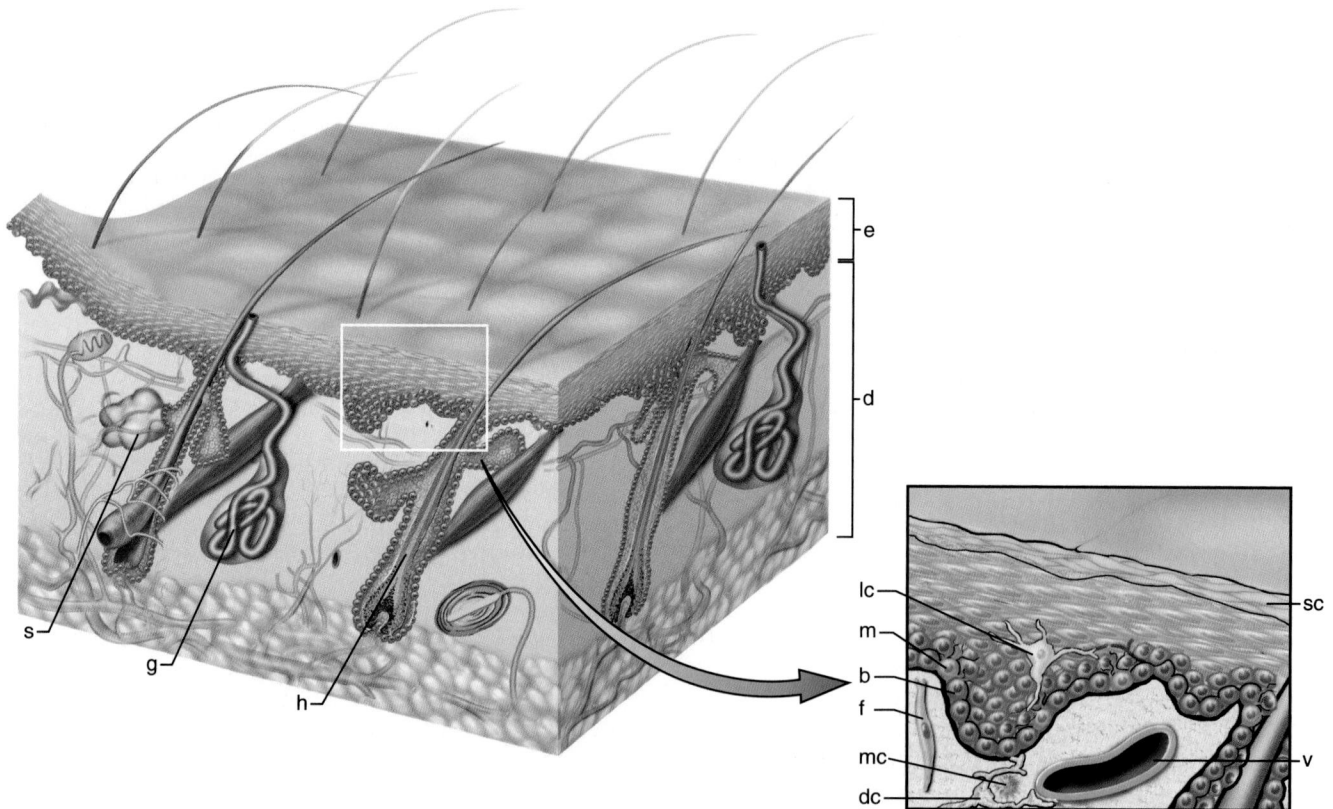

FIGURE 25–1 **A,** The skin is composed of an epidermal layer (e) from which specialized adnexa (hair follicles, h; sweat glands, g; and sebaceous glands, s) descend into the underlying dermis (d). **B,** This projection of the epidermal layer (e) and underlying superficial dermis demonstrates the progressive upward maturation of basal cells (b) into cornified squamous epithelial cells of the stratum corneum (sc). Melanin-containing dendritic melanocytes (m) (and rare Merkel cells containing neurosecretory granules) and mid-epidermal dendritic Langerhans cells (lc) are also present. The underlying dermis contains small vessels (v), fibroblasts (f), perivascular mast cells (mc), and dendrocytes (dc), potentially important in dermal immunity and repair.

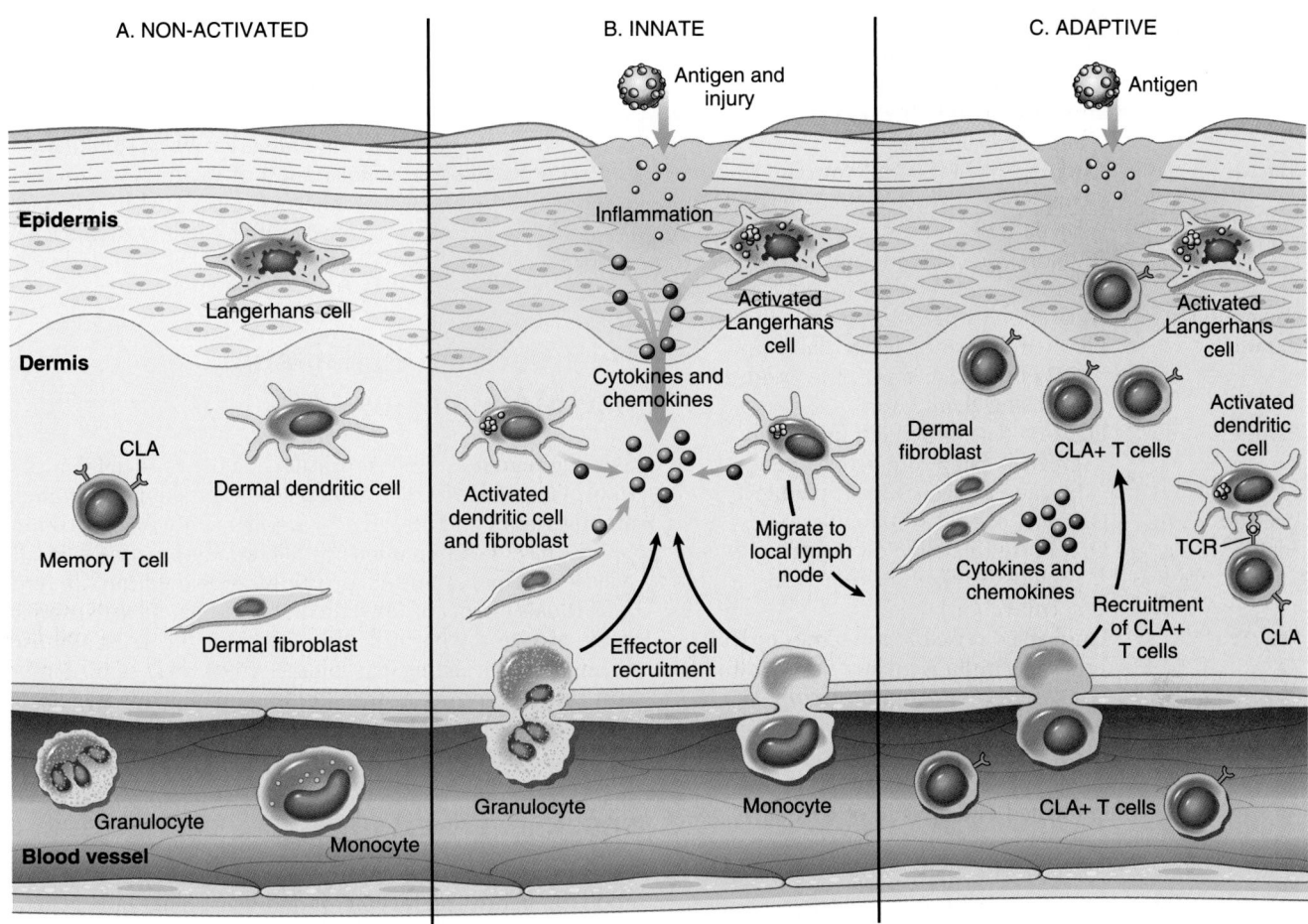

A. NON-ACTIVATED

Epidermis

Langerhans cell

Dermis

CLA

Dermal dendritic cell

Memory T cell

Dermal fibroblast

Granulocyte

Monocyte

Blood vessel

B. INNATE

Antigen and injury

Inflammation

Activated Langerhans cell

Cytokines and chemokines

Activated dendritic cell and fibroblast

Migrate to local lymph node

Effector cell recruitment

Granulocyte

Monocyte

C. ADAPTIVE

Antigen

Activated Langerhans cell

Activated dendritic cell

Dermal fibroblast

CLA+ T cells

TCR

Cytokines and chemokines

Recruitment of CLA+ T cells

CLA

CLA+ T cells

FIGURE 25–2 The cutaneous immune system. **A,** In the absence of inflammation, skin is populated by several immune cells, some stationary and others transitory, that survey the environment and are primed for response. **B,** The innate response to epithelial injury or antigen presentation activates the resident immune cells that then recruit nonspecific effector cells such as neutrophils and eosinophils. **C,** The adaptive response occurs when antigen presented in the context of the major histocompatibility complex is specifically recognized by T cells and as a result, additional antigen-specific skin-homing (CLA+) T cells are recruited. TCR, T-cell receptor.

tion to manufacturing hair shafts, harbor protected niches of epithelial stem cells capable of regenerating superficial epithelial skin structures that have been disrupted by various hostile external and internal agents (Chapter 3).[5]

Although the human integument may appear drab compared with the skin and pelage of certain other members of the animal kingdom, it is indeed extraordinarily vibrant with regard to the diversity and complexity of protective functions that it serves.

Imbalances in factors affecting the delicate homeostasis that exists among skin cells may result in conditions as diverse as wrinkles and hair loss, blisters and rashes, and life-threatening cancers and disorders of immune regulation. For example, chronic exposure to sunlight fosters premature cutaneous aging, blunting of immunological responses to environmental antigens, and the development of a variety of premalignant and malignant cutaneous neoplasms. Ingested agents, such as therapeutic drugs, can cause an enormous number of rashes or exanthems. Systemic disorders, such as diabetes mellitus, amyloidosis, and lupus erythematosus, may also have important manifestations in the skin.

Skin conditions are very common, affecting about one third of the United States population each year. Since skin is uniquely accessible to visual examination, for the experienced observer it can yield numerous insights into the functional state of the body, if not the soul, of a patient. Accurate description of the appearance of skin lesions is critical, since the gross appearance is often essential in formulating diagnoses and in understanding pathogenesis. To underscore the point, the appearance of skin lesions will be emphasized under each of the specific entities.

There are literally thousands of specific skin diseases. Only those that are common or that illustrate important pathologic mechanisms are described here. But first a brief primer of important clinical and histologic terms used in describing diseases of the skin is presented below.

DEFINITIONS OF MACROSCOPIC TERMS

| Excoriation | Traumatic lesion breaking the epidermis and causing a raw linear area (i.e., deep scratch); often self-induced |

Lichenification	Thickened and rough skin characterized by prominent skin markings (as lichen on a tree trunk); usually the result of repeated rubbing
Macule	Circumscribed lesion, 5 mm or smaller in diameter, characterized by flatness and distinguished by coloration (**patch** is greater than 5 mm)
Onycholysis	Separation of nail plate from nail bed
Papule	Elevated dome-shaped or flat-topped lesion 5 mm or less across (**nodule** is greater than 5 mm)
Plaque	Elevated flat-topped lesion, usually greater than 5 mm across (may be caused by coalescent papules)
Pustule	Discrete, pus-filled, raised lesion
Scale	Dry, horny, platelike excrescence; usually the result of imperfect cornification
Vesicle	Fluid-filled raised lesion 5 mm or less across (**Bulla** is greater than 5 mm. **Blister** is the common term for either.)
Wheal	Itchy, transient, elevated lesion with variable blanching and erythema formed as the result of dermal edema

DEFINITIONS OF MICROSCOPIC TERMS

Acantholysis	Loss of intercellular cohesion between keratinocytes
Acanthosis	Diffuse epidermal hyperplasia
Dyskeratosis	Abnormal, premature keratinization within cells below the stratum granulosum
Erosion	Discontinuity of the skin showing incomplete loss of the epidermis
Exocytosis	Infiltration of the epidermis by inflammatory cells
Hydropic swelling (ballooning)	Intracellular edema of keratinocytes, often seen in viral infections
Hypergranulosis	Hyperplasia of the stratum granulosum, often due to intense rubbing
Hyperkeratosis	Thickening of the stratum corneum, often associated with a qualitative abnormality of the keratin
Lentiginous	A linear pattern of melanocyte proliferation within the epidermal basal cell layer
Papillomatosis	Surface elevation caused by hyperplasia and enlargement of contiguous dermal papillae
Parakeratosis	Keratinization with retained nuclei in the stratum corneum. On mucous membranes, parakeratosis is normal.

Spongiosis	Intercellular edema of the epidermis
Ulceration	Discontinuity of the skin showing complete loss of the epidermis revealing dermis or subcutis
Vacuolization	Formation of vacuoles within or adjacent to cells; often refers to basal cell–basement membrane zone area

Disorders of Pigmentation and Melanocytes

Skin pigmentation has historically had major societal implications. Cosmetic desire for increased pigmentation (tanning) among whites and for fairness among normally dark-skinned people have both resulted in deleterious practices. Focal or widespread loss of normal protective pigmentation can render individuals targets of unwanted attention and extraordinarily vulnerable to the harmful effects of sunlight (as in albinism). Change in preexisting skin pigmentation may signify important primary events in the skin (e.g., malignant transformation of a mole) or disorders of internal viscera (e.g., in Addison disease, see Chapter 24).

FRECKLE (EPHELIS)

Freckles are the most common pigmented lesions of childhood in lightly pigmented individuals. They are generally small (1 to several mm in diameter), tan-red or light brown macules that appear after sun exposure. Once present, freckles fade and darken in a cyclic fashion during winter and summer, respectively. This is not because of changes in the number of melanocytes, but in the degree of pigmentation.

Morphology. Hyperpigmentation of freckles results from increased amounts of melanin pigment within basal keratinocytes; melanocytes may be slightly enlarged but are normal in density. It is unclear whether the freckle represents: (1) a focal abnormality in pigment production by a discrete field of melanocytes, (2) enhanced pigment donation to adjacent basal keratinocytes, or (3) both. The café au lait spots seen in neurofibromatosis (Chapter 5) are histologically indistinguishable from freckles, but the former evolve independently from sun exposure and can contain aggregated melanosomes (macromelanosomes) within the cytoplasm of melanocytes.

LENTIGO

The term *lentigo* (plural, *lentigines*) refers to a common benign localized hyperplasia of melanocytes occurring at all ages, but often initiated in infancy and childhood. There is no sex or racial predilection, and the cause and pathogenesis are unknown. These lesions may involve mucous membranes as well as the skin, and consist of small (5–10 mm across), oval, tan-brown macules or patches. Unlike freckles, lentigines do not darken when exposed to sunlight.

MELANOCYTIC NEVUS (PIGMENTED NEVUS, MOLE)

Most of us have at least a few moles and probably regard them as mundane and uninteresting. However, in truth moles (or nevi) are diverse, dynamic, and biologically intriguing. Strictly speaking, the term *nevus* denotes any congenital skin lesion (e.g., a birthmark). *Melanocytic nevus* refers specifically to any neoplasm of melanocytes and hence is somewhat of a misnomer, since most melanocytic nevi are acquired.

Common acquired melanocytic nevi are *tan to brown, uniformly pigmented, small (usually <6 mm across), solid regions of relatively flat (macules) to elevated skin (papules) with well-defined, rounded borders* (Figs. 25–3A and 25–4A). There are numerous clinical and histologic types of melanocytic nevi, with variable clinical appearance. Table 25–1 provides a comparative summary of salient features of some commonly encountered forms of melanocytic nevi. Acquired melanocytic nevi (Figs. 25–3 and 25–4) are probably the most common type and virtually universal. They may become more prominent during pregnancy, indicating a degree of hormone sensitivity.

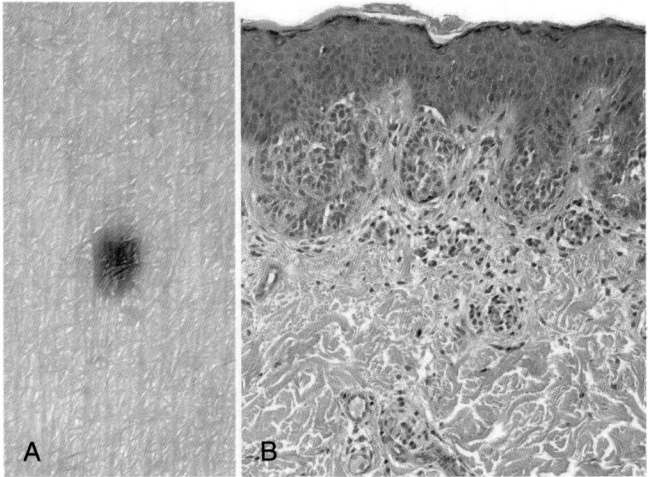

FIGURE 25–3 Melanocytic nevus, junctional type. **A,** In clinical appearance, lesions are small, relatively flat, symmetric, and uniform. **B,** On histologic examination, junctional nevi are characterized by rounded nests of nevus cells originating at the tips of rete ridges along the dermoepidermal junction.

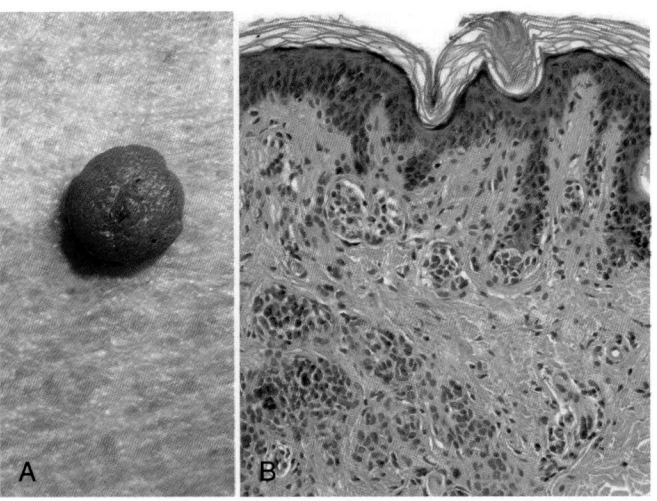

FIGURE 25–4 Melanocytic nevus, compound type. In contrast to the junctional nevus, the compound nevus (**A**) is more raised and dome-shaped. The symmetry and uniform pigment distribution suggest a benign process. Histologically (**B**), compound nevi combine the features of junctional nevi (intraepidermal nevus cell nests) with nests and cords of nevus cells in the underlying dermis.

Although melanocytic nevi are common, their clinical and histologic diversity necessitates thorough knowledge of their appearance and natural evolution, lest they be confused with other skin conditions, most notably melanoma. The biologic importance of some nevi, however, resides in their possible transformation to melanoma (see below).

TABLE 25–1 Representative Variant Forms of Melanocytic Nevi

Nevus Variant	Diagnostic Architectural Features	Cytologic Features	Clinical Significance
Congenital nevus	Deep dermal and sometimes subcutaneous growth around adnexa, neurovascular bundles, and blood vessel walls	Identical to ordinary acquired nevi	Present at birth; large variants have increased melanoma risk
Blue nevus	Non-nested dermal infiltration, often with associated fibrosis	Highly dendritic, heavily pigmented nevus cells	Black-blue nodule; often confused with melanoma clinically
Spindle and epithelioid cell nevus (Spitz nevus)	Fascicular growth	Large, plump cells with pink-blue cytoplasm; fusiform cells	Common in children; red-pink nodule; often confused with hemangioma clinically
Halo nevus	Lymphocytic infiltration surrounding nevus cells	Identical to ordinary acquired nevi	Host immune response against nevus cells and surrounding normal melanocytes
Dysplastic nevus	Coalescent intraepidermal nests	Cytologic atypia	Potential marker or precursor of melanoma

Pathogenesis. Proof that nevi are neoplasms has come from studies showing that many have acquired mutations in either *BRAF* or *NRAS*. *BRAF* encodes a serine/threonine kinase that is a positive mediator of RAS signals, and the mutations in *BRAF* and *NRAS* found in nevi both cause constitutive activation of the RAS/BRAF signaling pathway (described in more detail under melanoma).[6] Given that RAS lies in a potent transforming signaling pathway, it is reasonable to ask why nevi only rarely give rise to malignant melanomas. The answer appears to lie in the phenomenon referred to as oncogene-induced senescence. Expression of either activated RAS or BRAF in normal human melanocytes causes only a limited period of proliferation that is followed by a permanent growth arrest mediated by the accumulation of p16/INK4a,[7] which you will recall is a potent inhibitor of several cyclin-dependent kinases, including CDK4 and CDK6 (Chapter 7). This protective response is disrupted in melanoma and some melanoma precursor lesions.

DYSPLASTIC NEVI

The association of melanocytic nevi with melanoma was made more than 185 years ago,[8] but a precursor of melanoma was not clearly identified until 1978 when Clark and colleagues described the lesions that are now referred to as *dysplastic nevi.*[9] Several lines of evidence support the concept that *dys-*

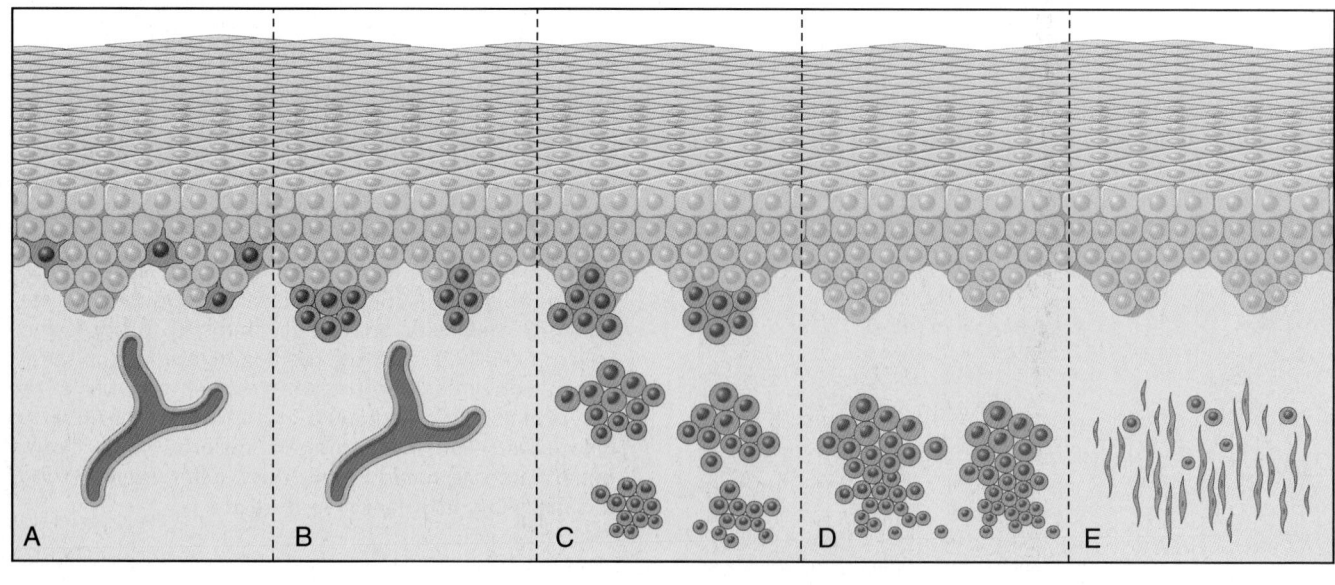

Time →

FIGURE 25–5 Maturation sequence of nondysplastic melanocytic nevi. **A,** Normal skin shows only scattered dendritic melanocytes within the epidermal basal cell layer. **B,** Junctional nevus. **C,** Compound nevus. **D,** Dermal nevus. **E,** Dermal nevus with neurotization (extreme maturation). Nevi may exist at any stage in this sequence for variable periods of time, although many are believed to progress through this sequence.

plastic nevi are precursors of melanoma. One of the most compelling pieces of evidence involves studies of families affected by *dysplastic nevus syndrome*,[10] in which a tendency to develop multiple dysplastic nevi and melanoma are co-inherited. The probability that a person with dysplastic nevus syndrome will develop melanoma is over 50% by age 60,[11] and at-risk individuals sometimes develop several melanomas at different sites. Even more directly, transformation of dysplastic nevi to melanoma has been documented histologically.

Although dysplastic nevi can give rise to melanoma, the vast majority of such lesions are clinically stable and never progress. Conversely, not all melanomas in individuals with dysplastic nevus syndrome arise from dysplastic nevi, suggesting that these lesions are best viewed as indicators or markers of increased melanoma risk. Dysplastic nevi may also occur as isolated lesions in otherwise normal individuals, in which case the risk of malignant change is very low.

Dysplastic nevi are *larger than most acquired nevi (often >5 mm across) and may number in the hundreds in those with the dysplastic nevus syndorme* (Fig. 25–6A). They are *flat macules, slightly raised plaques with a "pebbly" surface, or target-like lesions with a darker raised center and irregular flat periphery.* They can be recognized by their size, variability in pigmentation (variegation) and irregular borders, and seem to be acquired rather than congenital in most instances. Unlike ordinary moles, dysplastic nevi occur on both sun-exposed and protected body surfaces.

Morphology. Microscopically, dysplastic nevi are usually compound and exhibit both architectural and cytologic atypia (Fig. 25–6A, B). **Nevus cell nests within the epidermis may be enlarged and often fuse or coalescence with adjacent nests. As part of this process, single nevus cells begin to replace the normal basal cell layer along the dermoepidermal junction, producing lentiginous hyperplasia.** Cytologic atypia takes the form of nuclear enlargement, irregular, often angulated, nuclear contours, and hyperchromasia (Fig. 25–6C). Associated alterations in the superficial dermis include lymphocytic infiltrates (usually sparse); release of melanin from dead nevus cells into the dermis (melanin incontinence), where it is phagocytosed by dermal macrophages; and a peculiar linear fibrosis surrounding the epidermal rete ridges that are involved by the nevus. This constellation of features assists in the histologic diagnosis.

Pathogenesis. Clark and associates have proposed stages in the development of dysplastic nevi and their eventual progression to melanoma (Fig. 25–7),[12] presumably through stepwise acquisition of mutations or epigenetic changes. Dysplastic nevus syndrome is inherited in an autosomal dominant pattern. Several mutated genes have been discovered in affected families, including *CDKN2A* on chromosome 9p21 and *CDK4* (cyclin-dependent kinase 4) on chromosome 12q14, both of which are also associated with familial forms of melanoma (discussed later). However, linkage of these mutations to the dysplastic nevus phenotype is not straightforward, as not all patients with germline *CDKN2A* and *CDK4* mutations have dysplastic nevi, and not all familial dysplastic nevi are associated with mutations in these genes. It is suspected that other genetic modifiers determine whether *CDKN2A* and *CDK4* mutations cause dysplastic nevi in a particular individual; the identities of these modifier genes, as well as the other genes that are responsible for the syndrome, are being sought. Like conventional nevi, dysplastic nevi also frequently have acquired activating mutations in *NRAS* and *BRAF*.

MELANOMA

Melanoma is a relatively common neoplasm that remains deadly if not caught at its earliest stages. The great preponder-

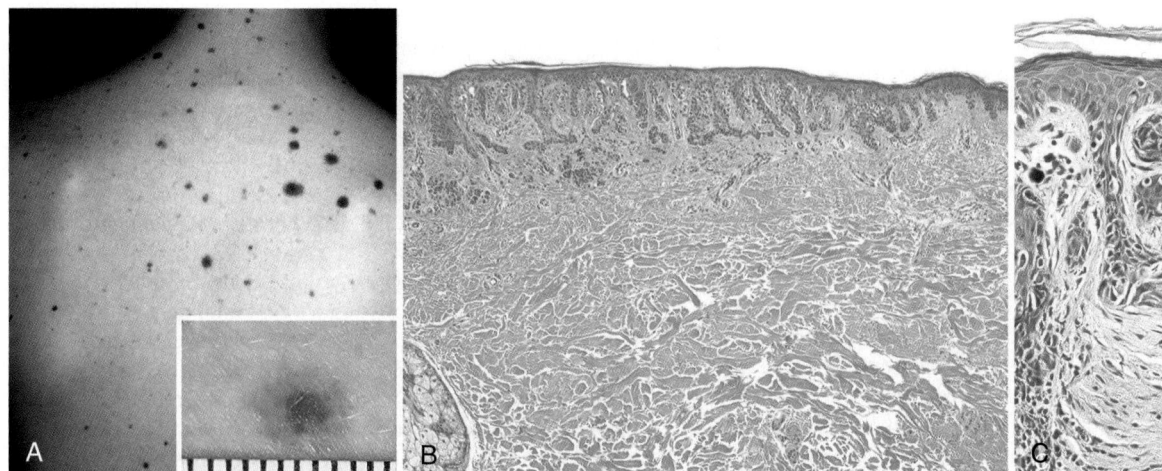

FIGURE 25–6 Dysplastic nevus. **A,** Numerous clinically atypical nevi on the back. **B,** One such lesion (*inset A*) has a compound nevus component (*left side* of scanning field) and an asymmetric junctional nevus component (*right side* of scanning field). The former correlates grossly with the more pigmented and raised central zone and the latter with the less pigmented, flat peripheral rim. **C,** An important feature is the presence of cytologic atypia (irregularly shaped, dark-staining nuclei). The dermis underlying the atypical cells characteristically shows linear, or lamellar, fibrosis.

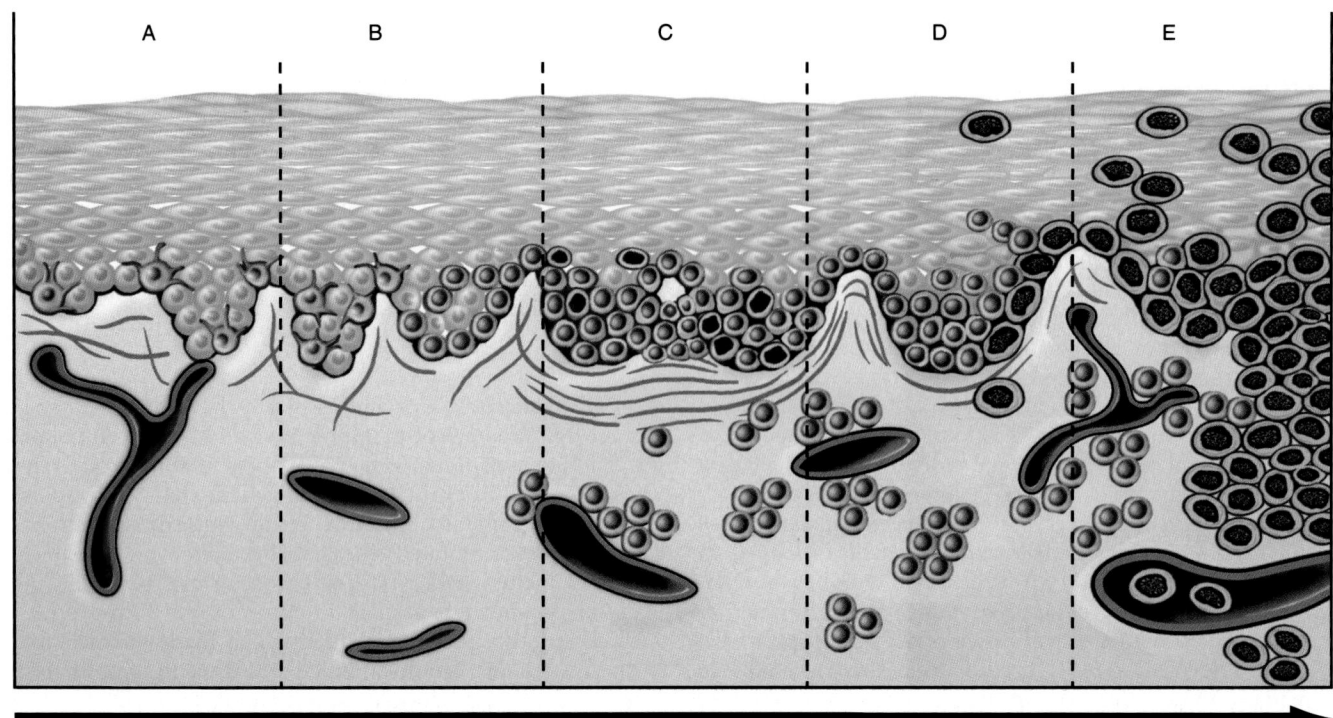

Time

FIGURE 25–7 Potential steps of tumor progression in dysplastic nevi. **A,** Lentiginous melanocytic hyperplasia. **B,** Lentiginous junctional nevus. **C,** Lentiginous compound nevus with abnormal architectural and cytologic features (dysplastic nevus). **D,** Early melanoma, or melanoma in radial growth phase (large dark cells in epidermis). **E,** Advanced melanoma (vertical growth phase) with malignant spread into the dermis and vessels. The risk of malignant transformation of any single dysplastic nevus is extremely low but can occur.

ance of melanomas arises in the skin; other sites of origin include the oral and anogenital mucosal surfaces, esophagus, meninges, and the eye (see Chapter 29). The following comments apply to cutaneous melanomas.

Today, as a result of increased public awareness of the signs of cutaneous melanoma, most are cured surgically.[13] Nevertheless, the reported incidence of melanoma is increasing; more than 60,000 cases and more than 8000 deaths are expected in the United States in 2008.[14]

Clinical Features. *Because melanomas evolve over time from localized skin lesions to aggressive tumors that metastasize and are resistant to therapy, early recognition and complete excision are critical.* Melanoma of the skin is usually asymptomatic, although itching or pain may be early manifestations. The majority of lesions are *greater than 10 mm in diameter* at diagnosis. The most consistent clinical signs are *changes in the color, size, or shape of a pigmented lesion.* Unlike benign nevi, melanomas show striking *variations in color,* appearing in shades of black, brown, red, dark blue, and gray (Fig. 25–8A). On occasion, zones of white or flesh-colored hypopigmentation also appear, sometimes due to focal regression of the tumor. The *borders of melanomas are irregular and often notched,* not smooth, round, and uniform as in melanocytic nevi. To reiterate, *the most important warning signs, sometimes called the ABCs of melanoma, are* (1) *asymmetry;* (2) *irregular borders;* and (3) *variegated color.* Other features of pigmented lesions that should raise concern are a diameter greater than 6 mm, any change in appearance, and new onset of itching or pain.

Morphology. Central to understanding the progression of melanoma is the concept of radial and vertical growth phases.[15] **Radial growth** describes the horizontal spread of melanoma within the epidermis and superficial dermis (Fig. 25–8B). During this initial stage the tumor cells seem to lack the capacity to metastasize. Tumors in radial growth phase fall into several clinicopathologic classes, including: **lentigo maligna,** usually presenting as an indolent lesion on the face of older men that may remain in the radial growth phase for several decades; **superficial spreading,** the most common type of melanoma, usually involving sun-exposed skin; and **acral/mucosal lentiginous** melanoma that is unrelated to sun exposure.

After a variable (and unpredictable) period of time, melanoma shifts from the radial phase to a **vertical growth phase,** during which the tumor cells invade downward into the deeper dermal layers as an expansile mass (Fig. 25–8C). **The vertical growth phase is often heralded by the appearance of a nodule and correlates with the emergence of a clone of cells with metastatic potential.** Unlike melanocytic nevi, maturation is absent from the deep invasive portion of melanoma. The probability of metastasis in such lesions correlates with the depth of invasion, which by convention is the distance from the superficial epidermal granular cell layer to the deepest intrader-

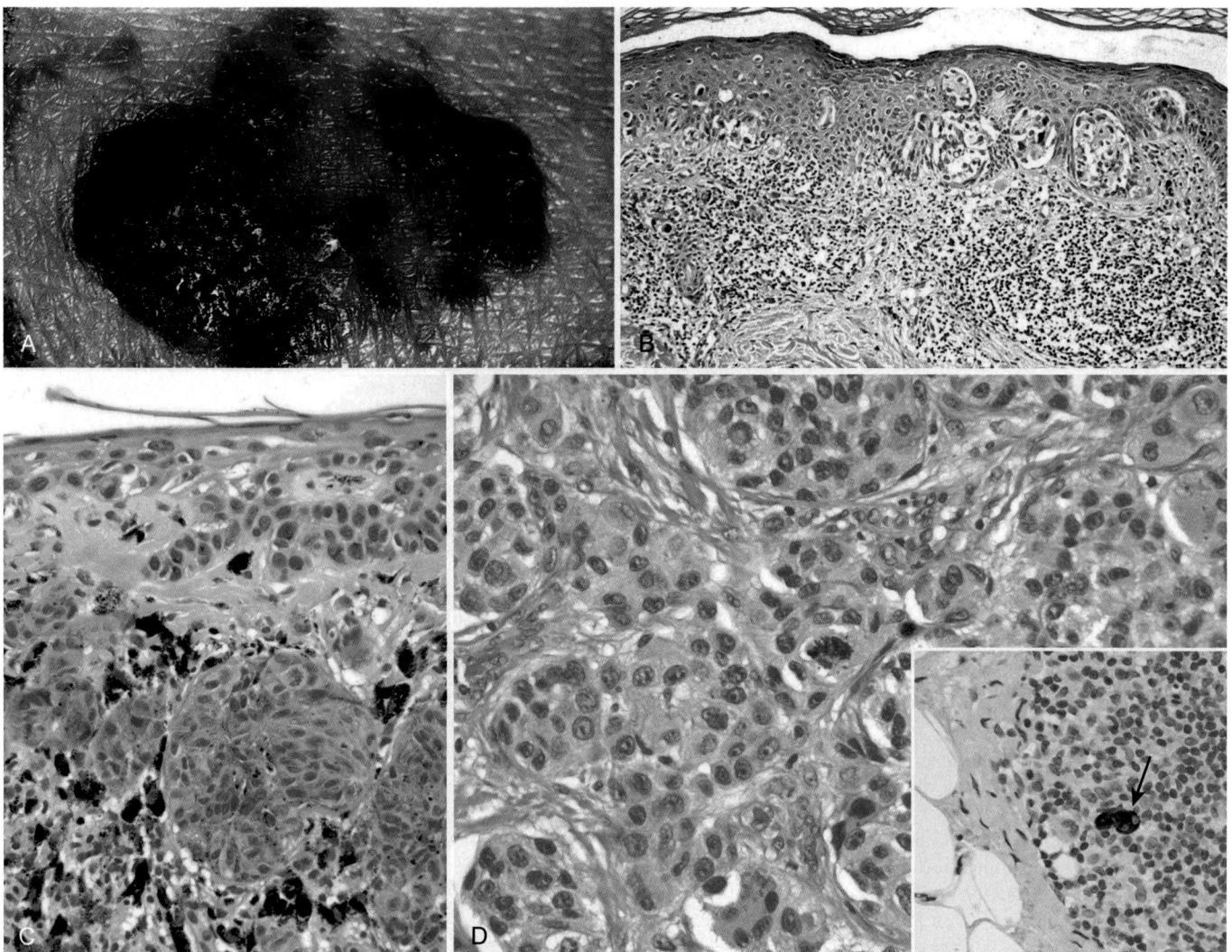

FIGURE 25–8   Melanoma. **A,** Typically, lesions are irregular in contour and pigmentation. Macular areas correlate with the radial growth phase, while raised areas usually correspond to nodular aggregates of malignant cells in the vertical phase of growth. **B,** Radial growth phase, showing irregular nested and single-cell growth of melanoma cells within the epidermis and an underlying inflammatory response within the dermis. **C,** Vertical growth phase, demonstrating nodular aggregates of infiltrating cells. **D,** High-power view of melanoma cells. The *inset* shows a sentinel lymph node with a tiny cluster of melanoma cells *(arrow)* staining for the melanocytic marker HMB-45. Even small numbers of malignant cells in a draining lymph node may confer a worse prognosis.

mal tumor cells; this measurement is known as the Breslow thickness.[16] Other histologic features that correlate with outcome include the number of mitoses and the presence of ulceration;[17,18] these and other prognostic factors are discussed further below.

Individual melanoma cells are usually considerably larger than normal melanocytes or cells found in melanocytic nevi. They contain large nuclei with irregular contours, chromatin that is characteristically clumped at the periphery of the nuclear membrane, and prominent red (eosinophilic) nucleoli (Fig. 25–8D). The appearance of the tumor cells is similar in the radial and vertical phases of growth. While most nevi and melanomas are easily distinguished based on their appearance, a minority of "atypical" lesions occupy a histologic gray zone and have been termed **melanocytic tumors of uncertain malignant potential**;[13,19] such lesions require complete excision and close clinical follow-up.

Prognostic Factors.   Once a melanoma is excised, a number of clinical and pathologic features are used to gauge the probability of metastatic spread and prognosis. One model predicts outcome based on the following variables:[20] (1) tumor *depth* (the Breslow thickness); (2) number of *mitoses*; (3) evidence of tumor *regression* (presumably due to the host immune response); (4) the presence and number of *tumor infiltrating lymphocytes* (TILs); (5) *gender*; and (6) *location* (central body or extremity). Determinants of a more *favorable prognosis* in this model include tumor depth of less than 1.7 mm, no or very few mitoses, a brisk TIL response, absence of regression, female gender, and location on an extremity. In a retrospective multivariate study by the American Joint Committee on Cancer (AJCC), tumor thickness and presence or absence of ulceration had prognostic significance independent of clinical stage.[21,22] Because most melanomas initially metastasize to regional lymph nodes, additional prognostic information may be obtained by performing a sentinel lymph node biopsy; as in breast cancer (Chapter 23), this involves the identification, removal, and careful examination of the lymph node (or nodes) that is the initial site of drainage of intratumoral lymphatic vessels. Microscopic involvement of a sentinel node by even a small number of melanoma cells (micrometastases) confers a worse prognosis (Fig. 25–8D, *inset*).[23] The degree of involvement and the total number of lymph nodes involved correlate well with overall survival.

Pathogenesis. *The two most important predisposing factors are inherited genes and sun exposure.* Melanomas most commonly arise on sun-exposed surfaces, particularly the upper back in men and the back and legs in women, and lightly pigmented individuals are at higher risk than are darkly pigmented individuals. However, the relationship between sun exposure and melanoma is not as straightforward as with other skin cancers (discussed later); some studies suggest that severe sunburns early in life are the most important risk factor. Since melanomas occur in dark-skinned individuals and at body sites that are not sun-exposed, sunlight is clearly not the only predisposing factor, and other environmental factors may also contribute to risk.[24]

It is estimated that 10% to 15% of melanomas are familial, and many (but not all) of those with familial melanoma also have dysplastic nevi. Several of the genes responsible for familial melanoma encode well-characterized tumor suppressors and are also mutated in sporadic tumors (discussed below). Other genetic variants linked to melanoma risk in fair-skinned populations control melanin production; these pigmentation genes have weak effects, conferring a slightly elevated risk. They include *MC1R*, which encodes the melanocortin-1 receptor; *ASIP* (agouti signaling protein), which encodes a regulator of melanocortin receptor signaling, and *TYR*, which encodes tyrosinase, a melanocyte-specific enzyme that is required for melanin synthesis.[25]

Mutations that diminish the activity of the retinoblastoma (RB) tumor suppressor proteins are common in both familial and sporadic melanomas. The *CDKN2A* gene (discussed earlier under dysplastic nevi) is mutated in approximately 40% of pedigrees with autosomal dominant familial melanoma. *CDKN2A* is a complex locus that encodes three different tumor suppressors, p15/INK4b, p16/INK4a, and p14/ARF. Of these, loss of p16/INK4a is clearly implicated in human melanoma, and experimental evidence also strongly supports a role for loss of p14/ARF. You will recall from Chapter 7 that p16/INK4a enhances the activity of tumor suppressor proteins of the RB family by inhibiting cyclin-dependent kinase 4 (CDK4) and cyclin-dependent kinase 6 (CDK6), while p14/ARF enhances the activity of the p53 tumor suppressor by inhibiting the activity of the MDM2 oncoprotein. *CDKN2A* is mutated in approximately 10% of sporadic melanomas,[26] and these mutations uniformly abolish the production of p16/INK4a and more variably affect p14/ARF. However, it is suspected that these mutations are the tip of the "oncogenic iceberg" with respect to molecular lesions affecting the function of RB proteins. For example, as many as 30% to 70% of

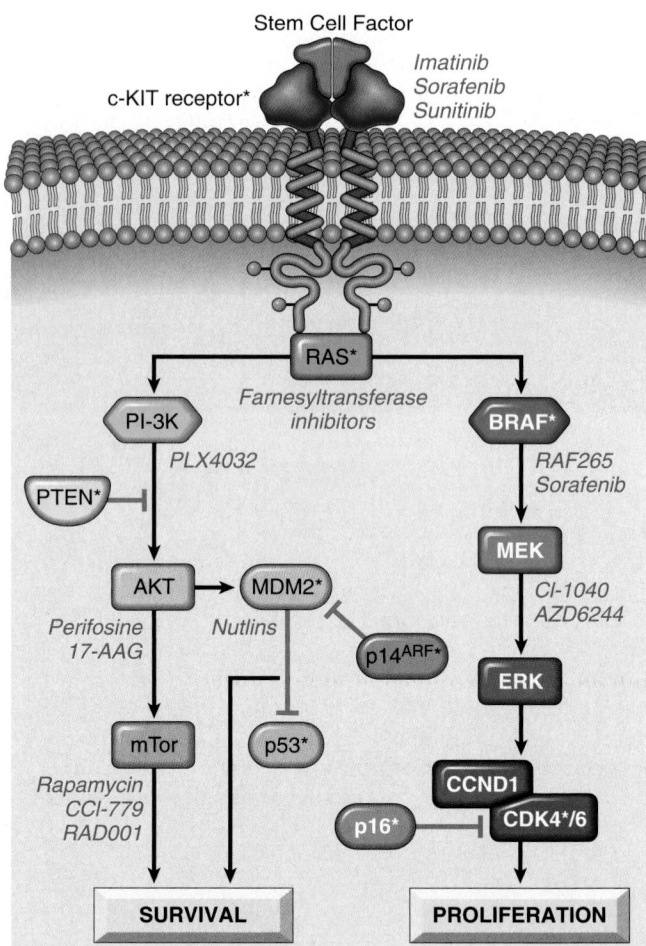

FIGURE 25–9 Pathways important in melanoma. The PI-3K/PTEN/AKT and BRAF/ERK pathways regulate cell survival and proliferation. Proteins altered in melanoma are indicated by asterisks. Inhibitors of these pathways are being studied as therapeutic agents; some specific examples are listed in red.

melanomas show loss of p16/INK4a expression though varied mechanisms,[27] and other uncommon familial and sporadic melanomas have mutations in CDK4 that prevent its inhibition by p16/INK4a. The net effect of all of these alterations is the same; increased melanocytic proliferation and escape from oncogene-induced cellular senescence.

The second common group of molecular lesions in sporadic melanoma leads to *aberrant increases in RAS and PI-3K/AKT signaling* (Fig. 25–9), which you will recall are pathways that promote cell growth and survival (Chapter 7). Activating mutations in *BRAF*, which encodes a serine/threonine kinase that is downstream of RAS, are seen in 60% to 70% of melanomas, while activating mutations in *NRAS* (which is upstream of BRAF) occur in additional 10% to 15% of tumors. For reasons that are unclear, melanomas arising in non-sun exposed sites are much more likely to have activating mutations in the c-KIT receptor tyrosine kinase,[28,29] which sits upstream of both RAS and PI-3K/AKT, than in *NRAS* or *BRAF*. *PTEN*, a tumor suppressor that acts by down-regulating PI-3K/AKT signaling, is epigenetically silenced in another 20% of melanomas.[30,31]

Molecular lesions of these two kinds are probably necessary, but not sufficient, for the development of melanoma. As discussed earlier, melanocytic nevi have the same activating mutations in *NRAS* and *BRAF* that are found in melanomas, yet become malignant very rarely, probably because unbridled RAS signaling leads to cellular senescence. p16/INK4a appears to be essential for the oncogene-induced cellular senescence,[31] and in its absence proliferation persists, placing melanocytes at risk for transformation into a melanoma. However, dysplastic nevi sometimes have lesions in both p16/INK4a and RAS or BRAF, yet transform into full-blown melanomas only somewhat more frequently than conventional nevi. Clearly, other pathways yet to be identified also contribute to the transformation process.

These molecular insights have spawned attempts to treat melanoma with new therapeutic agents that target the RAS and PI-3K/AKT pathways (Fig. 25–9). Such approaches are urgently needed, as metastatic melanoma is resistant to both conventional chemotherapy and radiation treatment. Ultimately, it is likely that these types of targeted therapies will be used in combinations tailored to the oncogenic leions found in individual tumors.[32] For example, a tumor with an activating mutation in c-KIT will require treatment with different inhibitors than a tumor with an activating mutation in RAS or BRAF. Immunotherapeutic approaches for melanoma in which host lymphocytes are "trained" to recognize and kill melanoma cells have also generated considerable interest, sparked in part by the recognition that spontaneous remissions of metastatic melanoma occur sporadically that are presumably mediated by the host immune response. Excellent responses are obtained on occasion,[33] but the general applicability of such treatments has yet to be demonstrated.

Benign Epithelial Tumors

Benign epithelial neoplasms are common and usually biologically inconsequential, although they may cause significant psychological discomfort for the affected individual. These tumors, derived from the keratinizing stratified squamous epithelium of the epidermis and hair follicles and the ductular epithelium of cutaneous glands, often recapitulate the structures from which they arise. They are sometimes confused clinically with malignancy, particularly when they are pigmented or inflamed, and histologic examination of a biopsy is frequently required to establish a definitive diagnosis. In rare instances they are a telltale sign of syndromes associated with potentially life-threatening visceral malignancies, such as multiple trichilemmomas in Cowden syndrome or multiple sebaceous neoplasms in Muir-Torre syndrome. Diagnosis of epithelial tumors in these instances may facilitate recognition of the underlying syndrome and implementation of appropriate clinical interventions.

SEBORRHEIC KERATOSES

These common epidermal tumors occur most frequently in middle-aged or older individuals. They arise spontaneously and are particularly numerous on the trunk, although the extremities, head, and neck may also be involved. In people of

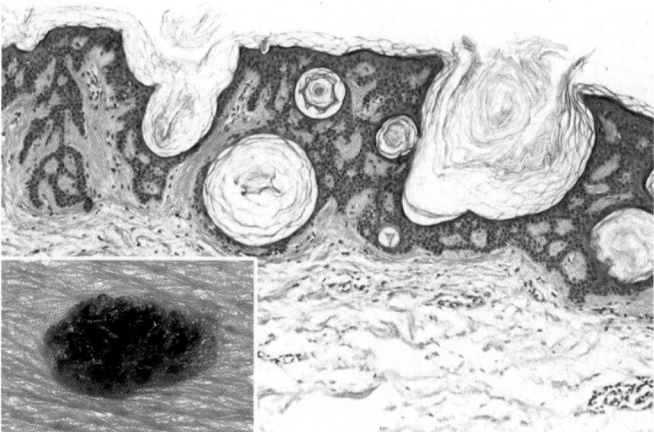

FIGURE 25–10 Seborrheic keratosis. A well-demarcated coinlike pigmented lesion containing dark keratin-filled surface plugs *(inset)* is composed histologically of benign basaloid cells associated with prominent keratin-filled "horn" cysts, some of which communicate with the surface (pseudo-horn cysts).

color, multiple small lesions on the face are termed *dermatosis papulosa nigra.*

Seborrheic keratoses characteristically appear as round, flat, coin-like, waxy plaques that vary in diameter from millimeters to several centimeters (Fig. 25–10, *inset*). They are uniformly tan to dark brown and usually have a velvety to granular surface. Inspection with a hand lens usually reveals small, round, porelike ostia impacted with keratin, a feature helpful in differentiating these pigmented lesions from melanomas.

> **Morphology.** On histologic examination, these neoplasms are exophytic and sharply demarcated from the adjacent epidermis. They are composed of sheets of small cells that most resemble basal cells of the normal epidermis (Fig. 25–10). Variable melanin pigmentation is present within these basaloid cells, accounting for the brown coloration. Exuberant keratin production (hyperkeratosis) occurs at the surface, and small keratin-filled cysts (horn cysts) and invaginations of keratin into the main mass (invagination cysts) are characteristic features. Interestingly, when seborrheic keratoses become irritated and inflamed, they develop whirling foci of squamous differentiation resembling eddy currents in a stream.[27]

Pathogenesis. Activating mutations in the fibroblast growth factor receptor-3 *(FGFR3)* gene are found in many sporadic seborrheic keratoses and are thought to drive the growth of the tumor.[34,35] Seborrheic keratoses may occur explosively in large numbers, as part of a paraneoplastic syndrome *(Leser-Trélat sign)*, possibly under the stimulation of transforming growth factor-α produced by tumor cells, most commonly carcinomas of the gastrointestinal tract.[36]

ACANTHOSIS NIGRICANS

Acanthosis nigricans is a condition marked by thickened, hyperpigmented skin with a "velvet-like" texture that most commonly appears in the flexural areas (axillae, skin folds of the neck, groin, and anogenital regions). *It can be an important cutaneous marker of benign and malignant conditions* and, accordingly, is divided into two types.[37] The *benign type*, which constitutes about 80% of all cases, develops gradually and usually occurs in childhood or during puberty. It may occur (1) as an autosomal dominant trait with variable penetrance, (2) in association with obesity or endocrine abnormalities (particularly with pituitary or pineal tumors and diabetes), and (3) as part of several rare congenital syndromes. As with seborrheic keratoses, acanthosis nigricans sometimes occurs as a paraneoplastic process resulting from the production of growth factors by a variety of tumors. The *malignant type* refers to lesions arising in middle-aged and older individuals in association with underlying cancers, most commonly gastrointestinal adenocarcinomas.

> **Morphology.** All forms of acanthosis nigricans have similar histologic features. The epidermis and underlying enlarged dermal papillae undulate sharply to form numerous repeating peaks and valleys. Variable hyperplasia may be seen, along with hyperkeratosis and slight basal cell layer hyperpigmentation (but no melanocytic hyperplasia).

Pathogenesis. Because lesions of acanthosis nigricans may precede clinical symptoms and signs of the underlying disorder, recognition of this entity may lead to early detection of covert systemic disease. The familial form is associated with germline activating mutations in FGFR3; depending on the mutation, acanthosis may be an isolated finding or be seen together with skeletal deformities, including achondroplasia and thanatophoric dysplasia.[38]

FIBROEPITHELIAL POLYP

The fibroepithelial polyp has many names (acrochordon, squamous papilloma, skin tag) and is one of the most common cutaneous lesions. It is generally detected as an incidental finding in middle-aged and older individuals on the neck, trunk, face, and intertriginous areas as a soft, flesh-colored, bag-like tumor often attached to the surrounding skin by a slender stalk. Rarely, fibroepithelial polyps and tumors of perifollicular mesenchyme (specialized fibroblasts associated with the hair bulb) are seen together in Birt-Hogg-Dubé syndrome, but the vast majority of polyps are sporadic.[39]

> **Morphology.** On histologic examination these tumors consist of fibrovascular cores covered by benign squamous epithelium. It is not uncommon for the polyps to undergo ischemic necrosis due to torsion, which may cause pain and precipitate their removal.

Fibroepithelial polyps are usually inconsequential, but can occasionally be associated with diabetes, obesity, and intestinal polyposis. Of interest, like melanocytic nevi and hemangiomas they often become more numerous or prominent during pregnancy, presumably related to hormonal stimulation.

EPITHELIAL CYST (WEN)

Epithelial cysts are common lesions formed by the invagination and cystic expansion of the epidermis or a hair follicle. The lay term, *wen*, derives from the Anglo-Saxon *wenn*, meaning a lump or tumor. These cysts are filled with keratin and lipid-containing debris derived from sebaceous secretions. Clinically, they are dermal or subcutaneous, well-circumscribed, firm, and often moveable nodules. When large, they may be subject to traumatic rupture, which can lead to inflammation and pain.

> **Morphology.** Epithelial cysts are divided into several histologic types. The **epidermal inclusion cyst** has a wall resembling normal epidermis and is filled with laminated strands of keratin. **Pilar** or **trichilemmal cysts** have a wall that resembles follicular epithelium, without a granular cell layer and filled by a more homogeneous mixture of keratin and lipid. The **dermoid cyst** is similar to the epidermal inclusion cyst, but also contains multiple appendages (such as small hair follicles) budding outward from its wall. Finally, **steatocystoma simplex** is a cyst with a wall resembling the sebaceous gland duct, and from which numerous compressed sebaceous lobules originate. The importance of recognition of this cyst derives from the often dominantly heritable nature of the lesion (**steatocystoma multiplex**), which can be caused by missense mutations in the gene encoding keratin 17. Interestingly, the same mutations are also associated with a syndrome called **pachyonychia congenital type 2**, which is associated with focal defects in skin, nails, and pilosebaceous cysts.[40,41] These phenotypes are consistent with the pattern of keratin 17 expression, which is restricted to nail bed and epidermal appendages.

ADNEXAL (APPENDAGE) TUMORS

There are literally hundreds of neoplasms arising from or showing differentiation toward cutaneous appendages. Their significance varies according to type and clinical context. Some are entirely benign, but may be confused with cutaneous cancers such as basal cell carcinoma. Other appendage tumors are associated with mendelian patterns of inheritance and occur as multiple disfiguring lesions. In some instances, these lesions warn of a predisposition for internal malignancy; such is the reationship between multiple *trichilemmomas* and Cowden syndrome, a disorder caused by germline mutations in the tumor suppressor gene *PTEN* that is associated with an increased risk of breast cancer and many other tumors.[42] Selected examples are provided here to illustrate neoplasms of hair follicles and sebaceous, eccrine, and apocrine glands.

Appendage tumors are often nondescript, flesh-colored solitary or multiple papules and nodules. Some have a predis-

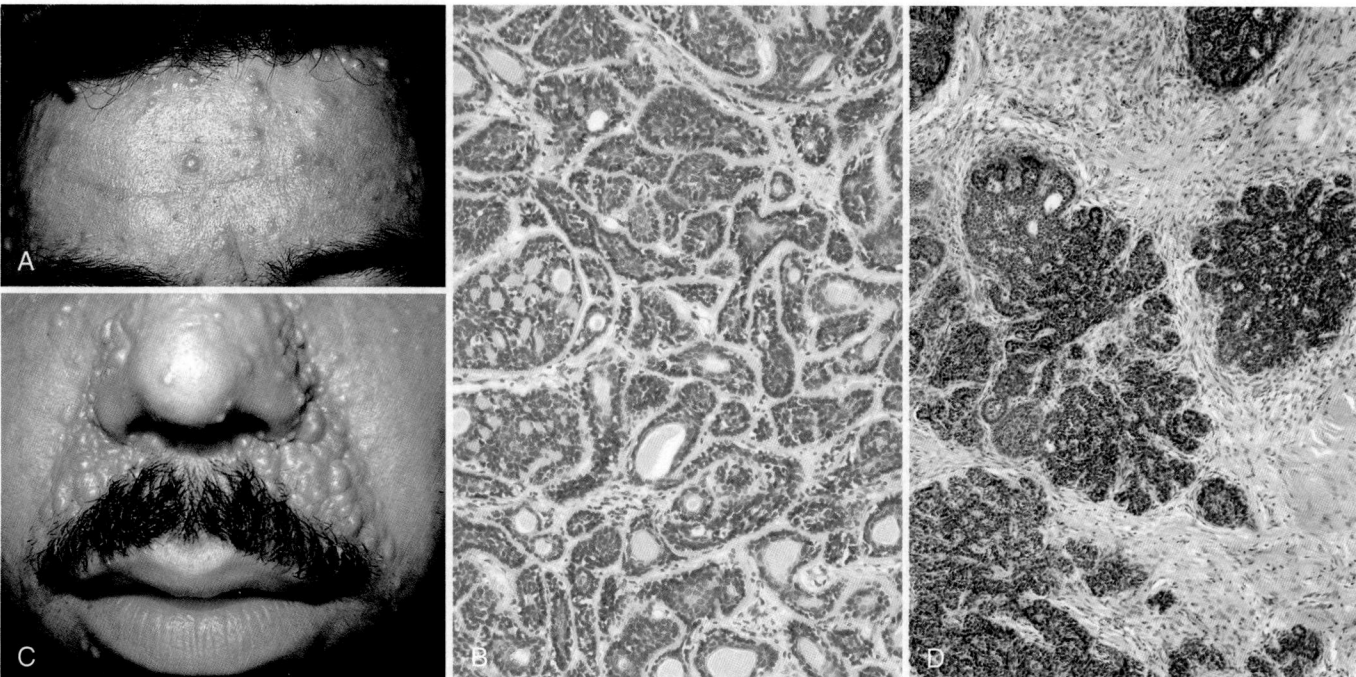

FIGURE 25–11 Adnexal tumors. **A,** Multiple cylindromas (papules) on the forehead are composed of islands of (**B**) basaloid cells containing occasional ducts that fit together like pieces of a jigsaw puzzle. **C,** Perinasal papules and small nodules of trichoepithelioma are composed of (**D**) buds of basaloid cells that resemble primitive hair follicles.

position for occurrence on specific body surfaces. For example, the *eccrine poroma* occurs predominantly on the palms and soles. *Cylindroma*, an appendage tumor with ductal (apocrine or eccrine) differentiation, usually occurs on the forehead and scalp (Fig. 25–11A), where coalescence of nodules with time may produce a hat-like growth, hence the name *turban tumor*. These lesions may be dominantly inherited; in such cases they appear early in life and are associated with inactivating mutations in the tumor suppressor gene *CYLD*, which encodes a deubiquitinating enzyme that regulates NF-κB and the cell cycle.[43,44] Germline mutations in this gene are associated with several related genetic syndromes including familial cylindromatosis, multiple familial trichoepithelioma (a follicular tumor), and Brooke-Spiegler syndrome (showing both tumor types).[45] *Syringomas,* lesions with eccrine differentiation, usually occur as multiple, small, tan papules in the vicinity of the lower eyelids. *Sebaceous adenomas* can be associated with internal malignancy in the Muir-Torre syndrome, a subset of the hereditary nonpolyposis colorectal carcinoma syndrome (Chapter 17) associated with germline deficits in DNA mismatch repair proteins; some of these have mutations in genes involved in WNT signaling.[46,47] *Pilomatricomas,* showing follicular differentiation, are associated with activating mutations in *CTNNB1*, the gene encoding β-catenin.[48] Mutations in this gene are seen in numerous neoplasms but are of interest here since WNT signaling through β-catenin is critical for early hair development and regulates the hair cycle. Adnexal tumors can also show primarily apocrine differentiation; these usually arise in body areas where apocrine glands are most prevalent, such as the axilla and scalp. Some skin adnexal tumors may arise from multipotent cutaneous stem cells,

which are believed to reside in a specialized niche associated with hair follicles.[49]

> **Morphology.** The **cylindroma** is composed of islands of cells resembling those of the normal epidermal or adnexal basal cell layer (basaloid cells). These islands fit together like pieces of a jigsaw puzzle within a fibrous dermal matrix (Fig. 25–11B). **Trichoepithelioma** is a proliferation of basaloid cells that forms primitive structures resembling hair follicles (Fig. 25–11C, D). **Sebaceous adenoma** shows a lobular proliferation of sebocytes with increased peripheral basaloid cells and more mature sebocytes in the central portion, characterized by frothy or bubbly cytoplasm due to lipid vesicle content (Fig. 25–12A). **Pilomatrixomas** are composed of basaloid cells that show trichilemmal or hairlike differentiation similar to that seen in the germinal portion of the normal hair bulb in the anagen growth phase (Fig. 25–12B). **Apocrine carcinoma** shows ductal differentiation with prominent decapitation secretion similar to that seen in the normal apocrine gland (Fig. 25–12C). The infiltrative growth pattern is a hint of malignancy in this otherwise well-differentiated tumor.

Although most appendage tumors are benign, malignant variants do exist. Apocrine tumors are unusual in that malignant forms seem to be more common than benign forms. *Sebaceous carcinoma,* for example, arises from the meibomian glands of the eyelid and may follow an aggressive course replete with systemic

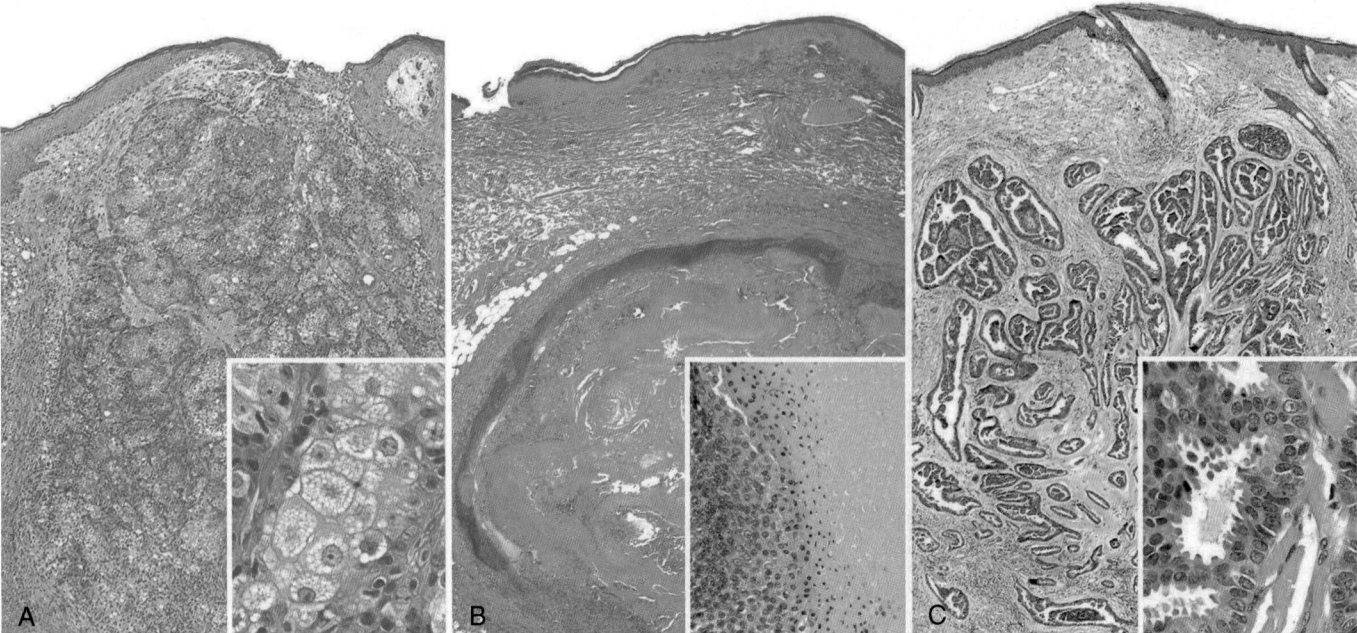

FIGURE 25–12 Adnexal tumors. **A,** Sebaceous adenoma; *inset* demonstrates sebaceous differentiation. **B,** Pilomatrixoma; *inset* shows hair matrical differentiation with characteristic maturation to anucleate "ghost cells." **C,** Apocrine carcinoma (well-differentiated); *inset* shows apocrine differentiation with characteristic luminal decapitation secretion.

metastases. *Eccrine* and *apocrine carcinomas* are often confused with metastatic adenocarcinomas to the skin because of their tendency for abortive gland formation.

Premalignant and Malignant Epidermal Tumors

ACTINIC KERATOSIS

The development of epidermal malignancy is typically preceded by a period of progressively worsening dysplastic changes, which are analogous to the precursor lesions that give rise to carcinoma of the squamous mucosa of the uterine cervix (Chapter 22). In the skin, these precursor lesions are called *actinic keratoses*; as the name implies, these usually occur in sun-damaged skin and exhibit hyperkeratosis. As would be expected, they occur with particularly high incidence in lightly pigmented individuals. Exposure to ionizing radiation, industrial hydrocarbons and arsenicals may induce similar lesions.

Actinic keratoses are usually less than 1 cm in diameter; are tan-brown, red, or skin-colored; and have a rough, sandpaper-like consistency. Some lesions may produce so much keratin that a "cutaneous horn" develops (Fig. 25–13A). Such horns may become so prominent that they actually resemble the horns of animals! Sun-exposed sites (face, arms, dorsum of hands) are most frequently affected. The lips may also develop similar lesions (termed *actinic cheilitis*).

> **Morphology.** Cytologic atypia is seen in the lowermost layers of the epidermis and may be associated with hyperplasia of basal cells (Fig. 25–13B) or, alter-

> natively, with atrophy that results in thinning of the epidermis. The atypical basal cells usually have pink or reddish cytoplasm due to dyskeratosis. Intercellular bridges are present, in contrast to basal cell carcinoma, in which they are not visible. The superficial dermis contains thickened, blue-gray elastic fibers (elastosis), a probable result of abnormal elastic fiber synthesis by sun-damaged fibroblasts[34]. The stratum corneum is thickened, and unlike normal skin, the cells in this layer often retain their nuclei (**parakeratosis**).

Whether all actinic keratoses would inexorably lead to skin cancer (usually squamous cell carcinoma), if given enough time, is conjectural. Studies indicate that lesions may regress or remain stable during a normal life span. However, enough become malignant to warrant local eradication. This can usually be accomplished by gentle curettage, freezing, or topical application of chemotherapeutic agents. More recently, a reagent called imiquimod, which activates the innate immune system through stimulation of Toll-like receptors (TLRs), has been used to eradicate the abnormal cells that compose this tumor.[50]

SQUAMOUS CELL CARCINOMA

Squamous cell carcinoma is the second most common tumor arising on sun-exposed sites in older people, exceeded only by basal cell carcinoma. Except for lesions on the lower legs, these tumors have a higher incidence in men than in women. Invasive squamous cell carcinomas are usually discovered while they are small and resectable. Less than 5% of these tumors

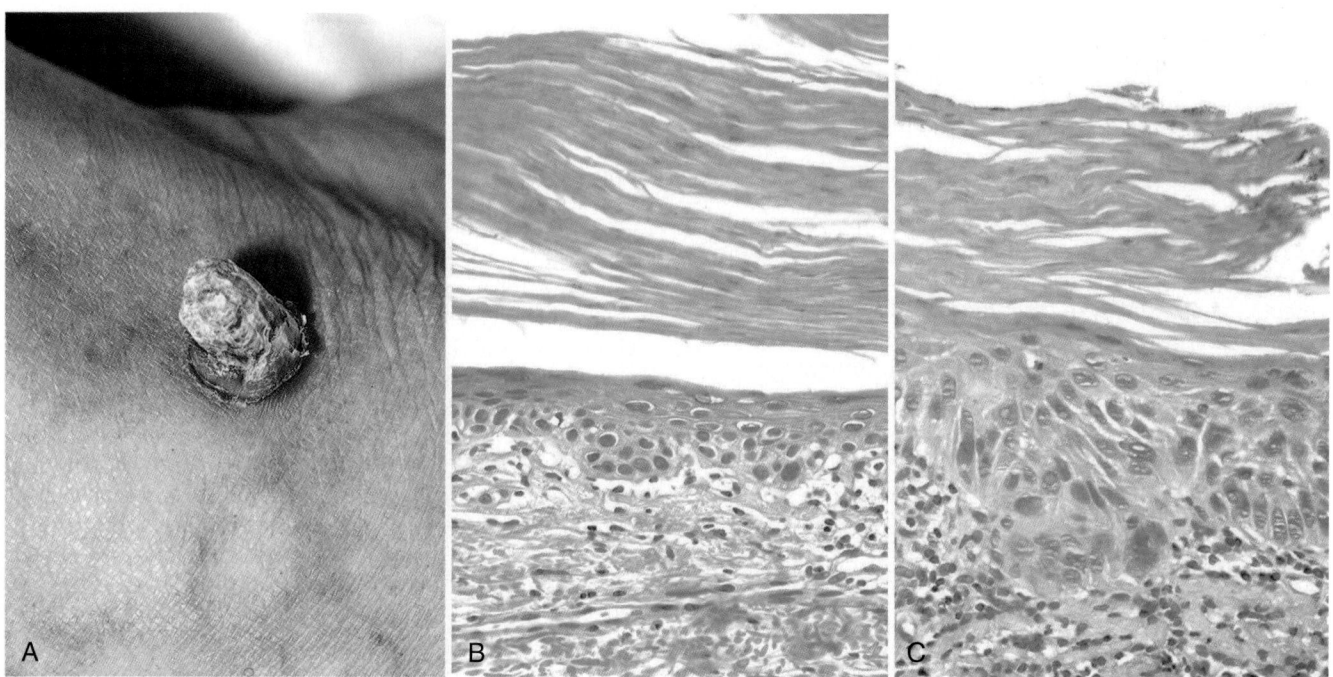

FIGURE 25–13   Actinic keratosis. **A,** Excessive scale formation in this lesion has produced a "cutaneous horn." **B,** Basal cell layer atypia (dysplasia) is associated with marked hyperkeratosis and parakeratosis. **C,** Progression to full-thickness nuclear atypia, with or without the presence of superficial epidermal maturation, heralds the development of squamous cell carcinoma in situ.

metastasize to regional nodes; these lesions are generally deeply invasive and involve the subcutis.

> **Morphology.** Squamous cell carcinomas that have not invaded through the basement membrane of the

dermoepidermal junction (termed **in situ carcinoma**) appear as sharply defined, red, scaling plaques. More advanced, invasive lesions are nodular, show variable keratin production (appreciated grossly as hyperkeratotic scale), and may ulcerate (Fig. 25–14A).

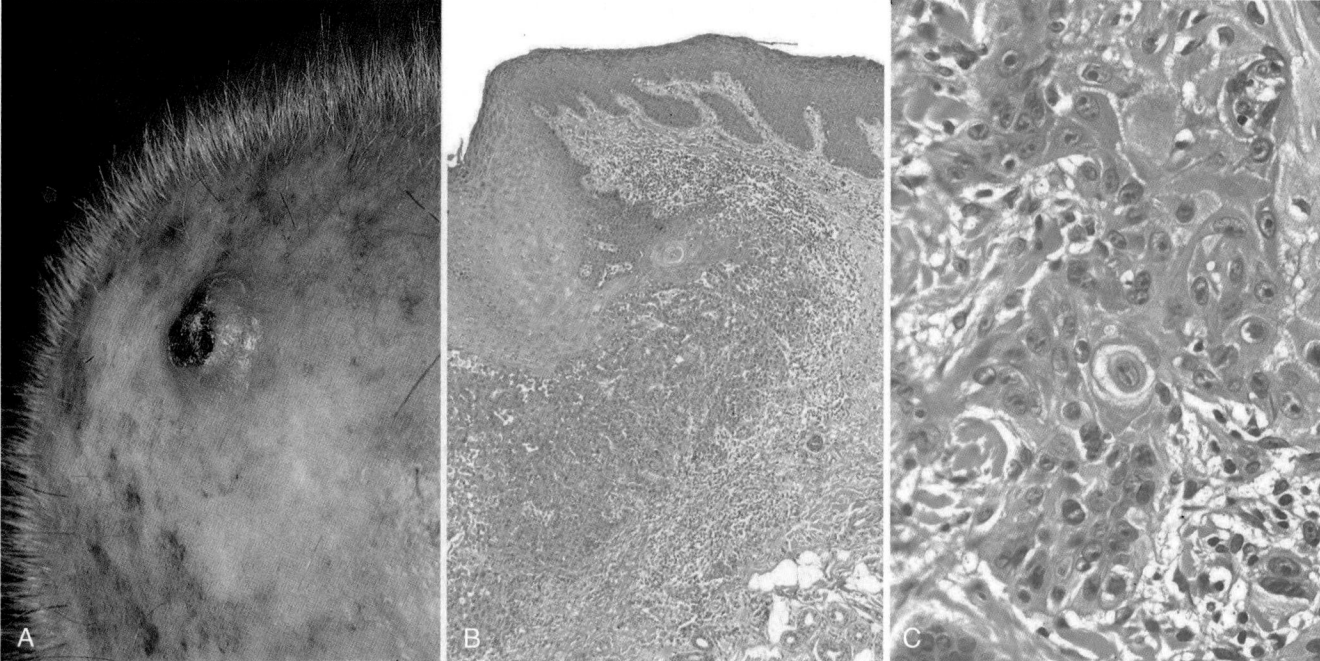

FIGURE 25–14   Invasive squamous cell carcinoma. **A,** Lesions are often nodular and ulcerated as seen in this scalp tumor. **B,** Tongues of atypical squamous epithelium have transgressed the basement membrane, invading deeply into the dermis. **C,** A magnified image reveals invasive tumor cells showing enlarged nuclei with angulated contours and prominent nucleoli.

Unlike actinic keratoses, in squamous cell carcinoma in situ, cells with atypical (enlarged and hyperchromatic) nuclei involve **all levels** of the epidermis (Fig. 25–13C). Invasive squamous cell carcinoma (Fig. 25–14B, C) shows variable degrees of differentiation, ranging from tumors composed of polygonal cells arranged in orderly lobules and having numerous large areas of keratinization, to neoplasms associated with geographic necrosis consisting of highly anaplastic cells that exhibit only abortive, single-cell keratinization (dyskeratosis). The latter tumors may be so poorly differentiated that immunohistochemical stains for keratins are needed to confirm the diagnosis.

Keratoacanthoma is a controversial lesion; some regard it as a variant of well-differentiated squamous cell carcinoma, while others consider it to be a distinct entity. It differs from conventional squamous cell carcinomas in that after a period of rapid growth, it usually regresses spontaneously. Grossly, it is a symmetric cup-shaped tumor with a central depression filled with keratin debris. Histologically, the tumor is composed of lobules of squamous cells with glassy cytoplasm that undergo kertinization without an intervening granular layer. Once established, keratoacanthomas elicit a brisk lymphocytic and eosinophilic host response.

Pathogenesis. *The most important cause of cutaneous squamous cell carcinoma is DNA damage induced by exposure to UV light.* Tumor incidence is proportional to the degree of lifetime sun exposure. A second common association is with immunosuppression, most notably chronic immunosuppression as a result of chemotherapy or organ transplantation.[51] Immunosuppression may contribute to carcinogenesis by reducing host surveillance and increasing the susceptibility of keratinocytes to infection and transformation by oncogenic viruses, particularly human papilloma virus (HPV) subtypes 5 and 8.[52] These same HPVs have been implicated in tumors arising in patients with a rare autosomal recessive condition, epidermodysplasia verruciformis, that is marked by a high susceptibility to cutaneous squamous cell carcinomas.[53] Sunlight, in addition to its damaging effect on DNA, seems to cause a defect in cutaneous immunity by dampening the immune surveillance function of epidermal Langerhans cells.[54] Other risk factors for squamous cell carcinoma include industrial carcinogens (tars and oils), chronic ulcers and draining osteomyelitis, old burn scars, ingestion of arsenicals, ionizing radiation, and (in the oral cavity) tobacco and betel nut chewing.

Most studies on the genetics of squamous cell carcinoma have focused on acquired defects in sporadic tumors and their precursors (actinic keratoses), and the relationships between these defects and sun-exposure. The incidence of *p53* mutations in actinic keratoses found in Caucasians is high, suggesting that p53 dysfunction is an early event in the development of tumors induced by sunlight. Normally, DNA damaged by UV light is sensed by checkpoint kinases such as ATM and ATR, which send out signals that upregulate the expression and stability of p53. p53 in turn arrests cells in the G_1 phase of the cell cycle and promotes either "high-fidelity" DNA repair or the elimination of cells that are damaged beyond repair by apoptosis (Chapter 7). When these protective functions of p53 are lost, DNA damage induced by UV light is more likely to be "repaired" by error-prone mechanisms, creating mutations that are passed down to daughter cells. Of note, the mutations that are seen in *p53* often occur at pyrimidine dimers, indicating that they, too, stem from damage caused by UV light. A similar story underlies the remarkable susceptibility of patients with xeroderma pigmentosum to squamous cell carcinoma. This disorder is caused by inherited mutations in genes in the nucleotide excision repair pathway, which is required for accurate repair of pyrimidine dimers; when this pathway is defective, error-prone repair pathways take over, leading to the rapid accumulation of mutations and eventual carcinogenesis.

As with all other forms of cancer, cutaneous squamous cell carcinoma stems from molecular lesions in multiple genes. In addition to defects in p53, studies of explanted human keratinocytes suggest that dysregulated RAS signaling plays an important role in the transformation process.[55]

BASAL CELL CARCINOMA

Basal cell carcinoma is the most common invasive cancer in humans, with nearly 1 million estimated cases per year in the United States.[56] These are slow-growing tumors that rarely metastasize. They have a tendency to occur at sun-exposed sites and in lightly pigmented people. As with squamous cell carcinoma, the incidence of basal cell carcinoma rises sharply with immunosuppression and in people with inherited defects in DNA repair such as xeroderma pigmentosum (Chapter 7).

These tumors present clinically as *pearly papules often containing prominent, dilated subepidermal blood vessels (telangiectasias)* (Fig. 25–15A). Some tumors contain melanin and thus appear similar to melanocytic nevi or melanomas. Advanced lesions may ulcerate, and extensive local invasion of bone or facial sinuses may occur after many years of neglect or in unusually aggressive tumors, explaining the archaic designation *rodent ulcers*. One common and important variant, the superficial basal cell carcinoma, presents as an erythematous, occasionally pigmented plaque that may resemble early forms of melanoma.

Morphology. Histologically, the tumor cells resemble those in the normal basal cell layer of the epidermis. They arise from the epidermis or follicular epithelium and do not occur on mucosal surfaces. Two patterns are seen: **multifocal growths** originating from the epidermis and sometimes extending over several square centimeters or more of skin surface (multifocal superficial type) and **nodular lesions** growing downward deeply into the dermis as cords and islands of variably basophilic cells with hyperchromatic nuclei, embedded in a mucinous matrix, and often surrounded by many fibroblasts and lymphocytes (Fig. 25–15B). The cells at the periphery of the tumor cell islands tend to be arranged radially with their long axes in parallel alignment **(palisading)**. In sections, the stroma retracts away from the carci-

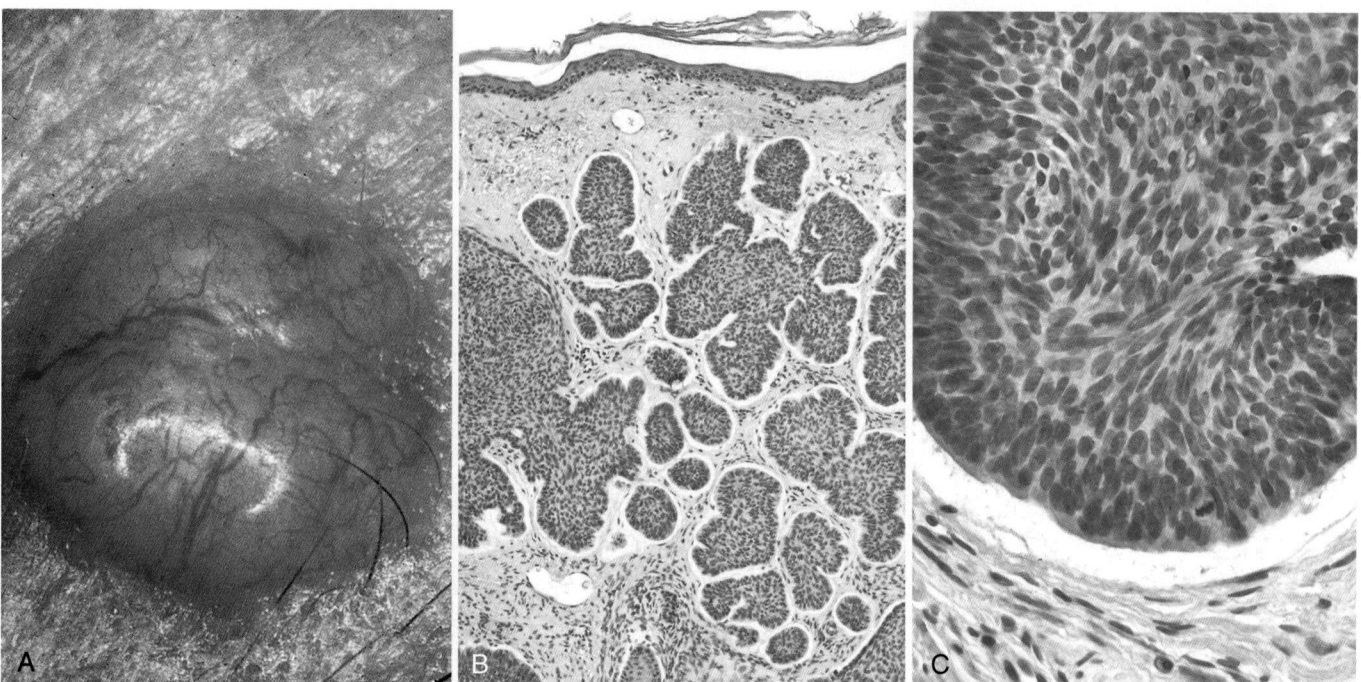

FIGURE 25–15 Basal cell carcinoma. Pearly, telangiectatic nodules (**A**) are composed of nests of uniformly atypical basaloid cells within the dermis (**B**) that are often separated from the adjacent stroma by thin clefts (**C**), an artifact of sectioning.

noma (Fig. 25–15C), creating clefts or separation artifacts that assist in differentiating basal cell carcinomas from certain appendage tumors that are also characterized by proliferation of basaloid cells, such as trichoepithelioma.

Pathogenesis. *Nevoid basal cell carcinoma syndrome* (NBCCS; also known as *basal cell nevus* or *Gorlin syndrome*) is an autosomal dominant disorder characterized by multiple basal cell carcinomas.[57] Most of these tumors develop before age 20 and are accompanied by various other conditions including tumors (especially medulloblastomas and ovarian fibromas), odontogenic keratocysts, and pits of the palms and soles. Multiple systemic manifestations such as intracranial calcification, cleft lip and palate, abnormal segmentation of the vertebra, and rib anomalies (bifid, fused, missing, splayed ribs) may also be present.[58] Though quite rare (incidence of 1 in 56,000), this syndrome has helped to elucidate the molecular genetics of basal cell carcinoma, including the common sporadic type. Examples of other genetic syndromes associated with skin tumors are listed in Table 25–2.

The gene associated with NBCCS, located on chromosome 9q22.3, is *PTCH*, the human homologue of the *Drosophila* developmental gene *patched*.[59] The pathogenesis of basal cell carcinomas in NBCCS fits the classical Knudson "two-hit" hypothesis for familial retinoblastoma (Chapter 7). Individuals with NBCCS are born with a germline mutation in one of the *PTCH* alleles; the second normal allele is inactivated in tumors by a mutation acquired by chance or due to exposure to mutagens (such as UV light).

The *PTCH* gene encodes a receptor for the protein product of the *sonic hedgehog gene (SHH)*, a member of the hedgehog *(HH)* family of genes that determine polarity during embryonic development.[60] The pathway is also involved in hair follicle formation and the hair cycle in skin.[5] The PTCH protein forms a receptor complex with another transmembrane protein, known as SMO (for "smoothened"). In the absence of its ligand, SHH, PTCH inactivates SMO and sequesters it from transducing a down-stream signal. Binding of SHH to PTCH releases the suppression of SMO, causing the up-regulation of hedgehog target genes through a signal cascade that involves the GLI1 transcription factor (Fig. 25–16). Experimental work in mice has shown that animals with defects in the *PTCH* signaling pathway, including overexpression of GLI1, develop skin tumors resembling basal cell carcinomas.[61,62] In NBCCS the absence of *PTCH* causes constitutive activation of SMO, leading to the development of basal cell carcinoma.

Mutations of genes belonging to the *PTCH* signaling pathway are also important for the development of the common sporadic form of basal cell carcinoma, as documented by the inactivation of *PTCH* and the presence of *SMO* activating mutations in these skin neoplasms.[63] *PTCH* mutations are found in approximately 30% of sporadic basal cell carcinomas, and of these about one third have mutations (C→T transitions) that are considered hallmarks of UV damage. Mutations in *p53* occur in 40% to 60% of basal cell carcinomas, and 60% of these have "UV signature."[64] Xeroderma pigmentosum, a disorder of DNA repair, presents a striking example of the connection between sun exposure and defects in *PTCH* and *p53*.[65] In these tumors the frequency of mutations in *PTCH* and *p53* are, respectively, 90% and 40%, and the majority of these bear the UV signature.

TABLE 25–2 Survey of Familial Cancer Syndromes with Cutaneous Manifestations

Disease	Inheritance	Chromosomal Location	Gene/Protein	Normal function/Manifestation of loss
Ataxia-telangiectasia	AR	11q22.3	*ATM*/ATM	DNA repair after radiation injury/neurologic and vascular lesions
Nevoid basal cell carcinoma syndrome	AD	9q22.3	*PTCH*/PTCH	Developmental patterning gene/multiple basal cell carcinomas; jaw cysts, etc.
Cowden syndrome	AD	10q23	*PTEN*/PTEN	Lipid phosphatase/benign follicular appendage tumors (trichilemmomas); internal adenocarcinoma (often breast)
Familial melanoma syndrome	AD	9p21	*CDKN2*/p16/INK4	Inhibits CDK phosphorylation of RB, promoting cell cycle arrest/melanoma; pancreatic carcinoma
			CDKN2/p14/ARF	Binds MDM2, promoting p53 function/ melanoma; pancreatic carcinoma
Muir-Torre syndrome	AD	2p22	*MSH2*/MSH2 *MLH1*/MLH1	Involved in DNA mismatch repair/sebaceous neoplasia; internal malignancy (colon and others)
Neurofibromatosis I	AD	17q11.2	*NF1*/neurofibromin	Negatively regulates RAS signaling/ neurofibromas
Neurofibromatosis II	AD	22q12.2	*NF2*/merlin	Integrates cytoskeletal signaling/ neurofibromas and acoustic neuromas
Tuberous sclerosis	AD	9q34 16p13.3	*TSC1*/hamartin *TSC2*/tuberin	Work together in a complex that negatively regulates mTOR/angiofibromas/mental retardation
Xeroderma pigmentosum	AR	9q22 and others	*XPA*/XPA and others	Nucleotide excision repair/melanoma and nonmelanoma skin cancers

AD, Autosomal dominant; AR, autosomal recessive.
From Tsai KY, Tsao H: The genetics of skin cancer. Am J Med Genet C Semin Med Genet 131C:82, 2004.

Tumors of the Dermis

The dermis contains a variety of elements such as smooth muscle, pericytes, fibroblasts, neural tissue, and endothelium. Neoplasms with differentiation toward all of these tissues occur not just in the skin, but also in soft tissues and viscera. In this section we consider two representative dermal neoplasms—one benign, one malignant—that arise primarily in the skin.

BENIGN FIBROUS HISTIOCYTOMA (DERMATOFIBROMA)

Benign fibrous histiocytoma refers to a heterogeneous family of morphologically and histogenetically related benign dermal neoplasms of uncertain lineage. These tumors are usually seen in adults and often occur on the legs of young to middle-aged women. Their biologic behavior is indolent.

These neoplasms appear as firm, tan to brown papules (Fig. 25–17A). Lesions are asymptomatic or tender and may increase and decrease slightly in size over time. Most are less than 1 cm in diameter, but actively growing lesions may reach several centimeters in diameter; with time they often become flattened. The tendency for fibrous histiocytomas to dimple inward on lateral compression can be helpful in distinguishing them from nodular melanomas, which protrude when squeezed.

The cause of fibrous histiocytomas remains a mystery. Many cases have a history of antecedent trauma, suggesting an abnormal response to injury and inflammation,[66] perhaps analogous to the deposition of increased amounts of altered collagen in a hypertrophic scar or keloid. These common yet curious tumors appear to be composed at least partially of factor XIIIa–positive dermal dendrocytes.

Morphology. The most common form of fibrous histiocytoma is referred to as a **dermatofibroma**. These tumors are formed by benign, spindle-shaped cells arranged in a well-defined, nonencapsulated mass within the mid-dermis (Fig. 25–17B, C). Extension of these cells into the subcutaneous fat is sometimes observed. Many cases demonstrate a peculiar form of overlying epidermal hyperplasia, characterized by downward elongation of hyperpigmented rete ridges (a pseudo-epitheliomatous pattern). Numerous histologic variants are noted, such as more cellular forms or tumors with pools of extravascular blood and hemosiderin (aneurysmal).

DERMATOFIBROSARCOMA PROTUBERANS

Dermatofibrosarcoma protuberans is best regarded as a well-differentiated, primary fibrosarcoma of the skin. These tumors

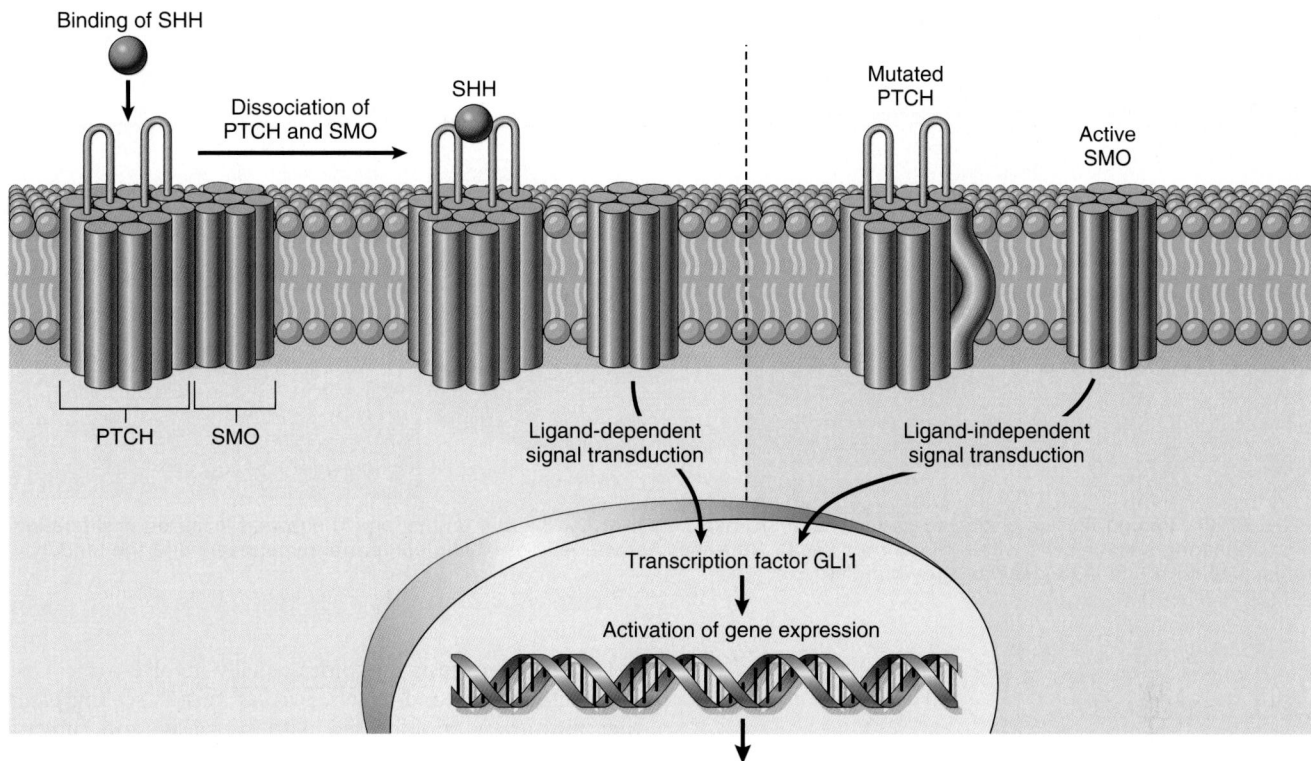

FIGURE 25–16 Normal and oncogenic hedgehog signaling. *Left*, Normally, PTCH and SMO form a receptor complex that binds sonic hedgehog (SHH). In the absence of SHH, PTCH blocks SMO activity. When SHH binds PTCH, SMO is released to trigger a signal transduction cascade that leads to activation of GLI1 and other transcription factors. *Right*, Mutations in *PTCH*, and less often in *SMO*, allow SMO to signal without ligand binding and underlie the nevoid basal cell carcinoma (Gorlin) syndrome.

are slow growing, and although they are locally aggressive and can recur, they rarely metastasize. Clinically they are firm, solid nodules that arise most frequently on the trunk. They often develop as aggregated "protuberant" tumors within a firm (indurated) plaque or nodule that may sometimes ulcerate.

> **Morphology.** On microscopic examination, these neoplasms are cellular, composed of fibroblasts arranged radially, reminiscent of blades of a pinwheel, a pattern referred to as **storiform**. Mitoses are rare. In contrast to that in dermatofibroma, the overlying epidermis is generally thinned. Deep extension from the dermis into subcutaneous fat, producing a characteristic "honeycomb" pattern, is frequently present (Fig. 25–18B, C). These tumors may extend down fibrous septae in the subcutis and thus require wider excision than would appear to be necessary to prevent local recurrence.

Pathogenesis. The molecular hallmark of dermatofibrosarcoma protuberans is a balanced translocation between genes encoding collagen 1A1 *(COL1A1)* and the platelet-derived growth factor-β *(PDGFB)*. It results in the juxtaposition of COL1A1 promoter sequences and the coding region of PDGFβ; this in turn leads to over-expression and secretion of PDGFβ, which drives tumor cell growth through an autocrine loop.[67,68] Such fusion genes are increasingly being recognized in a wide spectrum of tumors, including carcinomas.[69] While the primary mode of treatment is local wide excision, in cases not amenable to this approach the targeted tyrosine kinase inhibitor imatinib mesylate is used. This inhibits PDGF-β receptor activation and has marked antitumor activity.[70] Withdrawal of the drug allows tumor regrowth even after long-term treatment, so use of this agent is lifelong.

Tumors of Cellular Migrants to the Skin

Aside from tumors that arise directly from epidermal and dermal cells, several proliferative disorders of the skin involve cells whose progenitors arise elsewhere and home to the cutaneous microenvironment. The two examples discussed in this section—namely, cutaneous T-cell lymphoma and mastocytosis—are primary cutaneous disorders that arise from lymphocytes and mast cells, respectively.

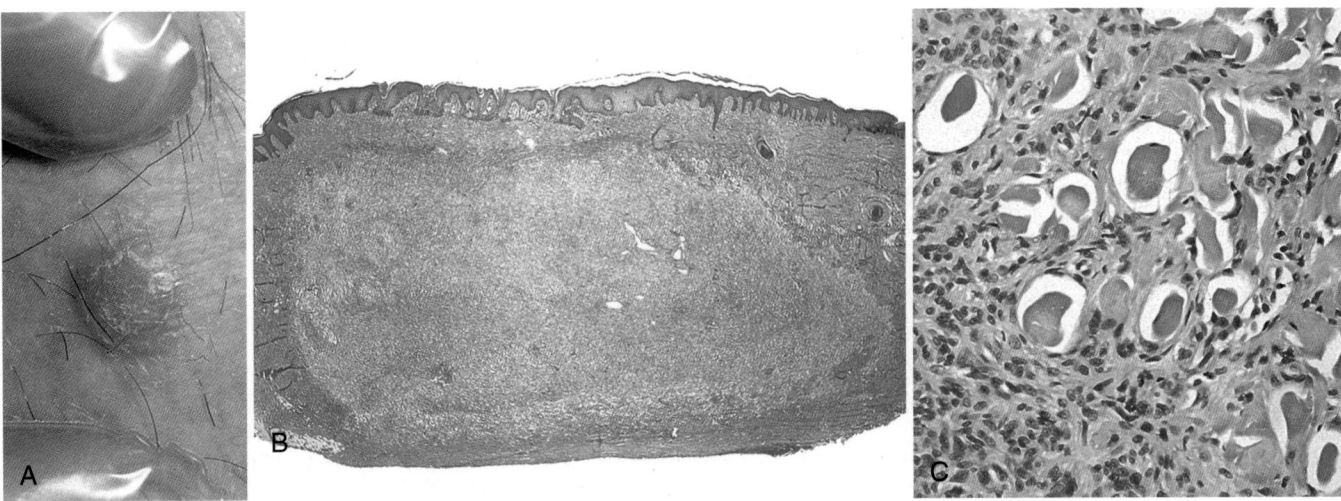

FIGURE 25–17 Benign fibrous histiocytoma (dermatofibroma). This firm, tan papule on the leg (**A**) shows a localized proliferation of benign-appearing spindle cells within the dermis (**B**). **C,** Note the characteristic overlying epidermal hyperplasia and the tendency of fibroblasts to surround individual collagen bundles.

MYCOSIS FUNGOIDES (CUTANEOUS T-CELL LYMPHOMA)

Cutaneous T cell lymphoma (CTCL) represents a spectrum of lymphoproliferative disorders affecting the skin (see also Chapter 13).[71] Two different clinical types of malignant T-cell disorders were originally recognized: *mycosis fungoides*, a chronic proliferative process; and a more aggressive nodular eruptive variant, *mycosis fungoides d'emblée*. It is now known that a variety of presentations of T-cell lymphoma occur in the skin, but this section will focus on mycosis fungoides.

Mycosis fungoides is a T-cell lymphoma that presents in the skin and may evolve into generalized lymphoma.[72] Most affected individuals have disease that remains localized to the skin for many years; a minority have rapid systemic dissemination. This condition may occur at any age, but most commonly it afflicts persons older than age 40.

Lesions of mycosis fungoides usually involve truncal areas and include scaly, red-brown *patches*; raised, scaling *plaques* that may even be confused with psoriasis; and fungating *nodules*. Prognosis is related to the percentage of body surface involved and progression from patch to plaque to nodular forms. Eczema-like lesions typify early stages of disease when obvious visceral or nodal spread has not occurred. Raised, indurated, irregularly outlined, erythematous plaques may then supervene. Development of multiple, large (≤10 cm or more in diameter), red-brown nodules correlates with systemic spread. Sometimes plaques and nodules ulcerate (Fig. 25–19A). Ultimately, lesions may affect numerous body surfaces, including the trunk, extremities, face, and scalp. In some individuals, seeding of the blood by malignant T cells is accompanied by diffuse erythema and scaling of the entire body surface (erythroderma), a condition known as *Sézary syndrome* (Chapter 13).

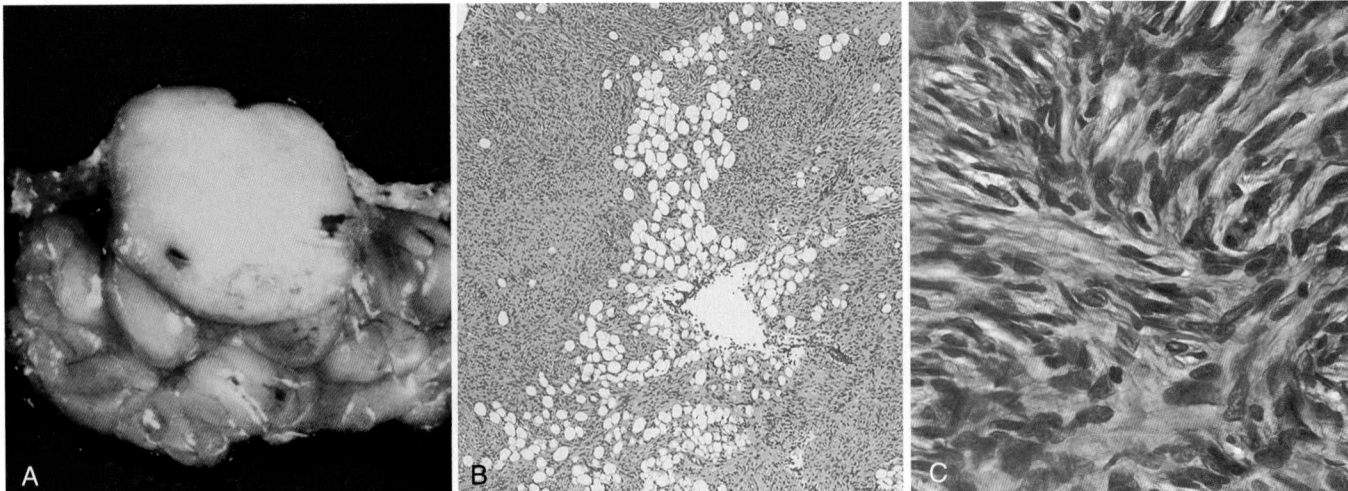

FIGURE 25–18 Dermatofibrosarcoma protuberans. **A,** The tumor usually presents as a flesh-colored to erythematous nodule, and has a fibrotic appearance on sectioning. **B, C,** Characteristic storiform cellularity is noted histologically, and the lesion often infiltrates the subcutis in a manner that resembles "Swiss cheese" to some afficianados.

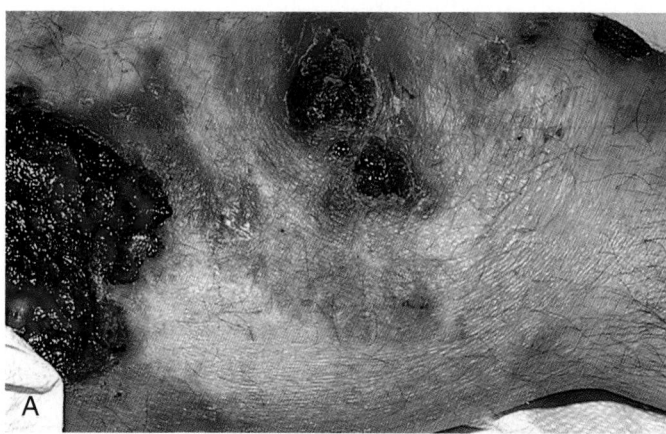
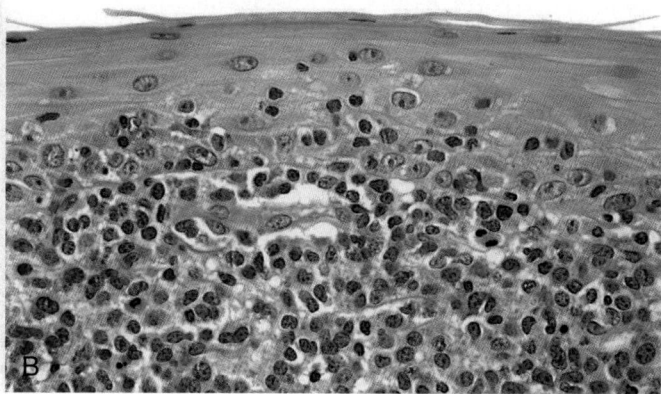

FIGURE 25–19 Cutaneous T-cell lymphoma. **A,** Several ill-defined, erythematous, often scaling, and occasionally ulcerated plaques. **B,** Microscopically, there is an infiltrate of atypical lymphocytes that show a tendency to accumulate beneath the epidermal layer and to invade the epidermis.

The proliferating cells in CTCL are clonal populations of lymphocytes of the CD4 subset.[2,73] The neoplastic cells are targeted to the skin by expression of CLA (see Fig. 25–2) and often express aberrant cell surface antigens as well as clonal T-cell receptor gene rearrangements. Detection of these features may be of diagnostic assistance in difficult cases. Topical therapy with steroids or UV light is often used for early lesions of CTCL, whereas more aggressive systemic chemotherapy is indicated for advanced disease.

> **Morphology.** The histologic hallmark of CTCL of the mycosis fungoides type is the presence of the **Sézary-Lutzner cells.** These are T-helper cells (CD4+) that characteristically form band-like aggregates within the superficial dermis (Fig. 25–19B) and invade the epidermis as single cells and small clusters **(Pautrier microabscesses).** These cells have markedly infolded nuclear membranes, imparting a hyperconvoluted or cerebriform contour. Although patches and plaques show pronounced epidermal infiltration by Sézary-Lutzner cells (epidermotropism), in more advanced nodular lesions the malignant T cells often lose this epidermotropic tendency, grow deeply into the dermis, and eventually spread systemically.

MASTOCYTOSIS

The term *mastocytosis* refers to a spectrum of rare disorders characterized by increased numbers of mast cells in the skin and, in some instances, in other organs. A localized cutaneous form of the disease that affects predominantly children and accounts for more than 50% of all cases is termed *urticaria pigmentosa.* These lesions are multiple, although solitary mastocytomas may also occur, usually shortly after birth. About 10% of individuals with mast cell disease have systemic disease, with mast cell infiltration of many organs. These individuals are often adults, and unlike localized cutaneous disease, the prognosis may be poor.

The pathologic findings in mastocytosis are highly variable. In urticaria pigmentosa, lesions are multiple and widely distributed, consisting of round to oval, red-brown, nonscaling papules and small plaques. Solitary mastocytomas present as one or several pink to tan-brown nodules that may be pruritic or show blister formation (Fig. 25–20A). In systemic mastocytosis skin lesions similar to those of urticaria pigmentosa are accompanied by mast cell infiltration of bone marrow, liver, spleen, and lymph nodes. Many of the signs and symptoms of mastocytosis are due to the effects of histamine, heparin, and other substances released as a result of mast cell degranulation. *Darier sign* refers to a localized area of dermal edema and erythema (wheal) that occurs when lesion skin is rubbed. *Dermatographism* refers to an area of dermal edema resembling a hive that occurs in normal skin as a result of localized stroking with a pointed instrument. In systemic disease, all of the following may be seen: pruritus and flushing triggered by certain foods, temperature changes, alcohol, and certain drugs (morphine, codeine, aspirin); watery nasal discharge (rhinorrhea); rarely, gastrointestinal or nasal bleeding, possibly due to the anticoagulant effects of heparin; and bone pain as a result of osteoblastic and osteoclastic involvement.

> **Morphology.** The histologic picture in urticaria pigmentosa or solitary mastocytoma varies from a subtle increase in the numbers of spindle-shaped and stellate mast cells around superficial dermal blood vessels, to large numbers of tightly packed, round to oval mast cells in the upper to mid-dermis (Fig. 25–20B). Variable fibrosis, edema, and small numbers of eosinophils may also be present. Mast cells may be difficult to differentiate from lymphocytes in routine, hematoxylin and eosin–stained sections, and special metachromatic stains (toluidine blue or Giemsa) must be used to visualize their granules (Fig. 25–20C). Even with these stains, extensive degranulation may result in failure to recognize these cells by light microscopy, but their identity can be readily confirmed with immunohistochemical stains for mast cell markers, such as mast cell tryptase.

Pathogenesis. The pathogenesis of many cases of mastocytosis involves acquired activating point mutations in

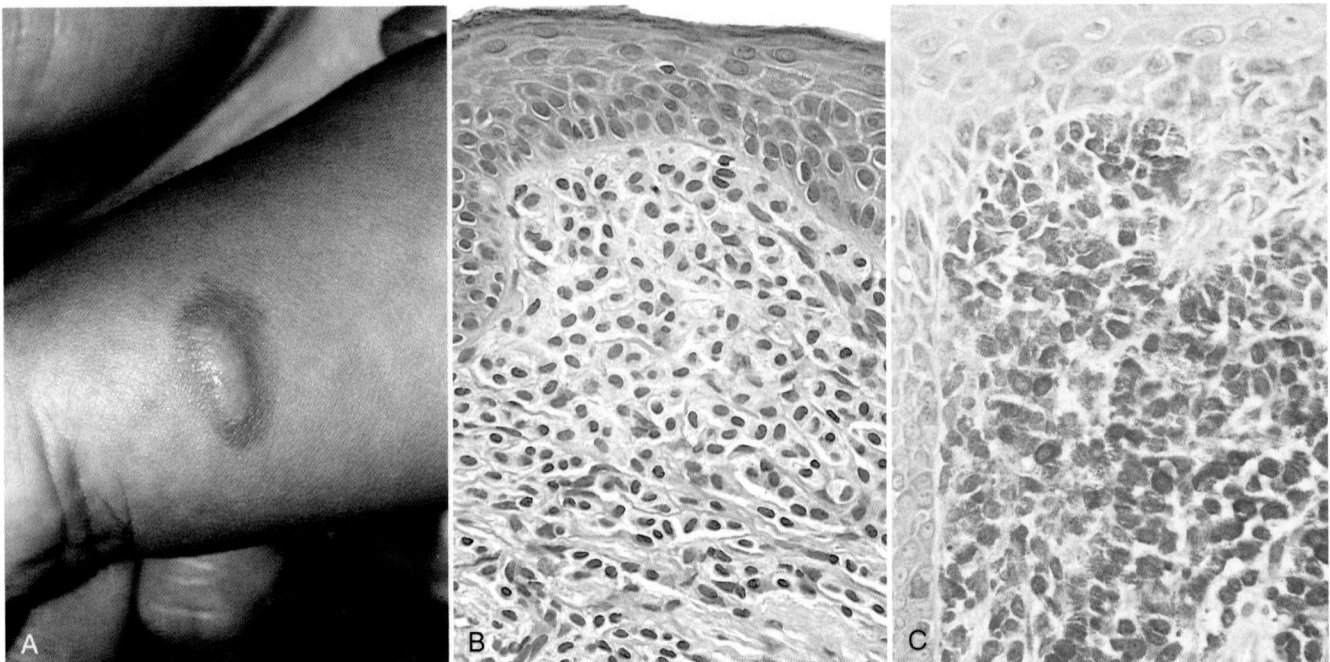

FIGURE 25–20 Mastocytosis. **A,** Solitary mastocytoma in a 1-year-old child. **B,** By routine histology, numerous ovoid cells with uniform, centrally located nuclei are observed in the dermis. **C,** Giemsa staining reveals purple, "metachromatic" granules within the cytoplasm of the cells.

the c-KIT receptor tyrosine kinase. The resulting increase in c-KIT signaling drives mast cell growth and survival.[74,75] Recognition of this etiology has led to attempts to treat this disorder with c-KIT inhibitors.

Disorders of Epidermal Maturation

ICHTHYOSIS

Of the numerous disorders that impair epidermal maturation, ichthyosis is perhaps one of the most striking. The term is derived from the Greek root *ichthy-*, meaning "fishy," and accordingly, this group of genetically inherited disorders is associated with chronic, excessive keratin buildup (hyperkeratosis) that results clinically in fish-like scales (Fig. 25–21A). Most ichthyoses become apparent either at or around the time of birth. Acquired (noninherited) variants also exist; in the acquired *ichthyosis vulgaris* in adults, there can be an association with lymphoid and visceral malignancies. The clinical types of ichthyosis vary according to the mode of inheritance, histology, and clinical features; the primary categories include *ichthyosis vulgaris* (autosomal dominant or acquired), *congenital ichthyosiform erythroderma* (autosomal recessive), *lamellar ichthyosis* (autosomal recessive), and *X-linked ichthyosis.*[76]

Morphology. All forms of ichthyosis exhibit a buildup of compacted stratum corneum that is associated with loss of the normal basket-weave pattern (Fig. 25–21B). There is generally little or no inflammation. Variations in the thickness of the epidermis and the stratum granulosum and the gross appearance and distribution of lesions are used to subclassify these disorders.

Pathogenesis. The primary abnormality in some forms of ichthyosis is defective desquamation, leading to retention of abnormally formed scale. For example, in X-linked ichthyosis, affected individuals have a deficiency of steroid sulfatase, an enzyme important for the removal of proadhesive cholesterol sulfate secreted into the intercellular spaces. Accumulation of cholesterol sulfate results in persistent cell-to-cell adhesion within the stratum corneum, hindering the desquamation process.

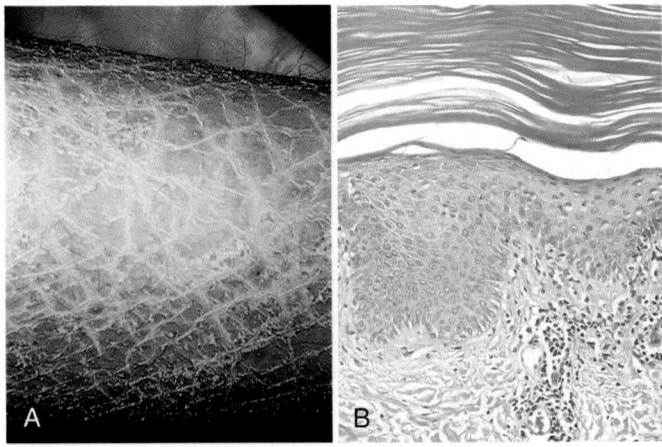

FIGURE 25–21 Ichthyosis. Note prominent fishlike scales (**A**) and compacted, thickened stratum corneum (**B**).

Acute Inflammatory Dermatoses

Literally thousands of inflammatory dermatoses have been described. In general, acute lesions last from days to weeks and are characterized by inflammatory infiltrates (usually composed of lymphocytes and macrophages rather than neutrophils), edema, and variable degrees of epidermal, vascular, or subcutaneous injury. Chronic lesions, on the other hand, persist for months to years and are often associated with changes in epidermal growth (atrophy or hyperplasia) or dermal fibrosis. The lesions discussed here are selected as examples of the more commonly encountered acute dermatoses.

URTICARIA

Urticaria (hives) is a common disorder of the skin characterized by localized mast cell degranulation and resultant dermal microvascular hyperpermeability. This gives rise to pruritic edematous plaques called *wheals*. Angioedema is closely related to urticaria and is characterized by deeper edema of both the dermis and the subcutaneous fat.

Urticaria most often occurs between ages 20 and 40, although all age groups are susceptible. Individual lesions develop and fade within hours (usually <24 hours), and episodes may last for days or persist for months. Lesions vary from small, pruritic papules to large edematous plaques (Fig. 25–22A). Individual lesions may coalesce to form annular, linear, or arciform configurations. Sites of predilection for urticarial eruptions include any area exposed to pressure, such as the trunk, distal extremities, and ears. Persistent episodes of urticaria may herald an underlying disease (e.g., collagen vascular disorders, Hodgkin lymphoma), but in the majority of cases no underlying cause can be identified.

> **Morphology.** The histologic features of urticaria may be very subtle. There is usually a sparse superficial perivenular infiltrate consisting of mononuclear cells and rare neutrophils. Eosinophils may also be present. Collagen bundles are more widely spaced than in normal skin, a result of superficial dermal edema (Fig. 25–22B). Superficial lymphatic channels are dilated due to increased absorption of edema fluid. Epidermal changes are typically absent.

Pathogenesis. In most cases, urticaria results from antigen-induced release of vasoactive mediators from mast cell granules through sensitization with specific IgE antibodies. This *IgE-dependent* reaction can follow exposure to many different antigens (pollens, foods, drugs, insect venom) (Chapter 6). *IgE-independent* urticaria may also result from substances that in certain individuals directly incite the degranulation of mast cells, such as opiates, certain antibiotics, curare, and radiographic contrast media. Another cause of IgE-independent urticaria is exposure to chemicals, such as aspirin, that suppress prostaglandin synthesis from arachidonic acid. *Complement-mediated urticaria* is seen in *hereditary angioneurotic edema* (Chapter 6), caused by an inherited deficiency of C1 inhibitor that results in uncontrolled activation of the early components of the complement system and production of vasoactive mediators.[77]

ACUTE ECZEMATOUS DERMATITIS

The Greek word *eczema*, meaning "to boil over," vividly describes the appearance of acute eczematous dermatitis. All forms of eczema are characterized by red, papulovesicular, oozing, and crusted lesions that, if persistent, develop into raised, scaling plaques due to reactive acanthosis and hyperkeratosis (Fig. 25–23). Based on initiating factors, eczematous dermatitis can be subdivided into the following categories: (1) allergic contact dermatitis, (2) atopic dermatitis, (3) drug-related eczematous dermatitis, (4) photoeczematous dermatitis, and (5) primary irritant dermatitis.

A striking example of eczema is an acute contact reaction to topical antigens such as poison ivy/oak *(Rhus toxicodendron)*, characterized by pruritic, edematous, oozing plaques,

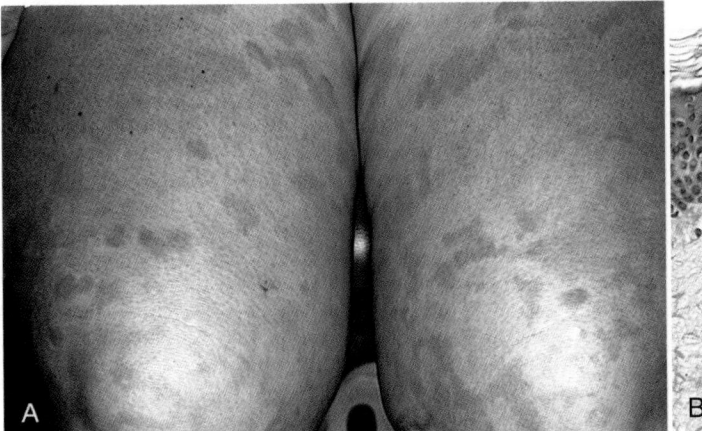
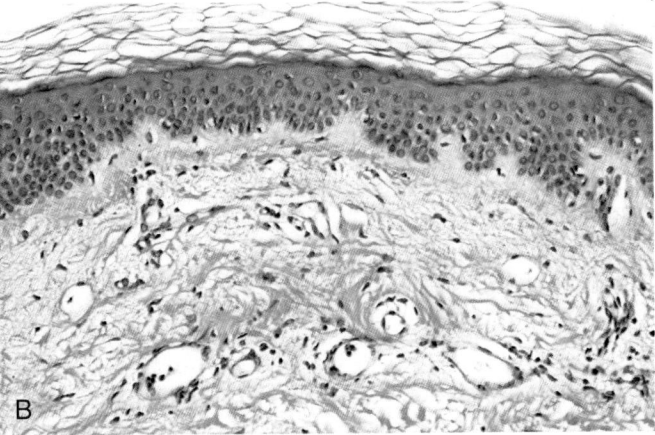

FIGURE 25–22 Urticaria. **A,** Erythematous, edematous, often circular plaques are characteristic. **B,** Histologically, there is superficial dermal edema, manifested by spaces between collagen bundles, and dilated lymphatic and blood-filled vascular spaces; the epithelium is normal.

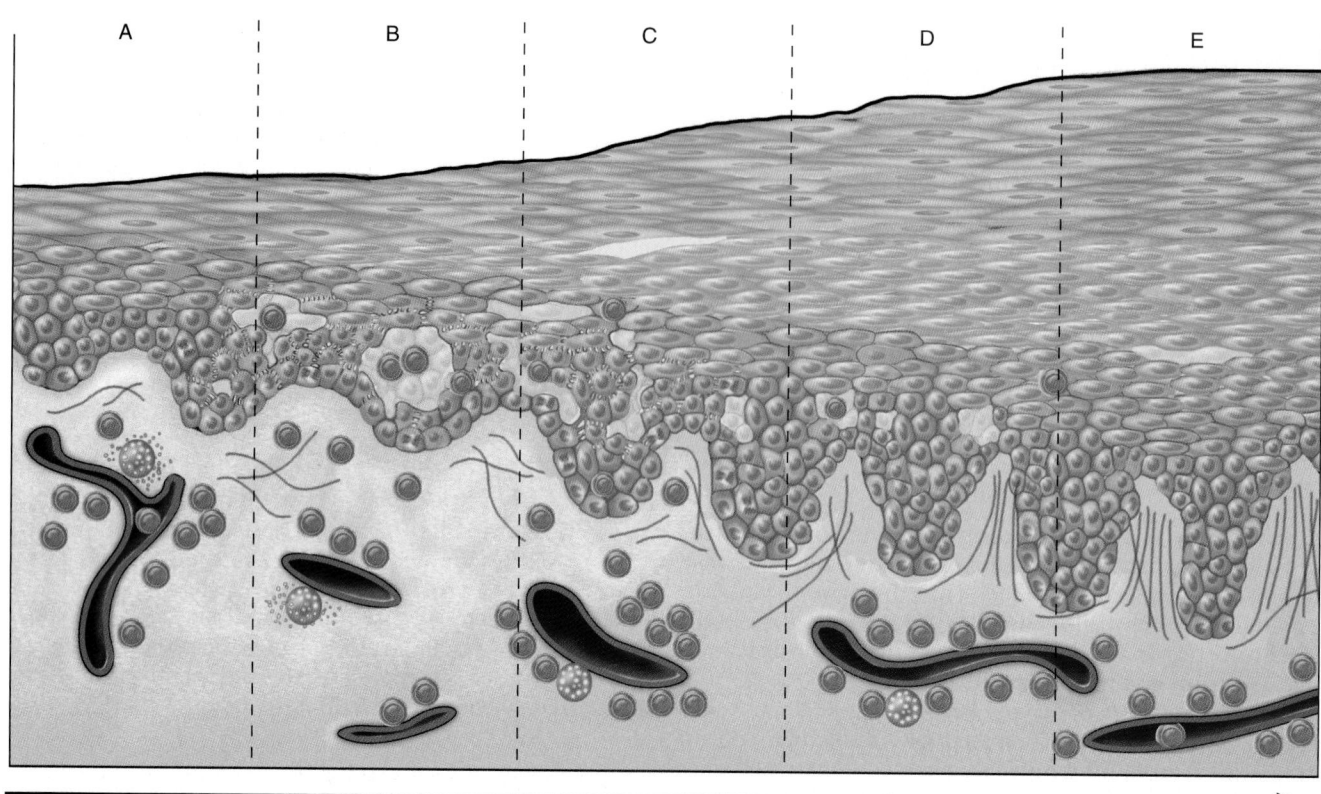

FIGURE 25–23 Stages of eczema development. **A,** Initial dermal edema and perivascular infiltration by inflammatory cells is followed within 24 to 48 hours by epidermal spongiosis and microvesicle formation (**B**). **C,** Abnormal scale, including parakeratosis, follows, along with progressive acanthosis (**D**) and hyperkeratosis (**E**) as the lesion becomes chronic.

often containing small and large blisters (vesicles and bullae) (Fig. 25–24A). Such lesions are prone to bacterial superinfection, which produces a yellow crust (impetiginization). With time, persistent lesions become less "wet" (fail to ooze or form vesicles) and become progressively scaly (hyperkeratotic) as the epidermis thickens (acanthosis). The clinical causes of eczema are sometimes broadly divided into "inside" and "outside" types: disease resulting from external application of antigen (such as poison ivy) or reaction to an internal circulating antigen (such as ingested food or drug).

Treatment of eczema involves a search for offending substances that can be removed from the environment. Topical steroids can also be used that nonspecifically block the inflammatory response. Such treatments are palliative and not curative, but are helpful in interrupting acute exacerbations of eczema that can become self perpetuating if unchecked.

Morphology. Spongiosis characterizes acute eczematous dermatitis, hence the histologic synonym spongiotic dermatitis. Unlike urticaria, in which edema is restricted to the superficial dermis, edema seeps into the intercellular spaces of the epidermis, splaying apart keratinocytes, particularly in the stratum spinosum. Mechanical shearing of intercellular attachment sites (desmosomes) and cell mem-

branes by progressive accumulation of intercellular fluid may result in the formation of intraepidermal vesicles (Fig. 25–24B).

During the earliest stages of eczematous dermatitis, there is a superficial, perivascular, lymphocytic infiltrate associated with papillary dermal edema and mast cell degranulation. The pattern and composition of this infiltrate may provide clues to the underlying cause. For example, eczema resulting from certain ingested drugs is marked by a lymphocytic infiltrate, often containing eosinophils, around deep as well as superficial dermal vessels. By contrast, eczematous dermatitis resulting from contact antigens tends to produce an inflammatory reaction that preferentially affects the superficial dermal layer.

Pathogenesis. This has been well studied in dermatitis triggered by contact antigens (e.g., poison ivy). Initially, antigens at the epidermal surface are taken up by dendritic Langerhans cells, which then migrate by way of dermal lymphatics to draining lymph nodes. Here, antigens, now processed by the Langerhans cell, are presented to naive CD4+ T cells, which are activated and develop into effector and memory cells (Chapter 6). On antigen re-exposure, these memory T cells migrate to affected skin sites of antigen localization, where

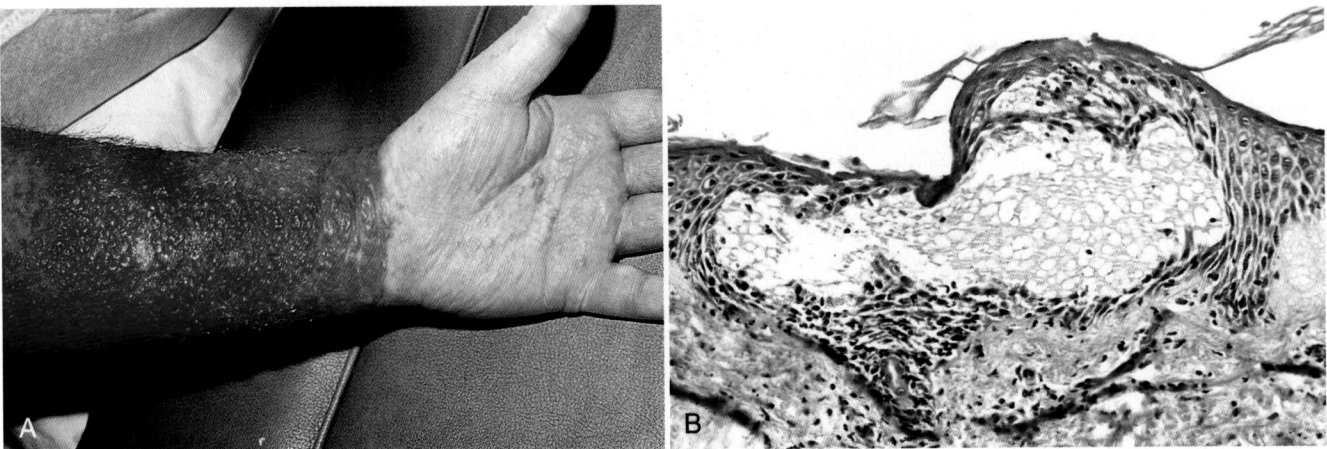

FIGURE 25–24 Eczematous dermatitis. **A,** Acute allergic contact dermatitis, with numerous vesicles on erythematous skin due to antigen exposure (in this case, laundry detergent in clothing). **B,** Histologically, intercellular edema within the epidermis creates small, fluid-filled intraepidermal vesicles.

they adhere to post-capillary venules, extravasate into tissues, and release cytokines and chemokines that recruit the numerous inflammatory cells characteristic of eczema. This process occurs within 24 hours and accounts for the initial erythema and pruritus that characterize cutaneous delayed hypersensitivity in the acute, spongiotic phase.[2]

Langerhans cells within the epidermis play a central role in contact dermatitis, and understandably factors that affect Langerhans cell function impact the inflammatory reaction. Chronic exposure to UV light is injurious to epidermal Langerhans cells and can prevent sensitization to contact antigens.[78] Other factors that modulate Langerhans cell function include neuropeptides released from nerve endings that terminate near the Langerhans cell body.[79]

ERYTHEMA MULTIFORME

Erythema multiforme is an uncommon, self-limited disorder that seems to be a hypersensitivity reaction to certain infections and drugs. This disorder affects individuals of any age and is associated with the following conditions: (1) infections such as herpes simplex, mycoplasmal infections, histoplasmosis, coccidioidomycosis, typhoid, and leprosy, among others; (2) administration of certain drugs (sulfonamides, penicillin, barbiturates, salicylates, hydantoins, and antimalarials); (3) malignant disease (carcinomas and lymphomas); and (4) collagen vascular diseases (lupus erythematosus, dermatomyositis, and polyarteritis nodosa).[80]

Affected individuals present with an array of "multiform" lesions, including macules, papules, vesicles, and bullae as well as the characteristic target lesion consisting of a red macule or papule with a pale, vesicular, or eroded center (Fig. 25–25A). Although lesions may be widely distributed, symmetric involvement of the extremities frequently occurs. An extensive and symptomatic febrile form of the disease, which is often but not exclusively seen in children, is called *Stevens-Johnson syndrome.* Typically, erosions and hemorrhagic crusts involve the lips and oral mucosa, although the conjunctiva, urethra, and genital and perianal areas may also be affected. Secondary infection of involved areas due to loss of skin integrity may result in life-threatening sepsis. Another variant, termed *toxic*

epidermal necrolysis, results in diffuse necrosis and sloughing of cutaneous and mucosal epithelial surfaces, producing a clinical situation analogous to an extensive burn when both infection and fluid loss are clinical concerns.[81]

Morphology. On histologic examination, early lesions show a superficial perivascular, lymphocytic infiltrate associated with dermal edema and accumulation of lymphocytes along the dermoepidermal junction, where they are intimately associated with degenerating and necrotic keratinocytes, a pattern termed *interface dermatitis* (Fig. 25–25B). With time there is upward migration of lymphocytes into the epidermis. Discrete and confluent zones of epidermal necrosis occur with concomitant blister formation. Epidermal sloughing leads to shallow erosions. The clinical **targetoid (target-like) lesion** shows central necrosis surrounded by a rim of perivenular inflammation (see Fig. 25–25A).

Pathogenesis. Erythema multiforme has similarities to other conditions characterized by immunologically mediated epidermal cell injury such as acute graft-versus-host disease, skin allograft rejection, and fixed drug eruptions.[82] In all these conditions epithelial cells are killed by skin-homing (CLA+) CD8+ cytotoxic T lymphocytes (CTLs). In erythema multiforme these cytotoxic cells are more prominent in the central portion of the lesions while CD4+ helper and Langerhans cells are more common in the raised, erythematous periphery. The precise target antigens within the epidermis that are recognized by CTLs in erythema multiforme remain unknown, but there is growing evidence that the basal cells that reside at the very tips of epidermal rete ridges may preferentially undergo apoptosis.[83]

Chronic Inflammatory Dermatoses

This category includes inflammatory skin disorders that persist for many months to years. The skin surface in some

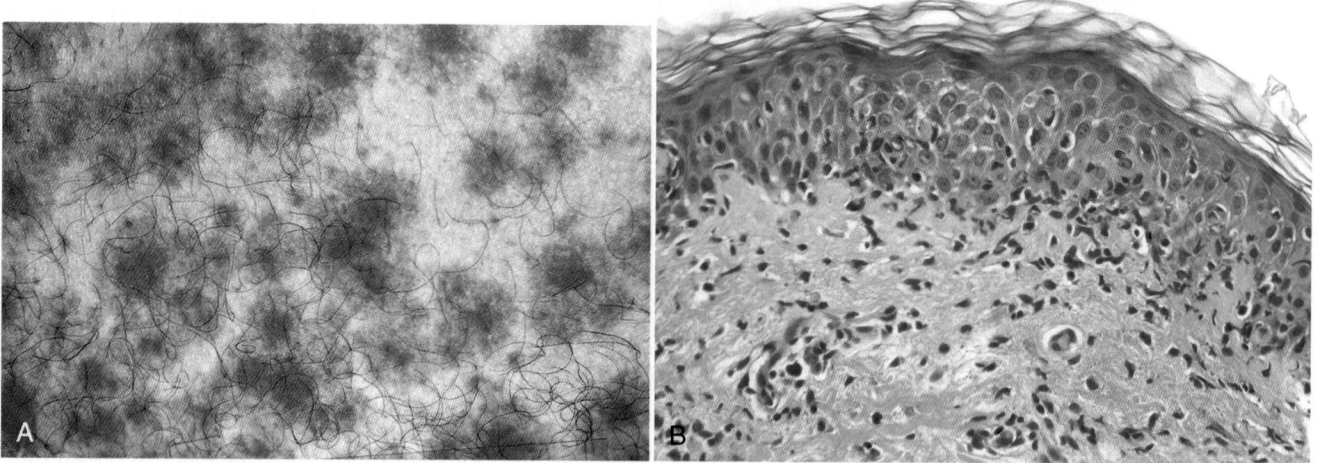

FIGURE 25–25 Erythema multiforme. **A,** The target-like clinical lesions consist of a central blister or zone of epidermal necrosis surrounded by macular erythema. **B,** Early lesions show lymphocytes collecting along the dermoepidermal junction where basal keratinocytes have begun to become vacuolated. With time, necrotic/apoptotic keratinocytes accumulate in the overlying epithelium.

chronic inflammatory dermatoses is roughened as a result of excessive or abnormal scale formation and shedding. However, not all scaling lesions are inflammatory; witness the hereditary ichthyoses, described above, with extensive scale due to defects in desquamation.

PSORIASIS

Psoriasis is a common chronic inflammatory dermatosis affecting as many as 1% to 2% of people in the United States. Persons of all ages may develop the disease. Psoriasis is sometimes associated with arthritis, myopathy, enteropathy, spondylitic joint disease, or the acquired immunodeficiency syndrome. Psoriatic arthritis may be mild or may produce severe deformities resembling the joint changes seen in rheumatoid arthritis.

Psoriasis most frequently affects the *skin of the elbows, knees, scalp, lumbosacral areas, intergluteal cleft, and glans penis.* The typical lesion is a well-demarcated, pink to *salmon-colored plaque* covered by loosely adherent scale that is characteristically *silver-white in color* (Fig. 25–26A). Variations exist, with some lesions occurring in annular, linear, gyrate, or serpiginous configurations. Psoriasis is one cause of total body erythema and scaling known as *erythroderma. Nail changes* occur in 30% of cases of psoriasis and consist of yellow-brown discoloration (often likened to an oil slick), with pitting, dimpling, separation of the nail plate from the underlying bed (onycholysis), thickening, and crumbling. In the rare variant called *pustular psoriasis* multiple small pustules form on erythematous plaques. This type of psoriasis is either benign and localized (hands and feet) or generalized and life-threatening, with associated fever, leukocytosis, arthralgia, diffuse cutaneous and mucosal pustules, secondary infection, and electrolyte disturbances.[84]

Morphology. Established lesions of psoriasis have a characteristic histologic picture. Increased epidermal

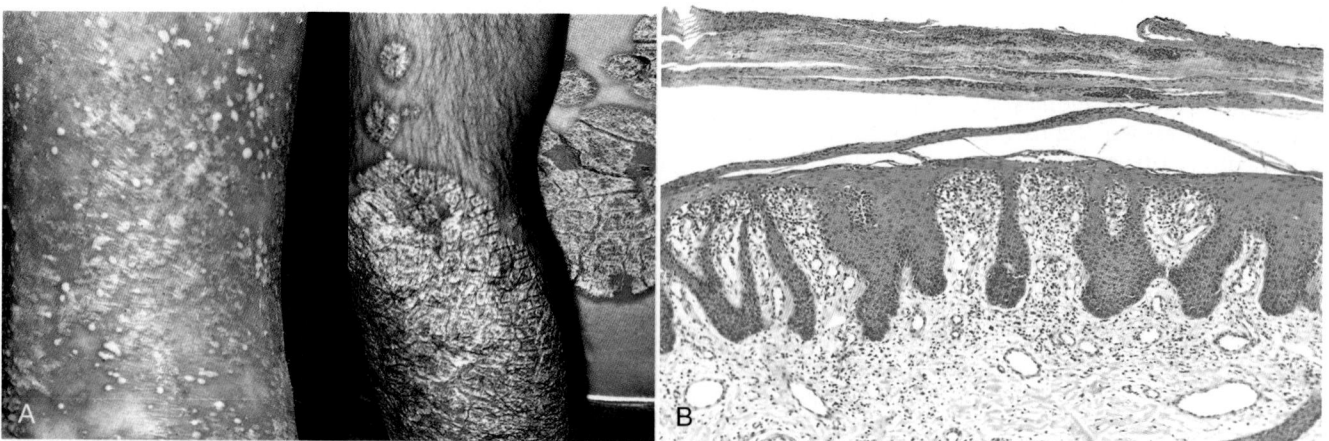

FIGURE 25–26 Clinical evolution of psoriasis. **A,** Early and eruptive lesions may be dominated by signs of inflammation, including small pustules and erythema *(left).* Established, chronic lesions demonstrate erythema surmounted by characteristic silver-white scale *(right).* **B,** Histologically, established lesions demonstrate marked epidermal hyperplasia, parakeratotic scale, and neutrophils within the superficial epidermal layers.

cell turnover results in marked epidermal thickening (acanthosis), with regular downward elongation of the rete ridges sometimes described as appearing like test tubes in a rack (Fig. 25–26B). Mitotic figures are easily identified well above the basal cell layer, where mitotic activity is confined in normal skin. **The stratum granulosum is thinned or absent, and extensive overlying parakeratotic scale is seen.** Typical of psoriatic plaques is thinning of the portion of the epidermal cell layer that overlies the tips of dermal papillae (suprapapillary plates) and dilated, tortuous blood vessels within these papillae. This constellation of changes results in abnormal proximity of vessels within the dermal papillae to the overlying parakeratotic scale, and accounts for the characteristic clinical phenomenon of multiple, minute, bleeding points when the scale is lifted from the plaque (**Auspitz sign**). Neutrophils form small aggregates within slightly spongiotic foci of the superficial epidermis (**spongiform pustules**) and within the parakeratotic stratum corneum (**Munro microabscesses**). In pustular psoriasis, larger abscess-like accumulations of neutrophils are present directly beneath the stratum corneum.

Pathogenesis. The pathogenesis of psoriasis seems to be multifactorial, with contributions from genetic and environmental factors. There is a strong association between psoriasis and HLA-C, particularly with the *HLA-Cw*0602* allele. About two thirds of affected individuals carry this allele; homozygotes for *HLA-Cw*0602* have a 2.5-fold higher risk of developing psoriasis than heterozygotes. Nevertheless, only 10% of individuals with *HLA-Cw*0602* develop psoriasis, indicating that other factors interact with this MHC molecule in causing disease susceptibility.[85] Sensitized populations of CD4+ T_H1 and T_H17 cells and activated CD8+ effector T cells enter the skin and accumulate in the epidermis. The culprit antigens remain elusive. T cell homing to the skin may create an abnormal microenvironment by inducing the secretion of cytokines and growth factors that induce keratinocyte proliferation, resulting in the characteristic lesions. The interactions between CD4+ T cells, CD8+ T cells, dendritic cells, and keratinocytes give rise to a cytokine "soup" dominated by T_H1-type and T_H17-type cytokines such as IL-12, interferon-γ, tumor necrosis factor (TNF), and IL-17.[2] The lymphocytes also produce growth factors for keratinocytes. Psoriatic lesions can be induced in susceptible individuals by local trauma, a process known as the *Koebner phenomenon*. The trauma may induce a local inflammatory response that promotes lesion development. There is much evidence that, as with rheumatoid arthritis, TNF is a major mediator in the pathogenesis of psoriasis. Indeed, anti-TNF therapies provide benefit and are currently in use.

SEBORRHEIC DERMATITIS

Seborrheic dermatitis is a chronic inflammatory dermatosis even more common than psoriasis, affecting 1% to 3% of the general population.[84] It classically involves regions with a high density of sebaceous glands, such as the scalp, forehead (especially the glabella), external auditory canal, retroauricular area, nasolabial folds, and the presternal area. However, it is important to note that seborrheic dermatitis is not a disease of the sebaceous glands. The individual lesions are macules and papules on an erythematous-yellow, often greasy base, typically in association with extensive scaling and crusting. Fissures may also be present, particularly behind the ears. Dandruff is the common clinical expression of seborrheic dermatitis of the scalp. In infants, seborrheic dermatitis presents as cradle cap but can also be part of a disorder known as *Leiner disease*, in which the condition is generalized and associated with diarrhea and failure to thrive. A severe form of seborrheic dermatitis that is difficult to treat is seen in many HIV–infected individuals with low CD4 counts.[86]

Morphology. Lesions of seborrheic dermatitis share histologic features with both spongiotic dermatitis and psoriasis, with earlier lesions being more spongiotic and later ones more acanthotic. Typically, mounds of parakeratosis containing neutrophils and serum are present at the ostia of hair follicles (so-called *follicular lipping*). A superficial perivascular inflammatory infiltrate generally consists of an admixture of lymphocytes and neutrophils. With human immunodeficiency virus infection, apoptotic keratinocytes and plasma cells may also be present.

Pathogenesis. The etiology of seborrheic dermatitis is unknown. However, therapeutic studies with ketoconazole, an antifungal agent, suggest that the lipophilic yeast *Malassezia furfur*, which is associated with tinea versicolor, may have a role in some cases.[87] Involvement of sebum is supported by clinical observations of people with Parkinson disease, who typically show increased sebum production secondary to dopamine deficiency and have a markedly increased incidence of seborrheic dermatitis.[88] Indeed, once treated with levodopa, the oiliness of the skin decreases and the seborrheic dermatitis improves. However, because other conditions associated with increased sebaceous activity such as acne (discussed below) do not show this association, sebum production is unlikely to be the sole or primary factor in the pathogenesis of seborrheic dermatitis.

LICHEN PLANUS

"Pruritic, purple, polygonal, planar papules, and plaques" are the tongue-twisting "six p's" of this disorder of skin and mucosa. Lichen planus is usually self-limited and most commonly resolves spontaneously 1 to 2 years after onset, often leaving zones of postinflammatory hyperpigmentation. Oral lesions may persist for years. Squamous cell carcinoma has been noted to occur in chronic mucosal and paramucosal lesions of lichen planus, but a direct pathogenetic relationship has not been established.[89,90]

Cutaneous lesions consist of itchy, violaceous, flat-topped papules that may coalesce focally to form plaques (Fig. 25–27A). These papules are often highlighted by white dots or lines called *Wickham striae*, which are created by areas of hypergranulosis. In darkly pigmented individuals, lesions may acquire a dark-brown color due to release of melanin into the dermis as the basal cell layer is destroyed. Multiple lesions are

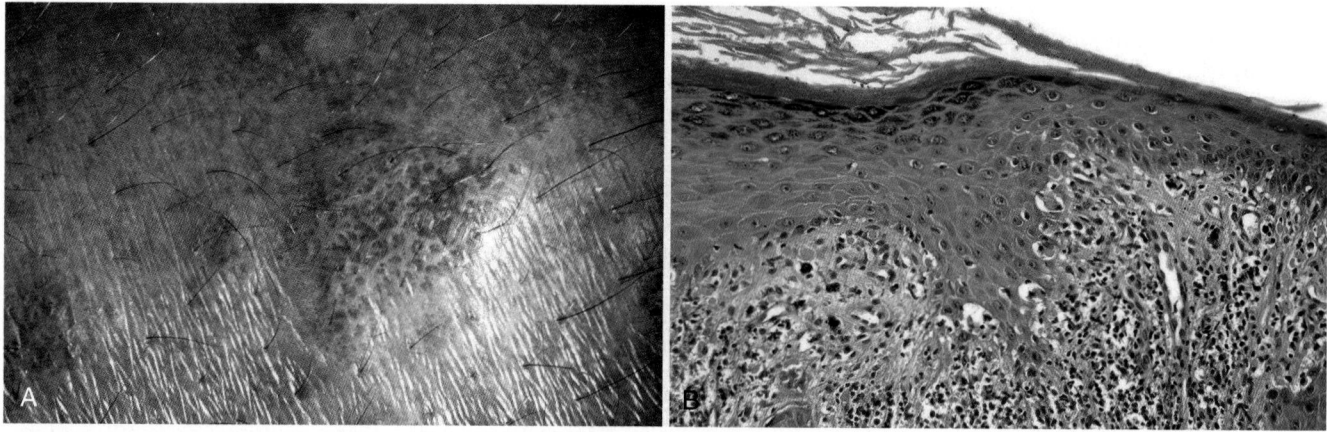

FIGURE 25–27 Lichen planus. **A,** This flat-topped pink-purple, polygonal papule has a white lacelike pattern that is referred to as Wickham stria. **B,** Biopsy specimen demonstrating a bandlike infiltrate of lymphocytes at the dermoepidermal junction, hyperkeratosis, hypergranulosis and pointed rete ridges (sawtoothing) as a result of chronic basal cell layer injury.

characteristic and are symmetrically distributed, particularly on the extremities, often about the wrists and elbows, and on the glans penis. In 70% of cases, oral lesions are present as white, reticulated, or netlike areas involving the mucosa. As in psoriasis, the Koebner phenomenon may be seen in lichen planus.[91]

> **Morphology.** Lichen planus is characterized histologically by a dense, continuous infiltrate of lymphocytes along the dermoepidermal junction, a prototypic example of *interface dermatitis* (Fig. 25–27B). The lymphocytes are intimately associated with basal keratinocytes, which show degeneration, necrosis, and a resemblance in size and contour to more mature cells of the stratum spinosum (squamatization). A consequence of this destructive infiltration of lymphocytes is a redefinition of the normal, smoothly undulating configuration of the dermoepidermal interface to a more angulated zigzag contour (sawtoothing). Anucleate, necrotic basal cells may become incorporated into the inflamed papillary dermis, where they are referred to as **colloid** or **Civatte bodies**. Though characteristic of lichen planus, these bodies may be detected in any chronic dermatitis in which basal keratinocytes are injured and destroyed. Although the lesions bear some similarities to those in erythema multiforme, lichen planus shows changes of chronicity, namely, epidermal hyperplasia (or rarely atrophy) and thickening of the granular cell layer and stratum corneum (hypergranulosis and hyperkeratosis, respectively). Lichen planus preferentially affecting the epithelium of hair follicles is referred to as **lichen planopilaris**.

Pathogenesis. The pathogenesis of lichen planus is not known. It is plausible that expression of altered antigens at the level of the basal cell layer and the dermoepidermal junction elicit a cell-mediated cytotoxic (CD8+/CLA+ T cell) immune response. In support of this notion, T lymphocyte infiltrates

and hyperplasia of Langerhans cells are characteristic features of this disorder.[92]

Blistering (Bullous) Diseases

Although vesicles and bullae (blisters) occur in several unrelated conditions such as herpesvirus infection, spongiotic dermatitis, erythema multiforme, and thermal burns, there exists a group of disorders in which blisters are the primary and most distinctive features. These *bullous diseases*, as they are called, produce dramatic lesions and in some instances are fatal if untreated. Blisters in the various disorders occur at different levels within the skin (Fig. 25–28); histologic assessment is essential for accurate diagnosis and provides insight into the pathogenic mechanisms. Knowledge of the molecular structure of the intercellular and cell-to-matrix attachments that provide the skin with mechanical stability is helpful in understanding these diseases (Fig. 25–29).

INFLAMMATORY BLISTERING DISORDERS

Pemphigus

Pemphigus is a blistering disorder caused by *autoantibodies that result in the dissolution of intercellular attachments within the epidermis and mucosal epithelium*. Though rare, without treatment it may be life-threatening, and its pathobiology provides important insight into the molecular mechanisms of keratinocyte adhesion. The majority of individuals who develop pemphigus are in the fourth to sixth decades of life, and men and women are affected equally. There are multiple variants: (1) pemphigus vulgaris, (2) pemphigus vegetans, (3) pemphigus foliaceus, (4) pemphigus erythematosus, and (5) paraneoplastic pemphigus.[93]

Pemphigus vulgaris, by far the most common type (accounting for more than 80% of cases worldwide), involves the mucosa and skin, especially on the scalp, face, axilla, groin, trunk, and points of pressure. It may present as oral ulcers that may persist for months before skin involvement appears. Primary lesions are superficial vesicles and bullae that rupture

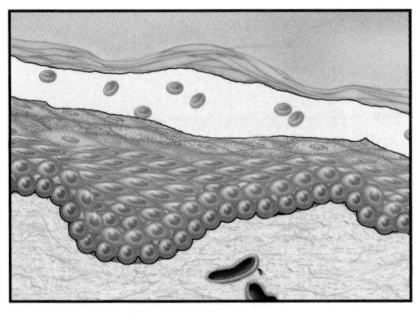 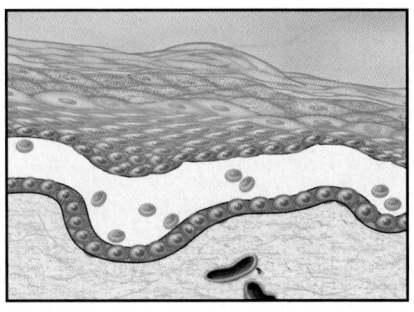 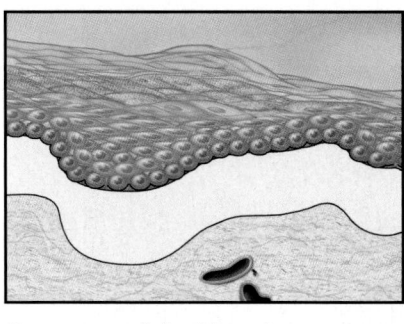

| A | Subcorneal | B | Suprabasal | C | Subepidermal |

FIGURE 25–28 Schematic representation of histologic levels of blister formation. **A,** In a subcorneal blister the stratum corneum forms the roof of the bulla (as in pemphigus foliaceus). **B,** In a suprabasal blister a portion of the epidermis, including the stratum corneum, forms the roof (as in pemphigus vulgaris). **C,** In a subepidermal blister the entire epidermis separates from the dermis (as in bullous pemphigoid).

easily, leaving shallow erosions covered with dried serum and crust (Fig. 25–30A). *Pemphigus vegetans* is a rare form that usually presents not with blisters but with large, moist, verrucous (wart-like), vegetating plaques studded with pustules on the groin, axillae, and flexural surfaces. *Pemphigus foliaceus* is a more benign form that is endemic in Brazil (where it is called *fogo selvagem*) and occurs sporadically in other geographic regions. Sites of predilection are the scalp, face, chest, and back, and the mucous membranes are only rarely affected. Bullae are so superficial that only zones of erythema and crusting, sites of previous blister rupture resulting in superficial erosions, are usually present on physical examination (Fig. 25–31A). *Pemphigus erythematosus* is considered to be a localized, less severe form of pemphigus foliaceus that may selectively involve the malar area of the face in a lupus erythematosus–like fashion. *Paraneoplastic pemphigus* occurs in association with various malignancies, most commonly non-Hodgkin lymphoma.

The mainstay of treatment is immunosuppressive agents, which decrease the titers of the pathogenic antibodies. In those with the most severe form of the disease, pemphigus vulgaris, this lowers but does not entirely prevent mortality.

Morphology. The common histologic denominator in all forms of pemphigus is **acantholysis**, the dissolu-

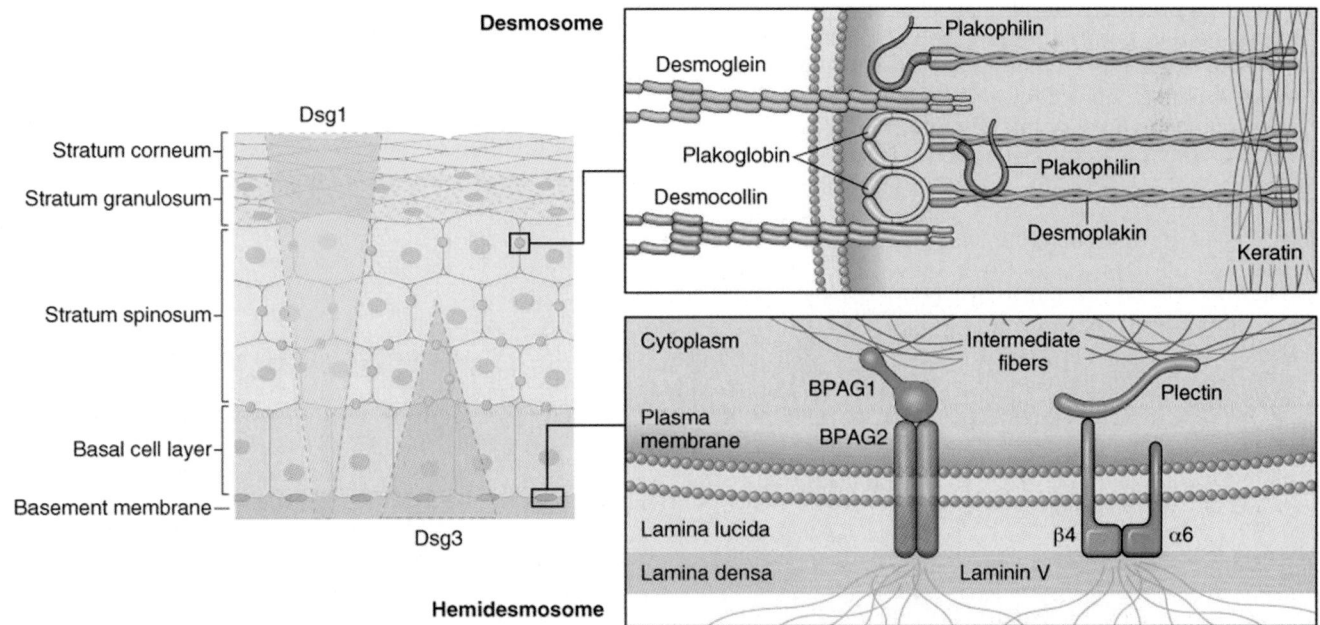

FIGURE 25–29 Squamous cell adhesion molecules. Knowledge of the proteins composing desmosomes and hemodesmosomes is key to understanding blistering disorders. Desmogleins 1 and 3 (Dsg1, Dsg3) are functionally interchangeable components of desmosomes, but have different distributions within the epidermis *(left panel)*. In pemphigus vulgaris, autoantibodies against Dsg1 and Dsg3 cause blisters in the deep suprabasal epidermis, whereas in pemphigus foliaceus, the autoantibodies are against Dsg1 alone, leading to superficial, subcorneal blisters. In bullous phemphigoid, autoantibodies bind BPAG2, a component of the hemidesomes, leading to blister formation at the level of the lamina lucida of the basement membrane. Dermatitis herpetiformis is caused by IgA autoantibodies to the fibrils that anchor hemidesmosomes to the dermis. The various forms of epidermolysis bullosa are caused by genetic defects in genes encoding proteins that either form or stabilize desmosomes or hemidesmosomes. α6/β4, α6/β4 integrin.

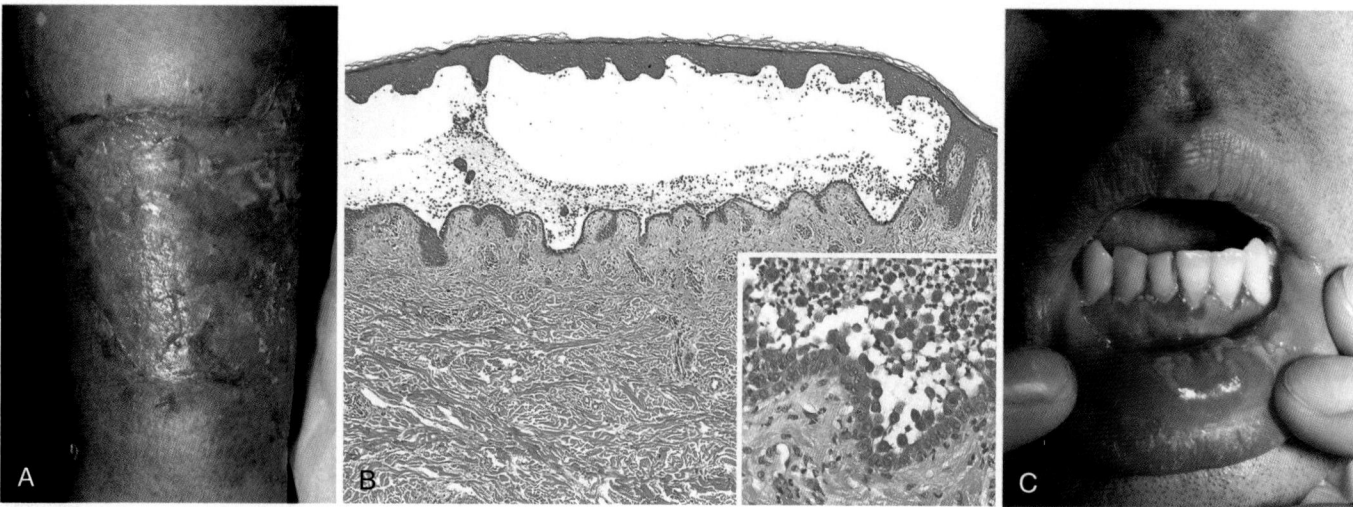

FIGURE 25–30 Pemphigus vulgaris. **A,** Eroded plaques are formed on rupture of confluent, thin-roofed bullae, here affecting axillary skin. **B,** Suprabasal acantholysis results in an intraepidermal blister in which rounded (acantholytic) epidermal cells are identified *(inset).* **C,** Ulcerated blisters in the oral mucosa are also common as seen here on the mucosal portion of the lip.

tion, or lysis, of the intercellular adhesions that connect squamous epithelial cells. Acantholytic cells dissociate from one another, lose their polyhedral shape and become rounded. In pemphigus vulgaris and pemphigus vegetans, acantholysis selectively involves the cells immediately above the basal cell layer. In the vegetans variant, there is also overlying epidermal hyperplasia. The **suprabasal acantholytic blister** that forms is characteristic of pemphigus vulgaris (see Fig. 25–30B). The single layer of intact basal cells that forms the blister base has been likened to a row of tombstones. In pemphigus foliaceus, a blister forms by similar mechanisms but, unlike the case with pemphigus vulgaris, selectively involves the superficial epidermis at the level of the stratum granulosum (Fig. 25–31B). Variable superficial dermal infiltration by

lymphocytes, histiocytes, and eosinophils accompanies all forms of pemphigus.

Pathogenesis. All forms of pemphigus are caused by IgG autoantibodies against desmogleins, and show linkage to specific HLA types.[94] By direct immunofluorescence, lesional sites show a characteristic net-like pattern of intercellular IgG deposits. IgG is usually seen at all levels of the epithelium in pemphigus vulgaris, but tends to be more superficial in pemphigus foliaceus (Fig. 25–32). The distribution of desmoglein 1 and 3 in the epidermis and the presence of autoantibodies to one or both proteins appear to explain the position and severity of the blisters (Fig. 25–29). The antibodies seem to function primarily by directly disrupting the intercellular adhesive function of the desmosomes and may activate intercellular proteases as well.[95] Paraneoplastic pemphigus most

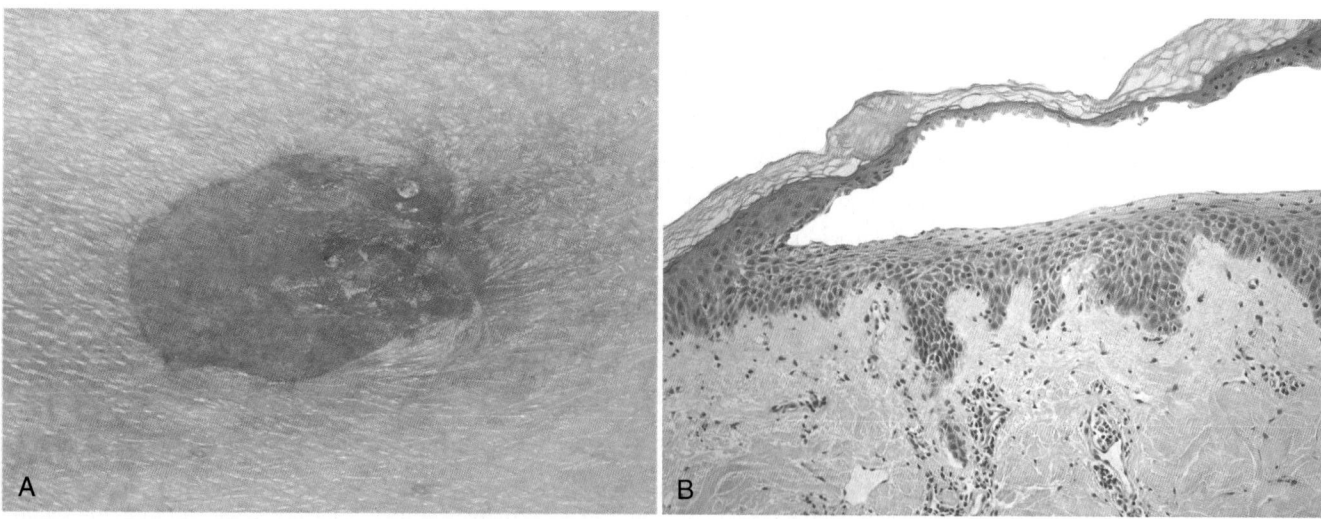

FIGURE 25–31 Pemphigus foliaceus. **A,** The delicate, superficial (subcorneal) blisters are much less erosive than seen in pemphigus vulgaris. **B,** Subcorneal separation of the epithelium is seen.

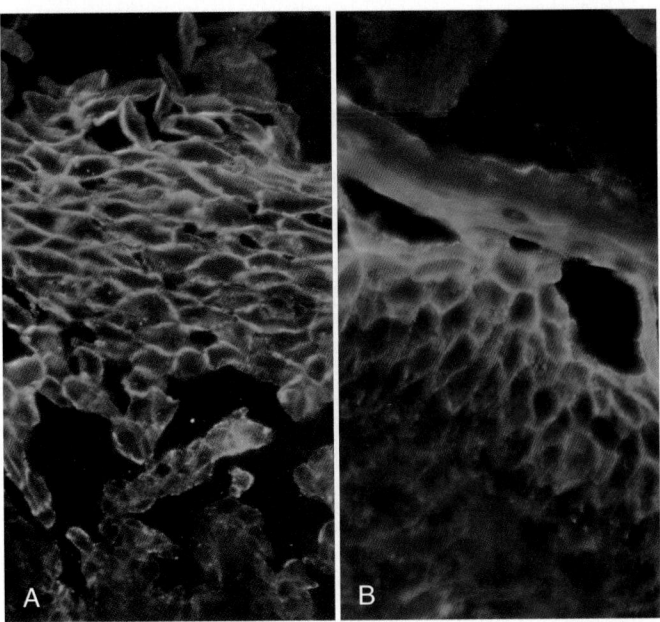

FIGURE 25–32 Direct immunofluorescence of pemphigus. **A,** In pemphigus vulgaris there is deposition of immunoglobulin along the plasma membranes of epidermal keratinocytes in a reticular or fishnet-like pattern. Also note the early suprabasal separation due to loss of cell-to-cell adhesion (acantholysis). **B,** In pemphigus foliaceus the immunoglobulin deposits are more superficial.

often arises in the setting of lymphoid neoplasms, and is caused by autoantibodies that may recognize desmogleins of other proteins involved in intercellular adhesion.[96]

Bullous Pemphigoid

Generally affecting elderly individuals, bullous pemphigoid shows a wide range of clinical presentations. It may involve only the skin, either locally or generally, or the skin and mucosal surfaces. Clinically, lesions are tense bullae, filled with clear fluid, on normal or erythematous skin (Fig. 25–33A). Lesions are usually up to 2 cm in diameter but occasionally may reach 4 to 8 cm in diameter. The bullae do not rupture as easily as do the blisters seen in pemphigus and, if they are not secondarily infected, heal without scarring. Sites of involvement include the inner aspects of the thighs, flexor surfaces of the forearms, axillae, groin, and lower abdomen. Oral lesions are present in 10% to 15% of affected individuals, usually appearing after the cutaneous lesions.[97] Some patients may present with urticarial plaques, with extreme associated pruritus.

> **Morphology.** The separation of bullous pemphigoid from pemphigus is based on the identification of **subepidermal, nonacantholytic** blisters. Early lesions show a superficial and sometimes deep perivascular infiltrate of lymphocytes and variable numbers of eosinophils, occasional neutrophils, superficial dermal edema, and associated basal cell layer vacuolization (Fig. 25–33B). Eosinophils showing degranulation are typically detected directly beneath the epidermal basal cell layer. The vacuolated basal cell layer eventually gives rise to a fluid-filled blister.

Pathogenesis. Bullous pemphigoid features *linear* deposition of immunoglobulin and complement in the basement membrane zone (Fig. 25–34A). Reactivity also occurs in the basal cell–basement membrane attachment plaques (hemidesmosomes), where most of the bullous pemphigoid antigen (BPAG) is located. This protein is involved normally in dermoepidermal bonding. There are two forms of the antigen recognized by auto-antibodies—BPAG1, a 230-kD plakin protein, and BPAG2, a 180-kD protein also known as collagen type XVIII. Both BPAG1 and BPAG2 are recognized as normal constituents of the hemidesmosomes that bind basal cells at the dermoepidermal junction (Figs. 25–34B and 25–29). Only antibodies to BPAG2 are proven to cause blistering.[98] Generation of auto-antibodies to this hemidesmosome component

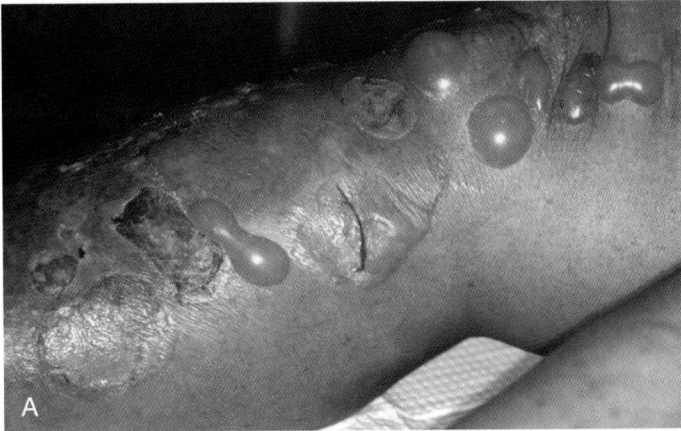
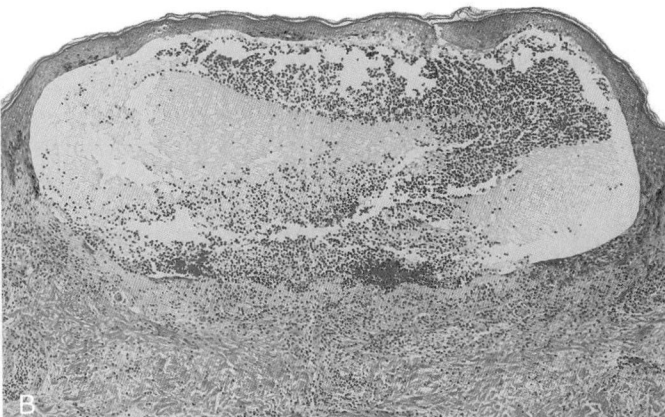

FIGURE 25–33 Bullous pemphigoid. **A,** Clinical bullae result from basal cell layer vacuolization, producing tense, intact subepidermal blisters that are difficult to rupture given the roof formed by the full thickness of the epidermis. Ulceration results upon rupture as the blisters are subepidermal. **B,** Histopathology shows an intact blister with eosinophils, as well as lymphocytes and occasional neutrophils, that may be intimately associated with basal cell layer destruction and the creation of the subepidermal cleft.

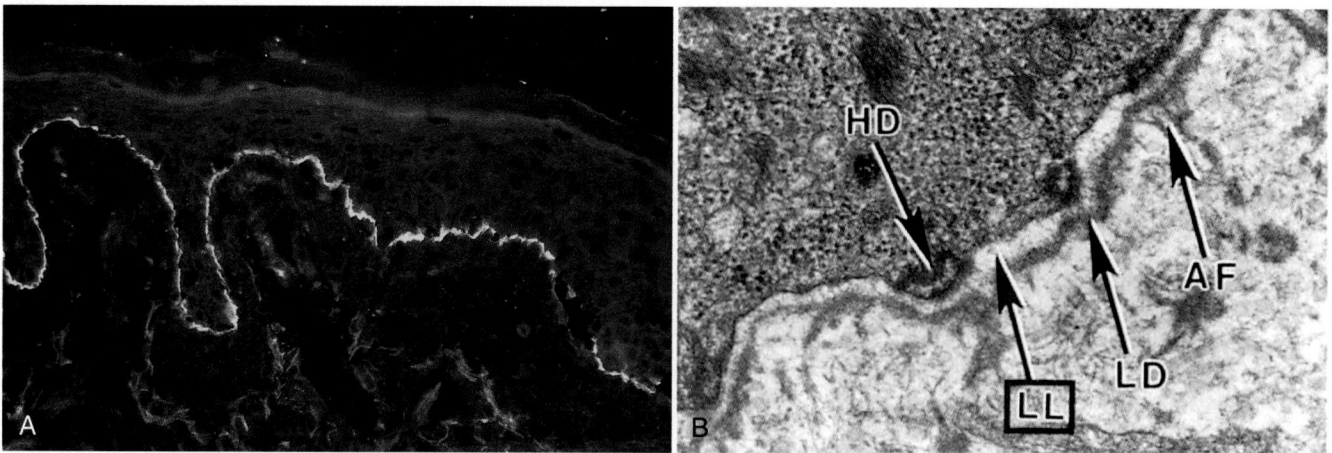

FIGURE 25–34   **A,** Linear deposition of complement along the dermoepidermal junction in bullous pemphigoid; the pattern has been likened to ribbon candy. **B,** Bullous pemphigoid antigen is located in the lowermost portion of the basal cell cytoplasm in association with hemidesmosomes (HD), with blister formation affecting the lamina lucida (LL) of the basement membrane zone. AF, anchoring fibrils; LD, lamina densa. (See also Fig. 25–31.)

results in continuous and linear deposition of IgG along the basement membrane and the fixation of complement with subsequent tissue injury by means of locally recruited neutrophils and eosinophils.

DERMATITIS HERPETIFORMIS

Dermatitis herpetiformis is a rare disorder characterized by *urticaria and grouped vesicles*. The disease affects predominantly males, often in the third and fourth decades. In some cases it occurs in association with intestinal celiac disease and responds to a gluten-free diet.

Pathogenesis. The association of dermatitis herpetiformis with celiac disease provides a clue to its pathogenesis. Genetically predisposed individuals develop IgA antibodies to dietary gluten (derived from the wheat protein gliadin). The antibodies cross-react with reticulin, a component of the anchoring fibrils that tether the epidermal basement membrane to the superficial dermis. The resultant injury and inflammation produce a subepidermal blister. Some people with dermatitis herpetiformis and gluten-sensitive enteropathy respond to a gluten-free diet.

> **Morphology.** As an early event, fibrin and neutrophils accumulate selectively at the **tips of dermal papillae,** forming small microabscesses (Fig. 25–35A). The basal cells overlying these microabscesses show vacuolization and focal dermoepidermal separation that ultimately coalesce to form a true **subepidermal blister.** By direct immunofluorescence, dermatitis herpetiformis shows discontinuous, **granular deposits of IgA** selectively localized in the tips of dermal papillae (Fig. 25–35B).

Clinical Features. The urticarial plaques and vesicles of dermatitis herpetiformis are extremely *pruritic*. The lesions are bilateral, symmetric and grouped, involving preferentially the extensor surfaces, elbows, knees, upper back, and buttocks (Fig. 25–35C).

NONINFLAMMATORY BLISTERING DISORDERS

Epidermolysis Bullosa and Porphyria

Some primary disorders characterized by vesicles and bullae are mediated by non-inflammatory mechanisms. Two such diseases are *epidermolysis bullosa* and *porphyria*.

Epidermolysis bullosa constitutes a group of disorders caused by inherited defects in structural proteins that lend mechanical stability to the skin. The common feature is a proclivity to form blisters at sites of pressure, rubbing, or trauma, at or soon after birth.[99] In the *simplex type,* defects of the basal cell layer of the epidermis result from mutations in the genes encoding keratins 14 or 5. These two proteins normally pair with one another to make a functional keratin fiber, thus explaining the similar phenotype resulting from mutation of either gene. In the *junctional type,* blisters occur in otherwise histologically normal skin at precisely the level of the lamina lucida (Figs. 25–36 and 25–29). In the scarring *dystrophic types,* blisters develop beneath the lamina densa, in association with rudimentary or defective anchoring fibrils. Dystrophic epidermolysis bullosa is an inherited disease resulting from mutations in the *COL7A1* gene that encodes type VII collagen (Chapter 3). Squamous cell carcinoma can sometime arise in these chronic blisters.[100] The histologic changes are so subtle that electron microscopy may be required to differentiate among these types in clinically ambiguous settings. Overall, approximately ten genes encoding structural proteins at the dermoepidermal junction have been implicated in the various forms of this disease.[101] One form, termed *non-Herlitz junctional epidermolysis bullosa* is caused by a genetic defect (usually a point mutation) in the *LAMB3* gene that encodes laminin Vβ3. Successful gene therapy has been carried out in one individual with this disease by inserting a normal LAMB3 gene into keratinocytes.

Porphyria refers to a group of uncommon inborn or acquired disturbances of porphyrin metabolism. Porphyrins are pigments normally present in hemoglobin, myoglobin, and cytochromes. The classification of porphyrias is based on both clinical and biochemical features. The five major types

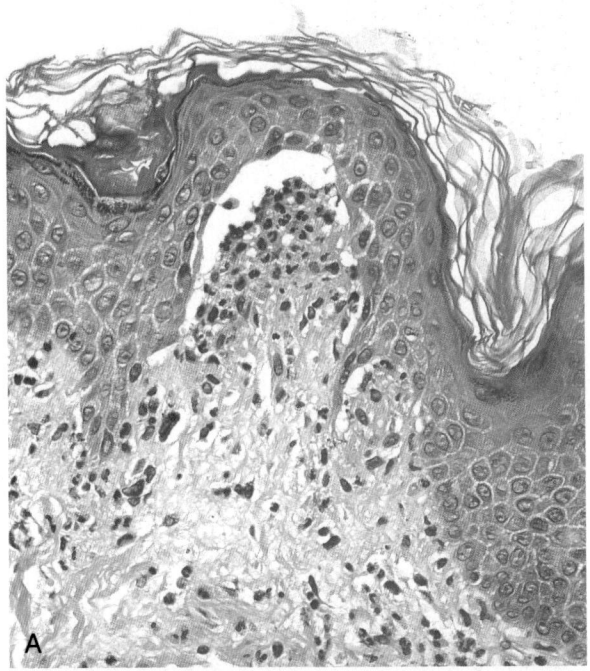

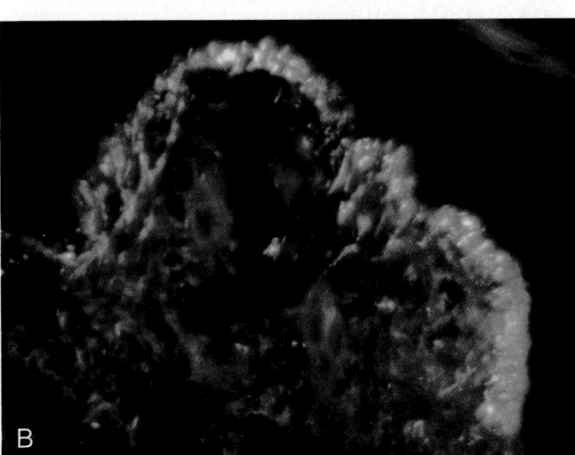

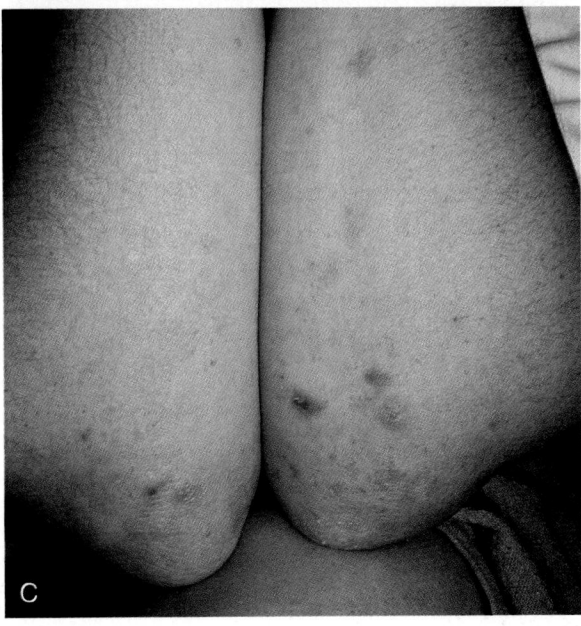

FIGURE 25–35 Dermatitis herpetiformis. **A,** The blisters are associated with basal cell layer injury initially caused by accumulation of neutrophils (microabscesses) at the tips of dermal papillae. **B,** Selective deposition of IgA autoantibody at the tips of dermal papillae is characteristic. **C,** Lesions consist of intact and eroded (usually scratched) erythematous blisters, often grouped (seen here on elbows and arms). (**B,** Courtesy of Dr. Victor G. Prieto, Houston, Texas.)

are (1) congenital erythropoietic porphyria, (2) erythrohepatic protoporphyria, (3) acute intermittent porphyria, (4) porphyria cutanea tarda, and (5) mixed porphyria. Cutaneous manifestations consist of urticaria and vesicles that heal with scarring and that are exacerbated by exposure to sunlight. The primary alterations by light microscopy are a *subepidermal vesicle* (Fig. 25–37) *with associated marked thickening of the walls of superficial dermal vessels.* The pathogenesis of these alterations is not well understood, although serum proteins, including immunoglobulins, typically form glassy deposits in the walls of superficial dermal microvessels.

Disorders of Epidermal Appendages

ACNE VULGARIS

Virtually universal in the middle to late teenage years, acne vulgaris affects both males and females, although males tend to have more severe disease. Acne is seen in all races but is usually milder in people of Asian descent. Acne vulgaris in adolescents is believed to occur as a result of physiologic hormonal variations and alterations in hair follicles, particularly the sebaceous gland. The clinical features of acne may be induced or exacerbated by drugs (corticosteroids, adrenocorticotropic hormone, testosterone, gonadotropins, contraceptives, trimethadione, iodides, and bromides), occupational contactants (cutting oils, chlorinated hydrocarbons, and coal tars), and occlusive conditions such as heavy clothing, cosmetics, and tropical climates. Some families seem to be particularly affected by acne, suggesting a hereditary component.

Acne is divided into noninflammatory and inflammatory types, although the types may coexist. The former consists of open and closed comedones. *Open comedones* are small follicular papules containing a central black keratin plug. This color is the result of oxidation of melanin pigment (not dirt). *Closed comedones* are follicular papules without a visible central plug. Because the keratin plug is trapped beneath the epidermal surface, these lesions are potential sources of follicular rupture and inflammation. Inflammatory acne is characterized by erythematous papules, nodules, and pustules (Fig. 25–38A). Severe variants (e.g., acne conglobata) result in sinus tract formation and physical scarring.

Morphology. Four key components contribute to the development of acne: (1) changes in keratinization of the lower portion of the follicular infundibulum with the development of a keratin plug blocking outflow of sebum to the skin surface; (2) hypertrophy of

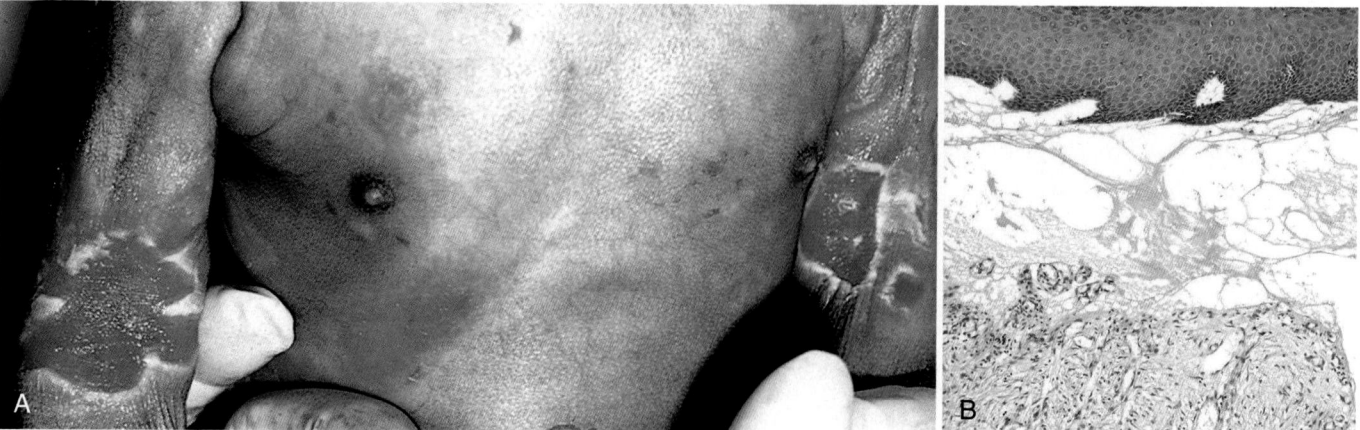

FIGURE 25–36   Epidermolysis bullosa. **A,** Junctional epidermolysis bullosa showing typical erosions in flexural creases. **B,** A noninflammatory subepidermal blister has formed at the level of the lamina lucida.

sebaceous glands with puberty or increased activity due to hormonal stimulation; (3) lipase-synthesizing bacteria *(Propionibacterium acnes)* colonizing the upper and midportion of the hair follicle, converting lipids within sebum to pro-inflammatory fatty acids; and (4) inflammation of the follicle associated with release of cytotoxic and chemotactic factors.[103] Depending on the stage of the disease, open or closed comedones, papules, pustules, or deep inflammatory nodules may develop. Open comedones have large, patulous orifices, whereas those of closed comedones are identifiable only microscopically (Fig. 25–38B,

C). Variable lymphohistiocytic infiltrates are present in and around affected follicles, and extensive acute and chronic inflammation accompanies follicular rupture. Dermal abscesses may form in association with rupture (see Fig. 25–38C), and gradual resolution, often with scarring, ensues.

Pathogenesis. The pathogenesis of acne is incompletely understood. Endocrine factors have been implicated (especially androgens) because, historically, young castrated males generally do not develop the condition (a questionable trade-off). It has been postulated that bacterial lipases of *Propionibacterium acnes* break down sebaceous oils, liberating highly irritating fatty acids and resulting in the earliest inflammatory phases of acne.[104] Inhibition of lipase production is a rationale for administration of antibiotics to individuals with inflammatory acne. The synthetic vitamin A derivative 13-*cis*-retinoic acid (isotretinoin) has brought about remarkable clinical improvement in some cases of severe acne through its strong anti-sebaceous action.[105,106]

ROSACEA

Rosacea is a common disease of middle age and beyond, affecting up to 3% of the US population, with a predilection for females. Four stages are recognized: (1) flushing episodes (pre-rosacea), (2) persistent erythema and telangiectasia, (3) pustules and papules, and (4) rhinophyma—permanent thickening of the nasal skin by confluent erythemaous papules and follicular prominence.[107]

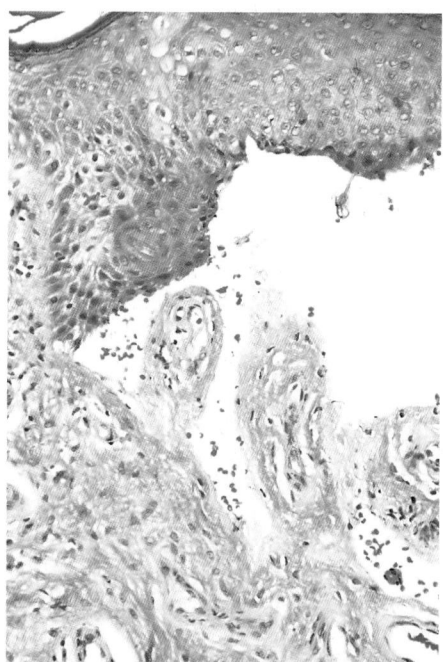

FIGURE 25–37   Porphyria. A noninflammatory blister is forming at the dermoepidermal junction; note the seemingly rigid dermal papillae at the base that contain the altered superficial vessels.

Morphology. Rosacea is characterized by a nonspecific perifollicular infiltrate composed of lymphocytes surrounded by dermal edema and telangiectasia. In the pustular phase neutrophils may colonize the follicles, and follicular rupture may cause a granulomatous dermal response. The development of rhinophyma is associated with hypertrophy of sebaceous glands and follicular plugging by keratotic debris.

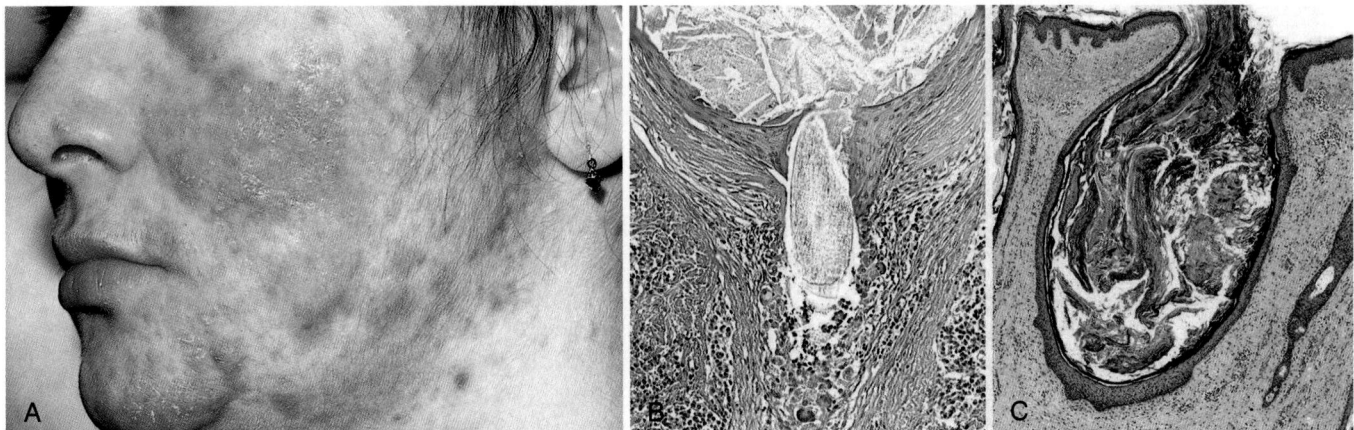

FIGURE 25–38   Acne. **A,** Inflammatory acne associated with erythematous papules and pustules. **B,** A hair shaft pierces the follicular epithelium, eliciting inflammation and fibrosis. **C,** Open comedone.

Pathogenesis. Individuals with rosacea have high cutaneous levels of the endogenous antimicrobial peptide cathelicidin, an important mediator of the innate immune response. The cathelicidin peptides present are qualitatively distinct from those seen in individuals without rosacea as a result of alternative processing by serine proteases such as stratum corneum tryptic enzyme.[108] While more study is needed, it seems that inappropriate activation of the innate immune system may play a role in this disorder.

Panniculitis

ERYTHEMA NODOSUM AND ERYTHEMA INDURATUM

Panniculitis is an inflammatory reaction in the subcutaneous adipose tissue that may preferentially affect (1) the connective tissue septa separating lobules of fat, or (2) the lobules of fat themselves. Panniculitis often involves the lower legs and usually has a subacute to chronic course. *Erythema nodosum* is the most common form and usually has an acute presentation. Its occurrence is often associated with infections (β-hemolytic streptococcal infection, tuberculosis and, less commonly, coccidioidomycosis, histoplasmosis, and leprosy), drug administration (sulfonamides, oral contraceptives), sarcoidosis, inflammatory bowel disease, and certain malignant neoplasms, but many times a cause cannot be identified.[109]

Erythema nodosum presents as poorly defined, exquisitely tender, erythematous plaques and nodules that may be more readily palpated than seen. Fever and malaise may accompany the cutaneous signs. Over the course of weeks, lesions usually flatten and become bruiselike, leaving no residual clinical scars, while new lesions develop. Biopsy of a deep wedge of tissue to generously sample the subcutis is usually required for histologic diagnosis.

Erythema induratum is an uncommon type of panniculitis that affects primarily adolescents and menopausal women. Although the cause is not known, most observers regard this as a primary vasculitis affecting deep vessels supplying lobules of the subcutis, with subsequent necrosis and inflammation within the fat. Erythema induratum presents as an erythematous,

slightly tender nodule that usually goes on to ulcerate. Originally considered a hypersensitivity response to tuberculosis, erythema induratum today most commonly occurs without an associated underlying disease.

> **Morphology.** The histopathology of **erythema nodosum** is distinctive. In early lesions, widening of the connective tissue septa is due to edema, fibrin exudation, and neutrophilic infiltration. Later, infiltration by lymphocytes, histiocytes, multinucleated giant cells, and occasional eosinophils is associated with septal fibrosis. Vasculitis is not present. In **erythema induratum**, on the other hand, granulomatous inflammation and zones of caseous necrosis involve the fat lobule. Early lesions show necrotizing vasculitis affecting small- to medium-sized arteries and veins in the deep dermis and subcutis.

Erythema nodosum and erythema induratum are but two of the many types of panniculitis. *Weber-Christian disease (relapsing febrile nodular panniculitis)* is a rare form of lobular, nonvasculitic panniculitis seen in children and adults. It is marked by crops of erythematous plaques or nodules, predominantly on the lower extremities, created by deep-seated foci of inflammation with aggregates of foamy histiocytes admixed with lymphocytes, neutrophils, and giant cells. *Factitial panniculitis* is a form of secondary panniculitis caused by self-inflicted trauma or injection of foreign or toxic substances. Rarely, T cell lymphomas (panniculitic T cell lymphoma) home to fat lobules, producing fat necrosis and superimposed inflammation that mimics panniculitis. Finally, disorders such as *lupus erythematosus* may occasionally have deep inflammatory components with associated panniculitis.[110] The etiologies for all of these except the self-inflicted form and the rare T cell lymphomas are not understood.

Infection

The skin frequently succumbs to the attack of microorganisms, parasites, and insects. We have already discussed the

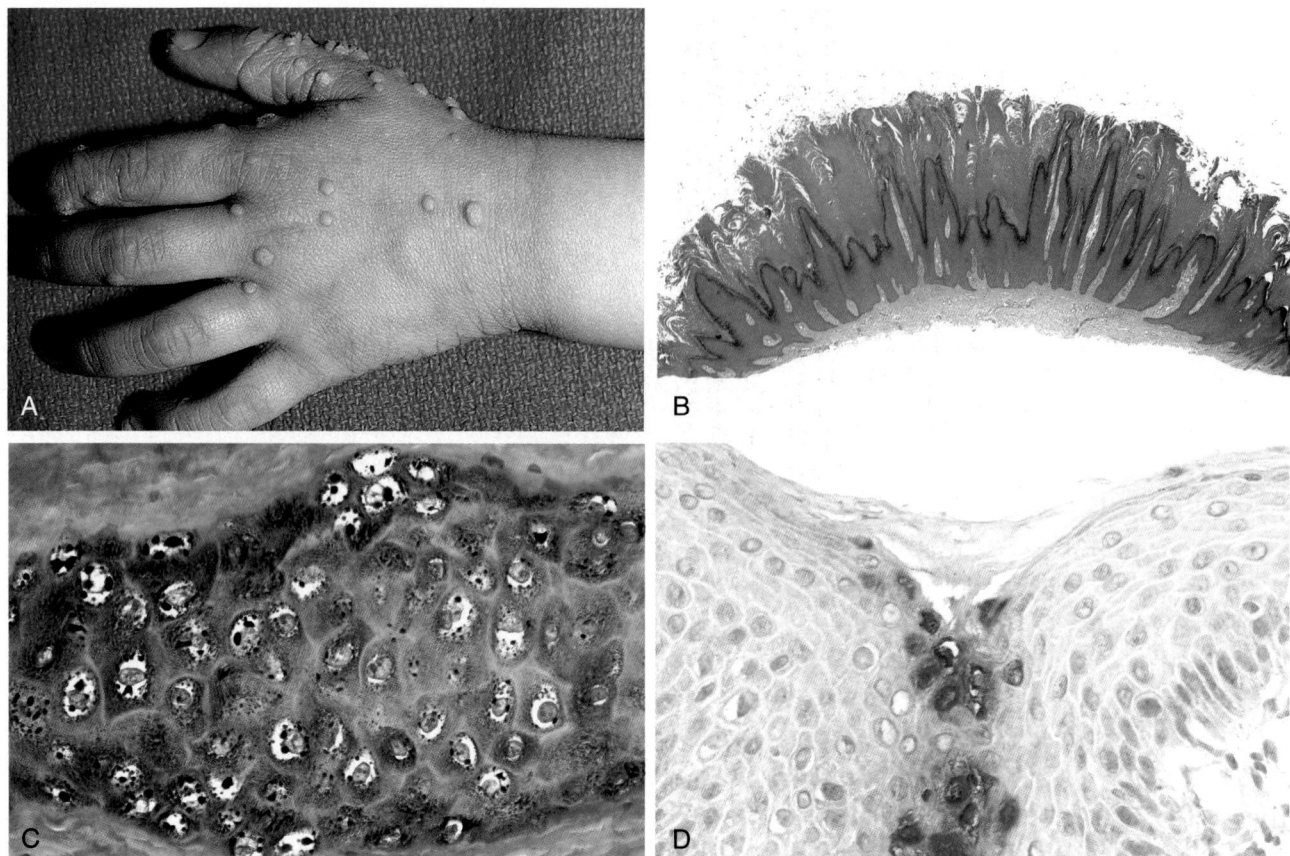

FIGURE 25–39 Verruca vulgaris. **A,** Multiple papules with rough pebble-like surfaces. **B** (low power) and **C,** (high power) histology of the lesions showing papillomatous epidermal hyperplasia and cytopathic alterations that include nuclear pallor and prominent keratohyaline granules. **D,** In situ hybridization demonstrating viral DNA within epidermal cells.

possible role of bacteria in the pathogenesis of common acne, and the dermatoses resulting from viruses are too numerous to list. In the setting of the immunocompromised individual, ordinarily trivial cutaneous infections may become life-threatening. Many disorders, such as herpes simplex and herpes zoster, the viral exanthems, deep fungal infections, and immune reactions in skin provoked by infectious agents, are discussed in Chapter 8. Here we cover a representative sampling of common infections whose primary clinical manifestations are in the skin.

VERRUCAE (WARTS)

Verrucae are common lesions of children and adolescents, although they may be encountered at any age. They are caused by human papillomaviruses. Transmission of disease usually involves direct contact between individuals or auto-inoculation. Verrucae are generally self-limited, regressing spontaneously within 6 months to 2 years.

The classification of verrucae is based largely on appearance and location.[111] *Verruca vulgaris* is the most common type of wart. The lesions of verruca vulgaris occur anywhere but most frequently on the hands, particularly on the dorsal surfaces and periungual areas, where they appear as gray-white to tan, flat to convex, 0.1- to 1-cm papules with a rough, pebble-like surface (Fig. 25–39A). *Verruca plana,* or *flat wart,* is common

on the face or the dorsal surfaces of the hands. The warts are slightly elevated, flat, smooth, tan papules that are generally smaller than verruca vulgaris. *Verruca plantaris* and *verruca palmaris* occur on the soles and palms, respectively. Rough, scaly lesions may reach 1 to 2 cm in diameter, coalesce, and be confused with ordinary calluses. *Condyloma acuminatum (venereal wart)* occurs on the penis, female genitalia, urethra, perianal areas, and rectum. Venereal warts appear as soft, tan, cauliflower-like masses that occasionally reach many centimeters in diameter.

> **Morphology.** Histologic features common to verrucae include epidermal hyperplasia that is often undulant in character, termed **verrucous or papillomatous epidermal hyperplasia** (Fig. 25–39B); and cytoplasmic vacuolization (koilocytosis) involving the more superficial epidermal layers, producing haloes of pallor surrounding infected nuclei. Electron microscopy of these zones reveals numerous viral particles within nuclei. Infected cells may also demonstrate prominent and apparently condensed keratohyaline granules and jagged eosinophilic intracytoplasmic keratin aggregates as a result of viral cytopathic effects (Fig. 25–39C). These cellular alterations are not as prominent in condylomas; hence, their diagnosis is based

primarily on hyperplastic papillary architecture containing wedge-shaped zones of koilocytosis.

Pathogenesis. More than 150 types of papillomavirus have been identified, many of them capable of producing warts in humans. The clinical variants of warts are often associated with distinct HPV subtypes. For example, anogenital warts are caused predominantly by HPV types 6 and 11. In contrast, there is a tendency for lesions induced by HPV type 16 to show some degree of dysplasia.[112] HPV type 16 has also been associated with in situ squamous cell carcinoma of the genitalia and with *bowenoid papulosis* (genital lesions of young adults with the histologic appearance of carcinoma in situ, but which usually regress spontaneously).[111] The relationship of HPV subtypes 5 and 8 to squamous cell carcinomas, particularly in individuals affected by the rare condition epidermodysplasia verruciformis, was mentioned earlier. These patients develop multiple flat warts that contain HPV genomes, some of which progress to carcinoma. Viral typing can be accomplished by either in situ hybridization (Fig. 25–39D) or polymerase chain reaction.

MOLLUSCUM CONTAGIOSUM

Molluscum contagiosum is a common, self-limited viral disease of the skin caused by a poxvirus. The virus is characteristically brick shaped, has a dumbbell-shaped DNA core, and measures 300 nm in maximal dimension, and thus represents the largest pathogenic poxvirus in humans and one of the largest viruses in nature. Infection is usually spread by direct contact, particularly among children and young adults.

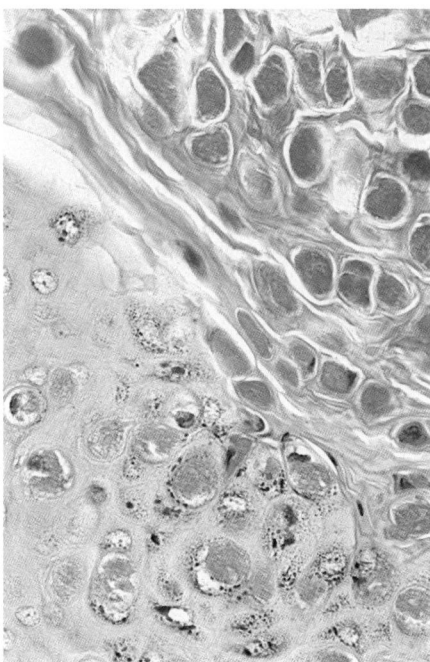

FIGURE 25–40 Molluscum contagiosum. A focus of verrucous epidermal hyperplasia contains numerous cells with ellipsoid cytoplasmic inclusions (molluscum bodies) within the stratum granulosum and stratum corneum.

Clinically, multiple lesions may occur on the skin and mucous membranes, with a predilection for the trunk and anogenital areas. Individual lesions are firm, often pruritic, pink to skin-colored umbilicated papules generally ranging in diameter from 0.2 to 0.4 cm. Rarely, "giant" forms occur measuring up to 2 cm in diameter. A curd-like material can be expressed from the central umbilication. Smearing this material onto a glass slide and staining with Giemsa reagent often shows diagnostic molluscum bodies.

Morphology. On microscopic examination, lesions show cuplike verrucous epidermal hyperplasia. The diagnostically specific structure is the **molluscum body,** which occurs as a large (up to 35 μm), ellipsoid, homogeneous, cytoplasmic inclusion in cells of the stratum granulosum and the stratum corneum (Fig. 25–40). In the H&E stain, these inclusions are eosinophilic in the blue-purple stratum granulosum and acquire a pale blue hue in the red stratum corneum. Numerous virions are present within molluscum bodies.

IMPETIGO

Impetigo is a common superficial bacterial infection of skin. It is highly contagious and is frequently seen in otherwise healthy children as well as occasionally in adults in poor health. Two forms exist, classically referred to as *impetigo contagiosa* and *impetigo bullosa*; they differ from each other simply by the size of the pustules. Over the past decade a remarkable shift in etiology has been observed. Whereas in the past impetigo contagiosa was almost exclusively caused by group A β-hemolytic streptococci and impetigo bullosa by *Staphylococcus aureus*, both are now usually caused by *Staphylococcus aureus*.[114]

The infection usually involves exposed skin, particularly that of the face and hands. It presents as an erythematous macule, but multiple small pustules rapidly supervene. As pustules break, shallow erosions form, covered with drying serum, giving the characteristic clinical appearance of *honey-colored crust.* If the crust is not removed, new lesions form about the periphery and extensive epidermal damage may ensue. A bullous form of impetigo mainly occurs in children.

Morphology. The characteristic microscopic feature of impetigo is accumulation of neutrophils beneath the stratum corneum, often producing a subcorneal pustule. Special stains reveal the presence of bacteria in these foci. Nonspecific, reactive epidermal alterations and superficial dermal inflammation accompany these findings. Rupture of pustules results in superficial layering of serum, neutrophils, and cellular debris to form the characteristic crust. Blistering lesions may show accumulation of fluid and neutrophils beneath the stratum corneum.

Pathogenesis. Bacterial species in the epidermis evoke an innate immune response that tends to be destructive within the epidermis leading to local serous exudate with

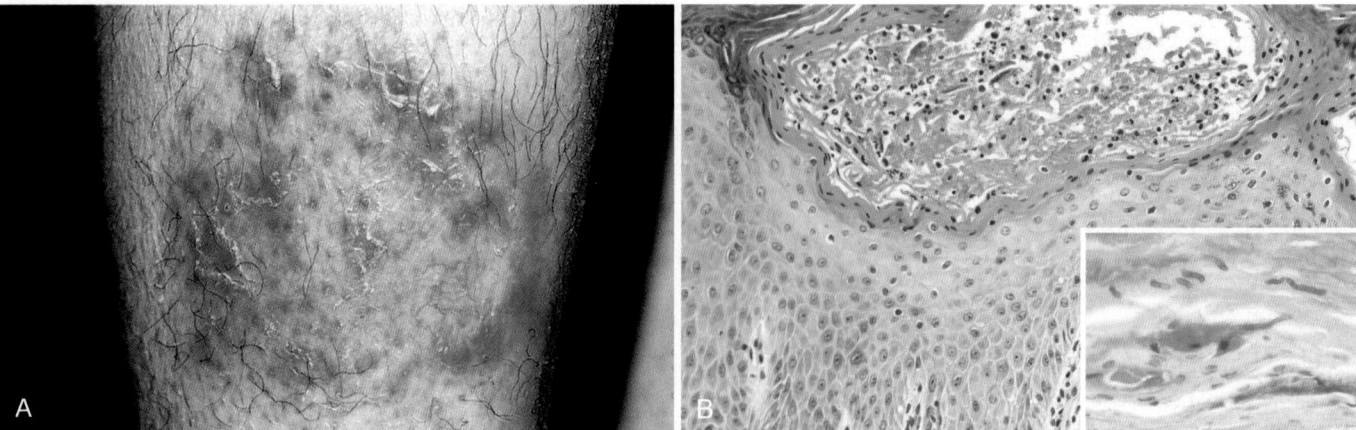

FIGURE 25–41   Tinea. **A,** Characteristic plaque of tinea corporis. Routine histology (**B**) shows a mild eczematous (spongiotic) dermatitis and focal neutrophilic abscesses. A periodic acid–Schiff stain (*inset*) reveals deep red hyphae within the stratum corneum.

formation of a scale crust (scab). The pathogenesis of blister formation in impetigo is related to bacterial production of a toxin that specifically cleaves desmoglein 1, the protein responsible for cell-to-cell adhesion within the uppermost epidermal layers.[115] Recall that in pemphigus foliaceus, which has a similar plane of blister formation, desmoglein 1 is compromised not by a toxin but by an autoantibody (see Fig. 25–29). Because there is virtually no involvement of the dermis, once the bacteria are eliminated the lesions heal without scarring.

SUPERFICIAL FUNGAL INFECTIONS

As opposed to deep fungal infections of the skin, where the dermis or subcutis is primarily involved, superficial fungal infections of the skin are confined to the stratum corneum, and are caused primarily by dermatophytes. These organisms grow in the soil and on animals and produce a number of diverse and characteristic clinical lesions.[116]

Tinea capitis usually occurs in children and is only rarely seen in infants and adults. It is a dermatophytosis of the scalp characterized by asymptomatic, often hairless patches of skin associated with mild erythema, crust formation, and scaling. *Tinea barbae* is a dermatophyte infection of the beard area that affects adult men; it is a relatively uncommon disorder. *Tinea corporis*, on the other hand, is a common superficial fungal infection of the body surface that affects persons of all ages, but particularly children. Predisposing factors include excessive heat and humidity, exposure to infected animals, and chronic dermatophytosis of the feet or nails. The most common type of tinea corporis is an expanding, round, slightly erythematous plaque with an elevated scaling border (Fig. 25–41A). *Tinea cruris* occurs most frequently in the inguinal areas of obese men during warm weather. Heat, friction, and maceration all predispose to its development. The infection usually first appears on the upper inner thighs, with gradual extension of moist, red patches that have raised, scaling borders. *Tinea pedis (athlete's foot)* affects 30% to 40% of the population at some time in their lives. There is diffuse erythema and scaling, often initially localized to the web spaces. Most of the inflammatory tissue reaction, however, has recently been shown to be the result of bacterial superinfection and not directly related to the primary dermatophytosis.[117] Spread

to or primary infection of the nails is referred to as *onychomycosis*. This produces discoloration, thickening, and deformity of the nail plate. *Tinea versicolor* usually occurs on the upper trunk and is highly distinctive in appearance. Caused by *Malassezia furfur*, a yeast rather than a dermatophyte, the lesions consist of groups of macules of all sizes, lighter or darker than surrounding skin, with a fine peripheral scale.[87]

> **Morphology.** The histologic features of dermatophytoses are variable, depending on the properties of the organism, the host response, and the degree of bacterial superinfection. There may be mild eczematous dermatitis associated with intraepidermal neutrophils (Fig. 25–41B). Fungal cell walls, rich in mucopolysaccharides, stain bright pink to red with periodic acid–Schiff stain. They are present in the anucleate cornified layer of lesional skin, hair, or nails (Fig. 25–41B, *inset*). Culture of material scraped from these areas will usually permit the identification of the offending species.

REFERENCES

1. Virchow R: Cellular Pathology. London, John Churchill, p 33, 1860.
2. Kupper TS, Fuhlbrigge RC: Immune surveillance in the skin: mechanisms and clinical consequences. Nat Rev Immunol 4:211, 2004.
3. Murphy GF: The secret of "NIN," a novel neural immunological network potentially integral to immunologic function in human skin. In Nickoloff BJ (ed): Dermal Immune System, Boca Raton, FL, CRC Press, 1993, p 227.
4. Johnson KO: The roles and functions of cutaneous mechanoreceptors. Curr Opin Neurobiol 11:455, 2001.
5. Fuchs E: Scratching the surface of skin development. Nature 445:834, 2007.
6. Pollock PM et al.: High frequency of *BRAF* mutations in nevi. Nat Genet 33:19, 2003.
7. Michaloglou C et al.: BRAFE600-associated senescence-like cell cycle arrest of human naevi. Nature 436:720, 2005.
8. Norris W: A case of fungoid disease. Edinburgh Med Surg J 16:562, 1820.
9. Clark WH, Jr. et al.: Origin of familial malignant melanomas from heritable melanocytic lesions. "The B-K mole syndrome." Arch Dermatol 114:732, 1978.
10. Tsai KY, Tsao H: The genetics of skin cancer. Am J Med Genet C Semin Med Genet 131C:82, 2004.

11. Greene MH et al.: High risk of malignant melanoma in melanoma-prone families with dysplastic nevi. Ann Intern Med 102:458, 1985.
12. Clark WH, Jr. et al.: A study of tumor progression: the precursor lesions of superficial spreading and nodular melanoma. Hum Pathol 15:1147, 1984.
13. Kim JC, Murphy GF: Dysplastic melanocytic nevi and prognostically indeterminate nevomelanomatoid proliferations. Clin Lab Med 20:691, 2000.
14. Geller AC et al.: Screening, early detection, and trends for melanoma: current status (2000–2006) and future directions. J Am Acad Dermatol 57:555, 2007.
15. Elder DE: Melanocytic tumors of the skin. In Atlas of Tumor Pathology, Third Series, Fascicle 1. Washington, DC, Armed Forces Institute of Pathology, 1991, p 183.
16. Breslow A: Prognosis in cutaneous melanoma: tumor thickness as a guide to treatment. Pathol Annu 15:1, 1980.
17. Kruper LL et al.: Predicting sentinel node status in AJCC stage I/II primary cutaneous melanoma. Cancer 107:2436, 2006.
18. Barnhill RL et al.: The importance of mitotic rate as a prognostic factor for localized cutaneous melanoma. J Cutan Pathol 32:268, 2005.
19. Elder DE, Xu X: The approach to the patient with a difficult melanocytic lesion. Pathology 36:428, 2004.
20. Clark WH, Jr. et al.: Model predicting survival in stage I melanoma based on tumor progression. J Natl Cancer Inst 81:1893, 1989.
21. Balch CM et al.: Prognostic factors analysis of 17,600 melanoma patients: validation of the American Joint Committee on Cancer melanoma staging system. J Clin Oncol 19:3622, 2001.
22. Balch CM et al.: The new melanoma staging system. Semin Cutan Med Surg 22:42, 2003.
23. Rousseau DL, Jr., Gershenwald JE: The new staging system for cutaneous melanoma in the era of lymphatic mapping. Semin Oncol 31:415, 2004.
24. Berwick M et al.: Sun exposure and mortality from melanoma. J Natl Cancer Inst 97:195, 2005.
25. Gudbjartsson DF et al.: ASIP and TYR pigmentation variants associated with cutaneous melanoma and basal cell carcinoma. Nat Genet 40:886, 2008.
26. Chin L: The genetics of malignant melanoma: lessons from mouse and man. Nat Rev Cancer 3:559, 2003.
27. Peters G: Tumor suppression for ARFicionados: the relative contributions of p16/INK4a and p14/ARF in melanoma. J Natl Cancer Inst 100:757, 2008.
28. Curtin JA et al.: Somatic activation of KIT in distinct subtypes of melanoma. J Clin Oncol 24:4340, 2006.
29. Curtin JA et al.: Distinct sets of genetic alterations in melanoma. N Engl J Med 353:2135, 2005.
30. Ibrahim N, Haluska FG: Molecular pathogenesis of cutaneous melanocytic neoplasms. Annu Rev Pathol Mech Dis 4:551, 2009.
31. Goel VK et al.: Examinations of mutations in BRAF, NRAS, and PTEN in primary cutaneous melanoma. J Invest Dermatol 126:154, 2006.
32. Chudnovsky Y et al.: Melanoma genetics and the development of rational therapeutics. J Clin Invest 115:813, 2005.
33. Hunder NN et al.: Treatment of metastatic melanoma with autologous CD4+ T Cells against NY-ESO-1. N Engl J Med 358:2698, 2008.
34. Hafner C et al.: High frequency of FGFR3 mutations in adenoid seborrheic keratoses. J Invest Dermatol 126:2404, 2006.
35. Ellis DL et al.: Melanoma, growth factors, acanthosis nigricans, the sign of Leser-Trelat, and multiple acrochordons. A possible role for alpha-transforming growth factor in cutaneous paraneoplastic syndromes. N Engl J Med 317:1582, 1987.
36. Logie A et al.: Activating mutations of the tyrosine kinase receptor FGFR3 are associated with benign skin tumors in mice and humans. Hum Mol Genet 14:1153, 2005.
37. Torley D et al.: Genes, growth factors and acanthosis nigricans. Br J Dermatol 147:1096, 2002.
38. Hafner C et al.: FGFR3 mutations in benign skin tumors. Cell Cycle 5:2723, 2006.
39. Leter EM et al.: Birt-Hogg-Dube syndrome: Clinical and genetic studies of 20 families. J Invest Dermatol 128:45, 2007.
40. Covello SP et al.: Keratin 17 mutations cause either steatocystoma multiplex or pachyonychia congenita type 2. Br J Dermatol 139:475, 1998.
41. McLean WH et al.: Keratin 16 and keratin 17 mutations cause pachyonychia congenita. Nat Genet 9:273, 1995.
42. Liaw D et al.: Germline mutations of the PTEN gene in Cowden disease, an inherited breast and thyroid cancer syndrome. Nat Genet 16:64, 1997.
43. Bignell GR et al.: Identification of the familial cylindromatosis tumour-suppressor gene. Nat Genet 25:160, 2000.
44. Trompouki E et al.: CYLD is a deubiquitinating enzyme that negatively regulates NF-kappaB activation by TNFR family members. Nature 424:793, 2003.
45. Young AL et al.: CYLD mutations underlie Brooke-Spiegler, familial cylindromatosis, and multiple familial trichoepithelioma syndromes. Clin Genet 70:246, 2006.
46. Barana D et al.: Spectrum of genetic alterations in Muir-Torre syndrome is the same as in HNPCC. Am J Med Genet A 125:318, 2004.
47. Takeda H et al.: Human sebaceous tumors harbor inactivating mutations in LEF1. Nat Med 12:395, 2006.
48. Chan EF et al.: A common human skin tumour is caused by activating mutations in β-catenin. Nat Genet 21:410, 1999.
49. Owens DM, Watt FM: Contribution of stem cells and differentiated cells to epidermal tumours. Nat Rev Cancer 3:444, 2003.
50. Jorizzo JL. Current and novel treatment options for actinic keratosis. J Cutan Med Surg 8 (Suppl 3):13, 2004.
51. Alam M, Ratner D: Cutaneous squamous-cell carcinoma. N Engl J Med 344:975, 2001.
52. Harwood CA, Proby CM: Human papillomaviruses and non-melanoma skin cancer. Curr Opin Infect Dis 15:101, 2002.
53. Ramoz N et al.: Mutations in two adjacent novel genes are associated with epidermodysplasia verruciformis. Nat Genet 32:579, 2002.
54. Beissert S, Schwarz T: Mechanisms involved in ultraviolet light-induced immunosuppression. J Investig Dermatol Symp Proc 4:61, 1999.
55. Khavari PA: Modelling cancer in human skin tissue. Nat Rev Cancer 6:270, 2006.
56. Rubin AI et al.: Basal-cell carcinoma. N Engl J Med 353:2262, 2005.
57. Gorlin RJ, Goltz RW: Multiple nevoid basal-cell epithelioma, jaw cysts and bifid rib. A syndrome. N Engl J Med 262:908, 1960.
58. Mirowski GW et al.: Nevoid basal cell carcinoma syndrome. J Am Acad Dermatol 43:1092, 2000.
59. Hahn H et al.: Mutations of the human homolog of Drosophila patched in the nevoid basal cell carcinoma syndrome. Cell 85:841, 1996.
60. Riobo NA, Manning DR: Pathways of signal transduction employed by vertebrate Hedgehogs. Biochem J 403:369, 2007.
61. Fan H et al.: Induction of basal cell carcinoma features in transgenic human skin expressing Sonic Hedgehog. Nat Med 3:788, 1997.
62. Nilsson M et al.: Induction of basal cell carcinomas and trichoepitheliomas in mice overexpressing GLI-1. Proc Natl Acad Sci U S A 97:3438, 2000.
63. Bale AE: The nevoid basal cell carcinoma syndrome: genetics and mechanism of carcinogenesis. Cancer Invest 15:180, 1997.
64. Kim MY et al.: Mutations of the p53 and PTCH gene in basal cell carcinomas: UV mutation signature and strand bias. J Dermatol Sci 29:1, 2002.
65. D'Errico M et al.: UV mutation signature in tumor suppressor genes involved in skin carcinogenesis in xeroderma pigmentosum patients. Oncogene 19:463, 2000.
66. Calonje E: Is cutaneous benign fibrous histiocytoma (dermatofibroma) a reactive inflammatory process or a neoplasm? Histopathology 37:278, 2000.
67. Simon MP et al.: Deregulation of the platelet-derived growth factor B-chain gene via fusion with collagen gene COL1A1 in dermatofibrosarcoma protuberans and giant-cell fibroblastoma. Nat Genet 15:95, 1997.
68. Patel KU et al.: Dermatofibrosarcoma protuberans COL1A1-PDGFB fusion is identified in virtually all dermatofibrosarcoma protuberans cases when investigated by newly developed multiplex reverse transcription polymerase chain reaction and fluorescence in situ hybridization assays. Hum Pathol 39:184, 2008.
69. Mitelman F et al.: The impact of translocations and gene fusions on cancer causation. Nat Rev Cancer 7:233, 2007.
70. Rubin BP et al.: Molecular targeting of platelet-derived growth factor B by imatinib mesylate in a patient with metastatic dermatofibrosarcoma protuberans. J Clin Oncol 20:3586, 2002.
71. Willemze R, Meijer CJ: Classification of cutaneous T-cell lymphoma: from Alibert to WHO-EORTC. J Cutan Pathol 33 (Suppl 1):18, 2006.
72. Duvic M, Edelson R. Cutaneous T-cell lymphoma. J Am Acad Dermatol 51:S43, 2004.

73. Zinzani PL et al.: Mycosis fungoides. Crit Rev Oncol Hematol 65:172, 2008.
74. Longley BJ et al.: Somatic c-KIT activating mutation in urticaria pigmentosa and aggressive mastocytosis: establishment of clonality in a human mast cell neoplasm. Nat Genet 12:312, 1996.
75. Longley BJ et al.: Chronically KIT-stimulated clonally-derived human mast cells show heterogeneity in different tissue microenvironments. J Invest Dermatol 108:792, 1997.
76. Oji V, Traupe H: Ichthyoses: differential diagnosis and molecular genetics. Eur J Dermatol 16:349, 2006.
77. Nettis E et al.: Clinical and aetiological aspects in urticaria and angiooedema. Br J Dermatol 148:501, 2003.
78. Murphy GF et al.: Topical tretinoin replenishes CD1a-positive epidermal Langerhans cells in chronically photodamaged human skin. J Cutan Pathol 25:30, 1998.
79. Steinhoff M et al.: Modern aspects of cutaneous neurogenic inflammation. Arch Dermatol 139:1479, 2003.
80. Lamoreux MR et al.: Erythema multiforme. Am Fam Physician 74:1883, 2006.
81. Parrillo SJ: Stevens-Johnson syndrome and toxic epidermal necrolysis. Curr Allergy Asthma Rep 7:243, 2007.
82. Murphy GF et al.: Cytotoxic T lymphocytes and phenotypically abnormal epidermal dendritic cells in fixed cutaneous eruptions. Hum Pathol 16:1264, 1985.
83. Gilliam AC et al.: Apoptosis is the predominant form of epithelial target cell injury in acute experimental graft-versus-host disease. J Invest Dermatol 107:377, 1996.
84. Schon MP, Reich K: Tumor necrosis factor antagonists in the therapy of psoriasis. Clin Dermatol 26:486, 2008.
85. Bowcock AM, Cookson WO: The genetics of psoriasis, psoriatic arthritis and atopic dermatitis. Hum Mol Genet 13 (Spec No 1):R43, 2004.
86. Schwartz RA et al.: Seborrheic dermatitis: an overview. Am Fam Physician 74:125, 2006.
87. Gupta AK et al.: Skin diseases associated with *Malassezia* species. J Am Acad Dermatol 51:785, 2004.
88. Fischer M et al.: Skin function and skin disorders in Parkinson's disease. J Neural Transm 108:205, 2001.
89. Mithani SK et al.: Molecular genetics of premalignant oral lesions. Oral Dis 13:126, 2007.
90. Patel GK et al.: Cutaneous lichen planus and squamous cell carcinoma. J Eur Acad Dermatol Venereol 17:98, 2003.
91. Katta R: Lichen planus. Am Fam Physician 61:3319, 2000.
92. Iijima W et al.: Infiltrating CD8+ T cells in oral lichen planus predominantly express CCR5 and CXCR3 and carry respective chemokine ligands RANTES/CCL5 and IP-10/CXCL10 in their cytolytic granules: a potential self-recruiting mechanism. Am J Pathol 163:261, 2003.
93. Edelson RL: Pemphigus—decoding the cellular language of cutaneous autoimmunity. N Engl J Med 343:60, 2000.
94. Tron F et al.: Immunogenetics of pemphigus: an update. Autoimmunity 39:531, 2006.
95. Gniadecki R: Desmoglein autoimmunity in the pathogenesis of pemphigus. Autoimmunity 39:541, 2006.
96. Wade MS, Black MM: Paraneoplastic pemphigus: a brief update. Australas J Dermatol 46:1, 2005.
97. Walsh SR et al.: Bullous pemphigoid: from bench to bedside. Drugs 65:905, 2005.
98. Blank M et al.: New insights into the autoantibody-mediated mechanisms of autoimmune bullous diseases and urticaria. Clin Exp Rheumatol 24:S20, 2006.
99. Fine JD et al.: Revised classification system for inherited epidermolysis bullosa: report of the Second International Consensus Meeting on diagnosis and classification of epidermolysis bullosa. J Am Acad Dermatol 42:1051, 2000.
100. Mallipeddi R et al.: Increased risk of squamous cell carcinoma in junctional epidermolysis bullosa. J Eur Acad Dermatol Venereol 18:521, 2004.
101. McGrath JA, Mellerio JE: Epidermolysis bullosa. Br J Hosp Med (Lond) 67:188, 2006.
102. Mavilio F et al.: Correction of junctional epidermolysis bullosa by transplantation of genetically modified epidermal stem cells. Nat Med 12:1397, 2006.
103. Harper JC, Thiboutot DM: Pathogenesis of acne: recent research advances. Adv Dermatol 19:1, 2003.
104. Miskin JE et al.: *Propionibacterium acnes*, a resident of lipid-rich human skin, produces a 33 kDa extracellular lipase encoded by gehA. Microbiology 143 (Pt 5):1745, 1997.
105. Goldsmith LA et al.: American Academy of Dermatology Consensus Conference on the safe and optimal use of isotretinoin: summary and recommendations. J Am Acad Dermatol 50:900, 2004.
106. Clarke SB et al.: Pharmacologic modulation of sebaceous gland activity: mechanisms and clinical applications. Dermatol Clin 25:137, 2007.
107. Diamantis S, Waldorf HA: Rosacea: clinical presentation and pathophysiology. J Drugs Dermatol 5:8, 2006.
108. Yamasaki K et al.: Increased serine protease activity and cathelicidin promotes skin inflammation in rosacea. Nat Med 13:975, 2007.
109. Requena L, Sanchez Yus E: Erythema nodosum. Semin Cutan Med Surg 26:114, 2007.
110. Ter Poorten MC, Thiers BH: Panniculitis. Dermatol Clin 20:421, 2002.
111. Lio P: Warts, molluscum and things that go bump on the skin: a practical guide. Arch Dis Child Educ Pract Ed 92:ep119, 2007.
112. de Villiers EM: Papillomavirus and HPV typing. Clin Dermatol 15:199, 1997.
113. Orth G: Genetics of epidermodysplasia verruciformis: insights into host defense against papillomaviruses. Semin Immunol 18:362, 2006.
114. Sladden MJ, Johnston GA: Current options for the treatment of impetigo in children. Expert Opin Pharmacother 6:2245, 2005.
115. Payne AS et al.: Desmosomes and disease: pemphigus and bullous impetigo. Curr Opin Cell Biol 16:536, 2004.
116. Schwartz RA: Superficial fungal infections. Lancet 364:1173, 2004.
117. Leyden JJ, Aly R: Tinea pedis. Semin Dermatol 12:280, 1993.

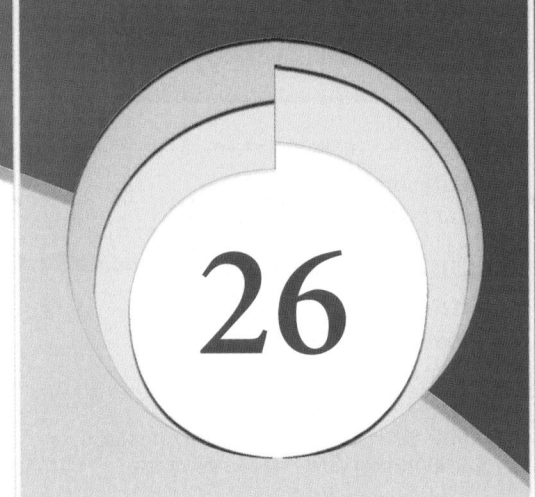

26

Bones, Joints, and Soft-Tissue Tumors

ANDREW E. ROSENBERG

■ BONES

Bone Modeling, Remodeling, and Peak Bone Mass

Bone Growth and Development

Developmental Abnormalities in Bone Cells, Matrix, and Structure
  Malformations and Diseases Caused by Defects in Nuclear Proteins and Transcription Factors
  Diseases Caused by Defects in Hormones and Signal Transduction Mechanisms
  Diseases Associated with Defects in Extracellular Structural Proteins
    Type 1 Collagen Diseases (Osteogenesis Imperfecta)
    Diseases Associated with Mutations of Types 2, 9, 10, and 11 Collagen
  Diseases Associated with Defects in Folding and Degradation of Macromolecules
    Mucopolysaccharidoses
  Diseases Associated with Defects in Metabolic Pathways (Enzymes, Ion Channels, and Transporters)
    Osteopetrosis
  Diseases Associated with Decreased Bone Mass
    Osteoporosis
  Diseases Caused by Osteoclast Dysfunction
    Paget Disease (Osteitis Deformans)

Diseases Associated with Abnormal Mineral Homeostasis
  Rickets and Osteomalacia
  Hyperparathyroidism
  Renal Osteodystrophy

Fractures

Osteonecrosis (Avascular Necrosis)

Infections—Osteomyelitis
  Pyogenic Osteomyelitis
  Tuberculous Osteomyelitis
  Skeletal Syphilis

Bone Tumors and Tumor-Like Lesions
  Bone-Forming Tumors
    Osteoma
    Osteoid Osteoma and Osteoblastoma
    Osteosarcoma
  Cartilage-Forming Tumors
    Osteochondroma
    Chondromas
    Chondroblastoma
    Chondromyxoid Fibroma
    Chondrosarcoma
  Fibrous and Fibro-Osseous Tumors
    Fibrous Cortical Defect and Non-Ossifying Fibroma
    Fibrous Dysplasia
    Fibrosarcoma Variants

Miscellaneous Tumors
  Ewing Sarcoma/Primitive Neuroectodermal Tumor
  Giant-Cell Tumor

Aneurysmal Bone Cyst
Metastatic Disease

■ **JOINTS**

Arthritis
  Osteoarthritis
  Rheumatoid Arthritis
  Juvenile Idiopathic Arthritis
  Seronegative Spondyloarthropathies
    Ankylosing Spondyloarthritis
    Reiter Syndrome
    Enteritis-Associated Arthritis
    Psoriatic Arthritis
  Infectious Arthritis
    Bacterial Arthritis
    Tuberculous Arthritis
    Lyme Arthritis
    Viral Arthritis
  Crystal-Induced Arthritis
    Gout and Gouty Arthritis
    *Calcium Pyrophosphate Crystal
    Deposition Disease (Pseudo-Gout)*
  Tumors and Tumor-Like Lesions
  Ganglion and Synovial Cyst
  **Tenosynovial Giant-Cell Tumor (Localized
  and Diffuse)**

■ **SOFT-TISSUE TUMORS AND
TUMOR-LIKE LESIONS**

Pathogenesis and General Features

Fatty Tumors
  Lipomas
  Liposarcoma

**Fibrous Tumors and Tumor-Like
Lesions**
  **Reactive Pseudosarcomatous
  Proliferations**
    Nodular Fasciitis
    Myositis Ossificans
  Fibromatoses
    *Superficial Fibromatosis (Palmar,
    Plantar, and Penile Fibromatoses)*
    *Deep-Seated Fibromatosis (Desmoid
    Tumors)*
  Fibrosarcoma

Fibrohistiocytic Tumors
  **Benign Fibrous Histiocytoma
  (Dermatofibroma)**
  Malignant Fibrous Histiocytoma

Tumors of Skeletal Muscle
  Rhabdomyosarcoma

Tumors of Smooth Muscle
  Leiomyomas
  Leiomyosarcoma

Synovial Sarcoma

BONES

Recognized by the bard for its persistence after death (Alas, poor Yorick!), the skeletal system is vital during life. It has an essential role in mineral homeostasis, houses the hematopoietic elements, provides mechanical support for movement, protects viscera, and determines body size and shape. As is well known, bones are largely made up of an organic matrix (osteoid) and the mineral calcium hydroxyapatite, which gives the bones strength and hardness. What is not obvious is that, despite its stony hard structure, bone is a dynamic tissue that is continuously resorbed, renewed, and remodeled. These processes are carried out by several different types of bone cells that are regulated by a number of transcription factors, cytokines, and growth factors[1-3] (Fig. 26–1).

- *Osteoprogenitor* cells are pluripotent mesenchymal stem cells that are found in the vicinity of all bony surfaces. When appropriately stimulated by growth factors they produce offspring that differentiate into osteoblasts, a process that is governed by the RUNX2/CBFA1 tran-

scription factor network and the WNT/β-catenin signaling pathway (Chapter 2).[2,3]

- *Osteoblasts and lining cells* are located on the surface of bones. These cells synthesize, transport, and arrange the many proteins of matrix detailed later (Fig. 26–2) and initiate the process of mineralization. Osteoblasts have receptors that bind regulatory hormones (parathyroid hormone, vitamin D, leptin, and estrogen), cytokines, growth factors, and extracellular matrix proteins,[2-6] and in turn express several factors that regulate the differentiation and function of osteoclasts (Fig. 26–2, described further below). If osteoblasts become surrounded by newly deposited organic matrix, they transform into *osteocytes*; alternatively, osteoblasts remaining on the bone surface may become flattened and quiescent bone lining cells.

- *Osteocytes* communicate with each other and with cells on the bone surface via an intricate network of cytoplas-

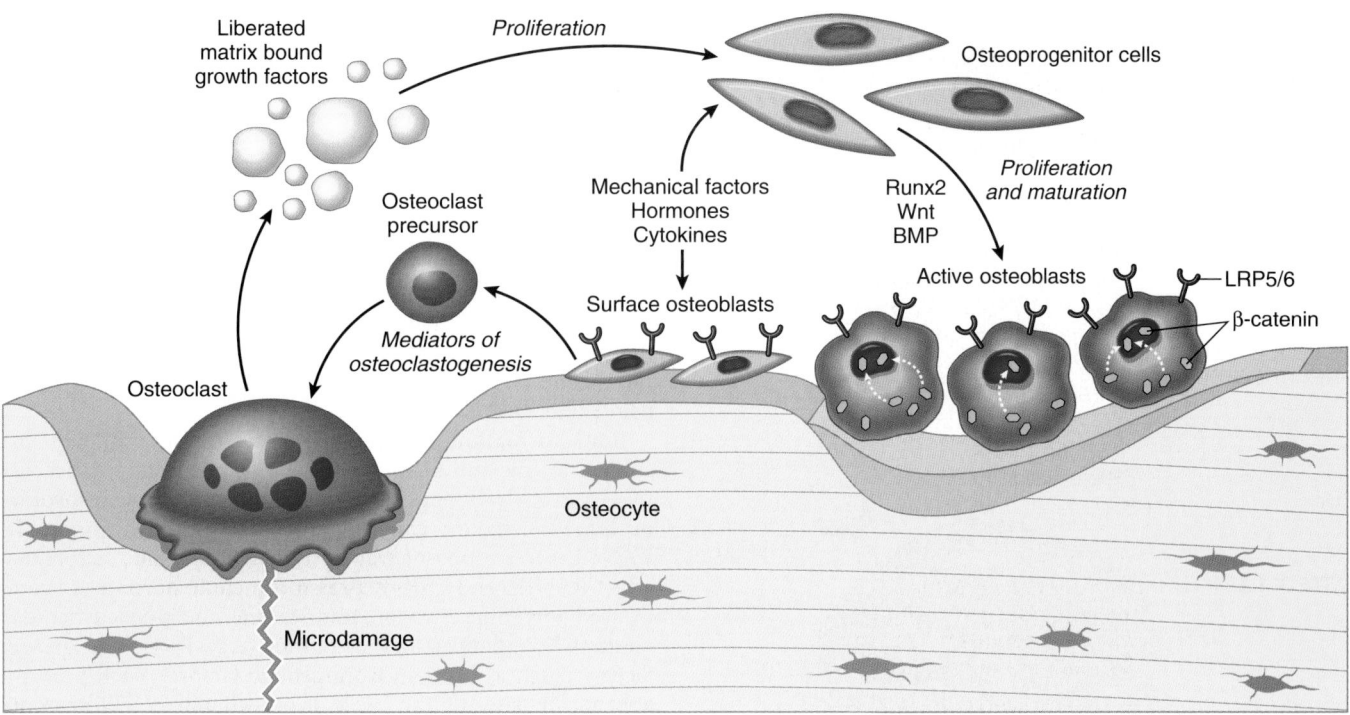

FIGURE 26–1 Bone cells and their interrelated activities. Hormones, cytokines, growth factors, and signal-transducing molecules are key in their formation and maturation, and allow communication between osteoblasts and osteoclasts. Bone resorption and formation in remodeling are coupled processes that are controlled by systemic factors and local cytokines, some of which are deposited in the bone matrix. BMP, bone morphogenic protein; LRP5/6, LDL receptor related proteins 5 and 6.

mic processes that traverse tunnels in the matrix known as *canaliculi*. Osteocytes help to control calcium and phosphate levels in the microenvironment, and detect mechanical forces and translate them into biologic activity—a process called *mechanotransduction*.[5,6]

● *Osteoclasts* are the cells responsible for bone resorption. They are derived from the same hematopoietic progenitor cells that also give rise to monocytes and macrophages. The cytokines and growth factors that regulate human osteoclast differentiation and maturation include macrophage colony-stimulating factor (M-CSF), interleukin-1 (IL-1), and tumor necrosis factor (TNF).[7,8] Mature multinucleated osteoclasts (containing 6 to 12 nuclei) form from the fusion of circulating mononuclear precursors and have a limited life span (approximately 2 weeks). They bind to the bone surface via integrins, where they form an underlying resorption pit—a self-contained extracellular space analogous to a secondary lysosome (Fig. 26–2). The cell membrane overlying the resorption pit is thrown into numerous folds (the *ruffled*

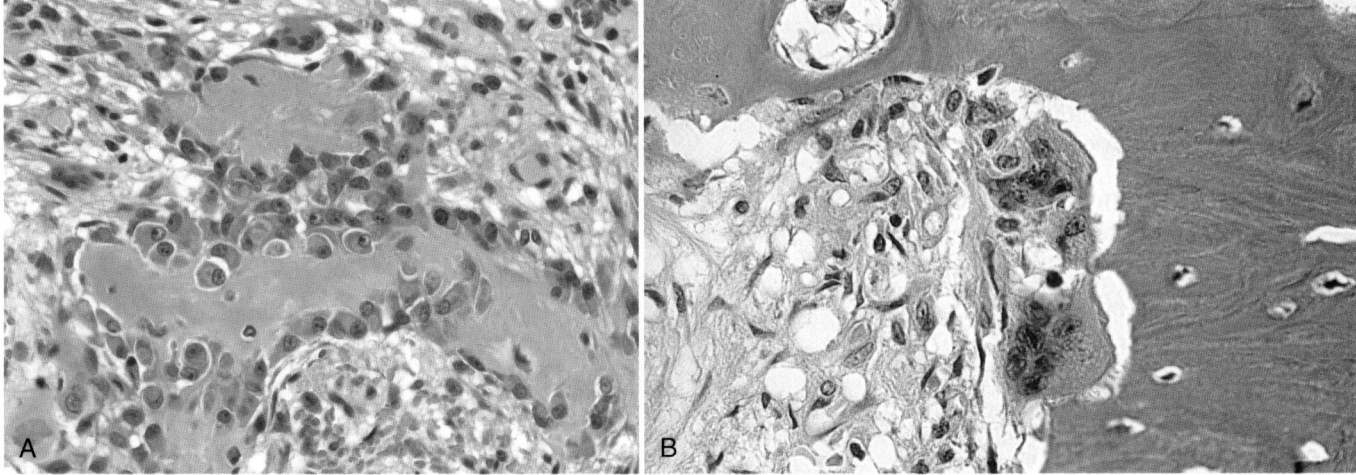

FIGURE 26–2 **A,** Active osteoblasts synthesizing bone matrix. The surrounding spindle cells represent osteoprogenitor cells. **B,** Two osteoclasts resorbing bone.

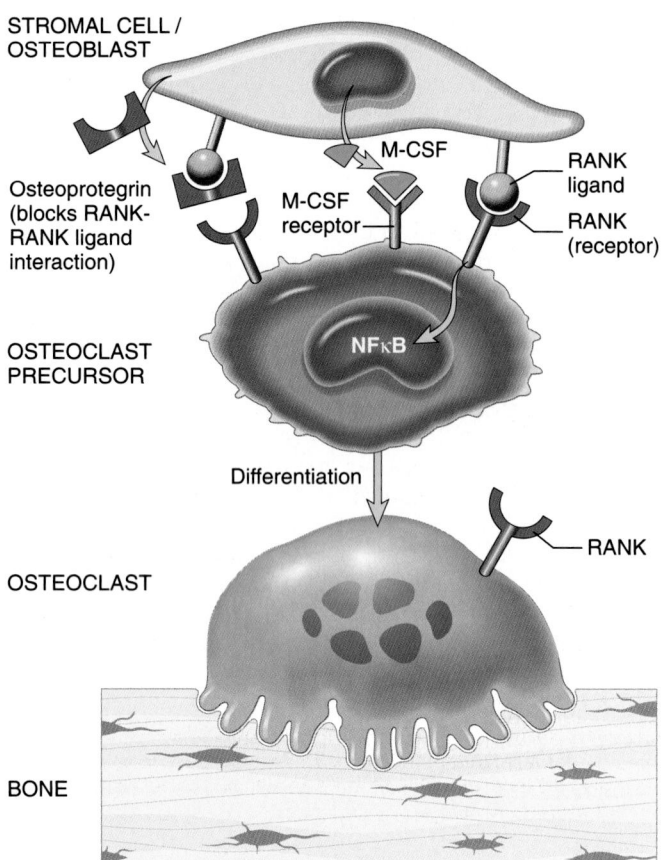

STROMAL CELL / OSTEOBLAST

Osteoprotegrin (blocks RANK-RANK ligand interaction)

M-CSF

M-CSF receptor

RANK ligand

RANK (receptor)

OSTEOCLAST PRECURSOR

NFκB

Differentiation

OSTEOCLAST

RANK

BONE

FIGURE 26–3 Paracrine molecular mechanisms that regulate osteoclast formation and function. Osteoclasts are derived from the same stem cells that produce macrophages. Osteoblast/stromal cell membrane–associated RANKL binds to its receptor RANK located on the cell surface of osteoclast precursors. This interaction in the background of macrophage colony-stimulating factor (M-CSF) causes the precursor cells to produce functional osteoclasts. Stromal cells also secrete osteoprotegrin (OPG), which acts as a decay receptor for RANKL, preventing it from binding the RANK receptor on osteoclast precursors. Consequently, OPG prevents bone resorption by inhibiting osteoclast differentiation.

border), increasing its surface area, while the adjacent cell surface forms a tight seal with the bone that prevents leakage of digestion products. The osteoclast removes the mineral by generating an acidic environment utilizing a proton pump system and digests the organic component by releasing proteases.

These cells and locally produced factors work together to regulate bone homeostasis. The control mechanisms are not known completely, but several signaling pathways of particular importance have emerged (Fig. 26–3). One such pathway involves three factors: (1) the transmembrane receptor RANK (receptor activator for NF-κB), which is expressed on osteoclast precursors; (2) RANK ligand, (RANKL) which is expressed on osteoblasts and marrow stromal cells; and (3) osteoprotegrin (OPG), a secreted "decoy" receptor made by osteoblasts and several other types of cells that can bind RANKL and thus short-circuit its interaction with RANK.[9] When stimulated by RANKL, RANK signaling activates the

transcription factor NF-κB, which is essential for the generation and survival of osteoclasts. A second important pathway involves M-CSF produced by osteoblasts and the M-CSF receptor, which is expressed by osteoclast progenitors. Activation of the M-CSF receptor stimulates a tyrosine kinase activity that is also crucial for the generation of osteoclasts. The other notable pathway is the WNT/β-catenin pathway. WNT proteins produced by marrow stromal cells bind to the LRP5 and LRP6 receptors on osteoblasts (see Fig. 26–1) and thereby trigger the activation of β-catenin and the production of OPG. The importance of these pathways is proven by rare but informative germline mutations in the *OPG, RANK, RANKL,* and *LRP5* genes, which cause severe disturbances of bone metabolism (described later).

Bone formation and resorption are tightly coupled and subject to fine-tuning at several levels. For example, because OPG and RANKL oppose one another, either bone resorption or bone formation can be favored by simply tipping the RANKL : OPG ratio one way or the other. Systemic factors that affect RANKL and OPG expression include hormones (parathyroid hormone, estrogen, testosterone, and glucocorticoids), vitamin D, inflammatory cytokines (e.g., IL-1), and growth factors (such as bone morphogenetic factors); each presumably acts by altering the levels of NF-κB and WNT/β-catenin signaling in osteoblasts. Another level of control involves paracrine crosstalk between osteoblasts and osteoclasts, and possibly osteocytes as well. We have seen that osteoblasts can enhance or inhibit osteoclast development and function by expressing OPG and RANKL in various proportions. As osteoclasts disassemble matrix proteins deposited by osteoblasts, growth factors, cytokines, and enzymes (such as collagenase) bound to the matrix are liberated and activated, including some that stimulate osteoblasts. *Thus, as bone is broken down to its elemental units, substances are released into the microenvironment that initiate its renewal* (see Fig. 26–1).

The *proteins of bone* include type 1 collagen and many noncollagenous proteins derived mainly from osteoblasts. Osteoblasts deposit collagen either in a random weave known as *woven bone* or in an orderly layered manner designated *lamellar bone* (Fig. 26–4). Normally, woven bone is seen in sites of

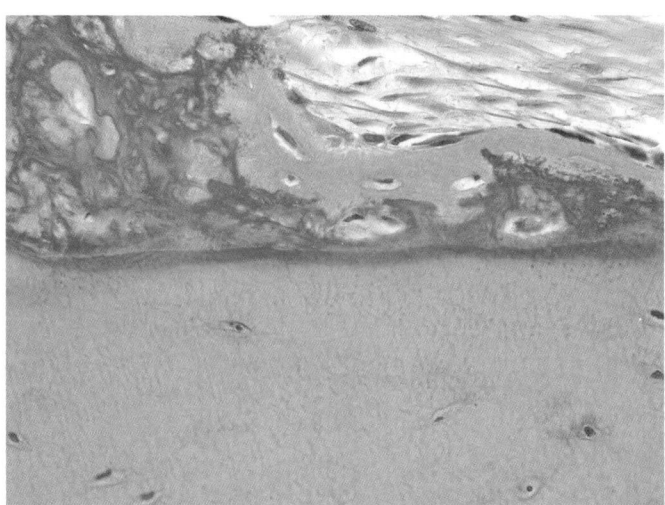

FIGURE 26–4 Woven bone *(top)* deposited on the surface of preexisting lamellar bone *(bottom)*.

TABLE 26–1 Proteins of Bone Matrix
OSTEOBLAST-DERIVED PROTEINS
Type 1 collagen
Cell adhesion proteins
Osteopontin, fibronectin, thrombospondin
Calcium-binding proteins
Osteonectin, bone sialoprotein
Proteins involved in mineralization
Osteocalcin
Enzymes
Collagenase, alkaline phosphatase
Growth factors
IGF-1, TGF-β, PDGF
Cytokines
IL-1, IL-6, RANKL
PROTEINS CONCENTRATED FROM SERUM
β₂-microglobulin
Albumin

IGF, insulin-like growth factor; TGF, transforming growth factor; PDGF, platelet-derived growth factor; IL, interleukin; RANKL, RANK ligand.

rapid bone formation such as the fetal skeleton and the base of growth plates. It is produced quickly and resists forces equally from all directions. The presence of woven bone in the adult is always abnormal; however, it is not diagnostic of a particular disease. We will see examples of this later in this chapter. *Lamellar bone, which gradually replaces woven bone during growth, is deposited much more slowly and is stronger than woven bone.*

The noncollagenous proteins of bone are bound to the matrix and grouped according to their function (Table 26–1).[8,10] Of these, only osteocalcin is unique to bone. It is measurable in the serum and used as a sensitive and specific marker for osteoblast activity. Cytokines and growth factors control bone cell proliferation, maturation, and metabolism, thereby playing a crucial role translating mechanical and metabolic signals into local bone cell activity and eventual skeletal adaptation.[8,11] In this fashion the skeleton is uniquely able to change its structure in response to new physical forces; witness the repositioning of teeth by braces.

Bone Modeling, Remodeling, and Peak Bone Mass

Local collections of osteocytes, osteoblasts, and osteoclasts work together to control bone formation and resorption, creating a functional unit referred to as the *basic multicellular unit* (BMU).[12,13] Early in life, as the skeleton grows and enlarges (modeling), bone formation predominates. Once the skeleton has reached maturity, the breakdown and renewal of bone that constitutes skeletal maintenance is called *remodeling* and is probably initiated at sites experiencing fatigue and microdamage. In adults, BMUs *remodel* or replace 10% of the skeleton annually.

Peak bone mass is achieved in early adulthood after the cessation of growth, and it is determined by a variety of factors, including polymorphisms in the receptors for vitamin D and LRP5/6, nutrition, physical activity, age, and hormonal status.

Beginning in the fourth decade, however, the amount of bone resorbed by the BMUs exceeds that formed, so that there is a steady decrement in skeletal mass.

Bone Growth and Development

Skeletal morphogenesis is determined by the *homeobox genes*, which encode transcription factors essential for the normal development of the skeleton.[12,14] Most bones are first formed as a cartilage model or anlage. Subsequently, around the eighth week of gestation the process of *enchondral ossification* begins, and the cartilage is removed by osteoclast-type cells forming the medullary canal. This process progresses along the length of the bone, while concurrently the periosteum in the midshaft generates osteoblasts that deposit the beginnings of the cortex; this region is known as the *primary center of ossification*. A similar sequence of events occurs in the epiphysis, resulting in the removal of cartilage and deposition of bone in a centrifugal fashion (*secondary center of ossification*), such that a plate of the cartilage anlage becomes entrapped between the expanding centers of ossification forming the *physis* or *growth plate* (Fig. 26–5). The chondrocytes within the growth plate are responsible for longitudinal growth as they undergo a series of changes, including proliferation, growth, maturation, and apoptosis—controlled by a number of signaling pathways, including those involving FGF receptors and bone morphogenetic protein, hedgehog protein, and parathyroid-hormone (PTH)-related protein.[15] In the region of apoptosis the matrix mineralizes and is resorbed by osteoclasts; however, remnant struts persist and act as scaffolding for the deposition of bone on their surfaces. These structures are known as primary spongiosa and are the first bony trabeculae. A similar

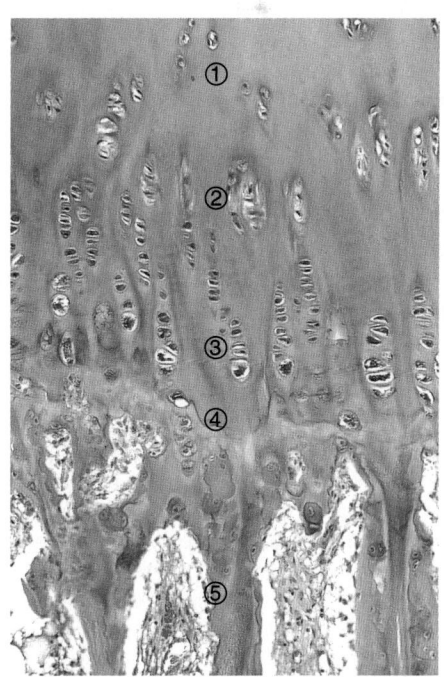

FIGURE 26–5 Active growth plate with ongoing enchondral ossification. 1, Reserve zone. 2, Zone of proliferation. 3, Zone of hypertrophy. 4, Zone of mineralization. 5, Primary spongiosa.

process occurs at the base of articular cartilage, and by this mechanism bones increase in length, and articular surfaces increase in diameter. In contrast, bones derived from *intramembranous formation*, such as the cranium and lateral portions of the clavicles, are formed by osteoblasts directly from a fibrous layer of tissue that is derived from mesenchyme. Because bone tissue is made only by osteoblasts, the enlargement of bones is achieved by the deposition of new bone on a preexisting surface. This mechanism of *appositional growth* is key to understanding bone growth and modeling.

The complexity of the skeleton's growth, development, maintenance, and relationships with other organ systems makes it unusually vulnerable to adverse influences. Not surprisingly, then, primary and secondary diseases of bone are varied and numerous. The spectrum of bone disorders is broad and the classification system is not standardized; here we will categorize the various disorders according to their perceived pathogenesis.

Developmental Abnormalities in Bone Cells, Matrix, and Structure

Developmental abnormalities of the skeleton are frequently genetically based; they first become manifest during the earliest stages of bone formation. In contrast, acquired diseases are usually detected in adulthood.[11] Developmental anomalies resulting from localized problems in the migration of the mesenchymal cells and the formation of the condensations are known as *dysostoses*. They are usually limited to defined embryologic structures and may result from mutations in certain transcription factors (e.g., *homeobox* genes). In contrast, mutations in the regulators of skeletal organogenesis, such as signaling molecules (e.g., growth factors and their receptors) and matrix components (e.g., types 1 and 2 collagen) affect cartilage and bone tissues globally; these disorders are known as *dysplasias*.[8,11,12,15–17] Table 26–2 shows a classification of developmental abnormalities of the bone based on the nature of the genetic abnormality. The classification of developmental and acquired abnormalities that follows is based on identified genetic defects and the skeletal manifestations of the disease processes. Many of the conditions can be classified in more than one category.

MALFORMATIONS AND DISEASES CAUSED BY DEFECTS IN NUCLEAR PROTEINS AND TRANSCRIPTION FACTORS

Congenital malformations or dysostoses of bone are relatively uncommon. The simplest anomalies include failure of a bone to develop (e.g., congenital absence of a phalanx, rib, or clavicle); the formation of extra bones (supernumerary ribs or digits); the fusion of two adjacent digits (syndactylism); or the development of long, spider-like digits. Some of these result from defects in the formation of the mesenchymal condensations and their differentiation into the cartilage anlage. They are caused by genetic alterations that affect transcription factors, especially those encoded by the *homeobox* genes, and certain cytokines.[8,11] One example of a defect in mesenchymal condensation is caused by a mutation in the homeobox

HOXD13 gene, which produces an extra digit between the third and fourth fingers as well as some degree of syndactyly.[12] Loss of function mutations in the *RUNX2* gene, which produces transcription factors important in osteoblastogenesis and some chondrocyte cell activity, results in *cleidocranial dysplasia*, an autosomal dominant disorder characterized by patent fontanelles, delayed closure of cranial sutures, Wormian bones, delayed eruption of secondary teeth, primitive clavicles, and short height.

DISEASES CAUSED BY DEFECTS IN HORMONES AND SIGNAL TRANSDUCTION MECHANISMS

Achondroplasia is the most common disease of the growth plate and is a major cause of dwarfism. It is caused by a mutation in the FGF receptor 3 (FGFR3).[11] Normally, FGF-mediated activation of FGFR3 *inhibits* cartilage proliferation; in achondroplasia, the mutations cause constitutive activation of FGFR3 and thereby suppress growth.

Achondroplasia is an autosomal dominant disorder; curiously approximately 80% of cases stem from new mutations, almost all of which occur in the paternal allele. Affected individuals have shortened proximal extremities, a trunk of relative normal length, and an enlarged head with bulging forehead and conspicuous depression of the root of the nose. The skeletal abnormalities are usually not associated with changes in longevity, intelligence, or reproductive status.

Thanatophoric dwarfism is the most common lethal form of dwarfism, affecting about one in every 20,000 live births. It is also caused by gain-of-function mutations in FGFR3 that differ from those in achondroplasia.[11] Affected individuals have micromelic shortening of the limbs, frontal bossing, relative macrocephaly, a small chest cavity, and a bell-shaped abdomen. The underdeveloped thoracic cavity leads to respiratory insufficiency, and these individuals frequently die at birth or soon after. The histologic changes in the growth plate show diminished proliferation of chondrocytes and poor columnization in the zone of proliferation.

Increased bone mass is a manifestation of a variety of diseases. Several are caused by caused by gain-of-function mutations in the gene that encodes LPR5, a cell surface receptor that is essential for the activation of the WNT/β-catenin pathway in osteoblasts. These diseases, namely endosteal hyperostosis, Van Buchem disease, and autosomal dominant osteopetrosis type 1, are characterized by increased bone mass including cortical thickening, enlarged and elongated mandible, and increased density and enlargement of the cranial vault; some affected individuals may develop torus palatinus.

Conversely, inactivating mutations in LPR5 cause *osteoporosis pseudoglioma syndrome*. In this disorder the skeleton is severely osteoporotic, resulting in fractures due to insufficient bone formation.

DISEASES ASSOCIATED WITH DEFECTS IN EXTRACELLULAR STRUCTURAL PROTEINS

The interaction of the organic components of bone matrix is complex and a focus of intense scientific investigation. The importance of the structural bone proteins is exemplified by

TABLE 26–2 Molecular Genetics of Diseases of the Skeleton			
Human Disorder	**Gene Mutation**	**Affected Molecule**	**Phenotype**
DEFECTS IN TRANSCRIPTION FACTORS PRODUCING ABNORMALITIES IN MESENCHYMAL CONDENSATION AND RELATED CELL DIFFERENTIATION			
Synpolydactyly	HOXD13	Transcription factor	Extra digit with fusion
Waardenburg syndrome	PAX3	Transcription factor	Hearing loss, abnormal pigmentation, craniofacial abnormalities
Greig syndrome	GLI13	Transcription factor	Synpolydactyly, craniofacial abnormalities
Campomelic dysplasia	SOX9	Transcription factor	Sex reversal, abnormal skeletal development
Oligodontia	PAX9	Transcription factor	Congenital absence of teeth
Nail-patella syndrome	LMX1B	Transcription factor	Hypoplastic nails, hypoplastic or aplastic patellas, dislocated radial head, progressive nephropathy
Holt-Oram syndrome	TBX5	Transcription factor	Congenital abnormalities, forelimb anomalies
Ulnar-mammary syndrome	TBX3	Transcription factor	Hypoplasia or absent ulna, third to fifth digits, breast, and teeth, delayed puberty
Cleidocranial dysplasia	CBFA1	Transcription factor	Abnormal clavicles, wormian bones, supernumery teeth
DEFECTS IN EXTRACELLULAR STRUCTURAL PROTEINS			
Osteogenesis imperfecta types I–IV	COL1A1, COL1A2	Type 1 collagen	Bone fragility, hearing loss, blue sclera, dentinogenesis imperfecta
Achondrogenesis II	COL2A1	Type 2 collagen	Short trunk, severely shortened extremities, relatively enlarged cranium, flattened face
Hypochondrogenesis	COL2A1	Type 2 collagen	Short trunk, shortened extremities, relatively enlarged, cranium, flattened face
Stickler syndrome	COL2A1	Type 2 collagen	Myopia, retinal detachment, hearing loss, flattened face, premature osteoarthritis
Multiple epiphyseal dysplasia	COL9A2	Type 9 collagen	Short or normal stature, small epiphyses, early-onset osteoarthritis
Schmid metaphyseal chondrodysplasia	COL10A1	Type 10 collagen	Mildly short stature, bowing of lower extremities, coxa vara, metaphyseal flaring
DEFECTS IN HORMONES AND SIGNAL TRANSDUCTION MECHANISMS PRODUCING ABNORMAL PROLIFERATION OR MATURATION OF CHONDROCYTES AND OSTEOBLASTS			
Brachdactyly type C	CDMP1	Signaling molecule	Shortened metacarpals and phalanges
Jansen metaphyseal chondroplasia	PTHrp receptor	Receptor	Short bowed limbs, clinodactyly, facial abnormalities, hypercalcemia, hypophosphatemia
Achondroplasia	FGFR3	Receptor	Short stature, rhizomelic shortening of limbs, frontal bossing, midface dificiency
Hypochondroplasia	FGFR3	Receptor	Disproportionately short stature, micromelia, relative macrocephaly
Thanatophoric dwarfism	FGFR3	Receptor	Severe limb shortening and bowing, frontal bossing, depressed nasal bridge
Crouzon syndrome	FGFR2	Receptor	Craniosynostosis
Osteoporosis-pseudoglioma syndrome	LRP5	Receptor	Congenital or infant-onset loss of vision, skeletal fragility

Modified from Mundlos S, Olsen BR: Heritable diseases of the skeleton. Part I: Molecular insights into skeletal development—transcription factors and signaling pathways. FASEB J 11:125–132, 1997; Mundlos S, Olsen BR: Heritable diseases of the skeleton. Part II: Molecular insights into skeletal development—matrix components and their homeostasis. FASEB J 11: 227–233, 1997; Superti-Furga A et al.: Molecular-pathogenetic classification of genetic disorders of the skeleton. Am J Med Genet 106:262–293, 2001.

the diseases associated with deranged metabolism of the collagens important in bone and cartilage formation (types 1, 2, 9, 10, and 11). Their clinical manifestations are highly variable, ranging from lethal disease to premature osteoarthritis.

Type 1 Collagen Diseases (Osteogenesis Imperfecta)

Osteogenesis imperfecta, or *brittle bone disease*, is a phenotypically diverse disorder caused by deficiencies in the synthesis of type 1 collagen. It is the most common inherited disorder of connective tissue. It principally affects bone, but also impacts other tissues rich in type 1 collagen (joints, eyes, ears, skin, and teeth). Osteogenesis imperfecta usually results from

autosomal dominant mutations (over 800 have been identified) in the genes that encode the α1 and α2 chains of collagen.[19] Many of these mutations involve the substitution of glycine residues in the triple-helical domain. The genotype-phenotype relationship underlying osteogenesis imperfecta is based on the location of the mutation within the protein. Mutations resulting in decreased synthesis of qualitatively normal collagen are associated with mild skeletal abnormalities. More severe or lethal phenotypes have abnormal polypeptide chains that cannot be arranged in the triple helix. Recently, mutations in the genes for cartilage-associated protein (CRTAP) and leucine proline-enriched proteoglycan 1 (LEPRE1) have been shown to be responsible for three rare variants of the disease.[20]

TABLE 26–3	Subtypes of Osteogenesis Imperfecta		
Subtype		**Inheritance**	**Collagen Defect**	**Major Clinical Features**

Subtype		**Inheritance**	**Collagen Defect**	**Major Clinical Features**
OI type I	Compatible with survival	Autosomal dominant	Decreased synthesis of pro-α1(1) chain Abnormal pro-α1(1) or pro-α2(1) chains	Postnatal fractures, blue sclera Normal stature Skeletal fragility Dentinogenesis imperfecta Hearing impairment Joint laxity Blue sclerae
OI type II	Perinatal lethal	Most autosomal recessive Some autosomal dominant ?New mutations	Abnormally short pro-α1(1) chain Unstable triple helix Abnormal or insufficient pro-α2(1)	Death in utero or within days of birth Skeletal deformity with excessive fragility and multiple fractures Blue sclera
OI type III	Progressive, deforming	Autosomal dominant (75%) Autosomal recessive (25%)	Altered structure of pro-peptides of pro-α2(1) Impaired formation of triple helix	Compatible with survival Growth retardation Multiple fractures Progressive kyphoscoliosis Blue sclera at birth that become white Hearing impairment Dentinogenesis imperfecta
OI type IV	Compatible with survival	Autosomal dominant	Short pro-α2(1) chain Unstable triple helix	Postnatal fractures, normal sclerae Moderate skeletal fragility Short stature Sometimes dentinogenesis imperfecta

OI, osteogenesis imperfecta.

Clinically, osteogenesis imperfecta is separated into four major subtypes that vary widely in severity (Table 26–3). The *type II variant* is at one end of the spectrum and is uniformly fatal in utero or during the perinatal period. It is characterized by extraordinary bone fragility with multiple intrauterine fractures (Fig. 26–6). In contrast, individuals with the *type I form* have a normal life span but experience childhood fractures that decrease in frequency following puberty. Other findings include *blue sclerae* caused by decreased collagen content, making the sclera translucent and allowing partial visualization of the underlying choroid; *hearing loss* related to both a sensorineural deficit and impeded conduction due to abnormalities in the bones of the middle and inner ear; and *dental imperfections* (small, misshapen, and blue-yellow teeth) secondary to a deficiency in dentin. *The basic abnormality in all forms of osteogenesis imperfecta is too little bone*, thus constituting a type of osteoporosis with marked cortical thinning and attenuation of trabeculae.

Diseases Associated with Mutations of Types 2, 9, 10, and 11 Collagen

Types 2, 9, 10, and 11 collagens are important structural components of hyaline cartilage. Although uncommon, mutations in the genes encoding them produce an array of disorders ranging from the fatal to those compatible with life but associated with early destruction of joints (see Table 26–2). In the severe disorders, the type 2 collagen molecules are not secreted by the chondrocytes, and insufficient bone formation occurs. In the milder disorders there is reduced synthesis of normal type 2 collagen.

DISEASES ASSOCIATED WITH DEFECTS IN FOLDING AND DEGRADATION OF MACROMOLECULES

Mucopolysaccharidoses

The mucopolysaccharidoses, as discussed earlier (Chapter 5), are a group of lysosomal storage diseases that are caused by deficiencies in the enzymes that degrade dermatan sulfate, heparan sulfate, and keratan sulfate. The affected enzymes are mainly acid hydrolases. Mesenchymal cells, especially chondrocytes, normally metabolize extracellular matrix mucopolysaccharides; hence, cartilage formation is severely affected. Consequently, many of the skeletal manifestations of the mucopolysaccharidoses result from abnormalities in hyaline cartilage, including the cartilage anlage, growth plates, costal cartilages, and articular surfaces. It is not surprising, therefore, that affected individuals are frequently of short stature and have chest wall abnormalities, and malformed bones.

DISEASES ASSOCIATED WITH DEFECTS IN METABOLIC PATHWAYS (ENZYMES, ION CHANNELS, AND TRANSPORTERS)

Osteopetrosis

Osteopetrosis, also known as *marble bone disease* and *Albers-Schönberg disease*, refers to a group of rare genetic diseases that are characterized by reduced bone resorption and diffuse symmetric skeletal sclerosis due to impaired formation or function of osteoclasts (Fig. 26–7). The term *osteopetrosis* reflects the stonelike quality of the bones; however, the bones are

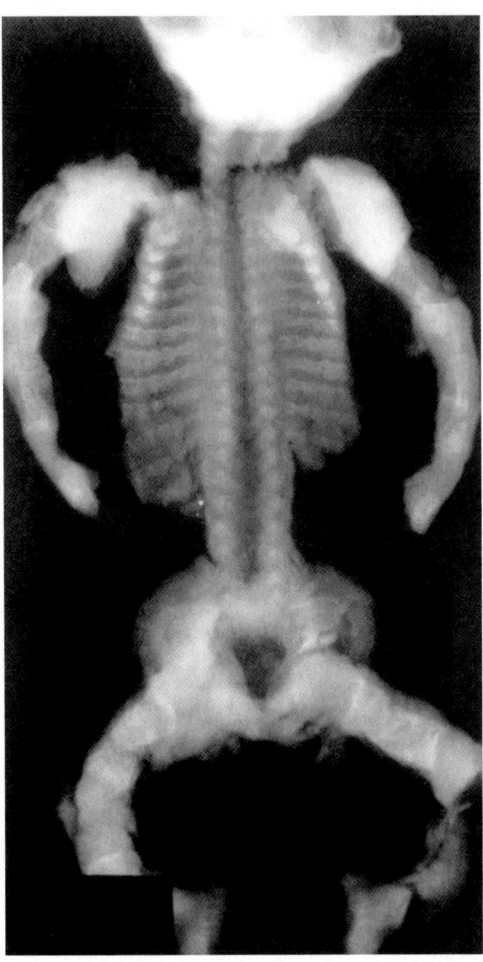

FIGURE 26–6 Skeletal radiogram of a fetus with lethal type II osteogenesis imperfecta. Note the numerous fractures of virtually all bones, resulting in accordion-like shortening of the limbs.

abnormally brittle and fracture easily, like a piece of chalk. Osteopetrosis is classified into variants based on both the mode of inheritance and the clinical findings. The two major groups include autosomal recessive and dominant forms. The autosomal recessive type is further divided into mild and severe variants. The autosomal recessive severe type and the autosomal dominant mild type are the most common variants.

Pathogenesis. Most of the mutations underlying osteopetrosis interfere with the process of acidification of the osteoclast resorption pit, which is required for the dissolution of the calcium hydroxyapatite within the matrix. Examples include autosomal recessive defects in the gene *CA2*, which encodes the enzyme carbonic anhydrase II.[21] Carbonic anhydrase II is required by osteoclasts and renal tubular cells to generate protons from carbon dioxide and water. Absence of CAII prevents osteoclasts from acidifying the resorption pit and solubilizing hydroxyapatite, and also blocks the acidification of urine by the renal tubular cells. In an autosomal recessive severe form of the disease, a mutation in the chloride channel gene *CLCN7* interferes with the function of the H⁺-ATPase proton pump located on the osteoclast ruffled border.[21] Another severe autosomal recessive form is caused by a muta-

tion in the gene *TCIRG1*, which encodes a component of the proton pump. A less severe autosomal recessive variant results from a mutation in the gene that encodes RANKL. Not surprisingly, these individuals have fewer osteoclasts than normal. In animals, osteopetrosis can also be caused by mutations in a large number of other genes, including M-CSF, RANK, and OPG, which you will recall regulate osteoclast formation and function.[21]

> **Morphology.** The morphologic changes of osteopetrosis are explained by deficient osteoclast activity. The bones lack a medullary canal, and the ends of long bones are bulbous (Erlenmeyer flask deformity) and misshapen. The neural foramina are small and compress exiting nerves. The primary spongiosa, which is normally removed during growth, persists and fills the medullary cavity, leaving no room for the hematopoietic marrow and preventing the formation of mature trabeculae (Fig. 26–8). Deposited bone is not remodeled and tends to be woven in architecture. In the end, these intrinsic abnormalities cause the bone to be brittle and predisposed to fracture. Histologically, the number of osteoclasts may be normal, increased, or decreased depending on the underlying genetic defect.

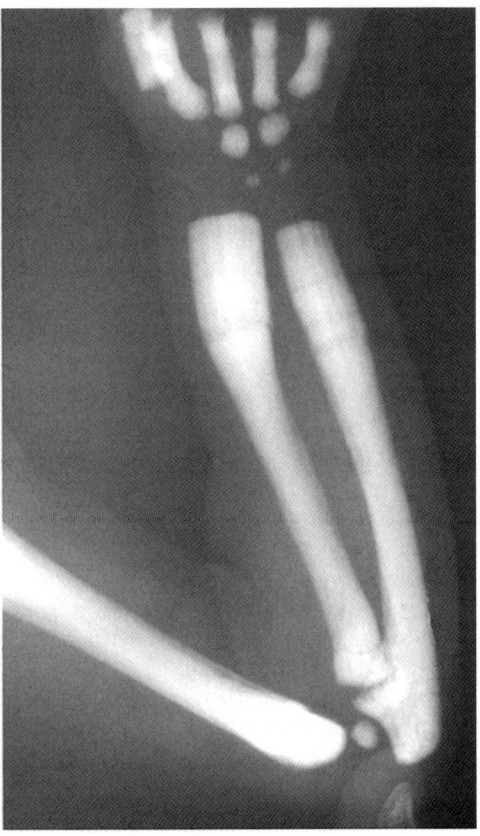

FIGURE 26–7 Radiogram of the upper extremity in an individual with osteopetrosis. The bones are diffusely sclerotic, and the distal metaphyses of the ulna and radius are poorly formed (Erlenmeyer flask deformity).

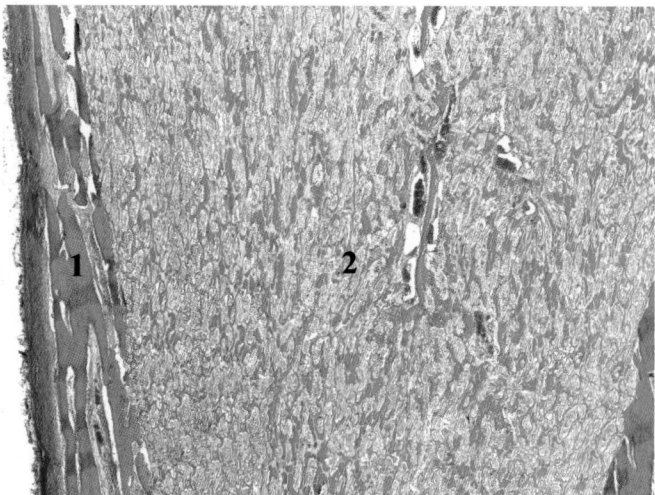

FIGURE 26–8 Section of proximal tibial diaphysis from a fetus with osteopetrosis. The cortex (1) is present, but the medullary cavity (2) is filled with primary spongiosa, which replaces the hematopoietic elements.

Clinical Features. Severe infantile malignant osteopetrosis is autosomal recessive and usually becomes evident in utero or soon after birth. Fracture, anemia, and hydrocephaly are often seen, resulting in postpartum mortality. Affected individuals who survive into their infancy have cranial nerve defects (optic atrophy, deafness, and facial paralysis) and repeated—often fatal—infections because of inadequacies of the marrow produced in extramedullary sites, which also causes prominent hepatosplenomegaly. The mild autosomal dominant benign form may not be detected until adolescence or adulthood, when it is discovered on x-rays performed because of repeated fractures. These individuals may also have mild cranial nerve deficits and anemia.

Osteopetrosis was the first genetic disease treated with bone marrow transplantation, since osteoclasts are derived from marrow monocyte precursors. The donor progenitor cells produce normal functioning osteoclasts, which reverse many of the skeletal abnormalities.

DISEASES ASSOCIATED WITH DECREASED BONE MASS

Osteoporosis

Osteoporosis is a disease characterized by porous bones and a reduced bone mass. The associated structural changes predispose the bone to fracture. The disorder may be localized to a certain bone or region, as in *disuse osteoporosis of a limb,* or may involve the entire skeleton, as a manifestation of a *metabolic bone disease.* Generalized osteoporosis, in turn, may be primary or secondary to a large variety of conditions (Table 26–4).

When the term osteoporosis is used in an unqualified manner, it usually refers to the most common forms, senile and postmenopausal osteoporosis, in which the loss of bone mass makes the skeleton vulnerable to fractures. It is estimated that one million Americans experience a fracture related to osteoporosis each year, at a cost of over 14 billion dollars. Effective treatment and prevention are imperative. The following discussion relates largely to these dominant forms of osteoporosis.

Pathogenesis. Peak bone mass is achieved during young adulthood. Its magnitude is determined largely by hereditary factors, especially polymorphisms in the genes that influence bone metabolism (discussed later).[22] Physical activity, muscle strength, diet, and hormonal state also make important contributions. Once maximal skeletal mass is attained, a small deficit in bone formation accrues with every resorption and formation cycle of each basic multicellular unit. Accordingly, age-related bone loss, which may average 0.7% per year, is a normal and predictable biologic phenomenon. Both sexes are affected equally and whites more so than blacks. Differences in the peak skeletal mass in men versus women and in blacks versus whites may partially explain why certain populations are prone to develop this disorder.

Although much remains unknown, discoveries in the molecular biology of bone have provided intriguing new hypotheses about the pathogenesis of osteoporosis (Fig. 26–9):

○ *Age-related changes* in bone cells and matrix have a strong impact on bone metabolism. Osteoblasts from elderly

TABLE 26–4 Categories of Generalized Osteoporosis
PRIMARY
Postmenopausal
Senile
Idiopathic
SECONDARY
Endocrine Disorders
Hyperparathyroidism
Hyperthyroidism
Hypothyroidism
Hypogonadism
Pituitary tumors
Diabetes, type 1
Addison disease
Neoplasia
Multiple myeloma
Carcinomatosis
Gastrointestinal
Malnutrition
Malabsorption
Hepatic insufficiency
Vitamin C, D deficiencies
Drugs
Anticoagulants
Chemotherapy
Corticosteroids
Anticovulsants
Alcohol
Miscellaneous
Osteogenesis imperfecta
Immobilization
Pulmonary disease
Homocystinuria
Anemia

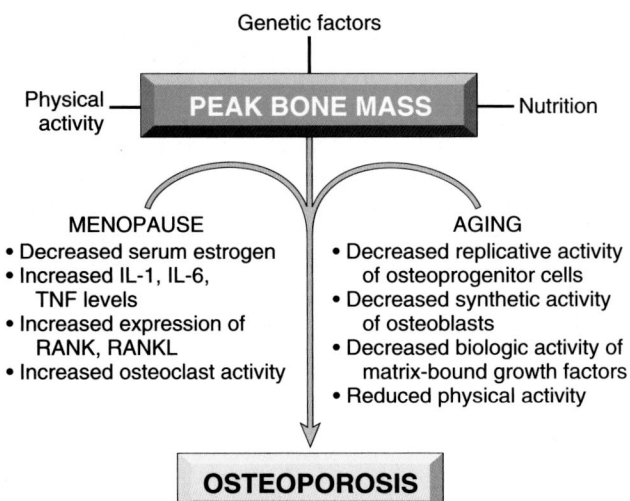

Genetic factors

Physical
activity — PEAK BONE MASS — Nutrition

MENOPAUSE
- Decreased serum estrogen
- Increased IL-1, IL-6,
  TNF levels
- Increased expression of
  RANK, RANKL
- Increased osteoclast activity

AGING
- Decreased replicative activity
  of osteoprogenitor cells
- Decreased synthetic activity
  of osteoblasts
- Decreased biologic activity of
  matrix-bound growth factors
- Reduced physical activity

OSTEOPOROSIS

FIGURE 26–9 Pathophysiology of postmenopausal and senile osteoporosis (see text).

individuals have reduced proliferative and biosynthetic potential when compared with osteoblasts from younger individuals.[23] Also, proteins bound to the extracellular matrix (such as growth factors, which are both mitogenic to osteoprogenitor cells and stimulate osteoblastic synthetic activity) lose their biologic punch over time. The net result is a diminished capacity to make bone. This form of osteoporosis, known as *senile osteoporosis*, is categorized as a *low-turnover variant*.

○ *Reduced physical activity* increases the rate of bone loss in experimental animals and humans, because mechanical forces stimulate normal bone remodeling. Bone loss in an immobilized or paralyzed extremity, the reduction of skeletal mass in astronauts in a zero gravity environment for prolonged periods, and the higher bone density in athletes exemplify the role of physical activity in preventing bone loss. The type of exercise is important, as load magnitude influences bone density more than the number of load cycles. Because muscle contraction is the dominant source of skeletal loading, resistance exercises such as weight training are more effective stimuli for increasing bone mass than repetitive endurance activities such as jogging. Certainly the decreased physical activity that is associated with aging contributes to senile osteoporosis.

○ *Genetic factors are also important*, as noted previously. It is estimated that 60% to 80% of the variation in bone density is genetically determined. In genome-wide association studies (GWAS), the top associated genes include *RANKL*, *OPG*, and *RANK*,[24] which you will recall encode key regulators of osteoclasts. Also associated are the MHC locus (perhaps reflecting the effects of inflammation on calcium metabolism) and the estrogen receptor gene (discussed below). Some studies have also implicated genetic variants of the vitamin D receptor and LRP5 as risk factors.

○ The body's *calcium nutritional state* is important. It has been shown that adolescent girls (but not boys) tend to have insufficient calcium intake in the diet. This calcium deficiency occurs during a period of rapid bone growth, stunting the peak bone mass ultimately achieved; thus,

these individuals are at greater risk of developing osteoporosis. Calcium deficiency, increased PTH concentrations, and reduced levels of vitamin D may also have a role in the development of senile osteoporosis.

○ *Hormonal influences.* In the decade after menopause, yearly reductions in bone mass may reach up to 2% of cortical bone and 9% of cancellous bone. Women may lose as much as 35% of their cortical bone and 50% of their trabecular bone within the 30 to 40 years after menopause. It is thus no surprise that post-menopausal women suffer osteoporotic fractures more commonly than men of the same age. *Postmenopausal* osteoporosis is characterized by a hormone-dependent acceleration of bone loss that occurs during the decade after menopause. *Estrogen deficiency plays the major role in this phenomenon, and estrogen replacement at menopause is protective against bone loss.* The effects of estrogen on bone mass are mediated by cytokines. Decreased estrogen levels appear to result in increased secretion of inflammatory cytokines by blood monocytes and bone marrow cells. These cytokines stimulate osteoclast recruitment and activity by increasing the levels of RANKL while diminishing the expression of OPG. Compensatory osteoblastic activity occurs, but it does not keep pace, leading to what is classified as a *high-turnover form* of osteoporosis.

Morphology. The entire skeleton is affected in postmenopausal and senile osteoporosis (Fig. 26–10), but certain regions tend to be more severely involved than others. In **postmenopausal** osteoporosis the increase in osteoclast activity affects mainly bones or portions of bones that have increased surface area, such as the cancellous compartment of vertebral bodies. The trabecular plates become perforated, thinned, and lose their interconnections, leading to progressive microfractures and eventual vertebral collapse. In senile osteoporosis the cortex is thinned by subperiosteal and endosteal resorption, and the haversian systems are widened. In severe cases the haversian systems are so enlarged that the cortex mimics cancellous bone. The bone that remains is of normal composition.

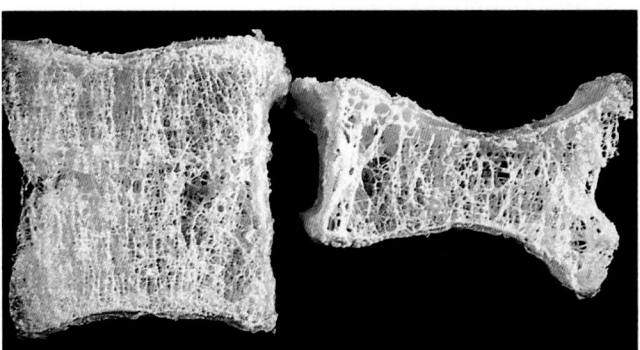

FIGURE 26–10 Osteoporotic vertebral body *(right)* shortened by compression fractures compared with a normal vertebral body. Note that the osteoporotic vertebra has a characteristic loss of horizontal trabeculae and thickened vertical trabeculae.

Clinical Course. The clinical manifestations of osteoporosis depend on which bones are involved. Vertebral fractures that frequently occur in the thoracic and lumbar regions are painful, and when multiple can cause significant loss of height and various deformities, including lumbar lordosis and kyphoscoliosis. Complications of fractures of the femoral neck, pelvis, or spine, such as pulmonary embolism and pneumonia, are frequent and result in 40,000 to 50,000 deaths per year.

Osteoporosis cannot be reliably detected in plain radiograms until 30% to 40% of the bone mass is lost, and measurement of blood levels of calcium, phosphorus, and alkaline phosphatase are not diagnostic. Osteoporosis is thus a difficult condition to diagnose accurately, since it remains asymptomatic until skeletal fragility is well advanced. The best procedures to accurately estimate the amount of bone loss, aside from biopsy, are specialized radiographic imaging techniques, such as dual-energy X-ray absorptiometry and quantitative computed tomography, which measure bone density.

The prevention and treatment of senile and postmenopausal osteoporosis includes exercise, appropriate calcium and vitamin D intake, and pharmacologic agents, most commonly bisphosphonates, which bind to bone and inhibit osteoclasts.

DISEASES CAUSED BY OSTEOCLAST DYSFUNCTION

Paget Disease (Osteitis Deformans)

This unique skeletal disease can be divided into three phases; *(1) an initial osteolytic stage, followed by (2) a mixed osteoclastic-osteoblastic stage, which ends with a predominance of osteoblastic activity and evolves ultimately into (3) a burnt-out quiescent osteosclerotic stage* (Fig. 26–11). The net effect is a *gain in bone mass*; however, the newly formed bone is disordered and architecturally unsound.

Paget disease usually begins in late adulthood (average age at diagnosis, 70 years) and becomes progressively more common thereafter. An intriguing aspect is the striking variation in its prevalence, both within certain countries and throughout the world. Paget disease is relatively common in whites in England, France, Austria, regions of Germany, Australia, New Zealand, and the United States. In contrast, Paget disease is rare in the native populations of Scandinavia, China, Japan, and Africa. The exact incidence is hard to determine because many affected individuals are asymptomatic; it is estimated that 1% of the US population over the age of 40 is affected and the prevalence rate in England is 2.5% for men and 1.6% for women 55 years or older. Recent surveys show that there has been a fall in new cases over the last 25–30 years, and a decline in its clinical severity.

Pathogenesis. The cause of Paget disease remains uncertain, and current evidence suggests both environmental and genetic factors. The risk of developing the disorder is approximately seven times greater in first-degree relatives of affected individuals than it is in normal controls,[25] and 15% to 40% of individuals with Paget disease have a family history that shows an autosomal dominant pattern of inheritance. Mutations in the *SQSTM1* gene are present in 40% to 50% of cases of familial Paget disease, and in 5% to 10% of patients without a family history. The *SQSTM* mutations enhance NF-κB acti-

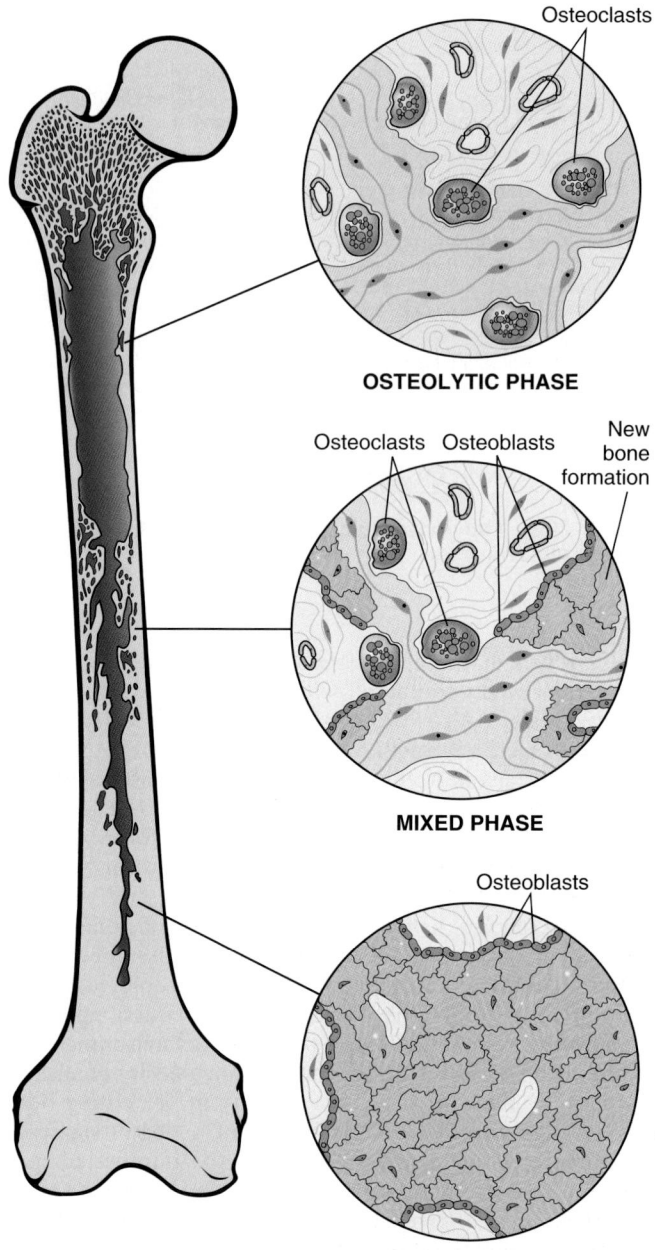

FIGURE 26–11 Diagrammatic representation of Paget disease of bone demonstrating the three phases in the evolution of the disease.

vation by RANK signaling, leading to increased osteoclast activity and an increased susceptibility to the disease. Mutations in *RANKL* and *RANK/OPG* have also been found in genetic diseases that have some phenotypic overlap with Paget disease; including familial expansile osteolysis, expansile skeletal hyperphosphatasia, early-onset Paget disease, juvenile Paget disease, and the syndrome of hereditary inclusion body myopathy, and frontotemporal dementia.

When Sir James Paget first described this condition in 1876, he attributed the skeletal changes to an inflammatory process, hence the term *osteitis deformans*. Support for this idea over the years has centered on a possible role for infection by a paramyxovirus, but this hypothesis remains unproven.

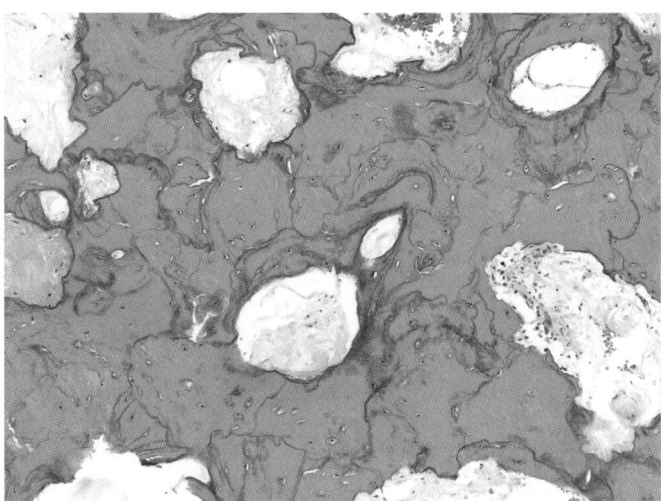

FIGURE 26–12 Mosaic pattern of lamellar bone pathognomonic of Paget disease.

Morphology. Paget disease is a focal process that shows remarkable histologic variation over time and from site to site. The hallmark is the **mosaic pattern** of lamellar bone. This pattern, which is likened to a jigsaw puzzle, is produced by prominent cement lines that anneal haphazardly oriented units of lamellar bone (Fig. 26–12). In the initial lytic phase there are waves of osteoclastic activity and numerous resorption pits. The osteoclasts are abnormally large and have many more than the normal 10 to 12 nuclei; sometimes 100 nuclei are present. Osteoclasts persist in the mixed phase, but now many of the bone surfaces are lined by prominent osteoblasts. The marrow adjacent to the bone-forming surface is replaced by loose connective tissue that contains osteoprogenitor cells and numerous blood vessels, which transport nutrients and catabolites to and from these metabolically active sites. The newly formed bone may be woven or lamellar, but eventually all of it is remodeled into lamellar bone. As the mosaic pattern unfolds and the cell activity decreases, the periosseous fibrovascular tissue recedes and is replaced by normal marrow. In the end, the bone becomes a caricature of itself: larger than normal and composed of coarsely thickened trabeculae and cortices that are soft and porous and lack structural stability. These aspects make the bone vulnerable to deformation under stress; consequently, it fractures easily.

Clinical Course. Clinical findings are extremely variable and depend on the extent and site of the disease. Most cases are mild and are discovered as an incidental radiographic finding. Paget disease is monostotic in about 15% of cases and polyostotic in the remainder. The axial skeleton or proximal femur is involved in up to 80% of cases. Even though no bone is immune, involvement of the ribs, fibula, and small bones of the hands and feet is unusual.

Pain localized to the affected bone is common. It is caused by microfractures or by bone overgrowth that compresses spinal and cranial nerve roots. Enlargement of the craniofacial skeleton may produce *leontiasis ossea* and a cranium so heavy that is difficult for the person to hold the head erect. The weakened pagetic bone may lead to invagination of the skull base *(platybasia)* and compression of the posterior fossa structures. Weight bearing causes anterior bowing of the femurs and tibiae and distorts the femoral heads, resulting in the development of *severe secondary osteoarthritis. Chalkstick-type* fractures are another frequent complication and usually occur in the long bones of the lower extremities. Compression fractures of the spine result in spinal cord injury and the development of kyphoses. The hypervascularity of pagetic bone warms the overlying skin, and in severe polyostotic disease the increased blood flow acts like an arteriovenous shunt, leading to high-output heart failure or exacerbation of underlying cardiac disease.

A variety of tumor and tumor-like conditions develop in pagetic bone. The benign lesions include giant-cell tumor, giant-cell reparative granuloma, and extra-osseous masses of hematopoiesis. The most dreaded complication is sarcoma, which occurs in 0.7% to 0.9% of all individuals with Paget disease, and in 5% to 10% of those with severe polyostotic disease. The sarcomas are usually osteosarcoma or fibrosarcoma, and they arise in Paget lesions in the long bones, pelvis, skull, and spine.

The diagnosis can frequently be made from the radiographic findings. Pagetic bone is typically enlarged with thick, coarsened cortices and cancellous bone (Fig. 26–13). Active

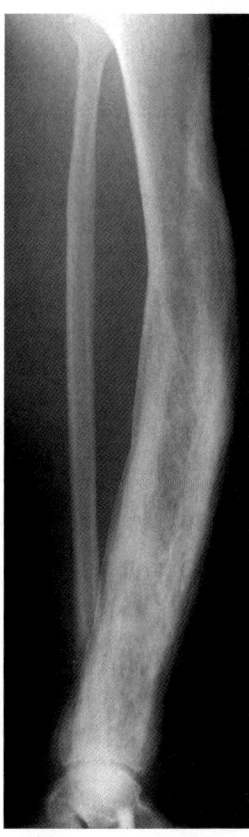

FIGURE 26–13 Severe Paget disease. The tibia is bowed and the affected portion is enlarged, sclerotic, and exhibits irregular thickening of both the cortical and cancellous bone.

disease has a wedge-shaped lytic leading edge that may progress along the length of the bone at a rate of 1 cm per year.[26] Many affected individuals have elevated serum alkaline phosphatase levels and increased urinary excretion of hydroxyproline.

In the absence of malignant transformation, Paget disease is usually not a serious or life-threatening disease. Most affected individuals have mild symptoms that are readily suppressed by calcitonin and bisphosphonates.

DISEASES ASSOCIATED WITH ABNORMAL MINERAL HOMEOSTASIS

Rickets and Osteomalacia

Rickets and osteomalacia are disorders characterized by a defect in matrix mineralization, most often related to a lack of vitamin D or some disturbance in its metabolism. The term *rickets* refers to the disorder in children in which deranged bone growth produces distinctive skeletal deformities. In the adult the disorder is called *osteomalacia*, because the bone that forms during the remodeling process is inadequately mineralized. This results in osteopenia and predisposition to insufficiency fractures. Both rickets and osteomalacia are discussed in Chapter 9.

Hyperparathyroidism

Hyperparathyroidism is classified into primary and secondary types as discussed in Chapter 24. Primary hyperparathyroidism results from autonomous hyperplasia or a tumor, usually an adenoma, of the parathyroid gland, whereas secondary hyperparathyroidism is commonly caused by prolonged states of hypocalcemia resulting in compensatory hypersecretion of PTH. Whatever the basis, the increased PTH concentrations are detected by receptors on osteoblasts, which then release factors that stimulate osteoclast activity. Thus, through a chain of signals, the skeletal manifestations of hyperparathyroidism are caused by unabated osteoclastic bone resorption. The following points should be noted:

- Similar to all metabolic bone disease, the entire skeleton is affected in hyperparathyroidism, even though some sites are more severely affected than others.
- The anatomic changes of severe hyperparathyroidism, known as *osteitis fibrosa cystica*, are now rarely encountered, because hyperparathyroidism is usually diagnosed and treated at an early asymptomatic stage detected on routine blood tests.
- Secondary hyperparathyroidism is usually not as severe or as prolonged as primary hyperparathyroidism, hence the skeletal abnormalities tend to be milder.

Morphology. For unknown reasons, the increased osteoclast activity in hyperparathyroidism affects cortical bone (subperiosteal, osteonal, and endosteal surfaces) more severely than cancellous bone. Subperiosteal resorption produces thinned cortices and the loss of the lamina dura around the teeth. X-rays reveal a pattern of radiolucency that is virtually diag-

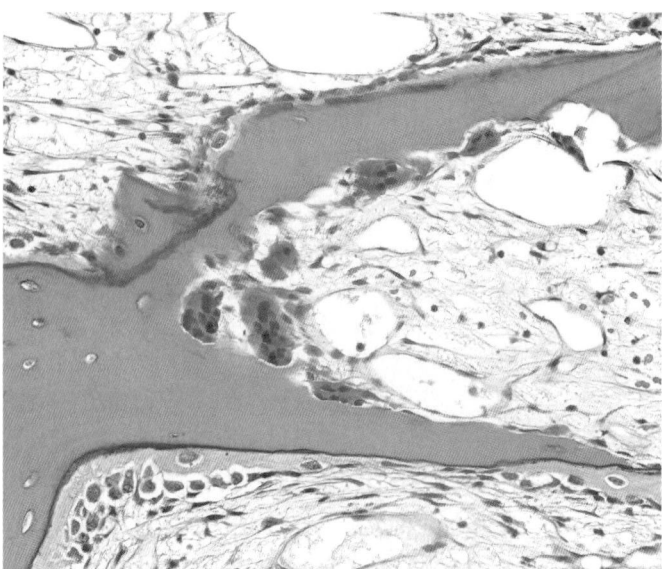

FIGURE 26–14 Hyperparathyroidism with osteoclasts boring into the center of the trabeculum (dissecting osteitis).

nostic of hyperparathyroidism. In cancellous bone, osteoclasts tunnel into and dissect centrally along the length of the trabeculae, creating the appearance of railroad tracks and producing what is known as **dissecting osteitis** (Fig. 26–14). The correlative radiographic finding is a decrease in bone density or osteopenia. Since bone resorption and formation are coupled processes, it is not surprising that osteoblast activity is also increased in hyperparathyroidism. The marrow spaces around the affected surfaces are replaced by fibrovascular tissue.

The bone loss predisposes to microfractures and secondary hemorrhages that elicit an influx of macrophages and an ingrowth of reparative fibrous tissue, creating a mass of reactive tissue, known as a **brown tumor** (Fig. 26–15). The brown color is the result of the vascularity, hemorrhage, and hemosiderin deposition, and it is not uncommon for the lesions to undergo cystic degeneration. The combined picture of increased bone cell activity, peritrabecular fibrosis, and cystic brown tumors is the hallmark of severe hyperparathyroidism and is known as **generalized osteitis fibrosa cystica (von Recklinghausen disease of bone).**

The decrease in bone mass predisposes to fractures, deformities caused by the stress of weight bearing, and joint pain and dysfunction as the lines of normal weight bearing are altered. Control of the hyperparathyroidism allows the bony changes to regress significantly or disappear completely.

Renal Osteodystrophy

The term *renal osteodystrophy* is used to describe collectively all of the skeletal changes of chronic renal disease, including (1) increased osteoclastic bone resorption mimicking osteitis

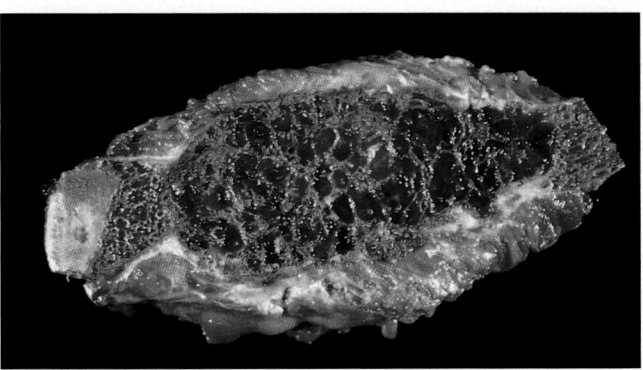

FIGURE 26–15 Resected rib, harboring an expansile brown tumor adjacent to the costal cartilage.

fibrosa cystica, (2) delayed matrix mineralization (osteomalacia), (3) osteosclerosis, (4) growth retardation, and (5) osteoporosis. As advances in medical technology have prolonged the lives of individuals with renal disease, its impact on skeletal homeostasis has assumed greater clinical importance.

The various histologic bone changes in individuals with end-stage renal failure can be divided into three major types of disorders.[27] *High-turnover osteodystrophy* is characterized by increased bone resorption and bone formation, with the former predominating. In contrast, *low-turnover or aplastic disease* is manifested by adynamic bone (little osteoclastic and osteoblastic activity) and, less commonly, osteomalacia. Many affected individuals have the third type, which is a mixed pattern of disease.

Pathogenesis. The pathogenesis of the various skeletal lesions can be summarized as follows:

○ Chronic renal failure results in *phosphate retention* and hyperphosphatemia.
○ Hyperphosphatemia, in turn, induces *secondary hyperparathyroidism*, because phosphate seems to regulate PTH secretion directly.
○ Hypocalcemia develops as the levels of vitamin D (1,25-dihydroxyvitamin D_3; 1,25-$(OH)_2D_3$) fall because of decreased conversion from the vitamin D metabolite 25-$(OH)D_3$ by damaged kidneys; inhibition of the renal hydroxylase involved in the conversion of 25-$(OH)D_3$ to the more active metabolite 1,25-$(OH)_2D_3$ by the high levels of phospate; and reduced intestinal absorption of calcium because of low levels of 1,25-$(OH)_2D_3$.
○ PTH secretion markedly increases at all levels of serum calcium. 1,25-$(OH)_2D_3$ suppresses *PTH* gene expression and secretion; in renal failure there is a decrease in the binding of 1,25-$(OH)_2D_3$ to parathyroid cells; and there is decreased degradation and excretion of PTH because of compromised renal function.
○ The resultant *secondary hyperparathyroidism* produces increased osteoclast activity.
○ *Metabolic acidosis* associated with renal failure stimulates bone resorption and the release of calcium hydroxyapatite from the matrix.
○ Other factors that are important in the genesis of adynamic renal osteodystrophy are diabetes mellitus, high dietary calcium ingestion, increasing age, and iron accumulation in

bone and aluminum deposition at the site of mineralization. *Aluminum deposition*, in particular, has received a great deal of attention in the past because of its iatrogenic origin. The sources of the aluminum include dialysis solutions prepared from water with a high aluminum content and oral aluminum-containing phosphate binders. Aluminum interferes with the deposition of calcium hydroxyapatite and hence results in osteomalacia. Aluminum is not only toxic to bone but also has been implicated as the cause of dialysis encephalopathy and microcytic anemia in individuals with chronic renal failure.

○ A complication that may be seen in association with hemodialysis is the deposition of *amyloid* in bone and periarticular structures. The amyloid is formed from β_2-microglobulin, which is increased in the blood of individuals who undergo long-term hemodialysis (Chapter 6).

Fractures

Traumatic and nontraumatic fractures are some of the most common pathologic conditions affecting bone. Fractures are classified as *complete* or *incomplete*; *closed (simple)* when the overlying tissue is intact; *compound* when the fracture site *communicates* with the skin surface; *comminuted* when the bone is splintered; or *displaced* when the ends of the bone at the fracture site are not aligned. If the break occurs in bone already altered by a disease process, it is described as a *pathologic fracture*. A *stress fracture* is a slowly developing fracture that follows a period of increased physical activity in which the bone is subjected to new repetitive loads—as in sports training or marching in military boot camp.

Bone is unique in its ability to repair itself; it can completely reconstitute itself by reactivating processes that normally occur during embryogenesis. This process involves regulated expression of a multitude of genes and can be separated into overlapping stages with particular molecular, biochemical, histologic, and biomechanical features, described next.

○ Immediately after fracture, rupture of blood vessels results in a hematoma, which fills the fracture gap and surrounds the area of bone injury. The clotted blood provides a fibrin mesh, which helps seal off the fracture site and at the same time creates a framework for the influx of inflammatory cells and ingrowth of fibroblasts and new capillary vessels. Simultaneously, degranulated platelets and migrating inflammatory cells release PDGF, TGF-β, FGF, and interleukins, which activate the osteoprogenitor cells in the periosteum, medullary cavity, and surrounding soft tissues and stimulate osteoclastic and osteoblastic activity.[28] Thus, by the end of the first week the hematoma is organizing, the adjacent tissue is being modulated for future matrix production, and the fractured ends of the bones are being remodeled. This fusiform and predominantly uncalcified tissue—called *soft-tissue callus or procallus*—provides some anchorage between the ends of the fractured bones but offers no structural rigidity for weight bearing.
○ Subsequently, the activated osteoprogenitor cells deposit subperiosteal trabeculae of woven bone that are oriented perpendicular to the cortical axis and within the medullary

cavity. In some cases the activated mesenchymal cells in the soft tissues and bone surrounding the fracture line also differentiate into chondroblasts that make fibrocartilage and hyaline cartilage. In an uncomplicated fracture, the repair tissue reaches its maximal girth at the end of the second or third week, which helps stabilize the fracture site. The newly formed cartilage along the fracture line undergoes enchondral ossification, such as normally occurs at the growth plate, forming a network of bone that connects to the reactive trabeculae deposited elsewhere in the medullary cavity and beneath the periosteum. In this fashion the fractured ends are bridged by a *bony callus*, and as it mineralizes the stiffness and strength of the callus increases to the point that controlled weight bearing can be tolerated (Fig. 26–16).

○ In the early stages of callus formation an excess of fibrous tissue, cartilage, and bone is produced. If the bones are not perfectly aligned, the volume of callus is greatest in the concave portion of the fracture site. As the callus matures and is subjected to weight-bearing forces, the portions that are not physically stressed are resorbed, and in this manner the callus is reduced in size until the shape and outline of the fractured bone have been re-established. The medullary cavity is also restored, and after this has been completed it may be impossible to demonstrate the site of previous injury.

The sequence of events in the healing of a fracture can be easily impeded or even blocked. For example, displaced and comminuted fractures frequently result in some deformity, and inadequate immobilization permits constant movement at the fracture site, so that the normal constituents of callus do not form, resulting in delayed union and nonunion. If a nonunion allows too much motion along the fracture gap, the central portion of the callus undergoes cystic degeneration, and the luminal surface can actually become lined by synovial-like cells, creating a false joint or *pseudoarthrosis*. A serious obstacle to healing is *infection* of the fracture site, which is a risk in comminuted and open fractures. The infection must be eradicated before bony union can be achieved.

Generally, with children and young adults, in whom most uncomplicated fractures are found, near perfect reconstitution is the norm. In older age groups in whom fractures tend to occur on a background of some other disease (e.g., osteoporosis and osteomalacia), repair is more often imperfect and may require mechanical immobilization (e.g., placement of stabilizing pins).

Osteonecrosis (Avascular Necrosis)

Infarction of bone and marrow is a relatively common event that can occur in the medullary cavity of the metaphysis or diaphysis and the subchondral region of the epiphysis. Ischemia underlies all forms of bone necrosis, which can occur in the setting of diverse predisposing conditions (Table 26–5) or as an isolated, idiopathic event. Aside from fracture, most cases of bone necrosis either are idiopathic or follow corticosteroid administration.

Morphology. Medullary infarcts are geographic and involve the cancellous bone and marrow. The cortex is usually not affected because of its collateral blood flow. In subchondral infarcts, a triangular or wedge-shaped segment of tissue that has the subchondral bone plate as its base undergoes necrosis. The overlying articular cartilage remains viable because it

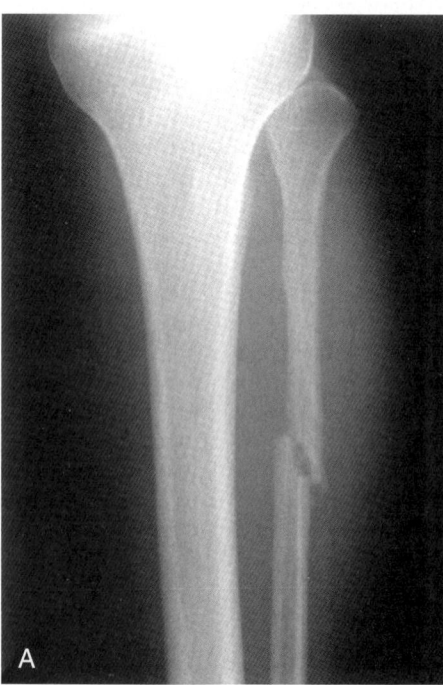
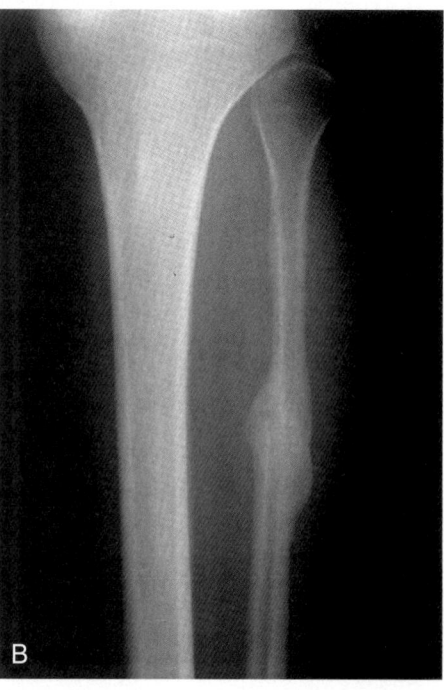

FIGURE 26–16 **A,** Recent fracture of the fibula. **B,** Marked callus formation 6 weeks later. (Courtesy of Dr. Barbara Weissman, Brigham and Women's Hospital, Boston, MA.)

TABLE 26–5 Conditions Associated with Osteonecrosis
Trauma
Corticosteroid administration
Infection
Dysbarism (e.g., the "bends")
Radiation therapy
Connective tissue disorders
Pregnancy
Gaucher disease
Sickle cell and other anemias
Alcohol abuse
Chronic pancreatitis
Tumors
Epiphyseal disorders

receives nutrition from the synovial fluid. The dead bone, recognized by its empty lacunae, is surrounded by necrotic adipocytes that frequently rupture, releasing their fatty acids, which bind calcium and form insoluble calcium soaps that may persist for life. In the healing response, osteoclasts resorb the necrotic trabeculae; however, those that remain act as scaffolding for the deposition of new bone in a process known as **creeping substitution**. In subchondral infarcts the pace of this substitution is too slow to be effective, so there is eventual collapse of the necrotic cancellous bone and distortion, fracture, and even sloughing of the articular cartilage (Fig. 26–17).

Clinical Course. The symptoms depend on the location and extent of infarction. Typically, subchondral infarcts cause chronic pain that is initially associated only with activity but then becomes progressively more constant as secondary changes supervene. In contrast, medullary infarcts are clinically silent except for large ones occurring in Gaucher disease, dysbarism, and sickle cell anemia. Medullary infarcts usually remain stable over time. Subchondral infarcts, however, often collapse and may predispose to severe, secondary osteoarthritis. More than 10% of the 500,000 joint replacements performed annually in the United States are for treatment of the complications of osteonecrosis.

Infections—Osteomyelitis

Osteomyelitis denotes inflammation of bone and marrow, and the common use of the term virtually always implies infection. Osteomyelitis may be a complication of any systemic infection but frequently manifests as a primary solitary focus of disease. All types of organisms, including viruses, parasites, fungi, and bacteria, can produce osteomyelitis, but infections caused by certain pyogenic bacteria and mycobacteria are the most

common. Currently in the United States, exotic infections in third world immigrants and opportunistic infections in immunosuppressed individuals have made the diagnosis and treatment of osteomyelitis quite challenging.

PYOGENIC OSTEOMYELITIS

Pyogenic osteomyelitis is almost always caused by bacteria. Organisms may reach the bone by (1) hematogenous spread, (2) extension from a contiguous site, and (3) direct implantation. In otherwise healthy children, most cases of osteomyelitis are hematogenous in origin and develop in the long bones.[30] The initiating bacteremia may stem from seemingly trivial injuries to the mucosa, such as may occur during defecation or vigorous chewing of hard foods, or minor infections of the skin. In adults, however, osteomyelitis more often occurs as a complication of open fractures, surgical procedures, and diabetic infections of the feet.[31]

Staphylococcus aureus is responsible for 80% to 90% of the cases of pyogenic osteomyelitis in which an organism is recovered. These organisms express receptors for bone matrix components such as collagen, which facilitates their adherence to bone tissue. *Escherichia coli*, *Pseudomonas*, and *Klebsiella* are more frequently isolated from individuals with genitourinary tract infections or who are intravenous drug abusers. Mixed bacterial infections are seen in the setting of direct spread or inoculation of organisms during surgery or open fractures. In the neonatal period, *Haemophilus influenzae* and group B streptococci are frequent pathogens, and individuals with sickle cell disease are predisposed to *Salmonella* infection. In almost 50% of cases, no organisms can be isolated.

The location of the infection within a bone is influenced by the osseous vascular circulation, which varies with age. In the neonate the metaphyseal vessels penetrate the growth plate, resulting in frequent infection of the metaphysis, epiphysis, or both. In children, localization of microorganisms in the metaphysis is typical. After growth plate closure, the metaphyseal vessels reunite with their epiphyseal counterparts and

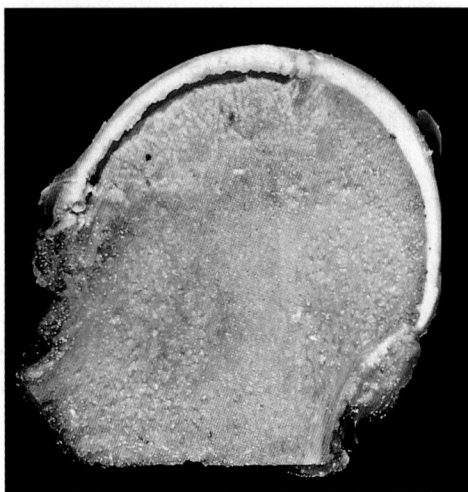

FIGURE 26–17 Femoral head with a subchondral, wedge-shaped pale yellow area of osteonecrosis. The space between the overlying articular cartilage and bone is caused by trabecular compression fractures without repair.

provide a route for the bacteria to seed the epiphyses and subchondral regions in the adult.

> **Morphology.** The morphologic changes of osteomy-elitis depend on the stage (acute, subacute, or chronic) and location of the infection. Once in bone, the bacteria proliferate and induce an acute inflammatory reaction. The entrapped bone undergoes necrosis within the first 48 hours, and the bacteria and inflammation spread within the shaft of the bone and may percolate throughout the haversian systems to reach the periosteum. In children the periosteum is loosely attached to the cortex; sizable **subperiosteal** abscesses may form that can track for long distances along the bone surface. Lifting of the periosteum further impairs the blood supply to the affected region, and both the suppurative and the ischemic injury may cause segmental bone necrosis; the dead piece of bone is known as a **sequestrum**. Rupture of the periosteum leads to a soft-tissue abscess and the eventual formation of a **draining sinus**. Sometimes the sequestrum crumbles and forms free foreign bodies that pass through the sinus tract.
>
> In infants, but uncommonly in adults, epiphyseal infection spreads through the articular surface or along capsular and tendoligamentous insertions into a joint, producing septic or suppurative arthritis, which can cause destruction of the articular cartilage and permanent disability. An analogous process involves the vertebrae, in which the infection destroys the hyaline cartilage end plate and intervertebral disc and spreads into adjacent vertebrae.
>
> After the first week chronic inflammatory cells become more numerous and their release of cytokines stimulates osteoclastic bone resorption, ingrowth of fibrous tissue, and the deposition of reactive bone in the periphery. When the newly deposited bone forms a sleeve of living tissue around the segment of devitalized infected bone, it is known as an **involucrum** (Fig. 26–18). Several morphologic variants of osteomyelitis have eponyms: **Brodie abscess** is a small intraosseous abscess that frequently involves the cortex and is walled off by reactive bone; **sclerosing osteomyelitis of Garré** typically develops in the jaw and is associated with extensive new bone formation that obscures much of the underlying osseous structure.

Clinical Course. Clinically, hematogenous osteomyelitis may manifest as an acute systemic illness with malaise, fever, chills, leukocytosis, and marked-to-intense throbbing pain over the affected region. The presentation may be subtler with only unexplained fever, particularly in infants, or only localized pain in the absence of fever in the adult. The diagnosis can be strongly suggested by the characteristic radiographic findings of a lytic focus of bone destruction surrounded by a zone of sclerosis. In many untreated cases blood cultures are positive, but biopsy and bone cultures are required to identify the pathogen in most instances. The combination of antibiotics and surgical drainage is usually curative. In 5% to 25% of

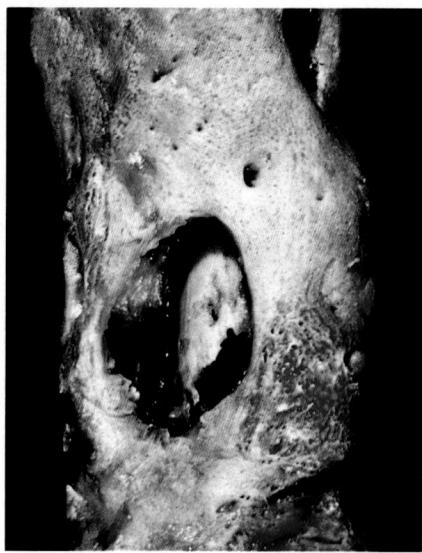

FIGURE 26–18 Resected femur in a person with draining osteomyelitis. The drainage tract in the subperiosteal shell of viable new bone (involucrum) reveals the inner native necrotic cortex (sequestrum).

cases, acute osteomyelitis fails to resolve and persists as chronic infection. Chronicity may develop when there is delay in diagnosis, extensive bone necrosis, inadequate antibiotic therapy or surgical debridement, and weakened host defenses. Acute flare-ups may mark the clinical course of chronic infection and are usually spontaneous, have no obvious cause, and may occur after years of dormancy. Other complications of chronic osteomyelitis include pathologic fracture, secondary amyloidosis, endocarditis, sepsis, development of squamous cell carcinoma in the sinus tract, and rarely sarcoma in the infected bone.

TUBERCULOUS OSTEOMYELITIS

A resurgence of tuberculous osteomyelitis is occurring in developed countries, attributed to the influx of immigrants from countries where tuberculosis is endemic, and the greater numbers of immunosuppressed people (Chapter 8). In developing countries the affected individuals are usually adolescents or young adults, whereas in the indigenous population of the United States they tend to be older, except for those who are immunosuppressed. Approximately 1% to 3% of individuals with pulmonary or extrapulmonary tuberculosis have osseous infection.

The organisms are usually blood borne and originate from a focus of active visceral disease during the initial stages of primary infection. Direct extension (e.g., from a pulmonary focus into a rib or from tracheobronchial nodes into adjacent vertebrae) or spread via draining lymphatics may also occur. The bony infection is usually solitary and in some cases may be the only manifestation of the disease that may fester for years before being recognized. Individuals with acquired immunodeficiency syndrome frequently have multifocal bone involvement.

The spine (40% of cases, especially the thoracic and lumbar vertebrae) followed by the knees and hips are the most common sites of skeletal involvement.[32] Tuberculous osteomyelitis tends to be more destructive and resistant to control than pyogenic osteomyelitis. In the spine *(Pott disease)* the infection breaks through intervertebral discs to involve multiple vertebrae and extends into the soft tissues forming abscesses. The histologic findings are typical of tuberculosis elsewhere (Chapter 8).

Typically, affected individuals present with pain on motion, localized tenderness, low-grade fevers, chills, and weight loss. Severe destruction of vertebrae frequently results in permanent compression fractures that produce severe scoliotic or kyphotic deformities and neurologic deficits secondary to spinal cord and nerve compression. Other complications of tuberculous osteomyelitis include tuberculous arthritis, sinus tract formation, psoas abscess, and amyloidosis.

SKELETAL SYPHILIS

Syphilis *(Treponema pallidum)* and yaws *(Treponema pertenue)* both can involve bone. Currently, syphilis is experiencing a resurgence; however, bone involvement remains infrequent because the disease is usually diagnosed and treated before this complication develops.

In congenital syphilis the bone lesions begin to appear about the fifth month of gestation and are fully developed at birth. The spirochetes tend to localize in areas of active enchondral ossification (osteochondritis) and in the periosteum (periostitis). In acquired syphilis bone disease may begin early in the tertiary stage, which is usually 2 to 5 years after the initial infection. The bones most frequently involved are those of the nose, palate, skull, and extremities, especially the long tubular bones such as the tibia. The syphilitic *saber shin* is produced by massive reactive periosteal bone deposition on the medial and anterior surfaces of the tibia.

> **Morphology.** Syphilitic bone infection is characterized by edematous granulation tissue containing numerous plasma cells and necrotic bone. Typical gummas may also form in both congenital and acquired syphilis (Chapter 8). The spirochetes can be demonstrated in the inflammatory tissue with special silver stains.

Bone Tumors and Tumor-Like Lesions

Bone tumors are diverse in their gross and morphologic features, and vary in their natural history from innocuous to the rapidly fatal. It is critical to diagnose these tumors correctly, stage them accurately, and treat them appropriately, so that affected patients not only survive, but also maintain optimal function of the affected body parts.

Most bone tumors are classified according to the normal cell or tissue type they recapitulate. Lesions that do not have normal tissue counterparts are grouped according to their distinct clinicopathologic features (Table 26–6). Overall, matrix-producing and fibrous tumors are the most common, and among the benign tumors, osteochondroma and fibrous cortical defect are most frequent. Excluding malignant neoplasms of marrow origin (myeloma, lymphoma, and leukemia), osteosarcoma is the most common primary cancer of bone, followed by chondrosarcoma and Ewing sarcoma.

The precise incidence of specific bone tumors is not known, because many benign lesions are not biopsied. Benign tumors greatly outnumber their malignant counterparts and occur with greatest frequency within the first three decades of life, whereas in the elderly a bone tumor is likely to be malignant. In the United States about 2400 new cases of bone sarcoma

TABLE 26–6 Classification of Major Primary Tumors Involving Bones		
Histologic Type	**Benign**	**Malignant**
Hematopoietic (40%)		Myeloma Malignant lymphoma
Chondrogenic (22%)	Osteochondroma Chondroma Chondroblastoma Chondromyxoid fibroma	Chondrosarcoma Dedifferentiated chondrosarcoma Mesenchymal chondrosarcoma
Osteogenic (19%)	Osteoid osteoma Osteoblastoma	Osteosarcoma
Fibrogenic	Fibrous cortical defect (fibroma) Non-ossifying fibroma Fibrous histiocytoma Desmoplastic fibroma	Fibrosarcoma
Unknown origin (10%)	Giant-cell tumor Unicameral cyst Aneurysmal bone cyst	
Neuroectodermal		Ewing sarcoma
Notochordal	Benign notochordal cell tumor	Chordoma

Data on percentage of each type from Unni KK: Dahlin's Bone Tumors, 5th ed. Philadelphia, Lippincott-Raven, 1996, p 4; by permission of Mayo Foundation.

are diagnosed annually, and approximately 1300 deaths from bone sarcoma occur each year.

As a group these neoplasms affect all ages and arise in virtually every bone, but most develop during the first several decades of life and have a propensity to originate in the long bones of the extremities. However, specific types of tumors target certain age groups and anatomic sites. Thus, the location of a tumor provides important diagnostic information.

Although the cause of most bone tumors is unknown, genetic alterations similar to those that occur in other tumors clearly play a role. For instance, bone sarcomas occur in the Li-Fraumeni and hereditary retinoblastoma cancer syndromes, which are linked to mutations in the genes encoding p53 and RB (Chapter 7). Bone infarcts, chronic osteomyelitis, Paget disease, radiation, and metal prostheses are also associated with a bone neoplasia. Such secondary neoplasms, however, account for only a small fraction of skeletal tumors.

Clinically, bone tumors present in various ways. The more common benign lesions are frequently asymptomatic and are detected as incidental findings. Many tumors, however, produce pain or are noticed as a slow-growing mass. In some circumstances the first hint of a tumor's presence is a sudden pathologic fracture. Radiologic imaging studies have an important role in diagnosing these lesions. In addition to providing the exact location and extent of the tumor, imaging studies can detect features that help limit diagnostic possibilities and give clues to the aggressiveness of the tumor. Ultimately, in most instances, biopsy and histologic study are necessary.

BONE-FORMING TUMORS

Common to all these neoplasms is the production of bone by the neoplastic cells. The tumor bone is usually deposited as woven trabeculae (except in osteomas) and is variably mineralized.

Osteoma

Osteomas are bosselated, round-to-oval sessile tumors that project from the subperiosteal surface of the cortex. They most often arise on or inside the skull and facial bones. They are usually solitary and are detected in middle age. Multiple osteomas are seen in the setting of *Gardner syndrome* (Chapter 17). They consist of a composite of woven and lamellar bone that is frequently deposited in a cortical pattern with haversian-like systems. Some variants contain a component of trabecular bone in which the intertrabecular spaces are filled with hematopoietic marrow.

Osteomas are generally slow-growing tumors of little clinical significance except when they cause obstruction of a sinus cavity, impinge on the brain or eye, interfere with function of the oral cavity, or produce cosmetic problems.

Osteoid Osteoma and Osteoblastoma

Osteoid osteoma and *osteoblastoma* are terms used to describe benign bone tumors that have identical histologic features but differ in size, sites of origin, and symptoms. *Osteoid osteomas* are by definition less than 2 cm in greatest dimension and usually occur in the teens and 20s. Seventy-five percent of

affected individuals are younger than 25 years old, and men outnumber women 2:1. They can arise in any bone but have a predilection for the appendicular skeleton and posterior elements of the spine. In 50% of cases the femur or tibia is involved, wherein they commonly arise in the cortex and less frequently within the medullary cavity. Osteoid osteomas produce severe nocturnal pain that is relieved by aspirin.[33] The pain is probably caused by excess prostaglandin E_2 (PGE_2) production by the proliferating osteoblasts. *Osteoblastoma* is larger than 2 cm and involves the spine more frequently; the pain is dull, achy, and unresponsive to salicylates, and the tumor usually does not induce a marked bony reaction.

Morphology. Osteoid osteoma and osteoblastoma are round-to-oval masses of hemorrhagic gritty tan tissue. They are well circumscribed and composed of randomly interconnecting trabeculae of woven bone that are prominently rimmed by osteoblasts (Fig. 26–19). The stroma surrounding the neoplastic bone consists of loose connective tissue that contains many dilated and congested capillaries. The relatively small size, well-defined margins, and benign cytologic features of the neoplastic osteoblasts help distinguish these tumors from osteosarcoma. Osteoid osteomas, especially those that arise beneath the periosteum, usually elicit a tremendous amount of reactive bone formation that encircles the lesion. The actual tumor, known as the **nidus**, manifests radiographically as a small round lucency that may be centrally mineralized (Fig. 26–20).

Osteoid osteoma is frequently treated by radioablation. Osteoblastoma is usually curetted or excised en bloc in a conservative fashion. The possibility of malignant transformation is remote except when osteoblastoma is treated with radiation (large tumors in the base of the skull and spine), which may promote this dreaded complication.

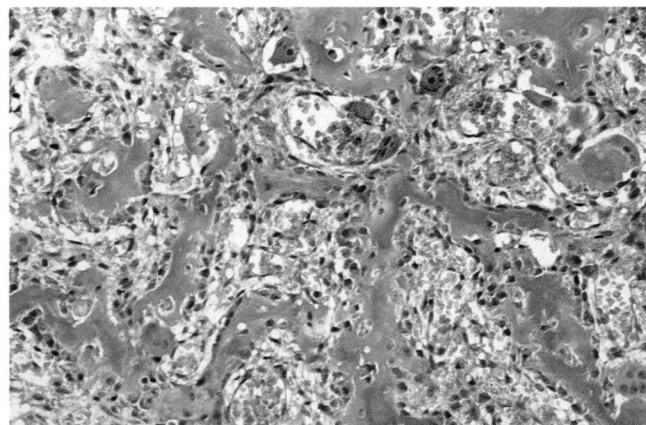

FIGURE 26–19 Osteoid osteoma composed of haphazardly interconnecting trabeculae of woven bone that are rimmed by prominent osteoblasts. The intertrabecular spaces are filled by vascularized loose connective tissue.

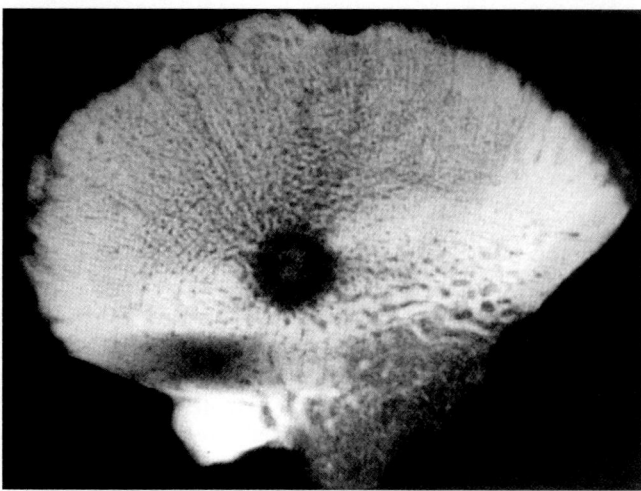

FIGURE 26–20 Specimen radiogram of intracortical osteoid osteoma. The round radiolucency with central mineralization represents the lesion and is surrounded by abundant reactive bone that has massively thickened the cortex.

Osteosarcoma

Osteosarcoma is a malignant mesenchymal tumor in which the cancerous cells produce bone matrix. It is the most common primary malignant tumor of bone, exclusive of myeloma and lymphoma, and accounts for approximately 20% of primary bone cancers. Osteosarcoma occurs in all age groups but has a bimodal age distribution; 75% occur in persons younger than 20 years of age.[34] The smaller second peak occurs in the elderly, who frequently suffer from conditions known to predispose to osteosarcoma—Paget disease, bone infarcts, and prior irradiation. Overall, men are more commonly affected than women (1.6 : 1). The tumors usually arise in the metaphyseal region of the long bones of the extremities, and almost 50% occur about the knee (Fig. 26–21). Any bone can be involved, however, and in persons beyond the age of 25, the incidence in flat bones and long bones is almost equal.

Pathogenesis. Approximately 70% of osteosarcomas have acquired genetic abnormalities such as ploidy changes and chromosomal aberrations, none of which are specific to this tumor. More telling is the presence of very frequent mutations that interfere with function of two genes: (1) *RB*, the retinoblastoma gene, a critical cell cycle regulator; and (2) *p53*, a gene whose product regulates DNA repair and certain aspects of cellular metabolism (Chapter 7). Although the basic mechanisms that cause the development of osteosarcoma are still unknown, it is clear that defects in RB and p53 play important roles in the process. This association is emphasized by rare patients with germline mutations in *RB*, who have a roughly 1000-fold increased risk of osteosarcoma; and similarly by patients with Li-Fraumeni syndrome (germline p53 mutations), who also have a greatly elevated incidence of this tumor. Abnormalities in *INK*4a, which encodes p16 (a cell cycle regulator) and p14 (which aids and abets p53 function), also are seen in osteosarcoma. It is also noteworthy that osteosarcomas tend to occur at sites of bone growth, presumably because proliferation makes osteoblastic cells prone to acquire mutations that could lead to transformation. The association may

contribute to the high incidence of osteosarcoma in large dog breeds, such as St. Bernards and Great Danes.

Morphology. Several subtypes of osteosarcoma are recognized and are grouped according to

- Site of origin (intramedullary, intracortical, or surface)
- Degree of differentiation
- Multicentricity (synchronous, metachronous)
- Primary (underlying bone is unremarkable) or secondary to preexisting disorders such as benign tumors, Paget disease, bone infarcts, previous irradiation
- Histologic features (osteoblastic, chondroblastic, fibroblastic, telangiectatic, small cell, and giant cell).

The most common subtype arises in the metaphysis of long bones and is primary, solitary, intramedullary, and poorly differentiated.

Grossly, osteosarcomas are big bulky tumors that are gritty, gray-white, and often contain areas of hemorrhage and cystic degeneration (Fig. 26–22). The

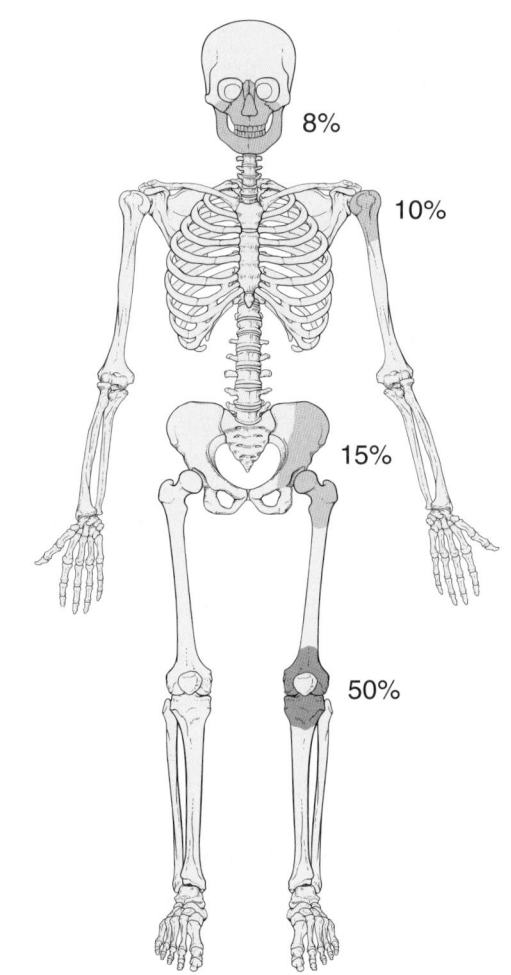

FIGURE 26–21 Major sites of origin of osteosarcomas. The numbers are approximate percentages arising at each site.

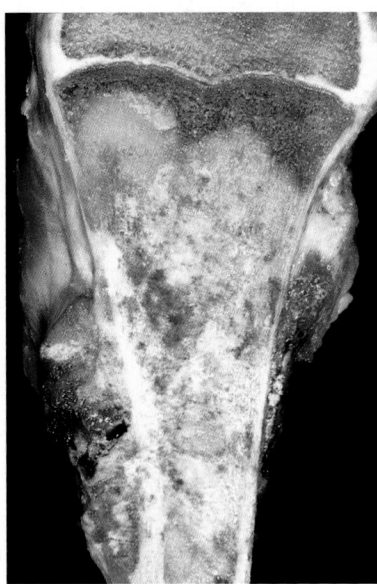

FIGURE 26–22 Osteosarcoma of the upper end of the tibia. The tan-white tumor fills most of the medullary cavity of the metaphysis and proximal diaphysis. It has infiltrated through the cortex, lifted the periosteum, and formed soft-tissue masses on both sides of the bone.

a coarse, lace-like architecture but also may be deposited in broad sheets or as primitive trabeculae. Other matrices, including cartilage or fibrous tissue, may be present in varying amounts. When malignant cartilage is abundant, the tumor is called **chondroblastic osteosarcoma**. Vascular invasion is usually conspicuous, and up to 50% to 60% of an individual tumor may be necrotic.

Clinical Course. Osteosarcomas typically present as painful, progressively enlarging masses. Sometimes a sudden fracture of the bone is the first symptom. Radiograms of the primary tumor usually show a large destructive, mixed lytic and blastic mass with infiltrative margins (Fig. 26–24). The tumor frequently breaks through the cortex and lifts the periosteum, resulting in reactive periosteal bone formation. The triangular shadow between the cortex and raised ends of periosteum is known radiographically as *Codman triangle* and is characteristic but not diagnostic of this tumor. These aggressive neoplasms spread hematogenously, and at the time of diagnosis approximately 10% to 20% of affected individuals have demonstrable pulmonary metastases, and it is likely that many more have occult metastases. In those who die of the neoplasm, 90% have metastases to the lungs, bones, brain, and elsewhere.

tumors frequently destroy the surrounding cortices and produce soft-tissue masses. They spread extensively in the medullary canal, infiltrating and replacing the marrow surrounding the preexisting bone trabeculae. Infrequently, they penetrate the epiphyseal plate or enter the joint. When joint invasion occurs, the tumor grows into it along tendoligamentous structures or through the attachment site of the joint capsule. The tumor cells vary in size and shape and frequently have large hyperchromatic nuclei. Bizarre tumor giant cells are common, as are mitoses. **The formation of bone by the tumor cells is characteristic** (Fig. 26–23). The neoplastic bone usually has

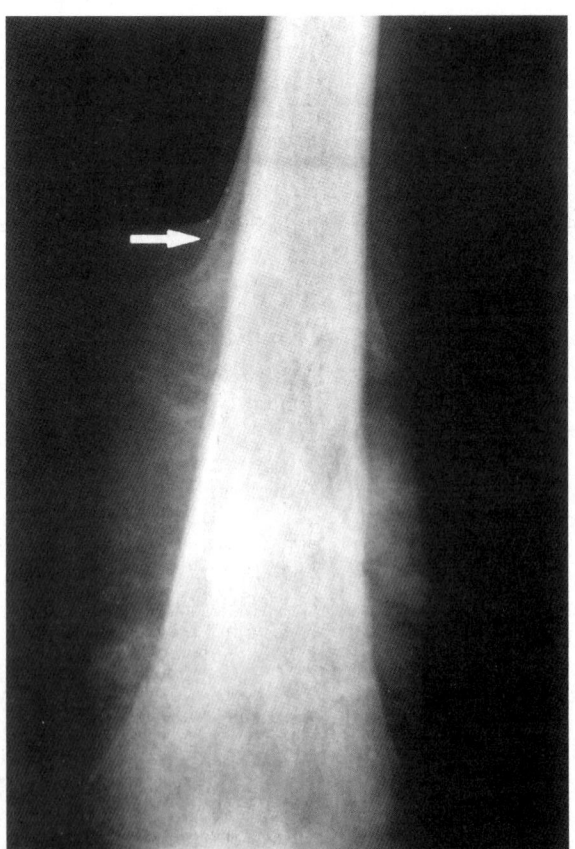

FIGURE 26–24 Distal femoral osteosarcoma with prominent bone formation extending into the soft tissues. The periosteum, which has been lifted, has laid down a proximal triangular shell of reactive bone known as a Codman triangle *(arrow)*.

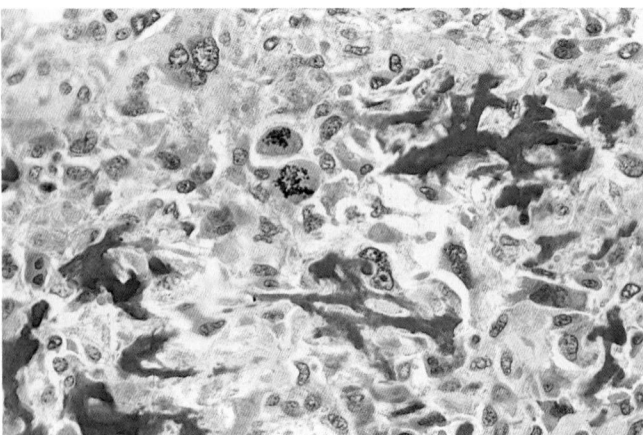

FIGURE 26–23 Coarse, lacelike pattern of neoplastic bone produced by anaplastic malignant tumor cells. Note the mitotic figures.

Osteosarcoma is treated with a multimodality approach that includes chemotherapy, which is given under the assumption that all patients at the time of diagnosis have metastases, which are usually too small to detect by imaging. The prognosis of patients without detectable metastases has improved substantially, with 5-year survival rates reaching 60% to 70% with aggressive chemotherapy and limb salvaging surgery. Unfortunately, the outcome for patients with overt metastases or recurrent disease is still poor (approximately 20% 5-year survival rate).

CARTILAGE-FORMING TUMORS

Cartilage tumors account for the majority of primary bone tumors and are characterized by the formation of hyaline or myxoid cartilage; fibrocartilage and elastic cartilage are rare components. As in most types of bone tumors, benign cartilage tumors are much more common than malignant ones.

Osteochondroma

Osteochondroma, also known as an *exostosis*, is a benign cartilage-capped tumor that is attached to the underlying skeleton by a bony stalk. It is the most common benign bone tumor; about 85% are solitary. The remainder are seen as part of the *multiple hereditary exostosis syndrome*, which is an autosomal dominant hereditary disease. Hereditary exostoses are caused by germline loss-of-function mutations in either the *EXT1* or *EXT2* genes, whereas inactivation of only *EXT1* has been detected in sporadic tumors. These genes encode proteins that function in the biosynthesis of heparin sulfate proteoglycans (Chapter 3). Reduced expression of *EXT1* and *EXT2* results in defective endochondral ossification, which somehow sets the stage for abnormal growth. Solitary osteochondromas are usually first diagnosed in late adolescence and early adulthood, but multiple osteochondromas become apparent during childhood. Men are affected three times more often than women. Osteochondromas develop only in bones of endochondral origin and arise from the metaphysis near the growth plate of long tubular bones, especially about the knee. Occasionally, they develop from bones of the pelvis, scapula, and ribs, and in these sites they are frequently sessile and have short stalks. Rarely, they involve the short tubular bones of the hands and feet.

Morphology. Osteochondromas are sessile or mushroom shaped, and range in size from 1 to 20 cm. The cap is composed of benign hyaline cartilage varying in thickness (Fig. 26–25) and is covered peripherally by perichondrium. The cartilage has the appearance of disorganized growth plate and undergoes enchondral ossification, with the newly made bone forming the inner portion of the head and stalk. The cortex of the stalk merges with the cortex of the host bone, so that the medullary cavity of the osteochondroma and bone are in continuity.

Clinically, osteochondromas present as slow-growing masses, which can be painful if they impinge on a nerve or if the stalk is fractured. In many cases they are detected as an incidental finding. In multiple hereditary exostosis the underlying bones may be bowed and shortened, reflecting an associated disturbance in epiphyseal growth. Osteochondromas usually stop growing at the time of growth plate closure. Rarely in sporadic cases, but more commonly in those with multiple hereditary exostosis, they give rise to a chondrosarcoma or some other type of sarcoma.

Chondromas

Chondromas are benign tumors of hyaline cartilage that usually occur in bones of enchondral origin. They can arise within the medullary cavity, where they are known as *enchondromas*, or on the surface of bone, where they are called *subperiosteal* or *juxtacortical chondromas*. Enchondromas are the most common of the intraosseous cartilage tumors and are usually diagnosed in individuals who are in their 20s to 40s. They are usually solitary metaphyseal lesions of tubular bones; the favored sites are the short tubular bones of the hands and feet. A syndrome of multiple enchondromas or enchondromatosis is known as *Ollier disease*. If the enchondromatosis is associated with soft-tissue hemangiomas, the disorder is called *Maffucci syndrome*.

Morphology. Enchondromas are usually smaller than 3 cm and grossly are gray-blue and translucent. They are composed of well-circumscribed nodules of cyto-

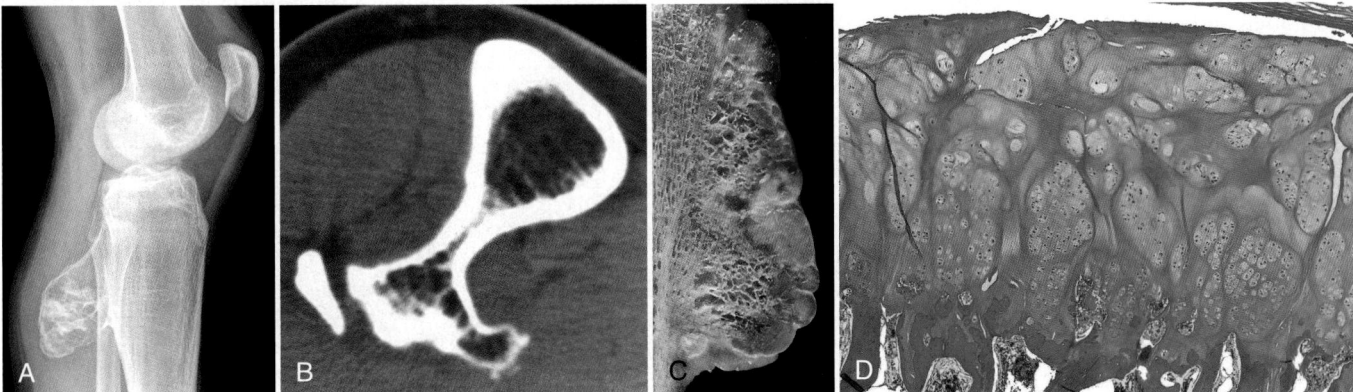

FIGURE 26–25 Osteochondroma. **A,** X-ray of an osteochondroma arising off the posterior surface of the tibia. **B,** Axial CT scan shows continuity of the cortex of the bone and the center of the osteochondroma. The fibula is adjacent to the mass. **C,** Gross specimen of sessile osteochondroma composed of a cap of hyaline cartilage undergoing enchondral ossification. **D,** The cartilage cap has the histologic appearance of disorganized growth plate-like cartilage.

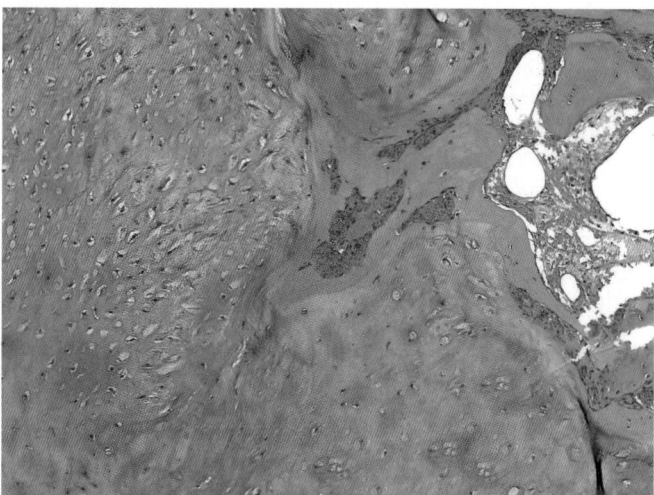

FIGURE 26–26   Enchondroma with a nodule of hyaline cartilage encased by a thin layer of reactive bone.

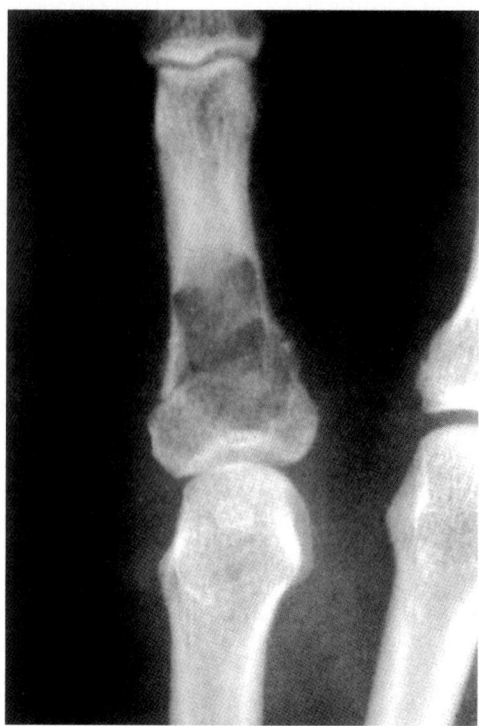

FIGURE 26–27   Enchondroma of the phalanx with a pathologic fracture. The radiolucent nodules of hyaline cartilage scallop the endosteal surface.

logically benign hyaline cartilage (Fig. 26–26). The peripheral portion of the nodules may undergo enchondral ossification, and the center can calcify and die. The chondromas in Ollier disease and Maffucci syndrome are sometimes more cellular and exhibit cytologic atypia, making it difficult to distinguish them from chondrosarcoma.

Clinical Features. Most enchondromas are asymptomatic and are detected incidentally. Occasionally they are painful and cause pathologic fracture. The tumors in enchondromatosis may be numerous and large, producing severe deformities. The radiographic features are characteristic; the unmineralized nodules of cartilage produce well-circumscribed oval lucencies that are surrounded by a thin rim of radiodense bone (*C or O ring sign*). If the matrix calcifies it is detected as irregular opacities. The nodules scallop the endosteum, but usually leave the cortex intact (Fig. 26–27). The growth potential of chondromas is limited, and most remain stable. Treatment depends on the clinical situation and is usually observation or curettage. Solitary chondromas rarely undergo sarcomatous transformation, but those associated with enchondromatoses do so more frequently. Individuals with Maffucci syndrome are also at risk of developing other types of malignancies, including ovarian carcinomas and brain gliomas.

Chondroblastoma

Chondroblastoma is a rare benign tumor that accounts for less than 1% of primary bone tumors. It usually occurs in young patients in their teens and has a male-to-female ratio of 2 : 1. Most arise about the knee; less common sites such as the pelvis and ribs are affected in older patients. Chondroblastoma has a striking predilection for epiphyses and apophyses (epiphyseal equivalents, i.e., iliac crest).[36]

Morphology. The tumor is composed of sheets of compact polyhedral chondroblasts that have well-defined cytoplasmic borders, moderate amounts of pink cytoplasm, and nuclei that are hyperlobulated

with longitudinal grooves (Fig. 26–28). Mitotic activity and necrosis are frequently present. The tumor cells are surrounded by scant amounts of hyaline matrix that is deposited in a lace-like configuration; nodules of well-formed hyaline cartilage are distinctly uncommon. When the matrix calcifies it produces a characteristic chicken-wire pattern of mineralization (see Fig. 26–28). Scattered through the lesion are non-neoplastic osteoclast-type giant cells. Occasionally the tumors undergo prominent hemorrhagic cystic degeneration.

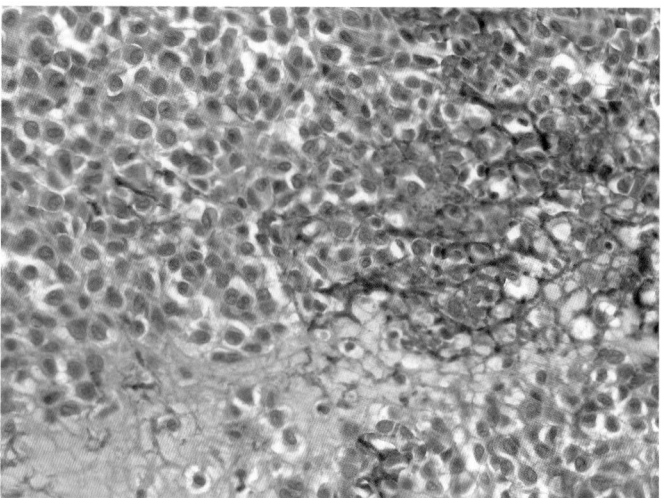

FIGURE 26–28   Chondroblastoma with scant mineralized matrix surrounding chondroblasts in a chicken wire–like fashion.

Chondroblastomas are usually painful, and because of their location near a joint they also cause effusions and restrict joint mobility. Radiographically, they produce a well-defined geographic lucency that commonly has spotty calcifications. Recurrences are not uncommon after curettage. Pulmonary metastases occur rarely in lesions that have undergone prior pathologic fracture or repeated curettage. Apparently in these circumstances the tumor cells are pushed into ruptured vessels, giving them access to the systemic circulation.

Chondromyxoid Fibroma

Chondromyxoid fibroma is the rarest of cartilage tumors and because of its varied morphology can be mistaken for sarcoma. It affects individuals in their teens and 20s and has a male preponderance. The tumors most frequently arise in the metaphysis of long tubular bones, but can involve virtually any bone of the body.

> **Morphology.** The tumors range from 3 to 8 cm in greatest dimension and are well-circumscribed, solid, and glistening tan-gray. Microscopically, there are nodules of poorly formed hyaline cartilage and myxoid tissue delineated by fibrous septae. The cellularity varies; the areas of greatest cellularity are at the periphery of the nodules. In the cartilaginous regions the tumor cells are situated in lacunae; however, in the myxoid areas, the cells are stellate, and their delicate cell processes extend through the mucinous ground substance and approach or contact neighboring cells (Fig. 26–29). In contrast to other benign cartilage tumors, the neoplastic cells in chondromyxoid fibroma show varying degrees of cytologic atypia, including the presence of large hyperchromatic nuclei. Other findings include small foci of calcification of the cartilaginous matrix and scattered non-neoplastic, osteoclast-type giant cells.

Individuals with chondromyxoid fibroma usually complain of localized dull, achy pain. In most instances, radiograms

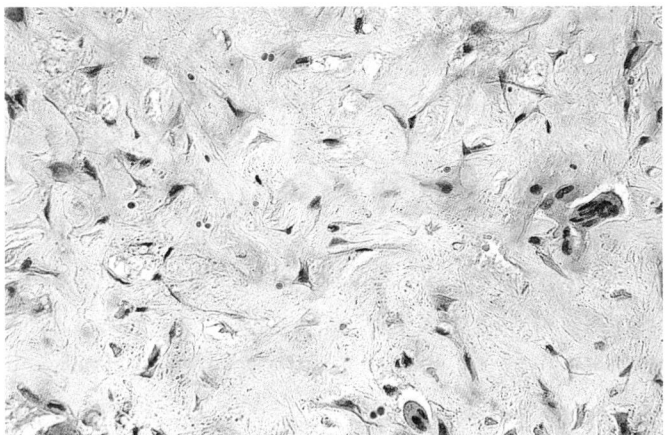

FIGURE 26–29 Chondromyxoid fibroma with prominent stellate and spindle cells surrounded by myxoid matrix. Occasional osteoclast-type giant cells are also present.

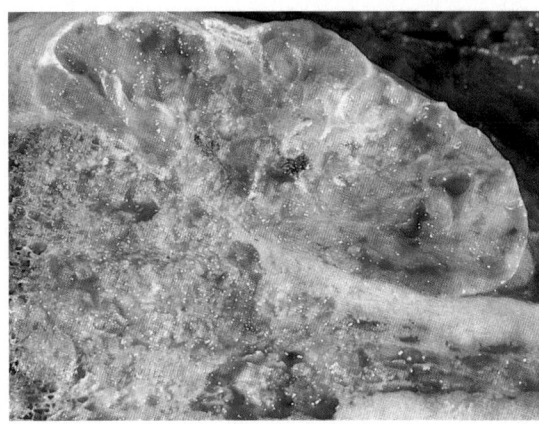

FIGURE 26–30 Chondrosarcoma with lobules of hyaline and myxoid cartilage permeating throughout the medullary cavity, growing through the cortex, and forming a relatively well-circumscribed soft-tissue mass.

demonstrate an eccentric geographic lucency that is well delineated from the adjacent bone by a rim of sclerosis. Occasionally the tumor expands the overlying cortex. The treatment of choice is simple curettage, and even though they may recur, they do not pose a threat for malignant transformation or metastasis.

Chondrosarcoma

Chondrosarcomas are a group of tumors that span a broad spectrum of clinical and pathologic findings. The feature common to all of them is the production of neoplastic cartilage. Chondrosarcoma is subclassified according to site as central (*intramedullary*) and peripheral (*juxtacortical* and *surface*). Histologically, they include *conventional (hyaline and/or myxoid), clear cell, dedifferentiated,* and *mesenchymal* variants. Conventional central tumors constitute about 90% of chondrosarcomas.

Chondrosarcoma of the skeleton is about half as frequent as osteosarcoma and is the second most common malignant matrix-producing tumor of bone. Individuals with chondrosarcoma are usually in their 40s or older. The clear cell and especially the mesenchymal variants occur in younger patients, in their teens or 20s. The tumor affects men twice as frequently as women. About 15% of conventional chondrosarcomas (usually peripheral tumors) arise from a preexisting enchondroma or osteochondroma.

> **Morphology.** Conventional chondrosarcoma is composed of malignant hyaline and myxoid cartilage. The large bulky tumors are made up of nodules of gray-white, somewhat translucent glistening tissue (Fig. 26–30). In predominantly myxoid variants, the tumors are viscous and gelatinous and the matrix oozes from the cut surface. Spotty calcifications are typically present, and central necrosis may create cystic spaces. The adjacent cortex is thickened or eroded, and the tumor grows with broad pushing fronts into the surrounding soft tissue. The malignant cartilage infiltrates the marrow space and surrounds pre-existing bony trabeculae. The tumors vary in degree of

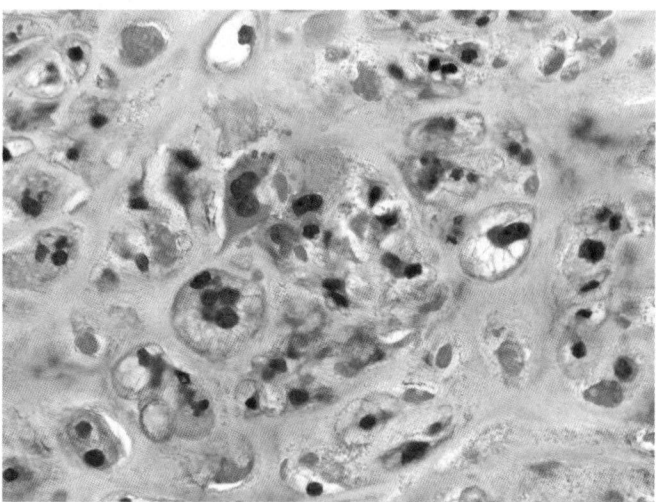

FIGURE 26–31 Anaplastic chondrocytes within a chondrosarcoma.

cellularity, cytologic atypia, and mitotic activity (Fig. 26–31). Low-grade or grade 1 lesions demonstrate mild hypercellularity, and the chondrocytes have plump vesicular nuclei with small nucleoli. Binucleate cells are sparse, and mitotic figures are difficult to find. Portions of the matrix frequently mineralize, and the cartilage may undergo endochondral ossification. By contrast, grade 3 chondrosarcomas are characterized by marked hypercellularity, extreme pleomorphism with bizarre tumor giant cells, and mitoses. Pure grade 3 chondrosarcomas are uncommon. Such malignant cartilage is more frequently a component of **chondroblastic osteosarcoma** (see earlier).

Approximately 10% of conventional low-grade chondrosarcomas have a second high-grade component that has the morphology of a poorly differentiated sarcoma; this combination defines **dedifferentiated chondrosarcomas**. The hallmark of **clear cell chondrosarcoma** is sheets of large malignant chondrocytes that have abundant clear cytoplasm, numerous osteoclast-type giant cells, and intralesional reactive bone formation, which often causes confusion with osteosarcoma. **Mesenchymal chondrosarcoma** is composed of islands of well-differentiated hyaline cartilage surrounded by sheets of small round cells, which can mimic Ewing sarcoma.

Chondrosarcomas commonly arise in the central portions of the skeleton, including the pelvis, shoulder, and ribs. The clear cell variant is unique in that it originates in the epiphyses of long tubular bones. *In contrast to enchondroma, chondrosarcoma rarely involves the distal extremities.* These tumors usually present as painful, progressively enlarging masses. The nodular growth pattern of the cartilage produces prominent endosteal scalloping radiographically. The calcified matrix appears as foci of flocculent densities. A slow-growing, low-grade tumor causes reactive thickening of the cortex, whereas a more aggressive high-grade neoplasm destroys the cortex and forms a soft-tissue mass. There is a direct correlation between the

grade and the biologic behavior of the tumor.[37] Fortunately, most conventional chondrosarcomas are indolent and fall into the range of grade 1 and grade 2. In one analysis, the 5-year survival rates were 90%, 81%, and 43% for grades 1 through 3, respectively. None of the grade 1 tumors metastasized, whereas 70% of the grade 3 tumors disseminated. Another prognostic feature is size; tumors greater than 10 cm are more aggressive than smaller tumors. When chondrosarcomas metastasize, they spread preferentially to the lungs and skeleton. The treatment of conventional chondrosarcoma is wide surgical excision. The mesenchymal and dedifferentiated tumors are also treated with chemotherapy, because of their aggressive clinical course.

FIBROUS AND FIBRO-OSSEOUS TUMORS

Tumors composed solely or predominantly of fibrous elements are diverse and include some of the most common lesions of the skeleton.

Fibrous Cortical Defect and Non-Ossifying Fibroma

Fibrous cortical defects are extremely common, being found in 30% to 50% of children older than 2 years. They are believed to be developmental defects rather than neoplasms. The vast majority arise eccentrically in the metaphysis of the distal femur and proximal tibia, and almost half are bilateral or multiple. Often they are small, about 0.5 cm in diameter. Those that grow to 5 or 6 cm in size develop into *non-ossifying fibromas*, which are usually not detected until adolescence.

Morphology. Both fibrous cortical defects and non-ossifying fibromas produce elongated, sharply demarcated radiolucencies that are surrounded by a thin rim of sclerosis (Fig. 26–32). They consist of gray to yellow-brown cellular lesions containing fibroblasts and macrophages (histiocytes). The cytologically bland fibroblasts are frequently arranged in a storiform (pinwheel) pattern, and the histiocytes are either multinucleated giant cells or clusters of foamy macrophages (Fig. 26–33).

Fibrous cortical defects are asymptomatic and are usually detected on radiography as an incidental finding. Most have limited growth potential and undergo spontaneous resolution within several years, being replaced by normal cortical bone. The few that progressively enlarge into non-ossifying fibromas may present with pathologic fracture or require biopsy and curettage to exclude other types of tumors.

Fibrous Dysplasia

Fibrous dysplasia is a benign tumor that has been likened to a localized developmental arrest; all of the components of normal bone are present, but they do not differentiate into their mature structures. The lesions arise during skeletal growth and development, and appear in three distinctive but sometimes overlapping clinical patterns: (1) involvement of a single bone (monostotic); (2) involvement of multiple bones

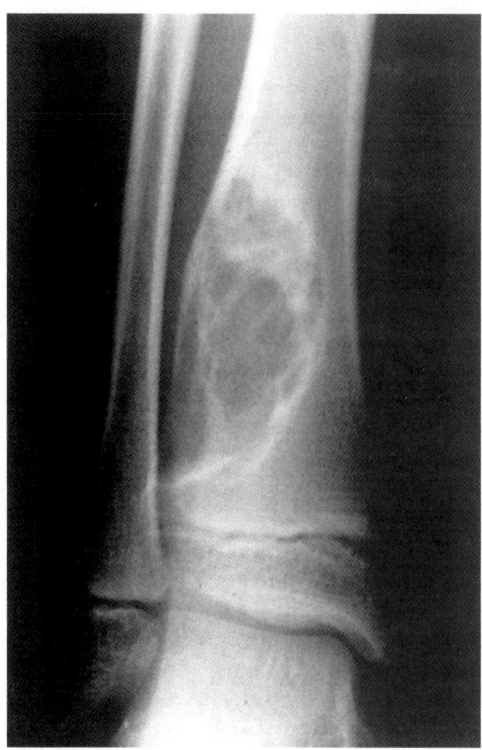

FIGURE 26–32 Non-ossifying fibroma of the distal tibial metaphysis producing an eccentric lobulated radiolucency surrounded by a sclerotic margin.

(polyostotic); and (3) polyostotic disease, associated with café-au-lait skin pigmentations and endocrine abnormalities, especially precocious puberty. The skeletal, skin, and endocrine lesions result from a somatic gain-of-function mutation occurring during embryogenesis in the *GNAS* gene, which you will recall is also mutated in pituitary adenomas (Chapter 24). The result of the mutations in both types of tumors is the same—the production of a hyperactive guanyl nucleotide binding protein, encoded by the *GNAS* gene, that drives abnormal growth.[38]

Monostotic fibrous dysplasia accounts for 70% of all cases. It occurs equally in boys and girls, usually in early adolescence, and often stops enlarging at the time of growth plate closure. The femur, tibia, ribs, jawbones, calvaria, and humerus are most commonly affected. The lesion is frequently asymptomatic and usually discovered incidentally but it may cause pain, fracture, and discrepancies in limb length. Fibrous dysplasia can cause marked enlargement and distortion of bone, so that if the craniofacial skeleton is involved, disfigurement, sometimes severe, can occur. Monostotic disease does not evolve into the polyostotic form.

Polyostotic fibrous dysplasia without endocrine dysfunction accounts for 27% of all cases. It manifests at a slightly earlier age than the monostotic type and may continue to cause problems into adulthood. The bones affected, in descending order of frequency, are the femur, skull, tibia, humerus, ribs, fibula, radius, ulna, mandible, and vertebrae. Craniofacial involvement is present in 50% of those who have a moderate number of bones affected and in 100% of those with extensive skeletal disease. Polyostotic disease has a propensity to involve the shoulder and pelvic girdles, resulting in severe, sometimes

crippling deformities (e.g., shepherd-crook deformity of the proximal femur) and spontaneous and often recurrent fractures.

Polyostotic fibrous dysplasia associated with café-au-lait skin pigmentation and endocrinopathies is known as the *McCune-Albright syndrome* and accounts for 3% of all cases. The endocrinopathies include sexual precocity, hyperthyroidism, pituitary adenomas that secrete growth hormone, and primary adrenal hyperplasia. The severity of manifestations in McCune-Albright syndrome depends on the number and cell types that harbor the mutation in the *GNAS* gene. The most common clinical presentation is precocious sexual development, which occurs most often in girls. The bone lesions are often unilateral but can be bilateral, and the skin pigmentation is usually limited to the same side of the body. The cutaneous macules are classically large; are dark to café-au-lait; have irregular serpiginous borders (coastline of Maine); and are found primarily on the neck, chest, back, shoulder, and pelvic region.

Morphology. The lesions of fibrous dysplasia are well circumscribed, intramedullary, and vary greatly in size. Larger lesions expand and distort the bone. The lesional tissue is tan-white and gritty and is composed of curvilinear trabeculae of woven bone surrounded by a moderately cellular fibroblastic proliferation. The shapes of the trabeculae mimic Chinese letters, and the bone lacks prominent osteoblastic rimming (Fig. 26–34). Nodules of hyaline cartilage with the appearance of disorganized growth plate are also present in approximately 20% of cases. Cystic degeneration, hemorrhage, and foamy macrophages are other common findings.

Clinical Course. The natural history of fibrous dysplasia is variable and depends on the extent of skeletal involvement. Individuals with monostotic disease usually have minimal symptoms, except if the tumor is strategically located, such as in the femoral neck. The lesion is readily diagnosed by radiology because of its typical ground-glass appearance and

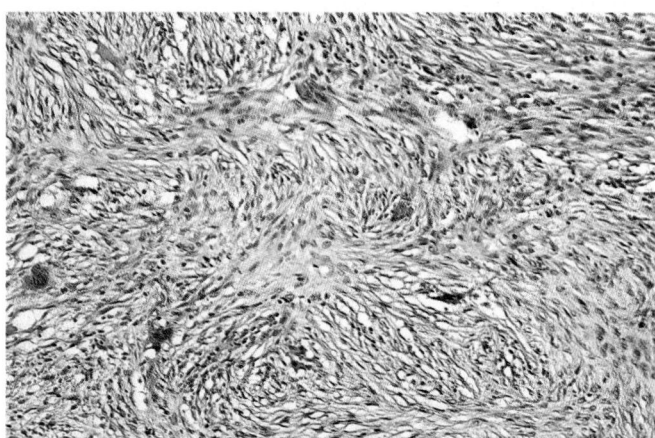

FIGURE 26–33 Storiform pattern created by benign spindle cells with scattered osteoclast-type giant cells characteristic of a fibrous cortical defect and non-ossifying fibroma.

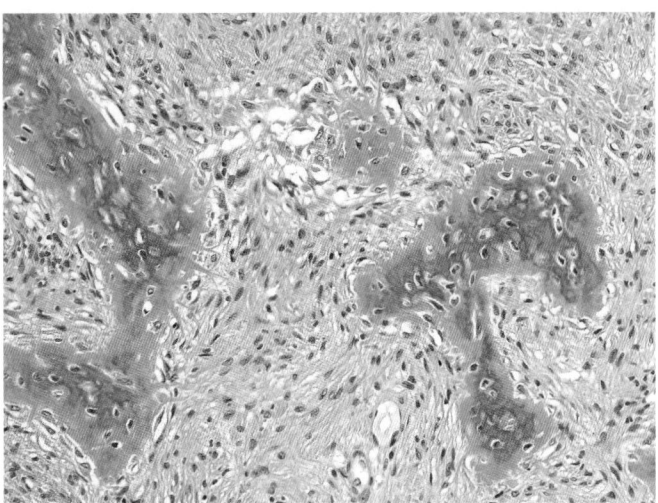

FIGURE 26–34 Fibrous dysplasia composed of curvilinear trabeculae of woven bone that lack conspicuous osteoblastic rimming and arise in a background of fibrous tissue.

well-defined margination. Lesions that fracture or cause significant symptoms are cured by conservative surgery. Polyostotic involvement is frequently associated with progressive disease. Those diagnosed at an earlier age are more likely to have severe skeletal complications, such as recurring fractures, long-bone deformities and persistent pain, and involvement and distortion of the craniofacial bones. These patients may require multiple corrective orthopedic surgical procedures. Bisphosphonates can be used to reduce the severity of the bone pain. A rare complication, usually in the setting of polyostotic involvement, is malignant transformation of a lesion into a sarcoma.

Fibrosarcoma Variants

Collagen-producing sarcomas with a fibroblastic phenotype occur at any age, but most affect the middle-aged and elderly. They have a nearly equal sex distribution and usually arise de novo; however, a few develop in preexisting benign tumors, bone infarcts, pagetic bone, and previously irradiated tissue.

> **Morphology.** Grossly these tumors are large, hemorrhagic, tan-white masses that destroy the underlying bone and frequently extend into the soft tissues. They are composed of cytologically malignant fibroblasts arranged in a herringbone storiform pattern. The level of differentiation determines the amount of collagen produced and degree of cytologic atypia. In the past, some of these tumors were called **malignant fibrous histiocytoma** because the pleomorphic cells resembled histiocytes (activated tissue macrophages).

Fibrosarcoma presents as an enlarging painful mass that usually arises in the metaphysis of long bones and pelvic flat bones. Pathologic fracture is a frequent complication. Radiographically it is permeative and lytic and often extends into the adjacent soft tissue. The prognosis depends on the size, location, stage, and grade of the tumor; large, high-grade tumors that are difficult to resect have a very poor prognosis.

Miscellaneous Tumors

EWING SARCOMA/PRIMITIVE NEUROECTODERMAL TUMOR

The Ewing sarcoma family of tumors encompasses Ewing sarcoma and primitive neuroectodermal tumor (PNET), which are primary malignant *small round-cell tumors* of bone and soft tissue (Chapter 10). Both Ewing sarcoma and PNET have a similar neural phenotype, and because they share an identical chromosome translocation they should be viewed as two variants of the same tumor that differ only in their degree of neural differentiation. Tumors that demonstrate neural differentiation are labeled PNETs, and those that are undifferentiated are diagnosed as Ewing sarcoma. This distinction has no clinical significance.

Ewing sarcoma and PNET together account for approximately 6% to 10% of primary malignant bone tumors and follow osteosarcoma as the second most common group of bone sarcomas in children. Of all bone sarcomas, Ewing sarcoma/PNET has the youngest average age at presentation, since most affected individuals are 10 to 15 years old, and approximately 80% are younger than 20 years. Boys are affected slightly more frequently than girls, and there is a striking predilection for whites; blacks are rarely afflicted. Most Ewing sarcoma/PNET have a translocation involving the *EWS* gene on chromosome 22 and a gene encoding an ETS family transcription factor; the most commonly involved *ETS* gene is *FLI1*, as part of a (11;22) (q24;q12) translocation. The fusion genes generated by these translocations produce chimeric transcription factors that alter the expression of a network of target genes, resulting in abnormal cell proliferation and survival.[39] Other recent evidence suggests that the precursor cell of Ewing sarcoma/PNET is a multipotent mesenchymal stem cell.[40]

> **Morphology.** Arising in the medullary cavity, Ewing sarcoma and PNET usually invade the cortex, periosteum, and soft tissue. The tumor is soft, tan-white, and frequently contains areas of hemorrhage and necrosis. It is composed of sheets of uniform small, round cells that are slightly larger than lymphocytes (Fig. 26–35). They have scant cytoplasm, which may appear clear because it is rich in glycogen. The presence of **Homer-Wright rosettes** (tumor cells arranged in a circle about a central fibrillary space) is indicative of neural differentiation. Although the tumor contains fibrous septae, there is generally little stroma. Necrosis may be prominent, and there are relatively few mitotic figures in relation to the dense cellularity of the tumor.

Clinical Features. Ewing sarcoma and PNET usually arise in the diaphysis of long tubular bones, especially the femur and the flat bones of the pelvis. They present as painful enlarging masses, and the affected site is frequently tender, warm, and swollen. Some affected individuals have systemic findings, including fever, elevated sedimentation rate, anemia, and leukocytosis, which mimic infection. Plain radiograms show a destructive lytic tumor that has permeative margins and

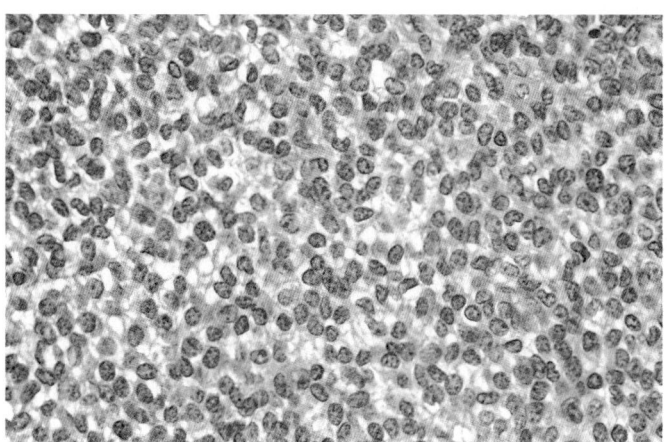

FIGURE 26–35   Ewing sarcoma composed of sheets of small round cells with small amounts of clear cytoplasm.

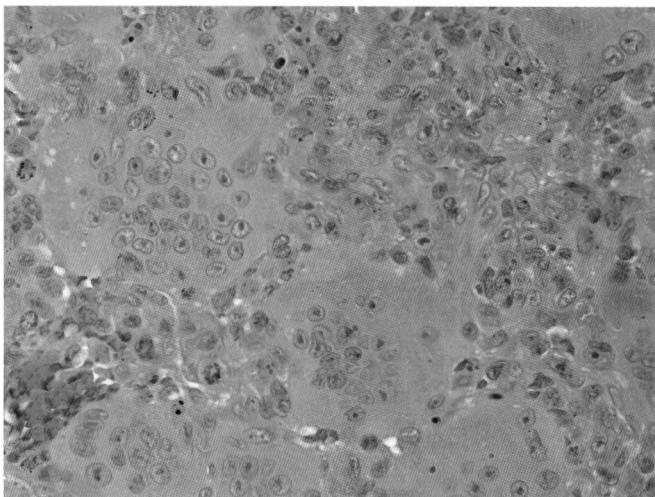

FIGURE 26–36   Benign giant-cell tumor illustrating an abundance of multinucleated giant cells with background mononuclear stromal cells.

extension into the surrounding soft tissues. The characteristic periosteal reaction produces layers of reactive bone deposited in an *onion-skin* fashion.

Treatment includes chemotherapy and surgical excision with or without irradiation. The advent of effective chemotherapy has markedly improved the prognosis from a dismal 5% to 15% to an approximately 75% 5-year survival; at least 50% have long-term cures. The amount of chemotherapy-induced necrosis is an important prognostic finding. Gene expression arrays of tumors appear to identify individuals with the most aggressive tumors.[41]

GIANT-CELL TUMOR

Giant-cell tumor is so named because it contains a mixture of mononuclear cells and a profusion of multinucleated osteo-clast-type giant cells, giving rise to the synonym *osteoclastoma*. This tumor is a relatively uncommon benign but locally aggressive neoplasm. It usually arises in individuals in their 20s to 40s. The mononuclear cells in giant-cell tumors express RANKL, and the giant osteoclast-like cells are believed to form via the RANK/RANKL signaling pathway.[42]

> **Morphology.** These are large, red-brown tumors that frequently undergo cystic degeneration. They are mostly composed of uniform oval mononuclear cells that constitute the proliferating component of the tumor. Scattered within this background are numerous osteoclast-type giant cells having 100 or more nuclei that resemble those of the mononuclear cells (Fig. 26–36). Necrosis, hemorrhage, hemosiderin deposition, and reactive bone formation are common secondary features.

Clinical Course. Giant-cell tumors in adults involve both the epiphyses and the metaphyses, but in adolescents they are confined proximally by the growth plate and are limited to the metaphysis. The majority arise around the knee (distal femur and proximal tibia), but virtually any bone can be involved. The typical location of these tumors near joints frequently causes arthritis-like symptoms. Occasionally, they present with

pathologic fractures. Most are solitary; however, multiple or multicentric tumors do occur, especially in the distal extremities. Giant-cell tumors often erode into the subchondral bone plate (Fig. 26–37) and destroy the overlying cortex, producing a bulging soft-tissue mass delineated by a thin shell of reactive bone. The margins with the adjacent bone are fairly circumscribed but seldom sclerotic. The biologic unpredictability of these neoplasms complicates their management. Conservative

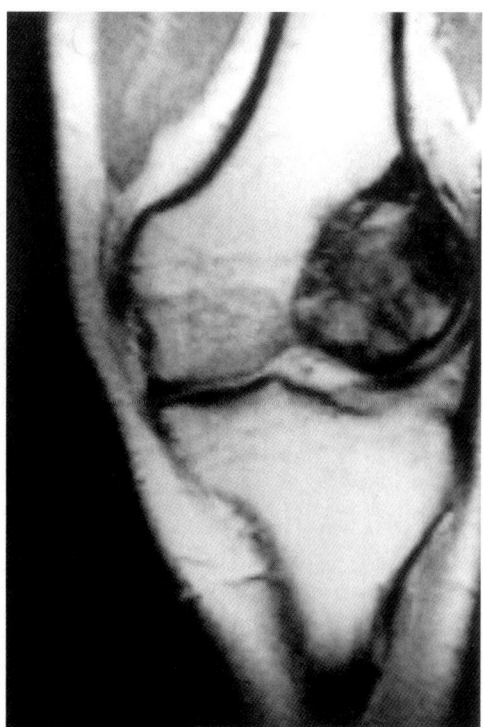

FIGURE 26–37   Magnetic resonance image of a giant-cell tumor that replaces most of the femoral condyle and extends to the subchondral bone plate.

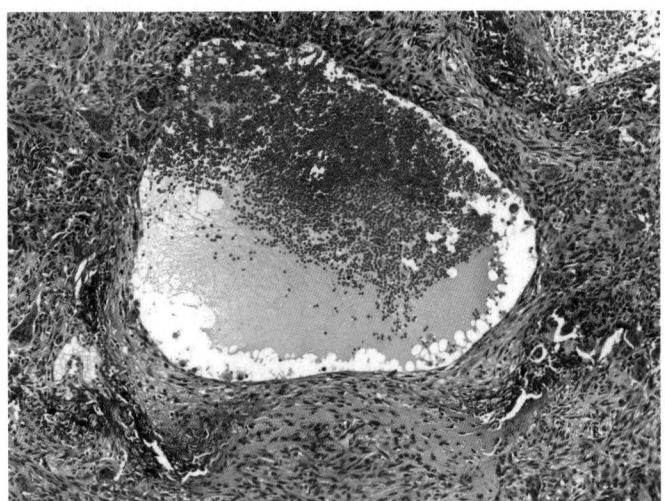

FIGURE 26–38 Aneurysmal bone cyst with blood-filled cystic space surrounded by wall containing proliferating fibroblasts, reactive woven bone, and osteoclast-type giant cells.

surgery such as curettage is associated with a 40% to 60% recurrence rate, and up to 4% metastasize to the lungs.

ANEURYSMAL BONE CYST

Aneurysmal bone cyst is a benign tumor of bone characterized by multiloculated blood-filled cystic spaces that may present as a rapidly growing expansile tumor. Despite its aggressive radiographic appearance, aneurysmal bone cyst behaves in a benign fashion. This tumor is associated with distinctive 17p13 translocations that result in up-regulation of USP6, a deubiquitinating enzyme.[43]

Morphology. Grossly, aneurysmal bone cyst consists of multiple blood-filled cystic spaces separated by thin, tan-white septa (Fig. 26–38). The walls are composed of plump uniform fibroblasts (which may be mitotically active), multinucleated osteoclast-like giant cells, and reactive woven bone. The bone is lined by osteoblasts, and its deposition typically follows the contours of the fibrous septa. Approximately one third of cases contain an unusual cartilage-like matrix, called "blue bone." Necrosis is uncommon unless there has been a previous pathologic fracture.

Clinical Course. Aneurysmal bone cyst affects all age groups but generally occurs during the first 2 decades of life and has no sex predilection. It most frequently develops in the metaphyses of long bones and the posterior elements of vertebral bodies. The most common signs and symptoms are pain and swelling. When an aneurysmal bone cyst involves the vertebrae, it can compress nerves and cause neurologic symptoms. Rarely, pathologic fractures occur.

Radiographically, aneurysmal bone cyst is usually an eccentric, expansile lesion with well-defined margins (Fig. 26–39A). Most lesions are completely lytic and often contain a thin shell of reactive bone at the periphery. Computed tomography and magnetic resonance imaging may demonstrate internal septa and characteristic fluid-fluid levels (Fig. 26–39B).

The treatment of aneurysmal bone cyst is surgical, usually in the form of curettage or, in certain situations, en bloc resection. The recurrence rate is low, and spontaneous regression may occur following incomplete removal.

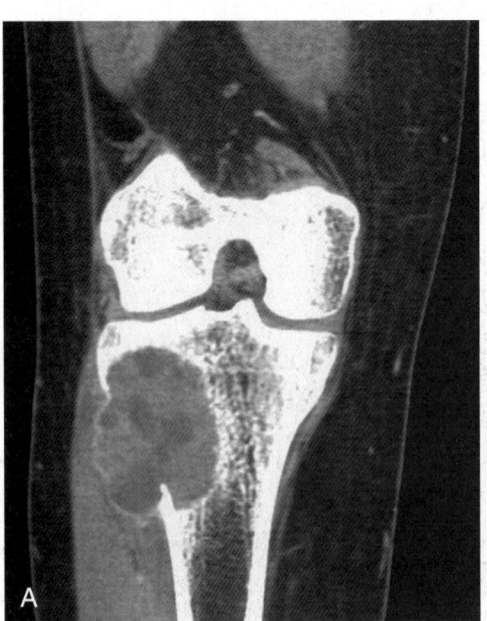
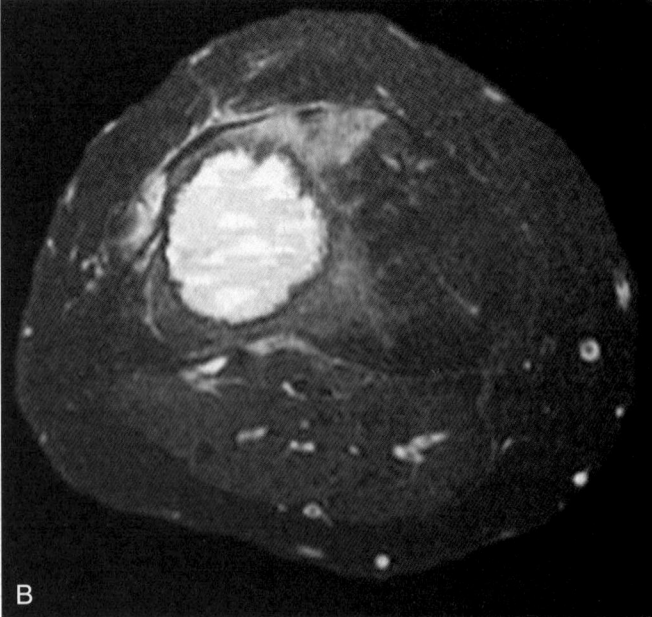

FIGURE 26–39 **A,** Coronal computed axial tomography scan showing eccentric aneurysmal bone cyst of tibia. The soft-tissue component is delineated by a thin rim of reactive subperiosteal bone. **B,** Axial magnetic resonance image demonstrating characteristic fluid-fluid levels.

METASTATIC DISEASE

Metastatic tumors are the most common form of skeletal malignancy. They usually develop in later stages of tumor progression. The pathways of spread include (1) direct extension, (2) lymphatic or hematogenous dissemination, and (3) intraspinal seeding (via the Batson plexus of veins). Any cancer can spread to bone, but in adults more than 75% of skeletal metastases originate from cancers of the prostate, breast, kidney, and lung. In children, metastases to bone originate from neuroblastoma, Wilms tumor, osteosarcoma, Ewing sarcoma, and rhabdomyosarcoma.

Skeletal metastases are typically multifocal; however, carcinomas of the kidney and thyroid are notorious for producing solitary lesions. The metastases may occur in any bone, but most involve the axial skeleton (vertebral column, pelvis, ribs, skull, sternum), proximal femur, and humerus in descending order of frequency. The red marrow in these areas, with its rich capillary network and slow blood flow, facilitates implantation and growth of the tumor cells. Metastases to the small bones of the hands and feet are uncommon and usually originate from cancers of the lung, kidney, or colon.

The radiographic manifestations of metastases may be purely lytic, purely blastic, or mixed lytic and blastic. In lytic lesions, the metastatic cells secrete substances such as prostaglandins, cytokines, and PTH-related protein that stimulate osteoclastic bone resorption; the tumor cells themselves do not directly resorb bone. Lysis of bone tissue rich in growth factors such as TGF-β, IGF-1, FGF, PDGF, and bone morphogenetic proteins, in turn helps create an environment conducive to tumor cell growth. Carcinomas of the kidney, lung, and gastrointestinal tract and malignant melanoma produce lytic bone destruction. Other metastases elicit a sclerotic response, particularly prostate adenocarcinoma, which may do so by secreting WNT proteins that stimulate osteoblastic bone formation. Most metastases induce a mixed lytic and blastic reaction.

JOINTS

Joints are constructed to provide both movement and mechanical stability. They are classified as solid (nonsynovial) and cavitated (synovial). The solid joints, known as *synarthroses*, provide structural integrity and allow for minimal movement. They lack a joint space and are grouped according to the type of connective tissue (fibrous tissue or cartilage) that bridges the ends of the bones; fibrous synarthroses include the cranial sutures and the bonds between roots of teeth and the jawbones; cartilaginous synarthroses (synchondroses) are represented by the symphyses (manubriosternalis and pubic). *Synovial joints*, in contrast, have a joint space that allows for a wide range of motion. Situated between the ends of bones formed via enchondral ossification, they are strengthened by a dense fibrous capsule reinforced by ligaments and muscles. The boundary of the joint space consists of the synovial membrane, which is firmly anchored to the underlying capsule and does not cover the articular surface. Its contour is smooth except near the osseous insertion, where it is thrown into numerous villous folds. Synovial membranes are lined by synoviocytes, cuboidal connective cells that are arranged one to four cell layers deep. Synoviocytes synthesize hyaluronic acid and various proteins. The synovial lining lacks a basement membrane, which allows for quick exchange between blood and synovial fluid. Synovial fluid is clear and viscous, and is a filtrate of plasma containing hyaluronic acid that acts as a lubricant and provides nutrition for the articular hyaline cartilage.

Hyaline cartilage is a unique connective tissue ideally suited to serve as an elastic shock absorber and wear-resistant surface. It lacks a blood supply and does not have lymphatic drainage or innervation. Hyaline cartilage is composed of type 2 collagen, water, proteoglycans, and chondrocytes, each of which has specific functions. The collagen fibers enable the cartilage to resist tensile stresses and transmit vertical loads. The water and proteoglycans give hyaline cartilage its turgor and elasticity and have an important role in limiting friction. The chondrocytes synthesize the matrix as well as enzymatically digest it, with the half-life of the different components ranging from weeks (proteoglycans) to years (type 2 collagen). Chondrocytes secrete the degradative enzymes in an inactive form and enrich the matrix with enzyme inhibitors. Diseases that destroy articular cartilage do so by activating the catabolic enzymes and decreasing the production of inhibitors, thereby accelerating the rate of matrix breakdown. Cytokines such as IL-1 and TNF trigger the degradative process; their sources include chondrocytes, synoviocytes, fibroblasts, and inflammatory cells. Destruction of articular cartilage by indigenous cells is an important mechanism in many joint diseases.

Arthritis

OSTEOARTHRITIS

Osteoarthritis, also called *degenerative joint disease*, is the most common type of joint disease and is one of the 10 most disabling conditions in developed nations. *It is characterized by the progressive erosion of articular cartilage.* It is estimated that more than 33 billion dollars are spent annually in the United States for its treatment and for lost days of work. The term *osteoarthritis* implies an inflammatory disease; however, even though inflammatory cells may be present (usually in small numbers), osteoarthritis is considered to be an intrinsic disease of cartilage in which biochemical and metabolic alterations in individuals with genetic susceptibility result in its breakdown.

In most instances osteoarthritis appears insidiously, without apparent initiating cause, as an aging phenomenon (idiopathic or primary osteoarthritis). In these cases the disease is usually oligoarticular (affects few joints) but may be generalized. In about 5% of cases, osteoarthritis may appear in younger individuals having some predisposing condition, such as previous injuries to a joint; a congenital developmental deformity of a joint(s); or some underlying systemic disease such as diabetes, ochronosis, hemochromatosis, or marked obesity. In these settings the disease is called *secondary osteoarthritis* and often involves one or several predisposed joints; witness the shoulder or elbow involvements in baseball players and knees in basketball players. Gender has some influence on distribution. The knees and hands are more commonly affected in women and the hips in men.

Pathogenesis. Osteoarthritis (OA) is a multifactorial disease that has genetic and environmental components. Studies of families and twins have suggested that the risk of OA is related to the net impact of multiple genes, each with a small effect. Genome-wide association studies (GWAS) are underway and it is likely that many risk-associated genes will be identified and validated shortly; a number of candidates have been identified, including genes involved in prostaglandin metabolism and WNT signaling.[44] The major environmental factors relate to aging and biomechanical stress, which is influenced by obesity, muscle strength, and joint stability, structure, and alignment. The association with aging is strong; the prevalence of OA increases exponentially beyond the age of 50, and about 80% to 90% of individuals have evidence of the disease by age 65. Thus, OA joins heart disease and cancer as one of the unfortunate dividends of growing older. However, it is an oversimplification to consider OA an inevitable consequence of cartilage wear and tear. The mechanisms leading to OA are complex and not yet clear, but chondrocytes are at the center of the process, which can be divided into several phases: (1) chondrocyte injury, which is related to aging and genetic and biochemical factors; (2) early OA, in which chondrocytes proliferate (cloning) and secrete inflammatory mediators, collagens, proteoglycans, and proteases, which act together to remodel the cartilaginous matrix and initiate secondary inflammatory changes in the synovium and subchondral bone; and (3) late OA, in which repetitive injury and chronic inflammation lead to chondrocyte drop out, marked loss of cartilage, and extensive subchondral bone changes.[45]

Morphology. In the early stages of osteoarthritis the chondrocytes proliferate, forming clusters. Concurrently, the water content of the matrix increases and the concentration of proteoglycans decreases. Subsequently, vertical and horizontal fibrillation and cracking of the matrix occur as the superficial layers of the cartilage and type 2 collagen molecules are degraded. Grossly this manifests as a granular soft articular surface. Eventually, chondrocytes die and full-thickness portions of the cartilage are sloughed. The dislodged pieces of cartilage and subchondral bone tumble into the joint, forming loose bodies (**joint mice**). The exposed subchondral bone plate becomes the new articular surface, and friction with the opposing degenerated articular surface smooths and bur-

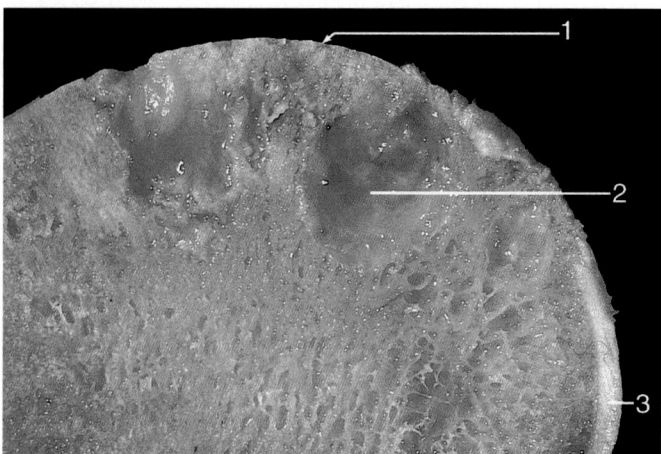

FIGURE 26–40 Severe osteoarthritis with small islands of residual articular cartilage next to exposed subchondral bone. 1, Eburnated articular surface. 2, Subchondral cyst. 3, Residual articular cartilage.

nishes the exposed bone, giving it the appearance of polished ivory (**bone eburnation**) (Fig. 26–40). Concurrently there is rebuttressing and sclerosis of the underlying cancellous bone. Small fractures through the articulating bone are common, and the fracture gaps allow synovial fluid to be forced into the subchondral regions in a one-way, ball valve–like mechanism. The loculated fluid collection increases in size, forming fibrous-walled cysts. Mushroom-shaped osteophytes (bony outgrowths) develop at the margins of the articular surface and are capped by fibrocartilage and hyaline cartilage that gradually ossify. The synovium is usually only mildly congested and fibrotic, and may have scattered chronic inflammatory cells.

Clinical Course. Osteoarthritis is an insidious disease. Patients with primary disease are usually asymptomatic until they are in their 50s. If a young person has significant manifestations of osteoarthritis, a search for some underlying cause should be made. Characteristic symptoms include deep, achy pain that worsens with use, morning stiffness, crepitus, and limitation of range of movement. Impingement on spinal foramina by osteophytes results in cervical and lumbar nerve root compression and radicular pain, muscle spasms, muscle atrophy, and neurologic deficits. Typically, only one or a few joints are involved except in the uncommon generalized variant. The joints commonly involved include the hips, knees, lower lumbar and cervical vertebrae, proximal and distal interphalangeal joints of the fingers, first carpometacarpal joints, and first tarsometatarsal joints of the feet (Fig. 26–41). *Heberden nodes*, prominent osteophytes at the distal interphalangeal joints, are common in women (but not men). The wrists, elbows, and shoulders are usually spared. There are still no satisfactory means of preventing primary osteoarthritis, and there are no effective methods of halting its progression. The disease may stabilize for years but more often is slowly progressive, and it is second only to cardiovascular diseases in causing long-term disability.

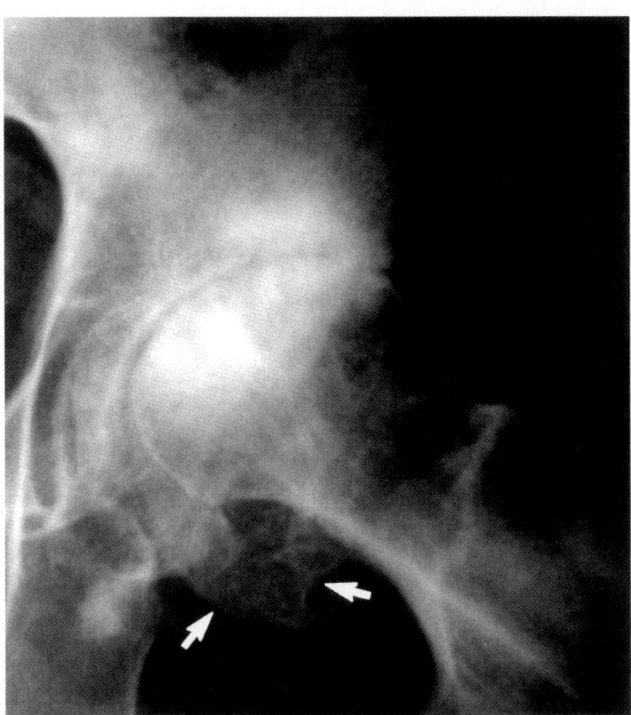

FIGURE 26–41 Severe osteoarthritis of the hip. The joint space is narrowed, and there is subchondral sclerosis with scattered oval radiolucent cysts and peripheral osteophyte lipping (arrows).

RHEUMATOID ARTHRITIS

Rheumatoid arthritis is a chronic systemic inflammatory disorder that may affect many tissues and organs—skin, blood vessels, heart, lungs, and muscles—but principally attacks the joints, producing a nonsuppurative proliferative and inflammatory synovitis that often progresses to destruction of the articular cartilage and ankylosis of the joints. Although the cause of rheumatoid arthritis remains unknown, genetic predisposition, environment, and autoimmunity have pivotal roles in the development, progression, and chronicity of the disease.

About 1% of the world's population is afflicted by rheumatoid arthritis, women three to five times more often than men. It is most common in those 40 to 70 years old, but no age is immune. We first consider the morphology as a background to discuss pathogenesis.

Morphology

Joints. Rheumatoid arthritis causes a broad spectrum of morphologic alterations; the most severe are manifested in the joints. Initially the synovium becomes grossly edematous, thickened, and hyperplastic, transforming its smooth contour to one covered by delicate and bulbous fronds (Fig. 26–42). The characteristic histologic features include (1) infiltration of synovial stroma by a dense perivascular inflammatory infiltrate composed of lymphoid aggregates (mostly CD4+ helper T cells), B cells, plasma cells, dendritic cells, and macrophages (Fig. 26–42C);

(2) increased vascularity due to vasodilation and angiogenesis, with superficial hemosiderin deposits; (3) aggregation of organizing fibrin covering portions of the synovium and floating in the joint space as rice bodies; (4) accumulation of neutrophils in the synovial fluid and along the surface of synovium but usually not deep in the synovial stroma; (5) osteoclastic activity in underlying bone, allowing the synovium to penetrate into the bone and cause juxta-articular erosions, subchondral cysts, and osteoporosis; and (6) **pannus** formation. The pannus is a mass of synovium and synovial stroma consisting of inflammatory cells, granulation tissue, and synovial fibroblasts, which grows over the articular cartilage and causes its erosion. In time, after the cartilage has been destroyed, the pannus bridges the apposing bones to form a **fibrous ankylosis**, which eventually ossifies and results in bony ankylosis. Inflammation in the tendons, ligaments, and occasionally the adjacent skeletal muscle frequently accompanies the arthritis.

Skin. **Rheumatoid nodules** are the most common cutaneous lesion. They occur in approximately 25% of affected individuals, usually those with severe disease, and arise in regions of the skin that are subjected to pressure, including the ulnar aspect of the forearm, elbows, occiput, and lumbosacral area. Less commonly they form in the lungs, spleen, pericardium, myocardium, heart valves, aorta, and other viscera. Rheumatoid nodules are firm, nontender, and round to oval, and in the skin arise in the subcutaneous tissue. Microscopically they have a central zone of fibrinoid necrosis surrounded by a prominent rim of epithelioid histiocytes (activated macrophages) and numerous lymphocytes and plasma cells (Fig. 26–43).

Blood Vessels. Affected individuals with severe erosive disease, rheumatoid nodules, and high titers of rheumatoid factor are at risk of developing vasculitic syndromes (Chapter 11). Rheumatoid vasculitis is a potentially catastrophic complication of rheumatoid arthritis, particularly when it affects vital organs. The involvement of medium- to small-size arteries is similar to that occurring in polyarteritis nodosa, except that in rheumatoid arthritis the kidneys are not involved. Frequently, segments of small arteries such as **vasa nervorum** and **digital arteries** are obstructed by an obliterating endarteritis resulting in peripheral neuropathy, ulcers, and gangrene. Leukocytoclastic venulitis produces purpura, cutaneous ulcers, and nail bed infarction.

Pathogenesis. Although much remains uncertain, it is currently believed that *rheumatoid arthritis is triggered by exposure of a genetically susceptible host to an arthritogenic antigen* resulting in a breakdown of immunological self-tolerance and a chronic inflammatory reaction. In this manner, an acute arthritis is initiated, but it is the continuing *autoimmune*

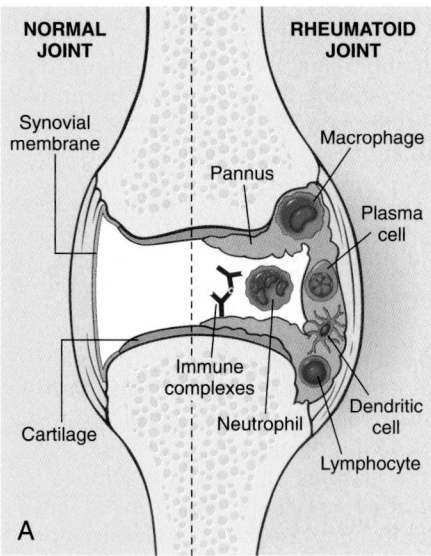
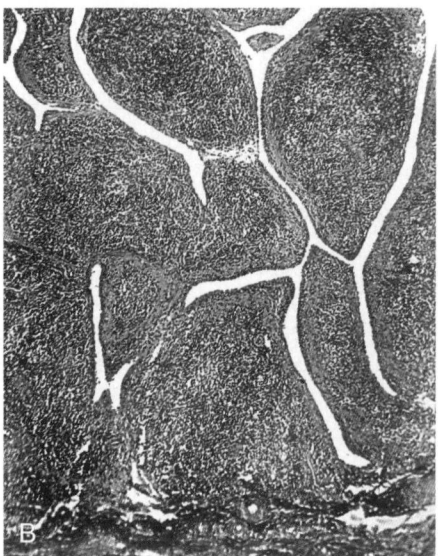
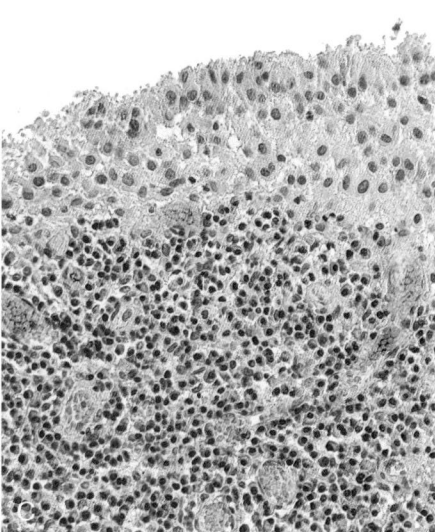

FIGURE 26–42 Rheumatoid arthritis. **A,** Schematic view of the joint lesion. (Modified from Feldmann M: Development of anti-TNF therapy for rheumatoid arthritis. Nat Rev Immunol 2:364, 2002.) **B,** Low magnification reveals marked synovial hypertrophy with formation of villi. **C,** At higher magnification, subsynovial tissue containing a dense lymphoid aggregate is seen.

reaction, the activation of CD4+ helper T cells, and the local release of inflammatory mediators and cytokines that ultimately destroys the joint (Fig. 26–44).

- *Genetic susceptibility* is clearly a major contributor to the pathogenesis of rheumatoid arthritis. Specific *HLA-DRB1* alleles have been shown to be associated with rheumatoid arthritis, and these alleles share a common sequence of amino acids in the third hypervariable region of the β chain, which is designated the shared epitope. The shared epitope is located in the antigen-binding cleft of the DR molecule. This location is presumably the specific binding site of the arthritogen(s) that initiates the inflammatory synovitis. Another gene associated with rheumatoid arthritis is *PTPN22*; it encodes a protein tyrosine phosphatase,

which participates in activation and control of inflammatory cells, including T cells.

- *Environmental arthritogen*: The environmental arthritogen thought to be the *initiator of the disease* remains uncertain. Microbial agents including Epstein-Barr virus, retroviruses, parvoviruses, mycobacteria, *Borrelia*, *Proteus mirabilis*, and *Mycoplasma* have all been implicated but none has been proved to be significant. Recently, *citrullinated proteins* (proteins modified by the enzymatic conversion of arginine to citrulline, many of which are fibrins) formed in the body (especially in the lungs of smokers) have been implicated in the pathogenesis of rheumatoid arthritis. The robust immune reaction to these autoantigens suggests that they are an important potential arthritogenic agent.[46]

- *Autoimmunity*: Once an inflammatory synovitis has been initiated, an *autoimmune reaction*—in which T cells have the pivotal role—is responsible for the chronic destructive nature of rheumatoid arthritis. The antigen inducing this reaction has not been identified with certainty; type 2 collagen and glycosaminoglycans have been implicated in animal models but may not be relevant in human disease. Regardless, activated CD4+ effector and memory T cells appear within affected joints early. T_H17 cells are important in the inflammatory reaction because they recruit neutrophils and monocytes. Interferon-γ-producing T_H1 cells may also contribute to the inflammatory reaction. *About 80% of individuals with rheumatoid arthritis have autoantibodies to the Fc portion of autologous IgG (rheumatoid factors).* These are mostly IgM antibodies but may be of other classes and they self-associate (RA-IgG) to form immune complexes in the sera, synovial fluid, and synovial membranes. Though not a causative factor of the disease, the circulating immune complexes are markers of disease activity. Rheumatoid factor, however, is not present in some individuals with the disease (seronegative), and is sometimes found in other disease states and even in otherwise healthy people. *Anti-*

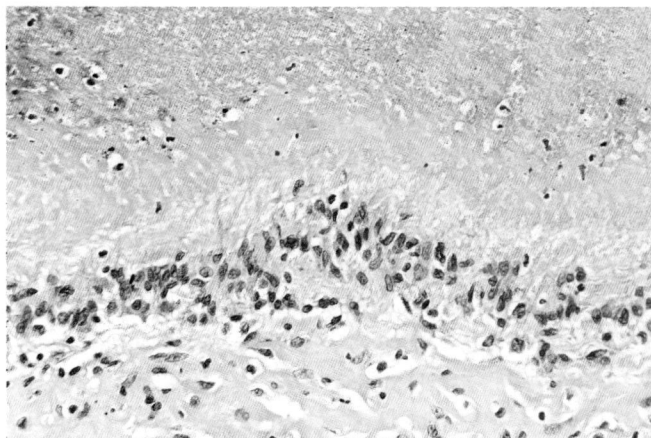

FIGURE 26–43 Subcutaneous rheumatoid nodule with an area of necrosis *(top)* surrounded by a palisade of macrophages and scattered chronic inflammatory cells.

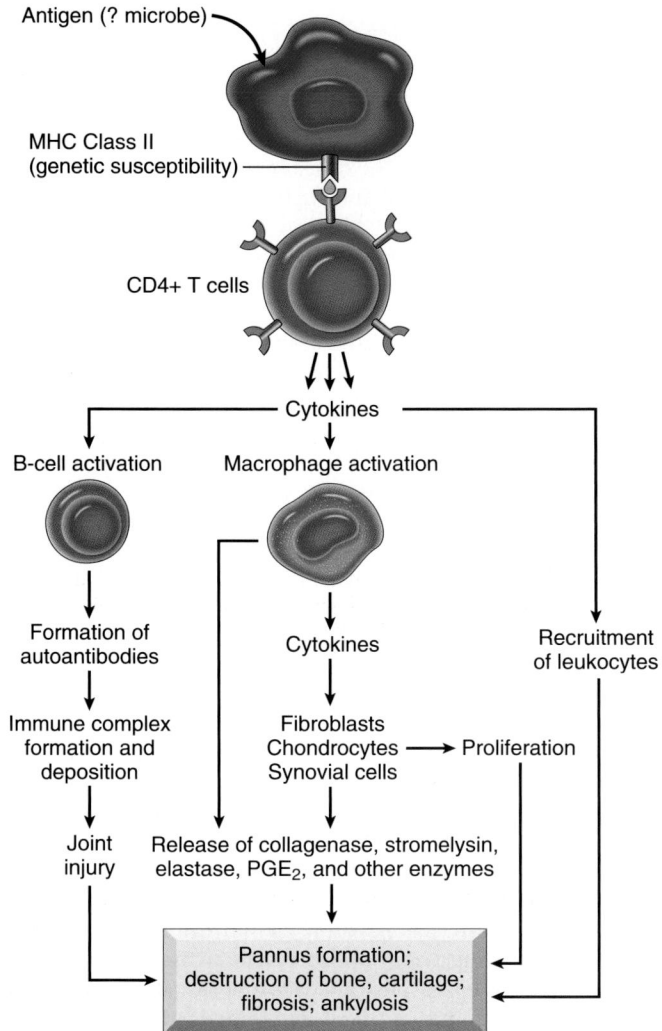

FIGURE 26–44   Immunopathogenesis of rheumatoid arthritis.

bodies to citrulline-modified peptides (anti-cyclic citrullinated peptide [CCP] antibodies) have been recently shown to be present in many people with rheumatoid arthritis and rarely in people with other inflammatory diseases or healthy individuals. These antibodies are produced at sites of inflammation and are recognized as being relatively specific for rheumatoid arthritis. Evidence suggests that the raised levels of anti-CCP antibodies in combination with a T-cell response to the citrullinated proteins contribute to the disease becoming chronic.[47,48]

What mediators then bring about the destructive proliferative synovitis? These represent the "usual suspects." The cytokines secreted by the T cells, such as interferon-γ and IL-17, act upon and stimulate synoviocytes and macrophages, which produce pro-inflammatory molecules such as IL-1, IL-6, IL-23, TNF, PGE$_2$, nitric oxide, and the growth factors granulocyte-macrophage colony-stimulating factor and TGF-β. The inflammatory mediators activate endothelial cells in the synovium and thus facilitate leukocyte binding and transmigration. They also cause an *increased production of cartilage matrix metalloproteinases*, which along with antigen-antibody

complexes, are important in the destruction of the articular cartilage. Additionally, they are potent stimulators of osteoclastogenesis and osteoclast activity by up-regulating the production of RANKL. RANKL is also expressed by the T cells and activated synoviocytes. Consequently the edematous, hyperplastic, and sticky (synoviocytes up-regulate vascular cell adhesion molecule) synovium rich in inflammatory cells becomes adherent to and grows over the articular surface, forming a pannus, and stimulates resorption of the adjacent bone. *In the end, the pannus produces sustained, irreversible cartilage destruction and erosion of subchondral bone.*

From this alphabet soup of mediators and cytokines, only one has been firmly implicated in the pathogenesis of rheumatoid arthritis—TNF. Happily, proof of its involvement has come from trials of specific TNF antagonists, which relieve swelling and pain, and appear to arrest disease progression (see below).

Clinical Course. The clinical course of rheumatoid arthritis is extremely variable. The disease begins slowly and insidiously in more than half of affected individuals. Initially there is malaise, fatigue, and generalized musculoskeletal pain, and only after several weeks to months do the joints become involved. The pattern of joint involvement varies, but it is generally *symmetrical and the small joints are affected before the larger ones.* Symptoms usually develop in the hands (metacarpophalangeal and proximal interphalangeal joints) and feet, followed by the wrists, ankles, elbows, and knees. Uncommonly the upper spine is involved, but the lumbosacral region and hips are usually spared.

Involved *joints are swollen, warm, painful, and particularly stiff on arising or following inactivity.* Approximately 10% of affected individuals have an acute onset over several days with severe symptoms and polyarticular involvement. The typical patient has progressive joint involvement over a period of months to years, with initial minimal limitation of motion that steadily becomes more severe. The disease course may be slow or rapid, and fluctuates over the years, with the greatest damage occurring in the first 4 or 5 years. Approximately 20% of affected individuals enjoy periods of partial or complete remission, but the symptoms inevitably return and involve previously unaffected joints.

The *radiographic hallmarks are joint effusions and juxta-articular osteopenia with erosions and narrowing of the joint space with loss of articular cartilage* (Fig. 26–45). Destruction of tendons, ligaments, and joint capsules produces characteristic deformities, including radial deviation of the wrist, ulnar deviation of the fingers, and flexion-hyperextension abnormalities of the fingers (swan neck, boutonnière). The end result is deformed joints that have no stability and minimal or no range of motion. Large synovial cysts, like the Baker cyst in the posterior knee, may develop as the increased intra-articular pressure causes outpunching of the synovium.

The presence of rheumatoid factor and anti-CCP antibody are laboratory indicators that together are sensitive and fairly specific for rheumatoid arthritis. As pointed out, rheumatoid factor may not be present and also appears in many other conditions. Analysis of synovial fluid confirms an inflammatory arthritis with neutrophils, high protein content, and low mucin content, but is nonspecific. The diagnosis is based primarily on the clinical features and includes the presence of four of the following criteria: (1) morning stiffness,

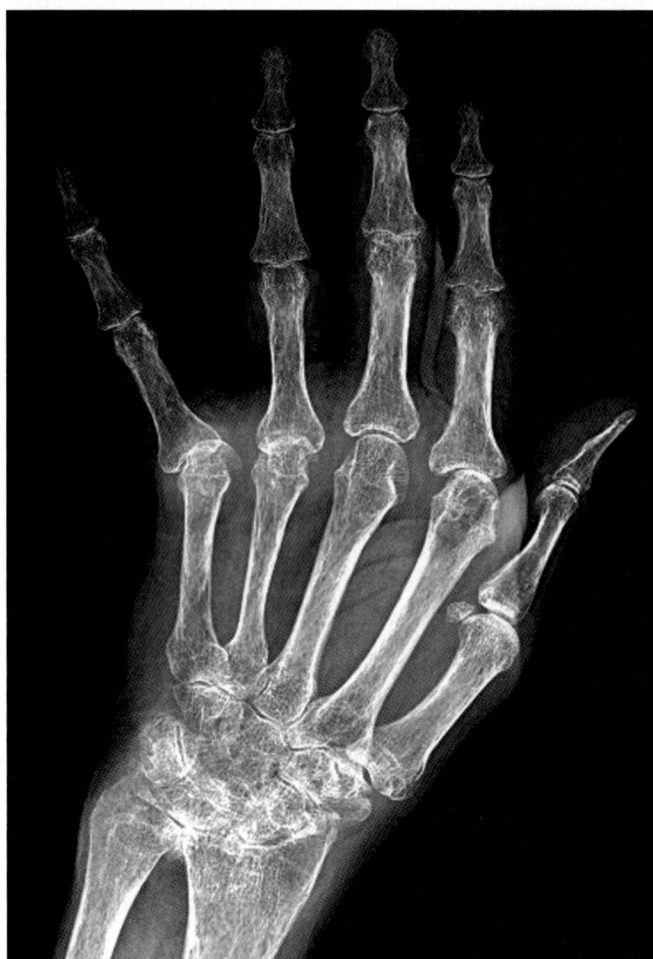

FIGURE 26–45 Rheumatoid arthritis of the hand. There is diffuse osteopenia, marked loss of the joint spaces of the carpal, metacarpal, phalangeal, and interphalangeal joints, periarticular bony erosions, and ulnar drift of the fingers.

(2) arthritis in three or more joint areas, (3) arthritis of hand joints, (4) symmetric arthritis, (5) rheumatoid nodules, (6) serum rheumatoid factor, and (7) typical radiographic changes.

The treatment of rheumatoid arthritis is aimed at relieving the pain and inflammation, and slowing or arresting the relentless joint destruction. Therapies include corticosteroids, and synthetic and biologic disease-modifying drugs such as methotrexate and, most notably, antagonists of TNF. As mentioned earlier, these are remarkably effective and now constitute the mainstay of treatment. Most importantly, they prevent or slow joint destruction, which is the greatest source of disability, and have altered the natural history of the disease for the better. However, anti-TNF agents are not curative, and patients must be maintained on TNF antagonists or other immunosuppressive drugs to avoid disease flares. Also, inhibiting the activity of a key inflammatory mediator comes with a price; patients treated with anti-TNF agents are susceptible to certain infections, particularly *M. tuberculosis*.

JUVENILE IDIOPATHIC ARTHRITIS

Juvenile idiopathic arthritis (JIA), previously known as juvenile rheumatoid arthritis, encompasses all forms of arthritis that develop before 16 years of age and that persist for a minimum of 6 weeks. JIA is one of the more common connective tissue diseases; it affects 30,000 to 50,000 children in the United States and is an important cause of functional disability. The etiology of JIA is unknown. It is classified into seven discrete clinical subsets that may correspond to separate diseases and genetic backgrounds; (1) systemic arthritis, (2) oligoarthritis, (3) rheumatoid factor–positive polyarthritis, (4) rheumatoid factor–negative polyarthritis, (5) enthesitis (inflammation of a point of attachment of skeletal muscle to bone)-associated arthritis, (6) psoriatic arthritis, and (7) undifferentiated arthritis.

JIA differs from rheumatoid arthritis in adults in the following ways: (1) oligoarthritis is more common, (2) systemic disease is more frequent, (3) large joints are affected more often than small joints, (4) rheumatoid nodules and rheumatoid factor are usually absent, and (5) antinuclear antibody (ANA) seropositivity is common. As in rheumatoid arthritis, risk is associated with genetic susceptibility (with particular HLA alleles) and environmental factors; the heterogeneity of the disease indicates that different factors may be at play in different individuals. The inflammatory synovitis and morphologic changes are similar to those in rheumatoid arthritis. There is evidence of abnormal immunoregulation and a prevalence of activated CD4+ memory T cells within involved joints; cytokine production is prominent and helps drive the process.

Systemic arthritis may have a rather abrupt onset, is associated with remitting, high spiking fevers, migratory and transient skin rash, hepatosplenomegaly, and serositis. Long-term follow-up shows that affected individuals may experience recurrent flares or persistent disease that may be associated with significant morbidity and serious complications.

Arthritis affecting four or fewer joints during the first 6 months of disease in the absence of psoriasis and an HLA-B27 genotype defines the *oligoarthritis variant*. The arthritis is asymmetric, develops at an early age (younger than 6 years), and is commonly associated with iridocylitis and a positive ANA.

Rheumatoid factor–positive polyarthritis is similar to the adult form of the disease and is mainly seen in teenage girls. Rheumatoid factor–negative polyarthritis involves more than five joints within the first 6 months and consists of several subtypes that have features that overlap with oligoarthritis and rheumatoid factor–negative arthritis in adults, and a subset that shows stiffness and contractions, but little swelling.

Enthesitis-related arthritis mainly affects male children younger than 6 years, and most affected individuals are HLA-B27 positive. The enthesitis and arthritis affects tendoligamentous insertion sites and joints of the lower extremities.

Undifferentiated arthritis encompasses patients who do not fulfill inclusion criteria of the other groups or have overlapping features.

Long-term prognosis of JIA is very variable. Although many affected individuals may have sustained disease activity, only about 10% develop serious functional disability.

SERONEGATIVE SPONDYLOARTHROPATHIES

The seronegative spondyloarthropathies are a group of diseases that develop in genetically predisposed individuals and are initiated by ubiquitous environmental factors, especially infectious agents. The manifestations are immune mediated and are triggered by a T-cell response presumably directed against an undefined antigen that may cross-react with native molecules of the musculoskeletal system. Clinically, the diseases produce inflammatory peripheral or axial oligoarthritis and enthesopathies. The seronegative spondyloarthropathies include *ankylosing spondylitis, reactive arthritis (Reiter syndrome and enteritis-associated arthritis), psoriatic arthritis, and arthritis associated with inflammatory bowel disease* (ulcerative colitis, Crohn disease). Many are associated with the HLA-B27 allele and a triggering infection but without specific autoantibodies (hence the term *"seronegative"*). They all have inflammation of synovial joints and share overlapping clinical features, with extra-articular involvement of the eyes, skin, and cardiovascular system being relatively commonplace.

Ankylosing Spondyloarthritis

Also known as *rheumatoid spondylitis* and *Marie-Strümpell disease*, ankylosing spondyloarthritis is a chronic synovitis that causes destruction of articular cartilage and resultant bony ankylosis, especially of the sacroiliac and apophyseal joints (between tuberosities and processes). Inflammation of tendinoligamentous insertion sites eventuates in their ossification, producing squaring and fusion of the vertebral bodies, and bony outgrowths, which together result in severe spinal immobility. It usually becomes symptomatic in the second and third decades of life, and men are affected two to three times more frequently than women. Affected individuals characteristically present with low back pain, which frequently follows a chronic progressive course. Involvement of peripheral joints, such as the hips, knees, and shoulders, occurs in at least one third of affected individuals. Fracture of the spine, uveitis, aortitis, and amyloidosis are other recognized complications. Approximately 90% of the risk of developing the disease and the severity of the clinical manifestations is determined genetically. Although 90% of affected individuals are HLA-B27 positive, it has been suspected the other genes also contribute. Recent genome-wide association studies have shown associations with *ARTS1*, a gene that encodes a peptidase that trims antigens being processed for presentation by class I HLA molecules; and *IL23R*, the gene for the IL-23 receptor, suggesting that IL-23 (which promotes T_H17 responses) may have a role in this disease.[49]

Reiter Syndrome

Reiter syndrome is a form of reactive arthritis and is defined by a triad of arthritis, nongonococcal urethritis or cervicitis, and conjunctivitis. Most affected individuals are men in their 20s or 30s, and more than 80% are HLA-B27 positive. This form of arthritis also affects individuals infected with the human immunodeficiency virus (HIV). The disease is probably caused by an autoimmune reaction initiated by prior infection of the gastrointestinal tract (*Shigella, Salmonella, Yersinia, Campylobacter*) and the genitourinary system (*Chlamydia*). Arthritic symptoms usually develop within several weeks of the inciting bout of urethritis or diarrhea. Joint stiffness and low back pain are common early symptoms. The ankles, knees, and feet are affected most often, frequently in an asymmetric pattern. Synovitis of a digital tendon sheath produces the sausage finger or toe, and ossification of tendoligamentous insertion sites leads to calcaneal spurs and bony outgrowths. Patients with severe chronic disease have involvement of the spine that is indistinguishable from ankylosing spondylitis. Extra-articular involvement manifests as inflammatory balanitis, conjunctivitis, cardiac conduction abnormalities, and aortic regurgitation. The natural behavior of Reiter syndrome is extremely variable. The episodes of arthritis usually wax and wane over a period of several weeks to 6 months. Almost 50% of affected individuals have recurrent arthritis, tendinitis, fasciitis, and lumbosacral pain that can cause significant functional disability.

Enteritis-Associated Arthritis

Enteritis-associated arthritis is caused by gastrointestinal infection by *Yersinia, Salmonella, Shigella,* and *Campylobacter,* among others. The outer cell membranes of these organisms have lipopolysaccharides as a major component, and they stimulate a host of immunological responses. The arthritis appears abruptly and tends to involve the knees and ankles but sometimes also the wrists, fingers, and toes. It lasts for about a year, then generally clears and only rarely is accompanied by ankylosing spondylitis.

Psoriatic Arthritis

Psoriatic arthritis is a chronic inflammatory arthropathy that affects peripheral and axial joints and entheses and is associated with psoriasis. Susceptibility to the disease is genetically determined and related to HLA-B27 and HLA-Cw6 alleles. It develops in more than 10% of the psoriatic population and has assorted phenotypic subtypes. Symptoms manifest between the ages of 30 and 50, and those involving the joints usually develop slowly but are acute in onset in one third of affected individuals. The patterns of joint involvement are diverse. The distal interphalangeal joints of the hands and feet are first affected in an asymmetric distribution in more than 50% of patients and may be associated with a sausage-like finger. The large joints such as the ankles, knees, hips, and wrists may be involved as well.[50] Sacroiliac and spinal disease occurs in 20% to 40% of affected individuals. Aside from conjunctivitis and iritis, extra-articular manifestations are uncommon. Histologically, psoriatic arthritis is similar to rheumatoid arthritis. Psoriatic arthritis, however, is usually not as severe, remissions are more frequent, and joint destruction is less frequent.

INFECTIOUS ARTHRITIS

Microorganisms of all types can seed joints during hematogenous dissemination. Articular structures can also become infected by direct inoculation or from contiguous spread from a soft-tissue abscess or focus of osteomyelitis. Infectious arthritis is potentially serious, because it can cause rapid destruction of the joint and produce permanent deformities.

Bacterial Arthritis

Bacterial infections almost always cause an acute suppurative arthritis. The bacteria usually seed the joint during an episode of bacteremia; however, in neonates there is an increased incidence of contiguous spread from underlying epiphyseal osteomyelitis. The most common organisms are gonococcus, *Staphylococcus*, *Streptococcus*, *Haemophilus influenzae*, and gram-negative bacilli (*E. coli*, *Salmonella*, *Pseudomonas*, and others). *H. influenzae* arthritis predominates in children under 2 years of age, *S. aureus* is the main causative agent in older children and adults, and gonococcus is prevalent during late adolescence and young adulthood. Individuals with sickle cell disease are prone to infection with *Salmonella* at any age. These joint infections affect the sexes equally except for gonococcal arthritis, which is seen mainly in sexually active women. Predisposing conditions include immune deficiencies (congenital and acquired), debilitating illness, joint trauma, chronic arthritis of any cause, and intravenous drug abuse.

The classic presentation is the sudden development of an acutely painful and swollen infected joint that has a restricted range of motion. Systemic findings of fever, leukocytosis, and elevated sedimentation rate are common. In disseminated gonococcal infection the symptoms are more subacute. In 90% of nongonococcal cases, the infection involves only a single joint, usually the knee, followed in frequency by the hip, shoulder, elbow, wrist, and sternoclavicular joints. Axial articulations are more commonly involved in drug addicts. Prompt recognition and effective therapy prevent rapid joint destruction.

Tuberculous Arthritis

Tuberculous arthritis (Chapter 8) is a chronic progressive monoarticular disease that occurs in all age groups, especially adults. It usually develops as a complication of adjoining osteomyelitis or after hematogenous dissemination from a visceral (usually pulmonary) site of infection. Onset is insidious and causes gradual progressive pain. Systemic symptoms may or may not be present. Mycobacterial seeding of the joint induces the formation of confluent granulomas with central caseous necrosis. The affected synovium may grow as a pannus over the articular cartilage and erode the bone along the joint margins. Chronic disease results in severe destruction with fibrous ankylosis and obliteration of the joint space. The weight-bearing joints are usually affected, especially the hips, knees, and ankles in descending order of frequency.

Lyme Arthritis

As previously discussed (Chapter 8), Lyme arthritis is caused by infection with the spirochete *Borrelia burgdorferi*, which is transmitted by the ticks of the *Ixodes ricinus* complex. The initial infection of the skin is followed within several days or weeks by dissemination of the organism to other sites, especially the joints.

Approximately 60% to 80% of untreated individuals with Lyme disease develop joint symptoms within a few weeks to 2 years after the onset of the disease. The arthritis is the dominant feature of late disease; it tends to be remitting and migratory, and primarily involves large joints, especially the knees, shoulders, elbows, and ankles in descending order of frequency. Usually one or two joints are affected at a time, and the attacks last for a few weeks to months. Infected synovium exhibits a chronic papillary synovitis with synoviocyte hyperplasia, fibrin deposition, mononuclear cell infiltrates (especially CD4+ T cells), and onion-skin thickening of arterial walls. The morphology in severe cases can closely resemble that of rheumatoid arthritis. Silver stains may reveal small numbers of organisms in the vicinity of blood vessels in approximately 25% of cases. Chronic arthritis that is antibiotic refractory develops in approximately 10% of affected individuals and results from infection-induced autoimmunity. It is hypothesized that specific HLA-DR molecules bind an epitope of *B. burgdorferi* outer surface protein A, which initiates a T-cell reaction to this epitope. The T-cells may cross-react with an unknown self-antigen (an example of "molecular mimicry"). The joints in these patients have synovial pannus, which causes articular cartilage destruction and permanent deformities.[51]

Viral Arthritis

Arthritis can occur in the setting of a variety of viral infections, including alphavirus, parvovirus B19, rubella, Epstein-Barr virus, and hepatitis B and C virus. The clinical manifestations of the arthritis are variable and range from acute to subacute symptoms. It is unclear whether the joint symptoms are caused by direct infection of the joint by the virus, as seen in rubella and some alphavirus infections, or whether the viral infection generates an autoimmune reaction as seen in other forms of reactive or post-infectious arthritides.[52] A variety of different rheumatic conditions, including reactive arthritis, psoriatic arthritis, and septic arthritis, have developed in individuals infected with HIV. The pathogenesis of some of these forms of HIV-associated chronic arthritis is probably autoimmune. The new effective antiretroviral therapies for HIV have ameliorated their severity.

CRYSTAL-INDUCED ARTHRITIS

Articular crystal deposits are associated with a variety of acute and chronic joint disorders. Endogenous crystals shown to be pathogenic include monosodium urate (gout), calcium pyrophosphate dihydrate, and basic calcium phosphate (hydroxyapatite). Exogenous crystals, such as corticosteroid ester crystals and talcum, and the biomaterials polyethylene and methyl methacrylate, may also induce joint disease. Silicone, polyethylene, and methyl methacrylate are used in prosthetic joints, and their debris that accumulates with long use and wear may result in local arthritis and failure of the prosthesis. Endogenous and exogenous crystals produce disease by triggering the cascade that results in cytokine-mediated cartilage destruction. Here we discuss the two most important crystal arthropathies: gout, caused by urates, and pseudo-gout, caused by calcium pyrophosphate.

Gout and Gouty Arthritis

Man is the only mammal to spontaneously develop hyperuricemia and gout, as only humans lack uricase, the enzyme responsible for the degradation of uric acid in other mammals. This, in combination with a high reabsorption rate of filtered urate, predisposes humans to hyperuricemia and gout, which is the common end point of a group of disorders that produce hyperuricemia.

Gout is marked by transient attacks of *acute arthritis* initiated by crystallization of urates within and about joints, leading eventually to *chronic gouty arthritis* and the appearance of *tophi.* Tophi represent large aggregates of urate crystals and the surrounding inflammatory reaction (see later). Most, but not all, individuals with chronic gout also develop urate nephropathy. Hyperuricemia (plasma urate level above 6.8 mg/dL) is necessary but not sufficient for the development of gout. More than 10% of the population of the Western hemisphere has hyperuricemia, and the prevalence is increasing; however, gout develops in fewer than 0.5% of these individuals. The various conditions producing hyperuricemia and gout (Table 26–7) are divided into those that produce primary gout (accounting for most idiopathic cases) and secondary gout (the cause of the hyperuricemia is known, and gout is not the main clinical expression of the disease). The role of hyperuricemia in the development of a variety of diseases, such as hypertension, chronic renal disease, cardiovascular disease, and the metabolic syndrome of hypertriglyceridemia, obesity, and insulin resistance, is controversial and remains a focus of investigation.

Pathogenesis. Uric acid is the end product of purine metabolism. Clinically, hyperuricemia develops from overproduction of urate in approximately 10% of cases (increased cell turnover—as in cancer, psoriasis, and during tumor lysis induced by chemotherapy) and reduced excretion in the remainder.

Plasma levels of uric acid are governed by a four-part renal transport system that involves glomerular filtration, reabsorption, secretion, and postsecretory reabsorption. Approximately 90% of the filtered urate is reabsorbed, and the urate transporter 1 gene *(URAT1)* has an important role in the reabsorption process. Decreased filtration and underexcretion of uric acid underlies most cases of primary gout. Two pathways are

involved in purine synthesis: (1) a de novo pathway in which purines are synthesized from non-purine precursors and (2) a salvage pathway in which free purine bases derived from the breakdown of nucleic acids of endogenous or exogenous origin are recaptured (salvaged) (Fig. 26–46). The enzyme hypoxanthine guanine phosphoribosyl transferase (HGPRT) is involved in the salvage pathway. A deficiency of this enzyme leads to increased synthesis of purine nucleotides through the de novo pathway and hence increased production of uric acid. A complete lack of HGPRT occurs in the uncommon X-linked *Lesch-Nyhan syndrome,* seen only in males and characterized by hyperuricemia, severe neurologic deficits with mental retardation, self-mutilation, and in some cases gouty arthritis. Less severe deficiencies of the enzyme may also induce hyperuricemia and gouty arthritis with only mild neurologic deficits, but together these causes of gout are uncommon.

As stated earlier, hyperuricemia does not necessarily lead to gouty arthritis. Many factors contribute to the conversion of asymptomatic hyperuricemia into primary gout, including the following:

- *Age* of the individual and *duration of the hyperuricemia.* Gout rarely appears before 20 to 30 years of hyperuricemia.
- *Genetic predisposition.* In addition to the well-defined X-linked abnormalities of HGPRT, primary gout follows multifactorial inheritance and runs in families.
- Heavy *alcohol* consumption predisposes to attacks of gouty arthritis.
- *Obesity* increases the risk of asymptomatic gout.
- Certain *drugs* (e.g., thiazides) reduce excretion of urate and predispose to the development of gout.
- *Lead toxicity* increases the tendency to develop saturnine gout (Chapter 9).

Central to the pathogenesis of the arthritis is precipitation of monosodium urate (MSU) crystals into the joints (Fig. 26–47). The solubility of MSU in a joint is modulated by temperature (the lower the less soluble) and by the intra-articular concentration of urate and cations. Crystallization is dependent on the presence of nucleating agents such as insoluble collagen fibers, chondroitin sulfate, proteoglycans, cartilage fragments, and other crystals. Since synovial fluid is a poorer solvent for monosodium urate than plasma, urates in the joint fluid become supersaturated more easily, particularly in the peripheral joints (ankles and toes), where temperatures are as low as 20°C. With prolonged hyperuricemia, crystals and microtophi of urates develop in the synovium and in the joint cartilage. Some unknown event, possibly trauma, causes the release of crystals into the synovial fluid, which begins a cascade of events that initiates, intensifies, and sustains a powerful inflammatory response that is the hallmark of the acute attack. MSU crystals are phagocytosed by macrophages and through an incompletely understood mechanism activate the NALP3 inflammasome, a multiprotein complex that includes the protease caspase 1. The inflammasome-activated caspase 1, in turn, cleaves and activates several cytokines, most notably IL-1β and IL-18. IL-1β induces the expression of adhesion molecules and the synthesis of the neurophil chemokine CXCL8, which is essential for the localization of neutrophils at the site of acute inflammation. The neutrophils pour fuel on the fire by

---

TABLE 26–7   Classification of Gout

PRIMARY GOUT (90% OF CASES)

Overproduction of uric acid
  Diet
  Unknown enzyme defects (80% to 90%)
  Known enzyme defects (e.g., partial HGPRT deficiency, rare)
Reduced excretion of uric acid with normal production

SECONDARY GOUT (10% OF CASES)

Overproduction of uric acid with increased urinary excretion
  Increased nucleic acid turnover (e.g., leukemias and other aggressive neoplasms)
  Inborn errors of metabolism (e.g., complete HGPRT deficiency)
Reduced excretion of uric acid with normal production
  Chronic renal disease

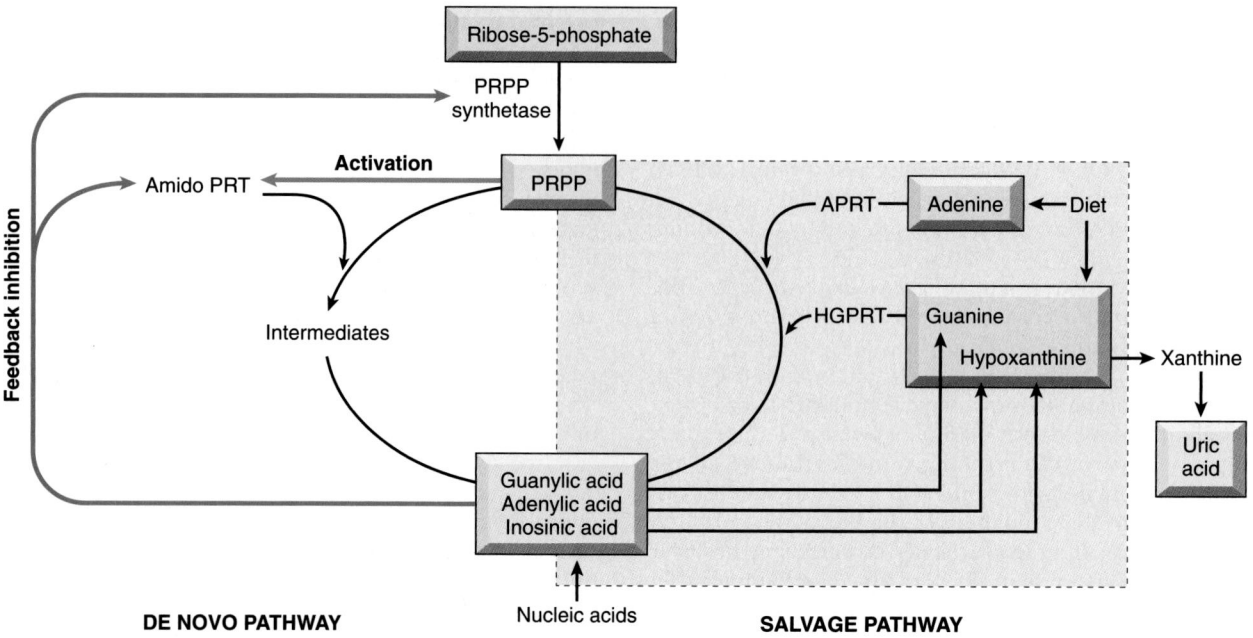

FIGURE 26–46 Purine metabolism. The conversion of PRPP to purine nucleotides is catalyzed by amido-PRT in the de novo pathway and by APRT and HGPRT in the salvage pathway. APRT, adenosine phosphoribosyltransferase; HGPRT, hypoxanthine-guanine phosphoribosyltransferase; PRPP, phosphoribosyl pyrophosphate; PRT, phosphoribosyltransferase.

releasing toxic free radicals, leukotrienes (leukotriene B4), and lysosomal enzymes. Thus comes about an acute arthritis, which typically remits spontaneously in days to weeks.[53] A scheme of these events is shown in Figure 26–47.

Repeated attacks of acute arthritis lead eventually to chronic arthritis and the formation of tophi in the inflamed synovial membranes and periarticular tissue, as well as elsewhere. In time, severe damage to the cartilage develops and the function of the joints is compromised. It is not known why the chronic arthritis is asymptomatic for intervals of days to months, even though crystals are undoubtedly present in abundance in the joints.

Morphology. The distinctive morphologic changes in gout are (1) acute arthritis, (2) chronic tophaceous arthritis, (3) tophi in various sites, and sometimes (4) gouty nephropathy. **Acute arthritis** is characterized by a dense neutrophilic infiltrate that permeates the synovium and synovial fluid. The MSU crystals are frequently found in the cytoplasm of the neutrophils and are arranged in small clusters in the synovium. They are long, slender, and needle shaped, and are negatively birefringent. The synovium is edematous and congested, and also contains scattered lymphocytes, plasma cells, and macrophages. When the episode of crystallization abates and the crystals are resolubilized, the acute attack remits.

Chronic tophaceous arthritis evolves from the repetitive precipitation of urate crystals during acute attacks. The urates may heavily encrust the articular surfaces and form visible deposits in the synovium (Fig. 26–48). The synovium becomes hyperplastic, fibrotic, and thickened by inflammatory cells and forms a pannus that destroys the underlying cartilage leading to juxta-articular bone erosions. In severe cases, fibrous or bony ankylosis ensues, resulting in partial to complete loss of joint function.

Tophi are the pathognomonic hallmark of gout. They are formed by large aggregations of urate crystals surrounded by an intense inflammatory reaction of macrophages, lymphocytes, and large foreign body giant cells, which may have completely or partially engulfed masses of crystals (Fig. 26–49). Tophi may appear in the articular cartilage of joints and in the periarticular ligaments, tendons, and soft tissues, including the olecranon and patellar bursae, Achilles tendons, and earlobes. Less frequently they may occur in the kidneys, nasal cartilages, skin of the fingertips, palms, soles, or elsewhere. Superficial tophi can ulcerate through the overlying skin.

Gouty nephropathy (Chapter 20) is associated with the deposition of MSU crystals in the renal medullary interstitium, sometimes forming tophi, intratubular precipitations, or free uric acid crystals, and the production of uric acid renal stones. Secondary complications, such as pyelonephritis, may ensue, particularly when the urates induce some urinary obstruction.

Clinical Course. The natural history of gout is said to have four stages: (1) asymptomatic hyperuricemia, (2) acute gouty arthritis, (3) intercritical gout, and (4) chronic tophaceous gout. *Asymptomatic hyperuricemia* appears around puberty in

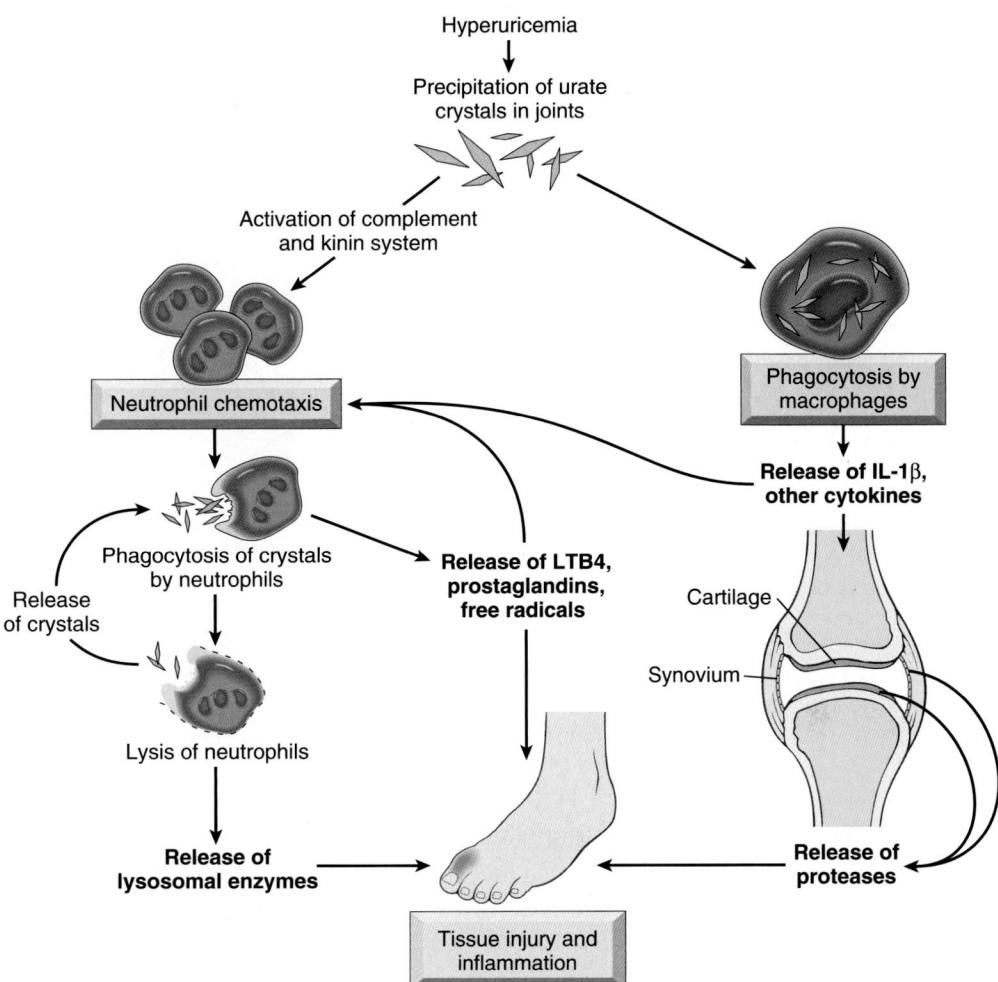

Hyperuricemia

Precipitation of urate
crystals in joints

Activation of complement
and kinin system

Neutrophil chemotaxis

Phagocytosis by
macrophages

**Release of IL-1β,
other cytokines**

Phagocytosis of crystals
by neutrophils

**Release of LTB4,
prostaglandins,
free radicals**

Release
of crystals

Cartilage

Synovium

Lysis of neutrophils

**Release of
lysosomal enzymes**

**Release of
proteases**

Tissue injury and
inflammation

FIGURE 26–47 Pathogenesis of acute gouty arthritis. LTB4, leukotriene B4.

males and after menopause in females. After many years *acute arthritis* appears in the form of the sudden onset of excruciating joint pain associated with localized hyperemia, warmth, and exquisite tenderness. Yet constitutional symptoms are uncommon except possibly mild fever. Most first attacks are monoarticular; 50% occur in the first metatarsophalangeal joint. Eventually, about 90% of affected individuals experience acute attacks in the following locations (in descending order of frequency): insteps, ankles, heels, knees, wrists, fingers, and elbows. Untreated, acute gouty arthritis may last for hours to

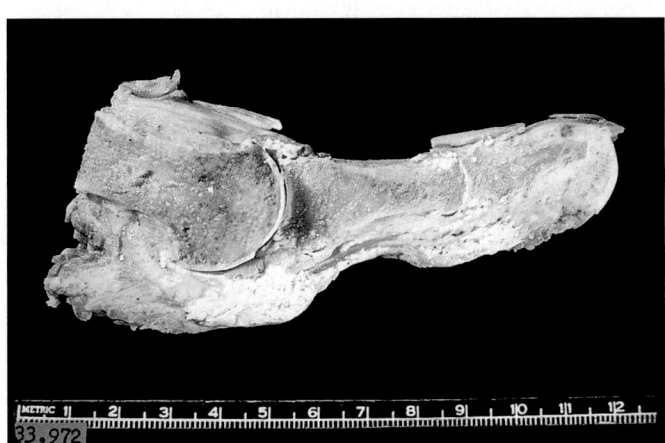

FIGURE 26–48 Amputated great toe with white tophi involving the joint and soft tissues.

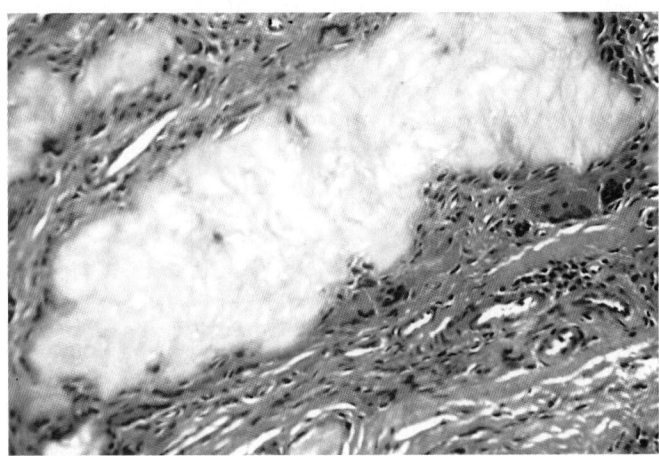

FIGURE 26–49 Photomicrograph of a gouty tophus. An aggregate of dissolved urate crystals is surrounded by reactive fibroblasts, mononuclear inflammatory cells, and giant cells.

weeks, but gradually there is complete resolution and the patient enters an *asymptomatic intercritical period*. Although some patients never have another attack, most experience a second acute episode within months to a few years. In the absence of appropriate therapy, the attacks recur at shorter intervals and frequently become polyarticular. Eventually, over the span of years, disabling *chronic tophaceous gout* develops. On average about 12 years pass between the initial acute attack and the appearance of chronic tophaceous arthritis. At this stage, radiograms show characteristic juxta-articular bone erosion caused by osteoclastic bone resorption and loss of the joint space. Progression leads to severe crippling disease.

Cardiovascular disease including atherosclerosis and hypertension is common in individuals with gout. Renal manifestations sometimes appear in the form of renal colic associated with the passage of gravel and stones and may proceed to chronic gouty nephropathy. About 20% of those with chronic gout die of renal failure. The diagnosis of gout should not be delayed, because numerous drugs are available to abort or prevent acute attacks of arthritis and mobilize tophaceous deposits. Their use is important, because many aspects of the disease are related to the duration and severity of the hyperuricemia. Generally, gout does not materially shorten the life span, but it may impair the quality of life.

Calcium Pyrophosphate Crystal Deposition Disease (Pseudo-Gout)

Calcium pyrophosphate crystal deposition disease (CPPD), also known as *pseudo-gout* and *chondrocalcinosis*, is one of the more common disorders associated with intra-articular crystal formation. It usually occurs in individuals over 50 years of age and becomes more common with increasing age, rising to a prevalence of 30% to 60% in those 85 years or older. The sexes and races are equally affected. CPPD is divided into sporadic (idiopathic), hereditary, and secondary types. In the hereditary variant the crystals develop relatively early in life and are associated with severe osteoarthritis. The autosomal dominant form of the disease is caused by germline mutations in the *ANKH* gene, which encodes a transmembrane pyrophosphate transport channel.[54] The secondary form is associated with various disorders, including previous joint damage, hyperparathyroidism, hemochromatosis, hypomagnesemia, hypothyroidism, ochronosis, and diabetes. The basis for crystal formation is not known; altered activity of the matrix enzymes that produce and degrade pyrophosphate is suspected.

> **Morphology.** The crystals first develop in the articular matrix, menisci, and intervertebral discs, and as the deposits enlarge they may rupture and seed the joint. Here, they are phagocytosed by macrophages, in which they activate the NALP3 inflammasome, eliciting a series of pro-inflammatory events similar or identical to those induced by urate crystals (Fig. 26–47). Neutrophils recruited by inflammatory media-

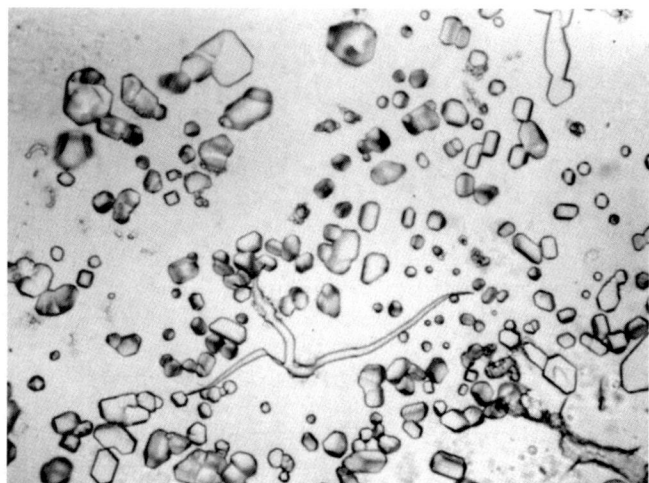

FIGURE 26–50 Smear preparation of calcium pyrophosphate crystals.

> tors are thought to produce damage through the release of reactive oxygen species, catabolic enzymes, and cytokines, calling forth the more chronic reactions associated with macrophages and fibrosis. The crystals form chalky white friable deposits, which are seen histologically in stained preparations as oval blue-purple aggregates. Individual crystals are generally 0.5 to 5 µm in greatest dimension, are weakly birefringent, and have geometric shapes (Fig. 26–50). Rarely the crystals are deposited in masslike aggregates simulating tophi.

CPPD is frequently asymptomatic; however, it also can produce acute, subacute, or chronic arthritis that can be confused with osteoarthritis or rheumatoid arthritis. The joint involvement may last from several days to weeks and may be monoarticular or polyarticular; the knees, followed by the wrists, elbows, shoulders, and ankles, are most commonly affected. Ultimately, approximately 50% of affected individuals experience significant joint damage. Therapy is supportive. There is no known treatment that prevents or retards crystal formation.

Tumors and Tumor-Like Lesions

Reactive tumor-like lesions, such as ganglions, synovial cysts, and osteochondral loose bodies, commonly involve joints and tendon sheaths. They usually result from trauma or degenerative processes and are much more common than neoplasms. Primary neoplasms are unusual and tend to recapitulate the cells and tissue types (synovial membrane, fat, blood vessels, fibrous tissue, and cartilage) native to joints and related structures. Benign tumors are much more frequent than their malignant counterparts, which are rare and discussed with the soft-tissue tumors.

GANGLION AND SYNOVIAL CYST

A *ganglion* is a small (1–1.5 cm) cyst that is almost always located near a joint capsule or tendon sheath. A common location is around the joints of the wrist, where it appears as a firm, fluctuant, pea-sized translucent nodule. It arises as a result of cystic or myxoid degeneration of connective tissue; hence the cyst wall lacks a true cell lining. The lesion may be multilocular and enlarges through coalescence of adjacent areas of myxoid change. The fluid that fills the cyst is similar to synovial fluid; however, there is no communication with the joint space.

Herniation of synovium through a joint capsule or massive enlargement of a bursa may produce a *synovial cyst*. A well-recognized example is the synovial cyst that forms in the popliteal space in the setting of rheumatoid arthritis (Baker cyst). The synovial lining may be hyperplastic and contain inflammatory cells and fibrin but is otherwise unremarkable.

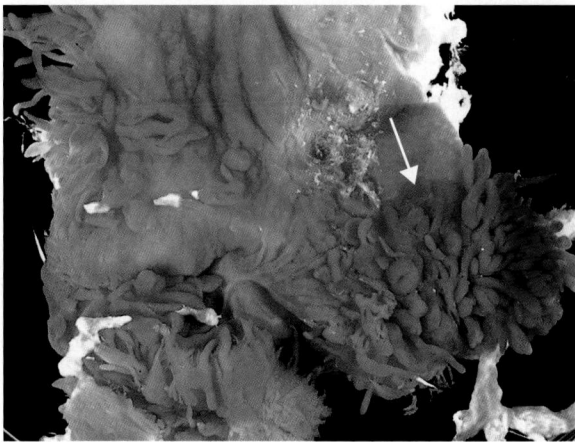

FIGURE 26–51 Excised synovium with fronds and nodules typical of pigmented villonodular synovitis *(arrow)*.

TENOSYNOVIAL GIANT-CELL TUMOR (LOCALIZED AND DIFFUSE)

Tenosynovial giant-cell tumor is the term for several closely related benign neoplasms that develop in the synovial lining of joints, tendon sheaths, and bursae. They harbor a consistent chromosomal translocation, t(1;2)(p13;q37), which fuses colony-stimulating factor 1 (CSF1) coding sequences to the promoter of the collagen type VI alpha-3 gene.[55] As a result, the tumor cells overexpress CSF1, a chemoattractant for macrophages, which infiltrate the tumor in large numbers. Variants of tenosynovial giant-cell tumor include the diffuse type (previously known as pigmented villonodular synovitis), and the localized type (also known as *giant-cell tumor of tendon sheath*). Whereas the diffuse form tends to involve one or more joints, the localized kind usually occurs as a discrete nodule attached to a tendon sheath, commonly of the hand. Both variants usually are diagnosed in the 20s to 40s and affect the sexes equally.

Diffuse tenosynovial giant-cell tumor usually presents in the knee in 80% of cases, followed in frequency by the hip, ankle, and calcaneocuboid joints. Affected individuals typically complain of pain, locking, and recurrent swelling. Tumor progression limits the range of movement of the joint and causes it to become stiff and firm. Sometimes a palpable mass is appreciated. Aggressive tumors erode into adjacent bones and soft tissues, causing confusion with other types of neoplasms. In contrast, the localized variant manifests as a solitary, slow-growing, painless mass that frequently involves the tendon sheaths along the wrists and fingers; it is the most common mesenchymal neoplasm of the hand. Cortical erosion of adjacent bone occurs in approximately 15% of cases. Surgery is the recommended treatment for both lesions; the diffuse tumors have a significant recurrence rate, because they are difficult to excise.

Morphology. Grossly, tenosynovial giant-cell tumors are red-brown to mottled orange-yellow. In diffuse tumors the normally smooth joint synovium is converted into a tangled mat by red-brown folds, finger-like projections, and nodules (Fig. 26–51). In contrast, localized tumors are well circumscribed and resemble a small walnut. The neoplastic cells, which account for only 2% to 16% of the cells in the mass, are polyhedral, moderately sized, and resemble synoviocytes (Fig. 26–52). In the diffuse variant they spread along the surface and infiltrate the subsynovial issue. In nodular tumors the cells grow in a solid aggregate that may be attached to the synovium by a pedicle. Both variants are heavily infiltrated by macrophages, which may contain hemosiderin and lipid-filled vacuoles, or coalesce into multinucleated giant cells.

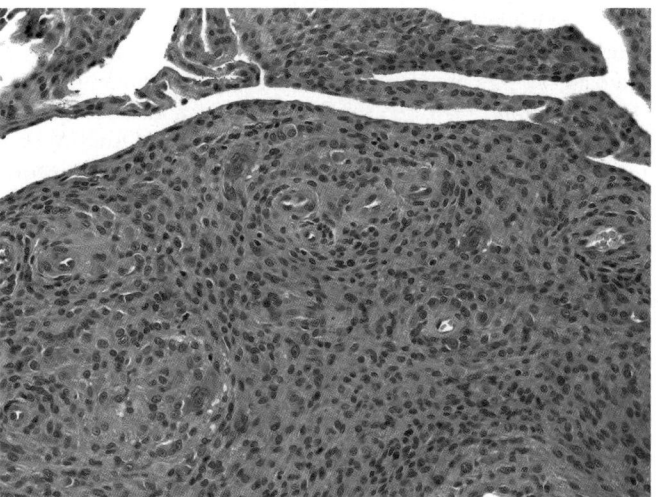

FIGURE 26–52 Sheets of proliferating cells in tenosynovial giant cell tumor bulging the synovial lining.

SOFT-TISSUE TUMORS AND TUMOR-LIKE LESIONS

Traditionally, soft-tissue tumors are defined as mesenchymal proliferations that occur in the extraskeletal, nonepithelial tissues of the body, excluding the viscera, coverings of the brain, and lymphoreticular system. They are classified according to the tissue they *recapitulate* (muscle, fat, fibrous tissue, vessels, and nerves) (Table 26–8), although there is little evidence that they actually arise from the normal differentiated counterpart. Some soft-tissue tumors have no normal tissue counterpart but have constant clinicopathologic features warranting their designation as distinct entities. The true frequency of soft-tissue tumors is difficult to estimate, because most benign lesions are not removed. A conservative estimate is that benign tumors outnumber their malignant counterparts (sarcomas) by a ratio of at least 100:1. In the United States, little more than 8000 sarcomas are diagnosed annually (0.8% of invasive malignancies), yet they are responsible for 2% of all cancer deaths, reflecting their lethal nature. In contrast to carcinomas, sarcomas usually metastasize via hematogenous routes, making the lung and skeleton common sites of dissemination.

Pathogenesis and General Features

The cause of most soft-tissue tumors is unknown. There are documented associations, however, with radiation therapy, and rare instances in which chemical burns, thermal burns, or trauma were associated with subsequent development of a sarcoma. Exposure to phenoxyherbicides and chlorophenols has also been implicated in some cases. Kaposi sarcoma is causally associated with the human herpesvirus 8; however, viruses are probably not important in the pathogenesis of most human sarcomas. The majority of soft-tissue tumors occur sporadically, but a small minority are associated with genetic syndromes, the most notable of which are neurofibromatosis type 1 (neurofibroma, malignant peripheral nerve sheath tumor), Gardner syndrome (fibromatosis), Li-Fraumeni syndrome (soft-tissue sarcoma), and Osler-Weber-Rendu syndrome (telangiectasia). Current evidence suggests that soft-tissue tumors develop due to mutations in mesenchymal stem cells that are widely distributed in the body. Some of the abnormalities, such as specific chromosomal translocations, produce fusion genes that encode chimeric transcription factors. How these abnormal transcription factors drive neoplastic transformation is not clear. These genetic events can be specific enough to serve as diagnostic markers in some tumors[56] (Table 26–9).

Soft-tissue tumors may arise in any location; approximately 40% occur in the lower extremity, especially the thigh, 20% in the upper extremities, 10% in the head and neck, and 30% in the trunk and retroperitoneum. Regarding sarcomas, males are affected more frequently than females (1.4:1), and the incidence generally increases with age. Fifteen percent arise in children, and they constitute the fourth most common malignancy in this age group, following brain tumors, hematopoietic cancers, and Wilms tumor in frequency. Specific sarcomas tend to appear in certain age groups (e.g., rhabdomyosarcoma in children, synovial sarcoma in young adulthood, and liposarcoma and fibrosarcoma in middle to late adult life).

Several features of soft-tissue tumors influence their prognosis:

● Accurate histologic classification is important in establishing the prognosis of a sarcoma. The cytologic appearance and the pattern of growth of tumor cells are helpful morphologic features (Tables 26–10 and 26–11), but these features are often not sufficient to arrive at a specific diagnosis. In such

TABLE 26–8   Soft-Tissue Tumors
TUMORS OF ADIPOSE TISSUE
Lipomas
Liposarcoma
TUMORS AND TUMOR-LIKE LESIONS OF FIBROUS TISSUE
Nodular fasciitis
Fibromatoses
Superficial fibromatoses
Deep fibromatoses
Fibrosarcoma
FIBROHISTIOCYTIC TUMORS
Fibrous histiocytoma
Dermatofibrosarcoma protuberans
Malignant fibrous histiocytoma
TUMORS OF SKELETAL MUSCLE
Rhabdomyoma
Rhabdomyosarcoma
TUMORS OF SMOOTH MUSCLE
Leiomyoma
Leiomyosarcoma
VASCULAR TUMORS
Hemangioma
Lymphangioma
Hemangioendothelioma
Angiosarcoma
PERIPHERAL NERVE TUMORS
Neurofibroma
Schwannoma
Granular cell tumor
Malignant peripheral nerve sheath tumors
TUMORS OF UNCERTAIN HISTOGENESIS
Synovial sarcoma
Alveolar soft-part sarcoma
Epithelioid sarcoma

TABLE 26–9 Chromosomal and Genetic Abnormalities in Soft-Tissue Sarcomas

Tumor	Cytogenetic Abnormality	Genetic Abnormality
Ewing sarcoma/Primitive neuroectodermal tumor	t(11;22)(q24;q12) t(21;22)(q22;q12) t(7;22)(q22;q12)	FLI1-EWS fusion gene ERG-EWS fusion gene ETV1-EWS fusion gene
Liposarcoma—myxoid and round-cell type	t(12;16)(q13;p11)	CHOP/TLS fusion gene
Synovial sarcoma	t(x;18)(p11;q11)	SYT-SSX fusion gene
Rhabdomyosarcoma—alveolar type	t(2;13)(q35;q14) t(1;13)(p36;q14)	PAX3-FKHR fusion gene PAX7-FKHR fusion gene
Extraskeletal myxoid chondrosarcoma	t(9;22)(q22;q12)	CHN-EWS fusion gene
Desmoplastic small round-cell tumor	t(11;22)(p13;q12)	EWS-WT1 fusion gene
Clear-cell sarcoma	t(12;22)(q13;q12)	EWS-ATF1 fusion gene
Dermatofibrosarcoma protuberans	t(17;22)(q22;q15)	COLA1-PDGFB fusion gene
Alveolar soft-part sarcoma	t(X;17)(p11.2;q25)	TFE3-ASPL fusion gene
Congenital fibrosarcoma	t(12;15)(p13;q23)	ETV6-NTRK3 fusion gene

cases other tests, particularly immunohistochemical stains and cytogenetic evaluation, are essential diagnostic aids.

○ For many types of soft-tissue sarcomas the histologic grade is important. Grading, usually I to III, is based on the degree of differentiation, the average number of mitoses per high-power field, cellularity, pleomorphism, and an estimate of the extent of necrosis (presumably a reflection of rate of growth).[57]

○ Staging helps determine the prognosis and chance of successful excision of a tumor. In the United States the American Joint Committee on Cancer (AJCC) staging system for soft-tissue sarcoma is utilized for treatment and is largely based on tumor size, location, depth, grade, and presence or absence of metastases.

○ In general, tumors arising in superficial locations (e.g., skin and subcutis) have a better prognosis than deep-seated lesions. In patients with deep-seated, high-grade sarcomas, metastatic disease develops in 80% of those with a tumor larger than 20 cm and 30% of those with a tumor larger than 5 cm. The overall 10-year survival rate for sarcomas is approximately 40%.

With this brief background, we now turn to the individual tumors and tumor-like lesions. Some of the soft-tissue tumors are presented elsewhere: tumors of peripheral nerve (Chapter 28); tumors of vascular origin, including Kaposi sarcoma (Chapter 11); and uterine tumors of smooth muscle origin (Chapter 22).

Fatty Tumors

LIPOMAS

Benign tumors of fat, known as lipomas, are the most common soft-tissue tumor of adulthood. They are subclassified according to particular morphologic features as conventional lipoma, fibrolipoma, angiolipoma, spindle cell lipoma, myelolipoma, and pleomorphic lipoma. Some of the variants have characteristic chromosomal abnormalities; for example, conventional lipomas often show rearrangements of 12q14–q15, 6p, and 13q, and spindle cell and pleomorphic lipomas have rearrangements of 16q and 13q.

Morphology. The conventional lipoma, the most common subtype, is a well-encapsulated mass of mature adipocytes that varies considerably in size. It

TABLE 26–10 Morphology of Cells in Soft Tissue Tumors

Cell Type	Features	Tumor Type
Spindle cell	Rod-shaped, long axis twice as great as short axis	Fibrous, fibrohistiocytic, smooth muscle, Schwann cell
Small round cell	Size of a lymphocyte with little cytoplasm	Rhabdomyosarcoma, primitive neuroectodermal tumor
Epithelioid	Polyhedral with abundant cytoplasm, nucleus is centrally located	Smooth muscle, Schwann cell endothelial, epithelioid sarcoma

TABLE 26–11 Architectural Patterns in Soft-Tissue Tumors

Pattern	Tumor Type
Fascicles of eosinophilic spindle cells intersecting at right angles	Smooth muscle
Short fascicles of spindle cells radiating from a central point like spokes on a wheel—storiform	Fibrohistiocytic
Nuclei arranged in columns—palisading	Schwann cell
Herringbone	Fibrosarcoma
Mixture of fascicles of spindle cells and groups of epithelioid cells—biphasic	Synovial sarcoma

arises in the subcutis of the proximal extremities and trunk, most frequently during middle adulthood. Infrequently, lipomas are large, intramuscular, and poorly circumscribed.

Lipomas are soft, mobile, and painless (except angiolipoma) and are usually cured by simple excision.

LIPOSARCOMA

Liposarcomas are one of the most common sarcomas of adulthood and appear in the 40s to 60s; they are rare in children. They usually arise in the deep soft tissues of the proximal extremities and retroperitoneum, and are notorious for developing into large tumors.

Morphology. Liposarcomas are histologically divided into well-differentiated, myxoid/round cell, and pleomorphic variants. The cells in well-differentiated liposarcomas are readily recognized as lipocytes, and the tumor cells frequently contain supernumerary rings and giant rod chromosomes due to amplification of the 12q14–q15 region containing the *MDM2* oncogene. This, you may recall, inhibits p53 (Chapter 7). In the other variants, most of the tumor cells are not obviously adipogenic, but some cells indicative of fatty differentiation are almost always present. These cells are known as **lipoblasts**; they mimic fetal fat cells and contain round clear cytoplasmic vacuoles of lipid that scallop the nucleus (Fig. 26–53). The myxoid/round cell variant of liposarcoma has a t(12;16)(q13;p11) chromosomal abnormality in most cases.

The well-differentiated variant is relatively indolent, the myxoid/round cell type is intermediate in its malignant behavior, and the pleomorphic variant usually is aggressive and frequently metastasizes. All types of liposarcoma recur locally and often repeatedly unless adequately excised.

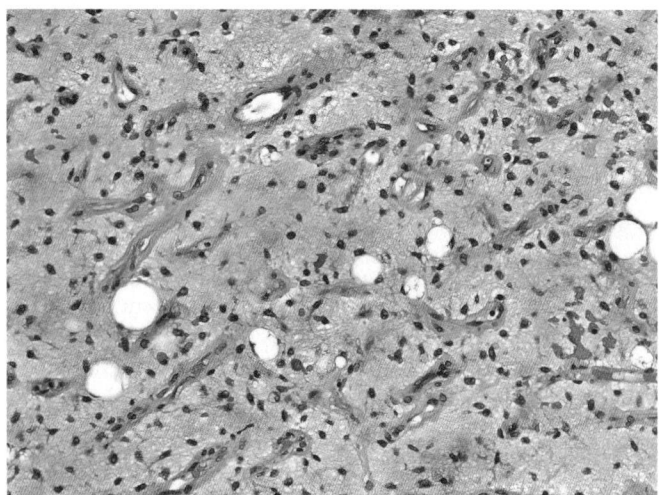

FIGURE 26–53 Myxoid liposarcoma with abundant ground substance in which are scattered adult-appearing fat cells and more primitive cells, some containing small lipid vacuoles (lipoblasts).

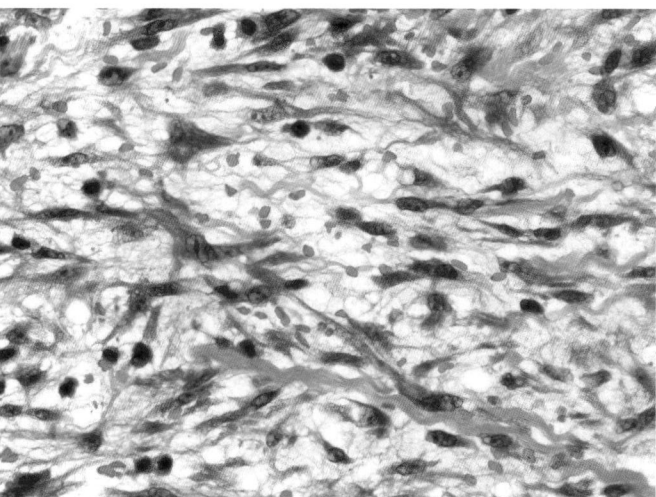

FIGURE 26–54 Nodular fasciitis with plump, randomly oriented spindle cells surrounded by myxoid stroma. Note the mitotic activity and extravasated red blood cells.

Fibrous Tumors and Tumor-Like Lesions

REACTIVE PSEUDOSARCOMATOUS PROLIFERATIONS

Reactive pseudosarcomatous proliferations are nonneoplastic lesions that either develop in response to some form of local trauma (physical or ischemic) or are idiopathic. They are composed of plump reactive fibroblasts and related mesenchymal cells. Clinically they are alarming, because they develop suddenly and grow rapidly. Histologically they cause concern, because their hypercellularity, mitotic activity, and primitive appearance mimic sarcoma. Representative of this family of lesions are *nodular fasciitis* and *myositis ossificans*.

Nodular Fasciitis

Nodular fasciitis, also known as *infiltrative* or *pseudosarcomatous fasciitis*, is the most common of the reactive pseudosarcomas. It most often occurs in adults on the volar aspect of the forearm, followed in order of frequency by the chest and back. Affected individuals typically present with a several-week history of a solitary, rapidly growing, and sometimes painful mass. Preceding trauma is reported in only 10% to 15% of cases.

Morphology. Nodular fasciitis arises in the deep dermis, subcutis, or muscle. Grossly the lesion is several centimeters in greatest dimension, is nodular in configuration, and has poorly defined margins. The lesion is richly cellular and contains plump, immature-appearing fibroblasts and myofibroblasts arranged randomly or in short intersecting fascicles (Fig. 26–54). The cells vary in size and shape (spindle to stellate) and have conspicuous nucleoli; mitotic figures are abundant. Frequently the stroma is myxoid and contains lymphocytes and extravasated red blood cells. The histologic differential is extensive, but important lesions that must be excluded are fibromatosis and spindle cell sarcomas. Nodular fasciitis rarely recurs after excision.

Myositis Ossificans

Myositis ossificans is distinguished from the other reactive fibroblastic proliferations by the presence of *metaplastic bone*. It usually develops in athletic adolescents and young adults and follows an episode of trauma in more than 50% of cases. The lesion typically arises in the musculature of the proximal extremities. The clinical findings are related to its stage of development; in the early phase the involved area is swollen and painful, and during the subsequent several weeks it becomes more circumscribed and firm. Eventually, it evolves into a painless, hard, well-demarcated mass.

> **Morphology.** Grossly the usual lesion is 3 to 6 cm in greatest dimension and well-demarcated. Initially, the lesion is cellular and consists of plump, elongated fibroblast and myofibroblast-like cells simulating nodular fasciitis (see earlier). In due course these cells are surrounded by an intermediate zone that contains osteoblasts, which deposit ill-defined trabeculae of woven bone. The most peripheral zone contains well-formed, mineralized trabeculae that closely resemble cancellous bone. Eventually the entire lesion ossifies, and the intertrabecular spaces become filled with bone marrow. The mature lesion is completely ossified.

The radiographic findings parallel the morphologic progression. Initially, X-rays may show only soft-tissue fullness, but at about 3 weeks patchy flocculent radiodensities form in the periphery. The radiodensities become more extensive with time and slowly encroach on the radiolucent center (Fig. 26–55). Myositis ossificans must be distinguished from extraskeletal osteosarcoma. The latter usually occurs in elderly patients, the proliferating cells are cytologically malignant, and the tumor lacks the zonation of myositis ossificans. Simple excision of myositis ossificans is usually curative.

FIBROMATOSES

Superficial Fibromatosis (Palmar, Plantar, and Penile Fibromatoses)

Palmar, plantar, and penile fibromatoses, lesions that are more bothersome than serious, constitute a small group of superficial fibromatoses. They are characterized by nodular or poorly defined broad fascicles of fibroblasts and myofibroblasts surrounded by abundant dense collagen. The molecular mechanisms underlying superficial fibromatoses are unknown, but they are different from their deep-seated counterparts.

In the palmar variant *(Dupuytren contracture)* there is irregular or nodular thickening of the palmar fascia either unilaterally or bilaterally (50%). Over a span of years, attachment to

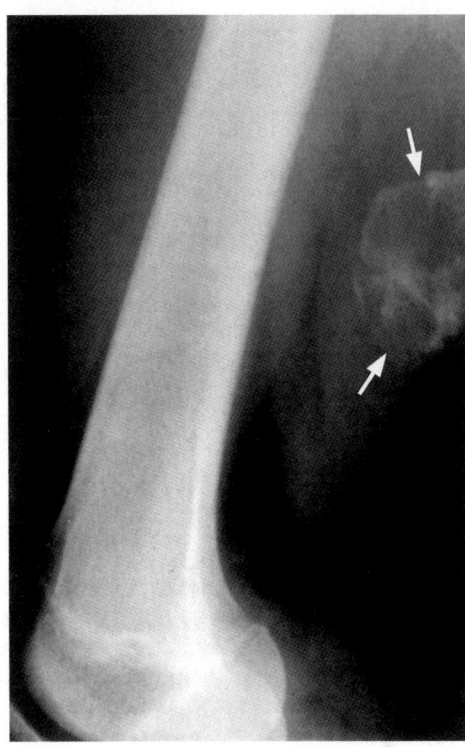

FIGURE 26–55 Peripherally mineralized myositis ossificans *(arrows)* involving the posterior thigh.

the overlying skin causes puckering and dimpling. At the same time a slowly progressive flexion contracture develops that mainly affects the fourth and fifth fingers of the hand. Essentially similar changes are seen with *plantar fibromatosis* except that flexion contractures are uncommon and bilateral involvement is infrequent. In *penile fibromatosis (Peyronie disease)* a palpable induration or mass appears, usually on the dorsolateral aspect of the penis. Eventually, it may cause abnormal curvature of the shaft, constriction of the urethra, or both.

All forms of superficial fibromatosis affect males more frequently than females. In about 20% to 25% of cases, the palmar and plantar fibromatoses stabilize and do not progress, in some instances resolving spontaneously. Some recur after excision, particularly the plantar variant.

Deep-Seated Fibromatosis (Desmoid Tumors)

Deep-seated fibromatoses lie in a gray zone between benign fibrous tumors and low-grade fibrosarcomas. On the one hand, they often present as large, infiltrative masses that frequently recur after incomplete excision; on the other, they are composed of banal well-differentiated fibroblasts that do not metastasize. They may occur at any age but are most frequent in the teens to 30s. Deep-seated fibromatosis is divided into *extra-abdominal, abdominal,* and *intra-abdominal* types, but all have similar gross and microscopic features. Extra-abdominal fibromatosis occurs in men and women with equal frequency and arises principally in the musculature of the shoulder, chest wall, back, and thigh. Abdominal fibromatosis generally arises in the musculoaponeurotic structures of the anterior abdominal wall in women during or after pregnancy. Intra-abdominal fibromatosis tends to occur in the mesentery

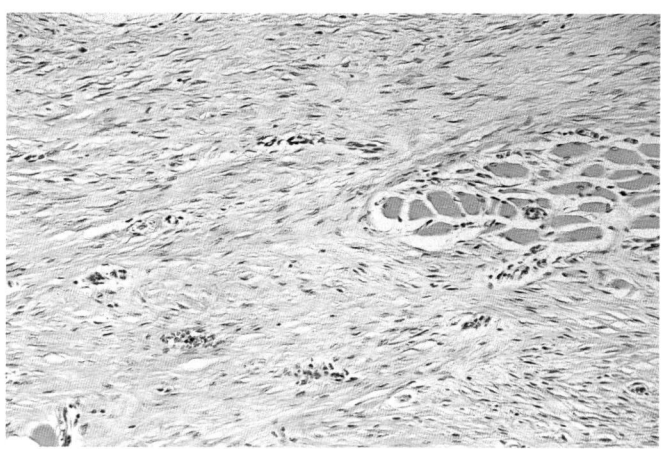

FIGURE 26–56 Fibromatosis infiltrating between skeletal muscle cells.

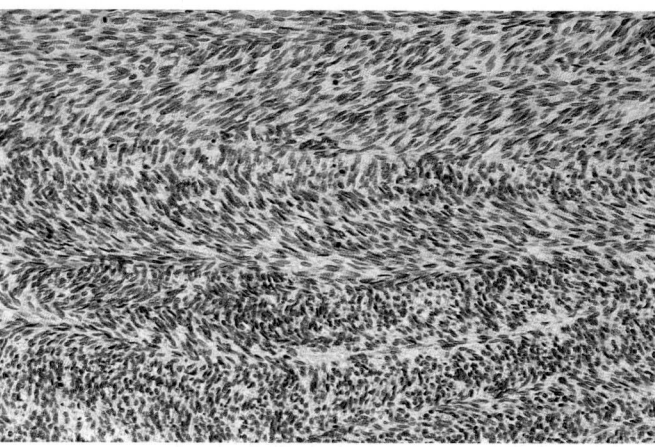

FIGURE 26–57 Fibrosarcoma composed of malignant spindle cells arranged in a herringbone pattern.

or pelvic walls, often in individuals having familial adenomatous polyposis (Gardner syndrome) (Chapter 17). Mutations in the *APC* or β-catenin genes are present in the majority of these tumors (whether or not the affected individuals have underlying Gardner syndrome) and have an important role in their genesis.

> **Morphology.** These tumors occur as gray-white, firm, poorly demarcated masses varying from 1 to 15 cm in greatest diameter. They are rubbery and tough, and infiltrate surrounding structures. Histologically deep-seated fibromatosis is composed of plump banal fibroblasts arranged in broad sweeping fascicles that infiltrate the adjacent tissue (Fig. 26–56). Mitoses may be frequent. Regenerative muscle cells when trapped within these lesions may take on the appearance of multinucleated giant cells.

In addition to possibly being disfiguring or disabling, deep-seated fibromatosis is occasionally painful. Although curable by adequate excision, these lesions frequently recur locally and persistently when incompletely removed. Some tumors have responded to treatment with tamoxifen, and in other cases chemotherapy or irradiation has been effective. The rare reports of metastasis of fibromatosis must be interpreted as misdiagnosis of fibrosarcoma.

FIBROSARCOMA

Fibrosarcomas occur anywhere in the body, but are most common in the deep soft tissues of the extremities. Many tumors previously considered fibrosarcoma have been reclassified based on immunohistochemistry or cytogenetic findings as fibromatosis (desmoid), malignant peripheral nerve sheath tumors, or monophasic synovial sarcomas.

> **Morphology.** Typically these neoplasms are unencapsulated, infiltrative, soft, fish-flesh masses often having areas of hemorrhage and necrosis. Better differentiated lesions may appear deceptively encapsu-

lated. Histologic examination discloses all degrees of differentiation, from slowly growing tumors that closely resemble cellular fibromatosis and sometimes having spindled cells growing in a herringbone fashion (Fig. 26–57), to highly cellular neoplasms dominated by architectural disarray, pleomorphism, frequent mitoses, and areas of necrosis (Fig. 26–58).

Fibrosarcomas are aggressive tumors, recurring in more than 50% of cases and metastasizing in more than 25%.

Fibrohistiocytic Tumors

Fibrohistiocytic tumors contain cellular elements that resemble both fibroblasts and histiocytes (macrophages). The phenotype of the neoplastic cells most closely resembles fibroblasts, and the term *fibrohistiocytic* should be viewed as descriptive in nature and not one that connotes the cell of origin.

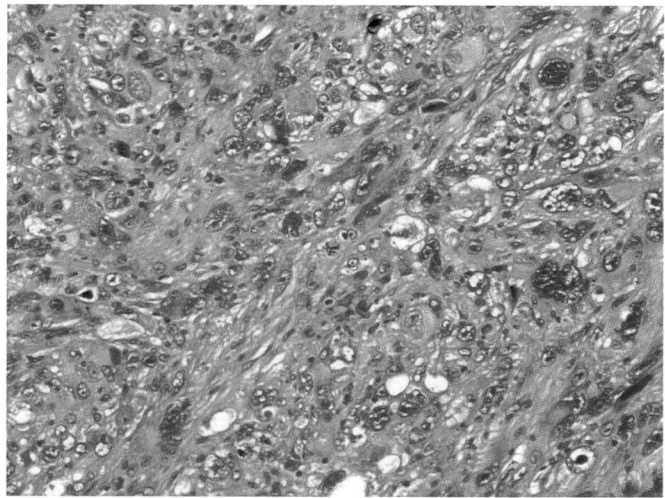

FIGURE 26–58 Pleomorphic fibrosarcoma revealing fascicles of plump spindled cells in a swirling (storiform) pattern, typical but not pathognomonic of this neoplasm.

BENIGN FIBROUS HISTIOCYTOMA (DERMATOFIBROMA)

Benign fibrous histiocytoma is a relatively common lesion that usually occurs in the dermis and subcutis. It is painless and slow growing, and most often presents in mid-adult life as a firm, small (≤1 cm) mobile nodule. Its morphologic features are described in Chapter 25.

MALIGNANT FIBROUS HISTIOCYTOMA

Once considered the most common sarcoma of adults, *malignant fibrous histiocytoma* referred to a group of soft-tissue tumors characterized by considerable cytologic pleomorphism, the presence of bizarre multinucleate cells, and storiform architecture. The phenotype of the neoplastic cell is now recognized to be fibroblastic and as a result malignant fibrous histiocytoma is being dropped as a diagnostic entity. Tumors previously diagnosed as malignant fibrous histiocytoma are currently classified as variants of fibrosarcoma (myxofibrosarcoma, pleomorphic fibrosarcoma, etc.) and other tumor types.

Tumors of Skeletal Muscle

Skeletal muscle neoplasms, in contrast to other groups of tumors, are almost all malignant. The benign variant, rhabdomyoma, is distinctly rare. The so-called cardiac rhabdomyoma is frequently seen in individuals with tuberous sclerosis and is discussed in Chapter 12.

RHABDOMYOSARCOMA

Rhabdomyosarcoma, the most common soft-tissue sarcoma of childhood and adolescence, usually appears before age 20. It may arise in any anatomic location, but most occur in the head and neck or genitourinary tract, where there is little if any skeletal muscle as a normal constituent. Only in the extremities do they appear in relation to skeletal muscle.

> **Morphology.** Rhabdomyosarcoma is histologically subclassified into **embryonal, alveolar**, and **pleomorphic** variants. The rhabdomyoblast—the diagnostic cell in all types—contains eccentric eosinophilic granular cytoplasm rich in thick and thin filaments. Rhabdomyoblasts may be round or elongate; the latter are known as tadpole or strap cells, and may contain cross-striations visible by light microscopy (Fig. 26–59). Ultrastructurally, rhabdomyoblasts contain sarcomeres, and immunohistochemically they stain with antibodies to the myogenic markers desmin, MYOD1, and myogenin.
>
> **Embryonal rhabdomyosarcoma** is the most common type, accounting for 60% of rhabdomyosarcomas. It includes the **sarcoma botryoides**, described in Chapter 22, as well as spindle cell and anaplastic variants. The tumor occurs in children younger than 10 years of age and typically arises in the nasal cavity, orbit, middle ear, prostate, and paratesticular region. This variant of rhabdomyosarcoma commonly has parental isodi-

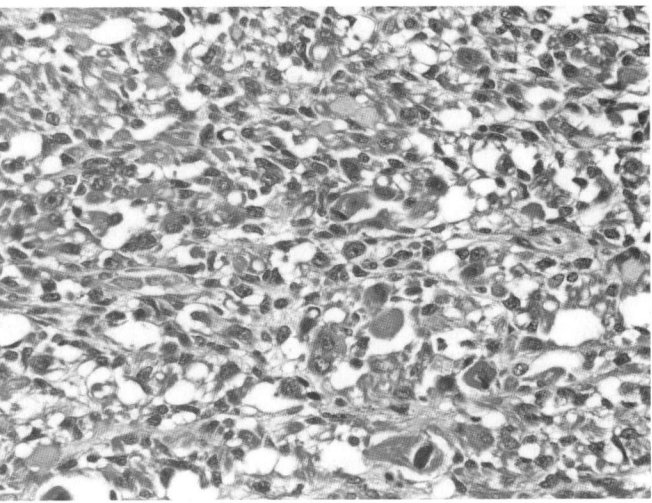

FIGURE 26–59 Rhabdomyosarcoma composed of malignant small round cells. The rhabdomyoblasts are large and round, and have abundant eosinophilic cytoplasm; no cross-striations are evident.

> somy of chromosome 11p15.5, which leads to overexpression of the imprinted *IGFII* gene.[58] The sarcoma botryoides subtype develops in the walls of hollow, mucosal-lined structures, such as the nasopharynx, common bile duct, bladder, and vagina. Where the tumors abut the mucosa of an organ, they form a submucosal zone of hypercellularity called the **cambium layer**.
>
> Most embryonal rhabdomyosarcomas present as a soft gray infiltrative mass. The tumor cells mimic skeletal muscle at various stages of embryogenesis and consist of sheets of both round and spindled cells in a myxoid stroma. Rhabdomyoblasts with visible cross-striations may be present.
>
> **Alveolar rhabdomyosarcoma** tends to develop in early to middle adolescence, commonly arises in the deep musculature of the extremities, and represents approximately 20% of rhabdomyosarcomas. Histologically the tumor is traversed by a network of fibrous septae that divide the cells into clusters or aggregates that creates a crude resemblance to pulmonary alveolae (Fig. 26–60). The tumor cells are moderate in size, and many have little cytoplasm. Those in the center of the aggregates are dyscohesive, while those at the periphery adhere to the septae. Cells with cross-striations are identified in about 25% of cases. Cytogenetic studies have shown that this variant of rhabdomyosarcoma has a chromosomal translocation that either fuses the *PAX3* to the *FOXO1a* gene, t(2,13)(q35;q14) or the *PAX7* to the *FOXO1a* gene, t(1;13)(p36;q14).[58] Tumors with the *PAX3-FOXO1a* fusion gene are more aggressive and associated with a worse prognosis.
>
> **Pleomorphic rhabdomyosarcoma** is characterized by numerous large, sometimes multinucleated, bizarre eosinophilic tumor cells. This variant is rare, has a tendency to arise in the deep soft tissue of adults, and can resemble other pleomorphic sarcomas histologically.

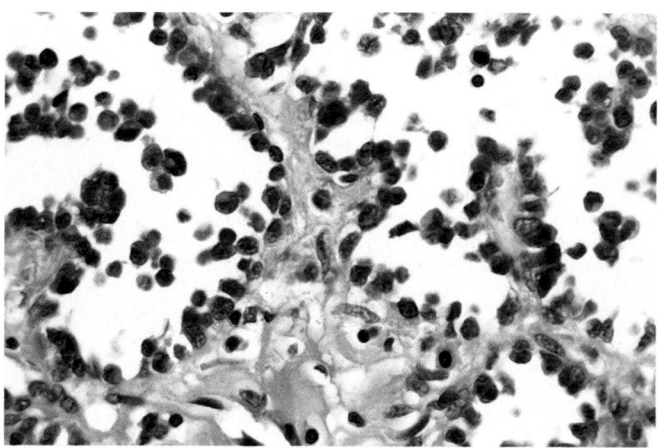

FIGURE 26–60 Alveolar rhabdomyosarcoma with numerous spaces lined by tumor cells.

Rhabdomyosarcomas are aggressive neoplasms that are usually treated with surgery and chemotherapy with or without radiation therapy. The histologic type and location of the tumor influence survival. The botryoid subtype has the best prognosis, while the anaplastic embryonal, pleomorphic, and alveolar variants are often fatal.

Tumors of Smooth Muscle

LEIOMYOMAS

Leiomyomas, the benign smooth muscle tumors, often arise in the uterus; in fact, uterine leiomyomas are the most common neoplasm in women (Chapter 22). They develop in 77% of women and, depending on their number, size, and location, may cause a variety of symptoms including infertility. Leiomyomas may also arise from the arrector pili muscles found in the skin, nipples, scrotum, and labia and less frequently develop in the deep soft tissues and the wall of the gut. Those arising in the arrector muscles (*pilar leiomyomas*) may be multiple and painful. The phenotype of multiple cutaneous leiomyomas, in some individuals, is transmitted as an autosomal dominant trait and is associated with uterine leiomyomas and a predisposition to develop renal cell carcinoma— hereditary leiomyomatosis and renal cell cancer syndrome. This disorder is associated with a germline loss-of-function mutation in the fumarate hydratase gene located on chromosome 1q42.3.

Leiomyomas are usually not larger than 1 to 2 cm in greatest dimension and are composed of fascicles of spindle cells that tend to intersect each other at right angles. The tumor cells have blunt-ended, elongated nuclei and show minimal atypia and few mitotic figures. Solitary lesions are easily cured; however, multiple tumors may be so numerous that complete surgical removal is impractical.

LEIOMYOSARCOMA

Leiomyosarcomas account for 10% to 20% of soft-tissue sarcomas. They occur in adults and afflict women more frequently than men. Most develop in the skin and deep soft tissues of the extremities and retroperitoneum.

Morphology. Leiomyosarcomas present as painless firm masses. Retroperitoneal tumors may be large and bulky and cause abdominal symptoms. Histologically they consist of malignant spindle cells with cigar-shaped nuclei arranged in interweaving fascicles. Ultrastructurally, malignant smooth muscle cells contain bundles of thin filaments with dense bodies and pinocytic vesicles, and individual cells are surrounded by basal lamina. Immunohistochemically, they stain with antibodies to smooth muscle actin and desmin.

Treatment depends on the size, location, and grade. Superficial or cutaneous leiomyosarcomas are usually small and have a good prognosis, whereas those of the retroperitoneum are large, cannot be entirely excised, and cause death by both local extension and metastatic spread.

Synovial Sarcoma

Synovial sarcoma is so named because it was once believed to recapitulate synovium, but the cell of origin is still unclear. In addition, although the term *synovial sarcoma* implies an origin from the joint linings, less than 10% are intra-articular. Synovial sarcomas account for approximately 10% of all soft-tissue sarcomas and rank as the fourth most common sarcoma. Most occur in the 20s to 40s. The majority develop in the deep soft tissue and about 60% to 70% involve the lower extremity, especially around the knee and thigh. Patients usually present with a deep-seated mass that has been noted for several years. Uncommonly, these tumors occur in the head and neck or in viscera.

Morphology. Synovial sarcomas are morphologically biphasic or monophasic. The histologic hallmark of biphasic synovial sarcoma is dual lines of differentiation (i.e., epithelial-like and mesenchymal-like). The epithelial cells are cuboidal to columnar and form glands or grow in solid cords or aggregates. The spindle cells are arranged in densely cellular fascicles that surround the epithelial cells (Fig. 26–61). Many synovial sarcomas are *monophasic*, being composed of only spindled cells or, very rarely, epithelial cells. Lesions composed solely of spindled cells are easily mistaken for fibrosarcomas or malignant peripheral nerve sheath tumors. A characteristic feature when present is calcified concretions that can sometimes be detected radiographically. Immunohistochemistry is helpful in identifying these tumors, since the tumor cells yield positive reactions for keratin and epithelial membrane antigen, differentiating them from most other sarcomas. In addition, most synovial sarcomas show a characteristic chromosomal translocation t(x;18)(p11;q11) producing *SS18-SSX1, SSX2*, or *SSX4* fusion genes that encode chimeric transcription factors.[59] The specific type of translocation in synovial sarcoma has not been shown to be related to prognosis.

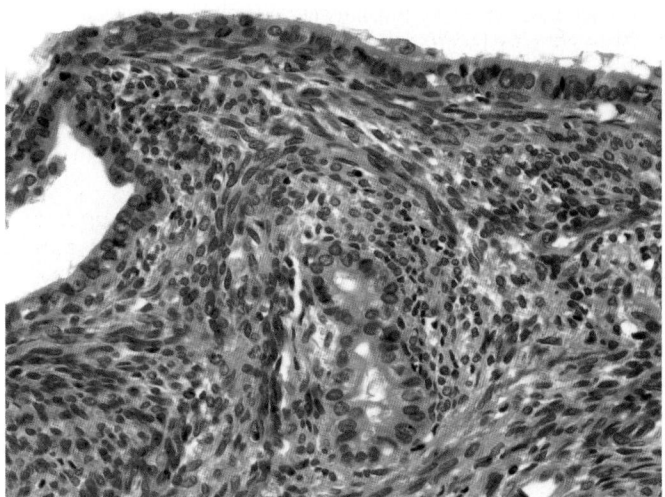

FIGURE 26-61 Synovial sarcoma revealing the classic biphasic spindle cell and glandular-like histologic appearance.

Synovial sarcomas are treated aggressively with limb-sparing therapy and frequently chemotherapy. The 5-year survival varies from 25% to 62%, and only 11% to 30% live for 10 years or longer. Common sites of metastases are the lung, skeleton, and occasionally the regional lymph nodes.

REFERENCES

1. Glimcher M: Metabolic Bone Disease and Clinical Related Disorders, 2nd ed. Philadelphia, WB Saunders, 1990.
2. Baron R, Rawadi G: Targeting the Wnt/beta-catenin pathway to regulate bone formation in the adult skeleton. Endocrinology 148:2635, 2007.
3. Day TF, Yang Y: Wnt and hedgehog signaling pathways in bone development. J Bone Joint Surg Am 90 (Suppl 1):19, 2008.
4. Cirmanova V et al.: The effect of leptin on bone—an evolving concept of action. Physiol Res 57 (Suppl 1):S143, 2008.
5. Kogianni G, Noble BS: The biology of osteocytes. Curr Osteoporos Rep 5:81, 2007.
6. Robling AG et al.: Mechanical stimulation of bone in vivo reduces osteocyte expression of Sost/sclerostin. J Biol Chem 283:5866, 2008.
7. Asagiri M, Takayanagi H: The molecular understanding of osteoclast differentiation. Bone 40:251, 2007.
8. Cohen MM: The new bone biology: pathology, molecular, and clinical correlates. Am J Med Genet 140A:2646, 2006.
9. Boyce BF, Xing L: Biology of RANK, RANKL, and osteoprotegerin. Arthritis Res Ther 9 (Suppl 1):S1, 2007.
10. Young MF et al.: Structure, expression, and regulation of the major noncollagenous matrix proteins of bone. Clin Orthop Relat Res 281:275, 1992.
11. Raisz LG: Physiology and pathophysiology of bone remodeling. Clin Chem 45:1353, 1999.
12. Olsen BR et al.: Bone development. Annu Rev Cell Dev Biol 16:191, 2000.
13. Zaidi M: Skeletal remodeling in health and disease. Nat Med 13:791, 2007.
14. Hartmann C: Skeletal development—Wnts are in control. Mol Cell 24:177, 2007.
15. Alman BA: Skeletal dysplasias and the growth plate. Clin Genet 73:24, 2008.
16. Mundlos S, Olsen BR: Heritable diseases of the skeleton. Part I: Molecular insights into skeletal development—transcription factors and signaling pathways. FASEB J 11:125, 1997.
17. Mundlos S, Olsen BR: Heritable diseases of the skeleton. Part II: Molecular insights into skeletal development—matrix components and their homeostasis. FASEB J 11:227, 1997.
18. Superti-Furga A et al.: Molecular-pathogenetic classification of genetic disorders of the skeleton. Am J Med Genet 106:282, 2001.
19. Marini JC et al.: Consortium for osteogenesis imperfecta mutations in the helical domain of type I collagen: regions rich in lethal mutations align with collagen binding sites for integrins and proteoglycans. Hum Mutat 28:209, 2007.
20. Martin E, Shapiro JR: Osteogenesis imperfecta:epidemiology and pathophysiology. Curr Osteoporos Rep 5:91, 2007.
21. Askmyr MK et al.: Towards a better understanding and new therapeutics of osteopetrosis. Br J Haematol 140:597, 2008.
22. Carbonell Sala S, Brandi ML: 2006 update on genetic determinants of osteoporosis. J Endocrinol Invest 30:2, 2007.
23. Mosekilde L: Mechanisms of age-related bone loss. Novartis Found Symp 235:150, 2001.
24. Styrkarsdottir U et al.: Multiple genetic loci for bone mineral density and fractures. N Engl J Med 358:2355, 2008.
25. Layfield R: The molecular pathogenesis of Paget disease of bone. Expert Rev Mol Med 9:1, 2007.
26. Whyte MP: Clinical practice. Paget's disease of bone. N Engl J Med 355:593, 2006.
27. Schwarz C et al.: Diagnosis of renal osteodystrophy. Eur J Clin Invest 36 (Suppl 2):13, 2006.
28. Giannoudis PV et al.: Fracture healing: the diamond concept. Injury 38 (Suppl 4):S3, 2007.
29. Lafforgue P: Pathophysiology and natural history of avascular necrosis of bone. Joint Bone Spine 73:500, 2006.
30. Kaplan SL: Osteomyelitis in children. Infect Dis Clin North Am 19:787, vii, 2005.
31. Calhoun JH, Manring MM: Adult osteomyelitis. Infect Dis Clin North Am 19:765, 2005.
32. Gardam M, Lim S: Mycobacterial osteomyelitis and arthritis. Infect Dis Clin North Am 19:819, 2005.
33. Lee EH et al.: Osteoid osteoma: a current review. J Pediatr Orthop 26:695, 2006.
34. Klein MJ, Siegal GP: Osteosarcoma: anatomic and histologic variants. Am J Clin Pathol 125:555, 2006.
35. Kansara M, Thomas DM: Molecular pathogenesis of osteosarcoma. DNA Cell Biol 26:1, 2007.
36. Ramappa AJ et al.: Chondroblastoma of bone. J Bone Joint Surg Am 82A:1140, 2000.
37. Chow WA: Update on chondrosarcomas. Curr Opin Oncol 19:371, 2007.
38. Weinstein LS: G(s)alpha mutations in fibrous dysplasia and McCune-Albright syndrome. J Bone Miner Res 21 (Suppl 2):P120, 2006.
39. Khoury JD: Ewing sarcoma family of tumors: a model for the new era of integrated laboratory diagnostics. Expert Rev Mol Diagn 8:97, 2008.
40. Ludwig JA: Ewing sarcoma: historical perspectives, current state-of-the-art, and opportunities for targeted therapy in the future. Curr Opin Oncol 20:412, 2008.
41. Nielson TO: Microarray analysis of sarcomas. Adv Anat Pathol 13:166, 2006.
42. Werner M: Giant cell tumour of bone: morphological, biological and histogenetical aspects. Int Orthop 30:484, 2006.
43. Oliveira AM et al.: Aneurysmal bone cyst variant translocations upregulate USP6 transcription by promoter swapping with the ZNF9, COL1A1, TRAP150, and OMD genes. Oncogene 24:3419, 2005.
44. Valdes AM, Spector TD: The contribution of genes to osteoarthritis. Med Clin North Am 93:45, 2009.
45. Goldring MB, Goldring SR: Osteoarthritis. J Cell Physiol 213:626, 2007.
46. Lundy SK et al.: Cells of the synovium in rheumatoid arthritis. T lymphocytes. Arthritis Res Ther 9:202, 2007.
47. Andersson AK et al.: Recent developments in the immunobiology of rheumatoid arthritis. Arthritis Res Ther 10:204, 2008.
48. Imboden JB: The immunopathogenesis of rheumatoid arthritis. Ann Rev Pathol Mech Dis 4:417, 2009.
49. Brown MA: Breakthroughs in genetic studies of ankylosing spondylitis. Rheumatology (Oxford) 47:132, 2008.
50. Turkiewicz AM, Moreland LW: Psoriatic arthritis: current concepts on pathogenesis-oriented therapeutic options. Arthritis Rheum 56:1051, 2007.
51. Drouin EE et al.: Human homologues of a Borrelia T cell epitope associated with antibiotic-refractory Lyme arthritis. Mol Immunol 45:180, 2008.
52. Rulli NE et al.: The molecular and cellular aspects of arthritis due to alphavirus infections: lesson learned from Ross River virus. Ann N Y Acad Sci 1102:96, 2007.

53. Choi HK et al.: Pathogenesis of gout. Ann Intern Med 143:499, 2005.

54. Rosenthal AK: Update in calcium deposition diseases. Curr Opin Rheumatol 19:158, 2007.

55. Moller E et al.: Molecular identification of *COL6A3-CSF1* fusion transcripts in tenosynovial giant cell tumors. Genes Chromosomes Cancer 47:21, 2008.

56. Riggi N et al.: Sarcomas: genetics, signalling, and cellular origins. Part 1: The fellowship of TET. J Pathol 213:4, 2007.

57. Rubin BP, Goldblum JR. Pathology of soft tissue sarcoma. J Natl Compr Canc Netw 5:411, 2007.

58. Paulino AC, Okcu MF. Rhabdomyosarcoma. Curr Probl Cancer 32:7, 2008.

59. de Bruijn DR et al.: The (epi)genetics of human synovial sarcoma. Genes Chromosomes Cancer 46:107, 2007.

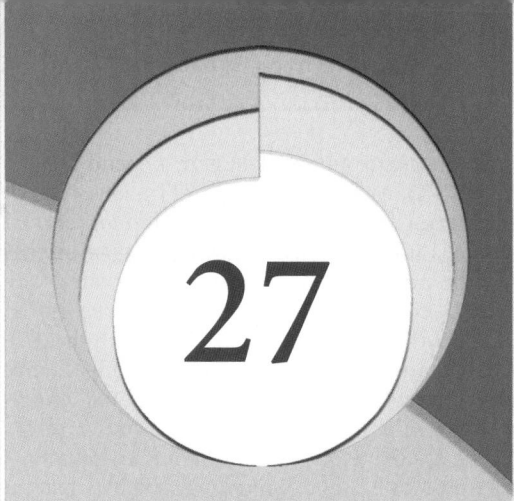

Peripheral Nerve and Skeletal Muscle

DOUGLAS C. ANTHONY · MATTHEW P. FROSCH · UMBERTO DE GIROLAMI

General Reactions of the Motor Unit
  Segmental Demyelination
  Axonal Degeneration and Muscle Fiber Atrophy
  Nerve Regeneration and Reinnervation of Muscle
  Reactions of the Muscle Fiber
Diseases of Peripheral Nerve
  Inflammatory Neuropathies
    Immune-Mediated Neuropathies
  Infectious Polyneuropathies
    Leprosy (Hansen Disease)
    Diphtheria
    Varicella-Zoster Virus
  Hereditary Neuropathies
    Hereditary Motor and Sensory Neuropathy Type I
    Other Hereditary Motor and Sensory Neuropathies
  Acquired Metabolic and Toxic Neuropathies
    Peripheral Neuropathy in Adult-Onset Diabetes Mellitus
    Metabolic and Nutritional Peripheral Neuropathies
    Neuropathies Associated with Malignancy
    Toxic Neuropathies
  Traumatic Neuropathies
  Tumors of Peripheral Nerve

Diseases of Skeletal Muscle
  Denervation Atrophy
    Spinal Muscular Atrophy (Infantile Motor Neuron Disease)
  Muscular Dystrophies
    X-Linked Muscular Dystrophy (Duchenne Muscular Dystrophy and Becker Muscular Dystrophy)
    Other Muscular Dystrophies
    Myotonic Dystrophy
  Ion Channel Myopathies (Channelopathies)
  Congenital Myopathies
  Myopathies Associated with Inborn Errors of Metabolism
    Lipid Myopathies
    Mitochondrial Myopathies (Oxidative Phosphorylation Diseases)
  Inflammatory Myopathies
    Noninfectious Inflammatory Myopathies
  Toxic Myopathies
    Thyrotoxic Myopathy
    Ethanol Myopathy
    Drug-Induced Myopathies
  Diseases of the Neuromuscular Junction
    Myasthenia Gravis
    Lambert-Eaton Myasthenic Syndrome
  Tumors of Skeletal Muscle

The functions of the neuromuscular system depend on the *motor units* (Fig. 27–1), each consisting of (1) a *lower motor neuron* in the anterior horn of the spinal cord or cranial nerve motor nucleus in the brain stem, (2) the *axon* of that neuron, and (3) the multiple *muscle fibers* it innervates. The principal structural component of peripheral nerve is the *nerve fiber* (an axon with its Schwann cells and myelin sheath). A nerve consists of numerous fibers that are grouped into fascicles by connective tissue sheaths. *Myelinated* and *unmyelinated* nerve fibers are intermingled within the fascicle. Peripheral nervous system axons are myelinated in segments (*internodes*) separated by *nodes of Ranvier*. A single Schwann cell supplies the myelin sheath for each internode. Unmyelinated axons are far more numerous than myelinated axons, and the cytoplasm of one Schwann cell envelops a variable number of unmyelinated fibers (5 to 20 axons in humans). The three major connective tissue components of peripheral nerve are the *epineurium*, which encloses the entire nerve; the *perineurium*, a multilayered concentric connective tissue sheath that encloses each fascicle; and the *endoneurium*, which surrounds individual nerve fibers. The motor and sensory fibers, which are separated within anterior and posterior roots, intermingle within the mixed sensorimotor nerve that exits the spinal canal.

General Reactions of the Motor Unit

Neuromuscular diseases are accompanied by weakness and are often due to disorders of the motor unit—either the motor neuron and axon, or the muscle fibers. The two main responses of peripheral nerve to injury are determined by the target of the injury: either the Schwann cell or the axon. Diseases that affect primarily the Schwann cell lead to a loss of myelin, referred to as *segmental demyelination*. In contrast, primary involvement of the neuron and its axon leads to *axonal degeneration*. In some diseases axonal degeneration may be followed by *axonal regeneration* and *reinnervation* of muscle.[1] The two principal pathologic processes seen in skeletal muscle are *denervation atrophy*, which follows loss of axons, and those due to a primary abnormality of the muscle fiber itself, referred to as *myopathy*.

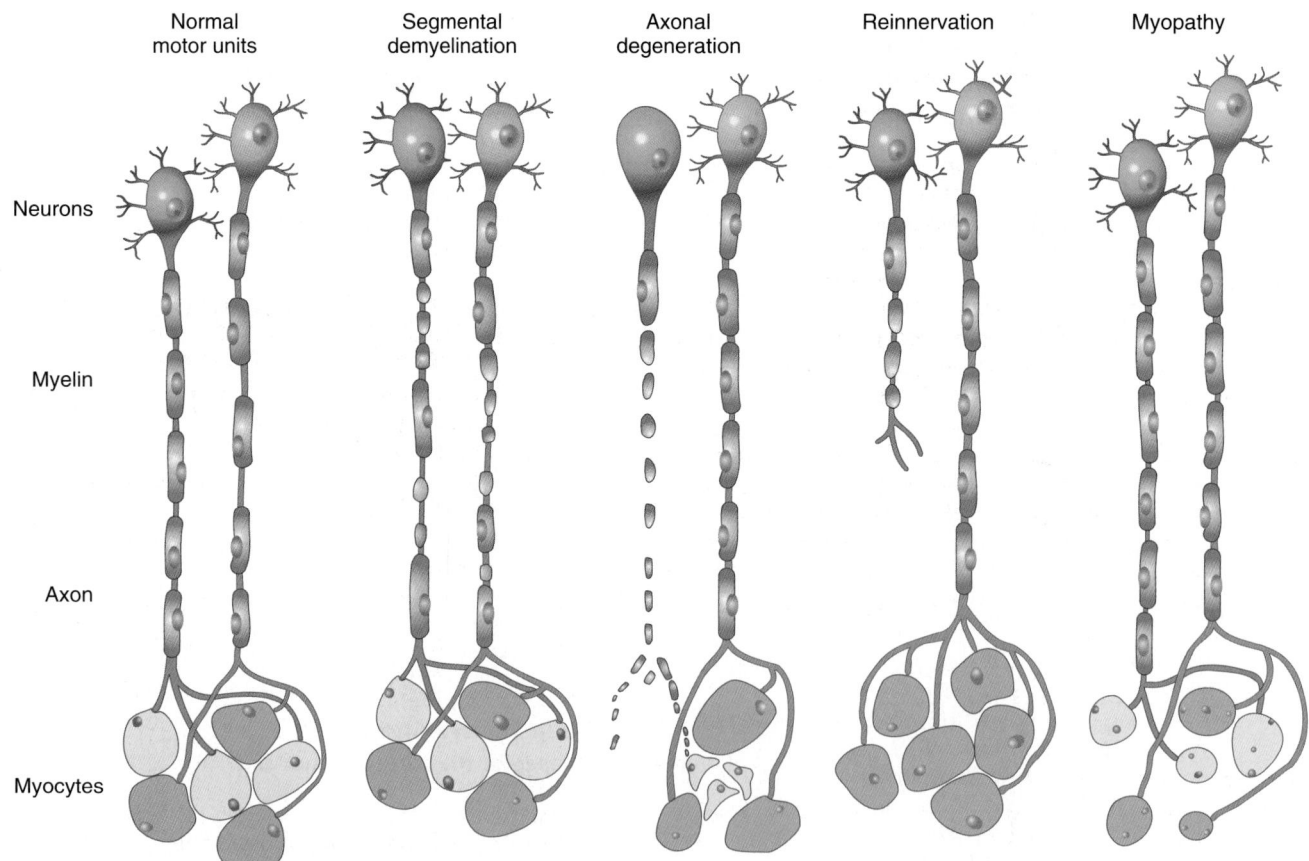

FIGURE 27–1 Normal and abnormal motor units. *Normal motor units*: Two adjacent motor units are shown (*red* and *green* neurons, *red* and *pale-pink* myocytes). *Segmental demyelination*: Random internodes of myelin are injured and are remyelinated by multiple Schwann cells, while the axon and myocytes remain intact. *Axonal degeneration*: The axon and its myelin sheath undergo anterograde degeneration (shown for the *green* neuron), with resulting denervation atrophy of the myocytes within its motor unit (*pale-pink* myocytes). *Reinnervation of muscle*: Sprouting of adjacent *(red)* uninjured motor axons leads to fiber type grouping of myocytes, while the injured axon attempts axonal sprouting. *Myopathy*: Scattered myocytes of adjacent motor units are small (degenerated or regenerated), whereas the neurons and nerve fibers are normal.

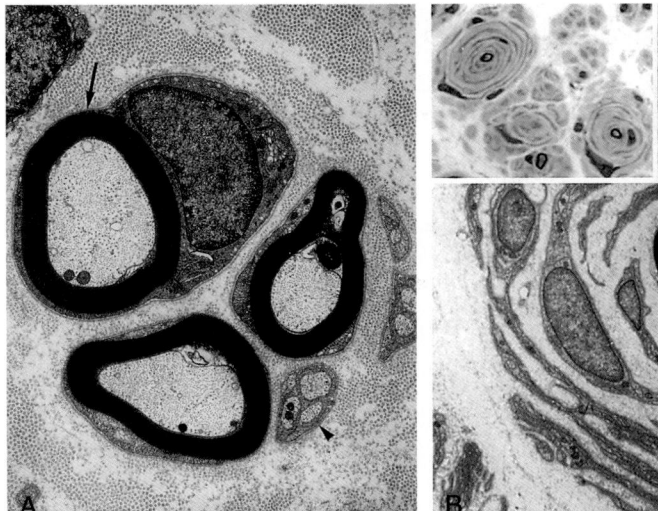

FIGURE 27–2 Compared with the normal ultrastructure of nerve (**A**), an "onion bulb" (**B**) is composed of a thinly myelinated axon *(arrow)* surrounded by concentrically arranged Schwann cells. *Inset*, Light-microscopic appearance of an onion bulb neuropathy, characterized by "onion bulbs" surrounding axons. (**B**, Courtesy of G. Richard Dickersin, MD, from Diagnostic Electron Microscopy: A Text Atlas. New York, Igaku-Shoin Medical Publishers, 2000, p 984.)

SEGMENTAL DEMYELINATION

Segmental demyelination occurs when there is dysfunction of the Schwann cell (as in hereditary motor and sensory neuropathy) *or damage to the myelin sheath* (e.g., in Guillain-Barré syndrome); there is no primary abnormality of the axon. The process may affect some Schwann cells and their corresponding internodes while sparing others (see Fig. 27–1). The disintegrating myelin is engulfed initially by Schwann cells and later by macrophages. The denuded axon provides a stimulus for remyelination. A population of precursor cells within the endoneurium has the capacity to replace injured Schwann cells. These cells proliferate and encircle the axon and, in time, remyelinate the denuded portion.[2] Newly formed myelinated internodes are shorter than normal, however, and several are required to bridge the demyelinated region (see Fig. 27–1). The new myelin sheath is also thin in proportion to the diameter of the axon.

With sequential episodes of demyelination and remyelination, there is an accumulation of tiers of Schwann cell processes that, on transverse section, appear as concentric layers of Schwann cell cytoplasm and redundant basement membrane surrounding a thinly myelinated axon *(called onion bulbs)* (Fig. 27–2). In time, many chronic demyelinating neuropathies give way to axonal injury. The specific conditions giving rise to demyelination are described later.

AXONAL DEGENERATION AND MUSCLE FIBER ATROPHY

Axonal degeneration is the result of primary destruction of the axon, with secondary disintegration of its myelin sheath (see Fig. 27–1). Damage to the axon may be due to a focal event occurring at some point along the length of the nerve (such as trauma or ischemia) or to a more generalized abnormality affecting the neuron cell body *(neuronopathy)* or its axon *(axonopathy)*. When axonal injury occurs as the result of a focal lesion, such as traumatic transection of a nerve, the distal portion of the fiber undergoes *Wallerian degeneration* (Fig. 27–3). Within a day the axon begins to break down, and

the affected Schwann cells begin to catabolize myelin and later engulf axon fragments, forming small oval compartments *(myelin ovoids).*[2] Macrophages are recruited into the area and participate in the phagocytosis of axonal and myelin-derived debris. The stump of the proximal portion of the severed nerve shows degenerative changes involving only the most distal two or three internodes and then undergoes regenerative activity. In the slowly evolving neuronopathies or axonopathies, evidence of axonal degeneration is scant because only a few fibers are actively degenerating at any given time.

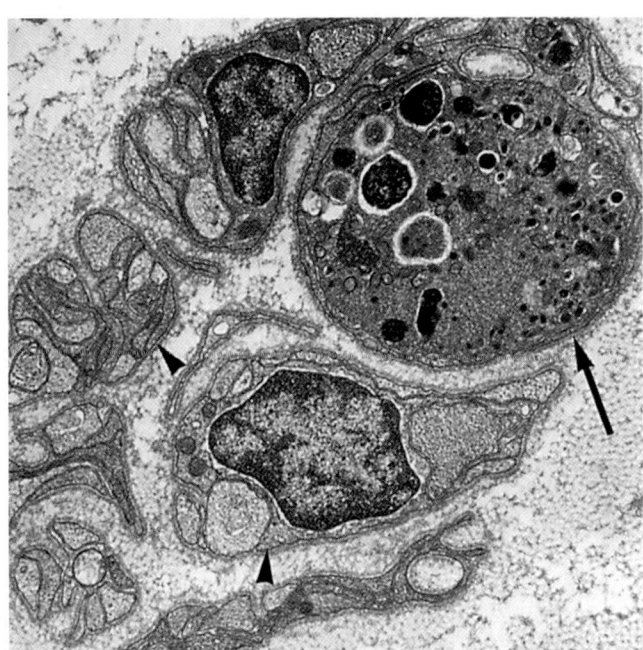

FIGURE 27–3 Electron micrograph of a degenerating axon *(arrow)* adjacent to several intact unmyelinated fibers *(arrowheads)*. The axon is markedly distended and contains numerous degenerating organelles and dense bodies.

TABLE 27–1	Muscle Fiber Types	
	Type 1	**Type 2**
Action	Sustained force	Sudden movements
Strength	Weight-bearing	Purposeful motion
Enzyme content	NADH-TR dark staining ATPase at pH 4.2, dark staining ATPase at pH 9.4, light staining	NADH light staining ATPase at pH 4.2, light staining ATPase at pH 9.4, dark staining
Lipids	Abundant	Scant
Glycogen	Scant	Abundant
Ultrastructure	Many mitochondria Wide Z-band	Few mitochondria Narrow-Z-band
Physiology	Slow-twitch	Fast-twitch
Color	Red	White
Prototype	Soleus (pigeon)	Pectoral (pigeon)

ATPase, adenosine triphosphatase; NADH-TR, nicotinamide adenine dinucleotide, reduced form, tetrazolium reductase.

When axonal degeneration occurs, the muscle fibers within the affected motor unit lose their neural input and undergo *denervation atrophy*. Denervation of muscle leads to breakdown of myosin and actin, with a decrease in cell size and resorption of myofibrils, but cells remain viable. In cross-section, the atrophic fibers are smaller than normal and have a roughly triangular ("angulated") shape. There is also cytoskeletal reorganization of some muscle cells, which results in a rounded zone of disorganized myofibers in the center of the fiber *(target fiber)*.

NERVE REGENERATION AND REINNERVATION OF MUSCLE

The proximal stumps of degenerated axons sprout and elongate, and they may develop new growth cones during the process of axonal regeneration. These growth cones use the Schwann cells vacated by the degenerated axons to guide them. The presence of multiple closely aggregated, thinly myelinated small-caliber axons is evidence of regeneration *(regenerating cluster)*. This regrowth of axons is apparently limited by the rate of the slow component of axonal transport, and the movement of tubulin, actin, and intermediate filaments, proceeding at about 1 mm per day. Despite its slow pace, axonal regeneration accounts for some of the functional recovery after nerve injury and can be accelerated with marrow stromal cell transplants.[4]

The reinnervation of skeletal muscle changes its composition, altering the distribution of the two major types of fibers, *type 1* and *type 2*. The fiber types, defined on the basis of histochemistry and physiology (Table 27–1), are determined by the neuron of the motor unit, and their properties are imparted through innervation. Type 1 fibers are high in myoglobin and oxidative enzymes and have many mitochondria, in keeping with their ability to perform tonic contraction; operationally, they are most often defined by their dark staining for adenosine triphosphatase (ATPase) at pH 4.2 but light staining at pH 9.4. Type 2 fibers are rich in glycolytic enzymes and are involved in rapid phasic contractions; they are dark staining

on ATPase stain performed at pH 9.4 but light staining at pH 4.2. *Since the motor neuron determines fiber type, all muscle fibers of a single unit are of the same type.* The fibers of a single motor unit are distributed across the muscle, giving rise to a checkerboard pattern of alternating fiber types, as is demonstrated especially well with staining for ATPase (Fig. 27–4A). Normally, there is some variability in the relative abundance of type 1 and type 2 fibers among different muscles. The mnemonic "*one* (type 1 fiber) *slow* (twitch) *fat* (lipid-rich) *red* (appearance) *ox* (oxidative)" is useful to keep the physiology and histochemistry of the fiber types in mind.

Reinnervation of the atrophic muscle fibers within an injured motor unit occurs when the axons belonging to an unaffected neighboring motor unit extend sprouts to reinnervate the denervated myocytes and incorporate them into the healthy motor unit. The number of muscle fibers within the healthy reinnervating motor unit can thus be increased. Furthermore, since muscle fiber type is imparted by the innervating neuron, the newly adopted reinnervated fibers assume the fiber type of their neighboring new siblings. The result of reinnervation is the loss of the checkerboard pattern and the occurrence of a patch of contiguous myocytes having the same histochemical type *(type grouping)* (Fig. 27–4B). *Group atrophy* ensues when a type group in turn becomes denervated, because it is affected in the course of disease progression (Fig. 27–4C).

Type-specific atrophy is characteristic of some disease states. Type 2 fiber atrophy is a relatively common finding and is associated with inactivity or disuse. This type of "disuse atrophy" may occur after fracture of a limb and application of a plaster cast, in pyramidal tract degeneration, or in neurodegenerative diseases. Type 2 fiber atrophy may also occur during therapy with glucocorticoids and is characteristic of "steroid myopathy."

REACTIONS OF THE MUSCLE FIBER

Although a wide spectrum of diseases may affect muscle, the pathologic reactions of myocytes are relatively limited. Patho-

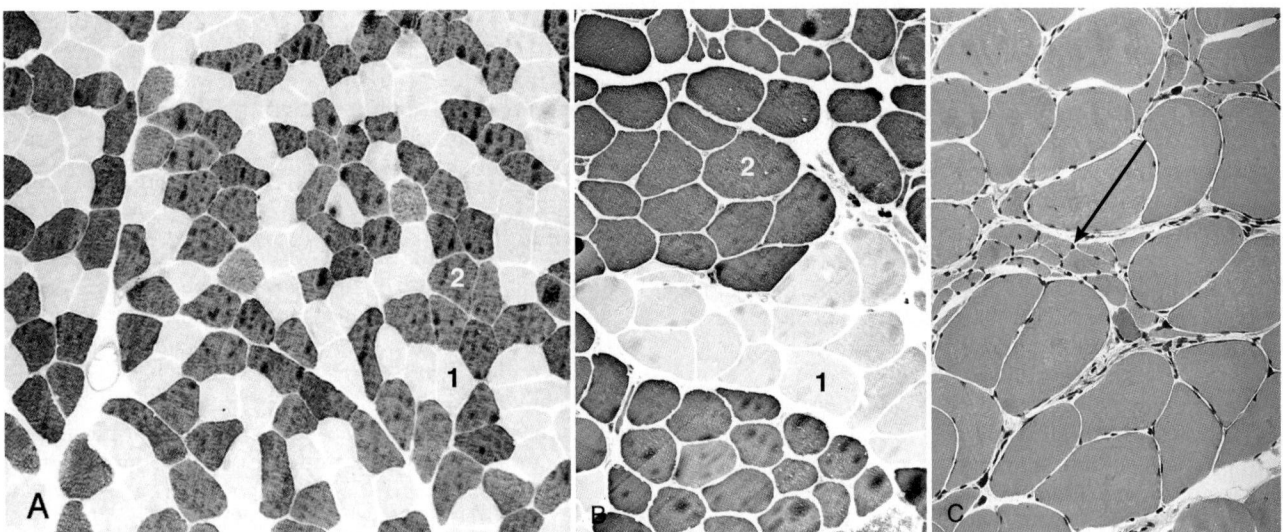

FIGURE 27–4 **A,** ATPase histochemical staining, at pH 9.4, of normal muscle showing checkerboard distribution of intermingled type 1 *(light)* and type 2 *(dark)* fibers. **B,** In contrast, fibers of both histochemical types are grouped together after reinnervation of muscle. **C,** A cluster of atrophic fibers (group atrophy) in the center *(arrow).*

logic changes may be seen in myopathies as well as in diseases that secondarily involve the muscle cells. The most common forms of reaction include the following:

- *Segmental necrosis,* destruction of a portion of the length of a myocyte, may be followed by *myophagocytosis* as macrophages infiltrate the region. The loss of muscle fibers in time leads to extensive deposition of collagen and fatty infiltration.
- *Vacuolation, alterations in structural proteins or organelles, and accumulation of intracytoplasmic deposits* may be seen in many diseases.
- *Regeneration* occurs when satellite precursor cells proliferate and reconstitute the destroyed portion of the fiber. The regenerating portion of the muscle fiber has large internalized nuclei and prominent nucleoli, and the cytoplasm, laden with RNA, is basophilic.
- Fiber *hypertrophy* occurs in response to increased load, either in the setting of exercise or in pathologic conditions in which muscle fibers are injured. Large fibers may divide longitudinally *(muscle fiber splitting)*, so that in cross-section, a single large fiber contains a cell membrane traversing its diameter, often with adjacent nuclei.

Diseases of Peripheral Nerve

Peripheral nerve is susceptible to the same wide range of categories of disease (inflammatory, traumatic, metabolic, toxic, genetic, neoplastic) as are other tissues. The pattern of disease, however, reflects the unique structure and function of nerves.

INFLAMMATORY NEUROPATHIES

These diseases are characterized by inflammatory cell infiltrates in peripheral nerves, roots, and sensory and autonomic

ganglia. In some, an infectious agent elicits the inflammatory responses; in others, immune mechanisms are presumed to be the primary cause of the inflammation.

Immune-Mediated Neuropathies

Guillain-Barré Syndrome (Acute Inflammatory Demyelinating Polyradiculoneuropathy)

Guillain-Barré syndrome is a life-threatening disease of the peripheral nervous system, with an overall annual incidence of one to three cases per 100,000 persons throughout the world.[5] The disease is characterized clinically by weakness beginning in the distal limbs but rapidly advancing to affect proximal muscle function ("ascending paralysis"), and histologically by inflammation and demyelination of spinal nerve roots and peripheral nerves (radiculoneuropathy).

Pathogenesis. Guillain-Barré syndrome is thought to be an acute-onset *immune-mediated demyelinating neuropathy*. Approximately two thirds of cases are preceded by an acute, influenza-like illness from which the affected individual has recovered by the time the neuropathy becomes symptomatic. Infections with *Campylobacter jejuni*, cytomegalovirus, Epstein-Barr virus, and *Mycoplasma pneumoniae*, or prior vaccination, have been shown to have a significant epidemiologic association with Guillain-Barré syndrome.[6] There has been no consistent demonstration of an infectious agent in peripheral nerves in these patients, and an immunological reaction is generally favored as the underlying cause. A similar inflammatory disease of peripheral nerves can be induced in experimental animals by immunization with a peripheral nerve myelin protein. A T cell–mediated immune response ensues, accompanied by segmental demyelination induced by activated macrophages. Transfer of these T cells to a naive animal results in comparable lesions. Moreover, lymphocytes from individuals with Guillain-Barré syndrome have been shown to produce demyelination in tissue cultures of myelinated nerve fibers. Circulating antibodies may also play a part, and plasmapheresis can be an effective treatment.[6]

> **Morphology.** The dominant histopathologic finding is **inflammation of peripheral nerve**, manifested as perivenular and endoneurial infiltration by lymphocytes, macrophages, and a few plasma cells. Inflammatory foci and demyelination are widely distributed throughout the peripheral nervous system, although their intensity is variable. The most intense inflammatory reaction is often localized in spinal and cranial motor roots and the adjacent parts of the spinal and cranial nerves. Segmental demyelination affecting peripheral nerves is the primary lesion, but damage to axons is also characteristic, particularly when the disease is severe. Electron microscopy has identified an early effect on myelin sheaths. The cytoplasmic processes of macrophages penetrate the basement membrane of Schwann cells, particularly in the vicinity of the nodes of Ranvier, and extend between the myelin lamellae, stripping away the myelin sheath from the axon. Ultimately, the remnants of the myelin sheath are engulfed by the macrophages. Remyelination follows the demyelination.

Clinical Course. The clinical picture is dominated by the ascending paralysis. Deep tendon reflexes disappear early in the process; although sensory involvement can often be detected, it is less troublesome than the weakness. The nerve conduction velocity is slowed because of the multifocal destruction of myelin segments involving many axons within a nerve. There is elevation of the CSF protein due to inflammation and altered permeability of the microcirculation within the spinal roots as they traverse the subarachnoid space. Inflammatory cells are contained within the roots, however, and there is little to no CSF pleocytosis. Many patients spend weeks in hospital intensive-care units before recovering normal function. With improved respiratory care and support, the mortality rate has fallen from 25% in the past but is still considerable; some 2% to 5% die of respiratory paralysis, autonomic instability, cardiac arrest, or the complications of treatment. Up to 20% of hospitalized patients have long-term disability.[5,6]

Chronic Inflammatory Demyelinating Polyradiculoneuropathy

In some patients, inflammatory demyelinating polyradiculoneuropathy follows a subacute or chronic course, usually with relapses and remissions over a period of several years, rather than the acute course of Guillain-Barré syndrome.[7] In these cases there is often a symmetric, mixed sensorimotor polyneuropathy, although some patients have predominantly sensory or motor impairment. Clinical remissions may occur with steroid treatment and plasmapheresis. Biopsies of sural nerves show evidence of recurrent demyelination and remyelination associated with well-developed onion bulb structures.[8]

INFECTIOUS POLYNEUROPATHIES

Many infectious processes affect peripheral nerve. Leprosy, diphtheria, and varicella-zoster cause unique and specific pathologic changes in nerves and are also discussed as systemic infectious diseases in Chapter 8.

Leprosy (Hansen Disease)

Peripheral nerves are involved in both lepromatous and tuberculoid leprosy (discussed in Chapter 8).[9] In lepromatous leprosy, Schwann cells are invaded by *Mycobacterium leprae*, which proliferate and eventually infect other cells. There is evidence of segmental demyelination and remyelination and loss of both myelinated and unmyelinated axons. As the infection advances, endoneurial fibrosis and multilayered thickening of the perineurial sheaths occur. Affected individuals develop a symmetric polyneuropathy affecting the cool extremities (due to lower temperatures favoring mycobacterial growth). The infection prominently involves pain fibers, and the resulting loss of sensation contributes to injury, since the patient is rendered unaware of injurious stimuli and damaged tissues. Thus, large traumatic ulcers may develop in the extremities. Tuberculoid leprosy shows evidence of active cell-mediated immune response to *M. leprae*, with nodules of granulomatous inflammation situated in the dermis. The inflammation injures cutaneous nerves in the vicinity; axons, Schwann cells, and myelin are lost, and there is fibrosis of the perineurium and endoneurium. In tuberculoid leprosy, affected individuals have much more localized nerve involvement.

Diphtheria

Peripheral nerve involvement results from the effects of the diphtheria exotoxin and begins with paresthesias and weakness[10]; early loss of proprioception and vibratory sensation is common. The earliest changes are seen in the sensory ganglia, where the incomplete blood-nerve barrier allows entry of the toxin. There is selective demyelination of axons that extends into adjacent anterior and posterior roots as well as into mixed sensorimotor nerves. The mechanism of action of diphtheria toxin is described in Chapter 8.

Varicella-Zoster Virus

Varicella-zoster virus is one of the most common viral infections of the peripheral nervous system.[11] Following chickenpox, a latent infection persists within neurons in the sensory ganglia of the spinal cord and brain stem, and reactivation leads to a painful, vesicular skin eruption in the distribution of sensory dermatomes (*shingles*), most frequently thoracic or trigeminal. The virus may be transported along the sensory nerves to the skin, where it establishes an active infection of epidermal cells. In a small proportion of patients, weakness is also apparent in the same distribution. Although the factors that give rise to reactivation are not fully understood, decreased cell-mediated immunity is of major importance in some cases.

Affected ganglia show neuronal destruction and loss, usually accompanied by abundant mononuclear inflammatory infiltrates; regional necrosis with hemorrhage may also be found.

TABLE 27–2	Hereditary Sensory and Autonomic Neuropathies (HSANs)	
Disease and Inheritance	**Gene and Locus**	**Clinical and Pathologic Findings**
HSAN I; autosomal dominant	Serine palmitoyl transferase, long-chain base, subunit 1 (*SPTLC1*) gene; 9q22.1–q22.3	Predominantly sensory neuropathy, presenting in young adults; axonal degeneration (mostly myelinated fibers)
HSAN II; autosomal recessive (some cases are sporadic)	*HSN2* gene; 12q13.3	Predominantly sensory neuropathy, presenting in childhood; axonal degeneration (mostly myelinated fibers)
HSAN III; (Riley-Day syndrome; familial dysautonomia; most often in Jewish children); autosomal recessive	IKAP histone acetyltransferase (*IKAP*) gene; 9q31	Predominantly autonomic neuropathy, presenting in infancy; axonal degeneration (mostly unmyelinated fibers); atrophy and loss of sensory and autonomic ganglion cells
HSAN IV; autosomal recessive dysautonomia, type II;	Neurotrophic tyrosine kinase receptor, type 1, or *NTRK1* gene; 1q21–q22	Congenital insensitivity to pain and anhidrosis; presentation in infancy; nearly complete loss of small myelinated and unmyelinated fibers
HSAN V; autosomal recessive	Nerve growth factor β subunit (*NGFB*) gene; 1p13.1	Congenital insensitivity to pain and temperature; presentation in infancy; nearly complete loss of small myelinated fibers

Peripheral nerve shows axonal degeneration after the death of the sensory neurons. Focal destruction of the large motor neurons of the anterior horns or cranial nerve motor nuclei may be seen at the corresponding levels. Intranuclear inclusions generally are not found in the peripheral nervous system.

HEREDITARY NEUROPATHIES

This is a group of heterogeneous, typically progressive, and often disabling syndromes that affect peripheral nerves. The genetic and molecular basis of many of the hereditary peripheral neuropathies is being elucidated,[12,13] and as they are further defined, adjustments in the current classification scheme can be anticipated. They can be divided into several groups:

- *Hereditary motor and sensory neuropathies* (HMSNs): The most common form of hereditary neuropathies, these disorders affect both strength and sensation (sensorimotor neuropathies). *They present as a spectrum of disorders, all caused by mutations in genes whose products are involved in peripheral nerve function.* Different mutations within the same gene may give rise to diseases with varying clinical features.[14] The different forms of HMSN are described below.
- *Hereditary sensory and autonomic neuropathies* (HSANs, summarized in Table 27–2): Symptoms in HSAN are usually limited to numbness, pain, and autonomic dysfunction such as orthostatic hypotension, but without weakness.
- *Familial amyloid polyneuropathies*: These are hereditary peripheral neuropathies characterized by the deposition of amyloid within the peripheral nervous system. Most kindreds show mutations of the *transthyretin* gene, located on chromosome 18q11.2–q12.1. Their clinical presentation is similar to that of HSAN. The amyloid fibrils are composed of transthyretin (Chapter 6), a protein involved in serum binding and transport of thyroid hormone.
- *Peripheral neuropathy accompanying inherited metabolic disorders*: Several hereditary metabolic disorders are accompanied by prominent peripheral neuropathy during the

course of the disease; the molecular basis and the clinico-pathologic characteristics of some of these are presented in Table 27–3.

The most common hereditary neuropathy, HMSN I, results in demyelination of peripheral nerve and slowing of the velocity of axonal conduction. The other hereditary neuropathies are axonal neuropathies that have fiber loss as their most prominent pathologic finding.

Hereditary Motor and Sensory Neuropathy Type I

HMSN I, also referred to as *Charcot-Marie-Tooth (CMT) disease, demyelinating type*, usually presents in childhood or early adulthood. A characteristic progressive muscular atrophy of the leg below the knee seen in these patients gives rise to the common clinical term *peroneal muscular atrophy*. Affected individuals may be asymptomatic, but when they present, it is often with symptoms such as distal muscle weakness, atrophy of the leg below the knee, or secondary orthopedic problems of the foot (such as *pes cavus*).

Pathogenesis and Molecular Genetics. The disease is genetically heterogeneous. The most common subtype (known as HMSN IA or CMT1A) has a duplication of a large region of chromosome 17p11.2, resulting in "segmental trisomy" of this region. The duplicated segment includes the gene that encodes peripheral myelin protein 22 (PMP22), a transmembrane protein expressed in compacted myelin. PMP22 and a set of related proteins are involved in the compaction of myelin in the peripheral nervous system (Fig. 27–5). Mutations affecting these myelin-associated genes result in demyelinating neuropathies of the HMSN I phenotype.[14] Mutations in another gene, on chromosome 1, which codes for myelin protein zero (MPZ), produce an identical clinical phenotype (HMSN IB). Additional pedigrees with hereditary demyelinating neuropathy show mutations in genes encoding structural proteins (connexin-32), protein degradation pathways (LITAF), and myelination induction genes (early growth response 2, EGR2).[12,14]

TABLE 27–3	Hereditary Neuropathies Accompanying Inherited Metabolic Disease			
Disease	**Genetic Defect**	**Inheritance**	**Clinical Findings**	**Pathologic Findings**
Adrenoleukodystrophy	ATP-binding cassette (ABC), transporter protein, subfamily D, member 1 (*ABCD1*); Xq28	X-linked; 4% of female carriers are symptomatic	Mixed motor and sensory neuropathy, adrenal insufficiency, spastic paraplegia; onset between 10 and 20 years for males with leukodystrophy, between 20 and 40 years for females with myeloneuropathy	Segmental demyelination, with onion bulbs; axonal degeneration (myelinated and unmyelinated); electron microscopy— linear inclusions in Schwann cells
Familial amyloid polyneuropathies	Transthyretin (*TTR*) gene (rarely other genes); 18q11.2–q12.1	Autosomal dominant	Sensory and autonomic dysfunction; age at onset varies with site of mutation	Amyloid deposits in vessel walls and endoneurium with axonal degeneration
Porphyria, acute intermittent (AIP) or variegate coproporphyria	Enzymes involved in heme synthesis (acute intermittent porphyria— porphobilinogen deaminase deficiency; 11q24.1–q24.2)	Autosomal dominant	Acute episodes of neurologic dysfunction, psychiatric disturbances, abdominal pain, seizures, proximal weakness, autonomic dysfunction; attacks may be precipitated by drugs	Acute and chronic axonal degeneration; regenerating clusters
Refsum disease	Peroxisomal enzyme phytanoyl CoA α-hydroxylase (*PAHX*) gene; 10pter–p11.2 (a rare genetically distinct infantile form also exists)	Autosomal recessive	Mixed motor and sensory neuropathy; palpable nerves; ataxia, night blindness, retinitis pigmentosa, ichthyosis; age at onset before 20 years	Severe onion bulb formation

ATP, adenosine triphosphate; CoA, coenzyme A.

Morphology. HMSN I is a demyelinating neuropathy. Histologic examination shows the consequences of repetitive demyelination and remyelination, with multiple onion bulbs, more pronounced in distal nerves than in proximal nerves (see Fig. 27–2). The axon is often present in the center of the onion bulb, and the myelin sheath is usually thin or absent. The redundant layers of Schwann cell hyperplasia surrounding individual axons are associated with enlargement of involved peripheral nerves that may become palpable, which has led to the term **hypertrophic neuropathy**. In the longitudinal plane, the axon may show evidence of segmental demyelination. Autopsy studies of affected individuals have shown degeneration of the posterior columns of the spinal cord.

Clinical Course. The disorder is most often autosomal dominant, and although it is slowly progressive, the disability of sensorimotor deficits and associated orthopedic problems such as pes cavus are usually limited in severity, and a normal life span is typical.

Other Hereditary Motor and Sensory Neuropathies

HMSN II

The axonal form of autosomal dominant CMT HMSN II (CMT-2) presents with signs and symptoms similar to those of HMSN I, although nerve enlargement is not seen and the

disease presents at a slightly later age. This form is less common than HMSN I. Some cases (designated HMSN IIA1 or CMT2A1) are caused by mutations in a gene encoding a kinesin family member, KIF1B.[15] Additional, less common mutations in other genes have been identified; these are classified as CMT2B to 2L.[23] Nerve biopsy specimens in HMSN II show loss of myelinated axons as the predominant finding. Segmental demyelination of internodes is infrequent. These findings suggest that the site of primary cellular dysfunction is the axon or neuron.

Dejerine-Sottas Neuropathy (HMSN III)

Dejerine-Sottas neuropathy is a slowly progressive, autosomal recessive disorder that begins in early childhood, and is manifested by delay in developmental milestones, such as the acquisition of motor skills. In contrast to HMSN I and HMSN II, in which muscular atrophy is limited to the leg, both trunk and limb muscles are involved in Dejerine-Sottas disease. On physical examination, *enlarged peripheral nerves* can be detected by inspection and palpation. The deep tendon reflexes are depressed or absent, and nerve conduction velocity is slowed. HMSN III is genetically heterogeneous, and arises from mutations in the same myelin-associated genes that are mutated in HMSN I. These include genes encoding PMP22, MPZ, periaxin (PRX), and EGR2.[16] Morphologically, the size of individual peripheral nerve fascicles is increased, often markedly, with abundant onion bulb formation as well as segmental demyelination. There is usually evidence of axonal loss, and the axons that remain are often of diminished caliber. Distal portions of peripheral nerves are most severely affected;

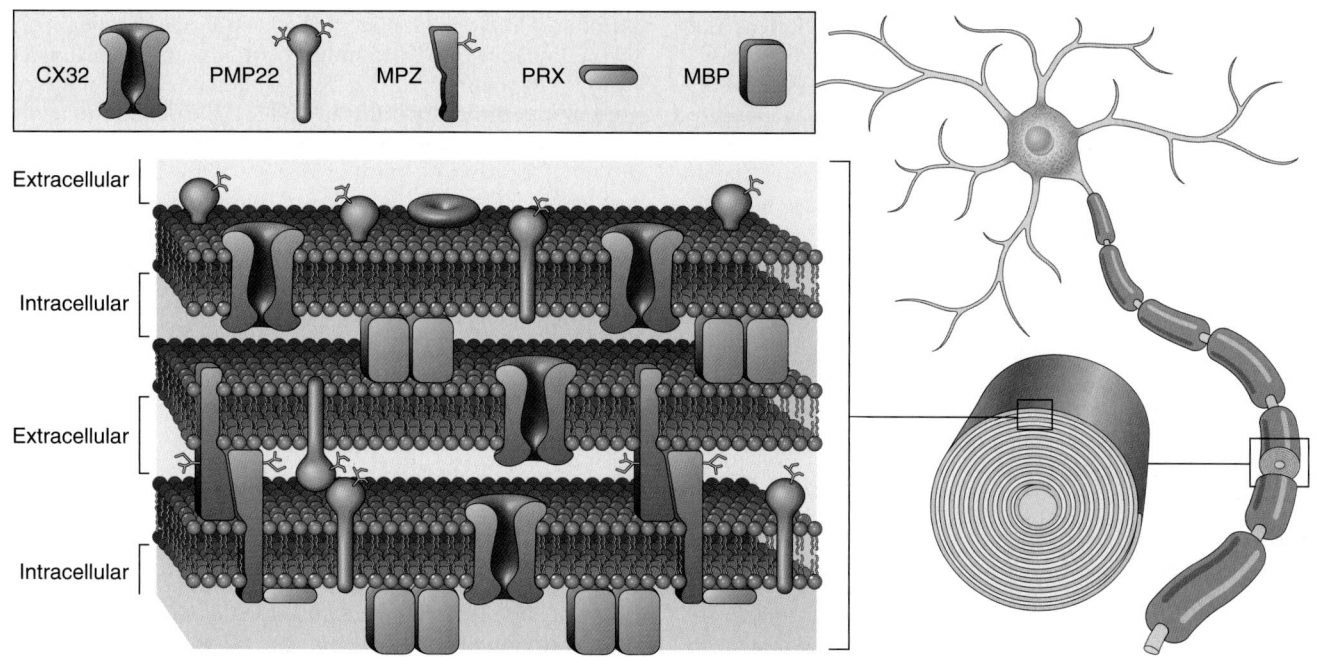

FIGURE 27–5 Relationship between the proteins of compacted myelin and the lipid bilayers. Myelin basic protein (MBP) is an intracellular protein that has a role in myelin compaction. Mutant forms of myelin protein zero (MPZ), peripheral myelin protein 22 (PMP22), and periaxin (PRX) cause hereditary demyelinating neuropathies of the Charcot-Marie-Tooth, type 1 category.

however, autopsy studies have shown that the spinal roots are also involved.

ACQUIRED METABOLIC AND TOXIC NEUROPATHIES

Functional and structural changes in peripheral nerves develop in response to various metabolic alterations—either from endogenous disorders or from exogenous agents. The most common of these processes are discussed here.

Peripheral Neuropathy in Adult-Onset Diabetes Mellitus

The prevalence of peripheral neuropathy in individuals with diabetes mellitus depends on the duration of the disease; up to 50% of diabetics overall have peripheral neuropathy clinically, and up to 80% of those who have had the disease for more than 15 years. Several distinct clinicopathologic patterns of diabetes-related peripheral nerve abnormalities have been recognized (Chapter 24). They are categorized as *distal symmetric sensory or sensorimotor neuropathy, autonomic neuropathy,* and *focal or multifocal asymmetric neuropathy*. Individuals may develop any combination of these lesions; in fact, the first two (sensorimotor and autonomic) are often found together. The mechanism of diabetic neuropathy is not completely resolved, but there is evidence for involvement of both the polyol pathway and the nonenzymatic glycation of proteins.[17]

Morphology. In individuals with a distal symmetric sensorimotor neuropathy, the predominant pathologic finding is an axonal neuropathy. As with other chronic axonal neuropathies, there is often some seg-

mental demyelination. There is a relative loss of small myelinated fibers and of unmyelinated fibers, but large fibers are also affected. Endoneurial arterioles show thickening, hyalinization, and intense periodic acid–Schiff positivity in their walls and extensive reduplication of the basement membrane[18] (Fig. 27–6).

Clinical Course. The most common peripheral neuropathy in type 2 diabetes mellitus is the symmetric neuropathy that involves distal sensory and motor nerves. Individuals with the neuropathy develop decreased sensation in the distal extremities with less evident motor abnormalities. The loss of pain sensation can result in the development of ulcers, which heal poorly because of the diffuse vascular injury in diabetes and are a major cause of morbidity. Another

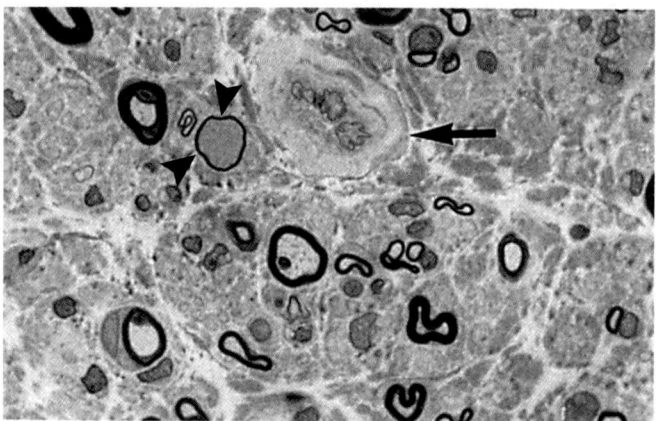

FIGURE 27–6 Diabetic neuropathy with marked loss of myelinated fibers, a thinly myelinated fiber *(arrowheads)*, and thickening of endoneurial vessel wall *(arrow)*.

manifestation of diabetic neuropathy is dysfunction of the autonomic nervous system; this affects 20% to 40% of individuals with diabetes mellitus, nearly always in association with a distal sensorimotor neuropathy.[17] Diabetic autonomic neuropathy has protean manifestations, including postural hypotension, incomplete emptying of the bladder resulting in recurrent infections, and sexual dysfuction. Some affected individuals, especially elderly adults with a long history of diabetes, develop a peripheral neuropathy that manifests itself as a disorder of single individual peripheral or cranial (oculomotor nerve) nerves (mononeuropathy), or of several individual nerves in an asymmetric distribution (multiple mononeuropathy or mononeuropathy multiplex). The pathogenesis of mononeuropathies in adult-onset diabetes is thought to involve vascular insufficiency, and ischemia of the affected peripheral nerve.[17]

Metabolic and Nutritional Peripheral Neuropathies

Most individuals with renal failure have a peripheral neuropathy (uremic neuropathy).[19] This is typically a distal, symmetric neuropathy that may be asymptomatic or may be associated with muscle cramps, distal dysesthesias, and diminished deep tendon reflexes. In these patients axonal degeneration is the primary event; occasionally there is secondary demyelination. Regeneration and recovery are common after dialysis.

Peripheral neuropathy can also develop in individuals with chronic liver disease, chronic respiratory insufficiency, and thyroid dysfunction. *Thiamine deficiency* is associated with axonal neuropathy, a clinical condition termed *neuropathic beriberi*. Axonal neuropathies also occur with deficiencies of vitamins B$_{12}$ (cobalamin), B$_6$ (pyridoxine), and E (α-tocopherol). Excessive chronic consumption of ethyl alcohol often leads to axonal neuropathy. There is a strong contribution of associated dietary deficiency, and affected individuals often have signs of thiamine deficiency. However, ethyl alcohol may have a direct toxic effect on peripheral nerve, since some affected individuals have adequate thiamine intake.[20]

Neuropathies Associated with Malignancy

Direct infiltration or compression of peripheral nerves by tumor is a common cause of mononeuropathy and may be the presenting symptom of cancer. These neuropathies include *brachial plexopathy* from neoplasms of the apex of the lung, *obturator palsy* from pelvic malignant neoplasms, and *cranial nerve palsies* from intracranial tumors and tumors of the base of the skull. A *polyradiculopathy* involving the lower extremity may develop when the cauda equina is involved by meningeal carcinomatosis.

In contrast, a diffuse, symmetric peripheral neuropathy may occur in individuals with a distant carcinoma as a *paraneoplastic* effect (Chapters 7 and 28). The most common type is a sensorimotor neuropathy characterized by weakness and sensory deficits that are often more pronounced in the lower extremities and that progress during months to years.[21] The neuropathy is most frequently associated with small-cell carcinoma of the lung; as many as 2% to 5% of people with lung cancer have clinical evidence of peripheral neuropathy. Patients with the less frequent pure sensory neuropathy present with

numbness and paresthesias that may precede the diagnosis of the malignancy by 6 to 15 months. An immunological mechanism for the neuropathy has been suggested based on the presence of inflammatory infiltrates within the dorsal root ganglia and the identification of IgG antibodies that bind a 35- to 38-kD RNA-binding protein expressed by neurons and the tumor.[22] The severity of clinical symptoms correlates with antibody titer, suggesting a causative relationship.

Paraneoplastic neuropathy may also develop in individuals with plasma cell neoplasms in one of two ways. The first is through the deposition of light-chain (AL type) amyloid in peripheral nerves (Chapter 6). The second is related to the production of monoclonal immunoglobulin that recognizes a major protein of myelin, myelin-associated glycoprotein.[23]

Toxic Neuropathies

Peripheral neuropathies can occur after exposure to industrial or environmental chemicals, biologic toxins, or therapeutic drugs.[24] Prominent among the environmental chemicals are heavy metals, including lead and arsenic (Chapter 9). In addition, many organic compounds are known to be toxic to the peripheral nervous system, leading to peripheral neuropathy.

TRAUMATIC NEUROPATHIES

Peripheral nerves are commonly injured in the course of trauma. *Lacerations* result from cutting injuries and can complicate fractures when a sharp fragment of bone lacerates the nerve. *Avulsions* occur when tension is applied to a peripheral nerve, often as the result of a force applied to one of the limbs. Regeneration of peripheral nerve axons following these types of injuries does occur, albeit slowly. Regrowth may be complicated by discontinuity between the proximal and distal portions of the nerve sheath as well as by the misalignment of individual fascicles. Axons, even in the absence of correctly positioned distal segments, may continue to grow, resulting in a mass of tangled axonal processes known as a *traumatic neuroma (pseudoneuroma* or *amputation neuroma)*. Within this mass, small bundles of axons appear randomly oriented; each, however, is surrounded by organized layers containing Schwann cells, fibroblasts, and perineurial cells (Fig. 27–7).

Compression neuropathy (entrapment neuropathy) occurs when a peripheral nerve is compressed, often within an anatomic compartment. *Carpal tunnel syndrome*, the most common entrapment neuropathy, results from compression of the median nerve at the level of the wrist within the compartment delimited by the transverse carpal ligament.[25] Women are more commonly affected than men, and the problem is frequently bilateral. The disorder may be observed in association with many conditions including tissue edema, pregnancy, inflammatory arthritis, hypothyroidism, amyloidosis (especially that related to β$_2$-microglobulin deposition in individuals on renal dialysis), acromegaly, diabetes mellitus, and excessive repetitive motions of the wrist. Symptoms are limited to dysfunction of the median nerve, including numbness and paresthesias of the tips of the thumb and first two digits. Other nerves prone to compression neuropathies include the ulnar nerve at the level of the elbow, the peroneal nerve at the level of the knee, and the radial nerve in the upper arm; the latter occurs from sleeping with the arm in an

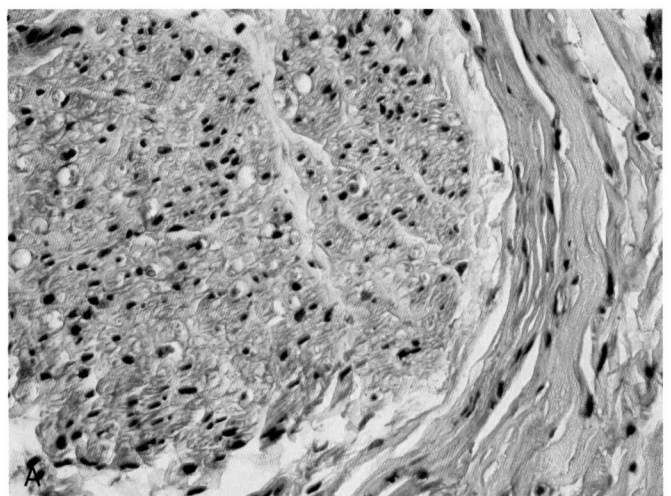

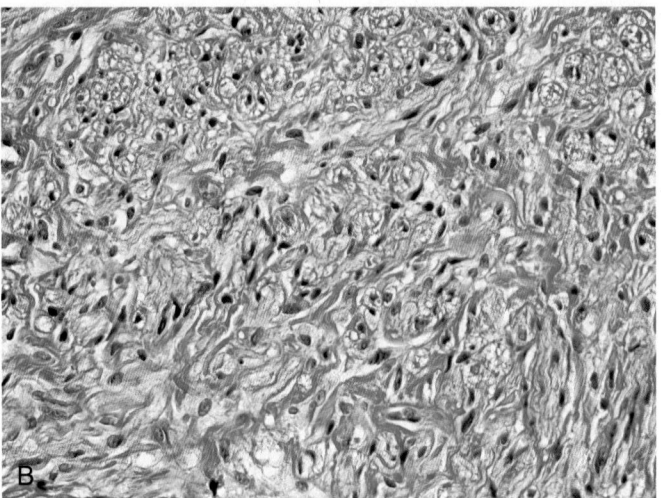

FIGURE 27-7 Normal appearance of peripheral nerve (**A**), with all the axons aligned in a single plane with sheaths of connective tissue, as compared with traumatic neuroma (**B**) showing disordered orientation of axons *(pale purple)* intermixed with connective tissue *(blue)*.

awkward position ("Saturday night palsy"). Another form of compression neuropathy is found in the foot, affecting the interdigital nerve at intermetatarsal sites. This problem, which occurs more often in women than in men, leads to foot pain (metatarsalgia). The histologic findings of the lesion *(Morton neuroma)* include evidence of chronic compression injury.

TUMORS OF PERIPHERAL NERVE

Both benign and malignant tumors can be derived from elements of the nerve sheath. These are discussed with tumors of the central nervous system (Chapter 28).

Diseases of Skeletal Muscle

DENERVATION ATROPHY

Neurogenic atrophy of muscle is caused by disorders that affect motor neurons (see Fig. 27-1). The response of muscle

to denervation and the histologic changes associated with reinnervation have been described earlier.

Spinal Muscular Atrophy (Infantile Motor Neuron Disease)

Motor neuron diseases are progressive neurologic illnesses that selectively destroy the anterior horn cells in the spinal cord and cranial nerve motor neurons. Motor neuron diseases in adults are discussed in Chapter 28. Spinal muscular atrophy (SMA) is a distinctive group of autosomal recessive motor neuron diseases that begin in childhood or adolescence. SMA is discussed here because the disease is commonly considered with the childhood myopathies and because the pathologic findings in skeletal muscle are characteristic.

Genetics. All forms of SMA are associated with mutations affecting survival motor neuron 1 (*SMN1*), a gene on chromosome 5 that is required for motor neuron survival. This region of chromosome 5 also contains variable numbers of copies of a second highly homologous gene, *SMN2*. Homozygous deletions of *SMN1* (or less commonly, intragenic mutations) cause SMA.[26] The number of copies of the homologous *SMN2* modifies the clinical phenotype, with more copies being associated with milder neurologic phenotype. *SMN* genes are expressed in all tissues, so why mutations or deletions of these genes cause only neuronal loss is not clear. It is postulated that the SMN protein is critical for normal axonal transport and integrity of neuromuscular junctions, and thus promotes survival of motor neurons.

Morphology. The typical histologic finding in muscle is large numbers of atrophic fibers, often only a few micrometers in diameter (Fig. 27-8). This is unlike the groups of angulated atrophic fibers seen in denervation atrophy of muscle in adults. In SMA the muscle fiber atrophy often involves an entire fascicle, a feature known as **panfascicular atrophy**. There are also scattered large fibers that are two to four times normal size.

Clinical Course. The most common form of SMA, Werdnig-Hoffmann disease (SMA type 1), has its onset at birth or within the first 4 months of life with severe hypotonia (lack of muscle tone and "floppiness"). It usually leads to death within the first 3 years of life. The other two forms (SMA

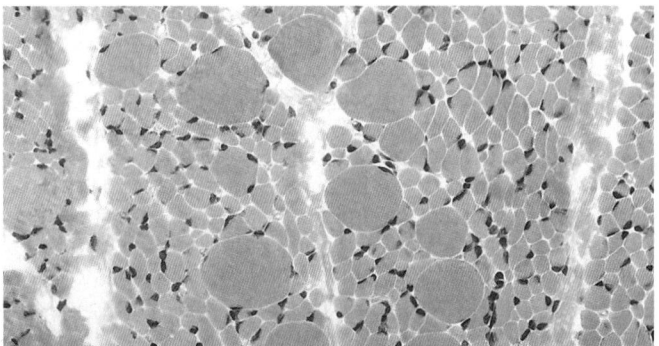

FIGURE 27-8 Spinal muscular atrophy with groups of round atrophic muscle fibers, or panfascicular atrophy, resulting from denervation atrophy.

2 and SMA 3) present at later ages, either in early childhood (between 3 and 15 months of age in SMA 2) or in later childhood (after 2 years of age in SMA 3). Those with SMA 2 usually die in childhood after age 4, whereas those with SMA 3 often survive into adulthood.

MUSCULAR DYSTROPHIES

The muscular dystrophies are a heterogeneous group of inherited disorders of muscle, often beginning in childhood, that lead to progressive weakness and muscle wasting. Histologically, in advanced cases muscle fibers undergo degeneration and are replaced by fibrofatty tissue and collagen. This feature distinguishes dystrophies from myopathies (described later), which also present with muscle weakness.

X-Linked Muscular Dystrophy (Duchenne Muscular Dystrophy and Becker Muscular Dystrophy)

The two most common forms of muscular dystrophy are X linked: *Duchenne muscular dystrophy* (DMD) and *Becker muscular dystrophy* (BMD). DMD is the most severe and common form of muscular dystrophy, with an incidence of about 1 per 3500 live male births. DMD becomes clinically manifest by the age of 5 years. It leads to wheelchair dependence by 10 to 12 years of age, and thereafter progresses relentlessly. Although BMD involves the same genetic locus, it is less common and much less severe than DMD.

Pathogenesis and Molecular Genetics. DMD and BMD are caused by abnormalities in *DMD*, a gene that is located in the Xp21 region. *DMD* is one of the largest human genes, spanning 2.3 million base pairs, and 79 exons. It encodes a 427-kD protein named *dystrophin*. A large proportion of the genetic abnormalities are deletions, with frameshift and point mutations accounting for the rest.[27] Approximately two thirds of the cases are familial, and the remainder represent new mutations. In the affected families females are carriers; they are clinically asymptomatic but often have elevated serum creatine kinase and show minimal histologic abnormalities on muscle biopsy. Female carriers and affected males who survive into adulthood are also at risk for developing dilated cardiomyopathy.[27]

Dystrophin is a cytoplasmic protein located adjacent to the sarcolemmal membrane in myocytes (Fig. 27–9). It is concentrated at the plasma membrane over Z-bands, where it forms a strong mechanical link to cytoplasmic actin. Thus, *dystrophin and the dystrophin-associated protein complex form an interface between the intracellular contractile apparatus and the extracellular connective tissue matrix.* The role of this complex of proteins in transferring the force of contraction to connective tissue has been proposed to be the basis for the myocyte degeneration that occurs in the absence of dystrophin[28] or various other proteins that interact with dystrophin (see later). Muscle biopsy specimens from individuals with DMD show little or no dystrophin by both staining and western blot analysis (Fig. 27–10). People with BMD, who also have mutations in the dystrophin gene, have diminished amounts of dystrophin, usually of an abnormal molecular weight, reflecting mutations that allow synthesis of an abnormal protein of smaller size (Fig. 27–10B).

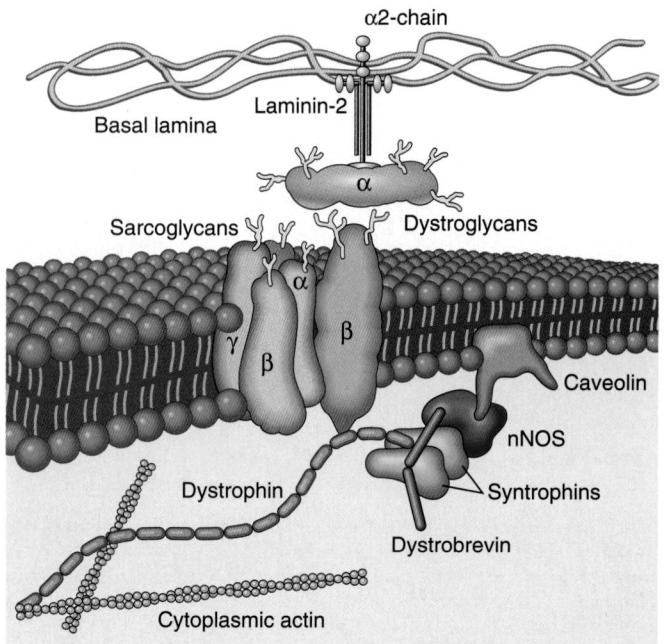

FIGURE 27–9 Relationship between the cell membrane (sarcolemma) and the sarcolemmal associated proteins. Dystrophin, an intracellular protein, forms an interface between the cytoskeletal proteins and a group of transmembrane proteins, the dystroglycans and the sarcoglycans. These transmembrane proteins have interactions with the extracellular matrix, including the laminin proteins. Dystrophin also interacts with dystrobrevin and the syntrophins, which form a link with neuronal-type nitric oxide synthetase (nNOS) and caveolin. Mutations in dystrophin are associated with the X-linked muscular dystrophies; mutations in caveolin and the sarcoglycan proteins with the limb-girdle muscular dystrophies, which can be autosomal dominant or recessive disorders; and mutations in the α2-laminin (merosin) with autosomal recessive congenital muscular dystrophy.

Morphology. Histopathologic abnormalities common to DMD and BMD include (1) **variation in fiber size** (diameter) due to the presence of both small and enlarged fibers, sometimes with fiber splitting; (2) **increased numbers of internalized nuclei** (beyond the normal range of 3% to 5%); (3) **degeneration, necrosis, and phagocytosis of muscle fibers**; (4) **regeneration of muscle fibers**; and (5) **proliferation of endomysial connective tissue** (see Fig. 27–10A). DMD cases also often show enlarged, rounded, hyaline fibers that have lost their normal cross-striations; such fibers, believed to be hypercontracted, are rare in BMD. Both type 1 and type 2 fibers are involved, and no alterations in the proportion or distribution of fiber types are evident. Histochemical reactions sometimes fail to identify distinct fiber types in DMD. In later stages **the muscles eventually become almost totally replaced by fat and connective tissue**. Cardiac involvement, when present, consists of interstitial fibrosis, which is more prominent in the subendocardium.

Clinical Course. Boys with DMD are normal at birth, and early motor milestones are met on time. Walking, however, is

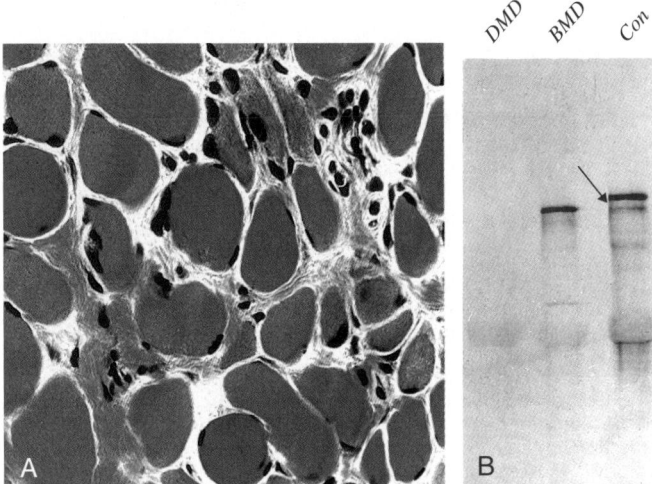

FIGURE 27–10 **A,** Duchenne muscular dystrophy (DMD) showing variation in muscle fiber size, increased endomysial connective tissue, and regenerating fibers *(blue hue).* **B,** Western blot showing absence of dystrophin in DMD and altered dystrophin size in Becker muscular dystrophy (BMD) compared with control *(arrow)* (Con). (Courtesy of Dr. L. Kunkel, Children's Hospital, Boston, MA.)

often delayed, and the first indications of muscle weakness are clumsiness and inability to keep up with peers. Weakness begins in the pelvic girdle muscles and then extends to the shoulder girdle. Enlargement of the muscles of the lower leg associated with weakness, a phenomenon termed *pseudohypertrophy,* is an important clinical finding. The increased muscle bulk is caused initially by an increase in the size of the muscle fibers and then, as the muscle atrophies, by an increase in fat and connective tissue. Pathologic changes are also found in the heart, and patients may develop heart failure or arrhythmias.[27] Although there are no well-established structural abnormalities of the central nervous system, cognitive impairment is a component of the disease and is sometimes severe enough to be considered a form of mental retardation. Serum creatine kinase is elevated during the first decade of life but returns to normal as muscle mass decreases. Death results from respiratory insufficiency, pulmonary infection, and cardiac decompensation. Gene therapy has received a great deal of attention but has been hampered by the size of the *DMD* gene. There has been success in experimental animals with two delivery systems: wild-type stem cell injections directly into muscle; and systemic injection of adeno-associated viruses carrying genes engineered to produce small, but functionally competent, portions of the dystrophin protein.[29] Induction of specific exon skipping using antisense RNA has been shown to restore the open reading in certain mutated *DMD* genes, and increase dystrophin expression in muscle biopsies.[30]

Boys with BMD develop symptoms at a later age than those with DMD. The onset occurs in later childhood or in adolescence, and is followed by a slower and more variable rate of progression, although there is considerable variation between pedigrees. Many patients have a nearly normal life span. Cardiac disease is frequently seen in these patients.

Other Muscular Dystrophies

Other less common forms of muscular dystrophy share many features of DMD and BMD, but have distinct clinical and pathologic characteristics. Some of these muscular dystrophies affect specific muscle groups, and the diagnosis is based largely on the pattern of muscle weakness (Table 27–4). Several autosomal muscular dystrophies, however, affect the proximal musculature of the trunk and limbs, similar to the X-linked muscular dystrophies, and are termed *limb girdle muscular dystrophies.*

Limb girdle muscular dystrophies (LGMDs) are inherited in either an autosomal dominant (type 1) or autosomal recessive (type 2) pattern (Table 27–5). Six subtypes of the dominant LGMDs (1A to 1F) and eleven subtypes of the recessive LGMDs (2A to 2K) have been identified. Mutations of the *sarcoglycan complex of proteins* have been identified in four of the limb girdle muscular dystrophies (2C, 2D, 2E, and 2F).[31,32] These membrane proteins interact with dystrophin through another transmembrane protein, β-dystroglycan (see Fig. 27–9).

Myotonic Dystrophy

Myotonia, the sustained involuntary contraction of a group of muscles, is the cardinal symptom in this disease. Patients often complain of "stiffness" and have difficulty in releasing their grip, for instance, after a handshake. Myotonia can often be elicited by percussion of the thenar eminence.

Pathogenesis. Inherited as an autosomal dominant trait, myotonic dystrophy is associated with a CTG trinucleotide repeat expansion on chromosome 19q13.2–q13.3. This expansion affects the mRNA for the dystrophia myotonia protein kinase (DMPK).[33] In normal subjects, fewer than 30 repeats are present; disease develops with expansion of this repeat, and several thousand repeats may be present in severely affected individuals. The mutation is not stable within a pedigree; with each generation more repeats accumulate, and the disease becomes more severe, a phenomenon called *anticipation* (Chapter 5). Expansion of the trinucleotide repeat influences the eventual concentration of protein product. However, it is not established if the disease is caused by abnormality of the protein affected by the trinucleotide repeat, or if this alters splicing of other RNAs.

Morphology. Skeletal muscle may show variation in fiber size. In addition, there is a striking increase in the number of internal nuclei, which on longitudinal section may form conspicuous chains. Another well-recognized abnormality is the **ring fiber**, with a subsarcolemmal band of cytoplasm that appears distinct from the center of the fiber. The rim contains myofibrils that are oriented circumferentially around the longitudinally oriented fibrils in the rest of the fiber. The ring fiber may be associated with an irregular mass of sarcoplasm **(sarcoplasmic mass)** extending outward from the ring. These sarcoplasmic masses stain blue with hematoxylin and eosin, red with Gomori trichrome, and intensely blue with the NAD–tetrazolium reductase histochemical reaction. Histochemical techniques have demonstrated a

TABLE 27-4	Other Selected Muscular Dystrophies		
Disease and Inheritance	**Gene and Locus**	**Clinical Findings**	**Pathologic Findings**
Fascioscapulohumeral muscular dystrophy; autosomal dominant	Type 1A—deletion of variable number of 3.3-kilobase subunits of a tandemly arranged repeat (*D4Z4*) on 4q35 Type 1B (*FSHMD1B*)—locus unknown	Variable age at onset (most commonly 10–30 years); weakness of muscles of face, neck, and shoulder girdle	Dystrophic myopathy, often associated with inflammatory infiltrates in muscle
Oculopharyngeal muscular dystrophy; autosomal dominant	Poly(A)-binding protein-2 (*PABP2*) gene; 14q11.2–q13	Onset in mid-adult life; ptosis and weakness of extraocular muscles; difficulty in swallowing	Dystrophic myopathy, but often including rimmed vacuoles in type 1 fibers
Emery-Dreifuss muscular dystrophy; X-linked	Emerin (*EMD1*) gene; Xq28	Variable onset (most commonly 10–20 years); prominent contractures, especially of elbows and ankles	Mild myopathic changes; absent emerin by immunohistochemistry
Congenital muscular dystrophies; autosomal recessive (also called muscular dystrophy, congenital, subtypes MDC1A, MDC1B, MDC1C)	Type 1A (merosin-deficient type)—laminin α2 (merosin) gene; 6q22–q23 Type 1B—locus at 1q42; gene unknown Type 1C; fukutin-related protein gene; 19q13.3	Neonatal hypotonia, respiratory insufficiency, delayed motor milestones	Variable fiber size and extensive endomysial fibrosis
Congenital muscular dystrophy with CNS malformations (Fukuyama type); autosomal recessive	Fukutin; 9q31	Neonatal hypotonia and mental retardation	Variable muscle fiber size and endomysial fibrosis; CNS malformations such as polymicrogyria
Congenital muscular dystrophy with CNS and ocular malformations (Walker-Warburg type)	Protein *O*-mannosyl transferases (*POMT1*, 9q34.1; *POMT2*, 14q24.3)	Neonatal hypotonia and mental retardation with cerebral and ocular malformations	Variable muscle fiber size and endomysial fibrosis; CNS and ocular malformations

CNS, central nervous system.

relative atrophy of type 1 fibers early in the course in some cases. Of all the dystrophies, only myotonic dystrophy shows pathologic changes in the intrafusal fibers of muscle spindles, with fiber splitting, necrosis, and regeneration.

Clinical Course. The disease often presents in late childhood with abnormalities in gait secondary to weakness of foot dorsiflexors and subsequently progresses to weakness of the hand intrinsic muscles and wrist extensors. Atrophy of muscles of the face and ptosis ensue, leading to the typical facial appearance. Cataracts, which are present in virtually every patient, may be detected early in the course by slit-lamp examination. Other associated abnormalities include frontal balding, gonadal atrophy, cardiomyopathy, smooth muscle involvement, decreased plasma IgG, and abnormal glucose tolerance. Dementia has been reported in some cases.

ION CHANNEL MYOPATHIES (CHANNELOPATHIES)

The *ion channel myopathies*, or *channelopathies*, are a group of familial diseases featuring myotonia, relapsing episodes of hypotonic paralysis (induced by vigorous exercise, cold, or a high-carbohydrate meal), or both. Hypotonia variants associated with elevated, depressed, or normal serum potassium levels at the time of the attack are called *hyperkalemic, hypokalemic, and normokalemic periodic paralysis*, respectively.

Pathogenesis. As their name indicates, these diseases are caused by mutations in genes that encode ion channels.[34] Hyperkalemic periodic paralysis results from mutations in the gene that encodes a skeletal muscle sodium channel protein (SCN4A), which regulates the entry of sodium into muscle during contraction. The gene for hypokalemic periodic paralysis encodes a voltage-gated L-type calcium channel.

Malignant hyperpyrexia (malignant hyperthermia) is a rare clinical syndrome characterized by a marked hypermetabolic state (tachycardia, tachypnea, muscle spasms, and later hyperpyrexia) triggered by anesthetics, most commonly halogenated inhalational agents and succinylcholine. The clinical syndrome may occur in predisposed individuals with hereditary muscle diseases, including congenital myopathies, dystrophinopathies, and metabolic myopathies. Mutations in several genes have been identified in families with susceptibility to malignant hyperthermia, including genes encoding L-type voltage-dependent calcium channel, notably the rynodine receptor (RyR1).[35] Upon exposure to anesthetic, the mutant receptor allows uncontrolled efflux of calcium from the sarcoplasm. This leads to tetany, increased muscle metabolism, and excessive heat production. Diagnosis can be made either by identifying the genetic mutation or by exposing

TABLE 27–5 Limb-Girdle Muscular Dystrophies (LGMDs)

Type	Locus	Protein	Clinicopathologic Features
AUTOSOMAL DOMINANT			
1A	5q31	Myotilin	Facial sparing, dysarthric speech
1B	1q21.2	Lamin A/C	Arrhythmias and cardiomyopathy
1C	3p25	Caveolin 3	Mild course
1D	7q	unknown	Adult onset
1E	6q23	unknown	Arrhythmias and cardiomyopathy
1F	7q32.1	unknown	No cardiac involvement
1G	4q21	unknown	Adult onset, lower limb/pelvic involvement
AUTOSOMAL RECESSIVE			
2A	15q15	Calpain 3	Slow progression
2B	2p13	Dysferlin	Mild clinical course
2C	13q12	γ-sarcoglycan	Severe course, Duchenne-like
2D	17q21	α-sarcoglycan	Severe course, Duchenne-like
2E	4q12	β-sarcoglycan	Severe course, Duchenne-like
2F	5q33	δ-sarcoglycan	Severe course, Duchenne-like
2G	17q12	Telethonin (titin cap)	Rimmed vacuoles
2H	9q31	TRIM 32	Sarcotubular myopathy
2I	19q13.3	Fukutin related protein (FKRP)	Cardiomyopathy
2J	2q24.3	Titin	Mild or severe, tibial myopathy
2K	9q34.1	Protein O-mannosyl transferase 1 (POMT1)	Childhood onset with mental retardation

biopsied muscle to the anesthetic agent and observing contraction.

CONGENITAL MYOPATHIES

The congenital myopathies are a group of disorders defined largely on the basis of the pathologic findings within muscle.[36] Most of these conditions share common clinical features, including onset in early life, nonprogressive or slowly progressive course, proximal or generalized muscle weakness, and hypotonia. Those affected at birth or in early infancy may present as "floppy infants" because of hypotonia or may have severe joint contractures (*arthrogryposis*); however, both hypotonia and arthrogryposis may also be caused by other neuromuscular dysfunction.

The best-characterized congenital myopathies are listed in Table 27–6. Figure 27–11 shows the structural characteristics of nemaline myopathy, one of the most distinctive types.

MYOPATHIES ASSOCIATED WITH INBORN ERRORS OF METABOLISM

Many of the myopathies associated with metabolic disease involve disorders of glycogen synthesis and degradation (Chapter 5). Combinations of clinical, pathologic, and molecular information are used to arrive at a specific diagnosis.[37] Myopathies can also result from disorders of mitochondrial function.

Lipid Myopathies

Abnormalities of carnitine transport or deficiencies of the mitochondrial dehydrogenase enzyme systems can lead to blocks in fatty acid oxidation and accumulation of lipid droplets within muscle (lipid myopathies).[38,39] Patients with these disorders develop muscle pain, tightness, and myoglobinuria following prolonged exercise or exercise during fasting states. Fatty acids provide energy for muscle contraction, especially when glycogen stores are depleted (as in fasting). With a metabolic block in fatty acid oxidation, the required energy is not available, resulting in symptoms. Concomitant cardiomyopathies and fatty liver may also occur.

Mitochondrial Myopathies (Oxidative Phosphorylation Diseases)

Approximately one fifth of the proteins involved in oxidative phosphorylation are encoded by the mitochondrial genome (mtDNA); additionally, this circular genome encodes 22 mitochondrial-specific transfer RNAs and 2 ribosomal RNA species. The remainder of the mitochondrial enzyme complexes are encoded in the nuclear genome. Mutations in both nuclear and mitochondrial genes cause the so-called *mitochondrial myopathies*.[40] Diseases that involve the mtDNA show maternal inheritance, since only the oocyte contributes mitochondria to the embryo (Chapter 5). There is a high mutation rate for mtDNA compared with nuclear DNA. The mitochondrial diseases may present in young adulthood and manifest with proximal muscle weakness, sometimes with severe involvement of the extraocular muscles involved in eye movements (external ophthalmoplegia). The weakness may be accompanied by other neurologic symptoms, lactic acidosis, and cardiomyopathy, so this group of disorders is sometimes classified as mitochondrial encephalomyopathies (Chapter 28).[41]

Morphology. The most consistent pathologic finding in skeletal muscle is aggregates of abnormal mitochondria that are demonstrable only by special techniques.[42] These occur under the sarcolemma in early

TABLE 27–6 Congenital Myopathies			
Disease and Inheritance	**Gene and Locus**	**Clinical Findings**	**Pathologic Findings**
Central-core disease; autosomal dominant	Ryanodine receptor-1 (*RYR1*) gene; 19q13.1	Early-onset hypotonia and weakness; "floppy infant"; associated skeletal deformities; may develop malignant hyperthermia	Cytoplasmic cores are lightly eosinophilic and distinct from surrounding sarcoplasm; found only in type 1 fibers, which usually predominate, best seen on NADH-TR stain
Nemaline myopathy (ENM)	AD NEM1—α-tropomyosin 3 (*TPM3*) gene; 1q22–q23 AR NEM2—nebulin (*NEB*) gene; 2q22 AR NEM3—α-actin-1 (*ACTA*) gene; 1q42 AR NEM4—tropomyosin-2 (*TPM2*) gene; 19p13.2–p13.1 AR NEM5—troponin T1 (*TNNT1*) gene; 19q13.4 AR NEM7—cofilin-2 (*CFL2*) gene; 14q12	Childhood weakness Hypotonia at birth; "floppy infant" Variable presentation; both infantile and adult onset Childhood-onset weakness Childhood onset in Amish families, with tremors Infant hypotonia; "floppy infant"	Aggregates of subsarcolemmal spindle-shaped particles (*nemaline rods*); occur predominantly in type 1 fibers; derived from Z-band material (α-actinin) and best seen on modified Gomori stain
Myotubular (centronuclear) myopathy	XL—myotubularin (*MTM1*) gene; Xq28 AD—dynamin-2 (and others) *DNM2* gene; 19p13.2 AR—amphiphysin-2(*BIN1*) gene; 2q14)	Severe congenital hypotonia, "floppy infant"; poor prognosis Childhood or young-adult weakness; slowly progressive weakness Childhood to adolescent presentation; severe weakness and hypotonia with survival into early adulthood	Abundance of centrally located nuclei involving the majority of muscle fibers; central nuclei are usually confined to type 1 fibers, which are small in diameter, but can occur in both fiber types

AD, autosomal dominant; AR, autosomal recessive; NADH, nicotinamide adenine dinucleotide, reduced-form; XL, X-linked.

stages, but with severe involvement, they may extend throughout the fiber. Since they are also associated with distortion of the myofibrils, the muscle fiber contour becomes irregular on cross-section, and the descriptive term **ragged red fibers** has been applied to them (Fig. 27–12A). Electron microscopy shows increased numbers of mitochondria with irregular shapes. Some contain paracrystalline **parking lot** inclusions or alterations in the structure of cristae (Fig. 27–12B). Cytochrome oxidase–negative fibers may be present in several mitochondrial myopathies, as assessed by histochemistry.

Clinical Course and Genetics. The relationship between clinical course and the genetic alterations in the mitochondrial disorders is not straightforward; however, three general types

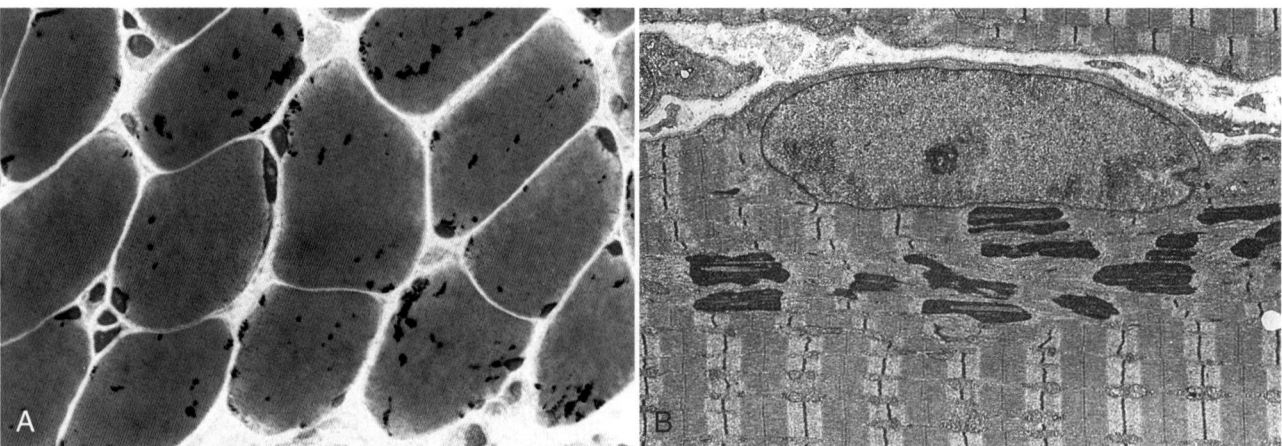

FIGURE 27–11 A, Nemaline myopathy with numerous rod-shaped, intracytoplasmic inclusions *(dark purple structures).* **B,** Electron micrograph of subsarcolemmal nemaline bodies, showing material of Z-band density located adjacent to nucleus, with normal sarcomeres (Z-band to Z-band) creating the typical cross-striation pattern of skeletal muscle.

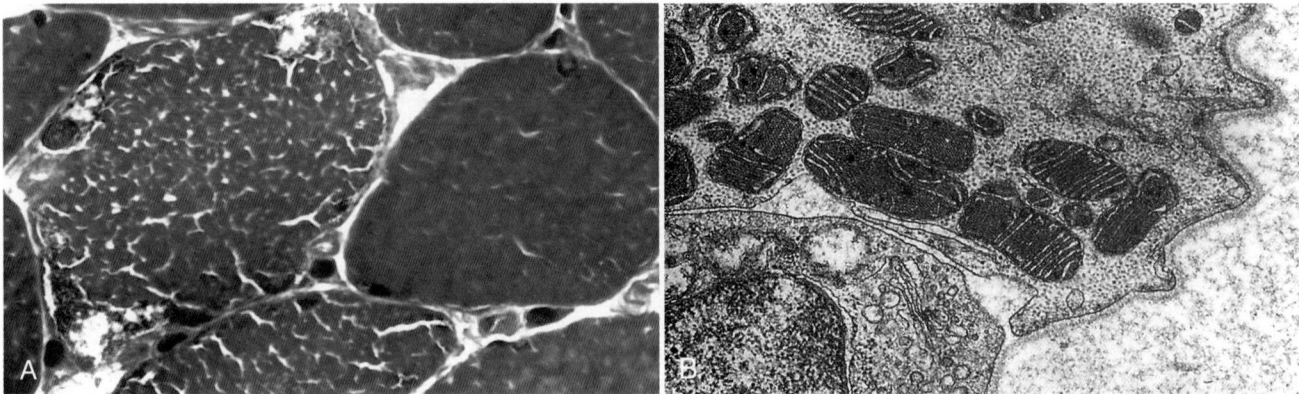

FIGURE 27–12 **A,** Mitochondrial myopathy showing an irregular fiber with subsarcolemmal collections of mitochondria that stain red with the modified Gomori trichrome stain *(ragged red fiber).* **B,** Electron micrograph of mitochondria from biopsy specimen in **A** showing "parking lot" inclusions.

of mutations have been defined. One consists of *point mutations in mtDNA*. Disorders associated with these show a maternal pattern of inheritance; some examples include myoclonic epilepsy with ragged red fibers, Leber hereditary optic neuropathy, and mitochondrial encephalomyopathy with lactic acidosis and strokelike episodes. As in other diseases caused by mutations in mtDNA, the expression of the disease is quite variable due to unequal distribution of mtDNA in affected cells (Chapter 5). A second set of mutations involves *genes encoded by nuclear DNA* and shows autosomal dominant or autosomal recessive inheritance. Some cases of subacute necrotizing encephalopathy (Leigh syndrome), exertional myoglobinuria, and infantile X-linked cardioskeletal myopathy (Barth syndrome) are due to mutations in nuclear DNA. The final subset of mitochondrial myopathies is caused by *deletions or duplications of mtDNA*. Examples include chronic progressive external ophthalmoplegia, characterized by a myopathy with prominent weakness of external ocular movements. Kearns-Sayre syndrome, another myopathy in this group, is also characterized by ophthalmoplegia but, in addition, includes pigmentary degeneration of the retina and complete heart block.

INFLAMMATORY MYOPATHIES

There are three subgroups of inflammatory muscle diseases: infectious, noninfectious inflammatory, and systemic inflammatory diseases that involve muscle along with other organs. Infectious myositis (Chapter 8) and systemic inflammatory diseases (Chapter 6) are discussed elsewhere.

Noninfectious Inflammatory Myopathies

Noninfectious inflammatory myopathies are a heterogeneous group of disorders that are most likely immune mediated and are characterized by injury and inflammation of skeletal muscle. Three relatively distinct disorders, *dermatomyositis, polymyositis,* and *inclusion body myositis,* are included in this category.[43] These may occur as an isolated myopathy or as one component of an immune-mediated systemic disease, particularly systemic sclerosis (Chapter 6). The clinical features of each disorder are presented first to facilitate discussion of pathogenesis and morphologic changes.

Dermatomyositis. As the name implies, individuals with dermatomyositis have an inflammatory disorder of the skin as well as skeletal muscle. It is characterized by a distinctive skin rash that may accompany or precede the onset of muscle disease. The *classic rash takes the form of a lilac or heliotrope discoloration of the upper eyelids associated with periorbital edema* (Fig. 27–13A). It is often accompanied by a scaling erythematous eruption or dusky red patches over the knuckles, elbows, and knees (Grotton lesions). *Muscle weakness is* slow in onset, bilaterally symmetric, and often accompanied by myalgias. *It typically affects the proximal muscles first.* As a result, tasks such as getting up from a chair and climbing steps become increasingly difficult. Fine movements controlled by distal muscles are affected only late in the disease. Dysphagia resulting from involvement of oropharyngeal and esophageal muscles occurs in one third of the affected individuals. Extramuscular manifestations, including interstitial lung disease, vasculitis, and myocarditis, may be present in some cases. Compared with the control populations, adults with dermatomyositis have a higher risk of developing visceral cancers. According to several studies, 20% to 25% of adults with dermatomyositis have cancer.[44]

Juvenile dermatomyositis[45] causes a similar onset of rash and muscle weakness but more often is accompanied by abdominal pain and involvement of the gastrointestinal tract. Mucosal ulceration, hemorrhage, and perforation may occur as the result of the dermatomyositis-associated vasculopathy. Calcinosis, which is uncommon in adult dermatomyositis, occurs in one third of youths with juvenile dermatomyositis.

Polymyositis. This inflammatory myopathy is characterized by symmetric proximal muscle involvement, similar to that seen in dermatomyositis. It *differs from dermatomyositis by the lack of cutaneous involvement and its occurrence mainly in adults.* Similar to dermatomyositis, there may be inflammatory involvement of heart, lungs, and blood vessels.

Inclusion Body Myositis. In contrast with the other two entities, inclusion body myositis begins with the *involvement of distal muscles,* especially extensors of the knee (quadriceps) and flexors of the wrists and fingers.[46] Furthermore, the weakness may be *asymmetric.* It is an insidiously developing disorder that typically affects individuals over the age of 50 years. Most cases are sporadic, but familial cases have been recognized as "inclusion body myopathy."

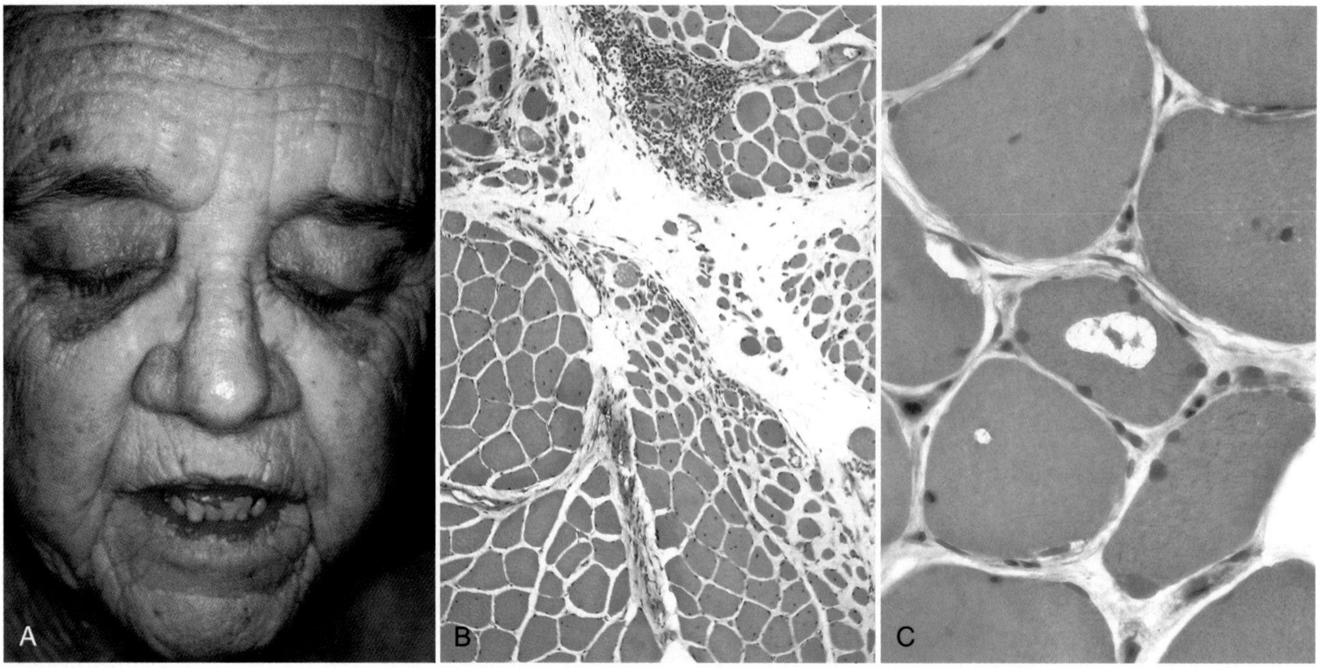

FIGURE 27–13 **A,** Dermatomyositis. Note the heliotrope rash affecting the eyelids. **B,** Dermatomyositis. The histologic appearance of muscle shows perifascicular atrophy of muscle fibers and inflammation. **C,** Inclusion body myositis showing a vacuole within a myocyte. (Courtesy of Dr. Dennis Burns, Department of Pathology, University of Texas Southwestern Medical School, Dallas, TX.)

Etiology and Pathogenesis. The cause of inflammatory myopathies is unknown, but the tissue injury is most likely mediated by immunological mechanisms. Capillaries seem to be the principal targets in dermatomyositis. Deposits of antibodies and complement are present in small blood vessels, and are associated with foci of myocyte necrosis. B cells and CD4+ T cells are present within the muscle, but there is a paucity of lymphocytes within the areas of myofiber injury. The perifascicular distribution of myocyte injury also suggests a vascular pathogenesis.

In contrast, polymyositis seems to be caused by cell-mediated injury of myocytes. CD8+ cytotoxic T cells and macrophages are seen near damaged muscle fibers, and the expression of HLA class I and class II molecules is increased on the sarcolemma of normal fibers. Similar to other immune-mediated diseases, antinuclear antibodies are present in a variable number of cases, regardless of the clinical category (Chapter 6). The specificities of autoantibodies are quite varied, but those directed against transfer RNA synthetases seem to be more or less specific for inflammatory myopathies.[47]

The pathogenesis of inclusion body myositis is less clear. As in polymyositis, CD8+ cytotoxic T cells are found in the muscle, but in contrast to the other two forms of myositis, immunosuppressive therapy is not beneficial. Intracellular deposits of β-amyloid protein, amyloid β–pleated sheet fibrils, and hyperphosphorylated tau protein, features shared with Alzheimer disease, have drawn attention to a possible relationship to aging. The protein deposition may result from abnormal protein folding. The two hereditary forms of inclusion body myopathy have a similar morphology. The autosomal recessive form is caused by mutations in the *GNE* gene (encoding UDP-N-acetylglucosamine 2-epimerase/N-acetylmannosamine kinase), and the autosomal dominant form is caused by mutations in the gene encoding myosin heavy chain IIa.[46,48]

Morphology. The histologic features of the individual forms of myositis are quite distinctive and are described separately.

Dermatomyositis. The inflammatory infiltrates in dermatomyositis are located predominantly around small blood vessels and in the perimysial connective tissue. Typically, groups of atrophic fibers are particularly prominent at the periphery of fascicles. This "perifascicular atrophy" is sufficient for diagnosis, even if the inflammation is mild or absent (Fig. 27–13B), and is most likely related to a relative state of hypoperfusion of the periphery of muscle fascicles. Quantitative analyses reveal a marked reduction in the intramuscular capillaries, believed to result from vascular endothelial injury and fibrosis. Necrotic muscle fibers and regeneration may also be seen throughout the fascicle, as in polymyositis.

Polymyositis. In this condition, the inflammatory cells are found in the endomysium. CD8+ lymphocytes and other lymphoid cells surround and invade healthy muscle fibers. Both necrotic and regenerating muscle fibers are scattered throughout the fascicle, without the perifascicular atrophy seen in dermatomyositis. There is no evidence of vascular injury in polymyositis.

Inclusion Body Myositis. The diagnostic finding in inclusion body myositis is the presence of rimmed vacuoles (Fig. 27–13C). The vacuoles are present within myocytes, and they are highlighted by basophilic granules at their periphery. In addition, the vacuolated fibers may also contain amyloid deposits that reveal typical staining with Congo red. Under the electron microscope, tubular and filamentous inclusions are seen in the cytoplasm and the nucleus that are composed of β-amyloid or hyperphosphorylated tau. The inflammatory cell infiltrate is similar to that seen in polymyositis.

The diagnosis of myositis is based on clinical symptoms, electromyography, elevated creatinine kinase in serum, and biopsy. Electromyography (EMG) is particularly informative; mixed neurogenic and myopathic changes on EMG are suggestive of inflammatory myopathy. As might be expected, muscle injury is associated with elevated serum levels of creatine kinase. Biopsy is required for definitive diagnosis. Immunosuppressive therapy is beneficial in adult and juvenile dermatomyositis and in polymyositis but not in inclusion-body myositis.

TOXIC MYOPATHIES

Thyrotoxic Myopathy

Thyrotoxic myopathy presents most commonly as an acute or chronic proximal muscle weakness that may precede the onset of other signs of thyroid dysfunction. *Exophthalmic ophthalmoplegia* is characterized by swelling of the eyelids, edema of the conjunctiva, and diplopia. In *hypothyroidism* there may be cramping or aching of muscles, and movements and reflexes are slowed. Findings include fiber atrophy, an increased number of internal nuclei, glycogen aggregates, and, occasionally, deposition of mucopolysaccharides in the connective tissue.

In thyrotoxic myopathy, there is myofiber necrosis, regeneration, and interstitial lymphocytosis. In chronic thyrotoxic myopathy, there may be only slight variability of muscle fiber size, mitochondrial hypertrophy, and focal myofibril degeneration; fatty infiltration of muscle is seen in severe cases. Exophthalmic ophthalmoplegia is limited to the extraocular muscles, which may be edematous and enlarged.

Ethanol Myopathy

Binge drinking of alcohol produces an acute toxic syndrome of rhabdomyolysis with accompanying myoglobinuria, which may lead to renal failure. Clinically, the affected individual may develop acute pain that is either generalized or confined to a single muscle group. Some patients have a complicated clinicopathologic syndrome consisting of proximal muscle weakness and electrophysiologic evidence of myopathy superimposed on alcoholic neuropathy. On histologic examination there is swelling of myocytes, fiber necrosis, myophagocytosis, and regeneration. There may also be evidence of denervation.

Drug-Induced Myopathies

Proximal muscle weakness and atrophy can occur as a result of the deleterious effects of steroids on muscle, whether in Cushing syndrome or during therapeutic administration of steroids, a condition known as *steroid myopathy*. The severity of clinical disability is variable and not directly related to the steroid level or the therapeutic regimen. It is characterized by muscle fiber atrophy, predominantly of type 2 fibers. When the myopathy is severe, there may be a bimodal distribution of fibers due to the presence of type 1 fibers of nearly normal caliber and markedly atrophic type 2 fibers. Electron microscopy has shown dilation of the sarcoplasmic reticulum and thickening of the basal laminae.

Chloroquine, originally used in the treatment of malaria but subsequently used in other clinical settings, can produce a proximal myopathy in humans. The most prominent finding is the presence of vacuoles within myocytes. Two types of vacuoles have been described: (1) autophagic membrane-bound vacuoles containing membranous debris; and (2) curvilinear bodies with short curved membranous structures with alternating light and dark zones. Vacuoles can be seen in as many as 50% of the myocytes, most commonly type 1 fibers, and with progression, myocyte necrosis may develop. A similar vacuolar myopathy occurs in some individuals treated with hydrochloroquine.

Statins are very frequently prescribed in the United States to reduce cholesterol and the risks of acute ischemic cardiac events and stroke. Myopathy is the most common complication of statins.[49] "Statin-induced myopathy" can occur with use of any of the statins (e.g., atorvastatin, simvastatin, pravastatin). The incidence is approximately 1.5% of users, and is unrelated to dose, cumulative dose, or statin subtype. Drug metabolism characteristics that can be predicted with pharmacogenetic predictors, on the other hand, may help to identify individuals at risk for myopathy.

DISEASES OF THE NEUROMUSCULAR JUNCTION

Myasthenia Gravis

Myasthenia gravis is a muscle disease caused by immune-mediated loss of acetylcholine receptor. It has a prevalence of about 30 in 100,000 persons.[50] When arising before age 40 years it is most commonly seen in women, but it occurs equally in both sexes in older patients. Thymic hyperplasia is found in 65% and thymoma in 15% of affected patients. Analysis of neuromuscular transmission in myasthenia gravis shows a decrease in the number of muscle acetylcholine receptors (AChRs), and circulating antibodies to the AChR are present in nearly all cases. The disease can be passively transferred to animals with serum from affected individuals.

Pathogenesis. In most instances the autoantibodies against the AChR lead to loss of functional AChRs at the neuromuscular junction by (1) fixing complement and causing direct injury to the postsynaptic membrane, (2) increasing the internalization and degradation of the receptors, and (3) inhibiting binding of acetylcholine. Electrophysiologic studies are notable for diminished motor responses after repeated stimulation; nerve conduction is normal. Sensory as well as autonomic functions are not affected. Despite the evidence that antibodies to AChR have a critical pathogenic role, there is not always a correlation between antibody titers and the neuromuscular deficit. Interestingly, in light of the immune-mediated etiology of the disease, thymic abnormalities are common in these patients, but the precise link between thymic function and autoimmunity is uncertain. Regardless of the type of thymic pathology, most affected individuals improve after thymectomy.

> **Morphology.** By light microscopic examination, muscle biopsy specimens are usually unrevealing. In severe cases type 2 fiber atrophy due to disuse may be found. By electron microscopy the postsynaptic membrane is simplified, and there is loss of AChRs from the region of the synapse. Immune complexes and the complement membrane attack complex (C5–C9) can be found along the postsynaptic membrane as well.

Clinical Course. Typically, weakness begins with the extraocular muscles; drooping eyelids (ptosis) and double vision (diplopia) cause the affected individual to seek medical attention. However, the initial symptoms may take the form of generalized weakness. The weakness fluctuates over days, hours, or even minutes, and intercurrent medical conditions can lead to exacerbations. Patients show improvement in strength in response to administration of anticholinesterase agents, which remains a useful clinical test. Respiratory compromise was a major cause of mortality in the past; 95% of affected individuals now survive more than 5 years after diagnosis because of improved methods of treatment and better ventilatory support. Effective forms of treatment include anticholinesterase drugs, prednisone, plasmapheresis, and thymectomy when thymic lesions are present.[50]

Lambert-Eaton Myasthenic Syndrome

Lambert-Eaton myasthenic syndrome is a disease of the neuromuscular junction that is distinct from myasthenia gravis. It is usually a paraneoplastic process, most commonly with small-cell carcinoma of the lung (60% of cases), but can occur in the absence of underlying malignant disease. Affected individuals develop proximal muscle weakness and autonomic dysfunction. Unlike myasthenia gravis, no clinical improvement is produced by anticholinesterase agents, and electrophysiologic studies show evidence of enhanced neurotransmission with repetitive stimulation. These clinical features allow this disorder to be distinguished from myasthenia gravis.

The content of anticholinesterase is normal in neuromuscular junction synaptic vesicles, and the postsynaptic membrane is normally responsive to anticholinesterase, but fewer vesicles are released in response to each presynaptic action potential. Some affected individuals have antibodies that recognize presynaptic PQ-type voltage-gated calcium channels, and a similar disease can be transferred to animals with these antibodies, suggesting that autoimmunity to the calcium channel causes the disease.

TUMORS OF SKELETAL MUSCLE

Skeletal muscle tumors are discussed with other soft-tissue tumors (Chapter 26).

REFERENCES

1. Navarro X et al.: Neural plasticity after peripheral nerve injury and regeneration. Prog Neurobiol 82:163, 2007.
2. Chen Z-L et al.: Peripheral regeneration. Annu Rev Neurosci 30:209, 2007.
3. Raivich G, Makwana M: The making of successful axonal regeneration: genes, molecules and signal transduction pathways. Brain Res Rev 53:287, 2007.
4. Chen C-J et al.: Transplantation of bone marrow stromal cells for peripheral nerve repair. Exp Neurol 204:443, 2007.
5. Chio A et al.: Guillain-Barré syndrome: a prospective, population-based incidence and outcome survey. Neurology 60:1146, 2003.
6. Hartung H-P et al.: Acute immunoinflammatory neuropathy: update on Guillain-Barré syndrome. Curr Opin Neurol 15:571, 2002.
7. French CSG: Recommendations on diagnostic strategies for chronic inflammatory demyelinating polyradiculoneuropathy. J Neurosurg Psychiatr 79:115, 2008.
8. Rentzos M et al.: Chronic inflammatory demyelinating polyneuropathy: a 6-year retrospective clinical study of a hospital-based population. J Clin Neurosci 14:229, 2007.
9. de Freitas MRG: Infectious neuropathy. Curr Opin Neurol 20:548, 2007.
10. Piradov MA et al.: Diphtheritic polyneuropathy: clinical analysis of severe forms. Arch Neurol 58:1438, 2001.
11. Weinberg JM: Herpes zoster: epidemiology, natural history, and common complications. J Am Acad Dermatol 57:S130, 2007.
12. Klein CJ: The inherited neuropathies. Neurol Clin 25:173, 2007.
13. Suter U, Scherer SS: Disease mechanisms in inherited neuropathies. Nat Rev Neurosci 4:714, 2003.
14. Nave K-A et al.: Mechanisms of disease: inherited demyelinating neuropathies—from basic to clinical research. Nat Clin Pract Neurol 3:453, 2007.
15. Zhao C et al.: Charcot-Marie-Tooth disease type 2A caused by mutation in a microtubule motor KIF1Bbeta. Cell 105:587, 2001. Erratum in: Cell 106:127, 2001.
16. Szigeti K et al.: Molecular diagnostics of Charcot-Marie-Tooth disease and related peripheral neuropathies. Neuromolecular Med 8:243, 2006.
17. Said G: Diabetic neuropathy—a review. Nat Clin Pract Neurol 3:331, 2007.
18. Zochodne DW: Diabetes mellitus and the peripheral nervous system: manifestations and mechanisms. Muscle Nerve 36:144, 2007.
19. Krishnan AV, Kiernan MC: Uremic neuropathy: clinical features and new pathophysiological insights. Muscle Nerve 35:273, 2007.
20. Koike H, Sobue G: Alcoholic neuropathy. Curr Opin Neurol 19:481, 2006.
21. Rudnicki SA, Dalmau J: Paraneoplastic syndromes of the peripheral nerves. Curr Opin Neurol 18:598, 2005.
22. Aguirre-Cruz L et al.: Clinical relevance of non-neuronal auto-antibodies in patients with anti-Hu or anti-Yo paraneoplastic diseases. J Neuro-Oncol 71:39, 2005.
23. Steck AJ et al.: Anti-myelin-associated glycoprotein neuropathy. Curr Opin Neurol 19:458, 2006.
24. London Z, Albers JW: Toxic neuropathies associated with pharmaceutic and industrial agents. Neurol Clin 25:257, 2007.
25. Bland JDP: Carpal tunnel syndrome [see comment]. BMJ 335:343, 2007.
26. Lunn MR, Wang CH: Spinal muscular atrophy. Lancet 371:2120, 2008.
27. McNally EM: New approaches in the therapy of cardiomyopathy in muscular dystrophy. Annu Rev Med 58:75, 2007.
28. Ervasti JM: Dystrophin, its interactions with other proteins, and implications for muscular dystrophy. Biochim Biophys Acta 1772:108, 2007.
29. Rodino-Klapac LR et al.: Gene therapy for Duchenne muscular dystrophy: expectations and challenges. Arch Neurol 64:1236, 2007.
30. van Deutekom JC et al.: Local dystrophin restoration with antisense oligonucleotide PRO051 [see comment]. N Engl J Med 357:2677, 2007.
31. Bonnemann CG: Limb-girdle muscular dystrophy in childhood. Pediatr Ann 34:569, 2005.

32. Guglieri M et al.: Molecular etiopathogenesis of limb girdle muscular and congenital muscular dystrophies: boundaries and contiguities. Clin Chim Acta 361:54, 2005.

33. Schara U, Schoser BGH: Myotonic dystrophies type 1 and 2: a summary on current aspects. Semin Pediatr Neurol 13:71, 2006.

34. Vicart S et al.: Human skeletal muscle sodium channelopathies. Neurol Sci 26:194, 2005.

35. Brandom BW: The genetics of malignant hyperthermia. Anesthesiol Clin North America 23:615, 2005.

36. Bruno C, Minetti C: Congenital myopathies. Curr Neurol Neurosci Rep 4:68, 2004.

37. Di Mauro S: Muscle glycogenoses: an overview. Acta Myol 26:35, 2007.

38. Wieser T et al.: Carnitine palmitoyltransferase II deficiency: molecular and biochemical analysis of 32 patients. Neurology 60:1351, 2003.

39. Vladutiu GD, Slonim AE: Combined biochemical and molecular diagnosis in blood of a common lipid myopathy. Muscle Nerve 23:1773, 2000.

40. DiMauro S, Gurgel-Giannetti J: The expanding phenotype of mitochondrial myopathy. Curr Opin Neurol 18:538, 2005.

41. DiMauro S, Hirano M: Mitochondrial encephalomyopathies: an update. Neuromuscul Disord 15:276, 2005.

42. Sarnat HB, Marin-Garcia J: Pathology of mitochondrial encephalomyopathies. Can J Neurol Sci 32:152, 2005.

43. Dalakas MC: Mechanisms of disease: signaling pathways and immunobiology of inflammatory myopathies. Nat Clin Pract Rheumatol 2:219, 2006. Erratum in: Nat Clin Pract Rheumatol 2:398, 2006.

44. Callen JP, Wortmann RL: Dermatomyositis. Clin Dermatol 24:363, 2006.

45. Griffin TA, Reed AM: Pathogenesis of myositis in children. Curr Opin Rheumatol 19:487, 2007.

46. Askanas V, Engel WK: Inclusion-body myositis, a multifactorial muscle disease associated with aging: current concepts of pathogenesis. Curr Opin Rheumatol 19:550, 2007.

47. Mimori T et al.: Autoantibodies in idiopathic inflammatory myopathy: an update on clinical and pathophysiological significance. Curr Opin Rheumatol 19:523, 2007.

48. Needham M et al.: Genetics of inclusion-body myositis. Muscle Nerve 35:549, 2007.

49. Antons KA et al.: Clinical perspectives of statin-induced rhabdomyolysis. Am J Med 119:400, 2006.

50. Conti-Fine BM et al.: Myasthenia gravis: past, present, and future. J Clin Invest 116:2843, 2006.

28

The Central Nervous System

MATTHEW P. FROSCH · DOUGLAS C. ANTHONY · UMBERTO DE GIROLAMI

Cellular Responses to Injury

Cerebral Edema, Hydrocephalus, and Raised Intracranial Pressure and Herniation
  Cerebral Edema
  Hydrocephalus
  Raised Intracranial Pressure and Herniation

Malformations and Developmental Diseases
  Neural Tube Defects
  Forebrain Anomalies
  Posterior Fossa Anomalies
  Syringomyelia and Hydromyelia

Perinatal Brain Injury

Trauma
  Skull Fractures
  Parenchymal Injuries
    Concussion
    Direct Parenchymal Injury
    Diffuse Axonal Injury
  Traumatic Vascular Injury
    Epidural Hematoma
    Subdural Hematoma
  Sequelae of Brain Trauma
  Spinal Cord Trauma

Cerebrovascular Diseases
  Hypoxia, Ischemia, and Infarction
    Hypotension, Hypoperfusion, and Low-Flow States (Global Cerebral Ischemia)
    Infarction from Obstruction of Local Blood Supply (Focal Cerebral Ischemia)

Hypertensive Cerebrovascular Disease
  Lacunar Infarcts
  Slit Hemorrhages
  Hypertensive Encephalopathy
Intracranial Hemorrhage
  Intracerebral (Intraparenchymal) Hemorrhage
  Subarachnoid Hemorrhage and Ruptured Saccular Aneurysms
  Vascular Malformations

Infections
  Acute Meningitis
    Acute Pyogenic (Bacterial) Meningitis
    Acute Aseptic (Viral) Meningitis
  Acute Focal Suppurative Infections
    Brain Abscess
    Subdural Empyema
    Extradural Abscess
  Chronic Bacterial Meningoencephalitis
    Tuberculosis
    Neurosyphilis
    Neuroborreliosis (Lyme Disease)
  Viral Meningoencephalitis
    Arthropod-Borne Viral Encephalitis
    Herpes Simplex Virus Type 1
    Herpes Simplex Virus Type 2
    Varicella-Zoster Virus (Herpes Zoster)
    Cytomegalovirus
    Poliomyelitis
    Rabies
    Human Immunodeficiency Virus
    Progressive Multifocal Leukoencephalopathy
    Subacute Sclerosing Panencephalitis
  Fungal Meningoencephalitis
  Other Infectious Diseases of the Nervous System

Transmissible Spongiform Encephalopathies (Prion Diseases)

Demyelinating Diseases

  Multiple Sclerosis

  Neuromyelitis Optica

  Acute Disseminated Encephalomyelitis and Acute Necrotizing Hemorrhagic Encephalomyelitis

  Other Diseases with Demyelination

Degenerative Diseases

  Degenerative Diseases Affecting the Cerebral Cortex
  Alzheimer Disease
  Frontotemporal Dementias
  Vascular Dementia

  Degenerative Diseases of Basal Ganglia and Brainstem
  Parkinsonism
  Parkinson Disease
  Dementia with Lewy Bodies
  Multiple System Atrophy
  Huntington Disease

  Spinocerebellar Degenerations
  Spinocerebellar Ataxias

  Degenerative Diseases Affecting Motor Neurons
  Amyotrophic Lateral Sclerosis (ALS; Motor Neuron Disease)
  Bulbospinal Atrophy (Kennedy Syndrome)
  Spinal Muscular Atrophy

Genetic Metabolic Diseases

  Neuronal Storage Diseases
  Neuronal Ceroid Lipofuscinoses
  Tay-Sachs Disease

  Leukodystrophies
  Krabbe Disease
  Metachromatic Leukodystrophy
  Adrenoleukodystrophy
  Pelizaeus-Merzbacher Disease
  Canavan Disease
  Alexander Disease
  Vanishing-White-Matter Leukodystrophy

  Mitochondrial Encephalomyopathies
  Mitochondrial Encephalomyopathy, Lactic Acidosis, and Strokelike Episodes
  Myoclonic Epilepsy and Ragged Red Fibers

Leigh Syndrome (Subacute Necrotizing Encephalopathy)
Kearn-Sayre Syndrome
Alpers Disease

Toxic and Acquired Metabolic Diseases

  Vitamin Deficiencies
  Thiamine (Vitamin B_1) Deficiency
  Vitamin B_{12} Deficiency

  Neurologic Sequelae of Metabolic Disturbances
  Hypoglycemia
  Hyperglycemia
  Hepatic Encephalopathy

  Toxic Disorders
  Carbon Monoxide
  Methanol
  Ethanol
  Radiation
  Combined Methotrexate and Radiation-Induced Injury

Tumors

  Gliomas
  Astrocytoma
  Oligodendroglioma
  Ependymoma and Related Paraventricular Mass Lesions

  Neuronal Tumors

  Poorly Differentiated Neoplasms
  Medulloblastoma
  Atypical Teratoid/Rhabdoid Tumor

  Other Parenchymal Tumors
  Primary CNS Lymphoma
  Germ Cell Tumors
  Pineal Parenchymal Tumors

  Meningiomas

  Metastatic Tumors

  Paraneoplastic Syndromes

  Peripheral Nerve Sheath Tumors
  Schwannoma
  Neurofibroma
  Malignant Peripheral Nerve Sheath Tumor

  Familial Tumor Syndromes
  Neurofibromatosis Type 1
  Neurofibromatosis Type 2
  Tuberous Sclerosis Complex
  Von Hippel–Lindau Disease

The principal functional unit of the central nervous system (CNS) is the neuron. Of all the cells in the body, neurons have a unique ability to receive, store, and transmit information. Neurons of different types and in different locations have distinct properties, including functional roles, distribution of their connections, neurotransmitters used, metabolic requirements, and levels of electrical activity at a given moment. A set of neurons, not necessarily clustered together in a region of the brain, may thus show *selective vulnerability* to various insults because it shares one or more of these properties. Since most mature neurons are incapable of cell division, destruction of even a small number of neurons essential for a specific function may leave the individual with a neurologic deficit. Stem cell populations in the brain may represent a potential mechanism for repair after injury.[1] The CNS is affected by a number of unique neurological disorders, and also responds to common insults (e.g., ischemia, infection) in a manner that is distinct from other tissues.[2,3]

Cellular Pathology of the Central Nervous System

Reactions of Neurons to Injury. Neurons vary considerably in structure and size throughout the nervous system and within a given brain region. Structural specializations associated with neuronal function include those related to synaptic transmission as well as axonal and dendritic differentiation. Neurons share pathways for response to injury, including apoptotic mechanisms, with cells in other tissues. During development, neuronal apoptosis has an important role in defining neuronal number; it comes into play in a variety of disease states as well, including certain neurodegenerative diseases. The principal patterns of neuronal injury are the following:

- *Acute neuronal injury ("red neurons")* refers to a spectrum of changes that accompany acute CNS hypoxia/ischemia or other acute insults and reflect cell death, either necrosis or apoptosis (see Fig. 28–13B). "Red neurons" are evident with hematoxylin and eosin (H&E) preparations at about 12 to 24 hours after an irreversible hypoxic/ischemic insult. The morphologic features consist of shrinkage of the cell body, pyknosis of the nucleus, disappearance of the nucleolus, and loss of Nissl substance, with intense eosinophilia of the cytoplasm.
- *Subacute and chronic neuronal injury ("degeneration")* refers to neuronal death occurring as a result of a progressive disease process of some duration, as is seen in certain slowly evolving neurologic diseases such as amyotrophic lateral sclerosis (ALS). The characteristic histologic feature is cell loss, often selectively involving functionally related groups of neurons, and reactive gliosis. When the process is at an early stage, the cell loss is difficult to detect; the associated reactive glial changes are often the best indicator of the pathologic process. For many of these diseases, there is evidence that cell loss is because of apoptosis. Neuronal *trans-synaptic degeneration* is seen when there is a destructive process that interrupts the majority of the afferent input to a group of neurons.
- *Axonal reaction* refers to the reaction within the cell body that attends *regeneration* of the axon; it is best seen in ante- rior horn cells of the spinal cord when motor axons are cut or seriously damaged. There is increased protein synthesis associated with axonal sprouting. This is reflected in enlargement and rounding up of the cell body, peripheral displacement of the nucleus, enlargement of the nucleolus, and dispersion of Nissl substance from the center to the periphery of the cell *(central chromatolysis)*.
- Neuronal damage may be associated with a wide range of subcellular alterations in the neuronal organelles and cytoskeleton. *Neuronal inclusions* may occur as a manifestation of aging, when there are intracytoplasmic accumulations of complex lipids *(lipofuscin)*, proteins, or carbohydrates. Abnormal cytoplasmic deposition of complex lipids and other substances also occurs in genetically determined disorders of metabolism in which substrates or intermediates accumulate (Chapter 5). Viral infection can lead to abnormal intranuclear inclusions, as seen in herpetic infection (Cowdry body), cytoplasmic inclusions, as seen in rabies (Negri body), or both nucleus and cytoplasm as in cytomegalovirus (CMV) infection.
- Some degenerative diseases of the CNS are associated with neuronal intracytoplasmic inclusions, such as neurofibrillary tangles of Alzheimer disease and Lewy bodies of Parkinson disease; others cause abnormal vacuolization of the perikaryon and neuronal cell processes in the neuropil (Creutzfeldt-Jakob disease). These aggregates are highly resistant to degradation, contain proteins with altered conformation, and may result from mutations that affect protein folding, ubiquitination, and intracellular trafficking (see discussion of protein folding in Chapter 1). The disorders may be referred to as *proteinopathies*. There is increasing evidence in many of these diseases that the visible aggregates are not the basis of cellular injuries; rather, small multimers of the proteins (oligomers) are the critical mediators of the damage.[4]

Reactions of Astrocytes to Injury. The astrocyte derives its name from its star-shaped appearance. These cells have multipolar, branching cytoplasmic processes that emanate from the cell body and contain the glial fibrillary acidic protein (GFAP), a cell type–specific intermediate filament (Fig. 28–1). Astrocytes act as metabolic buffers and detoxifiers within the brain. Additionally, through the foot processes, which surround capillaries or extend to the subpial and subependymal zones, they contribute to barrier functions controlling the flow of macromolecules between the blood, the cerebrospinal fluid (CSF), and the brain. *Gliosis* (or astrogliosis) is the most important histopathologic indicator of CNS injury, regardless of etiology, and is characterized by both hypertrophy and hyperplasia. In this reaction, the nuclei of astrocytes, which are typically round to oval (10 μm wide) with evenly dispersed, pale chromatin, enlarge, become vesicular, and develop prominent nucleoli. The previously scant cytoplasm expands to a bright pink, somewhat irregular swath around an eccentric nucleus, from which emerge numerous stout, ramifying processes; these cells are called *gemistocytic astrocytes*.

When directly injured, astrocytes can react with cytoplasmic swelling. This is seen in acute insults that cause the cell's ATP-dependent ion channels to fail, as occurs in hypoxia, hypoglycemia, and toxic injuries. The *Alzheimer type II astrocyte* is a gray-matter cell with a large (two to three times

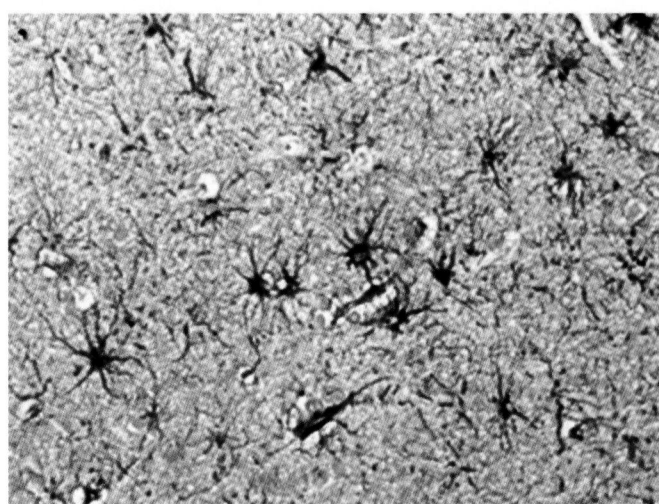

FIGURE 28-1 Astrocytes and their processes. Immunohisto-chemical staining for GFAP reveals astrocytic perinuclear cyto-plasm and well-developed processes *(brown)*.

normal) nucleus, pale-staining central chromatin, an intra-nuclear glycogen droplet, and a prominent nuclear membrane and nucleolus. Its name is a misnomer, as it is mainly seen not in Alzheimer disease but in individuals with long-standing hyperammonemia due to chronic liver disease, Wilson disease, or hereditary metabolic disorders of the urea cycle.

Astrocytes are not spared from processes that cause the formation of cytoplasmic inclusion bodies. *Rosenthal fibers* are thick, elongated, brightly eosinophilic, somewhat irregular structures that occur within astrocytic processes, and contain two heat-shock proteins (αB-crystallin and hsp27) as well as ubiquitin. Rosenthal fibers are typically found in regions of long-standing gliosis; they are also characteristic of one type of glial tumor, pilocytic astrocytoma. In *Alexander disease*, a leukodystrophy associated with a mutations in the gene encod-ing GFAP, abundant Rosenthal fibers are found in periven-tricular, perivascular, and subpial locations. More commonly seen are *corpora amylacea*, or polyglucosan bodies. These are round, faintly basophilic, periodic acid–Schiff (PAS)–positive, concentrically lamellated structures of 5 to 50 µm in diameter that are located wherever there are astrocytic end processes, especially in the subpial and perivascular zones. Though con-sisting primarily of glycosaminoglycan polymers, they also contain heat-shock proteins and ubiquitin. They occur in increasing numbers with advancing age and are thought to represent a degenerative change in the astrocyte. The *Lafora bodies* that are seen in the cytoplasm of neurons (as well as hepatocytes, myocytes, and other cells) in myoclonic epilepsy (Lafora body myoclonus with epilepsy) have a similar struc-ture and biochemical composition.

Reactions of Other Glial Cells to Injury. In contrast to astrocytes, oligodendrocytes and ependyma do not participate in the active response to CNS injury and show a more limited repertoire of reactions. Oligodendroglial cytoplasmic pro-cesses wrap around exons and form myelin. Each oligoden-drocyte myelinates numerous internodes on multiple axons. Injury or apoptosis of oligodendroglial cells is a feature of acquired demyelinating disorders and leukodystrophies. Oligodendroglial nuclei may harbor viral inclusions in pro-

gressive multifocal leukoencephalopathy. *Glial cytoplasmic inclusions*, primarily composed of α-synuclein, are found in oligodendrocytes in multiple system atrophy (MSA).

Ependymal cells, the ciliated columnar epithelial cells lining the ventricles, do not have specific patterns of reaction. When there is inflammation or marked dilation of the ventricular system, disruption of the ependymal lining is paired with proliferation of subependymal astrocytes to produce small irregularities on the ventricular surfaces *(ependymal granula-tions)*. Certain infectious agents, particularly CMV, may produce extensive ependymal injury, with viral inclusions in ependymal cells.

Reactions of Microglia to Injury. Microglia are meso-derm-derived cells whose primary function is to serve as a fixed macrophage system in the CNS. They share many surface markers with peripheral monocytes/macrophages (such as CR3 and CD68). They respond to injury by (1) proliferating; (2) developing elongated nuclei *(rod cells)*, as in neurosyphilis; (3) forming aggregates about small foci of tissue necrosis *(microglial nodules)*; or (4) congregating around cell bodies of dying neurons *(neuronophagia)*. In addition to resident microglia, blood-derived macrophages are the principal phagocytic cells present in inflammatory foci.

Cerebral Edema, Hydrocephalus, and Raised Intracranial Pressure and Herniation

The brain and spinal cord are protected by the rigid compart-ment defined by the skull, vertebral bodies, and dura mater. Generalized brain edema, increased CSF volume (hydroceph-alus), and focally expanding mass lesions may increase intra-cranial pressure. Depending on the degree and rapidity of this increase and the nature of the underlying lesion, the conse-quences range from subtle neurologic deficits to death.

CEREBRAL EDEMA

Cerebral edema or, more precisely, brain parenchymal edema, is of two principal types:

- *Vasogenic edema* is caused by blood-brain barrier disrup-tion and increased vascular permeability, allowing fluid to shift from the intravascular compartment to the intercel-lular spaces of the brain. The paucity of lymphatics greatly impairs the resorption of excess extracellular fluid. Vaso-genic edema may be either localized (e.g., adjacent to inflammation or neoplasms) or generalized.
- *Cytotoxic edema* is an increase in intracellular fluid second-ary to neuronal, glial, or endothelial cell membrane injury, as might be encountered in someone with a generalized hypoxic/ischemic insult or with metabolic damage.

In practice, conditions associated with generalized edema often have elements of both vasogenic and cytotoxic edema.

Interstitial edema (hydrocephalic edema) occurs especially around the lateral ventricles when an increase in intravascular pressure causes an abnormal flow of fluid from the intraven-tricular CSF across the ependymal lining to the periventricular

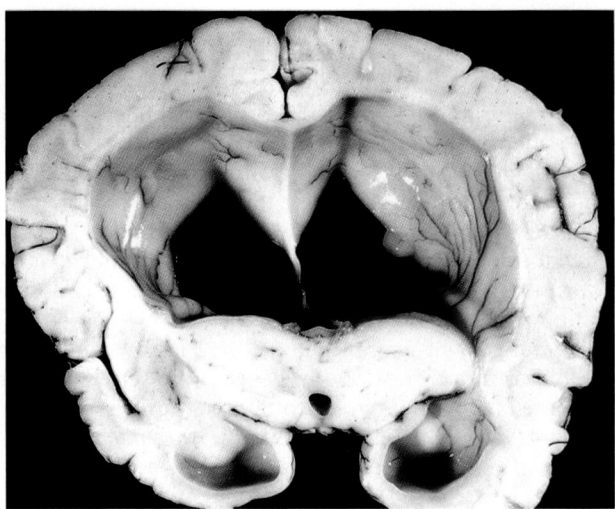

FIGURE 28–2 Hydrocephalus. Dilated lateral ventricles seen in a coronal section through the midthalamus.

white matter. In generalized edema, the gyri are flattened, the intervening sulci are narrowed, and the ventricular cavities are compressed. As the brain expands, herniation may occur.

HYDROCEPHALUS

The choroid plexus within the ventricular system produces CSF, which normally circulates through the ventricular system and enters the cisterna magna at the base of the brain stem through the foramina of Luschka and Magendie. Subarachnoid CSF bathes the superior cerebral convexities and is absorbed by the arachnoid granulations. *Hydrocephalus* refers to the accumulation of excessive CSF within the ventricular system (Fig. 28–2). Most cases occur as a consequence of impaired flow and resorption of CSF; only rarely is overproduction the cause of hydrocephalus (e.g., with tumors of the choroid plexus). An increased volume of CSF within the ventricles expands them and can elevate the intracranial pressure.

When hydrocephalus develops in infancy before closure of the cranial sutures, there is enlargement of the head, manifested by an increase in head circumference. Hydrocephalus developing after this period, in contrast, is associated with expansion of the ventricles and increased intracranial pressure, without a change in head circumference. If only a portion of the ventricular system is enlarged because of excess CSF, as may occur because of a mass in the third ventricle, the pattern is called *noncommunicating hydrocephalus*. In *communicating hydrocephalus* there is enlargement of the entire ventricular system. The term *hydrocephalus ex vacuo* refers to dilation of the ventricular system with a compensatory increase in CSF volume secondary to a loss of brain parenchyma.

RAISED INTRACRANIAL PRESSURE AND HERNIATION

When the volume of the brain increases beyond the limit permitted by compression of veins and displacement of CSF, the pressure within the skull will increase. Most cases are associated with a mass effect, either diffuse, as in generalized brain edema, or focal, as with tumors, abscesses, or hemorrhages. Elevated intracranial pressure may also reduce perfusion of the brain, further exacerbating cerebral edema. Because the cranial vault is divided by rigid dural folds (the falx and tentorium), localized expansion of the brain may cause it to be displaced in relation to these partitions. If the expansion is sufficiently severe, a *herniation syndrome* may occur (Fig. 28–3).

- *Subfalcine (cingulate) herniation* occurs when unilateral or asymmetric expansion of a cerebral hemisphere displaces the cingulate gyrus under the falx cerebri. This may lead to compression of branches of the anterior cerebral artery.
- *Transtentorial (uncinate, mesial temporal) herniation* occurs when the medial aspect of the temporal lobe is compressed against the free margin of the tentorium. With increasing displacement of the temporal lobe, the third cranial nerve is compromised, resulting in pupillary dilation and impairment of ocular movements on the side of the lesion. The posterior cerebral artery may also be compressed, resulting in ischemic injury to the territory supplied by that vessel, including the primary visual cortex. When the extent of herniation is large enough the contralateral cerebral peduncle may be compressed, resulting in hemiparesis ipsilateral to the side of the herniation; the change in the peduncle in this setting is known as *Kernohan's notch*. Progression of transtentorial herniation is often accompanied by hemorrhagic lesions in the midbrain and pons, termed *secondary brainstem*, or *Duret, hemorrhages* (Fig. 28–4). These linear or flame-shaped lesions usually occur in the midline and

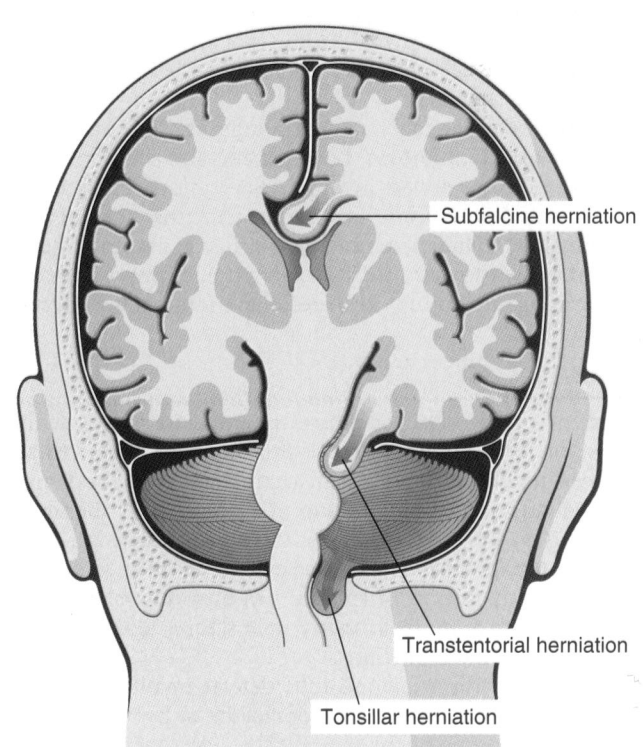

Subfalcine herniation

Transtentorial herniation

Tonsillar herniation

FIGURE 28–3 Major herniation syndromes of the brain: subfalcine, transtentorial, and tonsillar.

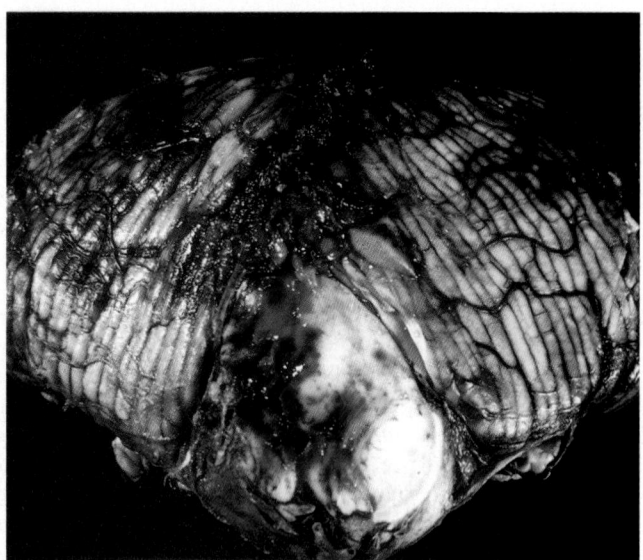

FIGURE 28–4   Duret hemorrhage involving the brainstem at the junction of the pons and midbrain.

paramedian regions and are believed to be due to distortion or tearing of penetrating veins and arteries supplying the upper brainstem.

○ *Tonsillar herniation* refers to displacement of the cerebellar tonsils through the foramen magnum. This pattern of herniation is life-threatening because it causes brainstem compression and compromises vital respiratory and cardiac centers in the medulla oblongata.

Malformations and Developmental Diseases

Although the pathogenesis and etiology of CNS malformations are largely unknown, both genetic and environmental influences appear to be involved. Aberrations of signaling molecules and mutations of homeotic genes that control body patterning are being increasingly identified as causes of developmental disorders of the CNS. Many toxic compounds and infectious agents are also known to have teratogenic effects.[5]

NEURAL TUBE DEFECTS

Failure of a portion of the neural tube to close, or reopening of a region of the tube after successful closure, may lead to one of several malformations.[6] All are characterized by abnormalities involving some combination of neural tissue, meninges, and overlying bone or soft tissues. An *encephalocele* is a diverticulum of malformed CNS tissue extending through a defect in the cranium. It most often occurs in the occipital region or in the posterior fossa. Collectively, neural tube defects account for most CNS malformations.

The most common neural tube defects involve the spinal cord and are caused by a failure of closure or by reopening of the caudal portions of the neural tube. *Spinal dysraphism* or *spina bifida* may be an asymptomatic bony defect (spina bifida occulta) or a severe malformation with a flattened, disorga-

nized segment of spinal cord, associated with an overlying meningeal outpouching. *Myelomeningocele* (or meningomyelocele) refers to extension of CNS tissue through a defect in the vertebral column; the term *meningocele* applies when there is only a meningeal extrusion. Myelomeningoceles occur most commonly in the lumbosacral region, and affected individuals manifest clinical deficits referable to motor and sensory function in the lower extremities as well as disturbances of bowel and bladder control from both the structural abnormality of the cord itself and superimposed infection that extends from the thin, overlying skin.

The frequency of neural tube defects varies widely among different ethnic groups. Both genetic and environmental factors are involved. The concordance rate is high among monozygotic twins, and the overall recurrence rate for a neural tube defect in subsequent pregnancies has been estimated at 4% to 5%. Folate deficiency during the initial weeks of gestation has been implicated as a risk factor; differences in rates of neural tube defects between populations can be attributed in part to polymorphisms in enzymes of folic acid metabolism. Folate deficiency may affect cell division during critical periods that coincide with closure of the neural tube. Antenatal diagnosis is based on imaging and the screening of maternal blood samples for elevation of α-fetoprotein.

Anencephaly is a malformation of the anterior end of the neural tube, with absence of the brain and calvarium. Forebrain development is disrupted at approximately 28 days of gestation, and all that remains in its place is the *area cerebrovasculosa*, a flattened remnant of disorganized brain tissue with admixed ependyma, choroid plexus, and meningothelial cells. The posterior fossa structures may be spared, depending on the extent of the skull deficit; descending tracts associated with disrupted structures are, as expected, absent.

FOREBRAIN ANOMALIES

The volume of brain may be abnormally large *(megalencephaly)* or small *(microencephaly)*. Microencephaly, by far the more common of the two, can occur in a wide range of settings, including chromosome abnormalities, fetal alcohol syndrome, and human immunodeficiency virus 1 (HIV-1) infection acquired in utero. It is postulated that the underlying anomaly is a reduction in the number of neurons that reach the neocortex and this leads to a simplification of the gyral folding—a model supported by experimental results in mouse models. The pool of proliferating precursor cells in the developing brain lies adjacent to the ventricular system. Neuronal number is determined by the fraction of proliferating cells that undergo transition into migrating cells with each cell cycle. Early on, most cell divisions yield two more progenitor cells, while as development progresses there are more asymmetric divisions yielding both a progenitor cell and a cell headed for the developing cortex. If excess cells exit the proliferating pool too early, then the overall generation of neurons is reduced; if too few exit during early rounds of division, then the geometric expansion of the proliferating population results in an eventual overproduction of neurons.[7-9]

Among the recognizable malformations[10] are conditions that can range from a noticeable decrease in the number of gyri to total absence, leaving a smooth-surfaced brain, *lissencephaly (agyria)* (Fig. 28–5). A variety of forms of lissenceph-

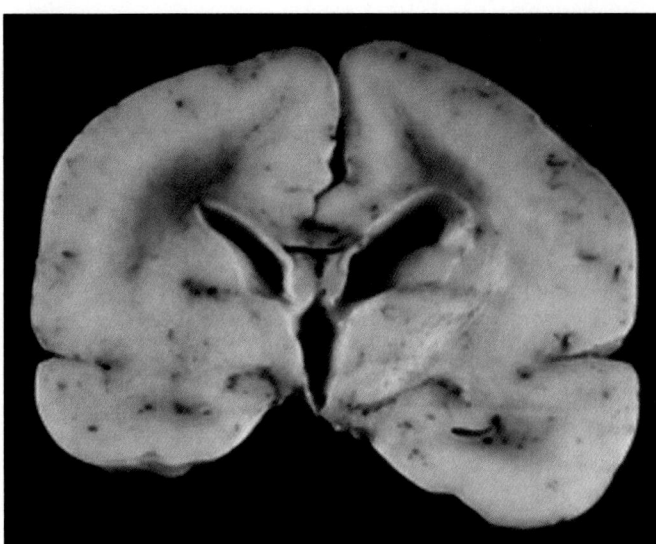

FIGURE 28–5 Lissencephaly. The absence of cortical gyri defines this abnormality, seen here in the brain from a full-term infant.

aly with distinct genetic causes have been described. One of the best understood causes is mutations in the gene encoding the microtubule-associated protein LIS-1, which complexes with dynein and affects the function of the centrosome in nuclear movement. Lissencephaly can also occur from a series of mutations in the genes encoding enzymes responsible for the glycosylation of α-dystroglycan; when this receptor for extracellular matrix components does not have appropriate post-translational modifications, its stability is diminished.

Polymicrogyria is characterized by small, unusually numerous, and irregularly formed cerebral convolutions. The gray matter is composed of four layers (or fewer), with entrapment of apparent meningeal tissue at points of fusion that would otherwise be the cortical surface. Polymicrogyria can be induced by localized tissue injury toward the end of neuronal migration, although genetically determined forms, which are typically bilateral and symmetric, are also recognized.[11]

Neuronal heterotopias are a group of migrational disorders that are commonly associated with epilepsy.[12] They consist of collections of neurons in inappropriate locations along the migrational pathways. As might be expected, one location in which heterotopias can be found is along the ventricular surface—as though the cells never managed to leave their place of birth. Periventricular heterotopias can be caused by mutations in the gene encoding filamin A, an actin-binding protein responsible for assembly of complex meshworks of filaments. This gene is on the X chromosome, and the mutant allele causes male lethality; in females the process of X inactivation separates neurons into those with a normal allele (in the correct location) and those with the mutant allele (in the heterotopia). Another microtubule-associated protein, doublecortin (DCX), is also encoded by a gene on the X chromosome; mutations in this gene result in lissencephaly in males and in subcortical band heterotopias in females. These heterotopias may consist of discrete nodules of neurons sitting in the subcortical white matter or complete ribbons that parody the overlying cortex.

Holoprosencephaly is a spectrum of malformations characterized by incomplete separation of the cerebral hemispheres across the midline. Severe forms manifest midline facial abnormalities, including cyclopia; less severe variants (arrhinencephaly) show absence of the olfactory cranial nerves and related structures. Intrauterine diagnosis of severe forms by ultrasound examination is now possible. Holoprosencephaly is associated with trisomy 13 as well as other genetic syndromes.[13] Sonic hedgehog is a member of a family of secreted proteins synthesized by the notochord and neural plate during neural development. Mutations affecting sonic hedgehog or its signaling pathway may result in holoprosencephaly.

In *agenesis of the corpus callosum*, a relatively common malformation, there is an absence of the white matter bundles that carry cortical projections from one hemisphere to the other (Fig. 28–6). Radiologic imaging studies show misshapen lateral ventricles ("bat-wing" deformity); on coronal wholemount sections of the brain, bundles of anteroposteriorly oriented white matter can be demonstrated. Agenesis of the corpus callosum can be associated with mental retardation or may occur in clinically normal individuals. It can be present in isolation or can be associated with a wide range of other malformations. Unlike patients with surgical callosal section, who show clinical evidence of hemispheric disconnection, individuals with this malformation can have minimal deficits.

POSTERIOR FOSSA ANOMALIES

The *Dandy-Walker malformation* is characterized by an enlarged posterior fossa. The cerebellar vermis is absent or present only in rudimentary form in its anterior portion. In its place is a large midline cyst that is lined by ependyma and is contiguous with leptomeninges on its outer surface. This cyst represents the expanded, roofless fourth ventricle in the absence of a normally formed vermis. Dysplasias of brainstem nuclei are commonly found in association with Dandy-Walker malformation.

The *Arnold-Chiari malformation* (Chiari type II malformation) consists of a small posterior fossa, a misshapen midline

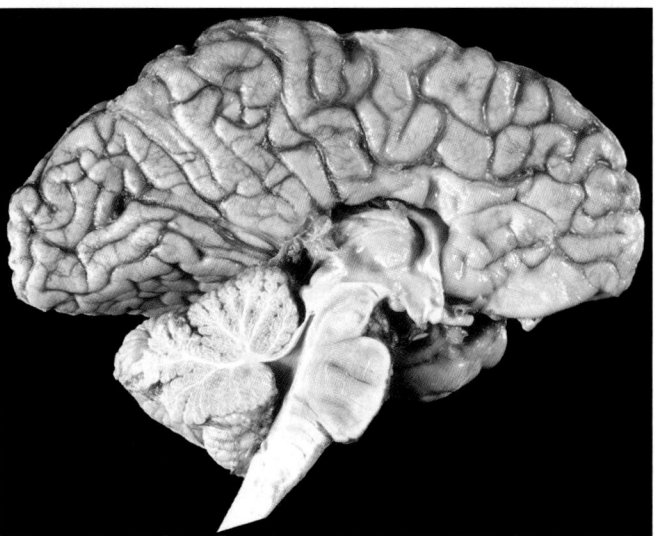

FIGURE 28–6 Agenesis of the corpus callosum. The midsagittal view of the left hemisphere shows the lack of a corpus callosum and cingulate gyrus above the third ventricle.

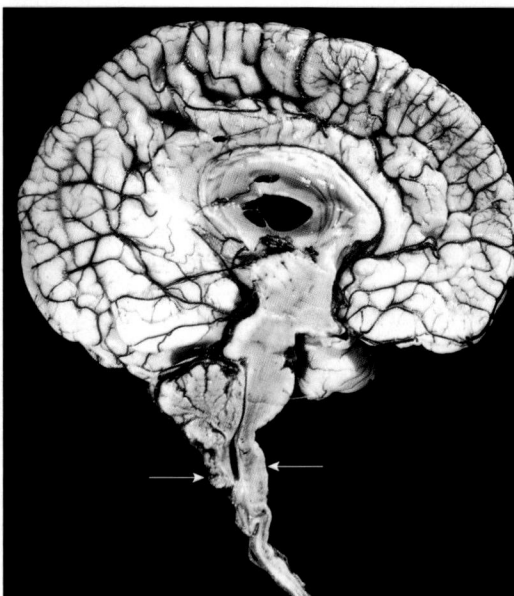

FIGURE 28–7 Arnold-Chiari malformation. Midsagittal section showing small posterior fossa contents, downward displacement of the cerebellar vermis, and deformity of the medulla (*arrows* indicate the approximate level of the foramen magnum).

cerebellum with downward extension of vermis through the foramen magnum (Fig. 28–7), and, almost invariably, hydrocephalus and a lumbar myelomeningocele. Other associated changes may include caudal displacement of the medulla, malformation of the tectum, aqueductal stenosis, cerebral heterotopias, and hydromyelia (see later). In the *Chiari I malformation*, low-lying cerebellar tonsils extend down into the vertebral canal. In contrast to the significant clinical consequences of the preceding two malformations, this may be a silent abnormality or may cause symptoms referable to obstruction of CSF flow and medullary compression; if present, these symptoms can usually be corrected by neurosurgical intervention.

SYRINGOMYELIA AND HYDROMYELIA

These are disorders characterized by a discontinuous multisegmental or confluent expansion of the ependyma-lined central canal of the cord *(hydromyelia)* or by the formation of a fluid-filled cleftlike cavity in the inner portion of the cord *(syringomyelia, syrinx)* that may extend into the brainstem *(syringobulbia)*.

Syringomyelia may be associated with the Chiari I malformation; it may also occur in association with intraspinal tumors or following traumatic injury. In general, the histologic appearance is similar in all these conditions, with destruction of the adjacent gray and white matter, surrounded by a dense feltwork of reactive gliosis. The disease generally becomes manifest in the second or third decade of life. The distinctive symptoms and signs of a syrinx are the isolated loss of pain and temperature sensation in the upper extremities because of the predilection for early involvement of the crossing anterior spinal commissural fibers of the spinal cord.

Perinatal Brain Injury

Brain injury occurring in the perinatal period is an important cause of childhood neurologic disability. Injuries that occur early in gestation may destroy brain tissue without evoking the usual "reactive" changes in the parenchyma and may be difficult to distinguish from malformations.

The broad clinical term *cerebral palsy* refers to a nonprogressive neurologic motor deficit characterized by combinations of spasticity, dystonia, ataxia/athetosis, and paresis attributable to insults occurring during the prenatal and perinatal periods. Signs and symptoms may not be apparent at birth and only later declare themselves, as development proceeds. Postmortem examinations of children with this syndrome have shown a wide range of neuropathologic findings, including destructive lesions traced to remote events that may have caused hemorrhage and infarction.

In premature infants there is an increased risk of *intraparenchymal hemorrhage* within the germinal matrix, often near the junction between the thalamus and the caudate nucleus. Hemorrhages may remain localized or extend into the ventricular system and thence to the subarachnoid space, sometimes leading to hydrocephalus.

Infarcts may occur in the supratentorial periventricular white matter *(periventricular leukomalacia)*, especially in premature infants. These are chalky yellow plaques consisting of discrete regions of white matter necrosis and calcification. When both gray and white matter are involved by extensive ischemic damage, large destructive cystic lesions develop throughout the hemispheres; this condition is termed *multicystic encephalopathy* (Fig. 28–8).

In perinatal ischemic lesions of the cerebral cortex, the depths of sulci bear the brunt of injury and result in thinned-out, gliotic gyri *(ulegyria)*. The basal ganglia and thalamus may also suffer ischemic injury, with patchy neuronal loss and

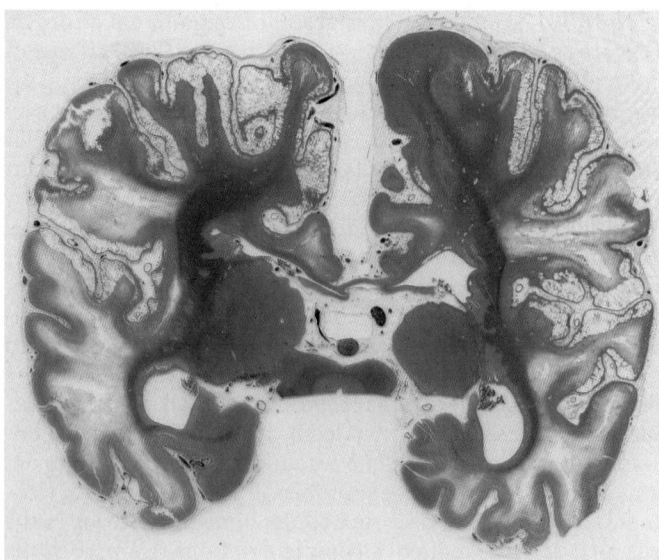

FIGURE 28–8 Multicystic leukoencephalopathy. Numerous cystic spaces representing the consequences of widespread ischemic injury are present.

reactive gliosis. Later, aberrant and irregular myelinization gives rise to a marble-like appearance of the deep nuclei: *status marmoratus*. Because the lesions are in the caudate, putamen, and thalamus, choreoathetosis and related movement disorders are common clinical sequelae.

Trauma

The anatomic location of the lesion and the limited capacity of the brain for functional repair are major determinants of the consequences of CNS trauma. Injury of several cubic centimeters of brain parenchyma may be clinically silent (e.g., in the frontal lobe), severely disabling (in the spinal cord), or fatal (in the brainstem).

The physical forces associated with head injury may result in *skull fractures*, *parenchymal injury*, and *vascular injury*; all three can coexist. The magnitude and distribution of a traumatic brain lesion depend on the shape of the object causing the trauma, the force of impact, and whether the head is in motion at the time of injury. A blow to the head may be *penetrating* or *blunt*; it may cause either an *open* or a *closed injury*.

SKULL FRACTURES

A fracture in which bone is displaced into the cranial cavity by a distance greater than the thickness of the bone is called a *displaced skull fracture*. The thickness of the cranial bones varies; therefore, their resistance to fracture differs greatly. Also, the relative incidence of fractures among skull bones is related to the pattern of falls. When an individual falls while awake, such as might occur when stepping off a ladder, the site of impact is often in the occipital portion of the skull; in contrast, a fall that follows loss of consciousness, as might follow a syncopal attack, commonly results in a frontal impact. Symptoms referable to the lower cranial nerves or the cervicomedullary region, and the presence of orbital or mastoid hematomas distant from the point of impact, raise the suspicion of a basal skull fracture, which typically follows impact to the occiput or sides of the head. CSF discharge from the nose or ear and infection (meningitis) may follow. The kinetic energy that causes a fracture is dissipated at a fused suture; fractures that cross sutures are termed *diastatic*. With multiple points of impact or repeated blows to the head, the fracture lines of subsequent injuries do not extend across fracture lines of prior injury.

PARENCHYMAL INJURIES

Concussion

Concussion is a clinical syndrome of altered consciousness secondary to head injury typically brought about by a change in the momentum of the head (when a moving head is suddenly arrested by impact on a rigid surface). The characteristic neurologic picture includes instantaneous onset of transient neurologic dysfunction, including loss of consciousness, temporary respiratory arrest, and loss of reflexes. Although neurologic recovery is complete, amnesia for the event persists. The pathogenesis of the sudden disruption of neurologic function is unknown; it probably involves dysregulation of the reticular

activating system in the brainstem. Postconcussive neuropsychiatric syndromes, typically associated with repetitive injuries, are well recognized.

Direct Parenchymal Injury

Contusion and *laceration* are lesions associated with direct parenchymal injury of the brain, either through transmission of kinetic energy to the brain and bruising analogous to what is seen in soft tissues (contusion) or by penetration of an object and tearing of tissue (laceration). As with any other organ, a blow to the surface of the brain, transmitted through the skull, leads to rapid tissue displacement, disruption of vascular channels, and subsequent hemorrhage, tissue injury, and edema (Fig. 28–9). The crests of gyri are most susceptible, since this is where the direct force is greatest. The most common locations for contusions correspond to the most frequent sites of direct impact and to regions of the brain that overlie a rough and irregular inner skull surface, such as the frontal lobes along the orbital ridges and the temporal lobes. Contusions are less frequent over the occipital lobes, brainstem, and cerebellum unless these sites are adjacent to a skull fracture (*fracture contusions*).

A person who suffers a blow to the head may develop a contusion at the point of contact (a *coup* injury) or a contusion on the brain surface diametrically opposite to it (a *contrecoup* injury). Since their macroscopic and microscopic appearance is indistinguishable, the distinction between them is based on forensic identification of the point of impact and the circumstances attending the incident. In general, if the head is immobile at the time of trauma, only a coup injury is found. If the head is mobile, both coup and contrecoup lesions may be found. Whereas the coup lesion is caused by the contact between brain and skull at the site of impact, the contrecoup contusion is thought to develop when the brain strikes the opposite inner surface of the skull after sudden deceleration.

Sudden impacts that result in violent posterior or lateral hyperextension of the neck (as occurs when a pedestrian is struck from the rear by a vehicle) may avulse the pons from the medulla or the medulla from the cervical cord, causing instantaneous death.

> **Morphology.** When seen on cross-section, contusions are wedge shaped, with the broad base lying along the surface, deep to the point of impact (Fig. 28–9B). The histologic appearance of contusions is independent of the type of trauma. In the earliest stages, there is edema and hemorrhage, which is often pericapillary. During the next few hours, the extravasation of blood extends throughout the involved tissue, across the width of the cerebral cortex, and into the white matter and subarachnoid space. Morphologic evidence of neuronal injury (pyknosis of the nucleus, eosinophilia of the cytoplasm, and disintegration of the cell) takes about 24 hours to appear, although functional deficits may occur earlier. Axonal swellings develop in the vicinity of damaged neurons or at great distances away. The inflammatory response to the injured tissue follows its usual

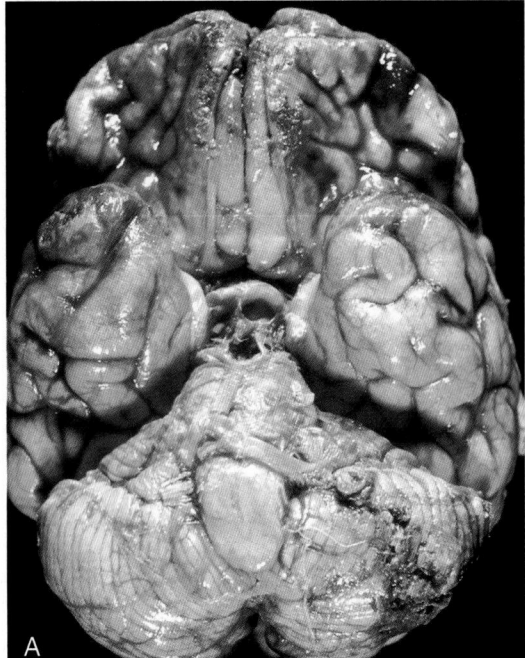

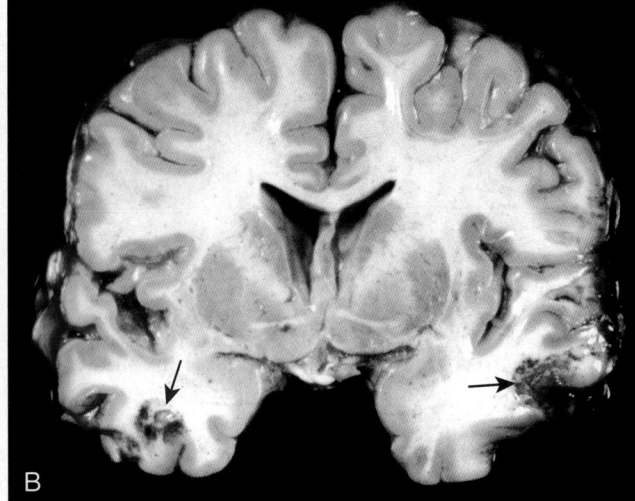

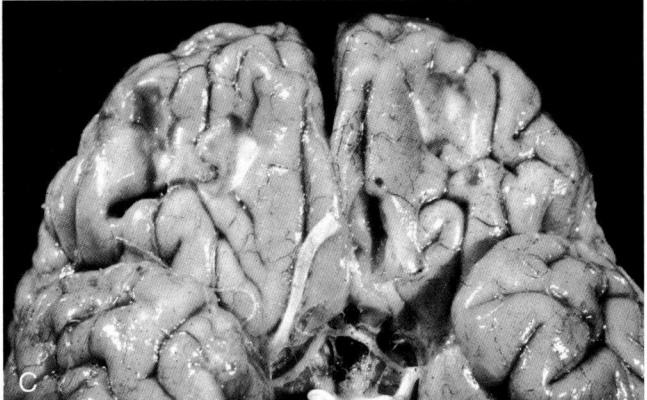

FIGURE 28-9 **A,** Multiple contusions involving the inferior surfaces of frontal lobes, anterior temporal lobes, and cerebellum. **B,** Acute contusions are present in both temporal lobes, with areas of hemorrhage and tissue disruption (*arrows*). **C,** Remote contusions are present on the inferior frontal surface of this brain, with a yellow color (associated with the term *plaque jaune*).

course, with the appearance of neutrophils followed by macrophages. Old traumatic lesions on the surface of the brain have a characteristic macroscopic appearance. They are depressed, retracted, yellowish brown patches involving the crests of gyri most commonly located at the sites of contrecoup lesions (inferior frontal cortex, temporal and occipital poles). The term **plaque jaune** is applied to these lesions (Fig. 28–9C); they can become epileptic foci. More extensive hemorrhagic regions of brain trauma give rise to larger cavitated lesions, which can resemble remote infarcts. In sites of old contusions, gliosis and residual hemosiderin-laden macrophages predominate.

Diffuse Axonal Injury

Although it is most often affected, the surface of the brain is not the only region of damage in traumatic injury. Also affected may be the deep white matter regions (the corpus callosum, paraventricular, and hippocampal areas in the supratentorial compartment), cerebral peduncles, brachium conjunctivum, superior colliculi, and deep reticular formation in the brainstem. The microscopic findings include axonal swelling, indicative of *diffuse axonal injury*, and focal hemorrhagic lesions. Angular acceleration alone, in the absence of

impact, can cause diffuse axonal injury as well as hemorrhage. As many as 50% of individuals who develop coma shortly after trauma, even without cerebral contusions, are believed to have diffuse axonal injury. The mechanical forces associated with trauma are believed to damage the integrity of the axon at the node of Ranvier, with subsequent alterations in axoplasmic flow.

Morphology. Diffuse axonal injury is characterized by the widespread but often asymmetric axonal swellings that appear within hours of the injury and may persist for much longer. These are best demonstrated with silver impregnation techniques or with immunoperoxidase stains for axonally transported proteins, including amyloid precursor protein and α-synuclein. Later, there are increased numbers of microglia in related areas of the cerebral cortex and, subsequently, degeneration of the involved fiber tracts.

TRAUMATIC VASCULAR INJURY

Vascular injury is a frequent component of CNS trauma. It results from direct trauma and disruption of the vessel wall, and leads to hemorrhage. Depending on the anatomic posi-

EPIDURAL HEMATOMA   SUBDURAL HEMATOMA

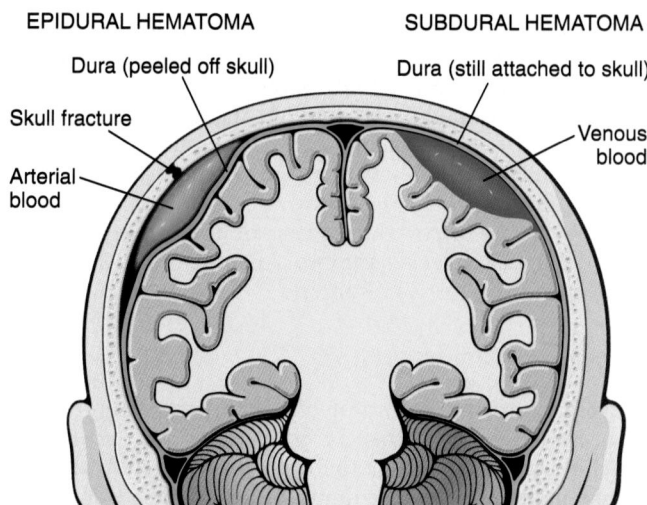

FIGURE 28–10 Epidural hematoma *(left)* in which rupture of a meningeal artery, usually associated with a skull fracture, leads to accumulation of arterial blood between the dura and the skull. In a subdural hematoma *(right)*, damage to bridging veins between the brain and the superior sagittal sinus leads to the accumulation of blood between the dura and the arachnoid.

tion of the ruptured vessel, hemorrhage may occur in the *epidural, subdural, subarachnoid,* and *intraparenchymal* compartments, sometimes in combination (Fig. 28–10). Subarachnoid and intraparenchymal hemorrhages most often occur concomitantly in the setting of brain trauma that also results in superficial contusions and lacerations. A traumatic tear of the carotid artery where it traverses the carotid sinus may lead to the formation of an arteriovenous fistula.

Epidural Hematoma

Normally the dura is fused with the periosteum on the internal surface of the skull. Dural arteries, most importantly the middle meningeal artery, are vulnerable to injury, particularly with temporal skull fractures in which the fracture lines cross the course of the vessel. In children, in whom the skull is deformable, a temporary displacement of the skull bones leading to laceration of a vessel can occur in the absence of a skull fracture.

Once a vessel has been torn, the extravasation of blood under arterial pressure can cause the dura to separate from the inner surface of the skull (Fig. 28–11). The expanding hematoma has a smooth inner contour that compresses the brain surface. When blood accumulates slowly patients may be lucid for several hours before the onset of neurologic signs. An epidural hematoma may expand rapidly and is a neurosurgical emergency requiring prompt drainage.

Subdural Hematoma

Between the inner surface of the dura mater and the outer arachnoid layer of the leptomeninges lies the subdural space. *Bridging veins* travel from the convexities of the cerebral hemispheres through the subarachnoid space and the subdural space to empty into the superior sagittal sinus. Similar anatomic relationships exist with other dural sinuses. These vessels are particularly prone to tearing along their course

through the subdural space and are the source of bleeding in most cases of subdural hematoma. It is thought that the brain, floating freely bathed in CSF, can move within the skull, but the venous sinuses are fixed. The displacement of the brain that occurs in trauma can tear the veins at the point where they penetrate the dura. In elderly individuals with brain atrophy, the bridging veins are stretched out and the brain has additional space for movement, hence the increased rate of subdural hematomas in these patients, even after relatively minor head trauma. Infants are also particularly susceptible to subdural hematomas because their bridging veins are thin-walled.

Morphology. On macroscopic examination, the **acute subdural hematoma** appears as a collection of freshly clotted blood along the brain surface, without extension into the depths of sulci (Fig. 28–12). The underlying brain is flattened and the subarachnoid space is often clear. Typically, venous bleeding is self-limited; breakdown and organization of the hematoma take place over time. This usually occurs in the following sequence:

- Lysis of the clot (about 1 week)
- Growth of fibroblasts from the dural surface into the hematoma (2 weeks)
- Early development of hyalinized connective tissue (1 to 3 months)

Typically, the organized hematoma is firmly attached by fibrous tissue only to the inner surface of the dura and is not adherent to the underlying smooth arachnoid, which does not contribute to its formation. The lesion can eventually retract as the granulation tissue matures, until there is only a thin layer of reactive connective tissue ("subdural membranes"). A common finding in subdural hematomas, however, is the occurrence of multiple

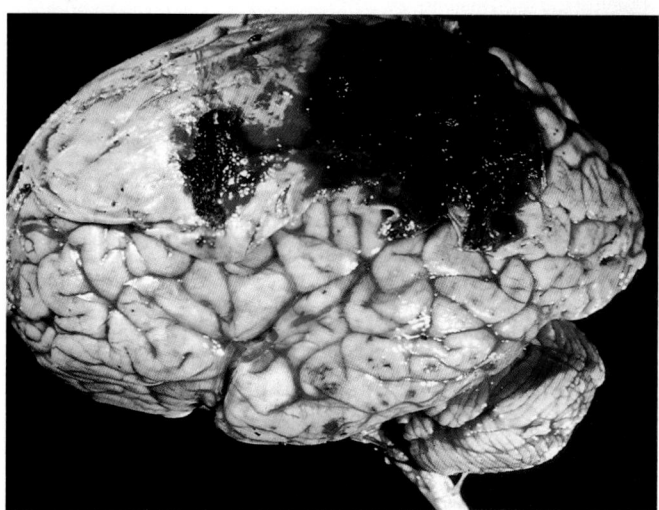

FIGURE 28–11 Epidural hematoma covering a portion of the dura. Also present are multiple small contusions in the temporal lobe. (Courtesy of the late Dr. Raymond D. Adams, Massachusetts General Hospital, Boston, MA.)

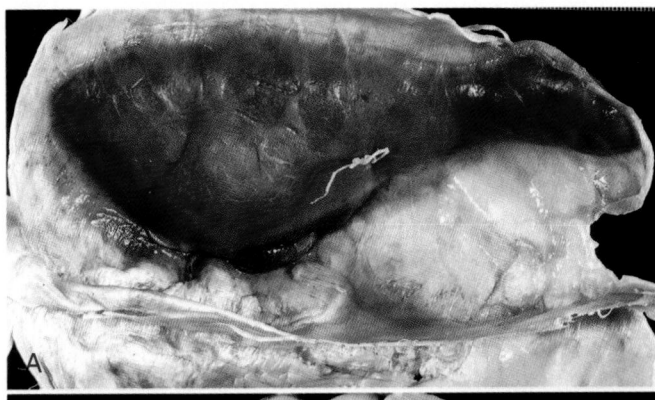

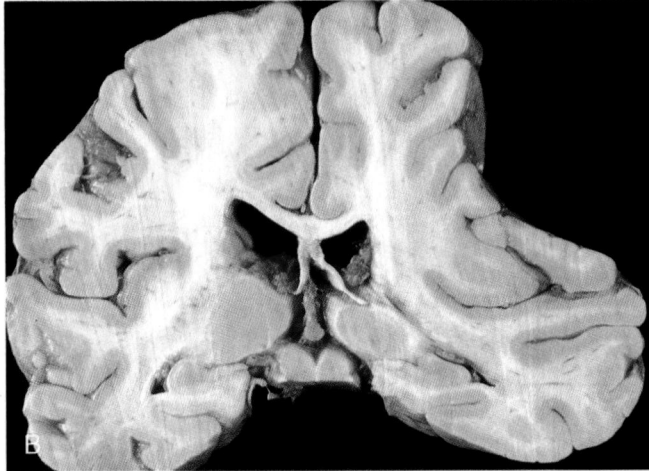

FIGURE 28–12 **A,** Large organizing subdural hematoma attached to the dura. **B,** Coronal section of the brain showing compression of the hemisphere underlying the subdural hematoma shown in **A.**

episodes of repeat bleeding (**chronic subdural hematomas**), presumably from the thin-walled vessels of the granulation tissue. The risk of repeat bleeding is greatest in the first few months after the initial hemorrhage.

Clinical Features. Subdural hematomas most often manifest within 48 hours of injury. They are most common over the lateral aspects of the cerebral hemispheres and are bilateral in about 10% of cases. Neurologic signs commonly observed are attributable to the pressure exerted on the adjacent brain. There may be focal signs, but often the clinical manifestations are nonlocalizing and include headache and confusion. Slowly progressive neurologic deterioration is typical, but acute decompensation may occur. The treatment of subdural hematomas is to remove the blood and associated organizing tissue.

SEQUELAE OF BRAIN TRAUMA

A broad range of neurologic syndromes may become manifest months or years after brain trauma of any cause. These have gained increasing notice in the context of legal medicine and litigation involving issues of compensation for those in the civilian work force and the military services. *Post-traumatic hydrocephalus* is largely due to obstruction of CSF resorption from hemorrhage into the subarachnoid spaces. *Post-traumatic dementia* and the *punch-drunk syndrome* (dementia pugilistica) follow repeated head trauma during a protracted period; the neuropathologic findings include hydrocephalus, thinning of the corpus callosum, diffuse axonal injury, neurofibrillary tangles (mainly in the medial temporal areas), and diffuse amyloid β (Aβ)-positive plaques (see "Alzheimer Disease"). Other important sequelae of brain trauma include post-traumatic epilepsy, tumors (meningioma), infectious diseases, and psychiatric disorders.[3]

SPINAL CORD TRAUMA

The spinal cord, normally protected within the bony vertebral canal, is vulnerable to trauma from its skeletal encasement. Most injuries that damage the cord are associated with displacement of the vertebral column, either rapid and temporary or persistent. The level of cord injury determines the extent of neurologic manifestations: lesions involving the thoracic vertebrae or below can lead to paraplegia; cervical lesions result in quadriplegia; those above C4 can, in addition, lead to respiratory compromise from paralysis of the diaphragm. Segmental damage to the descending and ascending white matter tracts isolates the distal spinal cord from its cortical connections with the cerebrum and brainstem; this interruption, rather than the segmental gray matter damage that may occur at the level of the impact, is the principal cause of neurological deficits.

Morphology. The histologic changes of traumatic injury of the spinal cord are similar to those found at other sites in the CNS. At the level of injury the acute phase consists of hemorrhage, necrosis, and axonal swelling in the surrounding white matter. The lesion tapers above and below the level of injury. In time the central necrotic lesion becomes cystic and gliotic; cord sections above and below the lesion show secondary ascending and descending wallerian degeneration, respectively, involving the long white-matter tracts affected at the site of trauma.

Cerebrovascular Diseases

Cerebrovascular disease is the third leading cause of death (after heart disease and cancer) in the United States; it is also the most prevalent neurologic disorder in terms of both morbidity and mortality. Cerebrovascular diseases include the expected three major categories, thrombosis, embolism, and hemorrhage, with patient management differing between groups. "Stroke" is the clinical designation that applies to all these conditions, particularly when symptoms begin acutely. From the standpoint of pathophysiology and pathologic anatomy, it is convenient to consider cerebrovascular disease as two processes:

- Hypoxia, ischemia, and infarction resulting from impairment of blood supply and oxygenation of CNS tissue
- Hemorrhage resulting from rupture of CNS vessels

The most common cerebrovascular disorders are global ischemia, embolism, hypertensive intraparenchymal hemorrhage, and ruptured aneurysm.

HYPOXIA, ISCHEMIA, AND INFARCTION

The brain requires a constant supply of glucose and oxygen, which is delivered by the blood. Although the brain accounts for only 1% to 2% of body weight, it receives 15% of the resting cardiac output and accounts for 20% of the total body oxygen consumption. Cerebral blood flow remains relatively constant over a wide range of blood pressure and intracranial pressure because of autoregulation of vascular resistance. The brain is a highly aerobic tissue, in which oxygen rather than metabolic substrate is limiting. The brain may be deprived of oxygen by several mechanisms: *hypoxia* caused by a low partial pressure of oxygen (Po_2), impairment of the blood's oxygen-carrying capacity, or inhibition of oxygen use in the tissue; or *ischemia*, either transient or permanent, after interruption of the normal circulatory flow. Cessation of blood flow can result from a reduction in perfusion pressure (as in hypotension), small- or large-vessel obstruction, or both.

When blood flow to a portion of the brain is reduced, the survival of the tissue at risk depends on the presence of collateral circulation, the duration of ischemia, and the magnitude and rapidity of the reduction of flow. These factors determine, in turn, the precise anatomic site and size of the lesion and, consequently, the clinical deficit. Two principal types of acute ischemic injury are recognized:

○ *Global cerebral ischemia* (ischemic/hypoxic encephalopathy) occurs when there is a generalized reduction of cerebral perfusion, as in cardiac arrest, shock, and severe hypotension.
○ *Focal cerebral ischemia* follows reduction or cessation of blood flow to a localized area of the brain due to large-vessel disease (such as embolic or thrombotic arterial occlusion, often in a setting of atherosclerosis) or to small-vessel disease (such as vasculitis or occlusion secondary to arteriosclerotic lesions seen in hypertension).

The general biochemical changes that attend cellular ischemia are discussed in Chapter 1. Here we describe several special responses to ischemia in the CNS.[14-16] The metabolic depletion of energy associated with ischemia can result in inappropriate release of excitatory amino acid neurotransmitters such as glutamate, initiating cell damage by allowing excessive influx of calcium ions through NMDA-type glutamate receptors. This elevation of cellular calcium ions can, in turn, trigger a wide range of processes including inappropriate activation of signaling cascades, free radical generation, and mitochondrial injury. All told, these together result in cell death, mostly through necrosis. In the region of transition between necrotic tissue and the normal brain, there is an area of "at-risk" tissue, referred to as the penumbra. This region can be rescued from injury in many animal models with a variety of anti-apoptotic interventions, implying that it may undergo damage by apoptosis as well.

Hypotension, Hypoperfusion, and Low-Flow States (Global Cerebral Ischemia)

The clinical outcome of a severe hypotensive episode that produces *global cerebral ischemia (diffuse hypoxic/ischemic encephalopathy)* varies with the severity of the insult. In mild cases there may be only a transient post-ischemic confusional state followed by complete recovery and no irreversible tissue damage. However, irreversible damage to CNS tissue may occur in some individuals who suffer mild or transient global ischemic insults. There is a hierarchy of sensitivity among CNS cells: neurons are the most sensitive, although glial cells (oligodendrocytes and astrocytes) are also vulnerable. There is also variability in the susceptibility of populations of neurons in different regions of the CNS *(selective vulnerability)*, based in part on differences in regional cerebral blood flow and cellular metabolic requirements. With severe global cerebral ischemia, widespread neuronal death occurs, irrespective of regional vulnerability. Patients who survive this injury often remain in a persistent vegetative state. Other patients meet the current clinical criteria for "brain death," including evidence of irreversible diffuse cortical injury (isoelectric, or "flat," electroencephalogram) and brainstem damage, such as absent reflexes and respiratory drive, and absent cerebral perfusion. When individuals with this pervasive form of injury are maintained on mechanical ventilation, the brain gradually undergoes an autolytic process—so-called "respirator brain."

Border zone ("watershed") infarcts occur in the regions of the brain or spinal cord that lie at the most distal reaches of the arterial blood supply, the border zones between arterial territories. In the cerebral hemispheres, the border zone between the anterior and the middle cerebral artery distributions is at greatest risk. Damage to this region produces a sickle-shaped band of necrosis over the cerebral convexity a few centimeters lateral to the interhemispheric fissure. Border zone infarcts are usually seen after hypotensive episodes.

Morphology. In the setting of global ischemia, the brain is swollen, the gyri are widened, and the sulci are narrowed. The cut surface shows poor demarcation between gray and white matter. The microscopic changes of irreversible ischemic injury (infarction) are grouped into three categories. **Early changes,** occurring 12 to 24 hours after the insult, include acute neuronal changes (red neurons; Figs. 28–13A and 28–13B) characterized at first by microvacuolization, then eosinophilia of the neuronal cytoplasm, and later nuclear pyknosis and karyorrhexis. Similar acute changes occur somewhat later in astrocytes and oligodendroglia. Pyramidal cells in CA1 of the hippocampus (Sommer sector), Purkinje cells of the cerebellum, and cortical pyramidal neurons are the most susceptible to global ischemia of short duration. After the acute injury, the reaction to tissue damage begins with infiltration by neutrophils (Fig. 28–13C). **Subacute changes,** occurring at 24 hours to 2 weeks, include necrosis of tissue, influx of macrophages, vascular proliferation, and reactive gliosis (Fig. 28–13D). **Repair,** robust after approximately 2

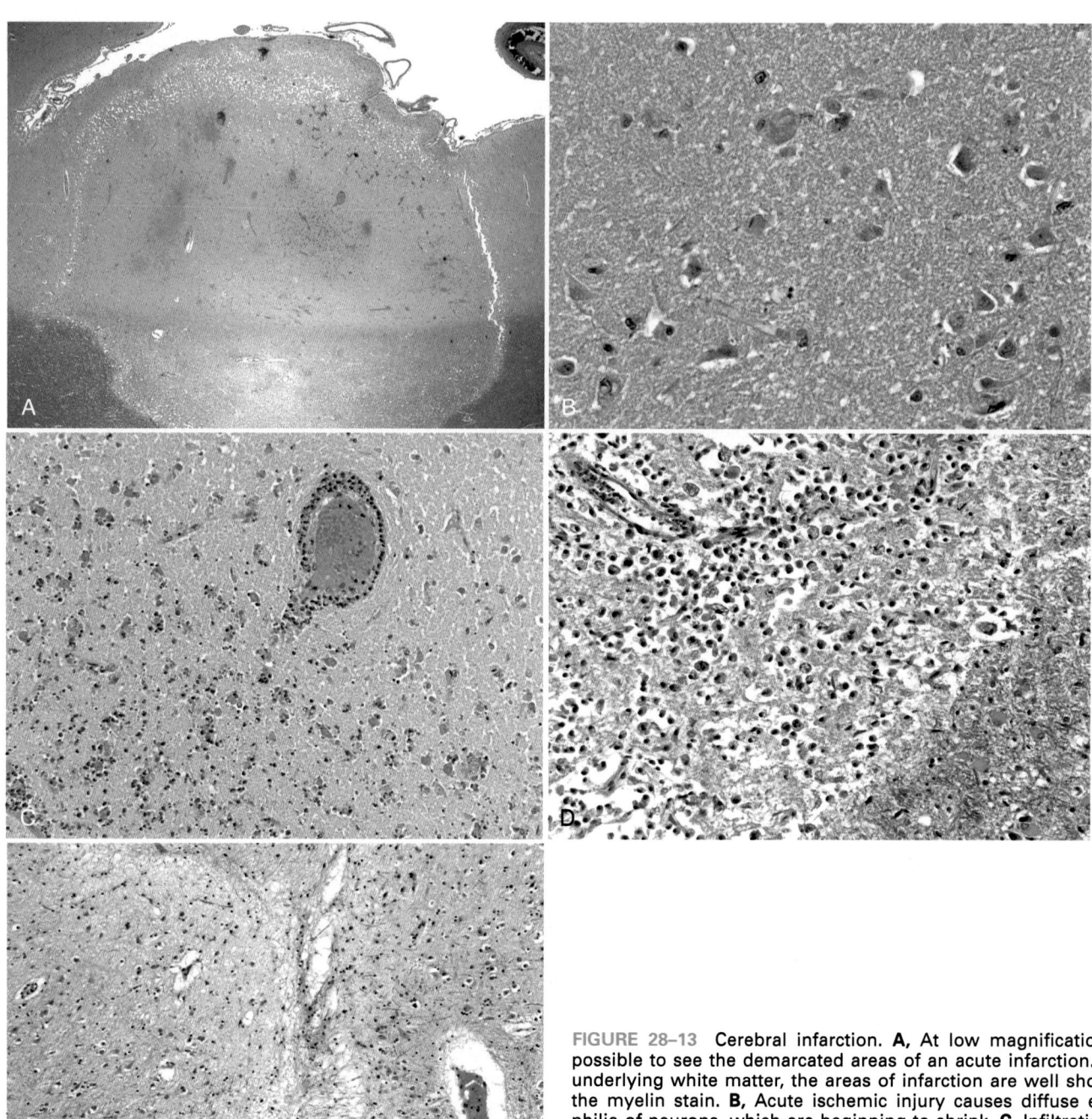

FIGURE 28–13 Cerebral infarction. **A,** At low magnification it is possible to see the demarcated areas of an acute infarction. In the underlying white matter, the areas of infarction are well shown by the myelin stain. **B,** Acute ischemic injury causes diffuse eosinophilia of neurons, which are beginning to shrink. **C,** Infiltration of a cerebral infarct by neutrophils begins at the edges of the lesion where vascular supply has remained intact. **D,** After about 10 days, an area of infarction is characterized by the presence of macrophages and surrounding reactive gliosis. **E,** Remote small intracortical infarcts are seen as areas of tissue loss with residual gliosis.

weeks, is characterized by eventual removal of all necrotic tissue, loss of normally organized CNS structure, and gliosis (Fig. 28–13E). In the cerebral cortex the neuronal loss and gliosis produce an uneven destruction of the neocortex, with preservation of some layers and involvement of others, a pattern termed **pseudolaminar necrosis.**

Infarction from Obstruction of Local Blood Supply (Focal Cerebral Ischemia)

Cerebral arterial occlusion may lead to focal ischemia and, if sustained, to infarction of a specific region within the territory of distribution of the compromised vessel. The size, location, and shape of the infarct and the extent of tissue damage that results are determined by modifying factors mentioned earlier, the most important being the adequacy of collateral flow. The major source of collateral flow is the circle of Willis (supplemented by the external carotid-ophthalmic pathway). Partial and inconstant reinforcement is available over the surface of the brain for the distal branches of the anterior, middle, and posterior cerebral arteries through cortical-leptomeningeal anastomoses. In contrast, there is little if any collateral flow for the deep penetrating vessels supplying structures such as the thalamus, basal ganglia, and deep white matter.

Occlusive vascular disease of severity sufficient to lead to cerebral infarction may be due to *in situ thrombosis, embolization* from a distant source, or various forms of vasculitides; the basic pathology of these conditions is discussed in Chapters 4 and 11.

The majority of thrombotic occlusions are due to atherosclerosis. The most common sites of primary thrombosis causing cerebral infarction are the carotid bifurcation, the origin of the middle cerebral artery, and either end of the basilar artery. The evolution of arterial stenosis varies from progressive narrowing of the lumen and thrombosis, which may be accompanied by anterograde extension, to fragmentation and distal embolization. Another important aspect of occlusive cerebrovascular disease is its frequent association with systemic diseases such as hypertension and diabetes.

Embolism to the brain occurs from a wide range of origins. Cardiac mural thrombi are among the most common sources; myocardial infarct, valvular disease, and atrial fibrillation are important predisposing factors. Next in importance are thromboemboli arising in arteries, most often originating over atheromatous plaques within the carotid arteries. Other sources of emboli include paradoxical emboli, particularly in children with cardiac anomalies; emboli associated with cardiac surgery; and emboli of other material (tumor, fat, or air). The territory of distribution of the middle cerebral artery—the direct extension of the internal carotid artery—is most frequently affected by embolic infarction; the incidence is about equal in the two hemispheres. Emboli tend to lodge where blood vessels branch or in areas of preexisting luminal stenosis. "Shower embolization," as in fat embolism, may occur after fractures; affected individuals manifest generalized cerebral dysfunction with disturbances of higher cortical function and consciousness, often without localizing signs. Widespread hemorrhagic lesions involving the white matter are characteristic of embolization of bone marrow after trauma (Fig. 28–14).

A variety of inflammatory processes that involve blood vessels may also lead to luminal narrowing and cerebral infarcts. While *infectious vasculitis* of small and large vessels was once most commonly associated with syphilis and tuberculosis, it is now more common in the setting of immunosuppression and opportunistic infection (such as aspergillosis or CMV encephalitis). *Polyarteritis nodosa* and other non-infectious vasculitides may involve cerebral vessels and cause single or multiple infarcts throughout the brain. *Primary angiitis of the CNS* is an inflammatory disorder that involves multiple small- to medium-sized parenchymal and subarachnoid vessels and is characterized by chronic inflammation, multinucleated giant cells, and destruction of the vessel wall. Granulomas may be found in association with the giant cells, leading to the alternative name of granulomatous angiitis of the nervous system. Affected individuals manifest a diffuse encephalopathic or multifocal clinical picture, often with cognitive dysfunction; patients improve with steroid and immu-

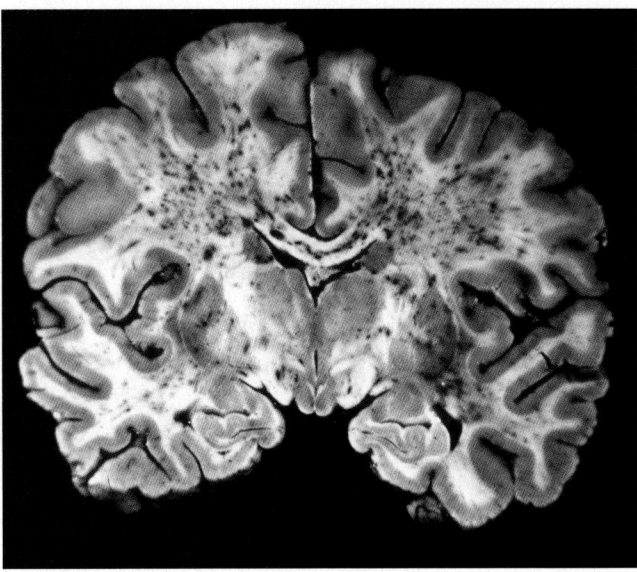

FIGURE 28–14 Widespread white-matter hemorrhages are characteristic of bone marrow embolization.

nosuppressive treatment. Other conditions that may cause thrombosis and infarction (and intracranial hemorrhage) include hypercoagulable states, dissecting aneurysm of extracranial arteries in the neck supplying the brain, and drug abuse (amphetamines, heroin, cocaine).

Infarcts are subdivided into two broad groups based on the presence of hemorrhage. *Hemorrhagic (red) infarction,* characterized by multiple, sometimes confluent, petechial hemorrhages, is typically associated with embolic events (Fig. 28–15A). The hemorrhage is presumed to be secondary to reperfusion of damaged vessels and tissue, either through collaterals or directly after dissolution of intravascular occlusive material. In contrast, *nonhemorrhagic (pale, bland, anemic) infarcts* are usually associated with thrombosis (Fig. 28–15B). The clinical management of patients with these two types of infarcts differs greatly as thrombolytic therapy may be used in cases of thrombosis but is contraindicated in hemorrhagic infarcts. Thrombolytic therapy is beneficial only during a narrow time window after onset of symptoms; therefore, rapid medical attention is essential.

Morphology. The macroscopic appearance of a **nonhemorrhagic infarct** varies with the time after loss of blood supply. During the first 6 hours of irreversible injury, little can be observed. By 48 hours the tissue becomes pale, soft, and swollen, and the corticomedullary junction becomes indistinct. From 2 to 10 days, the brain becomes gelatinous and friable, and the previously ill-defined boundary between normal and abnormal tissue becomes more distinct as edema resolves in the adjacent tissue that has survived. From 10 days to 3 weeks, the tissue liquefies, eventually leaving a fluid-filled cavity lined by dark gray tissue, which gradually expands as dead tissue is removed (Fig. 28–16).

On microscopic examination the tissue reaction evolves along the following sequence: *After the first*

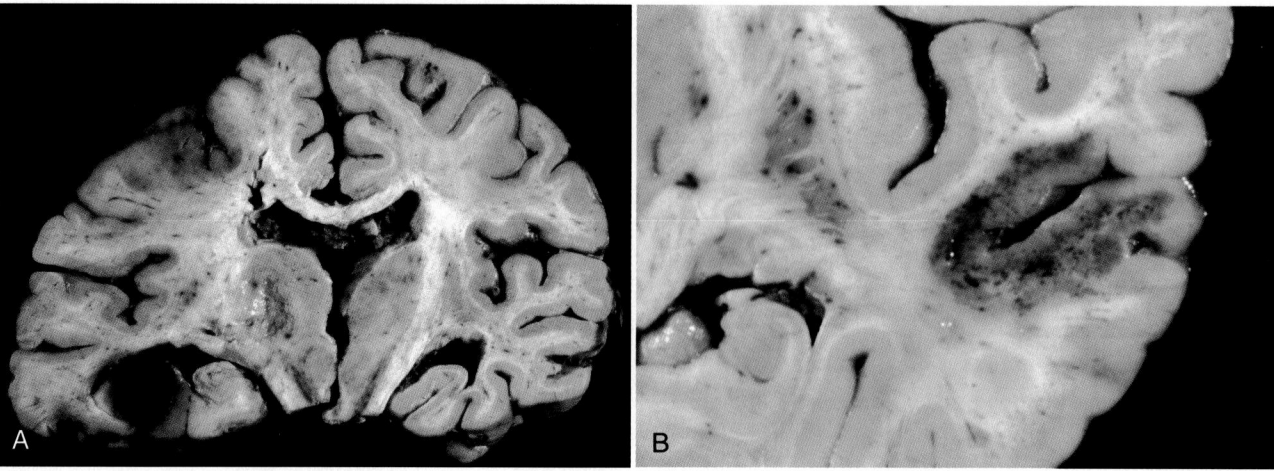

FIGURE 28–15   A, A hemorrhagic infarction is present in the inferior temporal lobe of the left side of this brain. **B,** A bland infarct with punctate hemorrhages, consistent with ischemia-reperfusion injury, is present in the temporal lobe.

12 hours, ischemic neuronal change (red neurons; see earlier) and both cytotoxic and vasogenic edema predominate. There is loss of the usual tinctorial characteristics of white- and gray-matter structures. Endothelial and glial cells, mainly astrocytes, swell, and myelinated fibers begin to disintegrate. *Up to 48 hours,* neutrophilic emigration progressively increases and then falls off. Phagocytic cells, derived from circulating monocytes and activated microglia, are evident at 48 hours and become the predominant cell type in the ensuing *2 to 3 weeks.* The macrophages become stuffed with the products of myelin breakdown or blood and may persist in the lesion for months to years. As the process of liquefaction and phagocytosis proceeds, astrocytes at the edges of the lesion progressively enlarge, divide, and develop a prominent network of cytoplasmic extensions. Reactive astrocytes can be seen as early as *1 week* after the insult.

After several months, the astrocytic response recedes, leaving behind a dense meshwork of glial fibers admixed with new capillaries and some perivascular connective tissue. In the cerebral cortex, the cavity is separated from the meninges and subarachnoid space by a gliotic layer of tissue, derived from the molecular layer of the cortex. The pia and arachnoid are not affected and do not contribute to the healing process. Infarcts undergo these reactive and reparative stages from the edges inward; thus, different areas of a lesion may look different, particularly during the early stages, revealing the natural progression of the response.

The microscopic picture and evolution of **hemorrhagic infarction** parallel ischemic infarction, with the addition of blood extravasation and resorption. In individuals receiving anticoagulant treatment, hemorrhagic infarcts may be associated with extensive intracerebral hematomas. Venous infarcts are often hemorrhagic and may occur after thrombotic occlusion of the superior sagittal sinus or other sinuses or occlusion of the deep cerebral veins. Carcinoma, localized infections, and other conditions leading to a hypercoagulable state increase the risk for venous thrombosis.

Spinal cord infarction may be seen in the setting of hypoperfusion or as a consequence of interruption of the feeding tributaries derived from the aorta. Occlusion of the anterior spinal artery is rarer and may occur as a result of embolism or vasculitis.

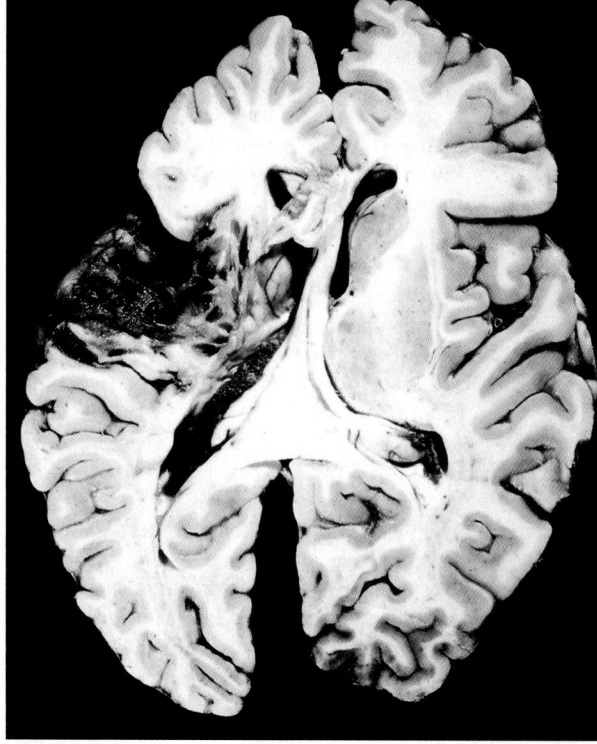

FIGURE 28–16   Old cystic infarct showing destruction of cortex with cavitation.

Clinical Features. Deficits associated with infarction are determined by the brain region involved rather than the underlying pathologic process. Neurologic symptoms referable to the area of injury often develop rapidly, over minutes, and may continue to evolve over hours. There can be improvement in severity of symptoms associated with reversal of injury in the ischemic penumbra as well as with resolution of associated local edema. In general, there is often a degree of slow improvement during a period of months. Because strokes are frequently associated with atherosclerosis, many of the genetic and lifestyle risk factors are the same as those for atherosclerotic disease.

HYPERTENSIVE CEREBROVASCULAR DISEASE

The most important effects of hypertension on the brain include lacunar infarcts, slit hemorrhages, and hypertensive encephalopathy, as well as massive hypertensive intracerebral hemorrhage. The incidence of these disorders is likely to decline with increased screening for hypertension and aggressive management of blood pressure.

Lacunar Infarcts

Hypertension affects the deep penetrating arteries and arterioles that supply the basal ganglia and hemispheric white matter as well as the brainstem. These cerebral vessels develop *arteriolar sclerosis* and may become occluded; the structural changes are similar to those described in the systemic vessels of individuals with hypertension (Chapter 11). An important clinical and pathologic consequence of CNS arterial lesions is the development of single or multiple, small, cavitary infarcts known as *lacunae* (Fig. 28–17). These are lake-like spaces, less than 15 mm wide, which occur in the lenticular nucleus, thalamus, internal capsule, deep white matter, caudate nucleus, and pons, in descending order of frequency. On microscopic examination they consist of areas of tissue loss with scattered lipid-laden macrophages and surrounding gliosis. Depending on their location in the CNS, lacunae can either be clinically silent or cause severe neurologic impairment. Affected vessels

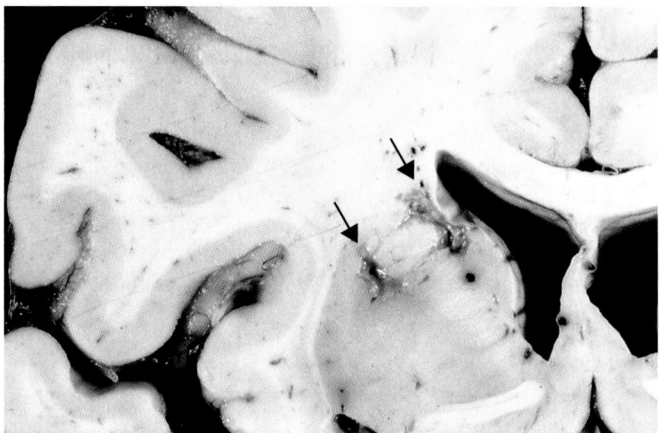

FIGURE 28–17 Lacunar infarcts in the caudate and putamen (*arrows*).

may also be associated with widening of the perivascular spaces but without tissue infarction (*état criblé*).

Slit Hemorrhages

Hypertension also gives rise to rupture of the small-caliber penetrating vessels and the development of small hemorrhages. In time these hemorrhages resorb, leaving behind a slitlike cavity (*slit hemorrhage*) surrounded by brownish discoloration; on microscopic examination, slit hemorrhages show focal tissue destruction, pigment-laden macrophages, and gliosis.

Hypertensive Encephalopathy

Acute hypertensive encephalopathy is a clinicopathologic syndrome arising in an individual with malignant hypertension, and is characterized by diffuse cerebral dysfunction, including headaches, confusion, vomiting, and convulsions, sometimes leading to coma. Rapid therapeutic intervention to reduce the accompanying increased intracranial pressure is required, since the syndrome often does not remit spontaneously. At postmortem examination such individuals may show an edematous brain with or without transtentorial or tonsillar herniation. Petechiae and fibrinoid necrosis of arterioles in the gray and white matter may be seen microscopically.

Individuals who, over the course of many months and years, suffer multiple, bilateral, gray matter (cortex, thalamus, basal ganglia) and white matter (centrum semiovale) infarcts may develop a distinctive clinical syndrome characterized by dementia, gait abnormalities, and pseudobulbar signs, often with superimposed focal neurologic deficits. The syndrome, generally referred to as *vascular (multi-infarct) dementia*, is caused by multifocal vascular disease of several types, including (1) cerebral atherosclerosis, (2) vessel thrombosis or embolization from carotid vessels or from the heart, and (3) cerebral arteriolar sclerosis from chronic hypertension. When the pattern of injury preferentially involves large areas of the subcortical white matter with myelin and axon loss, the disorder is referred to as *Binswanger disease*; this distribution of vascular white-matter injury must be distinguished clinically and radiologically from other diseases that affect the hemispheral white matter.

INTRACRANIAL HEMORRHAGE

Hemorrhages may occur at any site within the CNS. In some instances they may be a secondary phenomenon occurring, for example, within infarcts in arterial border zones or in infarcts caused by only partial or transient vascular obstruction. Primary hemorrhages within the epidural or subdural space are typically related to trauma and were discussed earlier with traumatic lesions. Hemorrhages within the brain parenchyma and subarachnoid space, in contrast, are more often a manifestation of underlying cerebrovascular disease, although trauma may also cause hemorrhage in these sites.

Intracerebral (Intraparenchymal) Hemorrhage

Spontaneous (nontraumatic) intraparenchymal hemorrhages occur most commonly in middle to late adult life, with a

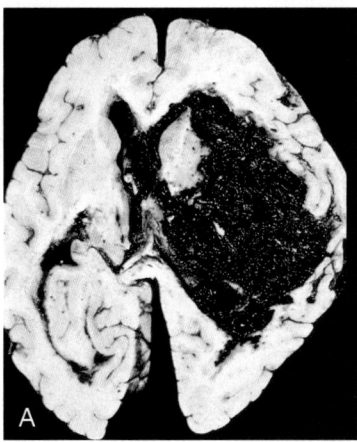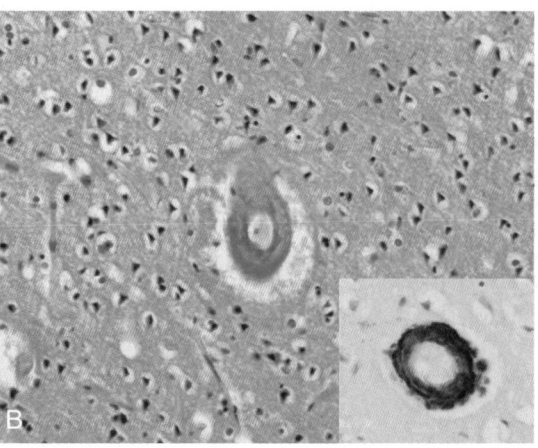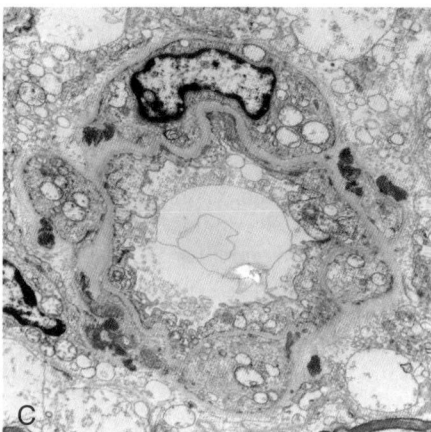

FIGURE 28–18 **A,** Massive hypertensive hemorrhage rupturing into a lateral ventricle. **B,** Amyloid deposition in a cortical arteriole in cerebral amyloid angiopathy; *inset*, Immunohistochemical staining for Aβ shows the deposited material in the vessel wall. **C,** Electron micrograph shows granular osmophilic material in a case of CADASIL.

peak incidence at about age 60 years. Most are caused by rupture of a small intraparenchymal vessel. When the hemorrhages occur in the basal ganglia and thalamus, they are designated ganglionic hemorrhages to distinguish them from those that occur in the lobes of the cerebral hemispheres, which are called lobar hemorrhages. The two major underlying etiologies of this form of cerebrovascular disease are hypertension and cerebral amyloid angiopathy (CAA). In addition, other local and systemic factors may cause or contribute to nontraumatic hemorrhage, including systemic coagulation disorders, neoplasms, vasculitis, aneurysms, and vascular malformations.

Hypertension is the most common underlying cause of primary brain parenchymal hemorrhage, accounting for more than 50% of clinically significant hemorrhages and for roughly 15% of deaths among individuals with chronic hypertension. Hypertension causes a number of abnormalities in vessel walls, including accelerated atherosclerosis in larger arteries; hyaline arteriolosclerosis in smaller vessels; and, in severe cases, proliferative changes and frank necrosis of arterioles. Arteriolar walls affected by hyaline change are presumably weaker than are normal vessels and are therefore more vulnerable to rupture. In some instances chronic hypertension is associated with the development of minute aneurysms, termed *Charcot-Bouchard microaneurysms,* which may be the site of rupture. Charcot-Bouchard aneurysms, not to be confused with saccular aneurysms of larger intracranial vessels, occur in vessels that are less than 300 μm in diameter, most commonly within the basal ganglia.

> **Morphology. Hypertensive intraparenchymal hemorrhage** may originate in the putamen (50% to 60% of cases), thalamus, pons, cerebellar hemispheres (rarely), and other regions of the brain (Fig. 28–18A). Acute hemorrhages, independent of etiology, are characterized by extravasation of blood with compression of the adjacent parenchyma. Old hemorrhages show an area of cavitary destruction of brain with a rim of brownish discoloration. On microscopic examination the early lesion consists of a central

> core of clotted blood surrounded by a rim of brain tissue showing anoxic neuronal and glial changes as well as edema. Eventually the edema resolves, pigment- and lipid-laden macrophages appear, and proliferation of reactive astrocytes is seen at the periphery of the lesion. The cellular events then follow the same time course that is observed after cerebral infarction.

CAA is a condition in which amyloidogenic peptides, nearly always the same one found in Alzheimer disease (Aβ$_{40}$; see the discussion below), deposit in the walls of medium- and small-caliber meningeal and cortical vessels. This deposition can result in weakening of the vessel wall and risk of hemorrhage. As with Alzheimer disease, in which there is a relationship between a polymorphism in the gene that encodes apolipoprotein E (ApoE) and risk of disease, there is an effect of the ApoE genotype on the risk of recurrence of hemorrhage from sporadic CAA. The presence of either an ε2 or ε4 allele increases the risk of repeat bleeding. While some mutations in the precursor protein for the Aβ peptide (amyloid precursor protein, APP) cause familial Alzheimer disease, others result in autosomal dominant forms of CAA.

> **Morphology.** The underlying vascular abnormality of CAA is typically restricted to the leptomeningeal and cerebral cortical arterioles and capillaries, although involvement of the molecular layer of the cerebellum can be observed as well. Involved vessels appear "stiff" on microscopic sections, remaining open with round lumens through tissue processing. Unlike with arteriolar sclerosis, there is no fibrosis; rather, dense and uniform deposits of amyloid are present (Fig. 28–18B).

Cerebral autosomal dominant arteriopathy with subcortical infarcts and leukoencephalopathy (CADASIL) is a rare hereditary form of stroke caused by mutations in the gene encoding the Notch3 receptor.[17] The disease is characterized clinically by recurrent strokes (usually infarcts, less often hemorrhages) and dementia. Histopathologic study has shown abnormalities of white matter and leptomeningeal arteries (also involving non-CNS vessels) consisting of concentric thickening of the media and adventitia. Basophilic, PAS-positive deposits, which appear as osmiophilic compact granular material by electron microscopy, have been consistently detected in the walls of affected vessels, as has loss of smooth muscle cells (Fig. 28–18C). The diagnosis can be made through the identification of these deposits in other tissues, such as skin or muscle biopsies, or through genetic approaches. Many of the causative mutations disrupt the normal folding of the extracellular domain of Notch3, and the characteristic deposits appear to be comprised of Notch3 ectodomains. How these deposits relate to the disease is not understood; a toxic gain-of-function mechanism affecting vascular smooth muscle has been proposed.[17]

Clinical Features. Intracerebral hemorrhage, independent of cause, can be clinically devastating if it affects large portions of the brain and extends into the ventricular system, or it can affect small regions and either be clinically silent or evolve like an infarct. Over weeks or months there is a gradual resolution of the hematoma, sometimes with considerable clinical improvement. Again, the location of the hemorrhage determines the clinical manifestations.

Subarachnoid Hemorrhage and Ruptured Saccular Aneurysms

The most frequent cause of clinically significant subarachnoid hemorrhage is rupture of a *saccular (berry) aneurysm*. Subarachnoid hemorrhage may also result from extension of a traumatic hematoma, rupture of a hypertensive intracerebral hemorrhage into the ventricular system, vascular malformation, hematologic disturbances, and tumors.

Saccular aneurysm is the most common type of intracranial aneurysm. Other aneurysm types include atherosclerotic (fusiform; mostly of the basilar artery), mycotic, traumatic, and dissecting. These latter three, like saccular aneurysms, are most often found in the anterior circulation, but differ in that they more often cause cerebral infarction rather than subarachnoid hemorrhage.

Saccular aneurysms are found in about 2% of the population according to recent data from community-based radiologic studies. About 90% of saccular aneurysms are found near major arterial branch points in the anterior circulation (Fig. 28–19); multiple aneurysms exist in 20% to 30% of cases in autopsy series.

Pathogenesis of Saccular Aneurysms. The etiology of saccular aneurysms is unknown. Although the majority occur sporadically, genetic factors may be important in their pathogenesis, since there is an increased incidence of aneurysms in first-degree relatives of those affected. There is also an increased incidence in individuals with certain mendelian disorders (such as autosomal dominant polycystic kidney disease, Ehlers-Danlos syndrome type IV, neurofibromatosis type 1 [NF1], and Marfan syndrome), fibromuscular dysplasia of extracranial arteries, and coarctation of the aorta. The predisposing factors include cigarette smoking and hypertension (estimated to be present in about half of these patients). Although they are sometimes referred to as congenital, the

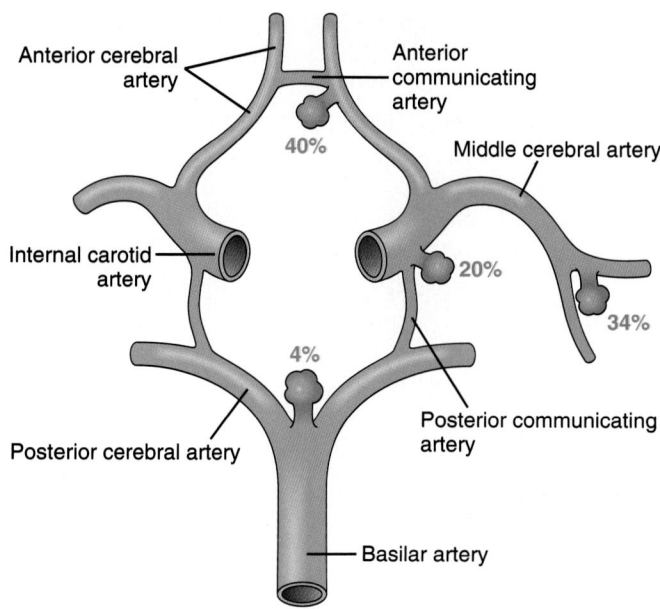

FIGURE 28–19 Common sites of saccular (berry) aneurysms in the circle of Willis.

aneurysms are not present at birth but develop over time because of an underlying defect in the media of the vessel.

Morphology. An unruptured saccular aneurysm is a thin-walled outpouching, usually at an arterial branch point along the circle of Willis or a major vessel just beyond. Saccular aneurysms measure from a few millimeters to 2 or 3 cm in diameter and have a bright red, shiny surface and a thin, translucent wall (Fig. 28–20). Atheromatous plaques, calcification, or thrombotic occlusion of the sac may be found in the wall or lumen of the aneurysm. Brownish discoloration of the adjacent brain and meninges is evidence of prior hemorrhage. The neck of the aneurysm may be either wide or narrow. Rupture usually occurs at the apex of the sac with extravasation of blood into the subarachnoid space, the substance of the brain, or both. The arterial wall adjacent to the neck of the aneurysm often shows some intimal thickening and gradual attenuation of the media as it approaches the neck. At the neck of the aneurysm, the muscular wall and intimal elastic lamina stop short and are absent from the aneurysm sac itself. The sac is made up of thickened hyalinized intima. The adventitia covering the sac is continuous with that of the parent artery.

Clinical Features. Rupture of an aneurysm with clinically significant subarachnoid hemorrhage is most frequent in the fifth decade and is slightly more frequent in females. Overall, the rate of bleeding is roughly 1.3% per year, with the probability of rupture increasing with the size of the lesion. Aneurysms greater than 10 mm in diameter have a roughly 50% risk of bleeding per year. Rupture may occur at any time,

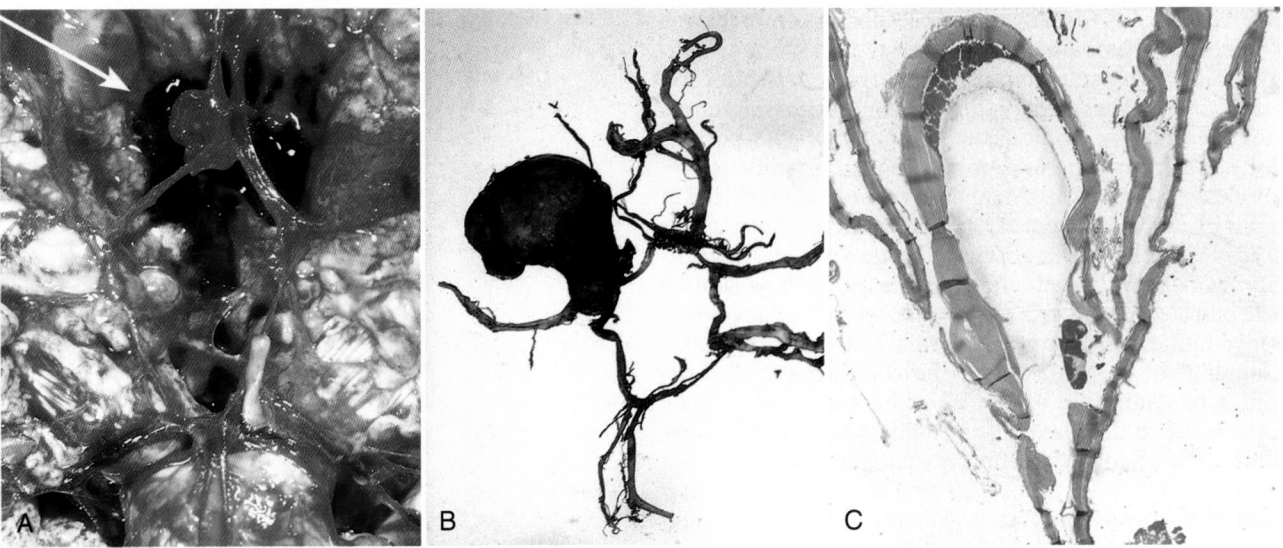

FIGURE 28–20   **A,** View of the base of the brain, dissected to show the circle of Willis with an aneurysm of the anterior cerebral artery *(arrow).* **B,** Dissected circle of Willis to show large aneurysm. **C,** Section through a saccular aneurysm showing the hyalinized fibrous vessel wall (H&E).

but in about one third of cases it is associated with acute increases in intracranial pressure, such as with straining at stool or sexual orgasm. Blood under arterial pressure is forced into the subarachnoid space and affected individuals are stricken with a sudden, excruciating headache ("the worst headache I've ever had"), rapidly losing consciousness. Between 25% and 50% of patients die with the first rupture, but patients who survive often improve and recover consciousness in minutes. Repeat bleeding is common in survivors, and it is currently not possible to predict in which patients repeat bleeding will occur. With each episode of bleeding, the prognosis is worse.

The clinical consequences of blood in the subarachnoid space can be separated into acute events, occurring within hours to days after the hemorrhage, and late sequelae associated with the healing process. In the first few days after a subarachnoid hemorrhage, regardless of the etiology, there is an increased risk of additional ischemic injury from vasospasm affecting vessels bathed in the extravasated blood. This problem is of greatest significance in cases of basal subarachnoid hemorrhage, in which vasospasm can involve major vessels of the circle of Willis. Various mediators have been proposed to have a role in this reactive process, including endothelins, nitric oxide, and arachidonic acid metabolites. In the healing phase of subarachnoid hemorrhage, meningeal fibrosis and scarring occur, sometimes leading to obstruction of CSF flow as well as interruption of the normal pathways of CSF resorption.

Vascular Malformations

Vascular malformations of the brain are classified into four principal groups: arteriovenous malformations, cavernous malformations, capillary telangiectasias, and venous angiomas. Of these, the first two are the types associated with risk of hemorrhage and development of neurologic symptoms.

Morphology. Arteriovenous malformations (AVM) involve vessels in the subarachnoid space extending into brain parenchyma or may occur exclusively within the brain. This tangled network of wormlike vascular channels has prominent, pulsatile arteriovenous shunting with high blood flow. They are composed of greatly enlarged blood vessels separated by gliotic tissue, often with evidence of prior hemorrhage. Some vessels can be recognized as arteries with duplication and fragmentation of the internal elastic lamina, while others show marked thickening or partial replacement of the media by hyalinized connective tissue.

Cavernous malformations consist of greatly distended, loosely organized vascular channels with thin, collagenized walls and are devoid of intervening nervous tissue (thus distinguishing them from capillary telangiectasias). They occur most often in the cerebellum, pons, and subcortical regions, in decreasing order of frequency, and have a low flow without arteriovenous shunting. Foci of old hemorrhage, infarction, and calcification frequently surround the abnormal vessels. **Capillary telangiectasias** are microscopic foci of dilated, thin-walled vascular channels separated by relatively normal brain parenchyma and occurring most frequently in the pons. **Venous angiomas** (varices) consist of aggregates of ectatic venous channels. **Foix-Alajouanine disease** (angiodysgenetic necrotizing myelopathy) is a venous angiomatous malformation of the spinal cord and overlying meninges, most often in the lumbosacral region, associated with ischemic myelomalacia and slowly progressive neurologic symptoms.

Clinical Features. Arteriovenous malformations are the most common type of clinically significant vascular malformation. Males are affected twice as frequently as females, and the lesion is often recognized clinically between the ages of 10 and 30 years, presenting as a seizure disorder, an intracerebral hemorrhage, or a subarachnoid hemorrhage. The most common site is the territory of the middle cerebral artery, particularly its posterior branches. Large arteriovenous malformations occurring in the newborn period can lead to congestive heart failure because of shunt effects, especially if the malformation involves the vein of Galen. Cavernous malformations are unique among this class of lesion in that familial forms are relatively common, with a variety of identified genetic loci.[18] Multiplicity of lesions is an additional hallmark of these autosomal dominant disorders with high penetrance.

Infections

With infection, damage to nervous tissue may be the consequence of direct injury of neurons or glia by the infectious agent or may occur indirectly through the elaboration of microbial toxins, destructive effects of the inflammatory response, or the result of immune-mediated mechanisms. There are four principal routes by which infectious microbes enter the nervous system. *Hematogenous spread* is the most common means of entry; infectious agents ordinarily enter through the arterial circulation, but retrograde venous spread can occur through anastomoses with veins of the face. *Direct implantation* of microorganisms is almost invariably traumatic or is associated with congenital malformations (such as meningomyelocele). *Local extension* can come from any of several adjacent structures (air sinuses, an infected tooth, cranial or spinal osteomyelitis). Transport along the *peripheral nervous system* occurs with certain viruses, such as rabies and herpes zoster. General aspects of the pathology of infectious agents are discussed in Chapter 8; here we focus on some of the distinctive forms of CNS infections.

ACUTE MENINGITIS

Meningitis refers to an inflammatory process of the leptomeninges and CSF within the subarachnoid space, while *meningoencephalitis* combines this with inflammation of the brain parenchyma. Meningitis is usually caused by an infection, but may also occur in response to a nonbacterial irritant introduced into the subarachnoid space *(chemical meningitis)*. Infectious meningitis is broadly classified into *acute pyogenic* (usually bacterial meningitis), *aseptic* (usually acute viral meningitis), and *chronic* (usually tuberculous, spirochetal, or cryptococcal) on the basis of the characteristics of inflammatory exudate on CSF examination and the clinical evolution of the illness.

Acute Pyogenic (Bacterial) Meningitis

The microorganisms that cause acute pyogenic meningitis vary with the age of the affected individual. In neonates, they include *Escherichia coli* and the group B streptococci; at the other extreme of life, *Streptococcus pneumoniae* and *Listeria monocytogenes* are more common. Among adolescents and in young adults, *Neisseria meningitidis* is the most common

pathogen, with clusters of cases causing frequent public health concerns. The introduction of immunization against *Haemophilus influenzae* has markedly reduced the incidence of meningitis associated with this organism in the developed world; the population that was previously at highest risk (infants) now has a much lower overall risk of meningitis, with *S. pneumoniae* being the most prevalent organism.

Affected individuals typically show systemic signs of infection superimposed on clinical evidence of meningeal irritation and neurologic impairment, including headache, photophobia, irritability, clouding of consciousness, and neck stiffness. A spinal tap yields cloudy or frankly purulent CSF, under increased pressure, with as many as 90,000 neutrophils per cubic millimeter, an increased protein concentration, and a markedly reduced glucose content. Bacteria may be seen on a smear or can be cultured, sometimes a few hours before the neutrophils appear. Untreated pyogenic meningitis can be fatal, while effective antimicrobial agents markedly reduce mortality. The Waterhouse-Friderichsen syndrome results from meningitis-associated septicemia with hemorrhagic infarction of the adrenal glands and cutaneous petechiae (Chapter 24). It occurs most often with meningococcal and pneumococcal meningitis. In the immunosuppressed individual, purulent meningitis may be caused by other agents, such as *Klebsiella* or an anaerobic organism, and may have an atypical course and uncharacteristic CSF findings, all of which make the diagnosis more difficult.

> **Morphology.** The normally clear CSF is cloudy and sometimes frankly purulent. In acute meningitis, an exudate is evident within the leptomeninges over the surface of the brain (Fig. 28–21). The meningeal vessels

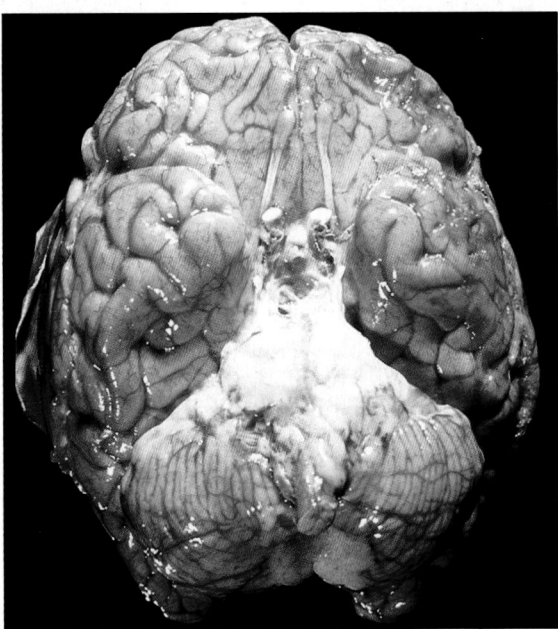

FIGURE 28–21   Pyogenic meningitis. A thick layer of suppurative exudate covers the brainstem and cerebellum and thickens the leptomeninges. (From Golden JA, Louis DN: Images in clinical medicine: acute bacterial meningitis. N Engl J Med 333:364, 1994.)

are engorged and stand out prominently. The location of the exudate varies; in *H. influenzae* meningitis, for example, it is usually basal, whereas in pneumococcal meningitis it is often densest over the cerebral convexities near the sagittal sinus. From the areas of greatest accumulation, tracts of pus can be followed along blood vessels on the surface of the brain. When the meningitis is fulminant, the inflammation may extend to the ventricles, producing ventriculitis.

On microscopic examination, neutrophils fill the subarachnoid space in severely affected areas and are found predominantly around the leptomeningeal blood vessels in less severe cases. In untreated meningitis, Gram stain reveals varying numbers of the causative organism, although they are frequently not demonstrable in treated cases. In fulminant meningitis, the inflammatory cells infiltrate the walls of the leptomeningeal veins and may extend into the substance of the brain (focal cerebritis). Phlebitis may also lead to venous thrombosis and hemorrhagic infarction of the underlying brain.

Leptomeningeal fibrosis may follow pyogenic meningitis and cause hydrocephalus. In some infections, particularly in pneumococcal meningitis, large quantities of the capsular polysaccharide of the organism produce a particularly gelatinous exudate that encourages arachnoid fibrosis, called **chronic adhesive arachnoiditis**.

Acute Aseptic (Viral) Meningitis

Aseptic meningitis is a clinical term referring to the absence of recognizable organisms in a patient with meningeal irritation, fever, and alterations of consciousness of relatively acute onset. The name is a misnomer, as the disease is generally of viral, and rarely of bacterial or other, etiology. The clinical course is less fulminant than that of pyogenic meningitis, and the CSF findings also differ; in aseptic meningitis there is a lymphocytic pleocytosis, the protein elevation is only moderate, and the glucose content is nearly always normal. The viral aseptic meningitides are usually self-limiting and are treated symptomatically. Remarkably, even with molecular methods for detection of pathogens, the etiologic agent is identified in only a minority of cases.[19] The spectrum of pathogens varies seasonally and geographically. An aseptic meningitis–like picture may also develop subsequent to rupture of an epidermoid cyst into the subarachnoid space or the introduction of a chemical irritant ("chemical" meningitis). In these cases the CSF is sterile, there is pleocytosis with neutrophils and an increased protein concentration, but the sugar content is usually normal.

ACUTE FOCAL SUPPURATIVE INFECTIONS

Brain Abscess

Brain abscesses may arise by direct implantation of organisms, local extension from adjacent foci (mastoiditis, paranasal sinusitis), or hematogenous spread (usually from a primary site in the heart, lungs, or distal bones or after tooth extraction). Predisposing conditions include *acute bacterial endocar-*

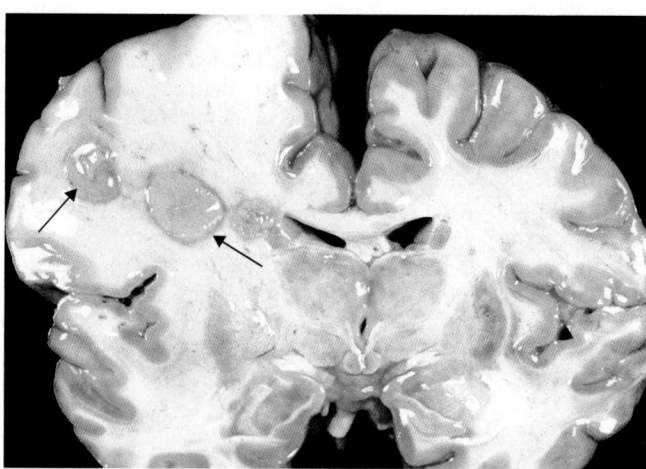

FIGURE 28–22 Frontal abscesses *(arrows)*.

ditis, which tends to produce multiple abscesses; *congenital heart disease* with right-to-left shunting and loss of pulmonary filtration of organisms; *chronic pulmonary sepsis*, as can be seen with bronchiectasis; and *immunosuppression*. Streptococci and staphylococci are the most common offending organisms identified in nonimmunosuppressed populations.

> **Morphology.** Grossly, abscesses are discrete lesions with central liquefactive necrosis surrounded by fibrosis and swelling (Fig. 28–22). On microscopic examination there is exuberant granulation tissue with neovascularization around the necrosis that is responsible for marked vasogenic edema. A collagenous capsule is produced by fibroblasts derived from the walls of blood vessels. Outside the fibrous capsule is a zone of reactive gliosis with numerous gemistocytic astrocytes.

Cerebral abscesses are destructive lesions and patients almost invariably present clinically with progressive focal deficits in addition to the general signs of raised intracranial pressure. The CSF is under increased pressure, the white cell count is raised, and protein concentration is increased, but the glucose content is normal. The source of infection may be apparent, or it may be a small systemic focus that is not symptomatic. The increased intracranial pressure and progressive herniation can be fatal, and abscess rupture can lead to ventriculitis, meningitis, and venous sinus thrombosis. With surgery and antibiotics, the otherwise high mortality rate can be reduced to less than 10%.

Subdural Empyema

Bacterial or occasionally fungal infection of the skull bones or air sinuses can spread to the subdural space, producing a subdural empyema. The underlying arachnoid and subarachnoid spaces are usually unaffected, but a large subdural empyema may produce a mass effect. Further, a thrombophlebitis may develop in the bridging veins that cross the subdural space, resulting in venous occlusion and infarction of the brain. With treatment, including surgical drainage, resolution of the empyema occurs from the dural side, and, if it is complete, a thickened dura may be the only residual finding. Symptoms include those referable to the source of the infection. In addition, most patients are febrile, with headache and neck stiffness, and, if untreated, may develop focal neurologic signs, lethargy, and coma. The CSF profile is similar to that seen in brain abscesses, because both are parameningeal infectious processes. If diagnosis and treatment are prompt, complete recovery is usual.

Extradural Abscess

Extradural abscess, commonly associated with osteomyelitis, often arises from an adjacent focus of infection, such as sinusitis or a surgical procedure. When the process occurs in the spinal epidural space, it may cause spinal cord compression and constitute a neurosurgical emergency.

CHRONIC BACTERIAL MENINGOENCEPHALITIS

Chronic bacterial infection of the meninges and the brain may be caused by *M. tuberculosis*, *T. pallidum*, and *Borrelia* species. Each of these is briefly described next.

Tuberculosis

Tuberculosis of the brain may be part of systemic disease or apparently isolated, the brain having been seeded from a silent, usually pulmonary, lesion. It may involve the meninges or the brain, often together.

> **Morphology.** On macroscopic examination, the subarachnoid space contains a gelatinous or fibrinous exudate, most often at the base of the brain, obliterating the cisterns and encasing cranial nerves. There may be discrete, white granules scattered over the leptomeninges. The most common pattern of involvement is a diffuse **meningoencephalitis**. On microscopic examination, there are mixtures of lymphocytes, plasma cells, and macrophages. Florid cases show well-formed granulomas, often with caseous necrosis and giant cells. Arteries running through the subarachnoid space may show **obliterative endarteritis** with inflammatory infiltrates in their walls and marked intimal thickening. Organisms can often be seen with acid-fast stains. The infectious process may spread to the choroid plexus and ependymal surface, traveling through the CSF. In cases of long-standing duration, a dense, fibrous adhesive arachnoiditis may develop, most conspicuous around the base of the brain. Hydrocephalus may result.
>
> Another manifestation of the disease is the development of a single (or often multiple) well-circumscribed intraparenchymal mass **(tuberculoma)**, which may be associated with meningitis. A tuberculoma may be as large as several centimeters in diameter, causing significant mass effect. On microscopic examination, there is usually a central core of caseous necrosis surrounded by a typical tuberculous granulomatous reaction; calcification may occur in inactive lesions.

Clinical Features. Patients with tuberculous meningitis usually have symptoms of headache, malaise, mental confusion, and vomiting. There is only a moderate CSF pleocytosis made up of mononuclear cells or a mixture of polymorphonuclear and mononuclear cells; the protein concentration is elevated, often strikingly so; and the glucose content typically is moderately reduced or normal. The most serious complications of chronic tuberculous meningitis are arachnoid fibrosis producing hydrocephalus, and obliterative endarteritis producing arterial occlusion and infarction of underlying brain. When the process involves the spinal cord subarachnoid space, nerve roots may also be affected. With tuberculomas, the symptoms are typical of space-occupying lesions of the brain, and have to be distinguished from CNS tumors.

Infection by *Mycobacterium tuberculosis* in individuals with acquired immunodeficiency syndrome (AIDS) is often similar to that in individuals not suffering from AIDS, but there may be less host reaction. HIV-positive individuals are also at risk for infection by *M. avium-intracellulare*, usually in the setting of disseminated infection. These lesions typically contain confluent sheets of macrophages filled with organisms, with little or no associated granulomatous reaction.

Neurosyphilis

Neurosyphilis is a manifestation of the tertiary stage of syphilis and occurs in only about 10% of individuals with untreated infection. The major patterns of CNS involvement are meningovascular neurosyphilis, paretic neurosyphilis, and tabes dorsalis; affected individuals often show incomplete or mixed pictures, most commonly the combination of tabes dorsalis and paretic disease (taboparesis). Individuals infected with HIV are at increased risk for neurosyphilis, particularly as an acute syphilitic meningitis or meningovascular disease, because of impaired cell-mediated immunity. The rate of progression and severity of the disease seem to be accelerated, possibly for the same reason.

> **Morphology. Meningovascular neurosyphilis** is a chronic meningitis involving the base of the brain and more variably the cerebral convexities and the spinal leptomeninges. In addition, there may be an associated obliterative endarteritis (Heubner arteritis) accompanied by a distinctive perivascular inflammatory reaction rich in plasma cells and lymphocytes. Cerebral gummas (plasma cell–rich mass lesions) may also occur in the meninges and extend into the parenchyma.
>
> **Paretic neurosyphilis** is caused by invasion of the brain by *Treponema pallidum* and is clinically manifested as insidious but progressive mental deficits associated with mood alterations (including delusions of grandeur) that terminate in severe dementia **(general paresis of the insane)**. On microscopic examination, inflammatory lesions are associated with parenchymal damage in the cerebral cortex (particularly the frontal lobe but also affecting other areas of the isocortex) characterized by loss of neurons, proliferations of microglia (rod cells), gliosis, and iron deposits. The latter are demonstrable with

the Prussian blue stain perivascularly and in the neuropil, and are presumably the sequelae of small bleeds stemming from damage to the microcirculation. The spirochetes can, at times, be demonstrated in tissue sections. There is often an associated hydrocephalus with damage to the ependymal lining and proliferation of subependymal glia, called **granular ependymitis**.

Tabes dorsalis is the result of damage by the spirochetes to the sensory nerves in the dorsal roots, which produces impaired joint position sense and resultant ataxia (locomotor ataxia); loss of pain sensation, leading to skin and joint damage (Charcot joints); other sensory disturbances, particularly the characteristic "lightning pains"; and absence of deep tendon reflexes. On microscopic examination there is loss of both axons and myelin in the dorsal roots, with corresponding pallor and atrophy in the dorsal columns of the spinal cord. Organisms are not demonstrable in the cord lesions.

Neuroborreliosis (Lyme Disease)

Lyme disease is caused by the spirochete *Borrelia burgdorferi*, transmitted by various species of *Ixodes* tick; involvement of the nervous system is referred to as neuroborreliosis. Neurologic symptoms are highly variable and include aseptic meningitis, facial nerve palsies and other polyneuropathies, as well as encephalopathy. The rare cases that have come to autopsy have shown a focal proliferation of microglial cells in the brain as well as scattered extracellular organisms (identified by Dieterle stain).

VIRAL MENINGOENCEPHALITIS

Viral encephalitis is a parenchymal infection of the brain almost invariably associated with meningeal inflammation (meningoencephalitis) and sometimes with simultaneous involvement of the spinal cord (encephalomyelitis).

Some viruses tend to infect the nervous system. Such neural tropism takes several forms: some viruses infect specific cell types (such as oligodendrocytes), while others preferentially involve particular areas of the brain (such as medial temporal lobes or the limbic system). *Latency* is an important facet of several viral infections of the CNS (e.g., herpes zoster, progressive multifocal leukoencephalopathy). Systemic viral infections in the absence of direct evidence of viral penetration into the CNS may be followed by an *immune-mediated disease*, such as perivenous demyelination (see "Acute Disseminated Encephalomyelitis and Acute Necrotizing Hemorrhagic Encephalomyelitis"). Intrauterine viral infection may cause *congenital malformations*, as occurs with rubella. A slowly progressive degenerative disease syndrome may follow many years after a viral illness; an example is *post-encephalitic parkinsonism* after the 1918 viral influenza pandemic.

Arthropod-Borne Viral Encephalitis

Arboviruses are an important cause of epidemic encephalitis, especially in tropical regions of the world, and they are capable of causing serious morbidity and high mortality. In the Western hemisphere the most important types are Eastern and Western equine, West Nile, Venezuelan, St. Louis, and La Crosse; elsewhere in the world, pathogenic arboviruses include Japanese B (Far East), Murray Valley (Australia and New Guinea), and tick-borne (Russia and Eastern Europe). All have animal hosts and mosquito vectors, except for the tick-borne type. Clinically, affected individuals develop generalized neurologic deficits, such as seizures, confusion, delirium, and stupor or coma, and often focal signs, such as reflex asymmetry and ocular palsies. Involvement of the spinal cord in West Nile encephalitis can lead to a polio-like syndrome with paralysis. The CSF is usually colorless but with a slightly elevated pressure and, initially, a neutrophilic pleocytosis that rapidly converts to lymphocytes; the protein concentration is elevated, but glucose content is normal.

Morphology. The encephalitides caused by various arboviruses differ in epidemiology and prognosis, but the histopathologic picture is similar, except for variations in the severity and extent of the lesions within the CNS. Characteristically, there is a lymphocytic meningoencephalitis (sometimes with neutrophils), and a tendency for inflammatory cells to accumulate perivascularly (Fig. 28-23A). Multiple foci of necrosis of gray and white matter are found; in particular, there is evidence of single-cell neuronal necrosis with phagocytosis of the debris (**neuronophagia**). Microglial cells form small aggregates around foci of necrosis, called **microglial nodules** (Fig. 28-23B). In severe cases there may be a necrotizing vasculitis with associated focal hemorrhages. While some viruses reveal their presence by inclusion bodies, the identification of viral pathogens is most often by a combination of ultrastructural, immunohistochemical, and molecular methods.[19]

Herpes Simplex Virus Type 1

Herpes simplex virus type 1 (HSV-1) encephalitis is most common in children and young adults. Only about 10% of the affected individuals have a history of prior herpes. The most commonly observed clinical presenting symptoms in herpes encephalitis are alterations in mood, memory, and behavior. Polymerase chain reaction (PCR)–based methods for virus detection in CSF samples have increased the ease of diagnosis and the recognition of a subset of patients with less severe disease. Antiviral agents now provide effective treatment in many cases, with a significant reduction in the mortality rate. In some individuals, HSV-1 encephalitis follows a subacute course with clinical manifestations (weakness, lethargy, ataxia, seizures) that evolve during a more protracted period (4 to 6 weeks).

Morphology. This encephalitis starts in, and most severely involves, the inferior and medial regions of the temporal lobes and the orbital gyri of the frontal lobes (Fig. 28-24). The infection is necrotizing and

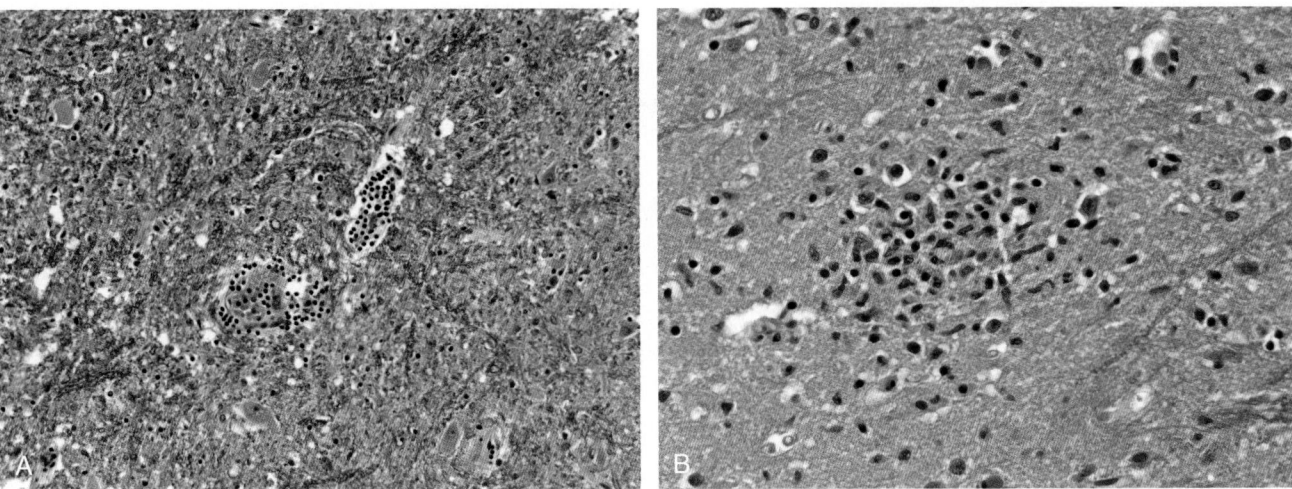

FIGURE 28–23   Characteristic findings of viral encephalitis include perivascular cuffs of lymphocytes (**A**) and microglial nodules (**B**).

often hemorrhagic in the most severely affected regions. Perivascular inflammatory infiltrates are usually present, and Cowdry type A intranuclear viral inclusion bodies may be found in both neurons and glia. In individuals with slowly evolving HSV-1 encephalitis, there is more diffuse involvement of the brain.

Herpes Simplex Virus Type 2

Herpes simplex virus type 2 (HSV-2) also infects the nervous system; in adults it causes meningitis, but as many as 50% of neonates born by vaginal delivery to women with active *primary* HSV genital infections acquire the infection during passage through the birth canal and develop severe encephalitis. In the face of active HIV infection, HSV-2 may cause an acute, hemorrhagic, necrotizing encephalitis.

Varicella-Zoster Virus (Herpes Zoster)

Primary varicella infection presents as one of the childhood exanthems (chickenpox), ordinarily without any evidence of neurologic involvement. Following the cutaneous infection, the virus enters a latent phase within sensory neurons of the dorsal root or trigeminal ganglia. Reactivation of infection in adults ("shingles") usually manifests as a painful, vesicular skin eruption in a single or limited dermatomal distribution. Herpes zoster reactivation is usually a self-limited process, but there may be a persistent postherpetic neuralgia syndrome particularly after age 60, including both persistent pain as well as painful sensation following nonpainful stimuli.

Overt CNS involvement with herpes zoster is much rarer but can be severe. Herpes zoster has been associated with a granulomatous arteritis; immunocytochemical and electron microscopic evidence of viral involvement has been obtained in a few of these cases. In immunosuppressed individuals, herpes zoster may cause acute encephalitis with numerous

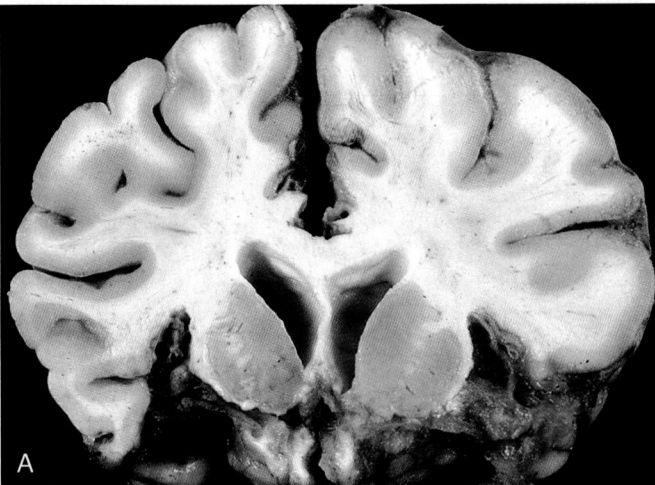
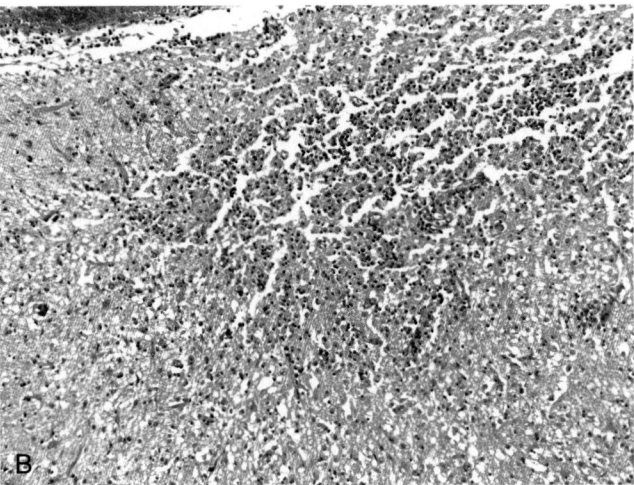

FIGURE 28–24   **A,** Herpes encephalitis showing extensive destruction of inferior frontal and anterior temporal lobes. **B,** Necrotizing inflammatory process characterizes acute herpes encephalitis. (**A,** Courtesy of Dr. T.W. Smith, University of Massachusetts Medical School, Worcester, MA.)

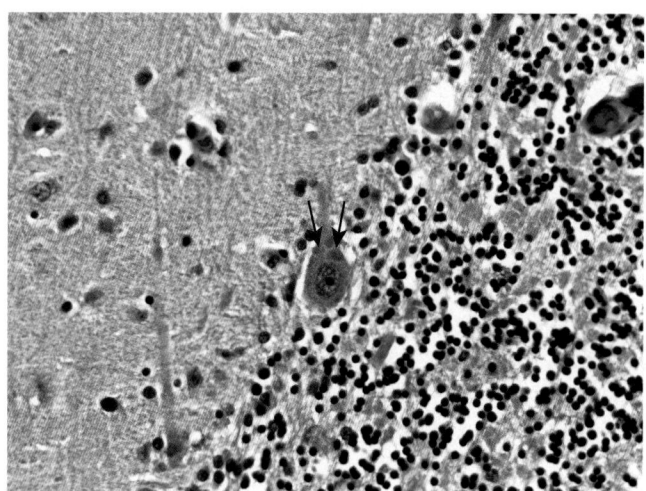

FIGURE 28-25 The diagnostic histologic finding in rabies is the eosinophilic Negri body, as seen here in a Purkinje cell *(arrows)*.

sharply circumscribed lesions characterized by demyelination followed by necrosis.

Cytomegalovirus

This infection of the nervous system occurs in fetuses and immunosuppressed individuals. The outcome of infection in utero is periventricular necrosis that produces severe brain destruction followed later by microcephaly and periventricular calcification. CMV is a common opportunistic viral pathogen in individuals with AIDS, with CNS involvement being common in this setting.

Morphology. In the immunosuppressed individual, the most common pattern of involvement is that of a subacute encephalitis, which may be associated with CMV inclusion-bearing cells (see Fig. 8-15). Although any type of cell within the CNS (neurons, glia, ependyma, endothelium) can be infected by CMV, there is a tendency for the virus to localize in the paraventricular subependymal regions of the brain. This results in a severe hemorrhagic necrotizing ventriculoencephalitis and a choroid plexitis. The virus can also attack the lower spinal cord and roots, producing a painful radiculoneuritis. Prominent cytomegalic cells with intranuclear and intracytoplasmic inclusions can be readily identified by conventional light microscopy and confirmed as CMV by immunohistochemistry.

Poliomyelitis

While paralytic poliomyelitis has been effectively eradicated by vaccination in many parts of the world, there are still regions where it remains a problem. In nonimmunized individuals poliovirus infection causes a subclinical or mild gastroenteritis, similar to that caused by other members of the picorna group of enteroviruses. In a small fraction of the vulnerable population, however, it secondarily invades the nervous system.

Morphology. Acute cases show mononuclear cell perivascular cuffs and neuronophagia of the **anterior-horn motor neurons of the spinal cord**. The inflammatory reaction is usually confined to the anterior horns but may extend into the posterior horns, and the damage is occasionally severe enough to produce cavitation. In situ reverse transcriptase–PCR has shown poliovirus RNA in anterior-horn cell motor neurons. The cranial motor nuclei are sometimes involved. Postmortem examination in long-term survivors of symptomatic poliomyelitis shows loss of neurons and gliosis in the affected anterior horns of the spinal cord, some residual inflammation, atrophy of the anterior (motor) spinal roots, and neurogenic atrophy of denervated muscle.

Clinical Features. CNS infection manifests initially with meningeal irritation and a CSF picture of aseptic meningitis. The disease may progress no further or advance to involve the spinal cord. When the disease affects the motor neurons of the spinal cord, it produces a flaccid paralysis with muscle wasting and hyporeflexia in the corresponding region of the body—the permanent neurologic residue of poliomyelitis. In the acute disease, death can occur from paralysis of the respiratory muscles, and a myocarditis sometimes complicates the clinical course. Because of the destruction of motor neurons, paresis or paralysis follows; when it involves the innervation of the diaphragm and intercostal muscles, severe respiratory compromise may occur and cause long-term morbidity. *Post-polio syndrome* can develop in patients 25 to 35 years after the resolution of the initial illness. It is characterized by progressive weakness associated with decreased muscle mass and pain, and has an unclear pathogenesis.

Rabies

Rabies is a severe encephalitis transmitted to humans by the bite of a rabid animal, usually a dog or various wild mammals that form natural reservoirs. Exposure to certain species of bats, even without a known bite, can also lead to rabies.

Morphology. On macroscopic examination the brain shows intense edema and vascular congestion. On microscopic examination there is widespread neuronal degeneration and an inflammatory reaction that is most severe in the brainstem. The basal ganglia, spinal cord, and dorsal root ganglia may also be involved. **Negri bodies,** the pathognomonic microscopic finding, are cytoplasmic, round to oval, eosinophilic inclusions that can be found in pyramidal neurons of the hippocampus and Purkinje cells of the cerebellum, sites usually devoid of inflammation (Fig. 28-25). The presence of rabies virus can be detected within Negri bodies by ultrastructural and immunohistochemical examination.

Clinical Features. Since the virus enters the CNS by ascending along the peripheral nerves from the wound site, the incubation period (commonly between 1 and 3 months) depends on the distance between the wound and the brain. The disease begins with nonspecific symptoms of malaise, headache, and fever, but the conjunction of these symptoms with local paresthesias around the wound is diagnostic. As the infection advances, the affected individual exhibits extraordinary CNS excitability; the slightest touch is painful, with violent motor responses progressing to convulsions. Contracture of the pharyngeal musculature on swallowing produces foaming at the mouth, which may create an aversion to swallowing even water (hydrophobia). There is meningismus and, as the disease progresses, flaccid paralysis. Periods of alternating mania and stupor progress to coma and death from respiratory center failure.

Human Immunodeficiency Virus

In the period before the availability of effective anti-retroviral therapy, neuropathologic changes were demonstrated at postmortem examination in as many as 80% to 90% of cases of AIDS. These included direct effects of virus on the nervous system, opportunistic infections, and primary CNS lymphoma. Since the early days, there has been a decrease in the frequency of these secondary effects of HIV infection, in those who receive intensive multidrug anti-retroviral therapy.[20,21]

HIV aseptic meningitis occurs within 1 to 2 weeks of seroconversion in about 10% of patients; antibodies to HIV can be demonstrated and the virus can be isolated from the CSF. The few neuropathologic studies of the early and acute phases of symptomatic or asymptomatic HIV invasion of the nervous system have shown a mild lymphocytic meningitis, perivascular inflammation, and some myelin loss in the hemispheres. Among the cell types of the CNS, only microglia have the appropriate combination of CD4 and a chemokine receptor (CCR5 or CXCR4) to allow for efficient infection by HIV.[22] During the chronic phase, an HIV encephalitis is commonly found when symptomatic individuals come to autopsy.

> **Morphology.** HIV encephalitis is best characterized microscopically as a chronic inflammatory reaction with widely distributed infiltrates of **microglial nodules**, sometimes with associated foci of tissue necrosis and reactive gliosis (Fig. 28–26). The microglial nodules are also found in the vicinity of small blood vessels, which show abnormally prominent endothelial cells and perivascular foamy or pigment-laden macrophages. These changes occur especially in the subcortical white matter, diencephalon, and brainstem. An important component of the microglial nodule is the macrophage-derived **multinucleated giant cell**. In some cases there is also a disorder of white matter characterized by multifocal or diffuse areas of myelin pallor, axonal swelling and gliosis. HIV can be detected in CD4+ mononuclear and multinucleated macrophages and microglia by immunoperoxidase and molecular methods.

Cognitive changes, both mild and florid enough to be termed *HIV-associated dementia*, appear to have persisted into the era of effective anti-HIV treatment regimens. Rather than having a specific pathologic lesion as its correlate, this disorder

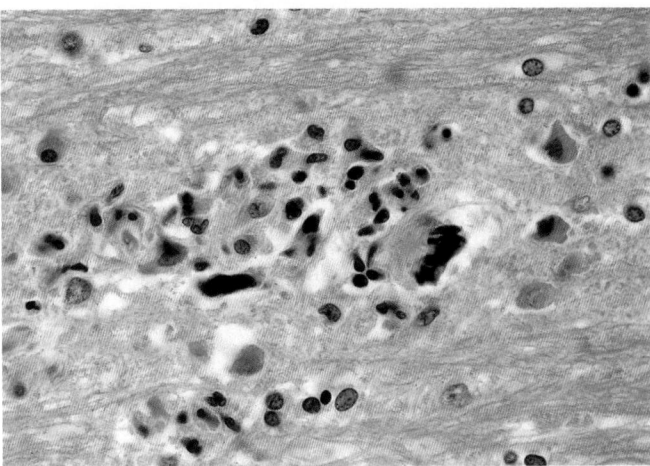

FIGURE 28–26 HIV encephalitis. Note the microglial nodule and multinucleated giant cells.

is most tightly related to the extent of activated microglia in the brain, not all of which are necessarily HIV-infected. A wide range of possible mechanisms for neuronal dysfunction and injury in this setting have been proposed, including actions of cytokines and activation of an inflammatory cascade as well as a cavalcade of toxic effects of HIV-derived proteins; in all probability, each of these pathways has a contributory role in the pathogenesis of neural injury (Chapter 6).

Progressive Multifocal Leukoencephalopathy

Progressive multifocal leukoencephalopathy (PML) is a viral encephalitis caused by the JC polyomavirus; because the virus preferentially infects oligodendrocytes, demyelination is its principal pathologic effect. The disease occurs almost exclusively in immunosuppressed individuals in various clinical settings, including chronic lymphoproliferative or myeloproliferative illnesses, immunosuppressive chemotherapy including monoclonal antibody therapy targeting integrins, granulomatous diseases, and HIV/AIDS.

Although most people have serologic evidence of exposure to JC virus by the age of 14 years, no clinical disease has been associated with primary infection by the virus. It is thought that PML results from the reactivation of virus in the setting of immunosuppression. Clinically, affected individuals develop focal and relentlessly progressive neurologic symptoms and signs, and imaging studies show extensive, often multifocal, lesions in the hemispheric or cerebellar white matter.

> **Morphology.** The lesions consist of patches of irregular, ill-defined destruction of the white matter ranging in size from millimeters to extensive involvement of an entire lobe of the brain (Fig. 28–27). On microscopic examination the typical lesion consists of a patch of demyelination, most often in a subcortical location, in the center of which are scattered lipid-laden macrophages and a reduced number of axons. At the edge of the lesion are greatly enlarged oligodendrocyte nuclei with glassy amphophilic viral inclusions (Fig. 28–27, *inset*), which contain viral antigens

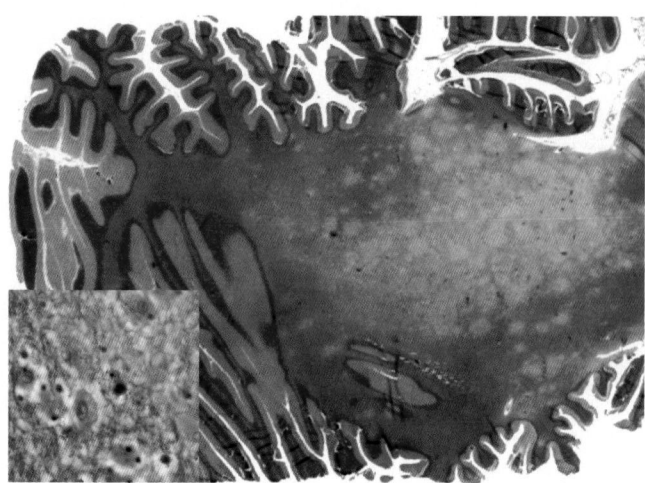

FIGURE 28–27 Progressive multifocal leukoencephalopathy. Section stained for myelin showing irregular, poorly defined areas of demyelination, which become confluent in places. *Inset,* Enlarged oligodendrocyte nucleus represents the effect of viral infection.

by immunohistochemistry. Within the lesions, there may be bizarre giant astrocytes with one to several irregular, hyperchromatic nuclei mixed with more typical reactive astrocytes.

Subacute Sclerosing Panencephalitis

Subacute sclerosing panencephalitis (SSPE) is a rare progressive clinical syndrome characterized by cognitive decline, spasticity of limbs, and seizures. It occurs in children or young adults, months or years after an initial, early-age acute infection with measles. The disease represents persistent, but nonproductive, infection of the CNS by an altered measles virus; changes in several viral genes have been associated with the disease. On microscopic examination, there are widespread gliosis and myelin degeneration; viral inclusions, largely within the nuclei, of oligodendrocytes and neurons; variable inflammation of white and gray matter; and neurofibrillary tangles. Ultrastructural study shows that the inclusions contain nucleocapsids characteristic of measles; immunohistochemistry for measles virus antigen is positive. The disease has largely disappeared with the spread of vaccination programs; however, there are still cases being reported from nonimmunized populations.

FUNGAL MENINGOENCEPHALITIS

Fungal disease of the CNS is encountered primarily in immunocompromised individuals. The brain is usually involved when there is widespread hematogenous dissemination of the fungus, most often *Candida albicans, Mucor species, Aspergillus fumigatus,* and *Cryptococcus neoformans.* In endemic areas, pathogens such as *Histoplasma capsulatum, Coccidioides immitis,* and *Blastomyces dermatitidis* may involve the CNS after a primary pulmonary or cutaneous infection; again, this often follows immunosuppression.

There are three main patterns of fungal infection in the CNS: chronic meningitis, vasculitis, and parenchymal invasion. Vasculitis is most frequently seen with *mucormycosis* and *aspergillosis,* both of which are characterized by direct fungal invasion of blood vessel walls, but it occasionally occurs with other infections such as *candidiasis.* The resultant vascular thrombosis produces infarction that is often strikingly hemorrhagic and that subsequently becomes septic from ingrowth of the causative fungus.

Parenchymal invasion, usually in the form of granulomas or abscesses, can occur with most of the fungi and often coexists with meningitis. The most commonly encountered fungi invading the brain are *Candida* and *Cryptococcus. Candidiasis* usually produces multiple microabscesses, with or without granuloma formation. Although most fungi invade the brain by hematogenous dissemination, direct extension may also occur, particularly in *mucormycosis,* most commonly in diabetics with ketoacidosis.

Cryptococcal meningitis, a common opportunistic infection in the setting of HIV/AIDS, may be fulminant and fatal in as little as 2 weeks or indolent, evolving over months or years. The CSF may contain few cells but usually has a high concentration of protein. The mucoid-encapsulated yeasts can be visualized in the CSF by India ink preparations and in tissue sections by PAS, mucicarmine, and silver stains.

Morphology. With cryptococcal infection, the brain shows a chronic meningitis affecting the basal leptomeninges, which are opaque and thickened by reactive connective tissue that may obstruct the outflow of CSF from the foramina of Luschka and Magendie, giving rise to hydrocephalus. Sections of the brain disclose a gelatinous material within the subarachnoid space and small cysts within the parenchyma ("soap bubbles"), which are especially prominent in the basal ganglia in the distribution of the lenticulostriate arteries (Fig. 28–28A). Parenchymal lesions consist of aggregates of organisms within expanded perivascular (Virchow-Robin) spaces associated with minimal or absent inflammation or gliosis (Fig. 28–28B). The meningeal infiltrates consist of chronic inflammatory cells and fibroblasts admixed with cryptococci.

OTHER INFECTIOUS DISEASES OF THE NERVOUS SYSTEM

Protozoal diseases (including malaria, toxoplasmosis, amebiasis, and trypanosomiasis), rickettsial infections (such as typhus and Rocky Mountain spotted fever), and metazoal diseases (especially cysticercosis and echinococcosis) may also involve the CNS and are discussed in Chapter 8.

Cerebral toxoplasmosis is another of the opportunistic infections commonly found in the setting of HIV-associated immunosuppression. The clinical symptoms of infection of the brain by *Toxoplasma gondii* are subacute, evolving during a 1- or 2-week period, and may be both focal and diffuse. Computed tomography and magnetic resonance imaging studies may show multiple ring-enhancing lesions; however, this radiographic appearance is not pathognomonic, since

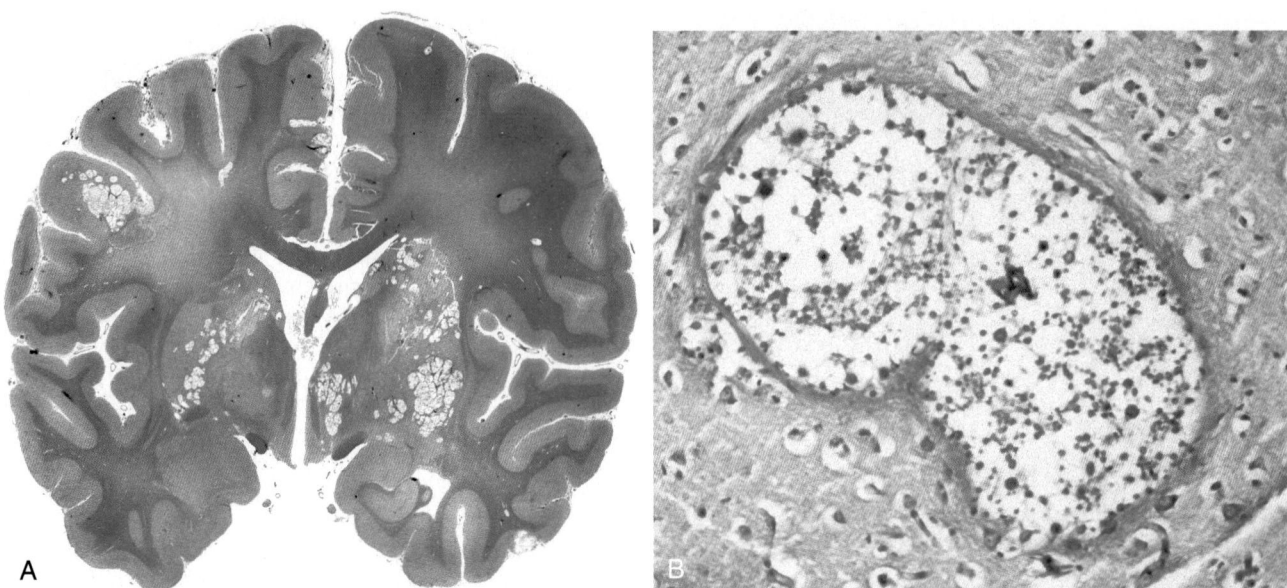

FIGURE 28–28 Cryptococcal infection. **A,** Whole-brain section showing the numerous areas of tissue destruction ("soap bubbles") associated with the spread of organisms in the perivascular spaces. **B,** At higher magnification it is possible to see the cryptococci in the lesions.

similar findings may be associated with CNS lymphoma, tuberculosis, and fungal infections. In nonimmunosuppressed hosts, the impact of toxoplasmosis on the brain is most often seen when primary maternal infection occurs early in the pregnancy. It may be followed by a cerebritis in the fetus, with the production of multifocal cerebral necrotizing lesions that may calcify, producing severe damage to the developing brain.

Morphology. Toxoplasmosis of the CNS produces brain abscesses, which are found most often in the cerebral cortex (near the gray-white junction) and deep gray nuclei, less often in the cerebellum and brainstem, and rarely in the spinal cord (Fig. 28–29). Acute lesions exhibit central foci of necrosis, petechial hemorrhages surrounded by acute and chronic inflammation, macrophage infiltration, and vascular proliferation. Both free tachyzoites and encysted bradyzoites (Fig. 28–29B) may be found at the periphery of the necrotic foci. The organisms are usually seen on routine H&E or Giemsa stains, but are more easily recognized by immunocytochemical methods. The blood vessels in the vicinity of these lesions may

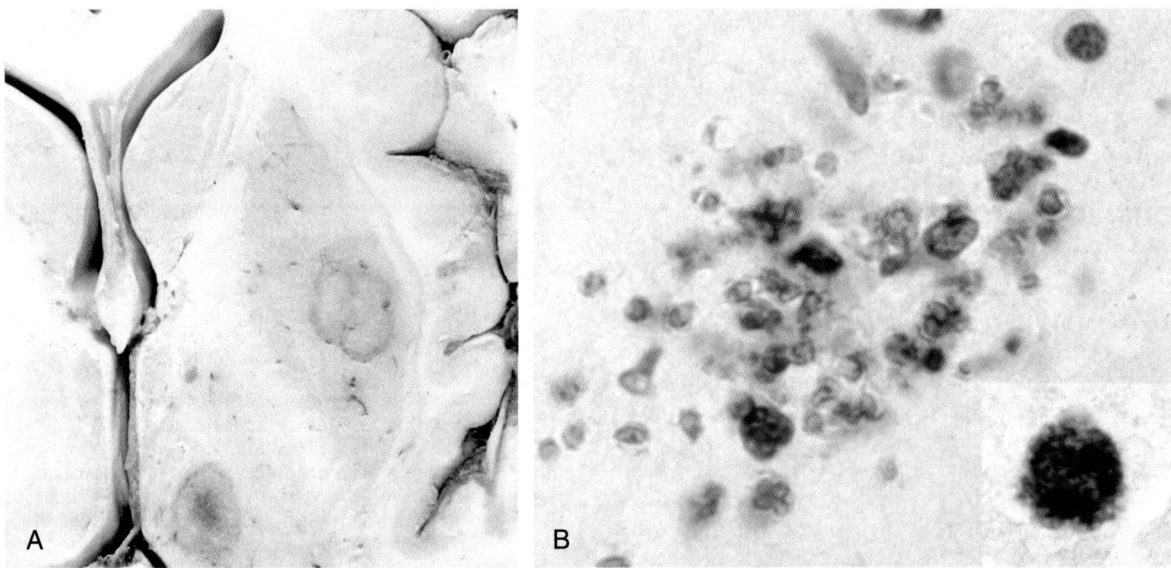

FIGURE 28–29 **A,** *Toxoplasma* abscesses in the putamen and thalamus. **B,** Free tachyzoites demonstrated by immunostaining; *inset:* *Toxoplasma* pseudocyst with bradyzoites highlighted by immunostaining.

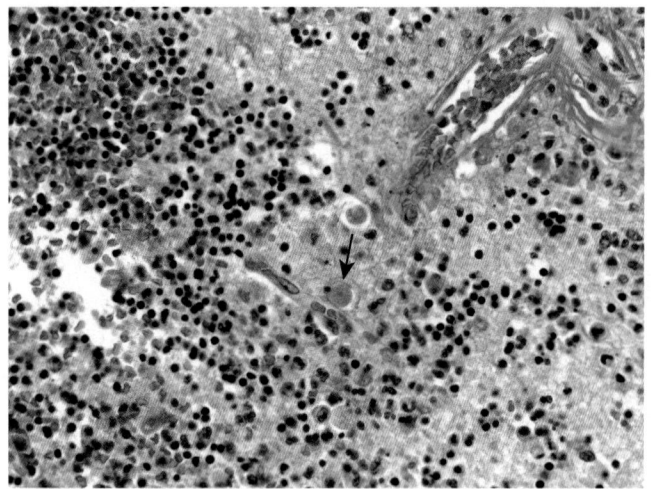

FIGURE 28–30 Necrotizing amebic meningoencephalitis involving the cerebellum (organism highlighted by *arrow*).

show marked intimal proliferation or even frank vasculitis with fibrinoid necrosis and thrombosis. After treatment, the lesions consist of large, well-demarcated areas of coagulation necrosis surrounded by lipid-laden macrophages. Cysts and free tachyzoites can also be found adjacent to these lesions but may be considerably reduced in number or absent if therapy has been effective. Chronic lesions consist of small cystic spaces containing scattered lipid- and hemosiderin-laden macrophages that are surrounded by gliotic brain. Organisms are difficult to detect in these older lesions.

Cerebral amebiasis. A rapidly fatal necrotizing encephalitis occurs with infection with *Naegleria* species, and a chronic granulomatous meningoencephalitis has been associated with infection with *Acanthamoeba*. The amebas may sometimes be difficult to distinguish from activated macrophages (Fig. 28–30). Methenamine silver or PAS stains are helpful in visualizing the organisms, although definitive identification ultimately depends on combined immunofluorescence studies, morphology, culture, and molecular methods.

Transmissible Spongiform Encephalopathies (Prion Diseases)

Prions are abnormal forms of a cellular protein that cause transmissible neurodegenerative disorders.[23,24] This group of diseases—which includes Creutzfeldt-Jakob disease (CJD), Gerstmann-Sträussler-Scheinker syndrome (GSS), fatal familial insomnia, and kuru in humans; scrapie in sheep and goats; mink-transmissible encephalopathy; chronic wasting disease of deer and elk; and bovine spongiform encephalopathy—share this etiologic basis that distinguishes them from other neurodegenerative and infectious diseases. While differences exist among these disorders, they are all associated with abnormal forms of a specific protein, termed *prion protein* (PrP),

that is both infectious and transmissible. As the name implies, they are predominantly characterized by "spongiform change" caused by intracellular vacuoles in neurons and glia. Clinically, most of the affected patients develop progressive dementia. The most common disorder is CJD. The sporadic form of CJD has an annual incidence of approximately 1 case per 1,000,000 population and accounts for about 90% of cases; familial and transmitted forms make up the rest.

Pathogenesis and Molecular Genetics. Normal PrP is a 30-kD cellular protein present in neurons. Disease occurs when the PrP undergoes a conformational change from its normal α-helix-containing isoform (PrP^c) to an abnormal β-pleated sheet isoform, usually termed PrP^{sc} (for scrapie) (Fig. 28–31). Associated with the conformational change, PrP acquires resistance to digestion with proteases, such as proteinase K. Accumulation of PrP^{sc} in neural tissue seems to be the cause of the pathology in these diseases, but how this material induces the development of cytoplasmic vacuoles and eventual neuronal death is still unknown. Western blotting of tissue extracts after partial digestion with proteinase K allows detection of PrP^{sc}, which is diagnostic.

The conformational change resulting in PrP^{sc} may occur spontaneously at an extremely low rate (resulting in sporadic cases) or at a higher rate if various mutations are present in PrP^c, such as occurs in familial forms of CJD and in GSS and fatal familial insomnia. PrP^{sc}, independent of the means by which it originates, then facilitates, in a cooperative fashion,

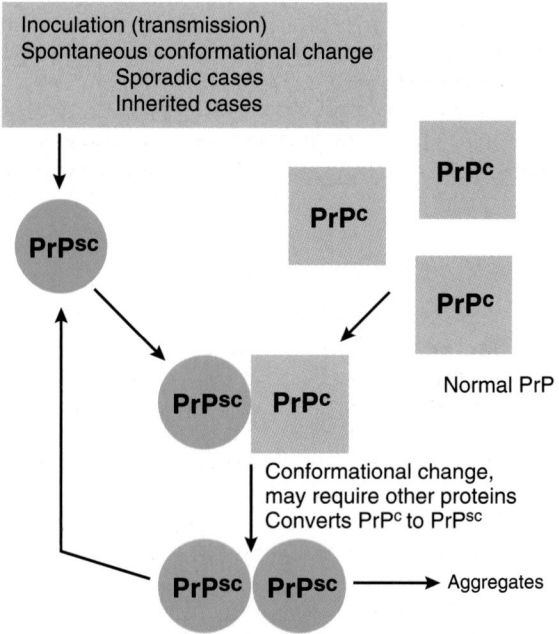

FIGURE 28–31 Proposed mechanism for the conversion of PrP^c through protein–protein interactions. The initiating molecules of PrP^{sc} may arise through inoculation (as in directly transmitted cases) or through an extremely low-rate spontaneous conformational change. The effect of the mutations in PrP^c is to increase the rate of the conformational change once PrP^{sc} is able to recruit and convert other molecules of PrP^c into the abnormal form of the protein. Although the model is drawn with no other proteins involved, it is possible that other proteins play critical roles in the conversion of PrP^c to PrP^{sc}.

the conversion of other PrP^c molecules to PrP^{sc} molecules. It is this activity of PrP^{sc} that accounts for the *infectious* nature of prion diseases.

The gene encoding PrP, termed *PRNP*, shows a high degree of conservation across species. A variety of mutations in *PRNP* have been found to underlie familial forms of prion diseases. In addition, a polymorphism at codon 129 that encodes either methionine (Met) or valine (Val) has been found to influence the disease: individuals who are homozygous for either Met or Val are over-represented among cases of CJD compared with the general population, implying that heterozygosity at codon 129 is protective against development of the disease. Interestingly, this protection also applies against iatrogenic CJD. It has been suggested that the amino-acid at this polymorphic site influences disease by altering the kinetics of aggregation and the conformations of PrP molecules.[25]

Creutzfeldt-Jakob Disease

CJD, the most common prion disease, is a rare disorder that manifests clinically as a rapidly progressive dementia. It is primarily sporadic (about 85% of cases) in its occurrence, and has a worldwide annual incidence of about 1 per million; familial forms also exist that are caused by mutations in *PRNP*. The disease has a peak incidence in the seventh decade. There are well-established cases of iatrogenic transmission, notably by corneal transplantation, deep implantation electrodes, and contaminated preparations of human growth hormone. The clinical onset is marked by subtle changes in memory and behavior followed by a rapidly progressive dementia, often with pronounced involuntary jerking muscle contractions on sudden stimulation (startle myoclonus). Signs of cerebellar dysfunction, usually manifested as ataxia, are present in a minority of affected individuals. The disease is uniformly fatal, with an average survival of only 7 months from the onset of symptoms, although a few patients have lived for several years. These long-surviving cases show extensive atrophy of involved gray matter.

Variant Creutzfeldt-Jakob Disease

Starting in 1995, a series of cases of a CJD-like illness came to medical attention in the United Kingdom. These new cases were different from typical CJD in several important respects: the disease affected young adults, behavioral disorders figured prominently in the early stages of the disease, and the neurologic syndrome progressed more slowly than in individuals with other forms of CJD. The neuropathologic findings and molecular features of these new cases were similar to those of CJD, suggesting a close relationship between the two illnesses. Pathologically, variant CJD (vCJD) is characterized by the presence of extensive cortical plaques with a surrounding halo of spongiform change. No alterations in the *PRNP* gene are present; nearly all affected patients are Met/Met homozygotes at codon 129. With the recent report of a case of vCJD arising in a Val/Val homozygote, the possibility of an influence of codon 129 on incubation period rather than susceptibility has emerged.[26] Several lines of evidence have linked vCJD with bovine spongiform encephalopathy, raising complex public health issues. There has also been documented transmission of vCJD by blood products.

Morphology. The progression of the dementia in CJD is usually so rapid that there is little if any grossly evident brain atrophy. On microscopic examination, the pathognomonic finding is a **spongiform** transformation of the cerebral cortex and, often, deep gray-matter structures (caudate, putamen); this multifocal process results in the uneven formation of small, apparently empty, microscopic vacuoles of varying sizes within the neuropil and sometimes in the perikaryon of neurons (Fig. 28–32A). In advanced cases there is severe neuronal loss, reactive gliosis, and sometimes expansion of the vacuolated areas into cystlike spaces ("status spongiosus"). No inflammatory infiltrate is present. Electron microscopy shows the vacuoles to be membrane-bound and located within the cytoplasm of neuronal processes. **Kuru plaques** are extracellular deposits of aggregated abnormal protein; they are Congo red- and PAS-positive and usually occur in the cerebellum (Fig. 28–32B) although they are present in abundance in the cerebral cortex in cases of vCJD, surrounded by the spongiform changes (Fig. 28–32C). In all forms of prion disease immunohistochemical staining demonstrates the presence of proteinase K–resistant PrP^{sc} in tissue.

Fatal Familial Insomnia

Fatal familial insomnia (FFI), named in part for the sleep disturbances that characterize its initial stages, is also caused by a specific mutation in the *PRNP* gene. The mutation, which leads to an aspartate substitution for asparagine at residue 178 of PrP^c, results in FFI when it occurs in a *PRNP* allele encoding methionine at codon 129, but causes CJD when present in tandem with a valine at this position. How these amino acids influence disease phenotype is not understood. In the course of the illness, which typically lasts fewer than 3 years, affected individuals develop other neurologic signs, such as ataxia, autonomic disturbances, stupor, and finally coma. A noninherited form of the disorder (fatal sporadic insomnia) has also been described.

Morphology. Unlike other prion diseases, FFI does not show spongiform pathology. Instead, the most striking alteration is neuronal loss and reactive gliosis in the anterior ventral and dorsomedial nuclei of the thalamus; neuronal loss is also prominent in the inferior olivary nuclei. Proteinase K–resistant PrP^{sc} can be detected by immunostaining or western blotting.

Demyelinating Diseases

Demyelinating diseases of the CNS are acquired conditions characterized by preferential damage to myelin, with relative preservation of axons. The clinical deficits are due to the effect of myelin loss on the transmission of electrical impulses along axons. The natural history of demyelinating diseases is determined, in part, by the limited capacity of the CNS to

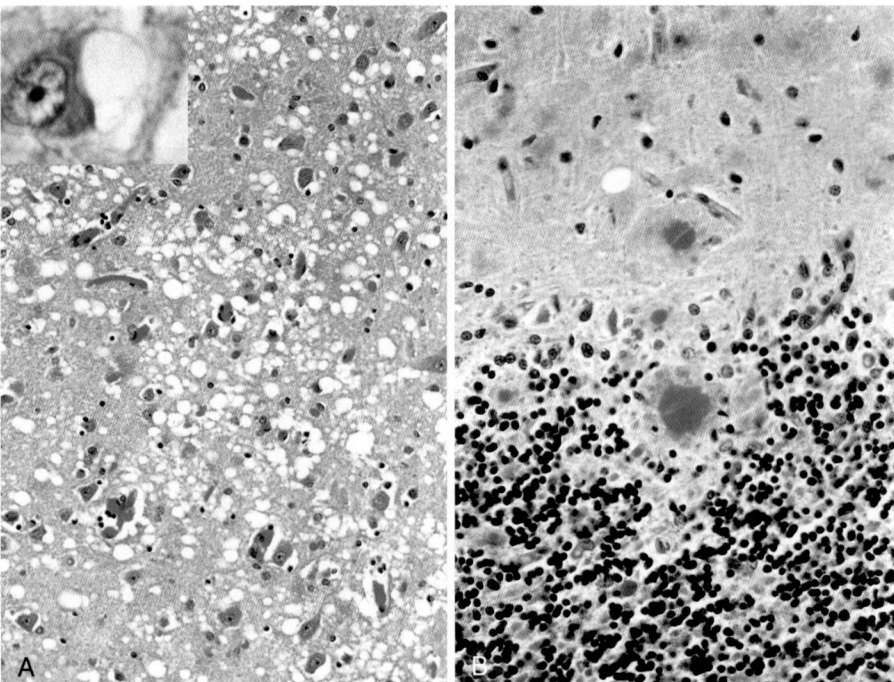

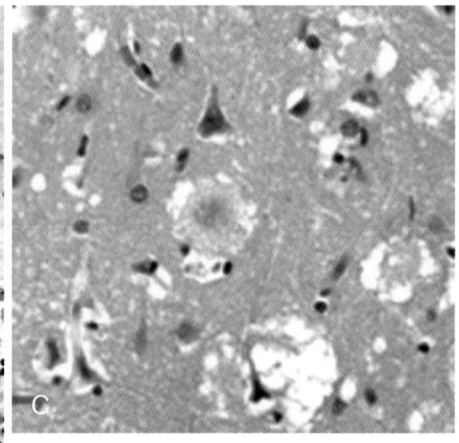

FIGURE 28–32 Prion disease. **A,** Spongiform change in the cerebral cortex. *Inset,* High magnification of neuron with vacuoles. **B,** Cerebellar cortex showing *kuru plaques* (PAS stain) representing aggregated PrPsc. **C,** Cortical plaques surrounded by spongiform change in vCJD.

regenerate normal myelin and by the degree of secondary damage to axons that occurs as the disease runs its course.

Several disease processes can cause loss of myelin. These include destruction of myelin by immunological reactions, as in multiple sclerosis, and by infections. In progressive multifocal leukoencephalopathy, JC virus infection of oligodendrocytes results in loss of myelin (described above). In addition, inherited disorders may affect synthesis or turnover of myelin components; these are termed *leukodystrophies* and are discussed with metabolic disorders.

MULTIPLE SCLEROSIS

Multiple sclerosis (MS) is an autoimmune demyelinating disorder characterized by distinct episodes of neurologic deficits, separated in time, attributable to white matter lesions that are separated in space. It is the most common of the demyelinating disorders, having a prevalence of approximately 1 per 1000 persons in most of the United States and Europe. The disease may become clinically apparent at any age, although onset in childhood or after age 50 years is relatively rare. Women are affected twice as often as are men. In most individuals with MS, the clinical course takes the form of relapsing and remitting episodes of variable duration (weeks to months to years) marked by neurologic defects, followed by gradual, partial recovery of neurologic function. The frequency of relapses tends to decrease during the course of time, but there is a steady neurologic deterioration in most affected individuals.

Pathogenesis. The lesions of MS are caused by an immune response that is directed against the components of the myelin sheath.[27,28] As in other autoimmune disorders, the pathogenesis of this disease involves both genetic and environmental factors (Chapter 6). The incidence of MS is 15-fold higher when the disease is present in a first-degree relative and

roughly 150-fold higher with an affected monozygotic twin. Genetic linkage of MS susceptibility to the DR2 extended haplotype of the major histocompatibility complex is also well established. A recent genome-wide screen supported this association and identified additional associations with single-nucleotide polymorphisms in IL-2 and IL-7 receptor genes.[29] The current thinking is that these cytokine receptor polymorphisms may influence the balance between pathogenic effector T cells and protective regulatory T cells. These genetic associations point to the importance of the immune system in the susceptibility to MS.

Given the prominence of chronic inflammatory cells within and around MS plaques as well as this genetic validation, immune mechanisms that underlie the destruction of myelin are the focus of much investigation. The available evidence indicates that the disease is *initiated by CD4+ T_H1 and T_H17 T cells that react against self myelin antigens and secrete cytokines.* T_H1 cells secrete IFNγ, which activates macrophages, and T_H17 cells promote the recruitment of leukocytes (Chapter 6). The demyelination is caused by these activated leukocytes and their injurious products. The infiltrate in plaques and surrounding regions of the brain consists of T cells (mainly CD4+, some CD8+) and macrophages. How the autoimmune reaction is initiated is not understood; a role of viral infection (e.g., EBV) in activating self-reactive T cells has been proposed but remains controversial.

Experimental autoimmune encephalomyelitis is an animal model of MS in which demyelination and inflammation occur after immunization of animals with myelin proteins.[30] Many of our concepts of MS pathogenesis have been derived from studies in this model. The experimental disorder can be passively transferred to other animals with T_H1 and T_H17 cells that recognize myelin antigens.

Based on the growing understanding of the pathogenesis of MS, therapies are being developed that modulate or inhibit T cell responses and block the recruitment of T cells into the brain. A potential contribution of humoral immunity has also been suspected for a long time, based on the early observation of oligoclonal bands of immunoglobulin in CSF.[31] The demonstration that B-cell depletion can decrease the incidence of demyelinating lesions lends support to this idea.[32]

Morphology. MS is a white matter disease that is best appreciated in sections of the brain and spinal cord. Lesions appear as multiple, well-circumscribed, somewhat depressed, glassy, gray-tan, irregularly shaped **plaques** (Fig. 28–33). In the fresh state these are firmer than the surrounding white matter **(sclerosis)**. Plaques can be found throughout the white matter and also extend into gray matter, since these have myelinated fibers running through them. The size of lesions varies considerably, from small foci that are only recognizable microscopically to confluent plaques that involve large portions of the centrum semiovale. The lesions often have sharply defined borders (Fig. 28–34). Plaques commonly occur adjacent to the lateral ventricles. They are also frequent in the optic nerves and chiasm, brainstem, ascending and descending fiber tracts, cerebellum, and spinal cord.

Microscopically, in an **active plaque** there is evidence of ongoing myelin breakdown with abundant

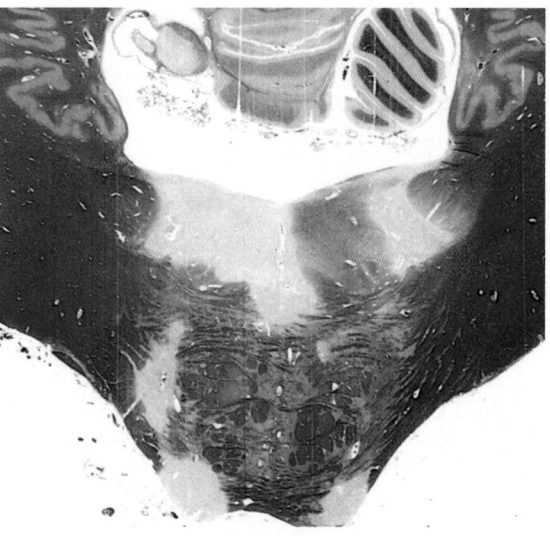

FIGURE 28–34 Multiple sclerosis (MS). Unstained regions of demyelination (MS plaques) around the fourth ventricle (Luxol fast blue PAS stain for myelin).

macrophages containing lipid-rich, PAS-positive debris. Inflammatory cells, including both lymphocytes and monocytes, are present, mostly as perivascular cuffs, especially at the outer edge of the lesion (Fig. 28–35A). Active lesions are often centered on small veins. Within a plaque there is relative preservation of axons (Fig. 28–35B) and depletion of oligodendrocytes. In time, astrocytes undergo reactive changes. As lesions become quiescent, the inflammatory cells slowly disappear. Within **inactive plaques**, little to no myelin is found, and there is a reduction in the number of oligodendrocyte nuclei; instead, astrocytic proliferation and gliosis are prominent. Axons in old gliotic plaques show severe depletion of myelin and are also greatly diminished in number.

Active plaques can also be grouped into four basic patterns: those that are sharply demarcated and centered on blood vessels, either with (pattern I) or without (pattern II) deposition of immunoglobulin and complement, and those that are less well demarcated and are not centered on vessels (patterns III and IV). These latter two are distinguished by the distribution of oligodendrocyte apoptosis (III, widespread; IV, central only). It has been observed that only one pair of patterns (I/II or III/IV) may be present in a given individual, suggesting that these may reflect distinct mechanisms rather than different stages of lesion.

In some MS plaques (**shadow plaques**) the border between normal and affected white matter is not sharply circumscribed. In this type of lesion some abnormally thinned-out myelin sheaths can be demonstrated, especially at the outer edges. This phenomenon is most commonly interpreted as evidence of partial and incomplete remyelination by surviving oligodendrocytes. Abnormally myelinated fibers have also been observed at the edges of typical plaques.

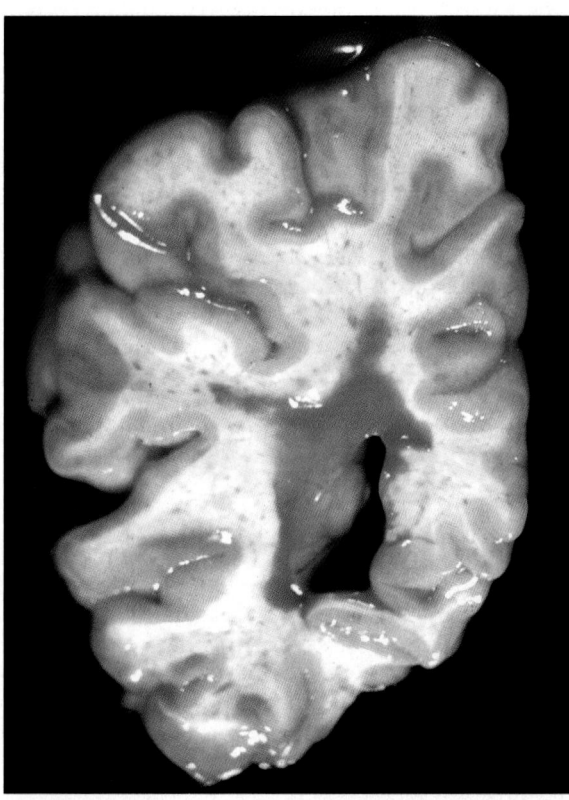

FIGURE 28–33 Multiple sclerosis. Section of fresh brain showing brown plaque around occipital horn of the lateral ventricle.

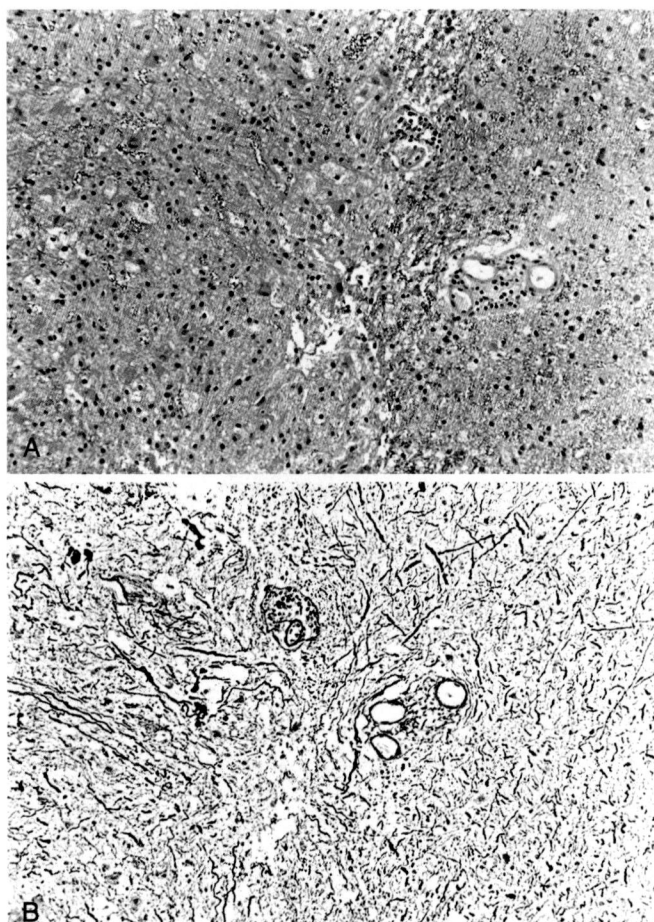

FIGURE 28–35 Multiple sclerosis. **A,** Myelin-stained section shows the sharp edge of a demyelinated plaque and perivascular lymphocytic cuffs. **B,** The same lesion stained for axons shows relative preservation.

Although these histologic findings suggest a limited potential for remyelination in the CNS, the remaining axons within most MS plaques remain unmyelinated; studies aimed at promoting remyelination are an important focus of research.[33]

Clinical Features. Although MS lesions can occur anywhere in the CNS and consequently may induce a wide range of clinical manifestations, certain patterns of neurologic symptoms and signs are commonly observed. Unilateral visual impairment, due to involvement of the optic nerve (*optic neuritis, retrobulbar neuritis*), is a frequent initial manifestation of MS. However, only some affected individuals (10% to 50%, depending on the population studied) with optic neuritis go on to develop MS. Involvement of the brainstem produces cranial nerve signs, ataxia, nystagmus, and internuclear ophthalmoplegia from interruption of the fibers of the medial longitudinal fasciculus. Spinal cord lesions give rise to motor and sensory impairment of trunk and limbs, spasticity, and difficulties with the voluntary control of bladder function. Examination of the CSF in individuals with MS shows a mildly elevated protein level, and in one third of cases,

there is moderate pleocytosis. IgG levels in the CSF are increased and oligoclonal IgG bands are usually observed on immunoelectrophoresis; these are indicative of the presence of a small number of activated B cell clones, postulated to be self-reactive, in the CNS. Radiologic studies using magnetic resonance imaging, typically based on identifying gadolinium-enhancing lesions, have taken on a prominent role in assessing disease progression; these studies, when correlated with autopsy studies as well as clinical findings, have indicated that some plaques may be clinically silent even in otherwise symptomatic patients.

NEUROMYELITIS OPTICA

The development of synchronous (or near synchronous) bilateral optic neuritis and spinal cord demyelination is referred to as *neuromyelitis optica* or *Devic disease.* White cells are common in the CSF, often including neutrophils. Within the damaged areas of white matter, there is typically necrosis, an inflammatory infiltrate including neutrophils, and vascular deposition of immunoglobulin and complement. These lesions have been suggested to be mediated by humoral immune mechanisms.[34] Many affected individuals show antibodies to aquaporins, which are in part responsible for maintenance of astrocytic foot process and thus the integrity of the blood-brain barrier.[35,36]

ACUTE DISSEMINATED ENCEPHALOMYELITIS AND ACUTE NECROTIZING HEMORRHAGIC ENCEPHALOMYELITIS

Acute disseminated encephalomyelitis (ADEM, perivenous encephalomyelitis) is a diffuse, monophasic demyelinating disease that follows either a viral infection or, rarely, a viral immunization. Symptoms typically develop a week or two after the antecedent infection and include headache, lethargy, and coma rather than focal findings, as seen in MS. The clinical course is rapid, and as many as 20% of those affected die; the remaining patients recover completely.

Acute necrotizing hemorrhagic encephalomyelitis (ANHE, acute hemorrhagic leukoencephalitis of Weston Hurst) is a fulminant syndrome of CNS demyelination, typically affecting young adults and children. The illness is almost invariably preceded by a recent episode of upper respiratory infection, most often of unknown cause. The disease is fatal in many patients, with significant deficits present in most survivors.

Morphology. In ADEM, macroscopic examination of the brain shows only grayish discoloration around white-matter vessels. On microscopic examination, myelin loss with relative preservation of axons can be found throughout the white matter. In the early stages, polymorphonuclear leukocytes can be found within the lesions; later, mononuclear infiltrates predominate. The breakdown of myelin is associated with the accumulation of lipid-laden macrophages. In contrast with MS, all lesions appear similar, consistent with the clinically monophasic nature of the disorder.

ANHE shows histologic similarities with ADEM, including a perivenular distribution of demyelination and widespread dissemination throughout the CNS (sometimes with extensive confluence of lesions). However, the lesions are much more severe than those of ADEM and include destruction of small blood vessels, disseminated necrosis of white and gray matter with acute hemorrhage, fibrin deposition, and abundant neutrophils. Scattered lymphocytes are seen in foci of demyelination.

The lesions of ADEM are similar to those induced by immunization of animals with myelin components or with early rabies vaccines that had been prepared from brains of infected animals. This has suggested that ADEM may represent an acute autoimmune reaction to myelin and that ANHE may represent a hyperacute variant, although no inciting antigens have been identified.

OTHER DISEASES WITH DEMYELINATION

Central pontine myelinolysis is characterized by loss of myelin (with relative preservation of axons and neuronal cell bodies) in a roughly symmetric pattern involving the basis pontis and portions of the pontine tegmentum but sparing the periventricular and subpial regions.[37] Lesions may be found more rostrally; it is extremely rare for the process to extend below the pontomedullary junction. Extra-pontine lesions occur in the supratentorial compartment, with similar appearance and apparent etiology. The condition is most commonly associated with rapid correction of hyponatremia, although it can be associated with other severe electrolyte or osmolar imbalance, as well as orthotopic liver transplantation. The clinical presentation of central pontine myelinolysis is that of a rapidly evolving quadriplegia; radiologic imaging studies localize the lesion to the basis pontis. Morphologically there is myelin loss without evidence of inflammation; neurons and axons are well preserved. Again, because of the monophasic nature of the disease all lesions appear to be at the same stage of myelin loss and reaction.

Degenerative Diseases

These are diseases of gray matter characterized by the progressive loss of neurons with associated secondary changes in white matter tracts. The pattern of neuronal loss is selective, affecting one or more groups of neurons while leaving others, sometimes immediately adjacent, intact. As genetic and molecular studies of these diseases have progressed certain shared features have emerged. A common theme among the neurodegenerative disorders is the *presence of protein aggregates that are resistant to degradation through the ubiquitin-proteasome system*. These aggregates are recognized histologically as inclusions, which often form the diagnostic hallmarks of these different diseases. The basis for aggregation varies across diseases. It may be directly related to an intrinsic feature of a mutated protein (e.g., expanded polyglutamine

repeats in Huntington disease), a feature of a peptide derived from a larger precursor protein (e.g., Aβ in Alzheimer disease), or an unexplained alteration of a normal cellular protein (e.g., α-synuclein in sporadic Parkinson disease).

Degenerative diseases differ in terms of the distribution of disease burden and in the specific neuropathologic findings (e.g., tangles, plaques, Lewy bodies). They can be grouped using two approaches:

- *Symptomatic/anatomic:* based on the anatomic regions of the CNS that are primarily affected, which is typically reflected in the clinical symptoms (e.g., neocortical involvement resulting in cognitive impairment and dementia)
- *Pathologic:* based on the types of inclusions or abnormal structures observed (e.g., diseases with inclusions containing tau or containing synuclein)

The discussion that follows is primarily based on the first approach (diseases of cortex, basal ganglia, etc.) with a few exceptions (all of the tau diseases and the synuclein diseases are considered together).

DEGENERATIVE DISEASES AFFECTING THE CEREBRAL CORTEX

The major cortical degenerative disease is Alzheimer disease, and its principal clinical manifestation is *dementia*, that is, progressive loss of cognitive function independent of the state of attention. There are many other causes of dementia, including the various forms of frontotemporal dementia, vascular disease, dementia with Lewy bodies (considered later in the context of Parkinson disease, the other Lewy body disorder), CJD, and neurosyphilis (both considered earlier). These diseases also involve subcortical structures, but many of the clinical symptoms are related to the changes in the cerebral cortex. Regardless of etiology, dementia is not part of normal aging and always represents a pathologic process.

Alzheimer Disease

Alzheimer disease (AD) is the most common cause of dementia in the elderly. The disease usually becomes clinically apparent as insidious impairment of higher intellectual function, with alterations in mood and behavior. Later, progressive disorientation, memory loss, and aphasia become manifest, indicating severe cortical dysfunction. Eventually, in 5 to 10 years, the affected individual becomes profoundly disabled, mute, and immobile. Patients rarely become symptomatic before 50 years of age, but the incidence of the disease rises with age, and the prevalence roughly doubles every 5 years, starting from a level of 1% for the 60- to 64-year-old population and reaching 40% or more for the 85- to 89-year-old cohort. This progressive increase in the incidence of the disease with age has given rise to major medical, social, and economic problems in countries with a growing number of elderly individuals. Most cases are sporadic, and although 5% to 10% are familial, the study of such familial cases has provided important insight into the pathogenesis of the more common sporadic form. While pathologic examination of brain tissue remains necessary for the definitive diagnosis of Alzheimer disease, the combination

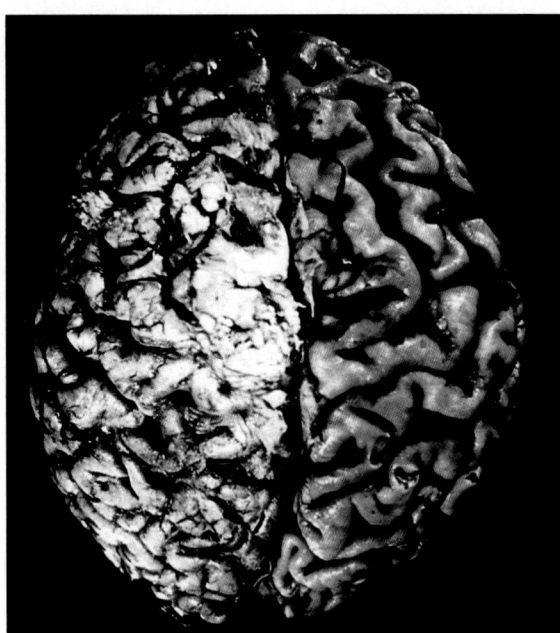

FIGURE 28–36 Alzheimer disease with cortical atrophy most evident on the right, where meninges have been removed. (Courtesy of the late Dr. E.P. Richardson, Jr., Massachusetts General Hospital, Boston, MA.)

of clinical assessment and modern radiologic methods allows accurate diagnosis in 80% to 90% of cases.

Morphology. Grossly, the brain shows a variable degree of **cortical atrophy** marked by widening of the cerebral sulci that is most pronounced in the frontal, temporal, and parietal lobes (Fig. 28–36). With significant atrophy, there is compensatory ventricular enlargement (hydrocephalus ex vacuo) secondary to loss of parenchyma and reduced brain volume. Structures of the medial temporal lobe, including hippocampus, entorhinal cortex and amygdala, are involved early in the course and are usually severely atrophied in the later stages. The major microscopic abnormalities of AD, which form the basis of the histologic diagnosis, are **neuritic (senile) plaques** and **neurofibrillary tangles**. There is progressive and eventually severe neuronal loss and reactive gliosis in the same regions that bear the burden of plaques and tangles.

Neuritic plaques are focal, spherical collections of dilated, tortuous, neuritic processes (dystrophic neurites) often around a central amyloid core, which may be surrounded by clear halo (Fig. 28–37A). Neuritic plaques range in size from 20 to 200 μm in diameter; microglial cells and reactive astrocytes are present at their periphery. Plaques are found in the hippocampus, amygdala, and neocortex, although there is usually relative sparing of primary motor and sensory cortices (this also applies to neurofibrillary tangles). The amyloid core, which can be stained by Congo Red, contains several abnormal proteins. The domi-

nant component of the amyloid plaque core is **Aβ**, a peptide derived through specific processing events from a larger molecule, amyloid precursor protein (APP) (Figs. 28–37 and 28–38). The two dominant species of Aβ, called $A\beta_{40}$ and $A\beta_{42}$, share an N-terminus and differ in length by two amino acids at the C-terminus. Other proteins are present in plaques in lesser abundance, including components of the complement cascade, pro-inflammatory cytokines, α_1-antichymotrypsin, and apolipoproteins. In some cases, there is deposition of Aβ peptides with staining characteristics of amyloid in the absence of the surrounding neuritic reaction. These lesions, termed **diffuse plaques**, are found in superficial portions of cerebral cortex as well as in basal ganglia and cerebellar cortex. Diffuse plaques appear to represent an early stage of plaque development. This conclusion is based primarily on studies of brains from individuals with trisomy 21. Recall that in patients with trisomy 21 (Down syndrome), early onset of Alzheimer disease is common (Chapter 5). In some brain regions (cerebellar cortex and striatum) these diffuse plaques represent a major manifestation of the disease, with other clear-cut findings of Alzheimer disease, or in isolation. While neuritic plaques contain both $A\beta_{40}$ and $A\beta_{42}$, diffuse plaques are predominantly made up of $A\beta_{42}$.

Neurofibrillary tangles are bundles of filaments in the cytoplasm of the neurons that displace or encircle the nucleus. In pyramidal neurons, they often have an elongated "flame" shape; in rounder cells, the basket weave of fibers around the nucleus takes on a rounded contour ("globose" tangles). Neurofibrillary tangles are visible as basophilic fibrillary structures with H&E staining (Fig. 28–37C) but are dramatically demonstrated by silver (Bielschowsky) staining (Fig. 28–37D). They are commonly found in cortical neurons, especially in the entorhinal cortex, as well as in other sites such as pyramidal cells of the hippocampus, the amygdala, the basal forebrain, and the raphe nuclei. Neurofibrillary tangles are insoluble and apparently resistant to clearance in vivo, thus remaining visible in tissue sections as "ghost" or "tombstone" tangles long after the death of the parent neuron. Ultrastructurally, neurofibrillary tangles are composed predominantly of paired helical filaments along with some straight filaments that appear to have a comparable composition. A major component of paired helical filaments is abnormally hyperphosphorylated forms of the protein **tau**, an axonal microtubule-associated protein that enhances microtubule assembly (Fig. 28–37E). Other components include MAP2 (another microtubule-associated protein) and ubiquitin. Paired helical filaments are also found in the dystrophic neurites that form the outer portions of neuritic plaques and in axons coursing through the affected gray matter as **neuropil threads**. Tangles are not specific to AD, being found in other diseases as well.

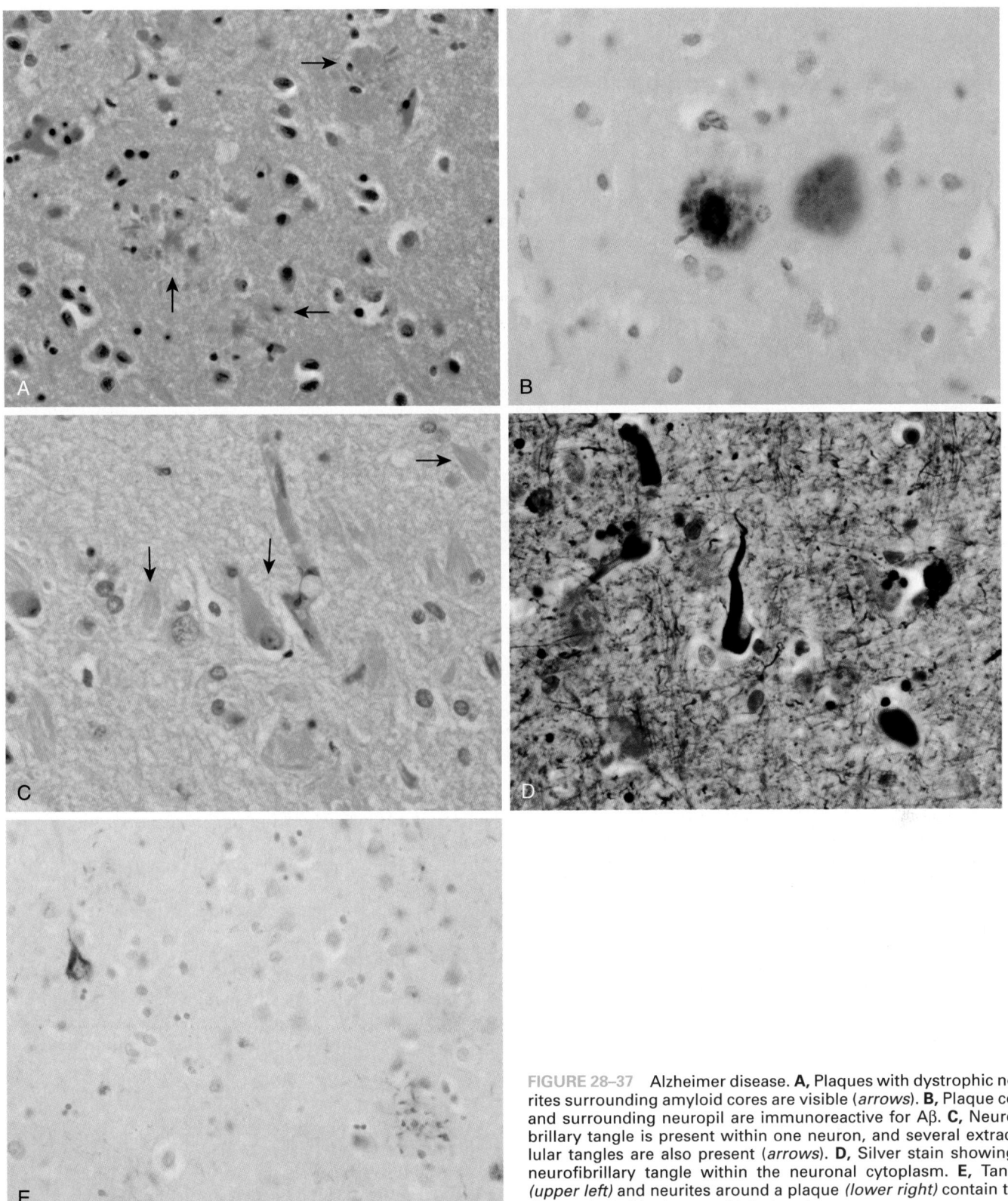

FIGURE 28–37   Alzheimer disease. **A,** Plaques with dystrophic neurites surrounding amyloid cores are visible (*arrows*). **B,** Plaque core and surrounding neuropil are immunoreactive for Aβ. **C,** Neurofibrillary tangle is present within one neuron, and several extracellular tangles are also present (*arrows*). **D,** Silver stain showing a neurofibrillary tangle within the neuronal cytoplasm. **E,** Tangle *(upper left)* and neurites around a plaque *(lower right)* contain tau, demonstrated by immunohistochemistry.

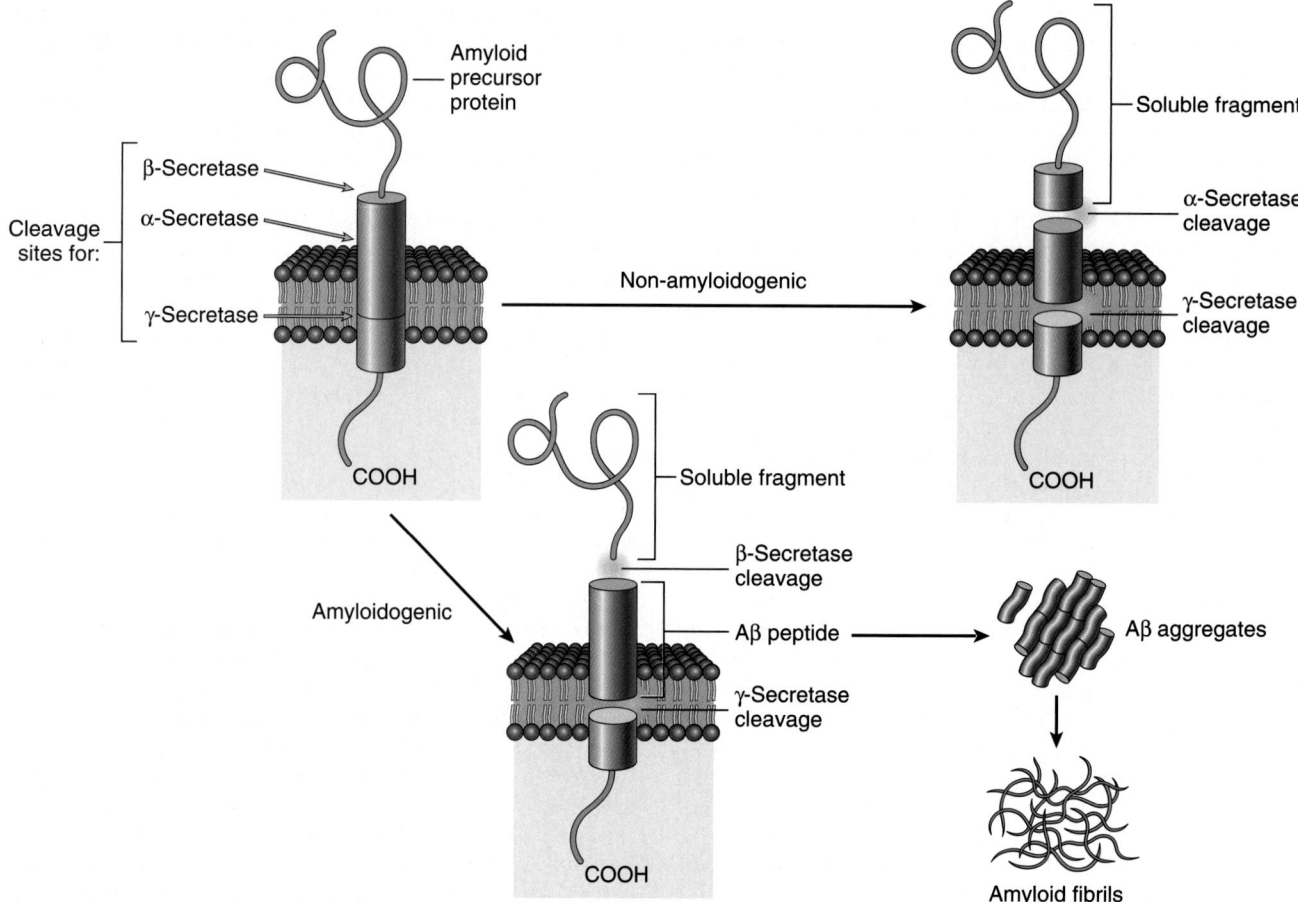

FIGURE 28–38 Mechanisms of processing of amyloid precursor protein (APP). APP can be processed by two pathways; sequential cleavage by β-secretase and γ-secretase is the pathway that results in the generation of Aβ and the formation of amyloid fibrils.

In addition to the diagnostic features of plaques and tangles, several other pathologic findings are seen in the setting of AD. **Cerebral amyloid angiopathy (CAA)** is an almost invariable accompaniment of Alzheimer disease; however, it can also be found in brains of individuals without AD (see Fig. 28–18B). Vascular amyloid is predominantly $A\beta_{40}$, as is also the case when CAA occurs without AD. **Granulovacuolar degeneration** is the formation of small (~5 µm in diameter), clear intraneuronal cytoplasmic vacuoles, each of which contains an argyrophilic granule. While it occurs with normal aging, it is most commonly found in great abundance in hippocampus and olfactory bulb in AD. **Hirano bodies**, found especially in AD, are elongated, glassy, eosinophilic bodies consisting of paracrystalline arrays of beaded filaments, with actin as their major component. They are found most commonly within hippocampal pyramidal cells.

Since both plaques and tangles may be present in low abundance in nondemented individuals, the diagnosis of Alzheimer disease is based on a combination of clinical and pathologic features. The progression of changes is fairly constant. Pathologic changes (specifically plaques, tangles, and the associated neuronal loss and glial reaction) are evident earliest in the entorhinal cortex, then spread through the hippocampal formation and isocortex, and then extend into the neocortex. Plaques are assessed semiquantitatively (absent, sparse, moderate, abundant) in each cortical area, while tangles are assessed based on how widespread they are in the brain.[38,39] These assessments are combined in the current NIA-Reagan criteria to provide an estimate of the likelihood that AD pathology caused a particular patient's dementia.[40,41]

Molecular Genetics and Pathogenesis. *The fundamental abnormality in AD is the deposition of Aβ peptides*, which are derived through processing of APP (Fig. 28–38). APP is a cell surface protein with a single transmembrane domain that may function as a receptor, although ligands have remained elusive. The Aβ portion of the protein extends from the extracellular region into the transmembrane domain. Processing of APP begins with cleavage in the extracellular domain, followed by an intramembranous cleavage. There are two potential pathways, determined by the type of initial proteolytic event. If the first cut occurs at the α-secretase site within the

Aβ sequence, then Aβ is not generated (the non-amyloidogenic pathway). This mostly occurs at the cell surface, since the various enzymes with α-secretase activity are involved in the shedding of surface proteins. Surface APP can also be endocytosed and may undergo cleavage by β-secretase, which cuts at the N-terminal region of the Aβ sequence (the amyloidogenic pathway). Following cleavage of APP at either of these sites, the γ-secretase complex performs an intramembranous cleavage. When paired with a first cut by α-secretase, it will produce a soluble fragment, but when paired with β-secretase cleavage, it generates Aβ. The variation in peptide length (Aβ$_{40}$ vs Aβ$_{42}$) arises from alterations in the exact location of the γ-secretase cleavage. The γ-secretase complex—containing presenilin, nicastrin, pen-2, and aph-1—is also responsible for processing of Notch, a cell fate-determining molecule, as well as many other membrane proteins.[42] Once generated, Aβ is highly prone to aggregation—first into small oligomers (which may be the toxic form responsible for neuronal dysfunction), and eventually into large aggregates and fibrils.

Familial forms of AD have provided support for the central role of Aβ generation as a critical step for at least initiation of AD pathogenesis. The gene encoding APP, on chromosome 21, lies in the Down syndrome region; AD pathology is an eventual feature of the cognitive impairment of these individuals. Histologic findings appear in the second and third decades followed by neurologic decline about 20 years later. A similar gene dosage effect is produced by localized chromosome 21 duplications that span the APP locus in some patients with familial AD.[44] Point mutations in APP are another cause of familial AD. Some mutations lie near the β-secretase and γ-secretase cleavage sites, and others sit in the Aβ sequence and increase its propensity to aggregate. The two loci identified as causes of the majority of early-onset familial AD encode the two presenilins (PS1 on chromosome 14 and PS2 on chromosome 1). These mutations lead to a gain of function, such that the γ-secretase complex generates increased amounts of Aβ, particularly Aβ$_{42}$. Thus, the genetic evidence strongly supports the notion that the underlying pathogenetic event in AD is the accumulation of Aβ.

The Aβ peptides readily aggregate, and can be directly neurotoxic. There are various lines of evidence indicating that the small aggregates of Aβ can result in synaptic dysfunction, such as blocking of long-term potentiation and changes in other membrane properties.[4] While aggregates are difficult to degrade, monomeric Aβ can be degraded by a variety of proteases. Both small aggregates and larger deposits elicit an *inflammatory response* from microglia and astrocytes. This response probably assists in the clearance of the aggregated peptide, but may also stimulate the secretion of mediators that cause damage.[43] Additional consequences of the activation of these inflammatory cascades may include alterations in tau phophosrylation, along with oxidative injury to the neurons.

The genetic locus on chromosome 19 that encodes apolipoprotein E (ApoE) has a strong influence on the risk of developing AD. Three alleles exist (ε2, ε3, and ε4) based on two amino acid polymorphisms. The dosage of the ε4 allele increases the risk of AD and lowers the age of onset of the disease, such that individuals with the ε4 allele are over-represented in populations of patients with AD. This ApoE isoform promotes Aβ generation and deposition, although the mechanisms have not been established. Overall, this locus has been estimated to convey about a quarter of the risk for development of sporadic AD. It is likely that other risk factor alleles will have much smaller population effects.[45] The newly evolving approach of genome-wide association screening may help locate these loci with weaker effects.[46]

Because neurofibrillary tangles contain the tau protein, there has been much interest in the role of this protein in AD. Tau is a microtubule-associated protein present in axons in association with the microtubular network. With the development of tangles in AD, it shifts to a somatic-dendritic distribution, becomes hyperphosphorylated, and loses the ability to bind to microtubules. It is, however, thought that the primary abnormality in AD is in Aβ and not in tau, because mutations affecting Aβ lead to the formation of tangles and AD but mutations in the gene encoding tau, *MAPT*, cause one of the frontotemporal demential (see below) but neither Aβ deposition nor AD. The mechanism of tangle injury to neurons remains poorly understood.

While there remains disagreement regarding the best correlate of dementia in individuals with AD, it is clear that the presence of a large burden of plaques and tangles is highly associated with severe cognitive dysfunction. The number of neurofibrillary tangles correlates better with the degree of dementia than does the number of neuritic plaques. Biochemical markers that have been correlated with the degree of dementia include loss of choline acetyltransferase, synaptophysin immunoreactivity, and amyloid burden.

Clinical Features. The progression of AD is slow but relentless, with a symptomatic course often running more than 10 years. Initial symptoms are forgetfulness and other memory disturbances; with progression of the disease other symptoms emerge, including language deficits, loss of mathematical skills, and loss of learned motor skills. In the final stages of AD, affected individuals may become incontinent, mute, and unable to walk. Intercurrent disease, often pneumonia, is usually the terminal event in these individuals. Discovery of biomarkers for AD is an area of continuing interest; the amyloid-binding positron emission tomography imaging agent PiB is beginning to be used for this purpose.[47,48]

Frontotemporal Dementias

Frontotemporal dementias (FTDs) are a group of disorders that were first classified together because they shared clinical features (progressive deterioration of language and changes in personality) corresponding to degeneration and atrophy of temporal and frontal lobes.[49] These entities have recently been better understood through a combination of immunohistochemical and biochemical, and genetic approaches. Several of the disorders to be considered share the accumulation of tau-containing deposits as their characteristic finding, giving rise to the term *tauopathy*.

Frontotemporal Dementia with Parkinsonism Linked to Tau Mutations

This is a genetically determined disorder in which the clinical syndrome of a FTD is often accompanied by parkinsonian symptoms.

Pathogenesis and Molecular Genetics. The study of families with FTD led to the recognition that in some, but not all, pedigrees there are mutations in the *MAPT* gene encoding tau. The mutations fall into several broad categories: coding-region mutations and intronic mutations. The tau protein has six splice forms. When exon 10 is present, the protein contains four microtubule-binding domains (called 4R), and in its absence there are three such domains (3R). Some of the intronic mutations influence the inclusion of this exon and thus determine the form of the protein that is produced. The ratio of the 4R to 3R form varies in different diseases but the basis of this effect is unknown and both forms can produce tangles. Coding-region mutations seem to have several different consequences, including alterations in the interaction of tau with microtubules and in the intrinsic tendency of tau to aggregate.

> **Morphology.** There is evidence of atrophy of frontal and temporal lobes in various combinations and to various degrees. The pattern of atrophy can often be predicted in part by the clinical symptomatology. The atrophic regions of cortex are marked by neuronal loss, gliosis, and the presence of tau-containing neurofibrillary tangles. These tangles may contain either 4R tau or a mixture of 3R and 4R tau. Nigral degeneration may also occur. Inclusions can also be found in glial cells in some forms of the disease.

Pick Disease

Pick disease (lobar atrophy) is a rare, distinct, progressive dementia characterized clinically by early onset of behavioral changes together with alterations in personality (frontal lobe signs) and language disturbances (temporal lobe signs). While most cases of Pick disease are sporadic, there have been some familial forms identified and linked to mutated tau protein.

> **Morphology.** The brain invariably shows a pronounced, frequently asymmetric, atrophy of the frontal and temporal lobes with conspicuous sparing of the posterior two thirds of the superior temporal gyrus and only rare involvement of either the parietal or occipital lobe. The atrophy can be severe, reducing the gyri to a wafer-thin ("knife-edge") appearance. This pattern of **lobar atrophy** is often prominent enough to distinguish Pick disease from AD on gross examination. In addition to the localized cortical atrophy there may also be bilateral atrophy of the caudate nucleus and putamen.
>
> Microscopically, neuronal loss is most severe in the outer three layers of the cortex. Some of the surviving neurons show a characteristic swelling **(Pick cells)**, while others contain **Pick bodies**, which are cytoplasmic, round to oval, filamentous inclusions that are only weakly basophilic but stain strongly with silver methods (Fig. 28–39). Ultrastructurally, these are composed of straight filaments, vesiculated endoplasmic reticulum, and paired helical filaments that are immunocytochemically similar to those found in

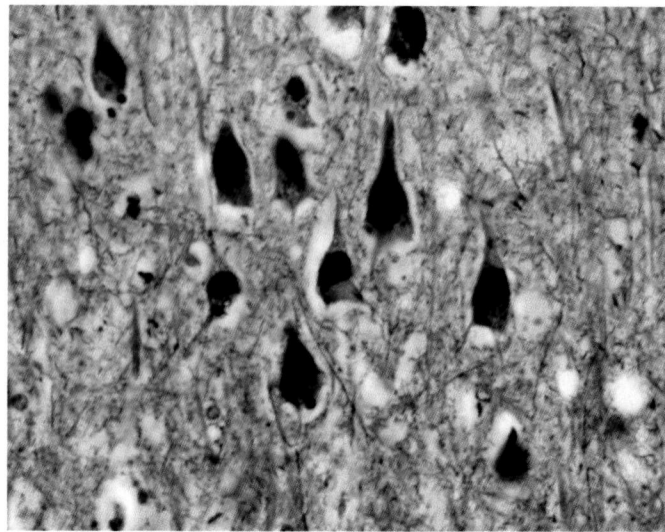

FIGURE 28–39 Pick disease. Pick bodies are round homogeneous neuronal cytoplasmic inclusions that stain intensely with silver stains.

> AD, and contain 3R tau. Unlike the neurofibrillary tangles of AD, Pick bodies do not survive the death of their host neuron and do not remain as markers of the disease.

Progressive Supranuclear Palsy

Progressive supranuclear palsy is an illness characterized clinically by truncal rigidity with dysequilibrium and nuchal dystonia; pseudobulbar palsy and abnormal speech; ocular disturbances, including vertical gaze palsy progressing to difficulty with all eye movements; and mild progressive dementia in most affected individuals. The onset of the disease is usually between the fifth and seventh decades, and males are affected approximately twice as frequently as are females. The disease is often fatal within 5 to 7 years of onset.

> **Morphology.** There is widespread neuronal loss in the globus pallidus, subthalamic nucleus, substantia nigra, colliculi, periaqueductal gray matter, and dentate nucleus of the cerebellum. Globose neurofibrillary tangles are found in these affected regions, in neurons as well as in glia. Ultrastructural analysis reveals 15-nm straight filaments that are composed of 4R tau.

Mutations in the *MAPT* gene have not been found in progressive supranuclear palsy. However, *MAPT* contains a series of polymorphisms in linkage dysequilibrium that fall into two haplotypes, one of which is highly over-represented in individuals with progressive supranuclear palsy. How this haplotype influences the risk of the disease is unknown.

Corticobasal Degeneration

This is a disease of the elderly, with considerable clinical and neuropathologic heterogeneity. Because of the extrapyramidal signs and symptoms in this disorder, it can also be grouped with syndromes of basal ganglia dysfunction.

Morphology. On macroscopic examination there is cortical atrophy, mainly of the motor, premotor, and anterior parietal lobes. These regions of cortex show severe loss of neurons, gliosis, and **"ballooned" neurons** (neuronal achromasia) that can be highlighted with immunocytochemical methods for phosphorylated neurofilaments. Tau immunoreactivity has been found in astrocytes ("tufted astrocytes"), oligodendrocytes ("coiled bodies"), basal ganglionic neurons, and, variably, cortical neurons. Clusters of tau-positive processes around an astrocyte ("astrocytic plaques") and the presence of tau-positive threads in gray and white matter may be the most specific pathologic findings of corticobasal degeneration. The substantia nigra and locus ceruleus show loss of pigmented neurons, neuronal achromasia, and tangles. Similar to progressive supranuclear palsy, the tau deposits in corticobasal degeneration contain predominantly 4R tau.

Clinical Features. The disease is characterized by extrapyramidal rigidity, asymmetric motor disturbances (jerking movements of limbs), and sensory cortical dysfunction (apraxias, disorders of language); cognitive decline occurs, and may be prominent in some cases. The same *MAPT* haplotype linked to progressive supranuclear palsy is also highly associated with corticobasal degeneration.

Frontotemporal Dementias without Tau Pathology

Some cases with clinical and pathologic findings involving the frontal and temporal lobes lack tau deposition; instead, usually tau-negative, ubiquitin-containing inclusions are found in superficial cortical layers in temporal and frontal lobes and in the dentate gyrus (giving rise to the term *FTD-U* for ubiquitin). Some of these cases are familial and show linkage to chromosome 17 but are caused by mutations in the gene for progranulin (an inflammatory modulator protein), which is close to the *MAPT* locus.[50] Similar pathology is seen accompanying the cognitive impairment that sometimes occurs with amyotrophic lateral sclerosis.[51]

Vascular Dementia

While some individuals with cognitive decline due to vasculitis show improvement with treatment, there is also an irreversible and progressive cognitive disorder associated with vascular injury to the brain.[52] Various etiologies include widespread areas of infarction (abundant cortical microinfarcts, multiple lacunar infarcts, cortical laminar necrosis associated with reduced perfusion/oxygenation), and diffuse white-matter injury (hypertension, cerebral autosomal dominant arteriopathy with subcortical infarcts and leukoencephalopathy). Additionally, dementia has been associated with so-called strategic infarcts, which are usually embolic and involve brain regions such as the hippocampus, dorsomedial thalamus, or the cin-

gulate gyrus of the frontal cortex. Many individuals, in fact, demonstrate a combination of pathologic changes. There is also a relationship between vascular injury and other dementing disorders, such as AD. It has been found that individuals with vascular changes above a certain threshold have a lower burden of plaques and tangles for their level of cognitive impairment than do those without vascular-based cerebral pathology.

DEGENERATIVE DISEASES OF BASAL GANGLIA AND BRAINSTEM

Diseases affecting these regions of the brain are frequently associated with movement disorders, including rigidity, abnormal posturing, and chorea. In general, they can be categorized as manifesting either a reduction of voluntary movement or an abundance of involuntary movement. The basal ganglia, especially the nigrostriatal pathway, play an important role in the system of positive and negative regulatory synaptic pathways that serve to modulate feedback from the thalamus to the motor cortex. The most important disorders in this group are those associated with parkinsonism and Huntington disease.

Parkinsonism

Parkinsonism is a clinical syndrome characterized by diminished facial expression, stooped posture, slowness of voluntary movement, festinating gait (progressively shortened, accelerated steps), rigidity, and a "pill-rolling" tremor. This type of motor disturbance is seen in a number of conditions that have in common damage to the nigrostriatal dopaminergic system. Parkinsonism may also be induced by drugs that affect this system, particularly dopamine antagonists and toxins. The principal diseases that involve the nigrostriatal system are as follows:

- Parkinson disease (PD)
- Multiple system atrophy, commonly associated with parkinsonism as well as other symptoms
- Postencephalitic parkinsonism, which was observed as a late consequence of the influenza pandemic of 1918
- Progressive supranuclear palsy and corticobasal degeneration, movement disorders that may also show cognitive impairment (discussed above with the FTDs)

Parkinson Disease

This diagnosis is made in individuals with progressive L-DOPA-responsive signs of parkinsonism (tremor, rigidity, and bradykinesia) in the absence of a toxic or other known underlying etiology. Familial forms of PD with autosomal dominant or autosomal recessive inheritance exist. Although these make up a limited number of cases, they have contributed to our understanding of the pathogenesis of the disease.

Morphology. The typical macroscopic findings are **pallor of the substantia nigra** (compare Fig. 28–40A and B) and locus ceruleus. On microscopic examination, there is loss of the pigmented, catecholaminergic neurons in these regions, associated with gliosis.

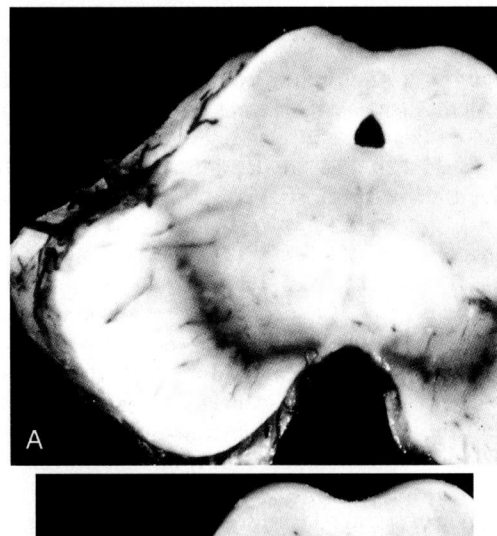

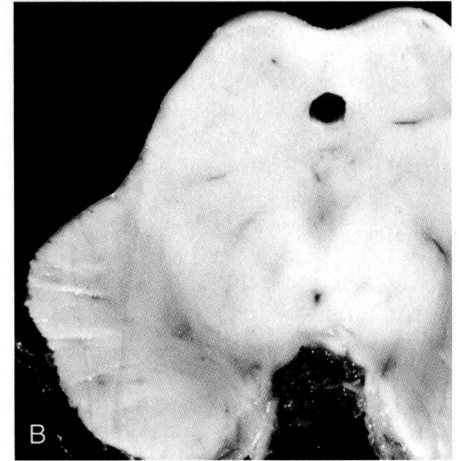

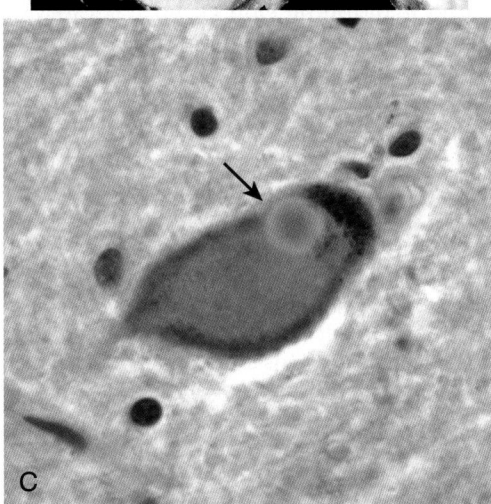

FIGURE 28–40 Parkinson disease. **A,** Normal substantia nigra. **B,** Depigmented substantia nigra in idiopathic Parkinson disease. **C,** Lewy body in a substantia nigra neuron, staining bright pink *(arrow).*

Lewy bodies (Fig. 28–40C) may be found in some of the remaining neurons. These are single or multiple, cytoplasmic, eosinophilic, round to elongated inclusions that often have a dense core surrounded by a pale halo. Ultrastructurally, Lewy bodies are com-

posed of fine filaments, densely packed in the core but loose at the rim; these filaments are composed of **α-synuclein**. Lewy bodies may also be found in the cholinergic cells of the basal nucleus of Meynert, which is depleted of neurons (particularly in patients with abnormal mental function), as well as in other brainstem nuclei including the locus ceruleus and the dorsal motor nucleus of the vagus.

Molecular Genetics. More than a dozen genetic loci for PD have been identified through linkage studies. The five genes currently known to be clearly associated with the disease point to a complex set of possible disease mechanisms.[53,54] The first gene to be identified as a cause of autosomal dominant PD encodes *α-synuclein*, an abundant lipid-binding protein normally associated with synapses that is also a major component of the Lewy body. Mutations in α-synuclein are rare; they take the form of point mutations and amplifications of the region of chromosome 4q21 that contains the gene. The occurrence of disease caused by changes in gene copy number implies a gene dosage effect, similar to what has been observed with APP in AD, and suggests that polymorphisms in the α-synuclein promoter that alter its expression may influence the risk of PD. Mutations in the gene encoding LRRK2 (leucine-rich repeat kinase 2) are a more common cause of autosomal dominant PD and are found in some sporadic cases of the disease. Several of these pathogenic mutations increase the kinase activity of LRRK2, suggesting that gains in LRRK2 function contribute to the development of PD.

A juvenile autosomal recessive form of PD is caused by loss of function mutations in the gene encoding *parkin*, an E3 ubiquitin ligase with a wide range of substrates. The pathology of parkin-linked PD is similar to that of α-synuclein–linked or sporadic PD except that Lewy bodies are absent in most cases. Other cases of autosomal recessive PD are the result of mutations in the gene encoding DJ-1, a protein involved in regulating redox responses to stress; or the gene encoding the kinase PINK1, which appears to regulate normal mitochondrial function.

Pathogenesis. No unifying pathogenic mechanism has emerged yet from these diverse genetic and biochemical clues, and many possibilities have been suggested, including a misfolded protein/stress response triggered by α-synuclein aggregation; defective proteosomal function due to the loss of the E3 ubiquitin ligase parkin; and altered mitochondrial function caused by the loss of DJ-1 and PINK1. Intriguingly, other lines of evidence also point to a role for mitochondrial dysfunction; for example, levels of mitochondrial complex I, a component of the oxidative phosphorylation cascade, are reduced in the brains of patients with sporadic PD, and some models of experimental PD are produced by the administration of mitochondrial inhibitors.

The dopaminergic neurons of the substantia nigra project to the striatum, and their degeneration in PD is associated with a reduction in the striatal dopamine content. The severity of the motor syndrome is proportional to the dopamine deficiency, which can, at least in part, be corrected by replacement therapy with L-DOPA (the immediate precursor of dopamine). Treatment does not, however, reverse the morphologic changes or arrest the progress of the disease; moreover, with progression, drug therapy tends to become less effective and symptoms become more difficult to manage. An acute parkinsonian syndrome and destruction of neurons in the substantia nigra follows exposure to MPTP (1-methyl-4-phenyl-1,2,3,6-tetrahydropyridine), discovered as a contaminant in the illicit synthesis of psychoactive meperidine analogues. The use of this toxin in experimental animals has proved highly useful in studies of therapeutic interventions for PD, including transplantation. Epidemiologic evidence has also suggested pesticide exposure as a risk factor for PD, while caffeine and nicotine may be protective.

Clinical Features. In addition to the signs of parkinsonism, autonomic dysfunction is common, as is some impairment of cognitive function. Parkinson disease is sometimes accompanied by a dementia, either early in the course of the illness or as a late additional morbidity. While L-DOPA therapy is often extremely effective in symptomatic treatment, it does not significantly alter the intrinsically progressive nature of the disease. Over time, L-DOPA becomes less able to help the patient through symptomatic relief and begins to lead to fluctuations in motor function on its own. Given the well-characterized biochemical defect in PD, it has been the focus of early therapeutic trials for neural transplantation and gene therapy.[55] Other current neurosurgical approaches to this disease include the strategic placement of lesions elsewhere in the extrapyramidal system to compensate for the loss of nigrostriatal function and placement of stimulating electrodes (deep brain stimulation).[56]

Dementia with Lewy Bodies

About 10% to 15% of individuals with PD develop dementia, with increasing incidence with advancing age. Characteristic features of this disorder include a fluctuating course, hallucinations, and prominent frontal signs. While some affected individuals have pathologic evidence of AD (or, less frequently, other degenerative diseases associated with cognitive changes) in combination with the findings of PD, in others the most prominent histologic correlate appears to be the presence of Lewy bodies in a wide range of cortical locations.[57,58] These inclusions are less distinct than those observed in the brainstem but similarly contain predominantly α-synuclein. Immunohistochemical staining for α-synuclein also reveals the presence of abnormal neurites, which contain aggregated protein—called *Lewy neurites* even though he never saw them! In this setting, the gross pathologic findings typically include depigmentation of the substantia nigra and locus ceruleus, paired with relative preservation of the cortex, hippocampus, and amygdala. The burden of cortical Lewy bodies is usually extremely low, and the mechanism by which this disease wreaks havoc on cognitive functioning is not clear. It has been suggested that Lewy body diseases represent a continuum; there is evidence that Lewy bodies and Lewy neurites are found first in the medulla, progress over time to reach the midbrain (when it becomes manifest as PD), and can eventually progress across the nervous system to reach the cortex (and manifest as dementia with Lewy bodies).[59]

Multiple System Atrophy

The designation multiple system atrophy (*MSA*) describes a group of disorders characterized by the presence of glial cytoplasmic inclusions, typically within the cytoplasm of oligodendrocytes, that can have different patterns of clinical presentation.[60] The dominant symptoms can be parkinsonism (MSA-P, historically known as striatonigral degeneration), or cerebellar dysfunction (MSA-C, previously known as olivopontocerebellar atrophy), or autonomic dysfunction (MSA-A, once known as Shy-Drager syndrome). Of these, MSA-C is the least frequently observed pure syndrome. These variants appear to stem from a single disease mechanism, and many affected individuals develop symptoms during the course of the illness that fall into more than one clinical pattern.

> **Morphology.** The gross pathology matches the clinical presentation. In cerebellar forms there is typically atrophy of the cerebellum, including the cerebellar peduncles, pons (especially the basis pontis), and medulla (especially the inferior olive), while in parkinsonian forms the atrophy involves both the substantia nigra and striatum (especially putamen). Since autonomic symptoms are related to cell loss from the catecholaminergic nuclei of the medulla and the intermediolateral cell column of the spinal cord, there are usually no specific gross findings. Atrophic brain regions show evidence of neuronal loss as well as variable numbers of neuronal cytoplasmic and nuclear inclusions.
>
> The diagnostic glial cytoplasmic inclusions were originally demonstrated in oligodendrocytes with silver impregnation methods and contain α-synuclein as well as ubiquitin and αB-crystallin. The inclusions are ultrastructurally distinct from those found in other neurodegenerative diseases and are composed primarily of 20- to 40-nm tubules. Similar inclusions may also be found in the cytoplasm of neurons, sometimes in neuronal and glial nuclei, and in axons.

Pathogenesis. As in PD, α-synuclein is the major component of the inclusions, but unlike PD, no mutations in the gene encoding this protein have been found in patients with MSA. Furthermore, unlike in PD, α-synuclein–containing inclusions are found in glial cells, notably oligodendrocytes. The relationship between glial cytoplasmic inclusions and disease is supported by the observation that the inclusions are present in low numbers at earliest stages of MSA and increase in abundance as the disease progresses, although they eventually disappear as cells die in the final stages. It appears that glial cytoplasmic inclusions can occur in the absence of neuronal loss, suggesting that they may represent a primary pathologic event; for example, glial cytoplasmic inclusions are consistently observed in the white matter projecting to and from the motor cortex. The origin of the α-synuclein in oligodendrocytes remains perplexing, since this is a neuronal protein associated with synaptic vesicles. Several studies have shown that there is no up-regulation of α-synuclein expression in white matter or in oligodendrocytes in MSA, suggesting that the protein may be acquired secondarily by oligodendrocytes from injured or dying neurons. It may be that the less conspicuous neuronal inclusions of α-synuclein, which are also present in MSA, are more closely linked to the disease process.[61]

Huntington Disease

Huntington disease (HD) is an autosomal dominant disease *characterized clinically by progressive movement disorders and dementia, and histologically by degeneration of striatal neurons.* Jerky, hyperkinetic, sometimes dystonic movements involving all parts of the body (chorea) are characteristic; affected individuals may later develop parkinsonism with bradykinesia and rigidity. The disease is relentlessly progressive, with an average course of about 15 years to death.

Molecular Genetics. Huntington disease is the prototype of the polyglutamine trinucleotide repeat expansion diseases (see Chapter 5).[62,63] The *HD* gene, located on chromosome 4p16.3, encodes a 348-kD protein known as *huntingtin*. In the first exon of the gene there is a stretch of CAG repeats, which encodes a polyglutamine region near the N terminus of the protein. Normal *HD* genes contain 6 to 35 copies of the repeat; when the number of repeats is increased beyond this level it is associated with disease. There is an inverse relationship between repeat number and age of onset, such that longer repeats are associated with earlier onset. Because other factors modify the effect of the repeats, determination of repeat length is not an accurate predictor of age of onset. Repeat expansions occur during spermatogenesis, so that paternal transmission is associated with early onset in the next generation, the phenomenon of anticipation. Newly occurring mutations are uncommon; most apparently sporadic cases can be related to non-paternity, the death of a parent before expression of the disease, or a father as yet unaffected but with a mild repeat expansion that further enlarged during spermatogenesis.

Morphology. Macroscopically, the brain is small and shows striking **atrophy of the caudate nucleus** and, less markedly at early stages, the putamen (Fig. 28–41). The globus pallidus may be atrophied secondarily, and the lateral and third ventricles are dilated. Atrophy is frequently also seen in the frontal lobe, less often in the parietal lobe, and occasional in the entire cortex. On microscopic examination, there is severe loss of striatal neurons; the most marked changes are found in the caudate nucleus, especially in the tail and portions nearer the ventricle. The putamen is involved in the later stages of disease. Pathologic changes develop in a medial-to-lateral direction in the caudate and from dorsal to ventral in the putamen. The nucleus accumbens is the best preserved portion of the striatum. Both the large and small neurons are affected, but loss of the small neurons generally occurs first. The medium-sized, spiny neurons that use γ-aminobutyric acid as their

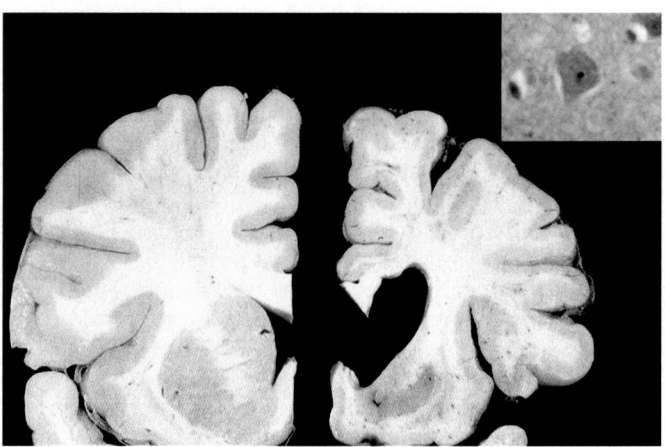

FIGURE 28–41   Huntington disease. Normal hemisphere on the *left*, compared with the hemisphere with Huntington disease on the *right* showing atrophy of the striatum and ventricular dilation. (Courtesy of Dr. J.-P. Vonsattel, Columbia University, New York, NY.) *Inset*, Intranuclear inclusions in neurons are highlighted by immunohistochemistry against ubiquitin.

neurotransmitter, along with enkephalin, dynorphin, and substance P, are especially affected. Two populations of neurons are relatively spared, the diaphorase-positive neurons that contain nitric oxide synthase and the large cholinesterase-positive neurons; both appear to serve as local interneurons. There is also fibrillary gliosis that is more extensive than in the usual reaction to neuronal loss. There is a direct relationship between the degree of degeneration in the striatum and the severity of clinical symptoms. Protein aggregates containing huntingtin can be found in neurons in the striatum and cerebral cortex (Fig. 28–41, *inset*).

Pathogenesis. The loss of medium spiny striatal neurons leads to dysregulation of the basal ganglia circuitry that modulates motor output. These neurons normally function to dampen motor activity; thus, their degeneration in HD results in increased motor output, often manifested as choreoathetosis. The cognitive changes associated with the disease are probably related to the neuronal loss from cerebral cortex.

The biologic function of normal huntingtin remains unknown, but there is little evidence to suggest that the disease is caused by haploinsufficiency related to a mutated allele. Rather, the expansion of the polyglutamine region seems to bestow a toxic gain of function on huntingtin. While the expanded polyglutamine repeat results in protein aggregation and formation of intranuclear inclusions as described above, it is not established that this is a direct pathway to cellular injury. Transcriptional dysregulation has been implicated in HD, with mutant forms of huntingtin binding important transcriptional regulators such as Sp1 and CBP (cyclic adenosine monophosphate response-element binding protein). A proposed consequence of this sequestration of critical transcription factors is the down-regulation of PGC-1α, itself a transcription factor involved in mitochondrial biogenesis and protection against oxidative injury.

Clinical Features. The age at onset is most commonly in the fourth and fifth decades and is related to the length of the CAG repeat in the *HD* gene. Motor symptoms often precede the cognitive impairment. The movement disorder of HD is choreiform, with increased and involuntary jerky movements of all parts of the body; writhing movements of the extremities are typical. Early symptoms of higher cortical dysfunction include forgetfulness and thought and affective disorders, but there is progression to a severe dementia. Although individuals with HD have an increased risk of suicide, intercurrent infection is the most common natural cause of death. Given the ability to screen for disease-causing mutations and the devastating nature of the disease, HD is often the focal point of discussion of ethical issues in genetic diagnosis.

SPINOCEREBELLAR DEGENERATIONS

This group of diseases affects, to a variable extent, the cerebellar cortex, spinal cord, peripheral nerves, and other regions of the neuraxis. The clinical spectrum includes cerebellar and sensory ataxia, spasticity, and sensorimotor peripheral neuropathy. This is a clinically and genetically heterogeneous group of illnesses, with differences in patterns of inheritance, age at onset, and signs and symptoms. Degeneration of neurons, sometimes without other distinctive histopathologic changes, occurs in the affected areas and is associated with gliosis. Genetic analysis continues to redefine and subclassify these illnesses.

Spinocerebellar Ataxias

This is a group of genetically distinct diseases characterized by signs and symptoms referable to the cerebellum (progressive ataxia), brainstem, spinal cord, and peripheral nerves, as well as other brain regions in different subtypes. Pathologically they are characterized by neuronal loss from the affected areas and secondary degeneration of white-matter tracts.

Molecular Genetics. The list of spinocerebellar ataxias (SCAs) has expanded to reach 29 distinct entities at this time. Three distinct types of mutations have been recognized: polyglutamine diseases linked to expansion of a CAG repeat, similar to HD; expansion of non–coding region repeats, similar to myotonic dystrophy; and other types of mutations.[64] Expanded polyglutamine repeats affecting different proteins underlie six forms of SCA (SCA1, 2, 3 [also known as Machado-Joseph disease], 6, 7, and 17). Intranuclear inclusions can be found in these forms of SCA, but just as in HD it remains unclear whether this contributes to or protects against neuronal injury. Putative disease mechanisms include sequestration and depletion of chaperone proteins by the formation of abnormal aggregates driven by the polyglutamine tracts as well as transcriptional dysregulation. In general, these forms of SCA show anticipation. The basis for the targeting of the cerebellar system for specific injury remains unknown.

In the diseases caused by non–coding region repeat expansions (SCA8, 10, and 12), the underlying mechanisms are even more obscure. Point mutations have been found in βIII spec-trin (SCA5), a voltage-gated potassium channel (Kv3.3 in SCA13), protein kinase Cγ (SCA14), and fibroblast growth factor 14 (SCA27). These have been linked to a wide range of potential disease mechanisms without any obvious shared pathways of neuronal injury.

Friedreich Ataxia

Friedreich ataxia, a distinctive spinocerebellar degeneration, is an autosomal recessive progressive illness, generally beginning in the first decade of life with gait ataxia, followed by hand clumsiness and dysarthria. Deep tendon reflexes are depressed or absent, but an extensor plantar reflex is typically present. Joint position and vibratory sense are impaired, and there is sometimes loss of pain and temperature sensation and light touch. Most affected individuals develop pes cavus and kyphoscoliosis. There is a high incidence of cardiac arrhythmias and congestive heart failure. Concomitant diabetes is found in about 10% of patients. Most patients become wheelchair-bound within about 5 years of onset; the cause of death is intercurrent pulmonary infections and cardiac disease.

Friedreich ataxia is caused by expansion of a GAA trinucleotide-repeat in the first intron of a gene on chromosome 9q13 that encodes a protein called *frataxin*.[65] Affected individuals have extremely low levels of the protein, which normally localizes to the inner mitochondrial membrane, where it may have a role in regulation of iron levels. Because iron is an essential component of many of the complexes of the oxidative phosphorylation chain, mutations in frataxin have been suggested to result in generalized mitochondrial dysfunction. Thus, Friedreich ataxia shares biologic features with other SCAs (anatomic distribution of pathology and trinucleotide-repeat expansion) as well as the mitochondrial encephalopathies.

Morphology. The **spinal cord** shows loss of axons and gliosis in the posterior columns, the distal portions of corticospinal tracts, and the spinocerebellar tracts. There is degeneration of neurons in the spinal cord (Clarke column), the brainstem (cranial nerve nuclei VIII, X, and XII), the cerebellum (dentate nucleus and the Purkinje cells of the superior vermis), and the Betz cells of the motor cortex. Large dorsal root ganglion neurons are also decreased in number; their large myelinated axons, traveling both in the dorsal roots and in dorsal columns, undergo secondary degeneration. The **heart** is enlarged and may have pericardial adhesions. Multifocal destruction of myocardial fibers with inflammation and fibrosis is detectable in about half the affected individuals who come to autopsy.

Ataxia-Telangiectasia

Ataxia-telangiectasia (Chapter 7) is an autosomal recessive disorder characterized by an ataxic-dyskinetic syndrome beginning in early childhood, with the subsequent development of telangiectasias in the conjunctiva and skin; and immunodeficiency. The ataxia-telangiectasia mutated (*ATM*) gene on chromosome 11q22–q23 encodes a kinase with a critical role in orchestrating the cellular response to double-stranded DNA breaks (Chapter 7). Cells from individuals with the disease show increased sensitivity to x-ray-induced chromosome abnormalities; these cells continue to replicate damaged DNA rather than stopping to allow repair or undergoing apoptosis. The carrier frequency of ataxia-telangiectasia has been estimated at 1%; in these individuals the mutated *ATM* allele may underlie an increased risk of cancer, specifically breast cancer. The link between DNA repair mechanisms and neurodegenerative disease is harder to understand than the connection to neoplasia. It has been suggested that mutations in *ATM* result in failure to remove cells with DNA damage from the developing nervous system, predisposing it to degeneration.[66]

> **Morphology.** The abnormalities are predominantly in the cerebellum, with loss of Purkinje and granule cells; there is also degeneration of the dorsal columns, spinocerebellar tracts, and anterior horn cells, and a peripheral neuropathy. Telangiectatic lesions have been reported in the CNS as well as in the conjunctiva and skin of the face, neck, and arms. Cells in many organs (e.g., Schwann cells in dorsal root ganglia and peripheral nerves, endothelial cells, pituicytes) show a bizarre enlargement of the nucleus to two to five times normal size and are referred to as amphicytes. The lymph nodes, thymus, and gonads are hypoplastic.

Clinical Features. The disease is relentlessly progressive, with death early in the second decade. Affected individuals first come to medical attention because of recurrent sinopulmonary infections and unsteadiness in walking. Later on, speech is noted to become dysarthric, and eye movement abnormalities develop. Many affected individuals develop lymphoid neoplasms, often T-cell leukemias; gliomas and carcinomas have been reported in some.

DEGENERATIVE DISEASES AFFECTING MOTOR NEURONS

These are a group of inherited or sporadic diseases that affect both lower motor neurons in the anterior horns of the spinal cord and brainstem motor nuclei and upper motor neurons in the motor cortex (also known as Betz cells).

These diseases occur in several age groups, and the course of the illnesses range from slowly progressive or nonprogressive to rapidly progressive and fatal in a period of months or a few years. Denervation of muscles from loss of lower motor neurons and their axons results in muscular atrophy, weakness, and fasciculations; the corresponding histologic changes in nerve and muscle are discussed in Chapter 27. The clinical manifestations of upper motor neuron loss include paresis, hyperreflexia, spasticity, and extensor plantar responses (Babinski sign). Sensory systems are unaffected, but some of these diseases may be associated with manifestations of cortical dysfunction, such as behavioral abnormalities and dementia.

Amyotrophic Lateral Sclerosis (ALS; Motor Neuron Disease)

ALS is characterized by loss of lower motor neurons in spinal cord and brainstem and upper motor neurons that project in corticospinal tracts. This relatively rare disease (incidence of about 2 cases per 100,000 population) affects men slightly more frequently than women and becomes clinically manifest in the fifth decade or later. Five to 10% of cases are familial (fALS), mostly with autosomal dominant inheritance.

Molecular Genetics. Close to a quarter of familial cases of ALS are caused by mutations in the gene encoding copper-zinc superoxide dismutase (*SOD1*) on chromosome 21.[67] A wide variety of mutations, nearly all missense mutations, have been identified throughout the gene; ALS seems to be caused by an adverse gain-of-function phenotype associated with mutant SOD1. A mutation resulting in an alanine to valine substitution in residue 4 is the most common in the United States; it is associated with a rapid course, and rarely has upper motor neuron signs. Other loci for ALS have been mapped, although none appears in linkage with as large a fraction of the patient population as *SOD1*. These mendelian loci include the genes encoding dynactin (a protein involved in retrograde axonal transport), VAMP-associated protein B (involved in regulation of vesicle transport), and alsin (containing guanine nucleotide exchange factor domains and associated with regulation of endosomal trafficking through interaction with Rab5b).

Pathogenesis. The pathogenesis of ALS is still not understood despite the identification of numerous genetic associations. The discovery of SOD1 mutations initially suggested that a reduced capacity to detoxify free radicals (the physiologic function of SOD) may account for neuronal death in ALS. However, this hypothesis has not been proved, and currently a more accepted idea is that the mutated SOD1 protein is misfolded and triggers an injurious unfolded protein response.[68] Mutated SOD1 in non-neuronal (glial and smooth muscle) cells may also contribute to the disease.[69] Alterations in axonal transport, neurofilament abnormalities, toxicity mediated by increased levels of the neurotransmitter glutamate, and aggregation of other proteins (such as one called TDP-43 that is sometimes found in cytoplasmic inclusions in neurons in ALS)[70], have all been suggested as mechanisms contributing to the progressive loss of motor neurons.

> **Morphology.** On gross examination, the anterior roots of the spinal cord are thin (Fig. 28–42A). The precentral gyrus may be atrophic in especially severe cases. Microscopic examination demonstrates a reduction in the number of anterior-horn neurons throughout the length of the spinal cord with associated reactive gliosis and loss of anterior-root myelinated fibers. Similar findings are seen in the hypoglossal, ambiguus, and motor trigeminal cranial nerve nuclei. Remaining neurons often contain PAS-positive cytoplasmic inclusions, called Bunina bodies, that appear to be remnants of autophagic vacuoles. Skeletal muscles innervated by the degenerated lower motor neurons show neurogenic atrophy. Loss of the upper motor neurons leads to degeneration of the corticospinal tracts, resulting in volume loss and

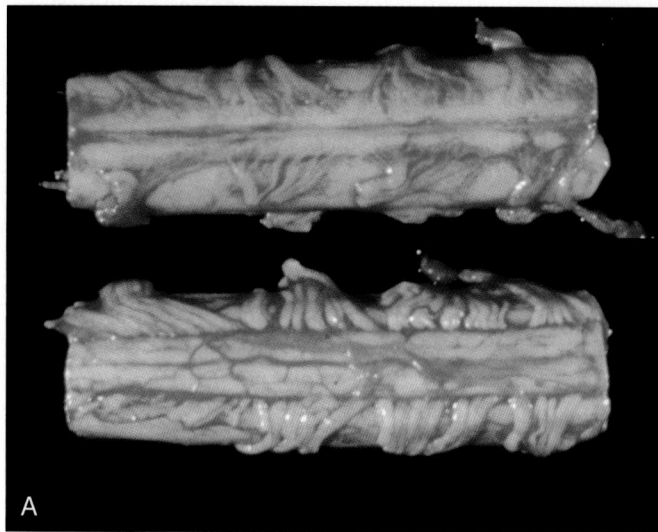

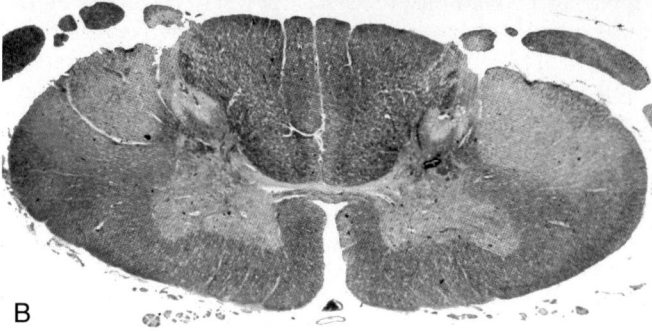

FIGURE 28–42 Amyotrophic lateral sclerosis. **A,** Segment of spinal cord viewed from anterior *(upper)* and posterior *(lower)* surfaces showing attenuation of anterior (motor) roots compared to posterior (sensory) roots. **B,** Spinal cord showing loss of myelinated fibers (lack of stain) in corticospinal tracts as well as degeneration of anterior roots.

absence of myelinated fibers, which may be particularly evident at the lower segmental levels (Fig. 28–42B).

Clinical Features. Early symptoms include asymmetric weakness of the hands, manifested as dropping objects and difficulty in performing fine motor tasks, and cramping and spasticity of the arms and legs. As the disease progresses, muscle strength and bulk diminish, and involuntary contractions of individual motor units, termed *fasciculations*, occur. The disease eventually involves the respiratory muscles, leading to recurrent bouts of pulmonary infection. The severity of involvement of the upper and lower motor neurons is variable; the term *progressive muscular atrophy* applies to those relatively uncommon cases in which lower motor neuron involvement predominates. In some affected individuals, degeneration of the lower brainstem cranial motor nuclei occurs early and progresses rapidly, a pattern referred to as *progressive bulbar palsy* or *bulbar ALS*. In these individuals, abnormalities of deglutition and phonation dominate, and the clinical course is inexorable during a 1- or 2-year period; when bulbar involvement is less severe, about half of affected individuals are alive 2 years after diagnosis. Although it has been suggested

that the motor neurons innervating extra-ocular muscles were spared in ALS, it is now clear that these cells are susceptible to the disease process when individuals survive longer. Familial cases develop symptoms earlier than most sporadic cases, but the clinical course is comparable.

Bulbospinal Atrophy (Kennedy Syndrome)

This X-linked adult-onset disease is characterized by distal limb amyotrophy and bulbar signs such as atrophy and fasciculations of the tongue and dysphagia. Affected individuals manifest androgen insensitivity, gynecomastia, testicular atrophy, and oligospermia. On microscopic examination there is degeneration of lower motor neurons in the spinal cord and brainstem. The gene defect is expansion of a CAG/polyglutamine repeat in the androgen receptor (40 to 60 for affected males as opposed to 11 to 33 for normals); nuclear inclusions containing aggregated androgen receptor can be found, although it remains unclear whether these inclusions are critical to cellular injury.[71]

Spinal Muscular Atrophy

This group of diseases affects mainly the lower motor neurons in children. As in ALS, there is a selective loss of anterior-horn cells and atrophy of anterior spinal roots. It includes several entities with distinct clinical courses (Chapter 27).

Genetic Metabolic Diseases

A subset of genetic metabolic diseases affects the nervous system preferentially and will be discussed here; other metabolic diseases are covered elsewhere in this book. Many of these disorders express themselves in children who are normal at birth but who begin to miss developmental milestones during infancy and childhood.

- *Neuronal storage diseases* are mostly autosomal recessive disorders caused by the deficiency of a specific enzyme involved in the catabolism of sphingolipids, mucopolysaccharides, or mucolipids. They are often characterized by the accumulation of the substrate of the enzyme within the lysosomes of neurons, leading to neuronal death. Cortical neuronal involvement leads to loss of cognitive function and may also cause seizures. The relationship between the accumulated material and cell injury and death is usually unclear.
- *Leukodystrophies* are characterized by myelin abnormalities (either abnormal synthesis or turnover) and generally lack neuronal storage defects. Some of these disorders involve lysosomal enzymes; others affect peroxisomal enzymes. Diffuse involvement of white matter leads to deterioration in motor skills, spasticity, hypotonia, or ataxia. Most are autosomal recessive disorders; adrenoleukodystrophy, an X-linked disease, is a notable exception. Subtypes, or variants, exist for many of these disorders. Variants are associated with an earlier age at onset, and generally follow a more severe clinical course.
- *Mitochondrial encephalomyopathies* are a group of disorders of oxidative phosphorylation, usually resulting from

mutations in the mitochondrial genome. They typically involve gray matter as well as skeletal muscle (Chapter 27).

NEURONAL STORAGE DISEASES

Neuronal Ceroid Lipofuscinoses

These are a set of inherited lysosomal storage diseases that are grouped because they share the accumulation of lipofuscin—an autofluorescent substance with a variety of ultrastructural appearances—in neurons. Neuronal dysfunction typically leads to a combination of blindness, mental and motor deterioration, and seizures. These disorders are classified based on age of onset into infantile (INCL), late infantile (LINCL), juvenile (JNCL), and adult neuronal ceroid lipofuscinoses (ANCL; Kuf disease), or on the pattern of inclusions by electron microscopy. Genetic studies indicate that there are likely eight causative loci, which encode a variety of proteins involved in the modification and degradation of proteins.[72] The *CLN1* locus, a common cause of INCL, encodes palmitoyl protein thioesterase 1 (PPT1), which removes palmitate residues from proteins; this is similar to *CLN3*, implicated in most cases of JNCL (also known as Batten disease), which encodes palmitoyl-protein Δ-9 desaturase, another enzyme related to regulation of membrane-associated palmitoylated proteins. How the abnormalities in protein modification lead to the accumulation of lipofuscin or the neuronal dysfunction is not understood.

Tay-Sachs Disease

This disease begins in early infancy with developmental delay, followed by paralysis and loss of neurologic function, and death after several years. It is discussed in Chapter 5 along with other lysosomal storage diseases.

LEUKODYSTROPHIES

Krabbe Disease

This disease is an autosomal recessive leukodystrophy resulting from a *deficiency of galactocerebroside β-galactosidase* (galactosylceramidase), the enzyme required for the catabolism of galactocerebroside to ceramide and galactose. More than 40 different mutations have been found in the gene encoding this enzyme, which is located on chromosome 14q31. While accumulation of galactocerebroside occurs, this is not the direct toxic agent in this disease. Instead, it seems that an alternative catabolic pathway removes a fatty acid from this molecule, generating galactosylsphingosine, which is a cytotoxic compound that may cause oligodendrocyte injury.

The clinical course is rapidly progressive, with onset of symptoms often between the ages of 3 and 6 months. Survival beyond 2 years of age is uncommon. The clinical symptoms are dominated by motor signs, including stiffness and weakness, with gradually worsening difficulties in feeding. The brain shows loss of myelin and oligodendrocytes in the CNS and a similar process in peripheral nerves (Fig. 28–43). Neurons and axons are relatively spared. A unique and diagnostic feature of Krabbe disease is the aggregation of engorged

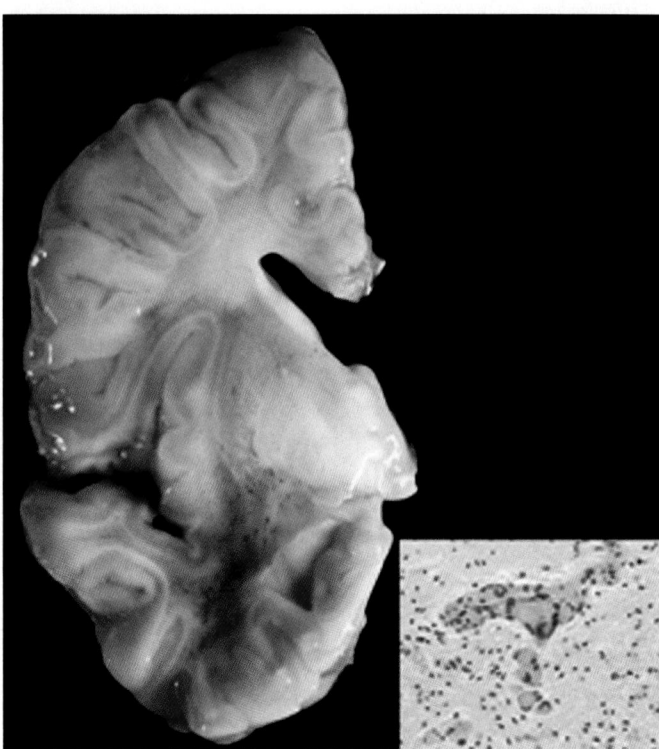

FIGURE 28–43 Krabbe disease. Much of the white matter is gray/yellow because of the loss of myelin. *Inset,* "Globoid" cells are the hallmark of the disease.

macrophages *(globoid cells)* in the parenchyma and around blood vessels (Fig. 28–43, *inset*). The potential exists for treatment with cord blood transplantation in the pre-symptomatic state.[73]

Metachromatic Leukodystrophy

This disorder is transmitted in an autosomal recessive pattern and results from a deficiency of the *lysosomal enzyme arylsulfatase A*. This enzyme, present in a variety of tissues, cleaves the sulfate from sulfate-containing lipids (sulfatides), the first step in their degradation. Enzyme deficiency leads to an accumulation of the sulfatides, especially cerebroside sulfate; how this leads to myelin breakdown is not known, although sulfatides are reported to inhibit differentiation of oligodendrocytes. The gene encoding arylsulfatase A has been localized to the distal end of chromosome 22q, and a wide range of mutations have been described. Recognized clinical subtypes of the disorder include a late infantile form (the most common), a juvenile form, and an adult form. The two forms with childhood onset often present with motor symptoms and progress gradually, leading to death in 5 to 10 years. In the adult form psychiatric or cognitive symptoms are the usual initial complaint, with motor symptoms coming later. Approaches using various types of bone marrow stem cell transplantation have been shown to provide benefit, most commonly when performed before the neurologic deficits appear.[74]

The most striking histologic finding is demyelination with resulting gliosis. Macrophages with vacuolated cytoplasm are scattered throughout the white matter. The membrane-bound vacuoles contain complex crystalloid structures composed of sulfatides; when bound to certain dyes such as toluidine blue, sulfatides shift the absorbance spectrum of the dye, a property called *metachromasia*. Similar changes in peripheral nerves are observed. The detection of metachromatic material in the urine is also a sensitive method of establishing the diagnosis.

Adrenoleukodystrophy

This disorder, which has several clinically and genetically distinct forms, is a progressive disease with symptoms referable to myelin loss from the CNS and peripheral nerves as well as adrenal insufficiency. In general, forms with earlier onset have a more rapid course. The X-linked form usually presents in the early school years with neurologic symptoms and adrenal insufficiency and is rapidly progressive and fatal. In individuals with later onset the course is more protracted; when it develops in adults it is usually a slowly progressive disorder with predominantly peripheral nerve involvement developing over a period of decades. The disease is associated with mutations in the *ALD* gene on chromosome Xq28, which encodes a member of the ATP-binding cassette transporter family of proteins, ABCD1. However, there is little correlation between clinical course and the underlying mutations. The disease is characterized by the inability to properly catabolize very-long-chain fatty acids (VLCFAs) within peroxisomes, with elevated levels of VLCFAs in serum. There is loss of myelin, accompanied by gliosis and extensive lymphocytic infiltration. Atrophy of the adrenal cortex is present, and VLCFA accumulation can be seen in remaining cells.

Pelizaeus-Merzbacher Disease

This is an X-linked, invariably fatal leukodystrophy beginning either in early childhood or just after birth, and characterized by slowly progressive signs and symptoms resulting from widespread white-matter dysfunction. Affected individuals present with pendular eye movements, hypotonia, choreoathetosis, and pyramidal signs early in the disease, followed later by spasticity, dementia, and ataxia. Although myelin is nearly completely lost in the cerebral hemispheres, patches may remain, giving a "tigroid" appearance to tissue sections stained for myelin. The disease has been shown to arise in most cases from mutations in a gene on the X chromosome that encodes two distinct myelin proteins, distinguished by alternative splicing: proteolipid protein (PLP) and DM20. Gene duplications are the most common mutation observed, although point mutations giving rise to null alleles are also observed; it remains unclear how these distinct mutations cause the disease.[75] This same genetic locus is also the site of one form of spastic paraplegia (SPG2).

Canavan Disease

This disease is characterized by megalocephaly, severe mental deficits, blindness, and signs and symptoms of white matter injury beginning in early infancy and relentlessly progressing to death within a few years of onset. Autopsy studies show spongy degeneration of the white matter. There is accumulation of *N*-acetylaspartic acid in this disorder as a consequence of loss-of-function mutations in the gene encoding the deacetylating enzyme aspartoacylase, located on chromosome 17. The mechanisms of myelin injury remain uncertain.[76]

Alexander Disease

This disease is characterized by megalencephaly, seizures, and progressive psychomotor retardation. There is white-matter loss, typically with a frontal-to-occipital gradient. The characteristic pathologic finding is the exuberant accumulation of Rosenthal fibers around blood vessels, in the subpial and subependymal zones and in the brain parenchyma. Even though Rosenthal fibers are primarily composed of various heat-shock proteins, including αB-crystallin, the basis of Alexander disease lies in mutations in the gene encoding glial fibrillary acid protein (GFAP).[77] The disease is believed to be caused by dominant gain-of-function mutations associated with decreased capacity to form filaments as well as induction of stress responses.

Vanishing-White-Matter Leukodystrophy

Vanishing-white-matter leukodystrophy, named for the characteristic progression of the disorder as revealed by imaging studies, is associated with mutations in the genes encoding any of the five subunits of eukaryotic initiation factor 2B (eIF2B).[78,79] The disease usually begins insidiously during the first few years of life, with ataxia and seizures as common symptoms. With a relentless downward course, sometimes exacerbated by intercurrent illnesses, affected individuals typically survive for a few years after onset of symptoms. Levels of eIF2B are reduced throughout the body; the basis for selective injury to the brain, with the primary burden falling on white matter, is not known.

MITOCHONDRIAL ENCEPHALOMYOPATHIES

While many of the inherited disorders of mitochondrial oxidative phosphorylation present as muscle diseases (Chapter 27), the CNS is the second most commonly affected tissue.[80,81] In addition to the diseases discussed below, Friedreich ataxia (considered above) is also recognized as a mitochondrial disorder associated with mutations in the frataxin gene.

Mitochondrial Encephalomyopathy, Lactic Acidosis, and Strokelike Episodes

Mitochondrial encephalomyopathy, lactic acidosis, and strokelike episodes (MELAS) is the most common neurologic syndrome caused by mitochondrial abnormalities. The syndrome is characterized by recurrent episodes of acute neurologic dysfunction, cognitive changes, and evidence of muscle involvement with weakness and lactic acidosis. The stroke-like episodes are often associated with reversible deficits that do not correspond well to specific vascular territories. Pathologically, areas of infarction are observed, often with vascular proliferation and focal calcification. The most prevalent mutations associated with MELAS occurs in tRNAs; coding-gene mutations have also been reported.

Myoclonic Epilepsy and Ragged Red Fibers

Myoclonic epilepsy and ragged red fibers (MERRF) is a maternally transmitted disease in which affected individuals have myoclonus, a seizure disorder, and evidence of a myopathy. Ataxia, associated with neuronal loss from the cerebellar system (including the inferior olive in the medulla, cerebellar cortex, and deep nuclei), is also a common component. Most cases of MERRF are associated with mutations in tRNA that are distinct from those in MELAS. In some affected individuals there seems to be an overlap between MERRF and MELAS.

Leigh Syndrome (Subacute Necrotizing Encephalopathy)

This disease of early childhood is characterized by lactic acidemia, arrest of psychomotor development, feeding problems, seizures, extra-ocular palsies, and weakness with hypotonia. Death usually occurs within 1 to 2 years. On histologic examination there are multifocal, moderately symmetric regions of destruction of brain tissue with a spongiform appearance and proliferation of blood vessels. The areas that are most commonly affected include the periventricular gray matter of the midbrain, the tegmentum of the pons, and the periventricular regions of the thalamus and hypothalamus. A wide spectrum of mutations has been identified as causing Leigh syndrome, including both nuclear and mitochondrial DNA mutations. Diverse mutations affecting mitochondrial genome–encoded components of oxidative phosphorylation complexes, as well as mitochondrial tRNA mutations, have been found; there does not seem to be a genotype-phenotype relationship. Interestingly, a point mutation in the mitochondrial gene for an ATPase subunit of complex V causes a maternally inherited form of Leigh syndrome when the cells contain a large proportion of the mutated mitochondrial DNA. However, when there is a higher fraction of normal mitochondria, the disease takes on a different clinical and pathologic appearance, as *neuropathy, ataxia, and retinitis pigmentosa* (NARP). Such unequal distribution of mitochondrial DNA among cells is called *heteroplasmy* (Chapter 5).

Kearn-Sayre Syndrome

Kearns-Sayre syndrome ("ophthalmoplegia plus") is a sporadic disorder most often associated with a large mitochondrial DNA deletion/rearrangement. The disorder presents with cerebellar ataxia, progressive external ophthalmoplegia, pigmentary retinopathy, and cardiac conduction defects. Pathologically, there is spongiform change in gray and white matter, with neuronal loss most evident in the cerebellum. The basis of the disease is large defects in the mitochondrial genome.

Alpers Disease

This disorder combines neurologic symptoms with evidence of hepatic dysfunction and pathologic findings including hepatitis and bile duct proliferation.[82] Alpers disease typically begins in the first few years of life with severe intractable seizures, followed by developmental delay, hypotonia, ataxia, and cortical blindness. There is neuronal loss in cerebral cortex and throughout deeper structures, and spongiform degeneration of gray matter. Mutations in the nuclear gene encoding DNA polymerase γ—the isoform of DNA polymerase responsible for replication of the mitochondrial genome—have been identified in Alpers disease.[83]

Toxic and Acquired Metabolic Diseases

Toxic and acquired metabolic diseases are relatively common causes of neurologic illnesses. These diseases were discussed in Chapter 9; only aspects that are relevant to CNS pathology are presented below.

VITAMIN DEFICIENCIES

Thiamine (Vitamin B$_1$) Deficiency

As was discussed in Chapter 9, thiamine deficiency may result in the slowly evolving clinical disorder *beriberi*, which is associated with cardiac failure. In certain affected individuals, thiamine deficiency may also lead to the development of psychotic symptoms or ophthalmoplegia that begin abruptly, a syndrome termed *Wernicke encephalopathy*. The acute stages, if unrecognized and untreated, may be followed by a prolonged and largely irreversible condition, *Korsakoff syndrome*, characterized clinically by memory disturbances and confabulation. Because the two syndromes are closely linked, the term *Wernicke-Korsakoff syndrome* is often applied. The syndrome is particularly common in the setting of chronic alcoholism, but it may also be encountered in individuals with thiamine deficiency resulting from gastric disorders, including carcinoma, chronic gastritis, or persistent vomiting. Treatment with thiamine may reverse the manifestations of Wernicke syndrome.

Morphology. Wernicke encephalopathy is characterized by foci of hemorrhage and necrosis in the mamillary bodies and the walls of the third and fourth ventricles. Early lesions show dilated capillaries with prominent endothelial cells. Subsequently, the capillaries become leaky, producing hemorrhagic areas. With time, there is infiltration of macrophages and development of a cystic space with hemosiderin-laden macrophages. These chronic lesions predominate in individuals with Korsakoff syndrome. Lesions in the dorsomedial nucleus of the thalamus seem to be the best correlate of the memory disturbance and confabulation.

Vitamin B$_{12}$ Deficiency

Deficiency of vitamin B$_{12}$ often causes anemia (Chapter 14) but can also have severe and potentially irreversible effects on the nervous system. The neurologic symptoms may present in the course of a few weeks, initially with numbness, tingling, and slight ataxia in the lower extremities, but may progress rapidly to include spastic weakness of the lower extremities. Complete paraplegia may occur, usually only later in the course. With prompt vitamin replacement therapy, clinical improvement occurs; however, if complete paraplegia has developed, recovery is poor. On microscopic examination vitamin B$_{12}$ deficiency is associated with a swelling of myelin layers, producing vacuoles. This begins segmentally at the midthoracic level of the spinal cord in the early stages. With time, axons in both the ascending tracts of the posterior columns and the descending pyramidal tracts degenerate.

While isolated involvement of descending or ascending tracts may be observed in a variety of spinal cord diseases, the combined degeneration of both ascending and descending tracts of the spinal cord is characteristic of vitamin B_{12} deficiency and has led to the designation *subacute combined degeneration of the spinal cord.*

NEUROLOGIC SEQUELAE OF METABOLIC DISTURBANCES

Hypoglycemia

Since the brain requires glucose and oxygen for its energy production, the cellular effects of diminished glucose resemble those of oxygen deprivation, as described earlier. Some regions of the brain are more sensitive to hypoglycemia than are others. Glucose deprivation initially leads to selective injury to large pyramidal neurons of the cerebral cortex, which, if severe, may result in pseudolaminar necrosis of the cortex, predominantly involving deep layers. The hippocampus is also vulnerable to glucose depletion and may show a marked loss of pyramidal neurons in Sommer sector (area CA1 of the hippocampus). Purkinje cells of the cerebellum are also sensitive to hypoglycemia, although to a lesser extent than to hypoxia. If the level and duration of hypoglycemia are of sufficient severity, there may be widespread injury to many areas of the brain.

Hyperglycemia

Hyperglycemia is most commonly found in the setting of inadequately controlled diabetes mellitus and can be associated with either ketoacidosis or hyperosmolar coma. The affected individual becomes dehydrated and develops confusion, stupor, and eventually coma. The fluid depletion must be corrected gradually; otherwise, severe cerebral edema may follow.

Hepatic Encephalopathy

The pathogenesis of hepatic encephalopathy is discussed in Chapter 18. The cellular response in the CNS is predominantly glial. Alzheimer type II cells are evident in the cortex and basal ganglia and other subcortical gray matter regions.

TOXIC DISORDERS

Cellular and tissue injury from toxic agents is discussed in Chapter 1. Aspects of several important toxic disorders that are of unique neurologic importance are discussed here.

Carbon Monoxide

Many of the pathologic findings that follow acute carbon monoxide exposure are the result of hypoxia from altered oxygen-carrying capacity of hemoglobin. Selective injury of the neurons of layers III and V of the cerebral cortex, Sommer sector of the hippocampus, and Purkinje cells is characteristic. Bilateral necrosis of the globus pallidus may also occur; it is more common in carbon monoxide–induced hypoxia than in hypoxia from other causes. Demyelination of white matter tracts may be a later event.

Methanol

Methanol toxicity preferentially affects the retina, where degeneration of retinal ganglion cells may cause blindness. Selective bilateral putamenal necrosis and focal white-matter necrosis also occur when the exposure is severe. Formate, a major metabolite of methanol, may have a role in the retinal toxicity.

Ethanol

Experience tells us that the effects of acute ethanol intoxication are reversible, but chronic alcohol abuse is associated with a variety of neurologic sequelae, including Wernicke-Korsakoff syndrome, considered above. The toxic effects of chronic alcohol intake may be either direct or secondary to nutritional deficits. Cerebellar dysfunction occurs in about 1% of chronic alcoholics, associated with a clinical syndrome of truncal ataxia, unsteady gait, and nystagmus. The histologic changes are atrophy and loss of granule cells predominantly in the anterior vermis (Fig. 28–44). In advanced cases there is loss of Purkinje cells and proliferation of the adjacent astrocytes (*Bergmann gliosis*) between the depleted granular cell layer and the molecular layer of the cerebellum. The fetal alcohol syndrome is discussed in Chapter 10.

Radiation

As discussed in Chapter 9, exposure to very high doses of radiation (>1000 rems) can cause intractable nausea, confusion, convulsions, and rapid onset of coma, followed by death. Delayed effects of radiation can also present with rapidly evolving symptoms, including headaches, nausea, vomiting, and papilledema that may appear months to years after irradiation. The pathologic findings consist of large areas of coagulative necrosis and adjacent edema. The typical lesion is restricted to white matter, and all elements within the area undergo necrosis, including astrocytes, axons, oligodendrocytes, and

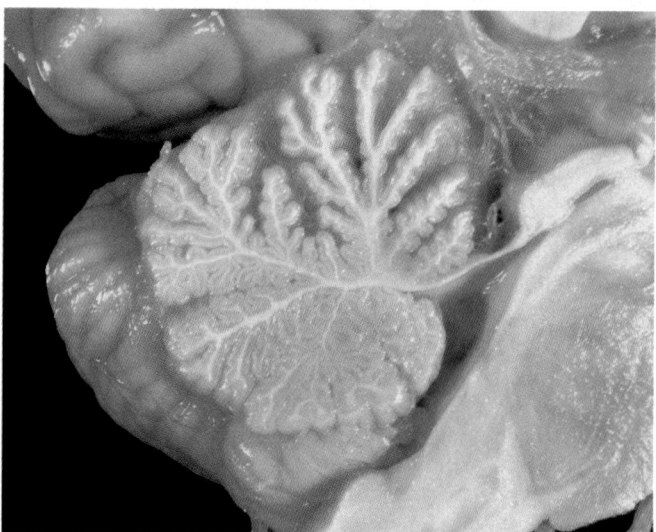

FIGURE 28–44 Alcoholic cerebellar degeneration. The anterior portion of the vermis *(upper portion of figure)* is atrophic with widened spaces between the folia.

blood vessels. Adjacent to the area of coagulative necrosis, proteinaceous spheroids may be identified, and blood vessels show thickened walls with intramural fibrin-like material. Radiation can also induce tumors, which usually develop years after radiation therapy and include sarcomas, gliomas, and meningiomas.

Combined Methotrexate and Radiation-Induced Injury

Methotrexate toxicity most commonly develops when the drug has been administered in association with radiation therapy, either together or at separate times. The interval between the inciting events and the onset of symptoms varies considerably but may be as long as months. Symptoms often begin with drowsiness, ataxia, and confusion, and may progress rapidly. While some affected individuals recover function, others may become comatose; rarely, methotrexate neurotoxicity may be responsible for the patient's death. The mechanisms of these delayed effects of methotrexate are unclear.

The pathologic basis of the symptoms are focal areas of coagulative necrosis within white matter, often adjacent to the lateral ventricles but at times distributed throughout the white matter or in the brainstem. Surrounding axons are often dilated and form axonal spheroids. Axons and cell bodies in the vicinity of the lesions undergo dystrophic mineralization, and there is adjacent gliosis.

Tumors

The annual incidence of tumors of the CNS ranges from 10 to 17 per 100,000 persons for intra-cranial tumors and 1 to 2 per 100,000 persons for intra-spinal tumors; about half to three quarters are primary tumors, and the rest are metastatic. Tumors of the CNS account for 20% of all cancers of childhood. Seventy percent of childhood CNS tumors arise in the posterior fossa; a comparable number of tumors in adults arise within the cerebral hemispheres above the tentorium. There is great interest in identifying tumor initiating (stem) cells that maintain tumor growth and, therefore, may be key targets of new therapies.[84,85]

While pathologists have developed classification schemes that distinguish between benign and malignant lesions on histologic grounds, the clinical course of disease is also influenced by relatively unique features of brain tumors. Thus, some glial tumors with benign histologic features (low mitotic rate, cellular uniformity, and slow growth) may infiltrate large regions of the brain and lead to serious clinical deficits and poor prognosis. Because of their infiltrative behavior, it is often not feasible to resect glial neoplasms completely without compromising neurologic function. Also, any neoplasm can have lethal consequences if it is located in a critical region, as when a benign meningioma, by compressing the medulla, causes cardiorespiratory arrest. Even the most highly malignant gliomas rarely metastasize outside the CNS. The subarachnoid space provides a pathway for spread, so seeding along the brain and spinal cord can occur in highly anaplastic as well as in well-differentiated neoplasms that extend into the CSF.

Classification of tumors is one of the arts of pathology, drawing on emerging molecular methods and the traditional recognition of histologic and biologic patterns.[86,87] Treatment protocols and experimental trials of glial tumors are usually based on the World Health Organization (WHO) grading scheme, which segregates tumors into one of four grades according to their biologic behavior, ranging from grade I to grade IV. Under the current classification scheme, lesions of different grade are always given distinct names. When tumors recur, they often show progression to a higher histologic grade and, thus, acquire a different name; this actually represents progression along a classification scheme rather than a new disease.

The major classes of primary brain tumors to be considered here include gliomas, neuronal tumors, poorly differentiated tumors, as well as a small collection of other tumors. In addition, we will discuss tumors of the meninges as well as tumors of peripheral nerves.

GLIOMAS

Gliomas, the most common group of primary brain tumors, include *astrocytomas*, *oligodendrogliomas*, and *ependymomas*.

Astrocytoma

The two major categories of astrocytic tumors are infiltrating astrocytomas and non-infiltrating neoplasms, of which the most common are the pilocytic astrocytomas. These tumor types have characteristic histologic features, distribution within the brain, age groups typically affected, and clinical course.

Infiltrating Astrocytomas

These account for about 80% of adult primary brain tumors in adults. Usually found in the cerebral hemispheres, they may also occur in the cerebellum, brainstem, or spinal cord, most often in the fourth through sixth decades. The most common presenting signs and symptoms are seizures, headaches, and focal neurologic deficits related to the anatomic site of involvement. Infiltrating astrocytomas show a spectrum of histologic differentiation that correlates well with clinical course and outcome; within this spectrum, tumors range from *diffuse astrocytoma* (grade II/IV) through *anaplastic astrocytoma* (grade III/IV) to *glioblastoma* (grade IV/IV). (The grade I/IV category is limited to pilocytic astrocytoma.)

Morphology. The gross appearance of **diffuse astrocytoma** is that of a poorly defined, gray, infiltrative tumor that expands and distorts the invaded brain (Fig. 28–45). These tumors range in size from a few centimeters to enormous lesions that replace an entire hemisphere. The cut surface of the tumor is either firm or soft and gelatinous; cystic degeneration may be seen. The tumor may appear well demarcated from the surrounding brain tissue, but infiltration beyond the outer margins is always present.

On microscopic examination, diffuse astrocytomas are characterized by a mild to moderate increase in glial cellularity, variable nuclear pleomorphism, and an intervening feltwork of fine, GFAP-positive astrocytic processes that give the background a fibrillary

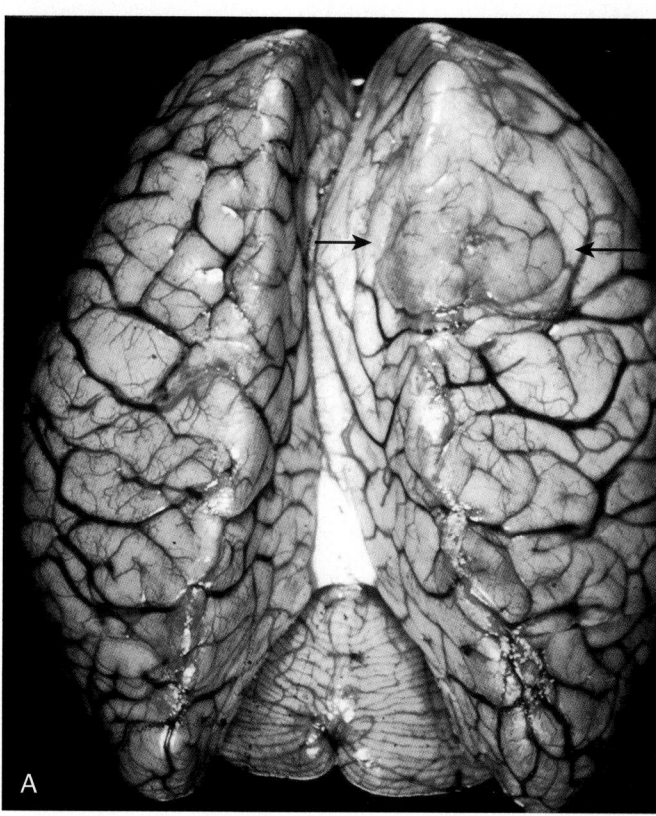

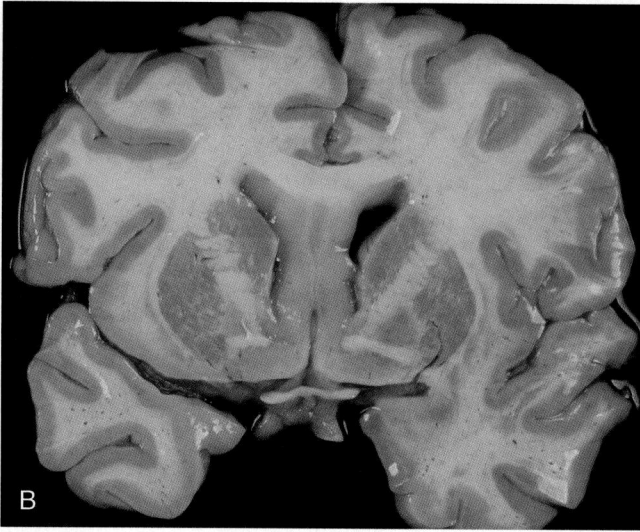

FIGURE 28–45   Diffuse astrocytoma. **A,** The right frontal tumor has expanded gyri, which led to flattening *(arrows)*. **B,** There is bilateral expansion of the septum pellucidum by gray, glassy tumor.

appearance. The transition between neoplastic and normal tissue is indistinct, and tumor cells can be seen infiltrating normal tissue at some distance from the main lesion.

Anaplastic astrocytomas show regions that are more densely cellular and have greater nuclear pleomorphism; mitotic figures are often observed. The term **gemistocytic astrocytoma** is used for tumors in which the predominant neoplastic astrocyte shows a brightly eosinophilic cell body from which emanate abundant, stout processes.

In **glioblastoma** (previously called *glioblastoma multiforme*) variation in the gross appearance of the tumor from region to region is characteristic (Fig. 28–46). Some areas are firm and white, others are soft and yellow due to necrosis, and yet others show regions of cystic degeneration and hemorrhage. The histologic appearance of glioblastoma is similar to anaplastic astrocytoma with the additional features of **necrosis** and **vascular or endothelial cell proliferation.** Necrosis in glioblastoma often occurs in a serpentine pattern in areas of hypercellularity. Tumor cells collect along the edges of the necrotic regions, producing a histologic pattern referred to as **pseudopalisading** (Fig. 28–47). Vascular cell proliferation is characterized by tufts of piled-up cells that bulge into the lumen; the minimal criterion for this feature is a double layer of endothelial cells. With marked vascular cell proliferation the tuft forms a ball-like structure,

the glomeruloid body (see Fig. 28–47). VEGF, produced by malignant astrocytes in response to hypoxia, contributes to this distinctive vascular change. Since histologic features can be extremely variable from one region of the neoplasm to another, a single small biopsy specimen might not be representative of the worst aspects of a tumor.

In the condition called **gliomatosis cerebri,** multiple regions of the brain, in some cases the entire brain, are infiltrated by neoplastic astrocytes. Because of the widespread infiltration, this process follows an aggressive course and is considered to be a grade III/IV lesion—independent of the appearance of the individual tumor cells.

Molecular Genetics. Certain genetic alterations correlate with the progression of infiltrating astrocytomas from low to high grade, which is part of the natural course of the disease in many patients.[86,88] Among the alterations that are most common in the low-grade astrocytomas are mutations affecting p53 and overexpression of platelet-derived growth factor α (PDGF-A) and its receptor. The transition to higher grade astrocytoma is associated with disruption of two well-known tumor suppressor genes, *RB* and *p16/CDKNaA*, and an unknown putative tumor suppressor on chromosome 19q.

It was recognized well before advances in genetic analyses that glioblastoma tends to occur in one of two clinical settings: most commonly as new onset disease, typically in older individuals *(primary glioblastoma)*, and in younger patients with

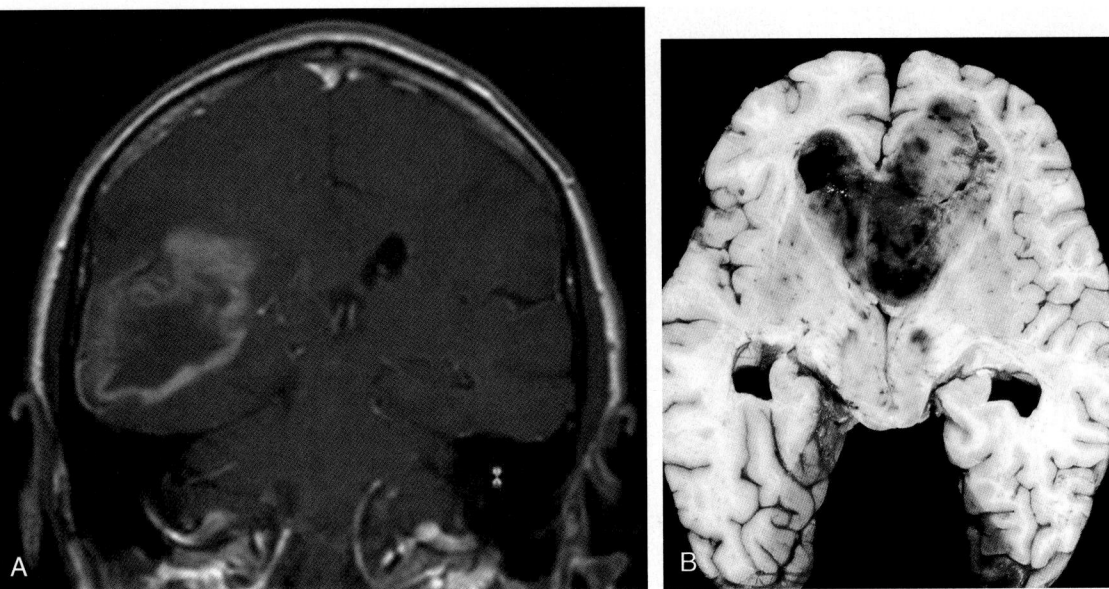

FIGURE 28-46 **A,** Post-contrast T1-weighted coronal MRI shows a large mass in the right parietal lobe with "ring" enhancement. **B,** Glioblastoma appearing as a necrotic, hemorrhagic, infiltrating mass.

a past history of lower-grade astrocytoma *(secondary glioblastoma).* While primary and secondary glioblastomas show some molecular distinctions, the molecular lesions found in the two types of glioblastoma tend to impinge on the same pathways. For example, whereas secondary glioblastomas usually have *p53* mutations, primary astrocytomas more commonly have amplification of *MDM2,* a gene that encodes an inhibitor of p53. Similarly, while secondary glioblastomas have increased signaling through the PDGF-A receptor, primary glioblastomas often have amplified, mutated epidermal growth factor receptor *(EGFR)* genes, which encode aberrant forms of EGFR known as EGFRvIII. Both types of mutations lead to increased receptor tyrosine kinase activity and the activation of the RAS and PI-3 kinase pathways, which

stimulate the growth and survival of tumor cells (Chapter 7). Based on whole genome sequencing, it is estimated that combinations of mutations that activate RAS and PI-3 kinase and inactivate p53 and RB are present in 80% to 90% of primary glioblastomas.[90]

Clinical Features. The presenting symptoms of infiltrating astrocytomas depend, in part, on the location and growth rate of the tumor. Well-differentiated diffuse astrocytomas may remain static or progress only slowly over a number of years; the mean survival is more than 5 years. Eventually, however, clinical deterioration occurs that is usually due to the appearance of a more rapidly growing tumor of higher histologic grade. Radiologic studies show mass effect as well as changes in the brain adjacent to the tumor, such as edema. High-grade astrocytomas have abnormal vessels that are "leaky" and therefore demonstrate contrast enhancement on imaging studies. The prognosis for individuals with glioblastoma is very poor, although the use of newer chemotherapeutic agents has provided some benefit.[92] Methylation of the promoter for the gene encoding the DNA repair enzyme MGMT predicts responsiveness to DNA alkylating drugs—as would be expected since MGMT is critical for the repair of the chemotherapeutically induced DNA modification.[91] Treatment of primary glioblastoma patients with tyrosine kinase inhibitors that target EGFR has produced some encouraging results.[89] With current optimal treatment, consisting of resection followed by radiation therapy and chemotherapy, the mean length of survival after diagnosis has increased to 15 months; 25% of such patients are alive after 2 years. Survival is substantially shorter in older patients, for those with lower performance status, and for large unresectable lesions.

Pilocytic Astrocytoma

Pilocytic astrocytomas (grade I/IV) are distinguished from the other types by their pathologic appearance and relatively

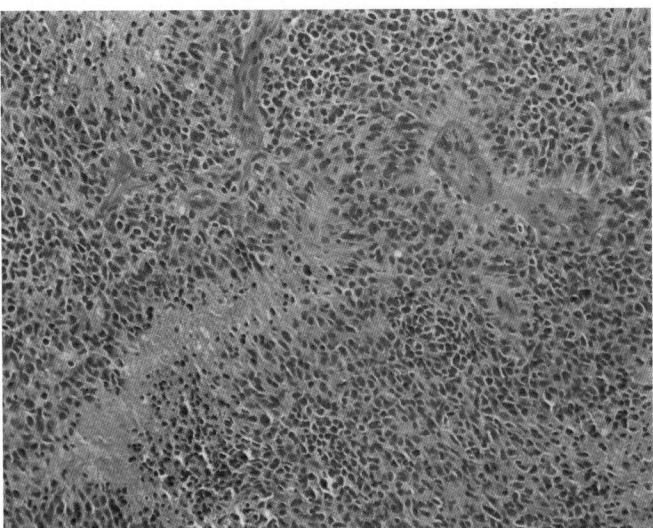

FIGURE 28-47 Glioblastoma. Foci of necrosis with pseudopalisading of malignant nuclei and endothelial cell proliferation.

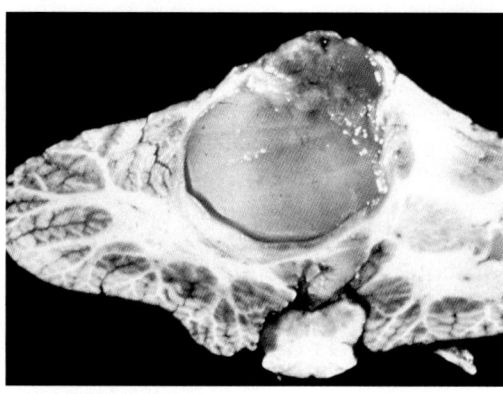

FIGURE 28–48 Pilocytic astrocytoma in the cerebellum with a nodule of tumor in a cyst.

benign behavior. They typically occur in children and young adults, and are usually located in the cerebellum but may also appear in the floor and walls of the third ventricle, the optic nerves, and occasionally the cerebral hemispheres.

Morphology. On macroscopic examination, a pilocytic astrocytoma is often cystic (Fig. 28–48); if solid, it may be well circumscribed or, less frequently, infiltrative. On microscopic examination the tumor is composed of bipolar cells with long, thin "hairlike" processes that are GFAP-positive and form dense fibrillary meshworks; Rosenthal fibers and eosinophilic granular bodies, are often present. Tumors are often biphasic with a loose microcystic pattern in addition to the fibrillary areas. An increase in the number of blood vessels, often with thickened walls or vascular cell proliferation, is seen but does not imply an unfavorable prognosis; necrosis and mitoses are uncommon. Unlike diffuse fibrillary astrocytomas of any grade, pilocytic astrocytomas have a narrow infiltrative border with the surrounding brain.

These tumors grow very slowly, and, in the cerebellum particularly, may be treated by resection. Symptomatic recurrence of incompletely resected lesions is often associated with cyst enlargement rather than growth of the solid component. Tumors that extend into the hypothalamic region from the optic tract can have a more ominous clinical course because of their location. The histologic separation of these tumors from other astrocytomas is supported by the rarity of *p53* mutations or other genetic changes that are found in infiltrating astrocytomas. Those pilocytic astrocytomas that occur in the setting of NF1 show functional loss of neurofibromin; this genetic alteration is not observed in sporadic forms.

Pleomorphic Xanthoastrocytoma

This is a tumor that occurs most often in the temporal lobe of children and young adults, usually with a history of seizures. The tumor consists of neoplastic, occasionally bizarre, astrocytes, which are sometimes lipidized; these cells often express neuronal and glial markers. The degree of nuclear atypia can be extreme and may suggest a high-grade astrocy-

toma, but the presence of abundant reticulin deposits, relative circumscription, and chronic inflammatory cell infiltrates, along with the absence of necrosis and mitotic activity, redirects the pathologist toward the diagnosis. This is usually a low-grade tumor (WHO grade II/IV), with a 5 year survival rate estimated at 80%. Necrosis and mitotic activity are indicative of a higher grade tumor and predict a more aggressive course.

Brainstem Glioma

A clinical subgroup of astrocytomas, brainstem gliomas occur mostly in the first two decades of life and make up about 20% of primary brain tumors in this age group. Several distinct anatomic patterns have been defined in the pediatric age group, each differing in clinical course: intrinsic pontine gliomas (the most common, with an aggressive course and short survival); tumors, often exophytic, arising in the cervicomedullary junction region (with a less aggressive course); and tectal gliomas (with an even more benign course). Among the rarer brainstem gliomas affecting adults, most are intrinsic pontine gliomas. These can be separated into low-grade diffuse fibrillary astrocytomas and glioblastoma, with the expected differences in clinical course and survival.

Oligodendroglioma

These tumors constitute 5% to 15% of gliomas and are most common in the fourth and fifth decades. Patients may have had several years of neurologic complaints, often including seizures. The lesions are found mostly in the cerebral hemispheres, with a predilection for white matter.

Morphology. On gross examination, oligodendrogliomas are well-circumscribed, gelatinous, gray masses, often with cysts, focal hemorrhage, and calcification. On microscopic examination, the tumors are composed of sheets of regular cells with spherical nuclei containing finely granular chromatin (similar to normal oligodendrocytes) surrounded by a clear halo of cytoplasm (Fig. 28–49). The tumor typically contains a delicate network of anastomosing capillaries. Calcification, present in as many as 90% of these tumors, ranges from microscopic foci to massive depositions. As the tumor cells infiltrate cerebral cortex, there is often formation of secondary structures, often with tumor cells arrayed around neurons (perineuronal satellitosis). Mitotic activity is usually very difficult to detect, and proliferation indices are low. Oligodendrogliomas are considered to be WHO grade II/IV lesions.

Anaplastic oligodendrogliomas (WHO grade III/IV) are characterized by increased cell density, nuclear anaplasia, increased mitotic activity, and necrosis. These changes can often be found in nodules within an otherwise grade II/IV oligodendroglioma. Also often present in these higher grade lesions are discrete round cells with cytoplasmic GFAP and nuclei that resemble the other elements of the tumor. These microgemistocytes differ from gemistocytic astro-

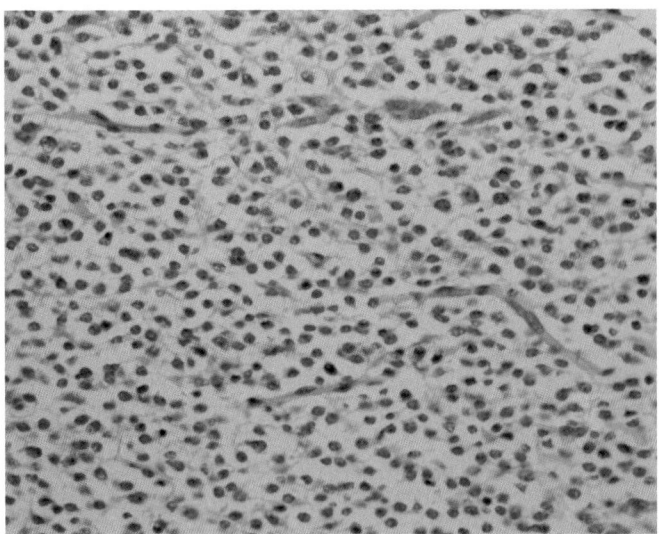

FIGURE 28–49 Oligodendroglioma. Tumor nuclei are round, with cleared cytoplasm forming "halos" and vasculature composed of thin-walled capillaries.

cytes in that they lack abundant processes; the intermediate filaments are restricted to a small lump of cytoplasm. Some of these high-grade oligodendroglial tumors also show patterns that are indistinguishable from glioblastoma. Because several studies have shown that such appearance correlates with worse behavior, these tumors are grouped with glioblastoma.

Molecular Genetics. The underlying molecular abnormalities, along with histologic appearance, distinguish oligodendrogliomas from astrocytic tumors. The most common genetic alterations in oligodendrogliomas are loss of heterozygosity for chromosomes 1p and 19q, seen in up to 80% of cases (depending on the level of histologic stringency in the study). The specific tumor suppressor loci that are involved in the generation of these tumors remain unknown. Additional genetic alterations tend to accumulate with progression to anaplastic oligodendroglioma. The more common of these include loss of 9p, loss of 10q, and mutation in *CDKN2A*. In contrast to high-grade astrocytic tumors, *EGFR* gene amplification is not seen in these tumors, but a significant proportion do show increased EGFR protein levels.

In addition to having implications for the biology of the tumors, the molecular alterations in anaplastic oligodendrogliomas impact treatment. Tumors with loss of 1p and 19q but without other alterations have consistent, long-lasting responses to chemotherapy and radiation.[91] Those with additional genetic changes have shorter-lived responses, and those without loss of 1p and 19q seem to be resistant to therapy.

Clinical Features. In general, individuals with oligodendrogliomas have a better prognosis than do those with astrocytomas. Current treatment with surgery, chemotherapy, and radiation therapy has yielded an average survival of 5 to 10 years. Individuals with anaplastic oligodendroglioma have an overall worse prognosis. Progression from low- to higher-grade lesions occurs, typically over about 6 years.

The terms *oligoastrocytoma* and *anaplastic oligoastrocytoma* refer to neoplasms consisting of distinct regions of oligodendroglioma and astrocytoma. The diagnostic criteria for these entities remain controversial. Despite their biphasic nature, these tumors are monoclonal, and show either 1p/19q deletion or *p53* mutations.

Ependymoma and Related Paraventricular Mass Lesions

Ependymomas, as would be expected, most often arise next to the ependyma-lined ventricular system, including the oft-obliterated central canal of the spinal cord. In the first two decades of life they typically occur near the fourth ventricle and constitute 5% to 10% of the primary brain tumors in this age group. In adults the spinal cord is the most common location; tumors in this site are particularly frequent in the setting of neurofibromatosis type 2 (NF2).

Morphology. In the fourth ventricle, ependymomas are typically solid or papillary masses extending from the floor of the ventricle (Fig. 28–50A). Although ependymomas are moderately well demarcated from adjacent brain, the proximity of vital pontine and medullary nuclei usually makes complete extirpation impossible. In the intra-spinal tumors this sharp demarcation sometimes makes total removal feasible. On microscopic examination ependymomas are composed of cells with regular, round to oval nuclei and abundant granular chromatin. Between the nuclei there is a variably dense fibrillary background. Tumor cells may form glandlike round or elongated structures (rosettes, canals) that resemble the embryologic ependymal canal, with long, delicate processes extending into a lumen (Fig. 28–50B); more frequently present are **perivascular pseudorosettes** (Fig. 28–50B), in which tumor cells are arranged around vessels with an intervening zone consisting of thin ependymal processes directed toward the wall of the vessel. GFAP expression is found in most ependymomas. While most ependymomas are well differentiated and behave as WHO grade II/IV lesions, anaplastic ependymomas (WHO grade III/IV) reveal increased cell density, high mitotic rates, areas of necrosis, and less evident ependymal differentiation.

Myxopapillary ependymomas are distinct but related lesions that occur in the filum terminale of the spinal cord and contain papillary elements in a myxoid background, admixed with ependymoma-like cells. Cuboidal cells, sometimes with clear cytoplasm, are arranged around papillary cores containing connective tissue and blood vessels. The myxoid areas contain neutral and acidic mucopolysaccharides. Prognosis depends on completeness of surgical resection; if the tumor has extended into the subarachnoid space and surrounded the roots of the cauda equina, recurrence is likely.

Molecular Genetics. Given the association of spinal ependymomas with NF2, it is not surprising that the *NF2* gene on

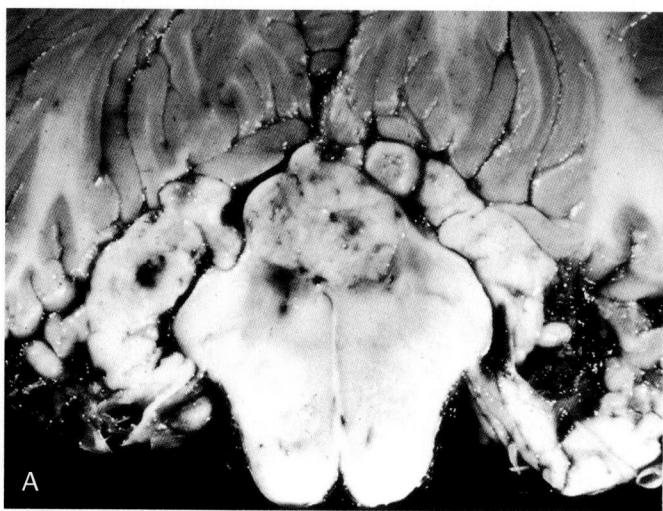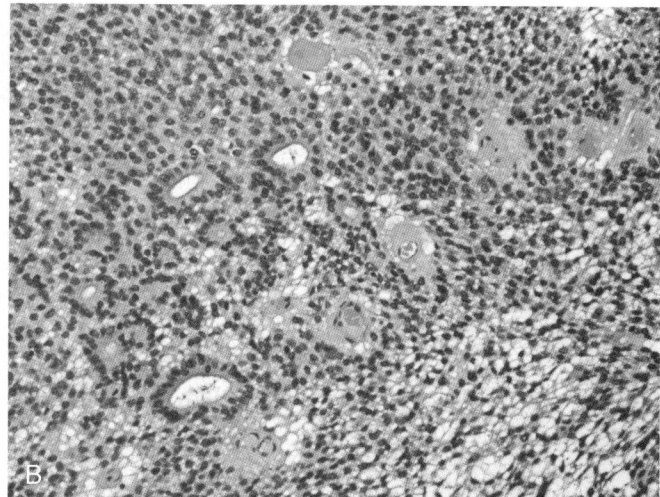

FIGURE 28–50 Ependymoma. **A,** Tumor growing into the fourth ventricle, distorting, compressing, and infiltrating surrounding structures. **B,** Microscopic appearance of ependymoma.

chromosome 22 is commonly mutated in ependymomas in the spinal cord but not at other sites. Supratentorial lesions are more likely to show alterations in chromosome 9. Ependymomas do not seem to share the genetic alterations that are found in other gliomas, such as mutations in *p53*.

Clinical Features. Posterior fossa ependymomas often manifest with hydrocephalus secondary to progressive obstruction of the fourth ventricle rather than invasion of the pons or medulla. Because of the relationship of ependymomas to the ventricular system, CSF dissemination is a common occurrence and portends a poor prognosis. Posterior fossa lesions have the worst overall outcome, particularly in younger children, with a 5-year survival of roughly 50%. The clinical outcome for completely resected supratentorial and spinal ependymomas is better.

Several other tumors occur either immediately below the ependymal lining of the ventricle or in association with the choroid plexus, which sits in continuity with the ependyma. With the exception of the rare choroid plexus carcinoma, these are benign to low-grade lesions; however, their location may cause clinical problems.

- *Subependymomas* are solid, sometimes calcified, slow-growing nodules attached to the ventricular lining and protruding into the ventricle. They are usually asymptomatic and are incidental findings at autopsy or imaging; if they are sufficiently large or strategically located, they may cause hydrocephalus. They are most often found in the lateral and fourth ventricles and have a characteristic microscopic appearance, with clumps of ependymal-appearing nuclei scattered in a dense, fine, glial fibrillar background.
- *Choroid plexus papillomas* can occur anywhere along the choroid plexus and are most common in children, in whom they are usually found in the lateral ventricles. In adults, they more often involve the fourth ventricle. These markedly papillary growths almost exactly recapitulate the structure of the normal choroid plexus. The papillae have connective tissue stalks covered with a cuboidal or columnar epithelium. Clinically, choroid plexus papillomas usually present with hydrocephalus due to obstruction of

the ventricular system by tumor or to overproduction of CSF. The far rarer *choroid plexus carcinomas* resemble adenocarcinoma. These tumors are usually found in children; in adults, they must be differentiated from the much more common metastatic carcinoma.

- *Colloid cyst of the third ventricle* is a non-neoplastic lesion that most often occurs in young adults. The cyst is attached to the roof of the third ventricle, where it can obstruct one or both of the foramina of Monro and, as a result, causes noncommunicating hydrocephalus, which may be rapidly fatal. Headache, sometimes positional, is an important clinical symptom. The cyst has a thin, fibrous capsule and a lining of low to flat cuboidal epithelium; it contains gelatinous, proteinaceous material.

NEURONAL TUMORS

The most common CNS tumor containing mature-appearing neurons (ganglion cells) is *ganglioglioma*, since there is usually an admixed glial neoplasm. Most of these tumors are slow growing, but the glial component occasionally becomes frankly anaplastic, and the disease then progresses rapidly. Lesions that contain mixtures of neuronal and glial elements often present as a seizure disorder; surgical resection of the tumor is usually effective in controlling the seizures.

> **Morphology.** Gangliogliomas are most commonly found in the temporal lobe and often have a cystic component. The neoplastic ganglion cells are irregularly clustered and have apparently random orientation of neurites. Binucleate forms are frequent. The glial component of these lesions usually resembles a low-grade astrocytoma, lacking mitotic activity and necrosis.

Dysembryoplastic neuroepithelial tumor is a rare, low-grade tumor of childhood that often presents as a seizure disorder, and has a relatively good prognosis after surgical resection. These lesions are typically located in the superficial temporal lobe, although other cortical sites are seen. There is often attenuation of the overlying skull, suggesting that the lesion has been present for a long time.

> **Morphology.** These lesions typically form multiple discrete intracortical nodules of small, round cells, arranged in columns around central cores of processes, and are associated with a myxoid background, known as the "specific glioneuronal element." There are well-differentiated "floating neurons" that sit in the pools of mucopolysaccharide-rich fluid of the myxoid background. The larger neurons and the small, round cells of the specific element express neuronal markers. Surrounding the nodules, there may be focal cortical dysplasia and sometimes low-grade astrocytoma. Lesions that show both the specific element and a glial component are termed **complex**.

Central neurocytoma typically is a low-grade neuronal neoplasm found within the ventricular system (most commonly the lateral or third ventricles), characterized by evenly spaced, round, uniform nuclei and often islands of neuropil. Although in pattern and shape the cells resemble oligodendroglioma, ultrastructural and immunohistochemical studies reveal the neuronal lineage of the tumor cells.

POORLY DIFFERENTIATED NEOPLASMS

Some tumors, though of neuroectodermal origin, express few if any of the phenotypic markers of mature cells of the nervous system and are described as poorly differentiated, or embryonal, meaning that they retain cellular features of primitive, undifferentiated cells. The most common is the *medulloblastoma*, which accounts for 20% of the brain tumors in children.

Medulloblastoma

This tumor occurs predominantly in children and exclusively in the cerebellum (by definition). Neuronal and glial markers may be expressed, but the tumor is often largely undifferentiated.

> **Morphology.** In children, medulloblastomas are located in the midline of the cerebellum, but lateral locations are more often found in adults. Rapid growth may occlude the flow of CSF, leading to hydrocephalus. The tumor is often well circumscribed, gray, and friable, and may be seen extending to the surface of the cerebellar folia and involving the leptomeninges (Fig. 28–51A). On microscopic examination medulloblastoma is extremely cellular, with sheets of anaplastic cells (Fig. 28–51B). Individual tumor cells are small, with scant cytoplasm and hyperchromatic nuclei that are frequently elongated or crescent shaped. Mitoses are abundant, and markers of cellular proliferation, such as Ki-67, are detected in a high percentage of the cells. The tumor may express neuronal (neurosecretory granules or

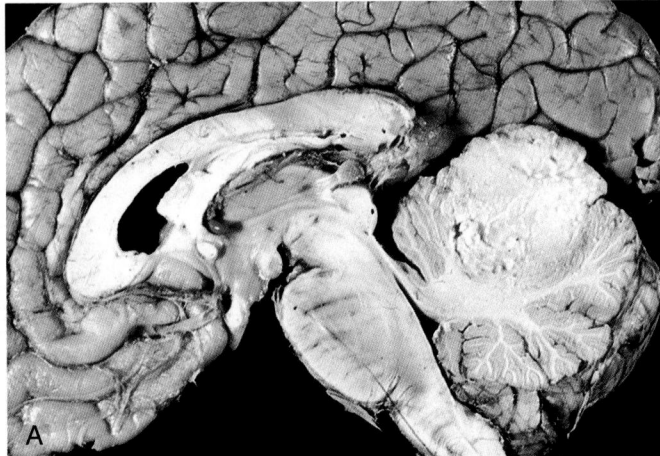
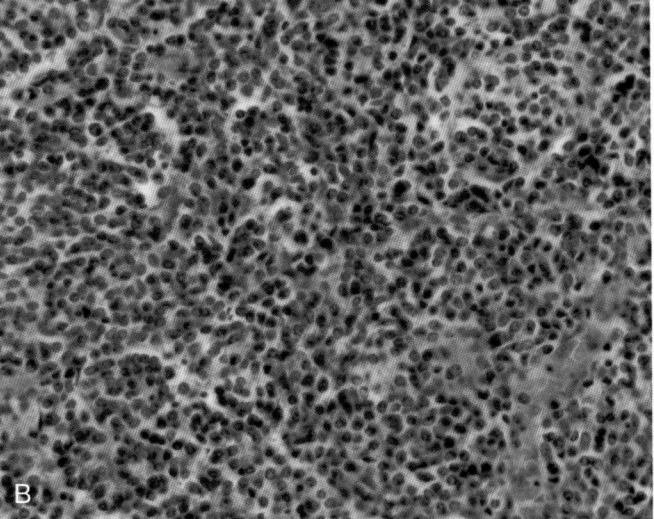

FIGURE 28–51 Medulloblastoma. **A,** Sagittal section of brain showing medulloblastoma destroying the superior midline cerebellum. **B,** Microscopic appearance of medulloblastoma.

> Homer Wright rosettes, as occur in neuroblastoma; Chapter 10) and glial (GFAP+) phenotypes. The **desmoplastic variant** is characterized by areas of stromal response, marked by collagen and reticulin deposition and nodules of cells forming "pale islands" that have more neuropil and show greater expression of neuronal markers.
>
> At the edges of the main tumor mass, medulloblastoma cells have a propensity to form linear chains of cells infiltrating through cerebellar cortex to aggregate beneath the pia, penetrate the pia, and seed into the subarachnoid space. Dissemination through the CSF is a common complication, presenting as nodular masses elsewhere in the CNS, including metastases to the cauda equina that are sometimes termed **drop metastases**.

Molecular Genetics. The most common genetic alteration is loss of material from 17p, with an abnormal chromosome derived from duplication of this chromosome's long arm (isochromosome 17q or i(17q)). Loss of 17p signals a poor prognosis. *MYC* amplification may also be found and is also associated with a more aggressive clinical course. Several other signaling pathways involved in normal cerebellar development are altered in subsets of medulloblastoma. These include the sonic hedgehog–patched pathway (involved in control of normal proliferation of cerebellar granule cells), the WNT signaling pathway (including APC and β-catenin), and Notch signaling pathway. Tumors that have increased levels of neurotrophin receptor TRKC have a better clinical outcome, as do those that show nuclear accumulation of β-catenin.

Clinical Features. The tumor is highly malignant, and the prognosis for untreated patients is dismal; however, it is exquisitely radiosensitive. With total excision and irradiation, the 5-year survival rate may be as high as 75%.

Tumors of similar histology and poor degree of differentiation, resembling medulloblastomas, can be found in the cerebral hemispheres. These lesions are known as CNS supratentorial primitive neuroectodermal tumors (CNS PNET). This term can lead to confusion with the peripheral lesion (peripheral neuroectodermal tumor), that shares a genetic alteration with Ewing sarcoma. In the CNS, PNET is genetically distinct from medulloblastoma and from the peripheral tumor.

Atypical Teratoid/Rhabdoid Tumor

This highly malignant tumor of young children occurs in the posterior fossa and supratentorial compartments in nearly equal proportions. The presence of rhabdoid cells, resembling those of a rhabdomyosarcoma, is the defining characteristic of the lesion.

> **Morphology.** Atypical teratoid/rhabdoid tumors tend to be large, with a soft consistency, and spread along the surface of the brain. The rhabdoid cells have eosinophilic cytoplasm, sharp cell borders and eccentrically located nuclei. When these cells are smaller the cytoplasm can take on an elongated appearance that mimics a rhabdomyosarcoma cell. The cytoplasm of the rhabdoid cell contains intermediate filaments and is immunoreactive for epithelial membrane antigen and vimentin. Some other markers that may be positive include smooth muscle actin and keratins. Other muscle markers such as desmin and myoglobin are not present. Rhabdoid cells are rarely a majority of the tumor; instead, islands of tumor with this pattern of differentiation are mixed with a small-cell component, as well as other histologic patterns (including mesenchymal and epithelial). Mitotic activity is extremely prominent.

Molecular Genetics. Consistent genetic alterations in chromosome 22 (>90% of cases) are a hallmark of rhabdoid tumor. The relevant gene is *hSNF5/INI1*, which encodes a protein that is part of a large complex involved in chromatin remodeling; functional deletions of the locus and loss of nuclear staining for INI1 protein are seen in the majority of tumors.

Clinical Features. These are highly aggressive tumors of the very young. Nearly all tumors occurr before the age of 5 and most patients live less than a year after diagnosis.

OTHER PARENCHYMAL TUMORS

Primary CNS Lymphoma

Primary CNS lymphoma accounts for 2% of extra-nodal lymphomas and 1% of intra-cranial tumors. It is the most common CNS neoplasm in immunosuppressed individuals, including those with AIDS and immunosuppression after transplantation. In non-immunosuppressed populations, the age spectrum is relatively wide, and the frequency increases after 60 years of age.

The term *primary* emphasizes the distinction between these lesions and secondary involvement of the CNS by lymphoma arising elsewhere in the body (Chapter 13). Primary brain lymphoma is often multifocal within the brain parenchyma, yet nodal, bone marrow, or extra-nodal involvement outside of the CNS is a rare and late complication. Conversely, lymphoma arising outside the CNS rarely involves the brain parenchyma; involvement of the nervous system, when it occurs in lymphoma, is usually manifested by the presence of malignant cells within the CSF and around intradural nerve roots, and occasionally by the infiltration of superficial areas of the cerebrum or spinal cord by malignant cells.

Most primary brain lymphomas are of B-cell origin. In the setting of immunosuppression, the cells in nearly all such tumors are latently infected by Epstein-Barr virus. Overall, primary lymphomas of the CNS are aggressive, with relatively poor response to chemotherapy compared with peripheral lymphomas.

> **Morphology.** Lesions are frequently multiple and often involve deep gray matter as well as white matter and cortex. Periventricular spread is common. The tumors are relatively well defined in comparison with glial neoplasms but are not as discrete as metastases and often show extensive areas of central necrosis. Diffuse large-cell B-cell lymphomas are the most common histologic group. Within the tumor malignant cells infiltrate the parenchyma of the brain and accumulate around blood vessels. Reticulin stains demonstrate that the infiltrating cells are separated from one another by silver-staining material; this pattern, referred to as "hooping," is characteristic of primary brain lymphoma. In addition to expressing B-cell markers, most of the cells also express BCL-6; when tumors arise in the setting of immunosuppression, various markers of Epstein-Barr viral infection can be used as an aid in diagnosis.

Intravascular lymphoma, an unusual lymphoid malignancy in which the tumor cells grow intraluminally within small vessels, often involves the brain along with other regions of the body.[93] Instead of presenting as a mass lesion, the occlusion of vessels by malignant cells can result in widespread microscopic infarcts. Affected individuals present with evidence of multifocal lesions, with the differential diagnosis usually including processes such as vasculitis and showers of emboli.

Germ Cell Tumors

Primary brain germ cell tumors occur along the midline, most commonly in the pineal and the suprasellar regions. They account for 0.2% to 1% of brain tumors in people of European descent but up to 10% in Japanese people. They are tumors of the young, with 90% occurring during the first two decades. Germ cell tumors, particularly teratomas, are among the more common congenital tumors. Germ cell tumors in the pineal region show a strong male predominance, which is not seen in suprasellar lesions.

The source of germ cells in the CNS is not clear; they may be "rests" that remain in the CNS or perhaps migrate there from other sites late in development. Germ cell tumors share many features with their counterparts in the gonads. In contrast to lymphomas, however, metastasis of a gonadal germ cell tumor to the CNS is not uncommon; thus, the presence of a non-CNS primary tumor must be excluded before a diagnosis of primary germ cell tumor is made. The histologic classification of brain germ cell tumors is similar to that used in the testis (Chapter 21), but the tumor that is histologically similar to the seminoma in the testis is referred to as germinoma in the CNS. The responses to radiation therapy and chemotherapy roughly parallel those of similar histologic lesions at other sites. As in the periphery, CSF levels of tumor markers including α-fetoprotein and β-human chorionic gonadotropin can be used to aid in diagnosis and track response to therapy.

Pineal Parenchymal Tumors

These lesions arise from specialized cells of the pineal gland (pineocytes) that have features of neuronal differentiation. The tumors range from well-differentiated lesions (*pineocytomas*, with areas of neuropil, cells with small, round nuclei, and no evidence of mitoses or necrosis) to high-grade tumors (*pineoblastomas*, with little evidence of neuronal differentiation, densely packed small cells with necrosis, and frequent mitotic figures). High-grade pineal tumors tend to affect children, while lower-grade lesions are found more often in adults. The highly aggressive pineoblastoma commonly spreads throughout the CSF space. It occurs with increased frequency in individuals with germline mutations in *RB* (so-called trilateral retinoblastoma). Gliomas are also found in the pineal region, arising from the glial stroma of the gland. Often low grade, these gliomas can be difficult to distinguish from the glial reaction that can accompany non-neoplastic pineal region cysts.

MENINGIOMAS

Meningiomas are predominantly benign tumors of adults, usually attached to the dura, that arise from the meningothelial cell of the arachnoid. Meningiomas may be found along any of the external surfaces of the brain as well as within the ventricular system, where they arise from the stromal arachnoid cells of the choroid plexus. Prior radiation therapy, typically decades earlier, is a risk factor for development of meningiomas. Other tumors such as metastases, solitary fibrous tumors, and a range of poorly differentiated sarcomas may also grow as dural-based masses.

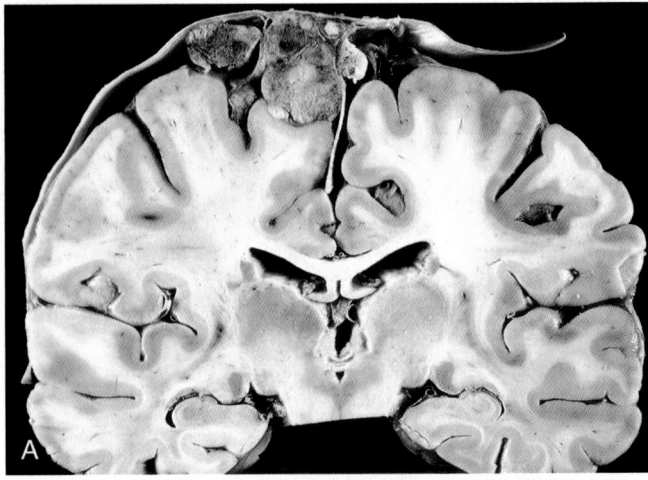
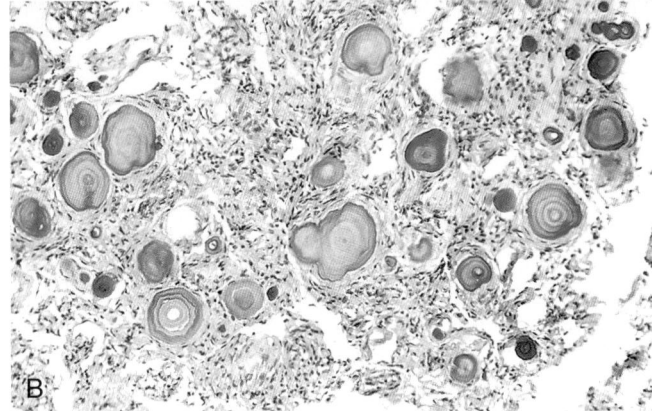

FIGURE 28–52 **A,** Parasagittal multilobular meningioma attached to the dura with compression of underlying brain. **B,** Meningioma with a whorled pattern of cell growth and psammoma bodies.

Morphology. Meningiomas are usually rounded masses with well-defined dural bases that compress underlying brain but are easily separated from it (Fig. 28–52A). Extension into the overlying bone may be present. The surface of the mass is usually encapsulated with thin, fibrous tissue and may have a bosselated or polypoid appearance. They may also grow **en plaque**, in which the tumor spreads in a sheetlike fashion along the surface of the dura. This form is commonly associated with hyperostotic reactive changes in the overlying bone. The lesions range from firm and fibrous to finely gritty, or they may contain numerous calcified psammoma bodies. Gross evidence of necrosis or extensive hemorrhage is not present.

Most meningiomas have a relatively low risk of recurrence or aggressive growth, and so are considered WHO grade I/IV. Various histologic patterns are observed, with no prognostic significance. These include **syncytial** ("meningothelial"), appropriately named for the whorled clusters of cells that sit in tight groups without visible cell membranes; **fibroblastic**, with elongated cells and abundant collagen deposition between them; **transitional**, which share features of the syncytial and fibroblastic types; **psammoma-**

tous, with psammoma bodies, apparently formed from calcification of the syncytial nests of meningothelial cells (Fig. 28–52B); **secretory**, with PAS-positive intracytoplasmic droplets and intracellular lumens by electron microscopy; and **microcystic**, with a loose, spongy appearance. Xanthomatous degeneration, metaplasia (often osseous), and moderate nuclear pleomorphism are common in meningiomas. Among these lesions, proliferation index has been shown to be a predictor of biologic behavior.

Atypical meningiomas (WHO grade II/IV) are lesions with a higher rate of recurrence and more aggressive local growth, and may require radiation therapy in addition to surgery. They are distinguished from lower grade meningiomas by the presence of either a mitotic index of four or more mitoses per 10 high power fields or at least three atypical features (increased cellularity, small cells with a high nuclear-to-cytoplasmic ratio, prominent nucleoli, patternless growth, or necrosis). Certain histologic patterns (**clear cell** and **chordoid**) are also considered to be grade II/IV because of their more aggressive behavior.

Anaplastic (malignant) meningioma (WHO grade III/IV) is a highly aggressive tumor with the appearance of a high-grade sarcoma, but retaining some histologic evidence of meningothelial origin. Mitotic rates are often extremely high (>20 mitoses per 10 high power fields). **Papillary** meningioma (with pleomorphic cells arranged around fibrovascular cores) and **rhabdoid** meningioma (with sheets of tumor cells with hyaline eosinophilic cytoplasm containing intermediate filaments) both have such a high propensity to recur that they are also considered to be WHO grade III/IV tumors.

While most meningiomas are easily separable from the brain even if they displace it, some tumors infiltrate the brain. This can occur with broad, pushing edges or as single cells. The presence of brain invasion is associated with increased risk of recurrence but does not alter the histologic grade of the lesion. Meningiomas are commonly immunoreactive for epithelial membrane antigen, in contrast to other tumors arising in this region, although with a higher grade, this may be less prominent. Keratin is restricted to lesions with the secretory pattern, and these tumors are also positive for carcinoembryonic antigen.

Molecular Genetics. The most common cytogenetic abnormality is loss of chromosome 22, especially the long arm (22q). The deletions include the region of 22q12 that harbors the *NF2* gene, which encodes the protein merlin; as expected, meningiomas are a common lesion in the setting of NF2 (see later). Of sporadic fibroblastic, transitional and psammomatous meningiomas, 50% to 60% harbor mutations in the *NF2* gene; most of these mutations are predicted to result in absence of functional merlin protein. Higher grade meningiomas often accumulate other genetic alterations as well; several studies have also supported the existence of a locus on chromosome 22 distinct from *NF2* as contributing to meningiomas.

Clinical Features. Meningiomas are usually slow-growing lesions that present either with vague nonlocalizing symptoms or with focal findings referable to compression of underlying brain. Common sites of involvement include the parasagittal aspect of the brain convexity, dura over the lateral convexity, wing of the sphenoid, olfactory groove, sella turcica, and foramen magnum. They are uncommon in children and generally show a moderate (3:2) female predominance, although the ratio is 10:1 for spinal meningiomas, which are also commonly psammomatous. Lesions are usually solitary, but when present at multiple sites, especially in association with acoustic neuromas or glial tumors, a diagnosis of NF2 should be considered. Clonality studies indicate that multiple lesions are much more likely to represent dissemination from a single tumor rather than distinct tumors. Meningiomas often express progesterone receptors and may grow more rapidly during pregnancy.

METASTATIC TUMORS

Metastatic lesions, mostly carcinomas, account for approximately a quarter to half of intra-cranial tumors in hospitalized patients. The five most common primary sites are lung, breast, skin (melanoma), kidney, and gastrointestinal tract, accounting for about 80% of all metastases. Some rare tumors (e.g., choriocarcinoma) have a high likelihood of metastasizing to the brain, whereas some more common tumors (e.g., prostatic carcinoma) almost never grow in the brain, even when they are metastatic to adjacent bone and dura. The meninges are also a frequent site of involvement by metastatic disease. Metastatic tumors present clinically as mass lesions and may occasionally be the first manifestation of the cancer. In general, there is a benefit to quality of life from localized treatment of solitary brain metastases. Metastases to the epidural or subdural space can cause spinal cord compression, which requires emergency treatment.

Morphology. Intraparenchymal metastases form sharply demarcated masses, often at the junction of gray matter and white matter, usually surrounded by a zone of edema. The boundary between tumor and brain parenchyma is well defined microscopically as well, although melanoma is one tumor that does not always follow this rule. Nodules of tumor, often with central areas of necrosis, are surrounded by reactive gliosis. Meningeal carcinomatosis, with tumor nodules studding the surface of the brain, spinal cord, and intradural nerve roots, is associated particularly with carcinoma of the lung and the breast.

PARANEOPLASTIC SYNDROMES

In addition to the direct and localized effects produced by metastases, *paraneoplastic syndromes* may involve the peripheral and central nervous systems, sometimes even preceding the clinical recognition of the malignant neoplasm.[94,95] A variety of specific clinical syndromes have been described.[96] The major underlying mechanism of paraneoplastic syndromes appears to be the development of an immune response against tumor antigens that cross-react with antigens in the central or peripheral nervous systems. The relationship among the underlying malignant process, the clinical features, and the target antigens is unclear. Some tumor types are associated with multiple types of autoantibodies, and the same antibodies can be present in different clinical syndromes. Among the well-recognized syndromes are various patterns of encephalomyelitis:

- *Subacute cerebellar degeneration,* with destruction of Purkinje cells, gliosis, and a mild inflammatory infiltrate, can be present.
- *Limbic encephalitis,* characterized by subacute dementia and marked by perivascular inflammatory cuffs, microglial nodules, some neuronal loss, and gliosis, most evident in the anterior and medial portions of the temporal lobe and resembling an infectious process. A comparable process involving the brainstem can be seen in isolation or together with limbic system involvement.
- *Eye movement disorders,* most commonly opsoclonus, may be found, often in association with other evidence of cerebellar and brainstem dysfunction. In children this is most commonly associated with neuroblastoma and is found along with myoclonus.

The peripheral nervous system can also be affected:

- *Subacute sensory neuropathy* may be found in association with limbic encephalitis or in isolation. It is marked by loss of sensory neurons from dorsal root ganglia, in association with lymphocytic inflammation.
- *Lambert-Eaton myasthenic syndrome,* caused by antibodies against the voltage-gated calcium channel in the presynaptic elements of the neuromuscular junction. This can be seen in the absence of malignancy as well.

For some disorders, such as limbic encephalitis associated with antibodies against voltage-gated potassium channels, there is evidence that therapies aimed at reducing the antibody titer result in clinical improvement. In other settings there remain questions as to how an immune response to intracellular proteins elicits disease, whether the antibodies are directly pathogenic or merely a marker of the disease, and even which components of the immune system are critically involved.

PERIPHERAL NERVE SHEATH TUMORS

These tumors arise from cells of the peripheral nerve, including Schwann cells, perineurial cells, and fibroblasts. Many express Schwann cell characteristics, including the presence of S-100 antigen as well as the potential for melanocytic differentiation. There is a transition between myelination by oligodendrocytes (central myelin) and myelination by Schwann cells (peripheral myelin) that occurs within several millimeters of the substance of the brain. Thus, peripheral nerve tumors can arise within the dura, as well as along the peripheral course of nerves. The various forms of peripheral nerve sheath tumors are also associated with the two forms of neurofibromatosis (discussed below with "Familial Tumor Syndromes").

Schwannoma

These benign tumors arise from the neural crest–derived Schwann cell and cause symptoms by local compression of the involved nerve or adjacent structures (such as brainstem or spinal cord). Schwannomas are a component of NF2, and even sporadic schwannomas are commonly associated with inactivating mutations in the *NF2* gene on chromosome 22. Loss of expression of the *NF2* gene product, *merlin,* is a consistent finding in all schwannomas. Merlin normally restricts the cell-surface expression of growth factor receptors, such as EGFR, through interactions involving the actin cytoskeleton; in its absence, cells hyperproliferate in response to growth factors.

Morphology. Schwannomas are well-circumscribed, encapsulated masses that are attached to the nerve but can be separated from it (Fig. 28–53A). Tumors form firm, gray masses that may have areas of cystic and xanthomatous change. On microscopic examination tumors show a **mixture of two growth patterns** (Fig. 28–53B). In the **Antoni A** pattern of growth, elongated cells with cytoplasmic processes are arranged in fascicles in areas of moderate to high cellularity and scant stromal matrix; the "nuclear-free zones" of processes that lie between the regions of nuclear palisading are termed **Verocay bodies.** In the **Antoni B** pattern of

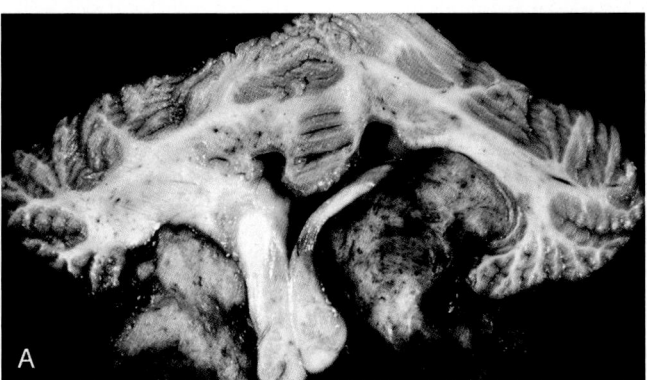
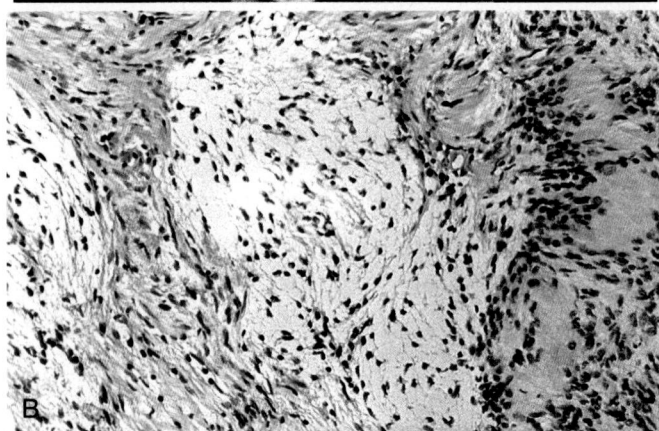

FIGURE 28–53 Schwannoma. **A,** Bilateral eighth-nerve schwannomas. **B,** Tumor showing cellular areas (Antoni A), including Verocay bodies *(far right),* as well as looser, myxoid regions (Antoni B, *center*). (**A,** Courtesy of the late Dr. K.M. Earle.)

growth, the tumor is less densely cellular and consists of a loose meshwork of cells, microcysts and myxoid stroma. In both areas the individual cells have an elongated shape and regular oval nuclei. Electron microscopy shows basement membrane deposits encasing single cells and collagen fibers. Because the lesion displaces the nerve of origin as it grows, silver stains or immunostains for neurofilament proteins demonstrate that axons are largely excluded from the tumor, although they may become entrapped in the capsule. The Schwann cell origin of these tumors is borne out by their S-100 immunoreactivity. A variety of degenerative changes may be found in schwannomas, including nuclear pleomorphism, xanthomatous change, and vascular hyalinization. Malignant change is extremely rare, but local recurrence can follow incomplete resection.

Clinical Features. Within the cranial vault most schwannomas occur at the cerebellopontine angle, where they are attached to the vestibular branch of the eighth nerve. Affected individuals often present with tinnitus and hearing loss; the tumor is often referred to as an "acoustic neuroma," although it actually is a vestibular schwannoma. Elsewhere within the dura, sensory nerves are preferentially involved, including branches of the trigeminal nerve and dorsal roots. When extradural, schwannomas are most commonly found in association with large nerve trunks, where motor and sensory modalities are intermixed.

Neurofibroma

Neurofibromas can present as discrete localized masses—most commonly as a *cutaneous neurofibroma* or in peripheral nerve as a *solitary neurofibroma*—or as an infiltrative lesion growing within and expanding a peripheral nerve *(plexiform neurofibroma)*. The presence of either multiple neurofibromas or plexiform neurofibromas strongly suggests the diagnosis of neurofibromatosis type 1 (NF1). Skin lesions grow as nodules, sometimes with overlying hyperpigmentation; they may become large and pedunculated. The risk of malignant transformation of these tumors is extremely small, and they are mostly of cosmetic concern. In contrast, plexiform tumors may result in significant neurologic deficits when they involve major nerve trunks, are difficult to remove because of their intraneural spread, and have a significant potential for malignant transformation.

Morphology

Cutaneous Neurofibroma. Present in the dermis and subcutaneous fat, these well-delineated but unencapsulated masses are composed of spindle cells. Although they are not invasive, the adnexal structures are sometimes enwrapped by the edges of the lesion. The stroma of these tumors is highly collagenized and contains little myxoid material. Lesions within peripheral nerves are of identical histologic appearance.

Plexiform Neurofibroma. These tumors may arise anywhere along a nerve, although the large nerve trunks are most commonly involved. They are frequently multiple. The affected nerves are irregularly expanded, as each of the fascicles is infiltrated by the neoplasm. Unlike schwannomas, it is not possible to separate the lesion from the nerve. The proximal and distal extremes of the tumor may have poorly defined margins, as fingers of tumor and individual neoplastic cells insert themselves between the nerve fibers. On microscopic examination, the lesion has a loose, myxoid background with a low cellularity. Several cell types are present, including Schwann cells with typical elongated nuclei and extensions of pink cytoplasm, larger multipolar fibroblastic cells, and a sprinkling of inflammatory cells, including mast cells. Although the myxoid stroma dominates, there are often areas of collagen bundles, which have a "shredded carrot" appearance. In contrast to schwannomas, axons can be demonstrated within the tumor.

Alterations in both copies of the *NF1* gene have been consistently observed in the Schwann cell components of plexiform neurofibromas, supporting a critical role for loss of NF1 function in the genesis of this tumor. The product of the *NF1* gene (*neurofibromin*) stimulates the activity of a GTPase that inhibits RAS activity (recall that RAS is active only when bound to GTP).

Malignant Peripheral Nerve Sheath Tumor

Malignant peripheral nerve sheath tumors are highly malignant tumors that are locally invasive, frequently with multiple recurrences and eventual metastatic spread. They are most commonly associated with medium to large nerves, rather than either cranial nerves or distal small nerves. While many occur sporadically, close to 50% of cases arise in the setting of NF1—either from transformation of a plexiform neurofibroma or following radiation therapy. *NF1* function is lost at an early stage of development of malignant peripheral nerve sheath tumors; subsequent alterations often disrupt both the p53- and RB-dependent pathways for regulation of cell proliferation.

Morphology

Morphology. The lesions are poorly defined tumor masses that frequently infiltrate along the axis of the parent nerve and invade adjacent soft tissues. On microscopic examination a wide range of histologic findings can be encountered. Patterns reminiscent of fibrosarcoma or pleomorphic sarcoma may be found. In other areas the tumor cells resemble Schwann cells, with elongated nuclei and prominent bipolar processes. Fascicle formation may be present. Mitoses, necrosis, and extreme nuclear anaplasia are common. Some but not all tumors are immunoreactive for S-100 protein. In addition, a wide variety of "divergent" histologic patterns may be admixed, including epithelial structures, rhabdomyoblastic differentiation (termed **Triton tumors**), cartilage, and even bone. **Epithelioid malignant schwannomas** are aggressive variants with tumor cells that have visible cell borders and grow in nests. They are immunoreactive for S-100 but not for keratin, allowing distinction from true epithelial tumors.

FAMILIAL TUMOR SYNDROMES

A variety of inherited diseases are associated with the occurrence of tumors. In most, the pattern of inheritance is autosomal dominant, with involvement of tumor suppressor genes.[97] In several of these syndromes, tumors of the nervous system are a prominent aspect of the disease and are discussed below. Other syndromes include tumors of the CNS as part of their spectrum, but the bulk of disease burden lies elsewhere. These include:

- *Cowden syndrome:* Dysplastic ganglioglicytoma of the cerebellum (Lhermitte-Duclos disease), caused by mutations in *PTEN* resulting in increased activity of AKT and mTOR pathways
- *Li-Fraumeni syndrome:* Medulloblastomas, caused by mutations in *p53* (Chapter 7)
- *Turcot syndrome:* Medulloblastoma or glioblastoma, caused by mutations in *APC* or mismatch repair genes (as for familial colon cancer; Chapter 17)
- *Gorlin syndrome:* Medulloblastoma, caused by mutations in the *PTCH* gene resulting in up-regulation of sonic hedgehog signaling pathways (Chapter 25).

Neurofibromatosis Type 1

This autosomal dominant disorder, one of the more common genetic disorders, having a frequency of 1 in 3000, is characterized by neurofibromas (plexiform and solitary), gliomas of the optic nerve, pigmented nodules of the iris *(Lisch nodules)*, and cutaneous hyperpigmented macules *(café au lait spots)*. In individuals with NF1 there is a propensity for the neurofibromas, particularly plexiform neurofibromas, to undergo malignant degeneration at a higher rate than that observed for comparable tumors in the general population. As described earlier under "Neurofibroma", the *NF1* gene, located at 17q11.2, encodes neurofibromin—a large protein with a GTPase-activating domain that inhibits RAS. The tumor cells in NF1-related tumors lack NF1 expression due to biallelic inactivation of the gene.

The course of the disease is highly variable; some individuals who carry a mutated gene have no symptoms, while others develop progressive disease with spinal deformities, disfiguring lesions, and compression of vital structures, including the spinal cord.

Neurofibromatosis Type 2 (NF2)

This is an autosomal dominant disorder resulting in a range of tumors, most commonly bilateral eighth-nerve schwannomas and multiple meningiomas. Gliomas, typically ependymomas of the spinal cord, also occur in these patients. Many individuals with NF2 also have non-neoplastic lesions, which include nodular ingrowth of Schwann cells into the spinal cord (schwannosis), meningioangiomatosis (a proliferation of meningeal cells and blood vessels that grows into the brain), and glial hamartia (microscopic nodular collections of glial cells at abnormal locations, often in the superficial and deep layers of cerebral cortex). This disorder is much less common than NF1, having a frequency of 1 in 40,000 to 50,000.

The *NF2* gene is located on chromosome 22q12, and the gene product, merlin, shows structural similarity to a series of cytoskeletal proteins; the *NF2* gene is also commonly mutated in sporadic meningiomas and schwannomas. The protein is believed to regulate membrane receptor signaling, including contact growth inhibition.[98] There is some correlation between the type of mutation and clinical symptoms, with nonsense and frameshift mutations causing a more severe phenotype than missense mutations.

Tuberous Sclerosis Complex

Tuberous sclerosis is an autosomal dominant syndrome, occurring at a frequency of approximately 1 in 6000 births. It is characterized by the development of hamartomas and benign neoplasms involving the brain and other tissues. Hamartomas within the CNS take the form of cortical tubers and subependymal nodules; subependymal giant-cell astrocytomas are low grade neoplasms that appear to develop from the hamartomatous nodules in the same location. Cortical tubers are often epileptogenic, and surgical resection can be beneficial when medical management of the seizures is difficult. Elsewhere in the body, lesions include renal angiomyolipomas, retinal glial hamartomas, pulmonary lymphangioleiomyomatosis and cardiac rhabdomyomas. Cysts may be found at various sites, including the liver, kidneys, and pancreas. Cutaneous lesions include angiofibromas, localized leathery thickenings (shagreen patches), hypopigmented areas (ash-leaf patches), and subungual fibromas.

One tuberous sclerosis locus (*TSC1*) is found on chromosome 9q34, and it encodes a protein known as hamartin; the more commonly mutated tuberous sclerosis locus (*TSC2*) is at 16p13.3 and encodes tuberin. These two proteins bind, forming a complex that inhibits the kinase mTOR, which is a key regulator of protein synthesis and other aspects of anabolic metabolism. Of note, mTOR is well-known to control cell size, and the tumors associated with tuberous sclerosis are remarkable for having voluminous amounts of cytoplasm, particularly giant-cell astrocytomas in the CNS, and cardiac rhabdomyomas. Cortical and subependymal tubers are associated with an intact copy of the wild-type allele, while in subependymal giant-cell astrocytomas there is biallelic loss. Treatment is symptomatic, including anticonvulsant therapy for control of seizures.

Morphology. Cortical hamartomas of tuberous sclerosis are firm areas of the cortex that, in contrast to the softer adjacent cortex, have been likened to potatoes, hence the appellation "tubers." These hamartomas are composed of haphazardly arranged neurons that lack the normal laminar organization of neocortex. In addition, some large cells have appearances intermediate between glia and neurons (large vesicular nuclei with nucleoli, resembling neurons, and abundant eosinophilic cytoplasm like gemistocytic astrocytes) and often express intermediate filaments of both neuronal (neurofilament) and glial (GFAP) types. Consistent with the preservation of the wild-type allele, these cells usually stain for both tuberin and hamartin. Similar hamartomatous features are present in the subependymal nodules, where the large astrocyte-like cells cluster beneath the ventricular surface. These multiple droplike masses that bulge into the ventricular system gave rise to the term *candle-guttering*. In subependymal areas a tumor unique to tuberous sclerosis, subependymal giant-cell astrocytoma, occurs, which is marked by having very large amounts of eosinophilic cytoplasm.

Von Hippel–Lindau Disease

This is an autosomal dominant disease in which affected individuals develop hemangioblastomas and cysts involving the pancreas, liver, and kidneys, and have a propensity to develop renal cell carcinoma and pheochromocytoma. Hemangioblastomas are most common in the cerebellum and retina. The disease frequency is 1 in 30,000 to 40,000.

The gene associated with von Hippel–Lindau disease (*VHL*), a tumor suppressor gene, is located on chromosome 3p25–p26 and encodes a protein (pVHL) that, among its other functions, is a component of a ubiquitin ligase complex that downregulates hypoxia-induced factor 1 (HIF-1), a transcription factor involved in regulating expression of vascular endothelial growth factor, erythropoietin, and other growth factors.[99] It is the dysregulation of erythropoietin that is responsible for the polycythemia observed in association with hemangioblastomas in about 10% of cases. There may be other targets of this ubiquitin ligase complex whose normal degradation is disrupted by loss of pVHL, explaining the other tumors associated with this syndrome. Missense mutations in *VHL*, but not other types of mutations, are highly likely to be associated with pheochromocytomas.

Morphology. Hemangioblastomas are highly vascular neoplasms that occur as a mural nodule associated with a large fluid-filled cyst. On microscopic examination, the lesion consists of a mixture of variable proportions of capillary-size or somewhat larger thin-walled vessels with intervening stromal cells of uncertain histogenesis characterized by vacuolated, lightly PAS-positive, lipid-rich cytoplasm and an indefinite immunohistochemical phenotype; nonetheless, studies have shown that these cells are the neoplastic element of the hemangioblastoma based on the presence of a second "hit" in the previously normal *VHL* allele.

Therapy is directed at the symptomatic neoplasms, including resection of the cerebellar hemangioblastomas and laser therapy for retinal hemangioblastomas.

REFERENCES

1. Alvarez-Buylla A, Garcia-Verdugo JM: Neurogenesis in adult subventricular zone. J Neurosci 22:629, 2002.
2. Love S et al. (eds): Greenfield's Neuropathology, 8th ed. London, Hodder Arnold, 2008.
3. Roper A, Samuels MA: Adams and Victor's Principles of Neurology, 9th ed. McGraw-Hill, Philadelphia, 2009.
4. Haass C, Selkoe DJ: Soluble protein oligomers in neurodegeneration: lessons from the Alzheimer's amyloid beta-peptide. Nat Rev Mol Cell Biol 8:101, 2007.
5. Golden J, Harding B (eds): Pathology and Genetics. Developmental Neuropathology. Basel, ISN Neuropath Press, 2004.
6. Copp A, Harding B: Neural tube defects. In Golden J, Harding B (eds): Pathology and Genetics. Developmental Neuropathology. Basel, ISN Neuropath Press, 2004, p 2.
7. Caviness VS et al.: Cell output, cell cycle duration and neuronal specification: a model of integrated mechanisms of the neocortical proliferative process. Cereb Cortex 13:592, 2003.
8. Ayala R et al.: Trekking across the brain: the journey of neuronal migration. Cell 128:29, 2007.
9. Bystron I et al.: Development of the human cerebral cortex: Boulder Committee revisited. Nat Rev Neurosci 9:110, 2008.
10. Guerrini R, Marini C: Genetic malformations of cortical development. Exp Brain Res 173:322, 2006.
11. Jansen A, Andermann E: Genetics of the polymicrogyria syndromes. J Med Genet 42:369, 2005.
12. Lian G, Sheen V: Cerebral developmental disorders. Curr Opin Pediatr 18:614, 2006.
13. Ming J, Golden J: Midline patterning defect. In Golden J, Harding B (eds): Pathology and Genetics. Developmental Neuropathology. Basel, ISN Neuropath Press, 2004, p 14.
14. Lo EH et al.: Exciting, radical, suicidal: how brain cells die after stroke. Stroke 36:189, 2005.
15. Mehta SL et al.: Molecular targets in cerebral ischemia for developing novel therapeutics. Brain Res Rev 54:34, 2007.
16. Lo EH et al.: Mechanisms, challenges and opportunities in stroke. Nat Rev Neurosci 4:399, 2003.
17. Monet M et al.: The archetypal R90C CADASIL-notch3 mutation retains Notch3 function in vivo. Hum Mol Genet 16:982, 2007.
18. Revencu N, Vikkula M: Cerebral cavernous malformation: new molecular and clinical insights. J Med Genet 43:716, 2006.
19. Debiasi RL, Tyler KL: Molecular methods for diagnosis of viral encephalitis. Clin Microbiol Rev 17:903, 2004.
20. Bell JE: An update on the neuropathology of HIV in the HAART era. Histopathology 45:549, 2004.
21. Vago L et al.: Pathological findings in the central nervous system of AIDS patients on assumed antiretroviral therapeutic regimens: retrospective study of 1597 autopsies. AIDS 16:1925, 2002.
22. Kramer-Hammerle S et al.: Cells of the central nervous system as targets and reservoirs of the human immunodeficiency virus. Virus Res 111:194, 2005.
23. Collinge J: Molecular neurology of prion disease. J Neurol Neurosurg Psychiatry 76:906, 2005.
24. Wadsworth JD, Collinge J: Update on human prion disease. Biochim Biophys Acta 1772:598, 2007.
25. Gambetti P et al.: Hereditary Creutzfeld-Jakob disease and fatal familial insomnia. Clin Lab Med 23:43, 2003.
26. Mead S et al.: Creutzfeldt-Jakob disease, prion protein gene codon 129VV, and a novel PrP^Sc type in a young British woman. Arch Neurol 64:1780, 2007.
27. Frohman EM et al.: Multiple sclerosis—the plague and its pathogenesis. N Engl J Med 354:942, 2006.
28. Lassmann H et al.: The immunopathology of multiple sclerosis: an overview. Brain Pathol 17:210, 2007.
29. Hafler DA et al.: Risk alleles for multiple sclerosis identified by a genome-wide study. N Engl J Med 357:851, 2007.
30. Baxter AG: The origin and application of experimental autoimmune encephalomyelitis. Nat Rev Immunol 7:904, 2007.
31. Owens GP et al.: The B cell response in multiple sclerosis. Neurol Res 28:236, 2006.
32. Hauser SL et al.: B-cell depletion with rituximab in relapsing-remitting multiple sclerosis. N Engl J Med 358:676, 2008.
33. Miller RH, Mi S: Dissecting demyelination. Nat Neurosci 10:1351, 2007.

34. Lucchinetti CF et al.: A role for humoral mechanisms in the pathogenesis of Devic's neuromyelitis optica. Brain 125:1450, 2002.

35. Misu T et al.: Loss of aquaporin 4 in lesions of neuromyelitis optica: distinction from multiple sclerosis. Brain 130:1224, 2007.

36. Roemer SF et al.: Pattern-specific loss of aquaporin-4 immunoreactivity distinguishes neuromyelitis optica from multiple sclerosis. Brain 130:1194, 2007.

37. Love S: Demyelinating diseases. J Clin Pathol 59:1151, 2006.

38. Mirra SS et al.: The Consortium to Establish a Registry for Alzheimer's Disease (CERAD). Part II. Standardization of the neuropathologic assessment of Alzheimer's disease. Neurology 41:479, 1991.

39. Braak H, Braak E: Neuropathological staging of Alzheimer-related changes. Acta Neuropathol 82:239, 1991.

40. Newell KL et al.: Application of the National Institute on Aging (NIA)–Reagan Institute criteria for the neuropathological diagnosis of Alzheimer disease. J Neuropathol Exp Neurol 58:1147, 1999.

41. Hyman BT, Trojanowski JQ: Consensus recommendations for the postmortem diagnosis of Alzheimer disease from the National Institute on Aging and the Reagan Institute Working Group on diagnostic criteria for the neuropathological assessment of Alzheimer disease. J Neuropathol Exp Neurol 56:1095, 1997.

42. Selkoe DJ, Wolfe MS: Presenilin: running with scissors in the membrane. Cell 131:215, 2007.

43. Heneka MT, O'Banion MK: Inflammatory processes in Alzheimer's disease. J Neuroimmunol 184:69, 2007.

44. Rovelet-Lecrux A et al.: APP locus duplication causes autosomal dominant early-onset Alzheimer disease with cerebral amyloid angiopathy. Nat Genet 38:24, 2006.

45. Bertram L et al.: Systematic meta-analyses of Alzheimer disease genetic association studies: the AlzGene database. Nat Genet 39:17, 2007.

46. Reiman EM et al.: *GAB2* alleles modify Alzheimer's risk in APOE epsilon4 carriers. Neuron 54:713, 2007.

47. Klunk WE et al.: Imaging brain amyloid in Alzheimer's disease with Pittsburgh Compound-B. Ann Neurol 55:306, 2004.

48. Pike KE et al.: Beta-amyloid imaging and memory in non-demented individuals: evidence for preclinical Alzheimer's disease. Brain 130:2837, 2007.

49. Cairns NJ et al.: Neuropathologic diagnostic and nosologic criteria for frontotemporal lobar degeneration: consensus of the Consortium for Frontotemporal Lobar Degeneration. Acta Neuropathol 114:5, 2007.

50. Eriksen JL, Mackenzie IR: Progranulin: normal function and role in neurodegeneration. J Neurochem 104:287, 2008.

51. Neumann M et al.: Ubiquitinated TDP-43 in frontotemporal lobar degeneration and amyotrophic lateral sclerosis. Science 314:130, 2006.

52. Hachinski V et al.: National Institute of Neurological Disorders and Stroke–Canadian Stroke Network vascular cognitive impairment harmonization standards. Stroke 37:2220, 2006.

53. Thomas B, Beal MF: Parkinson's disease. Hum Mol Genet 16 (Spec No. 2):R183, 2007.

54. Tan EK, Skipper LM: Pathogenic mutations in Parkinson disease. Hum Mutat 28:641, 2007.

55. Freed CR et al.: Transplantation of embryonic dopamine neurons for severe Parkinson's disease. N Engl J Med 344:710, 2001.

56. Perlmutter JS, Mink JW: Deep brain stimulation. Annu Rev Neurosci 29:229, 2006.

57. Bonanni L et al.: Diagnosis and management of dementia with Lewy bodies: third report of the DLB Consortium. Neurology 66:1455; author reply 1455, 2006.

58. McKeith IG: Consensus guidelines for the clinical and pathologic diagnosis of dementia with Lewy bodies (DLB): report of the Consortium on DLB International Workshop. J Alzheimers Dis 9:417, 2006.

59. Del Tredici K et al.: Where does Parkinson disease pathology begin in the brain? J Neuropathol Exp Neurol 61:413, 2002.

60. Yoshida M: Multiple system atrophy: alpha-synuclein and neuronal degeneration. Neuropathology 27:484, 2007.

61. Wakabayashi K, Takahashi H: Cellular pathology in multiple system atrophy. Neuropathology 26:338, 2006.

62. Greenamyre JT: Huntington's disease—making connections. N Engl J Med 356:518, 2007.

63. Orr HT, Zoghbi HY: Trinucleotide repeat disorders. Annu Rev Neurosci 30:575, 2007.

64. Soong BW, Paulson HL: Spinocerebellar ataxias: an update. Curr Opin Neurol 20:438, 2007.

65. Babady NE et al.: Advancements in the pathophysiology of Friedreich's ataxia and new prospects for treatments. Mol Genet Metab 92:23, 2007.

66. Rass U et al.: Defective DNA repair and neurodegenerative disease. Cell 130:991, 2007.

67. Pasinelli P, Brown RH: Molecular biology of amyotrophic lateral sclerosis: insights from genetics. Nat Rev Neurosci 7:710, 2006.

68. Kabashi E et al.: Oxidized/misfolded superoxide dismutase-1: the cause of all amyotrophic lateral sclerosis? Ann Neurol 62:553, 2007.

69. Lobsiger CS, Cleveland DW: Glial cells as intrinsic components of non-cell-autonomous neurodegenerative disease. Nat Neurosci 10:1355, 2007.

70. Kwong LK et al.: TDP-43 Proteinopathies: neurodegenerative protein misfolding diseases without amyloidosis. Neurosignals 16:41, 2008.

71. Adachi H et al.: Pathogenesis and molecular targeted therapy of spinal and bulbar muscular atrophy. Neuropathol Appl Neurobiol 33:135, 2007.

72. Haltia M: The neuronal ceroid-lipofuscinoses: from past to present. Biochim Biophys Acta 1762:850, 2006.

73. Escolar ML et al.: Transplantation of umbilical-cord blood in babies with infantile Krabbe's disease. N Engl J Med 352:2069, 2005.

74. Koc ON et al.: Allogeneic mesenchymal stem cell infusion for treatment of metachromatic leukodystrophy (MLD) and Hurler syndrome (MPS-IH). Bone Marrow Transplant 30:215, 2002.

75. Inoue K: PLP1-related inherited dysmyelinating disorders: Pelizaeus-Merzbacher disease and spastic paraplegia type 2. Neurogenetics 6:1, 2005.

76. Moffett JR et al.: *N*-Acetylaspartate in the CNS: from neurodiagnostics to neurobiology. Prog Neurobiol 81:89, 2007.

77. Quinlan RA et al.: GFAP and its role in Alexander disease. Exp Cell Res 313:2077, 2007.

78. Pronk JC et al.: Vanishing white matter disease: a review with focus on its genetics. Ment Retard Dev Disabil Res Rev 12:123, 2006.

79. van der Knaap MS et al.: Vanishing white matter disease. Lancet Neurol 5:413, 2006.

80. Finsterer J: Central nervous system manifestations of mitochondrial disorders. Acta Neurol Scand 114:217, 2006.

81. Wong LJ: Pathogenic mitochondrial DNA mutations in protein-coding genes. Muscle Nerve 36:279, 2007.

82. Gordon N: Alpers syndrome: progressive neuronal degeneration of children with liver disease. Dev Med Child Neurol 48:1001, 2006.

83. Hudson G, Chinnery PF: Mitochondrial DNA polymerase-gamma and human disease. Hum Mol Genet 15 (Spec No 2):R244, 2006.

84. Bao S, et al.: Glioma stem cells promote radioresistance by preferential activation of the DNA damage response. Nature 444:756, 2006.

85. Singh SK et al.: Identification of a cancer stem cell in human brain tumors. Cancer Res 63:5821, 2003.

86. Louis DN et al. (eds): WHO Classification of Tumours of the Central Nervous System. Lyon, International Agency for Research on Cancer, 2007.

87. Louis DN et al.: The 2007 WHO classification of tumours of the central nervous system. Acta Neuropathol 114:97, 2007.

88. Louis DN: Molecular pathology of malignant gliomas. Annu Rev Pathol 1:97, 2006.

89. Mellinghoff IK et al.: Molecular determinants of the response of glioblastomas to EGFR kinase inhibitors. N Engl J Med 353:2012, 2005.

90. The Cancer Genome Atlas Research Network. Comprehensive genomic characterization defines human glioblastoma genes and core pathways. Nature 455:1061, 2008.

91. Yip S et al.: Molecular diagnostic testing in malignant gliomas: a practical update on predictive markers. J Neuropathol Exp Neurol 67:1, 2008.

92. Stupp R et al.: Radiotherapy plus concomitant and adjuvant temozolomide for glioblastoma. N Engl J Med 352:987, 2005.

93. Ponzoni M, Ferreri AJ: Intravascular lymphoma: a neoplasm of "homeless" lymphocytes? Hematol Oncol 24:105, 2006.

94. Bataller L, Dalmau J: Paraneoplastic neurologic syndromes. Neurol Clin 21:221, 2003.

95. Graus F, Dalmau J: Paraneoplastic neurological syndromes: diagnosis and treatment. Curr Opin Neurol 20:732, 2007.

96. Graus F et al.: Recommended diagnostic criteria for paraneoplastic neurological syndromes. J Neurol Neurosurg Psychiatry 75:1135, 2004.

97. Farrell CJ, Plotkin SR: Genetic causes of brain tumors: neurofibromatosis, tuberous sclerosis, von Hippel–Lindau, and other syndromes. Neurol Clin 25:925, 2007.

98. Curto M, McClatchey AI: Nf2/Merlin: a coordinator of receptor signalling and intercellular contact. Br J Cancer 98:256, 2008.

99. Kaelin WG: Von Hippel–Lindau disease. Annu Rev Pathol 2:145, 2007.

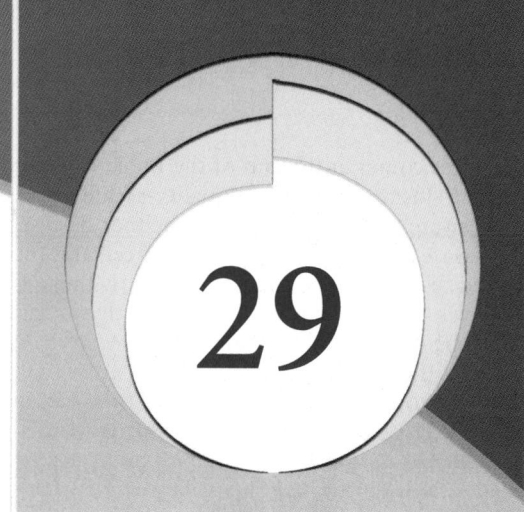

29

The Eye

ROBERT FOLBERG

Orbit
  Functional Anatomy and Proptosis
  Thyroid Ophthalmopathy
    (Graves Disease)
  Other Orbital Inflammatory Conditions
  Neoplasms

Eyelid
  Functional Anatomy
  Neoplasms

Conjunctiva
  Functional Anatomy
  Conjunctival Scarring
  Pinguecula and Pterygium
  Neoplasms

Sclera

Cornea
  Functional Anatomy
  Keratitis and Ulcers
  Corneal Degenerations and Dystrophies
    Band Keratopathies
    Keratoconus
    Fuchs Endothelial Dystrophy
    Stromal Dystrophies

Anterior Segment
  Functional Anatomy
  Cataract
  The Anterior Segment and Glaucoma
  Endophthalmitis and Panophthalmitis

Uvea
  Uveitis
  Neoplasms
    Uveal Nevi and Melanomas

Retina and Vitreous
  Functional Anatomy
  Retinal Detachment
  Retinal Vascular Disease
    Hypertension
    Diabetes Mellitus
    Retinopathy of Prematurity (Retrolental Fibroplasia)
    Sickle Retinopathy, Retinal Vasculitis, Radiation Retinopathy
    Retinal Artery and Vein Occlusions
  Age-Related Macular Degeneration
  Other Retinal Degenerations
    Retinitis Pigmentosa
  Retinitis
  Retinal Neoplasms
    Retinoblastoma
    Retinal Lymphoma

Optic Nerve
  Anterior Ischemic Optic Neuropathy
  Papilledema
  Glaucomatous Optic Nerve Damage
  Other Optic Neuropathies
  Optic Neuritis

The End-Stage Eye: Phthisis Bulbi

Although this chapter comes at the end of the book, it is not the least important. Vision is a major quality-of-life issue. Before the public awareness of AIDS and Alzheimer disease, the most feared disease among Americans was cancer, and the second most feared disease was blindness. So great is the fear of blindness that even today, people often tell their physicians, "Doctor, I'd rather be dead than be blind!"

In general, diseases that produce loss of vision do not attract as much of our attention as do many of the life-threatening conditions described in this book. For example, age-related macular degeneration (ARMD) is the most common cause of irreversible visual loss in the United States. Most individuals with ARMD do not even suffer from a total loss of vision—an immersion into total darkness. The histopathology is unspectacular: small scars develop in the macula. But consider the effect of these tiny scars perhaps in a retired schoolteacher with ARMD. The small macular scars make it impossible for this person to see anything clearly in the central portion of her or his vision. The faces of spouse or grandchildren are not visible. He or she cannot read a book or newspaper. Once a model of independence, this teacher can no longer drive a car and must be chauffered everywhere. True, his or her life is not threatened by the small scars in the eyes' macula, but the quality of life declines as this person is robbed of the common joys that most of us take for granted until they are lost.

To study the eye, one needs to comprehend all that has come before. For example, the pathology of the eyelids builds on knowledge of dermatopathology (Chapter 25), and the pathology of the retina and optic nerve extends what was learned in Chapter 28 about the brain and central nervous system. However, the study of ocular pathology does not merely repeat what has been presented thus far. The eye provides the only site in which a physician can easily visualize a variety of pathophysiologic disturbances in the microcirculation ranging from arteriosclerosis to angiogenesis in a clinical setting. Although there are conditions that are unique to the eye (such as cataract and glaucoma), many ocular conditions share similarities with disease processes elsewhere in the body that are modified by the unique structure and function of the eye (Fig. 29–1). Moreover, the eye has much to teach us about important mechanisms of disease that extend far beyond the visual system. For example, the tumor suppressor gene, *RB*, was described in retinoblastoma,[1] a quite uncommon ocular tumor of infants and very young children, but the discovery of *RB* opened an important pathway to the understanding of the regulation of cellular replication.

This chapter is organized on the basis of ocular anatomy. The discussion of each region of the eye begins with anatomic and functional considerations, and their impact on the understanding of ocular diseases.

Orbit

FUNCTIONAL ANATOMY AND PROPTOSIS

The orbit is a compartment that is closed medially, laterally, and posteriorly. Diseases that increase orbital contents there-

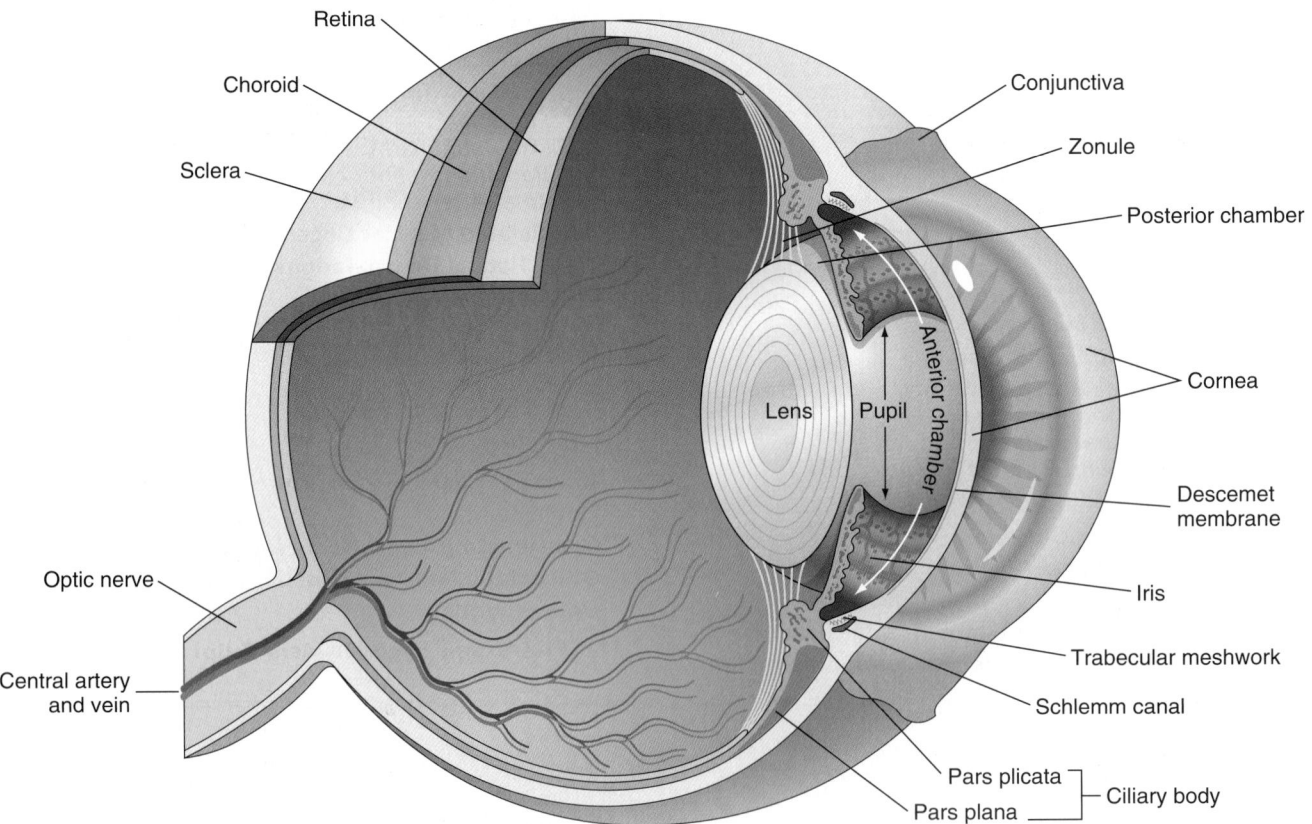

FIGURE 29–1   Anatomy of the eye.

fore displace the eye forward, a condition known as *proptosis*. Aside from the obvious cosmetic concerns, the proptotic eye might not be covered completely by the eyelids, and the tear film might not be distributed evenly across the cornea. Corneal exposure is painful and can predispose to corneal ulceration and infection. Proptosis may be axial (directly forward) or positional. For example, any enlargement of the lacrimal gland from inflammation (e.g., *sarcoidosis*) or neoplasm (e.g., *lymphoma, pleomorphic adenoma,* or *adenoid cystic carcinoma*) produces a proptosis that displaces the eye inferiorly and medially, because the lacrimal gland is positioned superotemporally within the orbit.

Masses contained within the cone formed by the horizontal rectus muscles generate axial proptosis: the eye bulges straight forward. The two most common primary tumors of the optic nerve (a tract of the central nervous system and not a peripheral nerve), *glioma* and *meningioma*, produce axial proptosis because the optic nerve is positioned within the muscle cone. The orbital contents are subject to the same disease processes that affect other tissues. Representative inflammatory conditions and neoplasms of the orbit are discussed briefly next.

THYROID OPHTHALMOPATHY (GRAVES DISEASE)

In the chapter on endocrine disorders (Chapter 24) it was noted that axial proptosis is an important clinical manifestation of Graves disease. Proptosis is caused by the accumulation of extracellular matrix proteins and variable degrees of fibrosis in the rectus muscles (Fig. 29–2). The development of thyroid ophthalmopathy may be independent of the status of thyroid function.[2]

OTHER ORBITAL INFLAMMATORY CONDITIONS

The floor of the orbit is the roof of the maxillary sinus, and the medial wall of the orbit—the lamina papyracea—

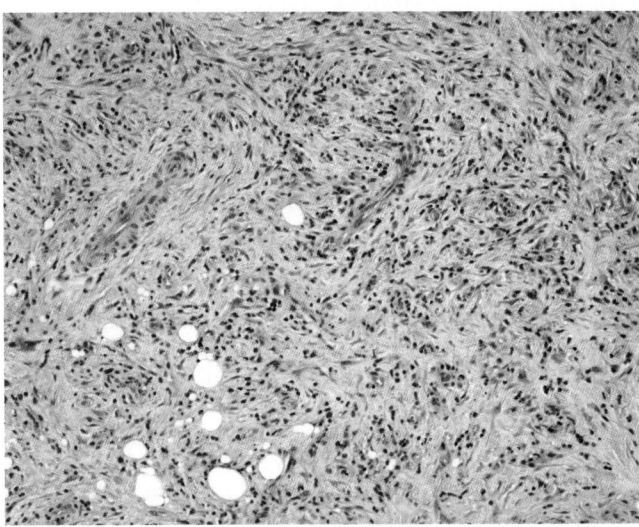

FIGURE 29–3 In idiopathic orbital inflammation (orbital inflammatory pseudotumor) the orbital fat is replaced by fibrosis. Note the chronic inflammation, accompanied in this case by eosinophils.

separates the orbit from the ethmoidal sinuses. Thus, uncontrolled sinus infection may spread to the orbit either as an acute infection (orbital *cellulitis*) or as a component of a fungal infection *(mucormycosis)* in immunosuppressed individuals, in patients with diabetic ketoacidosis, or, rarely, in persons without any predisposition. Systemic conditions such as *Wegener granulomatosis* (Chapter 11) may present first in the orbit and may be confined there for prolonged periods of time,[3] or alternatively, it may involve the orbit secondarily by extension from the sinuses.

Idiopathic orbital inflammation, also known as orbital inflammatory pseudotumor (Fig. 29–3), is another inflammatory condition affecting the orbit. This condition may be unilateral or bilateral, and may affect all orbital tissue elements or may be confined to the lacrimal gland *(sclerosing dacryoadenitis)*, the extra-ocular muscles *(orbital myositis)*, or the Tenon's capsule, the fascial layer that wraps around the eye *(posterior scleritis)*. In long-term follow-up a subset of individuals with idiopathic orbital inflammation may show evidence of systemic vasculitis or other forms of connective tissue diseases.

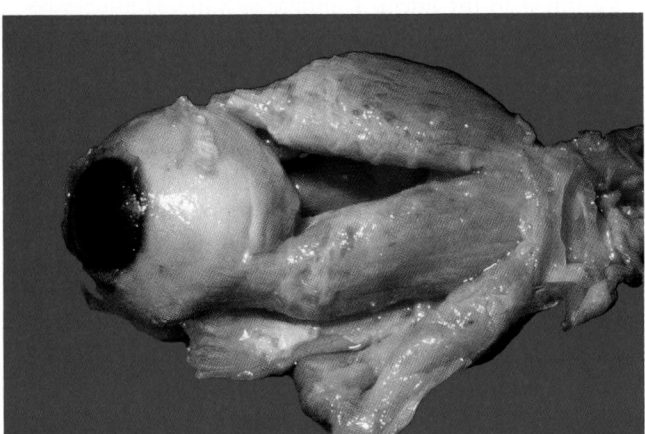

FIGURE 29–2 The extra-ocular muscles are greatly distended in this postmortem dissection of tissues from a patient with thyroid (Graves) ophthalmopathy. Note that the tendons of the muscles are spared involvement. (Courtesy of Dr. Ralph C. Eagle, Jr., Wills Eye Hospital, Philadelphia, PA.)

Morphology. Idiopathic orbital inflammation is characterized histologically by chronic inflammation and variable degrees of fibrosis. The inflammatory infiltrate typically includes lymphocytes and plasma cells and occasionally eosinophils. Germinal centers, when present, raise the suspicion of a reactive lymphoid hyperplasia. Vasculitis may be present, suggesting an underlying systemic condition. The presence of necrotic collagen along with vasculitis should raise the suspicion of Wegener granulomatosis. Idiopathic orbital inflammation is typically confined to the orbit but may develop concomitantly with sclerosing inflammation in the retroperitoneum, the mediastinum, and the thyroid.

NEOPLASMS

The most frequently encountered primary neoplasms of the orbit are vascular in origin: the capillary hemangioma of infancy and early childhood and the lymphangioma (both of which are unencapsulated) and the encapsulated cavernous hemangioma found typically in adults. These are described in other chapters. Only a handful of orbital masses are encapsulated (e.g., pleomorphic adenoma of the lacrimal gland, dermoid cyst, neurilemmoma), and the recognition of encapsulation on imaging studies allows the surgeon to anticipate pathologic findings.

Non-Hodgkin lymphoma, like idiopathic orbital inflammation, can affect the entire orbit or can be confined to compartments of the orbit such as the lacrimal gland. Orbital lymphomas are classified according to the WHO classification system (Chapter 13).

Primary orbital malignancies may arise from any of the orbital tissues and are classified according to the scheme used for the parent tissue. For example, the lacrimal gland may be considered a minor salivary gland, and tumors of the lacrimal gland are classified as salivary gland tumors are classified.

Metastases to the orbit may present with distinctive signs and symptoms that point to the origin of the tumor. For example, metastatic prostatic carcinoma may present clinically like idiopathic orbital inflammation; metastatic neuroblastoma and Wilms tumor—richly vascular neoplasms—may produce characteristic periocular ecchymoses. Neoplasms may also invade from the sinuses into the orbit.

Eyelid

FUNCTIONAL ANATOMY

The eyelid is composed of skin externally and mucosa (the conjunctiva) on the surface apposed to the eye (Fig. 29–4). In addition to covering and protecting the eye, elements within

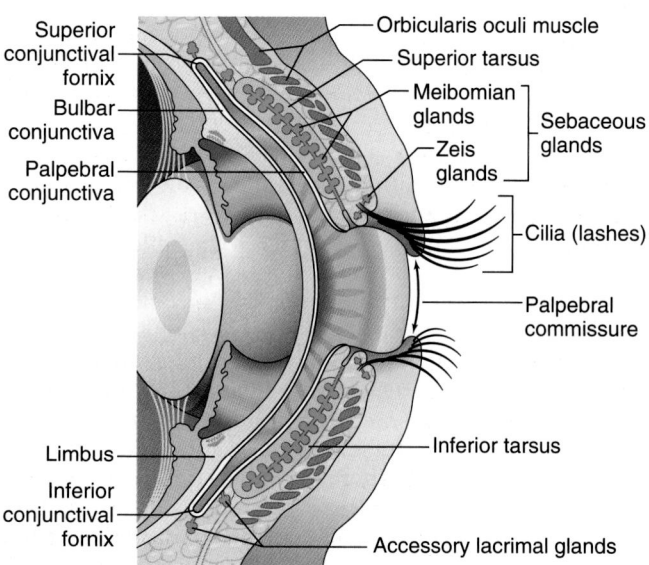

FIGURE 29–4 Anatomy of the conjunctiva and eyelids.

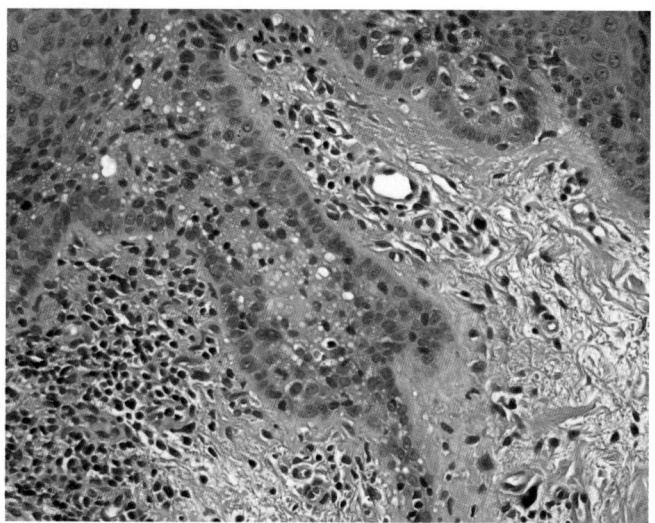

FIGURE 29–5 Pagetoid spread of sebaceous carcinoma. Neoplastic cells with foamy cytoplasm are detected within the epidermis. Invasive sebaceous carcinoma was identified elsewhere in this biopsy sample.

the eyelid generate critical components of the tear film. If the drainage system of the sebaceous glands is obstructed by chronic inflammation at the eyelid margin *(blepharitis)* or, less commonly, by neoplasm, then lipid may extravasate into surrounding tissue and provoke a granulomatous response producing a lipogranuloma, or *chalazion*.

NEOPLASMS

The most common malignancy of the eyelid is basal cell carcinoma. The second most common malignancy is sebaceous carcinoma, followed by squamous cell carcinoma. Surprisingly, primary melanomas of the eyelid skin are extremely rare. Regardless of histogenesis, eyelid neoplasms may distort tissue and prevent the eyelids from closing completely. Exposure of the cornea is not only painful but predisposes the individual to corneal ulceration. Therefore, prompt treatment of locally invasive basal cell carcinomas, which are typically not a threat to the affected individual's life, is imperative to preserve vision. *Basal cell carcinoma has a distinct predilection for the lower eyelid and the medial canthus.*

Sebaceous carcinoma may form a local mass that mimics *chalazion* or may diffusely thicken the eyelid. This neoplasm may also resemble inflammatory processes such as blepharitis or *ocular cicatricial pemphigoid* because of intraepithelial spread as occurs in Paget disease of the nipple (Chapter 23) or vulva. Sebaceous carcinoma tends to spread first to the parotid and submandibular nodes. The overall mortality rate can be as high as 22%.[4]

Morphology. In moderately differentiated or well-differentiated sebaceous carcinoma, vacuolization of the cytoplasm is present and helps in the diagnosis. This cancer may, however, resemble a variety of other malignancies histologically, including basal cell carcinoma, and establishing the correct diagnosis can be difficult. Pagetoid spread (Fig. 29–5) may mimic Bowenoid actinic keratosis in the eyelid and carcinoma in situ in the conjunctiva. Sebaceous carcinoma may spread through the conjunctival epithelium and the epidermis to the lacrimal drainage system and the nasopharynx. It may also extend into the lacrimal gland ductules and thereby into the main lacrimal gland.

In individuals with AIDS, *Kaposi sarcoma* may develop in either the eyelid or the conjunctiva. In the eyelid the lesion may appear clinically to have a purple hue because the vascular lesion is embedded in the dermis, but in the thin mucous membrane of the conjunctiva, Kaposi sarcoma appears bright red and may be confused clinically with a subconjunctival hemorrhage.

Conjunctiva

FUNCTIONAL ANATOMY

The conjunctiva is divided into zones (see Fig. 29–4), each with distinctive histologic features and responses to disease. The conjunctiva lining the interior of the eyelid, the *palpebral conjunctiva*, is tightly tethered to the tarsus and may respond to inflammation by being thrown into minute papillary folds as may occur in allergic conjunctivitis and bacterial conjunctivitis. The conjunctiva in the *fornix* is a pseudostratified columnar epithelium rich in goblet cells. The fornix also contains accessory lacrimal tissue, and the ductules of the main lacrimal gland pierce through the conjunctiva in the fornix superiorly and laterally. The lymphoid population of the conjunctiva is most noticeable in the fornix, and *in viral conjunctivitis, lymphoid follicles may enlarge sufficiently to be visualized clinically* by slit-lamp examination. *Granulomas* associated with systemic sarcoidosis may be detected in the conjunctival fornix, and the yield of granulomas from a nondirected conjunctival biopsy in individuals suspected of having sarcoid may be as high as 50%.[5] Primary lymphoma of the conjunctiva (typically indolent marginal zone B-cell lymphoma) is most likely to develop in the fornix. The *bulbar conjunctiva*—the conjunctiva that covers the surface of the eye—is a nonkeratinizing stratified squamous epithelium.

The conjunctiva, like the eyelid, is richly invested with lymphatic channels. Malignant neoplasms arising in the eyelid and conjunctiva tend to spread to regional lymph nodes (parotid and submandibular node groups).

CONJUNCTIVAL SCARRING

Many cases of bacterial or viral conjunctivitis cause redness and itching, but most heal without sequelae. However, infection with *Chlamydia trachomatis (trachoma)* may produce significant conjunctival scarring. Conjunctival scarring is also seen after exposure of the ocular surface to caustic alkalis or as a sequela to ocular cicatricial *pemphigoid* (Chapter 25). A reduction in the number of goblet cells due to conjunctival scarring leads to a decrease in surface mucin, which is essential for the adherence of the aqueous component of tears to the

corneal epithelium. Thus, even if the aqueous component of the tear film is adequate, the affected individual will suffer from a dry eye, a condition that, when severe, can be painful and can predispose to corneal opacification and ulceration. More commonly, however, dry eye results from a deficiency in the aqueous component of the tear film generated by the accessory lacrimal glands embedded within the eyelid and fornix.

The conjunctiva may be scarred iatrogenically through reaction to drugs or as a consequence of surgery. In other parts of the body, cancer surgery requires excision of the lesion with a margin of normal tissue to ensure complete removal. However, extensive surgical excision of even diseased conjunctiva can remove a large number of goblet cells or compromise lacrimal gland ductules that traverse the conjunctiva. Thus, removal of a conjunctival neoplasm or a precursor lesion may leave the affected individual with a painful dry eye that can compromise vision. Therefore, surgeons often remove only the invasive components of conjunctival neoplasms, and treat the intraepithelial components with tissue-sparing modalities such as cryotherapy or topical chemotherapy delivered as eyedrops.

PINGUECULA AND PTERYGIUM

Both pinguecula and pterygium appear as submucosal elevations on the conjunctiva. They result from actinic damage and are therefore located in the sun-exposed regions of the conjunctiva (i.e., in the fissure between both the upper and lower eyelids—the interpalpebral fissure). Pterygium typically originates in the conjunctiva astride the limbus. It is formed by a submucosal growth *of fibrovascular connective tissue that migrates onto the cornea*, dissecting into the plane occupied normally by the Bowman layer. Pterygium does not cross the pupillary axis and, aside from the possible induction of mild astigmatism, does not pose a threat to vision. Although most pterygia are entirely benign, it is worthwhile submitting the excised tissue for pathologic examination because, on occasion, precursors of actinic-induced neoplasms—squamous cell carcinoma and melanoma—are detected in these lesions.

Pinguecula, which, like pterygium, appears astride the limbus, is a small, yellowish submucosal elevation. Although the *pinguecula does not invade the cornea as pterygium* does, the presence of a focal conjunctival elevation near the limbus can result in an uneven distribution of the tear film over the adjacent cornea. As a consequence of focal dehydration, a saucer-like depression in the corneal tissue—a *dellen*—may develop.

NEOPLASMS

Both squamous neoplasms and melanocytic neoplasms and their precursors tend to develop at the limbus. Conjunctival squamous cell carcinoma may be preceded by intraepithelial neoplastic changes analogous to those seen in the evolution of cervical squamous cell carcinoma. In the conjunctiva the spectrum of changes from mild dysplasia through carcinoma in situ is designated as *conjunctival intraepithelial neoplasia*. Squamous papillomas and conjunctival intraepithelial neoplasia may be associated with the presence of human papillomavirus types 16 and 18.[6] Although conjunctival squamous cell carcinoma tends to follow an indolent course, *mucoepidermoid carcinoma* of the conjunctiva (reflecting the ability of conjunctival stem cells to differentiate into squamous epithelium and goblet cells) follows a much more aggressive course.

Conjunctival nevi are encountered commonly in clinical practice but seldom invade the cornea or appear in the fornix or over the palpebral conjunctiva.[7] Pigmented lesions in these zones of the conjunctiva most likely represent melanomas or melanoma precursors. Compound nevi of the conjunctiva characteristically contain subepithelial cysts lined by surface epithelium (Fig. 29–6A, B). In late childhood or adolescence, conjunctival nevi may acquire an inflammatory component rich in lymphocytes, plasma cells, and eosinophils. The resultant *inflamed juvenile nevus* is completely benign and not associated with vitiligo or halo nevus.

Conjunctival melanomas are unilateral neoplasms, typically affecting fair-complexioned individuals in middle age[8] (Fig. 29–6C, D). Most cases of conjunctival melanoma develop through a phase of intraepithelial growth termed *primary acquired melanosis with atypia*, which is roughly analogous to *melanoma in situ* but does not correspond neatly to the radial growth phase of cutaneous melanoma. Between 50% and 90% of individuals with incompletely treated primary acquired melanosis with atypia will develop conjunctival melanoma;

the best treatment of conjunctival melanoma is its prevention through extirpation of its precursor lesion. The lesions tend to spread first to the parotid or submandibular lymph nodes. The mortality for conjunctival melanoma is 25%.

Sclera

The sclera consists mainly of collagen and contains few blood vessels and fibroblasts; hence, wounds and surgical incisions tend to heal poorly. Immune complex deposits within the sclera, such as in *rheumatoid arthritis*, may produce a necrotizing *scleritis*.

The sclera may appear "blue" in a variety of conditions. It may become thin following episodes of scleritis, and the normally brown color of the uvea may appear blue clinically because of the optical Tyndall effect. Sclera may also be thinned in eyes with exceptionally high intraocular pressure and because this zone of scleral ectasia is lined by uveal tissue, the resulting lesion, known as a *staphyloma*, also appears blue. The sclera may appear blue in osteogenesis imperfecta. Finally, the sclera may appear blue because of a heavily pigmented congenital nevus of the underlying uvea, a condition known as *congenital melanosis oculi*. When accompanied by periocular cutaneous pigmentation, this condition is known as *nevus of Ota*.

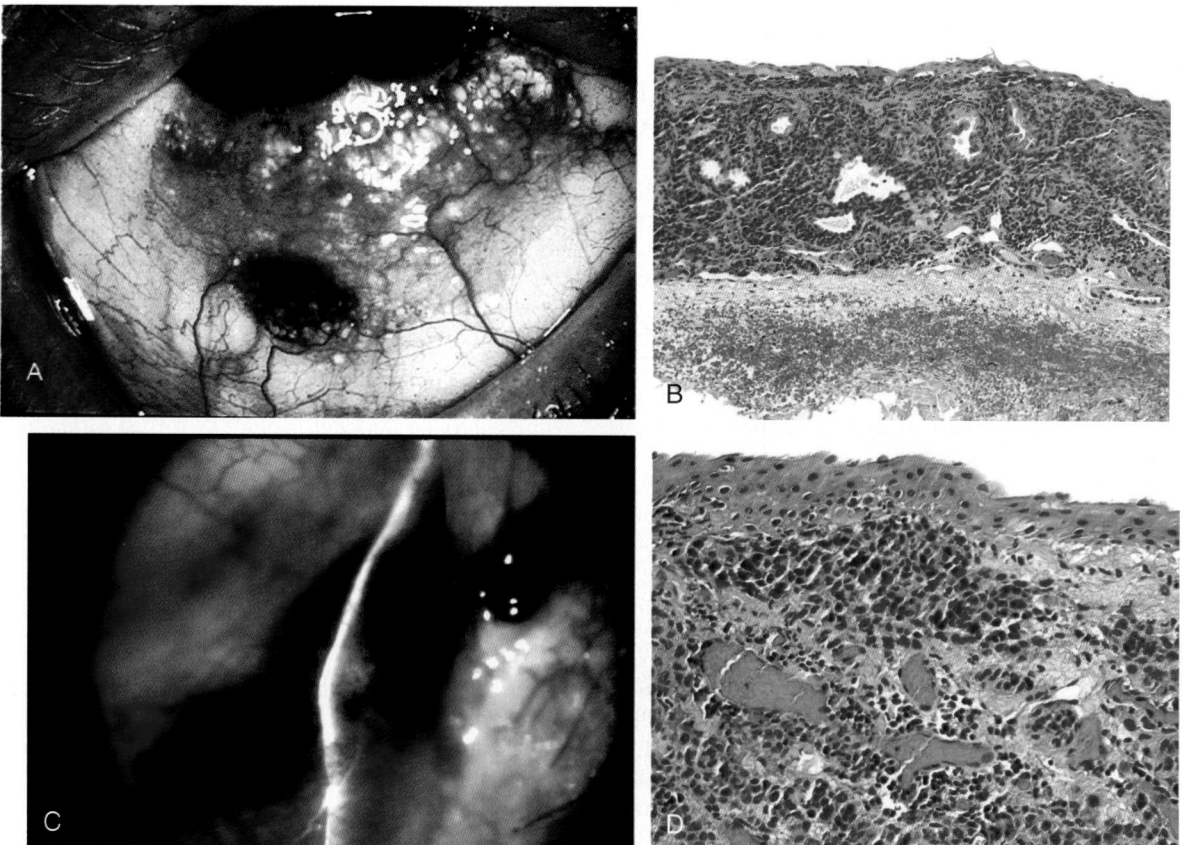

FIGURE 29–6   **A, B,** Cystic compound nevus of the conjunctiva. **C, D,** Conjunctival malignant melanoma. In **C**, note the deflection of the beam of the slit lamp over the surface of the lesion, indicative of invasion. (**A, B,** From Folberg R et al.: Benign conjunctival melanocytic lesions: clinicopathologic features. Ophthalmology 96:436, 1989.)

Cornea

FUNCTIONAL ANATOMY

The cornea and its overlying tear film—not the lens—make up the major refractive surface of the eye (Fig. 29–7). Parenthetically, myopia typically develops because the eye is too long for its refractive power, and hyperopia results from an eye that is too short. The popularity of procedures such as laser-assisted in situ keratomileusis (LASIK) to sculpt the cornea and change its refractive properties attests to the importance of corneal shape in contributing to the refractive power of the eye.

Anteriorly, the cornea is covered by *epithelium* that rests on a basement membrane. The *Bowman layer*, situated just beneath the epithelial basement membrane, is acellular and forms an efficient barrier against the penetration of malignant cells from the epithelium into the underlying stroma.

The *corneal stroma* lacks blood vessels and lymphatics, a feature that contributes not only to the transparency of the cornea, but also to high rate of success of corneal transplantation. Indeed, non-immunological graft failure (associated with loss of endothelial cells and subsequent corneal edema) is seen more commonly than is immunological graft rejection. The risk of corneal graft rejection increases with stromal vascularization and inflammation. A precise alignment of collagen in the corneal stroma also contributes to transparency. Scarring and edema both disrupt the spatial alignment of stromal collagen and contribute to corneal opacification. Scars may result from trauma or inflammation. Normally, the corneal stroma is in a state of relative deturgescence (dehydration), maintained in large part by active pumping of fluid from the stroma back into the anterior chamber by the corneal endothelium.

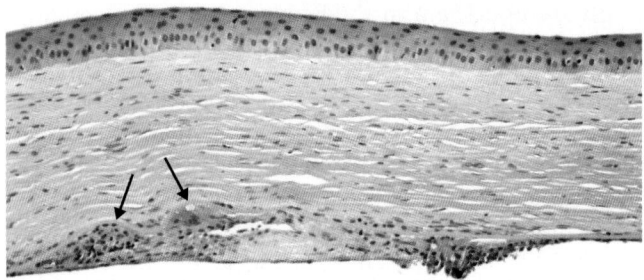

FIGURE 29–8 Chronic herpes simplex keratitis. The cornea is thin and scarred (note the increased number of fibroblast nuclei). Granulomatous reaction in the Descemet membrane, illustrated in this photomicrograph *(arrows)*, is a histologic hallmark of chronic herpes simplex keratitis.

The corneal *endothelium* is derived from neural crest and is not related to vascular endothelium. It rests on its basement membrane, Descemet membrane. A decrease in endothelial cells or a malfunction of endothelium results in stromal edema, which may be complicated by bullous separation of the epithelium *(bullous keratopathy)*. *Descemet membrane* increases in thickness with age. It is the site of copper deposition in the Kayser-Fleischer ring of Wilson disease (Chapter 18).

KERATITIS AND ULCERS

Various pathogens—bacterial, fungal, viral (especially herpes simplex and herpes zoster), and protozoal (*Acanthamoeba*)—can cause corneal ulceration. In all forms of keratitis, dissolution of the corneal stroma may be accelerated by activation of collagenases within corneal epithelium and stromal fibroblasts (also known as keratocytes). Exudate and cells leaking from iris and ciliary body vessels into the anterior chamber may be visible by slit-lamp examination and may accumulate in sufficient quantity to become visible even by a penlight examination *(hypopyon)*. Although the corneal ulcer may be infectious, the hypopyon seldom contains organisms and is an example par excellence of the vascular response to acute inflammation. The specific forms of keratitis may have certain distinctive features. For example, chronic herpes simplex keratitis may be associated with a granulomatous reaction involving the Descemet membrane (Fig. 29–8).

CORNEAL DEGENERATIONS AND DYSTROPHIES

Ophthalmologists have traditionally divided many corneal disorders into degenerations and dystrophies. Corneal degenerations may be either unilateral or bilateral and are typically nonfamilial. By contrast, corneal dystrophies are typically bilateral and are hereditary. Corneal dystrophies may affect selective corneal layers (e.g., *Reis-Bückler dystrophy* affects Bowman layer, and *posterior polymorphous dystrophy* affects the endothelium), or the changes may be distributed throughout multiple layers.

Band Keratopathies

Two types of band keratopathy serve as examples of corneal degenerations. *Calcific band keratopathy* is characterized by

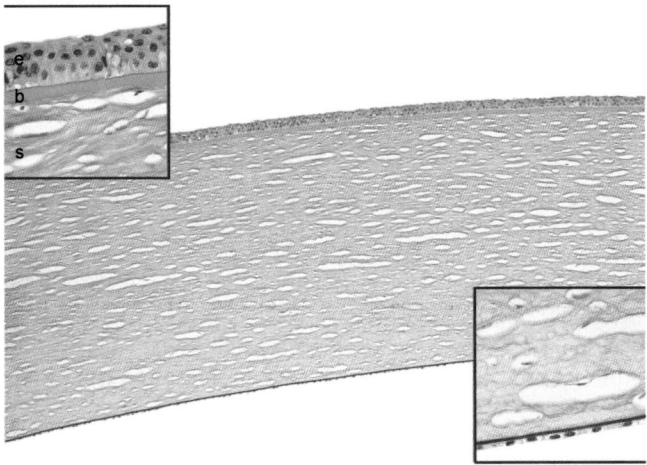

FIGURE 29–7 Normal corneal microarchitecture. The corneal tissue is stained by periodic acid–Schiff (PAS) to highlight basement membranes. The inset at the upper left is a high magnification of the anterior layers of the cornea: the epithelium *(e)*, Bowman layer *(b)*, and the stroma *(s)*. A very thin PAS-positive basement membrane separates the epithelium from the Bowman layer. Note that the Bowman layer is acellular. The *inset* at the *lower right* is a high magnification of the PAS-positive Descemet membrane and the corneal endothelium. The "holes" in the stroma are artifactitious spaces between parallel collagenous stromal lamellae.

deposition of calcium in the Bowman layer. This condition may complicate chronic uveitis, especially in individuals with chronic juvenile rheumatoid arthritis. *Actinic band keratopathy* develops in individuals who are exposed chronically to high levels of ultraviolet light. In this condition, extensive solar elastosis develops in the superficial layers of corneal collagen in the sun-exposed interpalpebral fissure, hence the horizontally distributed band of pathology. Similar to pinguecula, the sun-damaged collagen of the cornea appears clinically to be yellow to the point that this condition is sometimes erroneously called "oil-droplet keratopathy."

Keratoconus

With an incidence of 1 in 2000, *keratoconus* is a fairly common disorder characterized by progressive thinning and ectasia of the cornea without evidence of inflammation or vascularization. Such thinning results in a cornea that has a conical rather than spherical shape. This abnormal shape generates irregular astigmatism that is difficult to correct with spectacles. Rigid contact lenses generate a smooth, spherical surface to the cornea and may provide refractive relief for individuals with keratoconus. Patients whose vision cannot be corrected with spectacles or contact lenses are excellent candidates for corneal transplantation, which has a high degree of success in this condition. The etiology of keratoconus is unknown. Unlike many degenerations, it is typically bilateral. There is an association between keratoconus, Down syndrome, and Marfan syndrome, as well as with atopic disorders. Activation of collagenases, gelatinases, and matrix metalloproteinases has been implicated in the pathogenesis of this condition.

Morphology. Thinning of the cornea with breaks in the Bowman layer are the histologic hallmarks of keratoconus (Fig. 29–9). In some patients the Des-

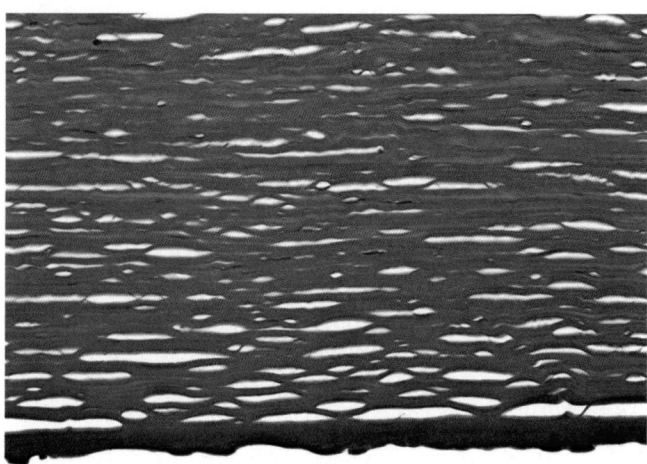

FIGURE 29–10 Fuchs dystrophy. This tissue section is stained by PAS to highlight the Descemet membrane, which is thick. Numerous droplike excrescences—guttata—protrude downward from the Descemet membrane. Endothelial cell nuclei are not seen. Epithelial bullae, not shown in this micrograph, were present, reflecting corneal edema.

cemet membrane may rupture precipitously, allowing the aqueous humor in the anterior chamber to gain access to the corneal stroma. The sudden effusion of aqueous humor through a gap in the Descemet membrane—corneal **hydrops**—may also cause vision to worsen suddenly. An episode of hydrops may be followed by corneal scarring that can also contribute to visual loss. Acute corneal hydrops can complicate Descemet membrane ruptures that develop secondary to extraordinary elevations of intraocular pressure in **infantile glaucoma (Haab's striae)** or following the now uncommon obstetric forceps injury to the eye.

Fuchs Endothelial Dystrophy

This condition, one of several dystrophies affecting the endothelium, is one of the principal indications for corneal transplantation in the United States. The two major clinical manifestations of Fuchs endothelial dystrophy—*stromal edema and bullous keratopathy*—are both related to a primary loss of endothelial cells. Early in the course of the disease endothelial cells produce droplike deposits of abnormal basement membrane material *(guttata)* that resemble the fetal component of the Descemet membrane ultrastructurally. Guttata can be visualized clinically by slit-lamp examination. With disease progression, there is a decrease in the total number of endothelial cells, and the residual cells are incapable of maintaining stromal deturgescence. Consequently the stroma becomes edematous and thickens; it acquires a ground-glass appearance clinically, and vision is blurred (Fig. 29–10). Because of chronic edema, the stroma may eventually become vascularized. On occasion the number of endothelial cells may decrease following cataract surgery even in individuals who do not have early forms of Fuchs dystrophy, and the condition is then known as *pseudophakic bullous keratopathy*.

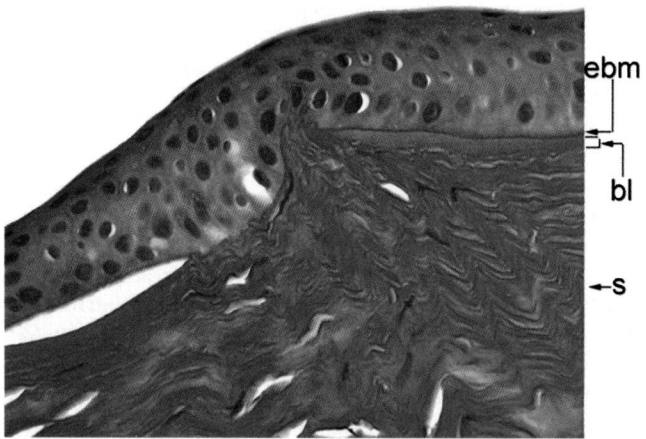

FIGURE 29–9 Keratoconus. The tissue section is stained by PAS to highlight the epithelial basement membrane (ebm), which is intact, the Bowman layer (bl), situated between the epithelial basement membrane, and the stroma (s). Following the Bowman layer from the *right side* of the photomicrograph toward the *center*, there is a discontinuity, diagnostic of keratoconus. The epithelial separation just to the *left* of the Bowman layer discontinuity resulted from an episode of corneal hydrops, caused by a break in the Descemet membrane (not shown).

With increasing stromal edema, the epithelium undergoes hydropic change, and the detachment of the epithelium from the Bowman layer produces epithelial bullae that may eventually rupture. Fibrous connective tissue may be deposited between the epithelium and Bowman layer (*degenerative pannus*) either by ingrowth from the limbus or perhaps through fibrous metaplasia of the corneal epithelium.

Stromal Dystrophies

In these conditions the *stromal deposits generate discrete opacities in the cornea* may eventually compromise vision. Deposits in the vicinity of the epithelium, its basement membrane, and Bowman layer may result in painful epithelial erosions. Scarring in the vicinity of Bowman layer may generate an irregular corneal surface, further compromising vision. *Macular corneal dystrophy* is so named because early in the disease, small nummular (macular) deposits of keratan sulfate develop in the corneal stroma. Later in the course of this autosomal recessive dystrophy, keratan sulfate is distributed diffusely throughout the stroma and may affect the endothelium.

The identification of specific mutations responsible for various stromal dystrophies is generating a new molecular classification of these disorders.[9] One example involves an autosomal dominant form of stromal dystrophy associated with mutations in the *TGFB1* gene, which encodes an extracellular matrix protein called *keratoepithelin*. Diverse mutations in *TGFB1* disrupt the folding of keratoepithelin, and depending on the exact mutation, lead to the deposition of various types of proteinaceous deposits in the cornea. These include needle-shaped deposits of amyloid (*lattice dystrophy*); chunky deposits of hyalin (*granular dystrophy*); and combinations of these opacities in the same person (*Avelino dystrophy*, named for the location of the first families with this condition).

Anterior Segment

FUNCTIONAL ANATOMY

The anterior chamber is bounded anteriorly by the cornea, laterally by the trabecular meshwork, and posteriorly by the iris (Fig. 29–11). Aqueous humor, formed by the pars plicata of the ciliary body, enters the posterior chamber, bathes the lens, and circulates through the pupil to gain access to the anterior chamber.

The lens is a closed epithelial system; the basement membrane of the lens epithelium (known as the lens capsule) totally envelops the lens. Thus, the lens epithelium does not exfoliate like the epidermis or a mucosal epithelium. Instead, the lens epithelium and its derivative fibers accumulate within the confines of the lens capsule, thus "infoliating." With aging, therefore, the size of the lens increases. Neoplasms of the lens have not been described.

CATARACT

The term *cataract* describes lenticular opacities that may be congenital or acquired. Systemic diseases (such as galactosemia, diabetes mellitus, Wilson disease, and atopic dermatitis),

drugs (especially corticosteroids), radiation, trauma, and many intraocular disorders are associated with cataract. Age-related cataract typically results from opacification of the lens nucleus (*nuclear sclerosis*). The accumulation of urochrome pigment may render the lens nucleus brown, thus distorting the individual's perception of blue color (the predominance of yellow hues in Rembrandt's paintings later in life might have been a consequence of nuclear sclerotic cataracts). Other physical changes in the lens may generate opacities. For example, the lens cortex may liquefy. Migration of the lens epithelium posterior to the lens equator may result in *posterior subcapsular cataract* secondary to enlargement of abnormally positioned lens epithelium. The technique that is most commonly used to remove opacified lenses extracts the lens contents, leaving the lens capsule intact (extracapsular cataract extraction). A prosthetic intra-ocular lens may be inserted into the eye. Residual lens epithelial cells may migrate over the lens capsule, contributing to opacification of the capsule and reduction in vision after surgery.

Inflammatory reactions to lens material may develop following exposure of the intact lens cortex caused by rupture of the capsule due to trauma or as a result of cataract extraction. It has been suggested that antigen-antibody complexes containing lens cortical material develop especially in the presence of *Propionibacterium acnes* (which acts as an adjuvant), generating a *lens-induced uveitis*.

Occasionally, the lens cortex may liquefy nearly entirely, a condition known as hypermature or *morgagnian cataract*. High-molecular-weight proteins from liquefied lens cortex may leak through the lens capsule (*phacolysis*). This phacolytic protein—either free or contained within macrophages—may clog the trabecular meshwork and contribute to elevation in intra-ocular pressure and optic nerve damage; phacolytic glaucoma is an example of secondary open-angle glaucoma.

THE ANTERIOR SEGMENT AND GLAUCOMA

The term *glaucoma* refers to a collection of diseases characterized by distinctive changes in the visual field and in the cup of the optic nerve. Most of the glaucomas are associated with elevated intra-ocular pressure, although some individuals with normal intra-ocular pressure may develop characteristic optic nerve and visual field changes (*normal* or *low-tension glaucoma*). The relationship between intra-ocular pressure and optic nerve damage is discussed later under "Optic Nerve."

To understand the *pathophysiology of glaucoma* it is useful to consider the formation and drainage of aqueous humor. As Figure 29–11 illustrates, aqueous humor is produced in the ciliary body and passes from the posterior chamber through the pupil into the anterior chamber. Although there are multiple pathways for the egress of fluid from the anterior chamber, most of the aqueous humor drains through the trabecular meshwork, situated in the angle formed by the intersection between the corneal periphery and the anterior surface of the iris. With this background, glaucoma can be classified into two major categories. In *open-angle glaucoma* the aqueous humor has complete physical access to the trabecular meshwork, and the elevation in intra-ocular pressure results from an increased resistance to aqueous outflow in the open angle. In *angle-closure*

ANTERIOR AND POSTERIOR CHAMBERS

MAJOR AQUEOUS OUTFLOW PATHWAY

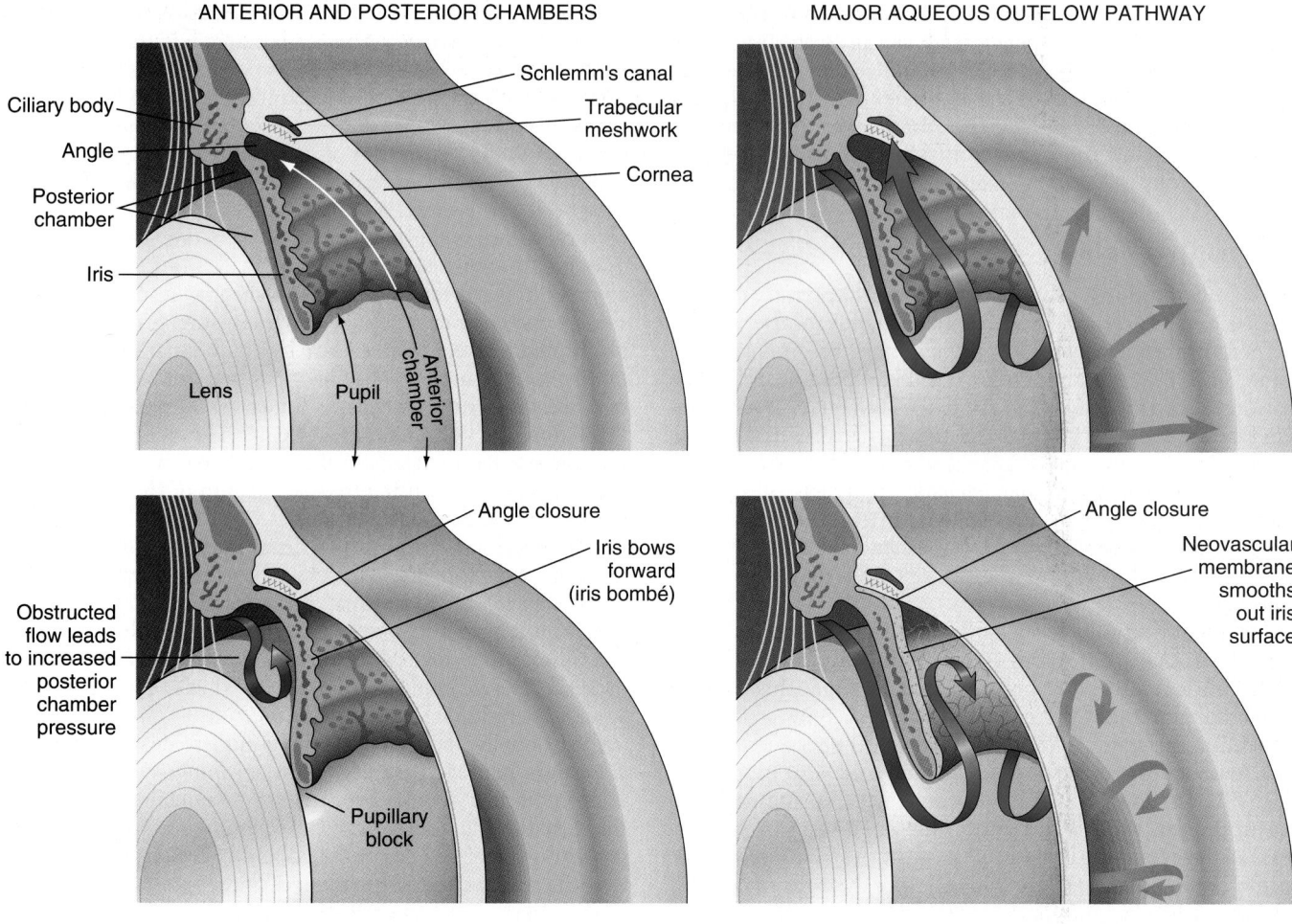

PRIMARY ANGLE-CLOSURE GLAUCOMA

NEOVASCULAR GLAUCOMA

FIGURE 29–11 *Upper left,* The normal eye. Note that the surface of the iris is highly textured with crypts and folds. *Upper right,* The normal flow of aqueous humor. Aqueous humor, produced in the posterior chamber, flows through the pupil into the anterior chamber. The major pathway for the egress of aqueous humor is through the trabecular meshwork, into the Schlemm canal. Minor outflow pathways (uveoscleral and iris, not depicted) contribute to a limited extent to aqueous outflow. *Lower left,* Primary angle-closure glaucoma. In anatomically predisposed eyes, transient apposition of the iris at the pupillary margin to the lens blocks the passage of aqueous humor from the posterior chamber to the anterior chamber. Pressure builds in the posterior chamber, bowing the iris forward (iris bombé) and occluding the trabecular meshwork. *Lower right,* A neovascular membrane has grown over the surface of the iris, smoothing the iris folds and crypts. Myofibroblasts within the neovascular membrane cause the membrane to contract and to become apposed to the trabecular meshwork (peripheral anterior synechiae). Outflow of aqueous humor is blocked, and the intra-ocular pressure becomes elevated.

glaucoma the peripheral zone of the iris adheres to the trabecular meshwork and physically impedes the egress of aqueous humor from the eye. Both open-angle and angle-closure glaucoma can be subclassified into *primary* and *secondary* types.

In *primary open-angle glaucoma,* the most common form of glaucoma, the angle is open, and few changes are apparent structurally. Mutations in the *MYOC* gene have been associated with a subset of individuals with juvenile and adult primary open-angle glaucoma. The function of the gene product, myocilin, is unclear. *MYOC* is present in the tracetabular meshwork, in other anterior segment tissues, and in the optic nerve. The pathogenesis of primary open-angle glaucoma may be related to several genes, but the genes identified thus far account for a small percentage of affected individuals with this condition.[10] The role of these genes in the pathogenesis of glaucoma is not clear.

There are multiple causes of *secondary open-angle glaucoma.* Particulate material such as high-molecular-weight lens proteins produced by phacolysis, senescent red cells after trauma *(ghost cell glaucoma),* iris epithelial pigment granules *(pigmentary glaucoma),* fragments of oxytalan fibers *(exfoliation glaucoma),* and necrotic tumors *(melanomalytic glaucoma)* can clog the trabecular meshwork in the presence of an open angle. Elevations in the pressure on the surface of the eye (episcleral venous pressure) in the presence of an open angle also contributes to secondary open-angle glaucoma. This type of glaucoma is associated with surface ocular vascular malformations seen in *Sturge-Weber syndrome* or as a consequence of arterialization of the episcleral veins following a spontaneous or traumatic carotid-cavernous fistula.

Primary angle-closure glaucoma typically develops in eyes with shallow anterior chambers, often found in individuals with hyperopia. Transient apposition of the pupillary margin of the iris to the anterior surface of the lens may result in obstruction to the flow of aqueous humor through the pupillary aperture *(pupillary block)*. Continued production of aqueous humor by the ciliary body thus elevates pressure in the posterior chamber and may bow the iris periphery forward *(iris bombé)*, apposing it to the trabecular meshwork. These anatomic changes provoke a marked elevation in intra-ocular pressure (see Fig. 29–11). Since the crystalline lens is avascular and the lens epithelium receives its nutrition from the aqueous humor, unremitting elevation in intra-ocular pressure in primary angle-closure glaucoma can damage the lens epithelium. This leads to minute anterior subcapsular opacities that are visible by slit-lamp examination *(glaukomflecken)*. Although the affected individual might have a normal complement of healthy corneal endothelial cells, sustained elevated intra-ocular pressure can produce corneal edema and bullous keratopathy.

There are many causes of *secondary angle-closure glaucoma*. Contraction of various types of pathologic membranes that form over the surface of the iris can draw the iris over the trabecular meshwork, occluding aqueous outflow. For example, chronic retinal ischemia is associated with the up-regulation of VEGF and other pro-angiogenic factors. The appearance of VEGF in the aqueous humor is thought to induce the development of thin, clinically transparent fibrovascular membranes over the surface of the iris. Contraction of myofibroblastic elements in these membranes leads to occlusion of the trabecular meshwork by the iris: *neovascular glaucoma* (see Fig. 29–11). Necrotic tumors, especially retinoblastomas, can also induce iris neovascularization and glaucoma. Secondary angle-closure glaucoma may be caused by other mechanisms as well; for example, tumors in the ciliary body can mechanically compress the iris onto the trabecular meshwork, closing off the major pathway of aqueous outflow.

ENDOPHTHALMITIS AND PANOPHTHALMITIS

In intra-ocular inflammation, vessels in the ciliary body and iris become leaky, allowing cells and exudate to accumulate in the anterior chamber. These changes can be visualized with a slit lamp; at times the inflammatory cells may adhere to the corneal endothelium, forming clinically visible *keratic precipitates*. The size and shape of these precipitates can provide clues to the underlying cause of the inflammation. For example, aggregates of macrophages on the endothelium in sarcoid produce characteristic "mutton-fat" keratic precipitates.

Just as pleural exudate in acute bronchopneumonia can lead to adhesions between the visceral and parietal pleura, the presence of exudate in the anterior chamber can facilitate the formation of adhesions between the iris and the trabecular meshwork or cornea *(anterior synechiae)* or between the iris and anterior surface of the lens *(posterior synechiae)*. Anterior synechiae can lead to elevation in intra-ocular pressure, which may lead to optic nerve damage. Prolonged contact between the iris and the anterior surface of the lens can deprive lens epithelium of contact with aqueous humor and can induce fibrous metaplasia of the lens epithelium: *anterior subcapsular cataract* (Fig. 29–12). The pharmacologic induction of pupillary dilation and cycloplegia in individuals with intra-ocular inflammation is intended in part to prevent the formation of synechiae and their sequelae.

Although inflammation confined to the anterior segment is technically intra-ocular inflammation, the term *endophthalmitis* is not applied clinically unless there is inflammation within the vitreous humor. The retina lines the vitreous cavity, and suppurative inflammation in the vitreous humor (endophthalmitis) is poorly tolerated by the retina; after only a few hours of exposure to acute inflammation, the retina may be irreversibly damaged. Endophthalmitis is classified as *exogenous* (originating in the environment and gaining access to the interior of the eye through a wound) or *endogenous* (delivered to the eye hematogenously). The term *panophthalmitis* is applied to inflammation within the eye that involves the retina, choroid, and sclera and extends into the orbit (Fig. 29–13).

Uvea

Together with the iris, the choroid and ciliary body constitute the uvea. The choroid is among the most richly vascularized sites in the body. As in the retina, there are no lymphatics within the uvea.

UVEITIS

The term *uveitis* can be applied to any type of inflammation in one or more of the tissues that compose the uvea. Thus, the

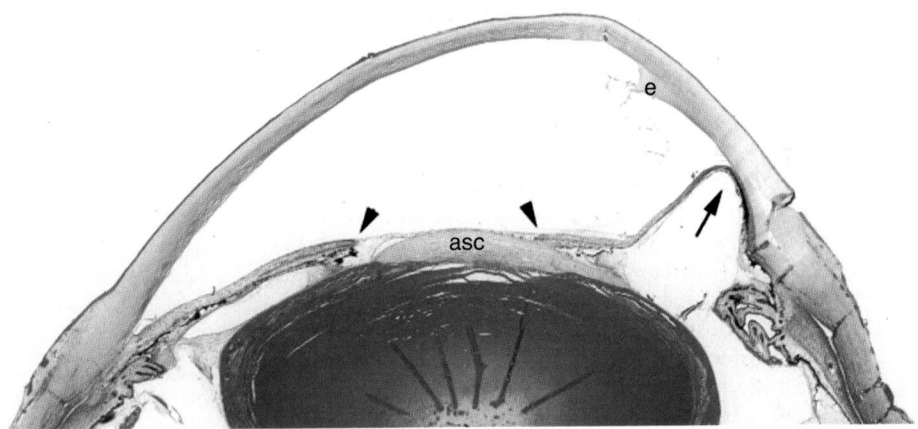

FIGURE 29–12 Sequelae of anterior segment inflammation. This eye was removed for complications of chronic corneal inflammation (not visible at this magnification). The exudate (e) present in the anterior chamber would have been visualized with a slit lamp as an optical "flare." The iris is adherent focally to the cornea, obstructing the trabecular meshwork (anterior synechia, *arrow*), and to the lens (posterior synechiae, *arrowheads*). An anterior subcapsular cataract (asc) has formed. The radial folds in the lens are artifacts.

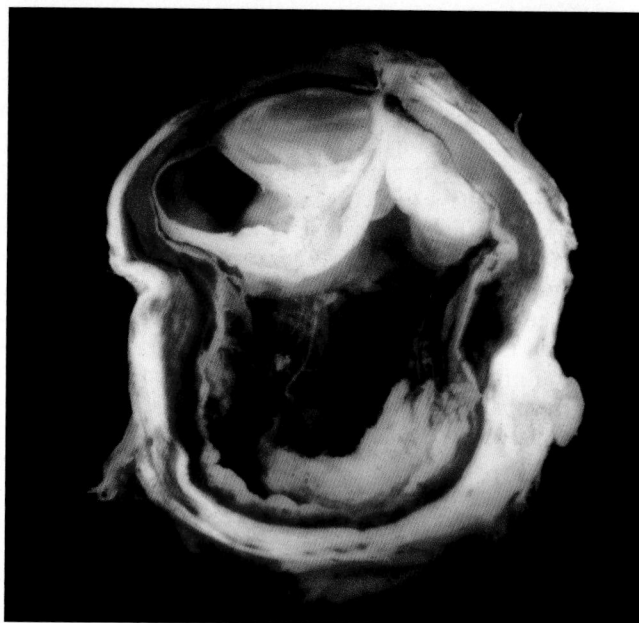

FIGURE 29–13 Exogenous panophthalmitis. This eye was removed after a foreign body injury. Note the suppurative inflammation behind the lens that is drawn up to the right of the lens to the cornea, the site of the wound. The central portion of the vitreous humor was extracted surgically (by vitrectomy). Note the adhesions to the surface of the eye at the eight o'clock position, indicating that the intra-ocular inflammation has spread through the sclera into the orbit: panophthalmitis. (From Folberg R: The eye. In Spencer WH (ed): Ophthalmic Pathology—An Atlas and Textbook, 4th ed. Philadelphia, WB Saunders, 1985.)

iritis that develops after blunt trauma to the eye or that accompanies a corneal ulcer is technically a form of uveitis. However, in clinical practice the term *uveitis* is restricted to a diverse group of chronic diseases that may be either components of a systemic process or localized to the eye. Uveal inflammation may be manifest principally in the anterior segment (e.g., in *juvenile rheumatoid arthritis*) or may affect both the anterior and posterior segments. The complications of chronic anterior segment inflammation were discussed earlier; the remainder of this discussion therefore focuses on the effects of uveal inflammation on the posterior segment of the eye. As will be described briefly, uveitis is frequently accompanied by retinal pathology. Uveitis may be caused by infectious agents (e.g., *Pneumocystis carinii*), may be idiopathic (e.g., sarcoidosis), or may be autoimmune in origin (sympathetic ophthalmia). Some examples are described below.

Granulomatous uveitis is a common complication of sarcoidosis (Chapter 15). In the anterior segment it gives rise to an exudate that evolves into "mutton-fat" keratic precipitates described earlier. In the posterior segment, sarcoid may involve the choroid and retina. Thus, granulomas may be seen in the choroid. Retinal pathology is characterized by perivascular inflammation; this is responsible for the well-known ophthalmoscopic sign of "candle wax drippings." Conjunctival biopsy can be used to detect granulomatous inflammation and confirm the diagnosis of ocular sarcoid.

Numerous infectious processes can affect the choroid or the retina. Inflammation in one compartment is typically associated with inflammation in the other. Retinal *toxoplas-mosis* is usually accompanied by uveitis and even scleritis. Individuals with AIDS may develop cytomegalovirus retinitis and uveal infection such as pneumocystis or mycobacterial choroiditis.[11–13]

Sympathetic ophthalmia is an example of noninfectious uveitis limited to the eye. This condition is characterized by bilateral granulomatous inflammation typically affecting all components of the uvea: a panuveitis. Sympathetic ophthalmia, which blinded young Louis Braille, may complicate a penetrating injury of the eye. In the injured eye, retinal antigens sequestered from the immune system may gain access to lymphatics in the conjunctiva and thus set up a delayed hypersensitivity reaction that affects not only the injured eye but also the contralateral, noninjured eye.[14] The condition may develop from 2 weeks to many years after injury. Enucleation of a blind eye (which can be the sympathizing eye rather than the directly injured eye) may yield diagnostic findings. Sympathetic ophthalmia is treated by the administration of systemic immunosuppressive agents. It is characterized by diffuse granulomatous inflammation of the uvea (choroid, ciliary body, and iris). Plasma cells are typically absent, but eosinophils may be identified in the infiltrate (Fig. 29–14).

NEOPLASMS

The most common intra-ocular malignancy of adults is metastasis to the uvea, typically to the choroid. The occurrence of metastases to the eye is associated with an extremely short survival, and treatment of ocular metastases, usually by radiotherapy, is palliative.

Uveal Nevi and Melanomas

Uveal melanoma is the most common primary intra-ocular malignancy of adults. Although it was formerly thought to be rare (7 per million per year), the incidence of this tumor increases with age, and by the seventh decade the incidence is

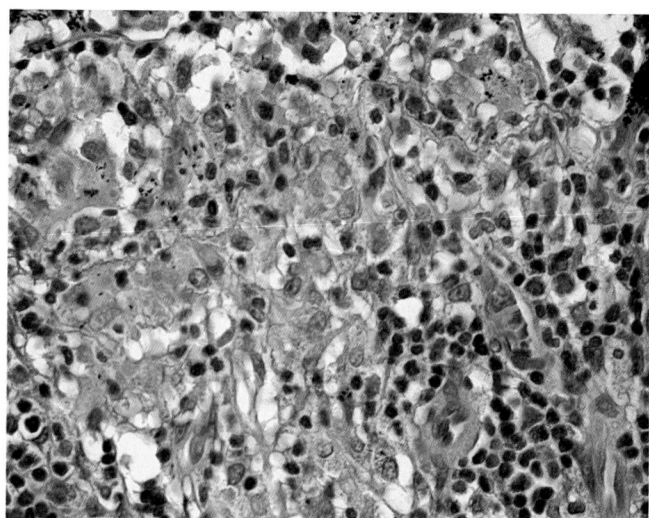

FIGURE 29–14 Sympathetic ophthalmia. The granulomatous inflammation depicted here was identified diffusely throughout the uvea. The uveal granulomas may contain melanin pigment and may be accompanied by eosinophils.

more than 20 per million per year. Unlike cutaneous melanoma, the occurrence of uveal melanoma has remained stable over many years.[15] Although excessive childhood exposure to ultraviolet radiation has been implicated, the link between ultraviolet light and uveal melanoma is not nearly as clear as it is for cutaneous melanoma. Therefore the etiology of uveal melanoma is still unresolved at this time. Uveal nevi, especially choroidal nevi, are rather common, affecting an estimated 10% of the Caucasian population but their progression to melanoma is exceptionally uncommon.

There are no lymphatics within the eye; hence, uveal melanomas, with very rare exception, spread exclusively by a hematogenous route (the only exception being the rare case of melanoma that spreads through the sclera and invades the conjunctiva, thereby gaining access to conjunctival lymphatics). Most uveal melanomas spread first to the liver, thereby providing an excellent example of organ-specific metastasis. Although the 5-year survival rate is approximately 80%,[16] the cumulative melanoma mortality rate is 40% at 10 years, increasing 1% per year thereafter.[17] Examples of metastases appearing many years after treatment are well known, making uveal melanoma a prime candidate for the investigation of tumor dormancy.

Morphology. Histologically, uveal melanomas may contain two types of cells, spindle and epithelioid, in various proportions (Fig. 29–15). Spindle cells are fusiform in shape and have little atypia, whereas epithelioid cells are spherical and have greater cytologic atypicality. Melanomas situated exclusively in the iris tend to follow a relatively indolent course, whereas melanomas of the ciliary body and choroid are more aggressive. The prognosis of choroidal and ciliary body melanomas is related to (1) size (in contrast to cutaneous melanoma, the lateral extent of the tumor rather than tumor depth is the size dimension related to adverse outcome); (2) cell type (tumors containing epithelioid cells have a worse prognosis than do those containing exclusively spindle cells); (3) and proliferative index. In contrast to cutaneous melanomas, large numbers of tumor-infiltrating lymphocytes are associated with an adverse outcome.[18] Extraocular extension is related to poor prognosis. Other features associated with poor prognosis include monosomy 3 and trisomy 8, and the presence of looping patterns rich in laminin that surround packets of tumor cells.[19] These "spaces" (which are not blood vessels) connect to blood vessels and serve as extravascular conduits for the transport of plasma and possibly blood.[20] In vitro studies and examination of human tissues suggest that these patterns are formed by aggressive tumor cells in a process termed vasculogenic mimicry.[21,22]

Uveal melanomas can have an adverse effect on vision, producing changes ranging from retinal detachment to glaucoma. There seems to be no difference in survival between tumors treated by removal of the eye (enucleation) and those treated by radiation treatment. It should be noted that patients treated by radiation and other vision-sparing modalities are diagnosed clinically without tissue removal for pathological examination. There is currently no effective treatment for metastatic uveal melanoma.

Retina and Vitreous

FUNCTIONAL ANATOMY

The neurosensory retina, like the optic nerve, is an embryologic derivative of the diencephalon. The retina therefore responds to injury by means of gliosis. As in the brain, there are no lymphatics. The architecture of the retina explains the ophthalmoscopic appearance of a variety of ocular disorders. Hemorrhages in the nerve fiber layer of the retina are oriented horizontally and appear as streaks or "flames;" the external retinal layers are oriented perpendicular to the retinal surface, and hemorrhages in these outer layers appear as dots (cross-sections of cylinders). Exudates tend to accumulate in the outer plexiform layer of the retina, especially in the macula (Fig. 29–16).

The retinal pigment epithelium (RPE), like the retina, is derived embryologically from the primary optic vesicle, an outpouching of the brain. Separation of the neurosensory retina from the RPE defines a *retinal detachment*. The RPE has an important role physiologically in the maintenance of the outer segments of the photoreceptors. Disturbances in the RPE-photoreceptor interface may play important roles in hereditary retinal degenerations such as *retinitis pigmentosa*.

The adult vitreous humor is avascular. Incomplete regression of fetal vasculature running through the vitreous humor can produce significant pathology as a retrolental mass *(persistent hyperplastic primary vitreous)*. The vitreous humor can be opacified by hemorrhage from trauma or retinal neovascularization. With age the vitreous humor may liquefy and collapse, creating the visual sensation of "floaters." Also, with aging, the posterior face of the vitreous humor—the posterior hyaloid—may separate from the neurosensory retina *(posterior vitreous detachment)*. The relationship between the posterior hyaloid and the neurosensory retina has a key role in the pathogenesis of retinal neovascularization and in some forms of retinal detachment.

RETINAL DETACHMENT

Retinal detachment (separation of the neurosensory retina from the RPE) is broadly classified by etiology based on the presence or absence of a break in the retina. *Rhegmatogenous retinal detachment is associated with a full-thickness retinal defect.* Retinal tears may develop after the vitreous collapses structurally, and the posterior hyaloid exerts traction on points of abnormally strong adhesion to the retinal internal limiting membrane. Liquefied vitreous humor then seeps through the tear and gains access to the potential space between the neurosensory retina and the RPE (Fig. 29–17). Re-attachment of the retina to the RPE generally requires relief of vitreous traction through indenting of the sclera by surgical procedures. This can be accomplished by the application of strips of silicon to the surface of the eye (scleral buckling) and possibly by

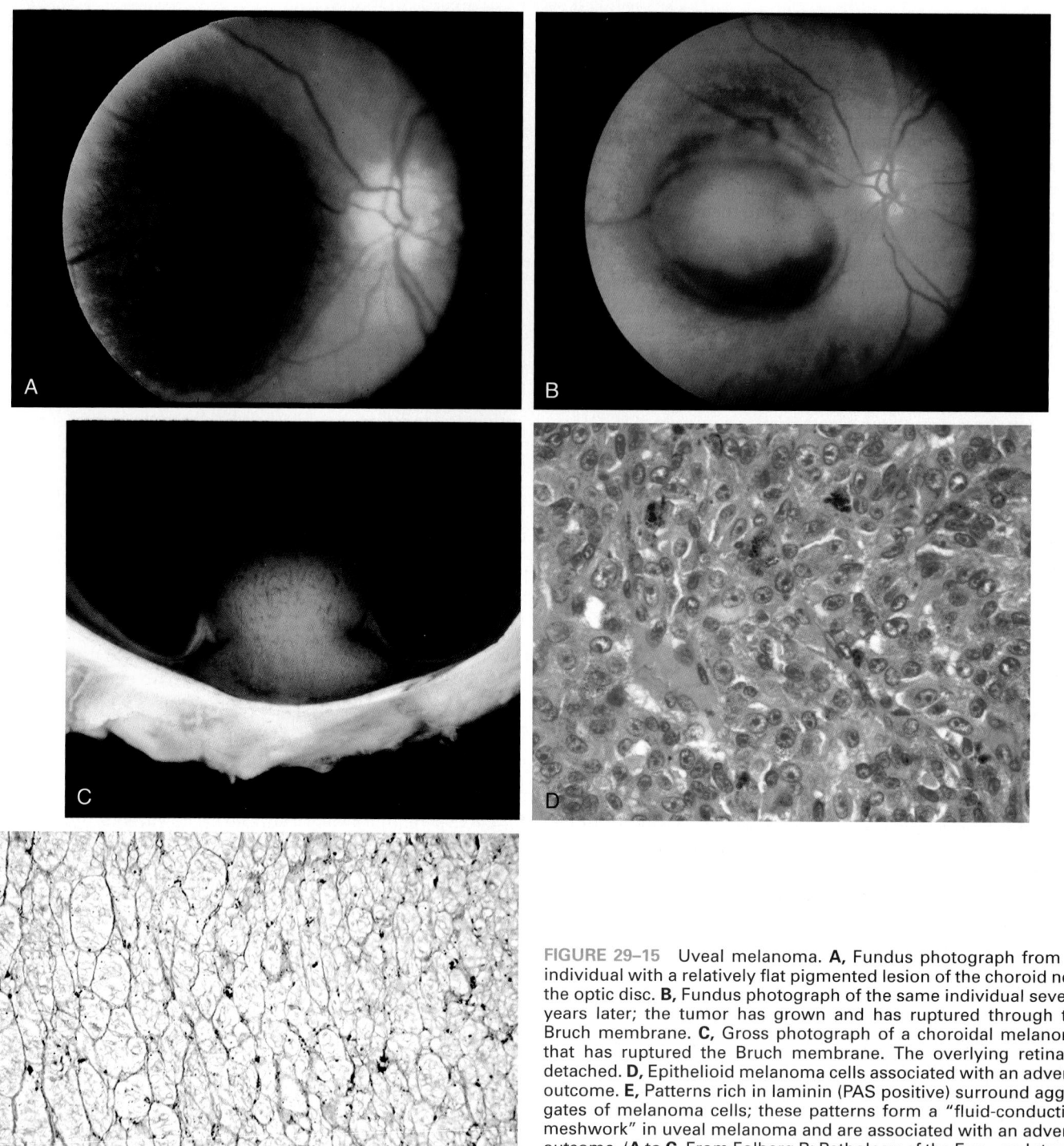

FIGURE 29–15 Uveal melanoma. **A,** Fundus photograph from an individual with a relatively flat pigmented lesion of the choroid near the optic disc. **B,** Fundus photograph of the same individual several years later; the tumor has grown and has ruptured through the Bruch membrane. **C,** Gross photograph of a choroidal melanoma that has ruptured the Bruch membrane. The overlying retina is detached. **D,** Epithelioid melanoma cells associated with an adverse outcome. **E,** Patterns rich in laminin (PAS positive) surround aggregates of melanoma cells; these patterns form a "fluid-conducting meshwork" in uveal melanoma and are associated with an adverse outcome. (**A** to **C,** From Folberg R: Pathology of the Eye—an Interactive CD-ROM Program. Philadelphia, Mosby, 1996; **E,** from Maniotis AJ et al.: Control of melanoma morphogenesis, endothelial survival, and perfusion by extracellular matrix. Lab Invest 82:1031, 2002.)

removal of vitreous material (vitrectomy). Rhegmatogenous retinal detachment may be complicated by *proliferative vitreoretinopathy*, the formation of epiretinal or subretinal membranes by retinal glial cells (Müller cells) or RPE cells.

Non-rhegmatogenous retinal detachment (retinal detachment without retinal break) may complicate retinal vascular disorders associated with significant exudation and any condition that damages the RPE and permits fluid to leak from the choroidal circulation under the retina. Retinal detachments associated with choroidal tumors and malignant hypertension are examples of non-rhegmatogenous retinal detachment.

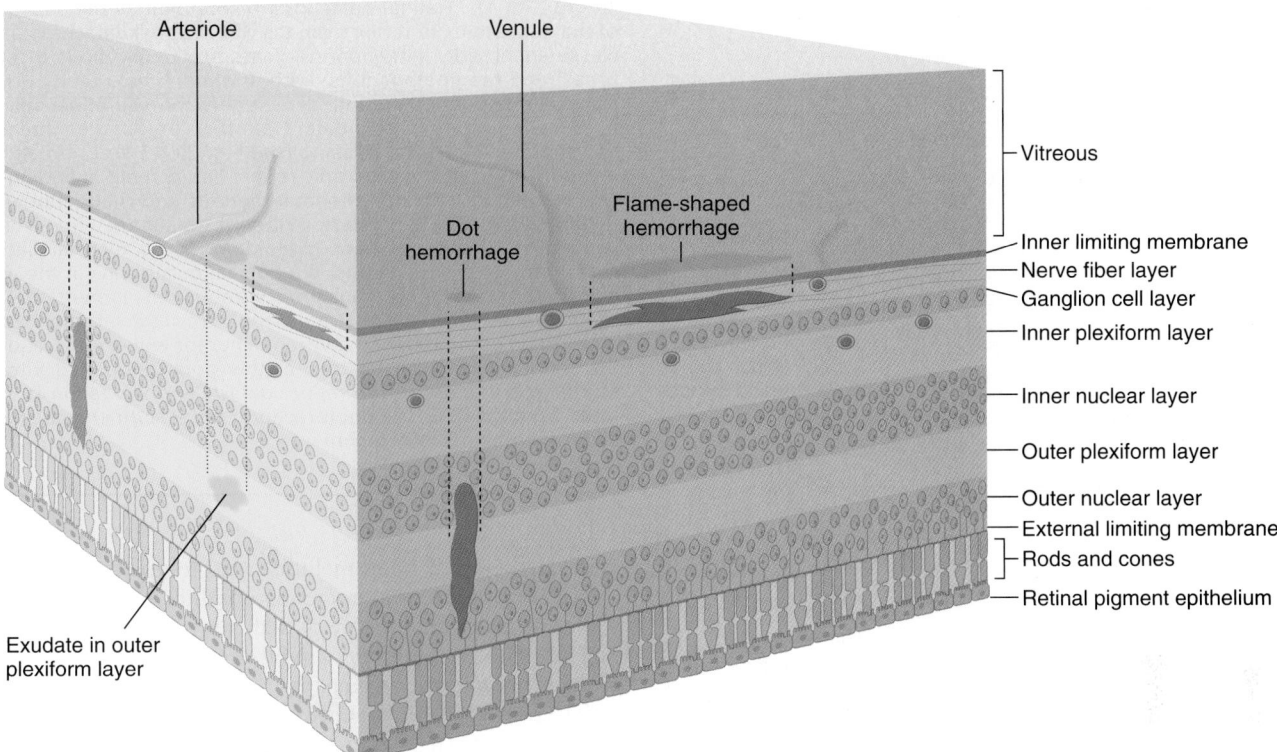

FIGURE 29–16 Clinicopathologic correlations of retinal hemorrhages and exudates. The location of the hemorrhage within the retina determines its appearance by ophthalmoscopy. The retinal nerve fiber layer is oriented parallel to the internal limiting membrane, and hemorrhages of this layer appear to be flame-shaped ophthalmoscopically. The deeper retinal layers are oriented perpendicular to the internal limiting membrane and hemorrhages in this location appear as cross-sections of a cylinder or "dot" hemorrhages. Exudates that originate from leaky retinal vessels accumulate in the outer plexiform layer.

RETINAL VASCULAR DISEASE

Hypertension

Normally, the thin walls of retinal arterioles permit a direct visualization of the circulating blood by ophthalmoscopy. In retinal arteriolosclerosis the thickened arteriolar wall changes the ophthalmic perception of circulating blood: vessels may appear narrowed, and the color of the blood column may change from bright red to copper and to silver depending on the degree of vascular wall thickness (Fig. 29–18A). Retinal arterioles and veins share a common adventitial sheath. Therefore, in pronounced retinal arteriolosclerosis the arteriole may compress the vein at points where both vessels cross (Fig. 29–18B). Venous stasis distal to arteriolar-venous crossing may precipitate occlusions of the retinal vein branches.

In malignant hypertension vessels in the retina and choroid may be damaged. Damage to choroidal vessels may produce focal choroidal infarcts, seen clinically as *Elschnig pearls*. Damage to the choriocapillaris, the internal layer of the choroidal vasculature, may, in turn, damage the overlying RPE and permit the exudate to accumulate in the potential space between the neurosensory retina and the RPE, thereby producing a retinal detachment. Exudate from damaged retinal arterioles typically accumulates in the outer plexiform layer of the retina (see Fig. 29–18A). The ophthalmoscopic finding of a macular star—a spokelike arrangement of exudate in the macula in malignant hypertension—results from exudate accumulating in the outer plexiform layer of the macula that is oriented obliquely instead of perpendicular to the retinal surface.

Occlusion of retinal arterioles may produce infarcts of the nerve fiber layer of the retina (axons of the retinal ganglion cell layer populate the nerve fiber layer). Axoplasmic transport in the nerve fiber layer is interrupted at the point of axonal damage, and accumulation of mitochondria at the swollen ends of damaged axons creates the histologic illusion of cells *(cytoid bodies)*. Collections of cytoid bodies populate the nerve fiber layer infarct, seen ophthalmoscopically as "cotton-wool spots" (Fig. 29–19). Although nerve fiber layer infarcts are described here in the context of hypertension, they may be detected in a variety of retinal occlusive vasculopathies. For example, retinal nerve fiber layer infarcts may develop in individuals with AIDS due to a retinal vasculopathy that is similar to the brain vasculopathy that may develop in this condition.

Diabetes Mellitus

The eye is profoundly affected by diabetes mellitus. The effects of hyperglycemia on the lens and iris have already been mentioned. Thickening of the basement membrane of the epithelium of the pars plicata of the ciliary body is a reliable histologic marker of diabetes mellitus in the eye (Fig. 29–20) and is reminiscent of similar changes in the glomerular mesangium. This discussion focuses on the retinal microangiopathy

**NON-RHEGMATOGENOUS
RETINAL DETACHMENT**

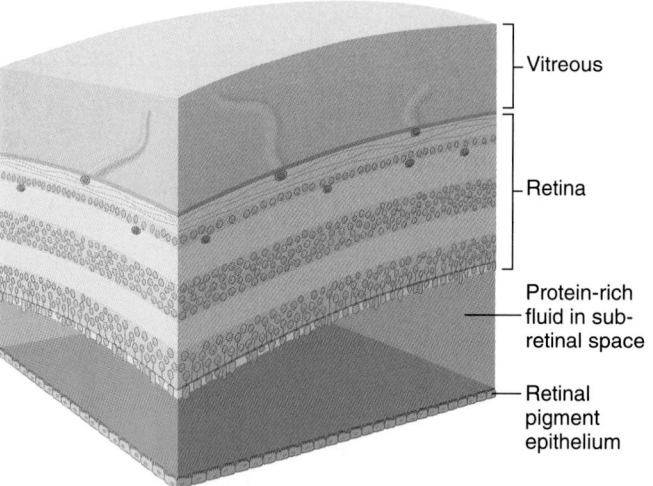

- Vitreous

- Retina

- Protein-rich
fluid in sub-
retinal space

- Retinal
pigment
epithelium

VITREOUS DETACHMENT

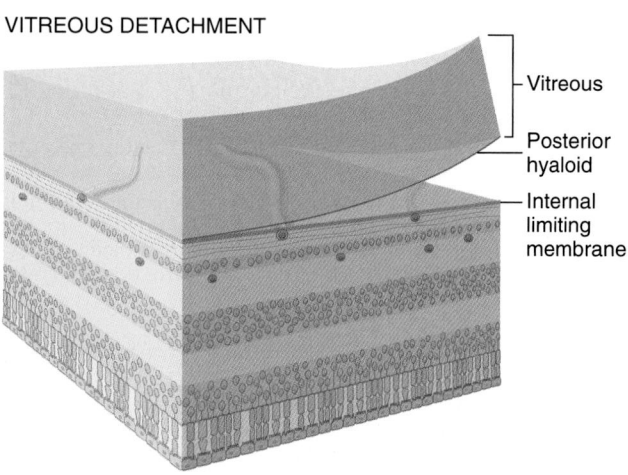

- Vitreous

- Posterior
hyaloid

- Internal
limiting
membrane

**RHEGMATOGENOUS
RETINAL
DETACHMENT**

Blood

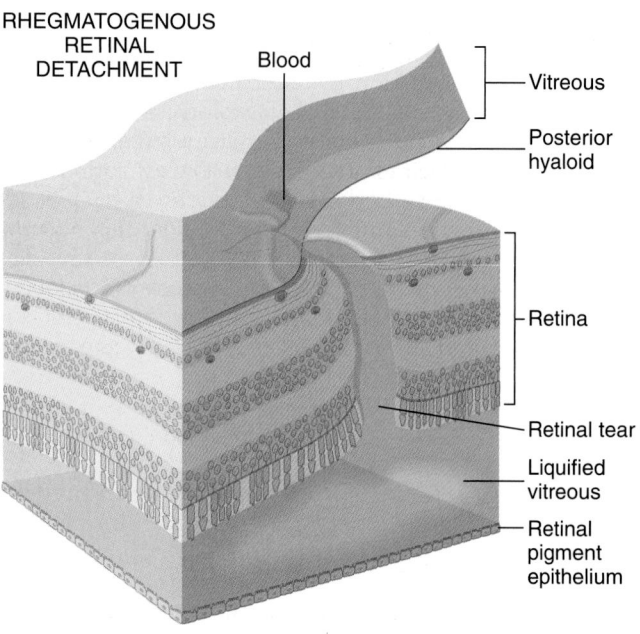

- Vitreous

- Posterior
hyaloid

- Retina

- Retinal tear

- Liquified
vitreous

- Retinal
pigment
epithelium

FIGURE 29–17 Retinal detachment is defined as the separation of the neurosensory retina from the RPE. Retinal detachments are classified broadly into non-rhegmatogenous (without a retinal break) and rhegmatogenous (with a retinal break) types. *Top,* In non-rhegmatogenous retinal detachment the subretinal space is filled with protein-rich exudate. Note that the outer segments of the photoreceptors are missing (see Fig. 29–16 for orientation of layers). This indicates a chronic retinal detachment, a finding that can be seen in both non-rhegmatogenous and rhegmatogenous detachments. *Middle,* Posterior vitreous detachment involves the separation of the posterior hyaloid from the internal limiting membrane of the retina and is a normal occurrence in the aging eye. *Bottom,* If, during a posterior vitreous detachment, the posterior hyaloid does not separate cleanly from the internal limiting membrane of the retina, the vitreous humor will exert traction on the retina, which will be torn at this point. Liquefied vitreous humor seeps through the retinal defect, and the retina is separated from the RPE. The photoreceptor outer segments are intact, illustrating an acute detachment.

associated with diabetes mellitus, a prototype for the consideration of other retinal microangiopathies.

The retinal vasculopathy of diabetes mellitus can be classified into *background (preproliferative) diabetic retinopathy* and *proliferative diabetic retinopathy.*[23]

Background (preproliferative) diabetic retinopathy includes a spectrum of changes ranging from structural and functional abnormalities of angiogenesis located within the retina (i.e., confined beneath the internal limiting membrane of the retina). As with diabetic microangiopathy in general, the *basement membrane of retinal blood vessels is thickened.* In addition, the number of pericytes relative to endothelial cells diminishes. *Microaneurysms* are an important manifestation of diabetic microangiopathy. They are typically smaller than the resolution of direct ophthalmoscopes, and findings customarily described as microaneurysms by ophthalmoscopy may in fact be retinal microhemorrhages. Structural changes in the retinal microcirculation have been associated with a physiologic breakdown in the blood-retinal barrier. Thus, the retinal microcirculation in diabetics may be exceptionally leaky, giving rise to *macular edema,* a common cause of visual loss in these patients. The vascular changes may also produce *exudates* that accumulate in the outer plexiform layer. Although the retinal microcirculation is often hyperpermeable, it is also subject to the effects of micro-occlusion. Both vascular incompetence and vascular micro-occlusions can be visualized clinically after intravenous injection of fluorescein.

Nonperfusion of the retina due to the microcirculatory change described above is associated with up-regulation of VEGF and retinal angiogenesis.[24] The development of intraretinal angiogenesis—new vessels confined within the retina beneath the internal limiting membrane—can be included with lesions termed *intraretinal microangiopathy.*

Clinically, *proliferative diabetic retinopathy* is defined by the appearance of new vessels that sprout from existing vessels—angiogenic vessels—on the surface of either the optic nerve head, which is termed *neovascularization of the disc,* or the surface of the retina, which is designated by the nebulous term *neovascularization elsewhere.* It is worth emphasizing that the term *retinal neovascularization* is not applied either clinically or pathologically unless the newly formed vessels breach the

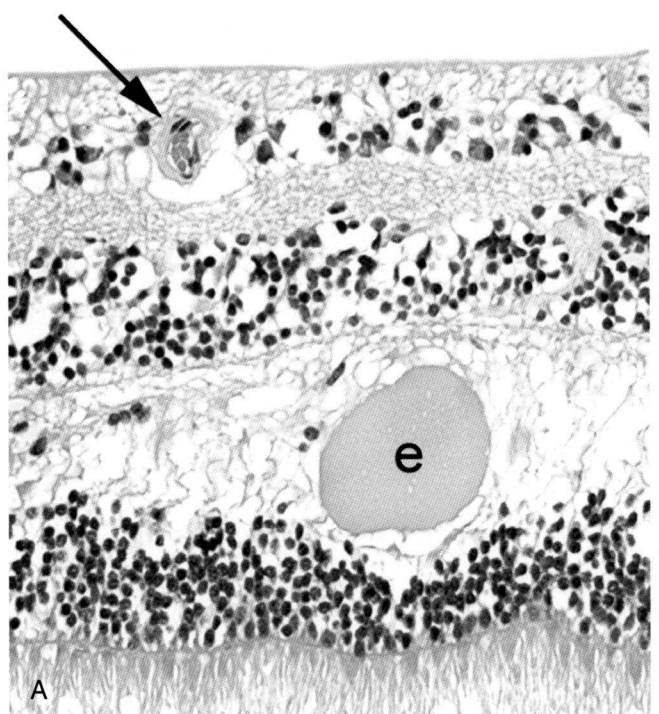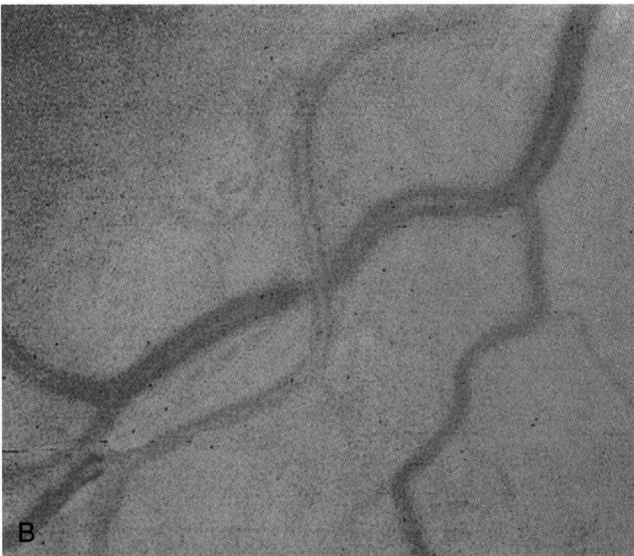

FIGURE 29–18 The retina in hypertension. **A,** The wall of the retinal arteriole *(arrow)* is thick. Note the exudate (e) in the retinal outer plexiform layer. **B,** The fundus in hypertension. The diameter of the arterioles is reduced, and the color of the blood column appears to be less saturated (copper wire–like). If the wall of the vessel were thicker still, the degree of red color would diminish such that the vessels might appear clinically to have a "silver-wire" appearance. In this fundus photograph, note that the vein is compressed where the sclerotic arteriole crosses over it. (**B,** Courtesy of Dr. Thomas A. Weingeist, Department of Ophthalmology and Visual Science, University of Iowa, Iowa City, IA.)

internal limiting membrane of the retina. The quantity and location of retinal neovascularization guide the ophthalmologist in the treatment of proliferative diabetic retinopathy. The web of newly formed vessels is called a *neovascular membrane* both clinically and histopathologically. It is composed of angiogenic vessels with or without a substantial supportive fibrous or glial stroma (Fig. 29–21).

If the vitreous humor has not detached and the posterior hyaloid is intact, neovascular membranes extend along the potential plane between the retinal internal limiting membrane and the posterior hyaloid. Thus, the separation of the vitreous humor from the internal limiting membrane of the retina *(posterior vitreous detachment)* after retinal neovascularization may precipitate massive hemorrhage from the disrupted neovascular membrane. Organization of the retinal neovascular membrane may wrinkle the retina, disrupting the orientation of retinal photoreceptors and producing visual distortion, and may exert traction on the retina, separating it from the RPE (retinal detachment). *Traction retinal detachment* may begin as a non-rhegmatogenous detachment, but severe traction may tear the retina, producing a traction rhegmatogenous detachment.

Retinal neovascularization may be accompanied by the development of a neovascular membrane on the iris surface, presumably secondary to increased levels of VEGF in the aqueous humor.[25] Contraction of the iris neovascular membrane may lead to adhesions between the iris and trabecular meshwork (anterior synechiae), thus occluding a major pathway for aqueous outflow and thereby contributing to elevation of the intra-ocular pressure *(neovascular glaucoma)*. Ablating nonperfused retina by laser photocoagulation or cryopexy triggers regression of both retinal and iris neovascularization.

Retinopathy of Prematurity (Retrolental Fibroplasia)

At term, the nasal (medial) aspect of the retina is vascularized, but the temporal (lateral) aspect of the retinal periphery is incompletely vascularized. In premature or low-birth-weight infants treated with oxygen, the immature retinal vessels in the temporal retinal periphery can constrict, rendering the retinal tissue distal to this zone ischemic. Retinal ischemia can result in up-regulation of pro-angiogenic factors such as VEGF and lead to retinal angiogenesis.[26] Contraction of a peripheral retinal neovascular membrane may result in "dragging" of the temporal aspect of the retina toward the temporal peripheral zone such that the macula (situated temporal to the optic nerve) is displaced laterally. With significant contraction the retina can detach.

Sickle Retinopathy, Retinal Vasculitis, Radiation Retinopathy

Retinopathy affecting individuals with sickle hemoglobinopathies (Chapter 14) has been divided into two types that roughly

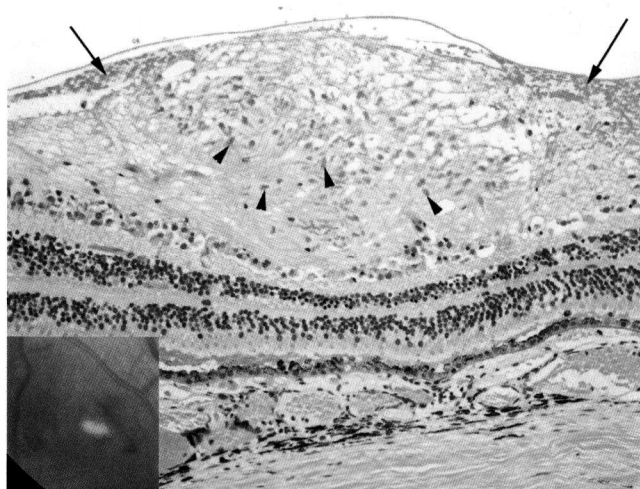

FIGURE 29–19 Nerve fiber layer infarct. A "cotton-wool spot" is illustrated in the *inset,* adjacent to a flame-shaped (nerve fiber layer) hemorrhage. The histology of a cotton-wool spot—an infarct of the nerve fiber layer of the retina—is illustrated in the photomicrograph. A focal swelling of the nerve fiber layer is occupied by numerous red to pink cytoid bodies *(arrowheads),* bulbous ends of severed axons. Hemorrhage *(arrows)* surrounding the nerve fiber layer infarct as illustrated here is a variable and inconsistent finding. (Fundus photograph, Courtesy of Dr. Thomas A. Weingeist, Department of Ophthalmology and Visual Science, University of Iowa, Iowa City, IA.)

parallel those used for diabetic retinopathy: nonproliferative (intraretinal angiopathic changes) and proliferative (retinal neovascularization). The final common pathway in both types is vascular occlusion.[27] Low oxygen tension within the blood vessels in the retinal periphery results in sickling and red cell deformation causing microvascular occlusions. In the nonproliferative form (which occurs in individuals with SS, and SC hemoglobins), *vascular occlusions* are thought to contrib-

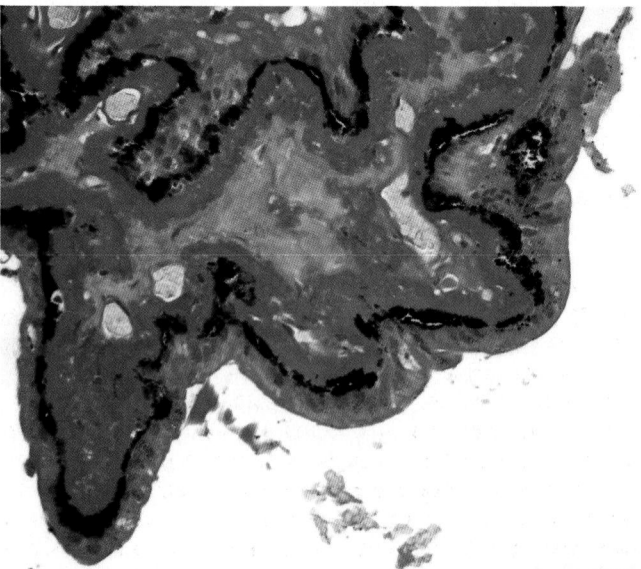

FIGURE 29–20 The ciliary body in chronic diabetes mellitus, PAS stain. Note the massive thickening of the basement membrane of the ciliary body epithelia, reminiscent of changes in the mesangium of the renal glomerulus.

ute to preretinal, intraretinal, and subretinal hemorrhages. The resolution of these hemorrhages may give rise to a variety of ophthalmoscopically visible changes, known as *salmon patches, iridescent spots,* and *black sunburst lesions.* Organization of pre-retinal hemorrhage may result in retinal traction and *retinal detachment.* Vascular occlusions may also contribute to angiogenesis secondary to up-regulation of both VEGF and basic fibroblast growth factor.[28] This can give rise to florid zones of retinal neovascularization in the periphery, described clinically as "sea-fans."

Neovascularization also occurs in a variety of other clinical settings such as peripheral retinal vasculitis, and in irradiation used to treat intra-ocular tumors. The feature common to these conditions is damage to retinal vessels, producing zones of retinal ischemia that drive retinal angiogenesis and its complications, hemorrhage and traction.

Retinal Artery and Vein Occlusions

The central retinal artery or its branches can be occluded by disorders that affect the vessels in general. For example, the lumen of the central retinal artery can be narrowed significantly by atherosclerosis, thus predisposing to thrombosis. Emboli to the central retinal artery can originate from thrombi in the heart or on ulcerated atheromatous plaques in the carotid arteries. Fragments of atherosclerotic plaques can lodge within the retinal circulation *(Hollenhorst plaques).* Total occlusion of a branch retinal artery can produce a segmental infarct of the retina. With sudden cessation of blood supply, the retina (an embryologic derivative of brain tissue) swells acutely and becomes optically opaque. By ophthalmoscopy the fundus in the affected area appears white instead of red or orange, because the retinal opacity blocks the view of the richly vascular choroid.

Total occlusion of the central retinal artery can produce a *diffuse infarct* of the retina. Following an acute occlusion, the retina appears relatively opaque by ophthalmoscopy. The fovea and foveola are physiologically thin; therefore, the normal orange-red of the choroid is not only visible but highlighted by the surrounding opaque retina—the origin of the *cherry-red spot* of the central retinal artery occlusion. The cherry-red spots seen in rare storage diseases such as *Tay-Sachs* and *Niemann-Pick* diseases also have their basis in the anatomic variations of the macula. The storage material accumulates in retinal ganglion cells: the ganglion cell layer of the macula surrounding the fovea is thick, but there are no ganglion cells in the center of the macula, the fovea. Thus, the fovea is relatively transparent to the underlying choroidal vasculature but is rimmed by relatively opaque retina, the result of storage material accumulating in the perifoveal macular ganglion cells (Fig. 29–22).

Retinal arterial occlusions are typically sudden events; therefore, they are not often complicated by prolonged ischemia to allow for up-regulation of pro-angiogenic factors. Hence, retinal arterial occlusions are seldom complicated by either retinal or iris neovascularization.

Retinal vein occlusion may occur with or without ischemia.[29] In ischemic retinal vein occlusion, VEGF and other pro-angiogenic factors are up-regulated in the retina, leading to neovascularization of the retina and surface of the optic nerve head as well as neovascularization of the iris and subse-

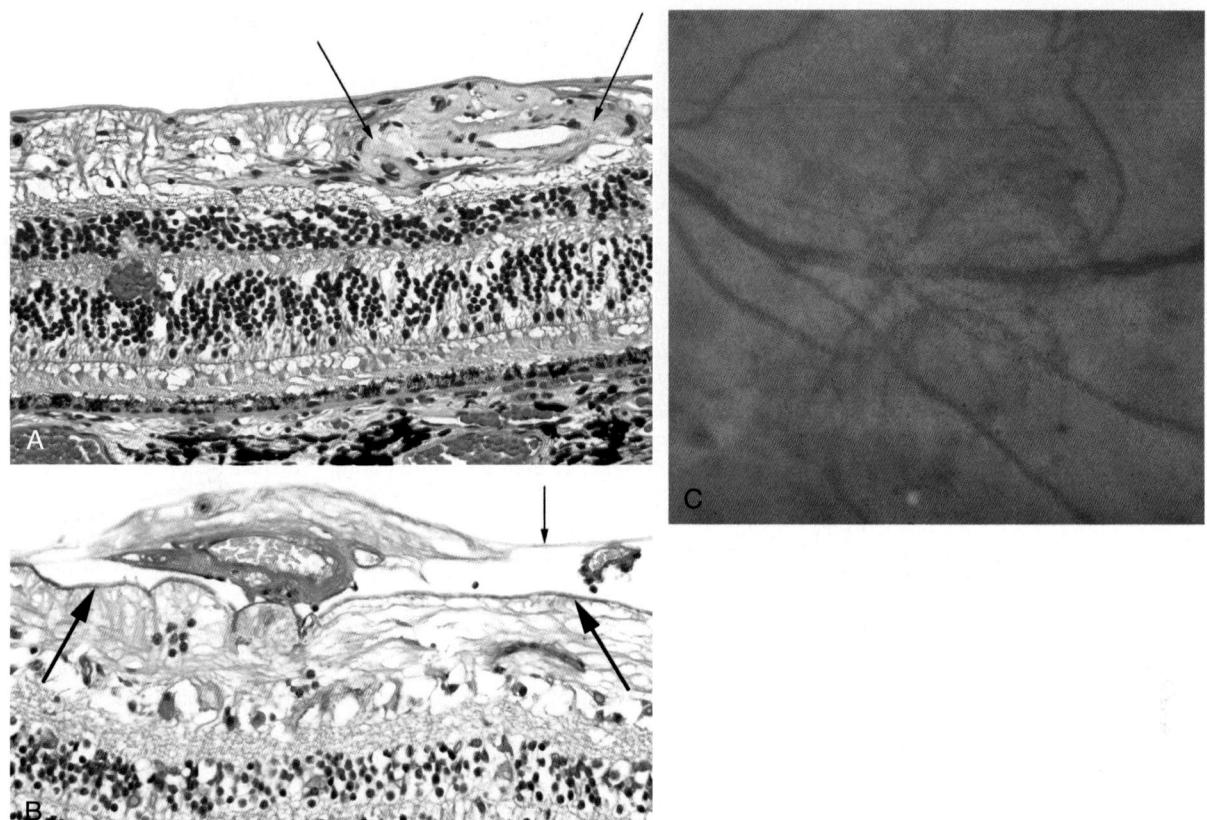

FIGURE 29–21 The retina in diabetes mellitus (see Fig. 29–16 for a schematic of retinal structure). **A,** A tangle of abnormal vessels lies just beneath the internal limiting membrane of the retina on the right half of the photomicrograph *(between arrows)*. This is an example of intraretinal angiogenesis known as intraretinal microangiopathy (IRMA). Note the retinal hemorrhage in the outer plexiform layer in the *left half*. The ganglion cell layer and the nerve fiber layer—the axons of the ganglion cells—are absent. The rarefied space beneath internal limiting membrane to the *left* of the focus of IRMA consists largely of elements of retinal glial (Müller) cells. Absence of the ganglion cell and nerve fiber layers is a hallmark of glaucoma. The chronic diabetes mellitus in this individual was complicated by iris neovascularization and secondary angle-closure glaucoma (neovascular glaucoma). **B,** In this section stained by PAS, the internal limiting membrane is indicated by the *thick arrows* and the posterior hyaloid of the vitreous by the *thin arrow*. In the potential space between these two landmarks, the vessels to the left of the *thin arrow* are invested with a fibrous-glial stroma and would appear ophthalmoscopically as a white neovascular membrane. The thin-walled vessel to the right of the *thin arrow* is not invested with connective tissue. A posterior vitreous detachment in an eye such as this might exert traction on these new vessels and precipitate a massive vitreous hemorrhage. **C,** Ophthalmoscopic view of retinal neovascularization (known clinically as neovascularization "elsewhere" in contrast with neovascularization of the optic disc) creating a neovascular membrane.

quent angle-closure glaucoma.[30] Non-ischemic retinal vein occlusion may be complicated by hemorrhages, exudates, and macular edema but is seldom complicated by retinal or iris neovascularization.

AGE-RELATED MACULAR DEGENERATION

From the name of this disorder, it is clear that advancing age is a risk factor. The cumulative incidence of age-related macular degeneration (ARMD) in individuals 75 years of age and older is 8%, and with increasing longevity ARMD is becoming a major health problem.[31]

Nearly 71% of cases are estimated to be heritable, but the identification of genetic risk factors has not yet contributed to therapeutic strategies that modulate the clinical course.[32] Attention is now focused on the roles of several genes, especially *CFH* (complement factor H) in the pathogenesis of this condition.[33] Individuals with the *CFH* CC genotype who have smoked at least 10 pack-years (i.e., at least 20 cigarettes per day for 10 years) have a 144-fold increase in developing the

neovascular form of ARMD than individuals with this genotype who have smoked for fewer than 10 pack-years.[34]

To understand the pathogenesis of ARMD it is important to appreciate the existence of a structural and functional unit composed of the retinal pigment epithelium (RPE), Bruch membrane (which contains the basement membrane of the RPE), and the innermost layer of the choroidal vasculature, the choriocapillaris. Disturbance in any component of this "unit" affects the health of the overlying photoreceptors, producing visual loss.

It is commonplace to describe ARMD as either non-neovascular (atrophic or dry) or neovascular (exudative or wet). Non-neovascular ARMD is identified ophthalmoscopically by diffuse or discrete deposits in the Bruch membrane (drusen) and geographic atrophy of the RPE. Approximately 10% to 20% of individuals with *non-neovascular* ARMD develop choroidal neovascular membranes. Loss of vision is substantially more severe in these individuals.

Choroidal neovascularization is defined by the presence of angiogenic vessels that presumably originate from the chorio-

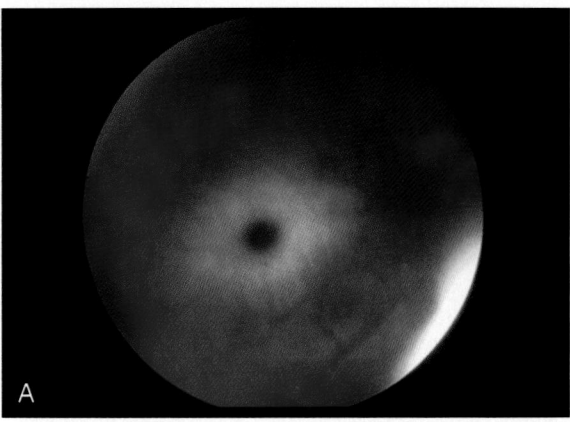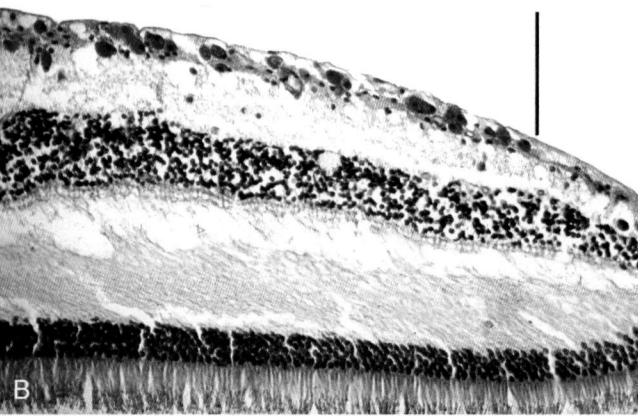

FIGURE 29–22 The cherry-red spot in Tay-Sachs disease. **A,** Fundus photograph of the cherry-red spot in Tay-Sachs disease. **B,** Photomicrograph of the macula in an individual with Tay-Sachs disease, stained with PAS to highlight the accumulation of ganglioside material in the retinal ganglion cells. The presence of ganglion cells filled with gangliosides outside the fovea blocks the transmission of the normal orange-red color of the choroid, but absence of ganglion cells within the fovea (to the right of the *vertical bar*) permits the normal orange-red color to be visualized, accounting for the so-called cherry-red spot. (**A,** Courtesy of Dr. Thomas A. Weingeist, Department of Ophthalmology and Visual Science, University of Iowa, Iowa City, IA; **B,** from the teaching collection of the Armed Forces Institute of Pathology.)

capillaris and penetrate through the Bruch membrane beneath the RPE (Fig. 29–23). This neovascular membrane may also penetrate the RPE and become situated directly beneath the neurosensory retina. The vessels in this membrane may leak, and the exuded blood may be organized by RPE cells into macular scars. Occasionally, hemorrhage from these neovascular membranes can be massive, leading to the localized suffusion of blood that may be mistaken clinically for an intra-ocular neoplasm, or may produce diffuse vitreous hemorrhage. Currently the mainstay of treatment for neovascular ARMD is the injection of VEGF antagonists into the vitreous of the affected eye.[35]

Choroidal neovascular membranes can develop in conditions that are unrelated to age, such as pathologic myopia (Fuchs spot), following traumatic disruption of the Bruch membrane, angioid streaks, or an immunological response to systemic histoplasmosis (presumed ocular histoplasmosis syndrome).

OTHER RETINAL DEGENERATIONS

Retinitis Pigmentosa

The term *"retinitis" pigmentosa* is an unfortunate relic that is used to describe a collection of inherited retinal disorders that were formerly incorrectly presumed to be inflammatory. The conditions that are grouped under the rubric of retinitis pigmentosa are fairly common and have an incidence of 1 in 3600. They may be inherited as X-linked recessive, autosomal recessive, or autosomal dominant (the age of onset correlates with the inheritance pattern, with autosomal dominant retinitis pigmentosa appearing later in life). Retinitis pigmentosa may be part of a syndrome such as *Refsum disease* or may develop in isolation (nonsystemic retinitis pigmentosa).

Retinitis pigmentosa is linked to mutations in genes that regulate the functions of either the photoreceptor cells or the RPE. These include genes that regulate the visual cascade and visual cycle, structural genes (transpanins), transcription

factors, retinal catabolic pathways, and mitochondrial metabolism.[36] *Typically, both rods and cones are lost to apoptosis,* though in varying proportions. Loss of rods may lead to early *night blindness* and constricted visual fields. As cones are lost, *central visual acuity* may be affected. Clinically, retinal atrophy is accompanied by constriction of retinal vessels and optic nerve head atrophy ("waxy pallor" of the optic disk) and the accumulation of retinal pigment around blood vessels, thus accounting for the "pigmentosa" in the disease's name. The electroretinogram reveals abnormalities characteristic of this disease.

RETINITIS

A variety of pathogens can contribute to the development of infectious retinitis. For example, *Candida* may disseminate to

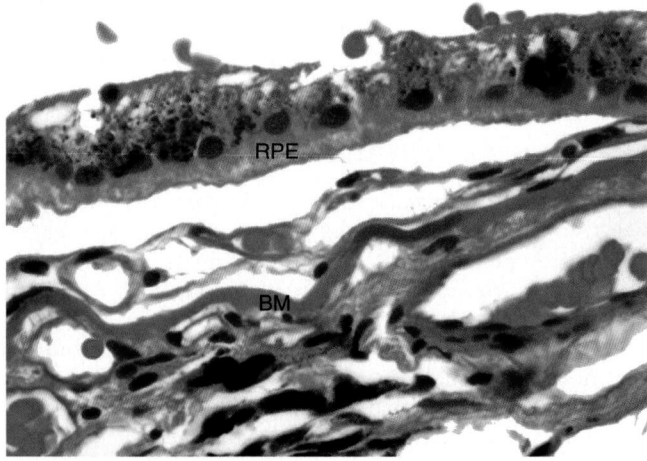

FIGURE 29–23 Age-related macular degeneration. A neovascular membrane is positioned between the RPE and Bruch membrane (BM). Note the blue discoloration of Bruch membrane to the right of the label, indicating focal calcification.

the retina hematogenously, especially in the setting of intravenous drug abuse or in systemic candidemia from other causes. Hematogenous dissemination of pathogens to the retina typically results in multiple retinal abscesses. As was mentioned previously, cytomegalovirus retinitis is an important cause of visual morbidity in immunocompromised individuals, especially those with AIDS.

RETINAL NEOPLASMS

Retinoblastoma

Retinoblastoma is the most common primary intra-ocular malignancy of children. The molecular genetics of retinoblastoma has been discussed in detail (Chapter 7). Although the name *retinoblastoma* might suggest origin from a primitive retinal cell that is capable of differentiation into both glial and neuronal cells, it is now clear that the cell of origin of retinoblastoma is neuronal. Recall that in approximately 40% of cases, retinoblastoma occurs in individuals who inherit a germline mutation of one *RB* allele. Retinoblastomas arising in the context of germline mutations not only may be bilateral but also may be associated with pinealoblastoma ("trilateral" retinoblastoma), which is associated with a dismal outcome.[37]

> **Morphology.** The pathology of retinoblastoma, both hereditary and sporadic types, is identical. Tumors may contain both undifferentiated and differentiated elements. The former appear as collections of small, round cells with hyperchromatic nuclei. In well-differentiated tumors there are Flexner-Wintersteiner rosettes and fleurettes reflecting photoreceptor differentiation. It should be noted, however, that the degree of tumor differentiation does not appear to be associated with the prognosis. As seen in Figure 29–24, viable tumor cells are found encircl-
>
> ing tumor blood vessels with zones of necrosis typically found in relatively avascular areas, illustrating the dependence of retinoblastoma on its blood supply. Focal zones of dystrophic calcification are characteristic of retinoblastoma.

In an effort to preserve vision and eradicate the tumor, many ophthalmic oncologists now attempt to reduce tumor burden by administration of chemotherapy; after chemoreduction, tumors may be obliterated by laser treatment or cryopexy. Retinoblastoma tends to spread to the brain and bone marrow and seldom disseminates to the lungs. Prognosis is adversely affected by extra-ocular extension and invasion along the optic nerve, and by choroidal invasion. A variant of retinoblastoma—retinocytoma or retinoma—has been reported and appears to be a pre-malignant lesion.[38] The appearance of retinoblastoma in one eye and retinocytoma in the other eye is characteristic of heritable retinoblastoma.

Retinal Lymphoma

Primary retinal lymphoma is analogous to primary large-cell lymphoma of the brain; therefore, it involves the two retinal layers derived from brain: the neurosensory retina and the RPE. The underlying choroid is typically filled with a cytologically benign lymphoid infiltrate. Primary intra-ocular lymphoma tends to occur in older individuals and may mimic uveitis clinically. The diagnosis depends on a demonstration of lymphoma cells in vitreous aspirates.[39]

Optic Nerve

As a sensory tract of the central nervous system, the optic nerve is surrounded by meninges, and cerebrospinal fluid circulates around the nerve. The pathology of the optic nerve is

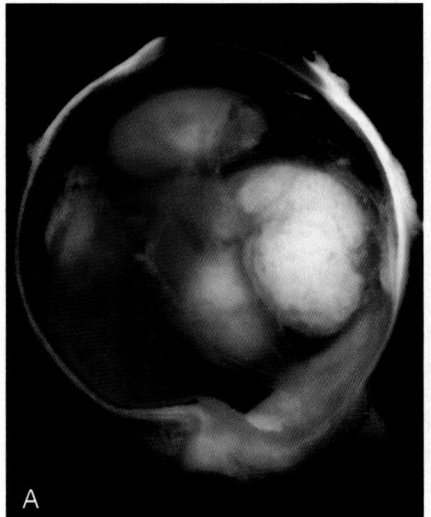
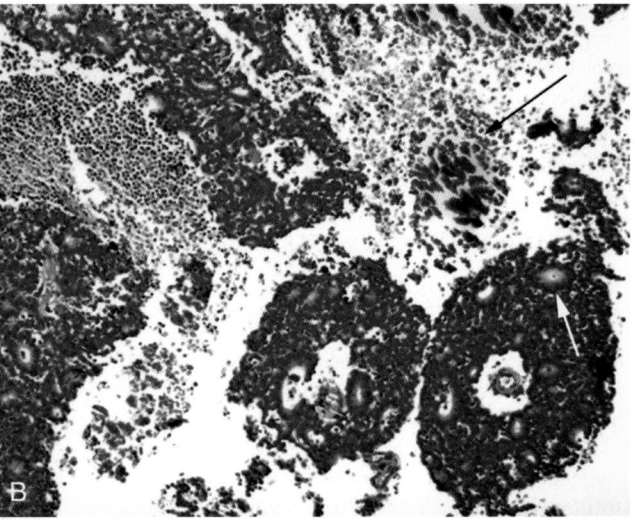

FIGURE 29–24   Retinoblastoma. **A,** Gross photograph of retinoblastoma. **B,** Tumor cells appear viable when in proximity to blood vessels, but necrosis is seen as the distance from the vessel increases. Dystrophic calcification *(dark arrow)* is present in the zones of tumor necrosis. Flexner-Wintersteiner rosettes—arrangements of a single layer of tumor cells around an apparent "lumen"—are seen throughout the tumor, and one such rosette is indicated by the *white arrow*.

similar to the pathology of the brain. For example, the most common primary neoplasms of the optic nerve are glioma (typically *pilocytic astrocytomas*) and meningioma.

ANTERIOR ISCHEMIC OPTIC NEUROPATHY

There are striking similarities between stroke and a condition known in ophthalmic terminology as *anterior ischemic optic neuropathy* (AION).[40] As used clinically, the term *AION* includes a spectrum of injuries to the optic nerve varying from ischemia to infarction. Thus, transient partial interruptions in blood flow to the optic nerve can produce episodes of transient loss of vision, whereas total interruption in blood flow can produce an optic nerve infarct, either segmental or total. Zones of relative ischemia may surround segmental infarcts of the optic nerve. Optic nerve function in these poorly perfused but not infarcted zones may recover. The optic nerve does not regenerate, and visual loss from infarction is permanent.

Interruption in the blood supply to the optic nerve can result from inflammation of the vessels that supply the optic nerve, known as *arteritic AION*, or from embolic or thrombotic events, known as *non-arteritic AION*. Bilateral total infarcts of the optic nerve resulting in total blindness have been reported in temporal arteritis (arteritic AION), adding urgency to the treatment of this condition with high doses of corticosteroids.

PAPILLEDEMA

Edema of the head of the optic nerve may develop as a consequence of compression of the nerve (as in a primary neoplasm of the optic nerve) or from elevations of cerebrospinal fluid pressure surrounding the nerve. The concentric increase in pressure encircling the nerve contributes to venous stasis both at the nerve head and in axoplasmic transport, leading to nerve head swelling. Swelling of the optic nerve head in elevated intra-cranial pressure is typically bilateral (unless the affected individual has experienced previous unilateral optic atrophy) and is commonly termed *papilledema*. Typically, acute papilledema from increased intra-cranial pressure is not associated with visual loss. Ophthalmoscopically, the optic nerve head is swollen and hyperemic; by contrast, the optic nerve head in the relatively acute phases of anterior ischemic optic neuropathy appears swollen and pale because of decreased nerve perfusion (Fig. 29–25). In papilledema secondary to increased intra-cranial pressure, the optic nerve may remain congested for a prolonged period of time.

GLAUCOMATOUS OPTIC NERVE DAMAGE

As discussed already, the majority of individuals with glaucoma have elevated intra-ocular pressure. However, there is a small group that develops the visual field and optic nerve changes typical of glaucoma with normal intra-ocular pressure: so-called *normal-tension glaucoma*. Interestingly, mutations in the optineurin gene are seen in individuals with normal-tension glaucoma but are not seen in individuals with primary open-angle glaucoma, in which pressure is elevated chronically.[41] Conversely, some individuals with elevated intra-ocular pressure who are followed over long periods of

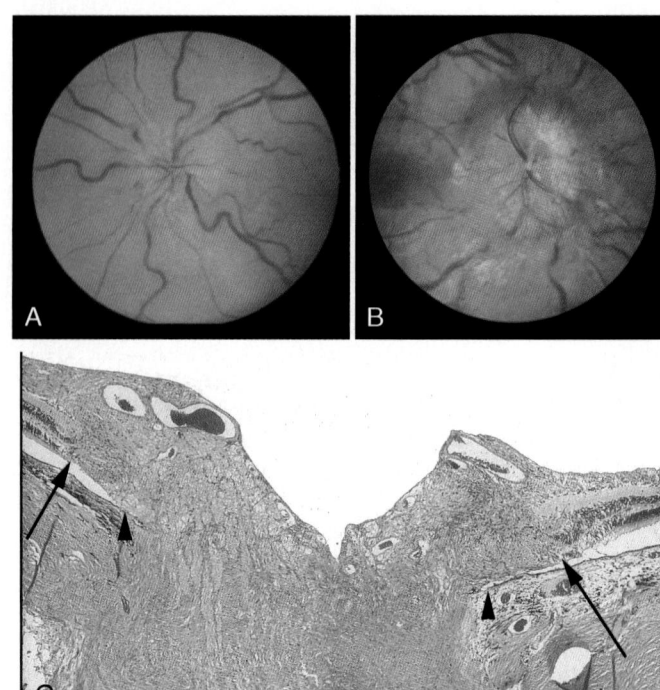

FIGURE 29–25 The optic nerve in anterior ischemic optic neuropathy (AION) and papilledema. **A,** In the acute phases of AION the optic nerve may be swollen, but it is relatively pale because of decreased perfusion. **B,** In papilledema secondary to increased intra-cranial pressure, the optic nerve is typically swollen and hyperemic. **C,** Normally, the termination of Bruch membrane *(arrowhead)* is aligned with the beginning of the neurosensory retina, as indicated by the presence of stratified nuclei *(arrow)*, but in papilledema the optic nerve is swollen, and the retina is displaced laterally. This is the histologic explanation for the blurred margins of the optic nerve head seen clinically in this condition. (**A** and **B,** Courtesy of Dr. Sohan S. Hayreh, Department of Ophthalmology and Visual Science, University of Iowa, Iowa City, IA; **C,** from the teaching collection of the Armed Forces Institute of Pathology.)

time never develop visual field changes or optic nerve cupping. Therefore, it is clear that whatever the mechanism of damage to the retinal ganglion cell—the axons of which populate the optic nerve—there is a spectrum of neuronal susceptibility to the effects of elevated intra-ocular pressure. Therefore, considerable research is now directed toward understanding mechanisms by which the optic nerve axons may be protected from injury.[42]

Morphology. Characteristically, there is a diffuse loss of ganglion cells and thinning of the retinal nerve fiber layer (Fig. 29–26), which can be measured by optical coherence tomography. In advanced cases, the optic nerve is both cupped and atrophic, a combination unique to glaucoma. Elevated intra-ocular pressure in infants and children can lead to diffuse enlargement of the eye **(buphthalmos)** or enlargement of the cornea **(megalocornea)**. Several mutations have been associated with the development of infantile glaucoma, but the mechanisms by which these genes produce glaucoma is unclear. After the eye reaches its adult size, prolonged elevation of intra-ocular pressure can lead to focal thinning of the sclera, and uveal tissue may line ectatic sclera **(staphyloma)**.

OTHER OPTIC NEUROPATHIES

Optic neuropathy may be inherited (as in Leber hereditary optic neuropathy) or may be secondary to nutritional deficiencies (as in so-called tobacco-alcohol amblyopia) or toxins such as methanol. Individuals may experience a severe visual disability if fibers in the optic nerve degenerate, especially if the central visual acuity is lost as a result of degeneration of the nerve fibers that originate from the macula.

The predilection for Leber hereditary optic neuropathy to develop in young men is explained by inheritance of mitochondrial gene mutations (Chapter 5). It is possible that these

mutations provide for a genetic susceptibility to a variety of environmental exposures that constitute the final trigger for optic nerve degeneration.[43] Since neuronal health is dependent on axoplasmic transport of mitochondria, mitochondrial dysfunctions give rise to neurologic disorders including optic neuropathy.[44]

OPTIC NEURITIS

Many unrelated conditions have historically been grouped under the heading of optic neuritis. Unfortunately, the term itself suggests optic nerve inflammation, which might not accurately describe the pathophysiologic changes. In common clinical usage the term *optic neuritis* is used to describe a loss of vision secondary to demyelinization of the optic nerve. One of the most important causes of optic neuritis is multiple sclerosis (Chapter 28). Indeed, optic neuritis may be the first manifestation of this disease. The 10-year risk of developing

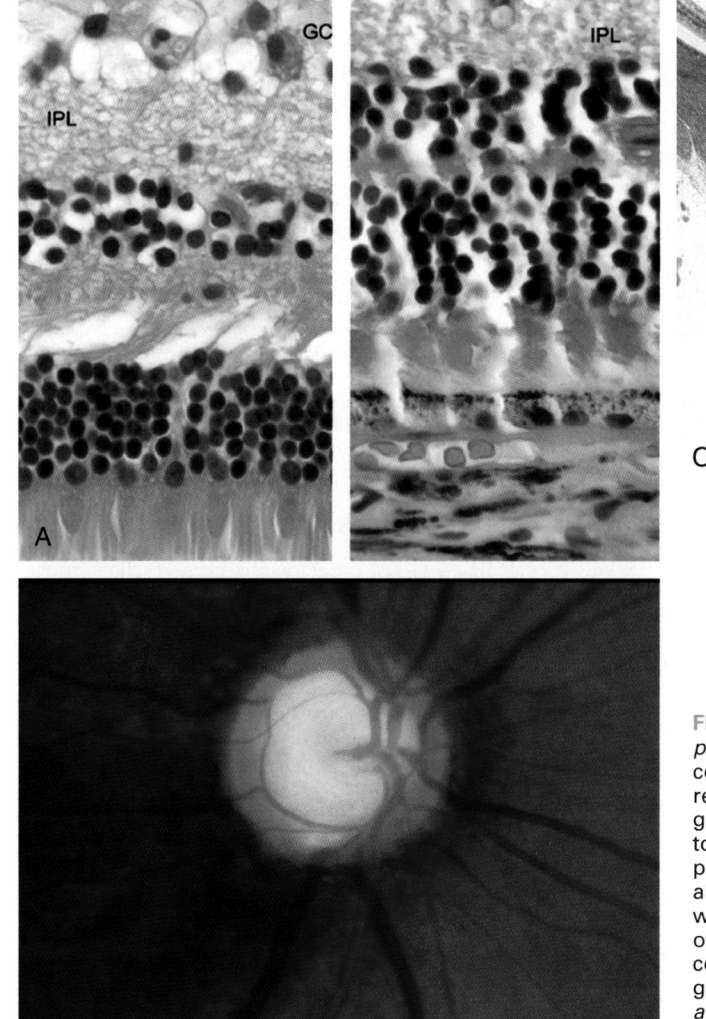

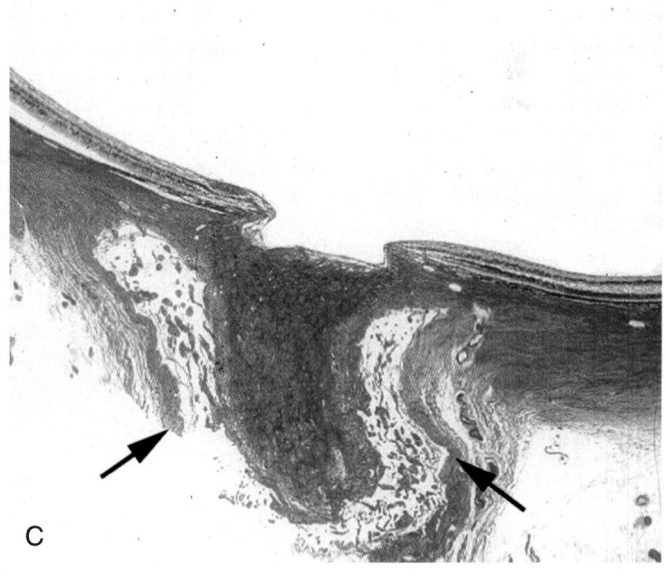

FIGURE 29–26 The retina and optic nerve in glaucoma. **A,** *Left panel*, normal retina; *right panel*, the retina in long-standing glaucoma (same magnification). The full thickness of the glaucomatous retina is captured *(right)*, a reflection of the thinning of the retina in glaucoma. In the glaucomatous retina, the areas corresponding to the nerve fiber layer (NFL) and ganglion cell layer (GC) are atrophic; the inner plexiform layer (IPL) is labeled for reference. Note also that the outer nuclear layer of the glaucomatous retina is aligned with the inner nuclear layer of the normal retina due to the thinning of the retina in glaucoma. See Figure 29-16 for orientation. **B,** Glaucomatous optic nerve cupping results in part from loss of retinal ganglion cells, the axons of which populate the optic nerve. **C,** The *arrows* point to the dura of the optic nerve. Notice the wide subdural space, a result of atrophy of the optic nerve. There is a striking degree of cupping on the surface of the nerve as a consequence of long-standing glaucoma.

multiple sclerosis after the first attack of optic neuritis increases if the affected person has concomitant evidence of brain lesions as detected by magnetic resonance imaging. However, even when brain lesions are detectable, the risk of progression to multiple sclerosis is only 40%.[45] Individuals with a single episode of optic nerve demyelinization may recover vision and remain disease free.

The End-Stage Eye: Phthisis Bulbi

Trauma, intra-ocular inflammation, chronic retinal detachment, and many other conditions can give rise to an eye that is both small (atrophic) and internally disorganized: *phthisis bulbi.* Congenitally small eyes—hypoplastic or *microphthalmic* eyes—are generally not disorganized internally. Phthisical eyes typically feature the following changes: the presence of exudate or blood between the ciliary body and sclera and the choroid and sclera *(ciliochoroidal effusion)*; the presence of a membrane extending across the eye from one aspect of the ciliary body to the other *(cyclitic membrane)*; chronic retinal detachment; optic nerve atrophy; the presence of intra-ocular bone, which is thought by many to originate from *osseous metaplasia* of the RPE; and a thickened sclera, especially posteriorly. Ciliochoroidal effusion is typically associated with the physiologic state of low intra-ocular pressure *(hypotony)*. The normal pull of the extra-ocular muscles on a hypotonous eye may render the appearance of the eye as square rather than round.

REFERENCES

1. Friend SH et al.: A human DNA segment with properties of the gene that predisposes to retinoblastoma and osteosarcoma. Nature 323:643, 1986.
2. Hatton MP, Rubin PA: The pathophysiology of thyroid-associated ophthalmopathy. Ophthalmol Clin North Am 15:113, 2002.
3. Ahmed M et al.: Diagnosis of limited ophthalmic Wegener granulomatosis: distinctive pathologic features with ANCA test confirmation. Int Ophthalmol 28:35, 2008.
4. Song A et al.: Sebaceous cell carcinoma of the ocular adnexa: clinical presentations, histopathology, and outcomes. Ophthal Plast Reconstr Surg 24:194, 2008.
5. Rose AS et al.: Hepatic, ocular and cutaneous sarcoidosis. Clin Chest Med 29:509, 2008.
6. Scott IU et al.: Human papillomavirus 16 and 18 expression in conjunctival intraepithelial neoplasia. Ophthalmology 109:542, 2002.
7. Folberg R et al.: Benign conjunctival melanocytic lesions: clinicopathologic features. Ophthalmology 96:436, 1989.
8. Jakobiec FA et al.: Clinicopathologic characteristics of premalignant and malignant melanocytic lesions of the conjunctiva. Ophthalmology 96:147, 1989.
9. Vincent AL et al.: Inherited corneal disease: the evolving molecular, genetic and imaging revolution. Clin Experiment Ophthalmol 33:303, 2005.
10. Wiggs JL: Genetic etiologies of glaucoma. Arch Ophthalmol 125:30, 2007.
11. Holland GN: AIDS and ophthalmology: the first quarter century. Am J Ophthalmol 145:397, 2008.
12. Zamir E et al.: Massive mycobacterial choroiditis during highly active antiretroviral therapy: another immune-recovery uveitis? Ophthalmology 109:2144, 2002.
13. Vrabec TR: Posterior segment manifestations of HIV/AIDS. Surv Ophthalmol 49:131, 2004.
14. Chu DS, Foster CS: Sympathetic ophthalmia. Int Ophthalmol Clin 42:179, 2002.
15. Singh AD, Topham A: Incidence of uveal melanoma in the United States: 1973–1997. Ophthalmology 110:956, 2003.
16. Singh AD, Topham A: Survival rates with uveal melanoma in the United States: 1973–1997. Ophthalmology 110:962, 2003.
17. Seddon JM et al.: A prognostic factor study of disease-free interval and survival following enucleation for uveal melanoma. Arch Ophthalmol 101:1894, 1983.
18. Folberg R et al.: Recommendations for the reporting of tissues removed as part of the surgical treatment of common malignancies of the eye and its adnexa. The Association of Directors of Anatomic and Surgical Pathology. Hum Pathol 34:114, 2003.
19. Kilic E et al.: Clinical and cytogenetic analyses in uveal melanoma. Invest Ophthalmol Vis Sci 47:3703, 2006.
20. Clarijs R et al.: Presence of a fluid-conducting meshwork in xenografted cutaneous and primary human uveal melanoma. Invest Ophthalmol Vis Sci 43:912, 2002.
21. Maniotis AJ et al.: Vascular channel formation by human melanoma cells in vivo and in vitro: vasculogenic mimicry Am J Pathol 155:739, 1999.
22. Folberg R, Maniotis AJ: Vasculogenic mimicry. APMIS 112:508, 2004.
23. Frank RN: Diabetic retinopathy. N Engl J Med 350:48, 2004.
24. Pe'er J et al.: Hypoxia-induced expression of vascular endothelial growth factor by retinal cells is a common factor in neovascularizing ocular diseases. Lab Invest 72:638, 1995.
25. Tolentino MJ et al.: Pathologic features of vascular endothelial growth factor–induced retinopathy in the nonhuman primate. Am J Ophthalmol 133:373, 2002.
26. Chen J, Smith LE: Retinopathy of prematurity. Angiogenesis 10:133, 2007.
27. Emerson GG, Lutty GA: Effects of sickle cell disease on the eye: clinical features and treatment. Hematol Oncol Clin North Am 19:957, 2005.
28. Mohan JS et al.: The angiopoietin/Tie-2 system in proliferative sickle retinopathy: relation to vascular endothelial growth factor, its soluble receptor Flt-1 and von Willebrand factor, and to the effects of laser treatment. Br J Ophthalmol 89:815, 2005.
29. Berker N, Batman C: Surgical treatment of central retinal vein occlusion. Acta Ophthalmol 86:245, 2008.
30. Funk M et al.: Intraocular Concentrations of Growth Factors and Cytokines in Retinal Vein Occlusion and the Effect of Therapy with Bevacizumab. Invest Ophthalmol Vis Sci 2008 Epub.
31. Klein R et al.: Fifteen-year cumulative incidence of age-related macular degeneration: the Beaver Dam Eye Study. Ophthalmology 114:253, 2007.
32. Scholl HP et al.: An update on the genetics of age-related macular degeneration. Mol Vis 13:196, 2007.
33. Maller J et al.: Common variation in three genes, including a noncoding variant in *CFH*, strongly influences risk of age-related macular degeneration. Nat Genet 38:1055, 2006.
34. DeAngelis MM et al.: Cigarette smoking, *CFH*, *APOE*, *ELOVL4*, and risk of neovascular age-related macular degeneration. Arch Ophthalmol 125:49, 2007.
35. Jager RD, Mieler WF, Miller JW: Age-related macular degeneration. N Engl J Med 358:2606, 2008.
36. Daiger SP et al.: Perspective on genes and mutations causing retinitis pigmentosa. Arch Ophthalmol 125:151, 2007.
37. Balmer A et al.: Diagnosis and current management of retinoblastoma. Oncogene 25:5341, 2006.
38. Sampieri K et al.: Genomic differences between retinoma and retinoblastoma. Acta Oncol 47:1483, 2008.
39. Choi JY et al.: Primary intraocular lymphoma: a review. Semin Ophthalmol 21:125, 2006.
40. Hayreh SS: Ischemic optic neuropathy. Prog Retin Eye Res, 2008 Epub.
41. Wiggs JL et al.: Lack of association of mutations in optineurin with disease in patients with adult-onset primary open-angle glaucoma. Arch Ophthalmol 121:1181, 2003.
42. Levin LA: Neuroprotection and regeneration in glaucoma. Ophthalmol Clin North Am 18:585, 2005.
43. Yen MY et al.: Leber's hereditary optic neuropathy: a multifactorial disease. Prog Retin Eye Res 25:381, 2006.
44. Mayorov VI et al.: Mitochondrial oxidative phosphorylation in autosomal dominant optic atrophy. BMC Biochem 9:22, 2008.
45. Beck RW et al.: High- and low-risk profiles for the development of multiple sclerosis within 10 years after optic neuritis: experience of the optic neuritis treatment trial. Arch Ophthalmol 121:944, 2003.

Index

Note: Page numbers followed by f indicate figures; those followed by t indicate tables.

A

A rings, 767

AA (arachidonic acid), in immediate hypersensitivity, 200

AA (arachidonic acid) metabolites, in inflammation, 50, 57t, 58–60, 58f, 59t

AA (amyloid-associated) protein, 250, 251f, 252–253

Aβ (β-amyloid) protein, 250–251
in Alzheimer disease, 1316–1317

ABCB4 gene, 843

ABCB11 gene, 843

ABCC8 gene, 1138

Abdominal abscesses, 378

Abdominal aortic aneurysm (AAA), 507–508, 508f

Abdominal striae, in Cushing syndrome, 1150, 1151f

Aberrantly expressed cellular proteins, as tumor antigens, 317

Abetalipoproteinemia, 797

ABL gene, 281t, 283–284, 283f

ABO incompatibility, fetal hydrops due to, 460–461

Abortion, spontaneous, 1053

Abrasion, 420

Abscess(es), 68, 69f
due to anaerobes, 378
biliary, 854
brain (cerebral), 1300, 1300f
Brodie, 1222
crypt
in *Campylobacter* enterocolitis, 799, 800f
in Crohn disease, 810
in ulcerative colitis, 812, 813f
extradural, 1301
liver, 854–855, 855f
amebic, 806
lung, 711t, 713, 716–717, 717f
staphylococcal, 359, 359f
Munro micro-, 1191
Pautrier micro-, 1185
perinephric, 941
pit, 778
ring, in infective endocarditis, 567
subareolar, recurrent, 1069, 1069f
subperiosteal, 1222
tubo-ovarian, 1010, 1010f

Absidia, 385

Acantholysis, 1168
in pemphigus, 1193–1194, 1194f

Acanthosis, 1168
nigricans, 1175–1176
due to cancer, 321t, 322
due to diabetes, 1138
due to lung carcinoma, 729

Accessory lacrimal glands, 1348f, 1349

Accessory spleens, 634–635

Acetaldehyde, metabolism of ethanol to, 413, 413f

Acetaldehyde dehydrogenase (ALDH), 413, 413f

Acetaminophen toxicity, 416–417, 417f

Acetylcholine receptors (AChRs), in myasthenia gravis, 1275–1276

Acetylsalicylic acid, adverse effects of, 417

Achalasia, 768

Achondrogenesis II, 1211t

Achondroplasia, 451, 1210, 1211t

Acid aerosols, as air pollutants, 404t

Acid hydrolases, 149

Acid maltase deficiency, 155, 157t

Acid phosphate deficiency, 151t

Acid proteases, in inflammation, 63

Acinar cell(s), 891–892, 892f

Acinar cell carcinoma, 903

Acinar cell injury, 895, 895f

Acinic cell tumor, 761

Acinus, 678

Acne vulgaris, 1197–1198, 1199f

Acquired immunity, 185

Acquired immunodeficiency syndrome (AIDS), 235–249. *See also* Human immunodeficiency virus (HIV).
abnormalities of immune function in, 241, 242t
acute retroviral syndrome in, 243–244, 243f
clinical features of, 245–248, 245t
CNS involvement in, 242–243, 248
defined, 235–236
effect of antiretroviral drug therapy on, 248
epidemiology of, 236–237
etiology of, 237–238, 237f, 238f
indicator diseases for, 245
Kaposi sarcoma associated with, 246–247, 247f, 523
morphology of, 249
Mycobacterium avium-intracellulare complex in, 246, 372, 373f
natural history of, 243–245, 243f, 244f, 244t
opportunistic infections in, 245t, 246, 346–347
pathogenesis of, 238–243
HIV infection of non–T cells in, 241–242

Acquired immunodeficiency syndrome (AIDS), pathogenesis of (Continued)
life cycle of HIV in, 239–240, 239f
mechanism of T-cell immunodeficiency in, 240–241, 241f, 242t
prognosis for, 249
progression to, 245
transmission of, 236–237
tuberculosis in, 246, 369–370
tumors in, 246–248, 247f

Acral lentiginous melanomas, 1169, 1172

Acrochordon, 1176

Acromegaly, 1104

ACTH (adrenocorticotropic hormone), ectopic secretion of, 1149

ACTH (adrenocorticotropic hormone) cell adenomas, 1100t, 1104, 1148

Actin, in myocardium, 531

Actinic band keratopathy, 1352

Actinic cheilitis, 1178

Actinic keratosis, 1178, 1179f

Actinomycetaceaea, 358t

Activation-induced cell death, 210f, 211, 240

Activation-induced cytosine deaminase (AID), 597

Active plaques, in multiple sclerosis, 1311

Acute cellular rejection, 228, 228f

Acute chest syndrome, in sickle cell disease, 648

Acute coronary syndromes, 546, 546f

Acute disseminated encephalomyelitis (ADEM), 1312–1313

Acute eczematous dermatitis, 1187–1189, 1188f

Acute fatty liver of pregnancy (AFLP), 875

Acute hemorrhagic leukoencephalitis of Weston Hurst, 1312–1313

Acute humoral rejection, 228–229, 228f

Acute illness, and malnutrition, 427

Acute inflammatory demyelinating polyradiculoneuropathy, 1261–1262

Acute intermittent porphyria (AIP), 1264t

Acute interstitial pneumonia (AIP), 680, 682–683

Acute kidney injury (AKI), 935–907
causes of, 936
clinical course of, 938
ischemic, 936, 937–938, 937f
morphology of, 937–938, 937f, 938f
nephrotoxic, 936, 937–938, 937f
pathogenesis of, 936–937, 936f

Acute lung injury (ALI), 680–683
  clinical course of, 682
  morphology of, 680
  pathogenesis of, 681–682, 682f
Acute lymphoblastic leukemia/lymphoma (ALL),
    600–603, 601t
  clinical features of, 603
  defined, 600–602
  epidemiology of, 602
  immunophenotype of, 602
  molecular pathogenesis of, 305t, 306, 602–603
  morphology of, 602, 602f
  prognosis for, 603
Acute myeloid leukemia (AML), 620, 621–624
  classification of, 622, 622t
  clinical features of, 624
  cytogenetics of, 623–624
  epidemiology of, 622
  genetic basis for, 305t, 306, 624
  immunophenotype of, 623
  morphology of, 622–623, 623f
  pathogenesis of, 621–622
  prognosis for, 624
Acute necrotizing hemorrhagic
    encephalomyelitis (ANHE), 1312–1313
Acute neuronal injury, 1281
Acute promyelocytic leukemia, 623, 623f, 624
Acute rejection, 228–229, 228f
Acute respiratory distress syndrome (ARDS),
    680–683
  clinical course of, 682
  conditions associated with development of,
    680, 681t
  morphology of, 680, 681f
  pathogenesis of, 681–682, 682f
Acute retroviral syndrome, 243–244, 243f
Acute tubular necrosis (ATN), 935–907
  causes of, 936
  clinical course of, 938
  ischemic, 936, 937–938, 937f
  morphology of, 937–938, 937f, 938f
  nephrotoxic, 936, 937–938, 937f
  pathogenesis of, 936–937, 936f
Acute-phase proteins, 74–75
Acute-phase responses, in inflammation, 62,
    74–75
Acylating agents, as carcinogens, 309t
AD. See Alzheimer disease (AD).
ADA (adenosine deaminase) deficiency, 143t,
    234
ADAM(s), in wound healing, 105
ADAM-33, in asthma, 691
Adamantinomatous craniopharyngioma,
    1106–1107, 1107f
ADAMTS13, in thrombotic microangiopathies,
    669, 952, 953
Adaptation(s), cellular, 6–11
  atrophy as, 9–10, 9f
  defined, 5, 6
  hyperplasia as, 8–9
  hypertrophy as, 6–8, 6f–8f
  metaplasia as, 10–11, 10f
  overview of, 5, 5f, 5t, 6f
Adapter proteins, in signal transduction
    pathways, 90
Adaptive immunity, 185
  cytokines of, 193
  peptide display system of, 190–192, 191f, 192f
ADCC (antibody-dependent cell-mediated
    cytotoxicity), 188, 202
Addison disease, 1155–1157, 1156f
Addison, Thomas, 1155
ADEM (acute disseminated encephalomyelitis),
    1312–1313

Adenocarcinoma, 261
  of bladder, 979
  of breast (See Breast carcinoma)
  of cervix, 1021, 1022f
  colorectal, 822–825
    chemoprevention of, 823
    clinical features of, 825
    diet and, 822–823
    epidemiology of, 822–823
    metastatic, 825, 826f
    morphology of, 264f, 824–825, 825f
    pathogenesis of, 823–824, 823f, 824f
    staging of, 825, 826t, 827t
  endometrioid, 1033, 1033f, 1045–1046
  esophageal, 772, 773f
    Barrett esophagus and, 770
  of fallopian tubes, 1039
  of gallbladder, 888–889, 888f
  gastric, 784–786, 785f, 786f
    chronic gastritis and, 781
    Helicobacter pylori and, 315–316
  of kidney, 964–967, 964f–966f
  of lung, 723–725, 726f, 734, 734f
    precursor lesions for, 725, 727f
  ovarian clear cell, 1046
  of prostate, 996–1002
    clinical course of, 1000–1002
    ductal, 1002
    etiology and pathogenesis of, 996–998
    genetic basis for, 305t, 306
    grading and staging of, 999–1000, 1000f,
      1001t
    incidence of, 996
    metastatic, 998, 998f
    morphology of, 998–999, 998f, 999f
  small-intestinal, celiac disease and, 796
Adenofibromas, endometrioid, 1045
Adenohypophysis, 1098–1099, 1099f
Adenoid cystic carcinoma, of salivary glands,
    760–761, 760f
Adenoma(s), 260, 261f
  adrenocortical, 1157–1158, 1157f, 1158f
    Cushing syndrome due to, 1149, 1150
    hyperaldosteronism due to, 1151,
      1152
  aldosterone-producing, 1151, 1152
  colorectal, 308f, 309, 819–820, 820f, 821f
  gastric, 782t, 784, 784f
  hepatic, 877, 877f
    oral contraceptives and, 415
  Hürthle cell (oxyphil), 1119, 1119f
  lactational, 1071
  liver cell, 877, 877f
  nephrogenic, 976
  oxyphil, 1119, 1119f, 1127
  parathyroid, 1127, 1127f, 1128f
  pituitary, 1100–1105
    ACTH cell (corticotroph), 1100t, 1104,
      1148
    atypical, 1102
    classification of, 1100, 1100t
    clinical course of, 1103
    epidemiology of, 1100
    functional, 1100
    genetic abnormalities in, 1101–1102, 1101t,
      1102f
    gonadotroph (LH- and FSH-producing),
      1100t, 1104–1105
    growth hormone cell (somatotroph),
      1100t, 1104
    invasive, 1102
    mammosomatotroph, 1100t, 1104
    micro- vs. macro-, 1100
    morphology of, 1102, 1102f, 1103f

Adenoma(s), pituitary (Continued)
    nonfunctioning (silent variant, null-cell),
      1100, 1102f, 1105
    prolactinomas (lactotroph), 1100t,
      1103–1104, 1103f
    thyrotroph (TSH-producing), 1100t, 1105
  pleomorphic, 261
    of salivary glands, 757–759, 758f
  renal papillary, 963
  sebaceous, 1177, 1178f
  of thyroid, 264f, 1118–1119, 1119f
    follicular, 1118–1119, 1119f, 1123, 1124f
Adenoma-carcinoma sequence, 308f, 309,
    823–824, 823f
Adenomatoid tumors
  of fallopian tubes, 1039
  paratesticular, 987
Adenomatous hyperplasia, of lung, 725, 727f
Adenomatous polyposis coli (APC) tumor
    suppressor gene, 274, 287t, 292–294, 293f
  in colorectal carcinoma, 308f, 309, 823–824,
    823f
    hereditary nonpolyposis, 821
  in familial adenomatous polyposis, 321
Adenomyosis, 1029, 1029f
  of gallbladder, 888
Adenosarcomas, of endometrium, 1035
Adenosine deaminase (ADA) deficiency, 143t,
    234
Adenosine phosphoribosyltransferase (APRT),
    in gout, 1244f
Adenosine triphosphate (ATP) depletion, cell
    injury due to, 17–18, 18f
Adenosis, of breast, 1071
  sclerosing, 1072, 1072f
Adenosquamous carcinoma, of cervix, 1021
Adenovirus
  gastroenteritis due to, 805
  structure of, 333f
ADH (alcohol dehydrogenase), 413, 413f
ADH (antidiuretic hormone), 1099
  syndrome of inappropriate secretion of, 1106
Adhesins, 343
Adhesions, intestinal, 790–791, 791f
Adhesive glycoproteins, in extracellular matrix,
    95f, 96–97, 97f
Adipocytes, in energy balance, 440f, 441
Adipokines, in insulin resistance, 1137
Adiponectin, in energy balance, 439, 441
Adipose tissue, in energy balance, 441
Adnexal components, of skin, 1166–1167,
    1166f
Adnexal tumors, of skin, 1176–1178, 1177f,
    1178f
ADPKD (autosomal-dominant polycystic kidney
    disease), 956–959, 957t, 958f
ADR(s). See Adverse drug reactions (ADRs).
Adrenal changes, due to shock, 132
Adrenal cortex, 1148–1159
  anatomy of, 1148
  disorders of (See Adrenocortical disorder(s))
Adrenal cysts, 1159
Adrenal glands, 1148–1161
  anatomy of, 1148
Adrenal hyperplasia, congenital, 1152–1154,
    1153f
Adrenal hypoplasia congenita, 1156
Adrenal incidentaloma, 1159
Adrenal medulla, 1159–1161
  anatomy of, 1148, 1159
  pheochromocytoma of, 1159–1161, 1160f,
    1160t, 1161f
Adrenal myelolipomas, 1159
Adrenal neuroblastoma, 449, 476f

Adrenal virilism, nonclassic or late-onset, 1153–1154
Adrenalitis
    autoimmune, 1155–1156, 1156f
    tuberculous, 1156
Adrenocortical adenomas, 1157–1158, 1157f, 1158f
    Cushing syndrome due to, 1149, 1150
    hyperaldosteronism due to, 1151, 1152
Adrenocortical atrophy, 1149
Adrenocortical carcinoma, 1158, 1158f
    Cushing syndrome due to, 1149, 1150
    hyperaldosteronism due to, 1151
Adrenocortical disorder(s), 1148–1159
    adrenocortical hyperfunction
        (hyperadrenalism) as, 1148–1154
        in adrenogenital syndromes, 1152–1154, 1153f
        in hypercortisolism (Cushing syndrome), 1148–1151, 1148t, 1149f–1151f, 1150t
        in primary hyperaldosteronism, 1151–1152, 1151f
    adrenocortical insufficiency as, 1154–1157
        causes of, 1154, 1154t
        primary
            acute, 1154–1155
            chronic (Addison disease), 1155–1157, 1156f
        secondary, 1157
        in Waterhouse-Friderichsen syndrome, 1155, 1155f, 1156f
    cysts as, 1159
    incidentalomas as, 1159
    myelolipomas as, 1159
    neoplastic, 1157–1158
        adenomas as, 1157–1158, 1157f, 1158f
        carcinomas as, 1158, 1158f
        Cushing syndrome due to, 1149, 1150
        hyperaldosteronism due to, 1151, 1152
Adrenocortical hyperfunction, 1148–1154
    in adrenogenital syndromes, 1152–1154, 1153f
    in hypercortisolism (Cushing syndrome), 1148–1151, 1148t, 1149f–1151f, 1150t
    in primary hyperaldosteronism, 1151–1152, 1151f
Adrenocortical hyperplasia
    Cushing syndrome due to, 1149–1150, 1149f, 1150f
    hyperaldosteronism due to, 1152
Adrenocortical insufficiency, 1154–1157
    causes of, 1154, 1154t
    primary
        acute, 1154–1155
        chronic (Addison disease), 1155–1157, 1156f
    secondary, 1157
    in Waterhouse-Friderichsen syndrome, 1155, 1155f, 1156f
Adrenocortical neoplasms, 1157–1158
    adenomas as, 1157–1158, 1157f, 1158f
    carcinomas as, 1158, 1158f
    Cushing syndrome due to, 1149, 1150
    hyperaldosteronism due to, 1151, 1152
Adrenocorticotropic hormone (ACTH), ectopic secretion of, 1149
Adrenocorticotropic hormone (ACTH) cell adenomas, 1100t, 1104, 1148
Adrenogenital syndromes, 1152–1154, 1153f
Adrenoleukodystrophy, 1156, 1264t, 1327
Adult hemoglobin (HbA), 645
Adult respiratory distress syndrome, 132
Adult T-cell leukemia/lymphoma, 601t, 615–616
    human T-cell leukemia virus type 1 and, 312–313

Advanced glycation end products (AGEs), 1138
Adventitia, of blood vessels, 488, 488f
Adverse drug reactions (ADRs), 414–417, 416t
    due to acetaminophen, 416–417, 417f
    due to anabolic steroids, 415–416
    due to aspirin (acetylsalicylic acid), 417
    defined, 414
    dermatologic, 415f
    epidemiology of, 414
    genetically determined, 144
    due to hormonal replacement therapy, 414–415
    due to oral contraceptives, 415
Aerobic glycolysis, in carcinogenesis, 303–304
Affected females, of fragile-X syndrome, 170
Affinity maturation, in humoral immunity, 196, 196f
Aflatoxin, and hepatocellular carcinoma, 311, 385, 443, 878
AFLP (acute fatty liver of pregnancy), 875
African trypanosomiasis, 390, 390f
AGA (appropriate for gestational age), 454
Agammaglobulinemia, X-linked (Bruton's), 231–233
Aganglionic megacolon, congenital, 766–767, 766f
Age, and cancer, 273
AGE(s) (advanced glycation end products), 1138
Agenesis, 450
Age-related macular degeneration (ARMD), 1346, 1363–1364, 1364f
Aging
    amyloid of, 252t, 253
    cellular, 6, 39–41, 39f, 40f
    and heart, 531–532, 532t
Agouti signaling protein (ASIP) gene, in melanoma, 1174
Agouti-related peptide (AgRP), in energy balance, 439, 440, 441f, 442
Agranulocytosis, 592–593
    antibody-mediated hypersensitivity in, 203
    oral manifestations of, 744t
Agricultural exposures, 408–410, 409t
Agyria, 1284–1285, 1285f
AID (activation-induced cytosine deaminase), 597
AIDS. See Acquired immunodeficiency syndrome (AIDS).
AION (anterior ischemic optic neuropathy), 1366, 1366f
AIP (acute intermittent porphyria), 1264t
AIP (acute interstitial pneumonia), 680, 682–683
AIP (aryl hydrocarbon receptor interacting protein) gene, in pituitary adenomas, 1101–1102
Air embolism, 127
Air pollution, 403–405, 404t
    and lung carcinoma, 722
    lung diseases caused by, 697t
Air-conditioner lung, 703
AIRE (autoimmune regulator) gene, 1130, 1156
AIRE (autoimmune regulator) protein, in immunological tolerance, 209
Airspace enlargement with fibrosis, 684
Airway remodeling, in asthma, 691
AKI. See Acute kidney injury (AKI).
AKT, 90, 294
AL (amyloid light chain) protein, 250, 251f, 252
Alagille syndrome, 870
Albers-Schönberg disease, 1212–1214, 1214f, 1215f
Albinism, 144

Alcohol
    blood level of, 412
    effects of, 412–414, 413f
    as teratogen, 452
Alcohol abuse
    and cancer, 273
    CNS toxicity of, 1329, 1329f
    and dilated cardiomyopathy, 573
    epidemiology of, 412
Alcohol consumption, during pregnancy, 414
Alcohol dehydrogenase (ADH), 413, 413f
Alcoholic cardiomyopathy, 414, 573
Alcoholic cerebellar degeneration, 1329, 1329f
Alcoholic cirrhosis, 857f, 858, 859f, 860
    and hemochromatosis, 863
Alcoholic hepatitis, 857f, 858, 858f, 860
Alcoholic hyaline, 35
Alcoholic liver disease, 414, 857–860
    clinicopathologic features of, 859–860
    epidemiology of, 857
    morphology of, 857–858, 858f, 859f
    pathogenesis of, 413, 858–859
Alcoholic pancreatitis, 414, 895, 896, 897f
Alcoholic steatohepatitis, 857f, 858, 858f
Alcoholic steatosis, 857–858, 857f, 859
Alcoholism
    acute, 413–414
    chronic, 414
    and malnutrition, 427
ALD gene, 1327
ALDH (acetaldehyde dehydrogenase), 413, 413f
ALDH2*2, 413
Aldosterone suppression test, 1152
Aldosterone-producing adenomas, 1151, 1152
Aldrin (dichlorodiphenyltrichlorethane), occupational exposure to, 409
Aleukemic leukemia, 623
Alexander disease, 1282, 1327
Alginate, in cystic fibrosis, 468
ALI. See Acute lung injury (ALI).
Alimentary tract. See Gastrointestinal tract.
ALK (anaplastic lymphoma kinase) gene, 475, 615
Alkaptonuria, 36, 155–156
Alkylating agents, as carcinogens, 309t
ALL. See Acute lymphoblastic leukemia/lymphoma (ALL).
Allele-specific polymerase chain reaction, 175, 175f
Allergen(s), 198, 198f, 199f
Allergen-induced asthma, 688, 689, 690f
Allergic alveolitis, 703–704, 703f
Allergic angiitis, 516
Allergic bronchopulmonary aspergillosis, 385, 693
Allergic contact dermatitis, 1187–1189, 1189f
Allergic diseases, chronic inflammation due to, 70
Allergic granulomatosis, 516
Allergic rhinitis, 749
Allergy, 197t, 198–201, 198f–200f, 201t
    non-atopic, 201
Allograft rejection, 226–230
    acute, 228–229, 228f
    chronic, 229, 229f
    hematopoietic stem cell, 230
    hyperacute, 227, 228, 228f
    kidney, 228–230, 228f, 229f
    mechanisms of, 226–228, 227f
    other solid organ, 230
    prevention of, 229–230
All-trans-retinoic acid, 431, 432
    in acute myeloid leukemia, 624
    and congenital anomalies, 453

Alpers disease, 1328
Alpha particles, 423
α cells, of pancreas, 1130, 1131f
$α_1$-antitrypsin ($α_1$-AT), 864–865
  in inflammation, 63
$α_1$-antitrypsin ($α_1$-AT) deficiency, 143t, 864–866
  clinical features of, 866
  in emphysema, 685, 685f, 686
  genetic basis for, 144, 864–865
  liver disease in, 864–866, 865f
  morphology of, 865, 865f
  pathogenesis of, 865
  protein accumulation in, 35
$α_2$-macroglobulin, in inflammation, 63
α-cell tumors, 1147
α-glucosidase deficiency, 155
α-granules, 117
α-methylacyl-coenzyme A-racemase (AMACR),
    in prostate cancer, 997, 999
α-thalassemia, 651–652, 652t
α-thalassemia trait, 651–652, 652t
Alport syndrome, 931–932, 932f
ALS (amyotrophic lateral sclerosis), 1324–1325,
    1325f
ALTE (apparent life-threatening event), 471–472
Aluminum deposition, in renal failure, 1219
Alveolar bone, 740f
Alveolar damage, diffuse, 680, 681f
  due to shock, 132
Alveolar ducts, 678
Alveolar epithelium, 678
Alveolar proteinosis, pulmonary, 705–706, 705f
Alveolar rhabdomyosarcoma, 1253, 1254f
Alveolar sacs, 678
Alveolar septa, 678–679, 678f
Alveolar soft-part sarcoma, genetic basis for,
    1249t
Alveolar walls, 678–679, 678f
Alveolitis
  allergic, 703–704, 703f
  cryptogenic fibrosing, 694–695, 694f, 695f
Alzheimer disease (AD), 1313–1317
  clinical features of, 1317
  epidemiology of, 1313
  familial, 1317
  molecular genetics and pathogenesis of,
      1316–1317
  morphology of, 1314–1316, 1314f–1316f
Alzheimer type II astrocyte, 1281–1282
AMACR (α-methylacyl-coenzyme A-racemase),
    in prostate cancer, 997, 999
Amastigote, of Leishmania, 389
Amebiasis, 805f, 806
  cerebral, 1308, 1308f
Amebic liver abscesses, 806
Ameboid migration, in metastasis, 300
Ameloblastoma, of oral cavity, 749
American trypanosomiasis, 391
Amides, as carcinogens, 309t
AML. See Acute myeloid leukemia (AML).
Ammonia, lung diseases due to, 697t
Amnion nodosum, 450
Amniotic bands, 448, 449f
Amniotic fluid embolism, 127, 128f
AMP-dependent protein kinase (AMPK), 304
Amphetamines, abuse of, 418t, 419
Amphiboles, 699–700
Ampulla of Vater, 891
Amputation neuroma, 1266, 1267f
Amylin, in energy balance, 442
Amyloid
  of aging, 252t, 253
  chemical nature of, 250–251
  defined, 249

Amyloid (Continued)
  endocrine, 252t, 253
  physical nature of, 249–250, 250f
  staining of, 249, 250f, 253–254
  of tongue, 254, 255
Amyloid deposition, in bone, 1219
Amyloid light chain (AL) protein, 250, 251f,
    252
Amyloid plaques, in Alzheimer disease, 1314
Amyloid polyneuropathies, familial, 253, 1263,
    1264t
Amyloid precursor protein (APP), 251
  in Alzheimer disease, 1314, 1316–1317, 1316f
Amyloid-associated (AA) protein, 250, 251f,
    252–253
Amyloidosis, 36, 249–255, 250f
  cardiac, 580, 580f
  classification of, 252–253, 252f
  clinical features of, 254–255
  diagnosis of, 255
  gastrointestinal, 255
  of heart, 254, 255
  hemodialysis-associated, 252t, 253
  heredofamilial, 252t, 253
  immunocyte dyscrasias with, 252, 609
  of kidney, 254, 254f, 255, 935
  and light-chain cast nephropathy, 948
  of liver, 254
  localized, 252t, 253
  morphology of, 253–254, 253f
  of pancreas, 1139, 1141f
  pathogenesis of, 251–252, 251f
  perivascular, 666
  primary, 252, 252t, 609
  prognosis for, 255
  properties of amyloid proteins and, 249–251,
      250f
  secondary, 75, 250, 252–253, 252t
  senile
    cardiac, 253
    systemic, 252t, 253
  of spleen, 254
  systemic (generalized), 252–253, 252t
    reactive, 252–253, 252t
    senile, 252t, 253
  of tongue, 254, 255
Amyotrophic lateral sclerosis (ALS), 1324–1325,
    1325f
ANA(s) (antinuclear antibodies)
  in systemic lupus erythematosus, 213,
      214–215, 214t, 217, 220
  in systemic sclerosis, 223
Anabolic steroids, adverse effects of, 415–416
Anaerobic bacteria, 378–379, 379f
Anal canal, tumors of, 825–826, 827f
Analgesic(s), and bladder cancer, 980
Analgesic nephropathy, 417, 945–946, 946f,
    947t
Anaphase lag, 159
Anaphylactic shock, 129
Anaphylatoxins, 57, 64, 199
Anaphylaxis, 64
  systemic, 201
Anaplasia, 263–264, 265f, 271t, 324
  in Wilms tumor, 481
Anaplastic astrocytoma, 1330, 1331
Anaplastic large-cell lymphoma, 601t, 615, 615f
Anaplastic lymphoma kinase (ALK) gene, 475,
    615
Anaplastic meningioma, 1339
Anaplastic oligodendroglioma, 1333–1334
Anaplastic seminoma, 989
Anaplastic thyroid carcinoma, 1121, 1124
Anasarca, in right-sided heart failure, 536

ANCAs (antineutrophil cytoplasmic antibodies)
  rapidly progressive glomerulonephritis due to,
      920–921, 920t
  vasculitis due to, 203t
Ancylostoma duodenale, enterocolitis due to, 806
Androblastomas, ovarian, 1051–1052, 1051f
Androgen(s), in prostate cancer, 997
Androgen insensitivity syndrome, complete, 167
Androgen receptors (ARs), in prostate cancer,
    997
Anemia(s), 639–665
  aplastic, 662–664, 663f, 663t, 664f
    oral manifestations of, 744t
  of blood loss, 640t, 641
  of chronic disease, 662
  due to chronic renal failure, 665
  classification of, 640, 640t
  clinical features of, 641
  defined, 639–640
  diagnosis of, 640
  of diminished erythropoiesis, 640t, 654–665
  due to endocrine disorders, 665
  Fanconi, 302–303, 663
  fetal hydrops and, 461, 461t
  of folate deficiency, 655t, 658–659
  hemolytic, 641–654
    autoimmune, 203, 203t
    classification of, 640t, 642
    clinical manifestations of, 642
    common features of, 641
    due to glucose-6-phosphate dehydrogenase
        deficiency, 644–645, 644f, 645f
    due to hereditary spherocytosis, 642–644,
        643f, 644f
    immuno-, 653–654, 653t
    microangiopathic, 654, 654f
    morphology of, 642, 642f
    due to paroxysmal nocturnal
        hemoglobinuria, 652–653, 653f
    pathogenesis of, 641–642
    due to red cell trauma, 654, 654f
    due to sickle cell disease, 645–648, 646f,
        647f
    due to thalassemia syndromes, 648–652,
        649f–651f, 652t
  due to hepatocellular liver disease, 665
  iron deficiency, 659–662, 659t, 660f–662f
    due to colorectal cancer, 825
    due to Crohn disease, 811
  macrocytic, 640
  megaloblastic, 654–659, 655f, 655t, 656f
  microcytic hypochromic, 640
    of iron deficiency, 661–662, 662f
  myelophthisic, 665
  normochromic, normocytic, 640
  pernicious (vitamin B_{12} deficiency), 655–658,
      655t, 656f, 657f
    antibody-mediated hypersensitivity in, 203t
    and autoimmune gastritis, 778, 779
  due to pure red cell aplasia, 664–665
  red cell indices for, 640–641, 641t
Anencephaly, 1284
Anergy, 209–210
Aneuploidy, 159
Aneurysm(s), 506–508
  aortic
    abdominal, 507–508, 508f
    pathogenesis of, 507, 507f
    thoracic, 508
  in atherosclerosis, 504
  defined, 506
  false (pseudo-), 506, 506f
  fusiform, 506, 506f
  inflammatory, 508

Aneurysm(s) (Continued)
  mycotic, 507, 508
  pathogenesis of, 506–507, 507f
  saccular (berry, developmental), 489, 506,
      506f, 507
    ruptured, 1297–1298, 1297f, 1298f
    and thrombosis, 122
  true, 506, 506f
  ventricular, due to myocardial infarction, 556f,
      557
Aneurysmal bone cyst, 1234, 1234f
Ang1 (angiopoietin 1), in angiogenesis, 101
Ang2 (angiopoietin 2), in angiogenesis, 101
Angelman syndrome, 172–173, 172f
Angiitis
  allergic, 516
  of CNS, primary, 1293
Angina pectoris, 545, 546–547, 546f
  preinfarction, 547
  Prinzmetal (variant), 547
  stable (typical), 546–547, 546f
  unstable (crescendo), 546, 546f, 547
Angioblasts, 99
Angiodysgenetic necrotizing myelopathy, 1298
Angiodysplasia, intestinal, 793
Angioedema, 1187
  hereditary, 235
Angiofibroma, nasopharyngeal, 751
Angiogenesis, 99–102, 489
  in carcinogenesis, 278, 297–298
  in chronic inflammation, 70
  from endothelial precursor cells, 99f, 100
  extracellular matrix proteins as regulators of,
      101–102
  growth factors and receptors in, 100–101,
      100t, 101f
  from preexisting vessels, 99–100, 99f
  sprouting, 101f
  in wound healing, 102, 103f, 105f
Angiogenic factors, in preeclampsia, 1056
Angiogenic switch, 297–298
Angiomas
  spider, due to liver failure, 836
  venous, of brain, 1298
Angiomatosis, 520
  bacillary, 520, 522, 523f
  encephalotrigeminal, 522
Angiomyolipoma, renal, 963
Angiopathy, cerebral amyloid, 1296, 1296f,
      1316
Angioplasty, pathology of, 526, 526f
Angiopoietin 1 (Ang1), in angiogenesis, 101
Angiopoietin 2 (Ang2), in angiogenesis, 101
Angiosarcoma(s), 524–525, 525f
  of breast, 1092–1093
  cardiac, 584
  hepatic, 524–525, 877
Angiotensin, in blood pressure regulation, 493,
      494f
ANHE (acute necrotizing hemorrhagic
      encephalomyelitis), 1312–1313
Anitschkow cells, in rheumatic fever, 566
ANKH gene, in calcium pyrophosphate crystal
      deposition disease, 1246
Ankylosing spondylitis, HLA alleles and, 192
Ankylosing spondyloarthritis, 1241
Ankyrin, 143t
  in hereditary spherocytosis, 642, 643f
Annexin V, in apoptosis, 27
Anoikis, in apoptosis, 295, 300
Anorexia nervosa, 430
Anovulatory cycle, 1026–1027
Anterior chamber, 1354f
Anterior compartment syndrome, 128

Anterior ischemic optic neuropathy (AION),
      1366, 1366f
Anterior segment, of eye, 1353–1355
  cataracts of, 1353
  endophthalmitis and panophthalmitis of,
      1355, 1355f, 1356f
  functional anatomy of, 1353, 1354f
  and glaucoma, 1353–1355
Anterior synechiae, of eye, 1355
Anthracosis, 36, 697–698
Anthrax, 337, 361–362, 362f
  cutaneous, 361
  gastrointestinal, 362
  inhalational, 361–362, 362f
Anti-angiogenic factors, in preeclampsia,
      1056
Antibiotic-associated colitis, 803, 803f
Antibiotic-associated diarrhea, 803, 803f
Antibodies, 185, 187, 187f
  antitumor effect of, 318–319
Antibody production, by spleen, 632
Antibody secretion, 196, 196f
Antibody-dependent cell-mediated (cellular)
      cytotoxicity (ADCC), 188, 202
Antibody-mediated diseases, 203t
Antibody-mediated glomerular injury, 911t,
      912–914, 913f, 914f
Antibody-mediated hypersensitivity, 197t, 198,
      201–204, 202f, 203t
Antibody-mediated reactions, in transplant
      rejection, 227–228
Anticipation, in fragile-X syndrome, 170
Anticoagulant effects, of endothelium, 116
Anti-cyclic citrullinated peptide (anti-CCP)
      antibodies, in rheumatoid arthritis, 1239
Antidiuretic hormone (ADH), 1099
  syndrome of inappropriate secretion of,
      1106
Anti-endothelial cell antibodies, vasculitis due
      to, 512
Antifibrinolytic effects, of endothelium, 117
Anti-GBM antibody–induced
      glomerulonephritis, 912, 913f, 920, 920t
Antigen(s), sequestered, 211
Antigen capture, 193, 194f
Antigen display, 191, 192f, 193–195, 194f
Antigen masking, in immune evasion, 320
Antigen processing, 191, 192f
Antigen recognition, 186, 186f, 193–195, 194f
Antigenic drift, with influenza virus, 715
Antigenic drugs, immunohemolytic anemia due
      to, 653
Antigenic shift, with influenza virus, 715
Antigenic variation, 345–346, 346t
Antigen-negative variants, selective outgrowth
      of, in immune evasion, 319
Antigen-presenting cells (APCs), 186f, 187
  in transplant rejection, 226, 227f
Anti-microsomal antibodies, 1110
Anti-myeloperoxidase (MPO-ANCA), 511
Antineutrophil cytoplasmic antibodies (ANCAs)
  rapidly progressive glomerulonephritis due to,
      920–921, 920t
  vasculitis due to, 203t
Antinuclear antibodies (ANAs)
  in systemic lupus erythematosus, 213,
      214–215, 214t, 217, 220
  in systemic sclerosis, 223
  vasculitis due to, 203t, 511–512
Antioxidant(s), 60
  free radical removal by, 21, 21f
  vitamins as, 437, 444
Antiphospholipid antibody(ies), in systemic
      lupus erythematosus, 215

Antiphospholipid antibody syndrome, 123
  and hemolytic-uremic syndrome, 953
  secondary, 215
Antiplatelet antibodies, 667–668
Antiplatelet effects, of endothelium, 116
Antiproteases, in inflammation, 63
Anti–proteinase-3 (PR3-ANCA), 511
Antiretroviral drug therapy, for HIV infection,
      248
Antithrombin III, 116, 117f, 120
Antithrombotic events, 115, 116f
Antithrombotic properties, of endothelium,
      115–116, 117f
Anti-thyroglobulin antibodies, 1110, 1112, 1114
Anti–thyroid peroxidase antibodies, 1110, 1112
Antitumor effector mechanisms, 318–319
Anti-viral defense, in innate immunity, 184
Anus, imperforate, 765
Aorta
  coarctation of, 544, 544f
  structure and function of, 488f
Aortic aneurysms
  abdominal, 507–508, 508f
  pathogenesis of, 507, 507f
  thoracic, 508
Aortic atresia, congenital, 544–545
Aortic dilation, in Marfan syndrome, 145
Aortic dissection, 508–510, 509f, 510f
Aortic regurgitation, 561t
Aortic stenosis, 561t
  calcific, 561–562, 562f
  congenital, 544–545
  rheumatic, 565f
  supravalvular, 545
  valvular, 544
Aortic valve, calcific stenosis of bicuspid,
      562–563, 562f
Aortic valve sclerosis, 562
Aorticosympathetic paraganglia, 1159
APC(s) (antigen-presenting cells), 186f, 187
  in transplant rejection, 226, 227f
APC (adenomatous polyposis coli) tumor
      suppressor gene, 274, 287t, 292–294, 293f
  in colorectal carcinoma, 308f, 309, 823–824,
      823f
  hereditary nonpolyposis, 821
  in familial adenomatous polyposis, 321
APC/β-catenin pathway, in colorectal carcinoma,
      823–824, 823f
Aphthous ulcers, 742, 742f
  in Crohn disease, 810
Aplasia, 450
Aplastic anemia, 662–664, 663f, 663t, 664f
  oral manifestations of, 744t
Aplastic crises
  in hereditary spherocytosis, 644
  in sickle cell disease, 648
APOBEC3G, in AIDS, 240
Apocrine carcinoma, 1177, 1178, 1178f
Apocrine cysts, of breast, 1071, 1071f
Apolipoprotein E (ApoE), in Alzheimer disease,
      1317
Apoptosis, 25–32
  biochemical features of, 27, 27f
  causes of, 25–26
  clinicopathologic correlations of, 30–32, 31f
  in control of normal cell proliferation, 80, 81f
  cytotoxic T lymphocyte–mediated, 31
  defined, 25
  disorders associated with dysregulated, 32
  due to DNA damage, 25, 30
  evasion of, in carcinogenesis, 278, 295–296,
      296f
  execution phase of, 30

Apoptosis (Continued)
    extrinsic (death receptor–initiated) pathway
        of, 28f, 29–30, 29f
    genes that regulate, in carcinogenesis, 277
    due to growth factor deprivation, 30
    in immune evasion, 320
    in immunological tolerance, 210f, 211
    intrinsic (mitochondrial) pathway of, 28–29,
        28f, 29f
    mechanisms of, 27–30, 28f, 29f
    morphologic changes in, 13f, 13t, 26–27, 26f
    overview of, 5, 5f, 11
    p53-induced, 292
    in pathologic conditions, 25–26
    in physiologic situations, 25
    due to protein misfolding, 25, 30–31, 31f
    removal of dead cells in, 30
    TNF receptor family–induced, 31
    in viral hepatitis, 851, 851f
Apoptosome, 29
Apoptotic bodies, 13f, 25, 26, 26f, 30
APP (amyloid precursor protein), 251
    in Alzheimer disease, 1314, 1316–1317, 1316f
Apparent life-threatening event (ALTE), 471–472
Appendage tumors, of skin, 1176–1178, 1177f,
    1178f
Appendicitis, acute, 826–827
    gangrenous, 827
    suppurative, 827
Appendix, tumors of, 828
Appositional growth, 1210
Appropriate for gestational age (AGA), 454
APRT (adenosine phosphoribosyltransferase), in
    gout, 1244f
APS1 (autoimmune polyendocrine syndrome
    type 1), 1130, 1155–1156
APS2 (autoimmune polyendocrine syndrome
    type 2), 1156
Aqueous humor, 1353, 1354f
AR(s) (androgen receptors), in prostate cancer,
    997
Arachidonic acid (AA), in immediate
    hypersensitivity, 200
Arachidonic acid (AA) metabolites, in
    inflammation, 50, 57t, 58–60, 58f, 59t
Arachnodactyly, congenital contractural, 145
Arachnoiditis, chronic adhesive, 1300
Arcuate nucleus
    in energy balance, 439, 441f
    hypoplasia of, in sudden infant death
        syndrome, 472
ARDS. See Acute respiratory distress syndrome
    (ARDS).
Area cerebrovasculosa, in anencephaly, 1284
ARF tumor suppressor gene, 294
Aristolochic nephropathy, 946
ARMD (age-related macular degeneration),
    1346, 1363–1364, 1364f
Arnold-Chiari malformation, 1285–1286, 1286f
Aromatic amines, as carcinogens, 309t, 311
ARPKD (autosomal-recessive polycystic kidney
    disease), 957t, 959
Array-based comparative genomic hybridization
    (array CGH), 179–180, 180f, 325–326.68f
Arrhythmias, 532
    due to myocardial infarction, 557
Arrhythmogenic right ventricular
    cardiomyopathy (ARVC), 575, 576f
Arrhythmogenic right ventricular dysplasia, 575,
    576f
Arsenic, as carcinogen, 274t
Arsenic poisoning, 408
Arterial dissection, 506, 506f
    aortic, 508–510, 509f, 510f

Arterial thrombosis, 124, 125
Arteriogenesis, 489
Arteriohepatic dysplasia, 870
Arteriolar sclerosis, in hypertensive
    cerebrovascular disease, 1295
Arterioles
    fibrinoid necrosis of, in malignant
        hypertension, 950–951, 950f
    structure and function of, 488f, 489
Arteriolitis
    hyperplastic, in malignant hypertension, 950f,
        951
    necrotizing, 496
Arteriolosclerosis, 496
    hyaline, 495, 495f
        in benign nephrosclerosis, 949, 950f
        due to diabetes mellitus, 1140, 1141f
    hyperplastic, 495f, 496
    renal, in diabetes mellitus, 1142
Arteriosclerosis, 496
    graft, 585, 585f
Arteriovenous fistulas, 489–490
Arteriovenous malformations (AVMs),
    1298–1299
Arteritis
    giant-cell (temporal), 512–513, 513f
    Huebner, 1301
    Takayasu, 513–514, 514f
Artery(ies), structure and function of, 488–489,
    488f
Arthritis, 1235–1246
    ankylosing spondylo-, 1241
    bacterial, 1242
    in calcium pyrophosphate crystal deposition
        disease, 1246, 1246f
    crystal-induced, 1242–1246
    enteritis-associated, 1241
    gouty, 1243–1246, 1243t, 1244f, 1245f
    immune complex, 205
    infectious, 1241–1242
    juvenile idiopathic, 1240–1241
    Lyme, 378, 1242
    osteo-, 1235–1236, 1236f, 1237f
    psoriatic, 1241
    reactive, 204t, 1241
    in Reiter syndrome, 1241
    due to rheumatic fever, 566
    rheumatoid, 1237–1240, 1238f–1240f
        heart disease associated with, 583
        juvenile, 1240–1241
        pulmonary involvement in, 696
        T cell–mediated hypersensitivity in, 206t
    seronegative spondyloarthropathies as,
        1241
    in systemic lupus erythematosus, 214t, 219
    tophaceous, 1243, 1244, 1245f, 1246
    tuberculous, 1242
    viral, 1242
Arthrochalasia, in Ehlers-Danlos syndrome, 146,
    146t
Arthrogryposis, 1271
Arthropod-borne viral encephalitis, 1302,
    1303f
Arthus reaction, 204t, 205
Articular changes, due to cancer, 321t, 322
Artificial heart valves, complications of,
    570–571, 571f, 571t
ARVC (arrhythmogenic right ventricular
    cardiomyopathy), 575, 576f
Aryl hydrocarbon receptor interacting protein
    (AIP) gene, in pituitary adenomas,
    1101–1102
Arylamines, and bladder cancer, 979
Arylsulfatase A deficiency, 1326

Asbestos
    as carcinogen, 274t
    and lung carcinoma, 722
    lung diseases due to, 697t
    and malignant mesothelioma, 733, 929
    pneumoconiosis due to, 410, 699–701
Asbestos bodies, 700, 700f, 733
Asbestosis, 699, 700
Asbestos-related diseases, 697t, 699–701,
    700f
Asbestos-related pleural plaques, 700–701, 700f,
    733
Ascaris lumbricoides, 336
    enterocolitis due to, 805, 805f
Ascending cholangitis, 887
Ascending infections, perinatal, 458
Aschoff bodies, 565–566, 565f
Ascites
    chylous, 520
    due to portal hypertension, 838–839, 838f
    in right-sided heart failure, 536
Ascorbic acid, 437–438
    deficiency of, 437–438, 437f, 438t
    function of, 437, 438t
    toxicity of, 438
ASD (atrial septal defect), 540f, 541
Aseptic meningitis, 1299, 1300
ASIP (Agouti signaling protein) gene, in
    melanoma, 1174
Aspartylglycosaminuria, 151t
Aspergilloma, 385
Aspergillosis, 384–385, 385f
    allergic bronchopulmonary, 385, 693
    of CNS, 1306
    invasive, 385, 385f
Aspergillus fumigatus, 384
Aspergillus spp, 384–385, 385f
Aspiration pneumonia, 711t, 716
Aspirin
    adverse effects of, 417
    bleeding disorder due to, 670
    mechanism of action of, 58f, 59–60
Aspirin-sensitive asthma, 689
Asplenia, 633, 634
Asthma, 683t, 688–692
    anatomic site of, 683t
    atopic, 688, 689, 690f
    clinical course of, 683t, 692
    defined, 688
    drug-induced, 689
    etiology of, 683t
    genetics of, 691
    major pathologic changes in, 683t
    morphology of, 691–692, 692f
    non-atopic, 688–689
    occupational, 689
    organic dusts that produce, 697t
    pathogenesis of, 689–691, 690f
Astrocyte(s), 1281, 1282f
    Alzheimer type II, 1281–1282
    gemistocytic, 1281
    reactions to injury of, 1281–1282, 1282f
Astrocytoma(s), 1330–1333
    anaplastic, 1330, 1331
    diffuse, 1330–1331, 1331f
    gemistocytic, 1331
    infiltrating, 1330–1332, 1331f, 1332f
    pilocytic, 1332–1333, 1333f
    pleomorphic xantho-, 1333
Astrogliosis, 1281
    in sudden infant death syndrome, 472
Ataxia(s)
    Friedreich, 168t, 1323
    spinocerebellar, 168t, 1323–1324

Ataxia-telangiectasia, 41, 275, 302–303, 1323–1324
Ataxia-telangiectasia and Rad3 related (ATR), 292
Ataxia-telangiectasia mutated (ATM) gene, 286t, 292, 302, 1324
Atelectasis, 679–680, 679f
ATG16L1, in Crohn disease, 809
Atheroembolic renal disease, 954, 954f
Atheroembolism, 504
Atheromas, 496, 496f, 502
    in pulmonary hypertension, 708, 709f
Atheromatous plaques. See Atherosclerotic plaques.
Atherosclerosis, 34–35, 496–506
    arterial thromboses due to, 125
    cerebral infarction due to, 1293
    chronic inflammation in, 70
    cigarette smoking and, 411
    consequences of, 504–506, 505f
    due to diabetes mellitus, 1139
    diet and, 444
    epidemiology of, 496–498, 497f, 497t, 498f
    hormone replacement therapy and, 415
    and ischemic heart disease, 545–546, 546f
    morphology of, 502–504, 502f–504f
        aneurysm formation in, 504
        atheroembolism in, 504
        atherosclerotic plaque in, 502–504
            anatomy of, 496, 496f
            calcification of, 503, 503f
            fibrous, 503
            gross features of, 502, 503f
            hemorrhage into, 504
            histologic features of, 502–503, 503f
            location of, 502
            rupture, ulceration, or erosion of, 503–504, 504f
            thrombosis of, 502–503, 506
            vulnerable vs. stable, 505, 505f
        fatty streaks in, 501, 502, 502f
    pathogenesis of, 498–502
        endothelial injury in, 499–500
        hemodynamic disturbances in, 500
        infection in, 500–501
        inflammation in, 500
        lipids in, 500
        overview of, 501–502, 501f
        response-to-injury hypothesis of, 499, 499f
        smooth muscle proliferation in, 501
    renal, in diabetes mellitus, 1142
Atherosclerotic ischemic renal disease, 954
Atherosclerotic plaques, 502–504
    anatomy of, 496, 496f
    calcification of, 503, 503f
    fibrous, 503
    gross features of, 502, 503f
    hemorrhage into, 504
    histologic features of, 502–503, 503f
    and ischemic heart disease, 546, 546f
    location of, 502
    rupture, ulceration, or erosion of, 503–504, 504f
    thrombosis of, 502–503, 506
    vulnerable vs. stable, 505, 505f
Atherosclerotic stenosis, 504
Athlete's foot, 1202
ATM (ataxia-telangiectasia mutated) gene, 286t, 292, 302, 1324
ATN. See Acute tubular necrosis (ATN).
Atopic asthma, 688, 689, 690f
Atopy, 200–201
ATP (adenosine triphosphate) depletion, cell injury due to, 17–18, 18f

ATP7B gene, 863, 864
ATR (ataxia-telangiectasia and Rad3 related), 292
Atrial fibrillation, in left-sided heart failure, 535–536
Atrial myxomas, 583, 583f
Atrial natriuretic peptide, in myocardium, 531
Atrial septal defect (ASD), 540f, 541
Atrioventricular (AV) canal defect, complete, 540f, 542
Atrioventricular (AV) node, 532
Atrioventricular septal defect (AVSD), 540f, 542
Atrophic glossitis, 779
    due to vitamin B$_{12}$ deficiency, 658
Atrophy, 9–10, 9f
    brown, 10
    causes of, 9–10, 9f
    defined, 9
    denervation, 9
    of disuse, 9
    mechanisms of, 10
    pathologic, 9
ATTR (transthyretin amyloid), 251, 251f, 252
Atypical ductal hyperplasia, 1073, 1074f
Atypical lobular hyperplasia, 1073, 1074f
Atypical teratoid/rhabdoid tumor, 1337
Auer rods, in acute myeloid leukemia, 623, 623f
Auspitz sign, 1191
Autoantibodies, in systemic lupus erythematosus, 204t, 213–215, 215t
Autocrine signaling, 89, 90f
Autoimmune adrenalitis, 1155–1156, 1156f
Autoimmune disease(s), 208–226, 208t
    clinical manifestations of, 209
    defective apoptosis in, 32
    epidemiology of, 208
    general features of, 212–213
    HLA alleles and, 193
    inflammation due to
        acute, 45
        chronic, 70
    inflammatory myopathies as, 215t, 225–226
    lupus erythematosus as
        chronic discoid, 221
        drug-induced, 215t, 216, 221
        subacute cutaneous, 221
        systemic, 213–221
            autoantibodies in, 204t, 213–215, 215t
            clinical features of, 204t, 217t, 220–221
            diagnostic criteria for, 213, 214t
            epidemiology of, 213
            etiology and pathogenesis of, 215–217, 216f
            morphology of, 217–220, 217t, 218f–220f
    mixed connective tissue disease as, 226
    organ-specific, 209
    polyarteritis nodosa and other vasculitides as, 204t, 226
    rheumatoid arthritis as (See Rheumatoid arthritis)
    Sjögren syndrome as, 215t, 221–223, 222f
    systemic or generalized, 209
    systemic sclerosis (scleroderma) as, 215t, 223–225, 223f–225f
Autoimmune encephalomyelitis, experimental, 1310
Autoimmune enteropathy, 794t, 796–797
Autoimmune gastritis, 778–779, 778t, 779f
Autoimmune hemolytic anemia, 203, 203t
Autoimmune hepatitis, 855–856, 855f
Autoimmune hypoparathyroidism, 1130
Autoimmune hypothyroidism, 1110
Autoimmune lymphoproliferative syndrome, 211

Autoimmune orchitis, 986
Autoimmune pancreatitis, 897
Autoimmune polyendocrine syndrome type 1 (APS1), 1130, 1155–1156
Autoimmune polyendocrine syndrome type 2 (APS2), 1156
Autoimmune regulator (AIRE) gene, 1130, 1156
Autoimmune regulator (AIRE) protein, in immunological tolerance, 209
Autoimmune thrombocytopenic purpura, 203t
Autoimmunity
    defined, 184, 208
    immunological tolerance and, 209–211, 210f
    infections in, 211f, 212, 213f
    mechanisms of, 211–212, 211f, 213f
    in rheumatoid arthritis, 1238–1239
    susceptibility genes in, 211f, 212
Autoinducer peptides, 343
Autoinflammatory syndromes, inherited, 61–62
Autonomic nervous system, in cardiac conduction system, 532
Autophagic vacuoles, 10, 32, 32f
Autophagolysosome, 32, 32f
Autophagy, 5, 10, 11, 32, 32f
    in tumor cells, 304
Autoregulation, of blood pressure, 492
Autosomal dominant inherited cancer syndromes, 274–275, 275t
Autosomal recessive inherited cancer syndromes, 275t
Autosomal dominant disorders, 140–141, 141t
Autosomal dominant hypoparathyroidism, 1130
Autosomal-dominant polycystic kidney disease (ADPKD), 956–959, 957t, 958f
Autosomal recessive disorders, 141–142, 142t
Autosomal recessive dysautonomia, 1263t
Autosomal-recessive polycystic kidney disease (ARPKD), 957t, 959
Autosomes, cytogenetic disorder involving, 161–164, 161f, 163f, 164f
Autosplenectomy, in sickle cell disease, 647, 647f
AV (atrioventricular) canal defect, complete, 540f, 542
AV (atrioventricular) node, 532
Avascular necrosis, 1220–1221, 1221f, 1221t
Avellino dystrophy, of cornea, 1353
Avian influenza, 715
AVMs (arteriovenous malformations), 1298–1299
AVSD (atrioventricular septal defect), 540f, 542
Avulsions, neuropathies due to, 1266
Axillary lymph node involvement, in breast carcinoma, 269f, 270, 1089
Axillary tail of Spence, 1067
Axonal degeneration, 1258, 1258f, 1259–1260, 1259f
Axonal injury, diffuse, 1288
Axonal processes, in skin, 1166
Axonal reaction, 1281
Axonopathy, 1259
Azo dyes, as carcinogens, 309t, 311
Azoospermia, in cystic fibrosis, 469, 470
Azotemia, 906–907
    postrenal, 907
    prerenal, 906–907
    in left-sided heart failure, 536
Azurophil granules, in inflammation, 63
Azzopardi effect, in small cell lung carcinoma, 726

B

B lymphocytes
    activation of, 195–196, 196f
    in AIDS, 242, 242t

B lymphocytes (Continued)
   antigen recognition by, 193
   in immune response, 185f, 187, 187f
   in immunological tolerance, 209–211
   in lymphoid organs, 189, 189f
   in X-linked agammaglobulinemia, 231, 232
B rings, 767–768
Babesia divergens, 388
Babesia microti, 388
Babesiosis, 388, 388f
Bacillary angiomatosis, 520, 522, 523f
Bacillus anthracis, 361–362, 362f
Bacillus Calmette-Guérin (BCG), for bladder
   cancer, 980
Back to Sleep campaign, 473
Backwash ileitis, 811
Bacteria, 333t, 334–335, 334f
   anaerobic, 378–379, 379f
   classification of, 334–335
   colonization by, 335
   enteropathogenic, 338
   flesh-eating, 360
   gram-negative, 334, 334f
   gram-positive, 334, 334f
   intracellular
      facultative, 335
      obligate, 335, 380–381, 381f, 382f
      virulence of, 344
   mechanisms of disease production by,
      343–344
   sexually transmitted, 341t
   structure of, 334–335, 334f
Bacterial adherence, to host cells, 343–344
Bacterial arthritis, 1242
Bacterial endocarditis, 566–567, 568f
Bacterial endocarditis–associated
   glomerulonephritis, 934
Bacterial exotoxins, 344
Bacterial gastroenteritis, 794t
Bacterial infection(s), 357–381, 358t
   abscesses due to, 378
   by Actinomycetaceaea, 358t
   in AIDS, 245t, 246
   anaerobic, 378–379, 379f
   anthrax as, 337, 361–362, 362f
   chancroid (soft chancre) as, 366
   chlamydial, 380
   clostridial, 358t, 378–379, 379f
   contagious childhood, 358t
   diphtheria as, 360–361, 361f
   enteric, 358t
   in Global Burden of Disease, 400
   gram-negative, 358t, 363–366, 364f, 365f
   gram-positive, 357–363, 359f–363f
   granuloma inguinale as, 366
   leprosy as, 372–374, 373f, 374f
   listeriosis as, 361
   of liver, 854
   Lyme disease as, 377–378, 378f
   myco-, 358t, 366–374, 367f, 369f–374f
   Mycobacterium avium-intracellulare complex
      as, 372, 373f
   neisserial, 363–364
   Nocardia as, 362–363, 363f
   obligate intracellular, 380–381, 381f, 382f
   plague as, 365
   Pseudomonas as, 364–365, 365f
   by pyogenic cocci, 357–360, 358t
   relapsing fever as, 377
   rickettsial, 380–381, 381f, 382f
   Rocky Mountain spotted fever as, 381, 382f
   scrub typhus as, 380, 381
   staphylococcal, 357–359, 359f
   streptococcal and enterococcal, 359–360, 360f

Bacterial infection(s) (Continued)
   syphilis as, 374–377, 374f–376f
   treponemal (spirochetal), 358t, 374–378,
      374f–376f, 378f
   tuberculosis as, 366–372, 367f, 369f–372f
   typhus fever as, 380, 381, 381f
   whooping cough as, 364, 364f
   zoonotic, 358t
Bacterial injury, mechanism of, 343–344
Bacterial meningitis, 1299–1300, 1299f
Bacterial meningoencephalitis, chronic,
   1301–1302
Bacterial pneumonia, 711–714, 712f, 713f
Bacterial toxins, 344
Bacterial vaginosis, 1009
Bacterial virulence, 343
Bactericidal/permeability increasing protein, in
   phagocytosis, 54
Bacteriophages, 343
Bacteroides fragilis, 378
BAFF, in systemic lupus erythematosus, 216
Bagasse, lung diseases due to, 697t
BAK, in apoptosis, 295, 296
Balanced reciprocal translocation, 160f, 161
Balanitis, 383
Balanoposthitis, 982
B-ALL (B-cell acute lymphoblastic leukemia/
   lymphoma), 601t, 602–603, 602f
Balloon angioplasty, pathology of, 526, 526f
Ballooned neurons, in corticobasal degeneration,
   1319
Ballooning, 1168
Ballooning degeneration, in viral hepatitis, 851,
   851f
Band keratopathies, 1351–1352
Bannayan-Ruvalcaba-Riley syndrome, 816t,
   818
Bare lymphocyte syndrome, 234
Barium sulfate, lung diseases due to, 697t
Baroreceptors, 1099
Barr body, 164
Barrett esophagus, 770–771, 770f, 771f
Bartholin cyst, 1011
Bartonella henselae, 522
Bartonella quintana, 522
Basal cell carcinoma
   of eyelid, 1348
   of skin, 1180–1181, 1181f, 1183f
   of vulva, 1014
Basal cell nevus, 1181, 1182t
Basal ganglia, degenerative diseases of,
   1319–1323, 1320f, 1322f
   dementia with Lewy bodies as, 1321
   Huntington disease as, 1322–1323, 1322f
   multiple system atrophy as, 1321–1322
   Parkinson disease as, 1319–1321, 1320f
   parkinsonism as, 1319
Basaloid vulvar carcinoma, 1012, 1013–1014,
   1013f
Basement membranes, 94, 95f
Basic fibroblastic growth factor (bFGF), in
   angiogenesis, 298
Basic multicellular unit (BMU), 1209
Basophil(s)
   adult reference range for, 592t
   differentiation of, 591f
   in immediate hypersensitivity, 199
Basophilia, 594t
Basophilic degeneration, of heart, 532
Basophilic leukocytosis, 594t
Batten disease, 1326
BAV (bicuspid aortic valve), calcific stenosis of,
   562–563, 562f
BAX, in apoptosis, 295, 296, 296f

B-cell acute lymphoblastic leukemia/lymphoma
   (B-ALL), 601t, 602–603, 602f
B-cell antigen receptor complex, 187, 187f
B-cell lymphomas
   AIDS-related, 248
   diffuse large, 601t, 606–607, 607f, 608
   Epstein-Barr virus in, 315
B-cell neoplasms
   origin of, 599f
   peripheral, 598t, 601t, 603–614
   precursor, 598t, 600–603, 601t, 602f
BCG (bacillus Calmette-Guérin), for bladder
   cancer, 980
BCL-2 gene
   in acute lymphoblastic leukemia/lymphoma,
      603
   in apoptosis, 28, 28f, 29f, 295–296, 296f
   in carcinogenesis, 308
   in diffuse large B-cell lymphoma, 607
   in follicular lymphoma, 305, 606, 606f
BCL-6 gene, 597, 607
BCL-10 gene, 597
BCL-XL, in apoptosis, 296, 296f
BCR gene, 283–284, 283f
BCR-ABL fusion gene
   in acute leukemia, 597f
   in chronic myeloid leukemia, 627, 627f, 628
BCR-ABL fusion protein, 283–284, 283f, 305
BCRAT (Breast Cancer Risk Assessment Tool),
   1076
BDNF (brain-derived neurotrophic factor), in
   energy balance, 440
Becker muscular dystrophy (BMD), 1268–1269,
   1268f
Beckwith-Wiedemann syndrome (BWS), Wilms
   tumor in, 480
Bellini duct carcinoma, 965, 966
Bence Jones protein(s)
   in amyloidosis, 252
   in plasma cell neoplasms, 609, 610
Bence Jones proteinuria
   and light-chain cast nephropathy, 948
   in multiple myeloma, 610–611
Bends, the, 127
Benign familial hematuria, 932
Benign fibrous histiocytoma, 1182, 1184f,
   1253
Benign fibrous mesothelioma, 732–733, 732f
Benign prostatic hyperplasia (BPH), 8, 994–996,
   995f, 996f
Benign tumor(s)
   characteristic(s) of malignant vs., 262–267,
      270, 271t
      cancer stem cells and cancer cell lineages as,
         267–268
      differentiation and anaplasia as, 262–265,
         264f–266f, 271t
      local invasion as, 268, 268f, 271t
      metastasis as, 269–270, 269f–271f, 271t
      rate of growth as, 265–267, 266f
   defined, 260
   in infants and children, 473–474, 474f
   nomenclature for, 260–261, 261f, 263t
Benzene
   as carcinogen, 274t
   lung diseases due to, 697t
   occupational exposure to, 409
Berger disease, 918t, 929–931, 931f
Bergmann gliosis, 1329
Beriberi, 1328
   neuropathic, 1266
Bernard-Soulier syndrome, 118f, 670
Berry aneurysms, 489, 506, 506f, 507
   ruptured, 1297–1298, 1297f, 1298f

Beryllium
  as carcinogen, 274t
  lung diseases due to, 697t
  pneumoconiosis due to, 410
Beta particles, 423
β cells, 1130, 1131f
β chemokines, 62
β2-microglobulin, in amyloidosis, 251
β-adrenergic receptor gene, in asthma, 691
β-amyloid (Aβ) protein, 250–251
  in Alzheimer disease, 1316–1317
β-carotene, 431
β-catenin gene, 281t, 287t, 292–294, 293f
  in colorectal carcinoma, 823–824, 823f
  in endometrial carcinoma, 1032, 1032f
  in Wilms tumor, 480
β-cell destruction, in type 1 diabetes mellitus, 1135, 1135f
β-cell dysfunction, in type 2 diabetes mellitus, 1137
β-cell function, genetic defects in, 1137–1138
β-cell tumors, 1146–1147, 1147f
β-globin synthesis, 648–649, 649f, 650f
β-thalassemia, 648–651
  clinical syndromes of, 649, 652t
  intermedia, 649, 652t
  major, 649–651, 650f, 651f, 652t
  minor, 651, 652t
  molecular pathogenesis of, 648–649, 649f, 650f
β-thalassemia trait, 649, 652t
bFGF (basic fibroblastic growth factor), in angiogenesis, 298
BH3-only proteins, in apoptosis, 28, 29f, 295, 296
BH4 (tetrahydrobiopterin), 463, 463f
Bicarbonate, in cystic fibrosis, 466
Bicuspid aortic valve (BAV), calcific stenosis of, 562–563, 562f
BID, in apoptosis, 295, 296f
Bile
  formation of, 839–840, 840f
  functions of, 839
Bile acid(s), 840
Bile acid malabsorption, primary, 794t
Bile canaliculi, 835
Bile duct(s)
  syndromatic paucity of, 870
  terminal, 835
Bile duct hamartomas, 869, 870f
Bile duct reactive changes, in viral hepatitis, 852
Bile ductules, 835
Bile plugs, 842, 843f
Bile salt(s), 840
Bile salt export pump (BSEP), 843
Biliary abscesses, 854
Biliary atresia, 887
Biliary cirrhosis
  in cystic fibrosis, 469, 470
  primary, 867–869, 867t, 868f
  secondary, 867, 867f, 867t
Biliary disease, intrahepatic, 866–870, 867t
  anomalies of biliary trees as, 869–870, 870f
  biliary cirrhosis as
    primary, 867–869, 867t, 868f
    secondary, 867, 867f, 867t
  polycystic, 869–870, 870f
  primary sclerosing cholangitis as, 867t, 869, 869f
Biliary excretory function, laboratory evaluation of, 835t
Biliary tract disorder(s), 882–889
  congenital anomalies as, 882, 882f
  of extrahepatic bile ducts, 887–888

Biliary tract disorder(s) (Continued)
  biliary atresia as, 887
  choledochal cysts as, 887–888
  choledocholithiasis and ascending cholangitis as, 887
  of gallbladder, 882–887
    cholecystitis as, 885–887, 886f
    cholelithiasis as, 882–884, 883f, 883t, 884f
  neoplastic, 888–889
    gallbladder carcinoma as, 888–889, 888f
Biliary trees, anomalies of, 869–870, 870f
Bilirubin
  defined, 839
  intracellular accumulation of, 38
  metabolism and elimination of, 839–840, 840f
  serum levels of, 840
  unconjugated vs. conjugated, 840
Bilirubin delta fraction, 840
Biliverdin, 839, 840f
Biliverdin reductase, 839, 840f
Binge eating, 430
Binswanger disease, 1295
Bioaerosols, as indoor air pollutant, 405
Bioinformatics, 136
Biopsy, for cancer, 323
Bioterrorism, agents of, 337–338, 337t
Biotin, function of, 438f
Birbeck granules, in Langerhans cell histiocytosis, 631, 631f
Bird droppings, lung diseases due to, 697t
Bird fancier's disease, 703
Birth defects. See Congenital anomaly(ies).
Birt-Hogg-Dubé syndrome, 1176
Bitot spots, 432, 432f
Black Death, 365
Black fever, 389
Black sunburst lesions, in sickle retinopathy, 1362
Bladder, 974–981
  anatomy of, 972
  congenital anomalies of, 974, 974f
  diverticula of, 974
  exstrophy of, 974, 974f
  inflammation of, 974–975, 975f, 976f
  metaplastic lesions of, 975–976
  obstruction of, 981, 981f
Bladder diverticula, 974
Bladder tumor(s), 976–981, 976t
  classification of, 976t
  mesenchymal, 980–981
  secondary, 981
  urothelial (transition), 976–980
    adenocarcinoma as, 979
    clinical course of, 980
    epidemiology and pathogenesis of, 976, 979–980
    grading of, 976–977, 977t
    high-grade, 978, 978f
    in situ, 978–979, 978f
    invasive, 979, 979f
    low-grade, 978, 978f
    morphology of, 977–979, 977f–979f
    precursor lesions to, 976
    squamous cell carcinoma as, 979
    staging of, 979, 979t
    variants of, 979
Blastema, and regeneration, 92
Blastomyces dermatitidis, chronic pneumonia due to, 718–719, 719f
Blastomycosis, 718–719, 719f
Bleeding disorder(s), 666–674
  due to abnormalities in clotting factors, 670–673, 671f
  due to defective platelet functions, 670

Bleeding disorder(s) (Continued)
  disseminated intravascular coagulation as, 673–674, 674f
  due to reduced platelet number, 667–670, 667t, 669f
  tests for evaluation of, 666
  due to vessel wall abnormalities, 666
Blepharitis, 1348
Blister, 1168
  formation of, 1193f
Blistering diseases, 1192–1197, 1193f
  inflammatory, 1192–1196
    bullous pemphigoid as, 1193f, 1195–1196, 1196f
    dermatitis herpetiformis as, 1193f, 1196, 1197f
    pemphigus as, 1192–1195, 1193f–1195f
  noninflammatory, 1196–1197
    epidermolysis bullosa as, 1193f, 1196, 1198f
    porphyria as, 1196–1197, 1198f
Blood alcohol level, 412
Blood cell(s)
  adult reference ranges for, 592t
  development and maintenance of, 590
  differentiation of, 591f
Blood cell disorders, due to adverse drug reactions, 416t
Blood cell progenitors, 590, 591f
Blood clots
  formation of, 102, 103f
  postmortem, 124
  in thrombosis, 115
Blood flow, alterations in, in thrombosis, 121–122
Blood group incompatibility, fetal hydrops due to, 460–461, 460f
Blood loss, anemias of, 640t, 641
Blood pressure, regulation of, 492–493, 494f
Blood supply, to heart, 532
Blood vessel(s), 487–527
  aneurysms and dissection of, 506–510, 506f–510f
  arteriosclerosis of, 496
  atherosclerosis of, 496–506
    anatomy of plaque in, 496, 496f
    consequences of, 504–506, 505f
    epidemiology of, 496–498, 497f, 497t, 498f
    morphology of, 502–504, 502f–504f
    pathogenesis of, 498–502, 499f, 501f, 502f
  congenital anomalies of, 489–490
  development, growth, and remodeling of, 489
  hypertensive disease of, 492–496, 493t, 494f, 495f
  in inflammation
    acute, 46–48, 46f, 47f
    chronic, 72
  pathology of vascular interventions for, 525–527, 526f, 527f
  Raynaud phenomenon of, 518, 518f
  responses to injury of, 490–492, 490f, 491f
  structure and function of, 488–489, 488f
  tumor(s) of, 520–525, 520t
    benign, 520–522, 520t
      bacillary angiomatosis as, 522, 523f
      glomus tumor (glomangioma) as, 522
      hemangioma as, 520–521, 521f
      lymphangiomas as, 522
      vascular ectasias as, 522
    intermediate-grade (borderline), 520t, 523–524
      hemangioendothelioma as, 524
      Kaposi sarcoma as, 523–524, 524f

Blood vessel(s) (Continued)
   malignant, 520t, 524–525
      angiosarcoma as, 524–525, 525f
      hemangiopericytoma as, 525
   vasculitis of, 510–518
      associated with other disorders, 517
      Churg-Strauss syndrome as, 516
      classification and characteristics of, 510,
         511t, 512t
      defined, 510
      giant-cell (temporal) arteritis as, 512–513,
         513f
      immune complex–associated, 510–511
      infectious, 517–518
      Kawasaki disease as, 515
      large-vessel, 511t, 512f
      medium-vessel, 511t, 512f
      microscopic polyangiitis as, 515, 516f
      noninfectious, 510–517
      polyarteritis nodosa as, 514–515, 514f
      small-vessel, 511t, 512f
      Takayasu arteritis as, 513–514, 514f
      thromboangiitis obliterans (Buerger
         disease) as, 517, 517f
      Wegener granulomatosis as, 516–517, 516f
   venous and lymphatic disorders of, 518–520,
      519f
Bloodstream expression sites, in African
   trypanosomiasis, 390
Bloom syndrome, 275, 302–303
Blue bloaters, 688
Blue nevus, 1170t
Blueberry muffin baby, 478
Blue-dome cysts, of breast, 1071, 1071f
BMD (Becker muscular dystrophy), 1268–1269,
   1268f
BMP (bone morphogenetic protein), 85
BMPR2 (bone morphogenetic protein receptor
   type 2) gene, in pulmonary hypertension,
   707–708, 708f
BMU (basic multicellular unit), 1209
β-myosin heavy chain (β-MHC), in
   hypertrophic cardiomyopathy, 577
Body mass index (BMI)
   and cancer, 443
   and malnutrition, 428
   and obesity, 438
Boerhaave syndrome, 768
Boil, 358
Bone(s), 1206–1235
   anatomy and physiology of, 1206–1209, 1207f,
      1208f, 1209t
   lamellar, 1208, 1208f
      mosaic pattern of, 1217, 1217f
   woven, 1208–1209, 1208f
Bone cells, 1206–1208, 1206f
   developmental and acquired abnormalities in,
      1210–1219
Bone cyst, aneurysmal, 1234, 1234f
Bone disease(s)
   with abnormal mineral homeostasis,
      1218–1219
   of collagen, 1211–1212, 1212t, 1213f
   with decreased bone mass, 1214–1216
   due to defects in extracellular structural
      proteins, 1210–1212, 1211t, 1212t, 1213f
   due to defects in folding and degradation of
      macromolecules, 1212
   due to defects in hormones and signal
      transduction mechanisms, 1210, 1211t
   due to defects in metabolic pathways,
      1212–1214
   due to defects in nuclear proteins and
      transcription factors, 1210, 1211t

Bone disease(s) (Continued)
   fractures as, 1219–1220, 1220f
   due to hyperparathyroidism, 1218, 1218f,
      1219f
   molecular genetics of, 1210, 1211t
   mucopolysaccharidoses as, 1212
   due to osteoclast dysfunction, 1216–1218
   osteogenesis imperfecta as, 1211–1212, 1211t,
      1212t, 1213f
   osteomyelitis as, 1221–1223
      pyogenic, 1221–1222, 1222f
      tuberculous, 1222–1223
   osteonecrosis (avascular necrosis) as,
      1220–1221, 1221f, 1221t
   osteopetrosis as, 1212–1214, 1213f, 1214f
   osteoporosis as, 1214–1216, 1214t, 1215f
   Paget disease (osteitis deformans) as,
      1216–1218, 1216f, 1217f
   renal osteodystrophy as, 1218–1219
   rickets and osteomalacia as, 1218
   skeletal syphilis as, 1223
   tumors and tumor-like lesions as,
      1223–1235
      aneurysmal bone cyst as, 1234, 1234f
      chondrogenic (cartilage-forming), 1223t,
         1227–1230
         chondroblastoma as, 1228–1229, 1228f
         chondromas as, 1227–1228, 1228f
         chondromyxoid fibroma as, 1229, 1229f
         chondrosarcoma as, 1229–1230, 1229f,
            1230f
         osteochondroma as, 1227, 1227f
      classification of, 1223, 1223t
      clinical presentation of, 1224
      epidemiology of, 1223–1224
      Ewing sarcoma as, 1232–1233, 1233f
      fibrogenic (fibrous and fibro-osseous),
         1223t, 1230–1232
         fibrosarcoma variants as, 1232
         fibrous cortical defects as, 1230, 1231f
         fibrous dysplasia as, 1230–1232, 1232f
         non-ossifying fibroma as, 1230, 1231f
      genetics of, 1224
      giant-cell, 1233–1234, 1233f
      hematopoietic, 1223t
      metastatic, 1235
      neuroectodermal, 1223t
      notochordal, 1223t
      osteogenic (bone-forming), 1223t,
         1224–1227
         osteoid osteoma and osteoblastoma as,
            1224, 1224f, 1225f
         osteoma as, 1224
         osteosarcoma as, 1225–1227, 1225f,
            1226f
      primitive neuroectodermal, 1232–1233
      of unknown origin, 1223t
Bone eburnation, 1236, 1236f
Bone formation, 1208–1210, 1209f
Bone growth and development, 1209–1210,
   1209f
Bone homeostasis, 1208, 1208f
Bone marrow, 590–592
   stem cells in, 85
Bone marrow disorders, due to adverse drug
   reactions, 416t
Bone marrow suppression, defects in leukocyte
   function due to, 55–56
Bone marrow transplantation, 230
   hepatic complications of, 874
Bone mass
   decreased, 1214–1216, 1214t, 1215f
   increased, 1210
   peak, 1209

Bone matrix
   developmental and acquired abnormalities in,
      1210–1219
   proteins of, 1208–1209, 1209t
Bone mineralization, vitamin D in, 435
Bone modeling, 1209
Bone morphogenetic protein (BMP), 85
Bone morphogenetic protein receptor type 2
   (BMPR2) gene, in pulmonary hypertension,
   707–708, 708f
Bone remodeling, 1209
Bone resorption, 1207–1208
Bone tissue, destruction of, hypercalcemia due
   to, 38
Bone tumors and tumor-like lesions, 1223–1235
   aneurysmal bone cyst as, 1234, 1234f
   chondrogenic (cartilage-forming), 1223t,
      1227–1230
      chondroblastoma as, 1228–1229, 1228f
      chondromas as, 1227–1228, 1228f
      chondromyxoid fibroma as, 1229, 1229f
      chondrosarcoma as, 1229–1230, 1229f,
         1230f
      osteochondroma as, 1227, 1227f
   classification of, 1223, 1223t
   clinical presentation of, 1224
   epidemiology of, 1223–1224
   Ewing sarcoma as, 1232–1233, 1233f
   fibrogenic (fibrous and fibro-osseous), 1223t,
      1230–1232
      fibrosarcoma variants as, 1232
      fibrous cortical defects as, 1230, 1231f
      fibrous dysplasia as, 1230–1232, 1232f
      non-ossifying fibroma as, 1230, 1231f
   genetics of, 1224
   giant-cell, 1233–1234, 1233f
   hematopoietic, 1223t
   metastatic, 1235
   neuroectodermal, 1223t
      primitive, 1232–1233
   notochordal, 1223t
   osteogenic (bone-forming), 1223t, 1224–1227
      osteoid osteoma and osteoblastoma as,
         1224, 1224f, 1225f
      osteoma as, 1224
      osteosarcoma as, 1225–1227, 1225f, 1226f
   of unknown origin, 1223t
Bone-forming tumor(s), 1223t, 1224–1227
   osteoid osteoma and osteoblastoma as, 1224,
      1224f, 1225f
   osteoma as, 1224
   osteosarcoma as, 1225–1227, 1225f, 1226f
Bony callus, 1220, 1220f
Border zone infarcts, 1291
Borderline serous tumors, of ovary, 1043–1044,
   1043f
Bordetella pertussis, 364, 364f
Borrelia burgdorferi, 334f, 377–378, 378f
Borrelia recurrentis, 377
Borreliosis, 377–378, 378f
Botulism, 379
Botulism toxin (Botox), 379
Bowel. See Intestine(s).
Bowel incarceration, 790, 791f
Bowel infarction, 792
Bowen disease
   of penis, 983, 984f
   of vulva, 1012–1014, 1013f
Bowenoid papulosis, 984, 1201
Bowman layer, of cornea, 1351, 1351f
BPAG (bullous pemphigoid antigen), 1195,
   1196f
BPD (bronchopulmonary dysplasia), in neonatal
   respiratory distress syndrome, 457–458

BPH (benign prostatic hyperplasia), 8, 994–996, 995f, 996f
Brachial plexopathy, 1266
Brachydactyly type C, 1211t
Bradykinin, in inflammation, 65, 65f
BRAF gene, 281t
  in colorectal carcinoma, 824, 824f
  in melanocytic nevi, 1170
  in melanoma, 1174, 1174f, 1175
  in ovarian carcinoma, 1042
  in papillary thyroid carcinoma, 1120, 1122
Braille, Louis, 1356
Brain
  respirator, 1291
  stem cells in, 85
  in Wilson disease, 864
Brain abscess, 1300, 1300f
Brain death, 1291
Brain edema, 113, 1282–1283
Brain herniation, 1283–1284, 1283f, 1284f
Brain injury, 1287–1290
  concussion as, 1287
  contusion as, 1287, 1288f
  coup and contrecoup, 1287
  diffuse axonal, 1288
  laceration as, 1287
  parenchymal, 1287–1288, 1288f
  perinatal, 1286–1287, 1286f
  sequelae of, 1290
  skull fractures as, 1287
  vascular, 1288–1290, 1289f, 1290f
Brain tumor(s), 1330–1343
  astrocytomas as, 1330–1333, 1331f–1333f
  atypical teratoid/rhabdoid, 1337
  ependymoma as, 1334–1335, 1335f
  epidemiology of, 1330
  familial syndromes of, 1342–1343
  germ cell, 1338
  gliomas as, 1330–1335, 1331f–1335f
  medulloblastoma as, 1336–1337, 1336f
  meningiomas as, 1338–1339, 1338f
  metastatic, 1339
  neuronal, 1335–1336
  neurorfibroma as, 1341
  other parenchymal, 1337–1338
  paraneoplastic syndromes due to, 1339–1340
  peripheral nerve sheath, 1340–1342, 1340f
  pineal parenchymal, 1338
  poorly differentiated, 1336–1337, 1336f
  primary lymphoma as, 1337
  schwannoma as, 1340–1341, 1340f
Brain-derived neurotrophic factor (BDNF), in energy balance, 440
Brainstem, degenerative diseases of, 1319–1323, 1320f, 1322f
  dementia with Lewy bodies as, 1321
  Huntington disease as, 1322–1323, 1322f
  multiple system atrophy as, 1321–1322
  Parkinson disease as, 1319–1321, 1320f
  parkinsonism as, 1319
Brainstem glioma, 1333
Brainstem hemorrhage, secondary, 1283–1284, 1284f
Branchial cyst, 755
Branchiomeric paraganglia, 1159
Brawny induration, 520
BRCA1, 275, 276, 287t, 303, 306
  and breast cancer, 1077–1078, 1078t, 1085
  and ovarian carcinoma, 1042
BRCA2, 275, 276, 287t, 303
  and breast cancer, 1077–1078, 1078t
  and ovarian carcinoma, 1042
  and prostate cancer, 997

Breast(s), 1065–1094
  anatomy of, 1066, 1066f
  developmental disorders of, 1067
  fibroadenoma of, 268f
  invasive ductal carcinoma of, 268f
  life cycle changes in, 1066–1067, 1067f
  male, 1093
  supernumerary, 1067
Breast Cancer Risk Assessment Tool (BCRAT), 1076
Breast carcinoma, 1073–1091
  basal-like, 1084–1085, 1086f
  classification of, 1079–1089
  comedo-, 1080, 1081f
  contralateral, 1077
  DNA content of, 1090
  ductal
    in situ, 1080–1082, 1081f, 1082f
    invasive (infiltrative), 1083–1085, 1085f
  epidemiology of, 1073–1077, 1075f
  estrogen receptors in, 1074, 1075, 1076, 1079, 1084, 1090
  etiology and pathogenesis of, 1077–1079, 1078t, 1080f
  fat intake and, 444
  gene expression profiling for, 1084–1085, 1086f, 1090
  genetic basis for, 303, 306
  grading of, 1089–1090
  HER2/neu-positive, 1085, 1086f, 1090
  hereditary, 1077–1078, 1078t
  hormone replacement therapy and, 415
  inflammatory, 1083, 1089
  in situ, 1080–1083, 1084t
    ductal, 1080–1082, 1081f, 1082f
    lobular, 1082–1083, 1083f
  invasive (infiltrative), 1083–1087, 1084t
    ductal (no special type), 1083–1085, 1085f
    lobular, 1085–1087
    papillary, 1088
  lobular
    in situ, 1082–1083, 1083f
    invasive, 1085–1087
  locally advanced, 1089
  luminal A, 1084, 1086f
  luminal B, 1084
  lymphovascular invasion by, 1090
  male, 1093–1094
  medullary, 1087, 1088f
  metaplastic, 1088–1089
  metastatic, 269f, 270, 301, 1087, 1089
  mucinous (colloid), 1087, 1088f
  neoadjuvant therapy for, 1090
  no special type, 1083–1085, 1085f
  occult, 1083
  papillary
    in situ, 1080, 1082f
    invasive, 1088
  prognostic and predictive factors in, 1089–1091, 1090t
  proliferative rate of, 1090
  risk factors for, 1076–1077
  screening for, 1068–1069, 1068f, 1074–1075
  sporadic, 1079
  staging of, 1089, 1090t
  susceptibility genes for, 275, 1077–1078, 1078t
  triple-negative, 1085, 1086f
  triple-positive, 1084
  tubular, 1087–1088, 1088f
  tumor size in, 1089
Breast changes, nonproliferative (fibrocystic), 1071, 1071f, 1074t
Breast cysts, 1071, 1071f
Breast density, and breast cancer, 1076

Breast disease
  benign epithelial, 1070–1073
    adenosis as, 1071
      sclerosing, 1072, 1072f
    atypical ductal hyperplasia as, 1073, 1074f
    atypical lobular hyperplasia as, 1073, 1074f
    clinical significance of, 1073, 1074t
    complex sclerosing lesion as, 1072, 1073f
    cysts as, 1071, 1071f
    epithelial hyperplasia as, 1071, 1072f
    fibrosis as, 1071
    lactational adenomas as, 1071
    nonproliferative (fibrocystic) changes as, 1071, 1071f, 1074t
    papillomas as, 1072, 1073f
    proliferative changes as
      with atypia, 1073, 1074f, 1074t
      without atypia, 1071–1073, 1072f, 1073f, 1074t
  calcifications due to, 1068
  carcinoma as (*See* Breast carcinoma)
  clinical presentations of, 1067–1069, 1068f
  densities due to, 1068
  inflammatory, 1069–1070
    fat necrosis as, 1070
    lymphocytic mastopathy as, 1070
    mammary duct ectasia as, 1070, 1070f
    mastitis as
      acute, 1069
      granulomatous, 1070
      periductal, 1069, 1069f
  lymphomas as, 1093
  male, 1093–1094
    carcinoma as, 1093–1094
    gynecomastia as, 1093, 1093f
  metastases as, 1093
  stromal tumors as, 1091–1093
    benign, 1092
    fibroadenoma as, 1091–1092, 1091f
    malignant, 1092–1093
    phyllodes tumor as, 1092, 1092f
Breast masses, 1068, 1068f
Breast milk, 1067
Breast pain, 1067
Breast tissue, accessory axillary, 1067
Breastfeeding, and breast cancer, 1077
Brenner tumor, 1046, 1046f
Bridge-fusion-breakage cycle, 296, 297, 297f
Bridging necrosis, in viral hepatitis, 851–852, 851f
Bridging veins, in subdural hematoma, 1289
Brittle bone disease, 1211–1212, 1211t, 1212t, 1213f
Brodie abscess, 1222
Bronchial carcinoids, 729–730, 729f
Bronchiectasis, 683t, 692–693, 693f
  in cystic fibrosis, 470
Bronchioalveolar carcinoma, 725, 727f
Bronchioles, 678
Bronchiolitis, 683t, 715–716
  obliterans, 688
    after lung transplantation, 720, 721f
Bronchiolitis obliterans organizing pneumonia, 696, 696f
Bronchiolitis-associated interstitial lung disease, 704–705
Bronchioloalveolar connections, in obstructive overinflation, 687
Bronchitis, chronic, 683t, 687–688, 687t
Bronchopneumonia, 712, 713, 713f
  herpes, 353
Bronchopulmonary dysplasia (BPD), in neonatal respiratory distress syndrome, 457–458

Brown atrophy, 10
  of heart, 532
Brown induration, 680
Brown tumors, 1128, 1218, 1219f
Brugia spp, 395
Brunn nests, 975
Bruton agammaglobulinemia, 231–233
Bruton tyrosine kinase (Btk), 231
BSEP (bile salt export pump), 843
Bubonic plague, 365
Budd-Chiari syndrome, 872–873, 873f
Buerger disease, 517, 517f
Buffalo hump, in Cushing syndrome, 1150
Bulbar conjunctiva, 1348f, 1349
Bulbospinal atrophy, 1325
Bulimia, 430
Bulla, 1168
Bullous diseases, 1192–1197, 1193f
  inflammatory, 1192–1196
    bullous pemphigoid as, 1193f, 1195–1196,
      1196f
    dermatitis herpetiformis as, 1193f, 1196,
      1197f
    pemphigus as, 1192–1195, 1193f–1195f
  noninflammatory, 1196–1197
    epidermolysis bullosa as, 1193f, 1196,
      1198f
    porphyria as, 1196–1197, 1198f
Bullous emphysema, 687, 687f
Bullous keratopathy, 1351
Bullous pemphigoid, 1193f, 1195–1196, 1196f
  oral manifestations of, 744t
Bullous pemphigoid antigen (BPAG), 1195,
  1196f
Bundle of His, 532
Buphthalmos, 1366
Burkholderia cepacia complex, in cystic fibrosis,
  469
Burkitt lymphoma, 601t, 607–608, 608f
  Epstein-Barr virus and, 314–315, 314f, 608
  genetic basis for, 283, 305, 305t, 608
Burn(s)
  full-thickness (third-degree), 421
  partial-thickness (second-degree), 421
  superficial (first-degree), 421
  thermal, 421–422
Burnet, Macfarlane, 316
1,3-Butadiene, occupational exposure to, 409
BWS (Beckwith-Wiedemann syndrome), Wilms
  tumor in, 480
Bystander effect, with radiation injury, 426

C

C cells, 1107–1108
C chemokines, 62
C ring sign, in enchondromas, 1228
C1 inhibitor deficiency, 235
C2 deficiency, 235
C3 convertase, 63
C3 deficiency, 235
C3 nephritic factor (C3NeF), 928–929
C3a, 64, 65, 65f, 66
C3b, 64
C4a, 64
C5 convertase, 63
C5a, 64, 65, 65f, 66
C282Y mutation, 862
CA2 (carbonic anhydrase II) gene, in
  osteopetrosis, 1213
CA-125
  in ovarian carcinoma, 1047
  as tumor marker, 327
CAA (cerebral amyloid angiopathy), 1296, 1296f,
  1316

Cachexia, 9, 62, 429
  due to cancer, 320–321
  epidemiology of, 429
  mechanisms of, 429, 430f
CAD. *See* Coronary artery disease (CAD).
CADASIL (cerebral autosomal-dominant
    arteriopathy with subcortical infarcts and
    leukoencephalopathy), 1296–1297, 1296f
Cadherins, in extracellular matrix, 96
Cadmium, as carcinogen, 274t
Cadmium toxicity, 408
Café au lait spots, 1168, 1342
Caisson disease, 127
Calcific aortic stenosis, 561–562, 562f
Calcific band keratopathy, 1351–1352
Calcification(s)
  of artificial heart valve, 571, 571f
  of breast, 1068
  dystrophic, 38, 38f
  metastatic, 38–39
  pathologic, 6, 24, 38–39, 38f
  valvular degeneration with, 561–563, 562f
Calciphylaxis, 1129
Calcitonin, 1108
Calcium, and osteoporosis, 1215
Calcium homeostasis
  loss of, cell injury due to, 18f, 19–20, 19f
  vitamin D in, 433–435, 435f, 436f
Calcium hydroxyapatite, in bone, 1206
Calcium influx, cell injury due to, 18f, 19–20,
  19f
Calcium oxalate stones, 962, 962t
Calcium phosphate stones, 962, 962t
Calcium pyrophosphate crystal deposition
  (CPPD) disease, 1246, 1246f
Calcium-sensing receptor gene *(CASR)*
  in hyperparathyroidism, 1127
  in hypoparathyroidism, 1130
Calculus, 741
Call-Exner bodies, in granulosa cell tumor, 1050,
  1050f
Callus
  bony, 1220, 1220f
  soft-tissue, 1219
Calor, 44, 69
Calorie restriction, 444
  and cellular aging, 41
Calymmatobacterium donovani, 366
CAM(s) (cell adhesion molecules), in
  extracellular matrix, 95f, 96–97, 97f
cAMP (3′,5′-cyclic adenosine monophosphate)
  pathway, 90–91, 91f
Campomelic dysplasia, 1211t
Campylobacter enterocolitis, 798t, 799–800, 800f
Campylobacter jejuni, 799–800, 800f
Canaliculi, 1208
Canals of Hering, 835
Canals of Lambert, in obstructive overinflation,
  687
Canavan disease, 1327
Cancer(s)
  alcohol consumption and, 414
  benign tumors *vs.,* 270, 271f, 271t
  cachexia due to, 320–321
  carcinogenic agent(s) in, 309–316
    chemical, 309–311, 309t, 310f
    microbial, 312–316
      Helicobacter pylori as, 315–316
      oncogenic DNA viruses as, 313–315,
        313f, 314f
      oncogenic RNA viruses as, 312–313
    radiation as, 311–312, 425–427
  categorization of undifferentiated, 324, 324f
  characteristic(s) of, 262–270, 271f, 271t

Cancer(s), characteristic(s) of *(Continued)*
    cancer stem cells and cancer cell lineages as,
      267–268
    differentiation and anaplasia as, 262, 264f,
      271t
    local invasion as, 268–269, 268f, 271t
    metastasis as, 269–270, 269f–271f, 271t
    rate of growth as, 265–267, 266f, 271t
  clinical aspect(s) of, 320–327
  defined, 260
  detection of molecules of prognostic or
    therapeutic significance in, 324
  diet and, 443–444
  epidemiology of, 270–276
    age in, 273
    genetic predisposition in, 273–276, 274t
    geographic and environmental factors in,
      272–273, 273f, 274f
    incidence in, 271–272, 272f
    nonhereditary predisposing conditions in,
      276, 277t
  genetic analysis for, 174
  grading and staging of, 322–323
  hereditary predisposition to, 325
  host defense against, 316–320
    antitumor effector mechanisms in, 318–319
    immune surveillance and escape as, 316,
      319–320, 319f
    tumor antigens in, 316–318, 317f
  in infants and children, 474–481
    incidence and types of, 475, 475t
    neuroblastic, 475–479, 476f, 477f, 477t, 479f
    Wilms tumor as, 479–481, 481f
  laboratory diagnosis of, 323–325, 323f, 324f
  local and hormonal effects of, 320
  molecular basis of, 276–308
    angiogenesis in, 297–298
    chromosomal changes in, 304–306, 305t
    clonality in, 260, 276–277, 278f
    dysregulation of cancer-associated genes in,
      304–308
    epigenetic changes in, 306–307
    essential alterations for malignant
      transformation in, 278–279, 280f
    evasion of apoptosis in, 295–296, 296f
    gene amplification in, 306
    genomic instability in, 302–303
    invasion and metastasis in, 298–302, 298f
      of extracellular matrix, 298–300, 299f
      metastatic development in, 301–302, 301f
      vascular dissemination and homing of
        tumor cells in, 300–301
    miRNAs in, 277, 307–308, 307f
    as multistep process, 277–278, 279f,
      308–309, 308f
    mutations in, 276
    oncogenes in, 279–286, 281t
      for cell cycle regulators, 281t
      for growth factor receptors, 280–281,
        281t
      for growth factors, 280, 281t
      for nonreceptor tyrosine kinases,
        283–286, 283f, 284f, 285f, 286t
      for nuclear-regulatory proteins, 281t
      for signal-transducing proteins, 281–283,
        281t, 282f
    regulatory genes in, 277
    stromal microenvironment in, 303
    telomerase in, 296–297, 297f
    tumor suppressor gene(s) in, 286–294, 287t
      in APC/β-catenin pathway, 292–294, 293f
      in *INK4a/ARF* pathway, 294
      NF1 as, 294–295
      NF2 as, 295

Cancer(s), tumor suppressor gene(s) in (*Continued*)
  p53 as, 290–292, 291f
  patched (*PTCH*) genes as, 295
  PTEN as, 287t, 294
  RB as, 287–290, 288f, 289f
  in TGF-β pathway, 294
  VHL disease, 295
  WT1 as, 295
  Warburg effects in, 303–304
  molecular profiles of, 325–326, 326f
  nomenclature for, 260, 261–262, 261f, 262f, 263t
  obesity and, 273, 442f, 443
  occupational, 274t
  oral contraceptives and, 415
  paraneoplastic syndromes due to, 321–322, 321t
  tumor markers for, 326–327, 327t
Cancer cell lineages, 267–268
Cancer immunoediting, 316
Cancer stem cells, 267–268
Cancer syndromes, inherited, 273–276, 275t
Cancer-testis antigens, 317
Candida albicans, 382, 383
Candida endocarditis, 384
Candida esophagitis, 383, 383f
Candida spp, 382–384, 383f
Candida vaginitis, 383
Candidate gene approach, 177, 178f
Candidiasis, 382–384
  in AIDS, 246
  of CNS, 1306
  cutaneous, 383
  of female genital tract, 1009
  invasive, 383–384
  morphology of, 383–384, 383f
  oral, 743
  pathogenesis of, 382–383
Canker sores, 742, 742f
Cannabinoids, abuse of, 418t, 419–420
Capillarization, of sinusoids, 837
Capillary(ies), structure and function of, 488f, 489
Capillary hemangiomas, 520–521, 521f
  in infants and children, 473, 474f
Capillary lymphangioma, 522
Capillary telangiectasias, 1298
Capsid, 332
Caput medusa, 520, 839
Car accident, mechanical injury due to, 420–421
Carbon dioxide (CO$_2$), in greenhouse effect, 401, 401f
Carbon dust, intracellular accumulation of, 36
Carbon monoxide (CO)
  as air pollutant, 405
  CNS toxicity of, 1329
Carbon tetrachloride, occupational exposure to, 409
Carbonic anhydrase II (*CA2*) gene, in osteopetrosis, 1213
Carboxyhemoglobin, 405
Carbuncle, 358
Carcinogen(s), 309–316
  chemical, 309–311, 309t, 310f
  in cigarette smoke, 411, 411t
  environmental, 273
  microbial, 309t, 312–316
    Helicobacter pylori as, 315–316
    oncogenic DNA viruses as, 313–315, 313f, 314f
    oncogenic RNA viruses as, 312–313
  occupational, 274t
  radiation as, 311–312, 425–427

Carcinogenesis, 276–308
  angiogenesis in, 278, 297–298
  chromosomal changes in, 304–306, 305f
  clonality in, 260, 276–277, 278f
  defects in DNA repair in, 277, 278, 302–303
  dysregulation of cancer-associated genes in, 304–308
  epigenetic changes in, 306–307
  essential alterations for malignant transformation in, 278–279, 280f
  evasion of apoptosis in, 278, 295–296, 296f
  gene amplification in, 306
  genomic instability in, 302–303
  insensitivity to growth-inhibitory signals in, 278, 286–295
  invasion and metastasis in, 278, 298–302, 298f
    of extracellular matrix, 298–300, 299f
    metastatic development in, 301–302, 301f
    vascular dissemination and homing of tumor cells in, 300–301
  limitless replicative potential in, 278, 296–297, 297f
  miRNAs in, 277, 307–308, 307f
  as multistep process, 277–278, 279f, 308–309, 308f
  mutations in, 276, 278, 308–309
  oncogenes in, 279–286, 281t
    for cell cycle regulators, 281t
    for growth factor receptors, 280–281, 281t
    for growth factors, 280, 281t
    for nonreceptor tyrosine kinases, 283–286, 283f, 284f, 285f, 286t
    for nuclear-regulatory proteins, 281t
    for signal-transducing proteins, 281–283, 281t, 282f
  regulatory genes in, 277
  self-sufficiency in growth signals in, 278, 279–286
  stromal microenvironment in, 303
  telomerase in, 296–297, 297f
  tumor suppressor gene(s) in, 286–294, 287t
    in APC/β-catenin pathway, 292–294, 293f
    in *INK4a/ARF* pathway, 294
    NF1 as, 294–295
    NF2 as, 295
    p53 as, 290–292, 291f
    patched (*PTCH*) genes as, 295
    PTEN as, 287t, 294
    RB as, 287–290, 288f, 289f
    in TGF-β pathway, 294
    VHL disease, 295
    WT1 as, 295
  Warburg effects in, 303–304
Carcinoid heart disease, 569–570, 570f
Carcinoid syndrome, 321t, 789
  malabsorption and diarrhea in, 794t
Carcinoid tumors
  of appendix, 828
  gastric, 787–789, 788f, 788t
  of lung, 729–730, 729f
  pancreatic, 1147
Carcinoma(s), 261. *See also under* Breast carcinoma; specific diseases, e.g., Basal cell carcinoma.
Carcinoma ex pleomorphic adenoma, of salivary glands, 759
Carcinoma in situ (CIS), 265, 266f
  of bladder, 976, 977f, 978–979, 978f
  of breast
    ductal, 1080–1082, 1081f, 1082f
    lobular, 1082–1083, 1083f
  of lung, 723, 724f
  of penis, 983, 984f

Carcinoma in situ (CIS) (*Continued*)
  of skin, squamous cell, 1179–1180
  of vulva, 1012–1014, 1013f
Carcinosarcomas, of endometrium, 1034–1035, 1036f
Cardiac amyloidosis, 254, 255
Cardiac arrhythmias, 532
  due to myocardial infarction, 557
Cardiac atrophy, 540
Cardiac cirrhosis
  due to centrilobular hemorrhagic necrosis, 872
  in right-sided heart failure, 536
Cardiac conduction system, 531
Cardiac dilation, 530
Cardiac disease. *See* Heart disease.
Cardiac effects, of noncardiac neoplasms, 584–585, 584t
Cardiac hypertrophy, 6, 6f, 7, 8f, 530, 533
  left ventricular, 534f
  physiologic (exercise-induced), 535
  pressure-overload, 533, 534f
  progression to heart failure from, 533–535, 534f, 535f
  volume-overload, 533
Cardiac hypoplasia, 540
Cardiac muscle, stem cells in, 86
Cardiac myocytes, 531
Cardiac output, and blood pressure, 492, 494f
Cardiac rupture syndromes, 556f, 557
Cardiac sclerosis
  due to centrilobular hemorrhagic necrosis, 872
  in right-sided heart failure, 536
Cardiac shunts, 539–540
  left-to-right, 540–542, 540f
    due to atrial septal defect, 540f, 541
    due to atrioventricular septal defect, 540f, 542
    due to patent ductus arteriosus, 540f, 541–542
    due to patent foramen ovale, 541
    due to ventricular septal defect, 540f, 541, 541f
  right-to-left, 540, 542–544, 542f
    due to persistent truncus arteriosus, 543
    due to tetralogy of Fallot, 542–543, 542f
    due to total anomalous pulmonary venous connection, 543–544
    due to transposition of the great arteries, 542f, 543, 543f
    due to tricuspid atresia, 543
Cardiac tamponade, 581
Cardiac thrombosis, 125
Cardiac transplantation, 585, 585f
Cardiac tumors
  metastatic, 584–585
  primary, 583–584, 583f
Cardiac valves, 531
  aging effect on, 532
  artificial, complications of, 570–571, 571f, 571t
Cardiogenic pulmonary edema, 680, 680t
Cardiogenic shock, 129, 130t
  due to myocardial infarction, 557
Cardiomegaly, 530
Cardiomyopathy(ies), 571–581
  alcoholic, 414, 573
  due to amyloidosis, 580, 580f
  arrhythmogenic right ventricular, 575, 576f
  due to cardiotoxic drugs, 579
  catecholamine, 579–580, 1161
  clinical manifestations of, 571
  conditions associated with, 573t

Cardiomyopathy(ies) *(Continued)*
  defined, 571
  dilated, 572–575
    clinical features of, 574–575
    functional patterns and causes of, 572t
    graphic representation of, 572f
    morphology of, 572–573, 574f
    pathogenesis of, 573–574, 574f, 575f
    X-linked, 573
  due to hyperthyroidism and hypothyroidism, 581
  hypertrophic, 575–577
    clinical features of, 577
    functional patterns and causes of, 572t
    graphic representation of, 572f
    morphology of, 575–576, 576f
    pathogenesis of, 574f, 575f, 577
  due to iron overload, 580
  ischemic, 546f, 558
  myocarditis as, 578, 578t, 579f
  peripartum, 573–574
  primary, 571
  restrictive, 572f, 572t, 577
  secondary, 571
Cardiorespiratory complications, of cystic fibrosis, 470
Cardiotoxic drugs, myocardial disease due to, 579
Cardiovascular causes, of hypertension, 493t
Cardiovascular defects
  fetal hydrops due to, 461, 461t
  prevalence of, 451t
Cardiovascular disease. *See* Heart disease.
Cardiovascular effects
  of cocaine, 417–418, 419f
  of noncardiac neoplasms, 584–585, 584t
Cardiovascular involvement, in systemic lupus erythematosus, 220
Cardiovascular syphilis, 375, 376
Carditis, acute rheumatic, 565, 565f, 566
Caries, 740
Carney syndrome, cardiac myxomas in, 584
Carney triad, gastrointestinal stromal tumors in, 789
Caroli disease, 870
Carotenoids, 431
Carotid body tumor, 755–756, 755f
Carpal tunnel syndrome, 1266
Carriers males, of fragile-X syndrome, 170
CART (cocaine and amphetamine-regulated transcripts), in energy balance, 439, 440, 441f
Cartilage, hyaline, 1235
Cartilage-forming tumor(s), 1223t, 1227–1230
  chondroblastoma as, 1228–1229, 1228f
  chondromas as, 1227–1228, 1228f
  chondromyxoid fibroma as, 1229, 1229f
  chondrosarcoma as, 1229–1230, 1229f, 1230f
  osteochondroma as, 1227, 1227f
Cartilaginous synarthroses, 1235
Caruncle, urethral, 981
Caseous necrosis, 16, 16f
  in immune granuloma, 74, 74f
Caspases, in apoptosis, 27, 28f, 29, 29f, 30, 295, 296, 296f
CASR (calcium-sensing receptor gene), in hyperparathyroidism, 1127
Catalase, 60
  in alcohol metabolism, 413, 413f
  free radical removal by, 21, 21f
Cataracts, 1353
  anterior subscapular, 1355, 1355f
  due to diabetes, 1145
  due to galactosemia, 464, 465

Catecholamine(s), 1148
  myocardial disease due to, 579–580
  due to neuroblastomas, 478
Catecholamine cardiomyopathy, 579–580, 1161
Catenins, in extracellular matrix, 96
Cathelicidins, 436
  in phagocytosis, 54
Cationic antigens, in poststreptococcal glomerulonephritis, 918
Cationic trypsinogen gene, in pancreatitis, 893–894
Cat-scratch disease, granulomatous inflammation in, 73t
Caveolin-1, in idiopathic pulmonary fibrosis, 694–695, 694f
Cavernous hemangiomas, 521, 521f
  of liver, 876, 876f
Cavernous lymphangioma, 522
Cavernous malformations, of brain, 1298, 1299
CBD (corticobasal degeneration), 1318–1319
CBF1α gene, in acute myeloid leukemia, 624
CBF1β gene, in acute myeloid leukemia, 624
C-C chemokine(s), 62
C-C chemokine receptors (CCR), 62
CCA (cholangiocarcinoma), 877, 880–881, 881f
C-cell hyperplasia, in medullary thyroid carcinoma, 1125–1126
CCND1 gene, 305
CCR5
  in AIDS, 239–240, 245
  in West Nile virus, 351
CCR7, in metastasis, 300
CD2, 186
CD4, 186
  in AIDS, 239
CD4+ helper T lymphocytes
  in delayed-type hypersensitivity, 205, 206f
  in HIV infection, 240–241, 241f, 243, 243f, 244–245, 244t
  in immune response, 185f, 186, 195, 195f
  proliferation and differentiation of, 206–207
CD8, 186
CD8+ cytotoxic T lymphocytes
  in cell-mediated cytotoxicity, 207–208
  in HIV infection, 243, 245
  in immune response, 185f, 186, 191
  in transplant rejection, 226, 227f
CD14 gene, in asthma, 691
CD16, 188
CD25
  in immunological tolerance, 211
  in type 1 diabetes mellitus, 1135
CD28, 186
  in anergy, 209
CD44 adhesion molecule, in metastasis, 300
CD56, 188
CD95, in apoptosis, 295, 296, 296f
CDH1 gene, in gastric carcinoma, 785
CDK(s) (cyclin-dependent kinases)
  in cell cycle, 86–87, 285, 285f
  functions of, 286t
  proto-oncogenes for, 281t, 284–286
CDK4 gene, 281t, 289f
  in dysplastic nevi, 1171
CDKIs (cyclin-dependent kinase inhibitors)
  in cell cycle, 87, 285, 285f
  functions of, 286t
CDKN1B gene, in pituitary adenomas, 1101
CDKN2A gene, 289f, 306
  in dysplastic nevi, 1171
  in melanoma, 1174
  in pancreatic carcinoma, 900
Celiac disease, 794t, 795–796, 795f, 796f
  IgA nephropathy with, 931

Cell adhesion molecules (CAMs), in extracellular matrix, 95f, 96–97, 97f
Cell adhesion proteins, in extracellular matrix, 95f, 96–97, 97f
Cell cycle, 86–87, 86f
Cell cycle regulators, proto-oncogenes for, 281t
Cell death
  activation-induced, 210f, 211, 240
  via apoptosis, 25–32
    biochemical features of, 27, 27f
    causes of, 25–26
    clinicopathologic correlations of, 30–32, 31f
    defined, 25
    execution phase of, 30
    extrinsic (death receptor–initiated) pathway of, 28f, 29–30, 29f
    intrinsic (mitochondrial) pathway of, 28–29, 28f, 29f
    mechanisms of, 27–30, 28f, 29f
    morphologic changes in, 13f, 13t, 26–27, 26f
    overview of, 5, 5f, 11
    in pathologic conditions, 25–26
    in physiologic situations, 25
    removal of dead cells in, 30
  morphologic alterations in, 12, 13f, 13t, 26–27, 26f
    via apoptosis, 13f, 13t, 26–27, 26f
    vs. necrosis, 13–14, 13f, 13t, 14f
  via necrosis
    caseous, 16, 16f
    clinicopathologic examples of, 23–25
    coagulative, 15, 16f
    fat, 16, 17f
    fibrinoid, 16–17, 17f
    gangrenous, 15–16
    liquefactive, 15, 16f
    morphologic changes in, 13–14, 13f, 13t, 14f
    overview of, 5, 5f, 11
    patterns of, 15–17, 16f, 17f
  overview of, 5, 5f, 6f, 11
  programmed, 25
Cell differentiation, vitamin A in, 431
Cell growth
  defects in proteins that regulate, 143t, 156
  signaling mechanisms in, 89–92, 90f–92f
  vitamin A in, 431
Cell injury
  causes of, 11–12
  chemical (toxic), 24–25
  clinicopathologic correlations of, 23–25
  irreversible
    events that determine, 23
    morphologic changes in, 13–14, 13f, 13t, 14f
    overview of, 5, 5f, 11
  ischemia-reperfusion, 24
  ischemic and hypoxic, 23–24
  mechanism(s) of, 17–23, 18f
    accumulation of oxygen-derived free radicals (oxidative stress) as, 18f, 20–22, 20t, 21f
    damage to DNA and proteins as, 18f, 23
    defects in membrane permeability as, 18f, 22–23, 22f
    depletion of ATP as, 17–18, 18f
    influx of calcium and loss of calcium homeostasis as, 18f, 19–20, 19f
    mitochondrial damage as, 18–19, 18f, 19f
  morphologic alterations in, 12–17, 12f, 13f–17f, 13t
    irreversible, 13–14, 13f, 13t, 14f
    reversible, 12–14, 14f, 15f

Cell injury *(Continued)*
  overview of, 5, 5f, 5t, 11
  reversible
    morphologic alterations in, 12–14, 14f, 15f
    overview of, 5, 5f, 11
Cell lysis, complement system in, 64, 64f
Cell proliferation
  control of normal, 80–86, 81f
  radiation effect on, 423–424, 423f
  in wound healing, 102–104
Cell replication, regulation of, 86–92
  growth factors in, 87–89, 87t
  signaling mechanisms in, 89–92, 90f–92f
Cell shrinkage, in apoptosis, 26, 26f
Cell surface receptors, 89–91, 91f
Cell turnover, in tumors, 266
Cell type–specific differentiation antigens, 318
Cell-derived mediators, of inflammation, 57–63,
    57t
  arachidonic acid metabolites (prostaglandins,
      leukotrienes, and lipoxins) as, 57t, 58–60,
      58f, 59t
  cytokines and chemokines as, 57t, 61–63, 61t,
      62f
  lysosomal constituents of leukocytes as, 57t,
      63
  neuropeptides as, 57t, 64
  nitric oxide as, 57t, 60–61, 61f
  platelet-activating factor as, 57t, 60
  reactive oxygen species as, 57t, 60
  vasoactive amines (histamine and serotonin)
      as, 57–58, 57t
Cell-matrix interactions, 94–98, 95f, 95t, 97f, 98f
Cell-mediated cytotoxicity, 207–208
Cell-mediated hypersensitivity, 197t, 198,
    205–208, 206f–208f, 206t
Cell-mediated immunity, 185, 194f, 195, 195f
  in glomerulonephritis, 915
Cell-surface glycolipids, as tumor antigens, 318
Cell-surface glycoproteins, as tumor antigens,
    318
Cellular adaptation(s), 6–11
  atrophy as, 9–10, 9f
  defined, 5, 6
  hyperplasia as, 8–9
  hypertrophy as, 6–8, 6f–8f
  metaplasia as, 10–11, 10f
  overview of, 5, 5f, 5t, 6f
Cellular aging, 6, 39–41, 39f, 40f
Cellular dysfunction, antibody-mediated, 202f,
    203–204
Cellular immunity, 185, 194f, 195, 195f
Cellular proteins, overexpressed or aberrantly
    expressed, as tumor antigens, 317
Cellular rejection, 226–227, 227f
Cellular response(s), to stress and toxic insults,
    3–41
  apoptosis as, 25–32
    biochemical features of, 27, 27f
    causes of, 25–26
    clinicopathologic correlations of, 30–32, 31f
    defined, 25
    execution phase of, 30
    extrinsic (death receptor–initiated) pathway
        of, 28f, 29–30, 29f
    intrinsic (mitochondrial) pathway of,
        28–29, 28f, 29f
    mechanisms of, 27–30, 28f, 29f
    morphologic changes in, 13f, 13t, 26–27,
        26f
    overview of, 5, 5f, 11
    in pathologic conditions, 25–26
    in physiologic situations, 25
    removal of dead cells in, 30

Cellular response(s), to stress and toxic insults
    (Continued)
  autophagy as, 5, 10, 11, 32, 32f
  cell death as
    morphologic alterations in, 12, 13f, 13t
    overview of, 5, 5f, 6f, 11
  cell injury as
    causes of, 11–12
    chemical (toxic), 24–25
    clinicopathologic correlations of, 23–25
    irreversible, 5, 5f, 11, 13–14, 13f, 13t, 14f, 23
    ischemia-reperfusion, 24
    ischemic and hypoxic, 23–24
    mechanisms of, 17–23, 18f, 19f, 20t, 21f, 22f
    morphologic alterations in, 12–17, 12f,
        13f–17f, 13t
    overview of, 5, 5f, 5t, 11
    reversible, 5, 5f, 6f, 11, 12–14, 14f, 15f
  cellular adaptation(s) as, 6–11
    atrophy as, 9–10, 9f
    defined, 5, 6
    hyperplasia as, 8–9
    hypertrophy as, 6–8, 6f–8f
    metaplasia as, 10–11, 10f
    overview of, 5, 5f, 5t, 6f
  cellular aging as, 6, 39–41, 39f, 40f
  intracellular accumulations as, 5–6, 32–38, 33f
    of glycogen, 36
    hyalin change as, 36
    of lipids, 33–35, 34f, 35f
    of pigments, 36–38, 37f
    of proteins, 35–36, 35f
  necrosis as
    caseous, 16, 16f
    clinicopathologic examples of, 23–25
    coagulative, 15, 16f
    fat, 16, 17f
    fibrinoid, 16–17, 17f
    gangrenous, 15–16
    liquefactive, 15, 16f
    morphologic changes in, 13–14, 13f, 13t,
        14f
    overview of, 5, 5f, 11
    patterns of, 15–17, 16f, 17f
  overview of, 5–6, 5f, 5t
  pathologic calcification as, 6, 24, 38–39, 38f
Cellular swelling, in cell injury, 12, 13–14, 13f,
    14f
Cellulitis
  clostridial, 379, 379f
  orbital, 1347
Celsus, 44
Cementum, 740, 740f
Centigray (cGy), 423
Central chromatolysis, 1281
Central nervous system (CNS), primary angiitis
    of, 1293
Central nervous system (CNS) disorder(s),
    1279–1343
  due to adverse drug reactions, 416t
  in AIDS, 242–243, 248
  due to cancer, 321t
  cellular pathology in, 1281–1282, 1282f
  cerebral edema as, 1282–1283
  cerebrovascular diseases as, 1290–1299
    hypertensive, 1295, 1295f
    hypoxia, ischemia, and infarction as,
        1291–1295, 1292f–1294f
    intracranial hemorrhage as, 1295–1299,
        1296f–1298f
  due to cocaine, 418
  degenerative, 1313–1325
    Alzheimer disease as, 1313–1317,
        1314f–1316f

Central nervous system (CNS) disorder(s),
    degenerative *(Continued)*
    amyotrophic lateral sclerosis as, 1324–1325,
        1325f
    ataxia-telangiectasia as, 1323–1324
    of basal ganglia and brainstem, 1319–1323,
        1320f, 1322f
    bulbospinal atrophy (Kennedy syndrome)
        as, 1325
    of cerebral cortex, 1313–1319
    corticobasal degeneration as, 1318–1319
    dementia with Lewy bodies as, 1321
    Friedreich ataxia as, 1323
    frontotemporal dementias as, 1317–1319,
        1318f
    Huntington disease as, 1322–1323, 1322f
    of motor neurons, 1324–1325, 1325f
    multiple system atrophy as, 1321–1322
    Parkinson disease as, 1319–1321, 1320f
    parkinsonism as, 1319
    Pick disease as, 1318, 1318f
    progressive supranuclear palsy as, 1318
    spinal muscular atrophy as, 1325
    spinocerebellar, 1323–1324
    vascular dementia as, 1319
  demyelinating, 1309–1313
    central pontine myelinolysis as, 1313
    encephalomyelitis as
      acute disseminated, 1312–1313
      acute necrotizing hemorrhagic,
          1312–1313
    multiple sclerosis as, 1310–1312, 1311f,
        1312f
    neuromyelitis optica as, 1312
  hydrocephalus as, 1283, 1283f
  infectious, 1299–1308
    abscess as
      brain, 1300, 1300f
      extradural, 1301
    acute focal suppurative, 1300–1301,
        1300f
    acute meningitis as, 1299–1300, 1299f
    meningoencephalitis as
      chronic bacterial, 1301–1302
      fungal, 1306, 1307f
      viral, 1302–1306, 1303f–1306f
    protozoal, 1306–1308, 1307f, 1308f
    subdural empyema as, 1300–1301
  malformations and developmental diseases as,
      1284–1286
    of forebrain, 1284–1285, 1285f
    neural tube defects as, 1284
    of posterior fossa, 1285–1286, 1286f
    syringomyelia and hydromyelia as, 1286
  metabolic diseases as
    acquired, 1328–1330, 1329f
    Alexander disease as, 1327
    Alpers disease as, 1328
    Canavan disease as, 1327
    genetic, 1325–1328
    hepatic encephalopathy as, 1329
    due to hyperglycemia, 1329
    due to hypoglycemia, 1329
    Kearn-Sayre syndrome as, 1328
    Krabbe disease as, 1326, 1326f
    Leigh syndrome as, 1328
    leukodystrophies as, 1325, 1326–1327,
        1326f
    mitochondrial encephalomyopathies as,
        1325–1326, 1327–1328
    myoclonic epilepsy with ragged red fibers
        as, 1327–1328
    neuronal storage diseases as, 1325, 1326
    Pelizaeus-Merzbacher disease as, 1327

Central nervous system (CNS) disorder(s), metabolic diseases as (Continued)
Tay-Sachs disease as, 1326
due to vitamin deficiencies, 1328–1329
neoplastic, 1330–1343
astrocytomas as, 1330–1333, 1331f–1333f
atypical teratoid/rhabdoid tumor as, 1337
ependymoma as, 1334–1335, 1335f
epidemiology of, 1330
familial syndromes of, 1342–1343
germ cell tumors as, 1338
gliomas as, 1330–1335, 1331f–1335f
medulloblastoma as, 1336–1337, 1336f
meningiomas as, 1338–1339, 1338f
metastatic, 1339
neuronal, 1335–1336
neurofibroma as, 1341
other parenchymal, 1337–1338
paraneoplastic syndromes due to, 1339–1340
peripheral nerve sheath tumors as, 1340–1342, 1340f
pineal parenchymal tumors as, 1338
poorly differentiated, 1336–1337, 1336f
primary lymphoma as, 1337
schwannoma as, 1340–1341, 1340f
perinatal brain injury as, 1286–1287, 1286f
prevalence of, 451t
raised intracranial pressure and herniation as, 1283–1284, 1283f, 1284f
in systemic lupus erythematosus, 214t, 219–220
toxic, 1329–1330, 1329f
transmissible spongiform encephalopathies (prion diseases) as, 1308–1309, 1308f, 1310f
traumatic, 1287–1290
concussion as, 1287
diffuse axonal injury as, 1288
parenchymal injuries as, 1287–1288, 1288f
sequelae of, 1290
skull fractures as, 1287
spinal cord, 1290
vascular, 1288–1290, 1289f, 1290f
Central nervous system (CNS) lymphoma, primary, 1337
Central neurocytoma, 1336
Central pontine myelinolysis, 1313
Central tolerance, 209, 210t
Central-core disease, 1272t
Centric fusion, 160f, 161
Centrilobular hemorrhagic necrosis, of liver, 872, 872f
Centrilobular necrosis, in right-sided heart failure, 536
Centroblasts, 595, 605, 605f
Centrocytes, 595, 605, 605f
Centronuclear myopathy, 1272t
Cepacia syndrome, in cystic fibrosis, 469
Cerebellar degeneration
alcoholic, 1329, 1329f
subacute, in paraneoplastic syndrome, 1340
Cerebellum, dysplastic gangliocytoma of, 1342
Cerebral abscesses, 1300, 1300f
Cerebral amebiasis, 1308, 1308f
Cerebral amyloid angiopathy (CAA), 1296, 1296f, 1316
Cerebral autosomal-dominant arteriopathy with subcortical infarcts and leukoencephalopathy (CADASIL), 1296–1297, 1296f

Cerebral cortex, degenerative diseases of, 1313–1319
Alzheimer disease as, 1313–1317, 1314f–1316f
corticobasal degeneration as, 1318–1319
frontotemporal dementias as, 1317–1319, 1318f
Pick disease as, 1318, 1318f
progressive supranuclear palsy as, 1318
vascular dementia as, 1319
Cerebral edema, 113, 1282–1283
Cerebral gummas, 1301
Cerebral hypoxia, 1291
Cerebral infarction, 1291–1295, 1292f–1294f
due to global cerebral ischemia, 1291–1292, 1292f
hemorrhagic (red), 1293, 1294, 1294f
nonhemorrhagic (pale, bland, anemic), 1293–1294, 1294f
due to obstruction of local blood supply, 1292–1294, 1293f, 1294f
Cerebral ischemia, 1291–1294
focal, 1291, 1292–1294, 1293f, 1294f
global, 1291–1292, 1292f
Cerebral palsy, 1286
Cerebral toxoplasmosis, 1306–1308, 1307f
Cerebrovascular disease(s), 1290–1299
in Global Burden of Disease, 400
global warming and, 402
hypertensive, 1295, 1295f
hypoxia, ischemia, and infarction as, 1291–1295, 1292f–1294f
intracranial hemorrhage as, 1295–1299, 1296f–1298f
Ceruloplasmin, 60, 863–864
Cervical carcinoma, 1021–1024
clinical features of, 1023
epidemiology of, 1017
human papillomavirus and, 313–314, 313f
morphology of, 1021–1022, 1022f
Pap smears for, 323f, 324
pathogenesis of
cervical intraepithelial neoplasia in, 1019–1021, 1020f, 1020t, 1021f, 1021t
human papillomavirus in, 1018–1019, 1018f, 1019f, 1020–1021, 1021f
screening and prevention for, 1018, 1023–1024, 1023f
staging of, 1022
Cervical intraepithelial neoplasia (CIN), 1019–1021, 1020f, 1020t, 1021f, 1021t, 1023f
Cervical lymphoepithelial cyst, 755
Cervicitis, 1009, 1017
Cervix, 1017–1024
anatomy of, 1007, 1008f
development of, 1006, 1007f
endocervical polyps of, 1018, 1018f
inflammations of, 1017
premalignant and malignant neoplasms of, 1018–1024
cervical carcinoma as, 1021–1024, 1022f, 1023f
cervical intraepithelial neoplasia as, 1019–1021, 1020f, 1020t, 1021f, 1021t
pathogenesis of, 1018–1019, 1018f, 1019f
squamous metaplasia of, 1008
Cestodes, 392–393, 392f
intestinal, 806
CFH (complement factor H) gene, in macular degeneration, 1363

CFTR (cystic fibrosis transmembrane conductance regulator)
defect in, 143t, 466–468, 467f, 468f
normal structure and function of, 465–466, 466f
CFTR (cystic fibrosis transmembrane conductance regulator) gene, mutations of, 466–467
in pancreatitis, 896
CFUs (colony-forming units), 590, 591f
CGH (comparative genomic hybridization), array-based, 179–180, 180f, 325–326, 326f
cGy (centigray), 423
Chagas disease, 391
myocarditis of, 578, 579f
Chagoma, 391
Chalazion, 1348
Chalkstick-type fractures, 1217
Chancre
soft, 366
in syphilis, 374, 375–376, 376f
Chancroid, 366
Channelopathies, 1270
and sudden cardiac death, 559
Chaperones, in protein folding, 31f
Charcot joints, 1302
Charcot-Marie-Tooth (CMT) disease, 1263–1264, 1265f
Checkpoints, in cell cycle, 86, 86f, 87, 286
Chédiak-Higashi syndrome, 55, 56t
Cheilitis, actinic, 1178
CHEK2 gene, and breast cancer, 1078, 1078t
Chemical agents
cell injury due to, 11
congenital anomalies due to, 452
toxicity of, 402–403, 402f, 403f
Chemical carcinogens, 309–311, 309t, 310f
Chemical cell injury, 24–25
Chemical esophagitis, 768–769
Chemical fumes and vapors, lung diseases due to, 697t
Chemical injury, inflammation due to, 45
Chemical meningitis, 1299, 1300
Chemokines
in glomerular injury, 916
in inflammation, 49, 49f, 50, 57t, 61t, 62–63
in metastasis, 300
Chemotaxis, of leukocytes, 48f, 50–51, 50f, 51f, 66t
Chemotherapy
esophagitis due to, 768
white cell neoplasia due to, 598
Chenodeoxycholic acid, 840
Cherry-red spot, in Tay-Sachs disease, 151–152, 1362, 1364f
CHF. See Congestive heart failure (CHF).
Chiari type I malformation, 1286
Chiari type II malformation, 1285–1286, 1286f
Chickenpox, 353, 353f
Chief cells, 1126
Child mortality, in Global Burden of Disease, 400, 401f
Childbirth, cardiomyopathy after, 573–574
Childhood, contagious bacterial diseases of, 358t
Children, 447–481
cancer in, 273
causes of death of, 448, 448t
congenital anomalies in, 448–453
causes of, 450–452, 450t, 451t
pathogenesis of, 452–453, 453f
types of, 448–450, 449f, 450f
inborn error(s) of metabolism in, 462–465, 463t
cystic fibrosis as, 465–471

Children, inborn error(s) of metabolism in (*Continued*)
    clinical features of, 468f, 469–471, 470t
    environmental modifiers of, 468
    genetic basis for, 465–468, 466f, 467f
    morphology of, 468–469, 469f
    galactosemia as, 464–465, 464f, 465f
    phenylketonuria as, 463–464, 463f
    tumors and tumor-like lesions in, 473–481
        benign, 473–474, 474f
        malignant, 474–481
            incidence and types of, 475, 475t
            neuroblastic, 475–479, 476f, 477f, 477t, 479f
            Wilms tumor as, 479–481, 481f
ChIP (chromatin immunoprecipitation), 181, 326
Chlamydia, 335
    genital, 380
    sexual transmission of, 341t
Chlamydia pneumoniae pneumonia, 714
Chlamydia trachomatis, 335, 341t, 380, 1009
    conjunctival scarring due to, 1349
Chlamydial infections, 380
Chloracne, 409–410
Chloride channels
    in cystic fibrosis, 466–467, 467f
    normal structure and function of, 465–466, 466f
Chloroform, occupational exposure to, 409
Chloroquine, myopathy due to, 1275
Chokes, the, 127
Cholangiocarcinoma (CCA), 877, 880–881, 881f
Cholangitis
    ascending, 854, 887
        in secondary biliary cirrhosis, 867
    due to gallstones, 884
    primary sclerosing, 867t, 869, 869f
Cholecalciferol, 433
Cholecystitis, 885–887
    acute, 885
    calculus *vs.* acalculous, 885
    chronic, 885–887, 886f
    gangrenous, 885
    xanthogranulomatous, 886
Choledochal cysts, 887–888
Choledocholithiasis, 887
Cholelithiasis, 882–884
    clinical features of, 884
    morphology of, 884, 884f
    obesity and, 442
    pathogenesis of, 883–884, 883f
    prevalence and risk factors for, 882–883, 883t
Cholera, 797–799, 798t, 799f
Cholestasis, 839, 842–843
    drug- and toxin-induced, 856t
    intrahepatic, 843
        benign recurrent, 843
        of pregnancy, 875
        progressive familial, 843
    morphology of, 842–843, 842f, 843f
    neonatal, 866, 866f, 866t
    obstructive, 884
        in secondary biliary cirrhosis, 867
    in viral hepatitis, 851, 851f
Cholestatic hepatitis, drug- and toxin-induced, 856t
Cholesteatomas, 754
Cholesterol
    and atherosclerosis, 497, 500, 501f
    functions of, 148
    intracellular accumulation of, 34–35
Cholesterol emboli, 126
Cholesterol esters, intracellular accumulation of, 34–35

Cholesterol metabolism, 147–148, 147f, 148f
Cholesterol stones, 882–883, 883f, 883t, 884f
Cholesterolosis, 35, 35f
Cholic acid, 840
Chondroblastic osteosarcoma, 1226, 1230
Chondroblastoma, 1228–1229, 1228f
Chondrocalcinosis, 1246, 1246f
Chondrocytes, 1235
Chondrodysplasia, Schmid metaphyseal, 1211t
Chondrogenic tumor(s), 1223t, 1227–1230
    chondroblastoma as, 1228–1229, 1228f
    chondromas as, 1227–1228, 1228f
    chondromyxoid fibroma as, 1229, 1229f
    chondrosarcoma as, 1229–1230, 1229f, 1230f
    osteochondroma as, 1227, 1227f
Chondroitin sulfate, in extracellular matrix, 97, 98f
Chondromas, 1227–1228, 1228f
Chondromyxoid fibroma, 1229, 1229f
Chondroplasia, Jansen metaphyseal, 1211t
Chondrosarcoma, 1229–1230, 1229f, 1230f
    clear cell, 1230
    dedifferentiated, 1230
    extraskeletal myxoid, 1249t
    mesenchymal, 1230
Chorioamnionitis, 454
    acute, 1055f
Choriocarcinoma
    gestational (uterine), 1059–1061, 1060f
    ovarian, 1049
    testicular, 990, 990f
Chorionic villi, 1052, 1053f
Choristoma, 262, 473
Choroid, 1346f
Choroid plexus carcinomas, 1335
Choroid plexus papillomas, 1335
Choroidal infarcts, 1359
Choroidal neovascularization, 1363–1364, 1364f
Christmas disease, 672–673
Chromaffin cells, 1159
Chromatin changes, in carcinogenesis, 307
Chromatin condensation, in apoptosis, 26, 26f
Chromatin immunopreciptation (ChIP), 181, 326
Chromatolysis, central, 1281
Chromium, as carcinogen, 274t
Chromophobe renal carcinoma, 965, 966
Chromosomal disorder(s), 138, 158–167
    in carcinogenesis, 304–306, 305t
    chromosome 22q11.2 deletion syndrome as, 162–164, 164f
    fetal growth restriction due to, 455
    fetal hydrops due to, 461, 461t
    hermaphroditism and pseudohermaphroditism as, 167
    involving autosomes, 161–164, 161f, 163f, 164f
    involving sex chromosomes, 164–167, 166f
    Klinefelter syndrome as, 165
    normal karyotype and, 158–159, 159f
    other trisomies as, 162
    prevalence of, 451, 451t
    structural, 159–161, 160f
    trisomy 21 (Down syndrome) as, 161–162, 161f, 163f
    Turner syndrome as, 165–167, 166f
    white cell neoplasia due to, 596–597, 597f
Chromosomal rearrangements, 160–161, 160f
Chromosome 22q11.2 deletion syndrome, 162–164, 164f
Chronic bronchitis, 683t, 687–688, 687t
Chronic disease, anemia of, 662
Chronic eosinophilic leukemia, 626t
Chronic granulomatous disease, 55, 56t

Chronic illness, and malnutrition, 427
Chronic inflammatory demyelinating polyradiculoneuropathy, 1262
Chronic lymphocytic leukemia (CLL), 601t, 603–605, 604f
Chronic myelogenous (myeloid) leukemia (CML), 627–628
    clinical features of, 627–628
    genetic basis for, 283, 283f, 305, 305t, 626t
    molecular pathogenesis of, 627, 627f
    morphology of, 627, 627f, 628f
Chronic neuronal injury, 1281
Chronic obstructive pulmonary disease (COPD), 683–684, 683f, 683t
Chronic pelvic pain syndrome, 975
Chronic rejection, 229, 229f
Chronic renal failure, anemia due to, 665
Chrysotiles, 699, 700
Churg-Strauss syndrome, 516
Chvostek sign, due to hypocalcemia, 1130
Chylocele, 993
Chylopericardium, 520
Chylothorax, 520, 732
Chylous ascites, 520
Ci (curie), 423
Cicatricial pemphigoid, ocular, 1348, 1349
Cigarette smoke, as teratogen, 452
Cigarette smoking
    and atherosclerosis, 498
    and bladder cancer, 979
    and breast cancer, 1077
    and cancer, 273
    carcinogens in, 310, 311
    effects of, 410–412, 410f–412f, 411t, 412t
    and emphysema, 684, 685–686, 685f
    and head and neck squamous cell carcinoma, 746
    interstitial diseases due to, 704–705, 704f
    and lung cancer, 410, 411, 412f, 412t, 721–722
    and pancreatic carcinoma, 901
    white cell neoplasia due to, 598
Ciliary body, 1346f, 1354f
    in diabetes mellitus, 1359, 1362f
Ciliary dyskinesia, primary, 692
Ciliochoroidal effusion, 1368
CIN (cervical intraepithelial neoplasia), 1019–1021, 1020f, 1020t, 1021f, 1021t, 1023f
Cingulate herniation, 1283, 1283f
Circulatory disorders, of liver, 870–874, 871f
    hepatic venous outflow obstruction as, 872–874
        due to hepatic vein thrombosis and inferior vena cava thrombosis, 872–873, 873f
        due to sinusoidal obstruction syndrome, 873–874, 873f
    impaired blood flow into liver as, 870–871
        due to hepatic artery compromise, 870–871, 871f
        due to portal vein obstruction and thrombosis, 871
    impaired blood flow through liver as, 871–872
        due to disseminated intravascular coagulation, 872
        due to passive congestion and centrilobular necrosis, 872, 872f
        due to peliosis hepatis, 872
        due to sickle cell disease, 872, 872f
Circulatory status, and wound healing, 106
Cirrhosis, 837–838
    alcoholic, 857f, 858, 859f, 860
    and hemochromatosis, 863

Cirrhosis *(Continued)*
 biliary
   in cystic fibrosis, 469, 470
   primary, 867–869, 867t, 868f
   secondary, 867, 867f, 867t
 cardiac
   due to centrilobular hemorrhagic necrosis, 872
   in right-sided heart failure, 536
 causes of, 837
 clinical features of, 838
 congestive splenomegaly due to, 634
 cryptogenic, 853
 drug- and toxin-induced, 856t
 due to hemochromatosis, 862
 Laennec, 858
 morphologic characteristics of, 837
 in nonalcoholic fatty liver disease, 861
 pathogenesis of, 837–838, 837f
 due to viral hepatitis, 853, 853f
CIS. *See* Carcinoma in situ (CIS).
Citrullinated proteins, in rheumatoid arthritis, 1238, 1239
Civatte bodies, 1192
CJD (Creutzfeldt-Jakob disease), 1308, 1309, 1310f
CK (creatine kinase), in myocardial infarction, 555–556, 555f
c-KIT
 in gastrointestinal stromal tumors, 790
 in seminoma, 988
CK-MB (MB fraction of creatine kinase), in myocardial infarction, 555–556, 555f
Class switching, in humoral immunity, 196, 196f
Claudication, instep, 517
CLCN7 gene, in osteopetrosis, 1213
Clear cell adenocarcinoma, of ovaries, 1046
Clear cell carcinoma
 of kidney, 964–966, 964f, 966f
 of vagina, 1016, 1016f
Clear cell sarcoma, genetic basis for, 1249t
Cleft lip, 449f
Cleft palate, 449f
Cleidocranial dysplasia, 1210, 1211t
Climate change, health effects of, 401–402, 401f
Clinical manifestations, 4
CLL (chronic lymphocytic leukemia), 601t, 603–605, 604f
Cloacogenic carcinoma, 825
Clonal selection hypothesis, 193
Clonal selection process, 193
Clonality, of tumors, 260, 276–277, 278f
Cloning
 reproductive, 84
 therapeutic, 84, 84f
Clostridial cellulitis, 379, 379f
Clostridial infections, 358t, 378–379, 379f
Clostridium botulinum, 379
Clostridium difficile, 379, 803, 803f
Clostridium perfringens, 348, 379, 379f
Clostridium septicum, 379
Clostridium sordellii, 334t
Clostridium spp, 358t, 378–379, 379f
Clostridium tetani, 379
Clotting factor abnormalities, 670–673, 671f
Clotting system, in inflammation, 57t, 64–66, 65f
Clubbing, due to cancer, 321t, 322
c-MET, in lung carcinoma, 725
CML. *See* Chronic myelogenous (myeloid) leukemia (CML).
CMT (Charcot-Marie-Tooth) disease, 1263–1264, 1265f
CMV. *See* Cytomegalovirus (CMV).

c-MYC oncogene, 281t, 315
 in Burkitt lymphoma, 608
 in white cell neoplasia, 597
CNS. *See* Central nervous system (CNS).
CNVs (copy number variations), 136, 180
CO (carbon monoxide)
 as air pollutant, 405
 CNS toxicity of, 1329
CO_2 (carbon dioxide), in greenhouse effect, 401, 401f
Coagulation, disseminated intravascular, 125, 673–674, 674f
 impaired blood flow through liver due to, 872
 in septic shock, 130–131
Coagulation cascade, in hemostasis, 118–120, 120f, 121f
Coagulation factor abnormalities, 670–673, 671f
 in preeclampsia, 1057
Coagulation system
 in glomerular injury, 916
 in inflammation, 57t, 64–66, 65f
Coagulative necrosis, 15, 16f
Coagulopathy
 consumption, 125
 due to liver failure, 836
Coal dust
 intracellular accumulation of, 36
 lung diseases due to, 697t
 pneumoconiosis due to, 410
Coal macules, 698
Coal nodules, 698
Coal workers' pneumoconiosis (CWP), 36, 697–698, 697t, 698f
Coarctation of the aorta, 544, 544f
Coated pits, 147, 148f
Cobalamin. *See* Vitamin B_{12}.
Cocaine abuse, 417–418
Cocaine and amphetamine-regulated transcripts (CART), in energy balance, 439, 440, 441f
Cocci, pyogenic, infections by, 357–360, 358t
Coccidioides immitis, chronic pneumonia due to, 719, 719f
Coccidioidomycosis, 719, 719f
Codman triangle, 1226
Codominance, 140
Coin lesion, 730
COL1A1 gene, 146
 in dermatofibrosarcoma protuberans, 1183
COL1A2 gene, 146
COL4A3, in Alport syndrome, 932
COL4A4, in Alport syndrome, 932
COL4A5, in Alport syndrome, 932
COL5A1 gene, 146
COL5A2 gene, 146
COL7A1 gene, in epidermolysis bullosa, 1196
Cold, common, 749
Cold agglutinin type immunohemolytic anemia, 653t, 654
Cold hemolysin type immunohemolytic anemia, 653t, 654
Cold sores, 352, 743
Colitis. *See also* Enterocolitis.
 antibiotic-associated, 803, 803f
 collagenous, 814, 814f
 diversion, 813–814, 814f
 indeterminate, 812–813
 lymphocytic, 814, 814f
   in celiac disease, 796
 microscopic, 814, 814f
 pseudomembranous, 379, 798t, 803, 803f
 ulcerative, 811–813
   clinical features of, 812
   vs. Crohn disease, 807, 808f, 808t
   epidemiology of, 807–808

Colitis. *See also* Enterocolitis. *(Continued)*
 morphology of, 811–812, 812f, 813f
 pathogenesis of, 808–810, 809f
Colitis-associated dysplasia, 813, 814f
Collagen
 in bone formation, 1208
 in extracellular matrix, 94–96, 95f, 95t, 97f
 genetic defect in, 143t, 145–147, 146t
 in scar formation, 79
 in wound healing, 102–104, 105–106
Collagen 1A1 *(COL1A1)* gene, 146
 in dermatofibrosarcoma protuberans, 1183
Collagen diseases, 1211–1212
Collagen vascular diseases, 213
Collagenous colitis, 814, 814f
Collapsing glomerulopathy, 927, 927f
Collar-button lesion, 957–958
Collaterals, in obstructive overinflation, 687
Collecting duct carcinoma, 965, 966
Colloid bodies, 1192
Colloid carcinoma
 of breast, 1087, 1088f
 of prostate, 1002
Colloid cyst, of third ventricle, 1335
Colon. *See also* Intestine(s).
 angiodysplasia of, 793
 ischemic bowel disease of, 791–793, 792f
Colonic diverticula, 814–815, 815f
Colonic polyps, 261f, 815–820, 816t
 in Cowden syndrome and Bannayan-Ruvalcaba-Riley syndrome, 816t, 818
 in Cronkhite-Canada syndrome, 816t, 818
 in familial adenomatous polyposis, 816t, 820–821, 822f, 822t
 hamartomatous, 816–818, 816t, 817f, 818f
 hyperplastic, 818–819, 819f
 inflammatory, 815–816, 816f
 juvenile, 816–817, 816t, 817f
 neoplastic, 819–820, 820f, 821f
 pedunculated, 815
 in Peutz-Jeghers syndrome, 816t, 817–818, 818f
 retention, 817
 sessile, 815
 in tuberous sclerosis, 816t
Colony-forming units (CFUs), 590, 591f
Colony-stimulating factors, 193
Colorectal adenomas, 308f, 309, 819–820, 820f, 821f
Colorectal cancer
 adenocarcinoma as, 822–825
   chemoprevention of, 823
   clinical features of, 825
   diet and, 822–823
   epidemiology of, 822–823
   metastatic, 825, 826f
   morphology of, 264f, 824–825, 825f
   pathogenesis of, 823–824, 823f, 824f
   staging of, 825, 826t, 827t
 diet and, 443, 822–823
 familial adenomatous polyposis and, 820–821
 hereditary nonpolyposis, 274, 275, 302, 821–822, 822t
 intramucosal carcinoma as, 820, 821f
 metastatic, 269f
 molecular model for evolution of, 308f, 309
Colostrum, 1067
Coma, hyperosmolar nonketotic, 1143
Comedocarcinoma, of breast, 1080, 1081f
Comedones, 1197, 1198, 1199f
Common bile duct, congenital dilations of, 887–888
Common cold, 749
Common variable immunodeficiency, 233

Comparative genomic hybridization (CGH), array-based, 179–180, 180f, 325–326, 326f
Compensatory growth, 93
Compensatory hyperinflation, 687
Compensatory hyperplasia, 93
Complement
  in antibody-mediated hypersensitivity, 202f, 203
  in glomerular injury, 915–916
Complement cascade, in septic shock, 130
Complement factor H (CFH) gene, in macular degeneration, 1363
Complement pathway, alternative, in membranoproliferative glomerulonephritis, 915, 928–929, 928f
Complement system
  activation and functions of, 63–64, 64f
  in cell lysis, 64, 64f
  genetic deficiencies of, 235
  in inflammation, 50, 51–52, 57t, 64, 64f, 65, 65f, 66
  in innate immunity, 184–185
  in ischemia-reperfusion injury, 24
  in phagocytosis, 64, 64f
Complement-mediated urticaria, 1187
Complete androgen insensitivity syndrome, 167
Complete atrioventricular canal defect, 540f, 542
Complex multigenic disorders, 138, 157–158
Complex sclerosing lesion, of breast, 1072, 1073f
Compound nevus, 1169, 1169f
  lentiginous, 1172f
Compression atelectasis, 679, 679f
Compression neuropathy, 1266–1267
Concretio cordis, 582
Concussion, 1287
Conduction system, of heart, 532
Condyloma acuminatum, 826, 827f, 1200
  of penis, 982–983, 983f
  of vulva, 1012, 1012f
Condylomata lata, in syphilis, 374, 376
Cones, in retina, 1359f
Confined placental mosaicism, 455, 455f
Congenital adrenal hyperplasia (CAH), 1152–1154, 1153f
Congenital aganglionic megacolon, 766–767, 766f
Congenital anomalies, 140, 448–453
  of biliary tract, 882, 882f
  of bladder, 974, 974f
  of blood vessels, 489–490
  of breasts, 1067
  causes of, 450–452, 450t, 451t
  of central nervous system, 1284–1286
    of forebrain, 1284–1285, 1285f
    neural tube defects as, 1284
    of posterior fossa, 1285–1286, 1286f
    syringomyelia and hydromyelia as, 1286
  defined, 448
  epidemiology of, 448
  of gallbladder, 882, 882f
  of gastrointestinal tract, 1668–1671
    atresia, fistulas and duplications as, 764–765, 765f
    diaphragmatic hernia, omphalocele, and gastroschisis as, 765
    ectopia as, 765
    Hirschsprung disease as, 766–767, 766f
    Meckel diverticulum as, 765–766, 765f
    pyloric stenosis as, 766
  of kidney, 955–956
    agenesis as, 955
    ectopic kidneys as, 955
    horseshoe kidneys as, 955

Congenital anomalies, of kidney (Continued)
    hypoplasia as, 955
    multicystic renal dysplasia as, 955–956, 956f
  of lungs, 679
  of pancreas, 892–893
  pathogenesis of, 452–453, 453f
  of penis, 982
  of testes, 984–985, 985f
  of thyroid, 1126
  types of, 448–450, 449f, 450f
  of ureters, 972
  of vagina, 1016
Congenital contractural arachnodactyly, 145
Congenital duplication cysts, of gastrointestinal tract, 765
Congenital fibrosarcoma, genetic basis for, 1249t
Congenital heart disease, 537–545
  cardiac development and, 537–538, 538f
  clinical features of, 539–540
  cyanotic, 540
  etiology and pathogenesis of, 538–539, 539t
  incidence of, 537, 537t
  with left-to-right shunts, 540–542, 540f
    atrial septal defect as, 540f, 541
    atrioventricular septal defect as, 540f, 542
    patent ductus arteriosus as, 540f, 541–542
    patent foramen ovale as, 541
    ventricular septal defect as, 540f, 541, 541f
  obstructive, 544–545
    aortic stenosis and atresia as, 544–545
    coarctation of the aorta as, 544, 544f
    pulmonary stenosis and atresia as, 544
  with right-to-left shunts, 540, 542–544, 542f
    persistent truncus arteriosus as, 543
    tetralogy of Fallot as, 542–543, 542f
    total anomalous pulmonary venous connection as, 543–544
    transposition of the great arteries as, 542f, 543, 543f
    tricuspid atresia as, 543
Congenital hepatic fibrosis, 870, 959
Congenital infection, with cytomegalovirus, 354
Congenital lobar overinflation, 687
Congenital melanosis oculi, 1350
Congenital muscular dystrophies, 1270t
Congenital myopathies, 1271, 1272f, 1272t
Congenital nevus, 1170t
Congenital pulmonary alveolar proteinosis, 705–706
Congenital syphilis, 375, 376–377
Congenital-infantile fibrosarcomas, 474
Congestion, 113–114, 114f
Congestive heart failure (CHF), 533–537
  edema due to, 112, 113
  epidemiology of, 533
  left-sided, 535–536
  pathogenesis of, 533
  progression from cardiac hypertrophy to, 533–535, 534f, 535f
  right-sided, 536–537
  treatment of, 537
Congestive hepatomegaly, in right-sided heart failure, 536
Congestive splenomegaly, in right-sided heart failure, 536
Conidia, 335, 382
Conjunctiva, 1349–1350
  functional anatomy of, 1346f, 1348f, 1349
  neoplasms of, 1349–1350, 1350f
  pinguecula and pterygium of, 1349
  scarring of, 1349
Conjunctival intraepithelial neoplasia, 1349–1350

Conjunctival melanoma, 1350, 1350f
Conjunctival nevi, 1350, 1350f
Conjunctival scarring, 1349
Conjunctival squamous cell carcinoma, 1349–1350
Conjunctivitis, 1349
Conn syndrome, 1151
Connective tissue diseases
  mixed, 226
  pulmonary involvement in, 696
Connective tissue remodeling, in wound healing, 105
Consumption coagulopathy, 125
Contact dermatitis, 206t, 207, 208f
  allergic, 1187–1189, 1189f
Contact inhibition, in extracellular matrix, 96
Contagious childhood bacterial diseases, 358t
Continuously dividing tissues, 81
Contractile dysfunction, due to myocardial infarction, 556–557
Contraction atelectasis, 679, 679f
Contraction bands, after myocardial infarction, 553
Contracture, 107, 107f
Contrecoup injury, 1287
Contusion, 420, 420f
  of brain, 1287, 1288f
Coombs antiglobulin test
  direct, 653
  indirect, 653
COPD (chronic obstructive pulmonary disease), 683–684, 683f, 683t
Copper
  deficiency of, 439t
  functions of, 439t
Copper excess, 863–864
Coproporphyria, variegate, 1264t
Copy number variations (CNVs), 136, 180
Cor pulmonale, 536–537, 559–560
  acute vs. chronic, 560
  in cystic fibrosis, 470
  disorders predisposing to, 536, 560t
  morphology of, 536–537, 560, 560f
  due to pulmonary embolism, 126, 706
Cords of Billroth, 632, 633f
Cornea, 1351–1353
  degenerations and dystrophies of, 1351–1353, 1352f
  functional anatomy of, 1346f, 1351, 1351f, 1354f
  keratitis and ulcers of, 1351, 1351f
  stem cells in, 86
Corneal hydrops, 1352, 1352f
Corneal stroma, 1351, 1351f
Corneal stromal dystrophies, 1353
Corneal ulcers, 432f, 1351
Coronary arteries, epicardial, 532
Coronary arteriosclerosis, graft, 585, 585f
Coronary artery disease (CAD), 496, 497f. See also Ischemic heart disease (IHD).
  hormone replacement therapy and, 415
  obesity and, 442
  in systemic lupus erythematosus, 220
Coronary artery occlusion, and myocardial infarction, 547–549, 548f, 548t
Coronary heart disease. See Coronary artery disease (CAD); Ischemic heart disease (IHD).
Coronary syndromes, acute, 546, 546f
Corpora amylacea, 1282
Corpus callosum, agenesis of, 1285, 1285f
Corpus luteum, 1007, 1024, 1025
Cortical atrophy, in Alzheimer disease, 1314, 1314f

Cortical hamartomas, in tuberous sclerosis, 1342–1343
Cortical inclusion cysts, of ovary, 1042, 1042f
Cortical necrosis, diffuse, 954–955, 954f
Corticobasal degeneration (CBD), 1318–1319
Corticosteroids, for inflammation, 58f, 60
Corticotroph(s), 1098
Corticotroph adenomas, 1100t, 1104, 1148
Corticotroph cell hyperplasia, 1148
Corynebacterium diphtheriae, 360
Costimulation, lack of, in immune evasion, 319–320
Costimulators
    in autoimmunity, 212, 213f
    in immune response, 195
Cot death, 471–473, 471t
Cotinine, 412
Cotton dust, lung diseases due to, 697t
Cotton-wool spot, in retinal infarcts, 1359, 1362f
Coumadin (warfarin), 119
Coup injury, 1287
Cowden syndrome, 1182t
    CNS tumors in, 1342
    colonic polyps in, 816t, 818
    PTEN in, 294
COX. *See* Cyclooxygenase(s) (COX).
Coxiella burnetii pneumonia, 714
C-peptide, 1133
CpG island(s), 181
CpG island methylation, in colorectal carcinoma, 824
CPPD (calcium pyrophosphate crystal deposition) disease, 1246, 1246f
Crack cocaine, 417
Cranial nerve palsies, 1266
Craniopharyngiomas, 1106–1107, 1107f
Craniotabes, 436
C-reactive protein (CRP), 74
    and atherosclerosis, 498, 498f
Creatine kinase (CK), in myocardial infarction, 555–556, 555f
Creeping fat, in Crohn disease, 810, 810f
Creeping substitution, 1221
Crescentic glomerulonephritis, 907, 908t, 920–921, 920t, 921f
CREST syndrome, 215t, 223, 224, 225
Cretinism, 1110–1111
Creutzfeldt-Jakob disease (CJD), 1308, 1309, 1310f
Crib death, 471–473, 471t
Crigler-Najjar syndrome type I, 841, 841t
Crigler-Najjar syndrome type II, 841, 841t
Crohn disease, 810–811
    clinical features of, 811
    epidemiology of, 807–808
    granulomatous inflammation in, 73t
    historical background of, 810
    morphology of, 810–811, 810f, 811f
    pathogenesis of, 808–810, 809f
    skip lesions in, 808f, 810
    T cell–mediated hypersensitivity in, 206t
    vs. ulcerative colitis, 807, 808f, 808t
Cronkhite-Canada syndrome, 816t, 818
Crooke hyaline change, 1149
Croup, 752
Crouzon syndrome, 1211t
CRP (C-reactive protein), 74
    and atherosclerosis, 498, 498f
Cryoglobulinemia, essential mixed, glomerular lesions in, 935
Crypt abscesses
    in *Campylobacter* enterocolitis, 799, 800f
    in Crohn disease, 810
    in ulcerative colitis, 812, 813f

Cryptitis, in *Campylobacter* enterocolitis, 799, 800f
Cryptococcal meningitis, 1306, 1307f
Cryptococcosis, 384, 384f
    in AIDS, 246
Cryptococcus neoformans, 384
Cryptogenic cirrhosis, 853
Cryptogenic fibrosing alveolitis, 694–695, 694f, 695f
Cryptogenic organizing pneumonia, 696, 696f
Cryptorchidism, 984–985, 985f
Cryptosporidiosis, 805f, 807
Cryptosporidium, enterocolitis due to, 805f, 807
Cryptosporidium hominis, 807
Cryptosporidium parvum, 807
Crystal-induced arthritis, 1242–1246, 1243t, 1244f–1246f
CTCL (cutaneous T-cell lymphoma), 1184–1185, 1185f
CTL(s). *See* Cytotoxic T lymphocyte(s) (CTLs).
CTLA-4
    in anergy, 209–210
    in type 1 diabetes mellitus, 1135
CTLA4 (cytotoxic T lymphocyte–associated antigen-4) gene, 1111
Cunninghamella, 385
Curie (Ci), 423
Curling ulcers, 775
Curschmann spirals, in asthma, 691
Cushing disease, 1104, 1148
Cushing syndrome, 1148–1151
    ACTH-dependent, 1148–1149, 1148t
    ACTH-independent, 1148t, 1149
    due to cancer, 321t, 322
    clinical course of, 151f, 1150–1151, 1150t
    iatrogenic, 1148
    morphology of, 1149–1150, 1149f, 1150f
    pathogenesis of, 1104, 1148–1149, 1148t
Cushing ulcers, 775
Cutaneous disorders. *See* Skin disorders.
Cutaneous immune system, 1166, 1167f
Cutaneous neurofibroma, 1341
Cutaneous T-cell lymphoma (CTCL), 1184–1185, 1185f
Cutaneous ulcers
    healing of, 104f
    in systemic sclerosis, 224, 225f
Cutaneous wound healing, 102–106
    cell proliferation and collagen deposition in, 102–104
    connective tissue remodeling in, 105
    formation of blood clot in, 102, 103f
    formation of granulation tissue in, 102, 103f–105f
    growth factors and cytokines in, 102, 104t
    macrophages in, 102, 105f
    phases of, 102, 103f, 104f
    by primary union or first intention, 102
    recovery of tensile strength in, 105–106
    scar formation in, 103f, 104
    by secondary union or secondary intention, 102, 103f, 104f
    wound contraction in, 103f, 104–105, 104f
CWP (coal workers' pneumoconiosis), 36, 697–698, 697t, 698f
CX3C chemokines, 62
C-X-C chemokine(s), 62
C-X-C chemokine receptors (CXCR), 62
CXCR3, in metastasis, 300
CXCR4, in AIDS, 239–240, 245
Cyanide poisoning, 24
Cyanosis, 114
Cyanotic congenital heart disease, 540

3′,5′-Cyclic adenosine monophosphate (cAMP) pathway, 90–91, 91f
Cyclin(s)
    in cell cycle, 86, 87, 285, 285f
    proto-oncogenes for, 281t, 284–286
Cyclin D gene, 281t, 285, 289, 289f
Cyclin D1, in mantle cell lymphoma, 613
Cyclin D1 gene inversions, in parathyroid adenomas, 1127
Cyclin E gene, 281t, 285–286, 288–289
Cyclin-dependent kinase(s) (CDKs)
    in cell cycle, 86–87, 285, 285f
    functions of, 286t
    proto-oncogenes for, 281t, 284–286
Cyclin-dependent kinase inhibitors (CDKIs)
    in cell cycle, 87, 285, 285f
    functions of, 286t
Cyclitic membrane, 1368
Cyclooxygenase(s) (COX), in inflammation, 58f, 59
Cyclooxygenase 1 (COX-1), in inflammation, 59
Cyclooxygenase 1 (COX-1) inhibitors, mechanism of action of, 58f, 59–60
Cyclooxygenase 2 (COX-2)
    in cancer, 276
    in inflammation, 59
Cyclooxygenase 2 (COX-2) inhibitors, mechanism of action of, 58f, 59–60
Cyclophosphamide, and bladder cancer, 980
Cyclosporine, for transplantation, 229
Cylindroma, 1177, 1177f
CYP (cytochrome P-450 enzyme system), 403
CYP1A1, 311
CYP2E1, in alcohol metabolism, 413, 413f
CYP11B1 gene, 1151
CYP11B2 gene, 1151
CYP21A1 gene, 1153
CYP21A2 gene, 1152–1153
Cyst(s)
    adrenal, 1159
    aneurysmal bone, 1234, 1234f
    Bartholin, 1011
    branchial (cervical lymphoepithelial), 755
    breast, 1071, 1071f
        apocrine, 1071, 1071f
        blue-dome, 1071, 1071f
    choledochal, 887–888
    dentigerous, 748
    dermoid, 262, 262f
        ovarian, 1047–1048, 1048f
        of skin, 1176
    epithelial, 1176
        of ovary, 1042, 1042f
    follicle, 1039
    foregut, 679
    Gartner duct, 1007, 1016
    of gastrointestinal tract, congenital duplication, 765
    horn, 1175, 1175f
    inclusion
        epidermal, 1176
        of ovary, 1042, 1042f
    invagination, 1175
    liver, 869–870, 870f
    luteal, 1039
    odontogenic, 748–749
    of ovary
        dermoid, 1047–1048, 1048f
        epithelial (mesothelial, cortical, germinal) inclusion, 1042, 1042f
    pancreatic, 898
        congenital, 898
        pseudo-, 898, 898f
    paratubal, 1038

Cyst(s) *(Continued)*
  periapical, 749
  peritoneal, 829
  pilar (trichilemmal), 1176
  Rathke cleft, 1105
  renal, 957t, 960
  of skin, dermoid, 1176
  subchondral, 1236f
  synovial, 1247
  of third ventricle, colloid, 1335
  thymic, 635
  thyroglossal duct, 755, 1126
Cystadenocarcinoma
  mucinous
      of appendix, 828
      of ovary, 1044
  ovarian, 1041
      mucinous, 1044
      serous, 1043, 1043f
Cystadenofibroma, ovarian, 1046
Cystadenoma(s), 260
  mucinous
      of appendix, 828
      müllerian, 1044
      of ovary, 1045
      of pancreas, 899, 899f
  papillary, 260–261
  serous
      ovarian, 1043, 1043f
      of pancreas, 899, 899f
Cystic disease(s), of kidney, 956–960, 957t
  acquired, 957t, 960
  autosomal-dominant (adult) polycystic,
      956–959, 957t, 958f
  autosomal-recessive (childhood) polycystic,
      957t, 959
  medullary sponge kidney as, 957t, 959
  nephronophthisis and adult-onset medullary,
      957t, 959–960, 960f
  obstructive uropathy as, 960–962, 961f
  simple cysts as, 957t, 960
Cystic fibrosis, 465–471
  clinical features of, 467–468, 468f, 469–471,
      470t
  diagnostic criteria for, 470t
  epidemiology of, 465
  genetic and environmental modifiers of, 468
  genetic basis for, 139f, 144, 465–468, 466f,
      467f
  genotype-phenotype correlations in, 467–468,
      468f
  malabsorption and diarrhea in, 794, 794t
  morphology of, 468–469, 469f
Cystic fibrosis transmembrane conductance
      regulator (CFTR)
  defect in, 143t, 466–468, 467f, 468f
  normal structure and function of, 465–466,
      466f
Cystic fibrosis transmembrane conductance
      regulator *(CFTR)* gene, mutations of,
      466–467
  in pancreatitis, 896
Cystic follicles, 1039
Cystic hygroma, 460, 461, 462f, 522
Cystic medial degeneration, 507, 507f, 509
Cystic neoplasms, of pancreas, 899–900, 899f,
      901f
Cystic teratomas, 262, 262f
  ovarian, 1047–1048, 1048f
Cysticercosis, 392, 392f
Cystine stones, 962, 962t, 963
Cystitis
  acute and chronic, 974–975
  cystica, 975–976

Cystitis *(Continued)*
  eosinophilic, 975
  glandularis, 975–976
  hemorrhagic, 975
  interstitial, 975
  with malacoplakia, 975, 975f, 976f
  morphology of, 975
  pathogenesis of, 974
  polypoid, 975
  radiation, 974
  tuberculous, 974
Cystocele, 972
Cystosarcoma phyllodes, 1092
Cytochrome c, in apoptosis, 28f, 29, 29f
Cytochrome P-450 enzyme system (CYP), 403
Cytogenetic disorder(s), 138, 158–167
  in carcinogenesis, 304–306, 305t
  chromosome 22q11.2 deletion syndrome as,
      162–164, 164f
  fetal growth restriction due to, 455
  fetal hydrops due to, 461, 461t
  hermaphroditism and
      pseudohermaphroditism as, 167
  involving autosomes, 161–164, 161f, 163f,
      164f
  involving sex chromosomes, 164–167, 166f
  Klinefelter syndrome as, 165
  normal karyotype and, 158–159, 159f
  other trisomies as, 162
  prevalence of, 451, 451t
  structural, 159–161, 160f
  trisomy 21 (Down syndrome) as, 161–162,
      161f, 163f
  Turner syndrome as, 165–167, 166f
  white cell neoplasia due to, 596–597, 597f
Cytoid bodies, 1359, 1362f
Cytokine(s)
  in glomerular injury, 916
  in immediate hypersensitivity, 200
  in immune response, 193, 195, 195f
  in inflammation, 49, 49f, 50, 57t, 61–63, 61t,
      62f
  in tissue regeneration and wound healing, 89,
      102, 103, 104t
Cytokine receptors, in inflammation, 52, 52f
Cytologic methods, for diagnosis of cancer, 323f,
      324
Cytologic smears, for cancer, 323f, 324
Cytomegalic inclusion disease, 354
Cytomegalovirus (CMV), 353–355
  in AIDS, 246
  congenital infection with, 354
  encephalitis due to, 1304
  in immunocompromised individuals, 354–355
  intrauterine infection with, 452
  morphology of, 354, 354f
  perinatal infection with, 354
  transmission of, 354
Cytomegalovirus (CMV) esophagitis, 769, 769f
Cytomegalovirus (CMV) mononucleosis, 354
Cytopathic reaction, 348, 348f
Cytoplasmic blebs, in apoptosis, 26, 26f
Cytoplasmic changes, due to ionizing radiation,
      424–425
Cytoplasmic inclusions, 332
Cytoproliferative reaction, 348, 348f
Cytoskeletal abnormalities, cell injury due to, 22
Cytoskeletal proteins, accumulation of, 35
Cytotoxic edema, 1282
Cytotoxic T lymphocyte(s) (CTLs)
  antitumor effect of, 318
  in cell-mediated cytotoxicity, 207–208
  in immune evasion, 320
  in immune response, 185f, 186

Cytotoxic T lymphocyte(s) (CTLs) *(Continued)*
  in transplant rejection, 226, 227f
  tumor antigens recognized by, 316, 317f
Cytotoxic T lymphocyte (CTL)-mediated
      apoptosis, 31
Cytotoxic T lymphocyte–associated antigen-4
      (CTLA4) gene, 1111
Cytotrophoblast, 1053f

D

D1 cells, 1130
Dacryoadenitis, sclerosing, 1347
Dacryocytes, in primary myelofibrosis, 630
DAD (diffuse alveolar damage), 680, 681f
  due to shock, 132
DALY (disability-adjusted life year), 400
Dandy-Walker malformation, 1285
Danger-associated molecular patterns, in innate
      immunity, 184
Darier sign, 1185
D-binding protein (DBP), 433
DC(s). *See* Dendritic cells (DCs).
DCIS (ductal carcinoma in situ), 1080–1082,
      1081f, 1082f
DCM. *See* Dilated cardiomyopathy (DCM).
D-dimers, 120
DDT (dichlorodiphenyltrichlorethane),
      occupational exposure to, 409
de Quervain thyroiditis, 1113, 1113f
Dead cells, removal of, 30
Deafness, maternally inherited diabetes and,
      1138
Death domains, 29, 29f
  in apoptosis, 295
Death receptor(s), 29
Death receptor–initiated pathway, of apoptosis,
      28f, 29–30, 29f
Decompression sickness, 127
Deep venous thrombosis (DVT), 125, 520
  edema due to, 112
  pulmonary embolism due to, 126, 126f
Defective DNA-repair syndromes, 275
Defensins
  in Crohn disease, 809
  in phagocytosis, 54
Deformations, 448–449
Degenerative disease(s), 1313–1325
  Alzheimer disease as, 1313–1317, 1314f–1316f
  amyotrophic lateral sclerosis as, 1324–1325,
      1325f
  ataxia-telangiectasia as, 1323–1324
  of basal ganglia and brainstem, 1319–1323,
      1320f, 1322f
  bulbospinal atrophy (Kennedy syndrome) as,
      1325
  of cerebral cortex, 1313–1319
  corticobasal degeneration as, 1318–1319
  dementia with Lewy bodies as, 1321
  Friedreich ataxia as, 1323
  frontotemporal dementias as, 1317–1319,
      1318f
  Huntington disease as, 1322–1323, 1322f
  of motor neurons, 1324–1325, 1325f
  multiple system atrophy as, 1321–1322
  Parkinson disease as, 1319–1321, 1320f
  parkinsonism as, 1319
  Pick disease as, 1318, 1318f
  progressive supranuclear palsy as, 1318
  spinal muscular atrophy as, 1325
  spinocerebellar, 1323–1324
  vascular dementia as, 1319
Degenerative joint disease, 1235–1236, 1236f,
      1237f
7-Dehydrocholesterol, 433, 434f

Dejerine-Sottas neuropathy, 1264–1265
Delayed-type hypersensitivity (DTH), 205–207, 206f–208f
  chronic inflammation due to, 70
Deletions, 138f, 139, 139f, 160, 160f
  in carcinogenesis, 306
  in immunological tolerance, 209
Dellen, 1349
δ cells, 1130, 1131f
δ (dense) granules, 117
δ-cell tumors, 1147
Delta-like ligand (Dll), in angiogenesis, 100, 101f
Dementia(s)
  frontotemporal, 1317–1319, 1318f
  HIV-associated, 1305
  with Lewy bodies, 1321
  post-traumatic (pugilistica), 1290
  vascular (multi-infarct), 1295, 1319
Demyelinating disease(s), 1309–1313
  central pontine myelinolysis as, 1313
  encephalomyelitis as
    acute disseminated, 1312–1313
    acute necrotizing hemorrhagic, 1312–1313
  multiple sclerosis as, 1310–1312, 1311f, 1312f
  neuromyelitis optica as, 1312
Demyelinating radiculoneuropathy, inflammatory
  acute, 1261–1262
  chronic, 1262
Demyelination, segmental, 1258, 1258f, 1259, 1259f
Dendritic cells (DCs)
  in cell-mediated immunity, 193, 194f
  dermal, 1166, 1166f, 1167f
  HIV infection of, 242, 249
  in immune response, 187–188, 187f
  in innate immunity, 184
Dendrocytes, 1166, 1166f
Denervation atrophy, 9, 1260, 1267
Dense (δ) granules, 117
Dense-deposit disease, 915, 918t, 928–929, 928f, 930f
Dental caries, 740
Dental plaque, 740–741
Dentatorubral-pallidoluysian atrophy, 168t
Dentigerous cyst, 748
Dentin, 740, 740f
Denys-Drash syndrome, Wilms tumor in, 480
Deoxynucleotidyltransferase, terminal, in acute lymphoblastic leukemia/lymphoma, 602
Deoxyribonucleic acid. See DNA.
Dependent edema, 113
Dermatan sulfate, in extracellular matrix, 97, 98f
Dermatitis
  acute eczematous, 1187–1189, 1188f
  contact, 206t, 207, 208f
    allergic, 1187–1189, 1189f
  herpetiformis, 1193f, 1196, 1197f
    in celiac disease, 796
  interface, 1189, 1192, 1192f
  due to ionizing radiation, 426f
  seborrheic, 1191
  spongiotic, 1188
Dermatofibroma, 1182, 1184f
Dermatofibrosarcoma protuberans, 1182–1183, 1184f
  genetic basis for, 1249t
Dermatographism, 1185
Dermatologic disorders. See Skin disorders.
Dermatomyofibroma, 1253
Dermatomyositis, 1273, 1274, 1274f
  due to cancer, 321t
Dermatophytes, 335

Dermatosis(es)
  inflammatory
    acute, 1187–1189
      acute eczematous dermatitis as, 1187–1189, 1188f
      erythema multiforme as, 1189, 1190f
      urticaria as, 1187, 1187f
    chronic, 1189–1192
      lichen planus as, 1191–1192, 1192f
      psoriasis as, 1190–1191, 1190f
      seborrheic dermatitis as, 1191
  papulosa nigra, 1175
Dermatosparaxis, in Ehlers-Danlos syndrome, 146, 146t
Dermis, 1166f, 1167f
  tumors of, 1182–1183
    benign fibrous histiocytoma as, 1182, 1184f
    dermatofibrosarcoma protuberans as, 1182–1183, 1184f
Dermoid cysts, 262, 262f
  ovarian, 1047–1048, 1048f
  of skin, 1176
DES (diethylstilbestrol), and developmental anomalies of vagina, 1016
Descemet membrane, 1346f, 1351, 1351f
Desmin filaments, 35
Desmoglein 1 (Dsg1), 1193f, 1194
Desmoglein 3 (Dsg3), 1193f, 1194
Desmoid tumors, 107, 1251–1252
Desmoplasia, 260
Desmoplastic small round cell tumor
  genetic basis for, 1249t
  of peritoneum, 829
Desmosomes, in extracellular matrix, 96
Desquamative interstitial pneumonia (DIP), 704, 704f
Detoxification, 403
Developmental aneurysms, 489, 506, 506f, 507
  ruptured, 1297–1298, 1297f, 1298f
Developmental disorders. See Congenital anomalies.
Developmental plasticity, 85
Developmental rests, of gastrointestinal tract, 765
Devic disease, 1312
DHPR (dihydropteridine reductase), 463, 463f
DHT (dihydrotestosterone), in benign prostatic hyperplasia, 995, 995f
Diabetes
  lipoatrophic, 1138
  maturity-onset, of young, 1137
  permanent neonatal, 1138
Diabetes and deafness, maternally inherited, 1138
Diabetes insipidus, 1106
Diabetes mellitus, 1131–1146
  and atherosclerosis, 498
  causes of, 1132, 1132t
  classification of, 1132, 1132t
  clinical features of, 1143–1146, 1144f, 1145t
  complications of, 1138–1139, 1140f
  defined, 1131
  diagnosis of, 1131–1132
  epidemiology of, 1131
  gestational, 1137
  glucose homeostasis and, 1132–1134, 1133f, 1134f
  insulin-dependent, 1134
  insulin-resistant, antibody-mediated hypersensitivity in, 203t
  juvenile, 1134
  maternal, congenital anomalies due to, 452
  monogenic forms of, 1137–1138
  morphology of, 1139–1143, 1141f, 1142f

Diabetes mellitus (Continued)
  papillary necrosis due to, 947t
  pathogenesis of, 1134–1137, 1135f, 1136f
  pre-, 1131, 1132
  retinal vascular disease due to, 1359–1361, 1362f, 1363f
  type 1, 1132, 1132t, 1145t
    clinical features of, 1143, 1144f
    pathogenesis of, 1134–1135, 1135f
    T cell–mediated hypersensitivity in, 206t
  type 2, 1132, 1132t, 1145t
    clinical features of, 1143
    pathogenesis of, 1136–1137, 1136f
Diabetic dyslipidemia, 1144–1145
Diabetic embryopathy, 452
Diabetic ketoacidosis, 1143
Diabetic macrovascular disease, 1139–1140, 1141f, 1144–1145
Diabetic mononeuropathy, 1146
Diabetic nephropathy, 934–935, 1141–1143
  epidemiology of, 1145
  morphology of, 934, 1141–1143, 1141f, 1142f
  pathogenesis of, 934–935
Diabetic neuropathy, 1143, 1145–1146, 1265–1266, 1265f
Diabetic ocular complications, 1143, 1145
Diabetic retinopathy, 1145, 1359–1361, 1362f, 1363f
Dialysis, kidney changes due to, 933
Dialysis-associated cystic disease, 960
Diapedesis, of leukocytes through endothelium, 48f, 50
Diaper rash, 383
Diaphragmatic hernia, 765
Diarrhea, 793–797
  in abetalipoproteinemia, 797
  in AIDS, 246
  antibiotic-associated, 803, 803f
  in autoimmune enteropathy, 794t, 796–797
  in celiac disease, 794t, 795–796, 795f, 796f
  in cystic fibrosis, 794, 794t
  defined, 794
  exudative, 794
  in lactase (disaccharidase) deficiency, 794t, 797
  malabsorptive, 794
  mechanisms of, 793–794, 794t
  osmotic, 794
  secretory, 794
  traveler's, 802, 807
  in tropical sprue, 794t, 796
Diastolic dysfunction, 533
Diastolic failure, 536
Diatheses, hemorrhagic, 114. See Bleeding disorder(s).
DIC (disseminated intravascular coagulation), 125, 673–674, 674f
  impaired blood flow through liver due to, 872
  in septic shock, 130–131
Dicentric chromosomes, 296, 297f
Dichlorodiphenyltrichlorethane (DDT, Lindane, Aldrin, Dieldrin), occupational exposure to, 409
Diet
  and atherosclerosis, 444
  and breast cancer, 1077
  and cancer, 443–444
  and colorectal cancer, 443, 822–823
  for galactosemia, 465
  for phenylketonuria, 464
  and prostate cancer, 997
Dietary insufficiency, 427–428
Diethylstilbestrol (DES), and developmental anomalies of vagina, 1016

Differentiated cells, reprogramming of, 84, 84f
Differentiation, 80, 81f
  in neoplasia, 262–263, 264f, 271t
  stochastic, 82
Differentiation antigens, cell type–specific, 318
"Differentiation therapy," 432
Diffuse alveolar damage (DAD), 680, 681f
  due to shock, 132
Diffuse axonal injury, 1288
Diffuse cortical necrosis, 954–955, 954f
Diffuse esophageal spasm, 767
Diffuse hypoxic/ischemic encephalopathy, 1291–1292, 1292f
Diffuse large B-cell lymphoma (DLBCL), 601t, 606–607, 607f, 608
Diffuse plaques, in Alzheimer disease, 1314
Diffuse proliferative glomerulonephritis, in systemic lupus erythematosus, 218, 218f
Diffuse pulmonary hemorrhage syndromes, 709–710, 709f
DiGeorge syndrome, 162–164, 164f, 234
Digital arteries, in rheumatoid arthritis, 1237
Dihydropteridine reductase (DHPR), 463, 463f
Dihydrotestosterone (DHT), in benign prostatic hyperplasia, 995, 995f
1,25-Dihydroxyvitamin D [$1\alpha,25(OH)_2D_3$], 433, 434f
Dilantin (phenytoin) ingestion, oral manifestations of, 744t
Dilated cardiomyopathy (DCM), 572–575
  clinical features of, 574–575
  functional patterns and causes of, 572t
  graphic representation of, 572f
  morphology of, 572–573, 574f
  pathogenesis of, 573–574, 574f, 575f
  X-linked, 573
DILI (drug-induced liver injury), 856–857, 856t
Dioxin (TCDD, 2,3,7,8-tetrachlorodibenzo-p-dioxin), occupational exposure to, 409–410
DIP (desquamative interstitial pneumonia), 704, 704f
Diphtheria, 360–361, 361f
  oral manifestations of, 744t
  polyneuropathy due to, 1262
Diphtheritic myocarditis, 578
Diphyllobothrium latum, 392, 806
Direct Coombs antiglobulin test, 653
Disability-adjusted life year (DALY), 400
Disaccharidase deficiency, 794t, 797
Disc, neovascularization of, 1360
Discoid rash, in systemic lupus erythematosus, 214t
Disomy, uniparental, 172
Dispersin, in enteroaggregative *E. coli* infection, 802
Disruptions, 448, 449f
Dissecting osteitis, 1218, 1218f
Dissection, arterial, 506, 506f
  aortic, 508–510, 509f, 510f
Disseminated intravascular coagulation (DIC), 125, 673–674, 674f
  impaired blood flow through liver due to, 872
  in septic shock, 130–131
Disseminated peritoneal leiomyomatosis, 1037
Dissolution, of thrombi, 124
Disuse, atrophy of, 9
Divalent metal transporter 1 (DMT1), 660, 661f
Diversion colitis, 813–814, 814f
Diverticulitis, sigmoid, 814–815, 815f
Diverticulum(a)
  bladder or vesical, 974
  colonic, 814–815, 815f
  epiphrenic, 767

Diverticulum(a) (Continued)
  Meckel, 765–766, 765f
  traction, 767
  of ureters, 972
  Zenker (pharyngoesophageal), 767
DLBCL (diffuse large B-cell lymphoma), 601t, 606–607, 607f, 608
Dll (delta-like ligand), in angiogenesis, 100, 101f
DMD (Duchenne muscular dystrophy), 1268–1269, 1268f, 1269f
DMD gene, in X-linked muscular dystrophy, 1268, 1269
DMPK (dystrophia myotonia protein kinase), 1269
DMT1 (divalent metal transporter 1), 660, 661f
DNA, mitochondrial, 171
DNA breakdown, in apoptosis, 27, 27f
DNA damage
  apoptosis due to, 25, 30
  cell injury due to, 18f, 23
  in cellular aging, 41
  due to ionizing radiation, 423–424, 423f, 425–426
DNA methylation, in carcinogenesis, 306
DNA microarrays, 325, 326f
DNA mismatch repair, 302
DNA ploidy, of neuroblastomas, 478
DNA polymorphisms, 176–177, 177f
DNA repair
  defects in, in carcinogenesis, 277, 278, 302–303
  p53 in, 291–292, 291f
DNA sequence alterations, detection of, 174–176, 175f, 176f
DNA viruses, oncogenic, 313–315, 313f, 314f
Döhle bodies, in leukocytosis, 594, 594f
Dolor, 44, 69
Dominant negative allele, 141
Donovanosis, 366
Dopamine, in Parkinson disease, 1320–1321
Dormancy, of metastasis, 301
Double minutes, in carcinogenesis, 306
Double-stranded breaks (DSBs), due to radiation injury, 426
Down syndrome, 161–162, 161f, 163f
Draining sinus, 1222, 1222f
Drug(s)
  cardiotoxic, 579
  cell injury due to, 11
  congenital anomalies due to, 452
  genetically determined adverse reactions to, 144
Drug abuse, 417–420, 418t, 419f
  of amphetamines, 418t, 419
  of cocaine, 417–418
  of hallucinogens, 418t
  of heroin, 418–419, 418t
  of marijuana, 418t, 419–420
  of opioid narcotics, 418–419, 418t
  of phencyclidine, 418t
  of sedative-hypnotics, 418t
Drug reactions
  adverse (*See* Adverse drug reactions (ADRs))
  antibody-mediated hypersensitivity in, 203
  bleeding disorders due to, 666
Drug toxicity, agranulocytosis due to, 593
Drug-induced asthma, 689
Drug-induced interstitial nephritis, 944–946, 945f, 946f, 947f
Drug-induced liver injury (DILI), 856–857, 856t
Drug-induced lung diseases, 701, 701t
Drug-induced lupus erythematosus, 215t, 216, 221
Drug-induced myopathies, 1275

Drug-induced thrombocytopenia, 668–669
Drug-metabolizing enzymes, 403
DSBs (double-stranded breaks), due to radiation injury, 426
Dsg1 (desmoglein 1), 1193f, 1194
Dsg3 (desmoglein 3), 1193f, 1194
DTH (delayed-type hypersensitivity), 205–207, 206f–208f
  chronic inflammation due to, 70
DUB (dysfunctional uterine bleeding), 1026–1027, 1026f, 1027t
Dubin-Johnson syndrome, 841t, 842, 842f
Duchenne muscular dystrophy (DMD), 1268–1269, 1268f, 1269f
Duct of Santorini, 891, 892f
Duct of Wirsung, 891, 892f
Ductal carcinoma, invasive (infiltrative), 1083–1085, 1085f
Ductal carcinoma in situ (DCIS), 1080–1082, 1081f, 1082f
Ductal hyperplasia, atypical, 1073, 1074f
Ductular reaction, in fulminant hepatitis, 853
Ductus arteriosus, patent, 540f, 541–542
  coarctation of the aorta with, 544, 544f
Duncan disease, 319, 357
Duodenal ulcers, 68, 69f, 780
Duplication(s), gastrointestinal, 764–765
Duplication cysts, congenital, of gastrointestinal tract, 765
Dupuytren contracture, 1251
Dürck granulomas, 388
Duret hemorrhage, 1283–1284, 1284f
Dutcher bodies
  in lymphoplasmacytic lymphoma, 612
  in multiple myeloma, 610
DVT (deep venous thrombosis), 125, 520
  edema due to, 112
  pulmonary embolism due to, 126, 126f
Dwarfism
  pituitary, 1106
  thanatophoric, 1210, 1211t
Dysautonomia
  autosomal-recessive, 1263t
  familial, 1263t
Dysembryoplastic neuroepithelial tumor, 1335–1336
Dysentery
  due to *Campylobacter*, 799
  due to *Entamoeba histolytica*, 805f, 806
Dysfunctional uterine bleeding (DUB), 1026–1027, 1026f, 1027t
Dysgerminoma
  ovarian, 1048–1049, 1049f
  testicular, 988
Dyskeratosis, 1168
Dyslipidemia, diabetic, 1144–1145
Dyslipoproteinemias, in atherosclerosis, 500
Dysostoses, 1210
Dysphagia, in systemic sclerosis, 225
Dysplasia, 265, 450
Dysplastic gangliocytoma, 1342
Dysplastic nevi, 1170–1171, 1170t, 1171f, 1172f
Dysplastic nevus syndrome, 1171
Dyspnea
  in left-sided heart failure, 535
  paroxysmal nocturnal, 535
Dystrophia myotonia protein kinase (DMPK), 1269
Dystrophic calcification, 38, 38f
Dystrophin
  in cachexia, 429, 430f
  defect in, 143t
  in X-linked muscular dystrophy, 1268, 1268f, 1269f

E

EAEC (enteroaggregative *Escherichia coli*), 798t, 800f, 802
Ear disorders, 754
Eating disorders, 430
EB (elementary body), of *Chlamydia trachomatis*, 380
EBNA-2 gene, 314
EBV. *See* Epstein-Barr virus (EBV).
E-cadherin
    in gastric carcinoma, 785
    in invasive lobular carcinoma, 1087
    in metastasis, 299
E-cadherin gene, 287t
Ecchymoses, 114
Eccrine carcinoma, 1178
Eccrine poroma, 1177
Echinococcal infection, of liver, 854, 855f
Echinococcus granulosus, 392–393
Echinococcus multilocularis, 392
Echinococcus spp, 336
ECL (enterochromaffin-like) cells, 779
Eclampsia, 1055–1057, 1057f
    hepatic disease associated with, 872, 875, 875f
ECM. *See* Extracellular matrix (ECM).
ECM1, in ulcerative colitis, 809
Ecstasy (3,4-methylenedioxymethamphetamine), 419
Ectatic arteries, 489
Ecthyma gangrenosum, 365
Ectocervix, 1007
Ectoparasites, 336
Ectopia lentis, in Marfan syndrome, 145
Ectopic hormone production, due to cancer, 322
Ectopic pregnancy, 1053–1054
Eczema, 1187–1189, 1188f
    herpeticum, 352–353
    immunodeficiency with, 235
Eczematous dermatitis, acute, 1187–1189, 1188f
Edema, 111–113
    cerebral, 113, 1282–1283
    clinical consequences of, 113
    cytotoxic, 1282
    dependent, 113
    in inflammation, 46, 47, 47f
    interstitial, 1282–1283
    morphology of, 113
    in nephrotic syndrome, 922
    pathophysiology of, 111–113, 112f, 112t, 113f
    periorbital, 113
    pitting, 113
    pulmonary, 113, 680
        in heart failure
            left-sided, 535
            right-sided, 536
        hemodynamic (cardiogenic), 680, 680t
        due to microvascular injury, 680, 680t
        noncardiogenic (*See* Acute lung injury (ALI))
    subcutaneous, 113
    tissue, in right-sided heart failure, 536
    vasogenic, 1282
Edema factor (EF), in anthrax, 362
Edwards syndrome, 162, 163f
Effector cells, 194f, 195
Effector molecules, in signal transduction pathways, 90
Effector T lymphocytes, 190, 190f, 194f
    responses of differentiated, 207, 207f, 208f
Effusion, 67, 68f
EGF (epidermal growth factor), in tissue regeneration and wound healing, 87t, 88
EGFR (epidermal growth factor receptor), 88
    proto-oncogene for, 281t

EGFR (epidermal growth factor receptor) gene
    in glioblastoma, 1332
    in lung carcinoma, 724–725
EHEC (enterohemorrhagic *Escherichia coli*), 798t, 800f, 802
Ehlers-Danlos syndromes (EDSs), 145–147, 146t
    aneurysms in, 507
    bleeding disorders due to, 666
Ehrlichiosis, 380–381, 381f
EIC (endometrial intraepithelial carcinoma), 1034, 1034f, 1035f
Eicosanoids, in inflammation, 50, 57t, 58–60, 58f, 59t
EIDs (emerging infectious diseases), in Global Burden of Disease, 400
EIEC (enteroinvasive *Escherichia coli*), 798t, 802
Eisenmenger syndrome, 540
Elastic arteries, 488–489
Elastic fibers, in extracellular matrix, 96
Elastin, in extracellular matrix, 95f, 96
Electrical injury, 422
Electromechanical dissociation, 707
Elementary body (EB), of *Chlamydia trachomatis*, 380
Elephantiasis, 395, 395f
    edema due to, 113
Elschnig pearls, 1359
Embolism, 125–127
    air, 127
    amniotic fluid, 127, 128f
    cerebral infarction due to, 1293, 1293f
    fat and marrow, 126–127, 127f
    paradoxical, 126, 540, 547
    pulmonary, 126, 126f, 706–707, 706f
        septic, 717
Embolization, of thrombi, 124
Embolus(i)
    cholesterol, 126
    coronary artery occlusion due to, 547
    defined, 125–126
    from infective endocarditis, 567
    paradoxical, 126, 540, 547
    saddle, 126
Embryoid bodies, 1050
Embryonal carcinoma
    ovarian, 1050
    testicular, 989, 990f
Embryonal rhabdomyosarcoma
    of bladder, 981
    of vagina, 1017, 1017f
Embryonic stem (ES) cells, 82, 82f, 83
    in therapeutic cloning, 84, 84f
Embryopathy
    diabetic, 452
    retinoic acid, 453
    valproic acid, 453
Emerging infectious diseases (EIDs), in Global Burden of Disease, 400
Emery-Dreifuss muscular dystrophy, 1270t
Emphysema, 683t, 684–687
    anatomic site of, 683t
    bullous, 687, 687f
    centriacinar (centrilobular), 684, 684f, 685f
        in coal workers' pneumoconiosis, 698
    clinical course of, 683t, 686–687, 687t
    defined, 684
    distal acinar (paraseptal), 684
    etiology of, 683t
    incidence of, 684
    interstitial, 687
    irregular, 684
    major pathologic changes in, 683t
    morphology of, 685f, 686
    other forms of, 687, 687f

Emphysema *(Continued)*
    panacinar (panlobular), 684, 684f, 685f
    pathogenesis of, 684–686, 685f
    types of, 684, 684f, 685f
Empty sella syndrome, 1105
Empyema
    of gallbladder, 885
    of lung, 713, 731
    of sinus, 750
    subdural, 1300–1301
EMT (epithelial-to-mesenchymal transition), in metastasis, 302
ENaC (epithelial sodium channel), in cystic fibrosis, 465–466, 467f
Enamel, 740, 740f
Encephalitis
    HIV, 1305, 1305f
    limbic, in paraneoplastic syndrome, 1340
    mumps, 350
    viral, 1302–1306, 1303f–1306f
Encephalocele, 1284
Encephalomyelitis
    acute disseminated (perivenous), 1312–1313
    acute necrotizing hemorrhagic, 1312–1313
    experimental autoimmune, 1310
Encephalomyopathies, mitochondrial, 1325–1326, 1327–1328
Encephalopathy(ies)
    hepatic, 836, 1329
    hypertensive, 1295
    hypoxic/ischemic
        diffuse, 1291–1292, 1292f
        in left-sided heart failure, 536
    multicystic, 1286, 1286f
    subacute necrotizing, 1328
    transmissible spongiform, 1308–1309, 1308f, 1310f
    Wernicke, 1328
Encephalotrigeminal angiomatosis, 522
Enchondral ossification, 1209, 1209f
Enchondromas, 1227–1228, 1228f
Endarteritis, obliterative, in tuberculous meningoencephalitis, 1301
Endemic relapsing fever, 377
Endocannabinoids, 419–420
Endocardial fibroelastosis, 577
Endocarditis
    bacterial, 566–567, 568f
        glomerulonephritis due to, 934
    Candida, 384
    infective, 566–568
        acute *vs.* subacute, 567
        with artificial heart valve, 570–571
        clinical features of, 568
        diagnostic criteria for, 568f, 569t
        etiology and pathogenesis of, 567
        morphology of, 124, 567–568, 567f, 568f
    marantic, 568
    nonbacterial
        thrombotic, 124, 567f, 568–569, 570f
            due to cancer, 321t, 322
        verrucous, in systemic lupus erythematosus, 220, 220f
    prosthetic valve, 567
    rheumatic, 566, 567f
    subacute, 567
    valvular (Libman-Sacks, of systemic lupus erythematosus), 124, 220, 220f, 567f, 569
    vegetative, 124, 567f
Endocervical polyps, 1018, 1018f
Endocervix, 1007
Endocrine amyloid, 252t, 253

Endocrine disorders, 1097–1163
  of adrenal cortex, 1148–1159
    adrenocortical hyperfunction
        (hyperadrenalism) as, 1148–1154
      in adrenogenital syndromes, 1152–1154,
          1153f
      in hypercortisolism (Cushing syndrome),
          1148–1151, 1148t, 1149f–1151f,
          1150t
      in primary hyperaldosteronism,
          1151–1152, 1151f
    adrenocortical insufficiency as, 1154–1157
      causes of, 1154, 1154t
      primary acute, 1154–1155
      primary chronic (Addison disease),
          1155–1157, 1156f
      secondary, 1157
      in Waterhouse-Friderichsen syndrome,
          1155, 1155f, 1156f
    cysts as, 1159
    incidentalomas as, 1159
    myelolipomas as, 1159
    neoplastic, 1157–1158
      adenomas as, 1157–1158, 1157f, 1158f
      carcinomas as, 1158, 1158f
  of adrenal medulla, 1159–1161
    pheochromocytoma as, 1159–1162, 1160f,
        1160t, 1161f
  due to cancer, 321–322, 321t
  hypertension due to, 493t
  multiple endocrine neoplasia as, 1161–1163
    type 1, 1161–1162
    type 2, 1162–1163
  of pancreas, 1131–1147
    diabetes mellitus as, 1131–1146
      classification of, 1132, 1132t
      clinical features of, 1143–1146, 1144f,
          1145t
      complications of, 1138–1139, 1140f
      diagnosis of, 1131–1132
      epidemiology of, 1131
      glucose homeostasis and, 1132–1134,
          1133f, 1134f
      monogenic forms of, 1137–1138
      morphology of, 1139–1143, 1141f, 1142f
      pathogenesis of, 1134–1137, 1135f, 1136f
    neoplastic, 1146–1147
      α-cell tumors (glucagonomas) as, 1147
      carcinoid tumors as, 1147
      δ-cell tumors (somatostatinomas) as,
          1147
      hyperinsulinism (insulinoma) as,
          1146–1147, 1147f
      pancreatic polypeptide–secreting, 1147
      VIPoma as, 1147
      Zollinger-Ellison syndrome
          (gastrinomas) as, 1147
  of parathyroid glands, 1126–1130
    hyperparathyroidism as, 1126–1129
      primary, 1126–1129, 1127f, 1128f, 1129t
      secondary, 1129
    hypoparathyroidism as, 1129–1130
      pseudo-, 1130
  of pineal gland, 1163
  of pituitary gland, 1100–1107
    carcinoma as, 1105
    clinical manifestations of, 1100
    hypopituitarism as, 1100, 1105–1106
    due to hypothalamic suprasellar tumors,
        1106–1107, 1107f
    pituitary adenomas and hyperpituitarism
        as, 1100–1105
      ACTH cell (corticotroph), 1100t, 1104
      atypical, 1102

Endocrine disorders, of pituitary gland
    (Continued)
      classification of, 1100, 1100t
      clinical course of, 1103
      epidemiology of, 1100
      functional, 1100
      genetic abnormalities in, 1101–1102,
          1101t, 1102f
      gonadotroph (LH- and FSH-producing),
          1100t, 1104–1105
      growth hormone cell (somatotroph),
          1100t, 1104
      invasive, 1102
      mammosomatotroph, 1100t, 1104
      micro- vs. macro-, 1100
      morphology of, 1102, 1102f, 1103f
      nonfunctioning (silent variant, null-cell),
          1100, 1102f, 1105
      prolactinomas (lactotroph), 1100t,
          1103–1104, 1103f
      thyrotroph (TSH-producing), 1100t,
          1105
    posterior, 1106
      diabetes insipidus as, 1106
      SIADH as, 1106
  of thyroid gland, 1108–1126
    congenital anomalies as, 1126
    goiter as, 1107, 1116–1118
      diffuse nontoxic (simple), 1116, 1117f
      dyshormonogenetic, 1110
      multinodular, 1116–1118, 1117f
    Graves disease as, 1109, 1109f, 1114–1116,
        1115f
    hyperthyroidism as, 1108–1109, 1108t,
        1109f
    hypothyroidism as, 1109–1111, 1110t
      cretinism due to, 1110–1111
      myxedema due to, 1111
    neoplastic, 1118–1126
      adenomas as, 1118–1119, 1119f
      carcinomas as, 1119–1126, 1120f, 1121f,
          1123f–1125f
    thyroiditis as, 1111–1114
      defined, 1111
      Hashimoto, 1111–1113, 1112f
      infectious, 1111
      subacute (granulomatous, de Quervain),
          1113, 1113f
      subacute lymphocytic (painless),
          1113–1114
Endocrine neoplasm(s)
  of adrenal cortex, 1157–1158
    adenomas as, 1157–1158, 1157f, 1158f
    carcinomas as, 1158, 1158f
  G-protein signaling in, 1101, 1102f
  multiple endocrine neoplasia as, 1161–1163
    type 1, 1161–1162
    type 2, 1162–1163
  pancreatic, 1146–1147
    α-cell tumors (glucagonomas) as, 1147
    carcinoid tumors as, 1147
    δ-cell tumors (somatostatinomas) as,
        1147
    hyperinsulinism (insulinoma) as,
        1146–1147, 1147f
    pancreatic polypeptide–secreting, 1147
    VIPoma as, 1147
    Zollinger-Ellison syndrome (gastrinomas)
        as, 1147
  of thyroid gland, 1118–1126
    adenomas as, 1118–1119, 1119f
    carcinomas as, 1119–1126, 1120f, 1121f,
        1123f–1125f
Endocrine signaling, 89, 90f

Endocrine system, 1097–1163
  adrenal cortex in, 1148–1159
    anatomy of, 1148
  adrenal medulla in, 1159–1161
    anatomy of, 1148, 1159
  feedback inhibition in, 1098
  hormones in, 1098
  pancreas in, 1130–1147
    anatomy of, 1130, 1131f
  parathyroid glands in, 1126–1130
    anatomy of, 1126
  pineal gland in, 1163
  pituitary gland in, 1098–1107
    anatomy of, 1098–1099, 1099f
  thyroid gland in, 1107–1126
    anatomy of, 1107–1108, 1108f
Endodermal sinus tumor
  ovarian, 1049, 1049f
  testicular, 989–990
Endoglin, in preeclampsia, 1056–1057
Endolymphatic stromal myosis, 1035
Endometrial carcinoma, 1031–1034
  and breast carcinoma, 1077
  clinical course of, 1034
  epidemiology of, 1031
  molecular pathogenesis of, 1031, 1032t
  morphology of, 1032–1033, 1033f, 1034, 1035f
  type I, 1031–1033, 1032f, 1032t, 1033f
  type II, 1032t, 1033–1034, 1034f, 1035f
Endometrial changes, due to oral contraceptives,
    1027
Endometrial hyperplasia, 8, 1029–1031, 1031f
  and endometrial carcinoma, 1032, 1032f
Endometrial intraepithelial carcinoma (EIC),
    1034, 1034f, 1035f
Endometrial polyps, 1026f, 1029
Endometrioid adenocarcinoma, 1033, 1033f,
    1045–1046
Endometrioid adenofibromas, 1045
Endometrioid carcinoma, 1033, 1033f,
    1045–1046
Endometrioid tumors, ovarian, 1045–1046
Endometriosis, 1028–1029, 1028f
Endometritis, 1026f, 1027–1028
Endometrium
  adenosarcomas of, 1035
  anatomy of, 1024
  carcinoma of, 1031–1034
    clinical course of, 1034
    epidemiology of, 1031
    molecular pathogenesis of, 1031, 1032t
    morphology of, 1032–1033, 1033f, 1034,
        1035f
    type I, 1031–1033, 1032f, 1032t, 1033f
    type II, 1032t, 1033–1034, 1034f, 1035f
  dating of, 1024, 1025
  endometriosis and adenomyosis of,
      1028–1029, 1028f, 1029f
  functional disorders of (dysfunctional uterine
      bleeding), 1026–1027, 1026f, 1027t
  histology in menstrual cycle of, 1024–1026,
      1025f
  hyperplasia of, 1029–1031, 1031f
  inflammation of, 1027–1028
  malignant mixed müllerian tumors of,
      1034–1035, 1036f
  polyps of, 1029
  stromal tumors of, 1035
Endomyocardial fibrosis, 577
Endomyocarditis, Loeffler, 577
Endoneurium, 1258
Endophthalmitis, 1355
Endoplasmic reticulum (ER) stress, 25, 31
Endostatin, in angiogenesis, 102

Endothelial cell(s)
  retraction of, in inflammation, 47, 47f
  vascular, response to injury of, 490–491, 490t, 491f
Endothelial cell activation, 61, 490–491, 491f
  in septic shock, 130–131
Endothelial dysfunction, 491, 491f
Endothelial injury
  in atherosclerosis, 499–500, 501f
  disseminated intravascular coagulation due to, 673
  in inflammation, 47, 47f
  in septic shock, 130–131
  in thrombosis, 121
  in thrombotic microangiopathies, 952
Endothelial nitric oxide synthase (eNOS), 60
Endothelial precursor cells (EPCs), angiogenesis from, 99f, 100
Endothelial-leukocyte adhesion molecules, 49, 49f, 49t, 50
Endothelin, in hemostasis, 115, 116f
Endothelitis, in acute cellular rejection, 228
Endothelium
  anticoagulant effects of, 116
  antifibrinolytic effects of, 117
  antiplatelet effects of, 116
  antithrombotic properties of, 115–116, 117f
  fibrinolytic effects of, 116
  in hemostasis, 115–117, 116f–118f
  platelet effects of, 116
  procoagulant effects of, 117
  prothrombotic properties of, 116–117, 117f, 118f
Endotoxin, bacterial, 344
Endovascular stents, pathology of, 526, 526f
End-stage renal disease, 907
Energy balance, regulation of, 439–442, 440f, 441f
Engulfment, in phagocytosis, 53, 53f
eNOS (endothelial nitric oxide synthase), 60
Entamoeba histolytica, 335
  enterocolitis due to, 805f, 806
Enteric fever
  due to *Campylobacter*, 799
  typhoid, 798t, 801–802
Enteric infections, 358t
Enteritis-associated arthritis, 1241
Enteroaggregative *Escherichia coli* (EAEC), 798t, 800f, 802
Enterobacteriaceae, morphology of, 334f
Enterobius vermicularis, enterocolitis due to, 806
Enterochromaffin cells, of pancreas, 1130
Enterochromaffin-like (ECL) cells, 779
Enterococcal infections, 359–360
Enterocolitis
  infectious, 797–807, 798t
    Campylobacter, 798t, 799–800, 800f
    due to cholera, 797–799, 798t, 799f
    due to enteric (typhoid) fever, 798t, 801–802
    due to *Escherichia coli*, 798t, 800f, 802
    mycobacterial, 794t, 798t, 804, 804f
    parasitic, 794t, 805—807, 805f
    pseudomembranous, 798t, 803, 803f
    due to salmonellosis, 798t, 801
    due to shigellosis, 798t, 800–801
    viral, 805f, 1708–1709
    due to Whipple disease, 798t, 803–804, 804f
    due to *Yersinia* spp, 798t, 800f, 802
  necrotizing, 458, 459f, 793
  radiation, 793
Enterohemorrhagic *Escherichia coli* (EHEC), 798t, 800f, 802
Enterohepatic circulation, 840

Enteroinvasive *Escherichia coli* (EIEC), 798t, 802
Enteropathogenic bacteria, 338
Enteropathy
  autoimmune, 794t, 796–797
  gluten-sensitive, 794t, 795–796, 795f, 796f
    IgA nephropathy with, 931
Enteropathy-associated T-cell lymphoma, 796
Enterotoxigenic *Escherichia coli* (ETEC), 798t, 802
Environment, defined, 400
Environmental carcinogens, 273, 274t
Environmental causes, of congenital anomalies, 451–452
Environmental disease(s), 399–427
  adverse drug reactions as, 414–417, 415f, 416t, 417f
  due to alcohol, 412–414, 413f
  due to climate change, 401–402, 401f
  defined, 400
  drug abuse as, 417–420, 418t, 419f
  due to electrical injury, 422
  epidemiology of, 400
  Global Burden of Disease for, 400, 401f
  historical background of, 400
  due to mechanical trauma, 420–421, 420f
  due to occupational health risks, 408–410, 409t
  due to pollution, 403–408
    air, 403–405, 404t
    by metals, 406–408, 406f, 407f
  due to radiation injury, 423–427, 423f, 424f, 425t, 426f
  due to thermal injury, 421–422
  due to tobacco, 410–412, 410f–412f, 411t, 412t
  due to toxicity of chemical and physical agents, 402–403, 402f, 403f
Environmental factors, white cell neoplasia due to, 598
Environmental hazards, toxicity of, 402–403, 402f, 403f
Environmental toxins, and breast cancer, 1077
Enzyme(s)
  in immediate hypersensitivity, 199–200
  in phagocytosis, 54
Enzyme defect(s), 143–144, 143t, 144f, 149–156
  alkaptonuria due to, 155–156
  Gaucher disease due to, 151t, 153–154, 154f
  glycogen storage diseases due to, 155, 156f, 157t, 158f
  lysosomal storage diseases due to, 149–155, 150f, 151t
  mucopolysaccharidoses due to, 151t, 154–155
  Niemann-Pick disease due to
    type C, 153
    types A and B, 151t, 152–153, 153f
  Tay-Sachs disease due to, 139f, 150–152, 151t, 152f
Enzyme inhibitor defect, 143t
Eosinophil(s)
  adult reference range for, 592t
  in chronic inflammation, 72, 73f
  differentiation of, 591f
  in immediate hypersensitivity, 200
Eosinophilia, 594t
  in inflammation, 75
  in necrosis, 14
  pulmonary, 704
    tropical, 395
  secondary, 704
  tropical, 704
    pulmonary, 395
Eosinophilic cystitis, 975
Eosinophilic esophagitis, 769f, 770
Eosinophilic gastritis, 780

Eosinophilic granuloma, 632
Eosinophilic leukemia, chronic, 626t
Eosinophilic leukocytosis, 594t
Eosinophilic pneumonia
  acute, 704
  idiopathic chronic, 704
Eotaxin, 62
EPCs (endothelial precursor cells), angiogenesis from, 99f, 100
Ependymal cells, response to injury of, 1282
Ependymal granulations, 1282
Ependymitis, granular, in neurosyphilis, 1302
Ependymomas, 1334–1335, 1335f
  myxopapillary, 1334
Ephelis, 1168
Epicardial coronary arteries, 532
Epidemic relapsing fever, 377
Epidemic typhus, 380, 381, 381f
Epidermal appendages, diseases of, 1197–1199
  acne vulgaris as, 1197–1198, 1199f
  rosacea as, 1198–1199
Epidermal growth factor (EGF), in tissue regeneration and wound healing, 87t, 88
Epidermal growth factor receptor (EGFR), 88
  proto-oncogene for, 281t
Epidermal growth factor receptor *(EGFR)* gene
  in glioblastoma, 1332
  in lung carcinoma, 724–725
Epidermal inclusion cyst, 1176
Epidermal maturation, disorders of, 1186
Epidermal tumors, premalignant and malignant, 1178–1181
  actinic keratosis as, 1178, 1179f
  basal cell carcinoma as, 1180–1181, 1181f, 1183f
  squamous cell carcinoma as, 1178–1180, 1179f
Epidermis, 1166f, 1167f
  stem cells in, 85
Epidermolysis bullosa, 1193f, 1196, 1198f
  junctional, 1196, 1198f
Epididymis, inflammation of, 986–987, 986f
Epididymitis, 986–987, 986f
Epidural hematoma, 1289, 1289f
Epigenetic changes, in carcinogenesis, 306–307
Epigenetics, 136, 180–181, 306
Epineurium, 1258
Epiphrenic diverticulum, 767
Epiploic appendices, 815
Epispadias, 982
Epithelial cell injury, in glomerular disease, 915, 915f
Epithelial cyst, 1176
Epithelial hyperplasia, of breast, 1071, 1072f
Epithelial inclusion cysts, of ovary, 1042, 1042f
Epithelial sodium channel (ENaC), in cystic fibrosis, 465–466, 467f
Epithelial tumors
  benign, 1175–1178
    acanthosis nigricans as, 1175–1176
    adnexal (appendage) tumors as, 1176–1178, 1177f, 1178f
    epithelial cyst (wen) as, 1176
    fibroepithelial polyp as, 1176
    seborrheic keratoses as, 1175, 1175f
  ovarian, 1040t, 1041–1047, 1041f
Epithelial-to-mesenchymal transition (EMT), in metastasis, 302
Epithelioid cells, 207, 207f
Epithelioid hemangioendothelioma, 524
Epithelioid malignant schwannomas, 1342
Epithelioid mesothelioma, 733–734, 733f
Epithelium, in innate immunity, 184
Epitope spreading, 212–213

Epstein-Barr virus (EBV), 355–357
  in AIDS, 248
  in Burkitt lymphoma, 314–315, 314f, 608
  clinical features of, 357
  in extranodal NK/T-cell lymphoma, 616
  in Hodgkin lymphoma, 620
  morphology of, 356–357, 356f
  oncogenic potential of, 314–315, 314f, 597
  pathogenesis of, 355–356, 356f
  structure of, 333f
ER(s) (estrogen receptors), in breast carcinoma,
    1074, 1075, 1076, 1079, 1084, 1090
ER (endoplasmic reticulum) stress, 25, 31
ERB-1, 88
ERB-2, 88
ERBB1 gene, 281, 281t
ERBB2 gene, 281, 281t, 306, 324
Erlenmeyer flask deformity, 1213
Erosion, 1168
Erysipelas, 360, 360f
Erythema, 113
  chronicum migrans, 378
  induratum, 1199
  infectiosum, perinatal infection with, 459,
    459f, 461
  multiforme, 1189, 1190f
    oral manifestations of, 744t
  nodosum, 1199
Erythroblastosis fetalis, 202, 461, 462f, 840
Erythrocyte(s)
  adult reference range for, 592t
  differentiation of, 591f
Erythrocyte sedimentation rate, 75
Erythroderma, 1190
Erythroid precursors, in hemolytic anemia, 642,
    642f
Erythromelalgia, in essential thrombocytosis,
    630
Erythroplakia, of oral cavity, 744–745, 745f
Erythropoiesis, anemias of diminished, 640t,
    654–665
  aplastic, 662–664, 663f, 663t, 664f
  of chronic disease, 662
  due to chronic renal failure, 665
  of folate deficiency, 655t, 658–659
  due to hepatocellular liver disease, 665
  iron deficiency, 659–662, 659t, 660f–662f
  megaloblastic, 654–659, 655f, 655t, 656f
  myelophthisic, 665
  pernicious (vitamin B_{12} deficiency), 655–658,
    655t, 656f, 657f
  due to pure red cell aplasia, 664–665
ES (embryonic stem) cells, 82, 82f, 83
  in therapeutic cloning, 84, 84f
Escherichia coli
  abscesses due to, 378
  enterocolitis due to, 798t, 800f, 802
  morphology of, 334f
  O157:H17, 798t, 800f, 802
  thrombotic microangiopathies due to, 953
E-selectin, in inflammation, 49, 49t
Esophageal adenocarcinoma, 772, 773f
  Barrett esophagus and, 770
Esophageal atresia, 765, 765f
Esophageal dysmotility, 767
Esophageal dysplasia, in Barrett esophagus, 771,
    771f
Esophageal lacerations, 768
Esophageal metaplasia, in Barrett esophagus,
    770–771, 770f
Esophageal mucosal webs, 767
Esophageal obstruction, 767–768
Esophageal rings, 767–768
Esophageal spasm, diffuse, 767

Esophageal stenosis, 767
Esophageal tumors, 772–774
  adenocarcinoma as, 772, 773f
    Barrett esophagus and, 770
  benign, 774
  squamous cell carcinoma as, 773–774, 773f
  uncommon, 774
Esophageal varices, 519–520, 771, 772f
Esophagitis, 768–770
  Candida, 383, 383f
  chemical and infectious, 768–769, 769f
  eosinophilic, 769f, 770
  herpes, 353
  due to lacerations, 768, 768t
  pill-induced, 768
  reflux, 769–770, 769f
Esophagus, 767–774
  achalasia of, 768
  agenesis of, 765
  anatomy of, 767
  Barrett, 770–771, 770f, 771f
  ectopia of, 765
  nutcracker, 767
Essential thrombocytosis (ET), 626t, 629–630,
    630f
Esthesioneuroblastoma, 751
Estrogen, in menstrual cycle, 1024, 1025
Estrogen exposure, and breast cancer, 1076, 1079
Estrogen receptors (ERs), in breast carcinoma,
    1074, 1075, 1076, 1079, 1084, 1090
État criblé, 1295
ETEC (enterotoxigenic Escherichia coli), 798t,
    802
Ethanol
  CNS toxicity of, 1329, 1329f
  effects of, 412–414, 413f
  metabolism of, 412, 413, 413f
Ethanol myopathy, 1275
Etiology, 4
ETS family transcription factors, in prostate
    adenocarcinoma, 306
ETS genes
  in Ewing sarcoma, 1232
  in prostate cancer, 997
ETV6-NTRK3 fusion transcript, 474
Euploidy, 159
Euthyroid metabolic state, 1116
Evelyn, John, 404
Ewing sarcoma, 1232–1233, 1233f
  genetic basis for, 305t, 306, 1249t
EWS-FL11 protein, 306
EWSR1 gene, 306
Excoriation, 1167
Executioner caspases, 30
  in apoptosis, 295
Exercise, and breast cancer, 1077
Exercise-induced cardiac hypertrophy, 535
Exocytosis, 1168
Exophthalmic ophthalmoplegia, 1275
Exostosis, 1227, 1227f
Exotoxins, bacterial, 344
Experimental autoimmune encephalomyelitis,
    1310
Exstrophy, of bladder, 974, 974f
EXT1 gene, in osteochondroma, 1227
EXT2 gene, in osteochondroma, 1227
External elastic lamina, of blood vessels, 488
External herniation, 790
External limiting membrane, of retina, 1359f
External os, of cervix, 1007
Extracellular matrix (ECM)
  in angiogenesis, 101–102
  components of, 94–98, 95f, 95t, 97f, 98f
  functions of, 94

Extracellular matrix (ECM) (Continued)
  invasion of, in metastasis, 298–300, 299f
  in regeneration and repair, 80, 81f, 98
Extracellular matrix (ECM) proteins, in
    angiogenesis, 101–102
Extradural abscess, 1301
Extrahepatic bile duct disorder(s), 887–888
  biliary atresia as, 887
  choledochal cysts as, 887–888
  choledocholithiasis and ascending cholangitis
    as, 887
Extralobar sequestrations, 679
Extranodal NK/T-cell lymphoma, 601t, 616
Extravascular hemolysis, 641
  in β-thalassemia major, 649, 650f
Exudate, 46, 46f
  fibrinous, 68, 68f
Eye(s), 1345–1368
  anatomy of, 1346, 1346f
  anterior segment of, 1353–1355
    cataracts of, 1353
    endophthalmitis and panophthalmitis of,
      1355, 1355f, 1356f
    functional anatomy of, 1353, 1354f
    and glaucoma, 1353–1355
  conjunctiva of, 1349–1350
    functional anatomy of, 1346f, 1348f, 1349
    neoplasms of, 1349–1350, 1350f
    pinguecula and pterygium of, 1349
    scarring of, 1349
  cornea of, 1351–1353
    degenerations and dystrophies of,
      1351–1353, 1352f
    functional anatomy of, 1346f, 1351, 1351f
    keratitis and ulcers of, 1351, 1351f
  end-stage (phthisis bulbi), 1368
  eyelid of, 1348–1349
    functional anatomy of, 1348, 1348f
    neoplasms of, 1348–1349, 1348f
  hypoplastic, 1368
  microphthalmic, 1368
  optic nerve of, 1346f, 1365–1368
    anterior ischemic optic neuropathy of,
      1366, 1366f
    glaucomatous damage to, 1366–1367,
      1367f
    Leber hereditary neuropathy of, 1367
    neuritis of, 1367–1368
    papilledema of, 1366, 1366f
  orbit of, 1346–1348
    cellulitis of, 1347
    functional anatomy and proptosis of,
      1346–1347
    idiopathic inflammation of, 1347, 1347f
    mucormycosis of, 1347
    neoplasms of, 1348
    thyroid ophthalmopathy of, 1347, 1347f
    Wegener granulomatosis of, 1347
  retina and vitreous of, 1357–1365
    age-related macular degeneration of, 1346,
      1363–1364, 1364f
    detachment of, 1357–1358, 1360f
    functional anatomy of, 1346f, 1357, 1359f
    neoplasms of, 1365, 1365f
    retinitis of, 1364–1365
    retinitis pigmentosa of, 1364
    vascular disease of, 1358–1363
      due to diabetes mellitus, 1359–1361,
        1362f, 1363f
      due to hypertension, 1359, 1361f, 1362f
      radiation retinopathy as, 1361–1362
      retinal artery and vein occlusions as,
        1362–1363, 1364f
      retinal vasculitis as, 1361–1362

Eye(s) *(Continued)*
  retinopathy of prematurity as, 1361
  sickle retinopathy as, 1361–1362
  in sarcoidosis, 702–703
  sclera of, 1346f, 1350
  uvea of, 1355–1357
    neoplasms of, 1356–1357, 1358f
    uveitis of, 1355–1356, 1356f
Eye movement disorders, in paraneoplastic
    syndrome, 1340
Eyelid, 1348–1349
  functional anatomy of, 1348, 1348f
  neoplasms of, 1348–1349, 1348f
EZH2
  in carcinogenesis, 307
  in prostate cancer, 997

F

FAB (French-American-British) classification, of
    acute myeloid leukemia, 622, 622t
Fabry disease, 151t
Factitial panniculitis, 1199
Factor III, in hemostasis, 115
Factor V Leiden mutation, and thrombosis, 122,
    123
Factor VIII, 670–671, 671f
Factor VIII deficiency, 143t, 672
Factor VIII-vWF complex, 670–671, 671f
Factor IX deficiency, 672–673
Factor XII, in inflammation, 64, 65, 65f, 66
Facultative intracellular bacteria, 335
FADD (Fas-associated death domain), in
    apoptosis, 30, 295, 296f
Fallopian tubes, 1038–1039
  anatomy of, 1007
  development of, 1006, 1007f
  inflammations of, 1038
  tumors and cysts of, 1038–1039
Familial adenomatous polyposis (FAP), 274,
    816t, 820–821, 822f, 822t
Familial amyloid polyneuropathies, 253, 1263,
    1264t
Familial cancers, 275, 275t
Familial disorders, 140
Familial dysautonomia, 1263t
Familial hematuria, benign, 932
Familial hypercholesterolemia, 144, 147–149,
    147t–149f
Familial hypocalciuric hypercalcemia, 1127
Familial isolated hypoparathyroidism (FIH),
    1130
Familial Mediterranean fever, 253
Familial mental retardation 1 *(FMR1)* gene, 139,
    169, 170
Familial mental retardation protein (FMRP),
    170–171, 170f
Familial mild fasting hyperglycemia, 1137
Fanconi anemia, 302–303, 663
FAP (familial adenomatous polyposis), 274,
    816t, 820–821, 822f, 822t
Farmer's lung, 703
Fas ligand (FasL), in apoptosis, 29–30, 31,
    211
Fas-associated death domain (FADD), in
    apoptosis, 30, 295, 296f
Fasciculations, in amyotrophic lateral sclerosis,
    1325
Fasciitis, nodular (infiltrative,
    pseudosarcomatous), 1250–1251, 1250f
Fascioscapulohumeral muscular dystrophy,
    1270t
FASDs (fetal alcohol spectrum disorders),
    452
Fat embolism, 126–127

Fat intake
  and atherosclerosis, 444
  and breast cancer, 444
  and colon cancer, 443
Fat necrosis, 16, 17f
  of breast, 1070
Fat saponification, 16, 17f
Fatal familial insomnia (FFI), 1308, 1309
Fatty change, 13, 33–34, 34f
  due to alcohol consumption, 857–858, 857f,
    859–860
  in Wilson disease, 864
Fatty liver, 33–34, 34f
  due to alcohol consumption, 857–858, 857f,
    859–860
  of pregnancy, 875
Fatty liver disease, nonalcoholic, 860–861, 861f
Fatty streaks, in atherosclerosis, 501, 502, 502f
Fatty tumors, 1249–1250
Favism, 644
FBN-1 (fibrillin-1) gene, 144–145, 563
FBN-2 (fibrillin-2) gene, 144–145
Fc receptor, in antibody-mediated
    hypersensitivity, 202f, 203
Feathery degeneration, in cholestasis, 842
Fecalith, 827
Feedback inhibition, 1098
Felons, 359
Female genital tract, 1005–1061
  anatomy of, 1007–1008, 1008f
  cervix in, 1017–1024
    endocervical polyps of, 1018, 1018f
    inflammations of, 1017
    premalignant and malignant neoplasms of,
      1018–1024
      cervical carcinoma as, 1021–1024, 1022f,
        1023f
      cervical intraepithelial neoplasia as,
        1019–1021, 1020f, 1020t, 1021f,
        1021t
      pathogenesis of, 1018–1019, 1018f, 1019f
  development of, 1006–1007, 1007f
  endometrium in
    adenosarcomas of, 1035
    anatomy of, 1024
    carcinoma of, 1031–1034, 1032f–1035f,
      1032t
    endometriosis and adenomyosis of,
      1028–1029, 1028f, 1029f
    functional disorders of (dysfunctional
      uterine bleeding), 1026–1027, 1026f,
      1027t
    histology in menstrual cycle of, 1024–1026,
      1025f
    hyperplasia of, 1029–1031, 1031f
    inflammation of, 1027–1028
    malignant mixed müllerian tumors of,
      1034–1035, 1036f
    polyps of, 1029
    stromal tumors of, 1035
  fallopian tubes in, 1038–1039
    inflammations of, 1038
    tumors and cysts of, 1038–1039
  gestational and placental disorders of,
    1052–1061
    choriocarcinoma as, 1059–1061, 1060f
    of early pregnancy, 1053–1054
    ectopic pregnancy as, 1053–1054
    gestational trophoblastic disease as,
      1057–1061
    hydatidiform mole as, 1057–1059, 1058f,
      1059f
    invasive mole as, 1059, 1060f
    of late pregnancy, 1054–1057

Female genital tract, gestational and placental
    disorders of *(Continued)*
    placental anatomy and, 1052–1053, 1053f,
      1054f
    of placental implantation, 1055
    placental infections as, 1055, 1055f
    placental-site trophoblastic tumor as, 1061,
      1061f
    preeclampsia and eclampsia as, 1055–1057,
      1056f, 1057f
    spontaneous abortion as, 1053
    twin placentas as, 1054, 1055f
  infections of, 1008–1010, 1009f, 1010f
  myometrium in
    anatomy of, 1024
    leiomyomas of, 264f, 271f, 1026f,
      1036–1037, 1037f
    leiomyosarcomas of, 1037–1038, 1038f
  ovaries in, 1039–1052
    cortical inclusion cysts of, 1042, 1042f
    follicle and luteal cysts of, 1039
    polycystic, 1039–1040, 1039f
    stromal hyperthecosis of, 1039f, 1040
    tumors of, 1040–1052
      Brenner, 1046, 1046f
      choriocarcinoma as, 1049
      classification of, 1040–1041, 1040t
      clear cell adenocarcinoma as, 1046
      cystadenofibroma as, 1046
      derivation of, 1041f
      dysgerminoma as, 1048–1049, 1049f
      endodermal sinus (yolk sac), 1049, 1049f
      endometrioid, 1045–1046
      epidemiology of, 1040
      fibromas, thecomas, and fibrothecomas
        as, 1051, 1051f
      frequency of, 1041t
      germ cell, 1040t, 1041f, 1047–1050, 1047t
      granulosa–theca cell, 1050, 1050f
      metastatic, 1040t, 1041f, 1052
      mucinous, 1044–1045, 1045f
      serous, 1042–1044, 1043f
      Sertoli–Leydig cell (androblastomas),
        1051–1052, 1051f
      sex cord–stromal, 1040t, 1041f,
        1050–1052
      of surface (müllerian) epithelium, 1040t,
        1041–1047, 1041f
      teratomas as, 1047–1048, 1048f
  vagina in, 1016–1017
    developmental anomalies of, 1016
    premalignant and malignant neoplasms of,
      1016–1017, 1016f, 1017f
  vulva in, 1011–1016
    Bartholin cyst of, 1011
    benign exophytic lesions of, 1012, 1012f
    condyloma acuminatum of, 1012, 1012f
    glandular neoplastic lesions of, 1015, 1015f
    lichen sclerosis of, 1011, 1011f
    malignant melanoma of, 1015–1016
    non-neoplastic epithelial disorders of,
      1011–1012, 1011f
    Paget disease of, 1015, 1015f
    papillary hidradenoma of, 1015, 1015f
    squamous cell hyperplasia of, 1011f, 1012
    squamous neoplastic lesions of, 1012–1014,
      1013f, 1014f
    vulvar carcinoma as, 1012–1014, 1013f,
      1014f
    vulvar intraepithelial neoplasia as,
      1012–1014, 1013f
Female pseudohermaphroditism, 167
Ferritin, 659–660
Ferroportin, 660, 661f

Ferruginous bodies, 700
Fetal alcohol spectrum disorders (FASDs), 452
Fetal alcohol syndrome, 414, 452
Fetal anemia, fetal hydrops due to, 461, 461t
Fetal growth restriction (FGR), causes of,
   454–456, 455f
Fetal hemoglobin (HbF), 645
Fetal hydrops, 459–462
   clinical features of, 462
   defined, 459–460
   immune, 460–461, 460f
   morphology of, 461–462, 462f
   nonimmune, 460, 461, 461t
Fetal infection, 455
Fetal influences, on fetal growth restriction, 455
Fetal lung maturity, 457
Fetal macrosomia, 452
Fetor hepaticus, 836
Fever(s)
   black, 389
   familial Mediterranean, 253
   hay, 749
   in inflammation, 66t, 74
   relapsing, 377
   rheumatic, 203t
   Rocky Mountain spotted, 381, 382f
   scarlet, 360
      oral manifestations of, 744t
   typhus, 380, 381, 381f
   viral hemorrhagic, 349t, 351
Fever blisters, 352
FFI (fatal familial insomnia), 1308, 1309
FGF (fibroblast growth factor)
   proto-oncogene for, 281t
   in tissue regeneration and wound healing, 87t,
      88
FGF3 gene, 281t
FGF-7 (fibroblast growth factor 7), in benign
   prostatic hyperplasia, 995
FGFR3 (fibroblast growth factor receptor 3), 451
   in achondroplasia, 1210
FGFR3 gene, in seborrheic keratosis, 1175
FGR (fetal growth restriction), causes of,
   454–456, 455f
FH₄ (tetrahydrofolic acid), 657, 657f, 658
Fiber intake, and colon cancer, 443
Fibrillar collagens, in extracellular matrix, 95,
   95f, 95t
Fibrillary glomerulonephritis, 935
Fibrillin
   in congenital heart disease, 539t
   defect in, 143t, 507
   in extracellular matrix, 96
   in mitral valve prolapse, 563
Fibrillin-1 (FBN-1) gene, 144–145, 563
Fibrillin-2 (FBN-2) gene, 144–145
Fibrin
   in coagulation cascade, 118, 119f
   in glomerular injury, 916
   in hemostasis, 115, 118
   in inflammation, 65f
Fibrin degradation products. See Fibrin split
   products (FSPs).
Fibrin split products (FSPs)
   in fibrinolysis, 120, 121f
   in hemostasis, 118
   in inflammation, 65, 65f
Fibrinogen, 74–75
   in coagulation cascade, 118, 119f
   in platelet aggregation, 118
Fibrinoid necrosis, 16–17, 17f
   of arterioles, in malignant hypertension,
      950–951, 950f
   in immune complex vasculitis, 205, 205f

Fibrinolysis, 120, 121f
Fibrinolytic cascade, 120, 121f
Fibrinolytic effects, of endothelium, 116
Fibrinolytic system, in inflammation, 65, 65f, 66
Fibrinous exudate, 68, 68f
Fibrinous inflammation, 67–68, 68f
Fibrinous pericarditis, 68f
Fibroadenoma, of breast, 268f, 1091–1092, 1091f
Fibroblast(s)
   in carcinogenesis, 303
   in wound healing, 102, 103, 103f
Fibroblast growth factor (FGF)
   proto-oncogene for, 281t
   in tissue regeneration and wound healing, 87t,
      88
Fibroblast growth factor 7 (FGF-7), in benign
   prostatic hyperplasia, 995
Fibroblast growth factor receptor 3 (FGFR3),
   451
   in achondroplasia, 1210
Fibrocystic changes, 1071, 1071f
Fibrocystin, 959
Fibroelastoma, papillary, cardiac, 584
Fibroelastosis, endocardial, 577
Fibroepithelial polyps, 1176
   of ureters, 973
   of vulva, 1012
Fibrogenic tumors, 1223t, 1230–1232
Fibrohistiocytic tumors, 1252–1253
Fibroids, uterine, 264f, 271f, 1026f, 1036–1037,
   1037f
Fibrolamellar carcinoma, of liver, 879, 880f
Fibroma(s)
   chondromyxoid, 1229, 1229f
   non-ossifying, 1230, 1231f
   of oral cavity
      irritation, 741, 741f
      peripheral ossifying, 742
   ovarian, 1051, 1051f
Fibromatosis(es)
   aggressive, 107
   of breast, 1092
   deep-seated, 1251–1252
   in infants and children, 474
   of soft tissue, 1251–1252, 1252f
   superficial (palmar, plantar, penile), 1251
Fibromuscular dysplasia, 490
   of renal artery, 951, 951f
Fibronectin, in extracellular matrix, 96, 97f
Fibro-osseous tumors, 1223t, 1230–1232
Fibrosarcoma(s), 1232
   congenital-infantile, 474
      genetic basis for, 1249t
   of ovaries, 1051
   of soft tissue, 1252, 1252f
Fibrosing disease, of lungs, 694–701
   cryptogenic organizing pneumonia as, 696,
      696f
   drug-induced, 701, 701t
   idiopathic pulmonary fibrosis as, 694–695,
      694f, 695f
   nonspecific interstitial pneumonia as, 695
   pneumoconioses as, 696–701, 697t, 698f–700f
   pulmonary involvement in connective tissue
      disease as, 696
   radiation-induced, 701
Fibrosis
   of breast, 1071
   in inflammation, 66, 67f, 70, 70f
   due to ionizing radiation, 424f, 425, 426f
   pipe-stem, 394, 394f
   in systemic sclerosis, 224
   in tissue repair, 80, 99, 107–108, 107f, 108f
Fibrothecomas, ovarian, 1051, 1051f

Fibrotic disorders, 108
Fibrous capsule, of tumor, 268, 268f
Fibrous cortical defects, 1230, 1231f
Fibrous dysplasia, 1230–1232, 1232f
Fibrous histiocytoma
   benign, 1182, 1184f, 1253
   malignant, 1253
Fibrous mesothelioma, benign, 732–733, 732f
Fibrous proliferative lesions, of oral cavity,
   741–742, 741f
Fibrous synarthroses, 1235
Fibrous tumors
   of bone, 1223t, 1230–1232
   of breast, 1092
   in infants and children, 474
   of soft tissue, 1250–1252
Fibrous union, in wound healing, 103f
Fibrovascular polyps, of esophagus, 774
Fifth disease of childhood, perinatal infection
   with, 459, 459f, 461
FIH (familial isolated hypoparathyroidism),
   1130
Filariasis
   edema due to, 113
   lymphatic, 395, 395f
Filtration slits, 910, 910f
Fine-needle aspiration, of tumors, 323
Fingertip regeneration, 92
Fish, methyl mercury in, 408
FISH (fluorescence in situ hybridization), 179,
   179f
Fish oil, for inflammation, 60
Fistulas
   arteriovenous, 489–490
   gastrointestinal, 764–765, 765f
   tracheoesophageal, 765, 765f
   vesicouterine, 974
Flame cells, in multiple myeloma, 610
Flax dust, lung diseases due to, 697t
Flesh-eating bacteria, 360
FLIP, and apoptosis, 30, 296
"Floaters," 1357
Flow cytometry, 324
FLT3 gene, 280, 281t
   in acute myeloid leukemia, 624
Fluorescence in situ hybridization (FISH), 179,
   179f
Fluoride deficiency, 439t
Fluorophore indicators, 175
FMR1 (familial mental retardation 1) gene, 139,
   169, 170
FMRP (familial mental retardation protein),
   170–171, 170f
FMS-like tyrosine kinase 3 receptor,
   proto-oncogene for, 280, 281t
Foam cells, 34, 35f
   in atherosclerosis, 500, 501f, 502, 502f
Focal adhesion complexes, in extracellular
   matrix, 97f
Focal cerebral ischemia, 1291, 1292–1294, 1293f,
   1294f
Focal nodular hyperplasia, hepatic, 876, 876f
Focal proliferative glomerulonephritis, in
   systemic lupus erythematosus, 217–218,
   218f
Focal segmental glomerulosclerosis (FSGS),
   918t, 926–928
   autosomal-recessive, 927
   due to chronic pyelonephritis, 943–944
   classification and types of, 926
   clinical course of, 928
   idiopathic, 926
   morphology of, 926–927, 927f
   pathogenesis of, 926–928

Focal segmental glomerulosclerosis (FSGS) (*Continued*)
  progressive nature of, 916–917, 917f
  renal ablation, 927–928
Fogo selvagem, 1193, 1193f
Foix-Alajouanine disease, 1298
Folate, function of, 438t
Folate deficiency, 438t
Folate deficiency anemia, 655t, 658–659
Folic acid, dietary sources of, 658–659
Folic acid antagonists, 659
Folic acid deficiency anemia, 655t, 658–659
Follicle cysts, 1039
Follicle-stimulating hormone (FSH)-producing adenomas, 1100t, 1104–1105
Follicular adenoma, of thyroid, 1118–1119, 1119f, 1123, 1124f
Follicular carcinoma, of thyroid, 1120–1121, 1123–1124, 1123f, 1124f
Follicular dendritic cells, 188
Follicular hyperplasia, 595, 596f
  in HIV infection, 249
Follicular lipping, 1191
Follicular lymphoma, 601t, 605–606, 605f, 606f
  genetic basis for, 305, 305t, 606
Follicular tonsillitis, 750
Folliculitis, 383
Foot processes, 910, 910f
  in minimal-change disease, 925, 925f
Foramen ovale, patent, 541
Forebrain anomalies, 1284–1285, 1285f
Foregut cysts, 679
Foreign bodies
  inflammation due to, 45
  and wound healing, 106
Foreign body granulomas, 74
Formaldehyde, as indoor air pollutant, 405
Formed blood elements, 590
  sequestration of, by spleen, 633
FOS, 90
Foveolar cells, 774
  hyperplasia of, 782, 783f
FOXE1 gene, 1110
Foxp3, in immunological tolerance, 211
FOXP3 gene, 796–797
Fractalkine, 62
Fracture(s), 1219–1220, 1220f
  chalkstick-type, 1217
  closed (simple), 1219
  comminuted, 1219
  complete or incomplete, 1219
  compound, 1219
  displaced, 1219
  pathologic, 1219
  skull, 1287
  stress, 1219
Fracture contusions, of skull, 1287
Fragile site, 169, 169f
Fragile-X syndrome, 139, 168t, 169–171, 169f, 170f
  polymerase chain reaction analysis of, 175–176, 176f
Frank-Starling mechanism, 533
Freckles, 1168
Free radicals
  cell injury due to, 18f, 20–22, 20t, 21f
    chemical (toxic), 25
    ischemia-reperfusion, 24
  defined, 20
  in emphysema, 685f, 686
  generation of, 20–21, 20t, 21f
  removal of, 20t, 21
French-American-British (FAB) classification, of acute myeloid leukemia, 622, 622t

Friedreich ataxia, 168t, 1323
Frontal bossing, 436
Frontotemporal dementias (FTDs), 1317–1319, 1318f
Frustrated phagocytosis, 55
FSGS. *See* Focal segmental glomerulosclerosis (FSGS).
FSH (follicle-stimulating hormone)-producing adenomas, 1100t, 1104–1105
FSPs. *See* Fibrin split products (FSPs).
Fuchs endothelial dystrophy, of cornea, 1352–1353, 1352f
Fucosidosis, 151t
Fukuyama muscular dystrophy, 1270t
Fulminant hepatic failure, 835, 853, 854f
Fulminant hepatitis, 835, 853, 854f
Functio laesa, 44
Functional derangements, 4
Functional endometrial disorders, 1026–1027, 1026f, 1027t
Functional regurgitation, 560–561
Fundic gland polyps, 782t, 783, 784f
Fungal infection(s), 382–386, 383f–386f
  in AIDS, 245t, 246
  aspergillosis as, 384–385, 385f
  candidiasis as, 382–384, 383f
  cryptococcosis as, 384, 384f
  deep, 335
    of oral cavity, 743
  of gastrointestinal tract, 338
  superficial, 335, 1202, 1202f
  zygomycosis (mucormycosis) as, 385–386, 386f
Fungal meningoencephalitis, 1306, 1307f
Fungi, 333t, 335
Funisitis, 454
Furuncle, 358
Fusion gene
  in chronic myeloid leukemia, 305
  in Ewing sarcoma, 306
Fusobacterium necrophorum, 378

G

G banding, 158–159, 159f
G protein–coupled receptors, 90–91, 91f
  in inflammation, 51, 52f
G_1 phase, of cell cycle, 86, 86f
G_1/S checkpoint, in cell cycle, 86, 86f, 87, 286
  role of RB in regulating, 288, 289f
G_2 phase, of cell cycle, 86, 86f
G_2/M checkpoint, in cell cycle, 86f, 87, 286
GAGs (glycosaminoglycans), in extracellular matrix, 97–98, 98f
Gain-of-function mutations, 141
Galactitol, 464
Galactocerebroside β-galactosidase deficiency, 1326
Galactokinase, 464, 464f
Galactonate, 464
Galactose metabolism, disorder of, 464–465, 464f, 465f
Galactose-1-phosphate, 464, 464f
Galactose-1-phosphate uridyl transferase (GALT), 464, 464f, 465
Galactose-1-phosphate uridyl transferase (GALT) deficiency, 143
Galactosemia, 464–465, 464f, 465f
  genetic basis for, 143
Galactosylceramidase deficiency, 1326
Gallbladder
  adenomyosis of, 888
  empyema of, 885
  hydrops of, 886

Gallbladder (*Continued*)
  inflammatory polyps of, 888
  porcelain, 886
Gallbladder carcinoma, 888–889, 888f
Gallbladder disorder(s), 882–887
  cholecystitis as, 885–887, 886f
  cholelithiasis as, 882–884, 883f, 883t, 884f
  congenital anomalies as, 882, 882f
Gallstones, 882–884
  clinical features of, 884
  morphology of, 884, 884f
  obesity and, 442
  pancreatitis due to, 893
  pathogenesis of, 883–884, 883f
  prevalence and risk factors for, 882–883, 883t
GALT (galactose-1-phosphate uridyl transferase), 464, 464f, 465
GALT (galactose-1-phosphate uridyl transferase) deficiency, 143
Gametocytes, of malaria, 387, 387f
Gamma rays, 423
γ chemokines, 62
Gangliocytoma, dysplastic, 1342
Gangliogliomas, 1335
Ganglion, 1247
Ganglion cell layer, of retina, 1359f
Ganglioneuroblastoma, 476
Ganglioneuromas, 476, 477f
  in MEN-2B, 1162
Gangliosides, as tumor antigens, 318
Gangrene, 128
  gas, 379
  of lower extremities, due to diabetes mellitus, 1140
  of lung, 717
  wet, 16
Gangrenous cholecystitis, 885
Gangrenous necrosis, 15–16
GAP(s) (GTPase-activating proteins), 283
Gap junctions, in myocardium, 531–532
Gardner syndrome, 816t, 821
  osteomas in, 1224
Gardnerella vaginalis, 1009
Garrod, Archibald, 462
Gartner duct cysts, 1007, 1016
Gas gangrene, 379
Gastric adenocarcinoma, 784–786, 785f, 786f
  chronic gastritis and, 781
  Helicobacter pylori and, 315–316
Gastric adenoma, 782t, 784, 784f
Gastric antral vascular ectasia (GAVE), 779
Gastric carcinoma, diet and, 443
Gastric dysplasia, 781–782
Gastric heterotopia, 765
Gastric lymphomas, 786–787, 787f
  Helicobacter pylori and, 316
Gastric perforation, 780–781, 781f
Gastric polyps, 783
  fundic gland, 782t, 783, 784f
  inflammatory and hyperplastic, 782t, 783, 784f
Gastric tumor(s), 784–790
  adenocarcinoma as, 784–786, 785f, 786f
  adenoma as, 782t, 784, 784f
  carcinoid, 787–789, 788f, 788t
  gastrointestinal stromal tumor as, 789–790, 789f
  lymphoma as, 786–787, 787f
Gastric ulcer(s), acute, 775–776, 776t
Gastrinomas, 782–783
  in MEN-1, 1162
  of pancreas, 1147

Gastritis
  acute, 774–776, 775f
    erosive hemorrhagic, 775
  autoimmune, 778–779, 778t, 779f
  chronic, 776–780
    complications of, 780–782
  cystica, 782, 782t
  eosinophilic, 780
  granulomatous, 780
  Helicobacter pylori, 776–778, 777f, 778t
  lymphocytic, 780
    in celiac disease, 796
  multifocal atrophic, 777
  uncommon forms of, 779–780
  varioliform, 780
Gastroenteritis
  bacterial, 794t
  global warming and, 402
  parasitic, 794t, 805—807, 805f
  viral, 794t, 804–805, 805f
Gastroesophageal reflux disease (GERD)
  Barrett esophagus due to, 770
  reflux esophagitis due to, 769–770, 769f
Gastrointestinal amyloidosis, 255
Gastrointestinal atresia, 764–765
Gastrointestinal disorders
  due to alcoholism, 414
  in cystic fibrosis, 470t
  due to occupational exposures, 409t
  prevalence of, 451t
Gastrointestinal ectopia, 765
Gastrointestinal stromal tumor (GIST), 789–790,
    789f
Gastrointestinal tract, 1667–1733
  congenital abnormalities of, 1668–1671
    atresia, fistulas and duplications as,
        764–765, 765f
    diaphragmatic hernia, omphalocele, and
        gastroschisis as, 765
    ectopia as, 765
    Hirschsprung disease as, 766–767,
        766f
    Meckel diverticulum as, 765–766, 765f
    pyloric stenosis as, 766
  esophagus in, 767–774
    achalasia of, 768
    Barrett, 770–771, 770f, 771f
    esophagitis of, 768–770
      chemical and infectious, 768–769,
          769f
      eosinophilic, 769f, 770
      due to lacerations, 768, 768t
      reflux, 769–770, 769f
    obstruction of, 767–768
    tumors of, 772–774
      adenocarcinoma as, 772, 773f
      benign, 774
      squamous cell carcinoma as, 773–774,
          773f
      uncommon, 774
    varices of, 771, 772f
  infections via, 338–339
  peritoneum of, 828–829
    cysts of, 829
    infection of, 828
    inflammatory disease of, 828–829
    sclerosing retroperitonitis of, 828–829
    tumors of, 829
  small intestine and colon in, 790–828
    acute appendicitis of, 826–827
    adenomas of, 819–820, 820f, 821f
    anal canal tumors of, 825–826, 827f
    angiodysplasia of, 793
    appendix tumors of, 828

Gastrointestinal tract *(Continued)*
  colitis of
    collagenous, 814, 814f
    diversion, 813–814, 814f
    and dysplasia, 813, 814f
    indeterminate, 812–813
    lymphocytic, 814, 814f
    microscopic, 814, 814f
    ulcerative, 808f, 808t, 811–813, 812f, 813f
  colorectal cancer of
    adenocarcinoma as, 264f, 822–825,
        823f–826f, 826t, 827t
    chemoprevention of, 823
    diet and, 443, 822–823
    familial adenomatous polyposis and,
        820–821
    hereditary non-polyposis, 274, 275, 302,
        821–822, 822t
    intramucosal carcinoma as, 820, 821f
    metastatic, 269f
    molecular model for evolution of, 308f,
        309
  familial syndromes of, 820–822
  graft-*versus*-host disease of, 814
  hemorrhoids of, 826
  infectious enterocolitis of, 797–807, 798t
    Campylobacter, 798t, 799–800, 800f
    due to cholera, 797–799, 798t, 799f
    due to enteric (typhoid) fever, 798t,
        801–802
    due to *Escherichia coli,* 798t, 800f, 802
    due to mycobacterial infection, 794t,
        798t, 804, 804f
    parasitic, 805–807, 805f
    due to pseudomembranous colitis, 798t,
        803, 803f
    due to salmonellosis, 798t, 801
    due to shigellosis, 798t, 800–801
    viral, 805f, 1708–1709
    due to Whipple disease, 798t, 803–804,
        804f
    due to *Yersinia* spp, 798t, 800f, 802
  inflammatory bowel disease of, 807–813
    colitis-associated dysplasia due to, 813,
        814f
    Crohn disease as, 808f, 808t, 810–811,
        810f, 811f
    epidemiology of, 807–808
    malabsorption and diarrhea in, 794t
    pathogenesis of, 808–810, 809f
    ulcerative colitis as, 808f, 808t, 811–813,
        812f, 813f
  irritable bowel syndrome of, 807
  ischemic disease of, 791–793, 792f
  malabsorption and diarrhea of, 793–797
    in abetalipoproteinemia, 797
    in autoimmune enteropathy, 794t,
        796–797
    in celiac disease, 794t, 795–796, 795f,
        796f
    in cystic fibrosis, 794, 794t
    in lactase (disaccharidase) deficiency,
        794t, 797
    mechanisms of, 793–794, 794t
    in tropical sprue, 794t, 796
  obstruction of, 790–791
    due to adhesions, 790–791, 791f
    due to hernias, 790, 791f
    due to intussusception, 791, 791f
    due to volvulus, 791, 791f
  polyps of, 815–820, 816t
    in Cowden syndrome and Bannayan-
        Ruvalcaba-Riley syndrome, 816t,
        818

Gastrointestinal tract, polyps of *(Continued)*
    in Cronkhite-Canada syndrome, 816t,
        818
    in familial adenomatous polyposis, 816t,
        820–821, 822f, 822t
    hamartomatous, 816–818, 816t, 817f,
        818f
    hyperplastic, 818–819, 819f
    inflammatory, 815–816, 816f
    juvenile, 816–817, 816t, 817f
    neoplastic, 819–820, 820f, 821f
    in Peutz-Jeghers syndrome, 816t,
        817–818, 818f
    in tuberous sclerosis, 816t
    sigmoid diverticulitis of, 814–815, 815f
  stomach in, 774–790
    acute ulceration of, 775–776, 776t
    adenomas of, 782t
    anatomy of, 774
    dysplasia of, 781–782
    gastritis of
      acute, 774–776, 775f
      autoimmune, 778–779, 778t, 779f
      chronic, 776–782
      cystica, 782, 782t
      eosinophilic, 780
      granulomatous, 780
      Helicobacter pylori, 776–778, 777f, 778t
      lymphocytic, 780
      uncommon forms of, 779–780
    hypertrophic gastropathies of, 782–783,
        782t, 783f
    Ménétrier disease of, 782, 782t
    mucosal atrophy and metaplasia of, 781
    peptic ulcer disease of, 780–781, 781f
    polyps of, 783
      fundic gland, 782t, 783, 784f
      inflammatory and hyperplastic, 782t,
          783, 784f
    reactive gastropathy of, 779
    tumors of, 784–790
      adenocarcinoma as, 784–786, 785f,
          786f
      adenoma as, 784, 784f
      carcinoid, 787–789, 788f, 788t
      gastrointestinal stromal tumor as,
          789–790, 789f
      lymphoma as, 786–787, 787f
      Zollinger-Ellison syndrome of, 780,
          782–783, 782t
  in systemic sclerosis, 224–225
Gastropathy(ies)
  hypertrophic, 782–783, 782t, 783f
  reactive, 779
Gastroschisis, 765
GATA4, in congenital heart disease, 539, 539t
Gaucher cells, 153–154, 154f
Gaucher disease, 151t, 153–154, 154f
GAVE (gastric antral vascular ectasia), 779
GB virus C (GBV-C), 849
GBD (Global Burden of Disease), 400, 401f
GBM (glomerular basement membrane),
    908–910, 909f, 910f
  thickening of, 911
    in diabetes mellitus, 1141, 1141f
GCK (glucokinase) gene, 1137
GDNF (glial-derived neurotrophic factor), in
    MEN-2A, 1162
Gemistocytic astrocyte, 1281
Gene(s), and human diseases, 137–140
Gene amplification, in carcinogenesis, 306
Gene chips, 174, 175f, 325, 326f
Gene expression profiling, for breast carcinoma,
    1084–1085, 1086f, 1090

General paresis
  of the insane, 1301
  due to syphilis, 375
Genetic analysis, 173–181
  for acquired genetic alterations, 174
  array-based comparative genomic
    hybridization in, 179–180, 180f
  detection of DNA sequence alterations in,
    174–176, 175f, 176f
  for epigenetic alterations, 180–181
  fluorescence in situ hybridization in, 179, 179f
  genome-wide, 138, 177, 178f
  for genomic alterations, 178–180, 179f, 180f
  for germ line genetic alterations, 173
  indications for, 173–174
  polymerase chain reaction in, 174–176, 175f,
    176f
  polymorphic markers in, 176–177, 177f, 178f
  postnatal, 173–174
  prenatal, 173
  RNA analysis in, 181
  Southern blotting in, 176, 176f, 178
Genetic architecture, 136–137, 137f
Genetic disorder(s), 135–181
  cell injury due to, 12
  chromosomal, 138, 158–167
    in carcinogenesis, 304–306, 305t
    chromosome 22q11.2 deletion syndrome
      as, 162–164, 164f
    fetal growth restriction due to, 455
    fetal hydrops due to, 461, 461t
    hermaphroditism and
      pseudohermaphroditism as, 167
    involving autosomes, 161–164, 161f, 163f,
      164f
    involving sex chromosomes, 164–167, 166f
    Klinefelter syndrome as, 165
    normal karyotype and, 158–159, 159f
    other trisomies as, 162
    prevalence of, 451, 451t
    structural, 159–161, 160f
    trisomy 21 (Down syndrome) as, 161–162,
      161f, 163f
    Turner syndrome as, 165–167, 166f
    white cell neoplasia due to, 596–597, 597f
  complex multigenic, 138, 157–158
  due to copy number variations, 136
  epidemiology of, 137
  molecular diagnosis of, 173–181
    for acquired genetic alterations, 174
    array-based comparative genomic
      hybridization in, 179–180, 180f
    detection of DNA sequence alterations in,
      174–176, 175f, 176f
    for epigenetic alterations, 180–181
    fluorescence in situ hybridization in, 179,
      179f
    genome-wide analyses in, 138, 177, 178f
    for genomic alterations, 178–180, 179f, 180f
    for germ line genetic alterations, 173
    indications for, 173–174
    polymerase chain reaction in, 174–176,
      175f, 176f
    polymorphic markers in, 176–177, 177f,
      178f
    postnatal, 173–174
    prenatal, 173
    RNA analysis in, 181
    Southern blotting in, 176, 176f, 178
  due to mutations, 138–140, 138f, 139f
  single-gene, 138
    mendelian, 140–158
      alkaptonuria as, 155–156
      autosomal dominant, 140–141, 141t

Genetic disorder(s) (Continued)
    autosomal recessive, 141–142, 142t
    biochemical and molecular basis of,
      142–144, 143t, 144f
    due to defects in proteins that regulate
      cell growth, 143t, 156
    due to defects in receptor proteins, 143t,
      144, 147–149, 147f–149f
    due to defects in structural proteins,
      143t, 144–147, 146t
    Ehlers-Danlos syndromes as, 145–147,
      146t
    due to enzyme defects, 149–156
    familial hypercholesterolemia as,
      147–149, 147t–149f
    Gaucher disease as, 151t, 153–154, 154f
    glycogen storage diseases as, 155, 156f,
      157t, 158f
    lysosomal storage diseases as, 149–155,
      150f, 151t
    Marfan syndrome as, 144–145
    mucopolysaccharidoses as, 151t, 154–155
    Niemann-Pick disease as, type C, 153
    Niemann-Pick disease as, types A and B,
      151t, 152–153, 153f
    Tay-Sachs disease as, 139f, 150–152, 151t,
      152f
    transmission patterns of, 140–142, 141t,
      142t
    X-linked, 142, 142t
  with nonclassic inheritance, 140, 167–173
    Angelman syndrome as, 172–173, 172f
    fragile-X syndrome as, 139, 168t,
      169–171, 169f, 170f
    due to genomic imprinting, 171–173,
      172f
    due to gonadal mosaicism, 173
    Leber hereditary optic neuropathy as,
      171, 171f
    due to mutations in mitochondrial genes,
      171, 171f
    Prader-Willi syndrome as, 172–173,
      172f
    due to triplet-repeat mutations, 139,
      167–171, 168f, 168t
  due to single-nucleotide polymorphisms, 136
Genetic heterogeneity, 140
Genetic polymorphisms, 176–177, 177f
Genetic predisposition, to cancer, 273–276, 275t
Genetic sex, 167
Genital chlamydia, 380
Genital herpes, 352, 1008–1009
Genital sex, 167
Genital tract. See Female genital tract; Male
    genital tract.
Genital warts, 826, 827f, 1012, 1012f, 1200
Genome-wide association studies (GWAS), 138,
    177, 178f
  of breast cancer, 1078
  of inflammatory bowel disease, 809
Genomic alterations, molecular analysis of,
    178–180, 179f, 180f
Genomic imprinting, 171–173, 172f
  in Beckwith-Wiedemann syndrome, 480
  loss of, 306, 480
Genomic instability, in carcinogenesis, 302–303
Genomics, 136
Genotoxic stress, apoptosis due to, 25, 30
GERD (gastroesophageal reflux disease)
  Barrett esophagus due to, 770
  reflux esophagitis due to, 769–770, 769f
Germ cell tumor(s)
  of brain, 1338
  ovarian, 1040t, 1041f, 1047–1050, 1047t

Germ cell tumor(s) (Continued)
    choriocarcinoma as, 1049
    dysgerminoma as, 1048–1049, 1049f
    embryonal carcinoma as, 1050
    endodermal sinus (yolk sac), 1049, 1049f
    mixed, 1050
    teratomas as, 1047–1048, 1048f
  testicular, 987–992
    choriocarcinoma as, 990, 990f
    classification and pathogenesis of, 987t, 988
    clinical features of, 991–992
    embryonal carcinoma as, 989, 990f
    environmental factors and genetic
      predisposition to, 987–988
    mixed, 991
    nonseminomatous, 992
    seminoma as, 988–989, 988f, 989f
      spermatocytic, 989
    teratoma as, 990–991, 991f
    yolk sac, 989–990
Germ line mosaicism, 173
Germinal center, of peripheral lymphoid organ,
    189
Germinal inclusion cysts, of ovary, 1042, 1042f
Germinomas, of pineal gland, 1163
Gerstmann-Sträussler-Scheinker (GSS)
    syndrome, 1308
Gestational choriocarcinoma, 1059–1061, 1060f
Gestational diabetes mellitus, 1137
Gestational disorder(s), 1052–1061
  choriocarcinoma as, 1059–1061, 1060f
  early, 1053–1054
  ectopic pregnancy as, 1053–1054
  gestational trophoblastic disease as,
    1057–1061
  hydatidiform mole as, 1057–1059, 1058f,
    1059f
  invasive mole as, 1059, 1060f
  late, 1054–1057
  placental anatomy and, 1052–1053, 1053f,
    1054f
  of placental implantation, 1055
  placental infections as, 1055, 1055f
  placental-site trophoblastic tumor as, 1061,
    1061f
  preeclampsia and eclampsia as, 1055–1057,
    1056f, 1057f
  spontaneous abortion as, 1053
  twin placentas as, 1054, 1055f
Gestational trophoblastic disease, 1057–1061
  choriocarcinoma as, 1059–1061, 1060f
  hydatidiform mole as, 1057–1059, 1058f,
    1059f
  invasive mole as, 1059, 1060f
  placental-site trophoblastic tumor as, 1061,
    1061f
GFAP (glial fibrillary acid protein), 85, 1281,
    1282f
  in Alexander disease, 1327
GH (growth hormone) cell adenomas, 1100t,
    1104
Ghrelin, in energy balance, 439, 440f, 441–442,
    441f
Giant cells, 74
Giant-cell arteritis, 512–513, 513f
Giant-cell myocarditis, 578, 579f
Giant-cell tumor
  of bone, 1233–1234, 1233f
  tenosynovial (of tendon sheath), 1247, 1247f
Giardia duodenalis, 806
Giardia intestinalis, 806
Giardia lamblia, 335
  enterocolitis due to, 805f, 806–807
Giardiasis, 805f, 806–807

Gigantism, 1104
Gilbert syndrome, 841–842, 841t
Gingiva, 740, 740f
Gingivitis, 740–741
Gingivostomatitis, 352
    acute herpetic, 742
GIST (gastrointestinal stromal tumor), 789–790, 789f
Glandular neoplastic lesions, of vulva, 1015, 1015f
Glanzmann thrombasthenia, 118, 118f, 670
Glaucoma, 1353–1355, 1354f
    angle-closure, 1353–1354
        primary, 1354–1355, 1354f
        secondary, 1355
    due to diabetes, 1145, 1363f
    exfoliation, 1354
    ghost cell, 1354
    infantile, 1352
    melanomalytic, 1354
    neovascular, 1354f, 1355, 1361, 1363f
    normal- or low-tension, 1353, 1366
    open-angle, 1353
        primary, 1354
        secondary, 1354
Glaucomatous optic nerve damage, 1366–1367, 1367f
Glaukomflecken, 1355
Gliadin, 795
Glial cells, reactions to injury of, 1282
Glial cytoplasmic inclusions, 1282
Glial fibrillary acid protein (GFAP), 85, 1281, 1282f
    in Alexander disease, 1327
Glial filaments, 35
Glial hamartia, 1342
Glial-derived neurotrophic factor (GDNF), in MEN-2A, 1162
Glioblastoma, 1330, 1331–1332, 1332f
    primary, 1331–1332
    secondary, 1332
Glioma(s), 1330–1335
    astrocytomas as, 1330–1333, 1331f–1333f
    brainstem, 1333
    ependymomas as, 1334–1335, 1335f
    hypothalamic suprasellar, 1106
    oligodendro-, 1333–1334, 1334f
Gliomatosis cerebri, 1331
Gliosis, 1281
    Bergmann, 1329
Global Burden of Disease (GBD), 400, 401f
Global cerebral ischemia, 1291–1292, 1292f
Global warming, health effects of, 401–402, 401f
Globoid cells, in Krabbe disease, 1326, 1326f
Glomangioma, 522
Glomerular basement membrane (GBM), 908–910, 909f, 910f
    thickening of, 911
        in diabetes mellitus, 1141, 1141f
Glomerular cells, antibodies to, 914
Glomerular crescent formation, 911
Glomerular disease, 907–935, 908t, 918t
    Alport syndrome as, 931–932, 932f
    in amyloidosis, 935
    clinical manifestations of, 908–911, 908t, 909f, 910f
    dense-deposit disease as, 915, 918t, 928–929, 928f, 930f
    due to diabetes mellitus, 934–935, 1141–1142, 1141f, 1142f
    in essential mixed cryoglobulinemia, 935
    focal segmental glomerulosclerosis as, 916–917, 917f, 918t, 926–928, 927f
    glomerulonephritis as

Glomerular disease (Continued)
    acute proliferative, 917–920, 918t, 919f
    bacterial endocarditis–associated, 934
    chronic, 918t, 932–933, 933f
    fibrillary, 935
    membranoproliferative, 915, 918t, 928–929, 928f–930f
    postinfectious, 918t, 920
    poststreptococcal, 917–920, 919f
    rapidly progressive (crescentic), 907, 908t, 920–921, 920t, 921f
    glomerulopathy as
        immunotactoid, 935
        membranous, 918t, 922–923, 924f
    in Goodpasture syndrome, 918t, 935
    in Henoch-Schönlein purpura, 934
    hereditary, 908t
    histologic alterations in, 911
    isolated urinary abnormalities as, 908t, 929–932
    in light-chain or monoclonal Ig deposition disease, 935
    lupus nephritis as, 934
    mechanisms of progression in, 916–917, 917f
    in microscopic polyangiitis, 935
    minimal-change disease as, 918t, 923–926, 925f
    in multiple myeloma, 935
    with nephritic syndrome, 908t, 917–920, 919f
    nephropathy as
        HIV-associated, 928
        IgA, 918t, 929–931, 931f
    with nephrotic syndrome, 908t, 921–929, 923t
    pathogenesis of injury in, 911–916, 911t, 913f–916f
    in plasma cell dyscrasias, 935
    primary, 908t
    in systemic diseases (secondary), 908t, 933–935
    thin basement membrane lesion as, 932
    in Wegener granulomatosis, 935
Glomerular filtration, 910–911, 910f
Glomerular filtration barrier, 910
Glomerular filtration rate, in blood pressure regulation, 493
Glomerular hyalinosis, 911
Glomerular hypercellularity, 911
Glomerular injury
    associated with systemic diseases, 933–935
    pathogenesis of, 911–916, 911t, 913f–916f
Glomerular sclerosis, 911
Glomeruloid body, in glioblastoma, 1331
Glomerulonephritis
    acute proliferative, 917–920, 918t, 919f
    anti-GBM antibody–induced, 912, 913f, 920, 920t
    bacterial endocarditis–associated, 934
    cell-mediated immunity in, 915
    chronic, 918t, 932–933, 933f
    circulating immune complex, 912–914, 913f, 914f
    fibrillary, 935
    immune complex, 205
    membranoproliferative, 918t, 928–929
        alternative complement pathway in, 915, 928–929, 928f
        clinical features of, 929
        morphology of, 929, 929f, 930f
        pathogenesis of, 928–929, 928f
        primary, 928
        secondary, 929
    membranous, in systemic lupus erythematosus, 218
mesangial lupus, 217

Glomerulonephritis (Continued)
    mesangiocapillary, 915, 918t, 928–929, 928f–930f
    postinfectious, 918t, 920
    poststreptococcal, 204t, 917–920, 919f
    proliferative, in systemic lupus erythematosus
        diffuse, 218, 218f
        focal, 217–218, 218f
    rapidly progressive (crescentic), 907, 908t, 920–921, 920t, 921f
    in systemic lupus erythematosus
        membranous, 218
        proliferative
            diffuse, 218, 218f
            focal, 217–218, 218f
Glomerulopathy(ies). See also Glomerular disease.
    collapsing, 927, 927f
    immunotactoid, 935
    membranous, 918t, 922–923, 924f
Glomerulosclerosis
    diffuse mesangial, in diabetes mellitus, 1141–1142, 1142f
    focal segmental, 918t, 926–928
        autosomal-recessive, 927
        due to chronic pyelonephritis, 943–944
        classification and types of, 926
        clinical course of, 928
        idiopathic, 926
        morphology of, 926–927, 927f
        pathogenesis of, 926–928
        progressive nature of, 916–917, 917f
        renal ablation, 927–928
    intercapillary, 1142, 1142f
    nodular, in diabetes mellitus, 1142, 1142f
Glomerulus, 908–910, 909f
Glomus tumor, 522
Glossitis, 742
    atrophic, 779
    due to vitamin B$_{12}$ deficiency, 658
Glucagon
    in glucose homeostasis, 1132–1133
    production of, 1130, 1131f
Glucagonomas, 1147
Glucocerebrosidase deficiency, 151t, 153–154, 154f
Glucocorticoid(s), 1148
    and wound healing, 106
Glucocorticoid-remediable hyperaldosteronism, 1151
Glucokinase (GCK) gene, 1137
Glucose, blood, 1131–1132, 1131f
Glucose homeostasis, 1132–1134, 1133f, 1134f
Glucose neurotoxicity, 1139, 1140t, 1142
Glucose-6-phosphatase deficiency, 155, 157t
Glucose-6-phosphate dehydrogenase (G6PD) deficiency, 142, 144, 644–645, 644f, 645f
Glue sniffing, 420
GLUT-2, 1133, 1133f
Glutathione peroxidase, 60
    free radical removal by, 21, 21f
Gluten, 795
Gluten-free diet, 796
Gluten-sensitive enteropathy, 794t, 795–796, 795f, 796f
    IgA nephropathy with, 931
Glycogen
    intracellular accumulation of, 36
    metabolism of, 155, 156f
Glycogen storage diseases, 36, 151t, 155, 156f, 157t, 158f
Glycogenoses, 36, 151t, 155, 156f, 157t, 158f
Glycolipids, altered cell surface, as tumor antigens, 318

Glycolysis, in carcinogenesis, 303–304
Glycoproteins
    adhesive, in extracellular matrix, 95f, 96–97, 97f
    altered cell surface, as tumor antigens, 318
Glycosaminoglycans (GAGs), in extracellular matrix, 97–98, 98f
Glycosylated hemoglobin (Hb$_{A1C}$), 1138
Glycosylphosphatidylinositol (GPI), 652
G$_{M1}$ gangliosidosis, 151t
G$_{M2}$ gangliosidosis, 139f, 150–152, 151t, 152f
GM-CSF (granulocyte-macrophage colony-stimulating factor), in pulmonary alveolar proteinosis, 705
GNAS gene
    in fibrous dysplasia, 1231
    in pituitary adenomas, 1101
Goblet cells, in Barrett esophagus, 770–771, 770f
Goiter, 1107, 1116–1118
    colloid, 1116, 1117f
    diffuse nontoxic (simple), 1116, 1117f
    dyshormonogenetic, 1110
    endemic, 1116
    intrathoracic or plunging, 1117
    multinodular, 1116–1118, 1117f
    sporadic, 1116
Goitrogens, 1107, 1116
Goitrous hypothyroidism, 1116
Gonadal mosaicism, 173
Gonadal sex, 167
Gonadoblastomas
    in Denys-Drash syndrome, 480
    ovarian, 1052
    testicular, 993
Gonadotroph(s), 1099
Gonadotroph adenomas, 1100t, 1104–1105
Gonococcal infection, pelvic inflammatory disease due to, 1009–1010
Gonococcal urethritis, 981
Gonorrhea, 334f, 341t, 363–364
    epididymitis and orchitis due to, 986
Goodpasture syndrome, 203t, 709–710
    anti-GBM antibodies in, 912, 920
    glomerular disease in, 918t, 935
Gorlin syndrome, 1181, 1182t, 1342
Gout, 1243–1246
    classification of, 1243, 1243t
    clinical course of, 1244–1246
    morphology of, 1244, 1245f
    pathogenesis of, 1243–1244, 1244f, 1245f
    primary, 1243, 1243t
    pseudo-, 1246, 1246f
        due to hemochromatosis, 862
    secondary, 1243, 1243t
    tophaceous, 1243, 1244, 1245f, 1246
Gouty arthritis, 1243–1246
    clinical course of, 1244–1246
    morphology of, 1244, 1245f
    pathogenesis of, 1243–1244, 1244f, 1245f
Gouty nephropathy, 907, 947, 1244
gp63, in leishmaniasis, 389
G6PD (glucose-6-phosphate dehydrogenase) deficiency, 142, 144, 644–645, 644f, 645f
GPI (glycosylphosphatidylinositol), 652
GpIIb-IIIa deficiency, 118, 118f
G-protein mutations, in pituitary adenomas, 1101, 1101t, 1102f
G-protein signaling, in endocrine neoplasia, 1101, 1102f
Graafian follicle, 1007
Grading, of cancer, 322
Graft arteriopathy, cardiac, 585, 585f

Graft-versus-host (GVH) disease, 230
    esophageal, 769
    intestinal, 814
    liver in, 874
Graft-versus-leukemia effect, 230
Gram-negative bacterial infections, 358t, 363–366, 364f, 365f
Gram-positive bacterial infections, 357–363, 359f–363f
Granular dystrophy, of cornea, 1353
Granular ependymitis, in neurosyphilis, 1302
Granulation tissue, formation of, 102, 103f–105f
    exuberant, 107
    inadequate, 106
Granulocyte(s), adult reference range for, 592t
Granulocyte count, radiation effect on, 425
Granulocyte-macrophage colony-stimulating factor (GM-CSF), in pulmonary alveolar proteinosis, 705
Granuloma(s), 16, 55, 73–74, 74f
    in cell-mediated hypersensitivity, 207, 208f
    eosinophilic, 632
    foreign body, 74
    gravidarum, 521
    hepatic, drug- and toxin-induced, 856t
    immune, 74
    inguinale, 366
    lethal midline, 750
    malarial (Dürck), 388
    noncaseating
        in Crohn disease, 811, 811f
        sarcoid, 701–703, 703f
    of oral cavity
        peripheral giant cell, 742
        pyogenic, 741–742, 741f
    periapical, 749
    peripheral giant cell, of oral cavity, 742
    pyogenic, 521, 521f
        of oral cavity, 741–742, 741f
    sarcoid noncaseating, 701–703, 703f
Granulomatosis
    allergic, 516
    Wegener, 516–517, 516f, 710
        glomerular lesions in, 935
        of orbit, 1347
Granulomatous disease
    chronic, 55, 56t
    of lungs, 701–704
        hypersensitivity pneumonitis as, 703–704, 703f
        sarcoidosis as, 701–703, 702f
Granulomatous gastritis, 780
Granulomatous inflammation, 73–74, 73t, 74f, 207, 207f, 347–348
Granulomatous lobular mastitis, 1070
Granulomatous mastitis, 1070
Granulomatous orchitis, 986
Granulomatous prostatitis, 994
Granulomatous thyroiditis, 1113, 1113f
Granulomatous uveitis, 1356
Granulosa–theca cell tumors, ovarian, 1050, 1050f
Granulovacuolar degeneration, in Alzheimer disease, 1316
Granzymes
    in apoptosis, 31
    in cell-mediated cytotoxicity, 208
Graves disease, 1114–1116, 1115f
    antibody-mediated hypersensitivity in, 203–204, 203t
    clinical findings in, 1114, 1115–1116
    epidemiology of, 1114
    morphology of, 1115, 1115f

Graves disease (Continued)
    ophthalmopathy in, 1109, 1109f, 1114–1115, 1347, 1347f
    pathogenesis of, 1114–1115
Gray (Gy), 423
Gray hepatization, 713
GRB-2, 90
Great arteries, transposition of, 542f, 543, 543f
Greenhouse effect, 401–402, 401f
Greig syndrome, 1211t
Grotton lesions, 1273
Ground-glass picture, due to neonatal respiratory distress syndrome, 456
Group atrophy, 1260
Growth, compensatory, 93
Growth factor(s)
    in angiogenesis, 100–101, 100t, 101f
    in cell replication, 87–89, 87t
    in glomerular injury, 916
    oncogenes for, 280, 281t
    in tissue regeneration, 87–89, 87t
    in wound healing, 87–89, 87t, 102, 103, 104t
Growth factor deprivation, apoptosis due to, 30
Growth factor receptors, oncogenes for, 280–281, 281t
Growth fraction, 266–267
Growth hormone (GH) cell adenomas, 1100t, 1104
Growth inhibition, insensitivity to, in carcinogenesis, 278, 286–295
Growth plate, 1209, 1209f
Growth rates, of tumors, 265–267, 266f, 271t
Growth signals, self-sufficiency in, in carcinogenesis, 278, 279–286
GSS (Gerstmann-Sträussler-Scheinker) syndrome, 1308
GSTP1, in prostate cancer, 997
GTP (guanosine triphosphate)-binding protein, proto-oncogene for, 281t
GTPase-activating proteins (GAPs), 283
Guanosine triphosphate (GTP)-binding protein, proto-oncogene for, 281t
Guillain-Barré syndrome, 1261–1262
    due to Campylobacter, 799
    T cell–mediated hypersensitivity in, 206t
Gull disease, 1111
Gull, William, 1111
Gummas
    cerebral, 1301
    syphilitic, 375, 376, 376f
Gut hormones, in energy balance, 441–442
Guttata, in Fuchs endothelial dystrophy, 1352, 1352f
GVH disease. See Graft-versus-host (GVH) disease.
GWAS (genome-wide association studies), 138, 177, 178f
    of breast cancer, 1078
    of inflammatory bowel disease, 809
Gy (gray), 423
Gynecomastia, 1093, 1093f
    due to liver failure, 836

H
H5N1 influenza virus, 715
HA (hyaluronan), in extracellular matrix, 95f, 97–98, 98f
Haab's striae, 1352
HAART (highly active antiretroviral therapy), for HIV infection, 248
HACEK group organisms, endocarditis due to, 567
Haemophilus ducreyi, 341t, 366
Haemophilus influenzae pneumonia, 711–712

Hageman factor
  in coagulation cascade, 119, 119f
  in inflammation, 64, 65, 65f, 66
Hair follicle(s), 1166, 1166f
Hair follicle bulge, stem cell sin, 85
Hairy cell leukemia, 601t, 614, 614f
Hairy leukoplakia, 743
Hallmark cells, in anaplastic large-cell
    lymphoma, 615, 615f
Hallucinogens, abuse of, 418t
Halo nevus, 1170t
Halogenation, in phagocytosis, 53, 53f
Hamartoma(s), 262
  bile duct, 869, 870f
  of breast, 1092
  cortical, in tuberous sclerosis, 1342–1343
  of infancy and childhood, 473
  PTEN, 818
  pulmonary, 730, 730f
Hamartomatous polyps, colonic, 816–818, 816t,
    817f, 818f
HAMP gene, 862
Hand-Schuller-Christian triad, 632
Hansen's disease, 372–374, 373f, 374f
  polyneuropathy due to, 1262
Haploinsufficiency, 277
Haplotypes, 177, 178f
HapMap project, 177, 178f
Haptoglobin, 642
Hashimoto thyroiditis, 1111–1113, 1112f
Hashitoxicosis, 1113
Hassall corpuscles, 635
HAV (hepatitis A virus), 844, 844t, 845f
Haw River syndrome, 168t
Hay, lung diseases due to, 697t
Hay fever, 749
HbA (adult hemoglobin), 645
Hb$_{A1C}$ (glycosylated hemoglobin), 1138
HbC (hemoglobin C), 645
HBcAg (hepatitis B core antigen), 846
HBeAg (hepatitis B "e" antigen), 846, 847f
HB-EGF (heparin-binding epidermal growth
    factor), in tissue regeneration and wound
    healing, 87t
HbF (fetal hemoglobin), 645
HbH (hemoglobin H) disease, 652, 652t
HBIG (hepatitis B immunoglobulin), 849
HbS (hemoglobin S), 140, 645
  and resistance to malaria, 387
HBsAg (hepatitis B surface antigen), 846,
    847f
HbSC (hemoglobin SC) disease, 645
HBV. See Hepatitis B virus (HBV).
HCC. See Hepatocellular carcinoma (HCC).
HCM. See Hypertrophic cardiomyopathy
    (HCM).
HCV. See Hepatitis C virus (HCV).
HD (Huntington disease), 168t, 1322–1323,
    1322f
HDL (high-density lipoprotein) cholesterol, and
    atherosclerosis, 497, 500
HDV (hepatitis D virus), 844t, 848–849
Head and neck disorder(s), 739–761
  of ears, 754
  of neck, 754–756, 755f
  of oral cavity, 740–749
    aphthous ulcers as, 742, 742f
    caries as, 740
    fibrous proliferative lesions as, 741–742,
      741f
    gingivitis as, 740–741
    glossitis as, 742
    hairy leukoplakia as, 743
    due to infections, 742–743

Head and neck disorder(s) (Continued)
    inflammatory/reactive tumor-like lesions as,
      741–742
    leukoplakia and erythroplakia as, 744–745,
      745f–747f
    odontogenic cysts and tumors as, 748–749,
      748f
    periodontitis as, 741
    squamous cell carcinoma as, 745–748, 747f
    due to systemic disease, 743, 744t
  of salivary glands, 756–761
    neoplasms as, 757–761, 757t, 758f–760f
    sialadenitis as, 756–757, 757f
    xerostomia as, 756
  of upper airways, 749–753, 750f–753f
Head and neck squamous cell carcinomas
    (HNSCCs), 745–748
Healing, 98–108
  angiogenesis in, 99–102, 99f, 100t, 101f
  cutaneous, 102–106, 103f–105f, 104t
  local and systemic factors that influence, 106
  pathologic aspects of, 106–108, 106f–108f
  regeneration and repair in, 79–80, 80f, 81f
Healthcare-associated infections, 342
Heart, 529–585
  aging effects on, 531–532, 532t
  amyloidosis of, 254, 255
  blood supply to, 531
  conduction system of, 531
  fatty change in, 34
  in hereditary hemochromatosis, 862
  myxedema, 581
  structure and specializations of, 530–531
  tumors of, 583–585
    cardiac effects of noncardiac, 584–585, 584t
    primary cardiac, 583–584, 583f
Heart attack. See Myocardial infarction (MI).
Heart disease
  due to adverse drug reactions, 416t
  due to alcoholism, 414
  carcinoid, 569–570, 570f
  cardiomyopathy(ies) as, 571–581
    alcoholic, 573
    due to amyloidosis, 580, 580f
    arrhythmogenic right ventricular, 575, 576f
    due to cardiotoxic drugs, 579
    due to catecholamines, 579–580
    conditions associated with, 573t
    dilated, 572–575
      clinical features of, 574–575
      functional patterns and causes of, 572t
      graphic representation of, 572f
      morphology of, 572–573, 574f
      pathogenesis of, 573–574, 574f, 575f
      X-linked, 573
    due to hyperthyroidism and
      hypothyroidism, 581
    hypertrophic, 575–577
      clinical features of, 577
      functional patterns and causes of, 572t
      graphic representation of, 572f
      morphology of, 575–576, 576f
      pathogenesis of, 574f, 575f, 577
    due to iron overload, 580
    myocarditis as, 578, 578t, 579f
    peripartum, 573–574
    restrictive, 572f, 572t, 577
  congenital, 537–545
    cardiac development and, 537–538, 538f
    clinical features of, 539–540
    cyanotic, 540
    etiology and pathogenesis of, 538–539, 539t
    incidence of, 537, 537t
    with left-to-right shunts, 540–542, 540f

Heart disease, congenital (Continued)
    atrial septal defect as, 540f, 541
    atrioventricular septal defect as, 540f, 542
    patent ductus arteriosus as, 540f,
      541–542
    patent foramen ovale as, 541
    ventricular septal defect as, 540f, 541,
      541f
    obstructive, 544–545
      aortic stenosis and atresia as, 544–545
      coarctation of the aorta as, 544, 544f
      pulmonary stenosis and atresia as, 544
    with right-to-left shunts, 540, 542–544,
      542f
      persistent truncus arteriosus as, 543
      tetralogy of Fallot as, 542–543, 542f
      total anomalous pulmonary venous
        connection as, 543–544
      transposition of the great arteries as,
        542f, 543, 543f
      tricuspid atresia as, 543
  epidemiology of, 530
  global warming and, 402
  hypertensive, 559–560
    pulmonary (right-sided), 559–560, 560f,
      560t
    systemic (left-sided), 559, 560f
  ischemic, 496–498, 545–559
    angina pectoris as, 545, 546–547, 546f
    chronic, 546f, 558
    epidemiology of, 545
    myocardial infarction as, 547–558
      clinical features of, 553–556, 555f
      completed, 549, 549f, 554f
      consequences and complications of,
        556–558, 556f, 558f
      expansion of, 556f, 557
      extension of, 553, 557
      healing of, 553
      incidence and risk factors for, 547
      microscopic features of, 552, 552f
      morphology of, 550–553, 550t, 551f, 552f
      pathogenesis of, 547–550, 548f, 548t,
        549f
      regions of, 549–550, 549f, 550–551, 551f
      reperfusion of, 553, 554f, 555f
      reversible vs. irreversible, 547–548, 548f,
        550t, 554f
      right ventricular, 557
      subendocardial, 550, 551f
      temporal evolution of, 550, 550t
      therapy for, 556
      transmural, 547, 550, 551f
      triphenyltetrazolium chloride staining in,
        551, 552f
    pathogenesis of, 545–546, 546f
    silent, 555
    sudden cardiac death due to, 546, 558–559
  due to occupational exposures, 409t
  oral contraceptives and, 415
  overview of pathophysiology of, 532
  pericardial, 581–583
    hemopericardium as, 581
    pericardial effusion as, 581
    pericarditis as, 581–583, 581t, 582f
    due to rheumatologic diseases, 583
  rheumatic, 565–566, 565f, 567f
  in systemic sclerosis, 225
  tumors as, 583–585
    cardiac effects of noncardiac, 584–585, 584t
    primary cardiac, 583–584, 583f
  valvular, 560–571
    with calcification, 561–563, 562f
    carcinoid, 569–570, 570f

Heart disease (Continued)
  causes of acquired, 561, 561t
  due to complications of artificial valves,
      570–571, 571f, 571t
  endocarditis as
    infective, 566–568, 567f, 568f, 569t
    Libman-Sacks, 567f, 569
    nonbacterial thrombotic, 567f, 568–569,
        570f
  mitral valve prolapse as, 563–565, 564f
  rheumatic, 565–566, 565f, 567f
Heart failure, 533–537
  epidemiology of, 533
  left-sided, 535–536
  pathogenesis of, 533
  progression from cardiac hypertrophy to,
      533–535, 534f, 535f
  right-sided, 536–537
  treatment of, 537
Heart failure cells, 114, 535, 680
Heart failure with normal ejection fraction
    (HFNEF), 536
Heart fields, in cardiac development, 537–538,
    538f
Heart transplantation, 585, 585f
Heart valves, 531
  aging effect on, 532
  artificial, complications of, 570–571, 571f,
      571t
  diseases of, 560–571
    with calcification, 561–563, 562f
    carcinoid, 569–570, 570f
    causes of acquired, 561, 561t
    endocarditis as
      infective, 566–568, 567f, 568f, 569t
      Libman-Sacks, 567f, 569
      nonbacterial thrombotic, 567f, 568–569,
          570f
    mitral valve prolapse as, 563–565, 564f
    rheumatic, 565–566, 565f, 567f
Heat cramps, 422
Heat exhaustion, 422
Heat stroke, 422
Heat-labile toxin (LT), 802
Heat-stable toxin (ST), 802
Heavy-chain disease, 609
Heberden nodes, 1236
Hedgehog signaling pathway, 451
Heinz bodies, 645, 645f
Helicobacter heilmannii, 777
Helicobacter pylori
  as carcinogen, 315–316
  and peptic ulcer disease, 780, 781
Helicobacter pylori gastritis, 776–778, 777f,
    778t
HELLP syndrome, 875, 1056, 1057
Helminth(s), 333t, 336
Helminthic infections
  in AIDS, 245t, 246
  of liver, 854
Helper T (T$_H$) lymphocytes
  in delayed-type hypersensitivity, 205, 206f
  in immediate hypersensitivity, 199, 199f
  in immune response, 185f, 186, 195, 195f
  proliferation and differentiation of, 206–207
Hemangioblast(s), 99
Hemangioblastomas, in von Hippel–Lindau
    disease, 1343
Hemangioendothelioma, 524
Hemangioma(s), 520–521, 521f
  capillary, 520–521, 521f
  cavernous, 521, 521f
    of liver, 876, 876f
  in infants and children, 473, 474f

Hemangioma(s) (Continued)
  pyogenic granuloma as, 521, 521f
  strawberry type (juvenile), 520, 521f
Hemangiopericytoma, 525
Hemangiosarcoma, 524
Hemarthrosis, 114
Hematemesis, esophageal causes of, 768, 768t
Hematocele, 993
Hematocrit, 640
  adult reference range for, 641t
Hematogenous spread, 270, 270f
Hematologic disorder(s)
  due to cancer, 321t, 322
  oral manifestations of, 744t
  in systemic lupus erythematosus, 214t
Hematologic infections, perinatal, 459, 459f
Hematoma, 114
  epidural, 1289, 1289f
  hepatic, due to eclampsia, 875, 875f
  pulsating, 506
  subdural, 1289–1290, 1289f, 1290f
Hematopoiesis, spleen in, 633
Hematopoietic disorders, 590
  due to occupational exposures, 409t
Hematopoietic stem cell(s) (HSCs), 84–85, 590
Hematopoietic stem cell (HSC) transplantation,
    230
Hematopoietic system
  components of, 589
  radiation effect on, 425
Hematopoietic tissues
  development and maintenance of, 590, 591f,
      592t
  morphology of, 590–592
Hematuria
  asymptomatic, 907
  benign familial, 932
Hemizygosity, 142
Hemochromatosis, 660
  clinical features of, 863
  hereditary (primary), 861–863, 861t, 863f
  liver disease due to, 861–863, 861t, 863f
  morphology of, 862–863, 863f
  myocardial disease due to, 580
  neonatal, 863
  pathogenesis of, 862
  secondary or acquired, 861t, 863
Hemodialysis-associated amyloidosis, 252t,
    253
Hemodynamic disorder(s), 111–115
  in atherosclerosis, 500
  edema as, 111–113, 112f, 112t, 113f
  hemorrhage as, 114–115, 115f
  hyperemia and congestion as, 113–114,
      114f
Hemodynamic pulmonary edema, 680, 680t
Hemoglobin
  adult reference range for, 641t
  defect in, 143t
  glycosylated, 1138
  mean cell, 640, 641t
Hemoglobin C (HbC), 645
Hemoglobin concentration, 640
  mean cell, 640, 641t
    in sickle cell disease, 645–646
Hemoglobin H (HbH) disease, 652, 652t
Hemoglobin S (HbS), 140, 645
  and resistance to malaria, 387
Hemoglobin SC (HbSC) disease, 645
Hemoglobinopathies, genetic basis for, 144
Hemoglobinuria, paroxysmal
  cold, 654
  nocturnal, 235, 652–653, 653f
Hemojuvelin (HJV), 862

Hemolysis
  extravascular, 641
    in β-thalassemia major, 649, 650f
  intravascular, 641–642
    in paroxysmal nocturnal hemoglobinuria,
        652–653
Hemolytic anemia(s), 641–654
  autoimmune, 203, 203t
  classification of, 640t, 642
  clinical manifestations of, 642
  common features of, 641
  due to glucose-6-phosphate dehydrogenase
      deficiency, 644–645, 644f, 645f
  due to hereditary spherocytosis, 642–644,
      643f, 644f
  immuno-, 653–654, 653t
  microangiopathic, 654, 654f
  morphology of, 642, 642f
  due to paroxysmal nocturnal hemoglobinuria,
      652–653, 653f
  pathogenesis of, 641–642
  due to red cell trauma, 654, 654f
  due to sickle cell disease, 645–648, 646f, 647f
  due to thalassemia syndromes, 648–652,
      649f–651f, 652t
Hemolytic disease of the newborn, 202, 461,
    462f, 840
Hemolytic-uremic syndrome (HUS), 669–670,
    669t, 952–954
  due to shigellosis, 801
Hemopericardium, 114, 581
Hemoperitoneum, 114
Hemophilia A, 672
Hemophilia B, 672–673
Hemorrhage(s), 114–115, 115f
  intracerebral (intraparenchymal), 1286,
      1295–1297, 1296f
  intracranial, 1295–1299, 1296f–1298f
  pulmonary, 30–31, 706f
    syndromes of diffuse, 709–710, 709f
  retinal, 1359f
  slit, 1295
  subarachnoid, 1297–1298, 1297f, 1298f
Hemorrhagic cystitis, 975
Hemorrhagic diatheses, 114. See also Bleeding
    disorder(s).
Hemorrhagic shock, 114, 129, 130t
  due to burn injury, 421
Hemorrhoids, 519–520, 826
Hemosiderin, 660
  in hereditary hemochromatosis, 862
  intracellular accumulation of, 36–38, 37f
Hemosiderosis, 37–38, 861t, 863
  in hemolytic anemia, 642
  idiopathic pulmonary, 710
  myocardial disease due to, 580
Hemostasis, 115–120
  coagulation cascade in, 118–120, 120f, 121f
  endothelium in, 115–117, 116f–118f
  general sequence of events in, 115, 116f
  genetic defects in, 143t
  and ischemic heart disease, 498
  platelets in, 115, 116f, 117–118, 119f
  primary, 115, 116f
  secondary, 115, 116f
  tests of, 666
Hemostatic clot, 115
Hemostatic plug, 115, 116f, 117
  secondary, 118
Hemothorax, 114, 732
Hemp dust, lung diseases due to, 697t
Henoch-Schönlein purpura, 666
  renal manifestations of, 934
Hepadnaviridae, 845–846

Heparan sulfate, in extracellular matrix, 97, 98f
Heparin-binding epidermal growth factor (HB-EGF), in tissue regeneration and wound healing, 87t
Heparin-induced thrombocytopenia (HIT), 123, 668–669
Heparin-like molecules, 116, 117f
Hepatic acinus, 834, 834f
Hepatic adenoma, 877, 877f
    oral contraceptives and, 415
Hepatic angiosarcomas, 524–525
Hepatic artery compromise, impaired blood flow into liver due to, 870–871, 871f
Hepatic complications, of organ or bone marrow transplantation, 874, 874f
Hepatic congestion, 114, 114f
Hepatic disease. See Liver disease.
Hepatic encephalopathy, 836, 1329
Hepatic failure, 835–836
    acute, 835–836
    chronic, 836
    fulminant, 835, 853, 854f
Hepatic fibrosis, 837, 837f
    congenital, 870, 959
    drug- and toxin-induced, 856t
Hepatic granulomas, drug- and toxin-induced, 856t
Hepatic hemangiomas, cavernous, 876, 876f
Hepatic hematoma, due to eclampsia, 875, 875f
Hepatic injury
    drug- and toxin-induced, 856–857, 856t
    patterns of, 835
Hepatic lobule, 834, 834f
Hepatic neoplasms, drug- and toxin-induced, 856t
Hepatic rupture, due to eclampsia, 875
Hepatic sclerosis, 871
Hepatic steatosis
    due to alcohol consumption, 857–858, 857f, 859–860
    in cystic fibrosis, 469
Hepatic stellate cells (HSCs), 835
Hepatic vein thrombosis, 872–873, 873f
Hepatic venous outflow obstruction, 872–874
Hepatitis
    alcoholic, 857f, 858, 858f, 860
    autoimmune, 855–856, 855f
    cholestatic, drug- and toxin-induced, 856t
    herpes, 353
    interface, 852, 853
    neonatal, 866, 866f
        due to α₁-antitrypsin deficiency, 865, 865f, 866
    viral, 843–853, 844t
        acute, 850, 851–852, 851f, 852f
        carrier state of, 850
        chronic, 850–851, 851f–853f, 852–853
        clinical course of, 853
        clinicopathologic syndromes of, 850–851
        defined, 844
        fulminant, 835, 853, 854f
        due to hepatitis A virus, 844, 844t, 845f
        due to hepatitis B virus, 844t, 845–847, 845f–847f
        due to hepatitis C virus, 844t, 847–848, 848f
        due to hepatitis D virus, 844t, 848–849
        due to hepatitis E virus, 844t, 849
        due to hepatitis G virus, 849
        HIV and, 850–851
        morphology of, 851–853, 851f–854f
    in Wilson disease, 864
Hepatitis A virus (HAV), 844, 844t, 845f
Hepatitis B core antigen (HBcAg), 846

Hepatitis B "e" antigen (HBeAg), 846, 847f
Hepatitis B immunoglobulin (HBIG), 849
Hepatitis B surface antigen (HBsAg), 846, 847f
Hepatitis B virus (HBV), 355, 844t, 845–847
    carrier state for, 850
    chronic, 850, 851, 852f
    clinical presentation of, 845
    epidemiology of, 845
    genomic structure of, 845–846, 846f
    and hepatitis D virus, 848–849
    and hepatocellular carcinoma, 878–879
    HIV and, 850–851
    natural course of, 846, 847f
    oncogenic potential of, 315
    potential outcomes of, 845, 845f
    serum markers for, 846, 847f
    transmission of, 845
    vaccine for, 846–847
Hepatitis C virus (HCV), 844t, 847–848
    carrier state for, 850
    chronic, 848, 848f, 850, 851, 852f
    clinical course of, 848
    epidemiology of, 847
    genomic structure of, 847, 848f
    HIV and, 850–851
    oncogenic potential of, 315
    quasispecies of, 847–848
    risk factors for, 847
    serologic markers for, 848, 848f
    transmission of, 847
Hepatitis D virus (HDV), 844t, 848–849
Hepatitis E virus (HEV), 844t, 849
Hepatitis G virus (HGV), 849
Hepatization
    gray, 713
    red, 713, 714f
Hepatoblastoma, 877–878, 878f
Hepatocavopathy, obliterative, 873
Hepatocellular carcinoma (HCC), 877, 878–880
    aflatoxin and, 311, 385, 443, 878
    clinical features of, 879–880
    epidemiology of, 878
    hepatitis B virus and, 315
    hepatitis C virus and, 315
    metastatic, 270
    morphology of, 879, 879f, 880f
    pathogenesis of, 878–879
Hepatocellular liver disease, anemia due to, 665
Hepatocellular necrosis, drug- and toxin-induced, 856t
Hepatocellular steatosis, alcoholic, 857–858, 857f, 859
Hepatocyte(s), anatomy of, 834–835
Hepatocyte function, laboratory evaluation of, 835t
Hepatocyte growth factor (HGF)
    proto-oncogene for, 281t
    in renal cell carcinoma, 965
    in tissue regeneration and wound healing, 87t, 88
Hepatocyte integrity, laboratory evaluation of, 835t
Hepatomegaly
    congestive, in right-sided heart failure, 536
    in cystic fibrosis, 470
    due to galactosemia, 464, 465f
Hepatopulmonary syndrome (HPS), 836
Hepatorenal syndrome, 836
Hepatotoxins, 856–857, 856t
Hepatotropic virus, 844
Hepcidin, 75
    in β-thalassemia major, 650
    in iron metabolism, 660, 661f, 862

HER2/neu, 88, 281
    in breast cancer, 1085, 1086f, 1090
Hereditary angioedema, 235
Hereditary disorders, 140
Hereditary hemochromatosis, 861–863, 861t, 863f
Hereditary hemorrhagic telangiectasia, 522, 666
Hereditary hyperbilirubinemias, 841–842, 841t, 842f
Hereditary motor and sensory neuropathies (HMSNs), 1263–1265, 1265f
Hereditary nephritis, 931–932, 932f
Hereditary neuropathies, 1263–1265, 1263t, 1264t, 1265f
Hereditary non-polyposis colorectal cancer (HNPCC), 274, 275, 302, 821–822, 822t
Hereditary predisposition, to cancer, 325
Hereditary sensory and autonomic neuropathies (HSANs), 1263, 1263t
Hereditary spherocytosis (HS), 642–644, 643f, 644f
Heredofamilial amyloidosis, 252t, 253
Hermaphroditism, 167
Hernia(s)
    diaphragmatic, 765
    hiatal, 770
    inguinal, 790, 791f
    intestinal, 790, 791f
Hernia sac, 790
Herniation
    of brain, 1283–1284, 1283f, 1284f
        subfalcine (cingulate), 1283, 1283f
        tonsillar, 1283f, 1284
        transtentorial (uncinate, mesial temporal), 1283–1284, 1283f
    external, 790
    internal, 791
Heroin, abuse of, 418–419, 418t
Herpes, genital, 352, 1008–1009
Herpes bronchopneumonia, 353
Herpes encephalitis, 1302–1303, 1303f
Herpes epithelial keratitis, 352
Herpes esophagitis, 353
Herpes hepatitis, 353
Herpes labialis, 743
Herpes simplex keratitis, 1351, 1351f
Herpes simplex virus (HSV), 341t, 352–353
    in AIDS, 246
    encephalitis due to, 1302–1303, 1303f
    genital infection with, 352, 1008–1009
    morphology of, 352–353, 352f
    of oral cavity, 742–743
Herpes stromal keratitis, 352
Herpes zoster, encephalitis due to, 1303–1304
Herpesvirus esophagitis, 769, 769f
Herpesvirus infections, 351–355
Herpetic gingivostomatitis, acute, 742
Herpetic stomatitis, recurrent, 743
5-HETE (5-hydroxyeicosatetraenoic acid), in inflammation, 58f, 59
Heterocyclic aromatic hydrocarbons, as carcinogens, 309t
Heterodimerization, 91–92
Heteroplasmy, 171, 1328
Heterotopia, 473
Heterotopic bone, in dystrophic calcification, 38
Heterotopic rest, 262
Heterozygosity, loss of, 288
HEV(s) (high endothelial venules), 190, 190f
HEV (hepatitis E virus), 844t, 849
Hexosaminidase, defect in, 143t
Hexosaminidase α-subunit deficiency, 139f, 150–152, 151t, 152f
Heymann nephritis, 912, 913f

HFE gene, 862
HFNEF (heart failure with normal ejection fraction), 536
HGF (hepatocyte growth factor)
 proto-oncogene for, 281t
 in renal cell carcinoma, 965
 in tissue regeneration and wound healing, 87t, 88
HGF gene, 281t
HGPRT (hypoxanthine guanine phosphoribosyl transferase), in gout, 1243, 1244f
HGV (hepatitis G virus), 849
HHD (hypertensive heart disease), 559–560
 pulmonary (right-sided), 559–560, 560f, 560t
 systemic (left-sided), 559, 560f
HHV-8 (human herpesvirus-8), 247, 523–524, 597
Hiatal hernia, 770
Hibernation, of myocardium, 553
Hidradenitis, 358–359
Hidradenoma, papillary, of vulva, 1015, 1015f
Hierarchical clustering, 325
HIF-1 (hypoxia-inducible factor-1), 24
 in renal cell carcinoma, 965
HIF-1α (hypoxia-inducible factor-1α), 45
High endothelial venules (HEVs), 190, 190f
High-density lipoprotein (HDL) cholesterol, and atherosclerosis, 497, 500
High-fiber diet, and colon cancer, 443
High-grade squamous intraepithelial lesion (HSIL), 1019–1021, 1020f, 1020t, 1021t, 1023f
Highly active antiretroviral therapy (HAART), for HIV infection, 248
Hilus cell(s), 1007
Hilus cell tumors, 1007, 1052
Hirano bodies, in Alzheimer disease, 1316
Hirschsprung disease, 766–767, 766f
Histamine
 in asthma, 689
 in immediate hypersensitivity, 199
 in inflammation, 57–58, 57t
Histiocytoma, fibrous
 benign, 1182, 1184f, 1253
 malignant, 1253
Histiocytosis(es), 596, 631
 Langerhans cell, 596, 631–632, 631f
 sinus, 596
Histologic methods, for diagnosis of cancer, 323
Histones, post-translational modifications of, in carcinogenesis, 306
Histoplasma capsulatum, chronic pneumonia due to, 717–718, 718f
Histoplasmosis, 717–718, 718f
 fulminant disseminated, 718, 718f
HIT (heparin-induced thrombocytopenia), 123, 668–669
HIV. *See* Human immunodeficiency virus (HIV).
HIV-associated nephropathy, 928
HJV (hemojuvelin), 862
HL. *See* Hodgkin lymphoma (HL).
HLA. *See* Human leukocyte antigen (HLA).
HMSNs (hereditary motor and sensory neuropathies), 1263–1265, 1265f
HNPCC (hereditary non-polyposis colorectal cancer), 274, 275, 302, 821–822, 822t
HNSCCs (head and neck squamous cell carcinomas), 745–748
H_2O_2 (hydrogen peroxide)
 cell injury due to, 20
 in inflammation, 60
 in phagocytosis, 53, 53f

Hodgkin lymphoma (HL), 616–620
 AIDS-related, 247
 classical forms of, 617
 classification of, 598, 598t, 617
 clinical features of, 620, 621t
 defined, 616
 epidemiology of, 617
 lymphocyte depletion type of, 618t, 619
 lymphocyte predominance type of, 618t, 619–620, 619f
 lymphocyte-rich type of, 618t, 619, 619f
 mixed-cellularity type of, 618t, 619, 619f
 molecular pathogenesis of, 620, 621f
 nodular sclerosis type of, 618–619, 618f, 618t
 non-Hodgkin *vs.,* 616–617, 617t
 Reed-Sternberg cells in, 616–620, 617f, 621f
 spread of, 600
 staging of, 620, 621t
 treatment of, 620
Hollenhorst plaques, 1362
Holoprosencephaly, 451, 1285
Holt-Oram syndrome, 1211t
Homan sign, 520
Homeobox genes
 in bone growth and development, 1209
 mutations in, 1210
Homeobox (HOX) proteins, 453
Homeostasis, 5
Homer-Wright pseudorosettes, in neuroblastomas, 476
Homing, of tumor cells, in metastasis, 300–301
Homocysteine, elevated levels of, and thrombosis, 122–123
Homocystinuria, and coronary artery disease, 498
Homogeneous staining regions, in carcinogenesis, 306
Homogentisic acid, intracellular accumulation of, 36
Homogentisic acid deficiency, 36, 155–156
Homologous recombination, 426
Honeycomb fibrosis, 695, 695f
Hookworms, 336
 enterocolitis due to, 806
Hormonal effects, of tumors, 320
Hormone(s), 1098
 ectopic production of, due to cancer, 322
 and wound healing, 106
Hormone replacement therapy (HRT), adverse effects of, 414–415
Hormone response elements, 91
Horn cysts, 1175, 1175f
Horner syndrome, due to lung carcinoma, 729
Horseshoe kidneys, 955
Hospital-acquired pneumonia, 711t, 716
Host cells, bacterial adherence to, 343–344
Host defenses
 against infections, 342
  injurious effects of, 344–345
 against tumors, 316–320
  antitumor effector mechanisms in, 318–319
  immune surveillance and escape as, 316, 319–320, 319f
  tumor antigens in, 316–318, 317f
Host resistance, to infections
 vitamin A in, 432
 vitamin D in, 436, 437f
Howell-Jolly bodies, in sickle cell disease, 646
HOX (homeobox) proteins, 453
HPS (hepatopulmonary syndrome), 836
HPV. *See* Human papillomavirus (HPV).
HRAS oncogene, 281t, 282
HRT (hormone replacement therapy), adverse effects of, 414–415

HS (hereditary spherocytosis), 642–644, 643f, 644f
HSANs (hereditary sensory and autonomic neuropathies), 1263, 1263t
HSC(s) (hepatic stellate cells), 835
HSC (hematopoietic stem cells), 84–85, 590
HSC (hematopoietic stem cell) transplantation, 230
HSIL (high-grade squamous intraepithelial lesion), 1019–1021, 1020f, 1020t, 1021t, 1023f
HST1 gene, 281t
HSV. *See* Herpes simplex virus (HSV).
5-HT (serotonergic) system, in sudden infant death syndrome, 472
HTLV-1 (human T-cell leukemia virus type 1), 312–313, 597, 615–616
Huebner arteritis, 1301
Human Genome Project, 136
Human herpesvirus-8 (HHV-8), 247, 523–524, 597
Human immunodeficiency virus (HIV), 235–249, 341t. *See also* Acquired immunodeficiency syndrome (AIDS).
 aseptic meningitis due to, 1305
 central nervous system involvement in, 242–243, 248, 1305, 1305f
 chronic infection with, 244–245
 clinical features of, 245–248, 245t
 effect of antiretroviral drug therapy on, 248
 encephalitis due to, 1305, 1305f
 epidemiology of, 236–237
 hairy leukoplakia with, 743
 and hepatitis, 850–851
 immune response to, 244f
 infection of non-T cells by, 241–242
 infection of T cells by, 239–240, 239f
 latency phase of, 243f, 244–245, 244f
 life cycle of, 239–240, 239f
 mechanisms of T-cell immunodeficiency in, 240–241, 241f, 242t
 morphology of, 249
 natural history of, 243–245, 243f, 244f, 244t
 opportunistic infections in, 245t, 246
 oral manifestations of, 744t
 pathogenesis of, 238–243
 pneumonia in, 719–720
 primary infection with, 243–244, 243f
 prognosis for, 249
 properties of, 237–238
 replication of, 239f, 240
 structure of, 237–238, 237f
 thrombocytopenia associated with, 669
 transmission of, 236–237
 tuberculosis in, 246, 369–370
 tumors in, 246–248, 247f
 types of, 237
Human immunodeficiency virus (HIV)-associated dementia, 1305
Human leukocyte antigen (HLA) alleles
 in rheumatoid arthritis, 1238
 in Sjögren syndrome, 221–222
 in transplant rejection, 227
Human leukocyte antigen (HLA) complex
 and disease association, 192–193, 193t
 in immune response, 190–192, 191f, 192f
Human leukocyte antigen (HLA) genes, in autoimmunity, 212
Human leukocyte antigen (HLA) haplotype, 192
Human leukocyte antigen (HLA) matching, for transplantation, 229
Human leukocyte antigen (HLA) molecules
 in immune response, 190–192, 191f, 192f
 in type 1 diabetes mellitus, 1134

Human papillomavirus (HPV), 341t
  in AIDS, 248
  and cervical carcinoma, 1018–1019, 1018f,
    1019f, 1020–1021, 1021f
  and condyloma acuminatum of penis,
    982–983
  and cutaneous squamous cell carcinoma,
    1180
  and head and neck squamous cell carcinoma,
    746
  laryngeal papillomatosis due to, 752
  oncogenic potential of, 313–314, 313f
  and penile carcinoma, 984
  and verrucae, 1201
  and vulvar intraepithelial neoplasia, 1013,
    1013f
Human papillomavirus (HPV) DNA testing,
    1024
Human papillomavirus (HPV) vaccine, 1023,
    1024
Human T-cell leukemia virus type 1 (HTLV-1),
    312–313, 597, 615–616
Humidifier lung, 703
Humoral immunity, 185, 195–196, 196f
Humoral rejection, 227–228
Hunner ulcers, 975
Hunter, John, 44
Hunter syndrome, 151t, 153, 154
Huntingtin, 1322
Huntington disease (HD), 168t, 1322–1323,
    1322f
Hurler syndrome, 151t, 154
Hürthle cell(s), 1112, 1112f
Hürthle cell adenoma, 1119, 1119f
Hürthle cell variant, of follicular thyroid
    carcinoma, 1123
HUS (hemolytic-uremic syndrome), 669–670,
    669t, 952–954
  due to shigellosis, 801
Hutchinson teeth, 377
Hyaline arteriolosclerosis, 495, 495f
  in benign nephrosclerosis, 949, 950f
  due to diabetes mellitus, 1140, 1141f
Hyaline cartilage, 1235
Hyaline change, 36
Hyaline membrane(s), in acute respiratory
    distress syndrome, 680, 681f
Hyaline membrane disease, 456–458,
    457f
Hyaluronan (HA), in extracellular matrix, 95f,
    97–98, 98f
Hydatid disease, 392–393
Hydatidiform mole, 1057–1059
  complete, 1058–1059, 1058f, 1059f
  partial, 1058, 1058f
Hydatids of Morgagni, 1039
Hydrocele, 993
Hydrocephalus, 1283, 1283f
  post-traumatic, 1290
Hydrogen peroxide (H_2O_2)
  cell injury due to, 20
  in inflammation, 60
  in phagocytosis, 53, 53f
Hydromyelia, 1286
Hydronephrosis, 961–962, 961f, 973
Hydropic change, in cell injury, 13
Hydropic swelling, 1168
Hydrops
  corneal, 1352, 1352f
  fetalis, 459–462
    due to α-thalassemia, 652, 652t
    clinical features of, 462
    defined, 459–460
    immune, 460–461, 460f

Hydrops, fetalis (Continued)
    morphology of, 461–462, 462f
    nonimmune, 460, 461, 461t
  of gallbladder, 886
Hydrosalpinx, 1010
Hydrostatic pressure, increased, edema due to,
    112, 112f, 112t
Hydrothorax, 732
Hydroureter, 972, 973
25-Hydroxycholecalciferol (25-OH-D), 433, 434f
5-Hydroxyeicosatetraenoic acid (5-HETE), in
    inflammation, 58f, 59
Hydroxyl radical
  cell injury due to, 20
  in inflammation, 60
21-Hydroxylase deficiency, 1152–1154, 1153f
5-Hydroxytryptamine, in inflammation, 57–58,
    57t
Hygiene hypothesis, 201
  of asthma, 691
  of inflammatory bowel disease, 808
Hygroma, cystic, 460, 461, 462f, 522
Hymenolepis nana, 806
Hyperacute graft rejection, 227, 228, 228f
Hyperadrenalism, 1148–1154
  in adrenogenital syndromes, 1152–1154,
    1153f
  in hypercortisolism (Cushing syndrome),
    1148–1151, 1148t, 1149f–1151f, 1150t
  in primary hyperaldosteronism, 1151–1152,
    1151f
Hyperaldosteronism
  bilateral idiopathic, 1151
  glucocorticoid-remediable, 1151
  primary, 1151–1152, 1151f
  secondary, 1151–1152
Hyperammonemia, due to liver failure, 836
Hyperbilirubinemia(s)
  due to hemolytic anemia, 642
  hereditary, 841–842, 841t, 842f
  unconjugated vs. conjugated, 841, 841t
Hypercalcemia, 1126
  causes of, 1128, 1129t
  familial hypocalciuric, 1127
  hypercalciuria without, 962
  incidental, 1126
  of malignancy, 321t, 322, 1126
  metastatic calcification due to, 38–39
  and nephrocalcinosis, 947
Hypercalciuria, without hypercalcemia, 962
Hypercholesterolemia
  and atherosclerosis, 497, 500, 501f
  familial, 144, 147–149, 147t–149f
Hyperchromatic nuclei, 263, 264, 265f
Hypercoagulability
  in systemic lupus erythematosus, 215
  in thrombosis, 122–123, 122t
Hypercortisolism, 1148–1151
  clinical course of, 151f, 1150–1151, 1150t
  morphology of, 1149–1150, 1149f, 1150f
  pathogenesis of, 1104, 1148–1149, 1148t
Hyperemia, 113
Hyperglycemia
  familial mild fasting, 1137
  intracellular, 1139
  neurologic sequelae of, 1329
  in septic shock, 131
Hypergranulosis, 1168
Hyperhomocystinemia, and coronary artery
    disease, 498
Hyper-IgM syndrome, 233–234
Hyperinflation, compensatory, 687
Hyperinsulinemia, obesity and, 442, 442f, 443
Hyperinsulinism, 1146–1147, 1147f

Hyperkeratinization, due to vitamin A
    deficiency, 433
Hyperkeratosis, 1168
Hyperlipidemia
  and atherosclerosis, 497, 500, 501f
  in nephrotic syndrome, 922
Hypermetabolic state, due to burn injury, 421
Hypermobility, in Ehlers-Danlos syndrome, 146,
    146t
Hypernephroma, 964
Hyperosmolar nonketotic coma, 1143
Hyperoxaluria, 962
Hyperparathyroidism, 1126–1129
  asymptomatic, 1128–1129
  brown tumors of, 1128
  causes of, 1127, 1127f
  clinical course of, 1128–1129
  epidemiology of, 1127
  hypercalcemia due to, 38
  in MEN-1, 1162
  morphology of, 1127–1128, 1128f
  primary, 1126–1129, 1127f, 1128f, 1129t
  in renal failure, 1219
  secondary, 1129
  skeletal disorders due to, 1218, 1218f, 1219f
  symptomatic, 1129
  tertiary, 1129
Hyperphenylalaninemia, 463–464, 463f
Hyperphosphatemia, in renal failure, 1219
Hyperpituitarism, 1100–1105
Hyperplasia, 8–9, 450
  compensatory, 8, 93
  hormonal, 8
  mechanisms of, 9
  pathologic, 8–9
  physiologic, 8
Hyperplastic arteriolitis, in malignant
    hypertension, 950f, 951
Hyperplastic arteriolosclerosis, 495f, 496
Hyperplastic polyps
  colonic, 818–819, 819f
  gastric, 782t, 783, 784f
Hyperprolactinemia, 1103–1104
Hyperpyrexia, malignant, 1270
Hypersensitivity myocarditis, 578, 579f
Hypersensitivity pneumonitis, 703–704, 703f
  organic dusts that produce, 697t
Hypersensitivity reactions, 197–208
  antibody-mediated (type II), 197t, 198,
    201–204, 202f, 203t
  cell-mediated (type IV), 197t, 198, 205–208,
    206f–208f, 206t
  defined, 197
  delayed-type, 205–207, 206f–208f
    chronic inflammation due to, 70
  immediate (type I), 197t, 198–201, 198f–200f,
    201t
  immune complex–mediated (type III), 197t,
    198, 204–205, 204f, 204t, 205f
  inflammation due to, 45
Hypersensitivity vasculitis, 515, 516f
Hypersplenism, 633
Hypertension, 492–496
  accelerated or malignant, 492, 949–951, 950f
    retina in, 1359
  and aortic dissection, 509
  and atherosclerosis, 497–498
  blood pressure regulation and, 492–493, 494f
  defined, 492
  in diabetes, 1144
  epidemiology of, 492
  essential (idiopathic), 492, 493–495
  due to hyperaldosteronism, 1152
  morphology of, 495–496

Hypertension *(Continued)*
pheochromocytoma and, 1159, 1161
portal, 838–839, 838f
idiopathic, 871
in right-sided heart failure, 536
during pregnancy, 455
pulmonary, 707–709, 708f, 709f
renovascular, 493t, 495
retinal disease due to, 1359, 1361f, 1362f
secondary, 492, 493t, 495
types and causes of, 492, 493t
vascular pathology in, 495, 495f
Hypertensive cerebrovascular disease, 1295,
1295f
Hypertensive encephalopathy, 1295
Hypertensive heart disease (HHD), 559–560
pulmonary (right-sided), 559–560, 560f, 560t
systemic (left-sided), 559, 560f
Hypertensive intraparencymal hemorrhage,
1296, 1296f
Hyperthermia, 422
malignant, 422, 1270
Hyperthyroidism, 1108–1109, 1108t, 1109f
antibody-mediated hypersensitivity in,
203–204, 203t
apathetic, 1109
myocardial disease due to, 581
Hypertrophic cardiomyopathy (HCM), 575–577
clinical features of, 577
functional patterns and causes of, 572t
graphic representation of, 572f
morphology of, 575–576, 576f
pathogenesis of, 574f, 575f, 577
Hypertrophic gastropathies, 782–783, 782t, 783f
Hypertrophic neuropathy, 1264
Hypertrophic osteoarthropathy, due to cancer,
321t, 322
Hypertrophic pulmonary osteoarthropathy, due
to lung carcinoma, 729
Hypertrophic scars, due to burn injury, 421
Hypertrophy, 6–8, 6f–8f, 450
mechanisms of, 7, 8f
myocardial, 6, 6f, 7, 8f
Hyperuricemia, 962
in gout, 1243, 1244–1245
Hyperuricosuric calcium nephrolithiasis, 962
Hyperviscosity, and thrombosis, 122
Hyperviscosity syndrome, in lymphoplasmacytic
lymphoma, 612
Hypervitaminosis A, 433
Hypervitaminosis C, 438
Hypervitaminosis D, 436
Hyphae, 335, 382
Hypnozoites, of malaria, 387
Hypoadrenalism, secondary, 1157
Hypoalbuminemia
due to liver failure, 836
in nephrotic syndrome, 922
Hypocalcemia, 1130
in renal failure, 1219
Hypocalcemic tetany, 433, 1130
Hypochlorite, in phagocytosis, 53, 53f
Hypochondrogenesis, 1211t
Hypochondroplasia, 1211t
Hypochromic microcytic anemia, 640
of iron deficiency, 661–662, 662f
Hypocitraturia, 962
Hypoglycemia
due to cancer, 321t
neurologic sequelae of, 1329
Hypogonadism, due to liver failure, 836
Hypoparathyroidism, 1129–1130
autoimmune, 1130
autosomal-dominant, 1130

Hypoparathyroidism *(Continued)*
familial isolated, 1130
pseudo-, 1130
Hypopituitarism, 1100, 1105–1106
Hypoplasia, 450
Hypoplastic left heart syndrome, 544
Hypoproteinemia, edema due to, 112, 112f, 112t
Hypopyon, 1351
Hypospasias, 982
Hypotension, 492
Hypothalamic suprasellar tumors, 1106–1107,
1107f
Hypothalamus-pituitary-thyroid axis,
homeostasis in, 1108f
Hypothermia, 422
Hypothyroidism, 1109–1111
acquired, 1110
autoimmune, 1110
causes of, 1109–1110, 1110t
congenital, 1110
cretinism due to, 1110–1111
epidemiology of, 1109
goitrous, 1116
myocardial disease due to, 581
myxedema due to, 1111
primary, 1109–1110, 1110t
secondary (central), 1110, 1110t
Hypotrophy, 450
Hypoventilation syndrome, obesity in, 442
Hypovolemic shock, 114, 129, 130t
due to burn injury, 421
Hypoxanthine guanine phosphoribosyl
transferase (HGPRT), in gout, 1243, 1244f
Hypoxia, 11
inflammation due to, 45
due to ionizing radiation, 424
Hypoxia-inducible factor-1 (HIF-1), 24
in renal cell carcinoma, 965
Hypoxia-inducible factor-1α (HIF-1α), 45
Hypoxic cell injury, 23–24
Hypoxic encephalopathy
diffuse, 1291–1292, 1292f
in left-sided heart failure, 536

I

IAPs (Inhibitors of Apoptosis Proteins), 296
Iatrogenic factors, white cell neoplasia due to,
598
IBD. *See* Inflammatory bowel disease (IBD).
IBS (irritable bowel syndrome), 807
I-cell disease, 151t
Ichthyosis, 1186, 1186f
Icterus, defined, 839
Idiopathic hyperaldosteronism (IHA), 1151
Idiopathic orbital inflammation, 1347, 1347f
Idiopathic pulmonary fibrosis (IPF), 694–695,
694f, 695f
Idiopathic pulmonary hemosiderosis, 710
Idiopathic retroperitoneal fibrosis, 828–829
IDL (intermediate-density lipoprotein),
metabolism of, 147, 147f
IE. *See* Infective endocarditis (IE).
IFN(s) (interferons), in systemic lupus
erythematosus, 216
IFN-γ (interferon-γ), in inflammation, 61t
Ig(s). *See* Immunoglobulin(s) (Igs).
IGF-1 (insulin-like growth factor-1), obesity
and, 442f, 443
IGF-2 (insulin-like growth factor-2), in
Beckwith-Wiedemann syndrome, 480
IGFBP-1 (insulin-like growth factor–binding
protein-1), obesity and, 442f, 443
IGFBP-2 (insulin-like growth factor–binding
protein-2), obesity and, 442f, 443

IHA (idiopathic hyperaldosteronism), 1151
IHD. *See* Ischemic heart disease (IHD).
IL(s). *See* Interleukin(s) (ILs).
IL13 gene, in asthma, 691
Ileitis, backwash, 811
Ileus, meconium, in cystic fibrosis, 469
Immediate hypersensitivity, 197t, 198–201,
198f–200f, 201t
local, 201
Immediate reaction, after allergen exposure, 198,
198f–200f
Immediate transient response, in inflammation,
47
Immune cell antigens, detected by monoclonal
antibodies, 599–600, 600t
Immune complex(es)
deposition of, 204f, 205
formation of, 204–205, 204f
in glomerular injury, 911t, 912–914, 913f, 914f
tissue injury caused by, 204f, 205
Immune complex deposition
rapidly progressive glomerulonephritis due to,
920, 920t
in systemic lupus erythematosus, 218, 218f,
219f
Immune complex disease
local, 204t, 205
systemic, 204–205, 204f
Immune complex–associated vasculitis, 205,
205f, 510–511
Immune complex–mediated hypersensitivity,
197t, 198, 204–205, 204f, 204t, 205f
Immune dysregulation, polyendocrinopathy,
enteropathy, X-linked (IPEX), 211, 796–797
Immune escape, 319–320, 319f
Immune evasion, 319–320, 319f
by microbes, 345–346, 345f, 346t
Immune granulomas, 74, 74f
Immune hydrops, 460–461, 460f
Immune inflammation, 72, 205–208, 206f
Immune mechanisms, of glomerular injury,
911–916, 911t, 913f–916f
Immune reactions, inflammation due to, 45
Immune reconstitution inflammatory syndrome,
248
Immune response, 184–197
adaptive immunity in, 185
antigen recognition in, 193–195, 194f
cell-mediated immunity in, 185, 195, 195f
cells of immune system in, 185–188,
185f–188f
cytokines in, 193
decline of, 196–197
humoral immunity in, 185, 195–196, 196f
innate immunity in, 184–185
lymphocyte activation in, 193–197, 194f–196f
major histocompatibility molecules in,
190–193, 191f, 192f, 193t
tissues of immune system in, 188–190, 189f,
190f
Immune stimulation, chronic, white cell
neoplasia due to, 598
Immune surveillance, 316, 319–320, 319f
Immune system, 183–255
cells of, 185–188, 185f–188f
cutaneous, 1166, 1167f
tissues of, 188–190, 189f, 190f
Immune system disorder(s)
amyloidosis as, 36, 249–255, 250f
classification of, 252–253, 252f
clinical features of, 254–255
endocrine, 252t, 253
hemodialysis-associated, 252t, 253
heredofamilial, 252t, 253

Immune system disorder(s), amyloidosis as (Continued)
immunocyte dyscrasias with, 252
localized, 252t, 253
morphology of, 253–254, 253f
pathogenesis of, 251–252, 251f
perivascular, 666
primary, 252
primary or immunocyte-associated, 609
properties of amyloid proteins and, 249–251, 250f
secondary, 75, 252–253, 252t
systemic, 252–253, 252t
reactive, 252–253, 252t
senile, 252t, 253
autoimmune, 208–226, 208t
chronic discoid lupus erythematosus as, 221
drug-induced lupus erythematosus as, 215t, 216, 221
general features of, 212–213
inflammatory myopathies as, 215t, 225–226
mixed connective tissue disease as, 226
polyarteritis nodosa and other vasculitides as, 226
rheumatoid arthritis as (See Rheumatoid arthritis)
Sjögren syndrome as, 215t, 221–223, 222f
subacute cutaneous lupus erythematosus as, 221
systemic lupus erythematosus as, 213–221
autoantibodies in, 213–215, 215t
clinical features of, 204t, 217t, 220–221
diagnostic criteria for, 213, 214t
epidemiology of, 213
etiology and pathogenesis of, 215–217, 216f
morphology of, 217–220, 217t, 218f–220f
systemic sclerosis (scleroderma) as, 215t, 223–225, 223f–225f
hypersensitivity reactions as, 197–208
antibody-mediated (type II), 197t, 198, 201–204, 202f, 203t
cell-mediated (type IV), 197t, 198, 205–208, 206f–208f, 206t
immediate (type I), 197t, 198–201, 198f–200f, 201t
immune complex–mediated (type III), 197t, 198, 204–205, 204f, 204t, 205f
inflammation due to, 45
immunodeficiency syndromes as, 230–249
infections in, 231t
primary, 230–235
common variable immunodeficiency as, 233
DiGeorge syndrome (thymic hypoplasia) as, 234
genetic basis for, 232f
genetic deficiencies of complement system as, 235
hyper-IgM syndrome as, 233
immunodeficiency with thrombocytopenia and eczema (Wiskott-Aldrich syndrome) as, 235
isolated IgA deficiency as, 233
mutations in, 232f
severe combined immunodeficiency as, 234–235
X-linked (Bruton's) agammaglobulinemia as, 231–233
secondary, 231, 235
AIDS as (See Acquired immunodeficiency syndrome (AIDS))
in systemic lupus erythematosus, 214t

Immune system disorder(s) (Continued)
transplant rejection as, 226–230
acute, 228–229, 228f
chronic, 229, 229f
hematopoietic stem cell, 230
hyperacute, 227, 228, 228f
kidney, 228–230, 228f, 229f
mechanisms of, 226–228, 227f
other solid organ, 230
prevention of, 229–230
Immune thrombocytopenia, 667
Immune thrombocytopenic purpura (ITP)
acute, 668
chronic, 667–668
Immune-mediated inflammatory diseases, 45, 70, 208–209, 208t
Immune-mediated neuropathies, 1261–1262
Immune-privileged sites, 211
Immunity
adaptive (acquired, specific), 185
cell-mediated (cellular), 185, 194f, 195, 195f
humoral, 185, 195–196, 196f
innate (natural, native), 75, 184–185
Immunocompromised individuals
cytomegalovirus in, 354–355
pneumonia in, 711t, 719–720, 720t
Immunocyte dyscrasias, with amyloidosis, 252, 609
Immunodeficiency
common variable, 233
severe combined, 234–235
with thrombocytopenia and eczema, 235
Immunodeficiency syndrome(s), 230–249
acquired (See Acquired immunodeficiency syndrome (AIDS))
infections in, 231t
primary, 230–235
common variable, 233
DiGeorge syndrome (thymic hypoplasia) as, 234
genetic basis for, 232f
genetic deficiencies of complement system as, 235
hyper-IgM syndrome as, 233
isolated IgA deficiency as, 233
mutations in, 232f
severe combined, 234–235
with thrombocytopenia and eczema (Wiskott-Aldrich syndrome) as, 235
X-linked (Bruton's) agammaglobulinemia as, 231–233
secondary, 231, 235
Immunodeficiency-associated large B-cell lymphoma, 607
Immunoglobulin(s) (Igs), 185, 187, 187f
Immunoglobulin A (IgA), in humoral immunity, 196
Immunoglobulin α (Igα), 187
Immunoglobulin A (IgA) deficiency
in celiac disease, 796
isolated, 233
Immunoglobulin A (IgA) nephropathy, 918t, 929–931, 931f
Immunoglobulin β (Igβ), 187
Immunoglobulin E (IgE)
in humoral immunity, 196
in immediate hypersensitivity, 199, 199f
Immunoglobulin E (IgE) dependent urticaria, 1187
Immunoglobulin E (IgE) independent urticaria, 1187
Immunoglobulin G (IgG), 187
in humoral immunity, 196
Immunoglobulin M (IgM), 187

Immunohemolytic anemia, 653–654, 653t
Immunohistochemistry, 324, 324f
Immunologic reactions, cell injury due to, 12
Immunological memory, 196–197
Immunological tolerance, 209–211, 210f
Immunosuppressed hosts, infections in, 346–347
Immunosuppression, in immune evasion, 320
Immunosuppression-associated Kaposi sarcoma, 523, 524
Immunosuppressive mediators, in septic shock, 131
Immunosuppressive therapy, for transplantation, 229–230
Immunotactoid glomerulopathy, 935
Imperforate anus, 765
Impetigo, 1201–1202
bullosa, 1201
contagiosa, 1201
Imprinting
genomic, 171–173, 172f
loss of, 306, 480
maternal, 171
paternal, 171, 1059
Inactive plaques, in multiple sclerosis, 1311
Inborn error(s) of metabolism, 462–465, 463t
cystic fibrosis as, 465–471
clinical features of, 468f, 469–471, 470t
environmental modifiers of, 468
genetic basis for, 139f, 144, 465–468, 466f, 467f
morphology of, 468–469, 469f
galactosemia as, 464–465, 464f, 465f
myopathies with, 1271–1273
phenylketonuria as, 463–464, 463f
Incarceration, bowel, 790, 791f
Incidentaloma, adrenal, 1159
Incised wound, 420
Inclusion bodies, 332
Inclusion body myositis, 1273, 1274, 1274f, 1275
Inclusion cysts
epidermal, 1176
epithelial (mesothelial, cortical, germinal), of ovary, 1042, 1042f
Incomplete penetrance, 140
Indirect Coombs antiglobulin test, 653
Indoor air pollution, 405
Induced pluripotent stem (iPS) cells, 82, 84, 84f
Inducible nitric oxide synthase (iNOS), 60
Industrial exposures, 408–410, 409t
and lung carcinoma, 722
Infant(s), 447–481
causes of death of, 448, 448t
congenital anomalies in, 448–453
causes of, 450–452, 450t, 451t
pathogenesis of, 452–453, 453f
types of, 448–450, 449f, 450f
fetal hydrops in, 459–462
clinical features of, 462
defined, 459–460
immune, 460–461, 460f
morphology of, 461–462, 462f
nonimmune, 460, 461, 461t
inborn error(s) of metabolism in, 462–465, 463t
cystic fibrosis as, 465–471
clinical features of, 468f, 469–471, 470t
environmental modifiers of, 468
genetic basis for, 465–468, 466f, 467f
morphology of, 468–469, 469f
galactosemia as, 464–465, 464f, 465f
phenylketonuria as, 463–464, 463f
perinatal infections in, 458–459, 459f
premature, 453–458
causes of, 454–456, 455f

Infant(s), premature (Continued)
  necrotizing enterocolitis in, 458, 459f
  neonatal respiratory distress syndrome in, 456–458, 457f
  sudden infant death syndrome in, 471–473, 471t
  tumors and tumor-like lesions in, 473–481
    benign, 473–474, 474f
    malignant, 474–481
      incidence and types of, 475, 475t
      neuroblastic, 475–479, 476f, 477f, 477t, 479f
      Wilms tumor as, 479–481, 481f
Infant mortality rate, 447–448
Infantile glaucoma, 1352
Infantile motor neuron disease, 1267–1268, 1267f
Infarct(s), 15, 16f
  defined, 127–128
  factors that influence development of, 129
  liver, 851, 871f
  red, 128, 128f
  renal, 955
  septic, 129
    in infective endocarditis, 567
  pulmonary, 707
  splenic, 634, 634f
    in sickle cell disease, 647, 647f
  white, 128, 128f
  of Zahn, 871
Infarction(s), 126, 127–129
  bowel, 792–793, 792f
  causes of, 128
  morphology of, 128–129, 128f, 129f
  myocardial, 547–558
    clinical features of, 553–556, 555f
    completed, 549, 549f, 554f
    consequences and complications of, 556–558, 556f, 558f
    expansion of, 556f, 557
    extension of, 553, 557
    healing of, 553
    incidence and risk factors for, 547
    microscopic features of, 552, 552f
    morphology of, 550–553, 550t, 551f, 552f
    oral contraceptives and, 415
    pathogenesis of, 547–550, 548f, 548t, 549f
    regions of, 549–550, 549f, 550–551, 551f
    reperfusion of, 553, 554f, 555f
    reversible vs. irreversible, 547–548, 548f, 550t, 554f
    right ventricular, 557
    silent, 555
    subendocardial, 550, 551f
    temporal evolution of, 550, 550t
    therapy for, 556
    and thrombosis, 122
    transmural, 547, 550, 551f
    triphenyltetrazolium chloride staining in, 551, 552f
  pulmonary, 30–31, 706f
  septic, 707
Infection(s)
  due to agranulocytosis, 593
  and asthma, 689–691
  and atherosclerosis, 500–501
  in autoimmunity, 212, 213f
  bacterial, 357–381, 358t
    by Actinomycetaceae, 358t
    anaerobic, 378–379, 379f
    chlamydial, 380
    clostridial, 358t, 378–379, 379f
    contagious childhood, 358t
    enteric, 358t

Infection(s), bacterial (Continued)
  gram-negative, 358t, 363–366, 364f, 365f
  gram-positive, 357–363, 359f–363f
  human treponemal (spirochetal), 358t, 374–378, 374f–376f, 378f
  myco-, 358t, 366–374, 367f, 369f–374f
  obligate intracellular, 380–381, 381f, 382f
  by pyogenic cocci, 357–360, 358t
  rickettsial, 380–381, 381f, 382f
  zoonotic, 358t
bleeding disorders due to, 666
due to burn injury, 421
cell death due to, 25–26
of central nervous system, 1299–1308
  abscess as
    brain, 1300, 1300f
    extradural, 1301
  acute focal suppurative, 1300–1301, 1300f
  acute meningitis as, 1299–1300, 1299f
  meningoencephalitis as
    chronic bacterial, 1301–1302
    fungal, 1306, 1307f
    viral, 1302–1306, 1303f–1306f
    protozoal, 1306–1308, 1307f, 1308f
  subdural empyema as, 1300–1301
in diabetes, 1146
of female genital tract, 1008–1010, 1009f, 1010f
fetal, 455
fungal, 382–386, 383f–386f
  superficial, 1202, 1202f
glomerulonephritis after, 918t, 920
healthcare-associated (nosocomial), 342
due to heroin use, 418–419
host defenses against, 342
  injurious effects of, 344–345
host resistance to
  vitamin A in, 432
  vitamin D in, 436, 437f
in immunodeficiencies, 231t
in immunosuppressed hosts, 346–347
inflammation due to
  acute, 45
  chronic, 60
intrauterine, 454
leukocytosis due to, 594
and malnutrition, 427
opportunistic, in AIDS, 245t, 246, 346–347
of oral cavity, 742–743
parasitic, 386–396
  metazoal, 391–396, 392f–396f
  protozoal, 386–391, 386f, 387f–390f
perinatal, 458–459, 459f
peritoneal, 828
pulmonary, 710–720
  lung abscess as, 711t, 713, 716–717, 717f
  after lung transplantation, 720
  pneumonia as
    aspiration, 711t, 716
    atypical, 711t, 714–716
    bacterial, 711–714, 712f, 713f
    broncho-, 712, 713, 713f
    chronic, 711t, 717–719, 718f, 719f
    classification of, 711, 711t
    community-acquired, 711–716, 711t, 713f, 714f
    complications of, 713–714
    due to Haemophilus influenzae, 711–712
    hospital-acquired, 711t, 716
    in immunocompromised host, 711t, 719–720, 720t
    due to Klebsiella pneumoniae, 712
    due to Legionella pneumophila, 712
    lobar, 712–713, 713f

Infection(s), pneumonia as (Continued)
  due to Moraxella catarrhalis, 712
  mycoplasmal, 714–715
  necrotizing, 711t, 716–1090, 717f
  due to Pseudomonas aeruginosa, 712
  due to Staphylococcus aureus, 712
  due to Streptococcus pneumoniae, 711
  viral, 714–716
sexually transmitted, 341–342, 341t
skin disorders due to, 1199–1202
  impetigo as, 1201–1202
  molluscum contagiosum as, 1201, 1201f
  superficial fungal, 1202, 1202f
  verrucae (warts) as, 1200–1201, 1200f
spectrum of inflammatory responses to, 347–348, 347f–349f
urinary tract, 907, 939–941, 940f
viral, 348–357, 349t
  acute (transient), 348–351, 350f
  chronic
    latent (herpesvirus), 351–355, 352f–354f
    productive, 355
    transforming, 355–357, 356f
and wound healing, 106
Infectious agent(s)
  bacteria as, 333t, 334–335, 334f
    mechanisms of disease production by, 343–344
  of bioterrorism, 337–338, 337t
  categories of, 332–336, 333t
  cell injury due to, 11
  ectoparasites as, 336
  fungi as, 333t, 335
  helminths as, 333t, 336
  immune evasion by, 345–346, 345f, 346t
  mechanisms of disease production by, 342–355
  prions as, 332, 333t
  protozoa as, 333t, 335–336
  routes of entry of, 338–339
  special techniques for diagnosing, 335t, 336
  spread and dissemination of, 339–340, 339f
  transmission of, 340–341
    sexual, 341–342, 341t
  viruses as, 332–333, 333f, 333t
    mechanisms of disease production by, 342–343, 343f
Infectious arthritis, 1241–1242
Infectious disease(s), 331–396
  bacterial, 357–381, 358t
    abscesses as, 378
    anthrax as, 337, 361–362, 362f
    chancroid (soft chancre) as, 366
    chlamydial, 380
    clostridial, 358t, 378–379, 379f
    diphtheria as, 360–361, 361f
    granuloma inguinale as, 366
    leprosy as, 372–374, 373f, 374f
    listeriosis as, 361
    Lyme disease as, 377–378, 378f
    with Mycobacterium avium-intracellulare complex, 372, 373f
    neisserial, 363–364
    Nocardia as, 362–363, 363f
    plague as, 365
    with Pseudomonas, 364–365, 365f
    relapsing fever as, 377
    rickettsial, 380–381, 381f
    Rocky Mountain spotted fever as, 381, 382f
    scrub typhus as, 380, 381
    staphylococcal, 357–359, 359f
    streptococcal and enterococcal, 359–360, 360f
    syphilis as, 374–377, 374f–376f

Infectious disease(s), bacterial *(Continued)*
tuberculosis as, 366–372, 367f, 369f–372f
typhus fever as, 380, 381, 381f
whooping cough as, 364, 364f
emerging, 400
fungal, 382–386
aspergillosis as, 384–385, 385f
candidiasis as, 382–384, 383f
cryptococcosis as, 384, 384f
zygomycosis (mucormycosis) as, 385–386, 386f
genetic analysis for, 174
in Global Burden of Disease, 400
global warming and, 402
of liver, 843–855
bacterial, parasitic, and helminthic, 854–855, 855f
viral hepatitis as, 843–853, 844t
acute, 850, 851–852, 851f, 852f
carrier state of, 850
chronic, 850–851, 851f–853f, 852–853
clinical course of, 853
clinicopathologic syndromes of, 850–851
fulminant, 835, 853, 854f
due to hepatitis A virus, 844, 844t, 845f
due to hepatitis B virus, 844t, 845–847, 845f–847f
due to hepatitis C virus, 844t, 847–848, 848f
due to hepatitis D virus, 844t, 848–849
due to hepatitis E virus, 844t, 849
due to hepatitis G virus, 849
HIV and, 850–851
morphology of, 851–853, 851f–854f
new and emerging, 336–337, 337t
oral manifestations of, 744t
parasitic, 386–396
African trypanosomiasis as, 390, 390f
babesiosis as, 388, 388f
Chagas disease as, 391
cysticercosis and hydatid disease as, 392–393, 392f
leishmaniasis as, 388–390, 389f
lymphatic filariasis as, 395, 395f
malaria as, 386–388, 387f, 388f
onchocerciasis as, 395–396, 396f
schistosomiasis as, 393–395, 394f
strongyloidiasis as, 391–392, 392f
trichinosis as, 393, 393f
pathogenesis of, 332–348
viral, 348–357, 349t
arboviral and hemorrhagic fevers as, 349t, 351
cytomegalovirus as, 353–355, 354f
Epstein-Barr virus as, 355–357, 356f
hepatitis B virus as, 355
herpes simplex virus as, 352–353, 352f
measles as, 349–350, 350f
mumps as, 350
poliovirus as, 350–351
varicella zoster virus as, 353, 353f
West Nile virus as, 351
Infectious enterocolitis, 797–807, 798t
Campylobacter, 798t, 799–800, 800f
due to cholera, 797–799, 798t, 799f
due to enteric (typhoid) fever, 798t, 801–802
due to *Escherichia coli*, 798t, 800f, 802
due to mycobacteria, 798t
parasitic, 805–807, 805f
pseudomembranous, 798t, 803, 803f
due to salmonellosis, 798t, 801
due to shigellosis, 798t, 800–801
viral, 805f, 1708–1709

Infectious enterocolitis *(Continued)*
due to Whipple disease, 798t, 803–804, 804f
due to *Yersinia* spp, 798t, 800f, 802
Infectious esophagitis, 768–769, 769f
Infectious mononucleosis, 355–357, 356f
oral manifestations of, 744t
Infectious polyneuropathies, 1262–1263
Infectious rhinitis, 749
Infectious vasculitis, 517–518
cerebral infarction due to, 1293
Infective endocarditis (IE), 566–568
acute *vs.* subacute, 567
with artificial heart valve, 570–571
clinical features of, 568
diagnostic criteria for, 568f, 569t
etiology and pathogenesis of, 567
morphology of, 124, 567–568, 567f, 568f
Inferior conjunctival fornix, 1348f
Inferior tarsus, 1348f
Inferior vena cava thrombosis, 873
Inferior vena caval syndrome, 519
Infertility, in cystic fibrosis, 469, 470
Infiltrative fasciitis, 1250–1251, 1250f
Inflammation, 43–75
acute, 45–56
components of, 45, 45f
defined, 45
due to foreign bodies, 45
due to immune reactions, 45
due to infections, 45
leukocytes in, 48–56
defects in function of, 55–56, 56t
other functional responses of activated, 54, 54f
recognition of microbes and dead tissues by, 51–52, 52f
recruitment to sites of infection and injury of, 48–51, 48f–51f, 49t
release of products of, 54–55
removal of offending agents by, 52–54, 53f
tissue injury mediated by, 54–55, 55t
vascular injury mediated by, 47f
outcomes of, 66, 67f
overview of, 44
reactions of blood vessels in, 46–48, 46f, 47f
stimuli for, 45
summary of sequence of events of, 68–70
termination of, 44, 56
due to tissue necrosis, 45
anemia of chronic disease due to, 662
in antibody-mediated hypersensitivity, 202f, 203
and atherosclerosis, 498, 498f, 500
of bladder, 974–975, 975f, 976f
cardinal signs of, 44, 69
in cell-mediated immunity, 194f
of cervix, 1017
chronic, 70–74
and cancer, 276, 277t
causes of, 70
defined, 70
granulomatous, 73–74, 73t, 74f
macrophages in, 71, 71f, 72f
morphologic features of, 70, 70f
other cells in, 72, 73f
overview of, 44
progression to, 66, 67f
and scarring, 348, 349f
consequences of defective or excessive, 44, 75
defined, 44
edema due to, 112t
of endometrium and myometrium, 1027–1028

Inflammation *(Continued)*
of fallopian tubes, 1038
fibrinous, 67–68, 68f
granulomatous, 73–74, 73t, 74f, 207, 207f, 347–348
historical highlights of, 44–45
immune, 72, 205–208, 206f
in innate immunity, 184
in insulin resistance, 1137
in ischemia-reperfusion injury, 24
mediator(s) of, 56–66, 57t
cell-derived, 57–63, 57t
arachidonic acid metabolites (prostaglandins, leukotrienes, and lipoxins) as, 57t, 58–60, 58f, 59t
cytokines and chemokines as, 57t, 61–63, 61t, 62f
lysosomal constituents of leukocytes as, 57t, 63
neuropeptides as, 57t, 64
nitric oxide as, 57t, 60–61, 61f
platelet-activating factor as, 57t, 60
reactive oxygen species as, 57t, 60
vasoactive amines (histamine and serotonin) as, 57–58, 57t
plasma protein–derived, 63–66
coagulation and kinin systems as, 57t, 64–66, 65f, 66t
complement system as, 57t, 63–64, 64f
mononuclear, 347, 347f
morphologic patterns of, 66–68, 67f–69f
overview of, 44
of penis, 982
of prostate, 993–994
and repair of damaged tissue, 44
salutary effect of, 44
serous, 67, 68f
suppurative or purulent, 68, 69f, 347, 347f
systemic effects of, 74–75
of testes and epididymis, 986–987, 986f
ulcers due to, 68, 69f
of ureters, 972, 973f
of urethra, 981
Inflammation phase, of cutaneous wound healing, 102
Inflammatory bowel disease (IBD), 807–813
colitis-associated dysplasia due to, 813, 814f
Crohn disease as, 808f, 808t, 810–811, 810f, 811f
defined, 807
epidemiology of, 807–808
granulomatous inflammation in, 73t
pathogenesis of, 808–810, 809f
ulcerative colitis as, 808f, 808t, 811–813, 812f, 813f
Inflammatory carcinoma, of breast, 1083, 1089
Inflammatory demyelinating radiculoneuropathy
acute, 1261–1262
chronic, 1262
Inflammatory dermatoses
acute, 1187–1189
acute eczematous dermatitis as, 1187–1189, 1188f
erythema multiforme as, 1189, 1190f
urticaria as, 1187, 1187f
chronic, 1189–1192
lichen planus as, 1191–1192, 1192f
psoriasis as, 1190–1191, 1190f
seborrheic dermatitis as, 1191
Inflammatory disorder(s)
of breast, 1069–1070
fat necrosis as, 1070
lymphocytic mastopathy as, 1070
mammary duct ectasia as, 1070, 1070f

Inflammatory disorder(s) *(Continued)*
mastitis as
acute, 1069
granulomatous, 1070
periductal, 1069, 1069f
HLA alleles and, 192, 193t
immune-mediated, 45, 70, 208–209, 208t
of peritoneum, 828–829
Inflammatory lymphadenitis, 48
Inflammatory mediators, in septic shock, 130
Inflammatory myofibroblastic tumor, of lung,
730
Inflammatory myopathies, 215t, 225–226,
1273–1275, 1274f
Inflammatory neuropathies, 1261–1262
Inflammatory polyps
colonic, 815–816, 816f
of esophagus, 774
of gallbladder, 888
gastric, 782t, 783
Inflammatory pseudotumors, of esophagus, 774
Inflammatory responses, to infection, 347–348,
347f–349f
Inflammatory/reactive tumor-like lesions, of oral
cavity, 741–742
aphthous ulcers as, 742, 742f
fibrous proliferative, 741–742, 741f
glossitis as, 742
Inflammosome, 61
Influenza virus, 715
Inguinal hernias, 790, 791f
Inherited autoinflammatory syndromes, 61–62
Inherited cancer syndromes, 273–276, 275t
Inherited genetic factors, white cell neoplasia
due to, 597
Inhibin, in granulosa cell tumor of ovaries, 1050
Inhibitors of Apoptosis Proteins (IAPs), 296
Initiation, of chemical carcinogenesis, 309, 310,
310t, 311
INK4a tumor suppressor gene, 287t, 294
in osteosarcoma, 1225
Inlet patch, 765
Innate immunity, 75, 184–185
cytokines of, 193
Inner limiting membrane, of retina, 1359f
Inner nuclear layer, of retina, 1359f
Inner plexiform layer, of retina, 1359f
iNOS (inducible nitric oxide synthase), 60
Insecticides, lung diseases due to, 697t
Insertions, 138, 139, 139f
Insomnia, fatal familial, 1308, 1309
Instep claudication, 517
Insulin
in energy balance, 439, 440f
in glucose homeostasis, 1132–1133
metabolic actions of, 1133–1134, 1133f
regulation of release of, 113f, 1133
synthesis and secretion of, 1130, 1131f, 1133,
1133f
Insulin action, genetic defects in, 1138
Insulin gene, 1133
in monogenic diabetes, 1138
in type 1 diabetes mellitus, 1135
Insulin receptor, 1134, 1134f
mutations in, 1138
Insulin receptor substrate (IRS) proteins, 1134,
1134f
Insulin resistance, 1136–1137, 1136f
defined, 1136
obesity and, 442, 442f, 443, 1136–1137, 1136f
in septic shock, 131
Insulin signaling pathway, 1134, 1134f
Insulin-like growth factor-1 (IGF-1), obesity
and, 442f, 443

Insulin-like growth factor-2 (IGF-2), in
Beckwith-Wiedemann syndrome, 480
Insulin-like growth factor–binding protein-1
(IGFBP-1), obesity and, 442f, 443
Insulin-like growth factor–binding protein-2
(IGFBP-2), obesity and, 442f, 443
Insulinoma, 1146–1147, 1147f
Insulin-resistant diabetes, antibody-mediated
hypersensitivity in, 203t
Insulitis, due to diabetes mellitus, 1139, 1141f
INT2 gene, 281t
Integrins
in angiogenesis, 101
in extracellular matrix, 95f, 96, 97f
in inflammation, 49–50, 49t
Intercalated discs, in myocardium, 531
Intercellular signaling, 89–91, 91f
Interdigitating dendritic cells, 187
Interface dermatitis, 1189, 1192, 1192f
Interface hepatitis, 852, 853
Interferon(s) (IFNs), in systemic lupus
erythematosus, 216
Interferon-γ (IFN-γ), in inflammation, 61t
Interfollicular stem cells, 85
Interleukin(s) (ILs), in immune response, 193
Interleukin-1 (IL-1)
in acute respiratory distress syndrome, 681,
682f
in inflammation, 57t, 61–62, 61t, 62t
Interleukin-2 (IL-2), in immunological
tolerance, 211
Interleukin-4 (IL-4) receptor gene, in asthma,
691
Interleukin-6 (IL-6)
in anemia of chronic disease, 662
in inflammation, 61t, 63
in multiple myeloma, 609
Interleukin-8 (IL-8), 62
in acute respiratory distress syndrome, 681,
682f
Interleukin-12 (IL-12), in inflammation, 61t
Interleukin-17 (IL-17), in inflammation, 61t, 63
Intermediate-density lipoprotein (IDL),
metabolism of, 147, 147f
Internal elastic lamina, of blood vessels, 488,
488f
Internal herniation, 791
Internodes, 1258
Interstitial cystitis, 975
Interstitial edema, 1282–1283
Interstitial emphysema, 687
Interstitial matrix, 94, 95f
Intertrigo, 383
Intervillositis, acute necrotizing, 1055f
Intestinal adhesions, 790–791, 791f
Intestinal cestodes, 806
Intestinal epithelium, stem cells in, 85
Intestinal flora, 335
Intestinal metaplasia
in autoimmune gastritis, 779, 779f
in Barrett esophagus, 770–771, 770f
due to chronic gastritis, 781
and gastric cancer, 784
Intestinal obstruction, 790–791, 791f
Intestinal strangulation, 790
Intestinal volvulus, 791, 791f
Intestinalization, due to vitamin B_{12} deficiency,
658
Intestine(s), 790–828
acute appendicitis of, 826–827
adenomas of, 819–820, 820f, 821f
anal canal tumors of, 825–826, 827f
angiodysplasia of, 793
appendix tumors of, 828

Intestine(s) *(Continued)*
colitis of
collagenous, 814, 814f
diversion, 813–814, 814f
and dysplasia, 813, 814f
indeterminate, 812–813
lymphocytic, 814, 814f
microscopic, 814, 814f
ulcerative, 808f, 808t, 811–813, 812f, 813f
colorectal cancer of
adenocarcinoma as, 822–825
chemoprevention of, 823
clinical features of, 825
epidemiology of, 822–823
metastatic, 825, 826f
morphology of, 264f, 824–825, 825f
pathogenesis of, 823–824, 823f, 824f
staging of, 825, 826t, 827t
chemoprevention of, 823
diet and, 443, 822–823
familial adenomatous polyposis and,
820–821
hereditary non-polyposis, 274, 275, 302,
821–822, 822t
intramucosal carcinoma as, 820, 821f
metastatic, 269f
molecular model for evolution of, 308f, 309
familial syndromes of, 820–822
graft-*versus*-host disease of, 814
hemorrhoids of, 826
infectious enterocolitis of, 797–807, 798t
Campylobacter, 798t, 799–800, 800f
due to cholera, 797–799, 798t, 799f
due to enteric (typhoid) fever, 798t,
801–802
due to *Escherichia coli,* 798t, 800f, 802
due to mycobacterial infection, 794t, 798t,
804, 804f
parasitic, 805–807, 805f
pseudomembranous, 798t, 803, 803f
due to salmonellosis, 798t, 801
due to shigellosis, 798t, 800–801
viral, 805f, 1708–1709
due to Whipple disease, 798t, 803–804, 804f
due to *Yersinia* spp, 798t, 800f, 802
inflammatory bowel disease of, 807–813
colitis-associated dysplasia due to, 813, 814f
Crohn disease as, 808f, 808t, 810–811, 810f,
811f
epidemiology of, 807–808
malabsorption and diarrhea in, 794t
pathogenesis of, 808–810, 809f
ulcerative colitis as, 808f, 808t, 811–813,
812f, 813f
irritable bowel syndrome of, 807
ischemic disease of, 791–793, 792f
malabsorption and diarrhea of, 793–797
in abetalipoproteinemia, 797
in autoimmune enteropathy, 794t, 796–797
in celiac disease, 794t, 795–796, 795f, 796f
in cystic fibrosis, 794, 794t
in lactase (disaccharidase) deficiency, 794t,
797
mechanisms of, 793–794, 794t
in tropical sprue, 794t, 796
obstruction of, 790–791
due to adhesions, 790–791, 791f
due to hernias, 790, 791f
due to intussusception, 791, 791f
due to volvulus, 791, 791f
polyps of, 815–820, 816t
in Cowden syndrome and Bannayan-
Ruvalcaba-Riley syndrome, 816t, 818
in Cronkhite-Canada syndrome, 816t, 818

Intestine(s) (Continued)
  in familial adenomatous polyposis, 816t,
    820–821, 822f, 822t
  hamartomatous, 816–818, 816t, 817f, 818f
  hyperplastic, 818–819, 819f
  inflammatory, 815–816, 816f
  juvenile, 816–817, 816t, 817f
  neoplastic, 819–820, 820f, 821f
  in Peutz-Jeghers syndrome, 816t, 817–818,
    818f
  in tuberous sclerosis, 816t
  sigmoid diverticulitis of, 814–815, 815f
Intima, of blood vessels, 488, 488f
Intimal thickening, in response to vascular
    injury, 491–492, 491f
Intra-amniotic infection, 454
Intracellular accumulations, 5–6, 32–38, 33f
  of glycogen, 36
  hyalin change as, 36
  of lipids, 33–35, 34f, 35f
  of pigments, 36–38, 37f
  of proteins, 35–36, 35f
Intracellular bacteria
  facultative, 335
  obligate, 335, 380–381, 381f, 382f
  virulence of, 344
Intracerebral hemorrhage, 1286, 1295–1297,
    1296f
Intracranial hemorrhage, 1295–1299
  intracerebral (intraparenchymal), 1286,
    1295–1297, 1296f
  subarachnoid (due to ruptured saccular
    aneurysms), 1297–1298, 1297f, 1298f
  due to vascular malformations, 1298–1299
Intracranial pressure, raised, 1283–1284
Intraductal carcinoma, 1080–1082, 1081f, 1082f
Intraductal papillary mucinous neoplasms
    (IPMNs), of pancreas, 899, 900f
Intraductal papilloma, of breast, 1072, 1073f
Intraepithelial lymphocytosis, in celiac disease,
    795, 796f
Intrahepatic biliary disease, 866–870, 867t
  anomalies of biliary trees as, 869–870, 870f
  biliary cirrhosis as
    primary, 867–869, 867t, 868f
    secondary, 867, 867f, 867t
  polycystic, 869–870, 870f
  primary sclerosing cholangitis as, 867t, 869,
    869f
Intrahepatic cholestasis, of pregnancy, 875
Intralobar sequestrations, 679
Intramembranous formation, of bone, 1210
Intramucosal carcinoma, colorectal, 820, 821f
Intramural arteries, 532
Intranuclear basophilic inclusions, in
    cytomegalovirus infection, 354, 354f
Intraparenchymal hemorrhage, 1286, 1295–1297,
    1296f
Intraretinal microangiopathy (IRMA), 1360,
    1363f
Intratubular germ cell neoplasia (ITGCN), 988
Intratubular germ cell neoplasia unclassified
    (ITGCNU), 988
Intrauterine growth retardation, 454–456, 455f
Intrauterine infection, prematurity due to, 454
Intravagal paraganglia, 1159
Intravascular hemolysis, 641–642
  in paroxysmal nocturnal hemoglobinuria,
    652–653
Intravascular lymphoma, 1337
Intrinsic factor, in vitamin B$_{12}$ metabolism, 656,
    656f
Intussusception, 791, 791f
Invagination cysts, 1175

Invasion, in carcinogenesis, 278, 298–300,
    299f
Invasive ductal carcinoma, of breast, 268f
Invasive mole, 1059, 1060f
Invasiveness, of neoplasm, 268–269, 268f, 271t
Inversin, 960
Inversion, 160–161, 160f
Inverted papillomas, sinonasal, 751, 751f
Involucrum, 1222, 1222f
Iodine, function of, 439t
Iodine deficiency, 439t
  hypothyroidism due to, 1110
Iodopsins, 431
Ion channel myopathies, 1270
Ion transport, defect in, 143t
Ionizing radiation
  carcinogenesis of, 311, 312
  defined, 423
  field size of, 423
  injury production by (See Radiation injury)
  and lung carcinoma, 722
  main determinants of biologic effects of,
    423–424, 423f, 424f
  rate of delivery of, 423
  sources of, 423
IPEX (immune dysregulation,
    polyendocrinopathy, enteropathy,
    X-linked), 211, 796–797
IPF (idiopathic pulmonary fibrosis), 694–695,
    694f, 695f
IPF1, in diabetes, 1137
IPMNs (intraductal papillary mucinous
    neoplasms), of pancreas, 899, 900f
iPS (induced pluripotent stem) cells, 82, 84,
    84f
IRGM, in Crohn disease, 809
Iridescent spots, in sickle retinopathy, 1362
Iris, 1346f, 1354f
  bombé, 1354f, 1355
IRMA (intraretinal microangiopathy), 1360,
    1363f
Iron
  dietary sources of, 659
  distribution in body of, 659, 659t
  functions of, 439t
  intracellular accumulation of, 36–38, 37f
  requirements for, 661
  total body pool of, 861
Iron absorption, 660, 661f
Iron deficiency, 439t
Iron deficiency anemia, 659–662, 659t,
    660f–662f
  due to colorectal cancer, 825
  due to Crohn disease, 811
Iron homeostasis, 862
Iron metabolism, 659–660, 660f, 661f
Iron overload, 861t
  in β-thalassemia major, 650
  in hereditary hemochromatosis, 862
  myocardial disease due to, 580
Iron oxide, lung diseases due to, 697t
Irritable bowel syndrome (IBS), 807
Irritation fibroma, of oral cavity, 741, 741f
IRS (insulin receptor substrate) proteins, 1134,
    1134f
Ischemia, 11
Ischemia-reperfusion injury, 24
Ischemic bowel disease, 791–793, 792f
Ischemic cardiomyopathy, 546f, 558
Ischemic cell injury, 23–24
Ischemic coagulative necrosis, 128
Ischemic encephalopathy
  diffuse, 1291–1292, 1292f
  in left-sided heart failure, 536

Ischemic heart disease (IHD), 496–498, 545–559
  angina pectoris as, 545, 546–547, 546f
  chronic, 546f, 558
  epidemiology of, 545
  in Global Burden of Disease, 400
  myocardial infarction as, 547–558
    clinical features of, 553–556, 555f
    completed, 549, 549f, 554f
    consequences and complications of,
      556–558, 556f, 558f
    expansion of, 556f, 557
    extension of, 553, 557
    healing of, 553
    incidence and risk factors for, 547
    microscopic features of, 552, 552f
    morphology of, 550–553, 550t, 551f, 552f
    pathogenesis of, 547–550, 548f, 548t, 549f
    regions of, 549–550, 549f, 550–551, 551f
    reperfusion of, 553, 554f, 555f
    reversible vs. irreversible, 547–548, 548f,
      550t, 554f
    right ventricular, 557
    silent, 555
    subendocardial, 550, 551f
    temporal evolution of, 550, 550t
    therapy for, 556
    transmural, 547, 550, 551f
    triphenyltetrazolium chloride staining in,
      551, 552f
  pathogenesis of, 545–546, 546f
  sudden cardiac death due to, 546, 558–559
Ischemic mitral regurgitation, 561
Islet cell hyperplasia, 1146
Islet cell tumors, 1146–1147
Islets of Langerhans, 1130, 1131f
Isochromosome, 160f, 161
Isolated IgA deficiency, 233
Itai-Itai, 408
ITGCN (intratubular germ cell neoplasia), 988
ITGCNU (intratubular germ cell neoplasia
    unclassified), 988
ITP (immune thrombocytopenic purpura)
  acute, 668
  chronic, 667–668

J
JAGGED1, in congenital heart disease, 539, 539t
JAK (Janus kinase) proteins, 90, 91f
JAK2
  in essential thrombocytosis, 629
  in myeloproliferative disorders, 284
  in polycythemia vera, 628, 629
  in primary myelofibrosis, 630
Jansen metaphyseal chondroplasia, 1211t
Janus kinase (JAK) proteins, 90, 91f
Jaundice, 38, 839–842
  causes of, 839, 840–841, 841t
  defined, 839
  due to fetal hydrops, 461
  due to hemolytic anemia, 642
  due to liver failure, 836
  neonatal, 841
  obstructive, due to pancreatic carcinoma, 903
  pathophysiology of, 840–842
JC virus, in AIDS, 246
JIA (juvenile idiopathic arthritis), 1240–1241
Joint(s), 1235–1247
  anatomy of, 1235
  arthritis of, 1235–1246
    ankylosing spondylo-, 1241
    bacterial, 1242
    in calcium pyrophosphate crystal
      deposition disease, 1246, 1246f
    crystal-induced, 1242–1246

Joint(s) (Continued)
  enteritis-associated, 1241
  gouty, 1243–1246, 1243t, 1244f, 1245f
  infectious, 1241–1242
  juvenile idiopathic, 1240–1241
  Lyme, 1242
  osteo-, 1235–1236, 1236f, 1237f
  psoriatic, 1241
  in Reiter syndrome, 1241
  rheumatoid, 1237–1240, 1238f–1240f
  seronegative spondyloarthropathies as, 1241
  tuberculous, 1242
  viral, 1242
  cavitated (synovial), 1235
  classification of, 1235
  solid (nonsynovial), 1235
  tumors and tumor-like lesions of, 1246–1247
    ganglion and synovial cyst as, 1247
    tenosynovial giant-cell tumor as, 1247, 1247f
Joint disease, degenerative, 1235–1236, 1236f, 1237f
Joint involvement, in systemic lupus erythematosus, 214t, 219
Joint mice, 1236
JUN, 90
Junctional epidermolysis bullosa, 1196, 1198f
Junctional nevus, 1169, 1169f
  lentiginous, 1172f
Juvenile hemangioma, 520, 521f
Juvenile idiopathic arthritis (JIA), 1240–1241
Juvenile laryngeal papillomatosis, 752
Juvenile polyp(s), colonic, 816–817, 816t, 817f
Juvenile polyposis, colonic, 816–817, 816t, 817f
Juvenile rheumatoid arthritis, 1240–1241
Juxtacortical chondromas, 1227

K

Kala-azar, 389
Kallikreins
  in coagulation cascade, 119f
  in inflammation, 65, 65f
Kaposi sarcoma (KS), 523–524
  AIDS-associated, 246–247, 247f, 523
  chronic (classic, European), 523, 524
  clinical features of, 524
  of eyelid, 1349
  lymphadenopathic (African, endemic), 523, 524
  morphology of, 524, 524f
  pathogenesis of, 523–524
  transplant-associated, 523, 524
Kaposi sarcoma herpesvirus (KSHV), 247, 523–524, 597
Kaposi varicelliform eruption, 352
Kartagener syndrome, 692
  sinusitis in, 750
Karyolysis, in necrosis, 14
Karyorrhexis
  in necrosis, 14
  in neuroblastomas, 476
Karyotyping, 158–159, 159f
  spectral, 325
Kawasaki disease, 515
Kayser-Fleischer rings, 864
KCNJ11 gene, 1138
Kearn-Sayre syndrome, 1328
Keloid, 106–107, 106f
Kennedy disease, 168t
Kennedy syndrome, 1325
Keratan sulfate, in extracellular matrix, 97, 98f
Keratic precipitates, 1355
Keratin filaments, 35

Keratinizing squamous cell carcinoma, of vulva, 1014, 1014f
Keratinocyte(s), 1166
Keratinocyte growth factor (KGF), in tissue regeneration and wound healing, 87t, 88
Keratitis, 1351, 1351f
  herpes
    epithelial, 352
    stromal, 352
  punctate, 396
Keratoacanthoma, 1180
Keratoconjunctivitis sicca, 756
  in Sjögren syndrome, 221, 222
Keratoconus, 1352, 1352f
Keratocyst, odontogenic, 748
Keratocytes, 1351
Keratoepithelin, 1353
Keratomalacia, 432, 432f
Keratopathy(ies)
  band, 1351–1352
  bullous, 1351
    pseudophakic, 1352
Keratosis(es)
  actinic, 1178, 1179f
  seborrheic, 1175, 1175f
Kernicterus
  due to erythroblastosis fetalis, 840
  due to fetal hydrops, 461–462, 462f
Kernohan's notch, 1283
Ketoacidosis, diabetic, 1143
Ketone bodies, 1143
Ketonemia, 1143
Ketonuria, 1143
KGF (keratinocyte growth factor), in tissue regeneration and wound healing, 87t, 88
Kidney(s)
  amyloidosis of, 254, 254f, 255
  in blood pressure regulation, 493, 494f
  ectopic, 955
  horseshoe, 955
  in left-sided heart failure, 536
  medullary sponge, 957t, 959
  myeloma, 610, 948, 948f
  in preeclampsia and eclampsia, 1057
  regeneration of, 92
Kidney disease. See Renal disease.
Kidney grafts, rejection of, 228–230, 228f, 229f
Kidney injury, acute, 935–907
  causes of, 936
  clinical course of, 938
  ischemic, 936, 937–938, 937f
  morphology of, 937–938, 937f, 938f
  nephrotoxic, 936, 937–938, 937f
  pathogenesis of, 936–937, 936f
Kidney stones, 907, 962–963, 962t, 963f
Killer T lymphocytes. See Cytotoxic T lymphocyte(s) (CTLs).
Kimmelstiel-Wilson disease, 1142, 1142f
Kinases, receptors that recruit, 90, 91f
Kinin(s), in inflammation, 57t, 65f, 66–66
Kininogens, in inflammation, 65
KIT gene, 281t
Klatskin tumors, 880
Klebsiella granulomatis, 341t, 366
Klebsiella pneumoniae
  morphology of, 334f
  pneumonia due to, 712
Klinefelter syndrome, 165
"Knock-in" mice, 83
Knockout mice, 83
Koebner phenomenon, 1191
Koilocytotic atypia
  of cervix, 1019, 1020, 1020f, 1021f
  in condyloma acuminatum, 1012, 1012f

Koplik spots, 350
Korsakoff syndrome, 1328
Krabbe disease, 151t, 1326, 1326f
KRAS gene, 281t, 282
  in colorectal carcinoma, 308f, 309, 823, 823f
  in endometrial carcinoma, 1032, 1032f
  in lung carcinoma, 724–725
  in ovarian carcinoma, 1042, 1044
  in pancreatic carcinoma, 900, 901f
Krukenberg tumor, 1052
KS. See Kaposi sarcoma (KS).
KSHV (Kaposi sarcoma herpesvirus), 247, 523–524, 597
Kuf's disease, 1326
Kupffer cells, 834
  in viral hepatitis, 852
Kuru, 1308
Kuru plaques, 1309, 1310f
Kwashiorkor, 428–429, 429f
Kyphoscoliosis, in Ehlers-Danlos syndrome, 146, 146t

L

Labile tissues, 81
Lacerations, 420, 420f
  of brain, 1287
  neuropathies due to, 1266
Lactase deficiency, 794t, 797
Lactation, breast during, 1067, 1067f
Lactational adenomas, 1071
Lactic acidosis, due to shock, 132
Lactiferous ducts, squamous metaplasia of, 1069, 1069f
Lactoferrin, in phagocytosis, 54
Lactotroph(s), 1098
Lactotroph adenomas, 1100t, 1103–1104, 1103f
Lactotroph hyperplasia, 1104
Lacunae, in hypertensive cerebrovascular disease, 1295
Lacunar infarcts, 1295, 1295f
LAD (left anterior descending) artery, 532
  in myocardial infarction, 549, 549f, 551, 551f
Laennec cirrhosis, 858
Lafora bodies, 1282
Lambert-Eaton myasthenic syndrome, 1276
  due to lung carcinoma, 729
  in paraneoplastic syndrome, 1340
Lambl excrescences, 532, 584
Lamellar bodies, 678
Lamellar bone, 1208, 1208f
  mosaic pattern of, 1217, 1217f
Laminar blood flow, 121
Laminin, in extracellular matrix, 95f, 96, 97f
Langerhans cell(s), 1166, 1166f
  in immune system, 187–188, 187f, 194f, 1167f
Langerhans cell histiocytosis(es), 596, 631–632, 631f
Lardaceous spleen, 254
Large cell carcinoma, of lung, 726f, 727
Large for gestational age (LGA), 454
Large granular lymphocytes. See Natural killer (NK) cells.
Large granular lymphocytic leukemia, 601t, 616
Large intestine. See Colon; Intestine(s).
Laryngeal carcinoma, 753, 753f
  cigarette smoking and, 411, 412f, 412t
Laryngeal chemoreceptors, in sudden infant death syndrome, 472
Laryngeal papillomatosis, 752
Laryngeal squamous papillomas, 752, 752f
Laryngitis, 752
Laryngotracheobronchitis, 715–716
Larynx, disorders of, 752–753, 752f, 753f
Laser capture microdissection, 325–326

Latent membrane protein-1 (LMP-1) gene, 314
Late-phase reaction, after allergen exposure, 198, 198f–200f
LCIS (lobular carcinoma in situ), 1082–1083, 1083f
LCX (left circumflex) artery, 532
  in myocardial infarction, 549, 549f, 551, 551f
LDL. See Low-density lipoprotein (LDL).
L-DOPA, for Parkinson disease, 1321
Lead poisoning, 406–407, 406f
Leber hereditary optic neuropathy, 171, 171f, 1367
Lectin pathway, in complement system, 63, 64f
Left anterior descending (LAD) artery, 532
  in myocardial infarction, 549, 549f, 551, 551f
Left bundle branch, 532
Left circumflex (LCX) artery, 532
  in myocardial infarction, 549, 549f, 551, 551f
Left ventricular hypertrophy, 534f
Left ventricular noncompaction, 571
Left-sided heart failure, 535–536
Left-sided hypertensive heart disease, 559, 560f
Left-to-right shunts, 540–542, 540f
  due to atrial septal defect, 540f, 541
  due to atrioventricular septal defect, 540f, 542
  due to patent ductus arteriosus, 540f, 541–542
  due to patent foramen ovale, 541
  due to ventricular septal defect, 540f, 541, 541f
Legionella pneumophila pneumonia, 712
Legionnaires disease, 712
Leigh syndrome, 1328
Leiomyoma(s)
  benign metastasizing, 1037
  of bladder, 981
  of esophagus, 774
  pilar, 1254
  of smooth muscle, 1254
  uterine, 264f, 271f, 1026f, 1036–1037, 1037f
Leiomyomatosis, disseminated peritoneal, 1037
Leiomyosarcomas, 271f
  of smooth muscle, 1254
  uterine, 1037–1038, 1038f
Leishmania, 335, 388–390
Leishmaniasis, 388–390, 389f
  cutaneous, 390
    diffuse, 390
  mucocutaneous, 390
  visceral, 389–390, 389f
Lemierre syndrome, 378
Lens, 1353, 1354f
  cataracts of, 1353
Lens-induced uveitis, 1353
Lentiginous, defined, 1168
Lentiginous compound nevus, 1172f
Lentiginous junctional nevus, 1172f
Lentiginous melanocytic hyperplasia, 1172f
Lentiginous melanomas, acral/mucosal, 1169, 1172
Lentiginous nevi, 1169
Lentigo, 1168–1169
Leontiasis ossea, 1217
Lepidic growth, of bronchioalveolar carcinoma, 725
Lepromin, 372
Leprosy, 372–374
  granulomatous inflammation in, 73t
  lepromatous (multibacillary, anergic), 373–374, 374f
  morphology of, 373–374, 373f, 374f
  pathogenesis of, 372–373
  polyneuropathy due to, 1262
  tuberculoid (paucibacillary), 373, 373f

Leptin, in energy balance, 439–440, 440f, 441f
Leptomeningeal fibrosis, 1300
LES (lower esophageal sphincter), relaxation of, 768
Lesch-Nyhan syndrome
  genetic basis for, 144
  X-linked, 1243
Leser-Trélat sign, 1175
Lethal factor (LF), in anthrax, 362
Lethal midline granuloma, 750
Letterer-Siwe disease, 631–632
Leukemia(s)
  acute
    lymphoblastic, 600–603, 601t
      clinical features of, 603
      defined, 600–602
      epidemiology of, 602
      genetic basis for, 305t, 306
      immunophenotype of, 602
      molecular pathogenesis of, 305t, 306, 602–603
      morphology of, 602, 602f
      prognosis for, 603
    molecular pathogenesis of, 597, 597f
    myeloid, 620, 621–624
      classification of, 622, 622t
      clinical features of, 624
      cytogenetics of, 623–624
      epidemiology of, 622
      genetic basis for, 305t, 306, 624
      immunophenotype of, 623
      morphology of, 622–623, 623f
      pathogenesis of, 621–622
      prognosis for, 624
      promyelocytic, 623, 623f, 624
  adult T-cell, 601t, 615–616
  aleukemic, 623
  chronic
    eosinophilic, 626t
    lymphocytic, 601t, 603–605, 604f
    myelogenous (myeloid), 627–628
      clinical features of, 627–628
      genetic basis for, 283, 283f, 305, 305f, 626t
      molecular pathogenesis of, 627, 627f
      morphology of, 627, 627f, 628f
  hairy cell, 601t, 614, 614f
  lymphocytic, 598
    chronic, 601t, 603–605, 604f
    large granular, 601t, 616
  vs. lymphoma, 598
  oral manifestations of, 744t
  plasma cell, 610
  stem cell, 626t
Leukemoid reactions, 595
  in inflammation, 75
  due to lung carcinoma, 729
Leukocyte(s), in inflammation, 48–56
  chemotaxis of, 48f, 50–51, 50f, 51f
  defects in function of, 55–56, 56t
  lysosomal constituents of, 63
  margination, rolling, and adhesion to endothelium of, 48–50, 48f, 49f, 49t
  migration through endothelium of, 48f, 50
  other functional responses of activated, 54, 54f
  recognition of microbes and dead tissues by, 51–52, 52f
  recruitment to sites of infection and injury of, 48–51, 48f–51f, 49t
  release of products of, 54–55
  removal of offending agents by, 52–54, 53f
  tissue injury mediated by, 54–55, 55t
  vascular injury mediated by, 47f

Leukocyte activation, in inflammation, 52, 54, 54f
Leukocyte adhesion, in inflammation, 48–50, 48f, 49f, 49t
Leukocyte adhesion deficiency, 50, 55, 56t
Leukocyte adhesion molecules, 49, 49f, 49t, 50
Leukocyte function, defects in, 55–56, 56t
Leukocyte infiltrate, in inflammation, 67f
Leukocyte products, release of, 54–55
Leukocyte receptors, in inflammation, 51–52, 52f
Leukocyte-mediated tissue injury, 54–55, 55t
Leukocytoclastic vasculitis, 515, 516f
Leukocytosis, 593–595, 594f, 594t
  in inflammation, 75
Leukodystrophy(ies), 1325, 1326–1327, 1326f
  adreno-, 1156, 1264t, 1327
  metachromatic, 151t, 1326–1327
  vanishing-white-matter, 1327
Leukoencephalitis, acute hemorrhagic, of Weston Hurst, 1312–1313
Leukoencephalopathy
  multicystic, 1286, 1286f
  progressive multifocal, 1305–1306, 1306f
Leukoerythroblastosis, in primary myelofibrosis, 630
Leukomalacia, periventricular, 1286
Leukopenia, 592–593
  in inflammation, 75
Leukoplakia
  hairy, 743
  of oral cavity, 744–745, 746f
  of vulva, 1011
Leukotriene(s) (LTs)
  in asthma, 689
  in immediate hypersensitivity, 200
  in inflammation, 57t, 58–60, 58f, 59t
Leukotriene B$_4$ (LTB$_4$), in inflammation, 50
Lewis, Thomas, 44
Lewy bodies, 1281
  dementia with, 1321
  in Parkinson disease, 1320, 1320f
Lewy neurites, 1321
Leydig cell tumors
  ovarian, 1051–1052
  testicular, 992
LF (lethal factor), in anthrax, 362
LGA (large for gestational age), 454
LGMDs (limb girdle muscular dystrophies), 1269, 1271t
LH (luteinizing hormone)-producing adenomas, 1100t, 1104–1105
Lhermitte-Duclos disease, 1342
Libman-Sacks endocarditis, 124, 220, 220f, 567f, 569
Lichen planopilaris, 1192
Lichen planus, 1191–1192, 1192f
  oral manifestations of, 744t
Lichen sclerosis, of vulva, 1011, 1011f
Lichen simplex chronicus, of vulva, 1011f, 1012
Lichenification, 1168
Liddle syndrome, 493
Life-threatening event, apparent, 471–472
Li-Fraumeni syndrome, 274, 290
  and breast cancer, 1078, 1078t
  CNS tumors in, 1342
  osteosarcoma in, 1225
Ligamentum arteriosum, in coarctation of the aorta, 544
Light-chain cast nephropathy, 610, 948, 948f
Light-chain deposition disease, 948
Light-chain Ig deposition disease, glomerular lesions in, 935

Limb girdle muscular dystrophies (LGMDs), 1269, 1271t
Limbal stem cells (LSCs), 86
Limbic encephalitis, in paraneoplastic syndrome, 1340
Limbus, 1348f
Limit dextrin, 155, 156f
Lindane (dichlorodiphenyltrichlorethane), occupational exposure to, 409
Lines of Zahn, 124
Lining cells, 1207
Linitis plastica, 786
Linkage analysis, 176–177, 177f, 178f
Linkage disequilibrium, 136, 176, 177
Lipid(s)
    in atherosclerosis, 500
    intracellular accumulation of, 33–35, 34f, 35f
Lipid mediators, in immediate hypersensitivity, 200
Lipid myopathies, 1271
Lipid peroxidation
    due to alcohol metabolism, 413
    in chemical (toxic) cell injury, 25
Lipid-mobilizing factor (LMF), 429
Lipiduria, in nephrotic syndrome, 922
Lipoatrophic diabetes, 1138
Lipoblasts, 1250, 1250f
Lipofuscin
    intracellular accumulation of, 36, 37f
    neuronal inclusions of, 1281
Lipofuscin granules, 10
Lipomas, 262, 1249–1250
    of breast, 1092
    cardiac, 584
    of esophagus, pedunculated, 774
    of spermatic cord, 987
Lipophosphoglycan, in leishmaniasis, 389
Lipoprotein (a), and ischemic heart disease, 498
Lipoprotein abnormalities, in atherosclerosis, 500, 501f
Liposarcoma, 1249t, 1250, 1250f
Lipoxins, in inflammation, 58f, 59
Lipoxygenase(s), in inflammation, 58f, 59
Lipoxygenase inhibitors, 60
Liquefactive necrosis, 15, 16f, 129
Lisch nodules, 1342
Lissencephaly, 1284–1285, 1285f
Listeria monocytogenes, 361
Listeriosis, 361
Liver
    amyloidosis of, 254
    anatomy of, 834–835, 834f
    fatty, 33–34, 34f
        due to alcohol consumption, 857–858, 857f, 859–860
        nonalcoholic, 860–861, 861f
        of pregnancy, 875
    nutmeg, 114, 114f, 872, 872f
    in preeclampsia and eclampsia, 1057
    in right-sided heart failure, 536
    in sarcoidosis, 702
    stem cells in, 85
    in syphilis, 376–377
Liver abscesses, 854–855, 855f
    amebic, 806
Liver cancer, 877–881
    cholangiocarcinoma as, 877, 880–881, 881f
    hepatitis B virus and, 315
    hepatoblastoma as, 877–878, 878f
    hepatocellular carcinoma as, 877, 878–880, 879f, 880f
    metastatic, 270, 270f, 881–882
Liver cell adenomas, 877, 877f
Liver cysts, 869–870, 870f

Liver disease, 835–882
    due to adverse drug reactions, 416t
    alcoholic, 414, 857–860
        clinicopathologic features of, 859–860
        epidemiology of, 857
        morphology of, 857–858, 858f, 859f
        pathogenesis of, 413, 858–859
    autoimmune hepatitis as, 855–856, 855f
    centrilobular hemorrhagic necrosis as, 872, 872f
    cholestasis as, 842–843, 842f, 843f
    circulatory, 870–874, 871f
        hepatic venous outflow obstruction as, 872–874
            due to hepatic vein thrombosis and inferior vena cava thrombosis, 872–873, 873f
            due to sinusoidal obstruction syndrome, 873–874, 873f
        impaired blood flow into liver as, 870–871
            due to hepatic artery compromise, 870–871, 871f
            due to portal vein obstruction and thrombosis, 871
        impaired blood flow through liver as, 871–872
            due to disseminated intravascular coagulation, 872
            due to passive congestion and centrilobular necrosis, 872, 872f
            due to peliosis hepatis, 872
            due to sickle cell disease, 872, 872f
    cirrhosis as, 837–838, 837f
    in cystic fibrosis, 469, 470
    drug- and toxin-induced, 856–860, 856t
    edema due to, 112
    end-stage, 835–836
    fatty, 33–34, 34f
        due to alcohol consumption, 857–858, 857f, 859–860
        nonalcoholic, 860–861, 861f
    general features of, 835–843
    IgA nephropathy with, 931
    infectious, 843–855
        bacterial, parasitic, and helminthic, 854–855, 855f
        viral hepatitis as, 843–853, 844t
            acute, 850, 851–852, 851f, 852f
            carrier state of, 850
            chronic, 850–851, 851f–853f, 852–853
            clinical course of, 853
            clinicopathologic syndromes of, 850–851
            fulminant, 835, 853, 854f
            due to hepatitis A virus, 844, 844t, 845f
            due to hepatitis B virus, 844t, 845–847, 845f–847f
            due to hepatitis C virus, 844t, 847–848, 848f
            due to hepatitis D virus, 844t, 848–849
            due to hepatitis E virus, 844t, 849
            due to hepatitis G virus, 849
            HIV and, 850–851
            morphology of, 851–853, 851f–854f
    intrahepatic biliary disease as, 866–870, 867t
        anomalies of biliary trees as, 869–870, 870f
        biliary cirrhosis as
            primary, 867–869, 867t, 868f
            secondary, 867, 867f, 867t
        polycystic, 869–870, 870f
        primary sclerosing cholangitis as, 867t, 869, 869f
    jaundice as, 839–842, 840f, 841t, 842f
    laboratory evaluation of, 835, 835t
    metabolic, 860–866

Liver disease, metabolic (Continued)
        due to α₁-antitrypsin deficiency, 864–866, 865f
        due to hemochromatosis, 861–863, 861t, 863f
        neonatal cholestasis as, 866, 866f, 866t
        nonalcoholic fatty, 860–861, 861f
        due to Wilson disease, 863–864
    neoplasms as
        benign, 876–877
            cavernous hemangiomas as, 876, 876f
            hepatic adenoma as, 877, 877f
        malignant, 877–881
            cholangiocarcinoma as, 877, 880–881, 881f
            hepatoblastoma as, 877–878, 878f
            hepatocellular carcinoma as, 877, 878–880, 879f, 880f
        metastatic, 270, 270f, 881–882
        nodular hyperplasias as, 875–876, 876f
        passive congestion as, 872
        polycystic, 869–870, 870f
            polycystic kidney disease and, 959
    portal hypertension as, 838–839, 838f
    in pregnancy, 874–875, 875f
Liver failure, 835–836
    acute, 835–836
    chronic, 836
    fulminant, 835, 853, 854f
Liver fibrosis, 837, 837f
Liver function, in infectious mononucleosis, 357
Liver infarct, 851, 871f
Liver injury
    drug- and toxin-induced, 856–857, 856t
    patterns of, 835
Liver metastases, 270, 270f, 881–882
Liver necrosis, in Wilson disease, 864
Liver regeneration, 93–94, 93f
Liver transplantation, complications of, 874, 874f
LKB1 gene, 304
LKB1/STK11 gene, in Peutz-Jeghers syndrome, 817, 818
LMF (lipid-mobilizing factor), 429
LMP-1 (latent membrane protein-1) gene, 314
L-MYC oncogene, 281t, 284
Lobar atrophy, 1318, 1318f
Lobar pneumonia, 712–713, 713f
Lobular carcinoma, invasive, 1085–1087
Lobular carcinoma in situ (LCIS), 1082–1083, 1083f
Lobular hyperplasia, atypical, 1073, 1074f
Local immune complex disease, 204t, 205
Local invasion, by neoplasm, 268–269, 268f, 271t
Loeffler endomyocarditis, 577
Loeys-Dietz syndrome, aneurysms in, 507
Löffler syndrome, 704
Long QT syndrome, and sudden cardiac death, 559
Loss of heterozygosity (LOH), 288
Loss-of-function mutations, 141
Low-density lipoprotein (LDL), metabolism of, 147, 147f
Low-density lipoprotein (LDL) cholesterol, and atherosclerosis, 497, 500
Low-density lipoprotein (LDL) receptor
    in cholesterol metabolism, 147–149, 147f, 148f
    defect in, 143t, 147–149, 147f–149f
Lower esophageal sphincter (LES), relaxation of, 768
Lower extremities, gangrene of, due to diabetes mellitus, 1140

Lower urinary tract, 972–982
  anatomy of, 972
  ureters in, 972–974
    congenital anomalies of, 972
    inflammation of, 972, 973f
    obstructive lesions of, 973–974, 973t
    tumors and tumor-like lesions of, 973, 973f
  urethra in, 981–982
    inflammation of, 981
    tumors and tumor-like lesions of, 981–982, 982f
  urinary bladder in, 974–981
    congenital anomalies of, 974, 974f
    inflammation of, 974–975, 975f, 976f
    metaplastic lesions of, 975–976
    neoplasms of, 976–981, 976t
      mesenchymal, 980–981
      secondary, 981
      urothelial, 976–980, 977f–979f, 977t, 979t
    obstruction of, 981, 981f
Low-grade squamous intraepithelial lesion
    (LSIL), 1019–1021, 1020f, 1020t, 1021f,
    1021t, 1023f
LSCs (limbal stem cells), 86
L-selectin, in inflammation, 49, 49t
LT(s) (leukotrienes)
  in asthma, 689
  in immediate hypersensitivity, 200
  in inflammation, 57t, 58–60, 58f, 59t
LT (heat-labile toxin), 802
LTB$_4$ (leukotriene B$_4$), in inflammation, 50
Lung(s), 677–734
  defense mechanisms of, 710
  development of, 678
  farmer's, 703
  gangrene of, 717
  humidifier or air-conditioner, 703
  in left-sided heart failure, 535
  metastasis to, 270
  microscopic structure of, 678–679, 678f
  pigeon breeder's, 703
  shock, 132
  in syphilis, 377
Lung abscess, 711t, 713, 716–717, 717f
  staphylococcal, 359, 359f
Lung carcinoma, 721–729
  adeno-, 723–725, 726f, 962, 962f
    precursor lesions for, 725, 727f
  air pollution and, 722
  asbestos exposure and, 701
  bronchioalveolar, 725, 727f
  clinical course of, 727–728, 728t
  combined, 727
  epidemiology of, 721
  etiology and pathogenesis of, 721–723
  histologic classification of, 723, 723t
  industrial hazards and, 722
  in situ, 723, 724f
  large cell, 726f, 727
  molecular genetics of, 722
  morphology of, 723–727, 724f–727f
  non–small cell, 722, 723
  paraneoplastic syndromes with, 728–729
  precursor lesions for, 722–723, 724f, 725, 727f
  secondary pathology due to, 727
  small cell, 722, 723, 726–727, 726f
  smoking and, 410, 411, 412f, 412t, 721–722
  squamous cell, 725–726, 725f, 726f
    precursor lesions for, 723, 724f
  staging of, 727, 728t
Lung disease(s)
  acute interstitial pneumonia as, 680, 682–683
  acute lung injury and acute respiratory
    distress syndrome as, 680–683

Lung disease(s) (Continued)
  clinical course of, 682
  conditions associated with development of,
    680, 681t
  morphology of, 680, 681f
  pathogenesis of, 681–682, 682f
  due to adverse drug reactions, 416t
  due to air pollutants, 697t
  atelectasis (collapse) as, 679–680, 679f
  chronic diffuse interstitial (restrictive),
    693–706, 694t
    fibrosing, 694–701
      cryptogenic organizing pneumonia as,
        696, 696f
      drug-induced, 701, 701t
      idiopathic pulmonary fibrosis as,
        694–695, 694f, 695f
      nonspecific interstitial pneumonia as,
        695
      pneumoconioses as, 696–701, 697t,
        698f–700f
      pulmonary involvement in connective
        tissue disease as, 696
      radiation-induced, 701
    granulomatous, 701–704
      hypersensitivity pneumonitis as,
        703–704, 703f
      sarcoidosis as, 701–703, 702f
    obstructive vs., 683, 683t
    pulmonary alveolar proteinosis as, 705–706,
      705f
    pulmonary eosinophilia as, 704
    smoking-related, 704–705, 704f
  congenital anomalies as, 679
  global warming and, 402
  due to infections, 710–720
    lung abscess as, 711t, 713, 716–717, 717f
    pneumonia as
      aspiration, 711t, 716
      atypical, 711t, 714–716
      bacterial, 711–714, 712f, 713f
      broncho-, 712, 713, 713f
      chronic, 711t, 717–719, 718f, 719f
      classification of, 711, 711t
      community-acquired, 711–716, 711t,
        713f, 714f
      complications of, 713–714
      due to Haemophilus influenzae,
        711–712
      hospital-acquired, 711t, 716
      in immunocompromised host, 711t,
        719–720, 720t
      due to Klebsiella pneumoniae, 712
      due to Legionella pneumophila, 712
      lobar, 712–713, 713f
      due to Moraxella catarrhalis, 712
      mycoplasmal, 714–715
      necrotizing, 711t, 716–1090, 717f
      due to Pseudomonas aeruginosa, 712
      due to Staphylococcus aureus, 712
      due to Streptococcus pneumoniae, 711
      viral, 714–716
  neoplastic, 721–731
    carcinoma as, 721–729
      adeno-, 723–725, 726f, 962, 962f
      bronchioalveolar, 725, 727f
      clinical course of, 727–728, 728t
      combined, 727
      epidemiology of, 721
      etiology and pathogenesis of, 721–723
      histologic classification of, 723, 723t
      large cell, 726f, 727
      morphology of, 723–727, 724f–727f
      paraneoplastic syndromes with, 728–729

Lung disease(s) (Continued)
      precursor lesions for, 722–723, 724f, 725,
        727f
      secondary pathology due to, 727
      small cell, 726–727, 726f
      squamous cell, 725–726, 725f, 726f
      staging of, 727, 728t
    hamartoma as, 730, 730f
    inflammatory myofibroblastic tumor as,
      730
    mediastinal, 730, 731t
    metastatic, 730–731, 731f
    miscellaneous, 730
    neuroendocrine, 729–730, 729f
  obstructive, 683–693, 683f
    asthma as, 683t, 688–692
      atopic, 688, 689, 690f
      clinical course of, 692
      drug-induced, 689
      genetics of, 691
      morphology of, 691–692, 692f
      non-atopic, 688–689
      occupational, 689
      pathogenesis of, 689–691, 690f
    bronchiectasis as, 683t, 692–693, 693f
    chronic bronchitis as, 683t, 687–688,
      687t
    emphysema as, 683t, 684–687
      bullous, 687, 687f
      centriacinar (centrilobular), 684, 684f,
        685f
      clinical course of, 686–687, 687t
      distal acinar (paraseptal), 684
      incidence of, 684
      interstitial, 687
      irregular, 684
      morphology of, 685f, 686
      other forms of, 687, 687f
      panacinar (panlobular), 684, 684f, 685f
      pathogenesis of, 684–686, 685f
      types of, 684, 684f, 685f
    restrictive vs., 683, 683t
  due to occupational exposures, 409t
  of pleura, 731–734
    neoplastic, 732–734, 732f–734f
    pleural effusion as, 731–732
    pneumothorax as, 732
  pulmonary edema as, 680, 680t
  in systemic lupus erythematosus, 220
  in systemic sclerosis, 225
  of vascular origin, 706–710
    diffuse pulmonary hemorrhage syndromes
      as, 709–710, 709f
    pulmonary embolism, hemorrhage, and
      infarction as, 706–707, 706f
    pulmonary hypertension as, 707–709, 708f,
      709f
Lung injury, acute, 680–683
  clinical course of, 682
  morphology of, 680
  pathogenesis of, 681–682, 682f
Lung transplantation, 720–721, 721f
Lupus anticoagulant, 215
Lupus anticoagulant syndrome, 123
Lupus erythematosus
  chronic discoid, 221
  drug-induced, 215t, 216, 221
  subacute cutaneous, 221
  systemic, 213–221
    autoantibodies in, 204t, 213–215, 215t
    clinical features of, 204t, 217t, 220–221
    diagnostic criteria for, 213, 214t
    endocarditis of, 124, 220, 220f, 567f, 569
    epidemiology of, 213

Lupus erythematosus *(Continued)*
    etiology and pathogenesis of, 215–217, 216f
    morphology of, 217–220, 217t, 218f–220f
Lupus nephritis, 214t, 217–219, 218f, 219f, 934
Lupus pneumonitis, 696
Lupus vasculitis, 517
Luteal cysts, 1039
Luteal phase, inadequate, 1027
Luteinizing hormone (LH)-producing
    adenomas, 1100t, 1104–1105
Luteoma, pregnancy, 1052
Lyme arthritis, 378, 1242
Lyme disease, 334f, 377–378, 378f
    nervous system involvement in, 1302
Lyme myocarditis, 578
Lymph node(s), 189, 189f, 595
    in infectious mononucleosis, 356
    in sarcoidosis, 702
Lymph node metastases, of breast carcinoma, 1089
Lymphadenitis, 48, 519, 595–596
    nonspecific
      acute, 595
      chronic, 595–596, 596f
    due to tuberculosis, 372
Lymphadenopathic Kaposi sarcoma, 523, 524
Lymphangiectasis, in infants and children, 473
Lymphangioma(s), 522
    cavernous, 522
    in infants and children, 473
    simple (capillary), 522
Lymphangiosarcoma, 525
Lymphangitis, 48, 519
Lymphatic filariasis, 395, 395f
Lymphatic obstruction, edema due to, 112t, 113
Lymphatic spread, 269–270, 269f
Lymphatic tumors, in infants and children, 473
Lymphatic vessels, in inflammation
    acute, 47–48
    chronic, 72
Lymphatics, structure and function of, 489
Lymphedema, 112t, 113, 519–520
Lymphoblast(s), 602, 602f
Lymphoblastic leukemia/lymphoma, acute, 600–603, 601t
    clinical features of, 603
    defined, 600–602
    epidemiology of, 602
    immunophenotype of, 602
    molecular pathogenesis of, 305t, 306, 602–603
    morphology of, 602, 602f
    prognosis for, 603
Lymphocyte(s). *See also* B lymphocytes; T lymphocytes.
    activation of, 193–196, 194f–196f
    adult reference range for, 592t
    antigen recognition by, 193–195, 194f
    atypical, in infectious mononucleosis, 355, 356, 356f
    in chronic inflammation, 72, 73f
    in immune response, 185–187, 185f–187f
    large granular (See Natural killer (NK) cells)
    in lymphoid organs, 189, 189f
    naïve, 185
    recirculation of, 190, 190f
    in skin, 1166, 1167f
Lymphocytic colitis, 814, 814f
    in celiac disease, 796
Lymphocytic gastritis, 780
    in celiac disease, 796
Lymphocytic leukemia(s), 598
    chronic, 601t, 603–605, 604f
    large granular, 601t, 616

Lymphocytic lymphoma, small, 601t, 603–605, 604f
Lymphocytic mastopathy, 1070
Lymphocytic myocarditis, 578, 579f
Lymphocytosis, 594t
    in inflammation, 75
    intraepithelial, in celiac disease, 795, 796f
Lymphoepithelioma, nasopharyngeal, 751
Lymphogranuloma venereum, 380
Lymphoid aggregates, in viral hepatitis, 851f, 852
Lymphoid neoplasm(s), 596, 598–620
    characteristics of, 599–600
    classification of, 598–600, 598t, 600t, 601t
    clinical presentation of, 598
    Hodgkin lymphoma as, 598, 598t, 616–620
    mucosa-associated, 613
      due to chromosomal translocations, 597
      Helicobacter pylori and, 316
    origin of, 599–600, 599f
    peripheral B-cell, 598t, 603–614
    peripheral T-cell and NK-cell, 598t, 614–616, 615f
    precursor B- and T-cell, 598t, 600–603, 602f
    terminology for, 598
Lymphoid organ(s)
    generative (primary, central), 188–189
    peripheral (secondary), 188f, 189–190
    tertiary, 72
Lymphoid organogenesis, 72
Lymphoid progenitor cells, 590, 591f
Lymphoid system, radiation effect on, 425
Lymphoid tissues, 589
Lymphoma(s)
    acute lymphoblastic, 600–603, 601t
      clinical features of, 603
      defined, 600–602
      epidemiology of, 602
      genetic basis for, 305t, 306
      immunophenotype of, 602
      molecular pathogenesis of, 305t, 306, 602–603
      morphology of, 602, 602f
      prognosis for, 603
    AIDS-related, 247–248
    anaplastic large-cell, 601t, 615, 615f
    B-cell
      AIDS-related, 248
      diffuse large, 601t, 606–607, 607f, 608
      Epstein-Barr virus in, 315
    of breast, 1093
    Burkitt, 601t, 607–608, 608f
      Epstein-Barr virus and, 314–315, 314f, 608
      genetic basis for, 283, 305, 305t, 608
    extranodal NK/T-cell, 601t, 616
    follicular, 601t, 605–606, 605f, 606f
      genetic basis for, 305, 305t, 606
    gastric, 786–787, 787f
      Helicobacter pylori and, 316
    Hodgkin, 616–620
      AIDS-related, 247
      classification of, 598, 598t, 617
      clinical features of, 620, 621t
      defined, 616
      epidemiology of, 617
      lymphocyte depletion type of, 618t, 619
      lymphocyte predominance type of, 618t, 619–620, 619f
      lymphocyte-rich type of, 618t, 619, 619f
      mixed-cellularity type of, 618t, 619, 619f
      molecular pathogenesis of, 620, 621f
      nodular sclerosis type of, 618–619, 618f, 618t
      Reed-Sternberg cells in, 616–620, 617f, 621f

Lymphoma(s) *(Continued)*
      staging of, 620, 621t
      treatment of, 620
    intravascular, 1337
    vs. leukemia, 598
    lymphoplasmacytic, 612, 612f
    MALTomas as, 613
      due to chromosomal translocations, 597
      gastric, 786–787, 787f
      Helicobacter pylori and, 316, 786
    mantle cell, 601t, 612–613, 613f
      genetic basis for, 305, 305t, 613
    marginal zone, 601t, 613–614
    Mediterranean, 609
    non-Hodgkin, 598
      Hodgkin *vs.*, 616–617, 617t
    of orbit, 1348
      staging of, 621t
    primary CNS, 1337
    retinal, 1365
    small lymphocytic, 601t, 603–605, 604f
    T-cell
      adult, 601t, 615—616
      cutaneous, 1184–1185, 1185f
      enteropathy-associated, 796
      extranodal, 601t, 616
      peripheral, unspecified, 601t, 614–615, 615f
    testicular, 993
Lymphopenia, 592
    in AIDS, 242t
Lymphoplasmacytic lymphoma, 612, 612f
Lymphoplasmacytic sclerosing pancreatitis, 897
Lymphopoiesis, 591f
Lynch syndrome, 274, 275, 302, 821–822, 822t
Lyon hypothesis, 164
Lysosomal constituents, of leukocytes, in inflammation, 63
Lysosomal enzymes, 149
    deficiency of, 149–150, 150f
    in inflammation, 63
    in leukocyte-mediated tissue injury, 55
    synthesis and intracellular transport of, 149, 150f
Lysosomal glucosidase deficiency, 157t
Lysosomal membranes, injury to, 23
Lysosomal storage disease(s), 149–155, 150f, 151t
    Gaucher disease as, 151t, 153–154, 154f
    mucopolysaccharidoses as, 151t, 154–155
    Niemann-Pick disease as
      type C, 153
      types A and B, 151t, 152–153, 153f
    Tay-Sachs disease as, 139f, 150–152, 151t, 152f
Lysosomes, 149
Lysozyme, in phagocytosis, 54

M

M component, in plasma cell neoplasms, 609
M phase, of cell cycle, 86, 86f
M protein, in multiple myeloma, 611, 611f
MAC (*Mycobacterium avium-intracellulare* complex), 372, 373f
    in AIDS, 246, 372, 373f
MAC (membrane attack complex), 63, 64, 64f
MacCallum plaques, 566
Machado-Joseph disease, 168t, 1323
Macroalbuminuria, in diabetic nephropathy, 1145
Macrocytic anemia, 640
Macroglobulinemia, Waldenström, 609, 612
Macrophage(s)
    activated, 54, 54f, 71, 71f, 72f
    antitumor effect of, 318

Macrophage(s) (Continued)
  in glomerular injury, 915
  HIV infection of, 241–242, 242t
  in immune response, 184, 188, 194f
  in inflammation
    acute, 56
    chronic, 71, 71f–73f, 72
  in metastasis, 303
  in phagocytosis, 53
  smokers', 704, 704f, 705
  in tuberculosis, 368
  in wound healing, 102, 103f, 105f
Macrophage aggregates, in viral hepatitis, 851, 851f
Macrophage colony-stimulating factor (M-CSF), in bone homeostasis, 1208, 1208f
Macrophage inflammatory protein-1α (MIP-1α), 62
Macrophage inhibitory factor (MIF), in acute respiratory distress syndrome, 682f
Macrosomia, fetal, 452
Macrovascular disease, diabetic, 1139–1140, 1140f, 1141f, 1144–1145
Macular corneal dystrophy, 1353
Macular degeneration, age-related, 1346, 1363–1364, 1364f
Macular edema, in diabetes, 1360
Macule, 1168
Maffucci syndrome, 1227, 1228
MAGE (melanoma antigen gene) family, 317
Magnesium ammonium phosphate stones, 962, 962t
Major basic protein
  in chronic inflammation, 72
  in phagocytosis, 54
Major histocompatibility complex (MHC)
  molecules
    in asthma, 691
    in autoimmunity, 212
    classification of, 190–192
    and disease association, 192–193, 193t
    in immune evasion, 319
    in immune response, 186, 186f, 190–192, 191f, 192f
    in transplant rejection, 226, 227f
Major histocompatibility complex (MHC) restriction, 186
Malabsorption, 793–797
  in abetalipoproteinemia, 797
  in autoimmune enteropathy, 794t, 796–797
  in celiac disease, 794t, 795–796, 795f, 796f
  in Crohn disease, 811
  in cystic fibrosis, 794, 794t
  in lactase (disaccharidase) deficiency, 794t, 797
  mechanisms of, 793–794, 794t
  in tropical sprue, 794t, 796
Malacoplakia, cystitis with, 975, 975f, 976f
Malar rash, in systemic lupus erythematosus, 214t, 219
Malaria, 386–388, 387f, 388f
  causative agents for, 386
  epidemiology of, 386
  host resistance to, 387
  life cycle and pathogenesis of, 386–387, 387f
  malignant cerebral, 388, 388f
  morphology of, 387–388, 388f
Malarial granulomas, 388
Malassezia furfur, 1202
Male breast, 1093
Male breast disease, 1093–1094
  carcinoma as, 1093–1094
  gynecomastia as, 1093, 1093f

Male genital tract, 982–1002
  penis in, 982–984
    congenital anomalies of, 982
    inflammation of, 982
    tumors of, 982–984, 983f, 984f
  prostate in, 993–1002
    benign enlargement of, 994–996, 995f, 996f
    inflammation of, 993–994
    normal anatomy and histology of, 993, 993f, 994f
    tumors of, 996–1002, 998f–1000f, 1001t
  testis and epididymis in, 984–993
    congenital anomalies of, 984–985, 985f
    inflammation of, 986–987, 986f
    regressive changes of, 985–986
    tumors of, 987–993, 987t
      germ cell, 987–992, 988f–991f
      gonadoblastoma as, 993
      lymphoma as, 993
      of sex cord–gonadal stroma, 992
      spermatic cord and paratesticular, 987
    tunica vaginalis of, 993
    vascular disorders of, 987, 987f
Male pseudohermaphroditism, 167
Male-specific Y (MSY) region, 164
Malformations, 448, 449f
Malignancy
  hypercalcemia of, 321t, 322, 1126
  neuropathies associated with, 1266
Malignant fibrous histiocytoma, 1253
Malignant hyperpyrexia, 1270
Malignant hypertension, 492, 949–951, 950f
  retina in, 1359
Malignant hyperthermia, 422, 1270
Malignant melanoma. See Melanoma(s).
Malignant mixed müllerian tumors (MMMTs), of endometrium, 1034–1035, 1036f
Malignant mixed tumor, of salivary glands, 759
Malignant peripheral nerve sheath tumor, 1341–1342
Malignant transformation. See Carcinogenesis.
Malignant tumor(s). See Cancer.
Mallory bodies, in alcoholic hepatitis, 858, 858f
Mallory-Weiss tears, 768
Malnutrition, 427, 428–429, 429f, 430f
  due to alcohol consumption, 859
  atrophy due to, 9
  criteria for, 428
  epidemiology of, 428
  global warming and, 402
  primary, 427
  secondary, 427
MALT (mucosa-associated lymphoid tissue), 778
MALT1 gene, 597
MALTomas (mucosa-associated lymphoid tumors), 613
  due to chromosomal translocations, 597
  gastric, 786–787, 787f
  Helicobacter pylori and, 316, 786
Mammalian chitinase family, in asthma, 691
Mammalian target of rapamycin (mTOR), 294
Mammary duct ectasia, 1070, 1070f
Mammographic screening, 1068–1069, 1068f
Mammosomatotroph adenoma, 1100t, 1104
Mammotrophs, 1098
Mannose receptors, in inflammation, 52
Mannose-binding lectin 2 (MBL2) gene, in cystic fibrosis, 468
Mannosidosis, 151t
Mantle cell lymphoma, 601t, 612–613, 613f
  genetic basis for, 305, 305t, 613
MAP kinase pathway, in papillary thyroid carcinoma, 1120

MAP kinase (mitogen-activated protein kinase) pathway, 90, 91f
MAPT gene, 1318
Marantic endocarditis, 568
Marasmus, 428–429, 429f
Marble bone disease, 1212–1214, 1214f, 1215f
Marfan syndrome, 96, 144–145
  aneurysms in, 506–507, 507f
  mitral valve prolapse in, 145, 563
Marfanoid habitus, in MEN-2B, 1162
Marginal zone lymphoma, 601t, 613–614
Marie-Strümpell disease, 1241
Marijuana, abuse of, 418t, 419–420
Marrow embolism, 126–127, 127f
Marrow stromal cells (MSCs), 85
MART gene, 1318
Mast cell(s)
  in immediate hypersensitivity, 198–199, 198f, 199f
  in inflammation, 56, 72
Mast cell mediators, in immediate hypersensitivity, 199–201, 200f, 201t
Mastalgia, 1067
Mastitis
  acute, 1069
  granulomatous, 1070
  periductal, 1069, 1069f
Mastocytosis, 1185–1186, 1186f
  systemic, 626t
Mastodynia, 1067
Mastopathy, lymphocytic, 1070
Masugi nephritis, 912
Maternal imprinting, 171
Maternal influences, on fetal growth restriction, 455–456
Maternal inheritance, 171
Matricellular proteins, in angiogenesis, 101–102
Matrix metalloproteinases (MMPs)
  in metastasis, 299–300
  in wound healing, 105
Maturation, of melanocytic nevi, 1169, 1170f
Maturation phase, of cutaneous wound healing, 102
Maturity-onset diabetes of the young (MODY), 1137
MB fraction of creatine kinase (CK-MB), in myocardial infarction, 555–556, 555f
MBL2 (mannose-binding lectin 2) gene, in cystic fibrosis, 468
MBP (myelin basic protein), 1265f
MC1R (melanocortin receptor 1) gene, in melanoma, 1174
MC4R (melanocortin receptor 4), in energy balance, 440, 441f
McArdle syndrome, 155, 157t
McBurney's point, 827
McBurney's sign, 827
McCune-Albright syndrome, fibrous dysplasia in, 1231
MCHC (mean cell hemoglobin concentration), 640, 641t
  in sickle cell disease, 645–646
MCKD1 gene, 960
MCKD2 gene, 960
MCP-1 (monocyte chemoattractant protein), 62
M-CSF (macrophage colony-stimulating factor), in bone homeostasis, 1208, 1208f
MCVs (molluscum contagiosum viruses), 1009
MDM2, 290–291
MDMA (3,4-methylenedioxymethamphetamine), 419
MDMX, 290
MDR1, in ulcerative colitis, 809

MDS (myelodysplastic syndrome), 620, 624–626, 625f
Mean cell hemoglobin, 640, 641t
Mean cell hemoglobin concentration (MCHC), 640, 641t
  in sickle cell disease, 645–646
Mean cell volume, 640
  adult reference range for, 641t
Measles, 349–350, 350f
  oral manifestations of, 744t
Mechanical factors, and wound healing, 106
Mechanical trauma, 420–421, 420f
Meckel diverticulum, 765–766, 765f
Meconium ileus, in cystic fibrosis, 469
Media, of blood vessels, 488, 488f
Medial hypertrophy, in pulmonary hypertension, 708, 709f
Median lobe hypertrophy, of prostate, 995
Mediastinal tumors, 730, 731t
Mediastinopericarditis, 582
  adhesive, 582
Mediterranean lymphoma, 609
Medullary carcinoma
  of breast, 1087, 1088f
  of thyroid, 1121, 1124–1126, 1125f
    in MEN-2, 1162–1163
Medullary cystic disease, adult-onset, 957t, 959–960, 960f
Medullary sponge kidney, 957t, 959
Medulloblastoma, 1336–1337, 1336f
Megacolon
  congenital aganglionic, 766–767, 766f
  toxic, 812
Megakaryocytes, in myelodysplastic syndrome, 625, 625f
Megalencephaly, 1284
Megalin, 912
Megaloblastic anemia(s), 654–659
  folate deficiency, 655t, 658–659
  morphology of, 655, 655f, 656f
  pernicious (vitamin B_{12} deficiency), 655–658, 655t, 656f, 657f
Megaloblastoid maturation, in myelodysplastic syndrome, 625
Megalocornea, 1366
Meibomian glands, 1348f
Melanin, intracellular accumulation of, 36
Melanin deficiency, 143–144
Melanocortin receptor 1 (MC1R) gene, in melanoma, 1174
Melanocortin receptor 4 (MC4R), in energy balance, 440, 441f
Melanocyte(s), 1166, 1166f
Melanocyte disorders, 1168–1175
  dysplastic nevi as, 1170–1171, 1170t, 1171f, 1172f
  freckles (ephelis) as, 1168
  lentigo as, 1168–1169
  melanocytic (pigmented) nevus (mole) as, 1169–1170, 1169f, 1170f, 1170t
  melanoma as, 1171–1175
    clinical features of, 1172, 1173f
    morphology of, 1172–1173, 1173f
    pathogenesis of, 1174–1175, 1174f
    prognostic factors for, 1173–1174
α-Melanocyte-stimulating hormone (MSH), in energy balance, 439
Melanocytic nevus, 1169–1170, 1169f, 1170f, 1170t
Melanocytic tumors of uncertain malignant potential, 1173
Melanoma(s), 1171–1175
  acral/mucosal lentiginous, 1169, 1172
  clinical features of, 1172, 1173f

Melanoma(s) (Continued)
  conjunctival, 1350, 1350f
  dysplastic nevi and, 1170–1171, 1172f
  epidemiology of, 1172
  familial, 275, 1174, 1182t
  morphology of, 1172–1173, 1173f
  pathogenesis of, 1174–1175, 1174f
  prognostic factors for, 1173–1174
  superficial spreading, 1172
  uveal, 1356–1357, 1358f
  of vulva, 1015–1016
Melanoma antigen gene (MAGE) family, 317
Melanotic pigmentation, of oral cavity, 744t
MELAS (mitochondrial encephalomyopathy, lactic acidosis, and strokelike episodes), 1327
Membrane alterations, in apoptosis, 27
Membrane attack complex (MAC), 63, 64, 64f
Membrane blebs, in cell injury, 13f, 23
Membrane permeability, defects in, cell injury due to, 18f, 22–23, 22f
Membranoproliferative glomerulonephritis (MPGN), 918t, 928–929
  alternative complement pathway in, 915, 928–929, 928f
  clinical features of, 929
  morphology of, 929, 929f, 930f
  pathogenesis of, 928–929, 928f
  primary, 928
  secondary, 929
Membranous glomerulonephritis, in systemic lupus erythematosus, 218
Membranous glomerulopathy, 918t, 922–923, 924f
Membranous nephropathy, 918t, 922–923, 924f
Memory cells, 185, 194f, 196, 196f, 197
MEN. See Multiple endocrine neoplasia (MEN).
MEN1 gene
  in hyperparathyroidism, 1127
  in MEN-1, 1162
  in pituitary adenomas, 1101
Mendelian disorder(s), 140–158
  alkaptonuria as, 155–156
  autosomal-dominant, 140–141, 141t
  autosomal-recessive, 141–142, 142t
  biochemical and molecular basis of, 142–144, 143t, 144f
  congenital anomalies due to, 451
  due to defects in proteins that regulate cell growth, 143t, 156
  due to defects in receptor proteins, 143t, 144, 147–149, 147f–149f
  due to defects in structural proteins, 143t, 144–147, 146t
  Ehlers-Danlos syndromes as, 145–147, 146t
  due to enzyme defects, 149–156
  familial hypercholesterolemia as, 147–149, 147t–149f
  Gaucher disease as, 151t, 153–154, 154f
  glycogen storage diseases as, 155, 156f, 157t, 158f
  lysosomal storage diseases as, 149–155, 150f, 151t
  Marfan syndrome as, 144–145
  mucopolysaccharidoses as, 151t, 154–155
  Niemann-Pick disease as
    type C, 153
    types A and B, 151t, 152–153, 153f
  Tay-Sachs disease as, 139f, 150–152, 151t, 152f
  transmission patterns of, 140–142, 141t, 142t
  X-linked, 142, 142t
Ménétrier disease, 782, 782t
Menin, 1162
Meningioangiomatosis, 1342

Meningioma(s), 1338–1339, 1338f
  anaplastic (malignant), 1339
  atypical, 1339
Meningitis
  acute, 1299–1300
    aseptic (viral), 1299, 1300
      HIV, 1305
    pyogenic (bacterial), 1299–1300, 1299f
  chemical, 1299, 1300
  chronic, 1299
  cryptococcal, 1306, 1307f
  defined, 1299
  tuberculous, 1301
Meningocele, 1284
Meningoencephalitis
  chronic bacterial, 1301–1302
  defined, 1299
  fungal, 1306, 1307f
  tuberculous, 1301
  viral, 1302–1306, 1303f–1306f
Meningomyelocele, 1284
Meningovascular neurosyphilis, 1301
Menopausal changes, 1027
Menstrual cycle
  anovulatory, 1026–1027
  breast changes during, 1066
  endometrial histology in, 1024–1026, 1025f
  inadequate luteal phase of, 1027
MEOS (microsomal ethanol-oxidizing system), 413
Mercuric chloride poisoning, 24
Mercury poisoning, 407–408
Merkel cells, 1166, 1166f
Merlin, 295, 1340
Merozoites, of malaria, 387, 387f
MERRF (myoclonic epilepsy and ragged red fibers), 1327–1328
Mesangial lupus glomerulonephritis, 217
Mesangiocapillary glomerulonephritis, 915, 918t, 928–929, 928f–930f
Mesenchymal tumors
  of bladder, 980–981
  of prostate, 1002
Mesial temporal herniation, 1283–1284, 1283f
Mesonephric duct, 1007, 1007f
Mesothelial inclusion cysts, of ovary, 1042, 1042f
Mesothelioma(s)
  asbestos exposure and, 701, 961
  benign fibrous, 732–733, 732f
  epithelioid, 733–734, 733f
  of fallopian tubes, 1039
  malignant, 733–734, 733f, 734f
  mixed, 961f, 962
  peritoneal, 734
  of peritoneum, 829
  sarcomatoid, 962
MET gene, in renal cell carcinoma, 965
Metabolic abnormalities, in septic shock, 131
Metabolic acidosis, due to shock, 132
Metabolic disease(s)
  of central nervous system
    acquired, 1328–1330, 1329f
    Alexander disease as, 1327
    Alpers disease as, 1328
    Canavan disease as, 1327
    genetic, 1325–1328
    hepatic encephalopathy as, 1329
    due to hyperglycemia, 1329
    due to hypoglycemia, 1329
    Kearn-Sayre syndrome as, 1328
    Krabbe disease as, 1326, 1326f
    Leigh syndrome as, 1328
    leukodystrophies as, 1325, 1326–1327, 1326f

Metabolic disease(s) *(Continued)*
   mitochondrial encephalomyopathies as, 1325–1326, 1327–1328
   myoclonic epilepsy with ragged red fibers as, 1327–1328
   neuronal storage diseases as, 1325, 1326
   Pelizaeus-Merzbacher disease as, 1327
   Tay-Sachs disease as, 1326
   due to vitamin deficiencies, 1328–1329
  neurologic sequelae of, 1329
  peripheral neuropathy with, 1263, 1264t
Metabolic liver disease, 860–866
  due to α$_1$-antitrypsin deficiency, 864–866, 865f
  due to hemochromatosis, 861–863, 861t, 863f
  neonatal cholestasis as, 866, 866f, 866t
  nonalcoholic fatty, 860–861, 861f
  due to Wilson disease, 863–864
Metabolic neuropathies
  acquired, 1265–1266, 1265f
  peripheral, 1266
Metabolic status, and wound healing, 106
Metabolic syndrome, 442, 442f, 1146
  and ischemic heart disease, 498
Metabolism
  inborn error(s) of, 462–465, 463t
   cystic fibrosis as, 465–471
    clinical features of, 468f, 469–471, 470t
    environmental modifiers of, 468
    genetic basis for, 139f, 144, 465–468, 466f, 467f
    morphology of, 468–469, 469f
   galactosemia as, 464–465, 464f, 465f
   myopathies with, 1271–1273
   phenylketonuria as, 463–464, 463f
  inherited errors of, HLA alleles and, 193
Metachromasia, 1327
Metachromatic leukodystrophy, 151t, 1326–1327
Metals, as environmental pollutants, 406–408, 406f, 407f
Metaphyseal chondrodysplasia, Schmid, 1211t
Metaphyseal chondroplasia, Jansen, 1211t
Metaplasia, 265
  causes of, 10–11, 10f
  on cervicovaginal smear, 323f
  columnar to squamous, 10, 10f
  connective tissue, 10–11
  defined, 10
  mechanisms of, 11
  squamous to columnar, 10
Metaplastic carcinoma, of breast, 1088–1089
Metaplastic lesions, of bladder, 975–976
Metaplastic theory, of endometriosis, 1028
Metapneumovirus (MPV), 716
Metastasis(es), 269–270, 269f–271f, 271t
  to bladder, 981
  to brain, 1339
  of breast cancer, 269f, 270, 301, 1087, 1089
  in carcinogenesis, 278, 298–302, 298f
  of colorectal cancer, 825, 826f
  determination of site of origin of, 324
  dormancy of, 301
  hepatic, 881–882
  invasion of extracellular matrix in, 298–300, 299f
  to lungs, 730–731, 731f
  molecular genetics of, 301–302, 301f
  myocardial, 584–585
  to orbit, 1348
  osteolytic, 1126
  to ovaries, 1040t, 1041f, 1052
  of prostate cancer, 998, 998f

Metastasis(es) *(Continued)*
  skeletal, 1235
  vascular dissemination and homing of tumor cells in, 300–301
Metastasis oncogenes, 302
Metastasis suppressors, 302
Metastatic calcification, 38–39
Metastatic cascade, 298, 298f
Metastatic signature, 301, 301f
Metastatic theory, of endometriosis, 1028
Metastatic variants, 301, 301f
Metazoal infections, 391–396, 392f–396f
Metchnikoff, Elie, 44
Methadone, 419
Methamphetamine (meth), abuse of, 419
Methane, in greenhouse effect, 401
Methanol, CNS toxicity of, 1329
Methemoglobin, 642
Methicillin-resistant *Staphylococcus aureus* (MRSA), 359
Methotrexate, CNS effects of, 1330
Methyl mercury poisoning, 408
Methylation-specific polymerase chain reaction, 181
Methylcobalamin, 657, 657f
3,4-Methylenedioxymethamphetamine (MDMA, Ecstasy), 419
Methylmalonic acid, in vitamin B$_{12}$ deficiency, 657
MGUS (monoclonal gammopathy of uncertain significance), 609, 611
MHC. *See* Major histocompatibility complex (MHC).
MI. *See* Myocardial infarction (MI).
Microabscesses
  Munro, 1191
  Pautrier, 1185
Microalbuminuria, in diabetic nephropathy, 1145
Microangiopathic hemolytic anemia, 654, 654f
Microangiopathy(ies)
  diabetic, 1140, 1140f
   intraretinal, 1360, 1363f
  thrombotic, 669–670, 669t
   renal disease due to, 952–954, 952f
Microarray-based DNA sequencing, 174, 175f
Microbe(s)
  bacteria as, 333t, 334–335, 334f
   mechanisms of disease production by, 343–344
  in bioterrorism, 337–338, 337t
  categories of, 332–336, 333t
  cell injury due to, 11
  ectoparasites as, 336
  fungi as, 333t, 335
  helminths as, 333t, 336
  immune evasion by, 345–346, 345f, 346t
  mechanisms of disease production by, 342–355
  prions as, 332, 333t
  protozoa as, 333t, 335–336
  release from body of, 340–341
  routes of entry of, 338–339
  special techniques for diagnosing, 335t, 336
  spread and dissemination of, 339–340, 339f
  transmission of, 340–341
   placental-fetal, 340
   sexual, 341–342, 341t
  viruses as, 332–333, 333f, 333t
   mechanisms of disease production by, 342–343, 343f

Microbial carcinogens, 309t, 312–316
  Helicobacter pylori as, 315–316
  oncogenic DNA viruses as, 313–315, 313f, 314f
  oncogenic RNA viruses as, 312–313
Microbial infections, pathogenesis of, 332–348
Microbiome, 335
Microbiota, in inflammatory bowel disease, 809–810
Microcephaly, 1284
Microcytic hypochromic anemia, 640
  of iron deficiency, 661–662, 662f
Microglia, reactions to injury of, 1282
Microglial nodules, 1282
  in arthropod-borne viral encephalitis, 1302, 1303f
  in HIV encephalitis, 1305, 1305f
Micropapillary carcinoma, ovarian, 1043f, 1044
Microphthalmia, 1368
MicroRNAs (miRNAs), 137, 137f
  in carcinogenesis, 277, 307–308, 307f
  in DNA repair, 291
  oncogenic, 307f–308
Microsatellite instability, 302
  in colorectal cancer, 822, 823, 824, 824f
Microsatellite repeats, 176
Microscopic colitis, 814, 814f
Microscopic polyangiitis, 515, 516f
  glomerular lesions in, 935
Microsomal ethanol-oxidizing system (MEOS), 413
Microsomal triglyceride transfer protein (MTP), 797
Microvascular disease, in systemic sclerosis, 223–224
Microvascular injury, pulmonary edema due to, 680, 680t
Microvascular occlusions, in sickle cell disease, 646, 646f
MIF (macrophage inhibitory factor), in acute respiratory distress syndrome, 682f
Migratory thrombophlebitis, 125, 520
  due to cancer, 321t, 322
  due to pancreatic carcinoma, 903
Mikulicz syndrome, 222–223
Milk of calcium, 1071
Milkline remnants, 1067
Millisieverts (mSv), 423
Milroy disease, 520
Minamata disease, 408
Mineral dusts
  inhalation of, 410
  lung diseases due to, 696–701, 697t
Mineralocorticoids, 1148
Minimal residual disease, detection of, 325
Minimal-change disease, 918t, 923–926, 925f
Mininutritional Assessment (MNA), 428
Minisatellite repeats, 176
Minocycline, skin pigmentation due to, 415f
MIP-1α (macrophage inflammatory protein-1α), 62
mir34, in DNA repair, 291, 291f
miRNAs (microRNAs), 137, 137f
  in carcinogenesis, 277, 307–308, 307f
  in DNA repair, 291
  oncogenic, 307f–308
Miscarriage, 1053
Misfolded proteins, accumulation of, apoptosis due to, 25
Mismatch repair, in colorectal cancer, 824, 824f
Mitochondrial damage, cell injury due to, 18–19, 18f, 19f
Mitochondrial DNA (mtDNA), 171

Mitochondrial encephalomyopathies, 1325–1326, 1327–1328
Mitochondrial encephalomyopathy, lactic acidosis, and strokelike episodes (MELAS), 1327
Mitochondrial genes, mutations in, 171, 171f
Mitochondrial membrane damage, 22
Mitochondrial myopathies, 1271–1273, 1274f
Mitochondrial pathway, of apoptosis, 28–29, 28f, 29f
Mitochondrial permeability transition pore, 19, 19f
Mitogen-activated protein kinase (MAP kinase) pathway, 90, 91f
Mitogillin, 385
Mitoses
    in neoplasia, 264, 265f
    in wound healing, 103f
Mitotic catastrophe, 296, 297f
Mitral annular calcification, 562f, 563, 564f
Mitral regurgitation, 561t
    ischemic, 561
Mitral stenosis, 561t
    rheumatic, 565, 565f
    and thrombosis, 122
Mitral valve, myxomatous degeneration of, 563–565, 564f
Mitral valve prolapse (MVP), 563–565, 564f
    in Marfan syndrome, 145, 563
    polycystic kidney disease and, 959
Mitral valvulitis, acute rheumatic, 565f
Mixed connective tissue disease, 226
Mixed tumors, 261, 261f
    of salivary glands, 757–759, 758f
    testicular, 991
ML(s) (mucolipidoses), 151t
MLH1 gene, 302, 306
    in colorectal carcinoma, 822, 824, 824f
MLL gene, 305, 603
MMMTs (malignant mixed müllerian tumors), of endometrium, 1034–1035, 1036f
MMPs (matrix metalloproteinases)
    in metastasis, 299–300
    in wound healing, 105
MNA (Mininutritional Assessment), 428
MODY (maturity-onset diabetes of the young), 1137
Molds, 382
Mole, 1169–1170, 1169f, 1170f, 1170t
    hydatidiform, 1057–1059
        complete, 1058–1059, 1058f, 1059f
        partial, 1058, 1058f
    invasive, 1059, 1060f
Molecular changes, 4
Molecular chaperone therapy, for lysosomal storage diseases, 150
Molecular diagnosis, 173–181
    for acquired genetic alterations, 174
    array-based comparative genomic hybridization in, 179–180, 180f
    detection of DNA sequence alterations in, 174–176, 175f, 176f
    for detection of minimal residual disease, 325
    for epigenetic alterations, 180–181
    fluorescence in situ hybridization in, 179, 179f
    genome-wide analyses in, 138, 177, 178f
    for genomic alterations, 178–180, 179f, 180f
    for germline genetic alterations, 173
    of hereditary predisposition to cancer, 325
    indications for, 173–174
    for infectious agents, 336
    of malignant neoplasms, 324–325
    polymerase chain reaction in, 174–176, 175f, 176f

Molecular diagnosis (*Continued*)
    polymorphic markers in, 176–177, 177f, 178f
    postnatal, 173–174
    prenatal, 173
    for prognosis of malignant neoplasms, 325
    RNA analysis in, 181
    Southern blotting in, 176, 176f, 178
Molecular mimicry, in autoimmunity, 212, 213f
Molecular profiles, of tumors, 325–326, 326f
Molluscum contagiosum, 1201, 1201f
Molluscum contagiosum viruses (MCVs), 1009
Mönckeberg medial sclerosis, 496
Monoblasts, in acute myeloid leukemia, 623, 623f
Monoclonal antibodies, immune cell antigens detected by, 599–600, 600t
Monoclonal gammopathy of uncertain significance (MGUS), 609, 611
Monoclonal immunoglobulin, in plasma cell neoplasms, 609
Monoclonal immunoglobulin (Ig) deposition disease, glomerular lesions in, 935
Monoclonal proliferations, 324
Monocyte(s)
    adult reference range for, 592t
    differentiation of, 591f
    in glomerular injury, 915
    HIV infection of, 242, 242t
    in inflammation
        acute, 50, 51f
        chronic, 71, 71f
    in innate immunity, 184
Monocyte chemoattractant protein (MCP-1), 62
Monocytic leukemia, oral manifestations of, 744t
Monocytosis, 594t
Mononeuropathy, diabetic, 1146
Mononuclear inflammation, 347, 347f
Mononuclear phagocyte system, in chronic inflammation, 71, 71f
Mononucleosis
    cytomegalovirus, 354
    infectious, 355–357, 356f
        oral manifestations of, 744t
Monosodium urate (MSU) crystals, in gouty arthritis, 1243, 1245f
Monosomy, 159
Monostotic fibrous dysplasia, 1231
Moon facies, in Cushing syndrome, 1150, 1151f
Moraxella catarrhalis pneumonia, 712
Morgagnian cataract, 1353
Morphologic changes, 4
Morton neuroma, 1267
Mosaicism, 160
    confined placental, 455, 455f
    gonadal, 173
Motor neurons, degenerative diseases of, 1324–1325, 1325f
Motor unit(s)
    in axonal degeneration, 1258, 1258f, 1259–1260, 1259f
    defined, 1258
    general reactions of, 1258–1261
    in myopathy, 1258, 1258f, 1260–1261
    in nerve regeneration and reinnervation of muscle, 1258, 1258f, 1260, 1260t, 1261f
    normal *vs.* abnormal, 1258f
    in segmental demyelination, 1258, 1258f, 1259, 1259f
Mott cells, 390
    in multiple myeloma, 610
Mouth disorders. *See* Oral cavity disorder(s).
MPGN. *See* Membranoproliferative glomerulonephritis (MPGN).

MPO (myeloperoxidase), in phagocytosis, 53, 53f
MPO (myeloperoxidase) deficiency, 56t
MPO-ANCA (anti-myeloperoxidase), 511
MPSs (mucopolysaccharidoses), 151t, 154–155
    skeletal manifestations of, 1212
MPV (metapneumovirus), 716
MPZ (myelin protein zero), 1263, 1265f
MRSA (methicillin-resistant *Staphylococcus aureus*), 359
MS (multiple sclerosis), 1310–1312, 1311f, 1312f
    T cell–mediated hypersensitivity in, 206t
MSA (multiple system atrophy), 1321–1322
MSCs (marrow stromal cells), 85
MSH (α-melanocyte-stimulating hormone), in energy balance, 439
MSH2 gene, 302
    in colorectal carcinoma, 822, 824, 824f
MSU (monosodium urate) crystals, in gouty arthritis, 1243, 1245f
mSv (millisieverts), 423
MSY (male-specific Y) region, 164
mtDNA (mitochondrial DNA), 171
mTOR (mammalian target of rapamycin), 294
MTP (microsomal triglyceride transfer protein), 797
Mucin(s), as tumor antigens, 318
Mucinous carcinoma, of breast, 1087, 1088f
Mucinous cystadenocarcinoma, of appendix, 828
Mucinous cystadenoma
    of appendix, 828
    of ovary, 1045
    of pancreas, 899, 899f
Mucinous cystic neoplasms, of pancreas, 899, 899f
Mucinous tumors, of ovaries, 1044–1045, 1045f
Mucocele
    of appendix, 828
    of salivary glands, 756, 757f
    of sinus, 750
Mucocutaneous lymph node syndrome, 515
Mucoepidermoid carcinoma, 759–760, 760f
    of conjunctiva, 1350
Mucolipidoses (MLs), 151t
Mucopolysaccharidoses (MPSs), 151t, 154–155
    skeletal manifestations of, 1212
Mucor, 385, 386f
Mucormycosis, 385–386, 386f
    of CNS, 1306
    of orbit, 1347
Mucosa-associated lymphoid tissue (MALT), 778
Mucosa-associated lymphoid tumors (MALTomas), 613
    due to chromosomal translocations, 597
    gastric, 786–787, 787f
    Helicobacter pylori and, 316, 786
Mucosal atrophy, due to chronic gastritis, 781
Mucosal bridges, in ulcerative colitis, 811, 812f
Mucosal infarction, of bowel, 792, 793
Mucosal lentiginous melanoma, 1172
Mucoviscidosis. *See* Cystic fibrosis.
Muir-Torre syndrome, 1182t
Müllerian ducts, 1006, 1007f
Müllerian mucinous cystadenoma, 1044
Müllerian tubercles, 1006, 1007f
Müllerian tumors, of ovaries, 1040t, 1041–1047, 1041f
Müllerian-inhibiting substance, in cryptorchidism, 985
Multicystic encephalopathy, 1286, 1286f
Multicystic renal dysplasia, 955–956, 956f
Multifactorial inheritance, congenital anomalies due to, 451
Multifocal atrophic gastritis, 777

Multigenic disorders, 138, 157–158
Multihormonal tumors, 1147
Multi-infarct dementia, 1295, 1319
Multinucleated giant cells, in HIV encephalitis, 1305
Multiple endocrine neoplasia (MEN) syndromes, 1161
Multiple endocrine neoplasia type 1 (MEN-1), 274, 1161–1162
    hyperparathyroidism due to, 1127
Multiple endocrine neoplasia type 2 (MEN-2), 274, 1162–1163
    hyperparathyroidism due to, 1127
    medullary thyroid carcinoma in, 1124, 1125
    pheochromocytomas in, 1160t
Multiple epiphyseal dysplasia, 1211t
Multiple hereditary exostosis syndrome, 1227
Multiple myeloma, 601t, 609–611, 610f, 611f
    glomerular lesions in, 935
Multiple sclerosis (MS), 1310–1312, 1311f, 1312f
    T cell–mediated hypersensitivity in, 206t
Multiple sulfatase deficiency, 151t
Multiple system atrophy (MSA), 1321–1322
Mumps, 350
    epididymitis and orchitis due to, 986
Munro microabscesses, 1191
Mural infarction, of bowel, 792, 793
Mural thrombus(i), 124, 124f, 546f
    due to myocardial infarction, 557
Muscle, reinnervation of, 1258, 1258f, 1260, 1260t, 1261f
Muscle fiber(s)
    reactions of, 1260–1261
    types of, 1260, 1260t, 1261f
Muscle fiber atrophy, 1259–1260, 1259f
Muscle fiber hypertrophy, 1261
Muscle fiber splitting, 1261
Muscle involvement, in sarcoidosis, 703
Muscle phosphofructokinase deficiency, 155
Muscle phosphorylase deficiency, 157t
Muscle syndromes, due to cancer, 321t, 322
Muscular arteries, 488f, 489
Muscular dystrophy(ies), 1268–1270
    congenital, 1270t
    Emery-Dreifuss, 1270t
    fascioscapulohumeral, 1270t
    limb girdle, 1269, 1271t
    oculopharyngeal, 1270t
    X-linked (Duchenne, Becker), 1268–1269, 1268f, 1269f
Musculoskeletal defects, prevalence of, 451t
Musculoskeletal system, in systemic sclerosis, 225
Mutated genes, products of, as tumor antigens, 316–317
Mutation(s), 138–140, 138f, 139f
    in carcinogenesis, 278, 308–309
    within coding sequences, 138, 138f
    defined, 138
    due to deletions and insertions, 138, 138f, 139, 139f
    frameshift, 138, 138f, 139, 139f
    full, 170
    gain-of-function, 141
    loss-of-function, 141
    missense, 138
    within noncoding sequences, 139
    nonsense, 138, 139f
    point, 138, 138f, 139f
    pre-, 170
    signature, 311
    trinucleotide-repeat, 139, 167–171, 168f, 168t

MVP (mitral valve prolapse), 563–565, 564f
    in Marfan syndrome, 145, 563
    polycystic kidney disease and, 959
Myasthenia gravis, 1275–1276
    antibody-mediated hypersensitivity in, 203, 203t
    due to cancer, 321t, 322
Myasthenia syndrome, Lambert-Eaton, 1276
MYC oncogene, 284, 284f, 305, 308, 309
Mycobacterial infection(s), 358t, 366–374, 367f, 369f–374f
    in AIDS, 246
    enterocolitis due to, 794t, 798t, 804, 804f
Mycobacterium avium-intracellulare complex (MAC), 372, 373f
    in AIDS, 246, 372, 373f
Mycobacterium leprae, 372–374, 373f, 374f
    granulomatous inflammation due to, 73t
    polyneuropathy due to, 1262
Mycobacterium tuberculosis, 366–372
    in AIDS, 246
    clinical features of, 368–370, 369f
    epidemiology of, 366–367
    granulomatous inflammation due to, 73t, 74, 74f
    morphology of, 370–372, 370f–372f
    pathogenesis of, 367–368, 367f
Mycoplasma, 335
    sexual transmission of, 341t
Mycoplasma hominis, 1009
Mycoplasma pneumoniae pneumonia, 714–715
Mycoplasmal pneumonia, 714–715
Mycosis(es). See also Fungal infection(s).
    fungoides, 601t, 616, 1184–1185, 1185f
        d'emblée, 1184
Mycotic aneurysm, 507, 508
Mycotic infections, of female genital tract, 1009
Myelin, compaction of, 1263, 1265f
Myelin basic protein (MBP), 1265f
Myelin figures, in cell injury, 13f, 14, 23
Myelin ovoids, 1259
Myelin protein zero (MPZ), 1263, 1265f
Myelin sheath, 1258
Myelinated nerve fibers, 1258
Myelinolysis, central pontine, 1313
Myeloblasts, in acute myeloid leukemia, 622–623, 623f
Myelodysplasia, 625, 625f
Myelodysplastic syndrome (MDS), 620, 624–626, 625f
Myelofibrosis, primary, 626t, 630–631, 631f
Myelogenous leukemia, chronic, 627–628, 627f, 628f
    clinical features of, 627–628
    genetic basis for, 283, 283f, 305, 305t, 626t
    molecular pathogenesis of, 627, 627f
    morphology of, 627, 627f, 628f
Myeloid blasts, in myelodysplastic syndrome, 625
Myeloid leukemia
    acute, 620, 621–624
        classification of, 622, 622t
        clinical features of, 624
        cytogenetics of, 623–624
        epidemiology of, 622
        genetic basis for, 305, 305t, 624
        immunophenotype of, 623
        morphology of, 622–623, 623f
        pathogenesis of, 621–622
        prognosis for, 624
    chronic, 627–628, 627f, 628f
        clinical features of, 627–628
        genetic basis for, 283, 283f, 305, 305t, 626t

Myeloid leukemia (Continued)
        molecular pathogenesis of, 627, 627f
        morphology of, 627, 627f, 628f
Myeloid neoplasm(s), 596, 620–631
    acute myeloid leukemia as, 620, 621–624, 622t, 623f
    myelodysplastic syndromes as, 620, 624–626, 625f
    myeloproliferative disorders as, 621, 626–631
Myeloid progenitor cells, 590, 591f
Myeloid tissues, 589
Myelolipomas, adrenal, 1159
Myeloma
    multiple (plasma cell), 601t, 609–611, 610f, 611f
        glomerular lesions in, 935
    smouldering, 609, 611
    solitary, 601t, 609, 611
Myeloma kidney, 610, 948, 948f
Myelomeningocele, 1284
Myelopathy, angiodysgenetic necrotizing, 1298
Myeloperoxidase (MPO), in phagocytosis, 53, 53f
Myeloperoxidase (MPO) deficiency, 56t
Myelophthisic anemia, 665
Myelopoiesis, 591f
Myeloproliferative disorder(s), 621, 626–631
    chronic myeloid leukemia as, 627–628, 627f, 628f
    common features of, 626
    essential thrombocytosis as, 626t, 629–630, 630f
    genetic basis for, 284, 626, 626t
    pathogenesis of, 626
    polycythemia vera as, 626t, 628–629, 629f
    primary myelofibrosis as, 626t, 630–631, 631f
MYOC gene, in glaucoma, 1354
Myocardial disease
    due to amyloidosis, 580, 580f
    due to cardiotoxic drugs, 579
    due to catecholamines, 579–580
    due to hyperthyroidism and hypothyroidism, 581
    due to iron overload, 580
Myocardial hypertrophy, 6, 6f, 7, 8f
    in hypertrophic cardiomyopathy, 575–576, 576f
Myocardial infarction (MI), 547–558
    clinical features of, 553–556, 555f
    completed, 549, 549f, 554f
    consequences and complications of, 556–558, 556f, 558f
    due to diabetes mellitus, 1139–1140
    expansion of, 556f, 557
    extension of, 553, 557
    healing of, 553
    incidence and risk factors of, 547
    microscopic features of, 552, 552f
    morphology of, 550–553, 550t, 551f, 552f
    oral contraceptives and, 415
    pathogenesis of, 547–550, 548f, 548t, 549f
    regions of, 549–550, 549f, 550–551, 551f
    reperfusion of, 553, 554f, 555f
    reversible vs. irreversible, 547–548, 548f, 550t, 554f
    right ventricular, 557
    silent, 555
    subendocardial, 550, 551f
    temporal evolution of, 550, 550t
    therapy for, 556
    and thrombosis, 122
    transmural, 547, 550, 551f
    triphenyltetrazolium chloride staining in, 551, 552f

Myocardial irritability, due to myocardial infarction, 557
Myocardial ischemia. *See also* Ischemic heart disease (IHD).
  causes of, 545
  consequences of, 546
  coronary artery occlusion due to, 547
  reversible *vs.* irreversible, 547–548, 548f, 550t, 554f
  temporal progression of, 547–548, 548f, 548t
Myocardial metastases, 584–585
Myocardial necrosis, progression of, 548–549, 549f, 554f
Myocardial response, to coronary artery obstruction, 547–549, 548f, 548t
Myocardial rupture, due to myocardial infarction, 556f, 557
Myocardial stunning, 553, 554f
Myocarditis, 578, 578t, 579f
  and dilated cardiomyopathy, 573
Myocardium, 530–531
  hibernation of, 553
  preconditioning of, 553
  stunned, 553, 554f
Myoclonic epilepsy and ragged red fibers (MERRF), 1327–1328
Myocyte(s), cardiac, 531
Myocyte proteins, in myocardial infarction, 555, 555f
Myocytolysis, in myocardial infarction, 552
Myofiber disarray, in hypertrophic cardiomyopathy, 576, 576f
Myofibroblast(s), in wound contraction, 104–105
Myofibroblastoma, of breast, 1092
Myometrium
  anatomy of, 1024
  leiomyomas of, 264f, 271f, 1026f, 1036–1037, 1037f
  leiomyosarcomas of, 1037–1038, 1038f
Myopathy(ies), 1258, 1258f, 1260–1261
  congenital, 1271, 1272f, 1272t
  drug-induced, 1275
  ethanol, 1275
  with inborn errors of metabolism, 1271–1273
  inflammatory, 215t, 225–226, 1273–1275, 1274f
  ion channel, 1270
  lipid, 1271
  mitochondrial, 1271–1273, 1274f
  myotubular (centronuclear), 1272t
  nemaline, 1272f, 1272t
  statin-induced, 1275
  steroid, 1275
  thyrotoxic, 1275
  toxic, 1275
Myopericarditis, 581
Myophagocytosis, 1261
Myosin, in myocardium, 531
Myositis
  inclusion body, 1273, 1274, 1274f, 1275
  orbital, 1347
  ossificans, 10–11, 1251, 1251f
Myotonia, 1269
Myotonic dystrophy, 168t, 1269–1270
Myotubular myopathy, 1272t
Myxedema, 1111
  pretibial, 1115
Myxedema heart, 581
Myxomas, cardiac, 583–584, 583f
Myxomatous degeneration, of mitral valve, 563–565, 564f

N
N-acetyaspartic acid, in Canavan disease, 1327
N-acetyl-*p*-benzoquinoneimine (NAPQI), in acetaminophen metabolism, 415
NAD (nicotinamide adenine dinucleotide), in alcohol metabolism, 413, 413f
NAFLD (nonalcoholic fatty liver disease), 860–861, 861f
Nail changes, due to psoriasis, 1190
Nail-patella syndrome, 1211t
2-Naphthylamine, and bladder cancer, 979
Narcotics, abuse of, 418–419, 418f
NARP (neuropathy, ataxia, and retinitis pigmentosa), 1328
Nasal disorders, 749–750, 750f, 751
Nasal polyps, 749, 750f
NASH (nonalcoholic steatohepatitis), 860, 861
Nasopharyngeal angiofibroma, 751
Nasopharyngeal carcinoma, 751, 752f
  Epstein-Barr virus in, 315
Nasopharynx
  disorders of, 750–751, 751f, 752f
  inflammations of, 750–751
  tumors of, 751, 752f
Native immunity, 75, 184–185
Natriuretic factors, in blood pressure regulation, 493
Natural immunity, 75, 184–185
Natural killer (NK) cell(s)
  antitumor effect of, 318
  in glomerular injury, 915
  in immune response, 184, 188, 188f
Natural killer (NK)-cell lymphoma, extranodal, 601t, 616
Natural killer (NK)-cell neoplasms, peripheral, 598t, 601t, 614–616, 615f
Natural killer T cells (NK-T cells), 186
Naxos syndrome, 575
NBCCS (nevoid basal cell carcinoma syndrome), 1181, 1182t
NBTE (nonbacterial thrombotic endocarditis), 124, 567f, 568–569, 570f
  due to cancer, 321t, 322
NEC (necrotizing enterocolitis), 458, 459f, 793
Necator duodenale, enterocolitis due to, 806
Neck disorders, 754–756, 755f
Necrosis
  caseous, 16, 16f
    in immune granuloma, 74, 74f
  clinicopathologic examples of, 23–25
  coagulative, 15, 16f
    ischemic, 128
  fat, 16, 17f
  fibrinoid, 16–17, 17f
  gangrenous, 15–16
  inflammation due to, 45
  liquefactive, 15, 16f, 129
  morphologic changes in, 13–14, 13f, 13t, 14f
  overview of, 5, 5f, 11
  patterns of, 15–17, 16f, 17f
Necrotizing arteriolitis, 496
Necrotizing enterocolitis (NEC), 458, 459f, 793
Necrotizing lesions, of nose and upper airways, 750
Necrotizing papillitis, in diabetes mellitus, 1143
NEFAs (nonesterified fatty acids), in insulin resistance, 1136–1137
Negative selection, in immunological tolerance, 209
Negri bodies, 1304, 1304f
Neisseria gonorrhoeae, 334f, 341t, 363–364
Neisseria meningitidis, 363–364
Neisserial infections, 363–364
Nelson syndrome, 1104

Nemaline myopathy, 1272f, 1272t
Neointima, 491–492
Neonatal atelectasis, 679
Neonatal cholestasis, 866, 866f, 866t
Neonatal hemochromatosis, 863
Neonatal hepatitis, 866, 866f
  due to α₁-antitrypsin deficiency, 865, 865f, 866
Neonatal jaundice, 841
Neonatal respiratory distress syndrome, 456–458, 457f
Neoplasia, 259–327. *See also* Tumor(s).
  basic components of, 260
  characteristic(s) of benign *vs.* malignant, 262–270, 271f, 271t
    cancer stem cells and cancer cell lineages as, 267–268
    differentiation and anaplasia as, 262–265, 264f–266f, 271t
    local invasion as, 268–269, 268f, 271t
    metastasis as, 269–270, 269f–271f, 271t
    rate of growth as, 265–267, 266f, 271t
  clinical aspect(s) of, 320–327
  clonality of, 260, 276–277, 278f
  defined, 260
  desmoplastic, 260
  host defense against, 316–320
    antitumor effector mechanisms in, 318–319
    immune surveillance and escape as, 316, 319–320, 319f
    tumor antigens in, 316–318, 317f
  local and hormonal effects of, 320
  malignant (*See* Cancer)
  molecular profiles of, 325–326, 326f
  nomenclature for, 260–262, 261f, 262f, 263t
  scirrhous, 260
  tumor markers for, 326–327, 327t
Neoplasm, defined, 260
Neoplastic polyps, colonic, 819–820, 820f, 821f
Neovascularization, 489
  in carcinogenesis, 297–298
  of disc, 1360
  retinal, 1360–1361, 1363f
Nephrin, 910, 910f
  in focal segmental glomerulosclerosis, 926
  in minimal-change disease, 925
Nephritic syndrome, 907, 908t, 917–920, 919f
Nephritis
  hereditary, 931–932, 932f
  Heymann, 912, 913f
  lupus, 214t, 217–219, 218f, 219f, 934
  Masugi (nephrotoxic), 912
  tubulointerstitial, 938–948, 939t
    due to acute phosphate nephropathy, 947–948
    acute *vs.* chronic, 938
    drug- and toxin-induced, 944–946, 945f, 946f
    due to hypercalcemia and nephrocalcinosis, 947
    due to light-chain cast nephropathy, 948, 948f
    due to pyelonephritis, 939, 941–944, 941f, 943f, 944f
    due to reflux nephropathy, 940, 940f, 942–944, 944f
    secondary, 938
    due to urate nephropathy, 947, 947f
    due to urinary tract infection, 939–941, 940f
Nephrocalcinosis, 947
Nephrocystins, 960
Nephrogenic adenoma, 976
Nephrogenic rests, in Wilms tumor, 480

Nephrolithiasis, 907, 947
  gouty, 907, 947
  hyperuricosuric calcium, 962
Nephronophthisis, 957t, 959–960, 960f
Nephropathy(ies)
  analgesic, 417, 945–946, 946f, 947t
  aristolochic, 946
  diabetic, 934–935, 1141–1143
    epidemiology of, 1145
    morphology of, 934, 1141–1143, 1141f,
      1142f
    pathogenesis of, 934–935
  gouty, 907, 947, 1244
  HIV-associated, 928
  IgA, 918t, 929–931, 931f
  light-chain cast, 610, 948, 948f
  membranous, 918t, 922–923, 924f
  phosphate, acute, 947–948
  polyomavirus, 942, 943f
  reflux, 940, 940f, 942–944, 944f
  sickle cell disease, 954
  urate, 947, 947f
  uremic, 1266
Nephrosclerosis, 495
  accelerated (malignant), 949–951, 950f
  benign, 949, 949f, 950f
  in diabetes mellitus, 1142, 1142f
Nephrotic syndrome, 907, 908t, 921–929
  due to cancer, 321t
  causes of, 922, 923t
  edema due to, 112
  due to focal segmental glomerulosclerosis,
    926–928, 927f
  due to HIV-associated nephropathy, 928
  due to membranoproliferative
    glomerulonephritis, 915, 918t, 928–929,
    928f–930f
  due to membranous nephropathy, 922–923,
    924f
  due to minimal-change disease, 923–926, 925f
  pathophysiology of, 922
Nephrotoxic nephritis, 912
Nerve fiber, 1258
Nerve fiber layer, of retina, 1359f
Nerve regeneration, 1258, 1258f, 1260, 1260t,
  1261f
Nerve syndromes, due to cancer, 321t, 322
Nesidioblastosis, 1146
Nestin, 85
Neural end organs, in skin, 1166
Neural precursor cells, 85
Neural stem cells (NSCs), 85
Neural tube defects, 1284
Neuritic plaques, in Alzheimer disease, 1314,
  1315f
Neuritis
  optic, 1367–1368
    in multiple sclerosis, 1312
  retrobulbar, in multiple sclerosis, 1312
Neuroblastic tumors, 475–479
  characteristic features of, 475
  clinical course and prognostic features of,
    477t, 478–479, 479f
  defined, 475
  epidemiology of, 475
  morphology of, 476–477, 476f, 477f, 477t
  staging of, 477–478
Neuroblastoma, 475–479
  clinical course and prognostic features of,
    477t, 478–479, 479f
  epidemiology of, 475
  genetic basis for, 284f, 306
  morphology of, 476–477, 476f, 477f, 477t
  olfactory, 751

Neuroblastoma (Continued)
  staging of, 477–478
  treatment for, 479
Neuroborreliosis, 1302
Neurocytoma, central, 1336
Neuroendocrine carcinoma, of cervix,
  1021–1022
Neuroendocrine tumors
  gastric, 787–789, 788f, 788t
  of lung, 729–730, 729f
Neurofibrillary tangles, 35, 1281, 1314, 1315f
Neurofibroma, 1341
Neurofibromatosis type 1 (NF1), 1342
  genetic basis for, 294–295, 1182t
  malignant peripheral nerve sheath tumors in,
    1341
  neurofibromas in, 1341
  pheochromocytomas in, 1160t
Neurofibromatosis type 2 (NF2), 1342
  genetic basis for, 295, 1182t
  meningiomas in, 1339
  schwannomas in, 1340
Neurofibromin, 143t, 295, 1341, 1342
Neurofibromin 2, 295
Neurofilaments, 35
Neurogenesis, from neural stem cells, 85
Neurogenic shock, 129
Neurohypophysis, 1098, 1099, 1106
Neurokinin A, in inflammation, 63
Neurolipin 1 (Nrp-1), 88
Neurolipin 2 (Nrp-2), 88
Neurologic causes, of hypertension, 493t
Neurologic disorders. See also Central nervous
  system disorder(s); Peripheral nerve
  disease(s).
  due to adverse drug reactions, 416t
  due to occupational exposures, 409t
  in systemic lupus erythematosus, 214t,
    219–220
Neurologic manifestations, of AIDS, 242–243,
  248
Neurologic sequelae, of metabolic disturbances,
  1329
Neuroma(s)
  in MEN-2B, 1162
  Morton, 1267
  traumatic (pseudo-, amputation), 1266, 1267f
Neuromuscular junction, diseases of, 1275–1276
Neuromyelitis optica, 1312
Neuromyopathic paraneoplastic syndrome, 321t,
  322
Neuron(s), red, 1281
Neuronal ceroid lipofuscinoses, 1326
Neuronal degeneration, 1281
Neuronal heterotopias, 1285
Neuronal inclusions, 1281
Neuronal injury
  acute, 1281
  reactions to, 1281
  subacute and chronic, 1281
Neuronal intracytoplasmic inclusions, 1281
Neuronal nitric oxide synthase (nNOS), 60
Neuronal storage diseases, 1325, 1326
Neuronal trans-synaptic degeneration, 1281
Neuronal tumors, of CNS, 1335–1336
Neuronopathy, 1259
Neuronophagia, 1282, 1302
Neuropathic beriberi, 1266
Neuropathy, ataxia, and retinitis pigmentosa
  (NARP), 1328
Neuropathy(ies), 1261–1267
  acquired metabolic, 1265–1266, 1265f
  compression, 1266–1267
  Dejerine-Sottas, 1264–1265

Neuropathy(ies) (Continued)
  diabetic, 1143, 1145–1146
    peripheral, 1265–1266, 1265f
  hereditary, 1263–1265, 1263t, 1264t, 1265f
  hypertrophic, 1264
  immune-mediated, 1261–1262
  inflammatory, 1261–1262
  optic
    anterior ischemic, 1366, 1366f
    Leber hereditary, 1367
  paraneoplastic, 1266
  peripheral
    acquired metabolic and toxic, 1265–1266,
      1265f
    diabetic, 1265–1266, 1265f
    hereditary, 1263–1265, 1263t, 1264t, 1265f
    immune-mediated, 1261–1262
    infectious poly-, 1262–1263
    inflammatory, 1261–1262
    with inherited metabolic disorders, 1263,
      1264t
    due to lung carcinoma, 729
    with malignancy, 1266
    metabolic and nutritional, 1266
    T cell–mediated hypersensitivity in, 206t
    traumatic, 1266–1267, 1267f
    subacute sensory, in paraneoplastic syndrome,
      1340
    toxic, 1266
    traumatic, 1266–1267, 1267f
Neuropeptide(s), in inflammation, 63
Neuropeptide Y (NPY), in energy balance, 439,
  440, 441f, 442
Neuropil, in neuroblastomas, 476
Neuropil threads, in Alzheimer disease, 1314
Neurosyphilis, 375, 376, 376f, 1301–1302
Neurotoxicity, glucose, 1139, 1140t, 1142
Neurotoxins, 344
Neurotransmission, cocaine effect on, 417–418,
  419f
Neurotrophic factors, receptor for,
  proto-oncogene for, 281t
Neurotrophin receptors, in neuroblastomas,
  479
Neutropenia, 592–593
Neutrophil(s)
  in acute respiratory distress syndrome, 681,
    682f
  adult reference range for, 592t
  differentiation of, 591f
  in glomerular injury, 915
  in inflammation
    acute, 50, 51f
    chronic, 72
  in innate immunity, 184
  in phagocytosis, 53
  in wound healing, 102, 103f
Neutrophilia, in inflammation, 75
Neutrophilic leukocytosis, 594f, 594t
Nevoid basal cell carcinoma syndrome
  (NBCCS), 1181, 1182t
Nevus(i)
  basal cell, 1181, 1182t
  blue, 1170t
  compound, 1169, 1169f
    lentiginous, 1172f
  congenital, 1170t
  conjunctival, 1350, 1350f
  dysplastic, 1170–1171, 1170t, 1171f, 1172f
  flammeus, 522
  halo, 1170t
  junctional, 1169, 1169f
    lentiginous, 1172f
  lentiginous, 1169

Nevus(i) *(Continued)*
 compound, 1172f
 junctional, 1172f
 melanocytic (pigmented), 1169–1170, 1169f, 1170f, 1170t
 of Ota, 1350
 spindle cell and epithelioid cell (Spitz), 1170t
 uveal, 1356–1357
Newborn
 hemolytic disease of, 202, 461, 462f, 840
 physiologic jaundice of, 841
Next-generation sequencing, 174
NF. *See* Neurofibromatosis (NF).
NF1 gene, 287t, 294–295, 1342
NF2 gene, 287t, 295, 1342
NF-κB. *See* Nuclear factor κB (NF-κB).
NGU (nongonococcal urethritis), 380, 981
NHEJ (nonhomologous end joining), 426
NHLs. *See* Non-Hodgkin lymphomas (NHLs).
Niacin
 deficiency of, 438t
 functions of, 438t
Nickel, as carcinogen, 274t
Nicotinamide adenine dinucleotide (NAD), in alcohol metabolism, 413, 413f
Nicotine, in cigarette smoke, 410–411
Nidus, in osteoid osteoma, 1224
Niemann-Pick disease type C (NPC), 35, 153
 cherry-red spot in, 1362
Niemann-Pick disease types A and B, 151t, 152–153, 153f
Night blindness, 432
Nipple(s)
 congenital inversion of, 1067
 Paget disease of, 1080–1081, 1082f
 supernumerary, 1067
Nipple discharge, 1068, 1068f
Nitric oxide (NO)
 cell injury due to, 21
 in inflammation, 57t, 60–61, 61f
 in phagocytosis, 53–54, 53f
Nitric oxide synthase (NOS), 60, 61f
Nitrites
 as carcinogens, 311
 and gastric carcinoma, 443
Nitrogen dioxide, as air pollutant, 404t
Nitrosamides, and gastric carcinoma, 443
Nitrosamines, and gastric carcinoma, 443
Nitrous oxide, lung diseases due to, 697t
NK cells. *See* Natural killer (NK) cells.
NKX2-5, in congenital heart disease, 539, 539t
N-MYC oncogene, 281t, 284, 284f, 306
 in neuroblastomas, 478, 479f
nNOS (neuronal nitric oxide synthase), 60
NO (nitric oxide)
 cell injury due to, 21
 in inflammation, 57t, 60–61, 61f
 in phagocytosis, 53–54, 53f
Nocardia, 362–363, 363f
Nocardia asteroides, 362–363, 363f
Nocardia brasiliensis, 362
NOD-2 gene
 in autoimmunity, 212
 in Crohn disease, 808–809, 810
Nodes of Ranvier, 1258
Nodular fasciitis, 1250–1251, 1250f
Nodular hyperplasia
 hepatic, 875–876, 876f
  regenerative, 876
 prostatic, 994–996, 995f, 996f
Nodule, 1168
Nonalcoholic fatty liver disease (NAFLD), 860–861, 861f

Nonalcoholic steatohepatitis (NASH), 860, 861
Nonbacterial thrombotic endocarditis (NBTE), 124, 567f, 568–569, 570f
 due to cancer, 321t, 322
Noncaseating granulomas, in Crohn disease, 811, 811f
Nonclassic inheritance single-gene disorder(s), 140, 167–173
 Angelman syndrome as, 172–173, 172f
 fragile-X syndrome as, 139, 168t, 169–171, 169f, 170f
 due to genomic imprinting, 171–173, 172f
 due to gonadal mosaicism, 173
 Leber hereditary optic neuropathy as, 171, 171f
 due to mutations in mitochondrial genes, 171, 171f
 Prader-Willi syndrome as, 172–173, 172f
 due to triplet-repeat mutations, 139, 167–171, 168f, 168t
Nondisjunction, 159
Nondividing tissues, 82
Nonesterified fatty acids (NEFAs), in insulin resistance, 1136–1137
Nongonococcal urethritis (NGU), 380, 981
Non-Hodgkin lymphomas (NHLs), 598
 Hodgkin *vs.,* 616–617, 617t
 of orbit, 1348
 staging of, 621t
Nonhomologous end joining (NHEJ), 426
Nonimmune hydrops, 460, 461, 461t
Noninfectious vasculitis, 226
Non-ossifying fibroma, 1230, 1231f
Nonproliferative breast changes, 1071, 1071f, 1074t
Nonreceptor tyrosine kinases, oncogenes for, 281t, 283–286, 283f, 284f, 285f, 286t
Nonseminomatous germ cell tumors (NSGCTs), 992
Non–small cell carcinoma, of lung, 722, 723
Nonspecific interstitial pneumonia (NSIP), 695
Nonsteroidal anti-inflammatory drugs (NSAIDs)
 bleeding disorder due to, 670
 mechanism of action of, 58f, 59–60
 nephropathy associated with, 946
Nonthrombocytopenic purpuras, 666
Nontreponemal antibody tests, 375
Normoblasts, in hemolytic anemia, 642, 642f
Normochromic, normocytic anemia, 640
Norovirus, gastroenteritis due to, 804, 805f
Norwalk-like virus, gastroenteritis due to, 804, 805f
NOS (nitric oxide synthase), 60, 61f
Nose
 disorders of, 749–750, 750f, 751
 inflammations of, 749–750, 750f
 necrotizing lesions of, 750
Nosocomial infections, 342
Notch pathway, in angiogenesis, 100, 101f, 298
NOTCH1, in congenital heart disease, 539t
NOTCH2, in congenital heart disease, 539, 539t
Noxious stimuli, cellular responses to. *See* Cellular response(s), to stress and noxious stimuli.
NPC (Niemann-Pick disease type C), 35, 153
 cherry-red spot in, 1362
NPC1, 147, 153
NPC2, 148, 153
NPH1 gene, 960
NPH2 gene, 960
NPH3 gene, 960
NPHS1 gene, 926
NPY (neuropeptide Y), in energy balance, 439, 440, 441f, 442

NRAS oncogene, 281t, 282
 in melanocytic nevi, 1170
 in melanoma, 1175
Nrp-1 (neurolipin 1), 88
Nrp-2 (neurolipin 2), 88
NSAIDs (nonsteroidal anti-inflammatory drugs)
 bleeding disorder due to, 670
 mechanism of action of, 58f, 59–60
 nephropathy associated with, 946
NSCs (neural stem cells), 85
NSGCTs (nonseminomatous germ cell tumors), 992
NSIP (nonspecific interstitial pneumonia), 695
NTRK1 gene, in papillary thyroid carcinoma, 1120
Nuclear budding abnormalities, in myelodysplastic syndrome, 625
Nuclear changes, in necrosis, 14, 14f
Nuclear factor κB (NF-κB)
 in acute respiratory distress syndrome, 681
 in AIDS, 240
 in hepatocellular carcinoma, 315
 in Hodgkin lymphoma, 620
 in innate immunity, 184
Nuclear inclusions, 332
Nuclear morphology, abnormal, 263–264
Nuclear sclerosis, of lens, 1353
Nuclear-regulator proteins, proto-oncogenes for, 281t
Nucleic acid amplification tests, for infectious agents, 336
Nurse cells, 592
Nutcracker esophagus, 767
Nutmeg liver, 114, 114f, 872, 872f
Nutrition, and wound healing, 106
Nutritional disease(s), 427–444
 anorexia nervosa and bulimia as, 430
 cachexia as, 429, 430f
 dietary insufficiency as, 427–428
 marasmus and kwashiorkor as, 428–429, 429f
 obesity as, 438–443, 440f–442f
 protein-energy malnutrition as, 427, 428–429, 429f, 430f
 trace element deficiencies as, 439t
 vitamin deficiencies as, 430–438, 438t
  of vitamin A, 430–433, 431f, 432f
  of vitamin C, 437–438, 437f
  of vitamin D, 433–436, 434f–437f
Nutritional imbalances, cell injury due to, 12
Nutritional peripheral neuropathies, 1266

O

O ring sign, in enchondromas, 1228
O_3 (ozone)
 as air pollutant, 404–405, 404t
 in greenhouse effect, 401
O_3 (ozone) layer, 404
OA. *See* Osteoarthritis (OA).
Obesity, 438–443
 and breast cancer, 1077
 and cancer, 273, 442f, 443
 central (visceral), 438
  in Cushing syndrome, 1150, 1151f
 criteria for, 438
 defined, 438
 epidemiology of, 438–439
 general consequences of, 442, 442f
 and insulin resistance, 442, 442f, 443, 1136–1137, 1136f
 pathogenesis of, 439–442, 440f, 441f
Obligate intracellular bacteria, 335, 380–381, 381f, 382f
Obligatory asymmetric replication, 82

Obliterative endarteritis, in tuberculous meningoencephalitis, 1301
Obliterative hepatocavopathy, 873
Obstructive lesions, of ureters, 973–974, 973t
Obstructive overinflation, 687
Obstructive uropathy, 960–962, 961f
Obturator palsy, 1266
OC(s) (oral contraceptives)
    adverse effects of, 415
    endometrial changes due to, 1027
Occlusive thrombus, 546f
Occupational asthma, 689
Occupational cancers, 274t
Occupational health risks, 408–410, 409t
Ochronosis, 36, 155–156
Ocular cicatricial pemphigoid, 1348, 1349
Ocular complications, diabetic, 1140f, 1143, 1145
Oculopharyngeal muscular dystrophy, 1270t
Odontogenic cysts, 748–749
Odontogenic keratocyst (OKC), 748
Odontogenic tumors, 748t, 749
Odontoma, 749
OGTT (oral glucose tolerance test), 1131–1132
25-OH-D (25-hydroxycholecalciferol), 433, 434f
OI (osteogenesis imperfecta), 1211–1212, 1211t, 1212t, 1213f
Oil-droplet keratopathy, 1352
Olfactory neuroblastoma, 751
Oligoastrocytoma, 1334
Oligodendrocytes, response to injury of, 1282
Oligodendroglioma, 1333–1334, 1334f
    anaplastic, 1333–1334
Oligodontia, 1211t
Oligohydramnios sequence, 449–450, 449f, 450f
Olivopontocerebellar atrophy, 1321
Ollier disease, 1227, 1228
Omphalocele, 765
Onchocerca volvulus, 395–396, 396f
Onchocerciasis, 395–396, 396f
Onchocercoma, 396
Oncocytic variant, of follicular thyroid carcinoma, 1123
Oncocytoma, renal, 964
Oncofetal antigens, 318, 327t
Oncogenes, 279–286, 281t
    for cell cycle regulators, 281t
    defined, 279
    for growth factor receptors, 280–281, 281t
    for growth factors, 280, 281t
    metastasis, 302
    for nonreceptor tyrosine kinases, 283–286, 283f, 284f, 285f, 286t
    for nuclear-regulatory proteins, 281t
    proto-, 277, 279, 281t
    for signal-transducing proteins, 281–283, 281t, 282f
Oncogenesis, two-hit hypothesis of, 287, 288f
Oncogenic DNA viruses, 313–315, 313f, 314f
Oncogenic RNA viruses, 312–313
Oncogenic viruses, tumor antigens produced by, 317–318
Oncology, 260
Oncomirs, 308
Oncoproteins, 279
    white cell neoplasia due to, 597, 597f
Onion bulbs, 1259, 1259f
Onion-skinning, in malignant hypertension, 950f, 951
ONOO- (peroxynitrite)
    cell injury due to, 20t, 21
    in phagocytosis, 53–54, 53f
Onycholysis, 1168
Onychomycosis, 383, 1202

OPG (osteoprotegerin), in bone homeostasis, 1208, 1208f
Ophthalmia, sympathetic, 1356, 1356f
Ophthalmopathy
    Graves, 1109, 1109f, 1114–1115
    thyroid, 1347, 1347f
Ophthalmoplegia
    exophthalmic, 1275
    plus, 1328
Opioid narcotics, abuse of, 418–419, 418t
OPN (osteopontin)
    in extracellular matrix, 96
    in fibrosis, 108
Opportunistic infections, in AIDS, 245t, 246
Opsonin(s), in inflammation, 51–53
Opsonin receptors, in inflammation, 51–53
Opsonization
    in antibody-mediated hypersensitivity, 202–203, 202f
    in inflammation, 51–53
Optic nerve, 1346f, 1365–1368
    anterior ischemic optic neuropathy of, 1366, 1366f
    glaucomatous damage to, 1366–1367, 1367f
    Leber hereditary neuropathy of, 1367
    neuritis of, 1367–1368
    papilledema of, 1366, 1366f
Optic neuritis, 1367–1368
    in multiple sclerosis, 1312
Optic neuropathy
    anterior ischemic, 1366, 1366f
    Leber hereditary, 1367
Oral candidiasis, 743
Oral cavity disorder(s), 740–749
    due to infection(s), 742–743
        deep fungal, 743
        with herpes simplex virus, 742–743
        oral candidiasis as, 743
    inflammatory/reactive tumor-like lesions as, 741–742
        aphthous ulcers as, 742, 742f
        fibrous proliferative, 741–742, 741f
        glossitis as, 742
    odontogenic cysts and tumors as, 748–749, 748t
    due to systemic disease, 743, 744t
        hairy leukoplakia as, 743
    of teeth and supporting structures, 740–741
        caries as, 740
        gingivitis as, 740–741
        periodontitis as, 741
    tumors and precancerous lesions as, 746–749
        leukoplakia and erythroplakia as, 744–745, 745f–747f
        squamous cell carcinoma as, 745–748, 747f
Oral contraceptives (OCs)
    adverse effects of, 415
    endometrial changes due to, 1027
Oral glucose tolerance test (OGTT), 1131–1132
Oral ulcers, in systemic lupus erythematosus, 214t
Orbicularis oculi muscle, 1348f
Orbit, 1346–1348
    cellulitis of, 1347
    functional anatomy and proptosis of, 1346–1347
    idiopathic inflammation of, 1347, 1347f
    mucormycosis of, 1347
    neoplasms of, 1348
    thyroid ophthalmopathy of, 1347, 1347f
    Wegener granulomatosis of, 1347
Orbital cellulitis, 1347
Orbital inflammation, idiopathic, 1347, 1347f
Orbital inflammatory pseudotumor, 1347, 1347f

Orbital myositis, 1347
Orchitis, 986–987
    mumps, 350
Orexigenic effect, 441
Orexin(s), 441f
Organ dysfunction, in septic shock, 131–132
Organ regeneration, mechanisms of, 92–94, 93f
Organ system failure, due to burn injury, 421
Organ transplantation, hepatic complications of, 874, 874f
Organ tropism, for metastasis, 300–301
Organic dusts, lung diseases due to, 697t
Organic solvents, occupational exposure to, 409
Organization
    of fibrinous exudate, 68
    of thrombi, 124–125, 125f
Organochlorines, occupational exposure to, 409
Organogenesis, 452, 453f
Organs of Zuckerkandl, 1159
Ormond disease, 828–829, 973–974
Orofacial defects, prevalence of, 451t
Orthopnea, in left-sided heart failure, 535
Osler-Weber-Rendu disease, 522
Osmoreceptors, 1099
Osseous changes, due to cancer, 321t, 322
Osseous metaplasia, of retinal pigment epithelium, 1368
Ossification
    enchondral, 1209, 1209f
    primary center of, 1209
    secondary center of, 1209
Osteitis
    deformans, 1216–1218, 1216f, 1217f
    dissecting, 1218, 1218f
    fibrosa cystica, 1218
        in hyperparathyroidism, 1128
Osteoarthritis (OA), 1235–1236
    clinical course of, 1236, 1237f
    idiopathic or primary, 1235
    morphology of, 1236, 1236f
    obesity and, 442
    due to Paget disease, 1217
    pathogenesis of, 1236
    secondary, 1235
Osteoarthropathy, hypertrophic
    due to cancer, 321t, 322
    pulmonary, 729
Osteoblast(s), 1206, 1207f
Osteoblastoma, 1224
Osteocalcin, 1209
Osteochondritis, syphilitic, 376
Osteochondroma, 1227, 1227f
Osteoclast(s), 1207–1208, 1207f
    dysfunction of, 1216–1218
Osteoclastoma, 1233–1234, 1233f
Osteocytes, 1206–1207, 1207f
Osteodystrophy, renal, 1129, 1218–1219
Osteogenesis imperfecta (OI), 1211–1212, 1211t, 1212t, 1213f
Osteogenic tumor(s), 1223t, 1224–1227
    osteoid osteoma and osteoblastoma as, 1224, 1224f, 1225f
    osteoma as, 1224
    osteosarcoma as, 1225–1227, 1225f, 1226f
Osteoid, in bone, 1206
Osteoid osteoma, 1224, 1224f, 1225f
Osteolytic metastases, 1126
Osteoma, 1224
    osteoid, 1224, 1224f, 1225f
Osteomalacia, 433, 435–436, 1218
Osteomyelitis, 1221–1223
    pyogenic, 1221–1222, 1222f
    sclerosing, of Garré, 1222
    tuberculous, 1222–1223

Osteonecrosis, 1220–1221, 1221f, 1221t
Osteonectin, in extracellular matrix, 96
Osteopetrosis, 1212–1214, 1214f, 1215f
Osteopontin (OPN)
    in extracellular matrix, 96
    in fibrosis, 108
Osteoporosis, 1214–1216
    categories of, 1214, 1214t
    clinical course of, 1216
    disuse, 1214
    morphology of, 1215, 1215f
    pathogenesis of, 1214–1215, 1215f
    postmenopausal, 1215
    primary, 1214t
    secondary, 1214t
    senile, 1215
Osteoporosis-pseudoglioma syndrome, 1210,
    1211t
Osteoprogenitor cells, 1206, 1207f
Osteoprotegerin (OPG), in bone homeostasis,
    1208, 1208f
Osteosarcoma, 1225–1227, 1225f, 1226f
    chondroblastic, 1226, 1230
Osteosclerosis, in primary myelofibrosis, 630
Otitis media, 754
Otosclerosis, 754
Outdoor air pollution, 404–405, 404t
Outer nuclear layer, of retina, 1359f
Outer plexiform layer, of retina, 1359f
Oval cells, 85
Ovarian carcinoma
    categories of, 1042
    chorio-, 1049
    clear cell, 1046
    clinical course, detection, and prevention of,
        1047
    endometrioid, 1045–1046
    mucinous, 1044–1045
    serous, 1042–1044, 1043f
    transitional cell, 1046
Ovarian pregnancy, 1053
Ovarian tumor(s), 1040–1052
    Brenner, 1046, 1046f
    choriocarcinoma as, 1049
    classification of, 1040–1041, 1040t
    clear cell adenocarcinoma as, 1046
    cystadenofibroma as, 1046
    derivation of, 1041f
    dysgerminoma as, 1048–1049, 1049f
    endodermal sinus (yolk sac), 1049, 1049f
    endometrioid, 1045–1046
    epidemiology of, 1040
    fibromas, thecomas, and fibrothecomas as,
        1051, 1051f
    frequency of, 1041t
    germ cell, 1040t, 1041f, 1047–1050,
        1047t
    granulosa–theca cell, 1050, 1050f
    metastatic, 1040t, 1041f, 1052
    mucinous, 1044–1045, 1045f
    serous, 1042–1044, 1043f
    Sertoli–Leydig cell (androblastomas),
        1051–1052, 1051f
    sex cord–stromal, 1040t, 1041f,
        1050–1052
    of surface (müllerian) epithelium, 1040t,
        1041–1047, 1041f
    teratomas as, 1047–1048, 1048f
Ovaries, 1039–1052
    anatomy of, 1007
    cortical inclusion cysts of, 1042, 1042f
    development of, 1006, 1007f
    follicle and luteal cysts of, 1039
    polycystic, 1039–1040, 1039f
    in pregnancy, 1052

Ovaries (Continued)
    streak, 166
    stromal hyperthecosis of, 1039f, 1040
Overexpressed cellular proteins, as tumor
    antigens, 317
Overinflation, obstructive, 687
Ovotestes, 167
Oxidant drugs, G6PD deficiency due to, 645,
    645f
Oxidant-antioxidant imbalance, in emphysema,
    685f, 686
Oxidative phosphorylation disease, 1271–1273,
    1274f
Oxidative stress, cell injury due to, 18f, 20–22,
    20t, 21f
Oxygen deprivation, cell injury due to, 11
Oxygen effects, of ionizing radiation, 424
Oxygen intermediates, in phagocytosis, 53, 53f
Oxygen toxicity, in neonatal respiratory distress
    syndrome, 457–458
Oxygen transport, defect in, 143t
Oxygen-derived free radicals, accumulation of,
    cell injury due to, 18f, 20–22, 20t, 21f
Oxyphil adenoma, 1119, 1119f, 1127
Oxyphil cells, of parathyroid glands, 1126
Oxytocin, 1099
Oxyuriasis vermicularis, 827
Ozone (O_3)
    as air pollutant, 404–405, 404t
    in greenhouse effect, 401
Ozone (O_3) layer, 404

P

p14 gene, 287t, 294
p14/ARF gene, in melanoma, 1174
P16 tumor suppressor gene, 287t
p16/CDKN2A gene, in pancreatic carcinoma,
    900, 901f
p16/INK4a gene, in melanoma, 1174, 1175
p53 tumor suppressor gene, 287t, 290–292, 291f
    in apoptosis, 30, 32, 296
    in breast cancer, 1078, 1078t
    in cancer, 290–292, 291f
    in colorectal cancer, 308f, 309, 823f, 824
    in cutaneous squamous cell carcinoma, 1180
    functions of, 286t
    in hepatocellular carcinoma, 311
    in lung carcinoma, 726, 727
    in nevoid basal cell carcinoma syndrome, 1181
    in osteosarcoma, 1225
    in pancreatic carcinoma, 900–901, 901f
    as tumor marker, 327
p57/KIP2 gene, in hydatidiform mole, 1059,
    1059f
p63, 292
p73, 292
PA(s) (plasminogen activators), in fibrinolysis,
    120, 121f
Pachyonychia congenita type 2, 1176
PAF. See Platelet-activating factor (PAF).
Paget disease
    of bone, 1216–1218, 1216f, 1217f
    of nipple, 1080–1081, 1082f
    of vulva, 1015, 1015f
Paget, James, 1216
Pagetoid spread, of urothelial carcinoma in situ,
    978
PAH (phenylalanine hydroxylase), defect in,
    143t, 463–464, 463f
Pain, in inflammation, 66t
Pain crises, in sickle cell disease, 647–648
Paired box-6 (PAX-6) gene, in Wilms syndrome,
    480
Paired box-8 (PAX-8) gene, 1110
    in follicular thyroid carcinoma, 1120–1121

Palmar erythema, due to liver failure, 836
Palmar fibromatoses, 1251
Palpebral commissure, 1348f
Palpebral conjunctiva, 1348f, 1349
Palsy
    cerebral, 1286
    obturator, 1266
    progressive supranuclear, 1318
    Saturday night, 1267
PAN (polyarteritis nodosa), 204t, 226, 514–515,
    514f
    cerebral infarction due to, 1293
Pancarditis, due to rheumatic fever, 566
Pancoast tumors, 729
Pancolitis, 811, 812f
Pancreas, 891–903
    agenesis of, 892
    anatomy and function of, 891–892, 892f
    annular, 893
    congenital anomalies of, 892–893
    development of, 891
    diabetes mellitus of, 1131–1146
        classification of, 1132, 1132t
        clinical features of, 1143–1146, 1144f, 1145t
        complications of, 1138–1139, 1140f
        diagnosis of, 1131–1132
        epidemiology of, 1131
        glucose homeostasis and, 1132–1134, 1133f,
            1134f
        monogenic forms of, 1137–1138
        morphology of, 1139–1143, 1141f, 1142f
        pathogenesis of, 1134–1137, 1135f, 1136f
    divisum, 892, 892f
    ectopic, 893
    endocrine, 1130, 1131f
    exocrine, 891–892, 892f
    in hemochromatosis, 862
    in MEN-1, 1162
    non-neoplastic cysts of, 898
        congenital, 898
        pseudo-, 898, 898f
    regeneration of, 92
Pancreatic abnormalities, in cystic fibrosis,
    468–469, 469f, 470, 470t
Pancreatic carcinoma, 900–903
    acinar cell, 903
    clinical features of, 903
    epidemiology, etiology, and pathogenesis of,
        901–902, 902t
    inherited predisposition to, 902, 902t
    molecular carcinogenesis of, 900–901, 901t
    morphology of, 902–903, 902f
    precursors to, 900, 901f
Pancreatic cysts, 898
    congenital, 898
    pseudo-, 898, 898f
Pancreatic duct
    accessory, 891, 892f
    main, 891, 892f
Pancreatic duct obstruction, 893, 894–895, 895f,
    896
Pancreatic endocrine neoplasm(s), 1146–1147
    α-cell tumors (glucagonomas) as, 1147
    carcinoid tumors as, 1147
    δ-cell tumors (somatostatinomas) as, 1147
    hyperinsulinism (insulinoma) as, 1146–1147,
        1147f
    pancreatic polypeptide–secreting, 1147
    VIPoma as, 1147
    Zollinger-Ellison syndrome (gastrinomas) as,
        1147
Pancreatic enzymes, 892
    in pancreatitis, 894–895, 895f
Pancreatic fibrosis, due to hemochromatosis, 862
Pancreatic insufficiency, in cystic fibrosis, 470

Pancreatic intraepithelial neoplasias (PanINs), 900, 901f
Pancreatic neoplasm(s)
  endocrine, 1146–1147
    α-cell tumors (glucagonomas) as, 1147
    carcinoid tumors as, 1147
    δ-cell tumors (somatostatinomas) as, 1147
    hyperinsulinism (insulinoma) as, 1146–1147, 1147f
    pancreatic polypeptide–secreting, 1147
    VIPoma as, 1147
    Zollinger-Ellison syndrome (gastrinomas) as, 1147
  exocrine, 898–903
    carcinoma as (See Pancreatic carcinoma)
    cystic, 899–900, 899f, 900f
    pancreatoblastoma as, 903
Pancreatic polypeptide (PP) cells, 1130
Pancreatic polypeptide (PP)-secreting tumors, 1147
Pancreatic pseudocysts, 898, 898f
Pancreatic tissue, ectopic, 765
Pancreatitis, 893–898
  acute, 893–896
    causes of, 893, 893t
    clinical features of, 895–896
    defined, 893
    epidemiology of, 893
    morphology of, 894, 894f
    necrotizing, 894, 894f
    pathogenesis of, 894–895, 895f
  alcoholic, 414, 895, 896, 897f
  autoimmune, 897
  chronic, 896–898
    causes of, 896
    clinical features of, 897–898
    in cystic fibrosis, 470
    defined, 896
    epidemiology of, 896
    malabsorption and diarrhea in, 794t
    morphology of, 896–897, 897f
    pathogenesis of, 896, 897f
  defined, 893
  hemorrhagic, 894
  hereditary, 893–894, 896
  idiopathic, 893
  lymphoplasmacytic sclerosing, 897
  tropical, 896
Pancreatoblastoma, 903
Pancytopenia, oral manifestations of, 744t
Panencephalitis, subacute sclerosing, 1306
Paneth cell granules, in Crohn disease, 809
Paneth cell metaplasia, in Crohn disease, 810
Panfascicular atrophy, 1267, 1267f
PanINs (pancreatic intraepithelial neoplasias), 900, 901f
Panniculitis, 1199
Pannus
  in Fuchs endothelial dystrophy, 1353
  in rheumatoid arthritis, 1237, 1238f
Panophthalmitis, 1355, 1356f
Pantothenic acid, function of, 438t
Panuveitis, 1356
PAP (pulmonary alveolar proteinosis), 705–706, 705f
Papanicolaou (Pap) smears, 323f, 324, 1017, 1018, 1023–1024, 1023f
Papilla of Vater, 891, 892f
Papillary carcinoma
  of breast
    in situ, 1080, 1082f
    invasive, 1088
  of kidney, 964, 964f, 965, 966, 966f
  of thyroid, 1120, 1121–1122, 1121f

Papillary craniopharyngioma, 1106, 1107
Papillary cystadenoma(s), 260–261
  lymphomatosum, 759, 759f
Papillary fibroelastoma, cardiac, 584
Papillary hidradenoma, of vulva, 1015, 1015f
Papillary microcarcinoma, of thyroid, 1122
Papillary muscle dysfunction, due to myocardial infarction, 556f, 557
Papillary necrosis
  in acute pyelonephritis, 941, 941f
  due to analgesic nephropathy, 945, 946f
  causes of, 946, 947t
  in diabetes mellitus, 1143
Papillary serous cystadenocarcinoma, of ovary, 1043f
Papillary transitional cell carcinoma, of ureters, 973f
Papillary urothelial neoplasms of low malignant potential (PUNLMPs), 977–978
Papilledema, 1366, 1366f
Papillitis, necrotizing, in diabetes mellitus, 1143
Papilloma(s), 260
  of bladder, 976, 977, 977f
  of breast, 1072, 1073f
  choroid plexus, 1335
  sinonasal (Schneiderian), 751, 751f
  squamous, 1176
    of esophagus, 774
    of vulva, 1012
Papillomatosis, 1168
Papillomatous epidermal hyperplasia, 1200–1201, 1200f, 1201f
Papule, 1168
Papulosis, bowenoid, 984, 1201
PAR(s) (protease-activated receptors), 120, 121f
  in inflammation, 64–65
Paracentric inversion, 160–161, 160f
Paracortical hyperplasia, 595–596
Paracrine signaling, 89, 90f
Paradoxical embolism, 126, 540, 547
Parafollicular cells, 1107–1108
Paraganglioma, 755–756, 755f
  extra-adrenal, 1160t
  familial, 1160t
Paraganglion system, 1159
Parakeratosis, 1168, 1178
Paramyxovirus, structure of, 333f
Paraneoplastic neuropathy, 1266
Paraneoplastic syndromes, 321–322, 321t
  with lung carcinoma, 728–729
  neurologic effects of, 1339–1340
Parasitic enterocolitis, 794t, 805—807, 805f
Parasitic infection(s), 386–396
  African trypanosomiasis as, 390, 390f
  babesiosis as, 388, 388f
  Chagas disease as, 391
  cysticercosis and hydatid disease as, 392–393, 392f
  leishmaniasis as, 388–390, 389f
  of liver, 854
  lymphatic filariasis as, 395, 395f
  malaria as, 386–388, 387f, 388f
  metazoal, 391–396, 392f–396f
  onchocerciasis as, 395–396, 396f
  protozoal, 386–391, 386t, 387f–390f
  schistosomiasis as, 393–395, 394f
  strongyloidiasis as, 391–392, 392f
  trichinosis as, 393, 393f
Paratesticular tumors, 987
Parathyroid adenoma, 1127, 1127f, 1128f
Parathyroid carcinomas, 1128
Parathyroid disorder(s)

hyperparathyroidism as, 1126–1129
  primary, 1126–1129, 1127f, 1128f, 1129t
  secondary, 1129
hypoparathyroidism as, 1129–1130
  pseudo-, 1130
in MEN-1, 1162
Parathyroid glands, 1126–1130
  anatomy of, 1126
  congenital absence of, 1130
Parathyroid hormone (PTH), 1126
  and hypercalcemia, 1128–1129, 1129t
Parathyroid hormone–related protein (PTHrP), 1126
  in hypercalcemia of malignancy, 322
  and hyperparathyroidism, 1128–1129
Parathyroid hyperplasia, 1127–1128
  in MEN-2A, 1162
Paratubal cysts, 1038
Parenchymal injuries, of central nervous system, 1287–1288, 1288f
Parent-of-origin effects, 172
Paresis, general, due to syphilis, 375
Paretic neurosyphilis, 1301–1302
Parkin, 1320
Parking lot inclusions, 1272, 1273f
Parkinson disease (PD), 1319–1321, 1320f
Parkinsonism, 1319
  frontotemporal dementia with, 1317–1318
Paronychia, 359, 383
Parotid gland, mixed tumor of, 261f
Parotitis, mumps, 350
Paroxysmal cold hemoglobinuria, 654
Paroxysmal nocturnal dyspnea, in left-sided heart failure, 535
Paroxysmal nocturnal hemoglobinuria (PNH), 235, 652–653, 653f
Partial thromboplastin time (PTT), 120, 666
Particulates
  as air pollutants, 404t, 405
  occupational exposure to, 409
Parvovirus B19
  perinatal infection with, 459, 459f, 461
  red cell aplasia due to, 665
Passive congestion, of liver, 872
Passive smoke inhalation, 410, 411–412
Patau syndrome, 162, 163f
Patch, 1168
Patched (PTCH) tumor suppressor genes, 295
  in nevoid basal cell carcinoma syndrome, 1181, 1183f
Patent ductus arteriosus (PDA), 540f, 541–542
  coarctation of the aorta with, 544, 544f
Patent foramen ovale, 541
Paternal imprinting, 171, 1059
Paterson-Brown-Kelly syndrome, 767
Paterson-Kelly syndrome, 742
Pathogen-associated molecular patterns, in innate immunity, 184
Pathogenesis, 4
Pathogenicity islands, 343
Pathology
  defined, 4
  etiology or cause in, 4
  functional derangements and clinical manifestations in, 4
  general, 4
  introduction to, 4–5
  molecular or morphologic changes in, 4
  pathogenesis in, 4
  systemic, 4
Pattern recognition receptors, in innate immunity, 184

Pauci-immune injury, in microscopic polyangiitis, 515
Pauci-immune rapidly progressive glomerulonephritis, 920–921, 920t
Pautrier microabscesses, 1185
Pawn ball megakaryocytes, in myelodysplastic syndrome, 625
PAX-6 (paired box-6) gene, in Wilms syndrome, 480
PAX-8 (paired box-8) gene, 1110
  in follicular thyroid carcinoma, 1120–1121
PBC (primary biliary cirrhosis), 867–869, 867t, 868f
PBDEs (polybrominated diphenyl ethers), occupational exposure to, 409
PBGFB gene, 281t
PCA3, in prostate cancer, 997
PCBs (polychlorinated biphenyls), occupational exposure to, 409–410
PCOD (polycystic ovarian disease), 1039–1040, 1039f
PCP (phencyclidine), abuse of, 418t
PCR. *See* Polymerase chain reaction (PCR).
PCV (polycythemia vera), 626t, 628–629, 629f, 665
PD (Parkinson disease), 1319–1321, 1320f
PD-1, in anergy, 209–210
PDA (patent ductus arteriosus), 540f, 541–542
  coarctation of the aorta with, 544, 544f
PDGF. *See* Platelet-derived growth factor (PDGF).
PDGFRB gene, 281t
PDX1, in diabetes, 1137
PE (pulmonary embolism), 126, 126f, 706–707, 706f
  septic, 717
Peak bone mass, 1209
Peau d'orange, 520, 1083
Pedicels, 910, 910f
Pedunculated adenomas, colorectal, 819, 820f
Pedunculated lipomas, of esophagus, 774
Pedunculated polyps, colonic, 815
Peliosis hepatis, 872
Pelizaeus-Merzbacher disease, 1327
Pelvic inflammatory disease (PID), 1009–1010, 1010f
Pelvic pain syndrome, chronic, 975
PEM (protein-energy malnutrition), 427, 428–429, 429f, 430f
Pemphigoid
  bullous, 1193f, 1195–1196, 1196f
  cicatricial, ocular, 1348, 1349
Pemphigus, 1192–1195
  erythematosus, 1193
  foliaceus, 1193, 1193f–1195f, 1194
  morphology of, 1193–1194, 1194f
  oral manifestations of, 744t
  paraneoplastic, 1193, 1194–1195
  pathogenesis of, 1194–1195, 1195f
  vegetans, 1193
  vulgaris, 203t, 1192–1193, 1193f–1195f, 1194
Pendred syndrome, 1110
Penetrating injury, 420
Penile fibromatoses, 1251
Penis, 982–984
  Bowen disease of, 983, 984f
  bowenoid papulosis of, 983
  carcinoma of
    in situ, 983, 984f
    invasive, 984, 984f
  congenital anomalies of, 982
  inflammation of, 982
  tumors of, 982–984, 983f, 984f

Peptic ulcer(s), 68, 69f
  due to Meckel diverticulum, 766
  due to Zollinger-Ellison syndrome, 1147
Peptic ulcer disease (PUD), 780–781, 781f
Peptide display system, of adaptive immunity, 190–192, 191f, 192f
Peptide YY (PYY), in energy balance, 439, 441f, 442
Peptostreptococcus spp, 378
Percutaneous transluminal coronary angioplasty, pathology of, 526, 526f
Perforating injury, 420
Perforins
  in apoptosis, 31
  in cell-mediated cytotoxicity, 208
Periampullary carcinoma, of liver, 880
Periapical cyst, 749
Periapical granuloma, 749
Periaxin (PRX), 1265f
Pericardial disease, 581–583
  hemopericardium as, 581
  pericardial effusion as, 581
  pericarditis as, 581–583, 581t, 582f
  due to rheumatologic diseases, 583
Pericardial effusion, 581
Pericardial space, in right-sided heart failure, 536
Pericarditis, 581–583, 582f
  acute, 581–582, 582f
  adhesive, 582
  caseous, 582
  causes of, 581, 581t
  chronic or healed, 582–583
  constrictive, 582–583
  fibrinous, 68f, 556f, 581–582, 583
  hemorrhagic, 582
  mediastino-, 582
  myo-, 582
  due to myocardial infarction, 556f, 557
  purulent or suppurative, 582, 582f
  serofibrinous, 581–582
  serous, 581
  in systemic lupus erythematosus, 214t, 220
Pericentric inversion, 160f, 161
Periductal mastitis, 1069, 1069f
Perihilar tumors, of liver, 880
Perinatal brain injury, 1286–1287, 1286f
Perinatal infection(s), 458–459, 459f
  with cytomegalovirus, 354
Perinephric abscess, 941
Perineural invasion, in prostate cancer, 998, 999f
Perineurium, 1258
Periodontal ligament, 740, 740f
Periodontitis, 741
Periorbital edema, 113
Periostitis, syphilitic, 376
Peripartum cardiomyopathy, 573–574
Peripheral B-cell neoplasms, 598t, 601t, 603–614
Peripheral giant cell granuloma, of oral cavity, 742
Peripheral myelin protein 22 (PMP22), 1263, 1265f
Peripheral nerve, anatomy of, 1258
Peripheral nerve disease(s), 1261–1267
  acquired metabolic and toxic neuropathies as, 1265–1266, 1265f
  due to cancer, 321t
  hereditary neuropathies as, 1263–1265, 1263t, 1264t, 1265f
  immune-mediated neuropathies as, 1261–1262
  infectious polyneuropathies as, 1262–1263
  inflammatory neuropathies as, 1261–1262

Peripheral nerve disease(s) *(Continued)*
  neoplastic, 1267
  traumatic neuropathies as, 1266–1267, 1267f
Peripheral nerve sheath tumors, 1340–1342, 1340f
Peripheral neuropathy(ies)
  acquired metabolic and toxic, 1265–1266, 1265f
  diabetic, 1265–1266, 1265f
  hereditary, 1263–1265, 1263t, 1264t, 1265f
  immune-mediated, 1261–1262
  infectious poly-, 1262–1263
  inflammatory, 1261–1262
  with inherited metabolic disorders, 1263, 1264t
  due to lung carcinoma, 729
  with malignancy, 1266
  metabolic and nutritional, 1266
  T cell–mediated hypersensitivity in, 206t
  traumatic, 1266–1267, 1267f
Peripheral NK-cell neoplasms, 598t, 601t, 614–616, 615f
Peripheral ossifying fibroma, of oral cavity, 742
Peripheral T-cell lymphoma, unspecified, 601t, 614–616, 615f
Peripheral T-cell neoplasms, 598t, 601t, 614–616, 615f
Peripheral tolerance, 209–211, 210f
Peripheral vascular resistance, and blood pressure, 492, 494f
Peritoneal cysts, 829
Peritoneal infection, 828
Peritoneal mesotheliomas, 734
Peritoneal space, in right-sided heart failure, 536
Peritoneum, 828–829
  cysts of, 829
  infection of, 828
  inflammatory disease of, 828–829
  sclerosing retroperitonitis of, 828–829
  tumors of, 829
Peritonitis, 828–829
  bacterial, 828
    spontaneous, 828
  sterile, 828
Perivascular amyloidosis, 666
Perivascular pseudorosettes, in ependymomas, 1334
Perivenous encephalomyelitis, 1312–1313
Periventricular leukomalacia, 1286
Permanent tissues, 82
Pernicious anemia, 655–658, 655t, 656f, 657f
  antibody-mediated hypersensitivity in, 203t
  and autoimmune gastritis, 778, 779
Peroneal muscular atrophy, 1263
Peroxisome proliferator-activated receptor(s) (PPARs), 432
Peroxisome proliferator-activated receptor γ (PPARγ), in insulin resistance, 1137
Peroxynitrite (ONOO⁻)
  cell injury due to, 20t, 21
  in phagocytosis, 53–54, 53f
Persistent hyperplastic primary vitreous, 1357
Persistent truncus arteriosus (PTA), 543
PET (positron emission tomography), of tumors, 303–304
Petechiae, 114, 115f
  in sudden infant death syndrome, 472
Peutz-Jeghers syndrome, 816t, 817–818, 818f
Peyronie's disease, 981, 1251
PFIC (progressive familial intrahepatic cholestasis), 843
PH (pulmonary hypertension), 707–709, 708f, 709f

Phacolysis, 1353
Phagocyte oxidase, 53, 53f
    defects in, 55
Phagocytosis
    in antibody-mediated hypersensitivity,
        202–203, 202f
    in apoptosis, 13f, 26, 30
    complement system in, 64, 64f
    discovery of, 44
    frustrated, 55
    in inflammation, 52–54, 53f
    spleen in, 632
Phagolysosome, 53, 53f
Phagolysosome function, inherited defects in,
    55
Phagosome, 53, 53f
Pharmacogenetics, 144
Pharyngitis, 750–751
    streptococcal, 359, 360
        rheumatic fever due to, 566
Pharyngoesophageal diverticulum, 767
Phencyclidine (PCP), abuse of, 418t
Phenotypic sex, 167
Phenylalanine hydroxylase (PAH), defect in,
    143t, 463–464, 463f
Phenylalanine metabolism, abnormalities of,
    463–464, 463f
Phenylketonuria (PKU), 463–464, 463f
Phenytoin (Dilantin) ingestion, oral
    manifestations of, 744t
Pheochromocytoma(s), 1159–1161
    bilateral, 1159
    clinical course of, 1161
    defined, 1159
    extra-adrenal, 1159
    in familial syndromes, 1159, 1160t
    and hypertension, 1159, 1161
    malignant, 1159
    in MEN-2, 1162
    morphology of, 1159–1161, 1160f, 1161f
    myocardial disease due to, 579
    rule of 10s for, 1159
Philadelphia chromosome, 305, 603
Phimosis, 982
Phlebothrombosis, 124, 125, 519
Phosphate nephropathy, acute, 947–948
Phosphatidyl inositol-3 kinase (PI3K) pathway,
    90, 91f
Phosphatidylinositol glycan complementation
    group A gene (PIGA), 652
Phosphatonins, 435
Phospholipase Cγ (PLCγ), in signal transduction
    pathway, 90, 91f
Phospholipid breakdown, increased, cell injury
    due to, 22
Phospholipid synthesis, decreased, cell injury
    due to, 22
Phosphoribosyl pyrophosphate (PRPP), in gout,
    1244f
Phosphorus homeostasis, vitamin D in, 433–435,
    435f, 436f
Photosensitivity, in systemic lupus
    erythematosus, 214t, 219
Phrygian cap, of gallbladder, 882, 882f
Phthalates, occupational exposure to, 410
Phthisis bulbi, 1368
Phycomycosis, 385–386, 386f
Phyllodes tumor, of breast, 1092, 1092f
Physical agents
    injury by, 420–427
        cell, 11
        electrical, 422
        inflammation due to, 45
        mechanical, 420–421, 420f

Physical agents, injury by (Continued)
        radiation, 422–426, 422f, 423f, 424t, 425f
        thermal, 421–422
    toxicity of, 402–403, 402f, 403f
Physiologic jaundice of the newborn, 841
Physis, 1209, 1209f
PI3K (phosphatidyl inositol-3 kinase) pathway,
    90, 91f
PI3K/AKT signaling pathway, 294
    in follicular thyroid carcinoma, 1120
    in melanoma, 1174, 1174f
Pick bodies, 1318, 1318f
Pick cells, 1318
Pick disease, 1318, 1318f
Pickwickian syndrome, 442
PID (pelvic inflammatory disease), 1009–1010,
    1010f
PIF (proteolysis-inducing factor), 429, 430f
PIGA (phosphatidylinositol glycan
    complementation group A gene), 652
Pigeon breast deformity, 436
Pigeon breeder's lung, 703
Pigment(s), intracellular accumulation of,
    36–38, 37f
    endogenous, 36–37, 37f
    exogenous, 36
Pigment stones, 882, 883–884, 883t, 884f
Pigmentation disorders, 1168–1175
    dysplastic nevi as, 1170–1171, 1170t, 1171f,
        1172f
    freckles (ephelis) as, 1168
    lentigo as, 1168–1169
    melanocytic (pigmented) nevus (mole) as,
        1169–1170, 1169f, 1170f, 1170t
    melanoma as, 1171–1175
        clinical features of, 1172, 1173f
        morphology of, 1172–1173, 1173f
        pathogenesis of, 1174–1175, 1174f
        prognostic factors for, 1173–1174
Pigmented nevus, 1169–1170, 1169f, 1170f,
    1170t
Pigmented villonodular synovitis, 1247, 1247f
PIK3CA gene
    in endometrial carcinoma, 1032, 1032f
    in follicular thyroid carcinoma, 1120
Pilar cyst, 1176
Pilar leiomyomas, 1254
Pili, 343–344
Pill-induced esophagitis, 768
Pilomatricomas, 1177, 1178f
PIN (prostatic intraepithelial neoplasia),
    997–998, 999
Pineal gland, 1163
Pineal parenchymal tumors, 1338
Pinealoma, 1163
Pineoblastomas, 1338
Pineocytes, 1163, 1338
Pineocytomas, 1338
Pinguecula, 1349
Pink puffers, 686
Pink tetralogy, 543
Pinworms, 806
Pipe-stem fibrosis, 394, 394f
Pit abscesses, 778
PIT-1 gene, 1105–1106
Pitting edema, 113
Pituicytes, 1099
Pituitary adenomas, 1100–1105
    ACTH cell (corticotroph), 1100t, 1104, 1148
    atypical, 1102
    classification of, 1100, 1100t
    clinical course of, 1103
    epidemiology of, 1100
    functional, 1100

Pituitary adenomas (Continued)
    genetic abnormalities in, 1101–1102, 1101t,
        1102f
    gonadotroph (LH- and FSH-producing),
        1100t, 1104–1105
    growth hormone cell (somatotroph), 1100t,
        1104
    invasive, 1102
    mammosomatotroph, 1100t, 1104
    micro- vs. macro-, 1100
    morphology of, 1102, 1102f, 1103f
    nonfunctioning (silent variant, null-cell),
        1100, 1102f, 1105
    prolactinomas (lactotroph), 1100t, 1103–1104,
        1103f
    thyrotroph (TSH-producing), 1100t, 1105
Pituitary apoplexy, 1100, 1103, 1105
Pituitary disorders, 1100–1107
    carcinoma as, 1105
    clinical manifestations of, 1100
    hypopituitarism as, 1100, 1105–1106
    due to hypothalamic suprasellar tumors,
        1106–1107, 1107f
    in MEN-1, 1162
    pituitary adenomas and hyperpituitarism as,
        1100–1105
        ACTH cell (corticotroph), 1100t, 1104
        atypical, 1102
        classification of, 1100, 1100t
        clinical course of, 1103
        epidemiology of, 1100
        functional, 1100
        genetic abnormalities in, 1101–1102, 1101t,
            1102f
        gonadotroph (LH- and FSH-producing),
            1100t, 1104–1105
        growth hormone cell (somatotroph),
            1100t, 1104
        invasive, 1102
        mammosomatotroph, 1100t, 1104
        micro- vs. macro-, 1100
        morphology of, 1102, 1102f, 1103f
        nonfunctioning (silent variant, null-cell),
            1100, 1102f, 1105
        prolactinomas (lactotroph), 1100t,
            1103–1104, 1103f
        thyrotroph (TSH-producing), 1100t, 1105
    posterior, 1106
        diabetes insipidus as, 1106
        SIADH as, 1106
Pituitary dwarfism, 1106
Pituitary gland, 1098–1107
    anatomy of, 1098–1099, 1099f
    anterior, 1098–1099, 1099f
    posterior, 1098, 1099, 1106
PKC (protein kinase C), activation of, 1139
PKD (polycystic kidney disease)
    autosomal-dominant (adult), 956–959, 957t,
        958f
    autosomal-recessive (childhood), 957t, 959
PKD1 gene, 956–957, 958
PKD2 gene, 956, 957, 958
PKHD1 gene, 959
PKU (phenylketonuria), 463–464, 463f
Placenta(s)
    accreta, 1055
    anatomy of, 1052–1053, 1053f, 1054f
    in preeclampsia and eclampsia, 1057, 1057f
    previa, 1055
    twin, 1054, 1055f
Placental growth factor (PlGF), 88
Placental implantation abnormalities, 1055
    and preeclampsia, 1056, 1056f
Placental infections, 1055, 1055f

Placental influences, on fetal growth restriction, 455, 455f
Placental-fetal transmission, 340
Placental-site trophoblastic tumor (PSTT), 1061, 1061f
Plague, 365
Plant products, as carcinogens, 309t
Plantar fibromatoses, 1251
Plaque(s), 1168
  in Alzheimer disease, 1314, 1315f
  asbestos-related pleural, 700–701, 700f, 733
  atheromatous (atherosclerotic)
    (See Atherosclerotic plaques)
  dental, 740–741
  Hollenhorst, 1362
  jaune, 1288, 1288f
  kuru, 1309, 1310f
  MacCallum, 566
  in multiple sclerosis, 1311–1312, 1311f, 1312f
Plasma cell(s)
  in chronic inflammation, 72
  in immune response, 185f, 187, 196, 196f
Plasma cell dyscrasias, glomerular lesions in, 935
Plasma cell leukemia, 610
Plasma cell myeloma, 601t, 609–611, 610f, 611f
  glomerular lesions in, 935
Plasma cell neoplasms, 609–612, 610f–612f
Plasma membrane damage, 22–23
Plasma oncotic pressure, reduced, edema due to, 112, 112f, 112t
Plasma protein–derived mediators, of inflammation, 63–66
  coagulation and kinin systems as, 57t, 64–66, 65f, 66t
  complement system as, 57t, 63–64, 64f
Plasmablasts, in multiple myeloma, 610
Plasmacytomas, 601t, 609, 611
Plasmids, 343
Plasmin
  in fibrinolysis, 120, 121f
  in inflammation, 65, 65f
Plasminogen, in fibrinolysis, 120, 121f
Plasminogen activators (PAs), in fibrinolysis, 120, 121f
Plasmodium falciparum, 386–388, 387f, 388f
Plasmodium malariae, 386
Plasmodium ovale, 386, 387
Plasmodium spp, 335, 386–388
  epidemiology of, 386
  host resistance to, 387
  life cycle and pathogenesis of, 386–387, 387f
  morphology of, 387–388, 388f
Plasmodium vivax, 386, 387
Platelet(s)
  adult reference range for, 592t
  decreased production of, 667, 667t
  decreased survival of, 667, 667t
  defined, 117
  differentiation of, 591f
  in glomerular injury, 915
  in hemostasis, 115, 116f, 117–118, 119f
  radiation effect on, 425
  sequestration of, 667
  in wound healing, 102, 103f
Platelet adhesion, 117, 118f
Platelet aggregation, 117, 118, 118f
  in thrombotic microangiopathies, 952
Platelet contraction, 118
Platelet counts, 666
Platelet effects, of endothelium, 116
Platelet functions
  defective, bleeding disorders due to, 670
  tests of, 666

Platelet number, reduced, bleeding disorders due to, 667–670, 667t, 669f
Platelet secretion, 117–118
Platelet-activating factor (PAF)
  in acute respiratory distress syndrome, 682f
  in asthma, 689
  in immediate hypersensitivity, 200
  in inflammation, 57t, 60
  in necrotizing enterocolitis, 458
Platelet-derived growth factor (PDGF)
  in angiogenesis, 101
  oncogenes for, 280, 281t
  in tissue regeneration and wound healing, 87t, 88
Platelet-derived growth factor (PDGF) receptor, proto-oncogene for, 281t
Platelet-derived growth factor receptor α (PDGFRA), in gastrointestinal stromal tumors, 790
Platelet-derived growth factor-β (PDGFB) gene, in dermatofibrosarcoma protuberans, 1183
Platelet-endothelial cell interactions, 118
Platybasia, 1217
PLCγ (phospholipase Cγ), in signal transduction pathway, 90, 91f
Pleomorphic adenoma, 261
  of salivary glands, 757–759, 758f
Pleomorphic rhabdomyosarcoma, 1253
Pleomorphic xanthoastrocytoma, 1333
Pleomorphism, in neoplasia, 263
Pleotropism, 140
Pleural disease, 731–734
  pleural effusion as, 731–732
  pleural tumors as, 732–734, 732f–734f
  pneumothorax as, 732
Pleural effusions, 731–732
  inflammatory, 959–960
  noninflammatory, 960
  in right-sided heart failure, 536
Pleural plaques, asbestos-related, 700–701, 700f
Pleural space, in right-sided heart failure, 536
Pleural tumors, 732–734, 732f–734f
Pleuritis, 713, 731
  in systemic lupus erythematosus, 214t
Plexiform lesion, in pulmonary hypertension, 708–709, 709f
Plexiform neurofibroma, 1341
PlGF (placental growth factor), 88
Ploidy, of neuroblastomas, 478
Plummer syndrome, 1117–1118
Plummer-Vinson syndrome, 662, 742, 767
Pluripotency, of hematopoietic stem cells, 590
PMF (progressive massive fibrosis), due to coal workers' pneumoconiosis, 697, 698, 698f
PML (progressive multifocal leukoencephalopathy), 1305–1306, 1306f
PML-RARα fusion protein, in acute myeloid leukemia, 624
PMP22 (peripheral myelin protein 22), 1263, 1265f
PNET (primitive neuroectodermal tumor)
  of bone, 1232–1233
  genetic basis for, 306, 1249t
Pneumatosis intestinalis, in necrotizing enterocolitis, 458, 459f
Pneumococcal pneumonia, 711
Pneumoconiosis(es), 410, 696–701, 697t
  asbestos-related, 697t, 699–701, 700f
  coal workers', 36, 697–698, 697t, 698f
  defined, 696
  pathogenesis of, 696–697
  silicosis as, 697t, 698–699, 699f
Pneumocystis jiroveci pneumonia, 246
Pneumocytes, 678, 678f

Pneumonia
  aspiration, 711t, 716
  bronchiolitis obliterans organizing, 696, 696f
  chronic, 711t, 717–719, 718f, 719f
  classification of, 711, 711t
  community-acquired, 711–716, 711t, 713f, 714f
    atypical, 711t, 714–716
    bacterial, 711–714, 712f, 713f
    broncho-, 712, 713, 713f
    complications of, 713–714
    due to *Haemophilus influenzae*, 711–712
    due to *Klebsiella pneumoniae*, 712
    due to *Legionella pneumophila*, 712
    lobar, 712–713, 713f
    due to *Moraxella catarrhalis*, 712
    mycoplasmal, 714–715
    due to *Pseudomonas aeruginosa*, 712
    due to *Staphylococcus aureus*, 712
    due to *Streptococcus pneumoniae* (pneumococcal), 711
    viral, 714–716
  cryptogenic organizing, 696, 696f
  eosinophilic
    acute, 704
    idiopathic chronic, 704
  hospital-acquired, 711t, 716
  in immunocompromised host, 711t, 719–720, 720t
    due to *Pneumocystis jiroveci*, 246
  interstitial
    acute, 680, 682–683
    desquamative, 704, 704f
    nonspecific, 695
    usual, 694, 695f
  necrotizing, 711t, 716–1090, 717f
  pathogenesis of, 710–711
Pneumonic plague, 365
Pneumonitis
  hypersensitivity, 703–704, 703f
    organic dusts that produce, 697t
  lupus, 696
  radiation, 701
Pneumothorax, 679, 732
  spontaneous idiopathic, 732
PNH (paroxysmal nocturnal hemoglobinuria), 235, 652–653, 653f
Podocin
  in focal segmental glomerulosclerosis, 927
  in minimal-change disease, 925
Podocytes, 909f, 910
  in minimal-change disease, 925, 925f
Poison(s)
  cell injury due to, 11
  defined, 402
Polarity, loss of, in neoplasia, 264
Poliomyelitis, 1304
Poliovirus infection, 350–351
Pollutants, toxicity of, 402–403, 402f, 403f
Pollution, 403–408
  air, 403–405, 404t
  by metals, 406–408, 406f, 407f
Polonium, as carcinogen, 427
Polyangiitis, microscopic, 515, 516f
  glomerular lesions in, 935
Polyarteritis nodosa (PAN), 204t, 226, 514–515, 514f
  cerebral infarction due to, 1293
Polybrominated diphenyl ethers (PBDEs), occupational exposure to, 409
Polychlorinated biphenyls (PCBs), occupational exposure to, 409–410
Polyclonal proliferations, 324

Polycyclic aromatic hydrocarbons, as carcinogens, 309t, 310, 311
Polycyclic hydrocarbons, occupational exposure to, 409
Polycystic kidney disease (PKD)
  autosomal-dominant (adult), 956–959, 957t, 958f
  autosomal-recessive (childhood), 957t, 959
Polycystic liver disease, 869–870, 870f
  polycystic kidney disease and, 959
Polycystic ovarian disease (PCOD), 1039–1040, 1039f
Polycystin-1, 956–957
Polycystin-2, 957
Polycythemia, 665
  absolute, 665, 665t
  due to cancer, 321t
  defined, 665
  pathophysiologic classification of, 665t
  primary, 665, 665t
  relative, 665, 665t
  secondary, 665, 665t
Polycythemia vera (PCV), 626t, 628–629, 629f, 665
Polydactyly, 449f
Polydipsia, due to diabetes, 1143
Polyglucosan bodies, 1282
Polyglutamine diseases, 168
Polykaryons, 348
Polymerase chain reaction (PCR), 174–176, 175f, 176f
  allele-specific, 175, 175f
  for diagnosis of cancer, 324–325
  for infectious agents, 336
  methylation-specific, 181
Polymicrogyria, 1285
Polymorphic markers, 176–177, 177f, 178f
Polymorphic reticulosis, 750
Polymorphisms, 157, 176
  and genome-wide analysis, 177, 178f
  repeat-length, 176, 177f
  single-nucleotide, 136, 176, 177, 178f
Polymyositis, 1273, 1274
Polyneuropathy(ies)
  familial amyloid, 253, 1263, 1264t
  infectious, 1262–1263
Polyol pathways, disturbances in, 1139
Polyomavirus nephropathy, 942, 943f
Polyostotic fibrous dysplasia, 1231
Polyp(s), 261, 261f
  colonic, 261f, 815–820, 816t
    in Cowden syndrome and Bannayan-Ruvalcaba-Riley syndrome, 816t, 818
    in Cronkhite-Canada syndrome, 816t, 818
    in familial adenomatous polyposis, 816t, 820–821, 822f, 822t
    hamartomatous, 816–818, 816t, 817f, 818f
    hyperplastic, 818–819, 819f
    inflammatory, 815–816, 816f
    juvenile, 816–817, 816t, 817f
    neoplastic, 819–820, 820f, 821f
    pedunculated, 815
    in Peutz-Jeghers syndrome, 816t, 817–818, 818f
    retention, 817
    sessile, 815
    in tuberous sclerosis, 816t
  endocervical, 1018, 1018f
  endometrial, 1026f, 1029
  esophageal, 774
  fibroepithelial, 1176
    of ureters, 973
    of vulva, 1012

Polyp(s) (Continued)
  gastric, 783
    fundic gland, 782t, 783, 784f
    inflammatory and hyperplastic, 782t, 783, 784f
  inflammatory
    colonic, 815–816, 816f
    of esophagus, 774
    of gallbladder, 888
    gastric, 782t, 783
    nasal, 749, 750f
    vocal cord, 752
Polyphagia, due to diabetes, 1143
Polypoid cystitis, 975
Polyposis, colonic
  familial adenomatous, 274, 816t, 820–821, 822f, 822t
  juvenile, 816–817, 816t, 817f
Polyradiculoneuropathy, inflammatory demyelinating
  acute, 1261–1262
  chronic, 1262
Polyradiculopathy, with malignancy, 1266
Polyuria, due to diabetes, 1143
POMC (pro-opiomelanocortin), in energy balance, 439, 440, 441f
Pompe disease, 151t, 157t
Porcelain gallbladder, 886
Pores of Kohn, 679
  in obstructive overinflation, 687
Porphyria, 1196–1197, 1198f, 1264t
  acute intermittent, 1264t
Porphyromonas spp, 378
Port wine stain, 522
Porta hepatis, 834
Portal fibrosis, noncirrhotic, 871
Portal hypertension, 838–839, 838f
  idiopathic, 871
  in right-sided heart failure, 536
Portal system, in right-sided heart failure, 536
Portal tracts, 834, 834f
  in primary biliary cirrhosis, 868, 868f
  in viral hepatitis, 852
Portal vein obstruction, 871
Portal vein thrombosis, 871
  congestive splenomegaly due to spontaneous, 634
Portosystemic shunting
  due to liver failure, 836
  due to portal hypertension, 839
Port-wine stains, 473
Positron emission tomography (PET), of tumors, 303–304
Postcapillary venules, 488f, 489
Posterior chamber, of eye, 1346f, 1354f
Posterior fossa anomalies, 1285–1286, 1286f
Posterior polymorphous dystrophy, of cornea, 1351
Posterior scleritis, 1347
Posterior synechiae, of eye, 1355
Posterior vitreous detachment, 1357, 1360f, 1361
Postinfectious glomerulonephritis, 918t, 920
Postmenopausal changes, 1027
Postmortem clots, 124
Postnatal genetic analysis, 173–174
Postpartum cardiomyopathy, 573–574
Postpartum renal failure, 953
Postpolio syndrome, 1304
Poststreptococcal glomerulonephritis, 204t, 917–920, 919f
Post-term, 454
Post-traumatic dementia, 1290
Post-traumatic hydrocephalus, 1290
Pott disease, 1223

Pott, Percival, 309
Potter sequence, 449–450, 449f, 450f
POU1F1 gene, 1105–1106
Poverty, and malnutrition, 427
PP (pancreatic polypeptide) cells, 1130
PP (pancreatic polypeptide)-secreting tumors, 1147
PPAR(s) (peroxisome proliferator-activated receptors), 432
PPARγ (peroxisome proliferator-activated receptor γ), in insulin resistance, 1137
PPARG gene
  in diabetes, 1138
  in follicular thyroid carcinoma, 1120–1121
PPD (purified protein derivative), 207, 207f
PPROM (preterm premature rupture of placental membranes), prematurity due to, 454
PR3-ANCA (anti–proteinase-3), 511
Prader-Willi syndrome, 172–173, 172f
  peptide YY in, 442
Precancerous conditions, 276
Preconditioning, of myocardium, 553
Precursor B-cell neoplasms, 598t, 600–603, 601t, 602f
Precursor T-cell neoplasms, 598t, 600–603, 601t, 602f
Pre-diabetes, 1131, 1132
Preeclampsia, 455, 1055–1057, 1057f
  hepatic disease associated with, 874–875
Pregnancy
  alcohol consumption during, 414
  and breast cancer, 1076
  breast during, 1067, 1067f
  cocaine during, 418
  ectopic, 1053–1054
  hepatic disease associated with, 874–875, 875f
  oral manifestations of, 744t
  ovaries in, 1052
  smoking during, 411
  theca lutein hyperplasia of, 1040
  toxemia of, 455
  twin, 1054, 1055f
Pregnancy disorder(s), 1052–1061
  choriocarcinoma as, 1059–1061, 1060f
  early, 1053–1054
  ectopic pregnancy as, 1053–1054
  gestational trophoblastic disease as, 1057–1061
  hydatidiform mole as, 1057–1059, 1058f, 1059f
  invasive mole as, 1059, 1060f
  late, 1054–1057
  placental anatomy and, 1052–1053, 1053f, 1054f
  of placental implantation, 1055
  placental infections as, 1055, 1055f
  placental-site trophoblastic tumor as, 1061, 1061f
  preeclampsia and eclampsia as, 1055–1057, 1056f, 1057f
  spontaneous abortion as, 1053
  twin placentas as, 1054, 1055f
Pregnancy luteoma, 1052
Pregnancy tumor, 521
Pregnancy-related cardiomyopathy, 573–574
Prekallikrein
  in coagulation cascade, 119f
  in inflammation, 65, 65f
Premature rupture of placental membranes (PROM), 454
Prematurity, 453–458
  causes of, 454–456, 455f
  classification of, 454

Prematurity *(Continued)*
  defined, 454
  epidemiology of, 454
  hazards of, 454
  necrotizing enterocolitis with, 458, 459f
  neonatal respiratory distress syndrome with,
    456–458, 457f
  retinopathy of, 457, 1361
Pre-miRNA, 137, 137f
Premutations, in fragile-X syndrome, 170
Prenatal genetic analysis, 173
Preproinsulin, 1133
Prerenal azotemia, in left-sided heart failure, 536
Pressure atrophy, 9–10
Pressure ulcers, healing of, 104f
Pressure-overload hypertrophy, 533, 534f
Preterm, 454
Preterm infants, respiratory distress syndrome
  in, 456–458, 457f
Preterm premature rupture of placental
  membranes (PPROM), prematurity due to,
  454
Pretibial myxedema, 1115
Prevotella spp, 378
Primary biliary cirrhosis (PBC), 867–869, 867t,
  868f
Primary ciliary dyskinesia, 692
Primary CNS lymphoma, 1337
Primary myelofibrosis, 626t, 630–631, 631f
Primary sclerosing cholangitis (PSC), 867t, 869,
  869f
Primary spongiosa, 1209, 1209f
Primitive neuroectodermal tumor (PNET)
  of bone, 1232–1233
  genetic basis for, 306, 1249t
Primum atrial septal defect, 541
Prinzmetal angina, 547
Prion(s), 332, 333t
Prion diseases, 1308–1309, 1308f, 1310f
Prion protein (PrP), 332, 1308–1309, 1308f
  in amyloidosis, 251
PRKAR1A (protein kinase A regulatory subunit
  1α) gene, in pituitary adenomas, 1101
PRNP gene, in prion diseases, 1309
Procallus, 1219
Procaspase 8, in apoptosis, 295, 296f
Procoagulant effects, of endothelium, 117
Proctitis, ulcerative, 811
Proctosigmoiditis, ulcerative, 811
Progenitor cells, 84
Progesterone, in menstrual cycle, 1024, 1025
Progesterone receptors, in breast carcinoma,
  1090
Proglottids, 806
Programmed cell death, 25
Progressive bulbar palsy, in amyotrophic lateral
  sclerosis, 1325
Progressive familial intrahepatic cholestasis
  (PFIC), 843
Progressive massive fibrosis (PMF), due to coal
  workers' pneumoconiosis, 697, 698, 698f
Progressive multifocal leukoencephalopathy
  (PML), 1305–1306, 1306f
Progressive muscular atrophy, in amyotrophic
  lateral sclerosis, 1325
Progressive supranuclear palsy (PSP), 1318
Prolactinemia, 1103
Prolactinomas, 1100t, 1103–1104, 1103f
  in MEN-1, 1162
Proliferation centers, in chronic lymphocytic
  leukemia/small lymphocytic lymphoma,
  603, 604
Proliferation phase, of cutaneous wound
  healing, 102

Proliferative breast disease
  with atypia, 1073, 1074f, 1074t
  without atypia, 1071–1073, 1072f, 1073f,
    1074t
Proliferative restenosis, 526, 526f
Proliferative vitreoretinopathy, 1358
Prolymphocytes, in chronic lymphocytic
  leukemia/small lymphocytic lymphoma,
  604f, 605
PROM (premature rupture of placental
  membranes), 454
Promastigote, of *Leishmania,* 389
Promotion, of chemical carcinogenesis, 309–310,
  310t, 311
Promyelocytic leukemia, acute, 623, 623f, 624
Pro-opiomelanocortin (POMC), in energy
  balance, 439, 440, 441f
Proptosis, 1346–1347, 1347f
Propylthiouracil, 1107
Propionibacterium acnes, 1198
Propagation, of thrombi, 124
Prostacyclin
  in hemostasis, 118
  in inflammation, 58f, 59
Prostaglandin(s), in inflammation, 57t, 58–60,
  58f, 59t
Prostaglandin D_2, in immediate hypersensitivity,
  200
Prostate, 993–1002
  benign enlargement of, 994–996, 995f, 996f
  colloid carcinoma of, 1002
  inflammation of, 993–994
  normal anatomy and histology of, 993, 993f,
    994f
  tumors of, 996–1002, 998f–1000f, 1001t
Prostate adenocarcinoma, 996–1002
  clinical course of, 1000–1002
  ductal, 1002
  etiology and pathogenesis of, 996–998
  genetic basis for, 305t, 306
  grading and staging of, 999–1000, 1000f,
    1001t
  incidence of, 996
  metastatic, 998, 998f
  morphology of, 998–999, 998f, 999f
Prostate specific antigen (PSA), 327,
  1001–1002
Prostatic hyperplasia, benign or nodular, 8,
  994–996, 995f, 996f
Prostatic intraepithelial neoplasia (PIN),
  997–998, 999
Prostatitis, 993–994
  acute bacterial, 993–994
  chronic
    abacterial, 994
    bacterial, 994
  granulomatous, 994
Prosthetic valve(s), complications of, 570–571,
  571f, 571t
Prosthetic valve endocarditis, 567
Protease(s), in inflammation, 57t
Protease-activated receptors (PARs), 120, 121f
  in inflammation, 64–65
Protease-antiprotease imbalance hypothesis, of
  emphysema, 685, 685f
Proteasomes, in atrophy, 10
Protective antigen, in anthrax, 362
Protein(s)
  damage to, cell injury due to, 18f, 23
  intracellular accumulation of, 35–36, 35f
Protein 4.1, defect in, 143t
Protein breakdown, in apoptosis, 27
Protein C, 120
Protein folding, 31f

Protein kinase A regulatory subunit 1α
  (PRKAR1A) gene, in pituitary adenomas,
  1101
Protein kinase C (PKC), activation of, 1139
Protein malnutrition, edema due to, 112
Protein misfolding, apoptosis due to, 25, 30–31,
  31f
Protein reabsorption droplets, in proximal renal
  tubules, 35, 35f
Protein S, 120
Protein tyrosine phosphatase-22 *(PTPN-22)*
  gene, 1111
  in autoimmunity, 212
  in rheumatoid arthritis, 1238
  in type 1 diabetes mellitus, 1135
Protein-aggregation diseases, 36
Proteinases, in angiogenesis, 102
Protein-energy malnutrition (PEM), 427,
  428–429, 429f, 430f
Proteinopathies, 36, 1281
Proteinosis, pulmonary alveolar, 705–706, 705f
Proteinuria
  asymptomatic, 907
  in nephrotic syndrome, 922
  in systemic lupus erythematosus, 214t
Proteoglycans
  in extracellular matrix, 95f, 97–98, 98f
  in immediate hypersensitivity, 200
Proteolysis-inducing factor (PIF), 429, 430f
Proteolytic cascade, 118
Proteomics, 326
Prothrombin, in coagulation cascade, 119f
Prothrombin gene mutation, and thrombosis,
  122, 123
Prothrombin time (PT), 119–120, 666
Prothrombotic properties, of endothelium,
  116–117, 117f, 118f
Proto-oncogenes, 277, 279, 281t
Protozoa, 333t, 335–336
  intestinal, 338–339
  sexual transmission of, 341t
Protozoal infections, 386–391, 386t, 387f–390f
  in AIDS, 245t, 246
  of CNS, 1306–1308, 1307f, 1308f
Proud flesh, 107
PrP (prion protein), 332, 1308–1309, 1308f
  in amyloidosis, 251
PRPP (phosphoribosyl pyrophosphate), in gout,
  1244f
PRSS1 gene, in pancreatitis, 893–894
PRX (periaxin), 1265f
PSA (prostate specific antigen), 327, 1001–1002
Psammoma bodies, 38
  in papillary thyroid carcinoma, 1122
PSC (primary sclerosing cholangitis), 867t, 869,
  869f
P-selectin, in inflammation, 49, 49f, 49t
Pseudoaneurysm, 506, 506f
Pseudoangiomatous stromal hyperplasia, of
  breast, 1092
Pseudoarthrosis, 1220
Pseudocysts, pancreatic, 898, 898f
Pseudoepitheliomatous hyperplasia, 366
Pseudo-gout, 1246, 1246f
  due to hemochromatosis, 862
Pseudohermaphroditism, 167
Pseudo-Hurler polydystrophy, 151t
Pseudohypertrophy, in X-linked muscular
  dystrophy, 1269
Pseudohypoparathyroidism, 1130
Pseudolaminar necrosis, 1292
Pseudomembranous colitis, 379, 798t, 803, 803f
Pseudomonas aeruginosa, 364–365, 365f
  in cystic fibrosis, 468, 469, 470

Pseudomonas aeruginosa pneumonia, 712
Pseudomonas infection, 364–365, 365f
Pseudomyxoma peritonei, 269, 828, 1045, 1045f
Pseudoneuroma, 1266, 1267f
Pseudopalisading, in glioblastoma, 1331, 1332f
Pseudo-Pelger-Hüet cells, in myelodysplastic
    syndrome, 625, 625f
Pseudophakic bullous keratopathy, 1352
Pseudopolyps, in ulcerative colitis, 811, 812f
Pseudopyloric metaplasia
    in Crohn disease, 810
    in ulcerative colitis, 812, 813f
Pseudosarcomatous fasciitis, 1250–1251, 1250f
Psoriasis, 1190–1191, 1190f
Psoriatic arthritis, 1241
PSP (progressive supranuclear palsy), 1318
PSTT (placental-site trophoblastic tumor), 1061,
    1061f
Psychosis, in systemic lupus erythematosus,
    214t
Psychostimulants, abuse of, 418t, 419
PT (prothrombin time), 119–120, 666
PTA (persistent truncus arteriosus), 543
PTCH (patched) tumor suppressor genes, 295
    in nevoid basal cell carcinoma syndrome,
        1181, 1183f
PTEN gene, 287t, 294, 304
    in Cowden syndrome and Bannayan-
        Ruvalcaba-Riley syndrome, 818
    in endometrial carcinoma, 1032, 1032f
    in endometrial hyperplasia, 1030
    in endometrioid carcinoma, 1045, 1046
    in melanoma, 1174
PTEN hamartoma syndrome, 818
Pterygium, 1349
PTH (parathyroid hormone), 1126
    and hypercalcemia, 1128–1129, 1129t
PTHrP (parathyroid hormone–related protein),
    1126
    in hypercalcemia of malignancy, 322
    and hyperparathyroidism, 1128–1129
PTPN-22 (protein tyrosine phosphatase-22)
        gene, 1111
    in autoimmunity, 212
    in rheumatoid arthritis, 1238
    in type 1 diabetes mellitus, 1135
PTT (partial thromboplastin time), 120, 666
PUD (peptic ulcer disease), 780–781, 781f
Pulmonary abscess, 711t, 713, 716–717, 717f
    staphylococcal, 359, 359f
Pulmonary alveolar proteinosis (PAP), 705–706,
    705f
Pulmonary atresia, congenital, 544
Pulmonary changes, in cystic fibrosis, 469, 470t
Pulmonary congestion, 114
Pulmonary disease. *See* Lung disease(s).
Pulmonary edema, 113, 680, 680t
    in heart failure
        left-sided, 535
        right-sided, 536
    hemodynamic (cardiogenic), 680, 680t
    due to microvascular injury, 680, 680t
    noncardiogenic (*See* Acute lung injury (ALI))
    in sudden infant death syndrome, 472
Pulmonary embolism (PE), 126, 126f, 706–707,
    706f
    septic, 717
Pulmonary eosinophilia, 704
Pulmonary fibrosis, idiopathic, 694–695, 694f,
    695f
Pulmonary hemorrhage, 30–31, 706f
Pulmonary hemorrhage syndromes, diffuse,
    709–710, 709f
Pulmonary hemosiderosis, idiopathic, 710

Pulmonary hypertension (PH), 707–709, 708f,
    709f
Pulmonary hypoplasia, 679
Pulmonary infarction, 30–31, 706f
Pulmonary injury, due to heroin, 418
Pulmonary interstitium, 678, 678f
Pulmonary lobule, 678
Pulmonary sequestration, 679
Pulmonary stenosis, congenital, 544
Pulmonary vascular engorgement, in sudden
    infant death syndrome, 472
Pulmonary venous connection, total anomalous,
    543–544
Pulp chamber, 740f
Pulsating hematoma, 506
Pulseless disease, 513–514, 514f
Pump failure, due to myocardial infarction, 557
Punch-drunk syndrome, 1290
Punctate keratitis, 396
Puncture wound, 420
PUNLMPs (papillary urothelial neoplasms of
    low malignant potential), 977–978
Pupil, 1354f
Pupillary block, 1354f, 1355
Pure red cell aplasia, 664–665
Purified protein derivative (PPD), 207, 207f
Purine metabolism, 1243, 1244f
Purkinje network, 532
Purpura(s), 114
    Henoch-Schönlein, 666
    nonthrombocytopenic, 666
    thrombocytopenic
        autoimmune, 203t
        immune
            acute, 668
            chronic, 667–668
        thrombotic, 669–670, 669t
            renal disease in, 952, 953–954
Purulent inflammation, 68, 69f, 347, 347f
Pus, 15, 46, 68, 69f
Pustular psoriasis, 1190
Pustule, 1168
Pyelonephritis, 939–944
    acute, 939, 941–942, 941f, 943f
    chronic, 939, 942–944, 944f
    due to diabetes mellitus, 1143
    due to ureteral obstruction, 973
    urinary tract infection and, 939–941, 940f
    xanthogranulomatous, 943
Pyemic lung abscess, 717
Pyknosis, in necrosis, 14
Pylephlebitis, 634
Pyloric stenosis, 766
Pyogenic bacteria, 68
Pyogenic cocci, infections by, 357–360, 358t
Pyogenic granuloma, 521, 521f
    of oral cavity, 741–742, 741f
Pyogenic meningitis, 1299–1300, 1299f
Pyogenic osteomyelitis, 1221–1222, 1222f
Pyonephrosis, 941
Pyosalpinx, 1010, 1010f
Pyridoxine
    deficiency of, 438t
    functions of, 438t
Pyrogens, 74
PYY (peptide YY), in energy balance, 439, 441f,
    442

Q
Q fever, 714
Quasispecies, of hepatitis C virus, 847–848
Quick-frozen section, for cancer, 323
Quiescent tissues, 81
Quorum sensing, 343

R
R (roentgen), 423
Rabies, 1304–1305, 1304f
Rachitic rosary, 436
Rad, 423
Radial scar, of breast, 1072, 1073f
Radial sclerosing lesion, of breast, 1072, 1073f
Radiation, defined, 423
Radiation carcinogenesis, 311–312, 425–427
Radiation cystitis, 974
Radiation enterocolitis, 793
Radiation exposure
    and breast cancer, 1076–1077
    CNS effects of, 1329–1330
    congenital anomalies due to, 452
    and lung carcinoma, 722
Radiation injury, 423–427
    carcinogenesis due to, 425–427
    DNA damage due to, 423–424, 423f, 425–426
    fibrosis due to, 425, 426f
    to hematopoietic and lymphoid systems, 425
    main determinants of, 423–424, 423f, 424f
    morphologic consequences of, 424–425, 424f,
        425t
    skin disorders due to, 426f
    due to total-body irradiation, 425, 425t
    vascular changes due to, 426f
Radiation pneumonitis, 701
Radiation retinopathy, 1361–1362
Radiation therapy
    and bladder cancer, 980
    esophagitis due to, 768
    white cell neoplasia due to, 598
Radiation units, 423
Radiation-induced lung diseases, 701
Radon
    as carcinogen, 274t, 427
    as indoor air pollutant, 405
    and lung carcinoma, 722
RAG-1 (recombination activating gene 1), 186
RAG-2 (recombination activating gene 2), 186
Ragged red fibers, 1272, 1273f
    myoclonic epilepsy and, 1327–1328
RANK (receptor activator of nuclear factor κB),
    in bone homeostasis, 1208, 1208f
RANKL (receptor activator of nuclear factor κB
    ligand), 1126
    in bone homeostasis, 1208, 1208f
RANTES (regulated and normal T-cell expressed
    and secreted), 62
Ranula, of salivary glands, 756
Rapid plasma reagin test, 375
Rapidly progressive glomerulonephritis (RPGN),
    907, 908t, 920–921, 920t, 921f
RAR(s) (retinoic acid receptors), 431
RARα (retinoic acid receptor-α), in acute
    myeloid leukemia, 624
RAS oncogene, 281t, 282–283, 282f, 308, 309
    in follicular thyroid carcinoma, 1120
    in melanocytic nevi, 1170
    in melanoma, 1174, 1175
Rathke cleft cyst, 1105
Raynaud's phenomenon, 518, 518f
    in systemic sclerosis, 225
RB pocket, 289
RB protein, 87, 143t, 288–290, 289f
RB tumor suppressor gene, 274, 287–290, 287t,
    288f, 289f
    in osteosarcoma, 1225
    in retinoblastoma, 1365
RB1 gene, in lung carcinoma, 727
RBP (retinol-binding protein), 431, 431f
RCA (right coronary artery), in myocardial
    infarction, 549, 549f, 551, 551f

RDS. *See* Respiratory distress syndrome (RDS).
Reabsorption droplets, in proximal renal
tubules, 35, 35f
Reactive arthritis, 204t, 1241
Reactive gastropathy, 779
Reactive lymphadenitis, 48
Reactive nitrogen species
ischemia-reperfusion injury due to, 24
in leukocyte-mediated tissue injury, 55
in phagocytosis, 53, 53f
Reactive nodules, of vocal cords, 752
Reactive oxygen species (ROS)
in alcohol metabolism, 413
in cell injury, 18f, 20–22, 20t, 21f, 22
ischemia-reperfusion, 24
in cellular aging, 40–41
in emphysema, 685f, 686
in inflammation, 57t, 60
in leukocyte-mediated tissue injury, 55
in phagocytosis, 53, 53f
in toxicology, 403
Reactive pseudosarcomatous proliferations,
1250–1251, 1250f, 1251f
Recanalization, of thrombi, 124–125, 125f
Receptor(s)
cell surface, 89–91, 91f
defects in, 143t, 144, 147–149, 147f–149f
with intrinsic tyrosine kinase activity, 90,
91f
without intrinsic tyrosine kinase activity that
recruit kinases, 90, 91f
and signal transduction pathways, 89–91, 91f
Receptor activator of nuclear factor κB (RANK),
in bone homeostasis, 1208, 1208f
Receptor activator of nuclear factor κB ligand
(RANKL), 1126
in bone homeostasis, 1208, 1208f
Receptor editing, in immunological tolerance,
209
Receptor-mediated signal transduction, in cell
growth, 89–92, 90f–92f
Recombination activating gene 1 (RAG-1), 186
Recombination activating gene 2 (RAG-2), 186
Rectal ulcer(s), solitary, 815–816, 816f
Red cedar dust, lung diseases due to, 697t
Red cell(s)
adult reference range for, 592t
differentiation of, 591f
Red cell aplasia
due to cancer, 321t
pure, 664–665
Red cell count, adult reference range for, 641t
Red cell distribution width, 640, 641t
Red cell enzyme defects, hemolytic disease due
to, 644–645, 644f, 645f
Red cell indices, 640–641, 641t
Red cell trauma, hemolytic anemia due to, 654,
654f
Red hepatization, 713, 714f
Red infarcts, 128, 128f
Red neurons, 1281
Red pulp, of spleen, 632, 633f
Red thrombi, 124
Red wine, resveratrol in, 414
Reed-Sternberg cells, 616–620, 617f, 621f
Re-epithelialization, 102, 103, 104f
Reflux esophagitis, 769–770, 769f
Reflux nephropathy, 940, 940f, 942–944, 944f
Refsum disease, 1264t, 1364
Regenerating cluster, 1260
Regeneration, 44, 92–94, 93f
Regenerative medicine, 82
Regulated and normal T-cell expressed and
secreted (RANTES), 62

Regulatory genes, in carcinogenesis, 277
oncogenes as, 279–286, 281t
for cell cycle regulators, 281t
for growth factor receptors, 280–281, 281t
for growth factors, 280, 281t
for nonreceptor tyrosine kinases, 283–286,
283f, 284f, 285f, 286t
for nuclear-regulatory proteins, 281t
for signal-transducing proteins, 281–283,
281t, 282f
tumor suppressor gene(s) as, 286–294, 287t
in APC/β-catenin pathway, 292–294, 293f
in INK4a/ARF pathway, 294
NF1 as, 294–295
NF2 as, 295
patched (PTCH) genes as, 295
PTEN as, 287t, 294
RB as, 287–290, 288f, 289f
in TGF-β pathway, 294
TP53 as, 290–292, 291f
VHL disease, 295
WT1 as, 295
Regulatory T cells, 210–211, 210f
Reid index, in chronic bronchitis, 688
Reinnervation, of muscle, 1258, 1258f, 1260,
1260t, 1261f
Reis-Bückler dystrophy, of cornea, 1351
Reiter syndrome
arthritis in, 1241
due to shigellosis, 801
urethritis in, 981
Rejection vasculitis, 228–229, 228f
Relapsing febrile nodular panniculitis, 1199
Relapsing fever, 377
Rem, 423
Renal ablation focal segmental
glomerulosclerosis, 927–928
Renal agenesis, 955
Renal arteriolosclerosis, in diabetes mellitus,
1142
Renal artery, fibromuscular dysplasia of, 951,
951f
Renal artery stenosis, 951–952, 951f
Renal atherosclerosis, in diabetes mellitus, 1142
Renal calculi, 907, 962–963, 962t, 963f
Renal cell carcinoma, 964–967
classification of, 964–965, 964f
clinical features of, 966–967
epidemiology of, 964
familial forms of, 964
metastatic, 270
to lung, 731f
morphology of, 965–966, 965f, 966f
Renal cysts, 957t, 960
Renal disease, 905–967
due to adverse drug reactions, 416t
atheroembolic, 954, 954f
atherosclerotic ischemic, 954
clinical manifestations of, 906–907, 908t
congenital anomalies as, 955–956
agenesis, 955
ectopic kidneys as, 955
horseshoe kidneys as, 955
hypoplasia as, 955
multicystic renal dysplasia as, 955–956, 956f
cystic, 956–960, 957t
acquired, 957t, 960
autosomal-dominant (adult) poly-,
956–959, 957t, 958f
autosomal-recessive (childhood) poly-,
957t, 959
medullary sponge kidney as, 957t, 959
nephronophthisis and adult-onset
medullary, 957t, 959–960, 960f

Renal disease (Continued)
obstructive uropathy as, 960–962, 961f
simple cysts as, 957t, 960
due to diabetes mellitus, 1141–1143, 1141f,
1142f
end-stage, 907
epidemiology of, 906
glomerular, 907–935, 908t, 918t
Alport syndrome as, 931–932, 932f
in amyloidosis, 935
clinical manifestations of, 908–911, 908t,
909f, 910f
dense-deposit disease as, 915, 918t,
928–929, 928f, 930f
in essential mixed cryoglobulinemia,
935
focal segmental glomerulosclerosis as,
916–917, 917f, 918t, 926–928, 927f
glomerulonephritis as
acute proliferative, 917–920, 918t, 919f
bacterial endocarditis–associated, 934
chronic, 918t, 932–933, 933f
fibrillary, 935
membranoproliferative, 915, 918t,
928–929, 928f–930f
postinfectious, 918t, 920
poststreptococcal, 917–920, 919f
rapidly progressive (crescentic), 907,
908t, 920–921, 920t, 921f
glomerulopathy as
immunotactoid, 935
membranous, 918t, 922–923, 924f
in Goodpasture syndrome, 918t, 935
in Henoch-Schönlein purpura, 934
hereditary, 908t
histologic alterations in, 911
isolated urinary abnormalities as, 908t,
929–932
in light-chain or monoclonal Ig deposition
disease, 935
lupus nephritis as, 934
mechanisms of progression in, 916–917,
917f
in microscopic polyangiitis, 935
minimal-change disease as, 918t, 923–926,
925f
in multiple myeloma, 935
with nephritic syndrome, 908t, 917–920,
919f
nephropathy as
diabetic, 934–935
HIV-associated, 928
IgA, 918t, 929–931, 931f
with nephrotic syndrome, 908t, 921–929,
923t
pathogenesis of injury in, 911–916, 911t,
913f–916f
in plasma cell dyscrasias, 935
primary, 908t
in systemic diseases, 908t, 933–935
thin basement membrane lesion as, 932
in Wegener granulomatosis, 935
due to heroin use, 419
neoplastic, 963–967
benign, 963–964
angiomyolipoma as, 963
oncocytoma as, 964
renal papillary adenoma as, 963
malignant, 964–967
renal cell carcinoma as, 964–967,
964f–966f
urothelial carcinomas of renal pelvis as,
967, 967f
due to nonrenal neoplasms, 948t

Renal disease (Continued)
    in systemic lupus erythematosus, 214t,
        217–219, 218f, 219f
    in systemic sclerosis, 225
    tubular and interstitial, 935–948
        acute kidney injury as, 935–938, 936f–938f
        clinical manifestations of, 907
        tubulointerstitial nephritis as, 938–948,
            939t
            due to acute phosphate nephropathy,
                947–948
            acute vs. chronic, 938
            drug- and toxin-induced, 944–946, 945f,
                946f
            due to hypercalcemia and
                nephrocalcinosis, 947
            due to light-chain cast nephropathy, 948,
                948f
            due to pyelonephritis, 940, 941–944,
                941f, 943f, 944f
            due to reflux nephropathy, 940, 940f,
                942–944, 944f
            secondary, 938
            due to urate nephropathy, 947, 947f
            due to urinary tract infection, 939–941,
                940f
        urolithiasis as, 962–963, 962t, 963f
        vascular, 949–955
            atheroembolic, 954, 954f
            atherosclerotic ischemic, 954
            benign nephrosclerosis as, 949, 949f, 950f
            diffuse cortical necrosis as, 954–955, 954f
            malignant hypertension and accelerated
                nephrosclerosis as, 949–951, 950f
            renal artery stenosis as, 951–952, 951f
            renal infarcts as, 955
            sickle-cell disease nephropathy as, 954
            thrombotic microangiopathies as, 952–954,
                952f
Renal effects, of shock, 132
Renal failure, 907
    acute, 907
    chronic, 907, 908t
    hypercalcemia due to, 38
    hyperparathyroidism due to, 1129
    postpartum, 953
Renal hypoplasia, 955
Renal infarcts, 955
Renal insufficiency, 907
Renal medulla, cystic diseases of, 959–960, 960f
Renal osteodystrophy, 1129, 1218–1219
Renal papillary adenoma, 963
Renal pelvis, urothelial carcinomas of, 967, 967f
Renal reserve, diminished, 907
Renal stones, 907, 962–963, 962t, 963f
Renal vein occlusion, 1362–1363
Rendu-Osler-Weber syndrome, oral
    manifestations of, 744t
Renin-angiotensin system, in blood pressure
    regulation, 493, 494f
Renovascular hypertension, 493t, 495
Repeat-length polymorphisms, 176, 177f
Reperfusion, of myocardial infarction, 553, 554f,
    555f
Reperfusion injury, 553, 554f, 555f
Replication, obligatory asymmetric, 82
Replicative potential, limitless, in carcinogenesis,
    278, 296–297, 297f
Replicative senescence, 39, 40–41, 40f, 87
Reproductive cloning, 84
Reproductive disorders, due to occupational
    exposures, 409t
Reproductive system. See Female genital tract;
    Male genital tract.

Reprogramming, of differentiated cells, 84, 84f
Residual bodies, 10
Resorption atelectasis, 679, 679f
Respirator brain, 1291
Respiratory bronchioles, 678
Respiratory bronchiolitis-associated interstitial
    lung disease, 704–705
Respiratory burst, in phagocytosis, 53
Respiratory disease. See Lung disease(s).
Respiratory distress syndrome (RDS)
    acute, 680–683
        clinical course of, 682
        conditions associated with development of,
            680, 681t
        morphology of, 680, 681f
        pathogenesis of, 681–682, 682f
    adult, 132
    neonatal, 456–458, 457f
Respiratory injury, due to burns, 421
Respiratory tract, infections via, 339
Response-to-injury hypothesis, of
    atherosclerosis, 499, 499f
Restriction enzymes, 175
Restriction point, in cell cycle, 86, 86f
Restrictive cardiomyopathy, 572f, 572t, 577
Restrictocin, 385
Resveratrol, in red wine, 414
RET gene, 280, 281t
    in Hirschsprung disease, 766
    in hyperparathyroidism, 1127
    in medullary thyroid carcinoma, 1121
    in MEN-2, 1162
Retention polyps, colonic, 817
Reti ovarii, 1007
Reticular hyperplasia, 596
Reticulocyte count, adult reference range for,
    641t
Reticulocytosis, 641
    in hemolytic anemia, 642
Reticuloendothelial system, in chronic
    inflammation, 71, 71f
Reticulosis, polymorphic, 750
Retina, 1357–1365
    age-related macular degeneration of, 1346,
        1363–1364, 1364f
    detachment of, 1357–1358, 1360f
    functional anatomy of, 1346f, 1357, 1359f
    neoplasms of, 1365, 1365f
Retinal, 430, 431
Retinal artery occlusion, 1362, 1364f
Retinal detachment, 1357–1358, 1360f
    traction, 1361
Retinal exudates, 1359f
Retinal hemorrhage, 1359f
Retinal infarct, 1359, 1362, 1362f
Retinal lymphoma, 1365
Retinal neovascularization, 1360–1361, 1363f
Retinal pigment epithelium (RPE), 1357, 1359f
    osseous metaplasia of, 1368
Retinal tears, 1357, 1360f
Retinal vascular disease, 1358–1363
    due to diabetes mellitus, 1359–1361, 1362f,
        1363f
    due to hypertension, 1359, 1361f, 1362f
    radiation retinopathy as, 1361–1362
    retinal artery and vein occlusions as,
        1362–1363, 1364f
    retinal vasculitis as, 1361–1362
    retinopathy of prematurity as, 1361
    sickle retinopathy as, 1361–1362
Retinal vasculitis, 1361–1362
Retinal vein occlusion, 1362–1363
Retinitis, 1364–1365
    pigmentosa, 1357, 1364

Retinoblastoma, 1365, 1365f
    genetic basis for, 274, 287–290, 287t, 288f,
        289f
Retinoic acid, 430
Retinoic acid embryopathy, 453
Retinoic acid receptor(s) (RARs), 431
Retinoic acid receptor-α (RARα), in acute
    myeloid leukemia, 624
Retinoic X receptor (RXR), 403
Retinoids, 431–432
Retinol, 430–431, 431f
Retinol-binding protein (RBP), 431, 431f
Retinopathy
    diabetic, 1145, 1359–1361, 1362f, 1363f
    of prematurity, 457, 1361
    radiation, 1361–1362
    sickle, 1361–1362
RET/PTC fusion protein, in papillary thyroid
    carcinoma, 1120, 1122
Retrobulbar neuritis, in multiple sclerosis, 1312
Retrograde transport, of cholera toxin, 797, 799f
Retrolental fibroplasia, 1361
Retroperitoneal fibrosis, idiopathic, 828–829
Retroperitonitis, sclerosing, 828–829
Retroviral syndrome, acute, 243–244, 243f
Reye syndrome, 857
RF (rheumatic fever), 565–566
    acute, 203t
Rh incompatibility, fetal hydrops due to, 460,
    460f
Rh isoimmunization, 460, 460f
Rhabdomyoblasts, 1253, 1253f
Rhabdomyoma, cardiac, 584
Rhabdomyosarcoma, 265f
    alveolar, 1253, 1254f
    embryonal
        of bladder, 981
        of skeletal muscle, 1253
        of vagina, 1017, 1017f
    pleomorphic, 1253
    of skeletal muscle, 1249t, 1253–1254, 1253f,
        1254f
Rhesus immune globulin (RhIg), 460
Rheumatic fever (RF), 565–566
    acute, 203t
Rheumatic heart disease (RHD), 565–566, 565f,
    567f
Rheumatoid arthritis, 1237–1240
    autoimmunity in, 1238–1239
    clinical course of, 1239–1240, 1240f
    environmental arthritogen in, 1238
    epidemiology of, 1237
    genetic susceptibility to, 1238
    heart disease associated with, 583
    juvenile, 1240–1241
    morphology of, 1237, 1238f
    pathogenesis of, 1237–1239, 1239f
    pulmonary involvement in, 696
    T cell–mediated hypersensitivity in, 206t
Rheumatoid factors, 1238
Rheumatoid nodules, 1237, 1238f
Rheumatoid spondylitis, 1241
Rheumatoid valvulitis, 583
Rheumatoid vasculitis, 517, 1237
Rheumatologic diseases, heart disease associated
    with, 583
RhIg (rhesus immune globulin), 460
Rhinitis
    allergic, 749
    chronic, 749–750
    infectious, 749
Rhinocerebral mucormycosis, 386
Rhizopus, 385
Rhodopsin, 431

Riboflavin
    deficiency of, 438t
    functions of, 438t
Ribonucleic acid. See RNA.
Richter syndrome, 605
Rickets, 433, 435–436, 435f, 1218
Rickettsia spp, 335, 380–381, 381f, 382f
    in Global Burden of Disease, 400
Rickettsial infections, 380–381, 381f, 382f
Riedel thyroiditis, 1114
Right bundle branch, 532
Right coronary artery (RCA), in myocardial
        infarction, 549, 549f, 551, 551f
Right ventricular infarction, 557
Right-sided heart failure, 536–537
Right-sided hypertensive heart disease, 559–560,
        560f, 560t
Right-to-left shunts, 540, 542–544, 542f
    due to persistent truncus arteriosus, 543
    due to tetralogy of Fallot, 542–543, 542f
    due to total anomalous pulmonary venous
            connection, 543–544
    due to transposition of the great arteries, 542f,
            543, 543f
    due to tricuspid atresia, 543
Riley-Day syndrome, 1263t
Ring abscess, in infective endocarditis, 567
Ring chromosome, 160, 160f
Ring fiber, in myotonic dystrophy, 1269
Ringed sideroblasts, in myelodysplastic
        syndrome, 625, 625f
RISC (RNA-induced silencing complex), 137,
        137f
Ritter disease, 358
RNA analysis, 181
RNA viruses, oncogenic, 312–313
RNA-induced silencing complex (RISC), 137,
        137f
Robertsonian translocation, 160f, 161
Rocky Mountain spotted fever (RMSF), 381,
        382f
Rod(s), in retina, 1359f
Rod cells, 1282
Rodent ulcers, 1180
Roentgen (R), 423
Rokitansky-Aschoff sinuses, 886, 886f
ROM (rupture of membranes), preterm
        premature, 454
ROS. See Reactive oxygen species (ROS).
Rosacea, 1198–1199
Rose spots, in typhoid fever, 802
Rosenthal fibers, 1282
Rotavirus
    gastroenteritis due to, 804
    structure of, 333f
Rotor syndrome, 841t, 842
Rouleaux formation, in multiple myeloma, 610
RPE (retinal pigment epithelium), 1357, 1359f
    osseous metaplasia of, 1368
RPGN (rapidly progressive glomerulonephritis),
        907, 908t, 920–921, 920t, 921f
R-SMADs, 294
Rubella, intrauterine infection with, 451–452
Rubeola, 349–350, 350f
Rubor, 44, 69
Ruffled border, 1207
Rupture of membranes (ROM), preterm
        premature, 454
Russell bodies, 35
    in lymphoplasmacytic lymphoma, 612
    in multiple myeloma, 610
RXR (retinoic X receptor), 403
Ryanodine receptor type 1 (RYR1), in heat
        stroke, 422

S
S phase, of cell cycle, 86, 86f
SA (sinoatrial) node, 532
SA (sinoatrial) pacemaker, 532
SAA (serum amyloid A) protein, 74–75
SAA (serum amyloid-associated) protein, 250,
        251–252, 251f
Saber shin, 1223
Saccular aneurysms, 489, 506, 506f, 507
    ruptured, 1297–1298, 1297f, 1298f
Sacrococcygeal teratomas, in infants and
        children, 474, 474f
Saddle embolus, 126
Sago spleen, 254
Salicylate poisoning, 417
Salicylism, 417
Salivary glands
    in cystic fibrosis, 469
    in sarcoidosis, 703
Salivary glands disorder(s), 756–761
    neoplasms as, 757–761, 757t, 758f–760f
    sialadenitis as, 756–757, 757f
    xerostomia as, 756
Salivary origin, mixed tumor of, 261, 261f
Salmon patches, in sickle retinopathy, 1362
Salmonella enteritidis, 801
Salmonella paratyphi, 801
Salmonella typhi, 801
Salmonellosis, 798t, 801
Salpingitis
    chronic follicular, 1010
    suppurative, 1038
        acute, 1010, 1010f
    tuberculous, 1038
Salpingo-oophoritis, 1010, 1010f
Salt retention, edema due to, 112–113, 112t
Salt-wasting syndrome, 1153
San Joaquin Valley fever complex, 719
Sandhoff disease, 151t
SAP gene, 319
Sarcoglycan complex of proteins, in limb girdle
        muscular dystrophies, 1269
Sarcoidosis, 701–703, 702f
    granulomatous inflammation in, 73t
Sarcoma(s), 261
    alveolar soft-part, genetic basis for, 1249t
    of bladder, 981
    botryoides
        of bladder, 981
        of skeletal muscle, 1253
        of vagina, 1017, 1017f
    of breast, 1092–1093
    cardiac, 584
    clear cell, genetic basis for, 1249t
    Ewing, 1232–1233, 1233f
        genetic basis for, 305t, 306, 1249t
    Kaposi, 523–524
        AIDS-associated (epidemic), 246–247, 247f,
                523
        chronic (classic, European), 523, 524
        clinical features of, 524
        of eyelid, 1349
        lymphadenopathic (African, endemic), 523,
                524
        morphology of, 524, 524f
        pathogenesis of, 523–524
        transplant-associated, 523, 524
    soft-tissue, chromosomal and genetic
            abnormalities in, 1248, 1249t
    stromal, of endometrium, 1035
    synovial, 1249t, 1254–1255, 1255f
    translocations in, 324–325
Sarcomatoid mesothelioma, 962
Sarcomere, of myocardium, 531

Sarcoplasmic mass, in myotonic dystrophy,
        1269
SARS (severe acute respiratory syndrome), 716
Satellite cells, 82
Saturday night palsy, 1267
SCA(s) (spinocerebellar ataxias), 168t,
        1323–1324
Scab, formation of, 102, 103f
Scale, 1168
Scar formation, 79–80, 81f
    healing by, 98, 103f, 104
    hypertrophic, 106–107, 106f
        due to burn injury, 421
    inadequate, 106
    inflammation and, 44, 348, 349f
Scarlet fever, 360
    oral manifestations of, 744t
Scatter factor, in tissue regeneration and wound
        healing, 87t, 88
Scavenger receptors
    in atherosclerosis, 500, 501f
    in inflammation, 52
SCC. See Squamous cell carcinoma (SCC).
SCD (sudden cardiac death), 546, 558–559
Schatzki rings, 767–768
Schiller-Duval body, in endodermal sinus tumor,
        of ovary, 1049, 1049f
Schistosoma haematobium infections, and
        bladder cancer, 979–980
Schistosoma spp, 393–395, 394f
Schistosomiasis, 393–395, 394f
    enterocolitis due to, 805f, 806
Schizont, of malaria, 387, 387f
Schlemm canal, 1346f, 1354f
Schmid metaphyseal chondrodysplasia, 1211t
Schneiderian papilloma, 751, 751f
Schwann cells, 1258
    in neuroblastomas, 476–477, 477f
Schwannomas, 1340–1341, 1340f
    epithelioid malignant, 1342
Schwannosis, 1342
SCID (severe combined immunodeficiency),
        234–235
Scirrhous tumors, 260
Sclera, 1346f, 1350
Scleral buckling, 1357
Scleritis, posterior, 1347
Scleroderma, 215t, 223–225, 223f–225f
    pulmonary involvement in, 696
Sclerosing adenosis, of breast, 1072, 1072f
Sclerosing cholangitis, primary, 867t, 869, 869f
Sclerosing dacryoadenitis, 1347
Sclerosing lymphocytic lobulitis, 1070
Sclerosing osteomyelitis of Garré, 1222
Sclerosing retroperitoneal fibrosis, of ureters,
        973–974
Sclerosing retroperitonitis, 828–829
Scrub typhus, 380, 381
Scurvy, 437–438, 437f
    bleeding disorders due to, 666
SDHB gene, in pheochromocytoma, 1159
Sebaceous adenomas, 1177, 1178f
Sebaceous carcinoma, of eyelid, 1348–1349,
        1348f
Sebaceous glands, stem cells in, 85
Seborrheic dermatitis, 1191
Seborrheic keratoses, 1175, 1175f
Second signals, in immunological tolerance, 209
Second-hand smoke, 410, 411–412
Secreted protein acidic and rich in cysteine
        (SPARC), in extracellular matrix, 96
Secundum atrial septal defect, 541
Sedative-hypnotics, abuse of, 418t
Seeding, of body cavities and surfaces, 269, 269f

Segmental demyelination, 1258, 1258f, 1259, 1259f
Segmental necrosis, 1261
Seizures, in systemic lupus erythematosus, 214t
Selectins
    in extracellular matrix, 96
    in inflammation, 49, 49t
Selenium
    deficiency of, 439t
    functions of, 439t
Self-renewal, of hematopoietic stem cells, 590
Semilunar valves, 532
Seminoma, 988–989, 988f, 989f
    anaplastic, 989
    spermatocytic, 989
Senescence, 39, 40–41, 40f, 87
    escape from, in carcinogenesis, 278, 286–295
    p53-induced, 292
Senile cardiac amyloidosis, 253, 580
Senile plaques, in Alzheimer disease, 1314, 1315f
Senile systemic amyloidosis, 252t, 253
Sensory neuropathy, subacute, in paraneoplastic syndrome, 1340
Sentinel lymph node biopsy, for breast carcinoma, 270, 1089
Sepsis, 75
    due to burn injury, 421
    perinatal, 459
Septic infarcts, 129
    in infective endocarditis, 567
    pulmonary, 707
Septic pulmonary embolism, 717
Septic shock, 75, 129, 130t
    epidemiology of, 75
    pathogenesis of, 129–132, 131f
    severity and outcome of, 132
Septicemic plague, 365
Sequence, 449–450, 449f, 450f
Sequestration crises, in sickle cell disease, 648
Sequestrum, 1222, 1222f
Serine protease inhibitor Kazal type 1 (SPINK1) gene, in pancreatitis, 894
Seronegative spondyloarthropathies, 1241
Serositis, in systemic lupus erythematosus, 214t
Serotonergic (5-HT) system, in sudden infant death syndrome, 472
Serotonin, in inflammation, 57–58, 57t
Serous borderline tumors, of ovary, 1043–1044, 1043f
Serous carcinoma, ovarian, 1042–1044, 1043f
Serous cystadenomas
    ovarian, 1043, 1043f
    of pancreas, 899, 899f
Serous effusion, 67, 68f
Serous endometrial carcinoma, 1033–1034, 1034f, 1035f
Serous inflammation, 67, 68f
Serous tumors, of ovaries, 1042–1044, 1043f
Serpentines, 699, 700
Sertoli cell tumors, testicular, 992
Sertoli–Leydig cell tumors, of ovaries, 1051–1052, 1051f
Serum amyloid A (SAA) protein, 74–75
Serum amyloid-associated (SAA) protein, 250, 251–252, 251f
Serum sickness, 204, 204t, 205
Sessile adenomas, colorectal, 819
Sessile polyps, colonic, 815
Sessile serrated adenomas, colorectal, 820, 821f, 824f
Severe acute respiratory syndrome (SARS), 716
Severe combined immunodeficiency (SCID), 234–235

Sex chromosomes, cytogenetic disorder involving, 164–167, 166f
Sex cord–stromal tumors
    of ovaries, 1040t, 1041f, 1050–1052
    testicular, 992
Sex hormones, in systemic lupus erythematosus, 216
Sex steroids, 1148
Sex-determining region Y gene (SRY), 164
Sex-linked disorders, 142, 142t
Sexually transmitted infections (STIs), 341–342, 341t
Sézary syndrome, 601t, 616, 1184
Sézary-Lutzner cells, 1185
SF-B (surfactant protein B) deficiency, in pulmonary alveolar proteinosis, 705
sFlt1 (soluble fms-like tyrosine kinase), in preeclampsia, 1056–1057
SFTBC gene, 456
SFTPB gene, 456
SGA (small for gestational age), 454
Shadow plaques, in multiple sclerosis, 1311
Shaw, George Bernard, 44
Sheehan syndrome, 1105
SHH (sonic hedgehog gene), in nevoid basal cell carcinoma syndrome, 1181, 1183f
Shift to the left, in inflammation, 75
Shiga toxin, 800, 801
Shiga-like toxin, in thrombotic microangiopathies, 953
Shigella, 798t, 800–801
Shigellosis, 798t, 800–801
Shingles, 353, 353f, 1262–1263
Shock, 129–133
    anaphylactic, 129
    cardiogenic, 129, 130t
        due to myocardial infarction, 557
    causes of, 129, 130t
    clinical consequences of, 133
    hypovolemic (hemorrhagic), 114, 129, 130t
        due to burn injury, 421
    morphology of, 132
    neurogenic, 129
    septic, 75, 129, 130t
        epidemiology of, 129
        pathogenesis of, 129–132, 131f
        severity and outcome of, 132
    stages of, 132
Shock lung, 132
Short stature homeobox (SHOX) gene, in Turner syndrome, 167
Shower embolization, 1293
SI (syncytia-inducing) virus, 241
SIADH (syndrome of inappropriate antidiuretic hormone secretion), 1106
    due to cancer, 321t
Sialadenitis, 756–757, 757f
Sialolithiasis, 756–757
Sicca syndrome, in Sjögren syndrome, 221
Sick building syndrome, 405
Sickle cell anemia
    genetic basis for, 140
    and thrombosis, 122
Sickle cell crisis, in liver, 872, 872f
Sickle cell disease, 645–648
    clinical features of, 647–648
    diagnosis of, 648
    epidemiology of, 645
    genetic basis for, 144
    morphology of, 646–647, 647f
    papillary necrosis due to, 947t
    pathogenesis of, 645–646, 646f
    prognosis for, 648
Sickle cell disease nephropathy, 954

Sickle cell trait, 140, 645
Sickle hemoglobin, 140, 645
Sickle retinopathy, 1361–1362
Sideroblasts, ringed, in myelodysplastic syndrome, 625, 625f
SIDS (sudden infant death syndrome), 471–473, 471t
Sievert (Sv), 423
Sigmoid diverticulitis, 814–815, 815f
Sigmoid septum, 532
Signal transducers and activation of transcription (STATs), 90, 91f
Signaling lymphocytic activation molecule (SLAM), in measles, 349
Signaling mechanisms, in cell growth, 89–92, 90f–92f
Signal-transducing proteins, oncogenes for, 281–283, 281t, 282f
Signature mutation, 311
Signet-ring cell carcinoma, gastric, 785, 786f
SIL (squamous intraepithelial lesion), of cervix, 1019–1021, 1020f, 1020t, 1021f, 1021t, 1023f
Silica, lung diseases due to, 697t
Silicosis, 697t, 698–699, 699f
    chronic inflammation in, 70
Singers' nodules, 752
Single-gene disorder(s), 138
    mendelian, 140–158
        alkaptonuria as, 155–156
        autosomal-dominant, 140–141, 141t
        autosomal-recessive, 141–142, 142t
        biochemical and molecular basis of, 142–144, 143t, 144f
        congenital anomalies due to, 451
        due to defects in proteins that regulate cell growth, 156
        due to defects in receptor proteins, 143t, 144, 147–149, 147f–149f
        due to defects in structural proteins, 143t, 144–147, 146t
        Ehlers-Danlos syndromes as, 145–147, 146t
        due to enzyme defects, 149–156
        familial hypercholesterolemia as, 147–149, 147t–149f
        Gaucher disease as, 151t, 153–154, 154f
        glycogen storage diseases as, 155, 156f, 157t, 158f
        lysosomal storage diseases as, 149–155, 150f, 151t
        Marfan syndrome as, 144–145
        mucopolysaccharidoses as, 151t, 154–155
        Niemann-Pick disease as
            type C, 153
            types A and B, 151t, 152–153, 153f
        Tay-Sachs disease as, 139f, 150–152, 151t, 152f
        transmission patterns of, 140–142, 141t, 142t
        X-linked, 142, 142t
    with nonclassic inheritance, 140, 167–173
        Angelman syndrome as, 172–173, 172f
        fragile-X syndrome as, 139, 168t, 169–171, 169f, 170f
        due to genomic imprinting, 171–173, 172f
        due to gonadal mosaicism, 173
        Leber hereditary optic neuropathy as, 171, 171f
        due to mutations in mitochondrial genes, 171, 171f
        Prader-Willi syndrome as, 172–173, 172f
        due to triplet-repeat mutations, 139, 167–171, 168f, 168t

Single-nucleotide polymorphisms (SNPs), 136, 176, 177, 178f, 326
Sinoatrial (SA) node, 532
Sinoatrial (SA) pacemaker, 532
Sinonasal papilloma, 751, 751f
Sinonasal polyps, in cystic fibrosis, 470
Sinopulmonary disease, chronic, in cystic fibrosis, 470, 470t
Sinus
   empyema of, 750
   mucocele of, 750
Sinus histiocytosis, 596
Sinus venosus defect, 541
Sinusitis, 750
Sinusoidal obstruction syndrome, 873–874, 873f
Sinusoids, capillarization of, 837
Sipple syndrome, 1162
siRNAs (small interfering RNAs), 137
Sirtuins, and cellular aging, 41
SIS gene, 281t
Sister Mary Joseph nodule, 786
Sjögren syndrome, 215t, 221–223, 222f
Skeletal metastases, 1235
Skeletal muscle, stem cells in, 86
Skeletal muscle disease(s), 1267–1276
   congenital myopathies as, 1271, 1272f, 1272t
   denervation atrophy as, 1267–1268, 1267f
   inflammatory myopathies as, 1273–1275, 1274f
   ion channel myopathies as, 1270
   muscular dystrophies as, 1268–1270, 1268f, 1269f, 1270t, 1271t
   myopathies associated with inborn errors of metabolism as, 1271–1273, 1273f
   of neuromuscular junction, 1275–1276
   toxic myopathies as, 1275
Skeletal muscle tumors, 1253–1254
   rhabdomyosarcoma as, 1249t, 1253–1254, 1253f, 1254f
Skin, 1165–1202
   anatomy and functions of, 1166–1167, 1166f, 1167f
   in immune system, 1166, 1167f
   infections via, 338
   stem cells in, 85
Skin cancer
   basal cell carcinoma as, 1180–1181, 1181f, 1183f
   melanoma as, 1171–1175
      clinical features of, 1172, 1173f
      morphology of, 1172–1173, 1173f
      pathogenesis of, 1174–1175, 1174f
      prognostic factors for, 1173–1174
   radiation and, 311–312
   squamous cell carcinoma as, 1178–1180, 1179f
Skin disorders, 1167–1202
   due to adverse drug reactions, 415f, 416t
   benign epithelial tumors as, 1175–1178
      acanthosis nigricans as, 1175–1176
      adnexal (appendage) tumors as, 1176–1178, 1177f, 1178f
      epithelial cyst (wen) as, 1176
      fibroepithelial polyp as, 1176
      seborrheic keratoses as, 1175, 1175f
   blistering (bullous), 1192–1197, 1193f
      inflammatory, 1192–1196
         bullous pemphigoid as, 1193f, 1195–1196, 1196f
         dermatitis herpetiformis as, 1193f, 1196, 1197f
         pemphigus as, 1192–1195, 1193f–1195f
         noninflammatory, 1196–1197

Skin disorders (Continued)
      epidermolysis bullosa as, 1193f, 1196, 1198f
      porphyria as, 1196–1197, 1198f
   due to cancer, 321t, 322
   of epidermal appendages, 1197–1199
      acne vulgaris as, 1197–1198, 1199f
      rosacea as, 1198–1199
   of epidermal maturation, 1186
      ichthyosis as, 1186, 1186f
   familial cancer syndromes with cutaneous manifestations as, 1182t
   due to heroin use, 419
   due to infections, 1199–1202
      impetigo as, 1201–1202
      molluscum contagiosum as, 1201, 1201f
      superficial fungal, 1202, 1202f
      verrucae (warts) as, 1200–1201, 1200f
   inflammatory dermatoses as
      acute, 1187–1189
         acute eczematous dermatitis as, 1187–1189, 1188f
         erythema multiforme as, 1189, 1190f
         urticaria as, 1187, 1187f
      chronic, 1189–1192
         lichen planus as, 1191–1192, 1192f
         psoriasis as, 1190–1191, 1190f
         seborrheic dermatitis as, 1191
   due to occupational exposures, 409t
   oral manifestations of, 744t
   panniculitis as, 1199
      erythema nodosum and erythema induratum as, 1199
   of pigmentation and melanocytes, 1168–1175
      dysplastic nevi as, 1170–1171, 1170t, 1171f, 1172f
      freckles (ephelis) as, 1168
      lentigo as, 1168–1169
      melanocytic (pigmented) nevus (mole) as, 1169–1170, 1169f, 1170f, 1170t
      melanoma as, 1171–1175
         clinical features of, 1172, 1173f
         morphology of, 1172–1173, 1173f
         pathogenesis of, 1174–1175, 1174f
         prognostic factors for, 1173–1174
   premalignant and malignant epidermal tumors as, 1178–1181
      actinic keratosis as, 1178, 1179f
      basal cell carcinoma as, 1180–1181, 1181f, 1183f
      squamous cell carcinoma as, 1178–1180, 1179f
   in systemic lupus erythematosus, 214t, 219, 219f
   in systemic sclerosis, 224, 224f, 225f
   terminology for, 1167–1168
   tumors of cellular migrants to skin as, 1183–1186
      mastocytosis as, 1185–1186, 1186f
      mycosis fungoides as, 1184–1185, 1185f
   tumors of dermis as, 1182–1183
      benign fibrous histiocytoma as, 1182, 1184f
      dermatofibrosarcoma protuberans as, 1182–1183, 1184f
Skin lesions, in sarcoidosis, 702
Skin tags, 1176
   of vulva, 1012
Skin ulcers
   healing of, 104f
   in systemic sclerosis, 224, 225f
Skip lesions, in Crohn disease, 808f, 810
Skull fracture(s), 1287
Skull fracture contusion, 1287

SLAM (signaling lymphocytic activation molecule), in measles, 349
SLC22A4, in Crohn disease, 809
SLE. See Systemic lupus erythematosus (SLE).
Sleeping position, for infants, 473
Slit hemorrhages, 1295
SLL (small lymphocytic lymphoma), 601t, 603–605, 604f
SMA (spinal muscular atrophy), 1267–1268, 1267f, 1325
SMAD(s), 89, 294
SMAD2 gene, 287t
   in colorectal carcinoma, 823, 823f
SMAD4 gene, 287t, 294
   in colorectal carcinoma, 823, 823f
   in pancreatic carcinoma, 900, 901f
Small airway disease, 683t
Small cell carcinoma
   of bladder, 979
   of lung, 722, 723, 726–727, 726f
Small for gestational age (SGA), 454
Small interfering RNAs (siRNAs), 137
Small intestinal adenocarcinoma, celiac disease and, 796
Small intestine. See also Intestine(s).
   ischemic bowel disease of, 791–793, 792f
   obstruction of, 790–791, 791f
Small lymphocytic lymphoma (SLL), 601t, 603–605, 604f
Small round blue cell tumors, 475
Small round-cell tumors, of bone, 1232, 1233f
Smallpox, 337–338
Smegma, 982
SMN1 gene, in spinal muscle atrophy, 1267
SMN2 gene, in spinal muscle atrophy, 1267
SMO protein, in nevoid basal cell carcinoma syndrome, 1181, 1183f
Smog, 404
Smokeless tobacco, 410
Smokers' macrophages, 704, 704f, 705
Smoking. See Cigarette smoking.
Smoking-related interstitial diseases, 704–705, 704f
Smooth muscle cells, vascular, response to injury of, 491
Smooth muscle proliferation, in atherosclerosis, 501, 501f
Smooth muscle tumors, 1254
   leiomyomas as, 1254
   leiomyosarcoma as, 1254
Smouldering myeloma, 609, 611
Smudge cells, in chronic lymphocytic leukemia/small lymphocytic lymphoma, 604, 604f
SNAIL, in metastasis, 302
SNPs (single-nucleotide polymorphisms), 136, 176, 177, 178f, 326
SOD(s) (superoxide dismutases), 60
   free radical removal by, 21, 21f
SOD1, in amyotrophic lateral sclerosis, 1324
Sodium excretion, and blood pressure, 493–495
Sodium retention, edema due to, 112–113, 112t
Soft chancre, 366
Soft tissue tumors and tumor-like lesions, 1248–1255
   architectural patterns in, 1249t
   chromosomal and genetic abnormalities in, 1248, 1249t
   classification of, 1248, 1248t
   defined, 1248
   epidemiology of, 1248
   fatty, 1249–1250
      lipomas as, 1249–1250
      liposarcoma as, 1249t, 1250, 1250f
   fibrohistiocytic, 1252–1253

Soft tissue tumors and tumor-like lesions
     (Continued)
  fibrous, 1250–1252
     fibromatoses as, 1251–1252, 1252f
     fibrosarcoma as, 1252, 1252f
     myositis ossificans as, 1251, 1251f
     nodular fasciitis as, 1250–1251, 1250f
     reactive pseudosarcomatous proliferations
        as, 1250–1251, 1250f, 1251f
  morphology of, 1249t
  pathogenesis and general features of,
     1248–1249, 1249t
  of skeletal muscle, 1253–1254
     rhabdomyosarcoma as, 1249t, 1253–1254,
        1253f, 1254f
  of smooth muscle, 1254
     leiomyomas as, 1254
     leiomyosarcoma as, 1254
  synovial sarcoma as, 1249t, 1254–1255, 1255f
Soft-tissue callus, 1219
Soft-tissue changes, due to cancer, 321t, 322
Soft-tissue sarcomas, chromosomal and genetic
     abnormalities in, 1248, 1249t
Solid-pseudopapillary neoplasm, of pancreas,
     900
Solitary fibrous tumor, of pleura, 732–733, 732f
Solitary myeloma, 601t, 609, 611
Solitary neurofibroma, 1341
Solitary rectal ulcer syndrome, 815–816, 816f
Solitary thyroid nodule, 1118, 1119f
Soluble fms-like tyrosine kinase (sFlt1), in
     preeclampsia, 1056–1057
Somatostatin, production of, 1130, 1131f
Somatostatinomas, 1147
Somatotroph(s), 1098
Somatotroph adenomas, 1100t, 1104
Sonic hedgehog gene (SHH), in nevoid basal cell
     carcinoma syndrome, 1181, 1183f
Soot
  as air pollutant, 404t, 405
  occupational exposure to, 409
SOS, 90
Southern blotting, 176, 176f, 178
Space of Disse, 834
SPARC (secreted protein acidic and rich in
     cysteine), in extracellular matrix, 96
Specific atrial granules, 531
Specific granules, in inflammation, 63
Specific immunity, 185
Spectral karyotyping, 325
Spectrin
  defect in, 143t
  in hereditary spherocytosis, 642, 643f
Speed, abuse of, 419
Spermatic cord, tumors of, 987
Spermatocele, 993
Spermatocytic seminoma, 989
Spherocytosis, hereditary, 642–644, 643f, 644f
Sphingolipidoses, 151t
Spider angiomas, due to liver failure, 836
Spider cells, in cardiac rhabdomyomas, 584
Spider telangiectasia, 522
Spina bifida, 1284
Spinal cord infarction, 1295
Spinal cord trauma, 1290
Spinal dysraphism, 1284
Spinal muscular atrophy (SMA), 1267–1268,
     1267f, 1325
Spindle cell and epithelioid cell nevus, 1170t
SPINK1 (serine protease inhibitor Kazal type 1)
     gene, in pancreatitis, 894
Spinobulbar muscular atrophy, 168t
Spinocerebellar ataxias (SCAs), 168t,
     1323–1324

Spinocerebellar degenerations, 1323–1324
Spirochetes, 358t, 374–378, 374f–376f, 378f
Spironolactone bodies, 1152
Spitz nevus, 1170t
Spleen, 632–635
  accessory, 634–635
  amyloidosis of, 254
  in chronic myeloid leukemia, 627, 628f
  congenital anomalies of, 634–635
  functions of, 632–633
  in infectious mononucleosis, 356
  lardaceous, 254
  neoplasms of, 634
  normal anatomy of, 632, 633f
  sago, 254
  in sarcoidosis, 702
  in sickle cell disease, 647, 647f
  in systemic lupus erythematosus, 220
Splenic cords, 632, 633f
Splenic infarcts, 634, 634f
  in sickle cell disease, 647, 647f
Splenic insufficiency, 633
Splenic rupture, 635
Spleniculi, 634–635
Splenitis, nonspecific acute, 633–634
Splenomegaly, 633–634
  congestive, 634
     in right-sided heart failure, 536
  disorders associated with, 633, 633t
  leukopenia due to, 593
  in polycythemia vera, 629, 629f
  due to portal hypertension, 839
Spondylitis, rheumatoid, 1241
Spondyloarthritis, ankylosing, 1241
Spondyloarthropathies, seronegative, 1241
Spongiform changes, in prion diseases, 1308,
     1309, 1310f
Spongiform pustules, 1191
Spongiosis, 1168
Spongiotic dermatitis, 1188
Spontaneous abortion, 1053
Sporozoite, of malaria, 386–387, 387f
Sprue
  celiac, 794t, 795–796, 795f, 796f
     IgA nephropathy with, 931
  refractory, 796
  tropical, 794t, 796
SQSTM1 gene, in Paget disease, 1216
Squamocolumnar junction, of cervix, 1007,
     1008f
Squamous cell adhesion molecules, 1193f
Squamous cell carcinoma (SCC), 261, 264f
  of bladder, 979
  of cervix, 1021, 1022f
  conjunctival, 1349–1350
  of esophagus, 773–774, 773f
  head and neck, 745–748
  of larynx, 753, 753f
  of lung, 725–726, 725f, 726f
     precursor lesions for, 723, 724f
  of oral cavity, 745–748, 747f
  of penis, 984, 984f
  of skin, 1178–1180, 1179f
  of vagina, 1016–1017
  of vulva, 1012, 1014, 1014f
Squamous cell hyperplasia, of vulva, 1011f,
     1012
Squamous dysplasia
  of esophagus, 773
  of lung, 723, 724f
Squamous epithelial cells, 1166
Squamous intraepithelial lesion (SIL), of cervix,
     1019–1021, 1020f, 1020t, 1021f, 1021t,
     1023f

Squamous metaplasia
  of bladder, 976
  of cervix, 1008, 1019, 1019f
  of lactiferous ducts, 1069, 1069f
  of lung, 723, 724f
  due to vitamin A deficiency, 432–433
Squamous neoplastic lesions, of vulva,
     1012–1014, 1013f, 1014f
Squamous papillomas, 1176
  of esophagus, 774
  laryngeal, 752, 752f
  of vulva, 1012
SRY (sex-determining region Y gene), 164
SSPE (subacute sclerosing panencephalitis), 1306
ST (heat-stable toxin), 802
Stable tissues, 81
Staghorn calculi, 962
Staging, of cancer, 323
Stalk cells, in angiogenesis, 100, 101f
Staphylococcal infections, 357–359, 359f
Staphylococcal scalded-skin syndrome, 358
Staphylococcus aureus, 357–359
  endocarditis due to, 567, 568f
  impetigo due to, 1201
  methicillin-resistant, 359
  morphology of, 334f, 358–359, 359f
  pyogenic osteomyelitis due to, 1221
Staphylococcus aureus pneumonia, 712
Staphylococcus epidermidis, endocarditis due to,
     567
Staphylococcus pyogenes, 357
Staphyloma, 1350, 1367
Starry sky pattern, in Burkitt lymphoma, 608,
     608f
Stasis thrombi, 124
STAT(s) (signal transducers and activation of
     transcription), 90, 91f
Statin(s), 497
Statin-induced myopathy, 1275
Status asthmaticus, 688, 691, 692
Status marmoratus, 1287
Steatocystoma
  multiplex, 1176
  simplex, 1176
Steatohepatitis
  alcoholic, 857f, 858, 858f
  drug- and toxin-induced, 856t
  nonalcoholic, 860, 861
     obesity and, 442
Steatorrhea, 794
Steatosis, 13, 33–34, 34f
  alcoholic, 857–858, 857f, 859–860
  in cystic fibrosis, 469
  drug- and toxin-induced, 856t
  nonalcoholic, 860–861, 861f
  in viral hepatitis, 852–853
  in Wilson disease, 864
Steel factor receptor, proto-oncogene for, 281t
Stein-Leventhal syndrome, 1039–1040, 1039f
Stellate cells, in cirrhosis, 837–838, 837f
Stem cell(s), 82–86
  adult (somatic), 84–85
  cancer, 267–268
  in control of normal cell proliferation, 81f
  embryonic, 82, 82f, 83
     in therapeutic cloning, 84, 84f
  generation and differentiation of, 82, 82f
  hematopoietic, 84–85
  interfollicular, 85
  limbal, 86
  lineage committed, 82f
  multipotent, 82f
  neural, 85
  niches for, 82, 83f

Stem cell(s) *(Continued)*
  pluripotent, 82, 82f
    induced, 82, 84, 84f
  in tissue homeostasis, 85–86
  in tissue proliferative activity, 81
  totipotent, 82f
Stem cell (steel) factor receptor, proto-oncogene for, 281t
Stem cell leukemia, 626t
Stem cell therapy, 84, 84f
Stenosis, of gastrointestinal tract, 765
Steroid(s), anabolic, adverse effects of, 415–416
Steroid hormone receptors, 91, 91f
Steroid myopathy, 1275
Stevens-Johnson syndrome, 1189
Stewart-Treves syndrome, 1093
STI(s) (sexually transmitted infections), 341–342, 341t
Stickler syndrome, 1211t
Stimulants, abuse of, 418t, 419
Stochastic differentiation, 82
Stomach, 774–790
  acute ulceration of, 775–776, 776t
  anatomy of, 774
  dysplasia of, 781–782
  gastritis of
    acute, 774–776, 775f
    autoimmune, 778–779, 778t, 779f
    chronic, 776–782
    cystica, 782, 782t
    eosinophilic, 780
    granulomatous, 780
    Helicobacter pylori, 776–778, 777f, 778t
    lymphocytic, 780
    uncommon forms of, 779–780
  hypertrophic gastropathies of, 782–783, 782t, 783f
  Ménétrier disease of, 782, 782t
  mucosal atrophy and metaplasia of, 781
  peptic ulcer disease of, 780–781, 781f
  polyps of, 783
    fundic gland, 782t, 783, 784f
    inflammatory and hyperplastic, 782t, 783, 784f
  reactive gastropathy of, 779
  tumors of, 784–790
    adenocarcinoma as, 784–786, 785f, 786f
    adenoma as, 782t, 784, 784f
    carcinoid, 787–789, 788f, 788t
    gastrointestinal stromal tumor as, 789–790, 789f
    lymphoma as, 786–787, 787f
    watermelon, 779
    Zollinger-Ellison syndrome of, 780, 782–783, 782t
Stomatitis, recurrent herpetic, 743
Stop codon, 138, 139f
Storage pool disorders, 670
Strangulation, intestinal, 790
Strategic infarcts, 1319
Strawberry type hemangioma, 520, 521f
Streak ovaries, 166
Streptococcal infections, 359–360, 360f
  glomerulonephritis after, 917–920, 919f
Streptococcal pharyngitis, 359, 360
  rheumatic fever due to, 566
Streptococcal sore throats, 750–751
Streptococcus agalactiae, 359
Streptococcus aureus, pharyngitis and tonsillitis due to, 750
Streptococcus mutans, 359, 360
Streptococcus pneumoniae, 359, 360
  morphology of, 334f
Streptococcus pneumoniae pneumonia, 711

Streptococcus pyogenes, 359–360
Streptococcus viridans, endocarditis due to, 567, 568f
Streptokinase, 120
Stress
  cellular responses to (*See* Cellular response(s), to stress and noxious stimuli)
  endoplasmic reticulum, 25, 31
  oxidative, cell injury due to, 18f, 20–22, 20t, 21f
Stress ulcers, 775, 776
Striatonigral degeneration, 1321
Stroke. *See* Cerebrovascular disease(s).
Stromal hyperthecosis, 1039f, 1040
Stromal microenvironment, and carcinogenesis, 303
Stromal nodule, of endometrium, 1035
Stromal sarcoma, of endometrium, 1035
Stromal tumors
  of breast, 1091–1093, 1091f, 1092f
  of endometrium, 1035
Strongyloides, enterocolitis due to, 805, 805f
Strongyloides stercoralis, 391–392, 392f
Strongyloidiasis, 391–392, 392f
Structural proteins, defects in, 143t, 144–147, 146f
Struma lymphomatosa, in Hashimoto thyroiditis, 1111
Struvite stones, 962, 962t
Stunned myocardium, 553, 554f
Sturge-Weber syndrome, 522
  glaucoma in, 1354
Subacute cerebellar degeneration, in paraneoplastic syndrome, 1340
Subacute endocarditis, 567
Subacute necrotizing encephalopathy, 1328
Subacute neuronal injury, 1281
Subacute sclerosing panencephalitis (SSPE), 1306
Subacute sensory neuropathy, in paraneoplastic syndrome, 1340
Subaortic stenosis, 545
Subarachnoid hemorrhage, 1297–1298, 1297f, 1298f
Subareolar abscess, recurrent, 1069, 1069f
Subchondral cyst, 1236f
Subcorneal blister, 1193f
Subcutaneous edema, 113
Subcutaneous tissues, in right-sided heart failure, 536
Subdural empyema, 1300–1301
Subdural hematoma, 1289–1290, 1289f, 1290f
Subendocardial infarction, 550, 551f
Subependymomas, 1335
Subepidermal blister, 1193f
Subfalcine herniation, 1283, 1283f
Subperiosteal abscesses, 1222
Subperiosteal chondromas, 1227
Substance P, in inflammation, 63
Substrate reduction therapy, for lysosomal storage diseases, 149–150
Subventricular zone (SVZ), stem cells in, 85
Sudden cardiac death (SCD), 546, 558–559
Sudden death, due to heroin, 418
Sudden infant death syndrome (SIDS), 471–473, 471t
Sulfatase deficiency, multiple, 151t
Sulfatidoses, 151t
Sulfonylurea receptor (SUR1), 1133, 1133f
Sulfur dioxide
  as air pollutant, 404t, 405
  lung diseases due to, 697t
Superantigens, 132, 344
Superior conjunctival fornix, 1348f, 1349

Superior tarsus, 1348f
Superior vena cava syndrome, 519, 585
Superoxide, in phagocytosis, 53, 53f
Superoxide anion
  cell injury due to, 20
  in inflammation, 60
Superoxide dismutases (SODs), 60
  free radical removal by, 21, 21f
Suppurative inflammation, 68, 69f, 347, 347f
Suprabasal blister, 1193f
  acantholytic, 1194, 1194f
Supravalvular aortic stenosis, 545
SUR1 (sulfonylurea receptor), 1133, 1133f
Surface epithelial tumors, of ovaries, 1040t, 1041–1047, 1041f
Surfactant
  composition of, 456
  exogenous, prophylactic administration of, 457
  synthesis of, 456
Surfactant deficiency, neonatal respiratory distress syndrome due to, 456
Surfactant protein B (SF-B) deficiency, in pulmonary alveolar proteinosis, 705
Surfactant-associated proteins, 456
Susceptibility phenotype, for congenital anomalies, 452
Sustentacular cells, in carotid body tumor, 755–756, 755f
Sv (sievert), 423
SVZ (subventricular zone), stem cells in, 85
Sweat glands, 1166, 1166f
  in cystic fibrosis, 466, 467f, 470–471
Swiss-cheese septum, 541
Sydenham chorea, in rheumatic fever, 566
Sympathetic ophthalmia, 1356, 1356f
Synarthroses, 1235
Synchondroses, 1235
Syncytia-inducing (SI) virus, 241
Syncytiotrophoblast, 1053f
Syndactyly, 449f
Syndecan, in extracellular matrix, 98f
Syndromatic paucity of bile ducts, 870
Syndrome, 450
Syndrome of inappropriate antidiuretic hormone secretion (SIADH), 1106
  due to cancer, 321t
Syndrome X, 1146
Synovial cyst, 1247
Synovial fluid, 1235
Synovial joints, 1235
Synovial membrane, 1235
Synovial sarcoma, 1249t, 1254–1255, 1255f
Synoviocytes, 1235
Synovitis
  due to hemochromatosis, 862
  pigmented villonodular, 1247, 1247f
Synpolydactyly, 1211t
α-Synuclein, 1320, 1321–1322
Syphilis, 374–377
  cardiovascular, 375, 376
  causative agent for, 374, 374f
  chancre in, 374, 375–376, 376f
  condylomata lata in, 374, 376
  congenital, 375, 376–377
  epidemiology of, 374
  epididymitis and orchitis due to, 986–987
  general paresis due to, 375
  granulomatous inflammation in, 73t
  gummas in, 375, 376, 376f
  morphology of, 375–377, 376f
  neuro-, 375, 376, 376f, 1301–1302
  osteochondritis and perichondritis in, 376
  pathogenesis of, 377

Syphilis (Continued)
  primary, 374, 375–376, 376f
  secondary, 374, 376
  serologic tests for, 375
  skeletal, 1223
  tertiary, 374–375, 376, 376f
    benign, 375, 376, 376f
Syringobulbia, 1286
Syringomas, 1177
Syringomyelia, 1286
Syrinx, 1286
Systemic disease, oral manifestations of, 743, 744t
Systemic immune complex disease, 204–205, 204f
Systemic lupus erythematosus (SLE), 213–221
  autoantibodies in, 204t, 213–215, 215t
  clinical features of, 204t, 217t, 220–221
  diagnostic criteria for, 213, 214t
  endocarditis of, 124, 220, 220f, 567f, 569
  epidemiology of, 213
  etiology and pathogenesis of, 215–217, 216f
  morphology of, 217–220, 217t, 218f–220f
Systemic mastocytosis, 626t
Systemic sclerosis, 215t, 223–225, 223f–225f
  pulmonary involvement in, 696
Systolic dysfunction, 533
Systolic failure, 536

T

T lymphocytes
  activation of, 186, 186f, 194f, 195, 195f
  anergy of, 209–210
  antigen recognition by, 186, 186f, 193–195, 194f
  in chronic inflammation, 72, 73f
  cytotoxic
    antitumor effect of, 318
    in cell-mediated cytotoxicity, 207–208
    in immune evasion, 320
    in immune response, 185f, 186
    in transplant rejection, 226, 227f
    tumor antigens recognized by, 316, 317f
  effector, 190, 190f, 194f
    responses of differentiated, 207, 207f, 208f
  in glomerular injury, 915
  helper
    in delayed-type hypersensitivity, 205, 206f
    in immediate hypersensitivity, 199, 199f
    in immune response, 185f, 186, 195, 195f
    proliferation and differentiation of, 206–207
  in immune response, 185f, 186–187, 186f
  in immunological tolerance, 209–211, 210f
  in lymphoid organs, 189, 189f
  naive, 190, 190f, 194f
  natural killer, 186
  proliferation and differentiation of, 194f
  recirculation of, 190, 190f
  regulatory, 210–211, 210f
T$_3$ (triiodothyronine), 1107, 1108f
T$_4$ (thyroxine), 1107, 1108f
TA (tricuspid atresia), 543
Tabes dorsalis, 1302
Taenia saginata, 392
Taenia solium, 392, 806
Taeniae coli, 815
Takayasu arteritis, 513–514, 514f
T-ALL (T-cell acute lymphoblastic leukemia/lymphoma), 601t, 602–603
  genetic basis for, 305t
Tapeworms, 392–393, 392f, 806
TAPVC (total anomalous pulmonary venous connection), 543–544

Target fiber, 1260
Target lesions, in aspergillosis, 385
Targeted therapy, 281
Targetoid lesion, 1189, 1190f
Tattooing, 36
Tau mutations, frontotemporal dementia with parkinsonism linked to, 1317–1318
Tau protein
  in Alzheimer disease, 1314, 1315f, 1317
  in corticobasal degeneration, 1319
Tay-Sachs disease, 139f, 150–152, 151t, 152f, 1326
  cherry-red spot in, 151–152, 1362, 1364f
TBX1, in congenital heart disease, 539, 539t
TBX5, in congenital heart disease, 539, 539t
TBX20, in congenital heart disease, 539, 539t
T-cell acute lymphoblastic leukemia/lymphoma (T-ALL), 601t, 602–603
  genetic basis for, 305t
T-cell immunodeficiency, in HIV infection, 240–241, 241f, 242t
T-cell leukemia, adult, 601t, 615—616
T-cell lymphoma
  adult, 601t, 615—616
  cutaneous, 1184–1185, 1185f
  enteropathy-associated, 796
  extranodal, 601t, 616
  peripheral, unspecified, 601t, 614–615, 615f
T-cell neoplasms
  origin of, 599f
  peripheral, 598t, 601t, 614–616, 615f
  precursor, 598t, 600–603, 601t, 602f
T-cell receptor (TCR), 186, 186f
T-cell–mediated hypersensitivity, 205–208, 206f–208f, 206t
T-cell–mediated reactions, in transplant rejection, 226–227, 227f
TCF7L2 (transcription factor 7–like-2), in type 2 diabetes mellitus, 1136
TCIRG1 gene, in osteopetrosis, 1213, 1213f
TDS (testicular dysgenesis syndrome), 988
TdT (terminal deoxynucleotidyltransferase), in acute lymphoblastic leukemia/lymphoma, 602
Teardrop-shaped red cells, in primary myelofibrosis, 630
Teeth
  anatomy of, 740, 740f
  disorders of, 740–741
  Hutchinson, 377
Telangiectasia(s), 522
  capillary, of brain, 1298
  hereditary hemorrhagic, 522, 666
  spider, 522
Telomerase, 40, 40f
  in aplastic anemia, 663
  in carcinogenesis, 296–297, 297f
Telomere(s), 40, 40f
  alternative lengthening of, 297
Telomere shortening, 40, 40f, 296, 297f
Temporal arteritis, 512–513, 513f
Tenascins, in extracellular matrix, 97
Tendon sheath, giant-cell tumor of, 1247, 1247f
Tenosynovial giant-cell tumor, 1247, 1247f
Tensile strength, recovery of, in wound healing, 105–106
Tension pneumothorax, 679
Teratogens, 452
Teratoid/rhabdoid tumor, atypical, 1337
Teratoma(s), 261–262, 262f
  cystic, 262, 262f
    of ovaries, 1047–1048, 1048f
  in infants and children, 474, 474f

Teratoma(s) (Continued)
  of ovaries, 1047–1048, 1048f
  testicular, 990–991, 991f
Terminal bile ducts, 835
Terminal bronchioles, 678
Terminal deoxynucleotidyltransferase (TdT), in acute lymphoblastic leukemia/lymphoma, 602
Terminal hepatic veins, 834, 834f
Terminally differentiated cells, 80
Testicular dysgenesis syndrome (TDS), 988
Testicular femininization, 167
Testicular lymphoma, 993
Testicular tumor(s), 987–993, 987t
  germ cell, 987–992, 987t
    choriocarcinoma as, 990, 990f
    classification and pathogenesis of, 987t, 988
    clinical features of, 991–992
    embryonal carcinoma as, 989, 990f
    environmental factors and genetic predisposition to, 987–988
    mixed, 991
    nonseminomatous, 992
    seminoma as, 988–989, 988f, 989f
    spermatocytic, 989
    teratoma as, 990–991, 991f
    yolk sac tumor as, 989–990
  gonadoblastoma as, 993
  lymphoma as, 993
  of sex cord–gonadal stroma, 992
  spermatic cord and para-, 987
Testis(es), 984–993
  atrophy of, 985–986
  congenital anomalies of, 984–985, 985f
  in hemochromatosis, 862–863
  inflammation of, 986–987, 986f
  regressive changes of, 985–986
  torsion of, 987, 987f
  tumors of, 987–993, 987t
    germ cell, 987–992, 988f–991f
    gonadoblastoma as, 993
    lymphoma as, 993
    of sex cord–gonadal stroma, 992
    spermatic cord and paratesticular, 987
  tunica vaginalis of, 993
  undescended, 984–985, 985f
  vascular disorders of, 987, 987f
Tetanus, 379
Tetany, hypocalcemic, 433, 1130
2,3,7,8-Tetrachlorodibenzo-p-dioxin TCDD, Dioxin), occupational exposure to, 409–410
Tetrahydrobiopterin (BH$_4$), 463, 463f
Δ^9-Tetrahydrocannabinol (THC), 419–420
Tetrahydrofolic acid (FH$_4$), 657, 657f, 658
Tetralogy of Fallot (TOF), 542–543, 542f
TFPI (tissue factor pathway inhibitor), 116, 117f, 119f, 120
TfR2 (transferrin receptor 2), 862
TGA (transposition of the great arteries), 542f, 543, 543f
TGF. See Transforming growth factor (TGF).
TGFA gene, 281t
T$_H$ (helper T) lymphocytes
  in delayed-type hypersensitivity, 205, 206f
  in immediate hypersensitivity, 199, 199f
  in immune response, 185f, 186, 195, 195f
  proliferation and differentiation of, 206–207
T$_H$1 cells
  in delayed-type hypersensitivity, 206–207, 206f
  in inflammatory bowel disease, 809
  in multiple sclerosis, 1310
  in tuberculosis, 368

T$_H$2 cells
  in asthma, 689, 690f
  in immediate hypersensitivity, 199, 199f, 200
T$_H$17 cells
  in delayed-type hypersensitivity, 206–207, 206f
  in inflammatory bowel disease, 809
  in multiple sclerosis, 1310
  in rheumatoid arthritis, 1238
Thalassemia(s), 648–652
  α-, 651–652, 652t
  β-, 648–651
    clinical syndromes of, 649, 652t
    intermedia, 649, 652t
    major, 649–651, 650f, 651f, 652t
    minor, 651, 652t
    molecular pathogenesis of, 648–649, 649f, 650f
  epidemiology of, 648
  genetic basis for, 144, 652t
Thalassemia trait
  α-, 651–652, 652t
  β-, 649, 652t
Thalidomide, as teratogen, 452
Thanatophoric dwarfism, 1210, 1211t
THC (Δ^9-tetrahydrocannabinol), 419–420
Theca lutein hyperplasia of pregnancy, 1040
Thecomas, ovarian, 1051, 1051f
Thermal burns, 421–422
Thermal injury, 421–422
Thermogenesis, leptin in, 440
Thiamine, functions of, 438t
Thiamine deficiency, 438t
  due to alcoholism, 414
  CNS effects of, 1328
  peripheral neuropathy due to, 1266
Thimerosal, 408
Thin basement membrane lesion, 932
Third ventricle, colloid cyst of, 1335
Thomas, Lewis, 316
Thoracic aortic aneurysm, 508
Thrombasthenia, Glanzmann, 118, 118f
Thrombin
  in cellular activation, 121f
  in coagulation cascade, 118, 119f, 673
  in hemostasis, 121f
  in inflammation, 65f, 120
Thromboangiitis obliterans, 517, 517f
Thrombocythemia, essential, 626t, 629–630, 630f
Thrombocytopenia
  due to antibody-mediated hypersensitivity, 203
  bleeding related to, 667–670, 669f
  causes of, 667, 667t
  dilutional, 667
  drug-induced, 668–669
  heparin-induced, 123, 668–669
  HIV-associated, 669
  immune, 667
  immunodeficiency with, 235
  petechiae due to, 114, 115f
Thrombocytopenic purpura
  autoimmune, 203t
  immune
    acute, 668
    chronic, 667–668
  thrombotic, 669–670, 669t
    renal disease in, 952, 953–954
Thrombocytosis, essential, 626t, 629–630, 630f
Thromboembolic complications, of artificial heart valves, 570, 571f
Thromboembolic disease, 115–129
  disseminated intravascular coagulation as, 125
  embolism in, 125–127, 126f–128f

Thromboembolic disease (Continued)
  infarction due to, 127–129, 128f, 129f
  normal hemostasis and, 115–120
  thrombosis in (See Thrombosis)
Thromboembolism, 126
  hormone replacement therapy and, 415
  oral contraceptives and, 415
  systemic, 126
Thrombomodulin, 116, 117f, 673
Thrombophilias
  during pregnancy, 455–456
  in thrombosis, 122–123, 122t
Thrombophlebitis, 519
  migratory, 125, 520
    due to cancer, 321t, 322
    due to pancreatic carcinoma, 903
Thromboplastin
  in coagulation cascade, 119, 119f
  in hemostasis, 115
Thromboplastin time, partial, 120, 666
Thrombosis, 121–125
  alterations in normal blood flow in, 121–122
  in antiphospholipid antibody syndrome, 123
  arterial, 124, 125
  of atherosclerotic plaque, 502–503, 506
  cardiac, 125
  defined, 115
  endothelial injury in, 121
  fate of thrombus in, 124–125, 125f
  in heparin-induced thrombocytopenia syndrome, 123
  hepatic vein, 872–873, 873f
  hypercoagulability in, 122–123, 122t
  inferior vena cava, 873
  morphology of, 123–124, 124f
  portal vein, 871
    congestive splenomegaly due to spontaneous, 634
  venous, 124, 125
  Virchow's triad in, 121, 122f
Thrombospondins, in extracellular matrix, 96
Thrombotic endocarditis, nonbacterial, 124
Thrombotic microangiopathies, 669–670, 669t
  renal disease due to, 952–954, 952f
Thrombotic occlusion, cerebral infarction due to, 1293
Thrombotic thrombocytopenic purpura (TTP), 669–670, 669t
  renal disease in, 952, 953–954
Thromboxane A$_2$ (TXA$_2$)
  in inflammation, 58f, 59
  in platelet aggregation, 118
Thrombus(i)
  arterial, 124
  clinical consequences of, 125
  fate of, 124–125, 125f
  formation of, 115, 116f
  morphology of, 123–124, 124f
  mural, 124, 124f, 546f
    due to myocardial infarction, 557
  in nonbacterial thrombotic endocarditis, 568
  occlusive, 546f
  red, 124
  stasis, 124
Thrush, 743
Thymic aplasia, 635
Thymic carcinoma, 636–637
Thymic cysts, 635
Thymic hyperplasia, 635–636
  follicular, 635
Thymic hypoplasia, 234, 635
Thymomas, 636–637, 636f

Thymus, 635–637
  developmental disorders of, 635
  embryology of, 635
  functions of, 635
  normal anatomy of, 635
Thyroglossal duct, 1126
Thyroglossal duct cyst, 755, 1126
Thyroid adenomas, 264f, 1118–1119, 1119f
Thyroid agenesis, 1110
Thyroid autonomy, 1107, 1118
Thyroid carcinoma, 1119–1126, 1120f
  anaplastic (undifferentiated), 1121, 1124
  epidemiology of, 1119
  follicular, 1120–1121, 1123–1124, 1123f, 1124f
  medullary, 1121, 1124–1126, 1125f
    in MEN-2, 1162–1163
  papillary, 1120, 1121–1122, 1121f
  pathogenesis of, 1120–1121
  subtypes of, 1119
Thyroid disorder(s), 1108–1126
  congenital anomalies as, 1126
  goiter as, 1107, 1116–1118
    diffuse nontoxic (simple), 1116, 1117f
    dyshormonogenetic, 1110
    multinodular, 1116–1118, 1117f
  Graves disease as, 1109, 1109f, 1114–1116, 1115f
  hyperthyroidism as, 1108–1109, 1108t, 1109f
  hypothyroidism as, 1109–1111, 1110t
    cretinism due to, 1110–1111
    myxedema due to, 1111
  neoplastic, 1118–1126
    adenomas as, 1118–1119, 1119f
    carcinomas as, 1119–1126, 1120f, 1121f, 1123f–1125f
  thyroiditis as, 1111–1114
    defined, 1111
    Hashimoto, 1111–1113, 1112f
    infectious, 1111
    subacute (granulomatous, de Quervain), 1113, 1113f
    subacute lymphocytic (painless), 1113–1114
Thyroid gland, 1107–1126
  anatomy of, 1107–1108, 1108f
Thyroid growth-stimulating immunoglobulins, in Grave disease, 1114
Thyroid hormone(s), mechanisms of action of, 1107, 1108f
Thyroid hormone receptor (TR), 1107, 1108f
Thyroid hormone resistance syndrome, 1110
Thyroid hormone response elements (TREs), 1107, 1108f
Thyroid hypoplasia, 1110
Thyroid nodule, solitary, 1118, 1119f
Thyroid ophthalmopathy, 1347, 1347f
Thyroid peroxidase (TPO) gene, 1110
Thyroid storm, 1109
Thyroid transcription factor (TTF-2) gene, 1110
Thyroiditis, 1111–1114
  defined, 1111
  Hashimoto, 1111–1113, 1112f
  infectious, 1111
  postpartum, 1114
  Riedel, 1114
  subacute
    granulomatous, de Quervain, 1113, 1113f
    lymphocytic (painless), 1113–1114
Thyroid-stimulating hormone (TSH), 1107, 1108f
  in hyperthyroidism, 1109
  in myxedema, 1111

Thyroid-stimulating hormone (TSH)-binding inhibitor immunoglobulins, in Grave disease, 1114
Thyroid-stimulating hormone (TSH)-producing adenomas, 1100t, 1105
Thyroid-stimulating immunoglobulin, in Grave disease, 1114
Thyrotoxic myopathy, 1275
Thyrotoxicosis, 1108–1109, 1108t, 1109f
Thyrotroph(s), 1098
Thyrotroph adenomas, 1100t, 1105
Thyrotropin (TSH), 1107, 1108f
    in hyperthyroidism, 1109
    in myxedema, 1111
Thyrotropin (TSH)-binding inhibitor immunoglobulins, in Grave disease, 1114
Thyrotropin (TSH)-producing adenomas, 1100t, 1105
Thyrotropin receptor (TSHR) gene, 1110
Thyrotropin-releasing hormone (TRH), 1107, 1108f
Thyroxine (T$_4$), 1107, 1108f
T-ICs (tumor-initiating cells), 267–268
Tie2, in angiogenesis, 101
Tigered effect, 34
Tiling arrays, 326
Tin oxide, lung diseases due to, 697t
Tinea, 335
    barbae, 1202
    capitis, 1202
    corporis, 1202, 1202f
    cruris, 1202
    pedis, 1202
    versicolor, 1202
Tingible bodies, 595, 596f
Tip cell, in angiogenesis, 100, 101f
Tissue damage, in inflammation, 66t, 71, 72f
Tissue factor
    in coagulation cascade, 119, 119f
    in hemostasis, 115, 117
Tissue factor pathway inhibitor (TFPI), 116, 117f, 119f, 120
Tissue growth, 80–86, 81f
Tissue homeostasis, stem cells in, 85–86
Tissue necrosis, 348
Tissue proliferative activity, 81–82
Tissue regeneration, 79–80, 80f, 81f
    mechanisms of, 92–94, 93f
Tissue repair, 79–80, 80f, 81f, 98–108
    angiogenesis in, 99–102, 99f, 100t, 101f
    cutaneous, 102–106, 103f–105f, 104t
    local and systemic factors that influence, 106
    pathologic aspects of, 106–108, 106f–108f
Tissue-type plasminogen activator (tPA), 115, 116, 116f, 120, 121f
TLRs. See Toll-like receptor(s) (TLRs).
TMPRSS2 gene, in prostate adenocarcinoma, 306
TNF. See Tumor necrosis factor (TNF).
TNM staging system, 323
Tobacco smoke, as indoor air pollutant, 405
Tobacco smoking. See Cigarette smoking.
Tolerance, immunological, 209–211, 210f
Tolerance-breaking drugs, immunohemolytic anemia due to, 654
Toll-like receptor(s) (TLRs)
    in inflammation, 45, 51, 52f
    in innate immunity, 184
    in septic shock, 130
    in systemic lupus erythematosus, 216
Toll-like receptor-4 (TLR-4), in preterm labor, 454
Tongue, tumor-forming amyloid of, 254, 255
Tonsillar herniation, 1283f, 1284

Tonsillitis, 750–751
    follicular, 750
Tooth
    anatomy of, 740, 740f
    disorders of, 740–741
Tooth decay, 740
Tophaceous arthritis, 1243, 1244, 1245f, 1246
Tophaceous gout, 1243, 1244, 1245f, 1246
Tophus(i), 1243, 1244, 1245f
TORCH infections, perinatal, 459
Torsion, testicular, 987, 987f
Total anomalous pulmonary venous connection (TAPVC), 543–544
Total-body irradiation, effects of, 425, 425t
Toxemia of pregnancy, 455
Toxic agents, chronic inflammation due to, 70
Toxic cell injury, 24–25
Toxic disorders, CNS effects of, 1329–1330, 1329f
Toxic epidermal necrolysis, 1189
Toxic granules, in leukocytosis, 594, 594f
Toxic megacolon, 812
Toxic metabolites, 403, 403f
Toxic myopathies, 1275
Toxic neuropathies, 1266
Toxic shock syndrome (TSS), 132, 357–358
Toxicity, of chemical and physical agents, 402–403, 402f, 403f
Toxicology, 402
Toxin(s)
    cell injury due to, 11
    and dilated cardiomyopathy, 573
Toxin-induced interstitial nephritis, 944–946, 945f, 946f, 947t
Toxin-induced liver disease, 856–857, 856t
Toxocara canis, 336
Toxoplasma gondii, 335
Toxoplasmosis
    in AIDS, 246
    cerebral, 1306–1308, 1307f
tPA (tissue-type plasminogen activator), 115, 116, 116f, 120, 121f
TPO (thyroid peroxidase) gene, 1110
TR (thyroid hormone receptor), 1107, 1108f
Trabecular meshwork, 1346f, 1354f
Tracheoesophageal fistula, 765, 765f
Trachoma, conjunctival scarring due to, 1349
Traction diverticulum, 767
Transcervical infections, perinatal, 458
Transcobalamin II, 656, 656f
Transcription factor(s)
    oncogenes for, 284
    in signal transduction systems, 90, 91–92, 91f
Transcription factor 7–like-2 (TCF7L2), in type 2 diabetes mellitus, 1136
Transcription factor mutations, acute leukemia due to, 597f
Transcriptional activators, proto-oncogenes for, 281t
Transcytosis, in inflammation, 47, 47f
Transdifferentiation, 82, 85
Transferrin, 60, 659
Transferrin receptor 2 (TfR2), 862
Transformation zone, of cervix, 1007, 1008f
Transforming growth factor α (TGF-α)
    in Ménétrier disease, 782
    proto-oncogene for, 281t
    in tissue regeneration and wound healing, 87t, 88
Transforming growth factor β (TGF-β)
    in angiogenesis, 101
    in fibrosis, 108
    in idiopathic pulmonary fibrosis, 694–695, 694f

Transforming growth factor β (TGF-β) (Continued)
    in Marfan syndrome, 145
    oncogenes for, 280
    in tissue regeneration and wound healing, 87t, 89, 103–104
Transforming growth factor β (TGF-β) pathway, tumor suppressor genes in, 294
Transforming growth factor β (TGF-β) receptor gene, 287t
    in colorectal carcinoma, 824, 824f
Transforming growth factor β1 (TGFB1), in cystic fibrosis, 468
Transfusion(s), thrombocytopenia due to, 667
Transfusion reactions, 202
Transit amplifying cells, 84
Transitional cell carcinoma, of ovaries, 1046
Translocations, 160f, 161
    in carcinogenesis, 305–306
    in diagnosis of cancer, 324–325
    white cell neoplasia due to, 596–597
Transmigration, of leukocytes through endothelium, 48f, 50
Transmissible spongiform encephalopathies, 1308–1309, 1308f, 1310f
Transmural infarction
    of bowel, 792, 793
    myocardial, 547, 550, 551f
Transplacental infections, 459, 459f
Transplant rejection, 226–230
    acute, 228–229, 228f
    cardiac, 585, 585f
    chronic, 229, 229f
    hematopoietic stem cell, 230
    hyperacute, 227, 228, 228f
    kidney, 228–230, 228f, 229f
    liver, 874, 874f
    lung, 720–721, 721f
    mechanisms of, 226–228, 227f
    other solid organ, 230
    prevention of, 229–230
Transplant-associated Kaposi sarcoma, 523, 524
Transport systems, genetic defects in, 143t, 144
Transposition of the great arteries (TGA), 542f, 543, 543f
Trans-synaptic degeneration, 1281
Transtentorial herniation, 1283–1284, 1283f
Transthyretin (TTR)
    in amyloidosis, 251, 251f, 252
    in familial amyloid polyneuropathies, 1263
Transthyretin amyloid (ATTR), 251, 251f, 252
Transudate, 46, 46f
Trauma
    central nervous system, 1287–1290
        concussion as, 1287
        diffuse axonal injury as, 1288
        parenchymal injuries as, 1287–1288, 1288f
        sequelae of, 1290
        skull fractures as, 1287
        spinal cord, 1290
        vascular, 1288–1290, 1289f, 1290f
    inflammation due to, 45
Traumatic neuroma, 1266, 1267f
Traumatic neuropathies, 1266–1267, 1267f
Traveler's diarrhea, 802, 807
TRE(s) (thyroid hormone response elements), 1107, 1108f
Trench foot, 422
Treponema pallidum, 341t, 374–377, 374f
    granulomatous inflammation due to, 73t
    skeletal infection with, 1223
Treponema pertenue, skeletal infection with, 1223
Treponemal antibody tests, 375

Treponemal infections, 358t, 374–378, 374f–376f, 378f

TRH (thyrotropin-releasing hormone), 1107, 1108f

Trichilemmal cyst, 1176

Trichilemmomas, 1176

Trichinella spiralis, 393, 393f

Trichinosis, 393, 393f

Trichoepithelioma, 1177, 1177f

Trichomonas vaginalis, 335, 341t, 1009

Trichuris trichiura, enterocolitis due to, 806

Tricuspid atresia (TA), 543

Triiodothyronine (T₃), 1107, 1108f

Trinucleotide-repeat mutations, 139, 167–171, 168f, 168t

Triphenyltetrazolium chloride staining, in myocardial infarction, 551, 552f

Triple stones, 962, 962t

Triplet-repeat mutations, 139, 167–171, 168f, 168t

Trisomy(ies), 159, 162

Trisomy 13, 162, 163f

Trisomy 18, 162, 163f

Trisomy 21, 161–162, 161f, 163f

Triton tumors, 1341

Tropheryma whippelii, 803–804

Trophozoites, of malaria, 387, 387f

Tropical eosinophilia, 704

pulmonary, 395

Tropical sprue, 794t, 796

Tropism, of viruses, 342

Troponins, in myocardial infarction, 555, 555f

Trousseau phenomenon, due to cancer, 321t, 322

Trousseau sign, 520

due to hypocalcemia, 1130

due to pancreatic carcinoma, 903

Trousseau syndrome, 125

Truncus arteriosus, persistent, 543

Trypanosoma, 335

Trypanosoma brucei gambiense, 390

Trypanosoma brucei rhodesiense, 390

Trypanosoma cruzi, 391

Trypanosomiasis

African, 390, 390f

American, 391

TSC1 gene, 1342

TSC2 gene, 1342

TSH. *See* Thyroid-stimulating hormone (TSH); Thyrotropin (TSH).

TSHR (thyrotropin receptor) gene, 1110

TSS (toxic shock syndrome), 132, 357–358

TTF-2 (thyroid transcription factor) gene, 1110

TTP (thrombotic thrombocytopenic purpura), 669–670, 669t

renal disease in, 952, 953–954

TTR (transthyretin)

in amyloidosis, 251, 251f, 252

in familial amyloid polyneuropathies, 1263

Tubal pregnancy, 1053

Tuberculin reaction, 207, 207f

Tuberculoma, 1301

Tuberculosis, 366–372

in AIDS, 246, 369–370

of brain, 1301

clinical features of, 368–370, 369f

diagnosis of, 369

endobronchial, endotracheal, and laryngeal, 371

epidemiology of, 366–367

epididymitis and orchitis due to, 986

granulomatous inflammation due to, 73t, 74, 74f

intestinal, 372, 794t, 798t, 804, 804f

Tuberculosis *(Continued)*

isolated, 371–372

lymphadenitis in, 372

miliary

pulmonary, 371

systemic, 371, 372f

morphology of, 370–372, 370f–372f

pathogenesis of, 367–368, 367f

primary, 367f, 368, 369f–371f, 370

progressive, 368, 369f, 370–371

pulmonary

miliary, 371

primary, 367f, 368, 369f–371f, 370

progressive, 368, 369f, 370–371

secondary, 368–369, 369f, 370, 372f

secondary, 368–369, 369f, 370, 372f

silicosis and, 699

Tuberculous adrenalitis, 1156

Tuberculous arthritis, 1242

Tuberculous cystitis, 974

Tuberculous granuloma, 73t, 74, 74f

Tuberculous meningitis, 1301

Tuberculous osteomyelitis, 1222–1223

Tuberculous salpingitis, 1038

Tuberous sclerosis, 1182t, 1342–1343

colonic polyps in, 816t

cortical hamartomas in, 1342–1343

Tubo-ovarian abscesses, 1010, 1010f

Tubular adenomas, colorectal, 819–820, 820f, 821f

Tubular basement membrane, thickening of, in diabetes mellitus, 1141, 1142f

Tubular carcinoma, of breast, 1087–1088, 1088f

Tubular necrosis, acute, 935–907

causes of, 936

clinical course of, 938

ischemic, 936, 937–938, 937f

morphology of, 937–938, 937f, 938f

nephrotoxic, 936, 937–938, 937f

pathogenesis of, 936–937, 936f

Tubulitis, 945

Tubuloglomerular feedback, 936f, 937

Tubulointerstitial fibrosis, 917

Tubulointerstitial nephritis, 938–948, 939t

due to acute phosphate nephropathy, 947–948

acute *vs.* chronic, 938

drug- and toxin-induced, 944–946, 945f, 946f

due to hypercalcemia and nephrocalcinosis, 947

due to light-chain cast nephropathy, 948, 948f

due to pyelonephritis, 939, 941–944, 941f, 943f, 944f

due to reflux nephropathy, 940, 940f, 942–944, 944f

secondary, 938

due to urate nephropathy, 947, 947f

due to urinary tract infection, 939–941, 940f

Tubulovillous adenomas, colorectal, 819–820

Tumor(s), 259–327. *See also* Neoplasia.

basic components of, 260

characteristic(s) of benign *vs.* malignant, 262–270, 271f, 271t

cancer stem cells and cancer cell lineages as, 267–268

differentiation and anaplasia as, 262–265, 264f–266f, 271t

local invasion as, 268–269, 268f, 271t

metastasis as, 269–270, 269f–271f, 271t

rate of growth as, 265–267, 266f, 271t

clinical aspect(s) of, 320–327

clonality of, 260, 276–277, 278f

defined, 260

desmoplastic, 260

host defense against, 316–320

Tumor(s) *(Continued)*

antitumor effector mechanisms in, 318–319

immune surveillance and escape as, 316, 319–320, 319f

tumor antigens in, 316–318, 317f

in infants and children, 473–481

benign, 473–474, 474f

malignant, 474–481

incidence and types of, 475, 475t

neuroblastic, 475–479, 476f, 477f, 477t, 479f

Wilms tumor as, 479–481, 481f

in inflammation, 44, 69

local and hormonal effects of, 320

malignant (*See* Cancer)

molecular profiles of, 325–326, 326f

nomenclature for, 260–262, 261f, 262f, 263t

scirrhous, 260

tumor markers for, 326–327, 327t

Tumor antigens, 316–318, 317f

Tumor cells, homing of, in metastasis, 300–301

Tumor giant cells, 264, 265f

Tumor immune surveillance, 316, 319–320, 319f

Tumor immunity, 316–320

antitumor effector mechanisms in, 318–319

immune surveillance and escape as, 316, 319–320, 319f

tumor antigens in, 316–318, 317f

Tumor markers, 326–327, 327t

Tumor necrosis factor (TNF)

in acute respiratory distress syndrome, 681, 682f

in cachexia, 320

in disseminated intravascular coagulation, 673

in inflammation, 57t, 61–62, 61t, 62t

in rheumatoid arthritis, 1239

in tissue regeneration and wound healing, 87t

in tuberculosis, 368

Tumor necrosis factor receptor 1 (TNFR1), in apoptosis, 29

Tumor necrosis factor receptor (TNFR) family, apoptosis induced by, 31

Tumor suppressor gene(s), 286–294, 287t

in APC/β-catenin pathway, 292–294, 293f

in INK4a/ARF pathway, 294

NF1 as, 294–295

NF2 as, 295

p53 as, 290–292, 291f

patched (*PTCH*) genes as, 295

PTEN as, 287t, 294

RB as, 287–290, 288f, 289f

in TGF-β pathway, 281t, 294

VHL disease, 295

WT1 as, 295

Tumor-associated antigens, 316

Tumorigenesis. *See* Carcinogenesis.

Tumor-initiating cells (T-ICs), 267–268

Tumor-specific antigens, 316

Tunica vaginalis, lesions of, 993

Turban tumor, 1177

Turcot syndrome, 816t, 821, 1342

Turner syndrome, 165–167, 166f

Twin placentas, 1054, 1055f

Twin-twin transfusion syndrome, 1054

TWIST, in metastasis, 302

Two-hit hypothesis, of oncogenesis, 287, 288f

TXA₂ (thromboxane A₂)

in inflammation, 58f, 59

in platelet aggregation, 118

Typhoid fever, 798t, 801–802

Typhoid nodules, 801

Typhus
  epidemic, 380, 381, 381f
  scrub, 380, 381
Typhus fever, 380, 381, 381f
Tyrosinase, as tumor antigen, 317
Tyrosinase (TYR) gene, in melanoma, 1174
Tyrosine kinase(s), nonreceptor, oncogenes for, 281t, 283–286, 283f, 284f, 285f, 286t
Tyrosine kinase activity
  receptors with, 90, 91f
  receptors without, 90, 91f
Tyrosine kinase mutations
  acute leukemia due to, 597f
  in myeloproliferative disorders, 626, 626t
Tzanck test, 743

U

UBE3A gene, 172–173, 172f
Ubiquitin-proteasome pathway, in atrophy, 10
UC. See Ulcerative colitis (UC).
UGT1 gene, 839
UGT1A1, 839
UIP (usual interstitial pneumonia), 694, 695f
Ulcer(s), 68, 69f
  aphthous, in Crohn disease, 810
  corneal, 432f, 1351
  Curling, 775
  Cushing, 775
  cutaneous
    healing of, 104f
    in systemic sclerosis, 224, 225f
  duodenal, 780
  gastric, acute, 775–776, 776t
  Hunner, 975
  oral, in systemic lupus erythematosus, 214t
  peptic, 68, 69f, 780–781, 781f
    due to Meckel diverticulum, 766
    due to Zollinger-Ellison syndrome, 1147
  rectal, solitary, 815–816, 816f
  rodent, 1180
  stress, 775, 776
Ulceration, defined, 1168
Ulcerative colitis (UC), 811–813
  clinical features of, 812
  vs. Crohn disease, 807, 808f, 808t
  epidemiology of, 807–808
  morphology of, 811–812, 812f, 813f
  pathogenesis of, 808–810, 809f
Ulcerative proctitis, 811
Ulcerative proctosigmoiditis, 811
Ulegyria, 1286
Ulnar-mammary syndrome, 1211t
Ultraviolet (UV) light
  carcinogenesis of, 312
  and cutaneous squamous cell carcinoma, 1180
  in systemic lupus erythematosus, 216
Uncinate herniation, 1283–1284, 1283f
Undernutrition, in Global Burden of Disease, 400
Undifferentiated carcinoma, of thyroid, 1121, 1124
Undifferentiated malignant tumors, categorization of, 324, 324f
Unfolded protein response, 18, 30–31, 31f
Uniparental disomy, 172, 480
Unmyelinated nerve fibers, 1258
u-PA (urokinase-like plasminogen activator), 120
UPJ (uteropelvic junction) obstruction, 972
Upper airway disorder(s), 749–753
  of larynx, 752–753, 752f, 753f
  of nasopharynx, 750–751, 751f
  necrotizing lesions as, 750
  of nose, 749–750, 750f

Upper airway disorder(s) (Continued)
  tumors of nose, sinuses, and nasopharynx as, 751, 751f, 752f
Urachal cysts, 974
Urachus, 974
Urate crystals, in gouty arthritis, 1243, 1245f
Urate nephropathy, 947, 947f
Urate transporter 1 gene (URAT1), in gout, 1243
Ureaplasma, 335
Ureaplasma urealyticum, 341t, 1009
Uremia, 907, 908t
  bleeding disorder due to, 670
  complications of, 933
Uremic nephropathy, 1266
Ureter(s), 972–974
  anatomy of, 972
  congenital anomalies of, 972
  dilation of, 972
  diverticula of, 972
  double and bifid, 972
  hydro-, 972, 973
  inflammation of, 972, 973f
  obstructive lesions of, 973–974, 973t
  sclerosing retroperitoneal fibrosis of, 973–974
  tumors and tumor-like lesions of, 973, 973f
Ureteral obstruction, 973, 973t
Ureteritis, 972, 973f
  cystica, 972, 973f
  follicularis, 972
Urethra, 981–982
  anatomy of, 972
  carcinoma of, 982, 982f
  inflammation of, 981
  tumors and tumor-like lesions of, 981–982, 982f
Urethral caruncle, 981
Urethritis, 981
  gonococcal, 981
  nongonococcal, 380, 981
Uric acid stones, 962, 962t
Urinary abnormalities, isolated, 908t, 929–932
Urinary bladder, 974–981
  anatomy of, 972
  congenital anomalies of, 974, 974f
  inflammation of, 974–975, 975f, 976f
  metaplastic lesions of, 975–976
  neoplasms of, 976–981, 976t
    mesenchymal, 980–981
    secondary, 981
    urothelial, 976–980, 977f–979f, 977t, 979t
  obstruction of, 981, 981f
Urinary tract, lower. See Lower urinary tract.
Urinary tract disorders, due to occupational exposures, 409t
Urinary tract infection, 907, 939–941, 940f
Urinary tract obstruction, 57f, 960–962
  papillary necrosis due to, 947t
Urinary tract stones, due to hyperparathyroidism, 1128
Urobilinogens, 839, 840f
Urogenital tract, infections via, 339
Urokinase-like plasminogen activator (u-PA), 120
Urolithiasis, 907, 962–963, 962t, 963f
Uropathy, obstructive, 960–962, 961f
Uroplakins, 972
Urothelial tumor(s), 976–980
  carcinoma as
    adeno-, 979
    clinical course of, 980
    epidemiology and pathogenesis of, 979–980
    high-grade, 978, 978f
    in situ, 79, 976, 977f, 978f
    invasive, 979, 979f

Urothelial tumor(s) (Continued)
  low-grade, 978, 978f
  mixed, 979
  papillary, 977f, 978, 978f
  precursor lesions to, 976
  of prostate, 1002
  of renal pelvis, 967, 967f
  small-cell, 979
  squamous cell, 979
  staging of, 979, 979t
  of ureters, 973, 973f
  variants of, 979
  grading of, 976–977, 977t
  morphology of, 977–979, 977f–979f
  non-invasive
    flat, 976, 977f, 978f, 979
    papillary, 976, 977
  pagetoid spread of, 978
  papillary
    carcinoma as, 977f, 978, 978f
    of low malignant potential, 977–978
    non-invasive, 976, 977
    papilloma as, 976, 977, 977f
Urothelium, 972
Urticaria, 1187, 1187f
  pigmentosa, 1185
Usual interstitial pneumonia (UIP), 694, 695f
Uterine bleeding, dysfunctional, 1026–1027, 1026f, 1027t
Uterine choriocarcinoma, 1059–1061, 1060f
Uterine fibroids, 264f, 271f, 1026f, 1036–1037, 1037f
Uterine leiomyomas, 264f, 271f, 1026f, 1036–1037, 1037f
Uterine leiomyosarcomas, 1037–1038, 1038f
Uterine spiral arteries, in preeclampsia, 1056, 1056f
Uteropelvic junction (UPJ) obstruction, 972
Uteroplacental insufficiency, 455
Uterus
  anatomy of, 1007–1008, 1008f
  development of, 1006, 1007f
  leiomyoma of, 264f, 271f, 1026f, 1036–1037, 1037f
  leiomyosarcoma of, 271f
  physiologic hypertrophy of, 6–7, 7f
UV (ultraviolet) light
  carcinogenesis of, 312
  and cutaneous squamous cell carcinoma, 1180
  in systemic lupus erythematosus, 216
Uvea, 1355–1357
  neoplasms of, 1356–1357, 1358f
  uveitis of, 1355–1356, 1356f
Uveal melanomas, 1356–1357, 1358f
Uveal nevi, 1356–1357
Uveitis, 1355–1356, 1356f
  lens-induced, 1353

V

Vacuolar degeneration, in cell injury, 13
Vacuolization, 1168
Vagina, 1016–1017
  anatomy of, 1007
  clear cell carcinoma of, 1016, 1016f
  development of, 1006, 1007f
  developmental anomalies of, 1016
  embryonal rhabdomyosarcoma of, 1017, 1017f
  premalignant and malignant neoplasms of, 1016–1017, 1016f, 1017f
  septate or double, 1016
  squamous cell carcinoma of, 1016–1017
Vaginal adenosis, 1016
Vaginal intraepithelial neoplasia, 1016–1017

Vaginal portio, 1007
Vaginitis, 1009
   Candida, 383
Vaginosis, bacterial, 1009
Valproic acid embryopathy, 453
Valvular endocarditis, 124, 220, 220f, 567f, 569
Valvular heart disease, 560–571
   aortic stenosis as, 544
   with calcification, 561–563, 562f
   carcinoid, 569–570, 570f
   causes of, 561, 561t
   due to complications of artificial valves,
      570–571, 571f, 571t
   endocarditis as
      infective, 566–568, 567f, 568f, 569t
      Libman-Sacks, 567f, 569
      nonbacterial thrombotic, 567f, 568–569,
         570f
   mitral valve prolapse as, 563–565, 564f
   rheumatic, 565–566, 565f, 567f
Valvular insufficiency, 560, 561
Valvular stenosis, 560, 561
Valvulitis, rheumatoid, 583
Vanishing-white-matter leukodystrophy, 1327
Variable expressivity, 140
Variant Creutzfeldt-Jakob disease (vCJD), 1309
Variant surface glycoprotein (VSG), in African
   trypanosomiasis, 390
Varicella-zoster virus (VZV), 353, 353f
   encephalitis due to, 1303–1304
   polyneuropathy due to, 353, 353f, 1262–1263
Varices
   of brain, 1298
   esophageal, 519–520, 771, 772f
Varicocele, 993
Varicose veins, 518–519, 519f
Variegate coproporphyria, 1264t
Varioliform gastritis, 780
Vas deferens, congenital bilateral absences of, in
   cystic fibrosis, 469
Vasa nervorum, in rheumatoid arthritis, 1237
Vasa vasorum, 488
Vascular caliber, in inflammation, 46–47, 46f
Vascular changes, due to cancer, 321t, 322
Vascular congestion, in inflammation, 47, 67f
Vascular damage
   due to ionizing radiation, 424, 424f, 425, 426f
   in systemic sclerosis, 223–224
Vascular dementia, 1295, 1319
Vascular disease, 487–527
   aneurysms and dissection as, 506–510,
      506f–510f
   arteriosclerosis as, 496
   atherosclerosis as, 496–506
      anatomy of plaque in, 496, 496f
      consequences of, 504–506, 505f
      epidemiology of, 496–498, 497f, 497t, 498f
      morphology of, 502–504, 502f–504f
      pathogenesis of, 498–502, 499f, 501f, 502f
   congenital anomalies as, 489–490
   hypertensive, 492–496, 493t, 494f, 495f
   of lungs, 706–710
      diffuse pulmonary hemorrhage syndromes
         as, 709–710, 709f
      pulmonary embolism, hemorrhage, and
         infarction as, 706–707, 706f
      pulmonary hypertension as, 707–709, 708f,
         709f
   Raynaud's phenomenon as, 518, 518f
   renal, 949–955
      atheroembolic, 954, 954f
      atherosclerotic ischemic, 954
      benign nephrosclerosis as, 949, 949f, 950f
      diffuse cortical necrosis as, 954–955, 954f

Vascular disease *(Continued)*
      malignant hypertension and accelerated
         nephrosclerosis as, 949–951, 950f
      renal artery stenosis as, 951–952, 951f
      renal infarcts as, 955
      sickle-cell disease nephropathy as, 954
      thrombotic microangiopathies as, 952–954,
         952f
   of testes and epididymis, 987, 987f
   vasculitis as (*See* Vasculitis)
   of veins and lymphatics, 518–520, 519f
Vascular dissemination, in metastasis, 300–301
Vascular ectasias, 522
Vascular endothelial growth factor (VEGF)
   in angiogenesis, 100–101, 100t, 101f, 298
   in tissue regeneration and wound healing, 87t,
      88
Vascular endothelium, response to injury of,
   490–491, 490t, 491f
Vascular flow, in inflammation, 46–47, 46f
Vascular grafts, pathology of, 526–527, 527f
Vascular injury
   of central nervous system, 1288–1290, 1289f,
      1290f
   leukocyte-mediated, in inflammation, 47f
Vascular interventions, pathology of, 525–527,
   526f, 527f
Vascular leakage, in inflammation, 47, 47f
Vascular lesions, hepatic, drug- and
   toxin-induced, 856t
Vascular malformations, of brain, 1298–1299
Vascular permeability, in inflammation, 47, 47f,
   66t
Vascular reactions, in inflammation, 46–48, 46f,
   47f
Vascular replacement, pathology of, 526–527,
   527f
Vascular stasis
   in inflammation, 46–47, 46f, 67f
   and thrombosis, 121–122
Vascular tumors and tumor-like conditions,
   520–525, 520t
   benign, 520–522, 520t
      bacillary angiomatosis as, 522, 523f
      glomus tumor (glomangioma) as, 522
      hemangioma as, 520–521, 521f
      lymphangiomas as, 522
      vascular ectasias as, 522
   intermediate-grade (borderline), 520t,
      523–524
      hemangioendothelioma as, 524
      Kaposi sarcoma as, 523–524, 524f
   malignant, 520t, 524–525
      angiosarcoma as, 524–525, 525f
      hemangiopericytoma as, 525
Vascular turbulence, and thrombosis, 121–122
Vascular wall cells, responses to injury of,
   490–492, 490f, 491f
Vascular wall weakening, and aneurysms,
   506–507, 507f
Vasculature
   development, growth, and remodeling of,
      489
   structure and function of, 488–489, 488f
Vasculitis, 114, 510–518
   due to ANCA, 203t, 511–512
   due to anti-endothelial cell antibodies, 512
   associated with other disorders, 517
   Churg-Strauss syndrome as, 516
   classification and characteristics of, 510, 511t,
      512t
   defined, 510
   giant-cell (temporal) arteritis as, 512–513,
      513f

Vasculitis *(Continued)*
   hypersensitivity or leukocytoclastic, 515, 516f
   immune complex–associated, 205, 205f,
      510–511
   infectious, 517–518
      cerebral infarction due to, 1293
   Kawasaki disease as, 515
   large-vessel, 511t, 512f
   lupus, 517
   medium-vessel, 511t, 512f
   microscopic polyangiitis as, 515, 516f
   noninfectious, 226, 510–517
   polyarteritis nodosa as, 514–515, 514f
   rejection, 228–229, 228f
   retinal, 1361–1362
   rheumatoid, 517, 1237
   small-vessel, 511t, 512f
   Takayasu arteritis as, 513–514, 514f
   thromboangiitis obliterans (Buerger disease)
      as, 517, 517f
   and thrombosis, 121
   Wegener granulomatosis as, 516–517, 516f
Vasculogenesis, 99, 489
Vasculogenic mimicry, 1357
Vasoactive amines
   in immediate hypersensitivity, 199
   in inflammation, 57–58, 57t
Vasoconstriction, 489
   in atherosclerosis, 506
   in blood pressure regulation, 494f, 495
   in hemostasis, 115, 116f
   intrarenal, 936f, 937
   due to shock, 132
Vasodilatation, 489
Vasodilation
   in inflammation, 46, 46f, 66t
   due to shock, 132
Vasogenic edema, 1282
Vasoocclusive crises, in sickle cell disease,
   647–648
Vasopressin, 1099
Vasospasm, coronary artery occlusion due to,
   547
vCJD (variant Creutzfeldt-Jakob disease), 1309
VDRL (Venereal Disease Research Laboratory)
   test, 375
Vector-borne infectious diseases, global warming
   and, 402
Vegetative endocarditis, 124, 567f
   infective, 566–568, 567f, 568f, 569t
   noninfected, 567f, 568–570, 570f
VEGF (vascular endothelial growth factor)
   in angiogenesis, 100–101, 100t, 101f, 298
   in tissue regeneration and wound healing, 87t,
      88
Vehicular accident, mechanical injury due to,
   420–421
Veins
   structure and function of, 488f, 489
   superior and inferior vena caval syndromes of,
      519
   thrombophlebitis and phlebothrombosis of,
      519
   varicose, 518–519, 519f
Velocardiofacial syndrome, 162
Venereal Disease Research Laboratory (VDRL)
   test, 375
Venereal warts, 826, 827f, 1012, 1012f, 1200
Veno-occlusive disease, of liver, 873–874, 873f
Venous angiomas, of brain, 1298
Venous thromboembolism, hormone
   replacement therapy and, 415
Venous thrombosis, 124, 125
   due to cancer, 321t

Ventricular aneurysm, due to myocardial infarction, 556f, 557
Ventricular remodeling, 533, 557
Ventricular septal defect (VSD), 540f, 541, 541f
   in tetralogy of Fallot, 542, 542f
   in transposition of the great arteries, 542f, 543
Ventricular septum
   hypertrophy of, 575–576, 576f
   rupture of, 556f, 557
Venules, structure and function of, 488f, 489
Verruca(e), 1200–1201, 1200f
   palmaris, 1200
   plana, 1200
   plantaris, 1200
   in rheumatic heart disease, 566, 567f
   vulgaris, 1200
Verrucous carcinoma
   of penis, 984
   vulvar, 1014, 1014f
Verrucous epidermal hyperplasia, 1200–1201, 1200f, 1201f
Very-long-chain fatty acids (VLCFAs), in adrenoleukodystrophy, 1327
Very-low-density lipoprotein (VLDL), metabolism of, 147, 147f
Vesical diverticulum, 974
Vesicle, 1168
Vesicoureteral reflux, 940, 940f, 942–944, 944f, 974
Vesicouterine fistulas, 974
Vesiculovacuolar organelle, in inflammation, 47
Vessel wall abnormalities, bleeding disorders due to, 666
VHFs (viral hemorrhagic fevers), 351
VHL disease. See Von Hippel-Lindau (VHL) disease.
Vibrio cholerae, 797–799, 798t, 799f
Vibrio parahaemolyticus, 797
Villous adenomas, colorectal, 819–820, 821f
Vimentin filaments, 35
VIN (vulvar intraepithelial neoplasia), 1012–1014, 1013f
Vinyl chloride
   as carcinogen, 274t
   occupational exposure to, 410
VIPoma, 1147
Viral arthritis, 1242
Viral esophagitis, 769, 769f
Viral gastroenteritis, 794t, 804–805, 805f
Viral hemorrhagic fevers (VHFs), 351
Viral hepatitis, 843–853, 844t
   acute, 850, 851–852, 851f, 852f
   carrier state of, 850
   chronic, 850–851, 851f–853f, 852–853
   clinical course of, 853
   clinicopathologic syndromes of, 850–851
   defined, 844
   fulminant, 835, 853, 854f
   due to hepatitis A virus, 844, 844t, 845f
   due to hepatitis B virus, 844t, 845–847, 845f–847f
   due to hepatitis C virus, 844t, 847–848, 848f
   due to hepatitis D virus, 844t, 848–849
   due to hepatitis E virus, 844t, 849
   due to hepatitis G virus, 849
   HIV and, 850–851
   morphology of, 851–853, 851f–854f
Viral infection(s), 348–357, 349t
   acute (transient), 348–351, 350f
   in AIDS, 245t, 246
   arboviral and hemorrhagic fevers as, 349t, 351

Viral infection(s) (Continued)
   of central nervous system, 349t
   chronic
      latent (herpesvirus), 351–355, 352f–354f
      productive, 355
   cytomegalovirus as, 353–355, 354f
   digestive, 349t
   Epstein-Barr virus as, 355–357, 356f
   hepatitis B virus as, 355
   herpes simplex virus as, 352–353, 352f
   latent, 333
      chronic, 351–355, 352f–354f
   measles as, 349–350, 350f
   mumps as, 350
   poliovirus as, 350–351
   respiratory, 349t
   systemic
      with hematopoietic disorders, 349t
      with skin eruptions, 349t
   transforming, 355–357, 356f
   varicella zoster virus as, 353, 353f
   warts due to, 349t
   West Nile virus as, 351
Viral injury, mechanism of, 342–343, 343f
Viral meningitis, 1299, 1300
Viral meningoencephalitis, 1302–1306, 1303f–1306f
Viral pneumonia, 714–716
Virchow, Rudolph, 4–5, 44, 126, 1166
Virchow's node, 786
Virchow's triad, 121, 122f
Virilism, nonclassic or late-onset adrenal, 1153–1154
Virilizing adrenogenital syndrome, simple, 1153
Virulence, bacterial, 343
   intracellular, 344
Virus(es), 332–333, 333t
   classification of, 332
   congenital anomalies due to, 451–452
   mechanisms of disease production by, 342–343, 343f
   sexually transmitted, 341t
   structure of, 332–333, 333f
   tropism of, 342
   white cell neoplasia due to, 597
Visceral epithelial cells, 909f, 910
Vision, vitamin A in, 431, 432, 432f
Visual impairment, due to diabetes, 1140f, 1143, 1145
Vitamin(s)
   essential, 430
   fat-soluble, 430
   water-soluble, 430
Vitamin A, 430–433
   deficiency of, 432–433, 432f, 438t
   forms of, 430–431
   functions of, 431–432, 438t
   metabolism of, 431, 431f
   sources of, 431
   toxicity of, 433
Vitamin B₁, functions of, 438t
Vitamin B₁ deficiency, 438t
   due to alcoholism, 414
   CNS effects of, 1328
   peripheral neuropathy due to, 1266
Vitamin B₂, functions of, 438t
Vitamin B₂ deficiency, 438t
Vitamin B₆, functions of, 438t
Vitamin B₆ deficiency, 438t
Vitamin B₁₂
   functions of, 438t, 657, 657f
   metabolism of, 656, 656f
Vitamin B₁₂ deficiency, 438t, 1328–1329

Vitamin B₁₂ deficiency anemia, 655–658, 655t, 656f, 657f
   antibody-mediated hypersensitivity in, 203t
   and autoimmune gastritis, 778, 779
Vitamin C, 437–438
   deficiency of, 437–438, 437f, 438t
   function of, 437, 438t
   toxicity of, 438
Vitamin D, 433–436
   in calcium and phosphorus homeostasis, 433–435, 435f, 436f
   deficiency of, 435–436, 435f–437f, 438t
   functions of, 433, 438t
   mechanism of action of, 433
   metabolism of, 433, 434f
   non-skeletal effects of, 436, 437f
   toxicity of, 436
Vitamin D receptor, defect in, 143t
Vitamin D₃, 433
Vitamin deficiency(ies), 430–438, 438t
   due to alcohol consumption, 859
   CNS effects of, 1328–1329
   primary *vs.* secondary, 430
   of vitamin A, 430–433, 431f, 432f
   of vitamin C, 437–438, 437f
   of vitamin D, 433–436, 434f–437f
Vitamin D–related disorders, hypercalcemia due to, 38
Vitamin E
   deficiency of, 438t
   functions of, 438t
Vitamin K
   deficiency of, 438t
   functions of, 438t
Vitreoretinopathy, proliferative, 1358
Vitreous humor
   anatomy of, 1357, 1359f
   posterior detachment of, 1357, 1360f, 1361
VLCFAs (very-long-chain fatty acids), in adrenoleukodystrophy, 1327
VLDL (very-low-density lipoprotein), metabolism of, 147, 147f
Vocal cord nodules and polyps, 752
Volume-overload hypertrophy, 533
Volvulus, 791, 791f
von Gierke disease, 155, 157t
von Hippel-Lindau (VHL) disease, 1343
   cavernous hemangiomas in, 521
   pheochromocytomas in, 1160t
   renal cell carcinoma in, 964, 965
von Hippel-Lindau (*VHL*) gene, 288, 295, 306, 1343
   in renal cell carcinoma, 965
von Meyenburg complexes, 869, 870f
von Recklinghausen disease, 1218
von Willebrand disease, 118f, 671–672
von Willebrand factor (vWF), 116, 118f, 670–671, 671f
VSD (ventricular septal defect), 540f, 541, 541f
   in tetralogy of Fallot, 542, 542f
   in transposition of the great arteries, 542f, 543
VSG (variant surface glycoprotein), in African trypanosomiasis, 390
Vulva, 1011–1016
   Bartholin cyst of, 1011
   benign exophytic lesions of, 1012, 1012f
   condyloma acuminatum of, 1012, 1012f
   glandular neoplastic lesions of, 1015, 1015f
   lichen sclerosis of, 1011, 1011f
   malignant melanoma of, 1015–1016
   non-neoplastic epithelial disorders of, 1011–1012, 1011f
   Paget disease of, 1015, 1015f
   papillary hidradenoma of, 1015, 1015f

Vulva *(Continued)*
squamous cell hyperplasia of, 1011f, 1012
squamous neoplastic lesions of, 1012–1014, 1013f, 1014f
vulvar carcinoma as, 1012–1014, 1013f, 1014f
vulvar intraepithelial neoplasia as, 1012–1014, 1013f
Vulvar carcinoma, 1012–1014, 1013f, 1014f
Vulvar intraepithelial neoplasia (VIN), 1012–1014, 1013f
vWF (von Willebrand factor), 116, 118f, 670–671, 671f
vWF metalloprotease, in thrombotic microangiopathies, 669
VZV (varicella-zoster virus), 353, 353f
encephalitis due to, 1303–1304
polyneuropathy due to, 353, 353f, 1262–1263

W
Waardenburg syndrome, 1211t
WAGR syndrome, 440
Wilms tumor in, 479–480
Waldenström macroglobulinemia, 609, 612
Walker-Warburg muscular dystrophy, 1270t
Wallerian degeneration, 1259, 1259f
Warburg effect, 303–304
Warfarin (Coumadin), 119
Warm antibody type immunohemolytic anemia, 653–654, 653t
Wart(s), 1200–1201, 1200f
flat, 1200
venereal (genital), 826, 827f, 1012, 1012f, 1200
Warthin tumor, 759, 759f
Warthin-Finkeldey cells, 350
Warty vulvar carcinoma, 1012, 1013f, 1014
WASP (Wiskott-Aldrich syndrome protein), 235
Water retention, edema due to, 112–113
Waterhouse-Friderichsen syndrome, 1155, 1155f, 1156f
in bacterial meningitis, 1299
in septic shock, 131
Watermelon stomach, 779
Watershed infarcts, in cerebral ischemia, 1291
Watershed zones, in ischemic bowel disease, 792
WDHA syndrome, 1147
Weber-Christian disease, 1199
Weber-Osler-Rendu syndrome, 666
Wegener granulomatosis, 516–517, 516f, 710
glomerular lesions in, 935
of orbit, 1347
Weibel-Palade bodies, 490
in inflammation, 49, 49f
Wen, 1176
Werdnig-Hoffmann disease, 1267
Wermer syndrome, 1161–1162
Werner syndrome, 39–40, 39f, 41
Wernicke encephalopathy, 1328
Wernicke-Korsakoff syndrome, 414, 1328
West Nile virus, 351
Wet gangrene, 16
Wheals, 1168, 1187
Whipple, Allen Oldfather, 803
Whipple disease, 794t, 798t, 803–804, 804f
Whipple, George Hoyt, 803
Whipworms, 806
White cell(s), adult reference range for, 592t
White cell disorder(s), 592–632
agranulocytosis as, 592–593
leukocytosis as, 593–595, 594f, 594t

White cell disorder(s) *(Continued)*
leukopenia as, 592–593
lymphadenitis as, 595–596, 596f
neoplastic, 596–632
etiology and pathogenesis of, 596–598, 597f
histiocytoses as, 596, 631–632, 631f
lymphoid, 596, 598–620
classification of, 598–600, 598t, 600t, 601t
definitions for, 598
Hodgkin lymphoma as, 616–620
origin of, 599–600, 599f
peripheral B-cell, 603–614
peripheral T-cell and NK-cell, 614–616, 615f
precursor B- and T-cell, 600–603, 602f
myeloid, 596, 620–631
acute myeloid leukemia as, 620, 621–624, 622t, 623f
myelodysplastic syndromes as, 620, 624–626, 625f
myeloproliferative disorders as, 621, 626–631
neutropenia as, 592–593
reactive (inflammatory), 593–596
White infarcts, 128, 128f
WHO (World Health Organization) classification
of acute myeloid leukemia, 622, 622t
of Hodgkin lymphoma, 617
of lymphoid neoplasms, 598–599, 598t
Whooping cough, 364, 364f
Wickham striae, 1191, 1192f
Williams-Beuren syndrome, 545
Wilms tumor, 295, 479–481
clinical features of, 481
epidemiology of, 479
morphology of, 480–481, 481f
pathogenesis and genetics of, 479–480
synchronous *vs.* metachronous, 479
Wilson disease, 863–864
Wire-loop lesion, in systemic lupus erythematosus, 218–219, 219f
Wiskott-Aldrich syndrome, 235
Wiskott-Aldrich syndrome protein (WASP), 235
WNT signal transduction
APC in, 293, 293f
proto-oncogene for, 281t
Wnt/β-catenin pathway
in bone homeostasis, 1208
in regeneration, 92
Wolbachia spp, 395
Wolman disease, 151t
Wood smoke, as indoor air pollutant, 405
World Health Organization (WHO) classification
of acute myeloid leukemia, 622, 622t
of Hodgkin lymphoma, 617
of lymphoid neoplasms, 598–599, 598t
Wound
incised, 420
puncture, 420
Wound contraction, 103f, 104–105, 104f
Wound contracture, 107, 107f
Wound healing, 98–108
angiogenesis in, 99–102, 99f, 100t, 101f
cutaneous, 102–106
cell proliferation and collagen deposition in, 102–104
connective tissue remodeling in, 105
formation of blood clot in, 102, 103f

Wound healing, cutaneous *(Continued)*
formation of granulation tissue in, 102, 103f–105f
growth factors and cytokines in, 102, 104t
macrophages in, 102, 103f, 105f
phases of, 102, 103f, 104f
by primary union or first intention, 102
recovery of tensile strength in, 105–106
scar formation in, 103f, 104
by secondary union or secondary intention, 102, 103f, 104f
wound contraction in, 103f, 104–105, 104f
local and systemic factors that influence, 106
pathologic aspects of, 106–108, 106f–108f
regeneration and repair in, 79–80, 80f, 81f
Woven bone, 1208–1209, 1208f
WT1 tumor suppressor gene, 287t, 295
in Wilms syndrome, 479–480
Wuchereria bancrofti, 395

X
X chromatin, 164
Xanthoastrocytomas, pleomorphic, 1333
Xanthogranulomatous cholecystitis, 886
Xanthogranulomatous pyelonephritis, 943
Xanthomas, 35
Xenobiotics, 402, 402f, 403, 403f
Xeroderma pigmentosum, 275, 302, 1182t
Xerophthalmia, 432
Xerostomia, 756
in Sjögren syndrome, 221, 222
X-inactivation, 164
XIST gene, 164
X-linked agammaglobulinemia, 231–233
X-linked disorders, 142, 142t
X-linked lymphoproliferative (XLP) syndrome, 319, 357
X-linked muscular dystrophy, 1268–1269, 1268f, 1269f
X-rays, as carcinogens, 312

Y
Yaws, skeletal infection with, 1223
Yeasts, 335, 382
Yersinia enterocolitica, 802
Yersinia pestis, 365, 802
Yersinia pseudotuberculosis, 802
Yersinia spp, enterocolitis due to, 798t, 800f, 802
Yolk sac tumor
ovarian, 1049, 1049f
testicular, 989–990

Z
Zeis glands, 1348f
Zellballen
in carotid body tumor, 755, 755f
in pheochromocytoma, 1160, 1160f
Zenker diverticulum, 767
Zinc
deficiency of, 439t
function of, 439t
Zollinger-Ellison syndrome, 780, 782–783, 782t
of pancreas, 1147
Zonula adherins, in extracellular matrix, 96
Zonule, of eye, 1346f
Zoonotic bacterial infections, 358t
Zuska disease, 1069, 1069f
Zygomycosis, 385–386, 386f